The Lippincott

Manual of Nursing Practice

Doris Smith Suddarth, R.N., B.S.N.E., M.S.N.

Resident Scholar
National Library of Medicine
Bethesda, Maryland

Contributors

Medical-Surgical Nursing

Brenda G. Bare
R.N., M.S.N.

Joyce A. Juliano Batcheller
R.N., M.S.N., C.C.R.N., C.N.A.

Elizabeth W. Bayley
R.N., M.S., Ph.D.

Carole E. Berkebile
R.N., B.S.H.S.

Sharon A. Bray
R.N., M.S.

Morag Ferguson Dahlstrom
R.N., M.S.N.

Joanne P. Finley
R.N., M.S., O.C.N.

David B. P. Goodman
M.D., Ph.D.

Leslie A. Hoffman
R.N., Ph.D.

Marilyn Hravnak
R.N., M.S.N., C.C.R.N., R.R.T.

Kathleen Jacobs-Irvine
R.N., M.A.

Christine Ashley Kessler
R.N., M.N., C.S.

Dorothy B. Liddel
R.N., M.S.N., O.N.C.

Susan Foster Marden
R.N., M.S., C.C.R.N.

Betty Temples-Mill
R.N., Ph.D.

M. Eletta Morse
R.N., M.S.N., C.A.N.P.,

Janet Nilsen Pavel
R.N.

Loretta Spittle
R.N., M.S., C.C.R.N., C.N.A.

Emma L. Witt
R.N.

Maternity Nursing

TINA WEITKAMP
R.N., M.S.N.

Pediatric Nursing

DONNAJEANNE BIGOS LAVOIE
R.N., M.S.N.

Beth M. Donaher
R.N., M.S.N.

Judith A. Farley
R.N., M.S.N., C.N.R.N.

Janice Selekman
R.N., M.S.N., D.N.Sc.

Donna Linthicum Shelly
R.N., M.S.

Christine Steinmuller
R.N., M.S.N., O.C.N.

Carol Jo Wilson
R.N., Ph.D.

5th
Edition

The Lippincott

Manual of
Nursing Practice

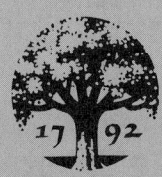

J.B. Lippincott Company   Philadelphia

New York   London   Hagerstown

Acquisitions/Sponsoring Editor	Diana Intenzo
Project Editor	Lorraine D. Smith
Copy Editors	Julie Gillman, Sue Reilly
Indexer	Ann Cassar
Design Coordinator	Doug Smock
Interior Designer	Eliz. Anne O'Donnell
Production Manager	Helen Ewan
Production Coordinator	Kathryn Rule
Compositor	Tapsco, Inc.
Printer/Binder	R. R. Donnelley & Sons Company

Fifth Edition

Library of Congress Cataloging-in-Publication Data

Suddarth, Doris Smith.
    The Lippincott manual of nursing practice.—5th ed./Doris
Smith Suddarth; contributors, Brenda Bare . . . [et al.]
        p.   cm.
    Rev. ed. of: The Lippincott manual of nursing practice/Lillian
Sholtis Brunner, Doris Smith Suddarth. 4th ed. c1986.
    Includes bibliographical references.
    Includes index.
    ISBN 0-397-54787-0 (hard cover)
    1. Nursing—Handbooks, manuals, etc.   I. Brunner, Lillian
Sholtis.   Lippincott manual of nursing practice.   II. Title.
III. Title: Manual of nursing practice.
    [DNLM: 1. Nursing Care—handbooks.   WY 39 S943L]
RT51.B78   1991
610.73—dc20
DNLM/DLC
for Library of Congress   90-13635
                                                               CIP

Any medical or nursing procedure or practice described in this book should be applied
by the health-care practitioner under appropriate supervision in accordance with
professional standards of care used with regard to the unique circumstances that apply
in each practice situation. Care has been taken to confirm the accuracy of information
presented and to describe generally accepted practices. However, the authors, editors,
and publisher cannot accept any responsibility for errors or omissions or for
consequences from application of the information in this book and make no warranty,
express or implied, with respect to the contents of the book. It is assumed that all
treatment is given under supervision of a physician.

Every effort has been made to ensure that drug selections and dosages are in
accordance with current recommendations and practice. Because of ongoing research,
changes in government regulations, and the constant flow of information on drug
therapy, reactions, and interactions, the reader is cautioned to check the package insert
for each drug for indications, dosages, warnings, and precautions, particularly if the
drug is new or infrequently used.

Contributors

Medical–Surgical Nursing

Brenda G. Bare, R.N., M.S.N.
Assistant Vice-President for Medical–Surgical Nursing
The Alexandria Hospital
Alexandria, Virginia
Chapter 1. Nursing Process and Patient Teaching
Chapter 2. Data Collection and History Taking

Joyce A. Juliano Batcheller, R.N., M.S.N., C.C.R.N., C.N.A.
Director, Nursing Special Projects
The Fairfax Hospital
Falls Church, Virginia
Chapter 22. Endocrine Disorders
Chapter 23. Diabetes Mellitus

Elizabeth W. Bayley, R.N., M.S., Ph.D.
Associate Professor, School of Nursing
Widener University
Chester, Pennsylvania
Chapter 33. Burns

Carole E. Berkebile, R.N., B.S.H.S.*
Advanced Clinical Nurse
National Institutes of Health
Bethesda, Maryland
Chapter 36. Allergy Problems

Sharon A. Bray, R.N., M.S.
Clinical Nurse Educator
Critical Care/Heart, Lung, and Blood Nursing Service
National Institutes of Health
Bethesda, Maryland
Chapter 18. Upper Gastrointestinal Disorders (Mouth, Neck, and Esophagus)
Chapter 21. Hepatic, Biliary, and Pancreatic Disorders

Morag Ferguson Dahlstrom, R.N., M.S.N.
Clinical Nurse Educator
Cancer Nursing Service
National Institutes of Health
Bethesda, Maryland
Chapter 6. Cancer Nursing

Joanne P. Finley, R.N., M.S., O.C.N.
Instructor
University of Maryland School of Nursing
Baltimore, Maryland
Chapter 28. Gynecologic Disorders
Chapter 29. Breast Conditions

David B. P. Goodman, M.D., Ph.D.
Professor and Department Chief, Department of Pathology and Laboratory Medicine
Hospital of the University of Pennsylvania
Philadelphia, Pennsylvania
Appendix I. Diagnostic Studies and Their Meaning

Leslie A. Hoffman, R.N., Ph.D.
Associate Professor, Pulmonary Medicine
University of Pittsburgh
Pittsburgh, Pennsylvania
Chapter 11. Respiratory Function and Therapy

Marilyn Hravnak, R.N., M.S.N., C.C.R.N., R.R.T.
Head Nurse, Cardiothoracic Surgical Intensive Care Unit
Presbyterian–University Hospital of Pittsburgh
Pittsburgh, Pennsylvania
Chapter 11. Respiratory Function and Therapy

Kathleen Jacobs–Irvine, R.N., M.A.
Head Nurse, Medical Cardiology
National Institutes of Health
Bethesda, Maryland
Chapter 19. Nutritional Assessment, Selected Problems, and Special Nutritional Management
Chapter 20. Gastrointestinal Disorders

Christine Ashley Kessler, R.N., M.N., C.S.
Clinical Nurse Specialist, Critical Care
The Mount Vernon Hospital
Alexandria, Virginia
Chapter 4. Care of the Surgical Patient
Chapter 5. IV Therapy

Dorothy B. Liddel, R.N., M.S.N., O.N.C.
Adjunct Instructor
Columbia Union College
Takoma Park, Maryland
Chapter 30. Musculoskeletal Trauma and Fractures
Chapter 31. Orthopedic Surgery and Musculoskeletal Problems

Susan Foster Marden, R.N., M.S., C.C.R.N.
Cardiac Clinical Specialist
National Heart, Lung, and Blood Institute
National Institutes of Health
Bethesda, Maryland
Chapter 14. Cardiac Disorders

Betty Temples–Mill, R.N., Ph.D.
Assistant Professor of Nursing
George Mason University
Fairfax, Virginia
Chapter 25. Eye Disorders
Chapter 26. Ear Disorders

M. Eletta Morse, R.N., M.S.N., C.A.N.P.
Geriatric Clinical Specialist
The Alexandria Hospital
Alexandria, Virginia
Chapter 7. Care of the Older Adult

Janet Nilsen Pavel, R.N.
Chief Nurse, Department of Transfusion Medicine
National Institutes of Health
Bethesda, Maryland
Chapter 13. Transfusion Therapy and Bone Marrow Transplantation

Loretta Spittle, R.N., M.S., C.C.R.N., C.N.A.
Adjunct Faculty
University of Virginia
Charlottesville, Virginia
Chapter 15. Electrocardiography
Chapter 16. Vascular Disorders
Chapter 17. High Blood Pressure

Emma L. Witt, R.N.*
Clinical Nurse
National Naval Medical Center
Bethesda, Maryland
Chapter 36. Allergy Problems

* The views expressed in this chapter are those of the author(s) and do not reflect the official policy or position of the Department of the Navy, Department of Defense, or the U.S. Government

Maternity Nursing

TINA WEITKAMP, R.N., M.S.N.
Assistant Professor of Clinical Nursing
Department of Parent–Child Nursing
College of Nursing and Health
University of Cincinnati
Cincinnati, Ohio

Pediatric Nursing

DONNAJEANNE BIGOS LAVOIE, R.N., M.S.N.
Assistant Professor, College of Nursing
Howard University
Neonatology Nurse Consultant; formerly
Neonatology Nurse Consultant, Children's Hospital
National Medical Center
Washington, D.C.

Beth M. Donaher, R.N., M.S.N.
Pediatric Clinical Nurse Specialist
Thomas Jefferson University
Philadelphia, Pennsylvania
Chapter 55. Metabolic Disturbances in Children

Judith A. Farley, R.N., M.S.N., C.N.R.N.
Clinical Nurse Specialist
Pediatric Neuroscience
Children's Hospital
Boston, Massachusetts
Chapter 58. Children With Neurologic and Neurosurgical Problems

Janice Selekman, R.N., M.S.N., D.N.Sc.
Associate Professor
Thomas Jefferson University
Philadelphia, Pennsylvania
Chapter 50. Blood Disorders in Children
Chapter 51. Children With Cardiovascular Disorders
Chapter 61. The Child at Risk—Special Pediatric Problems

Donna Linthicum Shelly, R.N., M.S.
Pediatric Clinical Nurse Specialist
Parent–Child Consultation
Gaithersburg, Maryland
Chapter 47. Pediatric Techniques

Christine Steinmuller, R.N., M.S.N., O.C.N.
Clinical Nurse III
Children's National Medical Center
Washington, D.C.
Chapter 60. Pediatric Oncology

Carol Jo Wilson, R.N., Ph.D.
Assistant Professor
Northern Illinois University
School of Nursing
DeKalb, Illinois
Chapter 53. Renal and Genitourinary Disorders in Children

Contents

List of Guidelines

Maternity Nursing

Pediatric Nursing

Health Education/Patient Education

Page numbers followed by f *indicate illustrations;* t *following a page number indicates tabular material.*
Page numbers in italics *deal with* pediatric *considerations and include parental teaching.*

Preface

As the 21st century approaches, nurses are faced with a vast amount of health care information, a constantly changing scientific database, and burgeoning technology. The purpose of *The Lippincott Manual of Nursing Practice* is to assist nurses to process and manage this knowledge in order to think critically, make sound clinical decisions, and administer quality health care in a variety of practice settings.

The focus of the *Manual* is clearly on the science and art of nursing. Relevant clinical content and guidelines are offered in a logical and readily accessible format. The use of the nursing process provides a *nursing* frame of reference and continuity. Scientific principles and rationale are offered to explain why and how something occurs and what may result. Included are the essential knowledge and understanding for monitoring the changing status of patients so that complications can be prevented or their effects minimized. The distinctive needs of older persons have been highlighted.

Every clinical problem has been reviewed, updated, or modified to reflect changes in therapy resulting from ongoing clinical research. Material is included to enhance the functions of nurses as discharge planners, case managers, and experts in quality assurance. The sections on "Patient Education" have been amplified to increase health-healing practices.

The writers acknowledge that nursing care interfaces with medical care plans. There are alternative management strategies and nursing approaches and these are included as far as space constraints permit.

Reviewing current literature, interpreting data, distilling information and presenting a balanced perspective are challenging tasks. The extensive bibliographies at the end of the chapters appropriately demonstrate scholarly research of recent publications. They have been selected to guide the reader to additional information and a wider experience in patient care. The bibliographic citations follow the format used by the National Library of Medicine for INDEX MEDICUS and MEDLINE, a database containing over six million references to health care journal articles.

For fresh perspective and insight, the scholarship and clinical expertise of a distinguished group of nursing colleagues, all actively engaged in patient care, have been enlisted. Their collaboration and wise counsel have contributed significantly to this volume.

Although the explosion of information and rapid progress occurring in biotechnology mandate change, nurses will continue to provide the "kinder, gentler" approach to our fellow humans whose lives we have the privilege of enhancing.

DSS

Acknowledgments

Jean DeVries, R.N.
Equipment Analyst
The Alexandria Hospital
Alexandria, Virginia

Sharon K. Hobson, R.N., M.S.
Certified Pediatric Nurse Practitioner
Baltimore City Health Department
Comprehensive School Health Services Program
Baltimore, Maryland

Michael A. Kaliner, M.D.
Chief, Allergic Diseases Section
National Institute of Allergy and Infectious Diseases
National Institutes of Health
Bethesda, Maryland

Susan F. Leitman, M.D.
Chief, Blood Services
Department of Transfusion Medicine
National Institutes of Health
Bethesda, Maryland

Research/Library

Mary Lou O'Brien, R.N., M.S.L.S.
Director, Health Science Library
The Mount Vernon Hospital
Alexandria, Virginia

Elizabeth A. Kayaian, R.N., M.S.L.S.
Medical Librarian; Clinical Information Specialist
National Institutes of Health
Bethesda, Maryland

Eve-Marie Lacroix
Chief of Public Services Division
National Library of Medicine
Bethesda, Maryland

Gladys L. Taylor and Staff
Head Monograph Processing Group
Circulation and Control Section
National Library of Medicine
Bethesda, Maryland

Jacqueline van de Kamp, M.L.S.
Technical Information Specialist
Biological Information Services Branch
Specialized Information Services Division
National Library of Medicine
Bethesda, Maryland

Reference Librarians, Reference Technicians

National Library of Medicine
Bethesda, Maryland

Art

Kathryn Born
Gary Lees
Art as Applied to Medicine
The Johns Hopkins University School of Medicine
Baltimore, Maryland

The following persons are acknowledged with special appreciation:

Lillian S. Brunner, my colleague who co-authored the first four editions of the *Manual,* with respect for her wisdom and affection for her friendship.

Members of the J.B. Lippincott staff:

Diana Intenzo, Editor-in-Chief of the Nursing Editorial Department, for her foresight and awesome grasp of nursing and publishing, whose knowledge and skills contributed significantly to this book.

Helen Ewan, Production Manager, for her care, efficiency, and dedication to the task of completing this project.

Lorraine D. Smith, Senior Project Editor, for her concern for excellence and her efficiency in creating continuity and consistency throughout this volume.

Susan Blaker, former Art Director and **Doug Smock**, Senior Designer, for their creative endeavors in directing the art program and coordinating design features for this edition.

Doris Wray, Administrative Assistant, Nursing Editorial Department, who smoothed the way with courtesy and competency.

And finally,

Hilton and **Barbara Hilton**, my husband and daughter, for their understanding, steadfast love, and support.

The Lippincott
Manual of Nursing Practice

Part I

Medical–Surgical Nursing

Components of Nursing Practice

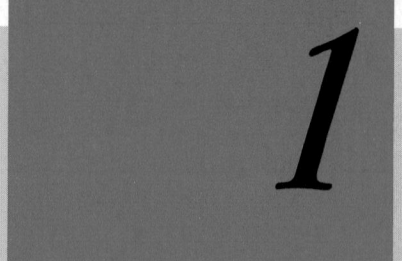

1 Nursing Process and Patient Teaching

The Nursing Process

The *nursing process* is a deliberate, problem-solving approach to meeting the health care and nursing needs of patients. It involves assessment (data collection), nursing diagnosis, planning, implementation, and evaluation, with subsequent modifications used as feedback mechanisms that promote the resolution of the nursing diagnoses. The process as a whole is cyclic, the steps being interrelated, interdependent, and recurrent.

Steps of the Nursing Process

A. *Assessment*—systematic collection of data to determine the patient's health status and to identify any actual or potential health problems. (Analysis of data is included as part of the assessment. For those who wish to emphasize its importance, analysis may be identified as a separate step of the nursing process.)
B. *Nursing Diagnosis*—identification of actual or potential health problems that are amenable to resolution by means of nursing actions.
C. *Planning*—development of goals and a plan of care designed to assist the patient in resolving the nursing diagnoses.
D. *Implementation*—actualization of the plan of care through nursing interventions or supervision of others to do the same.
E. *Evaluation*—determination of the patient's responses to the nursing interventions and of the extent to which the goals have been achieved.

Assessment

Assessment begins with the nurse's first encounter with the patient. It involves the systematic collection of data about the patient's nursing needs and the use of these data to formulate nursing diagnoses. Prehospital admission assessment is often conducted by nurses in physicians' offices, clinics, and outpatient departments. This assessment includes a nursing history and an appraisal of the patient's readiness for hospitalization or outpatient services. Any special instructions and preparation that the patient needs are given at this time.

A. The Nursing History (see details, p. 13)

1. Is carried out for the purpose of determining the patient's state of wellness or illness and is best accomplished as part of a planned interview.
2. Provides the nurse with the opportunity to collect data and also to convey interest, support, and understanding to the patient and to establish a relationship of mutual trust and respect.

B. The Physical Examination (see details, p. 18)

1. To determine the patient's physical alterations and limitations.
2. To determine the patient's assets, which may serve to offset his limitations.

C. Other Sources of Assessment Data

1. Patient's family and/or significant others.
2. Members of the health team.
3. Patient's health record.

Nursing Diagnosis

Those actual or potential health problems that are amenable to resolution by means of nursing actions.

1. Organize, analyze, synthesize, and summarize the collected data.
2. Identify the patient's health problem(s), its (their) particular characteristic(s) and etiology(ies).
3. State nursing diagnoses concisely and precisely.

Planning

See Example of a Nursing Care Plan, page 6.

1. Assign priorities to the nursing diagnoses. Highest priority is given to problems that are the most urgent and critical.
2. Establish goals for nursing interventions.
   a. Specify short-term, intermediate, and long-term goals as established by nurse and patient together.
   b. State goals in realistic and measurable terms.
3. Identify nursing interventions appropriate for goal attainment.
4. Establish expected-outcome criteria.
   a. State outcomes in terms of patient behaviors.
   b. Outcomes must be realistic and measurable.
   c. Identify critical time periods for the attainment of outcomes.
5. Formulate the nursing care plan (see sample nursing care plan, p. 6).
   a. Include nursing diagnoses in order of priority, goals, nursing interventions, outcome criteria, and critical time periods.
   b. Write entries precisely, concisely, and systematically.
   c. Keep the plan current and flexible to meet the patient's changing needs.
   d. Involve the patient, his family and/or significant others, nursing team members, other health team members, and community agencies in appropriate aspects of planning.

Implementation

1. Put the nursing care plan into action.
2. Coordinate the activities of the patient, his family and/ or significant others, nursing team members, and other health team members.
3. Delegate specific nursing interventions to other members of the nursing team, as appropriate.
   a. Consider the capabilities and limitations of the members of the nursing team.
   b. Supervise the performance of the nursing interventions.
4. Record the patient's responses to the nursing interventions.
   a. Record the responses precisely, concisely, and objectively.
   b. Recordings should be related to the nursing diagnoses.
   c. Include any additional pertinent assessment data.

Evaluation

1. Collect objective data.
2. Compare the patient's behavioral outcomes to the outcome criteria. Determine the extent to which the goals were achieved.
3. Include the patient, his family and/or significant others, nursing team members, and other health team members in the evaluation.
4. Identify alterations that need to be made in the goals and the nursing care plan.

Continuation of the Nursing Process

1. Continue all steps of the nursing process: assessment, nursing diagnosis, planning, implementation, and evaluation.
2. Continuous evaluation provides the means for maintaining the viability of the entire nursing process and for demonstrating accountability for the quality of nursing care rendered.

Health Education

Health education is an essential component of nursing care and is directed toward promotion, maintenance, and restoration of health, and toward adaptation to the residual effects of illness.

Objective:
To teach people to live life to its healthiest—that is, to strive toward achieving one's maximum health potential.

Principles of Teaching and Learning

1. The teaching–learning process requires the active involvement of both the teacher and the learner.
2. The desired outcome of the teaching–learning process is a change in the learner's behavior.
3. The teacher serves as a facilitator of learning.
4. Learning is facilitated by progressing from the simple to the complex and from the known to the unknown.
5. Learning is facilitated when the learner is aware of his progress toward the learning goals.

Variables That Affect Learning Readiness

A. Physical Readiness

1. Physical distress that absorbs the patient's attention prevents effective learning.
2. Readiness to learn can be promoted by alleviating or at least minimizing as much as possible the patient's physical distress.

B. Emotional Readiness

1. Motivation to learn depends upon
   a. Acceptance of the illness or acceptance of the fact that illness is a threat.
   b. Recognition of the need to learn.
   c. Values related to social and cultural background.
   d. A therapeutic regimen compatible with the patient's life-style or altered life-style.
2. Motivation to learn can be promoted by
   a. Creating a warm, accepting, positive atmosphere.
   b. Encouraging the patient to participate in the establishment of acceptable, realistic, attainable learning goals.
   c. Providing feedback about progress, that is, positive reinforcement when the patient is successful, constructive criticism when he is unsuccessful.

C. Experiential Readiness

1. The patient's previous experiences, especially learning experiences and experiences with illness and crisis, affect the learning process.
   a. Success in past learning experiences usually serves to motivate future learning.
   b. Failure in past learning experiences often causes the learner to be hesitant to make new attempts to learn; this learner must be helped to gain confidence in his ability to learn.
2. Learning is dependent upon attainment of those behaviors that are prerequisites to the specific learning task; for example, knowledge of the basics of normal nutrition is a prerequisite to understanding a special diet.

The Learning Atmosphere

1. The physical environment should be conducive to learning: quiet, uninterrupted, and comfortable. Consider the following variables:
   a. Temperature
   b. Lighting
   c. Noise level
   d. Traffic
   e. Seating facilities and arrangement
2. The time of the teaching–learning session should be scheduled to meet the patient's needs.
   a. Encourage the patient and his family to participate in the scheduling of the teaching–learning session.
   b. Select a time when the patient is most alert, most comfortable, and least fatigued.
   c. Select a time when the patient is not anticipating immediate diagnostic or therapeutic procedures.
   d. Select a time when family members who are to be included in the teaching plan are available.

Teaching Strategies

Learning is facilitated by selecting teaching techniques and methods that are most appropriate to meet the individual patient's needs.

Example of a Nursing Care Plan

Mr. John Preston, a 52-year-old businessman, was admitted to the hospital with a diagnosis of angina pectoris. He stated that he had experienced substernal chest pain and weakness in his arms and hands after having lunch with a business associate. The pain had lessened by the time he arrived at the hospital. The nursing history revealed that he had been hospitalized 5 months previously with the same complaints and had been told by his physician to go to the emergency department if the pain ever recurred. He had been placed on a low-fat diet and had stopped smoking. Physical examination revealed that Mr. Preston's vital signs were within normal ranges and that his chest pain had been relieved with nitroglycerin. He stated that he had feared he was having a "heart attack" until his pain subsided and until he was told that his ECG was normal. He verbalized that he wanted to find out how he could prevent the attacks of pain in the future. The physician's requests upon admission included activity as tolerated, low-cholesterol diet, and nitroglycerin 0.4 mg. ($\frac{1}{150}$ gr.) sublingually prn.

Nursing Diagnosis: Pain related to myocardial ischemia.

Goals:
Short-term: Relief of pain.
Long-term: Altered life-style to include measures that decrease myocardial oxygen demands.
            Compliance with therapeutic regimen.

Nursing Interventions	Outcome Criteria	Critical Time*	Outcome
Continue assessment of cardiac function:			
Monitor blood pressure (BP), pulse (P), respirations (R) q. 4 hr.	BP, P, R remain within normal limits.	24 hr.	BP: stable at 116–122/72–84. P: stable at 68–82. R: stable at 16–20.
Assess frequency of chest pain and precipitating events.	Free of chest pain.	24 hr.	Denies chest pain; able to walk length of hall, eat meals, and visit with family and friends without chest discomfort.
Encourage food and fluid intake that promotes normal nutrition, digestion, and elimination and that does not precipitate chest pain: light, regular meals; foods low in cholesterol; 1500–2000 ml. fluid/day.	Tolerates dietary regimen. Absence of chest pain after meals. Maintains normal bowel elimination. Intake of 1500–2000 ml. fluid/day.	48 hr.	Denies chest pain after meals; no constipation or diarrhea; fluid intake 1700–2100 ml./day.
Request consultation with dietitian—for diet teaching.	Identifies foods low in cholesterol and those foods that are to be avoided. Selects well-balanced diet within prescribed restrictions.	48 hr.	Selects and eats a balanced diet consisting of foods low in cholesterol; dietitian reviewed diet restrictions with patient and wife; wife counseled in meal planning.
Encourage alterations in activities and exercise that are necessary to prevent episodes of anginal pain.	Identifies activities and exercises that could precipitate chest pain: those that require sudden bursts of activity and heavy effort. Identifies emotionally stressful situations; explains the necessity for alternating periods of activity with periods of rest.	3 days	Patient and wife have identified activities and situations that should be avoided; patient and wife have studied their usual daily routine and have made plans to alter the routine to allow for rest periods; teenage son has volunteered to assist with strenuous home-maintenance chores.
Teaching: nitroglycerin regimen.	(See teaching plan, p. 8)		

* These times have not been standardized, but are individualized according to the patient's needs.

A. Lecture

1. Is most useful in teaching groups of patients who share the same learning needs.
2. Should always be accompanied by discussion, which allows the individual patient to
   a. Express his feelings and concerns.
   b. Ask questions.
   c. Clarify information.
3. Emphasize important (key) points; repeat these points to reinforce their importance.

B. Group Discussion

1. Is most useful for patients who relate well in groups.
2. Allows patients to experience feelings of security through being a member of a group of patients with similar problems or learning needs.
3. Provides patients with the opportunity to gain support, assistance, and encouragement from group members.

C. Demonstration and Practice

1. Are most useful when skills are to be learned.
2. Ample opportunity must be provided for practice sessions.
3. Equipment should be the same as that which the patient will use after leaving the hospital.

D. Teaching Aids

1. Are useful to supplement the resources of the nurse in helping the patient to learn.
2. Include books, pamphlets, pictures, films, slides, tapes, and models.
3. Must be reviewed prior to presentation to ensure that they are appropriate for meeting the patient's individual learning needs.

E. Reinforcement and Follow-up

1. Allow ample time for the patient to learn and to have his learning reinforced.
2. Follow-up sessions promote the patient's confidence in his ability to retain his newly learned behaviors.
3. It is imperative to evaluate the patient's progress and to plan additional teaching sessions as necessary.
4. Follow-up sessions after discharge may be needed to assist the patient in transferring what he has learned in the hospital to his home setting.

The Nursing Process in Patient Teaching

The teaching–learning process is an integral part of the nursing process. With a focus on learning and with regard for the principles, variables, techniques, and strategies of teaching and learning, the steps of the nursing process—assessment, nursing diagnosis, planning, implementation, and evaluation—are used for the purpose of meeting the teaching and learning needs of the patient and his family.

Assessment

1. Assess the patient's learning needs and his physical, emotional, and experiential readiness for health education.
   a. What are his health beliefs and behaviors?
   b. What psychosocial adaptations is he making?
   c. Is he ready to learn?
      (1) Is he able to learn these behaviors?
      (2) What are his expectations?
      (3) What additional information is needed about him?
2. Assess the patient's need for education and preparation related to the self-care activities for which he will be responsible after discharge.
3. Use appropriate assessment guides to facilitate data collection.
   Adapt such guides to the individual responses, problems, and needs of the patient.

Nursing Diagnosis

Formulate nursing diagnoses that relate to the patient's learning needs.

1. Organize, analyze, synthesize, and summarize the collected data.
2. Identify the patient's learning need(s), its (their) particular characteristic(s) and etiology(ies).
3. State nursing diagnoses concisely and precisely.

Planning

1. Assign priority to the nursing diagnoses.
2. Specify the short-term, intermediate, and long-term learning goals established by both the nurse and patient.
3. Identify teaching actions appropriate for goal attainment.
4. Establish expected-outcome criteria.
5. Identify critical time periods for the attainment of outcomes.
6. Develop a written teaching plan (see sample teaching plan, p. 8).
   a. Include diagnoses (in order of priority), goals, teaching strategies, outcome criteria, and critical time periods.
   b. Write entries precisely, concisely, and systematically.
   c. Include a topical outline of the information to be presented.
   d. Select appropriate teaching techniques and methods.
   e. Keep the plan current and flexible to meet the patient's changing learning needs.
7. Involve the patient, his family and/or significant others, nursing team members, and other health team members in all aspects of planning.

Implementation

1. Put the teaching plan into action.
2. Know the material to be presented.
3. Provide an atmosphere conducive to learning.
4. Use language the patient can understand.
5. Use appropriate teaching techniques and methods.
6. Use the same equipment that the patient will use after discharge.
7. Encourage the patient and his family to participate actively in learning.
8. Coordinate the activities of the patient, his family and/or significant others, nursing team members, and other health team members.
9. Emphasize the importance of learning to care for self after discharge.
10. Record the patient's responses to the teaching actions.

Example of a Teaching Plan *(For background information see Nursing Care Plan example, p. 6)*

Assessment of Mr. Preston's teaching and learning needs revealed the following: ● Basic knowledge about the etiology and pathology of angina pectoris ● Definitive plans for adherence to the dietary regimen ● Definitive plans for alteration of life-style to attempt to prevent episodes of anginal pain ● Inadequate knowledge about nitroglycerin therapy regimen.

Nursing Diagnosis: Potential altered health maintenance related to lack of knowledge of nitroglycerin therapy regimen.

Goals:
Short-term: Describe action, use, and correct administration of nitroglycerin.
Long-term: Complies with nitroglycerin therapy regimen.

Teaching Interventions	Outcome Criteria	Critical Time*	Outcome
Explain and discuss the action and use of nitroglycerin for treatment and prevention of anginal episodes.	Explains in his own words the action and use of nitroglycerin to treat anginal episodes.	3 days	Stated explanation accurately
	Identifies activities and exercises prior to which nitroglycerin should be taken for its prophylactic effects.	3 days	Accurately identified activities and exercises.
Explain and discuss the necessity for keeping a record of his use of nitroglycerin and providing the physician with this record.	Explains in his own words the necessity for recording the following data and reporting to his physician: Date and time of drug use Factors that precipitated pain Time required for relief of pain Amount of drug taken	3 days	Stated explanation accurately.
Explain and discuss the need to have nitroglycerin available at all times and the precautions to take to maintain its potency.	Explains in his own words the necessity to carry nitroglycerin with him at all times and the following precautions to take: Keep nitroglycerin in tightly capped, dark-colored glass bottle ("fresh" nitroglycerin produces a burning or tingling sensation under the tongue). Avoid carrying bottle in contact with body. Discard tablets after 6 months.	3 days	Stated explanation accurately.
Explain and discuss the procedure for use of nitroglycerin.	Explains in his own words the correct procedure for use of nitroglycerin: Place tablet under the tongue at first sign of chest discomfort. Rest in the upright position until all pain subsides. Take an additional tablet in 3 to 5 minutes. If pain is not relieved after the second tablet is taken, or if it recurs after a short interval, go to the nearest emergency facility.	3 days	Stated explanation accurately.
	Takes nitroglycerin according to procedure.	After discharge	
Encourage to wear Medic Alert bracelet and carry medication identification on his person.	Wears Medic Alert bracelet.	3 days	Obtained Medic Alert bracelet and wears it at all times.
	Carries medication identification on his person.	3 days	Filled out medication identification card and placed it in a visible place in his wallet.
Explain and discuss the necessity for keeping all physician appointments.	Explains in his own words the importance of keeping all appointments with physician.	3 days	Stated explanation accurately.
	Keeps all appointments with physician.	After discharge	

* These times have not been standardized, but are individualized according to the patient's needs.

Evaluation

1. Collect objective data.
   a. Observe the patient.
   b. Ask questions to determine if the patient understands.
   c. Use rating scales, checklists, anecdotal notes, and written tests when appropriate.
2. Compare the patient's behavioral outcomes with the outcome criteria. Determine the extent to which the goals were achieved.
3. Include the patient, his family and/or significant others, nursing team members, and other health team members in the evaluation.
4. Identify alterations that need to be made in the teaching plan.
5. Make referrals to appropriate resource persons or agencies for reinforcement of learning after discharge.
6. Continue all steps of the teaching–learning process: assessment, nursing diagnosis, planning, implementation, and evaluation.

Bibliography

Nursing Process

Books

Alfaro R. Applying Nursing Diagnoses and Nursing Process: A Step-by-Step Guide. Philadelphia, JB Lippincott, 1989

Carpenito LJ. Handbook of Nursing Diagnosis 1989–90. Philadelphia, JB Lippincott, 1989

Carpenito LJ. Nursing Diagnosis: Application to Clinical Practice. Philadelphia, JB Lippincott, 1989

Carroll–Johnson RM (ed). Classification of Nursing Diagnoses. Proceedings of the Eighth Conference North American Nursing Diagnosis Association. Philadelphia, JB Lippincott, 1989

Fitzpatrick JJ and Whall AL. Conceptual Models of Nursing: Analysis and Application. Norwalk, CT, Appleton and Lange, 1989

Gordon M. Manual of Nursing Diagnosis 1988–1989. St. Louis, CV Mosby, 1989

Gordon M. Nursing Diagnosis: Process and Application. New York, McGraw–Hill, 1987

Guzzeta CE et al. Clinical Assessment Tools for Use With Nursing Diagnoses. St. Louis, CV Mosby, 1989

McFarland GK and McFarlane EA. Nursing Diagnosis & Intervention: Planning for Patient Care. St. Louis, CV Mosby, 1989

Sundeen SJ et al. Nurse–Client Interaction: Implementing the Nursing Process. St. Louis, CV Mosby, 1989

Tucker SM. Patient Care Standards: Nursing Process, Diagnosis, and Outcome. St. Louis, CV Mosby, 1988

Wesorick B. Standards of Nursing Care: A Model for Clinical Practice. Philadelphia, JB Lippincott, 1989

Yura H and Walsh MB. The Nursing Process: Assessing, Planning, Implementing, Evaluating. Norwalk, CT, Appleton and Lange, 1988

Journals

Berry KN. Let's create diagnoses psych nurses can use. Am J Nurs 1987 May; 87(5):707–708

Clough JG and Hall K. Writing institutional criteria sets for nursing diagnoses: From idea to implementation. J Nurs Qual Assur 1987 Feb; 1(2):31–42

Creason NS. How do we define our diagnoses? Am J Nurs 1987 Feb; 87(2): 230–231

Curry K et al. Appropriate use of hospital monitoring capabilities. Nurs Manage 1989 May; 20(5):112I, 112L, 112P

Fitzpatrick JJ. Translating nursing diagnosis into ICD code. Am J Nurs 1989 Apr; 89(4):493–495

Herberth L and Gosnell DJ. Nursing diagnosis for oncology nursing practice. Cancer Nurs 1987 Feb; 10(1): 41–51

Johnson CF and Hales LW. Nursing diagnosis anyone? Do staff nurses use nursing diagnosis effectively? J Contin Educ Nurs 1989 Jan–Feb; 20(1):30–35

Kanar RJ. Standards of nursing practice assessed through the application of the nursing process. J Nurs Qual Assur 1987 Feb; 1(2):72–78

Krenz M, Karlik B, and Kiniry S. A nursing diagnosis based model: Guiding nursing practice. J Nurs Adm 1989; 19(5):32–36

Maas ML. Nursing diagnoses in a professional model of nursing: Keystone for effective nursing administration. J Nurs Adm 1986 Dec; 16(12):39–42

Moss AR. Determinants of patient care: Nursing process or nursing attitudes? J Adv Nurs 1988 Sep; 13(5):615–620

North American Nursing Diagnosis Association: 21 new diagnoses and a taxonomy. Am J Nurs 1986 Dec; 86(12):1414–1415

Popkiss-Vawter S et al. Should we diagnose strengths? Am J Nurs 1987 Sep; 87(9):1211–1212,1216

Rantz M and Miller TV. How diagnoses are changing in long-term care. Am J Nurs 1987 Mar; 87(3):360–361

Roberts SL. Physiologic nursing diagnoses are necessary and appropriate for critical care. Focus Crit Care 1988 Oct; 15(5):42–49

Santo-Novak DA. Seven keys to assessing the elderly. Nursing 1988 Aug; 18(8): 60–63

Schamel K. How to assess the patient on long-term care. RN 1987 Oct; 50(10): 65–68

Spatt L. Developing complex care plans: The nursing guide. Dimens Crit Care Nurs 1988 Jul–Aug; 7(4):236–242

Westfall UE. Standards of practice: Nursing values made visible. J Nurs Qual Assur 1987 Feb; 1(2):21–30

Woodtli A. Identification of nursing diagnoses and defining characteristics: Two research models. Res Nurs Health 1988 Dec; 11(6):399–406

Patient Teaching

Books

Haggard A. Handbook of Patient Education. Rockville, MD, Aspen Publishers, 1989

Pender NJ. Health Promotion in Nursing Practice. Norwalk, CT, Appleton and Lange, 1987

Redman B. The Process of Patient Education. St. Louis, CV Mosby, 1988

Journals

Armstrong ML. Orchestrating the process of patient education: Methods and approaches. Nurs Clin North Am 1989 Sep; 24(3):597–604

Bailey-Allen AM. Who is responsible for patient teaching? Orthop Nurs 1989 Jan–Feb; 8(1):53–54

Baker K, Kuhlmann T and Magliaro BL. Homeward bound. Discharge teaching for parents of newborns with special needs. Nurs Clin North Am 1989 Sep; 24(3):655–664

Barr WJ. Teaching patients with life-threatening illnesses. Nurs Clin North Am 1989 Sep; 24(3):639–644

Barron S. Documentation of patient education. Patient Educ Couns 1987 Feb; 9(1):81–85

Breeze W. Educational readiness in hospitalized adults. Today's OR Nurse 1987 Jul; 9(7):28–32

Brillhart B and Stewart A. Education as the key to rehabilitation. Nurs Clin North Am 1989 Sep; 24(3):675–680

Criteria for the development of health promotion and education programs. Am J Public Health 1987 Jan; 77(1): 89–92

DeMuth JS. Patient teaching in the ambulatory setting. Nurs Clin North Am 1989 Sep; 24(3):645–654

Dobberstein K. Computer-assisted patient ed. Am J Nurs 1987 May; 87(5): 697

Gessner BA. Adult education: The cornerstone of patient teaching. Nurs Clin North Am 1989 Sep; 24(3):589–595

Hicks S. The nurse and the patient: Partners in education. Can Crit Care Nurs J 1987 Sep–Oct; 4(3):18–22

Higgins MG. Learning style assessment: A new patient teaching tool? J Nurs Staff Dev 1988 Winter; 4(1):14–18

Hussey LC and Gilliland K. Compliance, low literacy, and locus of control. Nurs Clin North Am 1989 Sep; 24(3):605–611

Johnson EA and Jackson JE. Teaching the home care client. Nurs Clin North Am 1989 Sep; 24(3):687–693

Kick E. Patient teaching for elders. Nurs Clin North Am 1989 Sep; 24(3):681–686

Lemphers C. Adult education strategies important for nurses. AARN News Lett 1989 Jan; 45(1):14–15

Marchiondo K and Kipp C. Establishing a standardized patient education program. Crit Care Nurse 1987 May–Jun; 7(3):58, 60–64, 66

Oberst MT. Perspectives on research in patient teaching. Nurs Clin North Am 1989 Sep; 24(3):621–628

Ruzicki DA. Realistically meeting the educational needs of hospitalized acute and short-stay patients. Nurs Clin North Am 1989 Sep; 24(3):629–637

Siegel H. Nurses improve hospital efficiency through a risk assessment model at admission. Nurs Manage 1988 Oct; 19(10):38–40, 42, 44, 46

Smith CE. Overview of patient education: Opportunities and challenges for the twenty-first century. Nurs Clin North Am 1989 Sep; 24(3):583–587

Smith CE. Patient teaching: It's the law. Nursing '87 1987 Jul; 17(7):67–68

Tripp–Reimer T and Afifi LA. Cross-cultural perspectives on patient teaching. Nurs Clin North Am 1989 Sep; 24(3):613–619

Data Collection and History Taking

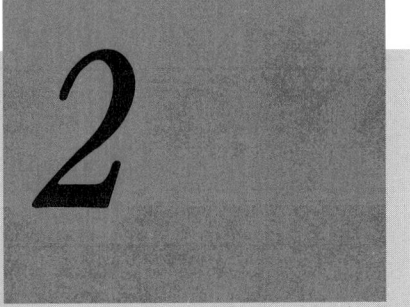

2

Data Collection

Purpose

1. Data collection is the first step in the process of defining problems.
2. A thorough and accurate assessment of a patient's problems or condition depends on the completeness and accuracy of the data collected.

Types of Data Collected

A. The Patient's History (see details, p. 13)

1. Is elicited in an interview.
2. The history, in final written form, logically presents the *patient's views* of:
   a. His health problems
   b. General health condition
   c. Past medical history
   d. Family health history
   e. A profile of the patient's personal and social life and well-being
3. The patient history will also reveal what the patient knows about his health, what is important in terms of health care, and expectations of the health care being sought.
   This may be supplemented by information from the patient's hospital record, conversations with other care-givers, significant others, parents (in the case of children and infants), or consultants.
4. The patient history is always *subjective* information in that it is presented from the point of view of the person reporting to the interviewer rather than directly observed by the interviewer.

B. The Physical Examination (see details, Chap. 3)— is performed by the practitioner for the following purposes:

1. To confirm the patient's history.
2. To observe any findings not reported in the history.
3. To obtain *objective* information about the individual's health state and/or status of a health problem.
   Objective information is that body of data about a person that can be perceived by another person.

C. Laboratory Data—from test results

It is important to know that laboratory data constitute another source of *objective data* that are important in assessing many health problems and conditions; these must be considered by all nurses engaged in caring for and understanding patients.

Principles of Data Collection

1. All data collection should be well-organized and should follow a format that promotes thoroughness.
2. There is no room for bias in data collection, since the practitioner's mind must be open to clues and cues that might otherwise be missed.
3. Understanding the techniques of interviewing is basic to collecting accurate data in the patient's history and to establishing the basis for a working relationship with the patient.
4. Information gathered must be organized and recorded so that it has meaning for members of the health care team and can guide patient assessment and care.

Recording the Data Gathered

General Guidelines

1. Keep in mind the purpose of recording the information and the audience for whom it is intended. These serve to guide the form and content of the record.
2. Remember that the patient's record is a legal document.
   The record must present the information about the patient as completely, concisely, and accurately as possible, without unnecessary duplication of material.
3. Avoid redundancy.
   Redundancy obscures important information and makes careful reading of the record unnecessarily time-consuming. As a result, the record is not read carefully.

General Principles

1. *When to record*
   As soon as the information is gathered—to minimize omission and distortion of facts.
2. *Organization*
   Information must be organized and recorded systematically. (This applies to complete history, physical examination, or progress notes.)

a. The history, or subjective information, is recorded first.
b. Then the physical examination, or objective data, is recorded.
c. From a systematic recording of the facts must stem a logical assessment of the subjective and objective data.
d. Therefore, facts must be reported so that their meaning is clear and they tell a connected story.

3. *Detail*
   Describe the data gathered, using the appropriate vocabulary.
4. *Language*
   a. The written record must be succinct, yet understandable to the reader.
   b. Avoid using abbreviations.
5. *Legal considerations*
   a. Since the patient's record is a legal document, facts must be identified and stated precisely and objectively.
   b. Both inaccuracy and interpretation must be avoided.
   c. Assessment or judgment can be made only after facts are obtained and recorded with great care.
   d. The document must be signed and dated.
6. *Ethical considerations*
   a. The patient should be fully informed of all aspects of the data-collection process.
   b. The patient's decision to participate in the data collection process must be made freely.
   c. The interview should be conducted in private, and confidentiality must be maintained.

Recording the History

(The general principles listed above apply to recording the history.)
1. The present illness must be recorded chronologically, beginning with the onset of the problem.
   Often it is helpful to think of a beginning phrase such as "The patient was well until. . . ." Each paragraph should then describe events in sequence up to the time that the patient is being interviewed.
2. Quantify anything related to measurement.
   For example: "The patient has *frequent* headaches" is less accurate than "The patient has an average of 3 headaches a week."

Recording the Physical Examination

(It is important to follow the above principles.) Other specific guidelines include the following:
1. Describe any abnormality in detail.
2. Carefully describe a normal finding in conditions where one might expect the normal to be abnormal.
   For instance, in the patient with hypertension, it would be important to report the absence of hemorrhages and exudates in the fundoscopic examination report.
3. If there are any laboratory results, they are recorded after the physical examination and before the assessment and plan.

Progress Notes

1. Progress notes are records of the patient's health status from visit to visit, day to day, or shift to shift, as the case may be.
2. They are usually written in relation to a specific problem or condition and report the relevant subjective (history) and objective (physical examination and laboratory results) data that bring the record up to date.
3. Progress notes also include an assessment of the data and a plan dealing with the problem.
   (The Problem Oriented Medical Record format developed by Dr. Lawrence Weed is an extremely useful and instructive guide in organizing and recording the initial data base and the progress notes.)

The Problem Oriented Record (POR)

A *problem oriented record* is a patient's health record organized so that specific problems are defined, numbered, and then referred to by number throughout the record. Problems are identified and numbered after the initial data base is collected.

Components of the POR

These may vary according to the particular setting in which the system is used. However, every system includes the following:

A. Initial Data Base

Consists of:
1. The patient's comprehensive health history
2. A complete physical examination
3. Nursing assessment
4. Patient profiles from other members of the health team
5. Available laboratory and radiologic data

B. Problem List

1. Consists of a numbered list of medical, social, environmental, and psychological problems and past problems derived from the initial data base.
2. Includes active and inactive problems, date of onset, and date of resolution when applicable.
   a. Often this list appears at the very beginning of the record and serves as an index.
   b. A number is never used twice even though new problems arise, some old ones are resolved, or several problems are found to be related to one common problem.
3. It is important to remember that the numbered problem list should serve as an index to the record, so that information can be systematically ordered around a problem and not get lost or be misinterpreted as the volume of the record grows in the course of many visits.

C. Progress Notes

See Sample Progress Note below.
1. Organization of the progress note varies, but the basic format remains the same.
2. The note begins with the problem and its number and then continues as follows:
   S = *Subjective* data (history, consultation) concerning the problem and covering the time interval since the last entry.
   O = *Objective data* (physical examination, laboratory reports) concerning the problem and covering the same time period.
   A = *Assessment* of the S and the O. Includes, as appropriate, statements about probable etiology; course of the problem; the patient's response to therapy and his coping ability; general diagnostic, therapeutic, and health education plans; and a rationale for the entire plan. It should include a statement

Sample Progress Note

Hypertension

S. The patient has felt well since he was seen 3 months ago. He has had no headaches, no visual or gastrointestinal problems, no chest pain or palpitations, no shortness of breath. His activity is unchanged, he sleeps on one pillow, has no nocturia or ankle swelling. He is taking his medications, knows their names and dosages. Drinks orange juice with fluid pill qd. He is following a diet that has "no added" salt, drinks 5 beers a week; lunchmeat sandwiches for lunch. He thinks he is gaining weight—his "clothes are tighter."

O. P 72 regular
Wt 82.5 kg. (182 pounds)
BP 148/95 right arm lying
140/100 right arm standing

Respiratory: Chest expands symmetrically; fremitus (perceptible vibration) normal bilaterally; bronchovesicular sounds present, no adventitious (unnatural) sounds.

Cardiovascular: No heaves or thrills; point of maximal impulse (PMI) at 5th intercostal space in midclavicular line; normal sinus rhythm without murmurs, gallops, or extrasystoles; trace of pedal edema.

A. BP is fairly well controlled. Weight is up 2.3 kg. (5 pounds). The patient is taking his medication. However, his diet contains a lot of sodium, even though none is "added." If he can cut out some of the high-salt foods and lose 2.3–4.5 kg. (5–10 pounds), his pressure will no doubt be under control. He seems motivated to lose some weight, since his clothes are tighter. He needs to know about sodium content of food, and his wife needs instruction, too, since she does the shopping. Will continue the same medications and try having the patient lose weight to bring BP under better control. The patient comprehends the consequences of uncontrolled hypertension and the need for sustained weight control and medical follow-up. His wife sounds very supportive. Patient will need routine yearly blood work and cardiogram by next visit.

P. 1. Diet instruction for patient and wife. Patient will call to suggest a convenient time and will set up appointment then.
2. Continue same medications: methyldopa 250 mg. tid, hydrochlorothiazide 50 mg. qd with dietary K^+ supplement.
3. Return visit in 3 months to check BP and weight.
4. Blood work before next visit (Na^+, K^+, CO_2, urea-N, glucose, creatinine).
5. Electrocardiogram before next visit.

I. Patient given the following instructions:
1. Dietitian's name and telephone number to make appointment for diet instruction.
2. Prescriptions for medications.
3. Appointment for return visit
4. Prescription for blood work and electrocardiogram

about the patient's participation in planning and his reaction to the plan.

P = *Plan*—This is a statement *specifying* what is to be done regarding the problem, who is to do it, and when it is to be done. A timetable is provided when possible. The plan stems directly from the rationale in the assessment and may include any or all of the following:
(1) *Diagnostic plan*—States what is to be done to make the data base more complete.
(2) *Therapeutic plan*—Indicates projected methods for curing, improving, or palliating the patient's problem.
(3) *Health education plan*—outlines content of health teaching concerning the problem and the diagnostic and/or therapeutic plan.

I = *Intervention*—Includes nursing actions done for or with the patient.

E = *Evaluation*—Patient outcomes are used as the basis for evaluation. The evaluation may appear in the next progress note because more time is needed to observe the patient's response to nursing interventions.

Computer Documentation

Purpose
1. Documentation of nursing care
2. Standardization of assessment and nursing care plans
3. Communication and information transferral
4. Facilitation of clinical and statistical data retrieval

General Guidelines
1. Computers are compatible with the problem oriented record system.
2. Computers do not replace nursing care and the nursing process—they are facilitators of care.
3. Computers facilitate the recording of the nursing care plan, but they do not exclude individualization of the plan.
4. The information processed and displayed by computers is only as reliable and as valuable as the data that have been entered into the computer.

The Patient History

General Principles

1. The first step in caring for a patient and in soliciting his active cooperation is to gather a careful and complete history.
   a. In *all* patient concerns and problems, an accurate history is the foundation on which data collection and the process of assessment are based.
   b. The comprehensiveness of the history elicited will depend on the information available in the patient's record.
2. Time spent early in the nurse–patient relationship gathering detailed information about what the patient knows, thinks, and feels about his problems will prevent time-consuming errors and misunderstandings later.
3. Skill in interviewing will affect both the accuracy of information elicited and the quality of the relationship established with the patient.
   This point cannot be overemphasized; the reader

is encouraged to consult other sources for detailed discussion of techniques of health interviewing.
4. The purpose of the interview is to encourage an interchange of information between the patient and the nurse.
The patient must feel that his words are understood and that his concerns are being heard and dealt with sensitively.

Interviewing Techniques

1. Provide privacy for the patient in as quiet a place as possible and see that he is comfortable.
2. Begin the interview with a courteous greeting and an introduction. Explain who you are and why you are there.
3. Be sure that facial expressions, body movements, and tone of voice are pleasant, unhurried, and nonevaluative, and that they convey the attitude of a sensitive listener, so that the patient will feel free to express his thoughts and feelings.
4. Avoid reassuring the patient prematurely (before you have adequate information about the problem). This only serves to cut off discussion; the patient may then be unwilling to bring up a problem causing concern.
5. At times a patient gives cues or suggests information, but does not tell enough. It may be necessary to probe for more information in order to obtain a thorough history; the patient must realize that this is done for his benefit.
6. Guide the interview so that the necessary information is obtained, without cutting off discussion. Controlling the rambling patient is often difficult, but with practice, it can be done skillfully, without jeopardizing the quality of the information gained.

Identifying Information

A. Purposes

1. To eliminate confusion about the patient's identity; to obtain the information required for contacting him if the need arises.
2. To provide an introduction to the patient and some indication of his habits, life-style, and beliefs, which may be explored in greater depth in the personal and social history.
3. To initiate a relationship based on recognition of the importance of the informant's role in sharing in the care of the patient (when this is the case).

B. Types of Information Needed

1. Date and time
2. Patient's name, address, telephone number, race, religion, birthdate, and age
3. Name of referring practitioner
4. Insurance data
5. Name of informant—the patient may be the person giving this history, if not, record the name, address, telephone number, and relationship to the patient of the person giving the history
6. Accuracy and reliability of informant—this is a judgment based on the consistency of responses to questions and on a comparison of information in the history with your own observations in the physical examination

C. Method of Collecting Data

1. Careful interviewing of the patient or his "care person" will provide most of the information.
2. The patient's hospital or clinic record may also be a valuable source.

3. Repeat information when necessary to verify accuracy (e.g., to ensure that there has been no change in address or telephone number).
4. Assume a direct and courteous manner.
5. Explain the reasons why the information is needed— to help put the patient at ease.

Chief Complaint

A. Purposes

1. To allow the patient to describe his own problems and expectations with little or no direction from the interviewer.
2. To identify the overriding problem for which the person is seeking help.
   a. Adults with chronic conditions often have numerous complaints.
   b. If possible, focus on a single problem or concern—the one most important to the patient.
3. To identify the patient's feelings about his symptoms. The patient may show fear, guilt, or defensiveness in this first statement.

B. Types of Information Needed

The patient's primary problem(s) or concern in his own words. A statement describing the duration of the complaint.

C. Method of Collecting Data

1. Ask the patient a direct question, for example, "How may I help you?" or "For what reason have you come to the hospital (clinic, etc.)?"
2. Avoid confusing questions, for example, "What brings you here?" ("The bus.") or "Why are you here?" ("That's what I came to find out.")
3. Ask how long the concern or problem has been present. If necessary, establish the time of onset precisely by offering such clues as "Did you feel this way a month (6 months or 2 years) ago?"
4. Let the patient speak freely without offering your opinion until he has had an opportunity to identify the problem as clearly as possible.
5. Write down what the patient says, using quotation marks to identify his words.

History of Present Illness

A. Purposes

1. To amplify the description of the chief complaint and to clarify its relationship to other symptoms and events.
2. To carefully describe a symptom or problem that may be a clue to future diagnosis.

B. Types of Information Needed

1. A *detailed chronological* picture beginning with the time the patient was last well (or, in the case of a problem with an acute onset, the patient's condition just prior to the onset of the problem) and ending with a description of the patient's current condition.
2. If there is more than one important problem, each is described in a separate, chronologically organized paragraph in the written history of present illness.
3. The outline for reporting the present illness will vary with each case.

C. Method of Collecting Data

1. For each problem investigate the following:
   a. Quality (e.g., sharp, dull, knife-like—referring to pain)
   b. Quantity (e.g., ½ cup sputum)

c. Location of symptoms, intensity, periodicity (e.g., epigastric area; daily; after meals)
d. Aggravating and alleviating factors (e.g., medications, prescribed and over-the-counter; rest; diet)
e. Associated phenomena (e.g., shortness of breath)

2. Date of onset of the problem as accurately as possible, since chronology is of the utmost importance (see Chief Complaint, p. 14).
3. Describe the character of the symptoms and state whether they have changed over time.
4. In the case of acute infections, inquire about possible exposure or an incubation period.
5. When the present illness has been characterized by attacks separated by free intervals, obtain the history of a typical attack:
   Onset, duration, and associated symptoms—pain; fever; chills; relation to any activity, either physical or emotional, or to such factors as diet, medication, etc.
6. In both acute and chronic illnesses, note whether and when the patient stopped working and/or went to bed.
7. Get the patient's subjective appraisal of whether the symptom or problem is getting better or worse.
8. When a particular organ or system is disturbed, ask for a review of that system and related systems so that important negative and positive information may be included in the written history.
   For instance, if a patient complains of chest pain, ask about both the respiratory and cardiac systems, as well as the musculoskeletal history of the chest.
9. Questioning may reveal that other systems must also be reviewed.
10. Ask about previous treatment, including medications, prescribing physician or practitioner, and place where treatment was obtained (name of hospital, clinic, etc.).
11. At the end, review the chronology and specifics with the patient and ask him to affirm or correct the information.
12. Organize the information for recording or presentation.

Past Medical History

A. Purposes

1. To determine any change in the patient's normal patterns of living that may or may not be caused by illness.
2. To identify clues that may aid in diagnosing the present illness.
3. To participate in gathering and recording information that may be helpful in making a diagnosis, even though the nurse may not have the final responsibility for diagnosing the patient's particular problem.

B. Types of Information Needed

1. *General health and strength*—sleeping patterns, appetite, stability of weight, usual activities.
2. *Acute infectious diseases*—measles, mumps, whooping cough, chickenpox, pneumonia, pleurisy, tuberculosis, scarlet fever, acute rheumatic fever, rheumatic heart disease, tonsillitis, hepatitis, polio, sexually transmitted disease, tropical or parasitic diseases, any other acute infectious problem the patient describes.
3. *Immunization*—polio, diphtheria, pertussis, tetanus, influenza, last PPD or other skin test, any abnormal or unusual reactions. Give date when possible.
4. *Operation*—indications, diagnosis, dates, hospital, surgeon, complications.
5. *Previous hospitalizations*—physician, hospital date (year), diagnosis, treatment.

6. *Injuries*—type; resulting disabilities.
7. *Major illnesses* (any prolonged illnesses not requiring hospitalization)—dates, symptoms, course, treatment.
8. *Allergies* (may appear in review of systems)—asthma, hay fever, hives, food allergies, drug reactions, previous treatment with penicillin and any reactions.
9. *Obstetrical history* (may appear in review of systems)
   a. Pregnancies, miscarriages, abortions.
   b. Describe course of pregnancy, labor, and delivery; date, place of delivery.
10. *Psychiatric history* (may appear in review of systems)—treatment by a psychiatrist or psychologist, indications, date, place, medications for "nerves."

C. Method of Collecting Data

1. Begin by explaining the purpose and type of questions you will be asking; for example, "I am now going to ask you some questions about your past health."
2. Explain that these questions are important in order to obtain an accurate picture of all the events that affected or that *did not* affect the patient's health in the past.
3. Use direct questions; for example, "How would you describe your general health?" and then proceed with more specific queries, such as "Has your weight been stable over the past 5 years?"

Family History

A. Purposes

1. To present a picture of the patient's family health, including specifically that of grandparents, parents, brothers, and sisters.
   It also involves the health of close relatives, since some diseases show a familial tendency or are hereditary.
2. To describe the health of the patient's spouse and children, since this may give clues about possible communicable disease problems.
   It also will be important in determining what sort of condition a family is in and how this affects the patient.

B. Types of Information Needed

1. Age and health status of (or age at and cause of death of) parent, sibling.
2. History, in immediate and close relatives, of heart disease, hypertension, stroke, diabetes, gout, kidney disease or stones, thyroid disease, asthma or other allergies, blood problems, cancer (types), epilepsy, mental illness, arthritis, alcoholism, obesity.
3. Hereditary diseases such as hemophilia or sickle cell disease.
4. Age and health status of spouse and children.

C. Method of Collecting Data

1. Begin with an explanation of what you are asking and why, since the patient may not understand the purpose of your questions. For example:
   "I am going to ask now about the health of your immediate family and relatives. It is important to know if there are any conditions which tend to or could occur in your family, or in you as a member of the family."
2. Ask direct questions.
   a. Begin with the patient's siblings.
      "Do you have any brothers and sisters?"
      "How old are they and what is the state of their health?"
   b. List each sibling separately, giving age and state of health.

Review of Systems

A. Purpose

To obtain detailed information about the current state of the patient and any past symptoms, or lack of symptoms, he may have experienced related to a particular body system.

B. Types of Information Needed

Subjective information about what the patient feels or sees with regard to the major systems of the body.

1. *Skin*—rash, itching, change in pigmentation or texture, sweating, hair growth and distribution, condition of nails.
2. *Skeletal*—stiffness of joints, pain, deformity, restriction of motion, swelling, redness, heat. If there are problems, ask the patient to specify any activities of daily life that he finds difficult or impossible to perform.
3. *Head*—headaches, dizziness, syncope, head injuries.
4. *Eyes*—vision, pain, diplopia, photophobia, blind spots, itching, burning, discharge, recent change in appearance or vision, glaucoma, cataracts, glasses/contact lenses worn, date of last refraction, infection.
5. *Ears*—hearing acuity, earache, discharge, tinnitus, vertigo.
6. *Nose*—sense of smell, frequency of colds, obstruction, epistaxis, postnasal discharge, sinus pain or therapy, use of nose drops or sprays (type and frequency).
7. *Teeth*—pain; bleeding, swollen or receding gums; recent abscesses, extractions; dentures; dental hygiene practices.
8. *Mouth and tongue*—soreness of tongue or buccal mucosa, ulcers, swelling.
9. *Throat*—sore throat, tonsillitis, hoarseness, dysphagia.
10. *Neck*—pain, stiffness, swelling, enlarged glands or lymph nodes.
11. *Endocrine*—goiter, thyroid tenderness, tremors, weakness, tolerance to heat and cold, changes in hat or glove size, changes in skin pigmentation, libido, bruisability, muscle cramps, polyuria, polydipsia, polyphagia, hormone therapy.
12. *Respiratory*
    a. Pain in the chest and relationship to respirations.
    b. Dyspnea, wheezing, cough, sputum (character, quantity), hemoptysis.
    c. Night sweats (Does the patient have to change his bedding?).
    d. Last chest x-ray and result; (indicate where obtained).
    e. Exposure to tuberculosis.
13. *Cardiac*
    a. Presence of pain or distress and location (have patient point to location); radiation of pain; precipitating/aggravating causes; alleviating measures; timing and duration.
    b. Palpitations, dyspnea, orthopnea (note number of pillows required for sleeping), edema, cyanosis.
    c. Exercise tolerance (determine in relation to patient's regular activities—how much can he do before stopping to rest?).
    d. Blood pressure (if known): last ECG and results (indicate where obtained).
14. *Hematologic*—anemia (if so, treatment received), tendency to bruise or bleed, thromboses, thrombophlebitis, any known abnormalities of blood cells.
15. *Lymph nodes*—enlargement, tenderness, suppuration, duration and progress of abnormality.
16. *Gastrointestinal*
    a. Appetite and digestion, intolerance to certain classes of foods.

b. Pain associated with hunger or eating, eructation, regurgitation, heartburn, nausea, vomiting, hematemesis.
c. Regularity of bowel movement (describe normal bowel habits and whether they have changed recently or not); diarrhea, flatulence, stools (color—brown, black, clay; tarry, fresh blood, mucus, etc.).
d. Hemorrhoids, jaundice, dark urine, use of laxatives—type; frequency. (This should be included under past medical history with medications, but may be repeated here.)
e. History of ulcer, gallstones, polyps, tumors.
f. Previous x-rays—where, when, results.

17. *Genitourinary*—dysuria, pain, urgency, frequency, hematuria, nocturia, polydipsia, polyuria, oliguria, edema of the face, hesitancy, dribbling, loss in size or force of stream, passage of stones, stress incontinence, hernias.
    a. Males
       (1) Puberty—onset, voice change, erections, emissions.
       (2) Libido—satisfaction with sexual relations.
    b. Females
       (1) Menses—onset, regularity, duration of flow, dysmenorrhea, last period, intermenstrual bleeding or discharge, dyspareunia.
       (2) Libido—satisfaction with sexual relations.
       (3) Pregnancies (see past medical history).
       (4) Methods of contraception.
       (5) Breasts—pain, tenderness, discharge, lumps, mammograms, breast self-examination—techniques and timing with regard to menstrual cycle.
18. *Neuromuscular*
    a. Mental status—orientation to time, place, person, and distance. "How far is your home from the hospital?" (Interviewer must be able to verify the answer.)
    b. Memory—distant memory shown by recalling past medical history.
       —recent memory shown by recalling what was eaten for breakfast.
    c. Cognition, or ability of patient to conceptualize (very useful information in determining a health education plan for the patient).
    d. Patient's description of his personality—how he views himself.
    e. Presence of tics, twitching, weakness, paralysis, tremor, wasting of muscles, incoordination, fatigue, sensory loss with respect to pain, temperature, touch, muscle pain, cramps.
    f. Psychiatric history may be entered here.
19. *General constitutional symptoms*—fever, chills, malaise, fatigability, recent loss or gain of weight.

C. Method of Collecting Data

1. Begin by explaining to the patient—"I am going to ask you many questions about your body which will help in understanding your present problem."
2. Ask direct questions about each system, using terms that the patient understands.
3. Whenever the patient complains or suggests a symptom, ask the questions outlined under method of collecting data about the present illness (onset, duration, etc.).
4. Never assume that things are "OK" if the patient fails to mention something.
    a. Ask about every aspect of the function of a particular system and be sure to record the patient's responses.

b. Often the fact that a body system has been free of any symptoms is as important as any symptoms that have been experienced.

5. If necessary, memorize a list of questions for each system or use a list when interviewing the patient.

Knowing what to ask about each system is based on knowledge of the function of each body system and of the way that normal function manifests itself.

Personal and Social History

A. Purposes

1. To describe the patient's life situation—may have bearing on the present condition and/or the patient's ability to cope with this problem.

2. To develop a plan of care that "fits" the patient.

Here the interviewer finds out the many personal and family resources an individual has to aid him in coping with the situation—both long-term and short-term.

3. To have some idea of how the patient patterns his life.
   a. Certain habits and patterns are more easily assimilated and changed, when necessary, than others.
   b. Knowing the patient's patterns is useful in helping to organize hospital routine in ways that will be least disruptive to the patient.

4. To help the patient develop a workable plan of care at home, based on knowledge of home conditions.

5. To determine if the patient's occupation is directly or indirectly related to his condition.

6. To determine if the patient's religious affiliation may affect therapy.

B. Types of Information Needed

1. *Personal status*—birth place, education, armed service affiliation, position in the family, satisfaction with life situations (home and job), personal concerns.

2. *Habits/patterns*
   a. Sleeping, activities/hobbies, nutrition/eating habits (diet for a typical day).
   b. Consumption of alcohol, coffee, tea, drugs (marijuana, over-the-counter medications).
   c. Tobacco (what form; how long).
   d. Sexual habits (can be part of GU history)—relationships, frequency, satisfaction.

3. *Home conditions*
   a. Marital status, nature of family relationships.
   b. Economic conditions—source of income; health insurance, Medicare, Medicaid.
   c. Living arrangements and housing (owning/renting, heating, sewage, pets, etc.).
   d. Involvement with agencies (name, case worker, etc.).

4. *Occupation*
   a. Past and present employment and working conditions, including exposure to stress/tension, noise, pollution.
   b. Working hours.
   c. Job satisfaction.

5. *Religion*—name, whether practicing or not, any stipulations with regard to health practices.

C. Method of Collecting Data

1. Begin by explaining that you are now going to ask questions about the patient's life situation in order to gain a clearer perspective of the patient's condition and of how you might help him.

2. Your manner should be matter-of-fact, yet concerned. If you are uncomfortable asking the questions, most likely the patient will sense that and be uneasy answering them.

3. A sensitive interviewer can ask most of the questions listed above in an initial interview without alienating the patient. For instance, ask "What has been your education?" instead of "How far have you gone in school?"

Ending the History

When you have completed the history, it is often helpful to say: "Is there anything else you would like to tell me?" or "What do you think is the matter with you?" This allows the patient to end the history by saying what is on his mind and what concerns him most.

Bibliography

Books

Bates B. A Guide to Physical Examination and History Taking. Philadelphia, JB Lippincott, 1991

Bowers AC and Thompson JM. Clinical Manual of Health Assessment. St. Louis, CV Mosby, 1988

Gordon M. Nursing Diagnosis: Process and Application. New York, McGraw-Hill, 1987

Guzzeta CE et al. Clinical Assessment Tools for Use with Nursing Diagnoses. St. Louis, CV Mosby, 1989

Jones DA. Health Assessment Manual. St. Louis, CV Mosby, 1986

Potter PA. Pocket Guide to Physical Assessment. St. Louis, CV Mosby, 1986

Seidel HM et al. Mosby's Guide to Physical Examination. St. Louis, CV Mosby, 1987

Sherman JL and Fields SK. Guide to Patient Evaluation: History Taking, Physical Examination, and the Nursing Process. New Hyde Park, NY, Medical Examination Publishing, 1988

Weber J. Nurses' Handbook of Health Assessment. Philadelphia, JB Lippincott, 1988

Weed L. Medical Records: Medical Education and Patient Care. Cleveland, Case Western Reserve University Press, 1968

Journals

Aimino PA. Perioperative nursing documentation. AORN J 1987 Jul; 46(1):73, 76–81, 84–86

Haller KB. Systematic documentation of practice. MCN 1987 Mar.–Apr.; 12(2): 152

Henson DK and Bresh C. Corporate standards for nursing care: An integral part of a computerized care plan. Comput Nurs 1988 Jul–Aug; 6(4):141–146

Rich PL. Make the most of your charting time. Nursing 1987 May; 17(5):68–73

Spillane RK. Assessment: Getting the patient's point of view—early. Nurs Manage 1987 May; 18(5):20, 22, 24, 27–28

Stanfield V. Perioperative documentation: Integrating nursing diagnoses on the patient record. AORN J 1987 Oct; 46(4):699–701, 703–704

Werley HH, Devine EC, and Zorn CR. Nursing needs its own minimum data set. Am J Nurs 1988 Dec; 88(12):1651–1653

3 Adult Physical Examination

General Principles

1. A complete or partial physical examination is conducted following a careful comprehensive or problem-related history.
2. It is conducted in a quiet, well-lit room with consideration for patient privacy and comfort.

Approach to the Patient

1. When possible, begin with the patient in a sitting position, so that both front and back can be examined.
2. Completely expose the part to be examined but drape the rest of the body appropriately.
3. Conduct the examination systematically from head to foot so as not to miss observing any system or body part.
4. While examining each region, consider the underlying anatomical structures, their function, and possible abnormalities.
5. Since the body is bilaterally symmetrical, for the most part, compare findings on one side with those on the other.
6. Explain all procedures to the patient while the examination is being conducted—to avoid alarming or worrying the patient and to encourage his cooperation.

Techniques of Examination and Assessment

Use the following techniques of examination as appropriate for eliciting findings.

Inspection

1. Begins with first encounter with the patient and is the most important of all the techniques.
2. Is an organized scrutiny of the patient's behavior and body.
3. With knowledge and experience, the examiner can become highly sensitive to visual clues.
4. The examiner begins each phase of the examination by inspecting the particular part with the eyes.

Palpation

1. Involves touching the region or body part just observed and noting what the various structures feel like.
2. With experience comes the ability to distinguish variations of normal from abnormal.
3. Is performed in an organized manner from region to region.

Percussion

1. By setting underlying tissues in motion, percussion helps in determining whether the underlying tissue is air-filled, fluid-filled, or solid.
2. Audible sounds and palpable vibrations are produced, which can be distinguished by the examiner.

There are five basic notes produced by percussion, which can be distinguished by differences in the qualities of sound, pitch, duration, and intensity.

	Relative Intensity	Relative Pitch	Relative Duration	Example Location
Flatness	Soft	High	Short	Thigh
Dullness	Medium	Medium	Medium	Liver
Resonance	Loud	Low	Long	Normal lung
Hyperresonance	Very loud	Lower	Longer	Emphysematous lung
Tympany	Loud	*	*	Gastric air bubble or puffed out cheek

* Distinguished mainly by its musical timbre.
(From Bates BL. A Guide to Physical Examination. 5th ed. Philadelphia, JB Lippincott, 1991)

3. The technique for percussion may be described as follows:
   a. Hyperextend the middle finger of your left hand, pressing the distal portion and joint firmly against the surface to be percussed.
      (1) Other fingers touching the surface will damp the sound.
      (2) Be consistent in the degree of firmness exerted by the hyperextended finger as you move it from area to area or the sound will vary.
   b. Cock the right hand at the wrist, flex the middle finger upwards, and place the forearm close to the surface to be percussed. The right hand and forearm should be as relaxed as possible.
   c. With a quick, sharp, relaxed wrist motion, strike the extended left middle finger with the flexed right middle finger, using the tip of the finger, not the pad. (A very short fingernail is a must!)
      Aim at the end of the extended left middle finger (just behind the nail bed) where the greatest pressure is exerted on the surface to be percussed.
   d. Lift the right middle finger rapidly to avoid damping the vibrations.
   e. The movement is at the wrist, not at the finger, elbow, or shoulder; the examiner should use the lightest touch capable of producing a clear sound.

Auscultation

1. Is a method that uses the stethoscope to augment the sense of hearing.
2. The stethoscope must be constructed well and must fit the user. Earpieces should be comfortable, the length of the tubing should be 25–38 cm. (10–15 inches), and the head should have a diaphragm and a bell.
   a. The bell is used for low-pitched sounds such as certain heart murmurs.
   b. The diaphragm screens out low-pitched sounds and is good for hearing high-frequency sounds such as breath sounds.
   c. Extraneous sounds can be produced by clothing, hair, and movement of the head of the stethoscope.

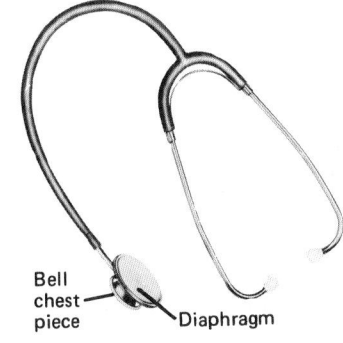

Bell chest piece

Diaphragm

Equipment

Thermometer
Sphygmomanometer
Oto-ophthalmoscope
Flashlight
Tongue depressor

Cotton applicator stick
Stethoscope
Reflex hammer
Tuning fork
Safety pin

Additional items include disposable gloves and lubricant for rectal examination and a speculum for examination of female pelvis.

Technique	Findings

Vital Signs

Importance—Many major therapeutic decisions are based on the vital signs; therefore, accuracy is essential.

Temperature

Routinely, where accuracy is not crucial, an oral temperature will suffice.

Temperature—may vary with the time of day.
Oral: 37°C. (98.6°F.) is considered normal

Technique	Findings

A rectal temperature is the most accurate,

Unless contraindicated (as in a patient with a severe cardiac dysrhythmia), a rectal temperature is often preferred.

May vary from 35.8°C. to 37.3°C. (96.4°F. to 99.1°F.).
Rectal: Higher than oral by 0.4°C. to 0.5°C. (0.7°F. to 0.9°F.).

Pulse

Palpate the radial pulse and count for at least 30 seconds.

If the pulse is irregular, count for a full minute and note the number of irregular beats/minute.

Note whether the beat of the pulse against your finger is strong or weak, bounding or thready.

Pulse—Normal adult pulse is 60–80 beats/minute; regular in rhythm. Elasticity of the arterial walls, blood volume, and mechanical action of the heart muscle are some of the factors that affect strength of the pulse wave, which normally is full and strong.

Respiration

Count the number of respirations taken in 15 seconds and multiply by 4.

Note rhythm and depth of breathing.

Respiration—Normally 16–20 respirations/minute.

Blood Pressure

Measure the blood pressure in both arms.

Palpate the systolic pressure before using the stethoscope in order to detect an auscultatory gap.*

Apply cuff firmly; if too loose, it will give a falsely high reading.

Use cuff in appropriate size: a pediatric cuff for children; a leg cuff for obese people.

The cuff should be approximately 2.5 cm. (1 inch) above the antecubital fossa.

Normal range
  Systolic—95–140 mm. Hg
  Diastolic—60–90 mm. Hg
A difference of 5–10 mm. Hg between arms is common.
Systolic pressure in lower extremities is usually 10 mm. Hg higher than reading in upper extremities.
Going from a recumbent to a standing position can cause the systolic pressure to fall 10–15 mm. Hg and the diastolic pressure to rise slightly (by 5 mm. Hg).

Height and Weight

Determine the patient's height and weight.

General Appearance

Begin observation on first contact with the patient (in the waiting room or while the patient is in bed); continue throughout the interview systematically—as the first step in the examination of each body part.

Inspection

Observe for: race, sex, general physical development, nutritional state, mental alertness, evidence of pain, restlessness, body position, clothes, apparent age, hygiene, grooming.

Careful observation of the general state of the individual provides many clues about a person's body image and how he behaves and also some idea of how well or ill he is.

Skin

1. Examination of the skin is correlated with the information obtained in the history and other parts of the physical examination.
2. Examine the skin as you proceed through each body system.

Inspection

Observe for: skin color, pigmentation, lesions (distribution, type, configuration, size), jaundice, cyanosis, scars, superficial vascularity, moisture, edema, color of mucous membranes, hair distribution, nails.

1. "Normal" varies considerably depending on racial or ethnic background, exposure to sun, complexion, pigmentation tendencies (e.g., freckles).

Palpation

Examine skin for temperature, texture, elasticity, turgor.

2. The skin is normally warm, slightly moist, and smooth and returns quickly to its original shape when picked up between two fingers and released. There is a characteristic hair distribution over the body associated with gender and normal physiologic function. Nails are present and smooth and cared for in some way.

---

* Auscultatory gap:
1. The first sound of blood in the artery is usually followed by continuous sound until nothing is audible with the stethoscope.
2. Occasionally the sound is not continuous and there is a gap after the first sound, after which the sound of blood in the vessel is heard again.
3. If one uses only the auscultatory method and pumps the cuff up until the sound is no longer heard, it is possible, when there is a gap in the sound or when the sound is not continuous, to get a falsely low systolic reading.

Technique	Findings

Head

Inspection

Observe for: symmetry of face, configuration of skull, hair color and distribution, scalp.

1. Normally, the skull and face are symmetrical, with distribution of hair varying from person to person. (However, determine by history if there has been any change.)

Palpation

Examine: hair texture, masses, swelling or tenderness of scalp, configuration of skull.

2. The scalp should be free of flaking, with no signs of nits (small, white louse eggs), lesions, deformities, or tenderness.

Eyes and Vision

Equipment

Ophthalmoscope

Anatomical Landmarks

Globes
Palpebral fissures
Lid margins
Conjunctivae
Sclerae
Pupils
Iris

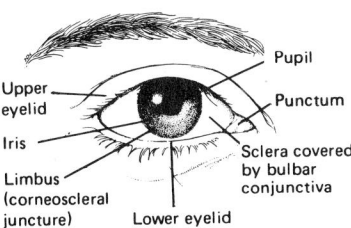

Inspection

1. *Globes*—for protrusion.
2. *Palpebral fissures* (longitudinal openings between the eyelids)—for width and symmetry.

3. *Lid margins*—for scaling, secretions, erythema, position of lashes.

4. *Bulbar and palpebral conjunctivae*—for congestion and color.

   Bulbar conjunctiva—membranous covering of the sclera (contains blood vessels).

   Palpebral conjunctiva—membranous covering of the inside of the upper and lower lids (contains blood vessels).
5. *Sclerae*—for color; *iris*—for color.
6. *Pupils*—for size, shape, symmetry, reaction to light and accommodation (ability of the lens to adjust to objects at varying distances).

7. *Eye movement*—extraocular movements, nystagmus, convergence.

   (Nystagmus: rapid, lateral, horizontal, or rotary movement of the eye.)
   (Convergence: ability of the eye to turn in and focus on a very close object.)
   (See neurologic examination, p. 41.)

8. *Gross visual fields*—by confrontation. (See neurologic examination, p. 41.)
9. *Visual acuity*
   Check with a Snellen chart (with and without glasses).

2. *Palpebral fissures*—appear equal in size when the eyes are open.
   Upper lid—covers a small portion of the iris and cornea.
   Lower lid—margin is just below the junction of the cornea and sclera (limbus).
   Ptosis—drooping of eyelids.
3. *Lid margins*—are clear; the lacrimal duct openings (puncta) are evident at the nasal ends of the upper and lower lids.
   Eye lashes—normally are evenly distributed and turn outward.
4. *Bulbar conjunctiva* (cover of sclera)—consists of transparent red blood vessels, which may become dilated and produce the characteristic "bloodshot" eye.
   Palpebral conjunctivae—are pink and clear.
   Conjunctivitis—inflammation of the conjunctival surfaces.
5. *Sclerae*—should be white and clear.
6. *Pupils*—normally constrict with increasing light and accommodation. Pupils are normally round and can range in size from very small ("pinpoint") to large (occupying the entire space of the iris).
7. *Extraocular movement*—movement of the eyes in conjugate fashion. (Six muscles control the movement of the eye.) Eyes normally move in conjugate fashion, except when converging on an object that is moving closer.
   Nystagmus—may be seen normally as a result of eye fatigue.
   Convergence—fails when double vision occurs, usually 10–15 cm. (4–6 inches) from nose.
8. *Peripheral vision*—is full (medially and laterally, superiorly and inferiorly) in both eyes.
9. *Normal vision*—20/20.
   Myopia—nearsightedness.
   Hyperopia—farsightedness.

Palpation

1. Determine strength of upper lids by attempting to open closed lids against resistance.
2. Palpate globes through closed lids for tenderness and tension.

1. The examiner should not be able to open the lids when the patient is squeezing them shut.
2. Globes normally are not tender when palpated.

Technique	Findings

Fundoscopic Examination (ends eye examination).

1. *Red retinal reflex*—check the transparency of the anterior and posterior chambers.

2. *Cornea*—check for transparency.
3. *Lens*—check for transparency.
4. *Retina*—check for color, pigmentation, hemorrhages, and exudates.
5. *Optic disc*—check for color, distinction of margins, pigmentation, degree of elevation, cupping.
6. *Macula*—check for color. (Lies at a distance of 2 optic disc diameters laterally from the optic disc.)
7. *Blood vessels*—check for diameter; arteriovenous (A/V) ratio; origin and course; venous–arterial crossings. (Both arteries and veins are present and move outward from the disc nasally and temporally.)

1. *Red retinal reflex*—can be spotted by the examiner while standing 30 cm. (12 inches) from the eye. The anterior and posterior chambers should be transparent.
2. *Cornea*—should be transparent.
3. *Lens*—should be transparent (i.e., retina can be seen).
4. *Retina*—color varies according to the amount of pigment present. There should be no hemorrhages or exudates.
5. *Optic disc*—is circular and has a yellowish-pink color. Although disc appearance may vary, the margins are normally distinct and regular, with varying amounts of pigment.
6. *Macula*—since it is free of blood vessels, it is lighter in color than the rest of the retina.
7. *Retinal arteries and veins*—arteries are approximately $\frac{4}{5}$ the size of the veins and lighter in color. Where arteries and veins cross, there is usually no disturbance in the course of either. Pulsations may occur in the vein near the optic disc.

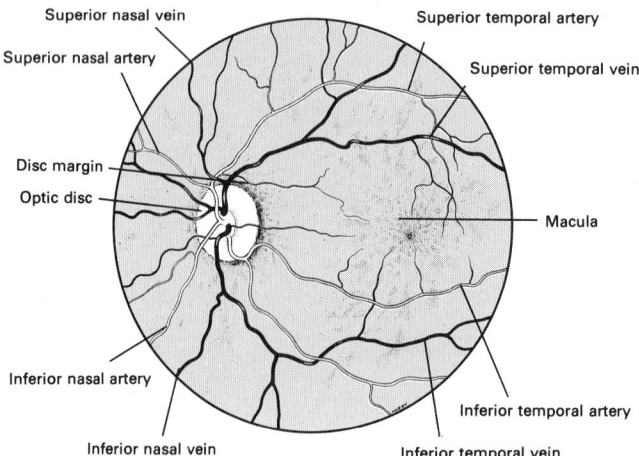

Superior nasal vein · Superior temporal artery · Superior nasal artery · Superior temporal vein · Disc margin · Optic disc · Macula · Inferior nasal artery · Inferior nasal vein · Inferior temporal vein · Inferior temporal artery

Use of the Ophthalmoscope

1. Hold the instrument in your right hand and use your right eye to examine the patient's right eye.
   a. Reverse the procedure to examine the patient's left eye.
   b. This approach allows you to get close to the patient without bumping noses.
2. Hold the instrument so that your last 2 fingers are straight, rather than curved around the handle.

   You can place these fingers against the patient's cheek to steady the instrument and to avoid hitting the patient with it.

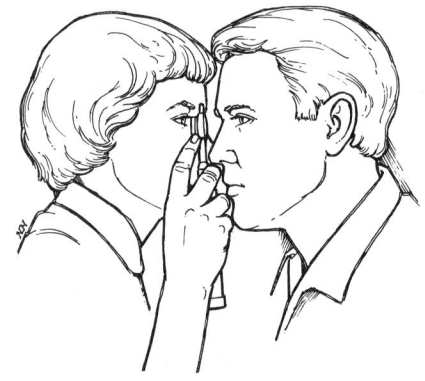

3. Begin the fundoscopic examination standing about 30 cm. (a foot) from the patient. The room should be darkened.
4. Turn the dial on the head of the ophthalmoscope to +8 or +10 (black numbers).
5. Turn on the ophthalmoscope light and place the eyepiece up to your eye.
   If you wear glasses or contact lenses, it is best to wear them during the examination so that you do not have to accommodate for your vision by turning the dial on the ophthalmoscope.
6. Aim the light at the pupil of the eye. You should see the red reflex immediately.
7. Slowly move in toward the patient, continuing to look through the eyepiece and keeping the light directed at the pupil, beyond which is the fundus.
8. With the index finger of the hand holding the ophthalmoscope, turn the dial toward zero as you move in.
   a. This allows you to focus on the various chambers of the eye.
   b. A way to find the eye and pupil is to put your hand on top of the patient's head and your thumb at the outer corner of the eye. If you lose the fundus, you can return to your thumb and get your bearings by moving medially from the thumb nail.

Technique	Findings

9. Once your hand is resting on the patient's cheek, continue to turn the dial until you can focus on the retina, and the blood vessels and the optic disc appear sharp.

10. Once you are focused on the optic disc, it is possible to follow the blood vessels out from the disc inferiorly and superiorly, medially and laterally. (See Chapter 25 [Eye Disorders] for visual fields, color vision tests, refraction, gonioscopy, tonometry.)

Ears and Hearing

Equipment

Tuning fork, otoscope

To Examine With Otoscope

1. Hold the helix of the ear and gently pull the pinna upward and back toward the occiput to straighten the external canal.
2. Gently insert the lighted otoscope, using an earpiece that is a comfortable size for the patient.
3. Once the otoscope is in place, put your eye up to the eyepiece and examine the external canal.

Techniques of Examination

Inspection

1. *Pinna*—examine for size, shape, color, lesions, masses.
2. *External canal*—examine with the otoscope for discharge, impacted cerumen, inflammation, masses, or foreign bodies.
3. *Tympanic membrane*—examine for color, luster, shape, position, transparency, integrity, and scarring.
4. *Landmarks*—note cone of light, umbo, handle and short process of the malleus, pars flaccida, and pars tensa.

   Gently move the otoscope to observe the entire drum. (Cerumen may obscure visualization of the drum.)

Palpation
Pinna—examine for tenderness, consistency of cartilage, swelling.

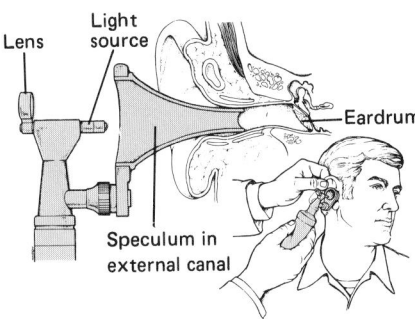

2. *External canal*—is normally clear with perhaps minimal cerumen.

3. *Tympanic membrane and landmarks*.

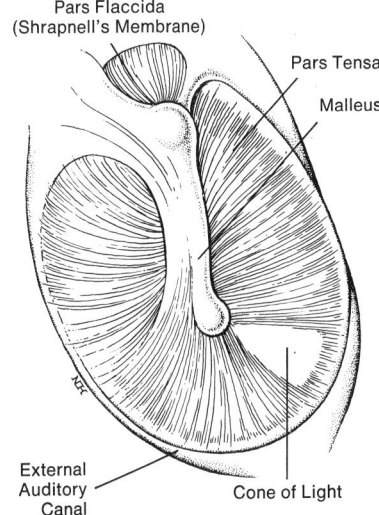

Mechanical Tests

1. Test each ear for gross hearing acuity using whispered word or watch. Cover the ear not being tested.

2. *Weber test*—test for lateralization of vibration. Place tuning fork in the center of the scalp near the forehead (*A*). (Also see Chapter 26 [Ear Disorders]).

1. A person with normal hearing can hear a whispered word from approximately 4.5 meters (15 feet) and a watch from 30 cm. (12 inches). The patient should hear the sound equally well in both ears, that is, there is no lateralization.

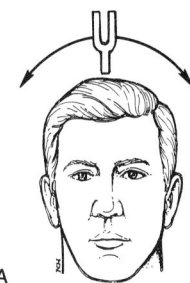

A

Technique	Findings

3. *Rinne Test*—compares air and bone conduction.
   a. Place vibrating tuning fork on the mastoid process behind the ear and have the patient tell you when the vibration stops (*B*).
   b. Then quickly hold the buzzing end of the tuning fork *near* the ear canal and ask if patient can hear it (*C*). (See p. 647 for Audiogram.)

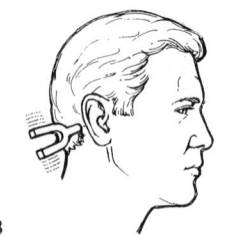 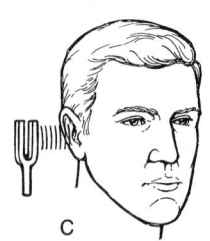

B   C

Normally, sound should be heard after vibration can no longer be felt, that is, air conduction is greater than bone conduction. Lateralization and conduction findings are altered by damage to the 8th cranial nerve and damage to the ossicles in the middle ear.

Nose and Sinuses

Equipment
Otoscope, nasal speculum

Techniques of Examination

Inspection
1. Observe for general deformity.
2. With nasal speculum (otoscope, if speculum is unavailable) examine for:
   a. Nasal septum (position and perforation).
   b. Discharge (anteriorly and posteriorly).
   c. Nasal obstruction and airway patency.
   d. Mucous membranes for color.
   e. Turbinates for color and swelling.

Nasal septum—is normally straight and not perforated.
Discharge—none should be present.
Airways—are patent.
Mucous membranes—are normally pink.
Turbinates—3 bony projections on each lateral wall of the nasal cavity covered with well-vascularized, mucus-secreting membranes. They serve to warm the air going into the lungs and may become swollen and pale with colds and allergies.

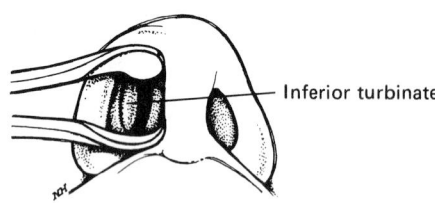

Inferior turbinate

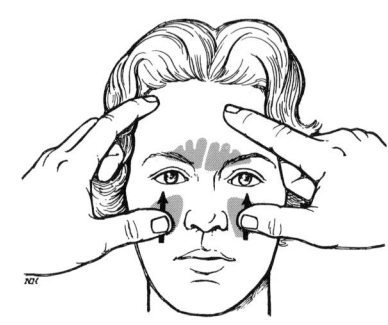

Palpation
Sinuses (frontal and maxillary)—for tenderness.
  Frontal—direct manual pressure upward toward wall of sinus. Avoid pressure on eyes.
  Maxillary—with thumbs, direct pressure upward over lower edge of maxillary bones.

Mouth

Equipment
Flashlight, tongue depressor, gloves, gauze sponges

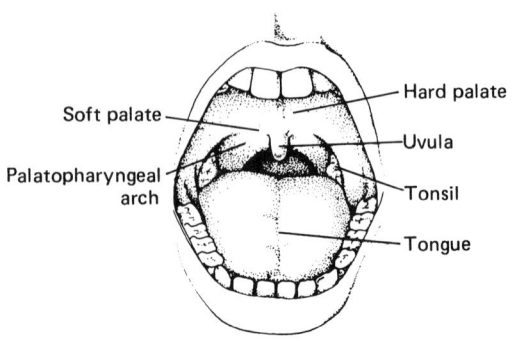

Soft palate — Hard palate
Uvula
Palatopharyngeal arch — Tonsil
Tongue

Technique	**Findings**

Techniques of Examination

Inspection

1. Observe lips for color, moisture, pigment, masses, ulcerations, fissures.
2. Use tongue depressor and penlight to examine:
   a. *Teeth*—number, arrangement, general condition.
   b. *Gums*—for color, texture, discharge, swelling, or retraction.

   c. *Buccal mucosa*—for discoloration, vesicles, ulcers, masses.
   d. *Pharynx*—for inflammation, exudate, and masses.
   e. *Tongue* (protruded)—for size, color, thickness, lesions, moisture, symmetry, deviations from midline, fasciculations.
   f. *Salivary glands*—for patency.
      Parotid glands

      Sublingual and submaxillary glands.

   g. *Uvula*—for symmetry when patient says "ah."
   h. *Tonsils*—for size, ulceration, exudates, inflammation.

   i. *Odor of breath.*

   j. *Voice*—for hoarseness.

Palpation

1. Examine oral cavity with gloved hand for masses and ulceration. Palpate beneath tongue and explore laterally the floor of the mouth (A).
2. Grasp tongue with gauze sponge to retract; inspect sides and undersurface of tongue and floor of mouth (B).

Teeth—the adult normally has 32 teeth.
Gums—commonly recede in adults.
Gums—bleeding is fairly common and may result from trauma, gingival disease, or systemic problems (less common).

Tongue—is normally midline and covered with papillae, which vary in size from the tip of the tongue to the back. (The circumvallate papillae are large and posterior.)

Parotid glands—open in the buccal pouch at the level of the upper teeth halfway back.
Sublingual and submaxillary glands—open underneath the tongue.

Lingual tonsils—can often be seen on the posterior portion of the tongue.

Odor of breath—may indicate dental caries.

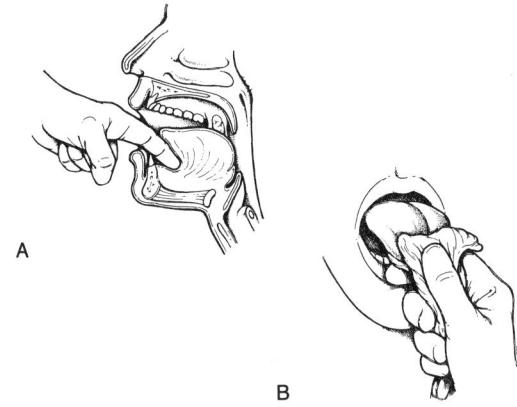

A

B

Neck

Equipment

Stethoscope

Techniques of Examination

Inspection

1. Inspect all areas of the neck anteriorly and posteriorly for muscular symmetry, masses, unusual swelling or pulsations, and range of motion.

2. *Thyroid*—ask the patient to swallow and observe for movement of an enlarged thyroid gland at the suprasternal notch.
3. *Muscular strength*
   a. *Cervical muscles*—have patient turn his chin forcefully against your hand.
   b. *Trapezius muscles*—exert pressure on the patient's shoulders while he shrugs his shoulders.

1. *Range of motion*—normally, the chin can touch the anterior chest, the head can be extended at least 45 degrees from the vertical position and can be rotated 90 degrees from midline to side.
2. *Thyroid*—is not usually visible, except in extremely thin persons.
3. *Strength*—see Findings, 11th cranial nerve, p. 42.

Technique	Findings

4. *External jugular veins*—observe with patient sitting and then lying at 30–40 degree angle; patient's neck should not be flexed.

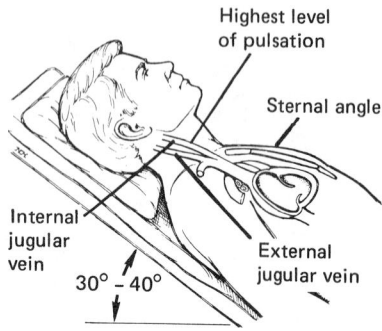

Jugular veins—when the patient is lying with head elevated 30–40 degrees, the jugular veins are approximately at the level of the right atrium, and pulsations that are transmitted from the right atrium can normally be seen with tangential lighting. Veins are not distended when the patient is sitting.

This serves as a fairly constant and therefore reliable landmark, when patient is supine or sitting, for estimating venous pressure, that is, the height in cm. measured from level of distended internal jugular veins to level of sternal angle.

Note the sternal angle, the point on the surface anatomy that is approximately 5–7 cm. (2–2.75 inches) above the right atrium.

Palpation

1. *Cervical nodes and salivary glands.*

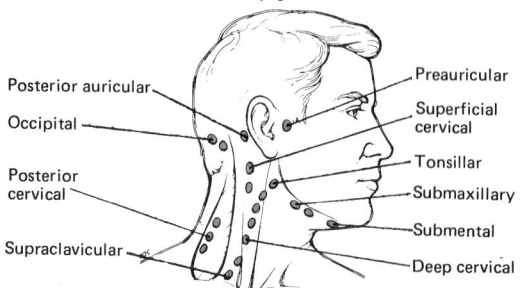

1. *Cervical nodes*—in the adult, the cervical lymph nodes are not normally palpable unless the patient is very thin, in which case the nodes are felt as small, freely movable masses.

2. *Trachea*—palpate at the sternal notch. Stand behind (or in front of) patient and allow the middle finger of each hand to glide off the head of the clavicle into the sternal notch. Palpate for deviation and tracheal tug.

2. *Trachea*—should be midline.
   Landmarks are easy to identify using this procedure.

   This is the downward pull synchronous with cardiac pulsation, usually the result of aneurysm of aorta.

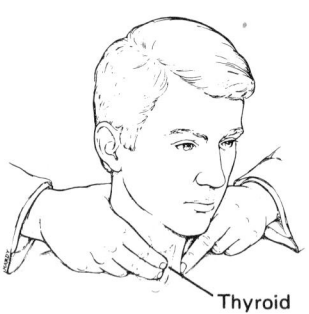

3. *Thyroid*
   a. Stand behind the patient and have him flex his neck to relax the cervical muscles.
   b. Place the fingertips of your left hand behind the left sternocleidomastoid muscle adjacent to the trachea just below larynx.
   c. Palpate the area over the trachea and to the left of the trachea.
   d. Note any enlargement, nodules, masses, consistency.
   e. Reverse the procedure and examine the right lobe of the thyroid.
   f. Since the thyroid gland moves upward upon swallowing, have the patient swallow to facilitate examination.

To discern the outline of the isthmus of the left lobe of the thyroid gland.

If the thyroid is palpable, it is normally smooth, without nodules, masses, or irregularities, or bruits (gushing sound produced by blood moving through a narrow vessel).

Technique	Findings

4. *Carotid arteries*
   a. Palpate the carotids 1 side at a time.
   b. The carotids lie anterolaterally in the neck—avoid palpating the carotid sinuses at the level of the thyroid cartilage just below the angle of the jaw, since this may cause slowing of heart rate.
   c. Note symmetry of pulsations, strength, and amplitude.

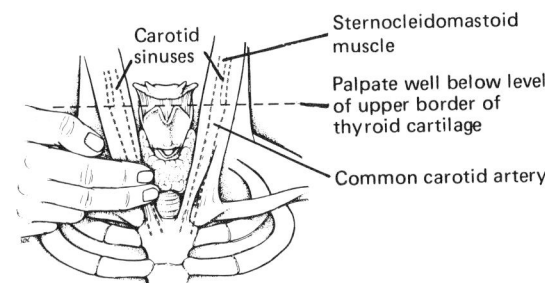

Lymph Nodes

1. It is important at some point in the examination to palpate all areas where lymphadenopathy might appear.
2. Often this is done as each region of the body is examined, for example, the cervical nodes are examined when the neck is examined.
3. However, in the record, the condition of the lymph nodes is described under a separate heading.

Techniques of Examination

Inspection
Note size, shape, mobility, consistency, tenderness, and inflammation.

Palpation
1. *Cervical, supra- and infraclavicular nodes.*

2. *Axillary nodes*
   a. Examine while the patient is sitting.
   b. Place the patient's arm at his side and insert the examining fingers to the apex of the patient's axilla. (Use the fingers of your right hand to examine the left axilla and vice versa.)
   c. Rotate the examining hand, so that the fingers can palpate the anterior and posterior axillary fossae pressing against the chest wall. Press against the humerus bone in the axilla to examine the lateral fossa for nodes. Conclude the axillary examination by moving the fingers from the apex of the axilla downward in the midline along the chest wall.

Cervical nodes and supra- and infraclavicular nodes—are not normally palpable.

Axillary nodes—are not normally palpable.

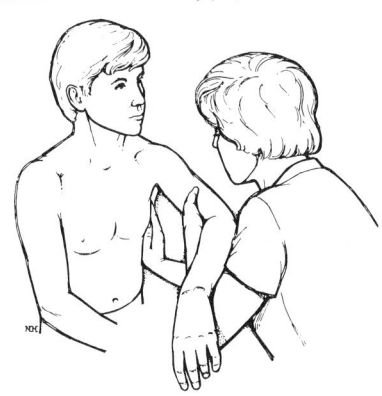

3. *Inguinal nodes*—are located in inguinal canal and are usually examined when the abdomen is examined.
4. *Epitrochlear nodes*—are palpated just above the olecranon process.

Inguinal nodes—a few may be felt, but are small, movable, and nontender.

Epitrochlear nodes—not usually palpable.

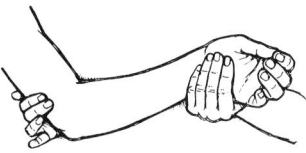

Breasts *(Male and Female)*

Female Breast

Inspection
(With the patient sitting, arms relaxed at sides.)
1. Inspect the areolae and nipples for position, pigmentation, inversion, discharge, crusting, and masses.

1. The *nipples* should be at the same level and protrude slightly. An *inverted nipple* (one that turns inward), if present since puberty, may be normal.

Technique	Findings

Extra, or supernumerary, nipples may occur normally, most commonly in the anterior axillary region or just below the normal breasts.

2. Examine the breast tissue for size, shape, color, symmetry, surface, contour, skin characteristics, and level of breasts. Note any retraction or dimpling of the skin.

3. Ask the patient to elevate her hands over her head; repeat the observation.

4. Have patient press her hands to her hips; repeat the observation.

Palpation

(This is best done with the patient recumbent.)

1. The patient with pendulous breasts should be given a pillow to place under the ipsilateral scapula of the breast being palpated so that the tissue is distributed more evenly over the chest wall.

2. The arm on the side of the breast being palpated should be raised above the patient's head.

3. Palpate one breast at a time, beginning with the "asymptomatic" breast if the patient complains of symptoms.

4. To palpate, use the palmar aspects of the fingers in a rotating motion, compressing the breast tissue against the chest wall. (This is done quadrant by quadrant until the entire breast has been palpated—including the "tail" of the breast tissue which extends into the axillary region in the upper outer quadrant of the breast.)

5. Note skin texture, moisture, temperature, or masses.

6. Gently squeeze the nipple and note any expressible discharge.

7. Repeat examination on the opposite breast and compare findings.

Male Breast

Examination of the male breast can be brief and should never be omitted.

1. Observe the nipple and areola for ulceration, nodules, swelling, or discharge.

2. Palpate the areola for nodules and tenderness.

A *supernumerary nipple* usually consists of a nipple and a small areola and may be mistaken for a mole.

2. *Breast size*—In the female it is not uncommon to find a difference in the size of the 2 breasts. Normal asymmetry has usually been present since puberty and is not a recent phenomenon.

3. If there is a mass attached to the pectoral muscles, contracting the muscles will cause retraction of the breast tissue.

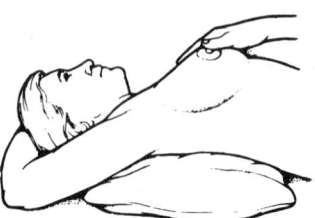

3. This allows the examiner to palpate the "normal" breast first and then compare the "symptomatic" breast to it.

4. *Breast texture*—varies according to the amount of subcutaneous tissue present.

   a. In young females, tissue is fairly soft and homogeneous; in postmenopausal women, tissue may feel nodular or stringy.

   b. Consistency also varies with menstrual cycle, being more nodular and edematous just prior to menstruation.*

5. *Masses*—If a mass is palpated, its location, size, shape, consistency, mobility, and associated tenderness are reported.

6. *Discharge*—In the normal nonpregnant or nonlactating female, there is no nipple discharge.

1. There should be no discharge.

Thorax and Lungs

General Information

1. Methodical inspection of the thorax requires reference to established "landmarks" in order to locate specific structures and to report significant findings.

2. The same structural landmarks are used in examining both the lung and the heart.

3. It is important to visualize the underlying structures and organs when examining the thorax.

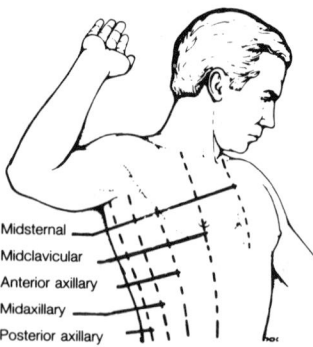

Midsternal
Midclavicular
Anterior axillary
Midaxillary
Posterior axillary

---

* In teaching women about breast self-examination, explain that the best time for performing the examination is a week after the menstrual period, when the breasts are least engorged and tender.

Technique	**Findings**

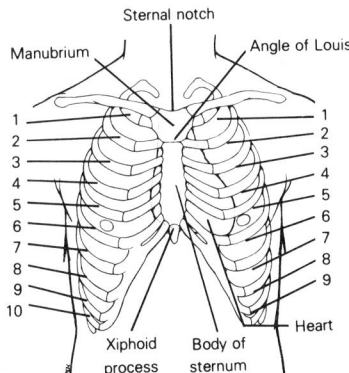

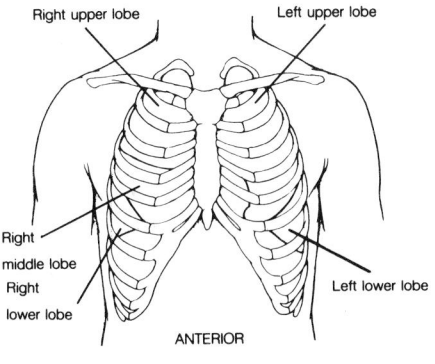

ANTERIOR

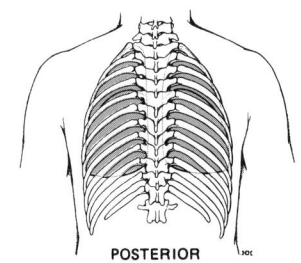

POSTERIOR

Techniques of Examination
Posterior Thorax and Lungs

Begin the examination with the patient seated; examine posterior chest and lungs.

Inspection

1. Inspect the spine for mobility and any structural deformity.
2. Observe the symmetry of the posterior chest and the posture and mobility of the thorax upon respiration. (Note any bulges or retractions of the costal interspaces upon respiration or any impairment of respiratory movement.)
3. Note the anteroposterior diameter in relation to the lateral diameter of the chest.

2. The thorax is normally symmetrical; it moves easily and without impairment upon respiration. There are no bulges or retractions of the intercostal spaces.

3. The anteroposterior (AP) diameter of the thorax in relation to the lateral diameter is approximately 1:2.

Palpation

1. Palpate the posterior chest with the patient sitting; identify areas of tenderness, masses, inflammation.
2. Palpate the ribs and costal margins for symmetry, mobility, and tenderness and the spine for tenderness and vertebral position.
3. To assess respiratory excursion—place the thumbs at the level of the 10th vertebra; with hands held parallel to the 10th ribs as they grasp the lateral rib cage, ask the patient to inhale deeply. Observe the movement of the thumbs while feeling the range, and observe the symmetry of the hands.
4. To elicit vocal and tactile *fremitus* (palpable vibrations transmitted through the bronchopulmonary system upon speaking).
   a. Ask the patient to say "99"; palpate and compare symmetrical areas of the lungs with the ball of one hand.

   b. Note any areas of increased or decreased fremitus.
   c. If fremitus is faint, ask the patient to speak louder and in a deeper voice.

2. On palpation there should be no tenderness; chest movement should be symmetrical and without lag or impairment.

4. Posteriorly, fremitus is generally equal throughout the lung fields.

   It may be increased near the large bronchi.

   It may be decreased or absent anteriorly and posteriorly when vocal loudness is decreased, when posture is not erect, or when excessive tissue or underlying structures are present.

   One must distinguish the various normal causes of increased or decreased fremitus from the pathologic causes.

Percussion

As with palpation, the posterior chest is percussed with the patient sitting.

1. Percuss symmetrical areas, comparing sides.
2. Begin across the top of each shoulder and proceed down between the scapulae and then under the scapulae, both medially and laterally in the axillary lines.
3. Note and localize any abnormal percussion sound.

Technique	Findings

4. For diaphragmatic excursion, percuss by placing the plex-imeter (stationary) finger parallel to the approximate level of the diaphragm below the right scapula.

  a. Ask the patient to inhale deeply and hold his breath; percuss downward to the point of dullness. Mark this point.

  b. Let the patient breathe normally and then ask him to exhale deeply; percuss upward from the mark to the point of resonance.

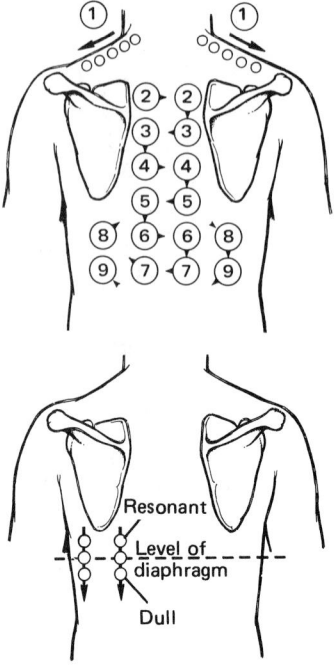

  c. Mark this point and measure between the 2 marks—normally 5–6 cm. (2–2.3 inches).

  d. Repeat this procedure medially and laterally on the right and left sides of the chest.

The lower border of the lungs on normal respiration is approximately at the level of the 10th thoracic spinous process.

Percussion normally reveals resonance over symmetrical areas of the lung.

Percussion sound may be altered by poor posture and/or presence of excessive tissue.

Breath Sounds

On auscultation, breath sounds vary according to proximity of the large bronchi.

  a. They are louder and coarser near the large bronchi and over the anterior.

  b. They are softer and much finer (vesicular) at the periphery over the alveolae.

Breath sounds also vary in duration with inspiration and expiration.

Sounds may normally decrease in obese individuals.

Pathology will alter the normal bronchial, bronchovesicular, and vesicular breath sounds. (Abnormal breath sounds or adventitious sounds are to be noted and localized.)

Auscultation

Aids in assessing air flow through the lungs, the presence of fluid or mucus, and the condition of the surrounding pleural space and lungs.

1. Have patient sit erect.*
2. With a stethoscope, listen to the lungs as the patient breathes somewhat more deeply than normally with mouth open. (Let the patient pause, as needed, to avoid hyperventilation.)
3. Place the stethoscope in the same areas on the chest wall as those percussed, and listen to a complete inspiration and expiration in each area.
4. Compare symmetrical areas methodically from the apex to the lung bases.
5. It should be possible to distinguish 3 types of normal breath sounds as indicated in the following table.

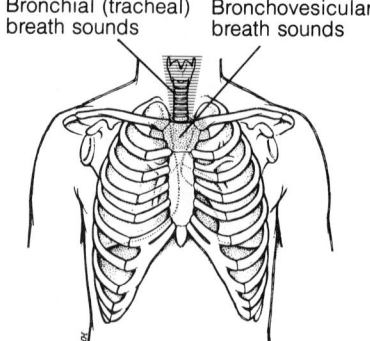

Bronchial (tracheal) breath sounds   Bronchovesicular breath sounds

Breath Sounds	Duration of Inspiration and Expiration	Pitch of Expiration	Intensity of Expiration	Normal Location
Vesicular	Insp. > Exp.	Low	Soft	Most of lungs
Broncho-vesicular	Insp. = Exp.	Medium	Medium	Near the main stem bronchi, *i.e.,* below the clavicles and between the scapulae, especially on the right
Bronchial or tubular	Exp. > Insp.	High	Usually loud	Over the trachea

(From Bates BL. A Guide to Physical Examination. 5th ed. Philadelphia, JB Lippincott, 1991)

* Note: if patient is unable to sit with or without assistance for examination of the posterior chest and lungs, position the patient first on one side and then on the other as you examine the lung fields.

Technique	Findings

Anterior Thorax and Lungs

(The patient should be recumbent with arms at sides and slightly abducted.)

Inspection

1. Inspect the chest for any structural deformity.
2. Note the width of the costal angle.

3. Observe rate and rhythm of breathing, any bulging or retraction of intercostal spaces on respiration, use of accessory muscles of respiration (sternocleidomastoid and trapezius on inspiration and abdominal muscles on expiration).
4. Note any asymmetry of chest wall movement on respiration.

2. The angle at the tip of the sternum is determined by the right and left rib margins at the xiphoid process. Normally, the angle is less than 90 degrees.
3. The thorax is normally symmetrical and moves easily without impairment on respiration. There are no bulges or retractions of the intercostal spaces.

Palpation

(Serves the same purposes in examining the anterior chest as in the posterior chest.)

1. To assess diaphragmatic excursion, place hands along the costal margins and note symmetry and degree of expansion as the patient inhales deeply.
2. Palpate for fremitus with the ball of the hand anteriorly and laterally.
    (Underlying structures, e.g., heart, liver, etc., may damp, or decrease, fremitus.)
3. Compare symmetrical areas.
4. If necessary, displace the female breast gently.

Percussion of anterior thorax

(1) Flat   (3) Resonant
(2) Dull   (4) Tympanic

Percussion

1. With patient's arms resting comfortably at his sides, examiner percusses the anterior and lateral chest.
   Begin just below the clavicles and percuss downward from one interspace to the next, comparing the sound from the interspace on one side with that of the contralateral interspace.
2. Displace the female breast, so that breast tissue does not damp the vibration. Continue downward, noting the intercostal space where hepatic dullness is percussed on the right and cardiac dullness on the left.
3. Note effect of underlying structures.

2. A tympanic sound is produced over the gastric air bubble on the left somewhat lower than the point of liver dullness on the right.

3. Percussion over heart will produce a dull sound. The upper border of the liver will be percussed on the right side, producing a dull note.

Auscultation

Listen to the chest anteriorly and laterally for the distribution of resonance and any abnormal or adventitious sounds.

Technique	Findings

Heart

General Approach

1. The examiner must visualize the position of the heart under the sternum and the ribs and know certain landmarks for identification of specific structures and significant findings.
2. It is also important to identify those "areas" on the chest wall that will yield the most information initially about the function of the heart and its valves.
   a. In locating the intercostal spaces, begin by identifying the angle of Louis, which is felt as a slight ridge approximately 2.5 cm. (1 inch) below the sternal notch, where the manubrium and the body of the sternum are joined.
   b. The 2nd ribs extend to the right and left of this angle.
   c. Once the 2nd rib is located, palpate downward and obliquely away from the sternum to identify the remaining ribs and intercostal spaces.

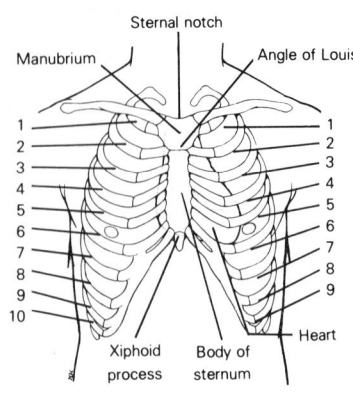

Inspection

1. Inspect the precordium for any bulging, heaving, or thrusting.
2. Look for the apical impulse approximately in the 5th or 6th intercostal space at or just medial to the midclavicular line.
3. Note any other pulsations. Tangential lighting is most helpful in detecting pulsations.

1. Normally there are no bulges.
2. An apical impulse may or may not be observable.
3. There should be no other pulsations.

Palpation

1. Use the ball of the hand to detect vibrations, or "thrills," which may be caused by murmurs. (Use the fingertips and/or palmar surface to detect pulsations.)

2. Proceed methodically through the examination so that no area is omitted. Palpate for thrills and pulsations in each area (aortic, pulmonic, tricuspid, mitral).
   a. Begin in the aortic area (2nd right intercostal space, close to the sternum) and proceed downward to the apex of the heart. (The mitral area is considered the apex of the heart.)
   b. In the tricuspid area, use the palm of the hand to detect any heaving or thrusting of the precordium (tricuspid area—5th intercostal space next to the sternum).
   c. In the mitral area (5th intercostal space, at or just medial to the midclavicular line) palpate for the apical beat; identify the point of maximal impulse (PMI) and note its size and force.

1. There should be no thrills or other pulsations. (Thrills are vibrations [caused by turbulence of blood moving through valves] that are transmitted through the skin—feels similar to a purring cat.)

Ordinarily, no heaving of the ventricle is felt, except, possibly, in the pregnant female.

The apical pulse should be felt approximately in the 5th intercostal space, at or just medial to the midclavicular line. In the young, thin person, it is a sharp, quick impulse no larger than the intercostal space. In the older person, the impulse may be less sharp and quick.

Percussion

1. Outline the border of the heart or area of cardiac dullness.
   a. The left border generally does not extend beyond 4, 7, and 10 cm. left of the midsternal line in the 4th, 5th, and 6th intercostal spaces, respectively.
   b. The right border usually lies under the sternum.
2. Percuss outward from the sternum with the stationary finger parallel to the intercostal space until dullness is no longer heard. Measure the distance from the midsternal line in centimeters.

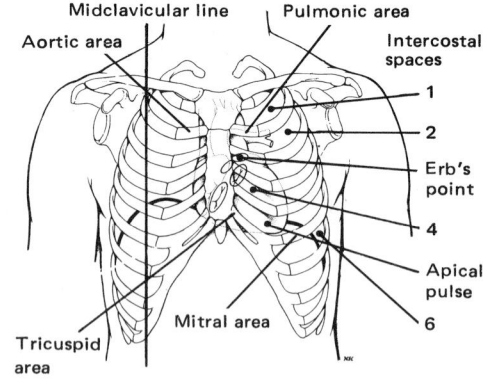

Auscultation

1. Place the stethoscope in the pulmonic or aortic area.
2. Begin by identifying the 1st (S_1) and 2nd (S_2) heart sounds.
   a. S_1 is caused by the closing of the tricuspid and mitral valves.
   b. S_2 results from the closing of the aortic and pulmonary valves.
   The 2 sounds are separated by a short systolic interval; each pair of sounds is separated from the next pair by a longer diastolic interval. Normally, 2 sounds are heard—"lub," "dub."

Technique	Findings

a. In the aortic and pulmonic areas, S_2 is usually louder than S_1. In this way, each of the paired sounds can be distinguished from the other.

b. In the tricuspid area, S_1 and S_2 are of almost equal intensity, and in the mitral area, S_1 is often slightly louder than S_2.

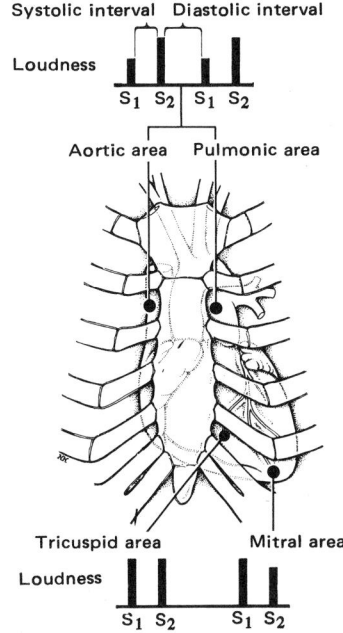

3. Once the heart sounds are identified, count the rate and note the rhythm as discussed under vital signs.

   If there is an irregularity, try to determine if there is any pattern to the irregularity in relation to the intervals, heart sounds, or respirations.

4. Once rate and rhythm are determined, listen in each of the 4 areas and at Erb's point (3rd left interspace, close to the sternum) systematically, first with the diaphragm (detects higher pitched sounds) and then with the bell (detects lower pitched sounds).

   a. In each area, listen to S_1 and then to S_2 for intensity and splitting.

   b. Listen to the intervals 1 at a time and note any extra sounds or murmurs.

Normally, the heart sounds are regular, with a rate of 60–80 beats/minute (in the adult). In the athlete or jogger, the resting pulse may be between 40 and 60 beats/minute.

a. Occasionally, there may be a splitting of S_2 in the pulmonary area. This is normal. Splitting of S_2 (2 contiguous sounds are heard instead of 1) is best heard at the end of inspiration, when right ventricular stroke volume is sufficiently increased to delay closure of the pulmonic valve *slightly* behind closure of the aortic valve.

b. There are usually no extra sounds.

Peripheral Circulation

Jugular Veins

Evaluation of jugular venous distention is most useful in patients with suspected compromise of cardiac function.

Inspection

1. Inspect neck for internal jugular venous pulsations.

1. Jugular venous pulsations can be distinguished from carotid pulsations by the following chart:

Internal Jugular Pulsations	Carotid Pulsations
Rarely palpable	Palpable
Soft, undulating quality, usually with 2 or 3 outward components (a, c, and v waves)	A more vigorous thrust with a single outward component
Pulsation eliminated by light pressure on the vein just above the sternal end of the clavicle	Pulsation not eliminated
Level of pulsation usually descends with inspiration	Pulsation not affected by inspiration
Pulsations vary with position	Pulsations are unchanged by position

(From Bates BL. A Guide to Physical Examination. 5th ed. Philadelphia, JB Lippincott, 1991)

Technique	Findings

2. Identify the highest point at which the pulsations can be seen and measure the vertical line between the point and the sternal angle.

   With the head raised to 45 degrees, the internal jugular venous pulsations should not be visible above 3 cm. (1.18 inch).

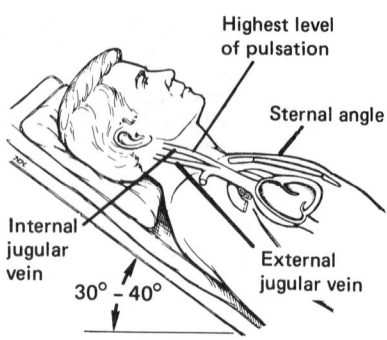

Extremities

Inspection

1. Observe skin over extremities for color, pallor, rubor, hair distribution.
2. Inspect for any superficial vessels.

1. Extremities should be symmetrically even in color, warmth, and moisture, without swelling.

   Swelling of feet may occur after prolonged standing or sitting, but will disappear readily when extremity is elevated.

Palpation

1. Note temperature of skin over extremities, comparing one side to the other.
2. Palpate pulses (radial, femoral, posterior tibial, dorsalis pedis), comparing symmetry from side to side.

2. There should be no arterial bruits.

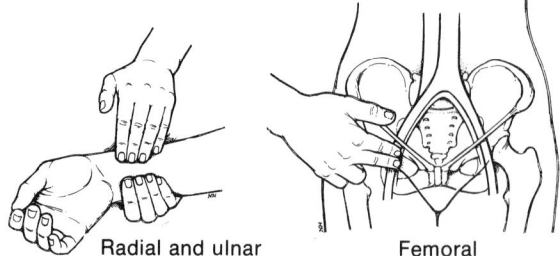

Radial and ulnar   Femoral

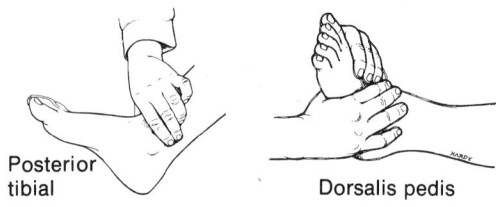

Posterior tibial   Dorsalis pedis

3. Palpate skin over the tibia for edema by pressing skin between thumb and index finger for 30 seconds to 1 minute.

   Then run pads of fingers over the area pressed and note indentation.

   If indentation is noted, repeat procedure, moving up the extremity, and note the point at which no more swelling is present.

3. Edema is usually graded from trace to 3+ or 4+ pitting (note scale used when recording data). Trace is a slight indentation that disappears in a short time. Grade 3+ or 4+, depending on the scale, is *deep* pitting that does not disappear readily. At best, these are subjective measurements, which are tried and confirmed through practice and comparison of findings with associates.

Abdomen

General Approach

1. Be sure the patient has an empty bladder.
2. The patient should be lying comfortably with arms at the side. Often, bending the knees slightly will help to relax the abdominal muscles and make palpation easier.
3. Expose the abdomen fully. Make sure your hands and the stethoscope diaphragm are warm.
4. Be methodical in visualizing the underlying organs as you inspect, auscultate, percuss, and palpate each quadrant or region of the abdomen.

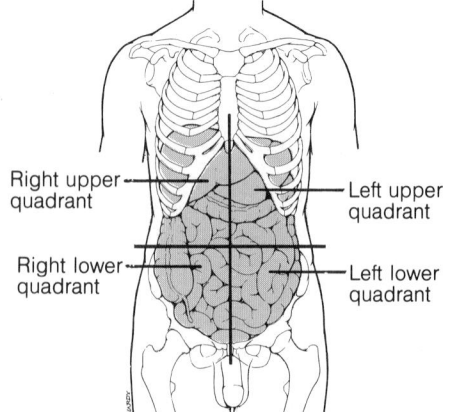

Technique	**Findings**

Inspection

1. Observe the general contour of the abdomen (flat, protuberant, scaphoid, or concave; local bulges). Also note symmetry, visible peristalsis, aortic pulsations.
2. Check the umbilicus for contour or hernia and the skin for rashes, striae, and scars.

1. The abdomen may or may not have any scars and should be flat or slightly rounded in the nonobese person.

Auscultation

1. This is done before percussion and palpation, since the latter may alter the character of bowel sounds.
2. Note the frequency and character of bowel sounds (pitch, duration).
3. Listen over the aorta and renal arteries (either side of the umbilicus) for bruits.

2. Anywhere from 5–35 bowel sounds/minute. May have familiar sound of "growling."
3. There should be no bruits or rubs.

Percussion

1. Percussion provides a general orientation to the abdomen.
2. Proceed methodically from quadrant to quadrant, noting tympany and dullness.
3. In right upper quadrant (RUQ) in the midclavicular line, percuss the borders of the liver.
   a. Begin at a point of tympany in the midclavicular line of the right lower quadrant (RLQ) and percuss upward to the point of dullness (the lower liver border); mark the point.
   b. Percuss downward from the point of lung resonance above the RUQ to the point of dullness (the upper border of the liver); mark the point.
   c. Measure in centimeters the distance between the 2 marks in the midclavicular line (the liver span).
   d. Tympany of the gastric air bubble can be percussed in the left upper quadrant (LUQ) over the anterior lower border of the rib cage.

2. Tympany should predominate.

3. Percussion of the liver should help guide subsequent palpation. The liver border in the midclavicular line should normally range from 6–12 cm. (2.3–4.6 inches).

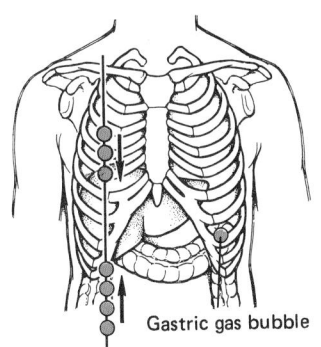

Gastric gas bubble

Midclavicular line

Kidney

1. Next palpate for the left and right kidneys.
2. Place the left hand under the patient's back between the rib cage and the iliac crest.
3. Support the patient while you palpate the abdomen with the right palmar surface of the fingers facing the left side of the body.
4. Palpate by bringing the left and right hands together as much as possible slightly below the level of the umbilicus on right and left.
5. If the kidney is felt, describe its size and shape, and any tenderness.
6. Costal vertebral angle (CVA) tenderness is palpated with the patient sitting—usually during the examination of the posterior chest. Locate the CVA in the flank region and strike firmly with the ulnar surface of your hand. Note any tenderness over the area.

4. The kidney is usually felt only in persons with very relaxed abdominal muscles (the very young, the aged, multiparous women). The right kidney is slightly lower than the left. The kidney is felt as a solid, firm, smooth elastic mass.

6. There should be no CVA tenderness.

Aorta

1. Next, palpate for the aorta with the thumb and index finger.
2. Press deeply in the epigastric region (roughly in the midline) and feel with the fingers for pulsations, as well as for the contour of the aorta.

1. The aorta is soft and pulsatile.

Other Findings

1. Palpation of the RLQ may reveal the part of the bowel called the cecum.

1. The cecum will be soft.

Technique	Findings
2. The sigmoid colon may be palpated in the LLQ.	2. The sigmoid colon is rope-like and vertical and, if filled with feces, may be quite firm.
3. The inguinal and femoral areas should be palpated bilaterally for lymph nodes.	3. Often small inguinal nodes are present; they are nontender, freely movable, and firm.

Male Genitalia and Hernias

This part of the examination, especially for hernias, is best done with the patient standing. (A *hernia* is the protrusion of a portion of the intestine through an abnormal opening.)

1. Drape the patient's chest and abdomen.
2. Expose the groin and genitalia.

Inspection

1. Inspect the pubic hair distribution and the skin of the penis.	
2. Retract or have the patient retract the foreskin, if present.	2. The foreskin of the penis, if present, should be easily retractable.
3. Observe the glans penis and the urethral meatus. Note any ulcers, masses, or scars.	3. The skin of the glans penis is smooth, without ulceration.
4. Note the location of the urethral meatus and any discharge.	4. The urethral meatus normally is located ventrally on the end of the penis. Normally, there is no discharge from the urethra.
5. Observe the skin of the scrotum for ulcers, masses, redness, or swelling. Note size, contour, and symmetry. Lift the scrotum to inspect the posterior surface.	5. The scrotum descends approximately 4 cm. (1.5 inches) in the adult; the left side is often larger than the right side.
6. Inspect the inguinal areas and groin for bulges (without and with the patient bearing down—as though having a bowel movement).	

Palpation

Wear gloves.

1. Palpate any lesions, nodules, or masses, noting tenderness, contour, size, and induration. Palpate the shaft of the penis for any induration (firmness in relation to surrounding tissues).	
2. Palpate each testis and epididymis separately between the thumb and first 2 fingers, noting size, shape, consistency, and undue tenderness (pressure on the testis normally produces pain).	2. The testes are usually rubbery and of equal size. The epididymis is located posterolaterally on each testis and is most easily palpable on the superior portion of the testis.
3. Also palpate the spermatic cord, including the vas deferens within the cord, from the testis to the inguinal ring. Note any nodules or tenderness.	
4. Palpate for inguinal hernias, using the left hand to examine the patient's left side and the right hand to examine the patient's right side. a. Insert the right index finger laterally, invaginating the scrotal sac to the external inguinal ring. b. If the external ring is large enough, insert the finger along the inguinal canal toward the internal ring and ask the patient to strain down, noting any mass that touches the finger.	4. Normally, there is no palpable herniating mass in the inguinal area. 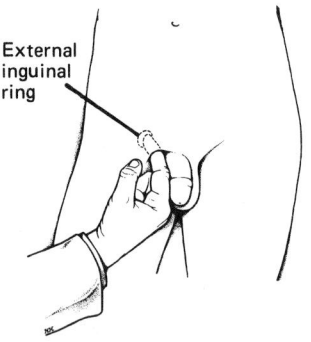 External inguinal ring
5. Also palpate the anterior thigh for a herniating mass in the femoral canal. Ask patient to strain down. (Femoral canal—not palpable, but is a potential opening in the anterior thigh, medial to the femoral artery below the inguinal ligament.)	5. Ordinarily, there is no palpable mass in the femoral area.

Female Genitalia

Equipment

Disposable gloves, lubricant, speculum of appropriate size, excellent direct lighting, cervical scraper, glass slide, fluid for fixing Papanicolaou smear, cotton tip applicator

Technique	**Findings**

General Approach

1. The patient's bladder should be empty.
2. The patient should lie in the lithotomy position with her buttocks extending slightly over the end of the examining table.
3. Her thighs are flexed and abducted; her feet are in the stirrups.
4. Her arms are at her side or crossed over her chest.
5. If a male is performing the examination, a female attendant must be present.
6. The examination will be most successful if the patient is relaxed. This can best be accomplished by draping the patient well so that the drape extends over the knees.
7. Explain each step of the procedure and avoid any quick, unexpected movements.
8. Be sure that your hands and the speculum are warm.

Inspection and Palpation

(These are performed almost simultaneously through the course of the examination.)

1. Begin with inspection of the pubic hair distribution.

2. Inspect the labia majora, the mons pubis, and the perineum (tissue between the anus and the vaginal opening).

3. With gloved hand, separate the labia majora and inspect the clitoris, urethral meatus, and vaginal opening. Note skin color, ulcerations, nodules, discharge, or swelling.

4. Note the area of the Skene's and Bartholin's glands. If there is any history of swelling of the latter, palpate the glands by placing the index finger in the vagina at the posterior end of the opening and the thumb outside the posterior portion of the vagina. Palpate between the finger and thumb for nodules, tenderness, or swelling. Repeat on each side of the posterior vaginal opening.

1. Normally, the pubic hair is distributed in an inverted triangle over the symphysis pubis.
2. In the virgin, the labia majora are full and rounded. They become thinner in older and multiparous women.
3. The labia minora and the prepuce around the clitoris are pinkish.

4. The hymen, or membranous fold that may partially occlude the vaginal opening, may or may not be present.

Speculum Examination

1. Have the appropriate size speculum available and lubricated with warm water. (Other lubricants may interfere with cytologic studies.)

2. Begin by inserting the first 2 fingers of the gloved hand into the vagina; locate the cervix, noting the angle of the fingers and the distance from the vaginal opening to the cervix.

3. Proceed by removing the 2 fingers to the edge of the vaginal opening. Press the 2 fingers downward against the perineum. Take the speculum in your other hand and, with the blades closed and held obliquely, guide the speculum past the 2 gloved fingers while exerting pressure downward. (This avoids putting painful pressure on the anterior urethral structures.) Avoid pinching the vagina with the speculum.

4. Once the speculum is inserted, remove the gloved fingers from the introitus (vaginal opening) and return the speculum blades to a horizontal position, maintaining pressure posteriorly.

5. Next, open the speculum blades and, with direct light, visualize the cervix. Maneuver the speculum, so that the cervix comes into full view.
(The cervix lies within the *fornix,* or posterior portion of the vagina, dividing the fornix into the anterior, posterior, right, and left fornices.)

2. Normally, the uterus is positioned forward with the cervix at almost a right angle to the vagina.

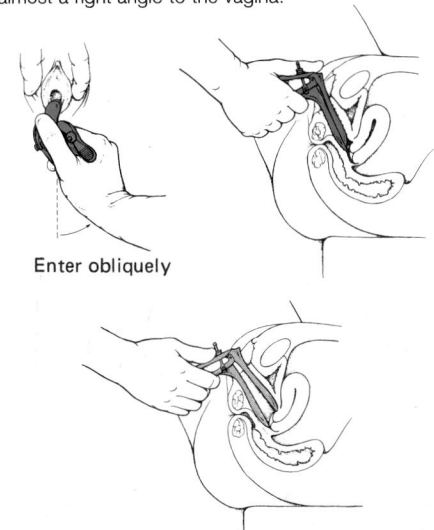

Enter obliquely

6. Inspect the cervix and its opening (os), noting position, color, and shape of the os, ulceration, nodules, bleeding, and discharge. (For Papanicolaou smear, see p. 719).

7. As you slowly pull the speculum out of the vagina, inspect the vaginal mucosa for color, inflammation, ulcers, masses, or discharge.

8. Close the blades before reaching the introitus, and remove the speculum without pinching the vaginal wall. (Also see Guidelines in Chap. 28, p. 718).

6. The cervix of the nonpregnant woman is pink and smooth.

7. A small amount of clear lubricating mucus is normal in the vagina. Normally, there is no bleeding from the nonmenstruating female.

Technique	Findings

Palpation *(Bimanual Examination)*

1. Lubricate the index and middle fingers of the gloved hand and insert them into the vagina, noting nodules, masses, or irregularities anteriorly and posteriorly.
2. Locate the cervix and fornices and note tenderness, shape, size, consistency, regularity, and mobility of the cervix.
3. Place the gloved finger in the posterior fornix and the ungloved hand on the abdomen approximately midway between the umbilicus and the symphysis pubis.

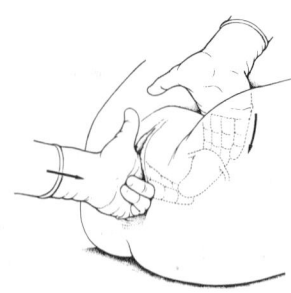

4. Press the 2 hands toward one another and palpate the uterus, noting its size, shape, regularity, consistency, mobility and tenderness, and any masses.
5. Next, place the gloved fingers in the right lateral fornix and the ungloved hand in the right lower quadrant. Palpate the ovaries, if possible, noting shapes, sizes, consistency, regularity, mobility, pain (the ovary is usually tender), or masses. Repeat the procedure on the left side.
6. Next, withdraw the gloved hand, leaving the index finger in the vagina and placing the middle finger in the rectum. Repeat the procedure of the bimanual examination.
7. If possible, press the uterus downward toward the rectal finger, so that as much of the posterior surface of the uterus as possible can be examined.
8. Proceed with the rectal examination (see below).
9. Upon completing the examination, wipe genitalia and perineum with a tissue or offer the patient one so that she may do it herself.

The cervix of the nonpregnant woman is smooth, firm, and slightly movable. It is nontender. The uterus is firm, smooth, and nontender.

5. The ovaries vary in size considerably, but average about 3.5 × 2 × 1.5 cm. (1.4 × 0.8 × 0.6 inches). The uterine (fallopian) tubes are generally not palpable.

6. Explain what you are doing, since this is uncomfortable for the patient and may produce the sensation of wanting to defecate.

Rectum

Equipment

Glove, lubricant

Techniques of Examination

Male

General Approach

1. If the patient is ambulatory, have him stand and bend over the edge of the table.
2. It is also possible to examine the anus and rectum with the patient lying on his left side, knees drawn up and buttocks close to the edge of the table. (This is generally an uncomfortable position, and the patient should be told that he may feel as though he wants to move his bowels.)
3. The patient should be draped so that only his buttocks are exposed.

Inspection

Spread the buttocks and inspect the anus, perianal region, and sacral region for inflammation, nodules, scars, lesions, ulcerations, or rashes. Ask the patient to bear down; note any bulges.

In males and females, the perianal and sacrococcygeal areas are dry, with varying amounts of hair covering them. In the sacrococcygeal region, it is not uncommon to find a small opening or sinus surrounded by a tuft of hair. This is a *pilonidal cyst;* it should be nontender and noninflamed.

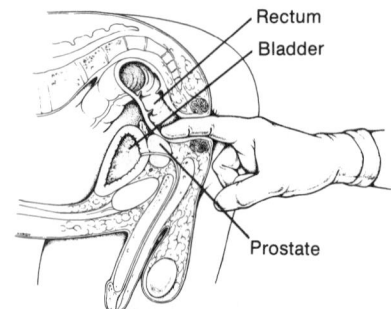

Palpation

1. Palpate any abnormal area noted on inspection.
2. Lubricate the index finger of the gloved hand. Rest the finger over the anus as the patient bears down and, as the sphincter relaxes, insert finger slowly into the rectum.

Technique	Findings

3. Note sphincter tone, any nodules or masses, or tenderness.

3. The anal canal is approximately 2.5 cm. (1 inch) long; it is bordered by the external and internal anal sphincters, which are normally firm and smooth.

4. Insert the finger further and palpate the walls of the rectum laterally and posteriorly while rotating your index finger. Note irregularities, masses, nodules, tenderness.

4. The wall of the rectum in males and females is smooth and moist.

5. Anteriorly, palpate the 2 lateral lobes of the prostate gland and its median sulcus for irregularities, nodules, swelling, or tenderness.

5. The male prostate gland is approximately 2.5 cm. (1 inch) long, smooth, regular, nonmovable, nontender, and rubbery.

6. If possible, palpate the superior portion of the lateral lobe, where the seminal vesicles are located. Note induration, swelling, or tenderness.

6. The seminal vesicles are generally not palpable unless swollen.

7. Just above the prostate anteriorly, the rectum lies adjacent to the peritoneal cavity. If possible, palpate this region for peritoneal masses and tenderness.

8. Continue to insert the finger as far as possible and have the patient bear down so that more of the bowel can be palpated.

9. Gently withdraw your finger. Any fecal material on the glove should be tested for occult blood.

9. There is normally no occult blood in the stools.

Female

General Approach

1. The examination is usually performed following the pelvic examination with the patient still in the lithotomy position.
2. If only the rectal examination is done, the patient may be positioned laterally, as for examination of the male.
    The lateral position permits better visualization of the sacral region.
3. The technique is basically the same for the female as for the male.
4. Anteriorly, the cervix, and perhaps a retroverted uterus, may be felt.

4. Anteriorly, the cervix is round and smooth.

Musculoskeletal System

General Approach

1. Examine the muscles and joints, keeping in mind the structure and functions of each.
2. This discussion will center on the technique for examining the patient who is asymptomatic and, therefore, will not present in detail the techniques for inspecting and palpating joints that are symptomatic or deformed.
3. It is important to ask in the history and to note in the examination whether the patient has difficulty performing activities of daily living:
    a. Bathing
    b. Dressing (buttoning, using zippers, tying shoelaces)
    c. Combing hair
    d. Brushing teeth
    e. Walking up and down stairs
    f. Bending
    g. Sitting
    h. Grasping and holding items without dropping them
    i. Standing from a sitting position, unaided
4. Once the above facts have been ascertained, the examination proceeds. Observe and palpate joints and muscles for symmetry and then examine each joint individually as indicated.
5. The examination is performed with the joints both at rest and in motion—moving through a full range of motion; joints and supporting muscles and tissues are noted.

Inspection

1. Inspect the upper and lower extremities for size, symmetry, any deformity, and muscle mass.

For the purpose of this text, it is sufficient to say that in the course of the history and examination, the examiner should not find any compromise or restriction of the patient's activities of daily living or any other normal activities. If any activity is restricted because of muscular or skeletal problems, the reader is referred to a more detailed text on physical examination.

2. Inspect the joints for range of motion (in degrees), enlargement, redness.
3. Note gait and posture; observe the spine for range of motion, lateral curvature, or any abnormal curvature.
4. Observe the patient for signs of pain during the examination.

Technique	Findings

Palpation

1. Palpate the joints of the upper and lower extremities and the neck for tenderness, swelling, temperature, and range of motion.
2. Hold the palm of the hand over the joint as it moves, or move the joint through the fullest range of motion and note any crepitation (crackling feeling within the joint).
3. Palpate the muscles for size, tone, strength, and tenderness.
4. Palpate the spine for bony deformities and crepitation. Gently hit the spine with the ulnar surface of your fist from the cervical to the lumbar region and note any pain or tenderness.

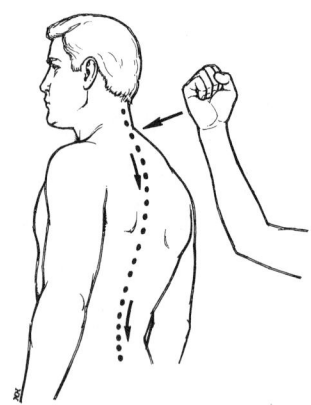

Neurologic System

Equipment

Safety pin, cotton, tuning fork, reflex hammer, flashlight, tongue blade

General Information

1. The examination described in this section is a screening neurologic examination.
   a. It is performed on individuals without specific neurologic complaints.
   b. There is a more detailed examination for patients with specific signs and symptoms.
   c. The student is referred to another text for the content and technique of a detailed neurologic examination.
2. The examination is performed with the patient in either the sitting or supine position.
3. Much of the neurologic examination can be performed as different regions of the body are being examined. This facilitates the flow of the entire examination.
   Example: The cranial nerves can be examined at the same time as the head and neck.
   A mental status evaluation can be done while the history is elicited and while the entire physical examination is performed.

Components of the Neurologic Examination

There are 6 components of the neurologic examination:
1. Mental status (cerebral function)
2. Cranial nerve function
3. Cerebellar function
4. Motor function
5. Sensory function
6. Deep tendon reflexes (DTRs)
The screening neurologic examination involves testing all of these components at least superficially. Learning these components in order will help in organizing the examination and in avoiding the omission of any part.

Basic Principles

1. Symmetry of function and findings on both sides of the body is important to note.
   Always compare one side of the body with the other side (e.g., compare degree of motor strength of the right biceps with that of the left biceps).
2. Integrating the neurologic examination into the examination of the various body regions is advisable, although the results of the neurologic findings should be recorded together as an entity.

Carrying Out the Examination

Mental Status

Components of the mental status examination include the following:
—State of consciousness (alert, somnolent, stuporous, comatose)
—Memory (short-term, long-term, intermediate)
—Cognition (calculations, current events)
—Affect (mood)
—Ideational content (hallucinations)

1. While recording the history ask the patient for identifying information (how to spell his name, where he lives), and ask what the date is. This tests orientation.

In a screening examination, mental status is evaluated by observing the patient's affect during the history and the content of what he or she says.

1. Normally the individual is alert, knows who he is and where he lives, and can tell you the date.

Technique   **Findings**

2. The patient's ability to remember is also evaluated as the history is taken—by asking for his past medical history (long-term memory) and dietary habits: "What did you eat for breakfast?" (intermediate memory).

3. Cognition and ideational content are evaluated throughout the history by what the patient says and by his articulateness, consistency, and reliability in reporting events.

4. Affect or mood is evaluated by observing the patient's verbal and nonverbal behavior in response to questions asked, to sudden noises, to interruptions—for example, does the patient laugh or smile when talking about normally sad events; is he easily startled by unexpected noises?

2. The patient remembers recent and past events consistently, and willingly admits forgetting something.
   Elderly people often have much better long-term memory than recent memory.

4. Mood should be appropriate to the content of the conversation.

Cranial Nerve Function

First (Olfactory) Nerve

(Is not usually tested unless the patient complains of a disturbance in sense of smell.)

1. The airway must be patent.
2. Occlude 1 nostril; ask the patient to close his eyes and then present various substances to smell (e.g., coffee, tobacco). Occlude the other nostril and repeat.
3. Use substances that do not have a lingering effect.

Second (Optic) Nerve

(Includes tests of visual acuity and of gross visual fields and examination of the optic disc with a fundoscope.)

Visual acuity:

   Is tested with the use of a Snellen chart (patient uses glasses if required).

1. Have the patient cover 1 eye at a time and read the smallest print possible on the chart from a distance of 6 meters (20 feet).

1. Normal vision and corrected vision should be 20/20.

Visual fields:

1. Measure by having patient cover his right eye with his right hand. (You cover your left eye with your left hand.)
2. Stand approximately 60 cm. (2 feet) from the patient and have him fix his gaze on your nose.
3. Bring 2 wagging fingers in from the periphery (in a plane equidistant from the patient and you) in all quadrants of the visual field and ask the patient to tell you when he sees your wagging fingers.

3. Assuming your visual fields are grossly normal, the patient and you should see the wagging fingers approximately simultaneously. (The patient's peripheral vision should approximate the examiner's, assuming that it is normal.)

Optic disc:

Is visualized as part of the fundoscopic examination (see p. 22).

Third (Oculomotor), Fourth (Trochlear), and Sixth (Abducens) Nerves

(Are tested together.) These nerves control the movements of the extraocular muscles of the eye—the superior and inferior oblique and the medial and lateral rectus muscles.

   The oculomotor nerve also controls pupillary constriction.

1. Hold your index finger approximately 30 cm. (1 foot) from the patient's nose. Ask the patient to hold his head steady.
2. Ask the patient to follow your finger with his eyes.
3. Move your finger to the right as far as the patient's eye moves. Before bringing your finger back to the center, move it up and then down, so that the patient glances up and peripherally and then down and peripherally.
4. Repeat the test, moving your finger to the left.

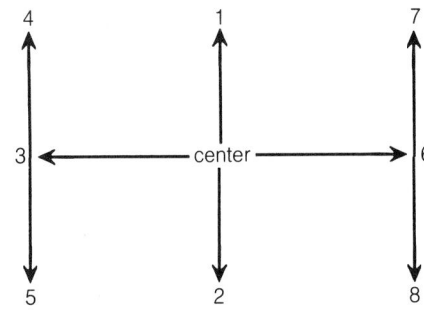

Fifth (Trigeminal) Nerve

(Has motor component that controls muscles of mastication and a sensory component that controls sensations of the face.)

Motor:

1. Have the patient bite down on a tongue depressor with one side of his mouth while you try to pull the blade out.
2. Repeat the test on the other side of the mouth and compare muscle strength of the 2 sides.

Muscle strength in the face should be present and should be symmetrical.

Technique	Findings

Sensory:

(Sensation to light touch.)

1. Have the patient close his eyes.
2. Touch first one side of the patient's face and then the other (forehead, cheek, and chin), asking the patient if the sensation is present and feels the same on both sides.

Sensation should be present and symmetrical. Always demonstrate to the patient how and with what you are testing sensation—to avoid startling the patient and to encourage cooperation.

3. Sensation to pain (pinprick) is tested similarly.

Seventh *(Facial)* **Nerve**

(Motor function is tested by observing facial expression and symmetry of facial movement.)

Ask the patient to frown, close his eyes, and smile.

The facial muscles should look symmetrical when the patient frowns, closes his eyes, and smiles. Notice particularly the symmetry of the nasolabial folds.

Eighth *(Acoustic)* **Nerve**

(Has 2 branches.)

Cochlear (mediates hearing). See ear examination, page 23.

Vestibular (helps control equilibrium).

Romberg test: Have the patient stand erect with his eyes closed and feet close together.

Slight swaying may occur, but the patient should not fall. (Stand close to the patient, so that you can assist if he begins to fall.)

Ninth *(Glossopharyngeal)* **and Tenth** *(Vagus)* **Nerves**

(Are tested together, since both have a motor portion innervating the pharynx.)

1. Ninth: Test the presence of the gag reflex.

2. Tenth: Ask the patient to say "ah" and observe the movement of the uvula and palate for deviation and asymmetry.

The gag reflex should be present, and there should be no difficulty in swallowing.

The palate and uvula should move symmetrically without deviation.

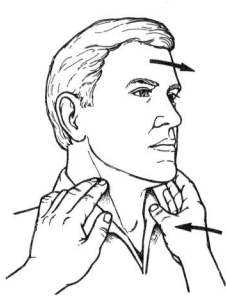

Eleventh *(Spinal Accessory)* **Nerve**

(Mediates the sternocleidomastoid and upper portion of the trapezius muscles.)

1. Ask the patient to turn his head to the side against resistance while your fingers apply pressure to the jaw.
2. Palpate the sternocleidomastoid muscle on the opposite side.
3. Then have the patient shrug his shoulders while you place your hands on his shoulders and apply slight pressure.

Neck and shoulder muscle strength should be symmetrical.

Twelfth *(Hypoglossal)* **Nerve**

(Innervates muscles of the tongue.)

Test by noting articulation and by having the patient stick out his tongue, noting any deviation or asymmetry.

The tongue should be symmetrical and should not deviate.

Cerebellar Function

(Purpose: to screen for coordination.)

1. Observe posture and gait.
2. Ask the patient to walk forward (and then backward) in a straight line.
3. To test for muscle coordination in the lower extremities, have the patient run his right heel down his left shin and vice versa.
4. To test coordination in upper extremities, have the patient close his eyes and touch his nose with his index finger (starting position: arms outstretched) first left, then right, in rapid succession.

The patient should be able to perform all the tests described with smooth, even movement and without losing balance.

The normal person can do this with rapid, smooth movements without undershooting or overshooting the target.

Motor Function

(Tested in conjunction with the skeletal system, since any bony deformity will affect motor function.)

Evaluate muscle mass, tone, strength, and any abnormal movements (tics, fasciculations, twitching).

Technique	Findings

Muscle mass: Note symmetry between sides of the body and distribution distally and proximally.

Tone: Test by noting the resistance the muscle offers to movement upon passive motion.

Strength:

Lower extremity—have the patient do deep knee bends; walk on his toes and then his heels; hop on 1 foot and then the other.

Upper extremity—have the patient squeeze your fingers with both hands; compare sides of the body.

Also, apply resistance (1) to the patient's outstretched arms and (2) when the patient flexes the wrist and elbow; compare sides.

Unusual muscle movements: If present, are noted both when muscle is at rest and when it is moving.

Muscle mass: Is usually considered in relation to sex and body build and to use of various muscle groups.

Tone: Generally there is slight resistance to passive movement of muscles as opposed to flaccidity (no resistance) or rigidity (increased muscle tone).

Strength: Will vary from person to person.

Normally, tremors, tics, or fasciculations are not present either at rest or with movement.

Sensory Function

(Should test sensitivity to light touch [cotton], pain [pinprick], vibration [tuning fork], and position.) Compare both sides of body.

Light touch: Ask the patient to close his eyes. Brush his skin with a piece of cotton (on back of hands, forearms, upper arms, dorsal portion of foot laterally and medially; and along the tibia and thigh laterally and medially). Ask the patient to indicate when he feels the cotton and to compare the sensation bilaterally.

Pain: Use a safety pin; touch the skin as lightly as possible to elicit a sharp sensation.

Vibration sense: Test by placing a vibrating tuning fork on a bony prominence (wrist, medial and lateral malleoli). Ask the patient to tell you when he no longer feels vibration. Stop the vibration with your hand.

The patient should normally feel no vibration within a very short time.

Position sense:

1. Have the patient close his eyes.
2. Move the patient's digit (finger, great toe) up or down and ask the patient to say in what direction his finger or toe is pointing.
3. Place your thumb and index finger on either side of the digit being moved, so that the patient will not sense any pressure from your finger in the direction in which you are moving the digit.

Normally the patient can tell you without hesitation in what direction his digit is pointing.

Deep Tendon Reflexes

1. Have the patient relax; provide support for the extremity being tested.
2. Compare reflex amplitude of the same tendons on either side of the body.

Amplitude of the reflex may vary for different tendons.

Upper Extremities

Biceps:

1. Place your right thumb on the patient's right biceps tendon (located in the antecubital fossa).
2. Rest the patient's forearm on your left hand and strike your thumb with the pointed end of the hammer head. (Hold the hammer loosely, so that it pivots in your hand when it is moved with a wrist action.)

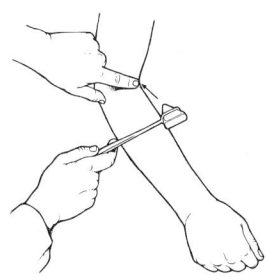

3. Strike your thumb with the least amount of pressure needed to elicit the reflex.

Triceps tendon:

1. Hold the patient's arm abducted and bent at the elbow.
2. Posteriorly, about 2.5 cm. (1 inch) above the olecranon process, strike the tendon directly, using the pointed end of the hammer.

The forearm may move, and your thumb should feel the tendon jerk.

The forearm should move slightly.

Technique	Findings

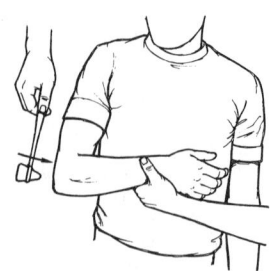

Brachioradialis tendon:
1. Strike the forearm with the hammer about 2.5 cm. (1 inch) above the wrist over the radius.
2. Be sure the forearm is supported and relaxed.

The thumb may be observed moving downward.

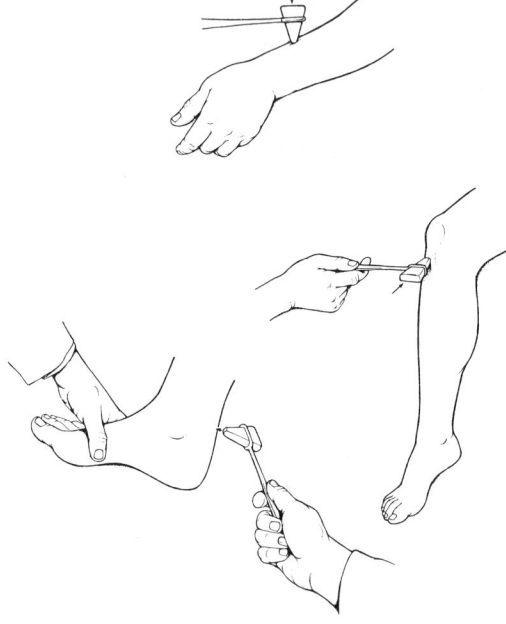

Lower Extremities

Quadriceps reflex:
1. Have the patient sitting with his legs hanging over the edge of the table or lying down while you support the legs at the knee (slightly bent).
2. Strike the tendon just below the patella.
3. If reflexes are difficult to elicit, have the patient interlace the fingers of both hands and then have him try to pull his hands apart. While he is thus distracted, inhibition of the quadriceps reflex is diminished, and the reflex can be elicited more easily. If such a distraction is used to elicit the reflex, record this fact with the physical findings.

Achilles reflex:
1. Support the foot in dorsiflexed position.
2. Tap the Achilles tendon with the hammer head.

The foot should move downward into your hand.

Nutritional Assessment—See Chapter 19

Suggested Bibliography

Books

Bates BL. A Guide to Physical Examination and History Taking. 5th ed. Philadelphia, JB Lippincott, 1991

Billings JA and Stoeckle JD. The Clinical Encounter. Chicago, Year Book Medical Pub, 1989

Block GH and Nolan JW. Health Assessment for Professional Nursing: A Developmental Approach. Norwalk, CT, Appleton–Century–Crofts, 1986

Bowers AC and Thompson JM. Clinical Manual of Health Assessment. 3rd ed. St Louis, CV Mosby, 1988

Clain A (ed). Physical Signs in Clinical Surgery. 17th ed. Littleton, MA, John Wright & Sons, 1986

Coulehan JL and Block MR. The Medical Interview: A Primer for Students of the Art. Philadelphia, FA Davis, 1987

DeGowin RL. DeGowin & DeGowin's Bedside Diagnostic Examination. New York, Macmillan, 1987

Gordon M. Manual of Nursing Diagnosis. 1988–1989. St Louis, CV Mosby, 1989

Grimes J and Burns E. Health Assessment in Nursing Practice. 2nd ed. Boston, Jones and Bartlett, 1987

Guckian JC (ed). The Clinical Interview and Physical Examination. Philadelphia, JB Lippincott, 1987

Guzzetta CE et al. Clinical Assessment Tools for Use with Nursing Diagnoses. St Louis, CV Mosby, 1989

Judge RD, Zuidema GD and Fitzgerald FT. Clinical Diagnoses. 5th ed. Boston, Little, Brown & Co, 1989

Kopf R. Handbook of Nursing Physical Assessment. Rockville, MD, Aspen Publishers, 1988

Levinson D. A Guide to the Clinical Interview. Philadelphia, WB Saunders, 1987

Lohman TG, Roche AF and Martorell R. Anthropometric Standardization Reference Manual. Champaign, IL, Human Kinetics Books, 1988

Lumsden CJ and Whiteside CI. Clinical Methods. New York, Alan R Liss, 1987

Magee DJ. Orthopedic Physical Assessment. Philadelphia, WB Saunders, 1987

Malasnos L et al. Health Assessment. 3rd ed. St Louis, CV Mosby, 1986

Morton PG (ed). Health Assessment in Nursing. Springhouse, PA, Springhouse Corp, 1989

Murray RB and Zenter JP. Nursing Assessment and Health Promotion Through the Life Span. 4th ed. Norwalk, CT, Appleton & Lange, 1989

Novey DW. Rapid Access Guide to the Physical Examination. Chicago, Year Book Medical Pub, 1988

Prout BJ and Cooper JG. An Outline of Clinical Diagnosis. 2nd ed. Littleton, MA, John Wright & Sons, 1987

Sandler G and Fry J. Early Clinical Diagnosis. Boston, MTP Press, 1986

Seidel HM et al. Mosby's Guide to Physical Examination. St Louis, CV Mosby, 1987

Sherman JL and Fields SK. Guide to Patient Evaluation. 5th ed. New Hyde Park, NY, Medical Examination Publishing, 1988

Swartz MH. Textbook of Physical Diagnosis: History and Examination. Philadelphia, WB Saunders, 1989

Weber J. Nurses' Handbook of Health Assessment. Philadelphia, JB Lippincott, 1988

Wilkins RL, Hodgkin JE and Lopez B. Lung Sounds: A Practical Guide. St Louis, CV Mosby, 1988

Journals

Andresen GP. A fresh look at assessing the elderly. RN 1989 Jun; 52(6):28–40

Becker KL and Stevens SA. Get in touch and in tune with cardiac assessment. Part 1. Nursing 1988 Mar; 18(3):51–55

Becker KL and Stevens SA. Performing in-depth abdominal assessment. Nursing 1988 Jun; 18(6):59–63

Caldroney RD. The periodic health examination. Hosp Pract 1987 Jul 15; 22(7):189, 194, 197 passim

Durham CF. The no-fault way to assess carotid arteries. Nursing 1988 Nov; 18(11):65–67

Handerham B. How to measure jugular venous distension. Nursing 1987 Sep; 17(9):48–49

Jess LW. Investigating impaired mental status: An assessment guide you can use. Nursing 1988 Jun; 18(6):42–49

Libow L. Evaluating the elderly patient: Some overlooked aspects. Geriatrics 1987 Nov; 42(11):18,20

Loudon RG. The lung exam. Clin Chest Med 1987 Jun; 8(2):265–272

McConnell EA. Getting the feel of lymph node assessment. Nursing 1988 Aug; 18(8):55–57

McConnell EA. Seeing your patient as a mosaic. Nursing 1988 Dec; 18(12):50–51

Merry JA. Take your assessment all the way down to the toes. RN 1988 Jan; 51(1):60–63

Miracle VA. Get in touch and in tune with cardiac assessment. Part 2. Nursing 1988 Apr; 18(4):41–47

Olsson HM et al. Role of the woman patient and fear of the pelvic examination. West J Nurs Res 1987 Aug; 9(3):357–367

Rudolph A and McDermott RJ. The breast physical examination: Its value in early cancer detection. Cancer Nurs 1987 Apr; 10(2):100–106

Smith CE. Assessing bowel sounds: More than just listening. Nursing 1988 Feb; 18(2):42–43

Stark JL. A quick guide to urinary tract assessment. Nursing 1988 Jul; 18(7):57–58

Stevens SA and Becker KL. A simple, step-by-step approach to neurologic assessment. Part 1. Nursing 1988 Sep; 18(9):53–56

Stevens SA and Becker KL. A simple, step-by-step approach to neurologic assessment. Part 2. Nursing 1988 Oct; 18(10):51–58

Stevens SA and Becker KL. How to perform picture perfect respiratory assessment. Nursing 1988 Jan; 18(1):57–63

Special Health Care Situations

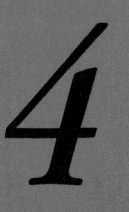

Care of the Surgical Patient

1: Perioperative Nursing

Introductory Information
Concept of Perioperative Patient Care

Perioperative nursing is a term used to describe the nursing functions in the total surgical experience of the patient: preoperative, intraoperative, and postoperative.

  Preoperative phase—from the time the decision is made for surgical intervention to the transference of the patient to the operating room.

  Intraoperative phase—from the time the patient is received in the operating room until he is admitted to the recovery room.

  Postoperative phase—from the time of admission to the recovery room to the follow-up home/clinic evaluation.

Types of Surgery

A. Types of Surgery

1. *Optional*
   Surgery is scheduled completely at the preference of the patient (e.g., cosmetic surgery).

2. *Elective*
   The approximate time for surgery is at the convenience of the patient; failure to have surgery is not catastrophic (e.g., superficial cyst).

3. *Required*
   The condition requires surgery within a few weeks (e.g., eye cataract).

4. *Urgent*
   Surgical problem requires attention within 24 to 48 hours (e.g., cancer).

5. *Emergency*
   Requires immediate surgical attention without delay (e.g., intestinal obstruction).

B. Surgical Procedures

1. Refer to appropriate system headings throughout manual for discussion of specific organ surgical procedures.

2. Common surgical incisions are pictured in Figure 4-1.

Ambulatory (Day) Surgery

Ambulatory surgery (day surgery, in-and-out surgery, outpatient surgery) is becoming a common occurrence for certain types of procedures. The office nurse is in a key role to assess patient status, plan perioperative experience, monitor, instruct, and evaluate the patient.

Advantages

1. Reduced cost to patient, hospital, and insuring and governmental agencies
2. Reduced psychological stress to the patient
3. Less evidence of hospital-acquired infection
4. Less time lost from work by patient; minimal disruption of patient's activities and family life

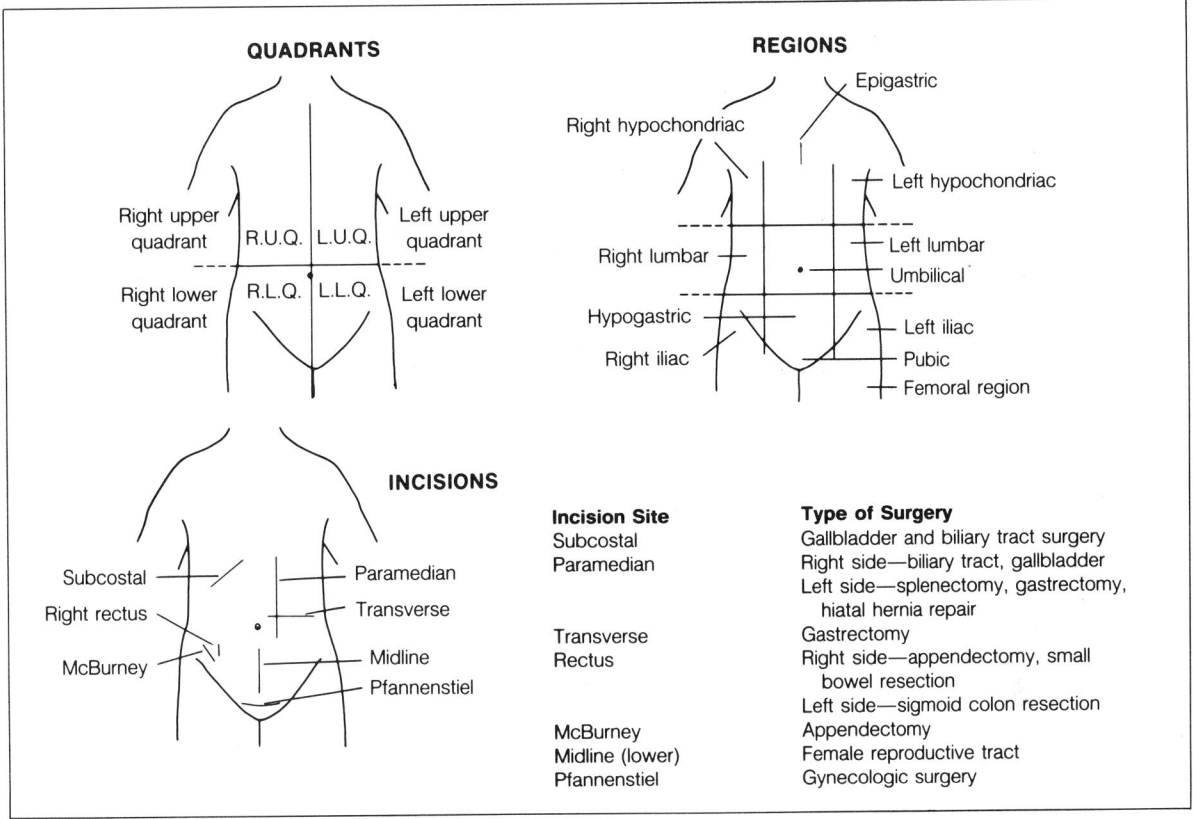

Figure 4-1. *Regions and incisions of the abdomen.*

Disadvantages

1. Less time to assess patient and perform preoperative teaching
2. Less time to establish rapport between patient and health personnel
3. No opportunity to assess for late postoperative complications (this is in the hands of the patient and lay individuals)

Patient Selection

Criteria for selection include:
1. Surgery of short duration (15–90 minutes)
2. Noninfected conditions
3. Type of operation in which postoperative complications are predictably low
4. Age is usually not a factor, although too risky in a premature infant
5. Types of frequently performed procedures:
   a. Dilatation and curettage (D & C)
   b. Tubal ligation
   c. Myringotomy
   d. Excision of skin lesions
   e. Oral surgery (T & A)
   f. Cystoscopy
   g. Diagnostic laparoscopy
   h. Vasectomy

Nursing Management

A. Initial Assessment

1. Develop a nursing history for the day surgical patient; this may be initiated in the physician's office.
2. Obtain signed informed consent form.
3. Explain what laboratory studies are needed and why.
4. Determine during initial assessment the patient's physical and psychological status
   Calm or agitated? Overweight? Disabilities or limitations? Clean or dirty? Allergies? Medications being taken? Condition of teeth (dentures, caps, crowns)? Blood pressure problems? Major illnesses? Other surgeries? Seizures? Severe headaches? Smoker?
5. Begin health education regimen. Instructions to patient:
   a. Notify physician and surgical unit immediately if you get a cold, have a fever, or have any illness before date of surgery.
   b. Arrive at specified time.
   c. Do not ingest food or fluid from midnight previous to day of surgery.
   d. Do not wear make-up or nail polish.
   e. Wear comfortable, loose clothing; low-heeled shoes.
   f. Leave valuables or jewelry at home.
   g. Brush teeth in morning, rinse, but do not swallow liquid.

Chart 4-1 Outpatient Postanesthesia and Post-surgery Instructions and Information

1. Although you will be awake and alert in the Recovery Room, small amounts of anesthetic will remain in your body for at least 24 hours and you may feel tired and sleepy for the remainder of the day. Once you are home, take it easy and rest as much as possible. It is advisable to have someone with you at home for the remainder of the day.

2. Eat lightly for the first 12–24 hours, then resume a well-balanced, normal diet. Drink plenty of fluids. Alcoholic beverages are to be avoided for 24 hours after your anesthesia or intravenous sedation.

3. Nausea or vomiting may occur in the first 24 hours. Lie down on your side and breathe deeply. Prolonged nausea, vomiting, or pain should be reported to your surgeon.

4. Medications, unless prescribed by your physician, should be avoided for 24 hours. Check with your surgeon and/or anesthesiologist for specific instructions if you have been taking a daily medication.

5. Your surgeon will discuss your postsurgery instructions with you and prescribe medication for you as indicated. You will also receive additional instructions specific to your surgical procedure prior to leaving the hospital.

6. Your family will be waiting for you in the hospital's waiting room area near the Outpatient Surgery Department. Your surgeon will speak to them in this area prior to your discharge.

7. DO NOT OPERATE A MOTOR VEHICLE OR ANY MECHANICAL OR ELECTRICAL EQUIPMENT FOR *24 HOURS* AFTER YOUR ANESTHESIA.

8. DO NOT MAKE ANY IMPORTANT DECISIONS OR SIGN LEGAL DOCUMENTS FOR *24 HOURS* FOLLOWING YOUR ANESTHESIA.

(Courtesy of Doctors' Hospital of Prince George's County, Lanham, Maryland)

---

   h. Shower the night before or day of surgery.
   i. Have a responsible adult accompany you and drive you home—have person stay with you for 24 hours after surgery.

B. Preoperative Preparation

1. Administer preanesthetic medication; check vital signs.
2. Escort the patient to surgery after he has emptied his bladder.

C. Postoperative Care

1. Check vital signs frequently until stable.
2. Administer oxygen if necessary; check temperature.
3. Change patient's position as he progresses in activity—head of bed elevated, dangling, ambulating with no dizziness or nausea.
4. Ascertain, using the following criteria, that the patient has recovered adequately to be discharged:
   a. Vital signs stable for at least 1 hour
   b. Stands without dizziness and nausea; begins to walk
   c. Comfortable and free of excessive pain or bleeding
   d. Able to drink fluids and void
   e. Oriented as to time, place, person
   f. No evidence of respiratory depression (2 hours after extubation)
   g. Has the services of a responsible adult who can escort patient home and remain with him at home
   h. Understands postoperative instructions and takes instruction sheet home (see Chart 4-1: Outpatient Postanesthesia and Post-surgery Instructions and Information.

Informed Consent *(Operative Permit)*

An *informed consent* (operative permit) is a form signed by the patient (and witnessed), granting permission to have the operation performed as described by the patient's physician; this is a medicolegal requirement. The consent form should be written using short words and brief, simple sentences. Such forms should be reviewed by patients and the hospital attorney prior to being adopted as a standard form.

Purposes

1. To ensure that the patient understands the nature of the treatment, including potential complications.
2. To indicate that the patient's decision was made without pressure.
3. To protect the patient against unauthorized procedures.
4. To protect the surgeon and hospital against legal action by a patient who claims that an unauthorized procedure was performed.

Informed Consent and the Adolescent Patient

1. An *emancipated minor* is usually recognized as one who is not subject to parental control or regulation.
   a. Married minor
   b. Those in military service
   c. College student who is under age 18 but living away from home
2. Most states have enacted *minor-treatment statutes.* This applies to persons 14 to 18 years of age (statutes vary widely).
3. Standards of informed consent are the same for adolescents and adults.
   If a patient of any age does not understand all material facts, the consent given will be held legally insufficient; no treatment should be given without parental consent except in an acute emergency.

Circumstances Requiring a Permit

1. Any surgical procedure where scalpel, scissors, suture, hemostats, or electrocoagulation may be used.
2. Entrance into a body cavity—paracentesis, bronchoscopy, cystoscopy.
3. General anesthesia, local infiltration, and regional block (e.g., for reduction of a fracture).

Obtaining Informed Consent

1. *Prior to signing an informed consent,* the patient should:
   a. Be told in clear and simple terms by the surgeon

what is to be done (drawings or audiovisual aids may help).

b. Be aware of the risks, possible complications, disfigurement, and removal of parts.

c. Have a general idea of what to expect in the early and late postoperative periods.

d. Have a general idea of the time frame involved from surgery to recovery.

e. Have an opportunity to ask any questions.

f. Sign a separate form for each operation.

2. *Written* permission is best and is legally acceptable.

3. Signature is obtained with the patient's complete understanding of what is to occur; it is obtained before he receives sedation and is secured without pressure or duress.

4. A witness is desirable—nurse, physician, or other authorized person.

5. In an emergency, permission via telephone or telegram is acceptable.

6. For a minor (or a patient who is unconscious or irresponsible), permission is required from a responsible member of the family—parent or legal guardian.

7. For a married minor, permission from the husband or wife is acceptable.

8. If the patient is unable to write, an "X" to indicate his sign is acceptable if there are two signed witnesses to his mark.

9. A separate consent form should be signed for each operation to be performed.

Surgical Risk Factors and Preventive Strategies

A. Obesity

1. Danger

a. Increases difficulty involved in technical aspects of performing surgery (e.g., sutures are difficult to tie because of fatty secretions); wound dehiscence is greater.

b. Increases likelihood of infection because of lessened resistance.

c. Increases postoperative pneumonia and other pulmonary complications because greatly obese patients chronically hypoventilate.

d. Increases demands on the heart, leading to cardiovascular compromise.

e. Increases possibility of renal, biliary, hepatic, and endocrine disorders.

f. Decreases ability to conserve heat due to radiant heat loss.

g. Has altered response to many drugs and anesthetics.

2. Therapeutic approach

a. Encourage weight reduction if time permits.

b. Consult with physician about obtaining preoperative pulmonary function test and arterial blood gases (to assess baseline pulmonary status).

c. Anticipate postoperative obesity-related complications.

d. Be extremely vigilant for respiratory complications.

e. Carefully splint abdominal incisions when moving or coughing; for large patients, sling a drawsheet around the patient's back and pull ends firmly together in front.

f. Be aware that some drugs should be dosed according to *ideal* body weight versus *actual* weight, or an overdose may occur (i.e., digoxin, lidocaine, aminoglycosides, and theophylline)

g. Avoid IM injections in morbidly obese individuals (IV or SQ routes preferred).

h. Never attempt to move impaired patient without assistance and using proper body mechanics.

i. Obtain dietary consultation early in patient's postoperative course.

B. Poor Nutrition

1. Danger

a. Preoperative malnutrition (especially protein and calorie deficits) greatly impairs wound healing.

b. Increases the risk of infection and shock.

2. Therapeutic approach

a. Any recent (within 4–6 weeks) weight loss of 10% of patient's normal body weight should alert health care staff of poor nutritional status.

b. Attempt to improve nutritional status prior to and after surgery. Unless contraindicated, provide diet high in proteins, calories, and vitamins (especially vitamins C and A); this may require enteral and parenteral feeding.

c. Recommend repair of dental caries and proper mouth hygiene to prevent respiratory tract infection.

C. Fluid and Electrolyte Balance

1. Danger

Dehydration and electrolyte imbalances can have adverse effects in terms of general anesthesia and the anticipated volume losses associated with surgery; this can cause shock and cardiac dysrhythmias.

> **NURSING ALERT:** Patients undergoing major abdominal operations (e.g., colectomies, aortic repairs, etc.) often experience a massive fluid shift into tissues around the operative site in the form of edema (as much as a liter may be lost from circulation). Watch for the fluid shift to reverse (from tissue to circulation) around the third postoperative day. Patients with heart disease may develop failure due to the excess fluid "load."

2. Therapeutic approach

a. Scrupulously assess patient's fluid and electrolyte status.

b. Rehydrate patient parenterally and orally as prescribed.

c. Monitor for evidence of electrolyte imbalance (Na^+, K^+, Mg^{++}, Ca^{++}, etc.)

d. Be aware of expected drainage amounts and composition; report excess and abnormalities.

e. Monitor the patient's intake and output; be sure to include all body fluid losses.

D. Aging

1. Danger

a. Recognize that reactions to injury are not as obvious and are slower in appearing.

b. Be aware that the cumulative effect of medications is greater in the older person than it is in younger people.

c. Note that medications such as morphine and barbiturates in the usual dosages may cause confusion

and disorientation; morphine may cause respiratory depression.
2. Therapeutic approach
   a. Consider using lesser doses for desired effect.
   b. Anticipate problems from long-standing chronic disorders such as anemia, obesity, diabetes, hypoproteinemia.
   c. Adjust nutritional intake to conform to higher protein and vitamin needs.
   d. When possible, cater to set patterns in older patients (sleeping and eating patterns).

E. Presence of Disease
1. *Cardiovascular*
   a. Increased diligence is required when a surgical problem is complicated by a cardiovascular problem.
   b. Avoid overloading the body with fluids (oral, parenteral, blood) because of possible myocardial infarction, angina, congestive failure, and pulmonary edema.
   c. Prevent prolonged immobilization, which results in venous stasis. Monitor for potential deep vein thrombosis or pulmonary embolus.
   d. Encourage change of position but avoid sudden exertion.
   e. Use antiembolic hose and pneumatic stockings intraoperatively and postoperatively.
   f. Note evidence of hypoxia and initiate therapy.
2. *Diabetes mellitus*
   a. Be aware that hyperglycemia is potentiated by increased catecholamines and glucocorticoids due to surgical stress
   b. Recognize the signs and symptoms of ketoacidosis and glucosuria (p. 564), which can threaten an otherwise smooth surgical experience.
   c. Reassure the diabetic patient that when his disease is controlled, the surgical risk may be no greater than it is for the nondiabetic person.
3. *Alcoholism*
   a. Anticipate the additional problem of malnutrition in the presurgical patient with alcoholism (increased tolerance to anesthetics).
   b. Be prepared to perform gastric lavage on the intoxicated patient if surgery cannot be postponed; this may lessen the chance of vomiting and aspiration during anesthesia induction.
   c. Note that risk due to surgery is greater for the individual who has chronic alcoholism.
   d. Anticipate the acute withdrawal syndrome (delirium tremens) within 72 hours of last alcoholic drink.
4. *Pulmonary and upper respiratory disease*
   a. Surgery may be contraindicated in the patient who has an upper respiratory infection because it might potentiate a more serious illness, such as pneumonia.
   b. Patients with chronic pulmonary problems such as emphysema, bronchiectasis, etc., should be treated for several days preoperatively with bronchodilators, aerosol medications, and conscientious mouth care, along with a reduction in weight and smoking, and methods to control secretions.
   c. Chronic pulmonary disease increases the risk of atelectasis and pneumonia and potentiates respiratory depression from narcotics.
5. *Concurrent or prior pharmacotherapy*
   a. Hazards exist when certain medications are given concomitantly with others; therefore, an awareness of prior drug therapy is essential. (Example: interaction of some drugs with anesthetics can lead to arterial hypotension and circulatory collapse.)
   b. Notify anesthesiologist if the patient is taking any of the following drugs:
      (1) Certain antibiotics*—may, when combined with a curariform muscle relaxant, interrupt nerve transmission, causing respiratory paralysis and apnea.
      (2) Antidepressants, particularly monoamine oxidase inhibitors (MAOs), increase hypotensive effects of anesthesia.
      (3) Phenothiazines increase hypotensive action of anesthetics.
      (4) Diuretics, particularly thiazides, cause electrolyte imbalance and respiratory depression during anesthesia.
      (5) Steroids inhibit wound healing.

Nursing Process Overview in the Preoperative Period

Preoperative Assessment

1. Assess the patient's reaction to and concerns about hospitalization and the forthcoming operation.
2. Take a nursing history and perform a general physical examination (see Chap. 3).
3. Assess nutritional status (weight-loss history, albumin and transferrin levels, total protein, mid-arm muscle circumference, triceps skin fold).
4. Prepare the patient for various diagnostic tests by explaining why and how they are done and how the patient may contribute to the success of the test. Record reactions to tests, as well as the outcome of such tests. (Diagnostic studies are specific for each patient and are presented in detail in each condition discussed in following chapters.)
5. Ascertain risk factors and develop individualized preventive strategies (see p. 51).
6. Determine the patient's level of understanding of his condition; develop a plan for preoperative patient education (see p. 53).

Nursing Diagnoses

1. Knowledge deficit regarding impending surgery and related preoperative and postoperative procedures.
2. Anxiety related to upcoming surgery, anticipated discomfort, and perceived significance of procedure.
3. Grief (anticipatory) related to altered body image and role performance as a result of surgery and postoperative care.

Nursing Interventions

1. Assist the patient in understanding the physical and psychosocial aspects of the surgical experience.
2. Acquaint the patient and his family with the perioperative environment, protocols, and expectations as surgery is anticipated.

---

* Neomycin, streptomycin, dihydrostreptomycin, polymyxin B, colistin, viomycin, paromomycin, kanamycin, tobramycin, and gentamicin.

3. Teach the patient certain procedures that will help in reducing postoperative complications and in increasing comfort and enhancing recovery.
4. Prepare the patient physically and psychologically for the anesthetic and operative procedure.
5. Collaborate with other members of the health team in coordinating all preoperative preparations.

Expected Outcomes

1. Approaches planned surgery with a positive attitude.
2. Demonstrates and explains the major postoperative activities he will be required to perform.
3. Reduces potential risks to acceptable levels.
4. Cooperates during immediate presurgical preparation and explains the reasons for receiving presurgical medication.

Preoperative Patient Education

Preoperative patient education may be offered through conversation, discussion, the use of audiovisual aids, demonstrations, and return demonstrations. It is designed to help the patient understand the surgical experience in order to minimize anxiety and promote full recovery from surgery and anesthesia.

Note: Parts of this program may be initiated before hospitalization by the physician or the office nurse practitioner. This is particularly important for patients who are admitted the day of surgery or undergo outpatient surgical procedures.

Teaching Strategies

A. Obtain Data Base and Plan Modus Operandi.

1. Determine what the patient already knows or wants to know. This can be accomplished by reading the patient's chart, by interviewing the patient, and by communicating with the physician, family, and other members of the health team.
2. Ascertain patient's psychosocial adjustment to impending surgery.
3. Determine cultural or religious health beliefs and practices that may impact the patient's surgical experience, such as refusal of blood transfusions, burial of amputated limbs within 24 hours, or special healing rituals.

B. Plan and Implement Teaching Program

1. Begin at the patient's level of understanding and proceed from there.
2. Plan this presentation, or series of presentations, for this individual patient or a group of patients.
3. Include family members and significant others in the teaching process.
4. Encourage active participation of patients in their care and recovery.
5. Demonstrate essential techniques; provide opportunity for patient practice and return demonstration.
6. Provide time for and encourage patient to ask questions and express concerns; make every effort to answer all queries truthfully and in basic agreement with the overall therapeutic plan.
7. Provide general information and assess the patient's level of interest in or reaction to it.
   a. Explain details of preoperative preparation.

b. Offer general information on the surgery. (Physician is the resource person.)
c. Tell when surgery is scheduled (if known) and how long it will take; explain that afterwards he will go to the recovery room.
d. Let patient know that family will be kept informed and that they will be told where to wait and when they can see him; note visiting hours.
e. Explain how a procedure or test may *feel* during or after.
f. Describe the recovery room; what personnel and equipment the patient may expect to see and hear (specially trained personnel, monitoring equipment, tubing for various functions, and a moderate amount of activity by nurses and physicians).
g. Stress the importance of active participation in postoperative recovery.
h. Utilize other resource persons: physicians, therapists, chaplain, interpreters, and so forth.
i. Document in outline form what has been taught, as well as the patient's reaction and level of understanding.

> **NURSING ALERT:** Touch is a useful modality in preoperative teaching of patients that appears to reduce anxiety significantly.

C. Utilize Audiovisual Aids if Available.

1. Videotapes with sound or film strips with narration are effective in giving basic information to a single patient or group of patients. Many hospitals provide a television channel dedicated to patient instruction.
2. Booklets, brochures, and models, if available, are helpful.
3. Demonstrate any equipment that will be specific for the particular patient. Examples:

Drainage equipment	Monitoring equipment
Side rails	Incentive spirometer
Ostomy bag	

> **NURSING ALERT:** The extent of preoperative patient teaching is determined on an individual basis; determinants are the patient's previous knowledge, his desire to learn and willingness to use this new knowledge, his emotional and physical condition, the amount of time available, and the quality of teaching. Effectiveness is greater when time is provided for patient participation and discussion.

Preoperative Practice of Postoperative Activities

Activities that the patient will practice and do postoperatively include the following:

A. Diaphragmatic Breathing

This is a mode of breathing in which the dome of the diaphragm is flattened during inspiration resulting in enlargement of the upper abdomen as air rushes into the chest. During expiration, abdominal muscles and the diaphragm relax (also see p. 172). It is an effective relaxation technique.

For the patient:
1. Assume bed position similar to that most likely to be used postoperatively (semi-Fowler's).
2. Place both hands over lower rib cage; make a loose fist and rest the flat surface of the fingernails against the chest (to feel chest movement).

3. Exhale gently and fully; ribs will sink downward and inward toward midline.
4. Inhale deeply through mouth and nose; permit abdomen to rise as lungs fill with air.
5. Hold this breath through a count of 5.
6. Exhale and let *all* air out through mouth and nose.
7. Repeat 15 times with a brief rest following each group of five.
8. Practice this twice each day preoperatively.

B. Incentive Spirometry

Preoperatively, the patient uses a spirometer to measure deep breaths (inspired air) while exerting maximum effort (see Guidelines, p. 229).

The preoperative measurement becomes the goal to be achieved as soon as possible after the operation.

1. Postoperatively, the patient is encouraged to use the incentive spirometer (available commercially) about 10–12 times an hour. (He does this on his own.)
2. Deep inhalations expand alveoli, which, in turn, prevents atelectasis and other pulmonary complications.
3. There is less pain with inspiratory concentration than with expiratory concentration, such as with coughing and using blow bottles.

C. Coughing

Coughing promotes the removal of chest secretions.

1. Interlace the fingers and place the hands over the proposed incision site; this will act as a splint during coughing and not harm the incision.
2. Lean forward slightly while sitting in bed.
3. Breathe, using the diaphragm as described under diaphragmatic breathing (see above, item A).
4. Inhale fully with the mouth slightly open.
5. Let out 3 or 4 sharp "hacks."
6. Then, with mouth open, take in a deep breath and quickly give 1 or 2 strong coughs.
7. Secretions should be readily cleared from the chest to prevent respiratory complications (pneumonia, obstruction, etc.).

Note: Certain position changes may be contraindicated following some surgeries (i.e., craniotomy and eye or ear surgery).

D. Turning

Changing positions from back to side-lying (and vice versa) stimulates circulation, encourages deeper breathing, and relieves pressure areas.

1. Assist the patient to move onto side if assistance is needed.
2. Place the uppermost leg in a more flexed position than that of the lower leg and place a pillow comfortably between the legs.
3. Ensure that the patient is turned from one side to back and onto the other side every 2 hours.

E. Foot and Leg Exercises

Moving the legs improves circulation and muscle tone.

1. Have the patient lie on back; instruct him to bend the knee and raise the foot—hold it a few seconds, extend the leg, and lower it to the bed.
2. Repeat above for about 5 times with 1 leg and then with the other. Repeat the set 5 times every 3–5 hours.
3. Then have the patient lie on side; exercise the legs by pretending to pedal a bicycle.
4. Suggest the following foot exercise: Trace a complete circle with the great toe.

F. Evaluation of Teaching Program

1. Observe patient for correct demonstration of expected postoperative behaviors, such as foot and leg exercises and special breathing techniques.
2. Ask pertinent questions to determine patient's level of understanding.
3. Reinforce information when necessary.

Preparation of Specific Operative Areas

Skin

1. Human skin normally harbors transient and resident bacterial flora, some of which are pathogenic.
2. Skin cannot be sterilized without destroying skin cells.
3. Friction enhances the action of detergent antiseptics; however, friction should *not* be applied over a superficial malignancy (causes seeding of malignant cells) or areas of carotid plaque (causes plaque dislodgement and emboli).
4. It is ideal for the patient to bathe or shower, using a bacteriostatic soap (e.g., povidone-iodine), on the day of surgery. The surgical schedule may require that the shower be taken the night before.
5. The Centers for Disease Control recommends that hair *not* be removed near the operative site unless it will interfere with surgery. Skin is easily injured during shaving and often results in a higher rate of postoperative wound infection.
6. If requested, shaving should be performed as close to the operative time as possible. The longer the interval between the shave and operation, the higher the incidence of postoperative wound infection.
   a. Use of electrical clippers are preferable. Hair should be removed within 1–2 mm. of the skin to avoid skin abrasion. Thorough cleaning of the clippers, after use, is essential.
   b. A sharp disposable razor, with a recessed blade, may be used as long as a "wet shave" is done. It is important that the shave be done in the direction of hair growth.
   c. Depilatory creams (hair-removing chemicals) offer the advantage of eliminating possible abrasions and cuts and producing clean, smooth, intact skin. Many patients even find this form of skin preparation relaxing. The depilatory creams may cause transient skin reactions in some patients, especially when used near the rectal and scrotal areas.
   d. Scissors may be used to remove hair greater than 3 mm in length.
7. For head surgery, obtain specific instructions from the surgeon concerning the extent of shaving.

Gastrointestinal Tract

1. Preparation of the bowel is imperative for intestinal surgery because escaping bacteria can invade adjacent tissues and cause sepsis.
   a. Cathartics and enemas remove gross collections of stool.
   b. Oral antimicrobial agents (e.g., neomycin, erythromycin) suppress the colon's potent microflora.
   c. Enemas "until clear" are prescribed the evening of elective surgery. Not more than three enemas

should be given because of negative effects on fluid and electrolyte balance. (It is also quite exhausting to the patient.) Notify the physician if the enemas never return clear.

2. Solid food is withheld from the patient for 8–10 hours prior to surgery. Patients having morning surgery are kept NPO overnight. Clear fluids (water) may be given up to 4 hours of surgery.

Genitourinary Tract

A medicated douche may be prescribed preoperatively if the patient is to have a gynecologic (e.g., hysterectomy) or urologic operation.

Immediate Presurgical Preparation of the Patient

Physical and Psychological Attention to the Patient

1. Provide patient with a short gown to be worn to the operating room.
2. Remove hairpins; braid long hair; cover hair with a cap.
3. Remove dentures or plates (unless anesthesiologist requests that they be left in to reduce respiratory tract obstruction); inspect mouth for foreign material such as chewing gum.
4. Remove jewelry, identify properly, and place in the hospital safe; if wedding ring cannot be removed, tie with gauze bandage fastened around wrist.
5. Remove contact lenses; have the patient place them in properly marked receptacle (left and right), identify properly, and deposit in the hospital safe.
6. Have the patient void before receiving preoperative medication and immediately before leaving for the operating room; measure amount and note time of voiding; document.
7. Continue to support the patient emotionally and correct any misconceptions he may have.
8. Permit the patient to relax as the medication becomes effective prior to his being called to the operating room; instruct the patient to call for assistance if necessary and not to be out of bed unassisted. Raise side rails.

Preanesthetic Medication

(Prescribed to meet individual needs)

A. Types

1. *Opiates*—such as morphine and meperidine (Demerol) are given to relax the patient and potentiate anesthesia.
2. *Anticholinergics*—such as atropine, scopolamine, and glycopyrrolate (Robinul) are given primarily to reduce respiratory tract secretions and to prevent severe reflex slowing of the heart during anesthesia. Typically given in conjunction with an opiate less than 1 hour prior to the patient's trip to the operating room.
3. *Barbiturates/tranquilizers*—such as pentobarbital (Nembutal) and other hypnotic agents are given the night prior to surgery to help ensure a restful night's sleep. It is important to note that reassurance from the nurse, anesthesiologist, and physician can do much to alleviate the patient's anxiety and insomnia.

4. *Prophylactic antibiotics*—are administered just prior to or during surgery when bacterial contamination is expected.

B. Goals

1. To facilitate the administration of any anesthetic
2. To minimize respiratory tract secretions and changes in heart rate
3. To relax the patient and reduce anxiety

NURSING ALERT: Administer preanesthetic medication precisely at the time it is prescribed. If given too early, the maximum potency will have passed before it is needed; if given too late, the action will not have begun before anesthesia is started.

"On Call" Medications

1. Have medication ready and administer as soon as call is received.
2. Proceed with remaining preparation activities.
3. Indicate on the chart or preoperative check list the time when medication was administered and by whom.

Transporting Patient to the Operating Room

1. Adhere to the principle of maintaining the comfort and safety of the patient.
2. Accompany operating room attendants to the patient's bedside for introduction and proper identification.
3. Assist in transferring the patient from bed to stretcher (unless bed goes to OR floor).
4. Complete chart and preoperative check list; include laboratory reports and x-rays as required by hospital policy or physician's directive.
5. Recognize importance of coordinating team effort to ensure arrival of the patient in the operating room at the proper time.

The Patient's Family

1. Direct the patient's family to the proper waiting room where magazines, television, and coffee may be available.
2. Inform the family that the surgeon will probably contact them there immediately after surgery to inform them of the operation.
3. Acquaint the family with the fact that a long interval of waiting does not mean the patient is in the operating room all the while; anesthesia preparation and induction take time, and after surgery the patient is taken to the recovery room.
4. Tell the family what to expect postoperatively when they see the patient—tubes, monitoring equipment, and blood transfusion, suctioning, and oxygen equipment.

Anesthesia and Related Complications
Anesthetic Drugs

The goals of anesthesia are to provide analgesia, sedation, and/or muscle relaxation appropriate for the type of operative procedure, as well as to control the autonomic nervous system.

Common Anesthetic Techniques

A. Conscious Sedation

1. Patient remains conscious with some alteration of mood, drowsiness, and sometimes analgesia.
2. Protective reflexes remain intact.

B. Deep Sedation

1. Patient asleep but easily arousable.
2. Protective reflexes minimally depressed.

C. General Anesthesia

1. Complete loss of consciousness, unarousable.
2. A reversible state that provides analgesia, muscle relaxation, and sedation.
3. Protective reflexes are partially or (more commonly) completely lost.
4. Produced by intravenous or inhaled anesthetics.

D. Regional Anesthesia

1. Production of analgesia in a specific body part.
2. Achieved by placing local anesthetics in close proximity (usually by injection) to appropriate nerves.

E. Spinal Anesthesia

1. Local anesthetic injected into lumbar intrathecal space.
2. Anesthetic blocks conduction in spinal nerve roots and dorsal ganglia; paralysis and analgesia occur below level of injection.

F. Epidural Anesthesia

1. Achieved by injecting local anesthetic into extradural space via a lumbar puncture.
2. Results similar to spinal analgesia.

G. Peripheral Nerve Blocks

1. Achieved by injecting local anesthetic at a specific site to render a defined area of anesthesia.

Intraoperative (Anesthesia) Complications

A. Hypoventilation (hypoxemia, hypercarbia)—inadequate ventilatory support following paralysis of respiratory muscles and ensuing coma.

B. Oral trauma (broken teeth, oropharyngeal, or laryngeal trauma)—due to difficult endotracheal intubation.

C. Hypotension—due to preoperative hypovolemia or untoward reaction to anesthetic agents.

D. Cardiac dysrhythmia—due to preexisting cardiovascular compromise, electrolyte imbalance, and/or untoward reactions to anesthetic agents.

E. Hypothermia—due to exposure to cool ambient operating room environment and loss of normal thermoregulation capability from anesthetic agents.

F. Peripheral nerve damage—due to improper positioning of patient (e.g., full weight on an arm) or restraints.

G. Malignant hyperthermia

1. *Cause*
   a. A rare reaction to anesthetic inhalants (notably cyclopropane, enflurane, ether, fluroxene, halothane, isoflurane) and muscle relaxants (e.g., succinylcholine).
   b. Such drugs as theophylline, aminophylline, epinephrine, and digitalis may also induce or intensify this reaction.
   c. This deadly complication is most prone in younger individuals with an inherited muscle disorder

(e.g., forms of muscular dystrophy) or a history of subluxating joints, scoliosis.
   d. Malignant hyperthermia is due to abnormal and excessive intracellular accumulations of calcium with resulting hypermetabolism and increased muscle contraction.

2. *Clinical manifestations*—tachycardia, pseudotetany, muscle rigidity, high fever, cyanosis, heart failure, and central nervous system damage.

3. *Treatment*—dantrolene sodium (Dantrium), oxygen, dextrose 50% (with extra insulin to enhance its utilization), diuretics, antidysrhythmics, sodium bicarbonate (for severe acidosis), and hypothermic measures (e.g., cooling blanket, iced IV saline solutions, or iced saline lavages of stomach, bladder or rectum).

The Nursing Process in the Immediate Postoperative Period

Assessment

Upon receiving a patient in the postanesthesia care unit (PACU) or Recovery Room from the anesthesiologist and circulating nurse, the following determinations are made:

1. Appraise the air-exchange status of the patient and note his skin color. Also note swallowing/gag reflexes and level of consciousness.
2. Verify the patient's identity, the operative procedure, and the surgeon who performed the procedure.
3. Request a briefing on problems encountered in the operating room and those that may arise in the recovery period.
4. Determine vital signs and establish with the anesthesiologist an agreement as to their meaning.
5. Determine and evaluate any lines, tubes, or drains, estimated blood loss, condition of the wound (open, closed, packed), medications used, infusions, and the patient's native language.
6. Perform safety checks to verify that padded side rails are in place and restraints properly applied, as needed, for infusions, transfusions, etc.
7. Review physician's orders and administer prescribed medications. Monitor signs related to nature of surgery.

Nursing Diagnoses

1. Ineffective airway clearance related to effects of general anesthesia.
2. Impaired gas exchange related to hypoventilation.
3. Fluid volume deficit, potential, related to blood loss, food and fluid deprivation, and vomiting.
4. Potential for hypothermia related to altered thermoregulatory ability and cool environment.
5. Alteration in sensory perception related to effects of medications and anesthesia.
6. Altered comfort, pain, related to surgical incision and tissue trauma.
7. Impairment of skin integrity related to operative incision.
8. Altered nutrition, less than body requirements, related to reduced intake preoperatively and during day of surgery.
9. Potential for injury related to sensory deprivation as a result of preanesthetic medications and anesthesia.

Nursing Interventions

A. Ensure the Maintenance of a Patent Airway and Adequate Respiratory Function.

1. Place the patient in the lateral position with neck extended (if not contraindicated)—this permits the best possible expansion of the lungs.
2. Allow metal, rubber, or plastic airway to remain in place until the patient begins to waken and is trying to eject the airway.
   a. The airway keeps the passage open and prevents the tongue from falling backward and obstructing the air passages.
   b. Leaving the airway in after the pharyngeal reflex has returned may cause the patient to gag and vomit.

Note: Many seriously ill patients return from the operating room with an endotracheal tube in place; this may be left in place for hours or days and requires special management.

3. When the patient is partially awake and the airway is removed, he may show signs of gagging, nausea, or vomiting; place him in the lateral position with the upper arm supported on a pillow.
   a. This will promote chest expansion.
   b. Turn the patient every hour or two to facilitate breathing and ventilation.
4. Aspirate excessive secretions when they are heard in the nasopharynx and oropharynx.
5. Encourage patient to take deep breaths to aerate lungs fully and prevent hypostatic pneumonia; use incentive spirometer to aid in this function (p. 54).
6. Administer humidified oxygen if required.
   a. Heat and moisture are normally lost during exhalation.
   b. Dehydrated patients may require oxygen and humidity because of higher incidence of irritated respiratory passages in these patients.
   c. Secretions can be kept moist to facilitate removal.
7. Employ mechanical ventilation to maintain adequate pulmonary ventilation if required (see p. 246).

B. Assess Status of Circulatory System.

1. Take vital signs (blood pressure, pulse, and respiration) frequently, as clinical condition indicates, until the patient is well stabilized. Then check every 4 hours thereafter.
   a. Know the patient's preoperative blood pressure in order to make significant comparisons.
   b. Report immediately a falling systolic pressure and an increasing heart rate.
   c. Variations in blood pressure and cardiac dysrhythmias are reportable.
   d. Respirations over 30 should be reported.
   e. Evaluate pulse pressure to determine status of perfusion. (A narrowing pulse pressure indicates impending shock.)
2. Closely monitor intake and output.
3. Recognize the variety of factors that may alter circulating blood volume.
   a. Reactions to anesthesia and medications
   b. Blood loss and organ manipulation during surgery
   c. Moving the patient from one position on the operating table to another on the stretcher
4. Monitor temperature hourly to be alert for hyperthermia and to detect hypothermia. A temperature over 37.7°C. (100°F.) or under 36.1°C. (97°F.) is reportable.
5. Be aware of early symptoms of shock or hemorrhage.
   a. Cool extremities, decreased urine output (less than 30 ml./hour), slow capillary refill (greater than 3 seconds), lowered blood pressure, narrowing of pulse pressure, and increased heart rate are often indicative of decreased cardiac output.
   b. Initiate oxygen therapy to increase oxygen availability from the circulating blood.
   c. Increase parenteral fluid infusion as prescribed.
   d. Place the patient in shock position with feet elevated (unless contraindicated).
   e. See page 61 for more detailed consideration of shock.

C. Assess Thermoregulatory Status.

1. Monitor temperature hourly to be alert for malignant hyperthermia (see p. 56) or to detect hypothermia.
2. A temperature over 37.7°C. (100°F.) or under 36.1°C. (97°F.) is reportable.
3. Monitor for *postanesthesia shivering (PAS)*. It is most significant in hypothermic patients 30–45 minutes after admission to the PACU. It represents a heat-gain mechanism and relates to regaining thermal balance.
4. Provide a therapeutic environment with proper temperature and humidity; when cold, provide the patient with warm blankets.

D. Promote Comfort and Maintain Safety.

1. Place side rails in protecting position until the patient is fully awake.
2. Protect the extremity into which intravenous fluids are running so that the needle will not become accidentally dislodged.
3. Turn the patient frequently and maintain good body alignment.
4. Avoid nerve damage and muscle strain by properly supporting and padding pressure areas.
5. Assess pain by observing behavioral and physiologic manifestations.
6. Administer analgesics (low blood pressure may be a result of pain) and document efficacy.

E. Continue Constant Surveillance of the Patient Until He Is Completely Out of Anesthesia.

NURSING ALERT: This phase of nursing care is geared to *recognizing* the significance of signs and *anticipating* and *preventing* postoperative difficulties. Carefully monitor the patient coming out of general anesthesia until:
1. Vital signs are stable for at least 30 minutes and are within *his* normal range.
2. He is breathing easily.
3. Reflexes have returned to normal.
4. He is out of anesthesia, responsive, and oriented to time and place.
For the patient who had regional anesthesia, observe carefully until:
1. Sensation has been recovered.
2. Reflexes have returned.
3. Vital signs have stabilized for at least 30 minutes.

1. Be aware of the fact that the patient cannot complain of injury such as the pricking of an open safety pin, or a clamp that is exerting pressure.
2. Check dressings for constriction.

3. Observe drainage tubes and catheters for proper connection and patency.
4. Note proper functioning of monitoring and suctioning devices, oxygen therapy equipment, etc.
5. Observe the patient for bladder distention (see Fig. 27-6, p. 671).
6. Inspect skin and tissue surrounding intravenous needles to detect early infiltration.
7. Evaluate periodically the patient's status of orientation—how he responds to being addressed by his name or performs simple movements upon receiving a command.

Note: Alterations in cerebral function may suggest impaired oxygen delivery to tissues.

8. Determine return of motor control following spinal anesthesia—indicated by how the patient responds to a pinprick or a request to move a part.

F. Recognize Stress Factors That May Affect the Patient in the Recovery Room and Attempt to Minimize These Factors.

1. Know that the ability to hear returns more quickly than other senses as the patient emerges from anesthesia.
2. Avoid saying anything in the patient's presence that may disturb him; he may appear to be sleeping but still consciously hears what is being said.
3. Explain procedures and activities at the patient's level of understanding.
4. Minimize the patient's exposure to emergency treatment of nearby patients by drawing curtains and lowering voice and noise levels.
5. Treat the patient as a person who needs as much attention as the equipment and monitoring devices.
6. Respect his feeling of sensory deprivation and simultaneous bombardment of sensory stimuli; make any necessary adjustments to minimize this problem.
7. Make every effort to demonstrate concern for and understanding of this patient—anticipate his needs and feelings.
8. Tell the patient repeatedly that the surgery is over and that he is in the recovery room.

G. Transfer the Patient From the Postanesthesia Care Unit to His Unit.

1. Relay appropriate information to the unit nurse regarding his condition; point out significant needs (e.g., drainage, fluid therapy, incision and dressing requirements, intake needs, urinary output).
2. Orient patient to room, attending nurse, call light, and therapeutic devices.

Expected Outcomes

(Criteria for leaving recovery unit)
1. Breathes easily with clear lung sounds noted via stethoscopic auscultation.
2. Reaches stable vital signs and achieves adequate circulatory perfusion.
3. Responds well to commands when asked to cough, breathe deeply, or move extremities.
4. Approaches a satisfactory level of awareness and consciousness.
5. Pain adequately controlled.
6. Maintains acceptable levels of urinary output (at least 30 ml/hr).
7. Appears to have vomiting well under control, if not absent.
8. Moves extremities following regional anesthesia.

Postoperative Discomforts

Most patients experience some discomforts postoperatively. These are usually related to the general anesthetic and/or the surgical procedure. The most common discomforts are nausea, vomiting, restlessness, sleeplessness, thirst, constipation, flatulence, and pain.

Nausea and Vomiting

Incidence

1. Occurs in many postoperative patients.
2. Most often related to inhalation (volatile) anesthetics, which may irritate the stomach lining and stimulate the vomiting center in the brain.
3. Results from an accumulation of fluid or food in the stomach before peristalsis returns.
4. May occur as a result of abdominal distention, which follows manipulation of abdominal organs.
5. Likely to occur if the patient believes preoperatively that he will vomit (psychological induction).
6. May be a side effect of narcotics.

Preventive Measures

1. Insert nasogastric tube preoperatively for operations on gastrointestinal tract to prevent abdominal distention, which triggers vomiting.
2. Determine whether patient is sensitive to morphine, meperidine (Demerol), or other narcotic, since they may induce vomiting in some patients.
3. Be alert for any significant comment such as, "I just know I will vomit under anesthesia." Report such a comment to the anesthesiologist, who may prescribe an antiemetic drug and also talk to the patient before the operation.

Nursing Interventions

1. Encourage patient to breathe deeply to facilitate elimination of anesthetic.
2. Support the wound during retching and vomiting; turn head to side to avoid aspiration.
3. Discard vomitus and refresh patient—mouthwash for mouth, clean linens for bed, etc.
4. Suspect idiosyncratic response to a drug if vomiting is worse when a medication is given (but diminishes thereafter).
5. Administer antiemetic medication such as prochlorperazine (Compazine) or promethazine (Phenergan); be aware that these drugs may potentiate the hypotensive effects of narcotics.
6. Offer hot tea with lemon or small sips of a carbonated beverage such as ginger ale, if tolerated or permitted.
7. Report excessive or prolonged vomiting so that the cause may be investigated.
8. Detect presence of abdominal distention, hiccups, suggesting gastric retention.

Thirst

Causes

1. Inhibition of secretions by preoperative medication with atropine.

2. Fluid lost via perspiration, blood loss, and dehydration due to preoperative fluid restriction.

Nursing Interventions

1. Administer fluids by vein or by mouth if tolerated.
2. Offer sips of hot tea with lemon juice to dissolve mucus.
3. Apply a moistened gauze square over lips occasionally to humidify inspired air.
4. Allow the patient to rinse mouth with mouthwash.
5. Obtain hard candies or chewing gum, if allowed, to help in stimulating saliva flow and in keeping the mouth moist.

Constipation and Gas Cramps

Causes

1. Trauma and manipulation of the bowel during surgery, as well as narcotic use, will retard peristalsis.
2. Local inflammation, peritonitis, or abscess.
3. Long-standing bowel problem; this may lead to fecal impaction.

Nursing Interventions and Preventive Measures

1. Encourage early ambulation to aid in promoting peristalsis.
2. Provide adequate fluid intake to promote soft stools and hydration.
3. Advocate proper diet to promote peristalsis.
4. Query patient as to his usual remedy for constipation and try it.
5. Encourage early use of non-narcotic analgesia, as many opiates increase chance of constipation.
6. Assess bowel sounds frequently.
7. Insert gloved finger and break up the fecal impaction manually, if necessary.
8. Administer an oil retention enema (180–200 ml.), if prescribed, to help soften the fecal mass and facilitate evacuation.
9. For gas cramps, administer a return-flow enema (if prescribed) or a rectal tube to decrease painful flatulence.
10. Administer gastrointestinal stimulants, laxatives, suppositories, and stool softeners if prescribed.

Pain

Pain is a subjective symptom in which the patient exhibits a feeling of distress caused by stimulation of, or trauma to, certain nerve endings as a result of surgery.

Incidence

1. Pain is one of the earliest symptoms that the patient expresses upon return to consciousness.
2. Maximal postoperative pain occurs between 12 and 36 hours after surgery and usually diminishes significantly by 48 hours.
3. Anesthetic agents that are soluble are slow to leave the body and therefore control pain for a longer time than agents that are insoluble; the latter produce rapid recovery, but the patient is more restless and complains more of pain.
4. Older persons seem to have a higher tolerance for pain than younger or middle-aged persons.

5. There is no documented proof that one sex tolerates pain better than the other.

Clinical Manifestations

1. Autonomic
   a. Outpouring of epinephrine
   b. Elevation of blood pressure
   c. Increase in heart and pulse rate
   d. Rapid and irregular respiration
   e. Increase in perspiration
2. Skeletal muscle
   Increase in muscle tension or activity
3. Psychological
   a. Increase in irritability
   b. Increase in apprehension
   c. Increase in anxiety
   d. Attention focused on pain
   e. Complaints of pain
   Patient's reaction depends upon:
1. Previous experience
2. Anxiety or tension
3. State of health
4. His ability to concentrate away from the problem or be distracted
5. Meaning that pain has for him

Nursing Interventions

A. Employ Basic Comfort Measures.

1. Provide therapeutic environment—proper temperature and humidity, ventilation, visitors.
2. Massage the patient's back and pressure points with soothing strokes—move him easily and gently and with prewarning.
3. Offer diversional activities, soft radio music, or favorite quiet television program.
4. Provide for fluid needs by giving a cool drink, offering a bedpan.
5. Investigate possible causes of pain such as bandage or adhesive that is too tight, full bladder, cast that is too snug, or elevated temperature suggestive of inflammation or infection.
6. Instruct patient to splint wound when moving.
7. Keep bedding clean, dry, and free of wrinkles and debris.

B. Recognize the Power of Suggestion.

1. Provide reassurance that the discomfort is temporary and that the medication will aid in pain reduction.
2. Clarify patient's fears regarding the perceived significance of pain.
3. Assist patient in maintaining a positive, hopeful attitude.

C. Assist in Relaxation Techniques
   Imagery, meditation, controlled breathing, self-hypnosis/suggestion (autogenic training), and progressive relaxation.

D. Apply Cutaneous Counterstimulation (Unless Contraindicated).

1. *Vibration*—a vigorous form of massage that is applied to a nonoperative site. It lessens patient's perception of pain. (Avoid applying this to calf, which may dislodge an unheralded thrombus.)
2. *Heat or cold*—apply to operative or nonoperative site as prescribed. This works best for well-localized pain. Cold has more advantages than heat and fewer un-

wanted side effects (e.g., burns). Heat works well with muscle spasm.

E. Give Analgesics as Prescribed in a Timely Manner

1. Instruct patient to request analgesic before the pain becomes severe.
2. If pain occurs consistently and predictably throughout a 24-hour period, analgesics should be given around the clock—avoiding the usual "demand cycle" of dosing that sets up eventual dependency and provides less adequate pain relief.
3. Administer prescribed medication to patient prior to anticipated activities and painful procedures (e.g., dressing changes).
4. Monitor for possible side effects of analgesic therapy (e.g., respiratory depression, hypotension, nausea, skin rash, etc.).

   Administer naloxone hydrochloride (Narcan) to relieve significant narcotic-induced respiratory depression.

> **NURSING ALERT:** Narcotic "potentiators," such as hydroxyzine (Vistaril) and promethazine (Phenergan), may further sedate the patient.

5. Assess and document efficacy of analgesic therapy.

Pharmacologic Interventions

A. Oral and Parenteral Analgesia

1. Surgical patients are often prescribed a parenteral analgesic for 2–4 days or until incisional pain abates. At that time an oral analgesic, narcotic or non-narcotic, will be prescribed.
2. While the physician is responsible for prescribing the appropriate medication, it is the nurse's responsibility to ensure the drug is given safely and assessed for efficacy.

B. Patient-Controlled Analgesia (PCA)

1. Benefits:
   a. Bypasses the delays inherent in traditional analgesic administration (the "demand cycle").
   b. Medication is administered intravenously, producing more rapid pain relief and greater consistency in patient response.
   c. The patient retains *control* over his pain relief (added placebo and relaxation effects).
   d. Decreased nursing time in frequent delivery of analgesics.
2. Contraindications
   a. Patients under 10–11 years of age.
   b. Patients with cognitive impairment (delirium, dementia, mental illness, hemodynamic or respiratory impairment).
3. A portable PCA device delivers a preset dosage of narcotic (usually morphine). An adjustable "lockout interval" controls the frequency of dose administration, preventing another dose from being delivered prematurely. An example of PCA settings might be a dose of 1 mg. of morphine with a lockout interval of 6 minutes (total possible dose is 10 mg. per hour).
4. Patient pushes a button to activate the device.
5. Instruction about PCA should occur preoperatively; some patients fear being overdosed by the machine and require reassurance.

C. Epidural Analgesia

1. Requires injections of narcotics into the epidural space via a catheter inserted by an anesthesiologist under aseptic conditions (see Fig. 4-2).
2. Benefits:
   a. Produces effective analgesia without sensory, motor, or sympathetic changes.
   b. Provides for longer periods of analgesia.
3. Disadvantages:
   a. The epidural catheter's proximity to the spinal nerves and spinal canal, along with its potential

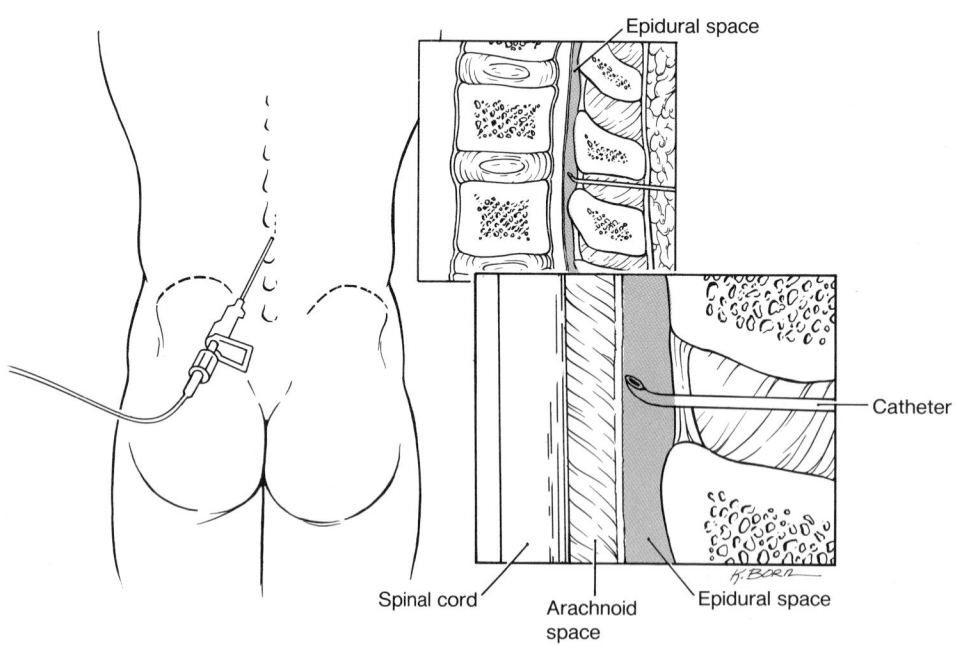

Figure 4-2. Epidural catheter placement.

for catheter migration, make correct injection technique and close patient assessment imperative.

   b. Requires specific hospital protocol for injection and verification of nursing staff's injection technique.

   c. Side effects include: generalized pruritus (common), nausea, urinary retention, respiratory depression, hypotension, motor block, sensory/sympathetic block. These side effects are related to the narcotic used (usually a morphine derivative [Duramorph] or fentanyl) and catheter position.

4. Strict asepsis is necessary when injecting the epidural catheter.
5. The catheter is initially aspirated gently; if blood or greater than 1 ml. clear fluid is aspirated, hold injection and notify physician of possible catheter migration into spinal column.
6. Narcotic-related side effects are reversed with naloxone hydrochloride (Narcan).
7. The nurse ensures proper integrity of both the catheter and the dressing.
8. Occasionally, concurrent use of low-dose anesthetics, e.g., bupivacaine (Marcaine) may be added to potentiate efficacy of epidural analgesia; this is most common following thoracic trauma.

Postoperative Complications

Shock

Shock is a response of the body to a decrease in the circulating volume of blood; tissue perfusion is impaired culminating, eventually, in cellular hypoxia and death.

Classification

1. *Hypovolemic* (hematogenic)—shock resulting from loss of plasma or whole blood; this may be external or internal. When 10% to 20% of the blood volume is lost, hypovolemic shock occurs.
2. *Septic* (bacteremic or toxic shock)—characterized by septic changes in the capillary endothelium, causing massive vasodilation and permitting loss of blood and plasma through capillary walls into surrounding tissues. Circulating volume decreases and tissues are underperfused.
3. *Cardiogenic*—observed when there is interference with the heart pumping action, as might occur in myocardial infarction or cardiac tamponade, which results in inadequate cardiac output and tissue hypoperfusion.
4. *Neurogenic* (vasogenic)—marked vasodilation and reflex inhibition, which results in a sluggish circulating system, depriving vital centers of proper blood supply.
5. *Anaphylactic shock*—an exaggerated form of hypersensitivity to an antigenic agent resulting in widespread vasodilation, increased vascular permeability, interstitial edema, and cardiovascular collapse.

Altered Physiology and Clinical Manifestations

1. In shock there is a loss of effective circulating blood volume and resultant hypoperfusion of tissue cells.
2. Compensatory mechanisms are activated:
   a. *Sympathetic nervous system stimulation*—results in arterial and venous vasoconstriction (except in early stages of septic shock where vasodilation predominates). There is accompanying tachycardia (except in neurogenic shock).
   b. *Renin–angiotensin–aldosterone system activation*—due to renal hypoperfusion, resulting in further vasoconstriction and enhanced sodium and water retention by kidneys as well as potassium excretion.
   c. *Pituitary gland stimulation*—results in release of adrenocorticotrophic hormone (ACTH), which stimulates increased release of glucocorticoids, resulting in increased blood glucose levels. Antidiuretic hormone (ADH) is also released by the pituitary gland, which increases water reabsorption by the kidneys.

3. Organ and metabolic changes:
   a. *Lactic acidosis*—ischemia enhances incomplete oxidation at the cellular level, resulting in lactic acid production and accumulation.
   b. *Heart*—increased cardiac workload and reduced coronary artery blood flow can result in cardiac ischemia, rhythm disturbances, and pump failure. Skin is cool and clammy (warm in early stages of septic shock), blood pressure falls (again, not so in early septic shock), pulse pressure narrows, and capillary refill is delayed.
   c. *Kidneys*—reduced urine output and acute tubular necrosis result.
   d. *Brain*—decreased cerebral perfusion with resultant restlessness, followed by confusion and coma.
   e. *Intestine*—splanchnic ischemia increases susceptibility for bacteria and toxins to cross the intestinal barrier and enter the circulation, leading to sepsis. There are decreased bowel tones and often an ileus.
   f. *Liver*—impaired hepatic cells have a decreased ability to detoxify circulating toxins and drugs.
   g. *Lungs*—release of vasoactive substances and proteolytic enzymes results in interstitial leakage and pulmonary congestion; tachypnea, hypoxemia, and cyanosis ensue.
   h. *Capillaries*—acidosis and circulating toxins damage capillary endothelial cells, allowing leakage of plasma proteins and fluid into interstitial tissues. Generalized edema may occur (especially in septic shock).
   i. *Platelets*—increased platelet aggregation and microthrombi may occur (with potential emboli), followed by intravascular coagulopathy (an increased bleeding tendency).
   j. *Cells*—total cellular deterioration occurs with hypoperfusion.
   k. *Temperature*—fever often manifests with hypovolemic shock and sepsis; it is often a finding in late shock stages.

Preventive Nursing Management

1. Prepare adequately the mental as well as the physical condition of the patient.
2. Anticipate any complications that may arise during and after surgery.
3. Have blood available if there is any indication that it may be needed.
4. Measure accurately any blood loss.
5. Anticipate progression of symptoms upon earliest manifestation.
6. Monitor vital signs frequently until they are stable.
7. Assess vital sign deviations; evaluate blood pressure in relation to other physiologic parameters of shock

and patient's premorbid values. Orthostatic hypotension is an important indicator of hypovolemic shock.
8. Prevent infection (e.g., indwelling catheter care, wound care, pulmonary care) as this will minimize septic shock.

Nursing Interventions

1. *Keep the airway patent.*
   a. May require an airway or endotracheal tube placement.
   b. Remove oral and tracheal secretions.
   c. Institute resuscitative measures if necessary.
2. *Arrest hemorrhage if present.*
3. *Place patient in most physiologically desirable position for shock* (Fig. 4-3).
   a. Elevate the head on a pillow.
   b. Keep the trunk horizontal.
   c. Elevate lower extremities about 20–30 degrees, keeping knees straight.

> **NURSING ALERT:** Do not use Trendelenburg position because (1) after initial increase in blood to the head, a reflex compensatory action takes place causing vasoconstriction and thereby decreasing blood supply to the brain; and (2) viscera tend to fall against the diaphragm, causing increased resistance to breathing and inadequate ventilation.

4. *Ensure an adequate venous return.*
   a. Insert one or more intravenous catheters for volume support.
   b. Assist with placement of a central venous pressure (CVP) catheter in or near the right atrium.
      (1) Monitor CVP measurements and note direction and degree of change from initial CVP reading.
      (2) Utilize central venous catheter for emergency fluid volume and electrolyte replacement.
   c. Increase rate of fluid infusion (preferably *isotonic* fluids).
   d. Start plasma expanders, if needed, until whole blood is available.
   e. Begin blood transfusion when blood is available.
5. *Monitor serum determinations* of blood gases, acid–base balance, and hematocrit.
   a. *p*H—may indicate acidosis resulting from anaerobic metabolism (lactic acidosis).
   b. PCO_2—assesses adequacy of ventilation.

c. PO_2—along with oxygen saturation determines adequacy of oxygenation.
d. Hematocrit—reveals plasma losses due to hemorrhage (low hematocrit) or dehydration (high hematocrit).
6. *Insert a urinary catheter* to monitor hourly urinary output. The objective is to maintain a 30 ml./hour urinary output to ensure adequate kidney perfusion.
7. *Administer antimicrobials* in order to offset infection, which may have precipitated (septic shock) or resulted from prolonged shock.
8. *Support the defense mechanisms of the patient.*
   a. Comfort and reassure the patient if he is conscious.
   b. Resort to sedation and analgesia with discriminating judgment.
   c. Keep the patient warm, but do not apply too much external covering, since it will produce unnecessary vasodilation, resulting in further reduced blood flow and tissue hypoperfusion.
9. Prepare to initiate other appropriate interventions specific to nature of shock (e.g., inotropic drugs in cardiogenic shock; glucocorticoids (i.e., Solu-Medrol) in anaphylactic shock).
10. During massive fluid resuscitation, monitor for signs of fluid overload and congestive heart failure—increasing CVP, heart gallop, pulmonary crackles, etc.
11. Throughout the entire panorama of impending shock, continue recording of vital signs, observations, and interventions on a flow sheet.
12. Septic shock is most often due to gram-negative infection; it may have direct toxic effects on the heart resulting in depressed cardiac function.

Hemorrhage

Hemorrhage is copious escape of blood from a blood vessel.

Classification

A. General

1. *Primary*—occurs at the time of operation.
2. *Intermediary*—occurs within the first few hours after surgery.
   Blood pressure returns to normal and causes loosening of some ligated sutures and flushing out of weak clots from unligated vessels.

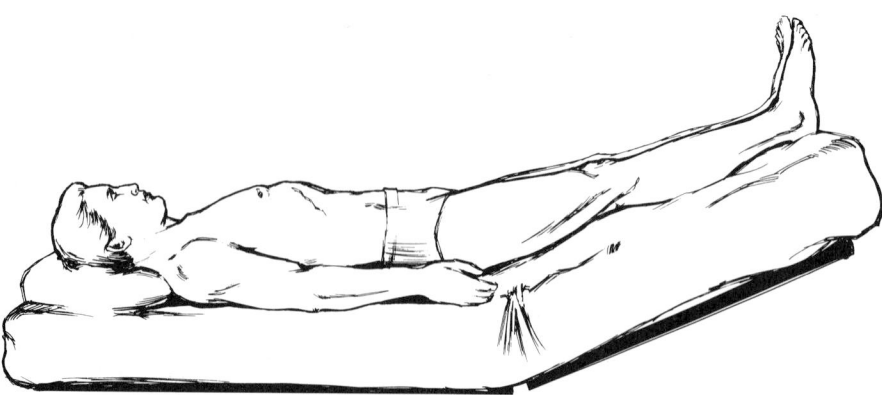

Figure 4-3. *Proper positioning of the patient who shows signs of shock. Elevate the lower extremities about 20 degrees, keeping the knees straight, trunk horizontal, and head slightly elevated.*

3. *Secondary*—occurs some time after surgery due to ligature slip from blood vessel and erosion of blood vessel.

B. According to Blood Vessels

1. *Capillary*—slow general oozing from capillaries.
2. *Venous*—bleeding that is dark in color and bubbles out.
3. *Arterial*—bleeding that spurts and is bright red in color.

C. According to Location

1. *Evident or external*—visible bleeding on the surface.
2. *Internal* (concealed)—bleeding that cannot be seen.

Clinical Manifestations

1. Apprehension, restlessness; thirst; cold, moist, pale skin and circumoral pallor.
2. Pulse increases, respirations become rapid and deep ("air hunger"), temperature drops.
3. With progression of hemorrhage:
   a. Decrease in cardiac output and narrowed pulse pressure.
   b. Rapidly decreasing blood pressure, as well as hematocrit and hemoglobin.
   c. Patient grows weaker until death occurs.

Nursing Interventions

1. Treat the patient as described for shock (p. 62).
2. Inspect the wound as a possible site of bleeding. Apply pressure dressing over external bleeding site.
3. Increase intravenous fluid infusion rate and administer blood as soon as possible.

NURSING ALERT: Numerous, rapid blood transfusions may induce coagulopathy and prolonged bleeding time. The patient should be monitored closely for signs of increased bleeding tendencies following such transfusions.

Deep Vein Thrombophlebitis

Deep vein thrombosis (DVT) occurs in pelvic veins or in deep veins of the lower extremities in postoperative patients. The incidence of DVT varies between 10% and 40% depending upon the complexity of the surgery or the severity of the underlying illness. DVT is most common following hip surgery, followed by retropubic prostatectomy, and general thoracic or abdominal surgery. Venous thrombi located above the knee are considered the major source of pulmonary emboli.

Causes

1. Injury to intimal layer of the vein wall.
2. Venous stasis.
3. Hypercoagulopathy, polycythemia.
4. High risks include obesity, prolonged immobility, cancer, smoking, advancing age, varicose veins, dehydration, splenectomy, and orthopedic procedures.

Clinical Manifestations

1. Majority of DVT are asymptomatic.
2. Pain or cramp in the calf or thigh, progressing to painful swelling of entire leg.
3. Slight fever, chills, perspiration.
4. Marked tenderness over anteromedial surface of thigh.

5. Intravascular clotting without marked inflammation may develop, leading to phlebothrombosis.
6. Circulation distal to the DVT may be compromised if sufficient swelling is present.

NURSING ALERT: A complaint of slight soreness of the calf is never ignored. The danger inherent in femoral thrombosis is that a clot may be dislodged and produce a pulmonary embolus.

Nursing Interventions

1. Hydrate the patient adequately postoperatively to prevent hemoconcentration.
2. Encourage leg exercises and ambulate the patient as soon as permitted by the surgeon. (Exercises are taught preoperatively—see p. 54)
3. Avoid any restricting devices such as tight straps that can constrict and impair circulation.
4. Avoid rubbing or massaging calves and thighs.
5. Instruct patient to avoid standing or sitting in one place for prolonged periods or crossing legs when seated.
6. Refrain from inserting IV catheters into legs or feet of adults.
7. Assess distal peripheral pulses, capillary refill and sensation of lower extremities.
8. Check for positive Homan's sign—calf pain upon dorsiflexion of the foot. This sign is present in nearly 30% of DVT patients.
9. Prevent the use of bed rolls or knee gatches in those patients at risk because there is danger of constricting the vessels under the knee.
10. Initiate anticoagulant therapy either intravenously, subcutaneously, or orally, as prescribed.
11. Prevent swelling and stagnation of venous blood by applying appropriately fitting elastic stockings or wrapping the legs from the toes to the groin with elastic bandage.
12. Apply pneumatic stockings, intraoperatively or postoperatively, to those patients at highest risk of DVT. In conjunction with elastic hose, pneumatic stockings can reduce the risk of DVT by 30% to 50% (see Fig. 4-4).

Pulmonary Complications

Preventive Measures

1. Report any evidence of upper respiratory infection to the surgeon.
2. Suction nasopharyngeal or bronchial secretions if patient is unable to clear own airway.
3. Prevent regurgitation and aspiration through proper patient positioning.
4. Recognize the predisposing causes of pulmonary complications:
   a. Infections—mouth, nose, sinuses, throat.
   b. Aspiration of vomitus.
   c. History of heavy smoking, chronic pulmonary disease.
   d. Obesity.

Complications

A. Atelectasis

1. Incomplete expansion of lung or portion of it occurring within 48 hours of surgery.

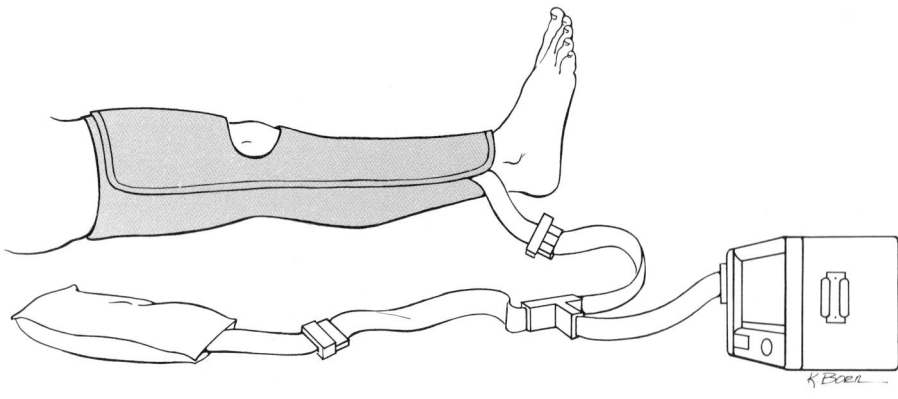

Figure 4-4. *Pneumatic hose. Pressures of 35 mm. Hg to 20 mm. Hg are sequentially applied from ankle to thigh, producing an increase in blood flow velocity and improved venous clearing.*

2. Attributed to absence of periodic deep breaths.
3. A mucous plug closes a bronchiole causing alveoli distal to plug to collapse.
4. Symptoms are often absent—may comprise mild to severe tachypnea, tachycardia, cough, fever, hypotension, and decreased breath sounds and chest expansion of affected side.

B. Aspiration

1. Caused by inhalation of food, gastric contents, water, or blood into the tracheobronchial system.
2. Anesthetic agents and narcotics depress the central nervous system causing inhibition of gag or cough reflexes.
3. Nasogastric tube insertion renders both upper and lower esophageal sphincters partially incompetent.
4. Gross aspiration has a 50% mortality.
5. Symptoms depend on severity of aspiration; it may be silent. Usually evidence of atelectasis occurs within 2 minutes of aspiration. Other symptoms include tachypnea, dyspnea, cough, bronchospasm, wheezing, rhonchi, crackles, hypoxia, and frothy sputum.

C. Pneumonia

1. An inflammatory response in which cellular material replaces alveolar gas.
2. In postoperative patient, most often caused by gram-negative bacilli due to impaired oropharyngeal defense mechanisms.
3. Predisposing factors include atelectasis, upper respiratory infection, copious secretions, aspiration, dehydration, prolonged intubation or tracheostomy, smoker, impaired normal host defenses (cough reflex, mucociliary system, alveolar macrophage activity).
4. Symptoms include dyspnea, tachypnea, pleuric chest pain, fever, chills, hemoptysis, cough (rusty or purulent sputum), and decreased breath sounds over involved area.

Nursing Interventions

1. Monitor the patient's progress very carefully on a daily basis for the first postoperative week to detect early signs and symptoms of respiratory difficulties.
   a. Slight temperature, pulse, and respiration elevations.
   b. Apprehension and restlessness or a decreased level of consciousness.
   c. Complaints of chest pain, signs of dyspnea or cough.
2. Promote full aeration of the lungs.
   a. Turn the patient frequently.
   b. Encourage the patient to take 10 deep breaths hourly, holding each breath to a count of 5 and exhaling.
   c. Utilize a spirometer or any device that encourages the patient to ventilate more effectively.
   d. Assist the patient in coughing in an effort to bring up mucous secretions. Have patient splint chest or abdominal wound to minimize discomfort associated with deep breathing and coughing.
   e. Assist the patient to ambulate as early as the physician will allow.
3. Initiate specific measures for particular pulmonary problems.
   a. Provide cool mist or heated nebulizer for the patient exhibiting signs of bronchitis or thick secretions.
   b. Encourage patient to take fluids to help "liquify" secretions and facilitate expectoration (in pneumonia).
   c. Elevate the head of bed and ensure proper administration of prescribed oxygen.
   d. Prevent abdominal distention—nasogastric tube insertion may be necessary.
   e. Administer prescribed antibiotics for pulmonary infections.

Pulmonary Embolism

Pulmonary embolism refers to the obstruction of one or more pulmonary arterioles by an embolus originating somewhere in the venous system or in the right side of the heart. Postoperatively, the majority of emboli develop in the pelvic or iliofemoral veins before becoming dislodged and traveling to the lungs.

Clinical Manifestations

1. Sharp, stabbing pains in the chest.
2. Anxiousness and cyanosis.
3. Pupillary dilation, profuse perspiration.
4. Rapid and irregular pulse becoming imperceptible—leads rapidly to death.
5. Dyspnea, tachypnea, hypoxemia.
6. Pleural friction rub (occasionally).

Nursing Interventions

1. Administer oxygen with the patient in an upright sitting position (if possible).
2. Reassure and quiet the patient.
3. Monitor vital signs, ECG, and arterial blood gases.

4. Treat for shock or heart failure as needed.
5. Give analgesics or sedatives to control pain or apprehension.
6. Prepare for thrombolytic therapy.

Urinary Retention

Causes

1. Occurs most frequently after operations of the rectum, anus, vagina, or lower abdomen.
2. Caused by spasm of bladder sphincter.
3. More common in males due to inherent increases in urethral resistance to urine flow.

Nursing Interventions

1. Assist patient to sit or stand (if permissible), since many patients are unable to void while lying in bed.
2. Provide the patient with privacy.
3. Use the psychological aid of running the tap water—frequently the sound or sight of running water relaxes spasm of the bladder sphincter.
4. Use warmth to relax sphincters (e.g., sitz bath, warm compresses).
5. Administer bethanechol chloride (Urecholine) intramuscularly if prescribed.
6. Catheterize only when all other measures are unsuccessful.

> **NURSING ALERT:** Recognize that when a patient voids small amounts (30-60 ml. every 15-30 minutes), this may be a sign of an overdistended bladder with "overflow" of urine.

Intestinal Obstruction

Bowel obstructions result in a partial or complete impairment to the forward flow of intestinal contents. Most obstructions occur in the small bowel, especially at its narrowest point—the ileum.

Causes

A. Mechanical

1. Adhesions (most common cause; occur long after operative healing).
2. Volvulus (twisting of bowel).
3. Intussusception (telescoping of bowel).
4. Malignancy.
5. Hernia.

B. Neurogenic

1. Paralytic ileus (due to intraoperative bowel manipulation, anesthetics, electrolyte imbalances, pneumonia, peritonitis, spinal cord injury, and wound dehiscence).

C. Vascular

1. Mesenteric arterial occlusion.
2. Shock.

Clinical Manifestations

1. Most commonly occurs between the third and fifth postoperative day. (Bowel obstructions, caused by adhesions, may occur months to years postoperatively.)
2. Sharp, colicky abdominal pains with pain-free intervals. Eating may intensify pain.
3. Pain is localized and should be noted, since it may become more generalized later; location may pinpoint source of difficulty.
4. Bowel sounds are absent or decreased in paralytic ileus; obstruction causes high-pitched, metallic tinkling bowel sounds above the level of obstruction.
5. The abdomen appears distended; peritonitis will cause the abdomen to become tender and rigid.
6. Pain-free intervals grow shorter as time advances.
7. With completion of obstruction, intestinal contents back up into stomach and cause vomiting. (Emesis is frequently comprised of fecal contents.)
8. Abdominal distention and perhaps hiccups occur, but no bowel movements, if obstruction is complete; if obstruction is partial or incomplete, diarrhea may occur.
9. Following simple enema, returns are clear, indicating very small amount of intestinal contents has reached large intestine.
10. If obstruction is not relieved, vomiting continues, distention becomes more pronounced, pulse increases, hypovolemic shock develops, and death occurs.

Management

1. Treat the cause.
2. Relieve abdominal distention by passing a nasoenteric suction tube.
3. Replace fluid and electrolytes.
4. Monitor fluid, electrolyte (especially potassium and sodium), and acid–base status.
5. Administer narcotics judiciously as these medications may further suppress peristalsis.
6. Consider preparing the patient for surgical intervention if obstruction continues unresolved.

Nursing Interventions

1. Closely monitor patient for signs of shock.
2. Provide medication judiciously for pain (opiates impair peristalsis).
3. Provide frequent reassurance to patient; use nontraditional methods to promote comfort (touch, relaxation, imagery).
4. Assess bowel tones and degree of abdominal distention (may need to measure abdominal girth); document these findings every tour of duty.
5. Monitor and document characteristics of emesis and nasogastric drainage.

Hiccups (Singultus)

Hiccups are intermittent spasms of the diaphragm causing the sound ("hic") that results from the vibration of closed vocal cords as air rushes suddenly into the lungs.

Cause

Irritation of the phrenic nerve between the spinal cord and terminal ramifications on undersurface of diaphragm.

1. *Direct*—distended stomach, peritonitis, abdominal distention, chest pleurisy, tumors pressing on nerves, or surgery performed near the diaphragm.
2. *Indirect*—toxemia, uremia.
3. *Reflex*—exposure to cold, drinking very hot or very cold liquids, intestinal obstruction.

Management

1. Remove the cause, if possible.
2. When removal of cause is not possible, favorite remedies may be tried.

a. Swallow a large glass of water.
b. Place tablespoon of coarse, granulated sugar on back of tongue and swallow it.
c. Medicate with a phenothiazine drug (e.g., Compazine, Thorazine)
d. Introduce a small catheter into the patient's pharynx (about 8–10 cm. [3–4 inches]); rotate gently and jiggle back and forth.
e. For rare, intractable hiccups, an extreme procedure is surgical crush of the phrenic nerve.

Wound Infection

Wound infections are the second most common nosocomial infection. The infection may be limited to the surgical site (60% to 80%) or may affect the patient systemically.

Cause

1. Drying tissues by long exposure, operations on contaminated structures, gross obesity, old age, chronic hypoxemia, and malnutrition are directly related to an increased infection rate.
2. The patient's own flora is most often implicated in wound infections (*Staphylococcus aureus*).
3. Other common culprits in wound infection include *Escherichia coli, Klebsiella, Enterobacter,* and *Proteus.*
4. Wound infections typically present 5–7 days postoperatively.
5. Factors affecting the extent of infection include:
   a. Kind, virulence, and quantity of contaminating microorganisms.
   b. Presence of foreign bodies or devitalized tissue.
   c. Location and nature of the wound.
   d. Amount of dead space or presence of hematoma.
   e. Immune response of the patient.
   f. Presence of adequate blood supply to wound.
   g. Presurgical condition of the patient, e.g., elderly, alcoholism, diabetes, malnutrition.

Clinical Manifestations

1. Redness, excessive swelling, tenderness.
2. Red streaks in the skin near the wound.
3. Pus or other discharge from the wound.
4. Tender, enlarged lymph nodes in axillary region or groin closest to wound.
5. Foul smell from wound.
6. Generalized body chills or fever.
7. Elevated temperature and pulse.

NURSING ALERT: Mild, transient fevers appear postoperatively due to tissue necrosis, hematoma, or cauterization. Higher sustained fevers arise with the following four most common postoperative complications: atelectasis (within the first 48 hours); wound infections (in 5–7 days); urinary infections (in 5–8 days); and thrombophlebitis (in 7–14 days).

Nursing Interventions

A. Preoperative

1. Encourage the patient to achieve an optimal nutritional level.
   Provide for enteral or parenteral alimentation if patient has hypoproteinemia with weight loss.
2. Reduce preoperative hospitalization to minimum to avoid acquiring nosocomial infections.
3. When the risk of developing an infection is high (or when infection would have grave consequences), antibiotic therapy is initiated preoperatively. Most commonly used antibiotics are the broad-spectrum cephalosporins.

B. Operative

1. Follow strict asepsis throughout the operative procedure.
2. When a wound has exudate, fibrin, desiccated fat, or nonviable skin, it is not approximated by primary closure but approximation is delayed (secondary closure).

C. Postoperative

1. Keep dressings intact, reinforcing if necessary, until prescribed otherwise.
2. Use strict asepsis when dressings are changed (see p. 72).
3. Monitor and document amount, type, and location of drainage. Ensure that all drains are working properly. (See Table 4-1 for expected drainage amounts from common types of drains and tubes.)

D. Postoperative Care of an Infected Wound

1. The surgeon removes one or more stitches, separates wound edges, and examines for infection using a hemostat as a probe.
2. A culture is taken and sent to the laboratory for bacterial analysis.
3. Wound irrigation may be done; have asepto syringe and saline available.
4. A drain may be inserted, or the wound may be packed with sterile gauze.
5. Antibiotics are prescribed.
6. Wet-to-dry dressings may be applied (see p. 70)

Table 4-1. *Expected Drainage From Tubes and Catheters*

Device	Substance	Daily Drainage
Foley catheter Ileal conduit Suprapubic catheter	Urine	500–700 ml./24 hours first 48 hours; then 1500–2500 ml./24 hours
Gastrostomy tube	Gastric contents	Up to 1500 ml./24 hours
Chest tube	Blood, pleural fluid, air	Varies: 500–1000 ml. first 24 hours
Ileostomy	Small bowel contents	Up to 4000 ml. in first 24 hours; then < 500 ml./24 hours
Miller-Abbott tube	Intestinal contents	Up to 3000 ml./24 hours
Nasogastric tube	Gastric contents	Up to 1500 ml./24 hours
T-tube	Bile	500 ml./24 hours

Wound Dehiscence *(Evisceration)*

Causes

1. Commonly occurs between fifth and eighth day postoperatively when incision has weakest tensile strength; greatest strength is found between the first and third postoperative day.
2. Chiefly associated with abdominal surgery.
3. This catastrophe is often related to the following:
   a. Inadequate sutures or excessively tight closures (the latter compromises blood supply)
   b. Hematomas; seromas
   c. Infections
   d. Excessive coughing, retching, distention
   e. Poor nutrition; immunosuppression
   f. Uremia; diabetes mellitus
   g. Steroid use

Preventive Measures

1. Apply abdominal binder for heavy or elderly patients or those with weak or pendulous abdominal walls.
2. Encourage patient to splint incision while coughing.
3. Monitor for and relieve abdominal distention.
4. Encourage proper nutrition with emphasis on adequate amounts of protein and vitamin C.

Clinical Manifestations

1. Heralded by sudden discharge of serosanguineous fluid from wound.
2. Patient complains that something suddenly "gave way" in his wound.
3. In an intestinal wound, the edges of the wound may part and the intestines may gradually push out—observe for drainage of peritoneal fluid on dressing (clear or serosanguineous fluid).

Nursing Interventions

1. Stay with the patient and have someone notify the surgeon immediately.
2. If intestines are exposed, cover with sterile moist saline dressings.
3. Monitor vital signs and watch for shock.
4. Keep the patient on absolute bed rest.
5. Instruct patient to bend his knees, with head of bed elevated in semi-Fowler's position to relieve tension on abdomen.
6. Assure the patient that his wound will be properly cared for; attempt to keep him quiet and relaxed.
7. Prepare the patient for surgery and repair of the wound.

Postoperative Psychological Disturbances

Classification

A. Depression

1. *Cause*—perceived loss of health or stamina, pain, altered body image, various drugs, and anxiety about an uncertain future.
2. *Clinical manifestations*—withdrawal, restlessness, insomnia, nonadherence to therapeutic regimens, tearfulness, and expressions of hopelessness.
3. *Management*
   a. Clarify misconceptions about surgery and its future implications.
   b. Listen to, reassure, and support patient.
   c. If appropriate, introduce patient to representatives of ostomy, mastectomy, or amputee clubs.
   d. Involve patient's partner and support persons in his care; psychiatric consultation is obtained for severe depression.

B. Delirium

1. *Cause*—prolonged anesthesia, cardiopulmonary bypass, drug reactions, sepsis, alcoholism (delirium tremens), electrolyte imbalances, and other metabolic disorders.
2. *Clinical manifestations*—disorientation, hallucinations, perceptual distortions, paranoid delusions, reversed day–night pattern, agitation, insomnia; delirium tremens often appears within 72 hours of last alcoholic drink and may include autonomic overactivity—tachycardia, dilated pupils, diaphoresis, and fever (see p. 956).
3. *Management*
   a. Treat the underlying cause (restore fluid and electrolyte balance).
   b. Reorient to environment and time.
   c. Keep surroundings calm.
   d. Explain every procedure done to patient in detail.
   e. Sedate patient to reduce agitation, prevent exhaustion, and promote sleep.
   f. Allow for extended periods of uninterrupted sleep.
   g. Reassure family members with clear explanations of patient's aberrant behavior.
   h. Apply restraints to patient if his safety is in question.

Postoperative Discharge Instructions

A. Rest and Activity

1. It is common to feel tired and frustrated about not feeling able to do all the things you want; this is quite normal.
2. Plan regular naps and quiet activities, gradually increasing your exercise over the following weeks.
3. When you begin to exercise more, start by taking a short walk 2 or 3 times a day. Consult your health care provider if more specific exercises are required.
4. Climbing stairs in your home may be surprisingly tiring at first. If you have difficulty with this activity, try going up stairs backwards ("scooching") on your "bottom" until your strength has returned.
5. Consult your health care provider to determine the appropriate time to return to work.

B. Eating

1. Follow dietary instructions provided at the hospital prior to your discharge.
2. It is not surprising to find that your appetite is limited at first, or that you may feel bioated after meals; this should become less a problem as you become more active. (Some prescribed medications can cause this.) If symptoms persist, consult your health care provider.
3. Eat small, regular meals and make them as nourishing as possible to promote wound healing.

C. Sleeping

1. If sleeping is difficult because of wound discomfort, try taking your pain medication at bedtime.
2. Attempt to get sufficient sleep to aid in your recovery.

D. Wound Healing

1. There are several stages of healing that your wound will go through. After initial pain at the site, the wound may feel tingling, itchy, numb, or tight (a slight pulling sensation) as healing occurs.
2. Do not pull off any scabs as they protect the delicate new tissues underneath. They will fall off without any help when ready.
3. Consult your health care provider if the amount of pain in your wound increases or if you notice increased redness, swelling, or discharge from wound.

E. Bowels

1. Irregular bowel habits can result from changes in activity and diet, or the use of some drugs.
2. Avoid straining, as it can intensify discomfort in some wounds; instead, use a rocking motion while trying to pass stool.
3. It may be helpful to take a mild laxative. Consult your health care provider if you have any questions.

F. Bathing, Showering

1. You may get your wound wet within 3 days of your operation (unless otherwise advised).
2. Showering is preferable, as it allows for thorough rinsing of the wound.

3. If you are feeling too weak, place a plastic or metal chair in the shower so that you may be seated during showering.
4. Be sure to dry your wound thoroughly with a very clean towel and dress it as instructed prior to discharge.

G. Clothing

1. Avoid tight belts, also underwear and other clothes with seams that may rub against the wound.
2. Wear loose clothing for comfort and to reduce mechanical trauma to wound.

H. Driving

1. It is important to ask your physician when you may resume driving. Safe driving may be affected by your pain medication. In addition, any violent jarring from an accident may disrupt your wound.

I. Bending and Lifting

1. How much bending, stretching, and lifting you are allowed depends upon the location and nature of your surgery.
2. Typically, for most major surgeries, you should avoid lifting anything heavier than 5 pounds for 4–8 weeks.
3. It is ideal to secure home assistance for the first 2–3 weeks after discharge.

2: Wound Care

Wounds and Wound Healing

A *wound* is a disruption in the continuity and regulatory processes of tissue cells; *wound healing* is the restoration of that continuity. Wound healing, however, may or may not restore normal cellular function.

Wound Classification

A. Mechanism of Injury

1. *Incised wounds*—made by a clean cut of a sharp instrument, e.g., a surgical incision with a scalpel.
2. *Contused wounds*—made by blunt force that typically does not break the skin but causes considerable tissue damage with bruising and swelling.
3. *Lacerated wounds*—made by an object that tears tissues producing jagged, irregular edges; examples include glass, jagged wire, and blunt knife.
4. *Puncture wounds*—made by a pointed instrument, such as an ice pick, bullet, and nail.

B. Degree of Contamination

1. *Clean*—an aseptically made wound, as in surgery, that does not enter the alimentary, respiratory, or genitourinary tracts.
2. *Clean–contaminated*—an aseptically made wound that enters the respiratory, alimentary, or genitourinary tracts. These wounds have a slightly higher probability of wound infection than do clean wounds.
3. *Contaminated*—wounds exposed to excessive amounts of bacteria. These wounds may be open (avulsive) or accidentally made, or the result of surgical operations in which there are major breaks in aseptic techniques or gross spillage from the gastrointestinal tract.
4. *Infected*—a wound that retains devitalized tissue or

involves preoperatively existing infection or perforated viscera. Such wounds are often left open to drain.

Physiology of Wound Healing

The phases of wound healing—inflammation, reconstruction (proliferation), and maturation—involve continuous and overlapping processes.

A. Inflammatory Phase (lasts 1–5 days)

1. Vascular and cellular responses are immediately initiated when tissue is cut or injured.
2. Transient vasoconstriction occurs immediately at the site of injury, lasting 5–10 minutes, along with deposition of a fibrinoplatelet clot to help control bleeding.
3. Subsequent dilation of small venules occurs; antibodies, plasma proteins, plasma fluids, leukocytes, and red blood cells leave the microcirculation to permeate the general area of injury, causing edema, redness, warmth, and pain.
4. Localized vasodilation is the result of direct action by histamine, serotonin, and prostaglandins.
5. Polymorphic leukocytes (neutrophils) and monocytes enter the wound to engage in destruction and ingestion of wound debris. Monocytes predominate during this phase.
6. Basal cells at the wound edges undergo mitosis; resultant daughter cells enlarge, flatten, and creep across the wound surface to eventually approximate the wound edges.

B. Proliferative Phase (lasts 2–20 days)

1. Fibroblasts (connective tissue cells) multiply and migrate along fibrin strands that are thought to serve as a matrix.
2. Endothelial budding occurs on nearby blood vessels forming new capillaries that penetrate and nourish the injured tissue.
3. The combination of budding capillaries and proliferating fibroblasts is called *granulation tissue.*
4. Active collagen synthesis by fibroblasts begins by the

fifth to seventh day and the wound gains tensile strength.

5. By 3 weeks, skin obtains 30% of its preinjury tensile strength, the intestinal tissue about 65%, and fascia 20%.

C. Maturation Phase (21 Days to Months and Even Years)

1. Scar tissue is composed primarily of collagen and ground substance (mucopolysaccharide, glycoproteins, electrolytes, and water).
2. From the start of collagen synthesis, collagen fibers undergo a process of lysis and regeneration. The collagen fibers become more organized, aligning more closely to each other and increasing in tensile strength.
3. The overall bulk and form of the scar continues to change once maturation has started.
4. Typically, collagen production drops off; however, if collagen production greatly exceeds collagen lysis, *keloid* (greatly hypertrophied, deforming scar tissue) will form.
5. Normal maturation of the wound is clinically observed as an initial red, raised, hard *immature scar* that molds into a flat, soft, and pale *mature scar.*
6. The scar tissue will never achieve greater than 80% of its preinjury tensile strength.

Types of Wound Healing (see Fig. 4-5)

A. First-intention Healing (Primary Union)

1. Wounds are made aseptic with a minimum of tissue damage and tissue reaction; wound edges are properly approximated with sutures.
2. Granulation tissue is not visible and scar formation is typically minimal (keloid may still form in susceptible individuals).

B. Second-intention Healing (Granulation)

1. Wounds are left open to heal spontaneously or surgically closed at a later date; they need not be infected.
2. Examples in which wounds may heal by second intention include burns, traumatic injuries, ulcers, and suppurative infected wounds.
3. The cavity of the wound fills with a red, soft, sensitive tissue (granulation tissue), which bleeds easily. A scar (cicatrix) eventually forms.
4. In infected wounds, drainage may be accomplished by use of special dressings and drains. Healing is thus improved.
5. In wounds that are later resutured, two opposing granulation surfaces are brought together.
6. Second-intention healing produces a deeper, wider scar.

Wound Management

Many factors promote wound healing, such as adequate nutrition, cleanliness, rest, and position, along with the patient's underlying psychological and physiologic state. Of added importance is the application of appropriate dressings and drains.

Dressings

A. Purpose Of Dressings

1. To protect the wound from mechanical injury.
2. To splint or immobilize the wound.

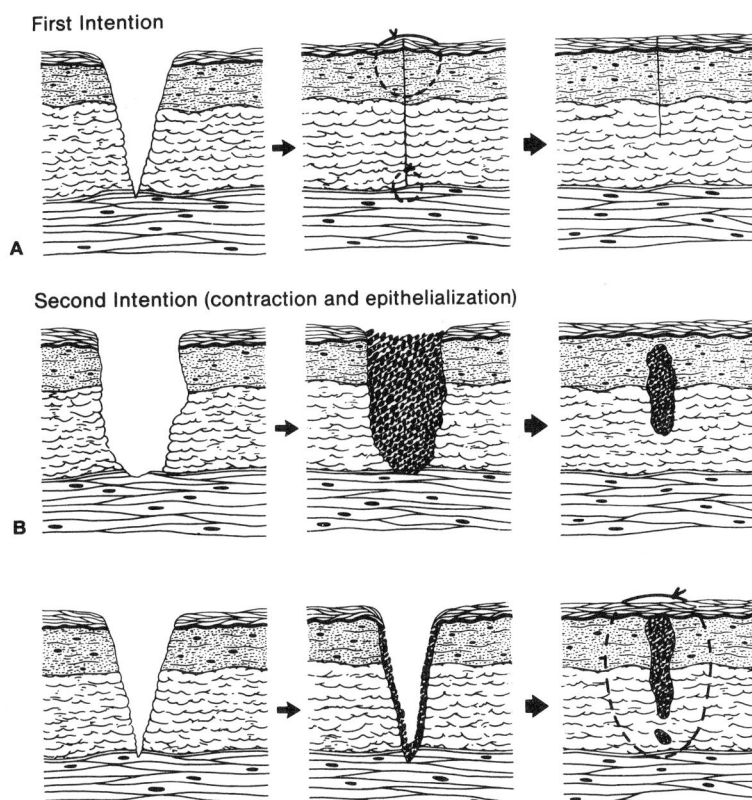

Figure 4-5. *Classification of wound healing. (A) First intention: A clean incision is made with primary closure; there is minimal scarring. (B and C) Second intention: The wound is left open so that granulation can occur; a large scar results, (B) or the wound is initially left open and later closed when there is no further evidence of infection (C).*

First Intention

A

Second Intention (contraction and epithelialization)

B

C

3. To absorb drainage.
4. To prevent contamination from bodily discharges (feces, urine).
5. To promote hemostasis, as in pressure dressings.
6. To debride the wound by combining capillary action and the entwining of necrotic tissue within its mesh.
7. To inhibit or kill microorganisms by using dressings with antiseptic or antimicrobial properties.
8. To provide a physiologic environment conducive to healing.
9. To provide mental and physical comfort for the patient.

B. Advantages for Not Using Dressings

When the initial dressing on a clean, dry, and intact incision is removed, it is often not replaced. This may occur within 24 hours following surgery.
1. Permits better visualization of wound.
2. Eliminates conditions necessary for growth of organisms (warmth, moisture, and darkness).
3. Minimizes adhesive tape reaction.
4. It is economical.

C. Types of Dressings

1. *Dry-to-dry dressings*
   a. Used primarily for wounds closing by primary intention.
   b. Offers good wound protection, absorption of drainage, esthetics for the patient and provides pressure (if needed) for hemostasis.
   c. Disadvantage—they adhere to the wound surface when drainage dries. Removal can cause pain and disruption of granulation tissue.
2. *Wet-to-dry dressings*
   a. Particularly useful for untidy or infected wounds that must be debrided and closed by secondary intention.
   b. Gauze saturated with sterile saline (preferred) or an antimicrobial solution is packed into the wound (eliminating dead space).
   c. The wet dressings are then covered by dry dressings (gauze sponges or absorbent pads).
   d. As drying occurs, wound debris and necrotic tissue are absorbed into the gauze dressing by capillary action.
   e. The dressing is changed when it becomes dry (or just before). If there is excessive necrotic debris on dressing, more frequent dressing changes are required.
3. *Wet-to-wet dressings*
   a. Used on clean open wounds or on granulating surfaces. Sterile saline or an antimicrobial agent may be used to saturate the dressings.
   b. Provide a more physiologic environment (warmth, moisture), which can enhance the local healing processes as well as assure greater patient comfort. Thick exudate is more easily removed.
   c. Disadvantage—surrounding tissues can become macerated, the risk of infection may rise, and bed linens become damp.

Types of Surgical Dressing Supplies

A. Purpose

1. *Hydrophobic* occlusive (petrolatum gauze)
   a. Impermeable, nonadhering dressing that protects wounds from air- and moisture-borne contamination.
   b. Used around chest tubes, and any fistula or stoma that drains digestive juices.
   c. It is relatively nonabsorptive.

2. *Hydrophilic,* permeable (oil-based gauze, Telfa pads)
   a. Allows drainage to penetrate dressing but remains somewhat nonadhering.
   b. For wounds with light to moderate exudate.
   c. Oil-based gauze used on abraded and open ulcerated or granulating wounds.
   d. May also be used to pack "caverns and sinuses" of large open wounds.
   e. Telfa pads are generally reserved for simple, closed, stable wounds.
3. *Dressing sponges* (Topper sponges or general-use gauze sponges)
   a. General-use gauze sponges come in various sizes (most commonly $2'' \times 2''$, $4'' \times 4''$) and may be used for simple dry dressings, wet-to-dry dressings, or wet-to-wet dressings. Large-pore mesh allows for better absorption of drainage and necrotic wound debris.
   b. Topper sponges are primarily used over stable surgical incisions. Their smaller pore size and cotton filling make them less suitable for debriding activities.
4. *All-absorbent combined dressing* (Surgipad, ABD)
   a. Large ($5'' \times 9''$ to $8'' \times 10''$) cotton-filled dressing that is typically used as an "over-dressing," covering gauze or hydrophilic dressings for added wound protection, stabilization of dressings, and drainage absorption.
   b. May also be used unaccompanied over intact surgical wounds.
5. *High-bulk gauze bandage* ("fluffs")
   Primarily used for packing of large wounds undergoing healing by secondary intention.
6. *Drain sponge*
   The drain sponge is similar to the Topper sponge except for the premade slit, which makes the dressing highly suitable for drain sites and tracheostomy sites.
7. *Transparent film dressing* (Tegaderm, Op-Site)
   a. Highly elastic dressing, adjusts exceptionally well to body contours. It is permeable to oxygen and water vapor but generally impermeable to liquids and bacteria.
   b. Controversies surrounding its use (related to incidence of infection) have reduced its once wide usage.
   c. Most common indications include covering arterial and venous catheter sites as well as protecting vulnerable skin exposed to shearing forces.
   d. It is not commonly used for surgical wounds.

Drains

A. Purpose of Drains

1. Drains are placed in wounds only when *abnormal fluid collections* are present or expected.
2. Drains are placed near the incision site; (a) usually in compartments (such as joints and pleural space) that are intolerant to fluid accumulation; (b) in areas with a large blood supply (such as the neck and kidney); (c) in infected draining wounds; and (d) in areas that have sustained large superficial tissue dissection (such as the breast).
3. Collection of body fluids in wounds can be harmful in the following ways:
   a. Provides culture media for bacterial growth.
   b. Causes increased pressure at surgical site, interfering with blood flow to area.
   c. Causes pressure on adjacent areas.

d. Causes local tissue irritation and necrosis (due to fluids such as bile, pus, pancreatic juice, and urine).

B. Wound Drainage

1. Drains are commonly made of soft rubber or plastic and placed either within wounds or body cavities.
2. Drains placed within wounds are typically attached to portable (or, rarely, wall) suction with a collection container.
    a. Examples include the Hemovac, Jackson-Pratt, and Surgivac drainage systems (see Guidelines, p. 75).
    b. The once popular Penrose drain, which opens directly into the dressing, is currently out of favor.
3. Drains may also be used postoperatively to form hollow connections from internal organs to the outside to drain a body fluid, such as the T-tube (bile drainage), nephrostomy, gastrostomy, jejunostomy, and cecostomy tubes.
4. Drains act as foreign bodies; granulation tissue forms around them, walling them off rapidly.
5. Drains within wounds are removed when the amount of drainage decreases over a period of days or rarely weeks.
6. Fistula-forming tubes are often left in for longer periods of time.
    a. Careful handling of these drains and collection bags is essential.
    b. Accidental early removal may result in caustic drainage leaking within the tissues.
    c. The risk is reduced within 7 to 10 days when a wall of fibrous tissue has been formed.
7. The amount of drainage will vary with the procedure. Most common surgical procedures (e.g., appendectomy, cholecystectomy, abdominal hysterectomy) have minimal wound drainage by the third to fourth postoperative day. Drains are not commonly used following these operations.

NURSING ALERT: The greatest amount of drainage is expected during the first 24 hours; closely monitor dressings and drains.

Nursing Process Overview

Assessment

The wound should be assessed every 15 minutes while the patient is in the recovery room. Thereafter, the frequency of wound assessment is determined by the nature of the wound, the degree of drainage, and the hospital protocol. Assessment and documentation of the wound's status should occur at least every tour of duty until patient discharge.

History and Physical Assessment

1. What type of surgery did the patient have?
2. Was hemostasis in the operating room effective?
3. Has the patient received blood to sustain an adequate hematocrit (and promote perfusion to wound)?
4. What is the patient's age?
5. What is his nutritional status? What was it preoperatively?
    a. Is his current intake of protein and vitamin C adequate?
    b. Is he obese or cachectic?
6. What underlying medical conditions does patient have,

and what medications is he taking that could affect wound healing (e.g., diabetes mellitus; steroids)?
7. How long has the patient been hospitalized preoperatively? (Longer preoperative hospital stays can increase complications.)
8. How is the wound held together?
    a. Staples, nylon sutures, adhesive strips, tension sutures?
    b. If the wound is left open, how is it being treated? Is there granulation tissue present?
9. Are there drains in place? What kind? How many?
    a. Is portable suction being used?
    b. Is the amount of drainage consistent with the nature of surgery?
10. What kind of dressings are being used?
    a. Are they saturated with exudate?
    b. Is the amount and type or drainage consistent with nature of the surgery?
11. How does the wound appear?
    a. Is there evidence of edema, irritation, inflammation?
    b. Are the wound edges well approximated?
    c. Is the wound clean and dry?
12. How does the patient appear?
    a. Are there signs of wound pain or discomfort?
    b. Is there fever or elevated white blood cell count present?
    c. Does patient express concern about the wound and potential disfigurement?
13. Does patient understand purpose of wound therapies, and can he or significant other effectively carry out discharge instructions about wound care?

Nursing Diagnoses

1. Pain related to incision site, drains, nature of surgery, dressing changes, etc.
2. Anxiety related to perceived future disfigurement or possibility of rupturing skin stitches.
3. Infection, potential for, at surgical site due to perioperative contamination.
4. Skin integrity, potential impairment of, related to delayed or inadequate wound healing.
5. Knowledge deficit regarding rationale for wound management during hospitalization and care of wound following discharge.

Nursing Interventions

1. Ensure asepsis during dressing changes.
2. Reinforce or change dressings promptly when saturated with drainage.
3. Give patient prescribed medication prior to painful dressing changes.
4. Minimize strain on incision site:
    a. Use appropriate tape, bandages, and binders.
    b. Have patient splint abdominal and chest incisions when coughing.
    c. Instruct patient in proper way to get out of bed while minimizing incision strain (e.g., for abdominal incision, turn on side and push self up with dependent elbow and opposite hand).
5. Keep drainage tubing away from actual incision site (to minimize wound trauma and contamination).
6. Clarify patient's misconceptions of surgery and surgical incision.
7. Instruct patient to avoid touching incision or "picking" at dressings in order to minimize wound contamination and injury.
8. Assess patient's nutritional intake; consult with pa-

tient's physician if supplemental nutritional intake is required.

9. Assess and accurately document condition of incision site each tour of duty.

10. Continue to monitor for signs of wound dehiscence (especially around the fifth day) and wound infection.

Patient Teaching

Prior to discharge, instruct patient and significant other on the techniques and rationale for wound care.

1. Report immediately to health care provider if the following signs of infection occur:
   a. Redness, marked swelling (beyond one half inch from incision site), tenderness, and increased warmth around wound.
   b. Pus or unusual discharge, foul odor from wound.
   c. Red streaks in skin near wound.
   d. Chills or fever (over 37.7°C. or 100°F.).
2. Follow directives of the nurse or physician regarding activity allowances.

3. Keep suture line clean (may shower unless contraindicated by physician; avoid tub bathing until wound heals); never vigorously rub near suture line, pat dry.

4. Report to health care provider if after 2 months the incision site continues to be red, thick, and painful to pressure (probable beginning of keloid formation).

Expected Outcomes

1. Relates improved comfort at incision site each day.
2. Verbalizes realistic expectations for wound recovery.
3. Displays no evidence of wound complications, such as infection (redness, increased pain, foul drainage) and dehiscence.
4. Demonstrates the correct skills for care of the wound after discharge.
5. Lists signs and symptoms that need to be reported: increasing incisional pain, redness, swelling; sudden increase in wound drainage; evidence of the incision "pulling apart"; unexplained fever.

Procedural Considerations in Wound Care

Guidelines Changing Surgical Dressings

General Considerations	1. The procedure of changing dressings, then examining and cleansing the wound, utilizes principles of asepsis.
	2. The initial dressing change is frequently done by the physician, especially for craniotomy, orthopedic, or thoracotomy procedures; subsequent dressing changes are the nurse's responsibility.
Equipment	*Sterile*
	Gloves—disposable
	Scissors, forceps (disposable packs available)
	Appropriate dressing materials
	Sterile saline
	Cotton-tipped swabs
	Culture tubes (if infection suspected)
	For draining wound: add extra gauze and packing material, absorbent pads, and irrigation set
	Unsterile
	Gloves
	Plastic bag for discarded dressings
	Tape, proper size and type
	Pads to protect patient's bed
	Gown for nurse if wound is purulent/infected
Procedure	*Preparatory Phase*
	1. Inform patient of dressing change. Explain procedure to him and have him lie in bed.
	2. Avoid changing dressings at mealtime.
	3. Ensure privacy by drawing the curtains or closing the door; expose the dressing site.
	4. Respect patient's modesty and prevent him from being chilled.
	5. Wash hands thoroughly.
	6. Place dressing supplies on a clean, flat surface (e.g., overbed table).
	7. If linen protection is needed, place clean towel or plastic bag under part of the body where wound is located.
	8. Cut (or tear) off pieces of tape to be used in dressing change.
	9. Place disposable bag nearby to collect soiled dressings.
	10. Determine how many and what types of dressings are necessary. Open each dressing by peeling apart the edges of package (MAINTAIN STERILITY OF DRESSING). Leave each dressing within the open package.

Nursing Action	Rationale
Removing Old Dressing	
1. Don disposable gloves.	1. Unsterile gloves are sufficient if care is used not to touch wound.

Procedure	Nursing Action	Rationale

Procedure
(continued)

2. Loosen all tape and gently pull tape ends toward the wound. It helps to hold skin taut with one hand while carefully peeling up an edge of the tape with the other hand. Wiping the back of tape with alcohol will hasten removal of "stuck" tape.
3. Remove old dressings, one layer at a time, and place in disposable bag.
4. Removal of adherent dressings may be facilitated by moistening dressing with sterile saline.

2. This process is less painful and less disturbing to the healing process (avoids pulling the wound edges apart and traumatizing sensitive skin).

3. Hasty removal of dressings can cause trauma to wound and dislodge existing drains.
4. This process is less painful and less traumatic to the delicate healing tissues.

Obtaining a Wound Culture

1. Use aseptic technique.

2. Open sterile package of gloves; open package containing sterile syringe and needle; open package containing cotton-tipped culture swab. Keep all products within their sterile open packages until use.
3. Don sterile gloves.
4. Aspirate generous amount of drainage liquid into syringe; inject into anaerobic tube. If liquid material is unobtainable, swab desired area with cotton-tipped culture swab, attempting to get maximum saturation.
5. See that specimen is properly labeled and sent to laboratory for study.

1. To prevent contamination of a clean wound or culture media, or to prevent further contamination of a "dirty" wound.
2. Preparation for septic procedure.

4. It is important to collect culture specimen before wound is cleansed. The swab is the more common approach to wound cultures.

Cleansing the Simple Surgical Wound

1. Use aseptic technique.
2. Open package of sterile gloves; open sterile cleaning supplies (e.g., cotton-tipped applicators, sterile gauze sponges, sterile solution cup, sterile saline).
3. Don sterile gloves.
4. Clean along wound edges using a small circular motion from one end of the incision to the other; be sure to clean each side of the wound separately. Repeat the process using another moistened gauze or swab until the entire incision is cleansed. DO NOT SCRUB BACK AND FORTH ACROSS THE INCISION LINE.
5. Sterile saline is the cleansing agent of choice. Topical antiseptics (e.g., povidone-iodine, hexachlorophene, alcohol, and boric acid) may be used on intact skin surrounding the wound but SHOULD NEVER BE USED WITHIN THE WOUND.
6. Repeat the same process with the drain site. Always clean the drain site separately from the primary incision site.
7. Discard used cleaning supplies in the disposable bag.
8. Pat the incision site and drain site dry with a sterile dressing sponge.

2. Preparation for aseptic procedure. Pour sterile cleansing solution (preferably saline) into the solution cup prior to donning sterile gloves.

4. To prevent contamination and mechanical trauma of wound.

5. Most of the antiseptic agents are caustic to tissues and impair healing. The old saying, "Never put anything in a wound that you couldn't put in your eye," is a truthful one.

6. Reduces chance of cross-contamination.

7. This will be incinerated later.
8. To prepare wound for final dressing.

Dressing the Wound

1. Maintain asepsis with use of sterile gloves.
2. After wound is dry, apply appropriate dressing, taking into consideration the nature of wound.
3. Tape dressing, using only the amount of tape required for secure attachment of dressing. Applying a "skin prep" on site to be taped can facilitate fixation and reduce irritation.
4. When *dressing the drain site:*
   a. Use premade drain sponge (can be prepared by making 5 cm. (2-inch) slit, with sterile scissors, in 4″ × 4″ gauze sponge).
   b. Gently slip sponge around drain; repeat process with second drain sponge, placing it at a right angle to the other sponge (see Fig. 4-6).

3. Excessive use of tape can cause irritation and trauma to intact skin.

a. The slit allows gauze to fit around the drainage tube.

b. Placement of the drain sponges in this manner allows for circumferential coverage of the drain site.

(continued)

Guidelines   Changing Surgical Dressings *(continued)*

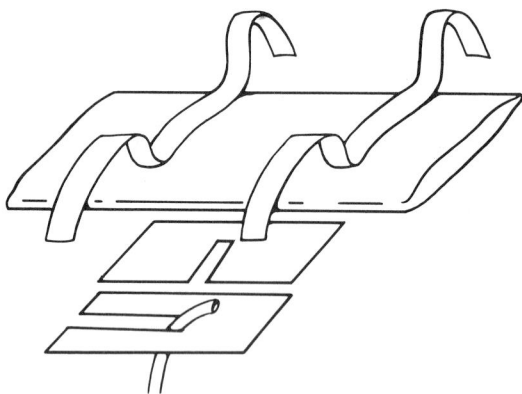

Figure 4-6. *Dressing the drainage tube insertion site. Be sure that one sponge is placed at a right angle to the second sponge so that the slits are going in different directions. If drainage is heavy, a sterile absorbent pad or extra gauze may be placed overall.*

Procedure *(continued)*	Nursing Action	Rationale

5. When *dressing an excessively draining wound:*
   a. Consider need for extra dressings and packing material.
   b. Use Montgomery straps if frequent dressing changes are required (see Fig. 4-7).

   a. More dressing materials are needed to absorb excess fluid.
   b. Frequent dressing changes can damage surrounding, intact skin due to the frequent application and removal of tape. Montgomery straps alleviate the problem.

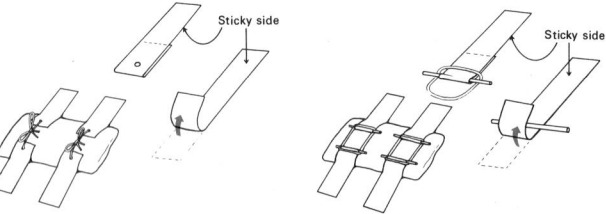

Figure 4-7. *Montgomery straps; two styles are shown.*

   c. Excessively draining wounds may be "pouched," much like an ostomy bag.
   d. Protect skin surrounding wound from copious or irritating drainage (e.g., gastrointestinal drainage), by applying some type of skin barrier.

   c. To protect surrounding skin, save nursing time, and facilitate accurate assessment of drainage.
   d. Maintaining the cleanliness and integrity of surrounding tissue is essential for successful overall wound healing.

Follow-up Care

1. Assess patient's tolerance to the procedure and help make him more comfortable.
2. Discard disposable items according to hospital protocol and clean equipment that is to be reused.
3. Wash hands.
4. Record nature of procedure and condition of wound, as well as patient reaction.

2. To prevent transmission of pathogenic organisms.

Skin Care Tips

1. Apply protective "screens" to skin surrounding wounds with copious or irritating secretions (e.g., gastrointestinal secretions):

   a. Hydrophobic gauze (e.g., vaseline gauze)
   b. Stomahesive (by Squibb)
   c. Skin Barrier (by Bard)
   d. Transparent film dressing

1. Some drainage can be quite damaging to normal or sensitive skin surrounding draining wound sites—adding another risk of infection. Acids and proteolytic enzymes from gastrointestinal drainage are especially caustic.

Guidelines Using Portable Wound Suction

Equipment   A calibrated collection container

Nonsterile gloves

Nursing Action	**Rationale**

1. When evacuator is full (200–800 ml.—depending on size of evacuator), it is time to empty. A good rule is to empty every 8 hours, or more frequently if necessary.
2. Carefully remove plug, maintaining its sterility.
3. Empty contents of evacuator into calibrated container.
4. Place evacuator on flat surface.
5. Cleanse opening, as well as plug, with an alcohol sponge.
6. Compress evacuator completely (see Fig. 4-8).

1. Negative pressure is dissipated as the evacuator fills.

2. Minimizes risk of wound infection.
3. Measure drainage.
4. To permit adequate compression.
5. To maintain cleanliness of outlet.
6. To remove air.

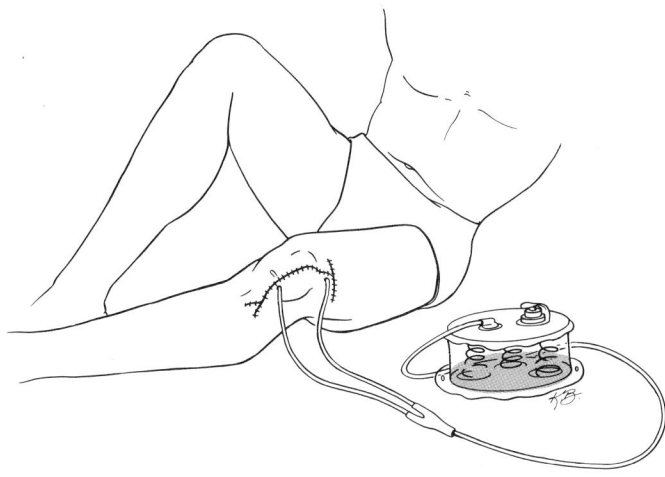

Figure 4-8. *Portable wound suction. Two perforated catheters are draining the incisional area following knee surgery. Drainage is drawn into the portable wound suction unit.*

7. Replace plug while evacuator is compressed.
8. As spring expands, a negative pressure of approximately 45 mm. Hg is produced.

9. Check system for proper operation.

10. Secure evacuator to patient's dressing; if patient is ambulatory, may fasten evacuator to his clothing.
11. Ensure that the drainage catheters are positioned off of incisional site.
12. Wash hands thoroughly.

13. Record character and amount of drainage.

7. To reestablish negative pressure (suction).
8. Any fluid and blood in tissues is sucked into evacuator. Negative pressure is not great enough to suck the soft tissues into the holes of the drainage catheter.
9. Look for fluid entering system; if none, look for disconnections.
10. This permits patient to move without disturbing closed suction.
11. Minimizes trauma and contamination of wound.
12. To prevent cross-contamination with other patients and staff.

Bibliography

Books

AORN. Standards and Recommended Practices for Perioperative Nursing. Denver, The Association of Operating Room Nurses, 1986

Atkinson L. Berry and Kohn's Introduction to Operating Room Technique. New York, McGraw–Hill, 1986

Barret J and Nyhus LM. Treatment of Shock. 2nd ed. Philadelphia, Lea & Febiger, 1986

Cameron J. Current Surgical Therapy. 2nd ed. St. Louis, CV Mosby, 1986

Demling RH and Wilson RF. Decision Making in Surgical Critical Care. Toronto, BC Decker, 1988

Fraulini KE. After Anesthesia: A Guide for PACU, ICU and Medical–Surgical Nurses. East Norwalk, CT, Appleton & Lange, 1987

Gruendemann BJ and Meeker MH. Alexander's Care of the Patient in Surgery. 8th ed. St. Louis, CV Mosby, 1987

Hardy JD. Hardy's Textbook of Surgery. Philadelphia, JB Lippincott, 1988

Hathaway RG. Nursing Care of the Critically Ill Surgical Patient.

Rockville, MD, Aspen Publishers, Inc, 1988

Julien RM. Understanding Anesthesia. Menlo Park, CA, Addison-Wesley, 1988

Kneedler JA and Dodge GH. Perioperative Patient Care: The Nursing Perspective. Boston, Blackwell Scientific Publications, 1987

Liechty RD and Soper RT (eds). Fundamentals of Surgery. St. Louis, CV Mosby, 1989

Miller TA. Physiologic Basis of Modern Surgical Care. St. Louis, CV Mosby, 1988

Rombeau JL and Caldwell MD. Parenteral Nutrition. Philadelphia, WB Saunders, 1986

Rothrock J. RN First Assistant: An Expanded Perioperative Nursing Role. Philadelphia, JB Lippincott, 1987

Sabiston D (ed). Handbook of Surgery. 13th ed. Philadelphia, WB Saunders, 1986

Schwartz SI. Principles of Surgery. 5th ed. New York, McGraw-Hill, 1989

Seymour G. Medical Assessment of the Elderly Surgical Patient. Rockville, MD, Aspen Publishers, Inc., 1986

Journals

Perioperative

Durrence C et al. Potential drug interactions in surgical patients. Am J Hosp Pharm 1985 Jul; 42(7):1553–1556

Fry DE. Antibiotics in surgery: An overview. Am J Surg 1988 May; 155(5A):11–15

Garner JS and Favero MS. CDC guidelines for handwashing and hospital environmental controls. Today's OR Nurse 1986 Apr; 8(4):26–37

Jackson MG. High risk surgical patients. J Gerontol Nurs 1988; 14(1):9–15

Johnson JE, Christman NJ and Stitt C. Personal control interventions: Short- and long-term effects on surgical patients. Res Nurs Health 1985 Jun; 8(2):131–146

Kaiser AB. Overview of cephalosporin prophylaxis. Am J Surg 1988 May; 155(5A):52–55

Keegan L. Holistic nursing: An approach to patient and self-care. AORN J 1987 Sep; 46(4):499–500, 502, 504

McConnell EA. Fluid and electrolyte concerns in intestinal surgical procedures. Nurs Clin North Am 1987 Dec; 22(4):853–860

Osis M. Drugs & geriatric surgery: Implications for pre-operative and post-operative care. Gerontion 1987 Summer; 2(2):8–10

Peterson KL. Perioperative vascular monitoring. Crit Care Q 1985 Sep; 8(2):1–8

Pollock AV. Surgical prophylaxis—The emerging picture. Lancet 1988 Jan 30; 1(8579):225–230

Reeder JM and Kapsar PP. Perioperative nursing competencies: The process and study. AORN J 1986 Jan; 43(1):220–222, 224–247

Stanfield V. Perioperative documentation: Integrating nursing diagnoses on the patient record. AORN J 1987 Oct; 46(4):699–701, 703–704

Tollerud L et al. A model for perioperative nursing practice. AORN J 1985 Jan; 41(1):188–194

Preoperative Nursing

Alverson E. The preoperative interview. AORN J 1987 May; 45(5):1158–1164

Aly R et al. Comparative antibacterial efficacy of a 2-minute surgical scrub with chlorhexidine gluconate, povidone-iodine, and chloroxylenol sponge-brushes. Am J Infect Control 1988 Aug; 16(4):173–177

Barron S. Preadmission made easy. Am J Nurs 1987 Dec; 87(12):1690–1691

Berron K. Transplant patients' perceptions about effective preoperative teaching. J Heart Transplant 1988 Mar–Apr; 5(2):162–165

Blackwood S. Back to basics—The preoperative examination. Am J Nurs 1986 Jan; 86(1):39–44

Brooke PS. Informed consent: An ethical dilemma having life/death and legal implications. Clin Nurse Spec 1988 Fall; 2(3):157–161

Brubakken KM. Preoperative antibiotic administration: A case for interdisciplinary monitoring. J Nurs Qual Assur 1989 Feb; 3(2):69–73

Cassidy VR and Oddi LF. Legal and ethical aspects of informed consent: A nursing research perspective. J Prof Nurs 1986 Nov–Dec; 2(6):343–349

Class P. PACU: Preanesthesia care unit? J Post Anesth Nurs 1988 Oct; 3(5):336–338

Cramer C et al. Preoperative care unit: An alternative to the holding room. AORN J 1987 Feb; 45(2):464, 466, 468

Douglas S and Larson E. There's more to informed consent than information. Focus Crit Care 1986 Apr; 13(2):43–47

El Guercio LRM. Preoperative exam for high-risk patients. Patient Care 1987 Nov; 6(6):37–42, 46–49

Evaluating the usefulness of routine preoperative tests. AORN J 1987 Mar; 45(3):696

Fay MF. Informed consent: A confusing concept. Today's OR Nurse 1986 Jul; 8(7):6–10

Garibaldi RA et al. The impact of preoperative skin disinfection on preventing intraoperative wound contamination. Infect Control Hosp Epidemiol 1988 Mar; 9(3):109–113

Goulart DT. Educating the cardiac surgery patient and family. J Cardiovasc Nurs 1989 May; 3(3):1–9

Goulart AE. Preoperative teaching for surgical patients. Perioper Nurs Q 1987 Jun; 3(2):8–13

Hathaway D. Effect of preoperative teaching on postoperative pain: A replication and explanation. Int J Nurs Stud 1985; 22(3):267–280

Hathaway D. An evaluation of a preoperative assessment program. Perioper Nurs Q 1987 Feb; 3(2):56–65

Hogue E. Informed consent. Nursing '86 1986 Jun; 16(6):47–48

Jackson CV. Preoperative pulmonary evaluation. Arch Intern Med 1988 Oct; 148(10):2120–2127

Johnson S. Preoperative teaching: A need for change. Nurs Manage 1989 Feb; 20(2): Or/Surg Procedure Ed: 80B, 90F, 80H

Knight CG et al. Assessing the preoperative adult. Nurs Pract 1988 Jan; 13(1):6, 8, 13

Leclair JM et al. Effect of preoperative shampoos on resident scalp flora. Today's OR Nurse 1988 Mar; 10(3):15–21

Leuze M et al. Preoperative assessment: Using the Roy Adaptation Model. AORN J 1987 Dec; 46(6):1122–1123, 1126, 1128–1129

Leirman J. Preoperative assessments: Can we afford to do without them? AORN J 1988 Feb; 47(2):586, 588–590

Lindeman CA. Patient education. Annu Rev Nurs Res 1988; 61:29–60

Lorenz RP et al. Skin preparation methods before cesarean section: A comparative study. J Reprod Med 1988 Feb; 33(2):202–204

Murphy EK. Informed consent: Part I. AORN J 1988 Apr; 47(4):1009, 1012–1013, 1016

Murray J et al. PACU preoperative visits make a difference. J Post Anesth Nurs 1987 Aug; 2(3):178–182

Nightingale K. The ideal and the actual: Preoperative visiting—revisited. Natnews 1988 Dec; 25(12):12–13

Proposed recommended practices: Preoperative skin preparation. AORN J 1987 Oct; 46(10):719–720, 722–724

Rathburn AM, Holland LA, Geelhoed GW. Preoperative skin decontamination. AORN J 1986 Jul; 44(1):62–65

Recommended practices: Preoperative skin preparation. AORN J 1988 Nov; 48(11):950–951, 953, 955

Rothrock JC. Perioperative nursing research: Preoperative psychoeducational interventions: Part I. AORN J 1989 Feb; 49(2):597, 599, 601–602

Smallwood SB. Preparing children for surgery: Learning through play. AORN J 1988 Jan; 47(1):177–178, 180–181, 183

Smith CC. Assessment of the preoperative visit by the postanesthesia nurse. J Post Anesth Nurs 1987 Feb; 2(2):32–35

Thomas EA. Preoperative fasting—A question of routine? Nurs Times 1987 Dec 9–15; 83(49):46–47

Vallejo BC. Is structured pre-surgical education more effective than non-structured education? Patient Educ Couns 1987 Jun; 9(3):14–18

Weikel C. Informed consent: An ethical dilemma. Today's OR Nurse 1987 Jan; 9(1):10–15

Day Surgery

Burden N. An ambulatory approach to ESWL. J Post Anesth Nurs 1988 Feb; 3(1):17–26

Domar AD. The preoperative use of the relaxation response with ambulatory surgery patients. Hosp Top 1987 Jul-Aug; 65(4):30–35

Fowler ME. Trends in ambulatory surgery. Preoperative preparation: The key to success in out-patient surgery. Plast Surg Nurs 1987; Spring; 7(1):21–23

Miller DK. The rationale and benefits of a required preadmission ambulatory surgery program. J Post Anesth Nurs 1988 Feb; 3(1):39–42

Preop visits help decrease cancellations and risks in SDS. Same Day Surg 1988 Jan; 12(1):1–5

Stanfield V. Perioperative education: Changing to meet short-stay needs—Education to the patient. J Post Anesth Nurs 1987 May; 2(2):74–77

Stewart SMB. Who is your same-day surgery learner?—Preoperative instruction. Perioper Nurs Q 1987 Jun; 3(2):14–18

Intraoperative Nursing

Aly R et al. Comparative antibacterial efficacy of a 2-minute surgical scrub with chlorhexidine gluconate, povidone-iodine and chlorxylenol sponge-brushes. Am J Infect Control 1988 Aug; 16(4):73–77

Crowley J. Innovative perineal draping for urological surgery. Urol Nurs 1988 Jul-Sep; 9(1):6–7

Erbstoesser M. Care of the patient with malignant hyperthermia. J Post Anesth Nurs 1989 Apr; 4(2):71–74

Garibaldi RA et al. Effects of preoperative shampoos on resident scalp flora. Today's OR Nurse 1988 Mar; 10(3):15–21

Glisson SN. Malignant hyperthermia. Compr Ther 1988 Oct; 14(10):33–41

Hardy JF. Large volume gastroesophageal reflux: A rationale for risk reduction in the perioperative period. Can J Anaesth 1988 Mar; 35(2):162–173

Larew RE. Malignant hyperthermia: Quick recognition and treatment to avoid death. Postgrad Med 1989 Jun; 70(6):1025–1026

Phillips R and Skov P. Rewarming and cardiac surgery: A review. Heart Lung 1988 Sep; 17(15):511–520

Masterson BJ. Skin preparation. Clin Obstet Gynecol 1988 Sep; 31(3):736–743

Piasecki P and Gitelis S. Use of a clean air system and personal exhaust suit in the orthopaedic operating room. Orthop Nurs 1988 Jul-Aug; 7(4):20–22

Radel TJ, Fallacaro MD, Sievenpiper T. The effects of a warming vest and cap during lower extremity orthopedic surgical procedures under general anesthesia. AANA J 1986 Dec; 54(6):486–489

Ritter MA and Marmion P. The exogenous sources and controls of microorganisms in the operating room. Orthop Nurs 1988 Jul-Aug; 7(4):23–28

Sebben JE. Sterile technique and the prevention of wound infection in office surgery: Part 2. J Dermatol Surg Oncol 1989 Jan; 15(1):38–48

Silo HM. Perioperative nursing research. Part V: Intraoperative recommended practices. AORN J 1989 Jun; 49(6):1627–1636

Stewart TP and Magnano SJ. Burns or pressure ulcers in the surgical patient? Decubitus 1988 Feb; 1(1):36–40

Taylor CA. Surgical hypothermia. Pharmacol Ther 1988; 38(2):169–200

Anesthesia

Boucher BA, Witt WO, and Foster TS. The postoperative adverse effects of inhalational anesthetics. Heart Lung 1986 Jan; 15(1):63–69

Milam SB. Intraoperative anesthetic complications. Dent Clin North Am 1987 Jan; 31(1):97–115

Matjasko MJ. Anesthesiology. JAMA 1989 May 19; 261(19):2826–2827

Montedonico J and Tarraze PM. Legal considerations of outpatient anesthesia. Anesthesiol Clin North Am 1987 Mar; 5(1):227–240

Scott NB and Kehlet H. Regional anaesthesia and surgical morbidity. Br J Surg 1988 Apr; 75(4):299–304

Tait AR and Knight PR. The effects of general anaesthesia on upper respiratory tract infections in children. Anesthesiology 1987 Dec; 67(6):930–935

Tiret L, et al. Complications related to anaesthesia in infants and children. Br J Anaesth 1988 Sep; 61(3):263–269

Postoperative Nursing Care

Consensus Conference. Prevention of venous thrombosis and pulmonary embolism. JAMA 1986 Aug 8; 256(6):744–749

Deitch EA. Infection in the compromised host. Surg Clin North Am 1988 Feb; 68(1):181–197

Dellinger EP. Use of scoring systems to assess patients with surgical sepsis. Surg Clin North Am 1988 Feb; 68(1):123–145

Johnson JC. Surgical assessment in the elderly. Geriatrics 1988 Dec; 43(suppl):83–90

Holtzclaw BJ. Postoperative shivering after cardiac surgery: A review. Heart Lung 1986 May; 15(3):292–302

Howe JN. How and when should I respond to postop fever? Nursing 1989 Jul; 19(7):984–986

Jermier BJ and Treloar DM. Bring your patient through gallbladder surgery. RN 1986 Nov; 49(11):18–20

Machiedo GW and Suval WD. Detection of sepsis in the postoperative patient. Surg Clin North Am 1988 Feb; 6(1):215–228

Nichols RR. Simple remedies for postoperative gas pain. RN 1986 Feb; 49(2):42–44

Rose SEM and MacKay RC. Postoperative stress: Do nurses accurately assess their patients? J Psychosoc Nurs Ment Health 1986 Apr; 24(4):16–22

Seckl J and Dunger D. Postoperative diabetes insipidus. Br Med J 1989 Jan 7; 298(6665):2–3

Schwartz SS and Yuska CM. Common patient care issues following surgery for head and neck cancer. Semin Oncol Nurs 1989 Aug; 5(3):191–194

Vaughan B. Discharge following surgery: Some helpful hints to aid your recovery. Nurs Times 1988 Apr 13; 84(15):32–33

Vaughn JB and Nemcek MM. Postoperative flatulence: Causes and remedies. Today's OR Nurse 1986 Oct; 8(10):19–23

Young ME. Fever in the postoperative patient. Focus Crit Care 1987 Apr; 14(2):13–18

Pain Control

American Pain Society. Relieving pain. An analgesic guide. Am J Nurs 1988 Jun; 88(6):815–826

Arnold C. Intraspinal analgesia: A new route for an old drug. J Neurosci Nurs 1989 Feb; 21(1):30–37

Berde CB. Pediatric postoperative pain management. Pediatr Clin North Am 1989 Aug; 36(4):921–940

Camp LD, Fernandez K, Reardon MB. Administering and monitoring epidural analgesia: Monitoring epidural morphine injections. Oncol Nurs Forum 1988 Nov-Dec; 15(6):817

Cornick P. A cry for help? Management of postoperative pain and discomfort in neonates. Prof Nurs 1989 Jun; 4(9):457–459

Dunajcik L. Controlling the dangers of epidural analgesics. RN Jan 1988; 48(1):41–45

Hadaway LC. Evaluation and use of advanced IV technology. Part 2: Patient controlled analgesia. J Intraven Nurs 1989 May-Jun; 12(3):184–191

Jackson D. A study of pain management: Patient controlled analgesia versus intramuscular analgesia. J Intraven Nurs 1989 Jan-Feb; 12(1):42–51

Kane NE. Patient-controlled analgesia. Va Med 1989 Apr; 116(4):71–72

Kearns PC. Exercises to ease pain after abdominal surgery. RN 1986 Jul; 49(7):45

Kleiman RL, Lipman AG, and Hare BD. PCA vs. regular IM injections for severe postoperative pain. Am J Nurs 1987 Nov; 87(11):1491–1492

King KB et al. Patient management of pain medication after cardiac surgery. Nurs Res 1987 May-Jun; 36(3):145–150

Olsson G and Parker G. A model approach to pain assessment. Nursing 1987 May; 17(5):52–56

Olsson GL, Leddo CC, and Wild L. Nursing management of patients receiving epidural narcotics. Heart Lung 1989 Mar; 18(2):130–138

Parish KA and Thompson GR. Epidural portals: Long-term management of intractable pain. AORN J 1989 Jul; 50(1):52–57, 60–64

Pasternak GW. Multiple morphine and enkephalin receptors and the relief of pain. JAMA 1988 Mar 4; 259(9):1362–1367

Power I and Douglas E. The nonsteroidal anti-inflammatory analgesics. Natnews 1989 Apr; 26(4):14–15

Rogers A. The nurse as acute pain specialist. Pain Manag 1988 Mar–Apr; 1(2):73–77

Rogers A. Analgesics: The physician's partner in effective pain management. VA Med 1989 Apr; 116(4):164–170

Shannon M and Berde CV. Pharmacologic management of pain in children and adolescents. Pediatr Clin North Am 1989 Aug; 36(4):855–871

Stewart SM. Controlling pain with epidural narcotics: Nursing implications. Crit Care Nurse 1986 May–Jun; 6(3):50–56

Thomas DW and Owen H. Patient-controlled analgesia—The need for caution: A case report and review of adverse incidents. Anaesthesia 1988 Sep; 43(9):770–772

Thorpe DM. Administering and monitoring epidural analgesia: Patient selection criteria. Oncol Nurs Forum 1988 Nov-Dec; 15(6):818–819

White PF. Use of patient-controlled analgesia for management of acute pain. JAMA 1988 Jan 8; 259(2):243–247

Wound Management

Bergamini TM and Polk HC Jr. Pharmacodynamics of antibiotic penetration of tissue and surgical prophylaxis. Surg Gynecol Obstet 1989 Mar; 168(3):283–289

Biblehimer HL. Dealing with a wound that drains 1.5 liters a day. RN 1986 Aug; 49(8):21

Calhoun JH and Mader JT. Antibiotic beads in the management of surgical infections. Am J Surg 1989 Apr; 157(4):443–449

Ceccio CM and Praiswater F. Keeping pin sites problem-free. RN 1988 Feb; 51(2):70

Czachor JS and Hawley HB. Anaerobic wound infection: Bacteroides and mediastinitis after cardiovascular surgery. Heart Lung 1988 Jul; 17(4): 335–338

Gustafsson G. Wound sepsis. Nurs RSA 1988 Jan; 3(1):27–29

Hadley SA and Black VL. Why use Dakin's solution for wound care? Am J Nurs 1988 Mar; 18(3):284–285

Krukowski ZH et al. Preventing wound infection after appendectomy: A review. Br J Surg 1988 Oct; 75(5): 1023–1033

Lange MP et al. Management of multiple enterocutaneous fistulas. Heart Lung 1989 Jul; 18(4):386–390

Larson E. Guidelines for use of topical antimicrobial agents. Am J Infect Control 1988 Dec; 16(6):253–266

Laufman H. Current use of skin and wound cleansers and antiseptics. Am J Surg 1989 Mar; 157(3):359–365

Lilienfeld DE et al. Obesity and diabetes as risk factors in postoperative wound infections after cardiac surgery. Am J Infect Control 1988 Feb; 16(1):3–6

Mancusi-Ungaro HR Jr and Rappaport NH. Preventing wound infection. Am Fam Physician 1986 Apr; 33(4):147–153

Mantanari J. Wound dehiscence. Nursing 1986 Feb; 16(2):33

Messer MS. Wound care. Crit Care Nurs Q 1989 Mar; 11(4):17–27

Morison MJ. How can the incidence of surgical wound infection be reduced? Prof Nurse 1988 Dec; 4(3):122–125

Oberg M and Lindsey D. Do not put hydrogen peroxide or povidone-iodine into wounds! Am J Dis Child 1987 Jan; 141(1):27–28

Pettengill C. Treatment of extraordinary wound: Ingenuity and cooperation. J Enterostomal Ther 1989 Jan-Feb; 16(1):29–33

Rodeheaver G. Controversies in topical wound management. Ostomy Wound Manage 1988 Fall; 20:58–68

Roth RA and Verbridge N. Surgical wound surveillance: Quality assurance approach. AORN J 1988 Mar; 47(3): 722–723, 726–729

Stradtman JC and Ballenger MJ. Nursing implications in sternal and mediastinal infections after open heart surgery. Focus Crit Care 1989 Jun; 16(3):178–183

Thomas C. Nursing alert—Wound healing halted with the use of povidone iodine. Ostomy Wound Manage 1988 Spring; 18:30–33

Troxler SH and Nichols RL. Surgical wound infections. Today's OR Nurse 1987 Mar; 9(3):16–22

Vitello-Cicciu J. Sternal wound management: A case study. Nursing grand rounds. J Cardiovasc Nurs 1989 May; 3(3):66–70

Wallace DM et al. Use of directional flow irrigation. Ostomy Wound Manage 1989 Spring; 22:34–40

Whitney JD. Physiologic effects of tissue oxygenation on wound healing. Heart Lung 1989 Sep; 18(5):466–467

IV Therapy

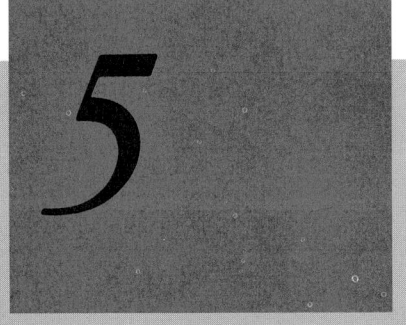

Goals and Principles

Goals

1. Maintain or replace body stores of water, electrolytes, vitamins, proteins, fats, and calories in the patient who cannot maintain an adequate intake by mouth.
2. Restore acid–base balance.
3. Restore volume of blood components.
4. Provide avenues for the administration of medications.
5. Monitor central venous pressure.

Physiologic Assimilation of Infusion Solutions

A. Principles

1. Tissue cells (e.g., erythrocytes, neurons, etc.) are surrounded by a semipermeable membrane.
2. *Osmotic pressure* is the "pulling" pressure demonstrated when water moves through the semipermeable membrane of tissue cells from an area of weaker concentration to stronger concentration of solute (e.g., sodium ions, blood glucose). The end result is dilution and equilibration between the intracellular and extracellular compartments.
3. Extracellular compartment fluids primarily include plasma and interstitial fluid.

B. Types of Fluids

1. *Isotonic*—a solution that exerts the same osmotic pressure as that found in plasma.
   a. Normal saline 0.9%
   b. Lactated Ringer's
   c. Blood components
2. *Hypotonic*—a solution that exerts less osmotic pressure than that of blood plasma. Administration of this fluid generally causes dilution of plasma solute concentration and forces water movement into cells to reestablish intracellular and extracellular equilibrium; cells will then expand or swell.
   a. Dextrose 5% and water
   b. Half-strength normal saline, 0.45%
   c. Quarter-strength normal saline, 0.2%
3. *Hypertonic*—a solution that exerts a higher osmotic pressure than that of blood plasma. Administration of this fluid increases the solute concentration of plasma, drawing water out of the cells and into the extracellular compartment to restore osmotic equilibrium; cells will then shrink.
   a. Dextrose 5% in normal saline
   b. Dextrose 5% in half-strength normal saline (only slightly hypertonic, as dextrose is rapidly metabolized and renders only temporary osmotic pressure)
   c. Dextrose 10% in water
   d. Dextrose 20% in water
   e. Normal saline, 3% and 5%
   f. Hyperalimentation fluids

C. Composition of Fluids (see Table 5-1)

1. Saline solutions—water and electrolytes (Na^+, Cl^-)
2. Dextrose solutions—water or saline and calories
3. Lactated Ringer's—water and electrolytes (Na^+, K^+, Cl^-, Ca^{++}, lactate)
4. Balanced isotonic—varies; water, electrolytes, some calories (Na^+, K^+, Mg^{++}, Cl^-, HCO_3^-, gluconate)
5. Whole blood and blood components
6. Plasma expanders—albumin, dextran, plasma protein fraction (Plasmanate), hetastarch (Hespan) (exert increased oncotic pressure, pulling fluid from interstitium into the circulation and temporarily increasing blood volume)
7. Parenteral hyperalimentation—fluid, electrolytes, amino acids, and calories

D. Uses and Precautions With Common Types of Infusions

1. Dextrose 5% in water:
   a. Used to replace water (hypotonic fluid) losses, supply some caloric intake, administer as carrying solution for numerous medications, or function as a slow "keep-vein-open" infusion.
   b. Cautious use in patients with water intoxication (hyponatremia, syndrome of inappropriate antidiuretic hormone release). Should not be used as concurrent solution infusion with blood or blood components. (See Table 5-2 for signs and symptoms of water excess or deficit.)
2. Normal saline:
   a. Used to replace saline (isotonic fluid) losses, administer with blood components, or treat patients in hemodynamic shock.
   b. Cautious use in patients with isotonic volume excess (e.g., heart failure, renal failure). (See Table 5-3 for signs and symptoms of isotonic fluid excess or deficit.)
3. Lactated Ringer's:
   a. Used to replace isotonic fluid losses, replenish

Table 5-1. *Composition of Selected Intravenous Solutions*

| Solution | Tonicity | Na⁺ | K⁺ | Cl⁻ | Ca⁺⁺ | pH | mOsm./liter | Calories |
		(mEq/liter)						
5% DW	Hypotonic	—	—	—	—	5.0	253	170
10% DW	Hypertonic	—	—	—	—	4.6	561	340
0.9% NS	Isotonic	154	—	154	—	5.7	308	—
0.45% NS	Hypotonic	77	—	77	—	5.3	154	—
5% D and 0.9% NS*	Slightly hypertonic	154	—	154	—	4.2	561	170
5% and 0.45% NS	Slightly hypertonic	77	—	77	—	4.2	407	170
5% and 0.2% NS†	Hypotonic	34	—	34	—	4.2	290	170
Lactated Ringer's†	Isotonic	148	4	156	4.5	6.7	309	9
5% D and lactated Ringer's	Slightly hypertonic	130	4	109	3.0	5.1	527	170
Normosol-R	Isotonic	140	5	96	—	6.4	295	—
Sodium lactate 1/6 molar	Slightly hypertonic	167	—	—	—	6.9	333	55
6% Dextran 75 and 0.9% NS	Isotonic	154	—	154	—	4.3	309	—

DW, dextrose in water; NS, normal saline

* 5% Dextrose metabolizes rapidly in the blood and, in reality, produces minimal osmotic effects.

† Lactate converts to bicarbonate in the liver.

specific electrolyte losses, and moderate metabolic acidosis (lactate converts to bicarbonate in the liver).

Nursing Process Overview: The Patient Undergoing IV Therapy

Assessment

﹒A. Assess Need for Infusion Therapy

1. How does the patient's illness affect his fluid balance? Are there obvious or subtle fluid and electrolyte losses? If so, how much, and what kind?
   a. Diarrhea and vomiting?
   b. Diuresis?
   c. Insensible losses such as diaphoresis, fever, hyperventilation?
   d. Fistula drainage? Ascites? Wound drainage? Signs of hemorrhage?
2. What is the patient's age? (The elderly and very young are more prone to fluid and electrolyte losses.)

3. What is the relation of his fluid intake to fluid output?
4. Is there any dietary restriction, or is the patient anorexic?
5. Is the patient immobile or confused (decreases patient's access to fluids)?
6. What prescribed medication or treatment could affect the patient's fluid and electrolyte status (e.g., diuretics, dialysis, nasogastric drainage)?
7. What is the physician's plan of treatment?

B. Evidence of Fluid and Electrolyte Imbalance in the Patient

1. It is important to observe the patient for both excesses or deficits in fluid and electrolytes.
2. Moderate to severe deficits are replenished with appropriate infusion therapy.
3. Patients receiving infusion therapy are at potential risk for fluid and electrolyte excesses.
4. Clinical manifestations of fluid and electrolyte imbalances are outlined in Tables 5-2 and 5-3.

Table 5-2. *Signs and Symptoms of Water Excess or Deficit*

Site	Hyponatremia (Water Intoxication)	Hypernatremia (Water Deficit)
CNS	Muscle twitching	Restlessness
	Hyperactive tendon reflexes	Weakness
	Convulsions	Delirium
	Increased intracranial pressure, coma	Coma
CV	Increased BP and pulse, if severe	Tachycardia
		Hypotension (if severe)
Tissues:	Increased salivation, tears	Decreased saliva and tears
	Watery diarrhea	Dry, sticky mucous membranes
	Fingerprinting of skin	Red, swollen tongue
		Flushed skin
Renal	Oliguria	Oliguria
Other	None	Fever

Table 5-3. *Signs and Symptoms of Isotonic Fluid Excess or Deficit*

Site	Deficit	Excess
CNS	Fatigue, apathy	Confusion (if severe)
	Anorexia	
	Stupor, coma	
CV	Orthostatic hypotension	Elevated venous pressure
	Flat neck veins	Distended neck veins
	Fast, thready pulse	Increased cardiac output
	Hypotension	Heart gallops
	Cool, clammy skin	Pulmonary edema
GI	Anorexia	Anorexia, nausea and vomiting
	Thirst	
	Silent ileus	Edema of stomach, colon, and mesentery
Tissues	Soft, small tongue with longitudinal wrinkling	Pitting edema
		Moist pulmonary crackles
	Sunken eyes	
	Decreased skin turgor	
Metabolism	Mild decrease in temperature	None

C. Inspection of Prescribed Fluid and Equipment to be Used for Infusion

1. Observe fluid for discoloration, foreign particles, cloudiness, film—if present, do not use.
2. *Fluid in a bag:* gently squeeze and observe for leakage.
3. *Fluid in a glass bottle:*
   a. Hold bottle up to light.
   b. Slowly rotate bottle in upright position and then on its side; carefully inspect for a flash of light that could indicate a crack.
4. Check IV tubing for discoloration or defects; if noted, secure new equipment.
5. Inspect the needle or catheter for signs of contamination, barbs on needle bevel, or frayed edges on the catheter tip.
6. Return defective equipment with a note describing defect to proper department.
7. Ensure that the prescribed medication is actually what is infusing or to be infused; determine that the appropriate volume is being delivered by calculating drip rate or checking rate setting on mechanical delivery system.

Nursing Diagnoses

1. Fluid volume deficit related to dehydration, hemorrhage, use of diuretics, etc.
2. Fluid volume excess related to overhydration by infusion therapy.
3. Knowledge deficit related to unfamiliarity with infusion procedures and rationale.
4. Pain related to needle insertion or discomfort associated with irritating infusions, or immobilization of arm or hand.
5. Other nursing diagnoses could include:
   a. Injury, potential for, related to IV infiltration, phlebitis, local and systemic infection, or (in central lines) air embolus.
   b. Anxiety related to fear of discomfort or perceived significance of infusion therapy.

Nursing Interventions

1. Acquaint the patient with the requirements and need for intravenous infusion.
2. Select a suitable vein for venipuncture to optimize benefits of infusion and minimize discomfort to patient.
3. Utilize best method of distending a vein to permit easiest access to a vessel (see p. 82).
4. Select appropriate needle/catheter suitable for type and location of infusion. For instance, if the solution is highly viscous (e.g., blood), a larger bore needle/catheter is required.
5. Consider local anesthesia for the unusually sensitive patient after verifying presence of allergies.
6. Thoroughly cleanse area of IV insertion according to hospital policy.
7. The use of arm boards is considered when IV devices are placed over or near areas of flexion to prevent injury to vein.
8. Adjust rate of flow of fluids appropriate to needs of patient as prescribed (see p. 84).
9. Monitor IV flow rates every 1–2 hours for accuracy.
10. Monitor patient at least every 4 hours for evidence of local IV-related complications (pain, tenderness, redness, or swelling).
11. Change infusion-site dressings and IV tubing every 48 hours or more frequently as hospital policy dictates. Label all tubing with initials, along with time and date initiated.
12. Check compatibility of all concurrently infused drugs and IV solutions with pharmacy prior to administration.
13. Accurately document time of insertion, location, needle/catheter description, and infusion type, volume, and rate on appropriate hospital records.

Evaluation

1. Receives adequate infusion therapy as prescribed.
2. Shows no untoward side effect of infusion therapy.
3. Communicates (if alert) an understanding of the reason for infusion therapy.
4. Expresses a reasonable degree of comfort throughout duration of infusion therapy.

Procedural Considerations in Intravenous Therapy

Criteria for Selecting a Vein Suitable for Venipuncture

A. Initial Considerations

1. Use distal branches of a large vein initially.

> **NURSING ALERT:** Select most distal vein on hand or arm initially for venipuncture or infusion. If, with subsequent venipunctures, this site is difficult to enter, move up higher on the arm; conversely, if the antecubital fossa area is used first, and if later there is difficulty entering at this site, the lower veins may not be usable.

2. Locate a vein that is not crooked, scarred (hardened), or inflamed.

B. Suitable Veins

1. Back of the hand—metacarpal vein (Fig. 5-1 *A*). Avoid digital veins if possible.
   a. The advantage of this site is that it permits arm movement.
   b. If later a vein problem develops at this site, another vein higher up the arm may be used.
2. Forearm—basilic or cephalic vein (Fig. 5-1*B*).
3. Inner aspect of elbow, antecubital fossa—median basilic and median cephalic for relatively short-term infusion.
   a. These veins are large and easily accessible.
   b. Note, however, that this site precludes arm movement.
   c. Choose site below elbow crease for patient's comfort.

C. In Adult Patients, Veins in Lower Extremities Are Used As a Last Resort.

1. Thigh—great saphenous and femoral veins.
2. Ankle—great saphenous; foot—venous plexus of dorsum, dorsal venous arch, medial marginal vein.
3. When varicose veins are present, the extremity must be carefully monitored.

> **NURSING ALERT:** Veins in lower extremities are avoided because of venous stasis, increased risk of thrombosis, and limitations imposed on ambulating patient.

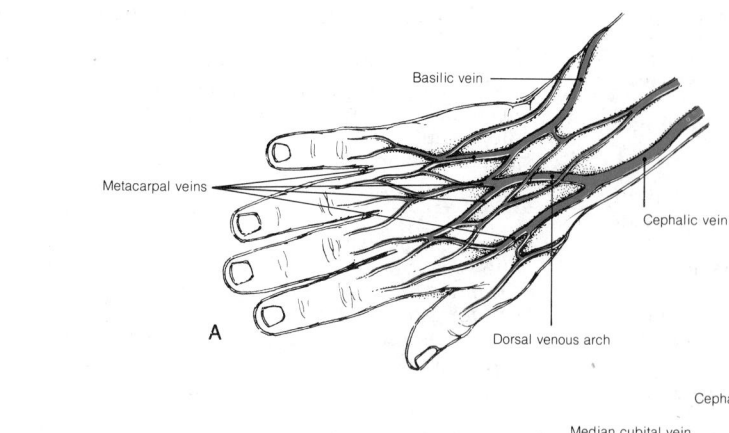

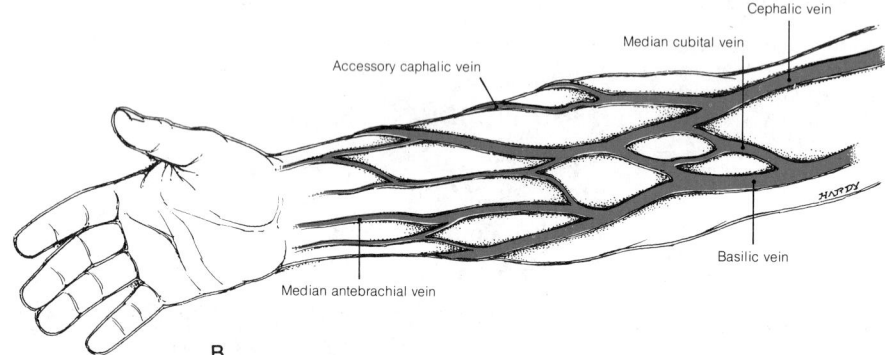

Figure 5-1. *(A) Superficial veins, dorsal aspect of hand. (B) Superficial veins, forearm.*

D. Instances When Central Veins Are Used (Fig. 5-2):

1. When medications and infusions are hypertonic or highly irritating, requiring rapid, high-volume dilution to prevent systemic reactions and local venous damage (e.g., chemotherapy, hyperalimentation).
2. When peripheral blood flow is diminished (e.g., shock) or when peripheral vessels are not accessible (e.g., obese patients).
3. When central venous pressure monitoring is desired.
4. When moderate or long-term fluid therapy is expected.

E. Other Considerations

1. Physicians or appropriately educated health care personnel are responsible for central venous catheter insertion.
2. Selection of infusion sites on infants or small children is discussed in Chapter 47.
3. Central lines may be percutaneously inserted (e.g., trilumen catheters), "tunneled" (Hickman, Groshong catheters), or "implanted." (See p. 111 for discussion of tunneled catheters.)
4. Management of central lines are similar to that described for Hickman catheters (p. 112).

Methods of Distending a Vein

1. Apply manual compression above site where cannula is to be inserted.
2. Have the patient periodically clench his fist (if arm is used).
3. Massage area in direction of venous flow.
4. Apply tourniquet (made of soft rubber tubing) at least 5–15 cm. (2–6 inches) above planned insertion site, fastening it with a slip knot or hemostat.

5. An alternative is to apply blood pressure cuff (keep pressure just below systolic pressure).
6. Lightly tap vein site; this is to be done gently so that the vein is not injured.
7. Allow extremity to be dependent (below heart level) for a few minutes.
8. Apply heat to a possible needle site by using a moist, warm towel or hand-operated blow dryer.

Cleansing Infusion Site

1. If skin is unusually soiled, cleanse infusion site thoroughly with a good surgical soap and rinse.
2. Cleanse IV site with effective topical antiseptic (according to hospital policy), working in a circular motion from the center outward to a diameter of 5–10 cm. (2–4 inches). Two techniques are as follows:
   a. Cleanse area with 1% to 2% tincture of iodine, allowing skin contact for at least 30 seconds. When dry, wipe with 70% alcohol. Iodine will cause skin discoloration if left in place.
   b. Cleanse skin with 70% alcohol, then prepare skin with vigorous scrub with iodophor (povidone-iodine) swab for 1 minute and allow to dry. Iodophor, an iodine compound, is less effective than regular iodine solutions.

NURSING ALERT: Iodine solutions and iodophors may cause allergic reactions in some patients. Patient should be assessed for iodine allergies prior to IV insertion. Iodine and iodophor (an iodine compound) should dry to facilitate their antimicrobial properties. Alcohol, an effective antiseptic, dries quickly.

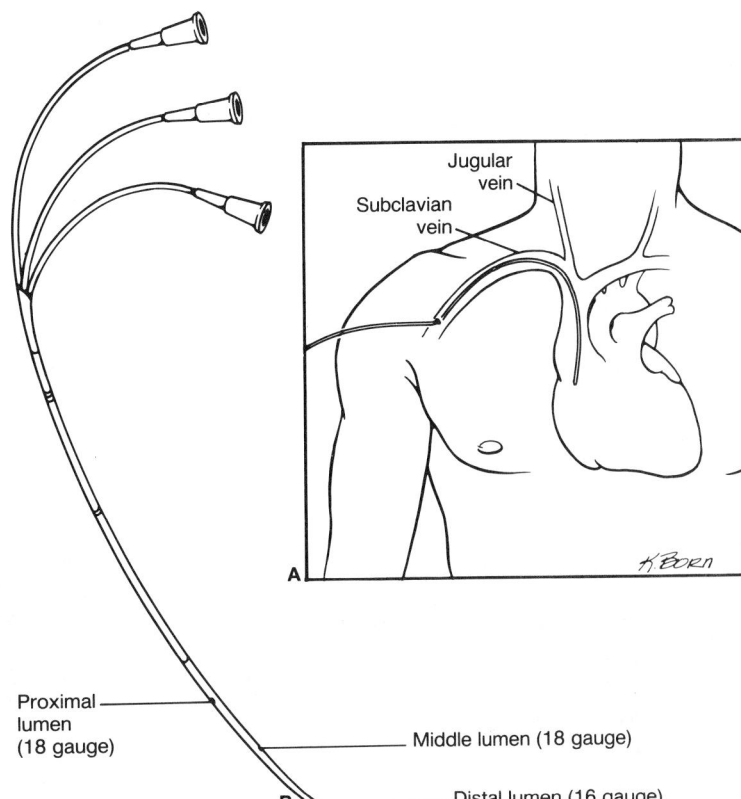

Figure 5-2. *(A) Placement of central venous catheter (subclavian approach). (B) Multilumen catheter.
Proximal lumen* used for venous sampling and
medication administration; middle lumen *used for
hyperalimentation infusion and medication administration; distal lumen* used for high volume infusions and blood products administration.

3. Wait until skin is dry before inserting needle; this is
   done to prevent carrying antiseptic solution into the
   vein.

Local Anesthesia Use

1. If large-bore needle (greater than 18 gauge) is being
   inserted in an unusually sensitive patient, 1% lidocaine
   (without epinephrine) may be infiltrated intradermally
   around the site to provide local anesthesia.
2. Local analgesia is best avoided because it may cause
   collapse of desired veins, allergic reactions, and increased cost of the procedure.

Equipment

A. Needle or Catheter

Peripheral infusion may be administered through a needle
(short-term) or through a catheter (long-term). Choice of
central line catheters is based on purpose for line and physician preference.

B. Bevel

To facilitate entering a vein with least injury to skin, the
bevel should face:
1. Upward—when entering a vein lumen that is larger
   than the needle.
2. Downward—when entering a small vein with lumen
   that approaches the size of the needle.

C. Solution Container

1. Soft polyvinylchloride containers are more convenient
   and easier to store than glass containers.
2. While plastic bags are the predominant containers

currently used for infusions, glass bottles are the choice
when delivering solutions containing drugs that are
absorbed into the polyvinyl walls of the bag (e.g., nitroglycerin, sodium nitroprusside)

D. Infusion Tubing

1. *Drip chambers*
   a. A "microdrip" system delivers 60 drops/ml. and
      is used when small volumes are being delivered
      (e.g., less than 50 ml./minute); this reduces the
      risk of clotting the IV line due to slow infusion
      rates.
   b. The "macrodrip" system delivers 10, 15, or 20
      drops/ml. and is used to deliver solution in large
      quantities or at fast rates.
2. *Vents*
   a. Vented tubing should be used with standard glass
      bottles; this permits air to enter the vacuum in the
      bottle and displace solution as it flows out.
   b. Nonvented tubing should be used for IV bags and
      glass bottles that have a built-in air vent.
3. *Filters*
   a. Help minimize the risk of contamination from
      certain microorganisms and particulate matter.
   b. Filters should be changed every 24–48 hours, as
      bacteria may become trapped in the filter and re-
      lease endotoxin, a small pyrogen capable of pass-
      ing through the filter.
   c. Filters must be added to the tubing and are indi-
      cated by hospital policy. They are recommended
      when administering parenteral nutrition and are
      contraindicated in some types of chemotherapy.

4. *Special Tubing*
   a. Most mechanical infusion pumps and controllers require specialized tubing to fit their particular pumping chamber. Need for such a device should be determined prior to initiating preparations for infusion therapy.
   b. If added tubing length is required (especially for children and restless patients), extension tubing is available; this should be added at the time of IV set-up.
   c. Secondary tubing is used for administration of intermittent "piggyback" medications that are connected to the port closest to the drip chamber.

Adjusting Rate of Flow of Fluid in Infusion Therapy

The physician prescribes the flow rate. However, the nurse is responsible for regulating and maintaining the proper rate.

A. Patient Determining Factors

1. Surface area of the patient—the larger the patient, the more fluid he may require and can tolerate.
2. Patient condition—a patient in hypovolemic shock requires greater amounts of fluids, while the patient with heart or renal failure should receive fluids judiciously.
3. Age of patient—fluids should be administered more slowly in the very young and elderly.
4. Tolerance to solutions—fluids containing medications causing potential allergic reactions or intense vascular irritation (e.g., potassium chloride) should be well diluted or given slowly.
5. Prescribed fluid composition—efficacy of some drugs are based on speed of infusion (e.g., antibiotics); other solutions are given at a rate titrated to the patient's response to them (e.g., dopamine, sodium nitroprusside, heparin).

B. Factors Affecting Rate of Flow

1. Pressure gradient—the difference between 2 levels in a fluid system.
2. Friction—the interaction between fluid molecules and surfaces of inner wall of tubing.
3. Diameter and length of tubing; gauge of cannula.
4. Height of column of fluid.
5. Size of opening through which fluid leaves receptacle.
6. Characteristics of fluid
   a. Viscosity
   b. Temperature—refrigerated fluids may cause diminished flow and vessel spasm; bring fluid to room temperature
7. Vein trauma, clots, plugging of vents, venous spasm, vasoconstriction, etc.
8. Flow-control clamp derangement
   a. Some clamps may slip and loosen, resulting in a very rapid, or "runaway," infusion.
   b. Plastic tubing may distort, causing "creep" or "cold flow"—the inside diameter of tubing will continue to change long after clamp is tightened or relaxed.
   c. Marked stretching of tubing may cause distortions of tubing and render clamp ineffective (may occur when patient turns over and pulls on a short tubing).
9. If there is any question regarding rate of fluid administration, check with the physician.

C. Calculation of Flow Rate

1. Most infusion rates are prescribed to be given at a certain volume per hour.
2. The delivery of the prescribed volume is determined by calculating the necessary drops per minute to deliver the volume.
3. Drops per ml. vary with commercial parenteral sets (e.g., 10, 15, 20, or 60 drops/ml.) Check directions on set.
4. Calculate infusion rate utilizing the following formula:

$$\text{Drops/minute} = \frac{\text{total volume infused} \times \text{drops/ml.}}{\text{total time for infusion in minutes}}$$

Example: Infuse 150 ml. of 5% D/W in 1 hour (set indicates 10 drops/1 ml.).

$$\frac{150 \times 10}{60 \text{ minutes}} = 25 \text{ drops/minute}$$

5. The nurse hanging a new IV solution should record date, time, and her initial on the container label.

NURSING ALERT: Never write directly on the IV bag. Write on label or tape using a regular pen. Do not use magic markers as they are absorbed into the plastic bag and perhaps into the solution.

6. Infusions with an established rate of 50 ml./hour or greater should be premarked to indicate the desired hourly fluid level. Minibag solutions, titrating solutions (e.g., dopamine), or rates less than 50 ml./hour need not have desired hourly fluid levels marked.

Intravenous "Push"

IV *"push" (or "IV bolus")* refers to the administration of a medication from a syringe and needle directly into an ongoing intravenous infusion. It may also be given directly into a vein or heparin lock.

Indications

1. For emergency administration of cardiopulmonary resuscitative procedures, allowing rapid concentration of a medication in the patient's bloodstream.
2. When quicker response to the medication is required (e.g., furosemide, digoxin).
3. To administer "loading" doses of a drug that will be continued via infusion (e.g., lidocaine).
4. To reduce patient discomfort by limiting need for IM injections.
5. To avoid incompatibility problems that may occur when several medications are mixed in one bottle.
6. To deliver drugs to patients unable to take them by mouth (e.g., coma) or IM (e.g., coagulation disorder).

Precautions and Recommendations

1. Prior to administration of the medication:
   a. Determine that the medication matches the physician's order.
   b. Dilute the drug as indicated by pharmacy references. Many medications are quite irritating to veins, requiring sufficient dilution.
   c. Determine the correct (safest) rate of administration. Consult pharmacy or pharmaceutical text.

Most medications are given slowly (rarely over less than 1 minute); sometimes as long as 30 minutes are required. Too rapid administration may result in serious side effects.

  d. If IV push is to be given with an ongoing IV infusion or to follow another IV push medication, check pharmacy for possible incompatibility. It is always wise to flush the IV tubing or cannula with saline prior to and following administration of a drug.

  e. Assess patient's condition and ability to tolerate the drug.

2. Watch patient's reaction to the drug.
  a. Are there major side effects, such as anaphylaxis, respiratory distress, tachycardia, bradycardia, seizures?
  b. What about minor side effects such as nausea, flushing, skin rash, confusion.
  c. Stop medication and consult physician if any such reactions occur.

3. Vesicants are always given through the side port of a running IV infusion.

4. Be familiar with hospital policies and guidelines regarding how, where, and by whom IV push medications can be given.

5. Medications should not be administered through a central line unless specifically ordered or the patient is in a critical care unit.

NURSING ALERT: Unusual dosages or unfamiliar drugs should always be confirmed with the physician and/or pharmacist prior to administration. The nurse is ultimately accountable for the drug that he or she administers.

Procedure

1. Directly into the vein (see Guidelines: Venipuncture, p. 87)
2. Into IV tubing
  a. As with venipuncture, aseptic technique is rigidly observed.
  b. The distal port is carefully swabbed with alcohol before it is punctured.
3. Via "piggyback" (see Guidelines: IV "piggyback," p. 91)
4. Into a "heparin lock" (see Guidelines: Heparin Lock, p. 91)
  a. All IV medications given via heparin locks are typically administered utilizing the *SASH* method. SASH is an acronym for:
    S—*S*aline flush
    A—*A*dminister medication
    S—*S*aline flush
    H—*H*eparin flush

Electronic Flow-Rate Regulators

Types

1. *Controller*—an electronic device that regulates flow of infusion by electronically monitoring drop rate (drops/minute) or monitoring volume passage (ml./minute); the latter is currently more commonly used because it is not affected by drop size, temperature, or fluid viscosity. The delivery of fluid will stop if the line is occluded or if infiltration is detected.
2. *Infusion pump*—an electronic device that exerts pressure (1) on the tubing or (2) on fluid. It continually pumps against a pressure gradient, providing a constant, accurate delivery of a preselected rate of fluid volume. The high-pressure pumping capability is particularly useful for arterial infusions.

Indications for Use

1. Intra-arterial infusions (the pump is required)
2. Critical care fluid and medication management
3. Parenteral nutrition (hyperalimentation)
4. Continuous heparin, insulin, aminophylline (etc.) infusions
5. Chemotherapy and oxytocic drugs
6. Small-volume infusions (less than 50 ml./minute)
7. Pediatric infusions

Advantages

1. Ability to infuse large and small volumes of fluid with accuracy.
2. An alarm warns of problem, such as air-in-line or occlusion.
3. Reduces nursing time in constantly readjusting flow rates.

Disadvantages

1. Requires special tubing.
2. There may be added cost to therapy.
3. Infusion pumps will continue to infuse despite presence of infiltration.

Nursing Considerations

1. Remember that a mechanical infusion regulator is only as effective as the nurse operating it.
2. Continue to check the patient regularly for complications, such as infiltration or infection.
3. Follow the manufacturer's instruction carefully when inserting the tubing.
4. Double-check the flow rate.
5. Be sure to flush all air out of the tubing before connecting it to the patient.
6. Explain purpose of the device and the alarm system. Added machines in the room can evoke greater anxiety in the patient and his family.

Complications of Intravenous Therapy

Infiltration

1. *Cause*—dislodgement of the IV cannula from the vein results in infusion of fluid into the surrounding tissues.
2. *Clinical manifestations*
  a. Swelling, blanching, and coolness of surrounding skin and tissues.
  b. Discomfort, depending on nature of solution.
  c. Fluid flows more slowly or stops.
  d. Absence of blood backflow in IV catheter and tubing.
3. *Preventive measures*
  a. Ensure that IV and distal tubing are secured sufficiently with tape to prevent movement.

b. Splint arm or hand as necessary.

c. Check IV site frequently for complications.

4. *Nursing interventions*

a. Stop infusion immediately and remove IV needle or catheter.

b. Restart IV in the other arm.

c. If infiltration is moderate to severe, apply warm, moist compresses and elevate limb.

d. If a vasoconstrictor agent (e.g., norepinephrine bitartrate [Levophed], dopamine) or a vesicant (e.g., various chemotherapy agents) have infiltrated, initiate emergency local treatment as directed; serious tissue injury, necrosis, and sloughing may result if actions are not taken.

e. Document interventions and assessments.

Thrombophlebitis

1. *Causes*

a. Injury to a vein during venipuncture, large-bore needle/catheter use, or prolonged needle/catheter use.

b. Irritation to vein due to rapid infusions or irritating solutions (e.g., hypertonic glucose solutions, cytotoxic agents, strong acids or alkalies, potassium, and others). Smaller veins are more susceptible.

c. Clot formation at the end of the needle or catheter due to slow infusion rates.

d. More often seen with synthetic catheters than steel needles.

2. *Clinical manifestations*

a. Tenderness at first, then pain along course of the vein.

b. Swelling, warmth, and redness at infusion site; the vein may appear as a red streak above insertion site.

3. *Preventive measures*

a. Anchor needle or catheter securely at insertion site.

b. Change insertion site at least every 72 hours.

c. Use large veins for irritating fluid because of higher blood flow which rapidly dilutes irritant.

d. Sufficiently dilute irritating agents prior to infusion.

4. *Nursing interventions*

a. Apply cold compresses immediately to relieve pain and inflammation.

b. Later follow with moist, warm compresses to stimulate circulation and promote absorption.

c. Document interventions and assessments.

Bacteremia

1. *Causes*

a. Underlying phlebitis increases risk 18-fold.

b. Contaminated equipment or infused solutions (see Fig. 5-3).

c. Prolonged placement of an IV device (catheter/needle, tubing, solution container).

d. Nonaseptic IV insertion or dressing change.

e. Cross-contamination by patient with other infected areas of body.

f. The critically ill or immunosuppressed patient is at greatest risk of bacteremia.

2. *Clinical manifestations*

a. Elevated temperature, chills

b. Nausea, vomiting

c. Malaise, increased pulse

d. Backache, headache

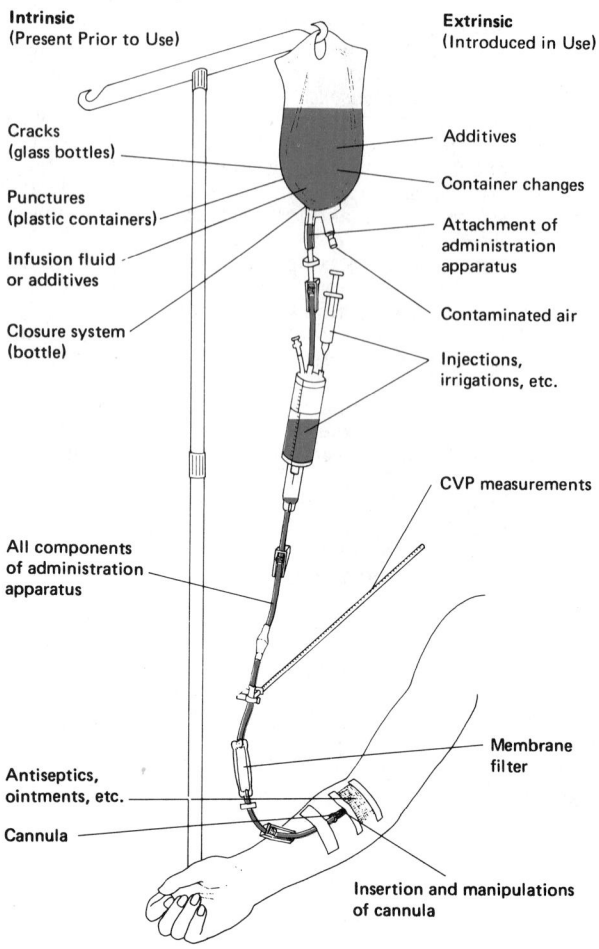

Figure 5-3. *Potential mechanisms for contamination of IV infusion systems.*

e. May progress to septic shock with profound hypotension.

f. Possible signs of local infection at IV insertion site (e.g., redness, pain, foul drainage)

3. *Preventive measures*

a. Follow same measures as outlined for thrombophlebitis.

b. Use strict asepsis when inserting IV or changing IV dressing.

c. Solutions should never hang longer than 24 hours.

d. Use filter (preferably 0.22 micron) with infusion unless contraindicated.

e. Change insertion site at least every 48 to 72 hours.

f. Change IV administration set every 24 to 48 hours.

g. Change IV dressing every 24 to 48 hours.

h. Maintain integrity of infusion system

4. *Nursing interventions*

a. Discontinue infusion and IV cannula.

b. IV device should be aseptically removed and the tip cut off with sterile scissors, placed in a dry sterile container, and immediately sent to the laboratory for analysis.

c. Check vital signs; reassure patient.

d. Obtain white blood cell count, as directed, and assess for other sites of infection (urine, sputum, wound).
e. Document interventions and assessments.

Circulatory Overload

1. *Cause*

   Delivery of excessive amounts of IV fluid (especially a risk for elderly patients, infants, or patient with cardiac or renal insufficiency).
2. *Clinical manifestations*
   a. Increased blood pressure and pulse.
   b. Increased central venous pressure (CVP), venous distention (engorged neck veins).
   c. Headache, anxiety
   d. Shortness of breath, tachypnea, coughing
   e. Pulmonary crackles
   f. Chest pain (if history of coronary artery disease)
3. *Preventive measures*
   a. Know whether patient has existing heart or kidney condition. Be particularly vigilant in the high-risk patient.
   b. Closely monitor infusion flow rate.
   c. Splint arm or hand if IV flow rate fluctuates too widely with movement.
4. *Nursing interventions*
   a. Slow infusion to a "keep-open" rate and notify physician.
   b. Monitor closely for signs of volume overload.
   c. Raise patient's head to facilitate breathing.
   d. Document interventions and assessments.

Air Embolism

1. *Causes*
   a. Greater risk in central venous lines, when air enters catheter during tubing changes (air sucked in during inspiration due to negative intrathoracic pressure).
   b. Air in tubing delivered by IV push or infused by infusion pump.
2. *Clinical manifestations*
   a. Drop in blood pressure, elevated heart rate
   b. Cyanosis, tachypnea

c. Rise in central venous pressure
d. Changes in mentation, loss of consciousness
3. *Preventive measures*
   a. Clear all air from tubing prior to infusion to patient.
   b. Change solution containers before they run dry.
   c. Ensure that all connections are secure.
   d. Use filter unless contraindicated.
4. *Nursing interventions*
   a. Immediately turn patient on his left side and lower head of bed; in this position, air will rise to right atrium.
   b. Notify physician immediately.
   c. Administer oxygen as needed.
   d. Reassure patient.
   e. Document interventions and assessments.

Mechanical Failure *(Sluggish IV Flow)*

1. *Causes*
   a. Needle may be lying against the side of the vein, cutting off fluid flow.
   b. There may be a clot at the end of the catheter or needle.
   c. Infiltration of IV cannula.
   d. Kinking of tubing or catheter.
2. *Nursing assessment and interventions*
   a. Assess for signs of local infiltration (swelling, coolness of skin).
   b. Remove tape and check for kinking of tubing or catheter.
   c. Pull back cannula because it may be lying against wall of vein, vein valve, or vein bifurcation.
   d. Elevate or lower needle to prevent occlusion of bevel.
   e. Move patient's arm to new position.
   f. Lower solution container below level of patient's heart and observe for blood backflow.
   g. If mechanical infusion regulator in use, check its integrity.
   h. If none of the preceding steps produces the desired flow, remove needle or catheter and restart infusion.

Intravenous Procedures

Guidelines Venipuncture Using Needle or Catheter

Equipment
Rubber tourniquet
Disposable gloves
Antiseptic swab (alcohol, iodine, povidone-iodine)
If continuous infusion:
    IV solution
    Tubing
    Filter (if appropriate)
If heparin lock:
    Heparin lock cap
    Heparin solution (1–2 ml.) in sterile syringe
Tape, 2 × 2-inch sterile gauze, antimicrobial ointment
         or

(continued)

Guidelines | Venipuncture Using Needle or Catheter *(continued)*

Equipment
(continued)

Transparent IV dressing
Covered armboard (if necessary)
Desired cannula:
    Catheter (Teflon, Silastic polyurethane, or polyvinylchloride) in chosen bore size (gauges 14 to 25)
    Winged ("butterfly") needle

Note: Thorough hand washing is required before handling sterile supplies and initiating venipuncture.

Procedure

Nursing Action	Rationale

Preparatory Phase

1. Explain procedure to patient. Have him lie in bed. Ascertain whether patient is left- or right-handed.

2. Clear all IV tubing of air; winged needle tubing as well (may clear air with fluid from infusion tubing by attaching needle to it, or by irrigating needle with saline in sterile syringe).

3. Don gloves.

4. Select site for insertion (see discussion on Site Selection, p. 81).

5. Apply tourniquet 5–15 cm. (2–6 inches) above desired insertion site and ascertain satisfactory distention of the vein. Distal pulses should remain palpable.

6. Have patient open and close first several times.

7. Cleanse the site:
    a. Cleanse the skin with an alcohol swab.
    b. Prepare skin with povidone-iodine (an iodophor) swab for 1 minute, working from the center of proposed site to the periphery until a circle of 5–10 cm. (2–4 inches) has been disinfected.
    c. Allow area to air dry.
    d. Clip hair if site is too obscured.

1. Helps alleviate patient anxiety about the procedure. Determining "handedness" of patient suggests the infusion be started in opposite arm if possible.

2. To prevent infusion of air and potential air embolus.

3. Complies with CDC requirements to minimize passing of blood-borne pathogens between the patient and nurse.

5. The vein must be visible or palpable before venipuncture is attempted. The tourniquet should not be applied too tightly as to interfere with arterial blood flow.

6. To increase blood supply in the area. Further techniques to aid in vein distention are discussed on p. 82. A tourniquet may not be necessary on greatly distended veins.

7. To reduce number of skin microorganisms and minimize risk of infection. If a 1% or 2% iodine solution is used, it should be used to prep the skin first (30–60 seconds), allowed to dry, then wiped with an alcohol swab.

Performance Phase: Catheter Insertion

1. Remove needle guard.

2. Grasp patient's arm so that the nurse's thumb is positioned approximately 5 cm. (2 inches) from the site. Exert traction on skin in direction of hand.

3. Insert the needle, bevel up, through the skin at a 45-degree angle. Use a slow, continuous motion.

4. If the vessel rolls, it may be necessary to penetrate the skin first at a 20-degree angle and then apply a second thrust parallel to the skin.

5. When the vein is entered, lower the catheter to skin level.

6. When inserting, always hold the catheter by the clear plastic flashback chamber and not by the colored hub.

7. Advance the catheter approximately 0.635–1.3 cm. (¼ to ½ inch) into the vein.

8. Pull back on needle to separate needle from catheter 0.635 cm. (about ¼-inch) and advance catheter into vein.

9. If resistance is met while attempting to thread catheter, stop, release tourniquet, and carefully remove both needle and catheter. Attempt another venipuncture with a *new* catheter.

10. Apply pressure on vein beyond catheter tip with the small or ring finger (Fig. 5-4); release tourniquet and slowly remove needle while holding catheter hub in place.

2. To stabilize the vein and facilitate successful cannulation.

3. Bevel up position allows for the smallest and sharpest point of the needle to enter the vein first.

4. Satisfactory penetration is evidenced by a sudden decrease in resistance and by appearance of blood coming back into syringe.

5. This will prevent puncturing through the vessel wall.

7. To ensure entry into the vein.

8. Pulling back on needle prevents inadvertent puncture of vein and provides stability of catheter for insertion.

9. The catheter may have become dislodged or encountered a turn or valve in the vein. It is better to start again than to cause further damage to vessel.

10. This will reduce blood leakage while removing needle and connecting tubing to infusion set.

Procedure
(continued)

| | **Nursing Action** | **Rationale** |

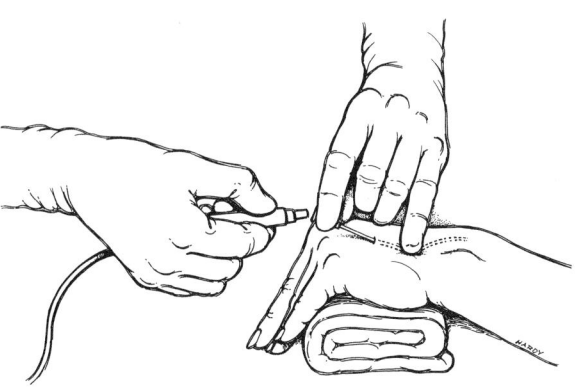

Figure 5-4. *Finger palpation of dorsal venous arch.*

11. *If an IV,* attach the cleared administration set to the hub of the catheter and adjust the infusion flow at the prescribed rate.

12. *If a heparin lock,* attach heparin lock cap, taking care to maintain sterility of the cap. Flush with 0.5 ml. of heparin solution.

13. Place one 1.3 cm (½–inch) strip of tape under hub of catheter (sticky side away from skin), criss-cross tape up over catheter hub, and secure to skin at an angle away from the direction of insertion site.

14. Apply antimicrobial ointment on insertion site and cover with sterile 2 × 2-inch gauze. Loop tubing and tape to dressing or arm.

13. It is important that the tape does not cross over the insertion site as this increases risk of infection and impairs visualization of site.

14. Efficacy of antimicrobial ointments is not conclusive; follow hospital policy. No ointment, gauze sponge, or tape is necessary if a transparent dressing is used (see Fig. 5-5).

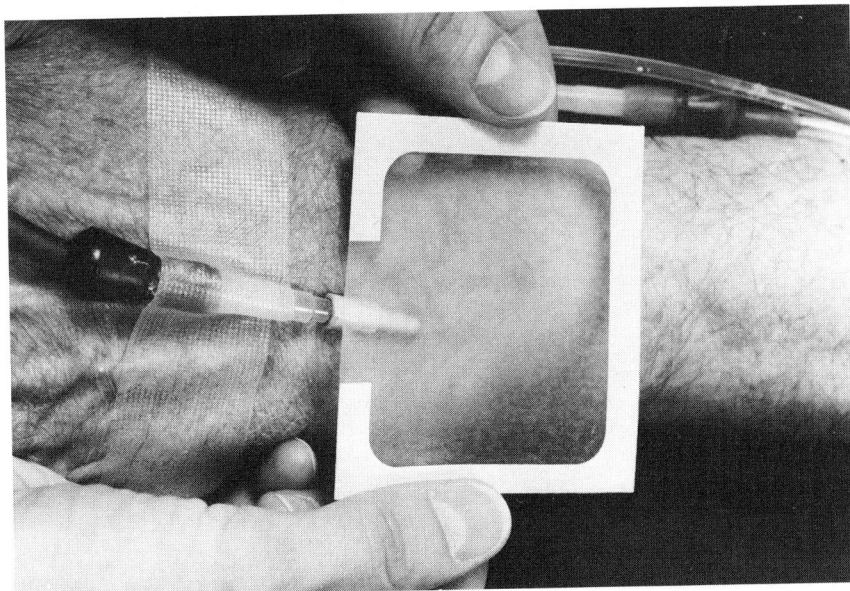

Figure 5-5. *Transparent IV dressing.*

15. Label strip of tape with an arrow indicating the path of the catheter, size of catheter, date, time of insertion and inserter's initials. Affix to dressing. Prepare similar label with each dressing change.

15. Labeling of dressing is dictated by hospital policy. Such a practice provides information useful in determining next dressing change and capability of needle to accommodate various types of infusion.

(continued)

Guidelines   Venipuncture Using Needle or Catheter *(continued)*

Procedure *(continued)*	**Nursing Action**	**Rationale**

Performance Phase: Winged Needle (Fig. 5-6)

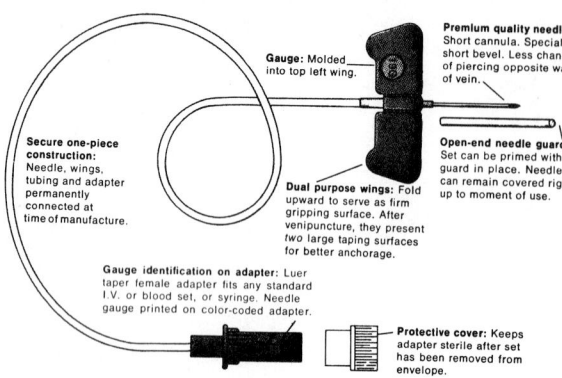

Figure 5-6. *"Butterfly" winged infusion set.*

Nursing Action

1. Position wing set so that bevel of needle is up. Note gauge of needle on the left wing.
2. Pinch wings firmly together between thumb and index finger.
3. Follow practice outlined for IV catheter in steps 1.–4. above.
4. Advance needle cautiously into vein; simultaneously, lift wings up slightly.
5. Once vein is entered, advance the needle to within about 0.32 cm. (⅛ inch) of the hub.
6. Release tourniquet and release wings; hold flat against patient's skin and permit fluid to flow as discussed in steps 12. and 13. above.
7. Apply tape parallel to needle on each side. Make a protective loop and fasten to arm with tape.
8. Apply dressing over site as discussed in steps 15. and 16. above.

Rationale

1. Most sets are marked for easy recognition of needle gauge. Needle length never varies—2.5 cm. (1 inch).
2. The needle is held firmly and comfortably for insertion.

4. To avoid piercing opposite vein wall.

6. This will anchor needle in vein and permit checking of flow of fluid.

7. To anchor needle position.

Follow-up Phase

Nursing Action

1. Engage in frequent inspection of venipuncture site for infiltration or infection. Ask patient if he is experiencing discomfort.
2. Record date of insertion, size, and type of catheter.
3. Change gauze dressing every 24–48 hours.
4. Change IV cannula every 48–72 hours; change transparent dressing at this time also.
5. Change IV tubing every 24–48 hours. Label tubing with date and initials whenever hung.

Rationale

1. To ensure proper functioning of and tolerance to infusion therapy.
2. This is done according to hospital policy.
3. Reduces risk of phlebitis and allows visualization of insertion site.
4. Increased potential for infection when use of IV site exceeds 72 hours.
5. Labeling reminds attending nurse of need for tubing change.

Discontinuance of IV Infusion

Nursing Action

1. If an infusion is discontinued due to complications at the site, the tubing is to be capped with a sterile needle and may be reused (if less than 24 hours old) following reinsertion of a new IV needle or catheter.
2. To remove the cannula:
   a. Turn off infusion.
   b. Place alcohol swab or 2 × 2-inch gauze sponge over insertion site and carefully remove the IV cannula.
   c. Apply pressure on insertion site until bleeding stops, generally less than 1 minute, unless patient has a bleeding disorder.
   d. Apply Bandaid or small gauze pad to site and tape.
3. Document time of discontinuance and status of insertion site on appropriate chart records.

Rationale

1. To maintain sterility of infusion set-up.

2. To safely discontinue infusion. Pressure and elevation of insertion site help restore hemostasis. A final dry dressing should be applied to protect site from mechanical trauma and contamination.

3. Follow hospital policy.

Guidelines | Heparin Lock

Heparin lock is an intermittent infusion reservoir that permits administration of periodic intravenous medications and solution without continuous fluid administration and aspiration of blood samples for laboratory analysis.

Equipment

Antiseptic swabs (usually alcohol)
Syringe containing prescribed 0.5–1 ml. heparin solution (100 units/ml.) or other prescribed amount of heparin
2 syringes containing 2 ml. sterile normal saline solution with 25-gauge needle.
Tape (if "piggy-back" medication is to be infused)

Procedure to Administer Medication

Nursing Action	Rationale/Amplification
1. Explain procedure to patient.	1. To minimize patient anxiety.
2. Cleanse injection port of the heparin lock with alcohol. Insert normal saline syringe needle into port and aspirate slightly.	2. When positive blood return is not obtained, monitor site carefully to detect infiltration. Small-gauge needle may not allow prominent blood return.
3. Inject normal saline solution slowly to flush reservoir of heparinized solution and blood.	3. Many drugs (especially antibiotics) are incompatible with heparin solutions. This also helps to further determine patency of IV cannula; resistance to injection may indicate a clot or infiltration. If that occurs, do not force injection. Replace cannula and heparin lock.
4. Insert medication syringe, administer drug, and remove syringe. If a piggyback solution is to be infused, insert needle into port and tape connection. Infuse it at prescribed rate.	
5. Following drug or solution administration, insert saline syringe and flush reservoir slowly; remove syringe.	5. Saline will clear the reservoir of medication and prepare the way to reheparinize the lock.
6. Inject heparin solution into the reservoir, ensuring total filling of reservoir and cannula.	6. To prevent blood clotting in the IV cannula. Central venous catheters require greater than 2.5 ml. of heparin solution to be effective.
7. Remove heparin syringe and needle from injection port.	7. Treatment is completed.

Follow-up Phase

1. Maintain patency of heparin lock by flushing it every 8–12 hours.	1. If resistance is met, device should not be flushed. Attempt to remove occlusion via aspiration. If unable to restore patency, remove IV device.
2. Record all actions and medications.	2. To ensure accurate account of patient's medications and to obtain charges for materials used in maintaining heparin lock patency.
3. IV administration set for intermittent therapy should be changed every 24 hours or immediately upon contamination. A new sterile needle should be used for each entry into the heparin lock. The tubing should only be used for the same medication.	3. Since the tubing is not maintained as a closed system, it poses a higher risk for infection.

Discontinuance of Heparin Lock

1. Remove immediately when IV therapy is no longer indicated.	1. To minimize risk of infection.

Guidelines | Setting Up an Automatic Intravenous "Piggyback"

"Piggyback" intravenous administration is a means of administering medication via the fluid pathway of an established primary infusion line.

Features and Advantages

1. Drugs may be given on an intermittent basis through a "keep-open" infusion.
2. The secondary bottle contains the medication; this may be single dose or multiple dose.
3. When desired, the primary infusion is clamped off, and the prescribed amount of medication from the secondary bottle is administered; or 2 solutions may run simultaneously depending on tubing design.
4. When a check-valve is present, it performs the following functions:
   a. Permits the primary infusion to flow after the medication has been administered.
   b. Prevents air from entering the system.
   c. Prevents secondary fluid from "running dry."
   d. Permits less mixing of primary fluid with secondary solution.
5. Higher flow rates can be achieved by elevating either of the receptacles.

(continued)

Guidelines Setting Up an Automatic Intravenous "Piggyback" *(continued)*

Equipment
Sterile infusion set (primary)
Sterile infusion set with admixture (secondary)
Sterile gauze squares and iodine-base antiseptic
Tourniquet
Tape

Procedure
Follow procedure of particular manufacturer of "piggyback" infusion set.
In general, most procedures are similar to the following:

Nursing Action	Rationale/Amplification
1. Wash hands thoroughly.	1. Minimizes possibility of infection.
2. Set up primary infusion set as described on p. 87; this may have a check-valve (Fig. 5-7A).	2. The primary set should be functioning effectively before the secondary (piggyback) set can be attached.
3. Lower the primary flask on the IV pole; usually, an extension hook accompanies the set.	3. This will permit the check-valve to function (Fig. 5-7A)

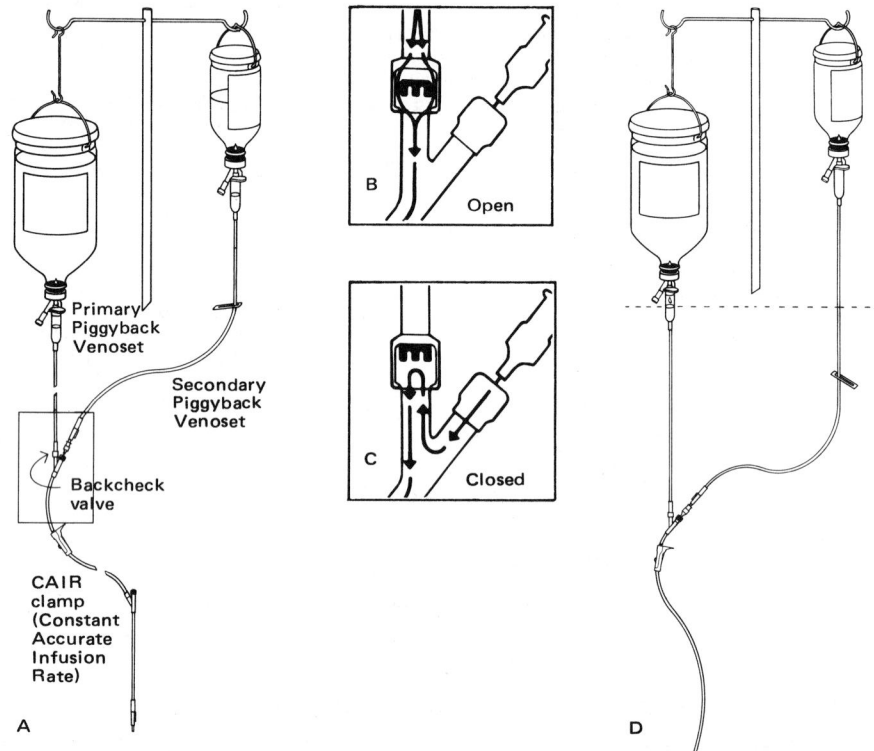

Figure 5-7. *(A) "Piggyback" IV. On left is the primary infusion flask. Note use of extension hook (hanging from IV pole) to suspend primary flask. Backcheck valve is seen more clearly in B and C. Secondary "piggyback" source is seen on the right. (B) Open check-valve. Fluid from primary source flows down on either side of movable disc. Fluid from secondary source is closed off with clamp (not visible). (C) Closed check-valve. Note that fluid source from secondary flask (where pressure is greater because flask source is higher) is forcing movable disc upward, thereby closing off fluid from primary source. (D) When last of fluid from secondary source reaches the level of the fluid in the primary set drip chamber (as indicated by broken line), hydrostatic pressure between both sets will equalize. This releases check-valve; flow will shift from secondary to primary source. (Adapted from Abbott Laboratories)*

4. Prime secondary set; hang it on IV pole. Ideally the system should be maintained as a closed system since each entry increases the risk of infection.	4. This may be a partial-fill bottle or special additive container. Priming allows all air to escape from the system.

Procedure *(continued)*	**Nursing Action**	**Rationale/Amplification**

5. Use antiseptic swab to carefully cleanse injection site.
6. Open clamp on secondary set; inspect the check-valve to ensure that it closes off the flow of solution from the primary source (Fig. 5-7C)

7. When fluid from secondary source reaches level of fluid in primary set drip chamber, hydrostatic pressure between the two sets equalizes (Fig. 5-7D).

Follow-up Phase

1. Follow specific instructions on manufacturer's set for secondary replacement.
2. Discontinuation of primary source is as for conventional infusion set.
3. Same as Follow-up Phase on page 90.

5. Usually this is a Y-connection on the primary set.
6. Pressure is greater from the secondary source, since it is more elevated; increased pressure forces the disc upward in the check-valve. This closes off the flow from the primary source.
7. This releases check-valve (Fig. 5-7B), and flow will then resume automatically from primary source.

3. NITA Standards of Practice; CDC Guidelines.

Bibliography

Infusion Management

Journals

Aly R, Bayles C and Maibach H. Restriction of bacterial growth under commercial catheter dressings. Am J Infect Control 1988 Jun; 16(3):95–100

Basil W. The use of heparin locks (PRN adapters) vs. intravenous therapy in outpatient surgery. Insight 1988 Feb; 13(1):13, 15

Bjeletich J. Declotting central venous catheters with urokinase in the home by nurse clinicians. NITA 1987 Nov-Dec; 10(6):428–430

Boykoff SL, Boxwell AO and Boxwell JJ. 6 ways to clear the air from an IV line. Nursing 1988 Feb; 18(2):46–48

Brismar B and Nystrom B. Thrombophlebitis and septicemia—Complications related to intravascular devices and their prophylaxis. A review. Acta Chir Scan 1986; 530(suppl):73–77

Brosnan KM et al. Stopcock contamination. Am J Nurs 1988 Mar; 88(3):320–324

Bryan CS. CDC says: The case of the IV tubing replacement. Infect Control 1987 Jun; 8(6):255–256

Coggins S. Evaluating and selecting IV equipment. NITA 1987 Jan-Feb; 10(1): 52–60

Cole MG. Flushing heparin locks: Is saline flushing really cost-effective? J Intraven Nurs 1989 Jan-Feb; 12(1 suppl):237–240

Dahl S. Sepsis rate and mechanical complications of triple lumen catheters. Nutr Support Serv 1988 Mar; 8(3):20–23

Dickey J. Effectiveness of intradermally injected lidocaine hydrochloride as a local anesthetic for intravenous catheter insertion. J Emerg Nurs 1988 May-Jun; 14(3):160–163

Donham JA et al. Heparin vs. saline in maintaining patency of intermittent infusion devices: Pilot study. Kans Nurse 1987 Nov 62(11):6–7

Duzak J. Not in vein: Declotting intravenous catheters. J Urol Nurs 1988 Jan-Mar; 7(1):380

Elliott TS. Intravascular-device infections. J Med Microbiol 1988 Nov; 27(3):745–752

Farber BF. The multi-lumen catheter: Proposed guidelines for its use. Infect Control Hosp Epidemiol 1988 May; 9(5):206–208

Fought SG. Venous access in burn injuries. Crit Care Nurse 1988 Jan-Feb; 8(1):12

Gardner C. Spartanburg General Hospital policy book on IV therapy administration. Part II. NITA 1986 Sep-Oct; 9(5):352–384

Garrelts JC et al. Comparison of heparin and 0.9% sodium chloride injection in the maintenance of indwelling intermittent IV devices. Clin Pharmacol 1989 Jan; 8(1):34–39

Hadaway LC. Evaluation and use of advanced IV technology: Central venous access devices. Part I. J Intraven Nurs 1989 Mar-Apr; 12(2):73–82

Hoffman KK et al. Bacterial colonization and phlebitis-associated risk with transparent polyurethane film for peripheral intravenous site dressings. Am J Infect Control 1988 Jun; 16(3): 101–106

Jones PM. Indwelling central venous catheter-related infections and two different procedures of catheter care. Cancer Nurs 1987 Jun; 10(3):123–130

Klass K. Troubleshooting central line complications. Nursing 1987 Nov; 17(11):58–61

Leff RD. Features of IV devices and equipment that affect IV drug delivery. Am J Hosp Pharm 1987 Nov; 44(11): 2530–253

Leibovici L. Daily change of an antiseptic dressing does not prevent infusion phlebitis: A controlled trial. Am J Infect Control 1989 Feb; 17(1):23–25

Messner RL and Gorse GL. Nursing management of peripheral intravenous sites. Focus Crit Care 1987 Apr; 14(2): 25–33

Miracle V et al. Normal saline vs. heparin lock flush solution: One institution's findings. Ky Nurse 1989 Jul-Aug; 37(3): 1; 6–7

Morris LL. Critical care's most versatile tool: A multilumen central venous catheter. RN 1988 May; 51(5):42–46

Mughal MM. Complications of intravenous feeding catheters. Br J Surg 1989 Jan; 76(1):150–151

Newman LN. A side-by-side look at two venous access devices. Am J Nurs 1989 Jun; 89(6):826–835

Petrosino B et al. Infection rates in central venous catheter dressings. Oncol Nurs Forum 1988 Nov-Dec; 15(6):709–717

Propp DA, Cline D and Hennenfent BR. Catheter embolism. J Emerg Med 1988 Jan-Feb; 6(1):17–21

Reilly KM. Problems in administration techniques and dose measurement that influence accuracy of IV drug delivery. Am J Hosp Pharm 1987 Nov; 44(11): 2545–2550

Rutherford C. Insertion and care of multiple lumen peripherally inserted central line catheters. J Intraven Nurs 1988 Jan-Feb; 11(1):16–19

Sadowski DA et al. The value of culturing central-line tips in burn patients. J Burn Care Rehabil 1988 Jan-Feb; 9(1): 66–68

Sawyer DL. Potential for infection: A nursing diagnosis for the patient with an indwelling catheter. Focus Crit Care 1989 Feb; 16(1):46–52

Scott WL. Complications associated with central venous catheters. Chest 1988 Dec; 94(6):1221–1224

Sharp PA et al. A new way to anchor central venous catheters. J Enterostomal Ther 1989 Mar-Apr; 16(2):86

Shearer J. Normal saline flush versus dilute heparin flush: A study of peripheral intermittent IV devices. NITA 1987 Nov-Dec; 10(6):425–427

Sherman RA. Multilumen catheter sepsis and an educational program to combat it. Am J Infect Control 1988 Aug; 16(4):31A–34A

Sohl L. Working with triple-lumen central venous catheters. Nursing 1988 Jul; 18(7):50–53

Stavrakis P. Central vein cannulation during CPR. Emerg Med 1988 Dec 15; 20(21):80, 91

The well-dressed peripheral IV site. Emerg Med 1988 Apr 15; 20(7): 63, 67

Thee KG and Bednarczyk L. Two-lumen peripheral IV catheter evaluation and overall clinical acceptance. J Intraven Nurs 1988 Nov-Dec; 11(6):368–371

Thompson DR et al. Potential of povidone-iodine antiseptic solution for the prevention of cannula-related thrombophlebitis. J Intraven Nurs 1989 Mar-Apr; 12(2):99–102

Wax PM and Talan DA. Advances in cutdown techniques. Emerg Med Clin North Am 1989 Feb; 7(1):65–82

What you should know about your at-home IV line, Patient Care 1989 Mar 15; 23(5):206–7

Yeung C et al. Infection rate for single lumen vs. triple lumen subclavian catheters. Infect Control Hosp Epidemiol 1988 Apr; 9(4):154–158

Young GP et al. Catheter sepsis during parenteral nutrition: The safety of long-term OpSite dressings. J Parenter Enteral Nutr 1988 Jul-Aug; 12(4):365–370

Cancer Nursing

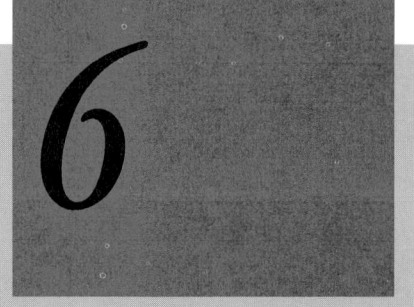

General Considerations

Etiology, Detection, and Prevention

The Optimistic Side of Cancer

1. Improved treatment modalities enable patients with cancer to live longer, more comfortably, and more productively.
2. Most cancer patients spend almost all their time away from hospitals and only come to the hospital intermittently for treatment.
3. More intense efforts at patient rehabilitation are proving effective.
4. Forty-nine percent of all patients with cancer can now be cured, according to the National Cancer Institute's Surveillance, Epidemiology, and End Results (SEER) Program.
5. Research continues unabated, and, as findings accumulate, prospects for specific cures are encouraging.

Cancer's Warning Signals

C hange in bowel or bladder habits
A sore that does not heal
U nusual bleeding or discharge
T hickening or lump in breast or elsewhere
I ndigestion or difficulty in swallowing
O bvious change in wart or mole
N agging cough or hoarseness

Metastasis

Metastasis is the transfer of disease cells from one organ or part to another not directly connected with it.
1. *Extension and invasion*—because they are not encapsulated, it is easy for cancer cells to invade other tissues and extend themselves rapidly via lymphatic and blood circulatory systems; cancer may also recur in treated areas.
2. *Lymph*—secondary growths of tumor cells are often caught in the lymph filter, the lymph node.
3. *Blood*—by invasion, tumor cells enter the blood vessels and are carried to organs where the venous blood passes through a capillary bed.

Epidemiology

1. The annual death toll from malignancy in the US is at least 500,000.
2. Cancer ranks second as the leading cause of death in the U.S.
3. Cancer strikes at any age. It affects children as well as adults, but it strikes with increasing frequency with advancing age.
4. No organ of the body is exempt. (See Fig. 6-1 for cancer death rates by site.)
5. The annual number of cases diagnosed in 1989 is estimated to be 1,010,000 in the U.S.
6. Five-year survival rates are increasing with improved therapy and earlier detection.

Nutrition and Cancer

> **GERONTOLOGIC ALERT:** Elderly patients, especially those who live alone, may be malnourished prior to the initiation of therapy. Dietary consultation may be *crucial prior to therapy*.

1. Diet does influence the risk of cancer.
2. The National Research Council recommends a diet moderate in total saturated fat, high in complex carbohydrates and fiber, low in sugars, and moderate in protein, especially animal proteins.
   a. High intake of fats is associated with breast, colon, and prostate cancer.
   b. Low intake of fruit, vegetables, complex carbohydrates, and fiber is linked with cancer of the colon, larynx, esophagus, prostate, bladder, stomach, and lung.
   c. Salt-cured foods may influence cancers of the esophagus and stomach.
   d. Alcohol use can increase the risk of cancer of the mouth, larynx, throat, esophagus, and liver.
   e. Obesity is linked to cancers of the breast, colon, uterus, and gallbladder.
   f. The role of heredity is also acknowledged.
3. See Table 6-1 for a comparison of the dietary guidelines for cancer prevention from the National Cancer Insti-

Table 6-1. *Dietary Guidelines for Cancer Prevention**

		NCI	ACS	NRC
Fats		30% or less of total calories	Decrease total fat	30% or less of total calories
Carbohydrates		20–30 grams of fiber daily		—
Breads, cereals, and legumes		3–5[†] servings	Increase foods high in fiber, and foods high in vitamins A and C, such as whole grain cereals, fruits, and vegetables. Include cruciferous vegetables.	6+ servings
Fruits		2–3 servings		5 + servings (especially citrus, and green and yellow vegetables)
Vegetables		3–5 servings		

* A comparison of the fat and carbohydrate recommendations from the dietary guidelines of the National Cancer Institute (NCI), American Cancer Society (ACS), and the National Research Council (NRC).
† Serving = 1 cup or 2 slices. **Note:** All other servings = ½ cup or 1 slice.
(J Nat'l Cancer Institute. 1989 Apr 5;81(7):4)

tute (NCI), the American Cancer Society (ACS), and the National Research Council (NRC).

Detection and Prevention

Early detection and prevention are very effective in decreasing mortality and morbidity of many cancers. The American Cancer Society (ACS) recommends specific screening measures to reduce an individual's risk of cancer (see Table 6-2).

Diagnosis of Cancer

Diagnostic Evaluation
1. Physical examination
2. Biopsy of tumor site to determine pathologic diagnosis
3. Laboratory tests including CBC with differential, platelet count, electrolytes, liver function tests, BUN, and creatinine to determine baseline laboratory values
4. Imaging procedures: chest X-ray, bone scan, CT scans, all to determine evidence and/or extent of metastasis

Differences Between Malignant and Benign Tumors

Characteristic	Benign	Malignant
Type of cell	Mature, differentiated	Embryonic characteristics; poorly differentiated
Growth	Controlled	Diffuse, no control
Invasion of local tissues	Has contact inhibition (recognizes boundaries)	Lacks contact inhibition (does not recognize boundaries)
Recurrence	Does not tend to recur	Has ability to recur
Metastasis	Usually localized	Has ability to spread to distant sites

Management: General Overview

1. The method of treatment depends upon the type of malignancy, the specific histologic cell type, stage, presence of metastasis, and condition of the patient.
2. Cancer is treated by surgery, chemotherapy, radiation, immunotherapy, or a combination of these modalities.

A. Surgery
1. *Biopsy*—surgical removal of a piece of tissue from the questionable area; the tissue sample is sent to the pathology laboratory for diagnostic verification.

2. *Preventive or prophylactic surgery*—removal of lesions which, if left in the body, are apt to develop into cancer. Example: polyps in rectum may lead to cancer of the colon.
3. *Palliative surgery*—a type of surgery that attempts to relieve the complications of cancer (e.g., obstruction of the gastrointestinal tract, pain produced by tumor extension into surrounding nerves).
4. *Curative surgery*—the removal of the primary site of malignancy and any lymph nodes to which the neoplasm has extended. Such surgery may be all that is required.

CANCER DEATH RATES* BY SITE, UNITED STATES, 1930-85

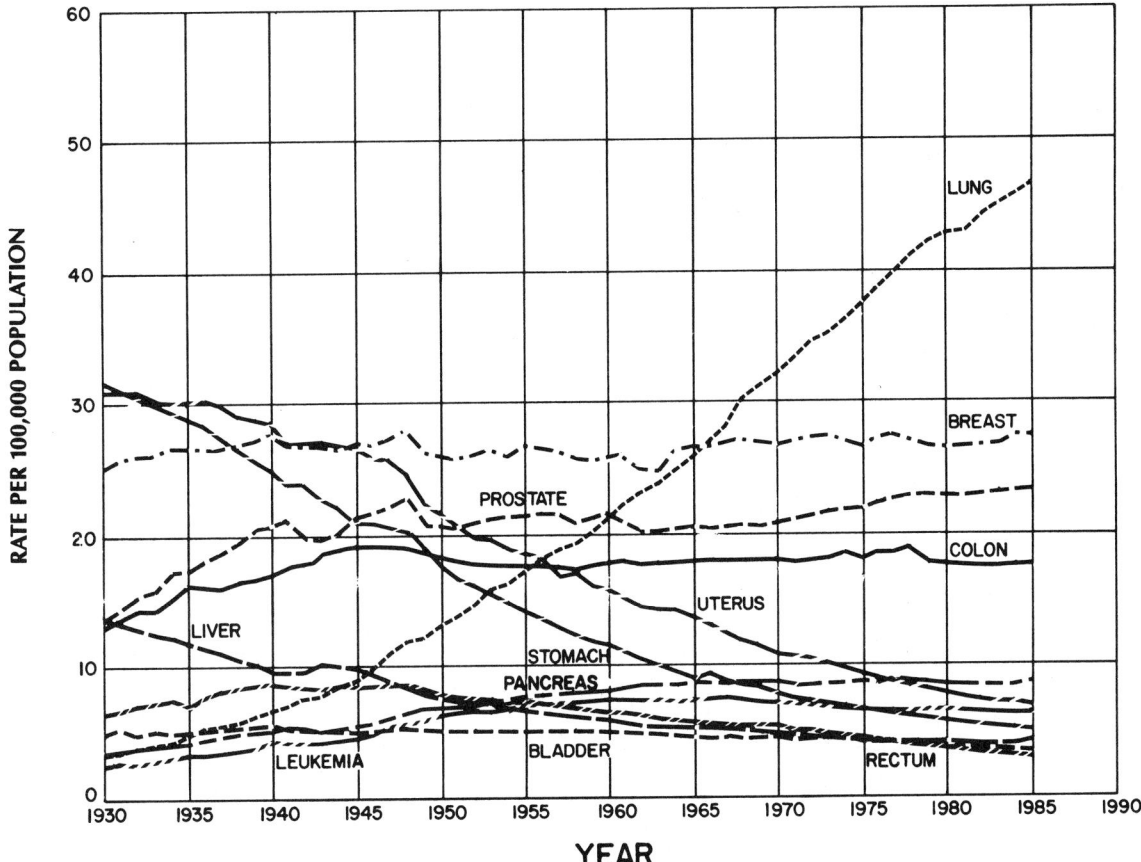

*Rate for the population standardized for age on the 1970 U.S. population.
Sources of Data: National Center for Health Statistics and Bureau of the Census, United States.
Note: Rates are for both sexes combined except breast and uterus female population only and prostate male population only.

Figure 6-1. *Cancer death rates. (From Cancer Facts and Figures, 1989. American Cancer Society)*

5. *Debulking surgery*—should be performed prior to the start of chemotherapy whenever possible.
6. *Surgery combined with radiation, chemotherapy, or immunotherapy*—combinations of treatment required to halt the spread of a malignancy.

Note: Details of surgical treatment are given in the sections relating to specific disease entities.

B. Chemotherapy—the use of antineoplastic drugs to promote tumor cell destruction by interfering with cellular function and reproduction. It includes the use of various chemotherapeutic agents and hormones.

C. Radiation—includes the use of external beam and radiation implants.

D. Immunotherapy—the newest modality for cancer therapy including interleukins, interferons, lymphokine-activated killer cells, tumor-infiltrating lymphocytes, and monoclonal antibodies.

Chemotherapy for Cancer

Overview

1. The goal of chemotherapy is to destroy as many tumor cells as possible with minimal effect on healthy cells.
2. Chemotherapy can be used for cure, control, or palliation.
   a. May be a curative for a patient with a small tumor and actively dividing cells. Dose kills a constant percentage of cells, not a constant number of cells.
   b. Also can be used as a palliative measure to ensure comfort and to relieve pain, such as seen in malignant ascites.
3. Many chemotherapeutic agents have associated toxicities that can be dose limiting and require nursing interventions (see Table 6-3).
4. Dosage can be accurately calculated in adults and children using body surface area (mg./m^2.).

Table 6-2. *Recommendations for the Early Detection of Cancer in Asymptomatic Persons*

Cancer Site	Test or Procedure	Sex	Age	Frequency
Colorectal	Sigmoidoscopy	M and F	50 and over	Every year until 2 satisfactory normal exams 1 year apart; thereafter, every 3–5 years
Colorectal	Stool blood test	M and F	50 and over	Every year
Colorectal	Digital rectal exam	M and F	40 and over	Every year
Cervical	Pap test and pelvic exam	F	Women who are or have been sexually active or have reached age 18	Every year; after 3 or more consecutive satisfactory normal annual exams, the Pap test may be performed less frequently at the discretion of the physician
Endometrial	Endometrial biopsy	F	At menopause; women at high risk*	At menopause
Breast	Breast self-exam	F	20 and over	Every month
Breast	Breast physical exam	F	20–40	Every 3 years
			40 and over	Every year
Breast	Mammography	F	35–39	Baseline
			40–49	Every 1–2 years
			50 and over	Every year
Other†	Health counseling and cancer checkup†	M and F	20 and over	Every 3 years
		M and F	40 and over	Every year

* History of infertility, obesity, failure to ovulate, abnormal uterine bleeding, or estrogen therapy.

† To include examination for cancers of the thyroid, testicles, prostate, ovaries, lymph nodes, oral region, and skin.

(Courtesy American Cancer Society)

5. Many types of cancers respond to chemotherapy, including specific types of leukemia and lymphomas, breast cancer, Hodgkin's disease, small cell lung cancer, Ewing's sarcoma, retinoblastoma, and Wilms' tumor.
6. Combinations of chemotherapeutic agents are often more effective and no more toxic than single agents.
7. Chemotherapy may be more effective in patients who have been treated successfully by surgery and/or radiation but in whom the recurrence risk may be high.
8. Combinations with immunotherapy appears promising. Precise scheduling of dosages is necessary to achieve effective results.
9. Toxicity is often the limiting factor when using chemotherapy; therefore, it is imperative that the toxicities be recognized by the nurse.

   Since many normal cells in the body also grow rapidly and have short life spans (e.g., bone marrow, gastrointestinal tract lining, hair follicles), many chemotherapeutic agents directly attack these normal cells. Herein lies the challenge for nurses.
10. Certain chemotherapeutic agents can be effective on 1 of the 4 phases of the cell cycle or during any phase of the cell cycle. The cell cycle is divided into 4 stages:
    a. G1 (Gap one) phase (Postmitotic): Enzymes for DNA synthesis are manufactured.
    b. S (Synthesis) phase: During a long time period the DNA component doubles for the chromosomes in preparation for cell division.
    c. G2 (Gap two) phase: This is a short time period; protein and RNA synthesis occurs, and also the formation of the mitotic spindle apparatus takes place.
    d. M (Mitosis) phase: In a very short time period, the cell actually divides into two identical daughter cells.
11. Cells not active in the cell cycle are designated as "resting" (G0).
12. Malignant cells may exhibit resistance to some antineoplastic agents, thus limiting their usefulness. The tumor can be resistant to certain drugs from the start of therapy (natural resistance) or become resistant after therapy has begun (acquired resistance).
13. Drugs may be given orally, intravenously, intramuscularly, or intra-arterially.

Intravenous Administration of Chemotherapy

Nursing Interventions

A. General Considerations

1. See page 81 for the techniques of intravenous therapy. If chemotherapy is administered for a prolonged period of time, a venous access device should be considered.
2. Chemotherapy should preferably be administered via the veins in the forearm. Second choice is the metacarpal veins. Third choice is the antecubital vein (see Fig. 5-1).

B. Administering Chemotherapeutic Agents

1. Select venipuncture site free of sclerosis, thrombosis, or scar formation if at all possible.
2. Avoid venipuncture in an arm where dissection of the axillary lymph nodes has been performed.
3. Avoid venipuncture in an arm where radiation therapy has caused marked fibrosis in the axillary area.
4. Use a running IV (flush solution) while administering a vesicant (blistering or necrotic) chemotherapeutic agent IV push.
5. If a small focal hematoma develops during insertion of the needle into the vein, DO NOT use this site for chemotherapeutic administration because of the increased risk for extravasation and/or infiltration.
6. Maintain constant supervision during administration of intravenous push vesicant chemotherapy.
7. If any doubt exists regarding vein patency or safety of chemotherapy administration, discontinue the administration and treat as an extravasation if a vesicant chemotherapeutic agent has been used.

Table 6-3. *Frequently Used Chemotherapeutic Agents*

Drug	Dose, Route, and Frequency	Where Drug Is Excreted	Major Side Effects			Other Side Effects or Comments
			Myelosuppression	*Thrombocytopenia*	*Risk for Nausea and Vomiting*	
Alkylators						
Cyclophosphamide (Cytoxan)	500–1500 mg./m.² IV every 3–4 weeks	Urine: 30% excreted unchanged in the urine	Marked	Mild	Moderate	Cystitis; alopecia. Monitor liver function Drink 3 L. fluids daily
	60–120 mg./m.² oral, daily, based on WBC		Moderate	Mild	Mild	
Busulfan (Myleran)	2–6 mg./m.² orally, daily	Renal	Marked	Marked	Mild	Pulmonary fibrosis; skin pigmentation
BCNU (Carmustine)	200–225 mg./m.² IV every 6 weeks 150–200 mg./m.² orally every 4–6 weeks	Renal: 60% to 70% excreted as metabolite in 24 hours	Marked	Marked	Marked	Mucositis; pulmonary fibrosis; renal failure; vesicant; crosses blood–brain barrier
CBCDA (Carboplatin)	200–400 mg./m.² IV every 4 weeks	Renal	Marked	Marked	Mild	Cumulative myelosuppression Thrombocytopenia can be severe and delayed
CCNU (Lomustine, CeeNU)	100–130 mg./m.² orally every 4–6 weeks	Primarily renal; <10% respiratory	Marked	Marked	Moderate	Myelosuppression can be cumulative and delayed Crosses blood–brain barrier Take at bedtime on empty stomach
Chlorambucil (Leukeran)	1–3 mg. orally, daily	Urine: <0.5% excreted unchanged after 24 hours	Moderate	Moderate	Mild	
Cisplatin	60–120 mg./m.² IV every 3–4 weeks	Urine	Moderate	Moderate	Severe	Nephrotoxicity; neuropathy; magnesium wasting; ototoxicity; anemia; anaphylaxis; vesicant
	15–40 mg./m.² IV daily for 5 days every 3–4 weeks		Mild	Mild	Moderate	
Ifosphamide (Ifex)	1200 mg./m.² IV for 5 days every 3 weeks 4 mg./m.² IV every 3 weeks	Renal: some is excreted unchanged in urine	Moderate	Moderate	Mild	Neurotoxicity; hemorrhagic cystitis; alopecia; concomitant uroprotection with Mesna
Mesna	1800–2400 mg./m.² with ifosphamide IV daily for 5.5 days		None	None	None	Not an antineoplastic agent. Binds to reactive metabolite of ifosphamide or cyclophosphamide without interfering with antitumor activity
MeCCNU (Semustine, Methyl CCNU)	150–200 mg./m.² every 4–6 weeks	Some is excreted in urine as a metabolite; biliary excretion accounts for remainder	Marked	Marked	Moderate	Delayed and cumulative myelosuppression; stomatitis; anorexia; renal failure and pulmonary fibrosis after prolonged administration
Mechlorethamine hydrochloride (nitrogen mustard)	0.4 mg./kg. IV every 4 weeks 0.2–0.4 mg./kg. (intracavitary)	Urine: small amount only	Marked	Marked	Severe	Vesicant; stomatitis; alopecia; chemical thrombophlebitis
Melphalan (L-Pam; Alkeran)	4 mg. orally, daily	Renal: approx. 50% Fecal	Moderate	Moderate	Mild	Leukemia; second malignancies Give on empty stomach
Streptozocin (Zanosar)	500 mg./m.² IV daily for 5 days every 3–4 weeks	Primarily renal Respiratory	Mild	Mild	Moderate–marked	Irritant; renal failure; reactivite hypoglycemia due to insulin release, diarrhea

(continued)

Table 6-3. *Frequently Used Chemotherapeutic Agents (continued)*

Drug	Dose, Route, and Frequency	Where Drug Is Excreted	Major Side Effects			Other Side Effects or Comments
			Myelosup-pression	Thrombocy-topenia	Risk for Nausea and Vomiting	
Antimetabolites						
Azacytidine	150–300 mg./m.^{2} IV for 5 days	Excreted primarily in urine	Marked	Marked	Severe	Diarrhea; neurotoxicity; mucositis
Cytarabine (Cytosar-U, ARA-C)	100 mg./m.^{2} every 12 hours subcutaneously or IV 7–21 days 100 mg./m.^{2} continuous infusion	Hepatic; unchanged in urine after 24 hours 70% excreted as metabolite	Marked	Marked	Moderate	Stomatitis; cholestasis; headaches
5-Fluorouracil (5-FU)	500 mg. IV every week or daily for 5 days 800 mg. IV for 5 days every 3–4 weeks	15% excreted in urine	Moder-ate–marked Mild	Moderate–marked Mild	Mild Moderate	Stomatitis; diarrhea; alopecia; vein discoloration; photosensitivity
5-FU with leucovorin rescue	375 mg. IV every week for 6 weeks 500 mg. IV every week for 6 weeks	Same as above	Marked	Marked	Mild	Diarrhea
Hydroxyurea (Hydrea)	1000 mg./m.^{2} orally, daily	50% renally excreted	Marked	Marked	Mild	Alopecia; diarrhea; stomatitis Crosses blood–brain barrier
6-Mercaptopurine (6-MP)	100 mg. orally, daily	Fraction excreted unchanged in urine	Moder-ate–marked	Moderate–marked	Mild	Stomatitis; hepatotoxicity Reduce dose if giving allopurinol concurrently
Methotrexate (Mexate)	20–80 mg./m.^{2} IV, IM, or orally	75% excreted unchanged in urine within 8 hours	Moder-ate–marked	Moderate–marked	Mild	Stomatitis; nephrotoxicity; diarrhea Crosses blood–brain barrier
High-dose methotrexate with leucovorin rescue	1–20 mg./m.^{2} IV every 3 weeks Leucovorin: 15 mg./m.^{2} every 6 hours for 7 days	Excreted in urine	Mild	Mild	Moderate	Renal failure; hepatic dysfunction
Thioguanine (6 TG, Tabloid)	100 mg./m.^{2} IV for 5 days every 3–4 weeks	Excreted in urine	Moder-ate–marked	Moderate–marked	Mild	Cholestasis; stomatitis; diarrhea; hepatotoxicity
Antibiotics						
Bleomycin (Blenoxane)	5–15 units/m.^{2} IV, IM, subcutaneously weekly Total dose not to exceed 400 units	50% to 80% excreted as active drug in renal system in 24 hours	Rare	Rare	Mild	Skin reaction; pulmonary fibrosis; fever; allergic reaction; alopecia; stomatitis
Dactinomycin (Actinomycin-D; Cosmegen)	0.6 mg./m.^{2} IV for 5 days every 3–4 weeks	50% excreted in urine unchanged	Marked	Marked	Moderate	Alopecia; stomatitis; skin rash; hepatic dysfunction; vesicant; radiation recall
Daunorubicin (Cerubidine)	30–60 mg./m.^{2} IV every 3–4 weeks 350 mg./m.^{2} total dose IV	15% excreted within 72 hours	Marked	Marked	Moderate	Cardiomyopathy; alopecia; red urine; radiation recall; vesicant

(continued)

Table 6-3. *Frequently Used Chemotherapeutic Agents (continued)*

Drug	Dose, Route, and Frequency	Where Drug Is Excreted	Major Side Effects			Other Side Effects or Comments
			Myelosuppression	*Thrombocytopenia*	*Risk for Nausea and Vomiting*	
Antibiotics						
Doxorubicin (Adriamycin)	30–75 mg./m.^{2} IV every 3 weeks Total dose: 550 mg	10% to 20% excreted as metabolite	Marked	Marked	Moderate	Alopecia; cardiomyopathy; radiation recall; red urine; hepatic dysfunction; vesicant
Plicamycin (Mithramycin)	1.75 mg./m.^{2} IV every other day until toxicity	Excreted in urine	Mild	Marked	Severe	Vesicant; hepatic dysfunction; coagulation abnormalities; dermatitis; neurologic excitability
Mitomycin (Mutamycin)	2 mg./m.^{2} IV daily for 3 days every 3 weeks 15–20 mg./m.^{2} IV every 6–8 weeks	Excreted in urine and small amount in bile	Marked	Marked	Moderate	Renal, pulmonary dysfunction; alopecia; stomatitis; vesicant
Plant Alkaloids						
Vinblastine (Velban)	4 mg./m.^{2} IV weekly 1.5–2 mg./m.^{2} daily IV for 5 days, every 4 weeks	70% excreted in feces as metabolite	Marked	Marked	Mild	Elevated uric acid; neurotoxicity; mucositis; alopecia
Vincristine (Oncovin)	0.5–2 mg./m.^{2} IV weekly	50% excreted as metabolite, the majority in feces; remainder in urine	Mild	Mild	Mild	Distal neuropathy; constipation; inappropriate ADH; vesicant
Vindesine (Eldisine)	2–4 mg./m.^{2} IV every 1–2 weeks	Excreted in bile; partially in urine	Moderate	Mild	Mild	Neurotoxicity—can be cumulative if administered with other plant alkaloids; vesicant
Teniposide (VM-26)	60–80 mg./m.^{2} IV weekly	Excreted in urine	Moderate	Mild	Mild	Distal neuropathy; can have cumulative neurotoxicity if administered with other plant alkaloids; alopecia; vesicant
Etoposide (Vepesid) (VP-16)	50–100 mg./m.^{2}/ day IV for 5 days 200–250 mg./m.^{2} IV weekly 125–240 mg./m.^{2} IV three times a week, every 4 weeks	40% to 60% excreted in urine unchanged	Moderate	Mild	Mild–moderate	Distal neuropathy; alopecia; hypotension can occur following rapid infusion; vesicant
Miscellaneous Drugs						
DTIC (Dacarbazine)	200 mg./m.^{2} IV daily for 5 days, every 3–4 weeks 800–1200 mg./m.^{2} IV every 4 weeks	Urine; 50% excreted unchanged	Mild	Mild	Marked	Flulike syndrome; alopecia; facial flushing and paresthesias; vesicant
Methenamine	150 mg orally, daily for 4 days	Bile/feces	Mild	Mild	Moderate	Neurotoxicity
Procarbazine (Matulane)	100–200 mg./m.^{2} orally, for 14 days	70% excreted in urine	Moderate	Moderate	Mild	Sensitive to amines; neurotoxicity Crosses blood–brain barrier

(Adapted from Goodman M. Managing the side effects of chemotherapy. Semin Oncol Nurs 1989 May; 5[2 suppl]:29–52 and Hubbard S and Jenkins J. Chemotherapy administration: Practical guidelines. In Chabner BA and Collins JM (eds): Cancer Chemotherapy: Principles and Practice. Philadelphia, JB Lippincott, 1989)

C. Monitoring and Managing an Extravasation (escape or leaking of the chemotherapeutic agent into the subcutaneous tissues from the vein)

1. *Symptoms of an extravasation*
   a. Monitor for pain, which the patient may describe as localized to severe burning and radiating along the vein.
   b. Examine the site for erythema or swelling. Over a period of days to weeks, the site can become mottled and lead to necrosis.
2. *Management of an extravasation*
   a. Stop the infusion of the chemotherapeutic agent.
   b. Aspirate all residual chemotherapeutic agent in the IV needle/catheter.
   c. Administer antidote (see Table 6-4)—inject intradermally in circular motion around the extravasation site to prevent leakage of drug to surrounding tissues (if appropriate) or inject via the IV catheter.

> **NURSING ALERT:** Do not inject an antidote via the catheter if unable to aspirate the chemotherapeutic agent.

   d. Apply ice or heat to the site, depending upon the chemotherapeutic agent that has extravasated.
3. *Follow-up after an extravasation*
   a. If only a small amount of drug extravasated and frank necrosis does not occur, phlebitis may still result, causing pain for several days and/or induration at the site that may last for weeks or months.
   b. Additional surgery for skin grafts may be needed.
   c. Patient may have reduced motor and sensory function due to extravasation and require rehabilitation.

D. Monitoring for Other Clinical Manifestations

1. Vein alterations
   a. Patient may describe sensations of pain, stretching, or pressure within the vessel, orginating near the venipuncture site or extending 7.5–12.5 cm. (3–5 inches) along the vein.
   b. Discoloration—red streak following the line of the vein (called a *flare reaction*). Seen most commonly with doxorubicin. May also see a darkening of the veins related to administration of 5-fluorouracil (5-FU).
2. Subcutaneous tissue
   Patient may complain of itching, urticaria, muscle cramps, or pressure in the arm.

Intra-arterial Infusion of Chemotherapy

Intra-arterial infusion is the introduction percutaneously of a catheter into a major artery under fluroscopic guidance. This does not require major surgery and can be repeated at intervals. The continuous administration of the chemotherapeutic agent into the artery leading to the tumor may last for several days or several weeks.

A. Routes

Brachial, carotid, femoral, or hepatic artery, determined by location of tumors.

B. Uses and Advantages

1. This method is used preferably when the tumor is completely encompassed by the vessels in question: to check this, fluoroscein may be injected into the catheter and the tumor observed under a special lamp for fluorescence.
2. Arterial infusion acts on the tumor over a longer period of time than is possible with systemic chemotherapy.
3. By increasing regional concentrations and using minimal systemic drug concentrations, systemic toxicity is limited.
4. This treatment is still considered investigational.

Nursing Management

A. Before Special Treatment

1. The patient needs concerned care; these are procedures (perfusion and arterial infusion) that are tried because the disease is advanced, although limited to an anatomic area.
2. Provide encouragement and enough information to acquaint the patient with the possible benefits as well as dangers of the procedure.
3. Give emotional support since the unpleasant side effects of chemotherapy can cause depression.

B. During Chemotherapy

1. Be familiar with the nature of the chemotherapeutic agent being used (toxic manifestations, etc.).
2. Observe arterial injection site to see that catheter is properly positioned. Guard against hemorrhage, leakage, sepsis, and tissue irritation.
3. Note any signs of malaise, nausea, vomiting, diarrhea, temperature elevation, changes in blood pressure and pulse.
4. Report intake and output accurately.
5. If necessary, administer fluids intravenously for first 48 hours to maintain general hydration as well as dilution of post-treatment antineoplastic drugs.

Table 6-4. *Guidelines for the Management of an Extravasation*

Chemotherapeutic Agent	Antidote	Administration	Comments
Doxorubicin hydrochloride	Decadron (has been used in the past)		Apply ice
Mechlorethamine hydrochloride	Isotonic sodium thiosulfate (1 gm./10 ml.)	Inject 5–6 ml. through IV line and multiple SQ injections into extravasated site	Apply ice
Vincristine Vinblastine	Hyaluronidase (150 units/ml.)	Inject 1–6 ml. SQ around the extravasated site by multiple injections	Apply heat

6. Record local or systemic changes in detail (e.g., diarrhea or melena).
7. Observe skin tissue in local area for reaction—erythema, blistering, edema, petechiae.
8. Check mucous membranes for signs of tissue breakdown, hemorrhage, or infection.
9. Turn the patient frequently because of increased possibility of pressure area breakdown.
10. See also Care of the Patient with a Venous Access Device (p. 111).

Safety Measures in Handling Cytotoxic Anticancer Drugs

Most cytotoxic drugs are irritating to the skin, eyes, and mucous membranes. If mishandled, these drugs can result in local toxic or allergic reactions.

A. Personal Safety to Minimize Exposure via Inhalation

1. The chemotherapeutic agents should be prepared in a Class II Biologic Safety Cabinet (vertical laminar flow hood).
2. If no Class II Safety Cabinet is available, prepare chemotherapy in a well-ventilated area while wearing gloves, goggles, and a gown of low-permeability fabric with cuffed long sleeves and closed front.
3. Vent vials with filter needle to equalize the internal pressure or use negative-pressure techniques.
4. Wrap gauze or alcohol pads around the neck of ampules when opening to decrease droplet contamination.
5. Wrap gauze or alcohol pads around injection sites when removing syringes or needles from IV injection ports.
6. Do not dispose of materials by clipping needles or removing needles from syringes.

B. Personal Safety to Minimize Exposure via Skin Contact

1. Wear latex gloves at all times when preparing or working with chemotherapeutic agents.
2. Wash hands before putting on gloves and after removing gloves.
3. Change latex gloves frequently (as often as every 30 minutes) since no conclusive data exist for permeability of chemotherapeutic agents via gloves.
4. Wear a gown of low-permeability fabric with a closed front and long cuffed sleeves.
5. Use syringes and IV tubing with Luer locks (which have a locking device to hold needle firmly in place).
6. Label all syringes and IV tubing containing chemotherapeutic agents as hazardous material.
7. Place an absorbent pad directly under the injection site to absorb any accidental spillage.
8. If any contact with the skin occurs, immediately wash the area thoroughly with soap and water.
9. If eye contact is made, immediately flush the eye with water and seek medical attention.

C. Personal Safety to Minimize Exposure via Ingestion

1. Do not eat, drink, chew gum, or smoke while preparing or handling chemotherapy.
2. Keep all food and drink away from preparation area.
3. Wash hands before and after handling chemotherapy.
4. Avoid hand-to-mouth or hand-to-eye contact while handling chemotherapeutic agents or body fluids of the person receiving chemotherapy.

D. Safe Disposal of Antineoplastic Agents

1. Discard gloves and gown into a leakproof container, which should be marked as contaminated or hazardous waste.
2. Use puncture- and leak-proof containers for noncapped, nonclipped needles and other sharp or breakable objects.

E. Safe Handling of Body Fluids and Excreta

1. Wear latex gloves for disposing of body excreta
2. Wear gloves and gowns for handling soiled linens
3. The literature pertaining to this topic has not been conclusive.

F. Special Safety Precautions for Administering Chemotherapy in the Home

1. Instruct the family to wash soiled linens twice and keep separate from family laundry.
2. Wear gloves while handling excreta.
3. Instruct family members to place disposable equipment in leakproof bags.
4. Use a sturdy cardboard container lined with plastic bag for disposal of needles or vials.
5. Instruct family members to wash hands and wear latex gloves when handling chemotherapeutic agents.
6. If chemotherapeutic agents are to be stored in the home, they should be stored out of reach of children. In addition, family members should be instructed regarding dangers of accidental ingestion or contamination with other items.

Nursing Process Applied to Patient Receiving Chemotherapy

Assessment

A. Side Effects and/or Toxicity

1. *Side effects* are usually not life-threatening but can be annoying (e.g., alopecia, change in taste sensation, skin reaction).
2. *Toxic effects* usually refer to a life-threatening reaction such as nephrotoxicity, severe bone marrow depression, or anemia. Medication dosage may have to be reduced or therapy may be postponed/discontinued.
3. Toxicities are usually graded on a scale of 0 to 4 with increasing severity (4 is life-threatening).

B. Integumentary System

1. Inspect for any open wounds on the skin surface. Assess for any signs of infection.
2. Assess for any areas that have undue pressure due to edema on bony prominences.
3. Determine if pressure sores exist on scapulae, elbows, iliac crests, vertebrae, ankles, knees, or heels.
4. Assess condition of gums, teeth, buccal mucosa, and tongue.
   a. Determine if any taste changes have occurred.
   b. Check for evidence of stomatitis, erythematous areas, or infection.
   c. Determine if the patient has any complaints of pain or burning of the oral mucosa.

C. Gastrointestinal System

1. *Nausea and vomiting*
   a. Assess for frequency, duration, and severity of nausea and vomiting episodes before and after chemotherapy.
   b. Determine the amount of emesis to prevent dehydration and electrolyte imbalance.

c. Assess if the patient is performing any interventions to relieve nausea and vomiting.

d. Assess if any particular stimulus increases nausea and vomiting, such as specific foods or aromas.

2. *Diarrhea or constipation*

a. Assess for hemorrhoids or potential areas for infection at anus.

b. Ascertain any changes in bowel patterns.

c. Discuss the consistency of stools.

d. Consider the frequency and duration of diarrhea (the number of stools each day for the number of days).

e. Evaluate any dietary changes that have had an impact on the diarrhea or constipation.

f. Discuss the use of stool softeners to minimize constipation.

3. *Anorexia*

a. Discuss taste changes and changes in food preferences.

b. Ask about daily food intake and normal eating patterns.

c. Evaluate if there are any changes in daily eating patterns.

d. Assess early satiety.

D. Hematopoietic System

1. *Neutropenia*—Absolute granulocyte count less than 500/mm³.

a. Assess for any signs of infection (pulmonary, integumentary, CNS, and urinary).

b. Auscultate lungs for any changes including crackles, wheezes, or rhonchi.

c. Determine if patient has productive cough or shortness of breath.

d. Ask if patient has experienced urinary frequency, pain, or odor.

e. Monitor for an elevation of a temperature >38.3°C (>101°F).

2. *Thrombocytopenia*—Platelet count less than 50,000/mm³ (mild risk); <20,000/mm³. (severe risk)

a. Assess skin and oral mucous membranes for petechiae.

b. Determine if patient has episodes of bleeding (including nose, urinary, rectal, or hemoptysis).

c. Assess if any blood in stools, urine, or emesis has been detected.

d. Remember that the patient is at risk for bleeding when platelet count is less than 50,000/mm³.

e. Assess for signs and symptoms of intracranial bleeding if platelet count is less than 20,000/mm³; monitor for changes in level of responsiveness, somnolence, coma. (See pp. 578–581 for assessment of the patient with increased intracranial pressure.)

3. *Anemia*

a. Assess skin color, turgor, and capillary refill.

b. Ascertain if patient has experienced dyspnea upon exertion.

c. Determine if patient complains of fatigue, weakness, or vertigo.

E. Respiratory and Cardiovascular Systems

1. Assess for pulmonary fibrosis evidenced by a dry, nonproductive cough with increasing dyspnea. Patients at risk include: >60 years old, a smoker, are receiving or had pulmonary radiation, receiving cumulative dose of bleomycin, or any pre-existing lung disease.

2. Assess for signs and symptoms of congestive heart failure and/or irregular apical or radial pulses.

F. Neuromuscular System

1. Ascertain if patient is having difficulty with fine motor activities, such as zipping pants, tying shoes, or buttoning a shirt.

2. Determine the presence of paresthesias (tingling, numbness).

3. Evaluate deep tendon reflexes.

4. Evaluate patient for weakness, ataxia, or slapping gait.

5. Determine impact on activities of daily living and discuss changes.

6. Discuss symptoms of urinary retention or constipation.

G. Genitourinary System

1. Assess if patient has increased urinary frequency.

2. Evaluate any changes in odor, color, or clarity of urine sample.

3. Assess for hematuria.

4. Monitor for the development of oliguria or anuria.

H. Sexuality, Body Image, and Self-Esteem

1. Discuss body image changes and the impact on the individual's life.

2. Be honest with the patient and listen closely.

3. Discuss risks to reproductive potential and the patient's emotions.

4. Consider and discuss changes in positions for sexual activity that are more comfortable.

Nursing Diagnoses

1. Knowledge deficit of purposes of chemotherapy, expected side effects, and patient role in management of side effects.

2. Potential for infection related to neutropenia (decreased WBC).

3. Potential for injury related to thrombocytopenia.

4. Fatigue related to anemia.

5. Potential for altered nutrition (less than body requirements) related to side effects of therapy, anorexia, and stomatitis.

6. Potential for altered oral mucous membranes related to stomatitis.

7. Potential for altered body image and self-esteem related to alopecia and weight loss.

8. Potential for altered bowel elimination related to effects of chemotherapeutic agent.

9. Potential for altered sexual patterns related to effects of chemotherapy.

Nursing Interventions

A. Acquiring Knowledge About Chemotherapy

1. Discuss the method of administration, expected side effects, and the overall goal of chemotherapy.

2. Instruct patient to report any discomfort, pain, or burning during administration of IV chemotherapy.

3. Write schedule on calendar of drug treatments, lab tests, and expected time period for neutropenia to develop.

4. Emphasize that side effects are usually temporary and are highly individualized.

5. Assist the patient to set realistic goals for work and activities.

6. Provide written information regarding the specific chemotherapeutic agents and side effects.

B. Avoiding Infections

1. Monitor vital signs every 4 hours; report any occurrence of fever >38.3°C. (101.0°F.).

2. Instruct patient about signs and symptoms of infection including:
   a. Mouth lesions, swelling, or redness.
   b. Redness, pain, or tenderness or hemorrhoids at rectum.
   c. Any change in bowel habits.
   d. Any areas of redness, swelling, induration, or pain on the surface of the skin.
   e. Any pain or burning when urinating or odor from urine.
   f. Any cough or shortness of breath.
3. Avoid performing invasive procedures—for example, rectal temperatures, enemas, or insertion of indwelling urinary catheters.
4. Reinforce good personal hygiene habits (routine bathing, preferably a shower, clean hair, nail, and mouth care).
5. Stress importance of strict handwashing.
6. Check for reduction in the number of leukocytes and differential count.
7. Calculate absolute neutrophil count (ANC) to determine the number of leukocytes capable of fighting an infection by:
   - Total WBC $\times$ (% polys + % bands) = ANC
   - Example: 700 $\times$ (10% + 5%) = 105
   - INTERPRETATION: 105 of the 700 WBCs are mature and capable of fighting an infection (indicates severe neutropenia).
8. Administer antibiotics as prescribed.
9. Change denture cleaning fluid, water for respiratory equipment, and other standing water every 24 hours to minimize a source of possible infections.

C. Avoiding Bleeding due to Thrombocytopenia

1. Avoid invasive procedures when platelet count <100,000 mm³, including IM injections, suppositories, enemas, and insertion of indwelling urinary catheters.
2. Apply pressure on injection sites for 5 minutes.
3. Avoid aspirin-containing products.
4. Monitor platelet count; administer platelets as prescribed.
5. Monitor and test all urine, stools, and emesis for blood.

D. Preventing/Coping With Fatigue From Anemia

1. Monitor blood counts (hemoglobin and hematocrit).
2. Explain why fatigue and shortness of breath may occur.
3. Plan frequent rest periods between daily activities.
4. Administer blood products as prescribed.
5. Caution the patient about physical overexertion; encourage him to rest frequently and to expect a tired feeling.
6. Explain that blood transfusions, if given, are a part of therapy and not necessarily an indication of a setback.
7. Observe skin color.

E. Minimizing Nausea and Vomiting to Increase Patient Comfort

1. Assess previous experiences with chemotherapy, if any.
2. Administer antiemetics on scheduled basis during 24-hour period of chemotherapy (not on a PRN basis) as prescribed. Some classes of antiemetics include phenothiazines (prochlorperazine), butyrophenones, (haloperidol, droperidol), benzamides (metoclopramide), cannabinoids (dronabinol), and glucocorticosteroids (dexamethasone and prednisone).
3. Schedule antiemetic(s) prior to chemotherapy (especially for cyclophosphamide, cisplatin, doxorubicin, mechlorethamine hydrochloride).

4. Monitor intake and output including emesis.
5. Encourage patient to eat bland, highly nutritious foods.
6. Encourage deep breathing and relaxation techniques.
7. Consult dietitian concerning patient's food preferences, intolerances, and individual dietary interventions.
8. Use antiemetics in combination as prescribed.
9. Offer soda crackers and ice chips—may relieve nausea.
10. Provide emesis basin and tissues; empty and clean basin after use.
11. Apply a cool, damp washcloth to forehead, face, and neck.
12. Administer an antiemetic; assess for dehydration.
13. Offer items for oral care after vomiting: mouthwash, toothbrush, and toothpaste.
14. Regulate temperature of fluids and foods coming in contact with the oral mucosa; avoid temperature extremes (too hot or too cold).
15. Serve high-protein and high-carbohydrate food; allow the patient to choose his foods; guide his selection so that a well-balanced diet of nutritionally desirable foods is served.
16. Present food as attractively as possible and serve it in a pleasant setting.
17. Ensure that the patient is physically comfortable; encourage having friends or family provide company during mealtime if this helps.
18. Encourage fluids because tissue metabolic rate is elevated and the patient needs to clear wastes from his body.
19. Entice the anorexic patient with refreshing mouth care before serving meals; a bad taste in the mouth discourages eating.
    a. Try giving the patient high-protein, high-calorie foods.
    b. Monitor weight loss.
20. Avoid highly seasoned foods, even if the patient ordinarily thrives on such foods.
21. Discourage smoking and use of alcoholic beverages since these irritate the mucous membranes.
22. Recognize that occasionally cancer and/or treatment may cause an alteration of taste perception, such as a keener taste of bitterness and loss of ability to detect sweet tastes.

F. Promoting Oral Comfort

1. *If no white patches are present:*
   a. Encourage prophylactic oral hygiene after meals and at night, more frequently if needed.
   b. Use soft toothbrush and remove dentures.
   c. Avoid spicy and hot foods; order bland, soft foods of moderate temperature.
   d. Assess need for oral antifungal or antibacterial agents.
   e. Avoid commercial mouthwashes that may irritate sensitive tissues.
2. If oral cavity *erythematous or white patches* are present:
   a. Monitor weight and encourage bland finger foods—less painful.
   b. Increase frequency of oral care.
   c. Use mild analgesic every 3–4 hours as prescribed, such as lidocaine HCL 2% as an oral swish.

> **GERONTOLOGIC ALERT:** The adult older than 80 years of age has a reduced gag reflex; assess for evidence of a gag reflex very carefully to prevent aspiration.

d. Use normal saline mouth rinses.
e. Combination mouth rinses may be used such as lidocaine, diphenhydramine HCL, and Maalox as prescribed.

G. Coping With Altered Body Image

1. Reassure patient that hair will usually grow back. It may grow back a different texture and/or different color.
2. Suggest wearing a turban, wig, or head scarf, preferably purchased prior to hair loss.
3. Scalp hypothermia 10–20 minutes prior to and 30 minutes after chemotherapy may minimize alopecia (for solid tumors only).
4. Encourage healthy scalp and hair care—use mild shampoo and avoid vigorous brushing.
5. Discourage use of permanents and hair coloring during treatment period.
6. Explain that hair loss is gradual.
7. Encourage patient to stay on therapeutic program.
8. Be honest with the patient.

Discharge Planning and Patient Education

A. Self-Monitoring for Neutropenia

1. Report any signs and symptoms of infection.
2. Take temperature.
3. Wash hands frequently.
4. Perform proper perineal/perianal care:
    a. Cleanse area after each urination or bowel movement.
    b. Cleanse from front to back.
5. Avoid crowds or persons with infections.

B. Self-Monitoring for Thrombocytopenia

1. Assess for areas of bleeding including urine, stool, and emesis.
2. Test urine, stools, and emesis for blood.
3. Use a nonabrasive toothbrush.
4. Use an electric razor rather than a blade to shave.
5. Avoid contact sports.
6. Prevent constipation and avoid use of Valsalva maneuver.
7. Report any episodes of increased bruising, excessive bleeding of gums, nosebleeds, black or tarry stools, coffee ground emesis, cloudy or reddish urine, or changes in mental status such as drowsiness.

C. Self-Monitoring and Coping for Anemia

1. Report shortness of breath and increasing fatigue.
2. Include frequent rest breaks in daily activities.

D. Coping With Nausea and Vomiting

1. Take antiemetics as prescribed.
2. Maintain adequate hydration.
3. Monitor amount of emesis and fluid intake.
4. Report inability to maintain adequate intake.

E. Self-Monitoring for Stomatitis

1. Perform good oral hygiene.
2. Check mouth for lesions or erythematous areas and report.
3. Use mouth rinses as prescribed.
4. Use antifungal or antibacterial agent as prescribed.
5. Eat bland diet of a moderate temperature.

F. Other Considerations

1. Report any changes in bowel or bladder habits.
2. Report any changes in sensations including numbness, weakness, and/or tingling in extremities.

Evaluation

1. Able to discuss plan, side effects, and patient interventions.
2. Is free of infection; maintains temperature within normal limits; no signs of infection.
3. No evidence of bleeding.
4. Maintains hemoglobin within acceptable limits.
5. Maintains body weight at acceptable level.
6. Demonstrates intact oral mucosa; reports lessening of discomfort.
7. Adapts to change in appearance; verbalizes self-acceptance.
8. Achieves satisfactory bowel elimination.
9. Seeks counseling for concerns about sexuality.

Radiation Therapy

Definitions

A. Radiation—frequently used in diagnosing and treating cancer. Newer advances are being added in ultrasonography, computed tomography, digital subtraction radiology, and magnetic resonance imaging.

B. Brachytherapy—the radiation source is used for surface, interstitial, or intracavity applications.

C. Teletherapy—the radiation source is exterior to the tumor such as the use of a linear accelerator.

D. Nuclide—any atomic entity capable of existing for a measurable lifetime, usually more than 10^{-9} seconds.

E. Radionuclide (radioactive nuclide)—one that disintegrates with the emission of particulate or electromagnetic radiations.

F. Radioactivity—the disintegration of the atom that gives up energy in the form of rays or particles.

G. Isotope—an element whose nucleus contains a fixed number of protons but has a differing number of neutrons, thereby changing its weight.

1. Optimal ratio between proton and neutron is stable.
2. By using nuclear reactors, it is possible to bombard a stable isotope with additional free neutrons.
3. Most radioisotopes emit:
    a. Particulate radiation—small fragments of the nucleus having mass and size (alpha and beta particles).
    b. Electromagnetic radiation—rays that have no mass (x-rays).

H. Radioactive Decay or Disintegration

1. The rate of decay varies from isotope to isotope.
2. "Half-life" or decay rate is the time required to reduce a particular radioactive substance by one half of its atoms, thereby reducing it to half of its initial activity. Example: ^{225}Radium—half-life of over 1600 years
3. A radioisotope administered to a patient in unsealed form has a relatively short life and is essentially inactive after therapeutic use has been completed. Example: ^{131}Iodine—half-life about 8 days

I. Units of Measurement (Activity)

1. Curie (c.)—basic unit for measuring amount of activity in a radioactive sample
2. Millicurie (mc.)—one thousandth of a curie
3. Microcurie (μc.)—one millionth of a curie
4. Picocurie (pc.)—one billionth of a curie

J. Units for Measuring Radiation Exposure or Absorption

1. *Gray* (Gy)—a unit to measure absorbed dose. 1 Gy equals 100 rads. (Rad—term used in the past to measure absorbed dose). Joules/kg. is also used to measure absorbed dose. 1 joule/kg. = Gy.
2. *Roentgen* (R)—standard unit of exposure (usually applied to x-ray or gamma rays)
3. *Milliroentgen* (mR)—one thousandth of a roentgen
4. *Rem*—unit of measure of radiation-dose equivalent that relates to biologic effectiveness (roentgen equivalent in humans).

   Standards were established by the International Committee on Radiation Protection (ICRP), which has continued its work in the United States through the National Council of Radiation, Protection, and Measurements. The ICRP recommends that the maximum permissible dose (MPD) for radiation workers is 5 rems for persons over age 18 and the maximum dose for women of reproductive capacity is 1.25 rems per quarter at an even rate.

Clinical Considerations

A. Nature and Indications for Use

1. Individualized to produce effective ionization within a tumor while avoiding unnecessary irradiation of normal structures.
2. Tissues most likely to respond to radiation exposure—those originating from reticuloendothelial tissues (leukemia, lymphomas) and those from embryonal tissues (teratomas).
3. Tissues least likely to respond—bone and muscle.

B. Factors Affecting the Benefit of Radiation Exposure vs. Risk of Tissue Damage

1. *Dose rate*—a prescribed dose causes less tissue destruction if given in small amounts over a long period of time rather than given all at once.
2. *Area of body exposure*—the larger the area exposed, the greater the effect.
3. *Cell susceptibility*
   a. Greater susceptibility—rapidly dividing cells with no specialized function (e.g., lymphocytes and germ cells); well-oxygenated.
   b. Lesser susceptibility—nondividing cells and highly differentiated cells (e.g., nerve or muscle cells); hypoxic.
4. *Biological variability*—individual differences play a role in human susceptibility.
   a. Healthy person more responsive than malnourished individual.
   b. Skin is especially vulnerable to radiation injury.
   c. Bone marrow is very radiosensitive; therefore, such damage is potentially the most lethal.
   d. Lung fibrosis may occur following radiation of chest.

Diagnostic Evaluation

A. Diagnostic Radiology

Ultrasonography—sound waves are reflected off points of variation in acoustic impedance.

Sonoendoscopy—utilizing high-frequency ultrasound transducers incorporated near tip of a flexible endoscope, such as for visualization of upper and lower gastrointestinal tract.

Computed tomography (CT)—density differences are revealed by passing a very narrow x-ray beam over tiny cubes of tissue. A computer reconstructs a transverse section of the body and displays the image on a television monitor.

Magnetic resonance imaging (MRI)—combines advantages of CT scan with ultrasound in using non-ionizing radiation and providing tomography in any desired plane.

Digital radiography

B. Roentgenologic Precautions During Radiography, Imaging, Fluoroscopy, or Radiotherapy

1. No one permitted in the room where the patient is undergoing x-ray therapy.
2. Equipment should not leak radiation.
3. Fluoroscopy room attendants should be protected from scattered radiation by wearing lead aprons and, if necessary, lead-impregnated gloves.
4. Appropriate lead shielding should be available to protect the patient's gonads during radiation exposure.

Management

1. Teletherapy radiopharmaceuticals:
   Cobalt-60 (^{60}Co)
   Cesium-137 (^{137}Ce)
2. Agents for management of side effects include antidiarrheals and antiemetic medications.
3. Brachytherapy radiopharmaceuticals:
   Temporary implants: ^{60}Co, ^{192}Ir, ^{137}Ce, ^{226}Ra, and ^{222}Rd
   Permanent implants: ^{198}Gold, ^{125}Iodine

Types of Brachytherapy

A. External Molds—a packaged and screened container in which a radioisotope can be placed and applied directly to the skin surface.

Examples:
1. ^{60}Co can be applied in this manner to small areas, as in the treatment of carcinoma of the lip, larynx, ear, etc.
2. ^{182}Ta (radioactive tantalum) can be applied in a flexible wire mold (e.g., to the external surface of a retinoblastoma involving eyeball and optic nerve).
3. ^{90}Sr (radioactive strontium) and ^{90}Y (radioactive yttrium) as in external molds used for shallow irradiation of eye neoplasms.

B. Intracavitary Isotope Therapy

Examples:
   Liquid radioisotopes:
   ^{198}Au (radioactive colloidal gold)
   ^{137}Ce

Used in the balloon of a catheter inside the bladder for internal bladder radiation of a few millimeters.

C. Interstitial Isotope Therapy

Examples:
1. Radioactive needles, seeds, tubes, or wires can be implanted directly into tumor tissue: ^{60}Co, ^{137}Ce, ^{198}Au, ^{125}I.
2. Implants may be temporary or permanent; they may be supplementary to surgery or to external beam irradiation.
3. Radioactive solutions may be injected directly into the tumor or surrounding tissue. Colloidal solution of radioactive colloidal gold (^{198}Au) is one of the most commonly used solutions.

D. Internal Irradiation

Examples:
1. Oral ingestion of solutions of radioiodine (^{131}I)—administered to patients with hyperthyroidism.
2. Intravenous injection of sodium phosphate (^{32}P)—used in the treatment of polycythemia vera.

Clinical action:
   In above instances, the target tissue has an affinity for the therapeutic agent; the isotope concentrates within the substance.

Complications

Complications are dependent upon site of radiation therapy, type of radiation therapy (brachytherapy or teletherapy), total radiation dose, daily fractionated doses, and overall health of the patient.

GERONTOLOGIC ALERT: Side effects may be prolonged due to decreased ability of the body to repair cellular damage.

A. Acute Side Effects (during treatment to 6 months after treatment) include:
1. Erythema at the site, possible dry-to-wet desquamation
2. Fatigue and malaise
3. Gastrointestinal effects: nausea and vomiting, diarrhea, and esophagitis
4. Oral effects: changes in taste, mucositis, dryness and xerostomia (dryness of mouth from lack of normal secretions)
5. Pulmonary effects: dyspnea, productive cough, pneumonitis
6. Renal and bladder effects: cystitis

B. Chronic Side Effects (after 6 months with a variability in time of expression) include:
1. Skin effects: fibrosis, telangiectasia, permanent darkening of the skin, and atrophy
2. Gastrointestinal effects: fibrosis, adhesions, obstruction, ulceration, and strictures
3. Oral effects: permanent xerostomia, permanent taste alterations, and dental caries
4. Pulmonary effects: fibrosis
5. Renal and bladder effects: radiation nephritis, fibrosis

Nursing Interventions for the Patient Receiving Teletherapy

A. Acquiring Knowledge About Teletherapy
1. Remove all opaque objects such as pins, buttons, and hairpins, and replace clothing with a gown for body x-rays.
2. Have the patient remain perfectly still; maintain position with the use of device made of foam, plastic, plaster, and/or variety of other materials that can conform to the patient's anatomy. It is vital that the patient be able to attain the same position readily from day to day.
3. Tell the patient that there will be no sensation or pain accompanying radiation therapy.
4. Advise the patient that he will be alone in the room for the protection of the technician, but that he will be in voice contact.
5. Determine from the physician what has been told to the patient about radiation therapy.
6. If a series of treatments is to be given, include the patient in the planning phase.

B. Maintaining Optimal Skin Care
1. Inform the patient that some skin reaction can be expected but that it varies from patient to patient. Examples: dry erythema, dry desquamation, wet desquamation, epilation, tanning.
2. Do not apply lotions, ointments, cosmetics, etc., to the site of radiation unless prescribed by the physician. Cornstarch may be used when the skin is dry and itchy.
3. Discourage vigorous rubbing, friction, or scratching because this can destroy skin cells. Apply ointments as instructed by health professionals.
4. Avoid wearing tight-fitting clothing over the treatment field; prevent irritation by not using rough fabric such as wool and corduroy.
5. Take precautions against exposure of radiation field to sunlight and extremes in temperature.
6. Do not apply adhesive or other tape to the skin.
7. Avoid shaving the skin in the treatment field.
8. Do not wash the area of radiation if possible.
9. If the area must be washed, use lukewarm water only.

C. See Other Nursing Interventions Under Chemotherapy, p. 104

Nursing Interventions for the Patient Receiving Brachytherapy

A. General
1. Identify the chart cover and doctor's and nurse's order sheets with the radioactive symbol.
2. For patients receiving the most minute quantities of tracer radioisotopes, such identification (see above) is not necessary.

B. Radiation Instruction Sheet
1. Type of radioactivity used
2. Time of insertion
3. Anticipated time of removal
4. Precautions to follow
5. Whom to notify when in doubt or in an emergency

C. Safety Precautions
The following are taken into consideration:
   1. The *distance* of the nurse from the patient

Note: The inverse square law applies: doubling the distance from a radiation source cuts intensity received to one fourth.

   2. Amount of *time* spent in actual contact with the patient
   3. Degree of *shielding* utilized
      Chosen according to type of radiation—alpha, beta, gamma

NURSING ALERT: During the period of greatest radioactivity (24–72 hours), limit amount of time spent with the patient to that required for essential care. Require the patient to remain in his bed or room during course of treatment.

   4. Personnel who may be exposed to penetrating radiation (x-ray or gamma rays) should wear film badges on front of the body.
   5. Take appropriate measures associated with *sealed sources of radiation* implanted within a patient (sealed internal radiation).
      a. Follow directives on precaution sheet that is placed on chart of all patients receiving radiotherapy.

b. Do not remain within 1 meter (3 feet) of the patient any longer than required to give essential care.
6. Know that the casing material absorbs all alpha radiation and most beta radiation, but that a hazard concerning gamma radiation may exist.
7. Do not linger longer than necessary in giving patient care, even though all precautions are followed.
8. Be alert for implants that may have become loosened (those inserted in cavities that have access to the exterior), for example, check the emesis basin following mouth care for a patient with an oral implant.
9. Notify the radiologist of any implant that has moved out of position.
10. Utilize long-handled forceps or tongs and hold at arm's length when picking up any accidentally dislodged radium needle, seeds, tubes, etc., that may appear on dressings, bed, or floor. *Never pick up a radioactive source with your hands.*
11. Do not discard any dressings or linens unless sure that no radioactive source is present.
12. Wash hands with soap and water after caring for a patient who is being treated with a radioisotope.
13. Upon discharge of a patient, it is a good policy for the radiologist to check the room with a radiograph or survey meter to be certain that all radioactive materials have been removed.
14. Continue radiation precautions when a patient has a permanent implant, until the radiologist declares precautions unnecessary.

Patient Education and Discharge Planning

1. Perform proper skin care.
2. Maintain adequate nutrition.

Cancer Immunotherapy or Adoptive Immunotherapy

Cancer immunotherapy, or adoptive immunotherapy, involves the transfer to the patient of previously sensitized immunologic substances that can directly or indirectly mediate an antitumor response (i.e., interleukin-2 or alpha interferon). Cancer immunotherapy is rapidly becoming a fourth modality for cancer treatment.

Underlying Principles

A. Function—The primary function of the immune system is to detect and eliminate substances that are recognized as "non-self."

B. The Immune System—has two major components: nonspecific (innate) and specific (acquired).

1. *Nonspecific or innate immunity* is inherent in all individuals. The largest component of the nonspecific system is the skin. Other nonspecific defense mechanisms include: mucous membranes, cilia, tears, sebaceous glands, and acidic urine.
2. *Specific immunity or acquired immunity* has two primary features—specificity and memory. It is composed of three groups: cell-mediated immunity, humoral immunity, and null cells.
   a. Cell-mediated immunity is the T cells: T4 (helper/inducer cells) and T8 (cytotoxic and suppressor).
   b. Humoral immunity is the B cells, which ultimately secrete antibodies.
   c. Null cells are cells that are neither T nor B cells. The principal function is still unknown. Natural killer (NK) cells and lymphokine activated killer (LAK) cells are included in this group.

C. Cytokines—are proteins produced by mononuclear cells of the immune system (usually the lymphocytes and monocytes) that have regulatory actions on other cells in the immune system or target cells involved in the immune reaction.

1. Cytokines include lymphokines (produced by lymphocytes) and monokines (produced by monocytes or macrophages).
2. Examples of cytokines include: interleukins, interferons, and colony stimulating factors (CSF). Six different Interleukins (1–6) have been identified, three types of interferon (alpha, beta, and gamma), and three different types of CSFs (granulocyte-macrophage CSF, granulocyte CSF, and macrophage CSF).

Management

1. Currently, clinical trials with high-dose interleukin-2 (IL-2) have been used most extensively. The most frequent regimen is a bolus of high-dose IL-2 via an IV infusion three times per day. The IL-2 is administered for 5 days, followed by a rest period of 7–10 days, then repeat the IL-2 for 5 more days.
2. Patients receive indomethacin, ranitidine, and acetaminophen prophylactically throughout the therapy.
3. Antiemetics and antidiarrheals are administered when needed.
4. Skin care is initiated prior to therapy and continued throughout. Skin care includes ointments, lotions, and mouth rinses.
5. Serum albumin is frequently given to minimize third spacing syndrome and urinary retention.

Nursing Process Applied to Patients Undergoing Immunotherapy

The administration of cytokines is investigational. Consequently, the toxicities vary depending upon the dose, frequency of administration, duration, and combination with other cytokines, chemotherapy, or radiation. The nursing process is based upon the assessment of side effects and toxicities associated with the administration of high-dose Interleukin-2. Similar side effects may be seen with other high-dose cytokines (interferon, colony stimulating factors, and other interleukins).

Nursing Assessment

1. Review patient's chart to determine site of cancer, previous cancer therapies, current medications, and other medical conditions.
2. Assess patient's understanding of immunotherapy and the associated toxicities.
3. Explain procedures and evaluate patient's understanding.

Nursing Diagnoses

1. Knowledge deficit of purpose of immunotherapy, expected side effects, and patient's role in management of side effects.
2. Potential for altered tissue perfusion (cardiopulmonary) related to capillary permeability leak syndrome (third spacing of fluid).

3. Potential for altered nutrition (less than body requirements) related to side effects of therapy and anorexia.
4. Potential for altered bowel elimination (diarrhea) related to immunotherapy.
5. Altered skin integrity related to immunotherapy.
6. Altered mucous membranes related to immunotherapy.
7. Altered pattern of urinary elimination related to oliguria secondary to immunotherapy.
8. Altered body temperature related to fever and chills secondary to immunotherapy.
9. Potential for altered thought processes related to immunotherapy.

Nursing Interventions

A. Acquiring Knowledge About Immunotherapy and the Side Effects

1. Discuss the overall goal of immunotherapy, expected side effects, and the method of administration.
2. Instruct the patient to report any discomfort including fever, chills, diarrhea, nausea and vomiting, itching, and/or weight gain.
3. Emphasize that the side effects are temporary and will usually cease within 1 week after treatment ends.

B. Avoiding Altered Tissue Perfusion
(Cardiopulmonary)

1. Monitor vital signs at least every 4 hours—including hypotension, tachycardia, tachypnea, and fever.
   a. Instruct patient to remain in bed if blood pressure is low.
   b. Monitor apical heart rate.
2. Assess respirations for rate, depth, and auscultate breath sounds for evidence of pulmonary edema.
3. Assess for signs of restlessness, apprehension, discomfort, or cyanosis, that may indicate respiratory distress.
4. Administer oxygen as prescribed.
5. Maintain patent IV line and administer serum albumin as prescribed.
6. Check extremities for warmth, color, and capillary refill.

C. Attaining and Maintaining Nutritional Requirements

1. Obtain baseline weight and measure abdominal girth.
2. Obtain daily weights; goal is to maintain weight within 2–5 kg. (5–10 lb.) of weight on admission to the hospital.
3. Assess for ascites in abdomen and edema of the extremities.
4. Measure intake and output.
5. Encourage patient to eat nutritious foods and drink fluids liberally.
6. Administer antiemetic medications as prescribed.
7. Facilitate a dietary consultation if required.

D. Minimizing Diarrhea and Maintaining Fluid Balance

1. Record amount and frequency of diarrhea.
2. Administer antidiarrheal agents as prescribed.
3. Inspect anal area for evidence of skin breakdown.
4. Offer sitz baths, warm compresses to irritated anal area.
5. Apply Tuck's or A & D ointment to alleviate tenderness of anal area.
6. Monitor intake and output; monitor laboratory values for electrolyte imbalances.

E. Minimizing Skin Reactions—rash, itching, dryness, desquamation, erythema, or infections

1. Wash skin with a mild soap or oil; avoid excessive towel drying.
2. Apply lotions and ointments to hydrate the skin—frequently.
3. Apply lubricant to lips.
4. Administer medications as prescribed to reduce itching.
5. Prevent skin irritation by wearing loose-fitting clothing or gowns.
6. Avoid using irritating deodorants or after-shave lotions.
7. Provide relief measures such as cool-water soaks or Aveeno baths.
8. Use relaxation techniques, if appropriate.

F. Achieving Oral Comfort

See nursing interventions for patient undergoing chemotherapy, p. 104.

G. Maintaining Adequate Urine Output

1. Document intake and output; weigh daily.
2. Maintain patent intravenous infusion lines.
3. Administer diuretics as prescribed, including serum albumin.
4. Monitor blood urea nitrogen and creatinine levels.
5. Insert indwelling urethral catheter as prescribed.

H. Maintaining Body Temperature Within Acceptable Range

1. Administer acetaminophen as prescribed to prevent chills.
2. Apply warm blankets at first sign of a chill.
3. Administer meperidine as prescribed for chills.
4. Monitor temperature every 4 hours.
5. Monitor patient closely for signs of infection.

I. Coping With Altered Thought Patterns

1. Monitor for signs of confusion including slow mentation, memory loss, restlessness, and agitation.
2. Observe patient closely during time period.
3. Reorient patient frequently.

Discharge Planning and Patient Education

Instruct the patient as follows:

A. Sleep Disturbances

1. May have difficulty falling asleep or may be unable to sleep for usual length of time.
2. Difficulty with sleep patterns will gradually cease in a month or so.

B. Thought Patterns

1. There may be difficulty in concentrating for prolonged time periods that will gradually diminish.
2. It is advised to avoid operating machinery (driving a car) until able to concentrate more effectively.

C. Skin Alterations—See above

D. Weight Gain and Activity Levels

1. Use medications as prescribed.
2. Eat nutritious foods.
3. Fluid accumulation should resolve after treatment ends.
4. Gradually increase activity level as fatigue decreases.

Evaluation

1. Able to discuss purpose of immunotherapy, side effects, and patient interventions.

2. No evidence of excess fluid in cardiopulmonary system.
3. Maintains body weight at an acceptable level.
4. Achieves satisfactory bowel elimination.
5. Demonstrates appropriate use of interventions for skin care, reports lessening of discomfort.
6. Demonstrates intact oral mucosa; reports lessening of discomfort.
7. Achieves satisfactory urinary elimination.
8. Maintains satisfactory body temperature.
9. Absence of abnormal thought patterns.

Special Considerations in Cancer Care
Care of the Patient With a Venous Access Device

Types of Devices *(Fig. 6-2)*

A *venous access device* (VAD) is an implanted catheter or device that remains in place for an extended period of time (weeks, months, or even years). It may be tunneled or implanted.

A. Tunneled Device

A tunneled catheter is inserted into a central vein (usually the subclavian, then the superior vena cava) and subcutaneously tunneled to an exit site approximately 10 cm. from the insertion site.

1. A Dacron cuff is located approximately 2–3 cm. from the exit site, providing a barrier against microorganisms.
2. Examples of the tunneled catheters in current use are Hickman, Broviac, and Groshong.

B. Implanted Device

A subcutaneous pocket is formed and a reservoir is placed; a catheter is attached to the reservoir and tunneled subcutaneously and inserted into a central vein (usually the catheter tip is in the superior vena cava). This device cannot be visualized exteriorly.

Examples of implanted devices in current use include the Port-A-Cath, Medi-Port, Infuse-A-Port, and Hickman Port.

Indications

1. Long-term therapy (e.g., chemotherapy, medication infusion, blood products and blood specimen collections).
2. Intravenous fluids in the home.
3. Limited peripheral venous access due to extensive previous IV therapy, surgery, and/or previous tissue damage.

Complications

1. Sepsis, especially when the patient is neutropenic.
2. Thrombus formation.
3. Dislodgement of catheter tip; catheter damage.

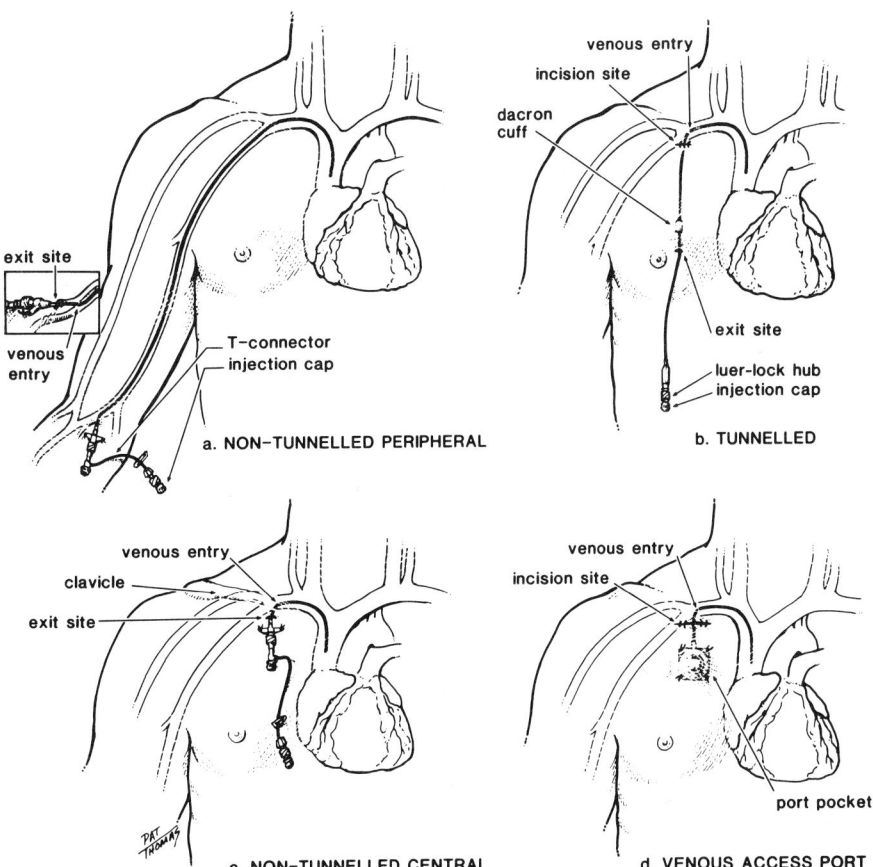

Figure 6-2. *Common sites for long-term venous access devices. (Courtesy American Cancer Society).*

a. NON–TUNNELED PERIPHERAL

b. TUNNELLED

c. NON–TUNNELLED CENTRAL

d. VENOUS ACCESS PORT

Management and Nursing Interventions (Table 6-5)

1. Assess patient and family's ability to handle medications, flush catheter, change dressings, monitor infusion and side effects, and handle complications.
2. Teach patient and family the above skills and ensure patient understanding. Give patient and family written materials.

Pain in the Patient With Cancer

Types of Pain

A. Acute Pain

1. Has a beginning and an end.
2. Duration—less than 6 months.
3. Can be readily described by the patient.
4. Can be controlled with medications.

B. Chronic Pain—most frequently seen in patients with cancer

1. Does not have a definitive beginning or end.
2. Duration—greater than 6 months.
3. Difficult for the patient to describe the type of pain.
4. Not always easily controlled; several different measures may be needed.

Causes

1. Caused by the cancer—pain due to bony involvement, visceral invasion. This accounts for approximately 75% to 80% of all pain problems.
2. Caused by the therapy—(e.g., peripheral neuropathies related to chemotherapy).
3. Unrelated to the cancer; for example, patient has concomitant or a history of rheumatoid arthritis.

Clinical Manifestations

1. Pain of varying degrees and severity including:
   a. Visceral pain—initially poorly localized and often referred to another area.
   b. Nerve pain—Symptoms can be diverse and range from pain to paresthesias to sensory loss. Patients may also experience referred pain.
   c. Bone pain—local bone pain can be manifested from a dull ache to a deep, boring, intense pain.
2. Fatigue from sleep disturbances; most patients may not have slept for extended periods of time.
3. Loss of appetite or weight gain from side effects of disease and/or therapy; anxiety and depression.
4. Change in self-concept from the impact of cancer, altered body image (e.g., weight loss, alopecia), change in life quality.

Management

A. Pharmacologic Management

1. Nonsteroidal anti-inflammatory drugs (NSAIDs)—act on the peripheral neurotransmitters.
2. Narcotic analgesics (morphine, methadone, hydromorphone)—bind to the opiate receptors and act on the central nervous system pathways.
3. Adjuvant analgesics—may enhance the narcotic analgesic effect or act independently and provide some analgesia.
4. Intraspinal opiates (see p. 587).

B. Surgical Management (See p. 587 for neurosurgical management of pain)

Stimulation procedures; transcutaneous electric nerve stimulation; cordotomy; rhizotomy.

Nursing Assessment

1. Evaluate objectively the nature of the patient's pain: location, duration, quality, and the manner in which the patient tolerates it or accepts it (behavioral responses to pain).
2. Use a pain intensity scale of 0 (for no pain) to 10 (worst possible pain).
3. Assess relief from medications and duration of relief. (Use the same measuring scale every time.)
4. Review recommendations and assessment of pain specialist.

Nursing Interventions

1. Convey the impression that patient's pain is understood and relief is forthcoming.
2. Explore pain interventions that have been used and their effectiveness.

Table 6-5. *Care of the Patient With a Venous Access Device*

Type	Flush	Dressing Change	Patient Education
Hickman/ Broviac	2.5 ml. heparin (1:100 units/ml. twice daily)	Change occlusive gauze or transparent dressing per agency policy; if not in use, site should be covered and a clamp available	Flush catheter Change cap weekly Change dressing if receiving infusion at home If catheter tears or breaks, instruct patient to clamp catheter and call health professional immediately
Groshong	5 ml. normal saline (NS) after each use and weekly Flush with 20 ml. NS after blood is drawn	Same as above	Flush catheter Change cap weekly Dressing change if receiving home infusion
Medi-Port or Port-A-Cath or Infusa-Port	Use noncoring needles only to access the port Flush every 4 weeks with 2.5–5 ml. of heparin if intravenous	No dressing necessary unless the port is accessed Sterile technique required during access Flush with 20 ml. NS after blood is drawn; then flush with heparin	Health professionals usually change dressings and flush the port Each port can be accessed between 1000 and 2000 times

3. Administer medications as specifically required:
   a. Analgesics—for discomfort and pain
   b. Narcotics—for more intense pain
   c. Muscle relaxants and antispasmodics—to relieve muscle spasm and/or tension
   d. Antiemetics—for nause and vomiting
   e. Stool softeners—to prevent constipation
   f. Anxiolytic drugs—for fear and apprehension
   g. Sedatives and hypnotics—to induce and promote analgesic effect and sleep
   h. Local anesthetics—for local pain
4. Administer medications around-the-clock (depending on drug in use) rather than PRN in order to maintain therapeutic level in the blood stream.
5. When changing from IV or IM to oral route, be sure of equivalency of doses between the different routes and also of half-life of medication.
6. Do not switch medications for at least 24 hours as it takes 24 hours to achieve a therapeutic blood level.
7. Monitor patient's comfort and pain level before and after pain medications.
8. Use alternative measures to relieve pain such as imaging, relaxation, and biofeedback.
9. Provide skilled nursing care; attend to concomitant problems promptly (e.g., nausea and vomiting, constipation, renal dysfunction)
10. Provide on-going support and open communication.
11. Monitor for complications.
    a. Constipation
    b. Nausea and vomiting
    c. Respiratory depression
    d. Liver dysfunction—difficulty metabolizing narcotics
    e. Cardiac alterations—decreased BP and pulse rate
    f. Renal dysfunction—difficulty excreting toxic wastes

Discharge Planning and Patient Education

1. Instruct patient regarding method of administration of medications and importance of maintaining prescribed schedule.
2. Instruct patient to call health professionals if pain has increased.
3. Instruct about side effects.
4. Be aware of changes in bowel pattern and report to health professionals.

Complications in Cancer

Septic Shock

Septic shock is a systemic disease associated with the presence and persistence of pathogenic microorganisms or their toxins in the blood.

A. Diagnostic Evaluation

1. Cultures: blood, urine, stool, sputum, central and peripheral intravenous lines, and any open wounds—to determine source and type of infection
2. Chest x-ray
3. Arterial blood gas evaluation
4. Electrolytes
5. CBC with differential

B. Management

1. Antibiotics started immediately; broad-spectrum antibiotics given until organism is cultured.
2. Intravenous fluids to restore circulating blood volume.
3. Administer oxygen.

4. Monitor vital signs frequently until stabilized, then every 4 hours.
5. Monitor lab counts, especially WBC, ANC (see chemotherapy, p. 105), and electrolytes.

Spinal Cord Compression (SCC)

Spinal cord compression is pressure on the spinal cord from a primary or metastatic tumor. The location of the compression can be either extradural or intradural.

A. Clinical Manifestations of Prodromal Phase

1. Progressive back pain for less than 6 months before diagnosis.
2. Pain is frequently accelerated with lower radicular thoracic pain.
3. Pain aggravated by coughing, lying down, or motion.
4. Pain pattern is diffuse or referred.

B. Clinical Manifestations of Compressive or Emergency Phase

1. Changes in sensation—paresthesias, numbness, tingling.
2. Loss of sphincter control.
3. Changes in motor function—foot drop, impaired ambulation.
4. Unsteadiness may be noted prior to weakness.

C. Diagnostic Evaluation

1. Ongoing neurologic examinations.
2. Myelogram—most useful test to determine precise level of spinal involvement.
3. MRI—useful in evaluating spinal cord lesions and spinal involvement.

D. Management

1. Corticosteroids—reduce inflammation and swelling at site, increase neurologic function and relieve pain.
2. Radiation to tumor on spinal cord, if applicable.
3. Immediate decompressive surgery (laminectomy—see p. 621), if applicable.

E. Complications

1. Respiratory impairment including pneumonia and atelectasis.
2. Mobility impairment including immobility, foot drop, skin impairment, postural hypotension.
3. Sensory losses creating safety concerns.
4. Bladder and/or bowel dysfunction.
5. Pain.

F. Patient Education and Discharge Planning

1. Facilitate referral to home care services for nursing assessment, nursing interventions, and rehabilitation for residual deficits.
2. Facilitate referral to appropriate outpatient services including physical therapy, occupational therapy, and psychosocial support.
3. Provide instructions regarding safety issues for residual sensory deficits (i.e., test bath water temperature, careful use of extreme heat or cold).

Hypercalcemia

Hypercalcemia is an elevated serum calcium level. Patients with tumors that frequently metastasize to the bone are at increased risk for hypercalcemia.

1. Some tumors (bronchogenic carcinoma and hypernephroma) can secrete parathormone (PTH)-like substance, which may also cause hypercalcemia.
2. An increase in prostaglandin from bony metastases can also cause hypercalcemia.

3. Stimulation of the osteoclasts by osteoclast activating factor (OAF) can cause bone remineralization, increasing the serum calcium.

A. Clinical Manifestations

1. Signs and symptoms may vary depending upon the severity of the hypercalcemia and the onset.
2. Symptoms may be nonspecific and insidious such as nausea and vomiting, anorexia, weakness, constipation, polyuria, polydipsia, and loss of memory.
3. A very rapid and life-threatening increase in calcium may cause dehydration, renal failure, and coma.

B. Diagnostic Evaluation

1. Serum calcium level
2. Electrolyte levels

C. Management

1. Hydration with intravenous normal saline (0.9% NaCl) is the initial treatment for patients with acute hypercalcemia and clinical symptoms.
2. Pharmacotherapy
   a. Diuretics may be used to promote further diuresis.
   b. Plicamycin or etidronate disodium is useful for patients who do not respond to normal saline diuresis. Plicamycin blocks PTH and may also inhibit bone resorption.
   c. Calcitonin inhibits osteoclast activity and causes hypocalcemia. It has a rapid onset of action.
   d. Oral phosphates used for chronic hypercalcemia, which can inhibit bone resorption.
   e. Diphosphonates used to stimulate osteoblast activity, which increases bone uptake of calcium.

D. Nursing Interventions

1. Prevent and detect hypercalcemia early.
   a. Recognize patients at risk and monitor for signs and symptoms such as nausea and vomiting, constipation, lethargy, and anorexia.
   b. Emphasize importance of mobility to minimize bone demineralization and constipation.
   c. Instruct patient on the importance of adequate hydration.
2. Administer normal saline infusions as prescribed.
3. Administer medications as prescribed.
4. Maintain accurate intake and output; observe for oliguria or anuria.
5. Take vital signs every 4 hours, especially apical pulse and blood pressure.
6. Monitor electrolyte values and renal function.
7. Assess mental status.
8. Assess cardiorespiratory status for signs of fluid overload.

Superior Vena Cava Syndrome (SVCS)

Superior vena cava syndrome is an obstruction of the superior vena cava resulting in multiple symptoms and physical findings. Patients at risk for SVCS are primarily those with mediastinal tumors.

A. Clinical Manifestations

1. Dyspnea and "tight collar" syndrome occurring for 2–4 weeks before diagnosis. Facial and neck swelling is frequently described by the patient as a "tight collar" feeling.
2. Chest pain, cough, and dysphagia.
3. Cyanosis and edema of the head and upper extremities may be apparent.
4. Progressive dyspnea, orthopnea, and neck vein distention occur.
5. CNS symptoms including headache, vertigo, irritability, lethargy, and visual disturbances.

B. Diagnostic Evaluation

1. Chest x-ray to confirm SVCS; CT scan

C. Management

1. Radiation therapy, if possible, to reduce tumor size and relieve pressure.
2. Chemotherapy may be used in conjunction with radiation. Specific chemotherapeutic agent(s) is dependent upon the tumor type.
3. Surgery (rarely used due to the associated high morbidity and mortality risks).
4. Oxygen for relief of dyspnea.
5. Analgesics and tranquilizers for discomfort and anxiety.
6. Fibrinolytic and anticoagulants may be employed if a thrombus is suspected or to prevent the formation of a thrombus.

D. Nursing Interventions

1. Administer oxygen as prescribed to relieve hypoxia.
2. Place patient in Fowler's position—facilitates gravity drainage and reduces facial edema.
3. Limit the patient's activity and provide a quiet environment.
4. Reassure patient that cyanotic color and facial edema will subside with treatment.
5. See nursing interventions for patient receiving chemotherapy and radiation, p. 104 and p. 108.

Psychosocial Components of Care

Nursing Assessment

1. Assess preillness life style. How did patient solve other problems?
2. Assess for signs of anxiety and coexistence of depression: agitation/restlessness, sleep disturbances, excessive autonomic activity, weight gain or loss, mood changes.
3. Review Mental Health Index (or other mental health evaluation) that measures global mental health, psychological well-being, or distress if done.
4. What activities of daily living can the patient perform?
5. What changes in life style have resulted from cancer and its treatment?
6. Ascertain the patient's perception of the disease/treatment.
7. Evaluate available social support; who is the most significant other?
8. Try to gain a sense of his emotional strengths and potential problem areas.

Nursing Interventions

A. Maintaining a Manageable Level of Anxiety

1. Establish and sustain an unhurried approach to give the patient time to organize his fears, thoughts, and feelings.
2. Allow patient to share his feelings about having cancer.
3. Reflect and amplify his insights and judgments; try to reduce anxiety through reflection and reorientation.
4. Recognize his feelings of losing control.
5. Discuss methods of stress reduction (imagery, relaxation, biofeedback).

6. Discuss the positive aspects of treatment.
7. Encourage expression of positive emotions—emphasis on living in the here and now, greater appreciation of life, etc.
8. Reinforce effective coping behaviors.
9. Encourage patient to join a support group—serves as a buffer against stress, decreases sense of isolation, helps provide insight, gives support in sympathetic, unhurried atmosphere.
10. Remain available as problems arise. Give patient telephone numbers of persons to call when needed—creates a sense of security.
11. Initiate referrals for additional rehabilitation and psychosocial services as appropriate.

B. Increasing Sense of Personal Worth

1. Encourage patient to enroll in a cancer education program.
2. Encourage patient to learn everything possible about his treatment as this promotes a sense of control.
3. Provide expert physical care.
4. Strengthen patient's support system (family, friends, visitors, health care personnel, volunteers, support group)—strengthens self-esteem through the experience of feeling accepted and valued.
5. Help patient readjust expectations and goals to promote ongoing adjustment.
6. Support family/friends as their contribution to the patient's well-being is significant.

Patient and Family Education

1. Be knowledgeable of the range of problems associated with cancer and its treatment.
2. Anticipate problems before they occur; forewarning assists patient/family to cope with different phases of illness/treatment.
3. Provide *ongoing* consistent information and teaching.
4. Help equip patient and family with skill and confidence to solve problems; learn and practice skills necessary in care.
5. Stress the importance of symptom monitoring and reporting changes early.
6. Encourage patient to talk to career counselor to locate resources (community, state, federal) to meet employment and insurance needs as appropriate.

Bibliography

Books

Billings JA. Outpatient Management of Advanced Cancer. Philadelphia, JB Lippincott, 1985

Brager B and Yasko J. Care of the Client Receiving Chemotherapy: A Self-Learning Module for the Nurse Caring for the Client with Cancer. Reston, VA, Reston Publishing, 1984

Casciato DA and Lowitz BB. Manual of Clinical Oncology. 2nd ed. Boston, Little, Brown, 1988

Cassileth BR. Caring for the Patient with Cancer at Home. Atlanta, American Cancer Society, 1988

Chabner B, Collins J and Myers C. Cancer Chemotherapy: Principles and Practice. Philadelphia, JB Lippincott, 1989

DeVita V, Hellman S and Rosenberg S. Cancer: Principles and Practice of Oncology. 3rd ed. Philadelphia, JB Lippincott, 1989

Dorr RT and Fritz WI. Cancer: Chemotherapy Handbook. 2nd ed. New York, Elsevier North Holland, 1989

Groenwald S. Cancer Nursing: Principles and Practice. 2nd ed.. Boston, Jones and Bartlett Publishers, 1990

Haskell CM. Cancer Treatment. 3rd ed. Philadelphia, WB Saunders, 1990

Johnson B and Gross J. Handbook of Oncology Nursing. Bethany, CT, CO, Fleschner Publishing, 1985

Morra M and Potts E. Choices: Realistic Alternatives in Cancer Treatment. 2nd ed. New York, Avon Books, 1987

Morra M and Potts E. Triumph: Getting Back to Normal When You Have Cancer. New York, Avon Books, 1990

Oncology Nursing Society. Biological Response Modifier Guidelines: Recommendations for Nursing Practice and Education. Pittsburgh, Oncology Nursing Society, 1989

Oncology Nursing Society. Safe Handling of Cytotoxic Drugs: Independent Study Module. Pittsburgh, Oncology Nursing Society, 1988

Oncology Nursing Society. Module I: Recommendations for Cancer Chemotherapy: Course Content and Clinical Practicum. Pittsburgh, Oncology Nursing Society, 1988

Oncology Nursing Society. Module III: Recommendations for Nursing Practice in the Outpatient Setting, Pittsburgh, Oncology Nursing Society, 1988

Oncology Nursing Society. Module IV: Recommendations for Nursing Practice in the Home Care Setting. Pittsburgh, Oncology Nursing Society, 1988

Oncology Nursing Society. Module V: Recommendations for the Management of Extravasation and Anaphylaxis. Pittsburgh, Oncology Nursing Society, 1988

Rosenthal S. Medical Care of the Cancer Patient. Philadelphia, WB Saunders, 1987

Ziegfeld CR. Core Curriculum for Oncology Nursing. Philadelphia, WB Saunders, 1987

Journals

Barry SA. Septic shock: Special needs of patients with cancer. Oncol Nurs Forum 1989 Jan/Feb; 16(1):31–38

Basch A. Changes in elimination. Semin Oncol Nurs 1987 Nov; 3(4):287–292

Beck S et al. The family high-risk program: Targeted cancer prevention. Oncol Nurs Forum 1988 May/Jun; 15(3):301–310

Blecke C. Home chemotherapy safety procedures. Oncol Nurs Forum 1989 Sep/Oct; 16(5):719–724

Bram PJ and Katz LF. Study of burnout in nurses working in hospice and hospital oncology settings. Oncol Nurs Forum 1989 Jul/Aug; 16(4):555–562

Bujorian GA. Clinical trials: Patient issues in the decision-making process. Oncol Nurs Forum 1988 Nov/Dec; 15(6): 779–784

Camp LD. Care of the Groshong catheter. Oncol Nurs Forum 1988 Nov/Dec; 15(6):745–754

Caruso-Herman D. Concerns for the dying patient. Semin Oncol Nurs 1989 May; 5(2):120–123

Chamorro T. Informed consent: Nursing issues and ethical dilemmas. Oncol Nurs Forum 1988 Nov/Dec; 15(6): 803–810

Chapman CR. Pain related to cancer treatment. J Pain Symptom Manage 1988 Fall; 3(4):188–193

Chernoff R and Ropka M. The unique nutritional needs of the elderly patient with cancer. Semin Oncol Nurs 1988 Aug; 4(3):189–197

Clark RA, et al. Antiemetic therapy: Management of chemotherapy-induced nausea and vomiting. Semin Oncol Nurs 1989 May; 5(2) Suppl 1:53–57

Collins C. Reverse isolation: What patients perceive. Oncol Nurs Forum 1989 Sep/Oct; 16(5):675–682

Coward DD. Hypercalcemia knowledge assessment in patients in risk of developing cancer-induced hypercalcimia. Oncol Nurs Forum 1988 Jul/Aug; 15(4):471–480

Curtis AE and Fernsler JI. Quality of life of oncology hospice patients: A comparison of patient and primary caregiver reports. Oncol Nurs Forum 1989 Jan/Feb; 16(1):49–56

Dalton JA. Nurses' preceptions of their pain assessment skills, pain management practices, and attitudes toward pain. Oncol Nurs Forum 1989 Mar/Apr; 16(2):225–236

d'Angelo TM and Gorrell CR. Breast reconstruction using tissue expanders. Oncol Nurs Forum 1989 Jan/Feb; 16(1):23–30

D'Angio G. Cure is not enough: Late consequences associated with radiation treatment. J Assoc Pediatr Oncol Nurses 1988; 5:20–23

Deininger H, Collins JL and Hubbard SM. Nurses and PDQ: What's in it for you? Oncol Nurs Forum 1989 Jul/Aug; 16(3):547–554

DeWolf MS. Ethical decision-making. Semin Oncol Nurs 1989 May; 5(2):77–81

Diekmann JM. Cancer in the elderly: Systems overview. Semin Oncol Nurs 1988 Aug; 4(3):169–177

Dillman JB. Toxicity of monoclonal antibodies in the treatment of cancer. Semin Oncol Nurs 1988 May; 4(2):107–111

Doig B. Adjuvant chemotherapy in breast cancer. Cancer Nurs 1988 Apr; 11(2):981–988

Donovan M. An historical view of pain management. Cancer Nurs 1989 Aug; 12(4):257–261

Edlund B and Sneed NV. Emotional responses to the diagnosis of cancer: Age-related comparisons. Oncol Nurs Forum 1989 Sep/Oct; 16(5):691–702

Ehlke G. Symptom distress in breast cancer patients receiving chemotherapy in the outpatient setting. Oncol Nurs Forum 1988 May/Jun; 15(3):343–348

Ferrell B et al. Effects of controlled-release morphine on quality of life for cancer pain. Oncol Nurs Forum 1989 Jul/Aug; 16(4):521–528

Fleck AE. Economic issues in the care of the elderly cancer patient. Semin Oncol Nurs 1988 Aug; 4(3):217–223

Foley MK. Children with cancer: Ethical dilemmas. Semin Oncol Nurs 1989 May; 5(2):109–113

Foltz AT. Nutritional factors in the prevention of gastrointestinal cancer. Semin Oncol Nurs 1988 Nov; 4(4):239–245

Foon KA. Advances in immunotherapy of cancer: Monoclonal antibodies and interferon. Semin Oncol Nurs 1988 May; 4(2):112–119

Foon KA. Biotherapy of cancer with interleukin-2, colony-stimulating factors, and monoclonal antibodies. Oncol Nurs Forum 1988 Nov/Dec; 15(6) Suppl 1:13–22

Frank–Stromborg M. Future projected trends in the care of the elderly individual with cancer, and implications. Semin Oncol Nurs 1988 Aug; 4(3):224–231

Frank–Stromborg M. The role of the nurse in cancer detection and screening. Semin Oncol Nurs 1986 Aug; 2(3):191–199

Fraser MC and Tucker MA. Host-susceptibility factors in cancer etiology. Semin Oncol Nurs 1986 Aug; 2(3):170–175

Fraser MC and Tucker MA. Second malignancies following cancer therapy.

Semin Oncol Nurs 1989 Feb; 5(1):43–55

Freeman J. Management of stomatitis symptoms. Dimens Oncol Nurs 1988 Fall; 2(3):14–17

Given BA and Given CW. Cancer nursing perspectives: Compliance among patients with cancer. Oncol Nurs Forum 1989 Jan/Feb; 16(1):97–103

Goodman M. Concepts of hormonal manipulation in the treatment of cancer. Oncol Nurs Forum 1988 Sep/Oct; 15(5):639–650

Goodman M. Managing the side effects of chemotherapy. Semin Oncol Nurs 1989 May; 5(2) Suppl 1:29–52

Grady C. Host defense mechanisms: An overview. Semin Oncol Nurs 1988 May; 4(2):86–94

Grant M. Nausea, vomiting, and anorexia. Semin Oncol Nurs 1987 Nov; 3(4):277–286

Grant MM. Nutritional interventions: Increasing oral intake. Semin Oncol Nurs 1986 Feb; 2(1):36–43

Graydon JE. Factors that predict patients' functioning following treatment for cancer. Int J Nurs Stud 1988; 25(2):117–124

Greene PE. The role of American Cancer Society in cancer public education. Semin Oncol Nurs 1986 Aug; 2(3):206–210

Gullo SM. Safe handling of antineoplastic drugs: Translating the recommendations into practice. Oncol Nurs Forum 1988 Sep/Oct; 15(5):595–602

Hadaway L. Evaluation and use of advanced I.V. technology—Part I: Central venous access devices. J Intraven Nurs 1989 Mar/Apr; 73–82

Haeuber D and DiJulio JE. Hemopoietic colony stimulating factors: An overview. Oncol Nurs Forum 1989 Mar/Apr; 16(2):247–262

Hagle ME. Implantable devices for chemotherapy: Access and delivery. Semin Oncol Nurs 1987 May; 3(2):96–105

Hahn MB and Jassak PF. Nursing management of patients receiving interferon. Semin Oncol Nurs 1988 May; 4(2):95–101

Haibeck SV. Intraoperative radiation therapy. Oncol Nurs Forum 1988 Mar/Apr; 15(2):143–150

Hanucharurnkul S. Predictors of self-care in cancer patients receiving radiotherapy. Cancer Nurs 1989 Feb; 12(1):21–27

Harnett S. Septic shock in the oncology patient. Cancer Nurs 1988 Aug; 12(4):191–201

Hassey KM. Principles of radiation safety and protection. Semin Oncol Nurs 1987 Feb; 3(1):23–29

Haughey BP et al. Breast self-examination: Reported practices, proficiency, and stage of disease at diagnosis. Oncol Nurs Forum 1988 May/Jun; 15(3):315–324

Haylock PJ. Breathing difficulty: Changes in respiratory function. Semin Oncol Nurs 1987 Nov; 3(4):293–298

Heiney SP. Assessing and intervening with dysfunctional families. Oncol

Nurs Forum 1988 Sep/Oct; 15(5):585–594

Herth KA. Relationship between level of hope and level of coping response and other variables in patients with cancer. Oncol Nurs Forum 1989 Jan/Feb; 16(1):67–74

Higgs D, Nagy C and Einhorn LH. Ifosfamide: A clinical review. Semin Oncol Nurs 1989 May; 5(2) Suppl 1:70

Hobbie WL and Schwartz CL. Endocrine late effects among survivors of cancer. Semin Oncol Nurs 1989 Feb; 5(1):14–21

Hoffman B. Cancer survivors at work: Job problems and illegal discrimination. Oncol Nurs Forum 1989 Jan/Feb; 16(1):39–48

Holden S and Felde G. Nursing care of patients receiving cisplatin-related peripheral neuropathy. Oncol Nurs Forum 1987 Jan/Feb; 14(1):13–20

Hymovich DP and Roehnert JE. Psychosocial consequences of childhood cancer. Semin Oncol Nurs 1989 Feb; 5(1):14–21

Jackson BS and Broadwell DC. Ostomy surgery: An overview of historical, current, and future perspectives. Semin Oncol Nurs 1986 Nov; 2(4):227–234

Jassak PF and Ryan MP. Ethical issues in clinical research. Semin Oncol Nurs 1989 May; 5(2):102–108

Jones LA. Superior vena cava syndrome: An oncologic complication. Semin Oncol Nurs 1987 Aug; 3(3):211–215

Jordan LN. Effects of fluid manipulation on the incidence of vomiting during outpatient cisplatin infusion. Oncol Nurs Forum 1989 Mar/Apr; 16(2):213–218

Kane NE et al. Use of patient-controlled analgesia in surgical oncology patients. Oncol Nurs Forum 1988 Jan/Feb; 15(1):29–32

Kaplan M. Investigation of age as a prognostic factor in early stage invasive cancer of the cervix: Implications for nursing. Cancer Nurs 1989 Jun; 12(3):177–182

Keller JF and Blausey LA. Nursing issues and management in chemotherapy-induced alopecia. Oncol Nurs Forum 1988 Sep/Oct; 15(5):603–610

Kramer J and Moore IM. Late effects of cancer therapy on the central nervous system. Semin Oncol Nurs 1989 Feb; 5(1):22–28

Kupchella CE. Environmental factors in cancer eitology. Semin Oncol Nurs 1986 Aug; 2(3):161–169

Lapin J et al. Guidelines for use of controlled-release oral morphine in cancer pain management: Correlation with clinical experience. Cancer Nurs 1988 Aug; 12(4):202–208

Leonard MA and Waskerwitz MJ. Late effects in adolescent survivors of childhood cancer. Semin Oncol Nurs 1986 May; 2(2):126–132

Lewis F and Levita M. Understanding radiotherapy. Cancer Nurs 1988 Jun; 11(3):174–185

Lierman LM. Phantom breast experiences after mastectomy. Oncol Nurs Forum 1988 Jan/Feb; 15(1):41–44

Lindsey AM. Cancer cachexia: Effects of

the disease and its treatment. Semin Oncol Nurs 1986 Feb; 2(1):19–29

Lisson EL. Ethical issues in pain management. Semin Oncol Nurs 1989 May; 5(2):114–119

Lydon J. Assessment of renal function in the patient receiving chemotherapy. Cancer Nurs 1989 Jun; 12(3):133–143

Lynch MT. The nurse's role in the biotherapy of cancer: Clinical trials and informed consent. Oncol Nurs Forum 1988 Nov/Dec; 15(6) Suppl 1:23–27

MacGeorge L, Steeves L and Steeves RH. Comparison of the mixing and reinfusion methods of drawing blood from a Hickman catheter. Oncol Nurs Forum 1988 May/Jun; 15(3):335–342

Maddock PG. Brachytherapy sources and applicators. Semin Oncol Nurs 1987 Feb; 3(1):15–22

Mahon S. Signs and symptoms associated with malignancy-induced hypercalcemia. Cancer Nurs 1989 Jun; 12(3):153–160

McCorkle R. The measurement of symptom distress. Semin Oncol Nurs 1987 Nov; 3(4):248–256

McMillan SC. The relationship between age and intensity of cancer-related symptoms. Oncol Nurs Forum 1989 Mar/Apr; 16(2):237–246

Meadows AT. Second malignant neoplasms in childhood cancer survivors. J Assoc Pediatr Oncol Nurses 1989; 6(1):7–11

Meeske K and Ruccione KS. Cancer chemotherapy in children: Nursing issues and approaches. Semin Oncol Nurs 1987 May; 3(2):118–127

Mioduszewski J and Zarbo AG. Ambulatory infusion pumps: A practical view at an alternative approach. Semin Oncol Nurs 1987 May; 3(2):106–111

Moldawer NP and Figlin RA. Tumor necrosis factor: Current clinical status and implications for nursing management. Semin Oncol Nurs 1988 May; 4(2):120–125

Monahan ML. Quality of life of adults receiving chemotherapy: A comparison of instruments. Oncol Nurs Forum 1988 Nov/Dec; 15(6):795–802

Morra ME. Choices: Who's going to tell the patients what they need to know? Oncol Nurs Forum 1988 Jul/Aug; 15(4):421–428

Moshang T Jr and Lee MM. Late effects: Disorders of growth and sexual maturation associated with the treatment of childhood cancer. J Assoc Pediatr Oncol Nurses 1988; 5(4):14–19

Mulvihill JJ and Byrne J. Genetic counseling of the cancer survivor. Semin Oncol Nurs 1989 Feb; 5(1):29–35

Nail LM and King KB. Fatigue. Semin Oncol Nurs 1987 Nov; 3(4):257–262

Northouse L. A longitudinal study of the adjustment of patients and husbands to breast cancer. Oncol Nurs Forum 1989 Jul/Aug; 16(4):511–520

Owen DC. Nurses' perspectives on the meaning of hope in patients with cancer: A qualitative study. Oncol Nurs Forum 1989 Jan/Feb; 16(1):75–86

Padavic-Shaller K. IL-2: Nursing applications in a developing science. Semin Oncol Nurs 1988 May; 4(2):142–150

Pape LH. Therapy-related acute leukemia: An overview. Cancer Nurs 1988 Oct; 11(5):295–302

Peters CAH. Myths of antiemetic administration. Cancer Nurs 1989 Apr; 12(2):102–106

Petrosino B, Becker H and Christian B. Infection rates in central venous catheter dressings. Oncol Nurs Forum 1988 Nov/Dec; 15(6):709–721

Poe CM and Taylor LM. Syndrome of inappropriate antidiuretic hormone: Assessment and nursing implications. Oncol Nurs Forum 1989 May/Jun; 16(3):373–386

Portenoy R. Practical aspects of pain control in the patient with cancer. CA 1988 Nov/Dec; 38(6):327–352

Quigley KM. The adult cancer survivor: Psychosocial consequences of cure. Semin Oncol Nurs 1989 Feb; 5(1):63–69

Reville B and Almadrones L. Continuous infusion chemotherapy in the ambulatory setting: The nurse's role in patient selection and education. Oncol Nurs Forum 1989 Jul/Aug; 16(4):529–538

Rose MA. Health promotion and risk prevention: Applications for cancer survivors. Oncol Nurs Forum 1989 May/Jun; 16(3):335–344

Rosenberg SA. Adoptive immunotherapy for cancer. Sci Am 1990 May; 262(5):62–69

Ruccione K and Weinberg K. Late effects in multiple body systems. Semin Oncol Nurs 1989 Feb; 5(1):4–13

Sansivero GE and Murray SA. Safe management of chemotherapy at home. Oncol Nurs Forum 1989 Sep/Oct; 16(5):711–718

Schulmeister L. Needle dislodgement from implanted venous access devices: Inpatient and outpatient experiences. J Intraven Nurs 1989 Mar/Apr; 12(2):90–92

Schwalb E and Crosson K. Helping you help your patients: The patient education program of the National Cancer Institute. Oncol Nurs Forum 1988 Sep/Oct; 15(5):651–661

Senn HJ, Glaus A and Schmid L (eds). Supportive care in cancer patients. Recent Results Cancer Res 1988; 108:1–342

Simon RC. Small gauge central venous catheters and right atrial catheters. Semin Oncol Nurs 1987 May; 3(2):87–95

Simpson C, Seipp CA and Rosenberg SA. The current status and future applications of interleukin-2 and adoptive immunotherapy cancer treatment. Semin Oncol Nurs 1988 May; 4(2):132–141

Souba WW and Copland EM III. Hyperalimentation in cancer. CA 1989 Mar/Apr; 39(2):105–114

Strohl RA. The nursing role in radiation oncology: Symptom management of acute and chronic reactions. Oncol Nurs Forum 1988 Jul/Aug; 15(4):429–438

Thomas CD. Insomnia: Identification and management. Semin Oncol Nurs 1987 Nov; 3(4):263–266

Thomasma DC. Ethics and professional practice in oncology. Semin Oncol Nurs 1989 May; 5(2):89–94

Thorne SE. Helpful and unhelpful communications in cancer care: The patient perspective. Oncol Nurs Forum 1988 Mar/Apr; 15(2):167–174

Varricchio CG and Jassak PF. Informed consent: An overview. Semin Oncol Nurs 1989 May; 5(2):95–98

Welch-McCaffery D and Dodge J. Acute confusional states in elderly cancer patients. Semin Oncol Nurs 1988 Aug; 4(3):208–216

Wickham R. Managing chemotherapy-related nausea and vomiting: The state of the art. Oncol Nurs Forum 1989 Jul/Aug; 16(4):563–578

Wilkie D et al. Cancer pain control behaviors: Description and correlation with pain intensity. Oncol Nurs Forum 1988 Nov/Dec; 15(6):723–734

Williams RD. Factors affecting the practice of breast self-examination in older women. Oncol Nurs Forum 1988 Sep/Oct; 15(5):611–624

Winningham ML et al. Effect of aerobic exercise on body weight and composition in patients with breast cancer on adjuvant chemotherapy. Oncol Nurs Forum 1989 Sep/Oct; 16(5):683–690

Woods NF, Lewis FM and Ellison ES. Living with cancer: Family experiences. Cancer Nurs 1989 Feb; 12(1):28–33

Workman ML. Immunologic late effects in children and adults. Semin Oncol Nurs 1989 Feb; 5(1):36–42

Yarbo CH. Carboplatin: A clinical review. Semin Oncol Nurs 1989 May; 5(2) Suppl 1:63–69

Yasko JM and Rust D. Trends in chemotherapy administration. Semin Oncol Nurs 1989 May; 5(2) Suppl 1:3–7

Zemore R and Shepel LF. Effects of breast cancer and mastectomy on emotional support and adjustment. Soc Sci Med 1989; 28(1):19–27

7
Care of the Older Adult

Health Maintenance and Preventive Care

Goals:
Maintain health and function.
Detect disease at an early stage.
Prevent deterioration of an existing condition.

A. Maintaining Health and Function.

1. Promote positive feeling about aging and health. Healthy elderly are those who are functionally independent and socially competent.
   a. Educate the older person about normal aging changes versus pathologic aging changes and atypical symptoms of disease, i.e., infection without fever, heart attack without chest pain.
   b. Foster independence by focusing on the individual's responsibility for own wellness and health promotion.
2. Encourage periodic health appraisal and counseling to give attention to health before illness develops, and to prevent deterioration of an existing condition. The principles of autonomy, minimal disruption of lifestyle, and avoidance of iatrogenic complications should be utilized in planning health promotion interventions.
3. Promote accident prevention among the elderly and their families.
   a. Inform elderly of high risk for falls and increased mortality from falls due to age, pathologic conditions, dysmobilities, decline in posture control, environmental risks, and medication.
   b. Clinically assess the patient using the functional model of health. Determine the patient's self-care abilities.
   c. Teach the older person and his family to periodically assess safety and environmental risks and to note major changes in functional ability.
4. Protect the patient against infectious diseases by immunization (especially against influenza and pneumonia).
5. Promote maintenance of preferred life-style, social interactions, and good mental health.
   a. Know risk factors—major losses of a sudden or unexpected nature, social isolation, relocation problems, dysmobility, and multiple drug use.
   b. Encourage to continue to take on intellectual challenges.
   c. Encourage a variety of interests and activities.
   d. Encourage and support interest in community and senior center activities aimed at prevention.

B. Detecting Disease at an Early Stage

1. Explain diagnostic tests available for early detection of problems, provide support and encouragement.
   a. Mammography—yearly screening x-ray of breasts to detect early cancers.
   b. Chest x-ray—for tuberculosis, lung cancer, heart size, changes in large blood vessels and bony structure of the chest.
   c. Testing the stool for blood (Hemoccult test)—to detect small, hidden amounts of blood in the stool.
   d. Sigmoidoscopy—periodic examination of the rectum and colon with a flexible tube that allows visualization. May be done in an outpatient setting.
   e. Tonometer test—to measure intraocular pressure for glaucoma.
   f. Blood glucose test—to detect diabetes mellitus.
   g. Papanicolaou smear—to detect cancer of the cervix.
   h. Hearing and vision tests.
   i. Assessment for alcoholism.
2. Emphasize accident prevention and safety in the environment.

C. Preventing Deterioration of an Existing Condition

Assess the patient's health habits and knowledge of disease.
1. Advise to remain as physically active as functionally possible.
2. Encourage to stop smoking.
3. Educate about proper foot care.
4. Ensure proper nutrition and monitor weight.
5. Educate about the risks of drug interactions and polypharmacy.
6. Provide education programs on specific health problems of the elderly.

D. Community Resources

1. Include preretirement counseling.
2. Ideally, every person over 70 who is living alone should be visited regularly by a health visitor (nurse, social worker, volunteer health aide).

3. Use comprehensive services available for elderly: diagnostic centers, extended care facilities, home care programs, homemaker services, "Meals on Wheels," day care centers, mental health services, vocational projects, continuing education, foster grandparents, social services, and congregate meal sites.

Health Problems of the Aged
Underlying Considerations

1. Although aging is not synonymous with illness, the aged are vulnerable to disease because of decreased physiologic reserve, less flexible homeostatic processes, and less effective defense mechanisms of the body.
2. An estimated 85% of elderly have some form of chronic illness, although the existence of chronic illnesses may or may not relate to the extent of functional impairment or disability.
3. Disease in the aged does not always present classic signs and symptoms; the usual clinical manifestations may be absent, attenuated, or disguised; atypical signs and symptoms may be present.
4. Depression and dementia often worsen health problems. Alterations in mental status often reflect an alteration in physical health.
5. Coping abilities and energies may be diminished when crises and readjustment demands are highest—causing increased stress.
6. Illnesses tend to cluster during the closing years of the very old person's life.

Disease Aspects

(Consult index for specific disease.)

Mental Health Aspects/ Psychological Needs

1. Basic psychological needs of all people include respect, security, self-esteem, and the need to feel appreciated and valued by others.
2. The maintenance of "self" (autonomy, integrity, identity) is important to the psychological survival of the elderly. A sense of self develops from one's life goals, values, and roles.
3. Personality traits tend to be stable throughout life—including old age.
4. The elderly person is vulnerable to emotional and mental stress from many losses.
   a. Losses through death of spouse, children, "significant others."
   b. Loss of social roles and resources—affects status and prestige.
   c. Socioeconomic losses—decreased income and inflation affect quality of health care, self-esteem, and position in society.
   d. Loss of work role produces sense of uselessness, feelings of nonparticipation. The role of the aging person in our society is not clear. Adaptation to role change is a major issue.
5. Successful aging depends on accommodation to the inevitable changes of growing older in our society.

Psychiatric and Cognitive Disorders

The psychiatric disorders of late life are a major cause of chronic ill health and disability. Disorders include depression, paranoid reactions, and dementias. An estimated 15% of elderly persons in the U.S. suffer from a psychiatric disorder. Only 3% of patients being treated for psychiatric problems are elderly. This age group is a very underserved population.

Depression

A. Basic Considerations

1. Most common emotional disorder of the aged, occurring in 10% of community-dwelling elderly and 10% to 20% of those in long-term care facilities. Major depression (as defined by DSM-R III criteria) is less prevalent in the aged and presents with the same symptom profile that identifies the younger depressed patient.
2. Late-life depression is characterized by apathy, sense of hopelessness and exhaustion, loss of interest, weight loss, and somatic or persecutory delusional themes. Less severe depressive symptoms are very prevalent in the elderly.
3. Several factors contribute to the underdiagnosing and poor treatment of depression in the aged. These factors include:
   a. Co-morbidity. Presence of neurologic or medical disease processes.
   b. Medications.
   c. Under-reporting of depressive symptoms by patient.
   d. The acceptance by family, physician, and other health care professionals of dysphoria as a manifestation of normal aging.
4. Depression may be masked as a cognitive disturbance in the elderly.
5. Older people (who make up 12% of the population) account for about 25% of reported suicides.

B. Assessment

1. Look for physical signs and symptoms that may manifest depression: weight loss, lethargy, sleep disorders, poor concentration.
2. Take a drug history (including over-the-counter preparations); many drugs can cause depression in the elderly.
3. Be aware of medical conditions associated with depression.

C. Nursing Interventions

1. Be aware that the depressed elderly may be mislabeled as "demented"—pseudodementia or depressive dementia. Assess mental status using an objective mental status evaluation tool.
2. Allow the patient to release anger, grief, feelings of hopelessness.
3. Treatment consists of drugs, psychotherapy, and occasionally electroconvulsive therapy (ECT). Reversibility is directly related to early recognition and intervention.

Paranoia

A. Basic Considerations

1. Paranoia is characterized by suspicion and ideas of persecution. Often accompanies first-time major depression in late life.

2. Frequently accompanied by concomitant neurologic disorder.
3. Highly correlated with sensory deficits and loneliness.

B. Management

1. Careful assessment of and treatment of underlying disorder.
2. Correction of sensory deficits.
3. Supportive counseling.

Senile Dementia of the Alzheimer's Type (Alzheimer's Disease)

Alzheimer's disease is an irreversible type of dementia characterized by progressive impairments of memory, cognition, language, judgment, and ability for self-care. Its cause remains unknown.

Alzheimer's disease is the most common form of dementia among the aged, affecting approximately 20% of the population at age 80. It is the major cause of institutionalization of the elderly.

Pathophysiology

1. Gross pathophysiologic changes include cortical atrophy, enlarged ventricles, and basal ganglia wasting. Biochemically, neurotransmitter systems have structural and functional impairments.
2. Microscopically, changes occur in the proteins of the nerve cells of the cerebral cortex and lead to accumulation of neurofibrillary tangles (abnormal) and characteristic senile plaques (deposits of protein and altered cell structures on the interneuronal junctions).
3. Research scientists report there is evidence of a significant and progressive decrease in the activity of the enzyme choline acetyltransferase (ChaT) in the brain tissue. Choline acetyltransferase is a crucial ingredient in the chemical process that produces acetylcholine, a neurotransmitter involved in *learning and memory*. This cholinergic deficit is the theoretical basis for several research studies into causes and treatments of Alzheimer's disease.
4. Other neurotransmitters, including norepinephrine, serotonin, and somatostatin, are affected by Alzheimer's disease and appear to have some relevance to memory function.

Theories of Causation

1. Genetic theory supported by:
   a. An increased prevalence of Alzheimer's disease in some families.
   b. Neuropathologic similarities between Alzheimer's disease and trisomy 21 (Down's syndrome).
2. Environmental theory
   a. Head injury—following a latency period of many years; pathologic findings include neurofibrillary tangles.
   b. Infectious agents—possible association between Alzheimer's disease histopathology and several viral agents, including herpes simplex and rabies.
   c. Neurotoxins—aluminum and silicon, two common elements, are found in the brains of Alzheimer's patients. These minerals can be neurotoxic, are found to be increased in the Alzheimer's diseased brain, but no connecting link has yet been found.

Clinical Manifestations

Early to terminal stages

1. *Intellectual*—forgetfulness, impaired judgment, memory loss, confusion, apraxia, amnesia, speech difficulty, muteness, no eye contact.
2. *Behavioral–Personality*—mood changes, withdrawal, depression, catastrophic behavioral reactions, aggression, agitation, inability to cooperate, unaware of environment.
3. *Functional*—work difficulties, poor hygiene, insomnia, wandering, gait disturbance, incontinence, perseveration, immobility, dysphagia.

Diagnostic Criteria

Diagnosis of probable Alzheimer's disease is based on clinically determined dementia confirmed by:
1. Two or more cognitive deficits.
2. Progressive worsening of memory and other cognitive functions.
3. No disturbances of consciousness.
4. Onset between 40 and 90 years of age.
5. Absence of systemic disorders or other brain disorders that could cause progressive deficits in memory and cognition.
6. Elimination of all potentially reversible causes of dementia.

Management Principles

1. Focus is on caring rather than cure.
2. Approach is multidisciplinary.
3. Family members must be involved in management and care plan.
4. Patients should be regularly assessed and monitored for signs of additional physical illness, sensory deficits, and functional impairments.
5. Emphasis is placed on patient's strengths and abilities and on preventing excess disability.

Nursing Process: The Person With Alzheimer's Disease

Nursing Assessment

1. Assess level of cognitive functioning using objective mental status examination.
2. Obtain history from family or significant other. Assess for progressive signs of short-term memory loss, impairment of judgment, loss of insight.
3. Assess for signs and symptoms of diseases that might affect level of cognition, e.g., delirium, hypothyroidism, folate deficiency.
4. Review patient record for medical history of reversible causes of dementia.

Nursing Diagnoses

1. Altered thought processes related to Alzheimer's disease.
2. Potential for injury related to impulsive behavior and confusion.
3. Ineffective individual coping related to catastrophic behaviors secondary to cognitive losses.
4. Self-care deficits related to inability to perform activities of daily living.
5. Sleep pattern disturbances related to anxiety, confusion, and activity/rest imbalance.

6. Altered nutrition (less than body requirements) related to confusion, lack of appetite, and imbalance of food intake and activity.
7. Altered family processes related to care of an ill family member.

Nursing Interventions

A. Maintaining Optimal Cognitive Function

1. Employ a calm, pleasant approach.
   a. Identify yourself, repeatedly if necessary. Call patient by name.
   b. Gain eye contact when speaking or working with patient.
   c. Touch the patient to reinforce contact.
   d. Assign same staff to patient as much as possible.
   e. Avoid changing patient's room if possible.
   f. Always approach patient in a consistent way.
2. Increase environmental cues.
   a. Color-code halls and doors; use labels and photos, name tags, etc.
   b. Use calendar, clock in patient's room.
   c. Encourage family to bring items from home familiar to patient.
   d. Keep personal items that patient uses in the same place.
   e. Use lists and written reminders and instructions.
   f. Keep a consistent schedule of daily activities.
3. Enhance communication.
   a. Speak slowly—use short clear statements.
   b. Avoid unnecessary decision-making situations.
   c. Don't move around when talking with patient.
   d. Use nonverbal cues to enhance verbal communication—gestures and touch.
   e. Listen to what the patient says and confirm message with patient.
   f. Ask yes–no questions.
4. See that activities maintain or reestablish normal social roles as much as possible.
   a. Assist patient to continue daily routine.
   b. Take patient outdoors.
   c. Conduct activities that have meaning for the patient.
   d. Encourage social encounters with family and friends.

B. Maintaining Physical Safety

1. Control the environment.
   a. Check for and control or eliminate obvious hazards.
   b. Prevent wandering outside of home or institution.
2. Reduce potential for injury.
   a. Use low bed, or put bed in low position when patient is left alone.
   b. Use night lights.
   c. Have patient wear sturdy slip-on shoes with firm soles for walking.
   d. Check patient's eyeglasses to see that they are clean and in good repair.
   e. Monitor all medications.
   f. Monitor all patients who smoke.
3. Promoting independence within safe environment.
   a. Avoid restraints.
   b. See that patient wears identification tag.

C. Promoting Coping and Orientation

1. Control environment to limit or prevent adverse behaviors.
   a. Avoid changing rooms.
   b. Don't move patient's personal belongings unnecessarily.
   c. Allow patient to "hoard" some things.
   d. Avoid excess stimulation.
   e. Maintain a regular routine.
   f. Accept forgetfulness—don't ask patient to "try harder to remember."
   g. Avoid attempting to reason with patient—reassure and be calm.
   h. Redirect patient—use distraction.
2. Enhance positive self-image and help to maintain dignity.
   a. Offer activities for patient—music, pets, exercise, simple chores.
   b. Don't talk about patient in his presence.
   c. Give positive direction and praise.

D. Promoting Maximum Independence in Activities of Daily Living

1. Prevent premature or excess disability.
   a. Use assistive devices.
   b. Use safety devices, i.e., tub bench, hand rails.
   c. Allow choices in clothing, foods, etc.
   d. Monitor all activities unobtrusively.
2. Facilitate independent ambulation.
   a. Encourage use of assistive device if needed.
   b. Avoid physical restraints.
   c. Avoid use of chemical restraints.
3. Promote continence.
   a. Provide privacy.
   b. Monitor fluid intake.
   c. Encourage fiber in diet.
   d. Monitor bowel movements to prevent constipation or impaction.
   e. Mark bathroom with color-coding or picture to facilitate remembering.
4. Monitor for signs and symptoms of illness.

E. Promoting a Balance of Sleep and Activity

1. Provide a schedule that promotes a balance of activity and sleep.
   a. Encourage regular exercise in daytime.
   b. Avoid daytime naps.
   c. Avoid use of hypnotics and sedatives that may have daytime "hangover" effect.
2. Reduce distractions and promote comfort at bedtime.
   a. Don't awaken patient for procedures or medications.
   b. Use night lights.
   c. Avoid restraints—provide safe environment instead.
   d. Provide comfort measures if patient wakens at night, i.e. toileting, back rub, blanket, drink.

F. Maintaining Optimal Nutrition and Stable Body Weight

1. Weigh patient weekly to monitor for weight change.
2. Monitor food and water intake—patient forgets to eat and drink.
   a. Remind patient to eat.
   b. Use "cueing" to promote independent feeding.
3. Provide pleasant environment for eating.
   a. Encourage feeding independently by using adaptive equipment, finger foods.
   b. Offer familiar foods that the patient likes.
   c. Offer high-protein snacks several times daily.
4. Encourage, monitor, and assist with regular mouth care.
5. Encourage use of dentures.

G. Promoting Family Coping and Support

1. Assess family's level of knowledge of disease.
2. Provide information as needed.
   a. Offer written material that family can read and refer to.
   b. Offer inservice programs on communication skills and home nursing skills.
   c. Encourage family to do legal and financial planning.
   d. Inform family of changes in patient's condition and level of functioning.
3. Encourage care-giver/family members to work through personal feelings about patient's disability and illness.
   a. Refer to family support groups.
   b. Have regular family meetings so that family actively participates in planning care.
   c. Encourage care-giver to maintain own physical and mental well-being.
   d. Support family decision for placement in an extended care facility if it becomes necessary.
4. Initiate referrals to community agencies.
   a. Refer to Alzheimer's Disease and Related Disorders Association.
   b. Encourage use of respite care.
   c. Refer to community case management service if available.

Evaluation

1. Shows reduction in confused behavior; demonstrates an awareness of environment and a gross orientation to time and place.
2. Does not wander out of home/institution; absence of accidents and falls.
3. Demonstrates fewer catastrophic reactions; participates in activities.
4. Demonstrates independence in performing activities of daily living; uses assistive devices.
5. Sleeps on a regular schedule.
6. Maintains weight within acceptable range; eats independently.
7. Family provides appropriate care and support; seeks help from community agencies and support group.

General Assessment of the Older Adult

In addition to the health history and physical examination, the nursing assessment involves an attempt to determine the functioning ability, strengths, and limitations of the patient.

Physiologic Assessment

1. How does the patient describe the activities of a "typical" day? (Assess for the usual level of functioning.)
2. How does he view his health?
3. How does he perform activities of daily living (ADLs) (dressing, feeding, bathing, toileting, transferring)?
4. How does he perform instrumental activities of daily living? (telephoning, shopping, cleaning, laundry, meal preparation, finances)?
5. How much physical capacity does the patient have? Has there been a recent change in capacity?
6. How much muscle strength and coordination does the patient have? Does he need assistive devices for safe ambulation?
7. How well does the patient see and hear? Does he have glasses or a hearing aid? What are dates of last vision and hearing tests?
8. What are the patient's usual eating, sleeping, elimination, and activity patterns? What constitutes a "normal" bowel movement? Does he use laxatives or enemas regularly?
9. How does the patient handle his sexual feelings?
10. Are there any recent changes in ADL ability?
11. What will the patient have to do to regain or maintain functioning ability?

Socioeconomic Assessment

1. What is the patient's background? Occupational history?
2. How many person-to-person contacts does the patient have in a day? Telephone contacts?
3. Who is the patient's significant other? (Include pet.) Are there good social supports (friends, family)?
4. Who visits the patient?
5. What is the patient's religion?
6. What are the patient's living arrangements? Are there stairs? Access to bathroom, bedroom, and kitchen on one level?
7. Is the patient in proximity to relatives or helping neighbors? Is there an emergency response in place for the patient who lives alone?
8. Are the patient's activities limited because of limited income? High-crime environment?
9. Does the patient drive? Are there transportation problems?
10. What are the patient's feelings about living independently?
11. Does the patient participate in any phase of community life?
12. How can the environment be adjusted to maintain independence?

Psychological Assessment

1. Is the patient alert and oriented?
2. Assess the patient's mental status using an established mental status assessment tool.
3. What does the patient identify as his major concerns and problems?
4. What are the patient's attitudes toward aging?
5. What are the patient's attitudes toward himself as he ages?
6. What psychological defenses does the patient use?
7. What are the patient's activities, interests, and hobbies?
8. What coping skills did the patient successfully use in the past? Can he still use those coping skills?
9. Is there dysphoria?
10. Assess patient's mood using established tool for depression screening.

Management of Special Needs and Problems

Nutritional Considerations for the Aged

A. **Nutritional Requirements of the Elderly**—are similar to those of other adults, although little information is actually available on nutritional requirements for the elderly.

1. It has been found that modest weight gain may be associated with decreased mortality in the elderly.

Calorie intake should be adjusted on an individual basis.
2. Health care providers often fail to recognize nutritional problems in elderly patients.
3. Loss of weight and vitamin deficiencies are common problems in the frail elderly.
4. Protein requirements are not reduced, but protein utilization may be less efficient in old age.
5. High-nutrient-density foods should be consumed to obtain adequate intake.

B. Risks for Malnutrition—Those elderly people most at risk are women, the poor, those with alcoholism, and elderly persons living alone.
1. Any recent weight change should be assessed—an unintentional weight loss of greater than 10% in 6 months is significant.
2. Protein calorie malnutrition is the most common type.
3. Obesity—defined as more than 20% above ideal body weight, can impede mobility and add to risk from cardiac disease.
4. Nutritional state of cognitively impaired individual must be carefully assessed and diet history confirmed with family member or care-giver.

C. Factors Affecting Nutritional Habits of the Elderly
1. Food habits of a life-time.
2. Social factors (eating alone).
3. Susceptibility to food fads (over-the-counter supplements, megavitamins).
4. Dental problems.
5. Mobility and sensory deficits that prevent shopping and/or preparation of food.
6. Reduced income.
7. Decreased appeal of food—loss of taste buds; less acute sense of smell.
8. Drug-induced malnutrition due to changes in appetite and taste.
9. Alcohol abuse.
10. Transportation problems.
11. Effects of chronic illness.

D. Assistance Programs
1. Community-based meal centers.
2. Multipurpose senior centers.
3. Supplemental Social Security income.
4. Home-delivered meals; "Meals on Wheels."
5. Friendly visitor program.
6. Nutritional counseling.
7. Food stamps.
8. Day care for the elderly.
9. Self-help eating devices.

Drug Therapy and the Aged

A. Factors Altering Drug Responses in the Elderly
1. Age-related changes predispose elderly to problems with medication side effects.
2. Absorption, distribution, metabolism, and excretion of many drugs are affected by aging.
   a. *Absorption*—affected by gastric *p*H, rate of gastric emptying, reduction in intestinal blood flow.
   b. *Distribution*—affected by alterations in body composition, protein binding, tissue permeability. There is a decline in lean body mass and total body water, and increase in total body fat.

   c. *Metabolism*—decreased metabolic capacity for detoxifying drugs and decreased number of receptors at which drug may act; diminished cardiac output.
   d. *Excretion*—renal clearance may be limiting factor. Age-related loss of function of liver and kidneys may contribute to decreased elimination of drugs.

B. Nursing Interventions to Improve Medication Use
1. Be aware that the potential for adverse reactions, interactions, and medication-induced disease is greater in older persons.
   a. Older persons may not be able to handle multiple medications due to cognitive or sensory deficits.
   b. They appear to be more sensitive to digoxin, diuretics, aspirin, long-acting oral antidiabetic drugs, sedatives, analgesics, psychotropics, etc.
   c. The more medications the patient takes, the greater is the risk for drug interactions and adverse reactions.
2. Obtain a nursing and drug history.
   a. Check nutritional status.
   b. Find out if the patient is taking drugs not currently prescribed.
   c. Ask what over-the-counter medications the patient is taking. The elderly use twice as many nonprescription preparations as those that are prescribed.
   d. Assess for alcohol usage.
3. Usually the physician will hold the dosage to the lowest effective amount. "Start low, go slow" is the guiding axiom.
   a. Reinforce verbal instructions with WRITTEN instructions. Use large print and simple wording.
   b. Have the patient repeat the instructions.
   c. Give instructions also to a relative/friend to reinforce patient education.
   d. Write what the drug is used for (e.g., "to thin the blood").
   e. Explain possible side effects.
   f. Be sure that the drug name and instructions for taking it are typed in large letters on the label. Bottles may have color-coded strips.
   g. Make sure that the patient can open medication container; child-proof container may not be appropriate.
   h. Arrange drug schedule to coincide with regular activity (arising, eating, retiring). Simplify the drug regimen.
   i. Arrange a check-off system, using a calendar or chart.
   j. Instruct patient to discard all old or unneeded drugs.
4. Carry out periodic drug review.
   a. Ask the patient to bring all medication on next visit to physician or clinic. Ask to see all medications on home care visits.
   b. Assess for patient compliance, response to therapy, possible side effects, drug interactions. Rate of noncompliance is high in elderly.
   c. Have the patient ask pharmacist to keep his drug profile on computer—used as a safeguard to detect potential drug interactions.
   d. Advise patient to ask for samples or two prescriptions (for short term and long term use) when a new drug is being prescribed. This is less expensive for the patient in the event of an adverse reaction or side effect.

e. Enlist help of all health care team members to reinforce proper drug use.

Hygienic Care

A. Skin Care

1. Aging skin is dry, thin, and inelastic; sweat gland and sebaceous gland activity and water-binding capacity of skin are decreased.
2. Bathe every other day using a mild, super-fatted soap.
3. After damp-drying the skin, use a nonocclusive emollient (a petrolatum or lanolin-based preparation) to prevent transepidermal water loss.
4. Avoid prolonged exposure to the sun.
5. Consult dermatologist if redness, pruritus, or new skin growths appear.

B. Oral Care

1. Common oral complaints include loss of teeth, dry mouth, abnormal taste, and burning sensations in mouth. Some of these can be side effects of medication and can seriously affect nutritional state.
2. Components of dental/oral care include proper diet, maintaining health of oral and denture-bearing structures, and using available dental services.
   a. Use electric toothbrush and WaterPic to remove retained food particles between teeth.
   b. Encourage increased fluid intake in persons with decreased salivary flow.

C. Elimination Problems (see p. 142)

D. Foot Care

1. One third of the elderly have foot disorders. Degenerative and systemic diseases, trauma, neglect, and misuse cause foot problems in the elderly.
2. Systemic diseases such as diabetes mellitus, arterial insufficiency, and the arthritides often are compounded by loss of sensation, abnormal gait patterns, and impaired vision; the assessment made by the nurse is of prime importance.
3. Nail disorders account for about one-fourth of foot complaints.
4. See p. 562 for assessment of feet.

Summary of Principles of Managing the Elderly

1. Understand the physiologic, psychological, and social changes of normal aging.
2. Conduct careful clinical assessment and identification of the patient's responses to illness and dysfunction.
3. Assess and adapt the environment to facilitate maximal functioning.
4. Individualize nursing care, taking into consideration the patient's past experiences, needs, and individual goals.
5. Set realistic and attainable goals with the patient; help him gain a sense of accomplishment and purpose and control over his own life.
6. Encourage active participation in plan of care.
   a. Learn something about the patient before the initial encounter. Help the patient identify his coping skills and patterns.
   b. Focus on strengths and abilities.
   c. Ask the patient's opinions.
   d. Encourage the patient to keep control over his own life and to make choices and decisions.
   e. Avoid making decisions for him; this promotes low self-esteem, dependency, and depression.
   f. Praise achievements.
   g. Support the patient during periods of anxiety; allow expression of troubles and difficulties.
   h. Urge the patient to remain active and continue preferred life-style. Direct attention to gains being made and to the controls the patient still retains.
7. Carry out nursing activities with the patient rather than for him.
8. Realize that necessary modifications and compromises imposed by the physiologic limits of normal aging must be made in the medical and nursing management of the patient.
9. Encourage elderly persons to remain in the mainstream of life to prevent physical, emotional, and mental deterioration.
10. Act as an advocate of the elderly.
11. Periodically and systematically evaluate the patient's progress toward attainment of goals.

Bibliography

Books

American Nurses Association. Standards and Scope of Gerontological Nursing Practice. Kansas City, MO, American Nurses Association, 1987

Bergener M and Reisberg B. Diagnosis and Treatment of Senile Dementia. New York, Springer–Verlag, 1989

Billig N. To Be Old and Sad: Understanding Depression in the Elderly. Lexington, MA, Lexington Books, 1986

Buchholz D. Sleep disorders. In Bayless TM, Brain MO and Cherniack RM. Current Therapy in Internal Medicine—2. Philadelphia, BC Decker, 1987

Burnside I. Nursing care. In Jarvik LF and Winograd EH (eds): Treatments for the Alzheimer's Patient. New York, Springer, 1988

Burnside IM. Nursing and the Aged: A Self Care Approach. 3rd ed. New York, McGraw–Hill, 1988

Callahan D. Setting Limits: Medical Goals in an Aging Society. New York, Simon & Schuster, 1987

Carnevali DL and Patrick M. Nursing Management for the Elderly. 2nd ed. Philadelphia, JB Lippincott, 1986

Cohen D and Eisdorfer C. The Loss of Self: A Family Resource for the Care of Alzheimer's Disease and Related Disorders. New York, WW Norton, 1986

Congress of the United States, Office of Technology Assessment. Losing a Million Minds: Confronting the Tragedy of Alzheimer's Disease and Others. Washington, DC, U.S. Government Printing Office, 1987

Eliopoulos C. Gerontological Nursing. 2nd ed. Philadelphia, JB Lippincott, 1987

Eliopoulos C. A Guide to the Nursing Care of the Aging. Baltimore, Williams & Wilkins, 1987

Esberger KK and Hughes S (ed). Nursing Care of the Aged. Norwalk, CT, Appleton & Lange, 1989

Gallo JJ, Reichel W and Anderson L. Handbook of Geriatric Assessment. Rockville, MD, Aspen Publishers, 1988

Golden S. Nursing a Loved One at Home. Philadelphia, Running Press, 1988

Holden VP and Woods RT. Reality Orientation. 2nd ed. New York, Churchill–Livingstone, 1988

Jarvik LF and Winograd CH (eds). Treatments for the Alzheimer's Patient. New York, Springer, 1988

Kalicki AC. Confronting Alzheimer's Disease. Owings Mills, MD, National Health Publishing, 1987

Kane R and Kane R. Assessing the Elderly. 2nd ed. Lexington, MA, Lexington Books, 1989

Kane RL, Ouslander JG and Abrass IB. Essentials of Clinical Geriatrics. 2nd ed. New York, McGraw-Hill, 1989

Kermis M. Mental Health in Late Life. Boston, MA, Jones & Bartlett Publishers, 1986

Lavizzo–Mourey R, et al. Practicing Prevention for the Elderly. Philadelphia, Hanley & Belfers, 1989

Levin NJ. How to Care for Your Parents. Washington DC, Storm King Press, 1987

Mourad L. Nursing Care of Adults with Orthopedic Conditions. 2nd ed. New York, John Wiley & Sons, 1988

National Institutes of Health Consensus Development Conference Statement. Differential Diagnosis of Dementing Diseases. U.S. Department of Health and Human Services, Public Health Service, July, 1987

Palmer M. Urinary Incontinence. Silver Spring, MD, National Gerontological Nursing Association, 1986

Reichel W. Clinical Aspects of Aging. 3rd ed. New York, Williams & Wilkins, 1989

Rossman I. Clinical Geriatrics. 3rd ed. Philadelphia, JB Lippincott, 1986

Surgeon General's Workshop, Health Promotion and Aging. Rockville, MD. U.S. Dept of Health and Human Services, Public Health Service, 1988

U.S. Dept of Health and Human Services, Public Health Service. Health Resources for Older Women. NIH Publication Number 87-2899, 1987

Volicer L, Fabiscewski K and Rheaume Y. Clinical Management of Alzheimer's Disease. Rockville, MD, Aspen Publishers, 1987

Walsh JR, Tsukuda RA, and Miller J. Management of the Frail Elderly by the Health Care Team. St. Louis, MO, Warren H. Green, 1989

Warne RW and Primsley DM. A Manual of Geriatric Care. New York, Williams & Wilkins, 1988

Zgola Y. Doing Things: A Guide to Programs and Organized Activities for Persons with Alzheimer's Disease and Related Disorders. Baltimore, MD, Johns Hopkins University Press, 1987

Journals

Barnes B and Donovan K. Functional outcomes after hip fractures. Phys Ther 1987 Nov; 67(11):1675–1679

Besdine RW, Wakefield KM and Williams TF. Assessing function in the elderly. Patient Care 1988 Jan; 22(2):69–79

Blazer D. Current concepts: Depression in the elderly. N Engl J Med 1989 Jan 19; 320(3):164–166

Bobb JK. Trauma in the elderly. J Gerontol Nurs 1987 Nov; 13(11):46–48

Boller F et al. Recording neurological symptoms and signs in Alzheimer's disease. Amer J Alzheimer's Care Res 1987 May-Jun 2(3):19–29

Brockenshire A. The "mini-mental state": A handy tool. Perspectives 1987 Winter; 11(4):7–8

Busse GC and Materson BJ. Geriatric hypertension: The growing use of calcium-channel blockers. Geriatrics 1988 Feb; 43(2):51–58

Consensus Conference, National Institutes of Health. Urinary incontinence. JAMA 1989 May 12; 261(18):2685–2690

Dreyfus JK. Depression assessment and interventions in the medically ill frail elderly. J Gerontol Nurs 1988 Sep; 14(9):27–36, 38–39

Escher JE, O'Dell C and Gambert SR. Typical geriatric accidents and how to prevent them. Geriatrics 1989 May; 44(5):54–69

Evans L and Strumpf N. Tying down the elderly: A review of the literature on physical restraint. J Am Geriatr Soc 1989 Jan; 37(1):65–75

Fabiszewski K. Caring for the Alzheimer's patient. Gerontologist 1987 Feb; 6(2):53–58

Fink A et al. Assuring the quality of health care for older persons. JAMA 1987 Oct 9; 258(14):1905–1908

Fitten L et al. Depression: UCLA geriatric grand rounds. J Am Geriatr Soc 1989 May; 37(5):459–472

Foreman MD. Reliability and validity of mental status questionaires in elderly hospitalized patients. Nurs Res 1987 Jul-Aug; 36(4):216–220

Gomez G and Gomez E. Dementia? Or delirium? Geriatr Nurs 1989 May-Jun; 10(3):141–142

Hall GR. Care of the patient with Alzheimer's disease living at home. Nurs Clin North Am 1988 Mar; 23(1): 31–46

Harper CM and Lyles YM. Physiology and complications of bed rest. J Am Geriatr Soc 1988 Nov; 36(11):1047–1054

Henderson V and Finch CE. The neurobiology of Alzheimer's disease. J Neurosurg 1989 Mar; 70:335–353

Jess LW. Investigating impaired mental status. Nursing 1988 Jun; 18(6):42–50

Johnson L and Keller KL. Staging Alzheimer's disease. Geriatr Nurs 1989 Jul-Aug; 10(4):196–197

Katz S and Stroud MW. Functional assessment in geriatrics: A review of progress and directions. J Am Geriatr Soc 1989 Mar; 37(3):267–272

Larson EB, Lo B and Williams ME. Evaluation and care of elderly patients with dementia. J Gen Intern Med 1986 Mar-Apr; 1(2):116–126

Lavizzo–Mourey R. Special skills for the clinical management of the older patient. Geriatrics 1988 Dec; 43(Suppl):3–10

Levy L. A practical guide to care of the Alzheimer's disease victim: The cognitive disability perspective. Top Geriatr Rehab 1986 Feb; 1(2):16–26

Linderborn KM. The need to assess dementia. J Gerontol Nurs 1988 Jan; 14(1):35–39, 40–42

Lipkin LV and Faude KJ. "Dementia"— Educating the caregiver. J Gerontol Nurs 1987 Nov; 13(11):23–27, 46–48

Mace NL. Principles of activities for persons with dementia. Phys Occup Ther Geriatr 1987 Spring; 5(3):13–27

MacKay S et al. Methods to assess aphasic stroke patients. Geriatr Nurs 1988 May-Jun; 9(3):177–179

McIntosh L. Hospital-based case management. Nurs Econ 1987 Sep-Oct; 5(5):232–236

Merriam AE et al. The psychiatric symptoms of Alzheimer's disease. J Am Geriatr Soc 1988 Jan; 36(1):7–12

O'Dell C. Atypical presentation of neurological illness in the elderly. Geriatrics 1988 Jan; 43(1):35–37

Parsons MT and Levy J. Nursing process in injury prevention. J Gerontol Nurs 1987 Jul; 13(7):36–40

Pinholt EM et al. Functional assessment of the elderly. Arch Intern Med 1987 Mar; 147(3):484–488

Rapp SR and Davis KM. Geriatric depression: Physicians' knowledge, perceptions and diagnostic practices. Gerontologist 1989 Feb; 29(2):252–257

Reisbery B. Dementia: A systematic approach to identifying reversible causes. Geriatrics 1986 Apr; 41(4):30–46

Ronsman KM. Pseudodementia—False confusion. Geriatr Nurs 1988 Jan-Feb; 9(1):50–52

Rosenthal MJ and Naliboff B. Postural hypotension: Its meaning and management in the elderly. Geriatrics 1988 Dec; 43(12):31–42

Seiler WC and Stahelin HB. Practical management of catheter-associated UTI. Geriatrics 1988 Aug; 43(8):43–48

Spellbring AM et al. Improving safety for hospitalized elders. J Gerontol Nurs 1988 Feb; 14(2):31–37, 46–47

Strumpf NE and Evans LE. Physical restraint of the hospitalized elderly: Perceptions of patients and nurses. Nurs Res 1988 May-Jun; 37(3):132–137

Teri L, Larson EB and Reifler BV. Behavioral disturbance in dementia of the Alzheimer's type. J Am Geriatr Soc 1988 Jan; 36(1):1–6

Weiler K and Buckwalter KC. Care of the demented client. J Gerontol Nurs 1988 Jul; 14(7):26–31, 37–38

Young SH, Muir-Nash J and Ninos M. Managing nocturnal wandering. J Gerontol Nurs 1988 May; 14(5):6–12, 38–39

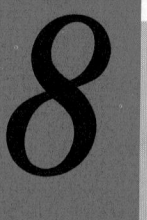

8 Rehabilitation Nursing

Rehabilitation Concepts

Rehabilitation involves an active, dynamic program and learning process aimed at enabling an ill or disabled person to achieve the highest level of physical, cognitive, psychological, social, educational, vocational, and economic functioning of which he is capable.

Goal of Rehabilitation

To enable an ill or disabled person to function optimally by the use of an individualized approach.

Rehabilitation Team

Rehabilitation is a creative process; it calls for a team of health care professionals working together and contributing their specialized services for a common goal for one person. In group sessions the team members evaluate the patient's progress and make necessary program changes.
  1. *Patient*—key member of the health care team; he participates in goal-setting, learning, and working on his individual rehabilitation program so that he eventually can control his own life.
  2. *Patient's family*—incorporated into the team; participating in problem-solving and care and in giving ongoing support.
  3. *Rehabilitation nurse*—responsible for developing a plan of patient care directed toward defined patient goals and for coordinating the actions of other team members toward these goals. Included in the rehabilitation nurse's responsibilities are the following:
      a. Prevention of further impairment/complications.
      b. Restoration and maintenance of optimal physical and psychosocial health.
      c. Application of the nursing process in skin care, positioning, transfer techniques, bladder and bowel management, nutrition, psychosocial support, and patient and family education.
  4. *Physician* (primary care practitioner)—makes the medical diagnosis, so that therapy can be directed toward realistic goals, designs the patient program, and directs the team.
  5. *Physiatrist*—a physician who is a specialist in physical medicine and rehabilitation.
      a. Tests the patient's physical functioning.
      b. Determines the potential functional goal.
      c. Prescribes treatment, especially for disorders of neuromuscular/musculoskeletal function.
      d. Supervises the rehabilitation program.
  6. *Psychologist*—determines the patient's cognitive, perceptual, and behavioral impairments as well as motivation, values, and attitudes toward his disability.
  7. *Physical therapist*—teaches and supervises the patient through prescribed exercise program designed to strengthen weak muscles and prevent deformities; also teaches new ways of locomotion, transportation, and daily activities.
  8. *Occupational therapist*—assists disabled person in adapting to challenges of daily living and interacting successfully with environment; uses activities to increase independent function, enhance development, and prevent further disability.
  9. *Social worker*—assesses the patient's social environment (life-style, coping patterns, resources, support system) and socioeconomic status; assists patient/family in adjusting to home and community. Advises on financial matters and disability benefits.
  10. *Vocational counselor*—tests the patient to determine his interests and aptitudes, so that vocational training can be instituted; plans job modifications and advises of employment opportunities.
  11. *Rehabilitation engineer*—uses science and technology in designing and constructing devices that help severely and multiply handicapped persons to function despite their disabilities.
  12. *Sex counselor*—is trained to diagnose and treat sexual dysfunctions of disabled persons. This role may also be assumed by a prepared health professional (social worker, nurse, psychologist).
  13. Other team members may include an orthotist, prosthetist, and speech-language pathologist.

Psychosocial Considerations

Psychological Reactions to a Disability

Disability has a tremendous impact on the patient's body image (physical appearance, bodily sensations, beliefs and emotions about the body). A patient with a disability has normal needs, which must sometimes be met in different ways. The mode of the patient's interpersonal relations will be altered by the changes he makes concerning his body image.

Stages of Psychological Reaction

A. Period of Confusion, Disorganization, and Denial

1. Is in a state of conflict; has to cope with problems of forced dependence, with loss of self-esteem, and with feeling that personal and family integrity is threatened.
2. Uses mechanisms of denial as a psychological defense against accepting information that is overwhelming. (Denial has a survival value.)
   a. Receives and processes only limited amounts of information; may have restricted problem-solving abilities.
   b. May have false hopes of a speedy and complete recovery.
   c. Likely to be self-centered and child-like.
   d. May attempt to remain "normal" and nondisabled.
   e. Denial is the mechanism used by those who have placed great value on strength and attractive appearance.

B. Period of Depression and/or Anxiety and Grief; a Period of Situational Reaction

1. Mourns for his lost function or missing body part
   a. Mourning for the loss of the old self is necessary before a new concept of self can develop.
   b. Clinical manifestations: preoccupation with loss, somatic distress, inappropriate behavior, hostility.
2. May have body-image distortions.
3. May be depressed because of sensory deprivation and restricted environmental stimulation.
4. Limited mobility and sensory stimulation may produce behavioral disruptions.
5. Behavior may further alienate family and health care personnel.

C. Period of Adaptation and Adjustment

1. Revises his body image and modifies his former picture of himself; has a reorientation of values.
2. Redirects energies toward coping with physical functioning, etc.
3. Accepts a degree of dependency.
4. Accepts limitations imposed by the disability.
5. Begins to develop realistic goals for the future.

D. Other Assessment Parameters

Assessment of self-concept, locus of control, hardiness, social support system—all of which enhance coping abilities.

Nursing Interventions

A. Providing Atmosphere of Acceptance

1. Develop a trusting relationship with patient and family.
2. Use open-ended questions to elicit and clarify information.

3. Allow open expression of feelings; assist the patient to identify sources of hostility/anger.
4. Avoid displaying value judgments regarding the patient's feelings.
5. Avoid discounting patient's coping methods.
6. Allow *time* for patient's coping and ego mechanisms.
7. Give emotional support to help patient work through shock, anger, and grief.
8. Clarify and validate reality.

B. Promoting Maximum Restoration

1. Determine the patient's resources for maintaining an effective life-style.
2. Do everything possible to help patient gain some control of his life—to enhance self-worth and foster independence.
3. Find out about previous interests, values, and goals.
4. Assist the patient in identifying positive coping patterns used in the past that can be used in present.
5. Work with the patient, emphasizing his assets, while, at the same time, listening, encouraging, and sharing his problems and triumphs.
6. Help the patient to think of substitutions and attaining goals of "being" (new joys, attitudes, perspectives, opportunities for fulfillment).
7. Help the patient to think about and resume previously rewarding activities.
8. Encourage the patient to assume increasing responsibility for his rehabilitation program.
9. Share responsibility for patient's appearance until patient can apply makeup, shave, etc.
10. Encourage socialization, participation in self-help groups.
11. Give positive reinforcement and feedback about progress.
12. Acknowledge that living with a disability *is* difficult, with physical, emotional, and financial stresses.
13. Reassure the patient that the support of other caring professionals/family/friends is available.

Family Support

Goals:
Total family health
To adapt to changes imposed by disability

Assessment

1. What is the current level of family functioning? Attitudes toward patient, his disability and his return home?
2. How did the family handle previous crises? How are they handling their present anxieties? Is there a perceived threat to family functioning related to the disability? Identify the problems the family feels are important.
3. What does the family need to know now? What information will the family need for future functioning?
4. What services will be needed at patient's discharge?
5. Assess for caregiver fatigue/burnout.

Nursing Interventions

A. Facilitating Family Coping

1. Listen to the concerns of the family. Develop a trusting relationship with them by treating them with respect and individuality.

2. Assist the family to face the reality of the patient's disability.
3. Provide information—to alleviate uncertainty and improve communication.
4. Involve the family in decision making and in the patient's care in order for them to develop and practice the skills necessary for the patient to reach his rehabilitation goals.
5. Encourage family to use their own initiative and to improvise in adapting equipment, environment, etc.
6. Point out the family's strengths and abilities.
7. Help place the concerns of the family into perspective.
8. Discuss ways in which family members can care for themselves. Give positive reinforcement and encourage them to return to their normal activities and interests.
9. Help extend and enlarge the needed family skills: problem solving, treatment needs of the disabled member, communicating with health professionals, using community resources.
10. Explore productive ways in which the disabled member can be involved in family life.
11. Give concrete information about services: community resources, respite care, programs for elderly, financial information, peer and support groups, counseling services.

Sexuality in Rehabilitation

Sexuality is part of a person's self-concept and involves feelings of self-worth, acceptance, sharing, affection, and intimacy, as well as feelings of masculinity or femininity. It includes physical, psychological, emotional, and social elements and is reflected in everything a person says and does.

The disabled person has the basic human need and capacity for intimacy.

Assessment

Includes assessment of patient's level of knowledge, predisability experience, effect of disability on functioning, availability of partner.

Nursing Interventions

A. Achieving a Satisfying Sexual Life-Style

1. Be comfortable with your own sexuality; avoid imposing your values on the patient.
2. Establish an atmosphere that is conducive to acceptance and open communication.
3. Let the patient know that sexuality is a legitimate concern and is part of the rehabilitation program.
4. Inform the patient that there is a breadth and depth of sexual expression possible and that he is a person of value.
5. Recognize that feelings of warmth, approval, and friendship, as well as sharing and touching, are important.
6. Be aware that patients with long-standing disabilities may need training in communication and assertiveness skills.

Note: Problems faced by the disabled include limited access to information about sexuality, lack of opportunity to form friendships and loving relationships, impaired self-image and low self-esteem, and lack of social skills.

7. Inform the patient of the availability of the following services:
   a. Social skills training
   b. Sex education/counseling services (individual, couples, and family)
   c. Genetic/contraceptive counseling
   d. Sex therapy
   e. Reading and audiovisual materials
   f. Group discussion.
8. See the Bibliography at the end of this chapter. The quarterly journal, *Sexuality and Disability* (Human Sciences Press, Inc., 72 Fifth Avenue, New York, NY 10011-8004), is devoted to the sexual implications of disability.

Preventing Complications and Deformities

Deformities and complications of illness or injury can often be prevented by *frequent changes of position, proper positioning in bed, exercise, and progressive ambulation.*

Positioning

Purposes for Changing Positions

1. To prevent contractures.
2. To stimulate circulation and to help prevent thrombophlebitis, pressure sores, and edema of the extremities.
3. To promote lung expansion and drainage of respiratory secretions.
4. To relieve pressure on a body area.

Patient Self-Care Activities

After receiving positioning instructions and turning schedules, the patient is encouraged to assume increasing responsibility for his positioning program.

Principles of Body Alignment in Body Positioning

A. Dorsal or Supine Position

1. The head is in line with the spine, both laterally and anteroposteriorly.
2. The trunk is positioned so that flexion of the hips is minimized.
3. The arms are flexed at the elbow with the hands resting against the lateral abdomen.
4. The legs are extended in a neutral position with the toes pointed toward the ceiling.
5. The heels are suspended in a space between the mattress and the footboard.
6. Trochanter rolls are placed under the greater trochanters in the hip joint areas.

B. Side-Lying or Lateral Position

1. The head is in line with the spine.
2. The body is in alignment and is not twisted.
3. The uppermost hip joint is slightly forward and supported by a pillow in a position of slight abduction.
4. A pillow supports the arm, which is flexed at both the elbow and shoulder joints.

C. Prone Position

1. The head is turned laterally and is in alignment with the rest of the body.
2. The arms are abducted and externally rotated at the shoulder joint; the elbows are flexed.
3. A small, flat support is placed under the pelvis, extending from the level of the umbilicus to the upper third of the thigh.
4. The lower extremities remain in a neutral position.
5. The toes are suspended over the edge of the mattress.

Therapeutic Exercise

Therapeutic exercise is the motion of the body or its parts to achieve symptom-free movement and function.

Goals:
To develop and retrain deficient muscles
To restore as much normal movement as possible to prevent deformity
To stimulate the functions of various organs and body systems
To build strength and endurance
To promote relaxation

Assessment

Functional evaluation is made by physiatrist and/or physical therapist: posture, goniometric measurements, manual muscle testing, range of motion testing, flexibility and endurance testing

Types of Exercises

1. Passive
2. Active assistive
3. Active
4. Resistive
5. Isometric or muscle-setting

A. Passive—an exercise carried out by the therapist or the nurse without assistance from the patient.

1. Purpose: to retain as much joint range of motion as possible; to maintain circulation.
2. Action
   a. Stabilize the proximal joint and support the distal part.
   b. Move the joint smoothly, slowly, and gently through its full range of motion (below).
   c. Avoid producing pain.

B. Active Assistive—an exercise carried out by the patient with the assistance of the therapist or the nurse.

1. Purpose: to encourage normal muscle function.
2. Action
   a. Support the distal part and encourage the patient to take the joint actively through its range of motion.
   b. Give only the amount of assistance necessary to accomplish the action.
   c. Short periods of activity are followed by adequate rest periods.

C. Active—an exercise accomplished by the patient without assistance.

1. Purpose: to increase muscle strength.
2. Action
   a. When possible, active exercise should be done against gravity.

   b. The joint is moved through the full range of motion without assistance.
   c. The patient should not substitute another joint movement for the one intended.
   d. Other active forms of exercise include turning from side to side, turning from back to abdomen, and moving up and down in bed.

D. Resistive—an active exercise carried out by the patient working against resistance produced by either manual or mechanical means.

1. Purpose: to provide resistance in order to increase muscle power.
2. Action
   a. The patient moves the joint through its range of motion while the therapist provides slight resistance at first and then progressively increases resistance.
   b. Sandbags and weights can be used and are supplied at the distal point of the involved joint.
   c. The movements should be done smoothly.

E. Isometric or Muscle-Setting—alternately contracting and relaxing a muscle while keeping the part in a fixed position. This exercise is performed by the patient.

1. Purpose: to maintain strength when a joint is immobilized.
2. Action
   a. The patient contracts or tightens the muscle as much as possible without moving the joint.
   b. He holds for several seconds, then "lets go" and relaxes.
   c. He breathes deeply during the contraction phase.

Range-of-Motion Exercises

Range of motion is the movement of a joint through its full range in all appropriate planes. It may be passive, active, or resistive.

Goals:
To prevent limitation of range of motion.
To maintain function and prevent deterioration.
To maintain or increase the maximal motion of a joint.

Underlying Principles

1. Range-of-motion testing is done by the physician or physical therapist to determine the movement that exists at the joint areas. Testing helps set realistic and positive goals.
2. The patient's range of motion is affected by his physical condition, the disease process, and his genetic make-up.
3. Each joint of the body has a normal range of motion (Table 8-1).
4. Joints may lose their normal range of motion, stiffen, and produce a permanent disability; frequently seen in neuromuscular conditions.
5. Range-of-motion exercises are individually planned, since there is wide variation in the degrees of motion of which patients of varying body builds and age-groups are capable.
6. Range-of-motion exercises should be carried out whenever there is physical inactivity, provided the patient's clinical status allows such activity.

Table 8-1. *Range of Motion*

SHOULDER

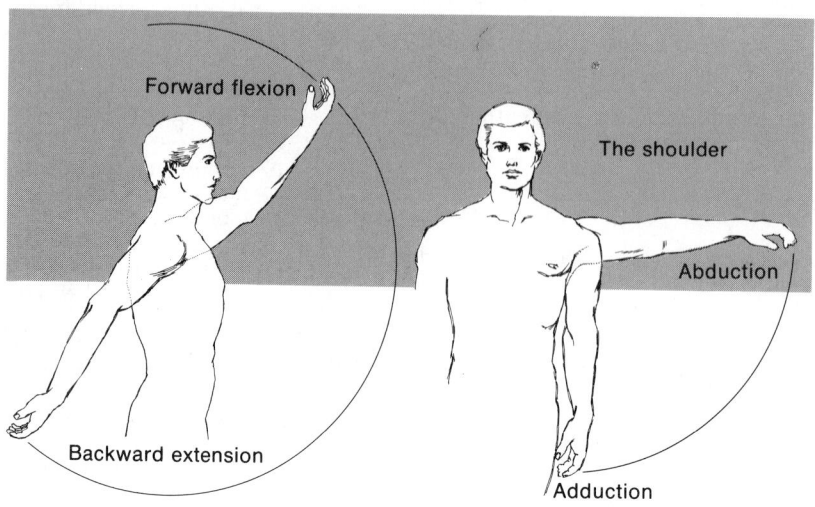

ELBOW

FOREARM

WRIST

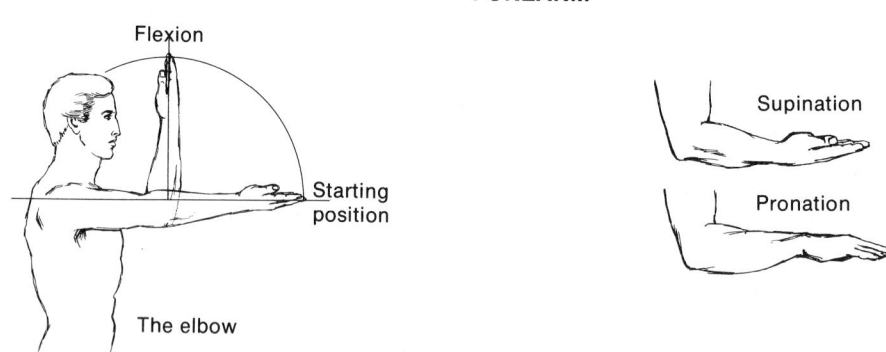

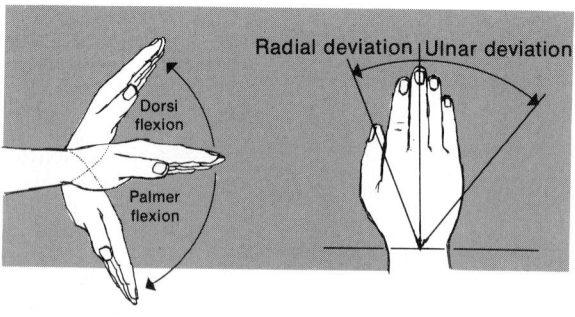

(continued)

Table 8-1. *Range of Motion (continued)*

THUMB

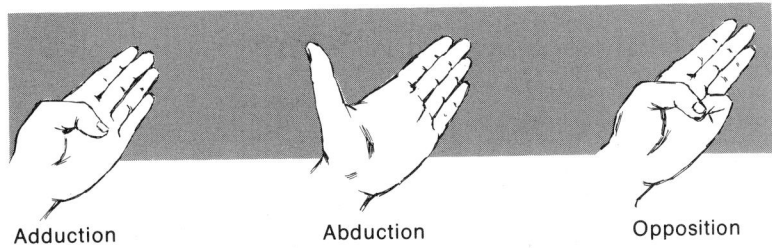

Adduction   Abduction   Opposition

FINGERS

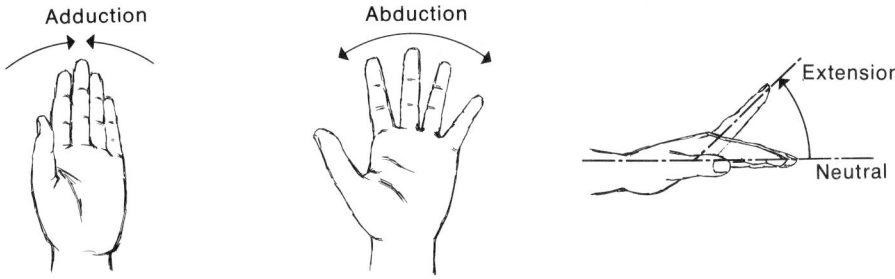

Adduction   Abduction   Extension / Neutral

ANKLE   **FOOT**

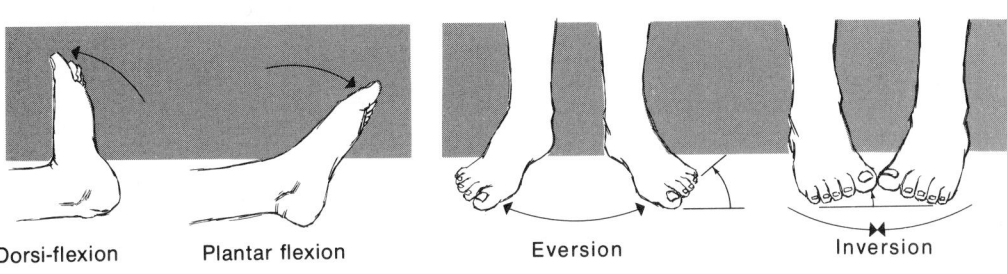

Dorsi-flexion   Plantar flexion   Eversion   Inversion

TOES

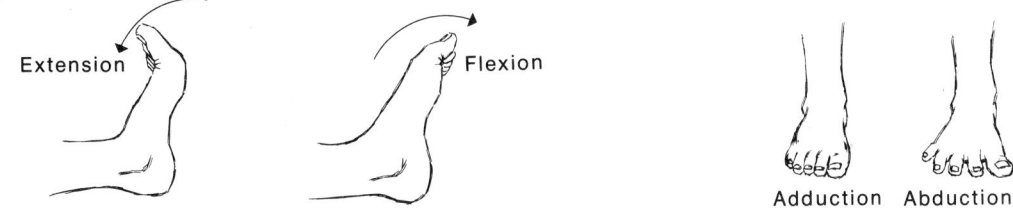

Extension   Flexion   Adduction Abduction

(continued)

Table 8-1. *Range of Motion (continued)*

HIP

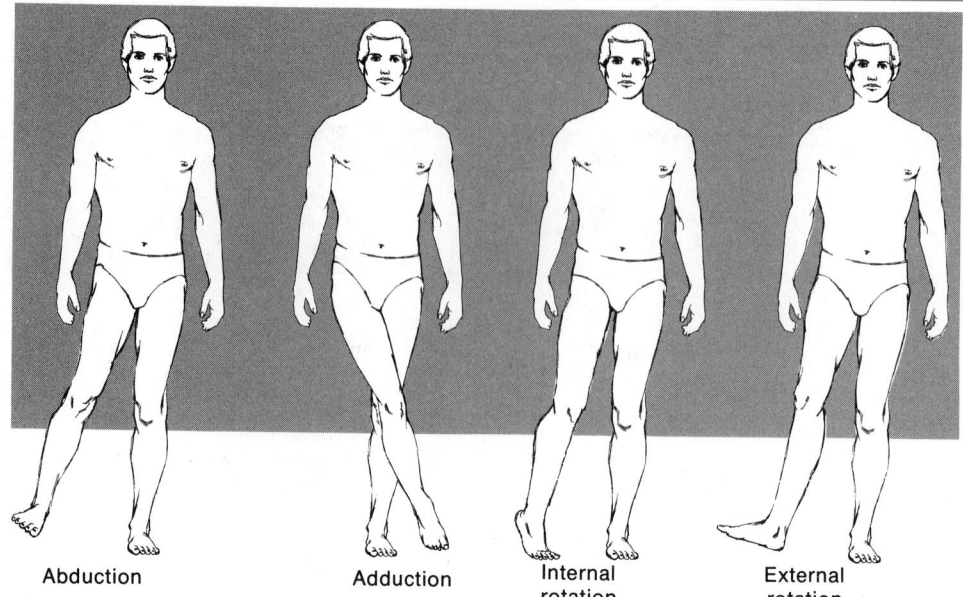

Abduction   Adduction   Internal rotation   External rotation

KNEE

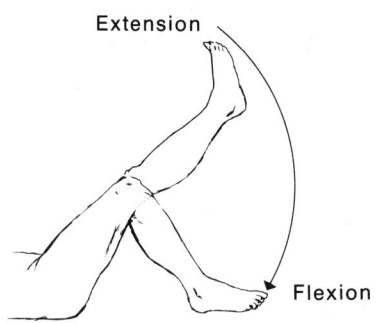

Extension

Flexion

CERVICAL SPINE

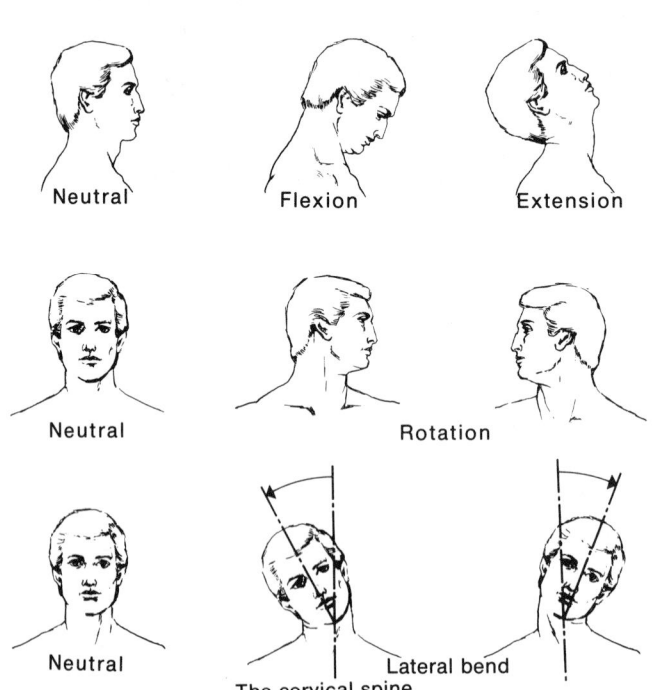

Neutral   Flexion   Extension

Neutral   Rotation

Neutral   Lateral bend
The cervical spine

Techniques of Range of Motion

1. Place the patient in a supine position with his arms to the side and the knees extended.
2. Hold the extremity at the joint (e.g., elbow, wrist, or knee) and move the joint smoothly, slowly, and gently through its range. If the joint is painful (as in arthritis), support the extremity in the muscular area.
3. Move each joint through its range of motion about 3–5 times, twice daily—smoothly, rhythmically, slowly.
4. Avoid moving a joint beyond its free range of motion; avoid forcing movement. The motion should be stopped at the point of pain.
5. When painful muscle spasm is present, move the joint slowly to the point of resistance. Then exert gentle, steady pressure until the muscle relaxes.
6. Refer to the figures in Table 8-1 for joint motion.

Definitions

Abduction—movement away from the midline of the body
Adduction—movement toward the midline of the body
Flexion—bending of a joint so that the angle of the joint diminishes
Extension—the return movement from flexion; the joint angle is increased
Inversion—movement that turns the sole of the foot inward
Eversion—movement that turns the sole of the foot outward
Dorsiflexion—flexing or bending the foot toward the leg
Plantar flexion—flexing or bending the foot in the direction of the sole
Pronation—rotating the forearm so that the palm of the hand is down
Supination—rotating the forearm so that the palm of the hand is up
Rotation—turning or movement of a part around its axis
    Internal: turning inward toward the center
    External: turning outward, away from the center

Preventing External Rotation of the Hip

Patients on prolonged bed rest may develop external rotation deformity of the hip. The hip, a ball-and-socket joint, has a tendency to rotate outward when the patient lies on his back.

Nursing Interventions

1. To prevent this deformity, use a trochanter roll extending from the crest of the ilium to the midthigh when the patient is lying on his back. A trochanter roll serves as a mechanical wedge under the projection of the greater trochanter.
2. Use a footboard when the patient is in the dorsal position.
3. To make and position a trochanter roll:
   a. Take both ends of a large Turkish towel and bring them to the center. The towel is now folded in half with the edges at the center.
   b. Turn the towel over so that the ends are facing downward.
   c. Turn the patient on his side with his upper leg flexed.
   d. Place one side of the towel in the midline of the buttock. The towel should extend from the crest of the ilium to the midthigh.
   e. Then place the patient in a dorsal position with his leg extended.
   f. Grasp the remaining side of the towel and roll inward in an underneath fashion until the entire roll is well under the patient's buttock. The roll should be kept taut and smooth.
   g. For the larger patient, a drawsheet or a bath blanket may be used.

Preventing Footdrop

Footdrop (plantar flexion) is a deformity caused by contraction of both the gastrocnemius and the soleus muscles; it may be produced by loss of flexibility of the Achilles tendon.

Causes

1. Prolonged bed rest and lack of exercise
2. Incorrect positioning in bed
3. Weight of bedding forcing the feet into plantar flexion (ankle bends in the direction of the sole of the foot)

Clinical Problem

If footdrop continues without correction, the patient will walk on his toes without the heel of his foot touching the ground.

Nursing Interventions

1. Use a footboard to keep feet at right angles to the legs when the patient is lying on his back.
   a. Position the feet with the entire plantar surface firmly against the footboard.
   b. Maintain the legs in a neutral position. Use a trochanter roll.
   c. Keep a space between the end of the bed and footboard to avoid pressure on the heels and to allow the patient to lie prone.
2. Do not allow the weight of the top bedding to force the feet into plantar flexion.
3. Encourage the patient to flex and extend (curl and stretch) his feet and toes frequently.
4. Have the patient rotate ankles clockwise and counterclockwise several times each hour.

Preventing Pressure Sores

Pressure sores (decubitus ulcers; bedsores) are localized ulcerations of the skin or deeper structures that occur when pressure greater than normal capillary pressure (32 mm. Hg) is applied to the skin for a prolonged period of time.

Altered Physiology

Pressure → compression of small nutrient vessels of skin and underlying tissue → tissue anoxia and ischemia → necrosis of tissue cells → sloughing and ulceration → invasion by microorganisms → infection → sepsis → involvement of underlying fascia, muscle, and bone → rapidly irreversible condition.

Causes

A. **Pressure**—exerted on skin and subcutaneous tissues by bony prominences and by the object on which the body part rests (mattress, cast, etc.); pressure interferes with the blood supply of the tissues and, if prolonged, will cause tissue death.

B. **Contributing Factors**
1. Immobility and lack of normal movement.
2. Shearing force—caused by sliding of adjacent surfaces producing a relative displacement and resulting in compression of capillary flow.
    a. Pulls tissues so that tissues and blood vessels are stretched and injured.
    b. Occurs when the patient is allowed to slide down in bed or chair, producing a shear in the sacral and coccygeal region.
3. Friction, moisture such as incontinence (increases the friction between two surfaces), and heat—irritate the skin, making it less resistant to injury.
4. Sensory and motor deficits
    a. Sensory loss—produces lack of awareness of pain and pressure.
    b. Motor paralysis with associated muscular atrophy—causes lack of movement and reduction in amount of padding between overlying skin and underlying bone.
5. Circulatory deficiencies
6. Nutritional deficits (obesity, underweight, protein deficiency; anemia; dehydration)—negative nitrogen, phosphorus, sulfur, and calcium balance will produce wasting of tissue, osteoporosis, and loss of weight.
7. Edema—impairs circulation and interferes with supply of nutrients to the cells.
8. Infection—lowers resistance of skin to breakdown; destroys tissue.
9. Age-related changes in the skin—loss of dermal vessels, thinning epidermis, flattening of dermal–epidermal junction, loss of elastic fibers—all increase susceptibility to skin breakdown.
10. Equipment—traction, casts, restraints, improper bedding and seats.

Sites (*See Fig. 8-1*)

A. **Weight-Bearing Bony Prominences Covered Only by Skin and Small Amounts of Subcutaneous Fat—** 75% of all pressure sores located at such sites.
1. Ischial tuberosities—especially in patients who sit for prolonged periods.
2. Trochanters
3. Sacrum
B. **Other Bony Prominences**—knees, malleoli, heels, and elbows.

Clinical Manifestations

1. Redness (a danger sign); redness will blanch on pressure; skin temperature is increased because of vasodilatation.
2. Dusky, cyanotic blue-gray area (fails to blanch on pressure)—shows capillary occlusion and subcutaneous weakening.
3. Vesiculation (blistering)
4. Break in skin, progressing to deep, penetrating necrosis; may involve deeper soft tissues, bursae, muscles, tendons, bone and/or joints.

Nursing Assessment

1. Inspect each pressure area for erythema.
    a. Press on the area; look for blanching; redness that does not disappear after finger pressure is applied indicates impending ulcer formation.
    b. Note how long hyperemia persists following removal of pressure.
2. Inspect for dry skin, moist skin, and breaks in the skin.
3. Palpate for warmth—compare with other parts of the body.
4. Palpate the peripheral pulses to evaluate circulatory status.
5. Check the patient's record for hematocrit, hemoglobin, and serum albumin levels.
6. Conduct a nutritional assessment.

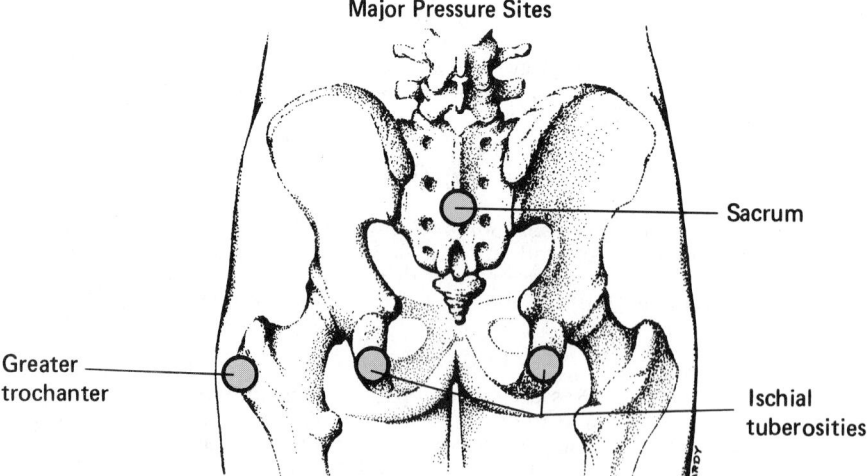

Major Pressure Sites

Sacrum

Greater trochanter

Ischial tuberosities

Figure 8-1. Sites of pressure sores.

Nursing Interventions

A. Relieving or Removing Pressure to Prevent Occurrence of Pressure Sore

1. Recognize those patients in whom pressure sores are likely to develop. *Pressure sores may appear in a matter of hours.*
2. Relieve pressure by encouraging the patient to keep active.
   a. Set up and adhere to a turning schedule.
   b. Turn the patient hourly or at 2-hour intervals—shifting of weight allows blood to flow back into tissues and helps tissues to recover from pressure.
3. Avoid shearing forces and friction.
   a. Avoid elevating head of bed more than 30 degrees—to reduce shearing forces.
   b. Avoid placing the patient in semi-recumbent positions; discourage activities that increase exposure to shearing forces.
   c. Avoid the use of rubber rings or doughnuts—they merely increase pressure around bony prominences and decrease blood flow to the area resting in the center of the device.
4. Use special devices (flotation pads, fleeces, egg-crate mattresses) to support specific areas of the body; the supporting medium should mold to the patient to ensure uniformly distributed pressure and should allow evaporation of perspiration.
5. Use an alternating pressure mattress or alternating pressure chair—alternating inflation and deflation of pad produce constriction of vessels followed by dilation of superficial blood vessels of the skin; pressure on any one part is reduced, and blood supply is increased.
6. Relieve pressure over bony prominences by correct positioning with pillows and bridging techniques.
7. Relieve pressure on bony prominences of patients sitting in wheelchairs for prolonged periods.
   a. Have wheelchair cushions fitted and adjusted on an individualized basis, using pressure-measurement techniques as a guide to selection and fitting.
   b. Teach the paraplegic patient to raise himself from his wheelchair for a few seconds every 20–30 minutes for intermittent relief of pressure from ischial tuberosities and prevention of ischial pressure sores.
   c. Encourage patient to shift weight frequently while sitting—redistributes blood flow in affected areas.
8. Inspect, adjust, and pad casts, braces, splints, and compression bandages.

B. Maintaining Skin in a Clean and Healthy Condition

1. Emphasize the importance of accepting responsibility for self-care.
2. Inspect the skin frequently for signs of pressure—especially for redness over bony prominences.
3. Maintain meticulous skin hygiene.
   a. Inspect the skin several times daily.
   b. Wash the skin with mild soap, rinse, and *blot* dry with a soft towel.
   c. Lubricate the skin with a bland lotion to keep the skin soft and pliable.
   d. Avoid placing the patient on a poorly ventilated mattress that is covered with plastic or impermeable material.

4. Employ active and passive exercises—to improve muscular, skin, and vascular tone.
5. Employ bladder and bowel programs in incontinent patient to prevent skin soilage.
6. Encourage mobility. Ambulate or use a tilt table whenever possible.

C. Ensuring Optimal Nutrition

1. Improve nutritional status and maintain a positive nitrogen balance—pressure sores develop more quickly and are more resistant to treatment in patients suffering from nutritional disorders.
   a. High-protein diet—adequate protein reserves are necessary to maintain tissue vitality.
   b. Vitamins and protein supplements.
   c. Iron preparations and transfusions of whole blood—hemoglobin level is a critical factor in the development of pressure sores.
   d. Zinc supplements—improve appetite and increase rate of wound healing.
2. Carry out frequent hemoglobin, hematocrit, and blood sugar determinations.

Managing the Patient With Pressure Sores

Assessment

1. See Assessment under "Prevention," page 134.
2. Document size, number, and location of pressure sores—for evaluation of treatment effects.
3. Look for surrounding erythema, purulent drainage, and foul odor—suggestive of infection.

Classification

> *Grade 1:* Defined area of soft-tissue swelling, erythema usually over a bony prominence (changes are reversible).
> *Grade 2:* Break in or blistering of epidermis surrounding erythema and induration.
> *Grade 3:* Ulcer extending into subcutaneous tissue but not into muscle.
> *Grade 4:* Deep ulceration extending through muscular tissue down to underlying bony prominence.
> *Grade 5:* An extensive ulcer penetrating underlying bone with widespread extension along bursae, into joints or body cavities (intestines, vagina, bladder).

Diagnostic Evaluation

1. Bacterial cultures from wound
2. Sinography and computed tomography—give information about deeper tissues and provide images showing complications

Complications

1. Abscesses; sepsis; bacteremia
2. Osteomyelitis; bone erosion

Management and Nursing Interventions

A. Eliminating Pressure

1. Relieve pressure from the area; a pressure ulcer will not heal when subjected to continuous pressure.

a. Continue preventive measures (See p. 135).
b. Develop a turning schedule—the patient must not sit or lie on the ulcer, even for a few minutes.

B. Systemic Management

1. Ensure good nutrition—to reverse catabolism, correct anemia and edema and increase tissue oxygenation and perfusion.
2. Implement prescribed treatment of any underlying disorder to allow ulcer healing.
3. Apply systemic antimicrobials (clindamycin; gentamicin) as prescribed when there is evidence of cellulitis, sepsis, or osteomyelitis.

C. Local Wound Care—to lower bacterial count so healing may occur.

1. Ulcer debridement—devitalized tissue promotes infection, delays granulation and impedes healing.
   Enzymatic debriding agents may be used during intervals between surgical debridement.
2. Mechanical cleansing of the ulcer—clears up sepsis and stimulates regeneration of epithelium.
   Deep ulcer may need irrigation with prescribed sterile solution or to be cleansed in a whirlpool.
3. Maintain moist wound environment to facilitate healing after the wound is cleaned—allows optimal epithelialization.
   a. Moisture-retaining occlusive dressings—may improve healing in superficial ulcers but not in deep or necrotic ulcers.
   b. Deep ulcers (after cleansing) may be dressed with fine-mesh gauze dressings moistened with normal saline or lactated Ringer's solution. This wet-to-dry dressing is changed every 6–8 hours to promote healing and is carried out until necrotic debris is removed and re-epithelialization begins.
4. Topical therapy.
   a. Role of topical agents is controversial.
   b. Wide variety of agents including enzymatic debriding agents, aerosol sprays, absorbable gelatin sponges, etc.

D. Controlling Infection

1. Monitor for purulent drainage and foul odor.
2. Assess for systemic infection, fever, lymphangitis, cellulitis.
3. Use gloves and mask when changing the dressing.
4. Administer prescribed antibiotics.

E. Other Management Modalities

1. Physical modalities
   a. Exposure of ulcer to air and sunlight.
   b. Using light stroking around lesion—promotes venous return and reduces edema.
   c. Ultraviolet irradiation.
   d. Whirlpool treatments—increase circulation and have disinfecting action.
   e. Hyperbaric oxygen therapy—oxygen under pressure applied directly on the ulcer directs more oxygen to tissues; hastens metabolic processes and reduces healing time.
2. Surgical procedures—for severe tissue loss, multiple large wounds.
   a. Excision and direct closure.
   b. Excision of ulcer, surrounding scar tissue, underlying bursae and infected bone.
   c. Grafting procedures used according to size of ulcer including skin grafts, skin flaps, muscle flaps, musculocutaneous flaps.

3. Postoperative nursing interventions.
   a. Continue to relieve pressure on surgical area by proper positioning and elimination of shearing forces for 4–6 weeks; special beds (Clinitron; Mediscus) may be used.
   b. Place patient in a prone position if there has been repair of ischia, sacrum, or trochanters.
   c. Allow controlled pressure on site (after 6 weeks) for 10–15 minutes, 2–3 times a day under close nursing surveillance; watch for redness or abrasion.

Promoting Function in Activities of Daily Living

Activities of Daily Living

Activities of daily living (ADL) are those self-care activities that must be accomplished each day in order for the patient to care for his own needs and the demands of daily life. They include:
   Mobility
   Personal hygiene and toilet management
   Dressing
   Getting in and out of bed (transfers)
   Eating
   Environmental management

Assessment

1. Physical examination; neurologic examination.
2. Evaluation of functional capacity—assessment of ability and energy for daily routine; determination of sitting balance, transfers, ADL skills, ambulation/mobility.

The Activities of Daily Living (ADL) Sheet

The ADL sheet is an information sheet for those who are caring for the patient. It is a guide to the assessment of the patient's functional capabilities.

Purposes:
   To inform each member of the rehabilitation team what activities the patient can perform.
   To serve as an index of progress.

Nurse's Responsibility in Using ADL Sheet
1. Review the ADL sheet periodically to know what the patient is capable of doing and what activities he is learning.
2. Avoid doing for the patient what he can do for himself.

Nursing Diagnosis

Self-care deficits related to general complex problems of disability, limited mobility and access, and potential for dependency.

Nursing Interventions

1. Define the goal with the patient.
2. Identify the patient's strengths and indications of wellness; point these out to the patient.
3. Determine how much the patient can do (and would like to do) for himself.
4. Study each component motion of the desired activity.
5. Ascertain what methods can be used to accomplish the task.
   Example: There are several ways of putting on a given garment.

6. Determine what the patient can do by watching him perform.
7. Encourage the patient to exercise the muscles used in performing the motions involved in the activity.
8. Select activities that encourage gross functional movements of the upper and lower extremities (e.g., bathing, holding larger objects).
9. Gradually include activities that use finer motions (e.g., buttoning clothes, eating with a spoon).
10. Set appropriate limits to allow the patient to move toward self-care.
11. Allow the patient to achieve mastery.
12. Extend the period of activity as much and as fast as the patient can tolerate.
13. Teach use of assistive devices.
14. Have the patient perform and practice the activity in a real-life situation.
15. Encourage the patient to perform every activity up to his maximal capabilities within the framework of his ability.
16. Support the patient by giving justifiable praise, reinforcement, and feedback for effort put forth and for acts accomplished.

Evaluation

Moves toward self-care in activities of daily living (as competently as residual functioning permits); shows progress in specific activities as indicated by ADL sheet.

Assisting the Patient With Mobility and Ambulation

Guidelines Using a Tilt Table

A *tilt table* is a board or table that can be tilted gradually from a horizontal to a vertical (upright) position.

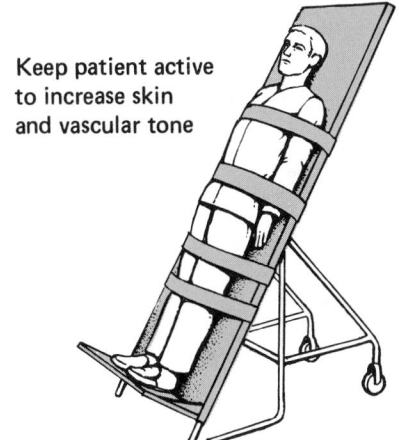

Keep patient active to increase skin and vascular tone

Purposes
1. To help the patient adjust gradually to varying degrees of the upright posture and ultimately to complete upright position.
2. To help the patient start weight-bearing activities.
3. To increase standing tolerance.
4. To prevent disuse syndrome.
5. To prevent demineralization of bone and development of urinary tract stones.
6. To condition the vascular system.

Clinical Usefulness
Spinal cord injuries
Orthostatic hypotension
Brain damage

Equipment
Tilt table with footboard
Straps
Sphygmomanometer and stethoscope
Abdominal binder, elastic stockings, or venous pressure gradient leotard*

*Jobst Venous Pressure Gradient Support

(continued)

Guidelines Using a Tilt Table *(continued)*

Procedure	Nursing Action	Rationale/Amplification

Preparatory Phase

1. Apply snug-fitting abdominal binder, elastic compression bandages from toes to groin on both legs, or a leotard (waist-high venous pressure gradient support*).

1. Compression of abdomen prevents pooling of blood in splanchnic area and subsequent postural hypotension and inadequate cerebral circulation. Compression of legs restricts the vascular walls of the blood vessels and prevents pooling of blood in the legs, with development of edema.

Performance Phase

1. Transfer the patient to the tilt table by 3-person carry method. Place the patient in a dorsal position with his feet placed firmly against the footboard. Position the body in correct alignment.
2. Fasten the straps across the pelvis, knees, chest, and abdomen.
3. Apply the blood pressure cuff to the arm and take and record the blood pressure while the patient is lying flat.
4. Tilt the table 15–30 degrees. Take the blood pressure every 3–5 minutes.
5. Evaluate the patient constantly and assess for a drop in blood pressure. If the patient feels dizzy and the blood pressure drops, return him to a flat position.
6. Observe for pallor, diaphoresis, tachycardia, and nausea.
7. Increase the standing tolerance by 5- to 10-degree increments.
8. Continue the procedure until the patient tolerates the desired tilt (usually between 45 degrees and 80 degrees).
9. Avoid allowing the patient to stand for prolonged periods.
10. Do not leave patient unattended.

3. This serves as a baseline recording for future comparisons.

4. Tilting the patient from a supine to an upright position causes a decrease in systolic pressure.

6. These are signs and symptoms of insufficient cerebral circulation.
7. The angle of tilt will be determined by the patient's tolerance, blood pressure stability, and the desired amount of weight-bearing.

9. Prolonged standing may cause pressure ulceration on plantar surfaces of feet.

Follow-up Phase

1. Place the patient back in bed at the end of the prescribed period or when his condition indicates.
2. Record degree of tilt, amount of time on tilt table, and reaction of patient.

Transfer Activities

A *transfer* is the movement of the patient from one piece of furniture or equipment to another (from bed to chair, bed to commode, bed to wheelchair).

Weight-bearing transfers—carried out by patients who have at least one stable lower extremity (hemiplegics, unilateral lower extremity amputees, patients with hip fractures).

Non-weight-bearing-transfers—done by double lower-extremity amputees, or paraplegics who are not wearing braces.

Preparation for Transfers

Goal:
Develop ability to raise and move the body in different positions.

A. Exercises to Strengthen Arm and Shoulder Extensors

1. Have the patient sit upright in bed.
2. Place a book under each hand.
3. Instruct the patient to push down on the book, thus raising his body weight.

B. Technique for Moving the Patient to the Edge of the Bed

1. Move the patient's head and shoulders toward the edge of the bed.
2. Move the patient's feet and legs to the edge of the bed. (The patient is now in a crescent position, giving good range of motion to the lateral trunk muscles.)
3. Place both of your arms well under the patient's hips. (Before the next maneuver, tighten or set the muscles of your back and abdomen.)
4. Straighten your back while moving the patient toward you.

C. Technique for Sitting the Patient on the Edge of the Bed

1. Place one arm and hand under the patient's shoulders.
2. Instruct the patient to push his elbow into the bed while you lift his shoulders with one arm and swing his legs over the edge of the bed with the other. (Gravity pulls the legs downward, which aids in raising the patient's trunk.)

D. Technique for Assisting the Patient to Stand

1. Place the patient's feet well under him.
2. Face the patient and firmly grasp each side of his rib cage.
3. Push your knee against one of the patient's knees.
4. Rock the patient forward as he comes to a standing position. (Your knee is pushed against the patient's knee as he comes to the standing position.)
5. Ensure that the patient's knees are "locked" (full extension) while he is standing. (Locking the patient's knees is a safety measure for those patients who are weak or who have been in bed for a period of time.)
6. Give the patient enough time to balance himself.
7. Pivot the patient, positioning him to sit in the chair.

E. Technique for Transfer by Sliding Board

1. A *sliding board* (or transfer board) is a polished lightweight board that is used to bridge the gap between two seats. It is polished to reduce friction.
2. When the muscles that the patient uses to lift himself off the bed are not strong enough to overcome the resistance of body weight, use the following technique:
   a. Place one side of the sliding board under the patient's buttocks and the other side on the surface of the chair, bed, toilet, etc., to which the transfer is being made.
   b. Instruct the patient to push up with his hands, to shift his buttocks, and to slide across the board to the other surface.

Crutch Walking

Crutches are artificial supports that assist patients who need aid in walking because of disease, injury, or a birth defect.

Preparation for Crutch Walking

Goals:
Develop power in the shoulder girdle and upper extremities that bear the patient's weight in crutch walking.
Strengthen and condition the patient.

A. To Strengthen the Muscles Needed for Ambulation

Instruct the patient as follows:
1. For *quadriceps setting*
   a. Contract the quadriceps muscle while attempting to push the popliteal area against the mattress and raise the heel.
   b. Maintain the muscle contracture for the count of 5.
   c. Relax for the count of 5.
   d. Repeat this exercise 10–15 times hourly.
2. For *gluteal setting*
   a. Contract or pinch the buttocks together for the count of 5.
   b. Relax for the count of 5.
   c. Repeat 10–15 times hourly.

B. To Strengthen the Muscles of the Upper Extremities and Shoulder Girdle

Instruct the patient as follows:
1. Flex and extend arms slowly while holding traction weights; gradually increase poundage of weight and number of repetitions to increase strength and endurance.
2. Do pushups while lying in a prone position.
3. Squeeze rubber ball—increases grasping strength.
4. Raise head and shoulders from bed; stretch hands forward as far as possible.
5. Sit up on bed or chair.
   a. Raise body from chair by pushing hands against chair seat (or mattress).
   b. Raise body out of seat. Hold. Relax.

C. To Measure for Crutches

1. When the patient is lying down (an approximate measurement)
   a. Instruct the patient to wear the shoes he will be using for walking.
   b. Measure from the anterior fold of the axilla to the sole of the foot. Then add 5 cm. (2 inches).
   c. Or subtract 40 cm. (16 inches) from the patient's height.
2. When the patient is standing erect.
   a. Stand the patient against the wall with feet slightly apart and away from the wall.
   b. The crutches should be fitted with large rubber suction tips.
   c. The elbow is flexed 30 degrees with the hand resting on the grip.
   d. There should be a 2-finger-width insertion between the axillary fold and the hand grip. A foam-rubber pad on the underarm piece will relieve pressure on the upper arm and thoracic cage.
   e. The tip of the crutch is placed 15–20 cm (6–8 inches) lateral to the forefoot.

D. Crutch Stance

1. Have the patient wear well-fitting shoes with firm soles.
2. Before using the crutches, have the patient stand by a chair on the unaffected leg to achieve balance.
3. Position the patient against a wall with his head in a neutral position.
4. *Tripod position*—basic crutch stance for balance and support
   a. Crutches rest approximately 20–25 cm. (8–10 inches) in front of and to the side of patient's toes (Fig. 8-2).
   b. Taller patient requires a wider base, whereas shorter patient needs a narrower base.
5. Teach the patient to support his weight on his hands; weight borne on the axillae can damage the brachial plexus nerves and produce "crutch paralysis."

Teaching the Crutch Gait

1. Crutch walking requires balance, coordination, and a high energy cost; these can be acquired with diligent and regular practice.
2. Practice balancing with crutches while leaning against the wall.
3. Practice shifting body weight in different positions, while standing with crutches.
4. The selection of the crutch gait depends on the type and severity of the disability and the patient's physical condition, arm and trunk strength, and/or body balance.

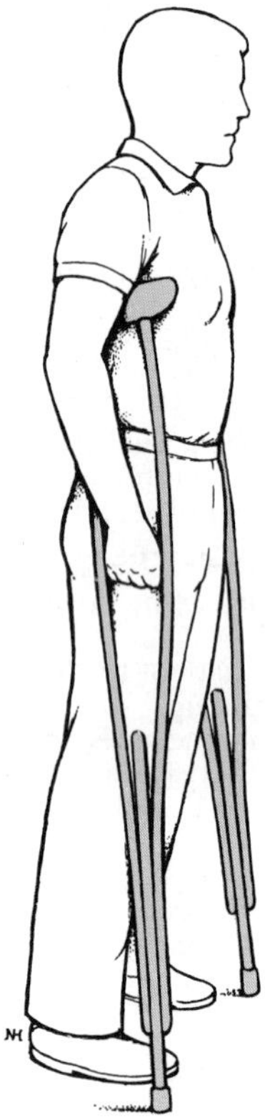

Figure 8-2. *The tripod position is the basic crutch stance for balance and support.*

5. Teach the patient at least 2 gaits—a faster gait to be used for making speed, and a slower one to be used in crowded places.
6. Instruct the patient to change from one gait to another—relieves fatigue, since a different combination of muscles is used.

Crutch Gaits

A. 4-Point Gait (4-point alternate crutch gait)
1. This is a slow but stable gait; the patient's weight is constantly being shifted.
2. 4-point gait can be used only by patients who can move each leg separately and bear a considerable amount of weight on each of them.

Crutch–foot sequence (Fig. 8-3):
1. Right crutch
2. Left foot
3. Left crutch
4. Right foot

B. 3-Point Gait (This is used when one leg is involved.)

Crutch–foot sequence (Fig. 8-4):
1. Both crutches and the involved lower leg are moved forward simultaneously.
2. Then the stronger lower extremity is moved forward, while putting most of the body weight on the crutches.

C. 2-Point Gait (This is a progression from the 4-point gait and allows faster ambulation.)

Crutch–foot sequence (Fig. 8-5):
1. Weight is borne on both lower extremities and both crutches.
2. Advance right foot and left crutch together.
3. Then advance left foot and right crutch together.

Crutch Maneuvering Techniques

A. To Stand Up
1. Move forward to the edge of the chair with the strong leg slightly under the seat.
2. Place both crutches in the hand on the side of the affected extremity.
3. Push down on the hand pieces while raising the body to a standing position.

B. To Sit in a Chair
1. Grasp the crutches at the hand pieces for control and bend forward slightly while assuming a sitting position.

C. To Go Up Stairs
1. Advance the stronger leg first up to the next step.
2. Then advance the crutches and the weaker extremity.

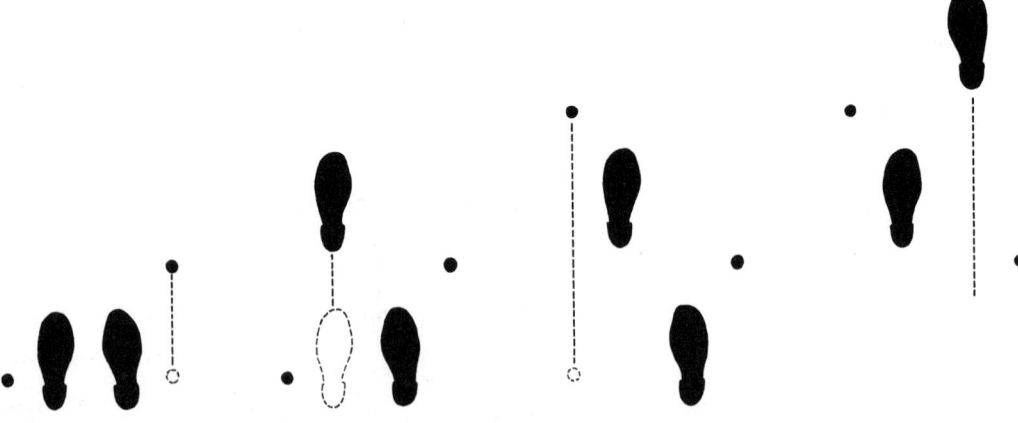

Right crutch forward   Advance left foot   Left crutch forward   Advance right foot

Figure 8-3. *Four-point gait.*

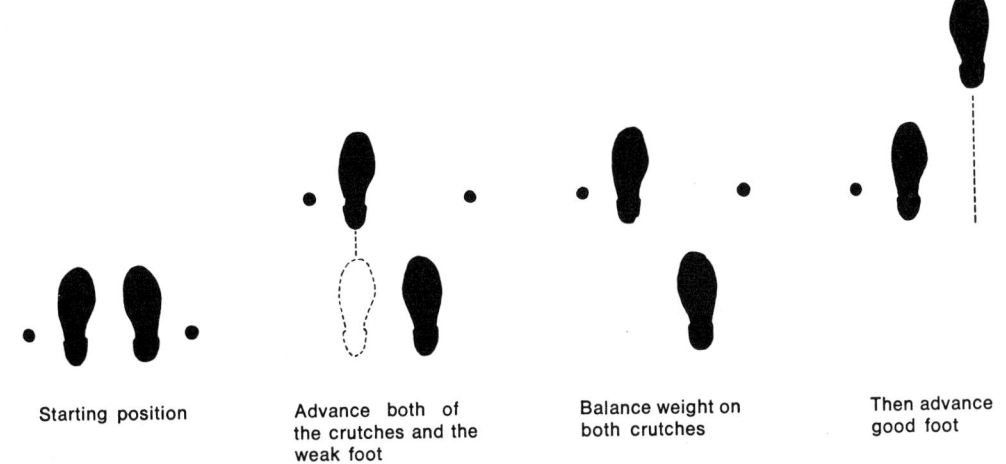

Figure 8-4. *Three-point gait.*

D. To Go Down Stairs

1. Place feet forward as far as possible on the step.
2. Advance crutches to the lower step. The weaker leg is advanced first and then the stronger one—the stronger extremity shares the work of raising and lowering the body weight with the patient's arms.

   Note: Strong leg goes up stairs first and down stairs last.

Ambulation With a Walker

A walker provides more support than crutches or a cane for the patient who has poor balance and cannot use crutches. It gives stability but does not permit a natural reciprocal walking pattern. Teach the following sequence:

1. Lift the walker, placing it in front of you while leaning your body slightly forward.
2. Take a step or two into the walker.
3. Lift the walker, and place it in front of you again.

Ambulation With a Cane

Purposes

A cane is used for balance and support:

1. To assist the patient to walk with greater balance and support and less fatigue.
2. To compensate for deficiencies of function normally performed by the neuromuscular skeletal system.
3. To relieve pressure on weight-bearing joints.
4. To provide forces to push or pull the body forward or to restrain the forward motion of the patient while walking.

Underlying Principles

1. An adjustable aluminum cane, fitted with a 3.75 cm. (1½-inch) rubber suction tip to provide traction while walking, gives optimal stability to the patient.
2. With bilateral disease, using 2 canes give better balance and weight relief.
3. To fit for a cane:
   a. Have patient flex his elbow at a 30-degree angle

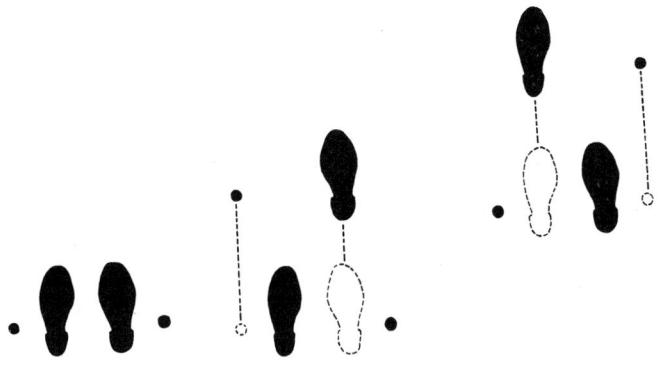

Figure 8-5. *Two-point gait.*

and hold the cane 15 cm. (6 inches) lateral to the base of his fifth toe.
  b. Adjust the cane so that the handle is approximately level with the greater trochanter.
4. OR while the patient is standing with his arms at his side, the handle of the cane should line up with the crease in his wrist.

Technique for Walking With a Cane

1. Hold the cane in the hand opposite to the affected extremity (i.e., the cane should be used on the good side)—allows partial weight-bearing relief as the cane is in contact with the floor at the same time as the affected extremity.
2. Advance the cane at the same time the affected leg is moved forward.
3. Keep the cane fairly close to the body to prevent leaning.
4. If the patient is unable to use the cane in the opposite hand, the cane may be carried on the same side and advanced when the affected leg is advanced.
5. To go up and down stairs
  a. Step up on *unaffected* extremity.
  b. Then place cane and affected extremity on the step.
  c. Reverse this procedure for descending steps.
  d. The strong leg goes up first and comes down last.

Orthotic or Prosthetic Devices

Orthotic Devices

An *orthosis* is a device added to the patient's body to provide support and alignment, prevent or correct deformities, immobilize a part, and improve the function of the body.
1. Orthotic devices include braces, splints, collars, corsets, supports, or calipers that may be designed and produced by an orthotist.
2. An orthosis may be static (no moving parts) or dynamic (allow movement in specific directions by the use of hinges, springs, or outriggers with elastic tension).
  a. Static orthoses are used to stabilize joints and to rest the splinted part.
  b. Dynamic orthoses are flexible and are used to improve functioning by assisting weak muscles.
3. Nursing interventions and patient education
  a. The major nursing functions are to work at attaining and maintaining a functional and pain-free range-of-motion for all joints and to prevent contractures.
  b. Reinforce the orthotist's instructions concerning the care of the skin under the device as pressure sores may develop.
  c. Teach the patient to examine the orthosis periodically to see that it has not slipped out of position or become distorted and that the padding distributes the pressure evenly.

Prosthetic Devices

A *prosthesis** is an artificial substitute for a missing part of the body (i.e., extremity, joint, eye, breast, tooth). A *prosthetist* is a limb maker or a maker of other prostheses.

---

* Specific prostheses are described in this volume under the clinical conditions requiring such devices. Information concerning prosthetic and orthopedic appliances may also be obtained from The American Orthotic and Prosthetic Association, 717 Pendleton Street, Alexandria, VA 22314.

1. Nursing Interventions
  a. Help the patient develop an attitude of realistic hopefulness and acceptance.
  b. Prevent deformities to limit the time between the healing of tissues and the fitting of the prosthesis.
  c. See page 798 for the preoperative and postoperative nursing interventions following an extremity amputation. The residual extremity (stump) must be bandaged correctly so that proper shrinkage and shaping occur for the patient to be fitted effectively for a prosthesis.

Overcoming Elimination Problems: Bladder and Bowel Training

Urinary Incontinence

Urinary incontinence is involuntary loss of urine severe enough to have social and/or hygienic consequences.

Types[†]

1. *Stress:* sudden losses of urine upon biomechanical provocation (straining; coughing) leading to leakage of urine; caused by dysfunction of bladder outlet.
2. *Urge:* involuntary loss of urine preceded by a strong desire to void; causes include CNS disorders (stroke, brain tumor), infection, uninhibited bladder contractions.
3. *Overflow:* leakage of small amounts of urine when bladder cannot empty normally and becomes overdistended; causes include neurologic abnormalities that impair detrusor contractile capacity or any factor that obstructs flow.
4. *Functional:* incontinence in which the function of the lower urinary tract is intact but other factors (immobility; severe cognitive impairment) cause the problem.

Diagnostic Evaluation

1. History and physical examination emphasizing genitourinary history, medications, pelvic and rectal examinations.
2. Laboratory tests to screen for diabetes and kidney disease.
3. Urodynamic evaluation—measurement of intravesical, intraurethral, and intra-abdominal pressures to define cause.
4. Determination of residual urinary volume.

Management

1. Behavioral interventions to manage urge, stress, and functional incontinence
  a. Scheduling regimens include bladder retraining, habit retraining, timed voiding, prompted voiding.
  b. Biofeedback approaches—techniques learned by patient to exert improved voluntary control over urine storage.
2. Pelvic floor muscle exercises (pubococcygeal/Kegal)—exercises to strengthen the voluntary periurethral and pelvic floor muscles, the contraction of which exert a closing force on the urethra.
3. Drug therapy: include bladder relaxants, smooth mus-

[†] Neurologic incontinence is discussed on page 692.

cle relaxants, calcium-channel blockers, bladder outlet stimulants, and estrogen.
4. Surgical approaches (depending on etiology) include insertion of artificial sphincter, bladder suspension surgery, transurethral resection of prostate.
5. Palliative and supportive interventions—catheter, environmental manipulation, prostheses (condom catheters, penile clamps), vaginal pessaries, incontinence pads, and briefs.

Nursing Assessment

1. Obtain a history of onset, duration, frequency, occurrence (diurnal, nocturnal, or both), precipitating circumstances (sneezing, position change) associated with symptoms.
2. Ask about environmental factors: accessible bathroom; available commode.
3. Determine how the patient perceives his incontinence. How is it interfering with lifestyle?
4. Assess patient's awareness/orientation and cognitive function (ability to follow directions). Assess mobility and energy levels.
5. Palpate over bladder area for signs of a distended bladder. Test for stress incontinence by asking patient to cough with a full bladder and monitor for incontinence.
6. Ask patient/family to keep a voiding record (incontinence monitoring record) to record frequency, timing, and circumstances of incontinence episodes.

Nursing Diagnoses

1. Incontinence (urge) related to deconditioned voiding reflexes.
2. Incontinence (functional) related to cognitive impairment, mobility problems. Other nursing diagnoses could include social isolation related to humiliation/embarrassment.

Nursing Interventions

A. Achieving Control of Voiding

1. Analyze the patient's voiding record.
2. Formulate a schedule of definite times for the patient to try to empty his bladder using a toilet or commode.
3. Instruct the patient to drink a measured amount of fluid at regularly scheduled times.
4. Have the patient wait 30 minutes and then ask him to attempt to void; *regularity is the key to success.*
   a. Position the patient with thighs flexed and feet and back supported; sufficient daily fluid intake (2500 ml.) is essential.
   b. Instruct him to press or massage over bladder area or increase intra-abdominal pressure by *leaning forward*—helps to initiate evacuation of bladder.
   c. Have the patient concentrate on voiding.
   d. Have the patient try to void every 2 hours; interval may be lengthened as control is gained.
5. Have the patient continue keeping a voiding schedule—a continuous record of time and amount of fluid ingested and time and amount of each voiding.
6. Encourage the patient to hold his urine until the specified voiding time if possible.
7. Assess for signs of urinary retention; test (catheterize) for residual urine as directed.

B. Nursing Interventions for Functional Incontinence (for patient with inability to recognize bladder and environmental cues)

1. Try prompted voiding; remind patient to void. Also, give positive reinforcement when patient remains dry.
2. Assist the patient to the bathroom at a regularly scheduled time—delay in responding is a common cause of incontinence.
3. Make sure that there is adequate intake of fluids.
4. Encourage the patient to continue self-care and exercise programs.
5. Encourage the patient to wear his own clothes—enhances self-esteem and is a strong deterrent to regressive behavior.
6. Avoid overt encouragement of incontinence such as the routine use of pads, diapers, and other depersonalizing procedures.
7. Create an environment that keeps sensory monotony to a minimum.
   Use orienting aids to discriminate day/night, seasons.
8. Stress the abilities (not the disabilities) of the patient.
9. Have a positive approach; the patient needs an atmosphere of encouragement and support.

Evaluation

1. Remains dry; fewer episodes of incontinence.
2. Empties bladder at specified times.

Bowel Elimination Problems

Clinical Manifestations

1. Irregularity
2. Fecal incontinence
3. Diarrhea
4. Fecal impaction

Nursing Assessment

1. Bowel history
2. Nutrition history
3. Assessment of physical status and functional ability

Nursing Diagnosis

1. Altered bowel elimination (incontinence) related to inactivity, CNS dysfunction, sphincter pathology, multifactorial causes (aging, confusional state)

Nursing Interventions

A. Bowel Training

1. Secure a bowel history; bowel schedule should be normal and comfortable for the patient.
2. Teach the patient to establish a specific and definite time for the bowel movement; regularity is necessary to establish reflex assistance.
   a. The exact time period depends on the patient's schedule.
   b. Attempts at evacuation should be made within 15 minutes of this same time daily.
   c. Establish bowel evacuation 20–40 minutes after a regularly scheduled meal—utilizes the stimulation of peristalsis and the gastrocolic and duodenocolic reflexes.
   d. Stimulate anorectal reflex if necessary by inserting a glycerin suppository or a gloved finger into rectum.
   e. Have the patient use a normal posture for defecation—a toilet seat or commode most nearly approximates the physiologic position for defecation.
   f. Instruct the patient to bear down and contract the abdominal muscles.

g. Have the patient lean forward to increase intra-abdominal pressure by compression against the thighs.

3. Ensure adequate fiber and fluid intake 2–4 liters (2.1–4.2 quarts) daily.
4. Encourage patient to exercise—good abdominal muscle tone and muscular activity is helpful in bowel training.

Evaluation

1. Achieves regular bowel functioning.
2. Is free of fecal soiling/incontinence.

Discharge Planning and Referral for Follow-up Care

Goals:

Improve the future quality of life.

Maintain continuity of care during transfer from the health care facility to another setting (home, extended care facility, or independent living arrangement).

1. Plan for care at home or in another setting as soon after hospital admission as possible.
2. Gather information about the patient's home environment (from patient, family, social worker, community health nurse, and other resources).
3. Plan, with the patient, ways and methods of coping with problems that may arise, and make realistic plans for the future.
4. Give the care-giver/family a written summary of the care plan, names of resource persons, lists of supplies and where these are obtained, and copies of equipment instructional booklets. (See Family Support, p. 127.)
5. Send referral form to local community health agency so nurse can evaluate the home environment.
   a. Review patient's ADL sheet with community health nurse—so community nurses will know exactly what activities patient can perform.
   b. Determine what modifications will be necessary in the home (for wheelchair, for self-care activities).
   c. Inquire how the patient expects to be transported for clinic visits, special therapy, etc.
6. Send referral to the State Vocational Rehabilitation Agency if the patient will require additional educational or job training.
7. Assist with transfer of the patient to extended-care facility if he is unable to return to home situation.
   a. Recognize that not all families can be expected to carry on the rehabilitation program that the patient may require.
   b. Send the ADL sheet to the extended-care facility with the patient to help orient staff to the patient's goals and programs.

Bibliography

Books

American Nurses Association and Association of Rehabilitation Nurses. Standards of Rehabilitation Nursing Practice. Kansas City, American Nurses Association, 1986

Bernstein LH, Grieco AJ, and Dete MK (eds). Primary Care in the Home. Philadelphia, JB Lippincott, 1987

Caplan B (ed). Rehabilitation Psychology Desk Reference. Rockville, MD, Aspen Publishers, 1987

Clarkson HM and Gilewich GB. Musculoskeletal Assessment: Joint Range of Motion and Manual Muscle Strength. Baltimore, Williams & Wilkins, 1989

DeLisa JA et al. Rehabilitation Medicine. Philadelphia, JB Lippincott, 1988

Dittmar SS. Rehabilitation Nursing: Process and Applications. St. Louis, CV Mosby, 1989

Goodgold J (ed). Rehabilitation Medicine. St. Louis, CV Mosby, 1988

Goodwill CJ and Chamberlain MA. Rehabilitation of the Physically Disabled Adult. London, Sheridan Medical Books, 1988

Granger CV, Seltzer GB, and Fishbein CF. Primary Care of the Functionally Disabled. Philadelphia, JB Lippincott, 1987

Hopkins HL and Smith HD. Willard and Spackman's Occupational Therapy. 7th ed. Philadelphia, JB Lippincott, 1988

Mosey AC. Psychosocial Components of Occupational Therapy. New York, Raven Press, 1986

Movrad LA and Droste MM. The Nursing Process in the Care of Adults with Orthopedic Conditions. New York, John Wiley & Sons, 1988

Musselwhite CR and St. Louis KW. Communication Programming for Persons with Severe Handicaps: Vocal and Augmentative Strategies. Boston, Little, Brown & Co., 1988

O'Sullivan SB. Physical Rehabilitation: Assessment and Treatment. Philadelphia, FA Davis, 1988

Payton OD et al (eds). Manual of Physical Therapy. New York, Churchill–Livingstone, 1989

Peat JM. Current Physical Therapy. Philadelphia, BC Decker, 1988

Pelosi T and Gleeson M. Illustrated Transfer Techniques for Disabled People. New York, Churchill–Livingstone, 1988

Power PW, Dell Orto AE, and Gibbons MB (eds). Family Interventions Throughout Chronic Illness and Disability. New York, Springer, 1988

Ringer SP. Neuromuscular Disorders: A Guide for Patient and Family. New York, Raven Press, 1987

Schover LR and Jensen SB. Sexuality and Chronic Illness: A Comprehensive Approach. New York, Guilford Press, 1988

Sinaki M. Basic Clinical Rehabilitation Medicine. Philadelphia, BC Decker, 1987

Trieschmann RB. Spinal Cord Injuries: Psychological, Social, and Vocational Rehabilitation. 2nd ed. New York, Demos Publications, 1988

Trieschmann RB. Aging with a Disability. New York, Demos Publications, 1988

Trombly CA. Occupational Therapy for Physical Dysfunction. 3rd ed. Baltimore, Williams & Wilkins, 1989

Van Husselt VB, Strain PS, and Hersen M. Handbook of Developmental and Physical Disabilities. New York, Pergamon Press, 1988

Weiss L. Access to the World: A Travel Guide for the Handicapped. New York, Henry Holt, 1986

Zarle N. Continuing Care. Rockville, MD, Aspen Publishers, 1987

Journals

General

Becker G and Kaufman S. Old age, rehabilitation and research: A review of the issues. Gerontol 1988 Aug; 28(4):459–468

Coburn J and Manderino MA. Stress innoculation: An illustration of coping skills training. Rehabil Nurs 1986 Jan-Feb; 11(1):14–17

Mulley GP. Walking sticks. Br Med J 1988 Feb 13; 296(6620):475

Painter P and Blackburn G. Exercise for patients with chronic disease. Postgrad Med 1988 Jan; 83(1):185–196

Selcher D. When your patient needs a cane, walker, or wheelchair. RN 1987 Dec; 50(12):60

Swanson B, Cronin–Stubbs D and Sheldon JA. The impact of psychosocial factors on adapting to physical disability: A review of the research literature. Rehabil Nurs 1989 Mar-Apr; 14(2):64–68

Vignos PJ Jr. Enhancing activities of daily living. Phys Med Rehabil 1988 Nov; 2(4):577–595

Family

Brillhart B. Family support for the disabled. Rehabil Nurs 1988 Nov-Dec; 13(6):316–319

Diehl LN. Client and family learning in the rehabilitation setting. Nurs Clin North Am 1989 Mar; 24(1):257–264

Murphy KE. The impact of home care on the family. Phys Med Rehabil 1988 Aug; 2(3):327–339

Power PW. Working with families: An intervention model for rehabilitation nurses. Rehabil Nurs 1989 Mar-Apr; 14(2):73–76

Incontinence Management

Andersson K-E. Current concepts in the treatment of disorders of micturition. Drugs 1988 Apr; 35(4):477–494

Consensus Conference (NIH). Urinary incontinence. JAMA 1989 May 12; 261(18):2685–2690

Hu T-W et al. A clinical trial of behavioral therapy to reduce urinary incontinence in nursing homes. JAMA 1989 May 12; 261(18):2556–2662

Kaplan SA and Blaivas JG. Practical approach to the diagnosis of urinary incontinence. Semin Neurol 1988 Summer; 8(2):131–136

Mathers S and Swash M. Faecal incontinence. Int Disabil Stud 1988; 10(4):164–168

Ouslander JG (ed). Urinary incontinence. Clin Geriatr Med 1986 Nov; 2(4):639–885

Parulkar BG and Barrett DM. Urinary incontinence in adults. Surg Clin North Am 1988 Oct; 68(5):945–963

Romanowski GL et al. Urinary incontinence in the elderly: Etiology and treatment. Drug Intell Clin Pharm 1988 Jul-Aug; 22(7–8):525–533

Solomon DH et al. New issues in geriatric care. Ann Intern Med 1988 May; 108(5):718–732

Wyman JF and Burgio KL. Advances in urinary incontinence management in the elderly. Adv Clin Rehabil 1988; 2: 82–107

Pressure Sores

Allman RM. Pressure sores among the elderly. N Engl J Med 1989 Mar 30; 320(13):850–853

Buntine JA and Johnstone BR. The contributions of plastic surgery to care of the spinal cord injured patient. Paraplegia 1988 Apr; 26(2):87–93

Conforti C. Pressure sores: Dressed for successful healing. Nursing 1989 Mar; 19(3):58–61

Crenshaw RP and Visnes LM. A decade of pressure sore research: 1977–1987. J Rehabil Res Dev 1989 Winter; 26(1): 63–74

Guralnik JM et al. Occurrence and predictors of pressure sores in the National Health and Nutrition Examination Survey follow-up. J Am Geriatr Soc 1988 Sep; 36(9):807–812

Knight AL. Medical management of pressure sores. J Fam Pract 1988 Jul; 27(1):95–100

Levine JM, Simpson M and McDonald RJ. Pressure sores: A plan for primary care prevention. Geriatrics 1989 Apr; 41(4): 75–76, 83–87, 90

Melcher RE, Longe RL and Gelbart AO. Pressure sores in the elderly: A systematic approach to management. Postgrad Med 1988 Jan; 83(1):299–308

Mondoux LCA (ed). Pressure ulcers. Nurs Clin North Am 1987 Jun; 22(2): 357–492

Moriarty M-B. How color can clarify wound care. RN 1988 Sep; 51(9):49–51, 54

Perdue RW and Wilson JL. Decubitus ulcers. J Am Board Fam Pract 1989 Jan-Mar; 2(1):43–48

Stotts NA. Predicting pressure ulcer development in surgical patients. Heart Lung 1988 Nov; 17(6) Part 1:641–647

Sexuality

Andrews S. Coping with the sexual health interview. J Nurse Midwifery 1988 Nov-Dec; 33(6):269–273

Bell N. Sexuality: Promoting fulfillment. Nurs Times 1989 Feb 8–14; 85(6):35–37

Bell N. Sexuality and the ostomist. Nurs Times 1989 Feb 1–7; 85(5):28–30

Berard EJ. The sexuality of spinal cord injured women: Physiology and pathophysiology. A review. Paraplegia 1989 Apr; 27(2):99–112

Blackmore C. The impact of orchidectomy upon the sexuality of the man with testicular cancer. Cancer Nurs 1988 Feb; 11(1):33–40

Csesko PA. Sexuality and multiple sclerosis. J Neurosci Nurs 1988 Dec; 20(6):353–355

Dewis ME and Thornton NG. Sexual dysfunction in multiple sclerosis. J Neurosci Nurs 1989 Jun; 21(3):175–179

Glass JC Jr and Dalton JA. Sexuality in older adults: A continuing education concern. J Contin Educ Nurs 1988 Mar-Apr; 19(2):61–64

Goddard LR. Sexuality and spinal cord injury. J Neurosci Nurs 1988 Aug; 20(4):240–244

Grant LM and Demetriou E. Adolescent sexuality. Pediatr Clin North Am 1988 Dec; 35(6):1271–1289

McKenzie F. Sexuality after total pelvic exenteration. Nurs Times 1988 May 18–24; 84(20):26–30

Pervin-Dixon L. Sexuality and the spinal cord injured. J Psychosoc Nurs Ment Health Serv 1988 Apr; 26(4):31–34

Pincus S. Sexuality in the mentally retarded patient. Am Fam Physician 1988 Feb; 37(2):319–323

Rieve JE. Sexuality and the adult with acquired physical disability. Nurs Clin North Am 1989 Mar; 24(1):265–276

Steinke EE. Older adults' knowledge and attitudes about sexuality and aging. Image J Nurs Sch 1988 Summer; 20(2): 93–95

Taylor MO. Teaching patients about their impaired adolescent's sexuality. MCN 1989 Mar-Apr; 14(2):109–112

White EJ. Appraising the need for altered sexuality information. Rehabil Nurs 1986 May-Jun; 11(6):6–9

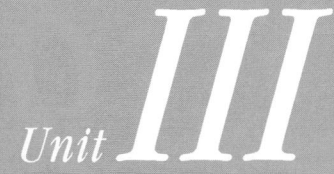

Respiratory Disorders

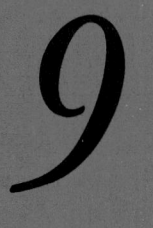

Upper Respiratory Disorders
(Conditions of the Nose and Throat)

Problems of the Nose and Sinuses

Rhinitis

Rhinitis is an inflammation of the mucous membrane of the nose, often producing excessive nasal secretions and obstruction.

Types

Allergic—IgE-mediated response causing release of vasoactive substances from mast cells

Infectious—viral (common cold) and bacterial (purulent)

Drug-induced (rebound rhinitis; rhinitis medicamentosa)—caused by excessive use of topical nasal decongestants

Nonallergic, noninfectious (vasomotor rhinitis)—unexplained autonomic nasal dysfunction as a result of overactivity of the parasympathetic nerve supply to the mucuous membranes of the nose and paranasal sinuses

Clinical Manifestations

1. Hypersecretion; wet running/dripping nose or post-nasal drip
2. Nasal obstruction symptoms: nasal congestion, pressure, or stuffiness
3. Headache

> **NURSING ALERT:** Instruct patient as follows:
> 1. Do not blow nose too frequently or too hard; doing so may cause infection to spread, sinuses to become infected, and an eardrum to be perforated.
> 2. Blow through both nostrils at the same time to equalize pressure.

Management

1. Treatment of underlying cause (allergy; infection)

Patient Education

1. Avoid irritating inhalants, especially smoke, aerosols, noxious fumes.
2. Do not over use topical nasal sprays/drops. Decongestant nasal sprays/drops should not be used for more than 3 consecutive days.

Nasal Obstruction

Causes

1. Deviated septum
2. Hypertrophy of turbinate bones
3. Nasal polyps
4. Tumors; scars; adhesions
5. Fractures; foreign bodies
6. Adenoid hypertrophy
7. Overuse of nose drops; drugs (rauwolfia; antithyroid drugs)

Related Problems

1. Chronic infection of nose
2. Sinusitis; pain in sinus regions
3. Recurrent otitis media

Management

1. Removal of cause, including surgical interventions (see Nasal Surgery)
2. Correction of infection

Epistaxis

Epistaxis refers to nose bleed or hemorrhage from the nose. It most commonly originates in the anterior portion of the nasal cavity. Posterior nasal bleeding usually originates from the turbinates or lateral nasal wall.

Causes

1. Local:
   a. Dryness leading to crust formation—bleeding occurs with removal of crusts by nose picking
   b. Trauma
2. Systemic: Hypertension, arteriosclerosis, renal and bleeding disorders

Diagnostic Evaluation

1. Inspection with nasal speculum to determine site of bleeding. Important to determine which side bled first.
2. Blood evaluation to exclude blood dyscrasias.

Management

(Depends on severity and source of bleeding in nasal cavity.)

1. Patient is placed in an upright posture, leaning forward to reduce venous pressure and instructed to breathe gently through the mouth to prevent swallowing of blood.
2. Patient is instructed to compress the soft part of nasal tip with index finger and thumb for 5–10 minutes to maintain pressure on the nasal septum.
3. A cotton pledget soaked with a vasoconstricting agent may be inserted into each nostril and pressure applied. After 5–10 minutes the cotton is removed, and the site of bleeding is identified.
4. The blood vessel may be cauterized.
5. If bleeding continues (posterior bleeding), packing may be layered into nasal cavity and the nasopharynx or balloon tamponade may be required to apply pressure over a larger area.

> **NURSING ALERT:** Monitor the patient for a vasovagal episode during insertion of nasal packing.

6. Surgical ligation of vessels may be required.

Complications

Rhinitis; maxillary and frontal sinusitis; hemotympanum; otitis media

Nursing Interventions/Patient Education

1. Be aware that packing is uncomfortable and painful.
2. Monitor patient with posterior packing for hypoxia (from aspiration of blood, sedation, and pre-existing pulmonary dysfunction).
3. Monitor for respiratory difficulty or obstruction—secondary to slippage of packing or balloon, swelling of palate, relaxation of tongue.
4. Instruct the patient as follows for self-management of minor bleeding episodes:
   a. Sit up and lean forward while compressing the soft part (tip) of nose between index finger and thumb.
   b. If bleeding continues, moisten a small piece of cotton with vasoconstricting nose drops (phenylephrine hydrochloride [Neo-Synephrine] or oxymetazoline hydrochloride [Afrin]) and place inside nose. Press against bleeding site 5–10 minutes.
5. Avoid blowing or picking nose after a nose bleed.
6. After a week or so, apply a lubricant to nasal septum twice daily to reduce dryness.
7. Use a humidifier if environmental air is dry.

Nasal Surgery

Submucous resection of the septum is an operation in which cartilaginous and/or osseous portions of the septum that lie between the flaps of the mucous membrane and perichondrium are removed or straightened—to establish an adequate partition between the right and left nasal cavities in order to provide a clear nasal airway.

Nasal septal reconstruction involves resection or removal of cartilaginous (or bony septum) followed by reconstruction of all parts of the septum that may produce nasal airway obstruction.

Nasal fracture results from direct trauma, for example, a blow inflicted by an object (ball or fist) or an injury sustained in an automobile collision.

Preoperative Interventions/Management

A. Control of Bleeding

1. Raise head of bed to promote drainage, lessen edema, and make patient more comfortable.
2. Apply intermittent cold compresses as directed.
3. With fracture:
   a. Prepare for reduction, which is usually done in ambulatory surgical setting.
   b. Following the procedure, the nose is taped near dorsum and a small cast may be applied to help reduce swelling and stabilize nasal bone fragments.

B. Give Adequate Explanations of What to Expect

1. Tell the patient that a pressure sensation may be felt in the nasal area during surgery.
2. Project that there may be short-term use of nasal packing to effect hemostasis.
3. Indicate that facial or periorbital ecchymosis (bruising) may be present, and that it will gradually subside.

Potential Complications Following Nasal Surgery

1. Hematoma/hemorrhage
2. Local infection—contaminated nasal packing an excellent culture medium for pathogens
3. Aspiration
4. Pressure necrosis (from packing)

Postoperative Nursing Interventions

Goal:
Promote comfort and prevent complications

1. Apply cold compresses or ice packs intermittently for 24 hours—to lessen edema and discoloration and to promote comfort.
2. Change the gauze pad under the nose as it becomes soaked with blood; this should gradually decrease in amount.
3. Notify surgeon if bleeding increases.
4. Reassure the patient about the sucking sound that will be experienced on swallowing; the nasal packing prevents air from moving through the nose, and a partial vacuum is created in the throat during swallowing.
5. Instruct the patient not to blow his nose but to blot secretions with tissue.
6. Administer frequent mouth care, as the patient is forced to breathe through the mouth; use flexible straw to sip mouthwash for rinsing purposes.

Patient Education

1. Keep head elevated (3–4 pillows) day and night to keep swelling down.
2. Use a vaporizer—helps relieve crusting of nasal mucosa from dryness.
3. Avoid aspirin and aspirin-containing products.
4. Remember that sneezing, straining, and nose blowing increase venous pressure and can result in bleeding/hematoma.
5. If unable to control sneezing, keep the mouth open while sneezing.
6. Do not remove adherent crusts; they will separate by themselves from underlying tissue.
7. Avoid environmental irritants, especially smoke.

8. Avoid strenuous activity and trauma to nose; the motion of bony fragments (following fracture) within soft tissue will produce laceration and bleeding.
9. Avoid excessive alcohol intake—dilates blood vessels.
10. If a nasal splint is present, avoid getting it wet; do not remove it.
11. Postoperative follow-up may need to continue for 6–12 months to monitor for excess callous formation or cosmetic deformity.

Sinusitis

Sinusitis is an inflammation of the mucous membranes of one or more paranasal sinuses. It is usually precipitated by congestion from a viral upper respiratory infection and/or nasal allergy. Obstruction of the ostia (resulting from mucosal swelling and/or mechanical obstruction), leads to retention of secretions and is the usual precursor to sinusitis.

Acute Sinusitis

A. Clinical Manifestations

1. Pain; stabbing or aching, over the infected sinus
   a. Frontal sinusitis—pain in forehead intensified by bending forward
   b. Maxillary sinusitis—aching pain in facial region and from inner canthus of the eye to the teeth
   c. Ethmoid sinusitis—frontal or orbital headache
   d. Sphenoid sinusitis—headache referred to top of head and deep to the eyes
2. Nasal congestion and discharge; may or may not be present
3. Anosmia (lack of smell): inspired or expired air cannot reach the olfactory groove
4. Red and edematous nasal mucosa

B. Diagnostic Evaluation

1. Clinical presentation and physical examination
2. Sinus radiographs
3. Antral puncture and lavage—provides culture material; also a therapeutic modality to clear sinus of bacteria, fluid, and inflammatory cells

C. Management

Goal:
To improve ostial patency

1. Topical decongestant spray or drops for mucosal shrinkage to encourage drainage from sinus. This should be limited to no more than 3 successive days of use.
2. Topical decongestant may be combined with oral decongestant.
3. Antibiotic (amoxicillin, cefaclor, etc.,) for purulent sinusitis
4. Analgesics—pain may be significant
5. Warm compresses; cool vapor humidity for comfort

D. Complications

(Depend on anatomic location of sinus involved)
1. Extension of infection to the orbital contents and eyelids

   Note: Watch for lid edema, edema of ocular conjunctiva, drooping lid, limitation of extraocular motion, visual loss.
2. Bone infection (osteomyelitis) may spread by direct extension or via blood vessels. Frontal bone commonly affected.

3. Central nervous system complications include meningitis, subdural and epidural purulent drainage, brain abscess, cavernous sinus thrombosis (acute thrombophlebitis originating from an infection in an area having venous drainage to cavernous sinus).

E. Patient Education

1. Acute sinus infection may lead to chronic sinus disease.
2. Swimming/diving may cause contaminated water to be forced into a sinus, usually the frontal sinus.

Chronic Sinusitis

Chronic sinusitis is a suppurative inflammation of the sinuses with chronic irreversible change in the mucosa and sinus bony area.

A. Clinical Manifestations

1. Persistent nasal obstruction; chronic nasal discharge, clear or purulent when infected
2. Cough—produced by constant dripping of discharge back into nasopharynx
3. Feeling of facial fullness/pressure
4. Headache, more noticeable in the morning

B. Diagnostic Evaluation

1. Sinus roentgenograms
2. Endoscopy of nose with computed tomographic imaging—reveals mucosal changes

C. Management

1. Vasoconstricting drugs to promote drainage.

   Note: Recognize danger of prolonged use of decongestants, which may lead to *rebound rhinitis* (rhinitis medicamentosa), a recurring cycle of nasal congestion, use of decongestants, rebound nasodilatation, nasal congestion, more decongestants, etc.
2. Antibiotics for infection
3. Surgical interventions (when conservative treatment is unsuccessful)
   a. Endoscopic sinus surgery—endoscopic removal of diseased tissue from affected sinus; used to treat chronic sinusitis of maxillary, ethmoid, and frontal sinuses
   b. Nasal antrostomy (nasal-antral window)—surgical placement of an opening under inferior turbinate to provide aeration of the antrum and to permit exit for purulent materials
   c. Caldwell–Luc operation—procedure provides for removal of diseased mucosal lining of maxillary sinus combined with development of nasal-antral window. Incision made along upper gumline above canine teeth.
   d. Surgical interventions for repair of structural abnormalities, deviated septum, polyps, etc.

D. Nursing Interventions/Patient Education

1. See Nasal Surgery, page 149.
2. Instruct patient about using careful oral hygiene. Use mouthwash with aid of flexible straw.
3. Avoid trauma to the nose.
4. Avoid smoke in the environment.
5. After Caldwell–Luc procedure:
   a. Provide cold compresses over lip to help reduce swelling.
   b. Advise patient that numbness in operative area may be present for several weeks to months.
   c. Instruct the patient to refrain from blowing nose after removal of packing, to avoid forcing nasal secretions back into maxillary sinus.

Specific Infections of the Upper Respiratory Tract

Viral Infections (Common Cold)

The *common cold* refers to a syndrome related to inflammation of the cells of the respiratory epithelium by any group of respiratory viruses.

Causes

Rhinoviruses (account for 50% of common colds; more than 100 serotypes), adenoviruses; myxoviruses; paramyxoviruses, coronaviruses

Clinical Manifestations

(Occur within 24–72 hours after viral inoculation)
1. Sneezing, scratchy sore throat, headache
2. Sensation of chilliness
3. Symptoms of nasal discharge and obstruction
4. Cough

Complications

1. Persons with asthma or chronic bronchitis may experience worsening of symptoms of chronic obstructive pulmonary disease.
2. Persistence of purulent nasal discharge after 10–14 days may indicate bacterial sinusitis.

Management

1. No single specific treatment
2. Symptomatic treatment includes:
   a. Aspirin to relieve systemic symptoms; does not shorten duration of infection
   b. Cold-water vaporization of immediate environment

Nursing Interventions/Patient Education

The following measures are intended to support body defenses and reduce susceptibility:
1. Observe careful handwashing to avoid person-to-person spread of virus-contaminated secretions.
2. Employ humidity measures indoors during winter months.
3. Minimize alcohol intake.
4. Avoid inhaling irritating substances: *smoke;* chemicals; dust; sprays.
5. Use health-enhancing behaviors, including good nutrition, regular exercise, adequate sleep, and positive coping strategies.

Herpes Simplex Infection (Type 1) (Cold Sores; Fever Blister)

The herpes simplex virus (HSV, type 1) is a DNA virus most often associated with lip and oral lesions (herpes labialis.) (Genital herpes is usually caused by herpes simplex virus, type 2).

Clinical Features

1. Following a primary infection, it is thought that the herpes simplex virus remains latent in the neural ganglia and is activated by some stimulus that triggers the migration of the virus to the oral epithelium, resulting in lesions commonly called a "cold sore" or "fever blister."
2. Recurrent herpes labialis may be precipitated by exposure to sunlight, fatigue, hormonal changes, gastrointestinal disturbances, and oral trauma (e.g., dental procedures).

Clinical Manifestations

1. Prodromal period: tautness, soreness, burning sensation, or swelling in area where lesions will develop.
2. Small vesicles appear, frequently in the mucocutaneous junction of the lips or adjacent skin.
3. Vesicles rupture: ulcerations fuse together and form larger weeping ulcers; lesions heal spontaneously in 7–14 days.

Management

1. Acyclovir may be useful in immunocompromised patients.
2. Topical anesthetic, lidocaine (Xylocaine), or dyclonine (Dyclone) may provide relief of painful lesions when applied to affected areas.
3. Applications of drying lotions/liquids may help dry lesions

Streptococcal Pharyngitis

Streptococcal pharyngitis is an acute bacterial infection of the throat caused by group A streptococci.

Clinical Manifestations

1. *Abrupt* onset of sore throat; fever above 38.2°C. (101°F.)
2. Throat pain aggravated by swallowing
3. Pharynx appears reddened with edema of uvula; tonsils enlarged and reddened; pharynx and tonsils may be covered with exudate
4. Swollen, palpable, and tender cervical lymph nodes

Diagnostic Evaluation

1. WBC—leukocytosis
2. Examination of oral cavity, oropharynx, hypopharynx, and neck
3. Throat culture for bacteriological diagnosis to determine presence/absence of streptococci.

Note: Rapid streptococcal antigen detection tests are now available for rapid detection of group A streptococci directly from a throat swab; results available while patient is in clinic/office

Management

1. Penicillin G orally for 10 days *or* benzathine penicillin G in a single IM dose—early antibiotic treatment appears to shorten duration of symptoms
2. Erythromycin—for patient who is allergic to penicillin

Complications

1. Suppurative complications—sinusitis; otitis media; mastoiditis
2. Nonsuppurative complications—acute rheumatic fever; acute glomerulonephritis

Note: Acute rheumatic fever, a complication of streptococcal pharyngitis, can be prevented if patient is treated adequately with penicillin. Unfortunately, there is no evidence that antibiotic therapy will prevent acute glomerulonephritis, also a complication of streptococcal pharyngitis.

Patient Education

Advise the patient to:
1. Rest in bed and drink liberal amounts of fluids.
2. Use local treatment for relief of throat soreness, including warm saline irrigations or gargles.
3. Monitor temperature.

Cancer of the Larynx

Incidence

1. Occurs predominantly in men over 60.
2. A majority of patients have a history of smoking; those with supraglottic laryngeal cancer frequently have a history of smoking and a high alcohol intake.
3. In North America, about ⅔ of carcinomas of the larynx arise in the glottis, almost ⅓ arise in the supraglottic region, and about 3% in the subglottic region of the larynx.

Clinical Expectations

1. When treated early, the likelihood of cure is great.
2. When limited to the vocal cords (intrinsic), spread is slow because of lessened blood supply.
3. When cancer involves the epiglottis (extrinsic), cancer spreads more rapidly because of abundant supply of blood and lymph and soon involves the lymph nodes of the neck.

Clinical Manifestations (Fig. 9-1)

(Depend on tumor location; sequence in appearance related to pattern and extent of tumor growth)

A. Supraglottic Cancer
1. Tickling sensation in throat
2. Dryness and fullness (lump) in throat
3. Painful swallowing (odynophagia)—associated with invasion of extra laryngeal musculature)
4. Coughing on swallowing
5. Pain radiating to ear (late symptom)

B. Glottic (Vocal Cord) **Cancer** (Most Common)
1. *Hoarseness or voice change*
2. Aphonia (loss of voice)
3. Dyspnea
4. Pain (in later stages)

C. Subglottic Cancer (Uncommon)
1. Coughing
2. Short periods of difficulty in breathing
3. Hemoptysis; fetid odor—results from ulceration and disintegration of tumor

Diagnostic Evaluation

1. Indirect mirror examination of larynx
2. Direct laryngoscopy and biopsy
3. CT scan and other special radiologic tests
4. Laryngography—contrast study of larynx to define blood vessels and lymph nodes

Management

(Depends on sites and stages of cancer)

A. Endoscopic Removal of Early Malignancy

B. Radiation
1. Singly or in combination with surgery

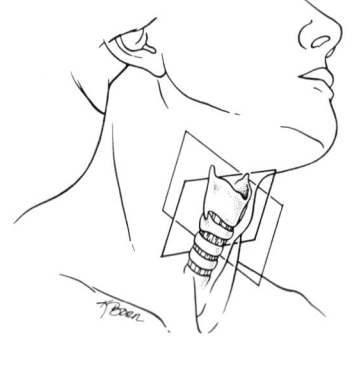 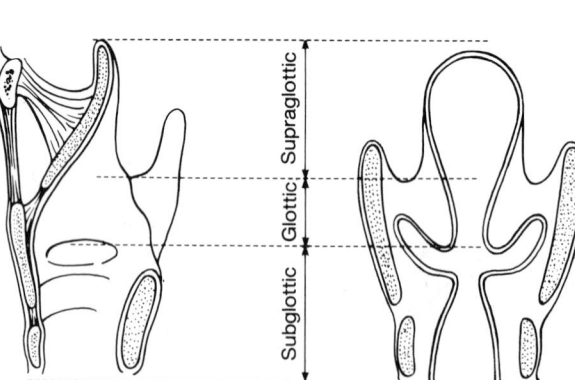

Figure 9-1. *Manifestations of cancer of the larynx. The larynx is divided into three regions: supraglottic, glottic, and subglottic. Clinical manifestations of cancer of the larynx depend on the tumor location and extent of tumor growth.*

2. Complications of radiation: edema of larynx; soft tissue and cartilage necrosis; chondritis (inflammation of cartilage)

C. Surgery

1. Carbon dioxide laser for early stage disease
2. Partial laryngectomy—removal of small lesion on true cord, along with a substantial margin of healthy tissue.
3. Supraglottic laryngectomy—removal of hyoid bone, epiglottis, and false vocal cords; tracheostomy may be done to maintain adequate airway; radical neck dissection may be done.
4. Hemilaryngectomy—removal of one true vocal cord, false cord, one half of thyroid cartilage, arytenoid cartilage.
5. Total laryngectomy—removal of entire larynx (epiglottis, false or true cords, cricoid cartilage, hyoid bone; 2 or 3 tracheal rings are usually removed when there is extrinsic cancer of the larynx [extension beyond the vocal cords]). A radical neck dissection may also be done because of metastasis to cervical lymph nodes.
6. Total laryngectomy with laryngoplasty—voice rehabilitation may be attempted through the *Asai operation.*
   a. A dermal tube is made from the upper end of the trachea into the hypopharynx.
   b. The tracheostomy opening is closed off with a finger.
   c. Then the patient expires air up the dermal tube into the pharyngeal cavity.
   d. The sound produced is transformed into almost normal speech.

Modes of Communication

1. Artificial larynx, using either neck or intraoral placement
   Electrolarynx—provides communication assistance in early postoperative period or later to those unable to learn alternate method
2. Tracheoesophageal puncture (TEP) with voice prosthesis. Puncture made between posterior wall of tracheostoma and underlying esophagus; a one-way valved voice prosthesis inserted through TEP that allows patient to shunt pulmonary air into esophagus for voice production (Fig. 9-2).
3. Esophageal speech—accomplished by training patient to force air down the esophagus and release it in a controlled manner
4. Surgical reconstructive procedures to restore voice

Preoperative Nursing Interventions

A. Preparation for Total Laryngectomy

1. Collaborate with the physician in preparing the patient; interpret and amplify what physician/speech–language pathologist have explained.
2. Inform patient that breathing will occur through an opening (tracheostoma) in the neck.
3. Apprise patient of the fact that speech will be altered by surgery.
   a. Expect reactions of anxiety and depression, as the psychosocial effects of voice loss are substantial.
   b. Practice a means of communication (pad and pencil, sign language, pictures, word cards, artificial larynx) that can be used until speech therapy begins.
   c. Arrange for patient to be visited by laryngectomee

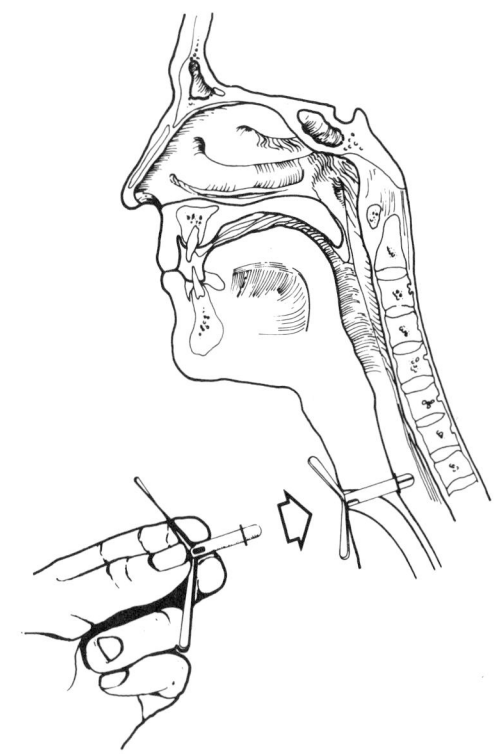

Figure 9-2. *Tracheoesophageal puncture for communication following laryngectomy. A one-way valved voice prosthesis can be placed in a surgically created tracheal–esophageal fistula to allow pulmonary air to be shunted into the esophagus for esophageal voice production. (From DeLisa JA. Rehabilitation Medicine: Principles and Practice. Philadelphia, JB Lippincott, 1988)*

(one who has had larynx removed) for hope and encouragement.
   d. Inform patient of available community services.

Nursing Assessment

1. Ask about smoking history, alcohol intake, drug history.
2. Ask about onset of hoarseness (duration and persistence), feeling of "lump" in throat, presence/absence of chronic irritative cough, weight loss.
3. Take a nutrition history and 24-hour food intake recall; review results of laboratory tests; weigh the patient.
4. Listen to the patient's voice—weak? muffled? clear?
5. Observe ability to swallow.
6. Review recommendations of speech-language pathologist and social worker.
7. Assess for independence, self-assuredness, and willingness to try new things; these are strengths on which to build.
8. Study patient's record to learn location of the lesion.
9. Assess reality of patient's expectations.
10. Find out about patient's social support system.

Nursing Diagnoses

1. Altered breathing pattern related to presence of artificial airway (tracheostomy or laryngectomy tube), accumulation of secretions, inability to cough secondary to surgical procedure

2. Altered nutrition (less than body requirements) related to impaired swallowing secondary to surgical alteration of pharynx and larynx; laryngeal edema and pain; radiation-induced mucositis; decrease in quantity and quality of sputum
3. Impaired verbal communication related to surgery/absence of larynx; presence of artificial airway
4. Knowledge deficit of stoma care and living with effects of laryngectomy
5. Anxiety related to fear of suffocation; inability to communicate
6. Potential impairment of skin integrity related to secretions from tracheostoma
7. Social isolation related to inability to express feelings, appearance of tracheostoma; unusual quality of esophageal speech
8. Disturbance in self-esteem related to feelings of inferiority, personal inadequacy, and frustration

Possible Complications

1. Salivary fistula—may develop following any surgical procedure that involves entering the pharynx or esophagus.
   a. Monitor for saliva collecting beneath the skin flaps or leaking through suture line or drain site.
   b. Management: Nasogastric tube feeding; meticulous local wound care with frequent dressing changes; promotion of drainage
2. Hemorrhage (carotid artery rupture) or hematoma formation
   a. A major postoperative complication such as skin necrosis or salivary fistula usually precedes carotid artery rupture.
   b. Management: Immediate wound exploration in operating room.
3. Stomal stenosis
4. Aspiration
5. *Long-Term Complications*
   a. Chest infections (from repeated aspiration)
   b. Recurrence of cancer in stoma

Nursing Interventions

A. Attaining and Maintaining Adequate Respirations

1. Monitor for signs of difficult breathing; suprasternal and intercostal retractions, tachypnea, dyspnea, tachycardia, changes in sensorium.
2. Auscultate trachea/chest for evidence of stridor, wheezing, and absence of breath sounds.
3. Be sure that the patient uses a specific signal to indicate need for suctioning; enter on nursing care plan.
4. Suction secretions as they accumulate to clean and protect the airway and prevent subsequent aspiration. (See page 173 for technique).
   a. Suction nasal secretions also as patient is unable to blow nose.
   b. Remove crusts from nares and apply ointment.
5. Employ chest physical therapy as necessary to remove secretions.
6. Remember that postoperative patient is unable to cough;
   a. Teach to bend forward until stoma is below lung level and to exhale rapidly—aids in secretion removal from lungs.
   b. Teach to wipe resultant secretions away from tracheostoma with a handkerchief.
7. Encourage breathing exercises, as most patients have been heavy smokers.

8. Supply *constant* humidification to moisten tracheostoma and avoid viscous secretions; tracheal air will require additional warmth and moisture.
9. Keep calm and maintain sense of security.
   a. Reassure patient that someone is always near to assist.
   b. Have call bell within reach.

B. Relearning Swallowing

1. Monitor intravenous fluids during first few postoperative days.
2. Administer fluids and nutrients by nasogastric or esophagostomy tube.
   a. Tube feedings started after bowel sounds are heard and continued until sufficient healing of pharynx has occurred (10–12 days) and patient is ready to resume oral feedings.
   b. Avoid manipulating nasogastric tube as it is resting on/near suture line.
   c. Cleanse nostrils and lubricate with water-soluble lubricant.
   d. Cleanse crusts on outside of tube.
   e. Give attention to oral hygiene, with regular tooth brushing and prescribed antiseptic mouthwashes.
3. Encourage patient as he relearns swallowing.
   a. Ensure quiet environment, as relearning how to swallow causes frustration and requires concentration. Have standby suction available.
   b. Place patient in sitting position, leaning slightly forward—allows larynx to move forward and hypopharynx to partially open.
   c. Explain that the epiglottis normally prevents fluid/food from entering larynx during swallowing.
   d. Training for swallowing:
      (1) Inhale before swallowing, swallow, cough gently while exhaling and re-swallow.
      (2) This ensures adequate air in lungs to cough out any food that has passed into the unguarded laryngeal region, thus preventing aspiration.

C. Mastering an Alternative Form of Communication

1. Advise patient to communicate by writing until voice work can begin with speech-language pathologist.
2. Discourage forced whispering, which increases pharyngeal tension.
3. Reassure that speech therapy will begin as soon as patient can swallow comfortably.
4. Encourage patient to join local laryngectomy support group (Lost Chord Club; New Voice Club)—gives opportunity to practice new speech and serves as a bridge between therapy and return to social life.

D. Learning About Tracheostoma Care and Living With Laryngectomy

1. Usually a laryngectomy or tracheostomy tube is worn until stoma heals (1–2 months); patient then starts gradual process of leaving tube out 1 hour at a time.
2. Demonstrate procedure for cleaning and changing tube.
   a. See page 239 for tracheostomy tube care.
   b. Place gauze dressing under tube to absorb secretions as prescribed. Change when it becomes soiled, to prevent skin irritation and odor.
   c. Encourage patient to practice changing tracheostomy tie tapes.
3. Tracheostoma care: Teach patient to:
   a. Wash hands before touching stoma to prevent infection.

b. Wet wash cloth with warm water; wring dry and gently wipe stoma.
   Do not use soap, tissues, or cotton balls, as these may enter airway.
c. Apply petrolatum around exterior of stoma to prevent skin irritation.
d. Report excessive redness, swelling, purulent secretions, or bleeding.

4. Stoma cover
   a. Stoma cover is necessary to filter air and increase humidity of air; also necessary for hygienic purposes.
   b. Stoma cover can be crocheted or made of cotton cloth
   c. For men: Ascot or turtle neck sweaters may be worn. When a regular shirt is worn, the second button from the top can be sewed over the buttonhole as though it were fastened—this leaves a wide opening through which a handkerchief can be inserted when coughing.
   d. For women: A variety of fashionable scarves, jewelry, high-neck dresses, and turtleneck sweaters can be worn.

5. Bowel care
   Discuss high-fiber diet and use of stool softener, as patient with tracheostoma is usually not able to hold breath to ''bear down'' for bowel movement.

Patient Education

Teach the patient the following:
1. Provide humidification at home; use pans of water in the rooms, a humidifier, or cool mist vaporizer, especially in bedroom.

2. Avoid cold air; cover tracheostoma with thin layer of foam rubber or other cover to warm and humidify air.
3. Drink fluids liberally (2–3 liters) to help liquefy secretions.
4. Always keep stoma covered for hygienic management of secretions and to keep dust/foreign matter from entering trachea.
5. Place a protective shield over stoma:
   a. Before bathing, showering, or shampooing hair and while getting a hair cut or shaving
   b. Use an electric razor instead of blade, as shaving cream can irritate.
   c. Swimming is not recommended.
6. Expect some loss of smell and impairment of taste sensation.
7. Check with physician before taking any medication, as many drugs tend to dry the mucous membranes of the stoma.
8. Seek immediate attention for the following: pain, difficulty in breathing or swallowing, the appearance of pus or blood-streaked sputum.
9. In the event of an obstruction to the stoma, see Guidelines: Emergency First Aid for the Laryngectomy, below.

Evaluation

1. Breathing quietly; no evidence of noisy secretions
2. Swallowing soft foods; maintaining weight
3. Able to make needs known; speech therapy has started
4. Able to manage tracheostomal care; has made provisions for home humidification and tracheostomal supplies

Guidelines Emergency First Aid for the Laryngectomee

Nature of the Problem

Clogging or obstruction of the neck stoma is a life-threatening problem.

Equipment (if available):

Suction equipment
Sterile disposable catheter
#14–16 Fr. (adult)
#8–10 Fr. (child)

Sterile gloves
Sterile saline
Portable mask and bag

Procedure for Total Neck Breather

One who breathes ONLY through the neck opening
1. There is no connection between lungs and nose or mouth.
2. A tracheostomy or laryngectomy tube may or may not be in the neck opening.

NURSING ALERT: No air can get through the mouth or nose of a total laryngectomee when stoma is clogged.

Nursing Action	Rationale/Amplification
1. PLACE PATIENT ON HIS BACK, on a firm surface, head straight, chin up. Bare the neck down to the sternum.	1. Access to the laryngeal stoma and observation of thoracic movement are facilitated.
2. Position a blanket or any article of clothing under the shoulders.	2. This promotes extension of the neck area, permitting access.

3. Make a rapid assessment of the situation:
   a. Is victim wearing a tracheostomy or laryngectomy tube?
	3.
	   a. In a laryngectomee, tube removal cannot cause immediate danger.

(continued)

Guidelines	Emergency First Aid for the Laryngectomee *(continued)*

Procedure for Total Neck Breather *(continued)*	**Nursing Action**	**Rationale/Amplification**
	b. Has he been operated on recently?	b. If so, tracheostomy tube cannot be removed.
	c. Check for tracheal obstruction. Clean stomal opening of mucus and encrusted matter.	c. Mucus, etc. may account for obstruction. Use a clean cloth or handkerchief—never tissue.
	4. START MOUTH-TO-NECK BREATHING PROMPTLY: Position yourself at side of victim. Place your mouth and lips tightly over neck opening or around the tracheal tube if the person is wearing one.	4. SECONDS COUNT Do not remove the tube.
	5. If suction equipment is available, insert a soft rubber tube 7.5–12.5 cm. (3–5 in.) into opening for a few seconds.	5. A partially open airway transporting air to the victim is infinitely better than a clean airway that does not supply air at this crucial time.
	6. Blow in a sufficient amount of air to see chest rise; then release and allow chest to fall.	
	7. For the first 5 seconds, repeat every 1–2 seconds; then slow down to a steady pace of every 4–5 seconds (12–20 times per minute).	
	8. Continue until spontaneous breathing returns.	

Follow-up Phase

1. When victim recovers, provide oxygen from a portable supply.	
2. If breathing fails again, resume mouth-to-neck breathing.	
3. You can also use mechanical resuscitation with the rubber or plastic inflatable bag and mask combination.	3. Attach baby-sized mask; be sure there is a tight seal against neck opening. Because a tight seal is difficult to maintain and because pressure of the mask on the major blood vessels of the neck may interfere with blood supply to the brain, mouth-to-neck breathing is safer and better.
4. Watch the chest rise	
5. Observe the patient constantly.	

Procedure for Partial Neck Breather

One who breathes MAINLY through the neck opening.
1. A connection between the lungs and the nose and mouth still exists.
2. The larynx may or may not be present.
3. A tracheostomy or laryngectomy tube may or may not be in the neck opening.

NURSING ALERT: With mouth-to-neck breathing, FAILURE OF THE CHEST TO RISE is reliable proof that the patient is a partial neck breather. The rescuer may hear or feel air escaping from the victim's nose or mouth, but it is not getting into the lungs.

1. a. Immediately place the palm of your hand (the one nearest to the patient's head) over the lips and mouth. b. Pinch the nose shut between your third and fourth fingers. c. Place your thumb in the soft space under the chin and firmly press upward and backward.	1. This will close the area between the trachea and throat and at the same time raise the base of the tongue against the palate and pharynx.
2. Remove the patient's dentures.	2. To ensure better lip closure and effective underchin thumb closure
3. Now mouth-to-neck breathing will fill the lungs and the chest will rise.	

Bibliography

Books

Browning GG. Updated ENT. 2nd ed. Boston, Butterworths, 1987

Collins SL (ed). Pharmacology in Otolaryngology—Head and Neck Surgery. Washington, DC, American Academy of Otolaryngology—Head and Neck Surgery Foundation, 1987

DeWeese DD et al. Otolaryngology—Head and Neck Surgery. 7th ed. St Louis, CV Mosby, 1988

Fried MP (ed). The Larynx: A Multidisciplinary Approach. Boston, Little, Brown & Co, 1988

Gates GA (ed). Current Therapy in Otolaryngology—Head and Neck

Surgery, 3. Philadelphia, BC Decker, 1987

Goldman JL, Blaugrund SM and Shugar JMA (eds). The Principles and Practice of Rhinology. New York, John Wiley & Sons, 1987

Goldstein JC, Kashima HK, and Koopmann CF Jr. Geriatric

Otorhinolaryngology. Philadelphia, BC Decker, 1987

Hall IS and Colman BH. Diseases of the Nose, Throat, and Ear: A Handbook for Students and Practitioners. New York, Churchill-Livingstone, 1987

Kerr AG and Groves J (eds). Scott-Brown's Otolaryngology. 5th ed. Vol 1–5. Boston, Butterworths, 1987

Kleinsasser O. Tumors of the Larynx and Hypopharynx. New York, Thieme Medical Publishers, 1988

Lucente FE and Sobol SM. Essentials of Otolaryngology. 2nd ed. New York, Raven Press, 1988

Marin AGD. Logan Turner's Diseases of the Nose, Throat, and Ear. 10th ed. Littleton, MA, John Wright & Sons, 1988

Marshall KG and Attia EL. Disorders of the Nose and Paranasal Sinuses: Diagnosis and Management. Littleton, MA, PSG Publishing, 1987

Meyer-Breiting E and Burkhardt A. Tumours of the Larynx: Histopathology and Clinical Inferences. New York, Springer-Verlag, 1988

Riley MAK. Nursing Care of the Client with Ear, Nose, and Throat Disorders. New York, Springer, 1987

Upchurch DT et al. Otolaryngology: Problems in Primary Care. Oradell, NJ, Medical Economics Books, 1989

Journals

Cancer of Larynx/Laryngectomy

Barratt GE and Coulthard SW. Upper airway obstruction: Diagnosis and management options. Contemp Anesth Pract 1987; 9:73–96

Biggs C. The cancer that can cost a patient his voice. RN 1987 Apr; 50(4):44–51

Blom ED, Singer MI and Hamaker RC. A prospective study of tracheoesophageal speech. Arch Otolaryngol Head Neck Surg 1986 Apr; 112(4):440–447

Chu ML. Continuing care of a total laryngectomy patient. Home Healthc Nurse 1985 Jul–Aug; 3(4):37–39

Demas PN and Sotereanos GC. The use of tracheotomy in oral and maxillofacial surgery. J Oral Maxillofac Surg 1988 Jun; 46(6):483–486

Feinstein D. What to teach the patient who's had a total laryngectomy. RN 1987 Apr; 50(4):53–57

Forastiere AA. Review: Management of advanced stage squamous cell

carcinoma of the head and neck. Am J Med Sci 1986 Jun; 291(6):405–415

Gardine RL et al. Predicting the need for prolonged enteral supplementation in the patient with head and neck cancer. Am J Surg 1988 Jul; 156(1):63–65

Griffin CW and Lockhart JS. Learning to swallow again. Am J Nurs 1987 Mar; 87(3):314–317

Harris LL and Kraege J. After the T-E puncture: Relearning to speak. Am J Nurs 1986 Jan; 86(1):55–58

Juarbe C et al. Primary tracheoesophageal puncture for voice restoration. Am J Surg 1986 Oct; 152(4):464–466

Lopez MJ et al. Voice rehabilitation practices among head and neck surgeons. Ann Otol Rhinol Laryngol 1987 May–Jun; 96(2 Pt 1):261–263

Mastropietro C. The anesthetic considerations for the patient undergoing total laryngectomy. AANA J (Am Assoc Nurse Anesthetists) 1987 Jun; 55(3):237–244

Romm S. Cancer of the larynx: Current concepts of diagnosis and treatment. Surg Clin North Am 1986 Feb; 66(1):109–118

Strong EW. Cancer of the larynx and hypopharynx. Probl Gen Surg 1988 Apr–Jun; 5(2):166–189

Herpex Simplex

Balciunas BA and Overholser CD. Diagnosis and treatment of common oral lesions. Am Fam Physician 1987 May; 35(5):206–220

Pazin GJ and Harger JH. Management of oral and genital herpes simplex virus infections: Diagnosis and treatment. Dis Mon 1986 Dec; 32(12):725–824

Young TB, Rimm EB and D'Alessio DJ. Cross-sectional study of recurrent herpes labialis: Prevalence and risk factors. Am J Epidemiol 1988 Mar; 127(3):612–625

Pharyngitis

DeNeef P. Role of rapid tests for streptococcal pharyngitis in hospital infection control. Am J Infect Control 1987 Feb; 15(1):20–25

DeNeef P. Selective testing for streptococcal pharyngitis in adults. J Fam Pract 1987 Oct; 25(4):347–353

Fisher PM. Rapid testing for streptococcal pharyngitis. Prim Care 1986 Dec; 13(4):657–665

Hillner BE and Centor RM. What a

difference a day makes: A decision analysis of adult streptococcal pharyngitis. J Gen Intern Med 1987 Jul–Aug; 2(4):244–250

Raz P and Bitnun S. Dilemmas of streptococcal pharyngitis. Am Fam Physician 1987 Apr; 35(4):187–192

Tanz RR and Shulman SS. Streptococcal pharyngitis. Postgrad Med 1988 Jul 84(1):203–206; 211–214

Telian SA. Sore throat and antibiotics. Otolaryngol Clin North Am 1986 Feb; 19(1):103–109

Rhinitis/Sinusitis

Buiter CT. Nasal antrostomy. Rhinology 1988 Mar; 26(1):5–18

Incaudo G, Gershwin ME and Nagy SM. The pathophysiology and treatment of sinusitis. Allergol Immunopathol (Madr) 1986 Sep–Oct; 14(5):423–434

Kimmelman CP and Ali GH. Vasomotor rhinitis. Otolaryngol Clin North Am 1986 Feb; 19(1):65–71

Lieberman P. Rhinitis: Allergic and nonallergic. Hosp Pract [Off] 1988 Jun 15; 23(6):117–145

Maisel RH and Kimberley BP. Treatment of chronic sinusitis with open drainage and cefaclor. Am J Otolaryngol 1988 Jan–Feb; 9(1):30–33

Middleton E Jr. Chronic rhinitis in adults. J Allergy Clin Immunol 1988 May; 81(5 Pt 2):971–975

Minor MW and Lockey RF. Sinusitis and asthma. South Med J 1987 Sep; 80(9):1141–1147

Togias A et al. Studies on the allergic and nonallergic nasal inflammation. J Allergy Clin Immunol 1988 May; 81(5 Pt 1):782–790

Weber AL. Inflammatory diseases of the paranasal sinuses and mucoceles. Otolaryngol Clin North Am 1988 Aug; 21(3):421–437

Surgery (Nasal)

Colton JJ and Beekhuis GJ. Management of nasal fractures. Otolaryngol Clin North Am 1986 Feb; 19(1):73–85

Holt GR, Garner ET and McLarey D. Postoperative sequelae and complications of rhinoplasty. Otolaryngol Clin North Am 1987 Nov; 20(4):853–876

Zinreich SJ et al. Paranasal sinuses: CT imaging requirements for endoscopic surgery. Radiology 1987 Jun; 163(3):769–775

Major Manifestations of Bronchopulmonary Disease

Cough and Sputum Production

A. Causes

1. Coughing is a protective mechanism that serves to clear the airways and protects the lungs from injury.
2. Cough-producing stimuli may be inflammatory, mechanical, chemical, or thermal.
3. Clinical problems producing cough are infection, inflammation, neoplasms, cardiovascular disorders, trauma, physical agents, and allergic disorders.
4. Severe coughing may lead to pneumothorax, pneumomediastinum, and interstitial emphysema.

B. Nursing Assessment

1. Evaluate the character of the cough.
   a. Throat-clearing cough—postnasal drip.
   b. Dry and hacking—may be due to nervousness, viral infections, bronchogenic carcinoma, early congestive heart failure.
   c. Loud and harsh—irritation in upper airway.
   d. Wheezing—associated with bronchospasm.
   e. Severe or changing in character or with position—may be bronchogenic cancer (cough, chest pain, hemoptysis).
   f. Loose—indicates problems in peripheral bronchi and lung parenchyma.
   g. Painful—may indicate pleural involvement, chest wall disease.
   h. Chronic, productive—sign of bronchopulmonary disease.
2. Note relationship of cough to time, to patient's position, and to environmental exposure.

   a. Recent onset of cough (hours or days) suggests infection.
   b. Cough most noticeable on awakening—suppurative lung disease; bronchitis.
   c. Coughing paroxysms at night—may indicate bronchial asthma or left-sided heart failure.
   d. Cough that worsens when patient is supine—may be due to postnasal drip from sinusitis, bronchiectasis.
   e. Cough associated with food intake—may be the result of aspiration into tracheobronchial tree.
   f. Cough of recent onset or gradually progressive over a period of weeks or months suggests tuberculosis or bronchogenic carcinoma.
3. Determine the patient's:
   a. Smoking history: Current? Past?
   b. Environmental or occupational exposure to dusts, fumes, or gases?
   c. Allergies, asthma, sinusitis, upper respiratory infection?
4. Observe character, quantity, and color of expectorated material and ability of patient to clear his secretions. Ask if there has been a change in the character or frequency of coughing.
   a. Clear or mucoid—stems from viral infection, chronic bronchitis, postnasal drip.
   b. Thick yellow or green sputum—due to primary or secondary bacterial infections.
   c. Rusty—may indicate bacterial pneumonia (if patient not receiving antibiotics).
   d. Malodorous—due to lung abscess, infection from fusospirochetal or anaerobic organisms.
   e. Frothy pink sputum—indicates acute pulmonary edema.
   f. Note amount of sputum produced daily. A sudden decrease in the quantity of sputum may indicate inspissation (drying and thickening) in tracheo-

bronchial tree and may lead to respiratory insufficiency and failure.

   g. Layering of sputum in sputum cup occurs in lung abscess or bronchiectasis.

C. Nursing Interventions

1. Give cough suppressants, expectorants, and mucolytic agents as prescribed.
2. Make sure the patient is adequately hydrated to liquefy sputum.
3. Assist the patient to cough productively by controlled coughing, postural drainage, and chest percussion.
4. Discourage smoking—interferes with lung defense mechanisms: interferes with ciliary action, increases bronchial secretions, causes inflammation and hyperplasia of mucous glands, reduces production of surfactant, impairs function of alveolar macrophages (scavenger cells).
5. Encourage oral hygiene—odor and taste of sputum depresses appetite.

Dyspnea

(Breathlessness or difficult breathing) May be acute, chronic, progressive, recurrent, or paroxysmal.

A. Causes

1. In lung disease, shortness of breath is due to change in lung rigidity or increased airway resistance.
2. Lung disease places strain on the right ventricle—may cause right ventricular failure.

B. Clinical Implications

1. In general, the acute lung diseases produce a more severe grade of dyspnea than do the chronic diseases.
2. Sudden dyspnea in a healthy person may indicate pneumothorax (air in pleural cavity).
3. Sudden dyspnea in ill or postoperative patient may indicate pulmonary embolus; pneumothorax.
4. Orthopnea—characteristic of cardiogenic pulmonary congestion.
5. Expiratory wheeze—arises from obstructive disease in peripheral airways (asthma, chronic bronchitis, emphysema).
6. Noisy respirations—related to localized obstruction of major branches, tumor, foreign body, or narrowing of smaller airways.
7. Inspiratory stridor—indicates partial obstruction at laryngeal or tracheal level.
8. Paroxysmal wheezing unrelated to exertion—may arise from bronchial (allergic) asthma or bronchitis.

C. Nursing Assessment

Ascertain circumstances that cause dyspnea.

1. Relation to exertion, position, or environmental exposure.
2. Quantify exertion and specify type producing dyspnea (housework, mowing lawn, walking a set distance).
3. Mode of onset? Sudden? Gradual?
4. Quantify change in dyspnea. (What could patient do a year ago, a month ago that he cannot do now?)
5. Can the patient take a deep breath?
6. Influenced by time of day/night? Seasons?
7. Is there associated cough? Sputum production?
8. Is there expiratory wheeze? Chest pain?
9. Is dyspnea associated with other symptoms?

D. Nursing Interventions

The treatment depends on alleviating the cause.

1. Place the patient at rest with his head elevated.
2. Administer oxygen as prescribed.
3. For chronic dyspnea, breathing re-training, exercise training, psychologic interventions, etc. may be helpful.

Hemoptysis

(Coughing up or expectoration of blood or bloodstained sputum from the respiratory tract)

A. Causes

1. Infection (bronchitis; pneumonia)
2. Neoplasm (bronchogenic carcinoma)
3. Pulmonary venous hypertension; thromboembolism
4. Cardiovascular conditions (mitral stenosis)

B. Nursing Assessment

1. Question the patient about ingestion of aspirin or aspirin-containing medication within the past 24 hours.
2. Ascertain whether blood is coming from nose or throat, gastrointestinal tract, or lungs.
   a. Nose (*epistaxis*)—usually there is a discharge of blood from nose.
     (1) During severe epistaxis, the patient may swallow or aspirate blood.
     (2) Look for dried blood in nose or nasopharynx.
   b. Gastrointestinal tract (*hematemesis*)
     (1) Usually preceded by nausea and accompanied by retching and vomiting.
     (2) Blood appears dark red in color; may contain food particles.
     (3) Blood is acid in reaction (pH less than 7.0).
   c. Lungs (*hemoptysis*)
     (1) Blood is *coughed* up; patient may have tickling in throat, salty taste, burning or bubbling sensation in chest.
     (2) Usually bright red and frothy; blood-tinged sputum may persist for days.
     (3) Blood is alkaline in reaction (pH greater than 7.0).

C. Nursing Interventions

1. Place the patient on bed rest and give mild sedation as prescribed.
   a. Place on affected side (if known)—to avoid flooding the contralateral lung.
   b. Maintain a calm reassuring approach—fright in a patient promotes hyperventilation.
2. Recognize the patient's fear and apprehension due to this threatening symptom and give him understanding and support.
3. Record quantity, color, and character (mixed with mucus, pure blood).
4. Save all coughed-up blood for inspection by physician.
5. Have equipment for emergency bronchoscopy/laryngoscopy in readiness—for removal of blood clots and identification of bleeding site.
6. In event of asphyxia or massive hemoptysis, prepare for balloon catheter insertion and inflation to occlude bleeding site and/or for surgical intervention.

Chest Pain

A. Causes

1. Parietal pleura has rich supply of sensory nerves coming from intercostal nerves to the diaphragm. These nerve endings may be stimulated by inflammation and stretching of membranes and by respiratory movements—produces a characteristic sharp, knife-like pain.

2. Pleuropulmonary pain—bacterial pneumonia, infarction, spontaneous pneumothorax.

B. Clinical Manifestations and Nursing Assessment

1. Pleural pain is a common manifestation of inflammatory and malignant disease, but also accompanies pneumothorax and pulmonary embolism.
2. Pleural pain (usually well localized, sharp, and stabbing); made worse by deep breathing and coughing.
3. Assess quality, intensity, and radiation of pain.
4. Note factors that precipitate pain.
5. Evaluate whether position of the patient changes character of pain.
6. Determine the effect of inspiration and expiration on the patient's pain.

C. Nursing Interventions

1. Should be directed toward relieving underlying causes.
2. Give prescribed analgesic, taking care not to depress respiratory center or productive cough.
3. Assist with regional anesthetic block—procaine is injected along the intercostal nerves that supply the painful area in cases where pain is intractable.

Hoarseness

A. Causes

1. Acute
   When associated with febrile episode, suggests viral laryngotracheobronchitis.
2. Persistent
   May indicate intrinsic neoplasm of vocal cord, bronchogenic cancer, mediastinal lesion.

Constitutional Manifestations of Bronchopulmonary Disease

A. Constitutional Symptoms of Bronchopulmonary Disease

1. Anorexia
2. Fever
3. Weight loss ⎤ related to duration and
4. Fatigue, malaise, weakness⎦ severity of disease
5. Sweats
6. Chills

B. Constitutional Signs of Bronchopulmonary Disease

1. Cyanosis
2. Clubbing of fingers
3. Wasting

Diagnostic Studies*

Radiography

A. Chest Roentgenogram

1. Normal pulmonary tissue is radiolucent. Thus, densities produced by tumors, foreign bodies, etc. can be detected.
2. Shows position of normal structures, displacement, and presence of abnormal shadows.
3. Chest x-rays may reveal extensive pathology in the lungs in the absence of symptoms.

* For physical examination of lungs and thorax, see page 28.

B. Tomography *(planigraphy)*

1. Provides films of sections of lungs at different levels within the thorax.
2. Useful in demonstrating presence of small, solid lesions, calcification, or cavitation within a lesion.

C. Computed Tomography

An imaging method in which the lungs are scanned in successive layers by a narrow beam x-ray. A computer printout is obtained of the absorption values of the tissues in the plane that is being scanned.

It may be used to define pulmonary nodules, small tumors adjacent to pleural surfaces (which may be invisible on routine roentgenograms), and to demonstrate mediastinal abnormalities and hilar adenopathy.

D. Positron Emission Tomography *(PET)*

Uses high-energy physics and computer techniques to study lung function; useful for quantitative measurements of regional pulmonary perfusion and for studying ventilation–perfusion relationships.

E. Fluoroscopy

Enables roentgenologist to view heart, lungs, and diaphragm in the dynamic (moving) state.

F. Barium Swallow

Outlines the esophagus and reveals displacement of esophagus and encroachment on its lumen by cardiac, pulmonary, and mediastinal abnormalities.

G. Bronchography

A radiopaque medium is instilled directly into the trachea and bronchi, and the entire bronchial tree or selected areas may be visualized. This is a diagnostic test for any disease that alters the caliber or patency of the bronchial tree or that causes its displacement. It is infrequently used since the advent of fiberoptics.

1. The patient is assessed for allergic reaction to anesthetic agent or contrast media before the test is started.
2. The patient is kept fasting—to avoid aspiration of gastric contents.
3. Preoperative medication may include atropine to decrease secretions and vagally mediated reflex bradycardia and diazepam (Valium) for sedation/tranquilization.
   a. Topical anesthesia is sprayed in the mouth, on tongue and posterior pharynx.
   b. Local anesthetic is injected into the larynx and tracheal tree to prevent gagging and coughing when the tube is passed.
      (1) Extreme caution is indicated in patients with respiratory insufficiency, as these patients may experience temporary problems with ventilation and diffusion.
      (2) Oxygen, antispasmodic agents, and cortisone should be available.
4. *Nursing Responsibilities after Bronchogram*
   a. Withhold fluids and food until patient demonstrates a cough reflex.
   b. Check vital signs as indicated.
   c. Encourage the patient to cough and clear his bronchial tree; postural drainage may be required. A slight elevation of temperature is common following a bronchogram.

H. Angiographic Studies of Pulmonary Vessels

Radiopaque medium is rapidly injected into vasculature of the lungs for radiographic study of pulmonary vessels and evaluation of pulmonary circulation.

1. It can be performed by
    a. Venous injection into one or both arms (or femoral vein) through a needle or catheter, OR
    b. Introducing a catheter into main pulmonary artery or its branches
2. Films are taken in rapid sequence after injection.

I. Aortography

Opacification studies of either thoracic aorta or abdominal aorta; taken when aneurysm of thoracic aorta is suspected.

Endoscopic Procedures

A. Bronchoscopy

The direct inspection and observation of the larynx, trachea, and bronchi through a flexible or rigid bronchoscope; has both diagnostic and therapeutic uses in pulmonary conditions.

1. *Diagnostic Uses*
    a. To collect secretions for cytologic/bacteriologic studies.
    b. To determine location and extent of a pathologic process and to obtain biopsy for diagnosis.
        (1) *Tissue biopsy*—use of small biopsy forceps to obtain sample of tissue for examination.
        (2) *Brush biopsy*—target bronchus is brushed using a small wire with brush on one end that is introduced through bronchoscope. Material (cells and secretions) can be examined cytologically or cultured for pathogenic organisms.
    c. To determine whether a tumor can be resected surgically.
    d. To diagnose bleeding sites (source of hemoptysis).
2. *Therapeutic Uses*
    a. To remove foreign bodies from tracheobronchial tree.
    b. To remove secretions obstructing the tracheobronchial tree when the patient is unable to clear them.
    c. To fulgurate and excise lesions.

B. Flexible Fiberoptic Bronchoscopy

Passage of thin, flexible bronchofiberscope that can be directed into segmental bronchi; by its smaller size, flexibility, and excellent optical system, it allows increased visualization of peripheral airways.

1. May be done transnasally, transorally, or through an endotracheal tube; allows for brush biopsy (see above).
2. Causes very little patient discomfort; better patient acceptance even under local anesthetic.
3. Clinical applications for flexible fiberoptic bronchoscopy: allows diagnostic visualization of airways to segmental bronchi; permits brushing for malignant cells/infecting agents; biopsy of lesions; therapeutic removal of secretions; localization of source of hemoptysis.

    Bronchoalveolar lavage—injection of saline through fiberoptic bronchoscope, which is immediately withdrawn; recovers alveolar cells, secretions, and pathogens by washing them from distal airways.
4. Possible complications: reaction to anesthetic agent, pneumothorax, dysrhythmias, bronchospasm.

C. Rigid Bronchoscopy

Hollow metallic tube with light at its end used for removal of foreign bodies, suctioning thick secretions, and investigating source of massive hemoptysis, or for endobronchial surgical procedures (resection of tumors, dilation of strictures, etc.). May be done under local or general anesthesia.

1. May be done under local or general anesthesia.
2. Rigid bronchoscope preferred in following instances: small children, endobronchial tumor resection, massive hemorrhage, foreign body retrieval; otherwise it is being replaced by flexible fiberoptic bronchoscopy.
3. Nursing interventions
    a. See that an informed consent form has been signed.
    b. Administer prescribed medication to reduce secretions and block the vasovagal reflex and relieve anxiety. Give encouragement and nursing support.
    c. Restrict fluid and food for 6 hours before procedure—to reduce risk of aspiration when reflexes are blocked.
    d. Remove dentures, contact lenses, and other prostheses.
    e. After the procedure.
        (1) Monitor cardiac rhythm
        (2) Withhold cracked ice/fluids until patient demonstrates that he can cough
    f. Following bronchoscopy watch patient for
        (1) Cyanosis
        (2) Hypotension
        (3) Tachycardia and dysrhythmia
        (4) Hemoptysis
        (5) Dyspnea
        (6) Confusion and lethargy in elderly

D. Mediastinoscopy (See p. 162.)

Radioisotope Diagnostic Procedures

Ventilation and perfusion scintigraphy—Refers to radioisotope imaging of ventilation and blood flow to the lungs. The camera may be interfaced to a computer to record, collate, and refine data.

A. Perfusion Lung Scan

Following injection of a radioactive isotope, scans are made with a scintillation camera.

1. Measures blood perfusion through the lungs; evaluates lung function on a regional basis.
2. Useful in perfusion (vascular) abnormalities—pulmonary embolism.

B. Ventilation Scan

1. Inhalation of radioactive gas (xenon, krypton), which diffuses throughout the lungs.
2. Useful in detecting ventilation abnormalities (emphysema).

C. Gallium Scan

Radioisotope lung scan used to detect inflammatory conditions of the lungs.

Examination of Sputum

A. Purpose

1. Sputum is obtained for evaluation of gross appearance, for microscopic examination, for gram staining and culture to identify the predominant organisms, and for cytologic examination.
    a. Direct smear—shows presence of white blood cells and intracellular (pathogenic) bacteria and extracellular (mostly nonpathogenic) bacteria.
    b. Sputum culture—to make diagnosis, to determine drug sensitivity, and to serve as a guide for drug treatment (choice of antibiotic).

c. Sputum cytology (exfoliative cytology)—used to identify tumor cells.
2. Patients receiving antibiotics, steroids, and immunosuppressive agents for prolonged periods may have periodic sputum examinations, as these agents may give rise to opportunistic pulmonary infections.

B. Methods of Obtaining Sputum

1. By deep breathing and coughing
   a. Secure early morning specimen—yields best sample of deep pulmonary material from all lung fields.
   b. Clear nose and throat and rinse mouth—to decrease sputum contamination.
   c. Instruct patient to take several deep breaths, exhale, and perform a series of short coughs.
   d. Cough deeply and expectorate the sputum into a sterile container.
   e. See that specimen is transported to laboratory immediately; allowing it to stand in a warm room will result in overgrowth of organisms, making identification of pathogen difficult; also alters cell morphology.
   f. Give oral hygiene frequently, especially if the patient has foul sputum.
2. By ultrasonic and/or heated hypertonic saline nebulization
   a. Patient inhales through mouth slowly and deeply for 10–20 minutes.
   b. Increases the moisture content of air going to lower tract; particles will condense on tracheobronchial tree and aid in expectoration.
3. Tracheal aspiration (see Guidelines, p. 173)
4. Bronchoscopic removal (p. 161)—provides sputum sampling by aspiration of secretions; brushing through a sterile catheter; bronchoalveolar lavage, and transbronchial biopsy.
5. Gastric aspiration (rarely necessary since advent of ultrasonic nebulizer).
   a. Nasogastric tube is inserted into the stomach to siphon out swallowed pulmonary secretions.
   b. This test is useful only for culture of tubercle bacilli, but not for direct examination.
6. Transtracheal aspiration (see Fig. 10-2). See Guidelines, page 166.

Examination of Pleural Fluid and Pleural Biopsy

A. Pleural Fluid

Pleural fluid is continuously produced and reabsorbed, with a thin layer of fluid normally in the pleural space; abnormal accumulation of pleural fluid (effusion) occurs in diseases of the pleura, heart, or lymphatics. The pleural fluid is studied along with other tests to determine underlying cause.
1. Pleural fluid is obtained by aspiration (thoracentesis) or by tube thoracotomy.
2. Pleural fluid is examined for cell count, differential, specific gravity, cytology, protein, glucose, pH, LDH, and amylase.
   a. Pleural fluid, usually light straw color
   b. Purulent fluid—suggests empyema
   c. Blood-tinged fluid—pulmonary infarction; neoplastic disease
   d. Milky fluid (chylothorax)—invasion of thoracic duct by tumor or inflammatory process; traumatic rupture of thoracic duct
3. Observe and record total amount of fluid withdrawn, nature of fluid, and its color and viscosity.

4. Prepare sample of fluid for laboratory evaluation if prescribed.

B. Pleural Biopsy

Accomplished via needle biopsy of pleura or via pleuroscopy (visual exploration of pleural space through a bronchofiberscope inserted into pleural space).

Biopsy Procedures of the Lung

Goal:
Obtain histologic material from lung to aid in diagnosis.

A. Transbronchoscopic Biopsy

Biopsy forceps inserted through bronchoscope and specimen of lung tissue obtained.

B. Transthoracic Needle Aspiration Biopsy *(Needle Biopsy Through Thoracic Wall)*

1. Skin site is cleansed and anesthetized.
2. Small skin incision is made, and a needle is advanced under fluoroscopic control to the desired site.
3. With the needle in the periphery of the lesion, the stylet is removed, the syringe attached, and suction applied while 2 or 3 short needle thrusts are made into mass.
4. Specimen is smeared and fixed on a slide for cytologic examination if neoplasm is suspected. Smears may also be made for bacteria, acid-fast organisms, and fungi.
5. A fluoroscopic survey is done to determine if a pneumothorax has developed that will require chest tube drainage.
6. Postbiopsy care
   a. Observe for possible complications: pneumothorax, hemoptysis, bacterial contamination of the pleural space.
   b. Encourage the patient to remain in bed for several hours with his aspirated lung in a dependent position.

C. Transcatheter Bronchial Brushing

D. Open Lung Biopsy

1. Used in making a diagnosis when other biopsy methods have been explored.
2. Usually done by a small anterior thoracotomy.
3. Subsequent pneumothorax controlled by chest tube connected to a drainage system.
4. Complications include pneumothorax and bleeding.

Lymph Node Biopsy *(Scalene or Mediastinal Nodes)*

Goal:
Detect lymph node spread of pulmonary disease. It is used as a diagnostic and prognostic measure.

1. Mediastinoscopy—endoscopic examination of the mediastinum for evaluation of tumor spread and biopsy of mediastinal nodes.
   a. Incision is usually made in suprasternal notch isthmus.
   b. The edges of incision are spread with forceps; the tissues overlying the trachea are dissected, and a channel is prepared for introduction of the mediastinoscope.
   c. Lymph nodes in the area are biopsied using a small forcep.
   d. Useful in diagnosing and staging bronchogenic

cancer to predict if tumor can be resected, and to obtain tissue for diagnosis in other conditions.
2. Percutaneous fine-needle aspiration biopsy of mediastinum—performed on selected mediastinal lesions under local anesthesia.
3. Mediastinotomy—surgical resection of second anterior costal cartilage for access to anterior mediastinum to evaluate lung lymphatic drainage.
     Procedure most frequently used to evaluate left upper lobe disease processes.
4. Scalene lymph nodes are enmeshed in deep cervical pad of fat; these nodes drain lungs and mediastinum and may show histologic changes from intrathoracic disease.

Pulmonary Function Studies

Pulmonary function studies (see Ventilatory Function Tests [Table 10-1]) are done to detect and measure abnormalities in respiratory function. Such tests include measurements of lung volumes, ventilatory function, diffusing capacity, gas exchange, lung compliance, airway resistance, and distribution of gases in the lung.

A. Ventilatory Studies *(Spirometry)*

1. Most commonly used test.
2. Requires water spirometer, electronic spirometer, or wedge spirometer that plots volume against time (*timed vital capacity*).
3. Patient is asked to take as deep a breath as possible and then to exhale into spirometer as completely and as forcefully as possible. Results are compared with normals for patient's age, height, and sex (see Table 10-1).
4. A reduction in the vital capacity *alone* may indicate a restrictive form of lung disease (disease due to increased lung stiffness).
5. A reduction in several parameters usually indicates an obstructive form of lung disease (obstruction to flow due to bronchial obstruction or loss of lung elastic recoil).

B. Lung Volumes

1. Are determined by asking the patient to inhale known concentration of inert gas such as helium or 100% oxygen and measuring concentration of inert gas or nitrogen in exhaled air (dilution method). May also be measured in plethysmograph.
2. Yields thoracic gas volume (total lung capacity, plus any unventilated blebs or bullae).
3. An increased residual volume is found in air-trapping due to obstructive lung disease.
4. A reduction in several parameters usually indicates a restrictive form of lung disease or chest wall abnormality.

C. Diffusing Capacity

1. Measures lung surface effective for the transfer of gas in the lung.
2. Requires the patient to inhale gas containing known low concentration of carbon monoxide.
3. Measures carbon monoxide concentration in exhaled air (difference between inhaled and exhaled concentrations is related directly to uptake of carbon monoxide across alveolar–capillary membrane).
4. Is reduced in parenchymal lung disease, possibly in severe anemia, and in some forms of heart disease.

Arterial Blood Gas Studies

A. Purpose

1. A measurement of partial pressure of oxygen and carbon dioxide in arterial blood, as well as the pH of the blood.
2. The partial pressure of oxygen, together with hemoglobin, is a measurement of the amount of oxygen in the arterial blood.
3. Provide a means of assessing the adequacy of oxygenation and ventilation (i.e., the lungs supplying O_2 to the body and removing CO_2).
4. Help assess the acid–base status of the body—whether acidosis or alkalosis is present and to what degree.

B. See Guidelines, p. 164.

Table 10-1. *Ventilatory Function Tests*

Term	Symbol	Description	Remarks
Vital capacity	V_C	Maximum volume of air exhaled after a maximum inspiration	VC < 10–15 ml./kg. suggests need for mechanical ventilation. VC > 10–15 ml./kg. suggests ability to wean.
Forced vital capacity	FVC	Vital capacity performed with a maximally forced expiratory effort	Reduced in obstructive disease (COPD) due to air trapping. Reflects airflow in large airways.
Forced expiratory volume in 1 second	FEV_1	Volume of air exhaled in the first second of the performance of a FVC	Reduced in obstructive disease (COPD) due to air trapping. Reflects airflow in larger airways.
Ratio of FEV_1/FVC	FEV_1/FVC	FEV_1 expressed as a percentage of the FVC	Decreased in obstructive disease. Normal in restrictive disease.
Forced midexpiratory flow	$FEF_{25\%-75\%}$	Average flow during the middle half of the FEV_1	Reflects airflow in small airways. Smokers may have change in this test before other symptoms develop.
Peak expiratory flow rate	PEFR	Most rapid flow during a forced expiration after a maximum inspiration	Used to measure response to bronchodilators, airflow obstruction in patients with asthma.

Guidelines   Assisting With Arterial Puncture for Blood Gas Analysis

Arterial blood gas levels are analyzed for oxygen tension, carbon dioxide tension, and hydrogen ion concentration. This gives important information regarding oxygenation by the lungs and the ability of the lungs to excrete CO_2.

Terminology   Partial pressure—pressure exerted by each type of gas in a mixture of gases.
The following is a list of symbols used in reference to arterial blood gas studies:
P = pressure
PO_2—partial pressure of oxygen
PCO_2—partial pressure of carbon dioxide
P_AO_2—partial pressure of alveolar oxygen
P_ACO_2—partial pressure of alveolar carbon dioxide
PaO_2—partial pressure of arterial oxygen
$PaCO_2$—partial pressure of arterial carbon dioxide
PvO_2—partial pressure of venous oxygen
$PvCO_2$—partial pressure of venous carbon dioxide
P_{50}—oxygen tension at 50% hemoglobin saturation

Equipment   Commercially available blood gas kit
2-ml. glass syringe with No. 25 gauge needle
10-ml. glass syringe with No. 20 gauge needle
Sodium heparin
Stopper or cap
Procaine
Sterile sponges and skin germicide
Basin containing ice
Gloves

Nursing Action	**Rationale/Amplification**
1. Record patient's inspired oxygen concentration.	1. Changes in inspired oxygen concentration alter the PaO_2. Degree of hypoxemia cannot be assessed without knowing the inspired oxygen concentration.
2. Take patient's temperature.	2. May be taken into consideration when results are evaluated. Hyperthermia and hypothermia influence oxygen release from hemoglobin at the tissue level.

Planning/Im-plementation   **Preparatory Phase**

1. Heparinize the syringe	
a. Withdraw a small amount of heparin into the syringe to wet the plunger and fill dead space in the needle.	a. This action coats the interior of the syringe with heparin to prevent blood from clotting.
b. Hold syringe in an upright position and expel excess heparin and air bubbles.	b. Air in the syringe may affect measurement of PaO_2. Heparin in the syringe may affect measurement of the *p*H.

Performance Phase (by physician, nurse, or respiratory therapist with special instruction)

1. Don gloves.	
2. Palpate the radial or femoral artery.	2. The radial artery is the preferred site of puncture. Arterial puncture is performed on areas where a good pulse is palpable.
3. If puncturing the radial artery, perform the Allen test. *In the conscious patient:*	3. The Allen test is a simple method for assessing collateral circulation in the hand. Ensures circulation if radial artery thrombosis occurs.
a. Obliterate the radial and ulnar pulses simultaneously by pressing on both blood vessels at the wrist.	a. Impedes arterial blood flow into the hand.
b. Ask patient to clench and unclench his fist until blanching of the skin occurs.	b. Forces blood from the hand.
c. Release pressure on ulnar artery (while compressing radial artery). Watch for return of skin color within 15 seconds.	c. Documents that ulnar artery alone is capable of supplying the hand, since radial artery is still occluded.

Note: If the ulnar artery does not have sufficient blood flow to supply the entire hand, another artery should be used.

**Planning/Im-
plementation**
(continued)

In the unconscious patient:

   a. Obliterate the radial and ulnar pulses simultaneously at the wrist.

   b. Elevate patient's hand above his heart and squeeze or compress his hand until blanching occurs.

   c. Lower patient's hand while compressing radial artery (release pressure on ulnar artery) and watch for return of skin color.

4. Place a small towel roll under the patient's wrist.

5. Feel along the course of the radial artery and palpate for maximum pulsation with the middle and index fingers. Prepare the skin with germicide. The skin and subcutaneous tissues may be infiltrated with a local anesthetic agent (lidocaine).

6. The needle is at a 45–60 degree angle to the skin surface (Fig. 10-1) and is advanced into the artery. Once the artery is punctured, arterial pressure will push up the hub of the syringe and a pulsating flow of blood will fill the syringe.

4. To make the artery more accessible.

5. The wrist should be stabilized to allow for finer control of the needle.

6. The arterial pressure will cause the syringe to be filled within a few seconds.

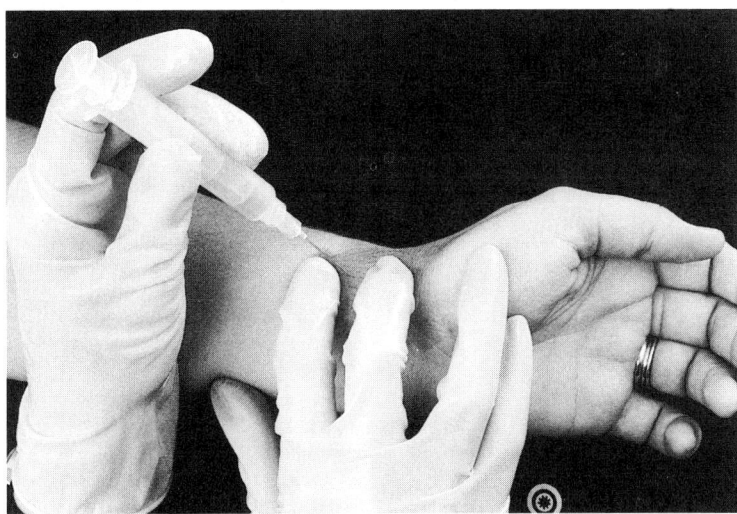

Figure 10-1. *Technique of arterial puncture for blood gas analysis.*

7. After blood is obtained, withdraw needle and apply firm pressure over the puncture with a dry sponge.

8. Cap the needle tightly or insert it into a rubber stopper.

9. Place the capped syringe in the container of ice.

10. Maintain firm pressure on the puncture site for up to 10 minutes (by the clock).

   If the patient is on anticoagulant medication, apply direct pressure over puncture site for 15 minutes and then apply a firm pressure dressing.

11. For patients requiring serial monitoring of arterial blood, an arterial catheter (connected to a flush solution of heparinized saline), is inserted into the femoral or radial artery.

7. Significant bleeding can occur because of pressure in the artery.

8. Immediate capping of the needle prevents room air from mixing with the blood specimen.

9. Icing the syringe will prevent a clinically significant loss of O_2.

10. Firm pressure on the puncture site prevents further bleeding and hematoma formation.

11. All connections must be tight to avoid disconnection and rapid blood loss. The arterial line also allows for direct pressure monitoring in the critically ill patient.

Follow-up Phase

1. Send the basin of ice with the syringe containing blood to the laboratory immediately.

2. Palpate the pulse (distal to the puncture site), inspect the puncture site and assess for cold hand, numbness, tingling, or discoloration.

1. Blood gas analysis should be done as soon as possible, as tension and *p*H can change rapidly.

2. Hematoma and arterial thrombosis are complications following this procedure.

(continued)

Guidelines — Assisting With Arterial Puncture for Blood Gas Analysis *(continued)*

Planning/Implementation *(continued)*	Nursing Action	Rationale/Amplification
	3. Change ventilator settings, inspired oxygen concentration, or type and settings of respiratory therapy equipment if indicated by the results.	3. The PaO_2 results will determine whether to maintain, increase, or decrease the F_1O_2. The $PaCO_2$ and *p*H results will detect if any changes are needed in tidal volume or rate of patient's ventilator.

Guidelines — Assisting With Transtracheal Aspiration

Transtracheal aspiration involves passing a needle and then a catheter through a percutaneous puncture of the cricothyroid membrane (Fig. 10-2). Transtracheal aspiration bypasses the oropharynx and avoids specimen contamination by mouth flora.

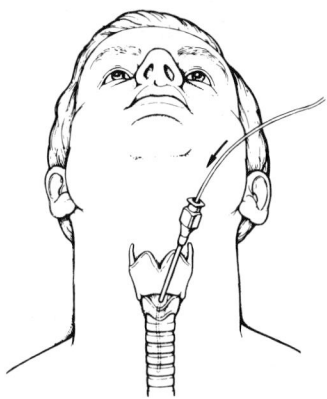

Figure 10-2. *Transtracheal aspiration. After the catheter is positioned into the trachea, the needle is withdrawn leaving the catheter in place.*

Purposes

1. To obtain an uncontaminated sputum specimen for culture and sensitivity studies.
2. To promote coughing in the patient with an absent cough reflex.

Equipment

Sterile transtracheal set:
  No. 14, No. 16, and No. 18 gauge needles
  Polyethylene catheter
  Syringe
  Skin preparation solutions
  Local anesthetic
  Sterile gloves; mask
  Specimen containers

Atropine
ECG monitoring equipment
Endotracheal tube
Suction apparatus with catheters
Cardiac resuscitation equipment

Procedure

Nursing Action	Rationale/Amplification
Preparatory Phase	
1. Explain the procedure and give reassurance by skilled and empathetic attention to the patient's needs. Instruct the patient to breathe quietly and to remain still.	1. Inform the patient that the procedure will cause coughing. There will be an unpleasant sensation of a foreign body in the lower airway.
2. Administer supplemental oxygen as directed during the procedure if the patient's arterial oxygen tension is below normal while the patient is breathing room air.	2. This prevents worsening of hypoxemia.

Procedure (continued)	**Nursing Action**	**Rationale/Amplification**
	3. Extend the patient's neck and place a pillow under his shoulders.	3. This is the optimum position for cricothyroid puncture.

Performance Phase (by the physician)

The cricothyroid membrane is identified by palpation.

Nursing Action	**Rationale/Amplification**
1. The skin over the cricothyroid area is cleansed and the area infiltrated with local anesthetic.	1. The cricothyroid membrane is less vascular and offers more safety in preventing posterior wall puncture than other areas.
2. A No. 14, 16, or 18 gauge needle is inserted through the cricothyroid membrane into the trachea, and a polyethylene catheter is threaded through the needle into the lower trachea.	2. Caution the patient against swallowing or talking while the needle is introduced through the cricothyroid membrane.
3. The needle is withdrawn, leaving the catheter in place.	3. The catheter's passage usually stimulates vigorous coughing.
4. A syringe is attached to the catheter and secretions may be aspirated back into the syringe as the patient coughs.	4. Request the patient to turn his head while coughing.
5. Air is removed from the syringe and the syringe is capped or the sample is injected into an anaerobic transfer vial. The specimen is sent to the laboratory for immediate processing.	5. This ensures anaerobic conditions. Cytologic, mycobacterial, and other studies are carried out.
6. The catheter is withdrawn and pressure applied over the puncture site.	6. Gentle firm pressure over the site for about 5 minutes helps prevent bleeding and reduces subcutaneous emphysema.

Follow-up Phase

1. Instruct the patient to rest quietly for an hour or so.	
2. Observe for the following complications: local bleeding, puncture of posterior tracheal wall, subcutaneous emphysema, vasovagal reactions, cardiac dysrhythmias.	2. Assess for hoarseness after the procedure; this may be from a submucosal tracheal hematoma, which can cause suffocation. Inform the patient that minor blood-streaking of sputum almost always occurs following this procedure.

Guidelines Assisting the Patient Undergoing Thoracentesis

Thoracentesis is the aspiration of fluid or air from the pleural space. It may be a diagnostic or a therapeutic procedure (Fig. 10-3).

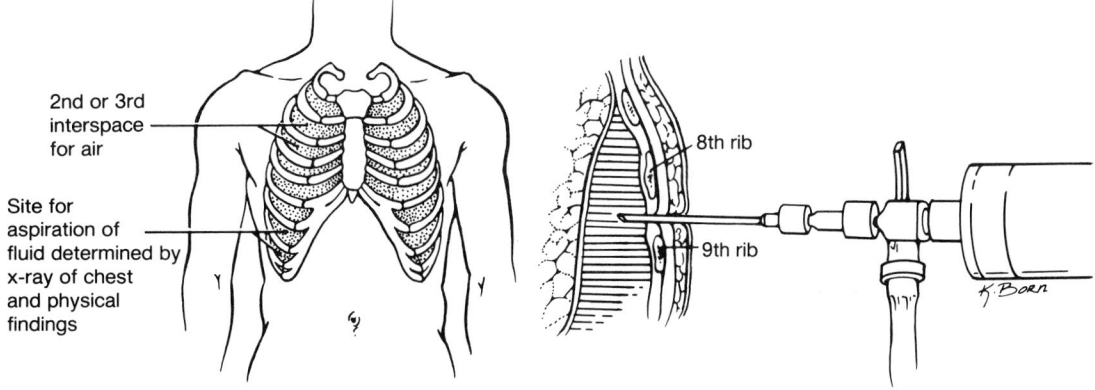

Site of insertion, and the needle/catheter in the pleural space

Figure 10-3. *Technique of thoracentesis.*

Purposes
1. To remove fluid and air from the pleural cavity (for diagnostic and therapeutic purposes).
2. To obtain diagnostic aspiration of pleural fluid.
3. To obtain pleural biopsy.
4. To instill medication into the pleural space.

(continued)

Guidelines Assisting the Patient Undergoing Thoracentesis *(continued)*

Equipment

Syringes: 5-, 20-, 50-ml. syringes
Needles: No. 22, No. 26, No. 16 (7.5 cm. long)
Stopcock and tubing
Hemostat
Biopsy needle
Germicide solution
Local anesthetic
Sterile gauze dressings
Sterile towels and drape
Sterile specimen containers
Sterile gloves

Or for ultrasound-directed thoracentesis:
  Needle–syringe assembly (needle, extension tubing, syringe)

Procedure

Nursing Action	Rationale/Amplification

Preparatory Phase

1. Ascertain in advance if chest roentgenograms and/or other tests have been prescribed and completed. These should be available at the bedside.
2. See if consent form has been explained and signed.
3. Determine if the patient is allergic to the local anesthetic agent to be used. Give sedation if prescribed.
4. Inform the patient about the procedure and indicate how he can be helpful. Explain:
   a. The nature of the procedure.
   b. The importance of remaining immobile.
   c. Pressure sensations to be experienced.
   d. That no discomfort is anticipated after the procedure.
5. Make the patient comfortable with adequate supports. If possible place him upright and in one of the following positions (Fig. 10-4):
   a. Sitting on the edge of the bed with feet supported and head on a padded over-the-bed table.
   b. Straddling a chair with his arms and head resting on the back of the chair.

1. Localization of pleural fluid is accomplished by physical examination, chest roentgenogram, ultrasound localization, or fluoroscopic localization.

4. An explanation helps orient the patient to the procedure, assists him to mobilize his resources, and gives him an opportunity to ask questions and verbalize anxiety.

5. The upright position ensures that the diaphragm is most dependent and facilitates the removal of fluid that usually localizes at the base of the chest. A comfortable position helps the patient to relax.

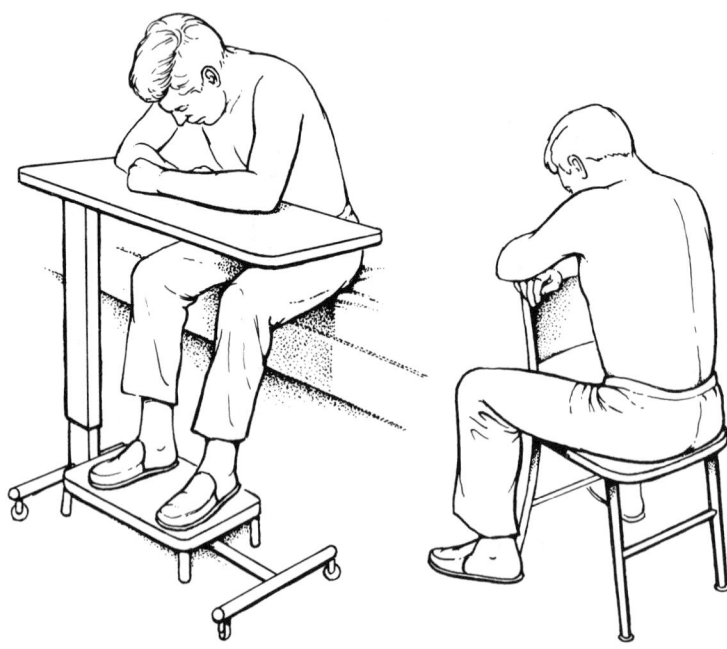

Over the bed table   **Straddling a chair**

Figure 10-4. *Positions for thoracentesis.*

Procedure
(continued)

Nursing Action	Rationale/Amplification

c. If patient is unable to sit in a chair or side of bed elevate head of bed 30–45° or place him on unaffected side and elevate head of bed.

6. Support and reassure the patient during the procedure.
   a. Prepare the patient for sensations of cold from skin germicide and for pressure and sting from infiltration of local anesthetic agent.
   b. Encourage the patient to refrain from coughing.

6. Sudden and unexpected movement by the patient can cause trauma to the visceral pleura with resultant trauma to the lung.

   A local anesthetic inhibits nerve conduction and is used to prevent pain during the procedure.

Performance Phase

1. The site for aspiration is determined from chest x-rays, by percussion, or by fluoroscopic or ultrasound localization. If fluid is in the pleural cavity, the thoracentesis site is determined by study of the chest x-ray and physical findings, with attention to the site of maximal dullness on percussion.

2. The procedure is done under aseptic conditions. After the skin is cleansed, the physician slowly injects a local anesthetic with a small caliber needle into the intercostal space.

3. The physician advances the thoracentesis needle with the syringe attached. When the pleural space is reached, suction may be applied with the syringe.
   a. A 20-ml. or 50-ml. syringe with a 3-way adapter (stopcock) is attached to the needle. (One end of the adapter is attached to the needle and the other to the tubing leading to a receptacle that receives the fluid being aspirated.)

   b. If a considerable quantity of fluid is to be removed, the needle is held in place on the chest wall with a small hemostat.

   c. A pleural biopsy may be performed.

4. After the needle is withdrawn, pressure is applied over the puncture site and a small sterile dressing is fixed in place.

1. If air is in the pleural cavity, the thoracentesis site is usually in the 2nd or 3rd intercostal space in the midclavicular line (Fig. 10-3). Air rises in the thorax because the density of air is much less than the density of liquid.

2. An intradermal wheal is raised slowly; rapid intradermal injection causes pain. The parietal pleura is very sensitive and should be well infiltrated with anesthetic before the thoracentesis needle is passed through it.

   a. When a larger quantity of fluid is withdrawn, a 3-way adapter serves to keep air from entering the pleural cavity. The amount of fluid removed depends on clinical status of the patient and absence of complications during the procedure.
   b. The hemostat steadies the needle on the chest wall and prevents too deep a penetration of pleural space. Sudden pleuritic pain or shoulder pain may indicate that the visceral or diaphragmatic pleura are being irritated by the needle point.

4. This is done to prevent air entry into pleural space.

Follow-up Phase

1. Place the patient on bed rest. A chest x-ray is usually obtained following thoracentesis.
2. Record vital signs every 15 minutes for 1 hour.
3. Administer oxygen as directed if patient has cardiorespiratory disease.
4. Record the total amount of fluid withdrawn and the nature of the fluid, its color and viscosity. If prescribed, prepare samples of fluid for laboratory evaluation (usually bacteriology, cell count and differential, determinations of protein, glucose, LDH, specific gravity). A small amount of heparin may be needed for several of the specimen containers to prevent coagulation. A specimen container with preservative may be needed if a pleural biopsy is to be obtained.
5. Evaluate the patient at intervals for increasing respirations, faintness, vertigo, tightness in the chest, uncontrollable cough, blood-tinged frothy mucus, and rapid pulse and signs of hypoxemia.

1. Chest x-ray verifies that there is no pneumothorax.

3. Pulmonary gas exchange may worsen after thoracentesis in patients with cardiorespiratory disease.
4. The fluid may be clear, serous, bloody, purulent, etc.

5. Pneumothorax, tension pneumothorax, hemothorax, subcutaneous emphysema, or pyogenic infection may result from a thoracentesis.

Chest Physical Therapy

Postural Drainage Exercises

Postural drainage is the use of specific positions so that the force of gravity can assist in the removal of bronchial secretions from the affected bronchioles into the bronchi and trachea by means of coughing or suctioning (Fig. 10-5).

Underlying Principles

1. The patient is positioned so that the diseased area(s) are in a near vertical position, and gravity is used to assist drainage of the specific segment(s).
2. The positions assumed are determined by the location, severity, and duration of mucus obstruction.
3. The exercises are usually performed 2 to 4 times daily, before meals and at bedtime.
4. Discontinue the procedure if tachycardia, palpitations, dyspnea, chest pain, or other symptoms occur—may indicate hypoxemia.

Nursing Interventions

1. Make the patient comfortable before the procedure starts and as comfortable as possible while he assumes each position.
   a. Bronchodilators, broncholytic agents, water, or saline may be nebulized and inhaled before postural drainage to reduce bronchospasm, decrease thickness of mucus and sputum, and combat edema of the bronchial walls.
   b. Use a folding cot to prop up patient to desired height if his bed is not adjustable; have an emesis basin ready for draining mucus.
2. Auscultate the chest to determine the areas of needed drainage.
3. Upper lobes are generally drained by upright positions; lower and middle lobes are drained by head-down positions.
4. Have patient assume left prone and left oblique positions (simultaneously)—this will give additional drainage to middle lobe and lateral segments of the right lower lobe; assuming the right prone and right

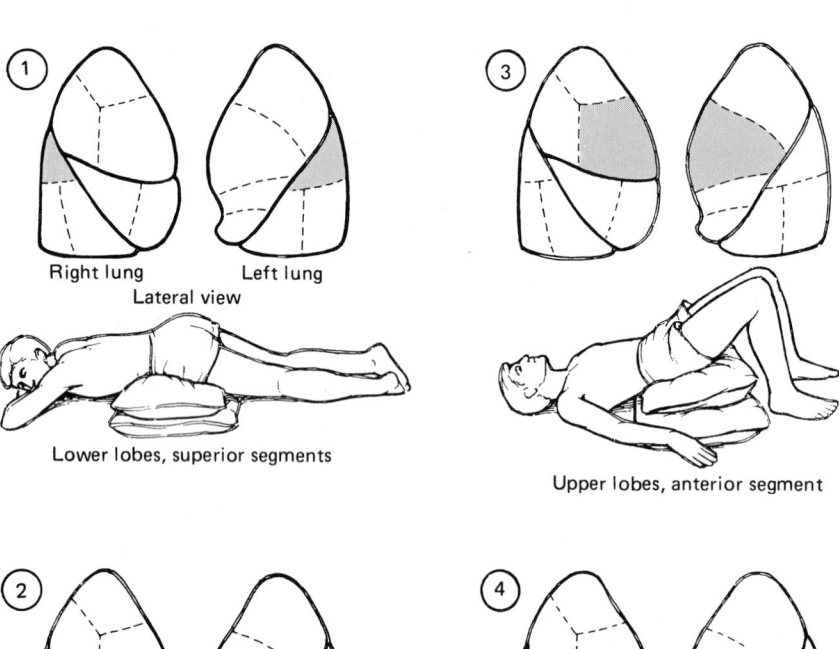

Right lung   Left lung
Lateral view

Lower lobes, superior segments

Upper lobes, anterior segment

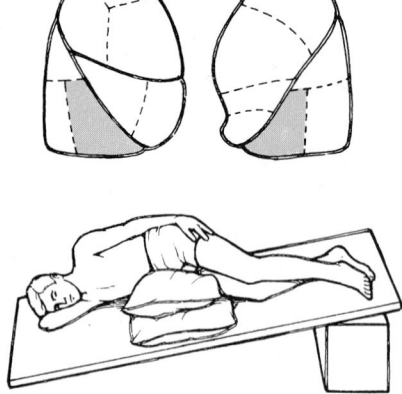

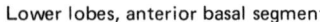

Lower lobes, anterior basal segment

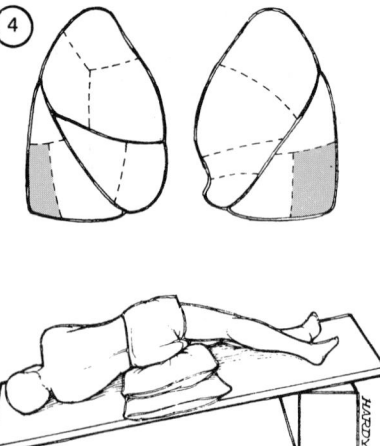

Lower lobe, lateral basal segment

Figure 10-5. *Postural drainage. The patient is positioned to allow the involved segments of the lung to drain by gravity.*

oblique position (simultaneously) will give additional drainage to middle lobe and lateral segments of the left lower lobe.
5. Encourage the patient to cough after he has spent the allotted time in each position.

6. Encourage diaphragmatic breathing (p. 172) throughout postural drainage exercises; this helps widen airways so that secretions can be drained.
7. Chest wall percussion may be desirable to loosen and propel sputum in the direction of gravity drainage.

Guidelines   Percussion (Clapping) and Vibration

Percussion and vibration are manual techniques designed to loosen secretions and promote drainage of mucus and secretions from the lungs while the patient is in the position of postural drainage indicated for his specific lung problem. The procedure requires trained personnel.
1. *Percussion*—movement done by striking the chest wall in a rhythmic fashion with cupped hands over the chest segment to be drained. The wrists are alternately flexed and extended so that the chest is cupped or clapped in a painless manner.
2. *Vibration*—technique of applying manual compression and tremor to the chest wall during the exhalation phase of respiration.

Purposes
1. To dislodge mucus adhering to the bronchioles and bronchi.
2. To help mobilize secretions.

Clinical Indications

Lung conditions that cause increased production of secretions:
  Bronchiectasis
  Empyema
  Cystic fibrosis
  Chronic bronchitis

Contraindications
1. Lung abscess or tumors
2. Pneumothorax
3. Diseases of the chest wall

4. Lung hemorrhage
5. Painful chest conditions
6. Tuberculosis

> **NURSING ALERT:** Postural drainage and chest percussion may result in hypoxia and should only be used if secretions are believed to be present.

Procedure

Nursing Action	Rationale/Amplification

Performance Phase

1. Instruct the patient to use diaphragmatic breathing (p. 172).

2. Position the patient in prescribed postural drainage position(s) (p. 170). The spine should be straight to promote rib cage expansion.

3. Percuss (or clap) with cupped hands over the chest wall for 1 or 2 minutes from:
   a. The lower ribs to shoulders in the back
   b. The lower ribs to top of chest in front
4. Avoid clapping over the spine, liver, kidneys, spleen, breast, scapula, clavicle, or sternum.
5. Instruct the patient to inhale slowly and deeply. Vibrate the chest wall as the patient exhales slowly through pursed lips.
   a. Place one hand on top of the other over affected area or place one hand on each side of the rib cage.
   b. Tense the muscles of the hands and arms while applying moderate pressure downward and vibrate hands and arms.
   c. Relieve pressure on the thorax as the patient inhales.
   d. Encourage the patient to cough, using his abdominal muscles, after 3 or 4 vibrations.

6. Allow the patient to rest several minutes.
7. Listen with a stethoscope for changes in breath sounds.

8. Repeat the percussion and vibration cycle according to the patient's tolerance and his clinical response; usually 15 to 20 minutes.

1. Diaphragmatic breathing helps the patient to relax and helps to widen airways.
2. The patient is positioned according to the area of the lung that is to be drained.

3. This action helps to dislodge mucus plugs and mobilize secretions toward the main bronchi and trachea. The air trapped between the operator's hand and chest wall will produce a characteristic hollow sound.

4. Percussion over these areas may cause injuries to the spine and internal organs.
5. This sets up a vibration that carries through the chest wall and helps free the mucus.

   b. This maneuver is performed in the direction in which the ribs move on expiration.

   d. Contracting the abdominal muscles while coughing increases cough effectiveness. Coughing aids in the movement and expulsion of secretions.

7. The appearance of moist sounds (crackles) indicates movement of air around mucus in the bronchi.

Guidelines Teaching the Patient Breathing Exercises

Breathing exercises are techniques used to compensate for respiratory deficits by increasing efficiency of breathing. They are aimed at conserving energy through controlled breathing.

Purposes
1. To relax muscles and relieve anxiety.
2. To eliminate useless uncoordinated patterns of respiratory muscle activity.
3. To slow the respiratory rate.
4. To decrease the work of breathing.

General Instructions

1. Clear the nasal passages before beginning breathing exercises.
2. Always inhale through the nose—permits filtration, humidification, and warming of air.
3. Breathe slowly in a rhythmic and relaxed manner—permits more complete exhalation and emptying of lungs; helps overcome anxiety associated with dyspnea and decreases oxygen requirement.
4. Avoid sudden exertion.
5. Practice breathing exercises in several positions, as air distribution and pulmonary circulation vary according to position of the chest.

Diaphragmatic Breathing

Purposes:
1. To strengthen the diaphragm—the main respiratory muscle
2. To decrease the use of the accessory muscles of respiration
3. To gain control over breathing pattern, especially during stressful situations

Teaching Procedure	Rationale/Amplification
Instruct the patient as follows:	
1. Place one hand on stomach just below the ribs and the other hand on the middle of the chest.	1. This helps the patient to become aware of the diaphragm and its function in breathing.
2. Breathe in slowly and deeply through the nose, letting the abdomen protrude as far as it will. The abdomen enlarges during inspiration and decreases in size during expiration.	2. Slow inhalation provides ventilation and hyperinflation of the lungs.
3. Breathe out through pursed lips while contracting (tightening) the abdominal muscles. Press firmly inward and upward on the abdomen while breathing out.	3. Contracting the abdominal muscles assists the diaphragm in rising to empty the lungs. The hand generates pressure on the abdomen to facilitate more complete expiration.
4. The chest should not move; attention is directed at the abdomen, not the chest.	4. Contraction of the abdominal muscles should take place during expiration.
5. Repeat for approximately 1 minute (followed by a rest period of 2 minutes). Work up to 10 minutes, 4 times daily.	
6. Learn to do diaphragmatic breathing while lying, then sitting, and ultimately standing and walking.	6. Diaphragmatic breathing helps the patient breathe in a controlled manner during activities that produce dyspnea. If the patient becomes short of breath, have him stop the exercises until his breathing pattern comes under control.
a. Coordinate diaphragmatic breathing with stair climbing, lifting, etc.	
b. Carry out activity (lifting) during the prolonged expiration phase.	

Pursed Lips Breathing

Purposes
1. To slow the respiratory rate
2. To assist in emptying the lungs
3. To combat dyspnea due to exertion.

Instruct the patient as follows:
1. Inhale through the nose.
2. Exhale slowly and evenly against pursed lips while contracting (tightening) the abdominal muscles.

    Count to 7 while prolonging expiration through pursed lips.

2. Pursing the lips increases intrabronchial pressure (helps maintain the bronchi in an open position) as well as intra-alveolar pressure. The pursed-lips maneuver also prolongs the expiratory phase of breathing, makes it easier to empty the air in the lungs, and promotes carbon dioxide elimination.

3. Sit in a chair. Fold the arms across the abdomen.
  a. Inhale through the nose.
  b. Bend over and exhale slowly through pursed lips while counting to 7.

    b. Leaning forward pushes the abdominal organs upward.

4. While walking:
  a. Inhale while walking 2 steps.
  b. Exhale through pursed lips while walking 4 steps.

4. Try any similar combinations according to breathing tolerance of patient.

Other Exercises

Lower Side Rib Breathing

1. Place hands on sides of lower ribs.
2. Inhale deeply and slowly while sides expand moving hands outward.
3. Exhale slowly through pursed lips and feel the hands and ribs move inward.
4. Rest.

Lower Back and Rib Breathing

1. Sit in a chair. Place hands behind back; hold flat against lower ribs.
2. Inhale deeply and slowly while rib cage expands backward; the hands will move outward.
3. Keep hands in place. Blow out slowly; hands will move in.

Segmental Breathing

1. Place hands on sides of lower ribs.
2. Inhale deeply and slowly while concentrating on moving the right hand outward by expanding the right rib cage.
3. Ensure that the right hand moves outward more than the left hand.
4. Keeping hands in place, exhale slowly, and feel the right hand and ribs moving in.
5. Repeat, concentrating on expanding left side more than the right side.
6. Rest.

Guidelines

Nasotracheal (NT) Suctioning

Suctioning of the tracheobronchial tree in a patient without an artificial airway is possible by inserting a suction catheter through the nares into the nasal passage, down through the oropharynx, past the glottis, and into the trachea (Fig. 10-6).

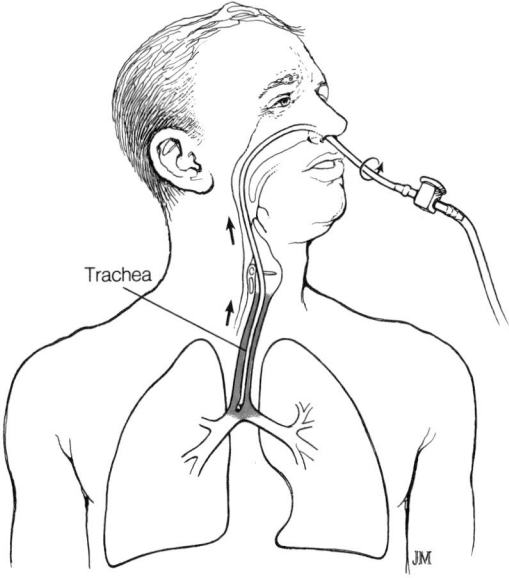

Trachea

Figure 10-6. Placement of nasotracheal tube for suctioning the tracheobronchial tree.

(a) In addition to direct removal of secretions, nasotracheal suctioning stimulates strong paroxysms of coughing, enabling mobilization of secretions.

(b) Nasotracheal suctioning may be indicated in patients who are mechanically capable of coughing but do not do so because of central nervous system (CNS) depression, in those who have an inadequate cough secondary to "splinting" as a result of pain, or in patients whose cough is ineffective.

(continued)

Guidelines Nasotracheal (NT) Suctioning *(continued)*

Contraindications	Bleeding disorder (disseminated intravascular coagulation [DIC], thrombocytopenia, leukemia, etc.)
	Laryngeal edema, laryngeal spasm
	Esophageal varices
	Tracheal surgery
	Gastric surgery with high anastomosis
	Myocardial infarction (check with physician)

Caution

1. Trauma to the nasal passages may occur. Do not attempt to force the catheter if resistance is met. Trauma to nasal membranes or polyps may occur. If significant bleeding occurs, notify the physician.
2. Repeated suctioning may produce irritation of the nasal passages, resulting in pain and swelling. Insertion of a nasal airway may help to protect the nasal passages from trauma.
3. Repeated NT suctioning may promote laryngeal edema due to irritation and trauma. Stop if suctioning becomes difficult or if the patient develops new upper airway noise or obstruction.

Equipment

Assemble the following equipment or obtain a prepackaged kit.
Disposable curved-tipped suction catheter
Sterile towel
Sterile disposable gloves
Sterile water
Anesthetic water soluble lubricant jelly
Suction source at −80 to −120 mm. Hg
Resuscitation bag with face mask—connect 100% O_2 source with flow 10 liters/min.

	Nursing Action	**Rationale/Amplification**

Assessment	1. Monitor heart rate, respiratory rate, color, ease of respirations. If the patient is on monitor, continue monitoring heart rate or arterial blood pressure. Discontinue the suctioning and apply oxygen if heart rate decreases by 20 beats per minute or increases by 40 beats per minute, if blood pressure decreases, or if cardiac dysrhythmia is noted.	1. Suctioning may cause the occurrence of:
		  a. Hypoxemia—initially resulting in tachycardia and increased blood pressure, and later causing cardiac ectopy, bradycardia, hypotension, and cyanosis.
		  b. Vagal stimulation resulting in bradycardia.

Planning/Implementation	**Preparatory Phase** 1. Ascertain that the suction apparatus is functional. Place suction tubing within easy reach.	1. The procedure must be done aseptically, as the catheter will be entering the trachea below the level of the vocal cords, and introduction of bacteria is contraindicated.

	2. Inform and instruct the patient regarding procedure.
	  a. At a certain interval the patient will be requested to cough to open the lung passage so that the catheter will go into the lungs and not into the stomach. He will also be encouraged to try not to swallow, as this will also cause the catheter to enter the stomach.
	  b. The postoperative patient can splint his wound to make the coughing produced by NT suctioning less painful.
		2. A thorough explanation will decrease patient anxiety and promote patient cooperation (which is necessary for successful implementation of this procedure).

	3. Place the patient in a semi-Fowler's or sitting position if possible.	3. NT suctioning should follow chest physical therapy, postural drainage, and/or ultrasonic nebulization therapy. The patient should not be suctioned after eating or after a tube feeding is given, unless absolutely necessary to decrease the possibility of emesis and aspiration.
	Performance Phase 1. Place sterile towel across the patient's chest. Squeeze small amount of sterile anesthetic water-soluble lubricant jelly onto the towel.	
	2. Open sterile pack containing curved-tipped suction catheter.	
	3. Aseptically glove both hands. Designate one hand (usually the dominant one) as "sterile" and the other hand as "contaminated."	3. The "contaminated" hand must also be gloved to ensure that organisms in the sputum do not come in contact with the nurse's hand, possibly resulting in infection of the nurse.
	4. Grasp sterile catheter with sterile hand.	

**Planning/Im-
plementation**
(continued)

5. Lubricate catheter with the anesthetic jelly and pass the catheter into the nostril and back into the pharynx.
6. Pass the catheter into the trachea. To do this, ask the patient to cough or say ''ahh.'' If he is incapable of either, try to advance the catheter on inspiration. Asking the patient to stick out his tongue, or hold his tongue extended with a gauze sponge, may also help to open the airway.

7. Specific positioning of catheter for deep bronchial suctioning:
   a. For left bronchial suctioning, turn the patient's head to the extreme right, chin up.
   b. For right bronchial suctioning, turn the patient's head to the extreme left, chin up.

5. If obstruction is met, do not force the catheter—remove it and try the other nostril.
6. These maneuvers may aid in opening the glottis and allowing passage of the catheter into the trachea. To evaluate proper placement, listen at the catheter end for air, or feel for air movement against the cheek. An increase in intensity of breath sounds or more air movement against cheek indicates nearness to the larynx. Gagging or sudden lessening of sound means the catheter is in the hypopharynx. Draw back and advance again. The presence of the catheter in the trachea is indicated by:
   a. Sudden paroxysms of coughing.
   b. Movement of air through the catheter.
   c. Vigorous bubbling of air when the distal end of the suction catheter is placed in a cup of sterile water.
   d. Inability of the patient to speak.

If a protracted amount of time is needed to position the catheter in the trachea, stop and oxygenate the patient with his face mask or the resuscitation bag–mask unit at intervals. If three attempts to place the catheter are unsuccessful, request assistance.

7. Turning the patient's head to one side elevates the bronchial passage on the opposite side, making catheter insertion easier. Suctioning of a particular lung segment may be of value in patients with unilateral pneumonia, atelectasis, or collapse.

Note: The value of turning the head as an aid to entering the right or left main stem bronchi is not accepted by all clinicians.

8. Never apply suction until catheter is in the trachea.
   a. Once correct position is ascertained, apply suction and gently rotate catheter while pulling it slightly upward. Do not remove catheter from the trachea.

9. Disconnect the catheter from the suctioning source after 5–15 seconds. Apply oxygen by placing a face-mask over the patient's nose, mouth, and catheter, and instruct the patient to breathe deeply.
10. Reconnect suction source. Repeat suction as necessary.

11. During the last suction pass, remove the catheter completely while applying suction and rotating the catheter gently. Apply oxygen when catheter is removed.

   a. Because entry into the trachea is often difficult, less change in arterial oxygen may be caused by leaving the catheter in the trachea than by repeated insertion attempts.
9. Be sure that adequate time is allowed to reoxygenate the patient, as oxygen is removed, as well as secretions, during suctioning.
10. No more than 3–4 suction passes should be made per suction episode.
11. Never leave the catheter in the trachea after the suction procedure is concluded, as the epiglottis is splinted open and aspiration may occur.

Follow-up Phase

Dispose of disposable equipment.
   1. Measure heart rate and blood pressure. Record the patient's tolerance of procedure, type and amount of secretions removed, and complications.

1. Notify physician of any patient intolerance of procedure (changes in vital signs, bleeding, laryngospasm, upper airway noise).

Clinical Conditions

The Pneumonias

Pneumonia is an inflammatory process, involving the terminal airways and alveoli of the lung, caused by infectious agents. (See Table 10-2.)

Predisposing Factors

1. The organism gains access to the lungs through aspiration of oropharyngeal contents, by inhalation of respiratory secretions from infected individuals, via the blood stream, or from direct spread to the lungs from surgery or trauma.
2. Patients with bacterial pneumonia usually have an underlying disease that impairs host defense; more often pneumonia arises from endogenous flora of the person whose resistance has been altered or from aspiration of oropharyngeal secretions.
3. When bacterial pneumonia occurs in a healthy person, there usually is a history of preceding viral illness.
4. Pneumonia may be divided into three groups:
   a. Community-acquired, due to a number of organisms, namely *Streptococcus pneumoniae;*
   b. Hospital or nursing home acquired (nosocomial)

Table 10-2. *Commonly Encountered Pneumonias*

Type	Organism Responsible	Manifestations	Clinical Features	Treatment	Complications
Bacterial					
Streptococcal pneumonia	*Streptococcus pneumoniae*	May be history of previous respiratory infection Sudden onset, with shaking and chills Rapidly rising fever; tachypnea Cough; with expectoration of rusty or green (purulent) sputum Pleuritic pain aggravated by cough Chest dull to percussion; crackles, bronchial breath sounds Confusion may be only presenting feature in elderly	Herpes simplex lesions often present on face or lips Usually involves one or more lobes	Penicillin G Alternate drug therapy: erythromycin, clindamycin, cephalosporins, other penicillins, trimethoprim-sulfa-methoxazole	Shock Pleural effusion Superinfections Pericarditis Otitis media
Staphylococcal pneumonia	*Staphylococcus aureus*	Often prior history of viral infection, especially influenza Insidious development of cough, with expectoration of yellow, blood-streaked mucus Onset may be sudden if patient is outside hospital Fever, pleuritic chest pain, progressive dyspnea Pulse varies; may be slow in proportion to temperature	Frequently seen in hospital setting; during influenza epidemics; in intravenous drug abuse These infections often lead to necrosis and destruction of lung tissue Treatment must be vigorous and prolonged owing to disease's tendency to destroy the lungs Organism may develop rapid drug resistance Prolonged convalescence usual	Penicillinase-resistant penicillins	Effusion/pneumothorax Lung abscess Empyema Meningitis
Pneumonia due to gram-negative enteric bacilli	*Klebsiella* species; *Pseudomonas* organisms, *Escherichia coli, Seratia, Proteus* species	Sudden onset with fever, chills, dyspnea Pleuritic chest pain and production of purulent sputum	Usually infection occurs from aspiration of pharyngeal flora into bronchioles Seen in persons with severe illness; among the more common causes of hospital-acquired pneumonia	Usually multiple drug regimens recommended; aminoglycoside antibiotic; cephalosporins	Early necrosis of lung tissue with rapid abscess formation High mortality rate
Legionnaires' disease	*Legionella pneumophila*	High fever, chills, cough, chest pain, tachypnea Respiratory distress	Peak incidence in persons over 50 who are cigarette smokers and have underlying diseases that increase susceptibility to infection	Erythromycin	Respiratory failure
Hemophilus influenza pneumonia	*H. influenzae*	Abrupt onset of coughing, fever, chills, chest pain	May affect healthy young adults	Depends on patient's previous or current use of antibiotic and on ampicillin-resistance rate in community	High mortality rate in patients with underlying disease (cancer; COPD) Pleural effusion common
Nonbacterial Pneumonias					
Mycoplasma pneumonia	*Mycoplasma pneumoniae*	Gradual onset; severe headache; irritating hacking cough producing scanty, mucoid sputum Anorexia; malaise Fever; nasal congestion; sore throat	Occurs most commonly in children and young adults, as well as in older adults in community hospital setting Rise in serum-complement-fixing antibodies to the organism	Erythromycin; tetracycline	Persisting cough, meningoencephalitis, polyneuritis, monoarticular arthritis, pericarditis, myocarditis
Viral pneumonia	Influenza viruses Parainfluenza viruses Respiratory syncytial viruses Rhinoviruses Adenovirus Varicella, rubella, rubeola, herpes simplex, cytomegalovirus, Epstein–Barr virus	Cough Constitutional symptoms may be pronounced (severe headache, anorexia, fever, and myalgia)	In majority of patients influenza begins as an acute coryza; others have bronchitis, pleurisy, etc., while still others develop gastrointestinal symptoms Risk of developing influenza related to crowding and close contact of groups of individuals	Treat symptomatically Amantadine relieves symptoms Prophylactic vaccination recommended for high-risk persons (over 65; chronic cardiac or pulmonary disease, diabetes, and other metabolic disorders)	Persons with underlying disease have increased risk of complications; primary influenzal pneumonia; secondary bacterial pneumonia Bacterial superinfection Pericarditis Endocarditis

(continued)

Table 10-2. *Commonly Encountered Pneumonias (continued)*

Type	Organism Responsible	Manifestations	Clinical Features	Treatment	Complications
Pneumocystis carinii pneumonia	*Pneumocystis carinii*	Insidious onset Increasing dyspnea and nonproductive cough Tachypnea; progresses rapidly to intercostal retraction, nasal flaring, and cyanosis Lowering of arterial oxygen tension Chest x-ray will reveal diffuse, bilateral interstitial pneumonia	Usually seen in host whose resistance is compromised; most common opportunistic infection in AIDS Organism invades lungs of patients who have suppressed immune system (from cancer, AIDS, leukemia) or following immunosuppressive therapy for cancer, organ transplant, or collagen disease Frequently associated with concurrent infection by viruses, (cytomegalovirus) bacteria, and fungi	Pentamidine methanesulfonate Trimethoprim-sulfamethoxazole	Patients are critically ill Prognosis guarded, since it usually is a complication of a severe underlying disorder
Fungal pneumonia	*Aspergillus fumigatus*	Fever, productive cough, chest pain, hemoptysis Chest x-ray reveals broad range of abnormalities from infiltration to consolidation, cavitation, and empyema	Neutropenic individual most susceptible May develop *Aspergillus* as a superinfection	Amphotericin B; ketoconazole	High fatality rate Invades blood vessels and destroys lung tissue by direct invasion and vascular infarction

due primarily to gram-negative bacilli and staphylococci; and
  c. In the immunocompromised person.
5. Immunocompromised patients (those receiving corticosteroids; those with cancer; those being treated with chemotherapy or radiotherapy; those undergoing organ transplantation) have an increased chance of developing overwhelming infection.
6. A wide variety of pulmonary infections may develop in patients receiving immunosuppressive drugs (aerobic and anaerobic gram-negative bacilli, *Staphylococcus, Nocardia,* fungi, *Candida,* viruses [including cytomegalovirus], *Pneumocystis carinii,* reactivation of tuberculosis, and others).
7. Any condition interfering with normal drainage of the lung will predispose the person to pneumonia (e.g., cancer of the lung).
8. Postoperative patients may develop bronchopneumonia, since anesthesia impairs respiratory defenses and decreases diaphragmatic movement.
9. Depression of the central nervous system (from drugs [including alcohol], head injury) predispose the patient to pneumonia.
10. Persons over 65 have a high mortality rate, even with appropriate antimicrobial therapy.

NURSING ALERT: Recurring pneumonia often indicates underlying disease (cancer of the lung, multiple myeloma).

Health Maintenance and Preventive Measures

1. Natural resistance should be maintained (adequate nutrition, rest, exercise).
2. Avoid contact with people who have upper respiratory infections.
3. Obliteration of cough reflex and aspiration of secretions should be avoided.
4. Adequate bronchial hygiene should be employed.
5. Immobilized patients should be turned every 2 hours and encouraged to breathe deeply, sigh, and cough.
6. Use every measure to reduce bacterial colonization and superinfection of the hospitalized patient.
7. Highly susceptible persons (elderly and chronically ill) should be immunized against influenza.
8. Pneumococcal vaccine should be given to those at greatest risk—chronically ill and elderly, particularly those in institutions.

Clinical Manifestations *(Bacterial Pneumonia)*

1. *Sudden* onset; shaking chill; rapidly rising fever (39.5°–40.5°C. [101°–105°F.])
2. Cough productive of purulent sputum
3. Pleuritic chest pain aggravated by respiration/coughing
4. Tachypnea (25–45/min) accompanied by respiratory grunting, nasal flaring, use of accessory muscles of respiration.
5. Rapid bounding pulse

Diagnostic Evaluation

1. Chest x-ray to show presence/extent of pulmonary disease
2. Gram stain, culture, and sensitivity studies of sputum
3. Blood culture to recover causative organism; bacteremia (blood stream invasion) occurs frequently with bacterial pneumonia
4. Immunologic test for detecting microbial antigens in serum, sputum, and urine

Management

1. Antimicrobial therapy—depends on laboratory identification of causative organism.
2. Oxygen therapy if patient has inadequate gas exchange.

Complications

1. Pleural effusion (see p. 180)
2. Sustained hypotension and shock, especially in gram-

negative bacterial disease, particularly in the elderly.
3. Superinfection; pericarditis, bacteremia, meningitis
4. Delirium—*this is considered a medical emergency*
5. Atelectasis—due to mucus plugs
6. Delayed resolution

Nursing Assessment

1. Take a careful history to help establish etiologic diagnosis.
   a. History of *recent* respiratory illness? Mode of onset?
   b. Number, frequency, and duration of chills.
   c. Description of chest pain.
   d. Any family illness?
   e. Any recent antimicrobial drugs? Alcohol? Tobacco? Drug abuse?
2. Observe for anxious, flushed appearance, shallow respirations, splinting of affected side, confusion, disorientation.
3. Auscultate for crackles overlying affected region, and for bronchial breath sounds when *consolidation* (filling of airspaces with exudate) is present.

Nursing Diagnoses

1. Impaired gas exchange related to decreased ventilation secondary to inflammation and infection involving distal airspaces; abnormal ventilation/perfusion ratios.
2. Ineffective airway clearance related to excessive tracheobronchial secretions
3. Pain related to inflammatory process and dyspnea.
4. Knowledge deficit of treatment regimen and preventive program

Nursing Interventions

A. Improving Gas Exchange

1. Observe the patient for cyanosis, dyspnea, hypoxia, and confusion.
2. Follow blood gas values to determine oxygen need and response to oxygen therapy.
3. Administer oxygen at concentration to maintain PaO_2 at acceptable level—hypoxemia may be encountered because of abnormal ventilation/perfusion ratios in affected lung segments.
4. Avoid high concentrations of oxygen in patients with chronic obstructive pulmonary disease (chronic bronchitis, emphysema)—*the use of high oxygen concentrations may worsen alveolar ventilation by removing the patient's only remaining ventilatory drive.*
5. Place patient in a fairly upright position to obtain greater lung expansion to improve aeration.

B. Improving Airway Clearance

1. Obtain freshly expectorated sputum for Gram stain and culture. Instruct the patient as follows:
   a. Rinse mouth with water to minimize contamination by normal flora.
   b. Breathe deeply several times.
   c. Cough deeply and expectorate raised sputum into sterile container.
2. Aspirate trachea with sterile catheter if patient is too ill to raise sputum. (See Guidelines, p. 173).
3. Encourage patient to cough—retained secretions interfere with gas exchange. Use tracheal aspiration in patient with poor cough response.
4. Encourage high level of fluid intake within limits of patient's cardiac reserve—adequate hydration thins

mucus and serves as an effective expectorant; replaces fluid losses due to fever, diaphoresis, dehydration, and dyspnea.
5. Humidify air to loosen secretions and improve ventilation.
6. Employ chest wall percussion and postural drainage when appropriate to loosen and mobilize secretions.
7. Auscultate the chest for crackles.
8. Control cough when coughing is nonproductive, debilitating, and when coughing paroxysms cause serious hypoxemia. Give codeine as prescribed.

C. Achieving Relief of Pleuritic Pain and Discomfort

1. Place in a comfortable position (semi-Fowler's) for resting and breathing; encourage frequent change of position to prevent pooling of secretions in lungs.
2. Demonstrate how to splint the chest while coughing.
3. Avoid suppressing a productive cough.
4. Administer prescribed analgesic agent to relieve pain.
   a. Evaluate patient's sensorium to assess for signs and symptoms suggestive of meningitis.

> **GERONTOLOGIC ALERT:** Sedatives, narcotics, and cough suppressants are generally contraindicated in the elderly, because of their tendency to suppress cough and gag reflexes and respiratory drive.

   b. Avoid narcotics in patients with a history of chronic obstructive pulmonary disease.

> **NURSING ALERT:** Restlessness, confusion, aggressiveness may be due to cerebral hypoxia. In such instances, sedatives are inappropriate.

5. Apply heat and/or cold to chest as prescribed.
6. Assist with intercostal nerve block for pain relief.
7. Maintain adequate hydration, as fluid loss is high from fever, dehydration, dyspnea, and diaphoresis.
8. Encourage modified bed rest during febrile period.
9. Treat abdominal distention or ileus, which may be due to swallowing of air during intervals of severe dyspnea.
   a. Pass nasogastric tube for acute gastric distention as prescribed.
   b. Use a rectal tube and give prescribed neostigmine methylsulfate to facilitate intestinal decompression.

D. Monitoring Response to Therapy

1. Remember that fatal complications may develop during the early period of antimicrobial treatment.
2. Monitor temperature, pulse, respiration, and blood pressure at regular intervals to assess the patient's response to therapy.
3. Listen to lungs and heart—heart murmurs or friction rub may indicate acute bacterial endocarditis, pericarditis, or myocarditis.
4. Employ special nursing surveillance for patients with the following conditions:
   a. Alcoholism or chronic obstructive pulmonary disease; these persons, as well as elderly patients, may have little or no fever.
   b. Chronic bronchitis; it is difficult to detect subtle changes in condition, as the patient may have seriously compromised pulmonary function.
   c. Epilepsy: pneumonia may result from aspiration following a seizure.

d. Delirium, which may be caused by hypoxia, meningitis, delirium tremens of alcoholism.
   (1) Prepare for lumbar puncture; meningitis may be lethal.
   (2) Ensure adequate hydration and give mild sedation.
   (3) Give oxygen.
   (4) Delirium must be controlled to prevent exhaustion and cardiac failure.
5. Assess these patients for *unusual behavior,* alterations in mental status, stupor, and congestive heart failure.
6. Assess for resistant fever or return of fever.

Patient Education

1. Fatigue, weakness, and depression may be prolonged after pneumonia.
2. Encourage chair rest after fever subsides; gradually increase activities to bring energy level back to pre-illness stage.
3. Encourage breathing exercises (p. 172) to clear lungs and promote full expansion and function after the fever subsides.
4. Explain that a chest x-ray is taken 4–6 weeks after discharge; should show clearing of lungs.
5. It is wise to stop smoking. Cigarette smoking destroys tracheobronchial cilial action, which is the first line of defense of lungs; also irritates mucosa of bronchi and inhibits function of alveolar scavenger cells (macrophages).
6. Advise the patient to keep up natural resistance with good nutrition, adequate rest—one episode of pneumonia may make the individual susceptible to recurring respiratory infections.
7. Instruct the patient to avoid fatigue, sudden extremes in temperature, and excessive alcohol intake, which lower resistance to pneumonia.
8. Encourage the patient to obtain influenza vaccine at prescribed times. Influenza increases susceptibility to secondary bacterial pneumonia.
9. Encourage the patient to seek medical advice about receiving pneumococcal vaccine against *Streptococcus pneumoniae,* which is effective against the majority of bacteremic pneumococcal diseases.

Evaluation

1. Shows improved gas exchange; color good; breathing normally
2. Demonstrates improved airway patency; coughing effectively; absence of crackles
3. Appears more comfortable; free of pain
4. Verbalizes at-home routine; has appointment for follow-up x-ray and smoking cessation counseling.

Aspiration Pneumonia

Aspiration is the inhalation of oropharyngeal secretions and/or stomach contents into the lungs. It may produce an acute form of pneumonia.

Etiology

Patients at risk and factors associated with risk:
1. Loss of protective airway reflexes—swallowing, laryngeal, cough
   a. Altered state of consciousness (general anesthesia, head injury, stroke, coma, convulsions)
   b. Alcohol; drug-overdose
   c. During resuscitation procedures
   d. Seriously ill, debilitated patients
   e. Abnormalities of gag and swallowing reflexes
2. Nasogastric tube feedings
3. Obstetrical patients—from general anesthesia, lithotomy position, delayed emptying of stomach from enlarged uterus, labor contractions
4. Esophageal disease—hiatal hernia
5. Delayed emptying time of stomach—intestinal obstruction, abdominal distention
6. Prolonged endotracheal intubation/tracheostomy—can depress glottic and laryngeal reflexes from disuse

Prevention

1. Be on guard constantly and monitor patients at risk as described above.
2. Elevate head of bed for debilitated patients, for those receiving tube feedings, and for those with motor diseases of the esophagus.
3. Place patients with impaired reflexes in a lateral position.
4. Be sure that nasogastric tube is patent.
5. Give tube feedings slowly, with patient sitting up in bed.
   a. Check position of tube in stomach before feeding.
   b. Check seal of cuff of tracheostomy or endotracheal tube before feeding.
6. Keep the patients in a fasting state before anesthesia (at least 8 hours).
7. Place the comatose patient on his side and elevate the foot of the bed 15–23 cm. (6–9 inches) unless medically contraindicated.

> **NURSING ALERT:** The morbidity and mortality rate of aspiration pneumonia remains high even with optimum treatment. Prevention is the key to the problem.

Clinical Manifestations

1. Depends on volume and character of aspirated material
   a. Particulate matter—mechanical blockage of airways and secondary infection
   b. Anaerobic bacterial aspiration—from oropharyngeal secretions
   c. Gastric juice—destructive to alveoli and capillaries; results in outpouring of protein-rich fluids into the interstitial and intra-alveolar spaces—impairs exchange of oxygen and carbon dioxide, producing hypoxemia, respiratory insufficiency and failure
2. Tachycardia/tachypnea
3. Dyspnea and cough; fever
4. Cyanosis
5. Crackles, rhonchi, wheezing
6. Pink, frothy sputum (may simulate acute pulmonary edema)

Diagnostic Evaluation

1. Appearance of patient
2. Chest x-ray shows abnormalities after period

Management

(Depends on the material aspirated)
1. Clearing the obstructed airway.
   a. If foreign body becomes lodged in the patient's throat, remove object with forceps.

b. Place the patient in tilted head-down position on right side (right side more frequently affected if patient has aspirated solid particles).
c. Suction trachea/endotracheal tube—to remove any particulate matter.
2. Laryngoscopy/bronchoscopy if patient is asphyxiated by solid material.
3. Fluid volume replacement for correction of hypotension.
4. Antimicrobial therapy if there is evidence of superimposed bacterial infection.
5. Correction of acidosis; respiratory acidosis and metabolic acidosis indicate a severe reaction due to aspiration of gastric contents.
6. Oxygen therapy and assisted ventilation if adequate blood gas values cannot be maintained.

Complications

1. Lung abscess; empyema
2. Necrotizing pneumonia

Nursing Interventions

A. Improving gas exchange

1. Monitor *trend* of arterial blood gas analyses
2. Administer oxygen as prescribed, when arterial blood gas evaluations demonstrate presence of hypoxemia.
3. Assist in placing on assisted ventilation if patient is unable to maintain an adequate PaO_2.

B. Monitoring for Infection

1. Observe for fever, purulent sputum, cough productive of foul-smelling sputum, and x-ray evidence of pulmonary infiltrate.
2. Administer prescribed antimicrobial drug.
3. Wash hands after each contact with respiratory secretions.

C. Restoring Fluid Balance

1. Assist with placement of Swan–Ganz flow-directed catheter to measure pulmonary capillary wedge pressure and cardiac output.
2. Measure intake and output as well as daily weight.
3. Give prescribed intravenous fluids.

D. Other Nursing Interventions

See *Pneumonia,* page 178.

Pleurisy

Pleurisy is a clinical term to describe *pleuritis,* (inflammation of the pleura).
Fibrinous pleurisy is deposition of a fibrinous exudate on the pleural surface.

Etiology

May occur in the course of many pulmonary diseases:
1. Pneumonia (bacterial, viral)
2. Tuberculosis
3. Pulmonary infarction, embolism
4. Pulmonary abscess
5. Upper respiratory tract infection
6. Pulmonary neoplasm

Clinical Manifestations

1. Chest pain—becomes severe, sharp, and knife-like on inspiration (pleuritic pain).

a. Pain may become minimal or absent when breath is held.
b. Pain may be localized or radiate to shoulder or abdomen.
2. Intercostal tenderness.
3. Pleural friction rub—grating or leathery sounds heard in both phases of respiration; heard low in the axilla or over the lung base posteriorly; may be heard for only a day or so.
4. Evidence of infection; fever, malaise, increased white cell count.

Diagnostic Evaluation

1. Chest x-ray
2. Sputum examination
3. Examination of pleural fluid obtained by thoracentesis for smear and culture
4. Pleural biopsy (selected patients)

Management and Nursing Interventions

1. Implement treatment for the underlying primary disease (pneumonia, infarction, etc.). Inflammation usually resolves when the primary disease subsides.
2. Relieve the pain.
   a. Give prescribed analgesics.
   b. Splint the rib cage when the patient coughs.
   c. Apply heat or cold—to provide symptomatic relief.
   d. Instruct the patient to lie on affected side occasionally—to splint chest wall.
   e. Assist with procaine intercostal block.
3. Watch for signs of development of pleural effusion (collection of fluid in pleural space): shortness of breath, pain, local decreased excursion of chest wall.

Pleural Effusion

Pleural effusion refers to a collection of fluid in the pleural space. It is almost always secondary to other diseases.

Etiology

Complication of:
1. Disseminated cancer (particularly lung and breast); lymphoma
2. Pleuropulmonary infections (pneumonia)
3. Congestive heart failure; cirrhosis; nephrosis
4. Others; sarcoidosis, systemic lupus erythematosus, peritoneal dialysis, etc.

Clinical Manifestations

1. Dyspnea, pleuritic chest pain, cough
2. Dullness or flatness to percussion (over areas of fluid) with decreased or absent breath sounds.

Diagnostic Evaluation

1. Physical findings of chest examination; chest x-ray
2. Thoracentesis—biochemical, bacteriologic, and cytologic studies of pleural fluid
3. Pleuroscopy (visual exploration of pleural space through a thoracoscope inserted into the pleural space); pleural biopsy

Management

A. General

Treatment is directed at underlying cause (heart disease, infection)

B. For Malignant Effusions

To relieve symptoms:
1. Thoracentesis (aspiration) for fluid removal and relief of dyspnea
2. Chest tube drainage, radiation, chemotherapy, surgical pleurodesis, pleuroperitoneal shunt, pleurodesis (see below)

> **NURSING ALERT:** In malignant conditions, thoracentesis may provide only transient benefits, as effusion may reaccumulate within a few days.

3. *Pleurodesis*—production of adhesions between the parietal and visceral pleura accomplished by tube thoracostomy, pleural space drainage, and intrapleural instillation of a sclerosing agent (tetracycline)
   a. Drug introduced through tube into pleural space; tube clamped
   b. Patient is helped to assume varying positions for 3–5 minutes each to allow drug to spread to all surfaces of the pleura.
   c. Tube is unclamped as prescribed.
   d. Chest drainage continued for 24 hours or longer.
   e. Resulting pleural irritation, inflammation, and fibrosis causes adhesion of the visceral and parietal surfaces when they are brought together by the negative pressure caused by chest suction.

Nursing Interventions Following Pleurodesis

1. Monitor for excessive pain from the sclerosing agent, which may cause hypoventilation.
2. Administer prescribed analgesic.
3. Assist patient undergoing instillation of intrapleural lidocaine if pain relief is not forthcoming.
4. Administer oxygen as required.
5. Observe patient's breathing pattern, and other vital signs, for evidence of improvement or deterioration.

Lung Abscess

A *lung abscess* is a localized, pus-containing, necrotic lesion in the lung characterized by cavity formation.

Etiology

1. Aspiration of vomitus or infected material from upper respiratory tract
2. Aspiration of foreign body into lung
3. Necrotizing pneumonia
4. Bronchial obstruction (usually a tumor) causes obstruction to bronchus, leading to infection distal to the growth.

Clinical Features

1. The right lung is involved more frequently than the left—owing to dependent position of the right bronchus, the less acute angle which the right main bronchus forms within the trachea, and its larger size.
2. In the initial stages, the cavity in the lung may or may not communicate with the bronchus.
3. Eventually the cavity becomes surrounded or encapsulated by a wall of fibrous tissue, except at 1 or 2 points where the necrotic process extends until it reaches the lumen of some bronchus or pleural space and establishes a communication with the respiratory tract, the pleural cavity (bronchopleural fistula), or both.

Clinical Manifestations

1. Cough
2. Fever and malaise—from segmental pneumonitis and atelectasis
3. Headache, anemia, weight loss
4. Pleuritic chest pain—from extension of suppurative pneumonitis to pleural surface
5. Production of mucopurulent sputum—often foul-smelling; blood streaking common; may become profuse after abscess ruptures into bronchial tree.

Diagnostic Evaluation

1. X-ray of chest—for diagnosis and location of lesion
2. Direct bronchoscopic visualization—to exclude possibility of tumor or foreign body; bronchial washings and brush biopsy may be done for cytopathologic study
3. Sputum culture and sensitivity—to determine causative organism(s) and antimicrobial sensitivity

Management

1. Administration of appropriate antimicrobial agent, usually by intravenous route, until clinical condition improves; then oral administration
2. Chest physical therapy and postural drainage to drain cavity
3. Surgical intervention only if patient fails to respond to medical management, sustains a hemorrhage, or has a suspected tumor

Complications

A. Hemoptysis—from an erosion of a vessel

1. Place patient on complete bed rest with bleeding site down (if known) or in head-down position if bleeding site is unknown.
2. Administer IV fluids as prescribed to correct hypotension.
3. Look for persistent flecks of blood in sputum after each acute episode.
4. Measure blood loss; more than 200 ml./24 hours has potential for life-threatening consequences related to asphyxiation from blood clotting in tracheobronchial tree.
5. Give antitussive (codeine) as directed; avoid total suppression of cough reflex, which may worsen gas exchange.
6. Prepare patient for bronchoscopy to localize bleeding site; prepare for intubation and/or balloon tamponade to obtain control of bleeding.
7. Continue to monitor for recurrent bleeding.

B. Empyema; Bronchopleural Fistula; Brain Abscess

Nursing Assessment

1. Examine oral cavity, as poor condition of teeth and gums increases number of anaerobes in oral cavity.
2. Auscultate chest for dullness; decreased breath sounds.
3. Monitor for foul-smelling sputum—indicates an anaerobic pulmonary infection.
4. Review results of laboratory and x-ray findings for location of abscess and identification of causative organism.

Nursing Diagnoses

1. Ineffective breathing pattern related to presence of suppurative lung disease
2. Pain related to infection
3. Altered nutrition (less than body requirements) related to catabolic state from chronic infection
4. Knowledge deficit of length of treatment and patient participation

Nursing Interventions

A. Relieving Respiratory Dysfunction

1. Monitor patient's response to antimicrobial therapy; take temperature at prescribed intervals.
2. Carry out drainage procedures to hasten resolution.
   a. Postural drainage positions to be assumed depend on location of abscess.
   b. Carry out percussion, coughing, and breathing exercises.
   c. Measure and record the volume of sputum—to follow patient's clinical course.
   d. Give adequate fluids to enhance liquefying of secretions.

B. Achieving Increasing Comfort

1. Use nursing measures to combat generalized discomfort; oral hygiene, positions of comfort, relaxing massage.
2. Take temperature, pulse, and respirations at regular intervals to determine type of fever and monitor the severity and duration of the infectious process.
3. Encourage rest and limitation of physical activity during febrile periods.
4. Monitor chest tube functioning.

C. Improving Nutritional Status

1. Give a high-protein and high-calorie diet.
2. Offer supplements for additional nutritional support when anorexia limits patient's intake.

Patient Education

1. Teach the patient that an extended course of antimicrobial therapy (4–8 weeks) is usually necessary; mixed infections are common and may require multiple antibiotics.
2. Encourage patient to have peridontal care, especially in presence of gingival lesions.
3. Stress importance of follow-up x-rays to monitor abscess cavity closure.
4. Remind family that patient may aspirate if weakness, confusion, alcoholism, seizures, and swallowing difficulties are present.
5. Encourage patient to assume responsibility for attaining/maintaining an optimal state of health through a planned program of nutrition, rest, and exercise.

Evaluation

1. Achieves improved respiratory function; temperature in normal range; less purulent sputum expectorated
2. Appears more comfortable
3. Demonstrates improving nutritional status; eating better
4. Has antibiotic prescription, appointment for follow-up x-ray, and appointment in dental clinic.

Bronchiectasis

Bronchiectasis is a chronic dilatation of the bronchi and bronchioles due to inflammation and destruction of their walls.

Causes

1. Pulmonary infections and obstruction of bronchi
2. Aspiration of foreign bodies, vomitus, or material from upper respiratory tract
3. Failure of immune system predisposes to infection.

Health Maintenance and Prevention

1. Treat all respiratory infections promptly.
2. Teach the family to seek medical treatment and on-going surveillance if child has recurrent respiratory infections; more than half of cases start in childhood.
3. All stuporous or comatose patients should be turned (prone position to lateral)—to drain all bronchial segments.
4. Encourage individual immunization program to prevent pertussis and measles (which can lead to bronchiectasis).

Clinical Manifestations

1. Persistent cough with production of purulent sputum
2. Intermittent hemoptysis; breathlessness
3. Recurrent fever and bouts of pulmonary infection
4. Crackles and rhonchi heard over involved lobes.

Diagnostic Evaluation

1. Chest roentgenogram (may reveal areas of atelectasis with widespread dilatation of bronchi)
2. Bronchogram (to map the entire bronchial tree to determine narrowing, dilatation, or obstruction of the bronchi)
3. Sputum examination

Complications

1. Progressive suppuration
2. Hemoptysis; major pulmonary hemorrhage
3. Emphysema; chronic respiratory insufficiency

Management

Goal:
Prevent progression of disease.

1. Infection controlled by:
   a. Smoking cessation
   b. Prompt antimicrobial treatment of exacerbations of infection
   c. Immunization against potential pulmonary pathogens (influenza and pneumonia)
2. Bronchodilators for selected patients with increased airway hyperreactivity
3. Surgical resection (segmental resection) when conservative management fails

Nursing Interventions

1. Use chest physical therapy to empty the bronchi of their accumulated secretions.
   a. Use postural drainage suitable to segment(s) involved to drain the bronchiectatic areas by gravity,

thus reducing degree of infection and amount of secretions.
  b. Employ percussion and vibration to assist in raising secretions.
  c. Encourage productive coughing to help clear secretions.
2. Encourage copious intake of fluids to reduce viscosity of sputum and make expectoration easier.
3. Use vaporizer to provide humidification and to keep secretions liquid.
4. Eliminate smoking and dusts, which are bronchial irritants that increase secretions.

Patient Education

1. Instruct the patient to avoid noxious fumes, dusts, and other pulmonary irritants (cigarette smoking).
2. Teach the patient to monitor sputum. Report to physician/clinic if change in quantity (increase/decrease) or character occurs.
3. Instruct the patient and family about importance of pulmonary drainage.
  a. Teach drainage exercises and chest physical therapy techniques.
  b. Encourage postural drainage before rising in the morning, as sputum accumulates during night.
  c. Engage in physical activity throughout day to help move mucus.
4. Encourage regular dental care.
5. Emphasize the importance of influenza and pneumonia immunizations.
6. See page 185 for other health teaching aspects (patient with emphysema).

Chronic Obstructive Pulmonary Disease (COPD)

Chronic obstructive pulmonary disease (COPD) is a term that refers to a group of conditions characterized by continued increased resistance to expiratory airflow.

COPD includes chronic bronchitis and pulmonary emphysema.

Altered Physiology

1. Basically, the person with COPD may have:
  a. Excessive secretion of mucus and chronic infection within the airways (bronchitis)
  b. An increase in size of air spaces distal to the terminal bronchioles, with loss of alveolar walls and elastic recoil of the lungs (emphysema)
  c. There may be an overlap of these conditions.
2. As a result of these conditions, there is a subsequent derangement of airway dynamics (e.g., obstruction to airflow).

Causes of COPD *(Emphysema–Bronchitis Complex)*

1. Cigarette smoking
2. Air pollution
3. Occupational exposure
4. Allergy
5. Autoimmunity
6. Infection
7. Genetic predisposition
8. Aging

Chronic Bronchitis

Chronic bronchitis is a chronic infection of the lower respiratory tract characterized by excessive mucus secretion, cough, and dyspnea associated with recurring infections of the lower respiratory tract.

Altered Physiology

Infection, irritation, hypersensitivity → local hyperemia → hypertrophy of mucous glands → increase in size and number of mucus-producing elements in bronchi (mucous glands and goblet cells) → inflammation and edema → narrowing and obstruction of airflow.

Clinical Features

1. A wide range of viral, bacterial, and mycoplasmal infections can produce acute exacerbations of bronchitis.
2. The course and prognosis are related to the degree of airflow obstruction, the age the abnormality was diagnosed, and the rate of change in ventilatory function.

Health Maintenance and Prevention

1. Smoking must be stopped, as this is the most frequent cause of chronic bronchitis.
2. Avoid all respiratory irritants.
3. Acute respiratory infections should be treated.

Clinical Manifestations

Usually insidious, developing over a period of years.
1. Presence of a productive cough lasting at least 3 months a year for 2 successive years
2. Production of thick, gelatinous sputum; greater amounts produced during superimposed infections
3. Wheezing and dyspnea as disease progresses

Diagnostic Evaluation

Pulmonary function and arterial blood gas studies

Management

  Goal:
  Reverse airflow obstruction
1. Bronchodilators; metered-dose inhalation of beta-adrenergic agonist (See Emphysema) or atropine-like agent, ipratropium bromide
2. Pulmonary rehabilitation to reduce symptoms that limit activity

For Nursing Process, nursing diagnoses, interventions, and health education, See Pulmonary Emphysema, page 184.

Pulmonary Emphysema

Pulmonary emphysema is a complex lung disease characterized by destruction of the alveoli, enlargement of distal airspaces, and a breakdown of alveolar walls. There is a slowly progressive deterioration of lung function for many years before the development of illness.

Causes

(See Causes of Chronic Obstructive Pulmonary Disease, opposite column.)

Clinical Manifestations

1. *Dyspnea;* slow in onset and steadily progressive
2. Cough—may be minimal, except with respiratory infection
3. Sputum expectoration

Diagnostic Evaluation

1. History of smoking, exertional dyspnea, cough, wheezing, expectoration, exposure to dust, fumes, and gases
2. Pulmonary (ventilatory) function tests to demonstrate airflow obstruction
3. Arterial blood gas analysis to detect hypoxemia
4. Alpha$_1$-antitrypsin assay useful in identifying genetically determined deficiency

Management

1. Smoking cessation
2. Bronchodilators, of which there are two main categories:
   a. Sympathomimetics: (metaproterenol; terbutaline; albuterol; bitolterol)—given to protect against bronchospasm
      (1) Aerosol formulations provide optimum therapy, because drug is applied directly to receptors in airways.
      (2) Bronchodilating aerosols delivered by metered-dose inhalers or hand-held or pump-driven devices
   b. Methylxanthines (theophylline) given orally as sustained-release formulation for chronic maintenance therapy
3. Antimicrobial agents for episodes of respiratory infection
4. Steroids—used in acute exacerbations for anti-inflammatory effect
5. Chest physical therapy, including postural drainage, breathing retraining
6. Low-flow oxygen therapy for patient with severe hypoxemia.

Nursing Assessment

1. Determine smoking history, positive family history of respiratory disease, onset of dyspnea.
2. Note amount, color, and consistency of sputum.
3. Inspect for use of accessory muscles of respiration and use of abdominal muscles during expiration; note increase of anteroposterior diameter of chest; distention of neck veins.
4. Auscultate for decreased/absent breath sounds, crackles, decreased heart sounds.
5. Review results of diagnostic tests.

Nursing Diagnoses

1. Ineffective airway clearance related to bronchoconstriction, increased mucus production, ineffective cough, possible bronchopulmonary infection
2. Ineffective breathing pattern related to chronic airflow limitation
3. Potential for respiratory infection related to compromised pulmonary function
4. Impaired gas exchanged related to chronic pulmonary obstruction; ventilation/perfusion abnormalities
5. Altered nutrition (less than body requirements) related to increased work of breathing, air swallowing, med-

ication effects, impaired gastrointestinal functioning (bloating; reflux), and depression
6. Activity intolerance related to compromised pulmonary function, resulting in shortness of breath and fatigue
7. Sleep pattern disturbance related to hypoxemia and hypercapnia
8. Impaired individual coping related to the stress of living with chronic disease
9. Knowledge deficit of how to live with chronic obstructive pulmonary disease

Complications

1. Respiratory failure
   a. Monitor for acute exacerbations of cough, change in sputum color/volume, breathlessness at rest, central cyanosis, increasing respiratory rate, drowsiness, and confusion.
   b. Obtain immediate blood gas analysis
2. Pneumonia; overwhelming respiratory infection
3. Right heart failure; dysrhythmias

Nursing Interventions

A. Improving Airway Clearance

1. Eliminate all pulmonary irritants, particularly cigarette smoking.
   a. Cessation of smoking usually results in less pulmonary irritation, sputum production, and cough.
   b. Keep patient's room as dust-free as possible.
   c. Add moisture (humidifier, vaporizer) to indoor environment.
2. Control bronchospasm to decrease the work of breathing—many patients with chronic obstructive pulmonary disease have some degree of bronchospasm.
   a. Administer prescribed bronchodilators.
   b. Assess patient for side effects—tremulousness, tachycardia, cardiac dysrhythmias, central nervous system stimulation, hypertension.
   c. Auscultate the chest after administration of aerosol bronchodilators to assess for improvement of air entry and reduction of adventitious breath sounds.
   d. Observe if patient has reduction in dyspnea.
3. Use postural drainage positions to aid in clearance of secretions, as mucopurulent secretions are responsible for airway obstruction.
   Employ percussion of thorax (p. 171) to assist in propulsion of sputum through the bronchi, when necessary.
4. Use controlled coughing.
   a. Inhale slowly and deeply.
   b. Exhale through pursed lips—empties lungs of residual volume.
   c. Cough in short bursts of "huffing" rather than vigorously forcing cough, which causes airways to collapse.
   d. Inhale slowly.
5. Keep secretions liquid.
   a. Encourage high level of fluid intake (8–10 glasses; 2–2½ liters daily) within level of cardiac reserve.
   b. Give inhalations of nebulized water to humidify bronchial tree and liquefy sputum.
   c. Avoid dairy products if these increase sputum production.

B. Improving Respiratory Pattern

1. Teach and supervise breathing retraining exercises to strengthen diaphragm and muscles of expiration to decrease work of breathing.
   a. Teach lower costal, diaphragmatic, and abdominal

breathing, using a slow and relaxed breathing pattern to reduce respiratory rate and decrease energy cost of breathing.
   b. Use pursed lips breathing at intervals and during periods of dyspnea to control rate and depth of respiration and improve respiratory muscle coordination.
2. Discuss and demonstrate relaxation exercises to reduce stress, tension, and anxiety.
3. Encourage patient to assume position of comfort to decrease dyspnea.

C. Controlling Infection

1. Recognize early manifestations of respiratory infection—increased dyspnea, fatigue; change in color, amount, and character of sputum; nervousness; irritability; low-grade fever.
2. Obtain sputum for smear and culture.
3. Give prescribed antimicrobials to control secondary bacterial infections in the bronchial tree, thus clearing the airways.

D. Improving Gas Exchange

1. Watch for excessive somnolence, restlessness, aggressiveness, anxiety, or confusion, which frequently is caused by acute respiratory insufficiency.
2. Review arterial blood gas analysis; record values on a flow sheet so that comparisons can be made over time.
3. Give low-flow oxygen to selected patients with severe, chronic, obstructive pulmonary disease—to correct hypoxemia in a controlled manner and thereby minimize CO_2 retention.
   a. In patients with COPD, poor exchange of gases may result in chronically elevated CO_2 (which is then a less effective stimulus to respiration). Giving a high concentration of oxygen may remove the hypoxic drive—leading to increased hypoventilation, respiratory decompensation, and the development of a worsening respiratory acidosis.
   b. Low-flow oxygen dosage is individualized and is given after analysis of arterial blood gases.

NURSING ALERT: Patients with acute respiratory failure along with acute ventilatory failure and rapid CO_2 retention will require mechanical ventilation.

E. Improving Nutrition

1. Take nutritional history and anthropometric measurements.
2. Encourage frequent small meals if patient is dyspneic; even a small increase in abdominal contents may press on diaphragm and impede breathing.
3. Offer nutritional supplements to improve caloric intake and counteract weight loss.
4. Avoid foods producing abdominal discomfort.
5. Employ good oral hygiene before meals to sharpen taste sensations.
6. Encourage pursed-lips breathing between bites if patient is very short of breath; rest after meals.
7. Give supplemental oxygen while patient is eating to relieve dyspnea, as directed.
8. Monitor body weight.

F. Increasing Activity Tolerance

1. Reemphasize the importance of graded exercise and physical conditioning programs (enhances delivery of oxygen to tissues; allows a higher level of functioning with greater comfort).
   a. Discuss walking, stationary bicycling, swimming.
   b. Portable oxygen system may be used for ambulation for patients with hypoxemia with marked disability.
2. Encourage patient to carry out *regular* exercise program to increase physical endurance.
3. Train patient in energy-saving methods.

G. Improving Sleep Patterns

1. Maintain a balanced schedule of activity and sleep.
2. Use nocturnal oxygen therapy when appropriate.

H. Psychosocial Support to Help Individual Coping

1. Understand that the constant shortness of breath and fatigue makes the patient irritable, apprehensive, anxious, and depressed, with feelings of helplessness/hopelessness.
2. Assess the patient for reactive behaviors (anger, depression, acceptance).
3. Demonstrate a positive and interested approach to the patient.
   a. Be a good listener and show that you care.
   b. Be sensitive to his fears, anxiety, and depression; helps give emotional relief and insight.
4. Strengthen the patient's self-image.
5. Allow the patient to express his feelings and retain (within a controlled degree) the mechanisms of denial and repression.
6. Be aware that sexual dysfunction is common in patients with COPD.
7. Support spouse/family members.

Patient Education

A. General Education

1. Give the patient a clear explanation of his disease, what to expect, how to treat and live with it.
   Reinforce by frequent explanations, reading material, demonstrations, and question and answer sessions.
2. Review with the patient the objectives of treatment and nursing management
3. Work with the patient to set goals (i.e., stair climbing, return to work, etc.).

B. Avoid Exposure to Respiratory Irritants—cigarette smoke, pollens, fumes, aerosols, dust, cold.

1. Stop smoking and avoid smoke-filled rooms.
2. Avoid sweeping, dusting, and exposure to paint, aerosols, bleaches, and other respiratory irritants.
3. Keep kitchen ventilated.
4. Stay out of extremely hot/cold weather to avoid aggravating bronchial obstruction and sputum production.
   a. Keep a warming mask or scarf over nose and mouth to warm inspired air in cold weather.
   b. Stay indoors with air conditioning when pollution level is high.
   c. Try to avoid abrupt environmental changes.
   d. Shower in warm (not too hot or too cold) water.
5. Humidify indoor air in winter; maintain 30%–50% humidity for optimal mucociliary function.
6. Consider the use of an air cleanser to remove dust, pollen, and other particulates.

C. Prevent and Treat Respiratory Infections.

1. Avoid exposure to persons with respiratory infections; a respiratory infection makes symptoms worse and can produce further irreversible damage.
2. Avoid crowds and areas with poor ventilation.

3. Obtain influenza and pneumococcal vaccines to decrease likelihood of developing these infections.
4. Recognize and report evidence of respiratory infection *promptly* to the physician/clinic—chest pain, changes in character of sputum (amount, color, or consistency), increasing difficulty in raising sputum, increasing cough/wheezing, increasing shortness of breath.
5. Take prescribed antimicrobial at first sign of infection.
    a. Have a home supply available.
    b. Have periodic sputum cultures when receiving long-term antimicrobial therapy.

D. Reduce Bronchial Secretions

1. Maintain an adequate fluid intake (8–10 glasses daily); mark down the amount of liquid consumed daily.
2. Take bronchodilators only as directed.
3. Follow postural drainage exercises as prescribed.
    a. Stay in each position 5–15 minutes.
    b. Use controlled cough after each position.

E. Improve Airflow

1. Use metered-dose inhaler properly to maximize aerosol deposition in the bronchial tree.
2. Breathe out normally; open mouth and let mouthpiece touch lip or place inhaler 2–4 inches in front of mouth.
3. Inhale slowly and activate cartridge to release spray.
4. Pause, holding breath for about 10 seconds; exhale slowly.

F. Try to Cough Productively With *Controlled Coughing*

1. Breathe slowly and deeply, using diaphragmatic breathing.
2. Hold breath several seconds.
3. Cough—2 short, forceful coughs with the mouth open; the first cough loosens mucus, and the second cough moves it.
4. Pause and inhale by sniffing quietly. (Inhaling vigorously may initiate unproductive coughing, which is energy consuming.)
5. Rest.

G. Do Breathing Exercises—to strengthen muscles of expiration, to strengthen and coordinate muscles of breathing, and to lessen fatigue and to help empty lungs more completely.

1. Learn the importance of slow and relaxed breathing (controlled breathing).
2. Practice diaphragmatic breathing and pursed-lips breathing.
3. Consciously use pursed-lips breathing during episodes of dyspnea and stress.
4. Maintain muscle tone of the body by regular exercise.

H. Maintain General Health at Highest Attainable Level

1. Follow good habits of nutrition—patients with COPD may have loss of muscle mass with poor nutritional status, poor appetite, potassium depletion, sodium retention, and dehydration.
2. Follow high-protein diet with adequate mineral, vitamin, and fluid intake.
3. Avoid excessive hot or cold fluids/foods that may provoke an irritating cough.
4. Avoid hard-to-chew foods (causes tiring) and gas-forming foods, which cause distention and restrict diaphragmatic movement.
5. Eat 5–6 small meals daily—to ease shortness of breath during and after meals.
6. Have rest periods before and after meals if eating produces shortness of breath.

7. Do not eat when upset/angry.
8. Avoid potassium depletion—patients with COPD tend to have low potassium levels; also patient may be taking diuretics.
    a. Watch for weakness, numbness, tingling of fingers, leg cramps.
    b. Foods high in potassium include bananas, dried fruits, dates, figs, orange juice, grape juice, milk, peaches, potatoes.
9. Restrict sodium as directed.
10. Use community resources (Meals on Wheels) if energy level is low.

I. Avoid Activities That Produce Excessive Shortness of Breath

1. Live within the limitations that emphysema imposes.
2. Learn to relax and work at a slower pace.
3. Enroll in a pulmonary rehabilitation program where available.
4. Obtain vocational counseling to secure a sedentary job if presently in a demanding manual job.
5. Avoid overfatigue, which is a factor in producing respiratory distress.
6. Adjust activities according to individual fatigue patterns.
7. Use pursed-lips breathing in a slow and relaxed manner during periods of breathlessness and physical exertion.
8. Try to cope with emotional stress as positively as possible—such stress triggers attacks of dyspnea.
9. Study individual life-style and avoid energy-wasting activities.
10. Exercise to improve physical condition.

J. Understand the Importance of Preserving Existing Function.

1. Become familiar with the nature of emphysema and reasons for a therapeutic program.
2. Accept the fact that therapy and health supervision must be continued for a lifetime.

Evaluation

1. Improves airway clearance; reduction in respiratory secretions
2. Breathing more effectively; performs breathing exercises at scheduled intervals
3. Avoids and seeks treatment for respiratory infection
4. Demonstrates improved gas exchange; arterial blood gas determinations improving; using low-flow oxygen
5. Improves nutritional status; times meals to coincide with periods of improved breathing
6. Increases activity level; walks longer distances without tiring
7. Reports better sleep; using low-flow oxygen at night
8. Demonstrates more effective coping; expresses feelings; seeking support group
9. Knows his drug regimen; demonstrates competence in use of metered-dose inhaler; recalls how to prevent infection

Pulmonary Heart Disease (Cor Pulmonale)

Pulmonary heart disease (*cor pulmonale*) is an alteration in the structure or function of the right ventricle resulting from disease affecting lung structure or function or its vasculature (except when this alteration results from disease of the left side of the heart or from congenital heart disease). Cor pulmonale refers to heart disease caused by lung disease.

Etiology

1. Pulmonary vascular disease; pulmonary embolism
2. Chronic obstructive pulmonary disease; chronic bronchitis; emphysema, most common

Pathophysiology

Chronic obstructive pulmonary disease → hypoxia → hypercapnia → acidosis → circulatory complications → pulmonary hypertension → right heart enlargement → right heart failure.

Clinical Manifestations

1. Increasing dyspnea and fatigue; progressive dyspnea (orthopnea, paroxysmal nocturnal dyspnea), chronic cough
2. Right heart enlargement
3. Peripheral edema
4. Manifestations of carbon dioxide narcosis—headache, confusion, somnolence, coma

Diagnostic Evaluation

1. Arterial blood gas analysis
2. Pulmonary function tests
3. Electrocardiogram

Management

1. Treatment of underlying lung disease
2. Long-term, low-flow oxygen to improve oxygen delivery to peripheral tissues, thus decreasing cardiac work and lessening sympathetic vasoconstriction.
    Liter flow individualized during activities, rest, and sleep
3. Diuretics to lower pulmonary artery pressure by reducing total blood volume and excess fluid in lungs
4. Pulmonary vasodilators (nitroprusside; hydralazine; calcium channel blockers) to dilate pulmonary vascular bed and reduce pulmonary vascular resistance; use is controversial

Nursing Interventions

A. Improving Ventilation and Correcting Hypoxemia

1. Monitor arterial blood gas values as a guide in assessing adequacy of ventilation.
2. Use continuous low-flow oxygen as directed to reduce pulmonary artery pressure.
3. Avoid central nervous system depressants (narcotics; hypnotics)—have depressant action on respiratory centers and mask symptoms of hypercapnia.
4. Combat respiratory infection, as infection causes carbon dioxide retention and hypoxemia.

B. Monitoring Patient and Response to Therapy

1. Watch alterations in electrolyte levels, especially potassium, which can lead to disturbances of cardiac rhythm.
2. Employ ECG monitoring when necessary, as there is a high incidence of dysrhythmias in these patients.
3. Limit physical activity until improvement is seen.
4. Restrict sodium intake if there is evidence of fluid retention.

Patient Education

1. Emphasize the importance of stopping cigarette smoking; cigarette smoking is a major cause of pulmonary heart disease.
    a. Query the patient about his smoking habits.
    b. Inform the patient of risks of smoking and benefits to be gained when smoking is stopped.
2. Teach the patient to recognize and treat infections immediately.
3. Inform the patient of interrelationship between infection, air pollution, and cardiopulmonary disease.
4. Explain to the patient/family that restlessness, depression, and poor sleeping, as well as irritable and angry behavior, may be characteristic; patient should improve with rise in O_2 and fall in CO_2 levels in arterial blood gas values.
5. Explain that if the patient has chronic lung disease it may be necessary to have continuous low-flow oxygen therapy at home.

Pulmonary Embolism

Pulmonary embolism refers to the obstruction of one or more pulmonary arteries by a thrombus (or thrombi) originating usually in the deep veins of the legs or in the right side of the heart, which becomes dislodged and is carried to the lungs.

Pulmonary infarction—necrosis of lung tissue that can result from interference with blood supply

Predisposing Factors

1. Stasis; prolonged immobilization
2. Concurrent clinical phlebitis
3. Previous heart (congestive failure; myocardial infarction) or lung disease
4. Injury to vessel wall
5. Coagulation disorders
6. Metabolic, endocrine, vascular, or collagen disorders
7. Malignancy
8. Advancing age; estrogen therapy

Health Maintenance and Prevention

1. Assess each patient with a high index of suspicion for pulmonary embolism.
2. Be aware of high-risk patients—immobilization, trauma to pelvis (especially surgical) and lower extremities (especially hip fracture), obesity, history of thromboembolic disease, varicose veins, pregnancy, congestive heart failure, myocardial infarction, malignant disease, postoperative patients, elderly.
3. Prevent stasis of blood in extremities due to dependent position of legs, prolonged sitting, immobility, constricting clothing.
    a. Encourage early mobilization and weight-bearing.
    b. Elevate legs 15–20 degrees at intervals—to minimize stasis and increase venous return.
    c. Apply fitted elastic stockings—to promote venous return and to maintain peripheral blood flow.
    d. Instruct the patient to wiggle toes, move feet, raise and lower legs frequently—to increase venous return.
    e. Do not allow the patient's legs and feet to dangle in a dependent position; have the patient place his feet on a chair when sitting on the edge of the bed (if bed is in a high position). Instruct the patient to avoid crossing the legs.
4. Encourage higher levels of fluid intake during periods of immobility; avoid hemoconcentration
5. Avoid leaving catheters in veins for prolonged periods.
6. Examine the patient's legs daily for evidence of venous thrombosis.

Clinical Manifestations

1. *Dyspnea*, pleuritic pain, tachypnea, apprehension
   Chest pain with apprehension and a sense of impending doom occurs when most of the pulmonary artery is obstructed.
2. Cyanosis, tachyarrhythmias, syncope, circulatory collapse encountered in patients with massive pulmonary embolism
3. Subtle deterioration in patient's condition with no explainable cause
4. Pleural friction rub
5. Presence of venous thrombosis in lower extremity

NURSING ALERT: Have a high index of suspicion if there is a subtle deterioration in the patient's condition and unexplained cardiovascular and pulmonary findings.

Diagnostic Evaluation

1. Physical findings: clinical signs and symptoms are elusive.
2. Arterial blood gases—systemic arterial hypoxemia is usually found, due to perfusion abnormality of the lung.
3. Radioisotope lung scans—perfusion scan investigates regional blood flow to determine presence of perfusion defects; ventilation scan may be done in patient with large perfusion defects.
4. Pulmonary angiogram (most definitive)—emboli seen as "filling defects."
5. Contrast phlebography or impedance phlebography—for detecting deep vein thrombosis of the legs.

Emergency Management (for massive pulmonary embolism)

NURSING ALERT: Massive pulmonary embolism is a medical emergency; the patient's condition tends to deteriorate rapidly. There is a profound decrease in cardiac output, with an accompanying increase in right ventricular pressure.

Goal:
To stabilize the cardiorespiratory system

1. Oxygen is administered to relieve hypoxemia, respiratory distress, and cyanosis.
2. An infusion is started to open an intravenous route for drugs/fluids.
3. Vasopressors, inotropic agents (dopamine) and/or antidysrhythmic agents may be indicated to support circulation if the patient is unstable.
4. The electrocardiogram is monitored continuously for right ventricular failure, which may have a rapid onset.
5. Small doses of intravenous morphine are given to relieve anxiety, to alleviate chest discomfort (which improves ventilation), and to ease adaptation to mechanical ventilator, if this is necessary.
6. Pulmonary angiography, hemodynamic measurements, arterial blood gas determinations, etc., are carried out.

Subsequent Management

A. Anticoagulation (for clinically stable patient)

1. Heparin (IV)—stops further thrombus formation and extends the clotting time of the blood; it is an anticoagulant and antithrombotic
   a. IV loading dose usually followed by continuous pump or drip infusion or given intermittently every 4–6 hours.
   b. Dosage adjusted to maintain the activated partial thromboplastin time at 1.5 to 2 times the pretreatment value (if the value was normal).
   c. Protamine sulfate may be given to neutralize heparin in event of severe bleeding.
2. Oral anticoagulation (warfarin) is usually used for follow-up anticoagulant therapy after heparin therapy has been established; interrupts the coagulation mechanism by interfering with the vitamin K–dependent synthesis of prothrombin and factors VII, IX, and X

Note: Dosage is controlled by monitoring serial tests of prothrombin time; desired prothrombin time is 1.2 to 1.5 times control value.

B. Thrombolytic Enzymes

1. Thrombolytic agents (urokinase; streptokinase) may be used in patients with massive pulmonary embolism; effective in lysing recently formed thrombi; improve circulatory and hemodynamic status.
   Administered intravenously in a loading dose followed by constant infusion
2. Newer clot-specific thrombolytics (tissue type plasminogen activator (t-PA), acylated plasminogen, streptokinase activator complex, single-chain urokinase)—activate plasminogen only within thrombus itself rather than systematically; minimize occurrence of generalized fibrinolysis and subsequent bleeding.

Surgical Intervention

Surgical intervention done when anticoagulation is contraindicated or patient has recurrent embolization or develops serious complications from drug therapy.

1. Interruption of vena cava—reduces channel size to prevent lower extremity emboli from reaching lungs. Accomplished by:
   a. Ligation, plication, or clipping of the inferior vena cava
   b. Placement of transvenously inserted intraluminal filter in inferior vena cava to prevent migration of emboli (Fig. 10-7).
2. Embolectomy (removal of pulmonary embolic obstruction)

Nursing Assessment

1. Take nursing history with emphasis on onset and severity of dyspnea and nature of chest pain.
2. Examine the patient's legs carefully. Assess for swelling of leg, duskiness, pain on pressure over gastrocnemius muscle, pain on dorsiflexion of the foot (positive Homan's sign).
3. Evaluate for dyspnea, pleuritic pain, tachypnea, and apprehension.
4. Monitor respiratory rate—may be accelerated out of proportion to degree of fever and tachycardia.
   a. Inspect rate of inspiration to expiration.
   b. Percuss for resonance, dullness, and flatness.
   c. Auscultate for abnormal breath sounds, friction rub, crackles, rhonchi, and wheezing.
5. Auscultate heart; listen for splitting of second heart sound.
6. Review results of physical examination, diagnostic studies, and laboratory tests.

Nursing Diagnoses

1. Ineffective breathing pattern (dyspnea) related to acute increase in alveolar dead space and possible changes in lung mechanics from embolism.

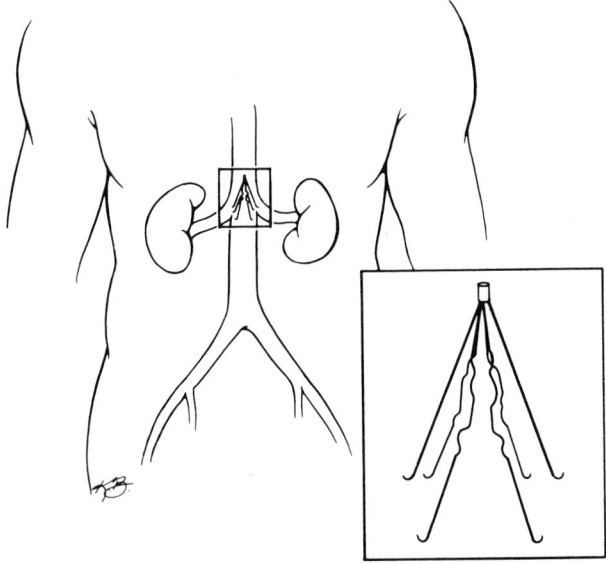

Figure 10-7. *Mechanical protection against pulmonary embolism. The vena cava filter is inserted transvenously with a special introducer system via the femoral or jugular vein. It traps emboli while preserving blood flow.*

2. Altered tissue perfusion related to decreased blood circulation
3. Pain (pleuritic) related to congestion, possible pleural effusion, possible lung infarction
4. Anxiety related to dyspnea, pain, and seriousness of condition
5. Knowledge deficit of condition and long-term treatment

Interventions for Complications

A. Shock—from low cardiac output secondary to resistance to right ventricular outflow or to myocardial dysfunction due to ischemia

1. Assess for skin color changes, particularly nail beds, lips, ear lobes, and mucous membranes.
2. Monitor blood pressure.
3. Measure urinary output.
4. Monitor IV infusion of isoproterenol or other prescribed agents.

B. Bleeding—related to anticoagulant or thrombolytic therapy

1. Assess patient for bleeding; major bleeding may occur from GI tract, brain, lungs, nose, and GU tract.
2. Perform stool guaiac test—to detect occult blood loss.
3. Monitor platelet count—to detect heparin-induced thrombocytopenia
4. Minimize risk of bleeding.
   a. Perform essential arterial blood gas studies on upper extremities; apply digital compression at puncture site for 30 minutes.
   b. Apply pressure dressing to previously involved sites; check site for oozing.
   c. Maintain patient on strict bed rest during thrombolytic therapy.
   d. Discontinue infusion in the event of uncontrolled bleeding.
   e. Avoid unnecessary handling; possibility of bruising is great.

Nursing Interventions

A. Restoring Pulmonary Function and Correcting Hemodynamic Consequences

1. Assess for hypoxia, headache, restlessness, apprehension, pallor, cyanosis, behavioral changes.
2. Monitor vital signs, ECG, and arterial blood gas levels for adequacy of oxygenation.
3. Monitor patient's response to IV fluids/vasopressors.
4. Monitor oxygen therapy—used to relieve hypoxemia.
5. Prepare patient for assisted ventilation when hypoxemia is due to local areas of pneumoconstriction and abnormalities of ventilation/perfusion ratios.

B. Improving Tissue Perfusion

1. Continue to monitor vital signs.
2. Monitor prescribed medications given to preserve right ventricular filling pressure and increase blood pressure.
3. Maintain patient on bedrest to reduce oxygen demands and risk of rebleeding.
4. Monitor urinary output hourly, as there may be reduced renal perfusion and decreased glomerular filtration.

C. Relieving Pain

1. Watch patient for signs of discomfort and pain.
2. Ascertain if pleuritic pain worsens with deep breathing and coughing; listen for friction rub.
3. Give prescribed morphine and monitor for pain relief and signs of respiratory depression.

D. Reducing Anxiety

1. Correct dyspnea and relieve physical discomfort.
2. Explain diagnostic procedures and the patient's role; correct any misconceptions.
3. Listen to the patient's concerns—attentive listening relieves anxiety and reduces emotional distress.
4. Speak calmly and slowly.
5. Do everything possible to enhance the patient's sense of control.

Health Education

1. See Preventive Measures, page 187.
2. Be aware of the possible need to continue taking anticoagulant therapy for 6 weeks up to an indefinite period.
3. Watch for signs of bleeding, especially of gums, nose, bruising, blood in urine and stools.
4. Avoid taking medications unless approved by physician, as many drugs interact with anticoagulants.
5. Notify dentist that you are taking an anticoagulant.
6. Avoid inactivity for prolonged periods or sitting with legs crossed.
7. Avoid sports/activities that may cause injury.
8. Avoid local injury to legs.
9. Wear a Medic-Alert bracelet identifying patient as anticoagulant user.
10. Lose weight if applicable; obesity is a risk factor for women.
11. Discuss contraceptive methods with patient if applicable; female patients are advised against taking oral contraceptives.

Evaluation

1. Achieves normal breathing pattern
2. Improved tissue perfusion evidenced by adequate urinary output
3. Patient reports freedom from pain
4. Appears more relaxed; sleeping at long intervals
5. Verbalizes reasons for taking anticoagulant/side effects

Occupational Lung Diseases

Diseases of the lungs can occur in a variety of occupations as a result of exposure to organic or inorganic (mineral) dusts and noxious gases.

Altered Physiology

1. Effects of inhaling noxious particles, gases, or fumes depends on composition of inhaled substance, its antigenic (precipitating an immune response) or irritating properties, the dose inhaled, the length of time inhaled, and the host's response.
2. Exposure to inorganic dusts stimulates pulmonary interstitial fibroblasts, resulting in pulmonary interstitial fibrosis.
3. Noxious fumes may cause acute injury to alveolar wall with increasing capillary permeability and pulmonary edema.
4. Occupational lung diseases usually develop slowly (20–30 years) and are asymptomatic in the early stages.
5. The most common occupational lung diseases are silicosis, asbestosis, and coal worker's pneumoconiosis.

Prevention and Health Maintenance

Goal:
Reduce exposure of workers to industrial products that may be hazardous to breathing.

1. Encourage smoking cessation.
2. Preserve, in every way possible, the general health of the worker/miner exposed to occupational dusts.
3. Enclose toxic substances, and reduce their concentration in the air.
   a. Engineering controls to reduce exposure
   b. Monitoring of air samples
4. Ventilate properly to reduce dust content of work atmosphere.
5. Have workers use protective devices (face masks, respirators, hoods, etc.).
6. Monitor workers who are exposed to high concentrations of industrial dusts.

Silicosis

Silicosis is a chronic pulmonary fibrosis caused by inhalation of silica dust.

A. Etiology and Altered Physiology

1. Exposure to silica dust is encountered in almost any form of mining because the earth's crust is composed of silica and silicates (gold, coal, tin, copper mining); also stone cutting, quarrying, manufacture of abrasives, ceramics, pottery, and foundry work.
2. When silica particles (which have fibrogenic properties) are inhaled, nodular lesions are produced throughout the lungs. These nodules undergo fibrosis, enlarge, and fuse.
3. Dense masses form in the upper portion of the lungs; restrictive and obstructive lung disease results.

B. Clinical Manifestations

1. Chronic productive cough
2. Dyspnea on effort
3. Susceptibility to lower respiratory tract infections

C. Management

1. There is no specific treatment; the patient is treated symptomatically.
2. Give prophylactic isoniazid to patient with positive tuberculin test, as silicosis is associated with tuberculosis.
3. *Prevention:* See Prevention and Health Maintenance.

Asbestosis

Asbestosis is a diffuse interstitial fibrosis of the lung caused by inhalation of asbestos dust and particles.

A. Etiology and Altered Physiology

1. Found in workers involved in manufacture, cutting, and demolition of asbestos-containing materials; there are over 4000 known uses of asbestos fiber (asbestos mining and manufacturing, construction, roofing, demolition work, brake linings, floor tiles, paints, plastics, shipyards, insulation).
2. Asbestos fibers are inhaled and enter alveoli, which in time are obliterated by fibrous tissue that surrounds the asbestos particles.
3. Fibrous pleural thickening and pleural plaque formation produce restrictive lung disease, decrease in lung volume, diminished gas transfer, and hypoxemia with subsequent development of cor pulmonale.

NURSING ALERT: Asbestosis is strongly associated with bronchogenic cancer, also with mesotheliomas of the pleura and peritoneal surfaces.

B. Clinical Manifestations (may develop 20–40 years after exposure)

1. Dyspnea on exertion; severe, progressive; irreversible
2. Severe nonproductive cough
3. Crackles heard at lung bases
4. Manifestations of respiratory failure and cardiac complications

C. Management

1. No treatment will affect the progressive fibrosis. Most of the asbestos fibers already in the lungs will remain there.
2. Persuade persons who have been exposed to asbestos fibers to stop smoking. The risk of developing lung cancer for an asbestos worker who smokes is greatly increased.
3. Keep worker under cancer surveillance; watch for changing cough, hemoptysis, weight loss, melena, etc.
4. *Prevention:* See Prevention and Health Maintenance, above.

Coal Worker's Pneumoconiosis

Coal worker's pneumoconiosis (CWP; "black lung") is a variety of respiratory disease found in coal workers in which there is an accumulation of coal dust in the lungs, causing a tissue reaction in its presence.

A. Altered Physiology

1. Dusts (coal, kaolin, mica, silica) are inhaled and deposited in the alveoli and respiratory bronchioles.
2. There is an increase of macrophages that engulf the particles and transport them to terminal bronchioles.
3. When normal clearance mechanisms no longer can handle the excessive dust load, the respiratory bronchioles and alveoli become clogged with coal dust, dying macrophages, and fibroblasts, which lead to the formation of the coal macule, the primary lesion of CWP.
4. As macules enlarge, there is dilation of the weakening bronchiole, with subsequent development of focal or centrilobular emphysema.

B. Clinical Manifestations

1. Progressive dyspnea
2. Cough and sputum production; expectoration of varying amounts of black fluid

C. Management

1. Effective management depends on *prevention*. See Prevention, page 190.
2. There is no specific treatment; the treatment is symptomatic. See also Management of Emphysema, page 184.

Cancer of the Lung
(Bronchogenic Cancer)

Bronchogenic cancer refers to a malignant tumor of the lung arising within the wall or epithelial lining of the bronchus. The lung is also a common site of metastasis from cancer elsewhere in the body via venous circulation or lymphatic spread.

Classification *(according to cell type)*

1. Epidermoid (squamous cell)—most common
2. Adenocarcinoma
3. Small cell (oat cell) carcinoma
4. Large cell (undifferentiated) carcinoma

Predisposing Factors

1. Cigarette smoking—amount, frequency, and duration of smoking have positive relationship to cancer of the lung.
2. Occupational exposure to asbestos, arsenic, chromium, nickel, iron, radioactive substances, isopropyl oil, coal tar products, petroleum oil mists alone or in combination with tobacco smoke

Health Maintenance and Prevention

1. Encourage patients to abstain from cigarette smoking.
   a. Teach by example.
   b. Refer patients to smoking cessation programs within the community.
   c. Continue efforts to discourage young people from starting smoking.
2. Maintain close watch of patients who are smokers—disease is insidious and exists before producing symptoms.

NURSING ALERT: Suspect cancer of the lung in patients who belong to a susceptible age-group and who have repeated unresolved respiratory infections.

Clinical Manifestations

Usually occur late and are related to size and location of tumor, extent of spread, and involvement of other structures.

1. Cough—especially a new type or changing cough—results from bronchial irritation.
2. Dyspnea; wheezing (suggests partial bronchial obstruction)
3. Chest pain (poorly localized and aching)
4. Excessive sputum production; repeated upper respiratory infections
5. Hemoptysis
6. Malaise, fever, weight loss, fatigue, anorexia
7. Paraneoplastic syndrome—metabolic or neurologic disturbances related to the secretion of substances by the neoplasm
8. Symptoms of metastases: bone pain, abdominal discomfort, nausea and vomiting from liver involvement, pancytopenia from bone marrow involvement, headache from CNS metastasis
9. Usual sites of metastases—lymph nodes, bones, liver

Diagnostic Evaluation

1. Roentgenogram of chest—including fluoroscopy and tomography; lung cancers may be partly or completely hidden by other structures.
2. Cytologic examination of sputum/chest fluids for malignant cells.
3. Fiberoptic bronchoscopy—for observation of location and extent of tumor; for biopsy
4. Computed tomography; sensitive in detecting small nodules and metastatic lesions
5. Lymph node biopsy; mediastinoscopy—to establish lymphatic spread; to plan treatment
6. Pulmonary function tests combined with split-function perfusion scan to determine if patient will have adequate pulmonary reserve to withstand surgical procedure

Management

The treatment depends on the cell type, stage of disease, and the physiologic status of the patient. It includes a multidisciplinary approach that may be used separately or in combination

1. Surgical resection
2. Radiotherapy
3. Chemotherapy
4. Immunotherapy

Nursing Assessment

1. Determine onset and duration of coughing, sputum production, and the degree of dyspnea. Ausultate for breath sounds. Observe symmetry of chest during respirations.
2. Take anthropometric measurements; weigh patient; review laboratory biochemical tests; conduct appraisal of 24-hour food intake.
3. Ask about pain; location, intensity, factors influencing pain.
4. Observe for weakness, fatigue, and dyspnea during activities of daily living.

Nursing Diagnoses

1. Ineffective breathing pattern related to obstructive and restrictive respiratory processes associated with lung cancer.
2. Altered nutrition (less than body requirements) related to hypermetabolic state, taste aversion, anorexia secondary to radtotherapy/chemotherapy
3. Pain related to tumor effects, invasion of adjacent structures, toxicities associated with radiotherapy/chemotherapy
4. Anxiety related to uncertain outcome and fear of recurrence.
5. Knowledge deficit of treatment protocol

Complications

1. Superior vena cava syndrome—oncologic complication caused by obstruction of major blood vessels draining the head, neck, and upper torso
   a. Look for facial and upper extremity edema, dyspnea/orthopnea, and cough.
   b. Observe for red florrid complexion, dilation of veins in neck, trunk, and upper extremities.
   c. Monitor for potential airway obstruction; other symptoms may include hoarseness, stridor, nausea, headaches, syncope.

2. Hypercalcemia (commonly from bone metastases)
   a. Observe for polyuria, nocturia, gastrointestinal symptoms, mental obtundation, profound weakness.
3. Syndrome of inappropriate antidiuretic hormone secretion with hyponatremia and abnormal water retention
4. Pleural effusion
5. Infectious complications, especially upper respiratory infections
6. Brain metastasis; spinal cord compression

Nursing Interventions

A. Relieving Respiratory Symptoms

1. Prepare patient physically, emotionally, and intellectually for prescribed therapeutic program.
2. Elevate head of bed to promote gravity drainage and prevent fluid collection in upper body (from superior vena cava syndrome).
3. Teach breathing retraining exercises to increase diaphragmatic excursion with resultant reduction in work of breathing.
4. Give prescribed treatment for productive cough (expectorant; antimicrobial agent) to prevent inspissated secretions and subsequent dyspnea.
5. Augment the patient's ability to cough effectively.
   a. Splint chest manually with hands.
   b. Instruct patient to inspire fully and cough 2–3 times in one breath.
   c. Provide humidifier/vaporizer to provide moisture to loosen secretions.
6. Support patient undergoing removal of pleural fluid (by thoracentesis or tube thoracostomy) and instillation of sclerosing agent (p. 181) to obliterate pleural space and prevent fluid recurrence.
7. Encourage energy conservation through decreasing activities.
8. Allow patient to sleep in a reclining chair if he is severely dyspneic.
9. Recognize the anxiety associated with dyspnea; teach relaxation techniques.

B. Improving Nutritional Status

1. Emphasize that nutrition is an important part of the treatment of lung cancer.
   a. Eat small amounts of high-calorie and high-protein foods frequently, rather than three daily meals.
   b. Eat major meal in the morning if rapidly becoming satiated and feeling full are problems.
   c. Be sure protein intake is adequate.
      (1) Substitute milk, eggs, chicken, fowl, fish, and oral nutritional supplements if aversion to meat is present.
      (2) Take prescribed vitamin supplement to avoid deficiency states, glossitis, and cheilosis
2. Change consistency of diet to soft or liquid if patient has esophagitis from radiation therapy.
3. Give enteral or total parenteral nutrition for malnourished patient who is unable or unwilling to eat.

C. Controlling Pain

1. Take a history of pain complaint; assess presence/absence of support system.
2. Administer prescribed drug, usually starting with nonsteroidal anti-inflammatory drugs and progressing to adjuvant analgesic and narcotic agents.
   a. Administer regularly to maintain pain at tolerable level.
   b. Titrate to achieve pain control.

3. Consider alternative methods: cognitive and behavioral training, biofeedback, relaxation—to increase patient's sense of control.
4. Discuss with physician problems of insomnia, depression, anxiety, etc. that may be contributing to patient's pain.
5. Initiate bowel training program, as constipation is a side effect of some analgesic/narcotic agents.
6. Facilitate referral to pain clinic/specialist if pain become refractory (unyielding) to usual methods of control.

D. Coping With Anxiety

See Patient Education (below) for emotional support of patient.

E. Other Nursing Interventions

1. Encourage sufficient hydration to thin secretions and to return calcium levels to normal if hypercalcemia is present.
2. Encourage patient to use muscles (range of motion and other exercises) to avoid complications of inactivity and disuse.
3. Use all known safeguards, including meticulous handwashing techniques, to reduce incidence of nosocomial infections, as the patient with lung cancer tends to be immunosuppressed.

Patient Education

A. Quality of Life

1. Focus on carrying on as normal a life as possible; an improved quality of life can be maintained.

B. Concerns About Pain

1. Realize that not every ache and pain is due to the results of lung cancer; some patients do not even experience pain.
2. Use nonsteroidal anti-inflammatory drugs or prescription medication as necessary. Do not be concerned about "addiction."
3. Radiation therapy may be used for pain control if tumor has spread to bone.
4. Report any new or persistent pain; it may be due to some other cause, such as arthritis.

C. Emotional Reactions

1. Shock, disbelief, denial, anger, and depression are all normal reactions to the diagnosis of lung cancer.
2. Try to have the patient express any concerns; share these concerns with health professionals.
3. Encourage the patient to communicate feelings to significant persons in his life.
4. Expect some feelings of anxiety and depression to recur during illness.
5. Encourage the patient to keep busy and remain in the mainstream. Continue with usual activities (work, recreation, sexual) as much as possible.
6. Secure services of a trained counselor if emotional stresses become overwhelming.
7. Talk to social worker about financial assistance, as money problems are a major concern to many.
8. Be aware that the American Cancer Society offers services and support modes to persons with cancer.

Evaluation

1. Copes with breathing difficulties; self-administers oxygen on occasion
2. Eats more frequently; monitors weight
3. States his pain is under control

4. Appears calmer; uses relaxation techniques
5. Verbalizes knowledge and acceptance of treatment protocol.

Chest Trauma

Chest trauma is an injury to the chest caused by any form of violence.
1. Chest injuries are potentially life-threatening because of (1) immediate disturbances of cardiorespiratory physiology and hemorrhage; and (2) later developments of infection, damaged lung, and thoracic cage.
2. Patients with chest trauma may have injuries to multiple organ systems.
3. The patient should be examined for intra-abdominal injuries, which must be treated aggressively.

Altered Physiology

1. In penetrating injuries, some air escapes into the pleural space. (Negative intrapleural pressure is replaced by atmospheric pressure.)
2. The loss of normal negative pressure within the pleural cavity causes collapse of the lung.

Clinical Manifestations

1. Dyspnea
2. Asymmetric chest movement
3. Pain with breathing
4. Cyanosis

Emergency Management

Goal:
Restore normal cardiorespiratory function as quickly as possible.
1. This is accomplished by performing effective resuscitation while simultaneously assessing the patient, restoring chest wall integrity, and reexpanding the lung. The order of priority is determined by the clinical status of the patient.
2. Complications of chest injuries: aspiration, atelectasis, pneumonia, mediastinal/subcutaneous emphysema, respiratory failure

Relief of Acute Respiratory Distress

A. Evaluate the Status of the Respiratory and Circulatory Systems

1. Examiner's ear is placed close to patient's mouth and nose, allowing him to listen at the airway, watch uncovered chest movements, and monitor pulse—this provides a rough estimate of the adequacy of ventilation.
2. Assess for signs of obstruction, sternal retraction, stridor, wheezing, and cyanosis.
3. Check neck for position of trachea, subcutaneous emphysema, and distended neck veins.

B. Establish and Maintain an Open Airway and Ventilation.

1. Aspirate secretions, vomitus, and blood from nose and throat via:
   a. Tracheal aspiration, if patient is unable to clear the tracheobronchial tree by coughing
   b. Use endotracheal tube if patient is bleeding from nasopharynx or if trachea is injured (short-term use).
   c. Employ bronchoscopic aspiration if necessary, if bronchial obstruction is suspected.
   d. Prepare for tracheostomy if necessary.
      (1) Tracheostomy helps to obtain clear, dry tracheobronchial tree, helps the patient breathe with less effort, decreases amount of dead air space in the respiratory tree, and helps reduce paradoxical motion.
      (2) The use of a cuffed tracheostomy tube permits a closed system for air exchange when connected to a ventilator.
2. Stabilize the chest wall.
3. Free the pleural cavity of blood and air.
4. Sucking chest wounds should be closed with an emergency dressing. The presence of lung injury and chest tube drainage also must be considered.

C. Control Hemorrhage

D. Treat for Shock. (Shock may be due to blood loss, impairment of cardiorespiratory function.)

1. Use one or more intravenous infusion lines; obtain blood for baseline studies.
2. Restore blood volume to adequate levels.
3. Give infusion rapidly.
4. Monitor serial central venous pressure readings to prevent hypovolemia and circulatory overload
5. Measure urinary output to monitor adequacy of circulation.

E. Apply Electrodes for ECG Monitoring—dysrhythmias are a frequent cause of death in chest trauma victims.

F. Ongoing Nursing Surveillance Includes:

1. Monitoring of arterial blood pressure, CVP, and respirations
2. Arterial blood gas measurements—to determine need for mechanical ventilation
3. Urinary output (hourly)—to evaluate tissue perfusion
4. Thoracic drainage—to provide information about rate of blood loss, whether or not bleeding has stopped, whether surgical intervention is necessary
5. ECG monitoring—for early detection and treatment of cardiac dysrhythmias

Types of Chest Injuries

Hemothorax

Blood in the pleural space as a result of penetrating or blunt chest trauma (accompanies a high percentage of chest injuries).

A. General Considerations

1. Blood in the pleural cavity produces a compression of the lungs and can result in hidden blood loss, causing signs and symptoms of shock.
2. Patient may be asymptomatic; or he may be dyspneic, apprehensive, or in shock.

B. Management

1. Blood and air are aspirated via needle thoracentesis
   or
2. An intercostal catheter (thoracotomy tube) is inserted and drainage instituted to accomplish more complete and continuous removal of blood and air—effects reexpansion of lung and permits monitoring of blood loss.
   The chest catheter is sutured in position and connected to a water-seal drainage-bottle.

3. Record the volume of fluid drained into the collection bottle hourly for the first several hours to alert for a sudden increase in drainage.
4. Prepare for immediate blood replacement and thoracotomy if bleeding continues.
5. Administer oxygen.

Pneumothorax

Air in the pleural space occurring spontaneously from injury or disease. In patients with chest trauma, it is usually the result of a laceration to the lung parenchyma, tracheobronchial tree, or esophagus.

The patient's clinical status depends on the rate of air leakage and size of wound.

A. Assessment

1. Hyperresonance; diminished breath sounds
2. Reduced mobility of affected half of thorax

B. Spontaneous Pneumothorax

1. May occur in healthy individuals; is usually due to rupture of a subpleural bleb of the lung.
2. Treatment is generally nonoperative if pneumothorax is not too extensive; needle aspiration or chest tube drainage may be necessary to achieve reexpansion of collapsed lung.
3. Surgical intervention (thoracotomy) is advised for patients with recurrent spontaneous pneumothorax.

C. Tension Pneumothorax—buildup of air under pressure resulting in interference with filling of both the heart and lungs

1. Clinical picture is one of air hunger, agitation, hypotension, and cyanosis; there is an *acute threat to life.*
2. Management
   a. Insert chest tube drain immediately to allow air to escape (chest tube then connected to underwater-seal suction).
   b. Use thoracentesis for emergency decompression of pleural space until tube thoracostomy can be accomplished.

Open Pneumothorax *(sucking wound of chest)*

Implies an opening in the chest wall large enough to allow air to pass freely in and out of thoracic cavity with each attempted respiration; the rush of air through the hole in the chest wall produces a "sucking sound." This represents an acute threat to life.

A. General Considerations

1. When there is a large open hole in the chest wall, the patient will have a "steal" in ventilation of other lung.
2. A portion of the tidal volume will move back and forth through the hole in the chest wall, rather than the trachea as it normally does.

B. Management

1. Close the chest wound immediately to restore adequate ventilation and respiration.
2. Instruct the patient to inhale and exhale gently against a closed glottis (Valsalva maneuver) as the pressure dressing (petrolatum gauze secured with elastic adhesive) is applied. (This maneuver helps to expand collapsed lung.)
3. Prepare for chest tube insertion and drainage to permit evacuation of fluid/air and produce reexpansion of the lung. Surgical intervention may be necessary.
4. If condition permits, place patient in semi-sitting position to permit greater ventilatory efficiency.

Fracture of Ribs and Sternum
(most common chest injury)

> **NURSING ALERT:** Rib fractures should be regarded as potentially serious because they may interfere with ventilation and may lacerate underlying lung. Atelectasis and pneumonia are common complications of rib fractures.

A. Clinical Manifestations

1. Localized tenderness or crepitus (crackling) over fracture site
2. Chest pain referred to the fracture site
3. Painful, shallow respirations (due to splinting of involved chest)

B. Management

1. Give analgesics (usually nonnarcotic) to assist in effective coughing and deep breathing.
2. Encourage deep breathing with strong inspiration; give local support to injured area with nurse's hands.
3. Assist with intercostal nerve block (see page 195)—to relieve pain so that coughing and deep breathing may be accomplished.
4. For multiple rib fractures, epidural anesthesia may be used.

Flail Chest

Loss of stability of chest wall, with subsequent respiratory impairment. This usually is the result of multiple rib fractures or combined fractures of the sternum and ribs.

A. Pathophysiology

1. When this occurs, one portion of the chest has lost its bony connection to the rest of the rib cage.
2. During respiration, the detached part of the chest will be pulled in on inspiration and blown out on expiration (paradoxical movement).
3. Normal mechanics of breathing impaired to a degree that seriously jeopardizes ventilation
4. Generally associated with other serious chest injuries; lung contusion, lung laceration, diffuse alveolar damage

B. Clinical Manifestations

1. Pain, dyspnea, cyanosis
2. Paradoxical (reverse of normal) movements of involved chest wall

C. Management

1. Stabilize the flail portion of the chest with the hands; apply a pressure dressing and turn the patient on his injured side, or place 10-pound sandbag at site of flail.
2. Thoracic epidural analgesia may be used for some patients to relieve pain and improve ventilation, *or*
3. If respiratory failure is present, prepare for immediate endotracheal intubation and ventilation therapy with mechanical ventilation—treats underlying pulmonary contusion and serves to stabilize the thoracic cage for healing of fractures, improves alveolar ventilation, and restores thoracic cage stability and intrathoracic volume by decreasing work of breathing.
4. Operative stabilization of chest wall in selected patients.

Pulmonary Contusion

Contusion is a bruise of the lung parenchyma that results in leakage of blood and edema fluid into the alveolar and interstitial spaces of the lung.

A. Clinical Manifestations (may not be fully developed for 24–72 hours)

1. Tachypnea, tachycardia
2. Crackles on auscultation
3. Pleuritic chest pain
4. Copious secretions
5. Cough—constant, loose, rattling

B. Management (for moderate lung contusion)

1. Employ mechanical ventilation to keep lungs inflated.
2. Administer diuretics—to reduce edema.
3. Correct metabolic acidosis with IV sodium bicarbonate.
4. Use pulmonary artery pressure monitoring.
5. Complication: pneumonia in contused segment

Cardiac Tamponade

Compression of the heart as a result of accumulation of fluid within the pericardial space

A. Clinical Manifestations

1. Falling blood pressure

2. Rising venous pressure/distended neck veins/elevated central venous pressure
3. Muffled heart sounds
4. Pulsus paradoxus (systolic blood pressure drops and fluctuates with respiration)
5. Dyspnea, cyanosis, shock

NURSING ALERT: A rapidly developing effusion interferes with ventricular filling and causes impairment of circulation. Thus, there is a reduced cardiac output and poor venous return to the heart. Cardiac collapse can result. In the patient with hypovolemia due to associated injuries, the venous pressure may not rise, thus masking the signs of cardiac tamponade.

B. Management (for penetrating injuries)

1. Emergency thoracotomy to control bleeding and to repair cardiac injury
2. Pericardial aspiration (pericardiocentesis), aspiration or drainage of the pericardium (see p. 310); to provide emergency relief and improve hemodynamic function until operation can be undertaken.

Guidelines   Assisting With an Intercostal Nerve Block (Fig. 10-8)

An *intercostal nerve block* is the injection of a local anesthetic into the area surrounding the intercostal nerves to relieve pain temporarily following rib fracture(s), chest wall injury, or thoracotomy.

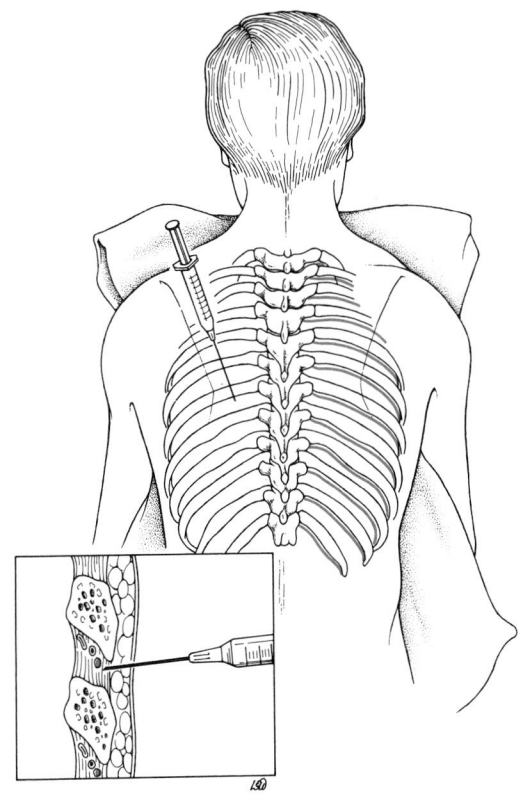

Figure 10-8. *Intercostal nerve block.*

Purpose   To decrease pain and improve the patient's ability to cough.

(continued)

Guidelines — Assisting With an Intercostal Nerve Block (Fig. 10-8) *(continued)*

Equipment

Syringes, 10 ml. Luer–Lok
Needles, No. 22–30 gauge
Anesthetic solution (lidocaine, bupivacaine, procaine)
Skin germicide; sterile gloves

Procedure

Nursing Action	Rationale/Amplification
Preparatory Phase	
1. Inform the patient that he will experience the prick of the needle and a slight sensation of pressure.	
2. Position the patient according to the physician's preference:	
a. Have the patient sit up, bend forward, and hug a pillow, OR	a. This posture moves the scapulae forward and out of the way.
b. Place the patient prone with pillow under his chest, OR	b. The prone position helps immobilize the patient.
c. Have the patient lie on his unaffected side with his upper arm hanging over the side of the table.	c. This pulls the scapula out of the way.
3. Ask the patient to identify the site of pain.	3. To determine which intercostal nerves are to be injected.
Performance Phase (by the physician)	
1. After the skin is prepared, the lower margin of the rib is palpated and a small skin wheal is raised, using a 25–30 gauge needle.	1. This is infiltration anesthesia.
2. Usually nerve blocks are done at the posterior angle of the ribs between the posterior axillary line and the spine.	2. The posterior angle is the most prominent and accessible, and an injection at this area produces a block of the entire distal nerve.
3. A fine needle is advanced through the wheal and directed downward so that it slips under the edge of the rib into the upper portion of the interspace.	3. The intercostal nerve runs in a groove along the undersurface of the above rib.
4. The syringe (needle in place) is aspirated.	4. To ensure that the needle has not punctured the lung or that an intercostal vessel has been entered.
5. The local anesthetic (usually 3–5 ml.) is injected into the area.	5. Usually the local anesthetic is injected above and below the painful rib to obtain complete relief of pain, as the sensory fields of intercostal nerves overlap.
Follow-up Phase	
1. Assess for relief of pain and less painful coughing.	1. This is the expected outcome.
2. Obtain a chest x-ray.	2. To ensure that a pneumothorax has not occurred.
3. Complications:	
a. Intravascular injection	
b. Puncture of the lung with pneumothorax	
c. Hypotension	

Guidelines — Assisting With Tube Thoracostomy (Chest Tube Insertion)

A *tube thoracostomy* is the insertion of one or more flexible tubes into the pleural space to evacuate air, blood, or fluid collections and to achieve full reexpansion of the lung. It also allows sclerosing agents to be placed in the pleural cavity for the treatment of malignant effusions.

Equipment

Tube thoracostomy tray:
  Syringes
  Needles/trocar
  Basins/skin germicide
  Sponges
  Scalpel/sterile drape/gloves
  Two large clamps

Suture material
Local anesthetic
Chest Tube (appropriate size); connector
Chest drainage system—connecting tubes and tubing,
    collection bottles or commercial system, vacuum pump
    (if required)

Sites for Chest Tube Placement	For pneumothorax—2nd or 3rd interspace along midclavicular or anterior axillary line
	For pleural effusion or hemothorax—6th–7th lateral interspace in the midaxillary line

Procedure	**Nursing Action**	**Rationale/Amplification**

Preparatory Phase

1. Assess patient for pneumothorax, hemothorax, presence of respiratory distress.
2. Obtain a chest x-ray. Other means of localization of pleural fluid include ultrasound and/or fluoroscopic localization.
3. Assemble drainage system.
4. Reassure the patient and explain the steps of the procedure. Tell the patient to expect a needle prick and a sensation of slight pressure during infiltration anesthesia.
5. Position the patient as for an intercostal nerve block, or according to physician preference.

2. To evaluate extent of lung collapse or amount of bleeding in pleural space

4. The patient can cope by remaining immobile and doing relaxed breathing during tube insertion.

5. The tube insertion site depends on the substance to be drained, the patient's mobility, and the presence/absence of coexisting conditions.

Performance Phase (by the physician)

Needle or IntraCath Technique

A needle or IntraCath catheter is used for removal of small amounts of air or a minimal air leak from the lung.

1. The skin is prepared and anesthetized using local anesthetic with a short 25 gauge needle. A larger needle is used to infiltrate the subcutaneous tissue, intercostal muscles, and parietal pleura.
2. An exploratory needle is inserted.

3. The IntraCath catheter is inserted through the needle into the pleural space. The needle is removed, and the catheter is pushed several centimeters into the pleural space.
4. The catheter is taped to the skin.

5. The catheter is attached to a connector/tubing and attached to a drainage system (underwater-seal or commercial system).

1. The area is anesthetized to make tube insertion and manipulation relatively painless.

2. To puncture the pleura and determine the presence of air/blood in the pleural cavity

4. To prevent it from being pushed out of the chest during patient movement or lung expansion

Trocar Technique for Chest Tube Insertion

A trocar catheter is used for the insertion of a large-bore tube for removal of a modest to large amount of air leak or for the evacuation of serous effusion.

1. A small incision is made over the prepared, anesthetized site. Blunt dissection (with a hemostat) through the muscle planes in the interspace to the parietal pleura is performed.
2. The trocar is directed into the pleural space, the cannula removed, and a chest tube inserted into the pleural space and connected to a drainage system.

1. To admit the diameter of the chest tube

2. There is a trocar catheter available equipped with an indwelling pointed rod for ease of insertion.

Hemostat Technique Using a Large-Bore Chest Tube (Fig. 10-9)

A large-bore chest tube is used to drain blood or thick effusions from the pleural space.

1. After skin preparation and anesthetic infiltration, an incision is made through the skin and subcutaneous tissue.

2. A curved hemostat is inserted into the pleural cavity and the tissue is spread with the clamp.
3. The tract is explored with an examining finger.

4. The tube is held by the hemostat and directed through the opening up over the rib and into the pleural cavity.
5. The clamp is withdrawn and the chest tube is connected to a chest drainage system.
6. The tube is sutured in place and covered with a sterile dressing.

1. The skin incision is usually made one interspace below proposed site of penetration of the intercostal muscles and pleura.

2. To make a tissue tract for the chest tube

3. Digital examination helps confirm the presence of the tract and penetration of the pleural cavity.

5. The chest tube has multiple openings at the proximal end for drainage of air/blood.

(continued)

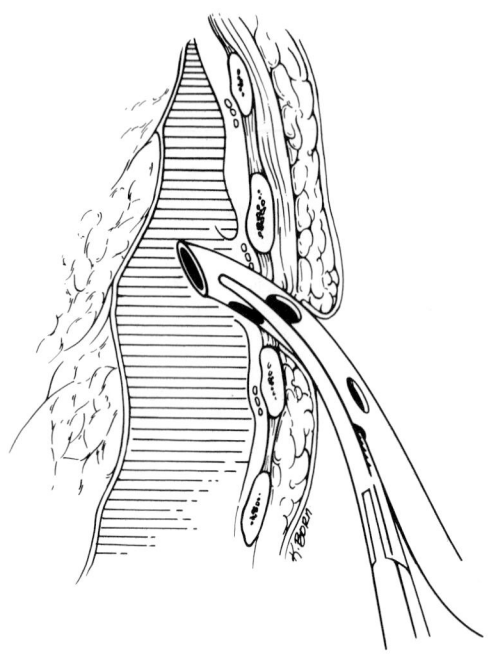

Figure 10-9. *Tube thoracostomy.*

Procedure *(continued)*	**Nursing Action**	**Rationale/Amplification**

Follow-up Phase

1. Observe the drainage system for blood/air.
   Observe that there is free fluctuation in the tube on respiration.
   (See water-seal drainage, p. 203)
2. Secure a follow-up chest x-ray.

3. Look for bleeding, infection, leakage of air and fluid around the tube.

1. If a hemothorax is draining through a thoracostomy tube into a bottle containing sterile normal saline, the blood is available for autotransfusion.

2. To confirm correct chest tube placement and reexpansion of the lung

---

Thoracic Surgery *(Fig. 10-10)*

> **NURSING ALERT:** Meticulous attention must be given to the preoperative and postoperative care of patients undergoing thoracic surgery. These operations are wide in scope and represent a major stress on the cardiorespiratory system.

Preoperative Care

Goal:
Ensure optimal condition for surgery.

A. Assess Preoperative Status

1. Assist the patient undergoing diagnostic studies.
   a. History and physical examination
   b. Chest roentgenograms
   c. Pulmonary function studies—to ascertain if patient will have adequate functioning lung tissue postoperatively
   d. Special diagnostic studies as required; radionuclide lung scanning may show if gas exchange will be affected by procedure
   e. Arterial blood gas studies to determine presence of hypoxemia
2. Nursing Assessment
   a. What signs and symptoms are present? (cough, expectoration, wheeze, hemoptysis, chest pain)
   b. What is smoking history (amount and duration)?
   c. What is the patient's cardiopulmonary tolerance while bathing, eating, walking, etc.?
   d. What is the "physiologic age" of the patient? (general appearance, mental alertness, behavior, degree of nutrition)
   e. What other medical conditions exist?

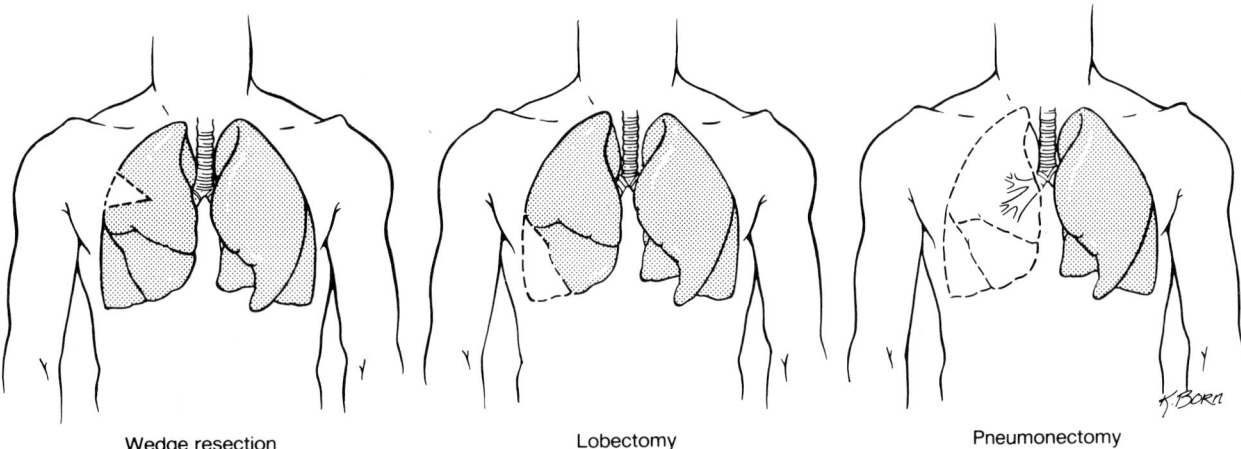

Wedge resection   Lobectomy   Pneumonectomy

Figure 10-10. *Thoracic surgery procedures. These are named for the extent of lung tissue removed. Wedge resection: Removal of a wedge of the lung. Lobectomy: Removal of a lobe of the lung. Pneumonectomy: Removal of the entire lung. Any lung resection results in the reduction of the pulmonary vascular bed and the patient's pulmonary reserve must be adequate to withstand the loss of lung volume and the thoracotomy incisions.*

   f. What is the breathing pattern?
   g. How much exertion is required to produce dyspnea?
   h. What are personal preferences and dislikes?

B. Improve Overall Respiratory Function

1. Encourage the patient to stop smoking to restore bronchial ciliary action and to reduce the amount of sputum and likelihood of postoperative atelectasis.
2. Teach an effective coughing technique.
   a. Sit the patient upright with knees flexed and body bending slightly forward.
   b. Splint the incision with your hands; show the patient how to splint the painful area with firm hand pressure or support it with a pillow or folded towel while coughing.
   c. Instruct the patient to take three short breaths, followed by a deep inspiration, inhaling slowly and evenly through the nose.
   d. Instruct patient to contract (pull in) abdominal muscles and cough twice forcefully with mouth open and tongue out.
   e. Have the patient lie on side with hips and knees flexed if unable to sit.
   f. Huffing and coughing—(a less painful technique)
     (1) Take a deep diaphragmatic breath and exhale forcefully against your hand; exhale in a quick distinct pant, or "huff."
     (2) Practice doing small "huffs" and progress to one strong "huff" while exhaling.
3. Employ all measures to reduce tracheobronchial secretions to a minimum.
   a. Measure sputum daily in patients with large volume of secretions to determine if volume of secretion is decreasing.
   b. Encourage patient to cough effectively (see above).
   c. Humidify the air to loosen secretions.
   d. Administor bronchodilators for bronchospasm.
   e. Give antimicrobials for infection.
   f. Encourage deep breathing with the use of incentive spirometer.
   g. Teach diaphragmatic breathing preoperatively.
   h. Set up a schedule of breathing exercises that encourage the use of abdominal muscles.
   i. Carry out postural drainage in patients having excessive tracheobronchial secretions.

C. Evaluate Cardiovascular and Pulmonary Status So That Complications May Be Anticipated and Prevented.

1. Study the results of diagnostic tests to learn of existing deviations from normal.
2. Observe the patient and his reactions to various activities of daily living.
3. Give cardiac drugs to patients with congestive heart failure.
4. Correct anemia, dehydration, and hypoproteinemia—intravenous infusions, tube feedings, blood transfusions as indicated.
5. Give prophylactic anticoagulant (low-dose heparin) as prescribed to reduce perioperative incidence of deep vein thrombosis and pulmonary embolism.

D. Teaching and Counseling

1. Orient the patient to events in the postoperative period.
   a. Coughing with chest support and breathing routine
   b. Suctioning (aspiration) of secretions
   c. Presence of chest tube and drainage bottles
   d. Oxygen therapy, ventilator therapy
   e. Measures used to control discomfort
   f. Leg exercises and range of motion exercises for affected shoulder
   g. Coping measures (breathing, turning, analgesics) for postoperative discomfort
2. Encourage expression of psychologic and safety needs.
3. See that consent form has been explained and signed.

Postoperative Care

Nursing Diagnoses

1. Ineffective breathing pattern related to altered physiology secondary to opening the pleural cavity and ineffective airway clearance.

2. Pain related to chest incision and presence of chest tubes.
3. Impaired mobility of affected shoulder and arm related to location of incision and presence of chest tubes.

Complications

1. Hypoxia—watch for restlessness, tachycardia, tachypnea, and elevated blood pressure.
2. Postoperative bleeding—monitor for restlessness, anxiety, pallor, tachycardia, and hypotension.
3. Pneumonia; atelectasis
4. Bronchopleural fistula from disruption of a bronchial suture or staple; bronchial stump leak
   a. Observe for sudden onset of cough productive of serosanguineous fluid; or sudden respiratory distress.
   b. Position with the operative side down.
   c. Prepare for immediate tube thoracostomy and/or surgical intervention.
5. Cardiac dysrhythmias; usually occurring 3–4th postoperative day; myocardial infarction; heart failure.

Nursing Interventions

A. Maintaining an Open Airway and Assuring Adequate Respiratory Function.

1. Auscultate chest for adequacy of air movement—to detect broncospasm, consolidation.
2. Look and listen at the patient's open mouth as he breathes for evidences of obstruction.
3. Monitor for adequacy of pulmonary function:
   a. Measure PaO_2, $PaCO_2$, and tidal volume.
   b. Use indwelling arterial line to facilitate drawing arterial blood samples and provide a continuous measurement of systemic arterial pressures.
4. Most patients have endotracheal tubes in place with ventilatory support until adequate respiratory function and stable cardiovascular status is attained. Ventilatory weaning is started as early as possible.

> **NURSING ALERT:** Tracheobronchial secretions are present in excessive amounts in post-thoracotomy patients because of trauma to the tracheobronchial tree during operation, diminished lung ventilation, and diminished cough reflex.

B. Aspirating all Secretions With Suctioning Until Patient Is Able to Cough Effectively (p. 173).

1. Listen for ineffective cough or "wet" cough.
2. Auscultate for crackles, rhonchi, and wheezing.
3. Listen for disappearance of breath sounds over area where previously heard; considered a danger signal.

> **NURSING ALERT:** Look for changes in color and consistency of aspirated sputum. Colorless, fluid sputum is not unusual; opacification or coloring of sputum may mean dehydration or infection.

C. Maintaining Continuing Nursing Surveillance of the Patient's Hemodynamic Status:

1. Take blood pressure, pulse, and respiration every 15 minutes or more frequently as indicated; extend the time intervals according to the patient's clinical status.
2. Evaluate *character* of respirations and patient's color—depth of respiration is an important criterion in evaluating whether lungs are being adequately expanded.

3. Auscultate and percuss chest frequently to determine adequacy of ventilation—detects early respiratory embarrassment.
4. Monitor heart rate and rhythm via auscultation and ECG, as dysrhythmias are more frequently seen after thoracic surgery.
   a. Dysrhythmias can occur anytime and contribute significantly to postoperative mortality rate.
   b. Rate of occurrence of dysrhythmias increases with patients over 50 and with those undergoing pneumonectomy or esophageal surgery.
   c. Begin antiarrhythmic measures immediately if indicated.
5. Monitor the central venous pressure for prompt recognition of hypovolemia and for evidence of excessive fluid administration.
6. Monitor cardiac output and pulmonary artery wedge or left atrial mean pressures.
7. Elevate the head of the bed 30–40 degrees when patient is oriented and his blood pressure stabilized—improves movement of diaphragm.

D. Assessing and Managing Chest Drainage System— which is used to drain fluid, blood, clots, and air from the pleura following a thoracotomy.

1. Check amount and character of chest tube drainage immediately postoperatively and at necessary intervals thereafter.
   a. Chest drainage should progressively decrease after first 12 hours.
   b. Prepare for blood replacement and possible reoperation to achieve hemostasis if bleeding persists.

   Note: A patient with a pneumonectomy usually does not have water-seal drainage, as it is desirable that the pleural space fill with an effusion, which eventually obliterates this space. Some surgeons do use a "modified" water seal system.
2. See page 203 for summary of nurse's role in the management of water-seal drainage.
3. Give humidified, warmed oxygen in immediate postoperative period—effective in decreasing ventilatory and myocardial work; warming and humidification of inspired gases prevents drying of secretions and loss of body heat.

E. Achieving Pain Relief

1. Provide intelligent pain relief—pain limits chest excursions, thereby decreasing ventilation.
   a. Severity of pain varies with type of incision and with the patient's reaction to and ability to cope with pain. Usually a posterolateral incision is the most painful.
   b. Give narcotics (usually by continuous IV infusion or by epidural catheter) for pain relief, as prescribed, to permit patient to breathe more deeply and cough more effectively.
   c. Avoid depressing respiratory and vascular systems with too much narcotic; patient should not be so somnolent that he does not cough.
   d. Assist patient having intercostal nerve block or cryoanalgesia (intercostal nerve freezing) for pain control.
2. Position in bed correctly.
   a. Position patient upright (15–30 degrees) if cardiovascular system is stable to facilitate optimal ventilation; allows diaphragm to descend and lung volume to increase; this also helps residual air to

rise in upper portion of pleural space, where it can be removed by the chest tube.

b. Patients with limited respiratory reserve may not be able to turn on unoperated side, as this may limit ventilation of the operated side.

c. Vary the position from horizontal to semi-erect; remaining in one position tends to promote the retention of secretions in the dependent portion of the lungs.

3. Encourage and promote an effective cough routine (Fig. 10-11); a persistent and ineffective cough exhausts the patient, may induce bronchospasm, and retained secretions lead to atelectasis and pneumonia.

a. Sit the patient on side of bed with feet supported on a chair if his condition permits.

b. Support the chest firmly over the operated side and against opposite chest to lessen incisional pain or support the thorax with one hand pressing on the midsternum and the other arm around the back if there is a median sternotomy incision.

c. Instruct the patient to take a deep breath (to increase cough pressure), to pull in his abdominal muscles, and to cough vigorously and expectorate secretions.

d. Assist the patient to cough at least every 1–2 hours during the first 24 hours and when necessary thereafter.

F. Maintaining Mobility of Affected Shoulder

1. Encourage breathing exercises to obtain full expansion of the chest wall.

2. Encourage skeletal exercises to promote abduction and mobilization of the shoulder.

3. Ambulate as soon as pulmonary and circulatory systems are compensated.

4. Encourage progressive activities.

G. Other Nursing Interventions

1. Administer blood and parenteral fluids at a slower rate after thoracic surgery—patient vulnerable to fluid overload because pulmonary vascular system has been reduced.

2. Continue to monitor blood gas and serum electrolyte values.

3. Monitor hourly urine output from indwelling catheter, as urine volume reflects cardiac output and organ perfusion.

Patient Education

1. There will be some intercostal pain for a time, which can be relieved by local heat and oral analgesia.

2. Weakness and fatigability are common during the first 3 weeks following a thoracotomy.

3. Range-of-motion exercises for the arm and shoulder on the affected side should be carried out several times daily to avoid ankylosis of the shoulder ("frozen shoulder").

4. Carry out deep-breathing exercises for the first few weeks at home—restoration of lung function is dependent on full expansion of residual lung tissue.

5. Consciously practice good body alignment, preferably in front of a full-length mirror.

6. The chest muscles may be weaker than normal for 3–6 months following surgery. Avoid lifting more than 20 pounds until complete healing has taken place.

7. Alternate walking and other activities with frequent

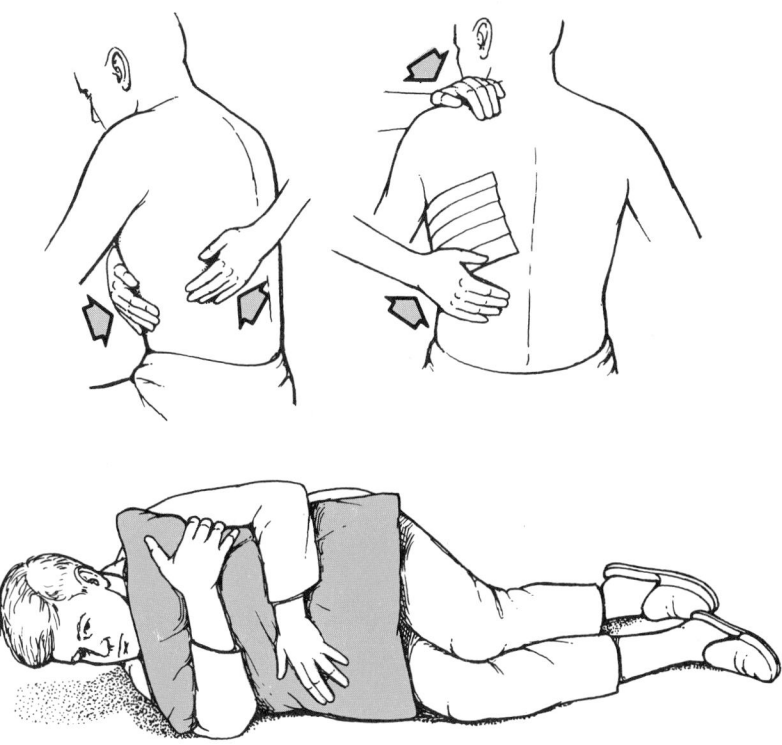

Figure 10-11. *Promotion of an effective cough. The patient is placed in a semi-Fowler's position.*

short rest periods. Walk at a moderate pace and gradually extend walking time and distance.

8. Stop any activity immediately that causes undue fatigue, increased shortness of breath, or chest pain.
9. Because all or part of one lung has been removed, stay away from respiratory irritants (smoke, fumes, high level of air pollution).
    a. Avoid anything that may cause spasms of coughing.
    b. Sit in nonsmoking areas in public places.
10. Have an annual influenza injection (pneumonectomy patients).
11. Report for follow-up care by the surgeon or clinic as necessary.

Evaluation

1. Maintains effective respiration: normal respiratory rate and blood gas measurements, absence of wheezes and crackles; able to cough up secretions
2. Achieves pain relief
3. Attains/maintains mobility of affected shoulder: extends arm at hourly intervals; checks posture; consciously tries to use affected arm; ambulates increasing distances
4. Recalls the features and rationale of postoperative program; breathing exercises, shoulder exercises, avoiding respiratory irritants

Chest Drainage

Pathophysiology

1. The normal breathing mechanism operates on the principle of negative pressure (the pressure in the chest cavity is lower than the pressure of the outside air, causing air to move into the lungs during inspiration).
2. Whenever the chest is opened, from any cause, there is loss of negative pressure, which can result in collapse of the lung. The collection of air, fluid, or other substances in the chest can compromise cardiopulmonary function and even cause collapse of the lung, because these substances take up space.
3. Pathologic substances that collect in the pleural space include: fibrin, or clotted blood, liquids (serous fluids, blood, pus, chyle) and gases (air from the lung, tracheobronchial tree, or esophagus).
4. Surgical incision of the chest wall almost always causes some degree of pneumothorax. Air and fluid collect in the intrapleural space, restricting lung expansion and reducing air exchange.
5. It is necessary to keep the pleural space evacuated postoperatively and to maintain negative pressure within this potential space. Therefore, during or immediately after thoracic surgery, chest tubes/catheters are positioned strategically in the pleural space, sutured to the skin, and connected to some type of drainage apparatus to remove the residual air and drainage fluid from the pleural or mediastinal space. This assists in the reexpansion of remaining lung tissue.

Principles of Chest Drainage

1. A chest drainage system must be capable of removing whatever collects in the pleural space so that a normal pleural space and normal cardiopulmonary function may be restored and maintained.
2. There are many types of commercial chest drainage systems in use, most of which use the water-seal principle. The chest catheter is attached to a bottle, using a one-way valve principle. Water acts as a seal and permits air and fluid to drain from the chest, but air cannot reenter the submerged tip of the tube (Fig. 10-12).
3. Chest drainage can be categorized into three types of mechanical systems (Fig. 10-12):

A. The Single-Bottle Water-Seal System

1. The end of the drainage tube from the patient's chest is covered by a layer of water, which permits drainage of air and fluid from the pleural space, but does not allow air to move back into the chest. Functionally, drainage depends on gravity, on the mechanics of respiration, and, if desired, on suction by the addition of *controlled* vacuum.
2. The tube from the patient extends approximately 2.5 cm. (1 inch) below the level of the water in the container. There is a vent for the escape of any air that may be leaking from the lung. The water level fluctuates as the patient breathes; it goes up when the patient inhales and down when the patient exhales.
3. At the end of the drainage tube, bubbling may or may not be visible. Bubbling can mean either persistent leakage of air from the lung or other tissues or a leak in the system.

B. The Two-Bottle System

1. The two-bottle system consists of the same water-seal chamber, plus a fluid-collection bottle.
2. Drainage is similar to that of a single unit, except that when pleural fluid drains, the underwater-seal system is not affected by the volume of drainage.
3. Effective drainage depends on gravity or on the amount of suction added to the system. When vacuum (suction) is added to the system from a vacuum source, such as wall suction, the connection is made at the vent stem of the underwater-seal bottle.
4. The amount of suction applied to the system is regulated by the wall gauge.

C. The Three-Bottle System

1. The three-bottle system is similar in all respects to the two-bottle system, except for the addition of a third bottle to control the amount of suction applied.
2. The amount of suction is determined by the depth to which the tip of the venting glass tube is submerged in the water.
3. In the three-bottle system (as in the other two systems), drainage depends on gravity or the amount of suction applied. The amount of suction in the three-bottle system is controlled by the manometer bottle. The mechanical suction motor or wall suction creates and maintains a negative pressure throughout the entire closed drainage system.
4. The manometer bottle regulates the amount of vacuum in the system. This bottle contains three tubes: (1) A short tube above the water level comes from the water-seal bottle; (2) another short tube leads to the vacuum or suction motor, or to wall suction; (3) the third tube is a long tube that extends below the water level in the bottle and opens to the atmosphere outside the

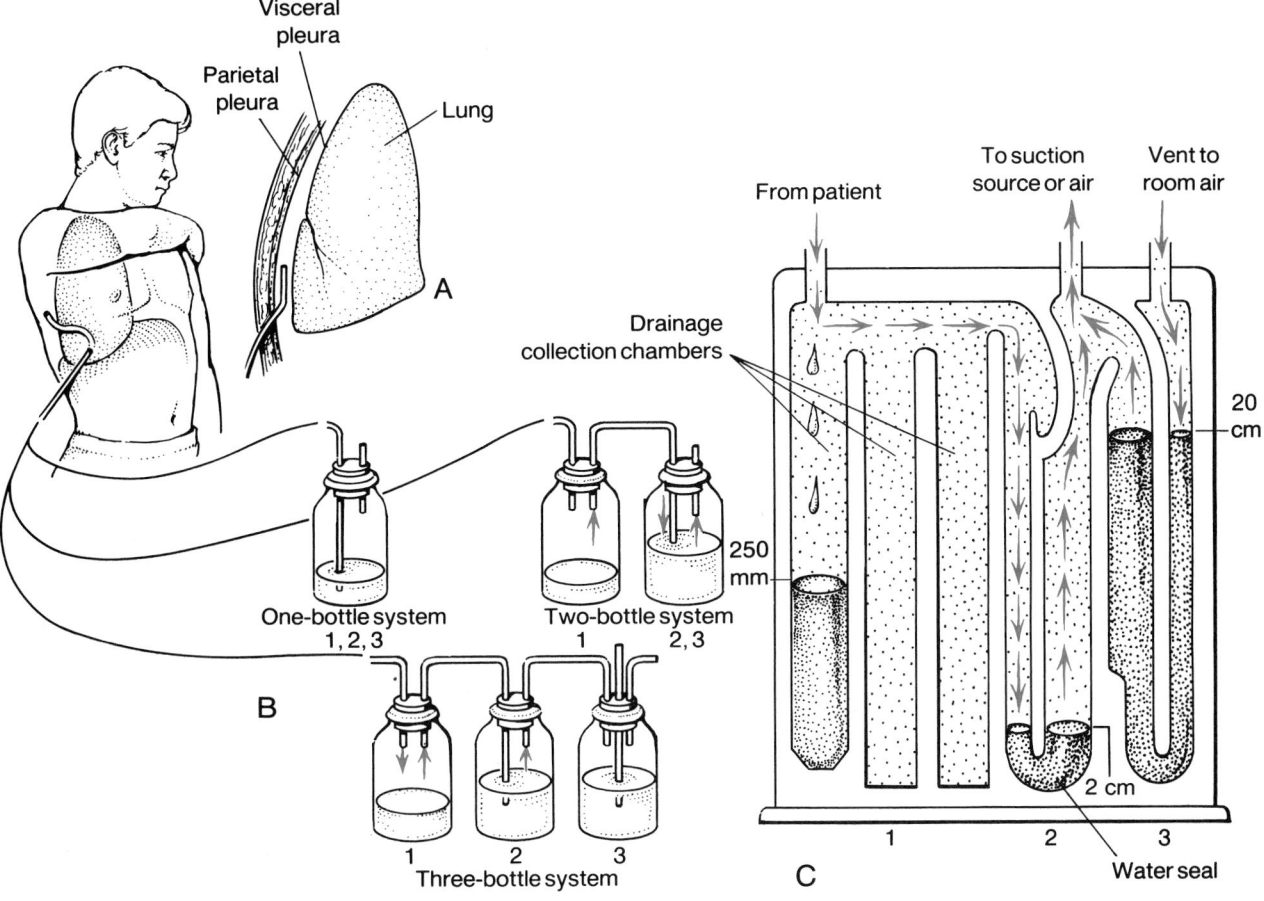

Figure 10-12. Chest drainage system. (A) Strategic placement of a chest catheter in the pleural space. (B) Three types of mechanical drainage systems. (C) A Pleur-Evac operating system: (1) the collection chamber, (2) the water seal chamber, and (3) the suction control chamber. The Pleur-Evac is a single unit with all three bottles identified as chambers. (From Brunner LS and Suddarth DS. Textbook of Medical–Surgical Nursing. 6th ed. Philadelphia, JB Lippincott, 1988)

bottle. This tube regulates the amount of vacuum in the system, depending on the depth to which the tube is submerged—the usual depth is 20 cm. (7.6 inches).
5. When the vacuum in the system becomes greater than the depth to which the tube is submerged, outside air is sucked into the system. This results in constant bubbling in the manometer bottle, which indicates that the system is functioning properly.

Note: When the motor or the wall vacuum is turned off, the drainage system should be open to the atmosphere so that intrapleural air can escape from the system. This can be done by detaching the tubing from the suction port to provide a vent.

6. In the commercially available systems, the three bottles are contained in one unit and identified as "chambers" (Fig. 10-12).

Guidelines Managing the Patient With Water-Seal Chest Drainage*

An intrapleural drainage tube is used after most intrathoracic procedures. One or more chest catheters are held in the pleural space by suture to the chest wall and are attached to a drainage system.

Purposes 1. To remove solids, liquids, and gas from the pleural space or thoracic cavity and the mediastinal space. (Liquids are serous fluid, blood, pus, and occasionally other fluids; gas and air from the lung, tracheobronchial tree, or esophagus.)
2. To bring about reexpansion of the lung and restore normal cardiorespiratory function after surgery, trauma, or medical conditions by establishing negative pressure in the pleural cavity.

* There are commercial disposable chest drainage devices available for collecting pleural fluid that use the water-seal principle.

(continued)

Guidelines   Managing the Patient With Water-Seal Chest Drainage *(continued)*

Equipment   Closed chest drainage system
Holder for drainage system (if needed)
Vacuum motor
Sterile connector for emergency use

Procedure

Nursing Action	Rationale/Amplification
1. Attach the drainage tube from the pleural space (the patient) to the tubing that leads to a long tube with end submerged in sterile normal saline.	1. Water-seal drainage provides for the escape of air and fluid into a drainage bottle. The water acts as a seal and keeps the air from being drawn back into the pleural space.
2. Check the tube connections periodically. Tape if necessary.	2. Tube connections are checked to ensure tight fit and patency of the tubes.
a. The tube should be approximately 2.5 cm. (1 inch) below the water level.	a. If the tube is submerged too deep below the water level, a higher intrapleural pressure is required to expel air.
b. The short tube is left open to the atmosphere.	b. Venting the short glass tube lets air escape from the bottle.
3. Mark the original fluid level with tape on the outside of the drainage-bottle. Mark hourly/daily increments (date and time) at the drainage level.	3. This marking will show the amount of fluid loss and how fast fluid is collecting in the drainage bottle. It serves as a basis for blood replacement, if the fluid is blood. Grossly bloody drainage will appear in the bottle in the immediate postoperative period and, if excessive, may necessitate reoperation. Drainage usually declines progressively after the first 24 hours.
4. Make sure that the tubing does not loop or interfere with the movements of the patient.	4. Fluid collecting in the dependent segment of the tubing will decrease the negative pressure applied to the catheter. Kinking, looping, or pressure on the drainage tubing can produce back pressure, thus possibly forcing drainage back into the pleural space or impeding drainage from the pleural space.
5. Encourage the patient to assume a position of comfort. Encourage good body alignment. When the patient is in a lateral position, place a rolled towel under the tubing to protect it from the weight of the patient's body. Encourage the patient to change his position frequently.	5. The patient's position should be changed frequently to promote drainage and his body kept in good alignment to prevent postural deformity and contractures. Proper positioning helps breathing and promotes better air exchange. Pain medication may be indicated to enhance comfort and deep breathing.
6. Put the arm and shoulder of the affected side through range-of-motion exercises several times daily. Some pain medication may be necessary.	6. Exercise helps to avoid ankylosis of the shoulder and assist in lessening postoperative pain and discomfort.
7. "Milk" the tubing in the direction of the drainage bottle as often as directed.	7. "Milking" the tubing prevents it from becoming plugged with clots and fibrin. Constant attention to maintaining the patency of the tube will facilitate prompt expansion of the lung and minimize complications.
8. Make sure there is fluctuation ("tidaling") of the fluid level in the long glass tube.	8. Fluctuation of the water level in the tube shows that there is effective communication between the pleural space and the drainage bottle, provides a valuable indication of the patency of the drainage system, and is a gauge of intrapleural pressure.
9. Fluctuations of fluid in the tubing will stop when: a. The lung has reexpanded b. The tubing is obstructed by blood clots or fibrin c. A dependent loop develops (see step 4) d. Suction motor or wall suction is not operating properly	
10. Watch for leaks of air in the drainage system as indicated by constant bubbling in the water-seal bottle. a. Report excessive bubbling in the water-seal chamber immediately. b. "Milking" of chest tubes in patients with air leaks should be done only if requested by surgeon.	10. Leaking and trapping of air in the pleural space can result in tension pneumothorax.
11. Observe and report immediately signs of rapid, shallow breathing, cyanosis, pressure in the chest, subcutaneous emphysema, or symptoms of hemorrhage.	11. Many clinical conditions may cause these signs and symptoms, including tension pneumothorax, mediastinal shift, hemorrhage, severe incisional pain, pulmonary embolus, and cardiac tamponade. Surgical intervention may be necessary.

Procedure (continued)	Nursing Action	Rationale/Amplification

12. Encourage the patient to breathe deeply and cough at frequent intervals. If there are signs of incisional pain, adequate pain medication is indicated.

13. If the patient has to be transported to another area, place the drainage bottle below the chest level (as close to the floor as possible) if he is lying on a stretcher.

    If the tube becomes disconnected, cut off the contaminated tips of the chest tube and tubing, insert a sterile connector in the chest tube and tubing, and reattach to the drainage system. Otherwise, do not clamp the chest tube during transport.

14. When assisting the surgeon in removing the tube:
    a. Instruct the patient to perform a gentle Valsalva maneuver or to breathe quietly.
    b. The chest tube is clamped and removed.
    c. Simultaneously, a small bandage is applied and made airtight with petrolatum gauze covered by 4 × 4-inch gauze and thoroughly covered and sealed with tape.

12. Deep breathing and coughing help to raise the intrapleural pressure, which allows emptying of any accumulation in the pleural space and removes secretions from the tracheobronchial tree so that the lung expands.

13. The drainage apparatus must be kept at a level lower than the patient's chest to prevent backflow of fluid into the pleural space.

14. The chest tube is removed as directed when the lung is reexpanded (usually 24 hours to several days). During tube removal avoid a large sudden inspiratory effort, which may produce a pneumothorax.

Bibliography

Books

Barnes HV et al. Clinical Medicine. Chicago, Year Book Medical Pub, 1988

Bates DV. Respiratory Function in Disease. 3rd ed. Philadelphia, WB Saunders, 1989

Benumof JL. Anesthesia for Thoracic Surgery. Philadelphia, WB Saunders, 1987

Birtran JD et al (eds). Lung Cancer: A Comprehensive Treatise. Orlando, Grune & Stratton, 1988

Brewis RAL. Lecture Notes on Respiratory Disease. Boston, Blackwell Scientific Publications, 1985

Cade JF and Pain MCF. Essentials of Respiratory Medicine. Boston, Blackwell Scientific Publications, 1988

Cherniack RM (ed). Drugs for the Respiratory System. Orlando, Grune & Stratton, 1986

Churg A and Green FHY. Pathology of Occupational Lung Disease. New York, Igaku-Shoin, 1988

Cotes JE and Steel J. Work-Related Lung Disorders. Boston, Blackwell Scientific Publications, 1987

Dantzker DR (ed). Cardiopulmonary Critical Care. Orlando, Grune & Stratton, 1986

DeVita VT, Hellman S, and Rosenberg SA. Cancer: Principles and Practice of Oncology. Philadelphia, JB Lippincott, 1989

Fishman AP. Pulmonary Diseases and Disorders, Vol 1, 2, and 3. 2nd ed. New York, McGraw–Hill, 1988

Fraser RG et al (eds). Diagnosis of Diseases of the Chest. 3rd ed. Philadelphia, WB Saunders, 1988

Hasse H. Surgical Treatment of Bronchial Carcinoma. New York, Springer-Verlag, 1986

Hodgkin JE and Petty TL. Chronic Obstructive Pulmonary Disease. Current Concepts. Philadelphia, WB Saunders, 1987

Hood RM et al. Surgical Diseases of the Pleura and Chest Wall. Philadelphia, WB Saunders, 1986

Hurt R and Bates M. Essentials of Thoracic Surgery. Boston, Butterworths, 1986

Kersten LD. Comprehensive Respiratory Nursing. Philadelphia, WB Saunders, 1989

Kirby RR and Taylor RW. Respiratory Failure. Chicago, Year Book Medical Pub, 1986

Marshall BE, Longnecker DE, and Fairley HB. Anesthesia for Thoracic Procedures. Boston, Blackwell Scientific Publications, 1988

Moghissi K. Essentials of Thoracic and Cardiac Surgery. London, William Heinemann Medical Books, 1986

National Heart, Lung and Blood Institute. Chronic Obstructive Lung Disease. Washington, DC, US Department of Health and Human Services, 1986

Pennington JE. Respiratory Infections: Diagnosis and Management. New York, Raven Press, 1989

Pierson DJ (ed). Respiratory Intensive Care. Dallas, Daedalus Enterprises, 1986

Roth JA, Ruckdeschel JC, and Weisenburger TH. Thoracic Oncology. Philadelphia, WB Saunders, 1989

Shields TW. General Thoracic Surgery. 3rd ed. Philadelphia, Lea & Febiger, 1989

Spagnolo SV and Medinger A. Handbook of Pulmonary Emergencies. New York, Plenum Medical Book Company, 1986

Stark JE et al. Manual of Chest Medicine. New York, Churchill-Livingstone, 1986

Stoll BA (ed). Coping with Cancer Stress. Boston, Martinus Nijhoff Publishers, 1986

Symbas PN. Cardiothoracic Trauma. Philadelphia, WB Saunders, 1989

von Hippel A. A Manual of Thoracic Surgery. 2nd ed. Anchorage, Stone Age Press, 1986

Weatherall DJ, Ledingham JGG, and Warrell DA. Oxford Textbook of Medicine, Vol 2. 2nd ed. New York, Oxford University Press, 1987

Weinberger SH. Principles of Pulmonary Medicine. Philadelphia, WB Saunders, 1986

Wilson JD. Drug Use in Respiratory Disease. Baltimore, Williams and Wilkins, 1987

Conditions of the Respiratory Tract

Journals

Diagnostic Procedures

Bartlett JG. The technique of transtracheal aspiration. J Crit Ill 1986 Jan; 1(1):43–49

Bramen SS (ed). Pulmonary signs and symptoms. Clin Chest Med 1987 Jun; 8(2):177–252

Loudon RG. The lung exam. Clin Chest Med Jun; 8(2):265–272

Shure D (ed). Diagnostic techniques. Clin Chest Med 1987 Mar; 8(1):1–64

Cancer of the Lung

Cella DF et al. The relationship of psychological distress, extent of disease, and performance status in patients with lung cancer. Cancer 1987 Oct 1; 60(7):1661–1667

Iannuzzi MC and Scoggin CH. Small cell lung cancer. Am Rev Respir Dis 1986 Sep; 134(3):593–608

Martini N (ed). Surgical treatment of lung carcinoma. Surg Clin North Am 1987 Oct; 67(5):909–1120

Maxwell MB and Ryan LS (eds). Nursing care of the patient with lung cancer. Semin Oncol Nurs 1987 Aug; 3(3): 163–236 (entire volume)

O'Rourke MA and Crawford J. Lung cancer in the elderly. Clin Geriatr Med 1987 Nov; 3(4):595–623

Saunders JM and McCorkle R. Social support and coping with lung cancer. West J Nurs Res 1987 Feb; 9(1):29–42

Watson PN and Evans RJ. Intractable pain with lung cancer. Pain 1987 May; 29(2):163–173

Lung Abscess

Bartlett JG. Anaerobic bacterial infections of the lung. Chest 1987 Jun; 91(6):901–909

Parker LA et al. Percutaneous small bore catheter drainage in the management of lung abscesses. Chest 1987 Aug; 92(2):213–218

Rice TW, Gisberg RJ and Todd TRJ. Tube drainage of lung abscesses. Ann Thorac Surg 1987 Oct; 44(4):356–364

Stavas J et al. Percutaneous drainage of infected and noninfected thoracic fluid collections. J Thorac Imaging 1987 Jul; 2(3):80–87

Chronic Obstructive Pulmonary Disease

American Thoracic Society. Standards for the diagnosis and care of patients with chronic obstructive pulmonary disease (COPD) and asthma. Am Rev Respir Dis 1987 Jul; 136(1):225–244

Anthonisen NR. Chronic obstructive pulmonary disease. Can Med Assoc J 1988 Mar 15; 138(6):503–510

Ipratropium. Med Lett Drugs Ther 1987 Jul 31; 29(745):71–72

Kronenberg RS (ed). Chronic bronchitis. Semin Respir Infect 1988 Mar; 3(1):1–80

Lareau S and Larson JL. Ineffective breathing pattern related to airflow limitation. Nurs Clin North Am 1987 Mar; 22(1):179–191

Make BJ et al. Pulmonary rehabilitation. Clin Chest Med 1986 Dec; 7(4):519–691 (entire volume)

Petty TL. Drug strategies for airflow obstruction. Am J Nurs 1987 Feb; 87(2):180–184

Skorodin MS. Pharmacologic management of obstructive lung diseases. Am J Med 1986 Nov; 14(81 suppl 5A):8–15

Stockley RA. Bonchiectasis—New therapeutic approaches based on pathogenesis. Clin Chest Med 1987 Sep; 8(3):481–494

Wilson DO et al. Nutritional intervention in malnourished patients with emphysema. Am Rev Respir Dis 1986 Oct; 134(4):672–677

Cor Pulmonale

deBoisblanc BP and Summer WR. Key steps in diagnosis and management of cor pulmonale. J Crit Ill 1986 Sep; 1(9):25–35

Michael JR et al. Pharmacologic therapy of cor pulmonale. Cardiovasc Clin 1987; 17(2):171–179

Peil ML and Rubin LJ. Therapy of secondary pulmonary hypertension. Heart Lung 1986 Sep; 15(5):450–456

Pleural Effusion

Lorch DG et al. Effect of patient positioning on distribution of tetracycline in the pleural space during pleurodesis. Chest 1988 Mar; 93(3): 527–529

Prakash VBS. Malignant pleural effusions. Postgrad Med 1986 Oct; 80(5):201–209

Sahn SA and Good JT Jr. Pleural fluid pH in malignant effusions. Ann Intern Med 1988 Mar; 108(3):345–349

Varkey B. Pleural effusions caused by infection. Postgrad Med 1986 Oct; 80(5):213–223

Pneumonia

Biller PL. Diagnosis and management of acute bronchitis and pneumonia in the ambulatory setting. Nurse Pract 1987 Oct; 12(10):12–15, 18, 23, passim

Gleckman RA and Bergman MM. Bacterial pneumonia: Specific diagnosis and treatment of the elderly. Geriatrics 1987 Sep; 42(9):29–36, 41

Joyce TH III. Prophylaxis for pulmonary acid aspiration. Am J Med 1987 Dec 18;83(6A):46–52

Niederman MS. (ed). Respiratory infections. Clin Chest Med 1987 Sep; 8(3):339–556

Palmer DL and Jones CC. Diagnosis of pneumococcal pneumonia. Semin Respir Infect 1988 Jun; 3(2):131–139

Pugliese G and Lichtenberg DA. Nosocomial bacterial pneumonia: An overview. Am J Infect Control 1987 Dec; 15(6):249–265

Roselle GA. Nosocomial and nursing home-acquired pneumonia. Postgrad Med 1987 Jan; 81(1):131–132; 135–136

Segreti J and Bone RC. Overwhelming pneumonia. DM 1987 Jan; 33(1):1–59

Pulmonary Embolism

Ansari A. Acute and chronic pulmonary thromboembolism: Current perspectives. Part III. Diagnosis. Clin Cardiol 1986 Oct; 9(10):512–524

Ansari A. Acute and chronic pulmonary thromboembolism: Current perspectives. Part VIII. Summary and references. Clin Cardiol 1987 Mar; 10(3):181–188

Consensus Conference: National Institutes of Health. Prevention of venous thrombosis and pulmonary embolism. JAMA 1986 Aug 8; 256(6): 744–749

Editorial. Preventing venous thrombosis and pulmonary embolism. Am Fam Physician 1987 Feb; 35(2):95, 98

Grassi CJ and Goldhaber SZ. Interruption of the inferior vena cava for prevention of pulmonary embolism: Transvenous filter devices. Herz 1989 Jun; 14(3):182–191

Greenfield LJ and Wakefield TW. Prevention of venous thrombosis and pulmonary embolism. Adv Surg 1989; 22:301–324

Hirsh J. Treatment of pulmonary embolism. Annu Rev Med 1987; 38:91–105

McCollum C. Vena caval filters: Keeping big clots down. Br Med J 1987 Jun 20; 294(6587):1566

Mohr DN et al. Recent advances in the management of venous thromboembolism. Mayo Clin Proc 1988 Mar; 63(3):281–290

Pais SO and Tobin KD. Percutaneous insertion of the Greenfield filter. AJR 1989 May; 152(5):933–938

Perry MO. Anticoagulation: A surgical perspective. Am J Surg 1988 Feb; 155(2):268–276

Roberts SL. Pulmonary tissue perfusion altered: Emboli. Heart Lung 1987 Mar; 16(2):128–139

Trulock EP. Approaches to deep venous thrombosis and pulmonary embolism in aging patients. Geriatrics 1988 Feb; 43(2):101–113

Valenzuela TD. Pulmonary embolism. Ann Emerg Med 1988 Mar; 17(3):209–213

Weinstein SM. Thrombolytic therapy. NITA 1986 Feb; 9(2):31–35

Surgery and Trauma

Bense L et al. Smoking and the increased risk of contracting spontaneous pneumothorax. Chest 1987 Dec; 92(6): 1009–1012

Cole PH and Wolfe WG. Mechanisms of healing in the injured lung treated with the Nd-YAG laser. Lasers Surg Med 1987; 6(6):574–580

Greene R. Lung alterations in thoracic trauma. J Thorac Imaging 1987 Jul; 2(3):1–11

Parker JG. Thoracic trauma. Nursing assessment and management. Nurs Clin North Am 1986 Dec; 21(4):685–692

Shorr RM et al. Blunt thoracic trauma. Ann Surg 1987 Aug; 206(2):200–205

Silver M and Bone RC. The technique of chest tube insertion. J Crit Ill 1986 Feb; 1(2):45–51

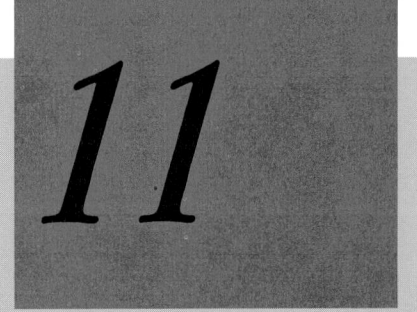
Respiratory Function

Basic Terminology

1. *Tidal volume* (V_T)—total volume of each breath. Normal = 500 ml. ± 100 ml. for a healthy adult.
2. *Minute ventilation* (V_E)—tidal volume (V_T) times the number of breaths per minute. Normal = 6–10 L./min. A V_E that is lower than normal predisposes to CO_2 retention. A V_E that is higher than normal increases the work of breathing.
3. *Vital capacity* (V_C)—maximum volume of air exhaled after a maximal inspiration. Indicates ability to take a sufficiently deep breath to prevent atelectasis. Normal = 65–75 ml./kg.
4. *Maximum voluntary ventilation (MVV)*—maximum volume of gas the patient can inspire and expire in 1 minute. Tests ability to maintain ventilation at greater than normal capacity for limited time.
5. *Negative inspiratory force (NIF)*—greatest negative pressure that can be generated when inspiring against an occluded external airway. Tests ability to generate sufficient force to cough effectively. Normal = ≥ -60 cm. H_2O.

   Note: Changes in these variables are used to monitor need for mechanical ventilation. Some indicators of the need for mechanical ventilation are: $V_C < 10$–15 ml./kg.; respiratory rate > 35/minute; $V_E > 10$ L/minute; or an NIF < -20–25 cm. H_2O.

6. *Hypoxemia*—less than normal arterial oxygen tension (PaO_2). May or may not be associated with symptoms depending on value. Normal PaO_2 = 80–100 mm. Hg on room air.
7. *Hypoxia*—insufficient oxygen at the cellular level. Causes symptoms reflecting decreased oxygen reaching the brain (i.e., irritability, anxiety, confusion, stupor, coma) and heart (i.e., tachycardia, dysrhythmias). Results from imbalance in oxygen delivery and oxygen consumption.
8. *Ventilation–Perfusion (V/Q) imbalance*—mismatch of ventilation and perfusion. Caused by: (1) blood perfusing an area of the lung where ventilation is reduced or absent, or (2) an excessive amount of blood flow for the amount of ventilation present. Cause of hypoxemia.
9. *Dead space* (V_D)—ventilation without perfusion.
   a. *Anatomical dead space*—portion of the respiratory tract (nose and mouth to bronchioles) that is ventilated but not perfused by the pulmonary circulation. Normal = 150 ml.
   b. *Alveolar dead space*—alveoli that are ventilated but not perfused as a result of the pulmonary capillaries receiving no blood flow (i.e., pulmonary embolism) or decreased blood flow (i.e., primary pulmonary hypertension, emphysema). Cause of hypoxemia.
10. *Shunt*—perfusion without ventilation.
    a. *Anatomic shunt*—results from deoxygenated blood that has nourished the bronchi mixing with oxygenated blood from the pulmonary capillaries. Anatomic shunt constitutes a small portion (2%–3%) of cardiac output.
    b. *Capillary shunt*—results from blood perfusing nonventilated alveoli. This blood cannot be oxygenated blood because no gas exchange occurs. Caused by conditions that lead to alveolar collapse (i.e., atelectasis) or fill the alveoli with fluid (i.e., adult respiratory distress syndrome, pneumonia, pulmonary edema). Intrapulmonary shunting is a major cause of hypoxemia in patients with acute lung disease.

Abbreviations

$PACO_2$—partial pressure of alveolar carbon dioxide
$PaCO_2$—partial pressure of arterial carbon dioxide
PAO_2—partial pressure of alveolar oxygen
PaO_2—partial pressure of arterial oxygen
FIO_2—fractional concentration of oxygen in the inspired air (ambient air 21% or 0.21)
For ventilatory function test symbols, see Table 10-1 page 163.
SaO_2—arterial oxygen saturation
SvO_2—venous oxygen saturation

Respiratory Failure and Insufficiency

Lung Function

The major function of the lung is to supply oxygen and remove carbon dioxide. When gas exchange becomes inadequate, changes occur in the amount of O_2 and CO_2 transported in the arterial blood. Changes in PaO_2 and $PaCO_2$ can be determined by analyzing a sample of the patient's arterial blood. Changes in SaO_2 and SvO_2 can be determined by oximetry. (See p. 212.) The degree of change (mild, moderate, severe), parameters that change (O_2, CO_2, or both), and rapidity of change (acute, chronic) define the type of respiratory failure experienced.

Pathophysiology

Development of respiratory failure can be conceptualized as a continuum, with progression from normal respiratory function → respiratory insufficiency → respiratory failure.

A. Respiratory Insufficiency

An alteration in the function of the respiratory system that produces clinical symptoms—usually includes dyspnea. The term signifies that respiratory function is abnormal but not sufficiently impaired to cause respiratory failure.

B. Respiratory Failure

An alteration in the function of the respiratory system that causes the PaO_2 to fall below 50 mm. Hg or the $PaCO_2$ to rise above 50 mm. Hg. Respiratory failure is determined by analysis of arterial blood. Patients may experience three types of respiratory failure:

1. *Oxygenation failure*
   a. Characterized by a decrease in PaO_2 and a normal or decreased $PaCO_2$.
   b. Primary problem is inability to adequately oxygenate the blood, resulting in hypoxemia.
   c. Hypoxemia occurs because damage to the alveolar–capillary membrane causes leakage of fluid into the interstitial space or into the alveoli and slows or prevents movement of oxygen from the alveoli to the pulmonary capillary blood. Typically this damage is widespread, resulting in many areas of the lung being poorly ventilated or nonventilated. Consequences are severe ventilation–perfusion imbalance and shunt.
   d. Hypocapnia results from hypoxemia and decreased pulmonary compliance. Fluid within the lungs makes the lung less compliant (stiffer). This change in compliance reflexively stimulates the juxtacapillary receptors (J reflex) to increase ventilation. Ventilation is also increased as a response to hypoxemia. Ultimately, if treatment is unsuccessful, the $PaCO_2$ will increase, and the patient

will experience both an increase in $PaCO_2$ and a decrease in PaO_2.

2. *Ventilatory failure with normal lungs*
   a. Characterized by an increased $PaCO_2$, a pH less than 7.35, and a decreased PaO_2 with normal or nearly normal lung function.
   b. Primary problem is insufficient respiratory center stimulation or insufficient chest wall movement, resulting in alveolar hypoventilation.
   c. Hypercapnia occurs because impaired neuromuscular function or chest wall expansion limits the amount of carbon dioxide removed from the lungs. In this type of respiratory failure, the primary problem is not the lungs. The patient's minute ventilation (tidal volume times the number of breaths per minute) is insufficient to allow normal alveolar gas exchange.
   d. The CO_2 not excreted by the lungs combines with H_2O to form carbonic acid (H_2CO_3). This predisposes to acidemia and a fall in pH.
   e. Hypoxemia occurs as a consequence of hypercapnia. When the $PaCO_2$ rises, the PaO_2 must fall unless increased amounts of oxygen are added to the inspired air.

3. *Ventilatory failure with intrinsic lung disease*
   a. Characterized by an increased $PaCO_2$, a pH less than 7.35, and a decreased PaO_2 with preexisting lung disease.
   b. Primary problem is acute exacerbation or chronic progression of previously existing lung disease, resulting in CO_2 retention.
   c. Hypercapnia occurs because damage to the lung parenchyma and/or airway obstruction limit the amount of carbon dioxide removed by the lungs. In this type of respiratory failure, the primary problem is preexisting lung disease—usually chronic bronchitis, emphysema, or severe asthma. This limits CO_2 removal from the lungs.
   d. The CO_2 not excreted by the lungs combines with H_2O to form carbonic acid (H_2CO_3). This predisposes to acidemia and a fall in pH.
   e. Hypoxemia occurs as a consequence of hypercapnia. In addition, damage to the lung parenchyma and/or airway obstruction limit the amount of oxygen that enters the pulmonary capillary blood.

Respiratory failure may develop within minutes or hours, or over months or years. A sudden further deterioration in respiratory function may also occur in patients with long-standing respiratory failure. Several additional terms are used to describe these conditions:

C. Acute Respiratory Failure

1. Characterized by hypoxemia (PaO_2 less than 50 mm. Hg) or hypercapnia ($PaCO_2$ greater than 50 mm. Hg) and acidemia (pH less than 7.35).
2. Occurs rapidly, usually in minutes to hours or days.

D. Chronic Respiratory Failure

1. Characterized by hypoxemia (decreased PaO_2) or hypercapnia (increased $PaCO_2$) with a normal pH (7.35–7.40).
2. Occurs over a period of months to years—allows for activation of compensatory mechanisms.

E. Acute and Chronic Respiratory Failure

1. Characterized by an abrupt increase in the degree of hypoxemia or hypercapnia in patients with preexisting chronic respiratory failure.
2. May occur following an acute upper respiratory infection or pneumonia, or without obvious cause.

3. Extent of deterioration is best assessed by comparing the patient's present arterial blood gases with previous arterial blood gases (patient "normals").

NURSING ALERT:

1. Arterial blood gases (ABG) should be obtained whenever the history or signs and symptoms suggest the patient is at risk for developing respiratory failure. Initial and subsequent values should be recorded on a flow sheet so that comparisons can be made over time.
2. Suspect a decrease in PaO_2 or SaO_2 if the patient has symptoms of hypoxia, i.e., irritability, agitation, confusion, stupor, coma, tachycardia or dysrhythmias. Suspect an increase in $PaCO_2$ with symptoms of morning headache, cognitive dysfunction, or confusion.
3. Monitor changes in the pH. Values < 7.35 or >7.45 indicate compensatory mechanisms are not able to keep acid–base balance within normal limits. A change in therapy may be indicated.
4. Need for ABG can be decreased by using an oximeter to continuously monitor the SaO_2. (See Monitoring Oxygen Therapy, p. 212.)
5. Frequent bedside measurements of respiratory rate, vital capacity, inspiratory force, and minute ventilation are helpful in following the progress of patients with ventilatory failure with normal lungs. These data should be recorded on a flow sheet and values compared over time.

Oxygenation Failure

Etiology

1. Cardiogenic pulmonary edema (left ventricular failure; mitral stenosis)
2. Adult respiratory distress syndrome or ARDS (shock of any etiology; infectious causes—gram-negative sepsis, viral pneumonia, bacterial pneumonia; trauma—fat emboli, head injury, lung contusion, aspiration—gastric fluid, near drowning; inhaled toxins—oxygen in high concentrations, smoke, corrosive chemicals; hematologic disorders—massive transfusions, postcardiopulmonary bypass; metabolic disorders—pancreatitis, paraquat ingestion, uremia).

Nursing Assessment

1. Note changes suggesting increased work of breathing (diaphoresis, intercostal muscle retraction) or pulmonary edema (fine, coarse crackles).
2. Determine PaO_2 and SaO_2 and compare with previous values. Typically, the SaO_2 will be $<90\%$ and PaO_2 < 50 mm. Hg on room air, and will increase minimally following administration of oxygen.
3. Determine pH and $PaCO_2$ and compare with previous values. Typically, the $PaCO_2$ will initially be low (25–35 mm. Hg). May become normal or increase if treatment is ineffective.
4. Determine hemodynamic status (blood pressure, pulmonary wedge pressure, cardiac output, SvO_2) and compare with previous values. Therapy (mechanical ventilation, positive end-expiratory pressure [PEEP]) may decrease venous return, resulting in decreased cardiac output.

Nursing Diagnoses

1. Impaired gas exchange related to interstitial edema and alveolar flooding.
2. Potential alteration in fluid volume (excess or deficit) related to underlying disorder (see above).

3. Potential alteration in cardiac output (decreased) related to left ventricular failure.

Nursing Interventions

1. Give specific treatment for underlying disorder (i.e., antibiotics for sepsis and pneumonia; cardiotonics and diuretics for pulmonary edema due to left ventricular failure).
2. Administer oxygen to maintain PaO_2 of 60 mm. Hg or $SaO_2 > 90\%$ using devices that provide increased oxygen concentrations (aerosol mask, partial rebreathing mask, nonrebreathing mask).
3. If these values cannot be achieved with devices described above or if inspired oxygen concentration required is greater than 60% for 24 hours, patient may require intubation and the use of positive end-expiratory pressure (PEEP) with mechanical ventilation.
4. Monitor fluid balance by direct measurement of pulmonary capillary wedge pressure to detect presence of hypo/hypervolemia.

Evaluation

1. Demonstrates reversal of symptomatology related to underlying disorder
2. Achieves normal PaO_2 and $PaCO_2$ without use of mechanical ventilation/supplemental oxygen
3. Maintains adequate cardiac output and fluid balance

Ventilatory Failure With Normal Lungs

Etiology

1. Insufficient respiratory center activity (drug intoxication—drug overdose, general anesthesia; vascular disorders—cerebral vascular insufficiency, cerebral tumor; trauma—head injury, increased intracranial pressure)
2. Insufficient chest wall function (neuromuscular disease—Guillain–Barré, myasthenia gravis, poliomyelitis, demyelinating disease, muscular dystrophy; trauma to the chest wall resulting in multiple fractures; spinal cord trauma; kyphoscoliosis)

Nursing Assessment

1. Assess breath sounds
   a. Diminished or absent sounds indicate inability to ventilate the lungs sufficiently to prevent atelectasis.
   b. Crackles indicate ineffective airway clearance.
2. Determine V_c, respiratory rate, V_E, and NIF and compare with values indicating need for mechanical ventilation:
   a. $V_c < 10–15$ ml./kg.
   b. Respiratory rate > 35/min
   c. $V_E > 10$ L./min
   d. NIF < -20 to -25 cm. H_2O.
3. Determine ABG and compare with previous values.
   a. If the patient cannot maintain a minute ventilation sufficient to prevent CO_2 retention, the pH will fall.
   b. Mechanical ventilation may be needed if the pH falls to <7.30.

Patient Problems/Nursing Diagnoses

1. Impaired gas exchange related to inadequate respiratory center activity or chest wall movement
2. Potential alteration in airway clearance related to inability to cough and breathe deeply

3. Impaired physical mobility related to underlying disorder (see above)

Nursing Interventions

1. Give specific treatment for cause of respiratory failure (i.e., narcotic antagonist for narcotic or narcotic analogue intoxication, pyridostigmine for myasthenia gravis).
2. Initiate measures to prevent atelectasis and promote chest expansion and secretion clearance (incentive spirometer, intermittent positive pressure breathing, out of bed, or head of bed elevated 30 degrees).
3. Monitor adequacy of alveolar ventilation by frequent measurement of respiratory rate, vital capacity, and inspiratory force and ABG.
4. If respiratory rate is >35/minute, vital capacity < 15 ml./kg. body weight, or inspiratory force is less than -25 cm. H_2O, the patient may require intubation and mechanical ventilation.
5. Compare monitored values with criteria indicating need for mechanical ventilation (See Nursing Assessment). Alert the physician and prepare to assist with intubation and initiation of mechanical ventilation, if indicated.

Evaluation

1. Demonstrates reversal of or no further deterioration in symptomatology related to underlying disorder.
2. Prevents development of atelectasis and secretion retention: coughs and breathes deeply at frequent intervals
3. Regains or maintains optimal physical mobility

Ventilatory Failure With Intrinsic Lung Disease

Etiology

1. Chronic obstructive pulmonary disease or COPD (chronic bronchitis, emphysema, cystic fibrosis)
2. Severe asthma

Nursing Assessment

1. Determine ABG and compare with previous values.
   a. If the patient cannot maintain a minute ventilation sufficient to prevent CO_2 retention, the pH will fall.
   b. Mechanical ventilation may be needed if the pH falls to <7.30.
2. Assess level of consciousness and ability to tolerate increased work of breathing.
   a. Confusion, rapid shallow breathing, abdominal paradox (inward movement of abdominal wall during inspiration), and intercostal retractions suggest inability to maintain adequate minute ventilation.
   b. Mechanical ventilation may be indicated.
3. Assess breath sounds.
   a. Wheezing indicates bronchospasm.
   b. Rhonchi and crackles indicate ineffective secretion clearance.

Nursing Diagnoses

1. Ineffective airway clearance related to increased or tenacious secretions.

2. Impaired gas exchange related to lung parenchyma damage and/or airway obstruction.
3. Alteration in fluid volume (excess) related to right ventricular failure.

Nursing Interventions

1. Administer oxygen at 24%–38% by Venturi mask, or 1–2 liters per minute by nasal cannula.
2. Initiate measures to increase alveolar ventilation—bronchodilators to reduce bronchospasm (Table 11-1), corticosteroids to reduce airway inflammation, chest physiotherapy to remove mucus, slow respiratory rate with pursed-lips breathing.
3. Give specific treatment for cause of the exacerbation (i.e., antibiotics for respiratory infection).
4. Administer intravenous fluids to reduce sputum viscosity.
5. If the patient becomes increasingly lethargic, cannot cough or expectorate secretions, cannot cooperate with therapy, or if pH falls below 7.30, despite use of the above therapy; intubation and mechanical ventilation may be required. Alert the physician and prepare to assist with intubation and initiation of mechanical ventilation, if indicated.

Evaluation

1. Demonstrates ability to clear airway of secretions (decrease in volume and tenacity of respiratory secretions)
2. Achieves blood gas values that are within the patient's normal limits
3. Demonstrates normal fluid balance

Oxygen Delivery

General Considerations

1. Oxygen is an odorless, tasteless, colorless, transparent gas that is slightly heavier than air.
2. Because oxygen supports combustion, there is always danger of fire when oxygen is being used.
   a. Avoid using oil or grease around oxygen connections.
   b. Post "NO SMOKING" signs on the patient's door and in view of the patient's visitors.
3. Oxygen can be dispensed from a cylinder, piped-in system, liquid oxygen reservoir, or oxygen concentrator. Oxygen is administered:
   a. At the prescribed flow rate or per cent, or
   b. According to previously written standards of care for patients at risk for hypoxemia.
4. Oxygen is given to relieve hypoxemia or hypoxia.
   a. *Hypoxemia*—present when the oxygen tension in arterial blood is below normal.
   b. *Hypoxia*—present when there is an insufficient amount of oxygen available in the tissue cells to meet the requirements of an organ or tissue at that moment.

Nursing Assessment

1. Suspect need for oxygen when patients predisposed to impaired gas exchange have:
   a. Tachypnea
   b. Tachycardia or dysrhythmias (premature ventricular contractions)
   c. A change in level of consciousness (symptoms of

Table 11-1. *Drugs Commonly Used to Prevent or Reverse Bronchospasm*

Drugs/Administration	Pharmacologic Effects	Indications	Undesired Effects	Nursing Implications
Bronchodilators				
Aminophylline (intravenous injection)	Methyl xanthine compound—relaxes smooth muscle by increasing level of cyclic adenosine monophosphate	Acute exacerbation of asthma or bronchitis	CNS—irritability, restlessness, insomnia CV—palpitations, tachycardia, hypotension GI—nausea, vomiting, diarrhea	Too rapid administration can cause hypotension, extra systoles, muscle tremors. Administer at prescribed rate with an intravenous infusion pump.
Theophylline preparations (oral)	Methyl xanthine compound—relaxes muscle by increasing cyclic adenosine monophosphate	Maintenance therapy for bronchospasm	CNS—irritability, restlessness, insomnia CV—palpitations, tachycardia, hypotension GI—nausea, vomiting, diarrhea	Teach patients to take at equal intervals throughout the day. To decrease GI irritation, take with milk or crackers.
Epinephrine (subcutaneous injection)	Sympathomimetic—acts on alpha (vasoconstrictor), $beta_1$ (cardiac stimulation), and $beta_2$ (bronchial smooth muscle relaxation) receptors	Acute exacerbation of asthma or bronchitis	Tachycardia, dysrhythmias, elevation of blood pressure, headache, nausea, vomiting, paradoxical increase in bronchospasm	Use with extreme caution in patients who are elderly or who have heart or thyroid disease; stop treatment and monitor pulse and blood pressure if undesired effects occur.
Terbutaline (oral, metered-dose inhaler, subcutaneous injection)	Sympathomimetic with selective $beta_2$ activity	Acute exacerbation of asthma or bronchitis (subcutaneous preparation) Maintenance therapy for bronchospasm (inhaled and oral preparation)	Nervousness, tachycardia, headache, nausea (subcutaneous preparation) Hand tremors (subcutaneous and oral preparations)	Caution patients that hand tremors may occur. Tremors decrease with prolonged oral use.
Metaproterenol (oral, metered-dose inhaler, inhalant solution)	Sympathomimetic with selective $beta_2$ activity	Maintenance therapy for bronchospasm	Rare	Observe inhalation by patient to be certain that correct technique is used.
Albuterol (oral, metered-dose inhaler)	Sympathomimetic with highly selective $beta_2$ activity	Maintenance therapy for bronchospasm	Rare	Observe inhalation by patient to be certain that correct technique is used.
Pirbuterol acetate (metered-dose inhaler)	Sympathomimetic with selective $beta_2$ activity	Maintenance therapy for bronchospasm	Rare	Observe inhalation by patient to be certain that correct technique is used.
Ipratopium bromide (metered-dose inhaler)	Anticholinergic	Maintenance therapy for bronchospasm	Rare. Can cause blurring of vision if sprayed into the eyes (atropine derivative)	Instruct patient to close lips around inhaler mouthpiece, close eyes during inhalation.
Corticosteroids				
Hydrocortisone/prednisone (intravenous injection, oral preparation)	Potent anti-inflammatory activity	Acute exacerbation of asthma or bronchitis (IV preparation) Maintenance therapy (oral preparation)	CNS—depression, euphoria GI—gastric irritation, peptic ulcer Metabolic—hypernatremia, hypokalemia	Should not be abruptly discontinued, as causes suppression of adrenal function.
Beclomethasone (metered-dose inhaler)	Synthetic corticosteroid with potent anti-inflammatory activity; effective only by inhalation	Asthma (alternative to use of oral steroids) COPD	Oral candidiasis Systemic side effects associated with oral steroids do not occur	Inhaled as a powder. May precipitate bronchospasm in acute exacerbation. Not used with status asthmaticus or acute asthma episodes.
Triamcinolone acetonide (metered-dose inhaler)	Anti-inflammatory steroid; effective only by inhalation.	Asthma COPD	Oral candidiasis No systemic side effects.	Packaged with a spacer. Decreases oral deposition and oral candidiasis.
Flunisolide (metered-dose inhaler)	Anti-inflammatory steroid; effective only by inhalation.	Asthma COPD	Oral candidiasis No systemic side effects.	Longer-acting. May be prescribed twice a day, rather than four times a day.
Miscellaneous				
Cromolyn sodium (solution for inhalation, powder used with special inhaler)	Inhibits release of histamine, from mast cells in the respiratory tract, *prevents* bronchospasm Not effective in acute attack; must be used for 2–4 weeks to show effectiveness	Maintenance therapy for asthma	Cough, bronchospasm	Should not be used with status asthmaticus or acute asthma episodes. May be given in combination with bronchodilator if administration causes bronchospasm.

decreased cerebral oxygenation are irritability, confusion, lethargy, and coma, if untreated)

2. Early use of oxygen therapy may prevent development of:
   a. Cyanosis—occurs as a late sign ($PaO_2 \leq 45$ mm. Hg)
   b. Labored respirations—indicates severe respiratory distress
   c. Myocardial stress—increase in heart rate and stroke volume (cardiac output) is the primary mechanism for compensation for hypoxemia or hypoxia.

3. Monitor response to oxygen therapy by oximetry.
   a. Oximeters function by passing a light beam through a vascular bed, such as the finger or earlobe. The oximeter determines the amount of light absorbed by oxygenated (red) and deoxygenated (blue) blood, calculates the SaO_2, and displays this as a digital value.
   b. Is indicated when
      (1) the patient is unstable and may experience sudden changes in blood oxygen level.
      (2) evaluating need for home oxygen therapy.
      (3) no conditions exist that alter light absorption, i.e., increased bilirubin, increased carboxyhemoglobin, low perfusion or $SaO_2 < 80\%$.

NURSING ALERT:

1. If the SaO_2 drops below 80%, the reading displayed by the oximeter may vary by $\pm 2\%$ from the actual SaO_2. Oximeters rely on differences in light absorption to determine SaO_2. At lower saturations, oxygenated hemoglobin appears more blue in color and is less easily distinguished from deoxygenated hemoglobin. ABG should be used in this situation.
2. If the blood is carrying carboxyhemoglobin (carbon monoxide inhalation), the reading will be falsely high. The oximeter cannot distinguish carboxyhemoglobin, which is cherry red in color, from well-oxygenated blood, which also is red in color. Arterial blood gases (ABG) should be used in this situation.
3. ABG require analysis of arterial blood and predispose the patient to risks associated with invasive monitoring. However, they are the most accurate method of assessing response to oxygen therapy.
4. Indicated when:
   a. the patient is at risk for CO_2 retention. Oximeters do not provide information about acid–base balance (pH, $PaCO_2$).
   b. conditions exist that may make oximetry inaccurate.

Nursing Interventions

1. Select the appropriate form of oxygen therapy after obtaining arterial blood gases (ABG) and assessing the patient's current oxygenation status and acid–base balance. Choices are:
   a. Low concentration (24%–28%)—appropriate for patients prone to retain carbon dioxide (chronic obstructive pulmonary disease, drug overdose). Such patients may be dependent on hypoxemia (hypoxic drive) to maintain respiration. If hypoxemia is suddenly reversed, hypoxic drive may be lost. Respiratory arrest may then occur.
   b. High concentration ($\geq 30\%$)—appropriate in patients not predisposed to carbon dioxide retention.
2. Monitor response to therapy by oximetry. If the patient has hypercapnia, ABG monitoring is needed to assess CO_2 retention.
3. Increase or decrease the inspired oxygen concentration (FiO_2), as appropriate.

Evaluation

Responds to oxygen therapy successfully by attaining desired SaO_2, PaO_2, and $PaCO_2$, adequate tissue oxygenation, decreased work of breathing.

Oxygen Delivery Systems

1. Oxygen may be administered by nasal cannula, transtracheal catheter, or various types of face masks. It also may be applied directly to endotracheal or tracheal tube via a mechanical ventilator, T-piece, or hyperinflation bag.
2. The method selected depends on the required concentration of oxygen, desired variability in delivered oxygen concentration (none, minimal, moderate), and required ventilatory assistance (mechanical ventilator, spontaneous breathing).

Guidelines Administering Oxygen by Nasal Cannula (Fig. 11-1)

Equipment

Oxygen source
Plastic nasal cannula with connecting tubing (disposable)
Humidifier filled with sterile distilled water to indicated level
Flowmeter
"NO SMOKING" signs

Assessment	Nursing Action	Rationale/Amplification
	1. Determine current vital signs, level of consciousness, and most recent ABG.	1. Provides a baseline for future assessment. Nasal cannula oxygen administration is often used for patients prone to CO_2 retention. Oxygen may depress the hypoxic drive of these patients (evidenced by a decreased respiratory rate, altered mental status, and further $PaCO_2$ elevation).
	2. Assess risk for CO_2 retention with oxygen administration.	2. **Note:** If $PaCO_2$ is decreased or normal, the patient is not experiencing CO_2 retention and can use oxygen without fear of the above consequences.
Planning/Implementation	1. Post "NO SMOKING" signs on the patient's door and in view of patient and visitors.	
	2. Show the nasal cannula to the patient and explain the procedure.	
	3. Make sure that the humidifier is filled to the appropriate mark.	3. Humidification may not be ordered if the flow rate is ≤ 4 L./min.

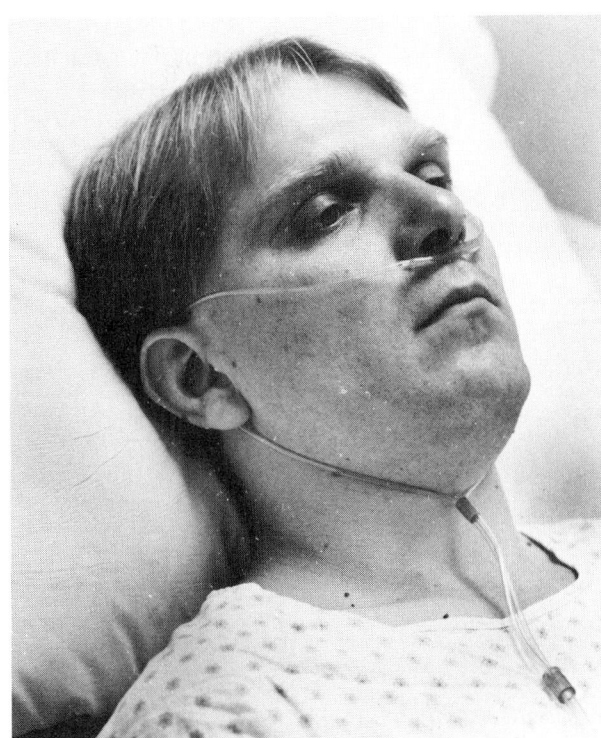

Figure 11-1. *Administering oxygen by nasal cannula. Patient's inspiration consists of a mixture of supplemental oxygen supplied via the nasal cannula and room air. Oxygen concentration is variable and depends on patient's tidal volume and ventilatory pattern. (Courtesy of Photography Department, Montefiore Hospital, Pittsburgh, PA)*

Planning/Implementation
(continued)

4. Attach the connecting tube from the nasal cannula to the humidifier outlet.
5. Set the flow rate at prescribed liters/minute. Feel to determine if oxygen is flowing through the tips of the cannula.

5. Because a nasal cannula is a low-flow system (patient's tidal volume supplies part of the inspired gas), oxygen concentration will vary, depending on the patient's respiratory rate and tidal volume. Approximate oxygen concentrations delivered are:

   1 liter = 24%–25%
   2 liters = 27%–29%
   3 liters = 30%–33%
   4 liters = 33%–37%
   5 liters = 36%–41%
   6 liters = 39%–45%

NURSING ALERT: Patients who require low, constant concentrations of oxygen and whose breathing pattern varies greatly may need to use a Venturi mask, particularly if they are carbon dioxide retainers.

6. Place the tips of the cannula in the patient's nose.

Evaluation/Outcome

1. Record flow rate used and immediate patient response.

2. Assess patient's condition, ABG or SaO_2, and the functioning of equipment at regular intervals.

3. Determine patient comfort with oxygen use.

1. Note the patient's tolerance of treatment. Notify the physician if intolerance is noted.

2. Depression of hypoxic drive is most likely to occur within the first hours of oxygen use. Monitoring of SaO_2 with oximetry can be substituted for ABG if the patient is not retaining CO_2.

3. Flow rates in excess of 4 liters/minute may cause irritation to the nasal and pharyngeal mucosa.

Guidelines Administering Oxygen by Transtracheal Catheter (Fig. 11-2)

Transtracheal oxygen delivery is accomplished via a small (8 Fr) catheter inserted between the second and third tracheal cartilage. The catheter does not interfere with talking, drinking, or eating and can be concealed under a shirt or blouse. Oxygen delivery is more efficient because all oxygen enters the lungs. Patients who meet criteria for continuous home oxygen therapy ($PaO_2 < 55$ mm. Hg on room air or <59 mm. Hg with evidence of right heart failure) may use this delivery method instead of nasal cannula delivery.

Equipment

Oxygen source
Transtracheal catheter with connecting tubing
Humidifier filled with sterile distilled water to indicated level
Flowmeter
"NO SMOKING" signs

Assessment

Nursing Action	Rationale/Amplification
1. Determine current vital signs, level of consciousness, and ABG, if patient is at risk for CO_2 retention.	1. Provides a baseline for future assessment.
2. Note evidence of infection (warmth, redness swelling at insertion site) or temperature elevation.	2. The transtracheal catheter provides a direct communication between the skin and trachea. If the insertion site is not kept clean and dry, infection can develop.
3. Assess catheter patency. Obstruction is indicated by a decreased SaO_2, whistling of the humidifier, high pressure in the delivery tubing, or stimulation of a cough.	3. Mucus can form on the end of the catheter and restrict oxygen delivery. This increases pressure in the delivery tubing and humidifier. The mucus may touch the back of the trachea, stimulating a cough.

Planning/Implementation

Stent Phase (Fig. 11-2A)

1. Instruct the patient in purpose of stent.	1. The stent is used to maintain a patent tract during the first week after catheter insertion. It facilitates tract healing and allows gradual adjustment to use of the catheter. It is not used for oxygen delivery.
2. Teach that care of stent involves daily cleaning of the site with cotton-tipped applicators and observation for signs of infection. A 4 × 4 may be placed over the stent.	2. Until the tract heals, the patient is at increased risk for infection. Because the stent is open to the trachea, mucus may be coughed from the stent.

Immature Tract (stent is removed and transtracheal catheter inserted) (Figs. 11-2B and 11-2C)

1. Instruct patient in cleaning and irrigation procedure. The patient should inject one half (1.5 ml.) ampule of NSS into the catheter, insert and remove the cleaning rod 3 times, and inject the remaining NSS 2–3 times a day (morning, noon, evening).	1. The catheter cannot be removed from the tract for cleaning until the tract completely heals (about 2 months). Cleaning in place helps to prevent mucus from forming on the end of the catheter and obstructing oxygen delivery.
2. Teach the patient use of the staged cough technique, i.e., sit with feet on floor, pillow over abdomen, inhale 3–4 times in through the nose and out through the mouth, on the last exhalation cough while bending forward with pillow against abdomen.	2. Use of this cough technique helps to increase airflow during coughing. Higher airflows help to dislodge any mucus that has formed on the outside of the catheter and cannot be removed by the cleaning technique.
3. Instruct the patient to clean the insertion site daily with cotton-tipped applicators and report signs of infection.	3. Mucus may form at the insertion site. Keeping the tract clean and dry decreases infection risk.
4. Teach the patient to place two small strips of transparent tape over the chain on either side of the catheter for the first 2 weeks of catheter use.	4. This helps to keep the catheter in place during the night when the patient is sleeping. Serves as a second security system to keep the catheter from being inadvertently pulled from the tract during the initial adjustment phase.
5. Instruct the patient to replace the nasal cannula and call for instructions if the catheter is displaced from the tract or if symptoms of subcutaneous emphysema develop (swelling at insertion site, tight chain, change in voice).	5. If the catheter comes out of the tract before it is mature, reinsertion may be difficult. If the tract is not completely healed, O_2 may enter the tissues around the insertion site. The patient may need to return to the clinic for assistance in replacing the catheter or delay using it until the tract is fully healed.

Mature Tract (catheter is removed for cleaning) (Fig 11-2D)

1. Instruct the patient in steps involved in removing the catheter from the tract for cleaning. Two catheters are used. The catheter in the tract is removed and replaced with a second catheter. The catheter removed from the tract is cleaned with antibacterial soap under warm running water. It then is air-dried and stored for reuse.	1. The catheter should easily enter the tract. Practicing while looking in a mirror helps to develop skill in removing and reinserting the catheter. This step should be performed twice daily if a catheter with multiple side holes (SCOOP 2) is used. Removal daily, or less often, is necessary with a single end hole catheter (SCOOP 1).

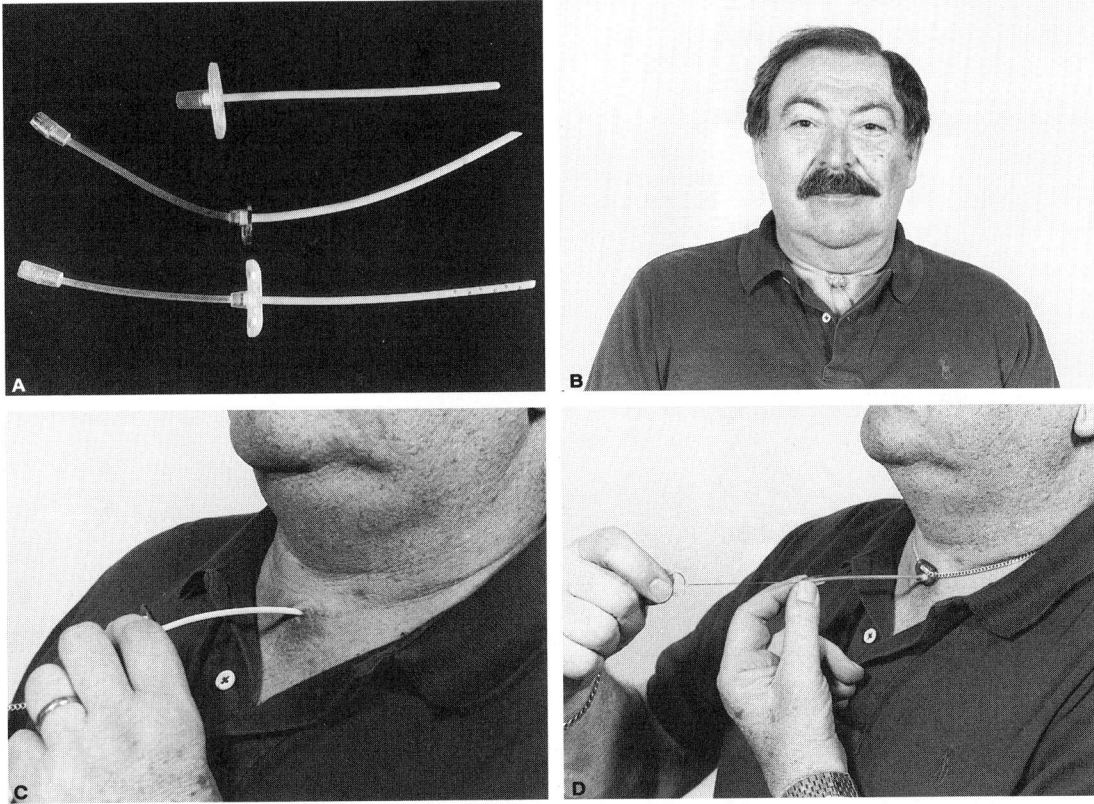

Figure 11-2. *Administering oxygen by transtracheal catheter. (A) Stent (upper), SCOOP 1 (middle), and SCOOP 2 (lower) catheter. (B) Transtracheal catheter in place. (C) While the tract is immature, the catheter is irrigated and cleaned 2 or 3 times a day with a cleaning rod. (D) When the tract is mature, the catheter can be removed from the tract for cleaning. (Courtesy of Medical Media Department, Veterans Administration Medical Center, Pittsburgh, PA)*

Planning/Im-plementation *(continued)*	2. Instruct the patient to report signs of infection and difficulty immediately replacing the catheter.	2. These problems are less common with a mature tract, but can still occur.
Evaluation/ Outcome	1. Record flow rate of oxygen used and patient response.	1. Transtracheal oxygen delivery is more efficient. The same SaO_2 is typically maintained at one half of the former flow rate.
	2. Determine patient ability to perform care independently.	2. Repeat demonstration of care may be required before the patient masters self-care skills.

Guidelines   Administering Oxygen by Venturi Mask (Figs. 11-3 and 11-4) (High air flow oxygen entrainment [HAFOE] system)

Underlying Principles

1. To ensure precise control of the oxygen concentration, total gas flow at the patient's face must meet or exceed peak inspiratory flow rate. When mask output does not meet inspiratory flow rate, room air (drawn through mask side holes) mixes with the gas mixture provided by the face mask, lowering the inspired oxygen concentration.
2. The Venturi mask mixes a fixed flow of oxygen with a high but variable flow of air to produce a constant oxygen concentration. Oxygen enters via a jet (restricted opening) at a high velocity. Room air also enters and mixes with oxygen at this site. The higher the velocity (smaller the opening), the more room air is drawn into the mask. Mask output ranges from approximately 97 liters/minute (24%) to approximately 33 liters/minute (50%).
3. Excess gas leaves through openings in the mask, carrying with it the expired carbon dioxide; this virtually eliminates rebreathing of carbon dioxide.

(continued)

Guidelines Administering Oxygen by Venturi Mask (Figs. 11-3 and 11-4) (High air flow oxygen entrainment [HAFOE] system) *(continued)*

Equipment Oxygen source
Flowmeter
Venturi mask for correct concentration (24%, 28%, 31%, 35%, 40%, 50%) or correct concentration adapter if interchangeable color-coded adapters are used
If high humidity desired:
    Compressed air source and flowmeter
    Nebulizer with sterile distilled water
    Large-bore tubing
"NO SMOKING" signs

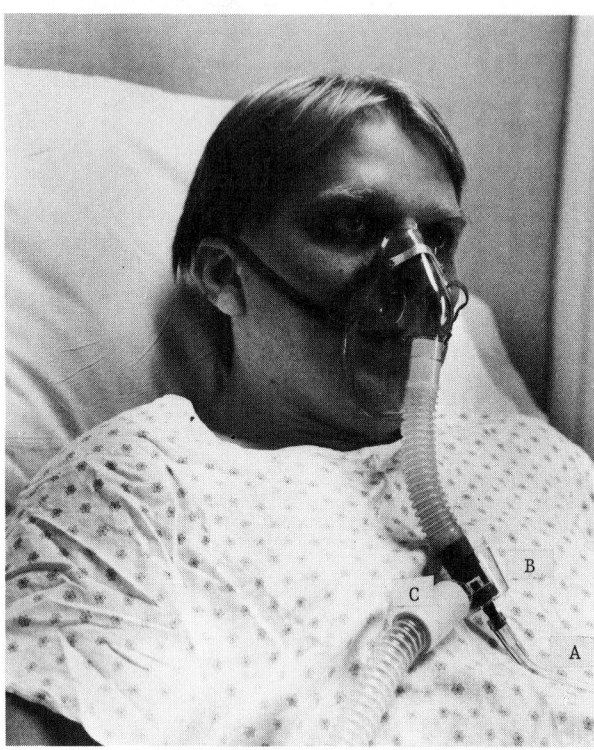

Figure 11-3. *Administering oxygen by Venturi mask. Oxygen (A) is diluted to a precise inspired oxygen concentration (24%–50%) by room air as it enters the specially constructed openings (B) of the mask. Additional humidity can be supplied via a humidification port (C), which is connected to a nebulizer and compressed air source. (Courtesy of Photography Department, Montefiore Hospital, Pittsburgh, PA)*

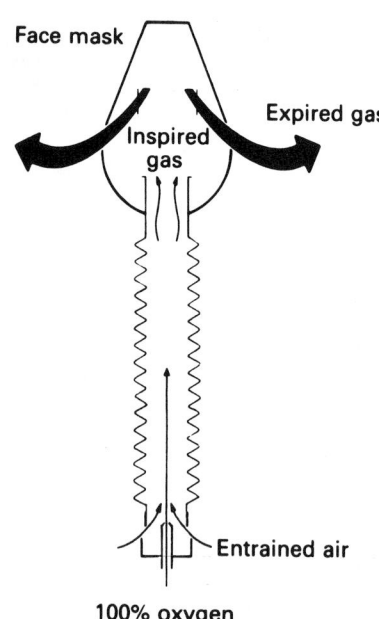

Figure 11-4. *Air flow diagram with Venturi mask. Arrows indicate direction of flow. (Burton GC and Hodgkin JE [eds]. Respiratory Care: A Guide to Practice. 2nd ed. Philadelphia, JB Lippincott, 1984)*

Assessment	Nursing Action	Rationale/Amplification
	1. Determine current vital signs, level of consciousness, and most recent ABG.	1. Provides a baseline for future assessment. Venturi masks are used for patients prone to CO_2 retention. Oxygen may depress the hypoxic drive of these patients (evidenced by a decreased respiratory rate, altered mental status, and further $PaCO_2$ elevation).
	2. Assess risk for CO_2 retention with oxygen administration.	2. Risk is greater if the patient is experiencing an exacerbation of his illness.
Planning/Im-plementation	1. Post "NO SMOKING" signs on the door of the patient's room and in view of patient and visitors.	
	2. Show the Venturi mask to the patient and explain the procedure.	

Planning/Implementation
(continued)

3. Connect the mask by lightweight tubing to the oxygen source.
4. Turn on the oxygen flowmeter and adjust to the prescribed rate (usually indicated on the mask). Check to see that oxygen is flowing out the vent holes in the mask.

5. Place Venturi mask over the patient's nose and mouth and under the chin. Adjust elastic strap.
6. Check to make sure holes for air entry are not obstructed by the patient's bedding.
7. If high humidity is used:
   a. Connect the nebulizer to a compressed air source.
   b. Attach large-bore tubing to the nebulizer and connect the tubing to the fitting for high humidity at the base of the Venturi mask.

4. To ensure the correct air/oxygen mix, oxygen must be set at the prescribed flow rate. Prescribed flow rates differ for different oxygen concentrations. Usually this information is printed on the mask or interchangeable color-coded adapter.

6. Proper mask function depends on mixing of sufficient amount of air and oxygen.
7. When a Venturi mask is used with high humidity, both an oxygen source and compressed air source are required. The compressed air source provides air for the air/oxygen mix. Excessive oxygen would be inspired if both tubings were connected to an oxygen source.

Evaluation/Outcome

1. Record flow rate used and immediate patient response.

2. If CO_2 retention is present, assess ABG every 30 minutes for 1–2 hours or until the PaO_2 is >50 mm. Hg and the $PaCO_2$ is no longer increasing. Monitor pH. Notify the physician if the pH decreases below the initial assessment value.
3. Determine patient comfort with oxygen use.

1. Note the patient's tolerance of treatment. Notify the physician if intolerance occurs. Depression of hypoxic drive is most likely to occur within the first hours of oxygen use.
2. A modest (5–10 mm. Hg) increase in $PaCO_2$ may occur after initiation of oxygen therapy. A decreasing pH indicates failure of compensatory mechanisms. Mechanical ventilation may be required.
3. Venturi masks are best tolerated for relatively short periods because of their size and appearance. They also must be removed for eating and drinking. With improvement in patient condition, a nasal cannula may often be substituted.

Guidelines — Administering Oxygen by Simple Face Mask With/Without Aerosol (Fig. 11-5)

Equipment

Oxygen source
Nebulizer bottle with sterile distilled water, if high humidity is desired
Plastic aerosol mask
Large-bore tubing (high humidity) or small-bore tubing
Flowmeter
"NO SMOKING" signs
For heated aerosol therapy:
   Nebulizer heating element

Assessment	**Nursing Action**	**Rationale/Amplification**
	1. Determine current vital signs, level of consciousness, and SaO_2 or ABG, if patient is at risk for CO_2 retention.	1. Because the aerosol face mask is a low-flow system (patient's tidal volume may supply part of inspired gas), oxygen concentration will vary depending on the patient's respiratory rate and rhythm. Oxygen delivery may be inadequate for tachypneic patients (flow does not meet peak inspiratory demand) or excessive for patients with slow respirations.
	2. Assess viscosity and volume of sputum produced.	2. Aerosol is given to assist in mobilizing retained secretions.
Planning/Implementation	1. Post "NO SMOKING" signs on patient's door and in view of the patient and visitors.	
	2. Show the aerosol mask to the patient and explain the procedure.	
	3. Make sure the nebulizer is filled to the appropriate mark.	3. If the nebulizer bottle is not sufficiently full, less moisture will be delivered.
	4. Attach the large-bore tubing from the mask to the nebulizer outlet.	
	5. Set desired oxygen concentration on nebulizer bottle and plug in the heating element, if used.	5. The inspired oxygen concentration is determined by the nebulizer setting. Usual percentages are 35%–50%.

(continued)

Guidelines Administering Oxygen by Simple Face Mask With/Without Aerosol (Fig. 11-5) *(continued)*

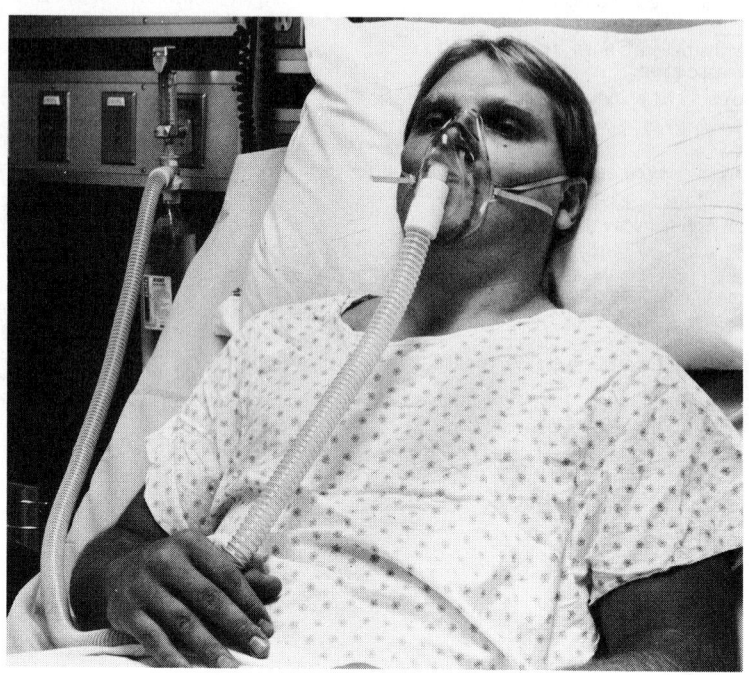

Figure 11-5. *Administering oxygen by simple face mask with aerosol. Simple face masks are inexpensive and relatively comfortable and often are used when the patient requires humidification or aerosol therapy with oxygen. (Courtesy of Photography Department, Montefiore Hospital, Pittsburgh, PA)*

Planning/Implementation *(continued)*	Nursing Action	Rationale/Amplification
	6. If the patient is tachypneic and a concentration of 50% oxygen or greater is desired, two nebulizers and flow-meters should be yoked together.	6. The aerosol mask is a low-flow system. Yoking two nebulizers together doubles nebulizer flow but does *not* change the inspired oxygen concentration.
	7. Adjust the flow rate until the desired mist is produced (usually 10–12 liters/minute).	7. This ensures that the patient is receiving flow sufficient to meet inspiratory demand and maintains a constant accurate concentration of oxygen.
	8. Apply the mask to the patient's face and adjust the straps so that the mask fits securely.	
	9. Drain the tubing frequently by emptying condensate into a separate receptacle, not into the nebulizer. If a heating element is used, the tubing will have to be drained more often.	9. The tubing must be kept free of condensate. Condensate allowed to accumulate in the delivery tube will block flow and alter oxygen concentration. If condensate is emptied into the nebulizer, bacteria may be aerosolized into the lungs.
	10. If a heating element is used, check the temperature. The nebulizer bottle should be warm, not hot, to touch.	10. Excessive temperatures can cause airway burns; patients with elevated temperatures should be humidified with an unheated device.
Evaluation/Outcome	1. Record inspired oxygen concentration and immediate patient response.	1. Note the patient's tolerance of treatment. Notify the physician if intolerance occurs.
	2. Assess the patient's condition and the functioning of equipment at regular intervals.	2. Assess the patient for change in mental status, diaphoresis, changes in blood pressure, and increasing heart and respiratory rates.
	3. If the patient's condition changes, assess SaO_2 or ABG.	3. If the patient has a high minute ventilation, flow from the mask may not be sufficient to meet inspiratory needs without pulling in room air. Room air will dilute the oxygen provided and lower the inspired oxygen concentration, resulting in hypoxemia. A change in mask or delivery system may be indicated.
	4. Record changes in volume and tenacity of sputum produced.	4. Indicates effectiveness of therapy

Guidelines Administering Oxygen by Partial Rebreathing or Nonrebreathing Mask (Figs. 11-6 and 11-7)

A *partial rebreathing mask* (Figs. 11-6 and 11-7*A*) has an inflatable bag that stores 100% oxygen. On inspiration, the patient inhales from the mask and bag; on expiration, the bag refills with oxygen. Perforations on both sides of the mask serve as exhalation ports. High concentrations of oxygen are indicated in the acute phase of some diseases (pneumonia, pulmonary edema, pulmonary embolism).

A *nonrebreathing mask* (Fig. 11-7*B*) has (1) an inflatable bag to store 100% oxygen, (2) a one-way valve between the bag and mask to prevent exhaled air from entering the bag (diverts it into the atmosphere), (3) one-way valves covering one or both exhalation ports to prevent entry of room air on inspiration, and (4) flap or spring-loaded valves to permit entry of room air should the oxygen source fail or patient needs exceed the available oxygen flow. Optimally, all the patient's inspiratory volume will be provided by the mask/reservoir, allowing delivery of nearly 100% oxygen.

Equipment

Oxygen source
Plastic face mask with reservoir bag and tubing
Humidifier with distilled water
Flowmeter
"NO SMOKING" signs

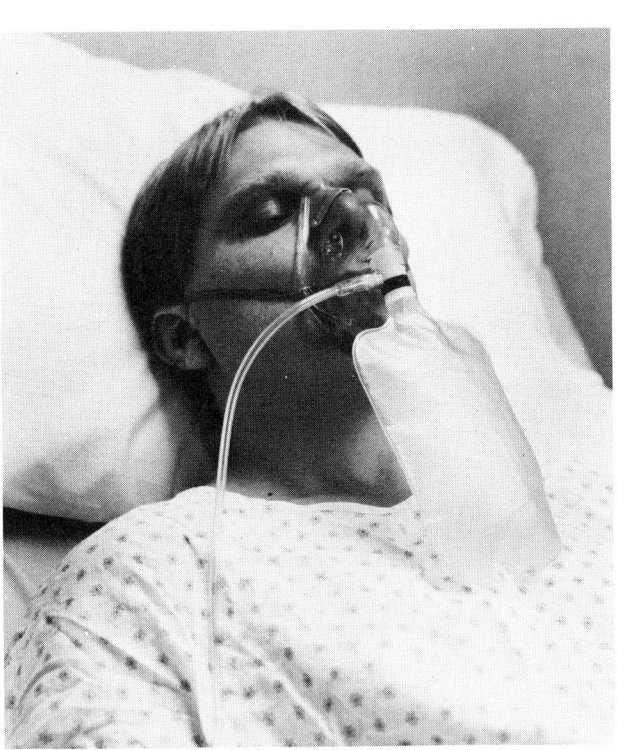

Figure 11-6. *Administering oxygen via a partial rebreathing mask. Liter flow is adjusted so that the rebreathing bag does not collapse even with deep inspiration. This prevents expired carbon dioxide from entering the bag. (Courtesy of Photography Department, Montefiore Hospital, Pittsburgh, PA)*

	Nursing Action	**Rationale/Amplification**
Assessment	1. Determine current vital signs, level of consciousness.	1. Provides a baseline for evaluating patient response. Typically used for short-term support of patients who require a high inspired oxygen concentration.
	2. Determine most recent SaO_2 or ABG.	2. Allows objective evaluation of patient response.
Planning/Implementation	1. Post "NO SMOKING" signs on the patient's door and in view of the patient and visitors.	
	2. Fill humidifier with sterile distilled water.	2. If the humidifier bottle is not sufficiently full, less moisture will be delivered.
	3. Attach tubing to outlet on humidifier.	

(continued)

Guidelines Administering Oxygen by Partial Rebreathing or Nonrebreathing Mask (Figs. 11-6 and 11-7) *(continued)*

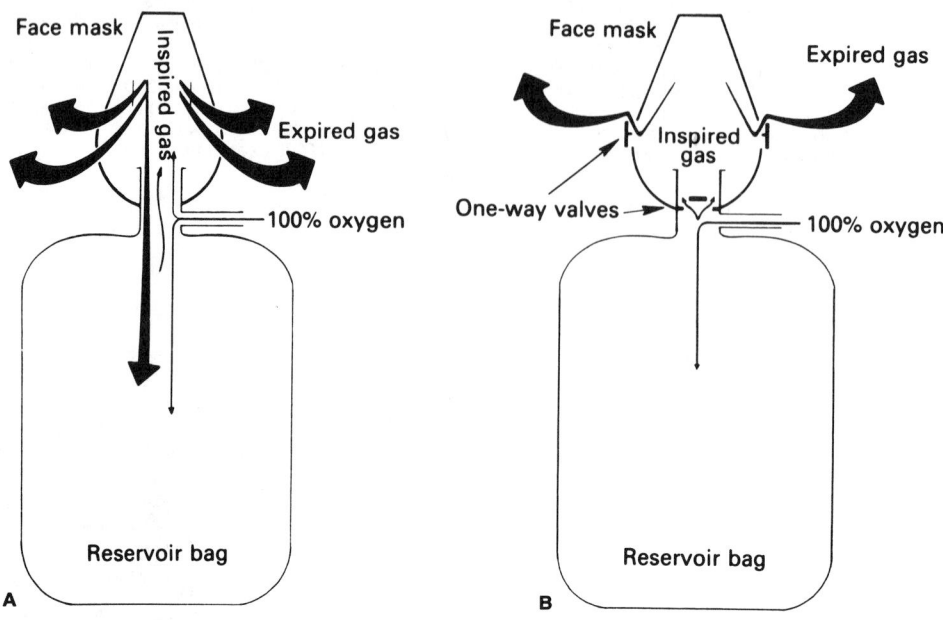

Figure 11-7. *(A) Air flow diagram with partial rebreathing mask. (B) Air flow diagram with nonrebreathing mask. Arrows indicate direction of flow. (Burton GC and Hodgkin JE [eds]. Respiratory Care: A Guide to Practice. 2nd ed. Philadelphia, JB Lippincott, 1984)*

Planning/Implementation *(continued)*

Nursing Action	Rationale/Amplification
4. Attach flowmeter.	
5. Show the mask to the patient and explain the procedure.	
6. Flush the reservoir bag with oxygen to inflate the bag and adjust flowmeter to 6–10 liters/minute.	6. Bag serves as a reservoir, holding oxygen for patient inspiration.
7. Place the mask on the patient's face.	7. Be sure that the mask fits snugly, as there must be an airtight seal between the mask and the patient's face.
8. Adjust liter flow so that the rebreathing bag will not collapse during the inspiratory cycle, even during deep inspiration.	8. With a well-fitting rebreathing bag adjusted so that the patient's inhalation does not deflate the bag, inspired oxygen concentration of 60%–90% can be achieved. Some patients may require flow rates higher than 10 liters/minute to ensure that the bag does not collapse on inspiration.

NURSING ALERT:
1. Adjust the flow to prevent collapse of the bag, even during deep inspiration.
2. A partial rebreathing mask does not have a one-way valve between the mask and reservoir bag. Exhaled air enters the bag very early (first ⅓ expiration). This is dead space ventilation and contains little CO_2. If the bag is allowed to collapse on inspiration, more exhaled air can enter the reservoir and the patient can inhale high concentrations of CO_2.
3. A nonrebreathing mask will deliver a lower concentration of O_2 if the bag is allowed to collapse on inspiration. O_2 from the bag will be diluted by room air drawn in through the side holes of the mask.

9. Stay with the patient for a time to make him comfortable and observe his reactions.	9. Be sure that oxygen is not escaping from the sides of the mask.
10. Remove mask periodically (if the patient's condition permits) to dry the face around the mask. Powder skin and massage face around the mask.	10. These actions reduce moisture accumulation under the mask. Massage of the face stimulates circulation and reduces pressure over the area.

Evaluation/Outcome

1. Record flow rate and immediate patient response.	1. Note the patient's tolerance of treatment. Notify the physician if intolerance occurs.
2. Observe the patient for change of condition. Assess equipment for malfunctioning and low water level in humidifier.	2. Assess the patient for change in mental status, diaphoresis, change in blood pressure, and increasing heart and respiratory rates.

**Evaluation/
Outcome**
(continued)

3. If the patient's condition changes, assess SaO_2 or ABG.

4. Determine patient comfort with oxygen use.

3. Inadequate oxygen concentration may cause hypoxemia or hypoxia. Rebreathing of CO_2 may cause CO_2 retention.

4. Moisture accumulation and tight fit of the mask predispose to skin breakdown, generally limiting mask to short-term use.

Guidelines Administering Oxygen by Continuous Positive Airway Pressure (CPAP) Mask (Fig. 11-8)

Continuous positive airway pressure (CPAP) provides expiratory and inspiratory positive airway pressure in a manner similar to positive end-expiratory pressure (PEEP) during mechanical ventilation but without endotracheal intubation. The mask has (1) an inflatable cushion and head strap designed to tightly seal the mask against the face, (2) a PEEP valve incorporated into the exhalation port to maintain positive pressure on exhalation, and (3) uses high inspiratory flow rates to maintain positive pressure on inspiration.

Equipment

Oxygen blender
Flowmeter
CPAP mask
Valve for prescribed PEEP (2.5, 5, 7.5, 10 cm. H_2O)
Nebulizer with sterile distilled water
Large-bore tubing
Nasogastric tube
Sealing pad to accommodate nasogastric tube

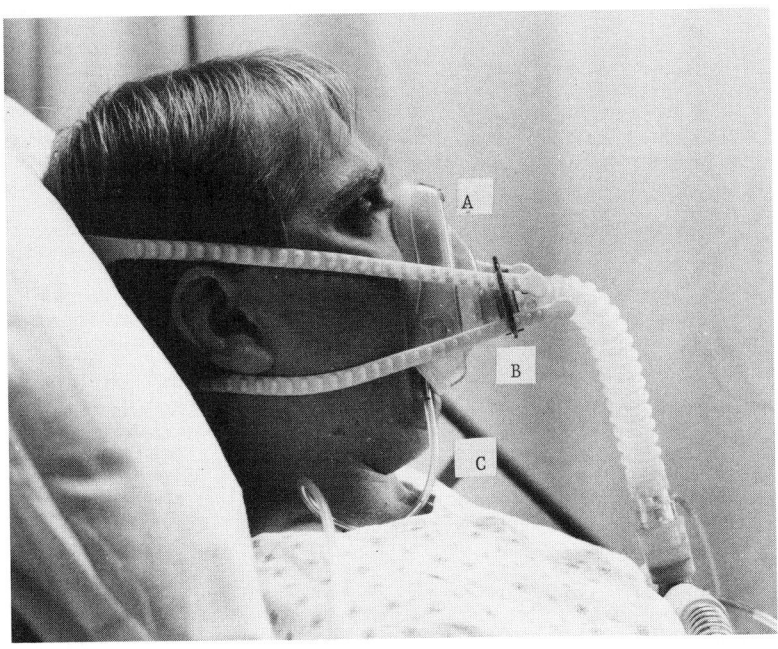

Figure 11-8. *Administering oxygen by face mask with continuous positive airway pressure (CPAP). The CPAP mask has a cushion (A), head strap (B), and positive end-expiratory pressure (PEEP) valve incorporated into the exhalation port (not shown). Nasogastric suction (C) diminishes the risk of gastric distention or emesis. (Courtesy of Photography Department, Montefiore Hospital, Pittsburgh, PA)*

(continued)

Guidelines   Administering Oxygen by Continuous Positive Airway Pressure (CPAP) Mask (Fig. 11-8) *(continued)*

Assessment	Nursing Action	Rationale/Amplification
	1. Assess the patient's level of consciousness and gag reflex.	1. Mask CPAP may lead to aspiration unless the patient is breathing spontaneously and is able to protect the airway.
	2. Determine current arterial blood gases.	2. Documents that patient meets criteria for use of this mask (normal or decreased $PaCO_2$) and provides baseline to evaluate whether therapy results in CO_2 retention.

> **NURSING ALERT:**
> 1. CPAP is used when patients have not responded to attempts to increase PaO_2 with other types of masks.
> 2. The patient will require frequent assessment to detect changes in respiratory status, cardiovascular status and level of consciousness.
> 3. If the patient's level of consciousness decreases or arterial blood gases deteriorate, intubation may be necessary.

Planning/Implementation	1. Post "NO SMOKING" signs on the patient's door and in view of the patient and visitors.	
	2. Show the mask to the patient and explain the procedure.	
	3. Make sure nebulizer is filled to the appropriate mark.	
	4. Insert nasogastric tube.	4. With CPAP, the patient may swallow air, causing gastric distention, emesis, and/or distention of gastric suture line. Prophylactic nasogastric suction diminishes this risk.

Note: Some clinicians do not believe a nasogastric tube is needed if the PEEP level is less than 10 cm. H_2O.

	5. Attach nasogastric tube adapter.	5. Use of adapter may decrease air leak around the mask.
	6. Set desired concentration of oxygen blender and adjust flow rate so that it is sufficient to meet the patient's inspiratory demand.	6. O_2 blenders are devices that mix air and O_2 using a proportioning valve. Concentrations of 21%–100% may be delivered at flows of 2–100 liters/minute, depending on the model. Because the patient will be receiving all of his minute ventilation from this "closed system," it is essential that the flow rate be adequate to meet changes in the patient's breathing pattern.
	7. Place the mask on the patient's face, adjust the head strap, and inflate the mask cushion to ensure a tight seal.	7. To maintain CPAP, an airtight seal is required. Head straps and the inflatable cushion help to ensure that difficult areas, such as the nose and chin, are sealed with greater comfort to the patient.
	8. Organize care to remove the mask as infrequently as possible.	8. If mask is removed (for coughing, suctioning), CPAP is not maintained and inspired oxygen concentrations drop.
Evaluation/ Outcome	1. Assess ABG, hemodynamic status, and level of consciousness frequently.	1. Provides objective documentation of patient response. CPAP may increase work of breathing, resulting in patient tiring and inability to maintain ventilation without intubation. CPAP may also decrease venous return (PEEP effect), resulting in decreased cardiac output.
	2. Immediately report any increase in $PaCO_2$ to the physician.	2. An increase in $PaCO_2$ suggests hypoventilation, resulting from tiring of the patient or inadequate alveolar ventilation. Need for intubation and mechanical ventilation should be evaluated.
	3. Assess patency of nasogastric tube at frequent intervals.	3. May become obstructed, causing gastric distention.
	4. Assess patient comfort and functioning of the equipment frequently.	4. Tight fit of the mask may predispose to skin breakdown. System may develop leaks, resulting in air escaping between the patient's face and mask.
	5. Record patient response. With improvement, oxygen therapy without positive airway pressure can be substituted. With deterioration, intubation and mechanical ventilation may be required.	5. Face mask CPAP is usually continued only for short periods (72 hours) because of patient tiring and the necessity to remove mask for suctioning and coughing. Note the patient's tolerance of treatment. Notify physician if intolerance occurs.

Guidelines   Administering Oxygen via Endotracheal and Tracheostomy Tubes With a T-Piece (Briggs) Adapter (Fig. 11-9)

Equipment	Oxygen	If oxygen blender is not used and precise O_2 concentrations
	Oxygen blender	If oxygen blender is not used and precise O_2 concentrations
	Flowmeter	are required:

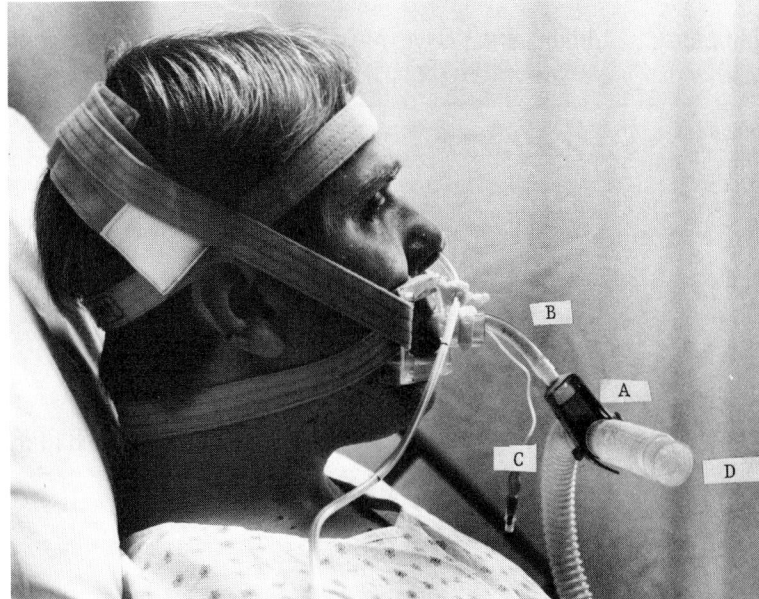

Figure 11-9. *Administering oxygen via endotracheal tube with a T-piece adapter. A T-piece adapter (A) is attached to the endotracheal tube (B) and large-bore tubing (C), which serves as a source of oxygen and humidity. On inspiration, aerosol mist should not be withdrawn into the reservoir tubing (D). (Courtesy of Photography Department, Montefiore Hospital, Pittsburgh, PA)*

| **Equipment** *(continued)* | Nebulizer and sterile distilled water (heating element may be used as described in aerosol masks)
Large-bore tubing
T-piece and reservoir tubing | Venturi tube
Humidity device and large-bore tubing
Compressed air source (as described in use of Venturi mask)
"NO SMOKING" signs |

Assessment	**Nursing Action**	**Rationale/Amplification**
	1. Assess patient's SaO$_2$, hemodynamic status, and level of consciousness frequently. If patient condition changes, assess ABG.	1. Provides baseline to assess response.
	2. Assess viscosity and volume of sputum produced.	2. Aerosol is given to assist in mobilizing retained secretions.
Planning/Implementation	1. Post "NO SMOKING" signs on the patient's door and in view of the patient and visitors.	
	2. Show the T-tube or Venturi tube to the patient and explain the procedure.	
	3. Make sure the nebulizer is filled to the appropriate mark.	3. If nebulizer is not sufficiently full, less aerosol will be delivered.
	4. Attach the large-bore tubing from the T-tube to the nebulizer outlet.	
	5. Set desired oxygen concentration of O$_2$ blender or nebulizer bottle and plug in heating element if used.	5. O$_2$ blenders are devices that mix air and O$_2$ using a proportioning valve. Concentrations of 21%–100% may be delivered at flows of 2–100 liters/minute, depending on the model. Used in situation when precise control is required.
	6. Adjust the flow rate until the desired mist is produced and meets the patient's inspiratory demand.	6. The aerosol mist in the reservoir tubing attached to the T-tube should not be completely withdrawn on patient inspiration. If mist is withdrawn (does not extend from reservoir tubing) on inspiration, room air may be inspired and O$_2$ concentration decreased.
	7. Drain the tubing frequently by emptying condensate into a separate receptacle, not into the nebulizer. If a heating element is used, the tubing will have to be drained more often.	7. The tubing must be kept free of condensate. Condensate allowed to accumulate in the delivery tube will block flow and alter oxygen concentration. If condensate is emptied into the nebulizer, bacteria may be aerosolized into the lungs.
	8. If a heating element is used, check the temperature. The nebulizer bottle should be warm, not hot, to touch.	8. Excessive temperatures can cause airway burns; patients with elevated temperatures will be better humidified with an unheated device.
Evaluation/Outcome	1. Record inspired oxygen concentration and immediate patient response.	1. Note the patient's tolerance of treatment. Notify physician if intolerance occurs.
	2. Assess the patient's condition and the functioning of equipment at regular intervals.	2. Assess the patient for change in mental status, diaphoresis, perspiration, changes in blood pressure, and increasing heart and respiratory rates.

(continued)

Guidelines Administering Oxygen via Endotracheal and Tracheostomy Tubes
With a T-Piece (Briggs) Adapter (Fig. 11-9) *(continued)*

Evaluation/ Outcome *(continued)*	Nursing Action	Rationale/Amplification
	3. If the patient's condition changes, assess SaO_2 or ABG and vital signs. Note changes suggesting increased work of breathing (diaphoresis, intercostal muscle retraction).	3. If the patient is being weaned, return to the ventilator if changes suggesting inability to tolerate spontaneous ventilation occur (See Weaning the Patient from Mechanical Ventilation, p. 251.)
	4. Record changes in volume and tenacity of sputum produced.	4. Indicates effectiveness of therapy

Guidelines Administering Oxygen by Manual Resuscitation Bag (Fig. 11-10 and 11-11)

A *manual resuscitation bag (MRB) and mask* are used to provide high oxygen concentrations when a patient is not intubated. The need to use an MRB and mask usually occurs during a cardiopulmonary arrest. The MRB also can be used to preoxygenate and hyperinflate ventilator patients during suctioning and when they are being transported.

Equipment
Oxygen source
Resuscitation bag and mask
Reservoir tubing or reservoir bag
O_2 connecting tubing
Nipple adapter to attach flowmeter to connecting tubing
Flowmeter
Gloves
Goggles or other eye protection.

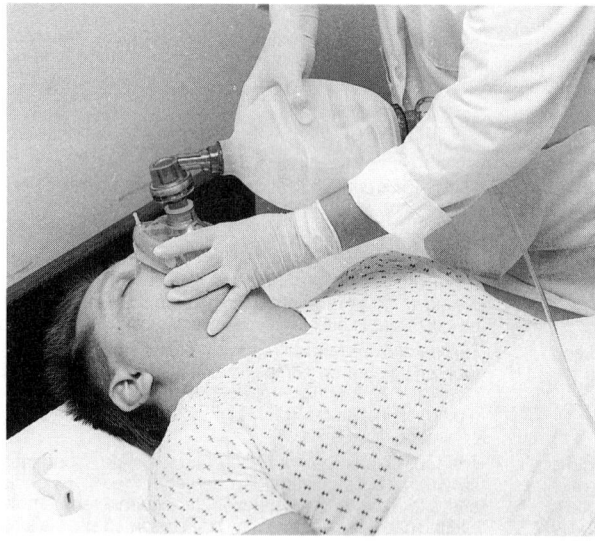

Figure 11-10. *Using a resuscitation bag with a mask. The patient's head is positioned to ensure an open airway. The mask is held tightly against the face to prevent an air leak; the bag is connected to an oxygen source and supplied with a reservoir tubing. (Courtesy of Photography Department, Montefiore Hospital, Pittsburgh, PA)*

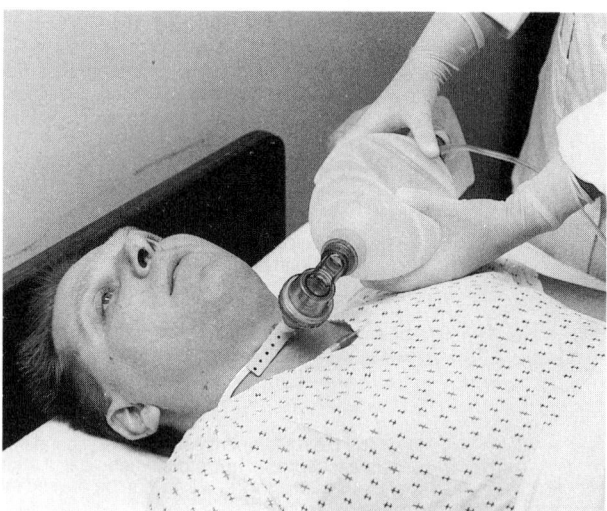

Figure 11-11. *Using a resuscitation bag connected to an artificial airway. This method is used to provide supplemental oxygen before, during, and after suctioning, during patient transport or during cardiopulmonary resuscitation. (Courtesy of Photography Department, Montefiore Hospital, Pittsburgh, PA)*

Assessment	Nursing Action	Rationale/Amplification

1. In cardiopulmonary arrest:
   a. Follow steps to establish that a cardiopulmonary arrest has occurred (See Guidelines: Cardiopulmonary Resuscitation, p. 931).

    a. These steps are: establish unresponsiveness; call for help; position the patient on a firm, flat surface; open the mouth and remove vomitus or debris, if visible; assess presence of respirations with the airway open; if apneic, ventilate; palpate the carotid pulse; if absent, deliver chest compressions.

   b. Use caution not to injury or increase injury to the cervical spine when opening the airway.

    b. If cervical spine injury is a potential, the modified jaw thrust should be used. In other situations, the head-tilt/chin-lift method can be used.
   These maneuvers lift the tongue off the back of the throat and, in some situations, may be all that is needed to restore breathing.

2. In suctioning or transport situation:
   Assess patient's heart rate, level of consciousness, and respiratory status.

    Provides a baseline to estimate patient's tolerance of procedure.

Planning/Implementation

1. Attach connecting tubing from flowmeter and nipple adapter to resuscitation bag.

    1. A humidifier bottle is not used, because the high flow rates of oxygen required would force water into the tubing and clog it.

2. Turn flowmeter to "flush" position.

    2. A high flow rate or "flush" position is necessary to meet the minute ventilation of the patient.

3. Attach reservoir tubing or reservoir bag to resuscitation bag.

    3. A high inspired O_2 concentration is required. Without a reservoir, inspired O_2 concentration will be low (.28–.56), because inspired gas will be air/O_2 mix. With a reservoir, manual resuscitation bags can achieve a F_1O_2 of >.96 at a flow rate of 15 liters/minute.

4. Put on goggles and gloves.

Cardiopulmonary Arrest

1. If respirations are absent after the airway is open, insert an oropharyngeal airway and ventilate twice with slow, full breaths of 1 to 1.5 seconds each. Allow 2 seconds between breaths.

    1. The airway helps prevent obstruction from prolapse of the tongue in an unconscious patient. If ventilation is difficult, confirm that airway is unobstructed.

NURSING ALERT: Airways are not appropriate in a conscious patient or patients with a gag reflex because stimulation of the oropharynx could cause vomiting and aspiration.

2. Breaths will have to be quickly interposed between cardiac compressions. If the patient needs only respiratory assistance, watch for chest expansion and listen with the stethoscope to ensure adequate ventilation.

    2. Squeeze resuscitation bag with sufficient force and at the rate necessary to maintain adequate minute ventilation.

3. A rate of approximately 12–15 breaths per minute is used unless the patient is being given external cardiac compressions (see p. 932).

    3. Continue squeezing bag at appropriate intervals until CPR (cardiopulmonary resuscitation) is no longer required.

Preoxygenation and Suctioning

If hyperinflation is being used with suctioning, ventilate the patient before and after each suctioning pass (*including* after the last suction pass). See Sterile Tracheobronchial Suction Via Tracheostomy or Endotracheal Tube, p. 241.

Hyperinflation prior to suctioning helps prevent hypoxemia. Hyperinflation after suctioning replaces O_2 removed during the procedure and helps to prevent atelectasis. The larger tidal volumes may also assist in mobilizing secretions and promote surfactant secretion.

Transport

If hyperinflation is used in transport, suction patient prior to disconnection for transport; monitor heart and respiratory rates and level of consciousness during procedure.

Establishes a patent airway before patient is moved. Provides information for assessing tolerance of transport.

Evaluation/Outcome

1. In cardiopulmonary arrest, verify return of spontaneous pulse and respirations. Initiate further support as needed.

    1. Establishes patient's need for definitive therapy (drugs, defibrillation, intensive care).

2. In suctioning or transport, return patient to previous support. Note patient tolerance of procedure.

    2. Note SaO_2, heart rate, rate and ease of respirations, arterial blood pressure (if monitored), level of consciousness. Notify physician if intolerance occurs.

Other Respiratory Therapeutic Modalities

Guidelines Assisting the Patient Undergoing Intermittent Positive Pressure Breathing (IPPB) (Fig. 11-12)

The *IPPB unit* is a piece of equipment that delivers air or oxygen to the airways under positive pressure (above atmospheric pressure) during inspiration (Fig. 11-12). The objective of the treatment is to open collapsed alveoli or deliver medicated aerosol therapy. It may be used when patients are unable to use incentive spirometry or a sidestream nebulizer.

Contraindica-tions
Untreated pneumothorax
Mediastinal and subcutaneous emphysema
Tracheoesophageal fistula
Use with caution in patients with gastrointestinal surgery, hemoptysis, bullous disease, cardiovascular insufficiency, active tuberculosis.

Hazards
Excessive ventilation
Excessive oxygenation
Decreased venous return
Gastric insufflation

Equipment
According to the type of machine used (each machine may have different controls and settings)
IPPB circuitry
Medication or fluid for aerosolization
''NO SMOKING'' signs if oxygen is used as the drive gas

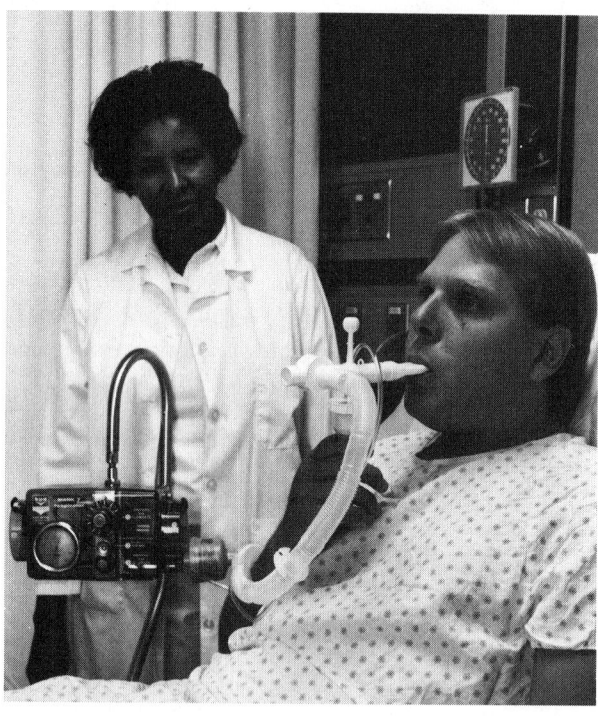

Figure 11-12. *Intermittent positive pressure breathing (IPPB) treatment. (Courtesy of Photography Department, Montefiore Hospital, Pittsburgh, PA)*

Assessment	Nursing Action	Rationale/Amplification
	1. Monitor the heart rate before and after the treatment, especially for patients using bronchodilator drugs.	1. Bronchodilators may cause tachycardia, palpitations, dizziness, nausea, or nervousness.
	2. Assess the patient's breath sounds.	2. This will help in evaluating post-treatment changes.
Planning/In-tervention	1. Post ''NO SMOKING'' signs if oxygen is used as the drive gas. Explain the procedure to the patient.	1. Proper explanation of the procedure helps to ensure the patient's cooperation.

Planning/
Intervention
(continued)

2. Place the patient in a comfortable sitting or semi-Fowler's position.

3. Plug the machine into the pressure source (oxygen or compressed air).

4. Place the prescribed medication or saline solution in the nebulizer.

5. Adjust all controls on tentative settings according to the machine directions or physician request.
   a. Sensitivity—adjusted to -1.5 cm./H_2O to -2 cm./H_2O.

   b. Flow—usually set at 15 cm./H_2O.

   c. Pressure—set at 10–15 cm./H_2O.

6. Check the nebulizer for mist.

7. Instruct the patient to bite down gently on the mouthpiece and seal the mouthpiece with his lips. Noseclips are sometimes used if the patient has difficulty breathing only through his mouth.

8. Tell the patient to breathe slowly and normally and let the machine do the work.

9. Observe expansion of the patient's chest and measure exhaled tidal volume to ensure adequate ventilation.

   a. The machine will exert the regulated pressure on inhalation, helping the patient to breathe more deeply.
   b. Instruct the patient to hold his breath 3–4 seconds at the end of each inspiration.

10. Remind the patient to exhale completely and slowly through the mouthpiece in a relaxed manner. The patient controls exhalation.

11. Monitor the treatment.

12. Encourage the patient to continue the treatment until all the medication is given.

---

2. Diaphragmatic excursion and lung compliance are greater in this position, and the upright position helps prevent air swallowing.

3. The machine is driven by pressure. No electricity is needed.

4. An IPPB treatment should not be given with dry gas.

5. Standard or individualized settings may be used for sensitivity, pressure, and flow.
   a. Must be adjusted to particular patient. A setting that is not sensitive enough may cause increased work of breathing.
   b. Adjustments may be needed to ensure that the patient's gas flow needs are met or exceeded. Insufficient flow will result in increased work of breathing, patient discomfort, and insufficient ventilation.
   c. The patient's chest should appear to have adequate expansion. Measured tidal volume should be 1½ times the baseline. Test the unit to make sure that the desired pressure is achieved before treating the patient.

6. Adequate fog and particle size is essential for effective distribution of medication and moisture.

7. The mouthpiece (or mask) must provide an airtight seal. This will enable the airway pressure to build and allow the unit to cycle properly. If air escapes through the patient's nose when the mouthpiece is used, the unit will be unable to attain the desired pressure.

8. A slight inspiratory effort will activate the positive pressure phase, and the lungs will be inflated with the flow of gas until the predetermined pressure is reached. Gas flow will then cease, and passive exhalation will occur.

9. Measurement of tidal volume is particularly important in the patient who has a high arterial PCO_2 and needs an adequate tidal volume to lower it.
   a. The patient should take 8–10 breaths per minute.

   b. This encourages settling of aerosal particles on bronchiolar mucosa.

10. This type of breathing encourages good diaphragmatic motion and reduces residual air volume.

11. Ensure that the patient is taking the treatment correctly:
   a. Make sure the patient has a good seal around the mouthpiece.
   b. Monitor for hyperventilation.
   c. Make sure the patient does not cycle the machine prematurely.

12. The treatment should last 10–15 minutes, depending on the clinical problem.

Evaluation/
Outcome

1. Record medication used, patient's respiratory rate and effort, pre- and post-treatment heart rate (if bronchodilator is used), pre- and post-treatment breath sounds, and description of secretions expectorated. Also record pressure limit and flow rate. Subjective comments may also be added.

2. Disassemble and clean the exhalation unit and nebulizer after each use. Keep this equipment in the patient's room. The equipment is changed every 24 hours.

---

1. Note the patient's tolerance of the treatment. Notify physician if intolerance is noted.

2. Each patient has his own breathing circuit (exhalation valve, nebulizer and tubing, mouthpiece or mask). Through proper cleaning, sterilization, and storage of equipment, organisms can be prevented from entering the lungs.

Guidelines

Assisting the Patient Undergoing Nebulizer Therapy Without Positive Pressure (Sidestream Jet Nebulizer) (Fig. 11-13)

A *nebulizer* is a device that produces a stable aerosol of fluid particles. The nebulizer most commonly used for medication administration to the spontaneously breathing patient is the *sidestream jet nebulizer*. The nebulizer is powered by compressed air. A specially designed nebulizer is used to deliver pentamidine aerosol therapy. All expired air enters a filter, which removes the drug and prevents environmental contamination.

Contraindications
Inability of patient to cooperate in taking deep breaths
Adverse reactions encountered with medication

Hazards
Swelling of dried, retained secretions
Precipitation of bronchospasm

Equipment
Air compressor
Connection tubing
Nebulizer manifold
Medication and saline solution

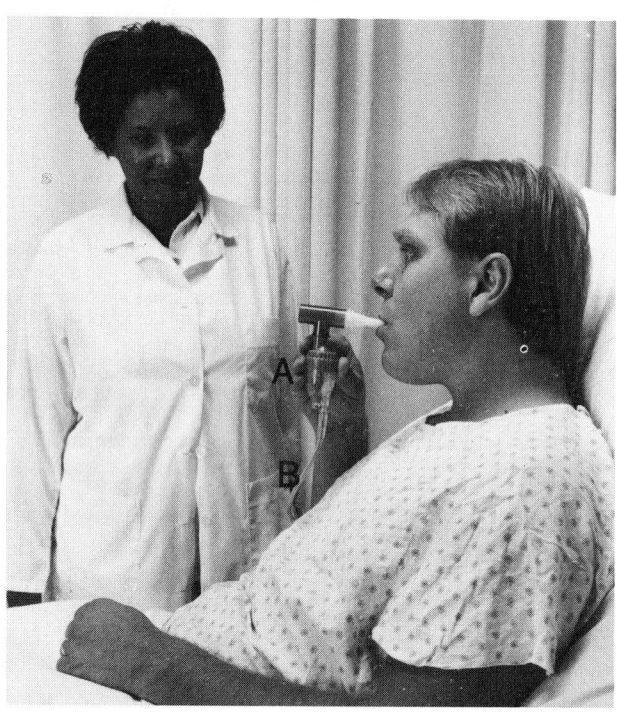

Figure 11-13. *A sidestream jet nebulizer. The nebulizer is filled with the prescribed amount of saline or medication (A) and attached to a compressed air source (B). (Courtesy of Photography Department, Montefiore Hospital, Pittsburgh, PA)*

	Nursing Action	Rationale/Amplification
Assessment	1. Monitor the heart rate before and after the treatment for patients using bronchodilator drugs.	1. Bronchodilators may cause tachycardia, palpitations, dizziness, nausea, or nervousness.
Planning/Implementation	1. Explain the procedure to the patient. *This therapy depends on patient effort.*	1. Proper explanation of the procedure helps to ensure the patient's cooperation and effectiveness of the treatment.
	2. Place the patient in a comfortable sitting or a semi-Fowler's position.	2. Diaphragmatic excursion and lung compliance are greater in this position. This ensures maximal distribution and deposition of aerosolized particles to basilar areas of the lungs.

Planning/Im-plementation
(continued)

3. Add the prescribed amount of medication and saline to the nebulizer. Connect the tubing to the compressor and set the flow at 6–8 liters/minute.
4. Instruct the patient to exhale.
5. Tell the patient to take in a deep breath from the mouthpiece, hold his breath briefly, then exhale.
6. Nose clips are sometimes used if the patient has difficulty breathing only through his mouth.
7. Observe expansion of the patient's chest to ascertain that he is taking deep breaths.
8. Instruct the patient to breathe slowly and deeply until all the medication is nebulized.
9. On completion of the treatment, encourage the patient to cough after several deep breaths.

3. A fine mist from the device should be visible.

5. This encourages optimal dispersion of the medication.

7. This will ensure that medication is deposited below the level of the oropharynx.
8. Medication will usually be nebulized within 15 minutes at a flow of 6–8 liters/minute.
9. The medication may dilate airways, facilitating expectoration of secretions.

Evaluation/Outcome

1. Record medication used, and description of secretions.

2. Disassemble and clean nebulizer after each use. Keep this equipment in the patient's room. The equipment is changed every 24 hours.

1. Note the patient's tolerance of the treatment. Notify physician of any intolerance.

2. Each patient has his own breathing circuit (nebulizer, manifold, tubing, and mouthpiece). Through proper cleaning, sterilization, and storage of equipment, organisms can be prevented from entering the lungs.

Guidelines Assisting the Patient Using an Incentive Spirometer (Fig. 11-14)

The *incentive spirometer* is a piece of equipment that encourages performance by the patient of active maximum sustained inspiration. Because this maneuver helps to open closed alveoli, it is used in the prevention and treatment of atelectasis. Patient self-administration is encouraged.

Equipment   According to the type of device used

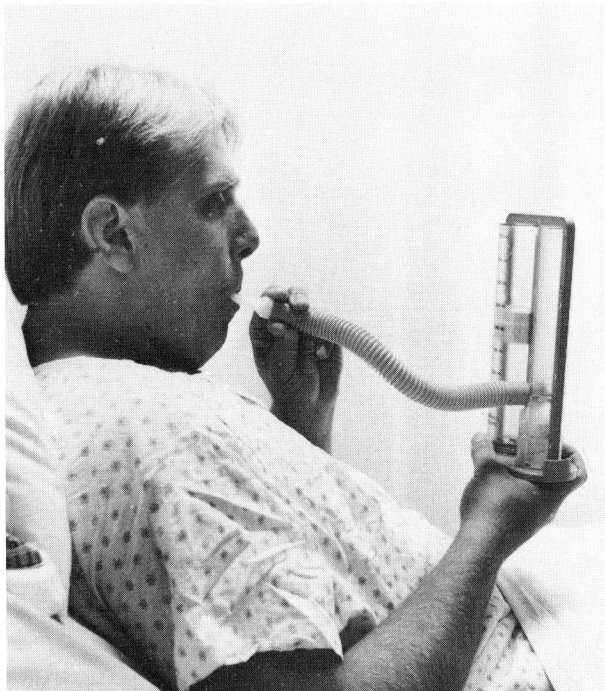

Figure 11-14. *An incentive spirometer, designed to encourage sustained maximum inspiration for patients who are predisposed to atelectasis. (Courtesy of Photography Department, Montefiore Hospital, Pittsburgh, PA)*

(continued)

Guidelines Assisting the Patient Using an Incentive Spirometer (Fig. 11-14) *(continued)*

Assessment	Nursing Action	Rationale/Amplification
	1. Measure the patient's normal resting tidal volume and auscultate the chest.	1. The patient's baseline is established.
Planning/Implementation	1. Explain the procedure and its purpose to the patient.	1. Optimal results are achieved when the patient is given pretreatment instruction. Preoperative instruction is also beneficial for the surgical patient.
	2. Place the patient in a comfortable sitting or semi-Fowler's position.	2. Diaphragmatic excursion is greater in this position; however, if the patient is medically unable to be in this position, the exercise may be done in any position.
	3. For the postoperative patient, try as much as possible to avoid discomfort with the treatment administration.	3. Try to coordinate treatment with administration of pain-relief medications. Instruct and assist the patient with splinting of incision.
	4. Set the incentive spirometer tidal volume indicator at the desired goal the patient is to reach or exceed (500 ml. is often used to start). The tidal volume is set according to the manufacturer's instructions.	4. The initial tidal volume may be prescribed by the physician, but the purpose of the device is to establish a baseline tidal volume and provide incentive to achieve greater volumes progressively.
	5. Demonstrate the technique to the patient.	
	6. Instruct the patient to exhale fully.	
	7. Tell the patient to take in a slow, easy deep breath from the mouthpiece.	7. Noseclips are sometimes used if the patient has difficulty breathing only through his mouth—this will ensure full credit for each breath measured.
	8. When the desired goal is reached (lungs fully inflated), ask the patient to continue the inspiratory effort for 3 seconds, even though he may not actually be drawing in more air.	8. Sustaining the inspiratory effort helps to open closed alveoli.
	9. Instruct the patient to remove the mouthpiece, relax, and passively exhale. He should take several normal breaths before attempting another one with the incentive spirometer.	9. Usually one incentive breath per minute minimizes patient fatigue. No more than 4–5 maneuvers should be performed per minute to minimize hypocarbia.
	10. Continue to monitor the patient's spirometer breaths, periodically increasing the tidal volume as the patient tolerates it.	
	11. At the conclusion of the treatment, encourage the patient to cough after a deep breath.	11. The deep lung inflation may loosen secretions and enable the patient to expectorate them.
	12. Instruct the patient to take 10 sustained maximal inspiratory maneuvers per hour and note the volume on the spirometer.	12. A total of 10 sustained maximal inspiratory maneuvers per hour during waking hours is a typical order. A counter on the incentive spirometer indicates the number of breaths the patient has taken.
Evaluation/Outcome	1. Auscultate the chest. Chart any improvement or variation, the volume attained, effectiveness of cough, description of any secretions expectorated.	1. Note the effectiveness and patient tolerance of the treatment.

Artificial Airway Management

An *artificial airway* is a tube that is inserted at the mouth or nose (endotracheal tube) or level of the second or third tracheal ring (tracheostomy tube) to permit mechanical ventilation and/or facilitate secretion removal. The distal end of the tube is located in the trachea below the vocal cords.

Indications

1. Acute respiratory failure, CNS depression, neuromuscular disease, pulmonary diseases, chest wall injury
2. Upper airway obstruction (tumor, inflammation, foreign body, laryngeal spasm)
3. Anticipated upper airway obstruction from edema or soft tissue swelling due to head and neck trauma, some postoperative head and neck procedures involving the airway, facial or airway burns, decreased level of consciousness
4. Aspiration prophylaxis
5. Fractured cervical vertebrae with spinal cord injury requiring ventilatory assistance

Route of Insertion

A. Endotracheal

The tube may be inserted through the nose or mouth. A cuff is always located at the distal end of the tube.
1. *Orotracheal*
   a. Insertion of an oral tube is technically easier, since it is done under direct visualization.
   b. Disadvantages are increased oral secretions, decreased patient comfort, difficulty with stabilization, and inability of patient to use lip movement as a communication means.

2. *Nasotracheal*
   a. May be more comfortable to the patient and is easier to stabilize
   b. Disadvantages are that blind insertion is required; possible development of pressure necrosis of the nasal airway, sinusitis, and otitis media.
3. *Tube types:*
   a. Vary according to length and inner diameter in millimeters. Usual sizes for adults are 6.0, 7.0, 8.0, and 9.0 mm.
   b. Vary according to cuff. Most are high volume, low pressure, with self-sealing inflation valves, or the cuff may be of foam rubber (Fome-Cuff)
   c. Vary according to number of lumens. Most tubes have a single lumen (Fig. 11-15*A*). Dual lumen tubes may be used to ventilate each lung independently (Fig. 11-15*B*).

B. Tracheostomy

Tube inserted into the trachea via an incision created at the level of the 2nd or 3rd cartilage ring; totally bypasses the upper airway. Tube types (Fig. 11-16):
1. Vary according to composition and cuff type. May or may not have inner cannula. Usually are cuffed.
   a. Tubes with high-volume, low-pressure cuffs, self-sealing inflation valves. With or without inner cannula.
   b. Fenestrated tube
   c. Foam-filled cuffs (Fome-Cuff)
   d. Speaking tracheostomy tube
   e. Tracheal button
   f. Silver (Silver tracheostomy tubes are rarely used.)
2. Vary according to length and inner diameter in millimeters. Usual sizes for an adult are 6.0, 7.0, 8.0, and 9.0 mm.

Nursing Interventions

1. Ensure adequate ventilation and oxygenation through the use of mechanical ventilation, continuous positive airway pressure (CPAP) device, Briggs T-piece adapter or tracheostomy mask.
2. Assess breath sounds every 2 hours. Note evidence of ineffective secretion clearance (rhonchi, crackles, which suggests need for suctioning.
3. Provide adequate humidity, as the natural humidifying pathway of the oropharynx is bypassed. Clear airway of secretions as needed with suctioning.
4. Use aseptic technique when entering the artificial airway. The artificial airway bypasses the upper airway, and the lower airways are sterile below the level of the vocal cords.
5. Elevate the patient to a semi-Fowler's or sitting position, when possible, because these positions result in improved lung compliance. The patient's position, however, should be changed at least every 2 hours to ensure ventilation of all lung segments and prevent secretion stagnation. Position changes are also necessary to avoid skin breakdown.
6. Confirm proper tube position by auscultating breath sounds (should be present bilaterally) and documenting that the distance from the proximal end of the tube to the teeth is unchanged.
7. Nutrition
   a. Endotracheal tube—recognize that the tube holds open the epiglottis. Therefore, only the inflated cuff prevents the aspiration of oropharyngeal contents into the lungs. *The patient must not receive oral feeding.* Nutrition must take the form of enteral tube feedings, or parenteral hyperalimentation.
   b. Tracheostomy—If the patient is unconscious, nutrition must take the form of enteral tube feedings, or parenteral hyperalimentation. Conscious patients may receive oral feedings with the cuff inflated. The inflated cuff prevents aspiration of food contents into the lungs, but causes the tracheal wall to bulge into the esophageal lumen, and may make swallowing more difficult. Patients who are not on mechanical ventilation and are awake, alert,

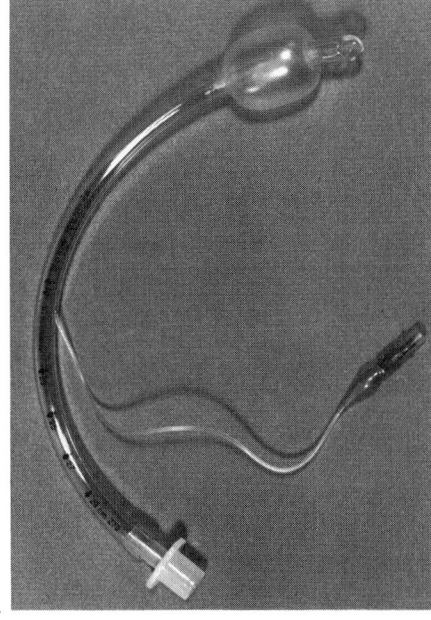 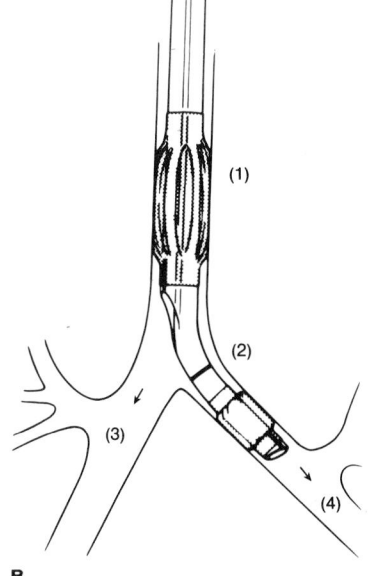

Figure 11-15. *(A) Single lumen endotracheal tube. (B) Double lumen endotracheal tube. When the double lumen tube is used, two cuffs are inflated. One cuff (1) is positioned in the tracks and the second cuff (2) in the left mainstem bronchus. After inflation, air flows through an opening below the tracheal cuff (3) to the right lung and through an opening below the bronchial cuff (4) to the left lung. This permits differential ventilation of both lungs, lavage of one lung, or selective inflation of either lung during thoracic surgery. (From Marshall BE, Longnecker DE and Fairley HB (eds). Anesthesia for Thoracic Procedures, p 381. Boston, Blackwell Scientific Publications, 1988. Used with permission)*

A   **B**

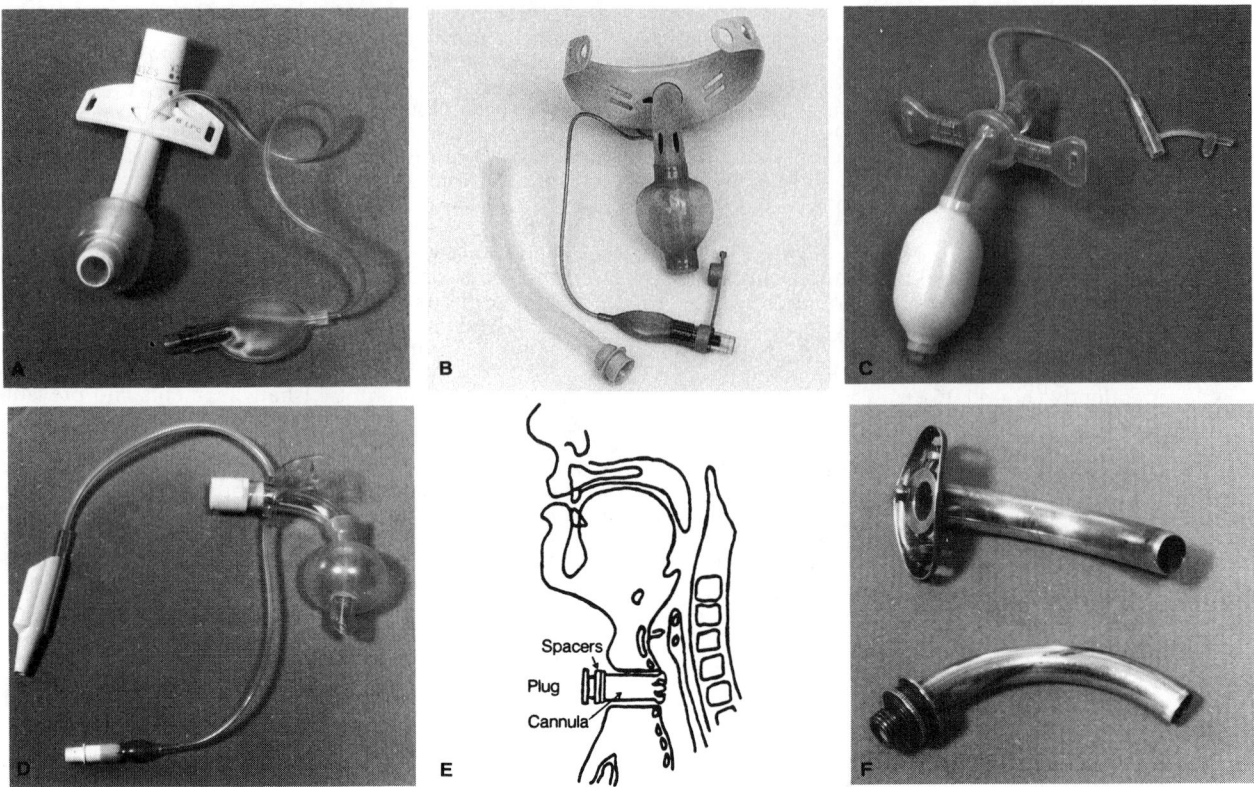

Figure 11-16. *Types of tracheostomy tubes. (A) Low pressure cuff (Shiley). (B) Fenestrated tube (Portex). (C) Polyurethane foam-filled cuff (FOME-Cuff). (D) Pitt speaking tube (National Catheter Corporation). (E) Tracheal button. (F) Silver tube. (Photographs courtesy of Photography Department, Montefiore Hospital, Pittsburgh, PA. Line drawing from Shelly RW. A post-insertion protocol for management of the olympic tracheostomy button. J Neurosurg Nurs 1981; 13(6):296)*

and able to protect the airway are candidates for eating with the cuff deflated.
  (1) To assess ability to protect the airway:
    (a) Sit the patient upright.
    (b) Feed the patient colored gelatin or juice.
    (c) If color from gelatin can be suctioned from the tracheostomy tube, aspiration is occurring, and the cuff must be inflated during feeding and for 1 hour afterward.
8. Monitor cuff pressure. Endotracheal tube cuffs should be inflated continuously and deflated only during intubation, extubation, and tube repositioning. The internal cuff pressure should be checked every 4 hours. Tracheostomy tube cuffs also should be inflated continuously in patients on mechanical ventilation or CPAP. Tracheostomized patients who are breathing spontaneously may have the cuffs inflated continuously (in the patient having suppressed levels of consciousness with an ability to protect airway), deflated continuously, or inflated only for feeding if the patient is at risk for aspiration. (See Cuff Inflation for technique.)
9. External tube site care
  a. Endotracheal tubes—patients with endotracheal tubes have mouth care every shift, or as frequently as needed. Oral secretions tend to stagnate, and

risk of oral infection is increased. An oral endotracheal tube may also stimulate an increase in the production of oral secretions. The tube must be secured at all times (see Endotracheal Intubation for technique), and the ventilator, CPAP, or T-piece tubing supported so that traction is not applied to the tube.
  b. Tracheostomy tube—the stoma should be cleaned once a shift or more frequently if needed, and the tracheostomy ties changed once a day (see Tracheostomy Site Care for technique). The ventilator, CPAP, or T-piece tubing must be supported so that traction is not applied to the tracheostomy tube.
10. Have available at all times at the patient's bedside a resuscitation bag, oxygen source, and mask to ventilate the patient in the event of accidental tube removal. Anticipate your course of action in such an event.
  a. Endotracheal tube—know location and assembly of reintubation equipment. Know method of contact of personnel capable of reintubation.
  b. Tracheostomy—have extra tracheostomy tube at bedside. Be aware of reinsertion technique, or know method to contact personnel capable of reinserting the tube.

Note: Remember that with tracheostomized patients, as long as the airway is patent (from upper to lower), it is possible to bag/mask ventilate with the resuscitation bag if the stoma is covered. Only patients with complete airway obstruction, an open stoma, or laryngectomy need have mouth-to-stoma ventilation performed.

Psychological Care of the Patient

1. Recognize that the patient is usually apprehensive, particularly about choking, inability to communicate verbally, being unable to remove secretions, difficulty in breathing, or mechanical failure.
2. Explain the function of the equipment carefully.
3. Inform the patient and his family that he will not be able to speak while the tube is in place, unless using a tracheostomy tube with a deflated cuff, a fenestrated tube, or a speaking tracheostomy tube. Develop with the patient the best method of communication (e.g., sign language, lip movement, letter boards, paper and pencil, magic slate, or coded messages). Patients with tracheostomy tubes or nasal endotracheal tubes may effectively use orally operated electrolarynx devices. Devise a means for the patient to get the nurse's attention when someone is not immediately available at the bedside, such as call bell, hand-operated bell, rattle, etc.

4. Anticipate some of the patient's questions by discussing "Is it permanent?" "Will it hurt to breathe?" "Will someone be with me?"

Complications

1. Mechanical
   a. Cuff leaks
   b. Cuff herniation
   c. Tube obstruction (biting, kinking, mucus plug,)
   d. Tube displacement
   e. Inadvertent extubation
   f. Right lung main stem bronchus intubation (endotracheal tube)
2. Laryngeal and tracheal
   a. Sore throat
   b. Hoarse voice
   c. Glottic edema
   d. Ulceration of tracheal mucosa
   e. Vocal cord ulceration, granuloma, or polyps
   f. Vocal cord paralysis
   g. Postextubation tracheal stenosis
   h. Tracheal dilatation
   i. Formation of tracheal–esophageal fistula
   j. Formation of tracheal–arterial fistula
   k. Inominate artery erosion
   l. See additional complications under specific procedures dealing with artificial airways.

Guidelines Endotracheal Intubation (Fig. 11-17)

An *endotracheal tube* may be inserted via the nose or the mouth. The indications for use are the same as those for any artificial airway.

Equipment

Laryngoscope with curved or straight blade and working light source (Check batteries and bulb periodically.)
Endotracheal tube with low-pressure cuff and adapter to connect tube to ventilator or resuscitation bag
Stylet to guide the endotracheal tube
Oral airway (assorted sizes) or bite block to keep patient from biting into and occluding the endotracheal tube
Adhesive tape or tube fixation system
Sterile anesthetic lubricant jelly (water-soluble)
Syringe
Suction source
Suction catheter and tonsil suction
Resuscitation bag and mask connected to oxygen source
Anesthetic spray
Sterile towel
Gloves
Goggles or other eye protection

Assessment	Nursing Action	Rationale/Amplification
	1. Monitor the patient's heart rate, level of consciousness, and respiratory status.	1. Provides a baseline to estimate patient's tolerance of procedure
Planning/Implementation	1. Remove the patient's dental bridgework and plates.	1. May interfere with insertion. Will not be able to remove easily from patient once intubated.
	2. Remove headboard of bed (optional).	
	3. Prepare equipment a. Ensure function of resuscitation bag with mask, and suction.	a. Patient may require ventilatory assistance during procedure. Suction should be functional, because gagging and emesis may occur during procedure.

(continued)

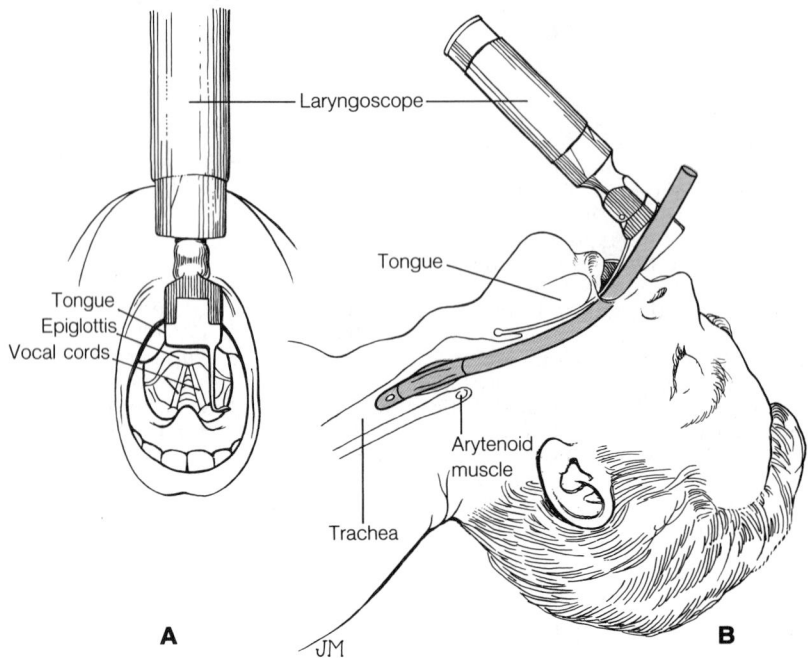

Figure 11-17. *Endotracheal intubation. (A) The primary glottic landmarks for tracheal intubation as visualized with proper placement of the laryngoscope. (B) Positioning the endotube.*

Planning/Implementation *(continued)*	Nursing Action	Rationale/Amplification
	b. Assemble the laryngoscope—make sure the light bulb is tightly attached and functional.	
	c. Select an endotracheal tube of the appropriate size (6.0–9.0 mm. for average adult).	
	d. Place the endotracheal tube on a sterile towel.	d. Although the tube will pass through the contaminated mouth or nose, the airway below the vocal cords is sterile, and efforts must be made to prevent iatrogenic contamination of the distal end of the tube and cuff. The proximal end of the tube may be handled, as it will reside in the upper airway.
	e. Inflate the cuff to make sure it assumes a symmetrical shape and holds volume without leakage. Then deflate maximally.	e. Malfunction of the cuff must be ascertained before tube placement occurs.
	f. Lubricate the distal end of the tube liberally with the sterile anesthetic water soluble jelly.	f. Aids in insertion.
	g. Insert the stylet into the tube (if oral intubation is planned—nasal intubation does not employ use of the stylet).	g. Stiffens the soft tube, allowing it to be more easily directed into the trachea.
	4. Aspirate stomach contents if nasogastric tube is in place.	
	5. If time allows, inform the patient of impending inability to talk and discuss alternate means of communication.	5. Discuss alternate means of communication (see Artificial Airway, Psychological Care, step 3).
	6. If the patient is confused, it may be necessary to apply soft wrist restraints.	6. Restraint of the confused patient may be necessary to promote patient safety and maintain sterile technique.
	7. Put on goggles and gloves or other eye protection system.	7. Prevents contact with patient's oral secretions.
	8. During oral intubation if cervical spine is not injured, place patient's head in a ''sniffing'' position, i.e., extended at the junction of the neck and thorax and flexed at the junction of the spine and skull.	8. Upper airway is open maximally in this position and mouth of the unconscious patient will often open.
	9. Spray the back of the patient's throat with an anesthetic spray if time is available.	9. Will decrease gagging

**Planning/Im-
plementation**
(continued)

10. Ventilate and oxygenate the patient with the resuscitation bag and mask before intubation.
11. Hold the handle of the laryngoscope in the left hand and hold the patient's mouth open with the right hand by placing crossed fingers on the teeth.
12. Insert the curved blade of the laryngoscope along the right side of the tongue, push the tongue to the left, and use right thumb and index finger to pull patient's lower lip away from lower teeth.
13. Lift laryngoscope forward (toward ceiling) to expose the epiglottis.
14. Lift laryngoscope upward and forward at a 45-degree angle to expose glottis and visualize vocal cords.
15. As the epiglottis is lifted forward (toward ceiling) the vertical opening of the larynx between the vocal cords will come into view (Fig. 11-17A).
16. Once vocal cords are visualized, insert tube into the right corner of the mouth and pass the tube—guided by blade, but keeping vocal cords in constant view.
17. Gently push the tube through the triangular space formed by the vocal cords and back wall of trachea.
18. Stop insertion just after the tube cuff has disappeared from view beyond the cords.

19. Withdraw laryngoscope while holding endotracheal tube in place. Disassemble mask from resuscitation bag and ventilate the patient.
20. Inflate cuff with the minimal amount of air required to occlude the trachea.

21. Insert bite block if necessary.

22. Ascertain expansion of both sides of the chest by observation and auscultation of breath sounds.

23. Record distance from proximal end of tube to the point where the tube reaches the teeth.
24. Secure tube to the patient's face with adhesive tape or apply a commercially available endotracheal tube stabilization device. The patient in Fig. 11-9 is wearing such a device.
25. Obtain chest x-ray to verify tube position.

10. Preoxygenation decreases the likelihood of cardiac dysrhythmias or respiratory distress secondary to hypoxemia.
11. Leverage is improved by crossing the thumb and index fingers when opening the patient's mouth (scissor-twist technique).
12. Rolling the lip away from teeth prevents injury by being caught between teeth and blade.

13. Do not use teeth as a fulcrum, which could lead to dental damage.
14. This stretches the hypoepiglottis ligament, folding the epiglottis upward and exposing the glottis.
15. Do not use wrist. Use shoulder and arm to lift epiglottis.

16. Make sure you do not insert tube into esophagus (Fig. 11-17B); the esophageal mucosa is pink and the opening is horizontal rather than vertical.
17. If the vocal cords are in spasm (closed), wait a few seconds before passing tube.
18. Advancing tube further may lead to its entry into a mainstem bronchus (usually the right bronchus) causing collapse of the unventilated lung.

20. Listen over the cuff area with a stethoscope. Occlusion occurs when no air leak is heard during ventilator inspiration or compression of the resuscitation bag (Fig. 11-21).
21. This keeps patient from biting down on the tube and obstructing the airway.
22. Observation and auscultation help in determining that tube remains in position and has not slipped into the right main stem bronchus.
23. This will allow for detection of any later change in tube position.
24. The tube must be fixed securely to ensure that it will not be dislodged. Dislodgement of a tube with an inflated cuff may result in damage to the vocal cords.

**Evaluation/
Outcome**

1. Record tube type and size, cuff pressure, and patient tolerance of the procedure. Auscultate breath sounds every 2 hours or if signs and symptoms of respiratory distress occur. Assess arterial blood gases after intubation if requested by the physician.
2. Measure cuff pressure with manometer; adjust pressure (see Cuff Inflation). Make adjustment in tube placement on the basis of the chest x-ray results.

1. Arterial blood gases may be prescribed to ensure adequacy of ventilation and respiration. Tube displacement may result in extubation (cuff above vocal cords), tube touching carina (causing paroxysmal coughing), or intubation of a mainstem bronchus (resulting in collapse of the unventilated lung).
2. The tube may be advanced or removed several centimeters for proper placement on the basis of the chest x-ray results.

Note: The previously described intubation technique may not be appropriate in certain cases. Glottic structures may be obscured due to vomitus, blood, foreign bodies, or trauma. If cervical spine injury is suspected, neck manipulation must be minimized. Alternate techniques of tracheal intubation that do not require direct visualization may be useful in these situations when employed by trained personnel. These techniques include:

1. *Tactile or "digital" intubation.* The patient is approached from the side, and the neck is maintained in the neutral position. The index and middle finger of the clinician's nondominant hand are slid along the patient's tongue and down into the oropharynx until the epiglottis is palpated. The endotracheal tube is then advanced. The index and middle finger of the nondominant hand are used to help guide the tip of the tube through the vocal cords and into the trachea.
2. *Transillumination intubation.* With this technique, a stylet is used that has a light at the tip. The tube and stylet are bent into a "J" shape at the distal end. The clinician's nondominant hand applies gentle traction on the patient's tongue, and the dominant hand slides the tube into the mouth. A "scooping" motion is used to hook the tube under the epiglottis and the tube then is passed into the trachea. If the tube is in the trachea, a bright, well-circumscribed glow is seen in the anterior neck at the level of the larynx. A diffuse, low-level glow, or no glow, indicates esophageal tube placement.

Guidelines Extubation

Extubation consists of removal of the oral or nasal endotracheal tube.

Note: Extubation may be performed only if personnel qualified to reintubate are available. The occurrence of laryngospasm or tracheal edema postextubation may require immediate tube replacement.

Equipment

Tonsil suction (surgical suction instrument)
10-ml. syringe
Resuscitation bag and mask with oxygen flow
Face mask connected to large bore tubing, nebulizer, and oxygen source.
Sterile towel
Suction catheter
Suction source
Gloves, goggles, or other eye protection device.

Assessment	**Nursing Action**	**Rationale/Amplification**
	1. Monitor heart rate, lung expansion, and breath sounds preextubation. Record tidal volume, vital capacity, and inspiratory force.	1. Tidal volume, vital capacity, and negative inspiratory force are measured to assess respiratory muscle function and adequacy of ventilation.
	2. Assess the patient for other signs of adequate muscle power.	2. Adequate muscle strength is necessary to ensure maintenance of a patent airway.
	a. Instruct the patient to tightly squeeze the index and middle fingers of your hand. Resistance to removal of your fingers from the patient's grasp must be demonstrated.	
	b. Ask the patient to lift his head from the pillow and hold for 2–3 seconds.	
Planning/Implementation	1. Obtain orders for extubation and postextubation oxygen therapy from the physician.	1. Do not attempt extubation until postextubation oxygen therapy is available and functioning at the bedside.
	2. Explain the procedure to the patient:	2. Increases patient cooperation.
	a. He will have the artificial airway removed.	
	b. He will be suctioned prior to extubation.	
	c. He will be asked to take deep breaths on command.	
	d. He will be asked to cough after extubation.	
	3. Prepare necessary equipment. Have ready for use tonsil suction, suction catheter, 10-ml. syringe, bag–mask unit, and oxygen via face mask.	
	4. Place patient in sitting or semi-Fowler's position (unless contraindicated).	4. Increases lung compliance and decreases work of breathing. Facilitates coughing.
	5. Put on goggles.	5. Spraying of airway secretions may occur.
	6. Suction endotracheal tube (see Sterile Tracheobronchial Suctioning).	
	7. Suction oropharyngeal airway above the endotracheal cuff as thoroughly as possible.	7. Secretions not cleared from above the cuff will be aspirated when the cuff is deflated.
	8. Put on gloves. Loosen tape or endotracheal tube-securing device.	
	9. Extubate the patient:	
	a. Ask the patient to take as deep a breath as possible (if the patient is not following commands, give a deep breath with the resuscitation bag).	a. At peak inspiration, the trachea and vocal cords will dilate, allowing atraumatic tube removal.
	b. At peak inspiration, deflate the cuff completely and pull the tube out in the direction of the curve (out and downward).	
	10. Once the tube is fully removed, ask the patient to cough or exhale forcefully to remove secretions. Then suction the back of the patient's airway with the tonsil suction.	10. Frequently, old blood is seen in the secretions of newly extubated patients. Monitor for the appearance of bright red blood due to trauma occurring during extubation.

Planning/Implementation
(continued)

11. Evaluate immediately for any signs of airway obstruction, stridor, or difficult breathing. If the patient develops any of the above problems, attempt to ventilate the patient with the resuscitation bag and mask and prepare for reintubation.

11. Immediate complications:

    a. Laryngospasm may develop, causing obstruction of the airway.

    b. Edema may develop at the cuff site. Signs of narrowing airway lumen are high-pitched crowing sounds, decreased air movement, and respiratory distress.

12. Administer oxygen as directed.

Evaluation/Outcome

1. Note patient tolerance of procedure, upper and lower airway sounds postextubation, description of secretions.

2. Observe patient closely postextubation for any signs and symptoms of airway obstruction or respiratory insufficiency.

3. Observe character of voice.

1. Establishes a baseline to assess improvement/development of complications.

2. Tracheal or laryngeal edema may develop postextubation (a possibility for up to 24 hours). Signs and symptoms include high-pitched, crowing upper airway sounds and respiratory distress.

3. Hoarseness is a common postextubation complaint. Observe for worsening hoarseness or vocal cord paralysis.

Guidelines ## Assisting With Tracheostomy Insertion (Fig. 11-18)

Tracheostomy is usually performed when the need for an artificial airway is protracted (usually greater than 14 days), when placement of an endotracheal tube is unsuccessful or contraindicated, or when surgical interruption of the airway is necessary (i.e., laryngectomy).

Equipment

Tracheostomy tube (sizes 6.0–9.0 mm. for most adults)
Sterile instruments: hemostat, scalpel and blade, forceps, suture material, scissors
Sterile gown and drapes, gloves
Cap and mask
Antiseptic prep solution

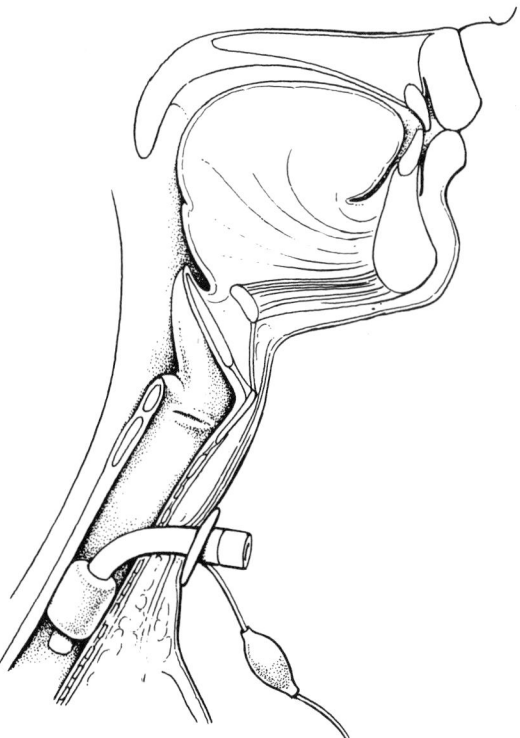

Figure 11-18. *Tracheostomy tube placement.*

(continued)

| **Guidelines** | Assisting With Tracheostomy Insertion (Fig. 11-18) *(continued)* |

Equipment
(continued)

Gauze sponges
Shave prep kit
Sedation
Local anesthetic and syringe
Resuscitation bag and mask with oxygen source
Suction source and catheters
Syringe for cuff inflation
Respiratory support available for post-tracheostomy (mechanical ventilation, tracheal oxygen mask, CPAP, T-piece)
Goggles or other eye protection device

Assessment	**Nursing Action**	**Rationale/Amplification**
	1. Monitor vital signs (heart rate, respiration, blood pressure, temperature) before insertion.	1. Provides baseline for assessment of progress or complications.
Planning/Implementation	1. Explain the procedure to the patient. Discuss a communication system with the patient.	1. Apprehension about inability to talk is usually a major concern of the tracheostomized patient.
	2. Obtain consent for operative procedure.	
	3. Shave neck region.	3. Hair and beard may harbor microorganisms. If beard is to be removed, inform the patient or family.
	4. Assemble equipment. Using aseptic technique, inflate tracheostomy cuff and evaluate for symmetry and volume leakage. Deflate maximally.	4. Ensures that the cuff is functional prior to tube insertion.
	5. Position the patient (supine with head extended, with a support under shoulders). Apply soft wrist restraints if the patient is confused.	5. This position brings the trachea forward. Restraint of the confused patient may be necessary to ensure patient safety and preservation of aseptic technique.
	6. Give medication per physician request.	
	7. Position light source.	
	8. Assist with antiseptic prep.	
	9. Assist physician with gowning and gloving.	
	10. Assist with sterile draping.	
	11. Put on goggles.	11. Spraying of blood or airway secretions may occur during this procedure.
	12. The physician performs the procedure with the nurse circulating. He or she or another designated nurse also monitors the patient's vital signs, suctions as necessary, gives medication as prescribed, or administers emergency care.	12. Bradycardia may result from vagal stimulation due to tracheal manipulation, or hypoxemia. Hypoxemia may also cause cardiac irritability.
	13. Immediately after the tube is inserted, inflate the cuff. The chest should be auscultated for the presence of bilateral breath sounds.	13. Ensures ventilation of both lungs.
	14. Secure the tracheostomy tube with twill tapes or other securing device (see Tracheostomy Care).	
	15. Apply respiratory assistive devices (mechanical ventilation, tracheostomy oxygen mask, CPAP, T-piece adapter).	
	16. Check the tracheostomy tube cuff pressure (see Cuff Inflation).	16. Excessive cuff pressure may cause tracheal damage.
	17. "Tie sutures" or "stay sutures" of 00 silk may have been placed through either side of the tracheal cartilage at the incision and brought out through the wound. Each is to be taped to the skin at a 45-degree angle laterally to the sternum.	17. Should the tracheostomy tube become dislodged, the stay sutures may be grasped and used to spread the tracheal cartilage apart, facilitating placement of the new tube.
Evaluation/Outcome	1. Assess vital signs and ventilatory status; note tube size used, physician performing procedure, type, dose, and route of medications given.	1. Provides baseline.
	2. Obtain chest x-ray.	2. Documents proper tube placement.
	3. Assess and chart condition of stoma: a. Bleeding	a. Some bleeding around the stoma site is not uncommon for the first few hours. Monitor and inform the physician of any increase in bleeding. Clean site aseptically when necessary (see Tracheostomy Care). Do not change tracheostomy ties for first 24 hours, since accidental dislodgment of the tube could result when the ties are loose, and tube reinsertion through the as yet unformed stoma may be difficult or impossible to accomplish.

**Evaluation/
Outcome**
(continued)

b. Swelling
c. Subcutaneous air

4. An extra tube, obturator, and hemostat should be kept at the bedside. In the event of tube dislodgment, reinsertion of a new tube may be necessary. For emergency tube insertion:

Spread the wound with a hemostat or stay sutures;
Insert replacement tube (containing the obturator) at an angle;
Point cannula downward and insert the tube maximally; remove the obturator.

c. When positive pressure respiratory assistive devices are used (mechanical ventilation, CPAP) before the wound is healed, air may be forced into the subcutaneous fat layer. This can be seen as enlargement of the neck and facial tissues and felt as crepitus or ''crackling'' when the skin is depressed. The physician is informed.

4. The hemostat will open the airway and allow ventilation in the spontaneously breathing patient. Avoid inserting the tube horizontally, as the tube may be forced against the back wall of the trachea.

Guidelines ## Tracheostomy Care (Routine)

Tracheostomy care keeps the area clean and dry, preventing skin irritation and infection. Secretions collected above the tracheostomy tube cuff ooze out of the surgical incision. The resultant wetness promotes irritation of the skin, and the wetness, coupled with the transmission of bacteria via the secretions, sets up a medium for infection to occur.

Equipment

Assemble the following equipment or obtain a prepackaged tracheostomy care kit:
Sterile towel
Sterile gauze sponges (12)
Sterile cotton swabs
Sterile gloves
Hydrogen peroxide
Sterile water
Antiseptic solution and ointment (optional)
Tracheostomy tie tapes
Goggles or other eye protection device

Assessment	**Nursing Action**	**Rationale/Amplification**
	1. Assess condition of stoma prior to tracheostomy care (redness, swelling, character of secretions, presence of purulence or bleeding).	1. The presence of skin breakdown or infection must be monitored. Culture of the site may be warranted by appearance of these signs.
Planning/Implementation	1. Suction the trachea and pharynx thoroughly prior to tracheostomy care.	1. Removal of secretions prior to tracheostomy care keeps the area clean longer.
	2. Explain procedure to the patient.	
	3. Wash hands thoroughly.	
	4. Assemble equipment:	
	a. Place sterile towel on patient's chest under tracheostomy site.	a. Provides sterile field
	b. Open 4 gauze sponges and pour hydrogen peroxide on them.	b. For removing mucus and crust, which promotes bacterial growth
	c. Open 2 gauze sponges and pour antiseptic solution on them.	c. May be applied to fresh stoma or infected stoma—not necessary for clean, healed stoma
	d. Open 2 gauze sponges, keep dry.	
	e. Open 2 gauze sponges and pour sterile water on them.	
	f. Place tracheostomy tube tapes on field.	
	g. Put on goggles and sterile gloves.	g. Goggles prevent spraying of secretions into the nurse's eyes. Sterile gloves prevent contamination of the wound by nurse's hands and also protect the nurse's hands from infection.

(continued)

Guidelines Tracheostomy Care (Routine) *(continued)*

Planning/Implementation *(continued)*	**Nursing Action**	**Rationale/Amplification**
	5. Clean the external end of the tracheostomy tube with 2 gauze sponges with hydrogen peroxide; discard sponges.	
	6. Clean the stoma area with 2 peroxide-soaked gauze sponges. Make only a single sweep with each gauze sponge before discarding.	6. Hydrogen peroxide may help loosen dry crusted secretions.
	7. Loosen and remove any crust with sterile cotton swabs.	
	8. Repeat step 2 using the sterile water-soaked gauze sponges.	8. Ensures that all hydrogen peroxide is removed.
	9. Repeat step 2 using dry sponges.	9. Ensures dryness of the area—wetness promotes infection and irritation.
	10. (Optional) An infected wound may be cleaned with gauze saturated with an antiseptic solution, then dried. A thin layer of antibiotic ointment may be applied to the stoma with a cotton swab.	10. May help clear wound infection.
	11. Change the tracheostomy tie tapes	
	a. Cut soiled tape while holding tube securely with other hand. Use care not to cut the pilot balloon tubing.	a. Stabilization of the tube helps prevent accidental dislodgement and keeps irritation and coughing due to tube manipulation at a minimum. Two persons may participate in the procedure at this point.
	b. Remove old tapes carefully.	
	c. Grasp slit end of clean tape and pull it through opening on side of the tracheostomy tube.	
	d. Pull other end of tape securely through the slit end of the tape.	
	e. Repeat on the other side.	
	f. Tie the tapes at the side of the neck in a square knot. Alternate knot from side to side each time tapes are changed.	f. To prevent irritation and rotate pressure site.
	g. Tape should be tight enough to keep tube securely in the stoma, but loose enough to permit two fingers to fit between the tapes and the neck.	g. Excessive tightness of tapes will compress jugular veins, decrease blood circulation to the skin under the tape, and result in discomfort for the patient.

Note: If only one clinician is available, the stoma is new (<2 weeks), or the patient's condition is unstable, follow steps c–f before removing old tapes. Two sets of ties will be in place at the same time. After completing step f, cut and remove the old tapes.

12. Some clinicians elect to place a gauze pad between the stoma site and the tracheostomy tube to absorb secretions and prevent irritation of the stoma (Fig. 11-19). Many clinicians feel that gauze should not be used around the stoma. In their opinion, the dressing keeps the area moist and dark, promoting stomal infection. They believe the stoma should be left open to the air and the surrounding area kept dry. A dressing is used only if secretions are draining onto subclavian or neck IV sites or chest incisions.

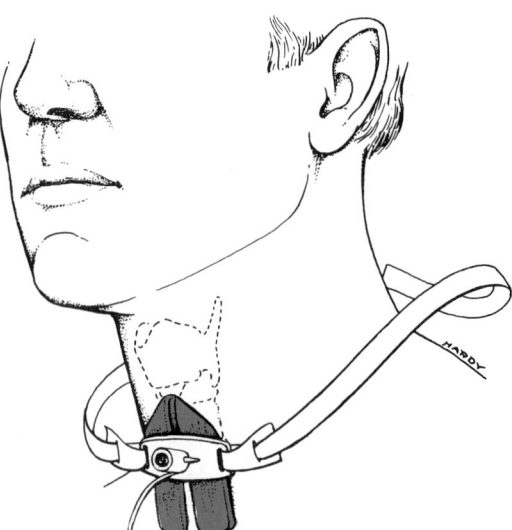

Figure 11-19. *Placement of tracheostomy tube tapes and elective gauze pad.*

Evaluation/Outcome	1. Document procedure performance, observations of stoma (irritation, redness, edema, subcutaneous air), and character of secretions (color, purulence).	1. Provides a baseline. Notify physician of changes in stoma appearance or secretions.
	2. Cleaning of the fresh stoma should be performed every 8 hours, or more frequently if indicated by accumulation of secretions. Ties should be changed every 24 hours, or more frequently if soiled or wet.	2. The area must be kept clean and dry to prevent infection or irritation of tissues.

Guidelines

Sterile Tracheobronchial Suction via Tracheostomy or Endotracheal Tube (Spontaneous or Mechanical Ventilation)

The patient with an ineffective cough cannot clear his secretions and requires suctioning. It is a sterile procedure. Secretion collection in the artificial airway or tracheobronchial tree may result in narrowing of the airway, respiratory insufficiency, increased work of breathing, and stasis of secretions.

Indications

1. When secretions can be seen or sounds resulting from secretions are heard with or without the use of a stethoscope
2. Following chest physiotherapy
3. Following bronchodilator treatments.
4. Following a sudden rise or the "popping off" of the peak airway pressure in mechanically ventilated patients that is not due to kinking of the artificial airway or ventilator tube, patient biting the tube, the patient coughing or struggling against the ventilator, or pneumothorax

Note: Patients with ineffective cough mechanisms do not require "routine" suctioning. The need for suctioning may be assessed by auscultation and chest x-ray findings. To aid in assessing need for suctioning, the patient may be ventilated with a resuscitation bag to increase ventilation and facilitate auscultation. Bagging may also stimulate the cough reflex, decreasing the need for suctioning.

Equipment

Assemble the following equipment or obtain a prepackaged suctioning kit:

Sterile suction catheters—No. 14 or 16 (adult), No. 8 or 10 (child). The outer diameter of the suction catheter should be no greater than one half the inner diameter of the artificial airway.

Two sterile gloves

Sterile towel

Suction source at 100–120 mm. Hg

Sterile water

Resuscitation bag with a reservoir connected to 100% oxygen source (if patient is on PEEP or CPAP, add positive end-expiratory pressure (PEEP) valve to exhalation valve on resuscitation bag in an amount equal to that on the ventilator or CPAP device).

Normal saline solution (in syringe or single-dose packet)

Sterile cup for water

Alcohol swabs

Sterile water-soluble lubricant jelly

Goggles or other eye protection device

Assessment	**Nursing Action**	**Rationale/Amplification**

	1. Monitor heart rate and auscultate breath sounds. If the patient is monitored, continuously monitor heart rate and arterial blood pressure. If arterial blood gases are done routinely, know baseline values. (It is important to establish a baseline because suctioning should be discontinued and oxygen applied or manual ventilation reinstituted if, during the suction procedure, the heart rate decreases by 20 beats per minute or increases by 40 beats per minute, blood pressure drops, or cardiac dysrhythmia is noted.)	1. Suctioning may cause:
		  a. Hypoxemia, initially resulting in tachycardia and increased blood pressure, progressing to cardiac ectopy, bradycardia, hypotension, and cyanosis.
		  b. Vagal stimulation, which may result in bradycardia.

Planning/Implementation	1. Instruct the patient how to "splint" surgical incision, as coughing will be induced during the procedure. Explain the importance of performing the suction procedure in an aseptic manner.	1. Thorough explanation lessens patient's anxiety and promotes cooperation.

(continued)

Guidelines   Sterile Tracheobronchial Suction via Tracheostomy or Endotracheal Tube
(Spontaneous or Mechanical Ventilation) *(continued)*

Planning/Implementation *(continued)*	Nursing Action	Rationale/Amplification
	2. Assemble equipment. Check function of suction and manual resuscitation bag connected to 100% O₂ source. Put on goggles.	2. Make sure that all equipment is functional before sterile technique is instituted to prevent interruption once the procedure is begun. Use of 100% O₂ will help to prevent hypoxemia.
	3. Wash hands thoroughly.	
	4. Open sterile towel—place in a bib-like fashion on patient's chest. Open alcohol wipes and place on corner of towel. Place small amount of sterile water-soluble jelly on towel.	
	5. Open sterile gloves—place on towel.	
	6. Open suction catheter package.	
	7. If the patient is on mechanical ventilation, test to make sure that disconnection of ventilator attachment may be made with one hand.	
	8. Don sterile gloves. Designate one hand as contaminated for disconnecting, bagging, and working the suction control. Usually the dominant hand is kept sterile and will be used to thread the suction catheter.	8. The hand designated as sterile must remain uncontaminated so that organisms are not introduced into the lungs. The contaminated hand must also be gloved to prevent sputum from contacting the nurse's hand, possibly resulting in an infection of the nurse.
	9. Use the sterile hand to remove carefully the suction catheter from the package, curling the catheter around the gloved fingers.	
	10. Connect suction source to the suction fitting of the catheter with the contaminated hand.	
	11. Using the contaminated hand, disconnect the patient from the ventilator, CPAP device, or other oxygen source. (Place the ventilator connector on the sterile towel and flip a corner of the towel over the connection to prevent fluid from spraying into the area).	11. Prevents contamination of the connection
	12. Ventilate and oxygenate the patient with the resuscitator bag, compressing firmly and as completely as possible approximately 4–5 times (try to approximate the patient's tidal volume). This procedure is called "bagging" the patient. In the spontaneously breathing patient, coordinate manual ventilations with the patient's own inspiratory effort.	12. Ventilation prior to suctioning helps prevent hypoxemia. When possible, two nurses work as a team to suction. Attempting to ventilate against the patient's own respiratory efforts may result in high airway pressures, predisposing the patient to barotrauma (lung injury due to pressure).
	13. Lubricate the tip of the suction catheter. Gently insert suction catheter as far as possible into the artificial airway without applying suction. Most patients will cough when the catheter touches the trachea.	13. Suctioning on insertion would unnecessarily decrease oxygen in the airway.
	14. Apply suction and quickly rotate the catheter while it is being withdrawn.	14. Failure to rotate catheter may result in damage to tracheal mucosa. Release suction if a pulling sensation is felt.
	15. Limit suction time to 10–15 seconds. Discontinue if heart rate decreases by 20 beats per minute or increases by 40 beats per minute, or if cardiac ectopy is observed.	15. Suctioning removes oxygen as well as secretions and may also cause vagal stimulation.
	16. Bag patient between suction passes with approximately 4–5 manual ventilations.	16. The oxygen removed by suctioning must be replenished before suctioning is attempted again.
	17. At this point, sterile nonbacteriostatic saline may be instilled into the trachea via the artificial airway if secretions are tenacious.	17. Some clinicians feel that secretion removal may be facilitated with saline instillation. Others feel that saline does not mix with mucus and that suctioning of the saline just instilled is the only effect produced by performing this step.
	a. Open prepackaged container and inject 3–5 ml. nonbacteriostatic saline into the artificial airway during spontaneous inspiration.	a. Instillation of the saline during inspiration will prevent the saline from being blown back out of the tube.
	b. Bag vigorously and then suction.	b. Bagging stimulates cough and distributes saline to loosen secretions.
	18. Rinse catheter between suction passes by inserting tip in cup of sterile water and applying suction.	
	19. Continue making suction passes, bagging the patient between passes, until the airways are clear of accumulated secretions. No more than 4 suction passes should be made per suctioning episode.	19. Repeated suctioning of a patient in a short time interval predisposes to hypoxemia, as well as being tiring and traumatic to the patient.
	20. Give the patient 4–5 "sigh" breaths with the bag.	20. Sighing is accomplished by depressing the bag slowly and completely with 2 hands to deliver approximately 1½ times the normal tidal volume to the patient, allowing for maximal lung expansion and prevention of atelectasis.

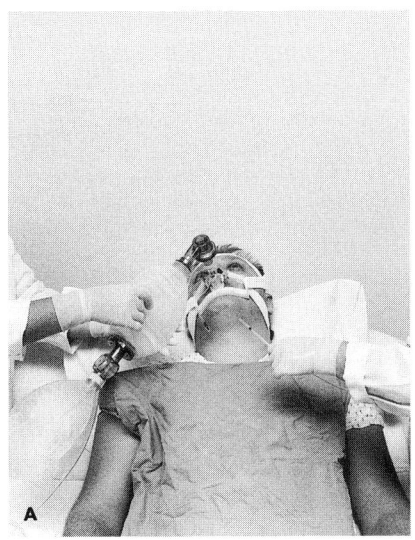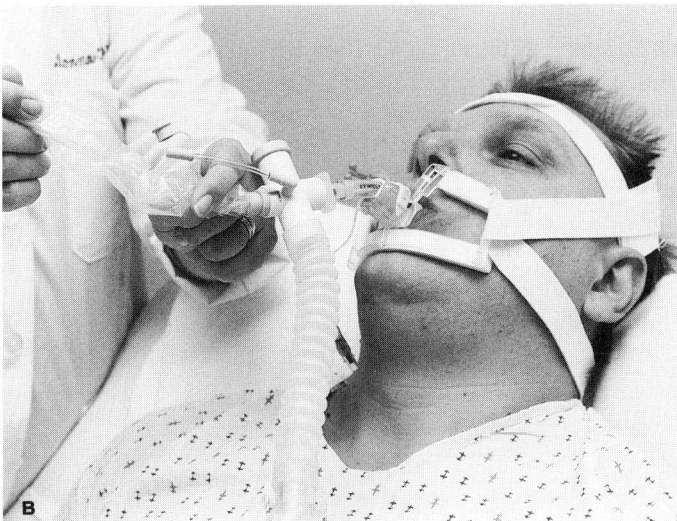

Figure 11-20. *Suctioning through an endotracheal or tracheostomy tube. (Courtesy of Photography Department, Montefiore Hospital, Pittsburgh, PA)*

Planning/Implementation
(continued)

21. Return the patient to the ventilator or apply CPAP or other oxygen-delivery device.
22. Suction oral secretions from the oropharynx above the artificial airway cuff.
23. Clean elbow fitting of resuscitation bag with alcohol; cover with a sterile glove or 4 × 4.

Evaluation/ Outcome

1. Note any change in vital signs or patient's intolerance to the procedure. Record amount and consistency of secretions.
2. Assess need for further suctioning at least every 2 hours, or more frequently if secretions are copious.

1. Evaluate the effectiveness of procedure and patient response.

Note: Two alternate approaches may be used for suctioning (Fig. 11-20):

1. *Ventilator reconnection.* The patient may be reconnected to the ventilator for 4–5 breaths of 100% oxygen between suction passes, rather than ventilating and oxygenating with a resuscitation bag.
2. *Closed system suctioning.* With closed systems, the suction catheter is contained in a tubing that is part of the ventilator circuitry, but is kept retracted and out of the airway when not in use. Closed suction systems allow suctioning without gloving or disconnecting the patient from the ventilator. Advantages include eliminating ventilator disconnection, decreased clinician exposure to body fluids, and time saving. A disadvantage is the added weight of the suction system, which increases traction on the artificial airway. Extra attention is required to secure and stabilize the endotracheal tube. Principles of suctioning are the same as previously described. Between suction passes, the patient is allowed to receive 4–5 breaths of 100% oxygen from the ventilator.

Guidelines Artificial Airway Cuff Inflation/Deflation (Cuff Pressure Measurement)

The cuffs of endotracheal and tracheostomy tubes must be inflated continuously when the patient is on mechanical ventilation or CPAP. The cuff is then deflated only for tube removal or repositioning. The cuffs of spontaneously breathing tracheostomized patients may require inflation at all times if the patient has a depressed level of consciousness or neuromuscular deficiency that does not permit the patient to protect his airway. The cuffs of spontaneously breathing tracheostomized patients not on mechanical ventilation or CPAP may be deflated:

1. When the patient can adequately protect the airway.
2. Between meals, if the patient is at risk for aspiration only during feeding. The cuff may be inflated prior to feeding and for 1 hour after feeding.

(continued)

Guidelines Artificial Airway Cuff Inflation/Deflation (Cuff Pressure Measurement) *(continued)*

Complications of Excessive Cuff Pressure	Tracheal swelling — Tracheoarterial fistula

Complications of Excessive Cuff Pressure

Tracheal swelling	Tracheoarterial fistula
Tracheal ulceration	Tracheal necrosis
Tracheoesophageal fistula	Tracheal malacia

Equipment

Suction catheter
Tonsil suction
Suction source
10-ml. syringe
Pressure manometer (mercury or anaeroid)
Manual resuscitation bag with reservoir, connected to 100% oxygen at 10–15 liters/minute.
Goggles or other eye protection device.

Assessment

Nursing Action	Rationale/Amplification
1. Note degree of air leakage around cuff by listening over the cuff area with a stethoscope.	1. Provides a baseline. Air leakage is heard as a crowing sound at peak airway pressure.
2. Auscultate breath sounds.	2. Provides baseline data

Planning/Implementation

1. Explain procedure to the patient.	1. Decreases the patient's anxiety and promotes cooperation
2. Put on goggles.	2. Spraying of secretions may occur.

Deflating the Cuff

1. Suction the trachea, then the oral and nasal pharynx. Then replace the catheter with a second sterile suction catheter.	1. Removes secretions collected above the cuff, which could be aspirated into the lungs when the cuff is deflated. Do not reenter the trachea with the same catheter used for suctioning the mouth.
2. Deflate the cuff slowly.	2. The small test balloon at the end of the tubing remains inflated as long as the cuff at the distal end of the tube is inflated. A vacuum within the syringe is sensed when no more air can be aspirated.
3. (Concomitant with step 2) Have the patient cough, or manually inflate the lungs with the resuscitation bag. Be ready to receive secretions in a tissue, or aspirate with a tonsil suction.	3. Positive pressure in the airways may help force secretions upward and prevent aspiration.
4. Suction through the tracheostomy or endotracheal tube.	4. Secretions that may have been present above the inflated cuff and around the exterior tube have now seeped downward. The coughing reflex may be stimulated, helping to mobilize secretions.
5. Provide adequate ventilation while the cuff is deflated.	
a. If the patient does not require assisted ventilation, maintain humidified oxygen as directed.	a. Continue observation of color, pulse, etc.
b. If the patient requires assisted ventilation, provide manual ventilation via a resuscitation bag. Leave cuff deflated for as long as the tube repositioning requires; then reinflate.	b. Monitor patient closely for tolerance. Loss of tidal volume or PEEP may promote hypoxemia and hypocarbia. Cuff should not be deflated for more than 30–45 seconds.

Inflating a Cuff

1. No leak technique:	1. Air leakage will be heard when the intra-airway pressure is most positive (maximum peak airway pressure). For the spontaneously breathing patient, air leakage will be heard on exhalation. For the patient on positive pressure ventilation, air leakage will be heard at maximum ventilator inspiration.
a. Attach air-filled syringe to cuff injection port.	
b. Slowly inject air until no air escapes from the patient's lungs around the cuff.	
c. Note amount of air injected to provide the seal.	
2. Minimal leak technique (for mechanical ventilation)	
a. Attach air-filled syringe to cuff injection port.	
b. Slowly inject air until no leak is heard at maximum peak airway pressure.	
c. Slowly remove air from cuff until a small air leak is heard at maximum peak airway pressure.	c. Adjustment in tidal volume setting may be necessary to compensate for the leak.
d. Note amount of air injected.	
3. Measurement of minimal occluding volume (Fig. 11-21)	
a. Inject sufficient air into the manometer tubing to raise the dial reading 1 cm. H_2O above the zero reading.	a. This "pressurizes" the tubing and prevents loss of air from the cuff to the tubing when the reading is taken.

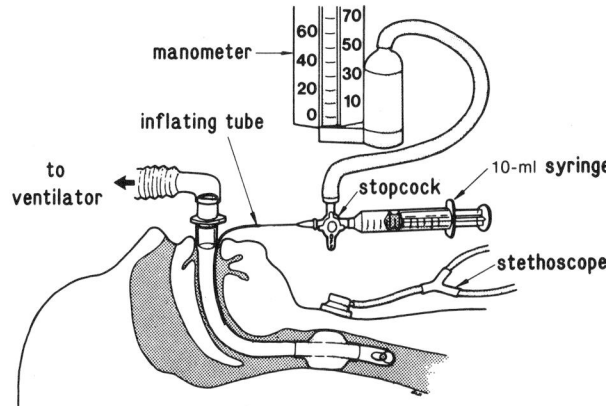

Figure 11-21. *Determination of minimal occluding volume and cuff inflation pressure. A stopcock is inserted into the cuff injection port. When the stopcock is opened to the manometer, cuff pressure is registered on the manometer. An aneroid manometer can also be used. (From Sills J. An emergency cuff inflation technique. Respiratory Care 1986 Mar; 31(3): 201)*

Planning/Implementation
(continued)

b. Insert male port of three-way stopcock into cuff injection port. One female port of stopcock holds the air-filled syringe, and one port holds the pressure manometer.

c. Inject air into cuff until desired intracuff pressure is reached at maximum peak airway pressure.

c. Anaeroid manometer measures cuff pressure in cm. H_2O: A pressure of 20–25 cm. H_2O is desired. Mercury manometer pressure should be 15–20 mm. Hg. Pressure greater than upper limit may cause compression of tracheal vessels, resulting in decreased blood flow to tissue. Pressure less than lower limit may allow aspiration of gastric or oral secretions.

d. Note amount of air needed to achieve the desired intracuff pressure.

e. Remove the stopcock from the injection port.

e. Most injection ports have self-sealing valves. If not, a cap or closed stopcock may be left in the injection port (clamping of the inflation tubing is discouraged, as it may result in cracking or kinking of the line permanently).

Monitoring Cuff Pressure

1. While the cuff is inflated, monitor cuff pressure every 4 hours. Maintain cuff pressure between 15–20 mm. Hg or 20–25 cm. H_2O.

2. Document the pressure required to maintain cuff pressure at this level.

1. Excessive pressure will decrease blood flow to the tissue, resulting in tracheal necrosis. Insufficient cuff pressure predisposes to aspiration.

2. Establishes a baseline for evaluation of change in pressure.

Inability to Maintain a Seal

1. Assess the degree of leakage and length of time elapsed since cuff volume was replenished.

1. If an inflated cuff leaks air within 10 minutes, assessment is necessary. Possibilities may be:
   a. Cuff positioned above the vocal cords (direct visualization necessary for repositioning)
   b. Incompetence of self-sealing valve on injection port
   c. Tracheal dilatation (requiring larger size tube)
   d. Cuff may be ruptured, requiring a new tube

2. Inflate the cuff to desired level.
3. Disconnect syringe (and manometer if used).
4. Assess for leakage.
5. If leakage recurs, place three-way stopcock between syringe and injection port, inflate cuff, close stopcock. Remove syringe (and manometer if used) leaving closed stopcock in injection port.
6. If air leak persists, tube repositioning or replacement may be necessary. Consult with appropriate personnel.

5. Closed stopcock left in injection port acts as "plug" if self-sealing valve is incompetent.

Evaluation/Outcome

1. Note and record amount of air used for adequate seal, intracuff pressure, and inability to achieve seal.

2. While the cuff is inflated, assess cuff pressure every 4 hours. The cuff pressure manometer is useful for this.

1. Notify physician or personnel qualified to intubate, or change tracheostomy tube if unable to achieve desired seal.

2. Leakage of air from the cuff or cuff injection port may occur. Assess the inflation status and adjust as needed.

Guidelines Insertion of a Tracheostomy Button

A *tracheostomy button* is a rigid cannula that is placed into the tracheostomy stoma following removal of a cuffed or uncuffed tracheostomy tube. When in proper position, the button does not extend into the tracheal lumen. The outer edge of the button is at the skin surface and the inner edge at the anterior tracheal wall.

Equipment

Tracheostomy button kit (includes cannula, solid closure plug, spacers, universal adapter)
Water-soluble lubricant
Syringe for deflation of tracheotomy cuff
Replacement tracheostomy tube

Assessment

1. Assess whether patient meets criteria for use of tracheostomy button. Criteria include: able to be adequately oxygenated with nasal cannula or face mask; able to swallow and protect the airway; able to cough up secretions; and a noninfected, nonirritated tracheal stoma.

2. Determine vital signs, level of consciousness, SaO_2 or ABG.

1. If patient does not meet these criteria, use of tracheostomy tube must be continued.

2. Provides baseline for future assessment

Planning/Implementation

1. Elevate the head of the bed 45 degrees, suction the airway, deflate the tracheostomy tube cuff, and remove the tube.

2. Determine the distance from anterior tracheal wall to the outer edge of the stoma (skin surface) using a probe with a right angle bend (contained in the kit).

3. Compare the length of the tracheostomy button cannula with this measurement. If the cannula is too long, it can be sized to fit by adding spacers included in the kit.

4. Coat the cannula with water-soluble lubricant. Ask the patient to relax and take several deep breaths. Insert the cannula into the stoma.

5. Insert the closure plug into the cannula. Ties may be used to hold the button in place until the stoma closes around the button.

6. Remove button 2 times a week, clean with antibacterial soap, and replace it.

1. See Guidelines: Artificial Airway Cuff Inflation/Deflation p. 243.)

2. Insert angled end of the probe into the stoma, pull gently until the probe touches the anterior wall, then mark the probe at the outer edge of the stoma (skin surface).

3. Spacer rings can be slipped over the cannula to size it for individualized patient requirements.

4. The cannula should pass easily into the stoma. If insertion is difficult, recheck cannula size. Several sizes are available.

5. A slight snap will be heard as the plug enters the cannula. The plug causes the proximal end of the cannula to flare, holding it in place.

6. Periodic removal helps to keep tissue from granulating into the distal portion of the cannula.

Evaluation/Outcome

1. Observe immediate patient response and obtain SaO_2 or ABG after insertion. Report changes to the physician.

2. Determine ability of patient to cough out secretions and swallow with button in place.

1. Use of the button increases dead space, which may increase work of breathing or cause a decrease in SaO_2.

2. Confirms patient will not retain secretions or be at risk for aspiration with use of this device.

Mechanical Ventilation

The *mechanical ventilator* is a device that functions as a substitute for the bellows action of the thoracic cage and diaphragm. The mechanical ventilator can maintain ventilation automatically for prolonged periods. It is indicated when the patient is unable to maintain safe levels of oxygen or carbon dioxide by spontaneous breathing even with the assistance of other oxygen delivery devices.

Types of Ventilators

A. Negative Pressure Ventilators

1. Applies negative pressure around the chest wall. This causes intra-airway pressure to become negative, thus drawing air into the lungs through the patient's nose and mouth.
2. No artificial airway is necessary—patient must be able to control and protect own airway.
3. Indications—may be used for selected patients with respiratory neuromuscular problems, or as adjunct to weaning from positive pressure ventilation.

B. Positive Pressure Ventilators

During mechanical inspiration, air is actively delivered to the patient's lungs under positive pressure. Requires use of a cuffed artificial airway. Exhalation is passive.
1. Pressure limited:
   a. Terminates the inspiratory phase when a preselected airway pressure is achieved
   b. Volume delivered is dependent on lung compliance (ml. volume/cm. H_2O airway pressure).
   c. Use of volume-based alarms are recommended because any obstruction between the machine and lungs that allows a buildup of pressure in the ventilator circuitry will cause the ventilator to cycle, but the patient will receive no volume.
2. Volume limited:
   a. Terminates the inspiratory phase when a designated volume of the gas is delivered into the ventilator circuit (12–15 ml./kg. body weight—usual starting volumes).
   b. Delivers the predetermined volume regardless of changing lung compliance (although airway pressures will increase as compliance decreases). Air-

way pressures vary from patient to patient and from breath to breath.

   c. Pressure-limiting valves, which prevent excessive pressure buildup within the patient–ventilator system, are used. Without this valve, pressure could increase indefinitely and pulmonary barotrauma could result. Usually equipped with a system that alarms when selected pressure limit is exceeded and vents excess inspired air to the atmosphere.

Modes of Operation

A. Controlled Ventilation (CV)

1. Cycles automatically at rate that is selected by operator.
2. Provides a fixed level of ventilation, but will not cycle or have gas available in circuitry to respond to patient's own inspiratory efforts. This typically increases work of breathing for patients attempting to breathe spontaneously.
3. Possibly indicated for patients whose respiratory drive is absent.

B. Assist/Control (A/C)

1. Inspiratory cycle of ventilator is activated by the patient's voluntary inspiratory effort.
2. Ventilator also cycles at a rate predetermined by the operator. Should the patient stop breathing, or breathe so weakly that the ventilator cannot function as an assistor, this mandatory baseline rate will prevent apnea. A minimum level of minute ventilation is provided.
3. Indicated for patients who are breathing spontaneously, but who have the potential to lose their respiratory drive or muscular control of ventilation. In this mode, the patient's work of breathing is greatly reduced.

C. Intermittent Mandatory Ventilation (IMV)

1. Allows patient to breathe spontaneously through ventilator circuitry.
2. Periodically, at preselected rate and volume, cycles to give a "mandated" ventilator breath. A minimum level of ventilation is provided.
3. Gas provided for spontaneous breaths usually flows continuously through the ventilator.
4. Indicated for patients who are breathing spontaneously, but at a tidal volume and/or rate less than adequate for their needs. Allows the patient to do some of the work of breathing.

D. Synchronized Intermittent Mandatory Ventilation (SIMV)

1. Allows patient to breathe spontaneously through the ventilator circuitry.
2. Periodically, at a preselected time, a mandatory breath is delivered. The patient may initiate the mandatory breath with his own inspiratory effort, and the ventilator breath will be synchronized with the patient's efforts, or will be "assisted." If the patient does not provide inspiratory effort, the breath will still be delivered, or be "controlled."
3. Gas provided for spontaneous breathing is usually delivered through a demand regulator, which is activated by the patient.
4. Indicated for patients who are breathing spontaneously, but at a tidal volume and/or rate less than adequate for their needs. Allows the patient to do some of the work of breathing.

E. Pressure Support

1. A positive pressure is set.
2. During spontaneous inspiration, ventilator circuitry is rapidly pressurized to the predetermined pressure and held at this pressure.
3. When the inspiratory flow rate decreases to a preset minimal level (20%–25% of peak inspiratory flow), the positive pressure returns to baseline. The patient may exhale, or complete inspiration without pressure support.
4. The patient ventilates spontaneously, establishing own rate, and inspiring the tidal volume that feels appropriate.
5. Pressure support may be used independently as a ventilatory mode, or used in conjunction with CPAP or SIMV.

Special Positive Pressure Ventilation Techniques

A. Positive End-Expiratory Pressure (PEEP)

1. Maneuver by which pressure during mechanical ventilation is maintained above atmospheric at end of exhalation, resulting in an increased functional residual capacity. Airway pressure is therefore positive throughout the entire ventilatory cycle.
2. Purpose—to increase functional residual capacity (or the amount of air left in the lungs at the end of expiration). This aids in:
   a. Increasing the surface area for gas exchange
   b. Preventing collapse of alveolar units and development of atelectasis
   c. Decreasing intrapulmonary shunt
3. Benefits
   a. Because a greater surface area for diffusion is available and shunting is reduced, it is often possible to use a lower fraction of inspired oxygen concentration (F_IO_2) than otherwise would be required to obtain adequate arterial oxygen levels. This reduces the risk of oxygen toxicity in conditions such as adult respiratory distress syndrome.
   b. Positive intra-airway pressure may be helpful in reducing the transudation of fluid from the pulmonary capillaries in situations where capillary pressure is increased (i.e., left heart failure)
   c. Increased lung compliance resulting in decreased work of breathing.
4. Hazards
   a. Because the mean airway pressure is increased by PEEP, venous return is impeded. This may result in a decrease in cardiac output (especially noted in hypovolemic patients).
   b. The increased airway pressure may possibly result in alveolar rupture. The likelihood is greater in patients with noncompliant lungs. This barotrauma may result in pneumothorax, tension pneumothorax, or development of subcutaneous emphysema.
   c. The decreased venous return may cause antidiuretic hormone formation to be stimulated, resulting in decreased urine output.
5. Precautions
   a. Monitor frequently for signs and symptoms of pneumothorax (increased pulmonary artery pressure, increased size of hemithorax, decreased lung movement, hyperresonant percussion note, diminished breath sounds).

b. Monitor for signs of decreased venous return:
(1) Decreased arterial blood pressure
(2) Decreased cardiac output
(3) Decreased urine output; formation of peripheral edema
c. Abrupt discontinuance of PEEP is not recommended. The patient should not be without PEEP for longer than 15 seconds. The manual resuscitation bag used for ventilation during suction procedure or patient transport should be equipped with a PEEP device. Some clinicians feel that loss of PEEP for short periods is not detrimental in the lower ranges (less than 10 cm. H₂O). An exception might be patients with increased intracranial pressure.
d. Intrapulmonary blood vessel pressure may increase because of compression of the vessels by increased intra-airway pressure. Therefore, CVP and PA pressures and wedge may be increased. The clinician must bear this in mind when determining the clinical significance of these pressures.

B. Continuous Positive Airway Pressure (CPAP)

1. Also provides for positive airway pressure during all parts of a respiratory cycle, but refers to spontaneous ventilation rather than mechanical ventilation.
2. May be delivered through ventilator circuitry when ventilator rate is at "0," or may be delivered through a separate CPAP circuitry that does not require the ventilator.
3. Indicated for patients who are capable of maintaining an adequate tidal volume, but have pathology preventing maintenance of adequate levels of tissue oxygenation.
4. CPAP has the same benefits, hazards, and precautions noted with PEEP. Mean airway pressures may be lower because of lack of mechanical ventilation breaths. This results in less risk of barotrauma and impedance of venous return.

Underlying Principles

1. Variables that control ventilation and oxygenation:
a. Ventilator rate—adjusted by rate setting.
b. Tidal volume—adjusted by tidal volume setting. Measured as inhaled volume.
c. Fraction inspired oxygen concentration (F_IO_2)—set on ventilator or with an oxygen blender. Measured with an oxygen analyzer.
d. Ventilator dead space—circuitry common to inhalation and exhalation. Tubing is calibrated.

e. PEEP—set within the ventilator or with the use of external PEEP devices. Measured at the proximal airway.
2. CO_2 elimination—controlled by tidal volume, rate, and dead space.
3. Oxygen tension—controlled by oxygen concentration and PEEP (also by rate and tidal volume).
4. The duration of inspiration should not exceed exhalation. Rate, tidal volume, gas flow in liters per minute, and inspiratory pause all control inspiratory time. Inverse inspiration: exhalation ratio results in "stacking" of breaths or buildup of pressure within the airway. Barotrauma and decreased cardiac output can result.
5. The inspired gas must be warmed and humidified to prevent thickening of secretions and decrease in body temperature. Sterile distilled water is warmed and humidified via a heated humidifier or nebulizer.

Clinical Indications

1. Mechanical failure of ventilation
a. Neuromuscular disease
b. Central nervous system disease
c. Central nervous system depression (drug intoxication, respiratory depressants, cardiac arrest)
d. Musculoskeletal disease
e. Inefficiency of thoracic cage in generating pressure gradients necessary for ventilation (chest injury, thoracic malformation)
2. Disorders of pulmonary gas exchange
a. Acute respiratory failure
b. Chronic respiratory failure
c. Left ventricular failure
d. Pulmonary diseases resulting in diffusion abnormality
e. Pulmonary diseases resulting in ventilation/perfusion mismatch

Complications

1. Airway obstruction (thickened secretions, mechanical problem with artificial airway or ventilator circuitry)
2. Tracheal damage (see artificial airway)
3. Pulmonary infection
4. Barotrauma (pneumothorax or tension pneumothorax)
5. Decreased cardiac output
6. Atelectasis
7. Alteration in GI function (dilation, bleeding)
8. Alteration in renal function
9. Alteration in cognitive-perceptual status.

Guidelines Managing the Patient Requiring Mechanical Ventilation

Equipment

Artificial airway
Mechanical ventilator
Ventilator circuitry
Humidifier
See manufacturer's directions for specific machine.

Assessment

Nursing Action	Rationale/Amplification
1. Obtain baseline samples for blood gas determinations (*p*H, PaO₂, PaCO₂, HCO₃) and chest x-ray.	1. Baseline measurements serve as a guide in determining progress of therapy.

Planning/Im-plementation

1. Give a brief explanation to the patient.

1. Emphasize that mechanical ventilation is a temporary measure. The patient should be prepared psychologically for weaning at the time the ventilator is first used.

2. Establish the airway by means of a cuffed endotracheal or tracheostomy tube (see Endotracheal Intubation, Tracheostomy, and Cuff Inflation).

2. A closed system between the ventilator and patient's lower airway is necessary for positive pressure ventilation.

3. Prepare the ventilator:
   a. Set up desired circuitry.
   b. Connect oxygen and compressed air source.
   c. Turn on power.
   d. Set tidal volume (usually 12–15 ml./kg. body weight)
   e. Set oxygen concentration.
   f. Set ventilator sensitivity.
   g. Set rate at 12–14 breaths per minute (variable).

   d. Adjusted according to pH and $PaCO_2$.
   e. Adjusted according to PaO_2.

   g. This setting approximates normal ventilation. These machines' settings are subject to change according to the patient's condition and response, and the ventilator type being used.

   h. Adjust flow rate (velocity of gas flow during inspiration). Usually set at 40–60 liters/minute. Is dependent on rate and tidal volume. Set to avoid inverse inspiratory:expiratory (I:E) ratio. Usual I:E ratio is 1:2.

   h. The slower the flow, the lower will be the peak airway pressure resulting from set volume delivery. This results in lower intrathoracic pressure and less impedance of venous return. However, a flow that is too low for the rate selected may result in inverse inspiratory:expiratory ratios.

   i. Select mode of ventilation.
   j. Check machine function—measure tidal volume, rate, I:E ratio, analyze oxygen, check all alarms.

   j. Ensures safe function

4. Couple the patient's airway to the ventilator.

4. Be sure that all connections are secure. Prevent ventilator tubing from "pulling" on artificial airway, possibly resulting in tube dislodgement or tracheal damage.

5. Assess patient for adequate chest movement and rate. Do not depend on digital rate readout of ventilator. Note peak airway pressure and PEEP. Adjust gas flow if necessary to provide safe I:E ratio.

5. Ensures proper function of equipment.

6. Set airway pressure alarms according to patient's baseline:
   a. High pressure alarm

   a. High airway pressure or "pop off" pressure is set at about 20 cm. H_2O above peak airway pressure. An alarm sounds if airway pressure selected is exceeded. Alarm activation indicates: decreased lung compliance (worsening pulmonary disease, decreased lung volume such as pneumothorax, tension pneumothorax, hemothorax, pleural effusion), increased airways resistance (secretions, coughing, breathing out of phase with the ventilator), loss of patency of airway (mucus plug, airway spasm, biting or kinking of tube).

   b. Low pressure alarm

   b. Low airway pressure alarm set at 5–10 cm. H_2O below peak airway pressure. Alarm activation indicates inability to build up airway pressure because of disconnection or leak, or inability to build up airway pressure because of insufficient gas flow to meet patient's inspiratory needs.

7. Assess frequently for change in respiratory status via arterial blood gas, spontaneous rate, use of accessory muscles, breath sounds, and vital signs. Other means of assessing are through the use of exhaled carbon dioxide or mixed venous oxygen saturation monitoring.

7. If change is noted, notify appropriate personnel. In emergency condition, disconnect from ventilator and ventilate with manual resuscitation bag.

8. Monitor and trouble-shoot alarm conditions. Ensure appropriate ventilation at all times.

8. Priority is ventilation and oxygenation of the patient. In alarm conditions that cannot be immediately corrected, disconnect the patient from mechanical ventilation and manually ventilate with resuscitation bag.

9. Positioning
   a. Turn patient from side to side every 2 hours, or more frequently if possible.

   a. For patients on long-term ventilation, this may result in sleep deprivation. Evolve a turning schedule best suited to a particular patient's condition.

(continued)

Guidelines Managing the Patient Requiring Mechanical Ventilation *(continued)*

Planning/Im-plementation *(continued)*	Nursing Action	Rationale/Amplification
	b. Lateral turns of 120 degrees are desirable; from right semi-prone to left semi-prone.	
	c. Sit the patient upright at regular intervals if possible.	c. Upright posture increases lung compliance.
	10. Carry out passive range of motion exercises of all extremities for patients unable to do so.	
	11. Assess for need of suctioning every 2 hours (see Suctioning).	11. Patients with artificial airways on mechanical ventilation are unable to clear secretions on their own. Suctioning may help to clear secretions and stimulate the cough reflex.
	12. Assess breath sounds every 2 hours:	
	a. Listen with stethoscope to the chest from bottom to top on both sides.	a. Auscultation of the chest is a means of assessing airway patency and ventilatory distribution. It also confirms the proper placement of the endotracheal or tracheostomy tube.
	b. Determine whether breath sounds are present or absent, normal or abnormal, and whether a *change* has occurred.	
	c. Observe the patient's diaphragmatic excursions and use of accessory muscles of respiration.	
	13. Humidification	
	a. Check the water level in the humidification reservoir to ensure that the patient is never ventilated with dry gas. Empty the water that condenses in the delivery and exhalation tubing into a separate receptacle, not into the humidifier. Humidifier and nebulizer must be changed every 24 hours.	a. Water condensing in the inspiratory tubing may cause increased resistance to gas flow. This may result in increased peak airway pressures. Warm, moist tubing is a perfect breeding area for bacteria. If this water is allowed to enter the humidifier, bacteria may be aerosolized into the lungs. Emptying the tubing also prevents introduction of water into the patient's airways. Always wash hands after emptying fluid from ventilator circuitry.
	14. Assess airway pressures at frequent intervals.	14. Monitor for changes in compliance, or onset of conditions that may cause airway pressure to increase or decrease (see step 3).
	15. Measure delivered tidal volume and analyze oxygen every 4 hours or more frequently if indicated.	
	16. Monitor cardiovascular function. Assess for depression.	
	a. Monitor pulse rate and arterial blood pressure; intra-arterial pressure monitoring may be carried out.	a. To accomplish intra-arterial pressure monitoring, a catheter is introduced into an artery, usually the radial or femoral, and the pressure at the catheter tip transmitted to a pressure transducer that converts the pressure wave into an electrical signal that is displayed for continuous visual observation on an oscilloscope and digital readout.
	b. Use Swan–Ganz catheter to monitor pulmonary capillary wedge pressure, mixed venous oxygen ($P\bar{v}O_2$), and cardiac output.	b. Intermittent and continuous positive pressure ventilation may increase the pulmonary artery pressures and decrease cardiac output.
	17. Monitor for pulmonary infection.	
	a. Aspirate tracheal secretions into a sterile container and send to laboratory for culture and sensitivity testing. This is done immediately after endotracheal intubation and in some instances on an every-other-day basis.	a. This technique allows the earliest detection of infection or change in infecting organisms in the tracheobronchial tree.
	b. Daily Gram staining of secretions may also be done in some institutions.	
	c. Monitor for systemic signs and symptoms of pulmonary infection (pulmonary physical examination findings, increased heart rate, increased temperature, increased WBC count).	
	18. Evaluate need for sedation or muscle relaxants.	18. Sedatives may be prescribed by the physician to decrease patient anxiety, or to relax the patient so that he is not "competing" with the ventilator. At times, pharmacologically induced paralysis may be necessary in order to permit mechanical ventilation. Paralysis is prescribed by the physician.

NURSING ALERT: Paralysis should not be administered by the nurse unless the patient is intubated and on mechanical ventilation.

| | 19. Report intake and output precisely and obtain an accurate daily weight to monitor fluid balance. | 19. Positive fluid balance resulting in increase in body weight and interstitial pulmonary edema is a frequent problem in |

Planning/Im-plementation
(continued)

20. Monitor nutritional status.

21. Monitor GI function.

    a. Test all stools and gastric drainage for occult blood.

    b. Measure abdominal girth daily.

22. Provide for care and communication needs of patient with an artificial airway (see Artificial Airway Management, Tracheobronchial Suctioning, Cuff Inflation/Deflation/Pressure Measurement, Tracheostomy Care).
23. Provide psychological support
    a. Assist with communication.
    b. Orient to environment and function of mechanical ventilation.
    c. Ensure that the patient has adequate rest and sleep.

patients requiring mechanical ventilation. Prevention requires early recognition of fluid accumulation. An average adult who is dependent on parenteral nutrition can be expected to lose 0.25 kg. (½ lb.)/day; therefore, constant body weight indicates positive fluid balance.

20. Patients on mechanical ventilation require inflation of artificial airway cuffs at all times. Patients with tracheostomy tubes may eat, if capable, or may require enteral feeding tubes or parenteral nourishment. Patients with endotracheal tubes are to be NPO (the tube splints the epiglottis open) and must be enterally tube fed or parenterally nourished.
21. Mechanically ventilated patients are at risk for development of stress ulcers.
    a. Stress may cause some patients requiring mechanical ventilation to develop GI bleeding.
    b. Abdominal distention occurs frequently with respiratory failure and further hinders respiration by elevation of the diaphragm. Measurement of abdominal girth provides objective assessment of the degree of distention.

23. Mechanical ventilation may result in sleep deprivation and loss of touch with surroundings and reality.

Evaluation/Outcome

1. Maintain a flow sheet to record ventilation patterns, arterial blood studies, venous chemical determinations, hemoglobin and hematocrit, status of fluid balance, weight, and assessment of the patient's condition. Notify appropriate personnel of changes in the patient's condition.
2. Change ventilator circuitry every 24 hours; assess ventilator's function every 4 hours or more frequently if problem occurs.

1. Establishes means of assessing effectiveness and progress of treatment.

2. Prevents contamination of lower airways.

Guidelines Weaning the Patient From Mechanical Ventilation

Weaning is the process by which the patient is gradually allowed to assume the responsibility for regulating and performing his own ventilation. Before weaning is instituted, the patient should have acceptable arterial blood gases while on the ventilator, have no evidence of acute pulmonary pathology, have an intrapulmonary shunt less than 20%, and be hemodynamically stable while on the ventilator.

Equipment

Varies according to technique used
Briggs T-piece (see earlier section)
IMV or SIMV (set up in addition to ventilator or incorporated in ventilator and circuitry)
Pressure Support

Assessment

Nursing Action	Rationale/Amplification

1. For weaning to be successful, the patient must be physiologically capable of maintaining spontaneous respirations. Assessments must ensure that:
  a. The underlying disease process is significantly reversed, as evidenced by pulmonary examination, arterial blood gas, chest x-ray.
  b. The patient can mechanically perform ventilation. Should be able to generate a negative inspiratory force (NIF) >-20 cm. H_2O, have a vital capacity >10–15 ml./kg;
	1. Provides baseline; ensures that patient is capable of having adequate neuromuscular control to provide adequate ventilation.

(continued)

Guidelines   Weaning the Patient From Mechanical Ventilation *(continued)*

Assessment *(continued)*	Nursing Action	Rationale/Amplification
	have a resting minute ventilation <10 liters/minute; and be able to double this; have a spontaneous respiratory rate of <25 breaths per minute; without significant tachycardia; not be hypotensive; have optimal hemoglobin for his condition.	
	2. Assess for other factors that may cause respiratory insufficiency.	2. Weaning is difficult when these conditions are present.
	a. Acid–base abnormality	
	b. Nutritional depletion	
	c. Electrolyte abnormality	
	d. Fever	
	e. Abnormal fluid balance	
	f. Hyperglycemia	
	g. Infection	
	h. Pain	
	i. Sleep deprivation	
	j. Decreased level of consciousness	
Planning/Implementation	1. Ensure psychological preparation. Explain procedure. Explain that weaning is not always successful on the initial attempt.	1. Explaining procedure to patient will decrease patient anxiety and promote cooperation. The patient should not be discouraged if weaning is unsuccessful on the first attempt.
	2. Prepare appropriate equipment.	
	3. Position the patient in sitting or semi-Fowler's position.	3. Increases lung compliance, decreases work of breathing.
	4. Pick optimal time of day, preferably early A.M.	4. The patient should be rested.
	5. Perform bronchial hygiene necessary to ensure that the patient is in best condition (postural drainage, suctioning) prior to weaning attempt.	5. The patient should be in best pulmonary condition for weaning to be successful.
	T-piece	
	This system provides oxygen enrichment and humidity to a patient with an endotracheal or tracheostomy tube while allowing completely spontaneous respirations (for set-up and function see oxygen delivery section).	
	1. Discontinue mechanical ventilation and apply T-piece adapter.	1. Stay with the patient during weaning time to decrease patient anxiety and monitor for tolerance of procedure.
	2. Time on T-piece may vary from 5–10 min./hr. to 15–30 min./hr.	
	3. Monitor the patient for factors indicating need for reinstitution of mechanical ventilation.	3. Indicates intolerance of weaning procedure.
	a. Blood pressure increase or decrease greater than 20 mm. Hg systolic or 10 mm. Hg diastolic	
	b. Heart rate increase of 20 beats/min. or rate greater than 110.	
	c. Respiratory rate increase greater than 10 breaths per minute or rate greater than 30.	
	d. Tidal volume less than 250–300 ml. (in adults)	
	e. Appearance of new cardiac ectopy, or increase in baseline ectopy	
	f. PaO_2 less than 60, $PaCO_2$ greater than 55, or pH less than 7.35 (may accept lower PaO_2 and pH, and higher $PaCO_2$ in patients with COPD)	
	4. Increase time off ventilator with each weaning attempt as the patient's condition indicates. Evaluate for toleration before moving to the next increment.	4. The patient will progress as he becomes mentally and physically able to perform adequate spontaneous ventilation.
	5. Institute other techniques helpful in encouraging weaning.	5. Provides motivation and positive feedback.
	a. Mental stimulation	
	b. Biofeedback	
	c. Participation in care	
	d. Provision of rewards	
	e. Contact with successfully weaned patients.	
	6. When the patient tolerates 40–60 min. of continuous weaning, weaning increments can increase rapidly.	
	7. When the patient can maintain spontaneous ventilation throughout day, begin night weaning.	

**Planning/Im-
plementation**
(continued)

CPAP Weaning

1. The principles and technique for CPAP weaning are the same as for T-piece weaning.
2. The patient breathes with CPAP at low levels (2.5–5 cm. H_2O), rather than with the T-piece, for periods that increase in length.
3. This weaning technique is preferred for patients prone to atelectasis when placed on a T-piece.

IMV or SIMV Weaning

1. Set ventilator to IMV or SIMV mode.
2. Set rate interval.

2. This determines the time interval between machine-delivered breaths, during which the patient will breathe on his own.

3. If the patient is on continuous flow IMV circuitry, observe reservoir bag to be sure that it remains mostly inflated during all phases of ventilation.

3. The gas flow rate into the bag must be adequate to prevent the bag from collapsing during inspiration. Flow rates of 6–10 liters per minute are usually adequate.

4. If gas for the patient's spontaneous breath is delivered via a demand valve regulator, ensure that machine sensitivity is at maximum setting.

4. Aids in decreasing work of breathing necessary to open demand valve

5. Evaluate for tolerance of procedure. Monitor for factors indicating need for increase or decrease of mandatory respiratory rate (see step 3 of T-piece adapter section above). In rapid weaning, changes may be made approximately every 20–30 minutes.

5. If the patient does not tolerate the procedure, the $PaCO_2$ will rise and *p*H will fall.

6. If $PaCO_2$ and *p*H levels remain stable, then continue to decrease mandatory rate as patient tolerates.

6. May be done as frequently as every 20–30 minutes with arterial blood gas monitoring, pulse or pulmonary artery (PA) oximetry, documentation of successful weaning

7. Institute other techniques helpful in encouraging weaning (see step 5, T-piece section above).

7. Provides motivation and positive feedback

Pressure Support

1. May be beneficial adjunct to IMV or SIMV weaning.
2. The amount of pressure support (cm. H_2O) provided to the airway is progressively decreased over time, allowing the patient to increase his role in supporting his spontaneous ventilation.
3. There is insufficient data available to define weaning protocols for this weaning mode at this time.

**Evaluation/
Outcome**

1. Record at each weaning interval: heart rate, blood pressure, respiratory rate, F_IO_2, arterial blood gas, pulse oximetry value, respiratory and ventilator rate (if IMV or SIMV), or length of time off ventilator (if T-piece weaning).

1. Provides record of procedure and assessment of progress

Note: It is not within the scope of this manual to establish criteria for the use of one weaning modality as opposed to another.

Bibliography

Books

Barnes TA (ed). Respiratory Care Practice. Chicago, Year Book Medical Pub, 1988

Bone RC, George RB, and Hudson LC (eds.). Acute Respiratory Failure. New York, Churchill-Livingstone, 1987

Kaczmarek RM and Stoller JK (eds). Current Respiratory Care. Philadelphia, BC Decker, 1988

Kersten LD. Comprehensive Respiratory Nursing: A Decision-Making Approach. Philadelphia, WB Saunders, 1989

Kirby RR and Taylor RW (eds). Respiratory Failure. Chicago, Year Book Medical Pub, 1986

Martin L. Pulmonary Physiology in

Clinical Practice: The Essentials for Patient Care and Evaluation. St. Louis, CV Mosby, 1987

Murray JF and Nadel JA (eds). Textbook of Respiratory Medicine. Philadelphia, WB Saunders, 1988

Rau JL. Respiratory Care Pharmacology. 3rd ed. Chicago, Year Book Medical Pub, 1989

Rippe JM (ed). Manual of Intensive Care Medicine. Boston, Little, Brown & Co, 1989

Scanlon CL, Spearman CB and Sheldon RL. Egan's Fundamentals of Respiratory Care. 5th ed. St Louis, CV Mosby, 1990

Shapiro BA et al. Clinical Application of

Respiratory Care. 3rd ed. Chicago, Year Book Medical Pub, 1985

Wilkins RL, Sheldon RL and Krider SJ. Clinical Assessment in Respiratory Care. St. Louis, CV Mosby, 1986

Journals

Acute Respiratory Failure

Bradley RB. Adult respiratory stress syndrome. Focus Crit Care 1987 Oct; 14(5):48–49

Petty TL. The use, abuse and mystique of positive end-expiratory pressure, Am Rev Respir Dis 1988 Aug; 138(2):475–478

Pingleton SK. Complications of acute

respiratory failure: State of the art. Am Rev Respir Dis 1988 Jun; 137(6):1463–1493

Airway Care

Bostick J and Wendelgass ST. Normal saline instillation as part of the suctioning procedure: Effects on PaO$_2$ and amount of secretions. Heart Lung 1987 Sep; 16(5):532–537

Carlon GC, Fox SJ, and Ackerman NJ. Evaluation of a closed-tracheal suction system. Crit Care Med 1987 May; 15(5):522–525

Chulay M. Hyperinflation/hyperoxygenation to prevent endotracheal suctioning complications. Crit Care Nurse 1987 Mar–Apr; 7(2):100–102

Heffner JE, Miller KS, and Sahn SA. Tracheostomy in the ICU. Part I. Indications, technique, management. Chest 1986 Aug; 90(2):269–274

Heffner JE, Miller KS and Sahn SA. Tracheostomy in the ICU. Part II. Complications. Chest 1986 Sep; 90(3):430–436

Hess D and Goff G. The effects of two-hand versus one-hand ventilation on volumes delivered during bag-value ventilation at various resistances and compliances. Respir Care 1987 Nov; 32(11):1025–1028

Hoffman LA and Maszkiewicz RC. Airway management for the critically ill patient. Am J Nurs 1987 Jan; 87(1):39–53

Hravnak M. Ventilator tubing stabilization for the tracheotomized patient. Crit Care Nurse 1984 Sep–Oct; 4(5):20–21

Snowberger P. Decreasing tracheal tissue damage due to excessive cuff pressures. Dimens Crit Care Nurs 1986 May–Jun; 5(3):136–142

Tasota FJ et al. Evaluation of two methods used to stabilize oral endotracheal tubes. Heart Lung 1987 Mar; 16(2):140–146

Yealy DM and Paris PM. Recent advances in airway management. Emerg Med Clin North Am 1989 Feb; 7(1):83–93

Arterial Blood Gases

Lindell KO and Wesmiller SW. Using arterial blood gases to interpret acid-base balance. Orthop Nurs 1989 May–Jun; 8(3):31–34

Milam DA. Mastering arterial punctures. Am J Nurs 1988 Sep; 88(9):1213–1224

Oxygen Delivery: Techniques and Monitoring

Ahrens TS. Concepts of oxygenation. Focus Crit Care 1987 Feb; 14(1):36–44

Briones TL. SvO$_2$ Monitoring. Part I. Clinical case application. Dimens Crit Care Nurs 1988 Mar–Apr; 7(2):70–78

Briones TL. SvO$_2$ Monitoring. Part II. Nursing research application. Dimens Crit Care Nurs 1988 Mar–Apr; 7(2):79–82

Campbell EJ, Baker MD, and Crites-Silver, P. Subjective effects of humidification of oxygen delivery by nasal cannula: A prospective study. Chest 1988 Feb; 93(2):289–293

Domigan–Wentz J. The CPAP Mask: A comfortable approach to ARDS. Am J Nurs 1985 Jul; 85(7):813–815

Hardy GR. SvO$_2$ monitoring techniques. Dimens Crit Care Nurs 1988 Jan–Feb; 7(1):8–17

Hoffman LA and Wesmiller SW. Home oxygen: Transtracheal and other options. Am J Nurs 1988 Apr; 88(4):464–469

Reischman RR. Review of ventilation and profusion physiology. Crit Care Nurse 1988 Oct; 8(7):24–28

Reischman RR. Impaired gas exchange related to intrapulmonary shunting. Crit Care Nurse 1988 Nov–Dec; 8(8):35–48

Schroeder CH. Pulse oximetry: A nursing care plan. Crit Care Nurse 1988 Nov–Dec; 8(8):50–67

Tobin MJ. Respiratory monitoring in the intensive care unit. Am Rev Respir Dis 1988 Dec; 138(6):1625–1642

Wesmiller SW and Hoffman LA. Interpreting your patient's oxygenation status. Orthop Nurs 1989; Nov–Dec; 8(6):56–60

Mechanical Ventilation: Initiation, Techniques, Weaning

MacIntyre NR. Symposium on pressure support ventilation. Respir Care 1988 Feb; 33(2):98–134

Nett LM, Morganroth ML and Petty TL. Weaning from mechanical ventilation. Am J Nurs 1987 Sep; 87(9):1173–1184

Norton LC and Neureuter A. Weaning the long-term ventilator-dependent patient: Common problems and management. Crit Care Nurse 1989 Jan; 9(1):42–52

Vasbinder–Dillon D. Understanding mechanical ventilation. Crit Care Nurse 1988 Oct; 8(7):42–56

Psychological Aspects

Estabrooks CA. Touch: A nursing strategy in the intensive care unit. Heart Lung 1989 July; 18(4):392–401

Gries ML and Fernsler J. Patient perceptions of the mechanical ventilation experience. Focus Crit Care 1988 Apr; 15(2):52–58

Stovsky G, Rudy E, and Dragonette P. Comparison of two types of communication methods used after cardiac surgery with patient with endotracheal tubes. Heart Lung 1988 May; 17(3):281–289

Cardiovascular Disorders

Cellular Components of Normal Blood

Erythrocytes (Red Blood Cells)

1. Constitute the vast majority of all blood cells; chiefly responsible for the color of blood.
2. Approximately 5 million erythrocytes per cubic millimeter of blood.
3. Normal red cell has no nucleus; it is a biconcave disc.
4. Mature red blood cells consist primarily of hemoglobin, which makes up 95% of cell mass.
    a. Presence of a large amount of hemoglobin enables the cell to perform its principal function, the transport of oxygen from the lungs to the tissues.
    b. Iron is present in the heme portion of the molecule and is necessary for oxygen transport.
5. Whole blood normally contains about 14–15 gm. of hemoglobin per 100 ml. of blood.
6. Red blood cells are produced in red bone marrow, which also provides most of the blood's leukocytes and all of its platelets.
7. For normal erythrocyte production, the bone marrow requires iron, vitamin B_{12}, folic acid, and other factors.
    If any of these factors is deficient during erythropoiesis (production of erythrocytes), decreased red blood cell production and anemia result.
8. Normal life expectancy of a red cell is between 115 and 130 days—then eliminated by phagocytosis in the reticuloendothelial system, predominantly in spleen and liver.

Leukocytes (White Blood Cells)

1. Normally the total leukocyte count is 5000 to 10,000 cells per mm³. Leukocytes can be differentiated from erythrocytes by the presence of a nucleus, their larger size, and different staining properties.

2. Leukocytes are divided into two general categories: granulocytes and mononuclear cells.
    a. *Granulocytes* (produced in marrow) account for 70% of all white cells.
        (1) Called *granulocytes* because of the abundant granules contained in their cytoplasm, or *polymorphonuclear leukocytes,* because their mature nuclei are of a highly irregular, multilobed configuration.
        (2) Granulocytes are divided into 3 subgroups according to their staining properties: eosinophils, basophils, neutrophils.
    b. *Mononuclear leukocytes* (lymphocytes and monocytes) are white blood cells with a single-lobed nucleus and a granule-free cytoplasm. In normal adult blood, lymphocytes account for approximately 30% and monocytes approximately 5% of the total leukocytes.
        (1) Mature lymphocytes are derived from marrow stem cells that undergo further differentiation in the lymph nodes and in the lymphoid tissue of the intestine, spleen, and thymus gland.
        (2) Monocytes are the largest of the blood leukocytes and are produced by the bone marrow.
3. Function of the leukocytes is to protect the body from invasion by foreign cells (e.g., bacteria)—provide protection by phagocytosis, production of antibodies, and rejection of foreign tissue.
    a. The chief function of some granulocytes is phagocytosis and intracellular kill of ingested organisms; others (eosinophils and basophils) function as reservoirs of potent biological materials such as histamine, serotonin, and heparin. Release of these compounds alters blood supply to the tissues and helps mobilize body defense mechanisms.
    b. Lymphocytes produce substances (interferon,

transfer factor, antibodies, etc.) that aid in attacking foreign material; responsible for the immunocompetence of an individual and for the long-term immunologic memory.
4. Reduction in leukocyte number or activity causes a patient to have decreased resistance to infections.

Platelets *(Thrombocytes)*

1. The smallest and most fragile of the formed elements; are small particles (devoid of nuclei) that arise as a result of budding from giant cells, called *megakaryocytes,* in the bone marrow.
2. Number approximately 150,000–450,000 platelets per mm^3 of blood.
3. Prime function is to control bleeding—important in the formation of clots at sites of injury to blood vessels; maintain the integrity of the vascular endothelium.
   a. Their granules contain adenosine diphosphate (ADP), calcium, serotonin, phospholipids, and other chemical substances.
   b. After tissue injury, circulating platelets stick to the damaged blood vessel walls, release their granules, and form a primary hemostatic plug.
   c. Platelet phospholipid metabolites such as thromboxane A_2 cause vasoconstriction at the site of injury, and ADP promotes platelet aggregation as well as the release of granules from other platelets.
   d. Additional substances released from platelets activate coagulation factors in the blood plasma.

Common Problems of Patients With Blood Disorders

Nursing Diagnoses and Interventions

A. Fatigue—related to effects of disease, anemia, stress of coping with disease and its treatment

1. Interventions
   a. Plan nursing care to conserve the patient's strength and emotional energy.
   b. Give frequent rest periods.
   c. Encourage ambulation activities as tolerated.
   d. Encourage conditioning exercises to increase endurance.
   e. Encourage optimal nutrition—high-protein and high-calorie foods and beverages.

B. Altered Oral Mucous Membranes—related to bacterial flora, presence of infections, cytotoxic action of chemotherapeutic agents on oral mucosal cells, and effects of radiation.

1. Manifestations
   a. Bleeding gums
   b. Pain/ulcerations
   c. Periodontal infection
   d. Pain with chewing and swallowing related to mucosal damage
   e. Xerostomia (dry mouth)
   f. Cheilitis; lip cracking
   g. Candidiasis (white curds, plaques, ulcerations)
   h. Herpes simplex (painful vesicles that rupture and become encrusted)

2. Interventions
   a. Develop and follow a plan for oral care based on oral assessment.
   b. Encourage regular dental visits—bleeding gums occur when there is gross tartar on the teeth.
   c. Use mechanical cleansing procedures to remove plaque and debris.
      (1) Use a soft, multitufted nylon toothbrush.
      (2) Employ careful flossing with short, delicate strokes to avoid damage to the gingiva; discontinue flossing if it causes pain.
   d. Offer mouthwash (normal saline solution or Cepacol diluted with water, 1:5) before and after meals.
   e. Moisten lips with water-soluble lubricant every 2–4 hours.
   f. For patients with mucositis, pain, periodontal infection, xerostomia:
      (1) Remove dentures.
      (2) Control moderate to severe pain of mucous membranes with topical anesthetic agents for mucous membranes.
      (3) Give systemic analgesics (acetaminophen; codeine) as directed for severe pain to allow pain relief for sleep and consumption of fluids.
      (4) Cleanse teeth with moistened gauze wrapped around finger; use Water Pik® on low setting.
      (5) Employ normal saline for mouth rinse every 2–4 hours; avoid alcohol-containing mouth washes.
      (6) Employ prophylactic nystatin rinses for candidiasis.
      (7) Offer a bland diet, avoiding temperature extremes.
      (8) Encourage a high intake (3000 ml.) of bland, chilled fluids.
      (9) Offer lemon drops, sugarless gum, ice chips, and saliva substitute (Salivart® Synthetic Saliva) to stimulate saliva and as a mouth moisturizer.

C. Ineffective Breathing Pattern—(dyspnea) related to reduction of oxyhemoglobin and possible bleeding into pulmonary system

1. Interventions
   a. Elevate the head of the bed.
   b. Use pillows to support the patient in the orthopneic position.
   c. Prevent unnecessary exertion.
   d. Administer oxygen when indicated.

D. Pain (Bone and joint pains)—related to proliferation of neoplastic cells; bleeding

1. Interventions
   a. Provide appropriate pain relief on a regular schedule.
   b. Relieve pressure of bedding by using a cradle.
   c. Provide for joint immobilization as prescribed.

E. Ineffective Thermoregulation—(fever) related to infection, hematologic malignancy

1. Interventions
   a. Assist in determining cause of fever (infection).
   b. Administer cool sponges.
   c. Give antipyretic (acetaminophen) drugs as prescribed.

d. Encourage liberal fluid intake unless contraindicated.

e. Maintain a cool environmental temperature.

F. Potential for Impaired Skin Integrity—(pruritus or skin eruptions) related to pathophysiologic process of hematologic malignancy, release of proteolytic enzymes by tumor, chemotherapy

1. Interventions
   a. Keep the patient's fingernails short.
   b. Use soap sparingly.
   c. Apply emollient lotions in skin care.
   d. Give antihistamines as prescribed.

G. Fear (of patient and family)—related to diagnosis, diagnostic procedures, therapy, and prognosis

1. Interventions
   a. Provide emotional support to facilitate the process of coping with the diagnosis and treatment of a hematologic disorder.
   b. Explain the nature, the discomforts, and limitations of activity associated with the diagnostic procedures and treatments.
   c. Offer the service of listening about anxieties, guilt, doubts, problems, etc.
   d. Provide an atmosphere of acceptance and understanding.
   e. Encourage the patient to verbalize his *feelings*.
   f. Give skilled care; promote relaxation and comfort.
   g. Promote a sense of independence and self-care within the patient's limitations.
   h. Teach the patient stress reduction techniques; progressive relaxation, distraction, guided imagery.
   i. Encourage the family to participate in the patient's care (as desired).

Hemorrhagic Tendencies

A. Examples

Bruising, petechiae, purpura, ecchymoses, menorrhagia, bleeding in mucous membranes of mouth, retina, GI tract related to thrombocytopenia, abnormalities of platelet function, thrombocytosis, blood vessel and connective tissue disease; depression of bone marrow from toxic effects of chemotherapy.

B. Interventions

1. Use measures to prevent bleeding.
2. Handle skin gently; avoid use of adhesive tape.
3. Use small-gauge needles when administering medication by injection; apply pressure to venipuncture site for 5 minutes with patient's arm extended above the level of his heart.

4. Give required IM injections with thin needles, Z-track technique, and pressure.
5. Rotate extremities for blood pressure measurement.
6. Use electric shaver instead of razor.
7. Avoid rectal instrumentation (thermometer; enemas; suppositories).
8. Avoid use of vaginal tampons.
9. Employ stool softeners to prevent rupture of blood vessels from straining.
10. Keep the patient at rest during the bleeding episodes.
11. Apply gentle pressure to the bleeding site.
12. Apply cold compresses to the bleeding site when indicated.
13. Avoid disturbing clots.
14. Offer a Popsicle to the patient who is bleeding orally— induces vasoconstriction; stop oral hygiene measures, including rinsing, during periods of active bleeding.
15. Measure blood loss; weigh linens, bandages, and note saturation of pads during menses.
16. Test urine, stool, and emesis for occult blood.
17. Monitor hematocrit and hemoglobin levels.
18. Observe for symptoms of internal bleeding.
19. Check supine and standing blood pressure and pulse; if pulse increases or BP goes down, patient is not stable.
20. Have a tracheostomy set available for the patient who is bleeding from the mouth or throat; observe for signs of asphyxiation.
21. Educate the patient to:
    a. Protect himself from injury.
    b. Avoid medications containing aspirin.
    c. Blow his nose gently with his mouth open.
    d. Avoid the Valsalva maneuver.

Blood and Bone Marrow Specimens

Blood may be obtained by (1) skin puncture (finger, toe, heel, or ear lobe) or (2) venipuncture.*

A *skin puncture* is performed when only a small amount of blood is needed (for red and white cell counts, hemoglobin and hematocrit determinations, reticulocyte counts, blood films for differential smear). However, the values for the red blood cells, hematocrit, hemoglobin, and platelets are lower in capillary blood than in venous blood.

A *venipuncture* is a puncture of a vein to obtain blood; used when larger amounts of blood are needed (preferred method).

---

* The most common hematologic tests are described in Appendix I.

Guidelines Obtaining Blood by Skin Puncture

Equipment

Disposable lancet
Pipette and tubing
Slides
Alcohol sponges and dry sterile gauze pads
or
Prepared alcohol prep pads

Procedure

Nursing Action	Rationale/Amplification

Performance Phase

Nursing Action	Rationale/Amplification
1. Cleanse site (preferably ball of finger) with alcohol and dry with sterile gauze square.	1. If any alcohol remains, it will alter red cell morphology; also, blood will not collect into a compact drop but will run down the patient's finger.
2. Create stasis by pressing on the distal joint of the finger to produce redness at the end of the finger.	
3. Use a sterile disposable lancet, or an automated lancet.	3. This avoids the possibility of the transference of blood-borne viral diseases.
4. Prick the skin sharply and quickly with the lancet.	4. Pricking the skin sharply and quickly minimizes pain and produces a free-flowing sample.
5. Release pressure on the finger. Wipe off the first drop of blood.	5. Epithelial or endothelial cells may be found in the first drop of blood and render the count inaccurate. Also, platelets will begin to clump immediately in the blood at the puncture site.
6. Allow the blood to flow freely with an adequate puncture.	6. Pressing out the blood dilutes it with tissue fluid.
7. Obtain the blood sample: 　a. Fill the pipette or microhematocrit tube. 　b. Make blood slides according to the study required.	b. Gently touch the drop of blood to glass slides or cover slip.
8. Apply pressure over the wound with a dry gauze sponge until bleeding stops.	

Guidelines Obtaining Blood by Venipuncture

Veins Used

Antecubital area
Wrist
Dorsum (back) of hand
Top of foot

Equipment

70% alcohol
Dry sterile sponges
5- and 10-ml. syringe
No. 20 gauge needle(s)
or
Vacutainer assembly

Procedure

Nursing Action	Rationale/Amplification

Performance Phase

Nursing Action	Rationale/Amplification
1. Reassure the patient. Explain that relatively little blood will be taken.	1. The patient is reassured when the nurse displays self-assurance and competence in relating to people and when performing technical skills.
2. Instruct the patient to extend his arm; the arm should be held straight at the elbow.	
3. Apply the tourniquet directly above the elbow with just sufficient pressure to prevent venous return.	3. A tourniquet increases venous pressure and makes the vein more prominent and easier to enter.

(continued)

Guidelines Obtaining Blood by Venipuncture *(continued)*

Procedure (continued)	**Nursing Action**	**Rationale/Amplification**
	4. Inspect the area to visualize the vein. Palpate the vein.	4. Select a vein that is visible, palpable, and well fixed to surrounding tissue so that it does not roll away. (Not all veins are visible; some may be deep and can only be palpated.)
	5. Cleanse the skin with iodine and alcohol. Dry.	5. Cleansing the skin reduces pathogens.
	6. Fix chosen vein with the thumb and draw the skin taut immediately below the site before inserting needle to stabilize the vein.	6. The vein may roll beneath the skin when the needle approaches its outer surface (especially in elderly and extremely thin patients).
	7. Hold the syringe between the thumb and last 3 fingers with the bevel up and directly in line with the course of the vein. Insert the needle quickly and smoothly under the skin and into the vein.	
	8. Obtain blood sample by *gently* pulling back on the plunger.	8. Use minimal suction to prevent hemolysis of blood and collapse of the vein.
	9. Release the tourniquet as soon as specimen is obtained.	
	10. Withdraw the needle slowly.	10. Slow withdrawal of the needle is less painful.
	11. Apply a sterile dry gauze to puncture site and request patient to apply gentle but firm pressure to site for 2–4 minutes.	11. Firm pressure over the puncture site prevents leakage of blood into surrounding tissues with subsequent hematoma development. Merely flexing the arm may not prevent a hematoma, as the vein can slip to the side of the area where pressure is applied.
	12. Make the blood smear from the needle as desired.	
	13. Remove the needle from the syringe. As soon as possible after drawing the blood, gently eject the blood sample into a test tube containing an anticoagulant.	13. Slowly transfer the blood into the test tube *without* forming bubbles.
	14. Place stopper on the test tube.	
	15. Invert the tube gently several times to mix blood with anticoagulant.	15. For some tests, the blood is allowed to coagulate in the test tube.
	16. Label specimens correctly and send to laboratory immediately.	16. Specimens should go to the laboratory with a minimum of delay for optimum reliability.
	17. Dispose needle and syringe in appropriate containers to avoid possible spread of blood-borne viral diseases. Clean all spills with 10% bleach solution.	

Guidelines Bone Marrow Aspiration and Biopsy

Bone marrow aspiration and/or *biopsy* is done so that specimens of bone marrow and bone can be obtained for establishing a diagnosis.

Purposes
1. To diagnose hematologic disorders—enables the precursors of cells in peripheral blood to be examined and their relative numbers determined; to evaluate for iron content.
2. To follow the course of disease and the patient's response to treatment.
3. To diagnose diseases other than pure hematologic disorders, such as primary and metastatic tumors, infectious diseases, and certain granulomas.
4. To isolate bacteria and other pathogenic agents by culture.

Complications
1. Bleeding and hematoma in patients with bleeding disorders

Equipment
Bone marrow aspiration tray
    Marrow aspiration needles with stylets
    Towels
    No. 25 and 22 gauge needles
    Two 20-ml. syringes
    Three 5-ml. syringes
Local anesthetic (1% procaine or xylocaine)
Sterile gauze squares
Sterile gloves, drape
Skin antiseptic

Equipment
(continued)

Laboratory equipment
    Coverslips
    Microscopic slides
    Test tubes (plain and heparinized)
Scalpel blade and handle

Procedure

Nursing Action	Rationale/Amplification

Preparatory Phase

1. Explain the procedure to the patient. Tell patient when the skin will be marked, antiseptic applied, and the needle puncture performed.
2. Give medication (meperidine) or tranquilizer as requested; usually not necessary for aspiration.
3. Place the patient in prone or supine position.
4. The following sites are most frequently used:
   a. Posterior superior iliac crest
   b. Anterior iliac crest (if patient is very obese)
   c. Sternum

1. An explanation helps the patient to cope with anticipated stress. Tactile sensations (pressure, cold) can be misinterpreted as pain unless the patient is forewarned.
2. Meperidine may be used as an analgesic and sedative for apprehension. Anxiety may produce excessive discomfort.

Iliac Crest Aspiration/Biopsy

Performance Phase (by physician)

1. Position the patient on his abdomen (prone) or on his side with top knee flexed.
   a. The posterior iliac crest is located and marked.

   b. The skin area is prepared and draped. The marked area is infiltrated with local anesthetic through the skin and subcutaneous tissue to the periosteum of the bone.
   c. A small incision may be made.

   d. The bone marrow needle, with stylet in place, is introduced through the incision.

   e. The needle is advanced and rotated by using firm and steady pressure. When the needle is felt to enter the outer cortex of the bone marrow cavity, the stylet is removed and the syringe attached. Negative pressure is applied, and a small volume of blood and marrow is aspirated.
   f. A biopsy is taken by using a special needle equipped with a sharp cutting edge and a hollow core.

   a. The iliac crest provides a large marrow cavity at the posterior superior iliac spine away from nearby abdominal organs.
   b. Tell the patient he will experience a needle prick followed by a burning sensation.
   The periosteum is the region of greatest sensitivity.
   c. The biopsy needle is large, and a small incision facilitates insertion.
   d. The needle is pointed toward the anterior superior iliac spine and brought into contact with the posterior iliac spine.
   e. There is usually decreased resistance when the bone marrow cavity is entered.
   The actual aspiration may cause brief pain, and the patient should be forewarned.
   Bone marrow appears rusty-red and normally has a thick, fluid-like consistency.

Sternal Aspiration

Performance Phase (by physician)

1. The skin is prepared and the site infiltrated with procaine or xylocaine.
2. The site selected is usually the midsternal line at the level of the 2nd interspace.
3. A small stab incision may be made before bone marrow needle insertion.
4. The marrow needle with stylet in place is inserted through the cortex of the bone with a slight rotating motion. The physician usually feels a ''give'' in the marrow needle when the marrow cavity has been penetrated.
5. The stylet is removed and a syringe attached to the hub of the needle. The plunger is withdrawn slowly until marrow appears in the syringe and is aspirated.
6. Warn the patient that he may feel a brief episode of sharp pain or pressure.
7. The syringe and needle are removed and passed to a technician for preparation of smears.

2. The sternum is thinner and marrow more plentiful between the sternal interspaces.
3. This technique avoids pushing the skin into the bone marrow.
4. A sternal puncture is considered more dangerous than other sites because of its proximity to vital structures in the mediastinum.
5. The marrow will appear as thick, dark reddish fluid.

6. The pain is caused by suction of the syringe and lasts only a few seconds.
7. Smears of aspirated marrow are made; technique is similar to that of preparing blood smears.

(continued)

Procedure *(continued)*	**Nursing Action**	**Rationale/Amplification**
	8. Pressure is applied over the puncture site for a brief period to ensure hemostasis.	8. If the patient has thrombocytopenia, pressure should be applied for 10–15 minutes.
	9. A small dressing is applied with pressure over the puncture site.	
	10. Remove dressing after 24 hours and inspect area for inflammation.	
	Follow-up Phase	
	1. Give mild analgesic if needed.	1. Most patients have no discomfort after aspiration, but the site of a biopsy may ache for a day or so.
	2. Assess the patient for discomfort, continued bleeding, and untoward symptoms.	

Anemia

Anemia is a laboratory definition that implies a low red cell count and a hemoglobin or hematocrit level that is below normal. Physiologically, anemia exists when there is an insufficient amount of hemoglobin to deliver oxygen to the tissues.

Altered Physiology

1. Anemia may result from
   (a) Increased destruction of red cells
   (b) Excessive blood loss
   (c) Decreased production of red cells
2. Vitamin B_{12} and folic acid are both essential to the maturing process of the red cell.
3. Marrow failure may occur as a result of nutritional deficiency, toxic exposure, tumor invasion, or unknown causes.
4. Red cells may be lost through hemorrhage or hemolysis (increased destruction).
   a. This problem may be rooted in an intrinsic red-cell defect that is incompatible with normal red-cell survival or is explainable on the basis of some factor extrinsic to the red cell that promotes red-cell destruction.
   b. Red-cell lysis occurs mainly within the phagocytic cells of the reticuloendothelial system, notably within the liver and spleen.
   c. As a by-product of this process, bilirubin, formed by the metabolism of hemoglobin within the phagocyte, enters the bloodstream, and an increase in hemolysis is promptly reflected by an increase in total plasma bilirubin.

Types of Anemia

Aplastic—anemia caused by aplasia (failure) of bone marrow or its destruction by chemical agents or physical factors
Autoimmune—acquired disorder characterized by premature erythrocyte destruction from abnormalities in the individual's own immune system
Hemolytic—anemia caused by increased destruction of erythrocytes resulting in a shortened life span

Iron deficiency—develops when the transport of iron by transferrin falls short of that required by erythropoietic cells
Megaloblastic—characterized by the presence of megaloblasts in the bone marrow; usually due to a deficiency of folic acid or vitamin B_{12}
Pernicious—a type of megaloblastic anemia due to a deficiency of vitamin B_{12} that is directly linked to the absence of intrinsic factor
Sickle—Hereditary chronic anemia in which abnormal sickle or crescent-shaped erythrocytes are present. It is due to the presence of hemoglobin S in the blood cells
Thalassemia—a group of hereditary anemias produced by either a defective production rate of alpha or the beta hemoglobin polypeptide. This disorder is inherited in homozygous or heterozygous state.

Clinical Manifestations

(Most manifestations are attributable to a decrease in the oxygen-carrying capacity of the blood, and are the same regardless of the cause of anemia.)
1. The more rapidly the anemia develops, the more severe its symptoms:
   a. Pallor of conjunctivae, nail beds, lips, oral mucosa, and palmar creases
   b. Susceptibility to fatigue
   c. Shortness of breath on exertion, palpitations, sweating
   d. Headache; disturbed cerebration; dizziness
   e. Symptoms of local ischemia from reduction of blood oxygen supply; angina pectoris
2. Severity of symptoms depends on rapidity of onset, duration, age, cardiovascular status, metabolic requirements and any complicating condition.

Diagnostic Evaluation

1. Variety of hematologic studies are done to determine type or cause of anemia:
   Measurements of hemoglobin and hematocrit, red cell indices, white cell studies, serum iron level, measurement of total iron-binding capacity, folate level, vitamin B_{12} level, platelet count, bleeding

time, prothrombin time, partial thromboplastin time
2. Bone marrow aspiration and biopsy

Management

1. Reversing/treating the underlying cause
2. See discussion of specific type of anemia.

Nursing Assessment

1. When taking the nursing history, ask about the family history, drug intake, blood loss, and any other symptoms.
2. Take a nutritional history, including recall of food intake over a 24-hour period.
3. Observe for weakness, fatigue, and general malaise.
4. Inspect the skin for pallor (hallmark of anemia), presence of jaundice, dryness of skin and hair. Examine nails for "spooning."
5. Assess cardiac status: tachycardia, palpitations, dyspnea, and exertional dyspnea.
6. Examine for evidence of congestive heart failure: cardiomegaly, pulmonary congestion, peripheral edema.

Nursing Diagnoses

1. Activity intolerance related to fatigue, weakness, and general malaise.
2. Potential decrease in cardiac output related to increased cardiac workload.
3. Altered nutrition related to inadequate intake of essential nutrients.

Nursing Interventions

(The following are general nursing interventions when anemia is one of the primary concerns of the patient with a hematologic disorder)

A. Normalizing Activity Tolerance

1. Explain that activities should be paced and spaced to conserve strength and physical and emotional energy.
2. Encourage frequent rest periods.
3. Assist in developing a schedule of activity, rest, and sleep.
4. Explain that conditioning exercises will increase strength and endurance.
5. Resume normal activities gradually as soon as blood studies show improvement.
6. Postpone activities that cause undue fatigue until greater endurance is achieved.

B. Attaining Normal Cardiac Output

1. Ask patient what activities cause palpitations and dyspnea; these should be avoided until condition improves.
2. Elevate the head of the bed and use pillow supports if patient is dyspneic.
3. Monitor for indications of fluid retention: crackles, peripheral edema, decreasing urinary output; neck vein distention.
4. Monitor vital signs.

C. Improving Nutritional Status

1. Discuss how to include sufficient vitamins and minerals, especially iron, in the diet.
2. Arrange dietitian referral; include family in teaching sessions.

Evaluation

1. Tolerates increasing activity
2. Attains/maintains normal cardiac output
3. Eats a nutritious diet

Iron Deficiency Anemia

Iron deficiency anemia is a condition in which the total body iron content is decreased below a normal level. (Iron is needed for synthesis of hemoglobin.) It is the most common type of anemia in all age groups and is a major health problem in developing countries.

Etiology

1. Chronic blood loss—gastrointestinal bleeding (e.g., from ulcers, malignancy), excessive menstrual bleeding, hookworm infestation
2. Malabsorption of iron—small bowel disease; gastroenterostomy
3. Increased iron requirements—during pregnancy, periods of rapid growth, menstruation (average of 20 mg. iron lost per menstrual cycle)
4. Insufficient intake (fad or weight-loss diets)

Iron Balance and Stores

1. Normal adult male has stores of 500–2000 mg.; adult female has 250 mg.
2. Adult male loses about 0.9 mg. iron per day; premenopausal woman loses about 1.5 mg. iron per day.
3. Approximately 6 mg. of iron is ingested per 1000 Kcal.; or 16–20 mg./day.
   The amount of iron ingested is related to the number of calories consumed.
4. Normally about 5%–10% of ingested iron is absorbed by the gastrointestinal mucosa, bound to transferrin (main iron-binding protein in plasma), and carried through the bloodstream to the bone marrow. In the marrow, iron is transported to red blood cells and reticuloendothelial cells.

Clinical Manifestations

Reduction in hemoglobin concentration decreases the capacity of the blood to transport and deliver oxygen to the tissues.
1. Easy fatigability
2. Headache, dizziness, tinnitus
3. Palpitations and dyspnea on exertion
4. Pallor of skin and mucous membranes
5. Smooth, sore tongue associated with a burning sensation
6. Cheilosis (lesions at corners of mouth)
7. Pica (craving to eat unusual substances)
8. Koilonychia (spoon-shaped fingernails)

Diagnostic Evaluation

1. Laboratory evaluation of iron status
   a. Red cell distribution width (RDW) elevated—earliest indication of iron depletion
   b. Decrease in serum ferritin
   c. Decrease in serum iron level
   d. Total iron-binding capacity normal or increased
2. Diagnosis of iron deficiency mandates a search for source of blood loss: sigmoidoscopy, colonoscopy;

upper and lower gastrointestinal studies; urine and stool specimens for occult blood examination

Management

A. Correction of Chronic Blood Loss

B. Oral Iron Therapy (Iron absorption occurs primarily in duodenum and upper jejunum)

1. Ferrous sulfate (preferred and least expensive); treatment continued until hemoglobin level normalizes and iron stores have been replaced (6 months or longer)
2. The dosage of iron may be gradually increased over a few days.

C. Parenteral Iron Therapy

1. Parenteral iron therapy is given only when the patient is unable to tolerate iron preparations orally, when the patient has severe gastrointestinal disorders, when there is continuing negative iron balance while patient is taking maximum oral dose tolerated, or when there is nonadherence by patient.
2. Parenteral iron preparations
   a. Iron dextran (Imferon)
   b. Iron sorbitex (Jectofer)—may cause patient's urine to turn black on standing, as about 50% of iron is excreted in the urine within 24 hours.

> **NURSING ALERT:** Extravasation of iron medication results in painful local induration. An anaphylactic reaction may occur following either intramuscular or intravenous injection of iron dextran.

3. Technique of parenteral iron administration:
   a. Discard needle that is used to draw medication into syringe; use a new needle for injection—to avoid tracking medication through subcutaneous tissue.
   b. Allow a small amount of air in syringe.
   c. Use a needle 5 cm. (2 inches) long—medication is injected deep into upper outer quadrant of buttock.
   d. Retract the skin over the muscle *laterally* before inserting needle (Z-track)—to prevent leakage along injection tract and staining of skin.
   e. Inject solution slowly followed by air in syringe. Wait a few seconds before withdrawing needle.

Nursing Interventions and Patient Education

Instruct the patient as follows:
1. Iron is usually taken on an empty stomach with a full glass of water or fruit juice with a 4-hour interval between doses to prevent reduced absorption by presence of food.
2. Anticipate a certain amount of dyspepsia (epigastric discomfort) from time to time. If side effects (epigastric distress, nausea, constipation, diarrhea) occur, iron may be taken with meals (which reduces absorption) and then shifted to a between-meal schedule.
3. Expect color changes (dark green to black) of the stools, as iron alters the color of stool. This is caused by unabsorbed iron and is harmless.
4. Liquid dosage forms of iron may stain teeth. Mix well with water/fruit juice. Use a straw to help keep medication away from teeth.
5. Take the iron faithfully and for the prescribed time.
6. Select a well-balanced diet: animal proteins, iron-fortified cereals and bread, green leafy vegetables, dried fruits, legumes, and nuts.

7. Arrange for nutritional counseling for adolescent girls, as fad diets limit amount of absorbable iron ingested.
8. Keep iron medications out of reach of small children—iron tablets are dangerous when ingested by small children.

Megaloblastic Anemias

1. A *megaloblast* is a nucleated red cell with delayed and abnormal nuclear maturation.
2. The most common megaloblastic anemias are caused by B_{12} deficiency (pernicious anemia) and/or folic acid deficiency.
3. Anemias due to deficiencies of vitamins B_{12} and folic acid show identical bone marrow and peripheral blood changes. This is because both vitamins are essential for normal DNA synthesis.

Pernicious Anemia

Pernicious anemia is a type of megaloblastic anemia due to deficiency of vitamin B_{12} that is directly linked to the absence of intrinsic factor. It is primarily a disorder of elderly persons.

(Vitamin B_{12} deficiency is seen also in diseases of the small intestine—malabsorption, blind loop syndrome, following gastrectomy.)

Altered Physiology

1. Pernicious anemia is produced by a defect in the gastric mucosa; the stomach wall becomes atrophic and fails to secrete intrinsic factor.
2. This substance ordinarily binds dietary vitamin B_{12} and travels with it to the ileum, where the vitamin is absorbed. Without intrinsic factor, orally administered B_{12} cannot be absorbed.
3. Therefore, after the body's store of B_{12} is used up, the patient begins to show signs of the anemia.
4. Vitamin B_{12} is necessary for normal DNA synthesis in maturing red cells.

Clinical Manifestations

A. Symptoms Due to Anemia

1. Pallor, fatigue, listlessness
2. Shortness of breath; palpitations on exertion
3. Angina pectoris; congestive heart failure

B. Symptoms Due to Gastrointestinal Tract Changes

1. Sore mouth with red, "beefy" tongue (glossitis)
2. Anorexia; nausea; vomiting; loss of weight
3. Indigestion and epigastric discomfort
4. Recurring diarrhea or constipation

C. Symptoms Due to Neurologic Changes (neuropathy occurs in high percentage of untreated patients)

1. Tingling and numbness or burning pain (paresthesia) involving hands and feet
2. Loss of position sense, leading to disturbances of gait
3. Disturbances of bladder and bowel function
4. Psychiatric symptoms—from cerebral dysfunction

Diagnostic Evaluation

1. Blood smear—reveals marked variation in size and shape of cells and a variable number of unusually large cells containing a normal concentration of hemoglobin.

2. Tests for serum and red cell folate levels and serum vitamin B_{12} level.
3. Gastric analysis—volume of gastric juice greatly diminished; the gastric juice lacks free hydrochloric acid (achlorhydria).
4. *Schilling Test*—a test for vitamin B_{12} absorption.
   a. The fasting patient is given a small dose of radioactive B_{12} orally followed in 2 hours by a nonradioactive IM injection (flushing dose) of vitamin B_{12}.
   b. A 24-hour urine specimen is collected and measured for radioactivity.
   c. If very little has been excreted, the test is repeated several days later (the "second stage"), with a capsule of oral intrinsic factor added to the oral vitamin B_{12}.
   d. If the patient has pernicious anemia, this time much more radioactivity will be found in the 24-hour urine specimen.

Management

Hydroxocobalamin or cyanocobalamin (vitamin B_{12} IM) as directed (daily for 7 days, weekly for 10 weeks, and then monthly for rest of life; many protocols for administration of B_{12} are in use).

1. Parenteral vitamin therapy is necessary, because most of these patients are unable to absorb the vitamin by mouth.
2. Reticulocytes begin to increase on 4th day after therapy is started; normal hemoglobin values are obtained in approximately 6 weeks.

Nursing Interventions/Patient Education

1. Impress on the patient that vitamin B_{12} must be continued for lifetime.
   a. Maintenance dose schedule—vitamin B_{12} IM every 4 weeks or at longer intervals, depending on patient's response.
   b. Teach patient and family or have community health nurse give maintenance therapy.
   c. Untreated pernicious anemia is fatal.
2. Instruct the patient to report for follow-up examinations every 6 months—for hematologic studies and gastric screening.
   a. Patient may develop hematologic or neurologic relapse if therapy is inadequate.
   b. Patients with pernicious anemia have a higher incidence of gastric cancer and thyroid problems; therefore, periodic stool examinations for occult blood and gastric cytology, along with thyroid function tests, are done.
3. Following total gastrectomy (and occasionally subtotal gastrectomy), patient should receive maintenance dose of vitamin B_{12} as often as indicated—removal of gastric fundus deprives the patient of all intrinsic factor; may take as long as 10 years for clinical symptoms to appear, because of the small amount of daily vitamin B_{12} required and the large body stores available for use.

Folic Acid Deficiency

Folic acid is necessary for normal red blood cell production. Folate depletion results in progressive anemia.

Causes of Folate Deficiency

1. Dietary deficiencies, malnutrition, marginal diets
   a. Common in alcoholism
   b. Almost universal among individuals who are elderly, poor, and those who overcook foods
2. Impaired absorption—most absorption of folic acid takes place in upper jejunum; seen in those with small bowel disease
3. Increased requirements—chronic hemolytic anemias, pregnancy, etc.
4. Impaired utilization—from folic acid antagonists (methotrexate) and other drugs (phenytoin; sulfamethoxazole; alcohol; oral contraceptives)

Clinical Manifestations

1. Symptoms of anemia—fatigue, weakness, pallor
2. Sore tongue; cracked lips

Diagnostic Evaluation

Determination of vitamin B_{12} and folate levels

Management

1. Oral folic acid replacement; vitamin B_{12} also may be prescribed.
2. Patient education concerns
   a. Proper diet will prevent most instances of folate deficiency: green vegetables (asparagus, broccoli, spinach); yeast, liver, organ meats, some fresh fruits.
   b. Avoid overcooking vegetables.

Aplastic Anemia

Aplastic anemia is a disorder characterized by bone marrow hypoplasia or aplasia (failure) resulting in pancytopenia (depression of each of normal bone marrow elements: white cells, red cells, and platelets).

Causes

1. Idiopathic
2. Drugs—anti-inflammatory, antibacterial, antiepileptic, antidiabetic, and miscellaneous drugs (chloramphenicol, indomethacin, phenylbutazone, diclofenac, gold therapy)
3. Chemical toxins
4. Viral infections, especially hepatitis
5. Congenital marrow aplasia (Fanconi's anemia)

Note: Secondary bone marrow aplasia is a predictable marrow suppression induced by antineoplastic agents and radiation therapy or bone marrow transplantation.

Clinical Course

1. The clinical course is variable, and the overall mortality rate is high; patients with severe pancytopenia with totally aplastic marrow have a poor prognosis.
2. Patients with aplastic anemia are at serious risk of infection, hemorrhage, and other complications of chronic anemia.

Clinical Manifestations

1. Abnormal bleeding—resulting from thrombocytopenia
   a. Bleeding from gums, nose, gastrointestinal and genitourinary tracts
   b. Purpura; petechiae; ecchymoses

2. Anemia—resulting from depression of hemoglobin; symptoms pronounced because of rapidity of blood cell change
   a. Pallor; weakness
   b. Exertional dyspnea, palpitations
3. Infections with high fever—resulting from granulocytopenia
   a. Pharyngitis and oropharyngeal mucositis
   b. Sepsis via gastrointestinal tract or genitourinary tract

Diagnostic Evaluation

1. Peripheral blood smear shows pancytopenia.
2. Bone marrow aspiration and biopsy—bone marrow is hypoplastic or aplastic; reduction of its cellular elements occurs, and there is an almost complete absence of hemopoietic activity.

Management

1. Removal of causative agent or suspected toxins from environment—gives marrow opportunity to recover before damaged too severely. Permanent damage often occurs.
2. Bone marrow transplant—treatment of choice for patient with severe aplastic anemia who has matched donor.
   a. Bone marrow transplantation should be carried out *early,* because subsequent blood and platelet transfusions can cause irreversible sensitization of patient and result in graft rejection.
   b. This modality of treatment is performed at specialized transplant centers.
   c. Drawbacks in bone marrow transplantation include immunologic problems (graft-versus-host disease) and marrow graft rejection.
3. Immunosuppressive therapy—antilymphocyte globulin (ALG), an antiserum to human lymphocytes; allows bone marrow recovery in high proportion of patients, but late complications (leukemia) may occur over time.
   • Other immunosuppressive agents in use include corticosteroids, cyclophosphamide, antithymocyte globulin (ATG).
4. Supportive treatment
   a. Platelet transfusions to arrest bleeding in patient hemorrhaging from thrombocytopenia
   b. Antibiotics administered for infection.
   c. Androgens (oxymetholone or testosterone enanthate) may stimulate bone marrow regeneration and bring about a remission; significant toxicity encountered.

Nursing Interventions

A. Monitoring for Infection

1. Maintain continuing surveillance for evidence of infection—infection is major cause of death.
   a. Organisms not usually pathogenic may become so, particularly those of the *Pseudomonas, Proteus,* and *Klebsiella* species.
   b. Sources of infection in these patients are endogenous bacteria from gastrointestinal and upper respiratory tracts, particularly in those patients hospitalized for prolonged periods.
2. Attempt to reduce potential endogenous pathogens in the hospitalized patient.

NURSING ALERT: Place the patient in a protected environment (private room) with handwashing precautions strictly enforced.

   a. Pay scrupulous attention to skin infections. Regard any small break in the skin as hazardous.
      (1) Use antibacterial agent (povidone-iodine solution) in bathwater—to diminish resident body flora.
      (2) Encourage the use of an electric rather than plain razor.
   b. Examine axillae and groin areas—apt to harbor pathogens and develop pustules.
   c. Monitor temperature—fever implies bacterial, fungal, or viral infection.

B. Supporting the Patient Receiving Transfusions

1. Monitor blood component therapy—to supply red cells, platelets, and granulocytes when bone marrow has ceased to produce them. See page 284.
   a. Keep veins open—patient may require frequent transfusions for long periods; monitor IV sites carefully.
   b. Give packed red cell transfusions carefully—to maintain hemoglobin level compatible with patient's activities and to relieve symptoms of dyspnea, palpitation, and weakness.
   c. Give platelet transfusions from histocompatible donors when necessary—to arrest bleeding in the patient hemorrhaging from thrombocytopenia. (Hemorrhagic complications occur with platelet counts below 20,000/mm.^{3})
   d. Keep patient who receives multiple transfusions over time under careful nursing surveillance—these patients may develop transfusion complications.
      (1) Eventually, patient may develop antibodies to minor red cell antigens and to platelet antigens, so that transfusions no longer raise the counts sufficiently.
      (2) Multiple transfusions decrease chance for successful bone marrow transplantation.
2. Make the patient comfortable during febrile episodes.
3. Support the patient who is bleeding (in skin, nose, GI tract, genitourinary tract, lungs, optic fundi, brain).
   a. See page 258.
   b. Exercise care with IM injections—use thin needle, Z-track technique, and pressure.
   c. Menses may be suppressed (hormonal manipulation) for females with excessive blood loss.

Patient Education

1. Avoid aspirin-containing drugs—aspirin interferes with platelet function and increases risk of thrombocytopenic bleeding.
2. Avoid solvents, sprays, paints, insecticides, and other potential bone marrow toxins.
3. Take only prescribed drugs.
4. Prevent minor infections. Any abrasion or wound of mucous membranes or skin is a potential site of infection.
5. Report any infection, no matter how trivial.
6. Report any fever >37.8°C. (100°F.).

Polycythemia Vera

Polycythemia vera (primary polycythemia) is a chronic myeloproliferative disorder involving all bone marrow elements, resulting in an increase in red blood cell mass and hemoglobin. The underlying cause is unknown. It is a multiple organ system disease.

Altered Physiology

1. Increased blood volume because of increase in red cell mass
2. Increased supply of precursor cells
3. Hyperplasia of all bone marrow elements
4. Striking increase in total blood volume; gradually increasing blood viscosity
5. Decreased marrow iron
6. Enlargement of spleen

Clinical Manifestations

(Clinical manifestations are referable to increased blood volume and viscosity from erythrocytosis [increased red cells].)
1. Plethoric appearance (reddish-purple hue of skin and mucosa)—from congestion causing distention of blood vessels
2. Pruritus, typically prickling in character induced by skin cooling (after showering/bathing)
3. Painful fingers and toes—from arterial and venous insufficiency
4. Bleeding tendency
5. Headache, dizziness, impaired mental ability, vertigo, visual abnormalities (scotomata; double or blurred vision)—from disturbed cerebral circulation
6. Splenomegaly, producing abdominal discomfort
7. Hepatomegaly
8. Hypertension
9. Hyperuricemia—from increased formation and destruction of erythrocytes and leukocytes and increased metabolism of nucleic acids
10. Weakness and easy fatigability

Diagnostic Evaluation

1. Increased red cell mass
2. Thrombocytosis; often abnormal platelet aggregation
3. Leukocytosis (in majority of patients)
4. Elevated granulocyte alkaline phosphatase activity
5. Increased serum B_{12}
6. Normal PO_2 (used to differentiate primary from secondary polycythemia)

Management

Goal:
To reduce blood viscosity
1. Phlebotomy (withdrawal of blood) to reduce red cell mass; frequency of phlebotomy determined by hematocrit.
   a. 250–500 ml. of blood removed every other day until hematocrit reaches desired level.
   b. Repeated phlebotomies may be performed to lower hemoglobin, hematocrit, and red cell mass.
2. Myelosuppressive therapy—radioactive phosphorus (^{32}P) either orally or intravenously—acts on hyperplastic bone marrow to suppress panmyelosis (proliferation of bone marrow elements)
3. Allopurinol—to control hyperuricemia (excess of uric acid in the blood)
4. Antihistamine drugs to give relief from pruritus

Nursing Interventions

1. Monitor for complications—the clinical course of polycythemia is determined by the development of complications.
   a. Thromboembolic complications—due to hyperviscosity, which leads to reduced blood flow and subsequent infarction.
      Includes deep vein thrombophlebitis, myocardial and cerebral infarction, and thrombotic occlusion of the splenic, hepatic, portal, and mesenteric veins.
   b. Hemorrhagic tendency—bleeding occurs spontaneously from increasing blood volume and capillary and venous distention. Platelets may also be qualitatively abnormal.
   c. Gout—from overproduction of uric acid (secondary to nucleoprotein turnover of marrow cells).
   d. Congestive failure—from increased blood volume and hypertension.
   e. Peptic ulcers
   f. Acute leukemia may be a terminal complication; myelofibrosis (replacement of marrow with fibrotic tissue) also may occur.
2. Keep the patient ambulatory, as the likelihood of thrombosis increases when the patient is on bed rest.

Patient Education

1. Report at prescribed intervals for follow-up blood (hematocrit) studies.
2. Avoid taking *hot* baths/showers, as skin cooling worsens pruritus.

The Leukemias

The *leukemias* are neoplastic disorders of the blood-forming tissues (spleen, lymphatic system, and bone marrow). The common features of the leukemias are an unregulated proliferation of white cells in the bone marrow with replacement of normal marrow elements. There also may be proliferation in the liver, spleen, and lymph nodes, and invasion of nonhematologic organs such as the meninges, gastrointestinal tract, kidney, and skin.

Predisposing Factors

Etiology unknown—several factors are associated with increase in incidence:
1. Environmental/industrial exposure to radiation or chemicals
2. Infectious agents—retroviruses
3. Hereditary aspects
   a. Family occurrence
   b. Chromosomal abnormalities (Down's syndrome)
4. Secondary to treatment administered for other diseases (e.g., Hodgkin's disease); therapy-related leukemia among patients treated with chemotherapy and/or radiotherapy for a neoplastic disease

Acute Leukemia*

The *acute leukemias* are a heterogenous group of hematopoietic (formation of blood cells) malignancies arising

* For discussion of acute leukemia in children, see page 1481.

in the bone marrow characterized by uncontrolled proliferation of immature cells. Lymphocytic, granulocytic (myelocytic), or monocytic cell types may be involved. The clinical course is similar for all types.

Clinical Manifestations

1. Easy fatigability and generalized malaise; pallor—secondary to anemia
2. Bleeding of gums, epistaxis, petechiae, prolonged bleeding following a surgical procedure—from thrombocytopenia (lowered platelet count)
3. Fever or infection—secondary to granulocytopenia
4. Enlarged lymph nodes and spleen; abdominal discomfort—from organ infiltration
5. Bone pain, arthralgia—from infiltration of bone by leukemic cells
6. Tachycardia, weight loss, dyspnea on exertion, intolerance to heat—from increased metabolism
7. Leukemic infiltration of the skin—tendency for leukemic cells to infiltrate other organs and tissues
8. Cerebral hemorrhage, cranial nerve paralysis, increased intracranial pressure—from neurologic complications (leukemic cells frequently invade the central nervous system)
9. Pain—from infarction, particularly the spleen

NURSING ALERT: Undiagnosed patients may appear in the emergency department for treatment of acute infections. Suspect leukemia.

Diagnostic Evaluation

1. Blood evaluation—total peripheral white count varies widely (1000–100,000/ml.^{3})
2. Bone marrow examination—characteristically large percentage of bone marrow's nucleated cells are immature leukocyte forms called "blasts"
3. Lymph node biopsy
4. Chest x-ray—to detect mediastinal node and lung involvement
5. Skeletal x-ray—to detect skeletal lesions
6. Immunologic methods used to detect cell lineage, stage of differentiation

Management

Goal:

To eradicate leukemia cells and restore normal hematopoiesis.

A. Types of Treatment

1. High doses of chemotherapy are given to obtain a *remission* (disappearance of all abnormal cell forms in bone marrow and blood) followed by cyclic readministration of chemotherapy to prevent relapse.
2. Central nervous system therapy—combined radiotherapy to the cranium with intrathecal methotrexate (given by lumbar puncture into the subarachnoid space) to prevent leukemic infiltration of the CNS.
3. Bone marrow transplantation (See p. 292)
   a. Patient's own bone marrow is treated in vitro to remove leukemic cells using monoclonal antibodies or drugs; bone marrow is cryopreserved and reinfused when needed.
   b. High-dose chemotherapy and total body irradiation is done to destroy all residual leukemic cells

and to suppress the immune function (prevent graft rejection), followed by rescue with bone marrow cells.
4. Hickman catheter may be implanted intravenously for administration of antibiotics and blood products and for parenteral nutrition.
5. Prompt treatment of infection

B. Underlying Principles of Chemotherapy

1. Chemotherapy inhibits growth of leukemic cells by destroying or inactivating nucleic acids or by interfering with their synthesis; causes bone marrow depression and depresses the patient's immunologic defense mechanism.
2. Drugs are usually given in combination (as they have different mechanisms of action) to maximize cell kill and minimize drug resistance. The treatment regimen is designed to affect cells in different phases of the mitotic cycle.
3. Commonly, there is intensive treatment with multiple agents at the beginning of therapy (induction) to induce a remission, followed by long-term continuation (maintenance) therapy. No one regimen produces successful responses in all patients.
4. The drugs used to treat leukemia produce major toxicity to the hematopoietic system, resulting in prolonged periods of pancytopenia.

C. Drugs Used for Acute Lymphocytic Leukemia

1. Combinations of vincristine, prednisone, daunorubicin, and asparaginase are used during the induction phase. Maintenance therapy employs combinations of 6-mercaptopurine, methotrexate, vincristine, and prednisone.
2. More recently, additional intensive chemotherapy is incorporated into some regimens, early or late in remission, in an attempt to eradicate residual leukemic cells and to prevent emergence of drug resistance.

Nursing Assessment

1. Take nursing history, focusing on weight loss, fever, incidence of frequent infections, progressively increasing fatigability, shortness of breath, palpitations, visual changes (retinal bleeding).
2. Ask about difficulty in swallowing, coughing, rectal pain.
3. Examine patient for enlarged lymph nodes and hepatosplenomegaly.
4. Examine eyegrounds—retina may reveal white-centered hemorrhages.
5. Inspect the skin for erythema and skin lesions; palpate for warmth and sweating.
6. Examine for evidences of bleeding: petechiae, especially on arms, legs, trunk, and back. Look for bruises and inspect IV sites for oozing. Check vital signs.
7. Examine lungs for abnormal breath sounds, crackles, rhonchi.
8. Look for evidence of infection: mouth, tongue, and throat for reddened areas/white patches. Examine for skin breakdown, which is a potential source of infection.
9. Examine rectal area for inflammation, point tenderness, induration, presence of ulceration. Ask about pain.
10. Observe body movements, including gait.
11. Review results of diagnostic studies.
12. Try to ascertain the emotional impact of the diagnosis/treatment.

Nursing Diagnoses

1. Potential for infection related to granulocytopenia secondary to leukemia or its treatment with cytotoxic drugs
2. Pain related to tumor growth and infection
3. Altered oral mucous membranes related to chemotherapy and/or viral and fungal infection
4. Knowledge deficit of disease, treatment, health care system, resources, remission/recovery, and coping with chronic disease
5. Anxiety related to gravity of diagnosis, treatment regimen, disease chronicity
6. Other possible nursing diagnoses:
   - Fluid volume deficit related to nausea, vomiting, and taste changes
   - Fatigue related to effects of disease and its treatment
   - Ineffective thermoregulation (fever) related to infection, possible widespread disease, reaction to drugs, or to transfusion of blood products
   - Activity intolerance related to anemia
   - Potential for impaired skin integrity related to malnutrition and immobility
   - Altered nutrition (less than body requirements) related to toxic effects of chemotherapy
   - Self-esteem disturbances related to alopecia, changes in appearance
   - Ineffective family coping related to physiological and psychological changes in patient's condition, family anxiety, and fatigue

Nursing Interventions

A. Preventing Infection

1. Monitor for infection, which is the major morbidity and mortality factor associated with leukemia.
2. Know the common types of infections associated with leukemia: pneumonia, pharyngitis, esophagitis, perianal cellulitis; urinary tract infections, and sinusitis
3. Monitor for *temperature elevation,* flushed appearance, chills, tachycardia, appearance of white patches in mouth, redness, swelling, heat or pain of eyes, ears, throat, skin, joints, abdomen, rectal and perineal areas; cough; changes in character and/or color of sputum, stool; skin rash.

   Remember that the usual manifestations of infection are altered in patients with leukemia. Prednisone may blunt the normal febrile response to infection.
4. Monitor the concentration of circulating granulocytes. Concentrations under 500/μl make the patient at serious risk of infection.
5. *Avoid mucosal and epithelial damage.*
   a. Avoid venipuncture, subcutaneous, and intramuscular injections unless absolutely necessary.
   b. Avoid urinary catheterization if possible.
   c. Avoid the use of vaginal tampons; use sanitary napkins.
6. Avoid rectal infections—from alteration in mucous membranes, neutropenia, changes in normal bowel flora from antibiotics, malnutrition, diarrhea, constipation, hemorrhoids, cytotoxic drugs.
   a. Maintain normal bowel function, as diarrhea and constipation can irritate rectal mucosa.
   b. Avoid rectal thermometers—perianal cellulitis and perirectal abscess are common complications.
   c. Avoid foods that increase bacterial colonization of gastrointestinal tract; these include fresh fruits and vegetables, rare meat, buttermilk.
   d. Keep perianal area clean.
7. Prevent infectious complications by control of environmental contamination.
   a. Use careful hand-washing techniques before and after every patient contact.
   b. Instruct patient to make sure that each individual washes his hands before coming into contact with him (e.g., hand-wash in his presence).
   c. Use intensive environmental cleaning procedures; double-bucket mopping; daily disinfecting of sink, toilet, horizontal surfaces in room, etc.
   d. Use ice that falls out of machine into container (without coming into hand contact), as ice is a source of contamination.
   e. Patient with greatly reduced granulocyte count may be maintained in a laminar air flow room (a unidirectional air flow "barrier" in which the infection-prone patient is free from contact with exogenous microorganisms).
8. Employ meticulous personal hygiene measures.
   a. Inspect all body sites that are at high risk for infection daily; orifices; perianal area; axilla and groin; IV sites; wounds.
   b. Bathe the patient daily.
   c. Establish and maintain oral hygiene regimen.
9. Treat infection promptly as directed.
   a. Obtain cultures (for both aerobes and anaerobes) of blood, urine, sputum, spinal fluid.
   b. Watch for development of fungal infection (especially *Candida* and *Aspergillus*)—from indwelling catheters, immunosuppressive effects of chemotherapy, bacterial suppression by antimicrobials, and decreased resistance of patient.

B. Preventing and Managing Bleeding Episodes

1. Assess the patient for signs of bleeding. Bleeding is usually secondary to severe thrombocytopenia caused by marrow failure.
   a. Monitor platelet count daily; major cause of hemorrhage is thrombocytopenia (decrease in platelets).
   b. Minor bleeding—petechiae, ecchymoses, conjunctival hemorrhage, epistaxis, bleeding gums; guaiac-positive emesis and stools; heme-positive urine, bleeding at puncture sites, vaginal spotting
   c. Serious bleeding—headache; change in responsiveness; blurred vision; hemoptysis; hematemesis; melena; hypotension with tachycardia; dizziness
   d. Check inside mouth for bleeding into mucous membranes of oral cavity, tonsilar bed and pharynx; check nose for bleeding.
   e. Monitor urine, feces, and emesis for occult bleeding.
   f. Monitor pad count/amount of saturation during menses.
2. Support the patient receiving blood component therapy.
3. Teach the patient to remain at rest during active bleeding episodes—helps to lower pulse rate and blood pressure and promotes clot formation.
4. Control bleeding—keep injections to a minimum; take blood samples and give analgesics through Hickman catheter.
   a. Control nose and mouth bleeding.

b. Intracranial bleeding
Avoid the Valsalva maneuver or activity that increases intracranial pressure.

C. Monitoring for Toxic Manifestations of Chemotherapy

1. Obtain baseline information before chemotherapy is started.
   a. Know the patient's "normal" TPR and BP.
   b. Follow the WBC, differential count, hemoglobin measurements, platelet counts—to be aware of the drug's effect on the body.
   c. Follow blood chemistry studies, electrolytes, urea nitrogen, creatinine, liver enzymes, bilirubin.
   d. Weigh the patient daily.
   e. Assist with bone marrow aspirations as directed (see p. 292).
2. Watch for toxic manifestations during chemotherapy.
   a. Modifications of the patient's chemotherapy regimen are based on laboratory and physical examinations before each course of treatment.
   b. Monitor intravenous infusion of drugs (see p. 98)—may cause local irritation in the veins; the patient may complain of burning sensations during infusions of methotrexate and prednisone.
      (1) Adjust infusion flow to a slower rate.
      (2) Change position of extremity to prevent muscle cramping.
      (3) The patient may complain of nausea, vomiting, and burning sensation along the gastrointestinal tract during or immediately after drug infusion.
      (4) Certain agents such as daunorubicin, mitomycin, and vincristine are "sclerosing" agents and cause extensive tissue damage and necrosis if infiltrated into subcutaneous spaces. These drugs should be given only by a physician or a specially trained oncology nurse.
      (5) Be sure infusion is finished within prescribed time; toxicities seem to be intensified by prolonged infusion.
   c. Watch for mouth ulcers—frequently occur when the patient is taking methotrexate. Offer prescribed medicated mouth rinses frequently to relieve oral discomfort.
   d. Expect the patient to experience loss of hair during antileukemic treatment—alopecia occurs in high percentage of patients receiving daunorubicin. Encourage the patient to experiment with wigs, hair pieces, head scarves.
   e. Check deep tendon reflexes. Assess patient for footdrop, weakening hand grasp, ptosis of eyelids—vincristine may cause neuropathy.
   f. Assess for constipation and abdominal pain—vincristine may produce adynamic ileus.
   g. Watch for personality changes, fluid retention, hypertension, gastric ulcers, and diabetes mellitus—occur with prednisone therapy.
   h. Watch for other drug side effects—diarrhea, maculopapular rash, stomatitis, phlebitis, bone marrow depression, evidences of cardiac toxicity (tachycardia, dysrhythmias, tachypnea, dyspnea).
   i. Take ECG readings as prescribed—cardiac toxicity is associated with certain chemotherapeutic agents.
   j. See page 103 for nursing management of the patient undergoing chemotherapy.
3. Encourage patient to endure discomfort associated with the treatment.

D. Promoting Oral Comfort and Healing

1. Examine oral mucosa—chemotherapeutic agents affect all rapidly proliferating tissue, including mucosa.
2. Watch for development of candidiasis and infective processes of the mouth—from corticosteroids and some antibiotics.
3. Give frequent and special mouth care to remove dried blood, combat odor, and soothe oral mucosa.

E. Relieving Pain and Discomfort

1. Control the pain and discomfort.
   a. Use milder analgesics when possible; change to a stronger narcotic as the patient's condition requires.
   b. Give tranquilizers as directed to enhance the effects of narcotics.
   c. Give antiemetic medication before meals—to help assuage the patient's nausea; sedatives may also be helpful.
2. Maintain oral intake between 3 and 4 liters daily—to prevent precipitation of uric acid crystals in the urine.
3. Control fever—employ cool sponges, increased fluid intake.

F. Promotion of Coping Mechanisms to Deal With Physiologic and Emotional Distress

1. Assist the patient to understand that the range of feelings about leukemia is normal—may help patient gain control.
   a. The patient may react with shock and anger when disease is first recognized; anger may be directed at health-care personnel.
   b. Anger is a defense mechanism; patient realizes that death is inevitable; anger is also a defense against anxiety.
   c. Develop ability to accept and deal with this anger—important for establishing a therapeutic patient–nurse relationship.
   d. Allow patient and family to ventilate their emotions.
   e. Patient may use mechanism of denial—denial may need to be supported or worked through.
2. Emphasize the positive aspects of modern treatment and the ability to resume a normal life-style when in remission.
3. Encourage participation in support group (American Cancer Society) to help diffuse anger and dependency and to provide support and education.
4. Pay attention to changing informational needs of patient.

Patient Education

1. Avoid possible sources of infection—crowds, unnecessary hospital visits, etc.
   a. Employ good, frequent hand-washing practices.
   b. Report any sign of infection to physician/clinic promptly.
   c. Report any exposure to varicella, measles, hepatitis, etc.
2. Pay careful attention to nutrition—undernourished person does not tolerate antileukemic drugs as well as well-nourished individual.
3. Follow instructions on proper Hickman catheter care.
4. Monitor weight to be certain a significant amount of weight is not lost.
5. See your dentist—oral disease is frequently present; request dentist to contact your physician before initiating dental examination.

6. Avoid rectal mucosal trauma by preventing constipation; use stool softeners, increase fluid intake, high-fiber foods; wash perineum with soap and water after each elimination.
7. Shower/bathe daily, paying attention to axillae, skin folds, groin, and perineum. Use an electric shaver.
8. Use a deodorant rather than an antiperspirant (antiperspirant blocks sweat glands and may cause infection).
9. Practice oral hygiene after each meal.
10. Watch for signs of bleeding—avoid use of sharp objects, straining at stool, forceful nose blowing, products containing aspirin.
11. Use birth control pills as directed to prevent breakthrough bleeding.
12. Remember that leukemia is a treatable disease, and that advances in treatment are continually being made; most side effects of antileukemic drugs are short-term and treatable.

Evaluation

1. No clinical or laboratory manifestations of leukemia; peripheral blood counts within normal limits; bone marrow appears within normal limits
2. Is free of infection
3. States that discomfort and pain are relieved
4. Demonstrates intact oral mucosa
5. Can recall signs and symptoms to report; knows how to report and manage bleeding episodes; asks questions
6. Copes with distress; adjusting to changing body image; uses support group; verbalizes feelings and concerns

Chronic Granulocytic Leukemia

Chronic granulocytic (myelocytic, myelogenous) leukemia is a chronic condition characterized by an increased proliferation of all myeloid cell lines, including granulocytes, monocytes, platelets, and occasionally red cells. It is often associated with great enlargement of the spleen and liver.

Clinical Features

1. Greatest incidence is in age range of 40 to 60 years.
2. Gradual, insidious onset; the disease runs a progressive course over several years.
3. The Philadelphia chromosome is present in cells of bone marrow origin in over 90% of patients.
4. Usually begins with a chronic phase when a complete or partial remission can be induced. After a variable period, it undergoes a metamorphosis to an accelerated phase that resembles acute leukemia.

Clinical Manifestations

1. Fatigue
2. Pallor, palpitations, dyspnea—from anemia
3. Dragging sensation or enlargement of left side of abdomen—from splenic enlargement
4. Hematologic features: elevated platelet count, elevated granulocyte count; blood smear shows predominance of granulocytes at all stages of maturation
5. Weakness, loss of weight, loss of appetite, night sweats—from increased metabolic rate due to high granulocyte turnover and anorexia from splenomegaly
6. Tenderness and pain in long bones (particularly tibia, ribs, lower part of sternum)—due to invasion by abnormal marrow

7. Thrombocytosis—manifested clinically as thromboembolic or hemorrhagic phenomena

Diagnostic Evaluation

1. Extremely elevated leukocyte count
2. Characteristic findings in peripheral blood
3. Demonstration of Philadelphia chromosome in bone marrow cells

Management

1. Chemotherapy—treatment with cytotoxic drugs will usually reduce size of spleen, restore leukocyte count to normal, and alleviate symptoms.
   a. Hydroxyurea or busulfan are the mainstays of treatment.
   b. Following initial treatment, the patient may be placed on long-term, low-dose maintenance therapy. This is known as the chronic phase of the disease.
   c. Interferon is currently being used to treat the chronic phase.
2. Eventually the patient will no longer respond; the acute exacerbation is termed myeloblastic or "blast" crisis, during which the disease resembles acute leukemia and is a terminal event in most patients.
3. See page 268 for the treatment of acute leukemia.
4. Bone marrow transplantation may produce prolonged disease-free survival if given early in chronic phase.
5. Leukapheresis (removal of white blood cells from whole blood; red blood cells transfused back into patient) may be used for the patient who needs white blood cell count reduced rapidly.

Nursing Interventions

1. See page 103 for nursing interventions for the patient receiving chemotherapy.
2. See page 269 for other nursing interventions for the patient with leukemia.

Chronic Lymphocytic Leukemia

Chronic lymphocytic leukemia (CLL) is a type of leukemia characterized by proliferation and accumulation of relatively mature-appearing lymphocytes in the circulation and in the lymphoid organs of the body. It is the most common type of leukemia in the Western countries.

Clinical Manifestations

1. Insidious onset affecting older populations (mean age greater than 60 years); the disease may run a protracted, relatively asymptomatic course over a number of years.
2. Symptoms and signs are related to infiltration of lymph nodes, bone marrow, liver, and spleen with lymphocytes.
   a. Increasing tiredness; decreasing exercise tolerance; excessive sweating or night sweats; weight loss
   b. Unexplained lymphocytosis
   c. Lymphadenopathy (enlarged nodes)—frequently in cervical, supraclavicular, and axillary regions
   d. Splenomegaly (may be painful)
   e. Anemia; thrombocytopenia—may be due to bone marrow infiltration, to immune dysfunction, or to hypersplenism

Diagnostic Evaluation

1. CBC—used also for following peripheral lymphocytosis
2. Bone marrow examination reveals lymphocytic infiltration of bone marrow
3. Lymph node biopsy

Management

A. Asymptomatic Patient With Chronic Lymphocytic Leukemia

1. May not require treatment for a period of years.
2. Support the patient with optimal nutrition, rest, exercise, recreation, and mental activity.

B. Symptomatic Patient (with symptomatic hepatosplenomegaly; bone marrow failure; hemolytic anemia; recurrent infections; persistent fever; progressive lymphocytosis).

1. Chemotherapy—brings symptomatic relief; decreases size of lymph nodes and spleen.
   a. Single-agent therapy—chlorambucil (Leukeran) or cyclophosphamide (Cytoxan)
   b. Combination drug therapy may be given to patients with advanced disease; reduces white cell count and improves constitutional symptoms.
2. Corticosteroids (prednisone)—given to enhance effect of chemotherapy. Usually produces decrease in lymphadenopathy; used to control leukocyte count and to treat immune-mediated hemolytic anemia and thrombocytopenia
3. Radiation therapy
   a. To shrink lymph nodes compromising vital organ function or causing disfigurement
   b. For relief of painful bone lesions
   c. To reduce size and relieve symptoms of splenomegaly; pain; anemia; thrombocytopenia
4. Transfusion therapy (leukocyte-depleted washed red cells) given for symptomatic anemia
5. Splenectomy—occasionally done for patient with hemolytic anemia, thrombocytopenia, pancytopenia, and painful splenomegaly

Complications

1. Infections (pneumonia; urinary tract infections) from immune impairment
2. Bruising and bleeding—from thrombocytopenia
3. Thrombophlebitis—from venous or lymphatic obstruction by enlarged lymph nodes.

Nursing Interventions/Patient Teaching

1. See page 103 for nursing support of the patient receiving chemotherapy, and page 269 for other aspects of management of patient with leukemia.
2. Instruct the patient to avoid aspirin and nonsteroidal anti-inflammatory drugs, as these interfere with normal platelet function and the patient is at increased risk of hemorrhage.
3. Advise patient to seek health care immediately for any evidence of infection in light of immunocompromised condition.
4. Keep in mind that patients with chronic lymphocytic leukemia appear to be at increased risk of developing skin cancer, Kaposi's sarcoma, and lung cancer.
5. Contact: Leukemia Society of America
   733 Third Ave., New York City 10017
   for information about patient education materials and support groups.

Malignant Lymphomas

The *lymphomas* are a group of neoplastic diseases of the lymphoreticular system and include Hodgkin's disease and the non-Hodgkin's lymphomas.

1. Lymphomas are classified both according to the predominant malignant cell type—as lymphocytic lymphomas, histiocytic lymphomas, or Hodgkin's disease—as well as by degree of malignant cell differentiation—well-differentiated, poorly differentiated, or undifferentiated.
2. These tumors usually start in lymph nodes, but can involve any lymphoid tissue in the spleen, gastrointestinal tract (tonsils, walls of stomach), liver, or bone marrow.
3. They may spread to all these areas and to extralymphatic tissues (lungs, kidneys, skin).
4. The etiology of these diseases is unknown.

Hodgkin's Disease

Hodgkin's disease is a malignant disease of unknown etiology that originates in the lymphoid system and involves predominantly the lymph nodes. It may occur in nearly any lymphoid tissue: spleen, bone marrow, liver.

Altered Physiology

1. The characteristic tumor cell of Hodgkin's disease is the "Reed–Sternberg" cell, which constitutes between 1% and 5% of all the cells in the tumor. The remaining cells are benign histiocytes, lymphocytes, eosinophils, and plasma cells.
2. Hodgkin's disease shows a highly predictable pattern of spread—usually via the lymphatic channels from one chain of lymph nodes to another, often to the spleen, and ultimately to extralymphatic sites.
3. Hodgkin's disease may also have a hematogenous mode of spread, as extra nodal sites involved include the gastrointestinal tract, bone marrow, skin, upper air passages, and other organs.

Clinical Manifestations

1. Painless enlargement of lymph nodes (usually on one side of neck)
2. Slight to high fever; chills, night sweats, weight loss
3. Pruritus (itching, either local or generalized)
4. Enlargement of lymph nodes in other regions of body: axillae, inguinal, femoral regions
5. Wide variety of symptoms may occur if there is pulmonary involvement, superior vena caval obstruction, hepatic or bone involvement, etc.

Diagnostic Evaluation

(The location and extent of the disease is determined before treatment.)

1. Biopsy of lymph node(s) to identify characteristic histologic features
2. Complete blood count
3. Chest x-ray and tomography—to detect mediastinal, hilar, or intrapulmonary disease
4. Computed tomography—to determine precise location of nodal involvement; used in treatment planning and follow-up
5. Bone marrow biopsy
6. Liver function tests and scan

7. Lymphangiogram
   a. Reveals size of lymph nodes
   b. Detects abdominal lymph node involvement, which may not be seen on tomography
8. Surgical staging (laparotomy with splenectomy, liver biopsy, multiple lymph node biopsies)—done in selected patients

Management

(Depends on anatomic extent of disease, histopathological findings, and prognostic indicators).

A. General Considerations

1. Hodgkin's disease is considered a potentially curable disorder.
2. More than one treatment strategy is currently available. Treatment protocols are being constantly evaluated and changed.
3. Radiotherapy or multiagent chemotherapy or a combination of these are used.

B. Radiotherapy (delivery of high-intensity radiation to the lymph nodes) is the treatment of choice in management of localized disease.

1. Areas of the body in which the lymph node chains are located can tolerate high doses without serious damage.
2. Males may wish to consider sperm banking before beginning therapy, as sterility is a complication. Females may wish to undergo oophoropexy (surgical placement of ovaries outside the radiation field).
3. Vital structures such as the heart, lungs, liver, kidney, and bone marrow are protected by lead shields.
4. *Complications* of intensive radiotherapy:
   a. Radiation pneumonitis and fibrosis, pericarditis and/or myocarditis, gastrointestinal injury (peptic ulceration, hemorrhage, chronic diarrhea, intestinal obstruction); thyroid dysfunction, sterility
   b. Acute reactions to irradiation—dryness of mouth; loss of taste; dysphagia; nausea and vomiting; apathy and lassitude; skin redness, dry peeling in treatment fields; loss of hair at back of neck and under areas treated; reduction of white blood cells.

C. Chemotherapy

1. Has many combinations in use; the response rate varies.
   a. Mechlorethamine hydrochloride, vincristine (Oncovin), procarbazine, and prednisone (MOPP).
      Many programs modify the MOPP combination with deletion of an agent, substitution of one or more drugs with agents from the same class, adding new agents in an attempt to overcome primary drug resistance.
   b. Doxorubicin (Adriamycin), bleomycin, and vinblastine is another combination used with MOPP
2. Three or four drugs may be given in intermittent or cyclical courses with periods off therapy to allow recovery of normal tissues.
   a. Doses of myelosuppressive agents adjusted according to pretreatment granulocyte and platelet count
   b. Toxic effects of these drugs often overlap, especially bone marrow depression.
   c. Late *complications:* cardiotoxicity, lung fibrosis, infertility, second neoplasms, avascular necrosis of bone
3. Combination chemotherapy in addition to extended field radiation may be used.

Nursing Interventions

1. Help the patient cope with unpleasant side effects of radiation.
   a. Esophagitis—bland soft foods at mild temperatures, anesthetic lozenges, pain medication before eating if patient unable to eat.
   b. Loss of taste—serve palatable meals.
   c. Anorexia—encourage patient to make the effort to eat.
   d. Nausea and vomiting—antiemetics given to cover peak time of nausea.
   e. Diarrhea—antidiarrheal medication.
   f. Skin reaction (sunburned/tanned appearance of treatment area)—avoid rubbing, heat, cold, application of lotions.
   g. Lethargy—rest/sleep to keep energy level up; diversional activities to prevent boredom.
   h. Tingling with numbness in hands, toes; weakness in knees, hands—use a cane for stability.
   i. See page 108 for nursing interventions for patient undergoing radiotherapy.
2. Support the patient having toxic effects from chemotherapy.
   a. Encourage the patient by saying that the therapy will end in "a period of time"—serves as an incentive for the patient to continue with therapy. Emphasize high likelihood of cure.
   b. Give stool softeners to control constipation that accompanies chemotherapy, or place on a bowel-conditioning program (see p. 143). Offer high-fiber foods (bran) to maintain intestinal tone.
   c. Anticipate that patients on chemotherapy will develop leukopenia, thrombocytopenia, and anemia.
   d. See page 103 for nursing management of patient undergoing chemotherapy.

NURSING ALERT: There is an apparent increase in second malignancies (primarily leukemia) of patients who are long-term survivors of Hodgkin's disease, especially in those who have received combination chemotherapy as well as radiation therapy.

Patient Education

The control of the disease requires continuing observation by the patient.

1. Report fever or any sign of infection (skin redness, tenderness, lesions, cough) immediately, as the disease and its treatment make one susceptible to infection.
   Herpes zoster occurs frequently; may become generalized in immunosuppressed patients.
2. Use humidifier/throat lozenges for dry throat and to control desire to cough.
3. Express feelings and anxieties; seek supportive persons and groups.
   a. Depression and fear are normal reactions to diagnosis, treatment, and stress of uncertain outcome.
   b. Expect to feel fatigued up to a year after therapy.
   c. Remain active and employed (if possible); seek to enjoy the present.
4. Expect some degree of hair loss if taking vincristine or mechlorethamine hydrochloride; almost always reversible after therapy is completed.
5. Avoid taking alcohol, narcotics, antihistamines, tran-

quilizers, or sympathomimetic agents when taking procarbazine.
6. Report for follow-up.

Non-Hodgkin's Lymphomas

The *Non-Hodgkin's lymphomas* are a group of disorders that can be defined as malignancies of lymphoid tissue other than Hodgkin's disease. They include a broad range of neoplasms derived from the T cells and B cells and their precursors in the lymphoid system.

Clinical Manifestations

1. Painless lymph node enlargement; multiple lymph node groups commonly involved
2. Splenomegaly
3. Fatigue (attributable to anemia); malaise, anorexia, weight loss
4. Fever and night sweats
5. Generalized pruritus
6. Abdominal and bone pain
7. Respiratory symptoms—from lymphoma involving the mediastinum, pulmonary parenchyma, pleura
8. Gastrointestinal symptoms (abdominal pain, intestinal obstruction, diarrhea)—from extranodal involvement

Diagnostic Evaluation

1. Biopsy of lymph node(s)
2. Bone marrow biopsy—for evidence of bone marrow involvement
3. Screening chest x-ray; computed tomography of chest/abdomen/pelvis to detect extent of abnormality
4. Blood tests; liver and renal function studies
5. Measurement of serum lactic acid dehydrogenase (LDH)—an indicator of extent of disease
6. Lymphogram—evaluates size and internal architecture of lymph nodes
7. Laparotomy—for staging

Management

The management approach depends on the stage of the disease, morphologic characteristics, and classification. Many of these patients have disseminated disease at the time of diagnosis.

A. **Radiation Therapy**—for early stage disease

B. **Chemotherapy**

1. Single-agent therapy (alkylating agent) for low-grade lymphomas
2. Combination chemotherapy may be used in advanced stage for cure. Variety of new drugs used with older drugs; more aggressive approaches being used.
3. *Complications*
   a. Administration of the agents used in non-Hodgkin's lymphoma (cyclophosphamide, vincristine, doxorubicin, methotrexate, bleomycin, etoposide, cytarabine) are associated with significant nausea and vomiting.
   b. Leukopenia and thrombocytopenia from myelosuppressive effects of chemotherapy.

Nursing Interventions

1. Be constantly vigilant for complications of non-Hodgkin's lymphoma:
   a. Infection—by bacteria, viruses, fungi; due to deficiencies of cellular immunity
   b. Anemia—from bone marrow invasion, hemorrhage, chemotherapy, hypersplenism, hemolysis
   c. Spinal cord compression—from lymphomatous meningitis
   d. Hyperuricemia
2. Bear in mind that patient may develop syndrome of anticipatory nausea that precedes actual chemotherapy.
3. See the discussion of nursing interventions for patient with Hodgkin's disease, page 273.

Mycosis Fungoides
(Cutaneous T-cell Lymphoma)

Mycosis fungoides is a T-cell lymphoma that usually begins in the skin and may involve the lymph nodes and other internal organs.

The term "mycosis fungoides" describes the mushroom-like appearance of the skin tumors. The late stage of the disease closely resembles malignant lymphoma.

Clinical Manifestations

1. Patch stage—nonspecific scaling, *itching,* erythematous eruption.
2. Plaque stage—lesions become indurated (hardened); plaques gradually increase in size.
3. Tumor stage—nodules or tumors appear in the skin as mushroom-like growths (scarlet or purplish in color), varying in size from 1–5 cm.; the body may become covered with these lesions. These tumors can ulcerate, become infected, and give rise to life-threatening septicemia.
4. Once the disease involves extracutaneous sites (nodes, liver, spleen), there is usually a progressively downward course

Diagnostic Evaluation

1. Biopsy of skin lesion—gives distinctive diagnostic pattern of mycosis fungoides
2. Biopsies of lymph nodes, bone marrow, liver
3. Liver scan

Management

(Selection of treatment depends on stage of disease)
1. Topical (local) therapy used for skin manifestations
   a. Skin lubrication
   b. Topical steroids
   c. Topical chemotherapy; mechlorethamine Allergic dermatitis may develop as a response to topical chemotherapy.
2. Radiation therapy (electron beam therapy, ultraviolet light, photochemotherapy [PUVA therapy]).
3. Systemic chemotherapy—used when visceral involvement is suspected, when skin tolerance limits further radiation therapy, or other methods fail to control the disease.
   a. A combination of topical therapy, radiotherapy, and systemic therapy may be used.
   b. Antimetabolites, cytotoxic antibiotics, alkylating agents and corticosteroids may be used.

Nursing Interventions

A. **Relieving Discomfort**

1. Support the patient who has painful open weeping lesions.
2. See care of burn patient, page 849.

3. Line pajamas and bed linens with Telfa®—to absorb drainage and prevent bedding from adhering to skin.
4. Give analgesics for discomfort.
5. Handle the patient with care.
6. Keep up nutritional status, as the patient loses protein and fluid from body surface.

B. Monitoring and Protecting From Infection

1. Bear in mind that infection is a major cause of death in these patients.
2. Wash hands before and after patient contact to reduce bacterial spread.
3. Continue with excellent skin care to keep bacterial levels low.
4. Use whirlpool therapy to aid in skin cleansing and debridement.
5. Apply prescribed topical cream—as prophylaxis against infection and to promote comfort by excluding air from exposed nerve endings.
6. Assist the patient to cope with foul odor from bacterial growth in lesions.

C. Other Nursing Interventions

1. See page 273 for nursing management of the patient with Hodgkin's disease.
2. See page 826 for management of exfoliative dermatitis.

Patient Education

1. Emphasize the importance of personal hygiene and skin care.
   a. Daily bathing with a mild superfatted soap and medicated bath oil
   b. Application of prescribed creams/ointments
2. Discuss modifications that may need to be made in life-style (role changes, sexual relations); psychotherapy may be helpful, especially for patient in terminal phase of illness.
3. Avoid using perfumes and after-shave lotion.
4. Wear nonrestrictive cotton clothing.
5. Report to the physician any flare-up in skin condition, fever, signs and symptoms of systemic illness; hospitalization is usually necessary.

Multiple Myeloma

Multiple myeloma (plasma cell myeloma; myelomatosis) is a malignant disorder of plasma cells that infiltrate bone marrow and soft tissues. The cause is not known. It is usually a disease of older people, which runs a progressive course.

Altered Physiology

1. The malignant cell is the plasma cell; a widespread proliferation of immature plasma cells infiltrate the bone marrow throughout the skeleton, causing bone destruction.
2. The bones most commonly affected are the vertebrae, skull, ribs, sternum, pelvis, upper ends of humerus. In later stages, the liver, spleen, and kidneys may become involved.
3. Plasma cells are derived from B lymphocytes and normally produce physiologic levels of immunoglobulins. Malignant plasma cells produce abnormal amounts of an immunoglobulin or parts of an immunoglobulin protein (Bence Jones protein) that usually can be de-

tected in the serum and in urine by immunoelectrophoresis.
4. There is a constant threat of hypercalcemia and hyperuricemia due to release of calcium from involved bones exceeding the excretory capacity of the kidneys.
5. Increased loss of bone substance leads to collapse of vertebral bodies and pathological or spontaneous fractures in areas of cortical thinning.
6. Renal dysfunction may be produced by Bence Jones proteinuria, hyperuricemia, hyperuricosuria, and dehydration.

Clinical Manifestations

1. Constant severe bone pain, especially on movement.
   a. Severe back, rib, or extremity pain—from loss of bone
   b. Osteolytic (punched out) skeletal lesions—producing swelling, tenderness, pain, and *pathological fractures*
2. Weakness from anemia—due to malignancy and/or replacement of marrow with myeloma cells. May be associated with thrombocytopenia and granulocytopenia—causes increased susceptibility to *infection* and *abnormal bleeding.*
3. Marked weight loss
4. Symptoms of renal failure—may be due to precipitation of the immunoglobulin in the tubules or to pyelonephritis, hypercalciuria, increased uric acid, infiltration of the kidney with plasma cells (myeloma kidney), renal vein thrombosis
5. Nausea, vomiting, constipation, lethargy (late stage)—these are symptoms of marked hypercalcemia.

Diagnostic Evaluation

1. Bone marrow aspiration and biopsy—reveal increased numbers and abnormal forms of plasma cells
2. Hematologic abnormalities—anemia (related to marrow replacement, accelerated erythrocyte destruction, blood loss, renal insufficiency, effects of radiotherapy and chemotherapy, associated infections and nutritional causes)
   • Malignant plasma cells produce abnormal globulins, which appear in serum electrophoresis as a monoclonal paraprotein "spike"—fragments of these globulins are excreted in urine as Bence Jones proteins.
3. Numerous osteolytic bone lesions may appear on x-ray.

Management

1. Chemotherapy—to reduce number of plasma cells
   a. Alkylating agent (melphalan or cyclophosphamide) combined with prednisone is frequently used.
   b. Combinations of vincristine, cyclophosphamide, doxorubicin, and prednisone and numerous other drugs are in current use.
   c. Patient eventually relapses or dies of other causes.
2. Radiation therapy—very helpful in palliating bone pain associated with lytic lesions and pathological fractures.
3. Treatment of concomitant anemia related to tumor burden of myeloma cells.
   a. Packed red cell transfusions for patients with severe anemia
   b. Chemotherapy administered to decrease degree of marrow infiltration may improve anemia.

4. Allopurinol and high fluid intake given to reduce serum calcium and uric acid levels
5. Dialysis may be required in severely hypercalcemic patients with advanced renal insufficiency.
6. Stabilization and fixation of pathologic fractures

Nursing Assessment

1. When taking the nursing history, question the patient about pain. Related to movement? Occur at night? Sudden onset? (suspect pathologic fracture) Bone tenderness? Has there been any change in height? (suspect vertebral collapse)
2. Examine for evidences of bone deformities and bone tenderness.
3. Review laboratory findings for evidence of anemia, hypogammaglobulinemia, and for monoclonal globulin peak in urine (Bence Jones proteinuria).
4. Find out about patient's support system; social services and other referrals may be indicated.

Nursing Diagnoses

1. Pain (bone) related to bone erosion and possible pathological fractures.
2. Fatigue related to anemia.
3. Potential for injury related to falling from vertebral collapse and/or fractures.
4. Ineffective individual coping related to change in lifestyle and body image.

Nursing Interventions

A. Monitoring for Complications

1. Pathological fracture—monitor for *sudden* severe pain.
2. Spinal cord compression—from extradural plasma cell tumors producing compression/paraplegia.
3. Bacterial infections—from a variety of immune deficits, including impaired capacity for antibody formation and defects in complement and granulocyte function.
   - Respiratory infections and urinary tract infections frequently seen.
4. Hypercalcemia. Monitor for nausea, drowsiness, confusion, and polyuria.
5. Renal failure from hypercalcemia and Bence Jones proteinuria.
6. Anemia
7. Acute leukemia—incidence increases in persons with multiple myeloma.

B. Relieving Pain

1. Control pain.
   Avoid excessive lifting and straining. Handle the patient with smooth, unhurried movements.
2. Administer pain-relieving medication at a scheduled time around the clock until pain control is attained.
3. Assess the effectiveness of pain intervention to decrease dosage or change medication until pain relief is achieved without sedation.
4. Radiation therapy to focal lesions, splinting, back brace, relaxation techniques—are other measures used for pain.

C. Coping With Fatigue

1. Determine methods to conserve energy; note these on patient's care plan.
2. Foster self-care and positive health behaviors.
3. Encourage good nutrition and regular physical exercise within limits of ability.
4. Teach stress management and relaxation techniques.

D. Preventing Injury

1. Keep the patient ambulatory and avoid immobilization unless lesions in spine (extradural plasmacytomas) produce danger of cord compression; ambulation prevents further bone resorption and hypercalcemia.
   a. Allow the patient to set own pace.
   b. Use walker and assistive devices to keep the patient active.
2. Recommend changes in physical environment when appropriate.

E. Monitoring for Renal Insufficiency—abnormal proteins may exert a nephrotoxic effect at tubular level; or renal failure may develop from hypercalcemia (from bony destruction and immobilization), amyloidosis, hyperuricemia, myeloma kidney.

1. Encourage liberal fluid intake and keep urine flow rate high—to prevent protein precipitation and to minimize hypercalciuria.
2. Monitor renal status through blood studies and urinalysis.
3. Watch for symptoms of hemorrhagic cystitis in patient taking cyclophosphamide; maintain on liberal fluid intake.
4. Avoid dehydration—can precipitate acute renal failure; IV fluids may be necessary.
5. Weigh patient daily to monitor fluid retention.

NURSING ALERT: Patients with multiple myeloma should *not* have their fluid intake restricted prior to diagnostic tests, as dehydrating procedures can precipitate acute renal failure.

F. Monitoring for Recurrent Infections—from decrease in normal circulating antibodies because of proliferation of abnormal plasma cells, which produce ineffective globulins; chemotherapy and radiotherapy cause marrow depression; steroids increase susceptibility to opportunistic infection.

1. Monitor temperature—patients on steroids may not have overt symptoms of infection. Assess for apathy, lethargy, and tachycardia.
2. Assess for symptoms of urinary tract and respiratory tract infections.
3. Secure cultures from skin lesions, blood, sputum, and urine as indicated.

G. Providing Psychosocial Support—Support the patient emotionally and demonstrate continuing interest.

1. Reinforce the patient's understanding of treatment and its possible side effects.
2. Take a positive approach, emphasizing the benefits of therapy.
3. Emphasize the patient's strengths.
4. Share and work through the patient's anxieties.
5. Explore precisely what the patient fears.
6. Allow the patient to talk about his problems. Give *specific* help (for pain, breathlessness, depression, etc.).
7. Anticipate the patient's anxieties after leaving the hospital.

Patient Education

1. Instruct the patient about proper body mechanics and avoiding heavy lifting.
2. Make the patient aware of potentially nephrotoxic factors such as *dehydration* or drugs.
3. Instruct the patient to wear a back brace as prescribed

and to use muscle-strengthening exercises to maintain performance status.
4. Report the presence of fever, bone pain, bleeding, or neurologic complications; report for regular follow-up.
5. Use nutritional supplement during periods of anorexia.

Evaluation

1. Reports relief of disabling bone pain
2. Increases activities
3. Uses walker; aware of hazards in environment that could precipitate a fall; avoids lifting heavy objects
4. Looks toward the future; making plans; says is coping better

---

Bleeding Disorders

Bleeding disorders may be classified as congenital or acquired and single or multifactorial.

Clinical Manifestations

1. Mucocutaneous bleeding—petechiae or ecchymosis on skin, nosebleeding, gum oozing while brushing teeth, hemorrhagic bullae in oral mucosa, gastrointestinal bleeding, lower urinary tract bleeding
2. Bleeding into soft tissue, joints, viscera
3. Palpable liver and spleen (hepatomegaly and splenomegaly)
4. Bleeding in central nervous system

Laboratory Evaluation

1. Falling hemoglobin/hematocrit levels
2. Thrombocytopenia
3. Prolonged prothrombin time (PT)
4. Prolonged partial thromboplastin time (PTT)
5. Prolonged bleeding time

Nursing Assessment

1. Is there a history of abnormal or excessive bleeding? Following previous surgery? Dental extraction? Tonsillectomy? Family history of bleeding tendencies?
2. What medications is the patient taking? (Many drugs impair platelet function.) Taking aspirin? (More than 250 preparations contain aspirin.)
3. Has there been occupational exposure to toxic agents? Ionizing radiation?

Nursing Interventions

1. Maintain integrity of skin.
   a. Use electric razor for shaving.
   b. Avoid intramuscular injections when possible.
   c. Handle the skin gently; try to avoid use of adhesive tape.
   d. Avoid the use of tourniquets.
   e. Rotate extremities for blood pressure measurement.
2. Promote integrity of mucous membranes.
   a. Lubricate lips.
   b. Cleanse mouth carefully (see Common Problems of Patients with Blood Disorders, p. 257).
   c. Encourage soft, bland, and nonirritating foods.
3. Monitor integrity of gastrointestinal tract.
   a. Avoid constipation by enhancing hydration and motility.
   b. Administer stool softeners to prevent rupture of blood vessels from straining.
   c. Avoid rectal instrumentation (rectal thermometers; enemas).
4. Measure blood loss.
   a. Weigh linens, bandages.
   b. Monitor the pad count/amount of saturation during menses.
   c. Measure drainage.
5. Evaluate hemoglobin and hematocrit levels.
6. Conserve the patient's strength during and after bleeding episodes.
7. See page 257 for other nursing interventions.

Vascular Purpuras

The term *purpura* refers to extravasation (escape) of blood into the skin and mucous membranes. Purpuric lesions may occur spontaneously as an isolated phenomenon or as an accompaniment of obvious disease.

Types of Purpura

1. *Petechiae*—small pinpoint hemorrhages under the skin
2. *Ecchymoses*—escape of blood into tissues; producing a large bruise
3. Petechiae and ecchymoses may occur as the result of vascular rupture, permitting the leakage of blood into the subcutaneous tissue of the mucous membranes.
4. *Symptomatic or secondary purpura*—certain types of bloodstream infections (e.g., meningococcemia and infective endocarditis) exhibit this phenomenon because of damage to the vascular walls by the infectious agent or by immune complexes.
5. Severe arterial hypertension—may cause the patient to bruise easily; Valsalva maneuver may cause petechiae.
6. *Anaphylactoid purpura*—generally regarded as an allergic disorder in which there are various skin lesions (purpuric and otherwise) and episodes of arthritis, abdominal pain, hematuria, gastrointestinal hemorrhages, and fever.
   a. Attacks last several weeks and recur for years.
   b. Steroid therapy is often effective.
7. *Familial hemorrhagic telangiectasia*—a hereditary disorder manifested by an abnormal tendency to bleed and bruise.
   a. Precise nature of defect is obscure.
   b. Condition does not respond to any proved method of treatment.
8. *Toxic purpura*—a condition observed after exposure to certain drugs and poisons
9. *Vitamin C deficiency*—a vascular purpura
10. Senile purpura
11. Rheumatic and collagen–vascular diseases—associated with *palpable purpura* caused by deposition of immune complexes in blood vessels of the skin.
12. Steroid purpura—associated with loss of capillary integrity.

Thrombocytopenia

Thrombocytopenia is a decrease in the circulating platelet count, which may result in bleeding or hemorrhage.

Altered Physiology and Causes

1. Decreased platelet production (infiltrative diseases of bone marrow, leukemia, myelosuppressive therapy, other tumors, myelofibrosis, radiation therapy, drug effect, aplastic anemia, etc.).
2. Increased platelet destruction (infection, idiopathic thrombocytopenic purpura, disseminated intravascular coagulation, drug-induced, etc.).
3. Abnormal distribution or sequestration—hypersplenism.
4. Loss of platelets from body (extracorporeal circulation, dilution due to blood loss and multiple blood transfusions).

Clinical Manifestations

When the platelet count drops below 20,000/mm.^{3}
1. Petechiae occur spontaneously.
2. Ecchymoses occur at sites of minor trauma (venipuncture, bruises).
3. Hematomas occur at sites of more significant trauma (surgical wounds).
4. Bleeding from mucosal surfaces, nose, GI, and genitourinary (GU) tracts, respiratory tract, and central nervous system may occur.
5. Menorrhagia is common.
6. Excessive bleeding after dental extractions is seen.

Management

1. Treatment of underlying cause (e.g., discontinue offending drugs, treat the leukemia, etc.)
2. Administration of steroids—may be helpful in selected patients
3. Platelet transfusions if platelet production is impaired; if excessive destruction of platelets is the problem, transfused platelets will also be destroyed and will not raise the count.
4. Hormonal control of menstrual periods is usually carried out.
5. Patient is instructed to avoid any maneuver that increases intracranial pressure when platelet count is <20,000/mm^3.
6. See Bleeding Disorders, opposite.

Idiopathic Thrombocytopenic Purpura (ITP)

The *immune thrombocytopenic purpura* are bleeding disorders due to immune destruction of platelets. Antiplatelet antibodies are produced for unknown reasons, so that the platelet life span is markedly shortened.

When no underlying condition can be found, the disorder is referred to as *idiopathic thrombocytopenic purpura* (ITP).

Clinical Manifestations

1. History of easy bruising
2. Bleeding—mild to severe (thrombocytopenia not usually accompanied by bleeding unless the platelet count falls below 20,000/mm.^{3}).
   a. Skin lesions—small red hemorrhages; do not blanch on pressure
   b. Purpuric lesions may occur in vital organ (brain)
   c. Bleeding may occur from nose, mouth, genitourinary tract

Diagnostic Evaluation

1. Platelets may be absent or only slightly decreased in number; abnormalities may be seen in platelet size or morphologic appearance.
2. Increased levels of immunoglobulins (IgG) or complement components on the platelet surface.
3. Bone marrow examination—bone marrow megakaryocytes are increased in number.

Management

(Management depends on severity of clinical situation.)
1. Corticosteroids (prednisone) given for acute bleeding; causes a decrease in the production of antibody and a decrease in the clearance of antibody-coated platelets by the spleen; also reduces capillary fragility.
2. Splenectomy, when patient does not respond to steroids—eliminates a major source of antibody production and the primary site for platelet destruction.
3. Immunosuppressive drugs (azathioprine; cyclophosphamide; vincristine)—reserved for those patients not responding to steroids and splenectomy.

Nursing Interventions

1. Keep the patient at bed rest during periods of active bleeding.
2. Support the patient receiving platelet transfusions (see p. 284)—given to patients with life-threatening hemorrhage.
3. See page 280 for nursing interventions following splenectomy.
4. See also page 258 for nursing interventions for the patient who is bleeding.

Patient Teaching

Instruct the patient as follows:
1. Employ self-monitoring for infectious complications if you are on long-term steroid therapy.
2. Avoid aspirin or aspirin-containing products.
3. Avoid potential sources of accidents; protect yourself from injury.

Bleeding Disorders Due to Coagulation Defects

Disseminated Intravascular Coagulation (DIC)

Disseminated intravascular coagulation is an acquired hemorrhagic syndrome in which there is widespread clotting in small vessels of the body, leading to consumption of the clotting factors and platelets so that bleeding and thrombosis are occurring simultaneously.

Clinical Features

1. Occurs most often as complication of an underlying disease.
   a. Overwhelming infections; bacterial and viral sepsis
   b. Obstetrical complications: abruptio placentae; eclampsia; amniotic fluid embolism; retention of dead fetus

c. Malignant diseases (lung, colon, stomach, pancreas) causes chronic DIC
d. Massive tissue injuries (burns and trauma; fractures; fat embolism)
e. Vascular and circulatory collapse; shock
f. Hemolytic transfusion reaction

2. Hemorrhagic tendency is the consequence of the acute activation of the clotting mechanism of the blood; results in intravascular consumption (or inactivation) of the plasma clotting factors
3. May lead to death as a result of hemorrhage or thrombosis or both

Clinical Manifestations

1. Unexplained bleeding or tendency to bleed—from occult internal bleeding to profuse hemorrhaging from all orifices
2. Acrocyanosis (cold, mottled fingers and toes)
3. Dyspnea, hemoptysis, crackles—from involvement of pulmonary circulation due to microcirculatory obstruction
4. Signs and symptoms of acute renal failure—from fibrin deposition in small vessels of kidneys

Diagnostic Evaluation

1. Platelet count
2. Clotting tests (prothrombin time; activated partial thromboplastin time, fibrin split products)
3. Fibrinogen level

Management of Acute DIC

1. Treatment of underlying disorder—to remove or treat pathological stimulus and correct conditions that exaggerate coagulopathy (disorder of coagulation), such as treatment of shock, acidosis, sepsis
2. Supportive measures (fluid replacement, oxygenation, maintenance of blood pressure and renal perfusion)—to restore circulatory volume and deliver oxygen to ischemic tissues
3. Replacement therapy for serious hemorrhagic manifestations:
   a. Fresh frozen plasma—given to bleeding patient, pending laboratory results
   b. Platelet transfusions—for marked thrombocytopenia and continuing bleeding
   c. Cryoprecipitate—for profound hypofibrinogenemia
4. Heparin therapy (controversial)—to inhibit formation of microthrombi

Nursing Assessment

1. Be aware that all severely ill persons are at risk.
2. Review patient's laboratory evaluations for abnormalities.
3. Examine patient's skin and mucous membranes for evidence of bleeding.
4. Look for secondary hemorrhage from puncture sites and surgical wounds.
5. Assess for changing level of responsiveness secondary to cerebral dysfunction.
6. See Nursing Interventions, below, for other assessment parameters.

Nursing Interventions

See page 284 for nursing interventions during blood component replacement.

A. Preventing and Controlling Hemorrhage

1. Give medications orally or through intravenous lines when possible; avoid IM injections.
2. Document all attempts at venipuncture.
   a. Use small-gauge needles.
   b. Use infusion control equipment to ensure constant, accurate flow rates.
   c. Avoid excessive skin handling and tape removal.
   d. Apply pressure to IV and IM sites.
3. Check and mark skin for progression of subcutaneous bleeding.
4. Check stools, urine, and emesis for occult blood.
5. Monitor vital signs.
6. Measure blood loss; weigh bandages and linen.
7. Stay calm during episodes of bleeding; help the patient control fear.

B. Monitoring for Occult Bleeding and Thromboembolic Occlusions

1. Look for bleeding from suture line, and oozing of blood from IV sites.
2. Assess color of skin and mucosa, petechiae, cold mottled hands and feet, gingival bleeding, nose-bleeding, bleeding/jaundice of conjunctivae and sclerae, hemoptysis.
3. Monitor for vascular occlusion, which produces circulatory obstruction and organ hypoperfusion.
   a. Kidneys—monitor for urine volume and hematuria.
   b. Skin—petechiae, purpura, ecchymoses—reflect bleeding into skin.
   c. Lungs (interstitial hemorrhage)—monitor for dyspnea, respiratory distress, hemoptysis, cyanosis; auscultate for crackles.
   d. CNS (cerebral thromboemboli/dysfunction)—assess level of responsiveness, orientation, sensory and motor dysfunction, convulsions, and coma.
4. Ask about bone and joint pain; changes in vision (retinal hemorrhage).
5. Evaluate cardiopulmonary function; assess for tachypnea, orthopnea, tachycardia, palpitations, orthostatic hypotension—reflect inadequacy of tissue oxygenation and/or fall in blood volume.
6. Examine for abdominal tenderness.
7. Monitor for falling platelet count, and prolonged prothrombin time and partial thromboplastin time.

Hemophilia

Hemophilia is a hereditary coagulation disorder (see p. 1307).

Von Willebrand's Disease

Von Willebrand's disease is a common bleeding disorder inherited as an autosomal dominant trait and characterized by a decreased level of factor VIII complex and a prolonged bleeding time. There are several types and subtypes.

Clinical Manifestations

1. Mucosocutaneous bleeding—bruising, epistaxis, and gingival bleeding.
2. Prolonged bleeding from cuts; excessive bleeding following dental procedures and common surgical procedures.

Diagnostic Evaluation

1. Prolonged bleeding time
2. Low level of factor VIII
3. Tests to define type of von Willebrand's disease

Management

1. Replacement therapy with infusions of cryoprecipitate—correct the defects of von Willebrand's disease.
2. Administration of antifibrinolytic therapy in form of aminocaproic acid (Amicar) to stabilize clot formation; given prior to dental extractions and minor surgery.
3. Desmopressin (DDAVP), a synthetic analogue of vasopressin, considered alternate therapy for mild to moderate bleeding.
4. See page 258 for nursing interventions for the patient who is bleeding.

Acquired Defects in Coagulation

Acquired defects in coagulation may be associated with many conditions, including:
1. Anticoagulant administration
2. Diseases of the liver
3. Disseminated intravascular coagulation
4. Renal disease
5. Massive transfusions (dilutional clotting factor deficiency)
6. Certain antibiotics—inhibit coagulation factors

Splenectomy/Splenic Repair

Splenectomy is surgical removal of the spleen.

Potential Indications for Splenectomy

1. Bleeding from trauma/rupture of the spleen
   a. History of blunt abdominal trauma; gunshot/stab wound
   b. Left upper quadrant pain made worse by deep inspiration
   c. Abdominal rigidity, rebound tenderness, shock
2. Staging procedure for lymphomas
3. Primary hematologic problems
   a. Hypersplenism (sequestration and premature destruction of red and white blood cells and of platelets by an enlarged spleen)
   b. Autoimmune hemolytic anemia, immune thrombocytopenia and/or immune neutropenia. Spleen is the major clearance site for antibody and/or complement-coated blood cells.

Underlying Consideration

In the event of trauma, management focuses on monitoring the patient in the intensive care unit and surgical repair or partial splenectomy when possible, as the spleen has a vital role in immunologic function.

Preoperative Management

1. Coagulation studies are carried out.
   a. Vitamin K may be administered for abnormalities of prothrombin time.
   b. Transfusion of packed red cells may be administered if patient has significant anemia.

2. Assist with preoperative pulmonary physical therapy—to reduce incidence of pulmonary complications; patient may be debilitated from hematologic disease, from immunosuppressants, etc.
3. Preoperative preparation for patient with rupture of spleen:
   a. Volume replacement
   b. Evacuation of stomach with nasogastric tube to prevent aspiration.
   c. Insertion of urinary catheter to monitor adequacy of circulating blood volume and renal perfusion.
   d. Monitoring for pneumothorax and/or hemothorax; thoracotomy tube may be in place before anesthesia is started.

Postoperative Nursing Interventions

A. General Aspects of Postoperative Nursing Management—See page 56
B. Monitoring for Complications

1. Respiratory complications
   Atelectasis of left lower lobe with pneumonia; pleural effusion—operations on left upper quadrant predispose to hypoventilation and limited diaphragmatic movement.
   a. Employ aggressive chest physiotherapy and incentive spirometry.
   b. Encourage early and progressive mobilization.
2. Bleeding
   a. Measure abdominal girth for persistent or recurring hemorrhage.
   b. Prepare for surgical reexploration after ensuring coagulation defects have been corrected with transfusions of platelets (for thrombocytopenia) or fresh frozen plasma (for abnormal clotting factors).
3. Infection
   Assess for persistent fever; may indicate subphrenic abscess/hematoma.

> **NURSING ALERT:** After splenectomy there is a significant risk of developing an opportunistic infection with a potentially fatal outcome. This risk is life-long.

4. Thrombocytosis (elevation of platelets above normal) may follow a few days after elective splenectomy; platelet count usually increases progressively during first 2 weeks; this postoperative physiologic thrombocytosis may be conducive to thromboembolic complications.
   Monitor daily platelet count to detect postsplenectomy thrombocytosis.
5. Postsplenectomy fever (not always the result of infection)
6. Postoperative pancreatitis and/or fistula formation— tail of pancreas is close to splenic hilum.

Patient Education

1. Seek *immediate* health care for any febrile illness. An antimicrobial agent is usually given at the first sign of infection and may be prescribed on a long-term basis in some circumstances.
2. Be alert to fact that there is a relatively high incidence of infections in splenectomized individuals.

3. Be aware that immunization with pneumococcal vaccine may be given several weeks prior to elective splenectomy because of risk of pneumococcal infections and sepsis.

Bibliography

Books

Brain MC and Carbone PP. Current Therapy in Hematology-Oncology. 3. Philadelphia, BC Decker, 1988

Brown BA. Hematology: Principles and Procedures. Philadelphia, Lea & Febiger, 1988

Burns ER. Clinical Management of Bleeding and Thrombosis. Boston, Blackwell Scientific Publications, 1987

Colman RW et al. Hemostasis and Thrombosis. 2nd ed. Philadelphia, JB Lippincott, 1987

Dutcher JP and Wiernik PH. Handbook of Hematologic and Oncologic Emergencies. New York, Plenum, 1987

Gale RP. Leukemia Therapy. Boston, Blackwell Scientific Publications, 1986

Jandl JH. Blood. Boston, Little, Brown & Co, 1987

Larcan A, Lambert H and Gerard A. Consumption Coagulopathies. New York, Masson Publishing USA, 1987

Matthas FR. Blood Coagulation Disorders. New York, Springer-Verlag, 1987

McKenzie SB. Textbook of Hematology. Philadelphia, Lea & Febiger, 1988

Piette WW. Cutaneous T cell lymphoma, pp. 154–163. In Callen JP et al. Dermatologic Signs of Internal Disease. Philadelphia, WB Saunders, 1988

Pittiglio DH and Sacher RA. Clinical Hematology and Fundamentals of Hemostasis. Philadelphia, FA Davis, 1987

Polliack A and Catovsky D. Chronic Lymphocytic Leukemia. New York, Harwood Academic Press, 1988

Selby P and McElwain TJ (eds). Hodgkin's Disease. Boston, Blackwell Scientific Publications, 1987

Whittaker JA and Delamore IW (eds). Leukaemia. Boston, Blackwell Scientific Publications, 1987

Wiernik PH et al (eds). Neoplastic Diseases of the Blood. Vol 1 and 2. New York, Churchill Livingstone, 1985

Wintrobe MM et al. Clinical Hematology. 9th ed. Philadelphia, Lea & Febiger, 1988

Journals

Anemias

Beissner RS and Trowbridge AA. Clinical assessment of anemia. Postgrad Med 1986 Nov 1; 80(6):83–95

Beutler E. The common anemias. JAMA 1988 Apr 22–29; 259(16):2433–2437

Doney K et al. Treatment of gold-induced aplastic anaemia with immunosuppressive therapy. Br J Haematol 1988 Apr; 68(4):469–472

English EC. Anemia. J Fam Pract 1987 May; 24(5):521–527

Howe RB. Current concepts of anemia in elderly patients. Compr Ther 1987 May; 13(5):30–36

International Agranulocytosis and Aplastic Anemia Study. Incidence of aplastic anemia: The relevance of diagnostic criteria. Blood 1987 Dec; 70(6):1718–1721

International Agranulocytosis and Aplastic Anemia Study. Risks of agranulocytosis and aplastic anemia: A first report of their relation to drug use with special reference to analgesics. JAMA 1986 Oct 3; 256(13):1749–1757

Kramer MS, Lande DA and Hutchinson TA. Analgesic use, blood dyscrasias, and case-control pharmacoepidemiology. J Chronic Dis 1987; 40(12):1073–1085

Marmont AM and Bacigalupo A. Aplastic anemia: Pathogenesis and treatment. Haematologica 1988 Mar–Apr; 73(2):133–141

Marsh JCW et al. Survival after antilymphocyte globulin therapy for aplastic anemia depends on disease severity. Blood 1987 Oct; 70(4):1046–1052

Parry TE. Megaloblastic anaemia in the elderly. Baillieres Clin Haematol 1987 Jul; 1(3):487–506

Rozman C et al. Criteria for severe aplastic anaemia. Lancet 1987 Oct 24; 2(8565):955–957

Stockman JA. Iron deficiency anemia: Have we come far enough? JAMA 1987 Sep 25; 258(12):1645–1647

Strobach RS et al. The value of the physical examination in the diagnosis of anemia. Arch Intern Med 1988 Apr; 148(4):831–832

Tichelli A et al. Late haematological complications in severe aplastic anaemia. Br J Haematol 1988 Jul; 69(3):413–418

Wallerstein RO Jr. Laboratory evaluation of anemia. West J Med 1987 Apr; 146(4):443–451

Bleeding Disorders

Carr ME Jr. Disseminated intravascular coagulation: Pathogenesis, diagnosis, and therapy. J Emerg Med 1987 Jul–Aug; 5(4):311–322

Dutcher JP. Hematologic abnormalities in patients with nonhematologic malignancies. Hematol Oncol Clin North Am 1987 Jun; 1(2):281–299

Fruchtman S and Aledort LM. Disseminated intravascular coagulation. J Am Coll Cardiol 1986 Dec; 8(6 Suppl B):159B–167B

Moroose R and Hoyer LW. Von Willebrand factor and platelet function. Annu Rev Med 1986; 37:157–163

Peltier LF. Fat embolism: A perspective. Clin Orthop 1988 Jul; 232:263–270

Ruggeri ZM and Zimmerman TS. von Willebrand factor and von Willebrand disease. Blood 1987 Oct; 70(4):895–904

Zimmerman TS and Ruggeri ZM. von Willebrand disease. Hum Pathol 1987 Feb; 18(2):140–152

Leukemia

Bortin MM. Allogeneic bone marrow transplantation in leukemia patients. Curr Probl Cancer 1986 Jan; 10(1):3–52

Brusamolino E, Pagnucco G and Bernasconi C. Acute leukemia occurring in a primary neoplasia (secondary leukemia). A review on biological, epidemiological and clinical aspects. Haematologica 1986 Jan–Feb; 71(1):60–83

Conrad JK. Cerebellar toxicities associated with cystosine arabinoside: A nursing perspective. Oncol Nurs Forum 1986 Sep–Oct; 13(5):57–59

Gale RP and Hoffbrand AV (eds). Acute leukaemia. Clin Haematol 1986 Aug; 15(3):567–904 (entire volume)

Gallagher MT and Wyland NL. Leukemia: When white cells run wild. RN 1986 Nov; 49(10):33–37

Johnson LE. Chronic lymphocytic leukemia. Am Fam Physician 1988 Dec; 36(6):167–176

Kim TH et al. Immunosuppressive techniques using radiation. Am J Clin Oncol 1988 Jan; 11(3):362–367

Moeller KI and Swartzendruber EJ. Suppressing the risks of bone marrow suppression. Nursing 1987 Mar; 17(3):52–54

Yeomans AC. Rectal infections in acute leukemia. Cancer Nurs 1986 Dec; 9(6):295–300

Malignant Lymphomas/Multiple Myeloma

Bonadonna G et al. Treatment strategies for Hodgkin's disease. Semin Hematol 1988 Apr; 25(2 Suppl 2):51–57

Bookman MA, Longo DL and Young RC. Late complications of curative treatment in Hodgkin's disease. JAMA 1988 Aug 5; 260(5):680–683

Clendenning WE. Perspectives on cutaneous T-cell lymphoma. Clin Exp Dermatol 1986 Mar; 11(2):109–126

Coia LR and Hanks GE. Complications from large field intermediate dose infradiaphragmatic radiation: An analysis of the patterns of care outcome studies for Hodgkin's disease and seminoma. Int J Radiat Oncol Biol Phys 1988 Jul; 15(1):29–35

Durie BGM. The biology of multiple myeloma. Hematol Oncol 1988 Apr–Jun; 6(2):77–81

Edelson RL. Cutaneous T cell lymphoma. J Dermatol 1987 Oct; 14(5):397–410

Epinette WW. Mycosis fungoides: Cutaneous T-cell lymphoma. Indiana Med 1986 Apr; 79(4):330–335

Hagemeister FB. Prognostic factor in decision-making in the clinical management of Hodgkin's disease. Hematol Oncol 1988 Jul–Sep; 6(3): 257–269

Hancock SL et al. Intercurrent death after Hodgkin disease therapy in radiotherapy and adjuvant MOPP trials. Ann Intern Med 1988 Aug 1; 109(3): 183–189

Hoppe RT. The non-Hodgkin's lymphomas: Pathology, staging and treatment. Curr Probl Cancer 1987 Nov–Dec; 11(6):363–434

Hopper KD et al. Hodgkin disease: Clinical staging and treatment. Radiology 1988 Oct; 169(1):17–22

Jacobson DR and Zolla-Pazner S. Immunosuppression and infection in multiple myeloma. Semin Oncol 1986 Sep; 13(3):282–290

Kilmo P and Connors JM. An update on the Vancouver experience in the management of advanced Hodgkin's disease treated with MOPP/ABV hybrid program. Semin Hematol 1988 Apr; 25(2 Suppl 2):34–40

Mundy GR and Bertolini DR. Bone destruction and hypercalcemia in plasma cell myeloma. Semin Oncol 1986 Sep; 13(3):289

Osserman EF, Merlini G and Bulter VP Jr. Multiple myeloma and related plasma cell dyscrasias. JAMA 1987 Nov 27; 258(2):2930–2937

Sporn JR and McIntyre OR. Chemotherapy of previously untreated multiple myeloma patients: An analysis of recent treatment results. Semin Oncol 1986 Sep; 13(3):318–325

van der Velden JW et al. Subsequent development of acute non-lymphocytic leukemia in patients treated for Hodgkin's disease. Int J Cancer 1988 Aug 15; 42(2):252–255

Willcox E. You're all right, Jack. Nurs Times 1988 Jul 20–26; 84(29):28–31

Polycythemia

Denman ST. A review of pruritus. J Am Acad Dermatol 1986 Mar; 14(3):375–392

Grotta JC et al. Red blood cell disorders and stroke. Stroke 1986 Sep–Oct; 17(5):811–817

Splenectomy

Kafidi KT and Rotschafer JC. Bacterial vaccines for splenectomized patients. Drug Intell Clin Pharm 1988 Mar; 22(3):192–197

Shatney Cl H. Complications of splenectomy. Acta Anaesthesiol Belg 1987; 38(4):333–339

Transfusion Therapy

Principles of Blood Compatibility

Because of the potentially life-threatening sequelae that may result from an incompatible transfusion, it is critical that the transfusionist have a clear understanding of basic immunohematology principles.

Antigens and Antibodies

A. Antigens

1. The surface membrane of the human red cell displays extensive *polymorphism,* or variability in expression. One of these polymorphic characteristics is the presence or absence of glycoproteins known as *antigens.*
   a. More than 400 different antigens have been identified on the red cell membrane.
   b. The clinically significant antigens number less than a dozen and, of these, only two antigenic systems, the ABO and the Rh systems, require routine prospective matching prior to the transfusion.
2. The ABO blood group system is the most important because the A and B antigens produce the strongest immune response.
   a. Antigens inherited from the parents determine blood group.
   b. An individual missing both A and B antigens is classified as group O.
   c. Antibody directed against the missing antigen(s) will be produced by the age of 3 months in neonates.
   d. Antibody formation in the absence of specific exposure is unique to the ABO system.

B. Antibodies

Antibodies are proteins that float freely in the plasma. They have a high degree of *specificity,* that is, they react only with the antigen that stimulated their production. They vary in size and molecular weight.

1. Anti-A and anti-B are large IgM molecules, which explains the potency of these two "naturally occurring" antibodies. Should anti-A or anti-B combine with A or B antigen on the red cell membrane surface, agglutination of red cells will occur.
2. These antibody–red cell complexes are capable of activating the complement cascade, resulting in massive and immediate intravascular hemolysis.
3. Alternatively, antibody-coated red cells may simply be trapped in the reticuloendothelial system and be removed from the circulation by the spleen.

C. Other Red Cell Antigens

Non-ABO red cell antigen–antibody reactions usually do not produce powerful immediate hemolytic reactions, but several do have clinical significance.

1. The second most immunogenic antigen is D, which is part of the Rhesus system (C,c,E,e,D,d).
2. D (Rh) negative individuals do not develop anti-D in the absence of specific exposure, but there is a high incidence of antibody development (alloimmunization) following exposure.
3. Two common methods of sensitization to red cell antigens are transfusion and fetomaternal hemorrhage during pregnancy.
4. Anti-D can complicate future transfusions and pregnancies and exposure should be avoided or treated with Rh immune globulin, which will prevent anti-D formation.
5. Exposure to red cell antigens from other antigenic systems (Kell, Kidd, Duffy) also can cause alloimmunization. These antibodies may or may not prove to be clinically significant, but the complex tests performed to determine specificity can result in transfusion delays.

Serologic Testing

Routine laboratory testing performed prior to transfusion requires approximately 1 hour and includes:

1. *Group and Type*—which determines the patient's ABO group and Rh type,
2. *Direct Coombs' test*—which detects the presence of antibody attached to the patient's red blood cells,
3. *Compatibility test*—(crossmatch) performed to detect agglutination of donor red cells caused by antibodies in the patient's serum,
4. *Indirect Coombs'*—which enhances crossmatch testing by identifying the presence of lower molecular weight antibodies (IgG) directed against blood group antigens.

Blood Transfusion Options

In recent years, the safety of blood transfusion has become a major public concern. In response to this concern, various transfusion options may be offered to patients. These options include:

1. *Homologous transfusion*—the standard transfusion, in which random donors are used for transfusion to other

individuals. Such units are labeled "Volunteer Donor" units.

2. *Autologous transfusion*—blood products donated by the patient for his own use.

Autologous red cells can also be salvaged during surgery or following trauma-induced hemorrhage by use of automated "cell saver" devices or manual suction equipment.

a. Autologous blood products must be clearly identified with "Autologous Blood" labels. If the signature of the donor appears on the label, ask the recipient to confirm the signature prior to transfusion.

b. Autologous transfusion eliminates the risks of alloimmunization, immune-mediated transfusion reactions, and transmission of viral diseases, making it by far the safest transfusion choice.

The nurse should encourage suitable candidates to consider this underutilized option.

3. *Directed transfusion*—blood products donated by an individual for transfusion to a *specified* recipient.

While there may be some medical indications for directed donation (a parent providing sole transfusion support for a child), in general there are no scientific data to confirm that directed donation decreases transfusion risks.

Whole Blood and Blood Components

General Considerations

1. A unit of whole blood is usually separated into its various component parts a short time after collection.
2. Less than 3% of the blood collected nationwide is transfused as whole blood.
3. The use of blood components conserves the limited supply of blood, provides optimal therapeutic benefit, and reduces the risk of circulatory overload.

Whole Blood

A. Composition

1. Consists of red blood cells, plasma, plasma proteins, and 63 ml. of anticoagulant/preservative solution.
2. Total volume is approximately 500 ml.

B. Indications

1. Transfusions are called for in the following circumstances
   a. When acute, massive blood loss occurs, requiring the oxygen-carrying properties of red cells as well as the volume expansion provided by plasma.
   b. When acute loss occurs of as much as one third of a patient's total blood volume (1000–1200 ml.)—can usually be safely replaced with crystalloid and/or colloid solutions.
2. The average adult dose is determined by the clinical situation.

C. Nursing Interventions

1. Gather necessary equipment (19 gauge needle, Y-type blood infusion set with 170-micron filter, 0.9% sodium chloride) and obtain adequate venous access.
2. For rapid infusion of large volumes of whole blood, include following equipment and precautions:
   a. *A small pore filter*—to remove microaggregates (platelets, white cells), which have been identified in the lungs of massively transfused patients. A

20–40-micron filter is recommended. Follow manufacturer's instructions for use.

b. *A blood warmer*—may be indicated to prevent hypothermia and cardiac dysrhythmias associated with the rapid infusion of refrigerated solutions.
   (1) Confirm that the warming apparatus has been tested and approved for blood products.
   (2) Blood warmers must have an audible alarm to warn of overheating (>39°C).

c. *Electromechanical infusion devices*—to deliver blood at high flow rates. These devices can hemolyze red blood cells and must be used with caution.
   • Check with the blood bank or the manufacturer to confirm that the device has been tested and approved for delivery of blood products.

3. Confirm ABO and Rh compatibility (Chart 13-1) and patient identity prior to administration.
4. Observe closely for the most common acute complication associated with whole blood transfusion—circulatory overload (rise in venous pressure, distended neck veins, dyspnea, cough, crackles at base of lungs).

Packed Red Blood Cells

A. Composition

Red blood cells (80%), plasma (20%) in a total volume of 250–350 ml./unit.

B. Indications and Adult Dose

1. Restoration or maintenance of adequate organ oxygenation with minimal expansion of blood volume.
2. Average adult dose is 2 units.

C. Nursing Interventions

1. Gather necessary equipment (19 gauge needle, blood infusion set with 170-micron filter, 0.9% sodium chloride) and obtain adequate venous access.
   a. Packed red cells may be viscous and require dilution with 0.9% sodium chloride solution.
   b. A Y-type administration set is recommended to facilitate the addition of saline.
2. Confirm ABO and Rh compatibility (Chart 13-1) and patient identity prior to administration.
3. Infuse at the rate prescribed by the physician.
   a. Usually, one unit is given over 2–3 hours.
   b. To reduce the risk of bacterial sepsis, do not exceed 4 hours per unit.

Platelet Concentrates

A. Composition

There are three basic types of platelet concentrates. Selection is based on clinical indications and availability.

1. *Single Unit Platelets*
   a. A minimum of 5.5×10^{10} (1 unit) platelets in 50–70 ml. of plasma.
   b. Obtained by separating platelet-rich plasma from one unit of fresh whole blood.
   c. *Indication:* To prevent or resolve hemorrhage in patients with thrombocytopenia or platelet dysfunction.

2. *Apheresis (Single Donor) Platelets*
   a. A minimum of 3.0×10^{11} platelets (6 units) in 200–400 ml. of plasma collected from a single donor, usually by automated cell separation techniques.
   b. *Indication:* To decrease the number of donor ex-

ABO & Rh Compatibility Chart

Whole Blood

Recipient	A	B	0	AB	Rh Positive	Rh Negative
					Donor	
A	●					
B		●				
O			●			
AB				●		
Rh Positive					●	●
Rh Negative						●

Red Blood Cells

Recipient	A	B	O	AB	Rh Positive	Rh Negative
					Donor	
A	●		●			
B		●	●			
O			●			
AB	●	●	●	●		
Rh Positive					●	●
Rh Negative						●

Plasma

Recipient	A	B	O	AB	Rh Positive	Rh Negative
					Donor	
A	●			●		
B		●		●		
O	●	●	●	●		
AB				●		
Rh Positive					●	●
Rh Negative					●	●

Chart 13-1. *The chart above identifies ABO and Rh compatibility when transfusing whole blood, red blood cells, and plasma. Components suspended in plasma, such as platelets and cryoprecipitate, usually follow plasma compatibility rules if the total volume exceeds 120 ml. for an adult patient.*

posures, which may reduce the risks of transfusion transmitted disease and HLA alloimmunization (formation of antibodies).

3. *HLA-Matched Platelets*
   a. Apheresis-derived platelets that have been collected from a donor with the same human leukocyte antigen (HLA) type as the recipient.
   b. *Indication:* HLA-matched platelets are indicated only if HLA antibodies are the primary cause of platelet destruction. A suboptimal increase or no increase at all in the peripheral platelet count 1 hour after transfusion may indicate the presence of HLA antibodies.

Note: Patients undergoing immunosuppressive treatment usually require intensive platelet therapy. HLA typing should be performed prior to the onset of leukopenia in the event that matched platelets are later required.

B. Dose

1. The adult platelet dose is based on the clinical situation and agency policy.
2. The recommended prophylactic dose for a nonbleeding, thrombocytopenic adult is 1 unit/10 kg. of body weight.
3. Surgical patients or those with active bleeding may require 8–10 additional units.

C. Nursing Interventions

1. Gather necessary equipment (19 gauge needle, component infusion set with 170-micron filter, 0.9% sodium chloride) and obtain adequate venous access.
2. Confirm plasma ABO and Rh compatibility (Chart 13-1) and patient identity prior to administration. Platelets contain few red blood cells and do not require ABO crossmatching.
3. Set flow at the prescribed rate, usually to complete infusion within 30–60 minutes.
   a. Sometimes platelets are suspended in a large volume of plasma (200–400 ml.).
   b. The volume may be reduced in the blood bank if fluid intake is restricted because of weight or clinical status.

Cryoprecipitate

A. Composition

1. Each unit contains approximately 80–120 units of factor VIII (antihemophilic and von Willebrand's factors), 250 mg. of fibrinogen, and 20%–30% of the factor XIII present in a unit of whole blood.
2. These proteins are suspended in 10–20 ml. of plasma.

B. Indications and Adult Dose

1. To correct deficiencies of factor VIII (i.e., hemophilia A and von Willebrand's disease), factor XIII, and fibrinogen.
2. The adult dose is 10 units, which may be repeated every 8–12 hours until the deficiency is corrected or the need to correct hemostasis is resolved.

C. Nursing Interventions

1. Gather necessary equipment (19–21 gauge needle, component infusion set with 170-micron filter, 0.9% sodium chloride) and obtain adequate venous access.
2. Confirm patient identity prior to administration. Because of the small plasma volume, ABO compatibility is preferred, but not required.
3. Allow 30–60 minutes for thawing and pooling. Cryoprecipitate must be transfused within 4 hours of the time it is prepared.
4. Infuse over 15–30 minutes.

Granulocyte Concentrates

A. Composition

1. A minimum of 1.0×10^{10} granulocytes, variable amounts of lymphocytes (usually less than 10% of the total number of white cells), 6–10 units of platelets, 30–50 ml. of red cells, and 200–400 ml. of plasma.
2. This product is usually obtained by granulocytapheresis.

B. Indications and Dosage

1. To treat patients with acquired severe neutropenia or congenital white cell dysfunction, who have infections unresponsive to conventional antibiotic therapy.
2. The long-term therapeutic benefits of granulocyte transfusions are still questionable and continue to be evaluated.
3. An average adult receives 1 unit daily for approximately 5–10 days.

C. Nursing Interventions

1. Gather necessary equipment (19 gauge needle, standard Y-type blood infusion set with 170-micron filter, 0.9% sodium chloride) and obtain adequate venous access.
2. Transfuse granulocytes as soon as possible. White blood cells have a short survival time, and therapeutic benefit is directly related to dose and viability.
3. Confirm ABO compatibility (See Red Blood Cells, Chart 13-1) and patient identity prior to administration. Granulocyte concentrates must be crossmatched because of the large number of red blood cells present.
4. Begin the transfusion slowly and increase to the prescribed rate if the patient exhibits no adverse symptoms. The recommended length of infusion is 1–2 hours.
5. Observe the patient closely throughout the transfusion because of the increased incidence of severe reactions, which sometimes progress to respiratory distress.
   a. Have emergency medications readily available.
   b. Premedication with an antihistamine, acetaminophen, steroids, and/or meperidine may be indicated to prevent adverse reactions.
6. DO NOT administer amphotericin B within 4 hours of granulocyte transfusion. Pulmonary insufficiency has been seen with the concurrent administration of amphotericin B and granulocytes.

Plasma

A. Composition

1. Liquid portion of the blood consisting primarily of water (91%), proteins (7%), and carbohydrate (2%).
2. One unit is the amount removed from a single unit of whole blood (200–250 ml.).

B. Methods for Preparing

There are two common methods of plasma preparation. Selection is based on the clinical situation and availability.
1. *Fresh Frozen Plasma (FFP)*
   a. Frozen within 6 hours of collection to preserve all clotting factors.
   b. Indications: To treat blood clotting disorders related to liver disease, DIC, over coagulation with warfarin (Coumadin), all congenital factor deficiencies, and dilutional coagulopathy resulting from massive blood replacement.
2. *Liquid Plasma*
   a. Stored in a liquid state, which results in the loss of labile clotting factors V and VIII.
   b. Indications: Same as above EXCEPT for the treatment of factor V and VIII deficiencies.

C. Dosage

Dosage will be determined by the clinical situation and assessment of the prothrombin time (PT), partial thromboplastin time (PTT), or specific factor assays.

D. Nursing Interventions

1. Gather necessary equipment (19–21 gauge needle, component infusion set with 170-micron filter, 0.9% sodium chloride) and obtain adequate venous access.
2. Confirm ABO compatibility (Chart 13-1) and patient identity. A crossmatch is not required because of minimal red blood cell content.

Fractionated Plasma Products

A. Composition

1. Highly concentrated plasma protein products, which are commercially prepared by pooling thousands of single plasma units and extracting the desired protein.
2. Most techniques include heat or chemical treatment, which eliminates the risk of transmitting blood-borne viruses (hepatitis and HIV).

B. Types

1. *Colloid Solutions*—Volume expanders, consisting of albumin, globulin, and other proteins. Two types of expanders are albumin and plasma protein fraction.
   a. Albumin is available as a 5% solution, which is oncotically equivalent to plasma and a concentrated 25% solution.
   b. Plasma protein fraction (PPF) is available only in a 5% solution. Hypotension has been associated with the rapid infusion of PPF.
   c. Colloids provide volume expansion in situations where crystalloid solutions are not adequate, such as therapeutic plasma exchange, shock, and massive hemorrhage.
      (1) Also used for the treatment of acute liver failure, burns, and hemolytic disease of the newborn.
      (2) Albumin and PPF are pasteurized and carry no risk of viral disease.
2. *Immune Serum Globulin (ISG)*—Concentrated aqueous solution of gamma globulin containing high titers of antibody. Can only be administered by intramuscular injection.
   a. *Nonspecific ISG* is prepared from random donor plasma and is used to increase gammaglobulin levels and enhance general immune response.
   b. *Specific ISG* is prepared from donors who have high antibody titers to known antigens. Hepatitis B immune globulin and Rh immune globulin are examples of specific immune globulins.
   c. Immune serum globulins carry no risk of hepatitis B or HIV.
3. *Intravenous Immune Gamma Globulin (IVIgG)*—Aqueous solution of immunoglobulins that is much more concentrated and is given in much larger volumes than ISG.
   a. Used as chronic replacement therapy in patients with congenital or acquired immunodeficiency syndromes.
   b. Also used in acute autoimmune disorders such as ITP (immune thrombocytopenic purpura).
   c. Intravenous gamma globulin solutions do not appear to transmit HIV, but have been reported to transmit non-A, non-B hepatitis.

4. *Factor VIII Concentrate*—Lyophilized concentrate containing large quantities of factor VIII used to treat moderate to severe congenital factor VIII deficiency (hemophilia A).
5. *Factor IX Concentrate*—Lyophilized concentrate containing large quantities of factor IX used to treat factor IX deficiency (Christmas disease).

Concentrated clotting factors are heat treated and carry minimal risk of viral disease.

C. Dosage

The recommended dosage of fractionated products is usually based on body weight and the clinical situation.

D. Nursing Interventions

1. Read the product insert and label to determine the method and rate of administration and potential complications.
2. As a result of extensive purification during fractionation, no additional testing or processing is required prior to administration. In many institutions, fractionated products are distributed by the pharmacy department, not the blood bank.

Modified Blood Products

To reduce the risk of specific transfusion complications, blood products may require further processing. Two common modified products are described below.

Leukocyte-Poor Blood Products

1. Are packed red cells and platelets with the majority of the leukocytes removed in an attempt to prevent reoccurrence of febrile, nonhemolytic transfusion reactions.

2. Leukocytes can be removed from packed cells using three standard techniques: filtration, washing, or freezing.
3. Leukocyte-poor platelets can be prepared by centrifugation, filtration, or washing.

A. Filtration—is a routine procedure required for all blood products.

1. The pore size of a standard blood administration set filter is 170 microns, which effectively removes gross fibrin clots.
2. Microaggregate filters remove microscopic aggregates of fibrin, platelets, and leukocytes, which accumulate in blood units during storage.
   a. Microaggregate filters are recommended for use during rapid, massive transfusion of whole blood or packed red cells to prevent pulmonary complications.
   b. They are also marginally effective in the removal of leukocytes to prevent febrile reactions.
3. Third-generation filters are available that remove virtually all leukocytes (Fig. 13-1).
4. Special leukocyte-depletion filters have also been developed for platelet concentrates (Fig. 13-1). These filters remove 80%–95% of the leukocytes and retain 80% of the platelets.
5. A product may be filtered prior to blood release and labeled "Leukocyte Poor." More commonly, the filter is issued with the product and must be attached to the standard infusion set at the bedside per manufacturer's or blood bank directives.

B. Washing

1. Washing red blood cells or platelets with a normal saline solution removes 80%–95% of the white blood cells and virtually all of the plasma.
2. Washing requires an additional hour of processing time, and the shelf life of the product is reduced to 24 hours.

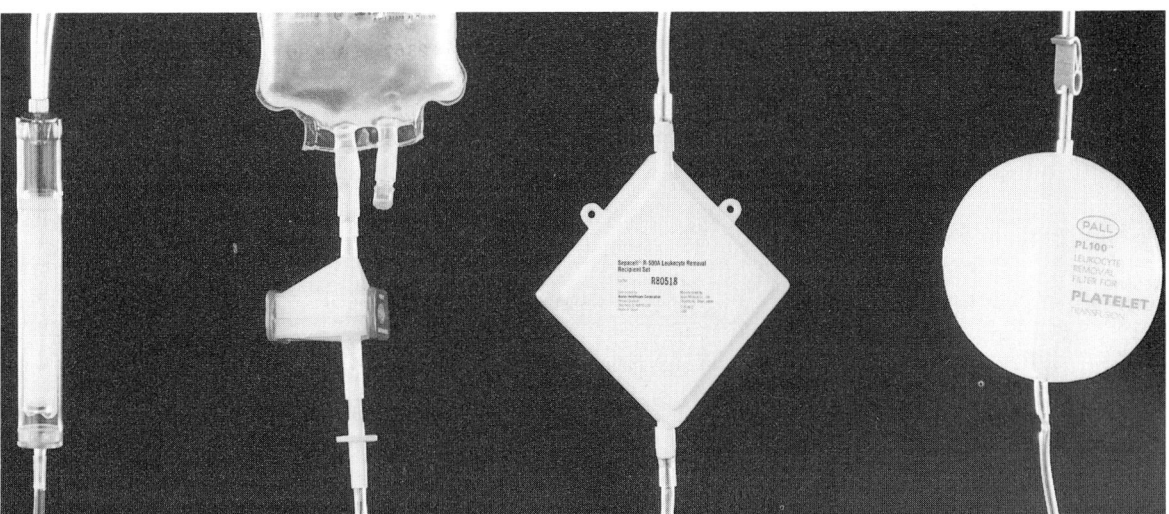

Figure 13-1. *Filters that effectively remove aggregates and white cells and are easy to use at the bedside are available from numerous manufacturers. Examples are (left to right): standard 170 micron filter (Baxter–Travenol Corp.); 40 micron microaggregate filter (Pall Biomedical Products); leukocyte-depleting filter (Baxter–Travenol Corp.); and platelet leukocyte-depleting filter (Pall Biomedical Products).*

C. Freezing

1. Freezing of red blood cells can be performed within 7 days of blood collection.
2. Red cells remain viable in the frozen state for 7–10 years.
3. Removal of the hypertonic freezing preservative (glycerol) prior to transfusion eliminates all plasma and 99% of the white blood cells.
4. This process extends preparation time by 90 minutes and reduces post-thaw shelf life to 24 hours.

Note: Freezing is also an effective means of storing rare blood types. In recent years, frozen red cell banks have gained popularity for long-term storage of autologous red cells.

Irradiated Blood Products

1. Consist of blood products that are exposed to a measured amount of ionizing radiation, which abolishes the mitotic capacity of the lymphocytes in the unit, but does not damage the red cells, platelets, or granulocytes.
2. Such treatment eliminates the ability of passenger lymphocytes to engraft and proliferate in the transfusion recipient, and thus prevents the possibility of transfusion-induced graft-versus-host reactions.
3. Patients at risk for post-transfusion graft-versus-host reactions include bone marrow transplant recipients, premature neonates, and patients with congenital immune deficiency syndromes, Hodgkin's disease, and non-Hodgkin's lymphoma.
4. Strong consideration should be given to irradiating all cellular blood products (red cells, whole blood, platelets, and granulocytes) given to such patients.

Transfusion Reactions

Every transfusion of blood or blood components can result in an adverse reaction. Reactions can be placed into two general categories: acute and delayed.

Acute Reactions

1. *Acute reactions* occur within minutes to hours after the blood product has been infused.
2. Acute reactions include allergic, febrile (nonhemolytic), septic, hemolytic, and circulatory overload.
3. Because reactions exhibit similar clinical manifestations, every symptom is considered potentially serious and the transfusion discontinued until the cause is determined.
4. When a reaction is suspected, blood bags with tubing from all products transfused within 4 hours are returned to the blood bank for evaluation. The following samples should be obtained if an acute reaction is suspected:
   a. A clotted blood sample is needed to examine serum for hemoglobin and confirm red cell group and type.
   b. An anticoagulated blood sample is used for a direct Coombs' test, to determine the presence of antibody on the red blood cells.
   c. A fresh urine sample is tested for hemoglobinuria.
5. Precautions must be taken to avoid the hemolysis of red cells during venipuncture and sample collection, as this could result in invalid testing. Whenever possible, blood samples should be drawn from a fresh venipuncture and not from existing needles or catheters.
6. If the only symptoms are those resulting from a mild allergic reaction (urticaria), extensive evaluation is not required. In the event of a severe reaction, more testing may be necessary.
7. See Table 13-1 for causes, clinical manifestations, management, and prevention of acute reactions.

Delayed Reactions

1. *Delayed reactions* occur days to years after the transfusion and include delayed hemolytic reactions, iron overload (hemosiderosis), graft-versus-host disease, and infectious diseases (hepatitis B, hepatitis C, cytomegalovirus, Epstein–Barr virus, malaria, and AIDS).
2. The symptoms of a delayed reaction vary from mild to very severe. Diagnosis can be complicated by the long incubation period between transfusion and symptoms and the complexity of diagnostic tests.
3. See Table 13-2 for causes, clinical manifestations, management, and prevention of delayed reactions.

Protection Measures Alert

The Centers for Disease Control requires health care workers to consider the body fluids of all patients potentially contaminated with communicable bloodborne organisms.
1. Reasonable precautions must be taken to reduce the risk of occupational accidents.

(Text continues on p. 290)

Table 13-1. *Acute Reactions to Blood Transfusion*

Acute Reaction	Cause	Clinical Manifestations	Management	Prevention
Allergic	Sensitivity to plasma protein or donor antibody, which reacts with recipient antigen	1. Flushing 2. Itching, rash 3. Urticaria, hives 4. Asthmatic wheezing 5. Laryngeal edema 6. Anaphylaxis	1. Stop transfusion immediately. Keep vein open (KVO) with normal saline. 2. Give antihistamine as directed (diphenhydramine). 3. Observe for anaphylaxis—prepare epinephrine if respiratory distress is severe. 4. If hives are the only clinical manifestation, the transfusion can sometimes continue at a slower rate.	Prior to transfusion, ask patient about past reactions. If patient has history of anaphylaxis, alert physician, have emergency drugs available, and remain at bedside for the first 30 minutes.

(continued)

Table 13-1. *Acute Reactions to Blood Transfusion (continued)*

Acute Reaction	Cause	Clinical Manifestations	Management	Prevention
Febrile, non-hemolytic	Hypersensitivity to donor white cells, platelets, or plasma proteins	1. Sudden chills and fever 2. Headache 3. Flushing 4. Anxiety	1. Stop transfusion immediately and KVO with normal saline. Notify physician and blood bank. 2. Send blood samples and blood bags to blood bank. Collect urine samples for testing. 3. Check temperature ½ hour after chill and as indicated thereafter. 4. Give antipyretics as prescribed—treat symptomatically.	Give antipyretic (acetaminophen or aspirin) before transfusion as directed. Leukocyte-poor blood products may be recommended for future transfusions.
Septic reactions	Transfusion of blood or components contaminated with bacteria	1. Rapid onset of chills 2. High fever 3. Vomiting; diarrhea 4. Marked hypotension	1. Stop transfusion immediately and KVO with normal saline. Notify physician and blood bank. 2. Obtain cultures of patient's blood and return blood bags with administration set to blood bank for culture. 3. Treat septicemia as directed—antibiotics, IV fluids, vasopressors, steroids.	Do not permit blood to stand at room temperature longer than necessary. Warm temperatures promote bacterial growth. Inspect blood for gas bubbles, clotting, or abnormal color before transfusion. Complete infusions within 4 hours. Change administration set after 4 hours of use.
Circulatory overload	Fluid administered at a rate or volume greater than the circulatory system can accommodate. Increased blood in pulmonary vessels and decreased lung compliance.	1. Rise in venous pressure 2. Distended neck veins 3. Dyspnea 4. Cough 5. Crackles at base of lungs	1. Stop transfusion and KVO with normal saline. Notify physician. 2. Place patient upright with feet in dependent position. 3. Administer prescribed diuretics, oxygen, morphine, and aminophylline.	Concentrated blood products should be given whenever possible. Transfuse at a rate within the circulatory reserve of the patient. Monitor CVP of patient with heart disease.
Hemolytic reaction	Infusion of incompatible blood products: 1. Antibodies in recipient's plasma attach to transfused red cells, hemolyzing the cells either in circulation or in the reticuloendothelial system. 2. Antibodies in donor plasma attach to recipient red cells, causing hemolysis (may result from infusion of incompatible plasma—less severe than incompatible red cells).	1. Chills; fever 2. Low back pain 3. Feeling of head fullness; flushing 4. Oppressive feeling 5. Tachycardia, tachypnea 6. Hypotension, vascular collapse 7. Hemoglobinuria, hemoglobinemia 8. Bleeding 9. Acute renal failure 10. Death	1. Stop transfusion immediately—KVO with 0.9% saline. 2. Notify physician and blood bank. 3. Treat shock, if present 4. Draw testing samples, collect urine sample. 5. Maintain BP with IV colloid solutions. Give diuretics as prescribed to maintain urine flow, glomerular filtration, and renal blood flow. 6. Insert indwelling catheter to monitor hourly urine output. Patient may require dialysis if renal failure occurs.	Meticulously verify patient identification—from sample collection to product infusion. Begin infusion slowly and observe closely for 30 minutes—consequences are in proportion to the amount of incompatible blood transfused.

Table 13-2. *Delayed Reactions to Transfusion Therapy*

Delayed Reaction	Cause	Clinical Manifestations	Management	Prevention
Delayed hemolytic reaction	The destruction of transfused red cells by antibody not detectable during crossmatch, but formed rapidly after transfusion. Rapid production may occur because of antigen exposure during previous transfusions or pregnancy.	1. Fever 2. Mild jaundice 3. Decreased hematocrit	Generally, no acute treatment is required, but hemolysis may be severe enough to cause shock and renal failure. If this occurs, manage as outlined under acute hemolytic reactions.	The crossmatch blood sample should be drawn within 3 days of blood transfusion. Antibody formation may occur within 90 days of transfusion and/or pregnancy.

(continued)

Table 13-2. *Delayed Reactions to Transfusion Therapy (continued)*

Delayed Reaction	Cause	Clinical Manifestations	Management	Prevention
Iron overload (hemosiderosis)	Deposition of iron in the heart, endocrine organs, liver, spleen, skin, and other major organs as a result of multiple, long-term transfusions (aplastic anemia, thalassemia).	1. Diabetes 2. Decreased thyroid function 3. Dysrhythmias 4. Congestive heart failure and other symptoms related to major organ failure	1. Treat symptomatically. 2. Deferoxamine (Desferal), which chelates and removes accumulated iron through the kidneys, may be administered IV, IM, or subcutaneously.	
Graft-versus-host disease	Engraftment of lymphocytes in the bone marrow of immunosuppressed patients setting up an immune response of the graft against the host.	(See p. 294)	(See p. 294)	Transfuse with irradiated blood products.
Infectious disease 1. Hepatitis B	Hepatitis B virus transmitted from blood donor to recipient via infected blood products.	1. Elevated liver enzymes (SGPT and SGOT) 2. Anorexia, malaise 3. Nausea and vomiting 4. Fever 5. Dark urine 6. Jaundice	Usually resolves spontaneously within 4–6 weeks. Can result in permanent liver damage. Treat symptomatically.	1. Screen blood donors, temporarily rejecting those who may have had contact with the virus. Those with a history of hepatitis after age 11 are permanently deferred. 2. Pretest all blood products (EIA).
2. Hepatitis C (formerly Non-A, Non-B hepatitis)	Hepatitis C virus transmitted from blood donor to recipient via infected blood products.	Similar to serum B hepatitis, but symptoms are usually less severe. Chronic liver disease and cirrhosis may develop.	Symptoms usually mild and require no treatment.	Pretest all blood donors (ALT, anti-HBc antibody, anti-hepatitis C antibody).
3. Epstein–Barr virus, cytomegalovirus, malaria	Transmitted through infected blood products.			Question prospective blood donors regarding colds, flu, foreign travel.
4. Acquired immunodeficiency syndrome	HIV virus transmitted from blood donor to recipient via infected blood products.	1. Night sweats 2. Unexplained weight loss 3. Lymphadenopathy 4. Pneumocystis pneumonia 5. Kaposi's sarcoma 6. Diarrhea	AZT may delay onset of AIDS symptoms. Active disease is treated symptomatically	Test each donor for HIV antibody. Reject prospective high-risk donors: 1. Males who have had sex with another male since 1977 2. Users of self-injected IV drugs 3. Male or female partners of prostitutes. 4. Hemophiliacs or their sexual partners 5. Sexual partners of those with AIDS 6. Immigrants from Haiti or sub-Saharan Africa
5. HTLV-I-associated myelopathy and tropical spastic paraparesis (HAM/TSP) Adult T-cell leukemia	Human T-lymphotropic virus type I (HTLV-I) transmitted from blood donor to recipient via blood products.	Signs of neuromuscular disease Signs of T-cell leukemia	HTLV-I–infected individuals have a low risk of developing disease (3%–5%). Incubation period 10–20 years. Should disease occur, treat symptomatically.	Screen all prospective blood donors for anti-HTLV-I antibody.
6. Syphilis	Spirochetemia caused by *Treponema pallidum.* Incubation 4–18 weeks	1. Presence of chancre 2. Regional lymphadenopathy 3. Generalized rash	Penicillin therapy	Test bood prior to transfusion (rapid plasma reagin—RPR). Organism will not remain viable in blood stored 24–48 hours at 4°C.

2. Gloves should be worn when performing venipunctures and all other procedures that may result in employee exposure to blood or body fluids.
3. Universal Precautions also call for the use of additional protective equipment (gowns, masks, goggles) in situations with potential for a large spill or body fluid spraying under pressure.
4. Contaminated areas should be cleaned with a 1:10 solution of sodium hypochlorite (bleach), which effectively destroys viruses and other organisms.

Guidelines Administering Blood/Blood Components

Purpose
1. To increase the amount of oxygen being delivered to the tissues and organs
2. To prevent or stop bleeding due to platelet defects or deficiencies or coagulation abnormalities
3. To combat infection due to decreased or defective white cells or antibodies

Equipment
Tourniquet
Iodine-containing skin antiseptic
Needle or venous catheter
Blood or component administration set
Normal saline
Blood product as described

Procedure

Nursing Action	Rationale/Amplification

Preparatory Phase

Nursing Action	Rationale/Amplification
1. Inform the patient of the procedure, blood product to be given, approximate length of time, and desired outcome of transfusion.	1. Instruct the patient to report unusual symptoms immediately.
2. Obtain and record baseline vital signs.	2. If the patient's clinical status permits, delay transfusion if baseline temperature is greater than 38.5°C.
3. Prepare infusion site. Select a large vein that allows patient some degree of mobility. Start the prescribed intravenous infusion.	3. Antecubital veins are not recommended for lengthy infusions. Prolonged restriction of arm movement is uncomfortable and inconvenient for the patient.
	In the event of an acute reaction, the intravenous catheter should be maintained with normal saline.

NURSING ALERT: Crystalloid solutions other than 0.9% saline and all medications are incompatible with blood products. They may cause agglutination and/or hemolysis.

Nursing Action	Rationale/Amplification
4. Obtain blood product from blood bank. Inspect for abnormal color, cloudiness, clots, and excess air. Read instructions on the product label regarding storage and infusion. Check expiration date.	4. Platelets are normally cloudy.
	If the transfusion cannot begin immediately, return product to blood bank. Blood out of proper storage for more than 30 minutes (above 10°C [50°F]) cannot be reissued. Never store blood in unauthorized refrigerators, such as those on the nursing unit.
5. Verify patient identification (Fig. 13-2).	5. The majority of acute fatal transfusion reactions are caused by clerical errors. Patient and product verification is the single most important function of the nurse. It is strongly recommended that two qualified individuals perform this task. Do not proceed with the transfusion if there is any discrepancy. Contact the blood bank immediately.
a. Ask the patient to state his full name and compare with name on the wrist band. If the patient is unable to state his name, verify identity with an individual familiar with the patient.	
b. Compare the name and ID number on the wristband with the bag tag, transfusion form, and medical order.	
c. Confirm ABO and Rh compatibility by comparing the bag label, bag tag, medical record, and/or transfusion form.	
d. Check bag labels for expiration date and satisfactory serologic testing.	

Performance Phase

Nursing Action	Rationale/Amplification
1. Start infusion slowly (i.e., 2 ml./minute). Remain at bedside 15–30 minutes. If there are no signs of an adverse reaction, increase flow to the prescribed rate.	1. Institutional policy may vary regarding flow rates and patient monitoring. Consult the Standard Operating Procedure manual for specific instructions.
	Signs of a severe transfusion reaction (i.e., acute hemolytic, anaphylactic) are usually manifested during infusion of the initial 50–100 ml.
2. Observe the patient closely and check vital signs at least hourly until 1 hour post-transfusion. Report signs and symptoms of adverse reaction to physician immediately.	2. Acute reactions may occur at any time during the transfusion.
3. Record the following information on the patient's chart:	3. Facts relating to the transfusion should be charted exactly.
a. Time and names of persons starting and ending the transfusion	

(continued)

Guidelines Administering Blood/Blood Components *(continued)*		
Procedure *(continued)*	**Nursing Action**	**Rationale/Amplification**

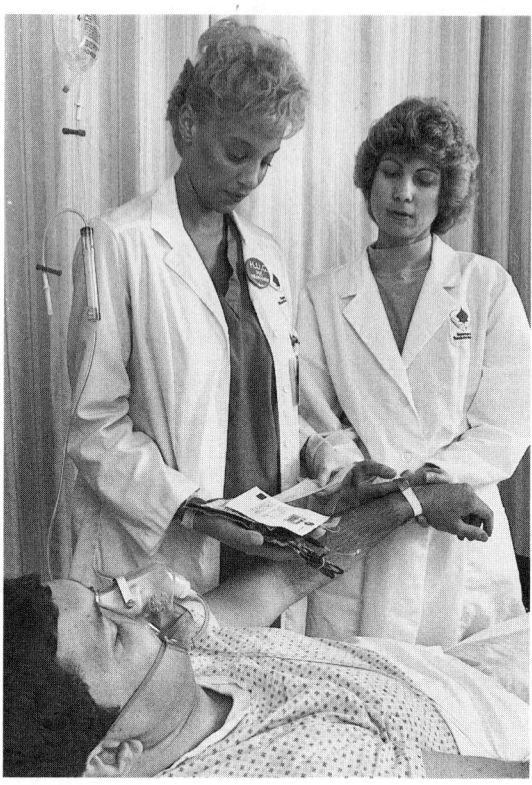

Figure 13-2. *The most important responsibility of the nurse is to confirm that the blood is given to the correct patient. Like other potentially lethal drugs, blood should be checked by two qualified individuals prior to administration.*

	b. Names of individuals verifying patient ID	
	c. Unique product identification number	c. It must be possible to trace each transfusion product to the original blood donor.
	d. Product and volume infused	
	e. Immediate response—for example, "no apparent reaction"	

Bone Marrow Transplantation

In the last 25 years, bone marrow transplantation (BMT) has progressed from a treatment of last resort to a viable therapeutic modality for a variety of malignant and non-malignant disorders. While the basic procedures involved in bone marrow transplant are well established, many of the medications given and techniques employed are still investigational. Recent scientific advances in marrow processing and supportive therapy have broadened BMT's potential uses and decreased morbidity and mortality.

Indications

Bone marrow transplant may be considered the treatment of choice in the following situations:

1. Aplastic anemia
2. Immunodeficiency disorders such as severe combined immunodeficiency disease (SCID) and Wiskott–Aldrich syndrome
3. Malignant disorders, specifically leukemia (certain types of acute, chronic, and preleukemic states), lymphoma, multiple myeloma, neuroblastoma, and selected solid tumors (metastatic breast cancer, small-

cell lung cancer, advanced ovarian cancer, poor-risk germ cell tumors)
4. Nonmalignant hematologic disorders such as Fanconi's anemia, thalassemia, and sickle cell anemia

Bone Marrow Harvesting

A. Bone Marrow Sources

There are three sources of donor bone marrow: autologous, syngeneic, and allogeneic. The disease being treated and compatibility are the deciding factors.

1. *Autologous marrow*—removed from the intended recipient, usually during the remission phase, for long-term storage in anticipation of later use.
   a. Autologous bone marrow may be harvested as a preventive measure in diseases having a high incidence of relapse.
   b. This will allow high-dose, cytotoxic therapy to be given, which may effectively destroy persistent tumor cells resistant to standard treatment.
   c. While autologous marrow eliminates the risk of adverse immunologic responses such as graft-versus-host disease (GVHD) and graft rejection, relapse following autologous bone marrow transplant is a frequent occurrence. This may be due to malignant cells contaminating the harvested bone marrow.
   d. Techniques to purge residual tumor cells from the marrow (i.e., chemotherapy, monoclonal antibodies) are currently under investigation.
2. *Syngeneic marrow*—obtained from an identical twin.
   a. While syngeneic marrow is a perfect histocompatible match, which eliminates the risks of marrow rejection and GVHD, the incidence of leukemic relapse is greater.
   b. This may be due to the absence of a graft-versus-leukemia effect.
3. *Allogeneic*—bone marrow is donated by a relative or unrelated person having an identical tissue type. This is the most common type of marrow transplant.

B. Histocompatibility Testing

Immunologic recognition of the differences in human leukocyte antigens (HLA) is the first step in host or transplant rejection.

1. *The HLA system antigens* are a complex set of protein structures found on the surface membrane of all human nucleated cells, solid tissues, and circulating blood cells, except red cells.
2. This genetically inherited mixture of antigens is considered representative of the *tissue type* of each individual.
3. While considerably more complex, determination of HLA type is similar to ABO testing:
   a. Lymphocytes are mixed with antibody directed against known HLA antigens. Lymphocytes will survive if the antigen is absent and will be inactivated if it is present. HLA-A-, -B, and -C antigens can be identified in this manner.
   b. A second test to determine compatibility of the HLA-D antigens is the mixed lymphocyte culture (MLC). Donor and recipient lymphocytes are combined in culture for several days. Survival of the cells indicates compatibility.

C. Compatibility Frequency

1. Siblings have a 1 in 4 chance of having identical sets of HLA antigens. This would provide the optimally matched preferred allogeneic bone marrow donor.
2. Because of the complexity of the HLA system, non-related persons have less than a 1 in 5000 chance of having identical HLA types. The establishment of the National Bone Marrow Donor Registry in 1987 has given hope to many patients who do not have a compatible donor. Ongoing recruitment efforts continue to enlarge the computerized list of potential HLA-typed unrelated bone marrow donors.
3. Investigational studies are also underway to purge donor marrow of T lymphocytes, which cause GVHD. This advancement would pave the way for mismatched marrow transplants. Unfortunately, removal of all T cells appears to significantly increase the rate of marrow rejection. Studies are currently aimed at determining the minimal number of T lymphocytes needed for marrow engraftment.

D. Donor Preparation

1. After confirming histocompatibility, an extensive workup is performed to assure the mental and physical well-being of the prospective donor.
   a. Histocompatibility testing
   b. Informed consent
   c. Thorough medical history and physical examination

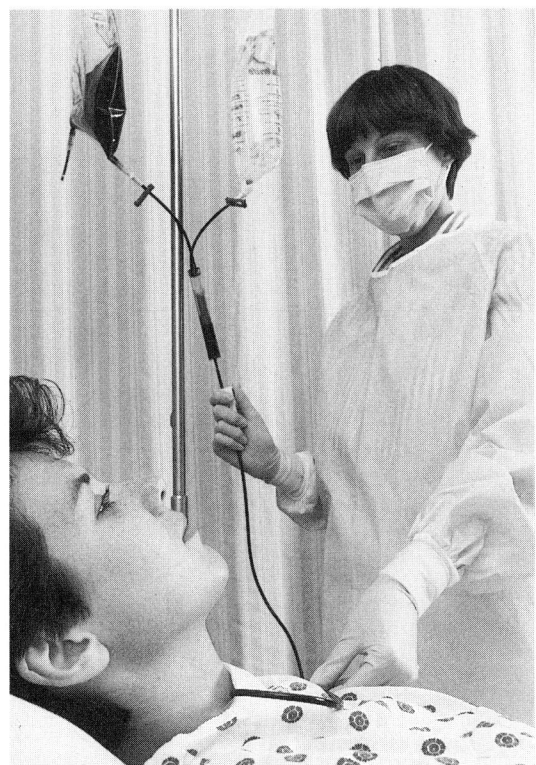

Figure 13-3. *Harvested marrow should be infused as rapidly as possible. Observe the patient closely for signs of an acute adverse reaction.*

d. Chest x-ray
e. Electrocardiogram
f. Laboratory evaluation (CBC, chemistry profile, viral testing, RPR [syphilis], ABO and Rh, coagulation studies, CMV status)
g. Psychological evaluation (may include psychiatric consult)

2. Prior to marrow harvest, an informed consent including potential donor complications must be obtained. While not usually life-threatening, the adverse affects may cause considerable pain and discomfort.
   a. Adverse affects of anesthesia
   b. Severe pain
   c. Hematoma
   d. Fever

3. Because of the significant loss of red blood cells during the harvest process, syngeneic and allogeneic donors are usually advised to give two units of autologous blood, which may be reinfused during marrow collection.

E. **Marrow Collection**

1. The donor is given general or spinal anesthesia in the operating room.

2. The marrow is obtained in 2–5-ml. aliquots from the marrow spaces of the posterior and occasionally anterior iliac crests and the sternum. Only two to three skin punctures are required, as the aspiration needle is redirected to various marrow spaces without withdrawing the needle. A total of 400–800 ml. of marrow is obtained.

3. The marrow is placed in heparinized tissue culture media and filtered to remove fat and bone particles.

4. Marrow can be infused immediately or frozen in a solution containing dimethylsulfoxide (DMSO), which preserves stem cells in the frozen state.

The Transplant

A. **Recipient Preparation**

1. The physical and psychological evaluation of the recipient is similar to that of the donor (Chart 13-1). Additional testing may be required to accurately stage existing disease.

2. The recipient must receive immunoablative therapy prior to transplant.
   a. This serves three purposes: malignant cells are destroyed, the immune system is inactivated,

Table 13-3. *Complications of Bone Marrow Transplantation*

Complication	Clinical Manifestations	Treatment/Nursing Interventions	Prevention
Infection	Fever, chills, hypotension, flushing, localized inflammation, cough, white patches in mouth, urinary frequency or burning	Broad-spectrum antibiotics until organism is identified, then more specific antibiotic. Antifungal agents for persistent fevers. Tepid sponge baths, hypothermia blankets, and acetaminophen may relieve symptoms.	"Sterilize" the alimentary tract with nonabsorbable antibiotics prior to the initiation of chemotherapy and/or radiation. Provide a pathogen-free environment (laminar flow room), if available. Otherwise, reverse isolation should be maintained until the peripheral polymorphonuclear count is >500/mm^3. In spite of precautions, infection is a major cause of death.
Bleeding	Petechiae, ecchymoses, epistaxis, bleeding gums, hematuria, guaiac-positive stools, uncontrolled menses, headache, and neurologic changes	Prophylactic platelet transfusions if peripheral platelet count less than 20,000/mm^3. Actively bleeding patients should be transfused if <50,000/mm^3. Provera is administered to control menses.	Avoid invasive procedures such as IM injections. Use Toothettes® to administer mouth care, rather than toothbrush. Instruct patient to avoid blowing the nose or straining with stools.
Stomatitis	Ulcerations, white plaques, red swollen gums, reduced salivation	Meticulous mouth care every 2–4 hours—including saline rinse and gentle swabbing. Antifungal rinses (nystatin) may be prescribed. Local and even IV analgesics may be required.	Stomatitis is usually an unpreventable side effect of both radiation and chemotherapy.
Venous occlusive disease (VOD)	Hepatomegaly, elevated bilirubin, heart failure, encephalopathy	Treat symptomatically	No measures prevent the occurrence of this complication in 25% of bone marrow transplant (BMT) patients; fatal in 40% of those patients.
Graft-versus-host disease (GVHD)	Acute—faint, red maculopapular rash 7–14 days posttransplant. Chronic—firm, inelastic skin, ulcerations, and/or contractures. Mucosal degeneration leading to guaiac-positive diarrhea, nausea, vomiting, ascites, and malnutrition. Hepatosplenomegaly	Apply creams and ointments to relieve itching and skin discomfort. Administer IV fluids and hyperalimentation. Parenteral analgesics may be required to relieve pain. ATG—antithymocyte globulin may be administered to reduce donor lymphocytes. Observe closely during administration. ATG is made from horse serum and can cause an anaphylactic response.	Select histocompatible donor. Irradiate all blood products prior to infusion. Administer chemotherapy agents and steroids to inhibit immune response. In spite of preventive measures, GVHD occurs in 30%–70% of the BMT patients—fatal in 20%–40% of those affected.

thereby reducing the risk of GVHD, and the marrow cavities are emptied to provide space for the transfused stem cells to implant.

b. Common protocols combine total body irradiation (TBI) and very high doses of a single chemotherapeutic agent or fractionated doses of multiple agents. (See p. 99 for a description of chemotherapy drugs.)

3. Strict isolation or a laminar flow room is required to prevent infection. Other pathogen-reduction measures include nonabsorbable oral antibiotics, medicated baths, douches, and a restricted cooked-food diet.

4. A central catheter is inserted, which will allow suitable access for marrow infusion as well as for antibiotics, blood products, hyperalimentation, and frequent blood sampling.

B. Bone Marrow Infusion

1. The infusion of the marrow is usually anticlimactic after the patient has undergone the rigorous preparatory chemotherapy and irradiation. The marrow is usually administered immediately after the conditioning regimen is complete.

2. Marrow is administered from a large blood infusion bag equipped with a standard blood filter (Fig. 13-3). Small volumes may also be prefiltered and given IV push by a physician.

Post-transplantation Care

1. Potential immediate adverse reactions are allergic (urticaria, chills, fever), volume overload, and pulmonary complications secondary to fat emboli.

2. The period immediately following transplant is critical.
   a. The life-threatening adverse effects of BMT are further complicated by the multisystem failure that may occur as a result of the ablative therapy given prior to transplant.
   b. Table 13-3 lists potential complications, clinical manifestations, treatment/nursing interventions, and prevention.

3. Intensive nursing care will be required for several weeks post-transplant.
   a. *Care is aimed at early diagnosis and treatment of complications.* The nurse should routinely assess all major organ systems.
   b. Abnormalities must be reported to the physician immediately.

4. Indications of successful engraftment are an increase in platelets and red blood cells in the peripheral blood count. This may occur as early as 14 days after marrow infusion.
   a. During the period of aplasia, blood component support is essential to control bleeding and treat symptoms of anemia.
   b. The infusion of granulocytes may also be considered to treat bacterial infection if conventional antibiotic therapy has failed.

5. The nurse must help the patient and family to deal with pain, isolation, altered body image, and fear.
   a. The financial resources required for transplant are substantial, which adds stress to a family unit already stretched to the limit.
   b. A multidisciplinary approach (social workers, nutritionist, clergy, community services) can improve quality of life for the patient and family.

Bibliography

Books

American Association of Blood Banks. Technical Manual of the American Association of Blood Banks: AABB Technical Manual. Arlington, Virginia, The Association, 1985

Mollison PL, Endelfriet C and Contreras M. Blood Transfusion in Clinical Medicine. 8th ed. Boston, Blackwell Scientific Publications, 1987

Moore SB (ed). Transfusion-Transmitted Viral Diseases. Arlington, VA, American Association of Blood Banks, 1987

Napier J. Blood Transfusion Therapy: A Problem-Oriented Approach. New York, John Wiley & Sons, 1987

Petz L and Swisher S. Clinical Practice of Transfusion Medicine. 2nd ed. New York, Churchill Livingstone, 1989

Rosvoll RV. Accreditation Requirements Manual of the American Association of Blood Banks. 2nd ed. Arlington, VA, American Assocation of Blood Banks, 1987

Snyder EL. Blood Transfusion Therapy: A Physician's Handbook. 2nd ed. Arlington, VA, American Association of Blood Banks, 1987

Journals

American Association of Blood Banks. Blood transfusions outside the hospital. Am J Nurs 1989 Apr; 89(4): 486–489

Armitage JO and Gale RP. Bone marrow autotransplantation. Am J Med 1989 Feb; 86(2):203–206

Berkman SA. Infectious complications of blood transfusion. Blood Rev 1988 Sep; 2(3):206–210

Blattner W. Human T-lymphocytic viruses and diseases of long latency. Ann Intern Med 1989 Jul; 111(1):4–5

Coffin CM. Current issues in transfusion therapy: Indications for use of blood components. Postgrad Med 1987 Jan; 81(1):343–346, 348–350

Ford R and Ballard B. Acute complications after bone marrow transplantation. Semin Oncol Nurs 1988 Feb; 4(1):15–24

Freedman SE. An overview of bone marrow transplantation. Semin Oncol Nurs 1988 Feb; 4(1):3–8

Levensky RJ. Recent advances in bone marrow transplantation. Clin Immunol Immunopathol 1989 Jan; 50(1 Pt 2): 124–132

Liwack K. Practical points for transfusion therapy. Journal of Post Anesthesia Nursing 1987 Nov; 2(4):257–261

Lonngvist B et al. Timing of marrow transplantation in secondary leukemia and myelodysplastic syndromes. Transplant Proc 1989 Feb; 21(1 Pt 3): 2958–2959

Miller JD, Rutman R and Silberstein L. Transfusion therapy in emergency medicine. Ann Emerg Med 1988 Apr; 17(4):327–335

Nims JW and Strom S. Late complications of bone marrow transplant recipients: Nursing care issues. Semin Oncol Nurs 1988 Feb; 4(1):47–54

O'Quin T and Moravec C. The critically ill bone marrow transplant patient. Semin Oncol Nurs 1988 Feb; 4(1):25–30

Peck NL. Blood transfusion reaction. Nursing 1987 Jan; 17(1):33

Peterman TA. Transfusion-associated acquired immunodeficiency syndrome. World J Surg 1987 Feb; 11(1):37–40

Phillips A. Are blood transfusions really safe? Nursing 1987 Jun; 17(6):63–64

Polesky HF and Hanson MR. Transfusion-associated hepatitis C virus (non-A, non-B) infection. Arch Pathol Lab Med 1989 Mar; 113(3):232–235

Popovsky MA. Autologous transfusion—Present practice and future trends. Journal of The National Intravenous Therapy Association 1986 Jul–Aug; 9(4):292–295

Sale GE and Buckner CD. Pathology of bone marrow in transplant recipients. Hematol Oncol Clin North Am 1988 Dec; 2(4):735–756

Sirchia J et al. Leukocyte depletion of red cell units at the bedside by transfusion through a new filter. Transfusion 1987 Nov; 27(5):402–405

Slavin S and Kedar E. Current problems and future goals in clinical bone marrow transplantation. Blood Rev 1988 Dec; 2(4):259–269

The latest protocols for blood transfusions. The Committee on Transfusion Practices. Nursing 1986 Oct; 16(10):34–42

Weir JA. Virus: A concern in transfusion therapy. Journal of The National Intravenous Therapy Association 1986 May–Jun; 9(3):234–236

Wenz B. Leukocyte poor blood. Crit Rev Clin Lab Sci 1986; 24(1):1–20

Cardiac Disorders 14

Manifestations of Heart Disease

Cardiovascular Assessment

Components of Cardiovascular Assessment

1. Health history
2. Physical examination

Health History

A. Chief Complaint/Problem—which prompted patient to seek health care

B. Family History—estimates the risk of cardiac disease for patient; ask if patient's family members (parents, grandparents, siblings, blood relatives) were diagnosed with coronary artery disease, hypertension, hyperlipidemia, diabetes.

C. Risk Factors—smoking, high serum cholesterol, hypertension, obesity, sedentary life-style, stress, male sex, alcohol; these factors increase risk of progression/development of disease.

D. Past Medical History

1. Past illnesses/hospitalizations: trauma to chest (possible myocardial contusion); sore throat/dental extractions (possible endocarditis); rheumatic fever (valvular dysfunction, endocarditis)
2. Allergies—particularly cardiac catheterization dye or shellfish (possible increase in sensitivity to dye).
3. Medications—many cardiac drugs must be tapered off to prevent a "rebound effect."

E. History of Present Illness—an overview of the patient's symptoms

Chest Pain

Most common complaint of patients with cardiac disease

A. Cardiac Causes of Chest Pain

1. Ischemia caused by an increase in demand for coronary blood flow and oxygen delivery, which exceeds available blood supply; due to coronary artery disease (angina pectoris, myocardial infarction).
2. Excruciating pain radiating to back and flanks—from acute dissecting aneurysm of the aorta.
3. Sharp precordial pain (over heart area) radiating to left shoulder and upper back, aggravated by respirations—indicates acute pericarditis.

B. Nursing Assessment of Chest Pain

1. *Nature and Intensity*
   a. Ask patient to describe in own words what the pain is like—dull, sharp, crushing, burning, heaviness, ache, pressure?
   b. Ask patient to rate pain relative to pain experienced in the past using a scale of 1–10. (10 being the most severe pain and 1 the least).
2. *Onset and Duration*
   a. When did the pain start?
   b. How long did the pain episode last?
3. *Location and Radiation*
   a. Ask patient to point to area where it hurts most. (Positive Levine's sign: clenched fist brought to patient's chest; indicative of diffuse visceral pain associated with unstable cardiac disease)
   b. Ask the patient if the pain seems to travel (most commonly radiates to left arm, jaw, back, and abdominal region).

4. *Precipitating and Relieving Factors*
    a. What activity was patient doing just prior to pain (rapid walking, exposure to cold, eating a spicy meal)?
    b. What relieves the pain (rest, medications, change of position)?
5. *Associated Signs/Symptoms*
    Observe for nausea, diaphoresis, dyspnea, fatigue, palpitations, disorientation.

Dyspnea

A. Description
1. *Dyspnea* is undue breathlessness, an awareness of discomfort associated with breathing.
2. It may be a sign of left ventricular failure or transient congestive heart failure.

B. Types of Cardiac Dyspnea
1. *Exertional*—breathlessness on moderate exertion that is relieved by rest.
2. *Paroxysmal nocturnal*—sudden dyspnea at night; awakens patient with feeling of suffocation; sitting up relieves breathlessness.
3. *Orthopnea*—shortness of breath when lying down. Patient must keep head elevated with more than one pillow to minimize dyspnea.

C. Nursing Assessment of Dyspnea
1. What precipitates or relieves dyspnea?
2. How many pillows does patient sleep with at night? (Several pillows is indicative of advanced heart failure.)

Palpitations

A. Description
1. *Palpitation* is a rapid, forceful, or irregular heartbeat felt by the patient.
2. Patient may complain of pounding, jumping sensations in chest (usually due to tachydysrhythmias) or sensation of skipped beats (usually due to premature atrial or ventricular beats).

B. Nursing Assessment of Palpitations
1. Do you ever feel your heart pound, beat too fast, or skip beats?
2. Do you feel dizzy or faint when you experience these sensations?
3. What do you do to relieve these sensations?

Weakness/Fatigue

A. Description
1. Fatigue is produced by low cardiac output. The heart is unable to provide sufficient blood to meet the increased metabolic needs of cells.
2. As heart disease advances, fatigue is precipitated by less effort.

B. Nursing Assessment of Weakness and Fatigue
1. What activities can you perform without becoming tired?
2. What activities cause you to become tired?

Dizziness and Syncope

A. Description
1. *Syncope* is a transient loss of consciousness due to a fall in cardiac output with resulting cerebral ischemia.

Near syncope refers to lightheadedness, dizziness, temporary confusion.
2. Dysrhythmias related to cardiac disease may cause syncope.

B. Nursing Assessment of Syncope
1. How many episodes of syncope/near syncope have been experienced?
2. Did a hot room, hunger, sudden position change, or pressure on your neck precipitate the episode (rules out incidents that may cause a vasovagal response)?

Physical Examination

Vital Signs

A. Determine Heart Rate
1. Time for 1 full minute; note regularity.
2. Compare apical and radial heart rate (pulse deficit).

B. Monitor Blood Pressure
1. Take pressure in both arms and note differences (5 mm. Hg difference is normal).
2. Determine *pulse pressure* (systolic pressure minus diastolic pressure) to evaluate cardiac output (30–40 mm. Hg normal, less than 30 mm. Hg indicates decreased cardiac output)
3. Note presence of *pulsus alternans*—loud sounds alternate with soft sounds with each auscultory beat (hallmark of left ventricular failure).
4. Note presence of *pulsus paradoxus*—abnormal fall in blood pressure during inspirations (cardinal sign of cardiac tamponade; see Pericardiocentesis p. 310.)

C. Assess for Postural/Orthostatic Hypotension
1. Autonomic compensatory factors for upright posture are inadequate due to volume depletion, bedrest, and/or neurological disease; prompt hypotension occurs with assumption of the upright position.
2. Note changes in heart rate and blood pressure in at least two of three positions: lying, standing, sitting; allow at least 3 minutes between position changes before obtaining rate and pressure.
3. Orthostatic changes evident if blood pressure decreases by 15 mm. Hg (systolic) or 5 mm. Hg diastolic and/or heart rate increases 15 beats with position changes.

Skin

A. Palpate for Temperature and Evidence of Diaphoresis
1. Warm/dry skin indicates adequate cardiac output.
2. Cool, clammy skin indicates compensatory vasoconstriction due to low cardiac output.

B. Observe for Cyanosis, Jaundice, and Fatty Skin Deposits (xanthomas).
1. *Cyanosis*—bluish discoloration of the skin and mucous membranes.
    a. *Central cyanosis*—low oxygen saturation of arterial blood. Noted on tongue, buccal mucosa, and lips. Indicative of cardiorespiratory disease; may be evident in heart failure or pulmonary edema.
    b. *Peripheral cyanosis*—reduced blood flow through extremities due to vasoconstriction. Noted on distal aspects of extremities, tip of nose, and ear lobes; due to cold exposure or obstructive peripheral vascular disease.

2. *Jaundice*—yellow discoloration of sclera of eyes and/ or skin; may be sign of right-sided heart failure or chronic hemolysis from prosthetic heart valve.
3. Yellow plaque (fatty deposits) evident on skin; associated with hyperlipidemia and coronary artery disease.

C. Inspect Nailbeds for Splinter Hemorrhages and Clubbing

1. Thin brown lines in nailbed are associated with endocarditis.
2. *Clubbing* (swollen nail base and loss of normal angle) is associated with congenital heart disease and cor pulmonale.

Edema

A. Description

1. *Edema* is an abnormal accumulation of serous fluid in soft tissue.
2. Location of edema is influenced by gravity—fluid collects bilaterally in lower parts of the body: sacral area (bedridden patients, ankles, and feet (ambulatory patients), and "pits" with pressure (dependent-pitting edema).
3. Weight gain occurs prior to clinical evidence of edema. Edema is a late sign of heart failure.

B. Nursing Assessment

1. Observe/palpate for edema.
2. Describe degree of edema in terms of depth of pitting that occurs with slight pressure; mild—0–¼″, moderate—½″, severe—¾″–1″.

Apical Impulse

A. General Assessment

1. Palpate the precordial area with palmar base of hand.
2. Note pulsation in apical area (fifth intercostal space—left of sternal border).
3. Pulsation (apical impulse) should be approximately 2 cm. in diameter; lateral displacement of greater than 7–9 cm. from sternal border indicates left ventricular hypertrophy.

B. Arterial Pulse

1. Examine the pulses bilaterally; peripheral pulses should be equal.
   a. Note amplitude (fullness), which depends on pulse pressure (difference between systolic and diastolic pressures); this gives an estimate of stroke volume.
   b. Small volume pulse may be from low stroke volume and peripheral vasoconstriction (myocardial infarction, shock, constrictive pericarditis, vasoconstrictive drugs).
   c. Large volume pulse produced by large stroke volume (aortic regurgitation, pregnancy, thyrotoxicosis, bradycardia, patent ductus arteriosus).
   d. Palpate carotid artery—reveals character of pulse in the proximal aorta and provides indication of any abnormality causing disease of left ventricle.

C. Respiration

Note rate, depth, and respiratory pattern.

D. Jugular Venous Pulse

1. Venous pulsation can be more easily seen than felt.
2. Identification of venous pulse permits assessment of height of venous pressure.
3. See page 33 for technique.

E. Heart Auscultation

1. Heart auscultation requires knowledge, experience, and a "listening ear" tuned to hear each event of the cardiac cycle.
2. Heart auscultation should be systematic, and the stethoscope should "inch" from one area to another.
3. Four main areas of auscultation: aortic area, pulmonary area, mitral area, and the tricuspid area.
4. Listen for rate and regularity of rhythm.
   a. Determine if an irregularity is related to respiratory movements.
   b. Evaluate the sequence in which an irregularity occurs.
5. During auscultation, the examiner assesses the venous pulse, feels the pulsation of the right carotid artery and the radial artery, feels precordial movement, and listens to the heart.
6. See Chapter 3 for a more complete discussion on heart examination and examination of abdomen and extremities.

Diagnostic Evaluation

Cardiographic Studies

A. Electrocardiogram (ECG)—a visual representation of the electrical activity of the heart as reflected by changes in electrical potential at the skin surface.

1. ECG is obtained by placing leads on various body parts and recording the electrical impulse as a tracing on a strip of paper or on the screen of an oscilloscope.
2. Clinical usefulness—evaluation of conditions that interfere with normal electrophysiological function—disturbances of rhythm, disorders of cardiac muscle, enlargement of chambers of heart, presence of myocardial infarction, electrolyte disturbances.
3. See page 362 for a more detailed account.

B. Echocardiography (Ultrasound Cardiography)—a record of high-frequency sound vibrations that have been sent into the heart through the chest wall. The cardiac structures return the echoes derived from the ultrasound. The motions of the echoes are traced on an oscilloscope and recorded on film.

1. The patient is placed in supine position, and the transducer is placed on his chest.
2. Transducer is applied (left sternal border) with ultrasonic gel to maintain airless contact between skin and transducer.
3. ECG is recorded simultaneously to time the events within cardiac cycle.
4. *Clinical usefulness*
   a. Demonstration of valvular and other structural deformities
   b. Detection of pericardial effusion
   c. Evaluation of prosthetic valve function
   d. Diagnosis of cardiac tumors; asymmetric thickening of interventricular septum
   e. Diagnosis of cardiomegaly (heart enlargement)

C. Ambulatory Electrocardiographic Monitoring—continuous recording of an ECG to monitor the heartbeat while the patient goes about his daily routine.

1. Patient wears miniaturized tape-recording device using a single- or double-lead system attached to belt or worn on a shoulder strap.
2. Patient keeps a diary—records his activities and any symptoms that are noted; useful when symptoms are

provoked by specific activities (jogging, stress); used for assessing patients who suffer from transient dizziness, syncope, or near syncope; detecting dysrhythmias; assessing response to therapy; and evaluating patients after myocardial infarction.

D. Exercise Stress Testing—exercise testing on a treadmill or a bicycle-like device carried out to identify ischemic heart disease, to evaluate patients with chest pain, to assess results of therapy, and to aid in developing individual physical fitness programs.

1. Obtain informed consent—patient advised of purpose and risks of test.
2. ECG electrodes applied to patient and tracings made before, during, and after exercise testing.
3. Patient is exercised by increasing walking speed and the incline of the treadmill or by increasing the load against which he pedals.
4. Instruct patient to avoid smoking, eating, and drinking for 4 hours prior to test, and to rest and avoid stimulants or extreme temperature changes after the test.

E. Phonocardiography—graphic recording of the heart sounds and pulse waves and their relation to time.

1. Helps to identify, to accurately time, and to differentiate various sounds and murmurs
2. Provides a permanent record for future comparison

F. Vectorcardiography—presents a three-dimensional view of the electrical forces of the heart.

1. Amplifies understanding of the ECG
2. Gives more specific information in certain situations than the standard electrocardiogram

G. Myocardial Imaging (Radionuclide imaging)

With the use of radionuclides and scintillation cameras, radionuclide angiograms can be used to assess left ventricular performance.

1. *"Hot spot" or positive imaging*
   a. Technetium-99m stannous pyrophosphate is a radionuclide most commonly used. Necrosed or ischemic myocardium takes up the phosphate and produces a "hot spot" indicative of a positive scan.
   b. Scans become positive within 12–36 hours and are usually negative after 7 days.
   c. Used when diagnosis of myocardial infarction (MI) is unclear. Not employed in routine workup for diagnostic evaluation of MI.
2. *"Cold spot" imaging*
   a. Thallium-201 most common isotope used. Thallium-201 concentrates in myocardial cells relative to blood flow. Areas of low concentration are termed "cold spots."
   b. Differentiation between old and new infarctions cannot be determined with this method, and no distinction can be made between areas of infarction and ischemia.
   c. A normal thallium scan is likely to rule out the diagnosis of myocardial infarction. Usually not employed in routine workup for diagnostic evaluation of MI.
3. *Radionuclide ventriculogram*
   a. A noninvasive method for accurate assessment of ventricular hemodynamics, and regional wall motion.
   b. Provides measurements of right and left ventricular ejection fraction, distinguishes regional from global ventricular wall motion, and allows for subjective analysis of cardiac anatomy to detect

intracardiac shunts, and valvular or congenital abnormalities.
   c. A radiopharmaceutical (usually Technetium-99m) is injected rapidly through a central venous catheter, Swan–Ganz catheter, or antecubital vein.
   d. Indices of ventricular performance are measured from the initial transit of the radiotracer through the heart.

Roentgenologic Studies

A. Chest X-Ray—shows heart size, contour, and position; reveals cardiac and pericardial calcifications and demonstrates physiologic alterations in pulmonary circulation.

B. Fluoroscopy—provides visual observation of the heart on a luminescent x-ray screen.

1. Shows heart and vascular pulsations; useful in the assessment of unusual cardiac contours and especially calcifications.
2. Useful in placement and positioning of intravenous electrodes and for guiding the catheter in cardiac catheterization.

C. Angiocardiography—injection of contrast medium into the vascular system (to outline the heart and blood vessels) accompanied by *cineangiograms* (rapidly changing films or movies on an intensified fluoroscopic screen), which record the passage of contrast media through the vascular tree.

Useful for providing information regarding coronary anatomy, structural abnormalities (occlusions, defects, fistulae) or abnormal heart valve function.

1. *Selective angiocardiography*—contrast medium is injected through a catheter directly into one of the heart chambers, coronary arteries, or greater vessels and the angiocardiogram is recorded by means of a rapid film changer or motion picture camera.
2. *Aortography*—a form of angiography that outlines the lumen of the aorta and major arteries arising from it.
3. *Coronary arteriography* (most common form of selective angiocardiography)—a radiopaque catheter is introduced into the right brachial artery via open arteriotomy (or femoral artery via percutaneous puncture), passed into the ascending aorta, and manipulated into appropriate coronary artery under fluoroscopic control.
   a. Used as an evaluation tool before coronary artery surgery or myocardial revascularization and after surgery to evaluate graft patency
   b. Used to study suspected congenital anomalies of the coronary arteries
4. Nursing implications in angiocardiography
   a. Before angiogram
      Keep the patient in a fasting state prior to examination—to minimize danger of pulmonary aspiration should emesis occur
   b. After angiogram
      (1) Record vital signs every 15 minutes × 4 (or more often as patient's condition indicates) until vital signs are stable.
      (2) Check for bleeding at puncture or cutdown site.
      (3) Check distal extremity for normal color and intact pulses.
      (4) The patient may complain of mild headache and/or discomfort in the groin or other site,

depending on route by which contrast medium was administered.

(5) Check for bedrest and special fluid directives from physician.

Cardiac Catheterization

Cardiac catheterization is a diagnostic procedure in which a catheter(s) is (are) introduced into the heart and blood vessels to (1) measure oxygen concentration, saturation, tension, and pressure in the various heart chambers; (2) detect shunts; (3) provide blood samples for analysis; and (4) determine cardiac output and pulmonary blood flow.

Angiography is usually combined with heart catheterization for coronary artery visualization.

A. Right-Heart Catheterization—a radiopaque catheter is passed from an antecubital or femoral vein into the right atrium, right ventricle, and pulmonary vasculature under direct visualization with a fluoroscope.

1. Right atrium and right ventricle pressures measured; blood samples taken for hematocrit and oxygen saturation.
2. After entering the right atrium, the catheter is then passed through the tricuspid valve, and similar tests are performed on blood within the right ventricle.
3. Finally the catheter is passed through the pulmonic valve and as far as possible beyond that point; capillary samples are obtained and "capillary pressures" (wedge pressure) are recorded.
4. Complications—cardiac dysrhythmias, venous spasm, thrombophlebitis, infection of cutdown site, cardiac perforation, and cardiac tamponade.

B. Left-Heart Catheterization—usually done by retrograde catheterization of the left ventricle or by trans-septal catheterization of the left atrium.

1. Retrograde approach—catheter inserted under direct vision into right brachial artery and advanced under fluoroscopic control into the ascending aorta and into the left ventricle; or, catheter may be introduced percutaneously by puncture of femoral artery.
2. Trans-septal approach—catheter is passed from the right femoral vein (percutaneously or by saphenous vein cutdown) into right atrium. A long needle is passed up through the catheter and is used to puncture the septum separating the right and left atria; needle is withdrawn and the catheter advanced under fluoroscopic control into left ventricle.
   a. Gives hemodynamic data—permits flow and pressure measurements of left heart.
   b. Most often performed to evaluate the function of the left ventricular muscle and mitral and aortic valves, or the patency of coronary arteries.
   c. Used to evaluate patients before and after cardiac surgery.
   d. Complications of left heart catheterization and implications for nursing assessment are
      (1) Dysrhythmias (ventricular fibrillation), syncope, vasospasm
      (2) Pericardial tamponade, myocardial infarction, pulmonary edema
      (3) Allergic reaction to contrast medium
      (4) Perforation of great vessels of heart; systemic embolization (stroke, MI)
      (5) Loss of pulse distal to arteriotomy and possible ischemia of lower arm and hand.

C. Nursing Management in Heart Catheterization

1. Preceding heart catheterization
   a. Know which approach is to be used in order to anticipate possible complications.
   b. Withhold food and fluid 6 hours before procedure—to prevent vomiting and aspiration.
   c. Ascertain history of previous allergies.
   d. Mark distal pulses—for easy reference after catheterization.
   e. Explain to the patient that he will be lying on an examining table for a prolonged period and that he may experience certain sensations:
      (1) Occasional thudding sensations in the chest—from extrasystoles, particularly when the catheter is manipulated in ventricular chambers.
      (2) Strong desire to cough—may occur during contrast medium injection into right heart during angiography.
      (3) Transient feeling of heat, particularly in the head—from injection of contrast medium.
   f. Remove dentures; give prescribed medication.
2. Following heart catheterization
   a. Record the blood pressure and apical pulse every 15 minutes (or more frequently) until vital signs are stable after the procedure—to discern dysrhythmias.
   b. Check peripheral pulses in affected extremity (dorsalis pedis, posterior tibial pulse in the lower extremity, and radial pulse in upper extremity); evaluate extremity temperature, color, and complaints of pain, numbness, or tingling sensation—to determine signs of arterial insufficiency.
   c. Watch puncture (cutdown) sites for hematoma formation. Question patient about increase in pain/tenderness at site.
   d. Assess for complaints of chest pain and report occurrence immediately—myocardial infarction may occur and is a serious complication of cardiac catheterization.
   e. See that the patient remains in bed with little movement of the involved extremity until the following morning.
   f. Evaluate complaints of back pain, thigh or groin pain (may indicate retroperitoneal bleeding).
   g. Be alert for signs/symptoms of vagal reaction (nausea, diaphoresis, hypotension, bradycardia); treat as directed with atropine and fluids.

Blood Studies

1. CBC
2. Blood electrolytes (potassium, sodium, chloride, carbon dioxide)—for patients treated with digitalis or diuretics
3. Blood urea nitrogen and creatinine—to evaluate cardiac output
4. Sedimentation rate, C-reactive protein, and antistreptolysin O titer—to rule out inflammatory heart disease
5. Blood culture—to exclude infective endocarditis

Enzyme and Isoenzyme Tests

A. Rationale of Tests—the release of enzymes from cells into body fluids and into the circulation provides an indication of tissue damage and of changes taking place within the cells.

B. Underlying Concepts

1. Heart muscle is rich in enzymes that promote different biochemical reactions.
2. When myocardial tissue is damaged (myocardial infarction) certain cardiac enzymes are released into the bloodstream and result in elevated peripheral blood enzyme levels:
   a. Creatine kinase (CK)
   b. Lactic dehydrogenase (LDH)
   c. Aspartate aminotransferase
3. However, these enzymes may be widely distributed in tissues and elevated in conditions not associated with myocardial infarction (i.e., damage to skeletal muscles, liver, brain, kidneys, and other organs).

C. Isoenzymes—forms of protein species that promote the same biochemical action as enzymes, but differ chemically, physically, and/or immunologically

1. Isoenzymes can be identified by laboratory methods to reveal the specific tissue that is damaged; creatine kinase can be separated into 3 isoenzymes, known as MM, MB, and BB.
2. An elevation of serum CK-MB activity signifies that an adverse effect on myocardial cells has taken place; thus, it is the most specific and sensitive enzymatic criterion of myocardial injury now available. CK-MB greater than 5 IU is significant.

(See Diagnostic Evaluation, Myocardial Infarction)

Hemodynamic Monitoring

Hemodynamic monitoring is the assessment of the patient's circulatory status; it includes measurements of heart rate, intra-arterial pressure, pulmonary artery, and pulmonary capillary wedge pressures (see below), central venous pressure (p. 307), cardiac output (p. 309), and blood volume.

Guidelines   Measuring Pulmonary Artery Pressure by Flow-Directed Balloon-Tipped Catheter (Swan–Ganz Catheter)

The Swan–Ganz catheter is a flow-directed, balloon-tipped, 4–5-lumen catheter that is percutaneously inserted at the bedside and allows for continuous hemodynamic monitoring of the critically ill patient. The precise hemodynamic data obtained is useful in evaluation of heart function and circulating volume. Based on the data, appropriate therapy for the patient with compromised cardiac dynamics can be selected, implemented, and the patient's response to the therapy evaluated continuously.

If monitoring of venous oxygen saturation (SvO_2) is desired, a PA catheter incorporating fiberoptics is used.

The catheter is 110 cm. long, marked at increments of 10 cm., and is available in varying diameters (Fig. 14-1).

Purposes
1. To monitor pressures in the right atrium (central venous pressure), right ventricle, pulmonary artery, and distal branches of the pulmonary artery (pulmonary capillary wedge pressure). The latter reflects the level of the pressure in the left atrium (or filling pressure in the left ventricle); thus, pressures on the left side of the heart are inferred from pressure measurements obtained on the right side of the circulation.
2. To measure cardiac output through thermodilution
3. To obtain blood for central venous oxygen saturation
4. To continuously monitor mixed venous oxygen saturation (SvO_2); (available on catheters with special fiberoptic sensors).
5. To provide for temporary atrial/ventricular pacing and intra-atrial electrocardiography (available only on special catheters).

Underlying Considerations
1. Left atrial pressure is closely related to left ventricular end diastolic pressure (LVEDP—filling pressure of the left ventricle) and is therefore an indicator of left ventricular function.
2. The pulmonary artery diastolic pressure (PAD) reflects the LVEDP in patients with normal lungs and mitral valve. The PAD can be continuously monitored as an approximation of LVEDP (limits excessive balloon inflation to obtain a pulmonary capillary wedge pressure and subsequent risk of balloon rupture).
3. If the amount of oxygen supplied to the tissues is inadequate to meet demands, more oxygen will be extracted from venous blood and the SvO_2 will decrease. If oxygen supply exceeds demand, the SvO_2 will increase.
4. The SvO_2 is affected by 4 factors: cardiac output, hemoglobin, arterial oxygen saturation (SaO_2), and tissue oxygen consumption.
5. Changes in SvO_2 alert the clinician to changes in these factors. More rapid detection of change facilitates interventions to correct problems before significant deterioration in patient's condition occurs.

Equipment
Swan–Ganz catheter set
ECG, monitor and display unit with paper recorder
For SvO_2 monitoring, fiberoptic PA catheter, optical module, and microprocessor unit.
Defibrillator
Pressure transducer (disposable/reusable)
Cutdown tray
Sterile saline solution
Pressurized bag
Heparin infusion in plastic bag
Continuous flush device
Local anesthetic
Skin antiseptic
Transparent/gauze dressing
Tape

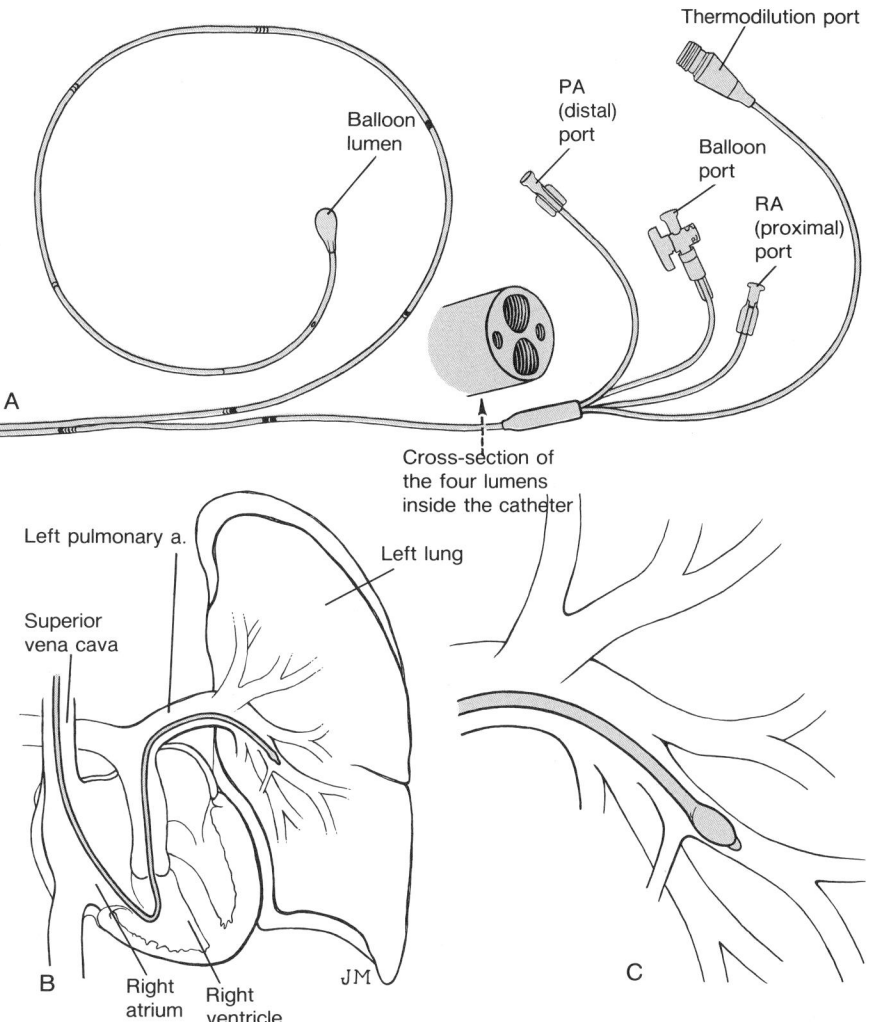

Figure 14-1. *(A) Swan–Ganz catheter. (B) Location of the Swan–Ganz catheter within the heart. The catheter enters the right atrium via the superior vena cava. The balloon is then inflated, allowing the catheter to follow the blood flow through the tricuspid valve, through the right ventricle, through the pulmonic valve, and into the main pulmonary artery. Waveform and pressure readings are noted during insertion to identify location of the catheter within the heart. The balloon is deflated once the catheter is in the pulmonary artery and properly secured. (C) Pulmonary capillary wedge pressure (PCWP). The catheter floats into a distal branch of the pulmonary artery when the balloon is in-flated, and becomes "wedged." The wedged catheter occludes blood flow from behind, and the tip of the lumen records pressures in front of the catheter. The balloon is then deflated, allowing the catheter to float back into the main pulmonary artery.*

Procedure (Fig. 14-1)	**Nursing Action**	**Rationale/Amplification**

Preparatory Phase (by nurses)

1. Explain procedure to the patient and family/significant other. Obtain informed consent.	1. Tell the patient he may feel the catheter moving through his vein, and this is normal.
2. Check vital signs and apply ECG electrodes.	
3. Place patient in a position of comfort; this is the baseline position.	3. Note the angle of elevation if patient cannot lie flat, as subsequent pressure readings are taken from this baseline position to ensure consistency.
4. Set up equipment according to manufacturer's directives: a. The pulmonary artery catheter requires a transducer; recording, amplifying, and flush systems (Fig. 14-1).	4. a. Monitoring systems may vary greatly. The complexity of equipment requires an understanding of the equipment in use. A constant microdrip of heparin flush solution is maintained to ensure catheter patency.

(continued)

Guidelines Measuring Pulmonary Artery Pressure by Flow-Directed Balloon-Tipped Catheter
(Swan–Ganz Catheter) *(continued)*

Procedure *(continued)*	**Nursing Action**	**Rationale/Amplification**
	b. Flush system according to manufacturer's directions.	b. Flushing of the catheter system ensures patency and eliminates air bubbles.
	5. Adjust transducer to level of patient's right atrium (phlebostatic axis–4th intercostal space, midaxillary line) (Fig. 14-2)	5. Differences between the level of the right atrium and the transducer will result in incorrect pressure readings; the phlebostatic axis is at the level of the right atrium.
	6. Calibrate pressure equipment.	6. A known quantity of pressure is applied to the transducer (usually by mercury manometer) to ensure accurate monitoring of pressure readings.

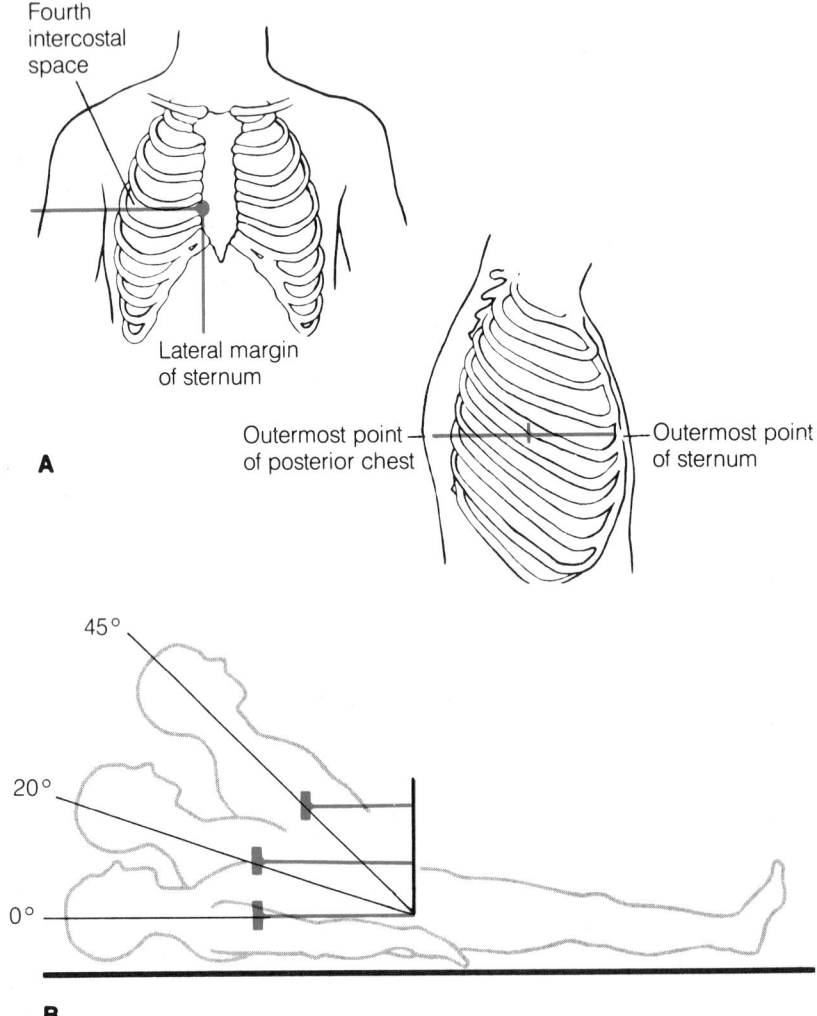

Figure 14-2. The phlebostatic axis and the phlebostatic level. (A) The phlebostatic axis is the crossing of two reference lines: (1) a line from the fourth intercostal space at the point where it joins the sternum, drawn out to the side of the body beneath the axilla; (2) a line midpoint between the anterior and posterior surfaces of the chest. (B) The phlebostatic level is a horizontal line through the phlebostatic axis. The transducer or the zero mark on the manometer must be level with this axis for accurate measurements. As the patient moves from the flat to erect positions, he moves his chest and therefore the reference level; the phlebostatic level stays horizontal through the same reference point. (After Shinn J et al: Heart Lung 8 [2]:324.

Procedure
(continued)

Nursing Action	**Rationale/Amplification**

7. Shave and prepare skin over insertion site.

7. The catheter is inserted percutaneously at the bedside under sterile conditions.

Performance Phase (by the physician)

1. Physician dons sterile gown and gloves, and places sterile drapes over patient.
2. The balloon is inflated with air under sterile water or saline to test for leakage (bubbles). The catheter may be flushed with saline at this time.
3. The Swan–Ganz catheter is inserted through the internal jugular, subclavian, or any easily accessible vein by either percutaneous puncture or venotomy.
4. The catheter is advanced to the superior vena cava. Oscillations of the pressure waveforms will indicate when the tip of the catheter is within the thoracic cavity. The patient may be asked to cough.
5. The catheter is then advanced gently into the right atrium and the balloon inflated with air.
6. The inflated balloon at the tip of the catheter will be guided by the flowing stream of blood through the right atrium and tricuspid valve into the right ventricle. From this position, it finds its way into the main pulmonary artery. The catheter tip pressures are recorded continuously by specific pressure wave forms as the catheter advances through the various chambers of the heart.
7. The flowing blood will continue to direct the catheter more distally into the pulmonary tree. When the catheter reaches a pulmonary vessel that is approximately the same size or slightly smaller in diameter than the inflated balloon, it cannot be advanced any further. This is the wedge position, called pulmonary capillary wedge pressure (PCWP) or pulmonary artery wedge pressure (PAWP).

1. Sterile field is established to prevent chance of infection.
2. To ensure that the balloon is intact and to remove air from catheter
3. The internal jugular vein establishes a short route into the central venous system.
4. Catheter placement may be determined by characteristic wave forms and changes. Coughing will produce deflections in the pressure tracing when the catheter tip is in the thorax.
5. The amount of air to be used is indicated on the catheter.
6. Watch ECG monitor for signs of ventricular irritability as catheter enters the right ventricle. Report any signs of dysrhythmia to the physician.
7. With the catheter in the wedge position, the balloon blocks the flow of blood from the right side of the heart toward the lungs. The sensor at the tip of the balloon detects pressures distally, which results in the sensing of retrograde left atrial pressures. The PCWP is thus equal to left atrial pressures.
   a. Normal PCWP is 8–12 mm. Hg. Optimal LV function appears to be at a wedge between 14–18 mm. Hg.
   b. Wedge pressure is a valuable parameter of cardiac function. Filling pressures less than 8–10 mm. Hg in an acutely injured heart are often associated with reduction in cardiac output, hypotension, and tachycardia. Filling pressures greater than 20 mm. Hg are associated with left ventricular failure, pulmonary congestion, and hypervolemia.

8. The balloon is deflated, causing the catheter to retract spontaneously into a larger pulmonary artery. This gives a continuous pulmonary artery systolic, diastolic, and mean pressure.

8. The normal systolic pulmonary pressure ranges are 20–30 mm. Hg, and the diastolic pulmonary pressure ranges are 8–12 mm. Hg. The normal mean pulmonary artery pressure (average pressure in pulmonary artery throughout the entire cardiac cycle) is 15–20 mm. Hg.

9. The catheter is then attached to a continuous heparin flush and transducer.

9. A low-flow continuous irrigation ensures that the catheter remains patent. The transducer converts the pressure wave into an electronic wave that is displayed on the oscilloscope.

10. The catheter is sutured in place and covered with a sterile dressing.
11. A chest x-ray is obtained after Swan–Ganz insertion.

11. To confirm catheter position and to provide a baseline for future reference

To Obtain a Wedge Pressure Reading

1. Note amount of air to be injected into balloon, usually 1 ml. Do not introduce more air into balloon than specified.
2. Inflate the balloon slowly until the contour of the pulmonary arterial pressure changes to that of pulmonary wedge pressure. As soon as a wedge pattern is observed, no more air is introduced.
   a. Note the digital pressure recordings on the monitor (an average of pressure waves is displayed, but these waves are not taken at end expiration).
   b. Obtain a strip of the pressure tracing.
   c. Determine PCWP from strip at end expiration.

2. The transducer converts the pressure wave into an electronic wave that is displayed on a screen.
   a. PCWP should be determined at end expiration because respiratory variation of the waveform occurs due to changes in intrathoracic pressures.
   b. A calibrated oscilloscope or graph paper is needed to read pressures at end expiration.

(continued)

Guidelines Measuring Pulmonary Artery Pressure by Flow-Directed Balloon-Tipped Catheter (Swan–Ganz Catheter) *(continued)*

Procedure *(continued)*	**Nursing Action**	**Rationale/Amplification**
	3. Deflate the balloon as soon as the pressure reading is obtained.	3. Segmental lung infarction may occur if the catheter balloon is left inflated for long periods. Pulmonary capillary wedge pressure is only measured intermittently. Do not allow catheter to remain in wedge position when patient is unattended or when not directly making the measurement.
	4. Record PCWP reading and amount of air needed to obtain wedge reading. Document recorded waveform by placing a strip of the waveform in patient's chart showing wedge tracing reverting to pulmonary artery waveform.	4. Overinflation of the balloon may cause a "superwedge" waveform, and data obtained will be inaccurate. Overinflation of balloon may cause balloon to lose elastic properties and rupture. The strip provides documentation that catheter was not left in wedge position.

To Obtain a SvO$_2$ Reading:

	1. Before insertion, perform a preinsertion calibration of the catheter.	1. This calibrates the catheter to light intensity in the environment.
	2. After insertion, perform a calibration for light intensity and an in vivo calibration every 8 hours.	2. The in vivo calibration insures that there is minimal difference, or "drift" between the actual SvO$_2$ value and the value displayed on the monitor. The light calibration adjusts for changes in light in the environment.

> **NURSING ALERT:** Also perform in vivo calibration if the optical module is disconnected at the catheter junction, if calibration data is lost, or if the SvO$_2$ is ±4% of the SvO$_2$ value calculated from mixed venous values obtained from the pulmonary artery catheter.

	3. Monitor SvO$_2$ at frequent intervals. Values of 60%–80% are normal.	3. Causes of an SvO$_2$ <60% include: a. Decrease in cardiac output b. Decrease in SaO$_2$ c. Decrease in hemoglobin d. Increase in O$_2$ consumption Causes of an SvO$_2$ > 80% include: a. Increase in SaO$_2$ b. Decrease in O$_2$ consumption
	4. If the SvO$_2$ changes ±10% from the prior value, confirm that the change reflects a change in patient condition.	4. The value displayed may not be accurate if fibrin or a clot is obstructing the catheter tip (low-intensity signal), if the catheter is touching the vessel wall or in a wedged position (high-intensity signal), or if the catheter is no longer calibrated accurately.
	5. If the catheter is not functioning properly, initiate steps to resolve the problem.	5. These steps may include aspiration to determine if a clot is obstructing the catheter or notifying the physician of the need to reposition the catheter.
	6. If no catheter malfunction is identified, report changes to the physician. Initiate therapy based on standards of care.	6. Prompt intervention can restore normal tissue oxygen delivery before untoward effects occur.

Follow-up Phase

	1. Inspect the insertion site daily. Look for signs of infection, swelling, and bleeding.	1. A foreign body (catheter) in the vascular system increases the risk of sepsis.
	2. Record date and time of dressing change and IV tubing change.	
	3. Assess the extremity for color, temperature, capillary filling, and sensation.	3. Ischemia (with possible loss of digits) may occur from inadequate arterial flow.
	4. Assess contour of waveform frequently and compare with previous documented waveforms.	4. Catheter may move forward and become lodged in wedge position or drift back into right ventricle. Turn patient to left side and ask him to cough (may dislodge catheter from wedge position). If not dislodged, notify physician.
	5. Assess for complications: pulmonary embolism, dysrhythmias, heart block, damage to tricuspid valve, intracardiac knotting of catheter, thrombophlebitis, infection, balloon rupture, rupture of pulmonary artery.	5. Blood coming back into syringe indicates balloon rupture. Notify physician immediately.

Postinsertion Phase (Physician)

	The catheter is removed without excessive force or traction; pressure dressing is applied over the site.	The site should be checked periodically for bleeding.

Guidelines Central Venous Pressure Monitoring

Central venous pressure monitoring refers to the measurement of right atrial pressure or the pressure of the great veins within the thorax.

1. Right-sided cardiac function is assessed through the evaluation of the central venous pressure.
2. Left-sided heart function is less accurately reflected by the evaluation of central venous pressure, but may be useful in assessing chronic right and left heart failure and/or differentiating right and left ventricular infarctions.

Technique

1. Central venous pressure monitoring requires the threading of a catheter into a large central vein (subclavian, internal/external jugular, median basilic, or femoral).
2. The catheter tip then is positioned in the upper portion of the superior vena cava or the inferior vena cava (femoral approach only).

Purposes

1. To serve as a guide for fluid replacement.
2. To monitor pressures in the right atrium and central veins.
3. To administer blood products, total parenteral nutrition, and drug therapy contraindicated for peripheral infusion.
4. To obtain venous access when peripheral vein sites are inadequate.
5. To insert a temporary pacemaker.
6. To obtain central venous blood samples.

Equipment

Venous pressure tray
Cutdown tray
Infusion solution/infusion set with CVP manometer
Heparin flush system/pressure bag (if transducer to be used)
IV pole
Arm board (for antecubital insertion)
Sterile dressing/adhesive tape
Gowns, masks, caps, and sterile gloves
ECG monitoring
Carpenter's level (for establishing zero point)

Procedure

Nursing Action	Rationale/Amplification

Preparatory Phase

1. Assemble equipment according to manufacturer's directions.	1. Evaluate patient's PT, PTT, CBC.
2. Explain the procedure to the patient and obtain informed consent.	2. Procedure is similar to an IV, and the patient may move in bed as desired after passage of catheter.
a. Explain to patient how to perform the Valsalva maneuver.	a. The Valsalva maneuver performed during catheter insertion and removal decreases chance of air emboli.
b. NPO 6 hours prior to insertion	
3. Position patient appropriately.	3. Provides for maximum visibility of veins.
a. Place in supine position.	
(1). Arm vein—extend arm and secure on armboard.	
(2). Neck veins—place patient in Trendelenburg position. Place a small rolled towel under shoulders (subclavian approach).	Trendelenburg position prevents chance of air emboli. Anatomic access and clinical status of the patient are considered in site selection.
4. Flush IV infusion set and manometer (measuring device) *Or,* prepare heparin flush for use with transducer.	4. Secure all connections to prevent air emboli and bleeding.
a. Attach manometer to IV pole. The zero point of the manometer should be on a level with the patient's right atrium.	a. The level of the right atrium is at the 4th intercostal space midaxillary line (see Fig. 14-2—phlebostatic axis).
b. Calibrate/zero transducer and level port with patient's right atrium.	b. Mark midaxillary line with indelible ink for subsequent readings.
5. Place patient on ECG monitor.	5. Dysrhythmias may be noted during insertion as catheter is advanced.

Insertion Phase (by physician)

1. Physician dons gown, cap, and mask.	1. CVP insertion is a sterile procedure.
2. The CVP site is surgically cleansed. The physician introduces the CVP catheter percutaneously or by direct venous cutdown.	2. Patient may be asked to perform Valsalva maneuver to protect against chance of air embolus.
3. Assist patient to remain motionless during insertion.	

(continued)

Guidelines Central Venous Pressure Monitoring *(continued)*

Procedure *(continued)*	**Nursing Action**	**Rationale/Amplification**
	4. Monitor for dysrhythmias as catheter is threaded to great vein or right atrium.	
	5. Connect primed IV tubing/heparin flush system to catheter and allow IV solution to flow at a minimum rate to keep vein open (25 ml. maximum).	5. Catheter placement must be verified before hypertonic or blood products can be administered.
	6. The catheter should be sutured in place.	6. Prevents inadvertent catheter advancement or dislodgement
	7. Place a sterile occlusive dressing over site.	
	8. Obtain a chest x-ray.	8. Verify correct catheter position.

To Measure the CVP

1. Place the patient in a position of comfort. This is the baseline position used for subsequent readings.
2. Position the zero point of the manometer at the level of the right atrium (Fig. 14-3).

2. The zero point or baseline for the manometer should be on a level with the patient's right atrium. The middle of the right atrium is the midaxillary line in the 4th intercostal space.

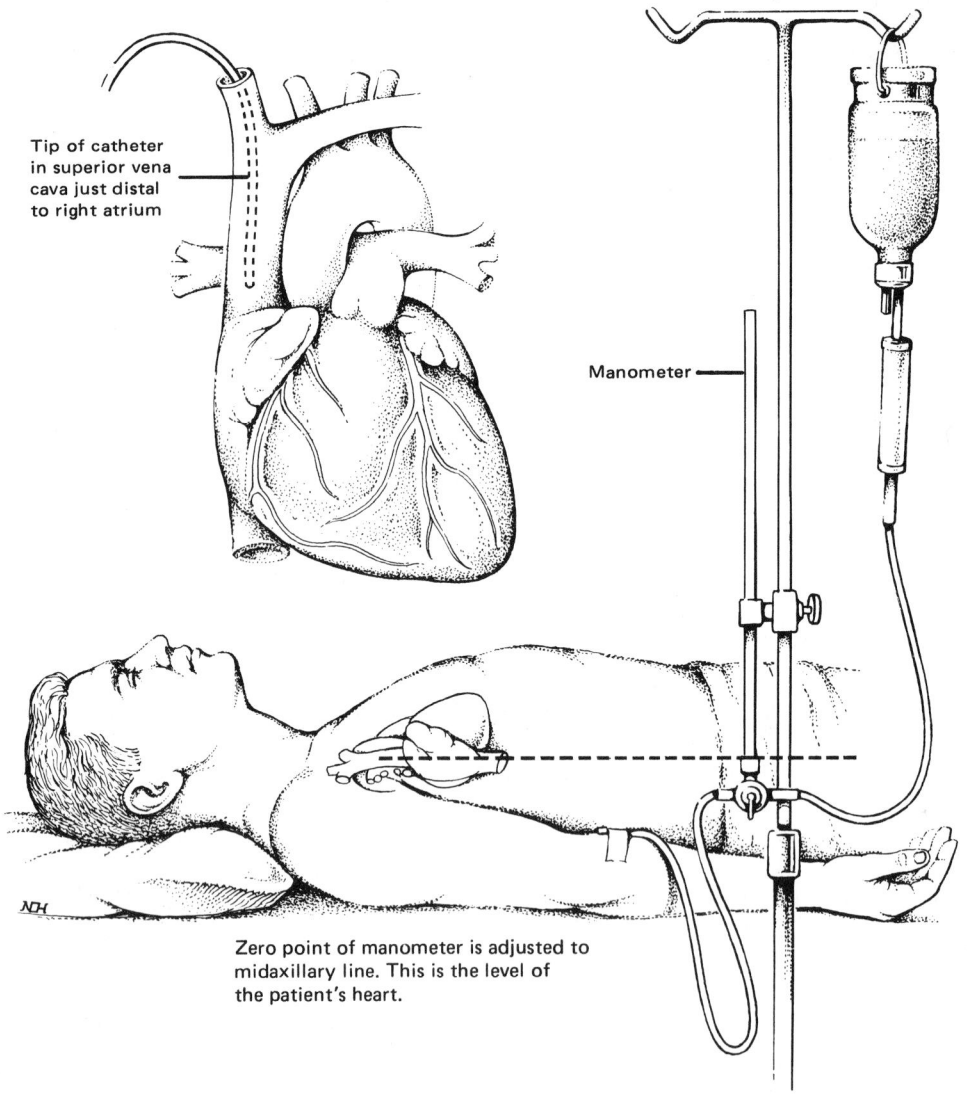

Tip of catheter in superior vena cava just distal to right atrium

Manometer

Zero point of manometer is adjusted to midaxillary line. This is the level of the patient's heart.

Figure 14-3. *Central venous pressure.*

Procedure *(continued)*	**Nursing Action**	**Rationale/Amplification**

Procedure *(continued)*

Nursing Action	Rationale/Amplification
3. Turn the stopcock so that the IV solution flows into the manometer, filling to about the 20–25 cm. level. Then turn stopcock so that solution in manometer flows into patient.	
4. Observe the fall in the height of the column of fluid in manometer. Record the level at which the solution stabilizes or stops moving downward. This is the central venous pressure. Record CVP and the position of the patient.	4. The column of fluid will fall until it meets an equal pressure (i.e., the patient's central venous pressure). The CVP reading is reflected by the height of a column of fluid in the manometer when there is open communication between the catheter and the manometer. The fluid in the manometer will fluctuate slightly with the patient's respirations. This confirms that the CVP line is not obstructed by clotted blood.
5. The CVP catheter may be connected to a transducer and an electrical monitor with either digital or calibrated CVP wave readout.	
6. The CVP may range from 5–12 cm. H_2O. (Absolute numerical values have not been agreed on.) Or, 2–6 mm. Hg.	6. The change in CVP is a more useful indication of adequacy of venous blood volume and alterations of cardiovascular function. The management of the patient is not based on one reading, but on repeated serial readings in correlation with patient's clinical status.
7. Assess the patient's clinical condition. Frequent changes in measurements (interpreted within the context of the clinical situation) will serve as a guide to detect whether the heart can handle its fluid load and whether hypovolemia or hypervolemia is present.	7. CVP is interpreted by considering the patient's entire clinical picture; hourly urine output, heart rate, blood pressure, cardiac output measurements. a. A CVP near zero indicates that the patient is hypovolemic (verified if rapid IV infusion causes patient to improve). b. A CVP above 15–20 cm. H_2O may be due to either hypervolemia or poor cardiac contractility.
8. Turn the stopcock again to allow IV solution to flow from solution bottle into the patient's veins.	8. When readings are not being made, flow is from a very slow microdrip to the catheter, bypassing the manometer.

Follow-up Phase

Nursing Action	Rationale/Amplification
1. Observe for complications. a. From catheter insertion: pneumothorax, hemothorax, air embolism, hematoma, and cardiac tamponade b. From indwelling catheter: infection, air embolism	1. Patient's complaints of new or different pain must be assessed closely. a. Signs/symptoms of air embolism include: severe shortness of breath, hypotension, hypoxia, rumbling murmur, cardiac arrest. b. If air embolism is suspected, immediately place patient in left lateral Trendelenburg position and administer oxygen. Air bubbles will be prevented from moving into the lungs and will be absorbed in 10–15 minutes in the right ventricular outflow tract.
2. Carry out ongoing nursing surveillance of the insertion site and maintain aseptic technique. a. Inspect entry site twice daily for signs of local inflammation/phlebitis. Remove immediately if there are any signs of infection. b. Change dressings as prescribed. c. Label to show date/time of change. d. Send the catheter tip for bacteriologic culture when it is removed.	

NURSING ALERT: A CVP line is a potential source of septicemia.

Cardiac Output

Cardiac output (CO) is the amount (volume) of blood ejected by the left ventricle into the aorta in 1 minute. The normal cardiac output is 4–8 liters/minute.

Underlying Concepts

Cardiac output is determined by stroke volume (SV) and heart rate (HR). The body alters CO by increases/decreases in one or both of these parameters. Cardiac output is maintained if the HR falls by an increase in SV. Likewise, a decrease in SV produces a compensatory rise in HR to keep the CO normal. Cardiac output will decrease if either of the determinants cannot inversely compensate for each other.

1. HR = number of cardiac contractions per minute. The integrity of the conduction system and nervous system innervation of the heart influence functioning of this determinant.
2. SV = amount of blood ejected from ventricle per beat. The amount of blood returning to the heart (preload), venous tone, resistance imposed on the ventricle prior to ejection (afterload), and the integrity of the cardiac muscle (contractility) influence the functioning of this determinant.

3. Adequacy of the CO to perfuse body tissues is evaluated by calculating the cardiac index (CI).

CI = CO divided by body surface area (BSA); BSA is determined through standard charts based on individual height and weight.

Assessment of Cardiac Output

Low cardiac output may be detected by:
1. Cyanosis or duskiness of buccal mucosa, nailbeds, and ear lobes
2. Cool, moist skin
3. Low urine output
4. Falling blood pressure
5. Changes in mental status
6. An increase in heart rate
7. Shortness of breath

Methods

1. Cardiac output is measured by a variety of techniques. In the clinical setting, it is usually measured by the thermodilution technique used in conjunction with a flow-directed balloon catheter. (Swan–Ganz catheter, p. 302).
2. The Swan–Ganz catheter is positioned in its final position in a branch of the pulmonary artery; it has a thermistor (external sensing device) situated 4 cm. from the tip of the catheter, which measures the temperature of the blood that flows by it.
3. Sterile dextrose or saline solution is injected through 1 lumen of the catheter. The solution mixes with the blood in the right side of the heart and flows to the pulmonary artery where blood temperature is detected by the thermistor.
4. A small computer converts the temperature changes into a direct reading of cardiac output.

Special Therapeutic Modalities

Guidelines Assisting the Patient Undergoing Pericardiocentesis

Pericardiocentesis is the puncturing of the percardial sac to aspirate fluid (Fig. 14-4). Excessive fluid within the pericardial sac can cause compression of the heart chambers, resulting in an acute decrease in cardiac output (cardiac tamponade).

Fluid accumulation can occur rapidly or slowly.

1. Acute—a rapid increase of fluid into pericardial space (as little as 200 ml.) causes a marked rise in intrapericardial pressure. Emergency intervention is required to prevent severe circulatory compromise.
2. Stable—slow accumulation of fluid into pericardial sac over weeks or months, causing pericardium to stretch and accommodate up to 2 liters of fluid without severe increases in intrapericardial pressure.

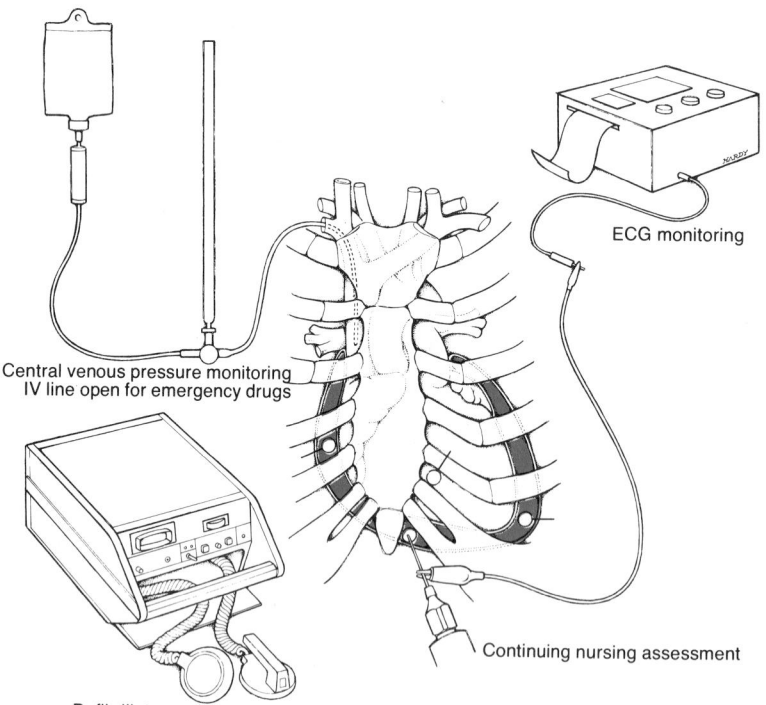

ECG monitoring

Central venous pressure monitoring
IV line open for emergency drugs

Continuing nursing assessment

Defibrillator and resuscitation equipment ready

Figure 14-4. *Nursing support of the patient undergoing pericardiocentesis. (Small circles indicate sites for pericardial aspiration.)*

Purpose

1. To remove fluid from the pericardial sac caused by:
   a. Infection
   b. Malignant neoplasm or lymphoma
   c. Trauma
      (1). Accidental—blunt or penetrating wounds
      (2). Iatrogenic—cardiac surgery; cardiopulmonary resuscitation; perforation of heart by catheter or transvenous pacemaker
   d. Drug reactions
   e. Radiation
   f. Myocardial infarction
   g. Chronic renal failure
2. To obtain fluid for diagnosis
3. To instill certain therapeutic drugs

Diagnostic Evaluation

Clinical Manifestations of Cardiac Tamponade

1. Rising venous pressure
2. Falling arterial blood pressure
3. Small, quiet heart, muffled heart sounds
4. Narrowing pulse pressure (difference between systolic and diastolic pressures)
5. Paradoxical pulse (abnormal degree of decline in systolic arterial blood pressure during inspiration). Assessment for paradoxical pulse (pulsus paradoxus) with cuff sphygmomanometry.
   a. Place the patient in recumbent position.
   b. Inflate cuff above the patient's palpated systolic pressure and the disappearance of Korotkoff sounds.
   c. Adjust the patient's position to enable reading of manometer and observation of patient's respiratory pattern.
   d. Slowly deflate cuff (2 mm. Hg per second) and listen for first Korotkoff sound at expiration; then observe the number of mm. the manometer falls while Korotkoff sounds cease on inspiration but are heard on expiration.
6. Decrease cuff until Korotkoff sounds are heard throughout respiratory cycle.
7. Record blood pressure and paradoxical pulse.
8. Palpation
   a. A decrease in amplitude during inspiration can be palpated at radial, femoral, or carotid arteries.
   b. Provides a gross assessment of paradoxical pulse and can be confirmed by cuff method. (Usually palpable if paradox is 15 mm. Hg.)
9. Distention of neck veins and inspiratory rise in venous pressure (Kussmaul's sign)
10. Apprehension; dyspnea
11. Tachypnea; pallor or cyanosis
12. Characteristic posture—sitting upright and leaning forward
13. Clinical shock

Clinical Manifestations of Pericarditis

1. Pleuritic chest pain
2. Tachycardia
3. Elevated temperature

ECG Manifestations—ST and T Wave Abnormalities

Echocardiogram—Determine Presence, Amount, and Distribution of Fluid

Equipment

Pericardiocentesis tray
Intracath set
Skin antiseptic
1%–2% lidocaine
Sterile gloves
ECG for monitoring purposes
Sterile ground wire—to be connected between pericardial needle and V lead of ECG (use alligator clip type connectors)
Equipment for cardiopulmonary resuscitation

Sites for Pericardiocentesis

1. Subxiphoid—needle inserted in the angle between left costal margin and xiphoid
2. Near cardiac apex, 2 cm. (0.8 inch) inside left border of cardiac dullness
3. To the left of the 5th or 6th interspace at the sternal margin
4. Right side of 4th intercostal space just inside border of dullness

(continued)

Guidelines Assisting the Patient Undergoing Pericardiocentesis *(continued)*

Procedure (Fig. 9-4)	**Nursing Action**	**Rationale/Amplification**

Preparatory Phase

1. Medicate the patient as prescribed.
2. Start a slow intravenous drip of saline or glucose.

3. Place the patient in a comfortable position with the head of the bed or treatment table raised to a 45-degree angle.
4. Apply the limb leads of the ECG to the patient.
5. Have defibrillator available for immediate use.
6. Have pacemaker available.
7. Open the tray using aseptic technique.

2. This preserves a route for intravenous therapy in the event of an emergency.
3. This position makes it easier to insert needle into pericardial sac.
4. The patient is monitored during the procedure by ECG.
5. In case the procedure has severe adverse effect.

Performance Phase (by physician)

1. The site is prepared with skin antiseptic; the area is draped with sterile towels and injected with anesthetic.
2. The pericardial aspiration needle is attached to a 50-ml. syringe by a 3-way stopcock. The V lead (precordial lead wire) of the ECG is attached to the hub of the aspirating needle by a sterile wire and alligator clips or clamp.
3. The needle is advanced slowly until fluid is obtained.

4. When the pericardial sac has been entered, a hemostat is clamped to the needle at the chest wall just where it penetrates the skin. Pericardial fluid is aspirated slowly.
5. Monitor the patient's ECG, blood pressure, and venous pressure constantly.

6. If a large amount of fluid is present, a polyethylene catheter may be inserted through a needle (an intracath) and left in the pericardial sac.
7. Watch for presence of bloody fluid. If blood accumulates rapidly, an immediate thoracotomy and cardiorrhaphy (suturing of heart muscle) may be indicated.

2. There is danger of laceration of myocardium/coronary artery and of cardiac dysrhythmias.

3. Fluid is generally aspirated at a depth of 2.5–4 cm. (1 to 1½ inches).
4. This prevents movement of the needle and further penetration while fluid is being removed. Aspirated fluid may be cloudy, clear, or bloody.
5. a. The ST segment rises if the point of the needle contacts the ventricle; there may be ventricular ectopic beats.
   b. The PR segment is elevated when the needle touches the atrium.
   c. Large, erratic QRS complexes indicate penetration of the myocardium.
6. An indwelling catheter left in the pericardial space permits further slow drainage of fluid and prevents recurrence of cardiac tamponade.
7. Bloody pericardial fluid may be due to trauma. Bloody pericardial effusion fluid does not clot readily, whereas blood obtained from inadvertent puncture of one of the heart chambers *does* clot.

Follow-up Phase

1. Monitor patient closely.
   a. Watch for rising venous pressure and falling arterial pressure.
   b. Auscultate the area over the heart.
2. Prepare for surgical drainage of pericardium if:
   a. Pericardial fluid repeatedly accumulates, or
   b. The aspiration is unsuccessful, or
   c. Complications develop
3. Assess for complications:
   Inadvertent puncture of heart chamber
   Dysrhythmias
   Puncture of lung, stomach, or liver
   Laceration of coronary artery or myocardium

1. Following pericardiocentesis, careful monitoring of blood pressure, venous pressure, and heart sounds will be necessary to indicate possible recurrence of tamponade. A repeated aspiration is then necessary.

2. In the presence of these signs, the patient is probably experiencing cardiac tamponade.

3. Listen for decrease in intensity of heart sounds indicating recurring cardiac tamponade.

Cardiac Pacing

A *cardiac pacemaker* is an electronic device that delivers direct stimulation to the heart. The purpose of the pacemaker is to initiate and maintain the heart rate when the heart's natural pacemaker is unable to do so.

Pacemaker Design

  A. Pulse Generator—contains the circuitry and batteries to generate the electrical signal.

  1. Pulse generators may be temporary (external) or permanently implanted (internal).

    a. Pulse generators are outside the body in temporary pacing systems and subcutaneously implanted in permanent systems.

    b. Temporary pacing systems are for short-term therapy; permanent pacing systems provide for long-term therapy.

    c. Temporary external pacemakers are used frequently during emergency situations requiring immediate cardiac pacing.

  2. The pulse generator in a permanent pacing system is encapsulated in a metal can, which protects the generator from electromagnetic interferences.

  3. A temporary pacing system generator is contained in a small box with dials for programming (see Fig. 14-5). The external box is attached to the patient with velcro straps.

    a. Transcutaneous external pacing systems house the generator in a piece of equipment similar to an ECG portable monitor. Dials for programming the unit and ECG monitoring are contained in the device.

    b. Electromechanical interference is more likely to occur with temporary systems.

    c. Temporary pacing systems use batteries, which need replacement based on use of device. The

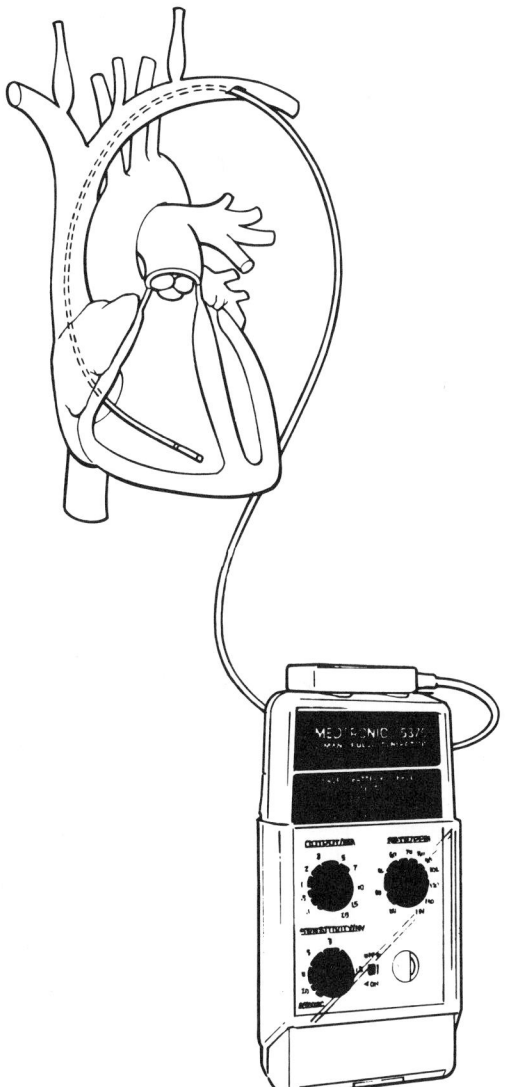
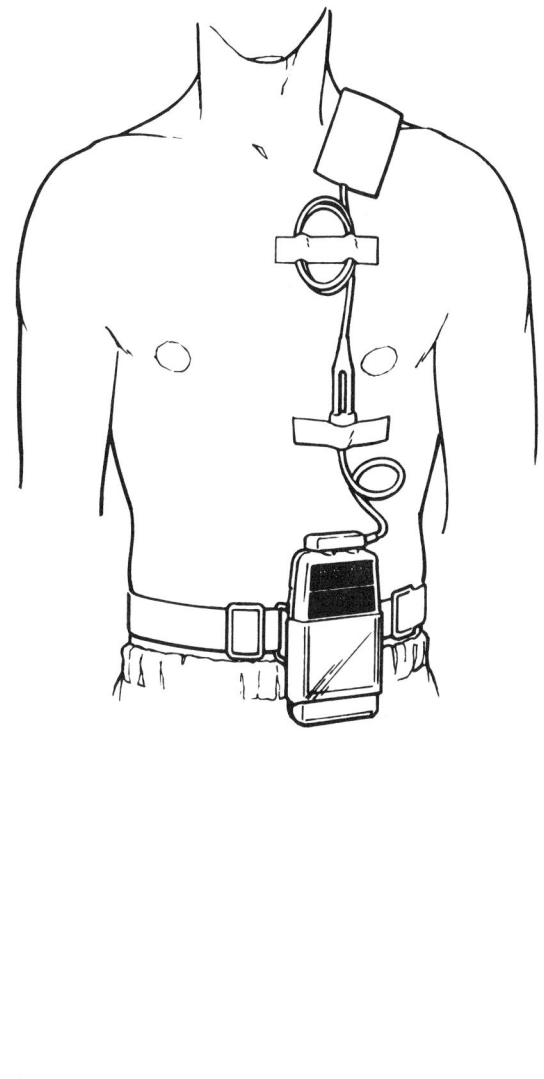

Figure 14-5. *Temporary external pacemaker. (Courtesy of MEDTRONIC, Inc.)*

transcutaneous system has rechargeable battery circuitry.

4. Permanent pacing systems use reliable power sources such as lithium or nuclear batteries. Lithium batteries have a projected life span of 8–12 years, whereas nuclear power sources, although used infrequently, offer a 20-year projected life span.

B. Pacemaker Lead—transmits the electrical signal from the pulse generator to the heart.

1. One or two leads may be placed in the heart.
   a. A "single-chamber" pacemaker has one lead in either the atrial or ventricular chamber. The sensing and pacing capabilities of the pacemaker are confined to the chamber where the lead is placed.
   b. "Dual-chamber" pacemakers have two leads. One lead is in the atrium and the other lead is located in the ventricle. Pacing and sensing can occur in both heart chambers, closely "mimicking" normal heart function (physiologic pacing).
   c. Pacemaker leads may be threaded through a vein into the right atrium and/or right ventricle (endocardial/transvenous approach) or introduced by direct penetration of the chest wall and attached to the left ventricle or right atrium (Fig. 14-6).
   d. Fixation devices located at the end of the pacemaker lead allow for secure attachment of the lead to the heart, reducing the possibility of lead dislodgement.
   e. Temporary lead(s) protrude from the incision and are connected to the external pulse generator; Permanent lead(s) are connected to the pulse generator implanted underneath the skin. (epicardial/transthoracic approach).

2. One (unipolar) or two (bipolar) electrodes are contained on the tip of the pacemaker lead in contact with the heart.

   a. A *unipolar* system better senses intrinsic cardiac signals, but the *bipolar* system is less affected by electromechanical interference.
   b. Unipolar leads produce a large spike on the ECG; bipolar leads produce a small, almost invisible spike.

3. Transcutaneous external pacing system noninvasively delivers electrical stimuli to the heart.
   a. The transcutaneous lead system consists of large pads containing electrodes.
   b. The pads or "leads" are applied to the anterior chest (V2, V3, or V5 position) and a second pad on the back (between the spine and left scapulae at heart level).
   c. The lead system then is connected to the external console.

Pacemaker Function

Cardiac pacing refers to the ability of the pacemaker to stimulate either the atrium, the ventricle, or both heart chambers in sequence and initiate electrical depolarization and cardiac contraction. Cardiac pacing is evidenced on the ECG by the presence of a "spike" or "pacing artifact."

A. Pacing Functions

1. *Atrial pacing*—direct stimulation of the right atrium producing a "spike" on the ECG preceding a P wave and normal ventricular conduction.
2. *Ventricular pacing*—direct stimulation of the right or left ventricle producing a "spike" on the ECG preceding a QRS complex.
3. *Atrioventricular pacing*—direct stimulation of the right atria and either ventricle in sequence; mimics normal cardiac conduction, allowing the atria to contract prior to the ventricles ("Atrial kick" received by the ventricles allows for an increase in cardiac output.).

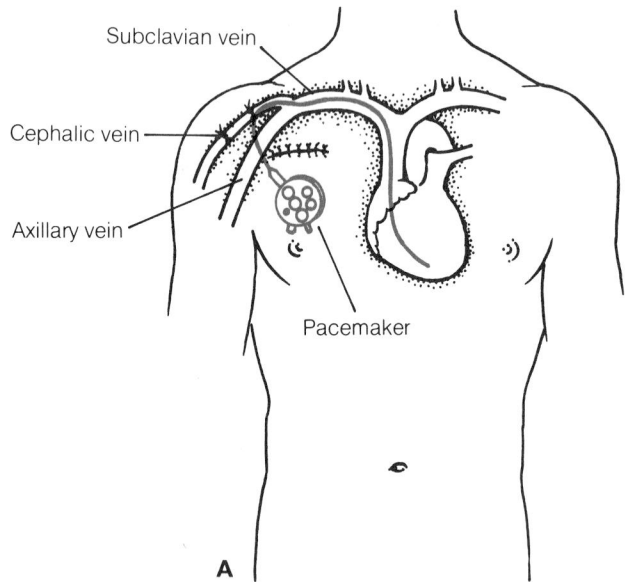

Transvenous installation of a permanent pacemaker.

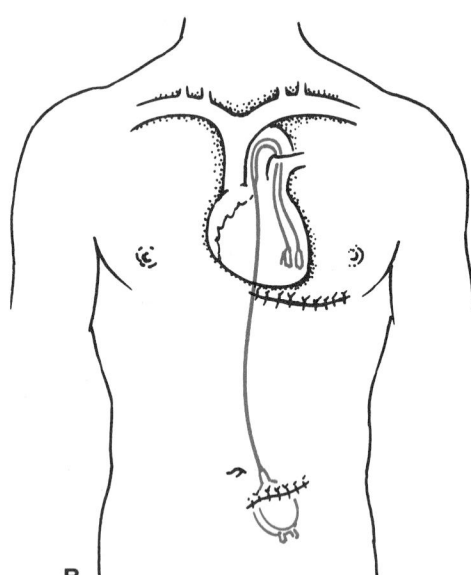

Transthoracic installation of a permanent pacemaker.

Figure 14-6. *(A) The catheter is unipolar and is threaded to the apical area of the right ventricle via a major vein. (B) The catheter is bipolar and is passed through an opening in the chest wall and is sutured to the external surface of the left ventricle.*

B. Sensing Functions

Cardiac pacemakers have the ability to "see" intrinsic cardiac activity when it occurs (sensing).

1. *Demand*—ability to "sense" intrinsic cardiac activity and deliver a pacing stimulus only if the heart rate falls below a preset rate limit.
2. *Fixed*—no ability to "sense" intrinsic cardiac activity; the pacemaker is unable to "synchronize" with the heart's natural activity and consistently delivers a pacing stimulus at a preset rate.
3. *Triggered*—ability to deliver pacing stimuli in response to "sensing" a cardiac event.
   a. "Sees" atrial activity (P waves) and delivers a pacing spike to the ventricle after an appropriate delay (usually 0.16 seconds, similar to PR interval).
   b. Maintains atrioventricular synchrony and increases heart rate based on increases in the body demands that occur with exercise or during stress.
   c. "Physiologic" sensors are currently being developed as alternatives to "trigger" a ventricular response, as many patients have atrial dysfunction.
   d. "Sensor-driven" rate-responsive pacemakers do not sense atrial activity; a triggered ventricular beat occurs when the pacemaker senses either increases in muscle activity, temperature, oxygen utilization, or changes in blood pH.

C. Capture Function

The pacemaker's ability to generate a response from the heart (contraction) after electrical stimulation is referred to as *capture*.

Pacemaker Codes

The Intersociety Commission for Heart Disease (ICHD) has established a five-letter code (1984) to describe the normal functioning of today's sophisticated pacemakers.

1. Letters 1, 2, 3
   a. The first letter of the code refers to the chamber paced.
   b. The second letter refers to the chamber sensed.
   c. The third letter refers to the response to sensing.
2. Letters 4 and 5
   a. The fourth and fifth letters refer to special functions of today's pacemakers.
   b. The fourth letter refers to the programmability of the pacemaker.
   c. The fifth letter refers to the various modes of operation for antitachycardic pacemakers.
3. These pacemakers are used to control tachydysrhythmias in patients who have failed conventional drug therapy.

Clinical Indications

1. Symptomatic bradydysrhythmias
2. Symptomatic heart block
   a. Mobitz II second-degree heart block
   b. Complete heart block
   c. Bifascicular and trifascicular bundle branch blocks
3. Prophylaxis
   a. Following acute MI: dysrhythmia and conduction defects
   b. Before or following cardiac surgery
   c. During diagnostic testing:
      (1) Cardiac catheterization
      (2) Electrophysiology studies
      (3) Percutaneous coronary angioplasty
      (4) Stress testing
      (5) Before permanent pacing
4. Tachydysrhythmias; to break rapid rhythm disturbances
   a. Supraventricular
   b. Ventricular

Nursing Assessment

1. Question patient about symptoms experienced.
2. Review findings on past and present health status.
3. Assess anxiety level of patient preoperatively and postoperatively: *mild*—increased alertness; *moderate*—decreased ability to communicate; *severe*—drastic decrease in ability to communicate; and *panic*—inability to communicate, distortion of reality. Learning cannot take place in severe or panic level of anxiety.
4. Assess patient's knowledge level of procedure: NPO prior to procedure; IV line insertion; performed in operating or special procedures room with fluoroscope and continuous ECG monitoring; local anesthetic to minimize discomfort; sedation.
5. Evaluate cognitive and behavioral status.
6. Evaluate patient's level of activity and those activities that patient engages in frequently for enjoyment.
7. Identify patient's social support network and potential caregivers.
8. Ask patient to verbalize his thoughts about receiving and living with a pacemaker.
9. Assess for verbal and nonverbal cues indicative of nonacceptance of pacemaker.
10. Assess patient's readiness to learn about his pacemaker.

Nursing Diagnoses

1. Altered cardiac output: (potential for decrease) related to pacemaker malfunction and pacemaker-induced dysrhythmias
2. Potential for injury related to pneumothorax, hemothorax, bleeding, microshock, and accidental malfunction
3. Potential for infection related to surgical implantation of pacemaker generator and/or leads
4. Anxiety related to pacemaker insertion, fear of death, lack of knowledge, and role change
5. Impaired physical mobility related to imposed restrictions of arm movement and bedrest
6. Pain related to surgical incision and transcutaneous external pacing stimuli
7. Self-concept, disturbance in body image, related to pacemaker implantation.

Nursing Interventions

A. Maintaining Optimal Cardiac Rhythm

1. Record the following information after insertion of the pacemaker:
   a. Pacemaker manufacturer, model, and lead type
   b. Operating mode (based on ICHD code, see opposite column)
   c. Programmed settings: lower rate limit; upper rate limit; AV delay; pacing thresholds
   d. Patient's underlying rhythm
   e. Patient's response to procedure
2. Attach ECG electrodes for continuous monitoring of heart rate and rhythm.
   a. Set alarm limits two beats below lower rate limit and two beats above upper rate limits (assures im-

mediate detection of pacemaker malfunction or failure).
  b. Keep alarms on at all times.
  c. Analyze ECG strip every 4 hours.
    (1) Identify presence/absence of pacing artifact.
    (2) Differentiate paced P waves and paced QRS complexes from spontaneous beats.
    (3) Measure AV delay (if pacemaker AV sequential).
    (4) Determine the paced rate.
    (5) Analyze the paced rhythm for presence and consistency of capture (every pacing spike is followed by atrial and/or ventricular depolarization).
    (6) Analyze the rhythm for presence and consistency of proper sensing. (After a spontaneous beat the pacemaker should not fire unless the interval between the spontaneous beat and the paced beat equals the lower pacing rate and/or the paced beat follows the programmed AV delay.)
3. Monitor vital signs every 15 minutes until stable; then as directed.
4. Monitor urine output and level of consciousness—ensures adequate cardiac output achieved with paced rhythm.
5. Observe for the presence of dysrhythmias (ventricular ectopic activity can occur because of irritation of ventricular wall by lead wire).
  a. Monitor for competitive rhythms such as runs of atrial fibrillation or flutter, accelerated junctional or idioventricular or ventricular tachycardia.
  b. Notify physician of all dysrhythmias.
  c. Administer antidysrhythmic therapy as directed.
6. Obtain 12-lead ECG daily as directed.
7. Transport patient to other parts of hospital with portable ECG monitoring and nurse. (Patients with temporary pacemakers should never be placed in unmonitored areas.)

B. Monitoring and Preventing Complications

1. Note that a postinsertion chest x-ray has been taken to ensure correct lead wire position and that no fluid is in lungs.
2. Monitor for signs/symptoms of hemothorax or pneumothorax.
  a. Hemothorax—inadvertent puncture of the subclavian vein or artery; can cause fatal hemorrhage; observe for diaphoresis, hypotension, and restlessness; immediate surgical intervention may be necessary.
  b. Pneumothorax—inadvertent puncture of the lung; observe for acute onset of dyspnea, cyanosis, chest pain, absent breath sounds over involved lung, acute anxiety, hypotension. Prepare for chest tube insertion.
3. Evaluate continually for evidence of bleeding.
  a. Check incision site frequently for bleeding.
    (1) Apply manual pressure and pressure dressing to control bleeding.
    (2) Palpate for pulses distal to insertion site. (Swelling of tissues from bleeding may impede arterial flow.)
4. Monitor for evidence of lead migration and perforation of heart.
  a. Observe for muscle twitching and/or hiccups (may indicate chest wall or diaphragmatic pacing).
  b. Evaluate patient's complaints of chest pain (may indicate perforation of pericardial sac).

  c. Auscultate for pericardial friction rub.
  d. Observe for signs/symptoms of cardiac tamponade: distant heart sounds, distended neck veins, pulsus paradoxus.
5. Provide an electrically safe environment for patient—stray electrical current can enter the heart through temporary pacemaker lead system and induce dysrhythmias.
  a. Protect exposed parts of electrode lead terminal in temporary pacing systems with a rubber glove. (Newer external generators have the lead terminals enclosed in a case; a rubber glove is not necessary.)
  b. Wear rubber gloves whenever touching temporary pacing leads. (Static electricity from your hands can enter the patient's body through the lead system.)
  c. Make sure all equipment is grounded with 3-prong plugs inserted into a proper outlet; biomedical engineer should routinely check room to assure safe environment.
  d. Temporary epicardial pacing wires (most common after cardiac surgery) should have the terminal needles protected by a plastic tube; place tube in rubber glove to protect it from fluids or electrical current.
6. Be aware of hazards in the hospital environment that can interfere with pacemaker function or cause pacemaker failure and/or permanent pacemaker damage.
  a. Avoid use of electric razors.
  b. Avoid direct placement of defibrillator paddles over pacemaker generator; anterior placement of paddles should be 4–5 inches away from pacemaker; always evaluate pacemaker function after defibrillation.
  c. Electrocautery devices and transcutaneous nerve stimulators (TENS units) pose a risk.
  d. Patients with permanent pacemakers should never be exposed to magnetic resonance imaging (MRI), because the strength of the magnetic field may alter or erase pacemaker program memory.
  e. Caution must be used if patient is to receive radiation therapy; the pacemaker should be repositioned if unit lies directly in the radiation field.
7. Prevent possible accidental pacemaker malfunctions.
  a. Use clear plastic covering over external temporary generators at all times (eliminates potential manipulation of programmed settings).
  b. Secure temporary pacemaker generator to patient's chest or waist; never hang on IV pole.
  c. Transfer of patient from bed to stretcher should only be attempted with an adequate number of personnel, so that patient can remain passive; caution personnel to avoid underarm lifts.
  d. Place a sign over patient's bed alerting personnel to presence of temporary pacemaker.
  e. Evaluate transcutaneous pacing electrodes every 2 hours for secure contact to chest wall; change electrode pads as directed or if patient is diaphoretic.
8. Monitor for electrolyte imbalances, hypoxia, and myocardial ischemia. (The amount of energy the pacemaker needs to stimulate depolarization may need adjustment if any of these are present.)

C. Avoiding Infection

1. Take temperature every 4 hours; notify physician of elevations. (Suspect pacemaker system for infection source if elevation occurs.)

2. Observe incision site for signs/symptoms of local infection: redness, purulent drainage, warmth, soreness.
3. Be alert to manifestations of bacteremia. (Patients with endocardial leads are susceptible to endocarditis; see Endocarditis, p. 337.)
4. Clean incision site as directed, using sterile technique.
5. Monitor vein through which the pacing lead wire was placed for evidence of phlebitis.
6. Evaluate patient's complaints of increasing tenderness and discomfort at incision site.
7. Administer antibiotic therapy as prescribed.

D. Alleviating Anxiety

1. Offer careful explanations regarding anticipated procedures and treatments and answer the patient's questions with concise explanations. Repeat as necessary. Information is geared to level of patient. (Patients have difficulty processing input—do not overload.)
   a. Preoperatively—reinforce explanation of procedure to the patient and family.
   b. Postoperatively—explain to the patient the nature and purpose of monitoring equipment (ECG), activity restrictions, and IV line. Monitoring will be continuous for several days, but the patient will be able to walk around in room and use bedside commode while being monitored.
   c. Explain to the patient that analgesics will be administered for pain at implantation site.
2. Explore with patient (preoperatively and postoperatively) those factors that evoke feelings of anxiety.
3. Converse with the patient frequently and convey willingness to listen.
4. Encourage the patient to use coping mechanisms to overcome anxieties—talking, crying, walking.
5. Encourage the patient to accept responsibility for care.
   a. Review plan of care with the patient.
   b. Encourage the patient to make decisions regarding a daily schedule of self-care activities.
   c. Engage the patient in goal-setting—establish with the patient priorities of care, time frames to accomplish goals up until discharge.
6. Encourage family members to offer support and understanding to the patient through a willingness to listen to the patient's concerns.
7. Monitor for unwarranted fears expressed by the patient (commonly, pacemaker failure) and provide explanations to alleviate fear. Explain to the patient life expectancy of batteries and the measures taken to check for failure (see Patient Education, below).
8. Talk to family members about their fears and offer explanations to help allay the fears (avoids the transmission of unwarranted fears to the patient).
9. Explore with the patient his feelings toward limitations secondary to illness.
   a. Discuss with the patient current life-style prior to need for pacemaker.
   b. Discuss with the patient areas of independence and dependence in his life.
   c. Discuss with the patient the importance of learning how to live with a pacemaker.
   d. Encourage family members to offer support and express to the patient their willingness to help.

E. Adhering to Activity Restrictions

1. Explain the purpose for bedrest (24–48 hours) and immobilization of extremity nearest to permanent or temporary pacemaker lead implant (allows for stabilization of lead in heart and prevents lead dislodgement).

2. Prevent complications of bedrest.
   a. Encourage patient to take deep breaths frequently each hour—promotes pulmonary function; caution against vigorous coughing (lead dislodgement may occur).
   b. Instruct patient in dorsiflexion exercises of ankles and tightening of calf muscles—promotes venous return and prevents venous stasis; exercises should be done hourly.

GERONTOLOGIC ALERT: Elderly patients require vigilant monitoring for evidence of altered skin integrity. Use foam or water mattresses and frequently position patient, to prevent skin breakdown and promote comfort.

3. Restrict movement of affected extremity.
   a. Place arm nearest to permanent pacemaker implant in sling as directed; extremity with temporary pacing wire should be immobilized and kept straight as prescribed.
   b. Instruct patient to gradually resume range of motion of extremity as directed (usually 24 hours for permanent implants); avoid over-the-head motions for approximately 5 days.
   c. Evaluate patient's arm movements to assure normal range of motion progression; assist patient with passive range of motion of extremity as necessary (prevents development of shoulder stiffness caused by prolonged joint immobility); consult physical therapy as directed if stiffness and pain occur.
4. Assist patients with ADLs as appropriate.

F. Minimizing Pain

1. Prepare patient for discomfort that may be experienced following pacemaker implant or initiation of transcutaneous pacing.
   a. Explain to patient that incisional pain will occur postprocedure; pain will subside after the first week, but some soreness will be experienced for up to 3–4 weeks.
   b. Explain to patient the potential for discomfort during transcutaneous pacing; assure patient that the lowest energy possible will be used and analgesics will be given.
2. Administer analgesics as directed; attempt to coincide peak analgesic effect with performance of range-of-motion exercises and ADLs.
3. Offer back rubs to promote relaxation.
4. Provide patient with diversional activities.
5. Evaluate effectiveness of pain-relieving modalities.

G. Maintaining a Positive Body Image

1. Encourage the patient to express concerns regarding self-image and pacer implant.
2. Reassure the patient that sexual activity and modes of dressing will not be altered by pacemaker implantation.
3. Offer the patient the opportunity to talk to others who have had a pacemaker implantation.
4. Encourage spouse of patient or significant other to discuss concerns of self-image with the patient.

Patient Education/Discharge Planning

A. General Principles

1. Patient teaching should be individualized, provide for active participation by patient, and if possible, include at least one significant other of patient.

2. To evaluate the patient's retention of material, the patient should be asked to repeat in his own words the concepts discussed and return a demonstration of the skills presented.

B. **Anatomy and Physiology of the Heart**—use diagrams to identify heart structure, conduction system, area where pacemaker is inserted, and why the pacemaker is needed.

C. **Introduction to Pacemaker**

1. Give the patient the manufacturer's instructions (for his particular pacemaker) and help him to become familiar with his pacemaker.
2. If available, give the patient a pacemaker to hold and identify unique features of patient's pacemaker; or show patient picture of pacemaker.
3. Explain to patient the purpose and function of the component parts of the pacemaker: generator and lead system.
4. Reassure patient that normal activities will be able to be resumed.
   a. Explain to patient that it takes about 2 months to develop full range-of-motion of arm (fibrosis occurs around the lead and stabilizes it in heart).
      (1) Instruct patient not to lift items over 3 lbs. or perform difficult arm maneuvers.
      (2) Caution patient against excessive stretching or bending exercises.
      (3) Avoid contact sports, tennis, golfing, bowling, and yardwork until resumption of these activities is permitted by physician.
      (4) Caution patient not to fire rifle with it resting over pacemaker implant.
      (5) Sexual activity may be resumed when desired.
   b. Instruct patient to gauge activities according to sensations of moderate pain in arm or site of implant and stretching sensation in and around implant site.

D. **Pacemaker Failure**

1. Teach the patient to check his own pulse rate at least every week for 1 full minute at rest to be certain that preset rate remains constant. (Patients may check pulse daily to assure all is well and promote a sense of control.)
2. Teach the patient to:
   a. Report *immediately* any slowing of pulse greater than 4–5 beats per minute, or any increase in pulse rate.
   b. Report signs and symptom of dizziness, fainting, palpitation, prolonged hiccups, and chest pain to physician immediately—indicative of pacemaker failure.
   c. Take pulse while these feelings are being experienced.
3. Encourage the patient to wear identification bracelet and carry pacemaker identification card that lists his pacemaker type, rate, physician's name, and the hospital where the pacemaker was inserted; encourage significant other to keep a card with patient's pacemaker information so that someone else will have it.

E. **Electromagnetic Interference**

Advise the patient that improvements in pacemaker design have reduced problems of electromagnetic interference (EMI).

1. High-energy radar, television and radio transmitters, industrial arc welders, electrocautery equipment, transcutaneous nerve stimulators (TENS), large motors (cars, boats), oversized magnets (magnetic resonance imaging equipment found at hospitals, junkyards where magnets lift cars), ultrasonic dental cleaning equipment, electric razors.
   a. Avoid direct contact and close proximity with these devices because they may affect the functioning of the pacemaker. (In many cases no damage to the generator will occur; devices may confuse the pacemaker and readjust the settings.)
   b. Teach the patient that if dizziness or sensations of a fast heart rate occur to move 4–6 feet away from source and check pulse. Pulse should return to normal.
2. Antitheft devices and airport security alarms will not affect pacemaker function, although the metal may trigger the alarm. Instruct patient to show his ID card.
3. Household and kitchen appliances will not affect pacemaker function. Microwave ovens are no longer a threat to pacemaker operation (old warning signs may still be near microwave ovens). Instruct patient to stand 4 feet away from oven if still concerned.

F. **Care of Pacemaker Site**

1. Advise patient to wear loose-fitting clothing around the area of pacemaker implantation until healing has taken place.
2. Watch for signs and symptoms of infection around generator and leads—fever, heat, pain, skin breakdown at implant site.
3. Advise patient to keep incision clean and dry. Encourage tub baths for the first 10 days after pacemaker implant rather than showers.
   a. Instruct patient not to scrub incision site or clean site with bath water.
   b. Teach patient to clean incision site with antiseptic as directed.
4. Explain to patient that healing will take approximately 3 months.
   a. Instruct patient to maintain a well-balanced diet to promote healing.

GERONTOLOGIC ALERT: Elderly patients may experience delayed wound healing because of poor nutritional status. Evaluate nutritional intake carefully and offer a balanced diet to ensure proper healing.

5. Instruct patient to inform dentist of pacemaker so that antibiotic prophylaxis can be administered prior to extractions or vigorous dental cleaning (prevents development of endocarditis (see Endocarditis, p. 337).

G. **Follow-up**

1. See that the patient has a copy of his ECG tracing (according to agency policy)—for future comparisons. Encourage patient to have regular pacemaker checkup (preferably at a pacemaker clinic) for monitoring function and integrity of his pacemaker.
2. Transtelephonic evaluation of implanted cardiac pacemakers for battery and electrode failure is available.
3. Review medications with the patient prior to discharge.
4. Inform the patient that the pulse generator will have to be surgically removed for a variety of reasons (battery depletion) and replaced; improved power sources and circuitry make reoperation less frequent.
   a. Relatively simple procedure performed under local anesthesia.

b. Incision made; old generator disconnected from electrode catheter.

c. New generator connected and placed in existing subcutaneous pocket; incision closed.

d. Prophylactic antibiotics usually administered.

e. Patient discharged from hospital 1–3 days postoperatively.

Evaluation

1. Maintains an optimal cardiac output; does not demonstrate signs and symptoms of pacemaker malfunction
2. Experiences no complications—exhibits no signs/symptoms of incisional or intrathoracic bleeding or pneumothorax; breath sounds audible bilaterally and throughout lung fields; absence of hematoma; blood pressure within normal limits; no pericardial friction rub; experiences no dysrhythmias.
3. Remains free of infection—exhibits no signs/symptoms of septicemia or phlebitis; temperature normal; incision free of redness
4. Achieves a reduction in anxiety—identifies sources of anxiety and communicates ability to cope with anxiety; recognizes factors causing fears—identifies fears related to pacemaker implant, uses family members for support, communicates ability to cope with fears; resumes previous roles and activities
5. Adheres to activity restrictions; absence of skin breakdown; range-of-motion of affected extremity normal
6. Maintains comfort level: verbalizes relief of incisional pain; engages in normal activities
7. Maintains a positive body image—expresses feelings of well-being

Automatic Implantable Defibrillator

The *automatic implantable defibrillator* is a device that delivers electrical shocks directly to the heart muscle (defibrillation) in order to terminate lethal dysrhythmias: ventricular fibrillation and ventricular tachycardia (Fig. 14-7). The automatic implantable defibrillator is surgically placed by one of four approaches: lateral thoracotomy, median sternotomy (in conjunction with cardiac surgery), subxiphoid, or subintercostal.

Design

The implantable defibrillator is slightly larger than a pacemaker and consists of two component parts:

1. *Pulse generator*—contains the circuitry and battery to detect dysrhythmias and generate the electrical shock. The generator is placed in a subcutaneous pocket in the upper abdominal quadrant.
   a. Battery life depends on usage. Longevity is estimated at 12–24 months or 100 shocks.
   b. The direct current electrical shock delivered is 25–32 joules.
2. *Lead system*—two sets of leads are used and can be placed in various positions on or in the heart.
   a. One set of lead electrodes senses lethal dysrhythmias in the heart.
   b. The other set of lead electrodes transmits the electrical shock from the pulse generator to the heart.
3. The implantable defibrillator is noninvasively turned on and off by a doughnut-shaped magnet.

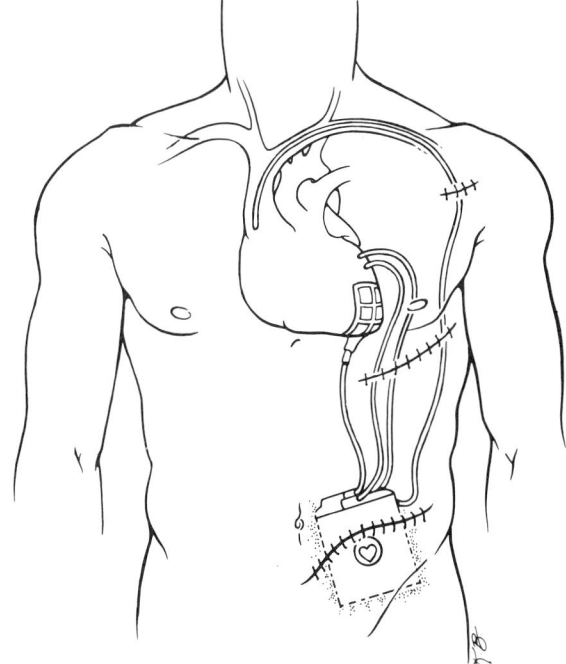

Figure 14-7. *Automatic implantable defibrillator.*

Function

Four electrical shocks are delivered in a programmed sequence:

1. The device allows 10–35 seconds to detect a lethal dysrhythmia, charge, and "defibrillate" the heart. The lethal dysrhythmia must meet two programmed criteria (rate and amount of time spent from the isoelectric line) to trigger the device to emit an initial 25-joule electrical shock.
2. Nontermination of the lethal dysrhythmia by the initial shock triggers the device to continue the sequence (detect, charge, and defibrillate) until a total of four or five shocks has been delivered (number of shocks depends on device model implanted).
   a. Subsequent shocks are slightly higher, at 30–32 joules.
   b. The total sequence lasts approximately 2 minutes.
3. Nontermination of the lethal dysrhythmia after the shock sequence signals the device to revert to the "detection" mode of operation and not to reinitiate the shocking sequence. The device will reinitiate the shocking sequence only if a rhythm other than the lethal dysrhythmia is detected and maintained for at least 35 seconds. If this criteria is met and another lethal dysrhythmia is detected, the device will cycle through the shocking sequence again.
4. Termination of a lethal dysrhythmia at any time during the shocking sequence signals the device to interrupt the sequence, return to a detection mode and reinitiate the shocking sequence if another lethal dysrhythmia is detected.

Indications

1. Failure of maximal conventional medical therapy to control ventricular fibrillation and/or ventricular

tachycardia (as determined by electrophysiology studies)
2. Survival of one episode of sudden cardiac death not associated with acute myocardial infarction.

Complications

1. Infection
2. Bleeding
3. Device failure
4. Pacemaker interaction
5. Constrictive pericarditis

Nursing Interventions

A. Decreasing Anxiety

1. Explain to patient and family reason for implant, surgical procedure, and pre- and postprocedure management:
   a. Performed in the operating room; anesthesia required.
   b. Incision location
   c. Endotracheal intubation; chest tubes
   d. Intravenous line; continuous ECG monitoring
   e. Early mobilization after procedure
   f. Cough and deep breathing exercises
   g. Management of incisional pain
   h. Turning on the device (usually 48–72 hours post-implantation)
2. Provide emotional support to patient and family.
   a. Encourage patient and family to verbalize fears and/or expectations of hospitalization, life-style adjustments, self-concept, body image, and device malfunction (misfiring/failure to fire).
   b. Reinforce to patient that daily activities will not increase the risk of the device misfiring.
   c. Explain the sensation that might be felt if the device fires and the patient is conscious. (Many patients will become unconscious before the device fires and therefore feel no sensations.) Sensations experienced in conscious patients vary, but are often described as a severe chest blow.
3. Allow patient to participate in his care as much as possible.
   a. Encourage patient to dress in street clothes during hospitalization (loose-fitting clothes are recommended to prevent chafing/irritation at implant site).
   b. Allow patient to look at incision site.
   c. Offer patient instructional booklets on the device.

B. Preventing Infection

1. Check temperature every 4 hours; notify physician of elevations (Suspect defibrillator system as infection source if elevation occurs; infections commonly occur within 5–10 days.).
2. Evaluate incision site every 4 hours; note redness, swelling, purulent/serous drainage; palpate around incision site for tenderness, warmth, and/or drainage.
3. Culture all drainage from incision.
4. Evaluate incision for tissue erosion.
5. Monitor WBC count and differential.
6. Cleanse incision and change dressing as directed, using aseptic technique.
7. Encourage a high-caloric/high-protein diet to promote wound healing and decrease chance of postoperative complications.

> **GERONTOLOGIC ALERT:** Elderly patients may not demonstrate abnormal temperature elevations with infections and experience prolonged wound healing.

C. Maintaining Hemodynamic Stability

1. Monitor vital signs frequently until stable.
2. Evaluate incision site for evidence of bleeding and/or hematoma.
3. Monitor chest tube drainage for excessive amount and note color.
4. Evaluate urine output.
5. Be alert to potential for dysrhythmias postoperatively. (Manipulation of heart and swelling may induce dysrhythmias 24–48 hours after implant.)
6. Treat dysrhythmias as directed—antidysrhythmic therapy and/or electrical countershock (standard anterior paddle placement or anterior/posterior paddle placement is recommended); correct underlying causes such as hypoxia and/or electrolyte disturbances.

> **NURSING ALERT:** CPR should be started immediately on any patient with an implantable defibrillator who becomes unconscious and has no pulse. A slight "buzz" sensation will be felt if the implanted device delivers a shock but it is not harmful. Gloves may be worn to minimize the sensation.

7. Evaluate carefully all complaints of chest pain (noncardiac pain may be due to lead fracture or dislodgement; pain may be noted along wire pathways).
8. Auscultate heart sounds every 4 hours for presence of friction rub.

D. Maintaining Pulmonary Function

1. Ask patient to take several deep breaths every hour to expand lung fields.
2. Encourage cough and deep breathing exercises frequently; medicate with analgesics prior to exercises and provide a pillow for splinting.
3. Monitor use of incentive spirometer.
4. Elevate head of bed to promote adequate ventilation.
5. Auscultate lung fields every 4 hours.
6. Assist with position changes every 2 hours while on bedrest.
7. Encourage early ambulation.

Patient Education/Discharge Planning

Goals:
Assist patient and family to understand the function of the device, impact of device on life-style, and follow-up evaluation.

A. Introduction to Implantable Defibrillator

1. Review anatomy of the heart with emphasis on the conduction system, using a diagram of the heart.
2. Give accurate explanations, using correct medical terminology (allows patient to interact with the health care team more effectively), regarding reason for device implantation, component parts of system, function of device.
   a. Use manufacturer's instructional booklet and video presentation about the device.
   b. Encourage family members to participate in education process.

B. Living With the Implantable Defibrillator

1. Instruct patient and family on actions to be taken should the device fire.
   a. Explain signs/symptoms that may be experienced if a lethal dysrhythmia occurs: palpitations, dizziness, shortness of breath, chest pain.
   b. If signs/symptoms are experienced, lie down and try to call "911" for help if alone.
   c. Family members should check for a pulse if patient becomes unconscious. CPR should be started immediately if no pulse is present and "911" has been called.
   d. Reinforce that shocks emitted from device are not harmful, and CPR should never be delayed to wait for the device to complete the shocking sequence.
   e. If patient remains conscious and/or is unconscious with a pulse, family members should monitor patient during episode, continually assessing for a pulse during shocking sequence. After the episode, follow instructions as directed by physician.
   f. Keep a diary of all episodes and shocks received from device. Include date, time, and associated symptoms.
2. Explore with patient/family fears regarding failure of device, sensation associated with a shock, and injury to others if a shock occurs.
   a. Sensations experienced vary, but most commonly described as a severe blow to the chest.
   b. No injury will occur to others if in contact with patient during a shock; a slight shock may be felt by your partner if the device fires during sexual intercourse.
   c. Battery life depends on frequency of use. The device is evaluated every 2 months for 1 year and every month thereafter.
3. Review sources of electromechanical interference that should be avoided (see Pacemakers, p. 313).
   a. The device will usually not become damaged, but may be turned off due to interference.
   b. A "beeping" sound may be audible if device is turned off by interferences.
   c. Airport security devices and hand-held airport security devices may affect device function. These devices must be avoided. Carry medic-alert card and show to security personnel.
   d. Areas/diagnostic tests using large magnets must be avoided.
   e. Notify physician as directed for contact with sources of potential interference.
4. Notify dentist of implanted device, as prophylaxis with antibiotics may be necessary prior to dental care (see endocarditis, p. 337).
5. Review with physician resumption of activities such as driving and sports.

C. Predischarge Instructions

1. Review care of incision site (see Pacemakers, p. 316).
2. Loose-fitting clothing should be worn until healing takes place.
3. Provide medic-alert card; encourage carrying card at all times and obtaining a corresponding medic-alert bracelet.
4. Reinforce how to keep diary of episodes and date of 2-month follow-up appointment.
5. Provide information to family members regarding CPR training courses.

Coronary Artery Disease

Coronary artery disease (CAD) is characterized by the accumulation of fatty deposits along the innermost layer of the coronary arteries. The fatty deposits may develop in childhood and progressively enlarge and thicken throughout the life span. The enlarged lesion (atheroma/plaque) can cause a critical narrowing (75% occlusion) of the coronary artery lumen, resulting in a decrease in coronary blood flow and an inadequate supply of oxygen to the heart muscle.

Pathophysiology

The most widely accepted cause of CAD is the accumulation of lipids (mainly cholesterol) and fibrous materials (smooth muscle cells) within the coronary artery lumen.

1. Increased blood levels of low-density lipoprotein (LDL— known as the "bad" cholesterol because it transports cholesterol to body tissues) irritate and damage the inner layer of the coronary vessels.
2. LDL enters the vessel after damaging the protective barrier, accumulates, and forms fatty streaks.
   a. Fatty streaks are yellow, flat, and cause no significant coronary artery obstruction.
   b. These lesions develop frequently between the ages of 8 and 18 years.
3. Smooth muscle cells (from the middle layer of the coronary artery) move to the inner layer to engulf the fatty substance, produce fibrous tissue, and stimulate calcium deposition.
4. This cycle continues, resulting in the transformation of the fatty streak into a fibrous plaque, and eventually a "complicated" CAD lesion evolves.
   a. A complicated lesion develops as small blood vessels grow into the fibrous plaque and the core of the lesion enlarges and calcifies.
   b. The complicated lesion can cause significant coronary obstruction by hemorrhage and ulceration of the plaque (see MI, p. 327).

Risk Factors

1. The three major risk factors include high blood cholesterol levels, hypertension, and cigarette smoking.
2. Unmodifiable risk factors include age, male sex, race, and family history of CAD.
3. Other risk factors include diabetes mellitus, obesity, sedentary life-style, stress, Type A personality.

Clinical Manifestations

A. Stable (Effort) Angina Pectoris—chest pain precipitated by physical exertion or emotional stress; increased oxygen demands are placed on the heart muscle, but the ability of the coronary artery to deliver blood to the muscle is impaired because of obstruction by a significant coronary lesion (75% narrowing of the vessel). Rest and nitroglycerin relieve the pain.

1. *Character*—substernal chest pain, pressure, heaviness, or discomfort. Other sensations include a squeezing, aching, burning, choking, strangling, and/or cramping pain.
   a. Pain may be mild or severe and typically presents with a gradual buildup of discomfort and subsequent gradual fading away.
   b. May produce numbness or weakness in arms, wrists, or hands.

c. Associated symptoms include diaphoresis, nausea, indigestion, dyspnea, tachycardia, and increase in blood pressure.
2. *Location*—behind middle or upper third of sternum; the patient generally will make a fist over the site of the pain (positive Levine sign; indicates diffuse deep visceral pain), rather than point to it with his finger.
3. *Radiation*—usually radiates to neck, jaw, shoulders, arms, hands, and posterior intrascapular area. Pain occurs more commonly on the left side than the right.
4. *Duration*—usually lasts 1–5 minutes after stopping activity; nitroglycerin relieves pain within 1 minute.
5. *Other precipitating factors*—exposure to hot or cold weather, eating a heavy meal, and sexual intercourse increase the workload of the heart and therefore increase oxygen demand.

B. Unstable (Preinfarction) **Angina Pectoris**—chest pain occurring at rest; no increase in oxygen demand is placed on the heart muscle, but an acute lack of blood flow to the muscle occurs because of coronary artery spasm aggravated by the presence of an enlarged plaque or hemorrhage/ulceration of a complicated lesion. Critical narrowing of the vessel lumen occurs abruptly in either instance.

1. A change in frequency, duration, and intensity of stable angina symptoms is indicative of progression to unstable angina.
2. Unstable angina pain lasts longer than 10 minutes, is unrelieved by rest or sublingual nitroglycerin, and mimics signs and symptoms of impending myocardial infarction (see MI, Clinical Manifestations, p. 328).

NURSING ALERT: Unstable angina can cause sudden death or result in a myocardial infarction. Early recognition and treatment are imperative to prevent complications.

C. Silent Ischemia—the absence of chest pain with documented evidence of an imbalance between myocardial oxygen supply and demand (ST depression of 1 mm. or more) as determined by ECG, exercise stress test, or ambulatory (Holter) ECG monitoring.

1. Silent ischemia most commonly occurs in the early morning hours (6:00 A.M.–10:00 A.M.).
2. Arousal causes an increase in sympathetic stimulation and blood viscosity, and coronary vessel tone increase in the morning causing silent ischemia episodes.

Diagnostic Evaluation

1. *Characteristic chest pain* and clinical history
2. *Nitroglycerin test*—relief of pain with nitroglycerin
3. *ECG stress testing*—progressive increases of speed and elevation of walking on a treadmill increase the workload of the heart. ST and T wave changes occur if myocardial ischemia is induced.
4. *Radionuclide imaging*—a radioisotope, thallium 201, injected during exercise is imaged by camera. Low uptake of the isotope by heart muscle indicates regions of ischemia induced by exercise. Images taken during rest show a reversal of ischemia in those regions affected.
5. *Radionuclide ventriculography* (gated blood pool scanning)—red blood cells tagged with a radioisotope are imaged by camera during exercise and at rest. Wall motion abnormalities of the heart can be detected and ejection fraction estimated.

6. *Cardiac catheterization*—coronary angiography performed during the procedure determines the presence, location, and extent of coronary lesions.

Management

Goals:

1. Reducing the work load of the heart to decrease oxygen demand
2. Remodeling or bypassing obstructive lesions to improve blood flow to the heart muscle
3. Preventing the progression of CAD to decrease incidence of myocardial infarction and sudden death

A. Drug Therapy

Antianginal medications (nitrates, beta-blockers, calcium channel blockers) are used to maintain a balance between oxygen supply and demand. Reduction of the work load of the heart decreases oxygen demand and consumption. Coronary vessel relaxation promotes blood flow to the heart muscle, thereby increasing oxygen supply.

1. *Nitrates*—cause generalized vasodilation throughout the body.
   a. Nitrates can be administered by various routes and provide short- or long-lasting effects.
   b. Short-acting nitrates provide immediate relief of acute anginal attacks or prophylaxis if taken prior to activity.
   c. Long-acting nitrates prevent anginal episodes and/or reduce severity and frequency of attacks.
2. *Beta-blockers*—inhibit sympathetic stimulation of receptors that are located in the conduction system of the heart and in heart muscle.
   a. Some beta-blockers inhibit sympathetic stimulation of receptors in the lungs as well as the heart ("nonselective" beta-blockers); vasoconstriction of the large airways in the lung occurs; generally contraindicated for patients with chronic obstructive lung disease.
   b. "Cardioselective" beta-blockers (in recommended drug ranges) affect only the heart and can be used safely in patients with lung disease.
3. *Calcium channel blockers*—inhibit the movement of calcium within the heart muscle and coronary vessels; promote vasodilation and prevent/control coronary artery spasm.
4. *Antilipid medications*—decrease blood cholesterol and triglyceride levels in patients with elevated levels. The progression of CAD may be prevented by this therapy.

B. Percutaneous Transluminal Angioplasty

1. A balloon-tipped catheter is placed in a coronary vessel narrowed by plaque.
2. The balloon is inflated and deflated to stretch the vessel wall and flatten the lesion (see PTCA, p. 325).
3. Blood flows freely through the unclogged vessel to the heart.

C. Coronary Artery Bypass Surgery

1. A graft is surgically attached to the aorta, and the other end of the graft is attached to a distal portion of a coronary vessel.
2. Bypasses obstructive lesions in the vessel and returns adequate blood flow to the heart muscle supplied by the artery

D. Life-style Modification

1. Cessation of smoking
2. Control of high blood pressure
3. Lowering of blood cholesterol level

Nursing Assessment

1. Ask patient to describe his anginal attacks.
   a. When do attacks tend to occur? Following a meal? After engaging in certain activities? After physical activities in general? After visits of family/others?
   b. Where is the pain located? Does it radiate?
   c. Was the onset of pain sudden? Gradual?
   d. How long did it last—seconds? minutes? hours?
   e. Was the pain steady and unwavering in quality?
   f. Is the discomfort accompanied by other symptoms? Sweating? Light-headedness? Nausea? Palpitations? Shortness of breath?
   g. How is the pain relieved? How long does it take for pain relief?
2. Evaluate patient's medical history for conditions that may influence choice of drug therapy (diabetes, heart failure, previous myocardial infarction, obstructive lung disease).
3. Discuss with patient current activity levels. (Effectiveness of antianginal drug therapy is evaluated by patient's ability to attain higher activity levels.)
4. Identify factors that may contribute to noncompliance with prescribed drug therapy.
5. Review renal/hepatic studies and complete blood count.
6. Obtain a baseline 12-lead ECG.
7. Assess patient's and family's knowledge of disease.
8. Gather information regarding the patient's cardiac risk factors.
9. Discuss with patient his beliefs regarding modification of risk factors and his willingness to change.
10. Identify patient's and family's level of anxiety and utilization of appropriate coping mechanisms.

Nursing Diagnoses

1. Pain related to an imbalance in oxygen supply and demand
2. Altered cardiac output: (potential for decrease) related to reduced preload, afterload, contractility, and heart rate secondary to hemodynamic effects of drug therapy.
3. Anxiety related to chest pain, uncertain prognosis, and threatening environment.

Nursing Interventions

A. Achieving Relief of Pain

1. Determine intensity of patient's angina.
   a. Ask patient to compare the pain with other pain he has experienced in the past, and on a scale of 1 (lowest) to 10 (highest), rate his current pain.
   b. Observe for other signs/symptoms: diaphoresis, shortness of breath, protective body posture, dusky facial color, and/or changes in level of consciousness.
2. Place patient in comfortable position.
3. Administer oxygen if prescribed.
4. Obtain blood pressure, apical heart rate, and respiratory rate.
5. Obtain a 12-lead ECG as directed.
6. Administer antianginal medication as prescribed.
7. Notify physician.

8. Monitor for relief of pain and note duration of anginal episode.
9. Take vital signs every 5–10 minutes until angina pain subsides.
10. Be alert to progression of stable angina to unstable angina: increase in frequency and intensity of pain, pain occurring at rest or at low levels of exertion, pain lasting longer than 15 minutes.
11. Determine level of activity that precipitated anginal episode.
12. Identify specific activities patient may engage in that are below the level at which anginal pain occurs.
13. Reinforce the importance of notifying nursing staff whenever angina pain is experienced.

B. Maintaining Hemodynamic Stability

1. Be aware of the physiologic effects, onset/duration of action of prescribed antianginal medications.
2. Monitor carefully the patient's response to drug therapy.
   a. Take blood pressure and heart rate in a sitting and lying position on initiation of long-term therapy (provides baseline data to evaluate for orthostatic hypotension that may occur with drug therapy).
   b. Recheck vital signs as indicated by onset of action of drug and at time of drug's peak effect.
   c. Note changes in blood pressure of more than 10 mm. Hg and changes in heart rate of more than 10 beats.
   d. Note patient complaints of headache (especially with use of nitrates) and dizziness.
      (1) Administer analgesics as directed for headache.
      (2) Place patient in supine position and elevate foot of bed for dizziness (usually associated with a decrease in blood pressure; preload is enhanced by this mechanism, thereby increasing blood pressure).
   e. Place patient on continuous ECG monitoring or obtain 12-lead ECG daily as directed.
      (1) Interpret rhythm strip every 4 hours for patients on continuous monitoring and measure PR intervals (beta-blockers and calcium channel blockers can cause significant bradycardia and various degrees of heart block).
   f. Evaluate for development of heart failure (beta-blockers and some calcium channel blockers decrease contractility, thus increasing the likelihood of heart failure).
      (1) Obtain daily weights.
      (2) Auscultate lung fields for crackles every 4 hours.
      (3) Monitor for the presence of edema.
3. Be sure to remove previous nitrate patch or paste before applying new paste/pad (prevents hypotension).
4. Be alert to adverse reaction related to abrupt discontinuation of beta-blocker and calcium channel blocker therapy. These drugs must be tapered to prevent a "rebound phenomenon": tachycardia, increase in chest pain, hypertension.
5. Notify physician of all untoward drug effects.

C. Decreasing Anxiety

1. Explain to the patient and family reasons for hospitalization, diagnostic tests, and therapies administered.
2. Encourage the patient to verbalize fears and concerns regarding illness through frequent conversations—conveys to the patient a willingness to listen.

3. Answer the patient's questions with concise explanations.
4. Administer drugs to relieve patient anxiety as directed. *Sedatives and tranquilizers*—may be used to prevent attacks precipitated by aggravation, excitement, or tension.
5. Explain to the patient the importance of anxiety reduction to assist in control of angina. (Anxiety and fear put an increased stress on the heart, requiring the heart to use more oxygen.)
6. Discuss measures to be taken when an anginal episode occurs. (Preparing patient decreases anxiety and allows patient to accurately describe his angina.)
   a. Review the questions that will be asked during anginal episodes.
   b. Review the interventions that will be employed to relieve anginal attacks.

Patient Education/Discharge Planning

Goals:
1. Comply with interventions to prevent angina episodes.
2. Adapt healthy life-style changes.

A. Instruct Patient and Family About CAD.

1. Review the chambers of the heart and the coronary artery system, using a diagram of the heart.
2. Show patient a diagram of a clogged artery; explain how the blockage occurs; point out on the diagram the location of the patient's lesions.
3. Explain what angina is (a warning sign from the heart that there is not enough blood and oxygen because of the blocked artery or spasm).
4. Review specific risk factors that affect CAD development and progression; highlight those risk factors that can be modified and controlled to reduce risk.
5. Discuss the signs/symptoms of angina, precipitating factors, and treatment for attacks. Stress to patient the importance of treating angina symptoms at once.
6. Distinguish for patient the different sign/symptoms associated with stable angina versus preinfarction angina.

B. Identify Suitable Activity Level to Prevent Angina.

1. Participate in a normal daily program of activities that do not produce chest discomfort, shortness of breath, and undue fatigue.
2. Avoid activities known to cause anginal pain—sudden exertion, walking against the wind, extremes of temperature, high altitude, emotionally stressful situations; may accelerate heart rate, raise blood pressure, and increase cardiac work.
3. Refrain from engaging in physical activity for 2 hours after meals. Rest after each meal if possible.
4. Do not undertake activities requiring heavy effort (carrying heavy objects).
5. Try to avoid cold weather if possible; dress warmly and walk more slowly. Wear scarf over nose and mouth when in cold air.
6. Reduce weight, if necessary, to reduce cardiac load.
7. Avoid overeating.
   a. Avoid excessive caffeine intake (coffee, cola drinks) that can increase the heart rate and produce angina.
   b. Do not use "diet pills," nasal decongestants, or any over-the-counter medications that can increase the heart rate or stimulate high blood pressure.
   c. Avoid the use of alcohol or drink alcohol only in moderation (alcohol can increase hypotensive side effects of drugs).

C. Instruct About Appropriate Use of Medications and Side Effects

1. Carry nitroglycerin at all times.
   a. Nitroglycerin is volatile and is inactivated by heat, moisture, air, light, and time.
   b. Keep nitroglycerin in original dark glass container, tightly closed—to prevent absorption of drug by other pills or pillbox.
   c. Do not carry nitroglycerin in a plastic or metal pillbox or mixed with other pills.
   d. Nitroglycerin should cause a slight burning or stinging sensation under the tongue when it is potent.
   e. Teach family member how to administer nitroglycerin and location of medication in case patient needs assistance.
2. Place nitroglycerin under tongue at first sign of chest discomfort.
   a. Stop all effort/activity; sit, and take nitroglycerin tablet—relief should be obtained in a few minutes.
   b. Bite the tablet between front teeth and slip under tongue to dissolve if quick action is desired.
   c. Repeat dosage in a few minutes for total of 3 tablets if relief is not obtained.
   d. Keep a record of number of tablets taken—to evaluate any change in anginal pattern.
   e. Take nitroglycerin prophylactically to avoid pain known to occur with certain activities.
3. Demonstrate for patient how to administer nitroglycerin paste correctly.
   a. Place paste on calibrated strip.
   b. Remove previous paste on skin by wiping gently with tissue.
   c. Rotate site of administration to avoid skin irritation.
   d. Apply paste to skin; use plastic wrap to protect clothing if not provided on strip.
   e. Have patient return demonstration.
4. Instruct patient on administration of transdermal nitroglycerin patches.
   a. Remove previous patch; wipe area with tissue to remove any residual medication.
   b. Apply patch to a clean dry nonhairy area of body.
   c. Rotate administration sites.
   d. Instruct patient not to remove patch for swimming or bathing.
   e. Have patient return demonstration of patch administration.
5. Instruct patient to eat a high-fiber diet and increase fluid intake to prevent constipation commonly associated with verapamil (calcium channel blocker).
6. Instruct patient to report increases in weight, shortness of breath, and difficulty sleeping if receiving beta- or calcium blockers (can precipitate heart failure).
7. Review the importance of not stopping beta- or calcium blockers abruptly, as serious withdrawal symptoms can occur.
8. Instruct patient to lie down and elevate feet or lower head between knees if dizziness occurs.

D. Describe Appropriate Action for Unusual Angina

Instruct patient to go to the nearest health facility if chest pain persists more than 15 minutes or is more intense and widespread than the usual angina episodes. (Do not drive yourself.)

E. Counsel on How to Modify Risk Factors

1. Inform patient of methods of stress reduction such as biofeedback and relaxation techniques.
2. Review information on low-fat/low-cholesterol diet with patient.
   a. Suggest to patient available cookbooks (American Heart Association) that may assist in planning and preparing foods.
   b. Have dietitian visit patient to design a menu plan for patient.
3. Inform patient of available cardiac rehabilitation pro-grams that offer structured classes on exercise, smoking cessation, and weight control.

Evaluation

1. Relief of pain; stops activity, calls nurse, experiences no chest pain
2. Maintains hemodynamic stability; blood pressure and heart rate within 10 mm. Hg or 10 beats of patient's normal limits; absence of edema; breathing rate and pattern normal; breath sounds normal; absence of dizziness; normal sensorium
3. Achieves decrease in anxiety; verbalizes lessening anxiety, verbalizes ability to cope

---

Percutaneous Transluminal Coronary Angioplasty *(PTCA)*

Percutaneous transluminal coronary angioplasty (PTCA) is a technique used for the treatment of coronary artery disease (CAD). A balloon-tipped catheter is introduced through a guidewire into a coronary vessel with a noncalcified atheromatous lesion. The balloon of the catheter is then inflated, causing disruption of the intima and changes in the atheroma. The result is an increase in the diameter of the lumen of the coronary vessel (as judged by angiographic criteria) and improvement of blood flow below the lesion. Balloon inflation/deflation may be repeated until satisfactory results are achieved (Fig. 14-8).

Indications

Patients meeting the following criteria are generally acceptable candidates for PTCA:

1. Stable angina (less than 1 year) or unstable angina (less than 6 months), despite optimal medical therapy
2. Single-vessel or multivessel disease (balloon dilatation of the most severe "culprit" lesion is initially attempted to determine if successful angioplasty can be achieved); surgery to bypass the lesion may be recommended if PTCA is unsuccessful.
3. Proximal, accessible noncalcified lesions; midvessel lesions may also be attempted with success.
4. Suitable candidate for heart surgery and has consented to heart surgery as an alternative treatment
5. Evolving myocardial infarction (may be in combination with thrombolytic therapy) and obstructed coronary bypass grafts

Contraindications

1. Patients with left main coronary artery disease
2. Patients with severe left ventricular dysfunction

Complications

1. Coronary occlusion, coronary dissection, myocardial infarction, coronary artery spasm, and prolonged angina may necessitate immediate coronary artery bypass graft surgery. *A cardiac surgical team must be on standby during all PTCA procedures.*
2. PTCA is associated with a restenosis rate of 30%–40%. Restenosis may occur acutely (within 24 hours) or within 6 months. A second angioplasty may be performed with improved long-term results.

Future Innovations

1. *Laser-assisted balloon angioplasty*
   a. A laser light is directed by a percutaneously inserted flexible fiber-optic catheter and is able to "vaporize" atheromatous lesions in the coronary vessels.
   b. Balloon angioplasty of the vessel may then be performed.
   c. This new technique may minimize damage to the intimal lining, open diseased vessels more effectively, prevent early and long-term restenosis, and expand the use to calcified, unusual lesions and total occlusions.
2. *Atherectomy*
   a. A burr-tipped high-speed rotating catheter is inserted percutaneously into a coronary vessel and "drills" through the atheromatous lesion, changing it to microscopic debris.
   b. This new technique may open diseased vessels more effectively, especially in patients who have coronary lesions not amenable to standard angioplasty.
3. *Intracoronary Stenting*
   a. A tiny coil or diamond mesh tubular device (stent) is placed in the coronary artery immediately following successful balloon angioplasty.
   b. The stent remains in the vessel to prevent restenosis.

Nursing Interventions

A. Decreasing Anxiety

1. Reinforce the reasons for the procedure.
   a. Describe the location of the coronary vessels using a diagram of the heart.
   b. Describe/draw the location of the patient's lesion using heart diagram.
2. Explain the events that will occur before, during, and after the procedure—preparation minimizes anxiety and increases compliance with care regimen.
   a. Performed in the cardiac catheterization laboratory; similar to the cardiac catheterization procedure (see Cardiac Catheterization, p. 301). Review auditory and tactile stimuli.
   b. Chest x-ray, ECG, blood tests (PT, PTT, CBC, electrolytes) prior to and after procedure
   c. Mild sedation given; patient remains alert throughout procedure to report any chest pain (indicates myocardial ischemia) and to cough when instructed (enhances catheter placement).
      (1) Medication (nitroglycerin) will be given prophylactically to prevent and relieve episodes of chest pain.

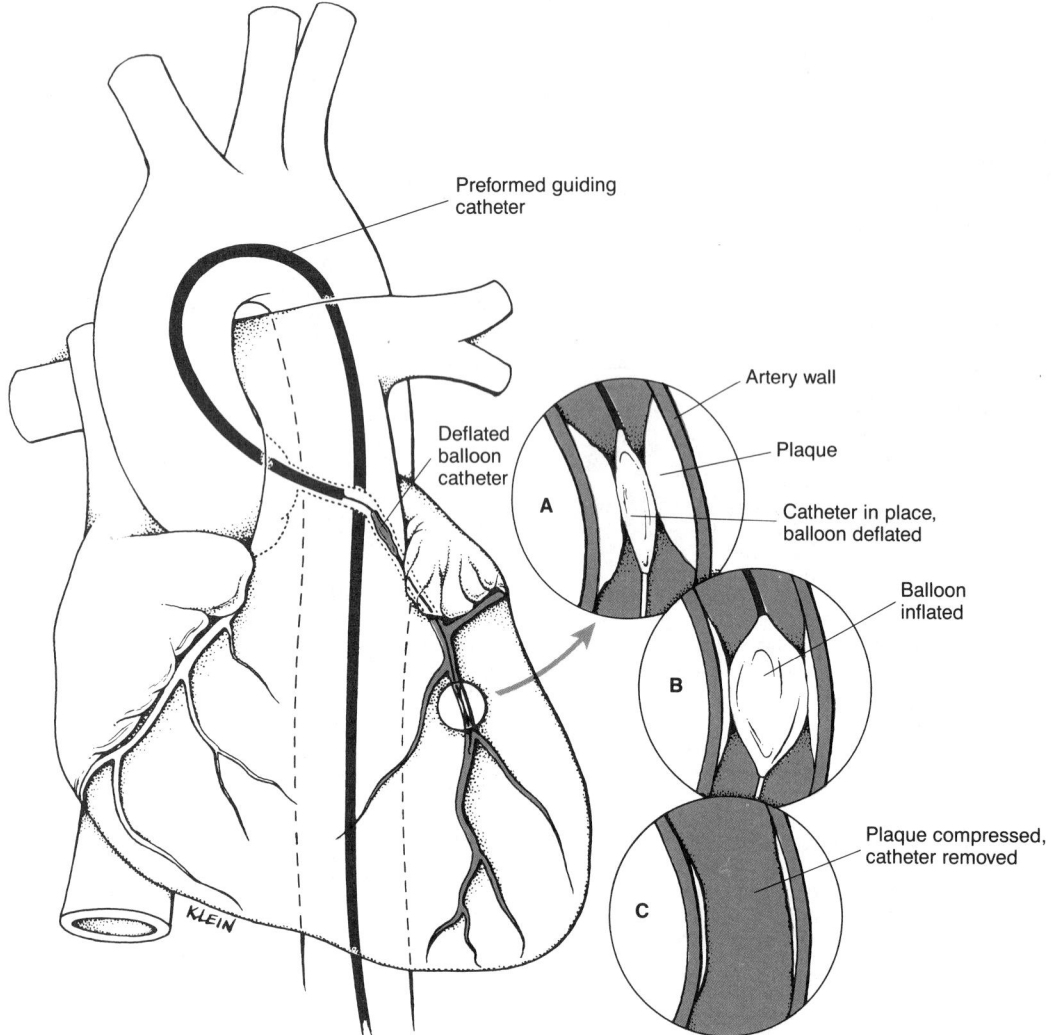

Figure 14-8. *Percutaneous transluminal coronary angioplasty. (A) The balloon-tipped catheter is passed into the affected coronary artery. (B) The balloon is then rapidly inflated and deflated with controlled pressure. (C) The balloon disrupts the intima and causes changes in the atheroma, resulting in an increase in the diameter of the lumen of the vessel and improvement of blood flow. (Redrawn after Purcell JA and Giffin PA. Percutaneous transluminal coronary angioplasty. Am J Nurs 1981 Sep; 9:1620–1626)*

(2) Heparin will be given to prevent clot formation.

(3) A temporary pacemaker may be inserted for emergency pacing if necessary.

d. Local anesthetic given at catheter insertion site.

(1) Catheter remains in the groin 4–6 hours postprocedure to avoid bleeding complications (patient remains anticoagulated after procedure).

(2) Bedrest maintained, affected extremity immobilized, and head of bed elevated no more than 30 degrees 12–24 hours postprocedure to prevent catheter dislodgement, bleeding, and prolonged healing of vessel lining.

(3) Analgesic medication given to prevent discomfort from catheter and bedrest.

e. IV line; continuous ECG monitoring; frequent vital sign checks

f. Peripheral pulses marked prior to procedure with indelible ink to facilitate frequent checks after procedure

g. NPO 24 hours prior to procedure; diet advanced as tolerated after procedure

3. Prepare patient for complications of procedure.

a. Provide preoperative teaching to patient and family regarding heart surgery (see Heart Surgery, p. 354).

B. Maintaining Hemodynamic Stability

1. Check vital signs every 15 minutes for 1 hour, then every half hour for 2 hours, and subsequently every 4 hours.

2. Continually evaluate for signs/symptoms of restenosis.
   a. Emphasize importance of reporting any chest discomfort or jaw, back, arm pain and/or nausea, abdominal distress.
   b. Take ECG for all complaints suspicious of possible myocardial ischemia.
   c. Administer oxygen and vasodilator therapy for pain as directed.
   d. Obtain CPK and isoenzymes as directed.
   e. Keep patient NPO if prolonged chest pain occurs (patient may return to catheterization laboratory).
3. Evaluate fluid and electrolyte balance.
   a. Record intake and output.
   b. Encourage fluid intake to prevent dehydration—contrast medium used during procedure causes diuresis.
   c. Observe for dysrhythmias possibly related to potassium imbalance—excessive diuresis causes potassium depletion.
   d. Administer potassium supplement as prescribed.
4. Be alert to potential of vasovagal reaction during removal of groin catheter.
   a. Observe for bradycardia, hypotension, diaphoresis, nausea.
   b. Administer IV atropine as directed.
   c. Place patient in Trendelenburg position to promote blood return to the heart and improve hypotension.
   d. Give fluid challenge as directed.

C. Preventing Bleeding and Thromboembolism

1. Check peripheral pulse of affected extremity and insertion site after each vital sign check.
2. Observe color, temperature, and sensation of affected extremity with each vital sign check.
3. Notify physician if extremities become cool and pale, and pulses become significantly diminished or absent.
4. Look for presence of hematoma and mark hematoma to note change in size.
   Notify physician if hematoma continues to enlarge.
5. Note petechiae, hematuria, and complaints of flank pain (vessel patency is maintained by not reversing intraprocedure heparinization; chance of bleeding is increased).
6. Hold direct pressure over insertion site if bleeding is observed and notify physician immediately.
7. Check bed linen under patient frequently for blood.
8. Ask patient to report any sensation of warmth at groin area.

D. Minimizing Discomfort

1. Administer analgesics/anxiolytic medication as directed.
2. Ensure a restful environment.
   a. Provide back rubs for muscle relaxation.
   b. Minimize noise and interruptions.
   c. Offer sleep medication as indicated.
3. Progress patient's diet as tolerated; (clear liquids/full liquid diet until catheters removed); assist patient with meals.

Patient Education/Discharge Planning

Instruct patient as follows:
1. Modification of cardiac risk factors as means of controlling progression of coronary artery disease
2. Name of medications, action, dosage, and side effects
   a. Common medications prevent clot formation (aspirin, dipyridamole [Persantine]); increase blood flow to heart (isosorbide dinitrate [Isordil]); or slow heart rate/decrease chest pain (propranolol [Inderal]); increase blood flow and prevent coronary artery spasm (diltiazem, nifedipine).
   b. Dates and importance of follow-up tests—exercise ECG, thallium-201 perfusion imaging. Symptoms for which patient should seek medical attention—side effects of medications, chest pain, or weight increases greater than 5 pounds.
      (1) Stenosis can recur within 6 months. Second angioplasty usually successful for more than 1 year.
      (2) Chest pain unrelieved with nitroglycerin and persisting longer than 15 minutes after rest is significant.

Myocardial Infarction

Myocardial infarction (MI) refers to a dynamic process by which one or more regions of the heart muscle experience a severe and prolonged decrease in oxygen supply because of insufficient coronary blood flow; subsequently, necrosis or "death" to the myocardial tissue occurs. The onset of the myocardial infarction process may be sudden or gradual and the progression of the event to completion takes approximately 3–6 hours.

Types of Heart Damage *(Fig. 14-9)*

Different degrees of damage occur to the heart muscle:
1. *Zone of necrosis*—death to the heart muscle caused by extensive and complete oxygen deprivation; irreversible damage
2. *Zone of injury*—region of the heart muscle surrounding the area of necrosis; inflamed and injured, but still viable if adequate oxygenation can be restored
3. *Zone of ischemia*—region of the heart muscle surrounding the area of injury, which is ischemic and viable; not endangered unless extension of the infarction occurs.

Causes

1. Acute coronary thrombosis (partial or total)—associated with 90% of MIs.
   a. Severe coronary artery disease (greater than 70% narrowing of the artery) precipitates thrombus formation.
   b. Intramural hemorrhage into atheromatous plaques causes the lesion to enlarge and occlude the vessel; dissecting hemorrhage can also occur.
   c. The plaque ruptures into the vessel lumen and a thrombus forms on top of the ulcerated lesion, with resultant vessel occlusion.
2. Other factors include: coronary artery spasm, coronary artery embolism, infectious diseases causing arterial inflammation, hypoxia, anemia, and severe exertion or stress on the heart in the presence of significant coronary artery disease (i.e., surgical procedures or shoveling snow).

Classification

1. According to the layers of the heart muscle involved
   a. Transmural (Q wave) infarction—area of necrosis occurs throughout the entire thickness of the heart muscle.

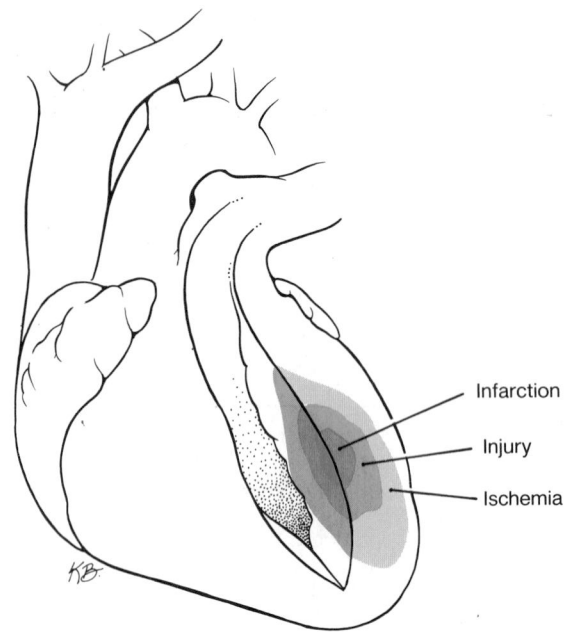

Infarction

Injury

Ischemia

Figure 14-9. Different degrees of damage occur to the heart muscle after a myocardial infarction. The diagram shows the zones of necrosis, injury, and ischemia.

b. Subendocardial (nontransmural/non-Q) infarction—area of necrosis is confined to the innermost layer of the heart lining the chambers.

NURSING ALERT: Patients with subendocardial infarctions should be considered as having an uncompleted MI; monitor carefully for signs/symptoms of extension of heart muscle damage.

2. According to the location of the damaged heart muscle within the left ventricle: inferior, anterior, lateral, and posterior.
   a. Left ventricle is the most common and dangerous location for an MI, as it is the main pumping chamber of the heart.
   b. Right ventricular infarctions commonly occur in conjunction with damage to the inferior and/or posterior wall of the left ventricle.
3. Region of the heart muscle that becomes damaged—determined by the coronary artery that becomes obstructed.
4. The amount of heart muscle damage and the location of the MI—determines prognosis.

Clinical Manifestations

1. Chest pain
   a. Severe, diffuse steady substernal pain of a crushing and squeezing nature
   b. Not relieved by rest or sublingual vasodilator therapy, but requires narcotics
   c. May radiate to the arms (commonly the left), shoulders, neck, back, and/or jaw
   d. Continues for more than 15 minutes
   e. May produce anxiety and fear, resulting in an increase in heart rate, blood pressure, and respiratory rate

2. Diaphoresis, cool clammy skin, facial pallor
3. Hypertension or hypotension
4. Bradycardia or tachycardia
5. Premature ventricular and/or atrial beats
6. Palpitations, severe anxiety, dyspnea
7. Disorientation, confusion, restlessness
8. Fainting, marked weakness
9. Nausea, vomiting, hiccups
10. Atypical symptoms: epigastric or abdominal distress, dull aching or tingling sensations, shortness of breath, extreme fatigue

NURSING ALERT: Many patients do not have symptoms; these are "silent myocardial infarctions." Nevertheless, there still is resultant damage to the heart.

GERONTOLOGIC ALERT: Elderly patients are more likely to experience silent MIs or have atypical symptoms: hypotension, low body temperature, vague complaints of discomfort, mild perspiration, strokelike symptoms, dizziness, change in sensorium.

Diagnostic Evaluation

A. General Findings

Characteristic chest pain, clinical history, and clinical findings

B. ECG Changes

1. Generally occur within 2–12 hours, but may take 72–96 hours
2. Necrotic, injured, and ischemic tissue alter ventricular depolarization and repolarization (see p. 365, ECG Interpretation of MI).

NURSING ALERT: A normal ECG does not rule out the possibility of infarction, as ECG changes can be subtle and obscured by underlying conditions (bundle branch blocks, electrolyte disturbances).

C. Elevation of Serum Enzymes

1. Lack of oxygen to the heart muscle for 30–60 minutes causes the release of intracellular enzymes; heart muscle damage can be assessed by evaluation of enzyme activity.
2. Enzymes spill into the blood at varying intervals characterized by a rise, peak, and return to normal levels within the first week of infarction.
3. Enzymes are drawn in a serial pattern, usually on admission and every 6–24 hours until three samples are obtained; enzyme activity then is correlated to the extent of heart muscle damage.
4. Normal values, rise, and peak of enzymes include:
   a. *Creatine kinase (CK)*—rise in 12 hours; peak in 36–72 hours; normalize (35–232 IU) in 3–5 days.
   b. *Lactic dehydrogenase (LDH)*—rise in 12 hours; peak in 12–24 hours; normalize (100–190 IU) in 10 days.
   c. *Aspartate aminotransferase (AST, formerly SGOT)*—rise in 8–12 hours; peak in 18–36 hours; normalize in 3–4 days.

NURSING ALERT: The greater the peak in enzyme activity and the length of time an enzyme remains at peak level correlates with serious damage of the heart muscle and a poorer prognosis for the patient.

5. CK, LDH, and AST are found in many other areas of the body such as the liver, kidneys, brain, skeletal muscle, bladder, and lungs; injuries to these areas can cause elevation of the enzymes.

D. Elevation of Serum Isoenzymes

1. CK and LDH can be broken down further into isoenzymes, which are more organ-specific.
2. CK-MB is specific to heart muscle and thus the most sensitive enzyme for determining heart muscle damage.
   a. Normal CK-MB activity is less than 5 IU
   b. Rise in 4–8 hours, peak in 24 hours, normalize in 72 hours
3. LDH1 and LDH2 are specific to heart muscle.
   a. LDH2 is normally greater than LDH1, except when the heart muscle is damaged a reversal occurs.
   b. A "flipped" pattern results, with LDH1 exceeding the value of LDH2, usually within 12–24 hours.

E. Other Findings

1. White blood cell count and sedimentation rate elevate due to inflammatory process associated with the damaged heart muscle.
2. Radionuclide imaging—allows recognition of areas of decreased perfusion (see p. 300).
3. Positron emission tomography—determines the presence of reversible heart muscle injury and irreversible or necrotic tissue; extent to which the injured heart muscle has responded to treatment also can be determined.

Management

Therapy is aimed at the protection of ischemic and injured heart tissue to preserve muscle function, reduce the infarct size, and prevent death. Innovative modalities provide early restoration of coronary blood flow, and the use of pharmacologic agents improve oxygen supply and demand, reduce/prevent dysrhythmias, and inhibit the progression of coronary artery disease.

A. Oxygen Therapy

Improves oxygenation to ischemic heart muscle

B. Pain Control

Endogenous catecholamine release during pain imposes an increased workload on the heart muscle, thus causing an increase in oxygen demand.

1. *Opiate analgesic therapy*
   a. Morphine is used to relieve pain, improve cardiac hemodynamics by reducing preload and afterload and to provide anxiety relief
   b. Meperidine (Demerol) is useful for pain management in those patients allergic to morphine or sensitive to respiratory depression.
2. *Vasodilator therapy*
   a. Nitroglycerin (sublingual, IV, paste) promotes venous (low-dose) and arterial (high-dose) relaxation as well as relaxation of coronary vessels and prevention of coronary spasm
   b. Myocardial oxygen demand is reduced with subsequent pain relief.
   c. Persistent chest pain requires IV nitroglycerin.
3. *Anxiolytic therapy*
   Benzodiazepines are used with analgesics when anxiety complicates chest pain and its relief.

C. Anticoagulation Therapy

1. Useful as an adjunct to thrombolytic therapy.
2. Also used in situations of prolonged bedrest, pulmonary embolism, deep vein thrombosis, mural thrombi, cardiogenic shock and patients with atrial fibrillation.

D. Beta-Adrenergic Blocking Agents

1. Improves oxygen supply and demand, decreases sympathetic stimulation to the heart, promotes blood flow in the small vessels of the heart, and has antidysrhythmic effects
2. Appears to lower mortality and decrease chance of reinfarction and sudden death post-MI.

E. Antidysrhythmic Therapy

Xylocaine (Lidocaine) decreases ventricular irritability commonly occurring post-MI.

F. Hemodynamic Monitoring

1. Evaluation of hemodynamic parameters guides the use of vasoactive drugs, diuretic therapy, and volume replacement.
2. Employed in patients with complicated infarctions (see Pulmonary Artery Catheter, p. 302).

G. Thrombolytic Therapy (intravenous or intracoronary)

1. Thrombolytic agents (tissue plasminogen activase, steptokinase, and urokinase) reestablish blood flow in coronary vessels by dissolving obstructing thrombus.
2. No effect on the underlying stenosis that precipitated the thrombus to form.
3. Intravenous route is preferred, as it allows for earlier initiation of therapy and decrease cost and risk benefit.

H. Percutaneous Transluminal Coronary Angioplasty (PTCA)

1. Mechanical opening of the coronary vessel can be performed during an evolving infarction.
2. PTCA can be used as an adjunct to thrombolytic therapy (see PTCA, p. 325).

I. Surgical Revascularization

1. Emergency coronary artery bypass surgery can be performed within 6 hours of evolving infarction.
2. Definite treatment of the stenosis and less scar formation on the heart is the benefit of this therapy.

J. Calcium Channel Blockers

1. Improve the balance between oxygen supply and demand by decreasing heart rate, blood pressure, and dilating coronary vessels.
2. Diltiazem has been shown to decrease the incidence of reinfarction in patients with non–Q-wave MIs and is currently the only calcium blocker proven to be beneficial.

Complications

1. Rhythm disturbances
2. Cardiac failure
   a. Infarct expansion (thinning and dilation of the necrotic zone)
   b. Infarct extension (additional heart muscle necrosis occurring after 24 hours of acute infarction).
   c. Congestive heart failure (20%–35% left ventricle damage)
   d. Right ventricular infarction
   e. Cardiogenic shock (see p. 333)
   f. Reinfarction
   g. Ischemic cardiomyopathy
3. Cardiac rupture
4. Ventricular mural thrombus
5. Thromboemboli

6. Ventricular aneurysm
7. Cardiac tamponade
8. Pericarditis (2–3 days post-MI)
9. Psychiatric problems—depression, personality changes

Nursing Assessment

1. Gather information regarding the patient's chest pain:
   a. Nature and intensity—describe the pain in his own words and compare it with pain experienced in the past.
   b. Onset and duration—exact time pain occurred, as well as the time pain relieved or diminished (if applicable).
   c. Location and radiation—point to the area where the pain is located and to other areas where the pain seems to travel.
   d. Precipitating and aggravating factors—describe the activity performed just prior to the onset of pain and if any maneuvers and/or medications alleviated the pain.
2. Question patient about other symptoms experienced associated with the pain. Observe patient for diaphoresis, facial pallor, dyspnea, guarding behaviors, rigid body posture, extreme weakness, confusion.
3. Evaluate cognitive, behavioral, and emotional status.
4. Question patient regarding his prior health status with emphasis on current medications, allergies (opiate analgesics, iodine, shellfish), recent trauma or surgery, aspirin ingestion, peptic ulcers, fainting spells, drug and alcohol use.
5. Analyze information for contraindications for thrombolytic therapy and/or PTCA.
6. Gather information on presence/absence of cardiac risk factors.
7. Identify patient's social support system and potential caregiver.
8. Identify significant other's reaction to the crisis situation.
9. Discuss with patient usual sleeping patterns and aids.
10. Discuss with patient usual stress and coping patterns.

Nursing Diagnoses

1. Pain related to an imbalance in oxygen supply and demand
2. Anxiety related to chest pain, fear of death, threatening environment, uncertain prognosis, and invasive therapies
3. Altered cardiac output (decreased): related to impaired contractility, tachy- and bradydysrhythmias, prolonged bedrest, volume depletion, reperfusion dysrhythmias, and complications
4. Activity intolerance related to insufficient oxygenation to perform activities of daily living (ADL), deconditioning effects of bedrest
5. Fluid volume deficit (potential for bleeding): related to dissolution of protective clots
6. Altered tissue perfusion (myocardial): related to coronary restenosis, extension of infarction
7. Potential for ineffective coping (individual): related to threats to self-esteem, disruption of sleep–rest pattern, lack of significant support system, and loss of control

Nursing Interventions

A. Maintaining Myocardial Oxygen Supply and Demand

1. Admit to cardiac care unit for constant monitoring.
   a. Lift patient from stretcher to bed and position comfortably.
   b. Obtain vital signs: heart rate, blood pressure, respiratory rate.
   c. Start an intravenous infusion to keep vein open for administration of IV medications in the event of dysrhythmias.
   d. Anticipate possible use of thrombolytic therapy: avoid noncompressible IV access sites; suggest the use of femoral or brachial site if central venous access is necessary.
2. Attach ECG monitoring electrodes to monitor heart rate.
   a. Set heart rate limit alarms 10–15 beats above and below patient's current rate. Leave alarms on at all times (brady- and tachydysrhythmias occur after acute MIs).
   b. A change in heart rate and/or rhythm must be detected and treated immediately.
3. Administer oxygen by nasal cannula if prescribed and encourage patient to take deep breaths—may decrease incidence of dysrhythmias by allowing the heart to be less ischemic and less irritable; may reduce infarct size, decrease anxiety, and resolve chest pain.
4. Take a 12-lead ECG to confirm clinical impression of MI; include right precordial leads (V4R, V5R, V6R) if right ventricular infarction suspected.
5. Offer support and reassurance to patient that relief of pain is a priority (reinforces to patient concern for pain relief).
6. Administer sublingual nitroglycerin as directed; recheck BP, heart rate (HR), and respiratory rate prior to administering nitrate therapy and 10–15 minutes after dose.
7. Administer narcotics as prescribed (morphine or meperidine)—decreases sympathetic activity and reduces heart rate, respirations, blood pressure, muscle tension, and anxiety.
   a. Use caution in administering narcotics to patients with chronic obstructive pulmonary disease, hypotension, dehydration, and to the elderly.
   b. Be alert that meperidine can have a vagolytic effect and cause tachycardia, thus increasing myocardial oxygen demands.

GERONTOLOGIC ALERT: Elderly patients are extremely susceptible to respiratory depression in response to narcotics. Analgesic agents with less profound effects on the respiratory center should be used. Anxiolytic agents also should be used with caution.

8. Obtain baseline vital signs prior to giving agents and 10–15 minutes after each dose. Place patient in a supine position during administration to minimize hypotension.
9. Give narcotic in small IV doses every 15–20 minutes (if vital signs are within safe limits) until pain is relieved (severe decreases in BP can be treated with IV naloxone [Narcan], IV fluid administration, and placing patient in Trendelenburg position as directed).
10. Give IV nitroglycerin as prescribed. Monitor BP con-

tinuously with automatic blood pressure machine or intra-arterially or every 5 minutes with auscultory method while titrating to pain relief.

> **NURSING ALERT:** Intravenous administration is the preferred route for analgesic medication, as intramuscular injections can cause elevations in serum enzymes, resulting in an incorrect diagnosis of myocardial infarction.

11. Review with patient frequently the importance of reporting any chest pain, discomfort, and/or epigastric distress without delay—patients may delay in reporting symptoms because of fear, denial, anxiety, and rationalization of atypical manifestations.

B. Alleviating Anxiety

1. Explain equipment, procedures, and need for frequent assessment to patient and significant others—minimizes anxiety due to threatening environment.
2. Discuss with patient and family member the anticipated nursing and medical regimen.
   a. Explain visiting hours and need to limit number of visitors at one time.
   b. Offer family members preferred times to phone unit to check on patient's status.
3. Observe for autonomic signs/symptoms of anxiety such as increases in heart rate, BP, respiratory rate, tremulousness—anxiety is associated with increased sympathetic stimulation, which puts more stress on the heart.
4. Administer antianxiety agents as prescribed.
   a. Explain to patient the reason for sedation: undue anxiety can make the heart more irritable and require more oxygen.
   b. Assure patient that the goal of sedation is to promote comfort and therefore should be requested if anxious, excitable, or "jittery" feelings occur—requesting medications can assist patient in managing his own anxiety and help regain a sense of control.
   c. Observe for adverse effects of sedation such as lethargy, confusion, and/or increased agitation.
5. Maintain consistency of care with one or two nurses regularly assisting patient, especially if severe anxiety is present.
6. Offer back massage to promote relaxation, decrease muscle tension, and improve skin integrity.

C. Maintaining Hemodynamic Stability

1. Monitor BP every 2 hours or as directed—hypertension increases afterload of the heart, elevating oxygen demand; hypotension causes reduced coronary and tissue perfusion.
   a. Calculate the difference between the systolic and diastolic pressures (pulse pressure) to estimate cardiac output (pulse pressure below 30 mm. Hg reflects a decrease in cardiac output).
   b. Be alert to presence of pulsus paradoxus if cardiac tamponade is suspected (see p. 311).
   c. Listen for the presence of pulsus alternans (hallmark of left ventricular failure).
2. Monitor respirations and lung fields every 2–4 hours or as prescribed.
   a. Auscultate for normal and abnormal breath sounds (crackles may indicate left ventricular failure; diffuse crackles indicate pulmonary edema).

> **NURSING ALERT:** Auscultation of clear lungs in the presence of cool, clammy skin, jugular venous distension, and hypotension may indicate right ventricular infarction.

   b. Observe for dypsnea, tachypnea, frothy pink sputum, orthopnea—may indicate left ventricular failure, pulmonary embolus, pulmonary edema.
3. Evaluate heart rate and heart sounds every 2–4 hours or as directed.
   a. Compare apical heart rate with radial pulse rate and determine the pulse deficit.
   b. Auscultate heart for the presence of a third heart sound (failing ventricle), fourth heart sound (stiffening ventricular muscle due to MI), friction rub (pericarditis), murmurs (valvular and papillary muscle dysfunction), intraventricular septal rupture.
4. Note presence of jugular venous distention and liver engorgement.
   a. Estimate right atrial pressure by determining jugular venous pressure.
   b. Observe for hepatojugular reflux.
5. Evaluate the major arterial pulses (weak pulse and/or presence of pulsus alternans indicates decreased cardiac output; irregularity results from dysrhythmias).
6. Take body temperature every 4 hours or as directed (most patients develop an increase in temperature within 24–48 hours due to tissue necrosis).
7. Observe for presence of edema (see Cardiac Assessment, p. 299).
8. Observe for evidence of cyanosis (see Cardiac Assessment, p. 298).
9. Monitor skin color and temperature (cool, clammy skin and pallor—associated with vasoconstriction secondary to decreased cardiac output.
10. Be alert to change in mental status such as confusion, restlessness, disorientation.
11. Employ hemodynamic monitoring for patients with complicated MIs (see Pulmonary Artery Catheter, p. 302).
    a. Monitor central venous, pulmonary artery, and pulmonary capillary wedge pressures and cardiac output.
    b. Calculate cardiac index and systemic vascular resistance (measurement of afterload).
    c. Titrate vasoactive drugs based on hemodynamic parameters.
12. Evaluate urine output (30 ml. per hour)—decrease in volume reflects a decrease in renal blood flow.
13. Monitor for life-threatening dysrhythmias (common within 24 hours following infarctions).
    a. Be vigilant for occurrence of any type of premature ventricular beats—may presage ventricular fibrillation or ventricular tachycardia.
    b. Anticipate possibility of reperfusion dysrhythmias following thombolytic therapy.
    c. Correct dysrhythmias immediately as directed (Lidocaine may be given prophylactically to protect against ventricular fibrillation and ventricular tachycardia.

D. Maximizing Cardiovascular Function

1. Promote rest with early gradual increase in mobilization—prevents deconditioning, which occurs with bedrest.

a. Minimize environmental noise.
b. Provide a comfortable environmental temperature.
c. Avoid unnecessary interruptions and procedures.
d. Structure routine care measures to include rest periods after activity.
e. Discuss with patient and family members the purpose of limited activity and visitors—to help the heart heal by lowering heart rate and blood pressure to maintain cardiac workload at lowest level and decrease oxygen consumption.
f. Promote restful diversional activities for patient (reading, listening to music, drawing, crossword puzzles, crafts).
g. Encourage frequent position changes while in bed.
2. Assist patient with prescribed activities (patient must be in stable condition: free of chest pain, heart failure, hypotension, and dysrhythmias).
a. Assist patient to rise slowly from a supine position.
b. Assist/instruct patient to sit on side of bed with feet on floor prior to getting out of bed—minimizes orthostatic hypotension.
c. Encourage passive and active range-of-motion exercise as directed for patient while on bedrest. Progress to performing exercises in bed or in chair, such as plantar and dorsiflexion of feet—prevents blood stasis.
d. Measure the length and width of the unit so that patients can gradually increase their activity levels with specific guidelines (walk one width [150 ft.] of the unit).
e. Elevate patient's feet when out of bed to chair to promote venous return.
f. Implement a step-by-step program for progressive activity as directed.

E. Preventing Bleeding

1. Take vital signs every 15 minutes during infusion of thombolytic agent and then hourly.
2. Observe for presence of hematomas or skin breakdown, especially in potential pressure areas such as the sacrum, back, elbows, ankles.
3. Be alert to verbal complaints of back pain indicative of possible retroperitoneal bleeding.
4. Observe all puncture sites every 15 minutes during infusion of thrombolytic therapy and then hourly for bleeding.
5. Apply manual pressure to venous or arterial sites if bleeding occurs. Use pressure dressings for coverage of all access sites.
6. Observe for blood in stool, emesis, urine, and sputum.
7. Minimize venipunctures and arterial punctures; use heparin lock for blood sampling and medication administration.
8. Avoid intramuscular injections.
9. Caution patient about vigorous tooth brushing, hair combing, or shaving.
10. Avoid trauma to patient by minimizing frequent handling of patient.
11. Monitor lab work: PT, PTT, Hct, Hgb.
12. Check for current blood type and crossmatch.
13. Administer antacids as directed to prevent stress ulcers.
14. Implement emergency interventions as directed in the event of bleeding: fluid, volume expanders, blood products.
15. Monitor for changes in mental status and headache.
16. Avoid vigorous oral suctioning.
17. Avoid use of automatic BP device above puncture sites or hematoma. Use care in taking BP; use arm not used for thrombolytic therapy.

F. Maintaining Tissue Perfusion

1. Observe for persistent and/or recurrence of signs and symptoms of ischemia: chest pain, diaphoresis, hypotension—may indicate extension of MI and/or reocclusion of coronary vessel.
2. Notify physician immediately.
3. Administer oxygen as directed.
4. Record a 12-lead ECG.
5. Prepare patient for possible emergency procedure: cardiac catheterization, bypass surgery, PTCA, thrombolytic therapy.

G. Developing Adaptive Coping Abilities

1. Listen carefully to patient and family members to ascertain their cognitive appraisals of stressors and threats.
2. Assist patient to establish a positive attitude toward his illness and progress adaptively through the grieving process.
3. Manipulate environment to promote restful sleep by maintaining patient's usual sleep patterns.
a. Implement patient's normal bedtime rituals such as snack, hygiene routines, lighting, and bedding.
b. Allow patient a minimum of 2 hours of uninterrupted sleep and avoid disruption during early morning hours.
c. Be alert to signs/symptoms of sleep deprivation—irritability, disorientation, hallucinations, diminished pain tolerance, aggressiveness.
d. Evaluate continually patient's sleep by asking patient about sleep quality.
4. Minimize possible adverse emotional response to transfer from the intensive care unit to the intermediate care unit.
a. Introduce the admitting nurse from the intermediate care unit to the patient before transfer.
b. Plan for the intermediate care nurse to answer questions the patient may have and to inform patient what to expect relative to physical layout of unit, nursing routines, and visiting hours.

Patient Education/Discharge Planning

Goals:
1. Restore patient to his optimal physiologic, psychological, social, and work level.
2. Aid in restoring confidence and self-esteem.
3. Develop patient's self-monitoring skills to assist him in managing his cardiac problems.
4. Modify risk factors.

1. Inform the patient and family member about what has happened to his heart.
a. Explain basic cardiac anatomy and physiology
b. Identify the difference between angina and MI.
c. Describe how the heart heals and that healing is not complete for 6–8 weeks following attack.
d. Discuss what the patient can do to assist in the recovery process and reduce the chance of future heart attacks.
2. Instruct patient on how to judge the body's response to activity.
a. Introduce the concept that different activities require varied expenditures of oxygen.
b. Emphasize the importance of rest and relaxation alternating with activity.

c. Instruct patient how to take his pulse prior to and after activity, as well as guidelines for the acceptable increases in heart rate that should occur.

d. Review signs/symptoms indicative of a poor response to increased activity levels: chest pain, extreme fatigue, shortness of breath.

3. Design an individualized activity progression program for patient as directed.

a. Determine activity levels appropriate for patient as prescribed and by predischarge low-level exercise stress test.

b. Encourage patient and family member to list activities they enjoy and would like to resume.

c. Establish the energy expenditure of each activity (i.e., which are most demanding on the heart) and rank activities from lowest to highest.

d. Instruct patient to move from one activity to another after the heart has been able to manage the previous workload as determined by signs/symptoms and pulse rate.

e. Give patient specific activity guidelines and explain activity guidelines will be reevaluated after his heart heals:

(1) Walk daily, gradually increasing distance and time as prescribed.

(2) Avoid activities that tense muscles, such as weight lifting, lifting heavy objects, isometric exercises, pushing/pulling heavy loads.

(3) Avoid working with arms overhead.

(4) Gradually return to work.

(5) Avoid extremes in temperature.

(6) Do not rush, avoid tenseness.

(7) Sexual relations may be resumed on advice of physician, usually after exercise tolerance is assessed.

If patient can walk briskly or climb two flights of stairs, he can usually resume sexual activity with familiar partner; resumption of sexual activity parallels resumption of usual activities.

Sexual activity should be avoided after eating a heavy meal, after drinking alcohol, or when tired.

(8) Get at least 7 hours of sleep each night and take 20–30-minute rest periods twice a day.

(9) Limit visitors to 3–4 daily for 15–30 minutes and shorten phone conversations.

(10) Eat 3–4 small meals per day rather than large heavy meals. Rest 1 hour after meals.

(11) Limit caffeine and alcohol intake.

(12) Driving a car, flying, use of public transportation, going out socially, climbing stairs should be resumed as prescribed.

4. Assist patient to participate in his medication regimen.

a. Teach patient purpose, dose, and side effect of each medication.

b. Encourage patient to establish cues that will remind him to take his medication.

c. Design a medication routine for home and begin routine while patient is still in hospital.

5. Instruct the patient to notify the physician when the following symptoms appear:

a. Chest pressure or pain not relieved in 15 minutes by nitroglycerin or rest

b. Shortness of breath

c. Unusual fatigue

d. Swelling of feet and ankles

e. Fainting, dizziness

f. Very slow or rapid heart beat

6. Assist patient to reduce his risk of another MI by risk factor modification.

a. Explain to patient the major risk factors that can increase his chances for having another MI: smoking, high blood cholesterol levels, and hypertension. Related risk factors include obesity, family history, diabetes, stress, and lack of exercise.

b. Instruct patient in strategies to modify risk factors.

7. Provide educational pamphlets on heart disease and risk factor modification for patient to read and take home. The American Heart Association provides excellent materials. Education materials can also be obtained from the National Heart, Lung and Blood Institute, Public Inquiries and Reports Office, Building 31, Bethesda, MD 20205.

8. Provide information to patient regarding support groups and clubs for cardiac patients (the local American Heart Association Affiliate sponsors these sessions).

Evaluation

1. Maintains balance between myocardial oxygen supply and demand; experiences no chest pain; calls nurse if experiencing pain

2. Experiences a decrease in anxiety; exhibits calm speech pattern, relaxed facial expression, verbalizes feelings about death

3. Maintains hemodynamic stability; exhibits no signs/symptoms of heart failure—diaphoresis, hypotension, change in mental status, cool, clammy skin, oliguria

4. Experiences no life-threatening dysrhythmias; heart rate 60–100 beats per minute; rhythm—normal sinus rhythm

5. Adheres to limited activity prescription; engages in gradual increase in activities; walks one flight of stairs.

6. Remains free of evidence of bleeding; blood pressure/heart rate within normal range for patient; absence of hematoma, ecchymosis, petechiae; absence of retroperitoneal pain; no oozing at puncture sites, urine clear.

7. Maintains tissue perfusion; absence of recurring chest pain; notifies nurse of any pain or discomfort.

8. Copes adaptively to illness; communicates self-confidence in future life-style; requests information regarding illness, environment, and routines; participates in self-care activities

Cardiogenic Shock

Cardiogenic shock occurs when the heart muscle loses its contractile power. Extensive damage of the left ventricle (40% or greater) due to myocardial infarction commonly initiates a perpetuating "shock cycle."

1. Impaired contractility causes a marked reduction in cardiac output.

2. Decreased cardiac output results in a lack of blood and oxygen to the heart as well as other vital organs (brain and kidneys).

3. Lack of blood and oxygen to the heart muscle results in continued damage to the muscle, a further decline in contractile power, and a continued inability of the heart to provide blood and oxygen to vital organs.

4. End-stage cardiomyopathy, severe valvular dysfunction,

and ventricular aneurysm can also precipitate cardiogenic shock.

Clinical Manifestations

1. Low systolic pressure (80 mm. Hg or 30 mm. Hg less than previous levels)
2. Oliguria—urine output less than 30 ml./hour for at least 2 hours—due to decreased perfusion of kidneys
3. Cold, clammy skin (blood is shunted from the peripheral circulation to perfuse vital organs)
4. Weak, thready peripheral pulses, fatigue, hypotension—due to inadequate cardiac output
5. Dyspnea, tachypnea, cyanosis (increased left ventricular pressures result in elevation of left atrial and pulmonary pressures, causing pulmonary congestion)
6. Confusion, restlessness, mental lethargy (due to poor perfusion of brain)
7. Dysrhythmias (due to lack of oxygen to heart muscle and as a compensatory mechanism for a decreased cardiac output)
8. Chest pain (due to lack of oxygen and blood to heart muscle)

Diagnostic Evaluation

1. Physical examination—signs/symptoms of decrease in cerebral, renal, and peripheral perfusion, pulmonary congestion, and hypotension
2. Medical history—reduction in cardiac output unrelated to hypovolemia, significant dysrhythmias, depressive drug therapy, arterial hypoxia, or acute pain
3. Diagnosis of MI—ECG, medical history, physical examination
4. Altered hemodynamic parameters (PCWP 18 mm. Hg or greater, cardiac index less than 2.2, systemic vascular resistance elevation)
5. Chest x-ray
6. Abnormal lab values (elevated BUN and creatinine, elevated liver enzymes).

Management

Goals:
Stimulating cardiac contractility, decreasing cardiac workload, preserving viable heart muscle to limit infarct size, and reducing total body fluid volume.

1. Cardiac glycosides (digoxin) and positive inotropic drugs (dopamine, dobutamine, amrinone) stimulate cardiac contractility.
2. Vasodilator therapy
   a. Decreases the workload of the heart by reducing venous return and lessening the resistance against which the heart pumps (preload and afterload reduction)
   b. Cardiac output improves, left ventricular pressures/pulmonary congestion decrease, and myocardial oxygen consumption is reduced.
3. Counterpulsation therapy (see p. 335)
   a. Improves blood flow to the heart muscle and reduces myocardial oxygen needs
   b. Results in improved cardiac output and preservation of viable heart tissue
4. Diuretic therapy
   a. Decreases total body fluid volume
   b. Relieves systemic and pulmonary congestion

Assessment

1. Identify patients at risk for development of cardiogenic shock.

2. Assess for early signs/symptoms indicative of shock:
   a. Increasing heart rate
   b. Decreasing pulse pressure (indicates impaired cardiac output)
   c. Presence of pulsus alternans (indicates left heart failure)
   d. Decreasing urine output, weakness, fatigue
3. Observe for presence of central and peripheral cyanosis (see Cardiac Assessment, p. 298).
4. Observe for development of edema (see Cardiac Assessment, p. 299).
5. Identify signs/symptoms indicative of extension of myocardial infarction—recurrence of chest pain, diaphoresis.
6. Identify patient's and significant other's reaction to crisis situation.

Nursing Diagnoses

1. Altered cardiac output (decreased) related to impaired contractility due to extensive heart muscle damage
2. Impaired gas exchange related to pulmonary congestion due to elevated left ventricular pressures
3. Altered tissue perfusion (renal, cerebral, cardiopulmonary, gastrointestinal and peripheral) related to decreased blood flow
4. Anxiety related to intensive care environment and threat of death

Nursing Interventions

A. Improving Hemodynamic Stability

1. Establish continuous ECG monitoring to detect dysrhythmias, which increase myocardial oxygen consumption.
2. Monitor hemodynamic parameters continually with Swan–Ganz catheter (see Swan–Ganz, p. 302) to evaluate effectiveness of implemented therapy.
   a. Obtain PAP, PCWP, and CO readings as indicated.
   b. Calculate the cardiac index (CI—cardiac output relative to body size) and systemic vascular resistance (SVR—measurement of afterload).
   c. Cautiously titrate vasoactive drug therapy according to hemodynamic parameters.
      (1) Be alert to adverse responses to drug therapy; dopamine may cause increases in heart rate; vasodilators (nitroglycerin and nitroprusside) may worsen hypotension; digoxin may result in dysrhythmias from toxicity; diuretics may cause hyponatremia, hypokalemia, and hypovolemia.
      (2) Administer vasoactive drug therapy through central venous access (peripheral tissue necrosis can occur if peripheral IV access infiltrates, and peripheral drug distribution may be lessened from vasoconstriction).
3. Monitor blood pressure and mean arterial pressure (MAP) with intra-arterial line (cuff pressures are difficult to ascertain and may be inaccurate) every 30 minutes and every 5 minutes during active titration of vasoactive drug therapy.
4. Maintain MAP greater than 60 mm. Hg (blood flow through coronary vessels is inadequate with a MAP less than 60 mm. Hg).
5. Measure/record urine output every hour from indwelling catheter and fluid intake.
6. Obtain daily weights.
7. Evaluate serum electrolytes for hyponatremia and hypokalemia.

8. Be alert to incidence of chest pain (indicates myocardial ischemia and may further extend heart damage).
   a. Notify physician immediately.
   b. Obtain a 12-lead ECG recording.
   c. Anticipate use of counterpulsation therapy.

B. Improving Oxygenation

1. Monitor rate and rhythm of respirations every hour.
2. Auscultate lung fields for abnormal sounds (coarse crackles indicate severe pulmonary congestion) every hour; notify physician.
3. Evaluate arterial blood gases.
4. Administer oxygen therapy to increase oxygen tension and improve hypoxia.
5. Elevate head of bed 20–30 degrees as tolerated (may worsen hypotension) to facilitate lung expansion.
6. Reposition patient frequently to promote ventilation and maintain skin integrity.
7. Observe for frothy pink-tinged sputum and cough (may indicate pulmonary edema); notify physician immediately.

C. Maintaining Tissue Perfusion

1. Perform a neurological check every 2 hours, using the Glasgow coma scale.
2. Report changes to physician immediately.
3. Obtain BUN and creatinine blood levels to evaluate renal function.
4. Auscultate for bowel sounds every 2 hours.
5. Evaluate character, rate, rhythm, and quality of arterial pulses every 2 hours.
6. Monitor temperature every 2–4 hours.
7. Employ sheepskin foot and elbow protectors to prevent skin breakdown.

D. Relieving Anxiety

1. Explain equipment and rationale for therapy to patient and family—increasing knowledge assists in alleviating fear and anxiety.
2. Encourage patient to verbalize fears concerning diagnosis and prognosis.
3. Explain sensations patient will experience prior to procedures and routine care measures.
4. Offer reassurance and encouragement.
5. Provide for periods of uninterrupted rest and sleep.
6. Assist patient to maintain as much control as possible over environment and care.
   a. Develop a schedule for routine care measures and rest periods with patient.
   b. Ensure that a calendar and clock are in view of patient.

Evaluation

1. Demonstrates improved cardiac output—CO greater than 4 liters/minute; CI greater than 2.2, PCWP less than 18 mm. Hg; Urine output greater than 30 ml./hour; heart rate 60–100 beats/minute; no dysrhythmias
2. Exhibits improvement in oxygenation—spontaneous respirations within normal limits for patient, unlabored and regular; normal breath sounds throughout lung fields; arterial blood gases within normal limits for patient
3. Demonstrates adequate tissue perfusion—normal sensorium; BUN and creatinine within normal limits; skin warm and dry
4. Achieves a reduction in anxiety—verbalizes a decrease in anxiety and fear; relaxed facial expressions; decreased tension

Intra-aortic Balloon Pump (IABP) Counterpulsation

Counterpulsation is a method of assisting the failing heart and circulation by mechanical support. The mechanism of counterpulsation therapy is opposite to the normal pumping action of the heart; counterpulsation devices pump while the heart muscle relaxes (diastole) and relax when the heart muscle contracts (systole).

A. Intra-aortic Balloon Pump (Fig. 14-10)

A balloon catheter is introduced into the femoral artery percutaneously or surgically, threaded to the descending thoracic aorta, and positioned distal to the subclavian artery.

1. The balloon catheter is attached to an external console, allowing for inflation/deflation of the balloon with gas (helium or carbon dioxide).
2. The external console integrates the inflation/deflation sequence with the mechanical events of the cardiac cycle (systole/diastole) by "triggering" gas delivery in sychronization with the patient's ECG and "timing" the duration of inflation and point of deflation in conjunction with the patient's arterial pressure waveform.

B. Counterpulsation With an Intra-aortic Balloon Pump (IABP)

1. Eases the workload of a damaged heart by increasing coronary blood flow (diastolic augmentation) and decreasing the resistance in the arterial tree against which the heart must pump (afterload reduction).
2. This results in an increase in cardiac output and a reduction in myocardial oxygen requirements.
3. The balloon is inflated at the onset of diastole; this results in an increase in diastolic pressure (diastolic augmentation), which increases blood flow through the coronary arteries.
4. The balloon is deflated just prior to the onset of systole, facilitating the emptying of blood from the left ventricle.
5. Clinical Uses
   a. Treatment of cardiogenic shock following myocardial infarction
   b. Low cardiac output states—following open heart surgery; life-threatening dysrhythmias
   c. High cardiac output states—sepsis, hemorrhage
   d. Myocardial ischemia unresponsive to medical therapy and external counterpulsation pressure

Nursing Interventions

A. Alleviating Fear

1. Explain IABP therapy to patient and family geared to their level of understanding.
   a. Review purpose of therapy and how the IABP functions.
   b. Reinforce mobility restrictions: flat in bed on back (head of bed elevated 15–30 degrees), no movement or flexing of leg with IABP catheter.
   c. Explain need for frequent monitoring of vital signs, rhythm, affected extremity, and pulses.
   d. Discuss the sounds associated with the functioning external console: balloon inflation/deflation and alarms.
2. Encourage family members to participate in care of patient.
   a. Allow family to visit patient frequently.
   b. Solicit family members' assistance in reinforcing

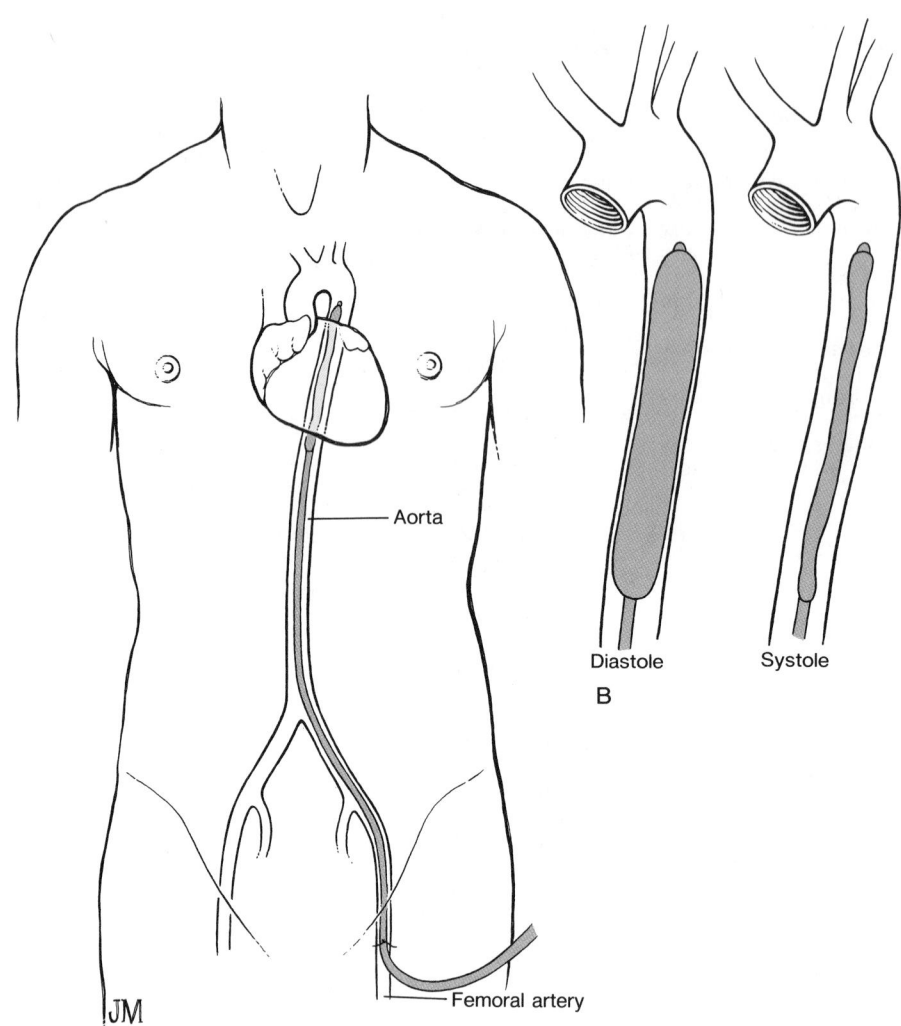

Aorta

Diastole   Systole

B

Femoral artery

JM

A

Figure 14-10. *Counterpulsation. (A) Introduction of the intra-aortic balloon catheter via the femoral artery. (B) The intra-aortic balloon pump augments diastole, resulting in increased perfusion of the coronary arteries and myocardium and a decrease in the left ventricular work load.*

mobility restrictions to patient and notifying nursing staff of patient comfort needs.
3. Allow patient to verbalize fears regarding therapy and illness.
4. Ensure informed consent is obtained from patient or authorized guardian/family member prior to IABP insertion.

B. Establishing Hemodynamic Stability

1. Assist patient and physician during insertion of IABP catheter.
   a. Offer patient reassurance and comfort measures (patient is only mildly sedated).
   b. Ensure strict aseptic environment during insertion.
   c. Establish ECG monitoring, choosing the lead with the largest R wave (external console senses R wave of the patient's ECG to trigger gas delivery) and without artifact (integration of the patient's cardiac cycle with the inflation/deflation balloon sequence is dependent on a continuous clear ECG tracing).

   d. Record date, time, and the patient's tolerance of procedure.
2. Start IABP immediately after insertion, as directed by physician; review manufacturer's manual for IABP equipment in use.
   a. Adjust the duration of balloon inflation/deflation by the arterial pressure waveform (inflation is "timed" to begin at the dicrotic notch of the arterial waveform, and deflation occurs prior to the next systole).
   b. Compare the patient's arterial pressure waveform with/without balloon augmentation to evaluate effectiveness of therapy.
      Note difference in patient's end diastolic pressure and balloon-assisted end diastolic pressure (the balloon-assisted end diastolic pressure should be lower, indicating a reduction in afterload).
   c. Monitor hemodynamic parameters with Swan–Ganz catheter (see hemodynamic monitoring, p. 302).

Record CVP, PAP, PCWP, and CO to evaluate overall effectiveness of therapy.

3. Monitor vital signs every 15–30 minutes for 4–9 hours and then hourly.
4. Monitor urine output from indwelling catheter every hour.
5. Maintain accurate intake/output.
6. Treat dysrhythmias as directed.
7. Report chest pain experienced by patient immediately to physician.
8. Check for blood oozing around IABP catheter every hour for 8 hours, then every 4 hours (anticoagulation therapy is used to prevent thrombus formation); apply direct pressure and notify physician if bleeding is noted.
9. See Cardiogenic Shock, page 333.

C. Maintaining Adequate Tissue Perfusion

1. Evaluate for ischemia of extremity with IABP catheter.
   a. Mark pulses with indelible ink to facilitate checks.
   b. Monitor peripheral pulses (dorsalis pedis, posterior tibial, and popliteal) for rhythm, character, and pulse quality every 15 minutes for 1 hour, then every 30 minutes for 1 hour, and then hourly.
   c. Use Doppler device for pulses difficult to palpate and to auscultate for bruits/hums.
   d. Observe skin temperature, color, sensation, and movement of affected extremity (dusky, cool, mottled, painful, numb/tingling extremity indicates ischemia).
2. Observe for possible indications of thromboemboli.
   a. Note decreases in urine output after initiation of therapy—may indicate renal artery emboli.
   b. Perform neurological checks every hour to evaluate for cerebral emboli.
   c. Auscultate bowel sounds to detect evidence of ischemia.
3. Recognize early signs/symptoms of compartment syndrome (increased pressure in tissue reduces blood flow).
   a. Note complaints of pain, pressure, and numbness of affected extremity induced by passive stretching.
   b. Palpate affected extremity for swelling and tension.
   c. Monitor CPK values (highly elevated CPKs may indicate compartment syndrome).

D. Maintaining Normal Skin Integrity and Joint Motion

1. Implement passive range of motion exercises with exception of extremity with IABP catheter.
2. Turn patient from side to side as a unit every 2 hours (patients are usually debilitated and prone to pressure sores).
3. Keep head of bed elevated 15–30 degrees or flat (catheter may migrate upward and obstruct left subclavian artery).

Endocardial Disease

Infective Endocarditis

Infective endocarditis (IE) (bacterial endocarditis) is an infection of the inner lining of the heart caused by direct invasion of bacteria or other organisms leading to deformity of the valve leaflets.

Altered Physiology

1. When the inner lining of the heart (endocardium) becomes inflamed, a fibrin clot (vegetation) forms.
2. The fibrin clot may become colonized by pathogens during transient episodes of bacteremia resulting from invasive procedures (venous/arterial cannulation, dental work causing gingival bleeding, GI tract surgery, liver biopsy, sigmoidoscopy, etc.), indwelling catheters, urinary tract infections, and wound/skin infections.
3. Platelets and fibrin surround the invading microorganisms, forming a protective covering and causing the infected vegetation to enlarge.
   a. The enlarged vegetation (the basic lesion of endocarditis) can deform, thicken, stiffen, and scar the free margins of valve leaflets, as well as the fibrous ring (annulus) supporting the valve.
   b. The vegetation(s) may also travel to various organs/tissues (spleen, kidney, coronary artery, brain and lungs) and obstruct blood flow.
   c. The "protective covering" surrounding the vegetation makes it difficult for white blood cells and antimicrobial agents to infiltrate and destroy the infected lesion.

Etiology

1. Bacteria
   a. *Streptococcus viridans*—bacteremia occurs after dental work or upper respiratory infection.
   b. *Staphylococcus aureus*—bacteremia occurs after cardiac surgery or parenteral drug abuse.
   c. *Enterococci* (penicillin-resistant group D streptococci)—bacteremia usually occurs in elderly (over 60) with genitourinary tract infection.
2. Fungi (*Candida albicans, Aspergillus*)
3. Rickettsiae

Characteristics

1. Infective endocarditis may develop on a heart valve already injured by rheumatic fever, congenital defects, on abnormally vascularized valves, normal heart valves, and mechanical/biological heart valves.
2. Infective endocarditis may be acute or subacute, depending on the microorganisms involved. Acute IE manifests rapidly with danger of intractable heart failure and occurs more commonly on normal heart valves.
3. Subacute IE manifests a prolonged chronic course with a lesser chance of complications and occurs more commonly on damaged/defective valves.
4. Infective endocarditis may follow cardiac surgery, especially when prosthetic heart valves are used; Foreign bodies such as pacemakers, patches, grafts, and dialysis shunts predispose to infection.
5. High incidence among drug abusers, in whom the disease mainly affects normal valves, usually the tricuspid.
6. Hospitalized patients with indwelling catheters, those on prolonged intravenous therapy or prolonged antibiotic therapy, and those on immunosuppressive drugs or steroids may develop fungal endocarditis.
7. Relapse due to metastatic infection is possible, usually within the first 2 months after completion of antibiotic regimen.

Clinical Manifestations

Severity of manifestations depends on invading microorganism.

A. General Manifestations

1. Fever, chills, sweats (fever may be absent in elderly or in patients with uremia)
2. Anorexia, weight loss, weakness
3. Cough; back and joint pain (especially in elderly over 60)
4. Splenomegaly

B. Skin and Nail Manifestations

1. Petechiae—conjunctiva, mucous membranes
2. Splinter hemorrhages in nail beds
3. Osler's nodes—painful red nodes on pads of fingers and toes; usually late sign of infection and found with a subacute infection
4. Janeway's lesions—light pink macules on palms or soles, nontender, may change to light tan within several days, fade in 1–2 weeks. Usually an early sign of endocardial infection

C. Heart Manifestations

1. New pathologic or changing murmur—no murmur with other signs/symptoms may indicate right heart infection
2. Tachycardia—related to decreased cardiac output

D. Central Nervous System Manifestations

1. Localized headaches
2. Transient cerebral ischemia
3. Altered mental status, aphasia
4. Hemiplegia
5. Cortical sensory loss

E. Pulmonary Manifestations

1. Usually occur with right-sided heart involvement
2. Pneumonitis, pleuritis, pulmonary edema, pulmonary infiltrates

F. Embolic Phenomena

1. Lung—hemoptysis, chest pain, shortness of breath
2. Kidney—hematuria
3. Spleen—pain in upper left quadrant of abdomen radiating to left shoulder
4. Heart—myocardial infarction
5. Brain—sudden blindness, paralysis, brain abscess, meningitis
6. Blood vessels—mycotic aneurysms
7. Abdomen—melena, acute pain

Diagnostic Evaluation

Varied clinical manifestations and similarities to other diseases make early diagnosis of IE difficult.

1. Blood cultures—at least two positive serial blood cultures isolating bacteria or fungi
2. Medical history—elicitation of a history of symptoms of disease
3. Physical examination—especially cardiac auscultation and funduscopic examination
4. Elevated sedimentation rate, tests indicative of anemia, mild leukocytosis, urine abnormalities indicating nephrosis
5. ECG
6. Echocardiography—identification of vegetations and assessment of location and size of lesions

Management

Goal:

Targeted at eradication of invading microorganism by parenteral antimicrobial therapy, treatment of symptoms of cardiac disease or failure, valve replacement relative to hemodynamic instability, and prevention of endocarditis in susceptible individuals.

1. Serial blood cultures to determine causative organism.
2. Antimicrobial therapy based on sensitivity of causative agent; penicillin G, nafcillin, vancomycin, gentamicin, rifampin alone or in combination for 4–6 weeks. Bactericidal serum levels of selected antibiotic are monitored by titering it against the causative organism; if serum lacks adequate bactericidal activity, more antibiotic or a different antibiotic is given.
3. Audiogram obtained before antibiotic regimen initiated
4. Urine cultures obtained after 48 hours to assess efficacy of drug therapy
5. Repeat blood cultures obtained after 48 hours to assess efficacy of drug therapy
6. Daily physical examination by cardiologist
7. Supplemental nutrition
8. Surgical intervention for:
   a. Acute destructive valvular lesion—excision of infected valves or removal of prosthetic valve
   b. Hemodynamic impairment
   c. Recurrent emboli
   d. Infection that cannot be eliminated with antimicrobial therapy
   e. Drainage of abscess/empyema—for patient with localized abscess or empyema
   f. Repair of peripheral or cerebral mycotic aneurysm

Complications

1. Severe heart failure due to valvular insufficiency
2. Uncontrolled/refractory infection
3. Embolic episodes (ischemia or necrosis of extremities and organs)
4. Conduction disturbances

Nursing Assessment

1. Identify factors that may predispose to endocarditis, such as rheumatic heart disease, congenital heart defects, idiopathic hypertrophic subaortic stenosis (IHSS), IV drug abuse, prosthetic heart valves, aortic/mitral stenosis, previous history of endocarditis.
2. Determine onset of signs/symptoms of endocarditis (early treatment of infection improves prognosis).
3. Identify potential incidents that may have precipitated a transient bacteremia capable of causing endocarditis.
4. Obtain blood cultures, complete blood count, renal/hepatic studies, and a baseline 12-lead ECG.
5. Assess patient for allergies, with special emphasis on untoward reactions to antibiotic therapy.
6. Note if patient is currently on antibiotic therapy (may affect blood culture results).
7. Identify patient's/family level of anxiety and utilization of appropriate coping mechanisms.

Nursing Diagnoses

1. Altered cardiac output (decreased) related to structural factors (incompetent valves)
2. Altered tissue perfusion (renal, cerebral, cardiopulmonary, gastrointestinal, and peripheral) related to interruption of blood flow
3. Hyperthermia related to illness, potential dehydration, and aggressive antibiotic therapy.

4. Altered nutrition (less than body requirements) related to anorexia.
5. Anxiety related to acute illness and hospitalization.

Nursing Interventions

A. Attaining Hemodynamic Stability

1. Auscultate heart to detect new murmur or change in existing murmur.
2. Monitor blood pressure and pulse.
   a. Note presence of pulsus alternans (indicative of left heart failure).
   b. Evaluate pulse pressure (30–40 mm. Hg normal; indicates adequate cardiac output).
3. Evaluate jugular venous distention.
4. Record intake and output.
5. Record daily weight.
6. Auscultate lung fields for evidence of crackles (rales).

B. Achieving Tissue Perfusion

1. Observe the patient for altered mentation, hemoptysis, hematuria, aphasia, loss of muscle strength, complaints of pain (see Clinical Manifestations, pp. 337–338).
2. Observe for splinter hemorrhages of nailbeds, Osler's nodes, and Janeway's lesions.
3. Notify physician of observed changes in the patient's status.

C. Maintaining Normothermia/Preventing Complications

1. Observe basic principles of asepsis, good handwashing techniques, and continuity of patient care by primary nurse.
2. Employ meticulous IV care for long-term antibiotic therapy.
   a. Note the date of needle or cannula insertion on nursing care plan.
   b. Rotate IV site every 72 hours or if site becomes tender, reddened, infiltrated, or has purulent drainage.
   c. Change gauze/transparent dressing every 24 hours to prevent infection.
3. Administer parenteral antibiotic therapy as directed.
   a. Develop chart for rotation of sites for intramuscular administration of antibiotic therapy.
   b. Observe for untoward reaction to antibiotic therapy (severe respiratory distress, rash, itching, fever).
   c. Observe for side effects of long-term antibiotic therapy—ototoxicity, renal failure.
4. Monitor temperature every 2–4 hours.
   a. Document results on graph.
   b. Note increases in heart rate/respirations with elevated temperatures.
   c. Provide cooling measures such as alcohol/tepid water sponge bath and/or cooling blanket as directed.
   d. Provide blankets and temperature-controlled comfortable environment if patient has shaking chills; change bed linens as necessary.
   e. Administer analgesic medications as directed.
5. Position patient frequently to prevent skin breakdown and pulmonary complications associated with bedrest.
6. Observe patient for a general "sense of well-being" within 5–7 days after initiation of therapy.
7. Monitor laboratory values—hematocrit, BUN, creatinine, WBC, antibiotic levels, blood cultures.
8. Promote adequate hydration, as diaphoresis and increased metabolic rate may cause dehydration.
   a. Encourage oral fluid intake.
   b. Administer IV fluids as directed.
   c. Observe skin turgor and mucous membranes.

D. Improving Nutritional Status

1. Assess the patient's daily caloric intake.
2. Discuss food preferences with the patient.
3. Consult with a dietitian regarding nutritional needs of patient and food preferences.
4. Encourage small meals and snacks throughout the day.
5. Record daily caloric intake and weight.
6. Educate family members about the patient's caloric needs.
7. Encourage family members to assist the patient with meals and bring in the patient's favorite foods.

E. Reducing Anxiety

1. Encourage the patient to verbalize fears regarding illness and hospitalization.
2. Explain all procedures to patient before initiation.
3. Offer the patient literature, if available, about his disease.
4. Encourage diversional activities for the patient such as television, reading, and interaction with other patients.
5. Encourage family members to interact with the patient as frequently as possible.

Patient Education/Discharge Planning

A. For Patients at Risk—develop in-depth formal program.

1. Discuss anatomy of heart and changes that occur during endocarditis, using diagrams of the heart.
2. Give the patient written literature on early signs and symptoms of disease; review these with the patient.
3. Discuss with individual the mode of entry of infection.
4. Indicate that antibiotic prophylaxis is recommended for persons at risk for the following:
   a. Congenital heart defects, prosthetic/biological heart valves, idiopathic hypertrophic subaortic stenosis (IHSS)
   b. Past history of endocarditis
   c. Mitral valve prolapse with insufficiency
   d. Rheumatic heart disease and valvular dysfunction
   e. Undergoing procedures most likely to cause bacteremia (dental procedures causing gingival bleeding, surgery on or instrumentation of GI tract, and certain genitourinary procedures, etc.)*
5. Identify individual steps necessary to prevent infection.
   a. Good oral hygiene, regular tooth brushing, and flossing
   b. Notification to health-care personnel of any history of congenital heart disease or valvular disease.
   c. Discuss importance of carrying emergency identification with information of medical history at all times.
   d. Take temperature if infection is suspected and notify physician of elevation.
   e. Teach individual to inspect soles of feet for Janeway's lesions indicative of possible relapse.
   f. Educate persons at risk to look for and treat symptoms of illness indicating bacteremia—injuries, sore throats, furuncles, etc.
6. Provide patient with American Heart Association Bacterial Endocarditis wallet card outlining recommended

---

* From the American Heart Association: Prevention of bacterial endocarditis. Circulation 70:1123A–1127A, 1984.

antibiotic prophylaxis for procedures (obtain at local American Heart Association chapter).

7. Encourage susceptible individuals to receive pneumococcal vaccine and influenza vaccine.
   Teach that vaccines reduce the risk of severe infections that could precipitate heart failure.
8. Teach women in childbearing years the risks of using IUDs for birth control (source of infection) and that antibiotic therapy is not necessary for individuals having normal deliveries.

B. For Individuals Who Have Had Endocarditis Regarding Possible Relapse

1. Discuss importance of keeping follow-up appointments after hospital discharge (infection can recur in 1–2 months).
2. Review the tests that will be performed after hospital discharge—blood cultures, physical examination.
3. Contact social worker to assist the patient with financial planning and home discharge arrangements if applicable.

Evaluation

1. Maintains hemodynamic stability—exhibits no symptoms of heart failure
2. Maintains satisfactory tissue perfusion—lack of signs/symptoms of embolic phenomena
3. Remains free of complications—normal temperature, negative blood cultures, normal WBC count, BUN, and creatinine, no hearing impairments
4. Achieves improved nutritional status—increases daily caloric intake compatible with height/weight/age
5. Demonstrates decrease in anxiety

Rheumatic Endocarditis (Rheumatic Heart Disease)

Rheumatic endocarditis is damage done to the heart, particularly the valves, resulting in valve leakage (regurgitation) and/or obstruction (narrowing or stenosis). There are associated compensatory changes in the size of the heart's chambers and the thickness of chamber walls.

Role of Streptococcal Infection

Rheumatic fever is a sequela to group A streptococcal infection. It is a preventable disease through the detection and adequate treatment of streptococcal pharyngitis.

Symptoms of Streptococcal Pharyngitis

1. Sudden onset of sore throat; throat reddened with exudate
2. Swollen, tender lymph nodes at angle of jaw
3. Headache and fever 38.9°–40°C. (101°–104°F.)
4. Abdominal pain (children)

NURSING ALERT: Some cases of streptococcal throat infection are relatively asymptomatic.

Clinical Manifestations of Rheumatic Fever

1. Polyarthritis; warm and swollen joints
2. Carditis
3. Chorea (irregular, jerky, involuntary, unpredictable muscular movements)

4. Erythema marginatum (wavy, thin red-line skin rash on trunk and extremities)
5. Subcutaneous nodules
6. Fever
7. Prolonged PR interval demonstrated by ECG
8. Heart murmurs; pleural and pericardial rubs

Diagnostic Evaluation

1. Throat culture—to determine presence of streptococcal organisms
2. Increased sedimentation rate; WBC count and differential and C-reactive protein—increase during acute phase of infection
3. Elevated antistreptolysin titer

Management

1. Antimicrobial therapy—to eradicate involved organism
2. Rest—to maintain optimal cardiac function
3. Salicylates—to control fever and pain
4. Prevention of recurrent episodes

Nursing Interventions

1. Limit physical activity during the acute phase—patient should rest in bed as long as there is fever or signs of active carditis.
2. Administer penicillin therapy as prescribed—to eradicate hemolytic streptococcus; erythromycin may be used if the patient is allergic to penicillin.
3. Give salicylates as prescribed—to suppress rheumatic activity by controlling toxic manifestations, to reduce fever, and to relieve joint pain.
4. Assess for effectiveness of drug therapy.
   a. Take and record temperature every 3 hours.
   b. Evaluate the patient's comfort level every 3 hours.
5. Monitor the patient's dietary intake (symptoms of disease inhibit the patient's ability to take in nutrients).
   a. Record the patient's daily caloric intake.
   b. Supplement diet with high-carbohydrate liquids if indicated.
6. Assess for signs/symptoms of acute rheumatic carditis.
   a. Be alert to the patient's complaints of chest pain, palpitations, and/or precordial "tightness."
   b. Monitor for tachycardia (usually persistent when the patient sleeps) or bradycardia.
   c. Be alert to development of second-degree heart block or Wenckebach's syndrome (acute rheumatic carditis causes PR interval prolongation).
7. Auscultate heart sounds every 4 hours.
   Document presence of murmur or pericardial friction rub (see Endocarditis, p. 337; Pericarditis, p. 344).
   b. Document extra heart sounds (S_3 gallop, S_4 gallop; see Congestive Heart Failure, p. 348).
8. See rheumatic fever in children, page 1327.
9. Be aware of the possible complication of chronic rheumatic endocarditis. Chronic rheumatic endocarditis is a complication of rheumatic fever that frequently produces progressive disability and a shortened life span. Every structural component of the heart is likely to be the site of an inflammatory reaction.
   a. Although the patient is symptom-free for a time, the damage to the valves (rigidity and deformity, thickening and fusion of the commissures, or shortening and fusion of chordae tendinae) will produce heart sounds that are characteristic of valvular stenosis, regurgitation, or both.

b. The myocardium will compensate for these valvular defects for a while, but in time it fails to compensate, and the patient develops symptoms of congestive heart failure.

c. See page 345 for treatment of valvular heart disease and page 349 for treatment of congestive heart failure.

Patient Education/Discharge Planning

A. Preventing Recurrence

1. Counsel the patient to maintain good nutrition.
   a. Provide teaching on basic food groups.
   b. Assist with planning several daily meal plans.
   c. Discuss proper preparation of food (clean utensils and kitchen area) and proper storage of food.
   d. Discuss with the patient his financial situation and home facilities relative to nutritional health maintenance. If appropriate, contact social services for the patient.
2. Counsel the patient on hygienic practices.
   a. Discuss proper hand-washing, disposal of tissues, laundering of handkerchiefs (decrease chance of exposure to microbes).
   b. Discuss importance of using patient's own toothbrush, soap, and washcloths when living in group situations.
3. Counsel the patient on importance of receiving adequate rest.
4. Counsel the patient to seek treatment immediately should sore throat occur.
   Explore with patient his ability to pay for medical treatment. If appropriate, contact social services for the patient. (Financial difficulties may inhibit the patient from seeking early treatment of symptoms.)

B. Other Points

1. Instruct the patient to use prophylactic penicillin therapy before undergoing surgery of genitourinary tract, lower intestinal tract, and respiratory tract.
2. See Patient Education, Endocarditis, page 339.

Myocarditis

Myocarditis is an inflammatory process involving the myocardium.

Etiology

1. Infectious process—viral (particularly Coxsackie group B, and may develop after influenza A or B, herpes simplex), bacterial, mycotic, parasitic, protozoal, rickettsial, and spirochetal infections
2. Following drug administration (doxorubicin [Adriamycin])
3. Other conditions—sarcoidosis, collagen diseases (rheumatic fever)
4. Immunosuppressive therapy

Clinical Manifestations

A. Symptoms

1. Depend on type of infection, degree of myocardial damage, capacity of myocardium to recover, and host resistance. Can be acute or chronic and occur at any age. Symptoms may be minor and go unnoticed.
   a. Fatigue and dyspnea
   b. Palpitations
   c. Occasional precordial discomfort

B. Clinical Findings

1. Cardiac enlargement
2. Cardiac murmur—abnormal heart sound; sounds like fluid passing an obstruction (due to papillary muscle dysfunction)
3. Pericardial friction rub
4. Gallop rhythm—a tripling or quadrupling of heart sounds (resembling the galloping of a horse) heard on auscultation
5. Pulsus alternans—a pulse in which there is a regular alternation of weak and strong beats
6. Fever with tachycardia
7. Evidence of development of congestive heart failure

Diagnostic Evaluation

1. History of recent infection
2. Transient ECG changes—ST segment flattened, T wave inversion, conduction defects, extrasystoles, supraventricular and ventricular ectopic beats
3. Elevated WBC count and sedimentation rate
4. Chest x-ray—may show heart enlargement and lung congestion
5. Elevated antibody titers (antistreptolysin-o [ASO titer] as in rheumatic fever)
6. Stool and throat cultures isolating bacteria or a virus

Management

Treatment objectives are targeted toward management of complications.

1. Diuretic and digoxin therapy for congestive heart failure and atrial fibrillation
2. Antidysrhythmic therapy (usually quinidine or procainamide)
3. Strict bed rest to promote healing of damaged myocardium
4. Antimicrobial therapy if causative bacteria is isolated

Nursing Interventions

A. Maintaining Hemodynamic Stability

1. Evaluate for clinical evidence that disease is subsiding—monitor pulse, auscultate for abnormal heart sounds (murmur or change in existing murmur), check temperature, auscultate lung fields, monitor respirations.
2. Record daily intake and output.
3. Record weight daily.
4. Check for peripheral edema.
5. Elevate head of bed, if necessary, to enhance respiration.
6. Treat the symptoms of congestive heart failure as prescribed (see p. 348).
   a. Digitalis—augments myocardial contractility and slows heart rate
   b. Diuretics—to control pulmonary or systemic congestion

> **NURSING ALERT:** Patients with myocarditis may be sensitive to digitalis—assess for toxic symptoms (see p. 373).

7. Evaluate the patient's pulse and apical rate for signs of tachycardia and gallop rhythm—indications that congestive heart failure is recurring.

8. Evaluate for evidences of dysrhythmias—*patients with myocarditis are prone to develop dysrhythmias.*
   a. Advocate that patient be placed in unit with continuous cardiac monitoring if evidences of a dysrhythmia develop.
   b. Have equipment for resuscitation, cardiac defibrillation, and cardiac pacing available in event of life-threatening dysrhythmia.

B. Ensuring Bed Rest

1. Ensure bed rest to reduce heart rate, stroke volume, blood pressure, and heart contractility; also helps to decrease residual damage and complications of myocarditis, and promotes healing.
   Prolonged bed rest may be required—until there is reduction in heart size and improvement of function.
2. Provide diversional activities for patient.
3. Allow the patient to use bedside commode rather than bedpan (reduces cardiovascular workload).

C. Coping Effectively With Illness

1. Explore with the patient his fears, anxieties, and concerns regarding illness and hospitalization.
2. Answer questions with a straightforward approach.
3. Discuss with the patient activities that can be continued after discharge.
   a. Discuss need to modify activities in immediate future.
   b. Explore with the patient life-style modifications and discuss adequacy of self-concept.
4. Emphasize the patient's strengths rather than limitations.
5. Encourage family members to support the patient and learn about his illness.
6. Discuss with family members their fears and anxieties relative to the patient's illness so that they will be able to communicate positively with the patient.

Patient Education/Discharge Planning

Instruct the patient as follows:
1. There is usually some residual heart enlargement; physical activity may be *slowly* increased; begin with chair rest for increasing periods; follow with walking in the room and then outdoors.
2. Report any symptom involving rapidly beating heart.
3. Avoid competitive sports, alcohol, and other myocardial toxins (doxorubicin).
4. Pregnancy is not advisable for women with cardiomyopathies (diseases that affect structure and function of myocardium).
5. Prevention—prevent infectious diseases by means of appropriate immunizations.

Cardiomyopathy

1. *Cardiomyopathy* refers to any disease of the heart muscle.
   a. *Primary cardiomyopathy*—The cause of the disorder is unknown.
   b. *Secondary cardiomyopathy*—The cause of the disorder is known or suspected (coronary artery disease can cause ischemic cardiomyopathy).
2. The cardiomyopathies are categorized into three major groups (dilated, hypertrophic, restrictive) to delineate

the variations in structural and functional abnormalities that can occur.

Dilated Cardiomyopathy

Pathophysiology and Causes

1. Both the right and left ventricle enlarge (dilate) significantly, causing a decrease in the ability of the heart to pump blood efficiently to the body.
2. Blood remaining in the ventricles after contraction causes increases in ventricular, atrial, and pulmonary pressures.
3. The increased pressures continue to diminish the ability of the heart to pump blood to the body, and heart failure occurs.
4. Alcohol abuse, chemotherapy, chemical agents, pregnancy (third trimester, postpartum), and infections can cause dilated cardiomyopathy.

Clinical Manifestations

1. Exertional dyspnea
2. Chest pain
3. Congestive heart failure (see Clinical Manifestations, Congestive Heart Failure, p. 348).
4. Pulmonary edema (see Clinical Manifestations, Pulmonary Edema, p. 351).
5. Dysrhythmias (frequent atrial/ventricular ectopic beats, sinus, atrial, and ventricular tachycardia).

Diagnostic Evaluation

1. History and physical examination
2. Chest x-ray (cardiomegaly)
3. ECG
4. Echocardiogram (detects abnormalities of heart wall movements)
5. 24-hour Holter monitoring (monitors for presence of dysrhythmias)
6. Radionuclide imaging (assess ventricular function)
7. Cardiac catheterization (assists to rule out coronary artery disease as etiology for dysfunction)

Management

The goal of therapy is to maximize ventricular function and prevent complications.
1. Effective management of heart failure by conventional therapy is of primary importance (see Management, Congestive Heart Failure, p. 349).
2. Oral anticoagulants may be instituted to prevent thrombus and pulmonary embolus.
3. Heart transplantation must be considered in the terminal disease phase.

> **NURSING ALERT:** Patients with dilated cardiomyopathy are susceptible to digoxin toxicity. Monitor patient carefully for evidence of nausea, vomiting, yellow vision, and dysrhythmias.

Complications

1. Mural thrombus (due to blood stasis in ventricles)
2. Severe heart failure
3. Sudden cardiac death
4. Pulmonary embolism

Hypertrophic Cardiomyopathy (HCM)

Pathophysiology and Causes

1. HCM is primarily due to the abnormal thickening of the ventricular septum of the heart.
2. The thickening of the heart muscle commonly occurs asymmetrically (septum is proportionately thicker than the other ventricular walls), but also may occur symmetrically (septum and the ventricular free wall both become equally thickened).
3. The ultrastructure of the heart is also disrupted by patches of myocardial fibrosis, disorganization of myocardial fibers, and abnormalities of the coronary microvasculature.
4. The thickened heart muscle and ultrastructure disruption change the shape, size, and distensibility of the ventricular cavity and alter the normal thickness and functioning of the mitral valve; as a result, the heart's ability to relax and contract normally is impaired.
   a. Muscle stiffness impairs the filling of the ventricle with blood during relaxation.
   b. Forceful contractions eject blood from the heart too rapidly, causing abnormal pressure gradients; mechanical narrowing of the passage by which the blood leaves the heart also may occur, acutely obstructing blood flow to the body.
5. HCM is a genetically transmitted disorder.

Clinical Manifestations

1. Chest pain (ischemia due to impaired relaxation of the ventricle)
2. Dyspnea (due to increased pulmonary pressures)
3. Palpitations, dizziness, and lightheadedness (due to dysrhythmias)
4. Syncope (due to dysrhythmias or obstruction of blood flow)
5. Dysrhythmias (bradycardia and tachycardias)

Diagnostic Evaluation

1. History and physical examination
   a. Familial occurrence prevalent
   b. Characteristic systolic murmur that changes intensity with various maneuvers (standing, squatting, Valsalva).
2. ECG
3. Echocardiography (septal thickening and abnormal mitral valve function can be detected)
4. Radionuclide imaging
5. Cardiac catheterization (detects pressure gradients if "obstruction" is present).

Management of Hypertrophic Cardiomyopathy

Treatment is directed toward improving cardiac function and preventing complications in an effort to provide symptom relief and avoid death.

1. *Beta adrenergic blockers*—reduce the force of the heart muscle's contraction, diminish obstructive pressure gradients, and decrease oxygen requirements. Propranolol is the agent of choice.
2. *Calcium channel blockers*—primarily improve the heart's ability to relax, but also have an effect on reducing the force of the heart muscle's contraction, thereby providing symptom relief. Verapamil is the agent of choice and is implemented after failure of beta adrenergic agents to control symptoms.
3. *Antidysrhythmic therapy*—Amiodarone is the agent of choice to prophylactically prevent lethal dysrhythmias.
4. *Myotomy and myectomy*—surgical resection of a portion of the septum to reduce muscle thickness and provide symptom relief
5. *Device implantation*—Pacemakers and automatic internal defibrillators may be implanted to treat severe bradycardias and lethal tachycardias.

NURSING ALERT: Chest pain experienced by HCM patients is managed by rest and elevation of the feet (improves venous return to the heart). Vasodilator therapy (nitroglycerin) may worsen chest pain by decreasing venous return to the heart and further increasing obstruction of blood flow from the heart; agents that increase contractility of the heart muscle (dopamine, dobutamine) should also be avoided or used with extreme caution.

Complications

1. Sudden cardiac death
2. Heart failure

Restrictive Cardiomyopathy

Pathophysiology

1. The heart muscle becomes infiltrated by various substances, resulting in severe fibrosis.
2. The heart muscle becomes stiff and nondistensible, impairing the ability of the ventricle to fill with blood adequately.
3. Amyloid and hemochromatosis (disorder of excess iron deposition) may cause restrictive cardiomyopathy.

Clinical Manifestations

1. Right-sided heart failure (see Clinical Manifestations, Congestive Heart Failure, p. 348).
2. Atrial fibrillation
3. Pericardial effusions

Diagnostic Evaluation

1. ECG
2. Echocardiography
3. Heart biopsy (may determine cellular infiltrate)
4. Magnetic resonance imaging (Pericardial imaging is useful to differentiate condition from constrictive pericarditis.)

Management

1. Therapy is palliative unless specific underlying process is established.
2. Heart failure can be controlled with fluid restriction and diuretic therapy alone
3. Digoxin is beneficial for controlling atrial fibrillation.
4. Oral anticoagulants are instituted to prevent emboli.

Complications

1. Severe heart failure
2. Systemic emboli

Pericarditis

Pericarditis is an inflammation of the pericardium, the membranous sac enveloping the heart. It is often a manifestation of a more generalized disease.

Pericardial effusion is an outpouring of fluid into the pericardial cavity.

Constrictive pericarditis is a condition in which a chronic inflammatory thickening of the pericardium compresses the heart so that it is unable to fill normally during diastole.

Etiology

1. Acute idiopathic—most common and typical form; etiology unknown
2. Infection
   a. Viral (influenza; Coxsackie virus)
   b. Bacterial—staphylococcus, meningococcus, streptococcus, pneumococcus, gonococcus, *Mycobacterium tuberculosis*
   c. Fungal
   d. Parasitic
3. Disorders of connective tissues and allergies—lupus erythematosus, periarteritis nodosa
4. Myocardial infarction; early, 24–72 hours; or late, 1 week to 2 years (Dressler's syndrome)
5. Malignant disease; thoracic irradiation
6. Chest trauma, heart surgery, including pacemaker implantation
7. Drug induced (procainamide; phenytoin)

Clinical Manifestations

1. Pain in anterior chest, aggravated by thoracic motion— may vary from mild to sharp and severe; located in precordial area (may be felt beneath clavicle, neck, scapular region)—may be relieved by leaning forward.
2. Pericardial friction rub—scratchy, grating, or creaking sound occurring in the presence of pericardial inflammation
3. Dyspnea—from compression of heart and surrounding thoracic structures
4. Fever, sweating, chills—due to inflammation of pericardium
5. Dysrhythmias

Diagnostic Evaluation

1. Echocardiogram—most sensitive method for detecting pericardial effusion
2. Chest x-ray—may show heart enlargement
3. ECG—to evaluate for myocardial infarction
4. WBC and differential
5. Antinuclear antibody serologic tests and lupus erythematosus cell preparation—to rule out lupus erythematosus
6. PPD test—for tuberculosis; ASO titers—for rheumatic fever
7. Pericardiocentesis—for examination of pericardial fluid for etiologic diagnosis
8. Serum urea nitrogen (BUN)—to evaluate for uremia

Management

The objectives of treatment are targeted toward determining the etiology of the problem, administering pharmacologic therapy for specified etiology, when known, and being alert to the possible complication of cardiac tamponade.

1. Bacterial pericarditis—penicillin or other antimicrobial agents
2. Rheumatic fever—procaine penicillin, prednisone
3. Tuberculosis—antituberculosis chemotherapy (see p. 910)
   (There is a high incidence of constriction in tuberculosis pericarditis.)
4. Fungal pericarditis—amphotericin B
5. Disseminated lupus erythematosus—adrenal steroids
6. Renal pericarditis—dialysis, indomethacin, biochemical control of end-stage renal disease
7. Neoplastic pericarditis—intrapericardial instillation of chemotherapy; radiotherapy
8. Postmyocardial infarction syndrome—bedrest, aspirin, prednisone
9. Postpericardiotomy syndrome (after open-heart surgery)—treat symptomatically

Nursing Assessment

A. Evaluate Complaint of Chest Pain.

1. Ask the patient if pain is aggravated by breathing, turning in bed, twisting body, coughing, yawning, or swallowing.
2. Elevate head of bed; position pillow on over-the-bed table so that the patient can lean on it.
   a. Assess if above intervention relieves the patient's chest pain (associated pleuritic pain of pericarditis is usually relieved by sitting up and/or leaning forward).
   b. Be alert to the patient's medical diagnoses when assessing pain. Postmyocardial infarction patients may experience a dull, crushing pain radiating to neck, arm, and shoulders, mimicking an extension of infarction.

B. Auscultate for Friction Rub.

1. Place the diaphragm of the stethoscope firmly on the chest wall along the mid-to-lower left sternal border or at the apex.
2. Listen to the heart with patient in different positions.
3. Listen carefully; friction rub may appear intermittently and briefly with respiratory movement.
4. Confirm auscultory findings with another staff nurse.

Nursing Diagnoses

1. Chest pain related to pericardial inflammation
2. Potential for injury related to cardiac tamponade and constrictive pericarditis

Nursing Interventions

A. Reducing Discomfort

1. Give prescribed drug regimen for pain and symptomatic relief.
   a. Nonsteroid anti-inflammatory drugs—suppress inflammatory symptoms of acute pericarditis
   b. Corticosteroids—for more severe symptoms
2. Relieve anxiety of the patient and family by explaining the difference between pain of pericarditis and pain of recurrent myocardial infarction. (Patients may fear extension of myocardial tissue damage.)
3. Explain to the patient and family that pericarditis does not indicate further heart damage.
4. Encourage the patient to remain on bedrest when chest pain, fever, and friction rub occur.

NURSING ALERT: Normal pericardial sac contains less than 25–30 ml. of fluid; pericardial fluid may accumulate slowly without noticeable symptoms. However, a rapidly developing effusion can produce serious hemodynamic alterations.

B. Avoiding Complications

1. Be alert to the possibility of cardiac tamponade (see Pericardiocentesis, p. 311).
   a. Assess for distant heart sounds, falling arterial pressures, and rising venous pressure.
   b. Note presence of paradoxical pulse.
   c. Prepare the patient for immediate pericardiocentesis (see Pericardiocentesis, p. 310).
2. Be cognizant of other complications of pericarditis—congestive heart failure, dysrhythmias, hemopericardium (complication in postmyocardial infarction patients on anticoagulation therapy).
3. Be alert for signs/symptoms of pericarditis when administering procainamide or phenytoin. (Agents may induce a lupuslike syndrome with pericarditis.)
4. Prepare the patient for surgical intervention (direct pericardial decompression)—for patient with cardiac embarrassment associated with constrictive pericarditis.

Patient Education/Discharge Planning

1. Teach patient the etiology of pericarditis.
2. Instruct patient about signs/symptoms of pericarditis and the need for long-term medication therapy to help relieve symptoms.
3. Review all medications with the patient—purpose, side effects, dosage, and special precautions.
4. Evaluate the patient's understanding by asking the patient to define pericarditis, the medications necessary for therapy, and the side effects and correct dosage of medications

Evaluation

1. Experiences minimal discomfort—no chest pain
2. Experiences no complications—respirations 14–18 times per minute, no dyspnea, no apprehension or acute anxiety

---

Acquired Valvular Disease of the Heart

Altered Physiology

1. The function of normal heart valves is to maintain the forward flow of blood from the atria to the ventricles and from the ventricles to the great vessels.
2. Valvular damage may interfere with valvular function by stenosis or by impaired closure that allows backward leakage of blood (valvular insufficiency, regurgitation, or incompetence).
3. Acquired valvular heart disease is often the result of previous rheumatic fever, which has damaged one or more heart valves; mitral valve is most commonly involved, followed by aortic, tricuspid, and pulmonary valves.
4. Patients with valvular disease usually develop congestive heart failure in time.

Types of Valvular Disease

1. Mitral stenosis
2. Mitral insufficiency
3. Aortic stenosis
4. Aortic insufficiency
5. Tricuspid stenosis
6. Tricuspid insufficiency

Mitral Stenosis

Mitral stenosis is the progressive thickening and contracture of valve cusps with narrowing of the orifice and progressive obstruction to blood flow. It is the most common of the late lesions produced by rheumatic fever.

Altered Physiology

1. Acute rheumatic valvulitis has "glued" the mitral valve flaps (commissures) together, thus shortening the chordae tendinae, so that the flap edges are pulled down, greatly narrowing the mitral orifice.
2. The left atrium has difficulty in emptying itself through the narrow orifice into the left ventricle; therefore, it dilates and hypertrophies. Pulmonary circulation becomes congested.
3. As a result of the abnormally high pulmonary arterial pressure that must be maintained, the right ventricle is subjected to a pressure overload and may eventually fail.

Clinical Manifestations

1. Progressive fatigue—result of low cardiac output
2. Dyspnea on exertion, cough, repeated respiratory infections, emotional stress
3. Hemoptysis—from pulmonary venous hypertension
4. Weak, irregular pulse; atrial fibrillation
5. Characteristic murmurs—increased first heart sound, opening snap, and low-pitched rumbling diastolic murmur heard at the apex
6. Chest pain (infrequent)
7. Hoarseness (due to compression of left recurrent laryngeal nerve)

Diagnostic Evaluation

1. ECG
2. Echocardiography—can demonstrate mitral valve thickening, calcification, and abnormal, slowed diastolic valve excursion
3. Cardiac catheterization and angiocardiography
4. Medical history, physical examination

Management

A. Medical Treatment

1. Prevent rheumatic recurrences with antimicrobial therapy.
2. Treat the developing congestive failure—vasodilators, digitalis, sodium restriction, limitation of activity (see p. 349).
3. Control dysrhythmias (especially atrial fibrillation).

B. Surgical Intervention

1. Closed mitral valvotomy—introduction of a dilator through the mitral valve to split its commissures
2. Open mitral valvotomy—direct incision of the commissures

3. Mitral valve replacement
4. See page 353 for the management of the patient undergoing heart surgery.

C. Balloon Valvuloplasty

1. A balloon-tipped catheter is percutaneously inserted, threaded to the affected valve, and positioned across the narrowed orifice.
2. The balloon is inflated/deflated, causing a "cracking" of the calcified commisures and enlargement of the valve orifice.

Mitral Insufficiency

Mitral insufficiency (regurgitation) is the result of incompetence and distortion of the mitral valve so that the free margins can no longer come into apposition during systole. The chordae tendinae may become shortened, preventing complete closure of the leaflets.

Mitral insufficiency may be caused by mitral valve prolapse, chronic rheumatic heart disease, postinfarction mitral regurgitation, infective endocarditis, and penetrating and nonpenetrating trauma.

Clinical Manifestations

(Mild mitral regurgitation may produce no symptoms.)
1. Palpitations; dysrhythmias
2. Shortness of breath on exertion; cough—due to pulmonary congestion
3. Murmur—soft first heart sound and a blowing pansystolic murmur heard at the apex and transmitted to the axilla (characteristic of mild regurgitation due to papillary muscle dysfunction of mitral prolapse)
4. Weakness/fatigue—result of low cardiac output

Diagnostic Evaluation

(Same as for mitral stenosis)

Management

1. Prophylaxis for infective endocarditis and rheumatic heart disease (see Infective Endocarditis, p. 339, and Rheumatic Endocarditis, p. 341)
2. Treat developing congestive heart failure (see Congestive Heart Failure, p. 349).
3. Surgical intervention—mitral valve replacement or annuloplasty (retailoring of the valve ring)

Aortic Stenosis

Aortic stenosis is a narrowing of the orifice between the left ventricle and the aorta. The obstruction to the aortic outflow places a pressure load on the left ventricle that results in hypertrophy and failure. In adults it may be congenital or from cusp calcification.

Clinical Manifestations

1. Loud, rough systolic murmur over aortic area; often associated with a palpable thrill
2. Exertional dyspnea and fatigue
3. Dizziness and fainting—from reduced blood supply to brain
4. Angina pectoris
5. Low blood pressure and low pulse pressure—from diminished blood flow, precipitating syncopal episodes

6. Dysrhythmias
7. Symptoms of congestive heart failure
8. Emboli

Diagnostic Evaluation

1. Chest x-ray—usually shows left ventricular enlargement
2. Cardiac catheterization
3. Angiocardiography
4. Echocardiography
} will reveal the pressures in the left ventricle and aorta

Management

1. Surgical replacement of aortic valve—prosthetic or tissue valve
   See page 353 for care of patient undergoing heart surgery.
2. Treat angina and congestive heart failure as dictated by the patient's condition. (Digitalis not indicated for treatment unless evidence of increased ventricular volume or decreased ejection fraction (see Angina, p. 321, and Congestive Heart Failure, p. 348).
3. Balloon valvuloplasty (see Management, Mitral Stenosis, p. 345 and opposite column).

Aortic Insufficiency

Aortic insufficiency (regurgitation) is caused by inflammatory lesions that deform the flaps so that they fail to completely seal the aortic orifice during diastole and thus permit a backflow of blood from the aorta into the left ventricle and by trauma.

It may be caused by rheumatic endocarditis, infective endocarditis, or congenital malformation, or by diseases that cause dilation or tearing of the ascending aorta (syphilitic disease, rheumatoid spondylitis, dissecting aneurysm).

Clinical Manifestations

1. Awareness of increased force of heartbeat, especially when lying down
   a. Arterial pulsations visible and palpable over precordium
   b. Arterial pulsations visible in neck
2. Exertional dyspnea; easy fatigability, progressing to paroxysmal nocturnal dyspnea and orthopnea
3. Widened pulse pressure
4. Water-hammer (Corrigan's) pulse—pulse strikes palpating finger with a quick, sharp stroke and then suddenly collapses
5. Murmur—high-pitched blowing decrescendo diastolic murmur audible along the left sternal edge
6. Nocturnal angina with diaphoresis
7. Tachycardia with exertion

Diagnostic Evaluation

1. ECG—shows pattern of left ventricular hypertrophy
2. Chest x-ray—reveals varying degrees of cardiomegaly from left ventricular enlargement
3. Echocardiography—estimates size and thickness of left ventricle
4. Cardiac catheterization and angiography

Management

1. *Surgical intervention*—replacement of damaged aortic valve. See page 353 for nursing management of patient undergoing heart surgery.

2. Prophylaxis for infective endocarditis and rheumatic heart disease (see Infective Endocarditis, p. 339 and Rheumatic Heart Disease, p. 341).

Tricuspid Stenosis

Tricuspid stenosis is restriction of the tricuspid valve orifice due to commissural fusion and fibrosis, usually following rheumatic fever. It is commonly associated with diseases of the mitral valve.

Clinical Manifestations

1. Dyspnea, nocturnal dyspnea, orthopnea
2. Visible pulsations of neck veins (may cause fluttering sensation)
3. Murmurs—similar to those of rheumatic mitral disease; blowing diastolic murmur along left sternal border
4. Symptoms of right-sided heart failure (late)—hepatomegaly, abdominal swelling, anasarca

Diagnostic Evaluation

1. ECG—may reveal atrial fibrillation
2. Cardiac catheterization and angiocardiography—to confirm diagnosis
3. Echocardiography—useful in estimating size of tricuspid orifice
4. Chest x-ray—marked cardiomegaly, enlarged right atrium

Management

1. The patient may have mitral and aortic disease, which must be corrected.
2. Surgical treatment of accompanying tricuspid valve disease may be carried out at the time of operation after correction of mitral valve disease.
3. Diuretics and sodium restriction to diminish hypervolemic symptoms

Tricuspid Insufficiency (Regurgitation)

Tricuspid insufficiency allows the regurgitation of blood from the right ventricle into the right atrium during ventricular systole. Common cause is dilation of right ventricle.

Clinical Manifestations

1. Right-sided heart failure—from overload of right ventricle
2. Edema—with congestion of liver and hepatic malfunction, ascites, hydrothorax
3. Elevated venous pressure
4. Pansystolic murmur in tricuspid area
5. Weakness, fatigue
6. Atrial fibrillation
7. Jugular venous distention

Diagnostic Evaluation

1. Chest x-ray—marked cardiomegaly
2. ECG—atrial fibrillation
3. Echocardiography

Management

Surgical treatment of associated mitral valve disease, tricuspid valvuloplasty, or tricuspid valve replacement

Nursing Process Overview: The Patient With Valvular Dysfunction

Assessment

A. General

1. Assess patient as often as necessary for complications and progression of valvular dysfunction (see Congestive Heart Failure, p. 348, Infective Endocarditis, p. 337, and Rheumatic Heart Disease, p. 340).
2. Auscultate for extra heart sounds and murmurs every tour of duty.

B. Mitral Stenosis

1. Auscultate for accentuated first heart sound, usually accompanied with an "opening snap" (due to sudden tensing of valve leaflets) at apex with diaphragm of stethoscope.
2. Place the patient in left lateral recumbent position. With bell of stethoscope at apex, auscultate for a low-pitched diastolic murmur (rumbling murmur). Note duration of murmur (long duration indicative of significant stenosis).

C. Mitral Insufficiency

1. Auscultate for diminished first heart sound.
2. Auscultate for systolic murmur (prominent finding), commencing immediately after first heart sound at apex, and note radiation of sound to axilla and left intrascapular area.
3. Mild insufficiency may produce a pansystolic murmur (little connection between severity of mitral insufficiency and intensity of murmur auscultated).

D. Aortic Stenosis

1. Auscultate for prominent fourth heart sound and possible paradoxical splitting of second heart sound (suggestive of associated left ventricular dysfunction). First heart sound is normal.
2. Auscultate for a midsystolic murmur at the base of the heart (heard best) and at the apex of heart. Note harsh and rasping quality at base of heart and a higher pitch at apex of heart.

E. Aortic Insufficiency

1. Auscultate for soft first heart sound.
2. Place the patient in sitting position leaning forward.
3. Place diaphragm of stethoscope along left sternal border at the third and fourth intercostal space and then along the right sternal border. Auscultate for a high-pitched diastolic murmur. To increase audibility of murmur, ask the patient to hold his breath at end of deep expiration. Re-auscultate for murmur.

F. Tricuspid Stenosis

1. Auscultate for a third heart sound (may be accentuated by inspiration).
2. Auscultate for a pansystolic murmur in the parasternal region at the fourth intercostal space. Murmur is usually high-pitched.

Nursing Diagnoses

1. Altered cardiac output (potential for decreased) related to mechanical factors (preload, afterload, and contractility
2. Activity intolerance related to reduced oxygen supply to perform activities of daily living.
3. Potential for ineffective coping (individual) related to acute/chronic illness.

Nursing Interventions

A. Maintaining Adequate Cardiac Output

1. Assess the patient for possible complications that would compromise cardiac function. Implement treatment protocols for these complications (congestive heart failure, infective endocarditis, rheumatic heart disease).
2. Prepare the patient for surgical intervention, or valvuloplasty if indicated (see Management of Patient for Heart Surgery, p. 353).

B. Improving Coping Ability

1. Instruct the patient regarding specific valvular dysfunction, possible etiology, and therapies implemented to relieve symptoms.
   a. Include family members in discussions with the patient.
   b. Stress the importance of adapting life-style to cope with illness.
2. Discuss with the patient surgical intervention as the treatment modality, if applicable (see Heart Surgery, p. 353).
3. Assess the patient's use of appropriate coping mechanisms to deal with illness.
   Spend some time daily with the patient, allowing him to express concerns and ask questions.
4. Refer the patient to appropriate counseling services, if indicated (vocational, social work, cardiac rehabilitation).

Patient Education/Discharge Planning

See Patient Education, Congestive Heart Failure, page 350, Infective Endocarditis, page 339, and Rheumatic Endocarditis, page 341.

Evaluation

1. Maintains adequate cardiac output—blood pressure and heart rate within normal limits for patient, respirations unlabored on exertion at 14–18 per minute, no cough or sputum production, no chest pain, fatigue minimal (rests between activities of daily living, verbalizes that fatigue has not worsened)
2. Copes adaptively to illness

Congestive Heart Failure

1. *Congestive heart failure* is a clinical syndrome that results from the heart's inability to pump the amount of oxygenated blood necessary to meet the metabolic requirements of the body.
2. Cardiac compensatory mechanisms (increases in heart rate, vasoconstriction, heart enlargement) occur to assist the failing heart.
   a. These mechanisms are able to "compensate" for the heart's inability to pump effectively and maintain sufficient blood flow to organs and tissue at rest.
   b. Physiologic stressors that increase the workload of the heart (exercise, infection) may cause these mechanisms to fail and precipitate the "clinical syndrome" associated with a failing heart (elevated ventricular/atrial pressures, sodium and water retention, decreased cardiac output, circulatory and pulmonary congestion).

Causes

1. Disorders of heart muscle resulting in decreased contractile properties of the heart; coronary heart disease leading to myocardial infarction; hypertension; valvular heart disease; congenital heart disease; cardiomyopathies; dysrhythmias
2. Pulmonary embolism; chronic lung disease
3. Hemorrhage and anemia
4. Anesthesia and surgery
5. Transfusions or infusions
6. Increased body demands (fever, infection, pregnancy, arteriovenous fistula)
7. Drug-induced
8. Physical and emotional stress
9. Excessive sodium intake

Clinical Manifestations

Initially there may be isolated left ventricular failure, but in time, the right ventricle fails because of the additional workload. Combined left and right ventricular failure is usual.

A. Left-sided Heart Failure (forward failure)

1. Congestion occurs mainly in the lungs from backing up of blood into pulmonary veins and capillaries
   a. Shortness of breath, dyspnea on exertion, paroxysmal nocturnal dyspnea (due to reabsorption of dependent edema that has developed during day), orthopnea, pulmonary edema
   b. Cough—may be dry, unproductive; often occurs at night
2. Fatigability—from low cardiac output, nocturia, insomnia, dyspnea, catabolic effect of chronic failure
3. Insomnia
4. Tachycardia—S_3 ventricular gallop
5. Restlessness

B. Right-sided Heart Failure (backward failure)

Signs and symptoms of elevated pressures and congestion in systemic veins and capillaries:
1. Edema of ankles; unexplained weight gain
   Pitting edema—is obvious only after retention of at least 4.5 kg. (10 pounds) of fluid
2. Liver congestion—may produce upper abdominal pain
3. Distended neck veins
4. Abnormal fluid in body cavities (pleural space, abdominal cavity)
5. Anorexia and nausea—from hepatic and visceral engorgement
6. Nocturia—diuresis occurs at night with rest and improved cardiac output
7. Weakness

Diagnostic Evaluation

1. Cardiovascular findings
   a. Cardiomegaly (enlargement of the heart)—detected by physical examination and chest x-ray
   b. Ventricular gallop—evident on auscultation; ECG
   c. Rapid heart rate
   d. Development of pulsus alternans (alternation in strength of beat)
   e. Distended neck veins
   f. Hepatomegaly (enlargement of the liver)
2. ECG, echocardiography
3. Chest x-ray—evaluate heart size, show lung fields (for pleural effusion) and vascular congestion
4. Arterial blood gas studies

5. Liver function studies—may be altered because of hepatic congestion

Management

Treatment is directed at eliminating excessive accumulation of body water, increasing the force and efficiency of myocardial contraction and reducing the work load of the heart. These goals are achieved through promoting rest and administering pharmacologic agents.

A. Diuretics

1. Eliminate excess body water and decrease ventricular pressures;
2. A low sodium diet and fluid restriction complement this therapy
3. Some diuretics may have slight venodilator properties.

B. Positive Inotropic Agents

1. Increase the heart's ability to pump more effectively by improving the contractile force of the muscle
2. Digoxin may only be effective in severe cases of failure
3. Dopamine also improves renal blood flow
4. Dobutamine in low dose range
5. Amrinone and milrinone are also potent vasodilators.

C. Vasodilator Therapy

1. Decreases the workload of the heart by dilating peripheral vessels.
2. By relaxing capacitance vessels (veins and venules), vasodilators reduce ventricular filling pressures (preload) and volumes.
3. By relaxing resistance vessels (arterioles), vasodilators can reduce impedance to left ventricular ejection and improve stroke volume.
4. Vasodilators used in congestive heart failure:
   a. Nitrates (nitroglycerin, isosorbide dinitrate, nitroglycerin ointment)—predominantly dilate systemic veins
   b. Hydralazine—predominantly affects arterioles; reduces arteriolar tone
   c. Prazosin—balanced effects on both arterial and venous circulation

D. Angiotensin-Converting Enzyme Inhibitors (ACE Inhibitors)

1. Inhibit the adverse effects of Angiotensin II (potent vasoconstrictor)
2. Decrease ventricular pressure with a subsequent decrease in heart rate associated with heart failure, thereby reducing the workload of the heart and increasing cardiac output
3. Captopril and enalapril are commonly used.

E. Heart Transplantation—Used in advanced heart failure

Complications

1. Intractable or refractory heart failure—patient becomes progressively refractory to therapy (not yielding to treatment)
2. Cardiac dysrhythmias
3. Myocardial failure
4. Digitalis toxicity—from decreased renal function, potassium depletion, etc.
5. Pulmonary infarction; pneumonia; emboli

Nursing Assessment

1. Ask the patient to recall how he felt when first becoming ill.

2. Discuss with patient the various daily activities that he can and cannot do without experiencing fatigue.
3. Ask patient about degree of fatigue experienced during/after activities.
4. Discuss with patient his response to rest; are his symptoms alleviated?
5. Assess peripheral arterial pulses; note quality, character, rhythm, and rate.
6. Inspect/palpate precordium for lateral displacement of point of maximum impulse.
7. Identify sleeping patterns and sleep aids commonly used by patient.
8. Identify normal coping mechanisms of patient.
9. Identify patient's social support system.

Nursing Diagnoses

1. Altered cardiac output (decreased) related to impaired contractility and increased preload/afterload
2. Impaired gas exchange related to alveolar edema due to elevated ventricular pressures
3. Fluid body excess related to sodium and water retention
4. Activity intolerance related to oxygen supply and demand imbalance

Nursing Interventions

A. Maintaining Adequate Cardiac Output

1. Place patient at physical and emotional rest to reduce work of heart.
   a. Provide rest in semirecumbent position or in armchair in air-conditioned environment—reduces work of heart, increases heart reserve, reduces blood pressure, decreases work of respiratory muscles and oxygen utilization, improves efficiency of heart contraction; recumbency promotes diuresis by improving renal perfusion.
   b. Provide bedside commode—to reduce work of getting to bathroom and for defecation.
   c. Provide for psychological rest—emotional stress produces vasoconstriction, elevates arterial pressure, and speeds the heart.
      (1) Promote physical comfort.
      (2) Avoid situations that tend to promote anxiety/agitation.
      (3) Offer careful explanations and answers to the patient's questions.
2. Evaluate frequently for progression of left ventricular failure.
   a. Take frequent blood pressure readings.
      (1) Observe for lowering of systolic pressure.
      (2) Note narrowing of pulse pressure.
      (3) Note alternations in strong and weak pulsations (pulsus alternans).
3. Auscultate heart sounds every 4 hours.
   a. Note for presence of S_3 or S_4 gallop (S_3 gallop is a significant indicator of congestive heart failure).
   b. Monitor for premature ventricular beats.
4. Observe for signs/symptoms of reduced peripheral tissue perfusion—cool temperature of skin, facial pallor, poor capillary refill of nailbeds.
5. Administer pharmacotherapy as directed.
6. Monitor clinical response of patient with respect to relief of symptoms (lessening dyspnea and orthopnea, decrease in crackles, relief of peripheral edema).

NURSING ALERT: Watch for sudden unexpected hypotension, which can cause myocardial ischemia and decrease perfusion to vital organs.

B. Achieving an Improved Ventilation/Perfusion Ratio

1. Raise head of bed 20–30 cm. (8–10 in.)—reduces venous return to heart and lungs; alleviates pulmonary congestion.
   a. Support lower arms with pillows—to eliminate pull of their weight on shoulder muscles.
   b. Sit orthopneic patient on side of bed with feet supported by a chair, head and arms resting on an over-the-bed table, and lumbosacral area supported with pillows.
2. Auscultate lung fields every 4 hours for crackles and wheezes in dependent lung fields (fluid accumulates in areas affected by gravity).
   a. Mark with water-soluble ink the level on the patient's back where adventitious breath sounds are heard.
   b. Use markings for comparative assessment during changes in tours of duty with other nursing personnel.
3. Observe for increased rate of respirations (could be indicative of falling arterial *p*H).
4. Observe for Cheyne–Stokes respirations (may occur in elderly because of a decrease in cerebral perfusion stimulating a neurogenic response).
5. Position the patient every 2 hours (or encourage the patient to change position frequently)—to help prevent atelectasis and pneumonia.
6. Encourage deep breathing exercises every 1 to 2 hours—to avoid atelectasis.
7. Offer small, frequent feedings—to avoid excessive gastric filling and abdominal distention with subsequent elevation of diaphragm that causes decrease in lung capacity.

C. Decreasing Excessive Body Fluid

Administer prescribed diuretic (agent that increases the rate of urine flow).
1. Type and dosage of diuretic administered depends on degree of heart failure and state of renal function.
2. Give diuretic early in the morning—nighttime diuresis disturbs sleep.
3. Keep input and output record—the patient may lose large volume of fluid after a single dose of diuretic.
4. Weigh the patient daily—to determine if edema is being controlled: weight loss should not exceed 0.45–0.9 kg. (1–2 pounds) per day.
5. Assess for weakness, malaise, muscle cramps—diuretic therapy may produce hypovolemia and electrolyte depletion, namely *hypokalemia.* Hypokalemia may cause weakening of cardiac contractions and may precipitate digitalis toxicity in the form of dysrhythmias.
6. Give oral potassium as prescribed.
7. Be aware that problems associated with diuretic administration include disorders of hyperuricemia, volume depletion, and hyponatremia, magnesium depletion, hyperglycemia, and diabetes mellitus.
8. Watch for signs of bladder distention in the elderly male with prostatic hyperplasia.
9. Observe for symptoms of electrolyte depletion—lassitude, apathy, mental confusion, anorexia, decreasing urinary output, azotemia.
10. Limit intravenous fluid administration through use of heparin lock (allows for periodic drug administration without increasing excessive fluid intake).
11. Monitor for pitting edema of lower extremities and sacral area.
    Use "egg crate" mattress and sheepskin to prevent pressure sores (poor blood flow and edema increase susceptibility).
12. Observe for the complications of bedrest—pressure sores (especially in edematous patients), phlebothrombosis, pulmonary embolism.
13. Be alert to complaints of right upper quadrant abdominal pain, poor appetite, nausea, and abdominal distention (may indicate hepatic and visceral engorgement).
14. Monitor the patient's diet. Diet may be limited in sodium—to prevent, control, or eliminate edema; may also be limited in calories.
15. Caution patients to avoid added salt in food and foods with high sodium content.

D. Establishing a Balance Between Oxygen Supply and Demand

1. Increase the patient's activities gradually.
    Alter or modify the patient's activities—to keep within the limits of his cardiac reserve.
    a. Assist the patient with self-care activities early in the day (fatigue sets in as day progresses).
    b. Be alert to complaints of chest pain or skeletal pain during or after activities.
2. Observe the pulse, symptoms, and behavioral response to increased activity.
    a. Monitor the patient's heart rate during self-care activities.
    b. Allow heart rate to decrease to preactivity level before initiating a new activity.
       (1) Note time lapse between cessation of activity and decrease in heart rate (decreased stroke volume causes immediate rise in heart rate).
       (2) Document time lapse and revise patient care plan as appropriate (progressive increase in time lapse may be indicative of increased left ventricular failure).
3. Relieve nighttime anxiety and provide for rest and sleep—patients with congestive heart failure have a tendency to be restless at night because of cerebral hypoxia with superimposed nitrogen retention.
    a. Give appropriate sedation—to relieve insomnia and restlessness.

Patient Education/Discharge Planning

1. Explain the disease process to the patient; the term "failure" may have terrifying implications.
    a. Explain the pumping action of the heart—"to move blood through the body to provide nutrients and aid in the removal of waste material."
    b. Explain the difference between "heart attack" and congestive heart failure.
2. Teach the signs and symptoms of recurrence.
    a. Watch for:
       (1) Gain in weight—report weight gain of more than 2–3 pounds (0.9–1.4 kg.) in a few days. Weigh at same time daily to detect any tendency toward fluid retention.
       (2) Swelling of ankles, feet, or abdomen
       (3) Persistent cough
       (4) Tiredness; loss of appetite
       (5) Frequent urination at night

3. Review medication regimen.
   a. Label all medications.
   b. Give written instructions concerning pharmacologic therapy.
      (1) Make sure the patient has a check-off system that will show that he has taken his medications.
      (2) Teach the patient to take and record his pulse rate and blood pressure.
      (3) Inform the patient of the signs and symptoms of adverse drug effects.
      (4) If the patient is taking oral potassium solution, it may be diluted with juice and taken after a meal.
   c. Tell the patient to weigh himself daily and log his weight if he is on diuretic therapy.
4. Review activity program.
   Instruct the patient as follows:
   a. Increase walking and other activities gradually, provided they do not cause fatigue and dyspnea.
   b. In general, continue at whatever activity level can be maintained without the appearance of symptoms.
   c. Avoid excesses in eating and drinking.
   d. Undertake a weight reduction program until optimal weight is reached.
   e. Avoid extremes in heat and cold—which increase the work of the heart; air conditioning may be essential in a hot, humid environment.
   f. Keep *regular* appointment with physician or clinic.
5. Restrict sodium as directed.
   a. Give patient a booklet containing sodium content of common foods from local chapter of American Heart Association.
   b. Give patient a written diet plan with lists of permitted and restricted foods.
   c. Advise patient to look at all labels to ascertain sodium content (antacids, laxatives, cough remedies, etc.).
      (1) Teach the patient to rinse the mouth well after using tooth cleansers and mouthwashes—some of these contain large amounts of sodium. Water softeners are to be avoided.
      (2) Teach the patient that sodium is present in alkalizers, cough remedies, laxatives, pain relievers, estrogens, etc.
6. Teach the patient the importance of adhering to the low-sodium diet.
   Sodium is present in many types of natural foods and in varying amounts in processed foods. Make the diet as palatable as possible.
   a. Use flavorings, spices, herbs, and lemon juice.
   b. Avoid salt substitutes in the presence of renal disease.

Evaluation

1. Maintains adequate cardiac output—normal blood pressure and heart rate (no hypotension, tachycardia, or cool clammy skin)
2. Exhibits improved ventilation/perfusion ratio—respiratory rate 16–20, arterial blood gases within normal limits, no signs of crackles or wheezes in lung fields
3. Demonstrates a decrease in body fluid—weight decrease of 1 pound (2.2 kg.) daily, no pitting edema of lower extremities and sacral area
4. Maintains balance between oxygen supply and de-

mand—heart rate within normal limits, rests between activities—checks heart rate after activities, if elevated more than 10 beats above preactivity heart rate, waits until heart rate decreases before next activity

---

Acute Pulmonary Edema

Acute pulmonary edema refers to the presence of excess fluid in the lung, either in the interstitial spaces or in the alveoli. It usually follows acute left ventricular failure.

Causes

1. Heart disease—acute left ventricular failure, myocardial infarction, aortic stenosis, severe mitral valve disease, hypertension, congestive heart failure
2. Circulatory overload—transfusions and infusions
3. Drug hypersensitivity; allergy; poisoning
4. Lung injuries—smoke inhalation, shock lung, pulmonary embolism, or infarct
5. Central nervous system injuries—stroke, head trauma
6. Infection and fever—infectious pneumonia (viral, bacterial, parasitic)
7. Postcardioversion, postanesthesia, postcardiopulmonary bypass
8. Narcotic overdose

Clinical Manifestations

1. Coughing and restlessness during sleep (premonitory symptoms)
2. Extreme dyspnea and orthopnea—patient usually uses accessory muscles of respiration with retraction of intercostal spaces and supraclavicular areas
3. Cough with varying amounts of white- or pink-tinged frothy sputum
4. Extreme anxiety and panic
5. Noisy breathing—inspiratory and expiratory wheezing and bubbling sounds
6. Cyanosis with profuse perspiration
7. Distended neck veins
8. Tachycardia
9. Precordial pain (if pulmonary edema secondary to myocardial infarction)

Diagnostic Evaluation

1. Medical history, physical examination
2. Chest x-ray
3. Echocardiogram (suspected valvular disease)
4. Measurement of pulmonary artery wedge pressure by Swan–Ganz catheter (differentiates etiology of pulmonary edema—cardiogenic or altered alveolar–capillary membrane)
5. Blood cultures (suspected infection)
6. Cardiac enzymes (suspected myocardial infarction)

Management

1. The immediate objective of treatment is to improve oxygenation and reduce pulmonary congestion.
2. Identification and correction of precipitating factors and underlying conditions is then necessary to prevent recurrence.
3. Increasing oxygen tension (oxygen therapy), reducing fluid volume (diuretics, vasodilators), improving the heart's ability to pump effectively (glycosides, beta ag-

onists), and decreasing anxiety guide therapeutic interventions.

4. *Oxygen therapy*—high concentrations of oxygen are used to combat hypoxemia. Intubation and ventilatory support may be necessary to improve hypoxemia and prevent hypercarbia.

5. *Morphine sulfate*—reduces anxiety, promotes venous pooling of blood in the periphery, and reduces resistance against which the heart must pump.

6. *Vasodilator therapy* (nitroglycerin and nitroprusside)—reduces the amount of blood returning to the heart and resistance against which the heart must pump.

7. *Diuretic therapy* (furosemide, ethacrynic acid)—reduces blood volume and pulmonary congestion by producing prompt diuresis.

8. *Contractility enhancement therapy* (digoxin, dopamine, and aminophylline)
   a. Improves the ability of the heart muscle to pump more effectively, allowing for complete emptying of blood from the ventricle and a subsequent decrease in fluid backing up into the lungs.
   b. Aminophylline also prevents bronchospasm associated with pulmonary congestion.

Nursing Assessment

1. Be alert to development of a new nonproductive cough.
2. Assess for signs/symptoms of hypoxia: restlessness, confusion, headache.
3. Auscultate lung fields frequently.
   Note inspiratory and expiratory wheezes, rhonchi, moist fine crackles appearing initially in lung bases and extending upward.
4. Auscultate for extra heart sounds.
   Note presence of third heart sound (may be difficult to hear because of respiratory sounds).
5. Identify patient/family level of anxiety and use of appropriate coping mechanisms.
6. Identify precipitating factors that place patient at risk for development of pulmonary edema (see Causes of Pulmonary Edema).

> **NURSING ALERT:** Acute pulmonary edema is a true medical emergency; it is a life-threatening condition.

Nursing Diagnoses

1. Impaired gas exchange related to excess fluid in the lungs
2. Anxiety related to sensation of suffocation and fear

Nursing Interventions

A. Improving Oxygenation

1. Give oxygen in high concentration—to relieve hypoxia and dyspnea.
2. *Take steps to reduce venous return to the heart.*
   Place patient in upright position; head and shoulders up, feet and legs hanging down—to favor pooling of blood in dependent portions of body by gravitational forces; to decrease venous return.
3. Give morphine in small titrated intermittent doses (IV) as directed.
   a. Morphine is *not* given if pulmonary edema is caused by stroke or occurs in the presence of chronic pulmonary disease or cardiogenic shock.
   b. Watch for excessive respiratory depression.
   c. Monitor blood pressure, as morphine may intensify hypotension.
   d. Have morphine antagonist available—naloxone hydrochloride (Narcan).
4. Give injections of diuretic (ethacrynic acid; furosemide) IV
   a. Insert an indwelling catheter—large urinary volume will accumulate rapidly.
   b. *Watch for falling blood pressure, increasing heart rate, and decreasing urinary output—indications that the total circulation is not tolerating diuresis and that hypovolemia may develop.*
   c. Check electrolyte levels, as potassium loss may be significant.
   d. Watch for signs of urinary obstruction in men with prostatic hyperplasia.
5. Administer vasodilator if patient fails to respond to therapy.
   a. Monitor by measuring pulmonary artery pressure and cardiac output
6. Aminophylline may be given when indicated.
   a. Monitor blood levels of drug.
   b. Evaluate for side effects of drug—ventricular dysrhythmias, hypotension, headache.
7. Administer cardiac glycosides (digitalis) per physician request.
8. Assist with cardioversion if indicated (pulmonary edema precipitates tachycardias).
9. Give appropriate drugs for severe, sustained hypertension.
10. Continually evaluate the patient's response to therapy. Reevaluate lung fields and cardiac status (see Assessment).

B. Decreasing Anxiety

1. Stay with the patient and display a confident attitude—the presence of another person is therapeutic, because the acute anxiety of the patient may tend to intensify the severity of his condition. (Arterial vasoconstriction diminishes as anxiety is relieved.)
2. Explain to the patient in a calm manner all therapies administered and the reason for their use.
   a. Give brief explanations related to goal of therapies (i.e., "Morphine will help you relax and ease your work of breathing.").
   b. Explain to the patient importance of wearing oxygen mask. Assure the patient that mask will not increase sensation of suffocation.
3. Inform the patient and family of progress toward resolution of pulmonary edema.
4. Allow time for the patient and family to ventilate concerns and fears.

Patient Education

During convalescence, instruct the patient as follows in order to prevent recurrences of pulmonary edema:
1. Ask: What symptoms did you have before the attack? (He should be aware of these.)
2. If coughing develops (a wet cough), sit with legs dangling over side of bed.
3. See Patient Education, Congestive Heart Failure, page 350.

Evaluation

1. Attains improved oxygenation—unlabored respirations at 14–18 times per minute, lungs clear on auscultation,

blood gases within normal limits for patient, no cough or sputum

2. Achieves decrease in anxiety—appears calm; rests comfortably

---

Heart Surgery

Open heart surgery is most commonly performed for coronary artery disease, valvular dysfunction, and congenital heart defects. The procedure requires temporary cardiopulmonary bypass (blood is diverted from the heart and the lungs and mechanically oxygenated and circulated) in order to provide a dry, bloodless field during the operation.

Types of Heart Surgery

1. *Coronary artery bypass surgery*
   a. A graft (leg and arm veins) is anastomosed to the aorta and the other end of the graft is secured to a distal portion of a coronary vessel.
   b. The graft "bypasses" the obstructive lesion in the vessel and adequate blood flow is restored to the heart muscle supplied by the artery.
   c. Multiple grafts can be placed to bypass lesions and the internal mammary artery may also be used for grafts.
2. *Valvular surgery*
   a. Prosthetic or biological valves are placed in the heart as definitive therapy for incompetent heart valves.
   b. Valve replacement can be done in conjunction with coronary artery bypass surgery.
3. *Congenital heart surgery*
   a. Defects of the heart can be surgically repaired and reconstructed.
   b. Temporary cardiopulmonary bypass is not always required.

Nursing Assessment

1. Review the patient's record to learn past history and present condition, paying close attention to pulmonary, renal, hepatic, hematologic, and metabolic systems.
   a. Cardiac history; *history of cardiac dysrhythmias.*
   b. Pulmonary health—patients with COPD may require prolonged postoperative respiratory support.
   c. Depression—can produce a serious postoperative depressive state and can affect postoperative morbidity and mortality.
   d. Ask about previous/present alcohol intake; smoking history.
2. Assess laboratory studies.
   a. Complete blood count; serum electrolytes; lipid profile; and nose, throat, sputum, and urine cultures
   b. Antibody screen
   c. Preoperative coagulation survey (platelet count, prothrombin time, partial thromboplastin time)—extracorporeal circulation will affect certain coagulation factors.
   d. Renal and hepatic function tests
3. Assess the patient's reactions to medications—these patients are usually on multiple drugs.
   a. Digitalis
      (1) Patient may be receiving large doses to improve myocardial contractility.
      (2) Drug may be stopped several days before sur-

gery—to avoid digitoxic dysrhythmias from cardiopulmonary bypass.
   b. Diuretics
      (1) Assess the patient for potassium depletion and volume depletion (weakness, postural hypotension)—diuretics may produce potassium loss, and severe diuresis may cause a decrease in blood volume.
      (2) Give potassium supplement if the patient is on prolonged diuretic therapy—to replenish body stores.
      (3) Diuretics may be omitted several days preoperatively to avoid electrolyte imbalance and consequent dysrhythmias postoperatively. Salt and water restriction may be advised.
   c. Beta-adrenergic blockers (propranolol)—continue as directed.
   d. Psychotropic drugs (diazepam; chlordiazepoxide)—postoperative withdrawal may cause extreme agitation.
   e. Antihypertensives (reserpine)—omitted as far in advance of procedure as possible to allow norepinephrine repletion.
   f. Alcohol—sudden withdrawal may produce delirium.
   g. Anticoagulant drugs—discontinued several days before operation to allow coagulation mechanism to return to normal.
   h. Determine if the patient has taken corticosteroids within the year prior to surgery—patients on steroids are given supplemental doses to cover stress of surgery.
   i. Prophylactic antibiotics may be given preoperatively.
   j. Determine whether the patient has any drug sensitivities.
4. Be aware of the preoperative conditions that predispose to postoperative respiratory complications.
   a. Pulmonary hypertension
   b. Pulmonary congestion or edema
   c. Preexisting lung disease
   d. Pulmonary sepsis
   e. Elderly or debilitated patient
5. Encourage the patient to stop smoking—smoking increases incidence of postoperative respiratory complications.
6. Surgical preparation:
   a. Shave anterior and lateral surfaces of trunk and neck; shave entire body down to ankles (for coronary bypass).
   b. Shower/bathe with Betadine soap.

Nursing Diagnoses

1. Anxiety related to fear of unknown, fear of death, and fear of pain
2. Potential for impaired gas exchange related to alveolar capillary membrane changes, immobility, altered blood flow
3. Potential for altered cardiac output: decreased, related to mechanical factors: decreased preload and impaired contractility
4. Potential for fluid volume deficit and electrolyte imbalance related to physiologic effects of heart–lung machine
5. Pain related to sternotomy and leg incisions
6. Potential for sensory/perceptual alterations related to intensive care environment, sleep deprivation, inability to speak, and immobility

7. Potential for injury related to postoperative complications (dysrhythmias, cardiac tamponade, myocardial infarction, embolization, bleeding, and infection)

Preoperative Nursing Interventions

A. Decreasing Anxiety

1. Evaluate the patient's emotional state and try to reduce his anxieties—patients undergoing heart surgery are more anxious and fearful than other surgical patients. (Moderate anxiety assists patient to cope with stresses of surgery. Low anxiety level may indicate that the patient is in denial. High anxiety may impair the patient's ability to learn and listen.)
   a. Offer support to patients in low- or high-anxiety states. Give support by being present, by listening, and by showing interest—patient is called on to deal with a stressful and life-threatening crisis.
   b. Encourage the patient to express what he feels and thinks—ventilation of feelings and fantasies relieves sense of isolation and facilitates a growing and supportive relationship.
   c. Help the patient and family to mobilize defenses and cope with fears.
   d. Clarify the information given the patient previously by the cardiovascular surgeon.
      (1) Ask the patient to state why surgery is necessary.
      (2) Give the patient pamphlet on heart surgery to reinforce discussions with health-team members and to review with family members.
   e. Anticipate and answer the patient's questions.
      (1) Ask the patient what he wants to know.
      (2) Establish a relationship of trust.
   f. Support the patient undergoing diagnostic studies to determine type and severity of specific lesions; tests also provide a baseline for postoperative evaluation.
      (1) Cardiac catheterization and angiography
      (2) Pulmonary function studies
      (3) ECG, echocardiogram, phonocardiogram
      (4) Exercise stress testing
      (5) Chest x-ray
   g. Expect some patients to have psychological and psychiatric problems from prolonged illness.

B. Preoperative Teaching

1. Prepare the patient for events in the postoperative period.
   a. Take the patient and family on tour of ICU—lessens anxiety about being in ICU.
      (1) Introduce the patient to staff personnel who will be caring for him.
      (2) Give family a schedule of visiting hours and times for phone contact.
   b. Teach chest physical therapy procedures—to optimize pulmonary function.
      (1) Have the patient practice with incentive spirometer.
      (2) Show and practice diaphragmatic breathing techniques.
      (3) Have the patient practice effective coughing, leg exercises.
   c. Prepare patient for presence of monitors, chest tubes, IVs, blood transfusion, endotracheal tube, nasogastric tube, pacing wires, arterial line, indwelling catheter.
      (1) Explain to the patient that two chest tubes will be inserted below incision into chest cavity for drainage and maintenance of negative pressure.
      (2) Explain to the patient that endotracheal tube will prevent speaking, but that he will be able to communicate through writing until tube is removed (usually within 24 hours).
      (3) Explain to the patient that his diet will consist of liquids until 24 hours after surgery.
      (4) Explain to the patient that monitoring equipment and intravenous lines will restrict movement, and nursing staff will position the patient comfortably every 2 hours and as necessary.
   d. Discuss with the patient the need to monitor vital signs frequently and the likelihood of frequent disturbances of the patient's rest.
   e. Discuss pain management with the patient; assure the patient that analgesics will be administered as necessary to control pain.
2. Tell the patient that both hands may be loosely restrained for a number of hours after surgery to eliminate possibility of pulling out tubes and intravenous lines inadvertently.
3. Discuss with the patient surgical preparation for the day of scheduled surgery and the night prior.
   a. Shave anterior and lateral surfaces of trunk and neck. (Shave entire body down to ankles for coronary bypass.)
   b. Explain to the patient that sedatives will be given before he goes to the operating room.
4. Encourage the patient to stop smoking—smoking increases chance of postoperative respiratory complications.
5. Document preoperative teaching done and the patient's behavior and level of understanding before and after teaching. Record specifically what the patient was taught.

Postoperative Nursing Interventions

1. Orient the patient to surroundings as soon as he awakens from surgical procedure. Tell the patient that operation is over, where he is, the time of day, and your name.
2. Allow family members to visit the patient as soon as his condition stabilizes. Encourage family members to talk to and touch the patient (Family members may be overwhelmed by critical care environment).
3. As the patient becomes more alert, remind him of the purpose of all the equipment in his environment. Continually orient the patient to time and place (Let the patient know if it is day or night).

A. Adequate Oxygenation

1. Ensure adequate oxygenation in early postoperative period; respiratory insufficiency is common following open-heart surgery.
2. Employ assisted or controlled ventilation (see p. 246)—respiratory support is used during first 24 hours to provide airway in the event of cardiac arrest, to decrease work of heart, to maintain effective ventilation.
   a. Adequacy of ventilation is assessed by the patient's clinical status and by arterial blood gases.
   b. Check endotracheal tube placement.
   c. Auscultate chest for breath sounds—crackles indicate pulmonary congestion; decreased or absent breath sounds indicate pneumothorax.
   d. Sedate patient adequately—to help him tolerate

endotracheal tube and cope with ventilatory sensations.
e. Use chest physiotherapy for patients with lung congestion to prevent retention of secretions and atelectasis.
   (1) Check chest x-ray and auscultate chest to determine problem areas.
   (2) Use percussion and vibrating techniques to loosen secretions.
   (3) Promote coughing, deep breathing, and turning—to keep airway patent, prevent atelectasis, and facilitate lung expansion.
f. Suction tracheobronchial secretions carefully (see p. 241)—prolonged aspiration leads to hypoxia and possible cardiac arrest.
g. Restrict fluids (per request) for first few days—danger of pulmonary congestion from excessive fluid intake.
h. Chest x-ray taken immediately after surgery and daily thereafter—to evaluate state of lung expansion and to detect atelectasis; to demonstrate heart size and contour, confirm placement of central line, endotracheal tube, and chest drains.
See page 251 for weaning process and endotracheal tube removal.

B. Adequate Cardiac Output

1. Employ hemodynamic monitoring* during immediate postoperative period, for cardiovascular and respiratory status and fluid and electrolyte balance—to prevent complications or to recognize them as early as possible.
2. Monitor cardiovascular status to determine effectiveness of cardiac output. Serial readings of blood pressure and arterial pressure, heart rate, CVP, and left atrial or pulmonary artery pressure from monitor modules are observed, correlated with the patient's condition, and recorded.
   a. Monitor arterial pressure every 15 minutes until stable and as directed thereafter
   b. Measure left atrial pressure or pulmonary artery wedge pressure—to determine the left ventricular end-diastolic volume; take central venous pressure readings.
      (1) Rising pressures may indicate congestive heart failure or pulmonary edema; or a pressure drop due to low blood volume
      (2) *Changes* in values are more important than isolated readings.
3. Check urine output every ½ to 1 hour (from indwelling catheter)—urine output is an index of cardiac output and renal perfusion.
4. Observe buccal mucosa, nail beds, lips, ear lobes, and extremities for duskiness/cyanosis—signs of low cardiac output.
5. Feel the skin; cool, moist skin reveals lowered cardiac output. Note temperature and color of extremities.
   a. Evaluate temperature.
6. Monitor neurologic status—the brain is dependent on a continuous supply of oxygenated blood and must rely on adequate and continuous perfusion by the heart.
   a. Hypoperfusion or microemboli (air debris) may produce CNS damage after heart surgery.

b. Observe for symptoms of hypoxia—restlessness, headache, confusion, dyspnea, hypotension, and cyanosis.
c. Note the patient's neurologic status hourly in terms of:
   (1) Level of responsiveness
   (2) Response to verbal commands and painful stimuli
   (3) Pupillary size and reaction to light
   (4) Movement of extremities; handgrasp ability
d. Treat postoperative convulsive seizures. Give medications according to therapeutic directives—coronary vasodilators, antibiotics, analgesics, anticoagulants (patients with prosthetic valves).

C. Fluid and Electrolyte Balance

1. Maintain fluid and electrolyte balance—adequate circulating blood volume is necessary for optimal cellular activity; metabolic acidosis and electrolyte imbalance can occur after use of pump oxygenator.
   a. Fluids may be limited to avoid overloading.
   b. Keep intake and output flow sheet—as a method of determining positive or negative fluid balance and the patient's fluid requirements.
      (1) IV fluids (including flush solutions through arterial and venous lines) considered intake.
      (2) Assess hydration status of patient—evaluation of pulmonary wedge, left atrial pressure, and CVP readings; weight, electrolyte levels, hematocrit readings, distention of neck veins, tissue edema, liver size, breath sounds.
      (3) Measure postoperative chest drainage—should not exceed 200 ml./hour for first 4–6 hours.
         (a) Watch for sudden cessation of chest drainage—from kinked or blocked chest tube.
         (b) See page 203 for management of patient with water-seal drainage.
2. Be alert to changes in serum electrolytes—a specific concentration of electrolytes is necessary in both extracellular and intracellular body fluids in order to sustain life.
   a. *Hypokalemia* (low potassium level)
      (1) May be caused by inadequate intake, diuretics, vomiting, excessive nasogastric drainage, stress from surgery
      (2) Effects of low potassium level—dysrhythmias, digitalis toxicity, metabolic alkalosis, weakened myocardium, cardiac arrest
      (3) Watch for specific ECG changes
      (4) Give IV potassium replacement as directed
   b. *Hyperkalemia* (high potassium level)
      (1) May be caused by increased intake, red cell breakdown from the pump, acidosis, renal insufficiency, tissue necrosis, and adrenal cortical insufficiency
      (2) Effects of high potassium level—mental confusion, restlessness, nausea, weakness, and paresthesia of extremities
      (3) Be prepared to administer an ion-exchange resin, sodium polystyrene sulfonate (Kayexalate), which binds the potassium.
   c. *Hyponatremia* (low sodium)
      (1) May be due to reduction of total body sodium or to an increased water intake, causing a dilution of body sodium.
      (2) Assess for weakness, fatigue, confusion, convulsions, and coma.

* Monitoring equipment is valuable only when it is understood and used correctly. The clinical assessment of the patient by the nurse is indispensable to patient care.

d. *Hypocalcemia* (low calcium level)
  (1) May be due to alkalosis (which reduces the amount of Ca^{++} in the extracellular fluid) and multiple blood transfusions
  (2) Signs and symptoms of reduced calcium levels—numbness and tingling in the fingertips, toes, ear, and nose, carpopedal spasm, muscle cramps, and tetany
  (3) Give replacement therapy as directed.
e. *Hypercalcemia* (high calcium level)
  (1) May cause dysrhythmias imitating those caused by digitalis toxicity
  (2) Assess for signs of digitalis toxicity.
  (3) Institute treatment as directed—this condition may lead to asystole and death.

D. Decrease in Discomfort

1. Examine sternotomy incision and leg dressings.
2. Relieve the patient's pain—cardiac surgical patients experience pain caused by sternotomy incision and irritation of pleura by chest tubes.
   a. Record nature, type, location, and duration of pain—pain and anxiety increase pulse rate, oxygen consumption, and cardiac work.
   b. Differentiate between incisional pain and anginal pain.
   c. Watch for restlessness and apprehension—may be from hypoxia or a low-output state; analgesics or sedatives do not correct this problem.
   d. Administer medication as often as prescribed—to reduce amount of pain and to aid the patient in performing deep breathing and coughing exercises more effectively.
     (1) Reassure the patient that staff understands that treatment is painful and that it is "OK to be angry."
     (2) Allow the patient to talk about his experience.

E. Mental and Psychological Orientation

Postcardiotomy delirium—may appear after a brief lucid period
1. Symptoms
   a. Psychic disturbances are more frequent after heart operations with extracorporeal circulation than after general surgery.
   b. Signs and symptoms include delirium (impairment of orientation, memory, intellectual function, judgment), transient perceptual distortions, visual and auditory hallucinations, disorientation, and paranoid delusions.
   c. Symptoms may be related to sleep deprivation, increased sensory input, disorientation to night and day, prolonged inability to speak because of endotracheal intubation, age, preoperative cardiac status, etc.
2. Keep the patient oriented to time and place; notify the patient of procedures and expectations of his cooperation. Give repeated explanations of what is happening.
3. Encourage family to come in at regular times—helps the patient regain sense of reality.
4. Plan care to allow rest periods, day–night pattern, and uninterrupted sleep.
5. Encourage mobility as soon as possible. Keep environment as free as possible of excessive auditory and sensory input. Prevent bodily injury.
6. Reassure the patient and his family that psychiatric disorders following cardiac surgery are usually transient.
7. Remove the patient from ICU as soon as possible. Allow patient to *ventilate* events of his psychotic episode—helps him deal with and assimilate experience.

Avoidance of Complications

A. Cardiac Dysrhythmias

Watch ECG monitor—cardiac dysrhythmias frequently occur after heart surgery.
1. Premature ventricular contractions occur most frequently following aortic valve replacement and coronary bypass surgery. May be treated with pacing, lidocaine, potassium.
2. Dysrhythmias also apt to occur with ischemia, hypoxia, alterations in serum potassium, edema, bleeding, acid–base or electrolyte disturbances, digitalis toxicity, myocardial failure.
3. Observe other parameters in correlation with monitor information—a low serum potassium level makes the heart susceptible to ventricular dysrhythmias.
4. See page 365 for discussion of cardiac dysrhythmias.

B. Cardiac Tamponade—results from bleeding into the pericardial sac or accumulation of fluids in the sac, which compresses the heart and prevents adequate filling of the ventricles.

1. Assess for signs of tamponade—arterial hypotension, rising CVP, rising left atrial pressure, muffled heart sounds, weak, thready pulse, neck vein distention, falling urinary output.
2. Check for diminished amount of drainage in the chest-collection bottle; may indicate that fluid is accumulating elsewhere.
3. Prepare for pericardiocentesis (see p. 310).

C. Myocardial Infarction

1. Check cardiac enzymes daily—elevations may indicate myocardial infarction.
2. Symptoms may be masked by the usual postoperative discomfort.
   a. Watch for decreased cardiac output in the presence of normal circulating volume and filling pressure.
   b. Obtain serial ECGs and isoenzymes to determine extent of myocardial injury.
   c. Assess pain to differentiate myocardial pain from incisional pain.
3. Treatment is individualized. Postoperative activity level may be reduced to allow heart adequate time for healing.

D. Cardiac Failure (low output syndrome)—causes deficient blood perfusion to different organs.

1. Observe for falling mean arterial pressure, rising filling pressures (CVP, PCW, or LAP), and increasing tachycardia
2. The patient may exhibit signs of restlessness and agitation, cold and blue extremities, venous distention, labored respirations, tissue edema, and ascites.

E. Persistent Bleeding—from cardiac incision, tissue fragility, trauma to tissues, clotting defects; blood clotting disturbances usually transitory following cardiopulmonary bypass; however, a significant platelet deficiency may be present.

1. Watch for steady and continuous drainage of blood; watch CVP and left atrial pressures.
2. Treatment—protamine sulfate, vitamin K, or blood components.
3. Prepare for potential return to surgery for bleeding persisting (over 300 ml. per hour) for 2 hours.

F. Hypovolemia (decreased circulating blood volume)

1. Assess for arterial hypotension, low CVP, increasing pulse rate, and low left atrial and pulmonary artery wedge pressures.
2. Prepare to administer blood, IV solutions.

G. Renal Failure—Urine output depends on cardiac output, blood volume, state of hydration, and condition of kidneys.

1. Renal injury may be caused by deficient perfusion, hemolysis, low cardiac output prior to and following open-heart surgery; use of vasopressor agents to increase blood pressure.
2. Measure urine volume; less than 20 ml./hour can indicate decreased renal function.
3. Carry out specific gravity tests to determine kidneys' ability to concentrate urine in renal tubules.
4. Watch BUN and serum creatinine levels, as well as urine and serum electrolyte levels.
5. Give rapid-acting diuretics and/or inotropic drugs (dopamine, dobutamine) to increase cardiac output and renal blood flow.
6. Prepare the patient for peritoneal dialysis or hemodialysis if indicated. (Renal insufficiency may produce serious cardiac dysrhythmias.)

H. Hypotension—May be caused by inadequate cardiac contractility and reduction in blood volume or by mechanical ventilation (when the patient "fights" the ventilator, or PEEP is used), all of which can produce a reduction in cardiac output.

1. Monitor vital signs, left atrial pressure, CVP, and arterial pressure.
2. Note chest tube drainage—hypotension may be caused by excessive bleeding.
3. Give blood as directed to maintain left atrial pressure at a level that will provide an adequate circulating volume for good tissue perfusion.

I. Embolization—may result from injury to the intima of the blood vessels, dislodgement of a clot from a damaged valve, venous stasis aggravated by certain dysrhythmias, loosening of mural thrombi, and coagulation problems.

1. Common embolic sites are lungs, coronary arteries, mesentery, extremities, kidneys, spleen, and brain.
2. Symptoms of embolization (vary according to site)—Midabdominal or midback pain; pain, cessation of pulses, blanching, numbness, coldness of extremity; chest pain and respiratory distress with pulmonary embolus or myocardial infarction; and, one-sided weakness, pupil changes, as in stroke.
3. Initiate preventive measures—antiembolic stockings; omit pressure on popliteal space (leg crossing, raising knee gatch); start passive and active exercises.

J. Postpericardiotomy Syndrome—a group of symptoms occurring following cardiac and pericardial trauma and myocardial infarction.

1. Cause is not certain—may be from anticardiac antibodies, viral etiology, etc.
2. Manifestations—fever, malaise, arthralgias, dyspnea, pericardial effusion, pleural effusion, friction rub.
3. Treatment is symptomatic (bed rest, aspirin), as condition is self-limiting but recurrence is not uncommon.

K. Postperfusion Syndrome

1. Signs and symptoms—fever, splenomegaly, lymphocytosis.

2. Draw blood for culture—postperfusion syndrome can mimic bacterial endocarditis or hepatitis.
3. Treatment is symptomatic, as syndrome is self-limiting.
4. Reassure patient that this is only a temporary setback in his convalescence.

L. Febrile Complications—probably from body's reaction to tissue trauma or accumulation of blood and serum in pleural and pericardial spaces.

1. Control higher degrees of fever by use of hypothermia mattress.
2. Evaluate for atelectasis, pleural effusion, or pneumonia if fever persists.
3. Evaluate for urinary tract infection/wound infection.
4. Bear in mind the possibility of infective endocarditis if fever persists (see p. 337).

M. Hepatitis

Patient Education, Discharge Planning, and Rehabilitation Following Cardiac Surgery

Goal:
Assume a normal life as promptly as possible.

A. Timing

1. Begin discussing long-range plans with patient during convalescence in order to help him make modifications in his life-style.

B. Written Guidelines

1. *Activities*
   a. Increase activities gradually within limits. Avoid strenuous activities until after exercise stress testing.
   b. Take short rest periods.
   c. Avoid lifting more than 20 pounds.
   d. Participate in activities that do not cause pain or discomfort.
   e. Increase walking time and distance each day.
   f. Stairs (1–2 times daily) the first week; increase as tolerated.
   g. Avoid large crowds at first.
   h. Driving—avoid driving until after first postoperative checkup. At this time ask physician when you may drive.
   i. Sexual relations—resumption of sexual relations parallels ability to participate in other activities. Usually may resume sexual activities 2 weeks after surgery. Avoid if tired or after heavy meal. Consult physician if chest discomfort, difficult breathing, or palpitations occur and last longer than 15 minutes after intercourse.
   j. Return to work—after first postoperative checkup, as advised by physician.
   k. Expect some chest discomfort.
2. Diet
   a. Some patients are placed on minimum salt restriction (e.g., no salt added at table); cholesterol may be limited.
   b. Weigh daily and report weight gain of more than 5 pounds per week.
3. Medications
   a. Label all medications; give purposes and side effects.
   b. Patients with prosthetic valves may continue warfarin regimen indefinitely.

C. Patients With Prosthetic Valves

1. Pregnancy usually discouraged in women with prosthetic valves.

2. Caution patient about need for antibiotic coverage following dental and surgical procedures.
3. Patients on anticoagulants should watch for bleeding and should avoid use of aspirin (and many other drugs)—interferes with action of warfarin.

D. Other

1. Advise the patient to carry an identification card stating cardiac condition and medications being taken.
2. The patient may be placed on rehabilitation and exercise program after exercise stress testing.
3. Inform the patient whom to contact (and how) in case of an emergency.
4. See also Patient Education After MI, page 332 and Patient Education, Infective Endocarditis, page 339.

Evaluation

1. Experiences a decrease in anxiety—verbalizes a lessening of anxiety, listens to and learns preoperative content taught (states reasons for operation, events to occur prior to and after surgery, need for follow-up rehabilitation after surgery)
2. Maintains adequate oxygenation—arterial blood gases within normal limits for patient, extubated 24 hours after surgery, spontaneous, unlabored respirations 14–18 per minute
3. Demonstrates adequate cardiac output—blood pressure and heart rate within normal limits for patient, skin warm and dry, urine output greater than 30 ml. per hour
4. Achieves fluid and electrolyte balance—serum electrolytes normal, lungs clear on auscultation, absence of edema
5. Adapts to intensive care environment—no hallucinations, oriented to time and place consistently when asked, sleeps 5 hours without interruption
6. Remains free of complications—absence of life-threatening dysrhythmias, heart sounds normal, cardiac enzymes normal, temperature within normal limits for patient, absence of bleeding
7. Experiences minimal discomfort; absence of incisional pain

Bibliography

Books

American Heart Association. Together Toward a Healthier Heart. Boston, American Heart Association, 1985

Andreoli KG et al. Comprehensive Cardiac Care. 6th ed. St. Louis, CV Mosby, 1987

Braunwald E. Heart Disease: A Textbook of Cardiovascular Disease. 3rd ed. Philadelphia, WB Saunders, 1988

Daily EK and Schroeder JS. Techniques in Bedside Hemodynamic Monitoring. 4th ed. St. Louis, CV Mosby, 1989

Frye SJ and Lounsbury P. Cardiac Rhythm Disorders: An Introduction Using The Nursing Process. Baltimore, Williams & Wilkins, 1988

Gillette PC and Griffin JC (ed). Practical Cardiac Pacing. Baltimore, Williams & Wilkins, 1986

Guzzetta CE and Dossey BM. Cardiovascular Nursing: Bodymind Tapestry, St. Louis, CV Mosby, 1984

Hathaway RG (ed). Nursing Care of the Critically Ill Surgical Patient. Rockville, Aspen Publisher, Inc., 1988

Hudak CM et al. Critical Care Nursing: A Holistic Approach. 4th ed. Philadelphia, JB Lippincott, 1986

Hurst JW (ed). The Heart. 7th ed. New York, McGraw-Hill, 1989

Kim MJ et al. Pocket Guide to Nursing Diagnoses. 2nd ed. St Louis, CV Mosby, 1987

Kinney M et al. AACN'S Clinical Reference for Critical Care Nursing. 2nd ed. New York, McGraw–Hill, 1988

Tarhan S. Cardiovascular Anesthesia and Postoperative Care. Chicago, Year Book Medical Pub, 1989

Tilkian AG and Daily EK. Cardiovascular Procedures: Diagnostic Techniques and Therapeutic Procedures. St. Louis, CV Mosby, 1986

Underhill SL et al. Cardiac Nursing. 2nd ed. Philadelphia, JB Lippincott, 1989

Vinsant MO and Spence MI. Commonsense Approach to Coronary Care: A Program. 5th ed. St Louis, CV Mosby, 1989

Vogel JH and King SB. Interventional Cardiology: Future Directions. St. Louis, CV Mosby, 1989

Weber J. Nurses' Handbook of Health Assessment. Philadelphia, JB Lippincott, 1988

Weeks LC (ed). Advanced Cardiovascular Nursing. Boston, Blackwell Scientific Publications, 1986

Yee BH and Zorb SL. Cardiac Critical Care Nursing. Boston, Little, Brown & Co, 1986

Journals

Myocardial Infarction

Altice NF and Jamison GB. Interventions to facilitate pain management in myocardial infarction. J Cardiovasc Nurs 1989 Aug; 3(4):49–56

Bauer WC and Dracup KA. Physiologic effects of back massage in patients with acute myocardial infarction. Focus Crit Care 1987 Dec; 14(6):42–52

Berron K. Role of the ventricular assist device in acute myocardial infarction. Crit Care Nurs Q 1989 Sep; 12(2):25–37

Blumenthal JA and Emery CF. Rehabilitation of patients following myocardial infarction. J Consult Clin Psychol 1988 Jun; 56(3):374–381

Brennan JJ and Cabin HS. The role of anticoagulation in acute myocardial infarction. Cardiol Clin 1988 Feb; 6(1):111–118

Brooks–Brunn JA. Formulating appropriate nursing diagnoses for the patient receiving tissue-type plasminogen activator. Heart Lung 1987 Nov; 16(6):792–794

Brewer-Senerchia C. Thrombolytic therapy: A review of the literature on streptokinase and tissue plasminogen activator with implications for practice. Crit Care Nurs Clin North Am 1989 Jun; 1(2):359–372

Cheitlin MD. Non-Q wave infarction: Diagnosis, prognosis, and treatment. Adv Intern Med 1988; 33:267–294

Conti CR. Drug therapy of patients with acute myocardial infarction in the era of thrombolysis. Mod Concepts Cardiovasc Dis 1989 Apr; 58(4):19–24

Cronin SN and Harrison B. Importance of nurse caring behaviours as perceived by patients after myocardial infarction. Heart Lung 1988 Jul; 17(4):374–380

Davenport J and Whittaker K. Secondary prevention in elderly survivors of heart attacks. Am Fam Physician 1988 Jul; 38(1):216–224

Erickson DE. Addendum: A standardized nursing care plan for the acute myocardial infarction patient receiving tissue-type plasminogen activator. Heart Lung 1987 Nov; 16(6):794–800

Gawlinski A. The challenge for evaluating the effects of salvaged myocardium. Heart Lung 1987 Nov; 16(6):756–759

Gibson RS. Non-Q-wave myocardial infarction: Diagnosis, prognosis and management. Curr Probl Cardiol 1988 Jan; 13(1):9–72

Haywood LJ. Treatment of myocardial infarction: A review. J Natl Med Assoc 1988 Apr; 80(4):459–461

Helfant RH and Klein LW. The Q-wave and non-Q wave myocardial infarction: Differences and similarities. Prog Cardiovasc Dis 1986 Nov–Dec; 29(3):205–220

Keeling AW. Health promotion in coronary care and step-down units: Focus on the family—Linking research to practice. Heart Lung 1988 Jan; 17(1):28–34

Kennedy JW. Thrombolytic therapy for acute myocardial infarction: A brief review. Heart Lung 1987 Nov; 16(6): 740–745

Kline EM. Recombinant tissue-type plasminogen activator in acute myocardial infarction: Role of the critical care nurse. Heart Lung 1987 Nov; 16(6):779–788

Kline EM. Comparison of thrombolytic agents: Mechanisms of action. Crit Care Nurs Q 1989 Sep; 12(2):1–7

Lynn-McHale DJ. Interventions for acute myocardial infarction: PTCA and CABGS. Crit Care Nurs Q 1989 Sep; 12(2):38–48

Mayberry–Tothe B and Landron S. Complications associated with acute myocardial infarction. Crit Care Nurs Q 1989 Sep; 12(2):49–63

McGlashan R. Strategies for rebuilding self-esteem for the cardiac patient. Dimens Crit Care Nurs 1988 Jan–Feb; 7(1):28–38

Misinski M. Role of conventional management and alternative therapies in limiting infarct size in acute myocardial infarction. Heart Lung 1987 Nov; 16(6):746–749

The Multicenter Diltiazem Postinfarction Trial Research Group. The effect of diltiazem on mortality and reinfarction after myocardial infarction. N Engl J Med 1988 Aug 18; 319(7):385–392

Niemyski P and Hellstedt LF. Patient selection and management in thrombolytic therapy: Nursing implications. Crit Care Nurs Q 1989 Sep; 12(2):8–24

Nowakowski JF. Use of cardiac enzymes in the evaluation of acute chest pain. Ann Emerg Med 1986 Mar; 15(3):354–360

Owen PM. Recovery from myocardial infarction: A review of psychosocial determinants. J Cardiovasc Nurs 1987 Nov; 2(1):75–85

Parchert MA and Creason N. The role of nursing in the rehabilitation of women with cardiac disease. J Cardiovasc Nurs 1989 Aug; 3(4):57–64

Puleo PR and Roberts R. An update on cardiac enzymes. Cardiol Clin 1988 Feb; 6(1):97–109

Roberts R. Preventing recurrent myocardial infarction. Use of calcium-channel blockers. Postgrad Med 1988 Jan; 83(1):249–256

Robison JS. Acute right ventricular infarction: Recognition, evaluation, and treatment. Crit Care Nurse 1987 Jul–Aug; 7(4):42–55

Runions J. A program for psychological and social enhancement during rehabilitation after myocardial infarction. Heart Lung 1985 Mar; 14(2):117–125

Sanders AB. Myocardial salvage: Pharmacological treatment. Emerg Med Clin North Am 1988 May; 6(2): 361–372

Schneider JR. Should patients with myocardial infarction receive

caffeinated coffee? Focus Crit Care 1988 Feb; 15(1):52–61

Siegel D et al. Risk factor modification after myocardial infarction. Ann Intern Med 1988 Aug 1; 109(3):213–218

Smucker DR and Burket MW. Thrombolytic therapy in acute myocardial infarction. Am Fam Physician 1988 Mar; 37(5):265–274

Sobel BE. Fibrinolysis and activators of plasminogen. Heart Lung 1987 Nov; 16(6):775–778

Thompson DR and Cordle CJ. Support of wives of myocardial infarction patients. J Adv Nurs 1988 Mar; 13(2):223–228

Topol EJ. Clinical use of streptokinase and urokinase therapy for acute myocardial infarction. Heart Lung 1987 Nov; 16(6):760–774

Valle GA et al. Circadian influence on coronary events. Heart Lung 1988 Sep: 17(5):586–593

Waller BF. The pathology of acute myocardial infarction: Definition, location, pathogenesis, effects of reperfusion, complications, and sequelae. Cardiol Clin 1988 Feb; 6(1): 1–28

Weisman H and Healy B. Myocardial infarct expansion, infarct extension, and reinfarction: Pathophysiologic concepts. Prog Cardiovasc Dis 1987 Sep–Oct; 30(2):73–110

Wilson BC and Cohn JN. Right ventricular infarction: Clinical and pathophysiologic considerations. Adv Intern Med 1988; 33:295–309

Assessment/Diagnostic Tests

Constant J. Jugular vein inspection to assess right atrial pressure. Med Times 1987 Jan; 115(1):45–50

Contrades S. Altered cardiac output: An assessment tool. Dimens Crit Care Nurs 1987 Sep–Oct; 6(5):274–282

Fahey VA and Riegel BJ. Advances in diagnostic testing for vascular disease. Cardiovasc Nurs 1989 May–Jun; 25(3): 13–16

Hill NE et al. Evaluating the use of a videotape in teaching the precardiac catheterization patient. J Cardiovasc Nurs 1988 May; 2(3):71–78

Vaughn P. Bedside assessment of the myocardial infarction patient. Crit Care Nurs 1984 Mar–Apr; 4(2):60–77

Watkins LO and Weaver L. Preparation for cardiac catheterization: Tailoring the content of instruction to coping style. Heart Lung 1986 Jul; 15(4):382–389

Pacemakers

Benditt DG. Sensor-triggered, rate-variable cardiac pacing. Ann Intern Med 1987 Nov; 107(5):714–724

Benditt DG et al. Sensor-triggered physiologic pacing. Cardiology 1987 Feb; 4(2):49–51, 69

Braun AE. Transthoracic pacing in the emergency department. JEN 1986 Nov–Dec; 12(6):354–359

Corey PL. Nursing care plan: Pacemaker insertion and intra-op care. Can Oper Room Nurs J 1986 Apr; 4(2):9–10

Dreifus LS. Expanding uses of pacemakers in the elderly. Drug Ther 1987 Apr; 17(4):60–70

Greenwood PV. Pacemakers: Who, when, what. Mod Med Can 1986 Oct; 41(10): 858–872

Guzy PM. Emergency cardiac pacing. Emerg Med Clin North Am 1986 Nov; 4(4):745–759

Hawthorne WJ. Cardiac pacemakers. Curr Probl Cardiol 1987 Nov; 12(11):649–693

Iscoff C. Understanding upper rate responses of DDD pacers. Heart Lung 1985 Jul; 14(4):327–334

Lanuza DM and Marotta SF. Endocrine and psychologic responses of patients to cardiac pacemaker implantation. Heart Lung 1987 Sep; 16(5):496–504

Pierce CD. Transcutaneous cardiac pacing: Expanding clinical applications. Crit Care Nurs North Am 1989 Jun; 1(2):423–435

Porterfield LM et al. Insertion of a permanent pacemaker. Crit Care Nurse 1987 Jul–Aug; 7(4):30–35

Stafford MJ. Monitoring patients with permanent cardiac pacemakers. Nurs Clin North Am 1987 Jun; 22(2):503–519

Wirtzfeld A et al. Physiologic pacing: Present status and future developments. Pace 1987 Jan–Feb; 10(1, Pt 1):41–57

Automatic Implantable Defibrillator

Chapman PD. The implantable defibrillator and the emergency physician. Ann Emerg Med 1989 May; 18(5):579–585

Cooper DK et al. Care of the patient with the automatic implantable cardioverter defibrillator: A guide for nurses. Heart Lung 1987 Nov; 6(6 pt 1):640–648

Furst E. (ed). Cardiovascular technology: Automatic implantable cardioverter-defibrillator. J Cardiovasc Nurs 1988 Nov; 3(1):77–81

Manolis AS et al. Automatic implantable cardioverter defibrillator: Current status. JAMA 1989 Sep 8; 262(10): 1362–1368

Messer MS. Wound care. Crit Care Nurs Q 1989 Mar; 11(4):17–27

Moser SA et al. Caring for patients with implantable cardioverter defibrillators. Crit Care Nurse 1988 Apr; 8(2):52–65

Noel DK et al. Challenging concerns for patients with automatic implantable cardioverter defibrillators. Focus Crit Care 1986 Dec; 13(6):50–58

Valladares BK and Lemberg L. Problem solving for complications with the AICD. Heart Lung 1987 Jan; 16(1): 105–108

Vitello-Cicciu J (ed). Nursing grand rounds: AICD implantation: Treatment for malignant ventricular dysrhythmias. J Cardiovasc Nurs 1988 Nov; 3(1):82–87

Wilson L and Miller PG. The automatic implantable cardioverter defibrillator: A lifesaving device. Am J Nurs 1986 Sep; 86(9):1004–1008

Cardiomyopathy/Congestive Heart Failure/Pulmonary Edema

Abelmann WH. Classification and natural history of primary myocardial disease. Prog Cardiovasc Dis 1984 Sep–Oct; 27(2):73–94

Allen SJ. Recent advances in pulmonary edema. Crit Care Med 1987 Oct; 15(10):963–970

Casey PE. Pathophysiology of dilated cardiomyopathy: Nursing implications. J Cardiovasc Nurs 1987 Nov; 2(1):1–12

Colucci WS. Usefulness of calcium antagonists for congestive heart failure. Am J Cardiol 1987 Jan 30; 59(3):53B–58B

Courtney-Jenkins, A. The patient with hypertrophic cardiomyopathy. J Cardiovasc Nurs 1987 Nov; 2(1):33–47

Cutillo AG. The clinical assessment of lung water. Chest 1987 Aug; 92(2):319–325

Jaeschke R and Guyatt GH. Medical therapy for chronic congestive heart failure. Ann Intern Med 1989 May 15; 110(10):758–760

Kopecky SL and Gersh BJ. Dilated cardiomyopathy and myocarditis: Natural history, etiology, clinical manifestations, and management. Curr Probl Cardiol 1987 Oct; 12(10):569–647

Maron BJ et al. Hypertrophic cardiomyopathy. Interrelations of clinical manifestations, pathophysiology and therapy (2). N Engl J Med 1987 Apr 2; 316(14):844–852

Maron BJ et al. Hypertrophic cardiomyopathy. Interrelations of clinical manifestations, pathophysiology, and therapy. (1) N Engl J Med 1987 Mar 26; 316(13):780–789

McElroy PA et al. Pathophysiology of the failing heart. Cardiol Clin 1989 Feb; 7(1):25–37

McHugh MJ. The patient with alcoholic cardiomyopathy. J Cardiovasc Nurs 1987 Nov; 2(1):13–22

Miniati M et al. Detection of lung edema. Crit Care Med 1987 Dec; 15(12):1146–1155

Parmley WW. Pathophysiology of congestive heart failure. Am J Cardiol 1985; 56:7A–11A

Parmley WW. Pathophysiology and current therapy of congestive heart failure. J Am Coll Cardiol 1989 Mar; 13(4):771–785

Sanzobrino B and Lember L. The cardiomyopathies. Heart Lung 1986 Jul; 15(4):416–419

Sica DA and Gehr T. Diuretics in congestive heart failure. Cardiol Clin 1989 Feb; 7(1):87–97

Silverman AT. Cardiac amyloidosis. Heart Lung 1987 Jan; 16(1):60–66

Szidon JP. Pathophysiology of the congested lung. Cardiol Clin 1989 Feb; 7(1):39–48

Weber LT and Kamoclo KS. Pathogenesis of heart failure. Cardiol Clin 1989 Feb; 7(10):11–24

Wigle ED. Hypertrophic cardiomyopathy 1988. Mod Concepts Cardiovasc Dis 1988 Jan; 57(1):1–6

Wingate S. Dilated cardiomyopathy: Part 2. Focus Crit Care 1984 Oct; 11(5):59–68

Zellis R et al. Vasoconstrictor mechanisms in congestive heart failure, part 1. Mod Concepts Cardiovasc Dis 1989 Feb; 58(2):7–12

Zellis R et al. Vasoconstrictor mechanisms in congestive heart failure: Part 2. Mod Concepts Cardiovasc Dis 1989 Mar; 58(3):13–18

Coronary Artery Disease/Percutaneous Transluminal Angioplasty

Cohen JA. Reducing cholesterol: Strategies for increasing patient awareness. Crit Care Nurse 1989 Mar; 9(3):25–36

Conti CR. Unstable angina before and after infarction: Thoughts on pathogenesis and therapeutic strategies. Heart Lung 1986 Jul, 15(4):361–367

Dix-Sheldon DK. Pharmacologic management of myocardial ischemia. J Cardiovasc Nurs 1989 Aug; 3(4):17–30

Eagen JS. Lasers: Applications in cardiovascular atherosclerotic disease. Crit Care Nurs Clin North Am 1989 Jun; 1(2):311–326

Eberts AE. Advances in the pharmacologic management of angina pectoris. J Cardiovasc Nurs 1986 Nov; 1(1):15–29

Enger EL and Schwertz DW. Mechanisms of myocardial ischemia. J Cardiovasc Nurs 1989 Aug; 3(4):1–16

Forrester JS et al. A perspective of coronary disease seen through the arteries of living man. Circulation 1987 Mar; 75(3):505–513

Galan KM et al. Significance of early chest pain after coronary angioplasty. Heart Lung 1985 Mar; 14(2):109–116

Guido BA. Hypercholesterolemia as a cardiovascular risk factor: Nursing implications. Crit Care Nurs Q 1989 Sep; 12(2):73–83

Halfman-Franey M and Levine S. Intracoronary stents. Crit Care Nurs Clin North Am 1989 Jun; 1(2):327–338

Kedas A et al. Nursing delivery of sublingual nifedipine. J Cardiovasc Nurs 1988 Aug; 12(2):31–38

Loan T. Nursing interaction with patients undergoing coronary angioplasty. Heart Lung 1986 Jul; 15(4):368–397

Miller CL. Medications in angina. Focus Crit Care 1988 Aug; 15(4):23–29

Perchalski DL and Pepine CJ. Patient with coronary artery spasm and role of the critical care nurse. Heart Lung 1987 Jul; 16(4):392–401

Radwin LE. Autonomous nursing interventions for treating the patient in acute pain: A standard. Heart Lung 1987 May; 16(3):258–265

Rentrop KP et al. Unstable angina and acute myocardial infarction. Cardiovasc Clin 1988 19(2):129–141

Ryan P. Strategies for motivating life-style change. J Cardiovasc Nurs 1987 Aug; 1(4):54–66

Savage M and Goldberg S. The high-risk patient. Cardiovasc Clin 1988; 19(2):169–180

Sipperly ME. Expanding role of coronary angioplasty: Current implications, limitations, and nursing considerations. Heart Lung 1989 Sep; 18(5):507–513

Topol EJ. Coronary angioplasty for acute myocardial infarction. Ann Intern Med 1988 Dec 15; 109(12):970–988

Wenger NK et al. The care of elderly patients with cardiovascular disease. Ann Intern Med 1988 Sep; 109(5):425–428

Cardiac Surgery

Alling-Berne L. The nurse's role: Early supervised exercise following coronary artery bypass surgery. Focus Crit Care 1987 Dec; 14(6):11–16

Artinian NT. Family member perceptions of a cardiac surgery event. Focus Crit Care 1989 Aug; 16(4):301–308

Blackshear GL and Blackshear PL. Extracorporeal blood pumping during heart-lung bypass. J Cardiovasc Nurs 1989 May; 3(3):71–73

Cuipylo KA. Sternal wound management: A case study. J Cardiovasc Nurs 1989 May; 3(3):66–70

Gortner SR et al. Elders' recovery from cardiac surgery. Prog Cardiovasc Nurs 1988 Apr–Jun; 3(2):54–61

Gortner SR et al. Expected and realized benefits from cardiac surgery: An update. Cardiovasc Nurs 1989 Jul–Aug; 25(4):19–22

Goulart D. Educating the cardiac surgery patient and family. J Cardiovasc Nurs 1989 May; 3(3):1–9

Jansen KJ and McFadden PM. Postoperative nursing management in patients undergoing myocardial revascularization with the internal mammary artery bypass. Heart Lung 1986 Jan; 15(1):48–54

Kern LS. Advances in the surgical treatment of coronary artery disease. J Cardiovasc Nurs 1986 Nov; 1(1):1–14

Ley SJ. Fluid therapy following intracardiac operation. Crit Care Nurs 1988 Jan–Feb; 8(1):26–37

Marshall JR and Hawrysio A. Inpatient recovery following myocardial infarction and coronary artery bypass graft surgery. J Cardiovasc Nurs 1988 May; 2(3):1–12

Newton KM and Killien MG. Patient and spouse learning needs during recovery from coronary artery bypass. Prog Cardiovasc Nurs 1988 Apr–Jun; 3(2):62–70

O'Brian-Norris S. Managing postoperative mediastinitis. J Cardiovasc Nurs 1989 May; 3(3):52–65

Philips R and Skov P. Rewarming and cardiac surgery: A review. Heart Lung 1988 Sep; 17(5):511–520

Schultz CK and Woodall CE. Using epicardial pacing electrodes. J Cardiovasc Nurs 1989 May; 3(3):25–33

Vitello-Cicciu JM et al. Profile of patients requiring the use of epicardial pacing wires after coronary artery bypass surgery. Heart Lung 1987 Mar; 16(3): 301–310

Young ME. Malnutrition and wound healing. Heart Lung 1988 Jan; 17(1): 60–68

Valvular Disease/Rheumatic Fever/ Myocarditis

Baddour LM and Bisno AL. Mitral valve prolapse: Multifactorial etiologies and variable prognosis. Am Heart J 1986 Dec; 112(6):1359–1362

Douglas PS. Rheumatic heart disease and other valvular disorders. Cardiovasc Clin 1989; 19(3):113–125

Grady KL and Costanzo-Nordin. Myocarditis: Review of a clinical enigma. Heart Lung 1989 Jul; 18(4): 347–354

Nichols L et al. Percutaneous aortic valvuloplasty procedure and implications for nursing. Heart Lung 1989 Aug; 18(4):356–363

Ohler L et al. Aortic valvuloplasty: Medical and critical care nursing perspectives. Focus Crit Care 1989 Aug; 16(4):275–288

Rahimtoola SH et al. Valvular and congenital heart disease. J Am Coll Cardiol 1987 Aug; 10(2):60a–62a

Rahimtoola SH. Perspective on valvular heart disease: An update. J Am Coll Cardiol 1989 Jul; 14(1):1–23

Virami R. Editorial: The tricuspid valve. Mayo Clin Proc 1988 Sep; 63(9):943–946

Hemodynamics/Intra-aortic Balloon Pump

Amin DK et al. The Swan–Ganz catheter: Insertion technique. J Crit Illness 1986 Apr; 1(4):38–45

Charette AL. Bridging the gap between hemodynamics and monitoring. Crit Care Nurs Clin North Am 1989 Sep; 1(3):539–546

Enger EL. Pulmonary artery wedge pressure. When it's valid, when it's not. Crit Care Nurs Clin North Am 1989 Sep; 1(3):603–618

Gardner PE. Cardiac output theory, technique, and troubleshooting. Crit Care Nurs Clin North Am 1989 Sep; 1(3):577–579

Goran SG. Vascular complications of the patient undergoing intra-aortic balloon pumping. Crit Care Nurs Clin North Am 1989 Sep; 1(3):459–458

Goran SF. Family perceptions of the intra-aortic balloon pumping experience. Crit Care Nurs Clin North Am 1989 Sep; 1(3):475–478

Gould KA. Perspectives on intra-aortic balloon-pump timing. Crit Care Nurs Clin North Am 1989 Sep; 1(3):469–474

Halfman–Franey M and Bergstrom D. Clinical management using direct and derived parameters. Crit Care Nurs Clin North Am 1989 Sep; 1(3):563–576

Mims BC. Physiologic rationale of SVO₂ monitoring. Crit Care Nurs Clin North Am 1989 Sep; 1(3):619–628

Schriner DK. Using hemodynamic waveforms to assess cardiopulmonary pathologies. Crit Care Nurs Clin North Am 1989 Sep; 1(3):563–576

Sitzmann JV. The technique of managing central venous lines. J Crit Illness 1986 Mar; 1(3):50–55

Cardiac Tamponade/Pericarditis

Kronick–Mest C. Postpericardiotomy syndrome: Etiology, manifestations, and interventions. Heart Lung 1989 Mar; 18(2):192–198

Randall EM. Recognizing cardiac tamponade. J Cardiovasc Nurs 1989 May; 3(3):42–51

Stechmiller J et al. Cardiac tamponade resulting from pneumopericardium: Case report and implications for the critical care nurse. Heart Lung 1987 Jul; 16(4):442–448

Sulzbach LM. Measurement of pulsus paradoxus. Focus Crit Care 1989 Apr; 16(2):142–145

Endocarditis

Birrer RB et al. Infective endocarditis. J Fam Pract 1987 Mar; 24(3):289–295

Burden LL and Rodger JC. Endocarditis: When bacteria invade the heart. RN 1988 Dec; 51(12):38–46

Karp RB. Role of surgery in infective endocarditis. Cardiovasc Clin 1987; 17(3):141–162

King K and Harkness JL. Infective endocarditis in the 1980's: Part 2. Treatment and management. Med J Aust 1986 May 26; 144(11):588–594

King K and Harkness JL. Endocarditis in the 1980's: Part 1. Etiology and diagnosis. Med J Aust 1986 May 12; 144(11):536–540

Lang S and Morris A. Infective endocarditis: Current recommendations for prophylaxis. Drugs 1987 Aug; 34(2):279–288

Robbins MJ et al. Infective endocarditis: A pathophysiologic approach to therapy. Cardiol Clin 1987 Nov; 5(4): 545–562

Trausch PA. Infective endocarditis: Nursing care and prevention. Prog Cardiovasc Nurs 1988 Apr–Jun; 3(2): 45–53

Weinstein L. Life-threatening complications of infective endocarditis and their management. Arch Intern Med 1986 May; 146(5):953–957

Nursing Diagnosis/Geriatrics

Burke LJ et al. Nursing diagnoses, indicators, and interventions in an outpatient cardiac rehabilitation program. Heart Lung 1986 Jan; 15(1): 70–86

Clark S. Nursing diagnosis: Ineffective coping I. A theoretical framework. Heart Lung 1987 Nov; 16(6, Pt 1):670–675

Clark S. Nursing diagnosis: Ineffective coping. II. Planning care. Heart Lung 1987 Nov; 16(6, Pt 1):677–683

Dougherty CM. The nursing diagnosis of decreased cardiac output. Nurs Clin North Am 1985 Dec; 20(4):787–798

Estbrooks CA. Touch: A nursing strategy in the intensive care unit. Heart Lung 1989 Jul; 18(4):392–402

Foreman MD et al. Impaired cognition in the critically ill elderly patient: Clinical implications. Crit Care Nurs Q 1989 Jun; 12(1):61–73

MacLean SL. The decision-making process in critical care of the aged. Crit Care Nurs Q 1989 Jun; 12(1):74–81

Rebenson–Piano M. The physiologic changes that occur with aging. Crit Care Nurs Q 1989 Jun; 12(1):1–14

Schwertz DW and Buschmann MT. Pharmacogeriatrics. Crit Care Nurs Q 1989 Jun; 12(1):26–37

Williams MA. Physical environment of the intensive care unit and elderly patients. Crit Care Nurs Q 1989 Jun; 12(1):52–60

15 Electrocardiography

The Electrocardiogram (ECG) and Heart Dynamics

Heart Anatomy and Physiology (Fig. 15-1)

1. Heart tissue is highly specialized muscle mass, which possesses the special properties of automaticity, rhythmicity, conductivity, and excitability.
2. The above properties make it possible for the heart to initiate a rhythmic wave of impulse with the subsequent conduction of that impulse resulting in a single heart contraction.
3. The site of normal impulse origin is referred to as the *sinoatrial* (SA) *node* and is located in the right atrium. The sinus node is the natural pacemaker of the heart because it possesses the fastest intrinsic rate above all other heart muscle. The SA node paces between 60 and 100 times per minute. The atrioventricular (AV) node has an intrinsic rate of between 40 and 60 times per minute; the ventricles' intrinsic rate is 20–40 times per minute.
4. Once excited by the sinoatrial node, the wave of impulse spreads over the thin walls of the atria to the atrioventricular node. The impulse is delayed at the AV node to allow for ventricular filling.
5. The AV node, as the name implies, lies at the junction of the atria and ventricles.
6. The wave of impulse then traverses the bundle of His and the left and right bundle branches of the ventricles and finally terminates in the Purkinje fibers of the ventricles. This electrical activity results in a single heart contraction and is referred to as *depolarization of the ventricles* (see Fig. 15-1).
7. The conduction system of the heart is under the control of the autonomic nervous system.
   a. Sympathetic—speeds the heart rate
   b. Parasympathetic—slows the heart rate (vagus nerve)
8. The relaxation phase, which follows contraction, is referred to as *repolarization*.

The ECG

1. Machine capable of transcribing to graph paper the electrical activity of the heart.

2. Electrical activity is generated by the cells of the heart as ions are exchanged across cell membranes.
3. Electrodes that are capable of conducting electrical activity from the heart to the ECG machine are placed at strategic positions on the extremities and chest precordium (Fig. 15-2).
4. The electrical energy sensed is then converted to a graphic display by the ECG machine. This display is referred to as the electrocardiogram.

Clinical Uses of ECG

The ECG is a useful tool in the diagnosis of those conditions that may cause aberrations in the electrical activity of the heart. Examples of these conditions are as follows:
1. Myocardial infarction and other types of coronary artery diseases, such as angina
2. Cardiac dysrhythmias
3. Cardiac enlargement
4. Electrolyte disturbances, especially of calcium and potassium levels
5. Inflammatory diseases of the heart
6. Drug effect(s)

The Normal ECG

1. Figure 15-3 represents the lead II of the normal ECG.
2. A heart contraction is represented by wave forms on the graph paper that are designated P, Q, R, S, and T waves.
3. Wave forms are referred to as deflections relative to an isoelectric line (e.g., a line that expresses no energy). The isoelectric line can be determined by looking at the T to P interval.
4. The P wave is the first positive deflection.
   a. The Q wave is the first negative deflection after the P wave; the R wave is the first positive deflection after the Q wave.
   b. The S wave is the negative deflection after the R wave.
   c. The T wave follows the S wave and is joined to the QRS complex by the ST segment.
   d. The QT interval is the time between the Q wave and the T wave.
5. The P wave represents atrial depolarization; the configuration of the P wave is useful in determining the

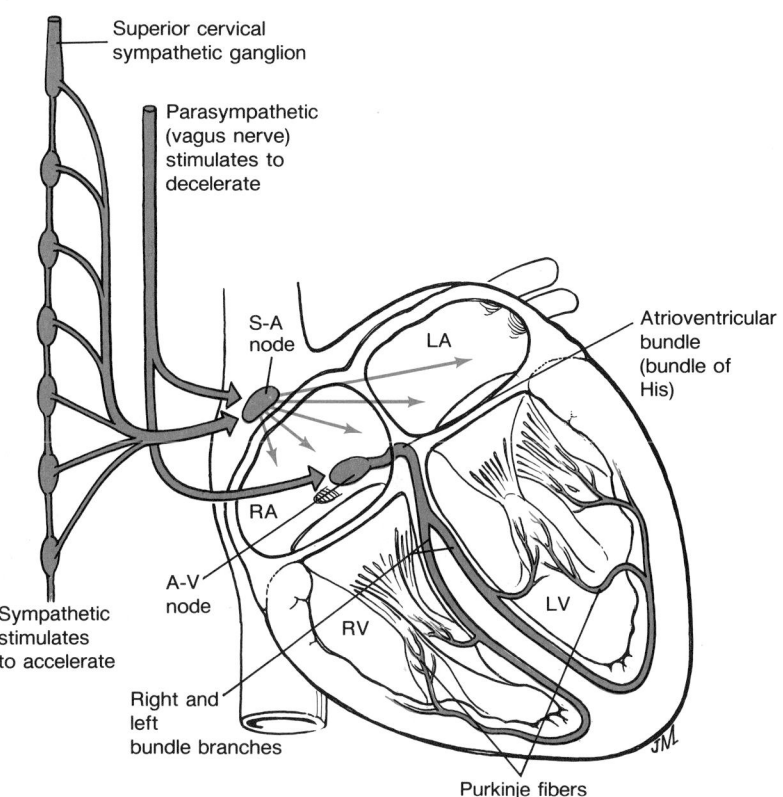

Figure 15-1. *Heart dynamics or wave of depolarization. Schematically represented is the pathway followed by a normal electrical impulse initiated at the sinus node. The electrical event is followed by a mechanical event that results in heart contraction. The influence of the autonomic nervous system is also depicted.*

source of impulse formation as being sinus node versus atrial muscle.

6. The QRS wave form is generally regarded as a unit and represents ventricular depolarization.
7. The T wave represents relaxation of the muscle fibers and is referred to as repolarization of the ventricles.

ECG Paper

1. ECG paper is graph paper with horizontal and vertical axes (Fig. 15-3).
2. Time is measured on the horizontal axis. There are 1500 1-mm. blocks in 60 seconds; therefore, a 1-mm. square equals 0.04 second (e.g., 1500 ÷ 60 = 0.04 second).
3. The superior margin of the ECG paper is marked by small vertical lines at 3-second intervals.
4. Amplitude is measured on the vertical axis; 1 small square equals 1 mm. of voltage.
5. Cardiac rate may be determined in a variety of ways using the time interval measurements.
6. The most expedient method for rate determination is to count the number of QRS complexes within a 6-second time interval (use the superior margin of ECG paper) and multiply the complexes by a factor of 10. (The factor of 10 is determined by dividing the 6-second interval into 60 seconds or 1 minute.) A gross estimate of rate may be determined in this manner.
   a. One must be cautioned that this method is accurate only for rhythms that are occurring at normal intervals and should not be used for determining rates in irregular rhythms.
   b. Irregular rhythms *are always* counted for 1 full minute for accuracy.
7. Another means of obtaining rate is to divide the number of large 5-square blocks between each two complexes into 300. Three hundred large blocks represent 1 minute on the ECG paper. Example: In Figure 15-3 the number of large square blocks between complexes #5 and #6 equals 5, or a rate of 60.

ECG Leads

1. The standard ECG consists of 12 leads (I, II, III, AVR, AVL, AVF, V_1, V_2, V_3, V_4, V_5, V_6).
2. Each lead records the heart's electrical activity from a different anatomical position.
3. Experience has rendered data confirming that certain leads give information about specific surfaces of the heart.
4. Identification of specific myocardial changes on certain leads assists in defining pathologic conditions.

Wave Form Analysis *(Fig. 15-4)*

A. P Wave

1. The P wave represents atrial depolarization.
2. The normal amplitude of the P wave is 3 mm. or less; the normal duration of the P wave is 0.04 to 0.11 seconds. P waves that exceed these measurements are considered to be a deviation from normal.

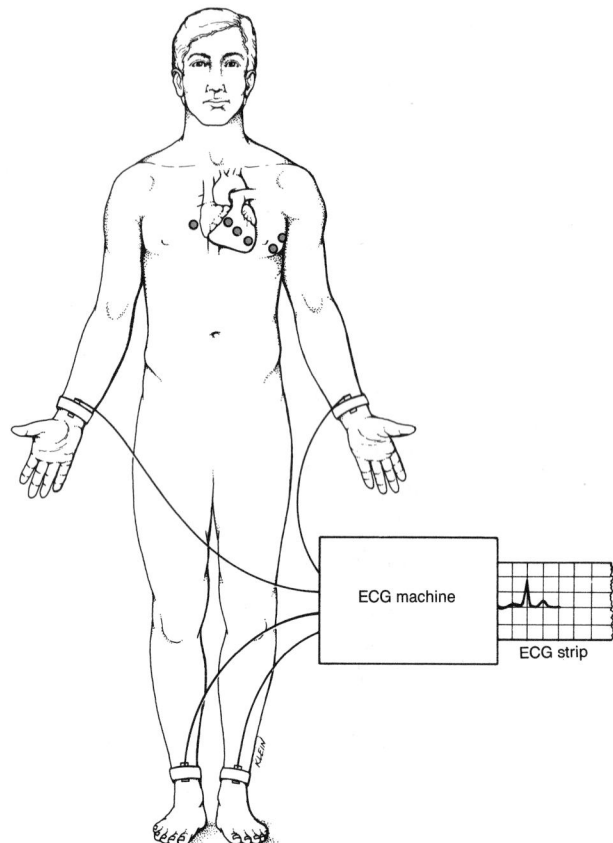

Figure 15-2. *Transmission of heart's impulse to a graphic display by ECG machine. The electrodes that are capable of conducting electrical activity from the heart to the ECG machine are placed at strategic positions on the extremities and chest precordium.*

3. Since the P wave represents atrial depolarization, enlargement of the atria may be inferred from ECG findings that exceed the normal limits.

a. For example, the increased workload imposed on the atria when mitral or tricuspid stenosis is present may cause the atria to enlarge.

b. The enlarged atria may be manifested as enlarged and distorted P waves.

B. P–R Interval

1. Is measured from the upstroke of the P wave to the QR junction.

2. The P–R interval is widely accepted to be between 0.12 and 0.20 seconds.

   a. The P–R interval represents the time of impulse transmission from the SA node to the AV node.

   b. There is a built-in delay in time at the AV node to allow for adequate ventricular filling to maintain normal stroke volume (the amount of blood ejected with each contraction).

C. Prolongation of the P–R Interval—may be a precursor to a variety of heart blocks; among the causes may be drug therapy and myocardial disease or ischemia.

D. The QRS Complex

1. First downward stroke after the P wave. A Q wave of significant deflection is not normally present in the healthy heart. A pathologic Q wave usually indicates an old myocardial infarction.

2. The R wave is the first positive deflection after the Q wave, normally 5 to 10 mm. in height. Increases and decreases in amplitude become significant in certain disease states. Ventricular hypertrophy produces very high R waves because the hypertrophied muscle requires a longer time to depolarize.

E. The S–T Segment

1. Begins at the end of the S wave, the first negative deflection after the R wave, and terminates at the upstroke of the T wave.

2. The S–T segment is elevated in states of acute injury; the S–T segment is depressed in ischemic states. Hypocalcemia will lengthen the S–T segment, whereas hypercalcemia will shorten the S–T segment. The S–T segment is also influenced by changes in potassium level.

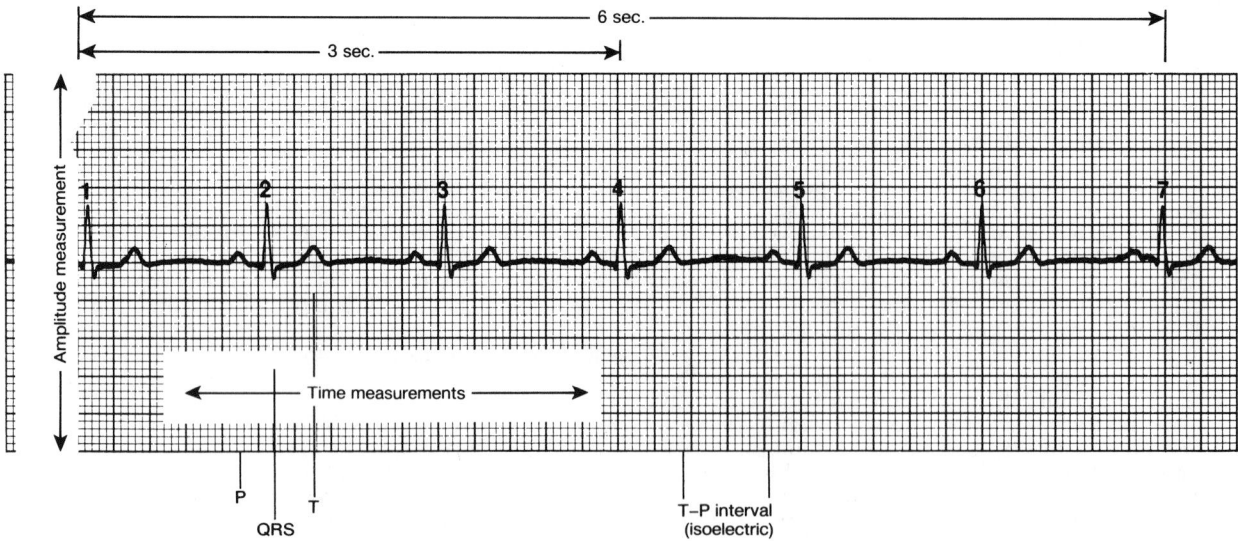

Figure 15-3. *Lead II normal sinus rhythm and ECG paper.*

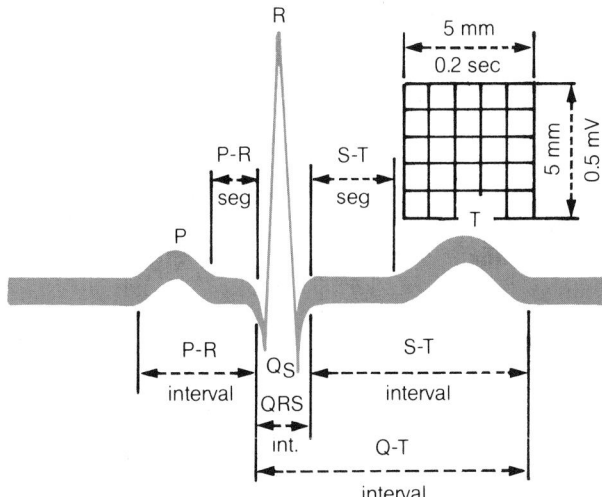

Figure 15-4. *Wave form analysis.*

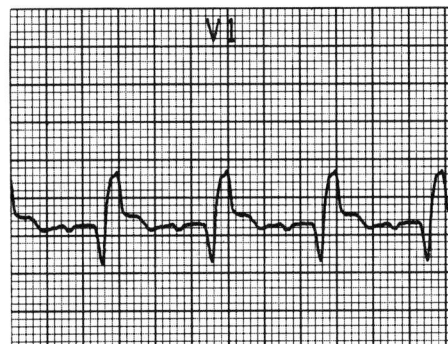

Figure 15-5. *Abnormal Q wave.*

F. The T Wave
1. Represents the repolarization of myocardial fibers or provides the resting state of myocardial work; the T wave should always be present.
2. Normally, the T wave should not exceed a 5-mm. amplitude in all leads except the precordial (V_1–V_6) leads, where it may be as high as 10 mm.
3. May invert during the evolution of myocardial infarction but will usually return to normal after the MI is resolved.
4. Is sensitive to potassium level changes.

ECG Interpretation of Myocardial Infarction

Note: The ECG is but one tool in diagnosing heart disease. The patient's history and serum enzymes are important for diagnosis of acute myocardial infarction. The noninvasive radionuclide studies are making it unnecessary to use the ECG beyond the initial onset of illness.

1. Elevation of the S–T segment heralds a pattern of injury and usually occurs as an initial change in acute MI.
2. T wave inversion may occur as the MI evolves. The T waves will return to the upright position after the MI resolves.
3. A pathologic Q wave will evolve as the patient's R waves diminish in amplitude or disappear. The evolution of Q waves is permanent. A pathologic Q wave is one that is greater than 0.04 seconds in time and greater than 3 mm. in depth or greater than ⅓ the height of the R wave (Fig. 15-5).

ECG Interpretation of Cardiac Dysrhythmias

1. Dysrhythmias (irregular rhythms) are a symptom of an underlying process and should be regarded as a symptom, not a diagnosis.

Note: All heart muscle tissue is capable of exciting impulses when the normal pacemaker is compromised. This fact serves as the basis for dysrhythmia formation.

2. Dysrhythmias are generally evaluated continuously by placing at-risk patients on a bedside monitor.
3. The rhythm strips obtained from the monitor should not be used for diagnostic purposes.

4. If a question should arise regarding a rhythm that requires diagnostic data, a standard 12-lead ECG is always done.

> **NURSING ALERT:** Cardiac output, which is defined as the volume of blood ejected from the ventricle with each heart beat, is a function of heart rate times the stroke volume. Dysrhythmias, which are alterations in rate or rhythm of heart contraction, can seriously alter cardiac output. This concept must be considered each time a patient experiences a dysrhythmia.

Approach for Assessment and Interpretation of Dysrhythmias

When reviewing a dysrhythmia, one should develop a systematic approach to assist in accurate interpretation. There is a variety of approaches that may be taken. One format that is particularly helpful is as follows:
1. Determine the rate. Is it fast, slow, or normal?
2. Determine the rhythm. Is it regular, irregular, regularly irregular, or irregularly irregular?
3. Find the P waves. Is one present for each QRS complex? Are they absent? Are they replaced by other wave forms? What is the configuration like? Are they identical, well-formed, or do they change shape?
4. Measure the P–R interval. The normal interval should be between 0.12 and 0.20 seconds.
5. Measure the QRS complex. The normal QRS complex should be between 0.06 and 0.10 seconds. Are they identical in configuration? Do they fall early? Does the configuration vary?
6. Look at the T wave. Is it positively or negatively deflected? Is it peaked?
7. Measure the Q–T interval. The normal Q–T interval should be less than ½ the R–R interval.

By following a format, one can, through deductive reasoning, arrive at a correct interpretation by associating each part of the format with anatomical and physiologic function of the heart.

Commonly Encountered Dysrhythmias

Dysrhythmias may be classified as disturbances in impulse formation or disturbances in conduction (heart blocks). The following dysrhythmias are considered disturbances of impulse formation. Heart blocks are treated in a separate section (see p. 378).

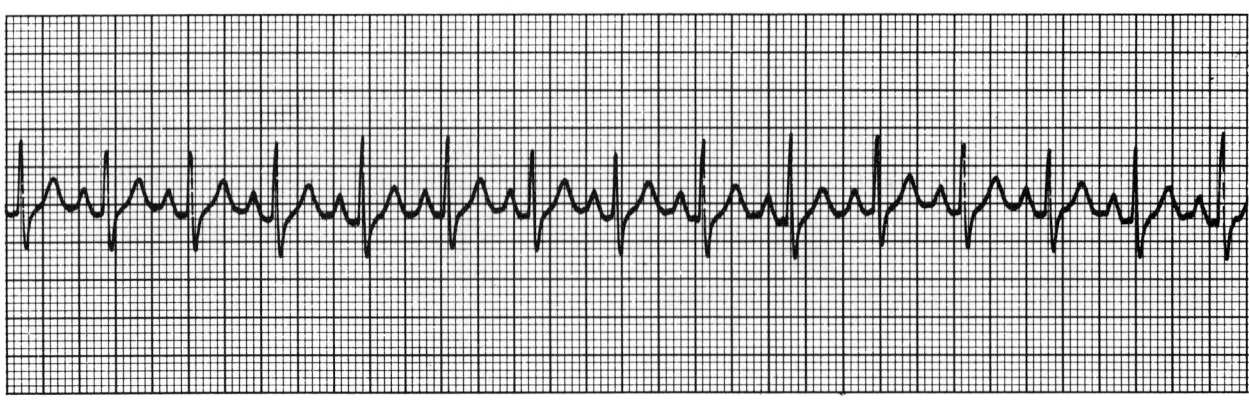

Figure 15-6. *Sinus tachycardia.*

Sinus Tachycardia *(Fig. 15-6)*

Sinus tachycardia is a dysrhythmia that is normal, except that the rate exceeds 100 beats per minute.

Etiology

The SA node is under the influence of the autonomic nervous system. The sympathetic fibers, which act to speed up excitation of the SA node, are stimulated by underlying causes.

Underlying Causes

1. Anxiety
2. Exercise
3. Fever
4. Shock
5. Drugs
6. Altered metabolic states, such as hyperthyroidism
7. Electrolyte disturbances

Mechanism of Sinus Tachycardia

The wave of impulse is transmitted through the normal conduction pathways; the rate of sinus stimulation is simply greater than normal.

Analysis of Rhythm Strip Depicting Sinus Tachycardia

Rate—130
Rhythm—R–R intervals are regular
P wave—present for each QRS complex, normal configuration, and each P wave is identical
P–R interval—falls between 0.12 and 0.20, or 0.16 seconds
QRS complex—normal in appearance, one follows each P wave
QRS interval—0.06 seconds
T wave follows each QRS complex and is positively conducted

Management

1. The urgency of treatment of sinus tachycardia is dependent on the effect of the rapid rate on the maintenance of adequate cardiac output. For example, sinus tachycardia is much more life-threatening to the individual with a new acute MI than it is to the person who experiences the dysrhythmia secondary to a fever.
2. Digitalis preparations may be required if the effect on cardiac output is negative; otherwise, treatment is directed to the cause of the tachycardia.

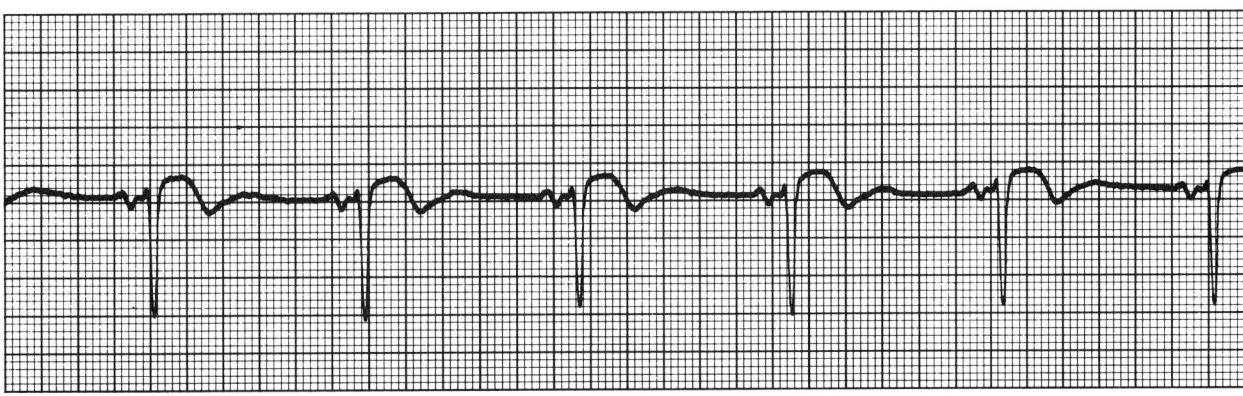

Figure 15-7. *Sinus bradycardia.*

Sinus Bradycardia *(Fig. 15-7)*

Sinus bradycardia is a dysrhythmia that is normal, except that the rate falls below 60 beats per minute.

Etiology

The parasympathetic fibers (vagal tone) are stimulated and cause the sinus node to slow.

Underlying Causes

1. Can be expected in the well-trained athlete
2. Drugs
3. Altered metabolic states, such as hypothyroidism
4. The process of aging, which causes increasing fibrotic tissue and scarring of the SA node
5. Certain cardiac diseases, such as acute MI

Mechanism of Sinus Bradycardia

The wave of impulse is transmitted through the normal conduction pathways; the rate of sinus stimulation is simply less than normal.

Analysis of Sinus Bradycardia

Rate—55
Rhythm—R–R interval is regular
P wave—present for each QRS complex, normal configuration, and each P wave is identical
P–R interval—falls between 0.12 and 0.20, or 0.18
QRS—normal in appearance, one follows each P wave
QRS interval—0.06
T wave follows each QRS and is positively conducted

Management

1. The urgency of treatment of sinus bradycardia is dependent on the effect of the slow rate on maintenance of cardiac output.
2. Atropine 0.5–1 mg. IV push blocks vagal stimulation to the SA node and therefore accelerates heart rate.
3. Isoproterenol hydrochloride may be used as a sympathetic stimulator if atropine is ineffective or contraindicated. (The accepted dilution is isoproterenol 1 mg./500 ml. D$_5$W.) The solution may be titrated to control the rate within parameters prescribed by the physician. Isoproterenol has a propensity for causing ventricular dysrhythmias and should be discontinued if this occurs.
4. If the bradycardia persists, a pacemaker may be required.

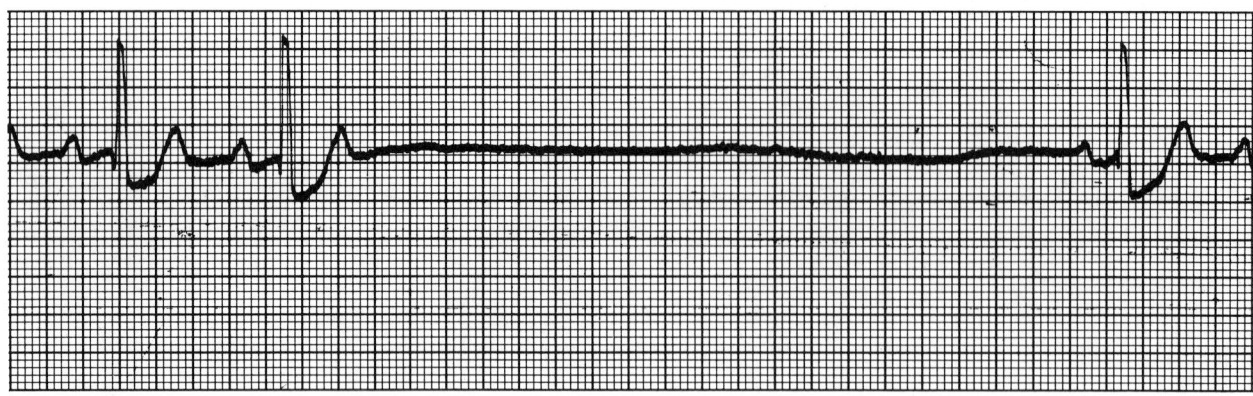

Figure 15-8. *Block or pause seen in sick sinus syndrome.*

Sick Sinus Syndrome *(Fig. 15-8)*

Sick sinus syndrome is a dysrhythmia that is caused by a diseased sinus node. The sinus node conducts at a slow rate or may fail to conduct at all, producing sinus block or pauses. Sometimes there is a related tachycardia, thus causing some to refer to this syndrome as brady–tachycardia syndrome. If the related tachycardia should stop abruptly, and the sinus node does not fire, all heart activity will cease (asystole).

Etiology

1. Arteriosclerotic heart disease
2. Acute MI

Mechanism of Sick Sinus Syndrome

1. When the sinus node fails to fire for whatever reason, the end result is a lack of impulse conducted to the atria or ventricles. Thus, there is a long pause before another impulse is discharged.

2. Whether or not the patient is affected depends on the length of the pause.
3. Ischemia is a common cause of sick sinus syndrome.

Analysis of Sick Sinus Syndrome

Rate—may be slow or within normal limits. Rhythm will be regular except when a pause occurs; when the rhythm resumes, it will be regular.

P wave—present before each QRS complex; normal configuration and identical, the P wave will suddenly not appear when expected. No QRS complex will follow.

P–R interval—within normal limits.

QRS complex—follows each QRS except where there is no P wave. The QRS will also be absent.

T wave—normally conducted in the normal complexes.

Management

A pacemaker will be required if the sick sinus syndrome does not abate with the treatment of ischemia.

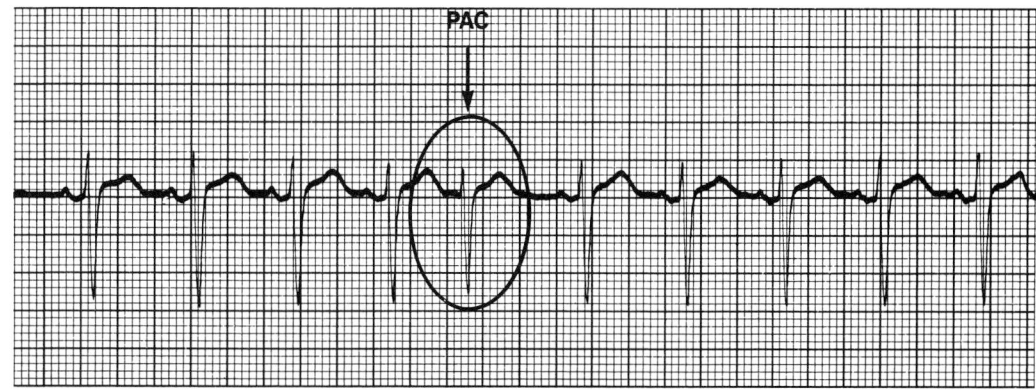

Figure 15-9. *Normal sinus rhythm with premature atrial contraction.*

Premature Atrial Contraction (PAC) (Fig. 15-9)

A *premature atrial contraction* (*PAC*) is an ectopic beat that originates in the atria and is discharged at a rate faster than that of the sinus node. The atrial beat occurs sooner than the next normal beat and is said to be early or premature.

Etiology

1. May occur in the healthy or diseased heart. It is of no particular significance in the healthy heart. In the diseased heart, it may represent ischemia and a resultant irritability.
2. The PAC may increase in frequency and be the precursor of more serious dysrhythmias in the diseased heart.

Mechanism of Premature Atrial Contraction

1. The wave of impulse of the PAC originates within the atria and outside the sinus node.
2. Because the impulse originates within the atria, the P wave will be present, but it will be different in appearance as compared with those beats originating within the sinus node.

3. The impulse traverses the remainder of the conduction system in a normal pattern; thus, the QRS complex is identical in configuration to the normal sinus beats.

Analysis of a PAC

Rate—may be slow or fast.
Rhythm—will be irregular; this is caused by the early occurrence of the PAC.
P wave—will be present for each normal QRS complex; the P wave of the premature contraction will be distorted in shape.
P–R interval—may be normal but can also be shortened, depending on where in the atria the impulse originated. The closer the site of atrial impulse formation to the AV node, the shorter the P–R interval will be.
QRS complex—within normal limits because all conduction below the atria is normal.
T wave—normally conducted.

Management

1. Generally requires no treatment.
2. PACs should be monitored for increasing frequency.
3. If treatment is required, quinidine or a calcium-channel blocker may be used.

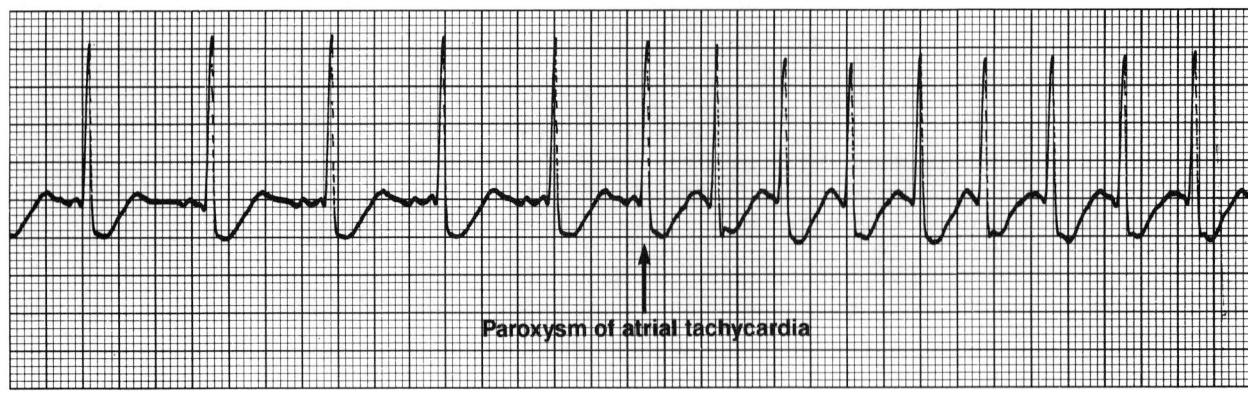

Figure 15-10. *Paroxysmal atrial tachycardia.*

Paroxysmal Atrial Tachycardia (PAT) (Fig. 15-10)

Paroxysmal atrial tachycardia (*PAT*) is a sudden onset of an atrial tachycardia with rates that vary between 140 and 250 beats per minute.

Etiology

1. Syndromes of accelerated pathways (e.g., Wolff–Parkinson–White syndrome
2. Syndrome of mitral valve prolapse
3. Ischemic coronary artery diseases
4. Excessive use of alcohol, cigarettes, caffeine
5. Drugs (digitalis is a frequent cause)

Mechanism of PAT

An ectopic atrial focus captures the rhythm of the heart and is stimulated at a very rapid rate; the impulse is conducted normally through the conduction system so that the QRS complex usually appears within normal limits. The rate is often so rapid that P waves are not obvious but may be "buried" in the preceding T wave.

Analysis of PAT

Rate—between 140 and 250 beats per minute
Rhythm—regular
P waves—are present before each QRS complex; however, the faster the rate, the more difficult it becomes to visualize P waves. The P waves can frequently be measured with calipers by observing the varying configuration of the preceding T wave.
P–R interval—usually not measurable
QRS complex—will appear normal in configuration and within 0.06–0.10 seconds
T wave—will be distorted in appearance as a result of P waves being buried in them

Management

1. Treatment is directed to first slowing the rate and second, reverting the dysrhythmia to a normal sinus rhythm.
2. Reducing the rate may be accomplished by having the patient perform a Valsalva maneuver. This stimulates the vagus nerve to slow the heart. A Valsalva maneuver may be done by having the patient gag himself or "bear down," as though attempting to have a bowel movement. The physician may choose to perform carotid massage. This should be performed by a *physician,* and only one side of the neck should be massaged at a time.
3. Digitalis preparations may also be used in varying doses as prescribed.
4. Beta-adrenergic blockers may also be used. Propranolol (by IV push) is an example of a commonly used beta-adrenergic blocker.
5. The calcium ion antagonists (e.g., verapamil) are effective in reverting this dysrhythmia.
6. If drug therapy is ineffective, elective electrical cardioversion can be used.
7. Other, less common drugs that may be used include morphine sulfate and diazepam.

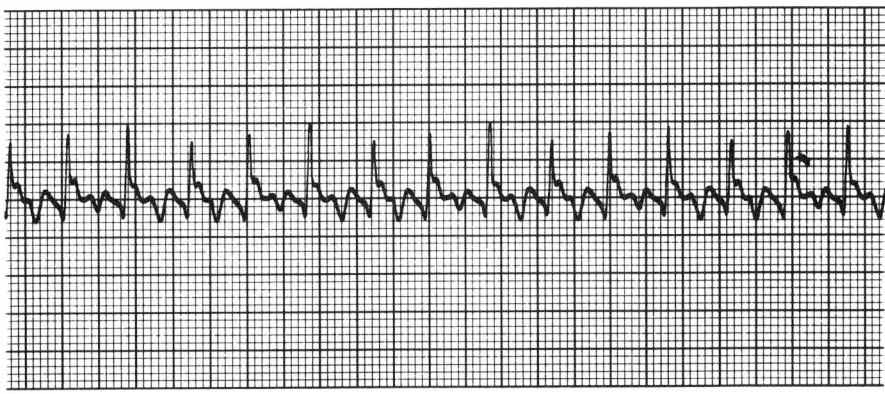

Figure 15-11. *Atrial flutter.*

Atrial Flutter (Fig. 15-11)

Atrial flutter is a dysrhythmia in which an atrial focus captures the heart rhythm and discharges impulses at a rate of between 200 and 400 times per minute.

Etiology

1. Atrial stretching or enlargement, as occurs in diseases of the atrioventricular valves
2. Myocardial infarction
3. Congestive heart failure

Mechanism of Atrial Flutter

1. An ectopic atrial focus captures the rhythm in atrial flutter and fires at an extremely rapid rate, with regularity.
2. Conduction of the impulse through the conduction system is normal; thus, the QRS complex is unaffected.
3. An important feature of this dysrhythmia is that the AV node sets up a therapeutic block, which disallows some impulse transmission.
   a. This can produce a varying block or a fixed block; that is to say, sometimes the AV node will transmit every second flutter wave, producing a 2:1 block, or the rhythm can be 3:1 or 4:1.
   b. This is an important feature of this rhythm; if the AV node conducted 1:1, then the outcome would be ventricular flutter, a life-threatening dysrhythmia.

Analysis of Atrial Flutter

Rate—atrial rate between 250 and 400 beats per minute; ventricular rate will depend on degree of block

Rhythm—regular or irregular, depending on kind of block (e.g., 2:1, 3:1, or a combination)

P wave—not present; instead, it is replaced by a saw-toothed pattern that is produced by the rapid firing of the atrial focus. These waves are also referred to as ''F'' waves.

P–R interval—not measurable

QRS complex—normal configuration and normal conduction time

T wave—present but may be obscured by flutter waves

Management

1. The standard treatment for atrial flutter is a digitalis preparation. This enhances the block at the AV node, thus slowing the rate.
2. Quinidine may also be given to control the ectopic focus. The concomitant use of digitalis and quinidine usually reverts the rhythm to sinus rhythm.
3. The calcium-channel blockers are being used for this dysrhythmia.
4. A beta-adrenergic blocking drug such as propranolol (Inderal) may also be used.
5. If drug therapy is unsuccessful, atrial flutter will often respond to electrical cardioversion. Small doses of electrical current are often successful.

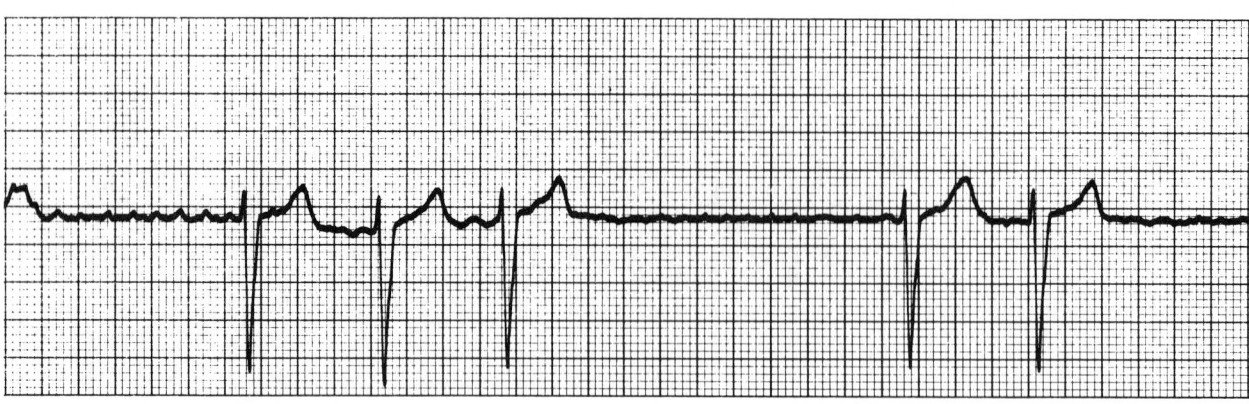

Figure 15-12. *Atrial fibrillation with slow ventricular response (controlled).*

Atrial Fibrillation (Fig. 15-12)

Atrial fibrillation is a dysrhythmia that is caused by the rapid and chaotic firing of atrial impulses by a multitude of foci. The AV node establishes a physiologic block so that only random foci are conducted to the ventricles. The rhythm of atrial fibrillation is a classic irregular irregularity.

Etiology

1. Fibrotic changes associated with the aging process
2. Acute MI
3. Valvular diseases
4. Digitalis preparations

Mechanism of Atrial Fibrillation

1. The atria fire impulses at rapid and disorganized rates.
2. The atria are not depolarized effectively; hence, there are no well-formed P waves.
3. Instead, the baseline between QRS complexes is filled with a "wiggly" line that is described as fine or coarse.
4. If the atrial rate is rapid enough, the line will appear almost flat. The atria are said to be firing at rates of between 300 and 500 times per minute.
5. The conduction of a QRS complex is so random that the rhythm is extremely irregular.
6. Atrial fibrillation may be described as *controlled* if the ventricular response is 100 beats per minute or less; the dysrhythmia is *uncontrolled* if the rate is above 100 beats per minute.

Analysis of Atrial Fibrillation

Rate—atrial fibrillation is usually immeasurable because fibrillatory waves replace P waves; ventricular rate may vary from bradycardia to tachycardia

Rhythm—classically described as an "irregular irregularity"

P wave—replaced by fibrillatory waves, sometimes called "little f" waves

P–R interval—immeasurable

QRS complex—a normally conducted complex

T wave—normally conducted

Management

1. Controlled atrial fibrillation of long-standing duration requires no treatment as long as the patient is experiencing no untoward effects. Most cardiologists agree that reversion of long-standing atrial fibrillation is hazardous because of the potential for a thrombus to be dislodged from the atria at the time of reversion.
2. Uncontrolled atrial fibrillation (ventricular responses of 100 beats per minute or greater) is treated with digitalis preparations. If the atrial fibrillation is of recent onset, the cardiologist may choose to revert the rhythm to a sinus rhythm.
3. Quinidine may be used in conjunction with digitalis if the rhythm is reverted to sinus. Quinidine is used to suppress ectopic foci.
4. Atrial fibrillation is treated less frequently with electrical cardioversion.
5. The beta-adrenergic blocking drugs or calcium ion antagonists may also be used if digitalis and quinidine prove ineffective.

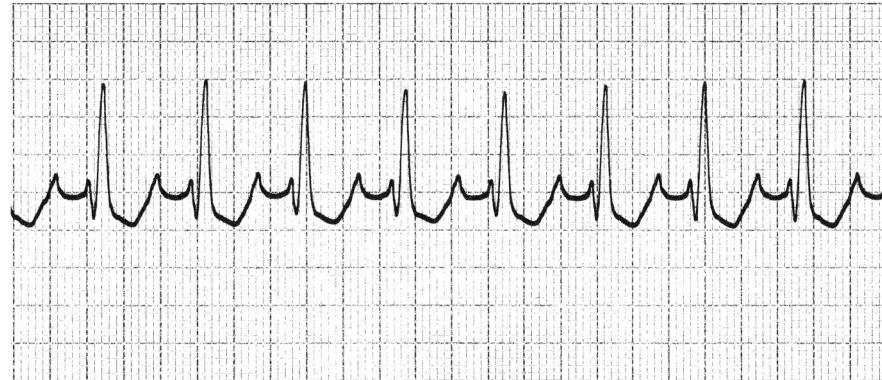

Figure 15-13. Digitalis toxicity.

Digitalis Toxicity (Fig. 15-13)

Digitalis toxicity is a dysrhythmia that results from excessive levels of serum digitalis. The two dysrhythmias that are most frequently associated with digitalis toxicity are ventricular bigeminy (every other beat is a ventricular complex) and PAT with block, although any dysrhythmia may occur.

Note: Digitalis effect, in contrast to toxicity, is a characteristic pattern of S–T depression. Digitalis toxicity and digitalis effect are not synonymous.

Analysis of Digitalis Effect

1. Therapeutic levels of digitalis will frequently be manifested by ECG.
2. A "drooping" of the S–T segment is apparent. The S–T segment depression that is manifest in myocardial ischemia is flatter in appearance. These wave form features are sometimes not distinguishing.
3. Measurement of the Q–T interval may be helpful.
   a. The Q–T interval in digitalis effect will be shortened.
   b. The Q–T interval in digitalis toxicity will be lengthened.

Analysis of Digitalis Toxicity

1. Digitalis toxicity should always be considered when the patient who has been taking the drug has a new onset of dysrhythmia, has excessive slowing of the heart rate, and complains of malaise, anorexia, and nausea and vomiting. This syndrome is frequently found in the poorly nourished population. Potassium level in the diet may be low, and hypokalemia tends to exaggerate the effect of digitalis.
2. Digitalis may be administered concomitantly with diuretics, which may contribute to potassium loss.
3. The dysrhythmias most commonly associated with digitalis are the ventricular ectopic beats; these usually, but not always, appear as bigeminy. Multifocal ventricular premature beats may also occur.
4. The next most common dysrhythmia is PAT with block.

Management

1. Obtain serum levels of digitalis and potassium.
2. Discontinue digitalis until excretion can take place and administer potassium if indicated by hypokalemia. This treatment usually resolves the problem.
3. Administer phenytoin (Dilantin) in a single dose as prescribed; this may be done as prophylaxis for ventricular dysrhythmia.
4. In more serious situations, when the patient may be hemodynamically threatened (cardiac output is severely compromised), a pacemaker may be required until the crisis is passed.
5. Cardioversion is extremely risky because of the potential for converting this dysrhythmia to a more lethal one; it is seldom done and only because no other therapies have been of benefit.

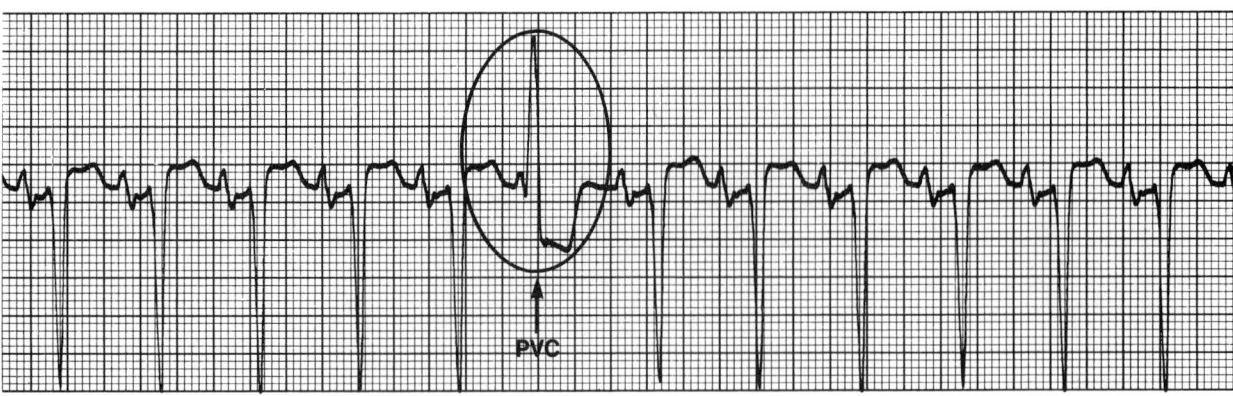

Figure 15-14. *Normal sinus rhythm with premature ventricular contraction.*

Premature Ventricular Contraction (PVC) (Fig. 15-14)

A *premature ventricular contraction* (*PVC*) is a dysrhythmia that is produced by an ectopic beat originating in the ventricle and is being discharged at a rate faster than that of the next normally occurring beat. The PVC is, by far, the most common dysrhythmia seen in the acute hospital setting.

Etiology

1. Acute MI
2. All other forms of heart disease
3. Pulmonary diseases
4. Electrolyte disturbances
5. Metabolic instability
6. Drug abuse

Mechanism of PVC

1. The wave of impulse originates within the ventricles.
2. Because the normal conduction pathway is bypassed, the configuration of the PVC is wider than normal and is distorted in appearance.
3. The PVC occurs early, and the P wave is absent.

Analysis of PVC

Rate—may be slow or fast
Rhythm—will be irregular because of the premature firing of the ventricular ectopic focus
P wave—will be absent, since the impulse originates in the ventricle, bypassing the atria and AV node.
P–R interval—immeasurable
QRS complex—the QRS of the PVC will be widened greater than 0.12 seconds, bizarre in appearance when compared with the normal QRS complex. The QRS of a PVC is often referred to as having a "sore thumb" appearance.
T wave—the T wave of the PVC is usually deflected opposite to the QRS.

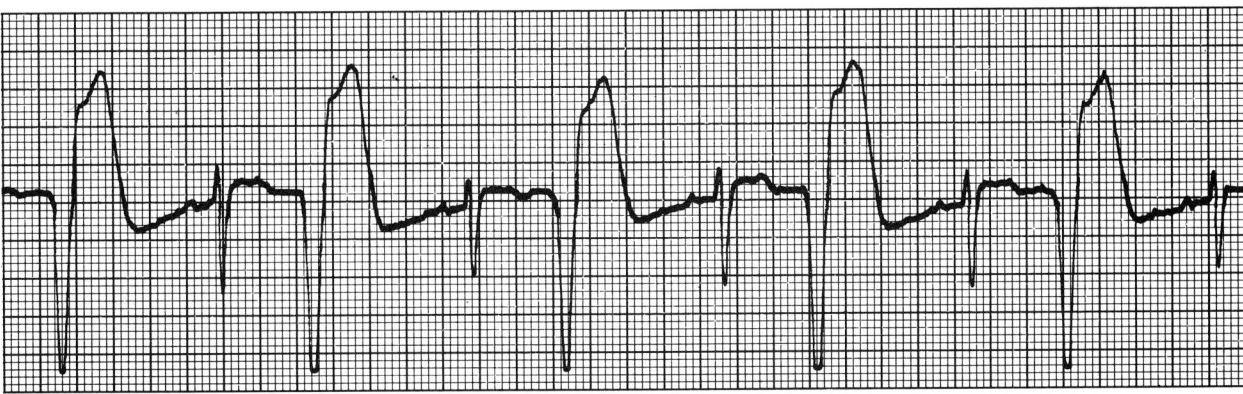

Figure 15-15. *Ventricular bigeminy.*

Management

1. PVCs are usually the precursors of more serious ventricular dysrhythmias. The following conditions involving PVCs require prompt and vigorous treatment:
   a. PVCs occurring at a rate exceeding 6 per minute.
   b. Occur 2 together (couplet).
   c. Occur 3 together (a salvo or ventricular tachycardia).
   d. Occur in a patterned sequence with the normal rhythm (e.g., every other beat is a PVC [bigeminy]) (Fig. 15-15).
   e. PVCs fall on the peak or down slope of the T wave (period of vulnerability).
   f. Are of varying configurations, indicating a multiplicity of foci.
2. The standard treatment of PVCs is with lidocaine hydrochloride by IV push.
   a. For effective treatment of PVCs, it is important to raise the serum level of lidocaine as rapidly as possible without causing toxic effects.
   b. An initial bolus of 75–100 mg. may be administered, followed by continuous drip of lidocaine in D_5W in a 4:1 concentration.
   c. The dosage may vary between 1 and 4 mg. per minute.
   d. If the dysrhythmia continues to "break through,"

another 50–100 mg. bolus of lidocaine may be given within 10–15 minutes.
3. Be alert to the development of confusion, slurring of speech, and diminished mentation, since lidocaine toxicity affects the central nervous system. Should these symptoms appear, slowing the lidocaine may cause them to abate.
4. If ventricular ectopy occurs concomitantly with a bradycardia, use lidocaine with caution, if at all. The ectopy may be compensation for the bradycardia. If lidocaine abolishes compensatory beats, the cardiac output may be seriously compromised, to the patient's detriment.
5. If ventricular premature beats occur in conjunction with a bradydysrhythmia, the physician may choose to use atropine to accelerate the heart rate and eliminate the need for ectopic beats.
6. Atropine should be used with caution in the acute MI. The injured myocardium may not be able to tolerate the accelerated rate.
7. If lidocaine proves to be ineffective in controlling PVCs, procainamide may be given (IV push), followed by a continuous drip. The average bolus dose is 300 mg. Procainamide may cause hypotension.
8. If lidocaine and procainamide prove ineffective, either alone or in combination therapy, bretylium tosylate may be used. Bretylium is administered in a continuous infusion.

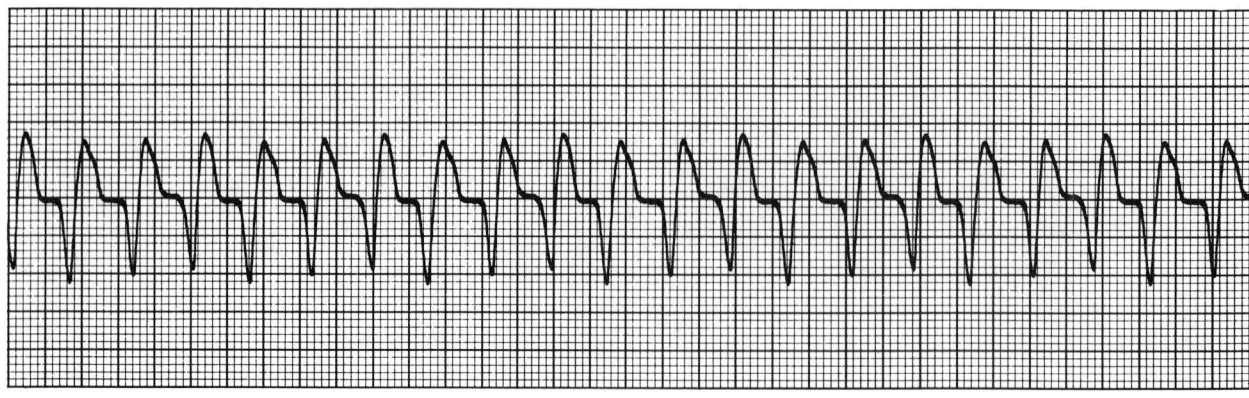

Figure 15-16. *Ventricular tachycardia.*

Ventricular Tachycardia *(Fig. 15-16)*

Ventricular tachycardia is a life-threatening dysrhythmia that originates from an irritable focus within the ventricle. It is an ineffective rhythm for maintaining cardiac output.

Etiology

1. Acute MI
2. Syndromes of accelerated rhythm that deteriorate (e.g., Wolff–Parkinson–White syndrome)
3. Metabolic acidosis, especially lactic acidosis
4. Electrolyte disturbances
5. Toxicity to certain drugs, such as digitalis or isoproterenol

Mechanism of Ventricular Tachycardia

The wave of impulse originates within the ventricles firing at a very rapid rate. Because the ventricles are capable of an inherent rate of 40 beats per minute or less, a ventricular rhythm at a rate of 100 beats per minute may be considered tachycardia.

Analysis of Ventricular Tachycardia

Rate—usually between 140 and 220 beats per minute
Rhythm—usually regular but may be irregular
P wave—not present
P–R interval—immeasurable
QRS complex—broad, bizarre in configuration, widened greater than 0.12 seconds
T wave—usually deflected opposite to the QRS complex.

Management

Ventricular tachycardia is life-threatening, and its presentation calls for immediate intervention by the nurse.

1. If the patient is alert and not hemodynamically decompensating, lidocaine hydrochloride is administered as a bolus. This is followed by continuous lidocaine infusion 4:1 drip from 1 to 4 mg./minute.
2. If the patient loses consciousness, immediate electrical defibrillation is indicated.
3. If the patient remains alert and drug therapy is not working, then synchronized defibrillation or cardioversion is applied. The purpose of electrical cardioversion is to abolish all cardiac rhythm and allow the normal pacemaker the opportunity to capture the rhythm.
4. In some cases, ventricular tachycardia may be refractory to drug therapy. Nonpharmacologic treatments such as endocardial resection, aneurysmectomy, antitachycardia pacemakers, cryoblation, automatic internal defibrillators, and catheter ablation are alternative treatment modalities.

NURSING ALERT: An atypical form of ventricular tachycardia, referred to as polymorphous ventricular tachycardia or Torsades de Pointes, can result as a consequence of quinidine therapy. It is important to differentiate this atypical form because its therapy differs from that of the more typical ventricular tachycardia.

1. Torsades de Pointes is characterized by a Q–T interval prolonged to greater than 0.60 seconds, varying R–R intervals, and polymorphous QRS complexes.
2. The treatment of choice is administration of isoproterenol, which shortens the Q–T interval. Propranolol and phenytoin may also be used if isoproterenol is ineffective.
3. Ventricular pacing to override the ventricular rate and hence capture the rhythm is also an acceptable treatment.
4. Lidocaine and procainamide are avoided, since their effect is to prolong the Q–T interval.

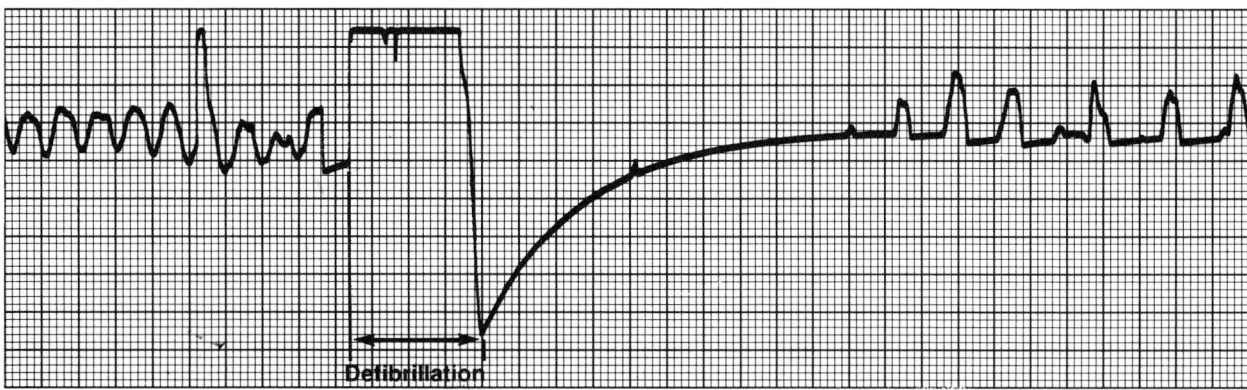

Figure 15-17. *Ventricular fibrillation with defibrillation.*

Ventricular Fibrillation (Fig. 15-17)

Ventricular fibrillation is a dysrhythmia that is characterized by the random and chaotic discharging of impulses within the ventricle at rates that exceed 300 beats per minute. Ventricular fibrillation produces clinical death and must be reversed immediately, or the patient will succumb.

Etiology

1. Deteriorating ventricular rhythms
2. Acute MI
3. Acidosis
4. Electrolyte disturbances

Mechanism of Ventricular Fibrillation

The ventricles are firing chaotically and so do not allow for effective impulse conduction. Cardiac output ceases, and the patient loses pulse, blood pressure, and consciousness.

Analysis of Ventricular Fibrillation

Rate—immeasurable because of absence of well-formed QRS complexes
Rhythm—chaotic
P wave—not present
P–R interval—not present
QRS complex—bizarre, chaotic, no definite contour
T wave—not apparent

Management

1. The only treatment for ventricular fibrillation is *immediate* electrical defibrillation. The current used may vary from 200 to 400 watt/second. See Guidelines, page 380.
2. Successful defibrillation will stop the heart and allow the heart to restart, controlled by the normal sinus pacemaker.
3. Unsuccessful defibrillation may be a result of lactic acidosis; therefore, it is important to administer sodium bicarbonate.
4. Epinephrine hydrochloride may also make the fibrillation more vulnerable to defibrillation.

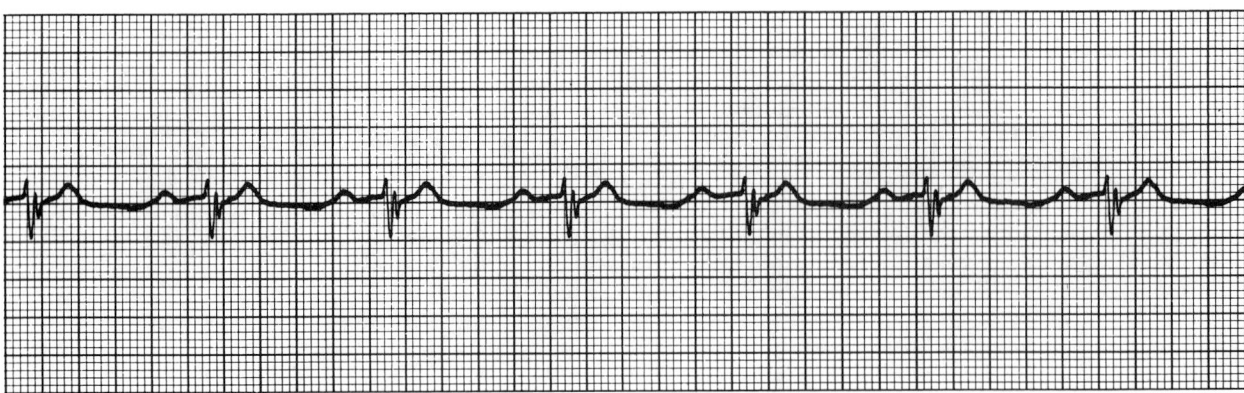

Figure 15-18. *First-degree AV block.*

The Heart Blocks

AV block implies that the transmission of the wave of impulse from the sinus node through the normal conduction pathway is altered at the level of the AV node. The altered state does not allow the impulse to be conducted on time or at all.

Types of AV Block

1. First-degree
2. Second-degree
3. Third-degree

Mechanisms of AV Blocks

1. Impaired tissue at the level of the AV node prevents the timely passage of the wave of impulse through the conduction system.
2. In first-degree AV block, the impulse is transmitted normally, but it is delayed longer at the level of the AV node. The P–R interval exceeds 0.20 seconds.
3. In second-degree AV block, the AV node becomes selective about which impulses are conducted to the ventricles.

4. In third-degree AV block, there is no relationship between the atrial activity recorded on the monitor and the ventricular activity. Both chambers are discharging impulses, but activity of the atria and activity of the ventricles bear no relationship to each other.

Analysis of First-Degree AV Block *(Fig. 15-18)*

Rate—usually normal but may be slow
Rhythm—regular
P wave—present for each QRS complex, identical in configuration
P–R interval—prolonged to greater than 0.20 seconds
QRS complex—normal in appearance and between 0.06 and 0.10 seconds
T wave—normally conducted

Analysis of Second-Degree AV Block *(Fig. 15-19)*

Rate—usually normal
Rhythm—may be regular or irregular
P wave—present but some may not be followed by a QRS complex. A ratio of 2, 3, or 4 P waves to 1 QRS complex may exist.
P–R interval—may be normal or prolonged
QRS complex—normally conducted
T wave—normally conducted

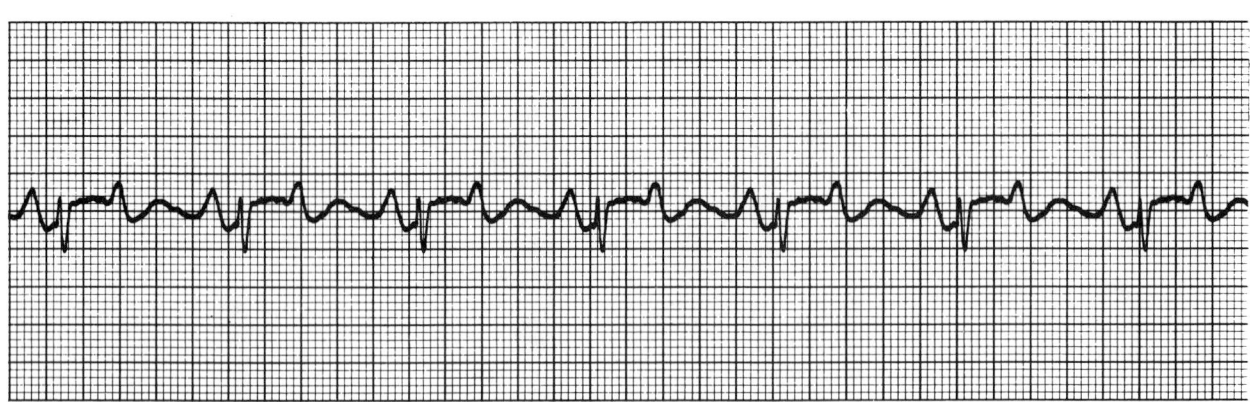

Figure 15-19. *Second-degree AV block.*

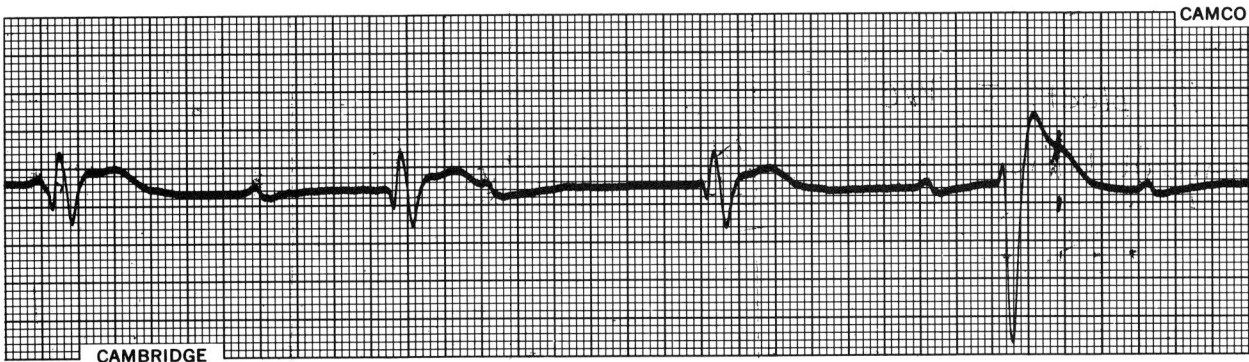

Figure 15-20. *Third-degree AV block.*

Analysis of Third-Degree AV Block
(Complete Heart Block) (Fig. 15-20)

Rate—atrial rate is measured independently of the ventricular rate. The ventricular rate is usually very slow.

Rhythm—each independent rhythm will be regular, but they will bear no relationship to each other

P wave—present before some QRS complexes; other P waves will fall at random

P–R interval—not really measurable

QRS complex—will be widened and distorted in appearance, but are usually all identical

T wave—normally conducted.

Management of AV Blocks

Like that of other dysrhythmias, the treatment of heart blocks depends on the effect the rate is having on cardiac output.

1. First-degree AV block requires no treatment.
2. Second-degree AV block may require treatment if the ventricular rate falls too low to maintain effective cardiac output.
3. Third-degree AV block may require treatment if cardiac output is compromised.
4. A ventricular pacemaker is the treatment of choice for an AV block requiring intervention.

5. Atropine may be given while awaiting the pacemaker, but it must be remembered that the effect of atropine is to block vagal tone, and the vagus acts on the sinus node. Since the AV node is the culprit in heart block, atropine may not be helpful.
6. A continuous infusion of isoproterenol 1 mg. in 500 ml. D_5W may also be attempted; however, the consequence of using isoproterenol may be ventricular tachycardia.
7. Persistent third-degree AV block will require a ventricular pacemaker. As in second-degree AV block, atropine and isoproterenol may be used, but their efficacy is questionable.

The Artificial Pacemaker

Ventricular Pacemaker *(Fig. 15-21)*

1. A *ventricular pacemaker* writes a pacing spike on the ECG paper just prior to the conduction of the QRS complex.
2. A QRS complex should follow each pacing spike.
3. On some occasions, a pacing catheter will fail to function normally.
4. The malfunctioning of a pacemaker can be caused by mechanical or electrical events.

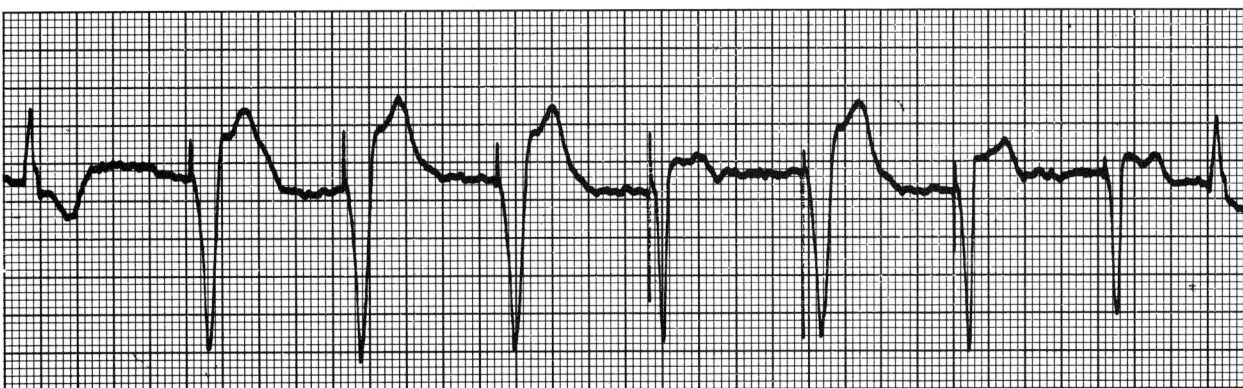

Figure 15-21. *Ventricular pacemaker.*

Guidelines Direct Current Defibrillation for Ventricular Fibrillation

Defibrillation (or countershock) is the passing of an electrical shock of short duration through the heart to terminate ventricular fibrillation or ventricular tachycardia without pulse.

A *defibrillator* is an instrument that delivers an electric shock to the heart to convert ventricular fibrillation to normal sinus rhythm. (Defibrillators are also used to convert other abnormal and rapid cardiac rhythms.)

Purpose To terminate ventricular fibrillation or ventricular tachycardia without pulse.

Equipment DC defibrillator with paddles
Interface material (saline-soaked gauze pads, electrode gels and pastes, disposable conductive gel pads)
Resuscitative equipment

Procedure

Nursing Action	Rationale/Amplification

Performance Phase (by nurse)

1. *Monitored patient*—if ventricular fibrillation recognized within 2 minutes, give precordial thump, assess rhythm and carotid pulse, and expose anterior chest.
   Unmonitored patient—expose anterior chest.

2. *Unmonitored patient*—START CARDIOPULMONARY RESUSCITATION IMMEDIATELY.
   Monitored patient—if within 2 minutes of detection of ventricular fibrillation, defibrillate before initiating cardiopulmonary resuscitation. Beyond 2 minutes, START RESUSCITATION EFFORTS IMMEDIATELY.

   2. This procedure should be carried out immediately after ventricular fibrillation is detected to minimize cerebral and circulatory deterioration.
   Cardiopulmonary resuscitation is essential before and after defibrillation to ensure blood supply to the cerebral and coronary arteries.

3. Apply interface material (gel, paste, saline pads) to the paddles. The electrode paddles should be in firm contact with the patient's skin.

   3. The interface material helps provide better contact and prevents skin burns. Do not allow any paste on the skin between the electrodes. If the paste areas touch, the current may short circuit (severely burning the patient) and may not penetrate the heart.

4. Disconnect the oxygen.

   4. Prevents danger of fire or explosion.

5. A second person should turn on the defibrillator to the prescribed setting. The American Heart Association recommends that initial defibrillation should be 200–300 watt-seconds of *delivered* energy. A second attempt at same level should be given if first attempt unsuccessful. A third attempt with an increase of energy level to 360 watt-seconds should be attempted only after assessment of arterial blood gases for presence of hypoxia and acidosis.

   5. The shock is measured in joules or watt-seconds (the dose is based on estimated body weight). The ideal energy dose for defibrillation remains controversial.

6. Apply one electrode just to the right of the upper sternum below the clavicle and the other electrode just to the left of the cardiac apex or left nipple (Fig. 15-22). About 20–25 lb. of pressure is applied to paddles to ensure good contact with the patient's skin.

   6. The paddles are placed so that the electrical discharge flows through as much myocardial mass as possible. If anteroposterior paddles are used, the anterior paddle is held with pressure on the middle sternum while the patient lies on the posterior paddle under the left infrascapular region. In this method the countershock more directly traverses the heart.

7. Grasp the paddles only by the insulated handles.

8. GIVE THE COMMAND FOR PERSONNEL TO STAND CLEAR OF THE PATIENT AND THE BED. Look quickly to make sure all are away from the patient and bed.

   8. If a person touches the bed, he may act as a ground for the current and receive a shock, especially if there are electrolyte solutions on the floor.

9. Push the discharge buttons in both paddles simultaneously.

10. Remove the paddles from the patient *immediately* after the shock is administered (unless monitoring leads are in the paddles).

11. Resume cardiopulmonary resuscitation efforts until stable rhythm, spontaneous respirations, pulse, and blood pressure return.

    11. After discharge of the countershock, CPR efforts should be resumed; total delay should be no more than 5 seconds in order to oxygenate the patient and restore circulation.

12. Look at the ECG monitor to determine the specific therapy for the resultant electrical mechanism. Further high-energy countershocks may be necessary.

(continued)

Procedure (continued)	Nursing Action	Rationale/Amplification

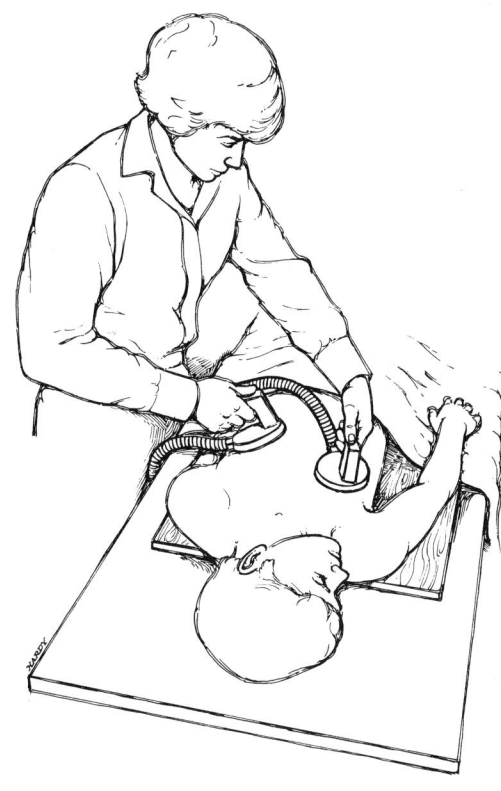

Figure 15-22. *Paddle placement in ventricular defibrillation.*

Follow-up Phase

1. After the patient is defibrillated and rhythm is restored, lidocaine is usually given to prevent recurrent episodes, and sodium bicarbonate administered to treat metabolic acidosis.
2. Continue with intensive monitoring/care.

1. Any resultant dysrhythmia may require appropriate drug intervention. Metabolic acidosis is due to accumulation of acidic products in blood because of cessation of respiration.

Guidelines — Synchronized Cardioversion

Synchronized cardioversion is a *timed* electrical shock to the heart for the purpose of terminating certain dysrhythmias. *Asynchronized cardioversion* is the same as defibrillation and is used principally for ventricular fibrillation.

Both types of cardioversion use the same type of electricity, but timed shock is not needed in ventricular fibrillation because there are no T waves. (Synchronized cardioversion is timed *not* to hit the T wave, since an electrical discharge during this phase of the cardiac cycle may cause ventricular fibrillation.)

Purpose
To stop the abnormal electrical activity of the heart and allow the SA node (heart's natural pacemaker) to resume normal sinus rhythm.

Contraindications
Synchronized cardioversion is generally *contraindicated* when a patient has been taking a significant amount of *digitalis*, since more lethal dysrhythmias may ensue after electrical discharge.

Equipment
Cardioverter and ECG machine
Conduction jelly and cardiac medications
Resuscitative equipment, including:
    Endotracheal tubes

(continued)

Guidelines Synchronized Cardioversion *(continued)*

Equipment
(continued)

Laryngoscopes
Suctioning equipment
Manual breathing bag
Pacing equipment

Procedure

Nursing Action	Rationale/Amplification
1. If the procedure is elective, it is advisable to have the patient "NPO" 12 hours before the cardioversion.	1. During sedation or the procedure, the patient may vomit and aspirate if the stomach is full.
a. Reassure the patient and see that informed consent has been obtained.	a. Do not use word "shock" since this will increase the patient's apprehension.
b. Make sure the patient has not been taking digitalis and that the serum potassium is normal.	b. Low potassium may precipitate post-shock dysrhythmias.
2. Make sure IV line is secure.	2. An IV line may be necessary for medications such as lidocaine and atropine.
3. Obtain a 12-lead ECG before and after cardioversion with the ECG machine. The ECG machine wires are best left on the patient, since the ECG printout is of much better quality than that of the monitor. This fact is especially important when one is trying to dissect complicated dysrhythmias.	3. An ECG is taken to ensure that the patient has not had a recent myocardial infarction (either just before or after the cardioversion).
4. a. Allow the patient to receive oxygen before and after cardioversion.	4. a. Oxygen will help prevent unwanted dysrhythmias after cardioversion.
b. Do *not* give oxygen during the procedure.	b. An explosion could occur if a spark from the paddles should ignite the oxygen during the procedure.

5. Place the paddles in one of the following 2 positions:
  a. *Anterior–posterior position*
    One paddle—left infrascapular area
    Other paddle—upper sternum at 3rd interspace
  b. *Anterior position*
    One paddle—just to right of sternum at 2nd interspace
    Other paddle—just under left nipple	

6. Determine if the machine's synchronization mechanism is working before applying the paddles.	
a. The discharge should hit near the peak of the R wave.	a. If the electrical discharge hits the T wave, ventricular fibrillation may occur.
b. The R wave usually must be of substantial height; if it is not, adjust the gain (sensitivity) or change the lead. On many machines, the R wave must be upright before there is synchronization.	b. Synchronization is not used for ventricular fibrillation. (The machine will not work for *defibrillation* if the synchronization mode is on.)
7. Apply electrode paste to all of the paddle surface, but make sure there is no excess around the edges of the paddles.	7. If there is excess paste around the paddles, the discharge may run onto the skin, causing a burn. If there is not firm contact between the paddle and skin, a burn may occur; also, electricity is lost from the heart.
a. The paste should be rubbed into the skin very thoroughly, since this allows more electricity to penetrate the body surface.	
b. Make sure paddles are clean because surface material will interfere with the flow of electricity.	
c. Apply firm pressure to the paddle.	
8. Set dial for lowest level of electrical energy that can be expected to convert the dysrhythmia. Some dysrhythmias (such as atrial flutter) can be converted with very low energies, such as 25 watt-seconds (joules).	8. Excessive energies may cause unnecessary discomfort to the patient.
9. Diazepam or a short-acting barbiturate should be given if the patient is conscious.	9. This helps produce amnesia concerning the cardioversion.
10. After the patient is in a light sleep from the IV medication and when no one is touching the bed or patient, discharge the cardioverter. If cardioversion does not occur, proceed to a higher energy level.	
11. Monitor the ECG after conversion occurs. Blood pressures should be recorded about every 15 minutes until the preshock blood pressure is reached.	11. The patient may revert to his previous dysrhythmias after conversion.

Bibliography

Books

Ahumada G. Cardiovascular Pathophysiology. New York, Oxford University Press, 1987

Andreoli K et al. Comprehensive Cardiac Care, 6th ed. St. Louis, CV Mosby, 1987

Brandenburg RO et al. Cardiology: Fundamentals and Practice. Chicago, Year Book Medical Pub, 1987

Braunwald E. Heart Disease: A Textbook of Cardiovascular Medicine, 3rd ed. Philadelphia, WB Saunders, 1988

Brunner LS and Suddarth DS. Textbook of Medical–Surgical Nursing, 6th ed. Philadelphia, JB Lippincott, 1988

Conover MB. Understanding Electrocardiography, 5th ed. St. Louis, CV Mosby, 1988

Conover MB and Marriott HJL. Advanced Concepts in Arrhythmias, 2nd ed. St. Louis, CV Mosby, 1989

Chung E. Principles of Cardiac Arrhythmias, 4th ed. Baltimore, Williams and Wilkins, 1989

Chung E. Quick Reference to Cardiovascular Diseases, 3rd ed. Baltimore, Williams & Wilkins, 1987

Davis D. How to Quickly and Accurately Master Arrhythmia Interpretation. Philadelphia, JB Lippincott, 1989

Dunn MI and Lipman BS. Lipman–Massie Clinical Electrocardiography, 8th ed. Chicago, Year Book Medical Pub, 1989

Edmonds JH. ECG STAT! Hospital Electrocardiography in Urgent Situations. Philadelphia, Lea & Febiger, 1988

Frye SJ and Lounsbury P. Cardiac Rhythm Disorders: An Introduction Using the Nursing Process. Baltimore, Williams & Wilkins, 1988

Grauer K and Curry WR. Clinical Electrocardiography: A Primary Care Approach. Oradell, NJ, Medical Economics Books, 1987

Hillis LD et al. Manual of Clinical Problems in Cardiology, 3rd ed. Boston, Little, Brown & Co, 1988

Kinny M et al. AACN's Clinical Reference Manual, 2nd ed. New York, McGraw–Hill, 1989

Khan MG. Manual of Cardiac Drug Therapy, 2nd ed. Philadelphia, WB Saunders, 1988

Mandel WJ. Cardiac Arrhythmias: Their Mechanisms, Diagnosis, and Management, 2nd ed. Philadelphia, JB Lippincott, 1987

Marriott HJL. Practical Electrocardiography, 8th ed. Baltimore, Williams & Wilkins, 1988

Meltzer LE, Pinneo R and Kitchell JR. Intensive Coronary Care: A Manual for Nurses, 4th ed. Bowie, MD, Prentice–Hall, 1983

Price SA and Wilson LM. Pathophysiology: Clinical Concepts of Disease Processes, 3rd ed. New York, McGraw-Hill, 1986

Underhill S et al. Cardiac Nursing, 2nd ed. Philadelphia, JB Lippincott, 1989

Journals

Andrews LK. ECG rhythms made easier with algorithms. Am J Nurs 1989 Mar; 89(3):365–369

Andrews LK. Tracking electrical impulses. Am J Nurs 1989 Mar; 89(3):370–371

Arrhythmias. Med Times 1989 Jan; 117(1):89–92

Bayless WA. The elements of cardiac pacing. Crit Care Nurse 1988 Aug; 8(7):31–41

Conover M. A common arrhythmia. Crit Care Nurse 1988 May; 8(5):112

Cook JR and Nieminski K. Ventricular tachycardia. Crit Care Nurse 1988 Oct; 8(7):15–17

Crisp CB. Calcium channel blockers in emergency medicine. Emerg Care Q 1987 Aug; 3(2):38–48

Dunnington CC et al. Patients with heart rhythm disturbances: Variables associated with increased psychologic stress. Heart Lung 1988 July; 17(4):381–389

Erickson SL. Wolff–Parkinson–White syndrome: A review and an update. Crit Care Nurse 1989 May; 9(5):28–35

Featherston RG. Care of sudden cardiac death survivors: The aberrant cardiac patient. Heart Lung 1988 May; 17(3):242–246

Heart Facts 1989. American Heart Association, Dallas, 1988

Jones S and Bagg A. L·E·A·D drugs for cardiac arrest. Nursing 1988 Jan; 18(1):34–42

Lazarus M et al. Cardiac arrhythmias: Diagnosis and treatment. Crit Care Nurse 1988 Jul; 8(7):57–65

Levy DB. Update on lidocaine. Emergency 1988 Sep; 20(9):15–18

Lunger DG. Potassium supplementations how and why? Focus Crit Care 1988 Oct; 15(5):56–60

Meola DR and Walker V. Responding quickly to tachydysrhythmias. Nursing 1987 Nov; 17(11):34–41

Miracle V. Idiopathic hypertrophic subaortic stenosis. Crit Care Nurse 1988 Mar; 8(3):102–111

Mutnik A, Fecitt S and Rogers B. Update on cardiac drugs: Inotropic and chronotropic agents. Nursing 1987 Oct; 17(10):58–61

Parker BM. Electrocardiography: Identifying diagnostic pitfalls. Consultant 1987 Aug; 27(8):34–38

Petrie JR. Distinguishing supraventricular aberrancies from ventricular ectopy. Focus Crit Care 1988 Jul; 15(4):15–21

Rhynsburger J. Action stat! Third-degree heart block. Nursing 1988 Oct; 18(10):33

Sargent RK. Advances in the treatment of ventricular dysrhythmias. Emerg Care Q 1987 Aug; 3(2):18–26

Schactman M. A case study of atrial fibrillation and mitral stenosis. Focus Crit Care 1987 May; 14(3):13–20

Teplitz L. Clinical close-up on lidocaine. Nursing 1989 Sep; 19(9):44–47

Teplitz L. Clinical close-up on epinephrine. Nursing 1989 Oct; 19(10):50–53

Teplitz L. Clinical close-up on atropine. Nursing 1989 Nov; 19(11):44–47

Valle GA and Lemberg L. Electrolyte imbalances in cardiovascular disease: The forgotten factor. Heart Lung 1988 May; 17(3):324–329

Waddell S. Vasovagal syncope. Crit Care Nurse 1989 Dec; 9(6):35–43

Walton J. Identification of patients at high risk for sudden cardiac death. Focus Crit Care 1987 Dec; 14(6):70–75

Weller DM and Noone J. Mechanisms of arrhythmias: Enhanced automaticity and reentry. Crit Care Nurse 1989 May; 9(5):42–62

16 Vascular Disorders

Vascular disorders is a term that refers to conditions of the blood vessels. *Peripheral vascular disease (PVD)* refers to disease affecting the blood vessels that supply the extremities: veins, arteries, and lymphatics. The terms vascular disorders and peripheral vascular disease (PVD) are used interchangeably.

Features and Terminology

Underlying Features

1. Results from an interruption in blood supply to the peripheral tissue causing hypoxia—local cell destruction, ulceration, and gangrene may result.
2. Impaired blood supply causes a slow and painful healing process.
3. The condition is often compounded by other medical problems such as diabetes, heart disease, and high blood pressure.
4. May appear minor but is very disabling while healing is taking place.
5. Recurrence of the condition is frequent.

Related Terminology

A. Thrombi

1. *Thrombus*—a blood clot that partially or completely occludes a blood vessel.
   a. Thrombosed vessel—an occluded vessel
   b. Thrombosis—the condition of having a thrombosed vessel
2. Spontaneous clotting of the blood will usually not occur unless there is damage to the intimal surface of the vessel wall.
   a. Injury by trauma
   b. Inflammation
   c. Degenerative changes due to arteriosclerosis
3. Injured intima—causes platelets to collect, fibrin to form, and thrombus to develop.

B. Embolus

Embolus—a fragment of a thrombus or a thrombus that has broken away from the point of formation.
1. *Embolism*—occurs when an embolus moving through a blood vessel arrives at a narrowing of the vessel and thus occludes it.
2. Air embolism—a bubble of air in the bloodstream.
3. Fat embolism—multiple droplets of fat in the bloodstream.

C. Ischemia

Ischemia—a lack of blood supply sufficient to meet tissue needs. This can develop as a result of:
1. Gradual occlusion of the lumen of the artery by encroachment of the thickened wall (atherosclerosis).
2. More rapid development of ischemia because of formation of a blood clot (thrombus) at the atherosclerotic site.
3. Rapid occlusion of an artery when a free-flowing clot (embolus) lodges at a bifurcation or narrowing of the vessel.

GERONTOLOGIC ALERT: The process of aging produces a stiffening of the peripheral vessels. Cellular proliferation and fibrosis cause intimal thickening, elastin fibers of the media calcify and become thin and fragmented, and collagen forms in the intima and media. The stiffening produced increases peripheral resistance, impairs blood flow, and increases the workload of the left ventricle. Pay particular attention to the signs and symptoms of peripheral vascular disease in the aged.

Clinical Manifestations

1. Severe cramplike pain in affected extremity(ies) usually associated with activity.
2. Changes in skin color and temperature. The skin may become pale, mottled, and shiny in appearance. The temperature will be cool to cold.

3. Diminished to absent pulses in the affected extremity(ies).
4. Scant or absent hair growth on affected extremity(ies).

Diagnostic Evaluation of Vascular Conditions

A. Doppler Ultrasound—a noninvasive test used to detect blood flow.

1. A beam of ultrasound is sent into the tissues through an acoustic gel on the skin. Reflected sound from moving blood cells is detected, amplified as audible sound, and recorded; velocity of blood flow has a direct effect on the waveforms (Figs. 16-1 and 16-2).
2. Usually, the posterior tibial, calf, popliteal, and common femoral veins are examined. Arterial flow can be detected by the pulsatile nature of the flow.
3. Signals are assessed for venous patency and valvular competence. Arterial flow is used as an indicator of patency, and the cuff pressure required to stop it indicates arterial pressure at that point.
4. Entire test takes about 5–10 minutes.
5. This technique, when checked with arteriography, has a reliability factor of 95% and thus qualifies as a simple, inexpensive, highly reliable, and noninvasive diagnostic tool.

B. Plethysmography (pulse volume recording, PVR)— a noninvasive measurement of changes in calf volume corresponding to changes in blood volume brought about by temporary venous occlusion with a high pneumatic cuff.

1. Variations of the above test are practiced in various clinics; some use a strain-gauge placed around the calf.
2. Temporary venous occlusion with a pneumatic cuff (50 mm. Hg) applied to the thigh results in an increase in circumference of the calf.
3. Sudden cuff deflation results in a decrease in calf circumference; this is proportional to rate of venous outflow from extremity.
4. Ocular pneumoplethysmography (OPG)—measures indirectly carotid artery blood flow; this is done by the application of pneumatic pressure on the eye to measure ophthalmic eye pressure.

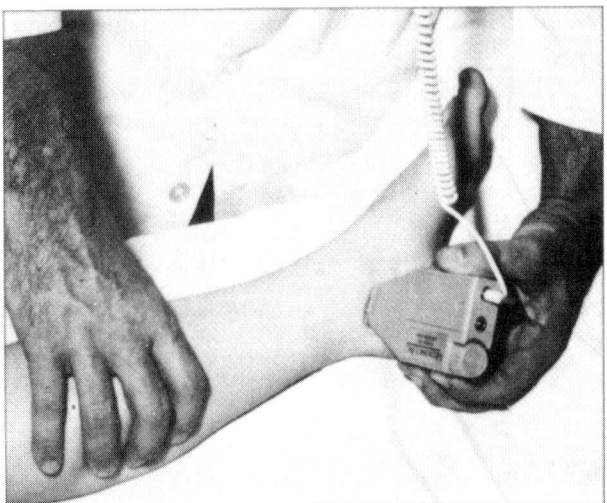

Figure 16-1. Doppler ultrasound transducer being used in screening for major deep-vein thrombosis.

C. Oscillometry

1. Degree of arterial occlusion may be measured by an oscillometer, which measures pulse volume. One extremity may be compared with the other.
2. An inflatable cuff is wrapped around the extremity, and the *oscillometric index* is determined by inflating the cuff and reading the dial.
3. Normal readings (points of pressure at which circulation ceases):

   a. Lower extremity

Midthigh	4–16 mm./Hg
Upper third of leg	3–12 mm./Hg
Above ankle	1–18 mm./Hg
Foot	0.2–1.0 mm./Hg

   b. Upper extremity

Upper arm	4–16 mm./Hg
Elbow	3–12 mm./Hg
Wrist	1–10 mm./Hg
Hand	0.2–2.0 mm./Hg

D. Phlebography (Venography)—an x-ray visualization of the vascular tree after the injection of a contrast medium (renografin).

1. Inform the patient that he may experience an intense burning sensation in the vessel where the solution is injected. This will last for only a few seconds.
2. Note any evidence of allergic reaction to the contrast medium; this may occur as soon as the contrast medium is injected, or it may be delayed and occur when the patient reaches his room.

   a. Perspiring, dyspnea, nausea, vomiting
   b. Rapid heart rate, numbness of extremities
   c. Hives
   d. Management
      (1) Notify physician.
      (2) Have epinephrine available for injection, as well as antihistamine drugs and oxygen.
3. Nursing Interventions

   a. Observe injection site for the following:
      (1) Signs of redness, swelling, bleeding; signs of thrombosis (loss of distal pulses)
         If above signs occur, notify physician.
      (2) Evidence of bleeding
         (a) Apply pressure dressing.
         (b) Notify physician.
   b. Check for arterial occlusion.
      (1) Note extremity pulses; check for quality.
      (2) Observe color (pallor or cyanosis).
      (3) Ask the patient about sensation of pain, numbness.
4. Chief disadvantages: It is an expensive and invasive diagnostic method and may cause painful side effects.

E. Treadmill Test

1. At a designated speed and incline, the patient walks for 5 minutes; he is stopped if:

   a. Symptoms of claudication occur.
   b. Other signs of intolerance, such as shortness of breath, develop.
2. Following the exercise, he is returned to the examining table, where ankle pressures, pulse volumes, and brachial systolic pressures are taken.
3. Normally, there is an increase in total extremity blood flow.

F. Intermittent Claudication Determination

1. At rest, blood supply is adequate—but an exercised muscle may require 10 times more blood.

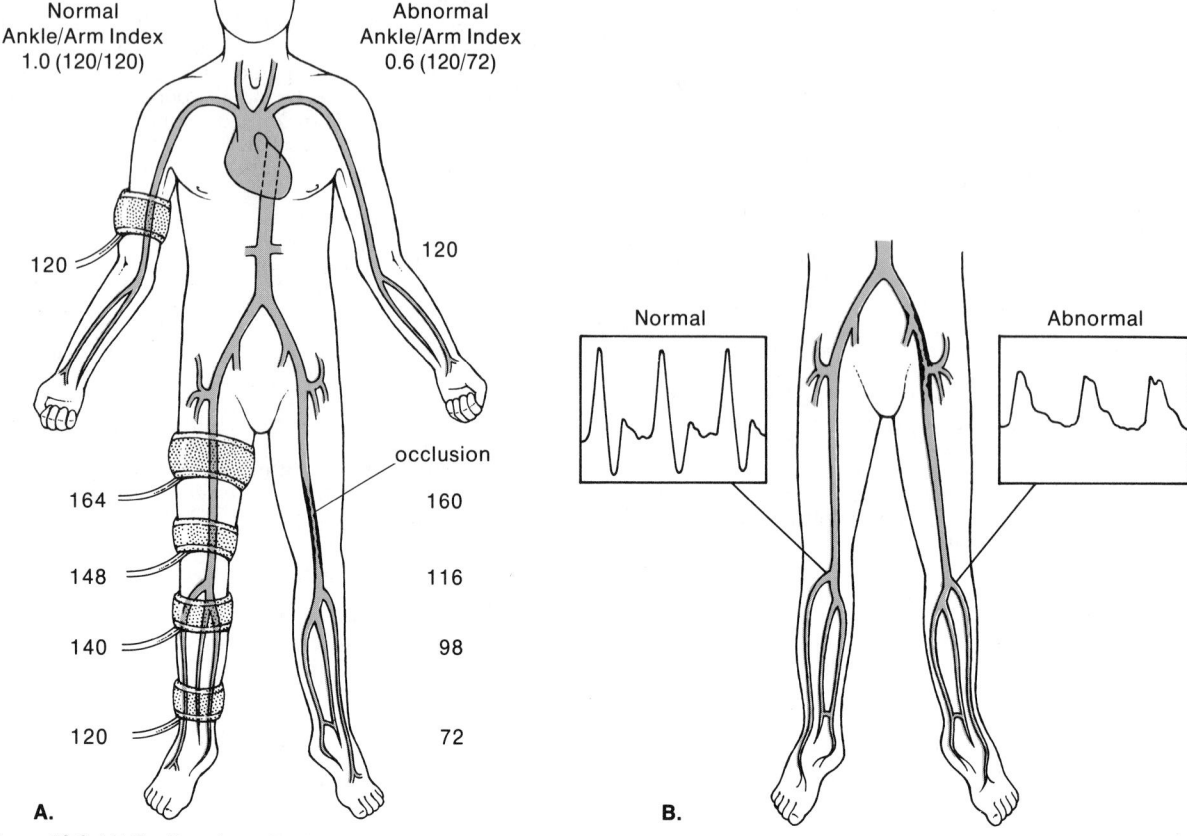

Figure 16-2. *(A) The Doppler probe determines pressures over the brachial and posterior tibial or dorsalis pedis arteries. The cuff is inflated until the arterial segment disappears; the cuff is then slowly deflated until the arterial velocity signal returns at systolic pressure. NOTE: Normally, ankle pressure is equal to or slightly above arm pressure. In the presence of occlusive arterial disease (right side of diagrammed person), ankle and lower leg pressures are lower by an amount proportional to the degree of circulatory impairment. (B) Diagram comparing the analogue wave tracings in a normal (left) and a diseased extremity (right). Note the lack of diastolic deflection and the protracted systolic components in the tracing of the abnormal extremity. (AbuRahma et al. Doppler testing in peripheral vascular occlusive disease. Surg Gynecol Obstet 1980 Jan; 150 [1]:27)*

2. Following exercise such as walking, running, or climbing stairs, a severe cramping pain or sensation of tiredness develops in those muscle areas not receiving an adequate blood supply.
3. Upon resting, pain is relieved; metabolites are carried away and normal blood-to-tissue demand ratio is restored.
4. Measurement
   a. Have the patient walk up steps, counting number of steps taken before pain occurs.
   b. Use a foot-pedal device, which lifts a weight when pressed.
      (1) Normally, fatigue occurs in 5–10 minutes.
      (2) The person with arterial occlusion usually complains of pain in less than a minute.

G. Digital Subtraction Angiography (DSA), or Digital Intravenous Angiography

A radiologic technique that uses an image-intensifier video system to display vessels on a television monitor. The images are received by a computer that translates them into numbers. By this conversion, it is possible to subtract the image obtained (before the injection of contrast medium) from the later images. Therefore, after computer subtraction, an enhanced image of the arterial system is presented.

1. Patient preparation
   a. No food intake within 2 hours of the test to prevent vomiting if there is a reaction to the contrast medium.
   b. The patient must be able to hold his breath and lie very still when directed.
   c. The patient is placed in supine position (appropriately centered) on a radiographic table.
   d. Brachial vein is prepared, and a large sterile drape is positioned to accommodate the guidewire and catheter.
   e. Fluoroscopy aids in moving the catheter properly; the catheter is moved over the guidewire and positioned near the superior vena cava/right atrial junction.
   f. The radiologist positions the area of interest under fluoroscopy.
   g. Study takes 20–40 minutes.
   h. Upon completion, the catheter is removed and pressure is applied to the puncture site for about 5 minutes; a sterile dressing is applied.

i. The patient is instructed to increase fluid intake over next 24 hours (1500–2000 ml.) to aid in excretion of contrast medium.

Management of Vascular Disorders

The goals of management are to improve the local blood supply and diminish injury to the involved tissue. This is accomplished by anticoagulant therapy, thrombolytic therapy, thermotherapy, pressure gradient therapy, surgical interventions, and ongoing patient education.

Anticoagulant Therapy

Anticoagulant therapy is the administration of medications to achieve the following:

Goals:
Disrupt the blood's natural clotting mechanism.
Prevent formation of a thrombus in postoperative patients.
Intercept the extension of a thrombus once it has formed.

Types of Anticoagulants

Oral

Coumarin derivatives: dicumarol, phenprocoumon, warfarin sodium, and warfarin potassium

Parenteral

Heparin sodium

Clinical Indications

1. *Venous thrombosis*—because of the danger of extension and the danger of emboli.
2. *Pulmonary embolism*—prophylactically, if patient is known to be suspect; also indicated during recovery phase to prevent further clot formation.
3. *Patient susceptible to embolism*—such as a surgical patient who has rheumatic heart disease, one who has had valve surgery.
4. *Coronary occlusion with myocardial infarction.*
5. *Stroke* caused by emboli or cerebral thrombi—to reduce sludging of blood: useful in prevention and treatment of strokes.

Contraindications

1. May cause spontaneous bleeding—therefore not used when there is likelihood of bleeding because of increased capillary fragility or an aneurysm.
2. Individuals with peptic ulcer and chronic ulcerative diseases are considered poor risks, because of the possibility of bleeding.
3. Should not be given following neurosurgery because of danger of hemorrhage in brain or spinal cord.
4. Liver disease may present a problem because of interference with plasma protein clotting factors.
5. Liver and kidney insufficiency diseases because of difficulty in metabolizing and eliminating them—resulting in toxicity and difficulty in responding to antidotal medication (not true of heparin).
6. Poor follow-up by patients; unless the patient cooperates by reporting for blood tests, he should not be on anticoagulants.

7. Severe diabetes, infections, or severe traumatic conditions are circumstances in which anticoagulant therapy may be contraindicated.

> **NURSING ALERT:** There is risk of bleeding in any patient receiving anticoagulants.

Nursing Interventions

1. The preferred method of heparin administration is continuous infusion (using a pump) because of the low incidence of hemorrhagic complications.
2. Check patient's weight, since dosage is calculated on the basis of weight.
3. Be sure clotting profiles are obtained before treatment is initiated, to detect hidden bleeding tendencies.
4. Place pump out of reach of patient to prevent interference with its proper functioning.
   Check frequently to ensure that system is working properly: exact dosage, no leaks, no kinks.
5. Note that periodic coagulation tests are done; these include hematocrit and partial thromboplastin time (PTT).
6. Recognize that heparin may be given by *intermittent intravenous injection.* This may be facilitated by the use of a "heparin-lock" (see p. 91).
7. *Minidose heparin* is used in certain patients preoperatively to reduce postoperative thromboembolism.
8. Since heparin may be given along with longer lasting hypoprothrombinemic agents, for the first few days of treatment, each day's medication orders should be checked *after* reports of daily prothrombin time tests are known.
9. Have on hand the antidotes to anticoagulants being used:
   Heparin—protamine sulfate
   Coumarin—phytonadione (vitamin K_1, Aquamephyton, Konakion, Mephyton)
10. Note that the relatively long duration of action of oral anticoagulants makes it easier to maintain low prothrombin levels for long periods.
11. Observe carefully for any possible signs of bleeding and report immediately so that anticoagulant dosage may be reviewed and altered if necessary:
    a. Urine—note evidence of hematuria; indandione derivatives may turn alkaline urine a red orange color—acidifying this urine causes this color to disappear.
    b. Stool—check for tarry color; use test tape for occult blood.
    c. Emesis basin following tooth brushing—note any pink or bloody return.
12. Be aware of the following with regard to sensitivity to coumarin derivatives:

May be intensified by	*May be decreased by*
Antibiotics	Antacids
Mineral oil	Barbiturates
Quinidine	Oral contraceptives
Salicylates	Adrenal corticosteroids
Tolbutamide (Orinase)	

> **NURSING ALERT:** Drug interactions can alter the effect of anticoagulants. Review with the physician the effect of other medications the patient may be taking during anticoagulant therapy.

Guidelines   Subcutaneous Injection of Heparin

Purpose   When prolonged therapy is indicated, heparin may be given subcutaneously into fatty tissues.

Equipment   1- or 2-ml. syringe or disposable tuberculin syringe
Fine sharp needle, No. 27, 1.6-cm. (⅝ inch) long (or premeasured Tubex cartridge-needle unit)
Skin antiseptic

Considera-   1. Most convenient sites are along lower abdominal fat pad—to avoid inadvertent intramuscular injection and hematoma formation.
tions   a. A common location site is the fatty area anterior to either iliac crest.
                 b. Avoid injection sites within 5 cm. (2 inches) of the umbilicus because of possibility of entering a larger blood vessel.
             2. Areas where subcutaneous layer is thin should be avoided.

> **GERONTOLOGIC ALERT:** The aging individual begins to lose subcutaneous fat padding. Examine patient for best site for subcutaneous administration of heparin.

Procedure

Nursing Action	Rationale/Amplification
Performance Phase	
1. Sponge the area gently with alcohol. Do not rub!	1. Rubbing or pinching skin might initiate damage to the tissue; heparin would aggravate any bleeding.
2. Attempt to stretch skin out, using palm of left hand. Some prefer to (gently) pick up a well-defined fold of skin.	2. Try to empty blood vessels in local area to lessen likelihood of their being pierced by needle—with subsequent hematoma formation.
3. Holding the shaft of the syringe in dart fashion, insert needle directly through the skin at a right angle just into the subcutaneous fatty layer.	
4. Move right hand into position to direct plunger.	4. Aspiration in a forcible manner can damage small blood vessels and frequently lead to bleeding and hematoma formation, especially in the presence of high local concentration of heparin.
a. Do not move needle tip once it is inserted.	
b. Do not pull back plunger for testing.	
5. Firmly push plunger down as far as it will go.	5. This ensures administration of total dose of heparin.
6. When injection has been made, withdraw needle gently at the same angle at which it entered, releasing skin roll upon withdrawal of needle.	6. To minimize tissue damage.
7. Press an alcohol sponge to the site for a few seconds.	7. To minimize oozing or bleeding.
Follow-up Care	
1. *Do not rub the area. Instruct patient not to rub area.*	1. Rubbing would increase the likelihood of bleeding.
2. *Site of injection*	
a. Change site of injection each time heparin is administered.	
b. A chart can be marked with time, date, and measured dosage so that rotation of sites can be ensured.	

Note: Low-dose heparin may be used to prevent deep vein thrombosis postoperatively

---

Patient Education *(Anticoagulant Therapy)*

1. Information to be relayed to the physician before anticoagulant therapy is initiated:
   a. What medications are currently being taken? Note that barbiturates increase metabolism of coumarin medications—therefore an increased dose of anticoagulants is in order.
   b. What treatments are being done for problems other than circulatory problems?
   c. If female, whether a pregnancy is planned or confirmed?
   d. If other treatments are anticipated, such as major dental work, hemorrhoidectomy?
2. During anticoagulant therapy:
   a. Follow instructions carefully and take medications exactly as prescribed.
   b. Take medications at the same time each day and do not stop taking them even though symptomless.
   c. Wear a bracelet or carry a card indicating that anticoagulants are being taken; include name, address, and phone number of physician.
3. Notify the physician:
   a. In case of accident, infection, or other significant illness that may affect blood clotting.

b. If surgical care by another physician or dentist is needed. Inform him that anticoagulants are being taken.

c. If a dose of anticoagulant is forgotten. Do not take extra pills to make up for a skipped dose.

d. In case of diarrhea, upset stomach, high fever.

4. Avoid:

a. Taking any other medications without first checking with physician, particularly

(1) Vitamins
(2) Aspirin
(3) Mineral oil
(4) Cold medicines
(5) Antibiotics
(6) Phenylbutazone (Butazolidin)

b. Excessive use of alcohol, since alcohol may affect clotting capacity; check on acceptable limits for social drinking.

c. Participation in activities in which there is high risk of injury.

d. Foods that may cause diarrhea or upset stomach.

5. Be alert for these warning signs:

a. Excessive bleeding that does not stop quickly (such as following shaving, a small cut, teeth brushing with gum injury, nose bleed)

b. Excessive menstrual bleeding

c. Skin discoloration or bruises that appear suddenly

d. Black or bloody bowel movements; for questionable stool discoloration, test for occult blood.

e. Blood in urine

NURSING ALERT: Patients taking phenindione produce orange or beige-colored urine; when the urine is acidified, this coloration disappears. With true hematuria, acid does not affect color.

---

f. Faintness, dizziness, or unusual weakness

6. A reminder:

Later, when anticoagulant medication is stabilized, the patient must be reminded to keep prothrombin test appointments as scheduled.

Thrombolytic Therapy

Thrombolytic therapy is administration of thrombolytic agents to dissolve any formed thrombus and inhibit the body's hemostatic function.

Types of Thrombolytics

Thrombolytic agents are available for parenteral use only. Commonly used thrombolytics include:

1. Streptokinase
2. Urokinase
3. Tissue-type plasminogen activator (tPA)

Clinical Indications

1. Acute myocardial infarction from coronary thrombosis
2. Pulmonary embolus
3. Occlusion of peripheral arteries

Contraindications

1. Generalized hemorrhage is a great risk because thrombolytic therapy inhibits the body's hemostatic system.

2. Individuals with peptic ulcer and chronic ulcerative diseases are poor risks.

3. Should not be given following any recent surgery.

4. Liver disease may be a contraindication because of interference with plasma protein clotting factors.

5. Thrombolytic agents are used for acute emergency management of thrombosis only and are usually administered in a very controlled setting such as cardiac catheterization laboratory or intensive care unit.

Nursing Interventions

1. Monitor clotting profiles; these are essential before the initiation of treatment to disclose any bleeding tendencies and to serve as a baseline for assessment of drug efficacy.

2. Observe for signs of bleeding and report immediately.

3. Monitor for allergic reaction. A small number of patients (less than 5%) may experience an allergic reaction.

a. Observe the patient for the onset of a new rash, fever, and chills.

b. Report any suspected allergic reaction immediately.

Nonpharmacologic Therapies

Thermotherapy

A. Dry Heat

1. Warm water bottles

a. Check temperature of water before filling bottle—not to exceed 48.8°C. (120°F).

b. Apply cover to bottle so that it does not come in direct contact with skin.

2. Heat cradle (thermostatically controlled or regulated with electric bulbs)

a. Pad metal edges of cradle to prevent injury to extremities.

b. Control temperature so that it will not exceed 32.2°C. (90°F.).

c. Ensure that bulbs are not likely to be touched by extremity (usually legs and feet).

d. Higher temperatures would stimulate metabolism (not desired).

e. Reduce temperature if patient complains of pain in extremity.

3. Ultrasound (acoustic vibration with frequencies beyond human ear perception)

a. Useful in small areas where deeper penetration of heat is desired and where circulation needs to be stimulated.

b. Application time is under 10 minutes.

c. Avoid areas where metal sutures may be present.

B. Moist Heat

1. Hydrotherapy

a. Sitz bath—used for perineal therapy.

b. Basin—for hands or feet, with prescribed temperatures and for prescribed times.

2. Whirlpool bath

a. In addition to moist heat, the effect of agitated water provides hydromassage.

b. May be used for 1 or 2 extremities or the whole body.

3. Warm compresses

a. Applied directly to the skin.

b. When hot, apply over toweling.

Put on supports early in the morning, before swelling occurs.

Always begin with supports "inside-out" . . . as they are when you receive them.

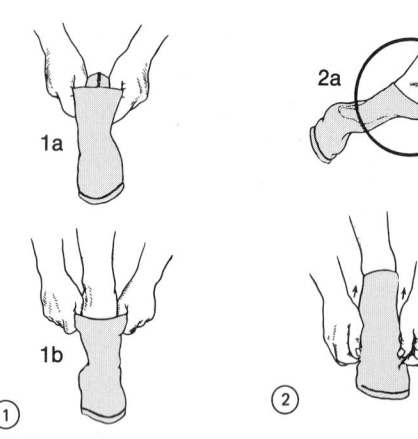

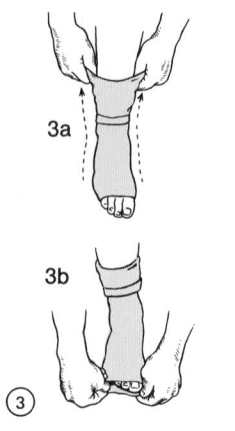

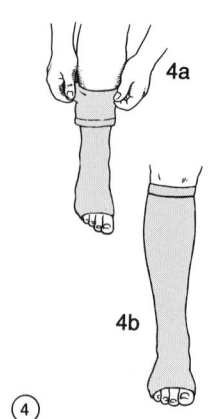

Sit with feet in easy reach. Support must be "inside out," with its foot inverted back to heel. Seam faces down (sketch 1a). Grasp each side firmly and pull onto foot (sketch 1b).

Pull past midpoint of heel (sketch 2a), so support will not slip back. Then, reach just beyond toes and grasp fabric between fingers and start pulling over foot. Pull from sides . . . never by seams.

Pull all the way up past ankle (sketch 3a). Seat heel in place. Pull foot portion of support out toward tips of toes (sketch 3b) to set fabric evenly on foot. Allow to settle back normally.

Using short (2 inches at a time) snappy pulls (sketch 4a) pull support up to point it was measured to end (sketch 4b). Smooth evenly down leg. **Never allow top to roll or turn down.**

Figure 16-3. *Method of applying supporting hose. (Courtesy of Jobst).*

Pressure Gradient Therapy to Promote Vasodilatation *(Compression Devices and Garments)*

A. Cuffs, Sleeves, or Boots

1. Circulator—electrically produced air pressure alternately inflates and deflates a boot in which the extremity is encased. Rhythm of occlusion and release as well as pressure can be regulated to correspond to pulse.
2. Pressor sleeve or boot—a plastic tube filled with air.
   a. Can be maintained at low pressure for several hours.
   b. Can be regulated to function intermittently (useful in lymphedema of arm following mastectomy.

B. Elastic Garments

1. Support for an extremity can be tailor-made: A unique measuring tape was devised by Jobst* so that exact "fabric pressures" are produced with their custom-made venous pressure gradient supports.
2. Method of applying supporting hose is demonstrated in Figure 16-3.
3. Any type of support hose, if applied incorrectly (such as permitting rolling at the top), can act as a tourniquet. This will produce stasis, rather than prevent it.
4. Many question the effectiveness of elastic stockings; the nurse will be guided by the preferences of the patient's physician.
5. Elastic stockings with inflatable pneumatic bladders connected to an automatic air pump are available to help prevent deep-vein thrombi from forming in the calf and lower leg.
   The bladders in this device, called the *Pulsatile Anti-Embolism System,* expand and contract and are designed to stimulate circulation.

* The Jobst Institute, 651–653 Miami Street, Toledo, OH 43694.

Surgical Interventions

1. Major vascular centers are reporting commendable results in vascular surgery as an alternative to amputation.
2. A second opinion is suggested if lower-extremity amputation is being considered.
3. Various synthetic graft materials are available for very specific vascular needs.
4. Microsurgery is adding a new dimension to very fine surgical repair.

Nursing Process Overview: The Patient With a Vascular Disorder

Nursing Assessment

Assessment begins with a patient history. The patient is then examined for the following signs and symptoms of vascular disorders:

A. Skin Color and Temperature.

Each extremity is palpated for skin temperature; extremities are compared with each other for temperature discrepancies. Observation of skin color is made simultaneously.

1. Coldness
   a. Due to deficient blood supply to a part even though the environment is warm.
   b. One extremity may be compared with another to note the difference.
   c. The patient notices that the part feels uncomfortably cold.
2. Pallor (Paleness)
   a. Normally, the pink hue of the skin is due to adequate superficial circulation.
   b. Diminished blood supply produces paleness, or lack of color.

c. Blanching occurs when the part is elevated above the level of the heart and the arterial pressure in that part is lower than normal.

3. Rubor (Redness)
    a. Instead of a normal rosy-pink, the part may be red or reddish-blue. This is due to injury of superficial capillaries, which causes them to remain dilated; it may also occur with chronic ischemia.
    b. Circulation is impaired.
    c. Anoxia or coldness may be the cause of rubor.
4. Cyanosis (Blueness)
    a. Indicates that less than a normal amount of oxygen is in the blood.
    b. When localized, it implies very slow circulation in that part.

B. Pain

1. Due to inadequate blood supply.
2. This is common, but varies with the condition. May be constant and severe (e.g., ulceration).
3. When it occurs only after a certain amount of exercise, it is called *intermittent claudication.* (This disappears after rest, but returns with exercise.)
4. When it occurs at rest (rest pain), it indicates a more severe degree of ischemia.

C. Necrosis

1. Loss of viability of tissue.
2. Noted first in most distal parts of the extremity.

D. Atrophy

1. The muscle shrinks, and there is loss of strength and joint mobility.
2. Due to chronic ischemia.

E. Exercise Tolerance

Measurement of the amount of exercise the involved part can tolerate before pain is experienced. The patient can usually define this explicitly.

F. Pulse Volume (Fig. 16-4)

A useful method for recording peripheral pulse volume, based on a scale from zero to +4, as follows:
    0 Not palpable—absent pulsations
    +1 Thready, weak, fades in and out—marked impairment of pulsations
    +2 Difficult to palpate; stronger than +1—moderate impairment
    +3 Easily palpable, not easily obliterated with pressure—slight impairment
    +4 Strong and bounding—normal pulsations

G. Bruits

1. An abnormal sound heard on auscultation as blood flows through a stenotic area of the artery.
2. This is heard most easily during systole; pitch is higher as stenosis becomes more marked.

H. Capillary Refill Time

The capillary bed contains arterial blood and is called *microcirculation.* Capillary refill time is an indicator of peripheral perfusion and cardiac output.

1. This test can be done at the same time that arterial pulses are checked.
2. Depress finger or toe nailbed until skin blanches.
3. Release pressure and note how rapidly color returns to the original appearance.
    a. Normally, capillaries fill within a fraction of a second.
        (1) Acceptable—less than 3 seconds
        (2) Abnormal or sluggish—more than 3 seconds

I. Blood Pressure

Serial blood pressure readings are taken with Doppler Ultrasound (see p. 385).

Nursing Diagnoses

1. Altered peripheral tissue perfusion related to compromised circulation.
2. Pain related to impaired ability of peripheral vessels to supply tissue with oxygen.
3. Potential impairment of skin integrity related to compromised circulation.
4. Knowledge deficit of self-care activities.

Nursing Interventions

A. Enhancing Arterial Blood Supply and Decreasing Venous Congestion

Teach the patient about the prescribed regimen as follows:
1. *Walking*—a simple but very effective exercise.
    a. A level surface is preferred.
    b. Encourage the patient to set realistic goals; each week these goals may be extended in keeping with his tolerance.
    c. Use assistive devices as necessary—walker, cane, etc.
    d. Evaluate the patient's ability to climb stairs.
2. *Jogging*—a means of stimulating collateral blood flow not only to legs, but also to the myocardium. Usually may be practiced as long as it is comfortable and pleasurable.
3. *Buerger's exercises*—prescribed according to condition of extremities and condition of patient.
    a. Elevate extremity for a minute.
    b. Place extremities in a dependent position until cyanosis or rubor becomes maximal.
    c. Lie with extremities horizontal for a minute.
    d. See Buerger—Allen exercises below.
4. *Buerger–Allen exercises*—exercises by which gravity alternately fills and empties the blood vessels (Fig. 16-5).
    a. Begin with the patient lying flat in bed. Elevate legs to above level of heart—2 minutes or until blanching takes place.
    b. Allow legs to be dependent; exercise feet—3 minutes or until legs are pink.
    c. Instruct the patient to lie flat—5 minutes.
    d. Repeat a, b, and c 5 times; do entire set 3 times a day.
5. *Activity tolerance and proper pacing.*
    a. Advise the patient to rest when he feels pain.
    b. Avoid chilly environment, since it causes vasoconstriction, which in turn further diminishes flow.
    c. Maintain stability, particularly if postural hypotension is a problem.
6. *Comfort*
    a. Improvise equipment that will provide comfortable support for the patient in the leg-elevated position.
    b. Well-padded straight-back chair can be placed on the bed so that the back of the chair supports the leg—top of chair is toward the top of the thigh.
    c. Overbed table may be used with a pillow.
7. *Discuss the advantages of the oscillating bed, if this has been prescribed;* provides postural exercises using a passive method.

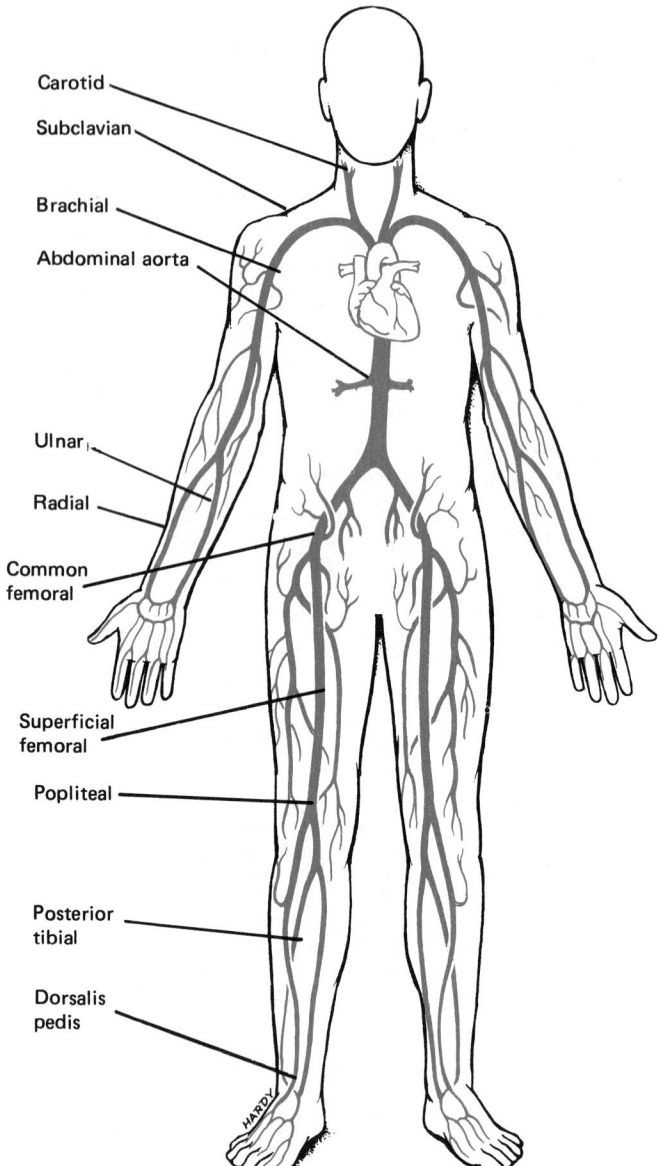

Carotid
Subclavian
Brachial
Abdominal aorta
Ulnar
Radial
Common femoral
Superficial femoral
Popliteal
Posterior tibial
Dorsalis pedis

Figure 16-4. *Salient points in evaluating peripheral arterial insufficiency: Reduced or absent femoral pulses indicate aortoiliac disease. Absent popliteal pulses indicate superficial femoral occlusion. Pulse deficits in one extremity, with normal pulses in contralateral extremity, suggest acute arterial embolus. Absent pedal pulses indicate tibioperoneal artery involvement.*

   a. Explain to the patient that the bed will assist in relieving his circulatory difficulty.
      (1) Explain how the bed is turned on, regulated, and stopped.
      (2) Advise the patient whether he can stop for meals, treatments, rest periods, etc.
   b. Introduce motion of bed gradually in order to eliminate the possibility of headache, dizziness, or nausea.
   c. Follow prescribed cycle for the individual patient.
      Cycle: Degree of angle and the length of time to be elevated
             Degree of angle and the length of time to be lowered
   d. Instruct the patient to use a padded footboard to prevent slipping downward in bed.

B. Relieving Pain Through Hygienic Measures and Activities to Increase the Blood Flow to the Extremities.

1. Maintain a warm and properly humidified environment.
2. Put on warm clothing before going out into cool air; protect hands and feet with lamb's wool lining in gloves and boots to prevent vasoconstriction.
3. Take a warm bath to offset chilling; replace vigorous rubbing of the skin after a bath with gentle patting.
4. Avoid excessive heat to extremities (using hot water bottle, electric pad, etc.)—increases metabolism, so that more oxygenated blood is demanded.
5. Sleep with the head of the bed elevated about 20.3 cm. (8 inches)—if patient has pain at rest; wear bedsocks to keep feet warm if necessary.
6. Walking is the best form of exercise; otherwise, active or passive exercise of the extremities is recommended.

POSITION 1
Place legs on a pillow-cushioned chair
for one minute to drain blood.

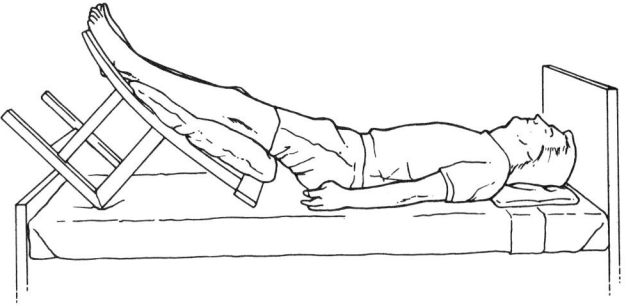

POSITION 2
Hold each of these
stretching positions
for 30 seconds
to enhance blood return.

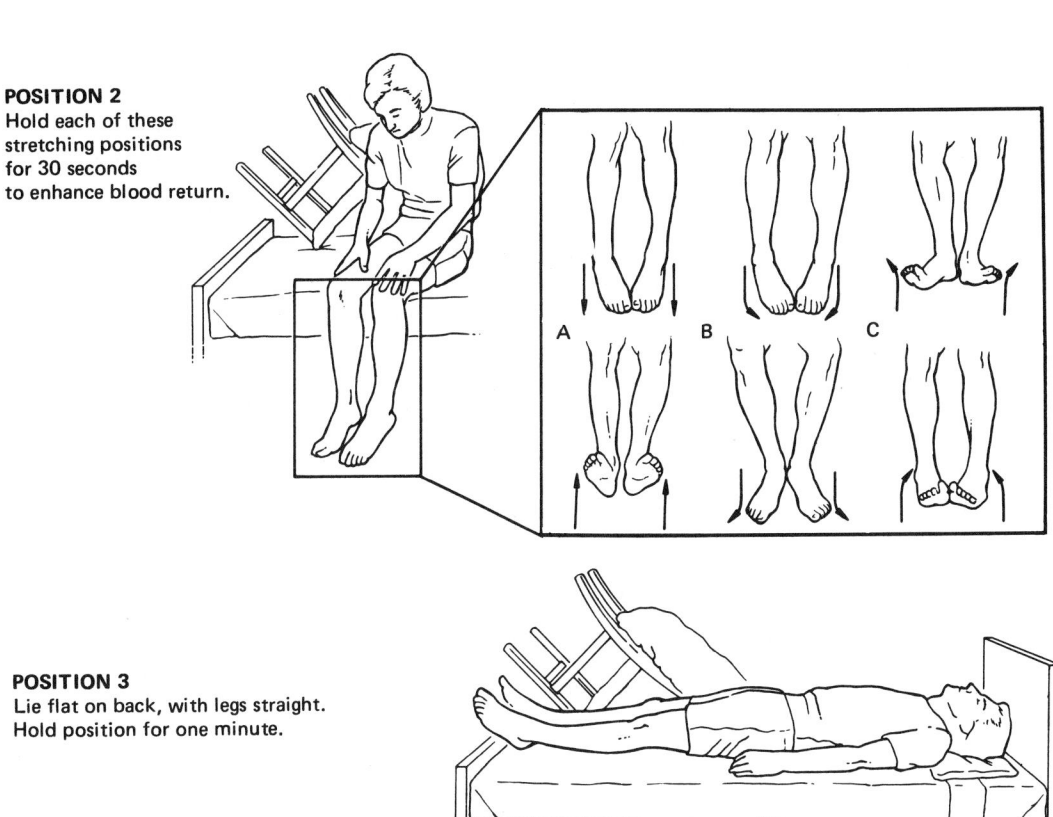

POSITION 3
Lie flat on back, with legs straight.
Hold position for one minute.

Figure 16-5. *Buerger-Allen exercises. Do exercise series 6 times, 4 times a day. (Forshee T and Minckley B: Lumbar sympathectomy. RN Vol. 39[2])*

7. Take analgesic and tranquilizing medications as required to keep comfortable.
8. Take prescribed vasodilating medications even though they may not appear to help; at times, they maintain the status quo and keep the problem from worsening.
9. Take prescribed antilipidic drugs to retard progress of concomitant atherosclerotic disease by reducing serum lipids.
10. Wear properly fitting and repaired hose and shoes.
11. Impress the patient with the *dangers of smoking.*
12. Promote an atmosphere that minimizes emotional tension; restrict those visitors who appear to upset the patient.
13. Advise the patient against wearing constrictive garments, such as panty girdles, garters, belts, jeans, and tight panty hose.

C. Attaining or Maintaining Tissue Integrity by Reducing Metabolic Demands on the Body.

1. Take precautions to prevent injury and infection, particularly of the extremities.
2. Practice daily hygienic cleanliness and care of the feet: trim nails properly, avoid strong medications, use lamb's wool for pressure areas, wear shoes and hosiery that fit correctly.
3. Avoid exposure to cold or excessive heat.
4. Exercise within recognized limits; set up a reasonable rest plan.

5. Remain in bed if there is evidence of necrosis, ulceration, or gangrene; consult physician.

Patient Education

Teach the patient the following:

A. Signs and Symptoms of Circulatory Disturbances Affecting Peripheral Tissues

1. Pain in the extremity—(Note whether this occurs at rest, with limited activity, or with more pronounced exercise.)
2. Color changes of the skin or nails—pallor, pinkness, rubor, cyanosis
3. Impaired or peculiar growth of nails
4. Shiny, taut skin
5. Discrepancy in size of one extremity when compared with contralateral (opposite) extremity
6. Enlarged veins or abnormal pulsations of veins
7. Temperature variations—abnormally cold or abnormally warm
8. Ulcerations, necrosis, or gangrene

B. Foot Care

1. Keep the feet clean to prevent irritation and infection.
   a. Wash daily with a bland soap and warm water.
   b. Dry thoroughly, paying particular attention to areas between the toes; pat rather than rub dry.
   c. Apply lanolin or petrolatum to prevent drying and cracking of skin.
   d. Wear clean hose daily: woolen socks for winter, cotton for summer.
2. Avoid injury, excessive pressure, or other irritants to the feet.
   a. Shoes
      (1) Wear properly fitting shoes with a comfortable heel.
      (2) Check inside of shoe; avoid wearing shoes with protruding seams, torn lining, piercing nails, or faulty lumps.
      (3) Wear shoes when out of bed; avoid going barefoot.
      (4) Break in new shoes gradually; alternate with an older pair.
      (5) Leather is preferred to rubber or synthetics because the latter interfere with proper circulation of air.
      (6) Allow wet or damp shoes to dry slowly on shoe trees to prevent misshaping.
   b. Hose
      (1) Wear proper length and size—if too short, toes are compressed; if too long, wrinkles form and exert pressure on skin.
      (2) Avoid seams, holes, or lumpy darned areas.
      (3) Use bedsocks rather than hot water bottle or heating pad if feet are cold in bed.
      (4) Use woolen or cotton hose; they absorb moisture; nylon is not as absorbent.
      (5) Avoid constricting garments—foundation garments, garters, and even support hose unless they are specifically prescribed.
   c. Pedicure
      (1) Trim toenails straight across after soaking the feet in warm water.
      (2) Place wisps of cotton under corner of great toenail if there is a tendency toward ingrown toenails.
      (3) Have a podiatrist cut corns and calluses; do not use corn pads or strong medications.
   d. Heat and cold
      (1) Keep feet warm; avoid exposure to cold for long periods of time.
      (2) Use heating devices only on advice of physician; excessive heat can be as damaging as insufficient warmth.
      (3) Rely on warm socks, fleece-lined boots or mitts, lightweight blankets, etc. rather than on heating extremities near a fire, oven, or radiator.
   e. General measures
      (1) Avoid areas where injury to feet is likely (e.g., crowded subways, construction areas, sports shows, etc.).
      (2) Prevent sunburn in the summer and avoid wading in very cold water.
3. Prevent pressure on feet; rest and exercise in moderation.
   a. Place a pillow under covers at end of bed to provide a footrest and prevent weight of top bedding from exerting pressure on toes.
   b. Avoid remaining in one position for long periods of time.
   c. Do not cross legs when sitting because of pressure on nerves and blood vessels.
   d. Elevate feet on a chair or footstool with proper support of leg; do this about 15 minutes every 2 hours.
4. If damage or injury occurs to any part of foot or leg, report to physician.
   a. Redness, swelling, irritation, blistering
   b. Itching, burning—athlete's foot
   c. Bruises, cuts, unusual appearance of skin

Evaluation

1. Demonstrates increased arterial blood supply to extremities—palpable pulses, warm extremities, reduced pain, normal color.
2. Is free of pain; uses measures to increase arterial supply to extremities.
3. Attains/maintains tissue integrity; avoids trauma and irritation to skin.
4. Performs self-management activities.

Conditions of the Veins

Phlebitis, Thrombophlebitis, Phlebothrombosis

Note: While the terms do not necessarily represent identical pathologies, for clinical purposes they are used interchangeably when discussing the same process.

Phlebothrombosis is the formation of a thrombus or thrombi in a vein; in general, the clotting is related to (1) stasis, (2) abnormality of the walls of the vein(s), and (3) abnormality of clotting mechanism. Deep veins of the lower extremities are most commonly involved.

Deep vein thrombosis (DVT) is the thrombosis of deep rather than superficial veins. Two serious complications are pulmonary embolism (p. 187) and postphlebitic syndrome (p. 398).

Phlebitis is an inflammation of the walls of a vein.

Thrombophlebitis is a condition in which a clot forms in a vein secondary to phlebitis or because of partial obstruction of the vein.

Etiology

A. General Points

1. Three antecedent factors are believed to play a significant role in the development of venous thromboses: (1) stasis of blood, (2) injury to the vessel wall, and (3) altered blood coagulation.
2. Usually two of the three factors occur before thrombosis develops.

B. Thrombosis-related Situations

1. Venous stasis—following operations, childbirth, or bedrest for any prolonged illness
2. Prolonged sitting or as a complication of varicose veins
3. Injury (bruise) to a vein; may result from direct trauma to veins from IV injections, indwelling catheters
4. Extension of an infection of tissues surrounding the vessel
5. Continuous pressure of a tumor, aneurysm, heavy pregnancy
6. Unusual activity in a person who has been sedentary
7. Hypercoagulability associated with malignant disease, blood dyscrasias

C. High-risk Factors

1. Malignancy
2. Previous venous insufficiency
3. Contraceptives (oral)
4. Conditions causing prolonged bedrest—myocardial infarction, congestive heart failure, sepsis, traction
5. Leg trauma—fractures, casts, joint replacements
6. General surgery—over 40 years of age
7. Obesity

Clinical Manifestations

1. For phlebothrombosis, there are no clinical signs, since there is no inflammation.
2. Slight swelling around ankle; obvious prominence of leg veins in affected leg.
3. Calf pain may be aggravated when foot is dorsiflexed with the knee flexed (Homan's sign) (Fig. 16-6A). Unfortunately, this is no clear sign of early or positive thrombosis. In some patients with obvious thrombophlebitis, this sign is not present, and in other kinds of involvement (irritation of sciatic nerve roots and myositis), the sign may be positive.
4. Muscle ache—may be falsely assumed to result from wearing flat bedroom slippers postoperatively.

Diagnostic Evaluation

A. Phlebography (Venography)—an x-ray visualization of the vascular tree after the injection of a contrast medium (renografin). See page 385 for a discussion of phlebography.

B. Plethysmography (Pulse Volume Recording [PVR])—a noninvasive measurement of changes in calf volume corresponding to changes in blood volume brought about by temporary venous occlusion with a high pneumatic cuff. See page 385 for a discussion.

C. ^{125}I Fibrinogen Uptake Test—an invasive radioactive test in which labeled fibrinogen, given before a thrombus forms, will be concentrated in the area of clot formation. Formation of clots may be detected with serial scanning and by comparing one leg with the other.

1. Advantages
   a. The most sensitive method to screen for acute calf vein thrombosis
   b. Preferred in detecting recurrent *active* venous thrombosis
2. Disadvantages
   a. Not sensitive to thrombi high in the iliofemoral region or to inactive thrombosis
   b. Costly and time-consuming

Management

Goals:

To prevent propagation of the thrombus and the risk of pulmonary embolus

To prevent recurrent thromboemboli

1. Anticoagulant and thrombolytic therapies (see pp. 387 and 389).

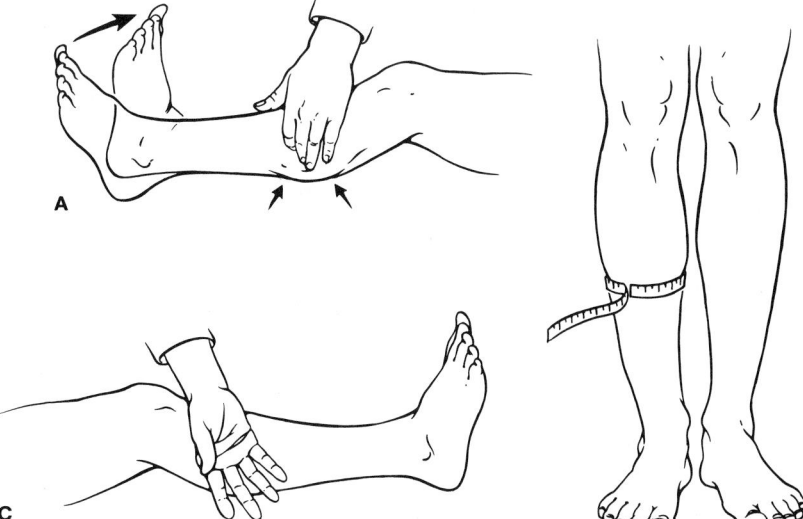

Figure 16-6. *Nursing assessment for deep-vein thrombosis. (A) Pain and tenderness in the calf of the affected extremity, especially on dorsiflexion of the foot (Homan's sign). (B) The affected extremity may have a larger circumference than the unaffected extremity caused by edema. (C) The affected extremity will be warm to touch compared to the unaffected extremity.*

2. Surgery may be considered in the following instances if:
   a. The patient cannot be given anticoagulants or thrombolytics.
   b. The danger of pulmonary embolism is extreme.
   c. Venous drainage is so severely compromised that permanent extremity damage will probably result.

Nursing Interventions

1. Inspect the lower extremities by removing top bedding from foot end up to the patient's groin (remove any temperature-controlling devices such as heavy wool socks, ice bag, at least 10 minutes before clinical inspection).
2. Note symmetry or asymmetry
   a. Measure and record leg circumferences daily (see Guidelines: Obtaining Leg Measurements to Detect Early Swelling)—mark on skin with felt-tip pen where the measuring tape is used so that the same area is measured each time.
3. Observe for evidence of venous distention or edema, puffiness, stretched skin, hardness to touch.
4. Hand-test extremities for temperature variations.
   a. Hands are placed simultaneously on each leg—first compare ankles, then move to the calf and up to the knee.
5. Examine for signs of obstruction due to occluding thrombus—swelling, particularly in loose connective tissue of popliteal space, ankle, or suprapubic area.
6. Avoid massaging or rubbing calf because of the danger of breaking up the clot, which can then circulate as an embolus.
7. Consult physician concerning proper position of the extremity, since there may be differences of opinion.
   a. Some recommend elevation—reduces venous congestion and edema.
   b. Others do not recommend elevation—because of the possibility of releasing emboli.
8. If prescribed, apply heat in the form of hot, wet dressings or a heat cradle to promote circulation and comfort.
9. Manage the patient's anticoagulant therapy (see p. 387).

> **NURSING ALERT:** Anticoagulation may not be prescribed pre-operatively because of fear of increasing possibility of hemorrhage during operation. Minidoses of heparin may be prescribed.

10. Encourage early ambulation of surgical patients—encourage leg exercises for the bedridden patient, to prevent venous stasis.
11. Suggest deep-breathing exercises that produce increased negative pressure in the thorax, which in turn assists in emptying large veins.
12. Recommend properly applied pressure gradient stockings to increase deep venous blood circulation. (Remove twice daily and check for skin changes or calf tenderness.)
13. Use electrical stimulation of calf and pneumatic compression of leg if prescribed.
14. Practice preventive measures for bedridden patients who are prone to develop thrombosis:
    a. Have the patient lie in bed in the slightly reversed Trendelenburg position because it is better for the veins to be full of blood than empty.
    b. Place a footboard across the foot of the bed.
    c. Instruct the patient to press the balls of the feet against the footboard, just as if he were rising up on his toes.
    d. Then have the patient relax the foot.
    e. Request that the patient do this many times a day.

Patient Education

Teach the patient as follows:
1. Prevent venous stasis by proper positioning in bed.
   a. Support full length of legs when they are to be elevated (Fig. 16-7).
   b. Prevent bony prominence of one leg from pressing on soft tissue of other leg (in side-lying position, place a soft pillow between legs).
   c. Avoid hyperflexion at knee as in jackknife position (head up, knees up, pelvis and legs down); this promotes stasis in pelvis and extremities.
2. Initiate active exercises, *unless contraindicated,* in which case use passive exercises.

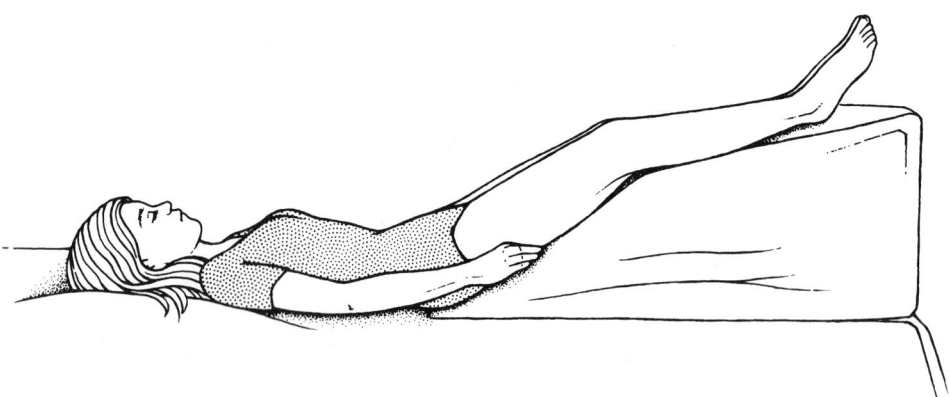

Figure 16-7. *This leg elevator is of foam construction with a removable cotton cover that may be machine washed. It is clamped to the lower end of the mattress. This position is anatomically correct and provides adequate support to all parts of the leg. Edema and stasis of the lower extremities can be controlled. (Courtesy of Jobst)*

a. If the patient is on bedrest:
   (1) Simulate walking if lying on back—5 minutes every 2 hours.
   (2) Simulate bicycle pedaling if lying on side—5 minutes every 2 hours.
b. If contraindicated, resort to passive exercises—5 minutes every 2 hours.
c. If permissible, have the patient sit up and move to side of bed in sitting position. Provide a foot support (stool or chair)—dangling of feet is not desirable, since pressure may be exerted against popliteal vessels and may cause obstruction to blood flow.
d. If the patient is permitted out of bed, encourage him to walk 10 minutes each hour; otherwise, carry out passive exercises.
e. Discourage crossing of legs because compression of vessels can restrict blood flow.

3. Promote circulation and prevent stasis by applying elastic hose.
   Apply elastic hose or elastic bandage from the toes up the leg; support must be consistent along entire leg.

> **NURSING ALERT:** Elastic hose have no role in the management of the acute phase of deep venous thrombosis, but are of value once ambulation has begun. Their use will minimize or delay the development of the postphlebitic syndrome.

4. Avoid straining or any maneuver that increases venous pressure in the leg. Eliminate the necessity to strain at stool by providing increased fiber in the diet and administer stool softeners if necessary.

Guidelines — Obtaining Leg Measurements to Detect Early Swelling

Purpose   To obtain leg measurements for serial data compilation that may detect swelling and thus indicate onset of thrombophlebitis.

Equipment   Flexible tape measure in centimeters/inches
Black felt-tip pen

Procedure   Preparatory Phase
1. Instruct patient to lie in dorsal recumbent position

Nursing Action	Rationale/Amplification

Performance Phase

Nursing Action	Rationale/Amplification
1. On admission of the patient, measure the circumference of the ankle, calf, and thigh.	1. This will provide baseline data.
2. Obtain measurements at the widest part of the ankle, calf, and thigh.	2. To provide a consistent anatomical place of measurement; some clinics have a predetermined starting point, such as 15 or 20 cm. from the knee cap.
3. Mark the leg with a black felt-tip pen.	3. To promote accuracy of measurements.
4. Thereafter, when measuring, place the measuring tape on the marked line.	
5. Repeat measurements taken on admission the next morning before any patient activity.	5. Otherwise, later measurements may give a false reading because of gravitational edema.
6. Thereafter, obtain measurements weekly unless there is evidence of swelling, in which case it is done daily.	6. Weekly—to detect swelling. Daily—to monitor swelling and its response to treatment.

7. Record measurements:

Leg Measurements
Date:
Time:

Right			Left		
Ankle_____		cm./inches	Ankle_____		cm./inches
Calf_____		cm./inches	Calf_____		cm./inches
Thigh_____		cm./inches	Thigh_____		cm./inches

8. Compare measurements:
   a. Check one leg with the other.

   b. Check each leg with baseline data.

Significant Findings:

1.5 cm. (males) difference between legs or compared with baseline.

1.2 cm. (females) difference between legs or compared with baseline.

Chronic Venous Insufficiency
(Postphlebitic Syndrome)

Postphlebitic syndrome is a form of chronic venous stasis; it may be a residual effect of phlebitis. It results from chronic occlusion of the veins or destruction of the valves.

Etiology

1. Smaller vessels have dilated because main channel for returning blood from the leg to the heart was blocked by a thrombus.
2. Valves of diseased veins can no longer prevent backflow, thereby → chronic venous stasis → swelling and edema → superficial varicose veins.
3. Lower leg becomes discolored because of venous stasis and pigmentation ulceration (postphlebitis).

Clinical Manifestations

1. Pressure in veins at ankle is much greater than normal when leg is dependent—leads to transudation of fluid from intravascular to interstitial space.
2. Stasis, intractable induration, chronic edema, discoloration, pain, venous congestion, ulceration, recurrent thrombosis → cellulitis.
3. The medial malleolus is the most common site.

Diagnostic Evaluation

1. Noninvasive screening—Doppler, plethysmography.

Management

1. Best treatment is prevention of phlebitis and constant use of compression if phlebitis has occurred.
2. After this syndrome has developed, only palliative and symptomatic treatment is possible because the damage is irreparable.

Nursing Interventions and Patient Education

Instruct the patient as follows:
1. Wear elastic stockings to prevent edema.
2. Avoid sitting or standing for long periods of time.
3. Elevate legs on a chair for 5 minutes every 2 hours.
4. Elevate legs above level of head by lying down (2–3 times daily).
5. Raise foot of bed 15–20 cm. (6–8 inches) at night to allow venous drainage by gravity.
6. Apply bland, oily lotions to prevent scaling and dryness of skin.
7. Avoid constricting bandages.
8. Prevent injury, bruising, scratching, or other trauma to skin of leg and foot.

Varicose Veins

Primary varicose veins—bilateral dilatation and elongation of saphenous veins; deeper veins are normal. As the condition progresses, because of hydrostatic pressure and vein weakness, the vein walls become distended, with asymmetrical dilatation, and some of the valves become incompetent. The process is irreversible.

Etiology

1. Dilatation of the vein prevents the valve cusps from meeting; this results in increased back-up pressure, which is passed into the next lower segment of the vein. The combination of vein dilatation and valve incompetence produces the varicosity (Fig. 16-8).
2. Varicosities may occur elsewhere in the body (esophageal and hemorrhoidal veins) when flow or pressure is abnormally high.
3. Predisposing factors
    a. Hereditary weakness of vein wall or valves
    b. Long-standing distention of veins brought about by pregnancy, obesity, or prolonged standing
    c. Old age—loss of tissue elasticity

Clinical Manifestations

1. Disfigurement due to large, discolored, tortuous leg veins
2. Easy leg fatigue, cramps in leg, heavy feeling, increased pain during menstruation, nocturnal muscle cramps

Complications

1. Leg edema, pain from superficial thrombosis
2. Hemorrhage due to the weakening of the vein wall and pressure upon it
3. Skin infection and breakdown, producing ulcers (rare in primary varices)

Diagnostic Evaluation

1. *Walking tourniquet test*—to demonstrate presence or absence of valvular incompetence of communicating veins.
    a. A penrose drain is snugly fastened around the lower extremity just above the highest noted varicosities.
    b. The patient is directed to walk briskly for 2 minutes.
    c. Failure of varicosities to empty suggests valvular incompetence of communicating veins distal to Penrose drain.

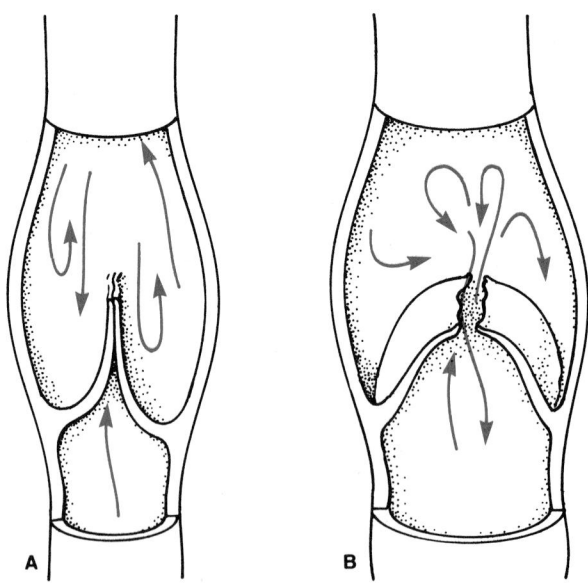

Figure 16-8. *Valve incompetence develops as dilatation of a vessel prevents effective approximation of valve cusps. (A) Closed venous valve. (B) Incompetent venous valve.*

2. *Photoplethysmography*—a noninvasive technique to observe venous flow hemodynamics by noting changes in the blood content of the skin. It can be done rapidly, is inexpensive and highly reproducible.
3. *Doppler ultrasound*—can detect accurately and rapidly the presence or absence of venous reflux in deep or superficial vessels.
4. *Venous outflow and reflux plethysmography*—able to detect deep venous occlusion.
5. *Ascending and descending venography*—an invasive technique that can also demonstrate venous occlusion and patterns of collateral flow.
    This test is expensive; it may not be required if a careful history, physical examination, and laboratory testing are done.

Management

A. Management of Varicose Veins

1. Conservative therapies such as encouraging weight loss if appropriate and avoiding activities that cause venous stasis by obstructing venous flow.
2. Surgery may be considered under the following conditions: progressively advancing varicosities, stasis ulceration, and cosmetic needs.

B. Surgical Procedures—a single method or combination of methods is tailored to meet the needs of the individual:

1. *Sclerosing injection*—not used as frequently today; may be combined with ligation or limited to treatment of isolated varicosities. The affected vessel may be sclerosed by injecting sodium tetradecyl sulfate or similar sclerosing agent. Compression bandage is then applied without interruption for 6 weeks; inflamed endothelial surfaces adhere by direct contact.
2. *Multiple vein ligation.*
3. *Ligation and stripping* of the greater and/or lesser saphenous systems. This is the most effective procedure.
4. *Laser therapy.*

Nursing Interventions

A. Conservative Management

The patient is instructed to:
1. Avoid activities that cause venous stasis by obstructing venous flow.
    a. Wearing tight garters, tight girdle
    b. Sitting or standing for prolonged periods of time
    c. Crossing the legs at knees for prolonged periods while sitting (reduces circulation by 15%)
2. Control excessive weight gain.
3. Wear firm elastic support as prescribed, from toe to thigh when in upright position.
    a. Put elastic stockings on in bed before getting up.
    b. Waist-high elastic support hose are available and may be useful.
4. Elevate foot of bed 15–20 cm. (6–8 inches) for night sleeping.
5. Avoid injuring legs.

B. Postoperative Nursing Care and Patient Support

1. At first, the legs are encased in pressure bandages from the toes to the groin; this is followed by knee-level elastic stockings for 3–4 weeks after surgery.
2. Elevate the legs about 30 degrees and provide adequate support of the entire leg.
3. Observe the patient for complaints of pain in specific areas of the foot or ankle; if the elastic bandage is too tight, loosen the bandage—later, have it reapplied.

4. Observe circulation to detect constriction or hemorrhage.
5. Activate the individualized therapeutic plan for the following:
    a. Permit ambulation according to the preoperative condition of the skin and subcutaneous tissues; if skin is healthy, bathroom privileges are usually permitted the day after surgery.
    b. Discourage dangling of the legs because it causes stasis of blood in the lower leg.
    c. Encourage the patient to walk with a normal gait; offer support if necessary; this activity should be progressive, depending on tolerance.
    d. If there are significant trophic changes in the leg due to long-term varicosities (past history), postoperative care requires more bedrest and slow ambulation; in this event, leg and foot exercises in bed are helpful.
    e. Note that complaints of patchy numbness can be expected but should disappear in less than a year.
    f. Recognize that varicosities may recur; therefore, conservative measures, learned preoperatively, should be continued.
    g. Follow-up visits as prescribed are urged.

Stasis Ulcers

Stasis ulcer is an excavation of the skin surface produced by sloughing of inflammatory necrotic tissue, usually caused by vascular insufficiency in the lower extremity.

Clinical Manifestations

Severity of symptoms depends upon the extent and duration of vascular insufficiency.
1. Open sore that is inflamed.
2. Drainage may be present or the area may be covered by a dark crust.
3. Patient may complain of swelling, heaviness, aching, and fatigue.
4. Postphlebitic syndrome and stasis are responsible for most leg ulcers.

GERONTOLOGIC ALERT: The occurrence of stasis ulcers is increasing, especially in the aging population.

Diagnostic Evaluation

1. Noninvasive screening—Doppler and plethysmography.

Management

Goals:
Healing the ulcer by removing devitalized tissue
Stimulating formation of granulation tissue and
Preventing recurrence.

A. Removal of Devitalized Tissue

1. Necrotic materials is flushed out with cleansing agents to dissolve slough. These agents are chemically or naturally derived enzymes that are proteolytic or fibrinolytic.
2. Surgical excision of slough.
    If necrotic tissue is loose, this procedure can be done without anesthesia; if the tissue is adherent, anesthesia will be required.

B. Stimulating Formation of Granulation Tissue

1. Dressing of choice—characteristics
   a. Nonadherent so removal is painless and does not damage newly forming tissue
   b. Highly absorbent
   c. Safe, nontoxic
   d. Sterile, accessible, and inexpensive
2. Application of compression over dressings generally through the use of bandages or elastic stockings. In some circumstances, inflatable pneumatic leggings may be appropriate.
3. Unna's boot, an effective treatment of choice, is an example of a combined dressing and compression bandage.
4. Bedrest with leg elevation
5. Systemic drug therapy.
   a. No single agent affects ulcer healing.
   b. Diuretic therapy through edema reduction may improve capillary circulation.
6. Application of skin grafts
   a. Skin grafts are used for ulcers that will not heal.
   b. Not recommended for first-line treatment.

C. Prevention of Recurrence.

1. Ligation of the sapheno–femoral or sapheno–popliteal vessels with stripping
2. Ligation of the lower leg communicating veins
3. Deep vein bypass or reconstruction
4. Injection compression sclerotherapy

Nursing Interventions

1. Elevate the leg and maintain bedrest.
2. Initiate proper dressing routine.
   a. Handle leg very gently.
   b. Be careful not to disturb healing tissue.
   c. When compression bandaging is used, be certain that pressure is maintained at the appropriate levels of the leg, that is, maximum compression at the ankle; minimum compression at the knee or thigh.

Patient Education

1. Stress the importance of following explicitly the recommendations of the physician–nurse team.
2. Explain the hazards of trying other remedies on his own at home.
3. Indicate that the treatment may be long but that patience is an important aspect.
4. Maintain healthy tissue when the ulcer is healed by continuing with the safeguards practiced before, because breakdown of healthy tissue, unfortunately, frequently occurs.
5. Encourage participation in physiotherapy and a regular exercise program.
6. Encourage weight control and proper dietary intake to insure adequate amounts of protein and vitamins.

Conditions of the Arteries
Arterial Embolism

Underlying Features

1. Arterial emboli usually (about 85%) originate from thrombi in the heart chambers.
2. Arteriosclerosis may cause roughening or ulceration of atheromatous plaques, which can lead to emboli.

Clinical Manifestations

May vary from:
1. The patient's being totally unaware of the event, to
2. Acute pain—severe to
3. Loss of function—motor and sensory
   a. Paralysis of part ⎫ Due to embolic block of
   b. Anesthesia of part ⎬ artery
   c. Pallor and coldness ⎭ Due to associated vasomotor reflex

Management and Nursing Interventions

Note: This is an emergency and is life-threatening; it requires immediate operative intervention if the embolus has major effect.

1. Heparin is administered intravenously to reduce tendency of emboli to form or expand—useful in smaller arteries.
2. Thrombolytic therapy (see p. 389).
3. Protect the extremity by keeping it at or below the horizontal plane; protect leg from hard surfaces and tight or heavy overlying bed linens.
4. Administer analgesics as prescribed for relief of pain.
5. Prepare the patient for surgery; surgical intervention (embolectomy) is essential when an embolus blocks a large artery, such as the iliac (Fig. 16-9).

Arteriosclerosis and Atherosclerosis

Arteriosclerosis is an arterial disease manifested by a loss of elasticity and a hardening of the vessel wall.

Atherosclerosis is the most common type of arteriosclerosis, manifested by the formation of atheromas (patchy lipoidal degeneration of the intima).

Underlying Features

1. Predisposition to arteriosclerosis is thought by many authorities to be inheritable (genetics).
2. Other etiologic factors include metabolic disturbances, arterial hypertension, platelet capability of initiating formation of atherosclerotic lesions.
3. Arteriosclerosis is the chief cause of death in the US.
4. One of the major clinical manifestations of arteriosclerosis is coronary heart disease (CHD).
5. Studies indicate that arteriosclerotic heart disease is partially preventable if attention is paid to "risk" factors.

Risk Factors

1. Heredity
2. Increasing age
3. Male sex
4. Cigarette smoking
5. Hypertension
6. Elevated blood cholesterol levels
7. Diabetes mellitus
8. Obesity
9. Physical inactivity
10. Stress

Clinical Manifestations

1. Arteriosclerosis is a generalized vascular disease; however, it varies from patient to patient in that it may affect one area more than another.
2. Often, it limits itself to a segment of the vascular tree.

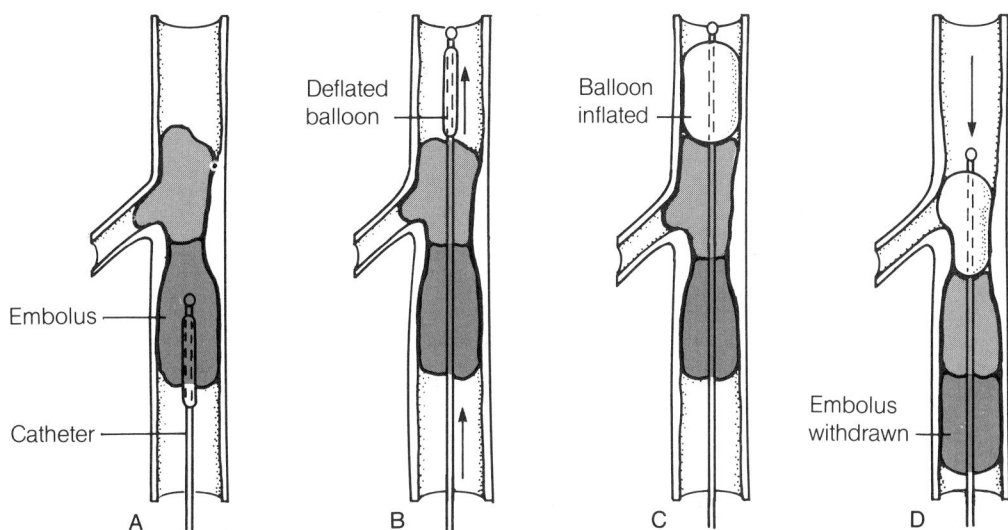

Figure 16-9. *Extracting an embolus from a vessel can be done with the use of a Fogarty embolectomy catheter. The catheter with a soft deflated balloon near the tip is threaded through the artery via an arteriotomy. (A and B) It is passed through the embolus and its thrombus; (C) it is then inflated. (D) A steady pull downward withdraws the embolus along with the catheter.*

3. Five areas that are the most dangerous and cause disturbing symptoms are:
   a. Brain—cerebroarteriosclerosis
   b. Heart—coronary artery disease
   c. Gastrointestinal tract—aneurysms eroding into the bowel
   d. Kidneys—renal artery stenosis
   e. Extremities—propensity for emboli
4. Prognosis depends on extent of pathology and area of involvement.

Management

1. Since arteriosclerosis and atherosclerosis affect many different parts of the body, treatment is described where the major condition occurs. For example: angina pectoris and myocardial infarction are brought about by atherosclerosis of coronary arteries; treatment is discussed under the disease entity.
2. Operative reconstruction of involved vessels.

Patient Education

Attention is directed to reducing risk factors by avoiding tension, reducing excess weight, giving up cigarette smoking, controlling diabetes, and adjusting diet to reduce cholesterol intake.

Percutaneous Transluminal Angioplasty

Percutaneous transluminal angioplasty (PTA) is a technique designed to relieve arterial stenosis when lesions are accessible, as in superficial femoral and iliac arteries, through the use of special inflatable balloon catheters).

A. Procedure

1. A balloon catheter is passed, usually via the common femoral artery, after a guidewire and angiographic catheter have been inserted under fluoroscopy. The balloon is then properly positioned.
2. The balloon is dilated with contrast material and inflated to exert pressure against the stenosed lesions of the arterial wall, thereby dilating the artery.

3. The catheter is then removed; heparin is injected through the angiographic catheter to prevent clots. Pressure is maintained at catheter entry site for 10–20 minutes.
4. The patient is instructed to lie flat for several hours.
5. After 8 hours, all restrictions are removed; aspirin and dipyridamole (Persantine) may be prescribed to reduce the possibility of recurrence by its vasodilating action.

B. Nursing Management Following PTA

1. Maintain adequate circulation through the site of the arterial repair.
2. Check and record status of pulses proximal and distal to the site of manipulation.
3. Check color and temperature of the extremity.
4. Monitor for signs of adequate circulating blood volume (e.g., urinary output, mental status, pulse rate and volume).

Occlusive Arterial Disease

Occlusive arterial disease is a form of arteriosclerosis in which the vascular system of the leg becomes blocked. Chronic occlusive arterial disease occurs much more frequently than does acute (which is the sudden and complete blocking of a vessel by a thrombus or embolus) (see Table 16-1).

Clinical Manifestations

Symptoms appear gradually:
1. Intermittent claudication
2. Coldness of extremity
3. Color change—pallor
4. Decrease in size of leg
5. Tingling, numbness of toes
6. Later—pain, even when leg is at rest; occurs at night, requiring patient to get out of bed to walk to relieve pain

Table 16-1. *Assessment of Acute Arterial Occlusion vs. Deep Vein Thrombosis*

Factor	Acute Arterial Occlusion	Deep Vein Thrombosis
Onset	Sudden	Gradual
Color	Pale; later—mottled, cyanotic	Slightly cyanotic; rubescent
Skin temperature	Cold	Warm
Leg size—diameter	May be reduced from normal	Enlarged
Superficial veins	Collapsed	Appear enlarged and prominent
Arterial pulsation	Pulse deficit noted	Normal and palpable (except in marked edema)
Effect of elevating leg	Condition worsens	Condition improves

7. Cramplike excruciating pain in calf muscles
8. Ulcers of toes and feet develop

Diagnostic Evaluation

1. Vascular physical examination, including brachial and ankle systolic pressures, before and after exercise
2. Doppler ultrasound probe
3. Segmental plethysmography
4. Angiography

Management

Goals
To preserve the extremity
To relieve intermittent claudication

1. Where conservative measures clearly are not enough, constructive arterial surgery (endarterectomy, arterial bypass grafting, or a combination) may be required.
2. Percutaneous transluminal angioplasty (PTA) may be used alone or with reconstructive surgery for dilatation of localized noncalcified segments of narrowed arteries (see Procedure, p. 401).
3. Microvascular surgery may be required for small-artery occlusive disease.
4. Following any surgery, a conservative program to manage intermittent claudication may be initiated (walking, weight reduction, no smoking, control of other conditions such as hypertension, diabetes mellitus).

Vasospastic Disorder—Raynaud's Phenomenon

Raynaud's phenomenon is a general term to describe a condition in which there is an increased or unusual sensitivity to cold or emotional factors, occurring primarily in the hands.

Underlying Features

1. Etiology unknown; there appears to be a hereditary predisposition.
2. Vasoconstriction appears to be mediated through release of catecholamines at the neuroarteriole junction.
3. An underlying problem such as a collagen vascular disease may exist as it is seen frequently in systemic lupus erythematosus.

4. The condition occurs most commonly in females between the ages 16 and 40 years.
5. It occurs more frequently in cold climates and during winter months.

Clinical Manifestations

1. Intermittent arteriolar vasoconstriction resulting in coldness, pain, pallor.
2. Involvement of the fingers appears to be asymmetric; thumbs are less often involved.
3. Characteristic color changes: blue–white–red
   a. Blue—cyanotic, relatively stagnant blood flow
   b. White—blanching, dead-white appearance if spasm is severe
   c. Red—a reactive hyperemia upon rewarming
4. Occasionally, there is ulceration of the finger tips.

Diagnostic Evaluation

The Allen test may provide clues to circulatory problems (Fig. 16-10).

Management: Drug Therapy

Goals:
To prevent pain and the deteriorating effects of Raynaud's phenomenon
To produce vasodilatation

Medication	Adverse Effects
1. Phenoxybenzamine hydrochloride (Dibenzyline)	Headache, tachycardia, nasal congestion, orthostatic hypotension
2. Cyclandelate (Cyclospasmol)	Headache, nausea, heavier than usual perspiration, vertigo, flushing, tingling
3. Tolazoline hydrochloride	Gastrointestinal upset, orthostatic hypotension, chilliness, tachycardia, palpitations
4. Nifedipine (Procardia)	None apparent

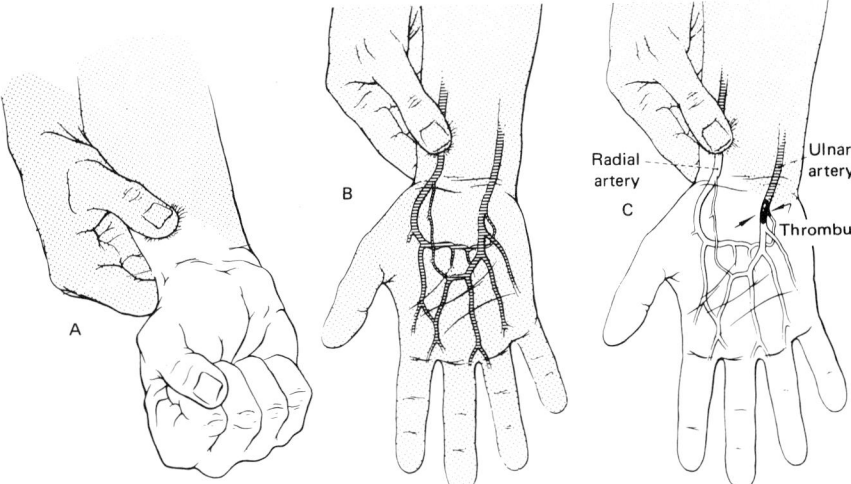

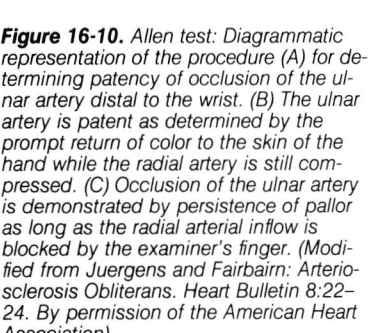

Figure 16-10. *Allen test: Diagrammatic representation of the procedure (A) for determining patency of occlusion of the ulnar artery distal to the wrist. (B) The ulnar artery is patent as determined by the prompt return of color to the skin of the hand while the radial artery is still compressed. (C) Occlusion of the ulnar artery is demonstrated by persistence of pallor as long as the radial arterial inflow is blocked by the examiner's finger. (Modified from Juergens and Fairbairn: Arteriosclerosis Obliterans. Heart Bulletin 8:22–24. By permission of the American Heart Association)*

Patient Education

1. Avoid whatever provokes vasoconstriction of vessels of hands.
2. Prevent injury to hands, which can aggravate vasoconstriction and lead to ulceration.
3. Minimize exposure to cold, since this precipitates a reaction.
4. Wear warm clothing—boots, gloves, hooded jackets, when going out in cold weather.
   a. Turn heat on in automobile during travel.
   b. Shop in heated stores; avoid unheated buildings.
5. Avoid placing hands in cold water, the freezer, or the refrigerator unless protective gloves are worn.
6. Use extra precautions to avoid injuries to fingers and hands from needle pricks, knife cuts.

Diseases of the Aorta*

Aortic Aneurysm

Aneurysm is a distention of an artery brought about by a weakening/destruction of the media of the arterial wall. It tends to enlarge, thereby producing serious complications by compressing surrounding structures or rupturing, causing a fatal hemorrhage.

Types of Aneurysms

Morphologically, they may be classified as follows:
1. Saccular—distention of a vessel projecting from one side
2. Fusiform—distention of the whole artery (i.e., entire circumference is involved)
3. Dissecting—hemorrhagic or intramural hematoma, separating the medial layers of the aortic wall

Etiology

1. Local infection, pyogenic or fungal (mycotic aneurysm)

---

* For aortic stenosis and aortic insufficiency, see page 346.

2. Congenital weakness of vessels
3. Arteriosclerosis
4. Syphilis
5. Trauma

GERONTOLOGIC ALERT: Because of vascular changes that occur as a natural process of aging, all patients over 65 years of age are assessed for the potential for aneurysms (Fig. 16-11)

Aneurysm of the Thoracoabdominal Aorta

(Lower descending thoracic aorta and upper abdominal aorta)

A. Clinical Manifestations

1. At first no symptoms; later symptoms may come from congestive heart failure or a pulsating tumor mass in the chest.
2. Pain and pressure symptoms
   a. Constant, boring pain because of pressure, or
   b. Intermittent and neuralgic pain because of infringement on nerves
3. Dyspnea, causing pressure against trachea
4. Cough, often paroxysmal and brassy in sound
5. Hoarseness, voice weakness, or complete aphonia, resulting from pressure against recurrent laryngeal nerve
6. Dysphagia due to impingement on esophagus
7. Edema of chest wall—infrequent
8. Dilated superficial veins on chest
9. Cyanosis because of vein compression of chest vessels
10. Ipsilateral dilatation of pupils due to pressure against cervical sympathetic chain
11. Pulse difference in two wrists if aneurysm interferes with circulation in left subclavian artery
12. Abnormal pulsation may be apparent on chest wall—due to erosion of aneurysm through rib cage—in syphilis

B. Management

1. The prognosis is poor for untreated patients.
2. Surgery—remove aneurysm and restore vascular continuity

   Aortic arch aneurysms are the most difficult to treat.

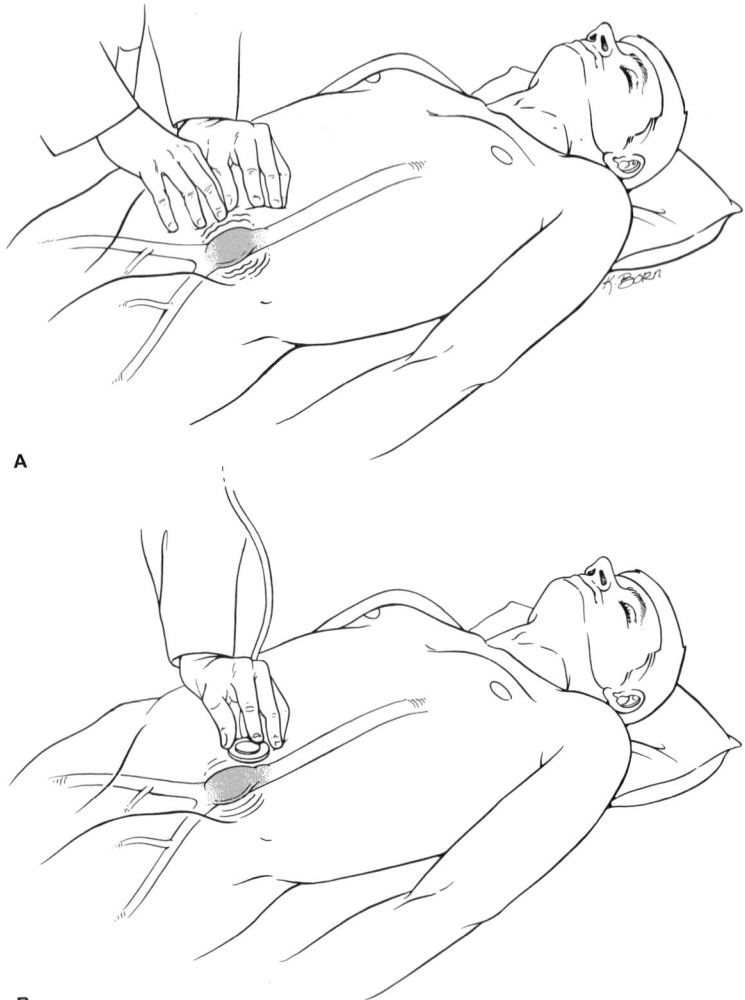

A

B

Figure 16-11. *Palpating and auscultating for an abdominal aortic aneurysm. (A) Hand applied over the aorta will feel a pulsatile rumbling referred to as a thrill (likened to the purring of a cat). (B) The stethoscope applied over the aorta will produce a murmurlike sound called a bruit.*

Abdominal Aneurysm

A. Clinical Manifestations

1. Many of these patients are asymptomatic; most are males (9:1) in their 6th or 7th decade.
2. Abdominal pain is most common; persistent or intermittent—often localized in middle or lower abdomen to the left of midline.
3. Low back pain.
4. Feeling of an abdominal pulsating mass, palpated as a thrill, auscultated as a bruit (Fig. 16-11).
5. Hypertension may be in evidence.

B. Diagnostic Evaluation

1. Ordinarily the systolic blood pressure of the thigh exceeds that in the arm; in many of these patients, the opposite is true.
2. A palpable pulsating abdominal mass; fluoroscopy will reveal pulsating tumor.
3. Angioaortogram allows visualization of vessels and aneurysm.
4. Ultrasound allows visualization of vessels and aneurysm. This is the best test to confirm the presence of and check the size of abdominal aortic aneurysms. It is less expensive than other tests.
5. Computed tomography allows visualization of vessels and aneurysm.

C. Management

1. If untreated, the prognosis is poor.
2. Types of surgical intervention.
   a. Excision of area affected
   b. Replacement of excised segment by a bypass (synthetic) graft

Dissecting Aneurysm of the Aorta

1. This is a type of aneurysm in which there is a tear in the intima of the aorta; as a result of pressure, blood splits the wall and may produce a large hematoma or may continue to rip the wall.
2. Symptoms may resemble coronary occlusion; diagnosis is confirmed by aortography.
3. Prognosis is poor, but surgical removal of involved aneurysm and replacement of segment with a graft may be effective.

Peripheral Vessel Aneurysms

1. May involve renal artery, subclavian artery, popliteal artery (knee), or any major artery.

2. These produce a pulsating mass and may cause pain or pressure on surrounding structures.
3. Replacement grafts are used to repair these aneurysms.

The Lymphatic System

The *lymphatic system* is a network of vessels and nodes that are interrelated with the circulatory system. It removes tissue fluid from intercellular spaces and protects the body from bacterial invasion. Lymph nodes are located along the course of the lymphatic vessels and filter lymph before it is returned to the bloodstream.

Significance of Lymphangiography

Radiologic visualization of the lymphatic system is possible when a contrast medium is injected into a lymphatic vessel of the hands or feet.

It is a means of detecting lymph node involvement due to metastatic carcinoma, lymphoma, or infection in otherwise inaccessible sites (except by surgery) such as the pelvis, retroperitoneum, deep axilla.

Lymphangitis

Lymphangitis is an acute inflammation of lymphatic channels, which most commonly arises from a focus of infection in an extremity.

Clinical Manifestations

1. Displays characteristic red streaks that extend up an arm or leg from an infection that is not localized and that can lead to septicemia.
2. Produces general symptoms—high fever, chills.
   Produces local symptoms—local pain, tenderness, swelling along involved lymphatics.
   Produces local lymph node symptoms—enlarged, red, tender (acute lymphadenitis).

Produces an abscess—necrotic, pus-producing (suppurative lymphadenitis).

Management and Nursing Interventions

1. Administer antimicrobial agents, since causative organisms usually are streptococci and staphylococci.
2. Treat affected part by rest, elevation, and the application of hot, moist dressings.
3. Incise and drain if necrosis and abscess formation take place.

Lymphedema

Lymphedema is a swelling of the tissues (particularly in the dependent position), produced by an obstruction to the lymph flow in an extremity.

Clinical Manifestations

1. Edema may be massive and is often firm.
2. Obstruction may be in lymph nodes, as well as in the lymphatic vessels.

   Observed in arm following radical mastectomy (see p. 756).

Management and Nursing Interventions

1. Apply elastic bandages or stocking.
2. Advise the patient to rest frequently with affected part elevated each joint higher than the preceding one.
3. Administer diuretics as prescribed to control excess fluid.
4. Give antimicrobials as prescribed.
5. Recommend isometric exercises with extremity elevated.
6. Suggest moderate sodium restriction in diet.
7. Advise the patient to avoid infection and trauma and to practice good hygiene to avoid superimposed infections.

Bibliography

Books

AbuRahma AF and Diethrich EB. Current Noninvasive Vascular Diagnosis. Littleton, MA, PSG Publishing, 1988

Browse NL, Burnand KG and Thomas ML. Diseases of the Veins. Baltimore, Edward Arnold, 1988

Brunner LS and Suddarth DS. Textbook of Medical–Surgical Nursing. 6th ed. Philadelphia, JB Lippincott, 1988

Comerota AJ. Thrombolytic Therapy. New York, Grune and Stratton, 1988

Fahey V. Vascular Nursing. Philadelphia, WB Saunders, 1988

Fronek A. Noninvasive Diagnostics in Vascular Disease. New York, McGraw–Hill, 1989

Gerlock AJ, Giyanani VL and Krebs C. Applications of Noninvasive Vascular Techniques. Philadelphia, WB Saunders, 1988

Giordano JM, Trout HH and DePalma R. The Basic Science of Vascular Surgery. New York, Futura Publishing, 1988

Kempczinski R and Yao J (eds.). Practical Noninvasive Vascular Diagnosis. 2nd ed. Chicago, Yearbook Medical Pub, 1987

Ogston D. Venous Thrombosis. New York, John Wiley and Sons, 1987

Price SA and Wilson LM. Pathophysiology: Clinical Concepts of Disease Processes. 3rd ed. New York, McGraw–Hill, 1986

Journals

Backhouse CM et al. Controlled trial of occlusive dressings in healing chronic venous ulcers. Br J Surg 1987 Jul; 74(7):626–627

Beaver BM. Health education and the patient with peripheral vascular disease. Nurs Clin North Am 1986 Jun; 21(2):265–272

Bondy B. An overview of arterial disease. J Cardiovasc Nurs 1987 Feb; 1(2):1–11

Briones TL. Tissue–plasminogen activator: Nursing implications. DCCN 1989 Jul–Aug; 8(4):200–209

Consensus Conference: Prevention of venous thrombosis and pulmonary emboli. JAMA 1986 Aug 8; 256(6):744–749

Cox JL and Jacobs CP. Laser-assisted angioplasty: Treating peripheral vascular disease. AORN J 1987 Nov; 46(5):835–841

Daeschner SA. Action STAT! Pulmonary embolism. Nursing 1988 Sep; 18(9):33

Dean E. Arterial assessment of the hand. Br J Occup Ther 1988 May; 51(5):163–167

Dickinson SP and Bury G. Pulmonary embolism—Anatomy of a crisis. Nursing 1989 Apr; 19(4):34–42

Doyle JE. Treatment modalities in peripheral vascular disease. Nurs Clin North Am 1986 Jun; 21(2):241–253

Ekers MA. Psychosocial considerations in peripheral vascular disease: Cause or effect? Nurs Clin North Am 1986 Jun; 21(2):255–263

Fahey V. An in-depth look at deep vein thrombosis. Nursing 1989 Jan; 19(1):86–93

Fahey V and Riegel BJ. Advances in diagnostic testing for vascular disease.

Cardiovasc Nurs 1988 Mar; 25(3):13–18

Gerdes L. Recognizing the multisystem effect of embolism. Nursing 1987 Dec; 17(12):34–42

Hopkins S. Prophylactic treatment for venous ulcers. Nurs Times 1987 Jul 1–7; 83(26):45–46

Kikta MJ et al. A prospective, randomized trial of Unna's boots versus hydroactive dressing in the treatment of venous stasis ulcers. J Vasc Surg 1988 Mar; 7(3):478–483

Kleven MR. Comparison of thrombolytic agents: Mechanisms of action, efficacy and safety. Heart Lung 1988 Nov; 17(6):750–755

Lachman T. Clinical aspects of peripheral neuropathy. Hosp Med 1987 Jul; 23(7):56–64

Menzoian JO and Doyle JE. Venous insufficiency of the leg. Hosp Pract 1989 May 30; 24(5a):109–116

Merry JA. Take your assessment all the way down to the toes. RN 1988 Jan; 51(1):60–63

Millam DA. Managing complications of IV therapy. Nursing 1988 Mar; 18(3):34–43

Miller RA and Evans WE. Nurse and patient: Allies preventing amputation. RN 1988 Jul; 51(7):38–42

Nemeth AJ, Eaglstein WH and Falanga V. Clinical parameters and transcutaneous oxygen measurements for the prognosis of venous ulcers. J Am Acad Dermatol 1989 Feb; 20(2):186–190

Olson AR. What you should know about thrombolytic therapy. Nursing 1987 Dec; 17(12):52–55

Osterman HM and Pinzur MS. Amputation: Last resort or new beginning? Geriatr Nurs 1987 Sep–Oct; 8(5):246–248

Robertson C. Caring for the diabetic with PAD. RN 1988 Jul; 51(7):42–44

Rosen BL and Brodkin RH. Cutaneous lesions in diabetic patients. Hosp Med 1987 Jan; 23(1):118–124

Silverberg SM. Trouble in the vascular periphery. Emerg Med 1987 Mar 15; 19(5):20–32

Stabile MJ and Warfield CA. The pain of peripheral vascular disease. Hosp Pract 1988 Mar 15; 23(3):99–107

Tretbar LL. Chronic venous insufficiency of the legs: Pathogenesis of venous ulcers. J Enterostomal Ther 1987 May-Jun; 14(3):105–108

Turner J. Nursing intervention in patients with peripheral vascular disease. Nurs Clin North Am 1986 Jun; 21(2):233–240

Vitello CJ. Thrombolytic therapy: Urokinase. J Cardiovasc Nurs 1987 Feb; 1(2):59–64

Webber M and Jenkins N. Laser treatment of peripheral vascular disease: Implications for nursing care. Prog Cardiovasc Nurs 1988 Jul-Sep; 3(3):81–88

High Blood Pressure

Physiologic Factors

Hypertension (high blood pressure) is a disease of vascular regulation in which the mechanisms that control arterial pressure within the normal range are altered. Predominant mechanisms of control are the central nervous system, the renal pressor system (renin–angiotensin–aldosterone system), and extracellular fluid volume. Why these mechanisms fail is not known. The basic explanation is that blood pressure is elevated when there is increased cardiac output plus increased peripheral vascular resistance.

Normal Physiology

1. Blood pressure is a function of total circulating volume (cardiac output) × peripheral vascular resistance.
2. Three mechanisms serve to regulate the above two variables to maintain normal blood pressure: neural, renal, and humoral control.
3. A short-term control of blood pressure is exercised through the autonomic nervous system.
4. Renal control is exercised through adjustment of sodium and fluid volume status.
5. Humoral control is more complicated and involves the following:
   a. Renin–angiotensin–aldosterone
   b. E_2 prostaglandins
   c. Kinins
   d. Corticosteroids
   e. Vasopressin (antidiuretic hormone)
6. Blood pressure readings measure pressures taken at two phases of the cardiac cycle: systole and diastole.
   a. *Systolic pressure* is the pressure the heart must pump against to force blood from the left side of the heart to the aorta and major arteries.
   b. *Diastolic pressure* is the pressure required to allow filling of the ventricles before the next systole.
   c. Blood pressure is reported as a biphasic number: a systolic numerical value over a diastolic numerical value. Normal ranges are 100/60 to 140/80.
   d. *Pulse pressure* represents the difference between the systolic and diastolic readings. A narrow pulse pressure may indicate a failing heart.
7. The *mean arterial pressure* is the average pressure attempting to push blood through the circulatory system.
8. See page 409 for blood pressure determination.

Causes of Blood Pressure Elevation

1. Cause of essential hypertension is unknown; however, there are several areas of investigation:
   a. Hyperactivity of sympathetic vasoconstricting nerves
   b. Presence of blood component containing a vasoconstrictor that acts on smooth muscle, sensitizing it to constrictor substances
   c. Increased cardiac output, followed by arteriole constriction
   d. Prostaglandins affect regulatory mechanisms, which include the renin–angiotensin system, renal sodium and water excretion, and vascular smooth muscle tone
   e. Familial (genetic) tendency
   f. Hypertensive vascular disease—modifications of both large elastic arteries (macroangiopathy) and small muscular arteries and arterioles (microangiopathy)
2. Individual tolerance of increased blood pressure varies; however, there is a direct correlation between increase in blood pressure and the rate at which atherosclerosis and arteriosclerosis develop.
3. Rising blood pressure adversely affects the brain, the heart, and the kidneys (Fig. 17-1).
   a. Heart—myocardial infarction, congestive heart failure
   b. Kidney—nephrosclerosis, kidney failure
   c. Brain—headache, encephalopathy, cerebral hemorrhage, stroke
4. Emotional stress affects the central nervous system, causing increased release of catecholamines, which may account for increased peripheral vascular resistance.

Prevalence and Risk Factors

1. Hypertension is one of the most prevalent chronic diseases for which treatment is available; however, most patients with hypertension are untreated.
2. There are no symptoms; thus it is termed "the silent killer."
3. Increase in incidence is associated with the following risk factors:
   a. Age—between 30 and 70
   b. Race—black
   c. Birth control pills
   d. Overweight
   e. Family history

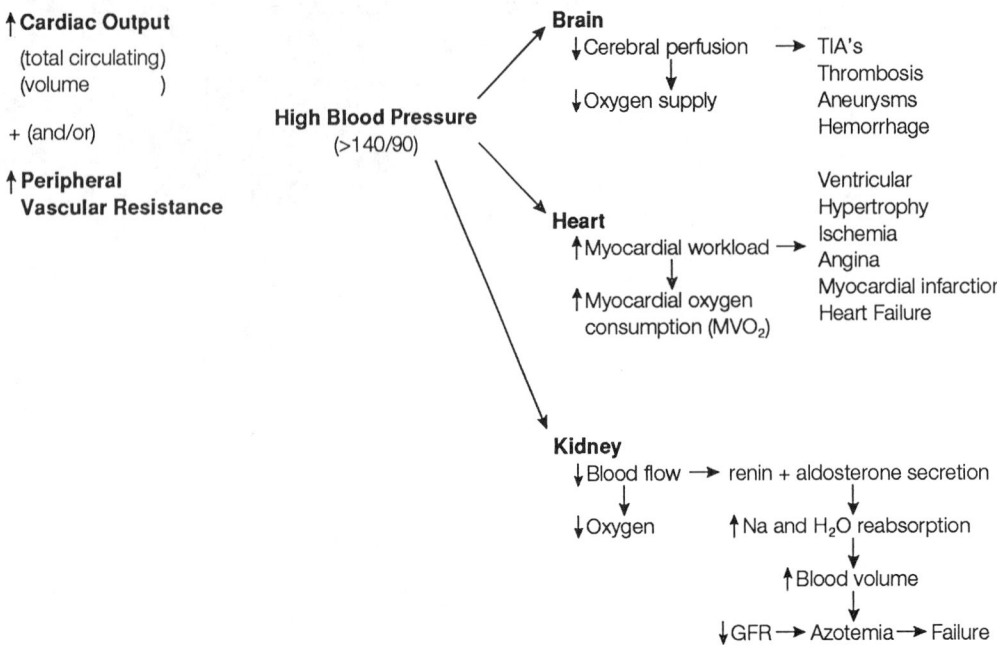

Figure 17-1. *Determinants and clinical effects of high blood pressure.*

f. Smoking
g. Sedentary life-style
h. Stress
i. Diabetes mellitus

Classification of Hypertension

Primary or Essential Hypertension

(Approximately 90% of patients with hypertension)
1. When the diastole pressure is 90 mm. Hg or higher and other causes of hypertension are absent, the condition is said to be *primary hypertension.* More specifically, an individual is considered hypertensive when the average of 3 or more blood pressure readings taken at rest several days apart exceeds the upper limits of the following chart:

Classification of Hypertension

Classification (Strata)		Diastolic Pressure (mm. Hg)	Percentage of Individuals
Mild	Stratum I	90–104	70%
Moderate	Stratum II	105–114	20%
Severe	Stratum III	115	10%

2. "Mild" is labeled such because of common usage; however, even for persons with so-called mild hypertension, the cardiovascular risk is twice that for individuals with normal blood pressure.
3. With the presence of target organ damage, the overall risk is increased.

4. Hypertension may be present for years *without any symptoms.*
5. *Labile* is a term used to indicate intermittently elevated blood pressure.
6. *Accelerated* refers to a sudden and severe escalation in arterial pressure, producing many symptoms and vascular damage.
7. *Resistant* is a reference to hypertension that is not responsive to usual treatment.

Secondary Hypertension

1. Occurs in approximately 5%–10% of patients with hypertension.
2. Follows other pathology.
3. *Renal pathology*—may lead to hypertension
   a. Congenital anomalies, pyelonephritis, renal artery obstruction, acute and chronic glomerulonephritis
   b. Reduced blood flow to kidney (such as atherosclerotic plaque)—release of *renin*
      (1) Renin reacts with serum protein in liver (alpha-2-globulin) → angiotensin I; this plus an enzyme → angiotensin II → leads to increased blood pressure.
      (2) Symptoms—proteinuria, polyuria, elevated blood pressure.
      (3) Correction of initial problem—endarterectomy, bypass graft, nephrectomy.
4. *Coarctation of aorta* (stenosis of aorta)
   a. Blood flow to upper extremities is greater than flow to lower extremities—hypertension of upper part of body.
   b. Correction—removal of stenosed section of vessel; anastomosis or graft to eliminate area.
5. *Endocrine disturbances*
   a. Pheochromocytoma—a tumor of the adrenal gland

that causes release of epinephrine and norepinephrine and a rise in blood pressure
   b. Adrenal cortex tumors lead to an increase in aldosterone secretion and an elevated blood pressure.
   c. Cushing's syndrome leads to an increase in adrenocortical steroids and hypertension
   d. Hyperthyroidism

Accelerated Hypertension—A Hypertensive Crisis

Blood pressure elevates very rapidly, threatening one or more of the target organs: brain, kidney, heart. (See p. 415.)

Management

"Stepped care" is an approach in which initial therapy is nonpharmacologic; however, if this is unsuccessful, it is followed with a pharmacotherapeutic approach, beginning with the mildest medication and progressing with additional drugs as determined by the needs of the patient.

Nonpharmacotherapy

1. Reduce weight if one is overweight, since there is a correlation between increases in body weight and increases in blood pressure.
2. Reduce dietary sodium consumption. Blood pressure response is monitored to determine individual sensitivity to sodium restriction.
3. Use alcohol moderately, as heavy alcohol consumption may elevate arterial blood pressure.
4. Reduce abnormal levels of blood cholesterol.
5. Avoid smoking.
6. Develop an exercise program after appropriate evaluation.
7. Consider relaxation and biofeedback therapies, as such behavioral modification methods may produce significant blood pressure reduction.

"Stepped Care" Regimen *(See Table 17-1)*

A. Step 1
1. Thiazide-type diuretics
   a. Favored for those over 50 years of age, black patients, those with peripheral vascular disease, asthma, or other chronic pulmonary disease
   b. Use smallest effective dose to minimize side effects.
   c. Potassium supplements are administered to avoid hypokalemia.
2. Calcium ion antagonists
   a. Gaining acceptance as drugs of choice for initial therapy
   b. Effective in reducing blood pressure with a minimal number of side effects

B. Step 2
Beta-adrenergic blockers
1. If step 1 does not produce a response, small doses of beta-adrenergic blockers can be added.
2. There are several drugs in this category, and it may be necessary to shift from one drug to another to find the best drug for a particular patient.
3. Favored for those under 50 years of age

4. May produce side effects
5. Sexual dysfunction may be experienced by patients taking these drugs.

C. Step 3
Vasodilators
1. If steps 1 and 2 are not effective in controlling blood pressure, then a third classification of drugs can be added—vasodilators.
2. May increase heart rate and myocardial contractility.
3. Use cautiously in patients with angina pectoris.
4. If dosages are increased too rapidly, the side effects can be headache, tachycardia, and palpitations.

D. Step 4
Guanethidine monosulfate
1. Added if first three steps are unsuccessful in controlling blood pressure.
2. May cause orthostatic hypotension, diarrhea, and retrograde ejaculation.

Nursing Process Applied to the Patient With High Blood Pressure

Nursing Assessment

A. Nursing History
Query the patient with regard to the following:
1. Family history of high blood pressure
2. Previous episodes of high blood pressure experienced by the patient
3. Excessive salt intake
4. Lipid abnormalities
5. Smoking (cigarette)
6. Episodes of headache, weakness, muscle cramps, tingling, palpitations, sweating, visual disturbances
7. Medication profile; note especially the taking of:
   a. Oral contraceptives, steroids
   b. Nonsteroidal anti-inflammatory drugs
   c. Nasal decongestants, appetite suppressants, tricyclic antidepressants
8. Other disease processes such as gout or diabetes, asthma, peptic ulcer

B. Blood Pressure Determination
1. Measure the blood pressure of the patient under the same conditions each time.
2. Avoid taking blood pressure readings immediately after stressful or taxing situations.
3. Place the patient in a position of comfort.
4. Support the bared arm; avoid constriction of arm by a rolled sleeve.
5. Use a blood pressure cuff of the correct size (Table 17-2 and Fig. 17-2).
   a. It is recommended that the width of the cuff be 20% greater than the width of the measured extremity.
   b. The length should be sufficient to encircle the measured extremity.
   c. The average dimensions for an adult cuff are 13 cm. wide by 24 cm. long.
6. Be aware that falsely elevated blood pressures may be obtained with a cuff that is too narrow; falsely low readings may be obtained with a cuff that is too wide.

Table 17-1. Pharmacotherapy for High Blood Pressure (Using Stepped Therapy Approach)

Purpose: To maintain blood pressure within normal ranges by the simplest and safest means possible with the fewest side effects for each individual patient

Medication	Major Action	Advantages	Contraindications	Effects and Nursing Considerations
STEP 1				
Diuretics and Related Drugs				
Thiazide Diuretics				
Chlorthalidone (Hygroton) Quinethazone (Hydromox) Chlorothiazide (Diuril) Hydrochlorothiazide (Esidrix; Hydro-DIURIL)	*At beginning of therapy* Decrease of blood volume, renal blood flow, and cardiac output Depletion of extracellular fluid Negative sodium balance (from natriuresis), mild hypokalemia Directly affect vascular smooth muscle	Effective orally Effective during long-term administration Mild side effects Enhance other antihypertensive drugs Counter sodium retention effect of other antihypertensive drugs	Gout Known sensitivity to sulfonamide-derived drugs Severely impaired kidney function	Dry mouth, thirst, weakness, drowsiness, lethargy, muscle aches, muscular fatigue, tachycardia, GI disturbance Postural hypotension may be potentiated by alcohol, barbiturates, or narcotics Because thiazides cause sodium loss, patient is instructed to watch for postural hypotension in the summer. (Eating salted pretzels in hot weather may avert this.) Administer supplementary potassium. *Gerontological Conditions:* Risk of postural hypotension is significant due to volume depletion; take blood pressure in three positions.
Loop Diuretics				
Furosemide (Lasix) Ethacrynic acid (Edecrin)	Volume depletion Block reabsorption of sodium and water in kidney Antagonize action of aldosterone	Action rapid Potent To be used only when thiazides fail	Same as for thiazides	Volume depletion is rapid—profound diuresis Electrolyte depletion—replacement is required. Thirst, nausea, vomiting, skin rash, postural hypotension Sweet taste noted; oral and gastric burning *Gerontological Conditions:* Same as Thiazides
Potassium-Sparing Diuretics				
Spironolactone (Aldactone) Triamterene (Dyrenium)	Competitive inhibitors of aldosterone Act on distal tubule independently of aldosterone	Spironolactone is effective in treating hypertension accompanying primary aldosteronism. Both spironolactone and triamterene retain potassium.	Renal disease Azotemia Severe hepatic disease	Drowsiness, lethargy, headache—decrease the dosage. Diarrhea and other GI symptoms—give drug after meals. Skin eruptions, urticaria Mental confusion, ataxia—perhaps dosage needs to be reduced. Gynecomastia (not for triamterene)
Calcium Antagonists				
Verapamil Diltiazem Nifedipine Nitrendipine	Act on vascular smooth muscle to produce vasodilation	Well absorbed orally Metabolic side effects are rare. Reduce left ventricular mass Absorbed rapidly	Known sensitivity to the drug	May produce headaches, tachycardia, palpitations. Observe for unusual form of peripheral edema that is not caused by sodium retention or fluid retention. Increased incidence of constipation because of effects on gastric smooth muscle

(continued)

Table 17-1. *Pharmacotherapy for High Blood Pressure (Using Stepped Therapy Approach) (continued)*

Purpose: To maintain blood pressure within normal ranges by the simplest and safest means possible with the fewest side effects for each individual patient

Medication	Major Action	Advantages	Contraindications	Effects and Nursing Considerations
STEP 2				
Adrenergic Inhibitors				
Reserpine (alkaloid of Rauwolfia serpentina)	Impairs synthesis and reuptake of norepinephrine	Slows pulse, which counteracts tachycardia of hydralazine	History of depression Psychosis Obesity Chronic sinusitis Peptic ulcer	May cause severe depression; report manifestations, as this may require that drug be omitted. Nasal stuffiness, which may require nasal vasoconstrictor Increases appetite—therefore, suggest stricter diet. Recurrence of peptic ulcer Administer with meals or milk. *Gerontological Conditions:* Depression and postural hypotension common in elderly
Methyldopa (Aldomet)	Dopa-decarboxylase inhibitor; displaces norepinephrine from storage sites	Effective in patients not controlled with thiazide-reserpine (with or without hydralazine) Useful in patients with renal failure Does not decrease cardiac output or renal blood flow Does not induce oliguria	Liver disease	Drowsiness, dizziness Dry mouth; nasal stuffiness (troublesome at first but then tends to disappear) Hemolytic anemia (a hypersensitization reaction)—positive Coombs' test; may not indicate drug discontinuance *Gerontological Conditions:* May produce mental and behavioral side effects in the elderly
Propranolol (Inderal)	Blocks the sympathetic nervous system (β-adrenergic receptors), especially the sympathetics to the heart, producing a slower heart rate and lowered blood pressure	Reduces pulse rate in patients with tachycardia and blood pressure elevation and is useful as an adjunctive drug with drugs that act at the neuroeffector site of the blood vessel	Bronchial asthma Allergic rhinitis Right ventricular failure due to pulmonary hypertension Congestive heart failure	Mental depression manifested by insomnia, lassitude, weakness, and fatigue Lightheadedness and occasional nausea, vomiting, and epigastric distress Blood dyscrasias such as agranulocytosis and thrombocytopenic purpura do occur but are uncommon. *Gerontological Conditions:* Risk of toxicity is increased for elderly with decreased renal and liver function. Take blood pressure in three positions and observe for hypotension.
Prazosin hydrochloride (Minipress)	Peripheral vasodilator acting directly on the blood vessel; similar to hydralazine	Acts directly on the blood vessel and is an effective agent in patients with adverse reactions to hydralazine	Angina pectoris and coronary artery disease. Induces tachycardia if not preceded by administration of propranolol and a diuretic	Occasional vomiting and diarrhea, urinary frequency, and cardiovascular collapse, especially if given in addition to hydralazine without lowering the dose of the latter. Patients occasionally experience drowsiness, lack of energy, and weakness.

(continued)

Table 17-1. *Pharmacotherapy for High Blood Pressure (Using Stepped Therapy Approach) (continued)*

Purpose: To maintain blood pressure within normal ranges by the simplest and safest means possible with the fewest side effects for each individual patient

Medication	Major Action	Advantages	Contraindications	Effects and Nursing Considerations
Clonidine hydrochloride (Catapres)	Exact mode of action not understood, but acts through the central nervous system, apparently through centrally mediated α-adrenergic stimulation in the brain, producing blood pressure reduction	Little or no orthostatic effect. Moderately potent, and sometimes is effective when other drugs fail to lower blood pressure	Severe coronary artery disease, pregnancy, children	Most common side effects are dry mouth, drowsiness, sedation, and occasional headaches and fatigue. Anorexia, malaise, and vomiting with mild disturbance of liver function have been reported. Skin rash, dreams and nightmares, insomnia, and anxiety have been reported but are not common.
Metoprolol (Lopressor)	Blocks access of norepinephrine to β_1-adrenergic receptors, especially in myocardium; decreases blood pressure by decreasing cardiac output and peripheral resistance	Rapid absorption	Cardiac failure Sinus bradycardia A-V conduction defects Diabetes mellitus	May cause bradycardia, congestive heart failure, intensification of heart block—take apical pulse before administration. May cause severe depression; report manifestations, as this may require that drug be omitted. Instruct patient to take radial pulse before each dose and report slow or irregular pulse to physician.

STEP 3

Vasodilators

Medication	Major Action	Advantages	Contraindications	Effects and Nursing Considerations
Hydralazine hydrochloride (Apresoline)	Decreases peripheral resistance but concurrently elevates cardiac output Acts directly on smooth muscle of blood vessels	Used as a third drug of choice when patient does not respond to thiazide-reserpine, thiazide-methyldopa, thiazide-guanethidine	Angina or coronary disease Congestive heart failure Hypersensitivity	Headache, tachycardia, flushing, and dyspnea may occur—can be prevented by pretreating with reserpine. Peripheral edema may require diuretics. May produce lupus erythematosuslike syndrome
Minoxidil	Direct vasodilating action on arteriolar vessels, causing decreased peripheral vascular resistance; reduces systolic and diastolic pressures	Hypotensive effect more pronounced than hydralazine No effect on vasomotor reflexes; thus does not cause postural hypotension	Pheochromocytoma	Tachycardia, angina pectoris, ECG changes, edema; take blood pressure and apical pulse before administration; monitor I&O and daily weights.
Nadolol (Corgard)	Blocks β-adrenergic receptors within the heart; reduces cardiac rate and output and decreases myocardial automaticity; exact mode of action for decreasing standing and supine blood pressures unknown	Can be used alone to treat hypertension, or in combination with a diuretic Long half-life; once daily administration	Cardiac failure Sinus bradycardia Bronchial asthma COPD	May cause bradycardia; instruct patient to take pulse before each dose and report slow pulse to physician. May cause dizziness, sedation, behavioral changes, depression; caution patient to avoid driving and other dangerous activities until response is known.

STEP 4

Medication	Major Action	Advantages	Contraindications	Effects and Nursing Considerations
Guanethidine (Ismelin)	Prevents release of sympathetic transmitter, norepinephrine. Is a depressant of adrenergic activity	Potency	Pheochromocytoma, because greatly enhances pressor effect of catecholamines	Severe postural hypotension accentuated by alcohol, exercise, hot weather Warn against suddenly standing or standing for a long time.

(continued)

Table 17-1. *Pharmacotherapy for High Blood Pressure (Using Stepped Therapy Approach) (continued)*

Purpose: To maintain blood pressure within normal ranges by the simplest and safest means possible with the fewest side effects for each individual patient

Medication	Major Action	Advantages	Contraindications	Effects and Nursing Considerations
	Depletes tissue stores			Diarrhea and nausea, nocturia
	Causes venous pooling, decreased venous return, and decreased cardiac output			Failure of ejaculation; counsel about possible sexual dysfunction.
	Decreases pulse rate, cardiac output, and renal blood flow			Fatigue and giddiness; blackout

Adapted from Brunner LS and Suddarth DS. Textbook of Medical–Surgical Nursing. 6th ed. Philadelphia, JB Lippincott, 1988.

C. Pressure Sounds

1. Systolic and diastolic pressures.
   a. When the blood pressure cuff is applied to an extremity, laminar flow of blood is obstructed.
   b. Turbulence of blood caused by the obstructing cuff produces Korotkoff sounds.
   c. These sounds correlate with the systolic and diastolic phases of the cardiac cycle and as such serve as markers for blood pressure measurement.
   d. As the cuff is deflated and arterial flow is reestablished, five phases of blood pressure measurement are referenced.
   e. The World Health Organization (WHO) and the American Heart Association (AHA) recommend the accurate reading of blood pressure to include identifying phases 1, 4, and 5 (see below).
2. Record precisely the systolic and diastolic pressures.
   a. Systolic—the pressure within the cuff indicated by the level of the mercury column at the moment when the first clear, rhythmic pulsatile sound is heard (phase 1).
   b. First diastolic—the pressure within the cuff indicated by the level of the mercury column at the moment when the sound becomes muffled (phase 4).
   c. Second diastolic—the pressure within the cuff at the moment the sound disappears, that is, the onset of silence (phase 5).

   d. Phases 2 and 3 are less distinct sounds produced between systolic and first diastolic and are not identified clinically nor recorded.
3. Document the blood pressure readings and indicate the patient's position and the arm used.

NURSING ALERT: The finding of an isolated elevated blood pressure does not necessarily indicate hypertension. However, the patient should be regarded at risk for high blood pressure until further assessment through history-taking and diagnostic testing either confirms or denies the diagnosis.

D. Physical Examination

1. Auscultate heart rate and palpate peripheral pulses; determine respirations.
2. If skilled in doing so, perform funduscopic examination of the eyes for the purpose of noting vascular changes. Look for edema, spasm, and hemorrhage of the eye vessels.
3. Examine the heart for a shift of the point of maximal impulse (PMI) to the left, which occurs in heart enlargement.
4. Auscultate for bruits over peripheral arteries to determine the presence of atherosclerosis, which may be manifested as obstructed blood flow.
5. Determine mentation status by asking patient about

Table 17-2. *Recommended Bladder Dimensions for Blood Pressure Cuffs*

Arm Circumference at Midpoint* (cm.)	Cuff Name	Bladder Width (cm.)	Bladder Length (cm.)
5–7.5	Newborn	3	5
7.5–13	Infant	5	8
13–20	Child	8	13
24–32	Adult	13	24
32–42	Wide adult	17	32
42–50[†]	Thigh	20	42

* Midpoint of arm is defined as half the distance from acromion to olecranon. Use nonstretchable metal tape.
† In persons with very large limbs, indirect blood pressure should be measured in leg or forearm.
From Recommendations for Human Blood Pressure Determination by Sphygmomanometers, American Heart Association, 1987.

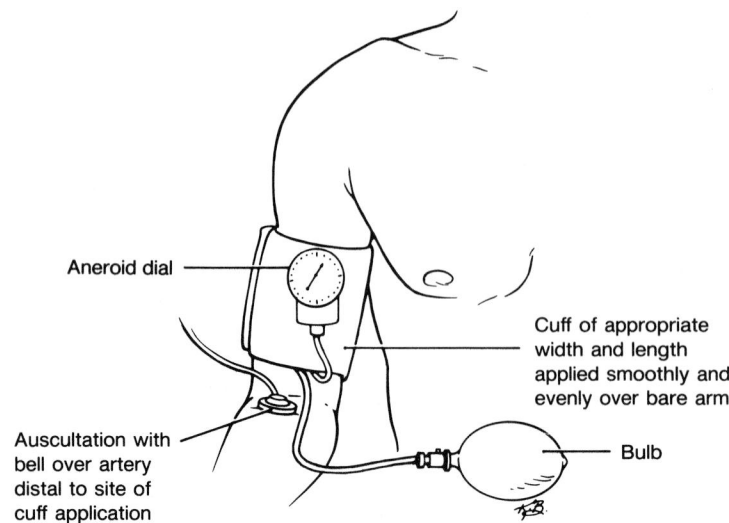

Aneroid dial

Cuff of appropriate
width and length
applied smoothly and
evenly over bare arm

Auscultation with
bell over artery
distal to site of
cuff application

Bulb

Figure 17-2. *Essentials for accurate blood pressure recording.*

memory, ability to concentrate, and ability to perform simple mathematical calculations.

Nursing Diagnoses

1. Knowledge deficit regarding the relationship between the treatment regimen and control of the disease process.
2. Potential nonadherence to the self-management program related to negative side effects of prescribed therapy and inability to believe that treatment is needed when symptoms are absent.

Patient Education

A. Basic Educational Program

1. Explain the meaning of high blood pressure, risk factors, and their influences on the cardiovascular, cerebral, and renal systems.
2. Stress that there can never be total cure, only control of essential hypertension; emphasize the consequences of uncontrolled hypertension.
3. Stress the fact that there may be no correlation between high blood pressure and symptoms; the patient cannot tell by the way he feels whether his blood pressure is normal or elevated.
4. Have the patient recognize that hypertension is chronic and requires persistent therapy and periodic evaluation; effective treatment improves life expectancy; therefore, follow-up health care visits are mandatory.
5. Present a coordinated and complementary plan of guidance.
   a. Inform the patient of the meaning of the various diagnostic and therapeutic activities to minimize his anxiety and to obtain his cooperation.
   b. Solicit the assistance of the patient's spouse/family/friend—provide information regarding the total treatment plan.
   c. Be aware of the dietary plan developed for this particular patient.
6. Explain the pharmacologic control of hypertension.
   a. Explain that the drugs used for effective control of elevated blood pressure will very likely produce side effects.

b. Warn the patient of the possibility that hypotension may occur following the intake of certain drugs.
   (1) Instruct the patient to get up slowly to offset the feeling of dizziness.
   (2) Encourage the patient to lie down immediately if he feels faint.
   c. Alert the patient to expect effects such as nasal congestion, asthenia (loss of strength), anorexia (loss of appetite), orthostatic hypotension (dizziness on changing position).
   d. Inform the patient that the goal of treatment is to control his blood pressure, reduce the possibility of complications, and use the minimum number of drugs with lowest dosage necessary to accomplish this.
7. Educate the patient to be aware of toxic manifestations and report them so that adjustments can be made in his individual pharmacotherapy.
   a. Note that dosages are individualized; therefore, they may need to be adjusted, since it is often impossible to predict reactions.
   b. Remember that certain circumstances produce vasodilation—a hot bath, hot weather, febrile illness, consumption of alcohol.
   c. Be aware that blood pressure is decreased when circulating blood volume is reduced—dehydration, diarrhea, hemorrhage.
   d. Suspect the presence of edema as a reportable symptom, particularly when guanethidine is taken; these medications are less effective in the presence of edema.

B. Self-Management Program

1. Enlist the patient's cooperation in redirecting his lifestyle in keeping with the guidelines of therapy.
   a. Present a written instructional program to fit individual requirements.
   b. Reassure the patient when encouragement is needed; the modifications required must appear meaningful to him.
   c. Encourage him in adapting and adjusting his activities in line with the prescribed therapeutic regimen.

2. Develop a plan of instruction to be practiced by the patient at home.
   a. Instruct the patient regarding proper method of taking his blood pressure at home and at work if his physician so desires. Inform him of the readings that are to be reported to the physician.
   b. Plan the patient's medication schedule so that the many medications are given at proper and convenient times; set up a daily checklist on which he can record the medication he has taken.
   c. Determine recommended dietary plans.

Evaluation

1. Demonstrates increased knowledge about high blood pressure, medication effects, and prescribed therapeutic activities.
2. Adheres to therapeutic regimen by limiting sodium intake, exercising, conscientiously taking medications, and keeping follow-up appointments.

> **GERONTOLOGICAL ALERT:** The multiple drugs required to control blood pressure may be difficult for the elderly patient to comprehend. The names of drugs are frequently difficult for the patient to pronounce. Color coding of medication bottles with an accompanying color-coded time of administration chart is one way to assist the patient in remembering when to take his medications. The elderly are also more sensitive to therapeutic levels of drugs and may demonstrate side effects while on an otherwise average dosage. The elderly may be more sensitive to postural hypotension and should be cautioned to change positions with great care.

Accelerated Hypertension

Accelerated Hypertension occurs when the blood pressure elevates very rapidly, threatening one or more of the target organs: brain, kidney, heart.

Pathophysiology

1. Elevated diastolic pressure → strain on arterial wall → thickening and calcification of arterial media (sclerosis) → narrowed blood vessel lumen.
2. Sclerosis of vessels → increased wall permeability → deposits placed on intima and media of vessels → cerebral, myocardial, or renal ischemia.

Clinical Effects

1. Brain effects
   a. Encephalopathy
   b. Stroke
   c. Progressive headache, stupor, seizures
2. Kidney effects
   a. Blood flow decreased, vasoconstriction
   b. BUN elevated
   c. Plasma renin activity increased
   d. Urine specific gravity lowered
   e. Proteinuria
3. Heart effects
   a. Left ventricular failure
   b. Acute myocardial infarction

Management

Goal:
Lower blood pressure to reduce the probability of permanent damage to a target organ: brain, heart, kidney.

Pharmacotherapy

1. If diastolic blood pressure exceeds 115–130 mm. Hg, hospitalization is recommended.
2. Immediate treatment if the following are present:
   a. Seizures
   b. Abnormal neurologic signs
   c. Severe occipital headache
   d. Pulmonary edema
3. The patient is hemodynamically monitored in the ICU.
4. Antihypertensive agents are administered parenterally.
5. Diuretics may be administered to maintain a sodium diuresis when the arterial pressure falls.
6. Vasopressor agents should be available if the blood pressure responds too vigorously to antihypertensive agents.

Nursing Interventions

1. Record blood pressure frequently. Some drugs necessitate the taking of blood pressure readings every 5 minutes or more frequently while titrating drug therapies.

> **NURSING ALERT:** The blood pressure should be reduced gradually and wide pressure variations avoided, as the patient's usual range may not be tolerated.

2. Measure urinary output accurately
3. Observe for hypokalemia, especially if patient is placed on diuretic therapy.
4. Observe for central nervous system complications.
   a. Note signs of confusion, irritability, lethargy, disorientation.
   b. Listen for complaints of headache, difficulty with vision; be alert for evidence of nausea or vomiting.
   c. Be alert to the possibility of seizure activity; provide for a safe environment, padded siderails, keep bed in lowest position.
5. Reduce the potential for activities or reactions that will increase arterial pressure.
   a. Avoid situations that may produce feelings of anxiety for the patient.
   b. Try to minimize alterations of daily routines of the patient.
6. Reinforce the value of rest by:
   a. Advising the patient to rest for a short time before and after eating
   b. Reminding the patient to rest each day for an amount of time appropriate for him
   c. Suggesting to the patient that he eat more frequently and in smaller amounts rather than 3 heavy meals

Bibliography

Books

Braunwald E. Heart Disease: A Textbook of Cardiovascular Medicine. 3rd ed. Philadelphia, WB Saunders, 1988

Brunner LS and Suddarth DS. Textbook of Medical–Surgical Nursing. 6th ed. Philadelphia, JB Lippincott, 1988

Drayer JI, Lowenthal DT and Weber MA.

Drug Therapy in Hypertension. New York, Marcel Dekker, 1987

Hurst JW (ed). The Heart. 7th ed. New York, McGraw–Hill, 1990

Kaplan NM. Clinical Hypertension. 4th ed. Baltimore, Williams & Wilkins, 1986

Kaplan NM, Brenner B and Laragh J. New Therapeutic Strategies in Hypertension. New York, Raven Press, 1989

Kinny M et al. AACN's Clinical Reference Manual for Critical Care Nursing. New York, McGraw-Hill, 1989

Page I. Hypertension Mechanisms. New York, Grune and Stratton, 1987

Price SA and Wilson LM. Pathophysiology: Clinical Concepts of Disease Processes. 3rd ed. New York, McGraw-Hill, 1986

Underhill S et al. Cardiac Nursing. 2nd ed. Philadelphia, JB Lippincott, 1989

Wollam G and Hall WD. Hypertension Management. Clinical Practice and Therapeutic Dilemmas. Chicago, Year Book Medical Pub, 1988

Journals

Adelman EM. When the patient's blood pressure falls . . . What does it mean? What should you do? Nursing 1987 Oct; 17(10):66–73

Beare PG. Calcium channel blockers: Nursing care for hypertension. Crit Care Nurse 1989 Feb; 9(2):37–44

Berenson GS, Ingelfinger JR and Jesse MJ. Identifying the young hypertensive. Patient Care 1988 Apr 15; 22(7):105–110

Brest AN. Antihypertensive therapy in perspective, part 1. Mod Concepts Cardiovas Dis 1988 Dec; 57(12):65–69

Brest AN. Antihypertensive therapy in perspective, part 2. Mod Concepts Cardiovas Dis 1989 Jan; 58(1):1–5

Brest AN. Antihypertensive therapy: Another look at the effects of cardioprotection. Consultant 1988 May; 28(5):46–48

Crisp CB. Calcium channel blockers in emergency medicine. Emerg Care Q 1987 Aug; 3(2):38–48

Cunningham SG. Nonpharmacologic management of high blood pressure. Cardiovasc Nurs 1987 Jul–Aug; 23(4):18–22

Frohlich ED. Calcium antagonists for initial therapy of hypertension. Heart Lung 1989 Jul; 18(4):370–376

Frohlich ED. Cardiac hypertrophy in hypertension. N Engl J Med 1987 Sep 24; 317(13):831–833

Hahn K. Think twice about borderline hypertension. Nursing 1988 Apr; 18(4):90–91

Hansson L. Current and future strategies in the treatment of hypertension. Am J Cardiol 1988 Feb 10; 61(5):2c–7c

Henneman E and Henneman PL. Intricacies of blood pressure measurement: Reexamining the rituals. Heart Lung 1989 May; 18(3):263–271

Hill MN and Cunningham S. The latest words for high blood pressure. Am J Nurs 1989 Apr; 89(4):504–508

Hill MN. Diuretics for mild hypertension: Still the best choice? Nursing 1987 Sep; 17(9):62–64

Hypertension. Med Times 1988 Sep; 116(9):57–60

Joint National Committee on Detection, Evaluation, and Treatment of High Blood Pressure. The 1988 Report of the Joint National Committee on Detection, Evaluation, and Treatment of High Blood Pressure. Arch Intern Med 1988 May; 148(5):1023–1038

Kirkendall WM, Weber MA and Weinberger MH. Which drug for the aging hypertensive? Patient Care 1988 Jan 15; 22(1):133–135, 139–140, 142–145

Nakagawa KH et al. Self-management of hypertension: Predictors of success in diastolic blood pressure reduction. Res Nurs Health 1988 Apr; 11(2):105–115

Trounson LW. Hypertensive crisis. J Post Anesth Nurs 1988 Apr; 3(2):102–106

Digestive and Gastrointestinal Disorders

18

Upper Gastrointestinal Disorders
(Mouth, Neck, and Esophagus)

Conditions of the Mouth

Psychosocial Considerations

1. Comfort, good nutrition, and general well-being are promoted by maintaining clean and well-cared-for teeth and gums.
2. Normal speech is dependent on the oral cavity for articulation and projection.
3. Personal attractiveness is enhanced.
4. Participation in routine dental health programs promotes prevention, early detection, and correction of dental and oral problems.

Assessment of the Mouth

A. History

1. Inquire regarding nutrition, dental care, normal mouth care habits, dental caries, use of partial or full dentures, stress-related grinding, clenching or clamping of teeth, bleeding gums, or injuries.
2. Assess common risk factors: smoking cigarettes or a pipe, using smokeless tobacco, consuming alcohol, diabetes, immunosuppression, and use of drugs that have oral reactions (e.g., phenytoin, diuretics).

B. Physical Assessment (see p. 24)

1. Remove dentures, if present.
2. Inspection
   a. Observe the lips for color, moisture, ulcers, lumps, localized discoloration, and cracking.
   b. Inspect the tongue for smoothness, moisture, condition of papillae, and color; note the presence of redness, swelling, lesions, or cracks (a thin white coat is normal). Note any deviation or tremor when the tongue is moved.
   c. Observe the palate and note any redness, fissures, cracks, abnormal coloring, or nodules.
   d. Inspect the teeth and gums for their number; note any missing, cracked, or discolored teeth; note obvious caries and local irritations; observe the gingiva for color, retraction, evidence of bleeding, or edema.
   e. Observe tooth-brushing and flossing technique, if possible.

3. Palpation
   a. With a tongue blade, depress the tongue and note the symmetry of the uvula when the soft palate rises as the patient says "ah"; note discoloration, enlargement, exudate, ulceration of the posterior pharynx.
   b. Wearing gloves, palpate the outer lips, the gingiva, the buccal mucosa, and the floor of the mouth for lesions, masses, or tenderness.

Candidiasis

Candidiasis is a fungal infection commonly caused by *Candida albicans,* usually occurring in the mouth and pharynx, but can become a source of systemic dissemination, particularly in high-risk individuals.

Risk Factors

1. Immunosuppression from disease states or treatment regimens (e.g., HIV infection, corticosteroids)
2. Altered oral environment from loss of epithelial layer, preexisting infections, poor oral hygiene or nutritional status, denture wearers

Clinical Manifestations

1. Oral discomfort, burning, altered taste, erythema
2. Possible pseudomembranous form (thrush) with adherent white plaques, which can be wiped off
3. Possible spread to the esophagus

Diagnostic Evaluation

1. Clinical signs and symptoms
2. Microbiological studies of the plaques
3. Occasionally, biopsy of lesions

Management

1. Topical antifungal agents in oral rinses, tablets, creams, or vaginal tablets (e.g., nystatin).
2. Systemic treatment is indicated if topical agents fail; amphotericin B is the drug of choice.
3. Analgesics for severe pain

Complications

1. Viral manifestations throughout the GI tract
2. Candida sepsis

Nursing Interventions

A. Alleviating the Infection

1. Administer antifungal agents as prescribed.
2. Observe for signs and symptoms of drug side effects: nausea, vomiting, diarrhea; renal, bone marrow, cardiovascular, or neurologic toxicities.
3. Follow prescribed suggestions for loosening encrustations with dilute hydrogen peroxide mouth rinses, followed by water rinses.

B. Attaining Comfort

1. Administer analgesics as prescribed.
2. Provide soft foods, soothing liquids; avoid extremes in temperature.
3. Provide gentle suctioning if pain becomes so severe that patient cannot handle secretions.

Patient Education

1. Instruct high-risk patients on daily oral examination and the signs and symptoms to observe.
2. Teach patient to avoid highly seasoned foods, extremes in temperature, alcoholic beverages, and smoking, all of which irritate the oral mucosa.
3. Encourage good oral hygiene.

Cancer of the Oral Cavity

Cancer of the oral cavity may rise from the lips, buccal mucosa, gums, hard palate, floor of the mouth, and anterior two thirds of the tongue.

Clinical Features

1. Most prevalent in men, 50–70 years of age; approximately 90% are squamous cell carcinoma.
2. High risk factors: use of tobacco and alcohol (particularly in combination); use of smokeless tobacco (snuff); and chronic sun exposure.
3. Overall 5-year survival rate is 30%–40%, depending on the stage of disease at diagnosis.

Clinical Manifestations

1. Often asymptomatic in early stages.
2. Mucosal erythroplasia—red inflammatory or erythroplastic mucosal changes; appears smooth, granular, and minimally elevated, with or without a white component (leukoplakia), persisting longer than 10–14 days.
3. Cancer of the lip—presence of a lesion that fails to heal.
4. Cancer of the tongue—swelling, ulceration, areas of tenderness or bleeding, abnormal texture, or limited movement of the tongue.
5. Floor of the mouth cancer—red, slightly elevated, mucosal lesion with ill-defined borders, leukoplakia, indurated, ulceration, or wartlike growth.
6. More advanced stages characterized by ulceration, bleeding, pain, induration, and/or cervical lymphadenopathy.

Diagnostic Evaluation

1. Careful inspection of the oral cavity with indirect mirror examination of pharynx
2. Staining of the oral lesion with toluidine blue—the lesion stains dark blue after rinsing with acetic acid (normal tissue does not absorb stain).
3. Excisional biopsy of suspected tissue
4. Radiologic studies: chest x-ray, computed tomography (CT) scans, to determine involvement

Management

(Selection of treatment depends on size and site of lesion and how extensively surrounding tissues are involved.)

1. Small lesions can be removed by wide excision or can be treated with radiotherapy or interstitial irradiation.
2. Large lesions may be excised widely or treated by radical neck dissection, followed by external irradiation.
3. Radiation therapy can be palliative, providing it has not been given previously.
4. Chemotherapy of previously untreated patients with locally advanced tumors has shown high response rates in recent clinical trials.

Complications

1. Second primary cancers of the larynx, hypopharynx, esophagus, and lungs.
2. Secondary to treatment:
   a. Surgery: transient salivary outflow obstruction, infection, voice changes, fistula formation, loss of swallowing, cosmetic defects
   b. Radiation: temporary loss of taste, xerostomia, radiation caries, osteoradionecrosis.

Nursing Assessment

1. Question the patient regarding changes in swallowing, smell or taste, salivation, discomfort when eating, or sore throat.
2. Note the quality of voice patterns.
3. Note and ask about breath odor, as some lesions produce a foul odor.
4. Inspect the oral cavity: erythema, red velvety areas; white patches; bleeding; swelling; record the size, location, and description.
5. Palpate the cervical lymph nodes for size, firmness, or tenderness.

Nursing Diagnoses

1. Pain related to malignant infiltration, lesion(s), difficulty swallowing, surgery, radiation therapy
2. Altered nutrition (less than body requirements) related to pain, difficulty in chewing or swallowing, history of alcohol abuse
3. Altered self-concept (disturbance in body image) related to changes in facial contour, cosmetic defect from surgery
4. Other Nursing Diagnoses, postoperatively could include:
   Anticipatory grieving related to the diagnosis of cancer
   Potential fluid volume deficit related to postoperative bleeding, inadequate intake
   Impaired communication (verbal) related to postoperative swelling, pain

Nursing Interventions

(See p. 423 if radical neck dissection has been performed)

A. Achieving an Acceptable Level of Comfort

1. Provide systemic analgesics or analgesic gargles as prescribed.
2. If the patient can tolerate it, provide mouth care with soft toothbrush and flossing between teeth.
3. If patient cannot tolerate brushing and flossing:
   a. Gently lavage oral cavity with a catheter inserted between the patient's cheek and gums with warmed, prescribed solution.
   b. Use power water spray to clean inaccessible areas if patient's comfort allows.
4. Encourage use of mouth washes that do not contain alcohol—may irritate the gums.
5. Management of excessive salivation and mouth odors:
   a. Insert a gauze wick in corner of mouth; place basin conveniently to catch drooling; replace frequently—to absorb and direct excess saliva.
   b. Suction secretions with a soft rubber catheter as needed; instruct patient on suctioning methods.
6. Management of decreased salivation
   a. Encourage intake of fluids, if not contraindicated.
   b. Instruct the patient to avoid dry, bulky, and irritating foods.
   c. Offer lemon lozenges or chewing gum to stimulate salivation.
7. Maintain a clean and odor-free environment by removing soiled dressings, tissues and gauzes, and providing room deodorants.

B. Improving Nutritional Status

1. Feeding problems may be handled in the following ways:
   a. Intravenously
   b. Nasogastric tube feedings or gastrostomy tube feedings
   c. Orally; serve meals high in protein and vitamin content, low in acidity and salt.
2. Provide mouth care before and after eating.
3. Allow the patient to have meals in privacy if so desired.
4. Offer easily chewed foods; mash or blenderize if necessary.
5. Add herbs or sweeteners to enhance flavor.
6. If swallowing difficulties persist, see Guidelines for Teaching the Patient with Dysphagia How to Swallow, page 430; or consult the occupational or swallowing therapist.

C. Improving Self-Concept

1. Assess the patient's reaction to his condition.
   a. Evaluate the patient's apprehension and offer emotional support.
   b. Correct any misinformation.
   c. Determine therapeutic plan of care for the patient's rehabilitation.
2. Recognize that face and neck surgery can be disfiguring and the patient often is embarrassed, withdrawn, and depressed.
3. Assist the patient in caring for his personal appearance.
4. Observe closely for indications of the patient's needs, which may be communicated in other ways.
5. Allow verbalization of fears, anger, distaste with body changes in a nondefensive manner.
6. Communicate acceptance of appearance in an honest manner.

7. Encourage the patient's family and friends to visit so that he is aware that others care about him.
8. Provide diversional activities.

Discharge Planning/Patient Education

1. Repeat the details of good mouth care and cleanliness of dressings.
2. Emphasize adequate nutrition—proper consistency, proper seasoning, and right temperature. Suggest the use of a blender if necessary.
3. If suctioning is required, instruct as to method, type of equipment, and where it can be obtained.
4. Provide detailed instructions to the patient and a member of his family on incisional care.
5. Review signs of obstruction, hemorrhage, infection, and depression and what to do about them if they are evident.
6. Refer to a speech–language pathologist, if indicated.
7. Encourage cessation of high-risk behaviors: smoking, alcohol consumption, use of smokeless tobacco, ingestion of highly spiced foods.
8. Emphasize the need for routine follow-up examinations.

Evaluation

1. Reports adequate comfort levels; is pain free; handles secretions adequately.
2. Achieves adequate nutritional status; able to eat prescribed diet.
3. Verbalizes acceptance of body image; demonstrates behaviors that reflect self-esteem (i.e., shaves, dresses, applies make-up).

Maxillofacial Fractures

Fractures of the maxillofacial bones may occur as the result of industrial, athletic, and vehicular accidents, violent acts, and falls; usually include soft tissue injury.

Clinical Manifestations

1. Malocclusion, asymmetry, abnormal mobility, crepitus (grating sound with movement), pain, or tenderness
2. Tissue injury: swelling; ecchymosis; bleeding

Diagnostic Evaluation

1. X-rays: posterioanterior; oblique; occlusal; panorex
2. CT scan

Management

1. Maintenance of adequate respiratory functioning; may include oxygen support, endotracheal intubation, or tracheostomy
2. Control of bleeding; usually accomplished with direct pressure
3. Reduction of the fracture—usually closed reduction
4. Immobilization—dependent on location, type, and severity of the fracture
   a. Barton's bandage with a Kling or stockinette bandage
   b. Interdental fixation with rubber bands or wiring
   c. Intermaxillary fixation with rubber bands or wiring
   d. Interosseous fixation with open reduction
5. Maintenance of adequate nutritional intake with liquid or soft diet—to maintain immobilization of fracture site.

6. Pain control to promote comfort.
7. Prevention of infection with antibiotics in the presence of positive cultures.

Complications

1. Airway obstruction
2. Aspiration
3. Infection
4. Disfigurement

Nursing Interventions

A. Monitoring and Preventing Complications

1. Maintain effective airway.
   a. Elevate head of bed 30–45 degrees, or position leaning over a bedside stand to reduce edema and improve handling of secretions.
   b. Assure readily accessible suctioning equipment; teach patient oral and nasal suctioning; position on side or upright during suctioning.
   c. Administer antiemetics as prescribed for nausea and vomiting to prevent aspiration.
   d. Assure the presence of wire cutters or scissors for immediate removal of the wires or rubber bands if the airway becomes obstructed. (Vertical rubber bands or wires should be cut.)
   e. Assure that a method for calling the nurse (call bell, bell) is within easy access to the patient at all times in case of emergency.
2. Monitor blood pressure, pulse, respirations, and temperature to note early onset of infection or aspiration.
3. Observe facial injuries for swelling, erythema, pain, or warmth to detect onset of infection.
4. Change facial dressings as needed to prevent soiling with secretions, food, or drainage, which may promote bacterial growth.

B. Maintaining Nutritional and Fluid Status

1. Administer fluids as prescribed; place straw against teeth or through any gaps in the teeth—teeth may initially be sensitive to hot and cold.
2. Position in upright position before, during, and for 45–60 minutes after all feedings.
3. Evaluate ongoing nutritional and hydration status; weight; intake, output, and specific gravity; laboratory values—24-hour urea nitrogen, transferrin level, electrolytes, and albumin.
4. Advance to blenderized diet as tolerated.
5. Make environment as pleasant as possible to enhance appetite—remove all sources of odor, decrease interruptions, position comfortably.

C. Increasing Comfort and Alleviating Pain

1. Administer liquid or a suspension of analgesics as prescribed—avoid narcotics, which may cause nausea and vomiting.
2. Administer diazepam (Valium) as prescribed to reduce anxiety and control reflex muscle spasm.
3. Apply paraffin wax to the ends of wire fixation devices to decrease irritation to the gums and oral mucosa.
4. Apply petrolatum jelly to the lips to decrease dryness and prevent cracking.

D. Maintaining Integrity of Oral Mucous Membranes

1. Provide mouth care every 2 hours while awake for the first several days, then 4–6 times per day.
2. Initially provide mouth care with warm normal saline mouth swishes.

3. As diet is progressed, remove collected debris with a pressurized water stream cleaner (Water Pik) and encourage the patient to brush teeth with a soft, child-sized toothbrush.

E. Supporting Body Image and Self-Concept

1. Provide firm reassurance regarding progress to reduce anxiety and allay fears.
2. Avoid unrealistic promises in relation to scars or disfigurement.
3. Allow the patient to choose the first time for looking in the mirror.
4. Provide privacy as requested—the patient may be sensitive to his appearance.

Discharge Planning/Patient Education

1. Encourage adequate nutrition—inform the patient and family that foods can be blenderized and thinned with juices or broths to a consistency that can be taken through a straw.
2. Explore with the patient options for maintaining proper oral care; encourage the patient to practice the options of choice.
3. Discuss the use of antiemetic medications to prevent nausea and vomiting, stressing the complications this could cause.
4. Make sure the patient has wire cutters or scissors and knows how to use them should airway obstruction occur.
5. Encourage follow-up health care visits.

Temporomandibular Joint (TMJ) Syndrome

TMJ Syndrome is a disorder of the temporomandibular joint structures or surrounding muscles, causing pain, muscle spasm, and changes in jaw movement.

Etiology

1. Malocclusion (uneven closure of the teeth)
2. Joint diseases—rheumatoid or osteoarthritis; lupus erythematosus, ankylosing spondylitis
3. Trauma
4. Teeth clenching or bruxism (teeth grinding)
5. Poor posture and its effect on the cervical spine
6. Psychological factors and tension—can induce or exacerbate symptoms.

Clinical Manifestations

1. Muscle spasm causing pain at the joint, temples, mandible, or masticatory muscles—worsens with jaw movement. Referred muscle spasm of the neck, trapezius, and sternocleidomastoid muscle causes discomfort (Fig. 18-1).
2. Clicking or crepitus—from grating or popping of the joint.
3. Limitation of movement, dislocation, or jaw locking.
4. Headaches, earaches, or tinnitus.

Diagnostic Evaluation

1. Radiographs of the head and neck to evaluate the bony components of the joint and determine cervical causes.
2. Occlusal analysis—evaluates the occlusion/malocclusion of the jaw and teeth in a bite position.

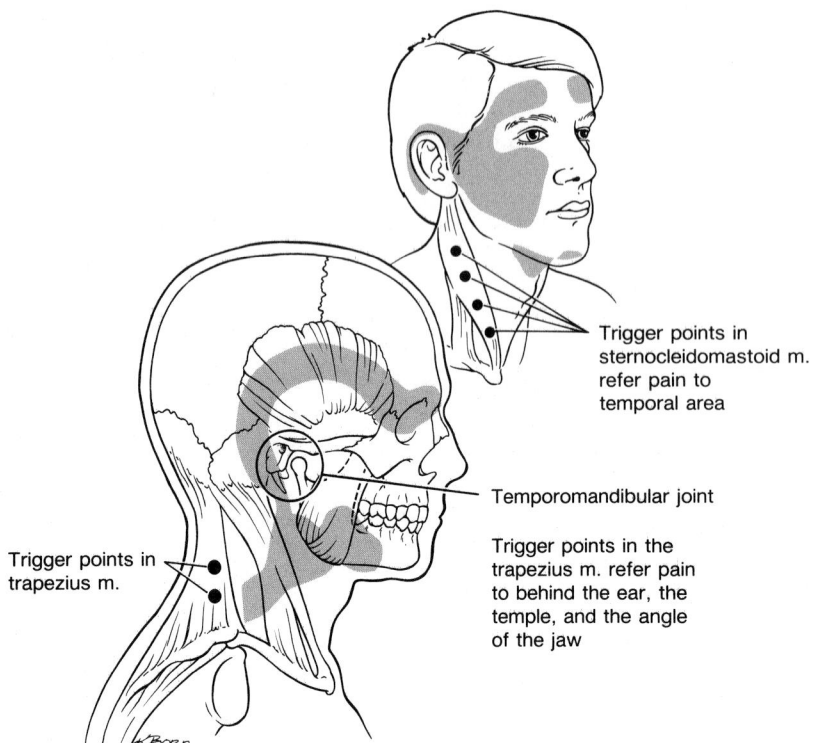

Trigger points in
sternocleidomastoid m.
refer pain to
temporal area

Temporomandibular joint

Trigger points in the
trapezius m. refer pain
to behind the ear, the
temple, and the angle
of the jaw

Trigger points in
trapezius m.

Figure 18-1. *TMJ syndrome.*

3. CT scan—to determine degenerative changes, fractures, or neoplasms.
4. Magnetic resonance imaging (MRI) demonstrates soft tissue abnormalities and disc displacement.
5. Mandibular kinesiograph to assess the degree of jaw dysfunction

Management

1. Therapeutic nightguard or splint—to realign malocclusion or joint disc and to optimize muscle relaxation
2. Moist heat or ultrasound (deep heat) therapy—to enhance analgesia, muscle relaxation, and to promote local tissue metabolism
3. Cold therapy—reduces inflammation, muscle spasms, and pain.
4. Transcutaneous electrical nerve stimulation (TENS)—reduces muscle spasm of head, neck, and back, and reduces pain.
5. Pharmacotherapy: analgesics and nonsteroidal anti-inflammatory drugs
6. Muscle stretching exercises—may use vapocoolant spray to the muscles prior to stretching—to reduce muscle spasm and optimize range of motion.
7. Arthroscopy—investigational procedure to visualize joint, reposition disc, lyse adhesions, or debride joint.
   a. Reserved for conditions not improved by medical management.
   b. Complications: seventh cranial nerve damage with facial paralysis and paresis; perforation of the external auditory canal; piercing of the middle cranial fossa.
8. Surgery—to remove the disc or reshape bony prominences.

   a. Complications: malocclusion, seventh cranial nerve damage, infection

Patient Education

1. Pain Management
   a. Assess the character, frequency, location, and duration of pain. Evaluate what triggers and relieves the pain. Determine how effective previous treatments have been.
   b. Explore the impact of the disorder on the patient's life-style.
   c. Instruct the patient on the indications, dosages, and side effects of analgesics and anti-inflammatory medications.
   d. Teach the patient proper use of heat and cold therapies.
2. Encourage the patient to perform active mouth opening, protrusion, and lateral movement exercises of the jaw for 5 minutes, 4–5 times per day, as prescribed.
3. Discuss the use of a therapeutic nightguard or splint as directed.
4. Explore tension-reducing modalities with the patient (e.g., relaxation exercises, biofeedback).
5. Encourage follow-up health care visits.

Head and Neck Malignancy

Head and neck cancer refers to a group of malignant tumors, most commonly squamous cell carcinoma, that may occur at any one or more anatomic locations in the upper digestive tract. Specific sites include ear, nasopharynx, nose and paranasal sinuses, palate, oral cavity, larynx, hypopharynx, and thyroid gland.

Clinical Manifestations

(Presence and severity dependent on location and stage of disease.)
1. Pain, dysphagia, dysphonia, persistent hoarseness, difficulty breathing
2. Hemoptysis, excessive salivation, loosening of teeth, dentures no longer fitting
3. Earache, nasal bleeding, infection
4. Neck swelling, weight loss

Diagnostic Evaluation

1. Close scrutiny of head and neck structures during physical examination; neurologic examination of cranial nerves.
2. Biopsy and histologic examination for confirming a diagnosis; direct and incisional biopsy, hypopharyngoscopy, laryngoscopy, bronchoscopy with bronchial washings, or esophagoscopy
3. Roentgenogram of head and chest, tomogram, CT scan, MRI—to determine size of lesion and presence of metastases or second primary lesion

Management

(Dependent on location, size, and metastases of lesion)
1. Treatment goal is to provide the best chance of cure while maintaining best possible aesthetics.
2. Nutritional supplementation to improve toleration of operative or radiation therapy, if nutritionally depleted.
3. Surgery
   a. Resection of lesion is the primary intervention; and/or removal of all tissue under the skin from the ramus of the jaw down to the clavicle; from midline back to the angle of the jaw. This includes sternocleidomastoid muscle, other smaller muscles, jugular vein in the neck.
   b. Many times resection is done with concomitant hemi- or total laryngectomy, and radical or modified neck dissection to assure removal of micrometastases.
   c. Often followed by postoperative radiation therapy. In some instances where resection is impossible, radical radiation therapy is the sole treatment.
   d. Surgical reconstruction may be performed with a rotational flap, skin graft, or free flap to promote healing and improve aesthetics.

Complications

1. Surgery: salivary incontinence, malocclusion, unintelligible speech, difficulty eating or swallowing, unacceptable deformity.
2. Radiation:
   a. Early: radiation mucositis, erythema, desquamation, dysphagia, secondary infection, oral pain
   b. Long-term: atrophy, fibrosis, salivary dryness, hoarseness, difficulty swallowing, bone pain, osteonecrosis, pathological fractures, limitation of movement

Nursing Assessment

Also see related activities under Cancer of the Mouth and Cancer of the Esophagus (p. 419, p. 432).
1. Assess nutritional status; eating habits, likes and dislikes, alcohol consumption.
2. Determine level of pain, dysphagia, difficulty breathing.
3. Evaluate patient's symptoms and laboratory tests, which may indicate concomitant cirrhosis, obstructive pulmonary or cardiovascular disease.
4. Assess condition of patient's mouth and ability to perform mouth care.
5. Assess level of understanding of disease process, treatment regimen, and follow-up care.
6. Evaluate the importance of body image in the patient's self-concept.

Nursing Diagnoses

1. Potential for altered breathing pattern (ineffective), related to laryngeal edema, secretions, presence of a tracheostomy
2. Potential for infection related to surgery, proximity of secretions to suture line, postoperative radiation
3. Altered nutrition (less than body requirements) related to anorexia, inability to swallow, pain on swallowing
4. Impaired communication (verbal) related to laryngeal edema, laryngectomy, tracheostomy
5. Potential for disturbance in body image related to surgical therapy, radiation changes

Nursing Interventions

A. Maintaining Effective Breathing Pattern

1. Place the patient in Fowler's position.
2. Observe for signs of respiratory embarrassment such as dyspnea, cyanosis, edema, hoarseness, or dysphagia.
3. Provide supplemental oxygen by face mask if necessary; if tracheostomy is present, provide oxygen by collar or T-piece, providing adequate humidification.
4. Auscultate for decreased breath sounds, crackles, wheezes; auscultate over the trachea in the immediate postoperative period to assess for stridor indicative of edema.
5. Encourage deep breathing and coughing.
6. Assist the patient in assuming a sitting position to bring up secretions (support the patient's neck with the nurse's hands).
7. Suction secretions orally or aseptically via tracheostomy if patient is unable to cough them up.

B. Preventing Infection

1. Assess vital signs for indication of infection: increased heart rate, elevation of temperature.
2. Inspect wound for hemorrhage, drainage, or tracheal constriction; reinforce dressings as needed.
3. Inspect incision for signs of infection; redness; warmth; swelling; drainage.
4. If portable suction is used, approximately 80–120 ml. of serosanguineous secretions are drawn off during the first postoperative day; this diminishes with each day.
5. Aseptically cleanse skin area around drain exit, using prescribed solution.
6. Assure the incision site remains clean and dry; cleanse away any secretions immediately.

C. Improving Nutrition

(See "Guidelines: Teaching the Patient with Dysphagia How to Swallow" if difficulty in swallowing is present.)
1. Postoperatively, feeding problems may be handled in the following ways:
   a. Intravenous feedings
   b. Tube feedings via nasogastric tube or gastrostomy tube
   c. Orally as soon as swallowing is established

2. Provide mouth care before and after meals.
3. If excessive or decreased salivation exists, see page 420.
4. Assure that emergency suctioning and airway equipment is available at the bedside during meals in the event of choking or aspiration
5. Position patient in an upright position, supporting shoulders and neck with pillows if necessary.
6. Inquire if the patient would prefer privacy during meals.
7. Provide an environment that is clean and free of interruptions and odor.
8. Assist with oral intake, providing easily chewed foods. Mash or blenderize meals if necessary.

D. Improving Ability to Communicate

1. If tracheostomy or laryngectomy has been performed, provide alternative methods of communication (letter board, chalk and slate, paper and pencil). If writing is a problem, it may be due to denervation of the trapezius muscle.
2. Allow adequate time for patient to communicate.
3. Place call bell and other articles that patient may need within easy access.
4. Recognize that patient may have difficulty nodding "yes" or "no" because of neck dissection.
5. Provide support and encouragement during communication attempts, recognizing that this patient often is depressed and frustrated even during limited communication.
6. Refer patient to speech–language pathologist if indicated.

E. Enhancing Self-Esteem

1. Respect the patient's desire for privacy during treatments, dressing change, and feedings.
2. Inform the patient's visitors of his appearance before they see him so that their expressions do not cause him to be upset.
3. Provide frequent aeration of the room and use deodorants to prevent unpleasant odors.
4. Observe for lower facial paralysis, as this may indicate facial nerve injury.
5. Watch for shoulder dysfunction, which may follow resection of spinal accessory nerves. (See Rehabilitation Exercises.)
   a. Use postoperative muscle exercises and muscle reeducation.
   b. Work with the patient to obtain good functional range of motion.
6. Consult with the surgeon and patient about decisions on future cosmetic surgery or in the use of a prosthetic device.
7. Encourage the patient to verbalize his concerns and feelings.
   a. Consult the physician to determine the nature and extent of explanation and prognosis that has been given to the patient.
   b. Encourage the patient to seek confirmation of his personal philosophy and religious beliefs because this may provide answers for him.
   c. Accentuate the positive.
   d. Encourage the patient to participate in his plan of care.
   e. Recognize that a great effort has to be made in behavior modification to change a life-style that included alcohol consumption and cigarette smoking. It is difficult to do.

Discharge Planning/Patient Education

A. Exercises—Instruct the patient and family regarding exercises to prevent limited range of motion and discomfort (Fig. 18-2).

1. Perform exercises morning and evening. At first exercises are done only once; then the number is increased by 1 each day until each exercise is done 10 times.
2. Following each exercise, the patient is instructed to relax.
3. For neck:
   a. Gently rotate head to each side as far as possible.
   b. Tilt head to the right side as far as possible; repeat for left side.
   c. Drop chin to chest and then raise chin as high as possible.
4. For shoulder:
   a. Standing beside bed, place hand from unoperated side on bed for support.
   b. Gradually swing arm on operated side up and back as far as is comfortable for the patient.
   c. Each day, work toward finishing a complete circle.

B. Follow-up Visits—Emphasize the need for frequent follow-up visits and completion of radiation therapy if prescribed.

C. For Permanent Tracheostomy—If patient has a permanent tracheostomy or laryngectomy, instruct the patient and family regarding:

1. Need for humidification
2. Protection measures
3. Activities to avoid that may cause aspiration
4. Referral for speech–language pathologist, social worker to meet ongoing communication needs

Evaluation

1. Maintains adequate breathing pattern; absence of dyspnea, shortness of breath; is able to handle secretions.
2. Is free of signs and symptoms of infection; vital signs stable; incision is clean, dry, without redness or drainage.
3. Is adequately hydrated, maintains stable nutritional status, is able to tolerate diet without choking or aspiration.
4. Able to communicate and make needs known.
5. Discusses concerns regarding condition; verbalizes comfort in the presence of others.

Conditions of the Esophagus
Diagnostic Evaluation of the Esophagus

Esophageal Endoscopy

This is the direct visualization of the mucosa of the esophagus using a rigid esophagoscope or a flexible esophagogastroduodenoscope to detect inflammation, ulceration, masses (tumors), or varices, and to obtain specimens for cytologic studies or biopsy.

A. Nursing Management and Patient Education

1. Give the patient nothing by mouth for 6 hours prior to test. This is done to decrease the possibility of aspiration and to be sure the esophagus is clear of particles that would block visibility.

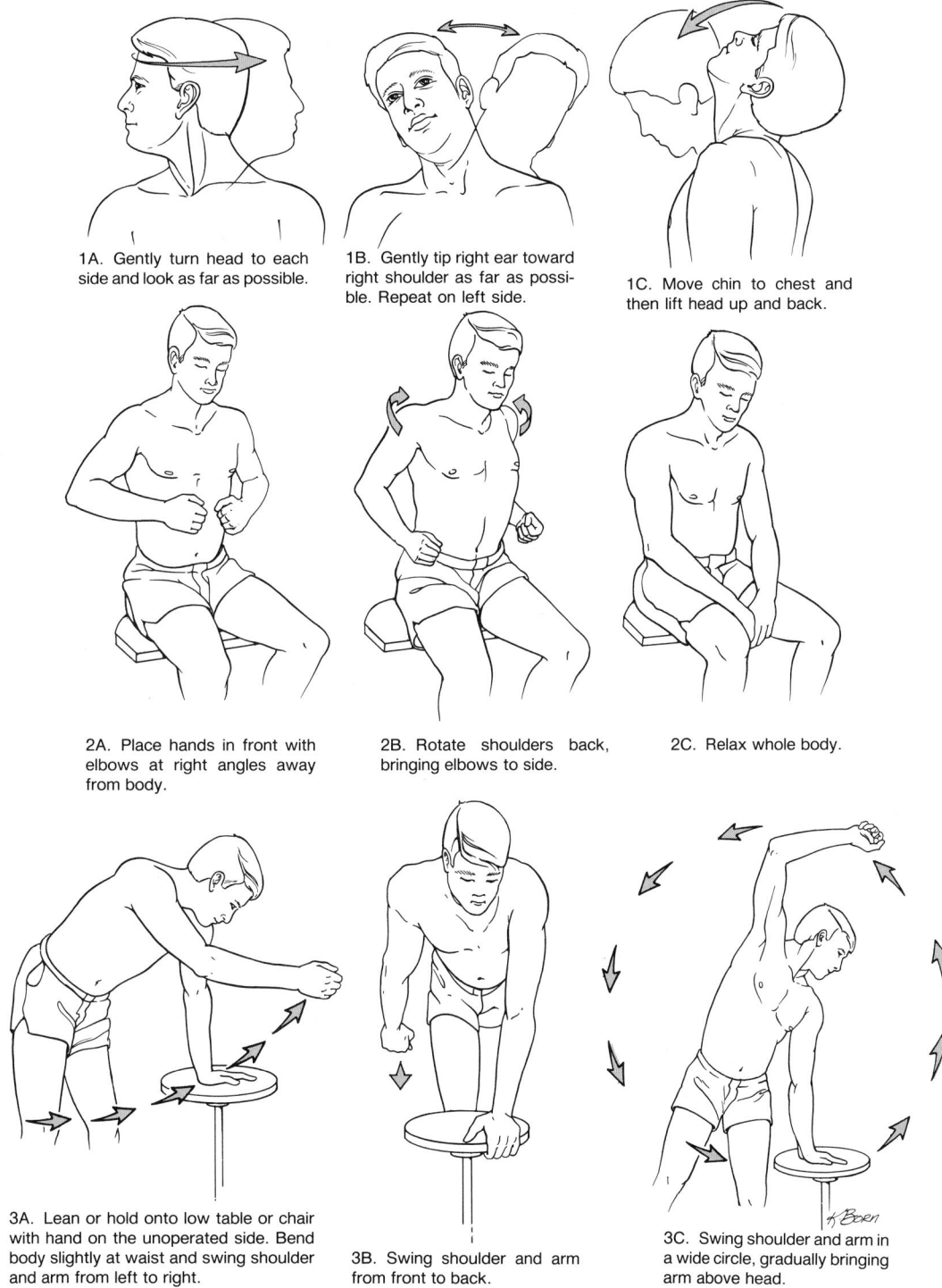

1A. Gently turn head to each side and look as far as possible.

1B. Gently tip right ear toward right shoulder as far as possible. Repeat on left side.

1C. Move chin to chest and then lift head up and back.

2A. Place hands in front with elbows at right angles away from body.

2B. Rotate shoulders back, bringing elbows to side.

2C. Relax whole body.

3A. Lean or hold onto low table or chair with hand on the unoperated side. Bend body slightly at waist and swing shoulder and arm from left to right.

3B. Swing shoulder and arm from front to back.

3C. Swing shoulder and arm in a wide circle, gradually bringing arm above head.

Figure 18-2. *Rehabilitation exercises following head and neck surgery to regain maximum shoulder function and neck motion.*

2. Explain the procedure to the patient before it is done, and explain the steps during the examination.
3. Administer diazepam (Valium) as a relaxant and meperidine (Demerol) as a narcotic as prescribed.

4. Spray the throat with local anesthetic (lidocaine spray) as prescribed to dull the effects of passing the esophagoscope and to reduce gagging.
5. If the esophagus is dilated (fluid-filled esophagus was

seen on x-ray), an Ewald tube may first be passed by the physician and then the esophagus is evacuated and irrigated.

> **NURSING ALERT:** For *all* endoscopies, have the following ready: oropharyngeal suction and emergency cardiopulmonary resuscitation equipment.

6. If a rigid scope is used, position the patient on his back. During insertion of esophagoscope, his neck is hyperextended and his head is tilted back and supported.
7. The flexible esophagofiberoscope is passed with the patient sitting; the examination is then completed with the patient lying on his left side.

B. Following Endoscopy

1. Withhold fluid and foods until the patient's gag reflex has returned (about 2 hours). Test the patient's swallowing with sips of water before foods or fluids are given.
2. Offer anesthetic lozenges or normal saline gargles for throat discomfort.
3. Observe the patient for 24 hours for symptoms such as bleeding, dysphagia, fever, and neck pain (cervical area) that are suggestive of perforation. Check also for substernal or epigastric pain (thoracic area); shoulder pain, dyspnea, abdominal pain (diaphragmatic area), and subcutaneous emphysema.

Esophageal Biopsy and Exfoliative Cytology

1. Biopsy of tissue may be taken during esophagoscopy: prepare tissue for laboratory examination.
2. Cytology
   a. Usually an overnight fast is required (no food or fluids).
   b. A No. 12 or No. 16 French nasogastric tube is passed to the cardioesophageal junction (45 cm.).
   c. Residual contents are aspirated.
   d. Physiologic saline (50 ml.) or Ringer's lactate solution is forcefully instilled with a syringe and is immediately aspirated below the cardia; this procedure is repeated at various levels of the esophagus (5-cm. intervals from 45 to 25 cm. from incisor teeth).
   e. Aspirated contents are collected in separate containers surrounded by ice; when all specimens are collected, they are to be taken *immediately* to the laboratory for analysis (must be centrifuged and pallet spread on slide as soon as possible after aspiration).

Esophagitis

Esophagitis is an acute or chronic inflammation of the esophagus. Severity of symptoms may be unrelated to the degree of inflammation seen at endoscopy.

Causative Factors

1. Gastroesophageal reflux associated with an incompetent lower esophageal sphincter—stomach contents reflux (flow backward) through the lower esophageal sphincter into the esophagus (most common cause); bending, stooping, and straining exacerbate symptoms.
2. Infections: fungal (*Candida*) and viral (herpes simplex)
3. Chemical—lye, ammonia, aerosols
4. Trauma—swallowing foreign body
5. Medications—pills, capsules
6. Malignancy associated with achalasia
7. Prolonged nasogastric intubation
8. Following gastric or duodenal surgery
9. Repeated vomiting (common in persons with bulimia)
10. Delayed gastric emptying

Clinical Manifestations

(Sudden or gradual onset)

1. Burning pain (heartburn or pyrosis), substernal or retrosternal, which may radiate to throat, jaw, arms, and back. *Pain may mimic "classic" chest pain of cardiac origin.*
2. Water brash phenomenon—a sensation of acidic or bitter regurgitation into the throat
3. Dysphagia—worse at onset of meal. Food "sticking" in throat or chest—produced by spasm, edema, or narrow lumen. While swallowing bolus of food, the patient may require "washing down" of food with liquids.
4. Pain on drinking citrus liquids, alcohol, or hot or cold fluids. Coffee often aggravates the pain.
5. Bleeding—acute or chronic; melena or hematemesis also occurs.
6. Respiratory symptoms, if reflux is present: chronic cough, asthma, bronchitis—due to aspiration of pharyngeal contents at night.
7. Symptoms aggravated by recumbency.
8. Symptoms may be precipitated by increases in intra-abdominal pressure, bending, lifting, straining.

Diagnostic Evaluation

1. Esophagoscopy with cytology and biopsy to visualize inflammation, lesions, strictures, or erosions and to delineate histologic changes
2. Cineradiographic esophagogram—identifies mass lesions, strictures, and abnormalities in peristalsis and esophageal clearing.
3. Esophageal manometry measures pressures and pH.
4. Acid perfusion test; onset of symptoms after ingestion of dilute hydrochloric acid and saline is considered positive.
5. Gastroesophageal scintiscanning
6. Ambulatory 24-hour pH monitoring may be done.

Management

(Depends on cause of esophagitis)

A. Life-style Changes:

1. Head of the bed raised 15 to 20 cm
2. No food or drink within 3 hours of bedtime
3. Bland diet, avoiding garlic, onion, alcohol, fatty foods
4. No coffee (even decaffeinated) or citrus juices
5. No tight-fitting clothes or smoking
6. Weight control

B. Pharmacologic

1. Antacids after each meal and before bedtime—used for acid-neutralizing ability.
2. Antisecretory agents (cimetidine or ranitidine) to decrease gastric acid secretion; results in a less irritating refluxant.
3. Metoclopramide hydrochloride—to augment sphincter tone and enhance gastric emptying; high incidence of

side effects (somnolence, nervousness, fatigue, dizziness)

C. Dilatation Therapy or Surgery—if necessary:

1. For strictures, dilatation therapy may be initiated; this may be done several times.
2. Surgery is indicated when conservative measures fail.
   a. Fundoplication for reflux to throat—severe stricture.
   b. Combined with vagotomy–pyloroplasty if associated with gastroduodenal ulcer.
   c. Stricture may need to be resected, and an esophagogastrostomy may be required.

Complications

1. Stricture formation
2. Ulceration of the esophagus, with or without fistula formation
3. Aspiration, may be complicated by pneumonia
4. Development of Barrett's esophagus—(presence of columnar epithelium above the gastroesophageal junction, which has been associated with adenocarcinoma of the esophagus)

Nursing Assessment

1. Assess for pain: Do you experience chest pain or heartburn?; Pain or discomfort when you eat?; Where?; How soon after eating?; Feel like food sticks in your throat or chest?; How long does the discomfort last?; How frequently does it occur?; What makes it better or worse?; Do you take over-the-counter antacids?.
2. Weight: How is your appetite?; Any signs of anorexia (loss of appetite)?; Weight loss?
3. Do you have to restrict the kinds of food you eat as determined by size or consistency (meat, for example), as determined by seasoning, or as determined by spiciness or acidity (citrus fruits)? Do you have to limit food because of temperature (hot or cold)?
4. Does the position of your body (bending, stooping, lying down) affect the problem? Do you lie flat when sleeping or do you have the head of the bed elevated? Does assuming a particular position help or make the problem worse?
5. Do you have belching, bloating, feeling of fullness, or difficulty finishing a meal?; Do you experience any vomiting, disagreeable taste in your mouth, intolerance for fatty foods?

GERONTOLOGIC ALERT: The strength of peristaltic esophageal contractions is significantly less, pain experience is diminished, and many medications diminish esophageal sphincter tone. Assessment in the elderly should include direct questions regarding symptomatology and use of antacids to elicit the possible presence of esophagitis.

Nursing Diagnoses

1. Pain related to inflammation of the esophagus, feeling bloated, nauseated
2. Potential for altered nutrition (less than body requirements) related to discomfort associated with eating, or with specific foods

Nursing Interventions

A. Attaining Comfort and Relief of Pain

1. Advise patient to take antacids, antisecretory agents as prescribed.

2. Place 15–20-cm. (6–8-in.) bed blocks under head of the bed—improves esophageal acid clearance and reflux of stomach contents. (Be sure to remove wheels from bed, if hospitalized.)
3. Advise patient not to eat food within 3 hours of bedtime to avoid nocturnal reflux.
4. Suggest patient try positional changes such as standing or walking to relieve pain.
5. Encourage patient to use meticulous oral hygiene.

B. Improving Nutrition

1. Encourage patient to eat small, bland, low-residue feedings—no bedtime meals or snacks.
2. Encourage to chew food well.
3. Provide a relaxing environment during meals.

NURSING ALERT: Milk is contraindicated for esophagitis because of high calcium content, which stimulates gastric acid secretion.

Discharge Planning/Patient Education

1. Teach the patient about prescribed medications, side effects, and when to notify the physician.
2. Inform the patient regarding medications that may exacerbate symptoms.
3. Advise the patient to sit or stand when taking any solid medication (pills, capsules); emphasize the need to follow the drug with at least 100 ml. of liquid.
4. Inform the patient and family what foods and activities to avoid: fatty foods, garlic, onions, alcohol, coffee and chocolate; straining, bending over, tight-fitting clothes, smoking.
5. Encourage the patient to sleep with the head of the bed elevated (not pillow elevation).
6. Encourage a weight-reduction program, if the patient is overweight—to decrease intra-abdominal pressure.

NURSING ALERT: Anticholinergics may further impair functioning of the lower esophageal sphincter, allowing reflux; antihistamines, antidepressants, antihypertensives, antispasmodics, and some neuroleptics and antiparkinson drugs decrease saliva production, which may decrease acid clearance from the esophagus.

Evaluation

1. Reports relief of symptoms and adequate rest.
2. Maintains adequate nutrition; is able to tolerate frequent small feedings.

Hiatal Hernia

A *hiatal hernia* is a protrusion of a portion of the stomach through the hiatus of the diaphragm and into the thoracic cavity. It results from muscle weakening due to aging or other conditions such as esophageal carcinoma, trauma, or following certain surgical procedures.

Types

1. Sliding hernia—the stomach and gastroesophageal junction slip up into the chest (most common).
2. Paraesophageal hernia (rolling hernia)—part of the greater curvature of the stomach rolls through the diaphragmatic defect.

Clinical Manifestations

1. May be asymptomatic
2. Heartburn (with or without regurgitation of gastric contents into the mouth)
3. Dysphagia; chest pain

Diagnostic Evaluation

1. Barium study of the esophagus
2. Endoscopic examination

Management

1. Elevation of head of bed (15–20 cm., 6–8 in.) to reduce night-time reflux.
2. Antacid therapy—to neutralize gastric acid
3. Histamine H$_2$-receptor antagonist (cimetidine; ranitidine)—if patient has esophagitis
4. Surgical repair of hernia if symptoms are severe

Patient Education

Prevent reflux of gastric contents into esophagus by:
1. Eating smaller meals
2. Avoiding stimulation of gastric secretions by omitting caffeine and alcohol
3. Refraining from smoking
4. Avoiding fatty foods—promote reflux and delay gastric emptying
5. Refraining from lying down for at least one hour after meals
6. Losing weight, if obese
7. Avoiding bending from the waist and/or wearing tight-fitting clothes
8. Reporting to health care facility immediately for the onset of acute chest pain—may herald incarceration of a large paraesophageal hernia.

Esophageal Trauma and Perforations

Esophageal trauma or perforations are injuries to the esophagus caused by external or internal insult.
1. External—stab or bullet wounds, crush injuries, blunt trauma
2. Internal—
   a. Swallowed foreign objects (coins, pins, bones, dental appliances, caustic poisons)
   b. Spontaneous or postemetic rupture—usually in the presence of underlying esophageal disease (reflux, hiatal hernia)

Clinical Manifestations

1. Pain at the site of injury or impaction, aggravated by swallowing; chest pain, may be severe
2. Dysphagia or odynophagia
3. Persistent foreign object sensation
4. Subcutaneous emphysema and crepitus of face, neck, or upper thorax—noted in cervical, thoracic, or esophageal perforations.
5. Temperature elevation occurring within 24 hours.
6. Blood-stained saliva or excessive salivation.
7. Respiratory difficulty if there is pressure on the tracheobronchial tree from injury or edema.

Diagnostic Evaluation

1. History of recent esophageal trauma
2. Chest x-ray.
3. Esophagogram.

Management

Goals:
Institute emergency life-saving treatment.
Restore continuity of esophagus.
Facilitate healing and prevent infection and constriction.

1. Maintenance of adequate respiratory functioning; may require oxygen support or endotracheal intubation—to assure an open airway in the presence of edema of the neck.
2. Control of bleeding and replacement of fluids, if indicated—to prevent shock.
3. Restoration of the continuity of the esophagus by removing the cause:
4. For external wound injury—emergency first aid wound care and surgical repair if indicated
5. For swallowed foreign bodies—
   a. Can usually be removed through esophagoscopy.
   b. When foreign body is made of metal, a magnet on the end of a retrieving instrument may remove the foreign body under fluoroscopic guidance.
   c. Meat impaction can be passed by having the patient slowly drink a glass of warm water containing unseasoned meat tenderizer.
6. For chemical ingestion, administer specific antidote.
   a. If lye or other caustic or organic solvent was swallowed, do NOT try to induce vomiting.
   b. A gastrostomy may be performed, either as a temporary or a permanent means of feeding the patient.
   c. Resulting strictures may be relieved by dilating the narrow esophagus.
      (See Guidelines: Esophageal Dilatation with Balloon-Tipped Catheter).
   d. Reconstructive surgery may be necessary to create a new passageway for food between pharynx and stomach.
7. Nasogastric tube intubation or esophagostomy—to allow the esophagus to heal
8. Administration of antibiotics to prevent infection

Complications

1. Airway occlusion
2. Shock
3. Perforation with mediastinitis or pleural effusion
4. Stricture formation
5. Abscess or fistula formation

Nursing Interventions

A. Monitoring and Preventing Complications

1. Auscultate the lungs and trachea for stridor, crackles, or wheezes. Assess respiratory rate, depth, use of accessory muscles, and skin color.
2. Position patient in semi-Fowler's position to facilitate breathing and reduce neck edema.
3. Monitor vital signs frequently for signs and symptoms of shock and infection.
4. Administer oxygen as prescribed.
5. Administer antibiotics as prescribed.
6. Replace fluid loss with parenteral crystalloid or colloid intravenous fluids as directed to prevent shock.

B. Reducing Pain and Enhancing Comfort

1. Administer analgesics as prescribed—intravenous analgesia may be required to control pain and allow the esophagus to rest.
2. Provide reassurance and support.

3. Assess and record pain relief.
4. Evaluate for symptoms that may indicate spillage of digestive contents into the mediastinum, pleura, or abdominal cavity—sudden onset of acute pain.

C. Maintaining Nutritional Status

1. Monitor daily weights and skin turgor.
2. Administer parenteral hyperalimentation as prescribed—to prevent gastric reflux into the esophagus, which may occur with enteral feedings.
3. Encourage progression of diet via nasogastric, esophagostomy, or oral feedings once esophagoscopy or esophagogram reveals healing of the esophagus.

Discharge Planning/Patient Education

1. Instruct the patient on the indications and side effects of analgesics.
2. Inform the patient on the signs and symptoms to report on possible complications: increase in severity or nature of pain; difficulty breathing or swallowing.

Motility Disorders of the Esophagus

Etiology/Pathophysiology

1. *Primary motility disorders* include achalasia, diffuse esophageal spasm, and those of nonspecific origin. *Secondary motility disorders* may be caused by neuromuscular, gastrointestinal, endocrine, and rheumatic diseases.
2. *Achalasia* refers to excessive resting tone of the lower esophageal sphincter (LES), incomplete relaxation of the LES with swallowing, and failure of normal peristalsis in the lower two thirds of the esophagus. The pathology is related to defective innervation of the myenteric plexus innervating the involuntary muscles of the esophagus.
3. *Diffuse esophageal spasm* is a motor disorder in which high-amplitude, nonpropulsive, nonperistaltic tertiary contractions (a form of aperistalsis) are present. LES functioning is frequently normal.

Clinical Manifestations

1. Dysphagia (difficulty in swallowing) liquids, solids, or both, exacerbated by stress or rapid ingestion.
2. Regurgitation of undigested foods; must be distinguished from vomiting.
3. Chest pain—rare in achalasia, but occurs in patients with vigorous achalasia types and diffuse esophageal spasm; may be associated with hot or cold food.
4. Heartburn is noticeably absent unless achalasia develops in patients with preexisting gastroesophageal reflux.
5. Halitosis and inability to eructate may be noticed.
6. Secondary pulmonary complications due to spillover of esophageal contents (aspiration pneumonia).
7. Weight loss is eventually noticed inasmuch as the patient has a decreased intake to avoid discomfort; eventually this can lead to emaciation.

Diagnostic Evaluation

1. Cineroentgenogram of esophagus with barium—to visualize the esophagus and peristaltic movement.
2. Esophagoscopy with cytologic studies and biopsy—may show dilated esophagus, aperistalsis, or mucosal inflammation secondary to food retention.
3. Esophageal manometry, conventionally or with balloon distention for 24-hour pressure and pH recording—to delineate motor function and reflux.

Management

1. Long-acting nitrates or calcium channel blockers to relax esophageal muscle tone; their efficacy is not well determined.
2. Esophageal dilatation with balloon-tipped catheter—to dilate the cardioesophageal sphincter.
3. Surgical esophagocardiomyotomy—to release muscle tension, with or without fundoplication to prevent subsequent reflux.

Complications

1. Malnutrition
2. Pneumonia, lung abscess, bronchiectasis
3. Esophagitis
4. Squamous cell carcinoma of the midsection esophagus.

Nursing Interventions

A. Monitoring and Preventing Complications

1. Incisional approach determines nature of postoperative care; thus, an incision through chest implies nursing care similar to that given to a patient with a thoracotomy (see p. 199).
2. Assess patient for discomfort, chest pain, regurgitation, and cough.
3. Assist with procedures, as necessary (see Guidelines: Esophageal Dilatation With Balloon-Tipped Catheter, p. 431).

B. Improving Nutritional Status

1. Direct patient to eat sitting in an upright position; eat slowly and chew food thoroughly.
2. Avoid food and beverages that precipitate symptoms.
3. Suggest that the patient sleep with his head elevated to avoid reflux or aspiration.
4. Provide a bland diet and tell the patient to avoid alcohol, as well as spicy, very hot, and very cold foods, to minimize symptoms.
5. Eliminate sources of tension as a precipitating factor producing stress during mealtime.
6. Administer pharmacologic agents, as prescribed.

Discharge Planning/Patient Education

1. Encourage life-style activity changes similar to those of patients with reflux (see p. 426).
2. See Guidelines: Teaching a Patient With Dysphagia How to Swallow (p. 430).
3. Provide information on drugs to avoid, i.e., anticholinergics.

Guidelines — Teaching the Patient With Dysphagia How to Swallow

Dysphagia—difficulty or discomfort in swallowing.

Purpose

To assist the patient who has difficulty swallowing after injury or surgical correction of the oropharynx or upper esophagus, or with neurologic deficit or stroke.

Clinical Manifestations

1. Sensation of food catching in throat or behind sternum
2. Coughing or choking during eating
3. Complains of difficulty controlling food in mouth; food escaping from lips during chewing
4. Weight loss

Nursing Assessment

1. Nursing history: Do you experience difficulty swallowing? Episodes of choking? Do you drool? Cough when you eat? Does food escape from your mouth or nose? Does food stick in your throat? If so, when does this occur? What foods or liquids are most difficult for you to swallow? Which are easier for you to swallow? Have you lost weight recently?
2. Observation: Is hoarseness present? Does the patient bring up food through the mouth or nose? Assess the cough, swallow, and gag reflexes.

Procedure

Nursing Action	Rationale/Amplification
Preparation	
1. Explain to the patient that you plan to work with him in developing an effective swallow.	1. The patient's cooperation, concentration, and directed participation are essential to the success of this learning experience.
2. Assure that emergency equipment is available at the bedside—suction, oxygen, face mask.	2. For use in the event that the patient chokes, vomits, or aspirates
3. Place the patient in an upright sitting position in a chair or support with pillows in high-Fowler's position if unable to get out of bed—for about 20 minutes before and 45–60 minutes after meals.	3. This will allow time to adjust and relax in this position prior to meals; allows gravity to assist the swallowing procedure during meals; helps prevent reflux or regurgitation after meals.
4. Provide mouth care before meals. Suction the patient if secretions are present. If the patient's mouth is dry, provide a lemon wedge or pickle to suck on.	4. This will increase patient's ability to taste and enjoy the sensation of eating.
5. Prepare an environment that is pleasant, peaceful, and without interruptions. Remove distractors, such as TV, radio.	5. Patient must be able to concentrate on the process of swallowing in a relaxed manner.
Food and Fluid Selection	
6. Foods should be chosen that hold some shape; moist enough to prevent crumbling but dry enough to hold a bolus shape—casseroles, custards, scrambled eggs.	6. Foods that crumble may be aspirated when they fall apart; foods that are too moist may be drooled through the lips.
7. Mugs and glasses with spouts or a straw should be used for liquids.	7. These utensils help prevent liquids from leaking out of corners of patient's mouth.
8. Avoid sticky foods—peanut butter, chocolate, milk, ice cream.	8. These foods stimulate thick mucous and will make swallowing more difficult.
9. Dry foods can be moistened with margarine, gravy, or broths. If liquids are a problem, juices can be thickened with sherbets.	9. Foods need to be of a consistency that will hold a bolus form until swallowed.
10. Avoid tepid or room temperature foods.	10. Hot and cold foods are thought to maximally stimulate receptors that activate swallowing mechanism.
Instructions During Meals	
11. Have patient position his head in the midline and forward, chin pointed toward chest.	11. Improves ability to consciously swallow without food falling down the posterior pharynx. Support patient's forehead with a hand if the patient lacks neck control.
12. Instruct the patient to smell the food before each bite; hold each bite for a few seconds; hold lips together firmly; concentrate on swallowing; then swallow.	12. Concentrating on each step before swallowing will increase the effectiveness of the swallow.
13. If the patient has an increase in saliva during the meal, instruct the patient to collect the saliva with the tongue and consciously swallow it between bites throughout the meal.	13. This will help prevent aspiration of saliva between mouthfuls.
14. If the patient complains of a dry mouth during meals, instruct the patient to move the tongue in a circular fashion against the insides of the cheeks.	14. This will help stimulate salivation.
15. Caution the patient against talking during the meal or with the mouth full of food.	15. Talking or laughing during eating is a common cause of airway obstruction.

Procedure (continued)	**Nursing Action**	**Rationale/Amplification**

Follow-up Care

16. Provide mouth care after meals.
17. Record the amount of intake, the patient's taste and food preferences, his progress, and any special tactics that were effective in helping the swallowing process.
18. Encourage family members to participate in the patient's feeding program.

16. Food particles may collect in the mouth or cheeks.
17. Progress notes will assist in moving toward self-care.

18. This will help provide continuity on discharge.

Feeding the Patient With an Affected Side of the Mouth (Facial Paralysis, Hemiplegia)

1. Turn the patient to the unaffected side.

2. Place food on the unaffected side of mouth rather than in the middle of the mouth.
3. Encourage the patient to form a bolus by moving the food around the mouth with the tongue.

1. This helps prevent food from falling down the weaker/paralyzed part of the oral cavity, a possible cause of aspiration.
2. Permits food to be managed more effectively.

3. This assists in placing food in a proper position for swallowing, rather than permitting food to collect near the cheek.

Guidelines ## Esophageal Dilatation With a Balloon-Tipped Catheter

Esophageal dilatation is the introduction of a balloon-tipped catheter into the esophagus. The balloon is inflated across the gastroesophageal sphincter to relieve stricture.

Equipment
Esophageal dilatation balloon-tipped catheters of various sizes
Guide wire or endoscope
Suctioning equipment

Procedure **Preparation**

1. Explain procedure to the patient; explain that some discomfort will be experienced, but that he will be given medication to control the pain.
2. Nothing is given by mouth after midnight prior to the treatment.
3. Medications are prescribed prior to treatment, usually meperidine (Demerol), atropine, and often diazepam (Valium).
4. A local anesthetic, throat spray, or gargle, is used to anesthetize the throat. General anesthesia with endotracheal intubation may be required for difficult strictures or in children.
5. Procedure is done with fluoroscopic control.

Medical Action	**Rational/Amplification/Nursing Support**

1. Place the patient in sitting position.
2. Balloon catheter is passed over a guide wire and positioned to straddle the stricture.
3. Balloon is inflated, gradually increasing the pressure, until the indentation produced by the stricture disappears. The balloon may be left inflated for 3–10 minutes.

1. Prevents aspiration
2. Done under fluoroscopic control

3. The patient may experience moderate to moderately severe pain. The nurse should observe the patient's response and provide support.

(Procedure may be repeated every few days when dilatation is incomplete or the stricture recurs.)

Nursing Action	**Rationale/Amplification**

Follow-up Phase

1. Continue to keep the patient in a fasting state.

2. Monitor vital signs frequently.

3. When the patient can take a few sips of water without choking or coughing, an esophagogram, using a water-soluble contrast medium, is performed.
4. Advance diet as tolerated.

1. To prevent aspiration prior to the return of the swallowing and gag reflexes
2. Observe for signs and symptoms that may indicate complications: pain; difficulty breathing; bleeding.
3. To rule out rupture or perforation of the esophagus

Esophageal Diverticulum

An *esophageal diverticulum* is an outpouching of the esophageal wall, usually in the cervical, posterior side, secondary to an obstructive or inflammatory process.

Types

1. Pharyngoesophageal (pulsion)—also called Zenker's diverticulum; upper end of esophagus protrudes through cricopharyngeal muscle.
2. Midesophageal (traction)—near tracheal bifurcation
3. Epiphrenic (traction–pulsion)—lower third of esophagus.

Clinical Manifestations

A. Pharyngoesophageal

1. Difficulty in swallowing, fullness in neck, a feeling that food stops before it reaches the stomach, and regurgitation of undigested food
2. Belching, gurgling, or nocturnal coughing brought about by diverticulum becoming filled with food or liquid, which is regurgitated and may irritate the trachea.
3. Halitosis and foul taste in mouth caused by food decomposing in a pouch (diverticulum).
4. Hoarseness, asthma, and pneumonitis may be the only signs in the very elderly.
5. Weight loss due to nutritional depletion

B. Midesophageal

1. Generally no symptoms
2. May experience mild retrosternal chest pain

C. Epiphrenic

At times associated with achalasia or diffuse esophageal spasm.

Diagnostic Evaluation

1. Roentgenograms using barium—to visualize esophagus and diverticulum.
2. Esophagoscopy is risky, because of danger of perforation of diverticulum, which may lead to mediastinitis.
3. Esophageal motility studies, cineradiography, and esophageal radionuclide scintigraphy—to determine underlying motility disorder.

Management

A. Pharyngoesophageal

1. Small diverticula may not be treated while the underlying cause is treated with dilatation or myotomy.
2. A transverse cervical diverticulectomy or diverticuloplexy with suspension and cricopharyngeal myotomy may be done.
   a. Caution is taken to avoid injury to common carotid artery and internal jugular vein.
   b. Sac is dissected free and then excised flush with esophageal wall.

B. Midesophageal

Therapy is usually not required because of absence of symptoms and rareness of complications.

C. Epiphrenic

1. Underlying primary condition must be treated.
2. Concomitant surgical resection of the diverticulum prevents further complications.

Complications

1. Aspiration pneumonia
2. Malnutrition

Nursing Interventions

A. Assessing and Preventing Complications

1. Preoperatively, or if the condition is nonoperative, implement nursing interventions similar to those for esophageal reflux or dysphagia (see p. 425).
2. Postoperatively, wound care is similar to that of other surgical incisions of the same anatomic position, i.e., thoracotomy or neck surgery.

B. Maintaining Adequate Nutritional Status

1. If a nasogastric tube is in place, institute nasogastric feedings using fluids.
   a. Irrigate tube carefully with water following each feeding.
   b. Record kind and amount of irrigating fluid.
2. Prepare the patient the morning after surgery for x-ray following ingestion of diatrizoate meglumine (Gastrografin) and diatrizoate sodium solution, or barium, to detect any leakage at mucosal closure site. If no leakage occurs, liquid diet is started, with diet increased to regular in the next 72 hours.

Esophageal Varices

See page 516.

Cancer of the Esophagus

Incidence and Clinical Features

1. Four types of esophageal carcinomas occur worldwide: squamous cell; adenocarcinoma; carcinosarcoma; and sarcoma.
2. Incidence of adenocarcinoma of the distal and middle third of the esophagus appears to be increasing in the Western world.
3. Squamous cell carcinoma, most often originating in the upper half of the esophagus, appears to have an equal incidence as adenocarcinoma.
4. Highest rate in the US. occurs in men, who are usually past the age of 60; more common in nonwhite males.

Risk Factors

Causative factors have not been proven; appears that Barrett's esophagus, linked to achalasia, may be a premalignant condition of the esophagus.

1. Chronic trauma—excessive use of alcohol, tobacco, spicy foods, hot liquid (tea) ingestion.
2. Alcohol consumption and smoking.
3. Genetic predisposition—nonwhite male population.
4. Lye ingestion.

Clinical Manifestations

1. Dysphagia is the usual presenting symptom, although it is a late sign by which time there often is regional or systemic involvement.
2. Mild atypical chest pain associated with eating precedes dysphagia, but is rarely significant enough for the patient to seek health care.
3. Pain on swallowing (odynophagia).

4. Possible hemorrhage—usually only occult bleeding.
5. Progressive weight loss.
6. Later symptoms—hiccup, respiratory difficulty, foul breath, regurgitation of food and saliva.

Diagnostic Evaluation

1. Brush cytology
2. Endoscopy—inspection, photography, and biopsy
3. Barium swallow; air contrast studies of esophagus
   A piece of bread or a marshmallow coated with barium may serve as a radiopaque bolus to locate the lesion.
4. Cineradiography
5. Computed tomography (CT) may be helpful in delineating the extent of the tumor, as well as in identifying presence of adjacent tissue invasion, and metastases.

Management

1. The goal of treatment may be cure or palliation, depending on the staging of the tumor and the patient's overall condition in relation to nutritional, cardiovascular, pulmonary, and functional status.
2. The wide variability in treatment reflects the overall poor results from any one approach.
3. Surgery
   a. Lesions of the middle and lower esophagus are excised via thoracotomy approach with esophagogastrectomy or colon interposition (A section of colon is used to replace the excised portion of the esophagus.).
   b. Lesions of the cervical esophagus are excised with a bilateral neck dissection and esophagogastrectomy; laryngectomy and thyroidectomy may be necessary.
   c. A two-step approach may be selected when resection with a cervical esophagostomy and feeding gastrostomy are performed initially; subsequent reconstructive surgery is carried out.
4. Additional procedures to improve the efficacy of surgery include radiation, chemotherapy, or their combination preoperatively and postoperatively.
5. The goal of palliative treatment is to reduce the complications of the tumor to improve quality of life. Any one or a combination of the aforementioned therapies can be used for palliative treatment.

Complications

1. Preoperatively: malnutrition; aspiration pneumonitis; hemorrhage; sepsis; tracheoesophageal fistula
2. Postoperatively: dumping syndrome; nutritional deficiencies; reflux esophagitis; anastomosis leakage

Preoperative Nursing Interventions

A. Monitoring and Preventing Complications

1. Promote the patient's nutritional status with a diet high in calories, vitamins, and protein. This may be by mouth, intravenous infusion, or hyperalimentation.
2. Place patient in semi-Fowler's position for feeding to avoid aspiration.
3. A nasogastric tube may be inserted prior to surgery.
4. Administer preoperative antibiotics as prescribed.

Postoperative Nursing Interventions

A. Monitoring for Complications

1. Monitor blood pressure, pulse, respiration, and temperature to note early onset of hemorrhage, infection, dysrhythmias, aspiration, or anastomosis leakage.
2. Observe drainage from incision and/or chest tube for bleeding or purulence.
3. Administer oxygen as prescribed.

B. Improving Nutritional and Fluid Status

1. Administer IV fluids as prescribed; initially the patient may require large volumes if extensive excision of lymph nodes was performed.
2. Assess for bowel sounds; administer fluids per nasogastric tube, as prescribed.
3. Encourage patient in advancing diet from liquids to soft foods after barium swallow indicates absence of anastomosis leakage.
4. Remind patient to remain in upright position after eating.

Discharge Planning/Patient Education

1. Encourage the patient to avoid overeating, take small bites, chew food well; avoid chunks of meat and stringy raw vegetables and fruit.
2. Encourage rest postoperatively, advancing activities as tolerated.

Bibliography

Books

Conditions of the Mouth and Esophagus

Brunner SL and Suddarth DS. Textbook of Medical–Surgical Nursing. 6th ed. Philadelphia, JB Lippincott, 1988

Friedman MH and Weisberg J. Temporomandibular Joint Disorders: Diagnosis and Treatment. Chicago, Quintessence Publishing, 1985

Hathaway RG. Nursing Care of the Critically Ill Surgical Patient. Rockville, MD, Aspen Publishers, Inc, 1988

Hill L et al. The Esophagus: Medical and Surgical Management. Philadelphia, WB Saunders, 1988

Kinney MR, Packa DR and Dunbar SB. AACN's Clinical Reference for Critical Care Nursing. 2nd ed. New York, McGraw–Hill, 1988

Okeson JP. Management of Temporomandibular Disorders and Occlusion. 2nd ed. St. Louis, CV Mosby, 1989

Regezi J and Scuibba J. Oral Pathology: Clinical–Pathologic Correlations. Philadelphia, WB Saunders, 1989

Skinner DB and Belsey RHR. Management of Esophageal Disease. Philadelphia, WB Saunders, 1988

Journals

Conditions of the Mouth

Bare VL. Temporomandibular joint arthroscopy. AORN J 1987 Jun; 45(6): 1368–1373

Blaney GM. Mouth care—Basic and essential. Geriatr Nurs 1986 Sep–Oct; 7(5):242–243

Blitzer A et al. Surgical management of aspiration. Otolaryngol Clin North Am 1988 Nov; 21(4):743–750

Campbell S. Mouth care in cancer patients. Nurs Times 1987 Jul; 83(29): 59–60

Danielson KH. Oral care and older adults. J Gerontol Nurs 1988 Nov; 14(11):6–10

DeConno F et al. Oral complications in patients with advanced cancer. J Pain Symptom Manage 1989 Mar; 4(1):20–30

Dibbets JMH and van der Weele LT. Prevalence of TMJ symptoms and x-ray findings. Eur J Orthod 1989 Feb; 11(1):31–36

Eilers J, Berger AM and Petersen MC. Development, testing, and application of the oral assessment guide. Oncol Nurs Forum 1988 May–Jun; 15(3):325–330

Epstein JB. Oral and pharyngeal candidiasis. Postgrad Med 1989 Apr; 85(5):257–258, 263–265, 268–269

Frank–Stromborg M. The role of the nurse in cancer detection and screening. Semin Oncol Nurs 1986 Aug; 2(3):191–199

Gale EN and Dixon DC. A simplified psychologic questionnaire as a treatment planning aid for patients with temporomandibular joint disorders. J Prosthet Dent 1989 Feb; 61(2):235–238

Gardner SS. Oral assessment. SGA J 1988 Winter; 11(3):161–165

Gerold KB. Special problems in posttrauma respiratory management: Maxillofacial, head, and chest injuries. Crit Care Nurs Q 1988 Sep; 11(2):59–62

Gordon SR and Jahnigen DW. Oral assessment of the edentulous elderly patient. J Am Geriatr Soc 1986 Apr; 34(4):276–281

Hay KD. Candidosis of the oral cavity: Recognition and management. Drugs 1988 Nov; 36(5):633–642

Herrera JL, Lyons MF and Johnson LF. Saliva: Its role in health and disease. J Clin Gastroenterol 1988 Oct; 10(5):569–578

Logemann JA. Swallowing physiology and pathophysiology. Otolaryngol Clin North Am 1988 Nov; 21(4):613–623

Lower J. Maxillofacial trauma. Nurs Clin North Am 1986 Dec; 21(4):611–628

Lundeen TF, George JM and Sturdevant JR. Stress in patients with pain in the muscles of mastication and the temporomandibular joints. J Oral Rehabil 1988 Nov; 15(6):631–637

Mashberg A and Samit AM. Early detection, diagnosis, and management of oral and oropharyngeal cancer. CA 1989 Mar–Apr; 39(2):67–88

Miller R and Rubinstein L. Oral health care for hospitalized patients: The nurse's role. J Nurs Educ 1987 Nov; 26(9):362–366

Pople J and Oliver D. Oral thrush in hospice patients. Nurs Times 1986 Nov; 82(45):34–35

Salazar M. Conquering cancer: Primary prevention and early detection. Am Assoc Occup Health Nurs J 1988 Aug; 36(8):303–313

Samaranayake LP. Nutritional factors and oral candidosis. J Oral Pathol 1986 Feb; 15(2):61–65

Schulmeister L. Join the fight against oral cancer. Nursing 1987 May; 17(5):66–67

Silverman S. Prevention, early detection and diagnosis of oral cancer. Dermatol Clin 1987 Oct; 5(4):675–680

Smith SD. Diagnosis and treatment of temporomandibular joint disorders. J Pain Symptom Manage 1987 Summer; 2(3):155–162

Suvine T and Reade P. Prognostic features of value in the management of temporomandibular joint pain–dysfunction syndrome by occlusal splint therapy. J Prosthet Dent 1989 Mar; 61(3):355–361

Vallerand AH, Russin MM and Vallerand WP. Taking the bite out of TMJ syndrome. AJN 1989 May; 89(5):688–690

Swallowing

Bruckstein AH. Dysphagia. Am Fam Physician 1989 Jan; 39(1):147–156

Buchin PJ. Swallowing disorders: Diagnosis and medical treatment. Otolaryngol Clin North Am 1988 Nov; 21(4):663–676

Campbell–Taylor I and Fisher RH. The clinical case against tube feeding in palliative care of the elderly. J Am Geriatr Soc 1987 Dec; 35(12):1100–1104

Carr EK and Hawthorn PJ. Lip function and eating after a stroke: A nursing perspective. J Adv Nurs 1988 Jul; 13(4):447–451

Choksi AJ, Dimery IW and Hong WK. Oral cancers, other head and neck tumors: Pitfalls and controversies in diagnosis and treatment. Consultant 1988 Aug; 28(8):100–102, 106–108

DiIorio C and Price ME. Swallowing: An assessment guide. Am J Nurs 1990 Jul; 90(7):38–41

Larson DL. Management of complications of radiotherapy of the head and neck. Surg Clin North Am 1986 Feb; 66(1):169–182

Merlo A and Cohen S. Swallowing disorders. Annu Rev Med 1988; 39:17–28

Price ME and DiIorio C. Swallowing: A practice guide. Am J Nurs 1990 Jul; 90(7):42–46

Prin J. New techniques in head and neck reconstruction . . . new nursing challenges. Plast Surg Nurs 1986 Spring; 6(1):21–23, 26

Prout MN. Early detection of head and neck cancer. Hosp Pract 1987 Nov; 22(11):111–112, 114, 118

Snow JB. Surgical management of head and neck cancer. Semin Oncol 1988 Feb; 15(1):20–28

Sonies BC and Baum BJ. Evaluation of swallowing pathophysiology. Otolaryngol Clin North Am 1988 Nov; 21(4):637–648

Esophagus

Ajani JA and Jackson DE. Gastric and esophageal cancers: Pitfalls and controversies in diagnosis and treatment. Consultant 1988 Dec; 28(12):93–96, 109

Backer CL and LoCicero J. Surgical management of esophageal disorders. Crit Care Q 1986; 9(3):12–19

Castell DO. Medical therapy for reflux esophagitis: 1986 and beyond. Ann Intern Med 1986 Jan; 104(1):112–114

Castell DO. Future medical therapy of reflux esophagitis. J Clin Gastroenterol 1986; 8(suppl 1):81–85

Crump WJ. Reflux esophagitis: Diagnosis,

pathophysiology, and management. Primary Care 1988 Mar; 15(1):13–30

DiPalma JA and Meyer GW. A rational clinical approach to esophageal motor disorders. Dysphagia 1987; 2(2):97–108

Evander A et al. Diverticula of the mid- and lower esophagus: Pathogenesis and surgical management. World J Surg 1986 Oct; 10(5):820–828

Feldman M. Southwestern Internal Medicine Conference: Esophageal achalasia syndromes. Am J Med Sci 1988 Jan; 295(1):60–81

Ferguson MK, Little AG and Skinner DB. Barrett's esophagus. Adv Surg 1987; 21:127–155

Gelfand MD and Botoman VA. Esophageal motility disorders: A clinical overview. Am J Gastroenterol 1987 Mar; 82(3):181–187

Goff JS. Infectious causes of esophagitis. Annu Rev Med 1988; 39:163–169

Goldsmith S and Juergen NH. Cancer of the esophagus. Hosp Med 1988 May; 24(5):148–165

Hawkins DB. Dilation of esophageal strictures: Comparative morbidity of antegrade and retrograde methods. Ann Otol Rhinol Laryngol 1988 Sep–Oct; 97(5 Pt. 1):460–465

Hill JW and Deluca SA. Achalasia. Am Fam Physician 1988 Mar; 37(3):201–203

Lieberman DA. Pathophysiology and management of reflux esophagitis. Compr Ther 1989 Feb; 15(2):36–41

Little AG and Skinner DB. Treatment of motility abnormalities of the esophagus. Adv Surg 1987; 20:265–277

Maran AGD, Wilson JA and Al Muhanna AH. Pharyngeal diverticula. Clin Otolaryngol 1986 Aug; 11(4):219–225

McCallum RW. The spectrum of esophageal motility disorders. Hosp Pract 1987 Dec; 22(12):71–83

Medvec BR. Esophageal cancer: Treatment and nursing interventions. Semin Oncol Nurs 1988 Nov; 4(4):246–256

Mold JW and Rankin RA. Symptomatic gastroesophageal reflux in the elderly. J Am Geriatr Soc 1987 Jul; 35(7):649–659

Kelsen DP, Hilaris B and Martini N. Neoadjuvant chemotherapy and surgery of cancer of the esophagus. Am J Gastroenterol 1988 Aug; 83(8):816–819

Nagrani M et al. Primary non-Hodgkin's lymphoma of the esophagus. Arch Intern Med 1989 Jan; 149(1):193–195

Ott DJ. Radiologic evaluation of esophageal dysphagia. Curr Probl Diagn Radiol 1988 Jan–Feb; 17(1):1–33

Pate JW. Tracheobronchial and esophageal injuries. Surg Clin North Am 1989 Feb; 69(1):111–123

Relief for gastroesophageal reflux. Patient Care 1987 Jul 15; 21(12):199–200

Peters LJ and Castell DO. Motility disorders of the esophagus. Compr Ther 1988 Jan; 14(1):19–23

Phaosawasdi K, Rice P and Lee B. Primary and secondary *Candida* esophagitis. IMJ 1986 Jun; 169(6):361–365

Reeders JWAJ and Tio TL. Diagnosis and preoperative staging of oesophageal malignancies. Baillieres Clin Gastroenterol 1987 Oct; 1(4):869–892

Robertson CS et al. Choice of therapy for achalasia in relation to age. Digestion 1988; Aug 40(4):244–250

Scarpignato C. Pharmacological bases of the medical treatment of gastroesophageal reflux disease. Dig Dis 1988; 6(3):117–148

Slaughter RL. The disabled esophagus. Emerg Med 1988 Sep 15; 20(15):99–102, 107–108

Sons HU. Etiologic and epidemiologic factors of carcinoma of the esophagus. Surg Gynecol Obstet 1987 Aug; 165(2):183–190

Spechler SJ and Goyal RK. Barrett's esophagus. N Engl J Med 1986 Aug; 315(6):362–371

Taylor RB. Esophageal foreign bodies. Emerg Med Clin North Am 1987 May; 5(2):301–311

Walsh TJ, Belitsos NJ and Hamilton SR. Bacterial esophagitis in immunocompromised patients. Arch Intern Med 1986 Jul; 146(7):1345–1358

Walsh TJ, Hamilton SR and Belitsos NJ. Esophageal candidiasis: Managing an increasingly prevalent infection. Postgrad Med 1988 Aug; 84(2):193–196, 201–205

Waterfall WE, Craven MA and Allen CJ. Gastroesophageal reflux: Clinical presentations, diagnosis and management. Can Med Assoc J 1986 Nov; 135(10):1101–1109

Westdorp ICE. Reflux oesophagitis: A review. Postgrad Med J 1986; 62(Suppl 2):43–55

Willis BL, Thompson LF and Howard JC. Esophageal perforation: A nursing diagnosis approach. Crit Care Nurs 1988 Jul–Aug; 8(5):20–30

19

Nutritional Assessment, Selected Problems, and Special Nutritional Management

Nutritional Assessment

Underlying Principles

1. Nutrition influences all body systems either favorably or unfavorably.
2. The nurse works cooperatively with the dietitian to teach the patient to select meals rich in the products that aid body maintenance, supply energy, repair tissues, aid in growth and development, and promote weight gain or loss, depending on the circumstances.
3. The four food groups—milk (milk and milk products), meat (meat, poultry, eggs, fish, dried beans, and peas), fruit and vegetables, and grain (cereals, breads and crackers) act as the *basis* for an adequate diet.
4. The calorie intake and the number of vitamins, proteins, carbohydrates, fats, and minerals also play an important role in providing appropriate nutrition.
5. Nutritional needs change in response to metabolic changes, age, sex, growth periods, stress (trauma, disease, pregnancy, lactation, increasing age), and physical condition.
6. Dietary supplements may be necessary in some instances.
7. See Appendix for Recommended Daily Dietary Allowances.

Nutritional Questionnaire

A. General Background Information

1. Name, age, sex, family, socioeconomic status, occupation
2. General health status. Any dietary restrictions (past and present)?
3. What cultural heritage/religious heritage factors influence eating habits?
4. Do you or anyone in your immediate family have diabetes?
5. Is anyone in your family obese?
6. Do you have any chronic illnesses? Describe.
7. List the medications taken.

B. Food Habits

1. What, if any, food fads?
2. How many meals and what time of day are these meals?
3. Describe a typical meal. Where eaten?
4. What foods are served most frequently?
5. Do you snack? How often? Describe.
6. How much alcohol do you drink? How often?
7. Describe all food and beverages you have consumed in the past 24 hours. Include amounts and how prepared.
8. What are your food likes? Dislikes?
9. Do you take any food supplements? Vitamins? Nutritional drinks?

C. Food Purchase and Preparation

1. Who purchases and prepares the food? Where is food purchased? How often?
2. What factors influence the kinds of food purchased?
3. Describe the facilities for food storage and preparation.

D. Nutritionally Related Problems

1. Have you lost or gained weight in the last month? How much? Intentional or unintentional?
2. Any food allergies? Describe the reaction.
3. Do you have problems chewing? Swallowing? Wear dentures?
4. Have you experienced any of the following gastrointestinal disturbances?
   a. Any change in sense of taste or smell? Unusual belching, eructations, flatus? How often?
   b. Loss of energy? Weakness? Change in muscle size?
   c. Abdominal pain? Describe onset, duration, location. Any changes in bowel habits? Constipation? Diarrhea?
   d. How are the above symptoms related to eating? How often do they occur?
   e. Do certain foods cause problems?

Food Intake Record (Calorie Counts)

1. Determine the amount of calories, protein, fats, and carbohydrates and other nutrients the patient is ingesting by keeping a food intake record.
2. Compare this record with the patient's calculated nutritional requirements. See Recommended Daily Dietary Allowances, Appendix III.
3. This is useful in determining the need for hyperalimentation, enteral feedings, or oral nutritional supplements.

Anthropometric Measurements

Anthropometry comes from the word anthropology and is the science that studies the size, weight, and proportions of the human body. These measurements are useful in determining nutritional status.

1. Height and weight—are determined on patient admission and later used as a baseline for comparisons in nutritional status.
   a. Height is the distance from the patient's feet to the top of the head.
   b. Weight is the measure of total body energy stores. See Table 19-1.
2. Skinfold thickness tests—provide information on the subcutaneous tissues and the amount of body fat.
   a. Triceps skinfold test: at the midpoint of the upper arm, grasp the skin and place the caliper over the skinfold (Fig. 19-1); the caliper jaws come toward one another when the pressure is released and the measurement is made. Do three readings and average them.
   b. Biceps skinfold test: lift the skinfold of the anterior aspect of the upper arm and follow the directions described above.
   c. Subscapularskinfold test: the skin is lifted under the inferior angle of the scapula and the measurement is taken with the calipers.
3. Circumferential tests—provide information on the amount of skeletal muscle and adipose tissue.
   a. Midarm circumference test—locate the midpoint of the patient's upper arm, using a tape measure, measure the circumference of this point.
   b. The midarm muscle circumference is calculated by multiplying the result of the triceps skinfold test (TSF) by 3.143 and subtracting this figure from the midarm circumference. (Adult standards are 16.5 mm. for women and 12.5 mm. for men)

Note: Keep in mind that edema will destroy the test results.

Selected Problems in Clinical Nutrition
Obesity

Obesity is usually defined as an overabundance of body fat, resulting in body weight 20%–30% over the average weight for the person's age, height, sex, and body frame. Contributing factors to obesity may include heredity, social pressures, psychological responses to stress, exercise level, and hormonal effects.

Types of Obesity

1. *Hyperplastic Obesity:* occurs in the first years of life through adolescence, resulting in an increase in the number and size of the fat cells.
2. *Hypertrophic Obesity:* occurs in adulthood and results in an increase in the size of the fat cells, but not in the number of the fat cells.
3. Exogenous—caused by excess calorie intake.
4. Endogenous—caused by a metabolic disorder

Clinical Manifestations

Body weight 20%–30% greater than normal.

Diagnostic Evaluation

1. Weight and height measurements
2. Body frame size
3. Skinfold measurements
4. Triceps skinfold measurement

Management

A. General Measures

1. Decreasing daily food intake, while increasing activity level. This will reduce the patient's weight so the adipose cells will have a normal (fat) lipid content.
2. Provision of a balanced, low-calorie diet containing few if any foods high in fats and sugars. Protein-sparing, modified fasting diets in which the patient eats 1–1.5 gm. protein/kg body weight per day are effective.
3. Teaching long-term modification of eating habits. (The low-carbohydrate diets offer no long-term weight reduction; remember rapid weight reduction is due to loss of water, not fat.)
4. Monitoring for signs of ketonemia, electrolyte imbalances, hypotension, and loss of lean body mass.
5. Hypnosis, behavior modification, and psychotherapy increase the patient's awareness and redirect behavior.

Table 19-1. *Height–Weight Tables*

Men					**Women**					
Height		*Small Frame*	*Medium Frame*	*Large Frame*	*Height*		*Small Frame*	*Medium Frame*	*Large Frame*	
Feet	*Inches*				*Feet*	*Inches*				
5	2	128–134	131–141	138–150	4	10	102–111	109–121	118–131	
5	3	130–136	133–143	140–153	4	11	103–113	111–123	120–134	
5	4	132–138	135–145	142–156	5	0	104–115	113–126	122–137	
5	5	134–140	137–148	144–160	5	1	106–118	115–129	125–140	
5	6	136–142	139–151	146–164	5	2	108–121	118–132	128–143	
5	7	138–145	142–154	149–168	5	3	111–124	121–135	131–147	
5	8	140–148	145–157	152–172	5	4	114–127	124–138	134–151	
5	9	142–151	148–160	155–176	5	5	117–130	127–141	137–155	
5	10	144–154	151–163	158–180	5	6	120–133	130–144	140–159	
5	11	146–157	154–166	161–184	5	7	123–136	133–147	143–163	
6	0	149–160	157–170	164–188	5	8	126–139	136–150	146–167	
6	1	152–164	160–174	168–192	5	9	129–142	139–153	149–170	
6	2	155–168	164–178	172–197	5	10	132–145	142–156	152–173	
6	3	158–172	167–182	176–202	5	11	135–148	145–159	155–176	
6	4	162–176	171–187	181–207	6	0	138–151	148–162	158–179	

Weight according to frame (ages 25–59) for men wearing indoor clothing weighing 5 lbs., shoes with 1-in. heels; for women, indoor clothing weighing 3 lbs., shoes with 1-in. heels.

(Courtesy Metropolitan Life Insurance Company)

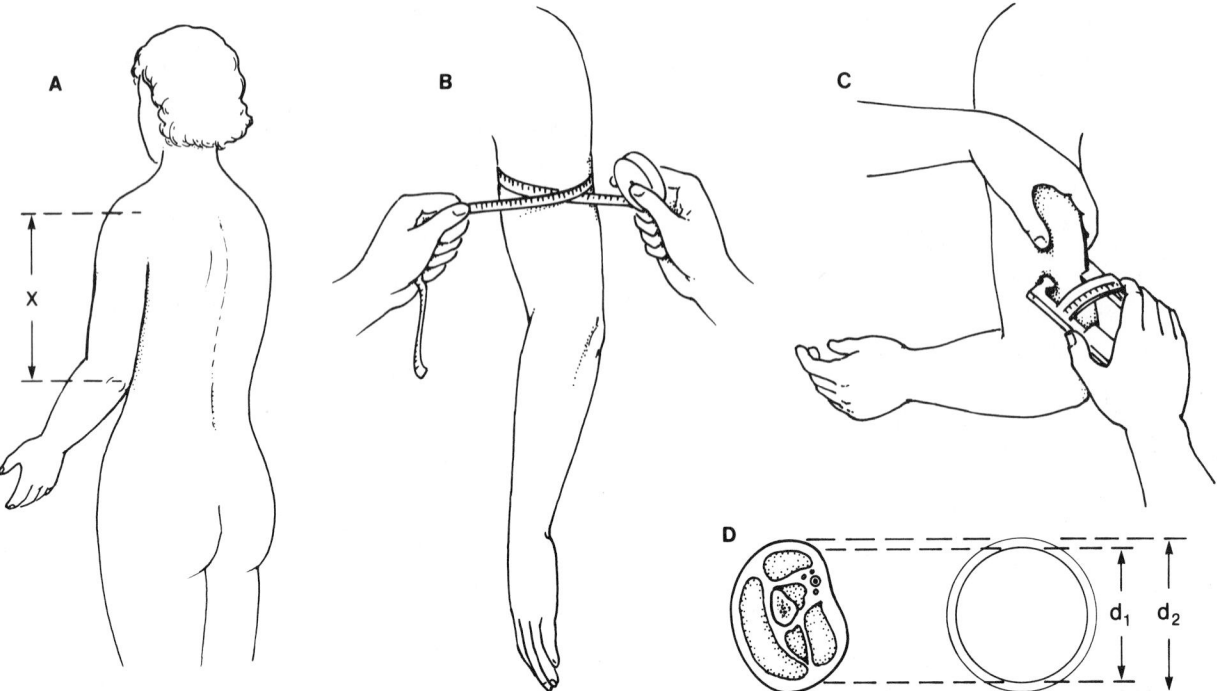

Figure 19-1. *Anthropometric measurements. Proper positioning of the patient is required: (A) for measuring the mid-upper arm, (B) to determine mid-arm circumference (AC); this position is also used to measure (C) the triceps skinfold (TSF) thickness which is measured with a caliper; (D) shows the relation between d_1 (AMC—arm muscle circumference) and d_2 (AC—arm circumference). Arm muscle circumference is a significant measurement in determining protein–calorie malnutrition. Formula for calculation: $AMC = AC - (0.314 \times TSF)$. (Adapted from Blackburn GL and Harvey KB. Nutritional assessment as a routine in clinical medicine. Postgrad Med 1982 May; 71(5):51)*

6. Appetite suppressants; however, use for long-term weight reduction is questionable, as they are habit forming.

B. Surgical Measures

1. Intestinal bypass operations
   a. Approximately 30–36 cm. of the jejunum is anastomosed to the ileum proximal to the ileocecal valve.
   b. These operations have fallen into disfavor due to their complications.
2. Gastric operations (Gastric partition, Gastroplasty)
   a. Stomach is partitioned, creating a small reservoir that empties into the larger distal portion of the stomach through a small channel
   b. Results in early satiety, and nausea and vomiting when overeating occurs.
3. Gastric balloon implantation (Garren Edwards gastric balloon)
   a. An inflated balloon is placed in the stomach via an orogastric feeding tube
   b. Reduces the space available for food.

Complications

1. Prolonged fasting or liquid protein diets have been associated with sudden death from cardiac dysrhythmias related to electrolyte imbalances.
2. Vitamin and nutrient deficiencies.
3. Gastric bypass complications: malnutrition, pancreatitis, electrolyte imbalances, gallstones, urinary calculi, and arthritis.

4. Garren Edwards gastric bubble complications: stomach perforation and ulceration and intestinal blockage.

Nursing Assessment

1. Obtain information on eating patterns, habits. See questionnaire for Nutritional Assessment, page 436.
2. Review past medical history for metabolic disorders, hereditary factors, and psychological factors.
3. Establish time of onset of obesity.
4. Monitor the following—daily weight; intake and output; calorie, protein, carbohydrate, fat, and nutrients in the diet; electrolytes; electrocardiogram abnormalities; vital signs—especially the blood pressure (watch for hypotension); activity level.

Nursing Diagnoses

1. Altered nutrition (more than body requirements) related to excessive intake of high-fat/high-calorie food, lack of exercise, psychosocial factors, and heredity.
2. Body image disturbance related to obesity.
3. Knowledge deficit of causes of obesity, nutrition, and effective eating habits.

Nursing Interventions

A. Achieving Normalization of Weight

1. Assess the patient's nutritional status, needs, food likes and dislikes.
2. Instruct the patient to weigh daily.
3. Measure and record intake of food and fluids.

4. Measure urinary output.
5. Review the patient's diet for the percentage of proteins, carbohydrates, fats, minerals, and nutrients.
6. Watch for signs of electrolyte imbalance (irregular pulse, cardiac dysrhythmias, muscle weakness, etc.).
7. Take blood pressure. Monitor for signs of hypotension.
8. Encourage increased physical activity to tolerance and cardiovascular status.

B. Enhancing Body Image

1. Encourage patient to ventilate feelings about body image, obesity, and eating habits.
2. Refer to support group: Weight Watchers, Overeaters Anonymous, Take Off Pounds Sensibly, etc.

Discharge Planning/Patient Education

Instruct the patient as follows:
1. Review the four food groups and the prescribed diet.
2. Identify the health hazards associated with obesity: diabetes, gallbladder disease, osteoarthritis, high blood pressure, stroke, shortness of breath, coronary artery disease, menstrual irregularities.
3. Weigh daily at the same time, with the same amount of clothing; record the weight.
4. Keep a record of what is eaten.
5. Avoid fad diets.
6. Expect a plateau period in which weight will not be lost for a period of time.
7. Take medications exactly as prescribed.
8. Monitor pulse; record any irregularities.
9. Report for follow-up health care as directed.

Evaluation

1. Continues to lose weight; free of electrolyte imbalances, vitamin or nutrient deficiencies.
2. Verbalizes a more positive self-concept.
3. Recalls the foods permitted on the prescribed diet.

Anorexia Nervosa

Anorexia nervosa is a disorder occurring most frequently in females between the stages of adolescence and young adulthood, in which the patient starves to the point of emaciation. The disease creates nutritional disorders. The cause of anorexia nervosa is not known, but it is presumed to be a disturbance in which the patient is preoccupied with being thin.

Clinical Manifestations

1. Excessive weight loss of 20% or more for no organic reason.
2. Intense fear of weight gain.
3. Emaciation, skeletal muscle atrophy, and loss of fatty tissue.
4. Excessive dieting and exercise.
5. Gorging, vomiting, purging, amenorrhea, lanugo (fine body hair), constipation, dental cavities, hypotension, and susceptibility to infections.
6. Self-administration of laxatives or diuretics without medical reason.

Diagnostic Evaluation

1. History of clinical signs or symptoms.
2. Loss of 20% of original body weight.
3. Studies to rule out malabsorption syndrome and malignancy.

4. Complete blood count (CBC), serum creatinine, BUN, uric acid, cholesterol, total protein, albumin, calcium, electrolyte panel, fasting blood glucose, liver function tests, urinalysis, and ECG.

Complications

1. Sudden death due to cardiac arrest from electrolyte imbalances.
2. Bradycardia, hypotension, decreased cardiac output, and dysrhythmias.
3. Amenorrhea, reduced bone mass, fluid abnormalities, increased liver enzymes, altered glucose, anemia, seizures, and dental cavities.

Management

1. Goal: Promote weight gain
   a. Treatment of complications requiring hospitalization (dysrhythmias, fluid and electrolyte imbalances).
   b. Dietary supplements such as Sustacal and Ensure orally, if able.
   c. Vitamin and nutrient supplements.
   d. Enteral feeding, if unable to take orally.
   e. Hyperalimentation may be necessary if patient is severely emaciated and dehydrated.
2. Behavior modification modalities
3. Psychotherapy and family therapy

Nursing Interventions

A. Promoting Weight Gain

1. Monitor weight daily before breakfast.
2. Monitor intake and output.
3. Offer small portions of food or drinks. (Nutritional drinks often work better because the anorectic patient often finds it difficult to choose between foods.)
4. If tube feedings or hyperalimentation are needed, explain these to the patient.
5. Discuss the patient's need for a balanced diet in a "matter of fact" tone.
6. Instruct the patient that edema and bloating may occur when eating is resumed. These will be temporary.

B. Maintaining Fluid Volume

1. Monitor fluids and electrolytes; report abnormal findings.
2. Watch for signs and symptoms of dehydration and electrolyte imbalance.
3. Monitor vital signs; watch for hypotension and bradycardia.

C. Enhancing Body Image

1. Encourage the patient to verbalize fears, feelings, and frustrations.
2. Facilitate and support recommendations made by psychotherapeutic personnel.
3. Advise family members to avoid discussing food with the patient.

Discharge Planning/Patient Education

Instruct the patient to:
1. Keep all appointments with both the physician and therapist.
2. Follow the prescribed diet.
3. Monitor weight (usually this is done by a person other than the patient).
4. Avoid laxatives and diuretics, which promote depen-

dency, diarrhea, constipation, and electrolyte disturbances.

5. Refer the patient and family to the Anorexia Nervosa and Associated Disorders Support Group.

Malabsorption Syndrome

Malabsorption occurs when there is inadequate absorption of nutrients (minerals and vitamins) from the intestinal tract. This can result in inadequate digestion and absorption of fats, carbohydrates, and proteins.

Causes

1. Small bowel disease
2. Enzyme deficiency.
3. Gastric or intestinal surface area loss
4. Injured vascular and lymphatic circulation
5. Antibiotics (neomycin)
6. Tropical sprue

Clinical Manifestations

1. Steatorrhea (excessive amount of fat in feces)
2. Anemia, weakness, fatigue
3. Diarrhea, abdominal distention, and flatulence occur because of impaired water and sodium absorption, unabsorbed fatty acids and bile salts, decreased carbohydrate absorption, and irritation from unabsorbed fatty acids.
4. Edema from protein depletion secondary to decreased absorption and intake
5. Malnutrition from decreased fat, carbohydrate, and protein absorption and calorie loss
6. Muscle wasting/atrophy from impaired protein metabolism, decreased protein absorption and intake, impaired protein synthesis, and increased protein loss
7. Muscle cramps and tetany occur due to decreased vitamin D and calcium levels.
8. Nitrogen imbalance from loss of protein
9. Dysrhythmias, muscle weakness, and flaccidity of muscles due to decreased potassium levels
10. Nocturia from delayed absorption and excretion of water

Diagnostic Evaluation

1. Fecal fat measurement detects steatorrhea in a 72-hour stool collection. Increased fecal fat in the stool indicates malabsorption.
2. D-xylose absorption—urine excretion of xylose after 5 hours; decreased excretion is indicative of malabsorption.
3. Biopsy of the small intestine differentiates malabsorption syndrome from small bowel disease.
4. Computed tomography, barium studies, and x-rays help to confirm the diagnosis.
5. Abnormal laboratory test results:
   a. Prothrombin time prolonged due to vitamin K malabsorption
   b. Serum cholesterol below normal due to decreased fat absorption and digestion
   c. Serum sodium, potassium, and chloride below normal due to electrolyte losses and diarrhea
   d. Serum calcium below normal due to vitamin D and amino acid malabsorption
   e. Serum protein and albumin below normal due to protein loss
   f. Serum vitamin A and carotene below normal due to bile salt deficiency and impaired fat absorption
   g. Altered blood coagulation due to vitamin K deficiency and decreased prothrombin level.

Management

1. Treatment of the cause (surgery, antibiotics)
2. Replacement of lost nutrients by oral, enteral, or parenteral means

Complications

1. Dehydration from lack of electrolyte absorption
2. Cardiac dysrhythmias from loss of potassium and other electrolytes
3. Anemia from lack of absorption of vitamin B_{12}, iron, and folic acid.
4. Blood clotting disorders due to decreased prothrombin levels and vitamin K deficiency

Nursing Interventions

A. Attending to Nutritional Needs

1. Provide a diet or supplement rich in carbohydrates, protein, fats, minerals, and vitamins if the patient is able to ingest food.
2. Encourage the patient to eat several smaller meals a day.
3. Monitor intake and output.

B. Achieving Normal Bowel Elimination

1. Monitor stools: number, character, consistency, color.
2. Monitor for abdominal distention.
3. Provide foods with bulk and restrict fluids and food that promote diarrhea.

C. Attaining and Maintaining Normal Fluid Volume

1. Fluid Volume Excess
   a. Monitor for edema.
   b. Ascultate lung sounds for crackles, rhonchi.
   c. Restrict fluids as prescribed; record intake and output.
2. Fluid Volume Deficit
   a. Watch the patient for signs and symptoms of dehydration—decreased skin turgor, muscle spasms, resting tachycardia, orthostatic hypotension, dry tongue, increased thirst, weight loss, oliguria, fever, and fatigue.
   b. Monitor the patient's vital signs. Watch for hypotension, increased and irregular pulse.
   c. Watch for signs and symptoms of electrolyte imbalance—nausea, vomiting, cardiac dysrhythmias, tremors and seizures, anorexia, malaise, weakness, and irregular pulse.
   d. Monitor laboratory electrolytes and report abnormalities.

D. Coping With Fatigue

1. Instruct the patient to rest before becoming too tired.
2. Monitor CBC results.
3. Encourage the patient to eat foods rich in iron and other nutrients.

Discharge Planning/Patient Education

1. Instruct the patient about malabsorption syndrome and what to expect.
2. Monitor stools—amount, type, consistency, color, and frequency.

3. Follow the prescribed diet—smaller meals, multiple times a day may be easier to digest.
4. Monitor pulse for irregularities and, if detected, call physician.
5. Weigh daily and chart weight.
6. Monitor for edema; call physician if any signs of shortness of breath.
7. Keep anal area clean and dry.
8. Keep all follow-up health care appointments to monitor progress and prevent complications.

Vitamin and Mineral Deficiencies

Vitamin Deficiencies

Vitamins are organic compounds found in natural foods and are needed for growth, reproduction, good health, and resistance to infection.
1. Types of vitamin deficiencies
   a. Fat-soluble
   b. Water-soluble
2. Vitamin requirements depend on activity, age, metabolic rate, excretion rate, absorption rate, and utilization.
3. Reasons for vitamin deficiency:
   a. Low intake
   b. Failure of absorption
   c. Liver disease—failure to store the vitamins or convert them to active vitamins

d. Increased demand or requirements (fever, pregnancy, lactation)
   e. Destruction or excretion in the GI tract by certain drugs (antibiotics)
   f. Lack of proper substance; certain amino acids need to be present for some vitamins to be effective.
4. See Table 19-2, below, for vitamin requirements, function, clinical manifestations, diagnostic evaluation, and management.

Mineral Deficiencies

1. Minerals are inorganic compounds occurring in nature.
2. Functions
   a. Form the hard parts of the body (bone, teeth, nails)
   b. Are essential components of all cells, respiratory pigments, and enzymes
   c. Regulate permeability of cell membranes and capillaries
   d. Regulate excitability of muscular and nervous tissue
   e. Essential for regulation of osmotic pressure
   f. Maintain proper acid–base balance
   g. Play a role in water metabolism
   h. Regulate blood volume
   i. Components of gland secretions
3. See Table 19-3 for mineral requirements and deficiency management.

Table 19-2. *Vitamin Requirements and Deficiency Management*

Vitamin, RDA Requirements	Function	Clinical Manifestations of Deficiency	Diagnostic Evaluation	Management
Vitamin A RDA: 4800–6000 IU Fat-soluble vitamin	1. Vitamin A is used by the body for tissue repair and maintenance. 2. Maintains normal epithelial tissues, especially those of the mucous membranes. 3. Plays a part in RNA synthesis and the production of rhodopsin (visual purple) for night vision. 4. Plays a role in tooth development and endocrine function (reproduction)	1. Bone growth is impaired 2. The patient is fatigued, loses appetite, has dry hair, blemishes, night blindness, itching and burning eyes, swelling and redness of lids, clouded cornea, rough and dry skin, teeth become soft, and the patient experiences sinus problems. 3. An infant with severe signs of vitamin A deficiency shows failure to thrive, dry skin, corneal changes, and apathy.	1. A dietary history with deficient vitamin A and ocular lesions. 2. Decreased carotene levels (less than 40 μg./1100 ml.) also suggest vitamin A deficiency. 3. Also serum levels of vitamin A below 20 μg./100 ml. suggest vitamin A deficiency.	1. Replacement therapy. 2. Good sources of vitamin A are fish, green and yellow fruits, green leafy vegetables, fish-liver oils (cod liver or halibut fish liver oil), yellow vegetables, and milk products. 3. Acute deficiency requires IM injections of aqueous vitamin A. 4. In patients with malabsorption of fat-soluble vitamins and patients with low dietary intake of vitamin A, IV supplements are required.
Vitamin B$_1$ (Thiamine) RDA: 1.0–1.5 mg. Water-soluble vitamin	1. Thiamine is important in the metabolism of carbohydrates. 2. Stimulates the appetite. 3. Promotes blood building, digestion, and HCl production, energy, growth, learning ability, pain inhibition, and muscle tone maintenance.	1. Appetite loss, constipation, dyspnea, fatigue, irritability, nervousness, memory loss, digestive problems, myocardial pain, numbness in hands and feet, pain and noise sensitivity. 2. Thiamine deficiency also causes an enlarged heart, palpitations, tachycardia, dyspnea, and circulatory collapse. Constipation and indigestion are common. 3. Alcoholics may develop cardiac beriberi with high-output congestive heart failure, neuropathy, and cerebral disturbances.	1. Thiamine serum levels drop less than 5 μg./100 ml. 2. Elevated levels of serum pyruvic and lactic acids occur, especially after exercise and the administration of glucose. 3. Low concentrations of thiamine in the urine. 4. Nonspecific changes in the ECG.	1. High protein diet with supplemental B complex vitamins. 2. Food sources rich in thiamine are molasses, brewer's yeast, poultry, wheat germ, brown rice, fish, eggs, meat, nuts, pork, peas, oatmeal, and liver.

(continued)

Table 19-2. *Vitamin Requirements and Deficiency Management (continued)*

Vitamin, RDA Requirements	Function	Clinical Manifestations of Deficiency	Diagnostic Evaluation	Management
B_2 (Riboflavin) RDA: 1.2–1.7 mg. Water-soluble vitamin	1. Helps to metabolize carbohydrates, fats, and proteins. 2. Assists in antibody and red blood cell formation 3. Aids in electron transport	1. Cracking of the mouth and lips, sore throat, cataracts, glossitis, dermatitis, burning, itching, light-sensitive eyes, tearing and vascularization of the corneas 2. Also neuropathy, anemia, and growth retardation occur in the late stages 3. The skin also becomes oily and the tongue develops redness and soreness.	1. Riboflavin levels drop to less than 2 μg./100 ml. 2. If the patient has a history of long periods of diarrhea, light sensitivity, and itching, burning, tearing eyes	1. Diet rich in foods that contain riboflavin: milk, meat, fish, green leafy vegetables, enriched flour, eggs, cereal. 2. Give patients with diarrhea riboflavin supplements. 3. Acute riboflavin deficiency requires daily oral doses of riboflavin alone or with other B-complex vitamins 4. Riboflavin supplements can also be given IV or IM.
B_6 (Pyridoxine) RDA: 2.0–2.2 mg.	1. Helps in the production of hydrochloric acid, antibody formation, RNA and DNA synthesis, hemoglobin production. 2. Maintenance of sodium and potassium balance in nerves, fat and protein utilization	1. Reddened lips and tongue, acne, depression, dizziness, hair loss, weakness, learning disabilities, irritability, dermatitis, abdominal pain, vomiting and CNS disturbances.	1. Elevated levels of xanthurenic acid indicate B_6 (pyridoxine) deficiency. 2. Decreased levels of serum and RBC transaminases. 3. Reduced excretion of pyridoxic acid in the urine	1. Provide foods rich in pyridoxine: bananas, molasses, brewer's yeast, fish, green leafy vegetables, meat, peanuts, raisins, walnuts, wheat germ, whole grains, liver, egg yolks. 2. Some women taking oral contraceptives may need to supplement their diets with pyridoxine.
B_{12} (Cyanocobalamin) RDA: 3.0 μg.	1. Aids in blood cell formation, iron absorption, the metabolism of proteins, fats, carbohydrates, neurological function, appetite stimulation 2. Functions in RNA and DNA synthesis and in erythrocyte formation	1. Pernicious anemia, memory impairment, confusion, depression, fatigue, weakness, nervousness, decreased reflex responses, walking and talking problems, demyelination of the large fibers of the spinal cord, anorexia, weight loss, yellowing of skin, abdominal pain, dyspnea, megaloblastic anemia, glossitis, peripheral neuropathy. 2. Also, anorexia, vomiting, and diarrhea 3. Bright red tongue 4. Cardiovascular changes; chest pain, and chronic congestive heart failure may be present.	1. Serum levels of B_{12} are less than 150 pg./ml. 2. Gastric analysis if used and hemoglobin studies 3. The Schilling test also measures absorption of radioactive B_{12}.	1. Parenteral B_{12} is given to patients with decreased gastric secretion of HCl, lack of intrinsic factor, some malabsorption syndromes or ileum resections. 2. Oral vitamin B_{12} is given to strict vegetarians 3. Parenteral B_{12} is given for 5–10 days, followed by monthly or daily B_{12} supplements. 4. Diet rich in foods containing B_{12}: beef, eggs, fish, organ meats, pork, milk products.
Biotin RDA: 100–200 μg.	1. Involved in lipid production and aids in cell growth. Also aids in the metabolism of fats, proteins, and carbohydrates. 2. Aids in the utilization of vitamin B.	1. Dry skin, fatigue, grayish skin color, muscle pain, depression, insomnia, and poor appetite.		1. Provide a diet rich in the foods that contain biotin—egg yolks, organ meats (liver, kidney), molasses, yeast, milk, grains, and nuts.
Folic acid RDA: 400 μg. Water-soluble vitamin	1. Stimulates the appetite. Aids in cell growth and reproduction. 2. Matures RBCs 3. Aids in hydrochloric acid production, DNA production, nucleic acid formation, liver function, and protein metabolism. 4. The coenzyme in amino acid metabolism, hematocrit and hemoglobin formation.	1. Graying of the hair, digestive problems, pallor, diarrhea, glossitis, megaloblastic anemia, growth problems, memory impairment, insomnia, and cardiac enlargement.	1. Serum value less than 100 mg./ml.	1. Provide with a diet rich in foods containing folic acid—citrus fruits, eggs, milk, vegetables, green leafy vegetables, milk products, organ meats, seafood, whole grains, yeast. 2. Folic acid is usually given as a nutritional supplement

(continued)

Table 19-2. *Vitamin Requirements and Deficiency Management (continued)*

Vitamin, RDA Requirements	Function	Clinical Manifestations of Deficiency	Diagnostic Evaluation	Management
Niacin RDA: 13–19 mg. Water-soluble vitamin	1. Aids the metabolism of carbohydrates, fats, and proteins. 2. Aids in the utilization of glucose for energy 3. Aids in cholesterol level reduction, hydrochloric acid production, tissue metabolism, and sex hormone production	1. Depression, fatigue, appetite loss, headaches, indigestion, muscle weakness, nervous disorders, nausea, insomnia, canker sores, dermatitis, diarrhea, reddened mouth, tongue and lips, confusion and disorientation, memory impairment	1. Serum niacin levels are less than 30 μg./100 ml. 2. Patient exhibits headaches, backaches, and sore mouth 3. Diminished or absent metabolites (in urine)	1. Provide patient with foods rich in niacin: eggs, lean meats, organ meats, poultry, seafood, milk products, peanuts, whole grains, enriched breads, brewer's yeast, fish, cereals. 2. Daily doses of niacinamide
Pantothenic acid RDA: 4–7 mg.	1. Pantothenic acids aid antibody formation 2. Conversion of carbohydrates, fats, and protein 3. Aids in cortisone production, growth stimulation, stress tolerance, vitamin utilization.	1. Diarrhea, hair loss, respiratory infections, nervousness, muscle cramps, premature aging, intestinal disorders, eczema, kidney problems		1. Provide patient with a diet rich in pantothenic acid; eggs, mushrooms, organ meats, salmon, wheat germ, whole grains.
Vitamin C (Ascorbic acid) RDA: 50–60 mg Water-soluble vitamin	1. Aids in healing of burns and wounds 2. Aids red blood cell formation, infection resistance, and vitamin protection 3. Aids in collagen production, digestion, iodine conservation, fine bone and tooth formation	1. Bleeding gums, tooth decay, nosebleeds, low infection resistance, dyspnea, bruising, swollen glands, pale, delayed wound and tissue healing, loose teeth, anemia, loss of appetite, pain in the joints—especially the knees, insomnia, weakness, ocular hemorrhaging, lethargy	1. Dietary history reveals an inadequate intake of ascorbic acid 2. Serum ascorbic acid levels of less than 0.4 mg./100 ml. 3. WBC ascorbic acid levels are less than 25 mg./100 ml.	1. Restore adequate vitamin C intake by daily doses of 100–200 mg. vitamin C and up to as much as 500 mg./day 2. Provide patient with a diet rich in vitamin C—fresh fruits and vegetables.
Vitamin D (Calciferol) RDA: 200–400 IU Fat-soluble vitamin	1. Regulates calcium and phosphate absorption and metabolism. 2. Aids in renal phosphate clearance, myocardial function, nervous system maintenance, and normal blood clotting.	1. Profuse sweating, restlessness, irritability, bone malformations, bow legs, knock knees, enlargement of wrists, burning sensation in the mouth and throat, pigeon breast, diarrhea, insomnia, softening of the skull, myopia 2. Pain in the back and legs may occur	1. Physical exam and dietary history 2. Calcium serum levels less than 7.5 mg./100 ml. 3. Inorganic phosphorus serum levels less than 3 mg./100 ml. 4. Alkaline phosphatase less than 4 Bodansky units/100 ml. 5. Serum citrate levels less than 2.5 mg./100 ml. 6. X-rays show bone deformities	1. Massive PO doses of vitamin D or cod liver oil or, in rickets accompanied by hepatic or renal disease, 25-hydroxycholecalciferol (active form of vitamin D). 2. Instruct the patient to eat foods rich in vitamin D—egg yolks, organ meats, vitamin D milk, fish liver oils, herring, sardines, liver. 3. Exposure to sunlight
Vitamin E (Tocopherol) RDA: 8–10 IU Fat-soluble vitamin	1. Aids in diuresis, fertility, lung protection, male potency, muscle and nerve maintenance, myocardial perfusion, serum cholesterol reduction, anticlotting factor, capillary wall strengthening, development of smooth skeletal, and vascular tissue, and erythrocyte protection	1. Dry or dull hair, edema, skin lesions, enlarged prostate gland, muscle weakness, GI problems, intermittent claudication in adults, hemolytic anemia, thrombocytosis, hair loss, impotency, sterility, muscle wasting, and miscarriage	1. Dietary and medical history 2. Serum alphatocopherol levels below 0.5 mg./100 ml. 3. Increased creatinuria, hemolytic anemia, phosphokinase, creatinine, and platelet counts	1. Replace vitamin E with water-soluble vitamin E supplement, either PO or parenteral. 2. Provide the patient with a diet rich in vitamin E foods—butter, eggs, fruits, vegetables, organ meats, vegetable oils, wheat germ, dark green vegetables, whole grains, nuts.
Vitamin K (Menadione) RDA: None stated	1. Blood clotting (coagulation). Formation of prothrombin and other clotting factors in the liver.	1. Abnormal bleeding times, hemorrhage, miscarriage, diarrhea, nosebleeds, prolonged prothrombin times	1. Prothrombin time longer than the normal range. 2. Rule out other causes of prolonged prothrombin time such as hepatic disease or anticoagulant therapy.	1. Administration of vitamin K. 2. Provide diet rich in the foods that contain vitamin K: molasses, green leafy vegetables, safflower oil, yogurt.

Table 19-3. *Mineral Requirements and Deficiency Management*

Mineral and RDA Requirements	Function	Clinical Manifestations of Deficiency	Diagnostic Evaluation	Management
Calcium RDA: 800–1200 mg.	1. Bone and tooth formation 2. Muscle growth and contraction 3. Coagulation of blood (blood clotting) 4. Nerve transmission 5. Cardiac rhythm 6. Activation of enzymes 7. Cell permeability 8. Ion balance 9. Lactation	1. Tooth decay 2. Muscle cramps, brittle fingernails, arm and leg numbness 3. Nervousness 4. Heart palpitations	1. Calcium levels below 8.9 mg./dl. or below 4.5 mEq./liter signify hypocalcemia 2. Calcium levels above 10.1 mg./ml. or above 5.5 mEq./liter signify hypercalcemia	1. Oral supplements of calcium such as calcitriol or IV supplements of calcium gluconate are given to raise serum calcium levels 2. If calcium levels are elevated, then treatment may include forcing fluids, limiting dietary intake of calcium, and promoting calcium excretion for forcing diuresis 3. To correct hypocalcemia, foods rich in calcium are: bone meal, cheese, milk, molasses, yogurt
Chromium RDA: 0.05–0.20 mg.	1. Aids in glucose metabolism 2. Maintains serum glucose levels 3. Aids in nucleic acid metabolism 4. Aids carbohydrate and lipid metabolism 5. Aids transport of amino acids to the liver and heart cells	1. Glucose intolerance, vertigo, abdominal pain, shock, convulsions, anuria, dermatitis	1. Volumes of serum chromium are 0.30–0.85 mg./ml. 2. High levels of chromium indicate chromium toxicity, which produces liver and kidney impairment 3. Low chromium levels decrease protein synthesis	1. Chromium supplements 250 mg. daily until symptoms improve and then daily doses of 20 mg. 2. Promote foods rich in chromium: brewer's yeast, clams, corn oil, whole grains
Copper RDA: 2–3 mg.	1. Hemoglobin synthesis, RBC formation 2. Bone formation 3. Hair and skin color 4. Healing processes 5. Mental thought processes	1. Weakness 2. Skin lesions 3. Altered respiratory status 4. Diarrhea (in infants)	1. 24-hour urine samples showing levels of urinary excretion of copper below 15–60 µg./24 hours indicate copper deficiency 2. Elevated copper levels indicate Wilson's disease—a rare inherited neurologic disorder 3. Serum or plasma copper levels	1. Copper supplementation such as cupric sulfate (oral copper is a potent emetic, with as little as 5–10 mg. causing nausea). The oral dose of 2 mg. 3–4 times daily has been used. 2. Patients on TPN are more susceptible to copper deficiency, should receive 0.25 mg. a day. Anything above this level is usually accumulated in the liver. Patients with liver problems should be given lower doses of copper. TPN patients with gastric fistula or gastric suction should be given more copper. 3. Promote foods rich in copper: molasses, nuts, organ meats, raisins, seafood (especially oysters)
Iodine RDA: 150 µg.	1. Physical and mental development 2. Metabolism 3. Energy production	1. Hypothyroidism 2. Nervousness, irritability 3. Obesity 4. Cold hands, feet, chills, dry hair 5. Fatigue, weakness 6. Bradycardia 7. Decreased cardiac output 8. Thick tongue, hoarseness 9. Poor memory 10. Hearing loss 11. Anorexia	1. Low T_4 with high iodine intake 2. Low 24-hour urine iodine 3. High TSH	1. Iodine supplements (potassium iodine SSKI) 2. Promote iodized table salt and foods rich in iodine such as seafood and dark green leafy vegetables
Iron RDA: 10–18 mg.	1. Hemoglobin production 2. Stress and disease resistance 3. Growth 4. Formation of RBCs 5. Transportation of oxygen needed for tissue respiration	1. Brittle nails 2. Tongue inflammation and soreness 3. Constipation 4. Respiratory problems and dyspnea 5. Decreased hemoglobin 6. Fatigue 7. Pallor 8. Inability to concentrate 9. Headache 10. Irritability 11. Susceptible to infection 12. Increased cardiac output and tachycardia	1. Low hemoglobin levels (males less than 12q/100 ml.; females less than 10q/100 ml.) 2. Low hematocrit levels (males less than 47 ml./100 ml. females less than 42 ml./100 ml.) 3. Low serum iron levels 4. Low serum ferritin levels 5. Low RBC count 6. Bone marrow studies show depleted or absent iron stores	1. Iron replacement therapy— a. Oral iron or iron with ascorbic acid (which enhances iron absorption) b. Parenteral iron c. IV iron infusion—iron dextron in normal saline given over 8 hours 2. Promote foods high in iron: molasses, eggs, fish, organ meats, poultry, wheat germ, almonds, asparagus, beans, celery, cauliflower, greens, beets, beef, cabbage, duck, goose, lamb, potatoes, peas

(continued)

Table 19-3. *Mineral Requirements and Deficiency Management (continued)*

Mineral and RDA Requirements	Function	Clinical Manifestations of Deficiency	Diagnostic Evaluation	Management
Magnesium RDA: 2.5–5.0 mg.	1. Protein structure 2. Acid–base balance 3. Activates enzymes 4. Associated with body temperature, neuromuscular contractions 5. Regulates skeletal muscles	1. Tetany, tremors 2. Confusion, disorientation, mental depression 3. Rapid pulse 4. Nervousness 5. Weakness	1. Decreased serum magnesium levels less than 1.5 mEq/L. confirms hypomagnesemia 2. Increased levels greater than 2.5 mEq/L. confirm hypermagnesemia	1. Daily magnesium supplements IM or PO or IV magnesium sulfate (10 to 40 mEq/L. diluted in IV fluid) 2. Magnesium intoxication is treated with calcium gluconate IV (10%) 3. Treatment of hypermagnesemia requires increased fluid intake, diuretics, and possibly peritoneal or renal dialysis if renal function fails. 4. Promote diet high in foods rich in magnesium for hypomagnesemia: nuts, bran, green vegetables, seafood

Phosphorus RDA: 800–1200 mg.	1. Nerve and muscle activity
	2. Vitamin utilization
	3. Kidney function
	4. Metabolism of carbohydrates, proteins, fats
	5. Cell growth and repair
	6. Myocardial contraction
	7. Energy production
	8. Bone and tooth formation
	9. Acid–base homeostasis
	10. Cell division
		1. Hypophosphatemia: anorexia, weakness, tremor, paresthesia, bone pain, hypoxia, weight loss, dental caries
		2. Hyperphosphatemia: hypocalcemia, tetany, convulsions, irritation of GI tract, cramps, headaches, GI bleeding, liver and kidney damage
			1. Serum phosphorus levels less than 1.7 mEq/L. confirm hypophosphatemia
			2. Urine phosphorus levels more than 1.3 g./24 hours indicate hypophosphatemia
			3. Serum phosphorus levels greater than 2.6 mEq/L. confirm hyperphosphatemia.
				1. Correct the underlying causes of the hypo- and hyperphosphatemia
				2. Hypophosphatemia
				  a. Replace phosphorus with a high phosphorus diet. Foods rich in phosphorus: eggs, fish, grains, meat, poultry, yellow cheeses, almonds, beans, cocoa, chocolate, liver, milk, peas, peanuts, walnuts, whole wheat, and rye
				  b. Administer phosphate salt tablets or capsules
				  c. IV infusion of potassium phosphate
				3. Severe hyperphosphatemia may require hemodialysis or peritoneal dialysis to lower the serum phosphate level
				4. Prolonged gastric lavage containing potassium permanganate to aid in the oxidizing of the phosphorus may be used.
				5. Blood transfusions

Potassium RDA: 1.875–5.625 mg.	1. Muscle contractions
	2. Heart beat
	3. Rapid growth
	4. Conduction of nerve impulses
	5. Maintains intracellular fluid
	6. Regulates osmotic pressure and acid–base balance
		1. Muscle weakness, fatigue, malaise, flaccidity
		2. Mental confusion, irritability, mental depression
		3. Thirst
		4. Dizziness
		5. Changes in ECG
		6. Hypotension
		7. Cardiac arrest
		8. Nausea, vomiting
		9. Diarrhea
		10. Anorexia
		11. Abdominal distention
		12. Leg cramps, numbness, tingling
		13. Polyuria, oliguria, anuria
		14. Metabolic alkalosis, acidosis
			1. Hypocalcemia: serum potassium levels below 3.5 mEq./L.; urine potassium level greater than 100 mEq./24 hours
			2. Hypercalcemia: serum potassium levels above 5.5 mEq./L. Urine potassium levels less than 40 mEq./24 hours.
				1. Hypocalcemia
				  a. Replace potassium—KCl IV or PO
				  b. If diuresis is necessary, spironolactone, a potassium diuretic, should be used
				  c. Foods rich in potassium: molasses, bananas, oranges, peaches, seafood, raisins
				2. Hypercalcemia:
				  a. Infuse calcium gluconate (10%); temporarily prevents cardiac arrest, but doesn't correct the serum potassium excess
				  b. Sodium bicarbonate causes potassium to shift back into the cells and increases the pH
				  c. Insulin and a 10%–50% glucose IV moves potassium back into the cells
				  d. K exalate enemas aid potassium excretion
				  e. Hemo- or peritoneal dialysis removes the K^+

(continued)

Table 19-3. *Mineral Requirements and Deficiency Management (continued)*

Mineral and RDA Requirements	Function	Clinical Manifestations of Deficiency	Diagnostic Evaluation	Management
Sodium RDA: 1100–3300 mg.	1. Maintains cellular fluid 2. Muscle contractions 3. Bioelectric potential of tissues—Ion balance 4. Maintains normal heart action 5. Produces buffer action in the blood	1. Hyponatremia: Weakness, weight loss, anxiety, headache, muscle twitching, convulsions, nausea, vomiting, oliguria, anuria, cyanosis, cold clammy skin, hypotension, tachycardia, abdominal cramps 2. Hypernatremia: Fever, dyspnea, respiratory arrest, flushed skin, dry mucous membranes, oliguria, agitation, dry tongue, thirst, excessive weight gain, restlessness, convulsions, pitting edema	1. Hyponatremia— a. Serum sodium less than 135 mEq./L. b. Urine sodium greater than 100 mEq./24 hours c. Low serum osmolality 2. Hypernatremia— a. Serum sodium more than 145 mEq./L b. Urine sodium less than 40 mEq./24 hours c. High serum osmolality	1. Hyponatremia a. Restrict free water intake b. Demeclocycline or lithium may be used to block ADH in the renal tubules, to promote water excretion c. Infusion of 3% or 5% saline and then Lasix (monitor venous pressure to prevent circulatory overload) 2. Hypernatremia a. Administer salt-free solutions like dextrose in water then use 0.45% sodium chloride to prevent hyponatremia b. Sodium-restricted diet c. Discontinue drugs that promote sodium retention
Zinc RDA: 15 mg.	1. Metabolism 2. Promotes synthesis of DNA, RNA 3. Maintains blood concentrations of vitamin A 4. Burn and wound healing 5. Prostate gland function 6. Reproductive organ growth and function	1. Hepatosplenomegaly 2. Fatigue 3. Loss of hair 4. Poor wound healing 5. Impaired growth, bone deformities 6. Loss of taste 7. Anorexia 8. Iron-deficiency anemia 9. Hypogonadism, dwarfism 10. Hyperpigmentation	1. Serum zinc levels below 121 μg./100 ml.	1. Correct underlying cause of deficiency. 2. Administer zinc supplements 3. Promote foods rich in zinc: liver, mushrooms, seafood, soybeans, spinach, oatmeal, wheat bran, eggs, dry yeast. 4. Avoid calcium supplements.

Special Nutritional Management

Overview of Enteral Feeding (Tube Feeding)

Enteral or *tube feeding* (Fig. 19-2) is the introduction of nutrients directly into the stomach or duodenum or jejunum. These feedings are indicated for the patient who cannot be fed orally but whose gastrointestinal tract is functional.

Clinical Indications

1. Gastrointestinal disease and surgery
2. Hypermetabolic states (burns; multiple trauma; sepsis; cancer)
3. Certain neurological disorders (stroke; coma)
4. Following certain types of surgery (head and neck; esophageal)

Sites

A. Short-Term Nutritional Support

1. *Nasogastric* (NG)—tube passed through the nose or mouth (orogastric) into the stomach and secured in place.
2. *Nasoduodenal* or *nasojejunal*—tube passed through the nose into duodenum or jejunum and secured in place.

B. Long-Term Nutritional Support

1. *Gastrostomy*—insertion of a tube, either surgically or via a percutaneous endoscopic procedure, into the stomach

2. *Jejunostomy*—insertion of tube directly into jejunum, either surgically or as a percutaneous endoscopic procedure.
   a. Jejunostomy feedings are by continuous infusion.
   b. Pump control is favored.

Types of Tubes

1. Small bore feeding tubes of nonreactive materials (polyurethane or silicone)
2. Tubes with weighted tips used for infusion of feeding solution into jejunum; ensures additional protection against aspiration as tube is passed beyond the intact pylorus.

Delivery Systems for Feeding Solution

1. Intermittent or continuous infusion of feeding solution by gravity—accomplished by hanging container of feeding solution from an IV pole and adjusting delivery rate by flow regulator
2. Continuous feeding by controller feeding pump—allows uniform flow, particularly of viscous solutions
3. Bolus—feeding solution poured into barrel of 60-ml. syringe attached to feeding tube and allowed to infuse by gravity.

Special Nursing Considerations

1. Elevate head of bed 30–45 degrees during bolus and intermittent feedings and continue elevation for 30–45 minutes after feedings to decrease likelihood of aspiration and to facilitate digestion.
2. Elevate head of bed at all times for patient receiving continuous drip or continuous pump feeding.

Table 19-4. *Potential Problems in Tube-Fed Clients and Examples of Corrective Measures*

Factors to Assess	Possible Causes of Problems	Corrective Measures
Gastrointestinal Function		
Vomiting	Feeding too soon after intubation	Allow patient time to relax and rest after tube is inserted.
	Improper location of tip of feeding tube	Qualified health professional should reposition tube.
	Rapid rate of infusion	Administer slowly.
	Excessive volume	
	Air	Be sure tube feeding container does not run dry before feeding is completed.
	Formula	Check with physician regarding number and size of feedings.
	Position of patient	Position on right side for 30 minutes following feeding—reverse Trendelenburg or semi-Fowler's position.
Applies to both vomiting and diarrhea	Food infection or poisoning	Check sanitation of formula and equipment.
	Anxiety	Explain procedures. Provide reassurance and other needed types of support. Provide privacy.
Diarrhea	Rapid rate of infusion	Administer slowly—very slowly if formula is cold.
	High osmolarity of formula or high concentration of formula	Adapt the patient to formula gradually.
	Lactose intolerance	Contact physician regarding change of formula.
Constipation	Lack of fiber	Contact physician regarding:
	Inadequate fluid intake	Change in formula / Laxatives / Increasing fluid
Fluid and Electrolyte Balance		
Dehydration	Rapid infusion of carbohydrate → hyperglycemia → osmotic diuresis → dehydration	Administer slowly. Exogeneous insulin is sometimes needed.
	Excess protein and electrolytes in formula	Change formula and/or increase fluid according to physician's requests.
	Inadequate fluid intake	
Edema	Excessive sodium in formula	Check with physician about change in formula
Nutritional Adequacy		
Undernutrition (gradual weight loss)	Inadequate number of calories to meet energy requirements	Check to see if the patient is receiving prescribed amount of formula. Estimate the patient's caloric intake. Check with physician regarding increasing the volume, concentration, or number of feedings given.
Overnutrition (gradual, undesirable gain of weight)	Excessive caloric intake	Check with physician regarding decreasing the volume, concentration, or number of feedings given.
Undernutrition (inadequate intake of protein and/or micronutrients leading to biochemical or clinical signs of deficiency)	Amount of standard formula needed to maintain weight is too low to meet requirements for essential nutrients.	Check with physician regarding providing appropriate nutrient supplements.

(Suitor CW and Crowley MF, Nutrition. 2nd ed. Philadelphia, JB Lippincott.)

3. Administer feeding solution at room temperature to prevent nausea and discomfort.
4. Do not allow feeding solution to hang longer than 6 hours; rinse and change subsequent equipment according to agency policy to prevent bacterial contamination.
5. Confirm tube placement and check for gastric residuals before administering feeding solution.
6. Flush tubing every 4 hours (or more frequently for patient with continuous infusion).
7. Monitor the patient receiving enteral therapy:
   a. Auscultate the chest at intervals.
   b. Examine the abdomen and auscultate for presence of bowel sounds.
   c. Keep an intake and output record, paying particular attention if patient has diarrhea.
   d. Weigh the patient daily.
   e. Monitor results of laboratory evaluations.
8. See Table 19-4 for problems that may be encountered.

Complications of Enteral Feeding

1. Gastrointestinal: *diarrhea*, nausea and vomiting, inadequate gastric emptying, steatorrhea, malabsorption
2. Mechanical: tube misplacement, tube migration, tube obstruction, tube coiling and knotting
3. Pulmonary: aspiration of gastric contents
4. Metabolic: hyperglycemia, electrolyte imbalances
5. Infectious; bacterial contamination of feeding solution

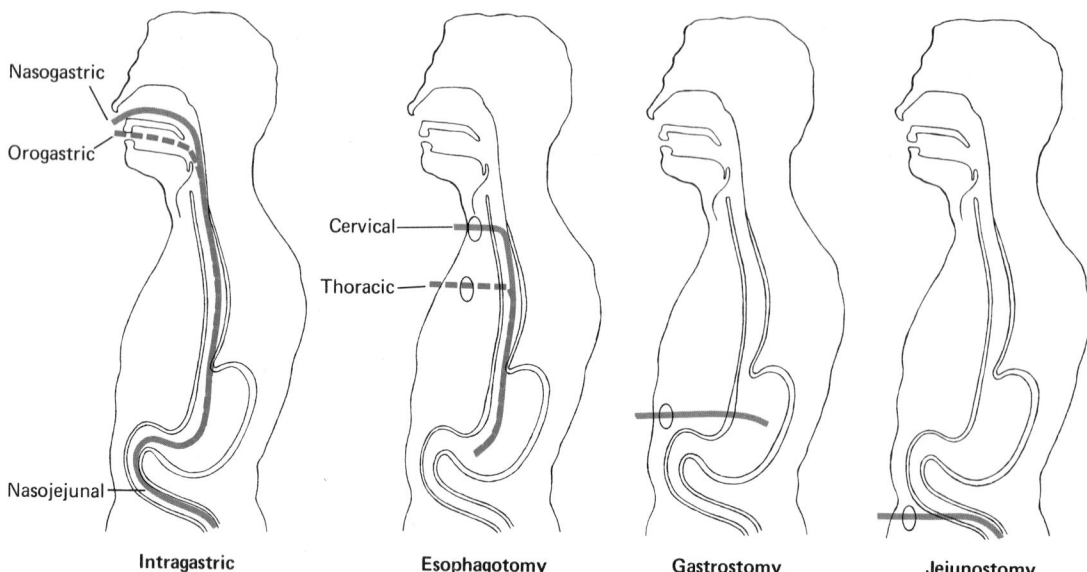

Nasogastric

Orogastric

Cervical

Thoracic

Nasojejunal

Intragastric	Esophagotomy	Gastrostomy	Jejunostomy

Figure 19-2. *Types and sites of enteral feeding.*

Intragastric (nasogastric, NG): *A tube is passed through the nose or mouth into the stomach and secured in place. (A tube passed through the mouth is more correctly called an orogastric tube. An orogastric tube is ordinarily inserted at mealtime and removed following the meal.) Intragastric tube preferred for short-term feeding; readily inserted by physician or nurse, remains in place between feedings. (Some clients are taught to insert their own tube; they may remove the tube between meals.) Variations include nasopharyngeal and nasojejunal feeding tubes.*

Esophagotomy: *A temporary or permanent opening (stoma) is constructed at one of several sites to allow a tube to be introduced through the skin into the esophagus. Feeding tube is usually removed between meals. Advantages—dependable for long-term feeding, allows concealment of apparatus, easy to handle.*

Gastrostomy: *A temporary or permanent stoma is constructed, allowing food to be introduced through the skin directly into the stomach. Preferred for long-term gavage feeding of children and for long-term feeding of adults when use of esophagus is contraindicated. Disadvantages—partial undressing necessary at mealtime, skin care may pose problems.*

Jejunostomy: *A stoma is constructed to give direct access to the jejunum. This method of feeding may be used when the stomach must be bypassed. Disadvantages—high incidence of dumping syndrome and diarrhea; adequate nutrient intake difficult to maintain. (Suitor CW and Crowley MF. Nutrition. Principles and Application in Health Promotion. Philadelphia, JB Lippincott)*

Guidelines Administration of Nasogastric Tube Feeding; Intermittent or Continuous

Goal   Administer specially prepared nutrients into a tube passed through the nose into the stomach.

Equipment

Feeding solution (formula)
Graduated containers
60-ml. catheter-tipped syringe
5–10-ml. syringe
Water
Stethoscope

Optional: Tube feeding bag, infusion controller, tubing set

Procedure

Nursing Action	Rationale/Amplification
1. See page 464 for technique of nasogastric tube insertion.	
2. Remove the feeding solution from refrigerator and allow it to reach room temperature.	2. Use prepared dietary formulas within 24 hours.
3. Shake container of prescribed solution or formula.	3. Shaking prevents separation of formula.
4. Using a syringe attached to the feeding tube, aspirate stomach contents, using gentle suction.	4. Aspiration determines amount of residual feeding and also confirms tube placement.
5. Using a 5–10-ml. syringe, instill 5–10 ml. of air through the feeding tube while auscultating the patient's stomach.	5. A "whooshing" sound or sharp loud gurgle helps confirm the tube's presence in the stomach.

NURSING ALERT: Tube feedings are contraindicated in patients with absent bowel sounds. Administration of feeding solution into an improperly placed tube may cause aspiration of the feeding into the lungs.

Procedure
(continued)

Nursing Action	Rationale/Amplification
6. Elevate the head of the bed 30–45 degrees.	6. This helps prevent aspiration and promotes digestion.
7. Attach the 60-ml. catheter-tipped syringe to the pinched-off feeding tube (for intermittent feeding) For continuous tube feedings, follow the manufacturer's directions.	7. Pinching the tube prevents excess air from entering the patient's stomach, causing distention. Be sure that all air is purged from the system before attaching tubing set to patient's feeding tube.
8. Fill catheter-tipped syringe with solution/formula, release the tubing, and allow solution to flow freely. For continuous tube feedings, set the prescribed flow rate according to manufacturer's directions. Open the regulator clamp on the feeding bag. Check tubing frequently to ensure patency. Squeeze the bag frequently.	8. The rate of flow is regulated by raising or lowering the syringe. Agitating the solution helps prevent tube clogging.
9. Pour additional formula into syringe when it is three-quarters empty.	9. This will prevent air from entering the patient's stomach.
10. Administer tube feeding slowly (200–350 ml. in 10–20-minute interval).	10. Feeding solution administered too rapidly may cause stomach distention, cramping, nausea, vomiting, and diarrhea.
11. After administering the prescribed amount of solution, flush the tubing with approximately 50 ml. of water. For an infusion pump, turn off the pump, close the regulator clamp on the tubing, and disconnect the tubing from the feeding tube.	11. This clears the tubing and prevents clogging.
12. Cover the end of the feeding tube with a plug or clamp.	12. This prevents leakage and contamination of the tube.
13. Allow the head of the bed to remain elevated for 30–45 minutes.	13. This decreases the potential for aspiration.
14. Aspirate the stomach contents 2–3 hours after the feeding. If more than 50–100 ml. of gastric contents is aspirated, notify the physician.	14. Aspiration of more than 50–100 ml. of stomach contents confirms delayed gastric emptying. Vomiting may occur if stomach becomes overdistended.
15. Rinse reusable equipment with warm water. Dry. Change the equipment according to agency policy.	15. This prevents contamination and infection.
16. Document the type and amount of feeding solution/formula, amount of water given, and the patient's tolerance of the procedure.	

Guidelines Assisting the Patient With a Gastrostomy Feeding

A *gastrostomy* is an opening into the stomach performed for the purpose of administering food and fluids. Gastrostomy tubes are placed surgically or by the percutaneous endoscopic technique.

Equipment

Feeding solution
Graduated containers
Large syringe (60-ml. catheter-tip)
Reservoir bag with tubing and regulator clamp
50 ml. water
Adapter to connect tubing
Sterile basin

4 × 4 gauze sponges
Towel/linen saver
Stethoscope
Tape measure
Optional: Infusion controller pump and tubing set for continuous feeding infusion

Note: The more recent tubes have a gastric balloon that prevents gastric leakage and tube migration. A gastrostomy feeding button may be used in a well-established gastrostomy site.

Preparatory Phase

1. Explain procedure to the patient. Give the patient a schedule of subsequent feedings if he is on intermittent feedings.
2. Administer the feeding at room temperature. Do not heat the formula, as heat could curdle the feeding solution, change the nutrients, or burn the patient.
3. Using clean technique, measure the prescribed amount of feeding solution into graduated container. (For continuous feeding, pour prescribed amount into reservoir bag).
4. Pour 50 ml. of water into another graduated container.
5. Remove air from the tubing by slowly opening the clamp.

(continued)

Guidelines Assisting the Patient With a Gastrostomy Feeding *(continued)*

Procedure	Nursing Action	Rationale/Amplification
	1. Provide privacy. Protect the patient from spillage.	
	2. Elevate the head of the bed 30–45 degrees during infusion of feeding and for 30–45 minutes after feeding stops.	2. Prevents aspiration by gastroesophageal reflux and also facilitates digestion.
	3. Remove the cap, plug, or clamp from the patient's gastrostomy tube.	
	4. Using a syringe, gently aspirate the stomach contents before each feeding.	4. A residual of 100 ml. or more indicates delayed gastric emptying. The risk of aspiration is increased with delayed gastric emptying. Vomiting will occur if stomach becomes distended.
	5. Connect the reservoir bag tubing to the gastrostomy tube. If a catheter-tip syringe is used, remove plunger and attach syringe to pinched-off end of feeding tube. Instill small amount of water into feeding tube.	5. Pinching the feeding tube will prevent excess air from entering stomach and causing distention. This verifies tube patency, moistens the tubing, and prevents feeding solution from adhering to the tubing.
	6. If an infusion controller pump is used, purge the air from the tubing according to the manufacturer's directions. Attach controller tubing to gastrostomy tube. Open the regulator clamp and adjust the flow rate.	
	7. If using a syringe, fill the syringe with feeding solution and release the feeding tube. When the syringe is almost empty, refill with feeding solution.	7. Do not allow air to enter the syringe; never allow the syringe to empty completely. The feeding infusion rate depends on the patient's condition and tolerance. Slower rates prevent nausea, vomiting, stomach distention, and diarrhea.
	8. Administer feeding slowly, usually 200–350 ml. over 10–15-minute period.	8. The height of the syringe will determine flow rate.
	9. Flush the tubing with 20–50 ml. of water after administering prescribed amount of feeding.	9. Clearing the tubing of solution maintains tube patency.
	10. Depending on the equipment in use, turn off the infusion controller; or, disconnect the syringe from the gastrostomy tube. Close the regulator clamp on the reservoir bag.	
	11. Cover the end of the feeding tube with a plug or cap and wrap it in gauze secured with a rubber band.	11. Securing the tube prevents leakage and contamination.
	12. Twist a thin strip of adhesive around the gastrostomy tube and attach firmly to abdomen, or coil on a dressing.	12. Prevents the tubing from being accidentally dislodged from the stomach.
	13. Allow patient to remain in a modified upright position for at least 30–45 minutes.	13. This helps prevent regurgitation and pulmonary aspiration, and aids digestion.
	14. Rinse reusable equipment with water. Dry.	14. The equipment is cleaned and changed according to agency policy.
	15. Document date, time feeding started and ended, type and amount of feeding solution administered, and the amount of water used. Record patient's tolerance to feeding. Record drugs given through the tube. Record and report cramping, abdominal distention, and diarrhea. Note results of laboratory tests.	15. Documentation of these findings provides information to alter rate, time, or type of future feeding solutions.

NURSING ALERT: Monitor skin status daily for signs of breakdown, irritation, or maceration. Wash skin around gastrostomy tube daily. Use a skin barrier when necessary.

Guidelines Hyperalimentation: Total Parenteral Nutrition (TPN)

Hyperalimentation (TPN) is the administration of nutrients through a catheter in a vein (usually the subclavian vein).

Purposes
1. To provide body nutrients by way of the intravenous route when it is impossible or inadvisable to use the normal digestive routes.
2. Total parenteral nutrition benefits the patient with severe burns, pancreatitis, inflammatory bowel syndrome, inflammatory bowel disease, ulcerative colitis, acute renal failure, hepatic failure, cardiac disease, surgery, and cancer.

Physiologic Basis
1. The intravenous route has heretofore not provided adequate nutrition; caloric and nitrogen deficiencies occurred.
2. Because of nutritional deficiencies, the process of gluconeogenesis takes place; this is the body's conversion of protein to carbohydrate.

Physiologic Basis
(*continued*)

3. Approximately 1500 calories/day are required by the average adult postoperative patient to prevent body protein from being used.
4. Caloric needs are increased when the patient has a hypermetabolic disease, fever, or injury—these needs may require up to 10,000 calories daily.
5. To meet the fluid volume necessary to provide so many additional calories would exceed fluid tolerance and lead to congestive heart failure/pulmonary edema.
6. This process provides desired calories in concentration directly into the intravenous system, which rapidly dilutes incoming nutrients to satisfactory levels of body tolerance.
   a. Hypertonic glucose—fulfills caloric requirement—permits amino acids to be released for protein synthesis (not energy).
   b. Potassium provides proper electrolyte balance—transports glucose and amino acids across cell membranes.
   c. Calcium, magnesium, and sodium chloride—meet cell requirements as determined by serum electrolyte needs.
   d. Other trace elements whose function is not known may be deficient in hyperalimentation, since they are not included.

Clinical Indications

1. As a substitute for oral or nasogastric intubation when these are ineffective, undesirable, or even hazardous. TPN is used under the following conditions:
   a. Chronic vomiting
   b. Cancer: chemotherapy or radiotherapy
   c. Stroke
   d. Anorexia nervosa
2. As a supplement for patients demonstrating large nitrogen losses (e.g., burn patients, those with metastatic cancer, and those who are receiving radiation and chemotherapy).
3. As a means of putting gastrointestinal tract at rest
   a. When there is evidence of gastrointestinal fistula
   b. With severe and extensive inflammatory bowel disease
   c. Following major intestinal resection
   d. For intestinal obstruction

Equipment

Skin detergent–germicide
Sterile drapes and gloves (2 pair)
20-ml. syringe
No. 14 (5 cm.) needle
No. 16 gauge 20-cm. radiopaque catheter
Tincture of benzoin spray
Organic solvent (10% acetone or 70% alcohol)
Antimicrobial solution (povidone–iodine)
Face mask
Sterile scissors
Optional: 0.22-micron cellulose filter

Sterile connecting tubing and adapters
Prescribed hyperalimentation solution
4 $\times$ 4 dressings—adhesive for occlusive dressing
Suture material
Antimicrobial ointment
Infusion pump
Hypoallergenic tape

Procedure

Preparatory Phase

Nursing Action	Rationale/Amplification
1. Remove the prescribed TPN solution from the refrigerator 30 minutes before procedure.	1. Delivery of a chilled solution can cause pain, hypothermia, venous spasm and constriction.
2. Compare the contents in the bottle with the physician's order.	2. Because multiple bottles of TPN are prescribed at one time, this is necessary for safety.
3. Observe the solution for cloudiness, turbidity, and particles in the container. If any are present, send the solution back to the pharmacy.	3. The solution is probably contaminated if these occur and should not be used.
4. Connect the pump tubing, filters, and extension tubing. Tape all connections.	4. This will prevent accidental separation and the potential for an air embolus.
5. Using strict aseptic technique, insert the pump tubing into the TPN container. Prime the tubing.	5. Aseptic technique is very important because the TPN solution is a medium for bacterial growth. Priming the tubing removes the air.
6. Gently tap the tubing.	6. This dislodges the air bubbles trapped in the Y injection sites.
7. Clean the patient's overbed table with isopropyl alcohol.	7. This promotes a clean environment.
8. Explain the procedure to the patient and why it is important for him not to touch the area where the catheter is inserted.	8. To provide reassurance; to prevent dislodging and contaminating catheter.
9. Tell the patient that he will probably be ambulatory during the extended time of therapy.	9. In the absence of other conditions requiring bedrest, ambulation is desirable.

(*continued*)

Guidelines Hyperalimentation: Total Parenteral Nutrition (TPN) *(continued)*

Procedure
(continued)

Nursing Action	Rationale/Amplification
10. Place patient in head-low position.	10. This position permits dilatation of neck and shoulder vessels, which makes catheter entry easier and prevents air embolus.
11. Suggest that the patient turn his face away from the area selected.	11. To prevent contamination of TPN site.
12. Put on a mask and gown, if applicable.	12. This is protection to ensure that the sterile drapes and area remain sterile.
13. Support the patient in proper position to permit extension of shoulder.	13. This position can be facilitated by placing a rolled sheet or towel vertically along spinal column.
14. Use depilatory or shave area if necessary and remove surface oils with acetone or ether.	14. To reduce probability of contamination.
15. Instruct the patient to remain still during the insertion of catheter.	15. To prevent the possibility of dislodging of catheter and perforation of subclavian vein.

Performance Phase (by physician)

Nursing Action	Rationale/Amplification
1. The area is prepared with detergent germicide by scrubbing a circular motion for 2 minutes, from the insertion site outward.	1. To prevent infection
2. A local anesthetic is injected into the skin and underlying tissues.	2. To promote comfort of patient and prevent patient movement
3. A No. 14 (5 cm.) needle with syringe attached is inserted beneath the clavicle and into the subclavian vein.	3. Subclavian vein is selected because it leads into the superior vena cava, which has a large volume of blood flow, and provides rapid dilution of hypertonic solution.
4. Instruct the patient to perform Valsalva maneuver.	4. By the patient's bearing down with mouth closed, positive pressure is produced when syringe and needle are replaced by catheter; thus preventing an air embolism.
5. The syringe is detached and a radiopaque catheter is threaded through the needle into the vein; the needle is withdrawn.	5. This permits the more flexible catheter to remain in position during subsequent feedings.
6. The catheter is attached to the tubing from the flask of prescribed hyperalimentation solution.	
7. The catheter is sutured in place.	7. This ensures against dislodgement.
8. Ensure the junction catheter tubing is secured.	8. This will prevent separation and the potential of an air embolus or exsanguination.
9. Cleanse the skin with the povidone—iodine solution again. Leave this solution on.	9. Its antimicrobial effects are long lasting and continue after drying.
10. According to agency policy, use a sterile swab, apply povidone–iodine ointment to the skin at the insertion site.	
11. Arrange the sterile dressing sponges to shield the insertion site and surrounding skin area. A precut drain sponge may be used around the catheter.	11. This shields the sterile area from airborne contaminants.

The Nurse Should:

Nursing Action	Rationale/Amplification
12. Apply the tincture of benzoin and an occlusive dressing to the patient's skin.	12. The dressing may be transparent or nontransparent, as long as it is occlusive.
13. Document the catheter size, date and time of insertion, and the solution infusing.	
14. Document the date and time of dressing change and the nurse's initials on the outside of the dressing. Document the condition of the catheter insertion site.	
15. Loop and tape the administration tubing over the intact dressing.	15. To prevent tension on the catheter and its accidental removal if the tubing is pulled
16. Remind the patient not to touch dressings.	16. Encourage the patient to turn in bed or to ambulate, but caution him against handling dressings, which causes contamination.
17. Check infusion rate every 30 minutes.	17. If infusion flow is too rapid, hyperosmolar diuresis occurs; excess sugar is excreted. Intractable seizures may occur; coma and death may ensue.
18. Weigh the patient daily; keep accurate intake and output records.	18. Comparison of daily weight changes are noted.
19. Check vital signs every 4 hours.	19. Note temperature rise, which may signify a complication.
20. Change dressing every 72 hours and as required.	20. Strict aseptic technique must be followed.

Procedure *(continued)*	**Nursing Action**	**Rationale/Amplification**
	21. IV tubing and filters must be changed daily or according to agency policy.	21. Procedure is done by a nurse especially trained in this technique.
	22. Encourage diversional therapy and activity during extended therapy.	22. This distracts the patient from the procedure.
	23. Observe the patient for signs of thrombophlebitis—edema and erythema at the catheter site. Also, unilateral swelling of the neck, arm, or face and pain along the vein are other signs and symptoms.	23. If these occur, notify the physician immediately.
	24. Watch for swelling at the catheter insertion site.	24. This indicates there is extravasation of the TPN solution that can cause necrosis.
	25. Check the catheter tubing for leaks.	
	26. Start the TPN slowly. If the patient tolerates it well the first day, the flow rate is usually increased to 1 liter every 12 hours for at least 2 days.	26. The solution is high in glucose content. A slow infusion rate allows the pancreatic beta cells to adapt by increasing insulin output.
	27. Collect a double-voided urine specimen every 6 hours and test for glucose and acetone.	27. Notify the physician if the glucose is greater than $\frac{1}{4}$% (2+).
	28. Record intake and output.	28. The I & O record is what is used for fluid replacement.
	29. Perform anthropometric measurements as required.	29. These measurements indicate whether or not the patient is gaining weight.
	30. Monitor the results of routine lab tests, and report abnormal findings to the physician (electrolytes, BUN, and glucose are usually requested 3 times a week. CBC, liver function studies, serum albumin, calcium, magnesium, and creatinine are done every week).	30. This will permit the physician to change the TPN solution as needed.
	31. Monitor for fluid and electrolyte disturbances. Watch for elevated glucose.	31. The patient may require supplementary insulin for the duration of TPN. The insulin can be added directly to the TPN solution by the pharmacist.
	32. When discontinuing TPN, decrease the rate slowly. Weaning usually takes place over 24–48 hours (it can be done in 4–6 hours if the patient receives adequate oral IV carbohydrates).	32. This will decrease the risk of hyperinsulinemia and hypoglycemia.

Possible Complications

A. Infection
   1. Patients receiving hyperalimentation are particularly susceptible to catheter-related infections.
   2. To minimize these complications:
      a. Solutions are prepared under a laminar flow hood.
      b. Solutions are prepared fresh daily and refrigerated until used.
   3. Preventive Measures
      a. Maintain sterility during procedure to prevent sepsis.
      b. Maintain consistent infusion rate, which is calculated on a 24-hour basis.
      c. Monitor patient carefully—including vital signs.
      d. Record data accurately.
      e. Provide emotional support to the patient.

B. Fever
   1. If the patient develops a fever, discontinue the TPN solution and replace it with 10% dextrose in water as prescribed.
   2. If temperature is reduced in 4–6 hours, the fever was probably due to the solution or the delivery device.
   3. If the fever persists, there may be catheter-related sepsis.
   4. Blood and urine cultures will help determine the cause of the infection.
   5. The catheter may be removed and fungal and bacterial cultures taken.
   6. The fever usually subsides in 12–24 hours after the catheter is removed.

C. Air Embolism
   1. Signs of air embolism—dyspnea, chest pain, tachycardia, hypotension, cyanosis, seizures, coma, and cardiac arrest.
   2. If an air embolus is suspected, position the patient on his left side in the Trendelenburg position, administer oxygen according to protocol.
   3. Call the physician.

Guidelines Intravenous Fat Emulsion

Intravenous fat emulsion is a form of essential fatty acids that can be administered to the patient intravenously when these essential nutrients are needed and cannot be acquired in any other way.

1. Lipid emulsions (10% and 20%) may be "piggybacked" onto the hyperalimentation solution and administered by this central line or they can be administered through a peripheral vein.
2. A concentrated amount of essential fatty acids and calories can be supplied in a relatively small volume of liquid.

Clinical Indications

Treatment or prevention of essential fatty acid deficiencies that may be due to:

1. Severe nutritional disorders and inability to take nourishment by mouth
2. Malignancies, burns, ulcerative colitis, severe renal disorders, nonfunctional gastrointestinal tracts
3. Extended semiconsciousness or unconsciousness
4. Specific preoperative and postoperative patients in whom it is necessary to increase caloric intake
5. Essential fatty acid deficiencies—characterized by sparse hair growth, eczematous scaly skin lesions, thrombocytopenia, and poor wound healing

Physiologic Action

1. Lipid emulsion is introduced into the blood: Protein in the blood acts as emulsifier (lipid–protein complex).
2. The lipid–protein complex carries nutrients to the liver, adipose tissue, etc., where they are degraded, synthesized, stored, mobilized, and oxidized for energy.
3. It is delivered with amino acid dextrose solution in order not to deplete the patient's protein resources.

Equipment

1. Amino acid dextrose solution
2. Fat emulsion
3. Y-type nonphthalate administration set
   Vented line for fat emulsion
   Nonvented line (with filter) for amino acid dextrose solution

NURSING ALERT: Use the administration set as recommended by the manufacturer, as some plastics in combination with lipids cause leaching of diethylhexyl phthalate (DEHP).

Procedure

Preparatory Phase

Nursing Action	Rationale/Amplification
1. Do not shake emulsion flask.	1. Agitation of emulsion may cause fat globules to aggregate.
2. Inspect flask of fat emulsion.	2. Look for signs of altered stability: a. Inconsistency in texture and color b. Separation of oil, or frothy solution
3. Wash hands. Wipe top of bottle with alcohol.	
4. Connect tubing to emulsion flask and clear tubing of all air (do not use the pump to prime tubing; use gravity only).	4. Air in system may cause an air embolus in the patient.
5. Connect IV tubing to Y-tube connection closest to insertion site; insert tubing primed with IV fat emulsion directly into this site.	5. This reduces length of time emulsion comes in contact with substances that may affect its stability.
6. Do not use in-line filters.	6. Particles are too large to go through a filter.
7. If infusion is to be administered by gravity drip, hang fat emulsion flask of amino acid solution.	7. This will prevent back-flow of fat emulsion (less density) into other amino acid flask (higher density).
8. Explain procedure to the patient; tell him that the milk-white solution is unlike other solutions he has received intravenously. Remind him that he is not to leave the unit while this emulsion is running.	8. Patient will have a better understanding of the reason for more frequent vital sign checks and other observations.
9. Document the patient's vital signs.	9. These will be used as a baseline comparison for later evaluation.
10. Start flow rate at 1 ml./minute for first 30 minutes; monitor vital signs every 10 minutes during this time.	10. Provides opportunity to assess patient for chills, fever, headache, dizziness, sleepiness, allergic reactions, back pain, chest pain, nausea, vomiting, pressure over eyes, etc.
11. If untoward signs occur, stop infusion and notify physician.	
12. If problems occur, heparin may be prescribed.	12. Heparin will hasten clearing of lipids from the patient's plasma.
13. If no complications occur, infusion rate may be increased—a good gauge is to administer 500 ml. in 4–6 hours.	13. Continue constant observation; monitor vital signs hourly.

Procedure (continued)	**Nursing Action**	**Rationale/Amplification**

14. At conclusion of infusion, detach emulsion flask and attach flask of 5% dextrose as per physician request.

14. Dextrose flushes out remaining fat emulsion from tubing.

Follow-up Phase

1. Examine the skin above the insertion site; watch for redness, warmth, and pain.

1. If the solution is infusing into a peripheral vein, the vein may become inflamed (phlebitis).

If These Occur

Discontinue the line and start in another vein.

2. Always use aseptic technique when handling equipment. Do not reuse a half-empty bottle of fat emulsion.

2. The emulsion is an excellent medium for bacterial growth.

3. Be alert for signs of sepsis: elevated temperature, lethargy, chills, elevated WBCs, altered level of consciousness.

3. The patient may report an unpleasant metallic taste.

4. Monitor triglyceride levels; these should return to normal within 18 hours after infusion of the fat emulsion. Monitor SGOT, SGPT, alkaline phosphatase, cholesterol, plasma free fatty acid and coagulation tests.

4. These tests monitor the patient's response to the fat emulsion. They provide indicators of the patient's ability to metabolize and clear the fat emulsion from the blood stream.

5. When dextrose has run in, clamp tubing securely until next lipid emulsion is to be given. If this is final treatment, disconnect as with any IV.

6. Continue to be alert for delayed adverse reactions.

6. Fat overload syndrome manifestations—headache, low-grade fever, nausea, abdominal pain, irritability, dyspnea, cyanosis, vomiting, flushing, diaphoresis, lethargy, syncope, chest and back pain, irritation at the insertion site. Prolonged administration of fat emulsion may cause hepatomegaly, splenomegaly, jaundice, thrombocytopenia, leukopenia, and increased values in liver function studies.

7. Record the nature of lipid emulsion given, amount, time, patient reactions, time of termination of procedure.

7. Include documentation of vital signs.

8. Monitor the patient for effectiveness of this treatment. Observe for changes in his clinical status.

8. This would determine effectiveness in treating an essential fatty acid (EFA) deficiency.

NURSING ALERT: Lipase synthesis increases insulin requirements in the patient with diabetes, and the insulin dose may need to be increased. The patient with hypothyroidism will need the thyroid-stimulating hormone to prevent intravascular accumulation of triglycerides.

Bibliography

Books

Burton BT and Foster WR. Human Nutrition. New York, McGraw–Hill, 1988

Cornatzer WE. Role of Nutrition in Health and Disease. Springfield, Charles C Thomas, 1989

Dintzis FR and Laszlo JA. Mineral Absorption in the Monogastric GI Tract. New York, Plenum Press, 1989

Johnston FE. Nutritional Anthropology. New York, Alan R. Liss, 1987

Linder MC. Nutritional Biochemistry and Metabolism With Clinical Applications. New York, Elsevier, 1985

Munro HN and Danford DE. Nutrition, Aging and the Elderly. New York, Plenum Press, 1989

National Research Council. Recommended Dietary Allowances. 10th ed. Washington, DC. National Academy Press, 1989

Paige DM. Clinical Nutrition. 2nd ed. St Louis, CV Mosby, 1988

Rombeau JL et al (eds). Atlas of Nutritional Support Techniques. Boston, Little, Brown & Co, 1989

Shils ME and Young VR. Modern Nutrition in Health and Disease. Philadelphia, Lea and Febiger, 1988

Winick M. Nutrition in the 20th Century. New York, John Wiley & Sons, 1984

Journals

Nasogastric Tubes

Beg MH and Reyazuddin. Distal esophageal stricture due to indwelling nasogastric tube. Indian J Chest Dis Allied Sci 1988 Jan–Mar; 30(1):64–66

Dodd CM et al. Hazards associated with passage of nasogastric tubes into the trachea. Can J Anaesth 1988 Sep; 35(5):541–542

Gibbons CL et al. Complications of nasogastric feeding. Br Med J [Clin Res] 1988 May 28; 296(6635):1537

Ikard RW and Federspiel CF. A comparison of Levin and sump nasogastric tubes for postoperative gastrointestinal decompression. Am Surg 1987 Jan; 53(1):50–53

Jones M. Removal of nasogastric tubes. Br Med J [Clin Res] 1988 May 7; 296(6632):1330

Levenson R et al. Do weighted nasoenteric feeding tubes facilitate duodenal intubations? JPEN (J Parenter Enteral Nutr) 1988 Mar–Apr; 2(2):135–137

Lie JT. On the positioning (or malpositioning) of a nasogastric tube. Am J Med 1988 Aug; 85(2):282

Marchard SP and Perkins AM. Clogging of feeding tubes. JPEN (J Parenter Enteral Nutr) 1988 Jul–Aug; 12(4):403–405

Metheny N. Measures to test placement of nasogastric and nasointestinal feeding tubes: A review. Nurs Res 1988 Nov–Dec; 37(6):324–329

Moore DM and Calcaterra TC. Inserting the nasogastric tube. Laryngoscope 1987 Dec; 97(12):1460

Taylor SJ. A guide to NG feeding

equipment. Prof Nurse 1988 Nov; 4(2): 91–94

Taylor SJ. A guide to nasogastric feeding. Prof Nurse 1988 Aug; 3(11):439–442

Maintaining a nasogastric tube. Nursing 1989 Feb; 19(2):25

Parenteral Nutrition

Bodoky A. Parenteral nutrition by peripheral vein, portal vein or central venous catheter? World J Surg 1986 Feb; 10(1):47–52

Driscoll DF and Bistrian BR. Clinical issues in the therapeutic monitoring of total parenteral nutrition. Clin Lab Med 1987 Sep; 7(3):699–714

Gutcher G and Cutz E. Complications of parenteral nutrition. Semin Perinatol 1986 Jul; 10(3):196–207

Muller JM et al. Indications and effects of perioperative parenteral nutrition. World J Surg 1986 Feb; 10(1):53–63

Murphy LM and Lipman TO. Central venous catheter care in parenteral nutrition: A review. JPEN (J Parenter Enteral Nutr) 1987 Mar–Apr; 11(2): 190–201

Robin AP and Greig PD. Basic principles of intravenous nutritional support. Clin Chest Med 1986 Mar; 7(1):29–39

Shanbhogue LK et al. Parenteral nutrition in the surgical patient. Br J Surg 1987 Mar; 74(3):172–180

Sim AJ. Practical aspects of intravenous nutrition. Contemp Issues Clin Biochem 1986; 4:221–231

Fat Emulsion

Bach AC et al. Medium-chain triglyceride-based fat emulsions: An alternative energy supply in stress and sepsis. JPEN (J Parenter Enteral Nutr) 1988 Nov–Dec; 12(Suppl 6):82S–88S

Carpentier YA et al. Fat emulsions are more than energy suppliers.

Infusionsther Elin Ernahr 1986 Aug; 13(4):182–184

Ekman L et al. New developments in lipid emulsions for parenteral nutrition. Infusionsther Klin Ernahr 1987 Sep; 14(Suppl 3):4–9

Nutrition

Bernstein MD et al. A technique for feeding jejunostomy. Surg Gynecol Obstet 1989 Feb; 168(2):173–174

Carpentier YA. Indications for nutritional support. Gut 1986 Nov; 27(Suppl 1): 14–17

Freeman B. The use of endoscopy after gastric partitioning for morbid obesity. Gastroenterol Clin North Am 1987 Jun; 16(2):339–347

Heymsfield SB et al. Physiologic response and clinical implications of nutrition support. Am J Cardiol 1987 Oct 30; 60(12):75G–81G

Koretz RL. Nutritional support: How much for how much? Gut 1986 Nov; 27(Suppl 1):85–95

Lembcke B and Caspary WF. Malabsorption syndromes. Baillieres Clin Gastroenterol 1988 Apr; 2(2):329–351

McConnell EA. Fluid and electrolyte concerns in intestinal surgical procedures. Nurs Clin North Am 1987 Dec; 22(4):853–860

O'Morain CA. Nutritional therapy in ambulatory patients. Dig Dis Sci 1987 Dec; 32(Suppl 12):95S–99S

Shaw JH. Recent advances in the nutritional and metabolic management of critically ill surgical patients. N Z Med J 1986 Sep 10; 99(809):665–667

Thomasma DC et al. Continuance of nutritional care in the terminally ill patient. Crit Care Clin 1986 Jan; 2(1): 61–71

Wahlqvist ML. Vitamin use in clinical medicine. Med J Aust 1987 Jan 5; 146(1):30–37

Enteral Nutrition

Allison SP. Enteral nutrition. Comtemp Issues Clin Biochem 1986; 4:204–220

Bastow MD. Complications of enteral nutrition. Gut 1986 Nov; 27(Suppl 1): 51–55

Farley JM. Current trends in enteral feeding. Crit Care Nurse 1988 Jun; 8(4):23–28

Heymsfield SB et al. Enteral nutritional support. Metabolic, cardiovascular, and pulmonary interrelations. Clin Chest Med 1986 Mar; 7(1):41–67

Jones BJ. Enteral feeding: Techniques of administration. Gut 1986 Nov; 27(Suppl 1):47–50

Silk DB. Diet formulation and choice of enteral diet. Gut 1986 Nov; 27(Suppl 1):40–46

Skipper A. Specialized formulas for enteral nutritional support. J Am Diet Assoc 1986 May; 86(5):654–658

Total Parenteral Nutrition

Anderson K. TPN: Total parenteral nutrition. Aust Nurses J 1988 Oct; 18(4):11–13

Benotti PN and Bristrian BR. Practical aspects and complications of total parenteral nutrition. Crit Care Clin 1987 Jan; 3(1):115–131

Johndrow PD. Making your patient and his family feel at home with T.P.N. Nursing 1988 Oct; 18(10):65–69

Kushner RF. Total parenteral nutrition-associated metabolic acidosis. JPEN (J Parenter Enteral Nutr) 1986 May–Jun; 10(3):306–310

Lemoyne M and Jeejeebhoy KN. Total parenteral nutrition in the critically ill patient. Chest 1986 Apr; 89(4):568–575

Michie B. Making sense of total parenteral nutrition. Nurs Times 1988 May 18–24; 84(20):46–47

Wolfram G. Medium-chain triglycerides (MCT) for total parenteral nutrition. World J Surg 1986 Feb; 10(1):33–37

Major Manifestations of Gastrointestinal Disturbance

Anorexia, Nausea, and Vomiting

Normal Physiology

A. Appetite—a desire for food, or an agreeable attitude toward ingesting food, often specific kinds of food.

1. The frontal and parietal areas of the cerebrum, but especially the hypothalamus, are known to be associated with appetite.
2. Desire for food is acutely associated with increased rates of gastric hydrochloric acid secretion, with gastric hyperemia, and hypermotility.

B. Hunger—a strong sensation or urge to eat following a period of fasting.

1. Hunger is temporarily associated with rhythmic contractions of the stomach.
2. The precise mechanisms by which hunger is produced are unknown; it is related to a low blood sugar level.

C. Satiety—a condition following consumption of an amount of food sufficient to meet present requirements; a feeling that one has had enough to eat.

Anorexia

Lack of appetite for food; lack of interest in all food.
1. Associated with a disinterest in consumption of even those foods that one ordinarily likes to eat
2. Associated with decreased secretion of gastric hydrochloric acid
3. Possible causes:
   a. Unpleasant or upsetting experiences
   b. Apprehension, fear, and anxiety
   c. Excitement, both pleasurable and undesirable
   d. Systemic and local diseases, such as hepatic failure and uremia

Dyspepsia (Indigestion)

Painful, difficult, or disturbed digestion. The person suffers from several of a group of symptoms—nausea, regurgitation, vomiting, heartburn, bloating, and stomach discomfort.

Nausea

A most unpleasant sensation usually associated with a distinct revulsion toward the ingestion of food; it may or may not precede vomiting.
1. Very often, anorexia is succeeded by nausea and vomiting. However, either of these states may occur without the others.
2. Associated with decreased motor activity of the stomach, pallor of gastric mucosa, and contraction of proximal duodenum.
3. Frequently associated with evidence of diffuse autonomic discharge—profuse watery salivation, sudden drenching perspiration, tachycardia.
4. Many patients find it difficult to describe:
   a. Vague unpleasantness in epigastrium
   b. Distressing feelings in the throat
   c. Vague unpleasantness spread diffusely in abdomen (must be distinguished from mild visceral abdominal pain)

Vomiting

Sudden forceful expulsion of stomach contents through the mouth.
1. Vomiting center is located in the medulla.
2. May or may not be preceded by nausea and retching.
3. Exaggerated and often extreme vasomotor activities may immediately precede and accompany the vomiting act; watery salivation, sweating, pulse rate change, vasoconstriction, and pallor.
4. Tachycardia prior to vomiting becomes bradycardia during process.
5. Incited by neuromuscular "reverse peristalsis" or mechanical obstruction.

Nature of Vomitus

Color/Taste/ Consistency	Possible Source
Yellowish or greenish	May contain bile
	Medication—senna
Bright red (arterial)	Hemorrhage, peptic ulcer
Dark red (venous)	Hemorrhage, esophageal or gastric varices
"Coffee grounds"	Digested blood from slowly bleeding gastric or duodenal ulcer
Undigested food	Gastric tumor?
	Ulcer obstruction?
"Bitter" taste	Bile
"Sour" or "acid"	Gastric contents
Fecal components	Intestinal obstruction

Constipation

Constipation is a decrease in the frequency, volume, or ease of stool passage.
Obstipation is absence of intestinal output (no stool).
1. Constipation is usually caused by altered routine in dietary and activity patterns; by drugs such as morphine, codeine, and atropine; by mechanical obstruction or surgery; by psychological factors resulting from restricted use of toilet facilities; and by old age. It may also occur as a result of chronic, strong-laxative abuse.
2. Manifestations of constipation include changes in color, consistency, and ease of expulsion of stools, which may be darker, harder, and difficult or painful to pass.

Diarrhea

Diarrhea is an increase in frequency, fluidity, and/or volume of stools.
1. It is a leading cause of death in developing countries, where sanitation is poor and dietary deficiency widespread.
2. Acute diarrhea can be a serious problem in elderly and debilitated persons.
3. Chronic diarrhea is associated with malabsorption, malnutrition, anemia, and increased susceptibility to other diseases.

Diagnostic Evaluation
Laboratory Studies

Stool Specimen

A. Description
1. The stool is examined for its amount, consistency, and color; a screening test for occult blood is also done. Normal color varies from light to dark brown. Special tests may be made for fecal urobilinogen, fat, nitrogen, parasites, food residue, and other substances.
2. Various foods affect stool color.
   a. Meat protein—dark brown
   b. Spinach—green
   c. Beets—red
   d. Cocoa—dark red or brown
   e. Licorice—black
3. Various medications affect stool color.
   a. Phenylbutazone (Butazolidin, Azolid)—black
   b. Oxyphenbutazone (Tandearil)—black
      Phenazopyridine (Pyridium)—orange–black
   c. Aluminum hydroxide—gray–white
   d. Pyrvinium pamoate (Povan)—red–orange
   e. Bismuth compounds—black
   f. Senna laxatives—yellow–green
   g. Hematinics (iron salts)—black
   h. Barium—white
4. Hemoglobin and bleeding affect the stool in the following way:
   a. *Occult* blood (not visible to the naked eye)—use occult stool testing kit for detection of bleeding.
   b. Upper GI bleeding—tarry black (melena)
   c. Lower GI bleeding—bright red blood
   d. Lower rectal or anal bleeding—blood streaking on surface of stool or on toilet paper
5. Characteristic clinical entities related to characteristics of stool:
   a. Bulky, greasy, foamy, foul in odor, gray in color with silvery sheen—steatorrhea
   b. Light gray "clay-colored" (due to absence of "acholic" bile pigments)—biliary obstruction
   c. Mucus or pus visible—chronic ulcerative colitis, shigellosis
   d. Small, dry, rocky-hard masses—constipation, obstruction, fecal obstruction
   e. Marble-sized stool pellets—spastic colon syndrome

B. Nursing Management
1. Use a tongue blade to place a small amount of stool in a disposable waxed container.
2. Save a sample of any fecal material if it is unusual in appearance, contains worms or blood, is blood-streaked, has unusual color or much mucus.
3. Send specimens to be examined for parasites to the laboratory immediately so that the parasites may be observed under microscope while viable, fresh, and warm.
4. Test for occult blood or to confirm grossly visible melena or blood—hemoccult guaiac slide test.

Hemoccult Guaiac Slide Test

Commercially available guaiac-impregnated slides present a simple, inexpensive, and aesthetically acceptable method of testing feces for blood.

A. Patient Preparation

(Preparation varies; therefore, check with physician.) Common practices are:

1. Diet should be high-residue during 48–72 hours before specimen is collected.
2. Similar diet is followed for next 3 days:
   a. Vegetables—particularly lettuce, spinach, and corn; cooked and raw
   b. Fruits—particularly prunes, grapes, plums, and apples
   c. Any product that is "all bran" for daily cereal
3. Any foods that cause severe diarrhea or severe abdominal pain are to be avoided.

B. Procedure

1. A wooden applicator is used to apply a stool specimen to the slide (for 3 successive days). Three samples are taken because:
   a. There may be intermittent bleeding.
   b. There is the possibility of false-negative results.
2. Slides inside a packet can be brought or mailed to the physician.
3. When hydrogen peroxide (denatured alcohol-stabilizing mixture) is added to samples, any blood cells present liberate their hemoglobin, and a bluish ring appears on the electrophoretic paper. Read precisely at 30 seconds, no more or less.
4. A single positive test is an indication for further diagnostic research for gastrointestinal lesions.
   a. False-positive results occur in about 10% of tests.
   b. Test may become false-negative in 10% of specimens tested 4 or more days after streaking on paper.

Radiographic and Imaging Studies

Upper Gastrointestinal Series and Small Bowel Series

A. Description

1. Upper gastrointestinal series and small bowel series are fluoroscopic x-ray examinations of the esophagus, stomach, and small intestine after the patient ingests barium sulfate.
2. As the barium passes through the gastrointestinal tract, fluoroscopy outlines the gastrointestinal mucosa and organs.
3. Spot films record significant findings.

B. Nursing Management and Patient Instruction

1. Explain procedure to patient.
2. Instruct patient to maintain low-residue diet for 2–3 days before test. A cathartic may be prescribed the night before the test.
3. Fast and avoid smoking after midnight before the test.
4. Tell patient the test takes up to 6 hours to complete.
5. The physician may prescribe all narcotics and anticholinergics to be held 24 hours before the test because they interfere with small intestine motility.
6. The patient will be instructed at various times throughout the procedure to drink the barium. (480–600 ml. [16–20 ounces])
7. A cathartic will be prescribed postprocedure to facilitate expulsion of barium.
8. Instruct the patient that his stool will be light in color for the next 2–3 days from the barium.
9. Instruct patient to notify physician if he hasn't passed

the barium in 2–3 days because retention of the barium may cause obstruction or fecal impaction.

> **NURSING ALERT:** An upper GI and small bowel series is contraindicated in patients with obstruction or perforation of the gastrointestinal tract. The barium may increase the obstruction.

Barium Enema

The fasting patient receives a rectal instillation of a barium sulfate suspension, which is viewed in the fluoroscope and then filmed. If the patient is adequately prepared, the fluoroscope will reveal:
   a. Colon—contour of entire colon is visible.
   b. Cecum and appendix—contour and motility observed.

Note: Air may be introduced to give air contrast studies.

Nursing Management and Patient Instruction

1. Explain to the patient:
   a. What the x-ray procedure involves
   b. That proper preparation provides a more accurate view of the tract
   c. That it is important to retain the barium so that all surfaces of the tract are coated with opaque solution
2. Two days before the examination, the patient may be given a minimal-residue diet.
3. The day before the examination, some physicians limit food intake to liquids; others advise liquids for the evening meal only.
4. The day before the examination, a cathartic may be prescribed.
5. The evening before and on the morning of the examination, a cleansing enema may be given. Food and fluids are restricted before the examination.
6. The above preparation varies, but the objective remains the same; to have the large intestine as clear of fecal material as possible.

> **NURSING ALERT:** Use nursing judgment regarding the administration of cathartics or enemas in the presence of acute abdominal pain or obstruction. For the patient with ulcerative colitis, cathartics or cleansing enemas may be too rigorous, and can possibly cause bleeding.

7. Administer an oil-retention enema or a cathartic following the barium enema to completely evacuate the barium.

> **NURSING ALERT:** Fecal impaction is a complication following barium studies.

8. Encourage the patient to eat following the examination, as he has been fasting and is undoubtedly hungry.

Computed Tomography (CT Scan)

Computed tomography (CT) is accomplished using a scanner that operates by detecting x-rays from a finely focused beam that rotates around a patient. The subtle differences in x-ray absorption by various tissues then are assembled by a computer and displayed on a screen as a radiologic image.

1. It provides precise anatomic and pathological information for a wide array of intra-abdominal and other conditions.
2. Abscesses can be drained using CT as a guide for catheter placement (obviating need for surgery).
3. By exactly noting the full extent (staging) of a malignancy, surgical intervention can be more precise.
4. In abdominal trauma, multiple organ involvement can be noted by CT, thereby reducing number of diagnostic tests.
5. Invasive vascular techniques may be reduced using CT scanner.

Ultrasonography (Ultrasound)

Ultrasonography is the focusing of a beam of high-frequency sound waves over an abdominal organ. This creates waves that vary with changes in tissue density.

Endoscopic Procedures

Upper Gastrointestinal Endoscopy

A. Description

Upper gastrointestinal fiberscopy is the direct visualization of the gastric mucosa through a lighted endoscope (gastroscope). Endoscopes are flexible scopes equipped with a fiberoptic lens through which colored photographs or motion pictures can be taken.

Primary diagnostic gastrointestinal endoscopy (PRIDGE) is a rapid, accurate, and safe method of examining the upper GI tract in selected patients and is an excellent initial examination.

B. Nursing Interventions

1. Explain the following to the patient:
   a. What is about to happen.
   b. That fasting is necessary before the examination to prevent aspiration of gastric contents and to permit complete visualization of the stomach.
   c. That dentures are removed to facilitate passing the scope and to prevent injury.
   d. That a sedative or tranquilizer may be given to help him to relax.
   e. That a topical anesthetic may be used for local comfort and to prevent gagging.
   f. That air will be pumped into the stomach during the procedure to permit visualization of the stomach.
2. Following a gastric examination:
   a. Check the gag reflex before offering food or fluids.
      (1) Tickle the back of the patient's throat with a tongue depressor or cotton swab; usually 2–4 hours after the examination, the reflex functions return to normal.
      (2) If fluids are handled normally, the patient may then be offered food.
   b. Check for signs of perforation—abdominal pain, subcutaneous emphysema, dyspnea, cyanosis, back pain, temperature elevation, hydrothorax, rigid abdomen.
   c. Offer throat lozenges or warm saline gargles to relieve throat soreness.
   d. Inform the patient that because of air pumped into the stomach, he may pass gas by belching or passing flatus.

Gastric Biopsy

A. Description

1. Obtaining tissue from the gastric mucosa can be done through a gastroscope during endoscopy or fiberscopy.
2. Forceps extended through the scope may be used to "bite" tissue, or tissue may be obtained via suction as it pulls mucosa to excising blades within the scope.
3. Tissue in one area may be representative of tissue in all sections of the stomach; however, by looking through the scope, the physician can be discriminating in selection of specific tissue.

B. Nursing Interventions

Similar to that for gastric endoscopy.

Guidelines Assisting With a Proctosigmoidoscopy

Proctosigmoidoscopy is the viewing of the sigmoid, rectum, and anal canal by means of a sigmoidoscope, a tubular fiberoptic or rigid instrument that can be illuminated. It is used to confirm radiologic findings, to obtain biopsies, cytologic and culture specimens, to locate and stop bleeding areas, and to perform a polypectomy.

Equipment

Fleet-type enema—used at least 1 hour before the sigmoidoscopy
Oral laxative
Water-soluble lubricant
Sigmoidoscope
Biopsy forceps
Culture swab
Long applicator sticks (cotton)
Drapes or sheets
Specimen bottles containing 10% formalin
Culture tubes
4 × 4 gauze sponges

Cytology brush
Glass eyepiece to fit on scope during insufflation of air
Disposable gloves for preliminary digital examination
Suction machine
Microscopic slides with fixative or 95% ethyl alcohol
Specimen labels

NURSING ALERT:
1. Emergency resuscitation equipment needs to be available, because the vagus nerve is often stimulated and can potentiate a vagal reaction (pallor, diaphoresis, dizziness, weakness, unconsciousness, decrease in blood pressure and pulse rate, sometimes causing these vital signs to be unobtainable).
2. If giving enemas before the procedure, do not advance the tube too high into the colon, and administer the fluid slowly. If rectal bleeding or abdominal pain occur, stop at once and call the physician.

Procedure   **Preparatory Phase**

1. Three to four hours before the procedure, give two Fleet enemas as prescribed. The enema should be retained at least 5–10 minutes before evacuation.
2. Some physicians request that the patient be on a light diet the evening before and the breakfast before the examination. Others prefer a cathartic the evening before the examination.
3. Ensure that all equipment is working properly.
4. Ensure that a consent form has been signed before the procedure.
5. Have the patient void and put on a hospital gown.

Procedure

Nursing Action	Rationale/Amplification
1. Record baseline vital signs. Leave the blood pressure cuff in place. An automatic blood pressure machine may be used; however, a manual cuff is preferred in the event the patient has a vagal reaction (see Nursing Alert above).	1. Monitoring of the blood pressure and pulse throughout the procedure will be necessary.

2. Have the patient assume the knee–chest or Sims' lateral position.
  a. Knee–chest position
    (1) Knees are spread comfortably apart
    (2) Thighs are perpendicular to table
    (3) Feet are extended over the edge
    (4) Head is turned sideways to right (head shares pillow with chest)
    (5) Left arm is flexed to side of chest
    (6) Right arm may rest above head
  b. Sims' lateral position
 	
    (1) Place patient on left side with left leg partially flexed at hip and knees; right leg should be fully flexed.
    (2) Pelvis to be perpendicular to table
	2. The position used depends on physician preference, patient condition, and nature of examining table (or bed).
	  a. This position permits the sigmoid to hang forward, diminishing the angle at the rectosigmoid junction.
	
	  b. Used for elderly, ill, or arthritic patients or those who are reluctant to assume the knee–chest position.

3. Drape the patient so that only perineum is visible.	3. A disposable large sheet with a circular opening is practical. This will minimize embarrassment.
4. Explain to the patient to take slow deep breaths as the physician examines the rectum by digital examination.	4. The physician is examining for tenderness, mucus, blood fistula, inflammation, ulceration, and feces. The digital examination also indicates the direction of the anal canal, its patency, and the presence of any abnormality; it promotes anal relaxation and helps to lubricate the orifice.
5. Warm sigmoidoscope in tap water or sterilizer to slightly above body temperature; lubricate tip of scope.	5. A cold scope would cause discomfort and promote contraction rather than relaxation of perianal muscles. Water-soluble lubricant permits easier passage of scope. It also minimizes the urge to defecate at tube insertion.
6. Physician spreads buttocks and anal margins with left hand and inserts instrument with right hand (or vice versa). Have the patient breathe deeply.	6. Keep instrument out of view of patient. Breathing slowly and deeply will help relax abdominal muscles and minimize cramping.
7. Nurse encourages relaxation and explains each step in advance.	7. Reassuring the patient promotes relaxation.
8. Physician may use a glass eyepiece over viewing end of scope; an insufflation bulb and tubing are attached. A small quantity of air may be pumped into the bowel. Tell patient as the air moves down the bowel he may experience flatulence. This is normal.	8. The purpose of inflating lower bowel with air is to expand the area viewed so that vision is not obstructed by mucosal folds and to facilitate passage into the sigmoid colon.
9. Examination of the sigmoid, rectum, and mucosa are done while the scope is being removed. If a rigid scope is used, passage of a large cotton swab through the scope may be done to remove blood, mucus, and feces. If a flexible scope is used, only suction is necessary to clear the field. Turn suction to lowest setting initially.	9. This clears the field of vision.
10. Passage of biopsy forceps, cytology brush, or culture swab through the scope is done to collect specimens.	10. Specimens will be placed in 10% formalin and labeled. A specimen for cytology is placed in a container of 95% ethyl alcohol or affixed to a microscopic slide with slide fixative. Specimens for cultures will be sent in specimen tubes.
11. Relay to the physician any expressions or complaints of pain by the patient.	11. Tenderness and pain may be experienced by the patient with a history of abdominal surgery; procedure may have to be terminated in order not to risk perforation.

(continued)

Assisting With a Proctosigmoidoscopy *(continued)*

Procedure *(continued)*	**Nursing Action**	**Rationale/Amplification**

Follow-Up Phase

1. On withdrawal of scope, assist patient in gradually assuming a relaxed position.
2. If disposable scope is used, rinse scope and discard in proper receptacle. Reusable scopes are thoroughly cleaned in soap and water.
3. Record the procedure, preparation of the patient, reaction of the patient, and patient's vital signs. Also note any collection of specimens.
4. Label all specimens and send to the laboratory.
5. Observe the patient for *complications:* hemorrhage (increased pulse rate, decreased blood pressure, weakness, pallor, rectal bleeding, and possible abdominal pain), perforation (sudden severe abdominal pain), fever, malaise, changes in vital signs, bloody or mucoid rectal drainage, and possible abdominal distention.

1. Wipe the perineal area to prevent soilage of garments and to promote comfort.
2. Sterilizable parts are sterilized before scope is stored.

Polypectomy and Postcare

1. Prepare intestinal tract meticulously; if there is any fecal matter in the field near the polyp, the procedure will be postponed and bowel preparation will have to be repeated.
2. When the tissue has been cut by cauterization, the snare-cautery device is removed, and the polyp tissue is withdrawn by suction.
3. Following polypectomy, the colonoscope may be reinserted, the inner bowel insufflated with air, and the operated area carefully examined for possible hemorrhage.

Postcare

1. Care following polypectomy depends on size of the polyps removed and the general condition of the patient. Usually the ambulatory patient can be discharged with no medication and no dietary restrictions.
2. For in-hospital patients, vital signs are checked for several hours, full liquid diet is given the day of surgery, and soft, low-residue diet is given for 2 weeks thereafter. Monitor for complications such as pain and bleeding.
3. Follow-up by complete colonoscopic examination usually is scheduled for 6–8 weeks later.
4. Inform the patient of dietary restrictions such as liquids for the first 24 hours post-polypectomy, then soft, low-residue food for the next 24 hours, and then regular, low-residue foods for a couple of weeks.

NURSING ALERT: Reminder: If a polypectomy is done through a sigmoidoscope or a colonoscope, barium enema should not be done until 7–10 days thereafter because of risk of perforation at the polypectomy site.

Assisting With a Colonoscopy

Colonoscopy is the direct visualization of the large intestine, descending transverse and ascending colon, cecum, sigmoid colon, rectum, and anal canal by means of a fiberoptic colonoscope.

Purposes

1. As a diagnostic aid to view and assess the status of the large intestine; used to diagnose such conditions as cancer, polyps, strictures, ulcerative colitis, and Crohn's disease.
2. As an operative instrument to remove polyps, to obtain tissue for biopsy, culture, and cytology specimens, and to remove foreign bodies.

Equipment

Complete colonoscope, possibly with sidearm second observer scope

Water-soluble lubricant
Suction apparatus
Air-insufflating equipment
Snare
Drapes or sheets
Fluoroscope
Specimen labels

Enema
Oral laxative
Specimen bottles containing 10% formalin; 95% ethyl alcohol
Microscopic slides with fixative
Culture tubes
4 × 4 gauze sponges

The Colonoscope

The *colonoscope* is an instrument consisting of a flexible 4-mm. glass bundle (containing about 250,000 glass fibers).

1. There is a lens at both ends equipped to focus and magnify.
2. Light is transmitted from an external source by way of a fiberoptic bundle to the tip of the scope; an image is transmitted regardless of the looping or twisting of the flexible bundle.
3. Accessory channels provide for
   a. Suction of fluid, blood, and mucus
   b. Insufflation of air or water
   c. Biopsy
4. There are two kinds of colonoscopes:
   a. To visualize left side of colon—105 cm.
   b. To visualize entire colon—165–185 cm.

NURSING ALERT:
1. Emergency resuscitation equipment needs to be available, because the vagus nerve is often stimulated and can potentiate a vagal reaction (pallor, diaphoresis, dizziness, weakness, unconsciousness, decrease in blood pressure and pulse rate, sometimes causing these vital signs to be unobtainable).
2. If giving enemas before the procedure, do not advance the tube too high into the colon, and administer the fluid slowly. If rectal bleeding or abdominal pain occur—stop at once and call the physician.
3. Keep narcotic antagonists handy to correct respiratory depression from the narcotics.

Procedure

Preparatory Phase

1. Explain the procedure to patient; his understanding and cooperation will promote his relaxation and facilitate his comfort during examination.
2. Limit the patient's intake to clear liquids for 24–48 hours before the procedure (as directed by the endoscopist).
3. Administer a cathartic as prescribed, in the evening for 2 days before the examination.
4. Give tap water or saline enemas, 1–2 liters, approximately 3 hours prior to the colonoscopy until the returns are clear.

Alternate Preparation

   a. GoLYTELY is an oral electrolyte solution given for bowel cleansing prior to colonoscopy.
   b. The preparation time is greatly reduced from usual procedure; the patient must understand the procedure and keep record of his intake, output, and any symptoms occurring during this time.
   c. Diarrhea is to be expected; mild cramps and transient feeling of fullness may be experienced.
5. Ensure that all equipment is working properly.
6. Ensure that a consent form has been signed prior to the procedure.
7. Have the patient void and put on a hospital gown.
8. Administer sedative or analgesic as prescribed; sedation is desirable, but the patient must be sensitive to any pain during the examination so that his response can be relayed to the endoscopist. Raise the side rails to prevent falls. Preferably, this procedure is performed where fluoroscopy is available.
9. Insert a heparin lock or start an IV infusion as prescribed to establish an open vein for administering a sedative or emergency medications. Observe the patient carefully for respiratory depression and bradycardia.

Procedure

Nursing Action	Rationale/Amplification
1. Record baseline vital signs. Leave the blood pressure cuff in place. An automatic blood pressure machine may be used; however, a manual cuff is preferred in the event the patient has a vagal reaction (see Nursing Alert above).	1. Monitoring the blood pressure and pulse throughout the procedure will be necessary.
2. Place patient in the left lateral position with knees flexed.	2. This position is assumed to follow the location of the sigmoid-rectum anatomically.
3. Warm the scope in tap water.	3. A warm scope promotes entrance. It also decreases the urge to defecate.
4. The lubricated scope is inserted and passed through the rectum.	4. This procedure is done under direct visualization; valvulae are prominent throughout the colon.
5. At apex of rectrosigmoid area, there is a red "blur-out."	5. Blur-out occurs because the tip of the colonoscope touches the sigmoid colon wall.
6. The instrument is steadily inserted, rotated, and flexed.	6. This will promote the sliding of the tip along the greater curvature of any loops in the sigmoid colon.
7. If mucosa does not appear red, but seems to blanch or become white, the scope is withdrawn until red mucosa appears.	7. Whitening or blanching is indicative of compression of bowel wall with danger of perforation.

(continued)

Guidelines Assisting With a Colonoscopy *(continued)*

Procedure *(continued)*	**Nursing Action**	**Rationale/Amplification**
	8. The endoscopist uses "maneuvers" to straighten difficult curves. A fluoroscope can also be used to monitor scope position and direction.	8. By various maneuvers, such as "alpha," "hooking," or "lifting," the endoscopist is able to continue with the insertion and examination of the walls of the colon.
	9. Maneuvers are resorted to at sharp turns such as the sigmoid-descending colon, the splenic flexure, the transverse colon, and the hepatic flexure.	9. Occasional withdrawal and appearance of a triangular configuration or a bluish color are techniques and observations to assist in advancing the scope.
	10. As the scope is advanced into the ascending colon, the nurse can position the patient on his back or on his right side.	10. This permits the maneuvering of the colonoscope into the cecum. It takes about 20–45 minutes to reach this point in the examination.
	11. If the physician directs, apply gentle pressure to the abdomen.	11. This facilitates passage of the scope.
	12. After the structures are viewed, a biopsy forceps, cytology brush, or culture swab may be passed through the scope to collect specimens. Specimens will be placed in 10% formalin and labeled.	12. Specimens for cytology are placed in containers of 95% ethyl alcohol or affixed to microscope slides, with slide fixative. Culture specimens will be sent in specimen tubes.
	13. The physician may prescribe atropine to control bowel spasms or glucagon to paralyze the bowel for a polypectomy. If either is used, monitor for hypotension and irregular pulse.	13. Relay to the physician any expressions or complaints of pain by the patient. Atropine increases the pulse rate.

Follow-Up Phase

1. Instruct the patient to remain on the examining table, stretcher, or in bed for 1–2 hours postprocedure until the sedative wears off.
2. Label all specimens and send to lab.
3. Monitor vital signs every 30 minutes postprocedure until stable.
4. Remove the heparin lock or IV infusion after the patient is stable.
5. Observe patient for *complications:* hemorrhage (increased pulse rate, decreased blood pressure, weakness, pallor, rectal bleeding, and possible abdominal pain), perforation (sudden severe abdominal pain), fever, malaise, changes in vital signs, bloody or mucoid rectal drainage, and possible abdominal distention.
6. Record the procedure, patient preparation, reaction of the patient, patient's vital signs, and any medications administered. Also, record collection of specimens.

Special Treatment Modalities

Guidelines Nasogastric Intubation and Removal—Levin Tube (Short Tube) or Salem Sump Tube

Goals

1. Remove fluid and gas from the GI tract (decompression).
2. Prevent or relieve nausea and vomiting after surgery or traumatic events by decompressing the stomach.
3. Determine the amount of pressure and motor activity in the GI tract (diagnostic studies).
4. Treat patients with mechanical obstruction and bleeding within the upper GI tract.
5. Administer medications and feeding (gavage) directly into the GI tract.
6. Obtain a specimen of gastric contents for laboratory studies (when pyloric or intestinal obstruction is suspected).

Equipment

Nasogastric tube—usually Levin (rubber or plastic, No. 12 to 18 French)—preferably disposable (plastic tubes are less irritating than rubber) or double-lumen Salem sump tube
Water-soluble lubricant
Suction equipment
Clamp for tubing
Towel, tissues, and emesis basin
Glass of water and straw, or perhaps ice chips
Tincture of benzoin
Hypoallergenic tape: ½" and 1"
Irrigating set with 20-ml. syringe or a 60-ml. catheter-tip syringe
Stethoscope
Tongue blade
Penlight
Disposable gloves

Follow-Up Equipment

Decongestant spray
Lip pomade
Mouth hygiene materials

Procedure

Preparatory Phase

1. Ask the patient if he has ever had nasal surgery, trauma, or a deviated septum.
2. Explain procedure to the patient and tell how mouth breathing, panting, and swallowing will help in passing the tube.
3. Place the patient in a sitting or high Fowler's position; place a towel across his chest.
4. Determine with the patient what sign he might use, such as raising his index finger, to indicate "wait a few moments" because of gagging or discomfort.
5. Remove dentures; place emesis basin and tissues within the patient's reach.
6. Inspect the tube for defects; look for partially closed holes or rough edges.
7. Place rubber tubing in ice-chilled water for a few minutes to make the tube firmer. Plastic tubing may already be firm enough; if too stiff, dip in warm water.
8. Determine the length of the tube needed to reach the stomach by placing the end of the tube at the tip of the patient's nose. Then extend it to the earlobe and down to the xiphoid process (Fig. 20-1). Mark this distance with hypoallergenic tape. (Measurement range for the average-size adult is 55–66 cm. [22–26 inches].)
9. Have the patient blow his nose to clear his nostrils.
10. Inspect the nostrils with a penlight, observing for any obstruction. Occlude each nostril and have the patient breathe. This will help determine which nostril is more patent.
11. Wash your hands. Put on disposable gloves.

Procedure

Nursing Action	Rationale/Amplification
1. Coil the first 7–10 cm. (3–4 inches) of the tube around your fingers.	1. This curves tubing and facilitates tube passage.
2. Lubricate the coiled portion of the tube with water-soluble lubricant. Avoid occluding the tube's holes with lubricant.	2. Lubrication reduces friction between the mucous membranes and tube and prevents injury to the nasal passages. Using a water-soluble lubricant prevents oil-aspiration pneumonia if the tube accidently slips into trachea.
3. Tilt back the patient's head before inserting tube into nostril and gently pass tube into the posterior nasopharynx, directing downward and backward toward the ear.	3. Passage of the tube is facilitated by following the natural contours of the body. The slower the advancement of the tube at this point, the less likelihood of putting pressure on the turbinates, which could cause pain and bleeding.
4. When tube reaches the pharynx, the patient may gag; allow him to rest for a few moments.	4. Gag reflex is triggered by the presence of the tube.
5. Have the patient hold his head in a partially flexed position; offer him several sips of water sipped through a straw or permit him to suck on ice chips, unless contraindicated. Advance tube as he swallows.	5. Flexed head position makes swallowing easier and the tube less likely to enter trachea. Swallowing facilitates passage of tube. Actually, once the tube passes the cricopharyngeal sphincter into the esophagus, it can be slowly and steadily advanced even if the patient does not swallow. Swallowing water or ice chips helps pass the tube into the esophagus.
6. Gently rotate the tube 180 degrees to redirect the curve.	6. This prevents the tube from entering the patient's mouth.
7. Continue to advance tube gently each time the patient swallows.	
8. If obstruction appears to prevent tube from passing, do not use force. Rotating tube gently may help. If unsuccessful, remove tube and try other nostril.	8. Avoid discomfort and trauma to patient.
9. If there are signs of distress such as gasping, coughing, or cyanosis, immediately remove tube.	
10. Continue to advance the tube when the patient swallows, until the tape mark reaches the patient's nostril.	10. This is the reference point where the tube was measured.
11. To check whether the Levin tube is in the stomach:	
a. Aspirate contents of stomach with a 20-ml. syringe or 50-ml. catheter-tip syringe. If stomach contents cannot be aspirated, place the patient on his left side and advance the tube 2.5–5 cm. (1–2 inches) and try again.	a. Aspirated stomach contents indicate that the tube is in the stomach.
b. Place a stethoscope over epigastrium; inject 5–15 ml. of air into Levin tube.	b. Air can be detected by a "whooshing" sound entering stomach rather than the bronchus. If belching occurs, the tube is probably in the esophagus.
c. Ask the patient to talk.	c. If the patient cannot talk, the tube may be coiled in his throat or passed through his vocal cords.
d. Use the tongue blade and pen-light to examine the patient's mouth—especially an unconscious patient.	d. If the patient is choking or has difficulty breathing, the tube has probably entered the trachea.
e. If unsure whether the tube is in the stomach, notify the physician.	e. X-rays may be done to confirm tube placement.

(continued)

Guidelines Nasogastric Intubation and Removal—Levin Tube (Short Tube) or Salem Sump Tube *(continued)*

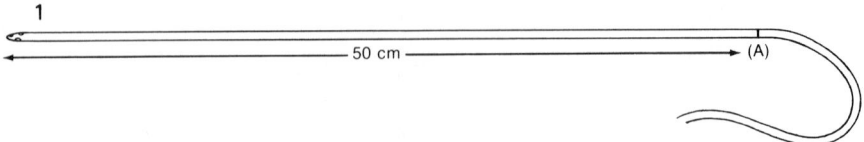

1. Mark the nasogastric tube at a point 50 cm. from the distal tip; call this point 'A'.

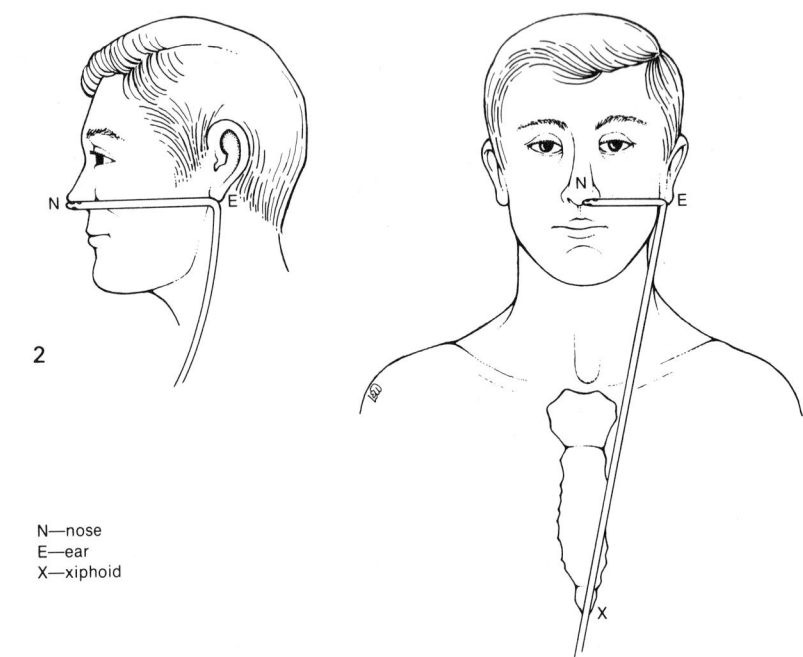

N—nose
E—ear
X—xiphoid

2. Have the patient sit in a neutral position with head facing forward. Place the distal tip of the tubing at the tip of the patient's nose (N); extend tube to the tragus (tip) of his ear (E), and then extend the tube straight down to the tip of his xiphoid (X). Mark this point 'B' on the tubing.

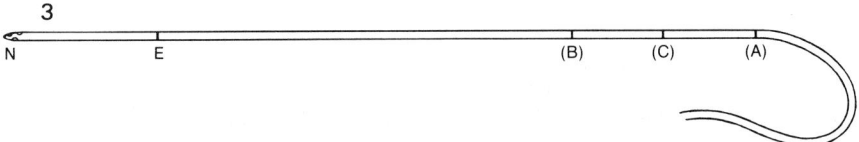

3. To locate point C on the tube, find the midpoint between points A and B. The nasogastric tube is passed to point C to ensure optimum placement in the stomach.

Figure 20-1. *The above diagram and steps (1, 2, 3) indicate how far a nasogastric tube is passed for optimal placement in the stomach (Hanson RL. Predictive criteria for length of nasogastric tube insertion for tube feeding. J Parenteral Enteral Nutr 1979 May–Jun; 3 [3]: 160–163)*

Procedure
(continued)

Nursing Action	Rationale/Amplification
12. After tube is passed and the correct placement is confirmed, attach the tube to suction or clamp the tube.	12. Clamping can be done using a metal clamp, plastic plug, or folding the tube over and slipping the bend into the tube end.
13. Apply tincture of benzoin to the area where the tape is placed.	13. This helps make the tube adhere, especially with diaphoretic patients.

Procedure
(continued)

Nursing Action	Rationale/Amplification

14. Anchor tube with hypoallergenic tape:
    a. Using (3″) hypoallergenic tape, split lengthwise and only half-way, attach unsplit end of tape to nose and cross split ends around tubing. Apply another piece of tape to bridge of nose.
15. Anchor the tubing to the patient's gown. Use a rubber band to make a slip-knot to anchor the tubing to the patient's gown. Secure the rubber band to the patient's gown using a safety pin.
16. Clamp the tube until the purpose for inserting the tube takes place.
17. Attach the tube to suction equipment if prescribed.
18. Assure the patient that most discomfort he feels will lessen as he gets used to the tube.
19. Irrigate the tube at regular intervals with small volumes of prescribed fluid.
    a. If the tube is a Salem sump, it will require periodic placing of 10–20 ml. of air through the vent port (blue port).
    b. Check the tube patency by placing the vent port next to your ear.

20. Administer oral hygiene every tour of duty.
    a. Cleanse tubing at nostril
    b. Use a decongestant spray, if necessary.
21. Apply cream or lip pomade to lips and nostril to prevent encrustation. Observe for necrosis.
22. If tube is to be in place for prolonged periods (beyond 12 hours), keep head of bed elevated at least 30 degrees.
23. Rotate tubing daily or more frequently.
24. Record the type, size of tube. Also note time and route of insertion. Document placement checks daily.

14. Prevents the patient's vision from being disturbed; prevents tubing from rubbing against nasal mucosa. This will ensure tape being secure.

15. To permit mobility of patient. This prevents tugging on the tube when the patient moves.

16. See #12.

19. **NURSING ALERT:** All enteric tubes must be irrigated at regular intervals using small volumes of fluid to ensure patency.
    a. This ensures patency of the Salem sump.
    b. A soft hissing sound is heard if the tube is patent.
    c. If the port hangs downward and the tube backs up, stomach contents will spill over the patient.

20. To promote patient comfort.

21. To keep tissue soft

22. To minimize gastroesophageal reflux

23. To prevent adherence to mucosa
24. This is to ensure proper placement at all times.

NURSING ALERT: If the patient has a nasal condition that prevents insertion through the nose, the tube is passed through the mouth. Remove dentures, slide the tube over the tongue, and proceed the same way as a nasal intubation. Make sure to coil the end of the tube and direct it downward at the pharynx.

Other Nursing Considerations

1. If the patient is unconscious, bend his head toward his chest. This will help close the trachea. Also advance the tube between respirations to make sure it does not enter the trachea. You will need to stroke the unconscious patient's neck to facilitate passage of the tube down the esophagus.
2. Watch for cyanosis while passing the tube in an unconscious patient. Cyanosis indicates the tube has entered the trachea.
3. Never place the end of the tube in a container of fluid while checking for placement. If the tube is in the trachea, the patient could inhale the water.
4. Do not tape the tube to the forehead; it can cause necrosis of the nostril.
5. Pain or vomiting after the tube is inserted indicates tube obstruction or incorrect placement.
6. Recognize the complications when the tube is in for prolonged periods: nasal erosion, sinusitis, esophagitis, esophagotracheal fistula, gastric ulceration, and pulmonary and oral infections (Fig. 20-2).

Removal of the Nasogastric Tube

Before Removing the Nasogastric Tubing
1. Be certain that gastric or small bowel drainage is not excessive in volume.
2. Ensure, by auscultation, that audible peristalsis is present.
3. Determine whether the patient is passing flatus; this indicates peristalsis.
4. There is a physician's order for removal.

Removing Nasogastric Tubing

(continued)

Guidelines   Nasogastric Intubation and Removal—Levin Tube (Short Tube) or Salem Sump Tube *(continued)*

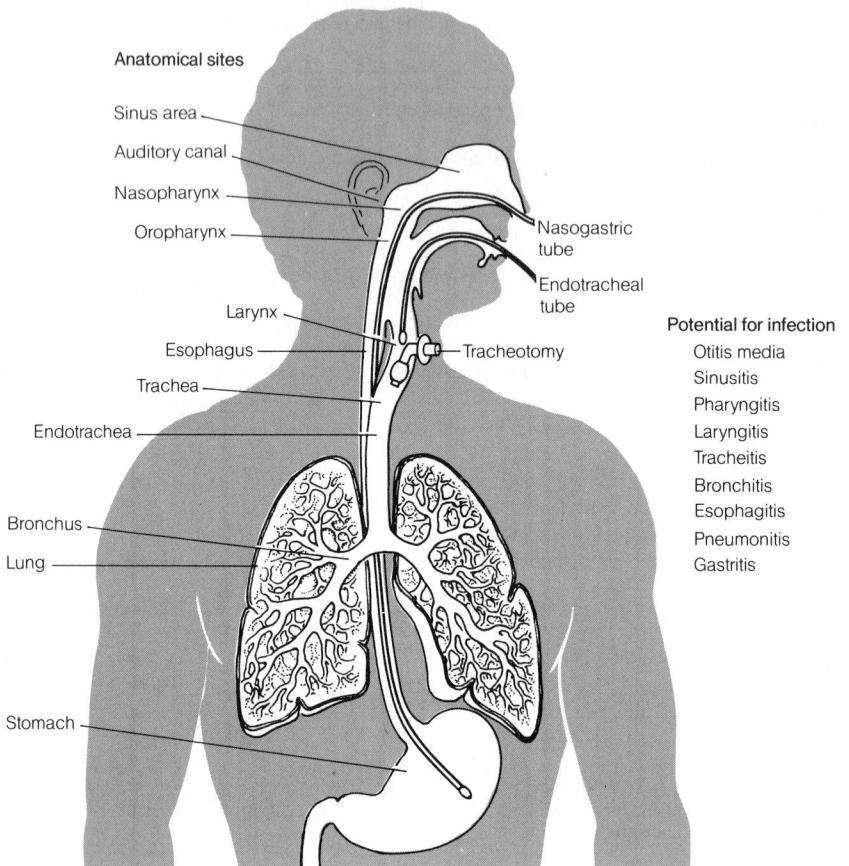

Anatomical sites

Sinus area

Auditory canal

Nasopharynx

Oropharynx

Nasogastric tube

Endotracheal tube

Larynx

Esophagus

Trachea

Tracheotomy

Endotrachea

Bronchus

Lung

Stomach

Potential for infection

Otitis media
Sinusitis
Pharyngitis
Laryngitis
Tracheitis
Bronchitis
Esophagitis
Pneumonitis
Gastritis

Figure 20-2. *All along the upper respiratory tract and upper digestive system, there is the potential for abnormal areas of colonization (infection) when various tubes are in place (e.g., tracheostomy, nasogastric or endotracheal tube). In addition, there is the potential for aspiration of secretions that may cause bronchitis and/or pneumonitis.*

Procedure *(continued)*	**Nursing Action**	**Rationale/Amplification**
	1. Place a towel across the patient's chest and inform him that the tube is to be withdrawn.	1. No doubt, the patient will be happy to have progressed to this stage.
	2. Rotate tubing and inject about 10 ml. of saline before clamping tubing.	2. Rotating the tube ensures mobility. The saline also clears the tube of any contents before clamping. Tubing is clamped to prevent drainage within tube from being aspirated.
	3. Remove the tape from the patient's nose.	
	4. Instruct the patient to take a deep breath and hold it.	4. This maneuver closes the epiglottis.
	5. Slowly but evenly withdraw tubing and cover it with a towel as it emerges. (As the tube reaches the nasopharynx, you can pull quickly.)	5. Covering the tubing helps dispel patient's nausea.
	6. Provide the patient with materials for oral care and lubricant for nasal dryness.	6. Mouthwash and a nasal lubricant will be appreciated by the patient.
	7. Document time of tube removal and the patient's reaction.	
	8. Continue to monitor the patient for signs of GI difficulties; changes in vital signs may suggest infection.	8. Recurrence of nausea or vomiting may require reinsertion of nasogastric tubing.
	9. Document tube removal and color, consistency, and amount of drainage in suction canister.	

NURSING ALERT: Recognize the potential for complications when intubation is prolonged—nasal erosion, sinusitis, esphogitis, and gastric ulceration. Pulmonary complications may occur postoperatively in patients with nasogastric intubation because of interference with coughing and clearing of the pharynx.

Guidelines Nasointestinal Intubation (Long Tube)

Purposes
1. To remove fluid and flatus from the intestinal tract (decompression)
2. To assess gastrointestinal bleeding
3. To treat intestinal obstruction
4. Used to prevent nausea, vomiting, and abdominal distention after gastrointestinal surgery

Equipment
(Choice made by physician)
1. Type of tube
    Single-lumen tube:
Suction equipment
Water-soluble lubricant
Gauze, tape, bulb syringe, rubber band, clamp, safety pin
Double-lumen tube:

Harris, Cantor
Distal end has a small rubber bag weighted with mercury; suction openings are proximal to bag.
Some single-lumen tubes use air to inflate balloon, or have a metal bulb at distal end.
Five to ten milliliters of mercury or water as prescribed
Miller–Abbott
  a. One outlet is for drainage
  b. The other outlet is for filling the small rubber bag near the distal end

2. Tube selection
    a. Miller–Abbott tube is used in presence of mechanical bowel obstruction with hyperactive bowel sounds.
    b. Other tubes are used for adynamic ileus (absent bowel sounds).

Procedure **Preparatory and Performance Phase**

NURSING ALERT: All tubes and endoscopes should be routinely pretested for patency and function before passage.

Physician Action—Nurse Assisted	Rationale/Amplification

1. Similar to passing a short nasogastric tube (see p. 464). Exception: Miller–Abbott. Carry out this procedure as follows:
    a. Pretest the bag volume; the proper amount of air will fill the bag to just less than fully distended (slightly compressible).
    b. Place 1 ml. mercury in the bag after it is in the stomach.
    c. After duodenum has been entered, instill 20–50 ml. air in bag according to pretested volume; place other opening on suction.
2. After the tube enters the stomach, it passes by peristalsis and gravity into the small intestine.
    a. Change patient's position from Fowler's to a position in which the patient is leaning forward.
3. On x-ray confirmation that the tubing is past the pylorus, permit the patient to ambulate.
	a. This will ensure that the bag is not leaky.
	
	b. This helps to pass tubing through the pylorus.
	c. This position checked by x-ray. Air-filled bag acts as a bolus and is carried distally by peristaltic action as suction evacuates retained air and fluid just ahead of bag.
	
	a. This will assist in advancing the tubing to and through the pylorus; tilting to the right is helpful.
	3. Passing the tube through the pylorus and into the duodenum under fluoroscopic guidance allows the entire procedure to be completed in less than 15 minutes with little patient discomfort.

Nursing Action 4. At specified time intervals, advance tubing 5–10 cm. (2–4 inches). 5. Tubing may be taped to the nose, and suction may be applied when the tubing tip has reached its destination. 6. Measure drainage; record its characteristics every 8 hours.	4. Physician may prescribe or suggest these times. 5. Once proper placement is confirmed, the physician injects the appropriate amount of mercury into the balloon lumen and prescribes x-rays to check for proper placement. The tubing is taped to the patient's nose to secure in place.

(continued)

Guidelines Nasointestinal Intubation (Long Tube) *(continued)*

> **NURSING ALERT:** If drainage is clear and up to 3000 ml. obtained per day, there is usually complete intestinal obstruction. If drainage is yellow with a fecal odor, the patient may have an obstruction of the small intestine.

Nursing Action	Rationale/Amplification
Follow-Up Phase	
1. Similar to short nasogastric tube.	1. See page 467.
2. Exception: in removing tubing, patient may feel tube resistance and become nauseated.	2. Due to action of sphincters through which the tube is withdrawn.
3. Deflate the balloon for a Miller–Abbott tube and slowly withdraw the tube 6–8 inches (15–20 cm) at a time. Withdraw a Cantor or Harris tube with mercury in the bag.	3. This avoids pulling on the intestines.
4. As tubing is drawn through posterior nasopharynx, have the patient open his mouth so that balloon or bag can be grasped with a clamp. Withdraw remaining tubing through the nose.	4. This permits balloon or bag to be removed through the mouth.
5. If tubing has advanced beyond the ileocecal valve, the physician may release it so that it can pass through the gastrointestinal tract. Peristalsis aids in passing the tubing.	5. After distal tube has been retrieved at the rectum, the proximal end can be released at the nose.

> **NURSING ALERT:** If strong resistance is felt during tube withdrawal, notify the physician.

Gastroduodenal Conditions

Gastrointestinal Bleeding

Bleeding is a symptom of a digestive or vascular problem or problems. It may be obvious in emesis or stool, or it may be occult (hidden).

Etiology and Causative Factors

1. Trauma anywhere along the gastrointestinal tract
2. Erosion of a blood vessel due to an ulcer, benign tumor, or malignancy
3. Rupture of an enlarged vein, such as a varicosity (esophageal varices)
4. Inflammation such as esophagitis, caused by acid or bile, gastritis, small intestine (Crohn's disease), polyps
5. Irritation of mucous membrane due to certain drugs—alcohol, aspirin-containing compounds, other drugs
6. Infection, such as intestinal (ulcerative colitis)
7. Diverticulosis

Clinical Manifestations

1. *Signs of blood*
   a. Bright red—vomited from high in esophagus (hematemesis); from rectum or distal colon (coating stool)
   b. Mixed with dark red—higher up in colon and small intestine; mixed with stool
   c. Shades of black ("coffee ground")—esophagus, stomach, and duodenum; vomitus from these areas
   d. Tarry stools (melena)—occurs in patient who accumulates excessive blood in the stomach
2. *Symptoms of massive bleeding*
   a. Weakness, dizziness, faintness, shortness of breath, crampy abdominal pain, diarrhea
   b. Rapid pulse, drop in blood pressure, shock
   c. Pale appearance, fatigue, lethargy
   d. Decreased hemoglobin and hematocrit

Diagnostic Evaluation

1. It is not difficult to diagnose bleeding, but it may be a problem to locate the source of bleeding.
2. History—change in bowel pattern, presence of pain or tenderness, recent intake of food and what kind (red beets?), alcohol consumption, drugs such as aspirin or steroids
3. Complete blood count
4. Endoscopy
5. Radioactive scanning
6. Test of stool for occult blood

Management

A. Symptomatic

1. Depends on cause and whether bleeding is acute or chronic
   a. If aspirin is the cause, eliminate aspirin and treat bleeding.
   b. If ulcer is the cause, an anti-ulcer drug is prescribed, along with life-style change and dietary change.
   c. If cancer is the cause, tumor to be removed (see Mouth Cancer, Esophageal Cancer, Gastric Cancer, Colon Cancer).
2. May required skilled endoscopist with a well-prepared diagnostic team.

B. Preparation for Emergency Intervention

1. Intravenous lines and oxygen therapy equipment to be available
2. If life-threatening bleeding occurs, treat shock, administer blood replacement as prescribed.

C. **Nasogastric Intubation** (See page 464 for procedure.)

1. Short tube (Levin, Salem sump, Ewald)
    a. Stomach irrigation of the patient with hemostasis using iced saline, tepid saline, or saline containing norepinephrine bitartrate (Levophed). All these methods are known to promote vasoconstriction
    b. Instillation of topical thrombin to clot blood at the site of bleeding by acting directly with fibrinogen

> **NURSING ALERT:** Because of the action of topical thrombin, it is used only on the surface of bleeding tissue and never is injected into the blood vessels, where intravascular clotting could take place.

2. Long Tube
    a. Sengstaken–Blakemore Tube, Miller–Abbott Tube, Minnesota Esophago-Gastric Tube, Harris Tube, and Cantor Tube
    b. Control the bleeding by placing pressure against the site.

D. **Other Measures**

1. Electrocoagulation and photocoagulation (laser) may be the treatment of choice
    Postlaser treatment requires careful monitoring for bleeding recurrence, nasogastric intubation, dependent drainage.
2. Pharmacotherapy depends on cause.
3. Surgery if conservative measures fail

Peptic Ulcer

A peptic ulcer is an excavation in the mucosal wall of the esophagus, stomach, pylorus, or the duodenum. It is frequently referred to as an esophageal, gastric, or duodenal ulcer (Fig. 20-3).

Types and Causes

A. **Gastric**

1. Increased gastric acidity
2. Decreased mucosal blood flow
3. Decreased secretions of mucus
4. Increased mucosal permeability
5. Stress
6. Chronic use of alcohol or aspirin

B. **Duodenal–Multifactorial Causes**

1. Hypersecretion of acid believed to be caused by an overactive vagus nerve, which stimulates the release of gastrin
2. Drugs: aspirin, anti-inflammatory drugs, and steroids
3. Methylxanthines (tea, coffee, cola, and chocolate)
4. Smoking
5. Genetic susceptibility to the erosion of the mucous lining of the stomach, pylorus, and the duodenum
6. Decreased mucosal blood flow, mucus, and mucosal resistance

Clinical Manifestations

A. **Gastric**

1. Pain occurring in the epigastric area radiating to the back
2. Pain increases when the stomach is empty, approximately ½–2 hours after eating.

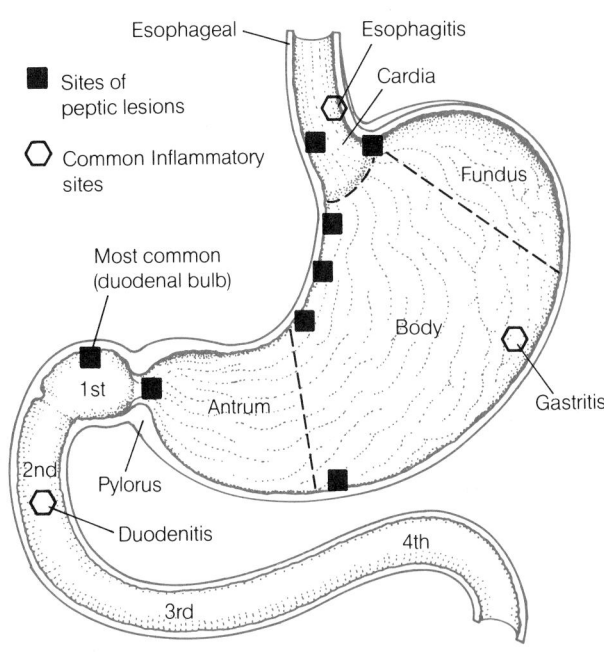

Figure 20-3. *The stomach is divided on the basis of its physiologic functions into two main portions. The proximal two thirds, the fundic gland area, acts as a receptacle for ingested food and secretes acid and pepsin. The distal third, the pyloric gland area, mixes and propels food into the duodenum and produces the hormone gastrin. "Peptic" lesions may occur in the esophagus (esophagitis), stomach (gastritis), or duodenum (duodenitis). Note peptic ulcer sites and common inflammatory sites.*

3. Pain or discomfort continuous in the daytime and increased by food
4. Pain is relieved after ingesting food or antacids.
5. Weight loss
6. Reflex vomiting
7. Gastrointestinal bleeding

B. **Duodenal**

1. Pain occurring in the epigastric area
2. Intermittent pain—occurring frequently at night when the stomach is empty
3. Pain increased by fatty foods, but relieved by other foods
4. Feeling of "hot water bubbling" in the back of the throat
5. May experience weight gain due to an increase in eating to relieve the pain
6. Pain occurring several times a year and then fading

Diagnostic Evaluation

1. Upper gastrointestinal series
2. Fiberoptic panendoscopy (Esophago-gastroduodenoscopy)—visualization of duodenal mucosa; identifies inflammatory changes, ulcers, lesions, bleeding sites, and malignancy
3. Serial stool specimens to detect occult blood

4. Gastric secretory studies (Gastric acid secretion test and the serum gastric level test)

Medical Management

1. Specific pharmacotherapy
   a. Acid-neutralizing agents (antacids)
   b. Anticholinergics (propantheline)—to inhibit vagus nerve stimulation, thus reducing gastrin production and gastric acidity; not used with gastric ulcers because anticholinergics prolong gastric emptying
   c. Histamine receptor antagonists (cimetidine; ranitidine)—inhibit action of histamine on the H_2 receptors of the parietal cells, thus reducing gastric acid output and concentration.
   d. Cytoprotective drug (sucralfate)—adheres to and protects the ulcer surface by forming a barrier
   e. Antisecretory/Cytoprotective (misoprostol)—prostoglandin having antisecretory and cytoprotective effects; inhibits hydrochloric acid production in the stomach
   f. Antisecretory (omeprazole)—inhibits the production of hydrochloric acid in the stomach. Can heal ulcers quickly—in 4–8 weeks.
2. Counseling to help cope with a stressful life-style
3. Sedatives/tranquilizers—for the patient with gastric ulcers, to provide rest and relaxation
4. Fluid, electrolyte, and blood needs monitored and replaced
5. Dietary management; food as tolerated; avoid whatever food causes discomfort; small frequent feedings*

Surgical Management

A. Gastrojejunostomy and Vagotomy (Fig. 20-4A).

1. The jejunum is anastomosed to the stomach to provide a second outlet of gastric contents.
2. The severed vagus nerve reduces secretions and movements of the stomach.

B. Antrectomy and Vagotomy (Fig. 20-4B)

1. The resected portion includes a small cuff of duodenum, the pylorus, and the antrum (about one half of the stomach).
2. The stump of the duodenum is closed by suture, and the side of the jejunum is anastomosed to the cut end of the stomach.

C. Subtotal Gastrectomy (Fig. 20-4C)

1. The resected portion includes a small cuff of the duodenum, pylorus, and from two thirds to three quarters of the stomach.
2. The duodenum or side of the jejunum is anastomosed to the remaining portion of the stomach.

D. Vagotomy and Pyloroplasty (Fig. 20-4D)

1. A longitudinal incision is made in the pylorus, and it is closed transversely to permit the muscle to relax and to establish an enlarged outlet.
2. This compensates for the impaired gastric emptying produced by the vagotomy.

---

* Whole milk, skim milk, and half-and-half have been used in the past as a dietary treatment for ulcers; however, recent studies have shown that protein and calcium, two milk components, stimulate acid production and secretion in the stomach. Milk also distends and leaves the stomach quickly, thus counteracting any extended buffering actions it was thought to have produced.

Complications

1. Hemorrhage
   a. Monitor for bright red blood or coffee ground material (blood that gastric acid has changed to acid hematin)
   b. Observe for black tarry stools (melena)
2. Perforation
   Monitor for acute upper abdominal pain, guarding, rebound tenderness, absent bowel sounds.
3. Obstruction
   Monitor for abdominal distention, tympany, and a splashing sound heard on abdominal auscultation.

Nursing Assessment

1. Determine location, character, radiation of pain, factors aggravating or relieving pain, how long it lasts, when it occurs (relieved by food? antacids? vomiting?).
2. Ask about eating patterns, regularity, types of food, eating circumstances.
3. Take a social history of alcohol consumption and smoking.
4. Ask about medications (especially aspirin, anti-inflammatory drugs, or steroids).
5. Determine if gastrointestinal bleeding has been experienced.
6. Take vital signs (lying, standing, and sitting blood pressures and pulses).
7. Ascultate bowel sounds; monitor intake and output; calorie intake; weight.

NURSING ALERT: A decrease in the blood pressure greater than 1 mm. Hg accompanied by an increase in the pulse by 20 beats per minute, in a standing or sitting position, indicates possible bleeding.

Nursing Diagnoses

1. Potential for fluid volume deficit secondary to hemorrhage
2. Pain related to epigastric distress secondary to hypersecretion of acid, muscosal erosion, or perforation
3. Diarrhea related to gastrointestinal bleeding or antacid therapy
4. Altered nutrition (less than body requirements) related to the disease process
5. Knowledge deficit of physical, dietary, and pharmacology treatment

Nursing Interventions: Acute GI Bleeding Episode

A. Avoiding Fluid Volume Deficit During Hemorrhage or Perforation

1. Monitor intake and output.
2. Observe stools for occult blood.
3. Monitor hemoglobin and hematocrit, and electrolytes.
4. Administer prescribed intravenous fluids.
5. Intubate (via nasogastric tube) as prescribed and monitor the tube drainage for signs of visible and occult blood.
6. Observe the patient for an increase in pulse and a decrease in blood pressure (signs of shock).
7. Replace blood via transfusion, as prescribed.

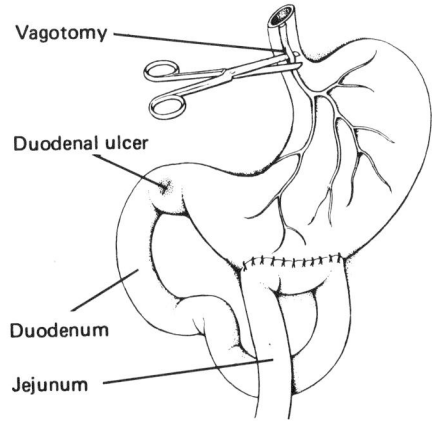

A. *Gastrojejunostomy and vagotomy. The jejunum is anastomosed to the stomach to provide a second outlet of gastric contents. The severed vagus nerve reduces secretions and movements of the stomach (90% good results).*

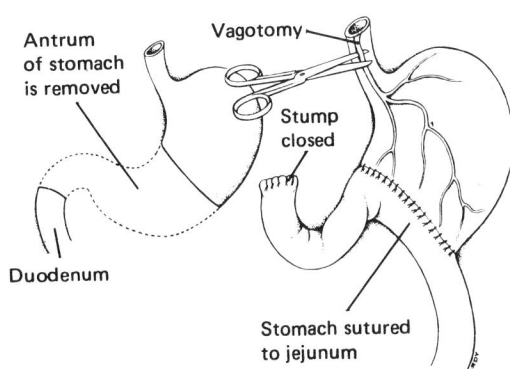

B. *Antrectomy and vagotomy. The resected portion includes a small cuff of duodenum, the pylorus, and the antrum (about one half of the stomach). The stump of the duodenum is closed by suture, and the side of the jejunum is anastomosed to the cut end of the stomach.*

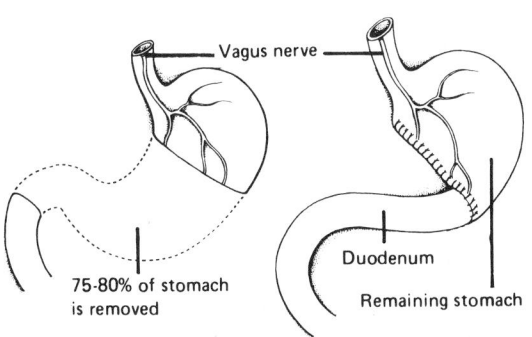

C. *Subtotal gastrectomy. The resected portion includes a small cuff of the duodenum, the pylorus, and from two thirds to three quarters of the stomach. The duodenum or side of the jejunum is anastomosed to the remaining portion of the stomach.*

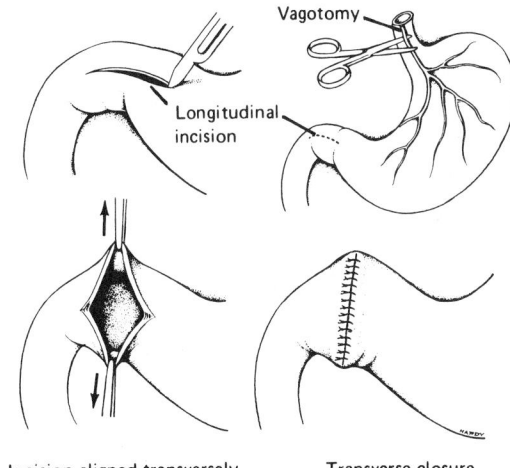

D. *Vagotomy and pyloroplasty. A longitudinal incision is made in the pylorus, and it is closed transversely to permit the muscle to relax and to establish an enlarged outlet. This compensates for the impaired gastric emptying produced by vagotomy.*

Figure 20-4. *Surgical procedures for peptic ulcer.*

8. If frank bleeding occurs, prepare patient for iced saline or tap water lavage as prescribed; the physician may prescribe norepinephrine to be added to lavage solution to promote vasoconstriction.
9. Administer vasopressin intravenously, as prescribed.
10. Administer antacids, if prescribed, through the nasogastric tube to neutralize acidity.
11. Prepare the patient for angiography or surgery to determine the source of bleeding.

B. Achieving Relief of Pain

1. Treat epigastric or "warning" pain by offering antacids as prescribed.
2. Administer prescribed medication.
   a. Anticholinergics, such as propantheline bromide, may be given to suppress gastric secretions and delay gastric emptying.

> **NURSING ALERT:** Anticholinergics are contraindicated in patients with glaucoma, urinary retention, gastric distention, and dysrhythmias.

   b. Encourage hydration to minimize the side effects of anticholinergic medicines.
   c. Give histamine receptor antagonists as prescribed.

> **NURSING ALERT:** Do not administer histamine receptor antagonists with antacids, because antacids block absorption of the histamine antagonists.

d. Offer prescribed antacids to decrease gastric acidity; antacids are given 1 hour after meals, at bedtime, and during the night as required for pain.

e. Offer prescribed sedatives or tranquilizers to lessen patient's response to stimuli and to promote relaxation and sleep.

3. Encourage bedrest to reduce physical activity and to separate patient from his usual environment if pain continues.
4. Provide small frequent meals to prevent gastric distention.
5. Teach the patient that caffeine, alcoholic beverages, and nicotine may increase gastric acidity and promote erosion of the gastric mucosa.
6. Alert the patient about the irritating effects on the gastric mucosa of certain drugs, especially aspirin-containing and anti-inflammatory drugs such as Alka-Seltzer, Pepto-Bismol, and ibuprofen.

C. Decreasing Diarrhea

1. Monitor patient's elimination patterns to determine effects of antacids.
2. Monitor vital signs; persistent diarrhea may be a sign of bleeding.
3. Watch for signs of hypovolemia.
4. Restrict foods and fluids that promote diarrhea: raw vegetables, fruits, whole grain cereals, carbonated drinks.
5. Administer antidiarrheal medication as prescribed.
6. Watch for signs of impaired skin integrity (erythema, soreness) around anus.

D. Achieving Adequate Nutrition

1. Eliminate foods that cause pain or distress; otherwise the diet is usually not restricted.
2. Provide meals on time.
3. Provide small, frequent feedings to decrease distention and the release of gastrin. Frequent feedings also help neutralize gastric secretions and dilute stomach contents. However, eating small frequent meals or snacks can lead to acid rebound, which occurs 2–4 hours after eating.
4. Advise the patient to avoid coffee and other caffeinated beverages, as well as carbonated drinks; these help to promote acid.
5. Advise the patient to avoid extremely hot or cold food or fluids, to chew thoroughly, and to eat in a leisurely fashion.

E. Understanding the Treatment Regimen

1. Explain all tests and procedures.
2. Review the physician's recommendations for diet, activity, medication, and treatment.
3. Give the patient a chart listing his medications, dosages, times of administration, and desired effects.
4. Instruct the patient to call if there is any evidence of bleeding, tarry stools, or dizziness.

Discharge Planning/Patient Education

Teach the patient the following:
1. Modify life-style to include health practices that will prevent recurrences of ulcer pain and bleeding.
2. Plan for rest periods and avoid or learn to cope with stressful situations.
3. Chew food thoroughly and eat in a leisurely manner and on a regular schedule.
4. Avoid large meals, as they tend to over-stimulate acid secretion.

5. Avoid irritating substances such as caffeine, carbonated drinks, alcohol, extremely spiced foods, tart fresh fruits, and rich pastries.
6. Avoid specific foods known to cause the individual patient distress and pain.
7. Avoid drugs known to cause ulcers.
8. Avoid fatigue. Recognize signs of potential problems (midepigastric pain). Reinstitute anti-ulcer medication if necessary.
9. Take antacids 1 hour after meals, at bedtime, and when needed. Warn the patient that antacids may cause changes in bowel habits.

Evaluation

1. Absence of complications; no signs of hemorrhage or perforation
2. Maintaining normal fluid and electrolyte balance
3. States he is free of pain
4. Decreased frequency of stools
5. Eating several meals a day; reports no loss of weight
6. Can describe peptic ulcer disease, its treatment and complications; complies with treatment regimen

Gastric Cancer

Cancer of the stomach accounts for about 14,000 deaths annually in the US—usually males of middle age. For unknown reasons, there has been a decrease in incidence in the US over the last 2 decades.

Clinical Manifestations

A. Early Manifestations

(Most often, patient presents with same symptoms as gastric ulcer; later, on evaluation, the lesion is found to be malignant.)
1. Progressive loss of appetite
2. Noticeable change in, or appearance of, gastrointestinal symptoms—gastric fullness (early satiety), dyspepsia lasting more than 4 weeks
3. Blood (usually occult) in the stools
4. Vomiting, which may indicate pyloric obstruction or cardiac-orifice obstruction
5. Occasionally, vomiting that has a coffee-ground appearance because of slow leaks of blood from ulceration of the cancer

B. Later Manifestations

1. Pain is a late symptom, often induced by eating and relieved by vomiting.
2. Weight loss, loss of strength, anemia, metastasis (usually to liver), hemorrhage, obstruction

Diagnostic Evaluation

1. History—weight loss and loss of strength over several months
2. Upper GI radiography
3. Fiberoptic endoscopy—affords direct visualization and provides means for obtaining tissue samples for histologic and cytologic review

Management

1. The only successful treatment of gastric cancer is surgical removal.
2. If tumor is localized to stomach and can be removed, chances are still poor that the patient can be cured.

3. If tumor has spread beyond the area that can be excised surgically, cure cannot be accomplished.
   a. Palliative surgery such as subtotal gastrectomy with or without gastroenterostomy may be performed to maintain continuity of the gastrointestinal tract.
   b. Surgery may be combined with chemotherapy to provide palliation and prolong life.

Gastric Resection

Gastric resection is the surgical removal of part of the stomach.

Management and Nursing Interventions

A. Promote Comfort and Wound Healing by Relieving the Patient of Pain and Discomfort.

1. Frequently turn the patient and encourage deep-breathing to prevent vascular and pulmonary complications.
2. Institute nasogastric suction to remove fluids and gas in the stomach.
3. Provide conscientious mouth care to prevent mouth dryness and ulceration.
4. Administer parenteral antibiotics to prevent infection.
5. See that the patient has nothing by mouth until prescribed (to promote gastric wound healing).

B. Meet Nutritional Needs of the Patient.

1. Give intravenous fluids to prevent shock and to provide adequate fluid and electrolytes.
2. Give fluids by mouth when audible bowel signs are present.
3. Increase fluids according to the patient's tolerance.
4. Offer a diet with vitamin supplements when the patient's condition permits.
5. Give protein–vitamin supplements to foster wound repair and tissue building.
6. Avoid high-carbohydrate foods, such as milk, that may trigger "dumping syndrome."

C. Anticipate Complications in Order to Prevent Them.

1. Shock and hemorrhage
   a. Evaluate status of blood pressure, pulse, and respiration.
   b. Observe the patient for evidence of apathy, apprehension, air hunger, pallor, or clammy skin.
   c. Check the dressings and drainage bottle frequently for evidence of bleeding.
   d. Administer intravenous infusions and blood as prescribed.
2. Cardiopulmonary complications
   a. Encourage the patient to cough and take deep breaths to promote ventilatory exchange and enhance circulation.
   b. Assist the patient to turn and move, thereby mobilizing secretions.
   c. Promote ambulation as prescribed to increase respiratory exchange.
3. Thrombosis and embolism
   a. Initiate a plan of self-care activities to promote circulation.
   b. Encourage early ambulation to stimulate circulation.
   c. Prevent venous stasis by use of elastic stockings if indicated.

d. Check for tight dressings or binder that might restrict circulation.

4. "Dumping syndrome"—a complex reaction, which may occur because of excessively rapid emptying of gastric contents.
   Manifestations—nausea, weakness, perspiration, palpitation, some syncope, and possibly diarrhea. Instruct the patient as follows:
   a. Eat small, frequent meals rather than three large meals.
   b. Suggest a diet high in protein and fat and low in carbohydrates, and avoid meals high in sugars, milk, chocolate, salt.
   c. Reduce fluids with meals, but take them between meals.
   d. Take anticholinergic medication before meals (if prescribed) to lessen gastrointestinal activity.
   e. Relax when eating; eat slowly and regularly.
   f. Take a rest after meals.
5. Phytobezoar formation (formation of a gastric concretion composed of vegetable matter)
   a. Avoid fibrous foods such as citrus fruits (skins and seeds), because they tend to form phytobezoars.
      (1) Following a gastric resection, the remaining gastric tissue is not able to disintegrate and digest fibrous foods.
      (2) This undigested fiber congeals to form masses that become coated by mucus secretions of the stomach.
   b. Stress the importance of adequate mastication.

Patient Education

(Adjustment to self-care and return to the community)

1. Emphasize the importance of coping with stressful situations.
2. Review nutritional requirements and regimen with the patient.
3. Stress the importance of vitamin B_{12} supplements.
4. Encourage follow-up visits with the physician.
5. Recommend annual blood studies and medical checkups for any evidence of pernicious anemia or other problems.
6. See above, C-4 "Dumping syndrome."

Intestinal Conditions

Nursing Process Overview: The Patient Undergoing Major Intestinal Surgery

Nursing Assessment

1. Have the patient describe his bowel pattern: frequency, color, consistency, and amount.
2. Assess the patient's bowel sounds. Observe for abdominal distention.
3. Assess patient's nutritional status: skin turgor, anthropometric measurements, etc. (See Nutrition, p. 434)
4. Observe patient for fluid and electrolyte imbalance.
5. Assess color, texture, turgor, and vascularity of skin. Ask patient about past history of wound healing; Any problems?
6. Have patient describe any allergies to antibiotics.
7. Ask patient to describe his understanding of the surgery or procedure.
8. Assess patient's previous experience with pain.

Patient Problems/Nursing Diagnoses

1. Altered bowel elimination related to surgical intervention
2. Altered nutrition, less than body requirements, related to dietary modification following surgery
3. Potential fluid volume deficit related to surgical procedure
4. Impaired skin integrity related to surgical wound and possible stoma placement
5. Potential for infection related to surgical wound
6. Knowledge deficit related to care and function of an ileostomy or colostomy
7. Pain related to surgical incision

Preoperative Nursing Interventions

A. Decreasing Colon Contents

1. Give low-residue diet and, when required, change to liquid diet.
2. Offer laxatives as prescribed. Saline catharsis may be preferred.
3. Administer enemas or colonic irrigations as prescribed.
4. Decompress gastrointestinal tract by means of indwelling gastrointestinal tube to control distention and vomiting as prescribed.
5. Monitor stools: frequency, consistency, color, and amount.

B. Attending to Nutritional Needs

1. Correct nutritional deficiencies—provide protein supplements, between-meal feedings, diet rich in carbohydrates, proteins, fats, minerals, and vitamins.
2. Monitor intake and output.

C. Attaining Normal Fluid Volume

1. Watch for signs of dehydration—decreased skin turgor, muscle spasms, resting tachycardia, orthostatic hypotension, dry tongue, increased thirst, weight loss, oliguria, fever, and fatigue.
2. Watch for signs and symptoms of electrolyte imbalance—nausea, vomiting, cardiac dysrhythmias, tremors, seizures, anorexia, malaise, weakness, and irregular pulse.
3. Monitor laboratory electrolytes and report abnormalities.
4. Administer parenteral therapy to correct fluid and electrolyte imbalance as prescribed.
5. Provide blood replacement to overcome losses sustained by bleeding, infection, and neoplasm as prescribed.

D. Obtaining Information About Procedure/Surgery

1. Explain all diagnostic tests, procedures, and the surgical process.
2. Assist with diagnostic studies as needed.
3. Encourage patient to ask questions.
4. Discuss preoperative and postoperative care.
5. Assess patient's understanding and expectations of surgical procedure. Identify fears and clarify misconceptions.
6. Teach the patient how to participate in preoperative and postoperative care and have him do return demonstrations (coughing, deep breathing, leg exercises, turning, splinting the incision).

Postoperative Nursing Interventions

A. Preventing Complications

1. Administer antibiotic agents as prescribed to suppress aerobic colon microflora.
2. Assist with general hygiene to promote cleanliness and to minimize skin and wound infection.
3. Monitor wound for signs of infection—redness, warmth, wound dehiscence.
4. Evaluate vital signs and recognize patterns of development that may suggest hemorrhage, infection, shock, obstruction, etc.
5. Stress preventive measures, such as turning frequently, maintaining fluid balance, encouraging coughing, and movement of legs.

B. Achieving Comfort

1. Administer prescribed analgesis when required by patient. Observe for effectiveness.
2. Turn the patient frequently to minimize discomfort.
3. Encourage coughing and deep breathing. Recommend splinting the incision to decrease the pain.

C. Maintaining Normal Fluid and Electrolyte Balance

1. Monitor intake and output.
2. Observe for signs of dehydration and electrolyte imbalance.
3. Administer intravenous or hyperalimentation therapy as prescribed to prevent fluid and electrolyte imbalances.

D. Increasing Knowledge About Stoma Care

1. Encourage the patient to express concerns and questions.
2. Show patient the appropriate procedures for taking care of the ileostomy or colostomy. See pages 483–485 or 497.
3. Encourage ambulation and self-care activities.
4. Help patient set progressive goals.
5. Emphasize the importance of follow-up visits to evaluate the healing process, general physical and psychological adjustment.
6. If needed, set up home health care referral to assist patient with the management of his stoma.

Evaluation

A. Preoperative Outcomes

1. Achieves an optimal nutritional state at the time of surgery.
2. Maintains appropriate fluid and electrolyte balance preoperatively.
3. Shows no evidence of infection when entering surgery.
4. Demonstrates turning, coughing, deep breathing, and leg exercises preoperatively.
5. Understands and cooperates with all preoperative procedures.
6. Able to explain the surgical procedure.

B. Postoperative Outcomes

1. Is free from complications
2. Attains level of comfort—verbalizes relief of pain
3. Regains regular pattern of elimination or learns to accommodate to intestinal diversion surgery (colostomy or ileostomy)
4. Modifies diet if needed in accordance with after-effects of surgery (colostomy, ileostomy)

5. Demonstrates ability to carry out stoma care if diversional surgery was performed

Appendicitis

Appendicitis is inflammation of the vermiform appendix caused by an obstruction of the intestinal lumen from infection, strictures, fecal masses, or barium ingestion.

Clinical Manifestation

1. Generalized or localized abdominal pain in the periumbilical area, and the upper right abdomen, moving to the right lower quadrant after 6–12 hours
2. Anorexia, nausea, and vomiting; "boardlike" rigidity in the right lower abdomen (McBurney's point) with increasing tenderness
3. Fever rising within several hours 37.2°C–38.9°C (99°–101°F)
4. Mild change in bowel habits (usually constipation)
5. Rebound tenderness (Rebound tenderness on the opposite side of the abdomen suggests peritoneal inflammation.)

> **NURSING ALERT:** If these clinical manifestations occur, encourage person to see a physician immediately. There is a tendency in the aging person to ignore aches and pains and to delay seeing a physician. Consequently, mortality in elderly persons with inflammatory bowel lesions is as high as 20%.

Diagnostic Evaluation

1. Physical examination, especially noting location and localization of pain, rebound tenderness, etc.
2. Blood studies, with particular attention to white blood cell count; urinalysis. A white blood cell count reveals a moderate leukocytosis (12,000 to 15,000/mm³).
3. Careful history to rule out other possibilities: gastritis, gastroenteritis, colitis, diverticulitis, pancreatitis, bladder infection, and ovarian cyst
4. Laparoscopy when appendicitis is difficult to diagnose

Management

A. Palliative Preoperative Care

1. Place the patient in a comfortable position to relieve abdominal pain and tension—usually Fowler's position.
2. See that the person takes nothing by mouth—to decrease peristalsis and to allow stomach to empty before surgery. Note time and nature of last meal.
3. Place ice bag to right lower quadrant—never heat because of the possibility of causing a rupture of appendix and peritonitis.
4. Do not administer cathartics—may cause rupture.
5. Evaluate vital signs frequently—to assess progression of infection.
6. When diagnosis of acute appendicitis is made, chemotherapy and/or antibiotics may be prescribed.

Note: Evidence of perforation and a generalized peritonitis increases the urgency for surgery (see below).

B. Surgical Management

1. If diagnosis of acute appendicitis is established, a simple appendectomy is performed.
2. Anesthetic may be general or spinal.

C. Postoperative Care

Without drainage
1. Measures following recovery from anesthetic
   a. Maintain Fowler's position.
   b. Give analgesic every 3 or 4 hours as needed.
   c. Give fluids and food as tolerated.
   d. Monitor vital signs, intake, and output.
   e. Encourage to cough and deep-breathe to prevent pulmonary complications.
2. Ongoing care
   a. Document bowel sounds and the passing of flatus or bowel movements (These are signs of the return of peristalsis.).
   b. Watch for surgical *complications* such as continuing pain or fever, which indicate an abscess or wound dehiscence.
   c. Stitches removed between fifth and seventh day (usually in physician's office).

Peritonitis

Peritonitis is an inflammation of the peritoneal cavity.

Etiology

A. General

1. Peritonitis indicates blunt or penetrating trauma to the peritoneum or inflammatory or neoplastic disease.
2. The point of origin may be the gastrointestinal tract, the ovaries, the uterus, or extraperitoneal organs (i.e., inflammation of the kidneys).

B. Primary Peritonitis—acute, diffuse

1. Occurs primarily in young females; often due to pathogenic bacteria (streptococci, pneumoccocci, gonococci) introduced through uterine tubes or through hematogenous spread.
2. In patients with nephrosis or cirrhosis, the offending organism is most often *E. coli.*

C. Secondary Peritonitis

1. Seen in surgical patients; caused by appendicitis, peptic ulceration, biliary tract disease, colonic inflammation.
2. May occur following gunshot wound, stab wounds, and motor vehicle accidents.

D. Postoperative

1. Theoretically preventable
2. Noted following ineffective preoperative preparation—inadequate nutrition and fluid and blood replacement, and technical problems
3. May occur in compromised patients who are diabetic, have malignancy, or are taking steroids

Altered Physiology

1. Any irritant, such as blood, bile, or pancreatic enzymes, causes an exudation of plasmalike, protein-rich fluid—"internal burn."
2. Secondary peritonitis often presents mixed flora, which include *E. coli* as well as the enterococci, *Clostridium, Klebsiella, Pseudomonas,* and *Bacteroides.*
3. If there is failure to seal the source of contamination (i.e., perforation along gastrointestinal tract), peritonitis will become progressively worse.
4. When the peritoneum is affected, the surface of the peritoneal cavity begins to exude a plasmalike fluid.

This process can account for losses of as much as 5 liters/day.

5. Paralytic ileus is usual, with fluid loss occurring into a dilated intestinal loop and stomach.
6. Individual is compromised because of fluid loss, abdominal distention with respiratory embarrassment; nutrients are not absorbed, leading to progressive rapid catabolism.

Clinical Manifestations

Depends on location and extension of the inflammation

1. Initially, local type of abdominal pain tends to become constant, diffuse, and more intense.
2. Abdomen becomes extremely tender, and muscles become rigid; rebound tenderness and ileus may be present; patient lies very still, usually with legs drawn up.
3. Nausea and vomiting often occur; peristalsis diminishes; anorexia is present.
4. Elevation of temperature and pulse, as well as leukocyte count
5. Fever, thirst occur, oliguria, dry swollen tongue, signs of dehydration
6. Percussion—resonance and tympany due to paralytic ileus; loss of liver dullness may indicate free air in abdomen.
7. Auscultation—decreased bowel sounds
8. Weakness, pallor, diaphoresis, and cold skin are a result of the loss of fluid, electrolytes, and protein into the abdomen
9. Hypotension and hypokalemia may occur
10. Shallow respirations may result from abdominal distention and upward displacement of the diaphragm

Diagnostic Evaluation

1. Blood studies—to show leukocytosis (leukopenia, if severe)
2. Urinalysis—may indicate urinary tract problems as primary source
3. Peritoneal aspiration (paracentesis)—to demonstrate blood, pus, bile, bacteria (gram staining), amylase
4. X-ray of abdomen—may indicate free air in abdomen under diaphragm or thorax—to rule out unexpected pneumonia
5. Severe abdominal pain with direct or rebound tenderness
6. Laparotomy—to identify the underlying cause

Management

1. Treatment of inflammatory conditions preoperatively and postoperatively with antibiotic therapy—prevents peritonitis
2. Antibiotic therapy using penicillin G, clindamycin, chloramphenicol, or streptomycin, depending on the infecting organisms
3. Replacement of fluid and electrolytes parenterally
4. Analgesics for pain
5. Nasogastric intubation to decompress the bowel
6. Rectal tube to facilitate passage of flatus
7. If localized, surgery is indicated to eliminate the source of infection by eliminating the spilled contents by inserting tubes for drainage
   a. If acutely inflamed appendix—an appendectomy is necessary.
   b. If ruptured duodenal ulcer—ulcer closed or plicated.
   c. Resection of diseased bowel; decompression (gastrostomy, colostomy, ileostomy)
8. Abdominal paracentesis may be done to remove accumulating fluid
9. Irrigation of the peritoneal cavity with antibiotic solutions also may be done

Complications

1. Spread of infection
2. Loss of fluid and electrolytes

Nursing Assessment

1. Assess for abdominal distention and tenderness, hypoactive or absent bowel sounds.
2. Ask patient if experiencing fever, chills, nausea, or vomiting. Does movement worsen the pain?
3. Observe for signs of shock—tachycardia and hypotension.
4. Watch for signs of guarding or rebound tenderness.
5. Monitor central venous pressure.
6. Record urinary output hourly.
7. Check vital signs frequently.
8. Obtain baseline and take frequent analyses of hematocrit, arterial blood gases, and electrolytes.

Nursing Interventions

A. Achieving Relief of Pain

1. Place the patient in semi-Fowler's position before surgery to enable less painful breathing.
2. After surgery, place the patient in Fowler's position to promote drainage by gravity.
3. After surgery, provide analgesics as prescribed.

B. Prevention of Infection and Promotion of Comfort

1. Give nothing by mouth—to reduce peristalsis; ensure meticulous oral hygiene.
2. Provide fluids by vein to establish adequate fluid intake and to promote adequate urinary output as prescribed.
3. Record accurately intake and output, including the measurement of vomitus and nasogastric drainage.
4. Administer antibiotics as prescribed.
5. Observe and describe symptoms accurately—pain and tenderness have a tendency to shift and must be reported precisely.
6. Reassure the patient.
7. Prevent nausea, vomiting, and distention by use of nasogastric suction; institute proper nursing measures for nasal and oral comfort.
8. Reduce parenteral fluids and give oral food and fluids when the following occur:
   a. Temperature and pulse return to normal.
   b. Abdomen becomes soft.
   c. Peristaltic sounds return (determined by abdominal auscultation).
   d. Flatus is passed and patient has bowel movements.
9. Be alert for possibility of *complications*—report immediately:
   a. Wound evisceration—"It feels as if something just gave way."
   b. Abscess formation—an area of abdomen is tender or painful, and fever increases.
10. Encourage and assist with ambulation as prescribed, usually the first postoperative day.

Discharge Planning/Patient Education

Instruct the patient in the following:
1. Avoid taking a laxative or applying heat to abdomen when abdominal pain of unknown cause is experienced.
2. Call your physician for increased pain at the incision site.
3. Wound care.

Abdominal Hernias

A *hernia* is a protrusion of an organ, tissue, or structure through the wall of the cavity in which it is normally contained. It is often called a "rupture."

Incidence

1. Results from congenital or acquired weakness of the abdominal wall.
2. Tends to increase in size and recurs with increase of intra-abdominal pressure brought about by coughing, straining, or pressure from a nearby tumor.

Classification

A. According to Area

1. *Inguinal*—hernia into the inguinal canal (more common in males)
   a. *Indirect inguinal hernia*—due to a weakness of the abdominal wall at the point through which the spermatic cord emerges in the male, and the round ligament in the female. Through this opening the hernia extends down the inguinal canal and often into the scrotum or the labia.
   b. *Direct inguinal*—passes through the posterior inguinal wall; more difficult to repair than indirect inguinal hernia
2. *Femoral*—hernia into the femoral canal, appearing below the inguinal ligament (Poupart's ligament), i.e., below the groin
3. *Umbilical*—protrusion of part of the intestine at the umbilicus due to failure of umbilical orifice to close. Occurs most often in obese women, in children, and in patients with increased intra-abdominal pressure from cirrhosis and ascites.
4. *Ventral or incisional*—hernia through the abdominal wall because of weakness in abdominal wall; may occur following impaired healing of incision due to infection, drainage, etc.

B. According to Severity

1. *Reducible*—the protruding mass can be placed back into abdominal cavity.
2. *Irreducible*—the protruding mass cannot be moved back into the abdomen.
3. *Incarcerated*—an irreducible hernia in which the intestinal flow is completely obstructed.
4. *Strangulated*—an irreducible hernia in which the blood and intestinal flow are completely obstructed.
   a. Develops when the loop of intestine in the sac becomes twisted or swollen and a constriction is produced at the neck of the sac.
   b. Clinical manifestations of strangulated hernia: pain, vomiting, swelling of hernial sac, lower abdominal signs of peritoneal irritation, fever

Clinical Manifestations

Signs and symptoms vary, depending on type and location.

Management

A. Surgery—*herniorrhaphy* (surgical repair of a hernia)

1. Surgical treatment is recommended to correct the hernia before strangulation occurs, in which case an emergency situation ensues.
2. Strangulated hernia requires resection of ischemic bowel in addition to repair of hernia.

B. Mechanical (reducible hernia only)

1. A *truss* is an appliance with a pad and belt that is held snugly over a hernia to prevent abdominal contents from entering the hernial sac.
2. Does not cure a hernia; used only when patient cannot withstand surgery, will not consent to surgery, etc.

Nursing Interventions

A. Preoperative

Make sure that the patient does not have an upper respiratory infection; if present, surgery is postponed, as coughing postoperatively may disrupt sutures.

B. Postoperative

1. Have the patient splint the incision site with hand or pillow when coughing to lessen pain and protect site from increased intra-abdominal pressure.
2. Monitor for urinary retention; a common problem postoperatively.
3. Encourage ambulation as soon as permitted. Young, healthy patients are usually discharged the day of surgery.
4. Bedrest, intermittent ice packs, and scrotal elevation are measures used for scrotal edema or swelling following repair of an inguinal hernia.

Patient Education

1. Pain and scrotal swelling may be present for 24–48 hours after repair of an inguinal hernia.
   a. Apply ice intermittently.
   b. Elevate scrotum and use scrotal support.
   c. Take medication prescribed to relieve discomfort.
2. Monitor self for signs of infection: pain, drainage from incision, temperature elevation. Also report difficulty in voiding.
3. Avoid heavy lifting for 4–6 weeks. Athletics and extremes of exertion are to be avoided for 8–12 weeks postoperatively.

Ulcerative Colitis

Ulcerative colitis is an inflammatory disease of the mucosa and, less frequently, the submucosa of the colon and rectum. Occasionally it involves the distal ileum as well.

Etiology and Incidence

1. Unknown (idiopathic); however, there are several unproven possibilities:
   a. A combination of causative factors—infection, stress, allergy, autoimmunity
   b. Emotional response alters blood supply to colon mucosa, but there is a question as to whether stress is a cause or effect of the disease process.

c. Unidentifiable organisms cause pathology.
d. Family history of the disease
e. Overproduction of enzymes that break down the mucous membranes

2. Most common in young adulthood and middle life; almost equal between sexes (slightly more in females); more prevalent among Jews; peak incidence at 20–40 years of age; familial incidence

Clinical Manifestations

1. Diarrhea (may be bloody or contain pus and mucus), tenesmus (painful straining), sense of urgency, and cramping
2. Multiple crypt abscesses of intestinal mucosa that may become necrotic and lead to ulceration
3. Increased bowel sounds; abdomen may appear flat, but as condition continues, abdomen may appear distended.
4. There often is weight loss, fever, dehydration, hypokalemia, anorexia, nausea and vomiting, iron-deficiency anemia, and cachexia.
5. Abdominal pain
6. The disease usually begins in the rectum and sigmoid and spreads upward, eventually involving the entire colon. Anal area may be excoriated and reddened; left lower abdomen may be tender on palpation.
7. There is a tendency for the patient to experience remissions and exacerbations.
8. Very high frequency of secondary and often multiple colon cancer.
9. It is a serious disease accompanied by systemic complications (see Complications below).

Diagnostic Evaluation

1. Stool examination to rule out bacillary or amebic dysentery; fecal analysis
2. Flexible proctosigmoidoscopy and/or colonoscopy/ with biopsy
3. Barium enema x-ray to assess extent of disease and detect pseudopolyps, carcinoma, and strictures
4. Decreased serum levels of potassium, magnesium, albumin, and hemoglobin
5. Leukocytosis and increased prothrombin time
6. Lactose–H_2 breath test

Management

A. General Measures

1. Bedrest
2. IV fluid replacement
3. Clear liquid diet
4. For patients with severe dehydration and excessive diarrhea, hyperalimentation is recommended to rest the intestinal tract and restore nitrogen balance.
5. Sulfasalazine—apparently has antibacterial and anti-inflammatory effects.
6. Corticosteroids—may be given systemically or by rectal instillation.
7. Antidiarrheal medications may be prescribed to control diarrhea, rectal urgency and cramping, abdominal pain; their use is not routine.
8. Treatment of anemia

B. Surgery

1. Surgery is recommended when patient fails to respond to medical therapy, if clinical status is worsening, for severe hemorrhage, or for signs of toxic megacolon.
2. Surgical procedures include subtotal colectomy and ileostomy; proctocolectomy and ileostomy; colectomy and ileorectal anastomosis; colectomy with rectal mucosectomy and ileoanal pouch procedure.

Complications

1. Perforation; hemorrhage; toxic megacolon
2. Abscess formation; stricture; anal fistula
3. Malnutrition; anemia; electrolyte imbalance
4. Skin ulcers
5. Arthritis; ankylosing spondylitis
6. Malignancy (cancer of colon)

Nursing Assessment

1. Review nursing history for patterns of fatigue and overwork; tension, family problems.
2. Assess behavioral manifestations indicative of emotional concerns.
3. Assess food habits that may have a bearing on triggering symptoms (milk intake may be a problem).
4. Determine number and consistency of bowel movements.
5. Listen for hyperactive bowel sounds.
6. Ask patient to describe abdominal pain.
7. Assess for low-grade fever, anorexia, nausea, vomiting, and weight loss.

Nursing Diagnoses

1. Pain related to disease process
2. Altered nutrition (less than body requirements) related to diarrhea, nausea, and vomiting
3. Potential fluid volume deficit related to diarrhea and loss of fluid and electrolytes
4. Ineffective individual coping related to fatigue, feeling of helplessness, and lack of support system (family and friends)

Nursing Interventions

A. Comfort Measures to Rest and Relax the Intestinal Tract

1. Follow prescribed treatment of reducing or eliminating food and fluid and instituting parenteral feeding or low-residue diets.
2. Give sedatives and tranquilizers, as prescribed, not only to provide general rest, but also to allow peristalsis to slow and afford rest to the inflamed bowel.
3. Be aware of the possibility of pressure sores because of malnourishment and enforced inactivity, especially if patient is thin.
   a. Cleanse the skin gently after each bowel movement.
   b. Apply a protective emollient such as petrolatum jelly, karaya gel, A&D ointment, or a similar agent.
4. Relieve painful rectal spasms (produced by frequent diarrheal stools) with anodyne suppositories as prescribed.
5. Report any evidence of *sudden* abdominal distention—may indicate toxic megacolon.
6. Reduce physical activity to a minimum or provide frequent rest periods.
7. Provide commode or bathroom next to bed, since urgency of movements may be a problem.

B. Achieving Nutritional and Fluid Requirements

1. Maintain acutely ill patient on parenteral replacement of vitamins, fluids, and electrolytes (potassium) as prescribed.

2. When resuming oral fluids and foods, select those that are nonirritating to the mucosa (mechanically, thermally, and chemically). If this fails, an elemental diet may be prescribed to provide low residue to rest the lower intestinal tract.
3. Avoid dairy products if patient is lactose intolerant—may ameliorate the diarrhea.
4. Provide a well-balanced, low-residue, high-protein diet to correct malnutrition.
5. Determine which foods agree with this patient and which do not. Modify diet plan accordingly.
6. Bolster with supplemental vitamin therapy, including vitamins C, B complex, and K, as prescribed.
7. Avoid cold fluids because they increase intestinal motility.
8. Administer prescribed electrolytes (especially potassium), which have been lost in diarrheal episodes.
9. Administer prescribed medications for symptomatic relief of diarrhea.
10. Discourage smoking because it also increases intestinal motility.
11. Maintain accurate intake and output records.
12. Weigh daily; rapid increase or decrease may relate to fluid imbalance.
13. Monitor serum electrolytes and report any abnormalities.
14. Observe for decreased skin turgor, dry skin, oliguria, decreased temperature, weakness, increased hemoglobin, hematocrit, BUN, and specific gravity, which all are signs of fluid loss leading to dehydration.

C. Interventions to Combat Infection, Toxicity, Anemia, and Hemorrhage

1. Give antibacterial drugs as prescribed—nonabsorbable sulfasalazine (Azulfidine) may be prescribed as an oral medication.
2. Administer corticosteroids as prescribed.
3. Provide conscientious skin care because excoriation is common following severe diarrhea.
4. For severe proctitis, instill rectal steroids as prescribed (dissolved in tap water, or as suppositories) to produce a remission of symptoms.
5. Administer prescribed therapy to correct existing anemia.
6. Observe for signs of colonic perforation and hemorrhage.

D. Coping and Psychological Adjustment

1. Recognize psychological needs of this patient:
   a. Fear, anxiety, and discouragement accompany diarrhea.
   b. Hypersensitivity may be evident.
   c. Acknowledge patient's complaints.
2. Encourage the patient to talk; listen and offer psychological support.
3. Answer questions about the permanent ileostomy if appropriate.
4. Initiate patient education about living with this chronic disease.
   a. Done on a long-range basis
   b. Patient should participate in the evaluation and planning of his care.
5. Contact National Foundation for Ileitis and Colitis, 444 Park Avenue South, New York, NY 10016, for educational brochures.
6. Plan all aspects of the patient's care in conference so that a team effort promotes the nursing process and ensures continuity of care, communication, and periodic evaluation.

7. Work with the family in helping to understand the patient.
   Note: Impotence occurs in males rather frequently after a colectomy because of damage to pudendal nerves.

Discharge Planning/Health Education

1. Teach patient about chronic aspects of ulcerative colitis and each component of care prescribed.
2. Encourage self-care in monitoring symptoms, seeking annual check up, and maintaining health.
3. Alert patient to possible postoperative problems with skin care, aesthetic difficulties, and surgical revisions.
4. Inform patients that any early indications of relapse, such as bleeding or increased diarrhea, should be reported immediately so that steroid treatment may be initiated.
5. If the patient has an ileostomy, facilitate referral to Ostomy Club.
6. Encourage patient to become a resource person for others undergoing similar procedure.

Evaluation

1. Reports lessening of pain; functions well without analgesics.
2. Demonstrates improved food and fluid intake; avoids roughage intake.
3. Diarrhea is controlled. Fluid and electrolyte balance is maintained.
4. Absence of complications.
5. Shows improved psychological outlook; appears to enjoy visits from family and friends.

Regional Enteritis (Crohn's Disease, Granulomatous Colitis, Transmural Colitis)

Regional enteritis is a chronic inflammatory disease of the small intestine, usually affecting the terminal ileum at the region just before the ileum joins the colon. The etiology is unknown.

Incidence

1. Affects both sexes equally.
2. Appears more often in Jewish persons of Eastern European origin.
3. A familial tendency exists.
4. May occur at any age, but occurs mostly in those between 15 and 35 years of age.

Clinical Features

1. Intestinal tissue thickens, first by edema and later by formation of scar tissues and granulomas.
2. At times, "skip lesions" occur with normal intestine in between.
3. This condition interferes with the ability of the intestine to transport the contents of upper intestine through the constricted lumen; this causes crampy pains after meals.
4. Inflammation and ulcers form in the lining membrane, producing a constant irritating discharge.
5. In some patients, the inflamed intestine may perforate and form intra-abdominal and anal abscesses.

Clinical Manifestations

These are characterized by exacerbations and remissions—may be abrupt or insidious:

1. Crampy pain after meals; this causes the patient to eat in small amounts or even to avoid eating, which then results in malnutrition, weight loss, and possible anemia (hypochromic or macrocytic).
2. Chronic diarrhea due to irritating discharge; usual consistency is soft or semi-liquid. Bloody stools may occur. Steatorrhea.
3. Milk products and chemically or mechanically irritating food may aggravate the problem.
4. Melena and malabsorption syndrome may occur.
5. Low-grade fever occurs if abscesses are present.
6. Lymphadenitis occurs in mesenteric nodes.
7. Abdominal tenderness occurs, especially in right lower quadrant.
8. Weight loss

Diagnostic Evaluation

1. Regional enteritis may simulate acute appendicitis.
2. Upper gastrointestinal barium studies—classic "string sign" is noted at terminal ileum that suggests a constriction of a segment of intestine.
3. Barium enema to permit visualization of lesions of large intestine and terminal ileum.
4. Proctosigmoidoscopy to note ulceration; biopsy
5. Laboratory findings show increased WBC and ESR; decreased potassium, magnesium, calcium, and hemoglobin.

Management

1. Parenteral hyperalimentation is instituted to maintain nutrition while allowing the bowel to rest.
2. Corticosteroids such as prednisone are given to decrease inflammation.
3. Tincture of opium and diphenoxylate are given to control diarrhea; however, these drugs are contraindicated in patients with intestinal obstruction.
4. Rest is prescribed.
5. Diet is restricted—containing no fruits or vegetables, low in fats to control steatorrhea, and free of dairy products to combat lactulose deficiencies.
6. Surgery may be necessary to correct hemorrhage, fistulas, bowel perforation, or intestinal obstruction. Colectomy and ileostomy are the surgical procedures most often performed.

Complications

1. Stricture and fistulae formation (ischiorectal, perianal—even to bladder or vagina)
2. Hemorrhage, bowel perforation, mechanical intestinal obstruction
3. Incidence of colorectal cancer is higher in these patients.

Nursing Assessment

1. Assess frequency and consistency of stools.
2. Have the patient describe the location, severity, and onset of abdominal cramping or pain.
3. Ask the patient if there has been recent weight loss.
4. Have the patient describe types of foods eaten.
5. Ask patient if there is a family history of inflammatory bowel disorders.

Nursing Diagnoses

1. Altered nutrition (less than body requirements) related to postprandial pain
2. Potential fluid volume deficit related to diarrhea

3. Pain related to the inflammatory disease of the small intestine.
4. Ineffective individual coping related to feelings of dejection and embarrassment.
5. Knowledge deficit about regional enteritis.

Nursing Interventions

A. Achieving Adequate Nutritional Balance

1. Monitor diet that is low in residue, fiber, and fat, and high in calories, protein, and carbohydrates, with vitamin supplements (especially vitamin K). Prepare for hyperalimentation if the patient is debilitated.
2. Monitor weight daily.
3. Provide small frequent feedings to prevent distention of the gastric pouch.
4. Have patient participate in meal planning.

B. Maintenance of Electrolyte and Fluid Balance

1. Monitor intake and output.
2. Provide fluids as prescribed to maintain hydration (1000 ml./24 hours is minimum intake to meet body fluid needs.).
3. Monitor stool frequency and consistency.
4. Monitor electrolytes, especially potassium. Monitor acid–base balance because diarrhea can lead to metabolic acidosis.
5. Watch for cardiac dysrhythmias and muscle weakness due to loss of electrolytes.

C. Controlling Pain

1. Administer antimicrobials and sulfonamides for control of inflammatory process as prescribed.
2. Observe and record changes in pain—frequency, location, characteristics, precipitating events, and duration.
3. Monitor for distention, increased temperature, hypotension, and rectal bleeding; all signs of obstruction due to the inflammation.
4. Clean rectal area and apply ointments as necessary to decrease discomfort from skin breakdown.
5. Prepare patient for surgery if response to conservative medical and pharmacotherapy is unsatisfactory.
   a. Surgery intended to relieve segmental obstruction. The involved segment may be resected with anastomosis; bypass procedures may be done.
   b. Surgery is determined specifically for each patient.
   c. Unfortunately, recurrence of the disease is possible following surgery.

D. Psychosocial Support

1. Offer understanding, concern, and encouragement—this person is often dejected, debilitated, embarrassed about frequent and malodorous stools, and even fearful of eating.
2. Facilitate supportive counseling if appropriate.

Evaluation

1. Attains improved nutritional intake; weight stabilized or weight gain noted.
2. Attains/maintains adequate fluid intake; prevents dehydration; maintains adequate electrolyte levels.
3. Achieves relief of pain after several days of dietary, pharmacologic, and psychological therapy.
4. Verbalizes improved mental attitude toward ways to live with the disease.
5. Demonstrates an understanding of the disease and the need for life-style changes.

Ileostomy

An *ileostomy* is an opening in the ileum for the purpose of treating intractable granulomatous, ulcerative colitis, regional enteritis, or of diverting intestinal contents in colon cancer, familial polyposis, congenital defects, or trauma. The opening (*stoma*) is brought out through the abdominal wall, usually the lower right section of the abdomen. This stoma becomes the outlet for discharge of intestinal contents.

Implications for the Patient

(See also Colostomy for Preoperative and Postoperative Nursing Management, p. 496)

A. Psychological Implications

1. Some patients welcome the ileostomy, because it means the removal of a long-standing incapacitating disease process.
2. However, many patients experience psychological problems that are often overwhelming.
3. Preoperative counseling by the health care team, as well as by a trained visitor from the local chapter of the United Ostomy Association, is helpful.
4. The patient appreciates the prospect of enjoying a normal diet, instead of the low-residue diet to which he has been restricted.

B. Postoperative Implications

1. Following surgery, the patient wears a soft vinyl or rubber pouch (appliance) with an open-end; a clamp fitted on the end of the pouch permits emptying. The pouch is emptied 4–5 times a day, usually when the patient goes to the bathroom to urinate.
2. The ileostomate requires instruction—first from the nurse in the hospital or an enterostomal therapist* and then from the community nurse.
   See Guideline: Changing an Ileostomy Appliance, p. 485
3. Appliances may be reusable or disposable. They are held in place in several ways—cement, double-faced adhesive discs, karaya rings.
4. Waterproof tape is effective in anchoring the appliance when the patient showers or swims.
5. At first the intestinal discharge will be liquid, but later the small intestine will begin to take on its water-absorbing function to permit a more semisolid, pasty discharge.
6. Because the drainage is rich in enzymes, it may cause skin irritation; therefore optimal skin care is a top priority consideration for the patient.
   a. Cleanse the skin thoroughly with mild soap and water; rinse well.
   b. Dry area thoroughly.

---

* An enterostomal therapist (ET) is a health care professional with special training in the rehabilitation of persons with ostomies and related problems. Enterostomal therapists are certified by the IAET.

The International Association of Enterostomal Therapy (IAET), 2081 Business Center Drive, Suite 290, Irvine, CA 92715.

The Journal of Enterostomal Therapy is the official publication of the IAET and is published 6 times yearly by CV Mosby, 11830 Westline Industrial Drive, St Louis, MO 63146-3318.

The United Ostomy Association (UOA) is a self-help group for ostomates and other interested persons. 36 Executive Park, Suite 120, Irvine, CA 92714.

c. Take baths or showers as soon after surgery as possible.
d. For elderly patients, soap may be too drying for skin; however, oil-base soaps may prevent adhesives from adhering.

Nutritional Management of the Ileostomate

1. Nutritional needs of the patient with an ileostomy are similar to those of a healthy individual.
2. With adequate diet, additional vitamins or food supplements are unnecessary.
3. Exceptions can be found under the Nursing Interventions section below.

Nursing Diagnoses

1. Altered nutrition (less than body requirements) related to negative nutritional balance during or after surgery; vomiting; diarrhea; inadequate absorption of nutrients; weight loss; loss of absorptive site for vitamin B_{12} and bile salts related to resection of terminal ileus
2. Potential fluid volume deficit related to diarrhea, dehydration
3. Impaired skin integrity related to irritating intestinal effluent; skin agents used to hold appliance in place; allergies; fungal or bacterial growth; poor stoma location; application of belt
4. Body image disturbance related to stoma, odor, diarrhea, expulsion of flatus

Nursing Interventions

A. Achieving Adequate Nutrition

1. Offer diet high in calories and protein, and additional vitamin and mineral supplements; fat restriction may be necessary.
2. Consider use of elemental diets (diet preparations already broken down to simple, easily digested forms) until ileum adapts to new shortened length.
3. Weigh and record weight daily.
4. Explain to the patient that ileostomy will continue to function even if oral intake is limited, and that adequate nutritional intake is essential for healing to occur.
5. Dietary supplements are appropriate (Ensure [Ross], Isocal, Sustacal [Mead–Johnson]).
6. Monitor blood for B_{12} levels. Give replacements by injection.
7. Restrict fat, as the patient may not be able to digest and absorb fats because of bile salt deficiency.
   a. Monitor carefully because a fat-restricted diet causes weight loss and restricts the absorption of fat-soluble vitamins: A, D, E, and K.
   b. Be aware that, with bile salt deficiency, formation of gallstones is a complication.
8. Restrict fibrous foods: whole-grain breads and cereals, fresh fruit skins, fresh vegetables, beans, corn, and nuts.
9. Increase salt intake.

Note: Increased intake of water does not increase effluent, because excess water is excreted in urine.

B. Maintaining Fluid and Electrolytes

1. Avoid salt tablets, which may act as cathartics.
2. Supplement fluids with beverages containing electrolytes and glucose (Gatorade, Sportade).
3. Monitor intake and output, including liquid stools.
4. Weigh patient daily.
5. Give fluids in amounts necessary to maintain hydration.

6. Monitor electrolytes and hematocrit.
7. Monitor vital signs.

C. Maintaining Skin Integrity

1. Evaluate for proper fit of appliance.
2. Use an appropriate skin barrier between skin and appliance; karaya (in powder, paste, rings, and sheet forms); Stomahesive (Squibb) or ReliaSeal (Davol).
3. Avoid products to which the patient may be sensitive. Patch test for any suspected allergy on patient's inner arm.
4. If large areas of skin are involved or ulcerated, avoid rubber cement-type adhesive.
5. Severe problems due to poor stoma location necessitate surgical revision.
6. If skin breakdown is present, use antacids on the skin to neutralize the enzymes and lessen irritation.
7. Refer to ostomy nurse or other resources.

D. Preventing Complications

1. *Stomal bleeding:*
   a. Mucosa is friable and easily injured.
   b. However, when handled gently, these tissues heal readily because of rich blood supply.
   c. Wipe stoma gently.
2. *Prolapsed stoma:*
   a. Remove appliance. Observe bowel for signs of compromised circulation (pale or dark color).
   b. Apply cold pads or packs to control edema.
   c. Notify surgeon. Bowel may be replaced manually or surgical intervention may be necessary.
3. *Obstruction:*
   a. Obstruction or stenosis may be due to edema or lymphatic blockage. More commonly, it is due to food blockage brought about by poor chewing habits and high-cellulose foods.
   b. Remove appliance.
   c. Have the patient lie down and apply warm compresses to abdomen, or relax in tub of warm water.
   d. Offer hot tea drinks. If this does not help within 2–3 hours, check with physician; it may be necessary to gently irrigate the ileostomy (physician prescribed) with a small volume of saline solution.
   e. Surgical correction may be required.
   f. Restrict fibrous foods; be alert to offenders such as celery, cabbage, nuts, and corn. Instruct the patient to chew food thoroughly.
4. *Kidney stones:*
   a. Increase the patient's fluid intake.
   b. If stones are urate crystals, sodium bicarbonate may be prescribed to alkalinize urine.
   c. If stones are calcium, ascorbic acid may be prescribed to acidify urine.
5. *Medication difficulties:*
   a. The various functions of the small and large bowel are interrupted or absent; therefore, drug action can be affected by altered transit time through the small intestine.
   b. Coated tablets may pass undissolved through bowel into ileostomy appliance. Suggest taking uncoated tablets or liquids.
   c. If medications do pass undissolved, thereafter crush them and take with water or applesauce. Check discharge to be sure pills are not being passed undissolved.
   d. Medications may not be absorbed. Do not use time- or sustained-release capsules or tablets.
   e. The terminal ileum is the absorptive site for B_{12}.

Administer B_{12} subcutaneously as prescribed if the distal ileum is removed.

E. Enhancing Positive Body Image

1. Odor:
   a. Be meticulous in cleaning procedure.
   b. Alternate reusable pouches; when not in use, allow pouch to hang in fresh air (not sun).
   c. If using disposable pouches, select odor-proof materials.
   d. Change medications when one is found to be odor-producing.
   e. Use oral deodorants: chlorophyll derivatives, bismuth subcarbonate, or bismuth subgallate.
   f. Insert deodorizer in appliance: charcoal, Banish (TM-United), or baking soda.
   g. Encourage foods such as spinach and parsley that act on the intestinal tract as deodorizers.
2. Diarrhea:
   a. Electrolyte imbalance may easily occur. Treat with clear liquids and antidiarrheal medications.
   b. Water, salts, and fluids can be replaced with commercial preparations (Gatorade, Quick Kick).
   c. Alternate a cup of salted broth and a cup of sweetened tea each hour.
   d. Water-absorbing drugs (hydrophilic colloids) such as Metamucil Powder are sometimes effective.
   e. If diarrhea does not resolve in 24 hours, the patient should seek medical care. IV fluids and electrolyte therapy may be necessary.
3. Expulsion of flatus:
   a. Limit gas-producing foods such as beans, cabbage, onions, beer.
   b. Try to avoid air-swallowing, which may occur during smoking, talking, eating, emotional upset.

Discharge Planning/Patient Education

Discharge from hospital for patient with ileostomy or colostomy.

A. Clothing

1. A girdle is permissible—a size larger is recommended to accommodate the pouch.
2. Swim suits (even 2-piece) can be worn; men prefer boxer-styled trunks; women may prefer a swim suit with a skirt.
3. For swimming, a rubber belt is preferred to elastic cloth, which sometimes loses elasticity when wet.

B. Medications

The ileostomate should not have laxatives, irrigations, enteric-coated, or time-release capsules.

C. Travel

1. Traveling by plane or any other vehicle is not contraindicated.
2. When traveling by plane, patient should carry ostomy kit (in the event that there is a delay in retrieving baggage).
3. Colostomates who irrigate should use only water suitable for drinking.
4. Bring along a suitable antidiarrheal medication.

D. Sports

1. All kinds of sports may be participated in, as reported by ostomates—tennis, water surfing, skin diving, water skiing, ice skating, horseback riding.
2. Problems may arise if the ostomate participates in contact sports such as football, ice hockey.

E. Sexual Functioning

1. Approximately 10%–20% of male ileostomates experience impaired sexual function; this may only be temporary.
2. Male colostomates vary from being fully potent to impotent.
3. In many instances, potency is regained, but this may take up to 2 years.

F. Pregnancy

1. An ostomy is not a contraindication to a successful pregnancy.
2. Careful medical supervision during pregnancy is required for a female ostomate.
3. The ostomy opening may change in size (stretch) as the pregnancy continues; thereafter, changes in the size of the appliance opening may be required.
4. Change in abdominal contour may necessitate the use of a very flexible appliance or faceplate.

G. Sleeping

1. Almost any position of comfort can be assumed if the pouch is properly fitted.
2. Sleeping on the stomach is comfortable when a small cushion is placed under the hip on the side of the stoma.

H. Obstruction or Blockage

1. Know signs and symptoms; notify enterostomal therapist or physician as necessary.

Evaluation

1. Achieves an acceptable weight gain.
2. Attains fluid balance; absence of signs and symptoms of dehydration.
3. Demonstrates healthy skin around stoma.
4. Copes with changed body image; manages care of stoma/appliance.

Guidelines Changing an Ileostomy Appliance

Goals
1. Prevent leakage (bag is usually changed every 2–4 days).
2. Permit examination of skin around stoma.
3. Assist in controlling odor if this presents a problem.

Time
1. Early in morning, before breakfast, or 2–4 hours after a meal, or just before bedtime when the bowel is least active.
2. Immediately, if patient is complaining of burning or itching underneath the disc or has pain around the stoma.

Equipment
Duplicate ileostomy appliance with or without belt (Fig. 20-5); pouch-closing device
Soap, water, and washcloth
Appropriate skin barrier
Gauze
Emesis basin
Tape (hypoallergenic)

Procedure

Nursing Action	Rationale/Amplification
Preparatory Phase	
1. Have the patient assume a relaxed position. Provide privacy.	1. Encourage patient participation and understanding so that eventually he will be able to change appliance himself.
2. Explain details of this activity.	2. Encourage questions.
3. Expose ileostomy area; remove ileostomy belt (if worn).	
4. Position lamp; wash hands.	
Performance Phase	
1. To remove appliance	
a. Sit or stand in a comfortable position.	a. Have the patient sit on toilet or on a chair facing toilet. If standing, face toilet.
b. Fill a container with prescribed solvent, then fill medicine dropper with solvent; apply a few drops of solvent between disc of appliance and skin. Do not pull off appliance.	b. As solvent works, pouch loosens and pulling is unnecessary. Solvent is often unnecessary when skin cement is not used. Pouch can be removed by gently pushing skin away from adhesive.
c. If adhesive residue builds up on skin, use very small amount of adhesive remover on gauze.	c. Do not use acetone, ether, or benzene because these are irritating to skin.
2. To cleanse skin:	
a. Remove any excess karaya with dry toilet tissue.	a. During this time, a gauze dressing or pieces of tissue may be used to cover the stoma to absorb excess drainage while skin is being cleaned.

(continued)

Guidelines   Changing an Ileostomy Appliance *(continued)*

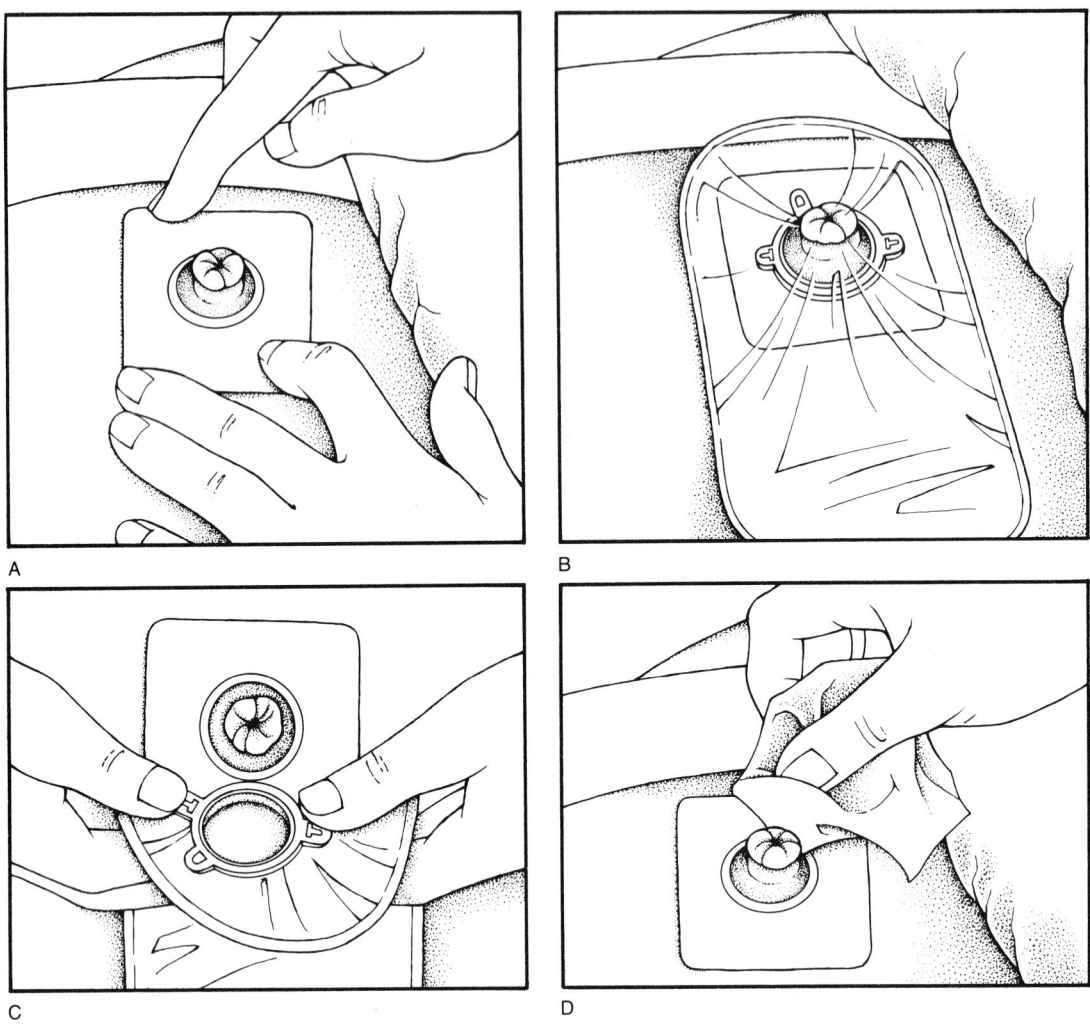

A

B

C

D

Figure 20-5. *Ileostomy care. (A) A Stomahesive wafer with flange (1½″, 1¾″, 2¼″, 2¾″) can be applied directly to the peristomal area after it has been thoroughly cleaned and dried. (B) An opaque or transparent drainable pouch is positioned at desired angle over stoma. (C) Pouch may be removed without removing wafer. (D) Stoma may be assessed without removing wafer. (Adapted by permission from ConvaTec, a division of ER Squibb & Sons, Inc.)*

Procedure
(continued)

Nursing Action	Rationale/Amplification
b. Wash skin gently with soft cloth moistened with tepid water and mild soap, or bathe before putting on clean appliance.	b. The patient may shower before removing appliance. Micropore or waterproof tape applied to sides of disc will keep it secure while bathing.
c. Rinse and dry skin thoroughly after cleansing.	c. Moisture or soap residue will interfere with appliance adhesion.
3. To put on appliance if no skin irritation:	
a. An appropriate skin barrier should be applied to peristomal skin before the pouch is applied.	a. There are many skin barriers available. Many disposable pouches have a built-in skin barrier to prevent peristomal skin erosion.
b. It is optional to apply tincture of benzoin or one of the many specially formulated skin preparations to help protect peristomal skin.	b. Note: Do not confuse with tincture of benzoin compound, which is too irritating.
c. Remove cover from adherent surface of disc of disposable plastic pouch and apply directly to skin.	c. Be sure skin is thoroughly dry.
d. Press firmly in place for 30 seconds.	d. To ensure adherence

Procedure *(continued)*	**Nursing Action**	**Rationale/Amplification**

4. To put on appliance if there is skin irritation:
   a. Cleanse skin thoroughly but gently; pat dry.
   b. Apply Kenalog spray; blot excess moisture with a cotton pledget and dust lightly with nystatin (Mycostatin) powder.

   (1) An alternate effective measure is to apply a wafer of Stomahesive (Squibb), which is available in 10 × 10 cm. (4″ × 4″) and 20 × 20 cm. (8″ × 8″) pieces. The stomal opening should be cut the same size as the stoma; use a cutting guide (supplied by Stomahesive). The wafer is applied directly to the skin.
   (2) A second alternative is to moisten a karaya gum washer and apply when it is tacky. If skin is "weepy," karaya powder may be applied first and any excess dusted off gently.
   c. The pouch is then applied to the treated skin.
5. Check the pouch bottom for closure; use rubber band or clip provided after pressing out air.
6. Attach belt if desired.

Follow-Up Phase

1. Dispose of waste materials.
2. Clean reusable ileostomy pouch by washing in soap and water.
3. Soak pouch in deodorant solution and hang to dry.

4. Instruct the patient how to perform the procedure. Allow him to take part and do more of the steps until he can complete the procedure himself.
5. To help control odor, a commercial deodorant can be placed in the pouch.
6. Instruct the patient to avoid odor-causing foods such as onions, cabbage, brussel sprouts, eggs, fish, and asparagus.
7. Instruct the patient to remove gas by releasing the closure clamp from the bottom.

Rationale/Amplification

a. To remove debris
b. The steroid preparation (Kenalog) helps decrease inflammation. The antifungal (nystatin) treats those types of infections that are common around stomas. A prescription is required for both medications.
   (1) Stomahesive is a substance that facilitates healing of excoriated skin. It adheres well even to "weepy" irritated skin.

   (2) Karaya also facilitates skin healing. Tackiness promotes adherence.

c. This will allow skin to heal while appliance is in place.
5. Proper closure controls leakage.

2. Preserves life of appliance and controls odor.

3. Deodorizing agents should be effective but not destructive to rubber or vinyl.

7. Never make a pinhole in the pouch to release gas because this destroys the odor-proof seal.

Guidelines Continent Ileostomy (Kock Pouch)

A *continent ileostomy* is the surgical creation of a pouch of small intestine that can act as an internal receptacle for fecal discharge; a nipple valve is constructed at the outlet to permit drainage from the abdomen. This kind of ileostomy may be done initially for selected patients when they present for an ileostomy, or it may be constructed from the conventional ileostomy (Fig. 20-6).

Preoperative Management

Essentially the same as for the patient having a traditional ileostomy.

Postoperative Management

1. A catheter will extend from the stoma and be attached to closed suction; drainage will be maintained about 10 days.
2. Catheter irrigation is done usually every 2 hours with 20–30 ml. saline solution to ensure patency; return flow is by gravity.
3. Nasogastric suction is used to relieve pressure on suture line by preventing a build-up of gastric contents.
4. Parenteral fluids are administered for 4–5 days; thereafter, clear liquids and diet as tolerated.
5. Monitor for nausea and abdominal distention.
6. Pain medication is given as required; early ambulation is encouraged.
7. In about 10–14 days, the catheter is removed from the stoma and the patient participates in the management of his ileostomy.
8. During initial postoperative period, pouch is kept empty to allow suture lines to heal and to prevent rapid pouch expansion.

Equipment

Catheter
Water-soluble lubricant
Gauze squares
Syringe
Irrigating solution in a bowl, emesis, or receiving basin
Urinary leg bag

Guidelines Continent Ileostomy (Kock Pouch) *(continued)*

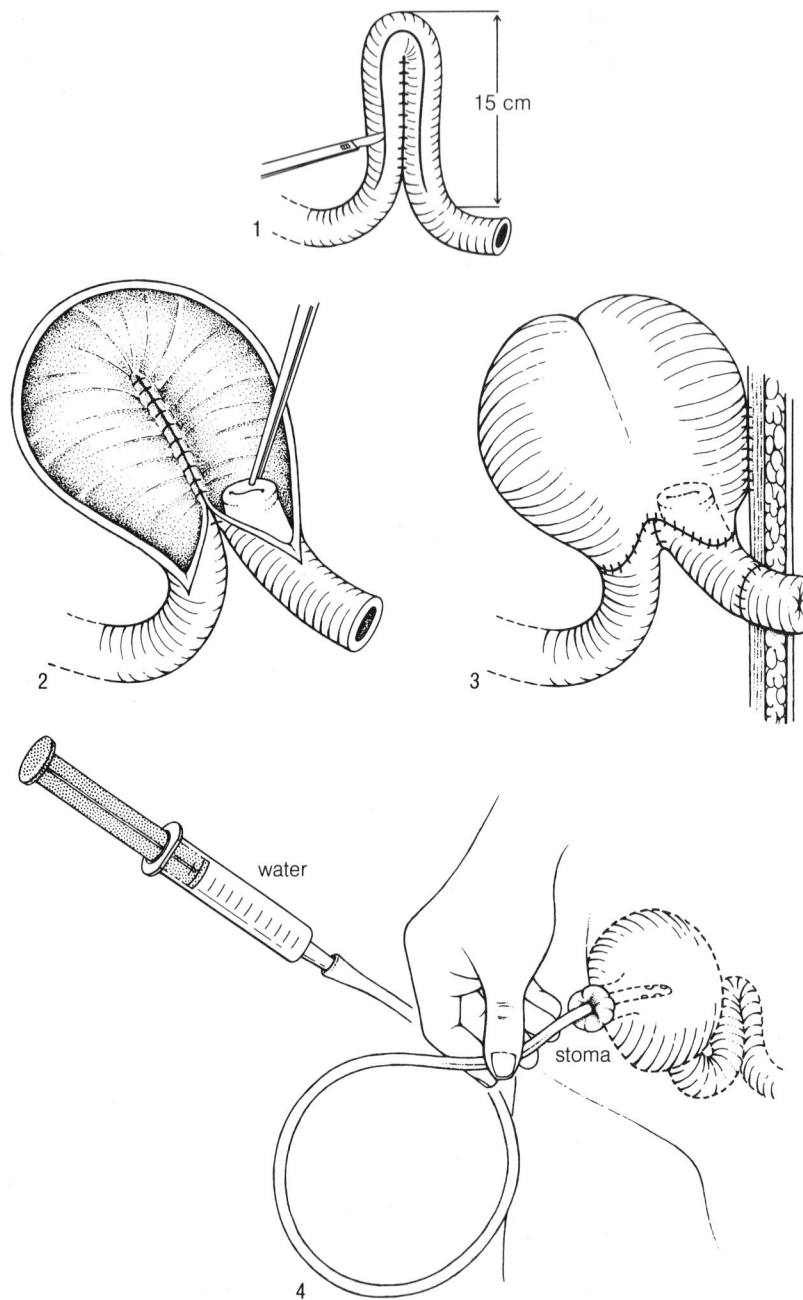

Figure 20-6. *Continent ileostomy (Kock pouch). 1. About 30 cm. of ileum will become an ileal pouch. By looping the ileum, there are about 15 cm. on each side as shown. The two sides are stitched together in the center. The surgeon then makes a U-shaped incision. 2. The ileum is opened, and the inner section is stitched, much like a seam, to make a smooth inner surface. After this, a valve or "nipple" is constructed on the right between pouch and stoma. Then the top of the ileum is folded to the bottom and stitched closed, as illustrated in part 3. This pouch is stitched to the inner wall for immobilization; likewise, the stoma is fixed to the abdominal wall. In part 4 a lubricated catheter is being gently inserted about 5 cm. into the ileal pouch for drainage. (Brunner LS and Suddarth DS. Textbook of Medical–Surgical Nursing. Philadelphia, JB Lippincott)*

Nursing Action	Rationale/Amplification
1. Lubricate catheter and gently insert about 5 cm. (2 inches).	1. Resistance may be felt at valve or "nipple."
2. If much resistance is encountered, fill syringe with 20 ml. air or water and inject through catheter; gently exert pressure on catheter.	2. This will permit catheter to enter pouch.
3. Place end of catheter in drainage basin (below level of stoma); later this can be done at toilet bowl.	3. Gravity facilitates drainage. Drainage may include flatus as well as effluent.
4. Following drainage, remove catheter. Wash area around stoma; dry and apply absorbent pad. Fasten with hypoallergenic tape.	4. Entire procedure requires about 5–10 minutes. At first, irrigation is done every 2 hours, then gradually extended to 3 times daily. If feces are not too thick, drainage through catheter may occur successfully without irrigation.
5. A urinary leg bag may be attached to the catheter to allow drainage while ambulating.	5. When gastrointestinal function first returns, output may exceed 2000 ml./day.
6. Monitor intake and output.	
7. Replace fluids as prescribed.	
8. Monitor bowel sounds.	8. To determine return of peristalsis and bowel function—usually 3–5 days after surgery.
9. When bowel function returns, administer clear liquids as prescribed. When fecal drainage appears in pouch, solid foods are prescribed. Check the catheter frequently.	9. Ensure the catheter is not plugged with mucus or undigested food.
10. If the catheter is clogged, rotate it gently to clear the catheter. If still blocked, try milking it. Remove, rinse and reinsert if still clogged. If all these fail, notify the physician.	
11. Measure output minus irrigation fluid.	
12. Instruct the patient to develop a schedule for drainage of pouch.	

Note: Patient may bathe or shower without the catheter, but it shouldn't be out for longer than 20 minutes, to prevent distention and fecal contents accumulating in the pouch.

Diverticulosis and Diverticulitis

A *diverticulum* is a pouch or saccular dilatation leading out from a tube or main cavity (Fig. 20-7).

Diverticulitis is an inflammation of diverticula.

Diverticulosis is the condition in which an individual has multiple diverticula.

Predisposing Factors

1. Probable congenital predisposition
2. Weakening and degeneration of muscular wall of the intestine, causing herniation of the lining mucous membrane through a muscle at site of artery penetration
3. Increased mechanical pressure due to abnormal high-pressure contractions of sigmoid colon in response to neurohumoral stimuli
4. Chronic overdistention of the large bowel
5. Diet low in roughage—reduces fecal residue, narrows the bowel lumen, and leads to higher pressure intra-abdominally during defecation

Incidence

1. Diverticulosis usually occurs in about 10% of individuals over 40 years of age and nearly 50% of persons over age 60; only a small percentage develop diverticulitis.
2. The condition is most common in sigmoid colon.
3. Small-bowel diverticula are unusual, but when they occur they are often multiple. They may act as areas of stasis and bacterial overgrowth, leading to malabsorption of fat and vitamin B_{12}.

Altered Physiology

(Colon diverticulosis and diverticulitis)
1. Constipation from spastic colon syndrome often precedes the development of diverticulosis by many years.
2. Following local inflammation of the diverticula, there may be narrowing of the colon with fibrotic stricture, which then leads to narrowed stools, cramps, and increasing constipation.
3. With the development of granulation tissue, occult bleeding may occur, producing iron-deficiency anemia; fatigue and weakness are then evident. However, massive bleeding is more common.
4. Abscess development causes a tender palpable mass; fever and leukocytosis also occur.
5. If the diverticulum perforates, local abscess or peritonitis results; peritonitis causes rigidity, abdominal pain, loss of bowel sounds, and eventually shock.
6. Uninflamed or minimally inflamed diverticula may erode adjacent arterial branches, causing acute massive rectal bleeding.

Clinical Manifestations

A. General Clinical Signs

1. May occur in acute attacks or may persist as a long, drawn-out smoldering infection.
2. Tends to spread to surrounding bowel wall, increasing the irritability and spasticity of the colon.
3. When infections are severe, perforation of the colon can occur, leading to peritonitis.
4. When infection is less acute but slowly progressive, extensive scarring and abscess formation involving the bowel wall may occur.

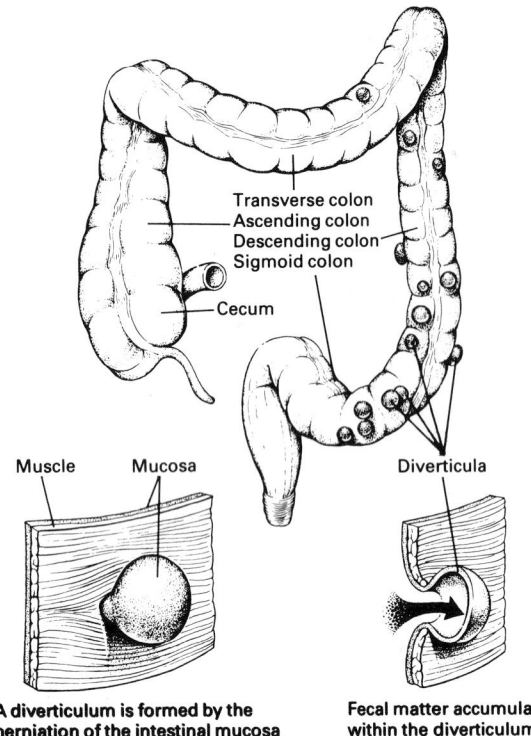

A diverticulum is formed by the herniation of the intestinal mucosa through the weakened muscular wall usually at site of arterial penetration on the mesenteric border of the colon.

Fecal matter accumulates within the diverticulum

Figure 20-7. Diverticula are most common in the sigmoid colon; they diminish in number and size as the colon approaches the cecum. Diverticula are rarely found in the rectum.

a. Lower bowel obstruction may occur
b. Sometimes, fistulae form with the bladder, the adjacent small bowel, the vagina, or even the skin.
5. Sepsis may spread via portal vein to liver, causing liver abscesses.

B. Specific Clinical Signs

1. Diverticulosis
   a. Bowel irregularity, constipation, and diarrhea
   b. Sudden massive hemorrhage
2. Milder forms of diverticulitis
   a. Bouts of soreness, mild lower abdominal cramps
   b. Bowel irregularity, constipation, and diarrhea
   c. Mild nausea, gas, low-grade fever, and leukocytosis
3. Moderately severe acute diverticulitis
   a. Crampy pain in lower left quadrant of abdomen
   b. Low-grade fever, chills, leukocytosis
   c. Ruptured diverticula produce abscesses or peritonitis
      (1) Abdominal rigidity
      (2) Signs of shock and sepsis (hypotension, chills, high fever)
      (3) Ruptured diverticulum near a blood vessel may cause massive hemorrhage
4. Chronic diverticulitis may cause adhesions that narrow the bowel's opening and can cause partial or complete bowel obstruction.

a. Constipation, "ribbonlike" stools, intermittent diarrhea
b. Abdominal distention leading to abdominal rigidity
c. Diminished or absent bowel sounds
d. Nausea, vomiting, and abdominal pain

Diagnostic Evaluation

1. History, physical examination, laboratory evaluation (for infection)
2. Flat film of abdomen, ultrasonography/CT scan
3. Sigmoidoscopy; possibly colonoscopy
4. Barium enema (after infection subsides)

NURSING ALERT: In patients with acute diverticulitis, a barium enema may rupture the bowel.

Management

1. Intestinal diverticulosis with pain usually responds to a liquid or bland diet and stool softeners to relieve symptoms, minimize irritation, and decrease the spread of the inflammation.
2. Some authorities prefer fiber content in the diet rather than a low-residue diet.
   a. With increased fiber, more bulk is added, to give the stool proper consistency.
   b. With a low-residue diet, the colon may work harder to propel contents, thereby producing high pressure on the intestinal walls, which in turn promotes diverticula formation.
3. Once the pain has stopped, high-residue diets and bulk medication such as psyllium hydrophilic mucilloid (Metamucil) is prescribed to counteract the tendency toward constipation.
4. Constipation is to be avoided. Stool softeners such as docusate sodium (Colace) are prescribed.
5. During acute episode, fluid and nutritional requirements may need to be maintained with intravenous therapy; nothing is given by mouth.
6. Antimicrobial therapy is prescribed to reduce infection.
7. For pain, meperidine (Demerol) is the analgesic of choice because it is less spasmogenic than other analgesics.
8. Antispasmodics such as propantheline are prescribed to control muscle spasm.
9. Warm-oil-retention enemas may be prescribed to treat inflammation locally by softening fecal mass.

NURSING ALERT: Ordinary enemas and laxatives may be harmful and should not be used.

Surgical Management

1. If there is little response to medical treatment, or if complications such as hemorrhage, obstruction, or perforation occur, surgery is necessary.
   a. Segment of intestine involved with diverticula is resected; two ends are reunited (anastomosis) to maintain continuity.
   b. Temporary colostomy is sometimes performed to divert fecal stream (see p. 495), with continuity restored in later second-stage procedure.

2. Preparation for surgery:
   a. Low-residue diet or nothing by mouth.
   b. Antimicrobials, systemic and intestinal surface-acting, to reduce bowel bacterial flora, diminish bulk of stool, and soften fecal mass for easier movement.
   c. Cleansing enemas may be prescribed.

Complications

1. Hemorrhage from colonic diverticula, usually in the right colon
2. Bowel obstruction
3. Intussusception (prolapse of one segment of the bowel into the lumen of another segment)
4. Volvulus (twisting of the bowel on itself) causing intestinal obstruction; pericolic abscess; peritonitis

Nursing Diagnoses

1. Pain related to intestinal discomfort, diarrhea, and/or constipation
2. Altered nutrition (less than body requirements) related to diarrhea, fluid and electrolyte loss, nausea, and vomiting
3. Altered bowel elimination (constipation/diarrhea) related to the disease process
4. Knowledge deficit of the relation between diet and diverticulosis

Nursing Interventions

A. Achieving Pain Relief

1. Observe for signs and location of pain, type and severity.
2. Ascultate bowel sounds.
3. Palpate abdomen to determine rigidity or tenderness due to perforation or peritonitis.
4. Administer nonopiate analgesics as prescribed (opiates may mask signs of perforation).
5. Administer anticholinergics as prescribed to decrease colon spasm.

B. Maintaining Adequate Nutrition

1. Follow prescribed diet that is high in soft residue and low in sugar.
   a. Provide lists of these foods to enhance familiarity with proper dietary control.
   b. Emphasize that proper food intake influences how well the intestinal tract functions.
2. Inform patient that bran products will add bulk to the stool and can be taken with milk or sprinkled over cereal.
3. Monitor intake and output.

C. Promoting Normal Bowel Elimination

1. Advise patient to establish regular bowel habits to promote regular and complete evacuation.
2. Observe color, consistency, and frequency of stools and record.
3. Encourage fluids if constipated.
4. Provide soft, high-residue, low-roughage, low-sugar diet to provide bulk and more consistency to the stool.

NURSING ALERT: Assess patient's response to diet. Increased bulk may result in increased symptoms; it may be necessary to reduce residue.

D. Increasing Understanding

1. Explain the disease process to the patient and its relationship to diet.
2. Have the patient continue periodic medical supervision and follow-up; report problems and untoward symptoms.

Evaluation

1. Expresses relief of pain and has a decrease in symptoms.
2. Consumes a prescribed diet and can relate what foods to include or avoid.
3. Reports near-normal bowel function; no diarrhea or constipation.
4. Delineates the general nature of diverticulosis and can list what helps or aggravates the condition.

Intestinal Obstruction

Intestinal obstruction is an interruption in the normal flow of intestinal contents along the intestinal tract.

The block may occur in the small or large intestine, may be complete or incomplete, may be mechanical or paralytic, and may or may not compromise the vascular supply. Obstruction most frequently occurs in the very young and the very old.

Types of Obstruction

A. Mechanical—a physical block to passage of intestinal contents without disturbing blood supply of bowel

1. Location
   a. Extrinsic (e.g., adhesion, hernia, intussusception)
   b. Intrinsic (e.g., hematoma, tumor)
   c. Intraluminal (e.g., foreign body, fecal or barium impactions, polyp)
2. Clinical pattern
   High small-bowel (jejunal) or low small-bowel (ileal) occurs 4 times more frequently than colonic obstruction.

B. Paralytic (adynamic, neurogenic) Ileus

1. Peristalsis is ineffective (diminished motor activity perhaps because of toxic or traumatic disturbance of the autonomic nervous system).
2. There is no physical obstruction and no interrupted blood supply.
3. Disappears spontaneously after 2–3 days.

C. Strangulation

Obstruction also compromises blood supply, leading to gangrene of the intestine.

Causes

A. Mechanical (extramural)

1. Adhesions—postoperative
2. Hernia
3. Malignancy
4. Volvulus (loop of intestine that has twisted)

B. Mechanical (intramural)

1. Carcinoma
2. Hematoma
3. Intussusception (telescoping of intestine)
4. Stricture or stenosis (scarring)

C. Paralytic

1. Spinal cord injuries; vertebral fractures
2. Postoperatively after any abdominal surgery
3. Peritonitis, pneumonia
4. Wound dehiscence (breakdown)
5. Gastrointestinal tract surgery
   Note:
1. In postoperative patients, approximately 90% of mechanical obstructions are due to adhesions.
2. In nonsurgical patients, hernia (most often inguinal) is the most common cause of mechanical obstruction.

Altered Physiology

1. Results in increased peristalsis, distention by fluid and gas, and increased bacterial growth proximal to obstruction. The intestine empties distally.
2. Increased secretions into the intestine are associated with diminution in the bowel's absorptive capacity.
3. The accumulation of gases, secretions, and oral intake above the obstruction causes increasing intraluminal pressure.
4. Venous pressure in the affected area increases, and circulatory stasis and edema result.
5. Bowel necrosis may occur because of anoxia and compression of the terminal branches of the mesenteric artery.
6. Bacteria and toxins pass across the intestinal membranes into the abdominal cavity; thereby leading to peritonitis.
7. *"Closed-loop" obstruction* is a condition in which the intestinal segment is occluded at both ends, preventing either the downward passage or the regurgitation of intestinal contents.

Clinical Manifestations

Fever, peritoneal irritation, increased white blood cell count, toxicity, and shock may develop with all types of intestinal obstruction.

1. Simple mechanical—high small bowel
   Colic (cramps) mid-to-upper abdomen, some distention, early bilious vomiting, increased bowel sounds (high-pitched tinkling heard at brief intervals), minimal diffuse tenderness
2. Simple mechanical—low small bowel
   Significant colic (cramps) midabdominal, considerable distention, vomiting—slight or absent—later feculent, increased bowel sounds and "hush" sounds, minimal diffuse tenderness
3. Simple mechanical—colon
   Cramps (mid-to-lower abdomen), later-appearing distention, then vomiting may develop (feculent), increase in bowel sounds, minimal diffuse tenderness
4. Partial chronic mechanical obstruction—may occur with granulomatous bowel (Crohn's) disease.
   Symptoms are cramping abdominal pain, mild distention, and diarrhea.
5. Strangulation
   Symptoms are initially those of mechanical obstruction, but later progress rapidly: Pain is severe, continuous, and localized. There is moderate distention, persistent vomiting, usually decreased bowel sounds and marked localized tenderness. Stools or vomitus become melenous or bloody or contain occult blood.

6. Paralytic ileus
   Gaseous distention is prominent; abdomen is tense; pain is dull, continuous, and diffuse; obstipation (intractable constipation) is rarely complete, as small amounts of flatus may be passed; peristalsis is usually depressed, and bowel sounds are infrequent or absent; vomiting occurs only after eating (Vomiting may later become fecal.).

Diagnostic Evaluation

1. X-rays—abdominal films show the presence and location of intestinal gas or fluid.
2. Barium enema shows a distended, air-filled colon or a closed loop of the sigmoid.
3. Laboratory results show decreased sodium, potassium, and chloride levels due to vomiting; elevated WBC counts with necrosis, strangulation, or peritonitis; increased serum amylase levels from irritation of the pancreas by the bowel loop.

Management

1. Correction of fluid and electrolyte imbalances
   a. Na^+, K^+, blood component therapy
   b. Ringer's lactate to correct interstitial fluid deficit
   c. Dextrose/water to correct intracellular fluid deficit
2. Long-tube decompression of intestine proximal to the blockage site (see p. 469); the tube can be passed more effectively with the patient lying on his right side.
3. Treatment of shock and peritonitis
4. Surgery to relieve complete small-bowel obstruction and colon obstruction. When tube suction therapy does not help after 12 hours, surgery is indicated.
   a. Resection of obstructing lesion and end-to-end anastomosis is done when no evidence of peritonitis and only minimal edema exist; this requires a proximal colostomy to decompress new anastomosis.
   b. Resection of all necrotic intestine is necessary.
   c. A tube enterostomy may be done by introducing a catheter into distended bowel; the other end of catheter is brought out through the abdominal wall via a separate incision. This is a palliative measure.
   d. A loop colostomy is done by drawing a proximal loop or segment of colon up to the skin surface and opening it as a colostomy; the distal portion of colon is treated later.
5. Hyperalimentation may be necessary to correct protein deficiency from chronic obstruction, paralytic ileus, or infection.
6. Analgesics and sedatives such as meperidine or phenobarbital, but not opiates because they inhibit GI motility.
7. Antibiotics for peritonitis

Complications

1. Dehydration due to loss of water, sodium, and chloride
2. Peritonitis
3. Shock due to loss of electrolytes and dehydration
4. Death due to shock

Nursing Assessment

1. In the nursing history, describe accurately the nature and location of the patient's pain, the presence of distention, the absence of flatus or defecation.

2. Monitor and record vital signs (including blood pressure) every 4 hours.
3. Watch for air–fluid lock syndrome in elderly, who often remain in the recumbent position for extended periods.
   a. Fluid collects in dependent bowel loops.
   b. Peristalsis is too weak to push fluid "uphill."
   c. Obstruction primarily occurs in the large bowel.
4. Conduct frequent checks of the patient's level of responsiveness; decreasing responsiveness may offer a clue to an increasing electrolyte imbalance.
5. Observe for evidence of postural hypotension as patient is moved from a low Fowler's position to an upright position; this may suggest circulatory insufficiency.
6. Compare the patient's state of orientation with his admission status; a lessening awareness of his environment may suggest the development of shock.

Nursing Diagnoses

1. Pain related to obstruction, distention, and strangulation
2. Potential fluid volume deficit related to impaired fluid intake, vomiting, and diarrhea from intestinal obstruction
3. Altered bowel elimination, diarrhea, related to obstruction
4. Anxiety and fear of death related to life-threatening symptoms of intestinal obstruction
5. Ineffective breathing pattern related to abdominal distention, which interferes with normal lung expansion

Nursing Interventions

A. Achieving Relief of Pain

1. Administer prescribed analgesics.
2. Provide supportive care during nasoenteral intubation, as this will help in relieving discomfort.
3. To relieve "air–fluid lock" syndrome, turn the patient from supine to prone position every 10 minutes until enough flatus is passed to decompress the abdomen. A rectal tube may help.

B. Maintaining Electrolyte and Fluid Balance

1. Measure and record all intake and output.
2. Administer IV's, hyperalimentation, and blood as prescribed.
3. Monitor electrolytes, urinalysis, hemoglobin, and blood cell counts and report any abnormalities.
4. Minimize those factors that would enhance gastric secretions to prevent fluid loss (via nasogastric suction); avoid conversation about enticing meals and eliminate meals being served within patient's range of seeing or smelling.
5. Monitor urinary output to assess renal function and to detect urinary retention due to bladder compression by the distended intestine.
6. Monitor vital signs; a drop in blood pressure may indicate decreased circulatory volume due to blood loss from strangulated hernia.
7. Postoperative nursing interventions
   For an enterostomy, connect tube to drainage bottle at side of bed; expect considerable amount of fecal drainage during the first 12–15 hours (500–1000 ml.).
   a. Observe frequently the patency of drainage equipment.

b. If there is difficulty with drainage, it may be necessary to inject 15 ml. of warm saline solution into the enterostomy tube every 2–4 hours, with approval of physician.
   c. Protect skin around enterostomy tube with a skin barrier such as Stomahesive or karaya preparations.
8. Follow additional postoperative management described in Major Intestinal Surgery on page 476.

C. Maintaining Normal Bowel Elimination

1. Save all stools to test for occult blood.
2. Maintain adequate fluid balance.
3. Record amount and consistency of stools.
4. Maintain nasogastric or Miller–Abbott tube as prescribed to decompress bowel.

D. Preventing Complications

1. Prevent infarction by carefully assessing the patient's status; pain that increases in intensity or becomes localized or continuous may herald strangulation.
2. Detect early signs of peritonitis, such as rigidity and tenderness, in an effort to minimize this complication.
3. Avoid enemas.
   a. An enema may distort an x-ray picture by introducing gas into the tract distal to the obstruction.
   b. An enema may make a partial obstruction worse.
4. Observe for signs of shock—pallor, tachycardia, hypotension.
5. Watch for signs of
   a. Metabolic alkalosis (slow, shallow respirations changes in sensorium, tetany)
   b. Metabolic acidosis (disorientation, deep rapid breathing, weakness, and shortness of breath on exertion).

E. Relieving Anxiety and Fears

1. Recognize the patient's concerns and initiate measures to secure his cooperation and confidence in the staff.
2. Ascertain the patient's specific anxieties and provide him with therapeutic responses.

F. Maintaining Proper Lung Ventilation

1. Keep the patient in Fowler's position to promote ventilation and relief from abdominal distention.
2. Monitor arterial blood gases.

Evaluation

1. Experiences minimal pain.
2. Takes food and fluid orally and exhibits no vomiting or diarrhea.
3. Demonstrates relief of bowel obstruction—passes flatus, has first bowel movement.
4. No signs of complications.
5. Appears relaxed and reports "feeling better."
6. Demonstrates improved breathing ability.

Cancer of the Colon

A neoplasm in the colon characterized by uncontrolled growth of anaplastic cells that tend to invade surrounding tissue and metastasize to other body sites.

Incidence

1. Cancer of the colon and rectum accounts for over 60,000 deaths annually—the second highest overall death rate in the US for any type of cancer. Colon can-

cer is diagnosed in approximately 107,000 Americans yearly.
2. Males and females are affected equally.
3. The highest incidence occurs in patients about 50 years of age.
4. Potentially curable in 80%–90% of patients if early diagnosis allows resection before node involvement.

Etiology and Risk Factors

1. *Familial polyposis*—numerous pedunculated growths or polyps arising from the mucosa and extending into the lumen of the intestine.
2. *Chronic ulcerative colitis*—definite risk of colon cancer (up to 20% after 20 years of age with active disease).
3. *Diverticulosis and cancer*—may be found together and simulate each other—no definite evidence that the presence of diverticula is significant in the development of cancer.
4. *Cultural Factors*
    a. Cancer of the colon occurs much more frequently in developed countries and rarely in underdeveloped countries.
    b. The increased incidence of colon cancer in developed countries is probably related to the relatively low fiber and excess animal fat (particularly beef) in the diet in these areas.
5. Unabsorbable fiber deficit appears to be related to intestinal transit time, stool bulk, and consistency.
6. The effect of diet on the colon bacterial flora is a factor possibly contributing to cancer.

Clinical Manifestations

1. Distribution of cancer in the colon is shown in Figure 20-8.
2. Most common symptoms:
    a. Blood in stools (usually occult)—causing anemia
    b. Partial obstruction—causing constipation alternating with diarrhea, lower abdominal pains (crampy), distention

c. Additional signs—progressive weakness, fatigue, anorexia, weight loss, shortness of breath, anginal pain, anemia, pallor, cachexia, ascites, hepatomegaly, lymphadenopathy, vertigo, vomiting, and other signs of intestinal obstruction
d. Progression of disease—"ribbon"-like stools, passing of stool or flatus relieves pain, bright red blood in the feces, and mucus in or on the stools

Diagnostic Evaluation

1. Digital rectal examination—half of all colon and rectal cancers are found this way.
2. Endoscopy (fiberoptic sigmoidoscopy/colonoscopy)—two thirds of all colon and rectal cancers can be seen and biopsies performed via proctoscope alone.
3. Barium enema
    a. Especially significant in unexplained abdominal mass.
    b. Napkin-ring-type outline clearly indicates obstruction and possible tumor.
4. Stool examination for blood
    a. Often reveals evidence of carcinoma when the patient is otherwise asymptomatic.
    b. Some recommend meat-free, high-residue diet prior to test with avoidance of peroxidase-producing vegetables (horseradish, turnips, and rutabagas), which produce false-positive results.
    c. Some prefer no dietary restriction except retesting those who have a positive test result.
5. Blood hemoglobin determination for anemia.
6. Intravenous pyelography and possible cystoscopy may be indicated to assess whether malignancy has spread locally to involve ureter or bladder.
7. Carcinoembryonic Antigen (CEA) cannot be used for early diagnosis, but it can detect metastasis or recurrence.

> **NURSING ALERT:** Giving a guaiac-impregnated slide kit to individuals over age 40 is an effective way of screening for colorectal cancer. Diet preparation prior to use of three slides is optional.

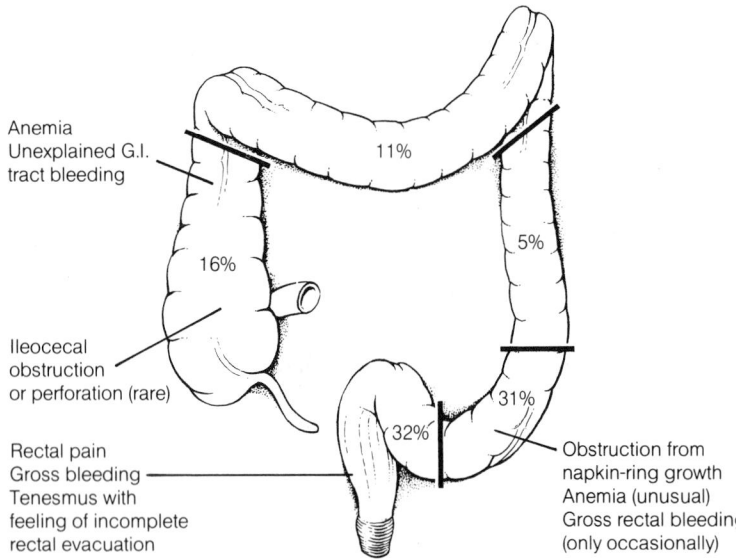

Anemia
Unexplained G.I. tract bleeding

11%

5%

16%

Ileocecal obstruction or perforation (rare)

Rectal pain
Gross bleeding
Tenesmus with feeling of incomplete rectal evacuation

32%

31%

Obstruction from napkin-ring growth
Anemia (unusual)
Gross rectal bleeding (only occasionally)

Figure 20-8. *Distribution of colorectal cancer.*

8. Diagnosis confirmed by
    a. Removing rectosigmoid polyps through sigmoidoscope for histologic study.
    b. Removing polyps above rectosigmoid by colonoscopy or laparotomy (if other symptoms are present) to verify diagnosis.

Management

A. Surgical Therapeutic Plan

1. Total colectomy for patient with familial history of polyposis or prolonged, universal, chronically active colitis, even before cancer is confirmed.
2. Most common operative procedures:
    a. Wide-segmented resection of colon and mesentery with anastomosis, or
    b. Abdominoperineal resection with colostomy (if lesion is in rectum). See Colostomy below.
    c. Even more extensive surgery involving removal of other organs if cancer has spread—such as to the bladder, uterus, small intestine, groin, etc.
    d. If cancer is extensive and it may not be in the patient's best interest to do radical surgery, palliative treatment may be done using radon seed implantation (combined surgery and preoperative radiation therapy is being done in several clinics) or local fulguration via colonoscope or proctoscope.
3. Colostomy
    a. This is a temporary or permanent opening of the colon through the abdominal wall.
    b. The placement of the colostomy will influence the nature of the discharge (Fig. 20-9).
    c. The *stoma* is that part of the colon that is brought above the abdominal wall in a colostomy and becomes the outlet for discharge of intestinal contents.
    d. Purposes are as follows:
        (1) It may be part of an abdominoperineal resection for cure or palliation of cancer.
        (2) It may be palliative when unresectable malignancy is present.
        (3) It can be a temporary measure to protect an anastomosis, such as after abdominal trauma.
        (4) It may be temporary to divert fecal stream during radiation or other therapy.

B. Drug Therapy

1. The National Cancer Institute (NCI) reports success with a combination drug therapy of levamisole (a medication used to treat worm infestations in farm animals) and 5-fluorouracil (a standard chemotherapeutic drug). However, this drug therapy is pending FDA approval, and NCI only recommends use after the obvious tumors have been removed surgically.
2. Chemotherapy is recommended for patients with metastasis or inoperable tumors. Drugs include 5-fluorouracil, mitomycin, vincristine, methotrexate, and lomustine.

C. Radiation Therapy

May be used before or after surgery to reduce the tumor.

Complications

1. Obstruction
2. Hemorrhage

Nursing Diagnoses

1. Altered nutrition (less than body requirements) related to malignant tumor effects and weight loss
2. Pain related to spread of malignancy, inflammation, and possible intestinal obstruction
3. Fear related to anesthesia, results of surgery, and potential for complications
4. Other possible nursing diagnoses
    • Knowledge deficit regarding diagnosis and treatment
    • Potential for infection
    • Body image disturbance related to colostomy
    • Impaired skin integrity
    • Altered sexuality patterns
    • Impaired home maintenance management

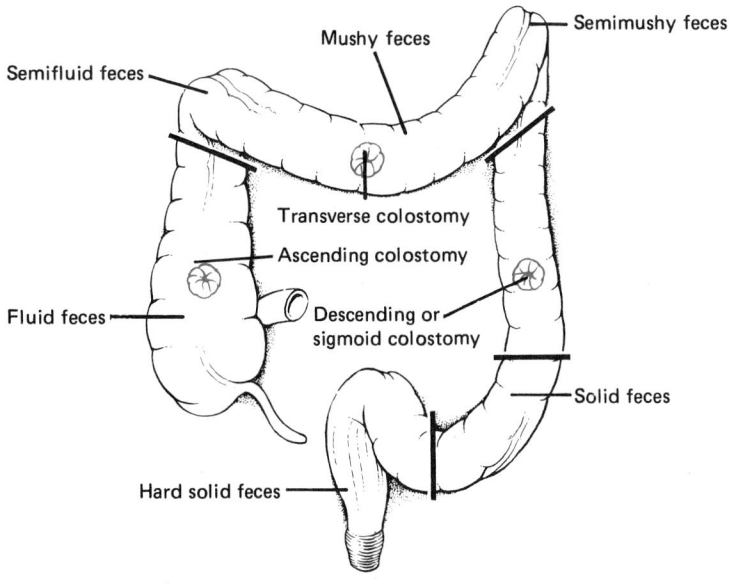

Figure 20-9. *A diagrammatic representation of the placement of permanent colostomies and the nature of the discharge at these sites.*

Nursing Interventions

A. Achieving Adequate Nutrition

When colostomy is not anticipated

1. Meet the patient's nutritional needs by serving a high-calorie, low-residue diet for several days before surgery, if condition permits.
2. Observe and record fluid losses, such as may be sustained by vomiting and diarrhea.
3. Maintain hydration by assisting with prescribed intravenous infusion, and observing and recording urinary output. Metabolic tissue needs are increased and more fluids are needed to eliminate waste products.
4. Reduce bacterial count of colon by mechanical cleansing and administering antimicrobials as prescribed—(orally and systemically).
   a. Whatever the choice, it should be effective against the full spectrum of aerobic and anaerobic fecal microbes.
   b. The degree of obstruction, acuteness, inflammation—all have a bearing on the nature of antimicrobial administration.
5. Assist the patient during nasoenteral intubation for decompression of intestinal tract.
6. Serve smaller meals spaced throughout the day to maintain adequate calorie and protein intake.
7. Encourage patient to participate in meal planning.
8. Adjust diet before and after treatments such as chemotherapy or radiation. Serve clear liquids, bland diet, or NPO as prescribed.
9. Instruct patient to take prescribed antiemetic every 4–6 hours as needed, especially if receiving chemotherapy.

B. Relieving Pain

1. Investigate different regimens such as relaxation techniques, repositioning, imaging, laughter, music, reading, and touch for control or relief of pain.
2. Administer prescribed analgesics.

C. Preoperative Preparation

1. Determine the nature of anticipated surgery
   a. The colostomy is positioned where the patient can see and care for it (this is determined by the surgeon and/or enterostomal therapist).
   b. The colostomy should not be placed in the laparotomy incision.
   c. It should be placed where it will not interfere with proper fitting and comfortable wearing of an appliance—away from iliac crest, costal margin, umbilicus, scars, deep folds.
2. Make specific plans for the patient's understanding and acceptance of a colostomy.
   a. Collaborate with the surgeon in ascertaining the nature of communication and information exchanged between surgeon and patient, including initial patient contact, in-hospital experience, plans for rehabilitation.
   b. Reinforce the patient's hope for a future that will be manageable and will lead to independent functioning.
   c. If possible, show the patient the intended appliance and have him try it on.
   d. Arrange a preoperative visit by a trained visitor from the local chapter of the United Ostomy Association.
   e. Develop a plan with the enterostomal therapist and patient to include short-term and long-term goals. Provide the patient with literature and information according to his level of understanding.

Take care not to overwhelm the patient with too much information.
   f. Preparation for surgery—follow usual preoperative procedures and modify to meet individual needs.

Postoperative Nursing Interventions

A. General Postoperative Care

(See pp. 56–58)

B. Initial Care of the Colostomy

1. Apply a temporary plastic colostomy bag to control odors and soiling.
   a. Tactfully try to have the patient look at colostomy and participate in its care.
   b. Evaluate learning readiness; never force independence.
   c. Emphasize that the stoma will be red and swollen. Explain that the swelling will eventually subside.
2. Begin to irrigate when the immediate postoperative period is past and bowel function has resumed
   a. Usually fifth or sixth day.
   b. (See Guidelines p. 497).
3. Use the treatment time of irrigating the colostomy as the learning time for the patient to begin to master the art of managing his colostomy independently. Recognize that some patients learn to control their colostomy without irrigation.
4. Although irrigation is widely used, recognize that there are some persons who cannot control the colostomy in this way (i.e., the patient with an ''irritable'' colon or with unpredictable bowel movements).
   a. Because of the nature of the contents, in various parts of the colon, only colostomies in the descending or sigmoid colon can be expected to be controlled by irrigation.
   b. Ascending and transverse colostomies have outputs that are too frequent and too liquid to facilitate control.
5. Often the recognition of a bowel movement occurs when the patient's pouch or dressing is checked; for others, it may be the awareness of the escape of flatus or the contact of stool on the skin.
6. For some, there is an awareness of motility, which enables them to get to the bathroom in time for discharging stool into the toilet.
7. Frequency and number of movements vary from person to person.
8. Irrigations for most persons are done every other day.
9. The cone-tip is excellent to prevent insertion of a catheter into insensitive mucosa with risk of perforating the bowel wall. The cone-tip is plugged into the stoma for about 2.5 cm. and permits irrigation without perforation or leakage.
10. Regulation is enhanced when there is systematic planning, balanced meals eaten at regular intervals, and a regular time for irrigation and evacuation.

C. Minimize Fear

1. Recognize and clarify fear.
2. Develop coping strategies for the fears.
3. Discuss results of surgery.
4. Explain all complications.

Patient Education

A. Skin Care

1. Contact enterostomal therapist who will evaluate the patient and suggest appropriate skin barrier.

2. Work with the enterostomal therapist to assess the patient's skin integrity and progress in adapting to appliance.
3. Coverings over the stoma may be a disposable pouch, gauze, facial tissue covered with petrolatum, Saran Wrap, or wax paper over a dressing. Hypoallergenic tape may be used.
4. For peristomal excoriation, corticosteroid aerosol sprays or nystatin powders are useful when used sparingly.
5. For allergic reactions, try other products until a compatible one is found; antacid suspensions are found to be practical for some patients.

B. Odor Control

1. Avoid foods known to cause odors—for example, onions, members of the cabbage family, eggs, fish, and beans.
2. Note that fecal odors are lessened with yogurt, cranberry juice, and buttermilk.
3. Odors can be controlled by taking one or two tablets of bismuth subcarbonate or bismuth subgallate at mealtimes and bedtime.

C. Control of Gas

1. Most gas is due to swallowed air (often taken in while chewing gum), highly spiced foods, and carbonated beverages, including beer.
2. Avoid gas-forming foods: beans, cabbage family, onions, radishes, cucumbers, and highly seasoned foods.

D. Diet

1. Avoid overeating and eating irregularly; chew food well.
2. Individualize the diet so that it is balanced and will not cause diarrhea and constipation. A daily diary is effective in determining what foods cause difficulty and can then be eliminated from the diet.
3. Note that fruits, fruit juices, and tomatoes may cause frequent bowel movements. Beer may be a laxative, as well as a gas-producer.

E. Enhanced Life-Style

1. Approximately 10%–12% of male ostomates suffer impairment of sexual function and potency:
   a. Is temporary in most cases
   b. Varies from full potency to complete impotence
   c. May take up to 2 years to regain potency
2. An ostomy in a woman does not preclude a successful pregnancy; close medical care is required.
3. There is no contraindication to any form of travel, including horseback riding.
4. Participation in any type of sport is possible.
5. Showering is possible with or without the appliance.
6. Girdles, swim trunks, and panty hose may all be worn, provided there is neither discomfort nor too much constriction.
7. Promote the patient's acceptance of the colostomy by building up self-esteem; encourage the family to assist the patient during the period of adjustment.
8. Contact the community nurse, who will serve as a liaison between hospital, physician, and home as a follow-up when the patient continues to adjust to the colostomy at home.
9. Inform the patient about the United Ostomy Association and encourage enrollment in the local support group.
10. Provide the patient with literature, addresses, and telephone numbers of the following organizations:
    a. Community Nursing Agencies:
    b. American Cancer Society
       1599 Clifton Road N.E., Atlanta, GA 30329
    c. Ostomy Quarterly—Official Publication of the United Ostomy Association, 36 Executive Park, Suite 120, Irvine, CA 92714
    d. The United Ostomy Association also has available many excellent booklets.
    e. Many manufacturers of ostomy supplies have free booklets available covering a wide variety of ostomy-related topics.

Evaluation

1. Exhibits weight gain trend and improved nutritional status as demonstrated by adequate dietary intake.
2. Has no pain and minimal discomfort following surgery for removal of colon cancer.
3. Is adjusting to changed life-style following surgery; no evidence of complications.
4. Discusses fears related to surgery, prognosis, and complications.
5. Demonstrates ability to care for colostomy.

Guidelines Irrigating a Colostomy

Purposes
1. To empty the colon of its contents: feces, gas, mucus
2. To cleanse the lower intestinal tract
3. To establish a regular pattern of evacuation so that normal life activities may be pursued

Equipment
Reservoir for irrigating fluids; enema bag, irrigating can
Irrigating fluid: 500–1500 ml. lukewarm water or other solution prescribed by physician
Tubing, connecting tubes, and clamp; preferable clamp—one that can be operated with one hand
Irrigating tip: cone tip for irrigation or soft rubber catheter—No. 22 or No. 24 with some type of shield to prevent backflow of irrigating solution
Irrigating sleeve or sheath: self-adhering (adhesive) or held in place with a belt (A plastic or rubber sheet can be used as a trough in place of a sheath.)
Newspaper or plastic bag: to collect soiled dressings and disposable pouch
Toilet tissue and water-soluble lubricant

(continued)

Guidelines Irrigating a Colostomy *(continued)*

Procedure **Preparatory Phase**

1. Select a suitable time, preferably after a meal, so that this hour fits into the patient's posthospital pattern of activity. Irrigation should be done at the same time each day.
2. Hang irrigating reservoir with solution 45–50 cm. (18–20 inches) above stoma (shoulder height with patient seated).
3. Have the patient sit in front of toilet commode on chair or on commode itself.
4. Remove dressings or pouch and place in bag.

Nursing Action	Rationale/Amplification

Performance Phase

1. Apply irrigating sleeve or sheath to stoma. Place end in commode.	1. Helps control odor and splashing. Allows feces and water to flow directly into commode.
2. Allow some of solution to flow through tubing and catheter/cone.	2. To release air bubbles in the setup so that air is not introduced into the colon, which would cause crampy pain.
3. Lubricate cone/catheter and gently insert into stoma. Insert catheter no more than 8 cm. (3 inches). Hold shield/cone gently, but firmly, against stoma to prevent backflow of water.	3. These steps are necessary to prevent intestinal perforation and to avoid irritating the mucous membranes.
4. If catheter does not advance easily, allow water to flow slowly while advancing catheter. NEVER FORCE CATHETER!	4. Slow rate of flow helps relax bowel and facilitates passage of catheter. Perforation of the bowel may occur if catheter is forced into stoma.
5. Allow fluid to enter colon slowly. If cramping occurs, slow down the flow rate or clamp off tubing and allow the patient to rest before progressing. Water should flow in over a 5–10-minute period.	5. Painful cramps are usually caused by too-rapid flow, water too cold, or too much solution. 500 ml. is usually sufficient for initial postoperative irrigation. Volume may be increased with subsequent irrigations to 1000 or 1500 ml., as patient needs for effective results.
6. Hold shield/cone in place 10 seconds after water has been instilled, then gently remove.	
7. Allow 10–15 minutes for most of return, then dry bottom of sleeve/sheath and attach it to top, or apply appropriate clamp to bottom of sleeve.	7. Most of water, feces, and flatus will be expelled in 10–15 minutes.
8. Leave sleeve/sheath in place about 20 minutes while patient gets up and moves around.	8. Ambulation stimulates peristalsis and completion of irrigation return.
9. Wait approximately 1 hour for the rest of the returns.	

Follow-Up Phase

1. Cleanse area with mild soap and water; pat dry.	1. Cleanliness and dryness will provide the patient with hours of comfort.
2. Apply a karaya preparation or other peristomal skin barrier; replace colostomy dressing or pouch.	2. The patient should use pouch until colostomy is sufficiently controlled. Karaya will protect skin from irritation.
3. Clean equipment with soap and water; dry before storing in well-ventilated area.	3. This will control odor and prolong life of equipment.
4. Inspect the skin and stoma for a change in appearance. Notify the physician for sustained dark color changes.	4. Stoma is usually pink to red, but some color changes may occur with the patient's emotions (fear—blanching; anger—red or purple). Sustained dark color changes are indicative of alterations in blood supply to the stoma.

Anorectal Conditions and Treatment
Nursing Process Overview

Assessment

1. Observe the stool for evidence of bleeding. Is stool mixed or coated with blood?
2. Determine presence of pain during and after evacuation. Is there associated abdominal pain? How long does it last?
3. When recording, describe the problem in the patient's words.
4. Note presence of a discharge. Is it purulent, bloody?

Nursing Diagnoses

1. Pain in rectal region related to pathology, infection, or surgery
2. Other diagnoses include: diarrhea/constipation related to discomfort during defecation
3. Diversional activity deficit related to discomfort
4. Self-care deficit (bathing/hygiene) related to difficulty in seeing or reaching anal area
5. Knowledge deficit of how to keep rectal area clean and reasons why this is important

Preoperative Nursing Interventions

1. Be an understanding and concerned listener when this patient relates problems of a personal nature.

2. Ensure and respect the patient's privacy when attending to personal hygiene, examinations, and treatments.
3. Do not minimize complaints of discomfort.

Postoperative Nursing Interventions

A. Promoting Comfort and Wound Healing

1. Be gentle in changing dressings, shaving, irrigating, or administering perineal care.
2. Use petrolatum gauze in protecting edges of wounds (e.g., following incision and drainage of ischiorectal abscess, excision of pilonidal sinus) to prevent crusting and the dressings from sticking to wound.
3. Provide sitz baths when recommended; adjust temperature of solution and provide a comfortable position for the patient.
4. Use caution in applying analgesic or anesthetic ointments, as this often leads to secondary skin rashes from allergy.
5. Keep the perineal area clean to minimize or eliminate infection; presence of *E. coli* demands meticulous cleanliness to prevent infection and promote healing.
6. Change the patient's position from side to side to prevent added discomfort on pressure sites.
7. Prevent constipation by proper attention to diet needs of patient; give mineral oil or mild cathartic only as prescribed; use stool softeners.
8. Encourage voluntary voiding to avoid catheterization; this may be facilitated by getting patient out of bed.
9. Observe vital signs and dressings for evidence of hemorrhage, particularly following hemorrhoidectomy.
10. Daily rectal sphincter dilatation may be needed to relieve pain from spasm, to ensure granulation of incisional wounds from bottom out, and to prevent postoperative stricture.

Patient Education

(To prepare patient for posthospital convalescence.)
1. Instruct the patient on perianal hygiene to minimize the possibility of infection; avoid rubbing area with toilet tissue; instead, pat the area dry.
2. Apply wet dressings (equal parts of witch hazel and water) to relieve edema.
3. Advise the patient regarding the effect of diet on stool formation.
   a. Plant fibers of leafy vegetables and the roughage of bran flakes, whole grains, and whole wheat bread add roughage to the diet to form cellulose.
   b. Cellulose absorbs water, swells, and softens stool, thereby stimulating peristalsis and aiding in intestinal elimination.
   c. Encourage the patient to eat fresh fruits, fruit juice, and fresh vegetables, except for seeds, skins, corn, and nuts.
4. Avoid cathartics so that stool is formed rather than being soft or liquid.
5. Recommend hot sitz baths or hot compresses to relieve painful sphincter spasm.
6. Suggest adequate fluid intake and daily exercise to prevent constipation; encourage the patient to have a regular time each day for having a bowel movement.
7. Stool softeners are often given until good bowel habits are established.
   a. "Wetting agents" contain docusate sodium, a substance that penetrates, moistens, and softens hard, dry stools.
   b. "Bulk producers" such as psyllium and agar preparations absorb water, add bulk, and add moisture to stool.

c. Mineral oil tends to destroy fat-soluble vitamins A, D, E, and K and interferes with absorption of calcium and phosphorus. It should be given at least 3 hours after the evening meal. (Do not give mineral oil to elderly patients because of possible aspiration pneumonia.)
8. Administer enemas only when absolutely necessary; rectal suppositories may be helpful.

Evaluation

1. Experiences decreased discomfort in rectal area.
2. Describes the dietary modification to be practiced to ensure regular and moderately soft stool.
3. Increases social contacts.
4. Practices hygienic health measures.
5. States explicitly how to clean perineal area after defecation/voiding.

Perianal Abscess, Anal Fistula/ Anal Fissure

A. Perianal Abscess

1. Description
   a. Localized infection in fatty tissue near rectum. Pain increases.
   b. Condition should raise suspicion of granulomatous bowel disease.
2. Management—Incision and drainage

B. Anal Fistula

1. Description
   a. Abnormal opening from the skin near the anus that winds tortuously into the anal canal.
   b. Because it is an infectious area, pus leaks outward.
   c. Condition should raise suspicion of granulomatous bowel disease.
2. Management
   a. Surgical identification of the path of a fistula.
   b. Fistulotomy or partial sphincterotomy.

C. Anal Fissure

1. Description
   Longitudinal ulcer (a crack that does not heal in the anal canal) frequently associated with constipation, as well as excruciating pain and blood streaking on defecation.
2. Management
   a. Stool softener (docusate sodium) or psyllium seed.
   b. If failure to heal with nonoperative therapy, dilatation of anal sphincter and sphincterotomy or fissurotomy.

Hemorrhoids

Hemorrhoids are varicosities in the lower rectum or anus resulting from congestion in the veins of the hemorrhoidal plexus; external hemorrhoids appear outside the external sphincter, whereas internal hemorrhoids appear above the internal sphincter. When blood within the hemorrhoids becomes clotted and infected, the hemorrhoids are referred to as *thrombosed*.

Predisposing Factors

1. Pregnancy
2. Straining at stool

3. Chronic constipation/diarrhea
4. Prolonged sitting/standing
5. Anal infection
6. Hereditary factor
7. Portal hypertension (cirrhosis)
8. Coughing; sneezing
9. Alcoholism
10. Loss of muscle tone due to old age
11. Rectal surgery or episiotomy
12. Anal intercourse

Clinical Manifestations

1. Sensation of incomplete fecal evacuation
2. Protrusion
3. Constipation
4. Bleeding during defecation
5. Infection or ulceration
6. Pain noted more in external hemorrhoids
7. Mucus discharge
8. Cosmetic deformity
9. Bright red blood on stool due to the injury of the mucosa covering the hemorrhoid
10. Anal itching
11. Sudden rectal pain due to thrombosis in external hemorrhoids

Diagnostic Evaluation

1. History and visualization by external examination and the use of an anoscope or proctoscope.
2. Barium enema, because hemorrhoids often are warning signs of more serious colonic lesions, which may be the actual source of observed rectal bleeding.

Management

Asymptomatic hemorrhoids require no treatment.

A. Medical Treatment

1. Patient should adhere to a low-roughage, high-fiber diet to keep stool soft.
2. Bowel habits should be regulated with nonirritating stool softeners to keep stools soft.
3. Frequent hot sitz baths to ease pain and combat swelling.
4. Insertion of soothing anal suppository 2–3 times daily.
5. Application of witch hazel compresses for comfort.
6. Control of itching by placement of a cotton pledget on folded soft tissue between the buttocks against the anus to absorb moisture.
7. Do not use topical anesthetics chronically on hemorrhoids or fissures, as they often produce hypersensitivity (allergic) perianal skin rashes with severe itching.
8. If hemorrhoids are prolapsed and the patient is unable to reduce them directly, the nurse may have to reduce them manually:
   a. Apply cold compresses to anal area.
   b. Gently apply anesthetic ointment with a gloved finger.
   c. Very gently manipulate hemorrhoids back through rectal sphincter.
   d. Apply an anesthetic ointment on a dressing to rectal area.
9. Injection of sclerosing solutions produces scar tissue, which decreases the prolapse.
10. Cryodestruction—freezing of hemorrhoids.
    a. Is claimed to be less painful
    b. Some patients have a foul-smelling discharge for about a week to 10 days following cryosurgery.

B. Surgical Treatment

1. Surgery may be indicated when the following conditions exist:
   a. Prolonged bleeding
   b. Disabling pain
   c. Intolerable itching
   d. General unrelieved discomfort
2. *Barron ligation with a rubber band* is considered "ideal" treatment.
   a. A large anoscope is used; the apex of the internal hemorrhoid is grasped and drawn through a double-sleeved cylinder.
   b. An elastic band is loaded on the inner cylinder and released by a trigger device so that the band encircles the base of the hemorrhoid.
   c. After a period of time, the hemorrhoid sloughs away.
3. *Dilatation*—dilatation of the anal canal and lower rectum under general anesthesia is another treatment.
   a. This procedure is not advocated for patients whose main complaints are prolapse or incontinence.
   b. It also is not recommended for aging patients with weak sphincters.
4. *Incision and removal of clot* from acutely thrombosed hemorrhoid.
5. *Excision of hemorrhoids*—includes the following procedures:
   a. Dilatation of rectal sphincter.
   b. Ligation and excision of hemorrhoid under local or spinal anesthesia
   c. Insertion of drainage tube to permit escape of flatus and blood
   d. Application of Gelfoam or oxycel gauze to control bleeding, if necessary.

Guidelines Manual Removal of Fecal Impaction

A *fecal impaction* is the retention of hardened feces in the rectum or lower sigmoid resulting from prolonged retention and accumulation of stool.

Manifestations and Occurrence

1. Complaints of constipation; patient often has a desire to defecate but is unable to do so.
2. Diarrhea or liquid fecal seepage—may occur around the obstructing impaction
3. Rectal pain
4. Patients at risk
   a. Elderly persons following chronic constipation, insufficient hydration or ingestion of fibrous foods
   b. Orthopedic patients who have been in traction or in body casts

Manifesta-tions and Oc-currence
(continued)

c. Occasionally, in patients following rectal surgery or when barium has not been adequately removed following radiologic examination

d. Common in patients with neurological or psychotic disorders.

Purpose of Fecal Disim-paction

To remove hardened feces in the rectum or lower sigmoid

Equipment

Clean (not necessarily sterile) rubber or plastic glove
Water-soluble lubricant
Bedpan
Plastic sheet with cloth protection
Soap, water, washcloth

Procedure

Nursing Action	Rationale/Amplification

Preparatory Phase

1. Explain procedure to the patient.
2. Position the patient on left side with upper knee flexed.
3. Drape the patient and place protecting pad under buttocks.
4. Place bedpan in a convenient place.
5. Put on glove and lubricate index finger generously (some prefer middle finger because it is longer).

2. To permit access to rectum and lower sigmoid
3. To prevent chilling and undue exposure
4. To serve as receptacle
5. To reduce friction during insertion; avoiding injury to tissue

Performance Phase (Fig. 20-10)

1. Insert gloved finger gently into rectum until impaction is felt. Instruct the patient to breathe deeply.
2. Gently remove or break fecal material within reach and deposit in bedpan; work finger around and into mass to break it up if possible. Work pieces to end of rectum.

1. This stimulation may increase peristalsis. Breathing deeply will promote relaxation.
2. The emphasis is on gentleness, as this may be painful.

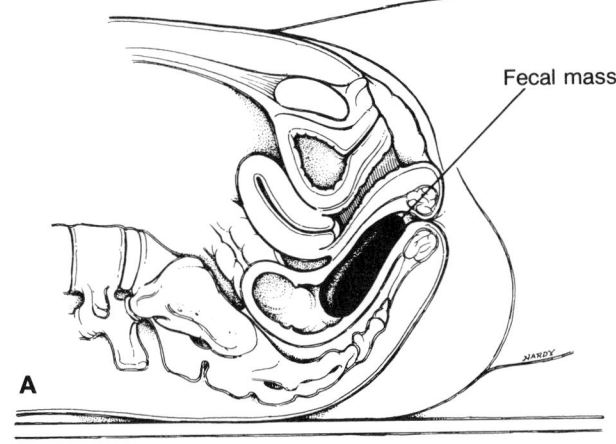

Fecal mass

A

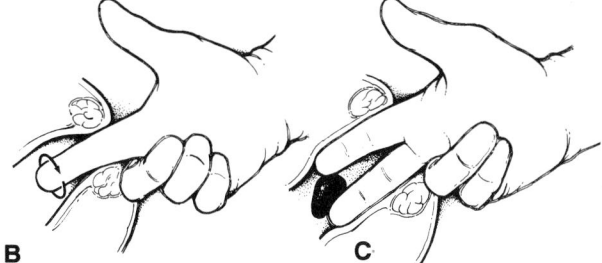

B   **C**

Figure 20-10. *Fecal impaction. (A) Note shaded area inside rectal sphincter—this indicates fecal impaction. (B) By gently stimulating the rectal wall with a gloved index finger, and using a circular motion, it is possible to loosen fecal material. (C) It may be necessary to gently insert two fingers in an attempt to crush the fecal mass. A scissorlike motion is used.*

(continued)

Guidelines   Manual Removal of Fecal Impaction *(continued)*

Procedure *(continued)*	Nursing Action	Rationale/Amplification
	3. Gently stimulate rectal sphincter by making a circular motion once or twice.	3. This may stimulate peristalsis and relax the sphincter.
	4. If step 3 does not result in removal of the impaction, it may be necessary to gently insert the middle and index finger and attempt to break up the mass by a scissorlike movement of the fingers. Repeat steps 2 or 4 until all easily reachable fecal masses are removed.	4. Greater leverage is afforded, and the mass may be more easily broken.
	5. Note any bleeding or pain; observe the patient for shortness of breath or perspiration; changes in pulse; diaphoresis.	5. Should any of these responses occur, stop the procedure.
	6. Offer patient the bedpan or commode.	6. Digital manipulation stimulates the urge to defecate.

Follow-Up Phase

	1. Gently wash and dry the rectal area; make the patient comfortable and have him rest.	1. Drying the area prevents skin excoriation and promotes comfort.
	2. Note bedpan contents and then empty.	
	3. Record color, consistency, and odor of stool.	3. These characteristics may provide clues to the nature of the problem.
	4. Plan health instruction measures in an effort to prevent a recurrence.	4. Investigate the possibility of using stool softeners; suggest periodic use of Fleet's enema.
	Explore nutritional and fluid needs of the patient; determine activity level and encourage suitable exercises to promote adequate elimination.	

NURSING ALERT:
1. Digital removal of fecal impaction can stimulate the vagus nerve and cause syncope and tachycardia.
2. This procedure is contraindicated in pregnancy, after genitourinary, rectal, perineal, abdominal, or gynecologic surgery. Also contraindicated in patients with myocardial infarction, coronary insufficiency, pulmonary embolus, congestive heart failure, heart block, gastrointestinal or vaginal bleeding, blood dyscrasias, hemorrhoids, and rectal polyps.

Bibliography

Books

Bayless TM. Current Therapy in Gastroenterology and Liver Disease—3. Toronto, BC Decker, 1990

Berk JE. Gastroenterology. Philadelphia, WB Saunders, vols 1–7, 1985

Caine RM and Bufalino PMcK. Nursing Care Planning Guides for Adults. Baltimore, Williams & Wilkens, 1987

Fazio VW. Current Therapy in Colon and Rectal Surgery. Philadelphia, BC Decker, 1990

Gomella LG. Clinicians Pocket Reference. Norwalk, CT, Appleton & Large, 1989

Johanson Brenda C et al. Standards for Critical Care. St. Louis, CV Mosby, 1988

Johnson Leonard R. Physiology of the Gastrointestinal Tract. New York, Raven Press, 1987

Kinney MR et al. AACN's Clinical Reference for Critical Care Nursing. New York, McGraw–Hill, 1988

Kirsner JB and Shorter RG. Diseases of the Colon, Rectum, and Anal Canal. Baltimore, Williams & Wilkins, 1988

McVan B. Disease and Disorders Handbook. Springhouse, PA, Springhouse Corporation, 1988

Newman SL. Critical Care Quarterly—Issues in Gastroenterology. Rockville, MD, Aspen Systems, 1982

Raffensperger EB et al. Clinical Nursing Handbook. Philadelphia, JB Lippincott, 1986

Sleisenger MH and Fordtran JS. Gastrointestinal Disease Pathophysiology, Diagnosis, and Management. Philadelphia, WB Saunders, 1989

Spiro HM. Clinical Gastroenterology. New York, Macmillan, 1983

Journals

Ulcers

Bardhan KD. Intermittent treatment of duodenal ulcer for long term medical management. Postgrad Med J 1988; 64(Suppl 1):40–46

Bright–Asare P et al. Prostaglandins, H2-receptor antagonists and peptic ulcer disease. Drugs 1988; 35(Suppl 3):1–9

Chiverton SG and Hunt RH. Medical regimens in short and long term ulcer management. Baillieres Clin Gastroenterol 1988 Jul; 2(3):655–676

Clouse RE. Anxiety and gastrointestinal illness. Psychiatr Clin North Am 1988 Jun; 11(2):399–417

de Paula CL. Antacids and duodenal ulcer: An update. Arq Gastroenterol 1988, 25 Spec No: 50–56

Elder JB. Surgical treatment of duodenal ulcer. Postgrad Med J 1988; 64(Suppl 1):54–59

Erwin WG. Common gastrointestinal disease in the elderly. Geriatrics 1988 Dec; 43(Suppl):75–82

Freston JW. The pathophysiology and pharmacological basis of peptic ulcer therapy. Toxicol Pathol 1988; 16(2): 260–266

Herrington JL Jr and Sawyers SL. Gastric ulcer. Curr Probl Surg 1987 Dec; 24(12):759–865

Hunt PS. Bleeding ulcer: Timing and technique in surgical management. Aust N Z J Surg 1986 Jan; 56(1):25–30

Johnston D and Blackett RL. A new look at selective vagotomies. Am J Surg 1988 Nov; 156(5):416–427

Lamers CB. The significance of gastrin in the pathogenesis and therapy of peptic ulcer disease. Drugs 1988; 35(Suppl 3):10–16

Marks IN. The efficacy, safety and dosage of sucralfate in ulcer therapy. Scand J Gastroenterol Suppl 1987; 140:33–38

Piper DW. Peptic ulcer. Aust N Z J Med 1988 May; 18(3):237–244

Pounder R. Histamine H2 receptor antagonists. Baillieres Clin Gastroenterol 1988 Jul; 2(3):593–608

Pounder R. Silent peptic ulceration: Deadly silence or golden silence. Gastroenterology 1989 Feb; 96(2 Pt 2 Suppl):626–631

Smejkal K. Gastroduodenal ulcer disease. Etiology, symptomatology, complications and diagnostics. Sb Ved Pr Lek Fak Karlovy Univerzity Hradci Kralove 1987; 30(3):413–482

Walan A. Omeprazole. Baillieres Clin Gastroenterol 1988 Jul; 2(3):629–640

Wormsley KG. Long-term treatment of duodenal ulcer. Postgrad Med J 1988; 64(Suppl 1):47–53

Enteritis

Morel P and Alexander–Williams J. Surgery for Crohn's disease. Gastroenterol Clin Biol 1988 Aug–Sep; 12(8–9):593–595

Nord HJ. Complications of inflammatory bowel disease. Hosp Pract [Off] 1987 Nov 30; 22(11A):65–67, 70–72, 75 passim

Payne–James JJ and Silk DB. Total nutrition as primary treatment in Crohn's disease—RIP? Gut 1988 Oct; 29(10):1304–1308

Routes J and Claman HN. Corticosteroids in inflammatory bowel disease. A review. J Clin Gastroenterol 1987 Oct; 9(5):529–535

Shiloni E et al. Role of total parenteral nutrition in the treatment of Crohn's disease. Am J Surg 1989 Jan; 157(1): 180–185

Zenilman ME and Becker JM. Emergencies in inflammatory bowel disease. Gastroenterol Clin North Am 1988 Jun; 17(2):387–408

Diverticulitis

Chappuis CW and Cohn I Jr. Acute colonic diverticulitis. Surg Clin North Am 1988 Apr; 68(2):301–313

Pohlman T. Diverticulitis. Gastroenterol Clin North Am 1988 Jun; 17(2):357–385

Ulcerative Colitis

Ament ME et al. Advances in ulcerative colitis. Pediatrician 1988; 15(1–2):45–57

Dozois RR and Rourke JS. Newer operations for ulcerative colitis and Crohn's disease. Surg Clin North Am 1988 Dec; 68(6):1339–1352

Farmer RG (ed). Inflammatory bowel disease. Med Clin North Am 1990 Jan; 74(1):1–227

Hawkey CJ and Hawthorne AB. Medical treatment of ulcerative colitis: Scoring the advances. Gut 1988 Oct; 29(10): 1298–1303

Appendicitis

Cooper G et al. Incidental appendectomy: The controversy. Md Med J 1987 Oct; 36(10):833–836

Pearson RH. Ultrasonography for diagnosing appenditis. Br Med J 1988 Jul 30; 297(6644):309–310

Hernia

Henderson RD et al. Review of the surgical management of recurrent hiatal hernia: 5 year follow up. Am J Gastroenterol 1988 Sep; 83(9):988–991

Wood RJ et al. Traumatic abdominal hernia: A case report and review of the literature. Am Surg 1988 Nov; 54(11): 648–651

Gastrointestinal Bleeding

Berstad A. Antacids, pepsin inhibitors, and gastric cooling in the management of massive upper gastrointestinal hemorrhage. Scand J Gastroenterol Suppl 1987; 137:33–38

Bianchi PG and Pace F. Ulcerogenic drugs and gastrointestinal bleeding. Baillieres Clin Gastroenterol 1988 Apr; 2(2):309–327

Langman MJ. Drug treatment of haematemesis and melaena. Scand J Gastroenterol Suppl 1987; 137:67–70

Pingleton SK. Recognition and management of upper gastrointestinal hemorrhage. Am J Med 1987 Dec 18; (6A):41–45

Potter GD and Sellin JH. Lower gastrointestinal bleeding. Gastroenterol Clin North Am 1988 Jun; 17(2):341–356

Schaffner J. Acute gastrointestinal bleeding. Med Clin North Am 1986 Sep; 70(5):1055–1066

Soehendra N. Endoscopic therapy of upper gastrointestinal bleeding. Endoscopy 1987 Sep; 19(5):205–206

Wara P. Endoscopic control of major ulcer bleeding. Scand J Gastroenterol Suppl 1987; 137:61–63

Wara P. Incidence, diagnosis, and natural course of upper gastrointestinal hemorrhage. Prognostic value of clinical factors and endoscopy. Scand J Gastroenterol Suppl 1987; 137:26–27

Colon Cancer

Bruce WR. Steps between diet and colon cancer. Prog Clin Biol Res 1988; 279: 123–130

Fazio VW. Cancer of the rectum-sphincter-saving operation. Stapling techniques. Surg Clin North Am 1988 Dec; 68(6):1367–1382

Fleischer DE et al. Detection and surveillance of colorectal cancer. JAMA 1989 Jan 27; 261(4):580–585

Otte DM. Nursing management of the patient with colon and rectal cancer. Semin Oncol Nurs 1988 Nov; 4(4): 285–292

Realini JP. Screening for colorectal cancer. Issues for primary care physicians. Prim Care 1988 Mar; 15(1): 63–77

Ross CC. Screening for colorectal cancer. Am Fam Physician 1988 Dec; 38(6): 105–114

Colostomy

Finan PJ. Stoma avoidance in rectal cancer. Br J Hosp Med 1987 Oct; 38(4):294–298

Harocopos C. Helping the stoma patient. Practitioner 1988 Mar 22; 232(1445): 318, 321–322, 326

Rolstad BS. Innovative surgical procedures and stoma care in the future. Nurs Clin North Am 1987 Jun; 22(2):341–356

Rubin GP and Devlin HB. The quality of life with a stoma. Br J Hosp Med 1987 Oct; 38(4):300–303, 306

Gastrostomy

Alltop SA. Teaching for discharge; Gastrostomy tubes. RN 1988 Nov; 51(11):42–46

Gauderer MW. Feeding gastrostomy or feeding gastrostomy plus antireflux procedure? J Pediatr Gastroenterol Nutr 1988 Nov–Dec; 7(6):795–796

Hahn JS et al. A case of vitamin B_{12} deficiency following megaloblastic anemia following total gastrectomy. Yonsei Med J 1988; 29(3):270–277

Huff JP et al. Complications of gastrostomy. South Med J 1988 Aug; 81(8):1050–1052

Sangster W et al. Percutaneous endoscopic gastrostomy. Am J Surg 1988 May; 155(5):677–679

Tom W et al. Prolapse of gastrostomy tube resulting in entero-enteric fistula and intussusception. Am Surg 1988 Apr; 54(4):245–247

Intestinal Obstruction

Brolin RE. Long tubes vs nasogastric tubes in the treatment of intestinal obstruction. Arch Surg 1987 Jan; 122(1):118

Canady J et al. Intestinal obstruction: Still a lethal clinical entity. J Natl Med Assoc 1987 Dec; 79(12):1281–1284

Colemont LJ and Camilier M. Chronic intestinal pseudo-obstruction: Diagnosis and treatment. Mayo Clin Proc 1989 Jan; 64(1):60–70

Holder WD Jr. Intestinal obstruction. Gastroenterol Clin North Am 1988 Jun; 17(2):317–340

Sigmoidoscopy/Colonoscopy

Rodney WM. Procedural skills in flexible sigmoidoscopy and colonoscopy for the family physician. Prim Care 1988 Mar; 15(1):79–91

Marks G and Borenstein BD. Complications of flexible fiberoptic sigmoidoscopy. A conceptual approach. Surg Endosc 1987; 1(1):59–62

Selby JV and Friedman GD. US Preventive Services Task Force. Sigmoidoscopy in the periodic health examination of asymptomatic adults. JAMA 1989 Jan 27; 261(4):594–601

Waye JD. Techniques of colonoscopy, hot biopsy forceps, and snare polypectomy. Prog Clin Biol Res 1988; 279:61–69

Hemorrhoids

Dennison AR et al. Hemorrhoids. Nonoperative management. Surg Clin North Am 1988 Dec; 68(6):1401–1409

Faulconer HT. Hemorrhoids—Alternative treatments. J Ky Med Assoc 1988 Nov; 86(11):617–620

Notaras MJ. Anal fissure and stenosis. Surg Clin North Am 1988 Dec; 68(6):1427–1440

Sanker MY and Joffe SN. Laser surgery in colonic and anorectal lesions. Surg Clin Am 1988 Dec; 68(6):1447–1469

Schussman LC and Lutz LJ. Outpatient management of hemorrhoids. Prim Care 1986 Sep; 13(3):527–547

Ileostomy

Francois Y et al. Small intestinal obstruction complicating ileal pouch—Anal anastomosis. Ann Surg 1989 Jan; 209(1):46–50

Myrvold HE. The continent ileostomy. World J Surg 1987 Dec; 11(6):720–726

Hepatic, Biliary, and Pancreatic Disorders

21

Hepatic and Biliary Disorders

Manifestations of Disorders of the Liver

Pathophysiology

Disorders of the liver result from direct damage to the liver cells (hepatocytes) or indirectly as a result of alterations in bile or blood flow through the liver.

Etiology

1. Viral infections and the effects of toxins may lead to hepatocellular dysfunction.
2. Chronic alcohol consumption, along with malnutrition, may cause toxic liver damage (cirrhosis).
3. Impairment of liver function may occur when flow of bile into the intestine is impeded (i.e., obstruction of the biliary tract by gallstones or a tumor).

Physical Assessment of Liver

1. Begin by placing the left hand under the patient's back at the level of the 11–12th rib. The liver border, if felt, should be firm and smooth.
   Place the right hand, with fingers angled and slightly facing the costal margin, just below the percussed lower border of the liver.
2. During palpation with the right hand, press upward with the left hand to move the liver anteriorly (to facilitate palpation).
3. Have the patient inspire, and on expiration press the fingers of the right hand inward. On deep inspiration by the patient, do not change the position of the right hand, feel for the liver edge moving over the fingers.

If nothing is felt on inspiration, palpate more deeply, then on each subsequent inspiration, move the finger upward toward the costal margin. With each new position of the fingers, have the patient breathe deeply and feel for the liver.
4. See also page 35.

Clinical Manifestations

A. Altered Skin Integrity Related to Jaundice and Edema

Jaundice is present when all tissues, including the sclerae and skin, assume a yellow or greenish–yellow tinge because of an increased concentration of bilirubin. Edema occurs when the liver is no longer able to synthesize adequate amounts of albumin. These changes impair normal skin integrity.
1. Normal bilirubin concentration in blood is 0.1–1.0 mg./100 ml. of blood.
2. Over 3.0 mg./100 ml. of blood—jaundice can be detected.
3. Normal albumin level is 3.5—5.5 gm./dl.
4. An albumin level below 3.0 gm./dl., with an increased serum globulin level, occurs with liver disease.

B. Bleeding Tendencies Related to Altered Clotting Mechanisms and Portal Hypertension

1. Because of blood coagulation defects, gastrointestinal hemorrhage, as well as bleeding gums, blood in urine, rectal bleeding, and tarry stool may occur.
2. Minor skin trauma may produce ecchymosis (bruising).
3. Following all types of intramuscular and intravenous injections and arterial punctures, it is necessary to apply pressure for longer than usual and to observe for hematoma.

Table 21-1. *Liver Diagnostic Studies*

Test and Purpose	Normal	Clinical and Nursing Significance
Bile Formation and Secretion		
1. *Serum bilirubin (van den Bergh reaction)* Measures bilirubin in the blood; this determines the ability of the liver to take up, conjugate, and excrete bilirubin. Bilirubin is a product of the breakdown of hemoglobin.		
Direct (conjugated)—soluble in water	0–5.1 μmol/L.	Abnormal in biliary and liver disease, causing jaundice clinically.
Indirect (unconjugated)—insoluble in water	0–14 μmol/L.	Abnormal in hemolysis and in functional disorders of uptake or conjugation.
Total serum bilirubin	1.7–20.5 μmol/L.	
2. *Urine bilirubin* Not normally found in urine, but if direct serum bilirubin is elevated, some spills into urine.	None (0)	Mahogany-colored urine; when specimen is shaken, yellow tinted foam can be observed. Confirm with Ictotest tablet or Dipstick. If phenazopyridine (Pyridium) is being taken, there may be a false-positive bilirubin result. (Mark laboratory slip if this medication is being taken.)
3. *Urobilinogen* Formed in small intestine by action of bacteria on bilirubin. Related to amount of bilirubin excreted into bile.	Urine urobilinogen up to 0.09–4.23 μmol/24 hr. Fecal urobilinogen 0.068–0.34 mmol/24 hr.	Urine specimen is collected over 2-hr. period after lunch. Place specimen in dark brown container and send it to laboratory immediately to prevent decomposition. If the patient is receiving antimicrobials, mark laboratory slip to this effect, as production of urobilinogen can be falsely reduced.
Protein Studies		
1. *Albumin and globulin measurement* Is of greater significance than total protein measurement		As one increases, the other decreases; hence,
Albumin—produced by liver cells	35–55 gm./L.	Albumin ↓ cirrhosis chronic hepatitis
Globulin—produced in lymph nodes, spleen, and bone marrow and Kupffer's cells of liver	15–30 gm./L.	Globulin ↑ cirrhosis chronic obstructive jaundice viral hepatitis
Total serum protein	60–80 gm./L.	
2. *Prothrombin time (PT)* Prothrombin and other clotting factors are manufactured in the liver; its rate is influenced by the supply of vitamin K.	100% of control	Prothrombin time may be prolonged in liver disease, in which case it will not return to normal with vitamin K. It may also be prolonged in malabsorption of fat and fat-soluble vitamins, in which case it will return to normal with vitamin K.
Fat Metabolism		
1. *Cholesterol* It is possible to measure lipid metabolism by determining serum cholesterol levels.	3.90–6.50 mmol/L. Esters = 60% of total	Serum cholesterol level is decreased in parenchymal liver disease. Serum lipid level is increased in biliary obstruction.
Liver Detoxification		
1. *Serum alkaline phosphatase* Because bile disposes this enzyme, any impairment of liver cell excretory function will cause an elevation. In cholestasis or obstruction, increased synthesis of enzyme causes very high levels in blood.	20–90 U/L. at 30°C	*Abnormalities:* The level is elevated to more than 3 times normal in obstructive jaundice, intrahepatic cholestasis, liver metastasis, or granulomas. Also elevated in osteoblastic diseases, Paget's disease, and hyperparathyroidism.
Enzyme Production		
Transaminase (SGOT) (Aspartate aminotransferase or AST)	4.8–19 U/L.	An elevation in these enzymes indicates liver cell damage.
Transaminase (SGPT) (Alanine aminotransferase or ALT)	2.4–17 U/L.	**Note:** Opiates may also cause a rise in SGOT and SGPT.
LDH	80–192 U/L.	Aspirin may cause an increase or decrease in SGOT and SGPT.
Gamma glutamyl transpeptidase (GGT)	0–30 U/L. at 30°C	Enzyme found in liver, kidney, heart, pancreas, spleen, brain. An elevation confirms hepatic involvement in the presence of an elevated alkaline phosphatase.
Ammonia (serum)	11.1–67.0 μmol/L.	Ammonia levels rise when the liver is unable to convert it to urea.
Bile acids radioimmunoassay (after cholecystokinin stimulation)		Elevated serum bile acids are seen in the presence of hepatic diseases.
Total	35.0–148.0 mmol/L.	
Chenodeoxycholic acid	10.0–61.4 mmol/L.	
Cholic acid	6.8–81.0 mmol/L.	
Deoxycholic acid	2.0–18.0 mmol/L.	
Lithocholic acid	0.8–2.0 mmol/L.	

C. Altered Fluid and Electrolyte Balance

1. Tissue edema and intra-abdominal fluid (ascites) are manifestations of sodium and water retention, combined with potassium excretion.
2. Hypoproteinemia, iron-decreased hepatic synthesis, and disturbed kidney function also contribute to fluid retention.

D. Altered Mental and Neurologic States Related to Deterioration of Liver Function

1. Pyridoxine deficiency can result in nervous irritability and convulsive seizures.
2. Thiamine deficiency may lead to polyneuritis and Wernicke–Korsakoff psychosis.
3. Failure to metabolize ammonia arriving from intestine in portal venous system and impaired metabolism of sedative drugs produce range of symptoms from irritability and confusion to stupor, somnolence, and coma.

E. Potential for Infection Related to Dysfunction of Kupffer Cells in the Liver

1. When portal hypertension is present, bacteria absorbed from the intestines bypasses the filtering reticuloendothelial system in the liver and can directly enter the systemic circulation, precipitating bacteremia.
2. High incidence of infections occur; bacteremia, pneumonia, spontaneous bacterial peritonitis, and meningitis

---

Diagnostic Evaluation of Liver Disease

Types of Liver Diagnostic Studies (Table 21-1)

1. Bile formation and secretion
2. Protein studies
3. Fat metabolism
4. Liver detoxification
5. Enzyme production

Liver Biopsy

1. Sample of liver tissue is obtained through needle aspiration.
2. See Guidelines: Assisting with Liver Biopsy.

Guidelines Assisting With Liver Biopsy

Liver biopsy is the sampling of liver tissue by needle aspiration.

Purpose To establish a diagnosis of liver disease by histologic study of liver tissue.

Equipment Sterile aspiration syringe and biopsy needle (Silverman)
Local anesthetic
Skin antiseptics, sterile fenestrated towel, gloves
Glass slides, specimen bottles containing fixative and/or test tubes

Procedure **Preparatory Phase**

1. See that consent form is signed.
2. Verify that the patient has had prothrombin tests and blood typing by checking the chart.
3. Determine availability of compatible blood, as these patients often have clotting defects.
4. Determine and record patient's pulse, respiration, blood pressure, and prothrombin time immediately before the biopsy to have a baseline of comparison with the postbiopsy condition of the patient.
5. Explain the steps of this procedure to the patient to reduce his concerns and gain his cooperation.

Nursing Action	Rationale/Amplification

Performance Phase

Nursing Action	Rationale/Amplification
1. Place the patient flat in bed with right arm under head and face turned left.	
2. Expose the upper abdomen in readiness for skin disinfection and local anesthetic injection.	2. For optimal exposure and comfort of patient, the right hypochondriac region is treated as a surgical area, to minimize danger of infection.
3. Give support to the patient during the procedure.	3. To enhance comfort and provide a sense of security
4. Physician will determine biopsy site—one interspace below upper border of liver dullness 2 cm. behind anterior axillary line.	
5. Physician anesthetizes the skin, intercostal tissues, and liver capsule with local anesthetic.	5. To promote local comfort
6. Physician introduces biopsy needle into intercostal tissues but not into liver.	6. To prevent tearing of diaphragm or liver

(continued)

Guidelines Assisting With Liver Biopsy *(continued)*

Procedure *(continued)*	**Nursing Action**	**Rationale/Amplification**
	7. Instruct the patient to inhale and exhale deeply 3 or 4 times, then to exhale and hold his breath.	7. Holding one's breath immobilizes the chest wall and diaphragm; this helps to prevent the needle from tearing the diaphragm or the liver.
	8. The physician rapidly introduces biopsy needle into the liver, aspirates tissue, and withdraws.	
	9. As soon as needle is withdrawn, inform the patient to resume normal breathing.	9. Actual insertion and withdrawal of needle takes about 10 seconds.
	Follow-up Phase	
	1. Following biopsy, assist the patient to turn on his right side, place a pillow under his lower rib cage, and instruct him to remain in this position for several hours.	1. Compressing the liver against the chest wall near the biopsy site reduces the possibility of bleeding.
	2. Determine and record the patient's pulse and respiratory rates and his blood pressure at frequent intervals until they stabilize. Observe biopsy site for bleeding or drainage.	2. The nurse needs to be aware of the possible complications of liver biopsy; hemorrhage and bile peritonitis. Anticipatory nursing includes early recognition of symptoms.
	3. Recognize that an increasing pulse and decreasing blood pressure may be indicative of hemorrhage; note any indication of pain or apprehension.	

Jaundice

Jaundice is a *symptom* of dysfunction or disease and not a disease itself. Dysfunction of several body organs or systems may be implicated when jaundice occurs.

Hemolytic Jaundice

Hemolytic jaundice is attributable to an abnormally high concentration of bilirubin in blood exceeding the capacity of liver cells to excrete it. This form is also referred to as *prehepatic jaundice;* liver function is usually normal.
1. Most common cause is massive hemolysis seen in hemolytic transfusion reactions, hereditary spherocytosis, autoimmune hemolytic anemia, erythroblastosis fetalis, and other hemolytic disorders.
2. Bilirubin in the blood is unconjugated (indirect-reacting).
3. In feces and urine, urobilinogen is increased; urine is free of bilirubin.
4. Prolonged jaundice leads to formation of "pigment stones" in gallbladder.

Hepatocellular Jaundice

Hepatocellular or *hepatic jaundice* is due to an inability of diseased liver cells to clear the normal amount of bilirubin from the blood.

A. Causes
1. Infection—hepatitis viruses
2. Drug or chemical toxicity—carbon tetrachloride, chloroform, phosphorus, arsenicals, ethanol, halothane, isoniazid, acetaminophen, mushroom poisoning

B. Clinical Manifestations
1. Mildly or severely ill patient
2. Lack of appetite, nausea, loss of vigor and strength, weight loss
3. Elevated aspartate aminotransferase (AST, transaminase or SGOT) and alanine aminotransferase (ALT, SGPT)—2 enzymes that are liberated with cellular necrosis.
4. Rise in bromsulphalein (BSP) and bilirubin. Alkaline phosphatase mildly elevated.
5. Abnormal serum proteins in prolonged illness; prothrombin time increased.
6. Headache and chills possible in infectious condition.
7. Bile acid radioimmunoassay tests are replacing BSP tests.

Cholestatic Jaundice *(posthepatic or obstructive jaundice)*

A. Causes
1. Extrahepatic obstruction—blockage of bile ducts by gallstone(s), tumor(s), an inflammatory process, or an enlarged pancreas pressing on the duct.
2. Intrahepatic cholestasis—caused by injury to bile canaliculi or blockage of intrahepatic ducts due to tumors or granulomas.
   Certain drugs may cause this, for example: phenothiazine derivatives (Thorazine), perphenazine (Trilafon), sulfonamides, tolbutamide (Orinase) and other antidiabetic drugs, thiouracil, and aminobenzoic acid.

B. Clinical Manifestations
Because of damming back of bile, it is reabsorbed by blood. The following responses may be noted:
1. Jaundice of skin and sclerae
2. Deep orange-colored urine
3. White or clay-colored stools
4. Itchy skin and dyspepsia due to impaired bile acid excretion
5. SGOT and SGPT (AST and ALT) rise only moderately.
6. Bilirubin and BSP are increased.
7. Alkaline phosphatase is strikingly elevated.
8. Cholesterol is elevated.

Fulminant Liver Failure *(FLF)*

Fulminant Liver Failure (FLF) is acute necrosis of the liver cells (hepatocytes) in the absence of preexisting liver disease, resulting in the inability of the liver to perform its many functions. Mortality rate is high, 50%–80%, depending on the etiology and age of the patient.

Etiologies

1. Viral hepatitis: hepatitis B most commonly
2. Poisons, chemicals, and drugs: acetaminophen, tetracycline, isoniazid, halothane and other halogenated anesthetics, monoamine oxidase inhibitors, valproate, amiodarone, methyldopa, and amanita mushrooms
3. Ischemia and hypoxia: hepatic vascular occlusion, hypovolemic shock, acute circulatory failure, septic shock, heat stroke
4. Miscellaneous causes: hepatic vein obstruction, Budd–Chiari syndrome, acute fatty liver of pregnancy, partial hepatectomy, reactivation of chronic hepatitis B, complication of liver transplantation

Clinical Manifestations

1. Malaise, anorexia, nausea, fatigue
2. Jaundice, especially mucous membranes; urine is tea-colored and frothy when shaken
3. Steatorrhea (gaseous, foul-smelling stool) and diarrhea—due to decreased fat absorption
4. Anorexia, nausea, vomiting, diarrhea
5. Pruritus—bile salts are deposited on the skin.
6. Peripheral edema—fluid moves from the intravascular to the interstitial spaces, secondary to hypoproteinemia.
7. Ascites—in the presence of hypoproteinemia or portal hypertension
8. Easy bruising, petechiae, prolonged prothrombin time (PT), overt bleeding from gums, needle punctures, or occult bleeding in urine or stool
9. Decreased platelet count
10. Altered levels of consciousness, ranging from irritability and confusion to stupor, somnolence, and coma
11. Portal systemic encephalopathy (PSE), also known as hepatic coma or hepatic encephalopathy, can occur in conjunction with cerebral edema.
12. Laboratory results
    a. Elevated ammonia, amino acid, and mercaptan levels
    b. Hypoglycemia or hyperglycemia
    c. Dilutional hyponatremia or hypernatremia, hypokalemia, hypocalcemia, hypomagnesemia
13. Cerebral edema is often the cause of death in FLF due to brainstem herniation or respiratory arrest.

Management

1. Maintenance of adequate respiratory functioning; may need oxygen support or endotracheal intubation
2. Monitoring fluid status and evaluation of renal function
3. Nasogastric tube placement for GI decompression
4. Pharmacotherapy:
    a. Oral or enema lactulose to minimize formation of ammonia and other nitrogenous byproducts
    b. Neomycin, (nonabsorbable antibiotic) to suppress urea-splitting enteric bacteria
    c. Low molecular dextran or albumin followed by a potassium-sparing diuretic (spironolactone [Aldactone]) to enhance fluid shift from interstitial back to intravascular spaces
    d. Pancreatin (if diarrhea and steatorrhea are present) to permit better tolerance of diet
    e. Mannitol for management of cerebral edema when indicated
    f. Cholestyramine (Questran) to promote fecal excretion of bile salts to decrease itching
    g. Antacids, H_2 antagonists, to reduce risk of bleeding from stress ulcers
5. Restriction of dietary protein and sodium while maintaining adequate caloric intake with diet or with hypertonic dextrose solutions
6. Augmentation of dietary intake with supplemental vitamins (A, B complex, C, and K) and folate
7. Fresh frozen plasma to maintain prothrombin time; cryoprecipitate as needed
8. Additional medical interventions, depending on patient's condition, include:
    a. Hemodialysis
    b. Hemofiltration
    c. Hemoperfusion
    d. Plasmapheresis
    e. Hepatic transplantation is becoming more standard medical therapy for FLF in patients who meet transplantation criteria.

Complications

1. Hypoglycemia
2. Fluid and electrolyte imbalance
3. Acid–base imbalance
4. Acute respiratory failure
5. Infections and sepsis
6. Cardiac dysrhythmias
7. Hypotension
8. Hepatorenal syndrome
9. Hemorrhage

Nursing Assessment

1. Assess results of arterial blood gas evaluations as well as hemoglobin and hematocrit determinations.
2. Observe for dyspnea, hyperventilation; auscultate for crackles.
3. Monitor vital signs frequently.
4. Evaluate for peripheral edema on a 0–4+ scale.
5. Observe for signs and symptoms of fluid overload or dehydration—may occur when large quantities of fluid have shifted to the interstitial spaces.
6. Observe for jaundice, petechiae, palmar erythema, bruising, overt bleeding.
7. Assess for presence and extent of pruritus.
8. Assess for history of diarrhea, anorexia, nausea, vomiting, altered elimination patterns, abdominal pain, GI bleeding.
9. Assess abdomen for size, shape, symmetry, and presence/absence of a fluid wave.
10. Note color, consistency, and frequency of stools.
11. Assess for signs and symptoms of malnutrition.
12. Monitor daily weight.
13. Assess orientation to person, place, and time, mental alertness, and fine muscle coordination.
14. Assess pattern of speech and cognitive abilities.
15. Evaluate pattern of sleep–wake cycle and history of sensory disturbances.

16. Assess for the presence of asterixis (a flapping tremor elicited when the arms are raised with forearms fixed and hands dorsiflexed).
17. Evaluate laboratory values for alterations.

Nursing Diagnoses

1. Fluid volume deficit related to hypoproteinemia, peripheral edema, ascites, increased circulating ADH and aldosterone, hemorrhage
2. Ineffective breathing pattern related to hypoxemia, anemia, hydrothorax, decreased lung expansion from ascites, pulmonary infection
3. Potential for altered tissue perfusion (peripheral) related to electrolyte disturbances, peripheral edema, hypovolemia, respiratory compromise, anemia, potential for infection
4. Altered nutrition (less than body requirements), related to nausea, vomiting, anorexia, decreased absorption of fats, decreased storage of vitamins and minerals, altered metabolism of carbohydrates, proteins, and fats
5. Potential for impaired skin integrity related to malnutrition, deposition of bile salts, peripheral edema, bedrest
6. Potential for infection related to decreased Kupffer cell activity, altered immune response, altered levels of alpha and beta globulins, malnutrition
7. Potential self-care deficit, feeding, bathing/hygiene, dressing/grooming, toileting, related to fatigue, altered level of consciousness

Nursing Interventions

A. Attaining Adequate Fluid Volume and Decreasing the Risk of Bleeding

1. Take and record vital signs frequently.
2. Weigh the patient daily and keep an accurate intake and output record; record frequency and characteristics of feces.
3. Measure and record abdominal girth daily.
4. Assess and record the presence of peripheral edema using a 0–4+ scale.
5. Restrict sodium and fluids; replace electrolytes as directed.
6. Administer low-molecular dextran or albumin and diuretics as prescribed.
7. Anticipate manifestations of hemorrhage, such as ecchymosis, petechiae, and epistaxis; initiate preventive measures.
8. Maintain a safe environment to prevent injury.
9. Avoid trauma such as forceful nose blowing, use of hard toothbrush, large-gauge needles for injection.
10. Apply prolonged pressure after arterial and venous punctures, and all injections.
11. Note and report signs of hematemesis and melena.
    a. Assess for anxiety, weakness, restlessness, and epigastric fullness as possibly heralding hemorrhage.
    b. Take and record vital signs frequently.
    c. Administer vitamin C as prescribed.
    d. Observe each stool for color, consistency, and amount. Test for occult blood.
    e. Record nature, amount, and time of vomiting.
12. Administer fresh frozen plasma and clotting factors, as prescribed.

B. Achieving Effective Breathing Pattern

1. Monitor respiratory rate, depth, use of accessory muscles, nasal flaring, and breath sounds.

2. Evaluate results of arterial blood gases and hemoglobin and hematocrit evaluations.
3. Elevate head of the bed to lower diaphragm and decrease respiratory effort.
4. Turn frequently to prevent stasis of secretions.
5. Administer oxygen therapy as directed.

C. Improving Nutritional Status

1. Evaluate nutritional status and needs.
2. Assist the patient in overcoming anorexia, weight loss, and fatigue.
    a. Encourage him to eat all meals and supplementary feedings by serving them with eye-catching appeal, in small servings, and in small frequent meals.
    b. Recognize the effect of esthetic factors—control odors, disturbing conversations, unpleasant situations.
    c. Avoid fatty, greasy, or heavy foods that patient will find unappealing.
    d. Offer hard candy, fruit juices, carbonated drinks— may be tolerated better than solid foods
3. Maintain adequate nutritional levels.
    a. Provide protein within ability of liver to handle it. Normal nutritious diet with vitamin supplements, especially B, C, and K and folate.
4. Encourage the patient to eat in a sitting position to decrease abdominal tenderness and feeling of fullness.
5. Conserve the patient's energy so that total food intake is not expended to replace energy requirements.
6. Provide special mouth care if the patient has bleeding from gums or fetor hepaticus.
7. Administer antiemetics as prescribed, ½-hour before meals.
8. Consider the patient's preferences in food. If the patient is severely anorexic or nauseated and eating poorly, tube feeding may be necessary.
9. Include milk and starch hydrolysate. Do not increase dietary protein if serum ammonia level is increased.
10. Adjust nutritional offerings if the patient has ascites or edema.
    a. Restrict sodium intake to 200–500 mg. daily (less than 10 mEq. daily).
    b. Maintain caloric and vitamin intake; give protein as tolerated.
    c. Avoid table salt, salty foods, salted margarine, and butter, as well as all ordinary frozen and canned foods, mouthwash, baking soda, and all other products containing large quantities of salt.
    d. Use "salt" substitutes such as lemon juice, oregano, thyme to enhance flavor; commercial salt substitute should be approved by physician.
    e. Encourage use of low-sodium milk and milk products.
11. If patient is unable to tolerate an oral diet, administer glucose intravenous fluids, as prescribed.

D. Attaining/Maintaining Skin Integrity

1. Observe skin and control pruritus.
    a. Provide good skin care; bathe without soap; apply soothing lotions.
    b. Use starch or baking soda, soothing lotions, such as calamine.
    c. Keep the patient's fingernails short to prevent him from scratching his skin.
    d. Administer medications as prescribed for pruritus; be alert for side effects of nausea, diarrhea, or constipation, and vitamin K depletion, which leads to bleeding.

2. Turn the patient frequently to prevent pressure sores.
3. Avoid trauma to skin, through gentle handling and prevention of falls.
4. Encourage intake of foods high in vitamin C.
5. Assist the patient in reducing the strong tendency to scratch his skin:
   a. Encourage activities to divert the patient's attention.
   b. Avoid excessive top bedding.
   c. Give soothing massages, particularly at night in preparing the patient for sleep, since this is a time when he is especially likely to scratch.
   d. Provide clean white gloves to use at night if the patient scratches during sleep.

E. Achieving Rest and Comfort

1. Promote rest during acute episodes to decrease demands on the liver.
2. Eliminate unnecessary stimuli to promote rest when indicated.
   a. Group nursing activities together to minimize disruption of the patient's rest.
   b. Limit visitors.
   c. Eliminate or reduce environmental noise and light.
3. Assist with bathing, feeding, toileting, when these activities become too fatiguing.
4. Assist the patient in planning periods of rest and activity when symptoms begin to subside.
5. Assess and record presence or absence of abdominal pain or tenderness, hepatomegaly, and splenomegaly.
6. Encourage the patient to maintain bedrest or restricted activities if abdominal pain or tenderness is present.
7. Notify the physician of sudden occurrence of or increase in pain or tenderness.
8. Encourage gradual resumption of activities and mild exercise during recovery.

F. Improving Neurological Status and Thought Processes

1. Evaluate neurological function
   a. Assess the patient's neurological status (i.e., his ability to do handwriting and perform simple arithmetic calculations). Keep daily record and note differences
   b. Observe and record extent and magnitude of characteristic tremor.
   c. Note and record the state of consciousness, including slight drowsiness, slight confusion, confused, or disoriented.
   d. Note response to painful stimuli.
   e. When the patient does not respond, note sucking and grasping abilities: check corneal reflex.
2. Recognize signs of increasing stupor, notify physician, and initiate nursing measures as follows:
   a. Be alert for evidence of mental changes, lethargy, hallucinations.
   b. Avoid giving the patient narcotics and barbiturates.
   c. Reduce and eliminate all unnecessary sedatives and analgesics. Administer only those specifically prescribed.
   d. Restrict dietary protein; offer small high-calorie feedings frequently.
   e. Protect the patient by keeping him in bed: pad siderails.
   f. Arouse the patient at intervals; orient to time, place, and person.
   g. Limit visitors.
   h. Provide constant nursing surveillance and emphasize sensitivity to the patient's changes and needs.
3. Remove factors that precipitate hepatic coma.
   a. Administer intestinal antibiotics (neomycin) as prescribed to reduce serum ammonia absorption from gastrointestinal tract.
   b. Administer lactulose (Cephulac) orally, by NG tube or by means of retention enema, as prescribed.
   c. Administer medications with caution.
   d. Promote bowel evacuation to reduce intestinal nitrogen load.

G. Preventing Infection

1. Monitor for signs and symptoms of infection.
2. Use sterile technique when caring for any break in the skin or mucous membranes, such as IV sites, indwelling catheter, etc.
3. Restrict visits with anyone who may have an infection.
4. Encourage patient to try not to scratch his itching skin.

H. Enhancing Self-Esteem

1. Encourage the patient to discuss concerns; accept the patient's concerns without minimizing them.
2. Instruct staff and the patient's visitors to avoid remarks or behaviors that indicate rejection or fear of the patient's altered appearance.
3. Explain cause of jaundice and altered appearance.
4. Reinforce the fact that change in appearance is usually temporary.
5. Place the patient's bed in a position where he cannot look at himself in a mirror.

Patient Education

Instruct the patient as follows:

A. Avoid Risks of Complications

1. Notify the nurse or physician if there is any incidence of increased difficulty breathing, evidence of overt bleeding, increased abdominal discomfort, incidence of hallucinations, or lapses in consciousness.
2. Avoid activities that increase the risk of bleeding: scratching, falling, forceful nose blowing, aggressive tooth brushing, use of a straight-edged razor.
3. Limit activities when fatigued and take rest periods.

Evaluation

1. Is adequately hydrated without bleeding; decreased peripheral edema, maintains stable vital signs; no evidence of overt or occult bleeding, laboratory values remain within normal limits
2. Maintains adequate breathing pattern; reports absence of dyspnea, shortness of breath
3. Achieves adequate nutritional status; consumes prescribed diet; reports absence of nausea, dyspepsia
4. Skin is clean, dry, and free of scratches, bruises; reports free of itching
5. Reports adequate rest and comfort
6. Maintains orientation to person, place, and time; denies loss of consciousness, tremors, and hallucinations
7. Is free of signs and symptoms of infection
8. Discusses concerns regarding condition

Hepatitis

Hepatitis is a viral infection of the liver associated with a broad spectrum of clinical manifestations from asymptomatic infection through icteric hepatitis to hepatic necrosis. Hepatitis is usually caused by one or more viruses; however, a less common form is toxic or drug-induced hepatitis.

Types of Hepatitis

1. Hepatitis A virus, HAV, infections; brief incubation period.
2. Hepatitis B virus, HBV; long incubation period, associated with several antigen and antibody systems.
3. Delta hepatitis, HDV, a defective RNA virus; only occurs with concomittant acute or chronic hepatitis B.
4. Hepatitis C virus.
5. Non-A non-B hepatitis, NANB; appears to be more than one type.

Type A Hepatitis (HAV)

Epidemiology

1. HAV is probably an RNA virus of the enterovirus family.
2. Mode of transmission
   a. Fecal–oral route
   b. Poor sanitation; person-to-person (epidemic-type prevalent in camps and overcrowded residences)
   c. Contaminated food, milk, polluted water, or shellfish
   d. Sexual contact
   e. Blood transfusion (rarely)
3. Incubation: 3–7 weeks; average, 4 weeks
4. Occurrence
   a. Worldwide
   b. Usually in children and young adults
5. Mortality—0.3% develop fulminating disease, which has a mortality rate of 75%–80%.
6. Most infectious for 2 weeks before the onset of jaundice, after which fecal excretion of the virus decreases.

Clinical Manifestations

1. May have no symptoms.
2. Prodromal symptoms: fatigue, anorexia, malaise, headache, low-grade fever, nausea and vomiting; highly contagious during this period.
3. Icteric phase: jaundice, amber-colored urine, pale stools, right upper quadrant tenderness.

Diagnostic Evaluation

1. Elevated serum transferase levels.
2. Radioimmunoassays that reveal the presence of IgM antibodies to hepatitis A virus in the acute phase.

Management

See General Management, p. 513

Type B Hepatitis (HBV)

Epidemiology

1. Causative agent—this particle is composed of:
   a. Antigenic material in an outer coat—hepatitis B surface antigen (HB_sAg)
   b. Antigenic material in an inner coat—hepatitis B core antigen (HB_cAg)
   c. An independent protein circulating in the blood—HB_eAg

2. Antibody—each antigen elicits a specific antibody:
   a. Anti-HB_s (produced early after hepatitis B infection). Its presence indicates immunity. Therefore, it is present if the patient has received hepatitis B vaccine.
   b. Anti-HB_c (noted late in acute phase or in convalescence)
   c. Anti-HB_e (noted later in convalescence)
3. Significance:
   a. HB_sAg—may be detected transiently in blood of 80%–90% of infected persons; may be noted in blood for months, and years, indicating that the patient has acute or chronic hepatitis B or is a carrier.
   b. HB_cAg—found only in liver cells, not serum
   c. HB_eAg—if absent, the patient is an asymptomatic carrier. If present, it indicates highly infectious period of acute, active hepatitis. If it persists, indicates progression to chronic state.
4. Modes of transmission (percutaneous or permucosal routes):
   a. Oral—via saliva (i.e., mother to child via breast feeding)
   b. Parenterally, or by intimate contact with carriers (Susceptible persons are surgeons, clinical laboratory workers, nurses, respiratory therapists.)
   c. Male homosexuals
   d. Blood, saliva, semen, vaginal secretions
5. Incubation—2–5 months
6. Occurrence—affects all ages, but mostly young adults, worldwide

Clinical Manifestations

1. Symptom onset usually more insidious and prolonged compared with HAV
2. May be asymptomatic
3. One week to 2 months of prodromal symptoms: fatigue, anorexia, malaise, transient fever, abdominal discomfort, nausea and vomiting, headache
4. Jaundice in addition to above symptoms
5. Extrahepatic manifestations may include: myalgias; photophobia; arthritis; angioedema; urticaria; maculopapular eruptions; skin rashes; vasculitis
6. May in rare cases progress to fulminant hepatic failure, also called *fulminant hepatitis*
7. May become chronic active or chronic persistent (asymptomatic) hepatitis

Diagnostic Evaluation

1. Elevated serum transferase levels.
2. Radioimmunoassays to include: HB_sAg, HB_eAg, Anti-HB_s, Anti-HB_c.

Management

See General Management, page 513

Hepatitis D Virus (HDV)

Hepatitis D virus is a defective RNA agent that appears to replicate only in the presence of the hepatitis B virus (HBV).

Epidemiology

1. Causative agent: RNA virus containing genetic material coded with hepatitis B surface antigen as a surface protein.

a. Coinfection occurs when the host is infected simultaneously with HBV and HDV, may be acute or chronic.
   b. Superinfection occurs when an acute HDV infection is superimposed on an HBV carrier.
2. Antibody
   a. Anti-hepatitis D (HD) may go undetected in coinfections as often only present temporarily.
   b. IgM anti-HD may persist in patients with chronic or progressive HDV.
3. Modes of transmission
   Same as for HBV

Clinical Manifestations

1. Not clinically distinguishable from other forms of hepatitis
2. Patients with acute coinfection may have a greater risk of developing fulminant hepatitis.
3. Patients with superinfection may have a greater risk of developing cirrhosis and its associated complications.

Management

See General Management, opposite column.

Hepatitis C (HCV)

This type of hepatitis accounts for the majority of blood-borne cases formerly classified as non-A, non-B hepatitis.

Epidemiology

1. Categories of transmission
   a. Post-transfusion of blood and blood products
   b. Intravenous drug use
   c. Heterosexual transmission
   d. Unknown in a percentage of cases
2. Incubation period varies from 1 week to several months

Clinical Manifestations

Similar to those associated with hepatitis B, but often less severe.

Diagnostic Evaluation

1. Radioimmunoassay anti-HCV.
2. Elevated serum transferase levels.

Non-A, Non-B Hepatitis (NANB)

This type of hepatitis is a viral infection that at present does not have an identified agent or antigenic markers.

Epidemiology

1. Types or categories
   a. Sporadic hepatitis
      These are cases of NANB hepatitis that occur in the general population with no identifiable mode of transmission.
   b. Epidemic hepatitis occurs in epidemic form in areas with fecal contamination of drinking water.
2. Incubation period varies depending on the type:
   a. Sporadic form remains undetermined.
   b. Epidemic water-borne type NANB hepatitis has an intermediate incubation period of about 40 days.

Clinical Manifestations

1. Similar to those associated with hepatitis B, but often less severe.
2. Epidemic type seems to be associated with higher frequency of fulminant hepatitis.

Diagnostic Evaluation

1. Rule out HAV, HBV, and HCV.
2. Elevated serum transferase levels as seen with other forms of hepatitis.

General Management (All types)

1. Rest according to patient's level of fatigue
2. Hospitalization with protracted nausea and vomiting or life-threatening complications
3. High-caloric, low-fat diet
4. Vitamin K injected subcutaneously if prothrombin time is prolonged
5. IV fluid and electrolyte replacement as indicated
6. Administration of metoclopramide hydrochloride, IV or IM for nausea

> **NURSING ALERT:** Prevention of infection for high-risk individuals with hepatitis B immune globulin (HBIG) after exposure is indicated. Active immunization is recommended for all high-risk populations, including health care workers, with either plasma-derived HB vaccine or recombinant DNA HB vaccine.

Complications of Acute Hepatitis Infection

1. Fluid and electrolyte imbalance
2. Chronic "carrier" hepatitis
3. Chronic active hepatitis
4. Cholestatic hepatitis
5. Fulminant hepatitis (see Fulminant Liver Failure, p. 509).
6. *HBV carriers have a higher risk of developing hepatocellular carcinoma (HCC).*

Nursing Interventions

A. Monitoring and Preventing Complications

1. Monitor for signs and symptoms of liver failure (see p. 509).
2. Use appropriate hand-washing, proper disposal of soiled linen, and needle precautions to minimize spread of the disease.
3. Strictly enforce Universal Precautions to protect patients and staff members from spread of the disease.

B. Maintaining Adequate Nutrition

1. Administer antiemetics as prescribed.
2. Encourage adequate high-calorie low-fat diet. Offer larger meals in the morning, as nausea tends to worsen throughout the day.
3. Encourage eating meals in a sitting position to decrease pressure on the liver—alleviating abdominal tenderness and feelings of fullness.
4. Provide aesthetically pleasing meals in an environment with minimal noxious stimuli (odors, noise, interruptions).

C. Attaining Comfort and Rest

1. Promote periods of rest during acute or symptomatic stage, according to level of fatigue.

2. Administer antihistamines as prescribed to reduce itching.
3. Assess and record presence of abdominal pain or tenderness, hepatomegaly, and splenomegaly.
4. Administer analgesics as prescribed.
5. Provide emotional support and diversional activities when recovery and convalescence are prolonged.
6. Encourage gradual resumption of activities and mild exercise during convalescent period.

Discharge Planning/Patient Education

1. Stress importance of proper public and home sanitation.
2. Instruct regarding the merits of conscientious surveillance in the proper preparation and dispensation of foods.
3. Instruct the patient and family members about transmission and prevention of transmission.

General Preventive Measures

1. Stress importance of proper public and home sanitation.
2. Emphasize importance of good personal hygiene.
3. Promote effective health supervision in schools, dormitories, and camps.
4. Initiate and support health education programs regarding hepatitis.
5. Identify individuals or groups of individuals at high risk.
6. Encourage administration of appropriate immune globulin or vaccine for high-risk individuals.
7. Screen blood donors to exclude carriers.
8. Employ proper safeguards to prevent use of blood and its components from infected donors.
9. Instruct all patients who have received a blood transfusion to refrain from donating blood for 6 months. This is necessary because of the long incubation period of hepatitis B.
10. Recognize merits of conscientious surveillance in the proper and safe preparation and dispensation of food.
11. Screen food handlers carefully.
12. Practice safe preparation and serving of food.

Hepatic Cirrhosis

Cirrhosis of the liver is a chronic disease in which there has been diffuse destruction of parenchymal cells followed by liver cell regeneration and an increase in connective tissue. These processes result in disorganization of the lobular architecture and obstruction of the hepatic venous and sinusoidal channels, causing portal hypertension.

Classification of Hepatic Cirrhosis

1. Laennec's cirrhosis (micronodular)
   a. Fibrosis—mainly around central veins and portal areas
   b. Most commonly due to chronic alcoholism and malnutrition
2. Postnecrotic (macronodular)
   a. Broad bands of scar tissue—due to collapse of necrotic lobules and confluence of portal areas
   b. Due to previous acute viral hepatitis or drug-induced massive hepatic necrosis

3. Biliary
   a. Scarring around bile ducts and lobes of liver
   b. Results from chronic biliary obstruction (with or without infection)
   c. Much more rare than Laennec's and postnecrotic cirrhosis

Etiology

1. Cirrhosis of the liver is characterized by repeated occurrences of death of the liver cells, replacement with scar tissue, and regeneration of liver cells.
2. Onset is insidious; it may be developing and progressing over many years.
3. Major causes in the US are excessive consumption of alcohol with nutritional deficiencies and chronic viral hepatitis.

Clinical Manifestations

A. Early Complaints—include fatigue, anorexia, edema of the ankles in evening, epistaxis and bleeding gums, and weight loss.

B. Later—chronic failure of liver function and obstruction of portal circulation.

1. Obstruction of portal circulation, causing portal hypertension with congestion of spleen, pancreas, and gastrointestinal tract.
   a. Chronic dyspepsia, change in bowel habits—diarrhea, constipation.
   b. Esophageal varices, dilated cutaneous veins around the umbilicus, internal hemorrhoids, ascites, splenomegaly, pancytopenia.
2. Chronic failure of liver function
   a. Plasma albumin is reduced, thereby leading to edema and contributing to ascites.
   b. Weakness increases, leading to depression, wasting, delirium, coma, and eventually death.
   c. Estrogen–androgen imbalance, causing spider angiomata and palmar erythema, amenorrhea develops in females; testicular and prostatic atrophy, gynecomastia, loss of libido, and impotence develop in males.
   d. Bleeding tendencies may be evident.

Diagnostic Evaluation

1. Liver biopsy (see p. 507)—determines abnormal hepatocyte structure and vascular arrangements; high risk of bleeding in the presence of clotting defects.
2. CT scan determines the size of the liver and its irregular nodular surface.
3. Radioisotopic liver scans—increased splenic and vertebral uptake of radioactive isotope with generalized decrease in liver uptake
4. Esophagoscopy—to determine the presence of esophageal varices
5. Paracentesis to examine ascitic fluid for cell count, for protein content, and for bacterial count
6. Test for serum hepatitis B surface antigen (HB_sAg)—an alternative etiology to alcohol toxicity.

Management

Medical management is directed toward minimizing further deterioration of liver function, correction of nutritional deficiencies and fluid and electrolyte imbalances, and relief of the patient's symptoms.

A. General Measures

1. Prevent further damage to the liver by withdrawing toxic substances, alcohol, and drugs.
2. Restrict sodium and water intake, depending on amount of fluid retention.
3. Restriction of water intake when significant hyponatremia and hypo-osmolality is present.
4. Bedrest—to aid in diuresis.

B. Treatment of Ascites

1. Diuretic therapy (spironolactone—potassium sparing and inhibits the action of aldosterone on the kidneys; furosemide).
2. Abdominal paracentesis usually accompanied by intravenous albumin
   a. To decrease extreme abdominal discomfort and prevent hypovolemia
   b. Ascitic fluid may be concentrated by ultrafiltration and reinfused into the central venous system
3. Peritoneovenous shunt
   a. May be performed in patients whose ascites is resistant to other forms of treatment
   b. Is associated with high-risk complications: bacterial infections, shunt obstruction, and intravascular coagulopathies

C. Additional Measures

1. Orthotopic liver transplantation may be considered.
2. Treatment of other problems associated with liver failure

Complications

1. Hyponatremia and water retention
2. Bleeding esophageal varices
3. Coagulopathies
4. Spontaneous bacterial peritonitis (SBP)
5. Hepatic encephalopathy—may be precipitated by use of sedatives, high protein diet, sepsis, or electrolyte imbalance.

Nursing Interventions

A. Monitoring and Preventing Complications

1. Observe for dyspnea, hyperventilation; auscultate lungs for crackles.
2. Assess abdomen for size, shape, presence/absence of a fluid wave, and abdominal girth at frequent intervals.
3. Monitor daily weight—to detect fluid retention/depletion.
4. Evaluate laboratory values for status of respiratory and liver function, as well as for coagulation abnormalities.
5. Elevate head of bed 30 degrees—to lower the diaphragm and increase lung expansion.

B. Maintaining Adequate Fluid Volume

1. Encourage bedrest during periods of necessary diuresis.
2. Restrict dietary sodium intake (40–60 mEq./day), as prescribed—to prevent additional water retention.
3. Administer diuretics as prescribed and assess for complications of therapy:
   a. Observe for signs and symptoms of intravascular volume depletion: tachycardia, hypotension, decreasing urine output with increased specific gravity.
   b. Assess for hyponatremia, hypokalemia, hypomagnesemia, metabolic acidosis.
   c. Monitor for the occurrence of hepatic encephalopathy.
4. Assist the patient undergoing a paracentesis and administer albumin as prescribed.

C. Achieving Rest and Comfort

1. Offer supportive care.
2. Position patient comfortably, supporting abdomen and back with pillows.
3. Encourage patient to limit activities when fatigued.
4. Assist the patient in planning activities to limit exertion.
5. Encourage gradual resumption of activities.

Discharge Planning/Patient Education

Instruct the patient regarding precautions and regimen to follow on discharge from the hospital.

1. Stress the necessity of giving up alcohol completely. Urge acceptance of skillful assistance from psychiatrist, Alcoholics Anonymous, or the alcohol treatment unit in the hospital.
2. Provide written dietary instructions, emphasizing the restriction of sodium (and protein, if necessary).
3. Discuss the side effects of diuretic therapy and when to seek medical attention.
4. Encourage daily weighing for self-monitoring of fluid retention or depletion.
5. Emphasize the significance of rest, a sensible life-style, and an adequate, well-balanced diet.
6. Involve the person closest to the patient (usually spouse) because recovery often is not easy and relapses are common; a close, trusted helper can help patient over the rough spots.

Guidelines   Assisting With Abdominal Paracentesis

Paracentesis is the withdrawal of fluid from the abdominal or peritoneal cavity.

Purposes
1. To withdraw fluid for diagnostic examination
2. To remove ascitic fluid when large accumulation of fluid causes severe symptoms and is resistant to other therapy
3. To prepare for other procedures (peritoneal dialysis, ascitic fluid reinfusion, surgery, etc.)

Danger and Complications
1. In chronic liver disease, paracentesis may precipitate hepatic coma.
2. Shock and hypovolemia rarely occur when fluid from general circulation shifts to abdomen to replace withdrawn fluid; lost fluid may be replaced by parenteral administration of albumin.

(continued)

Guidelines   Assisting With Abdominal Paracentesis *(continued)*

Equipment   Sterile paracentesis tray and gloves
Procaine hydrochloride 1%
Drape or cotton blankets
Collection bottle (vacuum bottle)
Skin preparation tray with antiseptic
Specimen bottles and laboratory forms

Procedure

Nursing Action	Rationale/Amplification
Preparatory Phase	
1. Explain procedure to the patient.	1. This may reduce the patient's fear and anxiety.
2. Record the patient's vital signs.	2. Provides baseline values for later comparison.
3. Have the patient void before treatment is begun. See that consent form has been signed.	3. This will lessen the danger of accidentally piercing the bladder with the needle or trocar.
4. Position the patient in Fowler's position with back, arms, and feet supported (sitting on the side of the bed is a frequently used position).	4. The patient is more comfortable, and a steady position can be maintained.
5. Drape the patient with sheet exposing abdomen.	5. Minimizes exposure of patient and keeps him warm.
Performance Phase	
1. Assist physician in preparing skin with antiseptic solution.	1. This is considered a minor surgical procedure, requiring aseptic precautions.
2. Open sterile tray and package of sterile gloves; provide anesthetic solution.	
3. Have collection bottle and tubing available.	
4. Assess pulse and respiratory status frequently during procedure; watch for pallor, cyanosis, or syncope (faintness).	4. Preliminary indications of shock must be watched for. Keep emergency drugs available.
5. Physician administers local anesthesia and introduces No. 20 needle or trocar.	
6. Needle or trocar is connected to tubing and vacuum bottle or syringe; fluid is drained from peritoneal cavity.	6. Drainage is usually limited to 1–2 liters to relieve acute symptoms and minimize risk of hypovolemia and shock.
7. Apply dressing when needle is withdrawn.	7. Elasticized adhesive patch is effective, serving as waterproof adhering dressing.
Follow-up Phase	
1. Assist the patient to be comfortable after treatment.	
2. Record amount and kind of fluid removed, number of specimens sent to laboratory, the patient's condition through treatment.	
3. Check blood pressure and vital signs every half hour for 2 hours, every hour for 4 hours, and every 4 hours for 24 hours.	3. Close observation will detect poor circulatory adjustment and possible development of shock.
4. Usually, a dressing is sufficient; however, if the trocar wound appears large, the physician may close the incision with sutures.	
5. Watch for leakage or scrotal edema after paracentesis.	5. If seen, notify physician at once.

Bleeding Esophageal Varices

Esophageal varices are dilated tortuous veins found in the submucosa of the lower esophagus; they may extend up in the esophagus and down into the stomach.

Pathophysiology

1. Increasing portal vein obstruction—venous blood returning to right atrium from intestinal tract and spleen seeks new pathways, through enlarging collateral esophageal veins.

2. Usually no symptoms are produced by dilated veins unless mucosa becomes ulcerated.
3. Hematemesis and melena, plus a history of alcoholism, tend to suggest esophageal varices; however, bleeding may result from associated gastritis or duodenal ulcer in 25% of patients with varices.
4. The strain of coughing or vomiting may precipitate variceal rupture, hemorrhage, and death.
5. Irritation of vessels by gastroesophageal reflux may cause esophagitis, esophageal rupture, hemorrhage, and death.
6. Has a high mortality rate due to further deterioration

of liver function (hepatic coma) and complications (e.g., aspiration pneumonia, sepsis, renal failure).

Etiology

1. Nearly always due to portal hypertension, which may result from obstruction of the portal venous circulation and cirrhosis of the liver.
2. Abnormalities of the circulation in splenic vein or superior vena cava.

Clinical Manifestations

A. Bleeding

1. Hematemesis (vomiting blood)—usually bright red
2. Melena (passage of black, tarry stools)
3. Bright red rectal bleeding—from hypermotility of the bowel. *Blood loss may be sudden and massive.*

B. Hypovolemia and Shock—from massive bleeding

C. Other—May present with other clinical manifestations of liver failure (see Fulminant Liver Failure, p. 509)

Diagnostic Evaluation

1. Gastrointestinal fiberoptic endoscopy (after hemodynamic stabilization of an acute hemorrhage)—to visualize the bleeding site
2. Liver diagnostic studies

Management

A. Restoration of Circulating Blood Volume

1. To replace blood loss and prevent shock
2. Involves use of blood products, crystalloids, and colloids

B. Pharmacotherapy

1. Vasopressin (intravenously) reduces portal pressure by decreasing splanchnic blood flow, and increases clotting and hemostasis.
2. Nitroglycerin (sublingually or intravenously) may be used to counter the systemic vasoconstrictive effects of vasopressin.

C. Gastric Lavage

1. To remove blood from the gastrointestinal tract, as it is a precipitator of encephalopathy in patients with liver disease
2. To enhance visualization for endoscopic examination

D. Endoscopic Sclerotherapy

1. Sclerosing agent injected directly into the varix with a flexible fiberoptic endoscope
2. To control bleeding and reduce the frequency of subsequent variceal hemorrhages
3. Complications: esophageal ulceration, stricture, and perforation
4. May be used as prophylactic measure to treat varices before bleeding has occurred
5. Repeated treatments may be required if bleeding recurs

E. Esophageal Balloon Tamponade

1. Inflation of balloons in the distal esophagus and the proximal stomach to collapse the varices and induce hemostasis
2. Examples: Sengstaken–Blakemore tube; Minnesota tube.
3. See Guidelines: Using Balloon Tamponade to Control Esophageal Bleeding, page 518.

F. Administration of Parenteral Feedings—to allow the esophagus to rest

G. Surgical Interventions

1. To lower portal pressure by shunting blood around the liver.
2. Portal–systemic shunts: portal vein is anastamosed to the inferior vena cava to reduce variceal blood flow and pressure.
3. Splenorenal shunt—a shunt is made between the splenic vein and the left renal vein; this is done when the portal vein cannot be used because of thrombosis or for other reasons.
4. Interposition mesocaval shunt: superior mesenteric vein is grafted to the inferior vena cava, also to reduce pressure.
5. Complications of surgery are acute hepatic failure and chronic portal systemic encephalopathy (PSE).
6. Care is similar to postabdominal surgery complicated by care required for a patient with severe cirrhotic liver.

H. Other Measures

1. Maintenance of adequate respiratory function and prevention of aspiration.
2. Prevention and management of complications related to liver failure (see Fulminant Liver Failure, p. 509).

Complications

1. Exsanguinating or recurrent hemorrhage
2. Portal systemic encephalopathy (PSE)
3. Complications of vasopressin therapy: hypertension, bradycardia, esophageal ulceration or perforation, aspiration pneumonitis, worsening variceal hemorrhage, water intoxication, cardiac ischemia in patients with preexisting cardiac disease.
4. Complications of esophageal tamponade: esophageal necrosis, perforation, aspiration, asphyxiation, stricture
5. Complications of acute shock syndrome

Nursing Interventions

> **NURSING ALERT:** The patient who experiences bleeding esophageal varices commonly has severe liver disease and, as a result, is subject to the problems encountered in fulminant liver failure (see p. 509).

A. Attaining Adequate Fluid Volume

1. Monitor vital signs frequently; arterial catheter may be inserted to monitor blood pressure directly. Use CVP, PCWP, or cardiac output, if available, to determine fluid replacement.
2. Assess urinary output; indwelling catheter may be required.
3. Monitor patient receiving transfusions of blood and blood products.
   a. Fresh whole blood: ammonia content is lower than in stored blood and coagulation effect is greater, particularly if the patient has severe liver disease.
   b. Administer required fresh frozen plasma—to replace clotting factors, if prescribed.
4. Administer vitamin K intramuscularly, as prescribed—deficiency of the vitamin K–dependent blood clotting proteins contributes to tendency to bleed.

B. Maintaining Effective Breathing Pattern

1. Assess respirations and monitor blood gas values to assess oxygenation of blood. An endotracheal tube may

be inserted to protect, control, and manage the patient's airway.
2. Note and report occurrence of signs of obstructed airway or ruptured esophagus from the esophageal balloon (e.g., changes in skin color, respirations, breath sounds, level of consciousness, presence of chest pain, vital signs, etc.).
3. Check location and inflation of esophageal balloon; maintain traction on tubes if applicable.
4. Have scissors readily available. Cut tubing and remove esophageal balloon immediately if the patient develops acute respiratory distress.
5. Keep head of bed elevated to avoid gastric regurgitation and aspiration of gastric contents.
6. When using the Sengstaken–Blakemore esophageal balloon tube, ensure removal of secretions above the esophageal balloon; position nasogastric tube in the esophagus for suctioning purposes. Or provide intermittent oropharyngeal suctioning.
7. Inspect nares for skin irritation; cleanse and lubricate frequently.

C. Reducing the Risk of Bleeding

1. Monitor patient having vasopressin infusion frequently for complications: hypertension, bradycardia, abdominal cramps, chest pain, or water intoxication.
2. Observe the patient for straining, gagging, or vomiting; these increase pressure in portal system and increase risk of further bleeding.
3. Note and report signs of hematemesis and melena.
4. Check all gastrointestinal secretions and feces for occult and frank blood.
5. Observe for signs of hypovolemia and shock.

6. Support the patient having lavage with saline if bleeding recurs.
7. Have an extra esophageal balloon tube available for reinsertion if bleeding occurs or recurs.
8. When bleeding has ceased, introduce nonirritating, soothing foods and fluids gradually.

D. Reducing Fear and Anxiety

1. Provide care in a concerned, nonjudgmental manner.
2. Explain all procedures to the patient.
3. Remain with the patient; place call bell within patient's reach.
4. Maintain close surveillance of the patient.
5. Avoid discussing the patient's condition or unrelated matters in the patient's vicinity.
6. Provide alternate means of communication if tubes or other equipment interfere with patient's ability to talk.
7. Use touch and other tactile stimuli to provide reassurance to patient.
8. Use protective restraints to prevent dislodging of tube in confused, combative patient.

Discharge Planning/Patient Education

1. Discuss with patient and family the signs and symptoms of recurrent bleeding and need to seek emergency medical treatment if these occur.
2. Instruct the patient to avoid behaviors that increase portal system pressure: straining, gagging, Valsalva maneuvers.
3. Encourage the patient, if appropriate, to abstain from alcohol consumption; discuss support organizations, e.g., Alcoholics Anonymous.

Guidelines   Using Balloon Tamponade to Control Esophageal Bleeding
(Sengstaken–Blakemore Tube Method; Minnesota Tube Method)

Purposes
1. To exert pressure on the cardiac portion of the stomach and against bleeding varices by a double balloon tamponade.
2. To prevent shock in the presence of acute esophageal bleeding.
3. To prevent blood accumulation in the gastrointestinal tract, which could precipitate hepatic encephalopathy.

Equipment
Esophageal balloon (Sengstaken–Blakemore or Minnesota)
Basin with cracked ice
Clamps for tubing
Water-soluble lubricant
Syringe (50 ml. with catheter tip)
Towel and emesis basin
Glass of water and straw
Adhesive tape
Device to apply traction (e.g., football helmet)
Large scissors (for emergency deflation)
Manometer (to measure balloon pressure)

Procedure
(Fig. 21-1)

Preparatory Phase

1. Provide support and reassure the patient that this procedure will help to control his bleeding.
2. Explain procedure to the patient and tell him how breathing through the mouth and swallowing can help in passing the tube.
3. Elevate head of bed slightly, unless the patient is in shock.

Nursing Action	Rationale/Amplification

Performance Phase

1. Check balloons by trial inflation to detect leaks.	1. This is best done under water because it is easier to see escaping air bubbles.

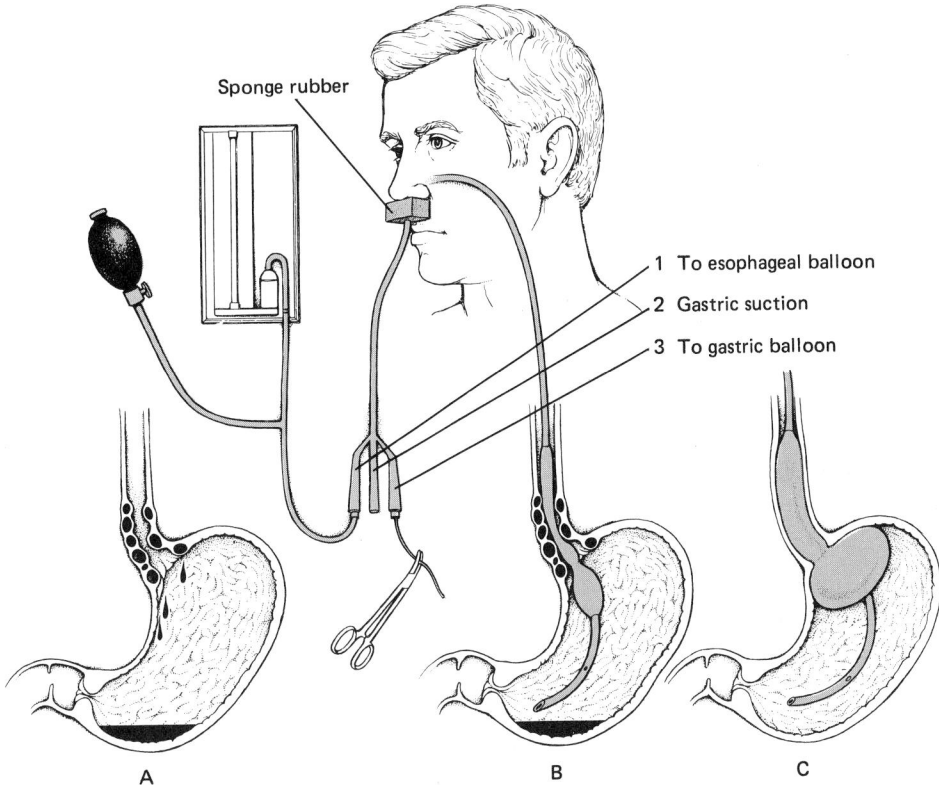

Sponge rubber

1 To esophageal balloon
2 Gastric suction
3 To gastric balloon

A   B   C

Figure 21-1. *Diagram showing esophageal varices and their treatment by a compressing balloon tube (Sengstaken-Blakemore). (A) Dilated veins of the lower esophagus. (B) The tube is in place in the stomach and the lower esophagus but is not inflated. (C) Inflation of the tube and compression of the veins, which can be obtained by inflation of the balloon. In some instances, it may be necessary to pass an additional tube through the other nostril for the purpose of aspirating secretions.*
Note: The Minnesota four-lumen esophagogastric tamponade tube has an additional outlet for aspiration of the esophagus.

Procedure
(continued)

Nursing Action	**Rationale/Amplification**
2. Chill the tube, then lubricate it before the physician passes it via mouth or nose (preferable).	2. Chilling makes the tube more firm and lubrication lessens friction.
3. Provide the patient with a few sips of water.	3. This will help pass the tube more easily.
4. After the tube has entered the stomach, verify its placement by irrigating the gastric tube with air while auscultating over the stomach.	4. It is imperative to be certain that the tube is in the stomach so that the gastric tube is not inflated in the esophagus.
5. After obtaining an x-ray film of the lower chest and upper abdomen to verify placement in the stomach, inflate gastric balloon (200–250 ml.) with air and gently pull tube back to seat balloon against gastroesophageal junction.	5. This is to exert force against the cardia.
6. Clamp gastric balloon; mark tube location at nares.	6. This prevents air leakage and tube migration. The mark on the tube allows for easy visualization of movement of the tube.
7. Apply gentle traction to the balloon tube and secure it with a foam rubber cube at the nares or tape it to the faceguard of a football helmet.	7. This prevents the tube from migrating with peristalsis and assists in exerting proper pressure.
8. Attach Y connector to esophageal balloon opening. Attach syringe to one arm of the Y connector and manometer to the other. Inflate esophageal balloon to 25–35 mm. Hg. Clamp esophageal balloon.	8. Maintains enough pressure to tamponade bleeding while preventing esophageal necrosis.
9. Apply suction to gastric aspiration opening. Irrigate at least hourly.	9. Suctioning and irrigating the tube can remove old blood from the stomach and prevent hepatic encephalopathy; allows monitoring of bleeding status.

(continued)

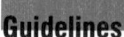 **Guidelines** Using Balloon Tamponade to Control Esophageal Bleeding
(Sengstaken–Blakemore Tube Method; Minnesota Tube Method) *(continued)*

Procedure *(continued)*	**Nursing Action**	**Rationale/Amplification**
	10. **[If using Senstaken–Blakemore tube]** Insert a nasogastric tube, positioning it above the esophageal balloon and attach to suction.	To suction saliva accumulated above the esophageal balloon, which may be aspirated, and to check for bleeding above the esophageal balloon
	[If using a Minnesota tube] Attach fourth port, esophageal suction port, to suction.	
	11. Label each port.	11. To prevent accidental deflation or irrigation.
	12. Tape scissors to head of bed.	12. Airway occlusion may occur if the esophageal balloon is pulled into the hypopharynx. If this occurs, the esophageal balloon tube must be cut and removed immediately.

Nursing Responsibilities

1. Maintain *constant* vigilance while balloons are inflated in the patient.
2. Keep balloon pressures at required level to control bleeding. (Clamps help to maintain pressure.)
3. Observe and record vital signs; monitor color and amount of nasogastric lavage fluid (subtracting lavage input) for evidence of bleeding.
4. Be alert for chest pain—may indicate injury or rupture of esophagus.
5. Irrigate suction tube as prescribed; observe and record nature and color of aspirated material.
6. Keep head of bed elevated to avoid gastric regurgitation and to diminish nausea and a sensation of gagging.
7. Maintain nutritional and electrolyte levels parenterally.
8. Maintain nasogastric suction or suction to esophageal suction port to aspirate any collected saliva.
9. Note nature of breathing; if counterweight pulls the tube into oropharynx, the patient may be asphyxiated.

NURSING ALERT: Keep a pair of scissors taped to the head of the bed. In the event of *acute respiratory distress*, use the scissors to cut across tubing (to deflate both balloons) and remove tubing.

Note: This procedure should be reserved for patients who are known, without a doubt, to be bleeding from esophageal varices, and in whom all forms of conservative therapy have failed.

Diseases of the Biliary *(Gallbladder)* System

Cholelithiasis, Cholecystitis, Choledocholithiasis

A. Cholelithiasis—stones in the gallbladder

1. Cholesterol gallstones
   a. Most common type found in the United States
   b. Occurs when cholesterol supersaturates the bile in the gallbladder, which crystallizes, eventually forming stones.
2. Pigment stones
   a. Composed primarily of calcium bilirubinate
   b. Occurs when free bilirubin combines with calcium.

B. Cholecystitis—inflammation of the gallbladder

1. Acute
   a. Most cases caused by gallstone obstruction of the cystic duct causing edema, inflammation, and frequently, bacterial invasion.
2. Chronic
   a. Gallbladder becomes thickened, rigid, fibrotic, and functions poorly.
   b. Results from repeated attacks of cholecystitis, presence of calculi, or chronic irritation.

C. Choledocholithiasis—stones in the common bile duct

Incidence

1. An estimated 25 million people in the United States have gallstones; one million new cases are discovered each year.
2. Women develop the disease more frequently than men; increases with age and multiparity.
3. More than one half million cholecystectomies are done annually.

Risk Factors

A. Cholesterol Gallstones

1. Obesity
2. Use of estrogen and oral contraceptives
3. Bile acid malabsorption (e.g., regional enteritis)
4. Genetic predisposition
5. Rapid weight loss
6. Cholesterol-lowering drugs (e.g., clofibrate)

B. Pigment Gallstones

1. Chronic hemolysis (e.g., hemolytic anemia)
2. Chronic liver disease

3. Biliary infection
4. Obstruction of the gallbladder or the bile ducts

Clinical Manifestations

1. Gallstones that remain in the gallbladder are usually asymptomatic.
2. Biliary colic
   a. Steady, severe aching pain or sensation of pressure in the epigastrium or right upper quadrant, which may radiate to the right scapular area or right shoulder
   b. Begins suddenly and persists for 1–3 hours until the stone falls back into the gallbladder or is passed through the cystic duct.
3. Acute cholecystitis
   a. Biliary colic pain that persists more than 4–6 hours, increases with movement, including respirations.
   b. Nausea and vomiting.
   c. Low-grade fever.
   d. Jaundice may be present with stones or inflammation of the common bile duct.
   e. Right upper quadrant guarding and Murphy's sign (inability to take a deep inspiration when examiner's fingers are pressed below the hepatic margin)
4. *Chronic cholecystitis*
   a. Heartburn, flatulence, indigestion
   b. Repeated attacks of symptoms resembling acute cholecystitis

Diagnostic Evaluation

1. Oral cholecystography—x-ray examination to determine those patients who are candidates for medical therapies.
   a. An initial film is obtained to determine the presence of calcium in stones—a condition that is less likely to respond to medical therapy.
   b. An iodized contrast media is administered orally or intravenously, increasing the density of bile, causing cholesterol stones to float to the top of the gallbladder—a criteria for medical management.

> **NURSING ALERT:** Cholecystography is ineffective in the jaundiced patient because the liver cells in this situation cannot transport contrast medium to the biliary tract.

   c. A fatty meal eaten during the procedure allows visualization of gallbladder contraction and emptying.
2. Ultrasonography—to detect the presence of gallstones and wall thickening
3. Cholescintigraphy—to determine filling of the gallbladder
4. Endoscopic retrograde cholangiopancreatography (ERCP) (shown in Fig. 21-3)
   a. Allows visualization of pancreatic ducts, bile ducts, and biopsy of the periampullary area
   b. Used to determine presence of common bile duct stones, and occasionally their removal
5. Laboratory values
   a. Elevated serum amylase—may indicate concomitant pancreatic involvement or stones in the common bile duct.
   b. Elevated white blood cell count—reflects inflammation.

Management

A. General Management

1. Nasogastric intubation—to decompress the gastrointestinal tract
2. Fluid and electrolyte replacement therapy—to correct dehydration and imbalances
3. Pain management—to promote comfort
4. Antibiotic therapy in the presence of a positive culture

B. Surgical Management

1. *Cholecystectomy*
   a. Removal of the gallbladder
   b. Done in situations of acute or chronic cholecystitis.
   c. The common bile duct may be explored in this procedure by either cholangiogram or choledochoscopy.
2. *Cholangiography*
   Contrast medium is injected directly into the biliary tree for vizualization.
3. *Choledochoscopy*
   a. A rigid or flexible scope is passed into the common bile duct to allow direct inspection for stones, tumors, strictures, or cholangitis.
   b. Stones can be removed with a wire basket or balloon.
   c. Endoscopic sphincterotomy may be performed on strictures.
   d. Biopsy obtained of suspicious tissue
4. A T-tube may be inserted through a choledochostomy
   a. To decompress the biliary tree and allow for postoperative T-tube cholangiogram.

C. Dissolution Therapy for Cholesterol Stones

1. Oral therapy with chenodeoxycholic acid, ursodeoxycholic acid, or a combination of both—to decrease the size of existing stones or dissolve small ones.
   a. Indicated for patients at high risk for surgery because of age or systemic disease.
   b. Major adverse effects include diarrhea, abnormal liver function tests, increases in serum cholesterol.
2. Direct contact therapy—a local cholelitholytic agent is repeatedly injected and aspirated from the gallbladder via a percutaneous transhepatic catheter.
   a. Indicated for symptomatic, high-risk patients whose gallbladder can be visualized on oral cholecystography.
   b. Side effects include pain from the catheter, nausea, transient elevations of liver function tests and white blood cell count.

D. Extracorporeal Shock Wave Lithotripsy—use of shock waves for noninvasive destruction of stones in the biliary system.

1. Indicated for symptomatic, high-risk patients with few noncalcified cholesterol stones
2. Patients lie prone on a water bag, interfaced with conductive gel, over a lithotriptor—ultrasound is used for stone localization and continuous monitoring of stone disintegration (Fig. 21-2).
3. Strong analgesics and sedatives are administered to reduce the pain and discomfort of the shock waves.
4. Treatment is followed with oral dissolution therapy to remove incompletely pulverized stone fragments.

Complications of Cholecystitis

1. Cholangitis
2. Necrosis, empyema, or perforation of the gallbladder

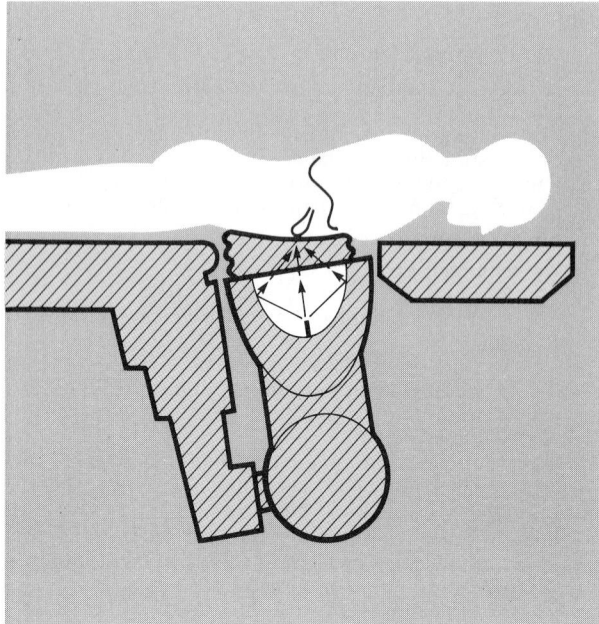

Figure 21-2. *Biliary lithotripsy. The patient lies on top of the machine. Water amplifies shock waves generated by the firing of a spark plug; waves then enter the body and crush the gallstone. (Reprinted with permission from the Summer 1989 issue of Helix, the University of Virginia Health Sciences Center quarterly magazine. Copyright 1989)*

3. Biliary fistula through the duodenum
4. Gallstone ileus
5. Adenocarcinoma of the gallbladder

Nursing Assessment

1. Assess patient's pain for location, description, intensity, relieving and exacerbating factors.
2. Assess for signs of dehydration: dry mucous membranes; poor skin turgor; low urine output with elevated specific gravity.
3. Monitor and record intake and output, including emesis and nasogastric drainage.
4. Monitor temperature and white blood cell count for indications of infection or perforation.
5. Evaluate serum electrolytes and bilirubin levels for abnormalities.

Nursing Diagnoses

1. Pain related to biliary colic or stone obstruction, surgical incision, extracorporeal shock wave lithotripsy.
2. Potential for fluid volume deficit related to preoperative nausea and vomiting, decreased intake, prolonged nasogastric intubation.
3. Potential for impaired skin integrity related to surgical incision, fluid and electrolyte changes, T-tube or drainage tube, jaundice.

Other nursing diagnoses could include:

4. Potential for infection related to inflammation, necrosis, or perforation of the gallbladder
5. Knowledge deficit of new procedures, surgery, or nonsurgical management.

Nursing Interventions

A. Promoting Comfort and Rest

1. Administer meperidine hydrochloride as prescribed (morphine sulfate may cause spasm of the sphincter of Oddi and exacerbate pain).
2. Evaluate and record response to pain medication.
3. Assist in attaining position of comfort.
4. Provide for uninterrupted rest.

B. Attaining Adequate Fluid and Electrolyte Status

1. Administer intravenous fluids during periods of restriction of oral intake as prescribed.
2. Administer electrolytes as necessary.
3. Administer prescribed antiemetics as necessary—to decrease nausea and vomiting; evaluate and record response.
4. Reintroduce food and fluids gradually, as tolerated, after acute symptoms subside or postoperatively.
5. Observe and record amount and character of T-tube drainage, if applicable.
6. Position drainage bottle from T-tube as directed. The bottle may be elevated to prevent total bile loss; allow bile drainage only as pressure develops in the biliary system, promoting normal bile flow through the common bile duct.

C. Maintaining Skin Integrity

1. Assist in changing position frequently.
2. Relieve pressure on pressure points: foam mattress; heel protectors; massage—to promote comfort and prevent skin breakdown.
3. Inspect cholecystectomy incision for warmth, erythema, drainage, or breakdown—to detect early any signs of infection.
4. Protect skin around incision site from bile seepage.
   a. Change the dressings frequently to provide for absorption of drainage; Montgomery straps may facilitate dressing changes.
   b. Apply protective skin pastes or use drainage pouches to prevent the bile drainage from contacting and excoriating the skin.
5. Position patient in low to semi-Fowler's position to enhance bile drainage.
6. Observe color changes in skin, sclerae, and stool, which will indicate whether bile pigment is disappearing from blood and draining again into the duodenum.
   a. Note color and consistency of all stools; chart an accurate description.
   b. Send specimens of urine and stool to the laboratory at frequent intervals for examination of bile pigments.
   c. Observe skin and sclerae for yellowish color, which would indicate bile-flow obstruction.

Discharge Planning/Patient Education

1. Discuss the importance of a high-protein, carbohydrate, low-fat diet.
2. Avoid foods that cause dyspepsia, flatulence, loose stools.
3. Review dosage, side effects, and implications of medications, particularly oral dissolution therapy.
4. Emphasize symptoms of complications to be reported: pain; fever; jaundice; pale-colored stools; dark urine; pruritus.
5. Encourage follow-up visits to the physician.

Evaluation

1. Reports decrease in level and frequency of pain; states adequate rest and comfort.
2. Achieves adequate hydration; skin turgor normal and mucous membranes moist; vital signs are stable; laboratory values are within normal limits.
3. Skin is dry and intact; no signs of erythema or breakdown around incision or drainage site; tube remains patent.

Guidelines   Endoscopic Retrograde Cholangiopancreatography (ERCP)

A fiberoptic endoscope (a side-viewing instrument) is placed in the descending duodenum so that the ampulla of Vater can be located and cannulated (Fig. 21-3).

In this examination, both the common and pancreatic ducts may be injected with contrast media to visualize the hepatobiliary tree and pancreatic ducts radiologically.

The clinician is able to diagnose abnormalities of the ductal system, detect disease processes, and obtain direct secretory information, as well as cells for cytologic examination.

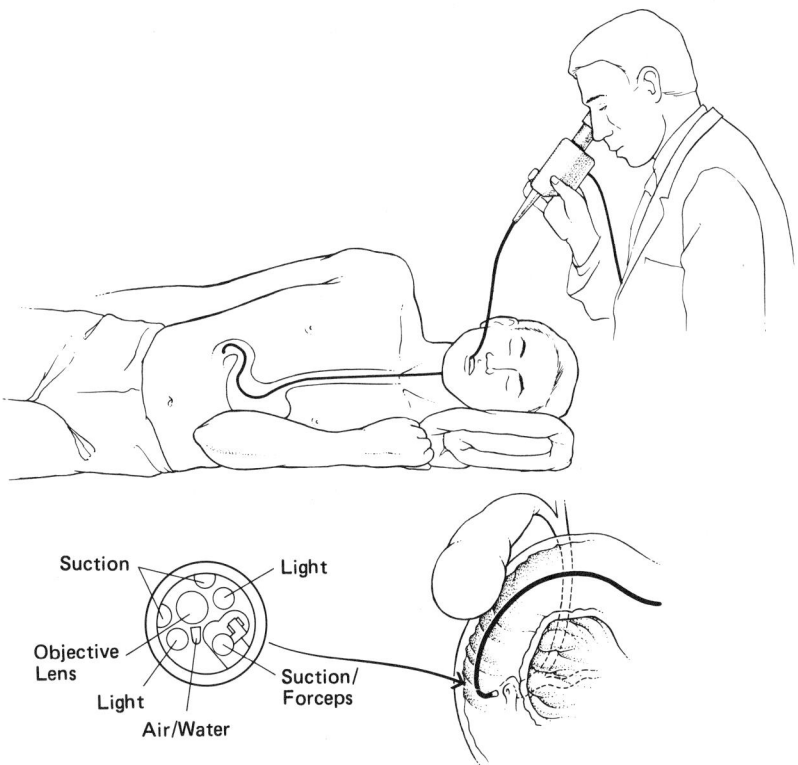

Figure 21-3. *Endoscopic retrograde cholangiopancreatography (ERCP). The patient is moved from left lateral to prone position as the flexible scope is passed. The circle on the left shows the tip of the scope; the objective lens is the viewing section assisted by two side lights. Air or water may be directed to an area, and suction is available. If a biopsy is to be taken, a separate channel is available. The lower right diagram shows the scope nearing the ampulla of Vater; the scope is in the duodenum; gallbladder is the topmost sac—note the biliary and common bile ducts.*

Indications

1. Biliary disease

2. Pancreatic disease

3. To diagnose:
   Cancer of the papilla
   Obstructive jaundice
   Calculus disease, pre- and postcholecystectomy
   Carcinoma of biliary ducts
   Carcinoma of pancreas
   Pancreatitis

(continued)

Guidelines Endoscopic Retrograde Cholangiopancreatography (ERCP) *(continued)*

Contraindications	1. Acute cardiorespiratory disease
	2. Acute recent attack of pancreatitis (within 3 weeks) because of risk of inducing another attack
	3. Stricture or obstruction of esophagus or duodenum
	4. Acute cholangitis
Equipment	A side-viewing duodenoscope*
	Sterilized cannula
Considerations	1. ERCP is not a simple endoscopic procedure; it must be done by a skillful, well-trained physician.
	2. There are certain risks, described below:
	a. After ERCP, a very small percentage of patients develop clinical pancreatitis, which may last 1–3 days.
	b. The patient may retain contrast material injected proximal to an obstructed duct; this may result in cholangitis or pancreatitis. Such a patient should be given broad-spectrum antibiotics; surgical drainage may be indicated.
	c. A very few patients are sensitive to iodinated compounds.
	d. The more experienced the team in performing ERCPs, the fewer the complications and the better the success rate.

Procedure

Nursing Action	Physician's Role	Rationale/Amplification
Preparatory Phase		
1. Be sure that consent form is signed and noted on the patient's chart.	1. Obtain informed consent.	
2. Remind the patient to take nothing by mouth after midnight.	2. Collaborate with nurse in patient preparation.	2. Limited intake produces a basal condition with reduced body secretions; this permits better visualization of tissues.
3. Explain contemplated examination to patient; discuss possibilities of after effects		
4. Determine the patient's sensitivity to iodine (or fish, which contains iodine) or any other medication.		4. A few patients are sensitive to iodine preparations (Hypaque sodium).
5. Take and record vital signs.		5. This information becomes a baseline for later comparison.
6. Offer the patient 3 ml. of tetracaine (Pontocaine) to be used as a gargle and swallow.	6. Prescribe topical anesthetic.	6. Tetracaine is an oropharyngeal topical anesthetic.
7. Intravenous infusion may be started, for administration of medications.	7. Start an intravenous infusion with normal saline.	7. This becomes the avenue for direct intravenous medications such as diazepam (Valium) and meperidine (Demerol) to promote relaxation; atropine to reduce oral secretions, prior to insertion of duodenoscope.
8. Instruct the patient to remove dentures; a mouthpiece is inserted.		8. To facilitate insertion of scope.
Performance Phase		
1. Place the patient in left lateral position.	1. Scope is passed through the patient's mouth into esophagus and stomach.	1. Anatomy is carefully examined as the scope advances.
2. Administer prescribed IV medication, which may include meperidine, diazepam, atropine, or glucagon.	2. Gently advance tip through pyloric ring into duodenal bulb and into descending duodenum.	2. Atropine will produce a hypotonic duodenum and relaxed sphincter at ampulla of Vater; secretion will be reduced.
	3. Minimal air insufflation used to search for the ampulla of Vater.	3. Unless this is obstructed by tumor, it can usually be identified with careful search.
4. Place the patient in prone position. (This provides the radiologist with a better position for fluoroscopy and radiography).	4. Administer glucagon.	4. Glucagon is given to further reduce duodenal motility.

* This duodenoscope is 125 cm. long and 1 cm. in diameter. Visual fields are oriented 90 degrees to its long axis. It includes a channel through which a cannula or biopsy forceps can be passed under direct vision.

Procedure *(continued)*	**Nursing Action**	**Physician's Role**	**Rationale/Amplification**
	5. Prepare a special radiopaque Teflon cannulation tube by filling it with contrast medium (to eliminate air).	5. When cannulation tubing is in correct position, contrast medium is slowly injected: 3–5 ml. for pancreatic ductal system; 15–20 ml. for biliary ductal system.	5. Cannulation tube is passed through biopsy channel of scope. Contrast medium is warmed to body temperature. Tube is advanced under fluoroscopy. X-ray pictures are taken while patient is in prone position following injection of contrast medium.
	6. Upon completion of film-taking, turn patient to lateral position. Draw blood sample for serum amylase determination. Use suction to remove oropharyngeal secretions.	6. Keep scope and cannula in place and patient in prone position until films are completed. If films are satisfactory any contrast dye spilled in the stomach and duodenum is removed by suction, and scope is carefully removed.	6. Await return and reading of films.
	Follow-up Phase		
	1. Check vital signs every 4 hours. Notify family as to when the patient will return to his room.		1. Postcannulation patient may experience a temperature rise, chills, abdominal pain. Report these responses to physician.
	2. In the absence of complications, permit the patient to eat in 2–4 hours (light diet); permit a full diet the next day.		2. A mild rise in serum amylase is observed in a high percentage of patients.
	3. Watch for palpitations related to atropine sulfate injection. Also watch for respiratory depression and transient hypotension.		3. Some patients experience mild to severe epigastric pain, nausea, and vomiting. These discomforts are usually transitory.

Conditions of the Pancreas

Acute Pancreatitis

Acute pancreatitis is an inflammation of the pancreas, ranging from mild edema to extensive hemorrhage, resulting from a variety of injuries.

Etiology

1. Excessive alcohol consumption—most common cause in the United States.
2. Biliary tract disease—cholelithiasis (gallstones), acute or chronic cholecystitis, or cholangitis.
3. Less common causes: hyperlipidemia; blunt abdominal trauma; hypercalcemia secondary to hyperparathyroidism or multiple myeloma; various infections; and some drug therapies (estrogens, thiazide diuretics, sulfonamides).

Pathology

1. Although exact mechanisms are not completely understood, autodigestion of all or part of the gland, provoked by premature activation of pancreatic enzymes from acinar cells, is involved.
2. Activation may be initiated by:
   a. Toxic effects of ethanol and its major metabolite, acetaldehyde, on acinar cells and ducts
   b. Obstruction of the ampulla of Vater or common bile duct
   c. Reflux of bile into the pancreatic duct
   d. Ischemia
   e. Stimulation of vasoactive substances—kallikrein, bradykinin, and prostaglandins

Clinical Manifestations

(Depends on severity of pancreatic damage)
1. Abdominal pain, usually constant in nature, midepigastric or periumbilical, radiating to back or flank
2. Nausea and vomiting
3. Low-grade fever
4. Involuntary abdominal guarding, epigastric tenderness to deep palpation, reduced or absent bowel sounds
5. Dry mucous membranes and tachycardia; may reflect mild to moderate dehydration from vomiting or capillary leak syndrome (third space loss)
6. Shock may be the presenting manifestation in most severe episodes
7. Purplish discoloration of the flanks (Turner's sign) or of the periumbilical area (Cullen's sign)—occurs in extensive hemorrhagic necrosis.

Diagnostic Evaluation

1. Laboratory determinations
   a. Serum amylase—often elevated 5–40 times upper limits of normal—increases early but declines to normal rapidly (24–72 hours).
   b. Urine amylase level—elevation persists longer than elevation of serum amylase.
   c. Serum lipase—elevation occurs in the same disorders that elevate serum amylase; its increase

persists longer than serum amylase in acute episodes of pancreatitis.
d. Elevations in the serum levels of the following occur in pancreatitis: glucose; bilirubin; alkaline phosphatase; lactic dehydrogenase; aspartate transferase/alanine transferase; potassium; and cholesterol—due to release of glucagon, low levels of insulin, and tissue damage.
e. Serum levels of the following are abnormally low in pancreatitis: albumin; calcium; sodium; and magnesium—due to dehydration, vomiting, and the binding of calcium in areas of fat necrosis.
2. Imaging studies
a. Radiographs of the chest and abdomen support the diagnosis with presence of pulmonary infiltrates, pleural effusion, pancreatic calcification, or peripancreatic gas of a pancreatic abscess.
b. Ultrasonography and computed tomography (CT) scan, with or without intravenous contrast injection, can determine some pancreatic changes and rule out alternative etiologies.

Management

(Depends on severity of episode; focused on alleviation of symptoms and support of patient to prevent complications)
1. Restoration of circulating blood volume with intravenous crystalloid or colloid solutions or blood products—to replace third space fluid loss or hemorrhage and prevent shock.
2. Maintenance of adequate oxygenation—reduced by pain, anxiety, acidosis, abdominal pressure, or pleural effusions.
3. Pain control with meperidine (Demerol)—to alleviate pain and anxiety, which increases pancreatic secretions.
4. Rest of the gastrointestinal tract
a. Withhold oral feedings to decrease pancreatic secretions
b. Nasogastric intubation and suction to relieve gastric stasis and distention, and ileus
5. Maintenance of gastric pH with H_2 antagonists and antacids to remove acid drive to pancreatic secretions and prevent stress ulcer complications of acute illness
6. Maintenance of adequate nutrition with parenteral feedings when on prolonged status of nothing by mouth and to reverse prior malnutrition states
7. Pharmacotherapy
a. Electrolyte replacements, if necessary
b. Sodium bicarbonate to reverse metabolic acidosis
c. Regular insulin to treat hyperglycemia
d. Antibiotic therapy in the presence of suspected infection or sepsis
8. Surgical intervention
a. Considered if all other therapy is ineffective, complications occur, or in the presence of gallstone-related pancreatitis
b. Procedures range from incision and drainage of infection and pseudocysts to extensive debridement or pancreatectomy to remove necrotic pancreatic tissue

Complications

1. Pancreatic abscess
2. Pancreatic pseudocyst
3. Respiratory compromise and adult respiratory distress syndrome
4. Hemorrhage with hypovolemic shock
5. Sepsis
6. Acute renal failure

Nursing Interventions

A. Attaining Adequate Fluid and Electrolyte Levels

1. Monitor and record vital signs, skin color and temperature, and urinary output for signs of decreased cardiac output.
2. Measure and record episodes of vomiting; administer antiemetics as prescribed.
3. Evaluate laboratory data; hemoglobin, hematocrit, albumin, calcium, potassium, sodium, and magnesium levels; administer replacement as prescribed.
4. Assess for behaviors reflective of hypocalcemia: neuromuscular irritability; nausea; vomiting; abdominal pain; or a positive Chvostek's sign—facial twitching after a tap over the facial nerve.
5. Assess for behaviors reflective of hypokalemia—potassium is a major cation in pancreatic juice: muscle weakness; hyporeflexia; hypotension; respiratory muscle weakness; ECG changes; apathy or irritability.

B. Maintaining Effective Breathing Pattern

1. Assess respirations and monitor arterial blood gas levels to determine effectiveness of respiration.
2. Monitor for signs of respiratory distress: tachypnea; dyspnea; intercostal retractions or use of accessory muscles; diminished breath sounds, particularly in lung bases; presence of crackles.
3. Position in upright or semi-Fowler's position to enhance diaphragmatic excursion.
4. Administer oxygen supplementation as prescribed to maintain adequate oxygen levels.

C. Attaining Comfort and Rest

1. Mild pain: Instruct the patient to sit up or lean over a bedside stand to alleviate visceral discomfort.
2. Administer meperidine (Demerol) as prescribed for episodes of pain, which cause increased metabolism, stimulating pancreatic enzymes.
3. Provide for periods of rest with a quiet environment and maximal time between nursing care activities to decrease metabolic rate.
4. Provide frequent oral care while NPO.

D. Assuring Adequate Nutrition

1. Assess nutritional status based on prior medical history and status of nothing by mouth.
2. Evaluate laboratory data to determine abnormalities that reflect pancreatitis and need for intervention.
3. Administer replacements of albumin and regular insulin therapy, as prescribed.
4. Administer prescribed total parenteral nutrition, using aseptic technique, closely monitoring blood glucose levels.
5. Administer H_2 antagonists and antacids as prescribed, monitoring gastric pH if nasogastric intubation is required—to prevent gastric acidity and ulcer formation.
6. Monitor frequently for the presence of bowel sounds; administer carbohydrate enteral feedings with supplementation, progressively adding proteins and fats, as indicated.
7. Monitor for recurrent signs of nausea and vomiting—early introduction of enteral feedings can result in a relapse.

Discharge Planning/Patient Education

1. Instruct the patient as follows:
   a. Gradually resume normal diet.
   b. Gradually increase normal activities, providing for daily rest periods.
2. If the pancreatitis resulted from excessive alcohol intake, discuss with the patient and family the benefits of abstinence; offer the names of support organizations (Alcoholics Anonymous).

Chronic Pancreatitis

Chronic Pancreatitis is defined as the persistence of pancreatic cellular damage and decreased pancreatic exocrine function.

Etiology

1. Alcohol abuse
2. Less common causes: hyperparathyroidism; hereditary pancreatitis; malnutrition; trauma to the pancreas

Clinical Manifestations

1. Pain
   a. Located in the epigastrium or left upper quadrant, often radiating to the back
   b. Similar to that observed in acute pancreatitis
   c. Pain is intense and constant, occurring at unpredictable intervals, often lasting for several days
2. Weight loss results from decreased intake secondary to anorexia and fear that eating will precipitate a painful attack.
3. Malabsorption, steatorrhea, and diarrhea—typically occurs late in the disease progression.
4. Diabetes with glucose intolerance

Diagnostic Evaluation

1. *Laboratory studies:* serum amylase and lipase—to determine decreased pancreatic enzyme excretion
2. *Pancreatic function tests*—evaluates direct decrease in exocrine functions and indirect abnormalities secondary to malabsorption.
   a. Secretin and CCK stimulatory tests to evaluate pancreatic exocrine function.
   b. Fecal fat analysis to evaluate steatorrhea, cause of weight loss, and need for pancreatic enzyme replacement.
3. *Computed tomography* (CT) or ultrasonography (US) to identify pancreatic structural changes—calcifications, masses, ductal irregularities, enlargement, and cysts
4. *Endoscopic retrograde cholangiopancreatography* (ERCP)—to define ductal anatomy and localize complications: pancreatic pseudocysts; ductal leaks

Management

1. Pain management—to promote comfort—with pancreatic enzyme replacement and analgesics
2. Maintenance of adequate nutrition with pancreatic enzyme replacement and nutritional supplementation with elemental preparations to reduce steatorrhea, enhance absorption, and reverse malnutrition.

3. Surgical interventions—to reduce pain, correct structural abnormalities, and manage complications
   a. Procedures range from sphincteroplasty to total pancreatectomy, depending on the extent of pathology and purpose of surgery.
   b. Postoperative complications include: fistula formation; abscess; common bile duct obstruction; and pseudocysts.

Complications

1. Pancreatic pseudocyst
2. Pancreatic ascites and pleural effusions
3. Gastrointestinal hemorrhage
4. Biliary tract obstruction

Nursing Interventions

A. Attaining Comfort

1. Assess and record the character, location, frequency, and duration of pain.
2. Determine precipitating and alleviating factors of the patient's pain.
3. Explore the impact of the pain on the patient's lifestyle and eating habits.
4. Administer analgesics as prescribed.
   - The patient may be drug dependent because of recurring episodes of severe pain, requiring careful assessment and management.

B. Assuring Adequate Nutrition

1. Assess nutritional status, history of weight loss and dietary habits, including alcohol intake.
2. Administer pancreatic enzyme replacement with meals, as prescribed. Administer antacids or H_2 receptor antagonists to prevent neutralization of enzyme supplements, as indicated.
3. Monitor daily weight.
4. Evaluate laboratory data reflecting pancreatic abnormalities.
5. Assess for diarrhea, bloating, steatorrhea, which may indicate inadequate enzyme replacement.
6. Monitor blood glucose levels and assess for signs and symptoms of onset of diabetes: polyuria; polydipsia; polyphagia; weakness.
7. Encourage intake of low-fat diet and prescribed nutritional supplementation.

Discharge Planning/Patient Education

1. Instruct the patient regarding use and side effects of analgesics and pancreatic enzyme replacement.
2. Inform the patient and family of the potential complications of chronic pancreatitis, signs and symptoms, and importance of health care follow-up.
3. Discuss with the patient and family the importance of abstinence from alcohol if it precipitated the chronic pancreatitis.

Pancreatic Pseudocysts and Abscesses

Pancreatic pseudocysts and abscesses are collections of inflammatory fluid located in or around the pancreas, resulting from local necrosis secondary to acute or chronic pancreatitis.

Clinical Manifestations and Pathophysiology

1. Abdominal pain.
2. History of chronic or acute pancreatitis.
3. Cysts may attain considerable size; they develop rapidly or slowly (within 72 hours or over several weeks or months).
4. Because they occur in the posterior peritoneum, they may exert pressure against the stomach or colon, visible on barium studies.
5. Persistent elevation of amylase (serum or urine) is the most common finding. Pain and vomiting may occur.
6. Leukocytosis and fever are common, but are usually mild with pseudocysts; these responses are more striking with abscess formation.

Diagnostic Evaluation

1. Abdominal ultrasound
2. Computed tomography (CT) scan
3. Endoscopic retrograde cholangiopancreatography (ERCP)

Complications

1. Infection
2. Rupture of pseudocyst
3. Hemorrhage

Management

1. Pseudocysts may occasionally subside spontaneously.
2. Drainage performed endoscopically (internal) or percutaneously (external) guided by ultrasound
3. Surgery may be required to evacuate pseudocysts or abscesses with external drain placement when size or location contraindicate other forms of drainage.
4. Antibiotic therapy in the presence of positive cultures to control infection

Nursing Interventions

A. Monitoring and Preventing Complications

1. Monitor vital signs and pain to identify onset of infection, rupture, or hemorrhage.
2. Administer analgesics and antibiotics as prescribed.
3. Should external drainage be done, recognize the irritating qualities of the pancreatic enzyme; meticulous skin care is required. Refer to enterostomal therapist to recommend skin protection.
4. Maintain adequate drainage, avoiding tube dislodgment.

Pancreatic Cancer

Cancer of the pancreas may arise in the head (70%) or body and tail (30%) of the pancreas (Fig. 21-4); ductal adenocarcinoma is the most common (80%); most cancers are in the exocrine portion of the pancreas (95%), whereas few occur in the islet cells.

Epidemiology

1. Incidence is increasing.
2. Occurs more frequently in males between the ages of 60 and 80.
3. Smoking and prolonged exposure to industrial chemicals are considered risk factors.
4. High-fat diet, excessive alcohol intake, diabetes mellitus, and chronic pancreatitis are associated with the incidence.

Clinical Manifestations

1. Symptoms are often vague and nonspecific, creating problems in early detection.
2. Weight loss, pain, anorexia, nausea, vomiting, and weakness
3. Pain usually occurs in upper abdomen, visceral in nature, gnawing or boring; may radiate to the back.
   a. Pain is often worse at night, aggravated in recumbent position, and relieved by lying with legs drawn up or by bending over while walking.
   b. Pain becomes more localized, severe, and unremitting as disease progresses.
4. Early satiety; feeling of bloating after meals
5. Jaundice, dark-colored urine, light-colored stool, and pruritus occur when pancreatic cancer in the head of the gland occludes the common bile duct.
6. Depression and lethargy
7. May report recent diagnosis of diabetes mellitus

Diagnostic Evaluation

1. Ultrasonography and computed tomography (CT) most useful noninvasive tests to determine tumors larger than 2 cm.
2. Endoscopic retrograde cholangiopancreatography (ERCP) with biopsy and secretin stimulation test
3. Laboratory studies: liver function tests; coagulation studies; and carcinoembryonic antigen (CEA) to determine liver and common bile duct involvement, and to verify presence of cancer
4. Percutaneous needle aspiration or biopsy via ultrasonography—tumor seeding can occur along the needle tract.

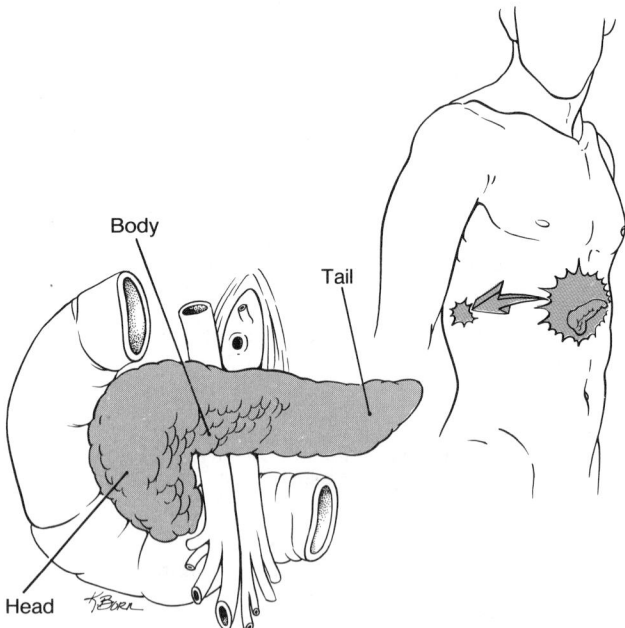

Figure 21-4. *Cancer may arise in the head or body and tail of the pancreas. Because the symptoms are often vague and nonspecific, the diagnosis is difficult. Pain in the midepigastrium radiating to the back and weight loss may be encountered.*

Management

1. The goal of treatment may be cure or palliation, depending on the staging of the tumor. Symptomatic patients are usually too advanced in their disease progression for cure.
2. Surgery
   a. Whipple procedure (pancreaticoduodenectomy)—removal of head (sometimes adjacent neck), adjacent stomach, distal portion of the common bile duct, and duodenum, possibly the gallbladder—for carcinoma of the head or periampullary area
   b. Total pancreatectomy—en bloc resection of the pancreas, duodenum, gastric antrum, bile duct, gallbladder, spleen, and peripancreatic nodes—for large or diffuse carcinoma
   c. Distal pancreatectomy—removal of the distal pancreas and spleen—for tumors localized in the body or tail
3. Radiation therapy—may be used alone palliatively or as adjuvant to surgery
   a. External beam irradiation—for local control, reduction of pain, and to palliate obstruction
   b. Intraoperative radiation therapy has been successful in some centers for palliation.
4. Chemotherapy may be used in combination with radiation therapy for unresectable lesions.
5. Endoscopic stent placement for relief of biliary obstruction
6. Chemical splanchnicectomy (excision of a section of the greater splanchnic nerve)—for relief of pain
7. Clinical investigations combining various treatments are aimed at improving the prognosis of pancreatic cancer.

Complications

1. Preoperatively: malnutrition; biliary obstruction with jaundice; gastroduodenal obstruction; metastases
2. Postoperatively: hyperglycemia; breakdown of surgical anastomoses; infection; pancreatic fistula; gastric retention; paralytic ileus; bowel obstruction; diabetes mellitus; malabsorption syndrome; injury by radiation to surrounding organs

Nursing Assessment

1. Assess for signs and symptoms of malnutrition, including diet history, anorexia, weight loss, nausea and vomiting, steatorrhea, skin turgor.
2. Evaluate laboratory values for alterations in glucose, liver function, and coagulation studies.
3. Assess patient's pain for location, description, duration, and palliative measures.
4. Note color, consistency, and frequency of stools.
5. Assess skin for color, ecchymosis, bleeding, and pruritus.
6. Assess psychosocial status to determine presence of depression, usual coping strategies, support systems, and experience with past serious illness.
7. Assess cognitive and psychomotor abilities to determine ability to provide self-care during a complex rehabilitation plan.

Nursing Diagnoses

1. Altered nutrition (less than body requirements) related to nausea, vomiting, anorexia, decreased absorption, pain, postoperative complications
2. Potential for fluid volume deficit related to preoperative hypoproteinemia, prolonged nasogastric intubation, leakage of anastomoses, or postoperative hemorrhage
3. Pain related to pancreatic tumor, surgical incision
4. Potential for impaired tissue integrity related to malnutrition, pruritus, postoperative pancreatic bile or gastric secretion leakage, bedrest, radiation therapy

Nursing Interventions

A. Improving Nutritional Status

1. Administer total parenteral nutrition (TPN) as prescribed preoperatively and postoperatively.
2. Assess for bowel sounds; administer fluids per nasogastric tube, gastrostomy, or jejunostomy, as indicated.
3. Monitor blood glucose levels and administer insulin as prescribed.
4. Assess for signs and symptoms of hypo- and hyperglycemia.
5. Encourage advancing diet from liquids to low-fat, high-caloric diet.
6. Observe for nausea and vomiting.
7. Administer pancreatic enzyme replacements as prescribed, observing for steatorrhea, which may indicate inadequate dosage.

B. Attaining Adequate Fluid Volume and Decreasing Risk of Bleeding

1. Monitor vital signs frequently; record accurate intake and output of fluid.
2. Evaluate serum albumin levels and replace as prescribed.
3. Evaluate laboratory values for hyponatremia, hypokalemia, hypochloremia, hypocalcemia, and metabolic alkalosis; replace electrolytes as prescribed.
4. Administer fluid replacement as indicated.
5. Evaluate coagulation studies, which may indicate high risk for bleeding.
6. Monitor for signs and symptoms of hypovolemia.
7. Monitor for bleeding from tubes and drains; assess for bluish–brown discoloration of one or both flanks (Turner's sign), indicating retroperitioneal bleeding.
8. Administer vitamin K as prescribed—to increase synthesis of clotting factors.

C. Achieving Rest and Comfort

1. Position in semi-Fowler's position to lower the diaphragm and ease respiratory effort.
2. Administer analgesics as prescribed, noting level of relief.
3. Provide additional means of pain relief (e.g., distraction, relaxation exercises, massage).
4. Administer adjuvant analgesics and medications (e.g., antidepressants) as prescribed.

NURSING ALERT: Recognize that if the patient has not had a vagotomy, pain and anxiety increase pancreatic secretions, increasing risk of leakage of anastomoses sites.

D. Attaining/Maintaining Tissue Integrity

1. Observe skin and control pruritus.
   a. Provide frequent skin care without soap.
   b. Apply soothing lotions such as calamine.
   c. Keep fingernails short to prevent scratching.
   d. Protect skin with skin barriers and ostomy bags

from leakage of enzymes and other fluids from drains and tubes.
 e. Contact enterostomal therapist for assistance.
2. Prevent tension on suture lines of anastamoses.
 a. Maintain patency of surgically placed tubes and drains.
 b. Position in semi-Fowler's to enhance drainage.
 c. Irrigate nasogastric tube with no more than 20 ml. of air to maintain patency while preventing stress on suture line.

Discharge Teaching/Patient Education

1. Instruct patient and family on self-care measures for pancreatic insufficiency: glucose monitoring; insulin administration; signs and symptoms of hypo- and hyperglycemia; pancreatic enzyme replacement.
2. Instruct patient and family on self-care measures for wound and drain care.

3. Inform patient of reportable signs and symptoms of late complications (e.g., gastrointestinal bleeding, ulcerations) and recurrence.
4. Explore the options for pain management.
5. Offer referral for home care follow-up or hospice care.

Evaluation

1. Achieves adequate nutritional status; tolerates prescribed diet without nausea, vomiting, steatorrhea; reports absence of signs and symptoms of hypo/hyperglycemia.
2. Is adequately hydrated without bleeding; maintains stable vital signs; no signs of overt or occult bleeding; laboratory values remain within normal limits
3. Reports adequate rest and comfort
4. Skin is clean, dry, and free of scratches; reports less itching; no evidence of erythema or breakdown around drainage sites; tubes and drains remain patent.

Bibliography

Books

Beger HG and Buchler M. Acute Pancreatitis. New York, Springer–Verlag, 1987

Boyer JL and Bianchi L (ed). Liver Cirrhosis. Lancaster, England, MTP Press Limited, 1987

Cass AS and Stahlgren LH. Principles of Biliary Lithotripsy. New York, Futura Publishing Company, 1989

Chopra S. Disorders of the Liver. Philadelphia, Lea & Febiger, 1988

Glazer G and Ranson JHC. Acute Pancreatitis: Experimental and Clinical Aspects of Pathogenesis and Management. London, Bailliere Tindall, 1988

Gitnick G. Modern Concepts of Acute and Chronic Hepatitis. New York, Plenum, 1989

Gitnick G et al (eds). Principles and Practice of Gastroenterology and Hepatology. New York, Elsevier, 1988

Hathaway RG. Nursing Care of the Critically Ill Surgical Patient. Rockville, MD, Aspen Publishers, 1988

Kinney MR, Packa DR and Dunbar SB. AACN's Clinical Reference for Critical Care Nursing, 2nd ed. New York, McGraw–Hill, 1988

Lygidakas NJ and Tytgat GNJ (eds). Hepatobiliary and Pancreatic Malignancies: Diagnosis, Medical and Surgical Management. New York, Thieme–Stratton, 1989

MacSween RNM, Anthony PP and Scheur PJ. Pathology of the Liver. New York, Churchill Livingstone, 1987

Preece PE, Cuschieri A and Rosin RD (eds). Cancer of the Bile Ducts and Pancreas. Philadelphia, WB Saunders, 1989

Schiff W and Schiff ER. Diseases of the Liver, 6th ed. Philadelphia, JB Lippincott, 1987

Journals

Liver Disorders

Adinaro D. Liver failure and pancreatitis: Fluid and electrolyte concerns. Nurs Clin North Am 1987 Dec; 22(4):843–852

Anthony PP. Liver tumours. Baillieres Clin Gastroenterol 1988 Apr; 2(2):501–522

Breimer DD. Pharmacokinetics in liver disease. Pharm Weekbl [Sci] 1987 Apr 24; 9(2):79–84

Cox EF et al. Blunt trauma to the liver. Ann Surg 1988 Feb; 207(2):126–134

Davis M. Alcoholic liver injury, Proc Nutr Soc 1988 Jul; 47(2):115–120

Dindzans VJ, Schade RR and Van Thiel DH. Medical problems before and after transplantation. Gastroenterol Clin North Am 1988 Mar; 17(1):19–31

Emond JC et al. Liver transplantation in the management of fulminant hepatic failure. Gastroenterology 1989 Jun; 96(6): 1583–1588

Flowerdew A and Taylor I. Treatment of liver metastases of colorectal cancer. Recent Results Cancer Res 1988; 110: 150–163

Friedman LS and Maddrey WC. Surgery in the patient with liver disease. Med Clin North Am 1987 May; 71(3):453–476

Gilmore IT. Modern methods of diagnosis in liver disease. J R Coll Physicians Lond 1986 Jul; 20(3):201–205

Greenway B. Hepatic metastases from colorectal cancer: Resection or not. Br J Surg 1988 Jun; 75(6):513–519

Hiyama DT and Fischer JE. Nutritional support in hepatic failure. Nutr Clin Pract 1988 Jun; 3(3):96–105

Kalra V and Murali MV. Fulminant hepatic failure and hepatic encephalopathy. Indian Pediatr 1986 Oct; 23(Suppl):139–146

Keith JS. Hepatic failure: Etiologies, manifestations, and management. Crit Care Nurse 1985; 5(1):60–86

Kelly DA and Summerfield JA. Hemostasis in liver disease. Semin Liver Dis 1987 Aug; 7(3):182–191

Koneru B et al. Postoperative surgical complications. Gastroenterol Clin North Am 1988 Mar; 17(1):71–91

Lotze MT. Surgical management of hepatocellular carcinoma. Gastroenterol Clin North Am 1987 Dec; 16(4):613–626

Martinez AJ, Estol C and Faris AA. Neurologic complications of liver transplantation. Neurol Clin 1988 May; 6(2):327–348

Millis JM et al. The management of liver transplant recipients treated with cyclosporine. Transplant Proc 1988 Jun; 20(3 Suppl 3):405–419

Munoz SJ and Maddrey WC. Major complications of acute and chronic liver disease. Gastroenterol Clin North Am 1988 Jun; 17(2):265–287

Nerenstone S and Friedman M. Medical treatment of hepatocellular carcinoma. Gastroenterol Clin North Am 1987 Dec; 16(4):603–612

Nerenstone SR, Ihde DC and Friedman MA. Clinical trials in primary hepatocellular carcinoma: Current status and future directions. Cancer Treat Rev 1988 Mar; 15(1):1–31

Roberts JP et al. Liver transplantation today. Annu Rev Med 1989; 40:287–303

Roberts J and Tumer N. Pharmacodynamic basis for altered drug action in the elderly. Clin Geriatr Med 1988 Feb; 4(1):127–149

Scott RB and Mitchell MC. Aging, alcohol, and the liver. J Am Geriatr Soc 1988 Mar; 36(3):255–265

Secor JW and Schenker S. Drug metabolism in patients with liver disease. Adv Intern Med 1987; 32:379–405

Sherlock S. Chronic portal systemic encephalopathy: Update 1987. Gut 1987 Aug; 28(8):1043–1048

Sherlock S. The spectrum of hepatotoxicity due to drugs. Lancet 1986 Aug 23; 2(8504):440–444

Van Thiel DH, Makowka L and Starzl TE. Liver transplantation: Where it's been and where it's going. Gastroenterol Clin North Am 1988 Mar; 17(1):1–18

Weinman MD and Chopra S. Tumors of the liver, other than primary hepatocellular carcinoma. Gastroenterol Clin North Am 1987 Dec; 16(4):627–650

Williams RL. Drug administration in hepatic disease. N Engl J Med 1983 Dec 29; 309(26):1616–1622

Williams R (ed). Fulminant hepatic failure. Semin Liver Dis 1986 May; 6(2):97–163

Wilson CB and Epenetos AA. Use of monoclonal antibodies for diagnosis and treatment of liver tumours. Baillieres Clin Gastroenterol 1987 Jan; 1(1):115–130

Zaloga GP and Prough DS. Monitoring hepatic function. Crit Care Clin 1988 Jul; 4(3):591–603

Hepatitis

Aach RD. The treatment of chronic Type B viral hepatitis. Ann Intern Med 1988 Jul; 109(2):89–91

Bastien MR and Smith JG. Prevention of hepatitis B. Arch Dermatology 1989 Feb; 125(2):212–215

Bruckstein AH. Immunoprophylaxis of viral hepatitis. Postgrad Med 1988 Jul; 84(1):85–94

Fagan EA and Williams R. Hepatitis B vaccination. Br J Clin Pract 1987 Jan; 41(1):569–576

Grieco MH. Prophylaxis of hepatitis B infection. Ration Drug Ther 1988 Feb; 22(2):1–6

Hepatitis B: The facts made simple. Lampada 1989 Spring; 11:23–26

Iwarson SA. Non-A, non-B hepatitis: Dead ends or new horizons? Br Med J 1987 Oct 17; 295(6604):946–948

Lee HS and Vyas GN. Diagnosis of viral hepatitis. Clin Lab Med 1987 Dec; 7(4):741–757

Lever AML. Non-A/non-B hepatitis. J Hosp Infect 1988 Feb; 11(Suppl A): 150–160

Maddrey WC. Alcoholic hepatitis: Clinicopathologic features and therapy. Semin Liver Dis 1988 Feb; 8(1):91–102

Mosley JW et al. Non-A, Non-B hepatitis an antibody to hepatitis C virus. JAMA 1990 Jan 5; 263(1):77–78

Rizzetto M, Bonino F and Verme G. Hepatitis Delta virus infection of the liver: Progress in virology, pathobiology and diagnosis. Semin Liver Dis 1988 Nov; 8(4):350–356

Schalm SW. Chronic hepatitis B: Diagnosis and treatment. Postgrad Med J 1986; 62(Suppl 2):11–20

Schreeder M. Viral hepatitis. Prim Care 1988 Mar; 15(1):157–173

Smith LG and Perez G. Viral hepatitis: The alphabet game. Postgrad Med 1988 Oct; 84(5):179–188

Stevens CE et al. Epidemiology of hepatitis C virus. JAMA 1990 Jan 5; 263(1):49–53

Wang JF. Hepatitis B viral infection: Issues in nursing practice. AAOHN J 1987 Oct; 35(10):430–438, 470–472

Zuckerman AJ. Hepatitis B vaccines. Postgrad Med J 1986; 62(Suppl 2):3–10

Esophageal Varices

Arroyo V et al. Management of patients with cirrhosis and ascites. Semin Liver Dis 1986 Nov; 6(4):353–369

Arroyo V et al. Pathophysiology of ascites and functional renal failure in cirrhosis. J Hepatol 1988 Apr; 6(2): 239–257

Bosch J et al. Diagnosis and evaluation of portal hypertension. Z Gastroenterol 1988 Sep; 26(Suppl 2):8–14

Brown MW. Gastroesophageal varices: Management of hemorrhage in the cirrhotic patient. Prim Care 1988 Mar; 15(1):175–186

Epstein O. Management aspects of cirrhosis. Practitioner 1987 Mar 22; 231(1426):395–401

Fleig WE. Pharmacological methods for the prevention of first and recurrent bleeding from esophagogastric varices. Z Gastroenterol 1988 Sep; 26(Suppl): 40–48

Infante-Rivard C, Esnaola S and Villeneuve JP. Role of endoscopic variceal sclerotherapy in the long-term management of variceal bleeding: A meta-analysis. Gastroenterology 1989; 96:1087–1092

Kirby DF. Management of esophageal varices: A review of treatment options and the role of the gastroenterology nurse and associate. Gastroenterol Nurs 1989 Summer; 12(1):10–14

Lebrec C. The medical prevention of variceal bleeding. Intensive Care Med 1988; 14(2):97–99

Management of acute variceal bleeding. Lancet 1988 Oct; 2(8618):999–1000

Reichen J. Etiology and pathophysiology of portal hypertension. Z Gastroenterol 1988 Sep; 26(Suppl):3–7

Ricci JA. Alcohol-induced upper GI hemorrhage: Case studies and management. Crit Care Nurs 1987 Jan–Feb; 7(1):56–63

Rice TL. Treatment of esophageal varices. Clin Pharm 1989 Feb; 8(2): 122–131

Rikkers LF. Current status of the management of patients with portal hypertension. Surg Annu 1988; 20:179–200

Rikkers LF. Variceal hemorrhage. Gastroenterol Clin North Am 1988 Jun; 17(2):289–302

Robertson D. Ruptured oesophageal varices. Nurs RSA 1988 Nov–Dec; 3(11/12):32–35

Van Stiegmann G. Endoscopic ligation of esophageal varices. Am J Surg 1988 Sep; 156(3Pt 2):9B–12B

Voiculescu M. Controversies and certitudes on the upper digestive hemorrhage through rupture of esophageal varices. Med Interne 1988 Jul–Sep; 26(3):179–190

Westaby D. Long-term injection sclerotherapy for the primary and secondary management of variceal haemorrhage. Gastroenterol 1988 Sep; 26(Suppl 2):36–39

Westaby D. The management of active variceal bleeding. Intensive Care Med 1988; 14(2):100–105

Disorders of the Biliary System

Bilhartz LE. Southwestern Internal Medicine Conference: Cholesterol gallstone disease: The current status of

nonsurgical therapy. Am J Med Sci 1988 Jul; 296(1):45–56

Classen M et al. Giant bile duct stones—non-surgical treatment. Endoscopy 1988 Jan; 20(1):21–26

Finlayson N. Cholecystectomy for gallstones. Br Med J 1989 Jan 21; 298(6667):133–134

Fromm H and Malavolti M. Dissolving gallstones. Adv Intern Med 1988; 33: 409–430

Hofmann AF. Pathogenesis of cholesterol gallstones. J Clin Gastroenterol 1988; 10(Suppl 2):S1–11

Keeffe EB. Sarcoidosis and primary biliary cirrhosis: Literature review and illustrative case. Am J Med 1987 Nov; 83(5):977–980

Levin B. Diagnosis and medical treatment of malignant disorders of the biliary tract. Semin Liver Dis 1987 Nov; 7(4):328–333

Lu SC. Frontiers of gallstone therapy: How far have we come with nonsurgical methods? Postgrad Med 1989 Feb 15; 85(3):90–92, 97, 100–104

May GR. Solvent dissolution of gallstones. Radiology 1988 Aug; 168(2):331–332

Nagorney DM and McPherson GAD. Carcinoma of the gallbladder and extrahepatic bile ducts. Semin Oncol 1988 Apr; 15(2):106–115

Paumgartner G. Fragmentation of gallstones by extracorporeal shock waves. Semin Liver Dis 1987 Nov; 7(4):317–321

Sackmann M et al. Gallstone treatment by extracorporeal shock-wave lithotripsy. J Hepatol 1988 Oct; 7(2): 283–287

Scher KS and Scott-Conner CEH. Complications of biliary surgery. Am Surg 1987 Jan; 53(1):16–21

Schoenfield LJ. Gallstones. Clin Symposia 1988; 40(2):2–32

Sharp KW. Acute cholecystitis. Surg Clin North Am 1988 Apr; 68(2):269–279

Sievert W and Vakil NB. Emergencies of the biliary tract. Gastroenterol Clin North Am 1988 Jun; 17(2):245–264

Taylor EL and Harrington TM. Cholecystitis and cholelithiasis. Prim Care 1988 Mar; 15(1):147–156

Thistle JL. Direct contact dissolution of gallstones. Semin Liver Dis 1987 Nov; 7(4):311–316

Pancreas

Axon ATR. Endoscopic retrograde cholangiopancreatography in chronic pancreatitis. Radiol Clin North Am 1989 Jan; 27(1):39–50

Bagg AM. Whipple's procedure: Nursing guidelines. Crit Care Nurs 1988 Jul–Aug; 8(5):34–45

Balthazar EJ. CT diagnosis and staging of acute pancreatitis. Radiol Clin North Am 1989 Jan; 27(1):19–37

Beazley RM and Cohn I. Update on pancreatic cancer. CA 1988 Sep–Oct; 38(5):310–319

Birdsall C and Fiore-Lopez N. How do you manage pancreatic sump tubes? Am J Nurs 1987 Jun; 87(6):770–771

Blake RL. Acute pancreatitis. Prim Care 1988 Mar; 15(1):187–199

Bourliere M and Sarles H. Pancreatic cysts and pseudocysts associated with acute and chronic pancreatitis. Dig Dis Sci 1989 Mar; 34(3):343–348

Boyd EJS, Rinderknecht H and Wormsley KG. Laboratory tests in the diagnosis of the chronic pancreatic diseases. Part 4. Tests involving the measurement of pancreatic enzymes in body fluid. Int J Pancreatol 1988 Jan–Feb; 3(1):1–16

Boyd EJS, Rinderknecht H and Wormsley KG. Laboratory tests in the diagnosis of the chronic pancreatic diseases. Part 6. Differentiation between chronic pancreatitis and pancreatic cancer. Int J Pancreatol 1988 May; 3(4):229–240

Boyd EJS and Wormsley KG. Laboratory tests in the diagnosis of the chronic pancreatic diseases. Part 1. Secretagogues used in tests of pancreatic secretion. Int J Pancreatol 1987 Jun; 2(3):137–148

Boyd EJS and Wormsley KG. Laboratory tests in the diagnosis of the chronic pancreatic diseases. Part 2. Tests of pancreatic secretion. Int J Pancreatol 1987 Aug; 2(4):211–221

Byrne JJ and Treadwell TL. Treatment of pancreatitis: When do antibiotics have a role? Postgrad Med 1989 Mar; 85(4): 333–334, 337–339

Cremer M, Deviere J and Engelholm L. Endoscopic management of cysts and pseudocysts in chronic pancreatitis: Long-term follow-up after 7 years of experience. Gastrointest Endosc 1989 Jan–Feb; 35(1):1–9

DiMagno EP. Early diagnosis of chronic pancreatitis and pancreatic cancer. Med Clin North Am 1988 Sep; 72(5): 979–992

Fain JA and Amato-Vealey E. Acute pancreatitis: A gastrointestinal emergency. Crit Care Nurs 1988 Jul–Aug; 8(5):47–61

Grimm H et al. New modalities for treating chronic pancreatitis. Endoscopy 1989 Mar; 21(2):70–74

Hennessy K. Nutritional support and gastrointestinal disease. Nurs Clin North Am 1989 Jun; 24(2):373–381

Ihse I and Lankisch PG. Treatment of chronic pancreatitis—current status. Acta Chir Scand 1988 Oct; 154(10): 553–558

Lebovits AH and Lefkowitz M. Pain management of pancreatic carcinoma: A review. Pain 1989 Jan; 36(1):1–11

Levy P et al. Mortality factors associated with chronic pancreatitis. Gastroenterology 1989 Apr; 96(4): 1165–1172

Mallory A and Kern F. Drug-induced pancreatitis. Baillieres Clin Gastroenterol 1988 Apr; 2(2):293–307

Mills AS. Pancreatitis: Disruption in structure and function. Gastroenterol Nurs 1989 Summer; 12(1):63–65

Moody FG. Pancreatitis as a medical emergency. Gastroenterol Clin North Am 1988 Jun; 17(2):433–443

Moorhouse MF, Geissler AC and Doenges ME. Patient care guidelines: Acute pancreatitis. J Emerg Nurs 1988 Nov–Dec; 14(6):387–391

Nealon WH, Townsend CM and Thompson JC. Preoperative endoscopic retrograde cholangiopancreatography (ERCP) in patients with pancreatic pseudocyst associated with resolving acute and chronic pancreatitis. Ann Surg 1989 May; 209(5):532–540

Potts JR. Acute pancreatitis. Surg Clin North Am 1988 Apr; 68(2):281–299

Reber HA. Pancreatic cancer: Presentation of the disease, diagnosis and surgical management. J Pain Symptom Manage 1988 Fall; 3(4):164–167

Rossi P, Allison DJ and Bezzi M. Endocrine tumors of the pancreas. Radiol Clin North Am 1989 Jan; 27(1): 129–161

Safrit HD and Rice RP. Gastrointestinal complications of pancreatitis. Radiol Clin North Am 1989 Jan; 27(1):73–79

Sarles H, Bernard JP and Johnson C. Pathogenesis and epidemiology of chronic pancreatitis. Annu Rev Med 1989; 40:453–468

Spross JA, Manolatos A and Thorpe M. Pancreatic cancer: Nursing challenges. Semin Oncol Nurs 1988 Nov; 4(4): 274–284

Stavas J. Pancreatic pseudocyst. Nebr Med J 1988 Oct; 73(10):313–315

Warshaw AL and Swanson RS. Pancreatic cancer in 1988: Possibilities and probabilities. Ann Surg 1988 Nov; 208(5):541–553

Wilson C et al. Hepatobiliary complications in chronic pancreatitis. Gut 1989 Apr; 30(4):520–527

Metabolic and Endocrine Disorders

Disorders of the Thyroid Gland

Physiology

1. The thyroid gland affects the rate at which all tissues metabolize.
   a. Speed of chemical reactions
   b. Volume of oxygen consumed
   c. Amount of heat produced
2. The stimulating effect is through the production and distribution of 2 hormones:
   a. Levothyroxine (T_4)—contains 4 iodine atoms; maintains body's metabolism in a steady state; it is believed that T_4 serves as a precursor of T_3.
   b. Triiodothyronine (T_3)—contains 3 iodine atoms; is approximately 5 times as potent as thyroxine; has a more rapid metabolic action and utilization than thyroxine. Most conversion of T_4 to T_3 occurs at the cellular level in the periphery. Some T_3 is produced in the thyroid gland.

Tests of Thyroid Function

A. T_4, Thyroxine, Free

1. Is a direct measurement of the concentration of total thyroxine in the blood
2. Is a good index of thyroid function when thyroxine-binding globulin (TBG) is normal
3. Used to diagnose hypo- and hyperfunction of thyroid and to guide and evaluate therapy
4. Interpretation
   a. Hypothyroidism—below normal
   b. Hyperthyroidism—above normal

B. Serum Triiodothyronine (T_3)

1. Directly measures concentration of triiodothyronine in the blood
2. T_3 is much less stable than T_4 and occurs in minute quantities in the active form.
3. Useful to rule out T_3 thyrotoxicosis, hypo- and hyperfunction of thyroid, to determine thyroid gland status, and to evaluate effects of thyroid replacement therapy
4. Interpretation
   a. Hypothyroidism—below normal
   b. Hyperthyroidism—above normal

C. T_3 Resin Uptake

1. Is an indirect measure of thyroid function based on the available protein-binding sites in a serum sample that can bind to radioactive T_3
2. The radioactive triiodothyronine is added to the serum sample in the test tube.
3. The effect of estrogen and pregnancy is to produce an increase in binding sites, causing a lowered percentage of binding by the available thyroid hormones.
4. This test is often used in conjunction with serum thyroxine (T_4).
5. Results may be altered if this patient has been taking estrogens, androgens, salicylates, or phenytoin.
6. Interpretation
   a. Hypothyroidism—below normal
   b. Hyperthyroidism—above normal

D. Radioactive (^{131}I) (^{99m}Tc)

^{131}I uptake:
1. A solution of sodium iodide-131 is administered orally to the fasting patient.
2. After a prescribed interval (anywhere from 2–48 hours, but frequently by 24 hours), measurements are taken with a scintillator of radioactive counts per minute that are detected above the isthmus of the thyroid gland.
3. Normal thyroid will remove 15%–50% of the iodine from the bloodstream.
4. Hyperthyroidism may result in the removal of as much as 90% of the iodine from the bloodstream.
5. Hypothyroidism—will be reflected in low uptake.

E. Thyroidal Iodide Clearance

1. Radioiodine clearance test measures the amount of circulating blood that is completely cleared of iodine per unit of time.
2. Radioiodine is injected intravenously; radioactivity over the thyroid gland is measured continuously for 30–60 minutes.
3. Total amount of ^{131}I concentrated in the gland per minute is computed.
4. Also, plasma ^{131}I content is measured in samples of blood collected 45–70 minutes after injection
5. These values are averaged.
6. Thyroid ^{131}I divided by the mean plasma ^{131}I equals thyroid clearance (i.e., ml. of plasma cleared of iodide per minute).

7. Interpretation
   a. Normal—25 ml./minute
   b. Hyperthyroidism—250 ml./minute
   c. Hypothyroidism—1.6 ml./minute

F. ^{131}I Excretion

1. Urinary output of radioiodine is measured during 6-hour and 24-hour periods after ingestion.
2. Interpretation
   a. Normal—40%–80% of ingested iodine in 24 hours
   b. Hyperthyroidism—less than 40%
   c. Hypothyroidism—greater than 90%

G. Thyroid "Scan" ^{131}I

1. The patient ingests sodium iodide-131 and is scanned the next day; if medium is given intravenously, the patient may be scanned within ½–1 hour.
2. The patient is supine; the detector head of the scintillation camera is centered over the patient's neck.
3. The thyroid images from the oscilloscope of the camera are recorded on film.
4. Benign adenomas may be visualized as "hot" nodules, indicating increased uptake of iodine, or as "cold" nodules, indicating decreased uptake.
5. Malignant nodules usually take the form of "cold" nodules.

H. Triiodothyronine (T_3) Suppression Test

1. Measures 24-hour radioactive iodine uptake.
2. Patient is placed on T_3 for 7 days.
3. 24-hour radioactive iodine uptake is measured.
4. Interpretation
   a. Normal—suppression to a radioactive iodine uptake below 20% at 24 hours (half original value).
   b. Graves disease—no suppression

NURSING ALERT: The use of radioactive substances is contraindicated in pregnancy. During pregnancy, thyroid testing is limited to blood testing.

Note: Thyroid tests must be scheduled carefully so that thyroid-blocking contrast agents for other x-rays, diagnostic tests, and medications do not interfere with interpretation of tests of thyroid function.

I. Thyrotropin-Releasing Hormone (TRH)

1. The patient fasts overnight.
2. Fifteen minutes prior to TRH injection, a blood specimen is drawn.
3. 500 μg synthetic TRH is injected into arterial system.
4. Blood specimen is drawn to determine thyroid-stimulating hormone (TSH) at 15, 30, 45, 60, 90, and 120 minutes.
5. Increased TSH should be seen. No rise in secondary hypothyroidism and no rise in hyperthyroidism.

J. Thyrotropin Radioimmunoassay (TSH)

1. Useful in differentiating between thyroid disorders due to disease of the thyroid gland itself and disorders due to disease of the pituitary or hypothalamus.
2. Blood sample is analyzed by radioimmunoassay.
3. Interpretation
   a. In primary hypothyroidism, TSH levels are elevated.
   b. In secondary hypothyroidism (failure of the pituitary gland), TSH levels are low.
   c. In hyperthyroidism, TSH levels are low.

K. Protein-Bound Iodine (PBI)

1. A conjugated molecule formed when thyroxine becomes attached to certain plasma protein fractions.
2. A reasonably accurate index of thyroid function is the concentration of PBI in the blood, but it is affected by many medications and conditions.
3. Interpretation
   a. Normal values: 3.5–8.0 μg. (0.0035–0.8880 mg./100 ml. of plasma)
   b. Over 8.0—thyroid overactivity
   c. Under 3.5—hypothyroidism
4. In many health-care facilities, this test has been replaced by tests for serum T_3 and serum T_4.

NURSING ALERT: Certain factors impair the PBI test:
1. Use of iodine skin antiseptic at venipuncture site
2. Ingestion of drugs or administration of dyes containing iodine:
   a. Expectorants, cough syrups, etc.
   b. Dyes used in arteriogram, bronchogram, etc.
3. Mercurial diuretics, estrogens, sulfonamides, steroids, phenylbutazone, thiocyanates
4. Pregnancy

Hypothyroidism

Hypothyroidism may be classified as primary, secondary, or tertiary.

Primary hypothyroidism is a condition resulting from the inability of the thyroid gland to secrete a sufficient amount of hormone.

Secondary hypothyroidism is caused by a failure of the pituitary gland to secrete an adequate amount of TSH (thyroid-stimulating hormone).

Tertiary hypothyroidism results from failure of the hypothalamus to release thyroid-releasing hormone (TRH).

Cretinism is a severe form of hypothyroidism resulting from deficiency of thyroid function during fetal life or shortly after birth. The mother has usually had deficiency of thyroid hormone function during pregnancy.

Etiology

1. Primary hypothyroidism is the most common form of this condition and is generally due to
   a. Removal, destruction, or suppression of all or some of the thyroid tissue by thyroidectomy.
   b. Use of radioactive iodine.
   c. Over-treatment with antithyroid drugs.
2. Hypothyroidism may also be idiopathic in origin or a result of chronic immunological dysfunction, as in Hashimoto's thyroiditis.

Pathophysiology

1. Inadequate secretion of thyroid hormone leads to a general slowing of all physical and mental processes.
2. There is a general depression of most cellular enzyme systems and oxidative processes.
3. The metabolic activity of all cells of the body decreases, reducing oxygen consumption, decreasing oxidation of nutrients for energy, and producing less body heat.
4. The signs and symptoms of the disorder range from vague, nonspecific complaints that make diagnosis difficult, to severe symptoms that may be life-threatening if unrecognized and untreated.

Clinical Manifestations

1. Fatigue and lethargy
2. Weight gain
3. Complaints of cold hands and feet
4. Temperature and pulse become subnormal; unable to tolerate cold and desires room temperature increased
5. Reduced attention span; impaired short-term memory
6. Severe constipation; decreased peristalsis
7. Generalized appearance of thick, puffy skin; subcutaneous swelling in hands, feet, and eyelids
8. Hair thins; loss of the lateral one third of eyebrow
9. Menorrhagia or amenorrhea; may have difficulty conceiving or experiences spontaneous abortion; decreased libido
10. Neurological signs (polyneuropathy, cerebellar ataxia); muscle aches or weakness, clumsiness
11. Hyperlipoproteinemia and hypercholesterolemia
12. Enlarged heart on chest x-ray
13. Increased susceptibility to all hypnotic and sedative drugs and anesthetic agents
14. In severe hypothyroidism—hypotension, unresponsiveness, bradycardia, hypoventilation, hyponatremia, (possibly) convulsions, hypothermia, cerebral hypoxia, and myxedema
15. High mortality rate

Diagnostic Evaluation

1. Low T_3 and T_4 levels
2. Elevated thyroid-stimulating hormone levels in primary hypothyroidism
3. Elevation of serum cholesterol
4. ECG—sinus bradycardia, low voltage of QRS complexes, and flat or inverted T waves
5. Prolonged deep tendon reflex response, especially ankle jerk
6. Possible previous treatment with radioactive iodine
7. Possible physical examination findings—subtle signs of hypothyroidism or a general suppression and depression of organs and systems

Management

A. Approach

1. The management depends on the severity of the patient's symptoms and may necessitate replacement therapy in mild cases or life-saving support and treatment in severe hypothyroidism and myxedema coma.
2. As thyroid hormone levels gradually return to normal, the patient is monitored closely to prevent complications resulting from sudden increases in metabolic rate and oxygen requirements.

B. Restoration of a Normal Metabolic State (Euthyroid) as Rapidly as Possible

1. Thyroid hormone—levothyroxine (Synthroid, Levothroid); thyroglobulin (Proloid); liotrix (Euthroid, Thyrolar).
   a. Because triiodothyronine acts more quickly than thyroxine, this is given via stomach tube if patient is unconscious.
   b. Sodium levothyroxine (Synthroid) is administered parenterally (until consciousness is restored) to restore thyroxine level.
   c. Later, the patient is continued on oral thyroid hormone therapy.
   d. With rapid administration of thyroid hormone, plasma thyroxine levels may initiate adrenal in-

sufficiency; hence, steroid therapy may be initiated.
2. Monitoring to anticipate treatment effects:
   a. Diuresis, decreased puffiness
   b. Improved reflexes and muscle tone
   c. Accelerated pulse rate
   d. A slightly higher level of total serum thyroxine
   e. All signs of hypothyroidism should disappear over a 3–12-week period.

> **GERONTOLOGIC ALERT:** Care must be taken with elderly patients and those with coronary artery disease when starting thyroid hormone replacement. It is preferable to start with much lower doses and increase very gradually, taking 1–2 months to reach full replacement doses.

Nursing Assessment

1. Identify patient at risk. Secure data about home medication program, post-treatment of thyroid disease, and presence of physical stress.
2. Secure data about signs and symptoms in patients at risk.
3. Perform frequent multisystem assessments, including cardiac, respiratory, neurological, and gastrointestinal systems.

Nursing Diagnoses

1. Potential altered cardiac output related to decreased metabolic rate, decreased cardiac conduction, elevated cholesterol levels, atherosclerosis, and coronary artery disease
2. Activity intolerance related to lethargy and fatigue, depressed neuromuscular status
3. Altered nutrition (less than body requirements) related to decreased metabolic rate, poor appetite, and depressed gastrointestinal function

Nursing Interventions

A. Improving Cardiac Output

1. Control factors that increase metabolic rate and threaten cardiovascular status:
   a. Monitor vital signs frequently to detect changes in cardiovascular status and ability to respond to stress.
   b. Monitor ECG tracings to detect dysrhythmias and deterioration of cardiovascular status.
   c. Implement prescribed measures intended to prevent and treat factors that increase metabolic rate (infection, stress, trauma).
   d. Prevent chilling to avoid increasing metabolic rate, which, in turn, places strain on the heart. Provide bed socks, bed jacket, warm environment.
   e. Even though hypothermia exists, do not apply external heat, as the resulting increased oxygen requirements and decreased peripheral vascular tone may compound the existing cardiac failure.
   f. Administer fluids cautiously, even though hyponatremia is present.
   g. Give prescribed glucose in concentrated amounts to prevent fluid overload if hypoglycemia is in evidence.
2. Administer all prescribed drugs with caution before and after thyroid replacement begins.
   a. Before treatment with thyroid hormone, the pa-

tient is susceptible to the effects of sedatives, narcotics, anesthetics, and other medications.
   b. After thyroid replacement is initiated, the thyroid hormones may increase the effects of digitalis and anticoagulants.
3. Report occurrence of angina, and the signs and symptoms of myocardial infarction and cardiac failure.
4. Monitor arterial blood gases to assess cardiopulmonary function.

B. Increasing Activity Tolerance and a Balance of Rest and Activity

1. Limit visitors during acute stage to prevent excessive stimulation.
2. Carry out activities, hygiene, and care for the patient during acute stage of illness.
3. Prevent pulmonary complications of immobility during acute stage by turning, and encouraging the patient to cough and take deep breaths.
4. Encourage resumption of activities as severe symptoms begin to subside and the patient begins to improve.
5. Assist the patient in planning activities to limit exertion and provide ample periods of rest.
6. Identify for the patient signs and symptoms indicating excessive exertion.
7. Provide good skin care to prevent skin breakdown secondary to immobility.
   a. Apply lubricant to the skin, as it is usually dry and scaly.
   b. Observe for pressure areas and initiate measures to relieve pressure.

C. Improving Nutritional Status

1. Assess return and gradual increase of gastrointestinal function (return of bowel sounds, absence of abdominal distention, occurrence and frequency of bowel movements).
2. Encourage frequent intake of fluids; include dietary fiber to prevent constipation.
3. Administer stool softeners if necessary.
4. Discourage straining at stool because of increased strain on the heart.
5. Work cooperatively with dietitian in offering appetizing, low-calorie meals; this patient is usually overweight, although his appetite is poor.

Discharge Planning and Patient Education

Instruct the patient about the following:
1. How and when to take medications
2. Signs and symptoms of insufficient and excessive medication; reinforce teaching by providing written instructions as well.
3. The necessity of having blood evaluations periodically to determine thyroid levels

Evaluation

1. Demonstrates improved cardiac status and output—normal blood pressure and pulse rate; normal ECG tracing (normal amplitude and return of normal T wave); normal cholesterol levels
2. Demonstrates increased activity tolerance and reports increased strength and well-being; decreased fatigue and lethargy
3. Demonstrates adequate nutritional intake—consumes low-calorie meals; avoids foods restricted in diet and reports loss of weight and absence of edema.

Hyperthyroidism

Hyperthyroidism (diffuse toxic goiter) is excessive activity of the thyroid gland.

Incidence

More common in women than in men; occurs in about 2% of the female population.

Types

1. Graves' disease (most prevalent)—diffuse hyperfunction of the thyroid gland associated with ophthalmopathy; most common in younger women; may subside spontaneously
2. Toxic nodular goiter (single or multiple)—more common in older females with preexisting goiter; will continue to be overactive unless eradicated or kept under suppressive therapy.

Etiology

1. Unknown; immunologic origin is likely.
2. Possible causes
   a. Thyroid-stimulating antibody (TSA_b)—long-acting thyroid stimulator correlates very closely with the clinical course of Graves' disease.
   b. TSA_b, an immunoglobulin found in the blood of patients with Graves' disease, is capable of reacting with the receptor for TSH on the thyroid plasma membrane and stimulating glandular function.
   c. May appear after an emotional shock, infection, or emotional stress
   d. Genetic predisposition, female sex
   e. B and T lymphocytes (immunologic factors) have been implicated.

Pathophysiology

1. Hyperthyroidism is characterized by hypertrophy and hyperplasia of the thyroid gland, which is accompanied by increased vascularity and blood flow and enlargement of the gland.
2. A hypermetabolic condition results from the excessive secretion of thyroid hormone, resulting in exaggeration of all metabolic processes.
3. The majority of cases of hyperthyroidism are thought to be due to an autoimmune reaction in which circulating autoantibodies mimic the action of TSH and increase the secretion of thyroid hormone.
4. Most of the clinical manifestations result from increased metabolic rate, excessive heat production, increased neuromuscular and cardiovascular activity, and hyperactivity of the sympathetic nervous system.
5. Hyperthyroidism ranges from a mild increase in metabolic rate to the severe hyperactivity known as thyrotoxicosis, thyroid storm, or thyroid crisis.
6. A patient with mild hyperthyroidism is not usually admitted to the hospital unless admitted for another problem and the hyperthyroidism is initially unsuspected.
7. The patient with severe thyrotoxicosis or thyroid crisis, however, is admitted to control the hypermetabolic state, prevent cardiac failure, or prepare for surgery.

Clinical Course and Manifestations

1. Nervousness, emotional lability, irritability, apprehension

2. Difficulty in sitting quietly
3. Rapid pulse at rest as well as on exertion (ranges between 90 and 160); palpitations
4. Heat intolerance; profuse perspiration; flushed skin (e.g., hands may be warm, soft, moist)
5. Fine tremor of hands; change in bowel habits—constipation or diarrhea
6. Increased appetite and progressive weight loss; frequent stools
7. Muscle fatigability and weakness; amenorrhea
8. Atrial fibrillation possible (cardiac decompensation common in elderly patients)
9. Bulging eyes (exophthalmos)—produces a startled expression
10. Course may be mild, characterized by remissions and exacerbations
11. It may progress to emaciation, extreme nervousness, delirium, disorientation, thyroid storm or crisis, and death.
12. *Thyroid storm* or *crisis,* an extreme form of hyperthyroidism, is characterized by hyperpyrexia, diarrhea, dehydration, tachycardia, dysrhythmias, extreme irritation, delirium, coma, shock, and death if not adequately treated (Fig. 22-1).
13. Thyroid storm may be precipitated by stress (surgery, infection, etc.), or inadequate preparation for surgery in a patient with known hyperthyroidism.

Diagnostic Evaluation

1. Elevated T_3 and serum thyroxine levels (T_4).
2. Elevated serum T_3 resin uptake.
3. Complete physical examination reveals a hypermetabolic state.
4. A bruit or thrill over the thyroid can often be detected because of the increased blood flow.
5. Thyroid gland may be palpable on examination.

Management

A. Types of Treatment

1. Antithyroid drug therapy
2. Radiation
3. Surgery

B. Factors Influencing Management Decision

1. Treatment depends on causes, age of patient, severity of disease, and complications.
2. According to causes:
   a. Remission of hyperthyroidism (Graves' disease) occurs spontaneously within 1–2 years; however, relapse can be expected in half of the patients. All three forms of therapy are appropriate.
   b. Nodular toxic goiter—excessive amounts of thyroid hormone secreted. Surgery or use of radioiodine is preferred.
   c. Thyroid carcinoma. Surgery or radiation.
3. According to age of patient:
   a. Radioiodine therapy may be used in all patients, regardless of age, when other forms of therapy are contraindicated.
   b. Radioiodine is used in older patients for whom surgery is contraindicated; surgery is recommended for younger patients.
   c. Radioiodine therapy is contraindicated in pregnancy and in women of childbearing age.
4. According to severity:
   Drug therapy is administered before proceeding with radioiodine or surgery.

5. According to patient preference:
   a. Radioiodine or surgery is suggested to the patient who does not take medication regularly.
   b. Surgery is recommended to those who prefer it.
6. According to social factors:
   Surgery indicated for patients living in remote areas without access to satisfactory medical care and those who wish to return to work as quickly as possible.
7. According to the size of the goiter:
   a. Surgery is indicated for patients with large or medium-sized goiters (>80 gm.).
   b. Antithyroid drugs are given to patients with a small goiter (<40 gm.).

C. Pharmacotherapy—Drugs That Inhibit Hormone Formation

1. **Goal:** To bring the metabolic rate to normal as soon as possible and maintain it at this level.
2. Thionamides
   a. Preparations:
      (1) Propylthiouracil
      (2) Methimazole (Tapazole)
          Carbimazole—a derivative of methimazole
   b. Action:
      (1) Depresses the synthesis of thyroid hormone by inhibiting peroxidase.
      (2) It has been standard practice to give these medications in divided daily doses (every 8 hours); experimental evidence appears to indicate that once-a-day dosage is effective for 24 hours or longer. Patient compliance is better with this latter medication schedule.
   c. Duration of treatment determined by clinical criteria:
      (1) Thyroid gland becomes smaller.
      (2) Measurement of T_4 and T_3 uptake to determine adequacy of dose
      (3) Treatment continued until patient becomes clinically euthyroid; this varies from 3 months to 1–2 years; if euthyroidism cannot be maintained without therapy, then another form of therapy (i.e., RAI or surgery) is recommended.
      (4) Therapy withdrawn gradually to prevent exacerbation.

D. Pharmacotherapy—to Control Peripheral Manifestations of Hyperthyroidism

1. *Propranolol* (Inderal)
   a. Acts as a beta-adrenergic blocking agent
   b. Abolishes tachycardia, tremor, excess sweating, nervousness
   c. Controls hyperthyroid symptoms until antithyroid drugs or radioiodine can take effect
2. *Glucocorticoids*
   Decreases the peripheral conversion of thyroxine to triiodothyronine.
3. *Radioactive iodine*
   a. Action:
      (1) Limits secretion of thyroid hormone by destroying thyroid tissue.
      (2) Dosage is controlled so that hypothyroidism does not occur.
   b. Advantages and disadvantages:
      (1) Chief advantage of radioiodine over thionamides is that a lasting remission can be achieved.

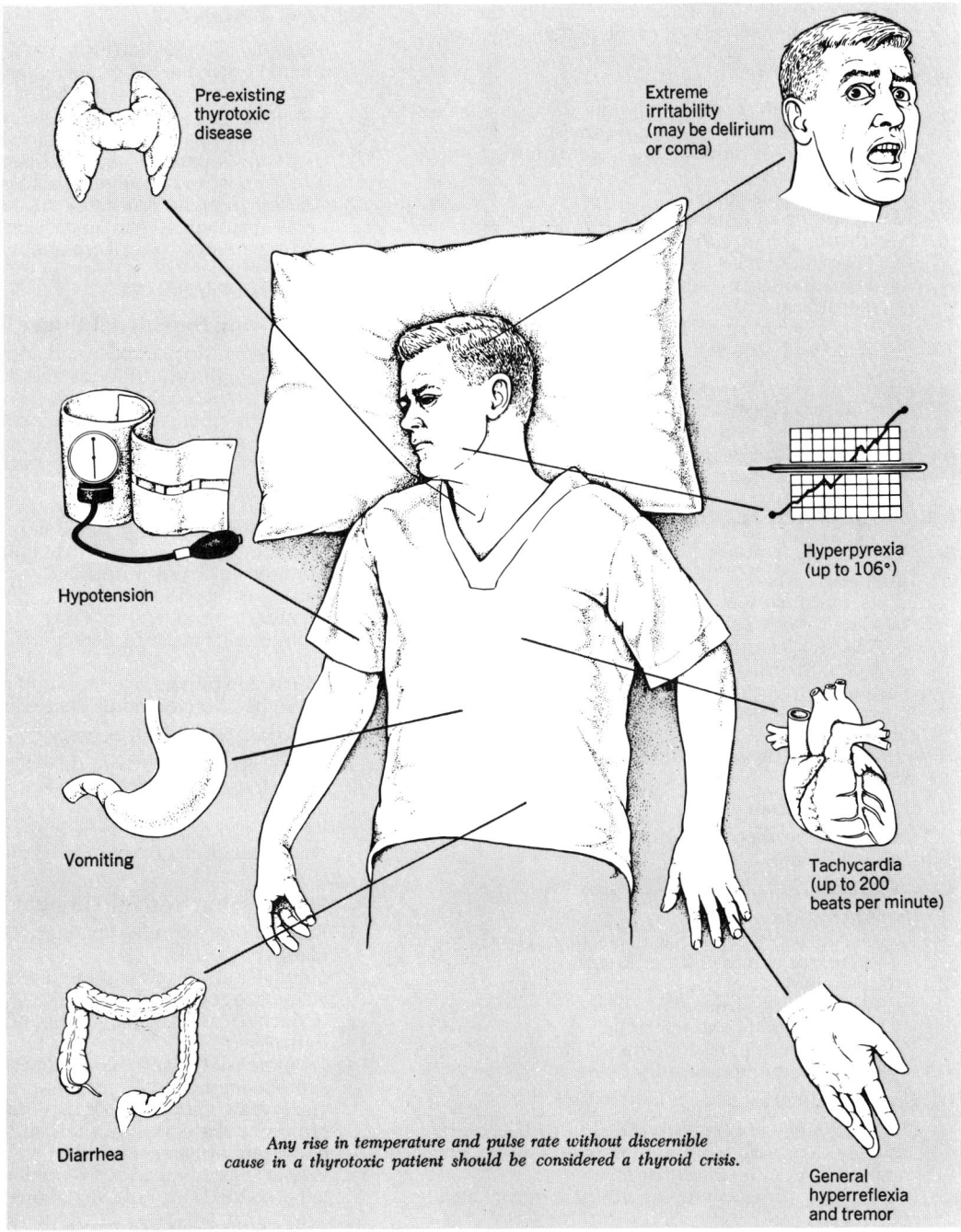

Figure 22-1. *Clinical picture of thyrotoxic crisis. (From Hospital Medicine 3[1]:39. Copyright Hospital Publications, Inc. Reprinted with permission.)*

(2) Chief disadvantage is that permanent hypothyroidism can be produced in patients treated with radioiodine.

(3) *Radiation thyroiditis* (a transient exacerbation of hyperthyroidism) may occur as a result of leakage of thyroid hormone into the circulation from damaged follicles.

E. Psychotherapy

1. Greater emphasis is being placed on the effect that psychogenic factors have on the severity of this disease.
2. A determination is made in caring for each patient of whether psychotherapy would be of value in preventing exacerbations.
3. The patient and family may require psychological sup-

port because of the disturbance caused by the irritability and outbursts related to the patient's hypermetabolic state.

F. Surgery

1. Surgery is an effective treatment modality in selected patients, those with very large goiters, or those for whom the use of radioiodine or thionamides is contraindicated.
2. *Subtotal thyroidectomy*
   Involves removal of most of the thyroid gland
3. *Preparation for surgery*
   a. The patient must be euthyroid at time of surgery.
   b. Thionamides are administered to control hyperthyroidism.
   c. Iodide is given to increase firmness of thyroid gland and reduce its vascularity.

NURSING ALERT: Observe the patient for evidence of iodine toxicity: swelling of buccal mucosa, excessive salivation, coryza, skin eruptions. If these occur, iodides are discontinued.

Complications of Hyperthyroidism

A. Thionamide toxicity

1. Agranulocytosis
   a. Is a most serious toxic condition.
   b. Occurs with a sudden onset.
   c. Patient to be apprised of this possibility and urged to report any signs of infection such as fever, sore throat, upper respiratory infection.
2. Skin rashes, fever, urticaria, inflammation of the salivary glands are other possible side effects.
3. An alternate drug is substituted if there are toxic manifestations.

B. Hypothyroidism

Radioactive iodine therapy causes patient to become hypothyroid with time.

C. Complications of Thyroidectomy

1. Hypothyroidism
   a. Occurs in 5% of patients in first postoperative year
   b. Increases at rate of 2%–3%/year
2. Hypoparathyroidism
   a. About 4% occurrence
   b. Usually is mild and transient
   c. Requires calcium supplements intravenously and orally when more severe

D. Eye Complications

1. *Exophthalmos*—abnormal protrusion of the eyeball, probably due to an autoimmune phenomenon; most commonly seen in Graves' disease
2. *Proptosis*—a forward bulging (displacement) of the eye
3. *Ophthalmoplegia*—paralysis of the eye muscle

Nursing Assessment

1. Identify patient at risk. Obtain data about home medication administration and presence of physical stress, particularly infection.
2. Secure data about signs and symptoms in patients at risk.
3. Perform frequent multisystem assessments, including cardiac, respiratory, neurological, and gastrointestinal systems.
4. Closely monitor the patient's temperature.

Nursing Diagnoses

1. Potential altered nutrition (less than body requirements) related to hypermetabolic state, increased fluid and calorie requirement, and fluid loss through diaphoresis.
2. Potential impaired skin integrity related to extreme diaphoresis, pyrexia, excessive restlessness, movement and tremor, and rapid weight loss
3. Altered thought processes related to insomnia, decreased attention span, and irritability
4. Anxiety related to concern about upcoming surgery

Nursing Interventions

A. Improving Nutritional Intake

1. Determine the patient's food and fluid preferences.
2. Provide high-calorie foods and fluids consistent with the patient's requirements.
3. Provide a quiet, calm environment at meals.
4. Restrict stimulants (tea, coffee, alcohol); explain rationale of requirements and restrictions to patient.
5. Encourage/permit the patient to eat alone if embarrassed or otherwise disturbed by voracious appetite.
6. Monitor intravenous infusion when prescribed to maintain fluid and electrolyte balance.
7. Monitor fluid and nutritional status by weighing the patient daily and keeping accurate intake and output records.
8. Monitor vital signs to detect changes in fluid volume status.
9. Assess skin turgor, mucous membranes, and neck veins for signs of increased or decreased fluid volume.

B. Maintaining Skin Integrity

1. Assess skin frequently to detect diaphoresis.
2. Bathe frequently with cool water; change linens when damp.
3. Protect and relieve pressure from bony prominences while immobilized or while hypothermia unit/mattress is used.

C. Encouraging Normal Thought Processes

1. Explain procedures to patient in an unhurried, calm manner.
2. Limit visitors; avoid stimulating conversations or television programs.
3. Reduce stressors in the environment; reduce noise and lights.
4. Promote sleep and relaxation through use of prescribed medications, massage, and relaxation exercises; draw the blinds for nap times.
5. Minimize disruption of the patient's sleep or rest by clustering nursing activities.
6. Employ safety measures to reduce risk of trauma or falls (padded side rails, maintain bed in low position).

D. Achieving Relief of Anxiety

1. Encourage the patient to verbalize concerns and fears about illness, treatment, and possible surgery.
2. Be selective in placing a suitable roommate with the patient (preferably one who is convalescing).
3. Gain the patient's confidence and attempt to assess factors that may cause aggravation or unhappiness, as an existing problem could thwart treatment efforts.

E. Other Nursing Interventions

1. Provide cool environment to prevent pyrexia; use fans or air conditioning.
2. Use prescribed hypothermia unit, antipyretics, cool

water, ice packs, or alcohol baths to reduce body temperature; avoid shivering.
3. Monitor rectal temperature frequently; report elevations in temperature.

Discharge Planning and Patient Education

1. Instruct the patient as follows:
   a. When to take medications
   b. Signs and symptoms of insufficient and excessive medication
   c. Necessity of having blood evaluations periodically to determine thyroid levels
   d. Signs and symptoms of thyroid storm (i.e., tachycardia, hyperpyrexia, extreme irritation) and predisposing factors to thyroid storm (i.e., infection, surgery, stress, abrupt withdrawal of antithyroid medications and adrenergic blocking agents).
2. Reinforce teaching by providing written instructions as well.

Evaluation/Expected Outcomes

1. Maintains adequate nutrition as measured by serum electrolyte levels and vital signs
2. Demonstrates normal skin integrity—skin is cool, dry, and intact without reddened, excoriated, or infected areas; normal temperature
3. Demonstrates improved thought processes—maintains concentration, follows conversation, and responds appropriately
4. Verbalizes concerns and fears about illness, treatment, and possible surgery; appears less anxious and reports an increased sense of well-being

The Patient Undergoing Thyroidectomy

Preoperative Nursing Interventions

1. Provide a restful and therapeutic environment. (See discussion, p. 540)
2. Promote adequate nutritional intake. (See discussion, p. 540)
3. Support the patient undergoing various diagnostic tests to determine nature of the endocrine problem or to ensure a euthyroid state prior to surgery.
   a. Explain the purpose and requirements of each prescribed test.
   b. Explain results of tests if unclear to the patient or questions arise.
4. Prepare the patient for surgery.
   a. Make a special effort to ensure that this patient has a good night's rest preceding surgery.
   b. Explain to the patient that speaking is to be minimized immediately postoperatively and that oxygen may be administered to facilitate breathing.
   c. Explain that postoperatively, fluids may be given intravenously to maintain fluid, electrolyte, and nutritional needs; glucose may also be given intravenously in the hours before the administration of anesthesia.

Postoperative Nursing Interventions

A. Providing Optimum Immediate Postoperative Care to Avoid Complications

1. Administer humidified oxygen as prescribed.
2. Move the patient carefully; provide adequate support to the head so that no tension is placed on the sutures.

3. Place the patient in semi-Fowler's position with the head elevated and supported by pillows; avoid flexion of neck.

B. Observing for Complications

1. *Damage of laryngeal nerve:*
   a. Observe for hoarseness or "whispery" voice, suggesting possible nerve damage.
   b. Recognize that a bilateral flaccid paralysis may lead to cord paralysis → closure of glottis → suffocation, months after operation.
2. *Hemorrhage*
   a. Be alert for this possibility between 12 and 24 hours postoperatively.
   b. Observe for bleeding at sides and back of the neck, as well as anteriorly, when the patient is in dorsal position.
   c. Note and report hypotension, tachycardia, and other signs of hypovolemia and shock.
   d. Watch for signs of irregular breathing, swelling, and choking—other signs pointing to the possibility of hemorrhage and tracheal compression.
   e. Watch for repeated clearing of the throat or complaint of smothering or difficulty swallowing, which may be early signs of hemorrhage.
   f. Reinforce dressing if indicated.
   g. Keep a tracheostomy set in the patient's room for 48 hours for emergency use.
3. *Tetany*
   a. The likelihood that tetany may develop depends on the number of parathyroid glands that have been removed or disturbed.
   b. Progression of signs:
      First—tingling of toes and fingers and around the mouth; apprehension.
      Second—positive *Chvostek's sign* (Tapping the cheek over the facial nerve causes a twitch of the lip or facial muscles.)
      Third—*Trousseau's sign* (carpopedal spasm induced by occluding circulation in the arm with a blood pressure cuff).

C. Collaborative Management of Tetany

1. Position the patient for optimal ventilation; pillow removed to prevent head from bending forward and compressing trachea.
2. Keep side rails in position and position the patient to prevent injury if a seizure occurs; do not use restraints, as they only aggravate the patient and may result in muscle strain or fractures.
3. Have equipment available to treat respiratory difficulties; provide tracheostomy and cardiac arrest equipment.
4. Monitor calcium levels: If in 48 hours, level falls below 7½ mg./100 ml. (3 mEq.), replacement of calcium (gluconate, lactate) is done intravenously.
5. Use caution in intravenous administration of calcium to the patient who has renal disease or who is receiving digitalis preparations.

Subacute Thyroiditis

Subacute thyroiditis is usually a self-limiting inflammation of the thyroid gland most likely due to viral infections.

Incidence

Affects younger women predominantly.

Clinical Manifestations

1. Pain, swelling, thyroid tenderness, which lasts several weeks or months, then disappears
2. Temperature elevation, sore throat
3. Pain referred to the ear, making swallowing difficult and uncomfortable
4. Fever, malaise, chills
5. May develop clinical manifestations of hyperthyroidism (irritability, nervousness, insomnia, and weight loss) or hypothyroidism

Diagnostic Evaluation

1. Low TSH level and low thyroid radioactive uptake levels are present.
2. Serum T_3 and T_4 levels are elevated.
3. Erythrocyte sedimentation rate is increased.

Management

1. Analgesics and mild sedatives
2. The patient may be placed on thyroid medications to maintain a normal level of circulating thyroid hormone.
3. Steroids may be administered for pain, fever, and malaise.
4. Aspirin may be indicated in mild cases to treat the symptoms of inflammation.

NURSING ALERT: Aspirin should be avoided if the patient exhibits signs of hyperthyroidism, because it displaces thyroid hormone from its binding sites, and it increases the amount of circulating hormone and the degree and severity of the symptoms of hyperthyroidism.

Complications

In about 10% of patients, permanent hypothyroidism occurs and long-term thyroxine therapy is needed.

Nursing Interventions

1. Assess for signs and symptoms of hyperthyroidism (see p. 537).
2. Provide for symptomatic relief of signs and symptoms.
3. Explain all tests and procedures to patient/family.

Discharge Planning/Patient Education

1. Explain all medications the patient is to continue at home.
2. Reassure patient that subacute thyroiditis usually resolves spontaneously over weeks to months.
3. Teach patient signs and symptoms of hypothyroidism (i.e., fatigue and lethargy, weight gain, cold intolerance) that he may experience and should report as the inflammation of the gland subsides.

Lymphocytic Thyroiditis (Hashimoto's Thyroiditis)

Lymphocytic thyroiditis (Hashimoto's thyroiditis) is a chronic progressive disease of the thyroid gland caused by infiltration of lymphocytes and resulting in progressive destruction of the parenchyma and hypothyroidism if untreated.

Cause

Unknown; believed to be an autoimmune disease, genetically transmitted and perhaps related to Graves' disease.

Incidence

1. Ninety-five percent of the cases affect women in their 40s or 50s
2. Possibly the most common cause of adult hypothyroidism
3. Appears to be increasing in incidence

Clinical Manifestations

1. Marked by a slowly developing, firm enlargement of the thyroid gland
2. Usually no gross nodules
3. Basal metabolic rate usually low
4. Normal or high concentration of protein-bound iodine

Diagnostic Evaluation

1. Twenty-four hour radioactive iodine (RAI) uptake
2. Thyroid scan
3. Resin T_3 uptake determination
4. Thyroid needle biopsy that shows heavy infiltrate of lymphocytes
5. T_3 and T_4 usually become subnormal as the disease progresses

Management

1. Thyroid medications to maintain a normal level of circulating thyroid hormone; this is done to suppress production of thyrotropin, to prevent enlargement of the thyroid, and/or to maintain an euthyroid state.
2. Propranolol to control symptoms of thyrotoxicosis if they occur
3. Resection of thymus if tracheal compression, cough, or hoarseness occur
4. Careful follow-up to detect and treat hypothyroidism and myxedema

Complications

1. Progressive hypothyroidism
2. Without treatment, Hashimoto's thyroiditis may progress from goiter and hypothyroidism to myxedema.

Nursing Interventions

Assess for signs and symptoms of hypothyroidism (see Hypothyroidism, p. 535).

Discharge Planning/Patient Education

1. Explain necessity of taking thyroid medications every day for the rest of his life.
2. Teach patient signs and symptoms of hyperthyroidism he may experience when the Hashimoto's thyroiditis goes through periods of activity, when large amounts of T_3 and T_4 are released into the system, resulting in signs and symptoms of thyrotoxicosis.

Cancer of the Thyroid

Incidence

1. Cancer of the thyroid occurs twice as frequently in females as in males and more frequently in whites than in blacks.

2. Incidence increases with age. The average age at time of diagnosis is 45.
3. There appears to be an association between external radiation to the head and neck in infancy and childhood and subsequent development of thyroid carcinoma. (Between 1949 and 1960, radiation therapy was often given to shrink enlarged tonsil and adenoid tissue, to treat acne, or to reduce an enlarged thymus.)

Types

1. Papillary and well-differentiated adenocarcinoma (most common)
   a. Growth is slow, and spread is confined to lymph nodes that surround thyroid area.
   b. Cure rate is excellent after removal of involved areas.
2. Follicular (rapidly growing, widely metastasizing type)
   a. Occurs predominantly in middle-aged and elderly persons.
   b. Brief encouraging response may occur with x-ray irradiation.
   c. Progression of disease is rapid; high mortality rate.
3. Parafollicular—medullary thyroid carcinoma (MTC)
   a. Rare, inheritable type of thyroid malignancy, which can be detected early by a radioimmunoassay for the hormone calcitonin.
   b. Screening of familial MTC suspects is done by measuring circulating plasma calcitonin levels.

Diagnostic Evaluation

1. History and physical examination are important. On palpation of the thyroid, there may be a firm, irregular, fixed, painless mass or nodule.
2. The occurrence of signs and symptoms of hyperthyroidism is rare.
3. A thyroid scan with ^{99m}technetium pertechnetate is preferred, as it delivers a much lower level of radiation than ^{131}I. ^{123}I is even better.
4. Surgical exploration

Management

1. Surgical removal is extensive, as required.
2. Thyroid replacement
   a. Thyroid hormone is administered to suppress secretion of TSH.
   b. Such treatment is continued indefinitely and requires annual checkups.
3. For unresectable cancer, patient is referred for treatment with ^{131}I, chemotherapy, or radiation therapy.

Disorders of the Parathyroid Glands
The Parathyroid Glands

The parathyroid glands are small, bean-sized structures embedded in the posterior section of the thyroid gland.

Functions

1. Produce, store, and secrete parathormone in response to the serum level of ionized calcium.
2. Increase plasma calcium ions by acting on
   a. The kidney—to decrease elimination of calcium ions in the urine
   b. The gastrointestinal tract—to increase absorption of calcium ions from chyme
   c. Bone—to increase its contribution of calcium ions to the plasma

Hyperparathyroidism

Hyperparathyroidism is overactivity of the parathyroids.

Cause

1. An overgrowth or hypertrophy of parathyroid glands, as a primary disorder of the parathyroid glands or as a secondary condition occurring with renal failure as a result of renal retention of phosphorus
2. Carcinoma of the parathyroid or secretion of parathyroid hormone by ectopic tissue in malignancy may produce manifestations of hyperparathyroidism.

Clinical Manifestations

1. Decalcification of bones
   a. Skeletal pain, backache, pain on weight-bearing, pathological fractures, deformities, formation of bony cysts
   b. Formation of bone tumors—overgrowth of osteoclasts
2. Depression of neuromuscular function
   a. The patient may trip, drop objects, show general fatigue, loss of memory for recent events, emotional instability, changes in level of consciousness with stupor and coma.
   b. Cardiac dysrhythmias, hypertension, cardiac standstill
   c. Formation of calcium-containing kidney stones

Diagnostic Evaluation

1. Persistently elevated serum calcium (11 mg./100 ml.); test is performed three times to determine consistency of results.
2. Exclusion of other causes of hypercalcemia—malignancy, vitamin D excess, multiple myeloma, sarcoidosis, milk–alkali syndrome, drugs such as thiazides, Cushing's disease, hyperthyroidism
3. Parathyroid hormone (PTH) levels are increased with hyperactivity of the parathyroid glands.
4. Serum calcium and alkaline phosphatase levels are elevated and serum phosphorus levels are decreased with increased parathyroid activity.
5. Skeletal changes are revealed by x-ray.
6. Diagnosis often is extremely difficult. (Complications may occur before this condition is diagnosed.)
7. Cineradiography will disclose parathyroid tumors more readily than x-ray.

Management

1. Hydration and diuretics—furosemide (Lasix) and ethacrynic acid (Edecrin)—to increase urinary excretion of calcium
2. Oral phosphate may be used as an antihypercalcemic agent.
3. Dietary calcium is restricted, and all drugs that might cause hypercalcemia (thiazides, vitamin D) are discontinued.
4. Reduction of digitalis, as patient with hypercalcemia is more sensitive to toxic effects of this drug.

5. Monitoring of daily serum calcium, BUN, potassium, and magnesium levels.
6. Surgery for removal of abnormal parathyroid tissue

Complications

1. Kidney involvement
   a. Formation of renal stones
   b. Calcification of kidney parenchyma
   c. Renal shutdown
2. Gastrointestinal problems
   Ulceration of upper gastrointestinal tract (stomach, duodenum), leading to hemorrhage and perforation
3. Skeletal problems
   a. Simple demineralization
   b. Cysts and fibrosis of marrow—leading to fractures
   c. Fractures of vertebral bodies and fractures of the ribs

Nursing Assessment

1. Perform frequent multisystem assessment.
2. Closely monitor patient's input and output and serum electrolytes, especially calcium level.
3. Observe for signs and symptoms of hypercalcemia.

Nursing Diagnoses

1. Potential fluid volume deficit related to effects of elevated serum calcium levels
2. Potential altered urinary elimination related to renal calculi and calcium deposits in the kidneys
3. Potential impaired physical mobility related to abnormal bone formation, weakness, bone pain, and pathological fractures
4. Anxiety related to potential complications of surgery and hypocalcemia

Nursing Interventions

A. Establishing Normal Fluid and Electrolyte Balance to Prevent or Counteract Life-Threatening Effects of Hypercalcemia

1. Assess fluid intake and output.
2. Provide adequate hydration—administer water, glucose, and electrolytes by mouth or intravenously as prescribed.

NURSING ALERT: A low specific gravity for urine does not necessarily mean adequate hydration.

3. Prevent or promptly treat dehydration by reporting vomiting or other sources of fluid loss promptly.
4. Assist patient in understanding why and how to avoid dietary sources of calcium.
5. Monitor ECG to detect changes secondary to hypercalcemia. (During moderate elevations of serum calcium, Q–T interval is shortened; with extreme hypercalcemia, widening of the T wave is seen).

B. Improving Urinary Elimination

1. Assess urinary output; strain all urine to observe for kidney stones (renal calculi).
2. Increase fluid intake to 3000 ml./day to maintain hydration and prevent precipitation of calcium and formation of stones.
3. Provide diet low in calcium; eliminate milk and milk products.

4. Instruct the patient about dietary recommendations.
5. Observe the patient for signs of urinary tract infection, hematuria, and renal colic.
6. Instruct the patient to avoid medications containing calcium (some antacids).
7. Assess renal function through serum creatinine and BUN levels.

C. Promoting Normal Physical Mobility

1. Assist the patient in hygiene and activities if bone pain is severe or if the patient experiences musculoskeletal weakness.
2. Protect the patient from falls or injury.
3. Turn the patient cautiously and handle extremities gently to avoid fractures.
4. Administer analgesia as prescribed.
5. Assess level of pain and the patient's response to analgesia.
6. Encourage the patient to participate in mild exercise gradually as symptoms subside.
7. Instruct and demonstrate correct body mechanics to reduce strain, backache, and injury.

D. Alleviating Anxiety and Promoting Postoperative Recovery Without Complications or Manifestations of Hypocalcemia

1. Encourage patient to verbalize fears and feelings about upcoming surgery.
2. Explain tests and procedures to the patient.
3. See page 541 for postoperative care—is similar to that after thyroidectomy.
4. Recognize that the patient will retain some fluid postoperatively.
   a. This will be manifested by a low urinary output.
   b. Therefore, avoid overhydration for first day or two.
5. Avoid giving calcium until the patient's calcium level is determined.
6. Evaluate signs and symptoms of hypocalcemia and onset of tetany.
   a. Observe calcium levels—if well below normal and if decline continues into the second week, the skeletal system is absorbing calcium.
   b. If some involvement was noted preoperatively (elevated alkaline phosphatase level), calcium may be prescribed by physician.
7. Reassure the patient about skeletal recovery.
   a. Bone pain diminishes fairly quickly.
   b. Fractures treated by orthopedic procedures.

Discharge Planning and Patient Education

1. Instruct the patient how and when to take medications.
2. Teach the most common signs and symptoms of tetany that the patient may experience and should report to physician (numbness and tingling in extremities or around mouth).

Evaluation

1. Attains/maintains adequate fluid and electrolyte balance as measured by balance of urine output and fluid intake, normal skin turgor, moist mucous membranes, normal calcium and BUN levels, no ECG changes.
2. Attains/maintains improved urinary elimination as measured by adequate urine output without signs of kidney stones, urine is acidic (low pH), dilute, and clear; is without signs and symptoms of urinary tract infection, and serum creatinine and BUN levels are normal.

3. Achieves improved physical mobility by having increased strength and well-being, less bone and joint pain, and by using correct body mechanics to move, turn, and carry out activities.
4. Recovers from surgery without complications or manifestations of hypocalcemia, as measured by normal fluid balance, normal serum calcium levels, no manifestations of hypocalcemia and tetany.

Hypoparathyroidism

Hypoparathyroidism results from a deficiency of parathyroid hormone and is characterized by hypocalcemia and neuromuscular hyperexcitability.

Etiology

1. The most common cause is accidental removal or destruction of parathyroid tissue or its blood supply during thyroidectomy or radical neck dissection for malignancy.
2. Decrease in gland function (idiopathic hypoparathyroidism); may be autoimmune or familial in origin
3. Malignancy or metastasis from a cancer to the parathyroid glands
4. Resistance to parathyroid hormone action

Pathophysiology

1. With inadequate parathyroid hormone (PTH) secretion, there is decreased resorption of calcium from the renal tubules, decreased absorption of calcium in the gastrointestinal tract, and decreased resorption of calcium from bone.
2. Blood calcium falls to a low level, causing symptoms of muscular hyperirritability, uncontrolled spasms, and hypocalcemic tetany.
3. In response to decreased serum calcium levels and in the absence of parathyroid hormone, there is a rise in serum phosphate level and decreased phosphate excretion by the kidneys.
4. If onset of hypocalcemia is acute, the major concerns are laryngeal spasm, acute airway obstruction, and cardiovascular failure.
5. Long-term effects of persistent hypoparathyroidism include calcium deposits in tissues.

Clinical Manifestations and Diagnostic Evaluation

1. Due to deficiency of parathormone
   a. Accumulation of phosphorus in blood
   b. Decrease in serum calcium level to a low level (7.5 mg./100 ml. or less)
2. *Tetany*—General muscular hypertonia; attempts at voluntary movement result in tremors and spasmodic or uncoordinated movements; fingers assume classic position.
   a. *Chvostek's sign*—A spasm of facial muscles that occurs when muscles or branches of facial nerve are tapped
   b. *Trousseau's sign*—Carpopedal spasm within 3 minutes after a blood pressure cuff is inflated 20 mm. Hg above the patient's systolic pressure
   c. Laryngeal spasm
3. Anxiety and apprehension are very marked.
4. Renal colic is often present if the patient has had stones; preexisting stones loosen and migrate into the ureter.

Management

A. Calcium Administration

1. A syringe and an ampule of a calcium solution are to be kept at the bedside at all times.
2. Most rapidly effective calcium solution is ionized calcium chloride (10%).
3. For rapid use to relieve severe tetany, infusion carried out every 10 minutes.
   a. Ionized calcium chloride (10%) is administered slowly. It is highly irritating, stings, and causes thrombosis; patient experiences unpleasant burning flush of skin and, more particularly, of the tongue. *Too rapid calcium administration may cause cardiac arrest.*
   b. Calcium is given intravenously; calcium carbohydrate combination also may be used—gluconate or heptonate (10%) are not irritating.
4. A slow drip of intravenous saline containing calcium gluconate is given until control of tetany is ensured; then intramuscular or oral administration of calcium is prescribed.
5. Later, vitamin D is added to calcium intake—increases absorption of calcium and also induces a high level of calcium in the bloodstream.

B. Control of Anxiety

1. Patient has a strong feeling of impending disaster.
2. Administration of intravenous calcium seems to bring about rapid relief of anxiety.

C. Other Measures

1. Renal colic treatment (see p. 689).
2. Patient monitored for hypercalciuria. Periodic 24-hour urinary calcium determinations are recommended.
3. Blood calcium monitored periodically; variations in vitamin D may affect calcium levels.
4. Patient education emphasizes symptoms of hypocalcemia and hypercalcemia; physician to be notified should these occur.

Nursing Interventions

1. Assess neuromuscular status in patients at risk for hypocalcemia (patients in the immediate postoperative period following thyroidectomy, parathyroidectomy, radical neck dissection).
2. Check for positive Trousseau's or Chvostek's sign.
3. Assess respiratory status frequently in postoperative recovery phase.
4. Monitor serum calcium and phosphorus levels.
5. Have tracheostomy set available at the patient's bedside.
6. Report indications of respiratory distress, laryngeal stridor, or cardiovascular failure.
7. Promote high-calcium diet if prescribed.
8. Instruct the patient about signs and symptoms of hypo- and hypercalcemia that should be reported.
9. Use caution in administering other drugs to the patient with hypocalcemia.
   a. The hypocalcemic patient is sensitive to digoxin; as hypocalcemia is reversed, the patient may rapidly develop digitalis toxicity.
   b. Cimetidine (Tagamet) interferes with normal parathyroid function, especially in the patient with renal failure, which increases the risk of hypocalcemia.
10. Institute seizure precautions (airway at bedside, padded siderails).

Disorders of the Adrenal Glands

The Adrenal Glands

Composition

A. Medulla

1. Is not necessary to maintain life, but enables a person to cope with stress
2. Secretes two hormones
   a. Epinephrine (adrenalin)
      (1) Acts on alpha- and beta-receptors
      (2) Increases contractility and excitability of heart muscle, leading to increased cardiac output
      (3) Facilitates blood flow to muscles, brain, and viscera
      (4) Enhances blood sugar by stimulating conversion of glycogen to glucose in liver
      (5) Inhibits smooth muscle contraction
   b. Norepinephrine (noradrenalin)
      (1) Acts primarily on alpha receptors
      (2) Increases peripheral vascular resistance, leading to increases in diastolic and systolic blood pressure

B. Cortex

1. Is essential to life
2. Secretes adrenocortical hormone—synthesized from cholesterol
   a. Glucocorticoids; cortisone and hydrocortisone
      (1) Enhance protein catabolism and inhibit protein synthesis
      (2) Antagonize action of insulin and increase blood sugar
      (3) Increase synthesis of glucose by liver
      (4) Influence defense mechanism of body and its reaction to stress
      (5) Influence emotional reaction
   b. Mineralocorticoids
      (1) Aldosterone—supplied by adrenal cortex
      (2) Desoxycorticosterone—usually not present in significant amounts
      (3) Regulate reabsorption of sodium cation
      (4) Regulate excretion of potassium cation by renal tubules
   c. Adrenosterones (adrenal androgens)

Pheochromocytoma

Pheochromocytoma is a catecholamine-secreting neoplasm associated with hyperfunction of the adrenal medulla. It may appear wherever chromaffin cells are located; however, most are found in the adrenal medulla. Pheochromocytoma can occur at any age, but is most common between the ages of 30 and 60; it is uncommon in individuals over the age of 65.

Pathophysiology and Clinical Manifestations

1. Most pheochromocytoma tumors are benign; 10% are malignant with metastasis.
2. These tumors produce increased secretion of epinephrine and norepinephrine; tumors located in the adrenal medulla produce both epinephrine and norepinephrine, and those located outside the adrenal gland tend to produce epinephrine only.
3. The excessive secretion of norepinephrine and epinephrine produces hypertension, hypermetabolism, and hyperglycemia.
4. Variation in symptoms depends on the predominance of norepinephrine or epinephrine secretion and on whether the hormones are secreted continuously or intermittently.
5. Hypertension may be paroxysmal (intermittent) or persistent (chronic). Chronic form may be difficult to differentiate from "essential hypertension"; however, drugs effective for essential hypertension are not effective in this patient. The hypertensive effects of pheochromocytoma produce headaches and visual disturbances.
6. The hypermetabolic and hyperglycemic effects of pheochromocytoma produce tachycardia, excessive perspiration, tremor, pallor or face flushing, nervousness, elevated blood glucose levels, polyuria, nausea, vomiting, diarrhea and abdominal pain, paresthesia in extremities.
7. Symptoms are often triggered by allergic reactions, physical exertion, emotional upset; they also can occur without identifiable stimulus.

Diagnostic Evaluation

1. If there is sympathetic overactivity, along with marked elevation of blood pressure, pheochromocytoma is strongly suspected.
2. Twenty-four hour urine tests:
   a. Vanillylmandelic acid (VMA) and metanephrine determinations in urine (VMA and metanephrine are metabolites of epinephrine and norepinephrine.)
   b. Determinations of catecholamines in urine and blood offer an effective test for overactivity of adrenal medulla.
   c. Normal urinary values:
      VMA, 0.7–6.8 mg./24 hours
      Metanephrines, less than 1.3 mg./24 hours
      Catecholamines, 0–275 μg./24 hours
3. Other tests—computed tomography (CT scan) and magnetic resonance imaging (MRI) of the adrenal glands may help in identifying the location of tumor.
4. Clonidine suppression test is useful to distinguish essential hypertension patients with increased plasma norepinephrine levels from those patients with hypertension due to pheochromocytoma. Clonidine will suppress plasma catecholamine secretion in patients with essential hypertension, but not in patients with pheochromocytoma.

Management

Goals:
Control blood pressure.
Diagnose the condition accurately.
Prepare the patient adequately for surgery.
Remove the cause surgically.

A. Preoperative Management

1. To accomplish blood pressure control, alpha-adrenergic blocking agents such as phentolamine (Regitine) or phenoxybenzamine hydrochloride (Dibenzyline) are prescribed to inhibit the effects of catecholamines (Effective control of blood pressure and blood volume may take 1 or 2 weeks.).
2. Catecholamine synthesis inhibitors also may be used—metyrosine (Demser).

3. Propranolol is helpful in controlling cardiac dysrhythmias or marked tachycardia.
4. Plasma volume is determined, as these patients are very sensitive to blood loss and therefore may benefit from preoperative volume expansion.
5. Adequate hydration is essential to minimize risk of intraoperative and postoperative hypotension.
6. For long-term maintenance of patients with inoperable tumors, metyrosine may be given.
   a. Moderate to severe sedation is a side effect when therapy is initiated; patients are cautioned against driving or participating in activities requiring alertness.
   b. Avoid concurrent use of alcohol or other CNS depressants.
   c. Maintain fluid intake as a precaution against crystalluria; maintain daily urinary output of at least 2000 ml.

B. Postoperative Management

1. Observe for complications
   a. Hypertension
   b. Hypotension
   c. Hyperglycemia
2. Maintain adequate fluid intake and blood volume.
3. Ensure that ventilation and oxygenation are adequate.
4. Alleviate postoperative pain.
5. Monitor blood glucose levels frequently for the first 24 hours postoperatively, as hyperglycemia commonly occurs.
6. Evaluate and document 24-hour urine specimens. The patient is considered surgically cured when 24-hour urine specimens are evaluated as "normal" when tested for catecholamines or catecholamine metabolites.

C. Familial Pheochromocytoma

Evaluation of the patient's family for pheochromocytoma and medullary carcinoma of the thyroid should be done.

Nursing Assessment

1. Secure data concerning history of signs and symptoms patient has been experiencing.
2. Assess for predisposing factors that may be triggering signs and symptoms (i.e., physical exertion, emotional upset, allergies).
3. Determine patient's/family's level of anxiety; reaction to illness.
4. Perform thorough physical assessment to gather objective information concerning signs and symptoms patient is currently exhibiting.
5. Review results of diagnostic studies to ascertain possible cause(s) of elevated blood pressure and other symptoms.

Nursing Diagnoses

1. Potential altered cardiac output related to severe hypermetabolism during preoperative and intraoperative period and to hypotension during the postoperative period
2. Anxiety related to the systemic effects of epinephrine and norepinephrine and preoperative anxiety

Nursing Interventions

A. Improving Cardiac Output

1. Monitor cardiovascular, neurological, and renal function closely.
2. Assess and record blood pressure, pulse, respiratory rate, intake and output, neurological signs, and serum creatinine and BUN levels.
3. Report changes in neurological, cardiovascular, and renal status and elevations in blood pressure.
4. Ensure bedrest and elevate the head of the bed to 45 degrees during episodes of severe hypertension.
5. Reduce environmental stressors by providing calm, quiet environment. Restrict visitors.
6. Explain all tests, procedures, and events to the patient.
7. Administer sedatives as prescribed to promote relaxation and rest.
8. Eliminate stimulants (coffee, tea, cola) from the diet.
9. Reduce events that precipitate episodes of severe hypertension—palpation of the tumor, physical exertion, emotional upset, anesthesia induction, and surgical intervention without adequate physical and emotional preparation.
10. Monitor ECG and arterial pressures postoperatively to detect cardiovascular changes and hyper- or hypotension.
11. Maintain intravenous infusion postoperatively.
12. Explain rationale for medications and necessity of taking medications for the rest of life if prescribed.

B. Alleviating Anxiety

1. Encourage the patient to verbalize fears and feelings about events and upcoming surgery.
2. Explain tests, procedures, and events to the patient.
3. Remain with the patient during acute episodes of hypertension.
4. Carry out tasks and procedures in calm, unhurried manner when with the patient.
5. Instruct the patient about use of relaxation exercises.

Discharge Planning/Patient Education

Instruct the patient how and when to take medications.

Evaluation

1. Maintains adequate cardiac output as measured by normal vital signs, adequate urine output, and normal serum creatinine and BUN levels.
2. Verbalizes concerns and fears about upcoming surgery and appears less anxious and reports an increased sense of well-being.

Primary Aldosteronism

Primary aldosteronism refers to excessive secretion of aldosterone by the adrenal cortex. Primary aldosteronism is usually caused by a cortical adenoma; secondary aldosteronism occurs in conjunction with heart failure, renal dysfunction, or cirrhosis of the liver.

Clinical Manifestations

1. Hypertension. (One to two percent of cases of hypertension are a result of primary aldosteronism, which usually can be treated successfully by surgical removal of the adenoma.)
2. A profound decline in blood levels of potassium (hypokalemia) and hydrogen ions (alkalosis) results in muscle weakness and inability of kidneys to acidify or concentrate urine, leading to excess volume of urine (polyuria).
3. A decline in hydrogen ions (alkalosis) results in tetany, paresthesia.

4. An elevation in blood sodium (hypernatremia) results in excessive thirst (polydipsia) and arterial hypertension.

Diagnostic Evaluation

1. Primary aldosteronism is suspected in all hypertensive patients with spontaneous hypokalemia; also in patients who become hypokalemic almost concurrently with the administration of diuretics and who remain so after the diuretics are discontinued.
2. Salt loading is a provocative screening test that can be used. Ingestion of sodium in excess of 200 mEq./day (approximately 12 gm. of salt) for 4 days does not influence the serum potassium level in the absence of aldosteronism, but will cause a decrease of serum potassium to less than 3.5 mEq./L. in a patient with aldosteronism.
3. CT scanning to determine and localize cortical adenoma

A. Primary Aldosteronism

Removal of adrenal tumor—adrenalectomy (see p. 551).

B. Secondary Aldosteronism

1. Management is dependent on treatment of the underlying disorder.
2. Spironolactone is usually effective in controlling both the hypertension and potassium-depleted stages; therapy is needed 4–6 weeks before the full effect on blood pressure is seen.

Cushing's Syndrome

Cushing's Syndrome is a condition in which the plasma cortisol levels are elevated, causing signs and symptoms of hypercortisolism.

Etiology

1. Pituitary Cushing's syndrome (Cushing's disease)—hyperplasia of both glands due to overstimulation of the adrenal cortex by ACTH, usually from a pituitary adenoma or hyperplasia.
   a. Most common cause of Cushing's syndrome
   b. Affects mostly women between 20 and 40 years of age.
2. Adrenal Cushing's syndrome
   a. Associated with tumors of the adrenal cortex—adenoma or carcinoma.
3. Ectopic
   a. Results from autonomous ACTH secretion by extrapituitary neoplasms
   b. Tumors elsewhere in body producing excess ACTH

Pathophysiology

1. The normal feedback mechanisms that control adrenocortical function are ineffective, resulting in secretion of adrenal cortical hormones despite adequate amounts of these hormones in the circulation.
2. The manifestations of Cushing's syndrome are the result of excess hormones (glucocorticoids, mineralocorticoids, and sex hormones).
3. Excess of one hormone or all the hormones can occur; the predominant hormone secreted in excess (usually glucocorticoids) determines the predominant symptoms.

Clinical Manifestations

Adult ("central-type obesity")

A. Manifestations Due to Excess Glucocorticoids

1. Weight gain/obesity
2. Heavy trunk; thin extremities
3. "Buffalo hump" in neck and supraclavicular area
4. Rounded face (moon face); plethoric, oily
5. Skin—fragile and thin; striae and ecchymosis, acne
6. Muscles—wasted due to excessive catabolism
7. Osteoporosis—characteristic kyphosis, backache
8. Mental disturbances—mood changes, psychosis
9. Increased susceptibility to infections

B. Manifestations Due to Excess Mineralocorticoids

1. Hypertension
2. Increased serum sodium level; low serum potassium level
3. Increased weight gain
4. Expanded blood volume
5. Edema

C. Manifestations Due to Excess Sex Hormones

1. Females (Cushing's syndrome occurs ten times more frequently in females than in males)
   a. "Virilism" or masculinization
      (1) Hirsutism—excessive growth of hair on the face and midline of trunk
      (2) Breasts—atrophy
      (3) Clitoris—enlarges
      (4) Voice—masculine
      (5) Loss of libido
   b. *In utero*—possible hermaphrodite
2. Males—loss of libido

Diagnostic Evaluation

1. Excessive plasma cortisol levels
2. An increase in blood glucose levels and glucose tolerance curve of diabetes mellitus
3. A decrease in serum potassium level
4. A reduction in the number of blood eosinophils
5. Elevation in the urine level of 17-hydroxycorticoids and 17-ketogenic steroids
6. Elevation of plasma ACTH in patients with pituitary tumors
7. Very low plasma ACTH levels in a patient with hypercortisolism are characteristic of an adrenal tumor
8. Loss of diurnal variation of cortisol secretion
9. X-rays of the skull to detect erosion of the sella turcica by a pituitary tumor
10. Adrenal angiography. (Procedure and preparation of the patient are similar to that of renal angiography, but the inferior adrenal artery, a branch of the renal artery, is injected with contrast medium for visualization.
11. Overnight dexamethasone suppression test
    a. Dexamethasone is administered the night before in the amount equivalent to the amount of cortisol normally produced by the patient in a day.
    b. Dexamethasone will normally suppress ACTH secretion and stop cortisol production.
    c. The next day, blood studies will be done; patients with Cushing's syndrome will not show suppression below a certain level.
12. If above test does not rule out the possibility of Cushing's syndrome, specific urinary excretion tests are performed with dexamethasone suppression.
13. Additional tests are done to determine whether the problem is due to hyperplasia or adrenocortical tumor.

14. Computed tomography (CT scan) and ultrasonography may be requested to detect the exact location of the tumor.

Management

A. Surgical Removal of Causative Factor

1. Tumor (adrenal or pituitary) is removed or treated with irradiation. The most recent development in the management of pituitary Cushing's syndrome in adults is transsphenoidal hypophysectomy (see p. 587).
2. Hyperplasia of adrenals—adrenalectomy

B. Replacement Therapy Postoperatively

1. Adrenalectomy patients require a lifelong replacement therapy with the following:
   a. A glucocorticoid—cortisone
   b. A mineralocorticoid—fludrocortisone (Florinef)
2. Following pituitary irradiation or hypophysectomy, patient may require adrenal replacement plus thyroid and gonadal replacement therapy.
3. Following transsphenoidal adenomectomy, patient requires hydrocortisone replacement therapy for periods of 12–18 months.
4. Protein anabolic steroids may facilitate protein replacement; potassium stores are usually depleted rapidly and may require replacement.

C. Medical Treatment

In patients unable to undergo surgery (e.g., because of myocardial infarction)
1. Mitotane, an agent toxic to the adrenal cortex (DDT derivative)—"medical adrenalectomy" (Nausea, vomiting, diarrhea, somnolence, and depression may occur with use of this drug.)
2. Metyrapone (Metopirone) to control steroid hypersecretion in patients who do not respond to mitotane therapy

Nursing Assessment

1. Observe patient for signs and symptoms of Cushing's disease.
2. Perform multisystem physical examination.
3. Monitor input and output, daily weights, and serum electrolytes.

Nursing Diagnoses

1. Altered skin integrity related to impaired healing, thin and fragile skin, and increased susceptibility to infection and edema
2. Potential self-care deficit (feeding, bathing/hygiene, dressing/grooming) related to muscle wasting, osteoporosis, weakness, and fatigue
3. Disturbance in self-concept (body image; self-esteem) related to altered physical appearance and emotional instability and role change

Nursing Interventions

A. Improving Skin Integrity

1. Assess skin frequently to detect reddened areas, breakdown or tearing of skin, excoriation, infection, or edema.
2. Handle skin and extremities gently to prevent trauma; protect from falls by use of siderails.
3. Avoid use of adhesive tape to reduce risk of trauma to skin on its removal.
4. Encourage the patient to turn in bed frequently or ambulate to reduce pressure on bony prominences and areas of edema.
5. Use meticulous skin care to reduce injury and breakdown.
6. Provide foods low in sodium to minimize edema formation.
7. Assess intake and output and daily weights to evaluate fluid retention.

B. Increasing Participation in Activities of Daily Living

1. Assist the patient with ambulation and hygiene when weak and fatigued.
2. Assist the patient in planning schedule to permit exercise and rest.
3. Encourage the patient to rest when fatigued.
4. Encourage gradual resumption of activities as the patient gains strength.
5. Identify for the patient signs and symptoms indicating excessive exertion.
6. Instruct the patient in correct body mechanics to avoid pain or injury during activities.
7. Use assistive devices during ambulation to prevent falls and fractures.
8. Provide foods high in potassium to counteract weakness related to hypokalemia.

C. Improving Body Image and Increasing Self-Esteem

1. Encourage the patient to verbalize concerns about illness, changes in appearance, and altered role functions.
2. Identify those situations that are disturbing to the patient; record these on the nursing care plan as situations to be avoided.
3. Be alert for evidence of depression; in some instances this has progressed to suicide; therefore, mood changes are most important.
4. Report if depression continues after surgery.
5. Recognize and accept the emotional stress in the female patient who manifests masculinization tendencies.
6. Explain to the patient who has benign adenoma or hyperplasia that, with proper treatment, evidence of masculinization can be reversed.
7. Recognize that weakness is a frustrating experience in a patient who heretofore has been active.
8. Provide a low-calorie, low-carbohydrate diet to reduce hyperglycemia and prevent obesity.

Evaluation

1. Demonstrates intact skin without evidence of breakdown or excoriation, infection, or evidence of trauma
2. Participates safely in activities of daily living as evidenced by ability to do own hygienic care; needs little to no assistance with ambulation
3. Experiences improved body image and self-esteem as evidenced by ability to verbalize concerns about illness/appearance, interacts appropriately with others, and is able to identify reasons for changes in appearance.

Adrenocortical Insufficiency

Adrenocortical insufficiency occurs when there is inadequate secretion of the hormones of the adrenal cortex, primarily the glucocorticoids and mineralocorticoids.

Etiology

A. **Primary Adrenocortical Insufficiency (or Addison's disease)**—occurs with destruction and subsequent hypofunction of the adrenal cortex, resulting in deficient production of the following adrenal steroids:
1. Glucocorticoids (principally cortisol)
2. Mineralocorticoids (principally aldosterone)

B. **Secondary Adrenocortical Insufficiency**—is a result of ACTH deficiency from
1. Pituitary disease with atrophy of adrenal cortex (a result of pituitary hypofunction)
2. Suppression or atrophy of hypothalamic–pituitary axis by corticosteroids (used in treating nonendocrine disorders)

Pathophysiology

1. The majority of the clinical manifestations of adrenocortical insufficiency result from deficiency of aldosterone, the chief mineralocorticoid, and deficiency of cortisol, the chief glucocorticoid; few symptoms related to deficiency of sex hormones, or androgens, occur.
2. Inadequate aldosterone produces disturbances of sodium, potassium, and water metabolism.
3. Cortisol deficiency produces abnormal fat, protein, and carbohydrate metabolism; absence of cortisol during a period of stress can precipitate Addisonian crisis, an exaggerated state of adrenal cortical insufficiency, and lead to death.

Clinical Manifestations

1. Decreased serum sodium and increased serum potassium levels
2. Water loss, dehydration, and hypovolemia
3. Muscular weakness, fatigue, weight loss
4. Gastrointestinal problems—anorexia, nausea, vomiting, diarrhea, constipation, abdominal pain
5. Low blood pressure, low blood sugar, low basal metabolic rate (BMR), increased insulin sensitivity
6. Mental changes occur—depression, irritability, anxiety, apprehension due to hypoglycemia and hypovolemia
7. Normal responses to stress lacking
8. Hyperpigmentation

Diagnostic Evaluation

1. *History*—Current or past use of corticosteroids
2. *Blood studies*
   a. Hypoglycemia—decrease in serum glucose level
   b. Hyponatremia—decrease in sodium concentration
   c. Hyperkalemia—increase in potassium concentration
   d. Lymphoid hyperplasia
   e. Low fasting plasma cortisol levels; low aldosterone levels
3. *Urine Studies*—Twenty-four–hour specimen for 17-ketosteroids, 17-hydroxycorticoids, and 17-ketogenic steroids—all values decreased
4. *Injection of a potent pituitary adrenocorticotropic hormone to artificially stimulate adrenals*
   a. Normal response—normal rise in plasma cortisol and urinary 17-ketosteroids.
   b. In Addison's disease

(1) Decrease in circulating eosinophils
(2) Increase in uric acid excretion in about 4 hours
(3) No rise in plasma cortisol and urinary 17-ketosteroids

Management

1. Restoration of normal fluid and electrolyte balance
   a. High-sodium, low-potassium diet and fluids
   b. Treatment of glucocorticoid deficiency with cortisone, cortisol, or prednisone. Mineralocorticoid deficiency treated with fludrocortisone

Note: Overtreatment may be manifested by hypertension, edema from sodium and water retention, weakness due to sodium loss.

2. Immediate treatment if Addisonian crisis or circulatory collapse is imminent:
   a. Intravenous administration of sodium chloride solution to replace sodium ions
   b. Hydrocortisone
   c. Injection of circulatory stimulants
3. Diagnosis and treatment of underlying cause of adrenocortical insufficiency or Addisonian crisis (e.g., antibiotic therapy to treat infection if this is a factor in crisis)
4. Cardiovascular support if indicated

Nursing Assessment

1. Review patient's record and results of physical examination and laboratory studies.
2. Maintain weight chart and monitor vital signs.
3. Observe patient during activities of daily living.
4. Monitor for signs of anxiety/depression; reactions to family and friends.

Nursing Diagnoses

1. Altered fluid and electrolyte balance related to renal losses of sodium and water and renal retention of potassium, gastrointestinal losses of fluid and electrolytes, and inadequate dietary intake
2. Potential ineffective individual coping related to inability to withstand stress secondary to decreased secretion of glucocorticoids and aldosterone.
3. Altered activity intolerance related to decreased cortisol production; fatigue

Nursing Interventions

A. **Establishing Normal Fluid and Electrolyte Balance**

1. Assess fluid intake and output and serial daily weights.
2. Monitor vital signs frequently; a drop in blood pressure may suggest an impending crisis.
3. Assess serum levels of sodium and potassium frequently.
4. Assess skin turgor and mucous membranes for signs and symptoms of dehydration.
5. Provide diet high in sodium and fluid content; administer potassium supplements if prescribed.
6. Administer prescribed glucocorticoids and mineralocorticoids; report response of patient.
7. Administer intravenous infusions of sodium, water, and glucose if prescribed and indicated by the patient's condition.

B. Promoting Increased Coping With Stressors

1. Minimize stressful situations in the patient with altered response to stressors.
2. Protect the patient from infection
   a. Control the patient's contacts so that infectious organisms are not transmitted.
   b. Protect the patient from drafts, dampness, exposure to cold.
   c. Prevent overexertion.
3. Observe carefully the emotional status of the patient.
   a. Control the temperature of the room to avoid sharp deviations in the patient's temperature.
   b. Maintain a quiet, peaceful environment; avoid loud talking and noisy radios.
4. Observe for early signs of Addisonian crisis, which may be indicative of ineffective coping
   a. Sudden drop in blood pressure
   b. Nausea, vomiting
   c. High temperature

C. Decreasing Activity Intolerance

1. Assist the patient with activities of daily living.
2. Provide for periods of rest and activity to avoid overexertion.
3. Provide for high-calorie, high-protein diet.

Discharge Planning and Patient Education

1. Instruct the patient about the necessity for long-term therapy for adrenocortical insufficiency and medical follow-up.
   a. Inform the patient that therapy must be continued throughout life.
   b. Emphasize the importance of taking more hormones when under stress.
   c. Suggest that the patient carry an identification card indicating the type of medication being taken and physician's telephone number.
2. Instruct the patient about manifestations of excessive use of medications and reportable symptoms.
3. Identify actions to take to avoid factors that may precipitate Addisonian crisis (infection, extremes of temperature, etc.).

Evaluation

1. Achieves/maintains adequate fluid and electrolyte balance as measured by balance of fluid intake and urine output, normal skin turgor, moist mucous membranes, normal sodium and potassium levels, normal vital signs
2. Demonstrates ability to cope with stressors as measured by normal vital signs, including temperature
3. Achieves/maintains normal activity tolerance as measured by ability to carry out ADL with minimal to no assistance

Management of the Patient Having an Adrenalectomy

Preoperative

1. Correct hyperglycemia by proper diet and insulin.
2. Administer high-protein diet to correct protein deficiency.
3. See page 52; care of patient is similar to that for general surgery of abdomen.

Postoperative Management

1. Similar to that for an abdominal operation (see p. 56)
2. Will require administration of hydrocortisone or similar compounds in large amounts; this should begin before surgery. If bilateral adrenalectomy is performed, life-long replacement is necessary.
3. For removal of pheochromocytoma
   a. Because of manipulation of tumor during surgery, there may be extreme fluctuations of blood pressure.
   b. On ligation of vessels from tumor, an abrupt fall of blood pressure may result. Administer large amounts of epinephrine intravenously.

> **NURSING ALERT:** Be prepared to monitor blood pressure frequently for 24–48 hours and to regulate vasopressor intravenous medications in order to stabilize the blood pressure.

4. Monitor vital signs, including blood pressure and central venous pressure, for up to 48 hours to detect early changes that may indicate impending cardiovascular collapse.
5. Anticipate stressful situations for the patient and avoid them; provide rest periods, anticipate the patient's needs, provide comfort measures.

Steroid Therapy

Classification of Steroids

(By major metabolic effects on body)
1. Mineralocorticoids
   a. Concerned with sodium and water retention and potassium excretion
   b. Example—aldosterone and 11-desoxycorticosterone
2. Glucocorticoids
   a. Concerned with metabolic effects, including carbohydrate metabolism
   b. Example—cortisol
3. Sex hormones
   a. Important when secreted in large amounts or when the growth of hormone-sensitive cancers is stimulated
   b. Examples:
      Androgens—testosterone
      Estrogens—estradiol
      Progestins—progesterone

Effects of Glucocorticoids
(corticosteroids, steroids)

1. Antagonize action of insulin—promote gluconeogenesis, which provides glucose
2. Increase breakdown of protein (inhibit protein synthesis)
3. Increase breakdown of fatty acids
4. Suppress inflammation, inhibit scar formation, block allergic responses
5. Decrease number of circulating eosinophils and leukocytes; decrease size of lymphatic tissue
6. Exert a permissive action (allow full expression of effects of another hormone) on all effects caused by catecholamines

7. Exert a permissive action on functioning of central nervous system
8. Inhibit release of adrenocorticotropin

IN SUMMARY: Glucocorticoids are necessary to resist noxious stimuli and environmental change.

Uses of Steroids

1. Physiologically—to correct deficiencies or malfunction of a particular endocrine organ or system (e.g., Addison's disease)
2. Diagnostically—to determine proper functioning of the endocrine system
3. Pharmacologically—to treat the following:
   a. Rheumatoid arthritis
   b. Acute rheumatic fever
   c. Blood conditions
      (1) Idiopathic thrombocytopenic purpura
      (2) Leukemia
      (3) Hemolytic anemia
   d. Allergic conditions—bronchial asthma, allergic rhinitis
   e. Dermatologic problems—drug rashes, giant hives, atopic dermatitis
   f. Ocular diseases—conjunctivitis, uveitis
   g. Connective tissue disorders—lupus erythematosus, periarteritis nodosa
   h. Gastrointestinal problems—ulcerative colitis
   i. Organ-transplant recipients—as an immunosuppressive agent
   j. Neurological—cerebral edema
   k. Other conditions—gout, multiple sclerosis
4. Emergency conditions
   a. Status asthmaticus
   b. Acute renal insufficiency
   c. Anaphylactic reaction (only after epinephrine has been given)

Preparing the Patient to Receive Steroid Therapy

1. Determine contraindications for such therapy
   a. Peptic ulcer
   b. Diabetes mellitus
   c. Viral infections
2. Administer a tuberculin test to determine need for antituberculin drugs. If this is not done prior to steroid therapy, the patient's hypersensitivity to tuberculin and response to the tubercle bacillus are suppressed.
3. Assess the patient's own level of steroid secretion, if possible.
4. Explain the nature of the therapy, what is required of the patient, how long he is to be on steroid medications, what adverse signs to watch for, and answer any questions.

Choice of Steroid and Method of Administration

1. May be given by a wide variety of methods—orally, parenterally, sublingually, rectally, by inhalation, or by direct application to skin or mucous membrane
2. Combinations of steroids with other drugs should be avoided.
3. To help avoid steroid side effects, alternate-day therapy should be used if at all possible, but is not always feasible.
4. Sometimes steroids are given in extremely high doses, then sharply reduced; if the patient has been taking steroids for a while, doses must be tapered gradually to prevent Addisonian crisis.

Nursing Interventions

A. Infection Control

1. Encourage the patient to avoid crowds and the possibility of exposure to infection.
   Steroids may affect the circulating blood—resulting in decreased eosinophils and lymphocytes, increased red cells, and increased incidence of thrombophlebitis and infection.
2. Use exercise schedules to prevent stasis.
3. Be aware that cardinal symptoms of inflammation may be masked.
4. Instruct all personnel coming in contact with this patient to wash hands thoroughly and practice meticulous asepsis.

B. Diet and Metabolism Considerations

1. Determine whether the patient needs assistance in dietary control.
   Steroids may cause weight gain and an increase in appetite.
2. Administer a high-protein, high-carbohydrate diet.
   Steroids affect protein metabolism; there may be negative nitrogen balance.
3. Encourage the patient to take steroids with milk or food.
   Steroids cause an increase in secretion of gastric hydrochloric acid and have an inhibiting effect on secretion of mucus in the stomach; they may aggravate an existing peptic ulcer.
4. Be on guard for early evidence of gastric hemorrhage such as melena, blood in vomitus.
5. Check urine for evidence of glucose.
   Steroids precipitate gluconeogenesis and insulin antagonism, which results in hyperglycemia, glucosuria, decreased carbohydrate tolerance.

C. Possible Bone Complications

1. Be on the alert for the possibility of pathological fractures. Stress safety measures to prevent injury.
   a. Steroids affect the musculoskeletal system, causing potassium depletion and muscular weakness.
   b. Steroids cause increased output of calcium and phosphorus, which may lead to osteoporosis.
2. Administer a diet high in calcium and protein.
3. Recommend a program of activities of daily living; normal range of motion for the bedridden.

D. Electrolyte Disturbance

1. Restrict sodium intake and increase potassium intake.
   a. Lemon juice is high in potassium and low in sodium.
   b. Avoid saline as a diluent in preparing injectable medications.
   c. Mineralocorticoid differs from other steroids, resulting in sodium retention and potassium depletion: edema, weight gain.
2. Check blood pressure frequently and weigh the patient daily.
3. Observe for evidence of edema.

E. Behavioral Reactions

1. Watch for convulsive seizures (especially in children).
   Steroids may alter behavior patterns, increase excitability, and affect the central nervous system.
2. Avoid overstimulating situations.

3. Recognize and report any mood deviating from the usual behavior patterns.
4. Report unusual behavior, haunting dreams, withdrawal, or suicidal tendencies.

F. Stress Reactions

1. Recommend that the patient carry at all times an identification card indicating that he is on steroid therapy and including the name of his physician and instructions for emergency care.

   Steroids affect the hypothalmic–pituitary–adrenal system; this in turn affects the individual's ability to respond to stress.

2. Advise the patient to avoid extremes of temperature, as well as infections and upsetting situations.

G. Safety Measures

1. Instruct the patient to avoid injury; stress safety precautions.

   Steroids interfere with fibroblasts and granulation tissue; there is altered response to injury, resulting in impaired growth and delayed healing.

2. Observe daily the healing process of wounds, particularly surgical wounds, to recognize the potential for wound dehiscence.

Patient Education

1. Recognize that steroids are valuable and useful medications, but if taken for longer than 2 weeks, they may produce certain side effects.
   a. "Acceptable" side effects may include weight gain (perhaps due to water retention), acne, headaches, fatigue, and increased urinary frequency.
   b. "Unacceptable" side effects that are to be reported to the physician are dizziness when rising from chair or bed (postural hypotension indicative of adrenal insufficiency), nausea, vomiting, thirst, abdominal pain, or pain of any type.
   c. Additional side effects that are reportable are convulsive seizures, feelings of depression or nervousness, or development of an infection.
   d. Patient and/or family member is/are instructed about the rationale for and side effects of steroid medication.
2. If the patient has a fall or is in an automobile accident, condition may precipitate adrenal failure—requires an immediate injection of hydrocortisone phosphate. (Long-term patients should wear a Medic-Alert tag and carry a kit with hydrocortisone.)
3. The patient is instructed to inform any physician, dentist, or nurse in future contacts that he is on steroid therapy.
4. Regular follow-up visits to physician are required.

Disorders of the Pituitary Gland

Diabetes Insipidus

Diabetes insipidus is a disorder of water metabolism caused by deficiency of vasopressin, the antidiuretic hormone (ADH) secreted by the posterior pituitary.

Etiology

1. Primary; idiopathic
2. Secondary; head trauma, neurosurgery tumors (intra-cranial or metastatic), vascular disease (aneurysms, infarct), infection (meningitis, encephalitis)

Clinical Manifestations

1. Marked polyuria—daily output of 5–20 liters of very dilute urine; appearance of urine like that of water, with a specific gravity of 1.000–1.005, corresponding to a urine osmolality of 50–200 mOsm./kg.
2. Polydipsia (intense thirst); 4–40 liters of fluid daily; patient has a craving for cold water
3. High serum osmolality (>295 mOsm.) and high serum sodium level (>145 mEq./L.)

Diagnostic Evaluation

1. Patient's history and clinical manifestations of polyuria and polydipsia, high serum osmolality and low urine osmolality.
2. Fluid deprivation test—water intake restricted and changes in urine volume and concentration noted
   a. Fluids usually withheld for 6–8 hours until urine osmolality of at least three consecutive urine specimens vary by <30 mOsm./kg.
   b. Once urine osmolality has stabilized, 5–10 U aqueous vasopressin is injected subcutaneously. One hour later, the urine osmolality is measured.
   c. Patients with diabetes insipidus will have an inability to increase specific gravity and osmolality of urine.
3. Measurements of serum and urine ADH

Management and Nursing Interventions

1. Diagnostic testing conducted to search for and correct underlying pathology; diabetes insipidus may occur in the course of many forms of intracranial pathology and systemic cancer.
2. Administration of antidiuretic hormone (ADH) or its derivative, the principal hormone controlling water balance. Available ADH preparations include:
   a. Vasopressin tannate (Pitressin tannate in oil)—effective for 24–72 hours.
      (1) Administered by IM injection
      (2) Vial should be warmed and shaken vigorously before administering, to ensure uniform dispersion, because active component settles at bottom of vial
   b. Lypressin (Diapid nasal spray)—drug absorbed through nasal mucosa into blood
      (1) Duration of action only a few hours
      (2) May cause chronic nasal irritation
   c. Desmopressin acetate (DDAVP)—a synthetic vasopressin derivative administered into the nose through a soft, flexible nasal tube
3. For patients who have some residual hypothalamic vasopressin
   a. Chlorpropamide (Diabinese)—potentiates action of vasopressin on renal-concentrating mechanism
   b. Clofibrate (Atromid-S)—probably acts by augmenting ADH secretion from neurohypophysis
   c. Carbamazepine (Tegretol)—stimulates endogenous ADH release

Patient Education

1. Inform the patient that metabolic status must be monitored on a long-term basis because the severity of diabetes insipidus changes from time to time.

2. Avoid limiting fluids to decrease urinary output; thirst is a protective function.
3. Wear an alerting device stating that the wearer has diabetes insipidus.
4. Weigh daily to monitor fluid retention/fluid loss.
5. Consider eliminating coffee and tea from diet—may have an exaggerated diuretic effect.
6. Give written instruction on vasopressin administration. Have the patient demonstrate injection technique.

Pituitary Tumors

Types of Pituitary Tumors

1. *Chromophobe adenoma*—tumor of the anterior pituitary gland of adults
   a. Most common pituitary tumor; does not secrete clinically significant amounts of hormones, but can destroy rest of pituitary gland.
   b. Produces failing vision, optic atrophy, bitemporal hemianopsia, enlargement of sella turcica, and endocrine disturbances.
2. *Eosinophilic adenoma*—endocrine secretion of tumor produces gigantism in children and acromegaly in adults.
3. *Basophilic adenoma*—gives rise to so-called Cushing's syndrome with features largely attributable to hyperadrenalism—masculinization and amenorrhea in females, girdle obesity, hypertension, osteoporosis, and polycythemia

Hypophysectomy

Hypophysectomy is removal of the pituitary gland.

Indications

1. Primary neoplasms (tumors) of the pituitary gland
2. Diabetic retinopathy
   a. Used to halt progress of hemorrhagic diabetic retinopathy and to prevent blindness
   b. Also reduces insulin requirements
3. Palliative measure for relief of bone pain secondary to metastasis of malignant lesions of breast and prostate; alters hormonal milieu of body to create a hormonal environment hostile to continued growth of neoplasm

Methods of Pituitary Ablation *(Removal)*

1. Surgery—done by transsphenoidal or frontal craniotomy approach
2. Cryogenic destruction or stereotaxic radiofrequency coagulation
3. Radiation therapy
4. Drug therapy

Management

The absence of the pituitary gland alters the function of many parts of the body.

1. The patient may need substitution therapy with adrenal steroids (hydrocortisone) and thyroid hormone.
2. Menstruation ceases and infertility occurs almost always after total or nearly total ablation.
3. See page 553 for treatment of diabetes insipidus; transient or permanent diabetes insipidus may follow surgery of pituitary gland.
4. See page 584 for nursing management of the patient undergoing cranial surgery and page 587 for nursing management of the patient undergoing transsphenoidal hypophysectomy.

Bibliography

Books

Carpenito LJ. Nursing Diagnosis. Application to Clinical Practice. 2nd ed. Philadelphia, JB Lippincott, 1987

DeGroot K and Damato M. Critical Care Skills. Norwalk, Appleton and Lange, 1987

DeGroot LJ. Endocrinology. Vol 1, 2nd ed. Philadelphia, WB Saunders, 1989

Greenspan FS and Forsham PH. Basic and Clinical Endocrinology. 2nd ed. Norwalk, Appleton–Century–Crofts, 1986

Hare JW. Signs and Symptoms in Endocrine and Metabolic Disorders. Philadelphia, JB Lippincott, 1986

Holloway NM. Nursing the Critically Ill Adult. Menlo Park, Addison–Wesley, 1988

Karb VB, Queener SF and Freeman JB. Handbook of Drugs for Nursing Practice. St Louis, CV Mosby, 1989

Krieger DK and Bardin CW. Current Therapy in Endocrinology and Metabolism 1985–1986. St Louis, CV Mosby, 1985

Loebl S, Spratto OR and Woods AL. The Nurse's Drug Handbook. Media, Harwal, 1989

Journals

Disorders of the Thyroid and Parathyroid Glands

Bagdade JD. Endocrine emergencies. Med Clin North Am 1986 Sep; 70(5): 1111–1128

Brown SL. Practical points in the postanesthesia assessment and care of the patient having a thyroidectomy. J Post Anesth Nurs 1986 Aug; 1(3):191–193

Daniels GH. Thyroid function testing. An approach to ordering and interpreting tests. Consultant 1986 Jan; 26(1):83–85, 88–89, 92, 94, 97, 98, 100–101, 105–106, 111

Drinka PJ. Subclinical hypothyroidism in the elderly: To treat or not to treat? Am J Med Sci 1988 Feb; 295(2):125–128

Ellyin F and Yow–Fuh C. Hypothyroidism with angina pectoris. Postgrad Med 1986 May; 79(7):93, 96–97

Feit H. Thyroid function in the elderly. Clin Geriatr Med 1988 Feb; 4(1):151–161

Kupperman HS. Hypothyroidism. Physician Assist 1986 Mar; 10(3):60, 65–71

Lennquist S. The thyroid nodule. Diagnosis and surgical treatment. Surg Clin North Am 1987 Apr; 67(2):213–231

Lockhart J and Griffin C. Action stat! Nursing 1988 Aug; 18(8):33

Mathewson M. Thyroid disorder. Crit Care Nurse 1987 Jan–Feb; 7(1):74–85

Mazzaferri EL. Adult hypothyroidism. Postgrad Med 1986 May; 79(7):64–71, 76–85, 89–90

McMillan JY. Preventing myxedema coma in the hypothyroid patient. Dimens Crit Care Nurs 1988 May–Jun; 7(3):136–145

Payne NR. Emergency care of the patient with myxedema coma. J Emerg Nurs 1986 Nov–Dec; 12(6):343–347

Raisz LG. Primary hyperparathyroidism. Physician Assist 1986 Apr; 10(4):143–151

Robuschi G and Safran M. Hypothyroidism in the elderly. Endocr Rev 1987 May; 8(2):142–153

Roher HD and Goretzki PE. Management of goiter and thyroid nodules in an area of endemic goiter. Surg Clin North Am 1987 Apr; 67(2):233–247

Santos E and Mazzaferri EL. Thyroid

function tests. Postgrad Med 1989 Apr; 85(5):333–352

Sarsany SL. Are you ready for this bedside emergency? Thyroid storm. RN 1988 Jul; 51(7):46–48

Sivula A and Ronni–Sivula H. Natural history of treated primary hyperparathyroidism. Surg Clin North Am 1987 Apr; 67(2):329–341

Spaulding SW. Age and the thyroid. Endocrinol Metab Clin North Am 1987 Dec; 16(4):1013–1025

Stoffer SS. Hypothyroidism. Postgrad Med 1986 May; 79(7):62–63

Thomas CG and Croom RD. Current management of the patient with autonomously functioning nodular goiter. Surg Clin North Am 1987 Apr; 67(2):315–328

Disorders of the Adrenal Glands

Burch WM. Cushing's disease. Arch Intern Med 1985 Jun; 145(6):1106–1111

Carpenter PC. Cushing's syndrome: Update of diagnosis and management. Mayo Clin Proc 1986 Jan; 61(1):49–58

Fuhrman SA. Appropriate laboratory testing in the screening and work-up of Cushing's syndrome. Am J Clin Pathol 1988 Sep; 90(3):345–350

Howlett TA and Rees LH. Is it possible to diagnose pituitary-dependent Cushing's disease? Ann Clin Biochem 1985 Nov; 22(6):550–558

Hull CJ. Phaeochromocytoma: Diagnosis, preoperative preparation and anesthetic management. Br J Anesth 1986 Dec; 58(12):1453–1468

Jeffcoate WJ. Treating Cushing's disease. Br Med J 1988 Jan; 296(6617):227–228

Larsen JL and Cathey WJ. Primary adrenocortical nodular dysplasia, a distinct subtype of Cushing's syndrome. Am J Med 1986 May; 80(5):976–984

Manger WM and Gifford RW. Pheochromocytoma: A clinical and experimental overview. Curr Probl Cancer 1985 May; 9(5):1–89

Melby JC. Diagnosis and treatment of primary aldosteronism and isolated hypoaldosteronism. Clin Endocrinol Metab 1985 Nov; 14(4):977–996

Nabarro J. Transsphenoidal surgery for Cushing's syndrome. J R Soc Med 1986 May; 79(5):253–254

Noth RH. Primary hyperaldosteronism. Med Clin North Am 1988 Sep; 72(5):1117–1131

Plouin PF and Chatellier G. Recent developments in pheochromocytoma diagnosis and imaging. Adv Nephrol 1988; 17:275–286

Pulleritis J. Anesthesia for phaeochromocytoma. Can J Anaesth 1988 Sep; 35(5):526–534

Schira MG. Steroid-dependent states and adrenal insufficiency. Nurs Clin North Am 1987 Dec; 22(4):837–841

Sheps SG and Jiang NS. Diagnostic evaluation of pheochromocytoma. Endocrinol Metab Clin North Am 1988 Jun; 17(2):397–414

Young WF and Klee GG. Primary aldosteronism. Diagnostic evaluation. Endocrinol Metab Clin North Am 1988 Jun; 17(2):367–389

Pituitary Disorders

Durr JA. Diabetes insipidus in pregnancy. Am J Kidney Dis 1987 Apr; 9(4):276–283

Geheb MA. Clinical approach to the hyperosmolar patient. Crit Care Clin 1987 Oct; 3(4):797–815

Germon K. Fluid and electrolyte problems associated with diabetes insipidus and syndrome of inappropriate antidiuretic hormone. Nurs Clin North Am 1987 Dec; 22(4):785–795

Robertson GL. Differential diagnosis of polyuria. Annu Rev Med 1988; 39:425–442

Weisberg LS and Szerlip HM. Disorders of potassium homeostasis in critically ill patients. Crit Care Clin 1987 Oct; 5(4):835–853

General Information and Management

Diabetes mellitus is a heterogeneous group of clinical syndromes characterized by hyperglycemia. There may be either a relative or absolute deficiency of insulin or ineffective insulin secretion. There are several types of diabetes with different causes, different clinical courses, and different treatment regimens; the common denominator is hyperglycemia.

Altered Physiology

1. In diabetes mellitus, there is excessive output of glucose from the liver via glycogenolysis and gluconeogenesis, and inadequate utilization of glucose by skeletal muscle, adipose tissue, and liver. Triglycerides are transported from the fat cells to the liver, where they are converted into ketones that can be utilized by the muscles for energy.
2. *Insulin* is a hormone secreted, when blood glucose rises, by the beta cells of the islets of Langerhans located in the pancreas.
   a. Insulin increases glycogen storage in the liver and the transport of glucose through the cell membrane of muscle and fat cells. Glucose passes into endothelial and nerve cells without the aid of insulin.
   b. The increased secretion of insulin following meals helps maintain the blood glucose at a normal level.
   c. The decreased secretion of insulin between meals facilitates the conversion of glycogen, amino acids, and triglycerides into glucose in the liver (gluconeogenesis).
3. In insulin-dependent diabetes mellitus (IDDM, type I), little or no insulin is secreted. In non–insulin-dependent diabetes mellitus (NIDDM, type II), there is an insensitivity of the glucose-sensing mechanism of the beta cells, and in obese patients with NIDDM, there is a decrease in the number of insulin receptors on the cell membrane of muscle and fat cells. Obese patients secrete an excessive amount of insulin, but it is ineffective because of the decreased number of receptors.

* See page 1397 for diabetes mellitus in children and page 1028 for diabetes during pregnancy.

4. When blood glucose is sufficiently high, the renal tubules are unable to reabsorb all of the glucose in the glomerulo-filtrate, and glucosuria occurs. This causes an osmotic diuresis accompanied by the loss of water, sodium, chloride, potassium, and phosphate.
5. Diabetic ketoacidosis is due to an absence of effective insulin. The ketone bodies are organic acids and cause acidemia. The patient compensates by hyperventilating and by excreting more water and salt in the urine.
6. Decompensated diabetes mellitus causes loss of fat stores, liver glycogen, cellular protein, electrolytes, and water, eventually resulting in death from ketoacidosis.
7. The sequelae of long-term poorly controlled diabetes (persistent hyperglycemia) are accelerated atherosclerosis in the larger arteries, thickened capillary basement membranes throughout the body, and degenerative changes in the peripheral nerves. These may lead to such complications as coronary thrombosis, stroke, gangrene of the feet, blindness, renal failure, and neuropathy.

Classification of Diabetes

A. Insulin-Dependent Diabetes Mellitus
(IDDM, type I)

1. These patients are unable to produce endogenous insulin. They require injections of insulin to prevent ketoacidosis and to stay alive.
2. Only 5% to 10% of all diabetic patients have IDDM. There may be a hereditary predisposition to this disease, but current evidence suggests that autoimmunity, viruses, and certain histocompatibility (HLA) antigens play a major role in the development of this type of diabetes. It may occur at any age but is most commonly seen in young people and generally has a sudden onset.

B. Non–Insulin-Dependent Diabetes Mellitus
(NIDDM, type II)

1. There may be a defect in insulin release from the beta cells of the islets of Langerhans, but most commonly there is resistance to the action of insulin in the peripheral tissues.
2. This type usually develops after age 40 but may be seen in obese children.
3. Eighty percent of these individuals are obese.
4. This type has an almost exclusive hereditary compo-

nent, and the onset may be prevented or postponed by calorie restriction and weight loss.

C. Diabetes Associated With Other Conditions

1. When the pancreas is damaged by inflammation or degeneration, it may be unable to produce sufficient insulin.
2. Several drugs, chemicals, hormones, and genetic syndromes are associated with decreased insulin activity and hyperglycemia.

D. Impaired Glucose Tolerance (IGT)

1. This stage of glucose intolerance was previously referred to as "latent diabetes" or "chemical diabetes."
2. Chief characteristic of the stage of glucose intolerance is a normal fasting glucose value with an abnormally high postprandial glucose or postglucose load value.
3. It is an asymptomatic stage of glucose intolerance, which may go on to overt diabetes or never progress to overt diabetes.
4. IGT that does not progress to overt diabetes rarely leads to microvascular complications, but there is a significant increase in atherosclerotic disease, a higher prevalence of ECG abnormalities, and hypertension.
5. The boundaries of this stage are not well-defined, but need to be so that proper recommendations can be made to these persons regarding treatment.

E. Gestational Diabetes (GDM)

This type of diabetes will be discussed in the section on diabetes in pregnancy (see p. 1028).

Clinical Manifestations

A. Insulin-Dependent Diabetes Mellitus (IDDM, type I)

1. The onset is usually abrupt, with polyuria (excessive urine), polydipsia (excessive thirst), and polyphagia (excessive ingestion of food), followed by weight loss, weakness, and fatigue.
2. The insulin deficiency causes hyperglycemia, which in turn causes glucosuria, osmotic diuresis, and the loss of water and electrolytes.
3. Increased gluconeogenesis from the mobilization of protein and fat stores results in weight loss and muscle wasting.
4. Excess ketogenesis leads to ketonemia and acidosis. Excessive diuresis leads to dehydration and hypovolemia (decreased blood volume).

B. Non–Insulin-Dependent Diabetes Mellitus (NIDDM, type II)

1. In the early stages there are no symptoms.
2. Later symptoms include any of those for type I diabetes, as well as the slow healing of cuts, fatigue, blurred vision, cramps in the legs, feet and fingers, itching, and drowsiness.
   a. The symptoms often are so obscure that the diagnosis is not made until a routine health examination or screening test reveals it.
   b. Frequently, a person presents with one of the long-term complications of diabetes (e.g., impotence resulting in a diagnosis of diabetes).

Diagnostic Evaluation

1. In the presence of classic symptoms (polydipsia, polyuria, polyphagia, and weight loss) a random glucose value over 200 mg./dl. is sufficient for diagnosis *or*
2. Fasting venous plasma glucose over 140 mg./dl. on two occasions *or*

3. Fasting plasma glucose level under 140 mg./dl. and a 2-hour plasma glucose value over 200 mg./dl. with one intervening value over 200 mg./dl. following a 75-gm. glucose load (oral glucose tolerance test—OGTT).
4. When unsuspected glucosuria is found, the plasma glucose should be determined immediately.
5. Impaired glucose tolerance—fasting plasma glucose level under 140 mg./dl. and 2-hour plasma glucose value between 140 mg./dl. and 200 mg./dl. with one intervening value over 200 mg./dl. following a 75-gm. glucose load.
6. Glucose tolerance test is rarely needed for diagnosis and is not accurate unless it is done properly:
   a. The patient should be on an unrestricted high-carbohydrate diet (150–300 gm. of carbohydrate) and participate in unrestricted physical activity for 3 days.
   b. The test is done in the morning after a 10- to 14-hour fast.
   c. A 75-gm. glucose load is given in adults; 100-gm. glucose load is given in pregnant women.
   d. The patient should remain seated and not smoke during the test; he should take no medication that affects blood glucose.
   e. Blood is drawn before the glucose is administered and every 30 minutes afterwards for 2 hours or more.

Management

Treatment will correct biochemical and metabolic abnormalities, attain and maintain the ideal body weight, and postpone the progression of the complications of diabetes by maintaining the plasma glucose level as close to normal as possible. *Every new patient requires intensive and extensive education in order to learn to eat properly, take prescribed insulin or oral agents, test blood, and exercise adequately. Reinforcement of diabetes education at every opportunity is an important part of the nursing management of the patient with diabetes mellitus.*

A. Dietary Management

Goal is to improve glucose control and promote well-being.

1. Controlling food portions and exercising are essential to prevent weight gain or to promote a slow, gradual weight loss.
2. Complex rather than simple carbohydrates should be used to help stabilize blood sugar. Meals should include more carbohydrate-rich foods such as starches and fibers, and fewer simple or refined sugars.
3. Less added fat, fewer fatty foods, and low-cholesterol items are recommended. Polyunsaturated (vegetable) fats should be used in place of saturated (mainly animal) fats.
4. Limitations are placed on salt and general sodium use.
5. The menu should be varied according to the patient's ethnic and cultural background, life-style, food preferences, exercise routine, and eating habits. The emphasis should be on what is allowed rather than on what is forbidden. The meal plan should be adapted to the diabetic, not the diabetic to the meal plan.
6. When insulin is taken, special consideration must be given to ensure adequate carbohydrate intake to correspond to the time when insulin is most effective and less carbohydrate when insulin is least effective.
7. Obese diabetics should be on a strict weight-control program. Many will have a normal plasma glucose after

they lose weight. (Remember that obese patients have an excessive amount of circulating insulin but are insulin resistant because of obesity).
8. The American Diabetes Association and American Dietetic Association have prepared exchange lists for patients that reflect these recommendations. EXCHANGE LISTS FOR MEAL PLANNING:
American Diabetes Association, Inc.
National Service Center
1660 Duke Street
Alexandria, VA 22314

American Dietetic Association
208 S. LaSalle Street
Suite 1100
Chicago, IL 60604–1003
9. A GUIDE FOR PROFESSIONALS: *The Application of "Exchange Lists for Meal Planning"* is also available to those health professionals who provide dietary counseling to individuals with diabetes and their families.
10. Each individual patient must be taught how to measure the correct portions at each meal and how to exchange one item for another on the list.
11. Routine blood glucose testing before each meal and at bedtime is necessary during initial control, in unstable patients, and during illness. Well-controlled, stabilized patients may be followed with fewer tests daily.
12. Intensive nutritional counseling by a professional diet counselor should be done initially and repeated several times with every patient.

B. Exercise

Exercise promotes the utilization of carbohydrates and enhances the action of insulin.
1. Insulin-treated patients may develop hypoglycemia after exercise unless they take extra carbohydrate beforehand.
2. Patients should be encouraged to exercise on a regular basis each day.
3. Because insulin is absorbed more quickly from an exercised extremity, many patients are more stable when injections are given in the abdomen on days when arms or legs are exercised.
4. The rate of insulin absorption varies with the site used—deltoid > anterior thigh > abdomen > buttocks. Site rotation should consist of rotation within a site and then use of another site, instead of daily rotation from one site to another.
5. Diabetics with blood glucose levels over 250 mg./dl., or who have ketones in their urine should not begin exercising until their blood glucose levels are in the normal range. Exercising with elevated blood glucose levels will cause increased secretions of glucagon, growth hormone, and catecholamines, resulting in high blood glucose levels.
6. Exercise in the diabetic with microangiopathy should be discussed with the physician because of potential harmful effects.

C. Insulin Therapy (see below)

Insulin Therapy

General Points

1. When the patient cannot produce an adequate amount of insulin, it is necessary to give it by injection.
2. Insulin lowers the blood glucose by decreasing the release of glucose from the liver and increasing the utilization of glucose by muscle and fat cells.

3. One or more insulin injections each day is required for patients with insulin-dependent diabetes.
4. Patients with non–insulin-dependent diabetes may require insulin during an acute illness, infection, stress, surgery, or pregnancy.
5. Obese patients can usually achieve a normal blood glucose by calorie restriction and weight loss.
6. Self-injection techniques are described in the Guideline on page 563.

Insulin Preparations

1. Insulin is extracted from the pancreas of slaughtered pigs and cows or is produced synthetically by amino acid substitution or by recombinant DNA techniques in bacteria. The latter two insulin production techniques result in an insulin identical in amino acid sequence to human insulin.
2. Indications for human insulin use include newly diagnosed insulin-dependent diabetes, diabetics using insulin temporarily (e.g., surgery, pregnancy), insulin allergy, and insulin resistance because of the likelihood of producing few if any insulin antibodies.
3. The available preparations vary in onset of action, time of peak effect, and duration of action (Table 23-1). It is important to know the action curve for each type of insulin in order to treat the patient properly.
4. Insulin is prescribed in units. U-100 insulin contains 100 units per milliliter.

Insulin Syringes and Needles

1. The insulin syringe is calibrated according to units (e.g., U-100 insulin should be given with a U-100 syringe).
2. Needles are numbered according to diameter; the higher the number the thinner the needle.
3. No. 27 or No. 28 needles are usually used; 1.2–2.5 cm. (½ to 1 inch).

Regulation of Insulin Doses

1. The dose of insulin is adjusted to maintain the blood glucose within normal range (65–130 mg./dl.) before each meal and at bedtime. Blood glucose tests obtained at this time give the blood glucose value.
2. Insulin activity curves vary from patient to patient and with the site of injection.
   a. Insulin acts more quickly when injected in the upper extremities than in the lower extremities.
   b. Insulin acts more quickly when injected intramuscularly than when injected subcutaneously.
   c. Insulin acts more quickly if there is vigorous exercise of the extremity that received the injection.
3. New patients with IDDM may be started on 20 units of Lente or NPH given before breakfast.
   a. The dose is increased each day until the blood glucose and urine glucose values are normal.
   b. When insulin requirements are changing rapidly, supplemental injections of regular insulin (crystalline zinc insulin) are given before each meal.

NURSING ALERT: There is a narrow margin between the amount of insulin needed to make the blood glucose normal and the amount that will cause hypoglycemia. Exercise and delayed meals decrease the need for insulin, whereas illness and emotional stress increase the need for insulin.

   c. The nurse should know when hypoglycemia is most likely to occur with the type of insulin that is being used.

Table 23-1. *Insulins Available in the United States*

Type*	Product Name—Manufacturer†	Appearance
Short Acting		
Onset 0.25–1 hour Peak 2–4 hour Duration 5–7 hour	Regular (Lilly; Squibb–Novo) Actrapid (Squibb–Novo) Velosulin (Nordisk) Humulin R (Lilly)† Actrapid Human (Squibb–Novo)‡	Clear
Intermediate Acting		
Onset 1–4 hour Peak 2–15 hour Duration 12–28 hour	Semilente (Lilly; Squibb–Novo) Semitard (Squibb–Novo) Protophane NPH (Squibb–Novo) NPH (Lilly, Squibb–Novo) Monotard (Squibb–Novo) Insulatard (Nordisk) Lente (Lilly; Squibb–Novo) Lentard (Squibb–Novo) Humulin N (Lilly)‡ Monotard Human (Squibb–Novo)‡	Turbid
Long Acting		
Onset 4–6 hour Peak 10–30 hour Duration 36+ hour	PZI (Lilly; Squibb–Novo) Ultralente (Lilly; Squibb–Novo) Ultratard (Squibb–Novo) Mixtard (Nordisk)	Turbid

* Consult individual manufacturer for exact time of onset, peak, and duration. Values given are approximate ranges.

† Some insulins are available in pure beef, pure pork, beef–pork, or human. Consult individual manufacturer for source.

‡ Lilly's human insulin is of recombinant DNA (biosynthetic) origin, while Squibb–Novo's human insulin is of semi-synthetic origin.

Note: Many insulins are available in either a standard or a purified form.

4. Patients are instructed to test blood for sugar before each meal and at bedtime.
5. The patient should keep a record of the blood tests and note on this record any changes in insulin dose, diet, or activities.
6. If blood glucose levels are elevated, urine should be tested for the presence of ketones.

Insulin Reactions

Hypoglycemic Reactions to Insulin

1. *Hypoglycemia* is an abnormally low blood glucose (usually below 50 mg./dl.).
2. Hypoglycemia results from too much insulin, not enough food, and/or excessive physical activity.
3. Hypoglycemia may occur 1–3 hours after regular (crystalline zinc) insulin, 4–18 hours after NPH or Lente insulin, or 18–30 hours after Protamine Zinc or Ultra-lente insulin.
4. Hypoglycemia may occur at any time, but it is most commonly seen before meals.
5. Patients at high risk for hypoglycemia are those with deficits of counter-regulatory hormones.

Evaluation of Signs and Symptoms of Hypoglycemia

1. Sweating, tremor, pallor, tachycardia, palpitation, nervousness—from release of adrenalin from the central nervous system when the blood glucose falls rapidly.
2. Headache, light-headedness, confusion, emotional changes, memory lapses, numbness of lips and tongue, slurred speech, lack of coordination, staggering gait, double vision, drowsiness, convulsions, coma—from depression of the central nervous system when the blood glucose level falls slowly.

NURSING ALERT: Patients with long-standing diabetes complicated by autonomic neuropathy may develop hypoglycemia without warning, as may patients taking certain beta blockers. Severe and prolonged hypoglycemia may cause brain damage and death. Any abnormal behavior in a patient taking insulin should be considered as resulting from hypoglycemia until proven otherwise.

Management of Hypoglycemia

1. Give some form of sugar orally if the patient is conscious and can swallow—orange juice, candy (6–7 Lifesavers), glucose tablets, lump sugar, or small box of raisins.
2. Give glucagon (subcutaneously or IM) if the patient cannot take sugar by mouth—this causes glycogenolysis in the liver if adequate glycogen stores are present.
3. As soon as the patient regains consciousness, he should be given carbohydrate by mouth.
4. If the patient does not respond to the above measures, he is given 50 ml. of 50% glucose intravenously (IV) or 1000 ml. of 5%–10% glucose in water IV. The recovery will be slow in patients who have had severe and prolonged hypoglycemia.

Preventing Hypoglycemic Reactions Due to Insulin

Instruct the patient as follows:
1. Hypoglycemia may be prevented by maintaining a regular regimen of diet, insulin, and exercise.
2. The early symptoms of hypoglycemia should be recognized and treated.
3. Some form of simple carbohydrate should be carried at all times and taken at the first symptoms of hypoglycemia.
4. Between-meal and bedtime snacks may be necessary to maintain a normal glucose level.
5. Extra food should be taken before unusual physical exertion.
6. Frequent blood tests may be necessary, especially in patients with fluctuating blood glucose levels.
7. An identification card or bracelet should be worn.
   a. Identification bracelet may be obtained from Medic-Alert Foundation, International, 2323 Colorado, Turlock, CA 95381.
   b. The card may be obtained from the American Diabetes Association, 1660 Duke Street, Alexandria, VA 22314.

Somogli Phenomenon

Hypoglycemia is followed by compensatory rebound hyperglycemia that lasts 12–72 hours or longer and is usually caused by an excessive dose of insulin.
1. The patient will have transient hypoglycemia, but most urine specimens will contain glucose.
2. Gradual reduction of the insulin dose and increase of the diet at the time of the hypoglycemia will help to stabilize the patient.

Local Allergic Reactions to Insulin

A. Local Reactions

Cause redness, stinging, and induration at the injection site.
1. The reaction may occur within 1 hour but may be delayed for 24 hours.
2. The reaction is usually seen in the early stages of therapy and disappears after a few weeks.
3. If local reactions persist, changing to purified pork insulin or human insulin will usually correct this problem.
4. A few patients have insulin resistance due to insulin allergy. These should be referred to a medical center for antibody testing and treatment.

B. Insulin Lipodystrophy

Causes either lipoatrophy (a loss of fat) or lipohypertrophy (an indurated fatty tumor) to appear at the site of insulin injection.
1. Insulin lipoatrophy causes pitting at the site of injection. It previously occurred in 25% of the women and children taking insulin but now occurs in only 2% or less of those who use purified pork or human U-100 insulin.
2. Lipohypertrophy can also be prevented by changing to either a purified pork insulin or human insulin.

C. Insulin Edema

Results from fluid retention after the sudden correction of prolonged hyperglycemia.

D. Insulin Resistant

Term applied to patients whose requirements exceed 200 units of insulin each day. This condition is rarely seen.

Oral Hypoglycemic Agents (Table 23-2)

1. Oral hypoglycemic agents may be effective for older, non–insulin-dependent (NIDDM), nonketotic patients who are normal in weight and have persistent hyperglycemia after treatment by only diet adjustment.
2. In the US, 6 sulfonylurea drugs are available as oral hypoglycemic agents. The initial effect of these drugs is to increase insulin release from the pancreas. There is a long-term effect of increasing the number of insulin receptors. (See package information for side effects and drug interactions.)
3. Patients usually are treated by diet and exercise alone before oral hypoglycemic drugs are used.
4. Insulin is required when ketosis or severe infection is present, or during surgery or periods of extreme stress.

Nursing Process Overview: The Patient With Diabetes Mellitus

Nursing Assessment

1. Obtain baseline information regarding history of:
   a. Polyuria, polydipsia, polyphagia and other symptoms of diabetes mellitus the patient may be experiencing.
   b. Number of years since diagnosis of diabetes.
   c. Family history of diabetes.

Table 23-2. *Oral Hypoglycemic Agents: Sulfonylurea Compounds*

Agent	Duration of Action (hr.)	How Given
"First Generation"		
Tolbutamide (Orinase)	6–10 hr.	Divided doses
Chorpropamide (Diabinese)	36–60 hr.	Single dose
Acetohexamide (Dymelor)	10–20 hr.	Single or divided doses
Tolazamide (Tolinase)	12–24 hr.	Single or divided doses
"Second Generation" (as of April 1984)		
Glyburide (Micronase or Diabeta)	12–24 hr.	Single or divided doses
Glipizide (Glibenese)	10–18 hr.	Single or divided doses

2. Perform physical assessment to evaluate and document signs and symptoms of diabetes mellitus.
3. Assess patient/family's knowledge and understanding of disease process, purpose of hospitalization, and planned therapy.
4. Determine patient/family's level of anxiety related to disease process and hospitalization.

Nursing Diagnoses

1. Potential fluid volume deficit related to osmotic diuresis (hyperglycemia), excessive gastric losses from nausea and vomiting.
2. Potential altered nutrition (less than body requirements) related to imbalance between insulin need and insulin dose.
3. Knowledge deficit of therapeutic regimen (dietary, weight control, insulin therapy, exercise program, potential complications) related to nonacceptance of disease and regimen or lack of understanding.
4. Other possible nursing diagnoses
   a. Potential nonadherence related to complexity of management regimen
   b. Self-care deficits related to lack of understanding, fatigue, etc.
   c. Potential sexual dysfunction (male) related to neuropathic complications of diabetes mellitus.
   d. Potential for injury related to decreased vision secondary to retinopathy.

Nursing Interventions

A. Preventing Ketoacidosis/Fluid Volume Deficit

1. Encourage patient to eat regularly spaced meals and snacks within prescribed caloric requirements.
2. Emphasize the importance of a daily exercise program in order to:
   a. Decrease blood glucose levels.
   b. Increase levels of high-density lipoproteins (HDL).
   c. Lower cholesterol and triglyceride levels.
   d. Reduce stress.
   e. Create a feeling of well-being.
3. Advise the patient to take insulin and/or oral hypoglycemic agents in the dose and time prescribed and use the appropriate method.
4. Monitor blood glucose levels daily.
5. Monitor urine for ketones if blood glucose levels are elevated.
6. Emphasize early recognition and treatment of hyperglycemia to avoid ketosis.
7. Advise the patient to contact physician for change in insulin dosage or additional insulin as indicated by elevated blood glucose and/or presence of urinary ketones.

B. Preventing Hypoglycemia/Maintaining Near-Normal Blood Glucose Levels

1. Encourage the patient to:
   a. Eat prescribed meal plan/snacks as scheduled.
   b. Eat extra food before periods of vigorous exercise.
   c. Take the prescribed insulin dose at same time each day.
   d. Monitor blood glucose levels daily.
2. Emphasize early treatment of hypoglycemia with a simple sugar.

C. Gaining Knowledge and Acceptance of Living With Diabetes

1. See Patient Education, opposite column.

Discharge Planning/Patient Education

The person with diabetes mellitus must play a major role in self-management. Patient education must be amplified, reinforced, and updated continually, since diabetes is a lifelong disease.

A. Become Familiar With Diabetes and How it Affects the Body

1. Visit the physician on a regular basis.
2. Study and review available literature from reputable sources.
3. Secure booklets and pamphlets from the American Diabetes Association, Inc., 1660 Duke Street, Alexandria, VA 22314.
4. Attend available classes.

B. Maintain Health at an Optimal Level

1. Maintain a consistent daily routine.
2. Get adequate rest and sleep.
3. Exercise regularly and consistently.
   a. Avoid "spurts" of arduous exercise before meals.
   b. Exercise 1½ hours after meals.
   c. Keep some form of carbohydrate (sugar, candy, orange juice) available during exercise periods.
4. Seek employment with regular hours.

C. Follow the Prescribed Dietary Regimen

1. Eat 3 or more measured meals each day. Plan ahead for prescribed meals and snacks.
2. Become thoroughly familiar with the food exchange lists.
3. Learn how to follow a calculated diet.
4. Know the caloric value of foods frequently eaten.
5. Use household measures or a gram scale until serving sizes can be judged accurately.
6. Avoid concentrated carbohydrates.
7. Avoid periods of fasting and feasting.
8. Keep weight at optimal level; normalize body weight.
   a. Weigh weekly.
   b. Keep a weight record.
9. If taking insulin, eat extra calories when unusual physical activity is anticipated.
10. Eat a bedtime snack when taking insulin (if permissible).

D. Be Aware of the Degree of Diabetes Control

1. Test blood for sugar.
2. Test blood before each meal and at bedtime while control is being attained or during periods of illness.
3. Test urine when blood sugar levels are high.
4. Keep a daily record of blood sugar tests (date, hour, value).
5. Test only freshly voided urine.
6. Take the record of blood tests to physician at appointed times.
7. Know that acetone in the urine indicates need for *more insulin.*
8. Protect all urine- and blood-testing equipment from light, moisture, and heat (to prevent false interpretation due to deterioration of test materials).
9. Monitor blood glucose when insulin requirements vary and during illness.
   a. Capillary blood is obtained from finger puncture and spread on enzyme strip.
   b. Reaction may be quantitated visually or with the use of a meter.

E. Become Familiar With all Aspects of Insulin Usage
(see p. 563 for guidelines for teaching self-injection of insulin)

1. Know when the prescribed insulin is having its peak action.
2. Adjust insulin dosage according to blood sugar tests as prescribed.
3. Rotate the sites of insulin injections in a systematic manner within sites and with attention to rates of insulin absorption.
4. Keep the syringe and needle in one particular place.
5. Keep a reserve supply of insulin in the refrigerator.
   a. Keep bottle in current use at *room temperature.*
   b. Avoid injecting cold insulin because it may contribute to tissue reaction.
6. Have an extra insulin syringe available.
7. Know the conditions that produce insulin reactions.
   a. Omission of a meal
   b. Unaccustomed or strenuous exercise
   c. Too much insulin
8. Know the symptoms of an insulin reaction.
   a. Any unfamiliar or peculiar sensation
   b. Hunger, perspiration, palpitation, tachycardia, weakness, tremor, pallor
9. Know how to treat an impending insulin reaction.
   a. Eat carbohydrates (orange juice, sugar, candy) when symptoms first occur.
   b. Test blood sugar.
   c. Carry extra carbohydrate at all times (sugar lumps, candy).
   d. Eat extra carbohydrate before strenuous exercise and during periods of prolonged exercise, or reduce insulin dosage.
   e. Eat a snack at bedtime.
10. Keep a check-off system to ensure taking insulin.
11. Wear identification bracelet or necklace. Carry more detailed information about insulin, etc., in wallet.
12. When traveling, carry diabetic supplies in hand luggage.
    a. Have letter from physician stating that you are a diabetic, as well as a prescription for insulin syringes and other medications.
    b. Keep your watch at the time of departure point until arrival at destination; do not change diabetic regimen en route.

F. Take Prescribed Oral Hypoglycemic Medication

1. Adhere faithfully to the prescribed diet.
2. Test urine or blood daily.
3. Take the medication exactly as directed.

G. Appreciate the Importance of Proper Foot Care to Prevent Infection, Ischemia, and Neuropathy, Which May Lead to Amputation and Death

1. Inspect the feet carefully and daily for calluses, corns, blisters, abrasions, redness, and nail abnormalities.
   a. Use a small mirror to check bottom of each foot.
   b. Use a magnifying glass under good light if eyesight is poor, or have someone else check feet.
2. Bathe the feet daily in warm (never hot) water.
   a. Do not soak the feet for prolonged periods. (Soaking is defatting.)
   b. Dry feet carefully, especially between the toes.
3. Massage the feet with an absorbable agent (vegetable oil, lanolin, Nivea cream) except between the toes—autonomically denervated foot loses its ability to sweat, and dries and cracks easily.
4. Prevent moisture between the toes to prevent maceration of the skin.
   a. Insert lamb's wool between overlapping toes.
   b. Use powder in the web spaces, especially if feet perspire.

5. Wear well-fitting, noncompressive shoes and socks—long enough, wide enough, soft, supple, and low-heeled.
   a. Buy shoes in the afternoon—feet are larger in the afternoon than in the morning.
   b. Have each foot measured before buying shoes—feet enlarge with age.
   c. Have the measurement taken while standing, since foot is larger in the standing position.
   d. Do not "break in" shoes all at one time.
   e. Avoid rubber- or plastic-soled, or vinyl shoes, which cause the feet to perspire and aggravate fungal infections.
   f. Avoid working in bedroom slippers or other casual footwear.
6. Go to a podiatrist on a regular basis if corns, calluses, and ingrown toenails are present.
   a. Cut toenails straight across to prevent ingrown toenails.
7. Avoid heat, chemicals, and injuries to the feet—do not go barefoot or expose feet to hot-water bottles, heating pads, caustic solutions, etc. Heat increases demand for blood, which cannot be met because of the reduction of vascular reserve. Diabetic neuropathy causes loss of cutaneous sensation, so that the patient may suffer burns or pressure lesions without being aware of them.
   a. Switch off electric blanket before going to bed; wear socks at night to keep feet warm if necessary.
   b. Avoid overheated baths and sitting too close to a fire.
8. Inspect inside of shoes for foreign objects, etc.
9. If an injury occurs to the foot:
   a. Wash the area with mild soap and water.
   b. Cover with a dry sterile dressing *without* adhesive.
   c. Wear white cotton socks; dye in colored socks and wool may serve as irritants when skin is already irritated.
   d. Call the physician.

H. Maintain Diabetes Control During Periods of Illness or Stress

1. Call physician immediately when any unusual symptoms become evident; *do not allow diabetes to get out of control.*
2. Make dietary adjustments during illness according to physician's directions.
3. Continue taking insulin; physician may increase dosage during illness.
4. Test blood for sugar and urine for acetone more frequently; keep records.
5. Monitor blood glucose.
6. Know the conditions that bring about diabetic acidosis.
   a. Nausea and vomiting
   b. Failure to increase insulin when blood sugar is increasing
   c. Failure to take insulin
   d. Stress
   e. Infections
   f. Menstrual periods
7. Know how to treat impending diabetic acidosis.
   a. Examine blood for sugar and urine for acetone and report results to physician.
   b. Take additional insulin as advised by physician.
   c. Go to bed and keep warm.
   d. Alert someone to be in attendance.
   e. Drink a glass of liquid hourly if possible. Replace calories needed with carbohydrate containing liquids.

I. Follow Other Health Directives

1. Avoid tobacco—nicotine constricts blood vessels, causing reduction in blood flow to feet.
2. Take only medications prescribed by physician—many drugs enhance effect of insulin and oral antidiabetic agents.

Evaluation

1. Prevents or reduces incidence of ketosis/ketoacidosis and subsequent fluid volume deficits.
2. Prevents or reduces incidence of hypoglycemia and maintains near-normal blood glucose level.
3. Gains knowledge and adheres to prescribed regimen.

Guidelines Teaching Self-Injection of Insulin

Underlying Considerations

1. Insulin injection should be taught as soon as the need for insulin treatment has been established.
2. A member of the patient's family should also be taught how to administer insulin.
3. An optimistic approach will offer the patient encouragement.
4. Teach insulin injection *first*, since this is the patient's major concern; then teach loading the syringe.

Equipment

Prescribed bottle of insulin
Disposable insulin syringe and needles
Absorbent cotton and alcohol or prepackaged alcohol swabs

Procedure

Teaching Action	Rationale/Amplification
1. Give the patient the prepared syringe containing the prescribed dose of insulin.	
2. Have patient wipe the skin with alcohol.	
3. Instruct the patient to hold the syringe as he would a pencil.	
4. Show the patient how to spread the skin taut on the anterior thigh (Fig. 23-1*A*). or Form a skin fold by picking up subcutaneous tissue between the thumb and forefinger if the patient is thin (Fig. 23-1*B*).	4. Either of the techniques ensures that the needle tip is inserted into subcutaneous tissue and outside the muscle. Avoid pressing the skin *tightly* between the fingers, since this is a common cause of local induration and infection.

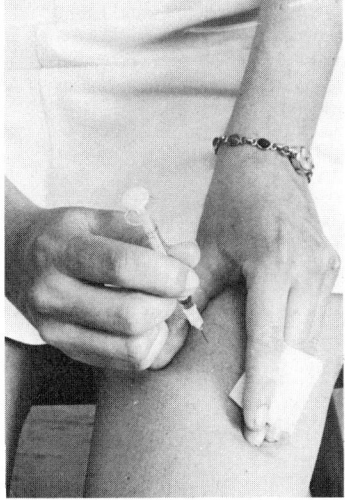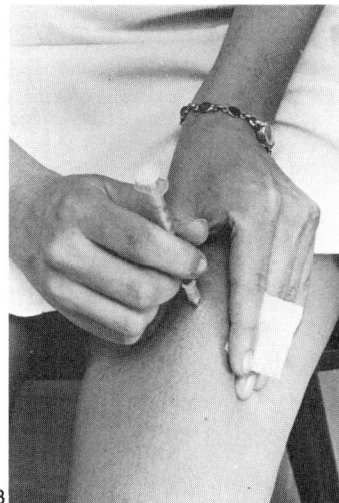

Figure 23-1. Self-injection of insulin. (A) The insulin syringe is held perpendicular to the stretched skin before the needle is thrust into the subcutaneous tissues. (B) Alternate method: If the patient has only a thin layer of subcutaneous fat, a fold of skin is pinched between the fingers to keep the needle from penetrating into the muscle.

A   B

5. Select areas of upper arms, thighs, flanks, and upper buttocks for injection after patient becomes proficient with needle insertion.	5. The skin is loose and there is more subcutaneous fat in these areas.
6. Assist the patient to insert needle with a quick thrust to the hub at a right angle to the skin surface (Fig. 23-1*B*).	6. The insulin is injected into deep subcutaneous tissue.
7. Instruct the patient to release the skin fold.	
8. Hold the alcohol sponge against the needle and gently withdraw the needle. Wipe area with alcohol sponge.	8. This maneuver prevents painful pulling of the skin as the needle is withdrawn.

(continued)

Guidelines Teaching Self-Injection of Insulin *(continued)*

Procedure *(continued)*	**Teaching Action**	**Rationale/Amplification**
	9. Develop a systematic plan for insulin administration (Fig. 23-2).	9. Systematic rotation of sites will keep the skin supple, and will favor uniform absorption of insulin.

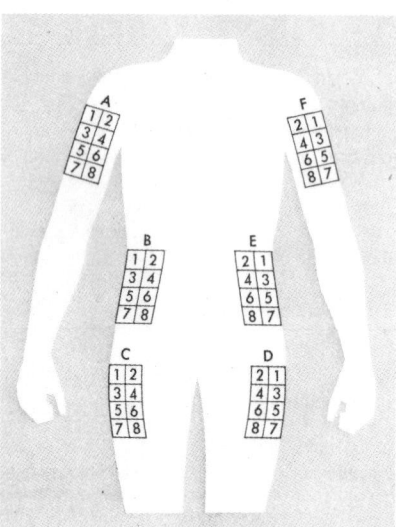

Figure 23-2. *Rotate within each site and keep in mind the various rates of absorption in different sites. Exercising an injected site will also hasten insulin absorption. (From ADA Forecast—the Diabetics' Own Magazine. Vol 4[1]. Courtesy of Becton, Dickinson.)*

To Load the Syringe:

1. Roll the bottle of insulin (Protamine Zinc, NPH and Lente) between the palms of the hands.	1. The rolling action mixes the insulin.
2. Wipe off the top of the insulin vial with an alcohol sponge.	
3. Inject approximately the same volume of air into the insulin vial as the volume of insulin to be withdrawn.	3. Air is injected into the vial to keep its contents under slight positive pressure and to make it easier to withdraw the insulin.

To Fill a Syringe With Long- and Short-Acting Insulin Mixture:

1. Wipe off the vial tops with an alcohol swab.
2. Inject air equal to the number of units to be injected into long-acting insulin first; withdraw needle.
3. Inject air into short-acting insulin bottle and withdraw prescribed amount of insulin.
4. Then withdraw prescribed amount of insulin from long-acting insulin bottle.

Acute Complications of Diabetes

The diabetic patient may become comatose because of hypoglycemia (see p. 559), diabetic ketoacidosis, and hyperosmolar–nonketotic coma, in addition to all of the conditions that can produce coma in the nondiabetic.

Diabetic Ketoacidosis

Diabetic ketoacidosis results from the absence of effective insulin, which causes hyperglycemia, ketonuria, dehydration, and acidosis. Glucose no longer enters muscle cells, and fat is metabolized to produce energy. Free fatty acids are converted to ketone bodies in the liver. The ketone bodies are organic acids that cause metabolic acidosis.

Precipitating Causes

1. Failure to take an adequate amount of insulin
2. Failure to increase the dose of insulin in the presence of acute infection
3. Failure to increase insulin to compensate for pregnancy, injury, surgery, or emotional stress

Clinical Manifestations

A. Early Manifestations

1. Polyuria, polydipsia, fatigue, malaise, drowsiness
2. Anorexia, headache, abdominal pains
3. Muscle cramps, nausea, vomiting, constipation

B. Later Manifestations

1. Kussmaul breathing—very deep respiratory movements

2. Sweetish odor of the breath due to ketonemia
3. Hypotension and weak, thready pulse
4. Stupor and coma

Diagnostic Evaluation

A. Blood
Glucose elevated, bicarbonate decreased, arterial pH decreased, strongly positive plasma ketone

B. Urine
Strongly positive for sugar and ketone, and moderately positive for protein

> **Goals:**
> Restore normal metabolism by supplying what the patient is missing—an adequate amount of insulin.
> Correct hypovolemia/fluid and electrolyte deficiencies.

Management and Nursing Interventions

1. Obtain blood and urine samples immediately:
   a. Test blood for glucose, ketone, BUN, electrolytes, complete blood count, arterial pH, PO_2, and PCO_2.
   b. Obtain urine specimen at prescribed time and measure sugar, acetone, and volume. Catheterize only if a voided specimen cannot be obtained.
   c. Set up a chronological flow chart that includes vital signs, clinical manifestations, laboratory data and therapy.
2. Carry out a rapid physical examination to look for infection, myocardial infarction, stroke, etc.
   a. Record vital signs, state of hydration, and mental status.
3. Start intravenous infusion of isotonic saline solution at a rate of about 500 ml. per hour to rehydrate the patient. Later the type of fluid and rate of administration are changed.
4. Give insulin as directed—to increase glucose utilization and decrease lipolysis. Insulin may be given by:
   a. Continuous infusion low-dose therapy. An infusion pump may be used, or insulin may be put into the bottle containing the intravenous solution. Because ⅓ of the solution adheres to the bottle and tubing, it is necessary to increase the dose as directed.
   b. Deep intramuscular injections of regular insulin into the deltoid may be used instead.
   c. Insulin may be administered via a bedside closed-loop insulin pump, which has a glucose sensor and an insulin reservoir. Only available in large medical centers. Used until the ketoacidosis has been resolved.
5. As the serum glucose falls, glucose is added to the infusion, and the insulin dose is reduced as directed.
6. Determinations of serum glucose, ketone, bicarbonate, and potassium are done every 3–6 hours.
7. One or more ECG tracings may be needed to rule out silent myocardial infarction, and to monitor intracellular potassium levels.
8. The rapid utilization of glucose under the influence of insulin causes potassium to migrate into the cells, and results in hypokalemia after 4–8 hours of treatment.
   a. This is corrected by administering buffered potassium phosphate (or chloride) at a rate of no more than 20 mEq. per hour. This is usually added to the infusion after 3 or 4 hours.
9. Hypotension will usually respond to adequate saline infusion.
10. If the patient is given nothing by mouth for 3 hours while rehydration takes place, nausea usually subsides, and the patient can usually be given clear liquids.
11. The recurrence of diabetic ketoacidosis can be prevented by adequate patient education. The patient should increase the dose of insulin when there is glucosuria and ketonuria, and seek medical advice when there are symptoms of diabetic ketoacidosis.

Nonketotic Hyperosmolar Coma

Nonketotic hyperosmolar coma is characterized by hyperglycemia, hyperosmolarity, severe dehydration, and stupor or coma, but there is no ketonemia or acidosis.

Altered Physiology

1. There is some, but not enough, insulin present. This condition occurs in older people who do not have diabetes but who have been given excessive carbohydrate without adequate fluid administration.
2. Hyperglycemia causes osmotic diuresis, resulting in severe loss of water and electrolytes.
3. Water shifts from the intracellular to the extracellular fluid and causes intracellular dehydration.

Clinical Manifestations and Diagnostic Evaluation

1. History of precipitating event—severe burns, pancreatitis, hemodialysis, hyperalimentation, and excessive use of diuretics may be factors.
2. Severe hyperglycemia with a negative serum acetone and a normal serum bicarbonate.
3. Severe dehydration with poor skin turgor, hypotension, fever, and decreased brain activity. Seizures may occur.
4. Serum osmolarity is greatly elevated.

Management

> **Goal:**
> To correct the volume depletion and hyperosmolar state.

1. Isotonic saline solution and low-dose insulin infusion is the primary treatment.
2. Potassium and glucose are added later as indicated by results of the blood chemistry tests.
3. As soon as the patient regains consciousness, liquids are given orally.

Infections

Underlying Considerations

Infections are more protracted and serious in diabetic individuals for the following reasons:
1. Hyperglycemia causes decreased leukocyte phagocytosis. Ketonemia causes decreased leukocyte migration.
2. Diabetes becomes more severe in the presence of infection.
3. Ketoacidosis may be precipitated by infection and inadequate insulin.

Types of Infection

1. Infections of the urinary tract may follow incomplete emptying of the bladder due to diabetic neuropathy or urethral obstruction. Bladder infections may spread to the kidney and cause pyelonephritis.
2. Infections of the extremities due to local injury may

occur in patients with diabetic neuropathy who cannot recognize pain. If the skin is dry and cracked, bacteria may penetrate the protective envelope and cause infection.
3. Dermatologic infections:
   a. Infections of the skin and vagina frequently found in poorly controlled diabetes.
   b. Furuncles and carbuncles due to staphylococcus.
   c. Gas-forming infections under the skin and in the genitourinary tract.

Management

1. The dose of insulin is increased enough to correct the ketonemia and hyperglycemia.
2. The blood is tested frequently for sugar to adjust the insulin dose.
3. Cultures of blood, urine, sputum, and pus are essential for determining the responsible organism and for selecting the correct antibiotic.

Long-Term Complications of Diabetes

Underlying Considerations

1. Diabetes is the most common cause of new blindness and new cases of end-stage renal disease in the US. Accelerated atherosclerosis causes an increased incidence of myocardial infarction, stroke, and gangrene.
2. Because diabetics are living longer, these complications are becoming more common.

Vascular Complications

1. The specific pathologic lesion (microangiopathy) of long-standing diabetes is thickening of the capillary basement membrane in every organ.
2. The prevalence of microangiopathy parallels the duration and severity of hyperglycemia.
3. Intercapillary glomerulosclerosis (Kimmelstiel–Wilson syndrome), the specific renal disease of diabetes, results from the thickening of the capillary basement membrane in the glomeruli.
4. Microangiopathy of the vessels supplying the skin, peripheral nerves, and walls of large arteries may be a factor in skin diseases, neuropathy, and atherosclerosis.
5. Major vessel occlusion (macroangiopathy) resulting from atherosclerosis causes stroke, myocardial infarction, intermittent claudication, and gangrene. The progress of atherosclerosis is accelerated in diabetics.

Diabetic Retinopathy

Diabetic retinopathy is a progressive impairment of retinal circulation that causes vitreous hemorrhage and loss of vision.
1. Incidence and severity of retinopathy are related to the duration and degree of control of diabetes; half of the patients who have had diabetes for more than 10 years have some evidence of retinopathy.
2. Impaired vision and blindness are caused by hemorrhage and neovascularization into the vitreous with the formation of scar tissue and eventual detachment of the retina.
3. Management
   a. Photocoagulation—produced when a narrow, intensive beam of light is directed into the eye and focused on the retina; the absorption of light produces heat, which coagulates the treated vessel and prevents it from bleeding.
      (1) Used when there are areas of newly formed blood vessels and proliferative retinopathy.
      (2) Photocoagulation must be done when proliferative changes first occur so that bleeding can be prevented.
   b. Vitrectomy—removal of blood and fibrous tissue through a small opening on the side of the eye and replacement with clear fluid that maintains the shape of the eye; may be tried for patients whose blindness is due to vitreous hemorrhage.

Diabetic Neuropathy

Diabetic neuropathy affects the peripheral and autonomic nervous system and produces a wide variety of syndromes.
1. Clinical manifestations
   a. Peripheral neuropathy—pain (dull, aching, burning, lancinating, or crushing), paresthesia (sensations of tingling or burning or coldness and numbness).
   b. Involvement of autonomic nervous system—orthostatic hypotension, sexual impotency, retrograde ejaculation, pupillary changes, abnormal sweating, bladder paralysis, nocturnal diarrhea.
2. Assessment of the feet of diabetic patients
   (The complications of neuropathy and vascular disease are most evident in the feet. Most amputations, other than those occurring from trauma, occur in diabetics.)
   a. Watch for lesions of the feet that do not heal.
   b. Compare the skin color of both feet and ankles. A blue-gray color is caused by diminution of the blood supply.
   c. Change the position of the extremity and note the color change. Pallor on elevation and dusky cyanosis on dependency indicate vascular insufficiency.
   d. Feel the temperature of the skin with the back of your hand and notice decreased temperature.
   e. Examine the toenails. Thick, ridged nails suggest circulatory impairment or fungus infection.
   f. Look for athlete's foot between the toes (epidermophytosis), and fungus infection of the nails (onychomycosis). Fungal infection is more serious in the diabetic and requires treatment.
   g. Look for calluses, corns, blisters, cracks, and abrasions; look between the toes and on the soles of the feet.
   h. Palpate the dorsalis pedis and posterior tibial arterial pulses; absence of a discernible pulse or diminution of the pulses indicate atherosclerosis.

Management of the Diabetic Patient Undergoing Surgery

Underlying Considerations

The diabetic patient must be followed closely at the time of surgery because stress, infection, and missed meals change insulin requirements.
1. The trauma of surgery causes hyperglycemia.
2. Infection causes the insulin requirements to rise.
3. Anesthesia may cause hyperglycemia and ketosis.

4. The patient's normal schedule of food intake is usually interrupted.

Management

Goal:
Achieve the best nutritional balance and best possible metabolic control of the diabetes preoperatively.

A. Preoperative Preparation
1. Essential preoperative evaluation studies are urinalysis, blood glucose, BUN, electrolyte, and CBC.
2. The usual diet is given, but the insulin dose may be reduced the day before surgery.

B. Day of Surgery
1. A fasting blood glucose is drawn and an intravenous infusion of 1000 ml. of 5% glucose may be given over a 4-hour period for each meal that is missed.
2. The patient is usually given ½ to ¾ his usual dose of insulin.

C. Postoperative Management
1. Maintain nutrition with intravenous glucose until patient is able to tolerate food by mouth.
2. Give insulin as directed. The usual dose of intermediate-acting insulin is started the day after surgery, and supplemental regular insulin may be given on a sliding scale according to blood glucose tests.

Bibliography

Books

Olson OC. Diagnosis and Management of Diabetes Mellitus. 2nd ed. New York, Raven Press, 1988

Rifkin H and Porte D Jr. (eds.). Ellenberg and Rifkin's Diabetes Mellitus: Theory and Practice. 4th ed. New York, Elsevier, 1990

Silverstein SR and Frommer D. Emergency Management of Metabolic and Endocrine Disorders. Rockville, MD, Aspen Publications, 1988

Sperling MA. Physician's Guide to Insulin-Dependent (Type I) Diabetes: Diagnosis and Treatment. Alexandria, VA, American Diabetes Association, 1988

Sperling MA. Physician's Guide to Insulin-Dependent (Type II) Diabetes: Diagnosis and Treatment. Alexandria, VA, American Diabetes Association, 1988

Journals

Ault K and Sheta M. Diabetic ketoacidosis and changing views of treatment. Indiana Med 1987 Aug; 50(8):719–725

Barmann KA and Domask ME. A multidisplinary approach: Assuring quality of care for the diabetic client. J Nurs Qual Assur 1989 Feb; (3)2:19–25

Bartlett EE. The step approach to patient education. Diabetes Educ 1988 Mar–Apr; 14(2):130–135

Bergenstal RM. Acute and chronic complications of diabetes. Caring 1988 Nov; 7(11):10–12, 14–15

Butts DE. Fluid and electrolyte disorders associated with diabetic ketoacidosis and hyperglycemic hyperosmolar nonketotic coma. Nurs Clin North Am 1987 Dec; 22(4):827–836

Cohen M and Field J. Managing diabetes complications. Patient Care 1988 Dec; 22(20):28–40

Cook GB. A computer program for teaching and auditing patient's knowledge of diabetes. Diabetes Educ 1987 Summer; 13(3):306–308

Cooper NA. Nutrition and diabetes: A review of current recommendations. Diabetes Educ 1988 Sep–Oct; 14(5):428–433

Gaffney JT and Singer GR. Diet needs of patients referred to home health. J Am Dietetic Assoc 1985 Feb; 85(2):109–202

Geheb MA. Clinical approach to the hyperosmolar patient. Crit Care Clin 1987 Oct; 5(4):797–815

Goodson JD et al. The limited value of home urine testing by diabetic patients. J Gen Intern Med 1986 Jul–Aug; 1(4):243–247

Guthrie RA. Self-monitoring of blood glucose. Patient Care 1987 Jul; 21(12):56–58, 60, 62–87

Haulin CE and Cryer PE. Hypoglycemia: The limiting factor in the management of insulin-dependent diabetes mellitus. Diabetes Educ 1988 Sep–Oct; 14(5):409–411

Hillman K. Fluid resuscitation in diabetic emergencies: A reappraisal. Intensive Care Med 1987 Apr; 13(1):4–8

Hollander P. Type II diabetes: More than "just a touch" of diabetes. Postgrad Med 1989 Mar; 85(4):215–221

Krane EJ. Diabetic ketoacidosis: Biochemistry, physiology, treatment and prevention. Pediatr Clin North Am 1987 Aug; 34(4):935–959

Kriesberg RA. Diabetic ketoacidosis: An update. Crit Care Clin 1987 Oct; 5(4):817–833

Malone JK and Meacham JE. The hyperglycemic hyperosmolar syndrome. Indiana Med 1988 Sep; 81(9):766–768

McFarland, K et al. Helping diabetic patients avoid guilt when "out of control." Diabetes 1989 Apr; 85(5):244–248

Molitch ME. Diabetes mellitus: Control and complications. Postgrad Med 1989 Mar; 85(4):182–199

Mullen L and Hollander P. A practical guide to using insulin. Postgrad Med 1989 Mar; 85(4):227–232

Patel DG and Kalhan SC. Diabetic ketoacidosis. Indiana J Pediatr 1986 Sep–Oct; 53(5):559–572

Rasaiah B et al. Committee on monitoring devices. Guidelines on the use of blood glucose meters and non-meter blood glucose reagent strips in hospitals. Can Med Assoc J 1988 Jan; 138(1):27–29

Reader D et al. Nutrition assessment and education for people with diabetes. Caring 1988 Nov; 7(11):22–24, 26

Spencer M. Type I diabetes: Control with individualized insulin regimens. Postgrad Med 1989 Mar; 85(4):201–206

Sperling MA. Outpatient management of diabetes mellitus. Pediatr Clin North Am 1987 Aug; 34(4):919–934

Stone MB. Questions that diabetes patients ask. Diabetes Educ 1987 Summer; 13(3):298–301

Teza SL, Davis WK and Hiss RG. Patient knowledge compared with national guidelines for diabetes care. Diabetes Educ 1988 May–Jun; 14(3):207–211

Neurological and Sensory Disorders

24 Neurological Disorders

Diagnostic Evaluation of Neurologic Disease

The neurologic examination involves history-taking, an assessment of the patient's mental status, speech, memory, and reasoning ability, as well as a physical examination in which special attention is given to examination of the nervous system. This involves testing of each cranial nerve, as well as assessment of functioning of peripheral nerves and the spinal cord.

Selected Imaging Procedures

A. Skull X-ray—reveals configuration, density, vascular markings, and intracranial calcification and tumor.

B. Computed Tomography (CT)—an imaging method in which the head is scanned in successive layers by a narrow beam of x-ray. It provides a cross-sectional view of the brain and distinguishes differences in the densities of various brain tissues. A computer printout is obtained of the absorption values of the tissues in the plane that is being scanned. The data are transformed into an image through a series of complex equations. The image is displayed on an oscilloscope or television monitor and photographed.

1. Lesions are seen as variations in tissue density differing from the surrounding normal brain tissue.
2. Abnormalities of tissue density indicate possible tumor masses, brain infarction, ventricular displacement; useful in patients with head trauma, suspected brain tumor, hydrocephalus. CT is also used for diseases of the spinal column and spinal cord and is commonly used in the evaluation of patients with herniated discs.
3. May be done with IV contrast medium enhancement to define boundaries of certain lesions and indicate presence of otherwise undetectable lesions.
4. *Patient preparation*
   a. Inquire about allergies and any previous adverse reaction to contrast agent.
   b. Be sure that a consent form has been signed.
   c. No special preparation is required; this is a noninvasive technique that can be done on an outpatient basis.
   d. Instruct the patient that he must lie perfectly still while the test is being carried out; he cannot talk or move his face as this distorts the image.

C. Magnetic Resonance Imaging (MRI)—a diagnostic imaging modality that uses a magnetic field and computers to produce images of the body. It is extremely sensitive in detecting abnormalities in the brain, especially chemical changes within cells, and for delineating the extent of intracranial tumors.

1. Patient removes all metallic objects (jewelry, including wedding ring and watch) and lies on a flat platform that will be moved into a table containing the magnet.
2. Explain that nothing will be felt during the scanning process but the thumping sound of the magnetic coils as the magnetic field is being pulsed will be heard.

D. Positron Emission Tomography (PET)—a computer-based imaging technique that permits study of the brain's metabolism and function; displays pictures of metabolic and biochemical activity within brain as thinking, speaking, hearing, and other activities occur.

1. Patient inhales a radioactive gas or is injected with a radioactive substance that emits positively charged particles.
2. When these positrons combine with negatively charged electrons (normally found in body cells), the resultant gamma rays can be detected by a scanning device.

E. Single Photon Emission Computed Tomography (SPECT)—a three-dimensional imaging technique using nuclear medicine procedures that employ radionuclides and instruments that emit and detect single photons.

1. Gamma photons are emitted from radiopharmaceutical in the patient and are detected by a rotating gamma camera; the image is sent to a microcomputer
2. Useful in detecting the extent and location of abnormally perfused areas of brain (following head injury, stroke; before and after neurosurgery) and localizing seizure foci in epilepsy.

Cerebral Angiography

Cerebral angiography is the x-ray study of the cerebral circulation following injection of contrast material into a selected artery.

A. General Points

1. The majority of cerebral angiograms are done by threading a catheter through the femoral artery in the groin and up to the desired vessel.
2. The procedure may also be accomplished by retrograde injection of contrast medium into the brachial artery.
3. After injection of selected artery, x-rays are made of arterial and venous phases of circulation through brain and head.
4. Useful in demonstrating position of arteries, intracranial aneurysms, presence or absence of abnormal vasculature, hematomas, or tumors, or to add specificity to a CT diagnosis.
5. *Digital subtraction angiography*—uses computerized radiographic techniques in the evaluation of vascular disease.
   a. Subtracts (masks out electronically) surrounding bony and soft tissue structures to give an unobstructed picture of blood vessels.

B. Nursing Support: Before Angiogram

1. Withhold meal preceding test, but clear liquids are usually permitted up to the time of the study.
2. The patient may be given sedation before test—may help minimize intensity of burning sensation felt along course of injected vessel.
3. Mark the appropriate peripheral pulses with a felt-tipped pen.
4. Instruct the patient as follows:
   a. Try to remain immobile during the film sequence.
   b. A brief feeling of warmth in the face, behind the eyes, or in the jaw, tongue, and lips and a metallic taste are likely to be experienced.

C. Nursing Support: Following Angiogram

1. Make repeated observations for neurologic sequelae—motor or sensory deterioration, alterations in level of responsiveness, weakness on one side, speech disturbances, dysrhythmias, blood pressure fluctuation.
2. Observe injection site for hematoma formation; apply an ice cap intermittently—to relieve swelling and discomfort.
3. Evaluate peripheral pulses—changes may develop if there is hematoma formation at puncture site or embolization to a distant artery.
4. Note color and temperature of involved extremity—to detect possible embolism.

Myelography

Myelography is an x-ray of the spinal subarachnoid space taken after an opaque medium or air is injected into the spinal subarachnoid space through a spinal puncture; outlines the spinal subarachnoid space and shows distortion of the spinal cord or dural sac by tumors, cysts, herniated intravertebral discs, or other lesions.

A. General Points

1. After injection of the contrast medium, the head of the table is tilted down and the course of the contrast medium is observed radioscopically. The contrast medium may be water soluble or oil based.
2. Metrizamide is a water-soluble contrast agent that is absorbed by the body and excreted by the kidneys; side effects include headache (probably due to CNS irritation by metrizamide).
3. Iophendylate (Pantopaque) is an oil-based iodine compound that the radiologist may remove by syringe and needle aspiration; patient may complain of sharp pain down the leg during aspiration if nerve root is affected.

B. Nursing Responsibilities: Before Test

1. Reinforce the physician's explanation of procedure.
2. Omit the meal preceding myelography.
3. Patient may be given a light sedative prior to procedure to help cope.

C. Nursing Support After the Test

1. If water-soluble medium (metrizamide) has been used, the patient lies with the head of the bed elevated 15–30 degrees—to reduce the upward dispersion of the medium.
2. If oil-based medium (Pantopaque) is used, the patient is instructed to lie in a recumbent position (12–24 hours) to reduce cerebrospinal fluid leakage and decrease the frequency of headache.
3. Encourage the patient to drink liberal quantities of fluid—for rehydration and replacement of cerebrospinal fluid and to decrease incidence of postlumbar puncture headache (thought to be due to escape of spinal fluid).
4. Assess neurologic and vital signs; note motor and sensory deviations from normal.
5. Check on patient's ability to void.
6. Watch for fever, stiff neck, photophobia (sensitivity to light), or other signs of chemical or bacterial meningitis.

Electroencephalography (EEG)

Records, by means of electrodes applied on the scalp surface (or by microelectrodes placed within brain tissue), the electrical activity that is generated in the brain.

1. Provides physiologic assessment of cerebral activity; useful in diagnosis of the epilepsies and as a screening

procedure for coma and organic brain syndrome; also serves as an indicator of brain death.

2. Electrodes are arranged on the scalp to record the electrical activity in various regions of the brain; the amplified activity of the neurons is recorded on a continuously moving paper sheet; this record is the encephalogram.
   a. For baseline recording, the patient lies quietly with his eyes closed.
   b. For activation procedures (done to elicit abnormal electrical discharges, especially seizure potentials), patient may be asked to hyperventilate for 3–4 minutes and then to look at a bright flashing light for photic stimulation.
   c. EEG may also be made during sleep and upon awakening—some abnormal brain waves are seen only during sleep.
3. Pharyngeal (electrode inserted through nose; rests on mucosa of pharyngeal roof) and sphenoidal (inserted transcutaneously with tips resting on sphenoid bone near foramen ovale) electrodes are used when epileptogenic area is inaccessible to conventional scalp preparation.
4. Depth recording of EEG is done by introducing electrodes stereotactically into a target area of the brain determined by the patient's seizure pattern and scalp EEG. Used to select patients who may benefit from surgical excision of epileptogenic foci.
5. Patient preparation for EEG.
   a. Tranquilizers and stimulants may be withheld 24–48 hours before EEG—may alter EEG wave patterns.
   b. Coffee, tea, or cola drinks are omitted in meal before test because of their stimulating effects.
   c. Do not omit meal because an altered blood sugar level can cause changes in brain wave patterns.
   d. Reassure the patient that he will not receive an electrical shock, that the EEG takes approximately 60–90 minutes (more for an EEG taken while sleeping), and that this is a *test,* not a form of treatment.

Evoked Potential Studies

These studies involve the changes and responses in brain waves recorded from scalp electrodes that are evoked (elicited) by the introduction of an external stimulus (visual, auditory, somatosensory).

1. These evoked changes are detected with the aid of computing devices, which extract, display the signal on an oscilloscope, and store the data on magnetic tape or disc.
2. These studies are based on the concept that any insult/dysfunction that can alter neuronal metabolism or disturb membrane function may change evoked responses in brain waves.
   a. Visual evoked responses—the patient looks at visual stimulus (flashing light; checkerboard pattern of a screen); the average of several hundred stimuli are recorded by EEG leads placed over the occiput; the transit time from the retina to the occipital area is measured (in milliseconds), using computer averaging methods.
   b. Auditory evoked responses—auditory stimulus (repetitive auditory click) is given and the transit time up the brain stem into the cortex is measured.

Specific lesions in auditory pathway will modify or delay the response.
   c. Somatosensory evoked response—peripheral nerves stimulated percutaneously. Transit time up the spinal cord to the sensory cortex of the brain is measured and recorded from scalp electrodes. Test is used to detect deficit in spinal cord, to measure conduction in spinal cord, and to monitor cord function during operative procedures.
   d. No special patient preparation other than reassurance and encouragement of relaxation.

Electromyography *(EMG)*

A technique that uses metal electrodes and an amplifier and oscilloscope to study electrical activity arising from muscles at rest and muscles that are contracted.

1. Useful in determining the presence of a neuromuscular disorder.

Nerve Conduction Studies

Performed by stimulating a peripheral nerve at several points along its course and recording the muscle action potential or the sensory action potential that results.

Other Neurologic Studies

A. Lumbar Epidural Venography—percutaneous insertion of a catheter into the femoral vein; catheter is guided into ascending lumbar vein and/or internal iliac veins. Contrast medium is injected to fill the epidural veins overlying the disc spaces and to opacify the epidural venous plexus.

1. Useful in diagnosis of herniated lumbar discs not demonstrated by myelography.
2. May be done as complementary diagnostic study with myelography.

B. Radionuclide Imaging Studies (brain scan)—following intravenous injection of radiopharmaceutical, the radioactivity subsequently transmitted through the skull is traced by a scanner that prints out a picture, or a gamma camera that prints out image without actually scanning may be used. CT scanning is replacing traditional radioisotope scanning.

1. This test is based on the principle that a radiopharmaceutical may diffuse through a disrupted blood-brain barrier into the abnormal cerebral tissue or areas where there is new vascularization. (Normal brain tissue is relatively impermeable.) There is an increased uptake of radioactive material at the site of pathology.
2. Brain scanning is useful in early detection and evaluation of intracranial neoplasms, stroke, abscess, follow-up of surgical or radiation therapy of brain.

C. Ultrasonography—the recording of echoes from the deep structures within the skull by means of ultrasound (high-frequency sound waves).

1. Ultrasound transducers are positioned over specified areas of the head while echoes are transcribed into images—monitors intracranial circulation.
2. Useful for detecting a shift of the cerebral midline structures caused by subdural hematoma, intracerebral hemorrhage, massive cerebral infarction, and neoplasms; can display dilation of ventricles; useful in evaluation of hydrocephalus.

D. Lumbar Puncture—see following Guideline.

Guidelines   Assisting the Patient Undergoing a Lumbar Puncture

Lumbar Puncture   Insertion of a needle into lumbar subarachnoid space and withdrawal of cerebrospinal fluid for diagnostic and therapeutic purposes.

Purposes
1. To obtain cerebrospinal fluid for examination (microbiologic, serologic, cytologic, or chemical analysis).*
2. To measure and relieve cerebrospinal pressure.
3. To determine the presence or absence of blood in the spinal fluid.
4. To detect spinal subarachnoid block.
5. To administer antibiotics intrathecally in certain cases of infection.
6. To administer anticancer drugs.

Equipment
Sterile lumbar puncture set
Sterile gloves
Xylocaine 1%–2%

Skin antiseptic
Band-Aid

Procedure

Nursing Action	Rationale/Amplification
Preparatory Phase	
1. Prior to the procedure, the patient should empty his bladder and bowel.	
2. Give a step-by-step summary of the procedure.	2. Reassures the patient and gains his cooperation.
For Lying Position: (Fig. 24-1).	
3. Position the patient on his side with a small pillow under his head and a pillow between his legs. He should be lying on a firm surface.	3. The spine is maintained in a horizontal position. The pillow between the legs prevents the upper leg from rolling forward.
4. Instruct the patient to arch the lumbar segment of his back and draw his knees up to his abdomen, clasping his knees with his hands.	4. This posture offers maximal widening of the interspinous spaces and affords easier entry into the subarachnoid space.
5. Assist the patient in maintaining this position by supporting him behind the knees and neck. Assist the patient to maintain the posture throughout the examination.	5. Supporting the patient helps prevent sudden movements, which can produce a traumatic (bloody) tap and thus impede correct diagnosis.
For Sitting Position:	
6. Have the patient straddle a straight-back chair (facing the back) and rest his head against his arms, which are folded on the back of the chair.	6. In obese patients and those who have difficulty in assuming an arched side-lying position, this posture may allow more accurate identification of the spinous processes and interspaces.
Performance Phase (by the physician)	
1. The skin is prepared with antiseptic solution, and the skin and subcutaneous spaces are infiltrated with local anesthetic agent.	
2. A spinal puncture needle is introduced at the L3–L4 interspace. The needle is advanced until the "give" of the ligamentum flavum is felt and the needle enters the subarachnoid space. The manometer is attached to the spinal puncture needle.	2. L3–L4 interspace is *below* the level of the spinal cord.
3. After the needle enters the subarachnoid space, help the patient to slowly straighten his legs.	3. This maneuver prevents a false increase in intraspinal pressure. Muscle tension and compression of the abdomen give falsely high pressures.
4. Instruct the patient to breathe quietly (not to hold his breath or strain) and not to talk.	4. Hyperventilation may lower a truly elevated pressure. Talking can elevate CSF pressure.
5. The initial pressure reading is obtained by measuring the level of the fluid column after it comes to rest.	5. With respiration there is normally some fluctuation of spinal fluid in the manometer. Normal range of spinal fluid pressure with the patient in the lateral recumbent position is 70–200 mm. H_2O.
6. About 2–3 ml. of spinal fluid is placed in each of 3 test tubes for observation, comparison, and laboratory analysis.	6. Spinal fluid should be clear and colorless. Bloody spinal fluid may indicate cerebral contusion, laceration, subarachnoid hemorrhage, or a traumatic tap.

* See Appendix for characteristics of normal cerebrospinal fluid.

(continued)

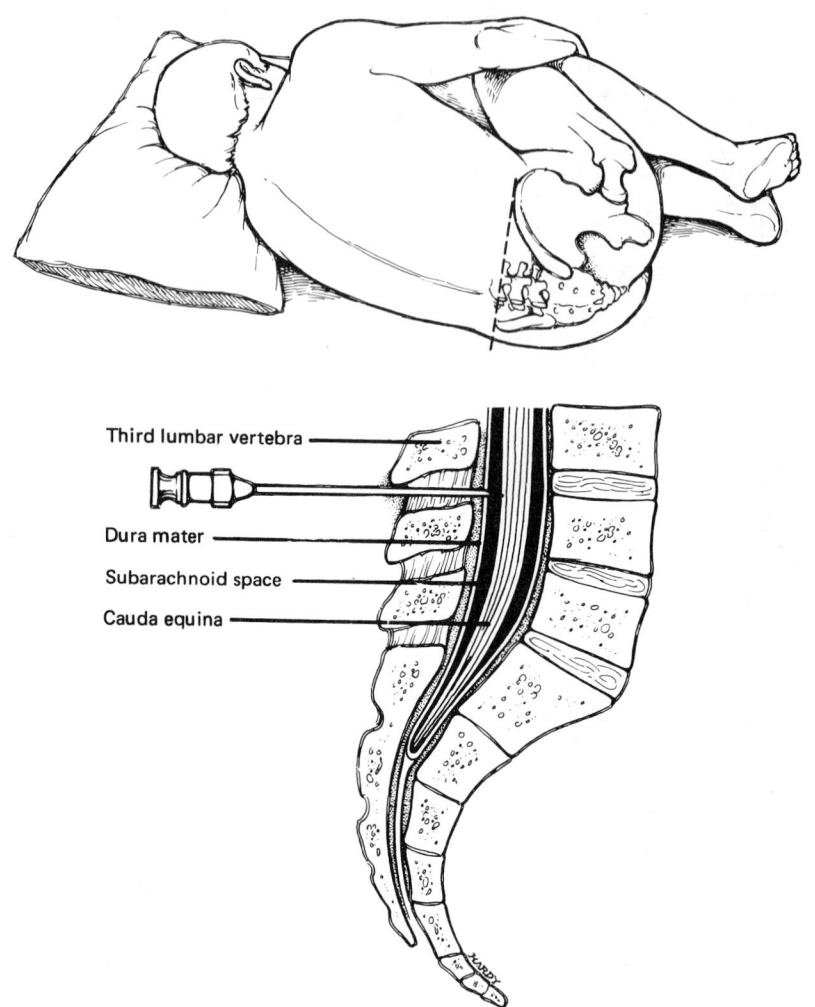

Figure 24-1. *Technique of lumbar puncture.*

Procedure *(continued)*	**Nursing Action**	**Rationale/Amplification**
	Lumbar Manometric Test (Queckenstedt Test)	
	1. A blood pressure cuff is placed around the patient's neck and inflated to a pressure of 20 mm. Hg (or an assistant compresses jugular vein or veins for 10 seconds).	This test is made when a spinal subarachnoid block is suspected (tumor; vertebral fracture or dislocation). In normal persons there is a rapid rise in pressure of CSF in response to jugular compression with rapid return to normal when the compression is released. If the pressure fails to rise or rises and falls slowly, there is evidence of a block due to a lesion's compressing the spinal subarachnoid pathways. This test is not done if an intracranial lesion is suspected.
	2. Pressure readings are made at 10-second intervals.	
	3. After the needle is withdrawn, a Band-Aid is applied to the puncture site.	
	Follow-up Phase	
	1. Following the procedure, the patient is asked to remain prone (on abdomen) for about 3 hours.	1. This allows the tissue surfaces along the needle track to come together to prevent cerebrospinal fluid leakage.

Procedure (continued)	**Nursing Action**	**Rationale/Amplification**

2. Encourage a liberal fluid intake.
3. Record (a) procedure, (b) appearance of spinal fluid, (c) whether or not specimens were sent to laboratory, (d) spinal pressure readings, and (e) condition and reaction of the patient.

Complications

Postlumbar puncture headache (throbbing, bifrontal or occipital headache that becomes severe when patient sits or stands, but lessens when he lies down in horizontal position); managed by bedrest, analgesics, and hydration

The cause is thought to be leakage of spinal fluid at the puncture site.

Herniation of intracranial contents
Traumatic complications (spinal epidural abscess; spinal epidural hematoma; meningitis).

Nursing Management of the Patient With an Altered State of Consciousness

Unconsciousness is a condition in which there is a depression of cerebral function ranging from stupor to coma.

Coma may be defined as no eye opening upon stimulation, absence of comprehensible speech, and failure to obey commands.

Causes of Unconsciousness

1. Head injury
2. Drug overdose
3. Diffuse cerebral disease
4. Metabolic dysfunction (hepatic or diabetic coma)

Assessment

Goals:

To assess arousal and awareness
To detect focal neurologic deficits and brain stem dysfunction

1. Assess the patient's level of responsiveness (arousal and awareness).
   a. Responds to command or stimulation (press pen against side of patient's nail bed for stimulation)
   b. Eye opening
   c. Verbal responses
   d. Motor responses
2. Assess motor function for strength and symmetry.
3. Record the patient's *exact* reactions. Use Glasgow coma scale for documentation (see p. 579).
4. Test brain stem reflexes to assess for brain stem dysfunction.
   a. Pupil size, symmetry, and reaction to light.
   b. Reflex eye movements elicited to head turning (oculocephalic response) or testing of oculovestibular response by medical staff.
5. Check respiratory rate and pattern (normal, Kussmaul, Cheyne-Stokes, apneic).
6. Check swallowing reflexes; deep tendon reflexes.
7. Examine head for signs of trauma, and mouth, nose, and ears for evidence of blood and cerebrospinal fluid (CSF).
8. Monitor any change in neurologic status over time.

Diagnostic Evaluation

1. Computed tomography of head.
2. Laboratory evaluation: CBC, blood glucose, electrolytes, creatinine, alcohol levels, toxicology screen.
3. EEG—provides information about depth of coma and degree of reactivity to stimulation.

Management

1. Specific treatment when cause is known (e.g., infection, drug overdose, CNS hemorrhage).
2. Oxygenation provided—is monitored through arterial blood gas evaluations.
3. Circulation is maintained and arterial pressure restored.
   a. Adequate pulse and blood pressure are essential to maintain cerebral circulation.
   b. Volume replacement to maintain blood pressure.
   c. Treatment of cardiac dysfunction.
4. Administration of intravenous glucose after blood is obtained for analysis.
5. Treatment of intracranial pressure (see p. 578).

Complications

1. Infectious complications: pulmonary, urinary tract, CNS; pressure sores.
2. Seizures.
3. Gastrointestinal bleeding.

Nursing Diagnoses

1. Ineffective airway clearance related to upper airway obstruction by tongue and soft tissues; inability to clear respiratory secretions.
2. Potential fluid volume deficit related to inability to ingest fluids, dehydration from osmotic therapy (when used to reduce intracranial pressure).
3. Altered oral mucous membranes related to mouth breathing, absence of pharyngeal reflex, inability to ingest fluid.
4. Potential impairment of skin integrity related to immobility or restlessness.
5. Impaired tissue integrity of cornea related to diminished/absent corneal reflex.
6. Potential hyperthermia related to potential damage to hypothalamic center.
7. Altered urinary elimination (incontinence or retention) related to unconscious state.

8. Altered bowel elimination (incontinence and/or constipation) related to unconscious state.
9. Other possible nursing diagnosis: altered family process related to sudden crisis of unconsciousness. See head injury, page 582.

Nursing Interventions *(Fig. 24-2)*

A. Maintaining an Effective Airway

1. Place the patient in a three-fourths prone or semi-prone or lateral position—prevents the tongue from obstructing the airway, encourages drainage of respiratory secretions, and promotes oxygen and carbon dioxide exchange.
2. Keep the airway free of secretions with efficient suctioning—in the absence of the cough and swallowing reflexes, secretions rapidly accumulate in the posterior pharynx and upper trachea and can lead to fatal respiratory complications.
   a. Insert oral airway if tongue is paralyzed or is obstructing the airway—an obstructed airway increases intracranial pressure. This is considered a short-term measure.
   b. Prepare for insertion of cuffed endotracheal tube to protect the airway from aspiration and to allow efficient removal of tracheobronchial secretions.
   c. See page 241 for technique of tracheal suctioning.
   d. Employ oxygen therapy as prescribed to deliver oxygenated blood to the central nervous system.
3. Evaluate pulses (radial, carotid, apical, and pedal); measure blood pressure—these parameters are a measure of circulatory adequacy/inadequacy.
4. Maintain circulation; support the blood pressure and treat life-threatening cardiac dysrhythmias.

B. Attaining and Maintaining Fluid and Electrolyte Balance

1. Monitor prescribed intravenous fluids carefully as a large volume of fluid may aggravate cerebral edema.
2. Or use hyperalimentation feedings.
3. Or initiate nasogastric feedings.
4. Measure urinary output and specific gravity.

C. Maintaining Healthy Oral Mucous Membranes

1. Remove dentures. Inspect patient's mouth for dryness, inflammation, and the presence of crusting.
2. Cleanse the mouth with prescribed solution every 2 hours—to prevent parotitis (inflammation of parotid gland).
3. Apply lip emollient to prevent angular stomatitis and cheilitis.

D. Maintaining Skin Integrity

1. Keep the skin clean, dry, and free of pressure—comatose patients are susceptible to the formation of pressure sores.
2. Clip the patient's nails to prevent excoriation.
3. Turn the patient from side to side on a regular schedule—relieves pressure areas and helps clear lungs by mobilizing secretions; turning also provides kinesthetic (sensation of movement), proprioceptive (awareness of position), and vestibular (equilibrium) stimulation.
4. Reposition carefully after turning to prevent ischemic necrosis over pressure areas and pressure on nerves that can lead to compression neuropathies.
5. Put all extremities through range-of-motion exercises at least 4 times daily; contracture deformities develop early in unconscious patients.

E. Maintaining Corneal Integrity

1. Protect the eyes from corneal irritation—the cornea functions as a shield. If the eyes remain open for long periods, corneal drying, irritation, and ulceration are likely to result.
   a. Make sure the patient's eye is not rubbing against bedding if blinking and corneal reflexes are absent.
   b. Inspect the size of the pupils and condition of eyes with a flashlight.
   c. Remove contact lenses if worn.
   d. Irrigate eyes with sterile prescribed solution to remove discharge and debris.
   e. Instill prescribed ophthalmic ointment in each eye—prevents glazing and corneal ulceration.
   f. Instill artificial tears as prescribed.
2. Prepare for temporary tarsorrhaphy (suturing of eyelids in closed position) if unconscious state is prolonged.

F. Reducing Fever

1. Look for possible sites of infections (respiratory, CNS, urinary tract, wound) when fever is present in an unconscious patient.
2. Control persistent elevations of temperature—increased metabolic demands will overburden brain circulation and oxygenation resulting in cerebral deterioration.
   a. Cool room to 18.3°C. (65°F.). However, an older patient requires a warmer temperature.
   b. Remove bedding over the patient except light sheet or loin cloth.
   c. Employ cool-water sponging and an electric fan blowing over the patient to increase surface cooling.
   d. Consider use of hypothermia blanket if hyperthermia is of neurogenic origin. Esophageal or other core temperature is monitored continuously.

G. Promoting Urinary Elimination

1. Palpate over the patient's bladder at intervals to detect urinary retention and an overdistended bladder.
2. Insert an indwelling urethral catheter for short-term management.
3. Use intermittent bladder catheterization for retention as soon as possible—to minimize risk of infection.
4. Monitor for fever and cloudy urine; inspect the urethral orifice for suppurative drainage.
5. Initiate a bladder training program (p. 142) as soon as consciousness is regained.

H. Promoting Bowel Function

1. Observe for constipation—from immobility and lack of dietary fiber.
   a. Stool softener may be prescribed and given with tube feeding.
   b. Glycerin suppository may be prescribed to stimulate bowel emptying.
2. Monitor for diarrhea—from infection, antibiotics, hyperosmolar fluids, and fecal impaction.
   a. Perform a rectal examination if fecal impaction is suspected.
   b. Use commercial fecal collection bags and meticulous skin care if patient has fecal incontinence.
3. Auscultate for bowel sounds; measure the girth of the abdomen with a tape measure for detection of abdominal distention.
4. Palpate lower abdomen for distention.

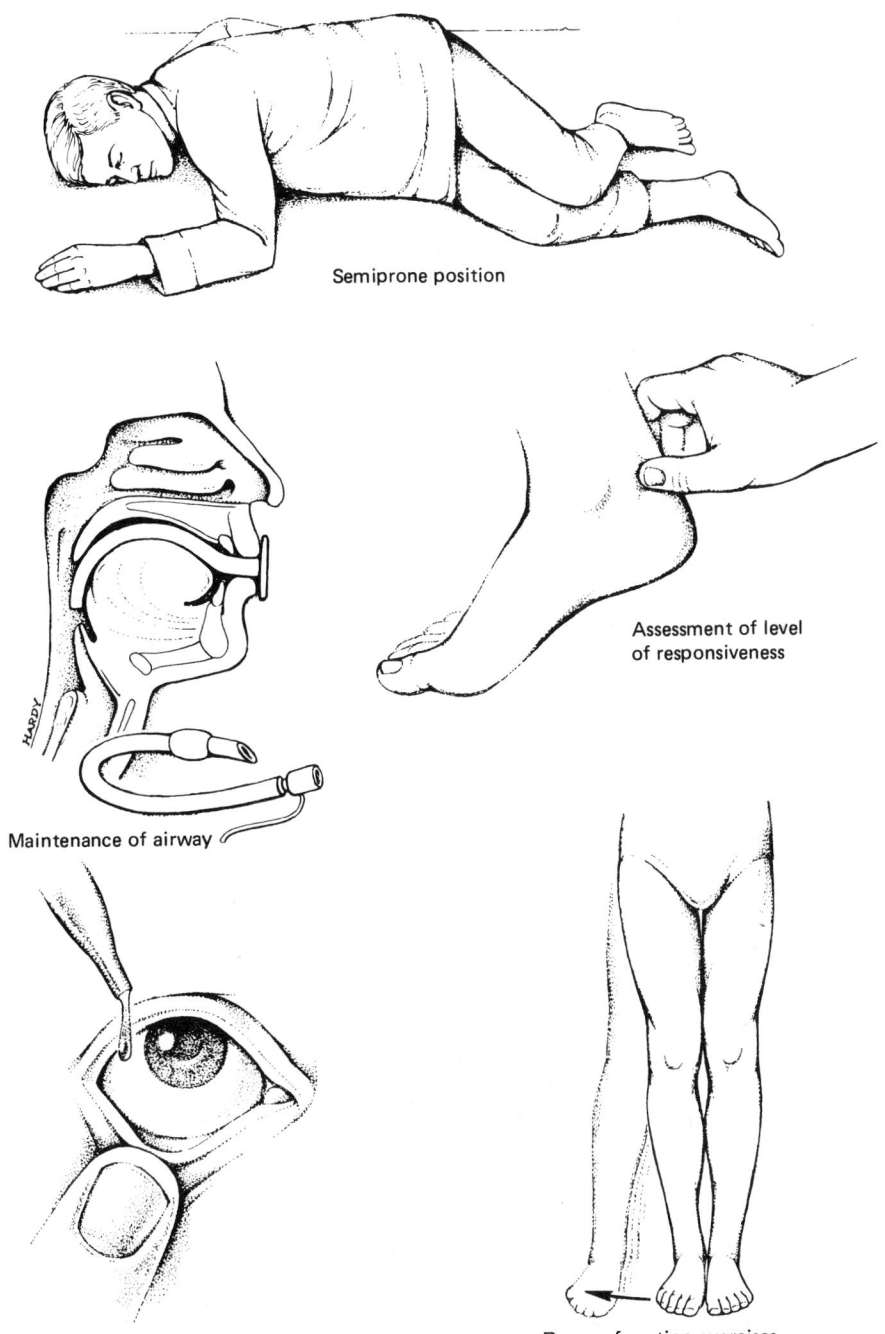

Semiprone position

Maintenance of airway

Assessment of level of responsiveness

Protection of eyes

Range of motion exercises

Figure 24-2. *Nursing priorities in the care of the patient with an altered state of consciousness.*

I. Other Nursing Interventions

1. Use every sensory avenue to stimulate the patient.
   a. Use physical touch and reassuring voice tone.
   b. Encourage family to talk in a meaningful way to the patient even when he is not responding.
   c. Orient to person, time, place, and situation.
2. Have adequate room lighting to prevent hallucinations as patient regains consciousness.
3. Be aware of the varying phases of restlessness—a certain degree of restlessness may be favorable. However, restlessness is seen in cerebral hypoxia or when there is a partially obstructed airway, distended bladder, etc.
4. Provide for social contacts and environmental enrichment—introducing meaningful sounds (conversation, music, taped sounds of patient's home and work environment) stimulates the cortical levels.

5. Be aware that the patient, after regaining consciousness, will feel uneasy concerning period of unconsciousness.
   a. Give an explanation of what has happened.
   b. Permit the patient to ask questions.

Evaluation

1. Maintains clear airway; coughs up secretions.
2. Attains/maintains adequate fluid volume status; absence of clinical signs of dehydration.
3. Has intact healthy appearing oral mucous membranes.
4. Absence of skin breakdown.
5. Absence of trauma to cornea.
6. Temperature within acceptable range.
7. Demonstrates bladder continence.
8. Maintaining normal bowel function.

Nursing Management of the Patient With Increasing Intracranial Pressure
(Intracranial Hypertension)

Intracranial pressure (ICP) is the pressure within the ventriculosubarachnoid space; in a "steady state," the intracranial compartments (blood, brain, cerebrospinal fluid [CSF]) are in a condition of pressure and volume equilibrium.

Increased ICP is defined as cerebrospinal fluid pressure greater than 15 mm. Hg.

Causes

1. Head injury/hematoma
2. Cerebral edema; stroke
3. Abscess, infection
4. Hemorrhage; impending aneurysmal rupture
5. Brain tumor
6. Intracranial surgery

NURSING ALERT: As intracranial pressure increases, the brain substance is compressed. A sudden increase may produce an emergency situation in a few minutes. This condition may lead rapidly to death or result in a vegetative existence for the patient.

Clinical Manifestations and Nursing Assessment

A. Change in Level of Responsiveness (consciousness)

1. *The level of responsiveness is the most important measure of the patient's condition.*
2. Look for lethargy, delay in response to verbal suggestions, slowing of speech.
3. Watch for sudden changes in condition—quietness to restlessness, orientation to confusion, increasing drowsiness, stupor, coma.
4. *Progressive deterioration is a serious sign* that may necessitate immediate surgical intervention.

B. Changes in Vital Signs

1. Rising blood pressure or widening pulse pressure (the difference between systolic and diastolic blood pressure).
2. Pulse changes—bradycardia changing to tachycardia as intracranial pressure rises.

3. Respiratory irregularities; tachypnea (early sign of intracranial hypertension); slowing of rate with lengthening periods of apnea; Cheyne-Stokes or Kussmaul breathing.
4. Moderately elevated temperature.

C. Pupillary Changes—increasing pressure or an expanding clot can displace the brain against the oculomotor or optic nerve, producing pupillary changes.

1. Inspect the pupils with a flashlight to evaluate size, configuration, and reaction to light. Compare both eyes for similarities/differences.
2. Evaluate gaze to determine if it is conjugate (paired, working together) or if eye movements are abnormal.
3. Evaluate ability of eyes to abduct and adduct.
4. Inspect the retina and optic nerve for hemorrhage and papilledema.

D. Other Changes

1. Headache—increasing in intensity; aggravated by movement/straining.
2. Vomiting—recurrent with little or no nausea; may be projectile.
3. Subtle changes—restlessness, headache, forced breathing, purposeless movements, and mental cloudiness.
4. Papilledema

Management

Increased intracranial pressure constitutes a true emergency and requires prompt treatment.

1. The airway is cleared and circulation ensured.
2. Administration of osmotic diuretics (mannitol; glycerol)—removes water from areas of the brain with an intact blood-brain barrier.
   a. Indwelling catheter inserted into bladder for management of subsequent diuresis.
3. Steroids (dexamethasone) administered—reduces edema surrounding brain tumor when brain tumor is the cause of ICP.
4. Hyperventilation with a volume ventilator—hyperventilation leads to respiratory alkalosis, which causes cerebral vasoconstriction and decreases cerebral blood volume and results in reduction of intracranial pressure.
   a. Neuromuscular paralyzing agents (pancuronium bromide)—may decrease ICP by preventing sudden changes from coughing, straining, and by preventing excess muscle activity.
5. Ventricular drainage of cerebrospinal fluid.
6. Treatment of fever as fever increases cerebral blood flow and cerebral blood volume; acute increases in ICP occur with fever spikes.
7. High-dose barbituates and other anesthetic agents—resultant comatose state suppresses brain metabolism, which in turn reduces cerebral blood flow, and the resultant fall in cerebral blood volume reduces the intracranial pressure.
   a. Requires a high level of nursing support.
   b. ICP, EEG, arterial pressure, and blood and serum barbituate levels are monitored.

Nursing Interventions

A. Reducing Intracranial Pressure and Preventing Irreversible Brain Damage

1. Provide continuing assessment of the patient's level of responsiveness (see opposite column).

2. Maintain a neurologic observation record.
   a. The Glasgow Coma Scale (Fig. 24-3) is a tool for objectively assessing the consciousness level by determining the patient's best response to stimulation in terms of eye opening, motor response, and verbal response.
   b. Know the patient's baseline (initial) condition; all observations should be compared with and evaluated accordingly.
   c. Carry out *repeated* nursing assessments—to determine clinical improvement or deterioration.
   d. Watch the patient carefully when changing his position; avoid compression of jugular veins (head falling to one side).
3. Use intracranial pressure monitoring when prescribed for sustained ICP; elevations (above 20 mm. Hg persisting 15 minutes or more or if there is a significant shift in pressure).

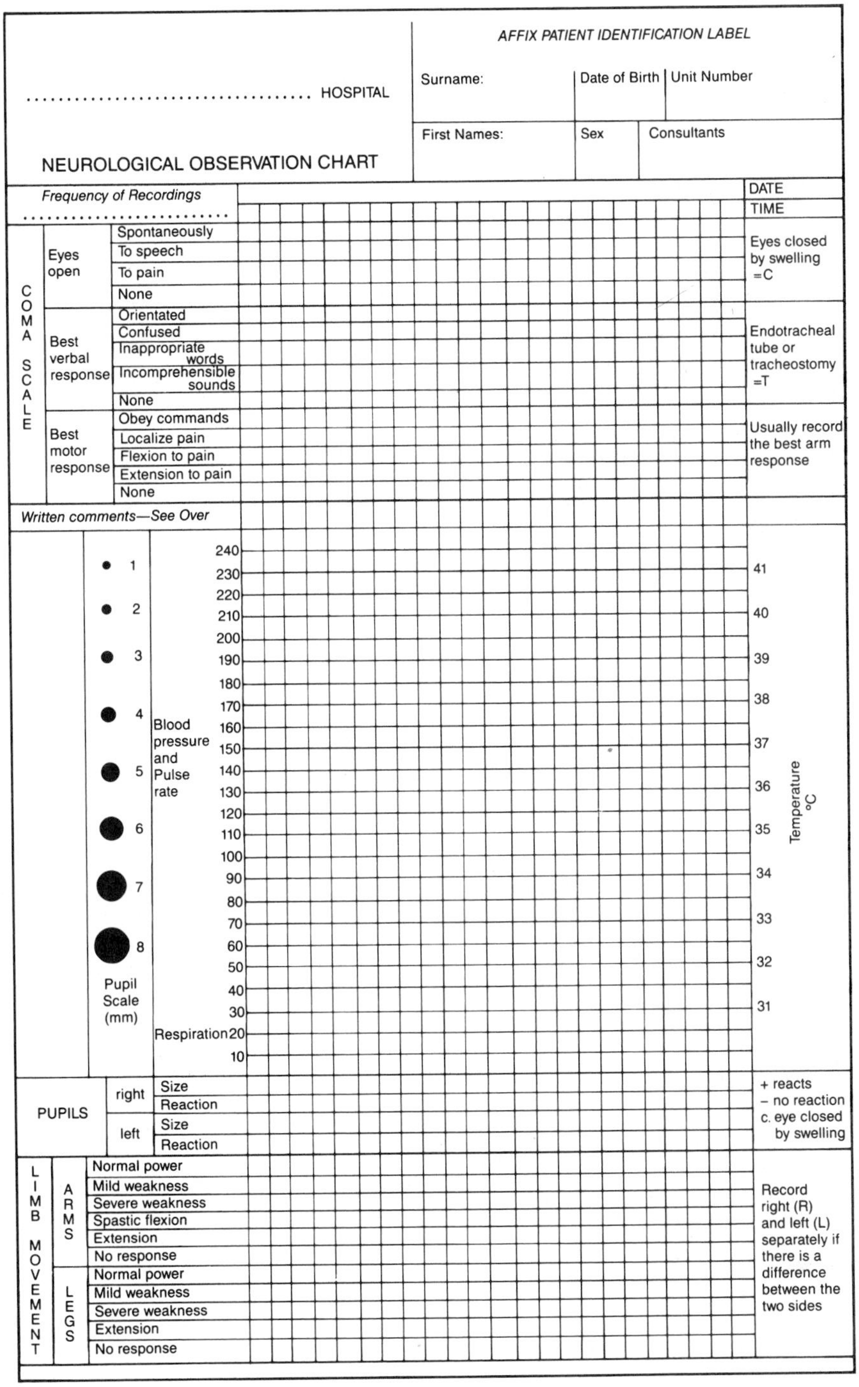

Figure 24-3. *Example of observation chart that includes the Glasgow Coma Scale. (Reproduced by courtesy of Butterworth and Company, London, from Campkin and Turner, Neurosurgical Anaesthesia and Intensive Care)*

4. Determine the nursing interventions (turning, suctioning, painful procedures) associated with ICP increases.
5. Monitor the patient's temperature.
   a. Avoid elevation of temperature since fever increases cerebral metabolism.
   b. Monitor cardiac output with Swan-Ganz catheter if measures are taken to reduce the patient's temperature.
6. Avoid activities or positions that produce a rise in intracranial pressure.
   a. Elevate head of bed to 30 degrees—encourages venous return, reduces jugular venous pressure, and lowers ICP (if CSF pathways are patent).
   b. The optimal head position for the individual patient is best determined by direct ICP monitoring.
   c. Avoid turning the head from side to side or allowing the head to fall to one side (this compresses the jugular veins and restricts venous return from the brain).
   d. Avoid the prone position, flexion of the neck, extreme hip flexion, the Valsalva maneuver, isometric muscle contractions, coughing and straining.
   e. Avoid any stimuli that can precipitate ICP.
   f. Watch ICP monitor during endotracheal suctioning; discontinue procedure if ICP rises precipitously.
   g. Remember that extracranial factors can elevate ICP, including motor posturing, use of PEEP, jugular compression, metabolic abnormalities, and various treatment modalities.
7. Prepare for surgical intervention if the patient's condition deteriorates.

Continuous Intracranial Pressure Monitoring

Intracranial pressure monitoring is the recording of the pressure exerted within the skull by the brain, cerebral blood, and cerebrospinal fluid. It gives a dynamic status of intracranial events.

Purpose

1. To provide immediate information for early detection and treatment of intracranial pressure to prevent brain deterioration
2. To guide therapy for control of intracranial pressure
3. To have access to cerebrospinal fluid for sampling and drainage
4. To serve as a prognostic indicator

Underlying Principles

A. Fluctuations

1. Intracranial pressure is not in a steady state, but fluctuates.
2. Fluctuations are indicated by waves of high pressure and troughs of relatively normal pressure.
3. These waves have been classified as A waves (plateau waves), B waves, and C waves.

B. A Waves

1. The plateau (A) waves have clinical significance:
2. They are characterized by rapid increases and decreases of pressure with recurring elevations of intracranial pressure that may last from 2–15 minutes and range in amplitude between 15–50 mm. Hg.
3. Plateau waves are usually related to cerebral dysfunction and caused by brain shift or distortion.
4. They may be accompanied by transient symptoms—headache, nausea, disturbances of consciousness.

C. B Waves

1. B waves are of shorter duration (½–2 minutes) with smaller amplitude (up to 50 mm. Hg)
2. They have less clinical significance than A waves.
3. But B waves occurring in runs tend to be associated with pathologic depressions of consciousness and may precede the appearance of A waves.

D. C Waves

1. C waves are small, rhythmic oscillations with frequencies of approximately 6 per minute.
2. They appear to be related to rhythmic variations of the systemic arterial blood pressure (Traube–Hering–Mayer waves).

Techniques for Measuring Intracranial Pressure*

A. Intraventricular Catheter

1. Insertion of a fine catheter into a lateral ventricle, using either a twist drill or burr hole opening.
2. It is connected by a fluid-filled system to a transducer.
3. It obtains continuous ICP recording and allows for drainage of CSF to reduce intracranial pressure.
4. *Complications:* Ventricular infection, meningitis; difficulty in cannulating the ventricles.

B. Subarachnoid Screw (Bolt)

1. Hollow metal or plastic screw is inserted through the skull and dura mater to the cranial subarachnoid space through a small twist drill hole in the skull.
2. It is attached to a pressure transducer, which converts mechanical pressure into an electrical signal that records intracranial pressure on an oscilloscope as pressure waves.
3. *Complications:* Blockage of screw by clot and/or brain substance; local and intracranial infections; technical complications.

C. Epidural Intracranial Pressure Monitoring

1. A miniature pressure sensor and a transmitter are implanted in epidural space.
2. A fiberoptic cable exists through the scalp and is attached to the bedside monitor.

Nursing Interventions

1. Note the pattern of wave forms.
   a. ICP is expressed by ventricular fluid pressures that normally fluctuate in the range of 0 to 12 mm. Hg.
   b. Sustained elevations above 15 mm. Hg are generally considered abnormal.
   c. The trend of ICP measurements over time is im-

---

* The direct measurement of intracranial pressure may be accomplished by a number of monitoring techniques that require complex sensors, transducers, recording devices, etc., each of which carries its own benefits and risks. The nurse needs a working knowledge of the system being used and its limitations. There is not a single ideal method of measuring ICP.

portant. Repeated neurologic checks and clinical examinations must be done.

2. Note the interventions/stimuli (suctioning, bathing, uncomfortable procedures) associated with increases in ICP.
3. Watch for developing/increasing frequency of plateau waves.

    Start immediate measures to reduce intracranial pressure (p. 578) since this signifies that brain function may be in disequilibrium.

4. Monitor the patient's arterial blood gases—a high $PaCO_2$ will cause vasodilation of the cerebral vessels, an increase in cerebral blood flow, and a rise in intracranial pressure.
5. Monitor blood pressure and respirations—intracranial pressure wave forms correlate with changes in blood pressure and the respiratory cycle.
6. Keep connections tight and the system closed—any leakage of the fluid column produces a gradual drift from the baseline.
    a. Recalibrate the system according to manufacturer's directions at regular intervals.
    b. Realign the transducer and recalibrate if the level of the bed is changed, i.e., the diaphragm of the transducer is positioned at the level of the lateral canthus of the eye, which roughly corresponds to the foramen of Monro.
    c. Avoid interrupting the integrity of the system.
    d. Handle system with sterile gloves; strict asepsis is maintained.
7. Avoid activities that can initiate a rise in intracranial pressure.
    a. Avoid excessive rotation or flexion of the patient's head—interferes with the outflow of blood from the cranial cavity; temporary occlusion causes a rise in intracranial pressure.
    b. Avoid the Valsalva maneuver (straining at stool; coughing), which impedes venous return from brain.
8. Monitor insertion site for redness, swelling, leakage.
9. Support the patient physically and emotionally—some monitoring systems limit patient mobility.

Nursing Management of the Patient With a Head Injury

Clinical Manifestations

1. Unconsciousness or disturbance in consciousness
2. Headache
3. Vertigo
4. Confusion or delirium
5. Restlessness
6. Changes in body temperature
7. Respiratory irregularities
8. Pupillary abnormalities
9. Sudden onset of neurologic deficit

Physical Assessment

1. Open brain injuries—recognized by inspection; patient taken to operating room
2. Depressed skull fracture—may/may not be recognized by gentle palpation
3. Basilar skull fracture—determined (in part) on basis of physical findings

NURSING ALERT: Regard every patient who has a head injury as having a potential spinal cord injury. A significant number of patients are under the influence of alcohol at the time of injury, which may mask the nature and severity of the injury.

Diagnostic Evaluation

1. Neurologic assessment
2. CT scanning of head—identifies and localizes lesions; detects bleeding, brain swelling, hydrocephalus, and infection
3. Skull and cervical spine films
4. Neuropsychological tests (during rehabilitation phase)—to determine cognitive, behavioral, and skill deficits

Management

Goals:

To preserve brain homeostasis
To prevent secondary brain damage from an expanding intracranial hematoma or physiologic dysfunction from raised intracranial pressure, hypoxia, seizures, hypoglycemia, hypotension, hyperthermia and infection

A. Maintaining Physiologic Functioning

1. Maintenance of airway and ventilation—hypoxia, ischemia, and hypercapnia can increase brain swelling and brain damage.
    a. Endotracheal intubation indicated for comatose patient to maintain airway and remove secretions and for hyperventilation to reduce cerebral edema.
    b. Adequate oxygenation—the injured brain tolerates hypoxia poorly.
2. Stabilization of cardiovascular and respiratory functions to maintain optimum perfusion of brain; cardiovascular autoregulation is often impaired in brain injury.
3. Establishment of appropriate vascular access (central venous or peripheral lines) for blood, blood products, isotonic solutions.
4. Repeated neurologic examinations for baseline information and determination of extent of brain damage and whether or not patient is progressing or deteriorating.

B. Limiting Extent of Intracranial Pressure Elevation

1. Intracranial pressure monitoring for patient with severe head injury (no eye opening, no verbal response, no purposeful motor responses)
2. Dehydration therapy (mannitol)—reduces brain water by osmotic diuresis
3. Diuretics (furosemide)—enhances renal excretion of water and promotes systemic dehydration
4. Controlled hyperventilation—induces hypocapnia, which constricts blood vessels and lowers blood flow to decrease cerebral blood volume.
5. Control of seizures (phenytoin)
6. Control of systemic arterial pressure elevations
7. See also Management of ICP, page 578

C. Surgery

Surgical intervention for evacuation of intracranial hematomas, debridement and elevation of depressed skull fractures, penetrating wounds, persistence of spinal fluid rhinorrhea/otorrhea, or for patient who is progressively deteriorating.

Nursing Assessment

1. Determine the cause of the injury, particularly the direction and force of the blow.
   Was there loss of consciousness? How long? Could the patient be aroused? Duration of coma is an index to the severity of brain injury.
2. Conduct a rapid examination. Is the patient comatose (no eye opening, no verbal responses, inability to follow commands)?

NURSING ALERT: A change in the level of responsiveness is the most sensitive indication of improvement or deterioration. The level of responsiveness may change from minute to minute.

   a. Make repeated and specific documentation of clinical findings including level of responsiveness (consciousness), eye opening, verbal response, quality of breathing, size and reaction of pupils, and vital signs.
   b. Describe stimuli administered.
   c. Keep neurologic flow sheet and Glasgow Coma Scale (p. 579).
3. Observe orifices for leakage of spinal fluid through the nose (rhinorrhea), and through the ear (otorrhea), a serious complication of head injury that carries the risk of meningitis.

NURSING ALERT: Cerebrospinal fluid leakage may mask the usual clinical signs of an expanding intracranial hematoma without evidence of increased intracranial pressure, changes in vital signs, or alternations in state of consciousness.

4. See Assessment of the Unconscious Patient, page 575.
5. See Assessment of the Patient with Increased Intracranial Pressure, page 578.

Complications

1. Increasing intracranial pressure—edema, diffuse brain swelling, cerebral herniation
2. Intracranial hemorrhage occurring in or extending into extradural, subdural, or subarachnoid spaces, into the brain, or into the ventricles
3. Infections—*systemic:* respiratory, urinary tract, septicemia; *neurologic:* wound, meningitis, ventriculitis, brain abscess
4. Posttraumatic epilepsy

NURSING ALERT: The risk for seizures following head injury includes severe injury, frontal and parietal depressed skull fractures, intracranial hematoma, occurrence of early seizures, and prolonged coma.

5. Physical deficits—paresis, abnormal muscle tone, ataxia, tremors
6. Sensory deficits—cranial nerve dysfunctions, impaired smell, diplopia, hearing disorder, vestibular dysfunction
7. Normal pressure hydrocephalus (expansion of ventricles due to posttraumatic atrophy of brain)
8. Organic psychosocial deficits—impulsiveness, emotional lability, uninhibited aggressive behaviors
9. Aphasia

Nursing Diagnoses

1. Potential ineffective breathing pattern related to cerebral hypoxia, obtunded laryngeal and pharyngeal reflexes.
2. Altered cerebral tissue integrity related to increased intracranial pressure.
3. Fluid volume deficit related to disturbance in consciousness, metabolic and hormonal dysfunction, hypovolemia, and results of dehydration therapy
4. Altered nutrition (less than body requirements) related to increases in basal metabolism with catabolism and weight loss.
5. Potential for injury related to disorientation and restlessness secondary to brain edema/damage.
6. Altered thought processes (deficits in cognitive function, communication, memory, information processing) related to results of brain injury.
7. Potential ineffective family coping related to unpredictability of outcome, prolonged recovery period, and patient's residual physical, cognitive, and personality changes.
8. The nursing diagnoses for the unconscious patient (p. 575) also are applicable.

Nursing Interventions

A. Establishing Effective Respiratory and Ventilatory Function

1. Prepare for endotracheal intubation and ventilatory assistance as indicated—to optimize arterial oxygenation and allow hyperventilation.
   a. Evaluate results of arterial blood gas studies to assess adequacy of ventilation.
   b. See page 251, managing the patient requiring mechanical ventilation.
   c. Ausculate the chest; review results of chest x-ray.
   d. Turn patient from side to side every 2 hours to encourage drainage from all lobes of the lungs.
   e. Employ *careful* tracheobronchial suctioning to remove secretions.
2. Elevate the head of the bed 20°–30° as directed—improves venous drainage and reduces jugular pressure, thus, lowering intracranial pressure.
3. Maintain normothermia with fever sponges, hypothermia blanket, etc., to lower metabolic requirements of the brain.

B. Maintaining Cerebral Perfusion

See page 586 (Surgical Intervention)

C. Attaining/Maintaining Fluid and Electrolyte Balance

1. Monitor results of serial blood and urine electrolyte and osmolality studies
   a. Head injuries may be accompanied by disorders of sodium regulation, water retention, and decreased serum potassium levels.
   b. Assess for apathy, headache, anorexia, nausea, vomiting, and in some instances, coma and seizures.
2. Weigh the patient daily
   Keep records of intake, output, and urinary specific gravity findings—to determine fluid loss and dehydration and to monitor for development of posttraumatic diabetes insipidus.
3. Test urine regularly for sugar and acetone.
4. Restrict fluid intake in patients with severe cerebral contusions to avoid increase in volume of extracellular space.

5. Monitor central venous pressure (CVP) for rational fluid replacement therapy.
6. Give intravenous solutions fairly slowly; overhydration can lead to cerebral edema.
7. Insert urethral catheter if patient is unconscious to measure urinary volume and to prevent restlessness from distended bladder.
8. Remove indwelling catheter as early as possible; place patient on intermittent catheterization schedule as required.

D. Ensuring Adequate Nutrition

1. Keep in mind that head injury results in metabolic changes that increase caloric consumption and nitrogen excretion.
2. Pass nasogastric tube through nose as directed (unless there is CSF rhinorrhea) if patient is unable to swallow after return of bowel sounds. See page 448 for technique of nasogastric feeding.

> **NURSING ALERT:** Gastric motility may cease after brain injury. Aspiration is an ever-present hazard.

3. Refer to health professional experienced in dysphagia treatment (speech–language pathologist, occupational or physical therapist) if swallowing problems persist.
4. Watch for gastrointestinal complications—gastric acid hypersecretion is common in patients with head injuries and may result in ulceration and hemorrhage of stomach and upper intestinal tract.

E. Preventing Injury

1. Support the patient during episodes of restlessness, agitation, and irrational behavior.
   a. Ask family/significant other to sit beside patient and calm him with their hands.
   b. Avoid sedation.
2. Make certain that the patient's airway is adequate and bladder is not distended; also, check bandages and casts for signs of constriction.
3. Avoid restraints, if at all possible, as straining increases intracranial pressure.
4. Pad the side rails and wrap hands in mitts if patient is agitated—to protect from self-injury and dislodgement of tubes.
5. Keep environmental stimuli to a minimum by speaking calmly and keeping room quiet.
6. Have adequate lighting if patient is hallucinating.
7. Avoid interrupting the patient's sleep–wake cycles.
8. Carry out rehabilitation nursing techniques.
   a. Position the patient correctly to prevent contracture deformities.
   b. Put all extremities through range-of-motion exercises.
   c. Begin program of graded exercises (when permitted)—exercise restores fitness and flagging motivation and helps elevate the patient's mood.
   d. Keep the skin clean, dry, lubricated, and free of pressure.

F. Improving Cognitive Functioning

1. Use every sensory avenue to provide psychic stimulation to the confused and disoriented patient.
   a. Keep in mind that the patient is easily exhausted and distracted.
   b. Have family and friends provide meaningful conversation, even when the patient's response is minimal.
2. Provide frequent orientation information.
3. Reassure the patient that amnesia regarding the injury impact is common.
4. Work cooperatively with neuropsychologist (specialist in evaluating and treating cognitive problems).
   Computer-assisted cognitive retraining softwear is available that deals with remediating problem solving, inductive reasoning, and abstract thinking as well as developing visual, motor, and memory skills.
5. Encourage patient gradually to increase physical and mental activities, including resumption of increasingly difficult mental tasks.

G. Promoting Family Coping: Discharge Planning/ Patient Education

1. If the patient is discharged from the hospital in a relatively short time, instruct the family to bring him to the Emergency Department *immediately* if the following occur: difficulty in awakening, difficulty in speaking, confusion, severe headache, vomiting, unequal pupils, or weakness of one side of the body.
2. Develop a therapeutic alliance with the family.
3. Keep family informed about progress, different stages in recovery from head injury, and defense mechanisms (denial, regression, progression) used by the patient.
   a. Remind them that there are fluctuations in orientation and memory.
   b. Discuss with them that irritability may be a reaction to limited cognitive, motor, and language abilities. Decreased inhibition and impaired judgment result in inappropriate behavior.
4. Help family to assist patient to recognize current limitations and not to focus on disability.
5. Reinforce the concept that retraining is carried on over an extended time period.
6. Counsel about the necessity of taking anticonvulsant drug to prevent posttraumatic seizures and subsequent epilepsy.
7. Arrange counseling for family for information regarding cognitive and personality deficits and how to cope with long-term realities of brain damage.
8. Encourage family to seek help to share responsibilities for caretaker burdens.
9. Encourage family to explore community resources and build a support network, e.g., National Head Injury Foundation, P.O. Box 567, Framingham, MA 01701.

Evaluation

1. Attains/maintains effective breathing, ventilation, and brain oxygenation.
2. Attains/maintains fluid and electrolyte balance.
3. Attains improved nutritional status; not losing weight; beginning to swallow soft foods.
4. Shows no evidence of new injuries.
5. Beginning to remember names and recognize faces.
6. Family developing own interests/goals while showing supportive commitment to the patient.

Nursing Management of the Patient Having a Seizure

Seizures are episodes of abnormal motor, sensory, autonomic, or psychic activity (or a combination of these) as a consequence of sudden excessive discharge from cerebral neurons.

Nursing Assessment

The following should be noted before and during the attack, as most seizures are diagnosed on the basis of focal or general motor activity:

1. Description of the circumstances before the attack (visual stimuli, auditory stimuli, olfactory stimuli, tactile stimuli, emotional or psychic disturbances, sleep, hyperventilation).
2. The first thing the patient does in an attack.
   a. Where the movements or the stiffness starts, position of the eyeballs and the head at the beginning of the attack.
   b. This information gives clues as to the location of the epileptogenic focus in the brain.
   c. In recording, always state whether or not the beginning of the attack was observed.
3. The type of movements of the part involved.
4. The parts involved. (Turn back bed covers and expose patient.)
5. The size of both pupils. Are the eyes open? Did the eyes/head turn to one side?
6. Whether or not automatisms (involuntary motor activity such as lip smacking or repeated swallowing) were observed.
7. Incontinence of urine or feces.
8. Did the patient bite his tongue?
9. Duration of each phase of the attack.
10. Unconsciousness, if present, and its duration.
11. Any obvious paralysis or weakness of arms or legs after the attack.
12. Inability to speak after the attack.
13. Movements at the end of the seizure.
14. Whether or not the patient sleeps afterward.
15. Whether or not the patient was confused following the attack.

Nursing Interventions During Seizure

A. Ensuring an Adequate Airway

1. If aura preceded seizure, insert a folded handkerchief between the teeth taking care not to injure your fingers as patient's jaw may go into spasm—to reduce possibility of tongue or cheek being bitten.
2. When jaws are clenched in spasm, do not attempt to pry open to insert a mouth gag.
3. When respiration returns following the seizure and the patient becomes flaccid, turn his head to the side to facilitate drainage of mucus and saliva and to prevent aspiration.
4. Try to hold the lower jaw forward when the patient is in flaccid stage.

B. Protecting the Patient From Injury.

1. If the patient is in bed, remove the pillows.
2. If the patient is ambulatory, ease him to the floor if there is enough time.
3. Protect his head with a folded blanket/pad to prevent head injury.
4. Loosen constrictive clothing.
5. Push aside any furniture that the patient may strike during the seizure.

C. Other Measures.

1. Give the patient privacy and protect him from curious onlookers; use a calm manner to defuse a potentially embarrassing event for the patient.
2. Stay with the patient until he is fully conscious.
3. Reorient him to his environment when he awakens.

4. Handle the patient with calm persuasion and gentle restraint when seizures are characterized by disturbed behavior.
5. Summon medical assistance if a second seizure follows before consciousness is regained. There is a risk of status epilepticus developing.
6. If the patient has severe postictal (following seizure) excitement, it may be necessary to bring him to the Emergency Department.
7. After the seizure, keep the patient turned on one side to prevent aspiration.

Family Education

Instruct the family as follows:
   No attempt should be made to restrain the patient during the seizure, since muscle contractions are strong and restraint can produce a fracture.

Nursing Management of the Patient Undergoing Intracranial Surgery

Craniotomy is the surgical opening of the skull to gain access to intracranial structures, remove a tumor, relieve intracranial pressure, evacuate a blood clot, or stop hemorrhage (Fig. 24-4).
   Craniectomy is excision of a portion of the skull.
   Cranioplasty is repair of a cranial defect by means of a plastic or metal plate.

Preoperative Management

1. Diagnostic neurologic tests to determine the precise location of the lesion (tumor, clot, aneurysm).
2. Steroids—to decrease brain edema.
3. Anticonvulsants—to prevent seizures.

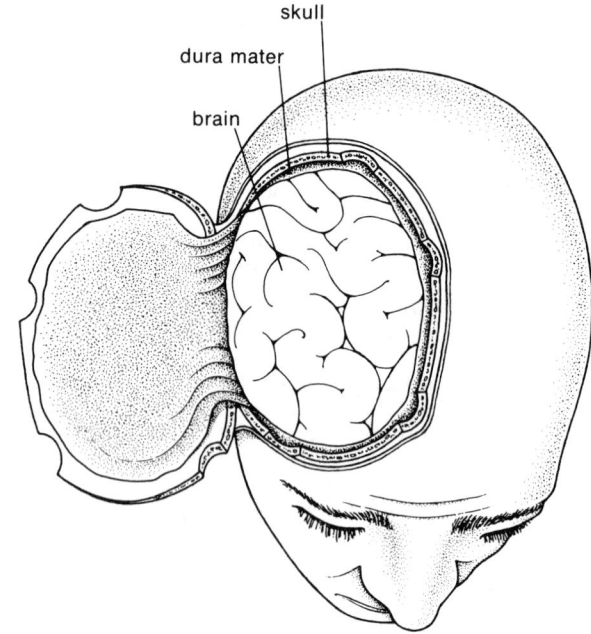

Figure 24-4. Craniotomy.

4. Hyperosmotic agent (mannitol) and a diuretic (furosemide) may be administered immediately preoperatively if patient tends to retain water.
5. Indwelling urethral catheter—to assess urinary volume during operative period.

Preoperative Nursing Interventions

1. Evaluate and record the patient's neurologic status, vital signs and clinical manifestations to establish a baseline for postoperative comparisons.
2. Explain the immediate postoperative care (monitoring devices, intubation, lines and catheters, dressings, and drains) and expected postoperative course.
3. Support the patient with neurologic motor and sensory defects.
   a. Position paralyzed extremities to prevent contracture deformities.
   b. Familiarize the blind patient with his environment.
   c. Assist the aphasic patient to communicate by means of picture cards, writing materials, gestures, etc.
   d. Protect the confused patient.
   e. Instruct and encourage the patient and family about the impending surgery—to relieve anxiety and tension.

Postoperative Management

1. Arterial and CVP lines for monitoring and careful control of central venous pressure.
2. Administration of oxygen
3. Pharmacotherapy:
   a. Mannitol—increases serum osmolality and drains free water from areas of brain
   b. Steroids—appears to decrease cerebral edema adjacent to brain tumors, continued through the expected period of maximum brain swelling (about 72 hours) and then tapered
   c. Acetaminophen—for fever and for pain
   d. Codeine—for headache
   e. Anticonvulsant (phenytoin) for patients undergoing supratentorial craniotomy to reduce incidence of seizures and the subsequent development of epilepsy
4. Management of ventricular catheter or other drainage—in patients with surgery of posterior fossa

Potential Complications

1. Intracranial bleeding/hematoma
2. Cerebral edema
3. Infections (postoperative meningitis; wound; pulmonary)
4. Seizures
5. Cranial nerve dysfunction

Nursing Assessment

1. Assess respiratory status—small degrees of hypoxia can aggravate cerebral ischemia.
   a. Monitor respiratory rate and pattern; alterations may be from anesthesia and/or increased intracranial pressure.
   b. Monitor vital signs; fluctuations may indicate increased ICP.
   c. Review results of arterial blood gas values.
   d. Take rectal temperature to evaluate for hyperthermia resulting from damage to hypothalamus which regulates body temperature.

2. Make frequent neurologic checks to detect increased intracranial pressure resulting from edema or bleeding following surgery.
   a. *Determine the level of responsiveness/consciousness* as measured by eye opening, motor responses, response to commands, and patient's spontaneous activity. See Glasgow Coma Scale, page 579.
   b. Determine if there is orientation to time, place, and person.
3. Watch for development of any neurologic deficit; diminished response to stimuli, speech problems, difficulty in swallowing, weakness or paralysis of an extremity, visual changes (diplopia; blurred vision), and paresthesias.
4. Keep a neurologic record flow sheet for sequentially assessing and documenting neurologic status, fluid administration, therapeutic agents, and laboratory data.
5. Inspect the head dressing for presence of bleeding and CSF drainage.

Nursing Diagnoses

1. Potential ineffective breathing pattern related to disruption of brain integrity, hypoxemia from residual anesthetic effects; postoperative cerebral edema; surgical involvement around respiratory centers.
2. Altered cerebral tissue perfusion related to cerebral edema.
3. Fluid volume deficit related to therapeutic attempts to reduce ICP; possible metabolic and hormonal dysfunction.
4. Potential for infection (intracranial) related to length and type of neurosurgical procedure.
5. Altered sensory perception (visual, auditory, possibly speech) related to periorbital edema, head dressings, endotracheal tube, and effects of increased intracranial pressure.

Nursing Interventions

A. Establishing Adequate Respiratory Exchange

1. Keep the patient in a lateral or a semi-prone position until consciousness returns unless otherwise indicated.
2. Employ tracheopharyngeal aspiration carefully to remove secretions—suctioning can raise intracranial pressure by stimulating an arousal response and by CO_2 accumulation during suction-induced apnea.
3. Maintain patient on controlled ventilation if indicated to maintain normal ventilatory status.
4. Monitor blood gas values to determine respiratory adequacy.
5. Elevate the head of the bed about 30.5 cm. (12 inches) after return of consciousness to aid venous drainage of brain.
   a. Keep the patient's head in a neutral position (in midline) to prevent jugular compression and facilitate venous drainage.
   b. Following a supratentorial operation, the patient is usually placed on back or side (unoperated side if large lesion was removed) with 1 pillow under head.
   c. Following an infratentorial operation, the patient is usually kept on side (off back) with head on a small firm pillow. Avoid flexing the head on chest.
   d. Use a turning sheet to prevent strain on the wound.
6. Evaluate vital signs to ensure cardiac stability.

B. Maintaining Cerebral Perfusion

1. Continue to assess patient's level of responsiveness/consciousness—the diminution of consciousness may be the first sign of increased intracranial pressure (ICP). Assess for:
   a. Eye opening (spontaneous, to sound, to noxious stimuli); pupillary reactions to light.
   b. Response to commands.
   c. Assessment of motor reflexes; press pen against side of patient's nail bed of finger for stimulation.
   d. Observation of patient's spontaneous activity.
2. Evaluate for signs and symptoms of increased intracranial pressure, which can lead to ischemia and further impairment of brain function.
   a. Diminished response to stimuli
   b. Fluctuations of vital signs
   c. Restlessness
   d. Weakness/paralysis of extremities
   e. Changes/disturbances in vision; pupillary changes
   f. Worsening of headache
4. Prepare to monitor ICP as indicated.
5. Keep the patient normothermic during postoperative period as a higher temperature increases the metabolic demands of the brain.
6. Modify nursing interventions to prevent further increase in intracranial pressure.
   a. Hyperventilate patient with resuscitator bag attached to 100% oxygen before suctioning is instituted.
   b. Avoid extreme rotation of neck and flexion of neck—these activities compress jugular veins and impede jugular venous drainage and increase ICP.
   c. Avoid extreme hip flexion, which causes an increase in intraabdominal and intrathoracic pressures, which can produce a rise in ICP.
   d. Avoid the Valsalva maneuver and isometric muscle contractions.
   e. Space nursing interventions to prevent transient increases in ICP. Avoid frequent arousal from sleep.
7. Prepare for CT scan if patient is deteriorating neurologically.

C. Attending to Fluid Volume Deficit

1. Ensure that patient has nothing by mouth until swallowing reflex is demonstrated and active bowel sounds are heard.
2. Record urinary specific gravity at intervals.
3. Evaluate electrolyte status—following certain intracranial procedures, patients have a tendency to retain water and sodium.
   a. Early postoperative weight gain indicates fluid retention.
   b. Loss of sodium and chlorides will produce weakness, lethargy, and coma.
   c. Low potassium will cause confusion and lower level of responsiveness.
4. Weigh patient daily; keep intake and output record.
5. Administer intravenous fluids with care.
6. Evaluate the patient having pituitary surgery for diabetes insipidus; monitor urine for sugar and acetone.

D. Preventing Infection

1. Know the patient at risk for infection after intracranial surgery.
   a. Those undergoing lengthy operations.
   b. Those with ventricular drains left in situ longer than 48–72 hours.
   c. Those with operations on the third ventricle.
2. Evaluate the dressings and contents of ventricular drainage system.
3. Inspect craniotomy site for redness, tenderness, bulging, separation, or foul odor.
4. Watch for leakage of cerebrospinal fluid since there is an ever-present danger of meningitis.
   a. Watch for *sudden* discharge of fluid from cranial or spinal wound; massive leak requires immediate surgical repair.
   b. Warn against coughing, sneezing, or nose blowing, which may aggravate CSF leakage.
   c. Assess for moderate elevation of temperature and neck rigidity.
   d. Note patency of ventricular catheter system.
   e. Keep head of bed elevated as prescribed.
5. Monitor and use appropriate interventions for pulmonary infection.
   a. Observe for signs of respiratory infection: rise in temperature, increase in pulse rate, respiratory changes.
   b. Auscultate lungs.
   c. Reposition the patient every 2 hours to mobilize secretions if ICP monitoring permits.
   d. Encourage yawning, sighing, and deep breathing to open up alveoli.
   e. Humidify room air.
   f. Continue to bear in mind that coughing and suctioning raise ICP.
6. Monitor intravenous line sites for evidence of sepsis.
7. Monitor for signs and symptoms of phlebitis (see p. 391).
8. Suspect drug fever if no other cause for temperature elevation can be found.

E. Compensating for Sensory Deprivation

1. Announce your presence upon entering patient's room.
2. Orient patient to time, place, and person frequently.
3. Employ measures to relieve periocular edema.
   a. Lubricate eyelids and around eyes with petrolatum.
   b. Apply light cold compresses over eyes at specified intervals to help reduce edema.
   c. Examine eyes for signs of keratitis if there is absence of corneal sensation.
   d. Reassure that puffiness about face and periorbital bruising are temporary.
4. Encourage interaction with family.

Discharge Planning/Patient Education

1. Devise a check-off system to make sure anticonvulsant medication is taken.
2. Advise the family to accompany the patient while walking in case of sudden attacks of dizziness or seizures.
3. Advise the patient to avoid getting scalp wet until sutures are removed; a clean scarf or cap may be worn until a wig/hairpiece can be purchased.
4. Discuss with family that following surgery patient is apt to be more sensitive to loud noises in environment.
5. Advise the family members that cognitive and behavioral deficits may occur after craniotomy and usually resolve more slowly than physical problems.
6. See Head Injury, page 581, for other aspects of patient teaching.

Evaluation

1. Demonstrates adequate breathing and respiratory exchange.
2. Shows improving neurologic function.
3. Attains/maintains acceptable fluid volume status.
4. Shows no signs of infection.
5. Copes with temporary postoperative sensory alterations.

Transsphenoidal Approach to the Pituitary

The transsphenoidal approach to the pituitary fossa is usually accomplished through an incision made beneath the upper lip with entry gained successively into the nasal cavity, sphenoid sinus, and sella turcica (saddle-shaped cavity at the base of the skull containing the pituitary gland).

Preoperative Management

1. CT or MR imaging
2. Endocrinologic, neurologic, and neuro-ophthalmologic evaluations
3. Administration of cortisone (source of ACTH is removed)

Postoperative Nursing Interventions

1. Monitor vital signs to evaluate hemodynamic, cardiac, and ventilatory status.
2. Check visual acuity by asking patient to count number of fingers held up by nurse—there is a close anatomic relationship of the pituitary gland to the optic chiasm.
3. Measure intake and output; transient diabetes insipidus may appear in 12–24 hours due to manipulation of posterior pituitary during surgery.
4. Promote patient comfort:
   a. Elevate head of bed to decrease pressure on sella turcica and to promote drainage.
   b. Use cool-mist vaporizer or room humidifier to help moisten mucous membranes; major discomfort is mouth dryness and thirst from mouth breathing secondary to nasal packing.
   c. Provide careful oral care as there is an incision above the teeth.
5. Caution patient against nose blowing, bending over, or straining during urination or defection—to prevent cerebrospinal fluid leakage.

Complications

1. CSF leakage
2. Transient diabetes insipidus
3. Syndrome of inappropriate secretion of antidiuretic hormone—thought to result from leakage of antidiuretic hormone from degradation of posterior lobe pituitary cells
4. Nasoseptal perforation; visual deterioration

Patient Education

1. Report any visible dripping of clear fluid from the nostrils (CSF leakage).
2. There is usually temporary numbness of upper lip and teeth following transsphenoidal surgery.
3. Have vision monitored by ophthalmologist—visual deterioration can occur in months to years after surgery; may be due to recurrent tumor.

Neurosurgical Management of Intractable Pain

Intractable pain is pain that causes incapacitation of function and that cannot be relieved satisfactorily by drugs short of drug addiction or incapacitating sedation.

Methods

1. Stimulation procedures
2. Administration of intraspinal opiates
3. Destructive or ablative (separation or detachment) procedures

Stimulation Procedures

1. Intermittent electrical stimulation is directed at a tract or center to inhibit the transfer of pain information.
2. Accomplished by
   a. Transcutaneous electrical nerve stimulation (TENS)
   b. Spinal stimulation
   c. Brain stimulation

A. Transcutaneous Electrical Nerve Stimulation (TENS)

1. Is the application of electrical stimulation through the skin using surface electrodes for the purpose of controlling pain.
2. Electrodes are placed over or around the painful area or on related paravertebral segments and their dermatomal distribution.
3. The patient operates the amplitude control until stimulation is detected by a vibration, buzzing, or tapping sensation felt within the deeper tissues.
4. The patients also controls the frequency and duration of the stimulation.
5. *Patient Education*
   a. Give the patient the instruction booklet provided by the manufacturing company for care of the skin, electrodes, and generator.
   b. Instruct him to keep a record evaluating the effectiveness of TENS.
   c. Watch for skin irritation or soreness.

B. Spinal Cord Stimulation

1. The spinal stimulating electrodes are placed in the epidural space through a needle guide; the receiver is implanted subcutaneously.
2. Used primarily for patients with chronic back and leg pain with varying degrees of success.

C. Brain Stimulation

1. A stimulating electrodes is implanted stereotactically into a target area deep within the brain—allows self-stimulation of periventricular gray matter to produce analgesia.
2. Used for severe pain that is bilateral, deep, and diffuse from metastases or of central origin.
3. Complications include infection, transient neurologic deficits, failure of system, development of tolerance.

Administration of Intraspinal Opiates

1. A catheter is placed into spinal epidural or subarachnoid (intrathecal) space for the management of acute or chronic pain.

2. Catheter may be placed percutaneously and sutured in situ or tunnelled subcutaneously to the abdominal wall and exteriorized, or the pump system may be implanted.
3. Catheter is positioned as near as possible to the spinal segment where the pain is projected.
4. Preservative-free sterile morphine or other analgesic/local anesthetic drug is injected into the system at specified intervals.
5. Spinally administered local anesthetics produce their effects predominantly by action on axons of spinal nerve roots; produce long-lasting pain relief with relatively low doses with little or no blunting of patient's level of responsiveness.
6. Complications include respiratory depression, urinary retention, pruritus, infection, leakage, technical problems, development of tolerance.
7. *Patient Education*
   a. The patient/family are taught drug administration, pump instruction, catheter and exit site care, monitoring of respiration, recognition of respiratory depression and its treatment.
   b. Arrange for home health care nurse to visit.

Destructive or Ablative Procedures

Interrupts a tract conducting pain between the periphery and the cerebral integration centers.

A. Rhizotomy
1. Is a surgical division of the spinal roots; used in controlling severe chest pain of lung cancer and for pain relief in head and neck malignancies.
2. Percutaneous rhizotomy—radiofrequency current is used to deliver heat selectively to coagulate the pain fibers, while the fibers concerned with touch and proprioception are preserved.

B. Cordotomy—interruption of the ascending spino-thalamic tract.
1. May be done with a radiofrequency current applied through a needle electrode inserted percutaneously or by an open surgical procedure.
2. Obliterates pain and temperature sensation below level of procedure but leaves motor function intact.

Nursing Interventions Following Cordotomy

1. Watch for respiratory complications following a cervical cordotomy. Observe for fatigue and weakening of the voice.
2. Monitor arterial blood gas values.
   a. Patients with reduced oxygen levels may require oxygen at night.
   b. They may ventilate adequately during the day but experience progressive hypercarbia and hypoxia while asleep.
3. Keep the neck in a neutral position following a cervical cordotomy.
4. Test motion, strength, and sensation of each extremity every few hours during the first 48 hours after surgery.
5. See page 621 for management of the patient following disc surgery for other nursing interventions relevant to this patient.
6. Potential complications include motor loss, dysesthesia (pins and needles sensations), loss of bladder and/or bowel control.
7. *Patient and Family Education*
   a. Protect against external temperature changes and extremes of weather; patient may not be aware of

sunburn or frostbite. Watch for skin trauma due to unnoticed injury.
   b. Test temperature of bath water before getting into tub.
   c. Avoid constricting clothing that impairs circulation.
   d. Sexual function may be impaired in males.

Cranial Nerve Disorders

Bell's Palsy

Idiopathic facial paralysis (Bell's palsy) is an acute peripheral facial paralysis involving the 7th cranial nerve on one side, producing weakness or paralysis of the facial muscles.

Clinical Features

1. The etiology of Bell's palsy is unknown. Possible causes include: viral infection, vascular ischemia, autoimmune disease, or a combination of these.
2. The majority of patients have a viral prodrome (upper respiratory infection) 1–3 weeks before onset of symptoms.

Clinical Manifestations

1. Distortion of face—from paralysis of facial muscles.
2. Facial numbness; diminished taste; and numbness of tongue.
3. Painful sensations in face, behind ear, and in the eye.
4. Eye problems
   a. Epiphora (overflow of tears down the cheek)—from keratitis caused by drying of cornea and lack of blink reflex; laxity of lower eyelids may alter proper drainage of tears.
   b. Lagophthalmos—inability to close eye.
   c. Decreased tear production—leads to a dry eye, predisposed to infection.
5. Speech difficulties—from facial paralysis.

Diagnostic Evaluation

1. Tests of cranial function and corneal sensation.
2. Electrophysiologic testing—to assess facial nerve functioning and prognosticate a return to function.

Management

1. Protection of involved eye: artificial tears (methylcellulose solution); ophthalmologic consultation.
2. Steroid therapy (prednisone)—to reduce inflammation and edema and relieve pain (controversial in terms of proven efficacy).
3. Physical therapy, including moist heat to face, facial massage, and exercises.
4. Non-narcotic analgesics.
5. Surgical intervention
   a. Surgical decompression of facial nerve to decrease edema—may prevent or arrest degeneration.
   b. Surgical procedures to correct eyelid deformities and protect the eye.

Complications

1. Corneal ulceration; corneal perforation.
2. Impairment of or loss of vision.

NURSING ALERT: Keratitis is a major threat to a patient with Bell's palsy.

Nursing Interventions/Patient Education

1. Reassure the patient that a stroke is not involved and that recovery will probably occur.
2. Protect the involved eye—facial paralysis may abolish blinking reflex, and inability to close eye results in corneal and conjunctival inflammation.
3. Keep cornea moist with prescribed artificial tears instilled into affected eye at regular intervals during the day.
   a. Use wrap-around goggles/wrap-around sunglasses to decrease normal evaporation from eye.
   b. Close eyelids periodically—this distributes tears across surface of eyes.
   c. Increase environmental humidity.
4. Avoid drying of cornea from sun, wind, or air conditioning.
5. Avoid eye irritants: fumes, aerosols, cosmetics.
6. Ensure eye protection during sleep.
   a. Use eye ointment at bedtime—helps to keep eyes closed during sleep by sticking the lashes together.
   b. Patient may tape upper lid closed by a strip of ¼-inch paper tape placed obliquely from the middle of the upper lid down to the malar eminence; *or*
   c. Wear a protective patch, making sure that the eye is completely closed, as the patch can eventually abrade the cornea if eyelids are open.
7. Report eye pain *immediately.*
8. Continue to use facial massage to maintain muscle tone.
9. Keep the face warm and free from drafts.
10. Do prescribed facial exercises to prevent facial muscle atrophy and to activate intact nerve fibers; helps maintain muscle tone. Do the following while looking in a mirror:
    a. Raise eyebrows.
    b. Squeeze eyes closed.
    c. Purse the lips.
    d. Move mouth from side to side.
    e. Blow out cheeks; smile.
    f. Whistle.

Trigeminal Neuralgia (Tic Douloureux)

Trigeminal neuralgia is a condition of the 5th cranial nerve, characterized by sudden paroxysms of sharp, stabbing, excruciating pain in the distribution of one or more branches of the trigeminal nerve (Fig. 24-5). The etiology is unknown.

Clinical Manifestations

1. Sudden and severe pain appearing without warning, alternating with pain-free intervals.
2. Numerous individual flashes of pain, ending abruptly; usually on one side.
3. Attacks predicted by pressure on a trigger point, the terminals of the affected branches. (Movement of the face, talking, chewing, yawning, swallowing, shaving, cold wind, may precipitate an agonizing attack.)

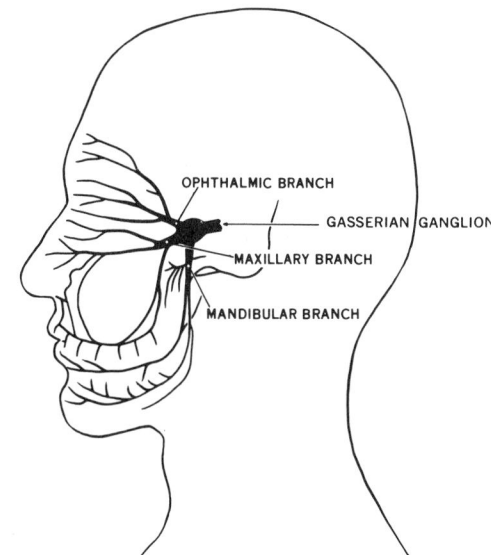

Figure 24-5. *The main divisions of the trigeminal nerve are ophthalmic, maxillary, and mandibular. Sensory root fibers arise in the Gasserian ganglion.*

Diagnostic Evaluation

Based on characteristic symptoms

Management: Pharmacotherapy

Carbamazepine (Tegretol) or phenytoin (Dilantin)—thought to relieve pain by reducing transmission of impulses at certain nerve terminals.

1. Produce drowsiness and ataxia.
2. Side effects of carbamazepine include bone marrow suppression, liver toxicity, and neurotoxicity.

Management: Surgical Interventions

Wide range, used after medical treatment fails to give relief.

A. Alcohol or Phenol Block

1. Injection into either the peripheral branches of the trigeminal nerve or directly into the ganglion
2. Offers pain relief, but pain recurs after months to 2 years due to nerve regeneration.

B. Percutaneous Radiofrequency Trigeminal Gangliolysis

Introduction of needle electrode through foramen ovale to the desired position of the trigeminal root; low-voltage stimulation applied to electrode, and a lesion is made. Carefully controlled electrical currents destroy enough of sensory portion of nerve to relieve pain without damaging touch sensation or motor function of face.

1. Root selection is made by the conscious patient's response to electrical stimulation.
2. Relief expected in most patients.
3. Complications include reduced corneal sensation, dysesthesia/paresthesia, masseter weakness.
4. Instruct the patient to:
   a. Instill artificial tears in eyes every 4 hours if there is a marked loss of corneal sensation.
   b. Restrict diet to soft foods for 2 weeks.
   c. Chew on unaffected side of mouth until he be-

comes accustomed to numbness; avoid biting lips, tongue, or inside of mouth.
   d. Do jaw-opening exercises as directed.

C. **Microvascular Decompression of Trigeminal Nerve**—an intracranial approach to decompress (remove pressure from) trigeminal nerve; postoperative nursing management is the same as for any intracranial operation.

D. **Open Surgical Retrogasserian Rhizotomy**—destruction of retrogasserian rootlets.

1. Gasserian ganglion lies in the middle fossa and may be reached by a subtemporal, intradural, or extradural route.
2. Following operation, the patient has a complete loss of sensation in the distribution of the divided nerve fibers.
3. See nursing management following craniotomy, page 585.
4. Complications—burning, stinging, numbness, discomfort in and around eye, herpetic lesions of the face, keratitis, and corneal ulceration.

Nursing Interventions/Patient Education

1. Recognize that certain factors may aggravate excruciating pain: touching face, cold air, ingestion of hot or cold fluids, etc.
2. Instruct the patient to:
   a. Take foods and fluids at room temperature; chew soft foods on unaffected side.
   b. Rinse mouth with room-temperature water after eating if tooth brushing precipitates pain.
   c. Use cotton pads with room-temperature water to wash face.
3. Be aware that anxiety, depression, and insomnia may accompany chronic, painful conditions; use appropriate nursing interventions and referrals.
4. Following surgical interventions, instruct the patient to:
   a. Instill artificial tears in eyes every 4 hours if there is a marked loss of corneal sensation.
   b. Chew on unaffected side of mouth until accustomed to numbness; avoid biting lips, tongue, or inside of mouth.
   c. Do jaw-opening exercises as directed.
   d. Report to dentist regularly—patient may not have pain in the event of dental caries.

Cerebrovascular Disease

Cerebrovascular disease refers to any functional abnormality of the central nervous system caused by interference with normal blood supply to the brain. The pathology may involve an artery, a vein, or both, when the cerebral circulation becomes impaired as a result of partial or complete occlusion of a blood vessel or hemorrhage resulting from a tear in the vessel wall.

Cerebrovascular Disease From Impairment of Cerebral Circulation

A. Transient Ischemic Attacks (TIAs)

Transient episodes of cerebral dysfunction commonly manifested by a sudden loss of motor, sensory, or visual function, lasting minutes up to an hour or more, but no longer than 24 hours.
   1. *Causes*—temporary impairment of blood flow to the brain from atherosclerosis of vessels supplying the brain, or obstruction of cerebral microcirculation by small embolus.

NURSING ALERT: A patient having transient ischemic attacks is at risk for subsequent stroke.

   2. *Management*
      a. Platelet aggregation inhibiting agents (aspirin; dipyridamole)—when problem is related to platelet aggregation.
      b. Anticoagulant therapy (heparin; warfarin).
      c. Surgical intervention—to increase blood flow to brain.
         (1) Carotid endarterectomy (p. 591); *or*
         (2) Extracranial/intracranial anastomosis—provides revascularization of brain. (See p. 584 for care of patient undergoing intracranial surgery.)

B. Reversible Ischemic Neurologic Deficit (RIND)

Episode producing neurologic deficits longer than 24 hours but followed by a return to the normal state.

C. Cerebral Thrombosis (from cerebral arteriosclerosis and slowing of cerebral circulation)

1. Usually produces transient loss of speech, visual disturbance, hemiplegia, or paresthesia in one half of the body, which may precede onset of severe paralysis.
2. See nursing management of the patient with a stroke, page 592.

D. Cerebral Embolism

Caused by heart disease (infective endocarditis, rheumatic heart disease, prosthetic heart valves, myocardial infarction), pulmonary emboli, arteriosclerotic plaque in carotid artery.
1. Embolism usually lodges in middle cerebral artery or its branches, where it disrupts circulation.
2. Symptoms—sudden onset of hemiparesis or hemiplegia, speech disturbances, visual disturbances.
3. See the nursing management of the patient with a stroke, page 592.

Cerebrovascular Disease From Hemorrhage

A. Extradural Hemorrhage

Hemorrhage occurring outside the dura mater
   1. This is considered a life-threatening emergency.
   2. See care of the patient with head injury for principles of immediate care, page 581.

B. Subdural Hemorrhage

Hemorrhage occurring beneath the dura mater. See care of the patient with a head injury, page 581.

C. Subarachnoid Hemorrhage

Hemorrhage occurring in the subarachnoid space—may result from leaking aneurysm, congenital arteriovenous malformation, hypertension, tumor, or trauma. See treatment of subarachnoid hemorrhage, page 598.

D. Intracerebral Hemorrhage

Hemorrhage occurring within the brain substance—usually from hypertension, cerebral atherosclerosis, aneurysm, etc.

Carotid Endarterectomy for Cerebrovascular Insufficiency

Carotid endarterectomy is the removal of atherosclerotic plaque(s) or thrombus from the carotid artery to prevent further transient ischemic attacks and to reduce the risk of stroke.

Clinical Manifestations of Carotid Occlusive Disease

1. History of transient ischemic attacks; headache, dizziness, blackout spells; brief loss of vision of 1 eye (anaurosis fugax) or homonymous visual field defects; numbness or weakness of extremity; temporary speech impairment
2. Bruit heard over carotid artery
3. Absent/diminished carotid pulsation in neck

Diagnostic Evaluation

1. *Cerebral angiography*—images the lumen of vessels to demonstrate degree of carotid stenosis and occlusion, adequacy of collateral blood flow, and presence of associated arterial lesions (ulcerative plaques); vascular malformation.
2. *Oculoplethysmography* (OPG)—gives direct measurement of central artery pressure and, therefore, pressure in the distal internal carotid artery.
3. *Carotid phonoangiography*—auscultation, direct visualization, and photographic recording of carotid bruits using a microphone, oscilloscope, and camera.
4. *Doppler ultrasound* technique—gives information about velocity of flow in the major intracranial anterior circulation.

Complications of Carotid Endarterectomy

1. Stroke
2. Myocardial infarction
3. Episodes of postoperative hypertension and hypotension
4. Cranial nerve injuries—many cranial nerves are in close proximity to carotid bifurcation and may be damaged during surgical dissection
5. Wound hematoma

Postoperative Nursing Interventions

A. Monitoring for Neurologic Deficits and Cardiac Function

1. Carry out frequent neurologic checks.
   a. Monitor equality, size, and reaction of pupils; handgrip, motor responses; mental status; symmetry of face; speech; presence of seizures and/or episodes of focal or sensory loss.
   b. Compare with preoperative status.
   c. Notify surgeon immediately if neurologic deficits occur; prepare for reoperation.
2. Monitor for cardiac function—high incidence of coexistent coronary artery disease.
   a. Monitor vital signs.
   b. Maintain blood pressure within individual patient's normal range—abrupt changes in blood pressure occur, presumably due to increased activity of the newly exposed baroreceptors.
   c. Control postoperative hypertension, as this may precipitate cerebral hemorrhage or new neurologic deficits.
      (1) Watch for sudden onset of severe hypertension, especially in patient with history of hypertension.
      (2) Monitor for agitation, confusion, and headache.
      (3) Administer prescribed antihypertensive medications.
   d. Monitor for hypotension and bradycardia—may be result of increased pressure waves reaching carotid sinus receptors after removal of plaque.
   e. Assist patient to assume upright posture cautiously—this activity can produce a significant drop in blood pressure.

B. Monitoring for Injuries to Cranial Nerves

1. Observe the patient for:
   a. Weakness of tongue muscles with tongue deviation to operated side—hypoglossal nerve injury.
   b. Upper airway obstruction; difficulty in swallowing and speaking—bilateral hypoglossal palsy.
   c. Facial weakness; asymmetry of face; drooping at corner of mouth; difficulty in managing saliva/fluids—facial nerve injury.
   d. Change in quality of voice; vocal cord paralysis—injury to vagus nerve or recurrent laryngeal nerve.

C. Other Nursing Interventions

1. Observe operative area closely for bleeding into neck and hematoma formation.
2. Prepare for immediate operation if hematoma is causing airway compromise and respiratory insufficiency.

Discharge Planning/Patient Education

1. Carotid artery disease is a manifestation of generalized atherosclerosis. The patient requires continuing health monitoring and care for subsequent stroke and coronary artery disease, particularly myocardial infarction.
2. Encourage patient to make life-style changes, including cessation of smoking, dietary restrictions of lipids, and correction of obesity.

Stroke

A *stroke* (*cerebral vascular accident*) is the onset of neurologic dysfunction resulting from disruption of the blood supply to the brain.

Causes

1. Thrombosis (blood clot within a blood vessel of the brain or neck)
2. Cerebral embolism
3. Ischemia (decrease of blood flow to an area of the brain)
4. Cerebral hemorrhage (rupture of a cerebral blood vessel with bleeding or pressure into the brain substance)

Risk Factors

1. Hypertension
2. Previous transient ischemic attacks
3. Heart disease (atherosclerotic/valvular disease; dysrhythmias)
4. Elevated cholesterol

5. Diabetes mellitus
6. Obesity
7. Carotid bruit; red blood cell disorders
8. Cigarette smoking

NURSING ALERT: Drug abuse (cocaine) is a cause of stroke, especially in young adults.

Clinical Manifestations

The result of interruption of blood supply to the brain may cause temporary or permanent loss of movement, thought, memory, speech, sensation.
1. Sudden severe headache
2. Numbness, weakness, or motor loss (hemiplegia) on either side of body.
3. Difficulty in speaking and/or swallowing
4. Visual field deficits (homonymous hemianopia—loss of half of the visual field)
5. Impairment of sensations
6. Impairment of mental activity and psychological affect
7. Depression

Diagnostic Evaluation

1. Computed tomography—distinguishes between hemorrhage and infarction
2. Angiography—demonstrates vascular pathology
3. Positron emission tomography—provides imaging of regional cerebral metabolism

Management

1. Close observation and monitoring of hemodynamic parameters
2. Management of increased intracranial pressure (see p. 578); initial measures to reduce ICP are similar regardless of underlying brain disorder.
3. Support of vital functions
4. Management of post-stroke rehabilitation program
5. Antispasmodic agents (diazepam; baclofen; dantrolene)
6. Treatment of post-stroke depression
   a. Tricyclic antidepressant agents
   b. Psychotherapy when indicated

Nursing Assessment

1. See Assessment of Unconscious Patient, page 575 and Assessment of Patient with Increased Intracranial Pressure, page 578.
2. Review the patient's record to determine the neurologic deficit.
3. Using nursing observation skills, work cooperatively with other members of rehabilitation team to evaluate patient's rehabilitation potential.
4. Assess quality of social support network.
5. Observe for manifestations of depression

Nursing Diagnoses

1. Impaired physical mobility related to hemiparesis (weakness or partial paralysis affecting one side of the body), loss of balance and coordination, spasticity, and brain injury.
2. Altered comfort (painful shoulder) related to hemiplegia, spasticity, and disuse.
3. Self-care deficits (hygiene, toileting, transfers, feeding, dressing) related to stroke sequelae (paresis, apraxia,

visual and sensory deficits, unilateral neglect, and decreased attention span).
4. Alteration in sensory perception (impairment/lack of awareness of one side of body, touch, proprioception, discrimination of size, shape, and texture) related to brain damage.
5. Altered patterns in urinary elimination (incontinence) related to damage to CNS, impaired motor function, and difficulty in communication.
6. Altered thought processes (impaired memory, judgment, concentration, confusion) related to brain damage.
7. Impaired verbal communication related to brain damage.
8. Altered family process related to catastrophic illness, cognitive and behavioral sequelae of stroke, and caregiving burdens.

Complications

1. Deep vein thrombosis; pulmonary embolism
2. Aspiration pneumonia
3. Spasticity; joint contractures with associated pain
4. Post-stroke depression
5. Recurrent stroke

Nursing Interventions

Improving Mobility and Preventing Deformities

A. Positioning

Position the patient in bed correctly—to prevent contractures, relieve pressure, and maintain good body alignment. (These principles of positioning are also carried out during the phase of altered consciousness.) See Figure 24-6.
1. Place a board under the mattress—to give the body firm support.
2. Encourage the patient to remain flat in bed except when engaged in activities of daily living—to prevent hip flexion deformities.

B. Measures to Avoid Contractures

1. Use a footboard during the flaccid period following a stroke to keep the feet dorsiflexed—prevents footdrop, heel cord shortening, and plantar flexion.
   a. Avoid use of a footboard after spasticity develops—it will promote spasticity and increase plantar flexion.
   b. Avoid excessive pressure on the ball of the foot after spasticity develops.
   c. Do not allow top bedding to pull affected foot into plantar flexion.
2. Use a night cast, splint, or brace to maintain proper joint position when necessary—by decreasing motion, the spastic muscles will receive less stimulation to their stretch reflex and spasticity may decrease.
3. Apply a trochanter roll from the crest of the ilium to the midthigh (Fig. 24-6B) to prevent external rotation of the hip joint when the patient is in a dorsal position.
4. Place a pillow in the axilla of the affected side when there is limited external rotation—to keep arm away from the chest and prevent adduction of the affected shoulder.
5. Place the affected upper extremity within its full range of motion (slightly flexed) on pillow supports with each joint positioned higher than the preceding one—to prevent edema and resultant fibrosis.
   Alternate upper extremity position by allowing periods of elbow extension.
6. Place the hand in slight supination with fingers slightly

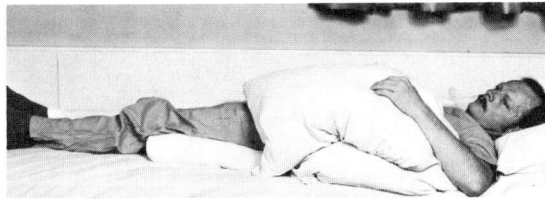

A. *A pillow is placed in the axilla to prevent adduction of the affected shoulder. Pillows are placed under the arm, which is in a slightly flexed position with each joint positioned higher than the preceding one.*

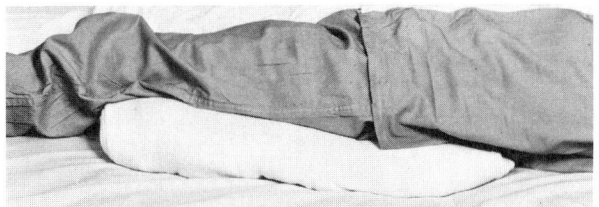

B. *The trochanter roll should extend from the crest of the ilium to the midthigh, since the hip joint lies between these 2 points. The trochanter roll acts as a mechanical wedge under the projection of the greater trochanter and prevents the femur from rolling.*

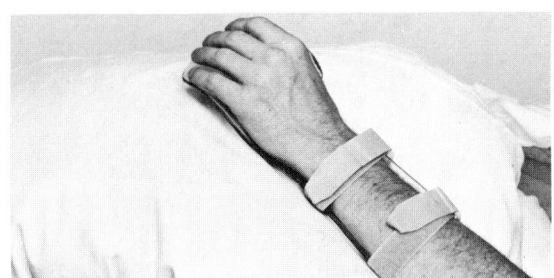

C. *A volar resting splint may be used to support the wrist and hand if the upper extremity is flaccid.*

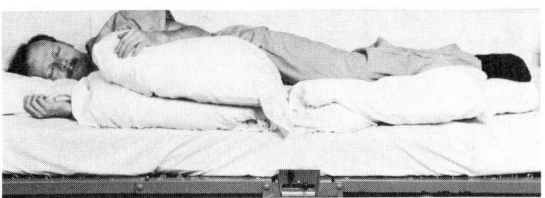

D. *Lateral or side-lying position. The patient should be turned on his unaffected side. The upper thigh should not be acutely flexed.*

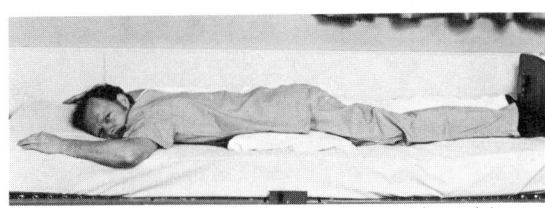

E. *Prone position. A pillow is placed under the pelvis to help promote hyperextension of the hip joints, which is essential for normal gait. Note position of arms.*

Figure 24-6. *Positioning for a patient following a stroke during the flaccid period. (Dark side of pajamas represents affected or hemiplegic side.)*

flexed; if upper extremity is flaccid, use a volar resting splint to support the wrist and hand in a functional position (Fig. 24-6C). If the upper extremity is spastic, use a dorsal cock-up splint to prevent pressure on the palm.
7. Place the patient in a prone position for 15 minutes to ½ hour 2–3 times daily (Fig. 24-6E)—to prevent knee and hip flexion contractures.

Exercise Program to Retrain Affected Extremities

A. Establishing Exercise Program

1. Exercise the affected extremities passively and carry out range-of-motion exercises 4–5 times daily—to maintain joint mobility, to prevent contracture development in the paralyzed extremity, to prevent further deterioration of neuromuscular system, to regain motor control, and to enhance circulation.
2. Involve family in exercise program since care of a stroke patient requires time and effort.
3. Remind the patient to exercise unaffected extremities regularly at intervals throughout the day—to prevent contracture development in the normal extremities.
4. Teach the patient to put his unaffected leg under the affected one in order to move and turn himself.

5. Instruct the patient to move his affected arm (and hand) with his good hand (Fig. 24-7).

B. Types of Exercises

1. *Quadriceps setting* (to each extremity)
   Instruct the patient as follows:
   a. Contract the quadriceps muscle (anterior portion of thighs) while raising the heel and attempting to push the popliteal space against the mattress.
   b. Hold the muscle contraction for the count of 5. Relax for the count of 5. Repeat.
2. *Gluteal setting*
   Instruct the patient as follows:
   a. Contract or "pinch" the buttocks together for the count of 5.
   b. Relax for the count of 5. Repeat.

C. Preventing Shoulder–Hand Syndrome

Maintain upper extremity joint mobility to prevent shoulder–hand syndrome.

1. Use a sling on the paralyzed arm when the patient is in upright position, if arm is flaccid, or if the patient complains of arm pain and heaviness. The sling is usually discarded when spasticity provides enough tone to prevent shoulder subluxation.
   a. Remove sling frequently and exercise arm.
   b. Instruct the patient to interlace his fingers, placing

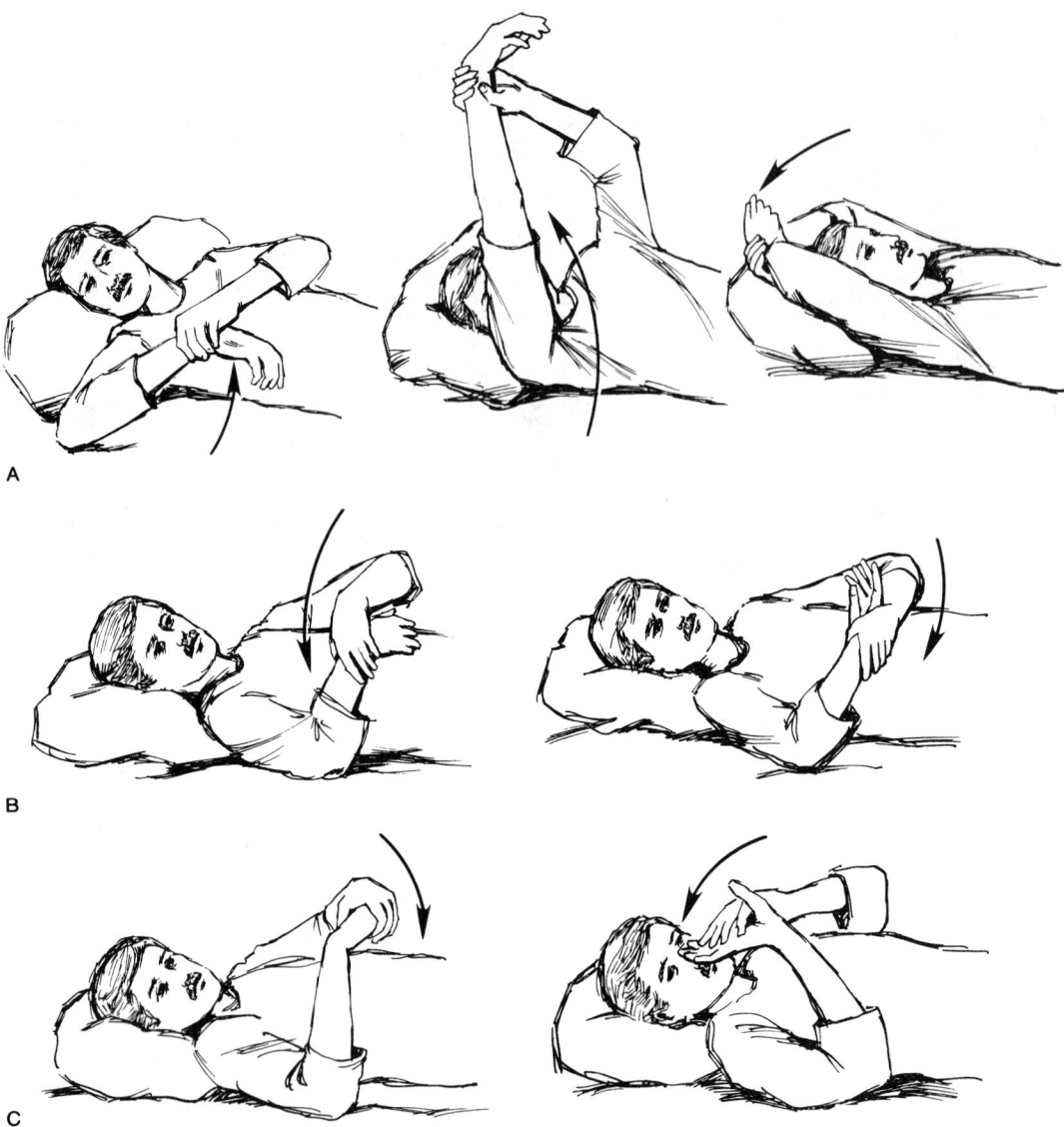

Figure 24-7. *(A) Exercise to maintain range of motion of the involved shoulder and the elbow in hemiplegia. (B) Exercise to maintain range of motion of pronation and supination in affected hand. (C) Exercise to maintain range of motion of the wrist and the finger in hemiplegia. (Hirschberg G, Lewis L and Vaughan P. Rehabilitation. 2nd ed. Philadelphia, JB Lippincott)*

the palms together. With elbows extended, lift both arms above head repeatedly throughout day.

2. When seated, keep the affected arm and hand elevated with a pillow to prevent dependent edema of the hand, or position the arm in a forearm trough attached to the armrest of wheelchair.
3. Instruct the patient to flex and extend his wrist and fingers with unaffected hand at frequent intervals.
4. Watch for shoulder–hand syndrome (painful shoulder and generalized swelling and pain of hand)—can cause atrophy of subcutaneous tissues and contractures.

Preparing for Ambulation

A. Preambulation Assessment

1. Check the blood pressure in both lying and sitting positions—a fall in blood pressure (orthostatic hypoten-

sion) may further damage the ischemic area of the brain.

2. Raise the bed to an upright position; instruct the patient to hold the bedrail with his good hand—helps to regain sense of balance.

B. Sitting on Edge of Bed

1. Adjust the bed to the low position.
2. Instruct the patient to place the strong leg beneath the weak leg and lift it toward the side of the bed.
3. Instruct the patient to press the strong elbow (which is flexed to a 90-degree angle) into the mattress and come to a sitting position by transferring weight to the forearm and then to the hand, while lifting the affected leg with the strong leg over the edge of the bed.
4. Extend the patient's strong arm with his hand flat on the bed behind him to assist in balancing.

5. Stand in front of the patient to observe and, if necessary, help him to maintain this posture.
6. A change in color, shortness of breath, increasing pulse rate, or profuse perspiration is an indication that the patient should be placed in bed again. The sitting time is increased as rapidly as the patient's condition permits.

C. Developing Standing Balance

1. Put walking shoes with strong shank on the patient for all ambulation activities.
2. Seat the patient on edge of bed and place a straight-back chair on each side of him.
   a. Tie affected hand to the chair if the patient lacks grasp strength.
   b. Assist the patient to a standing position by supporting his lower back with your hands and positioning your knees on the outside of the patient's knees.
   c. Encourage the patient to look upward briefly—facilitates lower extremity extension.
3. Assess the patient for dizziness, pallor, and increasing pulse rate. Have the patient practice standing and shifting weight from one leg to the other.
4. Assist the patient to achieve standing balance at frequent intervals throughout the day.
5. Help the patient begin walking as soon as standing balance is achieved (using parallel bars). Stand behind patient and stabilize him at waist level.
6. Encourage the patient to look at his feet occasionally—proprioceptive loss may accompany hemiplegia.

D. Using a "Hemiplegic" Wheelchair

1. Secure a wheelchair (seat lower than conventional wheelchair) for nonambulatory or minimally ambulatory patient.
2. Place wheelchair on the patient's unaffected side—allows him to see wheelchair and lead with the stronger leg.
3. Lock wheelchair brake and lift pedals out of the way.
4. To transfer from a chair to wheelchair, instruct the patient as follows:
   a. Move forward in chair, placing weight over strong leg. Push up with strong arm and foot.
   b. Place most of the weight on the strong leg while keeping weak knee locked.
   c. Pivot in the direction of the stronger leg; bring weak leg over to stronger leg. Maintain standing position a few moments.
   d. Lower body into chair gradually, using strong arm and leg.
5. Instruct patient to propel wheelchair by using the unaffected hand on the rim for steering and the unaffected foot on the floor for propulsion.

Preventing Shoulder Pain

1. Strive to avoid painful shoulder syndromes since shoulder function is essential to achieving balance and performing self-care and transfers.
2. Avoid lifting patient by the flaccid shoulder or pulling on the affected arm or shoulder.
   a. Position the flaccid arm on a table or pillows while the patient is seated.
   b. Use a properly applied sling when the patient first becomes ambulatory—to prevent paralyzed arm from dangling without support.
3. Continue to carry out range-of-motion exercises.
   a. Avoid over-strenuous exercise.
   b. Instruct patient to interlace his fingers, place palms together, and push his clasped hands slowly forward to bring the scapulae forward, and then raise his hands above his head. Repeat throughout the day.
   c. Instruct patient to flex affected wrist at intervals and move all the joints of affected fingers.
   d. Encourage him to touch, stroke, rub, and look at his hands.
   e. Elevate arm and hand at intervals—to prevent dependent edema of hand.

Other Nursing Interventions

A. Achieving Self-Care

1. Help patient set realistic goals and add a new task as soon as possible. Teach only one activity at a time.
2. Have the patient immediately transfer all self-care activities to the unaffected side. Teach one-handed methods and use assistive devices to make up for some deficits.
3. Be sure that the patient does not neglect his affected side.
4. Encourage the patient to dress himself for ambulatory activities; occupational therapist usually teaches dressing activities.
   a. Instruct the family to bring clothing that is one size larger than usually worn.
   b. Use clothing with front fasteners, Velcro closures, stretch fabric, etc.
   c. Have patient dress himself while seated—to achieve better balance.
5. Involve family in patient's care in order to develop and practice skills that help patient reach rehabilitation goal.

B. Developing Compensating Skills for Sensory Dysfunction

1. Test for hemianopia (defective vision in half of the visual field).
   a. Show the patient an object placed to one side and ask if he can identify it.
   b. Hemianopia is evident if the patient fails to see the object on the correct side, but responds by looking towards it on the other side. (Visual field is likely to be limited on the right if the patient has right hemiplegia.)
2. Place call light, bedside table, etc. on the side of his awareness.
3. Approach the bed from the uninvolved side.
4. Encourage the patient to turn his head from side to side to obtain the full view of a normal visual field.
5. Have the patient wear his eyeglasses.
6. Help the patient to relearn swallowing sequence (if capable of following instruction).
   a. Induce the sucking reflex.
      (1) Have the patient attempt to suck on gloved finger.
      (2) Place ice on tongue and encourage the patient to suck ice.
   b. Progress to popsicle, soft foods, and then regular diet.
   c. Give food and fluids from uninvolved side (if patient has droop of mouth).
   d. Remind the patient to chew on unaffected side.
   e. Inspect the patient's mouth for food collecting between cheek and gums on involved side; frequent oral hygiene is necessary.

C. Attaining Bladder Control

1. Remember that the patient with motor and proprioceptive deficits associated with visual neglect is more likely to be incontinent.

2. Analyze the patient's voiding pattern. Establish a schedule of voiding every 2–3 hours—prevents bladder capacity from reaching the point that uninhibited contractions occur.
3. Monitor for bladder infection.
4. See page 693 for management of patient with neurogenic bladder and page 142 for bladder retraining program.

D. Compensating for Altered Thought Processes

1. Review results of diagnostic procedures that delineate patient's cognitive, behavioral, and emotional deficits related to brain damage.
2. Have an awareness of the training program (cognitive–perceptual retraining, visual imagery, reality orientation, cueing procedures) that are used to compensate for patient's losses.
3. Focus on patient's strengths and what he still is able to do.
4. Observe patient's performance, and give positive feedback.
5. Use pictures of family members, clock, calendar; post the schedule of day's activities where patient can see it.

E. Achieving Communication

1. See page 597 for nursing interventions for helping the patient with aphasia.

F. Helping Family Coping

1. Encourage the family to have some type of counseling and/or support—to prevent caretaking responsibilities from taking toll on their health.
2. Advise of stress management techniques, personal health maintenance, respite care, day care programs, in-home services, etc.
3. Encourage family to maintain outside activities.
4. Advise of peer groups and stroke clubs—for information and social support.
5. Provide information about stroke and expected outcomes.
   a. Let family know what the patient can do.
   b. Work with occupational therapist in securing equipment and adaptive devices for patient's return home.

Discharge Planning/Patient Education

Instruct the family as follows:
1. Expect some emotional lability and some degree of brain damage if the patient has had a more severe stroke.
   a. The patient may have episodes of inappropriate crying/laughing and temper outbursts.
   b. Hemiplegic patients may be easily confused, forgetful, discouraged, hostile, uncooperative, withdrawn, and dependent.
   c. Post-stroke depression is *common* and should be treated, as depression can prevent sustained improvement.
   d. Support the patient psychologically; hemiplegia has a tremendous psychological impact on the patient (and his family).
2. Explain that the patient becomes easily fatigued.
   a. See that the patient has scheduled rest periods.
   b. Promote sense of progress and improvement.
3. Avoid doing those things for the patient that he can do for himself.
4. Be supportive and optimistic but firm and direct.
5. Maintain constancy of the environment without too many distractions.

6. Install handrails by the toilet and tub or shower and put safety rails on the bed.
7. Obtain self-help devices to assist in activities of daily living; modify and adapt devices and "gadgets" to encourage independence.
8. Encourage the patient to keep active and adhere to exercise program, and to remain as self-sufficient as possible.
9. Set realistic goals; make the best of what remains.
10. Have the patient medically evaluated from time to time.
11. Take advantage of community service agencies and the local or regional branch of the State Office of Vocational Rehabilitation.
12. Support and educational services:
    American Heart Association
    7320 Greenville Avenue
    Dallas, TX 75231

    National Stroke Association
    1420 Ogden Street
    Denver, CO 80218

Evaluation

1. Attains increasing mobility; exercises affected and unaffected extremities; shows beginning ability to walk with reciprocal pattern.
2. Absence of painful shoulder syndrome.
3. Acquiring increasing independence in self care.
4. Compensating for sensory deficits; turns head to compensate for visual field deficits.
5. Attains bladder control.
6. Copes with altered thought processes; using cues and memory aids.
7. Communicates needs and wants to others; uses gestures when word-finding is difficult.
8. Family seeking help and assistance from others.

Aphasia

Aphasia is an acquired disorder of communication resulting from brain damage. It may involve impairment of the ability to speak, understand the speech of others, read, write, calculate, and understand gestures. The majority of aphasic individuals have difficulty with expression and comprehension, albeit to different degrees.

Causes

1. Stroke (present in about one third of immediate survivors)
2. Head injury
3. Brain tumor

Aphasic Syndromes

A. Fluent Aphasias—patient retains verbal fluency but may have difficulty in understanding speech.

1. *Wernicke's aphasia*—the patient speaks readily, but speech lacks clear content, information, and direction; jargon frequently used.
2. *Anomic or amnesic aphasia*—speech is almost normal, but marred by word-finding difficulty.
3. *Conduction aphasia*—the patient's comprehension of language is good, but he has difficulty repeating spoken material.

B. Nonfluent Aphasia—sparse speech produced slowly and with effort and poor articulation; usually has a relative preservation of auditory comprehension.

C. Global Aphasia—severe disruption of all aspects of speech (reading, writing, speaking, understanding).

Diagnostic Evaluation/Assessment

Speech–language pathologist, using a comprehensive range of language and neuropsychological tests, determines the type of aphasia.

Management

1. Speech therapy—to help patient use remaining skills and to learn compensatory means of communication.
2. Bromocriptine (dopamine agonist)—may be given based on hypothesis that impaired initiation of speech may arise from reduced dopaminergic activity.

Nursing Diagnoses

1. Impaired communication (verbal) related to brain damage
2. Disturbance in self-concept related to inability to communicate
3. Impaired family coping related to frustration over communication deficit

Nursing Interventions

A. Improving Communication

1. Encourage the patient to listen; listening requires mental effort.
2. Give the patient plenty of *time* to speak and respond; he cannot sort out incoming messages and formulate a response under pressure.
   a. Speak slowly while making eye contact with the patient.
   b. Face the patient on the uninvolved side.
   c. Avoid talking too fast, too loudly, or too much.
   d. Use short sentences; pause; see if the patient indicates that he understands.
   e. Repeat or rephrase sentence.
   f. Provide visual clues (gestures, demonstration, pictures) if the patient has comprehension problems.
   g. Supplement speech with gestures when indicated.
   h. Talk to the patient while caring for him. Know his former interests.
   i. Be consistent—by using the same wording each time instructions are given and questions are asked.
3. Keep the environment relaxed and permissive.
4. Keep distractions at a minimum—damaged input pathways cannot sort out distracting stimuli in the environment.
5. Use as many sensory channels as possible.
   a. Supplement auditory stimulation with visual stimulation.
   b. Use visual aids (pictures); ask the patient to point to and name what he sees.
   c. Use games to stimulate the patient's mind and help organize thoughts.
   d. Use television, tape recorders, audio cassettes, electronic learning games, etc., to stimulate the patient's interest.
   e. Encourage the patient to use any form of communication—gestures, writing, drawing, etc., until his speech begins to return.
   f. Elicit responses from the patient (e.g., "Please nod your head if you understand"). Reinforce every correct response.
   g. Restate what you think the patient has said from time to time.

B. Enhancing Self-Concept

1. Give the patient as much psychological security as possible.
2. Give support by assuring the patient that there is nothing wrong with his intelligence.
   a. Treat the patient as an intelligent adult.
   b. Accept the patient as he is now; avoid artificial praise.
   c. Avoid forcing speech.
2. Maintain a calm, accepting, and deliberate manner, especially during periods of emotional lability.
3. Encourage the patient to socialize with his family and friends.
   a. Seek the help of other people to read aloud, play games, do puzzles.
   b. Have the patient's grandchildren visit and talk with him.
   c. Keep the patient in the social world.
   d. Be aware of support groups (stroke clubs) in the community.
4. Watch the patient for clues and gestures if his speech is unintelligible or jargon-like.
   a. Continue to listen to the patient.
   b. Nod and make neutral statements occasionally.
   c. Shift the topic when appropriate to provide another point of interest and frame of reference.
5. Observe the patient during the course of his daily schedule for clues to evaluate and assess his progress.

C. Promoting Family Coping/Family Education

1. See items **A** and **B**, above.
2. The patient's ability to speak may vary from day to day. Fatigue will have an adverse effect on speech.
3. The rate of recovery differs in different types of aphasia.
4. The patient is likely to become terribly frustrated by his inability to communicate; ignore swearing and abusive language.
5. Aphasia can also involve the patient's understanding.
6. Some persons cannot express themselves but can comprehend the spoken or written word; others can speak but do not understand; while some who do neither may respond to gesture and actions.
7. Seek information about aphasia: American Speech–Language–Hearing Association, 10801 Rockville Pike, Rockville, MD 20852
8. Seek support group (stroke club; group therapy for aphasic persons)—interaction with others decreases feelings of isolation. Encourage family to learn about electronic aids that are on the market for persons who are unable to speak.
9. Counsel family to continue life of their own and to seek counseling if necessary for dealing with frustration and pressures.

Evaluation

1. Communicates with others in accordance with his ability/deficit.
2. Demonstrates improvement in self-concept; tries to reduce isolation by social interactions.
3. Family learning about aphasia; making plans for future.

Rupture of Intracranial Aneurysm With Subarachnoid Hemorrhage (SAH)

An *intracranial aneurysm* is a dilation of the walls of a cerebral artery. Rupture of an intracranial aneurysm leads to subarachnoid hemorrhage (hemorrhage into the cranial subarachnoid space).

Etiology

1. Atherosclerosis—reflects an acquired defect in vessel wall with subsequent weakness of wall
2. Intracranial arteriovenous malformation
3. Hypertensive vascular disease
4. Head trauma
5. Unknown

Clinical Manifestations

1. Sudden onset of a new, atypical headache, often associated with a pain in the eye; "the worst headache I have ever had."
2. Loss of consciousness.
3. Visual disturbances—photophobia, blurred vision, diplopia (double vision).
4. Fever, neck stiffness—due to irritation of the basal meninges by the blood in the subarachnoid space.
5. Dizziness, nausea, and vomiting.
6. Hemiparesis (muscular weakness affecting one side of body) or hemiplegia (paralysis affecting one side of body).

Diagnostic Evaluation

1. CT scan of head—for presence of blood in the subarachnoid space and to rule out other lesions.
2. Lumbar puncture—to confirm presence of bloody spinal fluid.
3. Cerebral angiography—to determine presence and location of aneurysm and provide information about complications (vasospasm).

Management

1. Bedrest with sedation.
2. Cardiac monitoring—massive sympathetic discharge accompanying SAH is associated with life-threatening dysrhythmias.
3. Management of increased intracranial pressure—result of extensive SAH, hematoma, vasospasm, brain edema (see p. 578).
4. Control of hypertension
   a. Hydralazine hydrochloride, propranolol, nifedipine, labetalol, and nitroprusside are commonly used agents.
   b. Stool softeners—to prevent straining and subsequent rise of blood pressure.
5. Antifibrinolytic therapy (aminocaproic acid [Amicar])—to inhibit clot lysis in the wall of the aneurysm, thus reducing the likelihood of rebleeding.
6. Treatment of cerebral vasospasm with plasma volume expansion and possibly vasopressor agents—to increase cerebral perfusion pressure.
7. Calcium-channel blockers (nimodipine; nicardipine) used investigationally—to prevent ischemia secondary to vasospasm.
8. Prophylactic antiseizure therapy.
9. Surgical interventions to prevent further bleeding, by:
   a. Obliteration of aneurysm from the cerebral circulation by clipping or ligation; *or*
   b. Strengthening the arterial wall by wrapping.

Complications

1. Rebleeding or rerupture
   a. Incidence highest in first 3 weeks.

b. Monitor for sudden increase in headache.
   c. May be associated with nausea and vomiting.
2. Cerebral vasospasm (narrowing of cerebral arteries, leading to ischemic neurologic deficits)
   a. Generally develops from day 4–14.
   b. Monitor for increasing headache, drowsiness, increased meningismus (signs and symptoms of meningeal irritation), fever, and focal neurologic signs.
3. Hydrocephalus
   a. Related to obstruction and fibrosis of arachnoid villi by subarachnoid blood, thus inhibiting CSF absorption.
   b. Watch for insidious onset of impaired mentation and memory; gait disturbances.
4. Epilepsy
5. Psychiatric problems

Nursing Interventions

A. Modifying Activities to Prevent Recurrent Bleeding

> **NURSING ALERT:** There is a significant incidence of recurrent aneurysmal bleeding with a high mortality rate.

1. Place patient on immediate and absolute bed rest in a quiet, nonstressful setting—activity, pain, stress, anxiety may elevate blood pressure and potentiate bleeding.
   a. Restrict visitors except family who are counseled to ensure tranquility.
   b. Elevate head of bed 30–35 degrees—to facilitate venous drainage from brain and to lessen potential for cerebral edema.
2. Dim lighting, as photophobia is common.
3. Avoid any activity that increases blood pressure or obstructs venous return (Valsalva maneuver, straining, sneezing, pulling up in bed, acute flexion/rotation of head and neck [compromises jugular veins], cigarette smoking).
4. Instruct the patient to exhale through mouth during voiding/defecation to decrease strain.
5. Eliminate caffeinated beverages.
6. Avoid activities that cause a sudden increase in arterial blood pressure.
7. Use appropriate psychological interventions and reassurance to relieve fear and anxiety.

B. Monitoring for Complications

1. Monitor the patient continually to recognize neurologic deterioration (from recurrent bleeding, increasing intracranial pressure, vasospasm) and to determine optimum time for surgical intervention.
   a. Keep neurologic flow record of level of consciousness, blood pressure, pulse, temperature, respiration, pupillary size and reaction, movement of extremities.
   b. Monitor respiratory status—reduction in PO_2 in brain areas with impaired autoregulation potentiates cerebral infarction.
   c. Use intracranial pressure monitoring (p. 580) for patients who are unconscious or showing progressive neurologic deterioration.
2. Monitor for fluid and electrolyte disturbances—result from inappropriate secretion of antidiuretic hormone (common after subarachnoid hemorrhage).

C. Other Nursing Interventions

1. Institute protocols to reduce increased intracranial pressure if required (see p. 578).
2. See care of the unconscious patient, page 575.
3. See nursing management of the patient following stroke, page 592.

Patient Education

1. The risk of rebleeding, to a variable degree, remains for the rest of the patient's life.
2. Activities that cause a sudden increase in arterial blood pressure should be avoided.
3. See page 596 for patient and family teaching following a stroke, as many who survive SAH are left with major neurologic deficits.

Brain Abscess

A *brain abscess* is a localized collection of pus within the brain substance. It exists as a mass lesion.

Etiology

1. By direct invasion of the brain (intracranial trauma or surgery)
2. By spread of infection from nearby sites (ear, sinus, mastoid)
3. By spread of infection from elsewhere in the body (lung infections, infective endocarditis)

> **NURSING ALERT:** Have a high degree of suspicion of brain abscess when neurologic signs and symptoms develop in a person with a recent history of sinus or ear infection or lung abscess.

Clinical Manifestations

Caused by major alterations of intracranial mass dynamics (edema, brain shift), by infection, or by location of the abscess.
1. Headache—may be from increased intracranial pressure; worse in morning.
2. Focal neurologic signs (depending on site of abscess)—weakness of arm or leg, visual impairment, focal epileptic seizures, papilledema.
3. Fever and leukocytosis; temperature may be subnormal when there is a thick-walled abscess.
4. Change in the patient's mental alertness.

Diagnostic Evaluation

Computed tomography—demonstrates site(s) of abscess; used to follow evolution and resolution of suppurative lesion.

Management

1. Surgery (differing opinions of precise procedure)
    a. Drainage of abscess through burr holes; *or*
    b. Craniotomy with elevation of bone flap and excision of abscess.
2. Antibiotics—large intravenous doses necessary to penetrate brain tissue and abscess.
3. Steroids—to reduce cerebral edema around the abscess.

Complications

1. Meningitis.
2. Epilepsy.

3. Neurologic deficits (hemiparesis; visual deficits; cranial nerve palsies).
4. Relapse is common with a high mortality rate.

Nursing Interventions

1. See nursing interventions following intracranial surgery, page 585.
2. Monitor for increased intracranial pressure (p. 578)—cerebral edema surrounds an acute brain abscess and may produce a sudden increase in intracranial pressure.
3. Reinforce head dressings as soon as they become moist, using strict aseptic technique. Drainage may be copious.
4. Encourage patient to lie on the affected side, if permitted, to promote drainage.
5. Administer prescribed antimicrobial agent on exact time schedule as meningitis is a threat.
6. Monitor for retraction (drawing back) of head, neck stiffness, headache, chills, sweats.

Discharge Planning/Patient Teaching

1. Advise family that residual infection may surface again and that immediate health care should be sought.
2. Continue taking antimicrobial agent for entire length of prescribed time period.
3. Make sure that anticonvulsant medication is taken daily; have a check-off system.
4. Report for follow-up and serial CT scans.

Brain Tumor

A *brain tumor* is a localized intracranial neoplasm that occupies space within the skull and tends to cause a rise in intracranial pressure.

Incidence

1. A brain tumor may originate in the CNS (primary) or metastasize from tumors elsewhere in the body.
2. Tumors may be benign or malignant; however, any mass within the closed cranial vault may be lethal.
3. The greatest incidence of brain tumors in adults occurs between the ages of 50 to 70 years.

Classification

A. Tumors Originating in the Brain Tissue

1. Gliomas: infiltrating tumors that may invade any portion of the brain; most common type of brain tumor
2. Classification according to cell type
    a. Astrocytomas (grades 1 and 2)
    b. Glioblastomas (grades 3 and 4 astrocytomas)
    c. Ependymomas
    d. Medulloblastomas
    e. Oligodendrogliomas
    f. Colloid cysts

B. Tumors Arising from the Covering of the Brain

Meningioma: encapsulated, well-defined, growing outside the brain tissue; compresses rather than invades brain

C. Tumors Developing in or on the Cranial Nerves

1. Acoustic neuroma: derived from sheath of acoustic nerve
2. Optic nerve spongioblastoma polare

D. Metastatic Lesions (most commonly from lung and breast)

E. Tumors of the Ductless Glands

1. Pituitary
2. Pineal

F. Blood Vessel Tumors

1. Hemangioblastoma
2. Angioma

G. Congenital Tumors

Clinical Manifestations

(Depend on tumor location and biological nature of tumor)

A. Symptoms Due to Increased Intracranial Pressure—can lead to herniation of brain tissue and death.

1. Headache, persistent or recurrent—intensified by activity that increases intracranial pressure (stooping, straining); most common in morning.
2. Vomiting, unrelated to food intake—usually due to irritation of vagal centers in medulla
3. Papilledema (choked disc)—edema of optic nerve with associated blurring and impaired vision; diplopia
4. Mental clouding, lethargy; changes in behavior

B. Localized Neurologic Impairment—due to local effect of tumor's interference with specific regions of the brain.

1. Motor abnormalities—weakness, paralysis, lack of coordination, seizures
2. Sensory abnormalities—aberrations in smell, vision, hearing, and touch.

GERONTOLOGIC ALERT: Personality changes, confusion, speech dysfunction, and disturbances of gait are seen more frequently in elderly persons with intracranial tumors.

Diagnostic Evaluation

1. Clinical assessment of signs and symptoms.
2. CT scan—shows where tumor is located in a 3-dimensional fashion.
3. Magnetic resonance imaging—gives anatomical detail and allows visualization of areas poorly seen on CT scan; allows serial follow-up and provides data to assess growth rate.
4. EEG—detects abnormal brain waves in tumor-occupied region.
5. Stereotactic biopsy with CT scanning—tumor localized by CT scan with stereotactic apparatus employed to direct a needle/cannula to target area to obtain biopsy of lesion

Management

A. Problems Affecting Management

1. Effectiveness of treatment depends on type and site of tumor; many tumors are in vital or inaccessible areas (brain stem tumors); even biopsies in such locations can produce unacceptable disabilities.
2. Nonencapsulated and infiltrating tumors make complete removal almost impossible; resulting neurologic deficit (blindness, paralysis, mental impairment) would be too severe.
3. Cures may be obtained in certain tumors (meningiomas, acoustic neuromas, cystic astrocytomas of cere-

bellum, etc.) if treated early; complete removal of infiltrating gliomas not possible.

B. Principles of Management

1. Brain tumors require different therapeutic approaches, depending on cell type, tumor location, degree of invasiveness, and association with vital structures; and age and condition of the patient. Each patient (and his lesion) is evaluated individually, and the therapeutic program designed accordingly.
2. Treatment usually involves a multidisciplinary approach including surgery, radiation, and chemotherapy.

C. Preoperative Management

1. Corticosteroids (dexamethasone) given to reduce cerebral edema associated with brain tumor, thus lowering intracranial pressure.
2. Antacids or cimetidine administered with steroids to prevent gastric upset or gastrointestinal bleeding.
3. Anticonvulsant (phenytoin) usually given prophylactically to prevent seizures.

D. Surgery

Goal:

To excise the tumor for potential cure or as an adjuvant treatment to radiation or chemotherapy.

Surgical approaches include total removal of tumor when possible, decompression and cerebrospinal fluid–vascular shunt procedures.

E. Radiation Therapy

1. Whole-brain irradiation, usually started after scalp incision heals.
   a. Some headache and depression of mental status may appear after first week of radiation; possibly due to reactive edema formation.
   b. Nausea and fatigue may appear during latter part of radiation therapy.
   c. Some hair loss may be expected.
2. Radioisotope ^{125}I implanted directly into tumor to permit high doses of radiation to tumor (brachytherapy).
3. Complications of whole-brain irradiation:
   a. Brain edema
   b. Radiation necrosis (delayed), which may mimic recurrent tumor.

F. Chemotherapy (Neuro-oncology)

1. Chemotherapeutic drugs (BCNU, CCNU, procarbazine) may be given singly or in combination, or may be combined with surgery and radiation therapy.
2. Intravenous autologous bone marrow transplantation—fraction of patient's bone marrow aspirated from his iliac crest and stored.
   a. Patient exposed to large doses of chemoradiotherapy to destroy large numbers of malignant cells.
   b. Following completion of chemoradiotherapy, patient's marrow is reinfused intravenously.

G. Management of Patient with Brain Metastases from Systemic Cancer (lung, skin, breast)

1. Patients with systemic tumors may function well until tumor metastasizes to nervous system and rapidly produces frightening and disabling symptoms (motor loss, cranial neuropathies, intellectual impairment, convulsive seizures).
2. Metastases to brain are commonly multiple and often unresectable.

3. Therapeutic approach includes surgery, radiation, and chemotherapy; palliation more effective if treatment is started before major neurologic deficits develop.
4. Steroid doses may be increased in the patient with progression of tumor to decrease symptoms of increased intracranial pressure
5. Arrange for Nurse Clinician and/or Social Worker to meet with the patient and family to identify problems.
6. See Chapter 6 for nursing management of the patient with cancer.

Nursing Interventions

1. See page 584 for nursing interventions for the patient undergoing intracranial surgery.
2. See page 108 for nursing management of the patient undergoing radiation therapy and page 103 for the patient undergoing chemotherapy.
3. The nursing rehabilitation of a patient undergoing treatment for a brain tumor is similar to that of persons with like deficits resulting from stroke. See page 592.

Discharge Planning/Patient Education

1. Explain to the family that the patient may be more lethargic while undergoing postoperative radiation therapy; also, his condition may worsen temporarily after the first course of chemotherapy.
2. Keep in close contact with neurosurgeon and oncologist for directions and continuity of care.
3. Make the patient and family aware that discontinuing steroids may cause rapid deterioration and lapse into coma.
4. Encourage family to join a support group to provide psychological support, clarify attitudes and behaviors about the patient's illness, and provide education about the illness.

The Epilepsies

The *epilepsies* are a symptom-complex of several disorders of brain function characterized by recurrent seizures. There may be associated changes in behavior, mentation, and motor or sensory activity. The basic problem is thought to be an electrical disturbance (dysrhythmia) in the nerve cells in one section of the brain that causes them to give off abnormal, recurrent, uncontrolled electrical discharges.

Causes

The underlying disorder of the brain may be structural, chemical, or physiologic, or a combination of all three.
1. Genetic factors
2. Trauma—head/brain
3. Brain tumor/brain abscess; intracranial surgery
4. Circulatory disorder (stroke, arteriovenous malformation)
5. Metabolic disorder (hypoglycemia, hypocalcemia, anoxia)
6. Toxicity (drugs and alcohol)
7. CNS infection (encephalitis, meningitis, abscess)

Clinical Manifestations

(Seizures may range from simple staring spells to prolonged convulsive movements.)
1. Impaired consciousness
2. Excess or loss of muscle tone or movement

3. Disturbances of behavior, mood, sensation, and perception
4. Disturbances of the autonomic functions of the body

Diagnostic Evaluation

1. History of seizures (as noted by patient and observers)
2. Electroencephalograph (EEG)—finds and measures brain electrical discharge pattern; useful in locating the site where epileptic discharge begins, its spread, intensity, duration; helps classify seizure type.
3. EEG and closed circuit television monitoring of patients—split-screen techniques show the patient during a seizure with simultaneous EEG tracing.
4. Telemetering and computer equipment—the patient wears a device that holds electrodes on scalp and houses a small radio transmitter; EEG signals are picked up by receiver and tape-recorded; helps identify seizure patterns before and after they occur.
5. CT scan—to detect lesions in brain, focal abnormalities, cerebrovascular abnormalities, and degenerative changes.
6. Neuropsychological tests for epilepsy.

Management

A. Drug Therapy (regarded as a form of control, not cure)

See Table 24-1.
1. The drug(s) is (are) selected according to type of seizure; treatment is started with a single drug and the dosage adjusted until seizures are controlled or side effects appear.
2. All anticonvulsant drugs have side effects; there may also be long-term effects on cognition, behavior, and appearance.
3. Serum drug level monitoring is done to control drug levels and to improve patient compliance.

B. Biofeedback—patient is taught to control his brain wave activity

C. Surgical Interventions—for uncontrolled seizures
   Goal:
   To abolish/reduce seizures without introducing unacceptable neurologic deficits
1. Various resective and palliative operations are done for some forms of epilepsy.
2. Surgery may be done under local anesthesia; patient is awake so that cortex can be functionally mapped by electrical stimulation to identify motor and language areas.
3. See page 584 for nursing interventions for the patient undergoing intracranial surgery.

Nursing Assessment

1. Obtain information about seizure history: onset, pattern, precipitating events.
2. Are there any prodromal signs/symptoms? Insomnia? Irritability? Mood changes? etc.
3. How much alcohol intake?
4. Explore how epilepsy is affecting his life. Limitations imposed? Unemployed/underemployed? Recreation? Social interaction?
5. How is the patient coping? Are seizures socially/psychologically disabling?
6. See page 583 for nursing assessment during and after a seizure.

Table 24-1. *Drugs Commonly Used in Epilepsy*

Drug	Dose-Related Side Effects	Idiosyncratic Side Effects
Carbamazepine	Blurred vision; dizziness Tiredness Gastrointestinal disturbance	Skin rash Fever May produce hematologic toxicity, cardiovascular, hepatic, genitourinary and central nervous system effects
Phenytoin	Nystagmus; visual problems Tiredness Ataxia Gingival hyperplasia	Skin rash; hirsutism Hepatitis Peripheral neuropathy
Valproate	Gastrointestinal symptoms Sedation Ataxia; tremor	Hepatotoxicity Pancreatitis Bone marrow suppression
Ethosuximide	Gastrointestinal symptoms Sedation; unsteadiness Headache	Skin rash Psychotic behavior
Phenobarbital	Drowsiness; sedation Diplopia Dizziness	Skin rash
Primidone	(same as phenobarbital)	Skin rash

Patient Education

1. Take medication daily to keep the amount of drug in the body constant to prevent seizures.
2. Report to the laboratory for blood sampling before taking morning medication when testing is prescribed—testing is necessary to achieve the best control with the fewest side effects.
3. Do not stop taking the drug abruptly—sudden withdrawal of medication may cause seizures.
4. Avoid activities that require alertness and coordination until the effects of the drug have been evaluated.
5. Keep a calendar/record of the occurrence of seizures—this is the basis for evaluation of the therapeutic effect of the drug.
6. Carry a personal identification card stating the name of the drug you are taking.
7. Use good oral hygiene and have regular dental care.
8. Antiepileptic drugs must be regarded as potentially teratogenic.
9. Alcohol or substance abuse may precipitate loss of control.
10. Report any unusual symptoms immediately.

Nursing Diagnoses

1. Altered tissue perfusion (cerebral) related to occurrence of seizures.
2. Ineffective individual coping related to psychosocial and economic consequences and stress of having epilepsy.
3. Knowledge deficit of epilepsy and its control.
4. Other possible nursing diagnoses
   a. Fear relating to occurrence of seizures.
   b. Potential for injury related to sudden loss of consciousness.
   c. Potential noncompliance with therapeutic regimen related to side effects of medication, and taking medication for a prolonged time.

Nursing Interventions

A. Controlling Seizures and Preventing Occurrences

1. Emphasize the importance of *regularity* in taking the prescribed antiepileptic medication to reduce number and/or severity of seizures.

NURSING ALERT: The patient should not stop taking his antiepileptic medication without medical supervision, since sudden withdrawal can cause an increase in seizure frequency or precipitate the development of status epilepticus.

2. Instruct the patient to watch for toxic effects of antiepileptic medication
   a. Drowsiness, gingival hyperplasia, nervousness, visual difficulties, motor incoordination, staggering ataxia, bone marrow depression leading to blood dyscrasias.
   b. Advise the patient to avoid taking medication on an empty stomach; gastritis is apt to occur, especially with phenytoin (Dilantin).
   c. Instruct the patient to brush teeth frequently and massage gums to prevent gingival infection.
3. Encourage the patient to have periodic blood evaluations when taking antiepileptic drugs that may depress hemopoiesis.
4. Instruct the patient to keep a record of events surrounding his seizures (number, duration, time of occurrence, sleep/eating patterns)—to help determine proper therapy/patient compliance.
5. Follow a regular and moderate routine in lifestyle, diet, exercise and rest. See Patient Education, page 603.

B. Maximizing Coping Resources to Improve Quality of Life

1. Use a multidisciplinary approach to cope with social, emotional, and work-related pressures; involves health care professionals, teachers, rehabilitation counselors, social service providers, and family.
2. Learn stress-reduction techniques—anxiety and depression are often related to obstacles that epilepsy imposes on everyday living.
3. Secure individual/family counseling for insight and for coming to terms with epilepsy.
4. Attend a support group.
5. Refer for comprehensive services for patient with per-

sonality disorder, brain damage, and/or intractable epilepsy.

Patient Education

A. For Patient

1. Encourage the patient to study himself and his environment to determine what specific factors precipitate his seizures—illness, emotional stress, physical stress, hyperventilation, altered sleep patterns, photosensitivity, or other sensory stimuli, menses, etc.
2. The medication must be taken daily to prevent seizures; medication may have to be adjusted because of recurrent illness, weight change, increase in stress, etc.
3. Practice *regularity* and *moderation* in daily activities—diet, exercise, rest, avoidance of certain stimulating stresses.
   a. Have regular hours for sleep. *Avoid sleep deprivation.*
   b. Avoid emotional overstimulation (watching late television, etc.) or photic stimulation (flickering light).
   c. Eat a well-balanced diet—long-term antiepileptic therapy can cause deficiencies.
   d. Avoid alcohol when seizures are known to follow alcoholic intake.
   e. Avoid swimming alone or engaging in sports, occupations, or hobbies involving serious risks.
   f. Seek help and counseling (if necessary) during periods of crisis—death in family, divorce, etc.).
4. Report any changes in health status—easy bruising, purpura, bleeding gums, jaundice, fever, recurrent infections or dermatosis.
5. Have follow-up urinalysis and blood studies.
6. Stress the importance of activity, both physical and mental. Moderate amounts of physical and mental activity tends to reduce epileptic activity.

B. For Family

1. Help the family to perceive and cope with epilepsy in a positive manner as possible.
2. Provide written materials.
3. Encourage the patient or family to discuss feelings and attitudes about epilepsy.
   a. Help the patient/family toward self-acceptance; reinforce areas of strength.
4. Carry a wallet card and wear a medical-alert bracelet indicating that the wearer has epilepsy.
5. Patients having a combination of seizure types or atypical seizures may benefit from the resources of a comprehensive epilepsy center.
6. Learn of the services and publications of:
   a. Epilepsy Foundation of America
      4351 Garden City Drive
      Landover, MD 20785
   b. Comprehensive Epilepsy Program
      (Epilepsy Research Program)
      National Institutes of Health
      Bethesda, MD 20892

Evaluation

1. Maintains control of seizures; takes medication as prescribed.
2. Coping with stresses imposed by epilepsy; seeking counseling and a support group.
3. Knows seizure type and medication effects.

Status Epilepticus

Status epilepticus (acute, prolonged, repetitive seizure activity) is a series of generalized seizures without return to consciousness between attacks. The term has been broadened to include continuous clinical and/or electrical seizures lasting at least 30 minutes, even without impairment of consciousness.

Underlying Considerations

1. Status epilepticus is considered a serious neurologic emergency. It has a high mortality and morbidity rate (permanent brain damage; severe neurologic deficits).
2. Factors that precipitate status epilepticus include medication withdrawal, fever, metabolic or environmental stresses, alcohol withdrawal, sleep deprivation, etc., in patient with pre-existing seizure disorder.

Management

A. Ensuring Adequate Cardiorespiratory Function and Brain Oxygenation

1. Airway is established and blood pressure maintained.
2. Blood studies conducted for glucose, blood urea nitrogen, electrolytes, and anticonvulsant drug levels—to determine metabolic abnormalities and serve as a guide for maintenance of biochemical homeostasis.
3. Oxygen administered—there is some respiratory arrest at height of each seizure, which may produce venous congestion and hypoxia of brain.
4. IV lines established and kept open for blood sampling, drug administration, and infusion of fluids.

B. Controlling Seizures to Prevent Permanent Brain Damage and Death

1. Intravenous anticonvulsant (diazepam; phenytoin) given *slowly* to ensure effective brain tissue and serum concentrations.
   a. Additional anticonvulsants given as directed—effects of diazepam are of short duration.
   b. Anticonvulsant drug levels monitored regularly.
   c. Measures instituted to correct acidosis, electrolyte imbalance, and dehydration.
   d. Mechanical ventilation is employed as needed.
   e. If initial treatment is unsuccessful, general anesthesia may be required.

Nursing Interventions

1. Monitor the patient continuously; depression of respiration and blood pressure induced by drug therapy may be delayed.
2. Assist with stabilization of metabolic balance by monitoring for acidosis, electrolyte imbalance, and dehydration.
3. Assist with search for precipitating factors.
   a. Monitor vital and neurologic signs on a continuing basis.
   b. Employ electroencephalographic monitoring—to determine nature and abolition (after diazepam administration) of epileptic activity.
   c. Determine (from family member) if there is a history of epilepsy, alcohol/drug use, trauma, recent infection.
4. Support patient undergoing diagnostic work-up for meningitis, encephalitis, brain lesion, cerebral edema, etc.

5. Continue to monitor patient after seizures have been controlled; patient may succumb from cardiac involvement or respiratory depression.

Parkinson's Disease

Parkinson's disease is a progressive neurologic disorder affecting the brain centers responsible for control and regulation of movement. It is characterized by bradykinesia (slowness of movement), tremor, muscle rigidity, and impaired postural reflexes.

Pathophysiology

A deficiency of dopamine in the substantia negra of the brain is thought to be responsible for the symptoms of parkinsonism.

Etiology

1. Unknown
2. Viruses, encephalitis, cerebrovascular disease, and poisoning or toxicity (manganese, carbon monoxide) have been suspected.
3. Genetic susceptibility (positive family history)

Clinical Manifestations

1. Bradykinesia—dyskinesia, hypokinesia (gradual loss of spontaneous movement)—usually becomes the most disabling symptom
2. Tremor—usually worse at rest; disappears in sleep
3. Rigidity in performance of all movements
4. Muscle weakness—affecting eating, chewing, swallowing, and speaking
5. Mask-like facial expression with infrequency of blinking
6. Autonomic disorders—sleeplessness, salivation, sweating, orthostatic hypotension
7. *Depression;* psychiatric disturbances; dementia

Diagnostic Evaluation

Observation of characteristic signs and symptoms

Management: Pharmacotherapy

A. General

1. Based on a combination of drug therapy, physical therapy, rehabilitation techniques, and patient/family education.
2. Decreases symptoms but does not halt progression of disease.

B. Antihistamines

1. Diphenhydramine (Benadryl)—for anticholinergic and sedative effects.

C. Anticholinergics

1. Blocks the action of acetylcholine to reduce transmission of cholinergic pathways, which are thought to be overactive when there is dopamine deficiency.
2. Frequently used anticholinergics include trihexyphenidyl (Artane and others); benztropine mesylate (Cogentin), procyclidine hydrochloride (Kemadrin); biperiden hydrochloride (Akineton)
3. Assess for side effects of anticholinergic agents—dryness of mouth, blurred vision, urinary retention, constipation, confusion, forgetfulness.

D. Amantadine (Symmetrel)—An antiviral drug that may increase release of dopamine in the brain.

E. Combination of Levodopa and Decarboxylase Inhibitor (Sinemet)

1. Levodopa combined with decarboxylase inhibitor prevents destruction of levodopa in bloodstream and peripheral tissues, thus allowing a greater concentration of dopamine to enter the brain.
2. Beneficial effects most pronounced in first few years of treatment
3. Adverse effects may increase with continued use.
   a. Dyskinesias (abnormal involuntary movements)—facial grimacing, rhythmic jerking movements of hands progressing to head bobbing, chewing and smacking movements, jerking movements involving trunk and extremities
   b. Progressive shortening of levodopa's effect (reduced "on" time)
      On–off phenomena—sudden episodes of immobility ("off effect") lasting minutes to hours, followed by sudden return of effectiveness ("on effect")
   c. Psychiatric reactions—confusion, memory impairment, hallucinations, delusions
4. Deprenyl—has been shown to enhance and prolong action of levodopa and ameliorate the dose-related "wearing off."
5. Dopamine agonists
   a. Bromocriptine mesylate (Parlodel)—crosses blood-brain barrier and stimulates dopaminergic receptors.
   b. May be used in conjunction with levodopa.
   c. Adverse effects—confusion, delusions, hallucinations, gastrointestinal upset, abnormal involuntary movements.

Surgical Intervention

1. Implantation of autologous adrenal medullary tissue to the caudate nucleus of the brain.
2. Adrenal gland of patient removed via laparotomy; medullary fragments (dopamine-making cells) transplanted onto right caudate nucleus via craniotomy to restore nigrostriatal function.
3. Laparotomy and craniotomy done simultaneously.
4. Purported to relieve signs and symptoms, particularly tremor; considered investigational.

Complications of Parkinson's Disease

1. Slowing of mental processes; dementia
2. Aspiration with subsequent pulmonary infection

Nursing Assessment

1. Ask the patient about slowing of body movement, difficulty with equilibrium, muscle aching and soreness, weakness, fatigue, and insomnia.
2. Observe patient during daily activities; arising from bed/chair, walking, dressing, and eating.
3. Listen to patient's speech.
4. Ask the patient how Parkinson's disease is affecting the quality of life.
5. Assess for signs of depression.

Nursing Diagnoses

1. Impaired physical mobility related to slowness and weakness of voluntary movement, rigidity, and tremor.
2. Self-care deficits (feeding, hygiene, dressing, and toi-

leting) related to diminished motor function and tremor.

3. Altered bowel elimination (constipation) related to medication effects and reduced activity.

4. Altered nutrition (less than body requirements) related to tremor, slowness of eating, drooling, and difficulty in chewing and swallowing.

5. Potential for injury (falls) related to impaired balance, diminished postural reflexes, and slowed reactions.

6. Impaired verbal communication related to decreased speech volume, slowness of speech, inability to move facial muscles, and adverse effects of drugs.

7. Impaired social interaction related to depression and dysfunction due to disease progression.

Nursing Interventions

A. Improving Mobility and Functioning

1. Encourage the patient to continue on an exercise and physical therapy program to increase muscle strength, improve coordination and dexterity, treat muscular rigidity, prevent contractures, and compensate for lack of automatic movements.

2. Emphasize the importance of a *daily* exercise program (walk, ride stationary bike, swim, garden)—to maintain joint mobility.

3. Advise the patient to do stretching exercises (stretch–hold–relax) to loosen the joint structures.

4. Teach postural exercises and walking techniques to offset shuffling gait and tendency to lean forward
   a. Use a broad-based gait (feet wide apart).
   b. Make a conscious effort to swing arms, raise the feet while walking, use a heel–toe, heel–toe gait and increase the width of the stride.
   c. Practice walking to marching music or sound of ticking metronome—provides sensory reinforcement.
   d. Obtain a reciprocal walking frame if patient loses balance—allows patient to keep one part of frame in contact with floor at all times.

5. Encourage the patient to take warm baths, massage, and passive and active exercises—to help relax muscles and relieve painful muscle spasms that accompany rigidity.

6. Advise the patient to have frequent rest periods—the patient becomes fatigued and frustrated by his symptoms.

7. Encourage patient to be seen by a physical therapist on a regular basis to reinforce exercise program.

B. Gaining Independence in Self-Care

1. Teach the patient how to turn and get out of bed.
   a. Bend the knees (feet on mattress) and turn upper half of body; the lower half of the body will follow.
   b. To get out of bed, turn on side and then place feet over the edge of bed and push up with the arms.

2. Use assistive devices to help in bathing and grooming; electric razor, wash mitt, long-handled bath brush, soap-on-a-rope, Velcro clothing closures, button aids, dressing stick, elastic shoe laces, etc.

3. See also Patient Education.

C. Facilitating Bowel Elimination

1. Encourage patient to establish a regular bowel routine (p. 143)

2. Encourage intake of foods with a moderate fiber content.

3. Make a real effort to drink more water.

4. Secure a raised toilet seat.

D. Improving Nutritional Status

1. Help the patient think through swallowing sequence; close lips and with teeth together, place food on tongue, lift the tongue up—then back and swallow (up–back–swallow) while tilting the head forward.

2. Encourage the patient to make a conscious effort to chew and to chew first on one side and then the other.

3. Control the buildup of saliva by holding head in an upright position and making a conscious effort to swallow saliva often.

4. Secure a stabilized plate, nonspill cup, flexible plastic straw, built-up eating utensils, and an electrical warming tray as assistive devices and to keep food hot and allow the patient to rest during prolonged eating time.

5. Arrange for supplementary feedings to augment caloric intake.

6. Have patient/family keep a weekly weight chart.

7. Refer to occupational therapist (or dysphagia therapist) if patient is having severe swallowing problems.

E. Preventing Injury

1. Refer to physical therapist for postural and gait training, techniques in turning, rising from a chair, getting up from floor following a fall.

2. Consult with occupational therapist for selection of safety aids: grab rails on tub, raised toilet seat, handrails on both sides of steps, electric seat-lift chair.

3. Secure a knotted rope to foot of bed to allow patient to pull himself to a sitting position.

4. Minimize effects of orthostatic hypotension.
   a. Monitor blood pressure and pulse while lying and then standing.
   b. Elevate head of bed slightly.
   c. Encourage use of elastic stockings.

5. Be sure that patient has some form of call system.

F. Maximizing Residual Communication Ability

1. Encourage patient to take prescribed medication—levodopa appears to improve patient's overall speech intelligibility.

2. Refer to speech-language pathologist for assessment and therapy at an early stage. For list of approved speech and hearing centers and certified speech-language pathologists:
   American Speech-Language Hearing Association
   10801 Rockville Pike
   Rockville, MD 20852

3. Remind patient of the following:
   a. Take a deep breath before speaking—increases the volume of sound and number of words spoken per breath.
   b. Exaggerate pronunciation and speak in short sentences.
   c. Practice breathing exercises regularly—to increase thoracic and abdominal movement while speaking.
   d. Exercise facial muscles (smile, frown, grimace, pucker)—for facial mobility.

4. Advise the patient to practice reading aloud in front of a mirror to improve speech.

5. Have the patient speak into a tape recorder—to monitor progress.

6. Consider electronic devices for problem of weak voice (not beneficial for slurred speech, uneven speech rate).

G. Developing Positive Coping Abilities

1. Help the patient establish achievable goals (improvement of health and mobility, lessening of tremors).
2. Encourage the patient to be an *active* participant in his therapy and in social and recreational events—parkinsonism tends to lead to depression and withdrawal.
3. Have a planned program of activity throughout day—prevents daytime sleeping, disinterest, and apathy.
4. Reemphasize that disability can be prevented or delayed; offer realistic reassurance.
5. Try to dispel anxiety and fears of the patient that may be as disabling to him as his disease.
6. Provide caring and support for family who are vulnerable to emotional stresses and depression from living with a progressively disabled person.
   a. Allow expression of feelings of frustration, anger, depression, guilt, etc.
   b. Help family to identify problem areas and explore ways of coping and realistic alternatives.

Patient/Family Education

1. See A through C, page 605.
2. Explain that sudden changes in disability are encountered in Parkinson's disease.
3. Try the following routine when feet and legs seem to be "glued" to the floor.
   a. Raise head.
   b. Raise toes (eliminates muscle spasm).
   c. Rock from one foot to the other while bending knees slightly.
   d. Or raise arms in a sudden, short motion.
   e. Or take a small step backward; then start forward.
   f. Or step sideways; then start forward.
   g. Instruct the family not to pull patient during episodes of "freezing"—this increases the problem and may cause falling.
4. For the patient who has difficulty rising up from a chair:
   a. Choose straight-back wooden chairs with armrests (captain's chair); raise rear legs of chair 10 cm. (2 inches) to give chair a slight forward tilt.
   b. Move toward edge of seat, placing heels as far back under chair as possible.
   c. Lean forward from hips so that center of gravity is above feet.
      Another person may hold the patient's hand while pushing forward gently and firmly on his head with the other hand.
   d. Rise to a standing posture.
5. Establish a regular bowel routine, consciously increase fluid intake, and eat foods with a moderate fiber content—patients with parkinsonism have trouble with constipation because of muscle weakness, lack of exercise, inadequate fluid intake, and drug effects.
6. Eat a well-balanced diet—nutritional problems develop from slowness of movement, difficulties in chewing and swallowing, and dry mouth from medications.
7. Report for blood evaluations and tonometry (screening test for glaucoma) because levodopa or Sinemet can exacerbate blood disorders, GI bleeding, and glaucoma.
8. Avoid over-the-counter sedatives.
9. Learn all one can about Parkinson's disease. American Parkinson Disease Association, 116 John Street, New York, NY 10038, has illustrated booklets and a newsletter for patient education.

Evaluation

1. Working toward improved mobility; exercises and walks daily.
2. Achieving self-care; allows enough time.
3. Achieves improved bowel elimination.
4. Attains satisfactory nutritional status; eating slowly and without choking.
5. Absence of injuries.
6. Demonstrates improved verbal communication; practices speech exercises.
7. Maintaining some social contacts.

Multiple Sclerosis

Multiple Sclerosis (MS) is a chronic disease of the central nervous system characterized by the occurrence of small patches of demyelination of the central nervous system white matter, associated with inflammatory changes leading to eventual scarring of affected fiber tracts.

Pathophysiology

1. *Demyelination* refers to the destruction of myelin, the fatty and protein material that ensheaths certain nerve fibers in the brain and spinal cord.
2. Demyelination results in disordered transmission of nerve impulses.
3. Although the cause of MS is not known, evidence indicates a disordered immune system as part of the pathogenesis. An infectious process may contribute to the disease, and a certain genetic makeup influences susceptibility to MS.

Incidence

1. Multiple sclerosis is one of the most disabling of the neurologic diseases striking young adults during their most productive years (20–40 years of age).
2. MS maximizes the medical, psychological, social, and economic problems encountered by the patient and his family. However, a number of these patients have little or no disability for many years after diagnosis.

Clinical Manifestations

Note: The signs and symptoms reflect the location and areas of demyelination within the central nervous system. Patients have a wide range of clinical symptoms; there is great variability in the course of the disease, with many relapses and remissions.

1. Fatigue and weakness.
2. Abnormal reflexes, either absent or exaggerated.
3. Visual disturbances; impaired vision; diplopia; optic neuritis.
4. Tremor; ataxia; incoordination.
5. Sensory disturbances; paresthesias.
6. Bladder dysfunction with urinary frequency, nocturia, incontinence.
7. Impaired vibration and position sense.
8. Slurring, scanning speech (dysarthria)
9. Neurobehavioral syndromes; depression, cognitive impairment; emotional lability, pathologic laughing/weeping; euphoria.

Diagnostic Evaluation

1. Electrophoresis study of CSF—abnormal IgG antibody appears in CSF.

2. MRI—visualizes small plaques scattered throughout the nervous system; able to identify both total number of lesions and their size.
3. Visual, auditory, and somatosensory evoked potentials—slowed conduction time is evidence of demyelination.
4. Urologic evaluation—to document the type of bladder dysfunction.
5. Neuropsychologic testing—to detect cognitive changes.

Management

Although there is no specific treatment, the following is aimed at relieving symptoms and helping the patient function.

A. For Acute Attacks

1. Corticosteroids or adrenocorticotrophic hormone (ACTH)—used for anti-edema and anti-inflammatory properties to shorten duration of relapse/exacerbations.
2. Immunosuppressive agents (cyclophosphamide) may stabilize the course of disease.
3. Azathioprine—may be helpful in some patients.

B. Symptom Management

1. Spasticity—baclofen; dantrolene; diazepam; physical therapy; nerve blocks; surgical intervention.
2. Fatigue—amantadine (Symmetrel).
3. Depression and/or anxiety—antidepressant therapy; counseling.
4. Vertigo—bedrest; meclizine to suppress dizziness.
5. Bladder management
   a. Bladder drainage for flaccid/distended bladder.
   b. Anticholinergic drugs (propantheline; oxybutynin).
   c. Prompt treatment of urinary tract infection.
6. Bowel management—stool softeners; bulk supplements; laxatives, suppositories, enema.
7. Rehabilitation management—physical therapy; occupational therapy.

Complications

1. Respiratory problems.
2. Infection: sepsis; urinary tract infection; respiratory infection.
3. Complications from inactivity; pressure sores; contractures; deep vein thrombosis.

Nursing Assessment

1. Have an awareness of the potential/actual problems imposed by the disease, including neurologic problems, and the consequences of the disease on the patient and family.
2. Observe patient walking and moving before and after resting.
3. Determine his major problems—weakness? fatigue? spasticity? visual impairment? incontinence? speech disturbances?
4. Ask specifically about incontinence.
5. Take a brief sexual history to explore how MS has affected feelings about sexuality and ability to engage in sexual activity.
6. How is the patient coping? How did he handle other life crises or challenges? What adaptive capacities and mechanisms were used in the past?

7. Review results of physical and occupational therapist's evaluations to understand the goals and treatment regimens.

Nursing Diagnoses

1. Impaired physical mobility related to muscle weakness (secondary to impaired nerve conduction), spasticity, dizziness.
2. Fatigue related to disease process and stress of coping.
3. Potential for injury (falls) related to gait instability, sensory and visual impairment.
4. Alteration in sensory perception (visual) related to visual problems secondary to MS.
5. Altered urinary elimination (incontinence/retention) related to demyelination of nerves innervating the bladder.
6. Altered bowel elimination (constipation) related to spinal cord involvement.
7. Self-care deficits related to general weakness, spasticity, tremor, and fatigue.
8. Impaired skin integrity related to immobility.
9. Potential sexual dysfunction related to neurologic consequences of MS, and personal and partner and societal reactions to the condition.
10. Altered family process related to role reversal, disruption of life-style, financial obligations.
11. Other possible nursing diagnoses
    a. Diminished cognitive function
    b. Impaired verbal communication
    c. Pain
    d. Potential for infection
    e. Impaired home maintenance

Nursing Interventions

A. Improving Functioning Ability

1. Strengthen muscles and prevent and treat muscle spasticity—spasticity interferes with normal function.
   a. The patient should do muscle-stretching exercises daily—to minimize spasticity, joint contractures, and tightening and shortening of certain muscle groups.
   b. Teach the patient's family passive exercises and range-of-motion exercises for patients with severe spasticity.
   c. Teach the stretch–hold–relax routine and encourage the patient to do it throughout the day for relaxation.
   d. Apply ice packs (30 minutes) and give slow stretches to affected muscles; may reduce spasticity in early stages.
2. Advise the patient to avoid muscle fatigue; stop physical activity just short of fatigue and take frequent, short rest periods, preferably lying down.
3. Encourage general body-strengthening exercises for correcting and preventing specific muscle weakness of disuse and for balance and coordination.
4. Prevent muscle contractures and loss of muscle power from lack of use—diminishing motor power is a significant problem in multiple sclerosis.
5. Encourage the patient to sleep prone at intervals—to minimize flexor spasm at knees and hips.
6. Advise the patient to participate in walking exercises—to improve gait affected by loss of position sense in legs.
7. Utilize braces, canes, crutches, walker, when necessary—to keep the patient ambulatory.

B. Conserving Energy to Relieve Fatigue

1. Help patient to understand that fatigue is an integral part of MS and not to feel guilty.
2. Plan ahead. List priorities; plan time for rest and pace self throughout day.
3. Counsel with occupational therapist for help in planning time organization, energy conservation, and work simplification techniques.
4. Obtain publications on energy conservation.
5. Study self and use periods when energy is most readily available.
6. Avoid overheating (hot baths), overexertion, and infection.
7. Develop a life-style promoting wellness; use balanced diet, low in fat; balance rest and exercise, and avoid anything that aggravates symptoms.

C. Preventing Injury

1. Assist the patient to overcome effects of incoordination.
2. Teach the patient to walk with feet wider apart—to widen his base of support and increase his walking stability.
3. Inform the patient to avoid abrupt change in position and to be careful in turning, sitting, and standing.
4. Use weighted bracelets, wrist cuffs, eating utensils— to help overcome incoordination of upper extremities.

D. Compensating for Visual Impairment

1. Make the environment safe for the visually impaired patient.
2. Use eye patch; frosted lens—to block visual impulses of one eye when the patient has diplopia (double vision).
3. Prism glasses may be useful for the bedridden patient.
4. For the patient who has impaired eyesight or who is unable to hold a book, turn pages, or read regular print, secure books and magazines recorded on discs, tape cassettes, and open reel magnetic tape provided free of charge by: Division for the Blind and Physically Handicapped, Library of Congress, Washington, DC 20542.

E. Establishing Bladder Control

1. See page 693 for management of the patient with a neurogenic bladder.
2. Assess for bladder infection.
3. Assess for urinary retention, especially if patient is taking anticholinergic medications.
4. Ensure adequate fluid intake (3–5 liters daily)—to reduce urinary bacterial count and to minimize precipitation of urinary crystals, stone formation, and encrustation of the lumen of the indwelling urethral catheter.
5. Emphasize that bacterial urinary tract infection is common in MS; neurologic dysfunction increases when fever is present. Report immediately.
6. Support the patient who has urinary incontinence (or frequency and urgency).
   Female patient
   a. Set up a voiding-time schedule; every 1½ to 2 hours initially, with lengthening time intervals if regimen is successful.
   b. Encourage the patient to drink a measured amount of fluid every 2 hours.
   c. Have the patient try to void 30 minutes after drinking.
   d. Teach self-catheterization technique for patient with significant retention.
   e. Use low fracture bedpan at night; set alarm clock for patient with diminished warning sensation.
   f. For permanent urinary incontinence, urine may have to be diverted by means of ileal conduit (see p. 696).
   Male patient
   a. See a, b, c, and d under Female Patient, above.
   b. Use urinal at night.
   c. For permanent urinary incontinence, the patient may wear external sheath or condom appliance for urine collection.

F. Achieving Bowel Control

1. Establish a program of regularity.
   a. Have the patient eat regularly scheduled meals; include high-fiber foods.
   b. Establish bowel evacuation at same time each day.
2. Encourage the patient to drink 120 ml. (4 ounces) of prune juice at bedtime (same time each night).
3. Insert a glycerin or prescribed suppository into the rectum 30 minutes before scheduled bowel evacuation time—after eating a meal (preferably after breakfast).
4. Advise the patient to attempt to have a bowel movement within 30 minutes of eating, using as normal a position for defecation as possible.
   a. Instruct the patient to bear down and contract abdominal muscles.
   b. Teach the patient to apply pressure to abdomen with his hands—to assist with defecation.
   c. After routine is established, mechanical stimulation with a suppository may not be necessary.

G. Striving Toward Increased Independence in Self-Care Activities

1. Make occupational therapy referral for evaluation of structural arrangement of work place and home.
2. Secure proper wheelchair prescription (with input from entire rehabilitation team) with features that will maximize mobility.
3. Teach transfer activities (see p. 138).
4. Use assistive and self-help devices.
   a. Toilet facilities—raised toilet seat or bedside commode.
   b. Bathing facilities—use shower hose, stool in shower or tub, and handrails to compensate for weakness and to prevent falls.
   c. Self-care aids—prism glasses, telephone modifications, long-handled combs, tongs, and modified clothing.

H. Attaining/Maintaining Skin Integrity

1. Relieve pressure.
   a. Change position at least every 2 hours if the patient is in bed.
   b. Change position every 30 minutes if the patient is in a wheelchair.
   c. Use flotation pad, sheepskin, alternating air pressure mattress, and other modalities to distribute pressure away from bony points and over a wider area.
   d. Teach the patient to inspect pressure areas (using a long-handled mirror for posterior sites) for evidences of redness and heat.
2. Avoid skin trauma, heat, cold, and pressure.
3. Give careful attention to sacral and perineal hygiene.
4. See page 133 for discussion of prevention and treatment of pressure sores.

I. Adapting to Sexual Dysfunction

1. Encourage open communication between partners.
2. Discuss fertility control if childbearing is not a goal.
3. Arrange referral to a professional therapist for exploration of new ways to achieve sexual satisfaction, etc.
4. See Sexuality, a Part of the Rehabilitation Process, page 128.

J. Maintaining Family Integrity

1. See that the care-givers are maintaining their health and have some outside support and social life.
2. Help the family to learn of community resources.
3. Encourage them to rely on social worker and others to use available financial resources.
4. Encourage family to have family therapy if conflicts, psychosomatic conditions, and exhaustion threaten family stability.

Discharge Planning/Patient Education

1. Review A through J, above.
2. Help the family (and patient) understand the stresses imposed by multiple sclerosis.
   a. Situations may occur to which the person may respond "inappropriately."
   b. The patient may be depressed, or have brain damage with resultant denial of his disease, euphoria, or depressive and paranoid behavior.
   c. MS patients are often forgetful and easily distracted.
3. Understand that patients adapt to illness in many ways—frustration, anger, denial, depression, withdrawal, inactivity, resentment, etc.
4. Support the defense mechanisms of the patient, according to the patient's time table, when feasible.
   a. Avoid confronting him with stark reality.
   b. Answer questions honestly.
   c. Help the patient remain in control.
   d. Offer services of mental health professionals when advisable.
   e. Encourage the patient to keep up social interests and activities.
5. The patient may have feelings of alienation from family, others, work, and social life; he feels that his personal worth is lessened.
   a. Give opportunities for the patient to vent his feelings; suppressed anger is destructive.
   b. Try to keep him in the mainstream of life as much as possible.
   c. Seek support group to foster hope, for support, trust, and commitment based on shared and mutual experiences.
   d. Contact local chapter of the National Multiple Sclerosis Society, 205 East 42nd Street, New York, NY 10017, for services, publications, and contact with other MS patients.
6. Try to keep up the activities (physical, social, etc.) that the patient is able to do; once lost, certain abilities are almost impossible to regain.
   a. Physical abilities may vary from day to day.
   b. Devise modifications that will allow continuance of certain activities; obtain gadgets and adaptive devices for self-help (mail-order gift companies, medical supply catalogues, rehabilitation literature).
   c. Follow short periods of exertion with rest.
7. Try to avoid physical and emotional stresses—may worsen symptoms and impair performance.

a. Exposure to heat or cold—appears to increase fatigue.
   (1) Take tepid showers/baths.
   (2) Avoid becoming overheated, especially during the summer months.
   b. Overexertion—lessens motor power
   c. Fever
   d. Emotional upsets
8. Assist the patient to accept his new identity as a disabled person and cope with the disruption in his life.
9. See "Head Injury" for Management of Cognitive Impairment, page 583.
10. Keep channels of communication open.
11. Encourage meaningful and realistic short-term goals—to achieve a sense of purpose.

Evaluation

1. Demonstrates improved neurologic functioning; has increased mobility; uses techniques to improve coordination.
2. Trying to avoid fatigue by working out a realistic daily schedule.
3. Absence of injury.
4. Using aids to compensate for visual dysfunction.
5. Copes with bladder dysfunction; able to catheterize self.
6. Attains bowel control.
7. Achieves some independence in self-care.
8. Demonstrates intact skin.
9. Seeking counseling to cope with sexual dysfunction.
10. Family requesting and receiving help from community and professional resources.

Myasthenia Gravis

Myasthenia gravis is a disorder affecting the neuromuscular transmission of impulses in the voluntary muscles of the body; it is characterized by excessive fatigability of muscle function.

Pathophysiology

1. The basic defect is a reduction of acetylcholine receptors (AChRs) at neuromuscular junctions brought about by an autoimmune attack, which is thought to be antibody mediated.
2. The neuromuscular junction is the synapse between the motor axon and the muscle fiber.

Clinical Manifestations

1. Extreme muscular weakness and easy fatigability.
2. Diplopia (double vision); ptosis (drooping of one or both eyelids)—from ocular muscle weakness.
3. Sleepy, mask-like expression—from involvement of facial muscles.
4. Dysarthria (speaking difficulty) and dysphagia (difficulty in swallowing)—from weakness of laryngeal and pharyngeal muscles.
5. Problems with swallowing, choking, and aspiration—due to weakness of bulbar muscles.

Diagnostic Evaluation

1. Serum test for ACh receptor antibodies—positive in up to 90% of patients.

2. Edrophonium (Tensilon) test—intravenous injection of edrophonium may relieve muscle weakness markedly in 30 seconds.
3. Electrophysiologic testing—reveals decremental response to repetitive nerve stimulation.
4. CT scan—for thymoma or thymic hyperplasia; it is believed that the thymus gland may play a role in the initiation of the autoimmune response.

Management

A. Anticholinesterase Drugs—to enhance neuromuscular transmission. Neostigmine bromide (Prostigmin); pyridostigmine bromide (Mestinon; Regonol)

1. Drug scheduling is individualized and timed so that peak action coincides with patient's activities.
2. After initial medication adjustment has been made, the patient learns to take medication according to needs. Individual doses may vary with physical or emotional stress, intercurrent infection, etc.
3. Sedatives and tranquilizing drugs are given with caution; may aggravate hypoxia and hypercapnia and cause respiratory and cardiac depression.

NURSING ALERT: Watch for increase in muscle weakness within 1 hour after administering anticholinesterase drug; be alert for signs of respiratory embarrassment.

---

4. Toxicity or side effects of anticholinesterase—abdominal cramps, diarrhea, fasciculations (fine twitching), increasing weakness.

B. Immunosuppressive Drugs

Prednisone and azathioprine—commonly used Cyclosporine may be used as adjunctive therapy.

C. Plasmapheresis (plasma exchange)

1. Removal of the plasma containing acetylcholine receptor antibodies to improve muscle strength temporarily in patients with severe symptoms who do not respond to other treatment
2. Usually gives rapid clinical improvement

D. Surgical Intervention (thymectomy)—may give improvement or remission of the disease, especially in patients with tumor or hyperplasia of the thymus gland.

1. May be carried out by transcervical or sternal-splitting procedure.
2. Preoperative evaluation includes assessment of respiratory status (tidal volume, vital capacity), muscular strength, and the patient's chewing, swallowing, and ocular movements.
3. Monitoring for myasthenia crisis.
4. Postoperative nursing interventions (in intensive care unit) include:
   a. Monitoring and caring for the patient on mechanical ventilator, if needed.
   b. Continuing assessment of ventilatory function.
   c. Reassuring the patient that any weakness is usually temporary.

Crises in Myasthenia Gravis

A. Types of Crises

1. *Myasthenic crisis*
   a. May result from natural deterioration of disease, emotional upset, upper respiratory infection, sur-

gery, or trauma; or may be brought about by ACTH therapy.
   b. The patient may be temporarily resistant to anticholinesterase drugs or may need increased dosage.
2. *Cholinergic crisis*—from overmedication with anticholinergic drugs, which releases too much acetylcholine at the neuromuscular junction.
3. *Brittle crisis*
   a. Occurs when the receptors at the neuromuscular junction become insensitive to anticholinesterase medication.
   b. Not controlled by increasing or decreasing anticholinesterase therapy.

B. Clinical Manifestations of Impending Crisis

1. Sudden respiratory distress combined with varying signs of dysphagia (difficulty in swallowing), dysarthria (difficulty in speaking), eyelid ptosis, and diplopia.
2. Tachycardia; anxiety.
3. Rapidly increasing weakness of muscles of trunk and extremities.

C. Management and Nursing Interventions

1. Patient is placed in intensive care unit for constant monitoring—myasthenia gravis is a disease of rapidly fluctuating intensity and the patient is on the verge of respiratory arrest.
2. Ventilatory assistance is provided when muscles of respiration and swallowing become involved.
   a. Suction the patient as needed—*aspiration is a common problem.*
   b. See page 246 for management of the patient requiring ventilatory support.
3. Plasma exchange may be used as emergency treatment possibly to avoid need for ventilatory assistance.
4. Time of onset of symptoms is determined in relation to the last dose of anticholinesterase—may show whether patient is undermedicated or having a cholinergic reaction.
   a. Edrophonium may be given to differentiate type of crisis.
   b. Edrophonium (IV) improves the condition of the patient in myasthenic crisis, temporarily worsens that of the patient in cholinergic crisis, and is unpredictable in brittle crisis.
5. Appropriate drugs are administered as determined by the patient's status:
   a. For myasthenic crisis: neostigmine methylsulfate (Prostigmin) administered parenterally if the patient is in true myasthenic crisis.
   b. For cholinergic crisis: all anticholinesterase drugs are withdrawn. Atropine may be given to reduce excessive secretions.
6. Fluids, medication, and food are administered via nasogastric tube if the patient is unable to swallow.
7. Nursing Considerations
   a. Avoid giving enemas—may cause sudden respiratory problems.
   b. Develop a communication system for the patient on ventilator (or if he is too weak to speak).
   c. Give continuing psychological support since the patient is usually alert and anxious. Reassure that crisis will pass and that he will not be left alone.

Discharge Planning/Patient Education

Instruct the patient as follows:
1. Know the basic facts about anticholinergic drugs: ac-

tion, reason for and regulation of dose according to changing needs, importance of timing, dosage adjustment, symptoms of overdose, and toxic effects.
2. Know the drugs that interact with anticholinesterase drugs. Be aware that many drugs can aggravate the disease (antibiotics, antiarrhythmics, local and general anesthetics, muscle relaxants, analgesics).
3. Have mealtimes coincide with peak of anticholinesterase effect (when swallowing ability is best); have standby suction available in home if swallowing difficulties occur. (Use a blender when necessary.)
4. Wear an identification bracelet signifying that you have myasthenia gravis.
5. Try to prevent factors (emotional upset, infections) that may increase weakness and precipitate myasthenic crisis.
6. Wear an eyepatch over one eye (alternating from side to side) if diplopia occurs.
7. Avoid vigorous physical activity and other factors leading to fatigue.
8. Avoid contracting colds and influenza—respiratory infections are extremely dangerous to the myasthenic individual.
9. Avoid excessive heat and cold (hot baths, sun bathing); weak spells may follow long exposure to excessive heat/cold.
10. Advise the dentist that you are myasthenic, since Novocain is usually not well tolerated.
11. Rest before fatigue sets in; do not force yourself to continue with an activity.
12. Use adaptive and self-help devices to handle motion impairment problems.
13. Learn all you can about the condition; with good management, the patient should be able to live a relatively full life. The Myasthenia Gravis Foundation, Inc., 15 East 26th Street, New York, NY 10010.

Amyotrophic Lateral Sclerosis

Amyotrophic lateral sclerosis (ALS) is a progressively incapacitating and fatal disease of unknown cause in which there is degeneration of upper motor neurons (nerves leading from brain to medulla or to spinal cord) and to the lower motor neurons (nerves leading from spinal cord to muscles of body). There is loss of voluntary muscle function and subsequently the loss of functional capacity.

Clinical Manifestations

Depend on location of affected motor neurons, since specific neurons activate specific muscle fibers.
1. Progressive weakness and wasting of muscles of arms, trunk, and/or legs from degeneration of anterior horn cells in various segments of spinal cord.
2. Signs of spasticity, fasciculations (irregular twitching of muscles), and exaggerated reflexes.
3. Progressive difficulty in speaking, swallowing, and ultimately breathing—as a consequence of degeneration of the motor cranial nerve nuclei in the lower brain stem (or bulb, hence the ''bulbar'' symptoms).
   a. Drooling; pseudoptyalism (accumulation of saliva in mouth).
   b. Regurgitation of liquids through nose.
   c. Difficulty with swallowing with aspiration of food or fluid into trachea.
   d. Nasal and unintelligible speech.

Diagnostic Evaluation

1. Electromyography—demonstrates presence of denervation, muscle wasting, and atrophy.
2. Nerve conduction study.
3. Pulmonary function studies—to appraise respiratory function.
4. Barium swallow—to evaluate ability to achieve various phases of swallowing.

Management

No specific treatment available at present time to arrest or alter course of disease. The supportive treatment, determined by functional loss, includes:
1. Baclofen—for spasticity
2. Diazepam—for fasciculations
3. Antidepressant medication
4. Anticholinergic medication (atropine)—to control saliva
5. Feeding gastrostomy—when patient can no longer eat without risk of aspiration
6. Mechanical ventilation

Complications

1. Respiratory failure
2. Cardiopulmonary arrest

Nursing Interventions

A. Establishing Techniques to Cope With Impaired Physical Mobility and Lost Function
1. Encourage the patient to continue the usual activities as long as possible; avoid fatigue.
2. Work with physical therapist to teach patient and family exercises to strengthen unaffected muscles; carry out range-of-motion exercises.
3. Encourage stretching exercises (stretch–hold–relax) to avoid contractures.
4. Give special attention to shoulder joint as upper arm pain related to shoulder dysfunction is a major cause of discomfort.
5. Initiate referral to occupational therapist for instruction in use of orthoses (braces), splints, and supports for regions where weakness is disabling.
6. Instruct the patient to use energy conservation and work simplification methods.
7. Work cooperatively with occupational therapist to evaluate patient's needs and to advise on securing assistive devices (e.g., electrically powered wheelchair and bed, mechanical lift, etc.).
8. Teach family the techniques of positioning, turning, and transfers.
9. Teach pressure sore prevention (see p. 133).

B. Preventing Aspiration and Maintaining Nutritional Status
1. Observe patient swallowing fluids and look for regurgitation of fluid through nose—weakness of soft palate musculature prevents sealing off of nasopharynx during deglutition (swallowing).
2. Examine oral cavity—dysfunction of tongue indicated by food debris on lingual surface of teeth.
3. Look for food spillage from oral cavity—from weakness of lips, buccal muscles, and tongue.
4. Control saliva build-up as patient may be unable to move saliva to the back of his throat and swallow; use suctioning.

5. Encourage rest before meals to alleviate muscle fatigue.
6. Place patient in a bolt upright position with neck flexed (chin pointed toward the chest) to eat and drink—lessens risk of aspiration as in this position the airway is partially blocked by the esophagus.
7. Use a soft cervical collar if patient has difficulty holding his head up.
8. Give semi-solid foods—tend to hold together in a bolus form and are generally easier to swallow.
   a. Avoid easily aspirated, pureed foods and mucus-producing foods (milk).
   b. Offer very warm or very cold (not room temperature) food or drinks—makes use of temperature receptors in the mouth that are in part responsible for swallowing.
   c. Use soft foods that hold together (casseroles, stews, food with gravy).
   d. Do not wash down solids with fluids—may cause choking and aspiration.
9. Instruct patient to take a breath before swallowing, hold breath, exhale or cough after the swallow, and then swallow again.
   a. Turning the head to the side while swallowing may be helpful.
   b. Avoid talking while eating.
10. Look for signs and symptoms of chronic dehydration: malaise, decreased urine output, dry mouth, thick mucus, decreased skin turgor.
11. Advise patient/family to keep intake and output record to ensure adequate fluid intake; liquid intake is compromised as liquids fragment during swallowing and cause aspiration.
    a. Offer cold carbonated soft drinks—have more taste sensation than water.
    b. Offer Jello, popsicles, fruit sherberts, and fruit ices—help with liquid ingestion.
12. Make arrangements for home intravenous therapy as required.
13. Consider alternate feeding methods to maintain nutrition in patients with advanced dysphagia (nasogastric tube; feeding gastrostomy tube).

C. Monitoring and Managing Potential Respiratory Failure

1. Follow vital capacity measurements—vital capacity falling below 50 percent indicates considerable loss of muscular function.
2. Monitor for altered respiratory pattern during sleep: shallow respirations, fading in and out of sleep, nocturnal delirium, restlessness and anxiety—from chronic hypoxia.
3. Be attentive to complaint of inordinate fatigue in the absence of physical exertion—may herald the onset of respiratory failure.
4. Use techniques to enhance pulmonary function: upright position, suctioning of excessive secretions, chest physical therapy.
5. Work with respiratory therapist—incentive spirometry may be helpful in exercising respiratory muscles and keeping lungs inflated.
6. Prepare patient for intubation, tracheostomy, and mechanical ventilation when weakness of respiratory muscles leads to impaired gas exchange.
   Teach family the basic skills of ventilator therapy and other essentials of respiratory care.
7. If the patient decides against using a ventilator, he may consider making a "living will" to preserve his autonomy (not going on life-support; discontinuing life-support). Ideally, the patient should be made aware of options before ventilator use becomes necessary.

D. Enhancing Communication

1. *For patients with some speech abilities:*
   a. Refer to speech-language pathologist to maximize remaining potential for speech.
   b. Use mechanical speech aids; if possible the system should be tried before it is essential.
2. *When speech is lost:*
   a. Communication board (ALS Association newsletter [see 4., below] describes various communication devices), including eye-gaze communication boards.
   b. Use environmental control system—switch may be activated by slight movement of eyebrow, etc.
   c. Eye movement/eye blinks—may be the patient's only means of communication.
   d. Understand that the patient is alert and retains vision, ocular movement, intelligence, and consciousness, but he may be physically incapable of doing a solitary thing and cannot speak/swallow.
3. Have some type of signaling/alerting device. One possible source: National Association for Hearing and Speech Action, 10801 Rockville Pike, Rockville, MD 20852.

E. Enhancing Coping Abilities

1. Understand that the patient may have involuntary outbursts of forced laughing/crying unrelated to mood/surroundings (pseudobulbar affect).
2. Give the patient and family compassionate and caring support; problems are ever-changing.
3. Secure services of counselor, social worker, or ALS-experienced psychologist for family undergoing breakdown in communication.
4. Advise the family of helping services of the ALS Association, 15300 Ventura Boulevard, Suite 315, Sherman Oaks, CA 91403 (pamphlets, newsletter, patient care tips); and Muscular Dystrophy Association, 810 Seventh Avenue, New York, NY 10019 (services and equipment).

Guillain–Barré Syndrome
(Polyradiculoneuritis)

Guillain–Barré syndrome (polyradiculoneuritis) is an acute inflammatory demeylinating polyneuropathy of the peripheral nerves characterized by a rapid onset of weakness and often paralysis of extremities and respiratory muscles, abnormal sensations, and areflexia (loss of reflexes).

Pathophysiology

1. It is believed that Guillain–Barré syndrome (GBS) is an autoimmune disease of delayed hypersensitivity.
2. Viral infections may function as a trigger to set off the autoimmune response to damage the peripheral nerves.

Clinical Manifestations

1. Paresthesias—tingling, numbness, abnormal sensations, pain, vibrations, and "crawling" skin sensations.
2. Progressive muscle weakness, most often beginning

in legs; may progress to rapidly ascending paralysis involving the trunk, upper extremities, and facial muscles. Complete paralysis may develop.
3. Difficulty in chewing, swallowing and talking; facial paralysis—from cranial nerve involvement
4. Diminished or absent tendon reflexes; decrease in position and vibratory sense
5. Autonomic dysfunction—tachycardia, blood pressure changes (transient hypertension, orthostatic hypotension), bladder dysfunction
6. Pain, aching or cramping

Diagnostic Evaluation

1. Cerebrospinal fluid examination—shows elevated total protein
2. Electrodiagnostic testing—nerve conduction tests show slowing of conduction velocity in peripheral nerves

Management

1. Therapeutic plasmapheresis (plasma exchange)—produces temporary reduction in circulating antibodies
2. ECG monitoring and treatment of cardiac dysrhythmias
3. Analgesics and muscle relaxants—for joint and muscle pain and muscle spasms
4. Endotracheal intubation and mechanical ventilation—to prevent respiratory failure and minimize chance of aspiration and pneumonia
5. Rehabilitation

Nursing Assessment

1. Ask patient to identify most troubling difficulties: pain? dyspnea? burning sensations?
2. Take vital signs.
3. Inspect for paradoxic breathing (abdominal inversion during inspiration)—occurs secondary to diaphragmatic fatigue/impending paralysis.
4. Auscultate lungs for diminished breath sounds/crackles.
5. Determine if patient can cough and swallow.
6. Assess speech for effort, halting during conversation, and nasal quality.
7. Observe the patient swallowing.
8. Look for extremity weakness. Note facial expression and signs of facial weakness.

Nursing Diagnoses

1. Ineffective breathing pattern related to impending weakness/paralysis of respiratory muscles and neuromuscular respiratory failure.
2. Impaired physical mobility related to paralysis.
3. Impaired verbal communication related to cranial nerve dysfunction.
4. Altered nutrition (less than body requirements) related to inability to swallow secondary to cranial nerve dysfunction
5. Fear (of death, permanent disability, helplessness) related to sudden catastrophic illness and complete dependency.

Complications

1. Respiratory failure
2. Cardiac dysrhythmias
3. Complications of paralysis (pressure sores; contractures)
4. Urinary retention

Nursing Interventions

A. Maintaining Breathing When Rapidly Ascending Paralysis Develops

1. Anticipate the risk of respiratory failure; observe progression of patient's weakness and paralysis.
2. Monitor for pulse over 120 beats/minute or under 70 beats/minute. Evaluate respiratory rate > 30 breaths/minute—warning signals of impending respiratory failure.
3. Evaluate repeated measurements of vital capacity—gives warning that respiratory muscles are becoming weak
4. Watch for breathlessness while talking, shallow and irregular breathing, increasing pulse rate, and *change* in respiratory pattern.
5. Prepare patient for intubation and ventilatory support when signs of deteriorating respiratory function are noted.
6. Talk to the patient and explain what is being done—to alleviate patient's anxiety.

B. Compensating for Loss of Mobility

1. Position the patient correctly to avoid further damage to susceptible peripheral nerves, prevent contractures, and pressure sores.
2. Maintain joint mobility—range of motion exercises.
3. Place padding over patient's elbows and heads of fibula—patient has potential to develop compression neuropathies.
4. Elevate lower legs (35–40 degrees) periodically—to relieve edema.
5. Observe and encourage patient as he progresses from passive to active exercises, tilt table regimen, gait training, etc., depending on his clinical status.
6. Attend to bladder and bowel problems.

C. Coping With Communication Loss

1. Work cooperatively with speech-language pathologist to develop a communication plan as patient is often unable to talk, laugh, cry because of paralysis, tracheostomy. Cards, communication board, computer devices activated by eye movement, etc. are available.
2. Have some type of call or alarm system; check on patient frequently when he is unable to speak—fosters sense of well-being.
3. Maintain eye contact while speaking to patient.
4. Use diversional therapy (family visits, casette tapes, music) to alleviate frustration.

D. Maintaining Nutrition

1. Ausculate lower abdomen for bowel sounds.
2. Use nasogastric tube for feeding or total parenteral alimentation; reassure the patient that this is short-term management.
3. Be prepared to resume oral feedings when pharyngeal muscles are strong enough to prevent aspiration.

E. Relieving Fear

1. Offer continuing reassurance, explanations, and high-level care as the patient is alert, anxious, and has vision and hearing.
2. Encourage the patient to take a "day at a time"; patients generally stabilize for 1–4 weeks and then improve.
3. Help patient aim for specific goals during rehabilitation period.
4. Reassure him by pointing out gains being made. Chart improvements as this allows patient to assess progress.

Discharge Planning/Patient Education

1. Reinforce realization that convalescence may be lengthy and that recovery may continue from 3 months to 2 years.
2. Encourage breathing exercises to redevelop well-coordinated patterns of respiration.
3. Teach the patient to check feet for injuries as minor trauma may go unnoticed because of sensory impairment.
4. Avoid excessive weight gain—stresses an already compromised motor system.
5. Avoid overfatigue—decreases accuracy of motor coordination.
6. If indicated encourage career evaluation and counseling; career change may be indicated if recovery of neurologic function is prolonged.
7. Patient may need referral to rehabilitation center for neuromuscular re-education.
8. Contact: Guillain-Barre Syndrome Support Group, International, P.O. Box 262, Wynnewood, PA 19096, for educational materials, newsletters, and list of GBS chapters.

Evaluation

1. Achieves effective breathing pattern; no signs of aspiration or respiratory failure.
2. Demonstrates improved mobility; tries to participate during exercise sessions.
3. Able to communicate needs.
4. Able to swallow without choking.
5. Coping with fear; making plans for future.

Spinal Cord Injury

Spinal cord injury is a traumatic injury to the spinal cord that may vary from a mild cord concussion with transient numbness to immediate and permanent quadriplegia. The most common sites are the cervical areas C-5, C-6, and C-7 and the junction of the thoracic and lumbar vertebrae (T-12, L-1). Traumatic injury of the spinal cord may result in loss of function (paralysis) below the level of cord injury. There is usually a high frequency of associated injuries and medical complications. Ideally, patients should be admitted to regional spinal cord centers after condition has stabilized.

Pathogenesis of Spinal Cord Injury

1. Damage to the spinal cord ranges from transient concussion to contusion, laceration, and compression (either alone or in combination), to complete transection of the cord.
2. The cord's response to injury is ischemia, edema, and hemorrhage that lead to an irreversible cycle of progressive destruction unless there is appropriate intervention.

Causes

Trauma—automobile and motorcycle accidents; falls; stab wounds; diving injuries; sporting, industrial and agricultural accidents.

Clinical Manifestations

1. Acute pain or tenderness in neck and back
2. Numbness, tingling, burning, muscle weakness, twitching
3. Respiratory problems
4. Sensory loss and motor paralysis below the level of the lesion
5. Marked reduction of blood pressure—from loss of peripheral and vascular resistance
6. Loss of bladder and bowel control; usually urinary retention and bladder distention
7. Loss of sweating and vasomotor tone below level of cord lesion

Diagnostic Evaluation

1. X-ray of spinal column
2. Electrophysiologic monitoring methods (somotosensory evoked potentials)—reflect the function of neural pathways

Management

Requires a multidisciplinary approach; majority of patients have associated multisystem injuries.

1. Resuscitation, oxygenation and achievement of cardiovascular stability.
   a. Intubation and mechanical ventilation if patient is hypoventilting, unable to handle secretions or comatose—low O_2 and high CO_2 levels have detrimental effects.
   b. Diaphragmatic pacing (electric stimulation of phrenic nerve)—considered for patient with high cervical injury.
2. Ensuring perfusion of spinal cord with restoration of blood pressure, administration of naloxone, and local cooling of cord.
3. Realignment and stabilization of injured elements of vertebral column by traction and immobilization or by surgical decompression or reduction (see below).
4. Continuing neurologic assessment to determine level and severity of injury.
5. Insertion of nasogastric tube attached to low suction.
6. Insertion of urethral catheter for loss of bladder tone and areflexia leading to retention; intermittent catheterization instituted as early as possible.
7. Anticoagulant therapy (heparin; warfarin) if no contraindication—as prophylaxis of thromboembolism.

Complications

1. *Spinal shock*
   a. Represents a sudden loss of continuity between spinal cord and higher nerve centers.
   b. There is a complete loss of all reflex, motor, sensory, and autonomic activity below the level of the lesion.
2. Respiratory insufficiency; respiratory failure
3. Cardiac arrest
4. Thromboembolic complications
5. Infections: respiratory; urinary tract; pressure sores; osteomyelitis (usually from contiguous spread from an infected pressure sore)

Nursing Assessment

A. Motor and Sensory Function

1. Evaluate the patient constantly for motor and sensory changes below the level of injury.
   a. Motor and sensory loss occurs from cord edema, hemorrhage, etc., which may further compromise cord function.
   b. Document findings carefully.
2. Test motor ability by requesting the patient to spread fingers, squeeze examiner's hand, move toes, etc.

3. Test sensation by pinching the skin, starting at shoulder level and progressing down the sides of all extremities. Ascertain when the patient feels pinching sensation.
4. Note presence/absence of level of sweating.

B. General Neurological Function

1. Report immediately any decrease in neurologic function.
2. Keep a neurologic assessment record and flow sheet that includes grading of muscle function/strength.
3. Observe for symptoms of progressive neurologic damage.
   a. Symptoms of cord compression depend on level at which compression occurs.
   b. Clinical symptoms of cord compression are indistinguishable from those of cord edema.
   c. Loss of sensation.
   d. Inability to move extremities.
4. Look at functions that remain intact.

C. Other Assessment Parameters

1. Monitor vital signs—to observe for deteriorating cardiovascular status and presence of neurogenic shock.
2. Obtain psychosocial information: support system; behavior patterns of sleep, activities, work, recreation; coping methods; sexual concerns.

Nursing Diagnoses

1. Ineffective breathing pattern related to evolving diaphragmatic or intercostal or abdominal muscle paralysis; impairment of diaphragmatic function by gastric dilatation; and inability to cough and control secretions.
2. Impaired physical mobility related to motor and sensory dysfunction.
3. Potential impairment of skin integrity related to immobility and sensory loss.
4. Urinary retention related to inability to void spontaneously secondary to spinal shock; spinal cord lesion.
5. Altered bowel elimination (constipation) related to atonic bowel secondary to autonomic disruption.
6. Altered comfort related to prolonged immobility, presence of cervical tongs, traction.
7. Other possible nursing diagnosis—powerlessness related to losses incurred by the injury and forced dependency.

Nursing Interventions

A. Assessing for Complications

1. Spinal shock, respiratory insufficiency, cardiac arrest, thrombembolic complications, infections
2. Assess for signs of spinal shock
   a. Falling blood pressure
   b. Paralysis and lack of sensation below level of cord injury
   c. Bladder distention—from paralysis of bladder
   d. Bowel distention—caused by depression of reflexes; retroperitoneal hemorrhage may occur with fracture of low back, producing paralytic ileus
   e. Hyperthermia—during periods of spinal shock, the patient does not perspire on the paralyzed portions of his body since sympathetic activity is blocked.

B. Assuring Adequate Breathing

1. Assess the breathing pattern and maintain airway—patients with injuries at high levels are at risk for respiratory failure.
   a. Assess strength of cough; patient with expiratory muscle paralysis cannot develop enough pleural pressure for adequate cough.
   b. Measure vital capacity, tidal volume, and inspiratory force and monitor arterial blood gas values—guides to determine respiratory insufficiency.
2. Ensure proper hydration and humidification—to prevent secretions from becoming viscid and difficult to mobilize.
3. Suction secretions judiciously—can stimulate the vagus nerve, producing bradycardia, which can result in cardiac arrest.
4. Monitor for signs of respiratory infection: cough, fever, dyspnea.
5. Work with respiratory therapist when patient is placed on a ventilator.
6. Implement the following regimens when appropriate: change position every 2 hours, deep breathing exercises accompanied by incentive spirometry, chest percussion, and assisted cough.
7. For the halo patient, tape the wrench to halo vest in case the vest must be removed for cardiopulmonary resuscitation.

C. Attaining/Maintaining Mobility

1. See Cervical Traction for application of tongs/halo devices.
2. Transfer the patient to a turning frame (Stryker) or continuous horizontal rotating bed. If none is available, place the patient on a firm mattress with a bedboard under the mattress.
3. Maintain the patient in proper alignment to prevent deformities.
4. The patient may be placed on a kinetic treatment table, which rotates every 4–5 minutes, thus eliminating pressure on skin surface, providing access for patient care, and maintaining correct body alignment.
5. Turn patient as directed—patients with lesions above the midthoracic level have loss of sympathetic control of peripheral vasoconstrictor activity, leading to hypotension.
   a. Monitor blood pressure when positions are changed.
6. Employ care when placing the patient in the prone position—improper position on the headrest can cause pressure on the globe of the eye, resulting in retinal ischemia and blindness.
7. Work cooperatively with physical therapist to perform passive range-of-motion exercises as directed (usually within 48–72 hours)—to preserve joint motion and stimulate circulation and prevent contractures and other complications.

D. Preserving Skin Integrity

1. Maintain constant surveillance for pressure sores—inadequate peripheral circulation, loss of feeling, and immobility may cause pressure sores to develop within a few hours.
2. Turn every 2 hours (using turning frame) if patient can be turned—to obtain complete pressure relief; patients with initial vasovagal instability, as well as associated injuries may not tolerate positional changes.
3. Inspect the skin each time the patient is turned for redness, the perineum for soiling, and the catheter for drainage.
   a. Inspect the back of head periodically for signs of pressure.
   b. Assess for correct body alignment and comfort.
4. Wash the skin with mild soap
   a. Rinse well and blot dry.

b. Keep pressure-sensitive areas well-lubricated and soft with bland cream or lotion.

5. Teach patient to avoid uninterrupted sitting/lying, movements that generate shear forces (sliding across bed).

6. See page 133 for prevention and management of pressure sores.

E. Promoting Urinary Elimination

1. Monitor for urinary retention—from areflexic bladder.
2. Use intermittent catheterization early in acute phase, if possible.
    a. Avoid overdistention of bladder—after spinal injury, the bladder may lack functional nerve supply; overstretching of bladder may produce permanent damage.
    b. If intermittent catheterization is not feasible, insert an indwelling catheter.
3. Prevent urinary tract infection by meticulous attention to catheterization technique.
    a. Monitor temperature on routine basis—fever is most commonly caused by urinary tract infection.
    b. Obtain a urine culture; monitor urine for color change, cloudy appearance.
4. Remind patient to keep a record of fluid intake, voiding pattern, amounts of residual urine following catheterization, appearance of urine and any symptoms that may be occurring.
5. See page 693 for the management of the patient with a neurogenic bladder.

F. Acquiring Bowel Control

1. Observe for abdominal distention and auscultate for presence or absence of bowel sounds—immediately after spinal cord injury the patient usually has a paralytic ileus due to neurogenic paralysis of the bowel.
2. Monitor for fecal impaction—often presents as diarrhea, as stool proximal to the impaction is liquified and moves around the fecal mass.
3. After bowel activity returns:
    a. Encourage intake of high-calorie, high-protein and high-fiber diet—fiber increases bulk and speeds passage of formed stool through rectosigmoid colon, thus optimizing bowel function.
    b. Institute a bowel program (p. 143) as early as possible.

G. Increasing Mobility and Independence

1. Participate in program designed according to the patient's neurologic deficit.
2. An exercise conditioning regimen is started early.
3. Muscle-strengthening exercises for shoulder depressors, maintenance of sitting balance, getting in and out of wheelchair (or whatever is possible for the individual patient).
4. The period of immobilization is determined by the patient's condition. Mobilize only upon physician's request—if the patient has partial cord function, activity may produce further cord injury.
5. Anticipate that four-poster brace, neck brace, or molded collar is usually applied when the patient is mobilized after traction is removed.
6. Provide on-going support to enhance the patient's feelings of self-worth.
7. See page 618 for rehabilitation of the patient with a permanent spinal cord injury (paraplegic patient).

Evaluation

1. Maintains effective respiratory function
2. Demonstrates beginning adjustment to impaired physical mobility

3. Absence of skin breakdown
4. Absence of urinary retention or infection
5. Has attained bowel function
6. Is not complaining of discomfort

Management of the Patient With Cervical Spine Injury

1. To manage a cervical spine injury, there must be immediate immobilization, early reduction, and stabilization of the vertebral column.
2. To reduce the fracture dislocation and maintain alignment of the cervical spine, some form of skeletal traction (skeletal tongs/calipers; halo-vest technique) is used, or open reduction (surgery) may be required.

Cervical Traction (Fig. 24-8)

A. Skeletal Tongs

1. A variety of skeletal tongs are in use; spring-loaded Gardner-Wells and Heifitz tongs require no predrilled holes into the skull; Crutchfield and Vinke tongs are inserted through holes made with a special drill under local anesthesia.
2. Traction is applied to the tongs by weights (4.5–9 kg. [10–20 lbs.]) or more, depending on the patient's size.
3. The traction is gradually increased by addition of weights—as the amount of traction is increased, the spaces between the intervertebral discs widen, and the vertebrae slip back into position. Reduction will take place after correct alignment has been regained.
4. X-rays are taken after each addition of weight until reduction is obtained; monitor the patient carefully as weights are added.
5. When reduction is obtained, the weights are gradually removed until the amount of weight needed to maintain the alignment is obtained.
6. Keep traction tongs several inches from top of bed and allow weights to hang free—to prevent interference with traction.

B. Halo Devices

1. Halo devices consist of a stainless steel "halo ring," which is fixed to the skull by 4 pins. The ring is attached to a removable halo vest (lined with sheepskin or Kodel liner) which suspends the weight of the unit circumferentially around the chest. A metal frame connects the ring to the vest.
2. The halo ring may be used initially as a traction device or the ring and vest may be applied following removal of skull tongs/calipers.
3. Halo devices afford immobilization of the cervical spine while allowing early mobilization and participation in the rehabilitation program.

Nursing Interventions

A. Maintaining Skin Integrity

1. *For the patient in a halo device:*
    a. Inspect under halo vest; look for excessive perspiration, redness, skin blistering, especially on bony prominences (scapulae, ribs, shoulders, spinous processes).
    b. Have the patient lie prone for short periods to relieve pressure. Wash skin under vest; dry with dry washcloth. Open vests at sides to wash and dry skin; do not allow liner to become wet because this will cause skin problems.
    c. Avoid putting powder inside vest—may contribute to development of pressure sores.

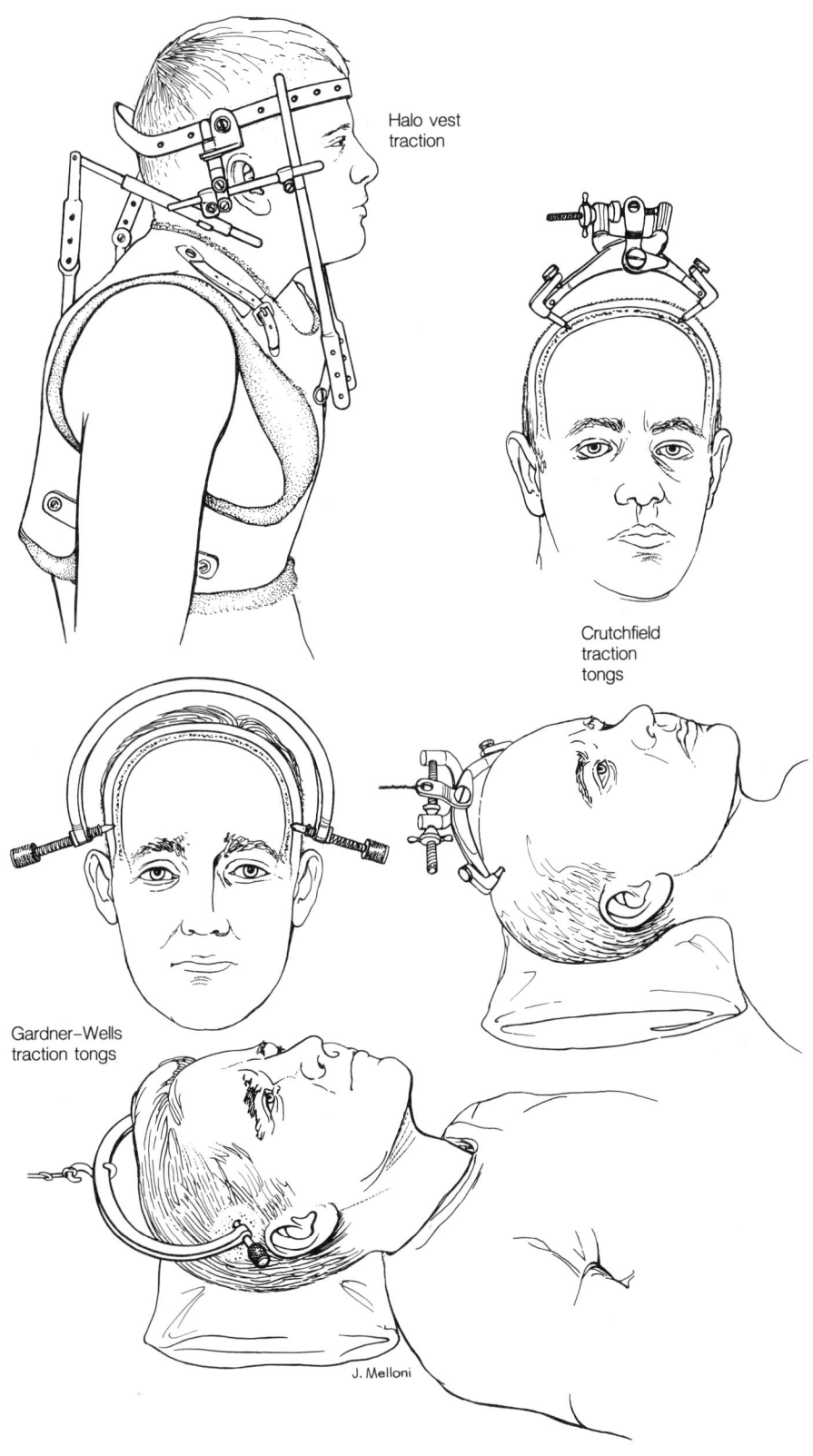

Halo vest traction

Crutchfield traction tongs

Gardner–Wells traction tongs

J. Melloni

Figure 24-8. *Methods of cervical traction.*

d. Turn the patient and his brace as a unit; do not use the halo or vest to turn, lift, or reposition the patient.
2. For the patients with skull tongs or callipers:
   a. Inspect tong sites for signs of infection.
      (1) Shave the hair around tongs.
      (2) Cleanse areas around the tong sites.
   b. Check back of head for signs of pressure; massage back of head at intervals, taking care not to move the neck.

B. Attaining Comfort—For the halo patient:
1. Be aware that the patient may be initially distressed by bizarre appearance of the halo but usually adapts readily to device.
2. Anticipate that the patient may experience a slight headache or minor pain around the skull pins for several days following application.
3. Cleanse areas around the pin sites daily; observe for redness, drainage, and pain.
   a. Observe for any loosening of pins; if one of pins become detached, stabilize the patient's head in a neutral position while another person notifies the surgeon.
   b. Have a torque screw driver available in case the screws on the frame need tightening.
4. Supervise the patient's activities (sitting, standing) initially because the weight of the halo may cause problems of balance, decreased peripheral field of vision, inability to see feet.

The Patient With Paraplegia

Paraplegia is loss of motion and sensation in the lower extremities.

Quadriplegia (tetraplegia) is loss of motion and sensation involving both upper and lower extremities.

Causes

1. Trauma—accidents, gunshot wounds
2. Spinal cord lesions (intervertebral disc, tumor, vascular lesions)
3. Multiple sclerosis
4. Infections and abscesses of spinal cord
5. Congenital defects

Long-Term Complications of Paraplegia

A. Autonomic Dysreflexia (autonomic hyperreflexia)
1. Syndrome occurring in patients with spinal cord lesions at or above T-6.
2. Characterized by exaggerated autonomic responses to local stimuli below level of injury.
   a. Distended bladder or bowel.
   b. Stimulation of skin (tactile, pain, thermal).
   c. Distention or contraction of visceral organs.
   d. Possible immediate and dangerous elevation of arterial blood pressure.
   e. Clinical syndrome characterized by pounding headache, profuse sweating, nasal congestion, piloerection (goose flesh), bradycardia, severe hypertension.

Management

Goal
To remove the triggering stimulus and avoid possible serious complications.

NURSING ALERT: Autonomic dysreflexia is considered an emergency.

1. Place patient in sitting position to help lower the blood pressure and diminish intracranial pressure.
2. Examine bladder for distention.
   a. Drain the bladder via catheter.
   b. Do not irrigate catheter with more than 30 ml. of irrigating solution.
   c. Obtain urine sample as urinary tract infection may be the cause.
3. Insert ointment containing a local anesthetic into rectum if fecal mass is present
   Mass is removed manually *after* symptoms subside.
4. Remove any other stimuli that may be triggering episodes; loosen tight clothing, leg straps, etc.
5. Give emergency antihypertensive medication as prescribed.
6. Monitor blood pressure every 3–5 minutes during episode.
7. Tag the patient's chart indicating he has had an episode of autonomic dysreflexia.

B. Spasticity
1. A syndrome characterized by an increase in the stretch reflex due to damage to the motor pathways in the nervous system.
2. Spasticity occurs 2 weeks to 3 months after injury starting with flexor activity followed by extensor spasticity—interferes with ADL, turning, transfers, sitting, and skin care.
3. Nursing interventions and patient education (for spasticity)
   a. Provide relaxed and calm environment.
   b. Correct any problems aggravating the spasticity (pressure sores; inadequate bladder/bowel emptying; apprehension). Teach the patient to search for cause of sudden increase of spasticity.
   c. Allow time for transfers and positioning.
   d. Maintain joint range of motion with slow, smooth movements.
   e. Avoid temperature extremes.
   f. Encourage patient to participate with prescribed regimen (diazepam, baclofen, dantrolene), relaxation training, biofeedback.
4. Surgical intervention includes epidural spinal cord stimulation or dorsal rhizotomy.

C. Other Long-Term Complications
1. Pressure sores
2. Urinary tract infection; urinary calculi; urethrocutaneous fistula
3. Heterotrophic ossification—formation of bone in abnormal anatomic location, usually soft tissues (most often in hips and knees)
4. Ankylosis of joints

Assessment

See Assessment of Spinal Cord Injury, page 614.

Nursing Diagnoses

1. Ineffective individual coping related to physical and psychological sequelae of paraplegia.
2. Compromised family coping related to care of permanently disabled member.

3. Impaired physical mobility related to permanent neurologic deficits.
4. Potential impaired skin integrity related to sensory deficits, lack of mobility, and spasticity.
5. Urinary incontinence/retention related to spinal cord injury.
6. Altered bowel elimination (constipation) related to effects of spinal cord injury.
7. Potential for sexual dysfunction related to neurologic deficit

Nursing Interventions

A. Promoting Coping Strategies

1. Allow the patient to work through his feelings about his disability at own pace (unless responses continue to be exaggerated or maladaptive).
2. Remember that learning to live with a disability is a life-long process.
3. Engage the family/significant other(s) as facilitators and collaborators.
4. See Psychological Reactions to a Disability, page 127.

B. Helping the Family Make Adaptive Changes

1. Remember that the family is faced with accepting the patient as "permanently different"; may cause frustration/isolation, alientation, resentment of family lifestyle changes, guilt-ridden death wishes for patient, overwhelmed and overburdened feelings.
2. Assess developmental needs of family members—at what developmental stage was each family member when patient became ill?
3. Focus on developmental issues and acquisition of strategies for long-term management of the patient.
4. Assist family to express feelings and to maintain their ego strengths.
5. Encourage family in making adaptive changes, in seeking social support, in personal health maintenance, stress management, respite care, counseling, and emotional support.

C. Establishing Optimum Functioning

1. Prepare for weight-bearing activities.
   a. The patient with complete cord severance should start early weight-bearing to decrease osteoporotic changes in long bones and to reduce incidence of urinary infections and the formation of renal calculi.
   b. Apply elastic hose from toes to thigh or a Jobst counterpressure leotard—to prevent pooling of blood in abdominal area.
   c. A patient with spinal cord paralysis lacks vasomotor tone in the lower extremities and will become hypotensive in the upright position.
   d. Use tilt table—to help the patient overcome vasomotor instability and tolerate upright posture.
   e. *Or* use high-back reclining wheelchair with extension leg rests; raise backrest slowly and lower leg rest gradually over a period of 7–10 days.
   f. Build the unaffected part of body to optimal strength, endurance, and coordination—to prepare for transfer and mobilization activities.
   g. Use assistive devices to allow fuller patient participation.

D. Maintaining Skin Integrity

> **NURSING ALERT:** The threat of pressure sores persists throughout the patient's life.

1. Emphasize that the patient is responsible for the health of his skin.
2. Teach the patient the following:
   a. Carry out regular skin inspection using a mirror for hard-to-see areas.
   b. Participate in weight shift and pressure-relieving liftoffs (usually every 15–30 minutes).
   c. Avoid uninterrupted sitting/lying.
   d. Avoid movements that generate shear forces (e.g., sliding across bed during transfers).
   e. Avoid obesity, which compounds risk of increased vertical pressure.

E. Promoting Bladder Control

1. Continue with bladder-training program. See Neurogenic Bladder, page 692.
2. Monitor for signs of infection: urine color changes, cloudy urine; fever.
3. Teach patient to monitor fluid intake, voiding patterns, quality of urine, changes in medication and diet, type of catheter used—to determine reason for infection.
4. Maintain adequate urine flow by drinking ample fluids; keep urine output at about 2000 ml./24 hours.
5. Teach patient to keep perineal area clean and dry; change cotton underwear daily.

F. Promoting Bowel Control

1. Start bowel-training program (see p. 143).
2. Promote regular habit time, sufficient fluid and fiber intake, use of glycerin suppositories, and digital stimulation (manual stimulation of anal sphincter) as part of bowel management.
3. Avoid fecal impaction.
   a. Insure total evacuation of fecal material from lower bowel.
   b. Employ regular digital examination of rectum—to determine presence of impacted fecal material.

G. Finding Sexual Expression

1. Most cord-injured persons can have some form of meaningful sexual expression and relationship, but some modifications will have to be made to cope with anxiety. Implantation of penile prosthesis may be considered.
2. The female patient may experience little sensation during intercourse, but fertility and ability to bear children are usually not affected.
3. Counseling and small group meetings provide an opportunity to share feelings, sexual concerns, give and receive information, and develop positive attitudes and adjustment.
4. See Sexuality in Rehabilitation, page 128

Discharge Planning/Patient Education

1. Help patient and family to continue to set collaborative goals reflecting individual priorities. The ultimate goal is to attain maximum function considering the neurologic deficit.
2. Emphasize that a patient with a spinal cord injury is at special risk during the first few weeks at home.
3. Reinforce that pressure sores, contractures, urinary tract infections, and deconditioning are life-long risks.
4. Support the services provided by other rehabilitation team members: rehabilitation engineering services, occupational therapy, vocational rehabilitation and counseling, social worker, recreational therapist, driver education, sex therapists, etc.
5. See that the patient and family have continuing access to counseling services to help cope with the impact of the disability.

6. The patient requires continuing life-long follow-up by the rehabilitation team—new problems can develop that take their toll in additional physical impairment, time, morale, and money.

Evaluation

1. Coping with altered life-style; expressing feelings
2. Family seeking professional and supportive services
3. Achieving modified mobility
4. Attains/maintains skin integrity
5. Attains/maintains bladder control
6. Has achieved reflex bowel functioning
7. Seeking counseling for sexual concerns

Herniation of Intervertebral Disc
(Ruptured Disc)

Herniation of the intervertebral disc is a protrusion of the nucleus of the disc into the annulus (fibrous ring around the disc), with subsequent nerve compression. The herniation may occur in any portion of the spine: cervical, lumbar, or thoracic (infrequent).

Causes

1. Degeneration
2. Trauma (accidents, strain, repeated minor stresses)
3. Congenital predisposition

Clinical Manifestations

Depend on location, size, rate of development (acute or chronic), and effect on surrounding structures

A. Cervical Disc

1. Pain and stiffness in neck, top of shoulders, and in region of scapulae
2. Pain in upper extremities and head
3. Paresthesia and numbness of upper extremities

B. Lumbar Disc

1. Low back pain accompanied by varying degrees of sensory and motor impairment
2. Pain radiating from the low back into the buttock and down the leg (sciatica)
3. Postural deformity of lumbar spine
4. Positive straight-leg raising test
   a. With the patient lying supine, the leg is raised with knee extended
   b. Test is positive if pain occurs in leg below the knee or if radicular (spinal nerve root) pain ensues
5. Weakness and asymmetric reflexes
6. Sensory loss

Diagnostic Evaluation

1. Myelogram—demonstrates area of pressure and localizes herniation of disc
2. CT or MRI scan
3. Electromyography—localizes specific spinal nerve involved

Management

A. Bedrest on a Firm Mattress—to reduce the weight load and gravitational forces, thereby freeing the disc from stress

B. Pharmacotherapy

1. Anti-inflammatory drugs (steroids [prednisone] or nonsteroidal anti-inflammatory drugs [ibuprofen; naproxen])—to counter inflammation of affected nerve roots and supporting tissues
2. Muscle relaxants; analgesics for pain

C. Physical Therapy—to reduce muscle spasm, increase soft tissue extensibility, and promote relaxation

D. Surgical Intervention

1. If significant neurologic deficit from nerve root compression occurs, for loss of bladder/bowel function, and for unremitting and recurrent pain
2. Operative removal of disc fragments. See Management of Patient Following Disc Surgery, page 621.

E. Chemonucleolysis (for lumbar disc)

1. Injection of chymopapain into herniated lumbar disc.
2. Has a proteolytic action that causes loss of water and proteolycans from the disc—reduces the size of the herniated material and relieves pressure on the nerve root.
3. Postinjection nursing care includes bedrest, monitoring for neurologic dysfunction, administration of analgesics, and gradual ambulation.
4. Complications of chemonucleolysis: anaphylaxis, paraplegia, subarachnoid hemorrhage.
5. Patient education
   a. Teach patient that injected disc will heal as any injured tissues, with inflammation lasting for several days, followed by deposition of collagen scar and its maturation—healing process may take up to 3–4 weeks.
   b. Restrict sitting until healing has taken place.
   c. Wear supportive shoes.
   d. Increase activities gradually.

Nursing Interventions: Cervical Disc Herniations

A. Immobilize and Rest the Cervical Spine—by one of the following methods:

1. *Bedrest*—reduces inflammation and edema in soft tissues around disc, relieving pressure on nerve roots; relieves cervical spine of supporting weight of head.
2. *Cervical collar*—allows maximal opening of intervertebral foramina.
   a. Collar should hold the head in a neutral or slightly flexed position.
   b. Inspect under the collar at intervals for skin rash.
   c. In acute herniation, the collar may have to be worn night and day until pain subsides (2–3 weeks).
   d. Cervical isometric exercises are started when the patient is pain-free—to strengthen neck musculature in preparation for "weaning" from collar.
3. *Cervical traction* (accomplished by head halter attached to a pulley and a weight)—increases vertebral separation and thus relieves pressure on the nerve roots.
   a. Cervical traction should be comfortable.
   b. Keep head of bed elevated and make sure that traction is in alignment.
   c. Inspect for skin burns from cervical halter; pad under the halter as necessary.
   d. Encourage male patient not to shave since beard offers a form of padding; shaving may cause irritation.
4. Brace.

B. Reducing Inflammation

1. Administer prescribed anti-inflammatory medications—to treat inflammatory response.
   Encourage food or antacid with anti-inflammatory agents to prevent gastrointestinal irritation.
2. Administer prescribed muscle relaxant
   a. To interrupt cycle of muscle spasm and allow for patient comfort.
   b. To increase range of motion of cervical spine.
3. Administer prescribed analgesic medications and sedatives—to control discomfort and anxiety often associated with cervical disc disease.
4. Teach family to apply moist hot compresses (10–20 minutes, several times daily) to back of neck—to increase blood flow to muscles and promote relaxation of the patient and spastic muscles.

C. Discharge Planning/Patient Education (cervical disc)

It may take 6 weeks to recuperate from disc herniation. Instruct the patient as follows:

1. Avoid extreme flexion, extension, and rotation of the neck while working.
2. Keep head in a neutral position while sleeping.
   a. Pillow should be filled with feathers or down.
   b. Sleep on side or back; do not sleep prone.
   c. Avoid excessive neck flexion—do not prop up in bed with several pillows.
3. Avoid excessive automobile riding during acute phase—vibration has adverse effect on spine.

Nursing Interventions: Lumbar Disc Herniations

Majority of disc herniations occur at L4–L5 or L5–S1 interspace because these are the levels of maximal movements between the lumbar spine and the pelvis

A. Reducing Pain

1. The patient is encouraged to remain on bedrest (usually at home with limited ambulation to bathroom)—recumbency reduces the pressure on the disc to half that of sitting.
   a. Encourage patient to assume a comfortable position, usually semi-Fowler's with moderate hip and knee flexion or side-lying position with knees flexed and a pillow between the legs.
   b. Ambulation is permitted when inflammatory reaction and edema have subsided; ambulation progressively increased if there are no symptoms.
   c. Encourage patient to continue taking prescribed muscle relaxant drugs (muscle spasm is prominent in acute phase), anti-inflammatory and analgesic agents.
2. Instruct family member in the use of heat and massage to relax muscle spasm and for analgesic and sedative effects.

B. Self-Monitoring for Neurologic Deficit

Instruct the patient to report immediately any of the following:

1. Diminishing or loss of neurologic function below level of disc, including loss of bladder/bowel control. Immediate surgery is required.
2. Unrelieved, acute pain.
3. Muscle weakness and atrophy.

C. Patient Education

1. Encourage the patient to do exercises after acute symptoms subside: (1) exercises to strengthen abdominal muscles and (2) gentle stretching exercises to improve the suppleness and elasticity of the paraspinal muscles and ligaments.
   a. Start exercises gently and gradually.
   b. Discontinue exercises if pain worsens.
2. Advise the patient to sleep on side with knees and hips flexed (pillow between knees).
   a. Do not sleep in prone position—hyperextends the spine.
   b. Pick up loads correctly (bend knees, keep back straight, avoid lifting anything above the elbows) and keep load close to body.
   c. Avoid lifting while back is in a flexed or rotated position.
3. Avoid lifting until healing has taken place—application of stress on the disc nucleus and annulus before complete healing causes chronicity and recurrence.
4. Encourage proper posture while standing, sitting, walking, and working.
5. Carry out a weight control program—the obese person with protruding abdomen and lordotic posture has chronic low back strain.
6. Undertake a formal conditioning program under supervision when permitted—to improve physical fitness and exercise tolerance.
7. See also patient education, low back pain, page 803, and management of the patient following disc surgery, below.

Management of the Patient Following Disc Surgery

Surgical excision of a herniated disc is performed when progressive neurologic deterioration occurs or if pain becomes unrelenting or incapacitating.

Types of Disc Surgery

1. *Discectomy*—excision of an intervertebral disc.
2. *Laminectomy* with excision of herniated disc material
   a. Removal of small amount of lamina (arch of bone covering the spinal canal) to expose nerve root.
   b. Allows inspection of the spinal canal and identification and removal of herniated material.
3. *Spinal fusion*
   a. Consolidation of two adjacent vertebrae to prevent movement.
   b. Bone graft is used to fuse the spinal vertebral process.
4. *Microsurgical discectomy*—involves use of microsurgical techniques with a small incision to excise herniated disc material.

Preoperative Nursing Assessment

1. Learn as much as possible about the patient who has the pain.
2. Note complaints of pain, paresthesia, and muscle spasm—to have a baseline for postoperative comparison.
3. Evaluate movement of extremities.
4. Determine if there is any bladder or bowel dysfunction.

Postoperative Nursing Interventions

A. Cervical Disc

1. Check neurologic and vital signs at frequent intervals—there is always the possibility of respiratory compro-

mise (from tracheal edema, pneumothorax, airway obstruction).
  a. Watch for hoarseness—from recurrent laryngeal nerve injury, resulting in inability to cough effectively and eliminate respiratory secretions.
  b. Observe for dysphagia (possibly from edema of the esophagus); offer a blenderized soft diet.
2. Promote patient comfort.
  a. Be aware that a sore throat will be a major complaint.
    (1) Give throat spray, throat lozenges as directed to relieve pain.
    (2) Do not give any spray or throat lozenges that numb the throat, since this may cause choking.
    (3) Humidify room air.
3. Protect bone graft (if fusion has been part of procedure).
  a. Prevent extremes of flexion and extension of neck.
  b. Use cervical collar to eliminate unnecessary movement.
4. Watch for sudden reappearance of radicular (root) pain—indicative of nerve root compression from slipping of bone graft or collapsing of disc space (if bone grafting has not been done).

B. Lumbar Disc

1. Carry out periodic neurologic examinations and check for any new deficit.
2. Assess sensation, motor power, color, and temperature of extremities—postoperative neurologic deficits may result from nerve root injury.
3. Check vital signs and inspect wound for evidence of hemorrhage—vascular injury is a complication of disc surgery.
4. Assess for signs of urinary retention.
5. Administer prescribed analgesics; discomfort in immediate postoperative period may vary from mild to severe pain.
6. Explain to the patient that there may be varying degrees of pain and sensory manifestations in the legs (sciatica-type pain) due to temporary inflammatory changes, edema, and swelling of compressed nerve.
7. Position the patient effectively.
  a. Use pillow under head and elevate the knee rest slightly—slight knee flexion relaxes muscles of the back.
  b. Encourage the patient to move and turn from side to side to relieve pressure.
  c. Instruct the patient to turn as a unit while keeping a pillow between the legs when turning.
  d. Place pillow between legs in side-lying position.
  e. Avoid sitting, except for defecation—to prevent compression.
8. Encourage ambulation as soon as patient is able (usually the day after surgery).
  a. Instruct the patient to lie on his side with his knees flexed, close to the edge of the bed.
  b. Push up with arms and swing legs over the edge of the bed in one smooth motion.
  c. Push up from sitting to standing while keeping back straight.
  d. Alternate walking with rest periods in bed.
9. Complications
  a. Nerve root injury
  b. Failed back syndrome
  c. Recurrent disc herniation
  d. Spinal stenosis; arachnoiditis (inflammation of arachnoidea covering the spinal cord)

Discharge Planning/Patient Education

Patient education is directed toward mobility, proper body mechanics, and prevention of further injury.
Instruct the patient as follows:
1. Increase activities *gradually;* the goal is progressive increase of activity without pain
2. Rest in a recumbent or semirecumbent position.
3. Keep sitting to a minimum; sitting in a car is discouraged initially. Avoid sitting in a soft chair.
4. Stop any activity that causes an increase in back pain or brings on leg pain.
5. Resume stretching exercises and continue on a daily basis.
6. A brace/corset may be worn for abdominal support (helps ambulation) for 6–8 weeks postoperatively.
7. Maintain ideal weight.
8. The following may be expected for a few weeks postoperatively: "pins and needles" sensations, calf cramping, and weakness. If leg, buttock, thigh and/or calf pain returns, restrict activities and return to physician for further evaluation.
9. See patient education for herniation of intervertebral disc, page 621, and management of low back pain, page 802.

Tumors of the Spinal Canal and Cord

Classification

1. *Extradural tumors* (outside the dural membrane): usually metastatic lesions (lung, breast, prostate, kidney), a majority of which spread to vertebral body, destroy bones, and compress spinal cord.
2. *Intradural–extramedullary tumors* (within the subarachnoid space): include meningiomas and schwannomas (usually benign and slow growing).
3. Intramedullary tumors (arise within the cord): majority are glial in origin and include astrocytomas, ependymomas, oligodendroglimomas.

Clinical Manifestations

(Depend on location and type of tumor)
1. Back pain
2. Weakness of extremities; reflex abnormalities
3. Numbness; sensory changes
4. Bladder dysfunction

NURSING ALERT: Patients with a rapid onset of signs and symptoms of spinal cord compression may deteriorate quickly and a mild neurologic deficit may become irreversible.

Diagnostic Evaluation

Myelography combined with magnetic resonance imaging.

Surgical Management

1. Surgical excision of tumor using microsurgical techniques (desirable unless associated with unacceptable neurologic consequences), *or*

2. Laminectomy and decompressive (removal of pressure) surgery followed by radiation therapy.

Complications

1. Spinal cord edema; spinal cord infarction
2. Persistent or recurrent tumor
3. Hydrocephalus (spinal cord astrocytomas)

Postoperative Nursing Management

1. See Nursing Interventions Following Disc Surgery, page 621.
2. Monitor for signs and symptoms of neurologic deficit; sudden onset of neurologic deficit is an ominous sign.
   a. Note that postoperative deficits are more likely to occur in patient with severe preoperative deficit.
   b. Check arm and leg movements, strength, and sensation.
   c. Check for loss of sensation.

3. Monitor vital signs. Be alert for signs of respiratory depression if tumor was in cervical area.
4. Palpate the area over the bladder for urinary retention.
5. Give prescribed analgesic in adequate amounts and at appropriate intervals—pain is the hallmark of spinal metastasis, sensory root involvement, or vertebral collapse.
6. Check bandage over operative area for signs of CSF leakage.

Discharge Planning/Patient Education

1. See Patient Education After Disc Surgery, page 622.
2. Recovery may be slow and incomplete if patient had a progressive neurologic deficit preoperatively.
3. Encourage patient with impaired motor function to use a cane or walker.
4. Caution the patient with sensory involvement about dangers of extremes in temperatures; be wary of heating devices (fireplaces, space heaters, etc.).

Bibliography

Books

Allan D (ed). Nursing and the Neurosciences. New York, Churchill Livingstone, 1988

Bernat JL and Vincent FM. Neurology: Problems in Primary Care. Oradell, NJ, Medical Economics Books, 1987

Bloch RF and Basbaum M. Management of Spinal Cord Injuries. Baltimore, Williams & Wilkins, 1986

Borenstein DG and Wiesel SW. Low Back Pain. Philadelphia, WB Saunders, 1989

Burns MS and Halper AS. Speech/Language Treatment of the Aphasias. Rockville, MD, Aspen Publishers, Inc., 1988

Caroscio JT. Amyotrophic Lateral Sclerosis: A Guide to Patient Care. New York, Thieme Medical Publishers, 1986

Cauthen JC (ed). Lumbar Spine Surgery. Baltimore, Williams & Wilkins, 1988

Chapey R (ed). Language Intervention Strategies in Adult Aphasia. 2nd ed. Baltimore, Williams & Wilkins, 1986

Cobble NE et al. Rehabilitation of the patient with multiple sclerosis. In DeLisa JA et al. Rehabilitation Medicine, pp 612–634. Philadelphia, JB Lippincott, 1988

Cooper PR (ed). Head Injury. 2nd ed. Baltimore, Williams & Wilkins, 1987

Cottrell JE and Turndorf H. Anesthesia and Neurosurgery. St Louis, CV Mosby, 1986

Crockard A, Hayward R and Hoft JT. Neurosurgery: The Scientific Basis of Clinical Practice. Boston, Blackwell Scientific Publications, 1985

Dalessio DJ. Wolff's Headache and Other Head Pain. 5th ed. New York, Oxford University Press, 1987

Dam M et al. Epilepsy: Progress in Treatment. New York, John Wiley & Sons, 1987

Ducker TB. New techniques of spinal injury management. In Cowley RA, Conn A and Dunham CM. Trauma Care: Surgical Management, Vol 1, pp 213–222. Philadelphia, JB Lippincott, 1987

Engel JJ Jr (ed). Surgical Treatment of the Epilepsies. New York, Raven Press, 1986

Fam BA et al. Spinal cord injuries. In Yalla SV et al. Neurourology and Urodynamics: Principles and Practice, pp 291–302. New York, Macmillan, 1988

Fromm GH (ed). The Medical and Surgical Management of Trigeminal Neuralgia. Mount Kisco, NY, Futura, 1987

Garrison SJ et al. Rehabilitation of the stroke patient. In DeLisa JA et al. Rehabilitation Medicine, pp 565–584. Philadelphia, JB Lippincott, 1988

Ghista DN and Frankel HL. Spinal Cord Injury: Medical Engineering. Springfield, Charles C Thomas, 1986

Granger CV, Seltzer GB and Fishbein CF. Primary Care of the Functionally Disabled. Philadelphia, JB Lippincott, 1987

Grundy D, Russell J and Swain A. ABC of Spinal Cord Injury. London, British Medical Journal, 1986

Heilbrun MP (ed). Stereotactic Neurosurgery. Baltimore, Williams & Wilkins, 1988

Hickey JB. The Clinical Practice of Neurological and Neurosurgical Nursing. Philadelphia, JB Lippincott, 1986

Horwitz NH and Rizzoli HV. Postoperative Complications of Extracranial Neurological Surgery. Baltimore, Williams & Wilkins, 1987

Jackson CG. Facial Nerve Paralysis. Washington, DC, American Academy of Otolaryngology, Head and Neck Surgery Foundation, 1986

Jankovic J and Tolosa E (eds). Parkinson's Disease and Movement Disorders. Baltimore, Urban & Schwarzenberg, 1988

Jenkins LC and Wong DHW. Anaesthetic Management of Carotid Endarterectomy. London, Lloyd-Luke Medical Books, 1987

Kaplan PE and Cerullo LJ. Stroke Rehabilitation. Boston, Butterworths, 1987

Kinney MR, Packa DR and Dunbar SB. AACN'S Clinical Reference for Critical Care Nursing. 2nd ed. New York, McGraw–Hill, 1988

Kirkaldy-Willis WH (ed). Managing Low Back Pain. 2nd ed. New York, Churchill Livingstone, 1988

Koller WC (ed). The Handbook on Parkinson's Disease. New York, Marcel Dekker, 1987

Kornblith PL and Walker MD. Advances in Neuro-Oncology. Mount Kisco, NY, Futura, 1988

Laidlaw J, Richens A and Oxley J. A Textbook of Epilepsy. 3rd ed. New York, Churchill Livingstone, 1988

Lundgren J. Acute Neuroscience Nursing Concepts and Care. Boston, Jones and Bartlett, 1986

Matthews PJ and Carlson CE. Spinal Cord Injury: A Guide to Rehabilitation Nursing. Rockville, MD, Aspen Publishers Inc., 1987

May M. The Facial Nerve. New York, Thieme, 1986

Meier MJ, Benton AL and Diller L (eds). Neuropsychological Rehabilitation. New York, Churchill Livingstone, 1987

Miller JD et al. Northfield's Surgery of the Central Nervous System. 2nd ed. Boston, Blackwell Scientific, 1987

Mitchell PH et al. AANN'S Neuroscience Nursing. Norwalk, Appleton & Lange, 1988

Moore WS (ed). Surgery for Cerebrovascular Disease. New York, Churchill Livingstone, 1987

Mori K. An Outline of Neurosurgery. New York, Springer–Verlag, 1988

Pansky B, Allen DJ and Budd GC. Review of Neuroscience. 2nd ed. New York, Macmillan, 1986

Post K et al. Acute, Chronic, and Terminal Care in Neurosurgery. Springfield, Charles C Thomas, 1987

Raimond J and Taylor JW. Neurological Emergencies: Effective Nursing Care. Rockville, MD, Aspen Publishers Inc., 1986

Ropper AH and Kennedy SF. Neurological and Neurosurgical Intensive Care. Rockville, MD, Aspen Publishers, 1988

Schapiro RT. Symptom Management in Multiple Sclerosis. New York, Demos, 1987

Schmidek HH and Sweet WH (eds). Operative Neurosurgical Techniques. 2nd ed, Vol 1 and 2. Orlando, Grune and Stratton, 1988

Sengupta RP and McAllister VL. Subarachnoid Haemorrhage. New York, Springer–Verlag, 1986

Simon RH and Sayre JT. Strategy in Head Injury Management. Norwalk, Appleton & Lange, 1987

Staas WE Jr. Rehabilitation of the spinal cord-injured patient. In DeLisa JA et al. Rehabilitation Medicine, pp 635–659. Philadelphia, JB Lippincott, 1988

Stern MB and Hurtig HI. The Comprehensive Management of Parkinson's Disease. New York, PMA, 1988

Tollison CD (ed). Handbook of Chronic Pain Management. Baltimore, Williams & Wilkins, 1989

Trimble MR and Reynolds EH. Epilepsy: Behaviour and Cognitive Function. New York, John Wiley & Sons, 1987

Trimble MR and Reynolds EH. What is Epilepsy: The Clinical and Scientific Basis of Epilepsy. New York, Churchill Livingstone, 1986

Weisberg LA, Strub RL and Garcia CA. Decision Making in Adult Neurology. Philadelphia, BC Decker, 1987

White AH, Rothman RH and Ray CD. Lumbar Spine Surgery: Techniques and Complications. St Louis, CV Mosby, 1987

Wirth FP and Ratcheson RA. Neurosurgical Critical Care. Baltimore, Williams & Wilkins, 1987

Ylvisaker M and Gobble EMR. Community Re-Entry for Head Injured Adults. Boston, Little, Brown & Co, 1987

Journals

Head Injury/Aneurysm/ICP Monitoring

Ampel L et al. An approach to airway management in the acutely head-injured patient. J Emerg Med 1988 Jan–Feb; 6(1):1–7

Anderson BJ. The metabolic needs of head trauma victims. J Neurosci Nurs 1987 Aug; 19(4):211–215

Biller J, Godersky JC and Adams HP Jr. Management of aneurysmal subarachnoid hemorrhage. Curr Concepts Cerebrovasc Dis Stroke 1988 May–Jun; 23(4):13–17

Brooks N. Behavioural abnormalities in head injured patients. Scand J Rehabil Med Suppl 1988; 17:41–46

Clifton GL. Controversies in medical management of head injury. Clin Neurosurg 1988; 34:587–603

Constantini S et al. Intracranial pressure monitoring after elective intracranial surgery. J Neurosurg 1988 Oct; 69(4): 540–544

Franges EZ and Beideman ME. Infections related to intracranial pressure monitoring. J Neurosci Nurs 1988 Apr; 20(2):94–103

Hassett JH, Sunby C and Flint LM. No elimination of aspiration pneumonia in neurologically disabled patients with feeding gastrostomy. Surg Gynecol Obstet 1988 Nov; 167(5):383–388

Hollingsworth-Fridlund P, Vos H and Daily EK. Use of fiber-optic pressure transducer for intracranial pressure measurements: A preliminary report. Heart Lung 1988 Mar; 17(2):111–120

Klingbeil GEG. Airway problems in patients with traumatic brain injury. Arch Phys Med Rehabil 1988 Jul; 69(7):493–495

Lee S-T. Intracranial pressure changes during positioning of patients with severe head injury. Heart Lung 1989 Jul; 18(4):411–414

Marshall LF. Intracranial pressure monitoring: Theory and practice. Adv Neurotraumatology 1986; 1:209–228

Mayberg MR, Dacey RG and Winn HR. Controversies in aneurysm surgery. Semin Neurol 1986 Sep; 6(3):299–308

Mollman HD, Rockswold GL and Ford SE. A clinical comparison of subarachnoid catheters to ventriculostomy and subarachnoid bolts: A prospective study. J Neurosurg 1988 May; 68(5):737–741

Sanguinetti M and Catanzaro M. A comparison of discharge teaching on the consequences of brain injury. J Neurosci Nurs 1987 Oct; 19(5):271–275

Springer MFB and Baker FJ. Cranial burr hole decompression in the emergency department. Am J Emerg Med 1988 Nov; 6(6):640–646

Starmark J-E, Holmgren E and Stalhammar D. Current reporting of responsiveness in acute cerebral disorders. J Neurosurg 1988 Nov; 69(5):692–698

Tosch P. Patients' recollections of their posttraumatic coma. J Neurosci Nurs 1988 Aug; 20(4):223–228

Treatment of brain abscess. Lancet 1988 Jan 30; 1(8579):219–220

Weir BK. The management of intracranial aneurysms: Prospects for improvement. Clin Neurosurg 1988; 34:154–160

Weiss MH. The technique of intracranial pressure monitoring. J Crit Illness 1987 Sep; 2(9):83–90

Pain/Neurosurgery

Adams CBT. The management of pituitary tumours and post-operative visual deterioration. Acta Neurochir 1988; 94(3–4):103–116

Amadio P Jr, Cummings DM and Amadio PB. A framework for management of chronic pain. Am Fam Physician 1988 Nov; 38(5):155–160

Bay JW and Sheeler LR. Results of transsphenoidal surgery for Cushing's disease. Cleve Clin J Med 1988 Jul–Aug; 55(4):357–364

Black PM et al. Management of large pituitary adenomas by transsphenoidal surgery. Surg Neurol 1988 Jun; 29(6): 443–447

Caplan LR and Pessin MS. Symptomatic carotid artery disease and carotid endarterectomy. Annu Rev Med 1988; 39:273–299

Conomy JP. The future of carotid endarterectomy: A neurologist's point of view. Clin Neurosurg 1988; 34:123–133

Cousins MJ. The spinal route of analgesia. Acta Anaesthesiol 1988; 39(3 Suppl 2):71–82

Cunha BA and Tu RP. Fever in the neurosurgical patient. Heart Lung 1988 Nov; 17(6 Pt 1):608–611

Downing JE, Busch EH and Stedman PM. Epidural morphine delivered by a percutaneous epidural catheter for outpatient treatment of pain. Anesth Anal 1988 Dec; 67(12):1159–1161

Dubuisson D and Warfeld CA. Neurosurgery for the pain of malignancy. Hosp Pract 1988 Jun 15; 23(6):41–60

Eisele DW. The sublabial transseptal transsphenoidal approach to sellar and parasellar lesions. Laryngoscope 1988 Dec; 98(12):1301–1308

Fahlbusch R and Buchfelder M. Transsphenoidal surgery or parasellar pituitary adenomas. Acta Neurochir 1988; 92(1–4):93–99

Gransden WR et al. Meningitis after trans-sphenoidal excision of pituitary tumours. J Laryngol Otol 1988 Jan; 102(1):33–36

Haight K. What you should know about epidural analgesia. Nursing 1987 Sep; 17(9):55–59

Hannegan L. Transient cognitive changes after craniotomy. J Neurosci Nurs 1989 Jun; 21(3):165–170

Iacono RP et al. Intraspinal opiates for the treatment of intractable pain in the terminally ill cancer patient. Int J Neurosci 1988 Jan; 38(1–2):111–119

Landolt AM (ed). Intensive care and monitoring of the neurosurgical patient. Prog Neurological Surg 1987; 12:1–193

Mampalam TJ, Tyrrell JB and Wilson CB. Transsphenoidal microsurgery for Cushing disease. Ann Intern Med 1988 Sep 15; 109(6):487–493

Miller E and Williams S. Alteration in cerebral perfusion: Clinical concept or nursing diagnosis? J Neurosci Nurs 1987 Aug; 19(4):183–190

Portenoy RK. Practical aspects of pain control in the patient with cancer. CA 1988 Nov–Dec; 38(6):327–352

Racz GB, McCarron RF and Talboys P. Percutaneous dorsal column stimulator for chronic pain control. Spine 1989 Jan; 14(1):1–4

Raney JP and Kirk KA. The use of an Ommaya reservoir for administration of morphine sulphate to control pain in select cancer patients. J Neurosci Nurs 1988 Feb; 20(1):23–29

Ross DA and Wilson CB. Results of transsphenoidal microsurgery for growth hormone-secreting pituitary adenoma in a series of 214 patients. J Neurosurg 1988 Jun; 68(6):854–867

Siegfried J. Electrostimulation and neurosurgical measures in cancer pain. Recent Results Cancer Res 1988; 108: 28–32

Theisen GJ and Grundy BL. Anesthesia and monitoring for carotid endarterectomy. Bull NY Acad Med 1987 Oct; 63(8):803–818

Williams A and Molitor RE. Epidural infusions of opiates and local anesthetic solutions for intractable cancer pain. Oncol Nurs Forum 1988 Nov–Dec; 15(6):819

Winslow CM et al. The appropriateness of carotid endarterectomy. N Engl J Med 1988 Mar 24; 318(12):721–727

Young HF and Salcman M. Early diagnosis of brain tumors. Am Fam Physician 1987 Jul; 36(1):149–157

Young RF. Brain and spinal stimulation: How and to whom. Clin Neurosurg 1989; 35:429–447

Youngberg JA and Neely CF. Perioperative anesthetic considerations for the carotid surgery patient. Adv Anesth 1988; 5:291–328

Zene M. Epidural opiates and nerve blocks. Recent Results Cancer Res 1988; 108:18–27

Cranial Nerve Involvement

Burchel KJ. Percutaneous retrogasserian glycerol rhizolysis in the management of trigeminal neuralgia. J Neurosurg 1988 Sep; 69(3):361–366

Dumitru D and Walsh NE. Electrophysiologic evaluation of the facial nerve in Bell's palsy. Am J Phys Med Rehabil 1988 Aug; 67(4):137–144

Fritz W, Schafer J and Klein JH. Hearing loss after microvascular decompression for trigeminal neuralgia. J Neurosurg 1988 Sep; 69(3):367–370

Gates GA. Facial paralysis. Otolaryngol Clin North Am 1987 Feb; 20(1):113–131

Sweet WH. The treatment of trigeminal neuralgia. N Engl J Med 1986 Jul 17; 315(3):174–177

Cerebrovascular Disease/Aphasia

Albert ML and Helm-Estabrooks N. Diagnosis and treatment of aphasia. I. JAMA 1988 Feb 19; 259(7):1043–1047

Albert ML and Helm-Estabrooks N. Diagnosis and treatment of aphasia. II. JAMA 1988 Feb 26; 259(8):1205–1210

Bolte MJ et al. Orthopaedic management of the stroke patient. I: Pathophysiology, limb deformity and patient evaluation. Orthopaedic Review 1988 Jun; 17(6):637–646

Bukowski L and Dudas S. (eds). Nursing care of the stroke patient. Nurs Clin North Am 1986 Jun; 21(2):273–374

Dombovy ML and Bach-y-Rita P. Clinical observations on recovery from stroke. Adv Neurol 1988; 47:265–276

Doolittle ND. Stroke recovery: Review of the literature and suggestions for future research. J Neurosci Nurs 1988 Jun; 20(3):169–173

Dupont RM, Cullum CM and Jeste DV. Poststroke depression and psychosis. Psychiatr Clin North Am 1988 Mar; 11(1):133–149

Ferido T and Habel M. Spasticity in head trauma and CVA patients: Etiology and management. J Neurosci Nurs 1988 Feb; 20(1):17–20

Goldberg G and Berger GG. Secondary prevention in stroke: A primary rehabilitation concern. Arch Phys Med Rehabil 1988 Jan; 69(1):32–40

Grotta JC. Post-stroke management concerns and outcomes. Geriatrics 1988 Jul; 43(7):40–48

Khan Z, Starr P and Singh VK. Neurologic basis of voiding disorders in patients with cerebrovascular accident. Semin Neurol 1988 Summer; 8(2):156–158

Koenig HG and Studenski S. Post-stroke depression in the elderly. J Gen Intern Med 1988 Sep–Oct; 3(5):508–517

Levine SR and Welch KMA. Cocaine and stroke. Curr Concepts Cerebrovasc Dis Stroke 1987 Sep–Oct; 22(5):25–30

Messner M and Messner E. Mood disorders following stroke. Compr Psychiatry 1988 Jan–Feb; 29(1):22–27

Sila CA and Furlan AJ. Drug treatment of stroke. Drugs 1988 Apr; 35(4):468–476

Starkstein SE and Robinson RG. Aphasia and depression. Aphasiology 1988 Jan–Feb; 2(1):1–19

Takolander R and Bergqvist D. Carotid endarterectomy as stroke prophylaxis. Eur J Vasc Surg 1987 Dec; 1(6):371–380

Wechsler LR and Ropper AH. Management of stroke in the intensive care unit. Semin Neurol 1986 Sep; 6(3):324–331

Winter JL and Rudansky MC. Poststroke neurobehavioral syndromes. Semin Neurol 1987 Dec; 7(4):361–364

Epilepsy

Blume HW and Schomer DL. Surgical approaches to epilepsy. Annu Rev Med 1988; 39:301–313

Brewer K and Sperling MR. Neurosurgical treatment of intractable epilepsy. J Neurosci Nurs 1988 Dec; 20(6):366–372

Chadwick D. The modern treatment of epilepsy. Br J Hosp Med 1988 Feb; 39(2):104–107, 110–111

Hauser WA, Ng SKC and Brust JCM. Alcohol, seizures, and epilepsy. Epilepsia 1988; 29(Suppl 2):S66–S78

Koch-Weser M et al. Prevalence of psychologic disorders after surgical treatment of seizures. Arch Neurol 1988 Dec; 45(12):1308–1311

Krall RL and Resor ST Jr. Drug treatment of epilepsy. Semin Neurol 1987 Jun; 7(2):128–138

Levin R, Banks S and Berg B. Psychosocial dimensions of epilepsy: A review of the literature. Epilepsia 1988 Nov–Dec; 29(6):805–816

Mahler ME. Seizures: Common causes and treatment in the elderly. Geriatrics 1987 Jul; 42(7):73–78

Neppe VM and Tucker GJ. Modern perspectives on epilepsy in relation to psychiatry: Classification and evaluation. Hosp Community Psychiatry 1988 Mar; 39(3):263–271

Neppe VM and Tucker GJ. Modern perspectives on epilepsy in relation to psychiatry: Behavioral disturbances of epilepsy. Hosp Community Psychiatry 1988 Apr; 39(4):389–396

Porter RJ and Theodore WH (eds). Epilepsy. Neurol Clin 1986 Aug; 4(3): 495–695

Santilli N and Sierzant TL. Advances in the treatment of epilepsy. J Neurosci Nurs 1987 Jun; 19(3):141–157

Stevens JR. Psychiatric aspects of epilepsy. J Clin Psychiatry 1988 Apr; 49(4 Suppl):49–57

Multiple Sclerosis/Myasthenia Gravis/ Parkinson's Disease

Aminoff MJ. Parkinson's disease of the elderly: Current management strategies. Geriatrics 1987 Jul; 42(7): 31–37

Berry P and Ward-Smith P. Adrenal medullary transplant as a treatment for Parkinson's disease: Perioperative considerations. J Neurosci Nurs 1988 Dec; 20(6):356–361

Blaivas JG and Kaplan SA. Urologic dysfunction in patients with multiple sclerosis. Semin Neurol 1988 Summer; 8(2):159–165

Consensus Conference. The utility of therapeutic plasmapheresis for neurologic disorders. JAMA 1986 Sep 12; 256(10):1333–1337

Csesko PA. Sexuality and multiple sclerosis. J Neurosci Nurs 1988 Dec; 20(6):353–355

Cummings JL and Benson DF. Psychological dysfunction accompanying subcortical dementias. Annu Rev Med 1988; 39:53–61

DeBaets MH, Oosterhuis HJGH and Toyka KV. Myasthenia gravis. Monogr Allergy 1988; 25:1–147

Delgado JM and Billo JM. Care of the patient with Parkinson's disease: Surgical and nursing interventions. J Neurosci Nurs 1988 Jun; 20(3):142–150

Drachman DB et al. Strategies for the treatment of myasthenia gravis. Ann NY Acad Sci 1988; 540:176–180

Grob D et al. The course of myasthenia gravis and therapies affecting outcome. Ann NY Acad Sci 1987; 505:472–479

Henderson JS. A pubococcygeal exercise program for simple urinary stress incontinence: Applicability to the female client with multiple sclerosis. J Neurosci Nurs 1988 Jun; 20(3):185–188

Jankovic J. Parkinson's disease: Recent

advances in therapy. South Med J 1988 Aug; 81(8):1021–1027

Jaretzki A et al. "Maximal" thymectomy for myasthenia gravis. J Thorac Cardiovasc Sur 1988 May; 95(5):747–757

Kelly B and Mahnon SM. Nursing care of the patient with multiple sclerosis. Rehabil Nurs 1988 Sep–Oct; 13(5): 238–243

Kierans CA. Parkinson's disease: A nursing challenge. Perspectives 1988 Summer; 12(2):10–14

Kleinfeld M and Corcoran AJ. Medicating the elderly. Compr Ther 1988 Jun; 14(6):14–23

Kurlan R. Practical therapy of Parkinson's disease. Semin Neurol 1987 Jun; 7(2): 160–166

Lichter DG et al. Cognitive and motor dysfunction in Parkinson's disease. Arch Neurol 1988 Aug; 45(8):854–860

Lieberman AN. The use of adrenal medullary and fetal grafts as a treatment for Parkinson disease. NY State J Med 1988 Jun; 88(6):287–289

Lisak RP. Overview of the rationale for immunomodulating therapies in multiple sclerosis. Neurology 1988 Jul; 38(7 Suppl 2):5–8

McFarland HF and Dhib-Jalbut S. Multiple sclerosis: Possible immunological mechanisms. Clin Immunol Immunopathol 1989 Jan; 50(Part 2):S96–105

Moore RY, Parkinson's disease: A new therapy. N Engl J Med 1987 Apr 2; 316(14):872–873

Nyberg-Hansen R and Gjerstad L. Immunopharmacological treatment in myasthenia gravis. Transplant Proc 1988 Jun; 20(3 Suppl 4):201–210

Ravits J. Myasthenia gravis. A well-understood disorder. Postgrad Med 1988 Jan; 83(1):219–233

Rhynsburger J. How to fight myasthenia's fatigue. Am J Nurs 1989 Mar; 89(3): 337–340

Rudick RA, Schiffer RB and Herndon RM. Drug treatment of multiple sclerosis. Semin Neurol 1987 Jun; 7(2):150–159

Sladek JR and Gash, JM. Nerve-cell grafting in Parkinson's disease. J Neurosurg 1988 Mar; 68(3):337–351

Strasberg PD and Brady SM. Sexual functioning of persons with neurologic disorders. Semin Neurol 1988 Summer; 8(2):141–144

Tulipan N. Brain transplants: A new approach to the therapy of neurodegenerative disease. Neurol Clin 1988 May; 6(2):405–420

Waxman SG. Clinical course and electrophysiology of multiple sclerosis. Adv Neurol 1988; 47:157–184

Weiner HL and Haffler DA. Immunotherapy of multiple sclerosis. Ann Neurol 1988 Mar; 23(3):211–222

Yahr MD and Bergmann KJ. Parkinson's disease. Adv Neurol 1987; 45:1–604

Amyotrophic Lateral Sclerosis

Beisecker AE, Cobb AK and Ziegler DK. Patients' perspectives of the role of care providers in amyotrophic lateral sclerosis. Arch Neurol 1988 May; 45(5):553–556

Brooks BR. Amyotrophic lateral sclerosis. Neurol Clin 1987 Feb; 5(1):1–192

Cesa-Bianchi M et al. Psychological aspects of ALS. Adv Exp Med Biol 1987; 209:311–322

Hudson AJ Jr. Outpatient management of amyotrophic lateral sclerosis. Semin Neurol 1987 Dec; 7(4):344–351

Mitsumoto H, Hanson MR and Chad DA. Amyotrophic lateral sclerosis: Recent advances in pathogenesis and therapeutic trials. Arch Neurol 1988 Feb; 45(2):189–202

Rose FC et al. Clinical management of ALS. Adv Exp Med Biol 1987; 209:167–252

Stone N. Amyotrophic lateral sclerosis: A challenge for constant adaptation. J Neurosci Nurs 1987 Jun; 19(3):166–173

Guillain–Barré Syndrome

Berger AR and Schaumburg HH. Rehabilitation of peripheral neuropathies. J Neurologic Rehabil 1988; 2(1):25–36

George MR. Neuromuscular respiratory failure: What the nurse knows may make a difference. J Neurosci Nurs 1988 Apr; 20(2):110–117

Guillain–Barré syndrome. Lancet 1988 Sep 17; 2(8612):659–661

Halls J, Bredkjaer C and Friis ML. Guillain–Barré syndrome: Diagnostic criteria, epidemiology, clinical course and prognosis. Acta Neurol Scand 1988 Aug; 78(2):118–122

Lisak RP and Brown MJ. Acquired demyelinating polyneuropathies. Semin Neurol 1987 Mar; 7(1):40–48

McKhann GM et al. Plasmapheresis and Guillain–Barré syndrome: Analysis of prognostic factors and the effect of plasmapheresis. Ann Neurol 1988 Apr; 23(4):347–355

Zelig G et al. The rehabilitation of patients with severe Guillain–Barré syndrome. Paraplegia 1988 Aug; 26(4): 250–254

Intervertebral Disc/Spinal Cord Injury/Spinal Tumors

Barolat G. Surgical management of spasticity and spasms in spinal cord injury: An overview. J Am Paraplegia Soc 1988 Jan–Apr; 11(1):9–13

Bell J and Hannon K. Pathophysiology involved in autonomic dysreflexia. J Neurosci Nurs 1988 Aug; 20(4):86–88

Bennett CJ et al. Sexual dysfunction and electroejaculation in men with spinal cord injury: Review. J Urol 1988 Mar; 139(3):453–457

Black KS (ed). Spinal cord injuries. Top Acute Care Trauma Rehabil 1987; 1(3): 1–94

Cohen AR et al. Malignant astrocytomas of the spinal cord. J Neurosurg 1989 Jan; 70(1):50–54

Di Marco A et al. Postoperative management of primary spinal cord ependymomas. Acta Oncol 1988; 27(4):371–375

Fam B and Yalla SV. Vesicourethral dysfunction in spinal cord injury and its management. Semin Neurol 1988 Summer; 8(2):150–155

Gilbert J. Critical management of the patient with acute spinal cord injury. Crit Care Clin 1987 Jul; 3(3):549–567

Goddard LR. Sexuality and spinal cord injury. J Neurosci Nurs 1988 Aug; 20(4):240–244

Heiss JD and Tew JM Jr. Diskogenic diseases of the spine: Clinical aspects. Semin Roentgenol 1988 Apr; 23(2):93–99

Hoffman LA. Ineffective airway clearance related to neuromuscular dysfunction. Nurs Clin North Am 1987 Mar; 22(1): 151–166

Janssen L and Hansebout RR. Pathogenesis of spinal cord injury and newer treatments: A review. Spine 1989 Jan; 14(1):23–32

Keppler JP. Rehabilitation in spinal cord injury. Crit Care Clin 1987 Jul; 3(3): 637–654

Mahon-Darby J et al. Powerlessness in cervical spinal cord injury patients. Dimens Crit Care Nurs 1988 Nov–Dec; 7(6):346–355

Neatherlin JS, Brillhart B and Henry JJ. Factors determining length of hospitalization for patients having laminectomy surgery. J Neurosci Nurs 1988 Feb; 20(1):39–41

Ozer MN and Schmitt JK (eds). Medical complications of spinal cord injury. Phys Med Rehabil 1987 Aug; 1(3):339–514

Pettibone KA. Management of spasticity in spinal cord injury: Nursing concerns. J Neurosci Nurs 1988 Aug; 20(4):217–222

Reed MA. Nursing considerations in acute spinal cord injury. Crit Care Clin 1987 Jul; 3(3):679–691

Schutz H and Watson CPN. Microsurgical discectomy: A prospective study of 200 patients. Can J Neurol Sci 1987 Feb; 14(1):81–83

Silby H. Conservative management of lumbar disk herniation. Postgrad Med 1988 Sep 1; 84(3):157–162, 167–172

Vijayakumar S et al. Ependymoma of the spinal cord and cauda equina: A review. Cleve Clin J Med 1988 Mar–Apr; 55(2):163–170

Zahrawi F. Microlumbar discectomy (MLD). Spine 1988 Mar; 13(3):358–359

Eye Disorders

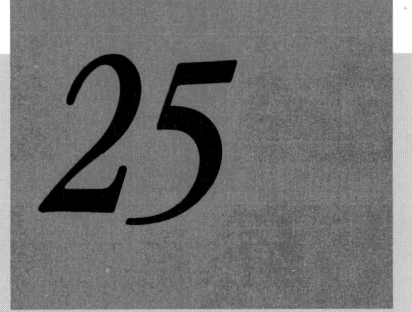

25

Normal Vision and Refractive Errors

Vision

Vision is the passage of rays of light from an object through the cornea, aqueous humor, lens, and vitreous humor to the retina, and its appreciation in the cerebral cortex.

A. Normal—emmetropia

Rays coming from an object at a distance of 6 meters (20 feet) or more are brought to a focus on the retina by the lens (Fig. 25-1*A*).

B. Abnormal—ametropia
1. Nearsightedness (myopia)
   a. Rays of light coming from an object at a distance of 6 meters (20 feet) or more are brought to a focus in front of the retina (Fig. 25-1*B*).
   b. Correction—concave lens.
2. Farsightedness (hyperopia)
   a. Rays of light coming from an object at a distance of 6 meters (20 feet) or more are brought to a focus in back of the retina (Fig. 25-1*C*).
   b. Correction—convex lens.

Accommodation

In *accommodation,* the focusing apparatus of the eye adjusts to objects at different distances by means of increasing the convexity of the lens (brought about by contraction of ciliary muscles).

Presbyopia—the elasticity of the lens decreases with increasing age; an emmetropic person with presbyopia will read a paper at arm's length and requires prescription lenses to correct the problem.

Curvature of Cornea

A. Normal—equal curvature of cornea

B. Abnormal—astigmatism
1. Uneven curvature of the cornea, causing the patient to be unable to focus horizontal and vertical rays on the retina at the same time
2. Correction—cylinder lenses

Examination and Diagnostic Procedures

(For history, physical examination, and assessment see pp. 13 and 21.)

External Examination

Includes examination of the eye and adnexa without the aid of special apparatus.

A. Visual Acuity

Snellen Chart and other methods.
1. Each eye is tested separately, with and without glasses.
2. Letters and objects are of a size that can be seen by the normal eye at a distance of 6 meters (20 feet) from the chart.
3. Letters appear in rows and are arranged so that the normal eye can see them at distances of 9, 12, 15 meters (30, 40, 50 feet), etc.
4. A person who can identify letters of the size 6 at 6 meters (20 at 20 feet) is said to have 6/6 (20/20) vision.
5. Additionally, if vision is less than 6/60 (20/200), tests may be recorded as follows:
   Counting fingers (C.F.) at __ meters (feet).
   Hand motion (H.M.)—ability to detect hand movement at a certain distance:

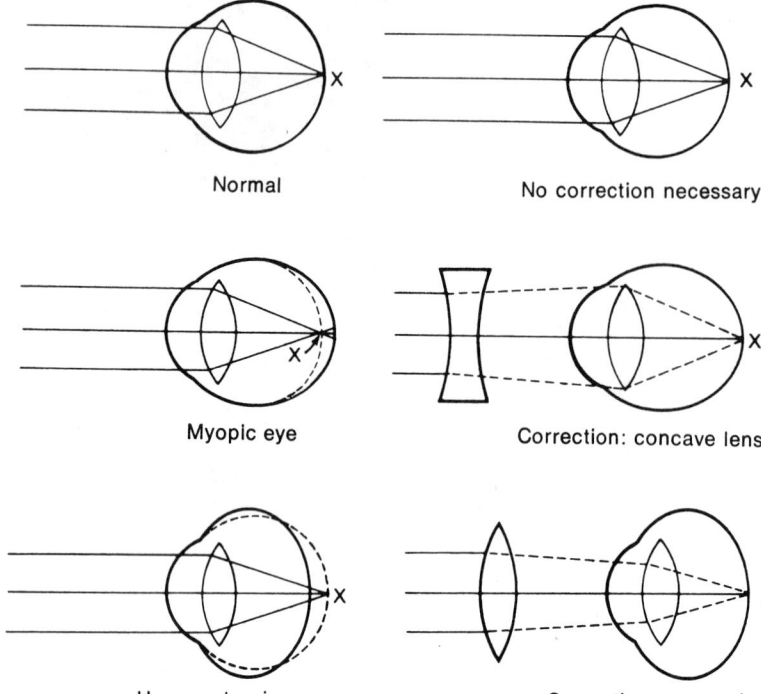

Normal

No correction necessary

Myopic eye

Correction: concave lens

Hypermetropic eye

Correction: convex lens

Figure 25-1. *Normal vision and refractory errors.*

Light perception and projection (L.P. & P.)
Light perception only (L.P.)
No light perception (N.L.P.)
6. Formula for converting meters to feet:

$$\frac{m.}{6/6 + 3} = \frac{ft.}{20/20 + 10}$$

Example: 6/6 = 20/20
6/9 = 20/30
.   .
.   .
6/60 = 20/200

B. Visual Fields

To determine function of optic pathways.
1. Equipment—light source and test objects.
2. Peripheral field—useful in detecting decreased peripheral vision in one or both eyes.
   a. Patient is seated 18–24 inches in front of the tester.
   b. The left eye is covered while the patient focuses with the right eye on a spot about 1 foot from the eye.
   c. A test object is brought in from the side at 15-degree intervals, through complete 360 degrees.
   d. The patient signals when he sees the test object and again when the object disappears through the 360 degrees.

C. Color Vision Tests

These tests are done to determine the person's ability to perceive primary colors and shades of colors; it is particularly significant for individuals whose occupation requires discerning colors: artists, interior decorators, transportation workers, surgeons, nurses.
1. Equipment
   a. Polychromatic plates: these are dots of primary colors printed on a background of similar dots in a confusion of colors.
   b. Individual colored discs: each disc is matched to its next closest color.
2. Procedure
   a. Various polychromatic plates are presented to the patient under specified illumination.
   b. The patterns may be letters or numbers that the normal eye can perceive instantly, but that are confusing to the person with a perception defect.
3. Outcome
   a. Color-blindness—person is unable to perceive the figures
   b. Red-green blindness—8% of males; 0.4% of females
   c. Blue-yellow blindness—extremely rare

D. Refraction

Refraction is a clinical measurement of the error of focus in an eye.
1. Usually this is accomplished by instilling a medication with cycloplegic and mydriatic properties into the conjunctiva of the eye.
   Tropicamide or cyclopentolate are two such medicines that cause ciliary muscle relaxation, pupil dilation (mydriasis), and lowered accommodative power (cycloplegia).
2. The refractive state of the eye can be determined as follows:
   a. Objectively—via retinoscopy
   b. Subjectively—trial of lenses to arrive at the best visual image

Note: In certain eye clinics an *auto-refractor* may provide automatic refraction of an individual's eyes as he sits in front of this special instrument. Findings are computed directly onto a printout sheet.

Internal Examination

A. Ophthalmoscopic Examination

The interior of the eye is examined when a beam of light is reflected through the pupil while the examiner looks through an ophthalmoscope. Clinical significance includes:
1. Detection of the clarity of the media: e.g., cataracts, vitreous opacities, corneal scars.
2. Close examination for the pathologic changes in retinal blood vessels: e.g., diabetes or hypertension.

3. Examination of choroid: e.g., tumors or inflammation.
4. Examination of retina: e.g., retinal detachment, scars, or diabetes.

B. Tonometry

Measurement of intraocular tension or pressure.
1. Air applanation tonometry—this requires no topical anesthesia and measures tension by sensing deformation of the cornea in reaction to a puff of pressurized air.

Ocular Procedures

Guidelines   Instillation of Eyedrops

Purposes
1. To dilate or contract the pupil
2. To relieve pain and discomfort
3. To act as an antiseptic in cleansing the eye
4. To combat infection; to relieve inflammation

Equipment   Sterile solution or medication (most containers have accompanying dropper)
Small gauze squares or cotton balls.

Procedure   **Preparatory Phase**

1. Inform the patient of the need and reason for instilling drops.
2. Allow the patient to sit with head tilted backward or to lie in a supine position.

Performance Phase

Nursing Action	Rationale/Amplification
1. Check the patient's name.	1. For proper patient identification.
2. Check physician's directives and bottle or vial for correct solution.	2. To avoid medication error.
3. Check physician's directives designating eye requiring drops. O.D. (oculis dexter)—right eye O.S. (oculis sinister)—left eye O.U. (oculis uterque)—both eyes	
4. Wash hand prior to instilling medication.	4. To prevent transfer of microorganisms to patient.
5. Fill eyedropper with medication but prevent medication from flowing back into bulb end.	5. Loose particles of rubber from bulb end may slip into medication.
6. Using forefinger, pull lower lid down gently (see Fig. 25-2A).	6. To expose inner surface of lid and cul-de-sac.
7. Instruct patient to look upward (see Fig. 25-2B).	7. Prevents medication from hitting sensitive cornea.
8. Drop medication into center of lower lid (cul-de-sac).	
9. Instruct patient to close eyes slowly but not to squeeze or rub them (Fig. 25-2C). Open eye (Fig. 25-2D).	9. Squeezing or rubbing would express medication from eye; closing allows medication to be distributed evenly over eye.
10. Wipe off excess solution with gauze or cotton balls.	10. Prevents possible skin irritation.
11. Wash hands after instilling medication.	11. Prevents transfer of microorganisms to self or other patients.

Follow-up Phase

Record time, type, strength, and amount of medication; and the eye into which medication was instilled.

Patient Education: Self-Instillation of Eyedrops

1. Tilt head back.	1. Places eye and lower lid in a horizontal plane.
2. Using forefinger, pull lower lid down.	2. Exposes inner surface of lower lid.

(continued)

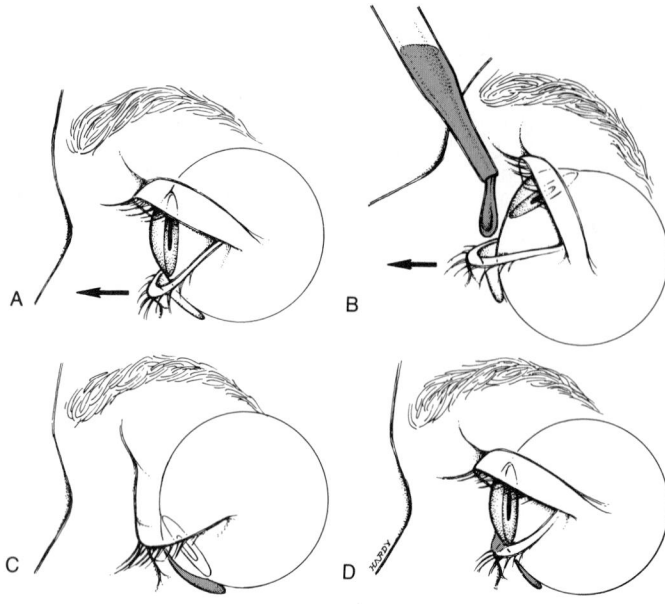

Figure 25-2. *Instillation of eyedrops.*

Guidelines   Instillation of Eyedrops *(continued)*

Nursing Action	Rationale/Amplification
3. With other hand, hold dropper horizontally and facing top of head.	3. Positions dropper outlet above receiving lid.
4. Look up and instill 1 drop onto lower lid. (Continue with steps 9–11 above.)	4. Prevents medication from hitting sensitive cornea.

Note: Eye ointments are frequently used—procedure is similar to instillation of eyedrops. Ointment from tube is gently squeezed as a ribbon of medication along inner lower lid with care taken not to touch eye with end of tube.

Guidelines   Irrigating the Eye (Conjunctival Irrigation)

Purposes
1. To remove secretions from the conjunctival sac.
2. To treat infections.
3. To relieve itching.
4. To provide moisture on the surface of the eyes of an unconscious patient.
5. To irrigate chemicals or foreign bodies from the eye.

Sterile Equipment   An eyedropper, asepto bulb syringe, or plastic bottle with prescribed solution depending on the extent of irrigation needed. For copious use, e.g., chemical burns: sterile normal saline or prescribed solution and IV set-up with attached tubing.

Procedure   **Preparatory Phase**

1. Verify that you have the right patient.
2. The patient may sit or lie in a supine position.
3. Instruct the patient to tilt head toward the side of the affected eye.

Nursing Action	Rationale/Amplification
1. Wash eyelashes and lids with prescribed solution at room temperature; a curved basin should be placed on the affected side of the face to catch the outflow.	1. Any materials on the lids and lashes can be washed off before exposing conjunctiva.

Nursing Action	Rationale/Amplification
2. Evert the lower conjunctival sac. (If feasible, have the patient pull down lower lid with his index finger).	2. Exposes inner surface of lower lid and conjunctival sac (involves the patient and gives a sense of control).
3. Instruct the patient to look up; avoid touching eye with equipment.	3. Prevents injury to the sensitive cornea.
4. Allow irrigating fluid to flow from the inner canthus to the outer canthus along the conjunctival sac.	4. Prevents solution from flowing toward the lacrimal sac, duct, and nose, possibly transmitting infection.
5. Use only enough force to flush secretions from conjunctiva. (Allow patient to hold curved basin near the eye to catch fluid.)	5. Prevents eye injury (involves the patient in the treatment).
6. Occasionally have patient close his eyes.	6. Allows upper lid to meet lower lid with the possibility of dislodging additional particles.

Follow-up Phase

1. Pat eye dry and dry the patient's face with a soft cloth.	1. Provides comfort.
2. Record kind and amount of fluid used, as well as its effectiveness.	2. Provides documentation for nursing actions.

Guidelines — ## Application of an Eye Patch, Eye Shield, and Pressure Dressings to the Eye

Purposes
1. To keep an eye at rest, thereby promoting healing.
2. To prevent the patient from touching his eye.
3. To absorb secretions.
4. To protect the eye.
5. To control or lessen edema.

Procedure

Nursing Action	Rationale/Amplification
Eye Patch	
1. Instruct patient to close both eyes.	1. It is difficult to close only the affected eye.
2. Place patch over the affected eye.	
3. Secure the patch with 3 or more strips of transparent tape diagonally from mid-forehead to below the ear.	3. Transparent tape is easy to remove—use hypoallergenic tape if patient has allergies to tape.
4. For unconscious patient, moisten the eye patch.	4. Dry patch can irritate cornea.
Eye Shield (Plastic or Metal)	
1. Apply over dressings or directly over the undressed eye, fastening with 2 strips of transparent tape.	1. Used primarily to protect the eye. Place tab or irregular extension toward the patient's ear.
2. For metal eye shields, a guard can be placed around flanged edges before use:	2. Protects skin from metal.
a. Cut 1.2–2.5-cm. (½–1-inch) strip from a rubber glove finger.	a. Covers metal edges of shield or guard.
b. Stretch it around perimeter of shield.	b. Two such pieces add cushioning and provide comfort.

Note: Check for patient allergies before applying rubber strips to guard and then to skin.

Nursing Action	Rationale/Amplification
Pressure Dressings	
1. Prepare 8–10 adhesive strips by cutting 2.5-cm. (1-inch) adhesive tape in 35-cm. (9-inch) lengths. Stretch tape (3M) may also be used.	1. Warming the tape may improve its adhesiveness.
2. Apply 2 eye patches to the affected eye.	2. Provides pressure dressing bulk.
3. Apply strips from forehead above unpatched eye across dressings to the cheek bone (maxillary prominence).	3. To secure dressing and apply pressure while permitting freedom of movement of the head.

NURSING ALERT: Prolonged use of pressure dressings may cause increased temperature in the interior of the covered eye since they act as a moisture chamber. Pressure dressings, also, may need to be removed periodically for a short time so that air can freely circulate over cornea.

Note: Check for allergies before using solution on skin.

Eye Injuries

Nursing Implications

1. Recognize that all ocular injuries are potentially serious.
2. Suspect a penetrating ocular injury with every eye wound until proved incorrect.
3. Protect the integrity of the visual system and prevent further damage to the injured part.
4. Evaluate the extent of injury; either refer the patient to an ophthalmologist or provide immediate treatment that will not extend damage.
5. Immediately refer all injuries of blunt trauma to an ophthalmologist.

NURSING ALERT: All patients with eye emergencies should have visual acuity checked in each eye as part of the history and preliminary examination and prior to any form of treatment.

Corneal Abrasion

1. An injury to the cornea that goes no deeper than the epithelium.
2. Is a common occurrence as a result of inadvertent contact with objects such as fingernails or tree branches, or overwearing of contact lenses (extended wear or nonoxygen-permeable).
3. Can lead to infection or ulcer formation.

Management

1. A solution is instilled to relieve pain and facilitate eye examination; systemic analgesics may be used.

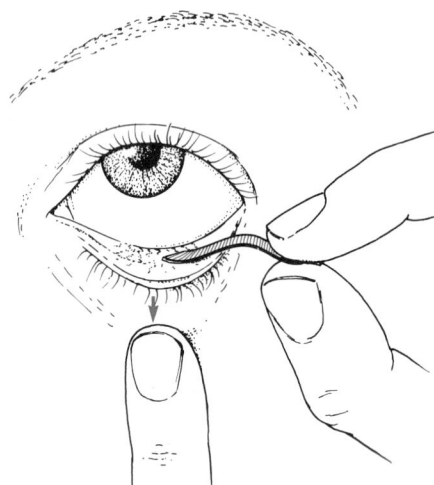

Figure 25-3. *Staining cornea with fluorescein strip.*
1. *After telling the patient what you plan to do, wet the distal end of a fluorescein strip with sterile normal saline solution. (Use sterile, individually wrapped fluorescein strip).*
2. *Pull lower eyelid down; gently touch the inner segment of the lower lid with the strip: a green stain will coat area of abrasion.*
3. *Have the patient blink several times to distribute the fluorescein dye.*
4. *The eye is now ready for examination.*

2. The cornea is stained with fluorescein—to detect existence of an abrasion and its extent (Fig. 25-3).
   a. The conjunctival surface of lower lid is touched with the fluorescein paper strip.
   b. The damaged corneal epithelium will take the stain and turn green; undamaged areas remain unstained. The stained area is viewed with a Wood's lamp, slit lamp, or a blue light.
   c. Following use of fluorescein, the eye is flushed since some patients react to fluorescein as an allergen.
   d. A drop of prescribed antibiotic is instilled since subsequent patching creates a moist environment conducive to flora growth.

Nursing Interventions

1. Advise the patient to rest his eyes for 24 hours for greater comfort; the corneal epithelium usually heals in 24–48 hours.
2. Apply dressing (as directed) firmly but gently over eye to put eye at rest and to prevent movement of the eyelid, with resultant irritation of abraded corneal area.
3. Give oral analgesic as directed—*abrasions of the cornea are very painful.*
4. Instruct patient to return to the ophthalmologist the following day for dressing change and inspection of eye for evidence of infection or ulcer formation.

Contusion

1. An injury in which the outer layer of tissue is intact but bruising takes place.
2. Internal injury may be minor or major.
3. *Black eye:* hemorrhage into the orbit from trauma.
   a. These contusions usually clear slowly and without treatment.
   b. Apply cold compresses intermittently for first 24 hours to control pain and swelling.
   c. Apply warm compresses (after 24 hours) intermittently to help healing process by promoting absorption of blood.
   d. Place the patient on bedrest with both eyes bandaged for *hyphema* (hemorrhage into anterior chamber of eye).
4. The patient is urged to consult an ophthalmologist if hemorrhage is severe or if pain and double vision are noted in order to rule out orbital fracture or hyphema.

Foreign Bodies Lodged in the Cornea

Immediate treatment by ophthalmologist or emergency department physician.
1. Sterile anesthetic is instilled into the conjunctival sac to facilitate examination.
2. Ophthalmologist will remove superficial particles with a moist cotton-tipped applicator; foreign body removed with a specialized instrument, using a slit lamp for magnification.

Nursing Interventions

1. Apply eye patch.
2. Reinforce instruction to return to ophthalmologist the following day to determine if healing is underway.

Penetrating Injuries to the Eye

1. Intraocular foreign bodies should be removed as soon as possible—they cause damage by disintegration or become encapsulated by fibrous tissue.
2. Aside from direct trauma, metallic foreign bodies may also release ions and cause toxicity.
3. Powerful magnets are still used; however, intraocular surgery through the posterior part of the ciliary body may be less traumatic.

Nursing Interventions

1. Protect eye and call ophthalmologist.
2. Give sedative–analgesic combination as directed; have patient lie quietly until ophthalmologist arrives.
3. Give prescribed tetanus prophylaxis, for any penetrating eye injury.
4. Give oral antimicrobials in high doses as prescribed— blood–aqueous barrier resists penetration.

Burns of the Eye

Disrupt integrity of cornea and cause drying of the cornea with resulting chronic conjunctivitis and corneal ulceration.

Management

A. Thermal burns

1. Associated with face and body burns.
2. Thermal burns are treated in the same way as burns of skin structures.
3. Call ophthalmologist.

B. Actinic trauma

1. Associated with damage to the cornea from ultraviolet rays; e.g., bright sun, sun lamp, snow.
2. Damage may be superficial and resolve in 48 hours; however, punctate keratitis may develop.
3. An ophthalmologist should be consulted immediately.
4. Reassure the patient and keep him quiet.
5. Apply patch to both eyes.
6. Instill anesthetic drops as prescribed.
7. Instill mydriatic–cycloplegic drugs as directed to relax ciliary muscles and iris sphincter spasms.
8. Instill emollient antibiotic ointment as prescribed.

C. Chemical Burns

1. Associated with either acid or alkali solutions.
2. Both cause intense pain and inflammation. *This is a true ocular emergency.*
3. *Irrigate eye with copious amounts of water*—hold patients's eye directly under running water with lids retracted by gauze pads when immediate irrigation is required.
4. Irrigate for at least 25 minutes.
5. Repeat irrigation in 15–20 minutes (using eye irrigation equipment) until the patient is seen by the ophthalmologist.
6. Instill prescribed topical anesthetic for pain and control severe pain thereafter with systemic analgesics as directed.
7. Check pH of tears with litmus paper and continue irrigations until pH is neutral.
8. Measure vision and intraocular pressure to determine status.
9. Alkali eye burns are more severe than acid burns; long-term management may require lavage, cycloplegics, and even collagenase inhibitors; contact lenses may be used to prevent ulcerations.

Patient Education and Preventive Measures

1. Eyeglasses and sunglasses should have impact-resistant lenses.
2. Appropriate glasses should be used for protection against very bright light, sun shining on snow, fumes of sprays, or chemicals.
3. Goggles or protective lenses should be worn if there is danger of flying gravel (power-mower lawn cutting), flying wood chips (chopping wood), flying metal or glass bits (machinery).
4. All students should use industrial-quality safety eyewear in shops and laboratories.
5. Protective lenses or goggles are highly recommended in various sports, e.g., racquet ball, handball, tennis, hockey, etc.
6. Children should be reminded of dangers of sling shots, BB guns, "sparklers," darts, arrows, etc.
7. Goggles must be worn when handling chemicals (anhydrous ammonia used as agricultural fertilizer) as these are very destructive agents. Sufficient water for irrigation should always be present.

Guidelines Removing a Particle From the Eye

Equipment	Local anesthesia	Cotton applicator sticks or tongue blades
	Hand lens	Irrigating saline
	Sterile fluorescein strips	Antibiotic solution

Procedure	**Nursing Action**	**Rationale/Amplification**
	1. As patient looks upward, evert lower lid to expose the conjunctival sac (see Fig. 25-4*A*).	1. Dust particles are often washed downward by the upper lid.
	2. With small cotton applicator dipped in saline, gently remove particle.	2. Wipe gently across lid—inner to outer aspect. Use hand magnifying lens if necessary.
	3. If offending particle is not found, proceed to examine upper lid.	
	4. Have the patient look downward while you stand in front of him.	4. Serves as a safety measure since cornea is away from area of activity.

(continued)

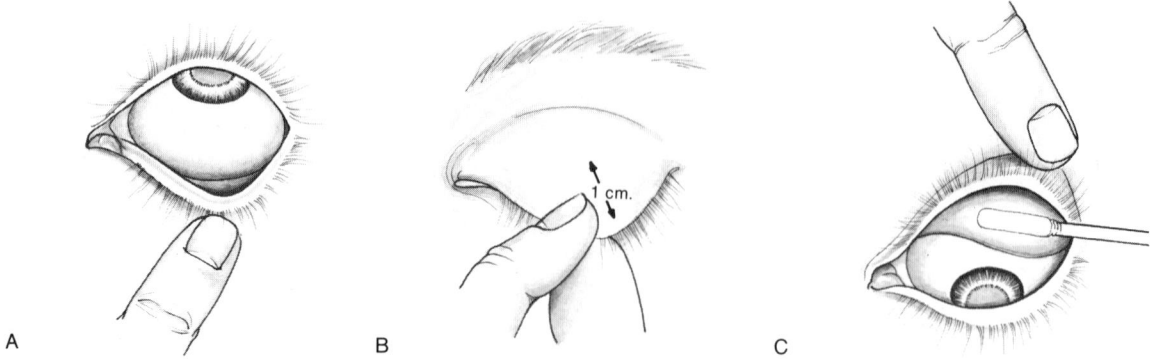

Figure 25-4. *Examining the eye for a foreign particle. (A) Evert lower lid. (B and C) Evert upper lid.*

Guidelines Removing a Particle From the Eye *(continued)*

Procedure *(continued)*	**Nursing Action**	**Rational/Amplification**
	5. Encourage the patient to relax; move slowly and reassure him that you will not hurt him.	5. Relaxation prevents squeezing the lids shut, a maneuver that contracts the obicularis muscle, making eversion of lid impossible.
	6. Place cotton applicator stick or tongue blade horizontally on outer surface of upper lid. Apply pressure about 1 cm. above lid margin (see Fig. 25-4*B*).	6. Since the upper tarsal plate extends 10–12 mm. above the lid margin, pressure must be applied at least 1 cm. above the lid margin for easy eversion of lid.
	7. Grasp upper eyelashes with fingers of other hand and pull the upper lid outward and upward over cotton applicator (Fig. 25-4*C*).	7. Particles may be washed under the lid; visual exposure assists in detection. Eyelid will remain everted by itself.
	8. Use fluorescein strip to detect corneal abrasion.	8. Green stain will so indicate if abrasion is present.

> **NURSING ALERT:** It is very important to take a patient history. Determine the nature of the particle—wood? metal? (What kind—magnetic? copper?) Was it projectile?
>
> If particle cannot be removed by the method described above, it may have become imbedded in lens or vitreous, in which case an ophthalmologist is required immediately.

Guidelines Removing Contact Lenses

Purpose: Since most contact lenses are designed to be worn while awake, if a person is injured and incapacitated because of an accident, sickness, or other cause, the lenses should be removed.

> **NURSING ALERT:**
> 1. If the injured person is unconscious or unable to remove his lenses, an optometrist or ophthalmologist is called.
> 2. If professional help is not available and the lenses must be removed, determine the type of lens.
>   a. Soft corneal lenses are widely used. The diameter covers the cornea plus a portion of the sclera of the eye. More than 75% of wearers in the US wear soft contacts.
>   b. Rigid or gas-permeable lenses are usually smaller than the cornea of the eye, although some are made to extend beyond the cornea onto the sclera of the eye.
> 3. *Do not remove lenses*—if the colored part of the eye is not visible upon opening the eyelids, await the arrival of an optometrist or ophthalmologist. If patient is to be transported, note that contacts are in the eyes. (Write out the message and tape it to the patient or send with transporter).

Procedure **Preparatory Phase**

1. Since the patient will undoubtedly be in the recumbent position, it is acceptable to remove the lens while he is in this position.
2. Wash your hands thoroughly.

Nursing Action	**Rationale/Amplification**

Performance Phase (See Fig. 25-5)

Corneal Lens (Hard type)

If an eye suction cup is available (as in Emergency Department), simply separate eyelids to expose lens fully; then, place cup over lens and apply slight pressure to cup. The suction produced will permit cup to lift contact lens from cornea.

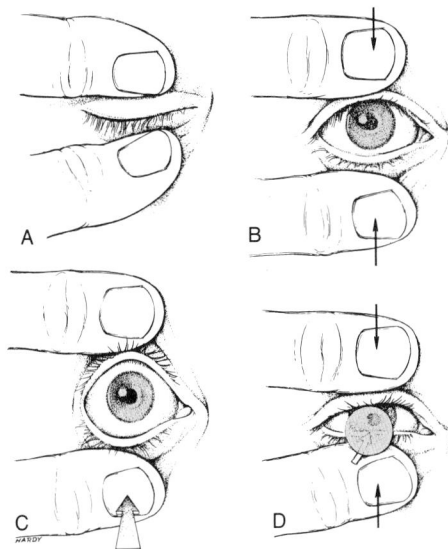

Figure 25-5. *Removing corneal contact lens.*

1. For right eye, stand on right side of patient so hands will have easier access to eye.
2. Lightly place left thumb on upper eyelid; right thumb on lower eyelid close to the edge and parallel with lids (Fig. 25-5*A*). Thumbs are placed in a leverage position on the eyelids.
3. Gently pull lids apart and observe if contact lens is visible (Fig. 25-5*B*). If contact lens is not visible, wait for an experienced practitioner.
4. If contact lens is visible, it should slide with the movement of the eyelids while thumbs are still kept at the edges of the eyelids.
5. Gently open the lids wider beyond the edge of the lens and maintain this position.
6. Press gently downward with right thumb on eyeball (Fig. 25-5*C*). This should cause the contact lens to tip up on the edge.
7. Then gently slide the eyelids and thumbs together (Fig. 25-5*D*). The contact lens should slide out between the lids where it can be taken off.
8. FORCE SHOULD NOT BE USED! Cornea may be irreparably damaged.
9. If contact lens can be seen but cannot be removed, gently slide it to the white sclera.
10. For left eye, move to left side of patient and repeat procedure.

Soft Contact Lenses

May be removed by gently grasping and pinching contact lens between thumb and forefinger. An ophthalmologist can be called to remove lenses if the patient is unable to do so. Also note, if a contact lens cannot be removed with relative ease, discontinue efforts and wait for the ophthalmologist to remove it.

Disposition of lenses

1. When lenses are found and removed, place in a case or bottle; label "right" and "left."
2. Store in normal saline solution to prevent drying.

1. Since right and left lenses are often different, storing them with proper labels will be appreciated.
2. Soft lenses must be kept moist.

Note: Extended-wear contacts or disposable contacts worn for more than 1 week may precipitate corneal damage.

Inflammation of the Eye

Superficial Lid Infections

Blepharitis—infection of eyelids, with crusting lids, redness, irritation, and mucopurulent secretion.
Hordeolum (sty)—infection of eyelash follicle.
Chalazion—infection of the meibomian gland.

Nursing Management

1. Cleanse lid margins by applying warm, moist compresses for 5 minutes 3 or 4 times daily.
2. Carefully wipe loose crusts away from lashes; apply ophthalmic antibacterial ointment and/or drops as directed.
3. Continue until infection clears.
4. Advise patient to keep his hands away from eyes and wash hands after eye care.
5. Chronic chalazion may require incision and curettage.

Conjunctivitis (Pinkeye)

An inflammation of the conjunctiva resulting from an allergy; a bacterial, viral, or chlamydial infection; or physical or chemical trauma.

Clinical Manifestations

1. Redness, pain, swelling, lacrimation; lids are frequently stuck together with crusting upon awakening.
2. Discharge according to offending organisms.
    a. Abundant purulence indicates infection caused by pneumococcus or gonococcus.
    b. In this country, chlamydia cause a subacute follicular conjunctivitis; also see *Trachoma,* below, caused by chlamydial agent (chronic keratoconjunctivitis).

Management and Nursing Interventions

1. Wear gloves to prevent dissemination of infection.
2. Instill chemotherapeutic ointments as prescribed following Gram stain for specific organism—infection will clear quicker if treatment is instituted for specific organism: 1–3 days versus 7–10 days.
3. Irrigate eye with saline to remove discharge.
4. Apply warm or cold compresses for 15 minutes, 3 or 4 times daily for comfort.
5. Avoid cross-contamination to unaffected eye by restricting use of washcloth and towel to infected eye.

Trachoma

1. A chronic, bilateral, contagious conjunctivitis caused by organism, *Chlamydia trachomatis,* that lives intracellularly.
2. If untreated, it leads to visual loss or blindness from entropion (inversion of the eyelid margin) with corneal scarring.
3. It is particularly severe and a leading cause of disability in developing countries.
4. It is a leading cause of preventable blindness.
5. The World Health Organization (WHO) has designed a scoring system to facilitate measurement of intensity of trachoma in any given area.

Clinical Manifestations

1. Onset is insidious with minimal discomfort.
2. Chemosis (swelling of conjunctiva), redness, velvety appearance of conjunctiva.
3. Later, photophobia, tearing, and pain.
4. By third week, follicles appear, and conjunctiva becomes congested due to papillary hypertrophy, engorgement, and inflammation of conjunctiva.
5. If treated, symptoms subside; if not treated, conjunctival scars appear in about 2 months.
    a. The scarred conjunctiva contracts, inverting the tarsal plate of eyelid, which causes lid to turn inward (entropion).
    b. Eyelashes rub against the cornea, causing further discomfort and pain. Corneal ulcers and synechial scars occur.

Management

1. Tetracycline topically (1% ointment) twice a day for 10 weeks.
2. Oral tetracycline twice a day may be prescribed for 2–3 weeks as a systemic treatment.
3. Erythromycin may be prescribed instead of tetracycline for nursing mothers, pregnant women, or small children.

Nursing Interventions

1. Instruct patient to use medications exactly as prescribed.
2. Emphasize importance of personal hygiene. (The WHO workers pass out packaged towelettes for washing the face, and this has been a deterrent to infection).
3. Provide health education—recognizing eye infection, controlling flies, practicing hand and face washing, using good water sources when available. Transmission is through direct contact, e.g., mother to child, child to child. Contamination is via insects (flies and gnats), fingers, and/or other vectors.

Uveitis

1. An inflammation of the uveal tract (iris, ciliary body, choroid).
2. It may involve any portion of the tract (anterior or posterior) or the entire tract (panuveitis).

Management

1. Emphasize goals of care.
    a. Patient comfort.
    b. Preservation of vision.
2. Give specific mydriatic—cycloplegics as prescribed (homatropine) to relieve discomfort caused by contraction of ciliary muscles.
3. Give prescribed anti-inflammatory agents to relieve inflammation.
    a. Corticosteroids in lowest effective dose.
    b. Topical steroids in high dosages are effective for anterior uveitis.

Sympathetic Ophthalmia

1. A severe granulomatous bilateral uveitis that may occur after any surgical or traumatic perforation involving the uveal tract.

2. A severe infection that appears to be an autoimmune reaction to uveal tissue may rarely occur.

Clinical Manifestations

1. Photophobia, blurring vision, and injection of conjunctiva ("bloodshot").
2. Injured (exciting) eye becomes inflamed, then the other eye (sympathizing) follows with an inflammation.

Management

1. Corticosteroids, locally and systemically, to reduce the amount of intraocular scarring.
2. Instillation of mydriatic medication locally to prevent adhesions between the iris and lens.
3. There is a possibility of preventive enucleation (removal of eyeball) of originally injured eye before sympathetic ophthalmia occurs.

Nursing Interventions

1. Assess the psychosocial implications of the individual situation.
2. Offer support, and collaborate with patient in planning immediate and long-term goals.
3. Recognize the difficult decision facing the patient if enucleation approach is suggested.
4. Allow time for patient to ask questions and voice concerns.

Corneal Ulcer

Keratitis is an inflammation of the cornea that, when accompanied by the loss of substance, results in corneal ulcer.

Clinical Manifestations

1. Severe pain, photophobia, increased lacrimation, and injected "bloodshot" eye.
2. If corneal ulcer progresses to involve the iris, iritis develops—pus formation in anterior chamber is seen as a white or yellow deposit (hypopyon) behind cornea.
3. If corneal ulcer perforates, iris may prolapse through the cornea.
4. Complications: Corneal destruction and perforation.

NURSING ALERT: Always question the patient about allergies to medications, whether topical or systemic, prior to institution of therapy.

Management and Nursing Interventions

1. Prevention
   a. Foreign bodies must be removed quickly.
   b. Corneal abrasions must be treated promptly.
2. Inform patient of medications to be used.
   a. Mydriatics are instilled prior to examination.
   b. Fluorescein is used to outline ulcer.
   c. Topical anesthetic is administered to relieve pain.
   d. Antibiotics or chemotherapeutic agents may be prescribed for specific infections.
3. Provide patient comfort.
   a. Apply warm compresses as prescribed.
   b. Administer prescribed therapeutics.
   c. Keep patient quiet in restful environment.

Ocular Surgery

Nursing Process Overview: The Patient Undergoing Eye Surgery

Nursing Assessment

1. Collect subjective and objective data during examination.
2. Ascertain sequence in which symptoms occurred. (For history, physical examination, and assessment, see pp. 13 and 21.)
3. Assess patient's mobility and self-care ability.
4. Assess visual impairments.
5. Gather data regarding usual support systems used by patient. Is family near? Do friends visit regularly?
6. Assess patient's daily schedule.
7. Record pertinent data in record.

Nursing Diagnoses

1. Sensory/perceptual alterations (visual) related to disease/trauma or postoperative eye condition.
2. Fear of blindness related to altered vision.
3. Self-care deficits related to reduced and/or altered vision.
4. Injury, potential, related to altered vision.
5. Knowledge deficit of postoperative expectations and discharge plans.
6. Other possible nursing diagnoses:
   a. Altered thought processes related to reduced external stimuli.
   b. Disturbances in self-concept (role performance) related to impaired vision.
   c. Social isolation related to reduced contacts with people due to impaired vision.

Nursing Interventions

A. Compensating for Altered Vision

1. Orient patient to any new environments—room arrangement and/or people.
2. Encourage self-care within the patient's limits.
3. Supervise attempts of patient to feed himself and in self-care activities.

B. Reducing Fear

1. Recognize that dependence on sight is exaggerated when one faces diminution or loss of sight.
2. Recognize that individual patient's concern of surgical outcome may be manifested differently, i.e., fear, depression, tension, resentment, anger, or rejection.
3. Encourage the patient to express his feelings.
4. Demonstrate interest and understanding.
5. Reassure the patient that rehabilitative programs and personnel are available.

C. Increasing Self-Care Activities

1. Provide diversional and occupational therapy to keep the patient occupied mentally within the limits of his decreased vision.
2. Provide rest periods as necessary.
3. Provide adequate diet and fluids to promote proper elimination.
4. Discourage patient's smoking, reading, and shaving self for safety reasons.
5. Caution the patient against rubbing his eyes or wiping them with soiled tissues.

6. Instruct patient to wear dark glasses if eyes are light-sensitive.
7. Maintain safe environment—doors should be completely open or closed; floors kept clear of articles.

D. Preparing for Surgery

1. Explain to the patient preoperative orders as well as postoperative expectations. (These will be specific for each type of surgery or physician.)
   a. Specific position in bed may be maintained for a few hours; e.g., patient may lie on unoperated side.
   b. Small pillow may be used while patient is in supine position.
2. Instruct patient to wash his hair the evening before surgery; long hair of female patients should be arranged so that it is off the face.
3. Check agency surgical policy regarding skin preparation. Patients may be requested to shower with antibacterial soap the evening prior to or morning of surgery.
4. Check that operative permit is correct and signed with specified eye having surgery noted.
5. Remove dentures, contact lenses, or artificial eye and any metal before patient goes to the operating room. (Wedding band can usually be taped in place).
6. Inform patient if any eye bandages are necessary postoperatively.
7. Administer any preoperative medications, analgesics, or tranquilizers as prescribed.
8. Position side rails (up) after administering any medications and place call bell next to patient.
9. Be available to answer any questions the patient may have relating to the surgery or postoperative period.

> **NURSING ALERT:** For eye patients requiring bedrest (e.g., following keratoplasty, injury, retinal detachment surgery), measures should be taken to prevent pulmonary and/or circulatory complications. This may include passive range-of-motion exercises, antiembolism stockings, special positioning, etc.

E. Preventing Injury Post-Surgery

1. Position the patient as permitted for specific surgery.
2. Position side rails (up) to offer patient a sense of security.
3. Place call bell next to patient; have him call the nurse rather than risk increased intraocular pressure from the stress and strain of attempting to be self-sufficient.
4. Instruct caregivers to tell the patient when they enter and leave the room.
5. Avoid activities such as combing hair that will disturb the patient's head or cause tension on sutures or operative site.

Patient Education

1. Advise patient to consult ophthalmologist before undertaking diversional or recreational therapy that is not fatiguing to the eyes—no reading; television in moderation.
2. Emphasize that lights should not be too bright or glaring.
3. Inform the patient before he leaves the hospital regarding medications, eye glasses, follow-up visits.
4. Instruct the patient and family on instillation of eye medications and proper cleansing of eyes.

a. Instillation of eye drops.
b. Application of an eye shield.
5. Inform the patient of "Talking Books" records, tapes, and machines available from most public libraries without charge.
6. Initiate follow-up visits with ophthalmologist.
7. Check the following with patient/family prior to discharge:
   a. Is a return appointment date with physician confirmed?
   b. Are patient's medications properly identified and labeled? Does the patient and family member know how to use the prescribed medications?
   c. Does the patient understand the restrictions placed on him and the reasons for them?
   d. Does patient/family know what signs/symptoms must be reported to physician between appointments (e.g., pain, temperature above 101°; discharge)?

Evaluation

1. Demonstrates improved vision in accordance with expectations of the surgery.
2. Appears relaxed and positive concerning outcome of surgery.
3. Manages self-care with minimal assistance.
4. Describes precautions that must be taken as safety measures, carries cane to prevent possible falls.
5. Enumerates symptoms that may occur if complications develop and the appropriate action to be taken for each symptom.

Corneal Transplantation *(Keratoplasty)*

The transplantation of a donor cornea, usually obtained at autopsy, to repair a corneal scar, burn, or deformity.

Types of Grafts

1. Full-thickness (6.5–8 mm.)—most common
2. Partial-thickness—lamellar

Corneal Graft

1. Fresh cornea is the preferred tissue; it is removed from the donor within 8–12 hours after death and used within 24 hours.
2. Special solutions for storage of fresh cornea are available that may extend storage up to 3 days.
3. *Cryopreservation* is the care and handling of corneal graft by freezing to retain its transparency.

Preoperative Nursing Interventions

1. Psychological preparation for surgery may be simplified because the patient is usually optimistic about the imminent transplant.
2. If cultural and spiritual concerns need to be discussed by the patient, the nurse and/or hospital chaplain should be available.
3. Soon after admission, the patient will have a thorough face cleansing with an antibacterial solution.
4. With local anesthesia, most discomfort will be alleviated with preoperative medication. (Momentary discomfort may be experienced during initial injection of local anesthesia.)
5. The patient is advised of the importance of remaining perfectly still during surgery.

Postoperative Nursing Interventions

A. Reducing Postoperative Anxiety

1. Following the procedure, an eye patch with shield is applied for protection. Daily changes follow examination by the ophthalmologist.
2. Recognize that healing is slow because of the avascularity of the cornea.
   a. Full-thickness (penetrating) type of transplant—emphasize the need for longer recovery.
   b. Lamellar-type transplant—activities resumed more rapidly.

B. Keeping Eye Pressure at Safe Level

This is to protect the eye from loss of aqueous humor or from injury because of the possibility of dislocating the newly transplanted cornea.

1. Prevent sudden turning of the head.
2. Minimize those activities or sources of irritants that may cause sneezing (dusting, sweeping, heavily scented flowers, sprays; no pepper on trays).
3. Avoid conversation that annoys or disturbs the patient; caution visitors not to upset the patient since emotional disturbances may increase intraocular pressure.

C. Preventing Complications Post-Surgery

1. Monitor for urinary retention; palpate over bladder area.
2. Prevent constipation or straining on defecation by avoiding constipating foods, maintaining adequate hydration, and administering stool softeners.
3. Administer prescribed analgesics as necessary to relieve pain.
4. Report unrelieved pain. It may indicate:
   a. Hemorrhage is occurring.
   b. Graft has slipped.
   c. Dressings are too tight.
   d. Possible early infection.
   e. Inflammation.
   f. Postoperative glaucoma.
5. Utilize measures that will prevent infection of the eye.
   a. Practice meticulous aseptic technique during dressing changes.
   b. Discourage the patient from touching the dressings.
6. Administer steroids, if prescribed, which will reduce likelihood of graft rejection (often retards wound healing).
7. Introduce additional activities gradually each day; avoid those that will require straining.
8. Be alert for signs of graft rejection (about 10–14 days postoperatively): decreased vision, ocular irritation, corneal edema, or redness of sclera.

Patient Education

1. Emphasize the importance of follow-up visits to the ophthalmologist.
2. Instruct the patient to monitor his eye for graft rejection daily for a period of months after surgery.
   a. Recommend assessment be done at the same time daily so comparisons can be made.
   b. Vision varies with individuals. Functional vision does not return until sutures are removed:
      (1) 6 weeks to 3 months for interrupted sutures.
      (2) About 1 year for continuous sutures.

Retinal Detachment

The detachment of the sensory retina (rods and cones) from the pigment epithelium of the retina (see Fig. 25-6A).

Clinical Manifestations

1. Retinal detachment occurs most commonly after age 40; it may occur slowly or rapidly.
2. The patient complains of flashes of light or blurred, "sooty" vision due to stimulation of the retina by vitreous pull.
3. The patient notes sensation of particles moving in his line of vision. (Normally, most individuals can see floating filaments when looking at a light background).
4. Delineated areas of vision may be blank; there is no pain.
5. A sensation of a veil-like coating coming down, coming up, or sideways in front of the eye may be present.
   a. This veil-like coating, or shadow, is often misinterpreted as a drooping eyelid or elevated cheek.

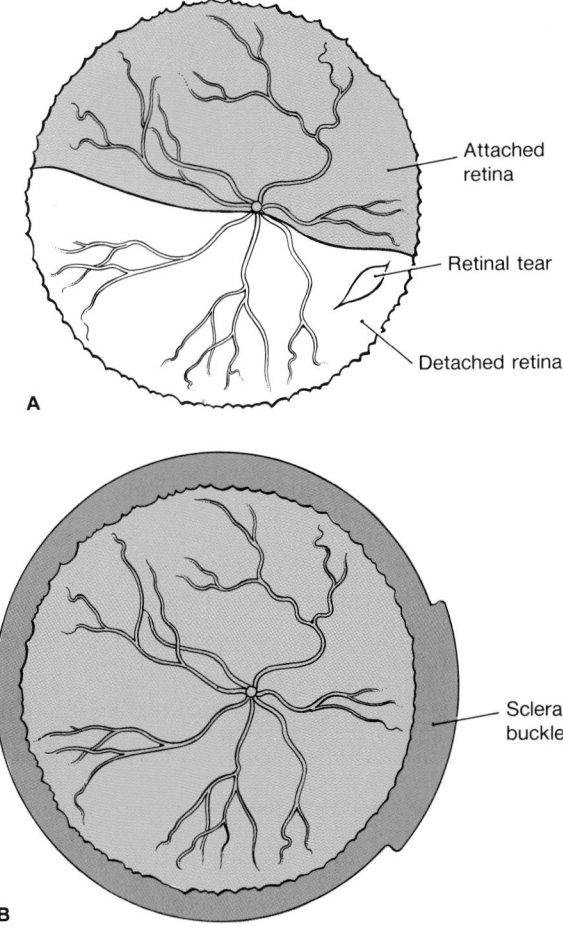

Figure 25-6. (A) Diagram shows area of attached retina, a retinal tear, and an area of retinal detachment. (B) The scleral buckling procedure is a surgical technique used to treat the detached retina.

b. Straight-ahead vision may remain good in early stages.
6. Unless the retinal holes are sealed, the retina will progressively detach, and ultimately there will be a loss of central vision as well as peripheral vision leading to legal blindness.

Management

1. The diagnosis is confirmed by the patient's history and binocular ophthalmoscopy. Surgical intervention is the only treatment.
2. The retinal hole is sealed, thereby ensuring that the retina will adhere to the choroid.
3. Return of visual acuity with a reattached retina depends on:
   a. Amount of retina detached prior to surgery.
   b. Whether the macula was detached.
   c. Length of time the retina was detached.
   d. Amount of external distortion caused by the scleral buckle.
   e. Possible macular damage as a result of diathermy of cryocoagulation.

   Note: If retina remains attached for 2 months postoperatively, the condition is likely to be corrected and unlikely to recur.
4. Surgical procedures that may be used include:
   a. Photocoagulation—a light beam (either laser or xenon arc) is passed through the pupil, causing a small burn and producing an exudate between the pigment epithelium and retina.
   b. Electrodiathermy—an electrode needle is passed through the sclera to allow subretinal fluid to escape. An exudate forms from the pigment epithelium and adheres to the retina.
   c. Cryosurgery or retinal cryopexy—a supercooled probe is touched to the sclera, causing minimal damage; as a result of scarring, the pigment epithelium adheres to the retina.
   d. Scleral buckling—a technique whereby the sclera is shortened to allow a buckling to occur, which forces the pigment epithelium closer to the retina (see Fig. 25-6*B*).

Complications

1. Surgical reattachment by scleral buckling, cryotherapy, or diathermy is successful in approximately 90% to 95% of cases. Secondary operations may be required.
2. Glaucoma and infection.

Preoperative Nursing Interventions

1. Provide emotional support during this time of stress and restriction.
2. Instruct the patient to remain quiet and in the prescribed position to prevent further detachment of the retina. (Proper position results in detached area remaining in dependent position.) Both eyes may be bandaged.
3. Explain preoperative orders and postoperative expectations.
   a. The circumorbital area may be black and blue, but will fade in a few weeks.
   b. The patient will have his eye(s) patched after surgery.
4. Wash patient's face gently preoperatively with an antibacterial solution to reduce possibility of eye infections.

5. Administer prescribed sedation and tranquilizers for comfort and relief or anxiety.

Postoperative Interventions

1. Proper positioning is important after the operation and is prescribed according to individual need.
   a. The patient may be permitted out of bed (on physician's directive) as long as straight-lined vision is maintained.
   b. Rapid eye movements from side to side should be avoided.
2. Take precautions to avoid the patient bumping his head, thus causing the retina to detach further.
3. Following general anesthesia, the patient is encouraged to breathe deeply but not to cough since this will increase eye pressure. Vomiting and sneezing must be avoided.
4. Allow additional activity as type of treatment permits.
5. Provide for diversional therapy, since the patient often becomes depressed.
   a. Moderate TV viewing (straight-lined vision).
   b. No handwork or reading until physician permits (rapid eye movements).
   c. "Talking Books," radio, and visitors permitted.
6. If local anesthesia is used, the patient is ambulatory postoperatively if condition permits (age, vision in other eye, other medical/physical problems).
7. Hospitalization for retinal detachment is usually minimal.

Patient Education

1. Self-care is possible at discharge, if done in an unhurried manner. (Avoid falls, jerks, bumps, or accidental injury.)
2. Instruct patient in following:
   a. Rapid eye movements should be avoided for several weeks.
   b. Driving is restricted.
      (1) Within 3 weeks light activities may be pursued.
      (2) Within 6 weeks heavier activities and athletics are possible. Define such activities for the patient.
   c. Avoid straining and bending head below the waist.
   d. Use meticulous cleanliness in giving eye medications.
   e. Apply a clean, warm, moist, washcloth to eyes and eyelids several times a day for 10 minutes—to provide soothing and relaxing comfort.
   f. Symptoms that indicate a recurrence of the detachment: floating spots, flashing light, progressive shadows. Recommend that the patient contact his physician if they occur.
3. The first follow-up visit to the ophthalmologist should take place in 2 weeks, with other visits scheduled thereafter.

Cataracts

An opacity or cloudiness of the crystalline lens.

Predisposing Factors

1. Most commonly a result of the aging process, after 70 years of age (senile cataracts).
2. Occurrence at birth (congenital cataract).

3. Occasionally a result of disease or following trauma in young individuals.

Clinical Manifestations

1. Alterations in vision:
   a. Objects are distorted and blurred.
   b. Glare annoys the patient when there are bright lights. There is no pain or eye redness.
   c. Visual loss is gradual.
2. Alterations in appearance:
   a. The pupil, usually dark, progresses to a milky-white color.
   b. Eventually opacity becomes complete.

Management

A. General

1. Surgical removal of the lens is indicated.
2. Usually a patient with one cataract can manage without surgery.
3. If cataract occurs in both eyes, surgery is recommended when vision in the better eye causes problems in daily activities. Surgery is done on only one eye at a time.
4. Cataract surgery is usually done under local anesthesia. Preoperative medications produce decreased response to pain and lessened motor activity (neuroleptanalgesia). Oral medications are given to reduce intraocular pressure.
5. Intraocular lens implants are usually implanted at the time of cataract extraction.
6. In some instances following lens extraction and the healing process, the patient may be fitted with appropriate eyeglasses or contact lenses to correct refraction.

B. Surgical Procedures

1. Two types of extractions:
   a. Intracapsular extraction—the lens as well as the capsule are removed through a small incision.
   b. Extracapsular extraction—the lens capsule is incised, and the nucleus, cortex, and anterior capsule are extracted.
      (1) The posterior capsule is left in place and is usually the base to which an intraocular lens (IOL) is implanted (see Fig. 25-7A and B).
      (2) A conservative procedure of choice, simple to perform, and usually done under local anesthesia.
2. Two types of procedures for extraction include:
   a. Cryosurgery—a special technique in which a pencil-like instrument with a metal tip is super-cooled (−35°C.), then is touched to the exposed lens, freezing to it so that the lens is easily lifted out.
   b. Phacoemulsification—the mechanical breaking up (emulsifying) of the lens by a hollow needle vibrating at ultrasonic speed. This action is coupled with irrigation and aspiration of the emulsified particles from the anterior chamber.

C. Intraocular Lens Implantation

1. The implantation of a synthetic lens (intraocular lens) is designed for distance vision; the patient may wear prescription glasses for reading and near vision.
   a. Intraocular lens implant is an alternative to sight correction with glasses or contact lenses for the aphakic (absence of lens) patient.
   b. Sophisticated calculations are required to determine the prescription for lens.

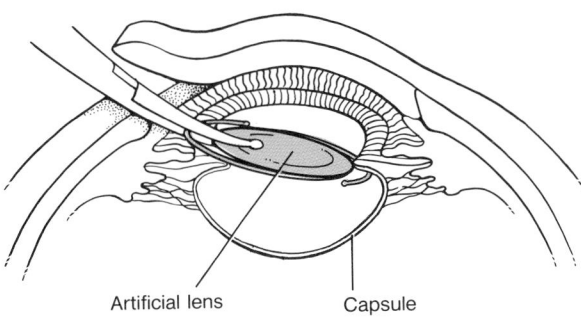

A Implantation of a posterior chamber lens

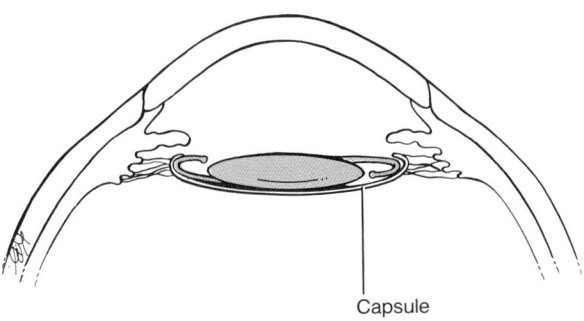

B Artificial lens in place

Figure 25-7. *Extracapsular cataract extraction with placement of an intraocular lens (IOL) after cataract surgery. (A) Placement of the intraocular lens in the posterior capsule. (B) Intraocular lens in place.*

   c. There are a number of types of intraocular lens available. Designs and materials change as new developments occur. Extended-wear contact lenses may replace intraocular lens.
2. Advantages of intraocular lens include:
   a. Provides an alternative for individual who cannot wear cataract glasses or contact lenses.
   b. Cannot be lost or misplaced like conventional glasses.
3. Complications (specific to implantation)
   a. Pain from inflammation of various eye structures—usually controlled by nonsteroidal anti-inflammatory drugs, but systemic antibiotics and immunosuppression may be required.
   b. Rosy vision (glare) due to keeping pupil from full constriction; excessive light enters pupil, causing a dazzling of macula.
   c. Degeneration of the cornea.
   d. Malpositioning or dislocation of lens.

Preoperative Nursing Interventions

A. Relieving Anxiety and Ensuring Safety

1. Explain the plan of care and postoperative expectations.
2. Orient patient to surroundings.
3. Assess patient's knowledge level regarding the surgery and anxiety level of postoperative expectations.
4. Administer tranquilizer(s) if prescribed.

B. Reducing the Conjunctival Bacterial Count and Minimizing the Chance of Postoperative Complications

1. Obtain a conjunctival culture if requested.
2. Employ aseptic technique when performing eye treatment.
3. Instruct the patient not to touch eyes.
4. Administer medications as prescribed.
   a. Antiemetics—prochlorperazine (Compazine), hydroxyzine (Vistaril)
   b. Narcotics—meperidine (Demerol) for pain control
   c. Ocular hypotensives
      (1) Cholinesterase inhibitors—acetazolamide (Diamox)
      (2) Osmotic hypotensives—glycerol (Glyrol), mannitol
   d. Mydriatics (Note whether pupil dilates after instillation of medication.)

Postoperative Nursing Interventions

A. Preventing Increased Intraocular Pressure

1. Caution the patient to refrain from coughing or sneezing.
2. Administer antiemetic drugs as prescribed and perhaps an osmotic agent—nausea may lead to vomiting.
3. Advise the patient to avoid rapid movements and caution him not to bend from the waist.

B. Promoting Comfort and Safety

1. Allow the patient to turn on unoperated side or on his back—provide a pillow or permit head elevation.
2. Offer analgesics as prescribed.
3. Monitor for sudden pain in the eye, which may be due to a ruptured vessel or suture and may lead to hemorrhage.
   a. Assess for restlessness and increasing pulse rate.
   b. Notify physician immediately.
4. Allow the patient to be ambulatory/go to the bathroom as soon as he has recovered from anesthesia (as prescribed).
5. Encourage the patient to wear shield at night to ensure protection of his eye from injury.

Patient Education

A. Promoting Independence

1. Orient the patient to his room and personal items.
2. Gradually increase the patient's activities each day— usually normal activities may be started a day after phacoemulsification.
3. Caution the patient to avoid any strain on the eye; heavy lifting (define weight); and straining on defecation.
4. Resumption of sexual activities may be discussed when the eye and suture line are examined.
5. Demonstrate to the patient and a responsible member of his family how to administer eye medications (see p. 629).

B. Convalescence Expectations

1. Apply plastic shield over the eye at night to avoid accidental injury during sleep.
2. Fitting for temporary corrective lenses for the first 6 weeks.
   a. Prescription for permanent lenses 6–12 weeks after surgery for intracapsular extraction.
   b. Prescription for contact lenses about 3–6 weeks after phacoemulsification.
3. Use dark glasses after eye dressings are removed to provide comfort.

C. Adjusting to the Eyeglasses

1. Stress the importance of patience in the coming weeks of adjustment—it is easy to become frustrated.
2. If glasses are to be worn, they will cause the perceived image to be about ⅓ larger than that seen by the patient before cataract formation. (Glass is usually heavier and thicker than the more expensive plastic cataract eyeglass lenses.)

Note: The patient can use only one eye at a time with glasses, if only one eye is operated for cataract, since the operated eye has a 30% increase in image size and the unoperated eye still has "normal" sized images, which cannot be superimposed.

3. Instruct the patient to look through the center of the corrective glasses and to turn head when looking to the side since peripheral vision is markedly distorted.
4. It is necessary to relearn space judgment—walking, using stairs, reaching for articles on the table (such as a cup of coffee), pouring liquids.
5. Use handrails while walking.

D. Becoming Familiar With Contact Lenses

1. With contact lenses, magnification is only about 5% to 10%; peripheral vision is not distorted.
2. Both eyes may be used together since the image difference between an aphakic eye with a contact lens and the unoperated eye is only 8% to 10%. Space judgment presents little difficulty.
3. If the patient has difficulty applying lenses, has a tremor of the hands, or if there are general hygienic problems that could cause soiling and infection, there may be complications. These patients are not prime candidates for contact lenses.

E. Becoming Familiar With Intraocular Lens

1. Recognize that with an intraocular lens, magnification problems are negligible. Both the operated eye and the unoperated eye can work together after cataract surgery with lens implantation.
2. No eyeglasses may be required for distance but may be needed for reading and writing.
3. Caution against straining of any type. Bend knees only if necessary to reach for something on the floor.
4. Sponge bath is recommended for bathing. Avoid getting soap in the eyes.
5. Avoid tilting head forward when washing hair; tilt head slightly backward. Vigorous shaking of the head is avoided.

F. Administering Eye Medications

1. Instill eye medications as directed (see p. 629).
2. Bring all eye medications to ophthalmologist appointment to permit adjustments in dosage and medications. What will not be used can then be discarded to prevent confusion.

Glaucoma

A condition in which an obstruction of outflow occurs within the travecular network and the canal of Schlemm leading to increased pressure within the eyeball. It is associated with progressive visual field loss and eventual blindness if allowed to progress.

Classification

1. Angle-closure (narrow angle)—acute or chronic
2. Open-angle (wide angle; simple; chronic single)—chronic
3. Congenital

Within these classifications, principal contributing factors may be primary or secondary.

Primary—genetically based
Secondary—result of ocular disease, injury, neoplasia, or surgery

Note: Because of the relative ease of developing glaucoma, unless a person past 40 years of age has a complete physical examination periodically, including measurement of eye pressure (tonometry), the disease may not be discovered until it is considerably advanced. Early detection and treatment will prevent loss of eyesight.

Acute (Angle-Closure) Glaucoma

A medical emergency that, if untreated, may lead to blindness within 3–5 days of onset.

Clinical Manifestations

1. Severe pain in and around eyes due to increased ocular pressure (often above 75 mm. Hg); transitory attacks.
2. Rainbow of color around lights.
3. Vision becomes cloudy and blurred.
4. Pupil dilates; nausea and vomiting may occur.
5. Although onset may have initial subclinical symptoms, severity of symptoms may progress to include systemic disturbances; (gastrointestinal, sinus, neurologic, and dental problems).

Management

1. Emergency pharmacotherapy is initiated to decrease eye pressure before surgery.
2. Medications are prescribed at the discretion of the ophthalmologist according to the patient's condition and needs.
3. Medication classifications prescribed include:
   a. Parasympathomimetic drugs used as miotic drugs—pupil contracts; iris is drawn away from cornea; aqueous humor may drain through lymph spaces (meshwork) into canal of Schlemm.

> **NURSING ALERT:** Dilatation of pupils is avoided if the anterior chamber is shallow. This is determined by oblique illumination of the anterior segment of the eye.

   b. Sympathomimetic drugs—decrease aqueous humor production rate.
   c. Carbonic anhydrase inhibitor—restricts action of enzyme that is necessary to produce aqueous humor.
   d. Beta blocker—nonselective—may reduce production of aqueous humor or may facilitate outflow of aqueous humor.
   e. Hyperosmotic agents—increase blood osmolarity.

Surgical Management

Surgery is indicated if:
1. Intraocular pressure is not maintained within normal limits by medical regimen.
2. There is progressive visual field loss with optic nerve damage.

Types

1. Peripheral iridectomy—excision of a small portion of the iris whereby aqueous humor can bypass pupil; treatment of choice.
2. Trabeculectomy—partial-thickness scleral resection with small part of trabecular meshwork removed and iridectomy. Necessary if peripheral anterior adhesions (synechiae) have developed due to repeated glaucoma attacks.

Chronic (Open-Angle) Glaucoma

Most common form of glaucoma, usually beginning around age of 40–45 with clinical symptoms appearing as late as age 60–65.

Clinical Manifestations

1. Mild, bilateral discomfort (tired feeling in eyes, foggy vision).
2. Slowly developing impairment of peripheral vision—central vision unimpaired.
3. Progressive loss of visual field.
4. Halos present around lights with increased ocular pressure.

Management

1. Often treated with a combination of miotic and carbonic anhydrase inhibitors.
2. Remission may occur; however, there is no cure. The patient should continue to see physician at 3–6-month intervals for control of intraocular pressure.
3. If medical treatment is not successful, surgery may be required, but is delayed as long as possible.

Surgery

1. *Laser trabeculoplasty* (LTP)
   a. An outpatient procedure, treatment of choice if increased ocular pressure unresponsive to medical regimen only.
   b. As many as 80–100 superficial surface burns are placed evenly at junction of pigmented and non-pigmented trabeculum meshwork for 360 degrees in anesthetized eye, which allows increased outflow of aqueous humor.
   c. Maximum decrease in intraocular pressure is achieved in 2–3 months, but intraocular pressure may rise again in 1–2 years.
2. *Iridencleisis* An opening is created between anterior chamber and space beneath the conjunctiva; this bypasses the blocked meshwork, and aqueous humor is absorbed into conjunctival tissues.
3. *Cyclodiathermy* or *cyclocryotherapy* The ciliary body's function of secreting aqueous humor is decreased by damaging the body with high-frequency electrical current or super-cooled probe applied to the surface of the eye over the ciliary body.
4. *Corneoscleral trephine* (rarely done) A permanent opening at the junction of the cornea and sclera is made through the anterior chamber so aqueous humor can drain.

Postoperative Nursing Interventions

(Glaucoma and cataracts, at times, are accompanying disorders.)

1. Nursing management is similar in the postoperative period (see p. 642).
2. Patient with glaucoma may be ambulatory quicker than patient with cataracts, and specific interventions depend on the type of surgery performed.
3. The head of the bed is elevated to promote drainage of aqueous humor after a trabeculectomy.
4. Medications (steroids and cycloplegics) are given as prescribed after peripheral iridectomy to decrease inflammation and to dilate the pupil.

Patient Education

1. The patient must remember that glaucoma cannot be cured, but it can be controlled.
2. Remind the patient that periodic eye check-ups are essential since pressure changes may occur.

3. Alert patient to avoid, if possible, circumstances that may increase intraocular pressure.
   a. Upper respiratory infections.
   b. Emotional upsets—worry, fear, anger.
   c. Exertion such as snow shoveling, pushing, heavy lifting.
4. Recommend the following:
   a. Continuous daily use of eye medications as prescribed.
   b. Moderate use of the eyes.
   c. Exercise in moderation to maintain general well-being.
   d. Fluid intake is not restricted: Alcohol and coffee may be permitted unless they are noted to cause increased intraocular pressure in the particular patient.
   e. Maintenance of regular bowel habits.
   f. Wearing a medical identification tag indicating the patient has glaucoma.

Bibliography

Books

Benson WE. Retinal Detachment Diagnosis and Management. 2nd ed. Philadelphia, JB Lippincott, 1988

Boyd–Monk H and Steinmetz CG. Nursing Care of the Eye. Norwalk, CT, Appleton & Lange, 1987

Call NB. Orbital surgery, pp 677–694. In Waltman SR et al. Surgery of the Eye, Vol 2. New York, Churchill Livingstone, 1988

Carroll DM. Management of ocular trauma, pp 1023–1052. In Waltman SR et al. Surgery of the Eye, Vol. 2. New York, Churchill Livingstone, 1988

Deutsch T and Feller D. Management of Ocular Injuries. Philadelphia, WB Saunders, 1985

Dowling JL Jr. Ambulatory cataract surgery, pp 97–117. In Waltman SR et al. Surgery of the Eye, Vol 1. New York, Churchill Livingstone, 1988

Doughman DJ et al. Long-term organ culture for corneal storage: Minnesota system, pp 84–92. In Brightbill FS (ed). Corneal Surgery: Theory, Technique, and Tissue. St. Louis, CV Mosby, 1986

Felt DP and Frueh BR. Ectropion, pp 459–470. In Waltman SR et al. Surgery of the Eye, Vol 1. New York, Churchill Livingstone, 1988

Flanagan JC, Kapustiak JF and Nowinski T. Orbital fractures, pp 695–718. In Waltman SR et al. Surgery of the Eye, Vol 2. New York, Churchill Livingstone, 1988

Frueh BR. Evaluation of blepharoptosis, pp 421–428. In Waltman SR et al. Surgery of the Eye, Vol 1. New York, Churchill Livingstone, 1988

Hargiss JL. Surgical correction of blepharoptosis, pp 429–446. In Waltman SR et al. Surgery of the Eye, Vol. 1. New York, Churchill Livingstone, 1988

Herschler J. Filtering surgery, pp 347–

359. In Waltman SR et al. Surgery of the Eye. Vol. 1. New York, Churchill Livingstone, 1988

Hilton G et al. Retinal Detachment. 5th ed. San Francisco, American Academy of Ophthalmology, 1989

Kaufman HE et al, (eds). The Cornea. New York, Churchill Livingstone, 1988

Kaufman HE et al. Intermediate-term storage medium (K-Sol), pp 78–84. In Brightbill FS (ed). Corneal Surgery: Theory, Technique, and Tissue. St. Louis, CV Mosby, 1986

Keates RH. Indications and techniques for removal of intraocular lenses, pp 173–184. In Waltman SR et al. Surgery of the Eye, Vol 1. New York, Churchill Livingstone, 1988

Keates RH. Lasers, pp 41–56. In Waltman SR et al. Surgery of the Eye, Vol 1. New York, Churchill Livingstone, 1988

McCammon RL. Ophthalmic anesthesia, pp 3–30. In Waltman SR et al. Surgery of the Eye. New York, Churchill Livingstone, 1988

McIntyre DJ. Manual extracapsular cataract extraction, pp 119–130. In Waltman SR et al. Surgery of the Eye, Vol 1. New York, Churchill Livingstone, 1988

Millodot M. Dictionary of Optometry. Boston, Butterworths, 1986

Nussenblatt RB. Nonsteroidal therapy for ocular inflammation, pp 1–18. In Duane TD et al. Biomedical Foundations of Ophthalmology. Philadelphia, Harper & Row, 1986

Okun E. The surgical treatment of retinal detachment, pp 839–888. In Waltman SR et al. Surgery of the Eye, Vol 2. New York, Churchill Livingstone, 1988

Shields MB. Textbook of Glaucoma. 2nd ed. Baltimore, Williams & Wilkins, 1987

Solish AM and Kass MA. Laser trabeculoplasty, pp 333–338. In Waltman SR et al. Surgery of the Eye. New York, Churchill Livingstone, 1988

Spaeth GL. Combined procedures for glaucoma and cataracts, pp 361–376. In Waltman SR et al. Surgery of the Eye, Vol. 1. New York, Churchill Livingstone, 1988

Sullivan JH. Trichiasis and distichiasis, pp 545–549. In Waltman SR et al. Surgery of the Eye, Vol 1. New York, Churchill Livingstone, 1988

Tennant JL. Intracapsular cataract extraction with intraocular lenses, pp 141–164. In Waltman SR et al. Surgery of the Eye, Vol. 1. New York, Churchill Livingstone, 1988

Vaughn D and Asbury T. General Ophthalmology, 11th ed, pp 132–136. Los Altos, CA, Lange Medical Publications, 1986

Waltman SR et al. Surgery of the Eye, Vols 1 and 2. New York, Churchill Livingstone, 1988

Watzke RC. Prophylaxis of retinal detachment, pp 829–838. In Waltman SR et al. Surgery of the Eye, Vol 2. New York, Churchill Livingstone, 1988

Wilenski J. Iridectomy, pp 323–331. In Waltman SR et al. Surgery of the Eye, Vol 1. New York, Churchill Livingstone, 1988

Wojno TH. Entropion, pp 447–458. In Waltman SR et al. Surgery of the Eye, Vol 1. New York, Churchill Livingstone, 1988

Journals

Retinal Detachment

Algrere P et al. Success and complications of pneumatic retinopexy. Am J Ophthalmol 1988 Oct 15; 106(4):400–404

Blumenkranz M et al. Vitrectomy for retinal detachment associated with acute retinal necrosis. Am J Ophthalmol 1988 Oct 15; 106(4):426–429

Bidwell AE et al. Macular halos and excellent visual acuity. Case report.

Arch Ophthalmol 1988 Oct; 106(10): 1350–1351

Cousins SW et al. Pseudophakic retinal detachments in the presence of various IOL types. Ophthalmology 1986 Sep; 93(9):1198–1208

Chang S et al. Giant retinal tears: Surgical techniques and results using perfluorocarbon liquids. Arch Ophthalmol 1989 May; 107(5):761–767

de Juan E Jr et al. Vitreous surgery for hemorrhagic and fibrosis complications of age-related macular degeneration. Am J Ophthalmol 1988 Jan 15; 105(1):25–29

Elkington AR and Khaw PT. ABC of eyes: Acute visual disturbances. Br Med J (Clin Res) 1988 Jul 23; 297(6643): 279–283

Engel JM et al. Use of the carbon dioxide laser in the drainage of subretinal fluid. Arch Ophthalmol 1989 May; 107(5):731–734

Fleischman JA et al. To admit or not to admit, that is the question. Arch Ophthalmol 1988 Nov; 106(11):1501

Goodlaw E. Role of the optometrist in age-related maculopathy. J Am Optom Assoc 1988 Jun; 59(6):472–479

Kingham JD. Macular hemorrhage in the aging eye: The effects of anticoagulants. N Engl J Med 1988 Apr 28; 318(17):1126–1127

Lawlor MC. Common ocular injuries and disorders: Acute loss of vision. J Emerg Nurs 1989 Jan–Feb; 15(1):32–36, 41–43

Olsen KR et al. Biodegradable mechanical retinal fixation: A pilot study. Arch Ophthalmol 1989 May; 107(7):735–741

Poliner LS, Grand MG and Schoch LH. New retinal detachment as a complication of pneumatic retinopexy. Ophthalmology 1987 Apr; 94(4):315–318

Roseman R et al. Limited retinal detachment: A retrospective analysis of treatment with transconjunctival retinocryopexy. Ophthalmology 1986 Jan; 93(1):216–223

Sergott RC et al. Acute retinal necrosis neuropathy: Clinical profile and surgical therapy. Arch Ophthalmol 1989 May; 107(5):692–696

Contact Lenses

Armitage BS et al. Overnight corneal swelling response in adapted and unadapted extended wear patients. Am J Optom Physiol Opt 1988 Mar; 65a(3):155–161

Carlson KH et al. Effects of long-term contact lens wear on corneal endothelial cell morphology and function. Invest Ophthalmol Vis Sci 1988 Feb; 29(2):185–193

Donnerfeld ED et al. Changing trends in contact lens associated corneal ulcers: An overview of 116 cases. CLAO J 1986 Jul–Sep; 12(3):145–149

Donzis PB et al. Microbial contamination of contact lens care systems. Am J Ophthalmol 1987 Oct 15; 104(4):325–333

Killingsworth DW et al. Pseudomonas keratitis associated with the use of disposable soft contact lenses: Case report. Arch Ophthalmol 1989 Jun; 107(6):795–796

Lane SL et al. Polysulfone corneal lenses. J Cataract Refract Surg 1986 Jan; 12(1): 50–60

Ludwig IH et al. Susceptibility of Acanthamoeba to soft contact lens disinfection systems. Invest Ophthalmol Vis Sci 1986 Apr; 27(4): 626–628

Riordan-Eav P et al. *Pseudomonas aeruginosa* corneal ulcer associated with an aerosol can of preservative-free saline. Arch Ophthalmol 1988 Nov; 106(11):1506–1507

Tsubota K. A contact lens for specular microscopic observation. Am J Ophthalmol 1988 Nov 15; 106(5):627–628

Glaucoma

Berger CM et al. Anterior lens capsule perforation and zonular rupture after Nd:YAG laser iridotomy. Am J Ophthalmol 1989 Jun 15; 107(6):674–675

Berlin O et al. Excimer laser photoablation in glaucoma filtering surgery. Am J Ophthalmol 1987 May 15; 103(5):713–714

Bishop KI et al. Bilateral argon laser trabeculoplasty in primary open-angle glaucoma. Am J Ophthalmol 1989 Jun 15; 107(6):591–595

Boyd-Monk H and Starita RJ. Surgical intervention to stop glaucoma. J Ophthalmol Nurs Tech 1985 May–Jun; 4(3):12–15

Elkington AR and Khaw PT. ABC of eyes: The glaucomas. Br Med J [Clin Res] 1988 Jun 25; 296(6639):1287–1290

Katz LJ et al. Reversible optic disk cupping and visual field improvement in adults with glaucoma. Am J Ophthalmol 1989 May 15; 107(5):485–492

Lewis JM et al. Intraocular pressure response to topical dexamethasone as a predictor for the development of primary open-angle glaucoma. Am J Ophthalmol 1988 Nov 15; 106(5):607–612

Poinoosawmy D et al. Glaucoma and race. Lancet 1989 May 20; 1(8647): 1134

Ticho U et al. Laser trabeculoplasty in glaucoma: Ten-year evaluation. Arch Ophthalmol 1989 Jun; 107(6):844–846

White GL Jr et al. Primary congenital glaucoma. Am Fam Physician 1989 May; 39(5):159–162

Yanazaki Y et al. Correlation between color vision and highest intraocular pressure in glaucoma patients. Am J Ophthalmol 1988 Oct 15; 106(5):607–612

Cataracts

Andrews CL. Nursing care of the cataract patient in an ambulatory surgery center. Ophthalmic Nurs Forum 1987 Mar; 3(3):1–8

Brown NA et al. The objective assessment of cataracts. Eye 1987 Feb; 1(2):234–236

Chylack LT Jr et al. Lens opacities classification system. Arch Ophthalmol 1988 Mar; 106(3):330–334

Elkington AR and Khaw PT. ABC of eyes: Cataracts. Br Med J [Clin Res] 1988 Jun 25; 296(6639):1787–1790

Guthauser U et al. Quantifying visual field damage caused by cataracts. Am J Ophthalmol 1988 Oct 15; 106(4):480–484

Hunt L. Use of Honan Intraocular Pressure Reducer. J Ophthal Nurs Technol 1988 Mar–Apr; 7(2):59–61

Koska MT. Hospitals big losers with new cataract rate. Hospitals 1989 Nov 5; 62(21):94

Kramer TR et al. Transscleral ND:YAG photo coagulation for cataract incision vascularization associated with recurrent hyphema. Am J Ophthalmol 1989 Jun 15; 107(6):681–682

Liu IY et al. The association of age-related macular degeneration and lens opacities in the aged. Am J Public Health 1989 Jun; 79(6):765–759

Taylor HR et al. Effect of ultraviolet radiation on cataract formation. N Engl J Med 1988 Dec 1; 319(22):1429–1433

Injuries

Arnold RW et al. Magnetized forceps for metallic corneal foreign bodies. Arch Ophthalmol 1988 Nov; 106(11):1502

Carroll ME. Retained glass foreign body in the eyelid. Am J Ophthalmol 1989 May 15; 107(5):555–556

Clark RB et al. Eye emergencies and urgencies. Patient Care 1989 Jan 15; 23(1):24–34, 36, 38+

Elkington AR and Khaw PT. Injuries around the orbit: More than meets the eye. Br Med J [Clin Res] 1987 Dec 19–26; 295(6613):1652–1654

Elkington AR and Khaw PT. Injuries to the Eye. Br Med J [Clin Res] 1988 Jul 9; 297(6641):122–125

Guy J et al. Surgical treatment of progressive visual loss in traumatic optic neuropathy: Report of two cases. J Neurosurg 1989 May; 70(5):799–801

Lubeck D. Penetrating ocular injuries. Emerg Med Clin North Am 1988 Feb; 6(1):127–146

Lubeck D and Greene JS. Corneal injuries. Emerg Med Clin North Am 1988 Feb; 6(1):73–94

Talley FM et al. Alkaline injuries to the eye. Ophthalmol Nurs Forum 1989; 5(1):1–4, 6–8

Corneal Ulcers

Cohen EJ et al. Corneal ulcers associated with cosmetic extended-wear soft contact lenses. Ophthalmology 1987 Feb; 94(2):109–114

Groden LR and Brinser JH. Outpatient treatment of microbial corneal ulcers. Arch Ophthalmol 1986 Jan; 104(1):84–86

Kershner RM. Infectious corneal ulcer with over extended wearing of disposable contact lenses. JAMA 1989 Jun 23–30; 261(24):3549–3550

Laibson PR and Donnenfeld E. Corneal ulcers related to contact lens use. Int Ophthalmol Clin 1986 Spring; 26(1): 3–14

Parker AV et al. Pseudomonas corneal ulcers after artificial fingernail injuries. Am J Ophthalmol 1989 May 15; 107(5):548–549

Surgery

Crawford R. Ambulatory surgery: The elderly patient. AORN J 1985 Feb; 41(2):356–359

Holland GN et al. Treatment of cytomegalovirus retinopathy with ganciclovir. Ophthalmology 1987 Jul; 94(7):815–823

Kalnins LY et al. Corneal decompensation after argon laser iridectomy. Arch Ophthalmol 1989 Jun; 197(6):792

Kersten RC et al. Selective approach to surgery for delayed enophthalmos. Arch Otolaryngol Head Neck Surg 1989 May; 115(5):634

Schwartz AL et al. Corneal decompensation after argon laser iridectomy. Arch Ophthalmol 1988 Nov; 106(11):1572–1574

Stern GA. Update on the medical management of corneal and external eye diseases, corneal transplantation, and keratorefractive surgery. Ophthalmology 1988 Jul; 95(6):842–854

Walker M. Growing old: Increased surgical risks in the elderly. AORN J 1986 Apr; 43(4):887–890

White GL Jr et al. Corneal transplantation. Am Fam Physician 1988 Nov; 38(5):135–138

General

Dimmett SB et al. Usefulness of ophthalmoscopy in mild to moderate hypertension. Br Med J [Clin Res] 1988, Aug 13; 297(6646):473–477

Deutsch TA. Ophthalmology. JAMA 1989, May 19; 261(19):2867–2868

Elkington AR and Khaw PT. ABC of eyes: The red eye. Br Med J [Clin Res] 1988 Jun 18; 296(6638):1720–1724

Elkington AR and Khaw PT. ABC of eyes: Refractive errors. Br Med J [Clin Res] 1988 Jul 16; 297(6642):192–195

Elkington AR and Khaw PT. ABC of eyes: History and examination. Br Med J [Clin Res] 1988 Jul 30; 296(6644):347–351

Elkington AR and Khaw PT. ABC of eyes: General medical disorders and the eye. Br Med J [Clin Res] 1988 Aug 6; 297(6645):412–416

Lichter PR. Controlling risks of the possible transmission of human immunodeficiency virus: Notice of American Academy of Ophthalmology. Clinical Alert. Ophthalmology 1989 Jan; 96(1):1–2

MacKay CJ. Color vision defects in retinal disease. Arch Ophthalmol 1989 Jun; 107(6):790–791

National Advisory Eye Council. Vision research: A national plan. 1987 Evaluation and Update. 1983–1987. NIH Publication #87-2755.

Noble KG et al. Progressive peripheral cone dysfunction. Am J Ophthalmol 1988 Nov 15; 106(5):557–560

Nussenblatt RB and Palestine AG. Cyclosporine: Immunology, pharmacology and therapeutic uses. Surg Ophthalmol 1986 Nov–Dec; 31(3):159–169

Intraocular Lens (IOL)

Hoffer KJ. Secondary intraocular lens implantation versus epikerataphakia for the treatment of aphakia. Ophthalmol 1987 Aug 15; 104(2):194–195

Smith PW et al. Complications of semiflexible, closed-loop anterior chamber intraocular lenses. Arch Ophthalmol 1987 Jan; 105(1):52–57

Inflammation

Mansir JH and Kin YJ. Intraocular inflammatory disease (uveitis). Ophthal Nurs Forum 1988 Jan; 4(1):1–8

Moore MB et al. Acanthamoeba keratitis: A growing problem in soft and hard contact lens wearers. Ophthalmology 1987 Dec; 94(12):1654–1661

Ear Disorders

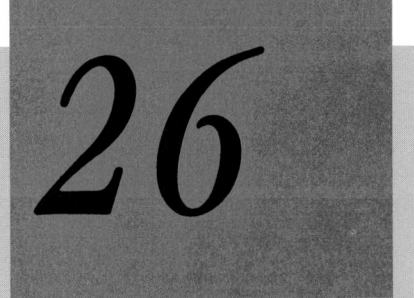

26

Hearing Problems

Problems with hearing rank high as a health disability.

Classification of Hearing Loss

1. *Conductive loss*—a hearing loss due to an impairment of the outer or middle ear or both. If causative problem cannot be corrected, a hearing aid may help.
2. *Sensorineural (perceptive) loss*—a hearing loss due to disease of the inner ear or nerve pathways; sensitivity to and discrimination of sounds are impaired. Hearing aids usually are helpful.
3. *Combined hearing loss*—a combination of the above.
4. *Psychogenic hearing loss*—usually a manifestation of an emotional disturbance and unrelated to evident structural changes in the hearing mechanisms. Loss is often total, but without physical basis; thus, the patient may suddenly recover.

Presbycusis

A progressive, bilaterally perceptive hearing loss of older individuals, usually involving high frequencies, that occurs with the aging process.

A. Treatment

There is no effective medical or surgical treatment.

B. Nursing Interventions

1. The patient should be counseled by an otologist in collaboration with an audiologist.
2. Helpful aids should be considered, such as a telephone amplifier, radio and television earphone attachments, buzzers instead of door bell.
3. Understanding and help from family members are important.

Assessment and Diagnostic Procedures

Nursing History

1. Designed to reveal status of adult hearing.
2. Question the patient about hearing loss, fullness/pain in the ear, dizziness, previous trauma, antibiotic use, aspirin use, smoking, exposure to loud noise.

Physical Examination

Examination techniques: Inspection, palpation, mechanical tests, and otoscopic examination.
1. Examine unaffected ear first in patient with ear pain.
2. If gentleness is demonstrated during examination of good ear, patient is more likely to submit to examination of painful ear.
3. If sensitive ear is hurt during examination, examiner risks not getting a good look at it or at the good ear.
4. Infection could be transmitted from painful ear to good ear.

Note: Tuning fork test (Weber's and Rinne tests) are mechanical tests and are used only for screening or confirmatory purposes (see Table 26-1).

Audiometry

Measurement of hearing.

Pure-Tone Audiometry

A. Test Principles

1. Sound stimulus consists of a pure (musical) tone presented in a variety of intensities and/or frequencies.
2. The louder the tone required for the patient to hear it, the greater the hearing loss.
3. Air conduction and bone conduction are tested by using ear phones and vibrating oscillator, respectively.
4. Noise level must be carefully controlled, usually by using acoustically shielded (sound-proof) booth.
5. An audiogram is the plotted results of the test.
6. Evaluation of the audiogram includes:
   a. Normal human ear perception—20–20,000 cps (Hz).
   b. Frequencies significant for speech range—500–2000 cps (Hz).
   c. Hearing is normally most astute near 1000 cps.

B. Examples of Hearing Impairment on an Audiogram

1. Conductive hearing loss
   a. A problem in the outer and middle ear may result in reduced sensitivity to tones received by air conduction.

Table 26-1. *Tuning Fork Tests*

Ear Condition	Weber's Test	Rinne Test
Normal, no hearing loss	No shifting of sounds laterally	Sound perceived longer by *air* conduction
Conductive loss	Shifting of sounds to poorer ear	Sound perceived as long or longer by *bone* conduction
Sensorineural loss	Shifting of sounds to better ear	Sound perceived longer by *air* conduction

    b. If the inner ear is unimpaired, bone conduction will be within normal range.
2. Sensorineural hearing loss
    a. A weakening of sound produced in some portion of the sensorineural mechanism (e.g., inner ear) results in reduced thresholds for air conduction.
    b. Usually it also causes a reduction in bone conduction.
3. Mixed hearing loss
    a. Weakening of sound in some portion of the sensorineural mechanism results in reduced bone conduction and air conduction.
    b. When there is also a lesion in the external auditory canal or middle ear, there will be additional weakening in thresholds for air conduction.

Speech Audiometry

A. Speech Reception Threshold (SRT)
1. This is the softest hearing threshold level at which a person can correctly repeat approximately 50% of very familiar two-syllable words.
2. This test provides only a gross estimate of the patient's ability to recognize and respond to speech.

B. Speech Discrimination Score (SDS)
1. This is a suprathreshold measure of speech discrimination.
2. The tester presents phonetically balanced monosyllabic words, which the patient is asked to repeat.
3. The percentage of correct responses is the SDS.

C. Acoustic Impedance Evaluation
1. This is an objective measurement (does not require direct patient response) relating to the function of the peripheral auditory mechanism.
2. A battery of acoustic impedance testing may be done.

Communicating With a Person Who Has a Hearing Impairment

When the Person Is Able to Lip-Read

1. Face the person as directly as possible when speaking.
2. Place yourself in good light so that he can see your mouth.
3. Do not chew, smoke, or have anything in your mouth when speaking.
4. Speak slowly and enunciate distinctly.
5. Provide contextual clues that will assist him in following your speech. For example, point to a tray if you are talking about the food on it.

6. To verify that he understands your message, write it for him to read (that is, if you doubt that he is understanding you).

When It Is Difficult to Understand the Person When He Speaks

1. Pay attention when the person speaks; his facial and physical gestures may help you understand what he is saying.
2. Exchange conversation with him when it is possible to anticipate his replies—this is particularly helpful in your initial contact with him and may help you become familiar with his speech peculiarities.
3. Anticipate context of his speech to assist in interpreting what he is saying.
4. If unable to understand him, resort to writing or include in your conversation someone who does understand him; request that he repeat that which is not understood.

Problems Affecting the External Ear

Otitis Externa

Otitis externa is an inflammation of the external ear canal that may occur 2–3 days after swimming and diving (swimmer's ear).

A. Prevention
1. Prevent or minimize by thoroughly drying the ear canal after coming into contact with water or moist environment.
2. Use of ear drops after swimming may assist in preventing swimmer's ear. Usually these solutions contain:
    a. Alcohol and glycerol to reduce moisture.
    b. Boric acid or acetic acid (vinegar) to limit growth of microorganisms and maintain normal acidity of the ear canal.

NURSING ALERT: Use of cotton-tipped applicators to dry the canal or remove ear wax should be avoided because:
a. Cerumen may be forced against the tympanic membrane.
b. The canal lining may be abraded, making it more susceptible to infection.
c. Cerumen that coats and protects the canal may be removed.

B. Management
1. Alcohol (dries moisture), acetic acid solution (restores acidity), and topical antibiotics (curb infection).
2. If canal is swollen and tender, topical corticosteroids may decrease inflammation and swelling.
3. Burow's solution (aluminum acetate solution) may decrease drainage caused by eczema.
4. When acute pain and swelling have subsided, a specially trained person can remove debris from ear canal with an applicator or by irrigation or suction.

Cerumen in Ear Canal

1. Accumulated cerumen (earwax) does not have to be removed unless it becomes impacted and interferes with hearing.
2. To irrigate ear canal, see Guidelines, below.

Foreign Bodies in External Canal

Note: Do not instill anything into external canal if eardrum may be perforated.

1. Insects
   a. Treat by instilling oil drops to smother insect, which then can be removed by health professional.
2. Vegetable foreign bodies (e.g., peas)
   a. Irrigation is contraindicated because vegetable matter absorbs water, which would further wedge it in the canal.
   b. Unskilled persons should not attempt to remove a foreign body because:
      (1) It may be forced into bony portion of the canal.
      (2) The canal skin may be perforated.
      (3) The eardrum may be perforated.
   c. Removal should be done skillfully with instruments; if the victim is very young, general anesthesia is required.

Guidelines Irrigating the External Auditory Canal

Purposes:
1. To remove discharge from the canal
2. To facilitate removal of cerumen or foreign body.
3. To apply heat or coolness to the tissues.

> **NURSING ALERT:** Ask if patient has a history of draining ears or has ever had a perforation or other complications from a previous ear irrigation. If the reply is "yes," check with the physician before proceeding with the irrigation.

Equipment and Solutions

Kind and amount of solution desired
Ear syringe or irrigating container with tubing, clamp, and catheter
Protective towels
Cotton balls and cotton-tipped applicators
Solution bowl and emesis basin
Bag for disposable items

Procedure

Preparatory Phase

1. After explaining procedure to the patient, place him in a position of sitting or lying with head tilted forward and toward affected ear.
2. Position protective towels.

Nursing Action	Rationale/Amplification

Performance Phase

Nursing Action	Rationale/Amplification
1. Use a cotton applicator to remove any discharge on outer ear.	1. To prevent carrying discharge deeper into canal.
2. Place basin close to the patient's head and under the ear.	2. To provide a receptacle to receive irrigating solution.
3. Test temperature of solution. It should be comfortable to the inner aspect of wrist area.	3. Solutions that are hot or cold are most uncomfortable and may initiate a feeling of dizziness.
4. Ascertain whether impaction is due to a foreign hydroscopic (attracts or absorbs moisture) body before proceeding.	4. If water contacts such a substance, it may cause it to swell and produce intense pain.
5. Gently pull the outer ear upward and backward (adult) or downward and backward (child).	5. To straighten the ear canal (see Fig. 26-1 *A–B*).
6. Place tip of syringe or irrigating catheter at opening of ear; gently direct stream of fluid against sides of canal (Fig. 26-1 *C*).	6. To decrease direct force of irrigation against eardrum and possibility of rupturing it.
7. If an irrigating container is used, elevate only high enough to remove secretions or no more than 15 cm. (6 inches) above patient's ear.	7. To provide safe and effective pressure of fluid; if height is more than 15 cm. (6 inches), pressure will be too great and may damage tissue.
8. Observe for signs of pain or dizziness.	8. Discontinue treatment if they occur.
9. If irrigating does not dislodge the wax, instill several drops of prescribed glycerin, carbamide peroxide (Debrox), or other solutions as directed 2 or 3 times daily for 2–3 days.	9. To soften and loosen impaction.

Guidelines   Irrigating the External Auditory Canal *(continued)*

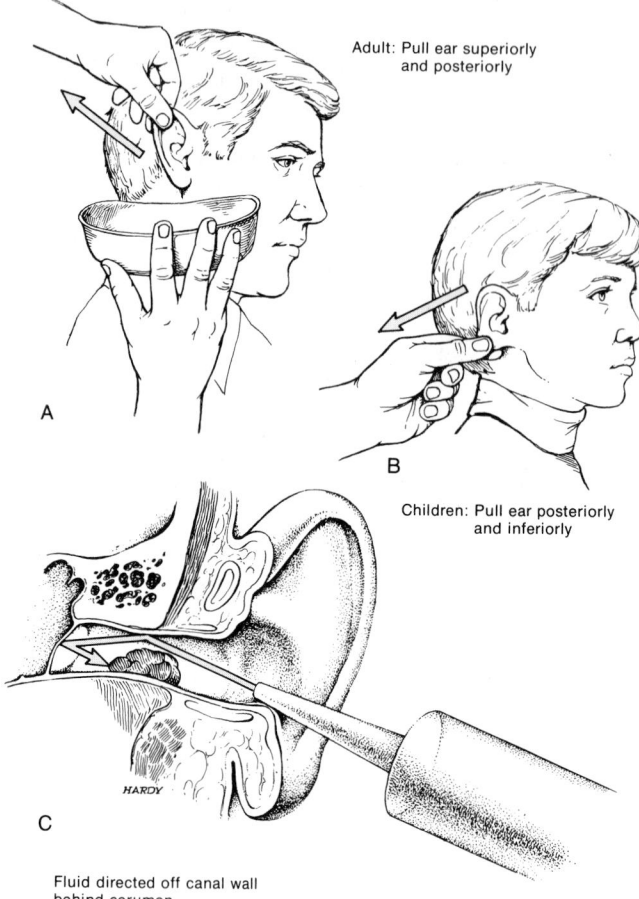

Adult: Pull ear superiorly and posteriorly

A

B

Children: Pull ear posteriorly and inferiorly

C

Fluid directed off canal wall behind cerumen

Figure 26-1. *Ear irrigation. (A) The external auditory canal in the adult can best be exposed by pulling the earlobe upward and backward. (B) The same exposure can be achieved in the child by gently pulling the auricle of the ear downward and backward. (C) An enlarged diagram showing the direction of irrigating fluid against the side of the canal. NOTE: This is more effective in dislodging cerumen than if the flow of solution were directed straight into the canal.*

Follow-Up Phase

1. Dry external ear.
2. Remove soiled equipment and make the patient comfortable.
3. Patient should lie on irrigated (affected) side for a few minutes after procedure to allow any remaining solution to drain out.
4. Record time of irrigation, kind and amount of solution, nature of return flow, and effect of treatment.

Acute Otitis Media

Acute otitis media is an inflammation, infection of the middle ear caused by the entrance of pathogenic organisms, with rapid onset of signs and symptoms. It is a major problem in children, but may occur at any age.

Clinical Manifestations

1. Pain is usually the first symptom.
2. Fever may rise to 40–40.6°C. (104°–105°F.).
3. Purulent drainage (otorrhea) is present if tympanic membrane is perforated.

4. Irritability may be noted in the young person.
5. Headache, hearing loss, anorexia, nausea, and vomiting may be present.
6. History may reveal prior upper respiratory infection, immunologic defect, or head injury (fractured skull).
7. Pneumatic otoscopy shows a tympanic membrane that is full, bulging, and opaque with impaired mobility.
8. Cultures of discharge may suggest causative organism.

Nursing Diagnoses

1. Pain related to infection.
2. Sensory/perceptual alteration (auditory) related to disease (infection) and hearing loss.

3. Knowledge deficit of preventive measures and treatment or possible surgery.

Management

1. Penicillin—the drug of choice for adults.
2. Administration of nasal decongestants and/or antihistamines.
3. Surgery—myringotomy
   a. An incision is made into the posterior inferior aspect of the tympanic membrane for draining purposes (to relieve pressure and drain pus from middle ear infection)
   b. Performed on selected patients to prevent recurrent episodes.
   c. May be done because of failure of patient to respond to antimicrobial therapy, for severe, persistent pain, and for persistent conductive hearing loss.

Nursing Interventions

A. Relieving Pain and Pressure; Preventing Infection From Spreading

1. Administer aspirin and other analgesics as prescribed. (Sedation is usually avoided because it may interfere with early detection of intracranial complications).
2. Give penicillin derivatives or broad-spectrum antibiotics, as prescribed.
3. Local cold compresses may promote comfort while heat may help resolve infectious process.

NURSING ALERT: With wide-spectrum antibiotic therapy, acute otitis media may become subacute with continued purulent discharge. Healing may take place, but the patient may be left with a residual deafness.

4. Recognize that symptoms such as headache, slow pulse, vomiting, and vertigo are significant and should be reported.
5. Sequelae may involve the mastoid or even the brain, producing meningitis or brain abscess.

B. Safety Measures to Prevent Falls

1. Utilize side rails when the patient is in bed.
2. Instruct the patient to call for assistance when getting out of bed or walking.
3. Tell the patient to move from one position to another *slowly* to decrease vertigo.

C. Preparing for Surgery

1. Explain to the patient preoperative orders as well as postoperative expectations.
2. Remind the patient not to touch ear.
3. Observe for drainage and monitor vital signs for possible evidence of bleeding.
4. Provide emotional support.

Patient Education

1. Instruct the patient on activities that are to be avoided until tympanic membrane heals (swimming, shampooing hair, showering).
2. Advise the patient of hygienic practices that will prevent reinfection (avoid ear-picking, inserting toothpick in ear to relieve itch, etc.).
3. Instruct patient of any symptoms that indicate recurrence (discomfort, pain, dizziness).

Chronic Otitis Media and Mastoiditis

Chronic otitis media and mastoiditis is a chronic inflammation of the middle ear and mastoid lasting more than 3 months from initial onset, accompanied by a nonintact tympanic membrane and discharge. It may be caused by an antibiotic-resistant organism or a particularly virulent strain of organism.

Clinical Manifestations

1. Painless discharge from the affected ear.
2. Air conductive hearing loss is present via audiometric tests.
3. Otorrhea may be odorless or foul-smelling.
4. Vertigo and pain may be present if central nervous system (CNS) complications have occurred.
5. History will indicate several episodes of acute otitis media, possible rupture of tympanic membrane.
6. X-rays may note mastoid pathology, e.g., cholesteatoma (soft ball of dead skin cells that erodes surrounding vital structures).

Management

Note: If advanced chronic ear disease is left untreated, inner ear and life-threatening CNS complications may develop because of erosion of surrounding structures.

A. Medical Therapy

1. Antibiotic and steroid eardrops may control infection and inflammation.
2. Frequent removal of epithelial debris and purulent drainage may protect tissue from damage.

B. Surgical Interventions

1. Indicated when cholesteatoma is present.
2. Indicated when there is pain, profound deafness, dizziness, sudden facial paralysis, or stiff neck (may lead to meningitis or brain abscess).
3. Types of procedures
   a. *Simple mastoidectomy*—removal of mastoid cells; indicated when there is persistent tenderness, fever, discharge from ear, or headache.
   b. *Radical mastoidectomy*—removal of all diseased tissue from mastoid area and middle ear.
   c. *Posteroanterior mastoidectomy*—combines simple mastoidectomy with tympanoplasty (reconstruction of middle ear structures).

Nursing Interventions

1. Provide for relief of pain postoperatively.
   a. Give aspirin or codeine sulfate as prescribed.
   b. Apply cold compresses to area.
   c. Position for comfort—may be specific to type of surgery or physician's preference.
2. Postoperatively, administer sedatives for restlessness.
3. Assist with dressing change since area is packed with gauze for drainage—this may be done daily or every other day; packing is removed on third or fourth day.
4. Instruct patient to observe for possible complications:
   a. Facial weakness or paralysis may indicate facial nerve injury.
   b. Infection
      (1) Observe for and teach clinical signs of inflammation.
      (2) Administer prescribed antibiotics.

c. Vertigo—may be apparent following radical mastoidectomy due to inner ear disturbance.
d. Spread of infection to brain—unusual rise in temperature, chills, stiff neck, nausea and vomiting (meningeal signs).

5. Note status of hearing.
   a. If stapes has been removed or dislodged, then hearing is lost.
   b. If stapes or cochlea has not been removed or disturbed, then hearing will probably be regained; a hearing aid may be required.

Perforation of the Eardrum

Etiology

1. Infection, followed by trauma, are the most frequent causes of permanent perforation of the tympanic membrane.

Management

A. Medical

1. Most accidental perforations of the eardrum heal spontaneously.
2. Cauterization of the perforation with application of a prosthesis (Gelfoam) will produce a healed membrane with scar tissue.

B. Surgical

Tympanoplasty is a reconstructive operation on the diseased or deformed components of the middle ear.

Goal

Improve or preserve the conductive mechanisms in an effort to salvage or improve hearing.

Types of Tympanoplasty *(Table 26-2)*

A. Type I (Myringoplasty)

1. Purpose—to close perforation by placing a graft over it in order to create a closed middle ear section, which in turn will improve hearing.

2. Perforation is closed using one of the following:
   a. Fascia from temporal muscle.
   b. Vein grafts from hand or forearm.
   c. Epithelium from auditory canal (eustachian tube).
3. Indications—to avoid risk of contamination when the patient bathes, swims, or dives; this in turn prevents recurrence of chronic otitis media or mastoiditis.
4. Contraindications
   a. Ossicular involvement.
   b. Presence of active infection.
   c. Presence of chronic middle ear infection, impairing or preventing drainage via auditory canal.
   d. Sinusitis or allergy that produces a chronic infectious discharge via nasopharynx.
   e. History of acute exacerbations of otitis media.

Note: Hearing improvement is achieved in inverse proportion to the amount of surgery required; the simpler the surgery, the better the chance for hearing to improve.

Nursing Interventions

1. Administer prescribed antibiotics for several days postoperatively to ensure freedom from infection.
2. Reinforce external dressings if they become soiled; otherwise, leave dressings intact.
   a. Do not add pressure to ear dressings.
   b. Gauze packing in canal may be removed at the end of a week.
   c. Do not apply suction or probe canal.
3. Do not use eardrops, because of danger of loosening graft.
   (Gentle capillary suction may be attempted by surgeon at end of second week to remove debris and crusts, but Gelfoam remains).
4. Dust lightly with antibiotic powder (Neosporin) as prescribed.

Patient Education

Instruct the patient to:
1. Avoid shampooing or showering, which may cause contamination of ear canal, until permission is obtained from physician.

Table 26-2. *Types of Tympanoplasty*

| Type | Middle Ear Damage | | Repair Process |
	Tympanic Membrane	*Ossicles*	
I	Perforated	Normal	Close perforation—myringoplasty
II	Perforated	Erosion of malleus and/or incus	Close perforation; graft against incus or whatever remains of malleus
III	Tympanic membrane destroyed or widely perforated	Rest of ossicular chain destroyed BUT stapes are intact and mobile	Grafts implanted to contact the normal stapes Tympanostapedopexy
IV	Tympanic membrane destroyed or widely perforated	Ossicular chain destroyed. Head, neck, and crura of stapes destroyed. Stapes footplate mobile	Expose mobile stapes footplate—graft implanted. Air pocket between graft and round window provides protection The Cavum minor operation
V	Tympanic membrane destroyed or widely perforated	Ossicular chain destroyed. Head, neck, and crura of stapes destroyed. Stapes footplate fixed	Make opening in horizontal semicircular canal; graft seals off middle ear to give sound protection for round window Tympanoplasty and fenestration of lateral semi-circular canal

2. Continue with antibiotics beyond first week if there is evidence of infection.
3. Use antihistamine with an ephedrine derivative as prescribed for at least 1 month postoperatively.
4. Continue using an antihistamine if rhinologic allergy is experienced.

B. Types II–V

1. Purpose (see Table 26-2)—these procedures are modifications used to correct various middle ear problems.
2. Preoperative and operative treatment.
   a. Topical and systemic antibiotics are administered when infection is present.
   b. Suitable replacement (polyethylene, stainless steel wire, bone, cartilage) is used to maintain continuity of conduction sound pathway.
3. The necessity of a two-stage procedure is determined.
   a. First stage—eradication of all diseased tissues; area is cleaned out to achieve a dry, healed middle ear.
   b. Second stage—performed 2–3 months after first stage; reconstruction, using grafts.
4. Postoperative nursing interventions
   a. Reinforce outer dressings as necessary, but keep inner dressings intact.
   b. Assist the patient in getting out of bed for the first time because he may become dizzy.

Otosclerosis

Otosclerosis is a pathologic condition in which there is formation of new spongy bone in the labyrinth, fixation of the stapes, and prevention of sound transmission through the ossicles to the inner fluids resulting in deafness.

Incidence

1. Cause is unknown.
2. Occurs more commonly in women than men.
3. Has a familial tendency.

Clinical Manifestations

1. Young adult presents a history of slow, progressive hearing loss of soft, spoken tones, with no middle ear infection.
2. A frequent complaint is tinnitus; both ears may be affected equally.
3. History reveals gradual hearing loss.
4. Audiometry findings substantiate hearing loss.
5. Bone conduction is much better than air conduction.

Management

1. No known medical treatment exists for this form of deafness, but amplification with a hearing aid may be helpful.
2. Surgery—stapedectomy
   a. The removal of otosclerotic lesions at the footplate of stapes and the creation of a tissue implant with prosthesis to maintain suitable conduction.
   b. To perform such delicate surgery, the otologic binocular microscope is used.

Nursing Interventions

1. Observe for the following:
   a. Fever—may indicate infection, external otitis, otitis media.
   b. Headache—may indicate infection, nerve encroachment.
   c. Vertigo—may indicate labyrinthitis or inner ear reaction.
   d. Ear pain—may indicate infection or irritation of auditory nerve.
2. Position the patient postoperatively as desired by physician.
   a. Some surgeons prefer that the patient be positioned with operated ear uppermost to maintain position of graft and stability.
   b. Others prefer that the patient be lying on operated ear to permit drainage.
   c. Still others advocate that the patient assume the most comfortable position.
3. Administer prescribed antimotion medications and sedatives if the patient experiences vertigo, nystagmus, or nausea.
4. Assist the patient when first ambulating—may feel dizzy for the first few days. Safety is of utmost importance.
5. Instruct the patient not to blow nose for a week; air may be forced up the auditory canal and disturb the operative site.
6. Encourage a restricted head position if the surgeon fears a misplacement of the prosthesis.
7. Administer prescribed pain medication for first several hours.

Patient Education

1. Advise the patient that there may be a temporary hearing loss for a few weeks after surgery because of tissue edema, packing, etc.
2. Packing is removed by surgeon in 5–6 days postoperatively. Patient should protect ear by placing cotton ball in outer ear (auditory meatus) and changing it twice daily.
3. Instruct the patient to:
   a. Avoid sudden pressure changes in the ear.
      (1) Do not blow nose.
      (2) Do not fly in a small plane.
      (3) Do not dive.
   b. Do not smoke.
   c. Protect ears when going outdoors for the first week.
   d. Avoid crowds or exposure to colds so that upper respiratory infection is prevented.
4. Instruct patient of signs and symptoms of complications.
   a. Return of tinnitus.
   b. Vertigo.
   c. Fluctuations of hearing ability.

Meniere's Disease

Meniere's disease (endolymphatic hydrops) is a chronic disease that involves the inner ear and causes a triad of symptoms: vertigo, hearing loss, and tinnitus. There is no specific cause, but there is fluid distention of the endolymphatic spaces of the labyrinth accompanied by destruction of cochlear hair cells.

Clinical Manifestations

A. During Attack

1. Dizziness, tinnitus, and reduced hearing occur on involved side.
2. Headache, nausea, vomiting, and incoordination are present.
3. Sudden attacks occur in which patient feels that the room is spinning around. Vertigo may last several hours or all day.
4. Sudden motion of the head may precipitate vomiting.
5. History often reveals ear trouble, vasomotor rhinitis, and allergies.
6. The most comfortable position for the patient is lying down.
7. Irritability; other personality changes.

B. After or Between Attacks

1. Patient behaves normally; may continue working.
2. Only complaint may be tinnitus or impaired hearing.

Diagnostic Evaluation

1. Caloric test/electronystagmography (ENG)
   a. Useful in differentiating Meniere's syndrome from intracranial lesion.
   b. Fluid, above or below body temperature, is instilled into the auditory canal.
   c. Results
      (1) Normal patient—complains of dizziness
      (2) Patient with acoustic neuroma—no reaction
      (3) Patient with Meniere's disease—severe attack as above
2. Audiogram
3. Allergy history and endocrine studies

Management

1. Patient can be asked to keep a diary noting presence of aural symptoms (e.g., tinnitus, distorted hearing) when episodes of vertigo occur—may help diagnose which ear is involved and if surgery will be needed.
2. Administration of vestibular suppressants such as oral acetazolamide when attacks are infrequent, in order to decrease symptoms.
3. Streptomycin (intramuscular) may be given to selectively destroy vestibular apparatus if vertigo is uncontrollable.
4. Administration of "vertigo sedatives" such a dimenhydrinate, meclizine, or diazepam.
5. Antiemetics to reduce nausea, vomiting, and vertigo.

Surgical

1. Conservative—simple sac decompression or sac "shunt."
2. Destructive surgery.
   a. *Labyrinthectomy*—recommended if the patient experiences progressive hearing loss and severe vertigo attacks so that he cannot perform normal tasks.
   b. *Vestibular nerve section*—neurosurgical suboccipital approach to the cerebellopontine angle for intracranial vestibular nerve neurectomy.

Nursing Interventions

A. Using Protective and Safety Measures

1. During attacks, position side rails "up" if patient is in bed; if patient is standing, help him to the floor to avoid injury.
2. Postoperatively, vertigo, nausea, and vomiting may be experienced; bedrest may be most comfortable for first 2 days.
3. Assist the patient out of bed since he may be unsteady—safety is of utmost importance.
4. Provide a "call system" for the patient if assistance is needed.
5. Help patient recognize aura so that he has time to prepare for an attack.

B. Employing Comfort Measures

1. Provide encouragement and understanding.
2. Remind the patient to move slowly since jerking or making sudden movements may precipitate an attack.
3. Avoid noises and glaring, bright lights, which may initiate an attack.

Patient Education

1. Eliminate smoking and the intake of coffee, tea, alcohol, and stimulating drugs—due to vasoconstriction effects.
2. Control environmental factors and personal habits that may cause stress or fatigue.
3. If there is a tendency to allergic reactions to foods, eliminate those foods from the diet.
4. Adhere to periodic use of diuretics, as prescribed, to relieve feeling of fullness in the ear, vertigo, and tinnitus.
5. Inform patient that the dizziness may last for varying lengths of time.

Cochlear Implant

A *cochlear implant* is a device that emits auditory signals for profoundly deaf individuals. The single-electrode system bypasses the damaged cochlear system and stimulates the remaining auditory nerve fibers. This results in the perception of sound.

Classification

Cochlear implants may be classified according to the following categories.

1. Location of electrodes
   a. Intracochlear (see Fig. 26-2)
   b. Extracochlear
2. Transmission of signals
   a. Single channel
   b. Multichannel
3. Features of speech signal
   a. Feature extraction—only certain features are transmitted.
   b. Nonfeature-specific—input signal is transmitted without extracting speech cues.
4. Types of electrodes
   a. Monopolar
   b. Bipolar
5. Method of stimulation
   a. Continuous
   b. Pulsatile

Patient Criteria

There are no standardized criteria for patient selection. Some data that are considered include:

1. Total hearing loss with no significant benefit from hearing aid.

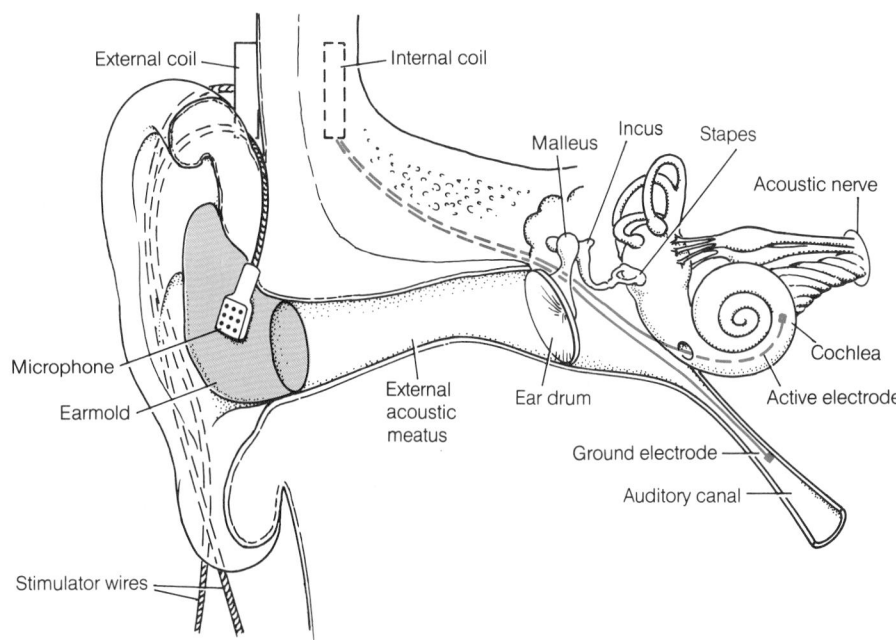

External coil — Internal coil

Malleus Incus Stapes

Acoustic nerve

Cochlea

Active electrode

Ear drum

Ground electrode

Auditory canal

External acoustic meatus

Microphone

Earmold

Stimulator wires

Figure 26-2. *Cochlear implant.*

2. Results of audiologic test show average hearing sensitivity at 500, 1000, 2000 Hz. to be no better than 90–100 db. hearing loss in either ear.
3. Zero percent correct on speech recognition.
4. Physically healthy, with adult-onset deafness. (Some surgery is being done on infants and children.)
5. No evidence of brain impairment, psychoses, or mental retardation.
6. Reasonable expectations and optimism—motivation must be present.

Nursing Interventions

A. Preoperative and Intraoperative Management

1. Encourage the prospective patient to talk with one who is currently using an implant to learn the positive and negative results of a cochlear implant.
2. Preoperative preparation will be specified.

3. Explain preoperative directives and postoperative expectations.

B. Postoperative Interventions

1. Provide care similar to that of a postmastoidectomy patient who has had general anesthesia (see p. 651).
2. Initiate rehabilitation—usually begins 2 months postsurgery. Included are:
   a. Adjustment of controls.
   b. Operation and maintenance of stimulator unit.
   c. Listening critically and learning lip reading.
   d. Learning discrimination of sounds through cochlear implant. Understanding speech through cochlear implant is not possible with this device alone.
   e. Many individuals trained with such an implant can lip read more easily and can distinguish voices and environmental sounds.

Bibliography

Books

Abel SM and Alberti PW. Noise and its effect on communication. In Alberti PW and Ruben RJ (eds). Otologic Medicine and Surgery, Vol 1, pp 943–953. New York, Churchill Livingstone, 1988

Adams GL, Boies LR Jr and Hilger PA. Boies Fundamentals of Otolaryngology: A Textbook of Ear, Nose, and Throat Diseases. 6th ed. Philadelphia, WB Saunders. 1989

Alberti PW. Noise and the ear. In Brown S (ed). Scott Brown's Diseases of the Ear, Nose and Throat, 5th ed. London, Butterworths, 1988

Alberti PW. Hearing conservation. In Alberti PW and Ruben RJ (eds).

Otologic Medicine and Surgery, Vol 2, pp 1739–1752. New York, Churchill Livingstone, 1988

Bluestone CD. Management and therapy of otitis media. In Alberti PW and Ruben RJ (eds). Otologic Medicine and Surgery, Vol 2, pp 1173–1202. New York, Churchill Livingstone, 1988

Brackmann DE, Benecke JE Jr and Stahl BA. Otologic instrumentation. In Alberti PW and Ruben RJ (eds). Otologic Medicine and Surgery, Vol 2, pp 957–994. New York, Churchill Livingstone, 1988

Brooks DN (ed). Adult Aural Rehabilitation. London, Chapman and Hall, 1989

Donlon JV Jr. Anesthesia for ear surgery.

In Alberti PW and Ruben RJ (eds). Otologic Medicine and Surgery, Vol 2, pp 995–998. New York, Churchill Livingstone, 1988

Eviatar A. Stapes surgery. In Alberti PW and Ruben RJ (eds). Otologic Medicine and Surgery, Vol 2, pp 1261–1275. New York, Churchill Livingstone, 1988

Farmer JC and Gillespie CA. Otologic medicine and surgery of exposures to aerospace, diving, and compressed gases. In Alberti PW and Ruben RJ (eds). Otologic Medicine and Surgery, Vol 2, pp 1753–1802. New York, Churchill Livingstone, 1988

Gibson WPR. Vestibular diagnostic tests. In Alberti PW and Ruben RJ (eds).

Otologic Medicine and Surgery, Vol 1, pp 487–507. New York, Churchill Livingstone, 1988

Gristwood RE. Otosclerosis (otospongiosis) treatment. In Alberti PW and Ruben RJ (eds). Otologic Medicine and Surgery, Vol 2, pp 1241–1259. New York, Churchill Livingstone, 1988

Gristwood RG. Otosclerosis (otospongiosis): general considerations. In Alberti PW and Ruben RJ (eds). Otologic Medicine and Surgery, Vol 1, pp 911–943. New York, Churchill Livingstone, 1988

Hazell JWP. Tinnitus. In Alberti PW and Ruben RJ (eds). Otologic Medicine and Surgery, Vol 2, pp 1605–1622. New York, Churchill Livingstone, 1988

Kruger B. Basic audiologic evaluation. In Alberti PW and Ruben RJ (eds). Otologic Medicine and Surgery, Vol 1, pp 365–397. New York, Churchill Livingstone, 1988

Lee KJ (ed). Textbook of Otolaryngology and Head and Neck Surgery. New York, Elsevier, 1989

Lim DJ and DeMaria TF. Pathogenesis and pathology of otitis media. In Alberti PW and Ruben RJ (eds). Otologic Medicine and Surgery, Vol 1, pp 779–803. New York, Churchill Livingstone, 1988

Lucente FE, Smith PG and Thomas JR. Diseases of the external ear. In Alberti PW and Ruben RJ (eds). Otologic Medicine and Surgery, Vol 2, pp 1073–1092. New York, Churchill and Livingstone, 1988

Michaels L. Pathology of the inner ear. In Alberti PW and Ruben RJ (eds). Otologic Medicine and Surgery, Vol 1, pp 615–712. New York, Churchill Livingstone, 1988

Michelson RP. Cochlear implants. In Alberti PW and Ruben RJ (eds). Otologic Medicine and Surgery, Vol 2, pp 1719–1737. New York, Churchill Livingstone, 1988

Neuman AC and Levitt H. Hearing aids. In Alberti PW and Ruben RJ (eds). Otologic Medicine and Surgery, Vol 2, pp 1637–1652. New York, Churchill Livingstone, 1988

Pfaltz CR. Sudden and fluctuant hearing loss. In Alberti PW and Ruben RJ (eds). Otologic Medicine and Surgery, Vol 2, pp 1577–1604. New York, Churchill Livingstone, 1988

Riko K and Alberti PW. Management of hearing-impaired adults. In Alberti PW and Ruben RJ (eds). Otologic Medicine and Surgery, Vol 2, pp 1695–1718. New York, Churchill Livingstone, 1988

Rybak L and Matz GJ. Ototoxicity. In Alberti PW and Ruben RJ (eds). Otologic Medicine and Surgery, Vol 2, pp 1623–1636. New York, Churchill Livingstone, 1988

Schein JD. Effects of hearing loss in adults. In Alberti PW and Ruben RJ (eds). Otologic Medicine and Surgery, Vol 1, pp 885–911. New York, Churchill Livingstone, 1988

Smyth GD. Surgical techniques of tympanoplasty. In Alberti PW and Ruben RJ (eds). Otologic Medicine and Surgery, Vol 2, pp 1277–1298. New York, Churchill Livingstone, 1988

Snow JB Jr. Management and therapy of trauma to the external ear and auditory and vestibular systems. In Alberti PW and Ruben RJ (eds). Otologic Medicine and Surgery, Vol 2, pp 1561–1576. New York, Churchill Livingstone, 1988

Suzuki J. Complications of ear surgery: Immediate and Delayed. In Alberti PW and Ruben RJ (eds). Otologic Medicine and Surgery, Vol 2, pp 1363–1388. New York, Churchill Livingstone, 1988

Weiss AD. Management and therapy of disequilibrium. In Alberti PW and Ruben RJ (eds). Otologic Medicine and Surgery, Vol 2, pp 1523–1534. New York, Churchill Livingstone, 1988

Welliver RC. Allergy and middle ear effusions: Fact or Fiction? In Bernstein JM and Ogra P (eds). Immunology of the Ear, pp 381–389. New York, Raven Press, 1987

Journals

General

Berger EH. Methods of measuring the attenuation of hearing protection devices. J Acoust Soc Am 1986 Jun; 79(6):1655–1687

Brummett RE et al. Potential hearing loss resulting from MR imaging. Radiology 1988 Nov; 169(2):539–540

Knecht J. Removing ceruminous ear impaction. Physician Assist 1989 Feb; 13(2):89

Marwick C. Information accumulating on how brain "hears." JAMA 1989 Jun 2; 261(21):3077

Page JC. Selecting a hearing protective device. AAOHN J 1988 Jan; 36(1):40–41

Wiet RJ. Help for the hearing impaired: Early evaluation, advanced technology, improved management. Postgrad Med 1988 Nov 1; 84(6):93–96, 101–103

Meniere's Disease

Meniere's disease. Mayo Clinic Health Letter 1988 May; 6(5):2–3

Vernon JA. Pathophysiology of tinnitus: A special case—hyperacusis and a proposed treatment. Am J Otol 1987 May; 8(3):201–202

Willatt DJ et al. Prognostic factors in labyrinthectomy. J Laryngol Otol 1988 Sep; 102(9):785–787

Xenellis J. HLA antigens in the pathogenesis of Meniere's disease. J Laryngol Otol 1986 Jan; 100(1):21–24

Otitis Media

Arola M et al. Rhinovirus in acute otitis media. J Pediatr 1988 Oct; 113(4):693–695

Cunha BA. Case studies in infectious disease: Otitis media. Emerg Med 1988 May 15;20(9):165, 166, 169, 172

Diamond C et al. Bacteriology of chronic otitis media with effusion. J Laryngol Otol 1989 Apr; 103(4):369–371

Eichenwald H. Developments in diagnosing and treating otitis media. Am Fam Physician 1985 Mar; 31(3):155–156

Feldman W et al. Trimethoprim-sulfamethoxazole vs. amoxicillin in the treatment of acute otitis media. Can Med Assoc J 1988 Nov 15; 139(10):961–964

Fireman P. Newer concepts in otitis media. Hosp Pract 1987 Nov 30; 22(11):85–91

Fireman P. Nasal allergy: A risk factor for middle ear disease. Ann Allergy 1987 Jun; 58(6):395–400

Fireman P. Allergy induced eustachian tube and middle ear pathophysiology. New Engl Reg Allergy Proc 1986 May–Jun; 7(3):246–252

Kurons Y et al. *Staphyloccoccus epidermidis* and *Staphylococcus aureus* in otitis media with effusion. Arch Otolaryngol Head Neck Surg 1988 Nov; 114(11):1262–1265

Ohaski Y et al. Mucociliary disease of the middle ear during experimental otitis media with effusion induced by bacterial endotoxin. Ann Otol Rhinol Laryngol 1989 Jun; 98(6):479–484

Otitis media due to contaminated ENT instruments. Nurses Drug Alert 1989 Jan; 13(1):3–4

Smith MA et al. *Pneumocystis carinii* otitis media. Am J Med 1989 Nov; 85(5):745–746

Takahashi H et al. Primary deficits in eustachian tube function in patients with otitis media with effusion. Arch Otolaryngol Head Neck Surg 1989 May; 115(5):581–584

Surgery

Tanz C. Quality patient care on surgery day. Today's OR Nurse 1988 Dec; 9(12):16–17, 34–35

Hearing Aids

DeBlase R and Kucler M. Assistive hearing device aids patient–staff communication. Geriatr Nurs Apr 1985; 6(4):223–224

Ear and Hearing (Official Journal of the American Auditory Society). Williams & Wilkins, 428 E. Preston Street, Baltimore, MD 21202

Harries ML et al. Hearing aids—A case for review. J Laryngol Otol 1989 Sep; 103(9):850–852

National Hearing Conservation Association. Selecting a hearing protective device. AAOHN J 1988 Jan; 36(1):40–41.

Wasson JH et al. The prescription of assistive devices for the elderly: Practical considerations. J Gen Intern Med 1990 Jan–Feb; 5(1):46–54

Cochlear Implants

Loeb GE. The functional replacement of the ear. Sci Am 1985 Feb; 252(2):104–111

National Institutes of Health (U.S. Department of Health and Human Services). Cochlear implants. Position paper 1988 May 4; 7(2)

Renal, Genitourinary, and Reproductive Problems

27 Renal and Genitourinary Conditions

Clinical Manifestations of Urinary Dysfunction

Changes in Micturition (Voiding)

A. Hematuria (red blood cells in urine)

1. Hematuria is considered a serious sign and requires evaluation.
2. Color of bloody urine dependent on pH of urine and amount of blood present.
   a. Acid urine is dark, smoky color.
   b. Alkaline urine is red color.
3. Hematuria may be due to systemic cause such as blood dyscrasias, anticoagulant therapy, neoplasms, trauma, extreme exercise.
4. Painless hematuria may indicate neoplasm in the urinary tract.
5. Hematuria from renal colic (stones in kidney).
6. Bloody spotting reveals bleeding from urethra, bladder neoplasms.
7. Hematuria also seen in renal tuberculosis, polycystic disease of kidneys, acute pyelonephritis, thrombosis and embolism involving renal artery or vein.

B Proteinuria (albuminuria)

1. Normal urine does not contain persistent protein in significant quantities.

2. Proteinuria characteristically seen in all forms of acute and chronic renal disease (more characteristic of glomerulonephritis than pyelonephritis).
   a. The protein is mainly albumin, but globulin is also present.
   b. Albumin and globulin escape through damaged glomerular capillaries in a greater amount than can be reabsorbed by the tubules, or damaged tubules fail to reabsorb normal amount filtered.
3. Proteinuria occurs in systemic diseases where there are varying degrees of renal anoxia, as in cardiac decompensation, diabetic glomerulosclerosis.
4. Mild proteinuria may occur from other sources—urethritis, prostatitis, cystitis.

C. Dysuria (painful or difficult voiding)—seen in wide variety of pathologic conditions.

D. Frequency—voiding occurs more often than usual, when compared with the patient's usual pattern (or with a generally accepted norm of once every 3–6 hours).

1. Determine if habits governing fluid intake have been altered—it is essential to know normal voiding pattern in order to evaluate frequency.
2. Increasing frequency can result from a variety of conditions—such as infection and diseases of urinary tract, metabolic disease, hypertension, medications (diuretics).

E. *Urgency* (strong desire to urinate—due to inflammatory lesions in bladder, prostate, or urethra, acute bacterial infections, chronic prostatitis in men, and chronic posterior urethrotrigonitis in women.

F. *Burning upon Urination*—seen in urethral irritation or bladder infections.

G. Other Changes

1. *Strangury* (slow and painful urination); only small amounts of urine voided; blood staining may be noted—seen in severe cystitis.
2. *Hesitancy* (undue delay and difficulty in initiating voiding)—may indicate compression of urethra, outlet obstruction, neurogenic bladder.
3. *Nocturia* (excessive urination at night)—suggests decreased renal concentrating ability or heart failure, diabetes mellitus, poor bladder emptying.
4. *Urinary incontinence* (involuntary loss of urine)—may be due to injury to external urinary sphincter, acquired neurogenic disease, severe urgency, etc.
5. *Stress incontinence* (intermittent leakage of urine due to sudden strain)—indicates weakness of sphincteric mechanism.
6. *Polyuria* (large volume of urine voided in given time)—demonstrated in diabetes mellitus, diabetes insipidus, chronic renal disease, diuretics.
7. *Oliguria* (small volume of urine; output between 100–500 ml./24 hours)—may result from acute renal failure, shock, dehydration, fluid–ion imbalance.
8. *Anuria* (absence of urine in the bladder; output less than 50 ml./24 hours)—indicates serious renal dysfunction requiring immediate medical intervention.
9. *Enuresis* (involuntary voiding during sleep)—may be physiologic to age of 3 years; thereafter, may be functional or symptomatic of obstructive disease (usually of lower urinary tract).
10. *Pneumaturia* (passage of gas in urine during voiding)—caused by fistulous connection between bowel and bladder, rectosigmoid cancer, regional ileitis, sigmoid diverticulitis (most common), and gas-forming urinary tract infections.

Urinary Tract Pain

1. Genitourinary pain is not always present in renal disease, but is generally seen in the more acute conditions.
2. Pain of renal disease is caused by sudden distention of the renal capsule; severity is related to how quickly the distention develops.
3. Kidney pain—may be felt as a dull ache in costovertebral angle; may spread to umbilicus.
4. Ureteral pain—felt in the back and radiates to the abdomen, upper thighs, testes, or labia.
5. Flank pain (side area between ribs and ilium)—radiates to lower abdomen or epigastrium and often is associated with nausea, vomiting, and paralytic ileus; most commonly secondary to a renal lesion (stone, tumor, or infection).
6. Bladder pain (low abdominal pain or pain over suprapubic area)—may be due to bladder infection or overdistended bladder.
7. Urethral pain from irritation of bladder neck, from foreign body in canal, or from urethritis due to infection or trauma.
8. Pain in scrotal area from inflammatory swelling of epididymis or testicle, or torsion of the testicle.
9. Testicular pain due to injury, mumps orchitis, torsion of spermatic cord.

10. Perineal or rectal discomfort from acute prostatitis, prostatic abscess.
11. Back and leg pain from cancer of prostate with metastases to pelvic bones.
12. Pain in glans penis is usually from prostatitis; penile shaft pain is from urethral problems.

Related Gastrointestinal Symptoms

1. Gastrointestinal symptoms related to urologic conditions include nausea, vomiting, diarrhea, abdominal discomfort, paralytic ileus, and gastrointestinal hemorrhage with uremia.
2. Occur with urologic conditions because the gastrointestinal and urinary tracts have common autonomic and sensory innervation and because of renointestinal reflexes.

Assessment of Urologic Function
History and Physical Assessment

Health History

Seek the following information related to urinary and renal function:

1. What is the patient's chief concern? Why is he seeking help?
2. What is (are) the patient's present and past occupation(s)? (Look for occupational hazards related to the urinary tract—contact with chemicals, plastics, pitch, tar, rubber.)
3. What is the patient's smoking history?
4. What is the past history, especially in relation to urinary problems?
5. Is there any family history of renal disease?
6. What childhood diseases did the patient have?
7. Is there a history of urinary infections?
8. Did enuresis continue beyond the usual age (past 3 years of age)?
9. Are there any voiding disorders?
   a. Dysuria? When does it occur? Where is it felt? Initial or terminal dysuria?
   b. Hesitancy? Straining? Pain during or after urination?
   c. Changes in color of urine? Diminished urine output?
   d. Incontinence? Stress incontinence? Urgency incontinence?
   e. Any history of hematuria?
   f. How often does the patient get up to void during the night? How much urine is passed? Date of onset?
10. Is pain present?
    Location? Character? Radiation? Duration? Related to voiding? What brings it on? What relieves it?
11. Has the patient had fever? Chills? Passage of stones?
12. Any history of genital lesions or sexually transmitted diseases?
13. For the female patient: Number of children? Their ages? Any forceps deliveries? Catheterizations? When? Why? Any signs of vaginal discharge? Vaginal/vulvar itch or irritation?
14. Does the patient have diabetes mellitus? Hypertension? Allergies?
15. Has the patient ever been hospitalized with a urinary tract infection?

a. Infection before the age of 12?
b. Cystoscopy? Indwelling catheter? Kidney x-ray procedures?

16. Is the patient receiving any prescription or over-the-counter drugs that may affect renal or urinary function? Have any drugs been prescribed for renal or urinary problems?

17. Is the patient at risk for urinary tract infection?

Diagnostic Tests

Radiologic Techniques

A. Plain Film—of the abdomen or KUB (kidneys, ureters, bladder)

1. Delineates size, shape, and position of kidneys.
2. Reveals any deviations, such as calcifications (stones), hydronephrosis, cysts, tumors, or kidney displacement.

B. Computed Tomography—provides a cross-sectional view of kidney and urinary tract to detect the presence and extent of urologic disease; a computer measures small changes in x-ray absorption and magnifies the differences from tissue to tissue so a display can be made and read. No preparation needed; noninvasive.

C. Magnetic Resonance Imaging (MRI)

1. Relies on magnets and computers to produce images. (see p. 570 for description).
2. In urology, provides excellent images of soft tissues.

D. Nephrotomogram—body section roentgenograms, which bring into focus the different layers of the kidney and the diffuse structures in that layer; done also as part of intravenous pyelogram study.

E. Infusion Drip Pyelography—an intravenous infusion of a large volume of dilute solution of contrast material to produce opacification of the renal parenchyma and complete filling of urinary tract. Films taken at intervals to demonstrate the filled and distended collecting system.

Patient preparation is same as for excretory urography *except that the patient is not dehydrated.*

F. Excretory Urography (intravenous urogram [IVU] or intravenous pyelogram [IVP])—introduction (IV) of a radiopaque contrast medium, which concentrates in the urine and thus facilitates visualization of the kidneys, ureter, and bladder. The contrast medium is cleared from the bloodstream by renal excretion.

> **NURSING ALERT:** Elderly patients with poor renal reserve or those with multiple myeloma may not tolerate dehydrating procedures and should be given water to drink. Persons with uncontrolled diabetes may be sensitive to fluid restriction.

G. Retrograde Pyelography—injection of opaque material through ureteral catheters, which have been passed up ureters into renal pelvis by means of cystoscopic manipulation. The opaque solution is introduced by gravity or syringe.

Retrograde pyelography may be done if intravenous urography provides inadequate visualization of the collecting system.

H. Renal Angiography—visualization of renal arterial supply.

1. A special needle is used to pierce the femoral (or axillary) artery and a catheter is threaded through the femoral and iliac arteries into the aorta or renal artery.
2. Contrast material is injected to opacify the renal arterial supply.
3. Angiography evaluates blood flow dynamics, demonstrates abnormal vasculature, and differentiates renal cysts from renal tumors.

I. Radionuclide Imaging

1. Radiopharmaceuticals (^{99}Tc-labeled compound or ^{131}I–hippurate) are injected intravenously.
2. Studies obtained with a scintillation camera placed posterior to the kidney with the patient in a supine, prone, or sitting position.
3. The resultant image (scan) indicates the distribution of the radiopharmaceutical within the kidney.
4. The Tc scan provides information about kidney perfusion and is useful when renal function is poor.
5. The hippurate scan provides information about kidney function.

J. Ultrasound (ultrasonic scan) uses sound waves that are passed into the body. Organs in the urinary system create characteristic ultrasonic images.

1. Abnormalities such as masses, malformations, or obstructions can be identified.
2. A noninvasive technique; no special patient preparation required.

Endourology (Urologic Endoscopic Procedures)

A. Cystoscopic Examination—is a method of direct visualization of the urethra, prostatic urethra, and bladder by means of a cystoscope that is inserted through the urethra into the bladder. It has a self-contained optical lens system that provides a magnified, illuminated view of the bladder.

1. *Uses*
   a. To inspect bladder wall directly for tumor, stone, or ulcer and to inspect urethra, especially the prostatic urethra prior to surgery.
   b. To allow insertion of catheters into the ureters to obtain a separate specimen from each kidney and evaluate renal function separately.
   c. To see configuration and position of ureteral orifices.
   d. To remove calculi from urethra, bladder, and ureter.
   e. To treat lesions of bladder, urethra, and prostate.
2. A sedative may be given prior to the procedure.
3. A local topical anesthetic is instilled into the urethra by the urologist before insertion of cystoscope.
4. *Nursing interventions following cystoscopic examination*
   a. Monitor for complications: urinary retention, urinary tract hemorrhage, infection within prostate or bladder.
   b. Expect the patient to have some burning upon voiding, blood-tinged urine, and urinary frequency from trauma to mucous membrane.
   c. Monitor patient with prostatic hyperplasia for urinary retention due to edema from instrumentation.
   d. Moist heat to lower abdomen or warm sitz baths (as prescribed) are helpful in relieving pain and promoting muscle relaxation.

e. An indwelling urethral catheter may be necessary if urinary retention persists.

B. Renal and Ureteral Brush Biopsy—after cystoscopy, introduction of catheter followed by a biopsy brush, which is passed through the catheter; suspected lesion is brushed back and forth to obtain cells and surface tissue fragments for histologic diagnosis.

1. Following procedure, the patient may be given an intravenous infusion to help clear the kidneys and prevent clot formation.
2. Urine may show blood (usually clearing in 24–48 hours) from oozing at brushing site.
3. Post-test renal colic occasionally occurs; responds to analgesics.

C. Renal Endoscopy, Nephroscopy—introduction of fiberoptic scope into the renal pelvis during an open renal operation (pyelotomy) or percutaneously to view interior of renal pelvis, remove calculi, biopsy small lesions, and diagnose renal hematuria and selected renal tumors.

Needle Biopsy of Kidney

Needle biopsy of the kidney is performed by percutaneous needle biopsy through renal tissue (Fig. 27-1*A*) or by open biopsy through a small flank incision. It is useful in evaluating the course of renal disease and in securing specimens for electron and immunofluorescent microscopy.

A. Prebiopsy Management

1. Coagulation studies are carried out to identify the patient at risk for postbiopsy bleeding; serum creatinine and urinalysis are done.
2. The patient may be placed on a fasting regimen for 3 hours before the procedure. An IV line may be established.
3. Secure and save a voided specimen before biopsy— for comparison with postbiopsy specimen.
4. Inform the patient that he may be asked to hold his breath (to stop movement of the kidney) during insertion of the biopsy needle.

B. Postbiopsy Nursing Interventions

Goal:
Observe the patient for evidence of bleeding.

1. Place the patient in a prone position immediately after biopsy and on bedrest for 24 hours to minimize bleeding.
2. Take the vital signs every 5–15 minutes for first hour and then with decreasing frequency if stable to assess for hemorrhage, which is a major complication.
   a. Watch for rise or fall in blood pressure, anorexia, vomiting, or development of a dull, aching discomfort in abdomen.
   b. Assess for flank pain (usually represents bleeding into the muscle) or colicky pain (clot in the ureter).
   c. Assess for backache, shoulder pain, or dysuria.
   d. Persistent bleeding may be suspected when there is an enlarging hematoma, which is palpable (Fig. 27-1*B*).
   e. If perirenal bleeding develops, avoid palpating or manipulating the abdomen after the first examination has determined that a hematoma exists.
3. Measure each voiding and inspect for bleeding. Compare samples with each other and with prebiopsy specimen.
4. Assess for any patient complaints, especially frequency and urgency.
5. Keep the fluid level at 3000 ml. daily if tolerated, unless the patient has renal insufficiency.
6. A hematocrit and hemoglobin study may be done within 8 hours to assess for anemia.
7. Prepare for transfusion and surgical intervention for control of hemorrhage, which may necessitate surgical drainage or nephrectomy (removal of kidney).

C. Discharge Planning and Patient Education

Instruct the patient as follows:

1. Avoid strenuous activity, strenuous sports, and heavy lifting for at least 2 weeks.
2. Notify physician if any of the following occur: flank pain, hematuria, light-headedness and fainting, rapid pulse, or any other signs and symptoms of bleeding.

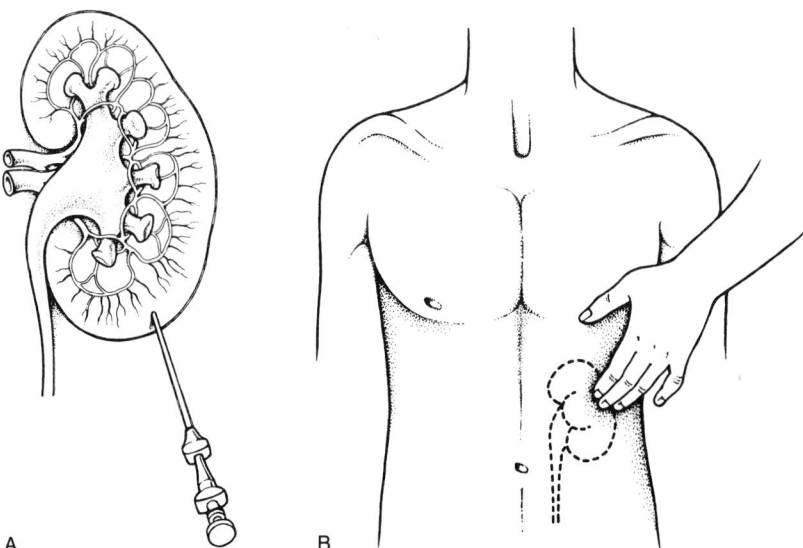

Figure 27-1. *(A) Percutaneous needle biopsy of the kidney. (B) Examining for enlarging hematoma.*

A   B

3. Report for follow-up 1–2 months after biopsy; the patient is checked for hypertension, and the biopsy area is auscultated for a bruit.

Urodynamic Measurements

Provide physiologic and structural tests to evaluate bladder and urethral function

1. Measure the rate of urine flow, bladder pressures during voiding and at rest, internal urethral resistance, and bladder contraction and relaxation.
2. Abdominal, bladder, and detrusor pressures, sphincter activity, bladder innervation, muscle tone, and sacral reflex are assessed.

A. Uroflowmetry (flow rate)—record of the volume of urine passing through the urethra per unit of time (ml./second).

B. Cystometrogram—graphic recording of the pressures exerted at varying phases of filling and emptying of the urinary bladder to assess its function. Intermittent filling of the bladder can be recorded and compared with changes in intravesical pressure.

1. The patient is requested to void. Physician observes the time it takes to initiate voiding; size, force, and continuity of urinary stream; degree of straining, hesitancy, intermittency of urination; presence of terminal dribbling.
2. A retention catheter is placed through urethra and into bladder. The residual volume is measured, and the catheter is left in place.
   The urethral catheter is connected to a water manometer, and water is allowed to flow into bladder, usually at the rate of 1 ml./second.
   a. The patient informs examiner when he feels the first desire to void and again when the bladder feels full. The degree of bladder filling at these points is recorded.
   b. The pressures above the zero level at the symphysis pubis are measured, and the pressures and volumes within the bladder are plotted and recorded.

C. Urethral Pressure Profile—graphic recording of the pressure within the urethra at each point along its length. Gas and fluid are instilled through a catheter that is withdrawn while pressures along the urethral wall are obtained.

D. Cystourethrogram—visualization of urethra and bladder either by retrograde injection or by voiding of contrast material.

E. Voiding Cystourethrogram—bladder is filled with contrast medium; patient then voids while rapid spot films are taken;

1. Demonstrates presence/absence of vesicoureteral reflux or congenital abnormalities in lower urinary tract.
2. Also used to investigate difficulty in bladder emptying and incontinence.

F. Electromyography—electrodes placed in the pelvic floor/musculature or anal sphincter to evaluate the neuromuscular function of the lower tract.

Tests of Renal Function

1. Renal function tests are used to determine effectiveness of the kidneys' excretory functioning, to evaluate the

severity of kidney disease, and to follow the patient's progress.
2. Renal function may be within normal limits until about 50% of renal function has been lost.
3. Best results are obtained by combining a number of clinical tests. Table 27-1 lists the more common tests of renal function.

Urine Examination

Amount

1. 1200–1500 ml./24 hours; less than 500 ml. is considered *oliguria*.
2. Day volume 2–3 times more than night volume.

Appearance

1. Normal urine is clear.
2. Turbid (cloudy) urine is not always pathologic. Normal urine may develop turbidity on refrigeration or from standing at room temperature; bacteria ferment urine quickly at room temperature.
3. Abnormally cloudy urine—due to pus, blood, epithelial cells, bacteria, fat, colloidal particles, phosphate, urates.

Odor

1. Normal—faint aromatic odor.
2. Characteristic odors produced by ingestion of asparagus, thymol.
3. Cloudy urine with ammonia odor—urea-splitting bacteria such as *Proteus,* causing urinary tract infections.
4. Offensive odor—bacterial action in presence of pus.

Color

1. Color shows degree of concentration and depends on amount voided.
2. Normal urine is clear yellow or amber because of the pigment urochrome.
3. Color varies with specific gravity:
   a. Dilute urine is straw-colored.
   b. Concentrated urine is highly colored; a sign of insufficient fluid intake.
4. Abnormally colored urine
   a. Turbid or smoky colored—may be from hematuria, spermatozoa, prostatic fluid, fat droplets, chyle.
   b. Red or red-brown—due to blood pigments, porphyria, transfusion reaction, bleeding lesions in urogenital tract, some drugs.
   c. Yellow-brown or green-brown—may reveal obstructive lesion of bile duct system or obstructive jaundice.
   d. Dark brown or black—due to malignant melanoma, leukemia.

Reaction (pH)

1. Reflects the ability of kidney to maintain normal hydrogen ion concentration in plasma and extracellular fluid; indicates *acidity* or *alkalinity* of urine.
2. The *p*H should be measured in fresh urine, since the breakdown of urine to ammonia causes urine to become alkaline.

Table 27-1. *Tests of Renal Function*

1. There is no single test of renal function; renal function is variable from time to time.
2. The rate of change of renal function is more important than the result of a single test.

Test	Purpose/Rationale	Test Protocol
Renal concentration test Specific gravity Osmolality of urine	Tests the ability to concentrate solutes in the urine. Concentration ability is lost early in kidney disease; hence, this test detects early defects in renal function.	Fluids may be withheld 12–24 hours to evaluate the concentrating ability of the tubules under controlled conditions. Specific gravity measurements of urine are taken at specific times to determine urine concentration.
Phenolsulfonphthalein excretion test (PSP)	A diagnostic agent (phenolsulfonphthalein) is given to determine the functional capacity of the kidney. (PSP test can also be used as a measure to assess residual urine.) Delayed excretion is seen in renal disease, cardiac failure, primary vascular disease.	Encourage fluids 1–1½ hours before the test. Phenolsulfonphthalein is given IV. (1) Record exact time dye is administered. (2) Collect urine in 15 minutes, 30 minutes, and 1 hour.
Creatinine clearance* (endogenous creatinine clearance)	Provides a reasonable approximation of rate of glomerular filtration. Measures volume of blood cleared of creatinine in 1 minute. Most sensitive indication of early renal disease. Useful to follow progress of the patient's renal status.	Collect all urine over 24-hour period. Draw one sample of blood within the period.
Serum creatinine	A test of renal function reflecting the balance between production and filtration by renal glomerulus. Most sensitive test of renal function.	Do test on blood serum.
Serum urea nitrogen (blood urea nitrogen [BUN])	Serves as index of renal excretory capacity. Serum urea nitrogen is dependent on the body's urea production and on urine flow. (Urea is the nitrogenous end-product of protein metabolism.) Affected by protein intake, tissue breakdown.	Do test on blood serum.

* Clearance is the amount of blood cleansed of a constituent per unit of time.

3. Normal *p*H is around 6 (acid); may normally vary from 4.6 to 7.5.
4. Urine acidity or alkalinity has relatively little clinical significance unless the patient is on special diet or therapeutic program or is being treated for renal calculous disease.
5. Alkaline urine is often cloudy because of phosphate crystals.

Specific Gravity

1. Reflects the kidney's ability to concentrate or dilute urine; may reflect degree of hydration or dehydration.
2. Normal specific gravity ranges from 1.005–1.025.
3. Specific gravity is fixed at 1.010 in chronic renal failure.

4. In a person eating a normal diet, inability to concentrate or dilute urine indicates disease.

Osmolality

1. *Osmolality* is an indication of the amount of osmotically active particles in urine (specifically, it is the number of particles per unit volume of *water*). It is similar to specific gravity, but is considered a more precise test; it is also easy to do—only 1–2 ml. of urine are required.
2. The unit of osmotic measure is the *osmole.*
   Average values:
       Females: 300–1090 mOsm./kg.
       Males: 390–1090 mOsm./kg.

Guidelines Technique for Obtaining Clean-Catch Midstream Voided Specimen

A *clean-catch midstream specimen* is the best clinically effective method of securing a voided specimen for urinalysis. It is not a simple procedure and requires patient education and active assistance of the female patient.

Equipment Antiseptic solution or liquid soap solution
Sterile water
4 × 4-inch sponges
Disposable gloves for nurse assisting female patient
Sterile specimen container

(continued)

Guidelines Technique for Obtaining Clean-Catch Midstream Voided Specimen *(continued)*

Procedure	Nursing Action	Rationale/Amplification

Male Patient

Nursing Action	Rationale/Amplification
1. Instruct the patient to expose glans and cleanse area around meatus. Wash area with mild antiseptic solution or liquid soap. *Rinse thoroughly.*	1. The urethral orifice is colonized by bacteria. Urine readily becomes contaminated during voiding. Rinse antiseptic solution or soap solution thoroughly because these agents can inhibit bacterial growth in a urine culture.
2. Allow the initial urinary flow to escape.	2. The first portion of urine washes out the urethra and contains debris.
3. Collect the midstream urine specimen in a sterile container.	3. The midstream sample reflects the status of the bladder.
4. Avoid collecting the last few drops of urine.	4. Prostatic secretions may be introduced into urine at the end of the urinary stream.
5. Send specimen to laboratory immediately.	5. A culture should be performed as soon as possible to avoid multiplication of urinary bacteria and lysis of cells.

Female Patient

Nursing Action	Rationale/Amplification
1. Ask the patient to separate her labia to expose the urethral orifice. If no one is available to assist the patient, she may sit backwards on the toilet seat facing the water tank or sit on (straddle) the wide part of the bedpan.	1. Keeping the labia separated prevents labial or vaginal contamination of the urine specimen. By straddling the toilet seat/bedpan, the patient's labia are spread apart for cleansing.
2. Cleanse the area around the urinary meatus with sponges soaked with antiseptic/soap solution. Rinse thoroughly. a. Wipe the perineum from the front to the back. b. Do not use sponges more than once.	2. The urethral orifice is colonized by bacteria. Urine readily becomes contaminated during voiding.
3. While the patient keeps the labia separated (Fig. 27-2), instruct her to void forcibly.	3. This helps wash away urethral contaminants.

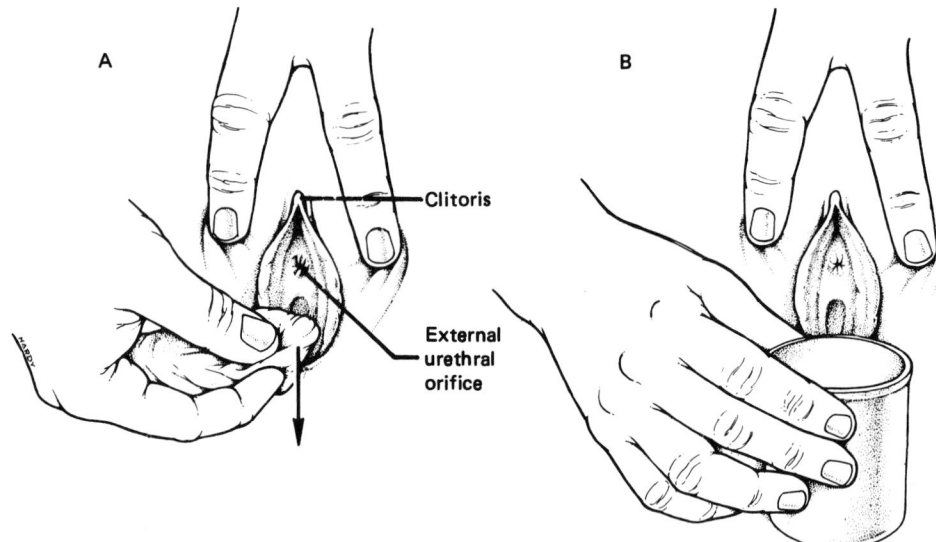

Figure 27-2. *Obtaining a clean-catch midstream urine specimen in the female. (A) Instruct the patient to hold the labia apart and wash from high up front toward the back with gauze soaked in soap. (B) The collection cup is held so that it does not touch the body, and the sample is obtained only while the patient is voiding with the labia held apart.*

Nursing Action	Rationale/Amplification
4. Allow initial urinary flow to drain into bedpan (toilet) and then catch the midstream specimen in a sterile container, making sure that the container does not come in contact with the genitalia.	4. The first portion of urine washes out the urethra. Have the patient remove the container from the stream while she is still voiding.
5. Send the specimen to the laboratory immediately.	5. Too long an interval between collection and analysis causes contaminants to multiply in the urine and cells to lyse.

Catheterization

Purpose
1. To relieve acute or chronic urinary retention.
2. For preoperative and postoperative urinary drainage.
3. To determine amount of residual urine after voiding.

Equipment
Sterile gloves
Disposable sterile catheter set with single-use packet of lubricant
Antiseptic solution for periurethral cleansing (sterile)
Gloves, drape, sponges
Sterile container for culture
Bath blanket/sheet for draping
Standing lamp (preferred) or flashlight

Selection of Catheter Size
Use the smallest size catheter capable of providing adequate drainage.

Procedure

Nursing Action	Rationale/Amplification
Female Patient	
Preparatory Phase	
1. Put the patient at ease.	1. The patient will feel reassured if the procedure is explained and if she is handled gently and considerately.
2. Open catheter tray using aseptic technique. Place waste receptacle in accessible place.	2. Catheterization requires the same aseptic precautions as a surgical procedure. The principle danger of catheterization is urinary tract infection, which is associated with increased morbidity and longer, more costly hospitalization.
3. Direct light for visualization of genital area.	
4. Place the patient in a supine position with knees bent, hips flexed, and feet resting on bed about 0.6 m. (2 feet) apart. Drape the patient.	
5. Position moisture-proof pad under the patient's buttocks.	
6. Wash hands. Put on sterile gloves.	
Performance Phase	
1. Separate labia minora so that urethral meatus is visualized; one hand is to maintain separation of the labia until catheterization is finished.	1. This maneuver helps prevent labial contamination of the catheter (Fig. 27-3).
2. Cleanse around the urethral meatus with a povidone-iodine solution.	2. Bacteria that normally colonize the distal urethra may be introduced into the bladder during or immediately after catheter insertion. Inadequate preparation of the urethral meatus is a major cause of infection.
a. Manipulate cleansing sponges with forceps, cleansing with downward strokes from anterior to posterior.	
b. Dispose of cotton sponge after each use.	
c. If the patient is sensitive to iodine, benzalkonium chloride or other cleansing agent is used.	
3. Introduce well-lubricated catheter 5–7 cm. (2–3 inches) into urethral meatus using strict aseptic technique.	3. A well-lubricated catheter reduces friction and trauma to the meatus. The female urethra is a relatively short canal, measuring 3–4 cm. in length.
a. Avoid contaminating surface of catheter.	
b. Ensure that catheter is not too large or too tight at urethral meatus.	b. Too large a catheter may cause painful distention of the meatus and cause damage to the uroepithelium.
4. Allow some bladder urine to flow through catheter before collecting a specimen.	4. This is a representative bladder aliquot.
5. Pinch off catheter and remove gently when urine ceases to flow.	5. Pinching off the catheter prevents air from entering the bladder as the catheter is removed.
Follow-Up Phase	
1. Dry area; make patient comfortable.	
2. Measure urine and dispose of equipment.	

(continued)

Procedure *(continued)*	**Nursing Action**	**Rationale/Amplification**

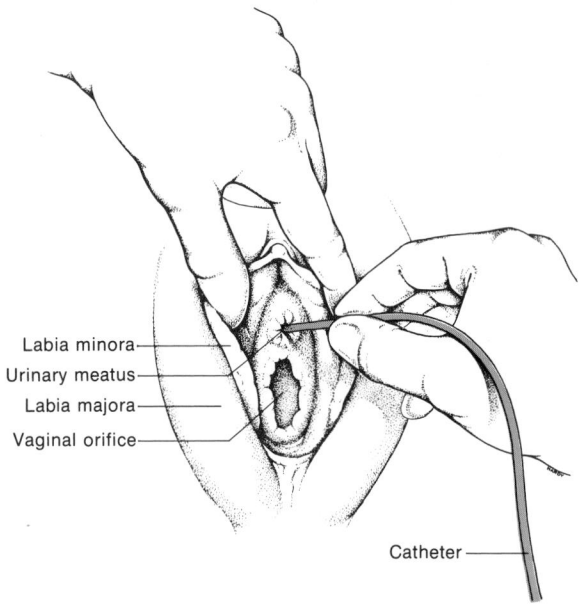

Labia minora
Urinary meatus
Labia majora
Vaginal orifice

Catheter

Figure 27-3. *Catheterization of urinary bladder in female.*

3. Send specimen to laboratory as indicated.
4. Record time, procedure, amount, and appearance of urine.

Male Patient

1. Carry out all of "preparatory phase" as for female patient except:
2. Place the patient in supine position with legs extended. Place the moisture-proof pad across upper thighs.
3. Position the perineal drape.
4. Lubricate the catheter well with lubricant or prescribed topical anesthetic.
5. Wash off glans penis around urinary meatus with an iodophor solution (Betadine) using forceps to hold cleansing sponges. Keep the foreskin retracted. Maintain sterility of dominant hand.

4. A well-lubricated catheter prevents urethral trauma (decreasing the opportunity for bacterial invasion).
5. Cleanse urethral meatus from tip to foreskin with downward stroke on one side. Discard sponge. Repeat as required.

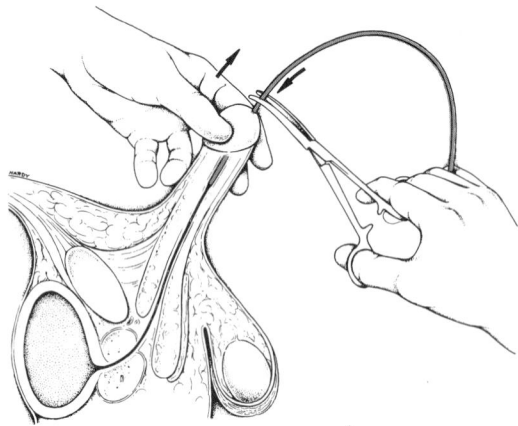

Figure 27-4. *Technique for catheterization in male.*

Procedure
(continued)

Nursing Action	Rationale/Amplification
6. Grasp shaft of penis (with nondominant hand and elevate it (Fig. 27-4). Apply gentle traction to penis while catheter is passed.	6. This maneuver straightens the penile urethra and facilitates catheterization. Maintaining a grasp of the penis prevents contamination and retraction of penis.
7. Using sterile gloves or forceps, insert catheter into the urethra; advance catheter 15–25 cm. (6–10 inches) until urine flows.	7. The male urethra is a canal extending from the bladder to the end of the glans penis. The length varies within wide limits; the average length is about 21 cm.
8. If resistance is felt at the external sphincter, slightly increase the traction on the penis and apply steady, gentle pressure on the catheter. Ask patient to strain gently (as if passing urine) to help relax sphincter.	8. Some resistance may be due to spasm of external sphincter. Inability to pass the catheter may mean that a urethral stricture or other forms of urethral pathology exist. The urethra may have to be dilated with sounds by a urologist.
9. When urine begins to flow, advance the catheter another 2.5 cm. (1 inch).	9. Advancing the catheter ensures its position in the bladder.
10. Reduce (or reposition) the foreskin.	10. Paraphimosis (retraction and constriction of the foreskin behind the glans penis), secondary to catheterization, may occur if the foreskin is not reduced.

Follow-Up Phase

Same as for female patient.

Guidelines

Management of the Patient With an Indwelling (Self-Retaining) Catheter and Closed Drainage System

Purpose

1. To empty urine from the bladder following bladder, prostate, or vaginal surgery.
2. To relieve urinary tract obstruction.
3. To permit urinary drainage in patients with neurogenic bladder dysfunction/urinary retention.
4. To determine accurate measurement of urinary drainage in critically ill patients.

Equipment

Completely closed system of urinary drainage
Catheter tray with triple-lumen catheter
Antibacterial solution for cleansing
Gauze squares
Single-use packet of lubricant

Procedure

Nursing Action	Rationale/Amplification
General Considerations	
1. Catheterize the patient (p. 665), using a catheter that is preconnected to a closed drainage system.	1. A closed drainage system is one that is closed to outside air.
a. Advance catheter almost to its bifurcation (for male patient).	a. This prevents the balloon from becoming trapped in the urethra.
b. Inflate the balloon according to manufacturer's directions. Be sure catheter is draining properly before inflating balloon, then withdraw catheter slightly.	b. Inadvertent inflation of the balloon within the urethra is painful and causes urethral trauma.
2. Secure the indwelling catheter.	2. Properly securing the catheter prevents catheter movement and traction on the urethra.
a. Female: Tape the catheter and drainage tubing to the thigh. Male: Tape the catheter to the lower abdomen and the tubing to the shaved thigh (Fig. 27-5).	This smooths out urethral curve and eliminates pressure on the urethra at the penoscrotal junction, which can eventually lead to the formation of a urethrocutaneous fistula.
b. Allow some slack of the tubing to accommodate the patient's movements.	
c. Keep the tubing over the patient's leg.	c. This tubing position helps prevent kinking or forming loops of stagnant urine.
Care of the Indwelling Catheter	
1. Cleanse around the area where catheter enters urethral meatus (meatal–catheter junction) with water during the daily bath to remove debris.	1. Suppurative drainage and encrustation occur at the exit of any tube. Infectious organisms can migrate to the bladder along the outside of any indwelling catheter.

(continued)

Guidelines Management of the Patient With an Indwelling (Self-Retaining) Catheter and Closed Drainage System *(continued)*

Procedure *(continued)*	**Nursing Action**	**Rationale/Amplification**

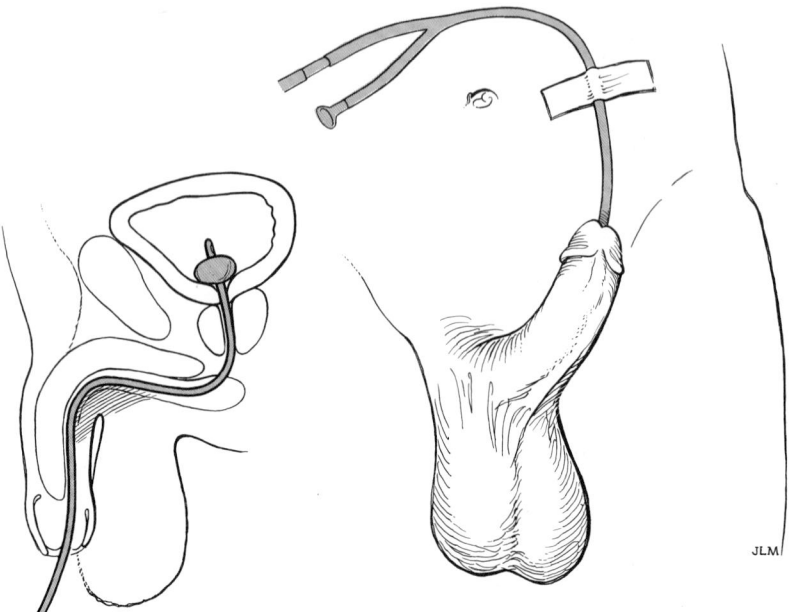

Figure 27-5. *In the male patient, the indwelling catheter is taped to the abdomen to straighten the angulation of the penoscrotal junction, thus reducing pressure on the ure-thra exerted by the catheter.*

Nursing Action	**Rationale/Amplification**
2. Avoid using powders and sprays on the perineal area.	2. Powder can encrust and cause soreness and infection.
3. Avoid pulling on the catheter during cleansing.	3. Pulling on the catheter may be painful. Backward and forward displacement of the catheter introduces contaminants into the urinary tract.
To Obtain Urine for Culture	
1. Clamp the drainage tubing below the aspiration (sampling) port for a *few minutes* to allow urine to collect.	1. Avoid separating catheter and connecting tube. Disconnection of the catheter and tubing is a major cause of urinary tract infection.
2. Cleanse the aspiration port with povidone-iodine or 70% alcohol.	
3. Insert a sterile No. 21 gauge needle (attached to a sterile syringe) into the aspiration port of the catheter.	3. Avoid inserting needle into the shaft of the catheter because this may cause balloon deflation.
4. Aspirate a small volume of urine for culture.	
5. Remove needle from syringe and release urine carefully into sterile specimen container.	
6. *Unclamp the drainage tube.*	
7. Send specimen to laboratory immediately.	7. The specimen should be marked as a ''catheterized specimen'' as the presence of any number of colonies of an organism indicates a urinary tract infection.
To Irrigate the Catheter	
Note: This is not done unless obstruction is anticipated (bleeding following bladder/prostate surgery).	
1. Wash hands. Don gloves.	
2. Using aseptic technique, pour sterile irrigating solution into sterile container.	
3. Cleanse around catheter/drainage tubing connection with sterile gauze pads soaked in povidone-iodine solution.	3. If frequent irrigations are necessary to keep the catheter open, change the catheter as the catheter itself is probably contributing to the problem.

Nursing Action	**Rationale/Amplification**
4. Disconnect catheter from drainage tubing. Cover tubing with a sterile cap or drainage-tubing adapter bag (sleeve).	
5. Place a sterile drainage basin under the catheter.	
6. Irrigate catheter using a large volume syringe and pre-scribed amount of sterile irrigant.	6. Instill about 30 ml. irrigating solution at a time. Avoid instilling the solution forcibly to prevent bladder irritation and spasms.
7. Remove syringe and place end of catheter over drainage basin, allowing returning fluid to drain into basin.	7. This provides gravitational flow.
8. Repeat irrigation procedure until fluid is clear or according to physician's directives.	
9. Disinfect the distal end of the catheter and end of drainage tubing; reconnect the catheter and tubing. Remove gloves. Wash hands.	
10. Document type and amount of irrigating solution, color and character of returning fluid, presence of sediment/blood clots, and patient's reaction.	10. Use irrigating equipment one time and then discard.

Changing the Catheter

Change catheter according to the needs of the patient.	An indwelling catheter should *not* be changed at arbitrarily fixed intervals.

Principles of Care When Managing a Closed Drainage System

1. Wash hands immediately before and after handling any part of the system. Wear clean disposable gloves when handling the drainage system.	1. Hands are the major route of transmission of gram-negative bacteria.
2. Maintain unobstructed urine flow.	2. Urine flow must be downhill.
a. Keep the drainage bag in a dependent position, below the level of the bladder.	a. Raising the bag will cause reflux of contaminated urine from the bag into the patient's bladder.
b. Urine should not be allowed to collect in the tubing, since a free flow of urine must be maintained to prevent infection.	b. Improper drainage occurs when the tubing is kinked or twisted, allowing pools of drainage to collect in the loops of tubing.
c. Keep the bag off the floor.	c. To prevent bacterial contamination.
3. To empty the drainage bag.	
a. Wash hands; don gloves.	a. Empty the bag at regular intervals, taking care to see that the drainage valve/spout is not contaminated.
b. Disinfect spigot. Empty the bag in a separate collecting receptacle for each patient. Disinfect spigot again.	b. Each patient should have his own collecting receptacle that is labeled with his name and kept in his bathroom, not on the floor—to prevent cross-contamination.
c. Avoid letting the drainage bag touch the floor.	
d. Change the drainage bag if contamination occurs, if the urine flow becomes obstructed, or if the connecting junctions start to leak.	

Measures to Prevent Cross-Contamination

1. Wash hands before and after handling the catheter/drain-age system and between patients.	1. Many urinary tract infections are due to extrinsically acquired organisms transmitted by cross-contamination.
2. Assign only one patient with an indwelling catheter to a room. If this is not possible, separate the infected patient with an indwelling catheter from an uninfected patient.	2. There appears to be a greater risk of microbial transmission between catheterized patients.
3. Know the patients at risk.	3. Female, elderly, debilitated, and critically ill patients, those in the postpartum state, and patients with obstructed or neurologically impaired bladders are at risk for infection.

Patient Education (Self-Care of Catheter at Home)

1. Wash hands before and after handling the catheter.
2. Wash around urinary opening daily, taking care to avoid pulling on the catheter during cleansing.
3. Drink 8–12 glasses of fluids daily; increase fluid intake if urine becomes dark and concentrated.
4. Wipe all connecting junctions with alcohol before changing from leg–bag drainage to overnight bottle drainage.
5. Keep the drainage bag at a lower level than the bladder; do not place the bag on your chair.
6. Avoid letting the bag lay on its side as urine may flow back into the drainage tube.
7. Usually the catheter is not changed except when obstruction or malfunction occurs.
8. Inspect the catheter upon removal for evidence of encrustation; if there are no signs of encrustation and blocking of lumen, the interval between catheter changes may be increased.
9. Call physician/clinic if fever and/or cloudy, bloody, or odoriferous urine develops.

Guidelines Assisting the Patient Undergoing Suprapubic Bladder Drainage (Cystostomy)

Suprapubic bladder drainage is a method of establishing drainage from the bladder by introducing a catheter percutaneously or by an incision through the anterior abdominal wall into the bladder.

Purpose

1. To drain the bladder when acute urinary retention is present and when urethral catheterization is not possible.
2. To divert the flow of urine from the urethra in event of urethral trauma, stricture, or fistula.
3. To obtain an uncontaminated urine specimen for culture.

Clinical Use-fulness

1. When urethral route is impassable—urethral stricture, injuries
2. Following gynecologic operations—vaginal hysterectomy, vaginal repair
3. Following bladder surgery
4. Pelvic fractures

Equipment

Sterile suprapubic drainage system package (disposable)
Skin germicide for suprapubic skin preparation; sterile gloves
Local anesthetic agent if needed

Procedure

Nursing Action	Rationale/Amplification

Preparatory Phase

1. Place the patient in a supine position with one pillow under head.
2. Expose the abdomen.

Performance Phase (by physician)

Nursing Action	Rationale/Amplification
1. The bladder is distended with 300–500 ml. of sterile saline via a urethral catheter, which is removed, or the patient is given fluids (oral or IV) before the procedure.	1. Distention of the bladder makes the bladder easier to locate by the suprapubic route.
2. The suprapubic area is surgically prepared. After the skin is dried, the needle entry point is located.	2. The needle entry point is in the midline, 2–3 cm. above the symphysis pubis and directly over the palpable bladder.
3. The skin and subcutaneous tissues are infiltrated with local anesthesia.	3. An adequate level of local anesthesia is achieved to facilitate catheter introduction.
4. A small stab wound (incision) may be made.	
5. The catheter* is introduced via a guidewire, needle, or cannula through the incision and advanced in a slightly caudal direction.	5. Entrance into the bladder is usually felt and can be verified by free flow of urine.
6. The catheter is advanced until the flange is against the skin where it is secured with tape, a body seal system, or sutures.	6. Another method is to advance a long needle into the bladder until urine flow verifies the needle is in the bladder.
7. The catheter is connected to a sterile drainage system.	7. Aseptic technique is employed in the area around the cystostomy tube.
8. Secure drainage tubing to lateral abdomen with tape.	8. Prevents undue tension on the catheter.
9. If the catheter is not draining properly, withdraw the catheter 2.5 cm. (1 inch) at a time until urine begins to flow. Do not dislodge catheter from bladder.	
10. The drainage is maintained continuously for several days.	
11. If a "trial of voiding" is requested, the catheter is clamped for 4 hours.	11. Usually, patients will void earlier after surgery with suprapubic drainage than with indwelling catheters.
a. Have the patient attempt to void while the catheter is clamped.	
b. After the patient voids, unclamp the catheter and measure residual urine.	
c. Usually, if the amount of residual urine is less than 100 ml. on 2 separate occasions (AM and PM), the catheter may be removed.	
d. If the patient complains of pain or discomfort, or if the residual urine is over the prescribed amount, the catheter is usually left open.	
12. The catheter is removed upon request, and a sterile dressing is placed over the site. Usually the tract will close within 48 hours.	12. Suprapubic drainage is considered more comfortable than an indwelling urethral catheter, it allows greater patient mobility, and there is less risk of bladder infection.
13. Monitor for complications.	13. Complications of this procedure: inadvertent peritoneal and bowel damage, leakage around catheter, kinking of catheter, hematuria, abdominal wall abscess.

* It is necessary to become familiar with the manufacturer's directions of the system being used.

Urinary Retention

Urinary retention is the inability to urinate despite a desire to do so. Retention may be acute or chronic. Chronic retention will often lead to overflow incontinence or residual urine (urine that remains in the bladder after voiding).

Etiology

A. Males

1. Benign prostatic hyperplasia
2. Stricture of urethra, calculus or foreign body in urethra, urethritis, tumor
3. Phimosis

B. Females

1. Urethral obstruction secondary to stricture, stones, vaginal cysts, carcinoma, edema
2. Retroverted gravid uterus

C. Both Sexes

1. Following any operation, particularly on anal or perineal region—due to reflex spasm of sphincters
2. Trauma
3. Neurogenic bladder dysfunction—spinal cord tumor, trauma, herniated intervertebral disc, multiple sclerosis
4. Certain drugs (anticholinergics, antihistamines)
5. Fecal impaction
6. Psychogenic urinary retention

Clinical Manifestations *(See Fig. 27-6)*

1. History of no voiding or frequent passing of small amounts of urine without relief.
2. Progressive slowing of urinary stream; hesitancy.
3. Lower abdominal discomfort and distress; severe pain. The patient may have little or no discomfort if bladder distends slowly.
4. Smooth, firm, oval-shaped mass that is palpable over bladder area.
5. Dullness to percussion above symphysis pubis (residual urine below 130 ml. is not usually percussible).
6. Visualization of a rounded swelling arising out of the pelvis.
7. Urine-stained clothing.

Management and Nursing Interventions

A. Retention Following Surgery

1. Use nursing measures to help patient void.
   a. Transport the patient to bathroom (or bedside

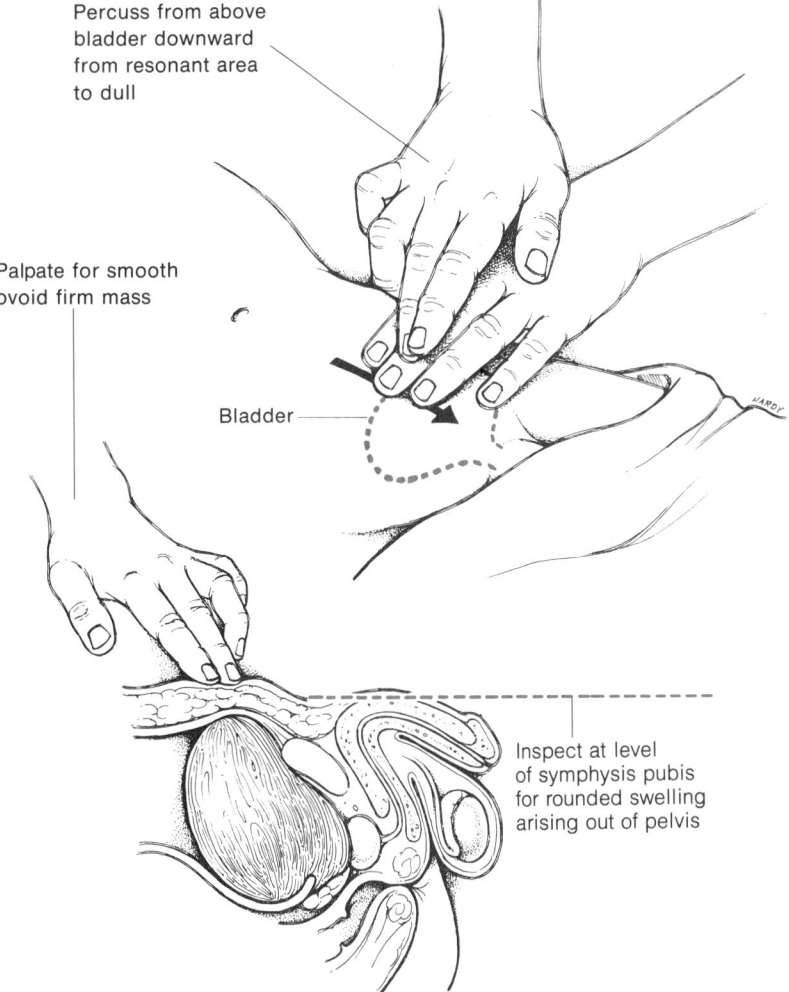

Percuss from above bladder downward from resonant area to dull

Palpate for smooth ovoid firm mass

Bladder

Inspect at level of symphysis pubis for rounded swelling arising out of pelvis

Figure 27-6. *Nursing assessment for urinary retention.*

commode) or allow to stand beside bed if possible—many patients are unable to void while lying in bed.
   b. Use warmth to relax sphincters—sitz bath, warm compresses to perineum, warm shower.
   c. Give hot tea to drink.
   d. Have patient listen to sound of running water; place hands in warm water.
   e. Administer bethanechol chloride (Urecholine) only if directed.
   f. Give psychological reassurance and support.
2. Give prescribed analgesic medication postoperatively.
   a. Voiding may be difficult because of pain in incisional area, especially in anterior vaginal operations.
   b. Sphincter spasm is generally present in patients with acute urinary retention.

B. For Urinary Retention From Obstruction

1. Decompress bladder before overdistention occurs—bladder mucosa that has been stretched from urinary retention is readily infected.
   a. Utilize indwelling catheter and closed drainage.
   b. Call urologist if unable to pass catheter readily; special instruments or operation may be necessary.
2. Monitor the hourly urine output; fluid loss may be replaced by intravenous infusions.
3. Evaluate the patient's biochemical status.
4. Monitor blood pressure, which may fluctuate; renal function may decline the first few days after bladder drainage is instituted.
5. Assist in determining the underlying cause.
   a. Carry out blood urea nitrogen tests and other renal function tests.
   b. Assist in carrying out diagnostic tests if obstructive uropathy (pathologic change in urinary tract from obstruction) is suspected.

Nursing Assessment for Fluid and Electrolyte Imbalance

The following manifestations of body fluid disturbances may occur in patients with renal disease.

Clinical Manifestations

A. Volume

1. Volume deficit—Acute weight loss (in excess of 5%), drop in body temperature, dry skin and mucous membranes, longitudinal wrinkles or furrows of tongue, oliguria or anuria.
2. Volume excess—acute weight gain (in excess of 5%), edema, moist crackles in lungs, puffy eyelids, shortness of breath.

B. Sodium

1. Sodium deficit—abdominal cramps, apprehension, convulsions, fingerprinting on sternum, oliguria or anuria.
2. Sodium excess—dry sticky mucous membranes, flushed skin, oliguria or anuria, thirst, rough and dry tongue.

C. Potassium

1. Potassium deficit—anorexia, gaseous distention of intestines, silent intestinal ileus, weakness, soft, flabby muscles.

2. Potassium excess—diarrhea, intestinal colic, irritability, nausea.

D. Calcium

1. Calcium deficit—abdominal cramps, carpopedal spasm, muscle cramps, tetany, tingling of ends of fingers.
2. Calcium excess—anorexia, nausea, vomiting, abdominal pain, abdominal distention, mental confusion.

E. Bicarbonate

1. Primary base bicarbonate deficit—deep, rapid breathing (Kussmaul), shortness of breath on exertion, stupor, weakness.
2. Primary base bicarbonate excess—depressed respiration, muscle hypertonicity, tetany.

F. Protein Deficit—chronic weight loss, emotional depression, pallor, ready fatigue, soft, flabby muscles.

G. Magnesium Deficit—positive Chvostek's sign, convulsions, disorientation, hyperactive deep reflexes, tremor.

Nursing Interventions

1. Observe the clinical course of the patient; record the data collected.
2. Keep an accurate intake and output record.
3. Check the vital signs every 4 hours. Weigh the patient daily.
4. Support the patient having repeated blood examinations for the surveillance of electrolyte balance.
5. Explain the purpose of these examinations.

Acute Renal Failure

Acute renal failure is a sudden decline in renal function caused by failure of the renal circulation or by glomerular or tubular dysfunction. The substances normally eliminated in the urine accumulate in the body fluids as a result of impaired renal excretion and lead to a disruption in homeostatic, endocrine, and metabolic functions. Renal failure is a disease affecting the entire body.

Causes and Clinical Manifestations

A. Prerenal Causes

1. Result from conditions that decrease renal blood flow (hypovolemia, shock, hemorrhage, burns, impaired cardiac output, diuretic therapy).
2. *Clinical manifestations:* nausea, vomiting, diarrhea, decreased tissue turgor, dryness of mucous membranes, somnolence.

B. Postrenal Causes

1. Arise from obstruction to urine flow (ureteral or urethral obstruction).
2. *Clinical manifestations:* difficulty in voiding; changes in urine flow.

C. Intrarenal Causes

1. Result from ischemic, toxic or immunologic mechanisms; from intrinsic disease of renal parenchyma including glomerular, tubo-interstitial, and vascular diseases.
2. *Clinical manifestations:* fever, skin rash, edema.

Preventive Measures

1. Identify patients with preexisting renal disease.
2. Initiate adequate hydration before, during, and after operative procedures.
3. Avoid exposure to various nephrotoxins. Be aware that the majority of drugs or their metabolites are excreted by the kidneys.
4. Avoid chronic analgesic abuse—causes interstitial nephritis and papillary necrosis.
5. Prevent and treat shock with blood and fluid replacement. Prevent prolonged periods of hypotension.
6. Monitor urinary output and central venous pressure hourly in critically ill patients to detect onset of renal failure at the earliest moment.
7. Schedule diagnostic studies requiring dehydration so that there are "rest days," especially in aged who may not have adequate renal reserve.
8. Pay special attention to draining wounds, burns, etc., which can lead to sepsis and progressive renal damage.
9. Avoid infection; give meticulous care to patients with indwelling catheters and intravenous lines.
10. Take every precaution to ensure that the right person receives the right blood—to avoid severe transfusion reactions, which can precipitate renal complications.

Clinical Phases of Acute Renal Failure

A. Period of Oliguria (urine volume less than 400 ml./24 hours)

1. Accompanied by rise in serum concentration of elements usually excreted by kidney (urea, creatinine, uric acid, organic acids, and the intracellular cations—potassium and magnesium).
2. There can be a decrease in renal function with increasing nitrogen retention even when the patient is excreting more than 2–3 liters of urine daily—called *nonoliguric* or *high-output failure*.

B. Period of Diuresis

Gradually increasing urinary output; glomerular filtration has started to recover but renal function is still abnormal.

C. Period of Recovery

1. Excretory and reabsorptive capabilities of kidneys gradually return; may take 1–2 years.
2. Usually there is some permanent loss of glomerular filtration and concentrating ability.

Diagnostic Evaluation

1. Urinalysis—reveals proteinuria, hematuria, casts.
2. Rising serum creatinine and blood urea nitrogen levels.
3. Urine chemistry examinations to distinguish various forms of acute renal failure.
4. Renal ultrasonography—for estimate of renal size and to exclude a treatable obstructive uropathy.

Management

1. Correction of any reversible cause of acute renal failure (e.g., improve renal perfusion; maximize cardiac output; surgical relief of obstruction)
2. Attention to and correction of underlying fluid excesses or deficits
3. Correction and control of biochemical imbalances—treatment of hyperkalemia
4. Restoration/maintenance of blood pressure
5. Maintenance of nutrition
6. Initiation of hemodialysis, peritoneal dialysis, or continuous hemodiafiltration for patients with progressive azotemia (abnormal retention of nitrogenous products in the blood) and other life-threatening complications

Nursing Assessment

1. Determine if there is a history of cardiac, malignancy, sepsis, or intercurrent illness.
2. Find out if patient has been exposed to potentially nephrotoxic drugs (antibiotics, nonsteroidal anti-inflammatory drugs, contrast agents, solvents).
3. Conduct an on-going physical examination for tissue turgor, pallor, alteration in mucous membranes, blood pressure, heart rate changes, and edema.
4. Monitor urine volume that may not correlate with severity of renal disease.
5. Study results of laboratory data for evidence of acid–base imbalances and electrolyte disorders.

Complications

1. Infection (see p. 684)
2. Hyperkalemia; dysrhythmias
3. Electrolyte (sodium, potassium, uric acid, calcium, phosphorus) abnormalities
4. Gastrointestinal bleeding; stress ulcerations
5. Multiple organ systems failure

Nursing Diagnoses

1. Fluid volume deficit related to failure of kidneys to maintain volume regulation, excrete waste products, maintain electrolyte and acid–base balance and endocrine activity
2. Potential for fluid volume excess related to fluid volume overload
3. Altered renal tissue perfusion related to kidney failure
4. Potential for infection related to alterations in the immunologic system and host defenses
5. Altered nutrition (less than body requirements) related to catabolic state, anorexia, and malnutrition associated with acute renal failure
6. Altered thought processes (changing mental status) related to progressive uremia

Nursing Interventions

A. Monitoring and Managing Hyperkalemia

1. Evaluate for hyperkalemia (potassium intoxication) by assessment of serum potassium levels (potassium values above 6 mEq./liter) correlated with ECG changes (peaking of T-waves and shortening of the QT interval).
2. Administration of sodium bicarbonate or glucose and insulin—causes temporary shift of potassium to the intercellular compartment.
3. Administer cation exchange resin (sodium polystyrene sulfonate [Kayexalate, given as a retention enema]) to provide more prolonged correction of elevated potassium.
4. Watch for cardiac dysrhythmias (cardiac arrest) and congestive heart failure from hyperkalemia, electrolyte imbalance, and/or fluid overload.
5. Control potassium balance.
6. Prepare for dialysis when rapid lowering of potassium is needed.

B. Providing Electrolyte Replacement

1. Acidosis
   a. Arises from inability of body to excrete normal acid load resulting from catabolism.
   b. Treatment: sodium bicarbonate.

2. Hyperphosphatemia
   a. Results from decreased renal clearance.
   b. Treatment: aluminum or calcium antacids given to bind phosphate in gastrointestinal tract to keep phosphate from being absorbed in blood stream.

C. Monitoring for Gastrointestinal Bleeding

1. Examine all stools for blood.
2. Administer H-2-receptor antagonist (cimetidine or ranitidine) and/or antacids as prophylaxis.
3. Prepare for endoscopy when gastrointestinal bleeding occurs.

D. Correcting Fluid Volume Deficits/Overload

1. Watch for signs and symptoms of hypovolemia (dehydration) or hypervolemia as regulating capacity of kidneys is inadequate.
   a. Hypovolemia: poor skin turgor, dryness of mucous membranes, hypotension, tachycardia.
   b. Hypervolemia: dyspnea, tachycardia, distended neck veins, crackles, peripheral edema, pulmonary edema.
2. Monitor the urinary output and urine specific gravity; measure and record intake and output including urine, gastric suction, stools, wound drainage, perspiration.
3. Monitor serum and urine electrolyte concentrations; fluid replacement tailored to match salt and water excretion.
4. Weigh the patient daily to provide an index of fluid balance; expected weight loss is 0.25–0.5 kg (½–1 lb. daily).
5. Record clinical events, fluid balance, daily laboratory values, and body weight on a flowchart to determine rate and trend of improvement or deterioration.
6. Measure and replace (as directed) sodium losses if large losses are anticipated from gastrointestinal tract via suction, vomiting, or diarrhea.
7. Monitor arterial blood gas values and prepare for ventilatory therapy if severe acidosis is present and/or respiratory problems develop.
8. Give only enough fluids to replace losses during oliguric phase (usually 400–500 ml./24 hours plus measured fluid losses).
9. Provide skin care as skin is dry or susceptible to breakdown because of edema and excoriation from pruritus.

E. Improving Renal Perfusion

1. Assist patient undergoing studies to diagnose and relieve obstructive uropathy.
2. Monitor fluid replacement in volume-depleted patient.
   a. Examine for signs and symptoms of hypovolemia or hypervolemia.
   b. Watch daily weight, input and output values.
   c. Examine presacral and pretibial areas several times daily for evidence of edema.

F. Avoiding Infection

1. Monitor for all signs of infection; renal failure patients do not always demonstrate fever and leukocytosis.
2. Remove bladder catheter as soon as possible; monitor for urinary tract infection.
3. Employ intensive pulmonary hygiene—high incidence of lung edema and infection.
4. Carry out meticulous wound care.

G. Improving Nutritional Status

1. Employ moderate protein restriction during oliguric phase to minimize accumulation of toxic end-products, etc., that result from digestion and metabolism of dietary protein.
2. Offer high-carbohydrate feedings, since carbohydrates

have a greater protein-sparing power and provide additional calories.
3. Restrict foods and fluids containing potassium and phosphorus (bananas, citrus fruits/juices, coffee).
4. Adjust sodium intake and sodium output as directed.
5. Prepare for hyperalimentation when adequate nutrition cannot be maintained through the gastrointestinal tract.
6. Be aware that nutrients can be added to dialysate.
7. Encourage a high-protein, high-caloric diet after diuretic phase.

H. Becoming More Oriented

1. Watch for mental status changes—somnolence, lassitude, lethargy, and fatigue progressing to irritability, disorientation, twitching, seizures.
2. Employ seizure precautions (p. 583).
3. Encourage and assist patient to turn and move, as drowsiness and lethargy may prevent activity.
4. Prepare for dialysis, which may help prevent neurologic complications.

Patient Education

1. Explain that the patient may experience residual defects in kidney function for long period of time after acute illness.
2. Report for routine urinalysis and follow-up examinations.
3. Avoid taking *any* medications unless specifically prescribed.
4. Resume activity gradually, as muscle weakness will be present from excessive catabolism.

Evaluation

1. Attains fluid and electrolyte balance; laboratory values show improvement
2. Excreting urine; weight in acceptable range
3. Absence of infection
4. Maintaining satisfactory nutritional status
5. Appears more alert; sleeping less during the day

Chronic Renal Failure
(End-Stage Renal Disease)

Chronic renal failure is a progressive deterioration of renal function, which ends fatally in uremia (an excess of urea and other nitrogenous wastes in the blood) and its complications unless dialysis or a kidney transplant is performed.

Causes

1. Hypertension; prolonged and severe
2. Diabetes mellitus
3. Glomerulopathies
4. Interstitial nephritis
5. Hereditary renal disease; polycystic kidney disease
6. Obstructive uropathy

Stages of Chronic Renal Failure

Decreased renal reserve → renal insufficiency → renal failure → uremia

Clinical Manifestations

1. Gastrointestinal manifestations—anorexia, nausea, vomiting, hiccoughs, ulceration of gastrointestinal tract, and hemorrhage.

2. Cardiopulmonary manifestations—hypertension, fibrinous pericarditis, pleuritis.
3. Neuromuscular disturbances—fatigue, sleep disorders, headache, lethargy, muscular irritability, peripheral neuropathy, seizures, coma.
4. Fluid and electrolyte disturbances.
5. Metabolic and endocrine alterations—glucose intolerance, hyperlipidemia, sex hormone disturbances.
6. Personality changes—emotional dullness, lability with impatient, demanding behavior.
7. Dermatologic disturbances—pallor, hyperpigmentation, pruritus, ecchymoses, uremic frost.
8. Skeletal abnormalities—renal osteodystrophy; hyperparathyroid bone disease.
9. Anemia.

Diagnostic Evaluation

1. Anemia (a characteristic sign)
2. Elevated serum creatinine or BUN
3. Elevated serum phosphorus
4. Decreased serum calcium
5. Low serum proteins, especially albumin
6. Usually, low CO_2 and acidosis (low blood pH)

Management

Goal:
Conservation of renal function as long as possible.

1. Detection and treatment of reversible causes of renal failure; e.g., bring diabetes under control; treat hypertension.
2. Dietary regulation—low-protein diet supplemented with essential amino acids or their keto-analogues to minimize uremic toxicity and to prevent wasting and malnutrition.
3. Treatment of associated conditions to improve renal dynamics.
   a. Anemia—with recombinant human erythropoietin, a synthetic kidney hormone.
   b. Acidosis—replacement of bicarbonate stores by infusion or oral administration of sodium bicarbonate.
   c. Hyperkalemia—restriction of dietary potassium; administration of potassium-binding agents.
   d. Phosphate retention—decrease dietary phosphorus (chicken, milk, legumes, carbonated beverages); administer phosphate-binding agents since they bind phosphorus in the intestinal tract.

> **NURSING ALERT:** Patients with impaired renal function may require major adjustments of common therapeutic agents. Give medications with caution.

4. Maintenance dialysis or kidney transplantation when symptoms can no longer be controlled with conservative management.

Nursing Assessment

1. See nursing assessment for acute renal failure, page 673.
2. Study degree of renal impairment by reviewing laboratory results.
3. Examine for edema, hypertension, neck vein distention.
4. Ask about bowel elimination: frequency, character, amount, sensations associated with constipation.
5. Assess for nutritional status using diet history (intake/recall records), height, weight, anthropometric measurements, and laboratory values. Consult with dietitian.
6. Inspect skin for paleness secondary to anemia. Ask about itching. Assess for scaling and excoriation.
7. Watch for symptoms of encephalopathy: confusion, lethargy, decreased memory, stupor, coma.
8. Evaluate for symptoms of depression: dysphoric mood, somatic symptoms (appetite changes, sleep disturbances), guilt, problems with concentration, loss of interest.
9. Assess for presence or absence and quality of social support system.

Nursing Diagnoses

1. Fluid volume deficit or excess related to impaired concentrating and diluting mechanisms of the kidneys.
2. Altered nutrition (less than body requirements) related to weight loss, muscle wasting, biochemical derangements, gastrointestinal effects of disease (anorexia, nausea, vomiting).
3. Impaired skin integrity related to itching, hyperpigmentation, peripheral neuropathy, and possible skin eruptions from drug reactions.
4. Altered elimination (constipation) related to fluid restriction, ingestion of phosphate-binding antacids, reduced intake of dietary fiber, medications, and lack of exercise.
5. Altered thought processes (shortened attention span, diminished cognitive ability, irritability, personality changes) related to altered central nervous system function from uremic toxins.
6. Ineffective individual coping related to frustration, dependency, and depression.
7. Potential for noncompliance with the therapeutic regimen related to restrictions imposed by chronic renal failure and its treatment.

Nursing Interventions

A. Monitoring for Potential Complications

Note: There is potential for complications of every organ system related to biochemical and physiologic dysfunction. The treatment of these complications is beyond the scope of this discussion.

1. Cardiovascular disease; congestive heart failure; pericarditis
2. Hypertension
3. Anemia
4. Chronic metabolic acidosis
5. Hyperlipidemia
6. Hyperuricemia
7. Renal osteodystrophy—renal bone disease, as uremia is associated with abnormal calcium metabolism, which causes bone pathology
8. Paresthesias; neurologic abnormalities

B. Achieving Fluid and Electrolyte Balance

1. Weigh the patient daily to assess fluid overload or depletion—weight should not increase or decrease more than 0.45 kg. (1 lb.) per day.
2. Carry out serial blood pressure measurements—indicator of vascular volume status. Hypertension also increases rate of renal deterioration and adversely affects the vascular system.
3. Adjust fluid intake to maintain adequate urinary volume and to avoid dehydration.
   a. Fluid restriction is not usually initiated until renal function is quite low.

b. Fluid allowance should be distributed throughout the day.

c. Avoid restricting fluids for prolonged periods for laboratory and radiologic examinations, since dehydrating procedures are hazardous to those patients who cannot produce concentrated urine.

d. Restrict salt and water intake if there is evidence of extracellular excess (congestive heart failure, pulmonary edema, hypertension).

4. Adjust sodium requirements as indicated by serum and urine measurements and daily weight evaluations—patients with chronic renal disease cannot tolerate severe sodium restriction or marked excess in sodium intake.

5. Monitor for acidosis, which commonly appears in chronic renal failure: stupor; deep, rapid breathing of Kussmaul type; shortness of breath on exertion; weakness; unconsciousness.

C. Maintaining Nutrition to Conserve Renal Function As Long As Possible

1. Work collaboratively with dietitian to regulate protein intake according to impaired renal function, since metabolites that accumulate in blood derive almost entirely from protein catabolism.

a. Protein should be of high biologic value, rich in essential amino acids (dairy products, eggs, meat), so that the patient does not rely on tissue catabolism for essential amino acids.

b. Low-protein diet may be supplemented with essential amino acids and vitamins.

c. As renal function declines, protein intake may be restricted proportionately.

d. Protein will be increased if the patient is on a dialysis program to allow for loss of amino acids occurring during dialysis.

2. Ensure high calorie intake—essential to spare protein for its own work, to provide energy, and to prevent wasting.

3. Encourage intake of hard candy, jelly beans, jellies, flavored carbohydrate powders.

4. Monitor nutritional state by measurement of body weight, anthropometric measurements, serum albumin and transferrin, and nitrogen balance.

D. Maintaining Skin Integrity

1. Use measures to produce vasoconstriction: cool environment, removal of excessive bedding.

2. Provide tepid, cooling baths or cool wet dressings—gradual evaporation of water from dressings cools skin and relieves pruritus.

3. Eliminate irritants; apply emollient lotions.

E. Relieving Constipation

1. Be aware that phosphate binders cause constipation that cannot be managed with usual interventions.

2. Encourage high-fiber diet, bearing in mind the potassium content of some fruits and vegetables.

a. Commercial fiber supplements (Fiberall; Fiber-Med) may be prescribed.

b. Employ stool softeners as prescribed.

c. Avoid laxatives and cathartics that cause electrolyte toxicities (compounds containing magnesium or phosphorus).

F. Preventing or Reducing Cognitive Distortions

1. Speak to the patient in simple orienting statements, using repetition when necessary.

2. Maintain predictable routine and keep change to a minimum.

3. Use close contact, nurturing voice, eye contact, and touch to establish rapport.

4. Correct cognitive distortions.

5. Use music tapes to promote relaxation.

6. Anticipate psychiatric intervention for acute changes in personality and cognition.

G. Enhancing Coping With Treatment Regimen

1. Prepare patient for dialysis or kidney transplantation.

2. Offer hope tempered by reality.

3. Enhance/improve (if possible) social support system of patient to lessen the impact of the stress of chronic kidney disease.

4. Encourage patient to share his thoughts and feelings with a confidant.

5. Encourage contact with family, friends, and work group.

6. Discuss option of supportive psychotherapy for depression.

H. Patient Education (to promote adherence to therapeutic program)

Teach the following:

1. Weigh every morning to avoid fluid overload.

2. Drink limited amounts *only* when thirsty.

3. Measure alloted fluids and save some for ice cubes; sucking on ice is thirst quenching.

4. Eat food before drinking fluids to alleviate dry mouth.

5. Use lemon wedges, hard candy, chewing gum—to moisten mouth.

Evaluation

1. Attains/maintains improved fluid balance.

2. Demonstrates improvement of nutritional status: improved laboratory values.

3. Free of skin excoriation: reports some relief of itching.

4. States that constipation is lessening.

5. Oriented to time, place, and person.

6. Verbalizes interest in dialysis/kidney transplantation.

7. Understands principles of treatment regimen: asks questions and shows interest in education materials.

Dialysis

Dialysis refers to the diffusion of solute molecules through a semipermeable membrane, passing from the side of higher concentration to that of lower concentration. The purpose of dialysis is to maintain the life and well-being of the patient until kidney function is restored. It is a substitute for some kidney excretory functions but does not replace the kidneys' endocrine and metabolic functions.

Methods

A. Peritoneal Dialysis

1. Intermittent peritoneal dialysis (short-term [see below] or chronic)

2. Continuous ambulatory peritoneal dialysis (see p. 679)

3. Continuous cycling peritoneal dialysis—uses automated peritoneal dialysis machine overnight with prolonged dwell time during day.

a. The patient is connected to cycler machine every evening, receiving 3–5 exchanges during night. In the morning, after infusing fresh dialysate, the catheter is capped.

b. Permits freedom from exchanges during day.

B. Hemodialysis (see p. 680)

C. Continuous Arteriovenous Hemofiltration—circulation of blood through a small-volume, low-resistance filter by the pressure of the patient's own arterial pressure rather than that of the blood pump used in hemodialysis; system used for temporarily replacing kidney function.

Guidelines Assisting the Patient Undergoing (Acute) Peritoneal Dialysis*

Peritoneal dialysis is a substitute for kidney function during renal failure. The peritoneum acts as a dialyzing membrane, and dialysate is delivered into the peritoneal cavity.

Purposes
1. Aids in the removal of toxic substances and metabolic wastes.
2. Establishes electrolyte balance.
3. Removes excessive body fluid.
4. Assists in regulating the fluid balance of the body.
5. Controls blood pressure.
6. Controls severe, intractable heart failure when diuretics no longer promote elimination of water and sodium.

Equipment
Dialysis administration set (disposable, closed system)
Peritoneal dialysis solution as requested
Supplemental drugs as requested
Local anesthesia
Central venous pressure monitoring equipment
ECG
Suture set
Sterile gloves
Skin antiseptic

Procedure

Nursing Action	Rationale/Amplification
1. Prepare the patient emotionally and physically for the procedure.	1. Nursing support is offered by explaining procedure mechanics, providing opportunities for the patient to ask questions, allowing him to verbalize his feelings, and giving expert physical care.
2. See that the consent form has been signed.	
3. Weigh the patient before dialysis and every 24 hours thereafter, preferably on an in-bed scale.	3. The weight at the beginning of the procedure serves as a baseline of information. Daily weight confirms ultrafiltration results and evaluates volume status.
4. Take temperature, pulse, respiration, and blood pressure readings prior to dialysis.	4. Measurement of vital signs at the beginning of dialysis is necessary for comparing subsequent changes in vital signs.
5. Have the patient empty his bladder.	5. If the bladder is empty, there is less likelihood of perforating it when the trocar is introduced into the peritoneum.
6. Assist with insertion of central venous pressure (CVP) catheter; ECG monitoring may also be employed.	6. CVP measurements may be carried out to assess fluid volume changes. Cardiac dysrhythmias may occur because of serum potassium changes and vagal stimulation.
7. Flush the tubing with dialysis solution.	7. The tubing is flushed to prevent air from entering the peritoneal cavity. Air causes abdominal discomfort and drainage difficulties.
8. Make the patient comfortable in a supine position. Have the patient and health-care personnel wear masks.	8. This helps protect the patient from airborne contamination.

Performance Phase (by the physician)

The following is a brief summary of the method of insertion of a temporary peritoneal catheter (*done under strict asepsis*).

1. The abdomen is prepared surgically, and the skin and subcutaneous tissues are infiltrated with a local anesthetic.	1. Surgical preparation of the skin minimizes or eliminates surface bacteria and decreases the possibility of wound contamination and infection.
2. A small midline stab wound is made 3–5 cm. below the umbilicus.	
3. The trocar is inserted through the incision with the stylet in place, or a thin stylet cannula may be inserted percutaneously.	

* Automated closed-system peritoneal cycling machines are available.

(continued)

Guidelines Assisting the Patient Undergoing (Acute) Peritoneal Dialysis *(continued)*

Procedure *(continued)*	**Nursing Action**	**Rationale/Amplification**
	4. The patient is requested to raise his head from the pillow after the trocar is introduced.	4. This maneuver tightens the abdominal muscles and permits easier penetration of the trocar without danger of injury to the intra-abdominal organs.

	5. When the peritoneum is punctured, the trocar is directed toward the left side of the pelvis. The stylet is removed, and the catheter is inserted through the trocar and maneuvered into position.
	  a. Dialysis fluid is allowed to run through the catheter while it is being positioned.
		
		  a. This prevents the omentum from adhering to the catheter, impeding its advancement or occluding its opening.

	6. After the trocar is removed, the skin may be closed with a purse-string suture. (This is not always done.) A sterile dressing is placed around the catheter.	6. The catheter is attached to the skin to prevent loss of the catheter in the abdomen.
	7. Attach the catheter connector to the administration set, which has been previously connected to the container of dialysis solution (warmed to body temperature, 37°C.)	7. The solution is warmed to body temperature for patient comfort and to prevent abdominal pain. Heating also causes dilatation of the peritoneal vessels and increases urea clearance.
	8. Drugs (heparin, potassium, antibiotic) are added in advance.	8. The addition of heparin prevents fibrin clots from occluding the catheter. Potassium chloride may be added on request unless patient has hyperkalemia. Antibiotics are added for the treatment of peritonitis.
	9. Permit the dialyzing solution to flow unrestricted into the peritoneal cavity (usually takes 5–10 minutes for completion). If the patient experiences pain, slow down the infusion.	9. The inflow solution should flow in a steady stream. If the fluid flows in too slowly, the catheter may need to be repositioned, since its tip may be buried in the omentum, or it may be occluded by a blood clot. Flushing may help.
	10. Allow the fluid to remain in the peritoneal cavity for the prescribed time period (20–30 minutes). Prepare the next exchange while the fluid is in the peritoneal cavity.	10. In order for potassium, urea, and other waste materials to be removed, the solution must remain in the peritoneal cavity for the prescribed time (dwell or equilibration time). The maximum concentration gradient takes place in the first 5–10 minutes for small molecules, such as urea and creatinine.
	11. Unclamp the outflow tube. Drainage should take approximately 20–30 minutes, although the time varies with each patient.	11. The abdomen is drained by a siphon effect through the closed system. Gravity drainage should occur fairly rapidly, and steady streams of fluid should be observed entering the drainage container. The drainage is usually straw-colored.
	12. Check outflow for cloudy appearance, blood, and/or fibrin.	12. May be an early sign of peritonitis.
	13. If the fluid is not draining properly, move the patient from side to side to facilitate the removal of peritoneal drainage. The head of the bed may also be elevated.	13. If the drainage stops, or starts to drip before the dialyzing fluid has run out, the catheter tip may be buried in the omentum. Rotating the patient may be helpful (or it may be necessary for the physician to reposition the catheter).
	14. Ascertain if the catheter is patent. Check for closed clamp, kinked tubing, or air lock. *Never push the catheter in.*	14. Pushing in the catheter introduces bacteria into the peritoneal cavity.
	15. When the outflow drainage ceases to run, clamp off the drainage tube and infuse the next exchange, using strict aseptic technique.	
	16. Take blood pressure and pulse every 15 minutes during the first exchange and every hour thereafter. Monitor the heart rate for signs of dysrrhythmia.	16. A drop in blood pressure may indicate excessive fluid loss from glucose concentrations of the dialyzing solutions. Changes in the vital signs may indicate impending shock or overhydration.
	17. Take the patient's temperature every 4 hours (especially after catheter removal).	17. An infection is more apt to become evident after dialysis has been discontinued.
	18. The procedure is repeated until the blood chemistry levels improve. The usual duration for short-term dialysis is 36–48 hours. Depending on the patient's condition, he will receive 24–48 exchanges.	18. The duration of dialysis depends on the severity of the condition and on the size and weight of the patient.

	19. Keep an exact record of the patient's fluid balance during the treatment.
	  a. Know the status of the patient's loss or gain of fluid at the end of each exchange. Check dressing for leakage and weigh on gram scale if significant.
	  b. The fluid balance should be about even or should show slight fluid loss or gain, depending on the patient's fluid status.
		19. Complications (circulatory collapse, hypotension, shock, and death) may occur if the patient loses too much fluid through peritoneal drainage. Large fluid losses around the catheter may not be noted unless the dressings are checked carefully.

Procedure *(continued)*	**Nursing Action**	**Rationale/Amplification**

	20. Promote patient comfort during dialysis.
	   a. Provide frequent back care and massage pressure areas.
	   b. Have the patient turn from side to side.
	   c. Elevate head of bed at intervals.
	   d. Allow the patient to sit in chair for brief periods if condition permits (only with surgically implanted catheter; with trocar, patient is usually on bedrest).
		20. The dialysis period is lengthy, and the patient becomes fatigued.

	21. Observe for the following: a. Abdominal pain—note the time of discomfort during exchange cycle and duration of symptoms.	a. Pain may be caused by the dialyzing solution's not being at body temperature, incomplete drainage of the solution, chemical irritation, pressure by the catheter, peritonitis, or air pressing on the diaphragm, causing referred shoulder pain.
	b. Dialysate leakage—change the dressings frequently, being careful not to dislodge the catheter; use sterile plastic drapes to prevent contamination. c. Place the patient in a more upright position and use smaller fluid volumes.	b. Leakage around the catheter predisposes the patient to infection at the exit site and peritonitis.

	22. Keep accurate records.
	   a. Exact time of beginning and end of each exchange: starting and finishing time of drainage
	   b. Amount of solution infused and recovered
	   c. Fluid balance
	   d. Number of exchanges
	   e. Medications added to dialyzing solution
	   f. Pre- and postdialysis weight, plus daily weight
	   g. Level of responsiveness at beginning, throughout, and at end of treatment
	   h. Assessment of vital signs and patient's condition	

	Complications
	1. Peritonitis
	   a. Watch for nausea and vomiting, anorexia, abdominal pain, tenderness, rigidity, and cloudy dialysate drainage.
	   b. Send specimen of dialysate for WBC count and full set of cultures.
		1. Peritonitis is the most common complication. Antibiotics may be added to dialysate and also given systemically.

	2. Bleeding a. A hematocrit of the drainage fluid may be taken to determine the amount of bleeding.	2. A small amount of bleeding around the catheter is not significant if it does not persist. During the first few exchanges, blood-tinged fluid from subcutaneous bleeding is not uncommon. Small amounts of heparin may be added to inflow solution to prevent the catheter from becoming clogged.

Continuous Ambulatory Peritoneal Dialysis (CAPD) (Fig. 27-7)

Continuous ambulatory peritoneal dialysis is a practical self-dialysis method that involves almost constant peritoneal contact with a dialysis solution for patients with end-stage renal disease.

1. A permanent indwelling catheter is implanted into the peritoneum; the internal cuff of the catheter becomes embedded by fibrous ingrowth, which stabilizes it and minimizes leakage.
2. A connecting tube is attached to the external end of the peritoneal catheter, and the distal end of the tube is inserted into a sterile plastic bag of dialysate solution.
3. The dialysate bag is raised to shoulder level and infused by gravity into the peritoneal cavity.
4. Then the plastic bag attached to the connecting tube is folded and placed in a pouch at the waist, under the patient's clothing.
5. At the end of the dwell time (approximately 4 hours) the bag is removed from the pouch, unfolded, and placed near the floor to allow the dialysate to drain by gravity over a 20- to 40-minute period.
6. After the dialysate is drained, a fresh bag of dialysate solution is attached under aseptic conditions, and the procedure is repeated.
7. The patient performs 4–5 exchanges daily, 7 days/week with an overnight dwell time allowing uninterrupted sleep; most patients become unaware of fluid in the peritoneal cavity.
8. Advantages
   a. Physical and psychological freedom and independence
   b. Free dietary intake; improvement of nutritional status
   c. Relatively simple and easy to use
   d. Satisfactory biochemical control of uremia
9. Complications
   a. Peritonitis and damage to peritoneal membrane

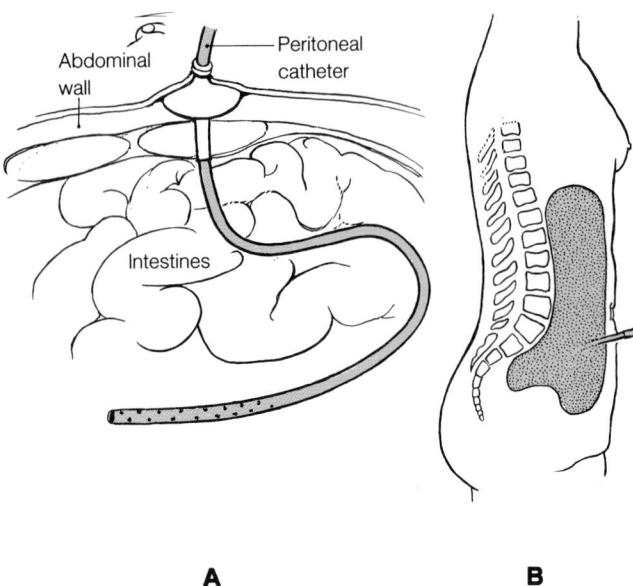

A   **B**

Figure 27-7. *Continuous ambulatory peritoneal dialysis. (A) The peritoneal catheter is implanted through the abdominal wall. (B) Fluid infusing into the peritoneal cavity.*

    b. Catheter-related problems; obstruction, leakage of fluid

Patient Education

1. The use of CAPD as a long-term treatment depends on prevention of recurring peritonitis.
   a. Use strict aseptic technique when performing bag exchanges.
   b. Perform bag exchanges in clean, closed-off area without pets and other activities.
   c. Wash hands before touching bag.
   d. Inspect bag, tubing for defects and leaks.
2. Do not omit bag changes—this will cause inadequate control of renal failure.
3. Some weight gain may accompany CAPD—the dialysate fluid contains a significant amount of dextrose, which adds calories to daily intake.
4. Report signs and symptoms of peritonitis—cloudy peritoneal fluid, abdominal pain or tenderness, malaise, fever.
5. Send sample of peritoneal fluid to laboratory for culture.

Hemodialysis

Hemodialysis is a process of cleansing the blood of accumulated waste products. It is used for patients with end-stage renal failure or for acutely ill patients who require short-term dialysis.

Underlying Principles

1. Heparinized blood passes down a concentration gradient through a semipermeable membrane by dialysis to the dialysate fluid.
2. The dialysate is designed to approximate the normal electrolyte structure of plasma and extracellular water.
3. Through the process of diffusion, the blood components equilibrate with those in the dialysate. By appropriate adjustment of the dialysate bath composition, noxious substances (urea, creatinine, uric acid, phosphate, and other metabolites) are transferred from the blood into the dialysate so that they can be discarded. Small pores of the membrane hold back desirable blood components.
4. Excess water is removed from the blood (ultrafiltration).
5. The body's buffer system is maintained by the addition and diffusion of acetate from the dialysate into the patient; it is metabolized to form bicarbonate.
6. Purified blood is returned to the body through one of the patient's veins.
7. At the end of the treatment, most poisonous wastes have been removed, electrolyte and water balances have been restored, and the buffer system has been replenished.

Requirements for Hemodialysis

1. Access to the patient's circulation
2. Dialyzer with semipermeable membrane
3. Appropriate dialysate bath
4. Time—approximately 4 hours, 3 times weekly, for a total of 12 hours
5. Place—home (if feasible) or at a dialysis center

Methods of Access to the Patient's Circulation

1. Arteriovenous fistula (AVF)—creation of a vascular communication by suturing a vein directly to an artery.
   a. Usually, radial artery and cephalic vein are anastomosed in nondominant arm; vessels in leg may also be used.
   b. Following the procedure, the superficial venous system of the arm dilates.
   c. By means of 2 large-bore needles inserted into the dilated venous system, blood may be obtained and passed through the dialyzer. The arterial end is used for arterial flow and the distal end for reinfusion of dialyzed blood.
   d. Healing of AVF requires several weeks; an external shunt (see below) is used in the interim.

2. Prosthetic arteriovenous fistula—vascular prosthesis (bovine; human umbilical vein; polytetrafluoroethylene [PTFE]).
3. Direct cannulation of veins (subclavian or femoral).
4. External arteriovenous shunt (cannula)
   a. Teflon–Silastic cannula sewn into radial artery and a forearm vein (or placed in leg). The two are connected by a Teflon bridge.
   b. During dialysis, the bridge is removed and the arterial and venous ends are connected to the flow lines of the artificial kidney.
   c. Used for temporary access while AVF is healing.

Complications Related to Vascular Access

1. Partial/complete obstruction (stenosis or thrombosis)
2. Infection
3. Bleeding
4. Aneurysm

Monitoring During Dialysis

The management of the patient on a dialyzer is a complex subject beyond the scope of this discussion. The reader is referred to the written protocol for the machine being used.

NURSING ALERT: Nurses attending patients undergoing hemodialysis are at risk of acquiring hepatitis B.

Life-Style Management by Patient on Chronic Hemodialysis

1. Dietary management involves restriction or adjustment of protein, sodium, potassium, and/or fluid intake.
2. On-going health care monitoring including careful adjustment of medications and surveillance for complications
   a. Arteriosclerotic cardiovascular disease; congestive heart failure; disturbance of lipid metabolism (hypertriglyceridemia); coronary heart disease; stroke
   b. Intercurrent infection
   c. Anemia and fatigue
   d. Gastric ulcers/gastrointestinal problems
   e. Bone problems (renal osteodystrophy; aseptic necrosis of hip)—from disturbed calcium metabolism
   f. Hypertension
   g. Disequilibrium syndrome
   h. Psychosocial problems: *depression,* suicide, sexual dysfunction
3. Helping agencies:
   American Association of Kidney Patients
   2111 E. 43rd Street, Suite 301
   New York, NY 10017

   National Kidney Foundation
   2 Park Avenue
   New York, NY 10003

Kidney Transplantation

Kidney transplantation is the transplantation of a kidney from a living donor or human cadaver donor to a recipient with end-stage renal failure who requires support from dialysis in order to maintain life.

Kidney transplants from well-matched related living donors are more successful than those from cadaver donors.

Postoperative Nursing Interventions

A. Monitoring for Complications

1. Infection (wound, urinary tract, pulmonary, central nervous system)
2. Renal graft failure and renal graft rejection (see below)
3. Vascular complications—thrombosis; hemorrhage
4. Urologic complications—stricture of grafted ureter; fistula
5. Gastrointestinal complications—GI ulceration, bleeding, perforation, sepsis, fungal colonization of GI tract

B. Maintaining Fluid and Electrolyte Balance

1. Patterns of urine output after kidney transplantation
   a. Oliguria with less than 30 ml./hour
   b. Normal urine output—30–100 ml./hour
   c. Polyuria—100–500 ml./hour
2. Keep accurate records on intake and output.
3. Monitor CVP, ECG, and skin temperature frequently to guard against occult volume depletion and electrolyte imbalance.
4. Monitor output from indwelling catheter, which has been connected to a closed drainage system.
   a. Measure urine every 30 minutes–1 hour.
   b. Irrigate catheter only on direct request.
   c. Palpate bladder to detect presence of distention.
   d. Instruct the patient to void frequently after catheter removal to avoid stressing the bladder closure.
5. Monitor serum and urine electrolytes to determine the patient's chemical balance.
   a. Anticipate adjustment of fluid replacement.
   b. Give IV fluids according to urine volume and serum electrolyte levels; serum and urine chemistries are measured at specified intervals.
   c. Avoid using dialysis access extremity for IV lines, intra-arterial monitoring, or restraints.
   d. Notify physician immediately if dysrhythmias or other cardiac symptoms develop.
6. Prepare for hemodialysis in postoperative period until transplanted kidney is functioning well.

C. Preventing Infection

1. Monitor and protect the patient from infection—kidney recipient is susceptible to faulty healing and infection because of both immunosuppressive therapy, which suppresses the immune response, and complications of renal failure.
2. Watch for fever and increased leukocyte count; search for pulmonary, wound, urinary tract, and vascular access sites for infection.
   a. Infection may be masked or confused with symptoms of rejection since impaired renal function and fever are evidences of both infection and rejection.
   b. Immunosuppressive drugs render the transplant recipient more vulnerable to infection, permitting opportunistic infections to occur (fungal, viral, bacterial infections).
3. Use aseptic precautions and strict handwashing; health care personnel and family may wear masks until immunosuppressive drug dosages are lowered.

4. Give aseptic care to wounds and puncture sites (central venous pressure [CVP] and IV lines, draining sites, etc.).
   a. Wound healing may be delayed because of effects of renal disease and immunosuppressive drugs.
   b. Change dressings promptly if drainage is present—drainage is an excellent culture medium for bacteria.
   c. Carry out bacteriologic testing of urine and all exit wounds. Catheter and drain tips are cultured on removal.
      (1) Before removing catheter, disinfect skin around entry site of catheter (or drain). Remove.
      (2) Using aseptic technique, cut off tip of catheter or drain and place in sterile container for laboratory culture.
5. Monitor vascular access to hemodialysis to ensure patency and watch for evidence of infection.
6. Give oral mycostatin mouthwash—to prevent mucosal candidiasis (fungal colonization occurs secondarily to steroid and antibiotic administration).
7. Give regular skin hygiene.

D. Monitoring for Threatened Rejection

1. Watch for signs of rejection—fever, chills, sweating, lassitude, hypertension, weight gain, peripheral edema, decrease in urine output.
   Graft may be enlarged, tender to palpation, associated with edema of overlying tissues.
   a. Acute rejection is common and usually reversible; often occurs in first weeks or months following transplant.
   b. If rejection is inevitable or when excessive immunosuppression is required, transplanted kidney is removed.
   c. The patient is placed back on maintenance dialysis; will require understanding and supportive emotional care.
2. Assist with various tests (biochemistry, hematology, bacteriology) to monitor recipient's immune status—tissue injury monitoring may be predictive of a rejection episode.
3. Give prescribed combinations of immunosuppressive agents to modify or suppress immune responses.
4. Be aware of complications of immunosuppressive protocols—infection or incomplete control of rejection.

E. Psychosocial Support

1. Be aware of the stresses associated with renal transplantation—difficulty in planning for uncertain future, fear of organ rejection, problems associated with immunosuppressants and steroids.
2. Keep the patient informed of his progress, proposed treatment plans, and short- and long-term goals.
3. Observe for changes in behavior, altered thought and feeling processes.
4. See page 676 for other aspects of psychological support.

Patient Education

1. The hospitalization period for a kidney transplant may be prolonged.
2. The patient receives individualized instruction about the following:
   a. Diet
   b. Medications (immunosuppressive drugs, antacids, vitamins, iron)
      (1) Review medications in detail, including color identification of pills, dose schedules, side effects, and the necessity for taking the medication.
   c. Fluids
   d. Daily weight
   e. Daily measurement of urine
   f. Management of intake and output
   g. Stool test for occult blood
   h. Prevention of infection
   i. Resumption of activity; exercise
3. Instruct the patient to report to the physician immediately if any of the following occur:
   a. Decrease in urinary output
   b. Weight gain (detectable edema means excess fluid)
   c. Malaise
   d. Fever
   e. Graft swelling and tenderness
   f. Changes in blood pressure readings
   g. Respiratory distress
   h. Anxiety, depression, changes in eating, drinking, or other habit patterns
4. Advise the patient to avoid strenuous contact sports after surgery.
5. The patient should know that follow-up care after transplantation is a lifelong necessity.
6. Encourage the patient to become active in renal self-help group:
   American Association of Kidney Patients
   2111 E. 43rd Street, Suite 301
   New York, NY 10017

Nursing Management of the Patient Undergoing Renal/Urologic Surgery

Diagnostic Evaluation

1. See page 52 for general preoperative evaluation.
2. Intravenous urogram to evaluate status of kidneys
3. Studies of renal function
4. Coagulation studies
5. ECG—serves as a baseline reference in event of postoperative cardiopulmonary complications
6. Pulmonary function studies/blood gas analysis—in patients with impaired respiratory function

Nursing Assessment

Note: Surgical approaches to the kidney predispose the patient to respiratory complications and paralytic ileus.

1. Review past and present health status and results of diagnostic tests.
2. Observe the functional status of the patient.
   a. Determine his ability to engage in physical activity without distress.
   b. Assess for alertness, appetite, and general well-being.
   c. Monitor for dyspnea, productive cough, other cardiac symptoms.
3. Assess status of vascular system of lower extremities, especially varicosities.
4. Inquire if there are any bleeding tendencies.
5. Assess fluid and electrolyte status.
   a. Weigh the patient daily to determine status of fluid balance.

b. Assess status of mucous membranes and skin turgor; maintain the hematocrit at optimal level.
c. Measure and record intake and output as an index of hydration.

Preoperative Nursing Interventions

1. Encourage liberal intake of fluids to promote excretion of waste products before surgery and to ensure that the patient is well-hydrated.
2. Give antimicrobial therapy as directed; kidney infection may be present preoperatively.
3. Teach the patient deep-breathing exercises and an effective cough routine.
4. Elevate patient's legs and apply elastic stockings to minimize stasis in superficial veins; encourage patient to perform leg exercises.
5. Encourage the patient to express feelings and concerns about impending surgery.
   a. Keep in mind that most patients entering the hospital with urologic conditions have pain, fever, hematuria, difficulty in voiding, etc.
   b. Obtain the patient's confidence by establishing a relationship of trust and by giving gentle and considerate care.
   c. Increase the patient's understanding of what to expect during the pre- and postoperative periods.
6. See page 52 for general preoperative nursing interventions

Nursing Diagnoses

1. Pain and discomfort related to the surgical procedure(s) and presence of drainage tubes and catheters.
2. Altered urinary elimination related to presence of drainage tubes and catheters.
3. Knowledge deficit of surgical procedure, postoperative management, and self-care.

Nursing Interventions

A. Preventing and Treating Complications

1. *Bleeding*
   Employ frequent and close observation of blood pressure, pulse, and respiration in order to recognize hemorrhage (and shock)—chief danger after renal surgery.
   a. Watch for pain, sanguineous drainage from drain site(s), mass over flank, shock.
   b. Prepare for rapid blood and fluid replacement and reoperation.
2. *Pulmonary complications*
   a. Assess for pulmonary complications: postoperative atelectasis, page 63, pneumothorax, page 194, and pneumonia, page 64.
   b. Use incentive spirometer to help maximize lung inflation; encourage coughing after each deep breath to loosen secretions.
3. *Postoperative ileus*
   a. Assess for abdominal distention, pain, and lack of intestinal peristalsis (determined by stethoscope auscultation).
   b. Resume oral feedings when active bowel sounds are heard.
   c. Give adequate and appropriate fluid and electrolyte replacement intravenously, as prescribed.
   d. Assist with decompression via nasogastric tube for relief of abdominal distention (p. 464). See page 65 for treatment of paralytic ileus.
   e. Keep record of fluid status.

4. *Thromboembolic episodes*
   a. Monitor for thrombophlebitis (p. 63) and pulmonary embolism (p. 64).
   b. Employ early ambulation as an aid in preventing thromboembolic episodes and improving patient endurance.

Note: Ambulation is contraindicated in prostatic patients with bleeding and with some types of reconstructive surgery.

   c. Encourage the patient to do leg exercises in bed.
5. Infection
Watch for elevation of temperature and monitor the drainage tube sites and urine output for evidences of infection.

B. Relieving Pain and Discomfort

1. Assess for pain similar to renal colic—caused by passage of clotted blood down the ureter; requires adequate doses of narcotics as prescribed for relief; *a flank incision is painful.*
2. Give postoperative sedation and pain control on an individual basis to reduce splinting of respiratory movements and to permit coughing, since incision is close to diaphragm; the patient will voluntarily tend to splint chest while breathing.
3. Use hands or pillow to splint incision during movement or during deep breathing and coughing exercises.
4. Use moist heat, massage, and analgesics as prescribed for muscular aches and pain resulting from position on operating table.
5. Assist with ambulation, while assuring placement of urinary drainage system, as soon as tolerated/prescribed.

C. Managing Patient With Drainage Tubes and Catheters

1. Assess adequacy of urinary output.
2. Use handwashing and asepsis when providing care and handling urinary drainage system.
3. Make certain that drainage tubes are functioning, since almost all urologic patients have drains, tubes, or catheters.
4. Make sure indwelling catheter is dependent and draining.
   a. Tape tubing to thigh to relieve traction on bladder. In supine male patient, tape catheter to lower abdomen. In women, anchor catheter to thigh, allowing enough slack for movement.
   b. Give meticulous catheter care.
5. Change dressings as indicated when the patient has profuse drainage.
6. Employ care with the patient with nephrostomy tube drainage (insertion of tube directly into kidney for temporary or permanent urinary diversion). It is attached to closed gravity drainage or to a urostomy appliance. A self-retaining U-tube or circular nephrostomy tube may be used.
   a. Purpose of nephrostomy drainage:
      (1) To provide drainage from kidney after surgery.
      (2) To conserve and permit physiologic restoration of renal tissue that has been traumatized by obstruction.
      (3) To provide drainage when ureter is no longer functioning.
   b. Evaluate for bleeding from nephrostomy site (main complication of nephrostomy); expect some bloody drainage for about 24 hours.
   c. Ensure that the nephrostomy tube is draining

freely—blocking of the tube by blood clot or debris causes pain in the flank, bursting of the suture line, and infection.
  (1) Call surgeon *immediately* if tube is inadvertently dislodged.
  (2) Do not clamp the nephrostomy tube.
  (3) Irrigate nephrostomy tube only by direct physician request. Use 10 ml. warm sterile saline solution—to avoid mechanical damage to kidney or infection from pyelorenal backflow.
  (4) Encourage adequate fluid intake—to produce effective mechanical flushing and to dilute urinary elements that cause calculous formation.
  (5) If there is a nephrostomy tube in each kidney, keep separate output records for each nephrostomy tube.
7. Assess the patient with indwelling ureteral catheter or stent (utilized to permit drainage from affected kidney or ureter).
  a. Ureteral catheters are inserted through a cystoscope and left in place for a period of time.
  b. Make notation on nursing care plan that catheter is an *ureteral* catheter.
  c. Do not irrigate a ureteral catheter; this is done by the urologist.
8. Watch for complications from ureteral stent; infection (from foreign body in genitourinary tract), bleeding or clot obstruction within the stent, dislodgement of the stent.

D. Other Nursing Interventions
1. See page 202 for management of chest tube drainage; thoracotomy tube drainage often seen with thoracoabdominal or high-flank incision.
2. Monitor vital signs for evidence of infection.

Patient Education
1. Teach the patient/family about care of catheters/tubes and management of dressings if the patient is to return home with indwelling tubes.
2. Continue a liberal intake of fluids.
3. Expect some muscle weakness in area of flank incision as a result of damage to its nerve supply.
4. Take frequent short rest periods and increase activities gradually.
5. Avoid straining or lifting heavy objects until permitted.

Evaluation
1. Achieves relief of pain and discomfort; moves freely.
2. Managing with drainage tubes and catheter; knows purpose; turning and moving freely.
3. Has a written protocol for home care; verbalizes who to call if assistance is needed.

Infections of the Urinary Tract

A *urinary tract infection* (UTI) is caused by the presence of pathogenic microorganisms in the urinary tract with or without signs and symptoms. Infection may predominate at the bladder (cystitis), urethra (urethritis), prostate (prostatitis), or kidney (pyelonephritis). Unfortunately, noninfectious conditions may generate symptoms that mimic those of urinary tract infection.

Bacteriuria refers to the presence of bacteria in the urine (10^5 bacteria/ml. of urine or greater generally indicates infection).
In *asymptomatic bacteriuria,* organisms are found in urine, but the patient has no symptoms.
Recurrent urinary tract infections may indicate the following:
1. *Relapse*—recurrent infection with an organism that has been isolated during a prior infection.
2. *Reinfection*—recurrent infection with an organism distinct from previous infecting organism.

Pathways of Infection Within Urinary Tract
Bacteria invade and spread within tract by the ascending (most common), bloodstream, and/or lymphatic pathways.
1. Urethra—from ascending bacteria
2. Bladder—from bacteria ascending from urethra (or, less commonly, descending from kidney)
3. Kidney—from ureterovesical reflux (incompetence of ureterovesical valve, which allows urine to regurgitate into ureters, usually at time of voiding); blood-borne
4. Prostate—from ascending urethral flora
5. Epididymis—from infected prostate
6. Testis—from bacteria via the bloodstream

NURSING ALERT: Infections in any part of the urinary tract may persist for months or years without symptoms and eventually cause serious kidney damage.

Predisposing Factors
1. Urinary stasis and obstruction (ureteral stenosis, stone, tumor)—slowing of urinary flow causes kidney to be more susceptible to bacterial infection.
2. Increasing intraluminal pressure or overdistended bladder
3. Reflux
  a. Urethrovesical reflux—flowing back of urine from urethra into bladder
  b. Vesicoureteral reflux (ureterovesical reflux)—flowing back of urine from bladder into one or both ureters
4. Fecal soiling of urethral meatus
5. Instrumentation—catheter, cystoscope
6. Pregnancy; old age.
7. Metabolic disorders (diabetes mellitus) and diseases of blood vessels (arteriosclerosis) may diminish blood supply to organs of urinary tract.
8. Neurologic abnormalities (neurogenic bladder dysfunction).

Lower Urinary Tract Infection(Cystitis, Acute Urethral Syndrome)

Cystitis is an inflammation of the urinary bladder.
Acute urethral syndrome is symptomatic urinary tract infection in women whose urine is either sterile or contains less than 10^5 bacteria/ml.

Etiology
1. Ascending infection after entry via the urinary meatus.
  a. Women seem to be more apt to develop acute cystitis because of shorter length of urethra, anatomic proximity to vagina, periurethral glands, and

rectum (fecal contamination), and the mechanical effect of coitus.
   b. Women with recurrent urinary tract infections often have gram-negative organisms at the vaginal introitus; there may be some defect of the mucosa of the urethra, vagina, or external genitalia of these patients that allows enteric organisms to invade the bladder.
   c. Poor voiding patterns cause increase in intravesical pressure, which tends to decrease blood flow to bladder mucosa.
   d. Acute infection in women most often from organisms of the patient's own intestinal flora (*Escherichia coli*).
2. In males, obstructive abnormalities (strictures, prostatism)—most frequent cause.
3. Upper urinary tract disease may occasionally cause recurrent bladder infection.

Clinical Manifestations

1. Dysuria, frequency, urgency, nocturia
2. Bearing-down sensation in region of bladder; suprapubic pain

Diagnostic Evaluation

Urine culture to detect presence of bacteria and for antimicrobial sensitivity testing

Management

Antimicrobial agent given according to sensitivity test.
1. A wide variety of antimicrobial drugs are available; urinary infections usually respond to drugs that are excreted in urine in high concentrations; a potentially effective drug should rapidly sterilize the urine and thus relieve the patient's symptoms.
2. For uncomplicated infection
   a. Single-dose antimicrobial therapy (trimethoprim-sulfamethoxazole or amoxicillin; however, a 3–4-day course may be necessary in some patients).
   b. Follow-up culture to prove treatment effectiveness.
   c. Side effects are nausea, diarrhea, drug-related rash, and vaginal candidiasis.
3. For acute urethral syndrome:
   a. Antimicrobial therapy for 10 days.
   b. Repeat urine culture in 7–10 days to ensure elimination of infection.
4. For recurrent infections with closely spaced episodes:
   a. The patient may require treatment for 6 months or more.
   b. Patients with recurring infections should have periodic urine cultures, since most recurrences are new infections with different organisms; relapses may occur with same organism.

Nursing Assessment

1. Determine if patient had a history of urinary tract infections in childhood, during pregnancy, or has had recurring infections; question about methods of contraception.
2. Ask if there are any associated symptoms of vaginal discharge, itching, or irritation—dysuria may be prominent symptom of vaginitis or infection from sexually transmitted pathogens.
3. Study results of urinalysis and urine culture.
4. Examine for suprapubic tenderness, abdominal tenderness, guarding, rebound, masses.

Nursing Diagnoses

1. Pain related to inflammation of the bladder.
2. Knowledge deficit of prevention of recurrence of urinary tract infection.

Nursing Interventions

A. Relieving Pain and Discomfort

1. Encourage the patient to take prescribed antimicrobial—eradication of infection is usually accompanied by rapid resolution of symptoms.
2. Encourage patient to take prescribed analgesics and antispasmodics; heat to the abdomen (if prescribed) relieves bladder spasms.
3. Encourage rest during the acute phase.
4. Encourage the patient to drink fluids sufficient to promote renal blood flow and to flush out bacteria in urinary tract.
5. Encourage the patient to void frequently (every 2–3 hours) and to empty bladder completely, since this enhances bacterial clearance, reduces urine stasis, and prevents reinfection. Infrequent voiding over-stretches the bladder wall, leading to hypoxia of bladder mucosa, which is then susceptible to bacterial invasion.

Patient Education

1. Encourage the patient to have follow-up urine studies to determine if there is resolution of infection or if asymptomatic infection is present; there is a marked tendency for infection to recur.
2. For women with repeated urinary tract infections, give the following instructions:
   a. Reduce vaginal introital concentration of pathogens by hygienic measures.
      (1) Wash in shower or while standing in bathtub—bacteria in bath water may gain entrance into urethra.
      (2) Cleanse around the perineum and urethral meatus after each bowel movement, with front to back cleansing to minimize fecal contamination of periurethral area.
   b. Drink liberal amounts of water to lower bacterial concentrations in the urine.
   c. Avoid irritants—coffee, tea, alcohol, cola drinks.
   d. Void every 2–3 hours during day and completely empty bladder.
   e. In certain women, sexual intercourse is the initiating event for the development of bacteriuria—urethral massage associated with intercourse facilitates entry of microorganisms into the bladder.
      (1) Void immediately after sexual intercourse.
      (2) A single dose of an oral antimicrobial agent may be prescribed following sexual intercourse.
   f. Avoid external irritants such as bubble baths and perfumed vaginal cleansers or deodorants.
   g. Patients with persistent bacteria may require long-term antimicrobial therapy to prevent colonization of periurethral area and recurrence of urinary tract infection.
      (1) Take drug the last thing at night after emptying bladder to ensure adequate concentration of drug during overnight period, since low rates of urine flow and infrequent bladder emptying predispose to multiplication of bacteria.

(2) Use self-monitoring tests (dip slides) at home to monitor for urinary tract infection.
3. Instruct patients who have had urinary tract infections during pregnancy to have follow-up studies.
4. Teach the patient that bacteriuria in young girls (under 5 years) increases the risk of developing a urinary tract infection as an adult.

Evaluation

1. Is free of urinary frequency, dysuria, and bacteriuria
2. Demonstrates no evidence of recurrence

Bacterial Pyelonephritis

Bacterial pyelonephritis is an acute inflammatory renal disease caused by bacteria.

Causes

1. Enteric bacteria (*E. coli*)
2. Secondary to vesicoureteral reflux (incompetence of ureterovesical valve, which allows urine to regurgitate into ureters, usually at time of voiding)
3. Urinary obstruction/infection
4. Trauma
5. Blood-borne infection
6. Renal disease
7. Pregnancy
8. Metabolic disorders

Clinical Manifestations

1. Fever, chills, costovertebral angle tenderness, flank pain (with or without radiation to groin)
2. Nausea, vomiting

NURSING ALERT: Elderly patients may exhibit gastrointestinal or pulmonary symptoms and not show the usual febrile response.

Diagnostic Evaluation

1. Identification of leukocytes, bacteria or pus in urine; gross or microscopic hematuria.
2. Identification of antibody-coated bacteria (ACB) in urine; bacteria invading kidney induce an antibody response that coats the bacteria—differentiates renal infection from bladder infection.
3. Other radiologic/urinary tests as necessary.

Management

1. Patient is monitored for complications: bacteremia and gram-negative sepsis (see p. 908); papillary necrosis, leading to renal failure; renal abscess/perinephric abscess.
2. Urine specimen collected for culture and sensitivity studies.
3. Organism-specific antimicrobial therapy is prescribed.
   a. Usually immediate treatment is started to cover the prevalent gram-negative pathogens; subsequently adjusted according to culture results.
   b. Acute pyelonephritis usually caused by *E. coli,* which is sensitive to many antimicrobial drugs.
   c. A 2-week or more treatment regimen is needed for bacteriuria of renal origin.
4. Parenteral antimicrobial therapy may be necessary if patient cannot tolerate oral intake and is dehydrated; usually admitted to hospital if patient is acutely ill.
5. Intravenous urogram and other diagnostic tests conducted—relief of obstructions is essential to save kidney from rapid destruction.
6. Urine cultured frequently to determine the patient's response to treatment, to search for secondary organisms, and to determine clinical and microbiologic resolution of infection.

A. For the Patient With Chronic or Recurring Infections—Preservation of Renal Function

1. Continuous treatment with urine-sterilizing agents after initial antibiotic treatment has been employed.
2. Patient to continue this regimen for months to years until there is no evidence of inflammation, causative factors have been treated or controlled, and there is evidence of stability of renal function.
3. Serial urine cultures and evaluation studies must be done for an indefinite period of time.
4. Blood counts and serum creatinine determinations are required during long-term therapy.

Acute Glomerulonephritis

Acute glomerulonephritis refers to a group of kidney diseases in which there is an inflammatory reaction in the glomeruli. It is not an infection of the kidney, per se, but rather the result of the immune mechanisms of the body. It is thought to involve an antigen–antibody reaction, which produces damage to the glomeruli, the filtering bed of the kidney.

Altered Physiology

Cellular proliferation, infiltration of glomerulus by leukocytes → glomerular trapping of circulating immune complexes → thickening of glomerular filtration membrane → scarring and loss of filtering surface → renal failure.

Clinical Manifestations

1. Mild disease is frequently discovered accidentally through a routine urinalysis.
2. History of infection: pharyngitis from group A streptococcus; hepatitis B virus; endocarditis
3. Proteinuria; oliguria
4. Puffiness of face; edema of extremities
5. Fatigue and anorexia
6. Hypertension (mild, moderate, or severe); headache
7. Anemia from loss of red blood cells into the urine

Diagnostic Evaluation

1. *Urinalysis*—hematuria (microscopic or gross), proteinuria, red cell casts, white cells, renal epithelial cells, and various casts in the sediment.
2. *Blood*—elevated blood urea nitrogen (BUN) and serum creatinine levels, low total serum protein level, increased antistreptolysin titre (from reaction to streptococcal organism).
3. *Needle biopsy* of the kidney reveals obstruction of glomerular capillaries from proliferation of endothelial cells.

Clinical Course

1. Diuresis usually starts 1–2 weeks after onset of symptoms.

2. Renal clearances and blood urea concentration return to normal.
3. Edema decreases and hypertension lessens.
4. Microscopic proteinuria or hematuria may persist many months.

Management

1. Management is symptomatic; in most patients spontaneous recovery is anticipated.
2. Antibiotic therapy is initiated to eliminate infection (endocarditis-associated glomerulonephritis).
3. Any concurrent infections are treated promptly.
4. Dietary protein is restricted moderately if there is oliguria and the BUN is elevated.
   a. Carbohydrates are increased liberally to provide energy and reduce catabolism of protein.
   b. Protein is restricted more drastically if acute renal failure develops (see p. 672).
   c. Sodium intake is restricted in presence of edema or signs of congestive heart failure.
5. Therapy for rapidly progressive glomerulonephritis may include:
   a. Plasma exchange
   b. Immunosuppressive therapy (corticosteroids; cyclophosphamide)
   c. Dialysis—may be considered if fluid retention and uremia cannot be controlled

Nursing Interventions

A. Prevention of Complications

1. Monitor for signs and symptoms of congestive heart failure: distended neck veins, tachycardia, gallop rhythm, enlarged and tender liver, crackles at bases of lungs.
2. Watch for symptoms of renal failure—nausea, fatigue, vomiting, diminished urinary output (see p. 672).
3. Observe for hypertensive encephalopathy.

B. Promotion of Kidney Function

1. Encourage bedrest during the acute phase until the urine clears and BUN, creatinine, and blood pressure normalize. (Rest also facilitates diuresis.)
2. Institute dietary restrictions as prescribed.
3. Measure and record intake and output.
4. Give fluids according to the patient's fluid losses (urine, respiration, feces) and daily body weight as prescribed.

Patient Education

Instruct the patient as follows:
1. Explain that the patient must have follow-up evaluations of blood pressure, urinary protein, and BUN concentrations to determine if there is exacerbation of disease activity.
2. Treat any infection promptly.
3. Call physician/clinic if symptoms of renal failure occur.

Nephrotic Syndrome

Nephrotic syndrome is a clinical disorder characterized by marked increase of protein in the urine (proteinuria), decrease in albumin in the blood (hypoalbuminemia), edema, and excess cholesterol in the blood (hypercholesterolemia). These occur as a consequence of excessive leakage of plasma proteins into the urine because of increased permeability of the glomerular capillary membrane.

Etiology

(Seen in any condition that seriously damages the glomerular capillary membrane)
1. Chronic glomerulonephritis
2. Diabetes mellitus with intercapillary glomerulosclerosis
3. Amyloidosis of kidney
4. Systemic lupus erythematosus
5. Renal vein thrombosis
6. Secondary to malignancy (older adults)

Clinical Manifestations

1. Insidious onset of edema; easily pitting edema
2. Marked proteinuria—leading to depletion of body proteins
3. Hypercholesterolemia—may lead to accelerated atherosclerosis

Diagnostic Evaluation

1. Renal function tests
2. Needle biopsy of kidney—for histologic examination of renal tissue to confirm diagnosis
3. Serum electrolyte evaluations (protein, albumin, etc.)
4. Triglyceride profile—to evaluate degree of hyperlipidemia
5. Urinary tests may show microscopic hematuria, urinary casts, other abnormalities

Management

1. Treatment of causative glomerular disease
2. General management of edema
   a. Sodium and fluid restriction
   b. Diuretics if renal insufficiency is not severe
   c. Steroids (prednisone) to reduce edema and proteinuria

Nursing Interventions

1. Monitor for complications—thromboembolic complications: renal vein thrombosis, extra renal thrombosis (venous and arterial thrombosis in extremities), pulmonary embolism, coronary artery thrombosis, cerebral artery thrombosis.
2. Encourage bedrest for a few days to help mobilize edema; however, some ambulation is necessary to reduce risk of thromboembolic complications.
3. Encourage patient to follow proposed dietary regimen to counteract hypoproteinemia.
   a. High protein diet to replenish wasted tissues and restore body proteins.
   b. Mild to moderate sodium restriction to control severe edema.
   c. Control of fluid intake as prescribed.
4. Monitor weight and blood pressure—to follow rate of diuresis and to determine that hypotension is not developing.
5. Protect patient from infection—thought to be due to loss of serum immune globulins into the urine.
6. See opposite column for nursing the patient with acute glomerulonephritis and page 675 for care of the patient with chronic renal failure.

Nephrolithiasis/Urolithiasis

Nephrolithiasis refers to renal stone disease, while *urolithiasis* refers to the presence of stones in the urinary system.

Stones are formed in the kidney by the deposit of crystalline substances. The majority of stones (70% to 80%), are composed mainly of calcium oxalate crystals; the rest are composed of calcium phosphate salts, uric acid, struvite (magnesium, ammonium, and phosphate), or the amino acid cystine.

Clinical Features

1. Stones may be found anywhere in the urinary system and vary in size from mere granular deposits (called sand or gravel) to bladder stones the size of an orange.
2. Four out of five patients with stones are men; in both sexes the peak age of onset is between 20 and 30 years.
3. Most stones migrate downward (causing severe colicky pain) and are discovered in the lower ureter. Spontaneous stone passage can be anticipated in 80% of patients with urolithiasis.
4. People who have had two stones tend to have recurrences.

Factors Favoring Stone Formation

1. Obstruction and urinary stasis facilitating precipitation of salts from the urine
2. Infection—particularly of urea-splitting organisms (*Proteus vulgaris*)
3. Dehydration and urine concentration—encourages precipitation of solids
4. Immobilization—produces slowing of renal drainage and altered calcium metabolism
5. Metabolic disorders
   a. Hypercalcemia (abnormally high concentration of blood calcium compounds) and hypercalciuria (abnormally large amounts of calcium in urine)

from dissolution of bone, excessive ingestion or excessive absorption of calcium from GI tract, or faulty renal reabsorption of calcium
   b. Hyperparathyroidism
   c. Excessive intake of vitamin D
   d. Excessive intake of milk and alkali
   e. Myeloproliferative disorders (leukemia, polycythemia vera) and chemotherapy for cancer—patients excrete increased amounts of uric acid
6. Excessive excretion of uric acid
7. Vitamin deficiency (especially vitamin A)
8. Foreign bodies in urinary tract
9. High intake of protein, calcium, excessive consumption of tea and fruit juices
10. Small bowel disease or small bowel surgery
11. Hereditary disease (cystinuria)
12. Idiopathic—no cause can be found

Clinical Manifestations

A. Pain—pattern depends on site of obstruction (Fig. 27-8)

1. Renal stones—produce an increase in hydrostatic pressure and distention of the renal pelvis and proximal ureter causing:
   Renal colic—pain of stone passage with sudden onset of extreme pain in flank with radiation down the abdomen toward the groin, associated with hematuria, dysuria, frequency, and urgency. Pain relief is immediate following stone passage.
2. Ureteral stones
   a. Acute colicky pain radiating down the thigh and to the genitalia (ureteral colic).
   b. Frequent desire to void but little urine is passed.

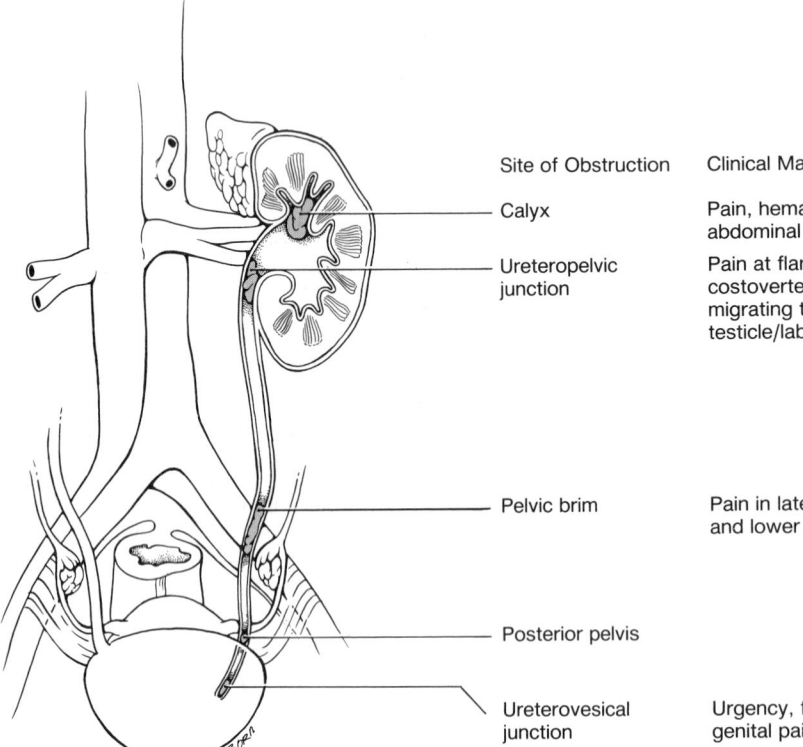

Site of Obstruction	Clinical Manifestations
Calyx	Pain, hematuria, abdominal distention
Ureteropelvic junction	Pain at flank or costovertebral angle, migrating to groin and testicle/labia minora
Pelvic brim	Pain in lateral flank and lower abdomen
Posterior pelvis	
Ureterovesical junction	Urgency, frequency, genital pain

Figure 27-8. *Areas where calculi may obstruct the urinary system. The ensuing clinical manifestations depend on the site of obstruction. Stones that have broken loose may obstruct the flow of urine, cause severe pain, and injure the kidney.*

3. Stones blocking flow of urine produce symptoms of urinary tract infection: chills, fever, dysuria.

B. Gastrointestinal Symptoms—include nausea, vomiting, diarrhea, abdominal discomfort—due to renointestinal reflexes and anatomic proximity of kidneys to stomach, pancreas, and large intestine; celiac ganglion serves both the kidneys and stomach.

Ileus is associated with retroperitoneal irritation and occurs frequently.

Diagnostic Evaluation

1. Intravenous urography—to determine site and evaluate degree of obstruction.
2. Analysis of available stone material—crystals can be identified by polarization microscopy, x-ray diffraction, and infrared spectroscopy.
3. Urine culture and drug sensitivity studies.

Management

A. Extracorporeal Shock Wave Lithotripsy (ESWL)—a noninvasive technique; treatment of choice for stones less than 2 cm. (¾ inch) in diameter (80% of stones fall into this category).

1. High-energy shock waves are directed at the kidney stone, disintegrating it into minute particles that pass in the urine. (A *shock wave* is a large condensed wave of energy produced by high-speed motion.)
2. Patient is placed on specially designed table and immersed in a water bath or placed on an adjustable stretcher positioned over a cushion of water.
   a. In water bath model, waves travel through water surrounding the patient.
   b. In cushion model, a layer of gel lies between the stretcher and water; shock waves move through the cushion and gel.
3. Position of the kidney stone is located by x-rays and the shock waves are targeted directly at the stone. The shock waves do not affect soft tissue.
4. Eliminates need for surgery in majority of patients in US and can be repeated for recurrent stones with no apparent risk to kidney structure.
5. *Complications* include pain, urinary infection, and temporary bleeding around kidney.
6. *Postprocedure patient teaching*
   a. Drink a large quantity of fluid to accelerate passing of stone particles.

b. Take prescribed analgesic; colicky pain sometimes accompanies passage of stone debris.
c. Expect some blood to appear in urine.

B. Percutaneous Nephrolithotomy (Fig. 27-9) for stones larger than 2 cm. in diameter.

1. Under fluoroscopic/ultrasound guidance, a needle is advanced into collecting system; guidewire is advanced into kidney, pelvis, or ureter.
2. Tract is dilated with dilators or high-pressure balloon dilator until nephroscope can be inserted up against stone.
3. Stones can be broken apart with hydraulic shock waves or a laser beam and can be removed using forceps, graspers, or basket.
4. May be combined with ESWL

C. Percutaneous Stone Dissolution (chemolysis, dissolution by chemical agents)

A multiholed nephrostomy tube (catheter) is placed in kidney; offers a pathway for introduction of solvent (depending on chemical composition of stone) to be infused into stone. A second catheter may be used for drainage.

1. Used for struvite, uric acid, and cystine stones.
2. May be used to shrink large stones before other retrieval methods or to irrigate debris after lithotripsy procedures.
3. Irrigating solution introduced at a continuous rate that patient can tolerate without flank pain or elevation of intrarenal pressure above 25 cm. H_2O.
4. The patient receives antimicrobial agents before, during, and after procedure to maintain sterile urine.
5. Complications include infection (renal and perirenal abscesses, pyelonephritis, septic shock) and thrombophlebitis and pulmonary embolism (associated with immobilization).

D. Surgical Procedures

1. *Pyelolithotomy*—removal of stones from kidney pelvis. *Coagulum pyelolithotomy*—intraoperative injection of certain coagulation factors into the renal pelvis, producing a coagulum that entraps the stones and expedites their removal.
2. *Nephrolithotomy*—incision into kidney for removal of stone.
3. *Nephrectomy*—removal of kidney; indicated when kidney is extensively and irreparably damaged and is no longer a functioning organ; partial nephrectomy sometimes done.

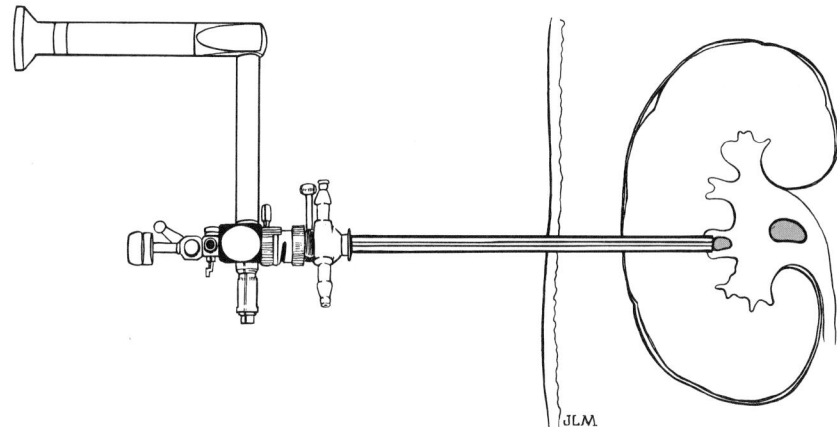

Figure 27-9. *A percutaneous nephrostomy tract permits access to the collecting system of the kidney for removal of kidney stones under direct vision via a nephroscope.*

4. *Ureterolithotomy*—removal of stone in ureter.
5. *Cystolithotomy*—removal of stone from bladder.

Preventive Management

1. Increased fluid intake (24-hour urinary output greater than 2 liters)—increases urinary output, thereby lowering the concentration of substances involved in stone formation.
2. For calcium oxalate stones
   a. Dietary excesses of calcium and phosphorus are to be avoided; low-sodium diet instituted—sodium restriction decreases amount of calcium absorbed in intestine.
   b. Drug therapy includes thiazide diuretics to reduce urine calcium excretion; allopurinol therapy to reduce uric acid excretion, as increased uric acid excretion is associated with calcium oxalate stones.
3. For uric acid stones
   a. Alkalinization of urine to enhance urate solubility.
   b. Allopurinol—to lower uric acid excretion.
   c. Reduction of dietary purine intake (low protein—red meat, fish, fowl).
4. Infection (struvite) stones—formed in the presence of infection by urea-splitting organisms. These may occur as large staghorn calculi and cause significant renal damage from infection and obstruction.
   a. Removal of stones (ESWL/percutaneous nephrolithotomy)
   b. Appropriate antibacterial therapy
5. For cystine stones—occur in *cystinuria,* a hereditary disorder of amino acid transport.
   a. Alkalinization to increase cystine solubility
   b. Drug therapy—*d*-penicillamine—to lower cystine concentration or dissolution by direct irrigation with thiol derivatives

Nursing Assessment

1. Take nursing history focusing on family history of stones, episodes of dehydration, prolonged immobility, urinary tract infection, dietary and medication history.
2. Assess pain location, area of radiation, and severity. Observe for presence of associated symptoms: nausea, vomiting, diarrhea, abdominal distention.
3. Monitor for signs and symptoms of urinary tract infection: chills, fever, dysuria, frequency.
4. Observe for signs and symptoms of obstruction: frequent urination of small amounts, oliguria, anuria.
5. Ascertain patient's knowledge about renal stones and the measures to take to prevent recurrence.

Nursing Diagnoses

1. Pain related to inflammation, obstruction, and abrasion of urinary tract by migration of stones
2. Altered urinary elimination related to blockage of urine flow by stones
3. Potential for infection related to obstruction of urine flow
4. Knowledge deficit regarding prevention of stone recurrence

Complications

1. Obstruction
2. Infection

Nursing Interventions

A. Relieving Pain

1. Give prescribed narcotic analgesic (IV or IM) until cause of pain can be removed. Monitor patient closely for *increasing* pain. Report this promptly.
2. Encourage patient to assume the position that brings relief.
3. Prepare for other treatment (lithotripsy, etc.) if severe pain is unresolved and stone is not passed spontaneously.

B. Maintaining Urine Flow

1. Encourage patient to maintain a high round-the-clock fluid intake (hourly when awake) to reduce concentration of urinary crystalloids and ensure a high urine output.
2. Monitor total output and patterns of voiding.
3. Strain all urine through gauze to harvest the stone; uric acid stones may crumble. Crush clots and inspect sides of urinal/bedpan for clinging stones.
4. Instruct patient to report decreased urine volume and bloody or cloudy urine.
5. Assist patient while walking, if necessary, as ambulation may help move the stone through the urinary tract.

Patient Education

1. Follow prescribed regimen to prevent stone formation.
2. Maintain a high fluid intake over a 24-hour period since stones form more readily in a concentrated urine.
   a. Drink enough fluids to achieve a urinary volume of 2000–3000 ml. or more/24 hours.
   b. Drink larger amounts during periods of strenuous exercise, if you perspire freely.
   c. Take fluids in evening to guarantee a high urine flow during the night.
   d. Set the alarm clock in order to drink water in middle of night.
   e. Avoid sudden increases in environmental temperatures that may cause a drop in urinary volume.
   f. Increase fluid intake when engaging in activities that produce excessive perspiration.
3. Report urinary infection immediately; must be treated vigorously.
4. Avoid prolonged periods of recumbency—slows renal drainage and alters calcium metabolism.
5. Avoid excessive ingestion of vitamins and minerals, especially vitamin D.
6. Test urine *p*H with a *p*H indicator if urine *p*H is a factor in causing a particular type of stone.
7. Follow a healthy eating pattern.
   a. Avoid excessive sugar and animal proteins—refined carbohydrates appear to lead to hypercalciuria and urolithiasis; animal proteins increase urine excretion of calcium, uric acid, and oxalate.
   b. Increase consumption of fiber—inhibits calcium and oxalate absorption.
8. Save any stone passed for analysis.

Evaluation

1. Achieves relief of pain; passes stone
2. Excretes clear urine without burning or discomfort
3. Is free of infection
4. Participating in educational program to avoid stone recurrence

Renal Tumors

General Considerations

1. Renal cell carcinoma is the most common malignant renal tumor, occurring more frequently in men.
2. There appears to be a link between cigarette smoking as well as a high consumption of fats and the development of renal cell carcinoma.

Clinical Manifestations

1. Many renal tumors produce no symptoms and are discovered on routine physical examination as a palpable abdominal mass.
2. Fatigue, malaise, anorexia, weight loss, fever—from paraneoplastic (remote humoral) effects of renal cancer; does not necessarily indicate presence of metastases.
3. Classic triad (late symptoms)
   a. Hematuria (intermittent, microscopic, or gross)—may be initial, terminal, or total, depending on location of tumor.
   b. Flank pain—from distention of renal capsule, invasion of surrounding structures.
   c. Palpable mass in flank.
4. Wide variety of metastatic sites (Fig. 27-10).

Diagnostic Evaluation

1. Intravenous urography—usually initial screening procedure
2. Ultrasonography—helpful in differentiating renal cyst from renal tumor; used as a complement to urography
3. Computed tomography or magnetic resonance imaging—for patients with urographic findings suggesting tumor; useful for detecting, categorizing, and staging a renal mass

Management

Goal:
To eradicate the tumor and prevent metastasis

A. Radical Nephrectomy (en bloc removal of kidney and associated tumor, adrenal gland, surrounding perirenal fat, Gerota's fascia, and possibly regional lymph nodes)—provides maximum opportunity for disease control.

1. Performed through a vertical midline, subcostal, thoracoabdominal, or flank incision.
2. See page 683 for care of patient following renal surgery.

B. Renal Artery Embolization (preoperative occlusion of renal artery) followed by nephrectomy—for patient with metastatic renal cancer.

1. Catheter is advanced into renal artery.
2. Embolizing material (Gelfoam, steel coils, blood clot) is injected into artery and carried with arterial blood flow to occlude the tumor vessels.
3. Procedure decreases tumor vascularity and minimizes blood loss, relieves pain, and devitalizes the tumor preoperatively, thereby decreasing the chance for tumor cell implantation at time of surgery.
4. Monitor for postinfarction syndrome—severe abdominal pain, nausea, vomiting, diarrhea, fever.
5. Complications—arterial obstruction, bleeding, diminution of renal function.

C. Pharmacotherapy

Renal cell carcinomas are generally refractory (unyielding) to chemotherapeutic agents, radiation, and hormonal manipulation. Interleukin-2 (a lymphokine that stimulates growth of T lymphocytes) may offer some benefit to patients with metastatic renal cancer; toxicity is severe.

D. Symptomatic Management—to promote comfort for patients with metastatic disease

1. Orthopedic prosthetic surgery for patients with painful bone metastases

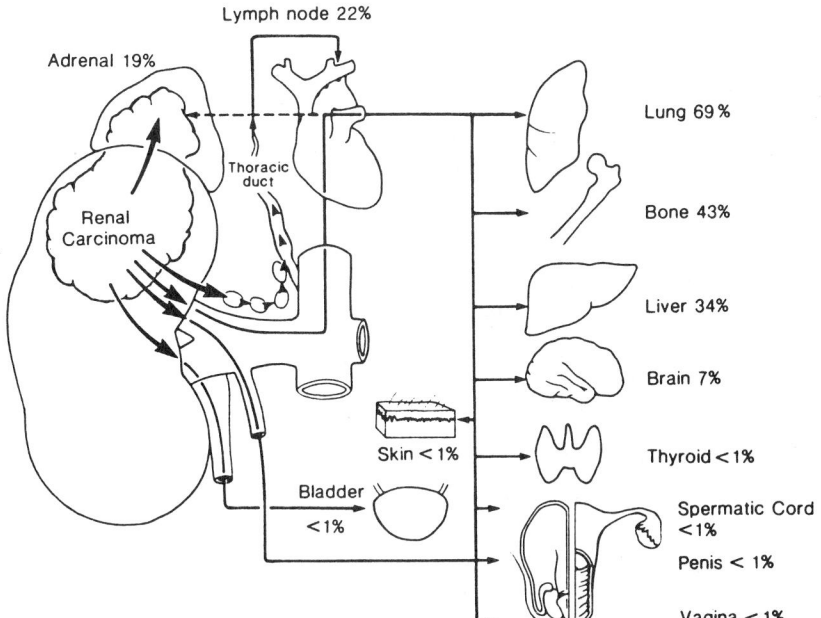

Figure 27-10. *Routes of common metastases from renal carcinoma. (From Semin Roentgenol 1987 Oct; 22[4]. Reproduced with permission.)*

2. Nutritional support
3. Psychological support

Patient Education

Have a yearly physical examination and x-ray examination of chest.

Injuries to the Kidney

Trauma to abdomen, flank, or back may produce renal injury. Suspicion is high in a patient with multiple injuries.

Types of Injuries

1. Contusion
2. Lacerations
3. Rupture
4. Renal pedicle injury

Major Problems Following Kidney Trauma

1. Control of hemorrhage—may be persistent or recurring
2. Injuries to other organs
3. Late complications are significant

Clinical Manifestations

1. Hematuria—degree of hematuria shows no correlation with severity of injury
2. Pain—costovertebral, flank, upper abdomen
3. Nausea, vomiting, abdominal rigidity—from ileus (seen when there is retroperitoneal bleeding)
4. Shock—from severe/multiple injuries

Diagnostic Evaluation

1. History of injury—determine if injury was caused by blunt or penetrating trauma (stab/gunshot wounds)
2. Serial urine studies for hematuria
3. Computed tomography—defines lacerations, hematomas; detects extravasation
4. Excretory urography (IVP)—to define extent of injury to involved kidney and the function of contralateral kidney

Management and Nursing Interventions

A. Monitoring for Complications

1. Place patient on bedrest to minimize bleeding.
2. Monitor blood pressure and pulse—to assess for bleeding and impending shock; perirenal hemorrhage may cause rapid exsanguination.
3. Save, inspect, and compare each urine specimen—to follow the course and degree of hematuria.
4. Monitor serial hematocrit determinations to be certain that continued bleeding is not occurring.
5. Evaluate the patient frequently during the first few days following injury.
   a. Assess for flank and abdominal pain, muscle spasm, and swelling over flank—suggests renal hemorrhage and extravasation.
   b. Outline original mass with marking pencil for future comparisons.
   c. Examine renal area for development of bruising and/or swelling.
   d. Watch for any *sudden* change in the patient's con-

dition. This may indicate hemorrhage, which requires surgical intervention.
6. Monitor for other complications: abscess; urinary fistula, urinary extravasation, and urinoma (cyst containing urine); hypertension.
   a. Avoid narcotic analgesia—may mask accompanying abdominal symptoms.
   b. Give antibiotics as directed to discourage infection from perirenal hematoma and/or urinoma, or severely contaminated wounds.

B. Restoring or Maintaining Renal Function

1. Maintain urinary drainage.
2. Prepare for surgical exploration if the patient has penetrating injury (laceration, rupture, pedicle injury), palpable mass and tenderness in flank, or shock.

Patient Education

1. Activity should be restricted for about 1 month following trauma to minimize incidence of delayed/secondary bleeding.
2. Encourage the patient to have follow-up examinations after discharge—to detect late-developing complications (post-traumatic hypertension, decreasing renal function).

Neurogenic Bladder

Neurogenic bladder refers to a bladder disturbance that results from a lesion of the nervous system.

Normal Physiology

1. Normal bladder action depends on intact sensory and motor nerve supply.
2. The bladder fills to approximately 300–500 ml.—triggers an emptying reflex.
3. This reflex initiates a contraction of the musculature inside the bladder wall, which forces urine out through the urethra until the bladder is empty.

Causes

1. Spinal cord injury; spinal tumor; herniated intervertebral disc
2. Certain neurologic diseases (multiple sclerosis)
3. Certain congenital anomalies (spina bifida, myelomeningocele)
4. Infection

Types of Neurogenic Bladder

A. Spastic (reflex, automatic or hypertonic)

1. Characterized by automatic, reflex, or uncontrolled expulsion of urine from the bladder with incomplete emptying.
2. Caused by any lesion of the spinal cord above the voiding reflex arc (upper motor neuron lesion); the result is a loss of conscious sensations and cerebral motor control.
3. Reduced bladder capacity and marked hypertrophy of bladder wall occurs, causing bladder to behave in reflex fashion with minimal or no controlling influence to regulate its activity (spontaneous uncontrolled voiding).

B. Flaccid (atonic, nonreflex or areflexic)

1. Characterized by loss of sensation of bladder fullness and thus overfilling, causing distention of the bladder; usually caused by a lower motor neuron lesion; most commonly due to trauma.
2. Bladder continues to fill until it becomes greatly distended—bladder musculature does not contract forcefully at any time.
3. When pressure reaches a breakthrough point, small amounts of urine dribble from urethra as bladder continues to fill (overflow incontinence).
4. Sensory loss may accompany flaccid bladder; the patient is not aware of discomfort.
5. Extensive distention causes damage to bladder musculature, infection of stagnant urine, and infection of kidneys by back pressure of urine.

C. Mixed (spastic/flaccid)

1. Generally associated with injuries occurring at the conus–cauda equina junctions.
2. Leads to a combination of upper motor neuron/lower motor neuron dysfunction.

Complications

1. *Infection*—from stasis of urine and subsequent catheterization.
2. *Vesicoureteral reflux*—backing up of urine from the bladder to the ureters.
3. *Hydronephrosis*—dilation of the internal structures of the kidney by increased pressure of the backed-up urine.
4. *Urolithiasis*—stones in the urinary tract from urinary stasis and infection and from demineralization of bone due to prolonged bedrest.
5. *Renal failure*—major cause of death of patients with neurologic impairment of the bladder.

Diagnostic Evaluation

1. Measurement of residual urine volume
2. Measurement of fluid intake and urinary output
3. Serial studies of BUN, serum creatinine, creatinine clearance—to determine status of renal function
4. Cystometry—to determine changes in bladder compliance; assess effectiveness of treatment
5. Urethrogram—for presence of urethral complications
6. IV urogram—to outline upper urinary tract
7. Pressure and flow studies
8. Cystoscopy—to assess for loss of muscle fibers and elastic tissues; gives opportunity for biopsy

Management: Initial Phase

A. Catheterization to Reduce Bladder Distention—following spinal cord injury, the syndrome of spinal shock is reflected in the bladder; sensation is not perceived, and the bladder usually cannot contract and empty itself. The bladder must be decompressed by either intermittent or continuous catheterization.

1. Intermittent catheterization (preferred)
   a. Bladder catheterized at designated intervals (4, 6, or 8 hours) with a small-caliber catheter; this intermittent emptying approximates physiologic function; circumvents complications usually seen with indwelling catheter.
      (1) Hourly fluid intake and output record is kept to assess individual output patterns.

(2) Catheterization technique requires strict asepsis and skilled personnel.
      (3) Patients with upper extremity function may be taught to catheterize themselves.
2. Continuous catheterization
   a. Bladder is catheterized using continuous drainage and irrigation system (p. 667) to avoid overdistention and risk of contracture from being constantly empty.
      (1) Tape catheter to abdomen (male) to remove sharp angulation and pressure at penoscrotal angle.

B. Maintaining a High Fluid Intake—to reduce urinary bacterial count, reduce stasis, decrease the concentration of calcium in the urine, and minimize the precipitation of urinary crystals and subsequent stone formation.

C. Promoting Mobility—to reduce incidence of calculosis (presence of calculi)

1. Turn, move, and exercise the patient.
2. Get the patient up on tilt table or in wheelchair as soon as possible.
3. Give low-calcium diet as directed—to prevent calculi.

Management: Chronic Phase

Each person with neurogenic bladder disease has a particular type of problem(s); it is difficult to assess what the rehabilitation potential and eventual urologic disability may be.

A. Establishing an Effective Spontaneous Reflex Voiding (for Spastic Bladder)

1. Have the patient drink a measured amount of fluid from 8 AM–8 PM; no fluids (except sips) taken after 8 PM to avoid bladder overdistention.
2. At specified time, the patient attempts to void by using pressure over bladder or stimulates reflex voiding by abdominal tapping or digital stretch of anal sphincter to trigger the bladder.
3. Estimate residual urine by comparing intake and output; palpate and percuss over bladder.
4. Palpate the bladder at repeated intervals to determine if bladder is being emptied.
5. Immediately following voiding attempt, catheterize the patient to determine urine residual.
   a. Measure all urine, voided and catheterized.
   b. Avoid *overdistention* of bladder.
   c. Caution patient to be alert for any sign that his bladder is full—perspiration, coldness of hands or feet, feelings of anxiety, etc.
6. *Intervals between catheterizations.*
   Catheterization intervals are lengthened and program is moved forward as residual urine decreases.
      Catheterization checks are usually discontinued when the volume of residual urine is at an acceptable level compatible with urine sterility and radiologic normalcy of upper urinary tract.

B. Establishing Complete and Regular Emptying of Bladder (for Flaccid Bladder)

1. The patient may be placed on bladder routine (outlined above); the fluid intake and output are adjusted to prevent bladder overdistention.
2. *Or,* if no reflex or only a partial reflex can be induced, the patient is maintained on intermittent catheteriza-

tion until he develops spontaneous reflex voiding; or surgical intervention may be required.

  a. Male patient—may use condom collecting device if bladder empties well and no residual remains.
  b. Female patient—may use pads, waterproof pants; or urinary diversion procedure may be required.

3. Electrical stimulation—application of electrical stimulation to bladder or reflex voiding center in spinal cord.

C. Surgical Intervention to Correct Condition—surgical intervention may be carried out to correct bladder neck contractures, correct vesicoureteral reflux, or perform some type of urinary diversion procedure (see p. 697).

Patient Education

1. Instruct the patient to do vaginal and rectal contractions to strengthen periurethral tissue.
   a. Tighten the rectum or vaginal vault.
   b. Hold the contraction while counting slowly to 6; relax.
   c. Continue relaxing and tightening for a 5-minute period.
   d. Perform these exercises twice daily for 5 minutes over a 6–8-week period—success or failure of exercise program is then evaluated.
2. Bladder rehabilitation may take weeks to months.
3. The patient with chronic problem should have kidney function studies and intravenous urogram annually.

Guidelines Intermittent Self-Catheterization—Clean (Nonsterile) Technique

---

Intermittent self-catheterization is the periodic drainage of urine from the bladder by the patient via catheterization; it is necessitated by temporary or permanent inability to empty the bladder (bladder-emptying dysfunction, neurogenic disease, obstructive uropathy, decompensated bladder).

Underlying Considerations

1. Intermittent catheterization is the treatment of choice following spinal cord injury. It is done under aseptic conditions by qualified health professionals until the patient is able to catheterize himself. After discharge from the hospital, the patient may be able to use a "clean" (nonsterile) technique.
2. The patient should be medically followed at regular intervals to prevent complications—reflux, hydronephrosis, external sphincter spasm, infection.
3. Advantages of self-catheterization: better patient acceptance; promotes independence; fewer complications; permits more normal sexual relations.
4. Goal: to decrease morbidity associated with long-term use of indwelling catheter and to achieve a catheter-free status, if possible.

Equipment

Soap and water towelettes for handwashing
Liquid cleansing agent
No. 14 Fr. catheter (several to be kept in reserve); water-soluble lubricant
Mirror (female patient)
Shallow pan
Irrigation tip syringe
Clear plastic bag or case—for carrying catheter

Procedure

Action (By Patient)	**Rationale/Amplification**
1. The patient must understand the importance of frequent catheterization and emptying of bladder at prescribed time regardless of circumstances.	1. An overdistended bladder slows the circulation of blood through the bladder walls and weakens its resistance to infection.
2. Try to void before catheterizing self using reflex triggering mechanisms—pressure on abdomen, thigh stroking, etc.	2. This may help to develop voluntary voiding without catheterization.
3. Wash hands with soap and water.	3. Do not forego catheterization if soap and water are not available. Catheterize at prescribed time regardless of circumstances.
4. Lubricate the catheter.	
Female	
1. Position mirror in line of vision with urinary meatus. Assume the most comfortable position with the knees as far apart as possible (sitting on the toilet seat or standing with one leg on toilet seat).	1. This position helps to expose the urethral meatus.
2. Spread labia apart and upward with the second and fourth fingers of one hand, thus freeing the middle finger to palpate/locate the meatus. Cleanse the urinary meatus.	2. The nurse points out the location of the clitoris, urethral meatus, and vaginal outlet (in the mirror). The patient is taught to confirm the position of the clitoris, urethral meatus, and vaginal outlet by palpation so that eventually a mirror will not be necessary.
3. With the dominant hand, direct the lubricated catheter toward this area, over the middle finger and into the meatus. Allow urine to flow into a shallow pan/toilet.	
4. When urine stops flowing, remove catheter.	

Procedure *(continued)*	**Nursing Action**	**Rationale/Amplification**

Male Patient

1. Assume sitting position until technique is learned.
2. Lubricate the catheter.

    2. A well-lubricated catheter is particularly necessary in the male to avoid traumatic urethritis.

3. Retract foreskin of penis with one hand; then grasp penis and hold it at right angle to body.

    3. This maneuver straightens the urethra and facilitates ease of catheter insertion.

4. Insert the cather 15–25 cm. (6–10 inches) until urine begins to flow.
5. Then advance catheter about 2.5 cm. (1 more inch) and allow urine to flow into shallow pan/toilet. When urine stops flowing, remove catheter.

    5. Measure or estimate volume of residual urine.

Follow-up Phase

1. Wash outside surface of catheter in warm soapy water. Rinse inside and outside with clear water.
2. Wrap catheter in plastic bag/paper towel.

    2. The catheter may be carried in a plastic bag or case. The emphasis is on availability and cleanliness.

Injuries to the Bladder *(and Urethra)*

Types of Bladder Injuries

1. Contusion of bladder
2. Intraperitoneal rupture
3. Extraperitoneal rupture   } or combination of both
4. Injury to urethra

Types of Urethral Injuries

1. Contusion
2. Partial or complete rupture

Problems Associated With Bladder Injury

1. Injuries to the bladder and urethra are commonly associated with pelvic fractures and multiple trauma. Certain surgical procedures (hysterectomy, surgery of lower colon and rectum) also carry a risk to the bladder.
2. With injury, there is a rise in intravesical (within bladder) pressure, which produces extravasation of urine into the peritoneal cavity or perivesical space.
3. Rupture of the bladder requires immediate treatment.

Clinical Manifestations

1. Failure to void
2. Hematuria; presence of blood at urinary meatus
3. Shock and hemorrhage—pallor, rapid and increasing pulse rate
4. Suprapubic pain and soreness
5. Rigid abdomen—indicates intraperitoneal rupture
6. Swelling/discoloration of penis, scrotum, and anterior perineum

Diagnostic Evaluation

1. Retrograde urethrogram—to detect any rupture of urethra. *Do first* (before catheterization).
2. Cystogram—to detect and localize perforation/rupture of bladder.
3. Plain film of abdomen—may show associated pelvic fracture.
4. Excretory urogram—to survey the kidneys for injury.

Management

A. Bladder Injury

1. Treatment instituted for shock and hemorrhage.
2. Retrograde urethrography is carried out in suspected injuries involving lower urinary tract.
3. Patient is catheterized only after urethrogram is done.
   a. Indwelling catheter serves as a means of continuous urinary drainage.
   b. Catheter also serves as a splint to urethra if urethra has been injured, but it may complete a partial rupture if urethral injury is not recognized with a urethrogram.
4. Surgical intervention carried out for bladder rupture
   a. Extravasated blood and urine will be drained and urine diverted with suprapubic cystostomy and indwelling catheter.
   b. Bladder tears will be sutured; urethral repairs may be postponed.
5. Drainage systems maintained after surgery.
   a. Suprapubic cystostomy drainage—until healing of bladder is complete.
   b. Indwelling urethral catheter drainage—to divert urine drainage and permit suprapubic incision to heal.
   c. Perivesical areas drained with Penrose drain (will be brought out through suprapubic incision).

B. For Urethral Injury *(management is controversial)*

1. Assist with cystostomy drainage (p. 670)—to provide urine drainage until reconstructive surgery is done.
2. Treatment modalities determined by level of urethral injury and its effect on bladder continence.

Patient Education

Urethral stricture, incontinence, and impotence may follow urethral injury.

Cancer of the Bladder

Cancer of the bladder includes a heterogenous (dissimilar) group of tumors with the ability to recur, transform histologically, and metastasize.

Clinical Features

1. Accounts for 2% of malignancies in adults; occurs 3 times more frequently in males; peak incidence occurs in the 6th decade.
2. Recurrences may develop years after last known tumor is treated.
3. Metastases occur in bladder wall and pelvis, para-aortic or supraclavicular nodes; in liver, lungs, and bone.

Etiology

It appears that multiple agents are responsible for the development of cancer of the bladder. The specific etiology is unknown.

1. Cigarette smoking.
2. Prolonged exposure to aromatic amines or their metabolites—generally dyes manufactured by the chemical industry and used by other industries.
3. Causal relationship may exist between excessive coffee drinking and consumption of excessive amounts of analgesics and bladder cancer.

Clinical Manifestations

1. Painless hematuria, either gross or microscopic—most characteristic sign
2. Dysuria, frequency, urgency—symptoms of bladder irritability
3. Flank pain, chills, fever—from progressive tumor growth, infiltration of bladder wall, ureteral obstruction, and bladder infection
4. Pelvic or back pain—from distant metastases
5. Leg edema—from invasion of pelvic lymph nodes

Diagnostic Evaluation

1. Intravenous urography (IVU)—to determine status of upper tracts
2. Endoscopic examination under anesthesia
   a. Cystoscopy for visualization of number, location, and appearance of tumors; for biopsy
   b. Urine and bladder washing for cytologic study
   c. Bimanual examination of pelvis to determine degree of mobility, fixation of tumor, degree of extravesical extension
3. Computed tomography (CT) scan—to evaluate extent of disease and tumor responsiveness
4. Quantitative fluorescence image analysis—uses a computer-controlled fluorescence microscope to scan and image the nucleus of each cell on a slide; based on the fact that cancer cells contain abnormally large amounts of DNA; a urine test

Management

A. Surgery

1. Transurethral resection and/or fulguration—endoscopic resection for superficial tumors; usually combined with intravesical chemotherapy to prevent tumor recurrence (see below).
2. Cystectomy (removal of bladder) or radical cystectomy for invasive or poorly differentiated tumors; may be combined with other treatment, including radiation or chemotherapy.
   a. Cystectomy requires diversion of the urinary stream (see this page, right-hand column).
   b. *In male,* includes removal of bladder, prostate and seminal vesicles, proximal vas deferens, and part of proximal urethra.
   c. *In female,* consists of anterior exenteration with removal of bladder, urethra, uterus, ovarian tubes, ovaries, and segment of anterior wall of the vagina.
   d. Complications: sepsis, wound dehiscence or evisceration, ileus, urine leakage, ureterointestinal obstruction, rectal fistula. Late complications include pyelonephritis, stone formation, progressive loss of renal function.

B. Intravesical (Within the Bladder) Chemotherapy

1. Instillation of antineoplastic agent (thiotepa; mitomycin C; doxorubicin; bacillus Calmette–Guerin) allows a high concentration of drug to come in contact with the tumor and urothelium with minimal systemic toxicity.
2. Patient is instructed as follows:
   a. Do not take fluids during instillation period to minimize dilution of drug during contact intervals.
   b. Change position as directed during instillation in an effort to have drug contact as much of urothelial surface as possible.
   c. Wash hands and perineal area after voiding the medication to prevent contact dermatitis.
   d. Void frequently after procedure to avoid chemical cystitis from residual drug in the bladder.
   e. Drink fluids liberally after procedure is completed.
3. Patient is monitored for allergic reaction during instillation period.
4. Patient is monitored for signs and symptoms of urinary infection.
5. Patient is encouraged to complete course of treatment; most involve weekly instillations for 6–8 weeks.

C. Systemic Chemotherapy—bladder cancer is a chemotherapeutically responsive tumor; cisplatin is widely used.

D. Radiation Therapy—may be internal or external.

Nursing Interventions

1. Give patient time to face fears and organize thoughts and feelings—helps establish a sense of organization and control.
2. Emphasize the positive aspects of the treatment.
3. Help patient to emphasize functional abilities.
4. See nursing management of the patient undergoing urinary diversion, page 697, chemotherapy, page 103, and radiation therapy, page 108.

Urinary Diversion

Urinary diversion refers to diverting the urinary stream from the bladder so that it exits via a new avenue. There is a great number of operative procedures.

Clinical Conditions Requiring Urinary Diversion

1. Malignancy of bladder or ureters; pelvic malignancy
2. Congenital abnormality of lower urinary tract
3. Neurogenic bladder

Methods of Urinary Diversion (Fig. 27-11)

A. Ileal Conduit (most common)—transplanting the ureters to an isolated section of the terminal ileum and bringing one end through the abdominal wall to create a stoma; urine flows from the kidney into a ureter, then through the ileal conduit, and exits through urinary stoma. The ureter may also be transplanted

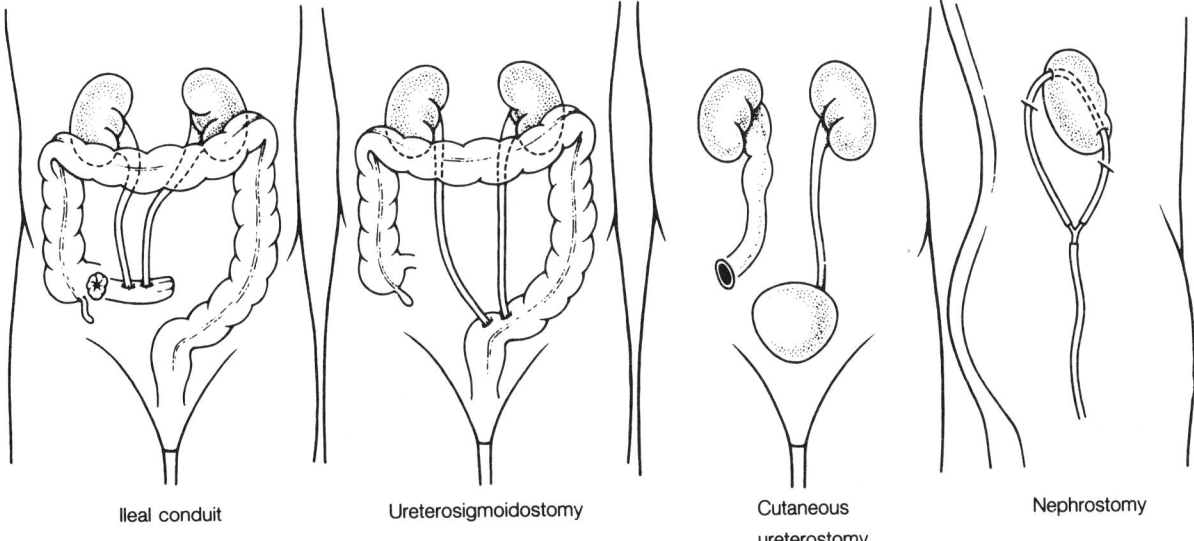

Figure 27-11. *Methods of urinary diversion.*

into the transverse colon (colon conduit) or proximal jejunum (jejunal conduit).

B. Ureterosigmoidostomy—introducing the ureters into the sigmoid, thereby allowing urine to flow through the colon and out the rectum.

C. Cutaneous Ureterostomy—bringing the detached ureter through the abdominal wall and attaching it to an opening in the skin.

D. Nephrostomy—inserting a catheter into the renal pelvis via an incision into the flank or by percutaneous catheter placement into the kidney.

E. Continent Urinary Diversion Procedures—creating a urinary reservoir from an intestinal segment that is either brought to the skin where a valve mechanism is created or is anastomosed to the proximal urethra.

1. *Continent ileal urinary reservoir* (Kock pouch)—transplanting the ureters into a segment of ileum where a pouch is created for urine with two intussuscepted nipple valves: one to provide the continence mechanism and the second to prevent reflux to the kidney (Fig. 27-12). Patient does not have to wear an external appliance, but the procedure does require intermittent self-catheterization

2. *Functional reservoir anastomosed to urethra (ileocystoplasty)*—using ileum shaped into "U," which is anastomosed directly to the urethral stump in men; voiding is through the urethra. Patient usually has nocturnal incontinence; not all patients are candidates for this procedure.

Preoperative Nursing Interventions

1. See page 682 for general aspects of preoperative care for the patient undergoing renal surgery.
2. Pay careful attention to cardiopulmonary status, since the patient is probably older and undergoing a lengthy, complex procedure.
3. Prepare the bowel for surgical intervention to prevent fecal contamination during surgery and the potential complication of infection.

For outpatient, instruct as follows:

  a. Take clear liquids and prescribed cathartic for mechanical cleansing of the bowel.

  b. Take prescribed antibiotic (nonabsorbable; active against enteric organisms) to reduce bacterial count in the bowel lumen.

4. Employ adequate hydration, including intravenous in-

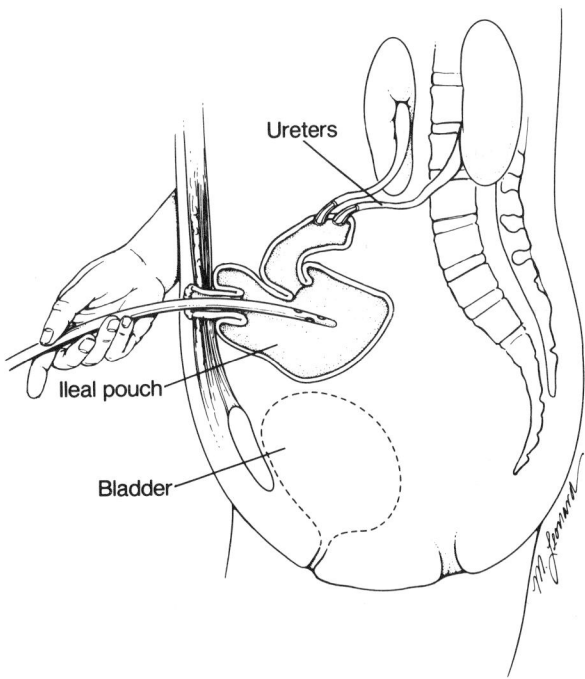

Figure 27-12. *Continent ileal urinary reservoir (Kock pouch). Insertion of a catheter through the valve to drain stored urine. (From Brunner LS and Suddarth DS: Textbook of Medical–Surgical Nursing. 6th ed. Philadelphia, JB Lippincott, 1988)*

fusions, to ensure urine flow during surgery and to prevent hypovolemia.

5. Reinforce the surgeon's and enterostomal therapist's explanations of the procedure. The following is for ileal conduit and cutaneous ureterostomy:
   a. The stoma site is planned preoperatively with the patient standing, sitting, and lying—to place the stoma away from bony prominences, skin creases, and scars, and where the patient can see it.
   b. Several types of skin adhesives or cement are applied to abdomen preoperatively to determine contact allergies and to facilitate management of ostomy appliance postoperatively.
   The patient wears the intended appliance preoperatively.
6. Assist with enteral or intravenous hyperalimentation—to give nutritional support, minimize toxicity, promote healing, and improve response to treatment.
7. Assist the patient undergoing nasogastric intubation before surgery (p. 464), or temporary gastrostomy may be done during surgery to facilitate gastric decompression.

Nursing Assessment

1. Review the patient's chart concerning past and present health status.
2. Review results of diagnostic tests.
3. Ascertain functional status: physical (including self-care), mental, emotional, and social.
4. Observe degree of manual dexterity and visual acuity—essential for stoma care.
5. Find out about patient's psychosocial resources: available support systems, including all significant others and community resources, education, occupation, economic resources, coping strengths, attitude.

Nursing Diagnoses

1. Knowledge deficit of proposed surgery and consequences of living with an ostomy.
2. Disturbances in body image related to change in toileting habits, presence of external stoma and collecting device, loss of independence.
3. Fear (of death, recurring disease, loss of body function) related to diagnosis of genitourinary cancer.

Postoperative Nursing Interventions

A. Monitoring for Complications

1. Monitor patient for evidence of wound infection, urinary or fecal leakage, peritonitis, paralytic ileus, pelvic thrombophlebitis, pulmonary embolism, and stenosis of stoma. These operations are extremely taxing and patients may have little or no reserve.
2. Late complications include stomal problems, pyelonephritis, and stone formation.

B. Immediate Postoperative Management for Urinary Diversion Procedures

1. See page 475 for nursing management of patient following intestinal surgery and page 683 for nursing interventions following renal/urologic surgery. The care related to the presence of the stoma is discussed below.
2. Keep nasogastric tube in place. Restrict oral fluids until bowel peristalsis is normal.
3. Be aware that ureteral stents may be used to protect ureteroconduit anastomoses; stents may emerge from stoma and are usually removed in 1 week.

4. Keep careful check of fluid balance including intake and output and daily weight.
5. Monitor suction drains placed in pelvis—sudden increase in drainage suggests a urine leak.
6. Monitor total parenteral nutrition (p. 450) if the patient is unable to return to oral feedings.

C. Nursing Interventions Related to Presence of Urinary Stoma

1. Immediately after surgery, a skin barrier and clear disposable urinary pouch are sealed around the stoma—allows visualization of stoma color and patency of stents as well as monitoring of urinary output.
2. The patient with a cutaneous ureterostomy or an ileal conduit diversion wears an appliance day and night. Urine (but not feces) drains constantly.
   a. Pouch has a urinary drain adapter and is connected to a drainage tube and bag; urine volume is recorded hourly.
   b. Urinary appliance remains in place as long as no leakage occurs. It is changed as necessary.
3. The stoma is inspected for color, size, whether it is flush, nippled, or retracted, and the condition of the skin around the stoma is noted; baseline information used for subsequent comparison.
   a. Stoma is red, wet with mucus, soft, and slightly rubbery to the touch.
   b. Cyanotic stoma indicates poor circulation.
   c. Necrotic stoma is blue/black or tan/brown.
4. Monitor stoma for bleeding, necrosis, sloughing, suture separation; check patency of stents.
5. Check urine in pouch; usually blood-tinged first few postoperative days.
6. Instruct patient in stoma care as described in following section.

D. Enhancing Coping Abilities to Adapt to Altered Body Image

1. Encourage the patient to express his feelings about situation; reflect and amplify.
2. Expect patient to go through adaptation process (shock, defensive retreat, acknowledgment, and adaptation/resolution) while resolution of loss occurs.
3. Help the patient talk about support network.
4. Include the family in caring for the patient; allow for verbalization of fear and anxiety.
5. Encourage membership in a self-help group (United Ostomy Association) and visits by an ostomy association visitor.
6. Help the patient and family gain a positive attitude and hope.

E. Reducing Fear

1. Accept the patient's depression, which usually follows any surgery that interferes with body integrity.
   a. Understand the patient's irritability and lack of motivation to learn.
   b. Give extra support until the patient can cope.
   c. Counsel the patient to take 1 day at a time.
   d. Reinforce the concept that the stoma will be manageable.
2. Acknowledge feelings of fear and anxiety as normal.
3. Help patient/family to gain independence through learning to manage the ostomy. Provide for demonstrations, supervised practice, and return demonstrations until patient is independent in self-care.
4. Provide written instructions to reinforce learning and confidence.

5. Teach techniques of stress reduction: progressive muscle relaxation; imagery.

Patient Education for Stoma Care

A. Appliance—the urinary appliance/pouching system may be disposable or permanent. The choice is determined by location of stoma, patient activity, body build, and economic status. The appliance consists of a face plate, disc, or mounting ring that fits over the stoma, a pouch to collect the urine, and some type of skin barrier to protect the skin from irritation from urine.

B. Determining Stoma Size (for ordering correct appliance)

1. The stoma will shrink considerably as edema subsides, and the opening is recalibrated every 3–6 weeks for the first few months postoperatively.
2. Measure the widest part of the stoma with a ruler.
3. The inside diameter of the faceplate should not be more than $^1/_{16}$ to $^1/_8$ inch larger than the diameter of the stoma:

C. Changing the Appliance

1. Change appliance early in morning before taking fluids or before evening meal—urine output is lower at these times.
2. Prepare the appliance according to manufacturer's directives.
3. Remove the faceplate with warm water. Instruct patient to bend over quickly and remain in that position for a minute to allow conduit to empty before the skin is washed and dried.
4. Wash the skin with noncream-based soap and water. Rinse and pat dry. *The skin must be dry or appliance will not adhere.*
5. A gauze or tissue wick may be applied over the stoma to absorb urine while the appliance is being changed. Keep the skin free from direct contact with urine.
6. Apply skin barrier around the stoma.
7. Center the appliance directly over the stoma and apply it carefully. Apply gentle pressure around appliance for secure adherence and to remove air bubbles and creases.
8. Apply hypoallergenic tape in a picture-frame effect around the pouch.
9. The skin under the appliance may be dusted with pure talcum powder and a cotton cover used to absorb perspiration and eliminate warmth from the pouch.
10. The use of a belt is optional, but follow manufacturer's directions, since an ill-fitting belt can cause abrasion of the stoma.

D. Odor Control

1. Instruct the patient to avoid foods and medication that produce strong odors.
2. Drink liberal amounts of fluids to flush the conduit free of mucus and reduce possibility of urinary infection.
3. Flush ostomy pouch with white vinegar solution daily if there is an odor problem.

E. Managing the Ostomy Appliance

1. Empty the appliance when it is $^1/_3$–$^1/_2$ full to prevent weight of urine from loosening adhesive seal—urinary ostomy appliances are closed with a drain valve (spigot) for periodic emptying.
2. Some patients prefer wearing a leg bag attached with an adapter to the drainage apparatus.

3. Attach outlet on appliance to a collecting bottle with plastic tubing for nighttime drainage; have at least 1.5 m. (5 ft.) of tubing to allow patient to turn in bed. The tubing may be threaded down the pajama leg to prevent kinking.
4. Position the drainage bottle lower than the level of the bed—to enhance flow by gravity.

F. Cleaning and Deodorizing the Appliance

1. Clean faceplate with solvent, and remove all adhesive. Rinse in clear water.
2. Wash appliance with warm, soapy water. A capful of white vinegar or commercial mouthwash may help deodorize the appliance. Rinse well.
3. Clean nighttime drainage equipment with soap and water. Rinse well.
4. Discard equipment that no longer can be cleaned adequately or when odor persists.

G. General Patient Instructions

1. Urinary stoma care is not difficult or complicated and should be regarded as part of personal grooming and dressing routine.
2. The stoma is normally red in color; it may protrude or be flush with the skin. It may bleed if it is bumped or rubbed. Report to your physician if it continues bleeding for several hours.
3. Mucus shreds in the urine are normal following an ileal conduit operation because the conduit lining and stoma are mucous membrane.
4. Choose an appliance that fits your needs. Successful urinary ostomy management requires a well-fitting appliance, meticulous skin care, and control of urinary odor.
5. Always carry spare pouches and cement in a small case in handbag or pocket.
6. The wearing time of an appliance varies. Experiment with your appliance; usually an appliance may be worn 5–7 days. See above for changing, cleaning, and management of appliance.
7. Before changing to a new skin adhesive, apply a test patch to the other side of the abdomen or forearm.
8. Wear cotton (rather than nylon) underwear. Avoid a heavy girdle because it may cause chafing of the stoma and leakage from pressure on the pouch.
9. Avoid heavy lifting for 6 weeks. Sexual activities, driving the car, returning to work, etc., may be resumed when energy level increases.
10. Get in touch with local medical supply distributor or enterostomal therapist or consult *Ostomy Quarterly* (address below) for manufacturer's advertisements of appliances, deodorizers, skin barriers, and other new products.
11. Call your physician or enterostomal therapist for instructions if skin problems develop or if one or more of the following symptoms of kidney complications occur: fever, chills, pain, change in color of urine (cloudy, bloody), diminishing urine output.
12. Contact local ostomy association for visits, reassurance, and practical information from ostomy visitor. For further information and valuable periodical materials:
United Ostomy Association, Inc.
36 Executive Park
Suite 120
Irvine, CA 92714

International Association Enterostomal Therapists
505 North Tustin Ave, Suite 219
Santa Ana, CA 92705

Evaluation

1. Demonstrates ability to care for ostomy: removes appliance, cleanses skin, changes appliance; has written instructions and telephone number of enterostomal therapist.
2. Demonstrates progress in adapting to change in body image; resuming social relationships.
3. Appears less fearful; discusses fears and feelings; sleeping better.

Problems Affecting the Urethra

Urethritis

Urethritis is inflammation of the urethra. It is usually an ascending infection.

Etiology

1. Nongonococcal urethritis—urethritis not caused by gonococcus. However, a large number of cases are sexually transmitted by:
   a. *Chlamydia trachomatis* and *Ureaplasma urealyticum*—cause approximately 80% of nongonococcal urethritis.
   b. Other sexually transmitted organisms causing acute urethritis include herpes simplex virus, *Candida albicans, Trichomonas vaginalis.*
2. Nonsexually transmitted:
   a. Bacterial urethritis—may be associated with urinary tract infection.
   b. From trauma—secondary to passage of urethral sounds, repeated cystoscopy, indwelling catheter.

Clinical Manifestations

1. May be asymptomatic
2. Itching and burning around area of urethra
3. Urethral discharge: may be scant or profuse; thin, clear, or mucoid; or thick and purulent
4. Dysuria and frequency
5. Penile discomfort

Diagnostic Evaluation

1. Gram stain of urethral discharge
2. Urine culture(s)

Management

1. Antimicrobial therapy (tetracycline or erythromycin) usually effective for nongonococcal urethritis); sulfa and high dose amoxicillin eliminates chlamydia.
2. Complications include epididymitis, conjunctivitis, proctitis.

Patient Education

1. Encourage the patient to stay on the antimicrobial regimen for the prescribed time period.
2. Advise the patient to temporarily discontinue sexual activity and ingestion of alcohol—these activities may prolong the acute phase of urethritis.
3. Urge treatment for sexual partner—in event of treatment failure and recurrence.
4. Advise that barrier methods of contraception (condom; diaphragm) will reduce transmission of chlamydia and *Ureaplasma.*

Urethritis From Gonorrhea

Etiology

1. *Neisseria gonorrhoeae*—the specific organism.
2. Transmitted through sexual contact.
3. More and more asymptomatic carriers are being recognized.

Clinical Manifestations

Male

1. Inflammation of meatal orifice; burning on urination; *may be asymptomatic*
2. Urethral discharge—scant and serous to thick, yellowish pus (4–10 days or longer after sexual exposure)

Female

1. Purulent urethral discharge
2. Frequency, urgency, nocturia
3. Red, swollen urinary meatus
4. Pelvic infection accompanied by abdominal pain
5. Often is asymptomatic

Complications (local)

1. Male—periurethritis, prostatitis, epididymitis, urethral stricture, sterility due to vasoepididymal duct obstruction
2. Female—pelvic infection, abscess of greater vestibular glands (Bartholin's glands), urethral stricture

Patient Education

1. See page 904 for management of gonorrhea.
2. Instruct the patient to avoid sexual activity with untreated previous sexual partners until they have been treated and examined to prevent reinfection.
3. Emphasize that the patient must return in 4–7 days to assess results and determine if there is need for further treatment and tests.
4. Urge the patient to have any sexual contacts present themselves for treatment.

Urethral Stricture

Urethral stricture is a narrowing of the lumen of the urethra due to scar tissue and contraction.

Etiology

1. Urethral injury
   a. Urethral instrumentation—transurethral surgical procedures, indwelling catheters, cystoscopic procedures
   b. Straddle injuries, automobile accidents, pelvic fractures, direct trauma to urethra
2. Untreated gonorrheal urethritis
3. Congenital abnormalities

Clinical Manifestations

1. Diminution in force and size of urinary stream
2. Urinary infection and retention—dysuria and urgency
3. Symptoms of complication from stricture—back pressure produces cystitis, prostatitis, pyelonephritis, etc.

Diagnostic Evaluation

1. Voiding cystourethrogram—to locate site and degree of stricture

2. Passing of catheter or sounds (bougies)—to determine the diameter and location of urethral narrowings

Prevention

1. Treat urethral infections promptly.
2. Use utmost care in urethral instrumentation (catheterization, etc.).
3. Avoid prolonged urethral catheter drainage.

Management

1. Gradual dilatation of the narrowed area with metal sounds or bougies
   a. Sounds of increasing size are used.
   b. Sounds are passed at lengthening intervals (2 weeks, 1 month, 3 months) for an indefinite period, depending on how long the strictured lumen is patent.
   c. Hot sitz baths and nonnarcotic analgesics are prescribed—to control pain after instrumentation.
   d. Antimicrobials may be given several days after dilatation—lessens discomfort and minimizes infectious reaction.
2. Other treatment measures
   a. Balloon catheter dilatation.
   b. Surgical interventions include internal urethrotomy; urethroplasty.
      (1) Suprapubic cystostomy may be necessary following surgery.
      (2) Complications: bleeding; recurrent strictures.

Conditions of the Prostate

Benign Prostatic Hyperplasia (Hypertrophy)

Benign prostatis hyperplasia is enlargement of the prostate. The etiology is uncertain but is presumably related to endocrine changes associated with aging that initiate hyperplasia of both glandular and cellular tissue of the prostate.

Clinical Manifestations

1. In early or gradual prostatic enlargement, there may be no symptoms, since the detrusor musculature can compensate for increased peripheral resistance.
2. Obstructive symptoms—hesitancy, diminution in size and force of urinary stream, postvoiding dribbling, sensation of incomplete emptying of the bladder.
3. Symptoms of recurring urinary infection and stasis—frequency, urgency, chills, fever.
4. Renal symptoms (prolonged obstruction)—ureteral dilatation, hydronephrosis, renal infection, azotemia, uremia.

Diagnostic Evaluation

1. Rectal examination—palpated for size, consistency, and shape of gland; hyperplasia usually produces a smooth, firm, symmetric enlargement of the prostate.
2. Catheterization after voiding—to determine amount of residual urine.
3. Intravenous urogram or abdominal ultrasound—to document upper urinary tract obstruction.
4. Uroflowmetry—measures peak urine flow rate, voiding time and volume.

5. Cystourethroscopy—to inspect urethra and bladder and evaluate prostatic size.
6. Serum creatinine and BUN—to evaluate renal function.

Management

The plan of treatment depends on the cause, the severity of obstruction, and the condition of the patient.
1. Surgery—usually transurethral resection of the prostate (TURP) when obstructive symptoms occur.
2. Cystostomy drainage of the bladder—for the poor-risk patient, or one acutely ill with retention, uremia, etc.

Patient Education

1. See page 704 for nursing management of the patient having a prostatectomy.
2. Advise patient that surgical procedures for benign enlargement usually do not result in impotence, but may cause retrograde ejaculation (passing back of fluid into the bladder during sexual intercourse).

Prostatitis

Prostatitis is an inflammation of the prostate gland.

Classification

Bacterial prostatitis (acute or chronic), nonbacterial prostatitis, prostatodynia.

Etiology *(Bacterial Prostatitis)*

1. Bacterial invasion of prostate
   a. From reflux of infected urine into ejaculatory and prostatic ducts
   b. From hematogenous (bloodstream) origin or lymphogenous spread
   c. Secondary to urethritis—from ascent of bacteria from urethra
2. Descending infection from kidneys

Clinical Manifestations

(From infection and local inflammation)
1. Sudden chills and fever (moderate to high fever)
2. Bladder irritability—frequency, dysuria, urgency, hematuria
3. Pain in perineum, rectum, lower back, lower abdomen, and penile head

Diagnostic Evaluation

1. Culture and sensitivity tests of urethral and prostatic fluid and urine.
   a. The pathogens in each specimen are identified by collection of divided urine specimens and expressed prostatic fluid (obtained by prostatic massage).
   b. The pH of the prostatic fluid is usually elevated.
2. Rectal examination—frequently reveals exquisitely tender, painful, swollen prostate, warm to the touch.

Management

A. Acute Bacterial Prostatitis

Antimicrobial therapy (10–14 days) based on drug-sensitivity studies of the organisms.

B. Chronic Bacterial Prostatitis

1. Specific therapy (doxycycline; trimethoprim–sulfamethoxazole)—chronic bacterial prostatitis is difficult

to cure because most antimicrobial agents diffuse poorly into prostatic fluid.
   a. Prolonged therapy may be necessary to control symptoms and prevent bacteriuria.
   b. Oral antispasmodic agents provide relief from urinary frequency and urgency.

C. Nonbacterial Prostatitis

1. Most common type; etiology obscure.
2. Therapy is directed toward control of symptoms and is individualized to meet specific needs; acute symptoms may be controlled with anticholinergic or anti-inflammatory drugs, hot sitz baths, etc.

D. Prostatodynia—the patient has symptoms of urinary irritation but no evidence of bacteria or inflamed prostatic fluid or tissue.

1. Treatment is symptomatic; psychological counseling may be helpful.

Nursing Interventions

1. Monitor for complications: urinary retention, persistence of fever, perineal pain or difficulty in voiding (may indicate prostatic abscess), recurring urinary tract infection, relapsing infection, epididymitis, bacteremia and septicemia.
2. Start prescribed parenteral antibiotic therapy as soon as urine and blood are obtained for culture.
3. Give supportive care
   a. Bedrest—to relieve perineal and suprapubic pain.
   b. Warm sitz baths—to promote muscular relaxation of pelvic floor and reduce potential for urinary retention.
   c. Keep the patient well hydrated.
   d. Administer stool softeners as prescribed.

Patient Education

Instruct the patient as follows:
1. Take antibiotic for the full time period.
2. Use hot sitz baths (10–20 minutes) several times daily.
3. Drink fluids to satisfy thirst, but avoid "forcing fluids," since an effective level of drug must be maintained in the urine.
4. Avoid food and drinks that have diuretic action or are prostatic irritants and increase prostatic secretions (alcohol, coffee, tea, chocolate, cola, spices).
5. Avoid sexual arousal/intercourse during period of acute inflammation; sexual intercourse may be beneficial in the treatment of chronic prostatitis; chronic prostatic infection is *not* sexually transmissible.
6. Be assured that the causative agent of prostatitis is not the type that causes sexually transmitted disease. (This may be an unspoken fear.)
7. Avoid sitting for long periods of time.
8. Prolonged follow-up is necessary, since recurrence of prostatitis due to the same or different organisms can occur.

Cancer of the Prostate

Cancer of the prostate is a malignant tumor of the prostate gland. It arises from the parenchyma of the prostate, usually in the most posterior part; therefore, most prostatic cancers are palpable on rectal examination.

Clinical Features

1. Cancer of the prostate is the second leading cause of cancer death among American men and is the most common carcinoma in men over 65 years of age.
2. It can spread by local extension, by lymphatics, or via the bloodstream.
3. Prostatic cancer is potentially curable at an early stage; however, the majority of patients present with obstructive symptoms or metastatic lesions.

> **NURSING ALERT:** Annual rectal examination of males over 40 is important for early diagnosis of prostatic cancer.

Clinical Manifestations

1. Symptoms due to obstruction of urinary flow
   a. Hesitancy and straining on voiding, frequency, nocturia
   b. Diminution in size and force of urinary stream
2. Symptoms due to metastases

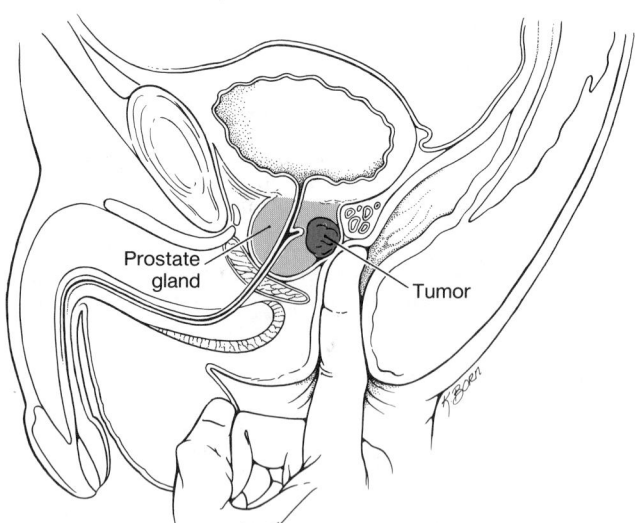

Figure 27-13. *The prostate gland can be felt through the wall of the rectum. The size of the gland, overall consistency, and the presence of any firm areas and nodules are noted.*

a. Pain in lumbosacral area radiating to hips and down legs (from bone metastases)
b. Perineal and rectal discomfort
c. Anemia, weight loss, weakness, nausea, oliguria (from uremia)
d. Hematuria (from urethral or bladder invasion, or both)
e. Lower extremity edema—occurs when pelvic node metastases compromise venous return.

Diagnostic Evaluation

1. Digital rectal examination—prostate can be felt through the wall of the rectum; cancer feels like a hard nodule instead of a fleshy gland (Fig. 27-13).
2. Needle biopsy (through anterior rectal wall or through perineum) for histologic study of biopsied tissue and/or aspiration for cytologic study.
3. Transrectal ultrasonography—a sonar probe placed in rectum emits ultrasound waves that are reflected differently by normal and abnormal tissue. Different densities between normal prostate tissue and cancer are seen as shadows on the ultrasound image.
4. Serologic markers of prostate cancer
   a. Prostate-specific antigen (PSA)—protein found on prostate cells (normal and malignant); sensitive in detection of prostate cancer and in staging and follow-up of treatment.
   b. Prostatic acid phosphatase—elevated in patients with prostatic cancer.
5. Excretory urogram—to demonstrate changes from ureteral obstruction
6. Metastatic work-up: chest x-ray, intravenous urography, and bone scan for detecting skeletal metastases

Management

A. Surgical Interventions (curative)

1. Transurethral resection of prostate (TURP) may be done for patients with very early stage disease.
2. Radical prostatectomy—removal of entire prostate gland, prostatic capsule, and seminal vesicles; may include regional lymphadenectomy.
3. A technique of surgical dissection has been refined that preserves the collection of nerves that control erection, thus preserving sexual potency.
4. Complications of radical prostatectomy: urinary incontinence, impotence, rectal injury.

B. Radiation (curative)

1. External beam radiation (using linear accelerator) focused on the prostate—to deliver maximum radiation dose to tumor and minimal dose to surrounding tissues.
2. Interstitial radiation—interstitial implantation of radioactive substances (brachytherapy) into prostate, which delivers doses of radiation directly to tumor while sparing uninvolved tissue.
3. Complications of radiation: radiation cystitis (urinary frequency, urgency, nocturia), urethral injury (stricture), radiation enteritis (diarrhea, anorexia, nausea), radiation proctitis (diarrhea, rectal bleeding), impotence.

C. Hormone Manipulation (palliative)

1. Prostate cancer is a hormone-sensitive cancer. The aim of hormonal treatment is to deprive tumor cells of androgens or their by-products and thereby alleviate symptoms and retard progress of disease.
2. Bilateral orchiectomy (removal of testes) results in reduction of the major circulating androgen, testoster-

one, which is released from the testis and is regulated by the hypothalamic–pituitary–gonadal axis. A small amount of androgen is produced by adrenal gland.
3. Estrogen therapy (diethylstilbestrol)—suppresses release of luteinizing hormone, thereby indirectly decreasing testosterone levels.
   a. Therapy with estrogens leads to water retention, cardiovascular side effects, and gynecomastia (soreness and enlargement of breasts).
   b. Pretreatment radiation therapy to breasts can prevent gynecomastia.
4. Other methods of achieving androgen deprivation
   a. LHRH analogs (leuprolide)—agonists of luteinizing hormone-releasing hormone appear to reduce testosterone levels as effectively as orchiectomy or estrogen.
   b. Antiandrogen drugs (megestrol acetate; flutamide)—drugs that can block androgen action directly at the target tissues (testes and adrenals) as well as androgens synthesized within the prostate gland.
   c. Ketoconazole—reduces testosterone production in both adrenals and testes.

D. Symptom Control for Advanced Prostatic Cancer

1. Pain
   a. Analgesics and narcotics to relieve pain
   b. Short course of radiotherapy for specific sites of bone pain
   c. Internal fixation for pathologic fractures
2. Bladder outlet obstruction (by tumor)
   a. Transurethral resection of prostate to remove obstructing tissue
   b. Suprapubic catheter placement

Nursing Assessment

1. Review patient's record to learn the severity and treatability of disease.
2. Listen to patient's complaints of pain: location, character, and whether it is influenced by activity or position.
3. Palpate lymph nodes, especially in supraclavicular and inguinal regions—may be first sign of metastatic spread.
4. Learn about patient's psychological support system, his coping mechanisms, etc.

Nursing Diagnoses

1. Pain related to tumor metastases to bone; subsequent pain due to infection or inflammatory processes, to bladder outlet obstruction
2. Sexual dysfunction (decrease or loss of libido, impotency) related to effects of therapy
3. Anxiety related to impact of living with uncertainty, relentless worry, and of being in pain

Complications of Metastatic Prostatic Cancer

Bone pain, spinal cord compression from vertebral collapse, pathologic fractures.

Nursing Interventions

A. Achieving Relief of Pain and Discomfort

1. Support patient undergoing radiation therapy—radiation therapy to bony lesions may give significant pain improvement.

2. Monitor catheter drainage, via either suprapubic or urethral catheter, when maintaining the patency of urethral passage becomes difficult.
3. See that the pain is effectively controlled.
   a. Encourage patient to take prescribed aspirin or nonsteroidal anti-inflammatory drugs for reduction of mild pain; oral narcotics require monitoring and adjustment.
   b. Be sure that patient is not undermedicated.
   c. Help family understand that addiction is not a concern.
   d. Teach family member how to administer drugs IM when patient cannot tolerate oral narcotics.
   e. Assist patient to use progressive relaxation techniques; use music tapes for relaxation.

B. Coping With Sexual Dysfunction

1. Be aware that the patient may be in ill health and suffering from pain, weight loss, and the effects of endocrine therapy or chemotherapy; in this event, the patient may not be much concerned with sexuality.
2. Give the patient permission to communicate his concerns and sexual needs.
3. Understand the stages (shock and denial, mourning, resolution) the patient goes through concerning sexual dysfunction.
4. Expect some patient feelings of depression, anxiety, anger, and regression.
5. Help the patient to use positive coping strategies (sexual counseling, learning other options of sexual expression, consideration of penile implant).

C. Attending to Anxieties

1. Develop a trusting relationship with patient. Avoid displaying value judgments regarding his feelings.
2. Be able to acknowledge the impact of the disease on the patient's existence.
3. Validate his feelings (anxiety, anger, helplessness, hopelessness).
4. Give repeated explanations of treatment; identify and correct misconceptions—this helps patient gain some feeling of control.
5. Try to address what patient is actually worried about; think about the patient from the patient's point of view.
6. Help patient/family set reachable small goals.
7. Comfort the patient with nurturing voice, touch, eye contact, and expert physical care.

Evaluation

1. Reports pain relief; requests medication when needed; is free of urinary symptoms.
2. Verbalizes coping strategies in dealing with sexual dysfunction.
3. Appears less anxious; sleeping at longer intervals; discusses his feelings and situation with family.

Management of the Patient Undergoing Prostatic Surgery

Surgical Procedures

A. Four Approaches for Prostatectomy

1. Transurethral removal of prostatic tissue by an instrument introduced through urethra.
2. Open surgical removal of prostate (procedures used are named for area of incision).

   a. Perineal
   b. Retropubic
   c. Suprapubic

B. Factors Influencing Choice of Surgical Approach

1. Size of gland and severity of obstruction
2. Age and condition of the patient
3. Presence of associated disease(s)

Preoperative Evaluation and Management

1. Renal function studies—to determine if there is renal impairment from prostatic back pressure and to evaluate renal reserve.
2. Hematologic investigation—to ascertain specific clotting defects since hemorrhage is a major postoperative complication.
3. Cardiac-supporting drugs—when indicated; also help alleviate renal symptoms.
4. Antibiotics—according to culture and sensitivity tests, to combat and control infection.
5. Intravenous fluids—according to patient's requirements as indicated by clinical status and serum electrolyte determinations.
6. Type and crossmatch for blood transfusions.

Preoperative Nursing Interventions

1. Maintain adequate bladder drainage via indwelling catheter or suprapubic cystostomy—renal function usually improves with reestablishment of drainage.
   a. Introduce indwelling catheter if the patient has continuing retention, if residual urine is more than 75–100 ml., or if renal function has been impaired by back pressure of urine into the upper tract.
   b. Assist with cystostomy if patient cannot tolerate urethral catheter.
2. Watch the patient closely after drainage is instituted—blood pressure fluctuates and renal function may decline first few days after drainage is established.
3. Ensure adequate hydration—the patient is frequently dehydrated from self-limitation of fluids because of frequency.
   a. Encourage fluid intake of 2500–3000 ml. daily (if cardiac reserve is adequate)—to help in overcoming azotemia.
   b. Weigh the patient daily and monitor fluid intake and output.
4. See page 52 for general preoperative nursing interventions.

Nursing Assessment

1. Review findings on past and present health status and results of laboratory evaluations.
2. Ask patient to describe presenting urinary problem: decreased force of urinary flow, decreased ability to initiate voiding, urgency, frequency, nocturia, dysuria, urinary retention, hematuria.
3. Question patient about back pain, flank pain, lower abdominal or suprapubic discomfort.
4. Observe the functional ability of the patient: how active is he?
5. Watch for any other clinical manifestations, as older individual may have atypical manifestations.
6. Evaluate cognitive, behavioral, and emotional status.
7. Find out about the patient's social support network: identify present and potential care-givers.

Nursing Diagnoses

1. Altered pattern of urinary elimination related to indwelling urethral catheter, bladder spasms, and nature of the surgery.
2. Pain and discomfort related to surgical procedure, bladder spasms, and catheter placement.
3. Potential for infection related to bacterial invasion of the incision.
4. Anxiety related to incontinence, difficulty in voiding, and sexual function.
5. Knowledge deficit of postoperative self-care and after-effects of surgery.

Nursing Interventions

A. Monitoring and Preventing Complications

1. Evaluate for shock and hemorrhage.
   a. Watch for evidence of hemorrhage in drainage bag, on dressings, and at incision site.
   b. Take blood pressure, pulse, and respiration as frequently as clinical condition indicates. Compare with preoperative vital sign readings to assess degree of hypotension present.
      (1) Observe for cold, sweating skin, pallor, restlessness, fall in blood pressure, increasing pulse rate.
      (2) Apply manual traction on the urethral catheter as directed to help stop bleeding; release traction intermittently and reassess the bleeding.
      (3) Irrigate the bladder as directed (see below).
      (4) Prepare patient for blood component therapy or transfusion.
      (5) Prepare for surgical intervention if bleeding persists.
2. Monitor for other postoperative complications.
   a. Monitor incision for induration, erythema, purulent drainage.
   b. Watch for signs of urinary infection, septic shock, urethritis (from catheter), urinary fistula, epididymitis.
   c. Deep vein thrombosis/pulmonary embolism.
   d. Late complications: urethral stricture, internal meatal stenosis.

B. Establishing Adequate Drainage of the Bladder

1. Utilize a closed sterile gravity system of drainage—3-way system is useful in controlling bleeding; irrigating system keeps clots from forming (does not correct the *cause* of bleeding).
2. Watch drainage for evidence of increased bleeding—bright red urine indicates arterial bleeding; dark red urine suggests venous bleeding.
3. Encourage oral fluids to ensure a high urine volume to discourage clot formation.
4. Watch for bladder distention, which stretches the prostatic urethra and may increase bleeding—usually caused by clots/retained prostate chips in bladder.
5. Irrigate bladder (amount and time prescribed by urologist) to avoid clot formation in the bladder.
   a. Frequency of bladder irrigation determined by amount of bleeding.
   b. Irrigation is adjusted to keep urine a light pink to straw color, free of clots, and transparent in appearance.
   c. Irrigate catheter *gently* if it is occluded—catheter opening may be obstructed by blood clot, tissue remnant, or by being in contact with the bladder wall.
      (1) Rotate catheter to move drainage eye of catheter away from bladder wall/clot.
      (2) Irrigate catheter with small amount of sterile fluid; too much force or fluid may damage recently operated area.
      (3) Apply *gentle* suction—strong suction on a recently occluded vessel can cause bleeding.
      (4) Avoid overdistending bladder—may produce secondary hemorrhage by stretching the coagulated vessels in the prostatic capsule.
6. Maintain an input and output record, including the amount of fluid used for irrigation.
7. Tape the drainage tubing (not the catheter) to shaved inner thigh—to prevent traction on bladder. (However, traction on the catheter by the urologist may control bleeding.)
8. Tape cystostomy catheter to lateral abdomen.
9. Note time and amount of each voiding after removal of catheter.
   a. May be urinary leakage around wound several days after removal of catheter in perineal, suprapubic, and retropubic surgery.
   b. Cystostomy tube may be removed before or after removal of urethral catheter.

C. Relieving Pain and Discomfort

1. Keep the patient quiet and comfortable during *immediate* postoperative period to prevent episodes of bleeding.
   When a patient experiences pain following prostatectomy, it may cause him to strain (from bladder irritability)—this causes pelvic vein engorgement and promotes venous hemorrhage and clot formation.
2. Administer prescribed analgesic or tranquilizer.
   a. Take blood pressure before administering tranquilizers and analgesics.
   b. Give pain medication before irrigation if bladder spasms are severe.
3. Explain again to the patient the purpose of the catheter.
   a. Tell the patient that the urge to void is caused by the presence of the catheter and bladder spasm (painful contractions of muscles of bladder wall and neck).
      (1) Watch catheter tubing—a column of urine moving between pain episodes or when patient coughs may indicate bladder spasms.
      (2) A frequent cause of spasm is the catheter touching (and stimulating) the posterior bladder wall.
      (3) Gently draw catheter back toward external meatus.
   b. Encourage him to refrain from pulling on catheter—will cause bleeding, clots, plugging of catheter, and distention.
   c. Tape catheter to lower abdomen (see Fig. 27-5) to prevent pressure on penoscrotal junction.
   d. Wash urethral meatus adjacent to catheter with water; rinse and apply an antibacterial ointment as directed.
4. Be alert for blockage of urinary drainage tube by kinking, mucus plugs, and blood clots.
5. Avoid rectal instrumentation (thermometers, rectal tubes, enemas) following prostatic surgery. Because the rectum is close to the prostatic fossa, instrumentation may be dangerous until healing has taken place.

6. Help the patient to ambulate as quickly as possible; avoid sitting for prolonged periods, since this increases intra-abdominal pressure and increases the possibility of bleeding.
7. Promote the comfort of the patient who has perineal sutures.
   a. Wash perineum with prescribed solution. Dry carefully.
   b. Use heat lamp to perineal area (cover scrotum with towel)—to promote healing.

Discharge Planning and Patient Education

Instruct the patient as follows:

A. Urinary Control

1. After the catheter is removed, there may be some burning on urination and/or frequent desire to void. These symptoms will disappear in a few weeks.
2. Expect urinary dribbling for a period of time (especially after catheter removal). Urinary incontinence may follow any type of prostatic surgery.
3. Exercises to gain urinary control.
   a. Perineal exercises
      (1) Tense the perineal muscles by pressing the buttocks together. Hold this position as long as possible; relax.
      (2) Perform this exercise 10–20 times each hour.
      (3) Continue with perineal exercises until full urinary control is gained.
   b. When starting to void
      (1) Shut off the stream for a few seconds.
      (2) Continue with full voiding.
      (3) Continue this exercise with each urination until control improves; may take many weeks.
4. Urinate as soon as the first desire to do so is felt.
5. The urine may be cloudy for several weeks after surgery. As the prostate area heals, the cloudiness will disappear.
6. Avoid activities that increase chance of postoperative bleeding: excessive physical activity; sitting for prolonged periods (e.g., long automobile rides); excessive use of alcohol.
7. Drink adequate fluids (8 glasses/day), since dehydration increases tendency for clot obstruction.
8. Do not take anticholinergics and diuretics unless by direct prescription of the physician.

B. Sexual Functioning

1. Prostatectomy does not usually cause impotence—penile erection depends on intact spinal cord, intact autonomic nerves to penis, normal erectile tissue/adequate blood supply, and psychological well-being; a simple prostatectomy does not affect these factors.
   a. Total prostatectomy (removal of entire prostatic contents and capsule) results in impotence, since the nerves and muscular tissue surrounding the capsule (which have a function in penile erection) have been severed.
   b. More recently, nerve-sparing radical prostatectomy is being done to prevent impotency.
   c. Penile prosthesis (inflatable, semi-rigid, and flexible types) may be surgically implanted—used to make the penis rigid for sexual intercourse.
2. In most instances sexual activity may be resumed in 6–8 weeks; this is the time required for healing of the prostatic fossa to take place.
3. Do not be alarmed if no fluid appears on ejaculation; following ejaculation, the fluid goes into the bladder and is voided at the next urination.
   a. This does not reduce the level of sexual performance or satisfaction.
   b. The urine voided after intercourse may have a milky appearance.

C. Other Considerations

1. Avoid straining and strenuous exercises.
2. Report to the physician any bleeding or a decrease in the size of the urinary stream.

Evaluation

1. Achieves improved pattern of urinary elimination; reports absence of frequency, urgency, or bladder fullness; displays no palpable suprapubic distention after voiding.
2. Is free of pain.
3. Is free of infection; demonstrates wound healing; no signs of inflammation; maintains vital signs within normal limits.
4. Shows lessening anxiety; gaining control in voiding; describes reasons for change in sexual functioning.
5. Responds positively to self-care; does exercises to promote bladder control.

Conditions Affecting the Testes and Adjacent Structures

Testicular Cancer

The majority of testicular cancers are of germ cell origin; the most common germinal tumors in adults are seminoma, embryonal carcinoma, teratocarcinoma, and choriocarcinoma.

Clinical Features

1. The etiology of testicular tumors is unknown, but there is a relationship between cryptorchidism (failure of the testes to descend into the scrotum) and tumor occurrence.
2. The majority of testicular tumors are malignant; men aged 20–34 years are at greatest risk.
3. Testicular tumors metastasize to the retroperitoneal lymph nodes with subsequent involvement of the mediastinal lymph nodes, lungs, and liver.
4. Testicular germ cell tumors are considered potentially curable.

Clinical Manifestations

1. Painless swelling or enlargement of the testis; accompanied by sensation of heaviness in scrotum
2. Pain in the testis (if patient has epididymitis or bleeding into tumor)

Diagnostic Evaluation

1. Elevated serum markers: human chorionic gonadotropins (HCG) and alpha-fetoprotein (AFP); assay of tumor markers also used for diagnosis, detection of early recurrence, staging, and monitoring response to therapy.

2. Scrotal ultrasonography—identifies location of lesion and differentiates between solid and cystic lesion.
3. Chest film—to seek pulmonary or mediastinal metastases.
4. CT scanning of chest, abdomen, and pelvis—to evaluate retroperitoneal lymph nodes and to follow progress of therapy.

Management

(Choice of treatment depends on tumor histology and stage of disease)

A. Surgery

1. Inguinal orchiectomy—removal of testis and its tunica and spermatic cord
2. Retroperitoneal lymph node dissection (RPLND) usually performed after orchiectomy for staging and therapeutic purposes (testicular cancer metastasizes to retroperitoneal lymph nodes)
   a. Long-term morbidity is infertility due to ejaculatory dysfunction; does not influence erections and orgasm; a modified nerve-sparing unilateral lymphadenectomy can be done on selected patients, thus preserving ejaculation.
   b. Unilateral orchiectomy eliminates half of germinal cells, thus reducing sperm count; chemotherapy and radiation may also affect fertility.

B. Radiation Therapy

Radiation therapy to lymphatic drainage pathways (after orchiectomy) is used in most patients with testicular cancer; may be curative or palliative, depending on circumstances.

C. Chemotherapy

1. Cisplatin combination therapy used in treatment of primary tumor and regional lymphatic metastases and in managing distant metastatic disease.
2. Discomforts of chemotherapy include significant nausea and vomiting, alopecia, myalgias, gastrointestinal cramping, and mucositis.

Nursing Interventions

1. See page 56 for care of the patient following surgery, page 108 for care of the patient undergoing radiation therapy, and page 103 for care of the patient undergoing chemotherapy.
2. Nursing interventions following retroperitoneal node dissection
   a. Monitor for paralytic ileus, which is common following extensive resection.
   b. Defer oral feedings until intestinal activity returns.
3. The younger patient should have the opportunity to discuss depositing sperm in sperm bank; however, he may be ineligible for sperm banking because of disease-impaired sperm production.
4. Inform the patient of the following:
   a. Genital cancer is not "punishment" for real/imagined sexual activity.
   b. Orchiectomy will not diminish virility.
   c. Radiotherapy to the abdomen will cause no change in sexual performance but may diminish semen volume.
5. Refer the patient to a social worker as required; frequent hospitalizations may be necessary with interruption of work/personal life.
6. Be aware of community resources that can be used to assist patient and family, e.g., American Cancer Society, Veteran's Administration, marriage counselor, Medicaid/Medicare, Make Today Count.

Patient Education

1. There is a risk of a second tumor; therefore, patient should be followed by health care team indefinitely.
2. Carry out periodic self-examinations of the testes (see Guidelines, below).

Guidelines Self-Examination for Testicular Tumor

1. The testis is easily accessible for self-examination. Most tumors are palpable and can be detected by self-examination.
2. The hormonally active years (15–35) are the tumor-prone years.

Procedure	Action (by Patient)	Explanation
	1. Examine for testicular tumor periodically, preferably while showering/bathing.	1. Detection of abnormalities is more readily accomplished after or during a warm shower or bath, when the scrotum wall is relaxed.
	2. Use both hands to palpate (feel). Carefully examine all scrotal contents (Fig. 27-14).	2. A small lump (nodule) can slip away from one hand. You can feel differences in weight between the testicles by using both hands.
	3. Locate the epididymis; this is the irregular cordlike structure on the top and at the back of the testicle that stores and transports sperm. The spermatic cord (and vas) extends upward from the epididymis.	3. It is important to know what the epididymis feels like so you will not confuse it with an abnormality.
	4. Feel each testis between the thumb and first 2 fingers of each hand.	4. The testes lie freely in the scrotum, are oval shaped, and measure 4–5 cm. in length, 3 cm. in width, and about 2 cm. in thickness.
	5. Note size, shape, abnormal tenderness.	5. An abnormality may be felt as a firm area on the front or side of the testicle.
	6. Stand in front of mirror and look for changes in size/shape of scrotum.	6. It is normal to find one testis larger than the other.

(continued)

Guidelines Self-Examination for Testicular Tumor *(continued)*

Procedure *(continued)*	**Nursing Action**	**Rationale/Amplification**

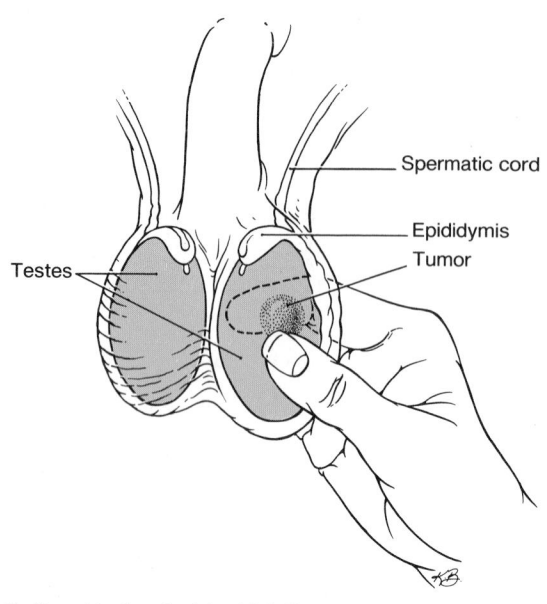

Spermatic cord

Epididymis
Tumor

Testes

Figure 27-14. *Palpation for testicular tumor. Using the fingertips and thumb, the epididymis, testes, and spermatic cord are located bilaterally.*

7. Report to the physician/clinic if there is any evidence of a small, pea-size lump or other abnormality.

Epididymitis

Epididymitis is an infection of the epididymis that usually descends from an infected prostate or urinary tract.

Causes

1. Complication of prolonged catheter drainage, bacterial prostatitis, gonococcal or nongonococcal bacterial urethritis
2. In men under 40, sexually transmitted organisms are the main etiologic agents: *Chlamydia trachomatis, Ureaplasma urealyticum, Neisseria gonorrhoeae*
3. In older men, the main causes are bladder outlet obstruction and urinary bacteria (*E. coli, Pseudomonas aeruginosa*)

Clinical Manifestations

1. Localized scrotal pain and tenderness
2. Edema, redness, and tenderness of scrotum
3. Chills and fever
4. Pyuria and bacteriuria

Diagnostic Evaluation

1. Examination of initial and midstream urine sample to detect bacteria
2. Examination of urethral discharge and expressed prostatic secretions to establish causative organism

Management

1. Antimicrobial therapy after collection of specimens
2. Analgesics for severe pain relief
3. Intermittent cold compresses to scrotum to control swelling and for pain relief
4. Local heat or sitz bath later—to hasten resolution of inflammatory process
5. Stool softeners

Nursing Interventions

1. Monitor for complications: possible abscess formation—look for fever, leukocytosis, scrotal erythema and edema, epididymal/testicular tenderness.
2. Encourage bedrest during the acute phase.
3. Apply scrotal support for enlarged testicle. Use rolled towel under scrotum or scrotal bridge—to relieve edema and discomfort, to improve venous drainage, and to take tension off the cord. A cotton-lined athletic supporter may promote comfort.

Patient Education

Instruct the patient as follows:
1. Avoid straining (lifting, defecation, and sexual activity) until infection is under control.
2. Sex partners of patients with chlamydial or gonorrheal urethritis or epididymitis should be examined and treated.
3. Reassure the patient that sexual performance should not be affected after the inflammation has subsided.
4. It may take 2–4 weeks or longer for epididymis to return to normal.
5. If patient does not respond to treatment, he should report for re-examination to make certain that there is no mass within the body of testicle.
6. Uncontrolled infection may impair fertility.

Hydrocele

Hydrocele is a collection of fluid generally in the tunica vaginalis of the testicle, although it may also occur within the spermatic cord.

Causes

(Caused by defective or inadequate reabsorption of normally produced hydrocele fluid)
1. Secondary to infection, trauma, or idiopathic
2. Secondary response to an intrascrotal lesion (tumor)

Clinical Manifestations/Diagnostic Evaluation

1. Enlargement of the scrotum
2. Usually painless until fluid accumulation is large enough to cause pressure
3. Transmits light when transilluminated
4. Ultrasonography differentiates between normal/abnormal testis within hydrocele

Management

1. No treatment is required unless there is significant underlying cause (tumor) or if the hydrocele is large, uncomfortable, and cosmetically unacceptable to the patient.
2. Surgical intervention—hydrocelectomy (excision of tunica vaginalis of testis) for removal of fluid and control of swelling

Nursing Interventions

1. Monitor for complications
   a. Formation of a hematoma in the loose tissues of the scrotum—keep surgical drains in place until bleeding has stopped.
   b. Scrotal edema—reassure patient that this is due to dissection and manipulation of scrotal skin during surgery.
2. Instruct the patient to apply ice pack intermittently to scrotum for the first few hours postoperatively to reduce pain.
3. Advise patient to apply scrotal support for comfort.

Varicocele

Varicocele is an abnormal dilation of the veins of the pampiniform venous plexus in the scrotum (network of veins from the testis and the epididymis, constituting part of the spermatic cord).

Clinical Manifestations

1. Subfertility may occur with varicocele.
2. A dragging sensation in the scrotum is usually the patient's chief complaint.
3. Varicocele on the right may indicate retroperitoneal tumor.

Diagnostic Evaluation

Palpation of intrascrotal mass (with patient in upright position) that disappears in a short time after he has been lying down.

Management

1. Scrotal support to relieve discomfort
2. Surgical intervention—ligation and excision of veins (varicocelectomy); may be performed on an outpatient basis

Nursing Interventions and Patient Education

1. Apply ice bag for first few hours postoperatively to relieve edema.
2. Apply scrotal support for comfort.
3. Advise patient of the following:
   a. Notify surgeon if temperature exceeds 38.3°C. (101°F.), if he bleeds from the operative site, or if his pain is not relieved by the prescribed analgesic.
   b. Avoid driving for about 1 week; avoid heavy labor or strenuous physical exertion until permitted by surgeon.

Vasectomy

Vasectomy is the surgical procedure of interrupting the continuity of the vas deferens to prevent passage of sperm or retrograde passage of bacteria. It is performed as a sterilization procedure or to prevent ascending infection that can result in epididymitis.

Underlying Considerations

1. A vasectomy interrupts the passage of the sperm. This procedure has no effect on sexual potency, erection, ejaculation, or production of male hormones.
2. Seminal fluid is mostly manufactured in the seminal vesicles and prostate, which are unaffected by vasectomy.
   a. There will be no noticeable decrease in the amount of ejaculated fluid; the sperm accounts for less than 5% of the volume. The sperm cells are reabsorbed into the body.
   b. Psychological problems have been noted in an occasional patient following this procedure.
3. A vasectomy can be done on an outpatient basis with local anesthesia.
4. A legal consent form must be obtained, usually from the patient and his partner.
5. The patient should be advised that he will be sterile but that potency will not be altered following a bilateral vasectomy. Rarely is there a spontaneous reanastomosis resulting in pregnancy.
6. A vasectomy may not be reversible and should be considered permanent; microsurgical techniques are being used for vasectomy reversal (vasovasotomy); success rates are promising.

Complications

1. Bleeding and hematoma
2. Sperm granuloma—due to extravasation of sperm
3. Infection: abscess, epididymitis
4. Recanalization of vas deferens

Nursing Interventions

1. Apply ice bags intermittently (10–15 minutes every 2–3 hours) to the scrotal area during the first day following procedure—to reduce swelling and relieve discomfort.
2. Advise the patient of the following:
   a. Remain in bed the rest of the day of the procedure.
   b. Discoloration of scrotal skin, swelling and edema are to be expected.
   c. Wear jockey shorts or an athletic supporter for added comfort and support.
   d. Use acetaminophen (Tylenol) for discomfort; avoid aspirin-containing products.

Patient Education

Instruct the patient as follows:

1. The primary function of the testicle(s) is the production of hormones and of sperm. A vasectomy will not interfere with these functions, but it will interrupt the descent of sperm from the testicle to the ejaculatory ducts.
2. Avoid strenuous activities for several days.
3. Avoid sexual activity for first week following surgery to allow healing.
4. Contraceptives should be used until the sperm stored distal to the point of interruption of the vas is evacuated (2 negative semen specimens 1 month apart). *The patient is still fertile for a variable period of time after vasectomy.*
5. Absence of sperm must be demonstrated microscopically; laboratory tests confirm that no sperm are present in the seminal fluid.
6. A vasectomy does not prevent sexually transmitted disease.
7. Report any inflammatory process such as increasing pain, swelling, redness, or fever.

Conditions Affecting the Penis

Infections

1. *Chancre*—venereal ulceration caused by *Treponema pallidum* (see Syphilis, p. 903)
2. *Chancroid*—a sexually transmitted disease caused by *Haemophilus ducreyi;* usually 1 or several penile ulcers are present, as well as enlarged lymph nodes
3. *Genital herpes* (herpes simplex virus [HSV])—a sexually transmitted disease that produces multiple bilaterally distributed vesicles on or near the penis.
4. *Gonorrhea*—see pages 904–908.

Clinical Manifestations

Ulceration of the penis should be suspected as being sexually transmitted until proved otherwise.

Management

Varies greatly, depending on the cause of ulceration

Other Conditions

Phimosis

A condition in which the foreskin is constricted so that it cannot be retracted over the glans.

Management consists of:

1. Antibacterial/antifungal ointment and warm baths
2. Debridement, circumcision, meatomy—in more advanced disease

Paraphimosis

A condition in which the foreskin is retracted behind the glans, and because of narrowness and subsequent edema, cannot be reduced back to its normal position.

Priapism

An uncontrolled persistent erection of the penis occurring from neural or vascular causes, including sickle cell thrombosis, spinal cord tumors, and tumor invasion of the penis or its vessels. This condition is considered a urologic emergency.

Management includes bedrest, sedation, and/or surgery.

Carcinoma of the Penis

Carcinoma of the penis occurs in the skin of the penis; appears as a painless, wart-like growth or ulcer on the glans or coronal sulcus under the prepuce.

A. Prevention

1. Instruct the patient about proper hygiene—cancer associated with poor hygiene leading to build-up of retained smegma.

B. Management

1. Surgery (Moh's surgery; partial penectomy; radical penectomy for more invasive cancer)
2. Radiation and chemotherapy also used

Circumcision

Circumcision is the excision of the foreskin (prepuce) of the glans penis.

Clinical Indications

1. Usually done in infancy for hygienic purposes
2. In adults—phimosis; paraphimosis; recurrent infection of the glans and foreskin; personal desire of the patient

Postoperative Nursing Interventions

1. Watch for bleeding.
2. Change petrolatum (Vaseline) gauze dressing as directed.
3. Give analgesia as the patient's condition indicates; circumcision can be quite painful in the adult male.

Bibliography

Books

Blandy J. Operative Urology. 2nd ed. Boston, Blackwell Scientific Publications, 1986

Brenner BM and Lazarus JM. Acute Renal Failure. New York, Churchill Livingstone, 1988

Brenner BM and Rector FC Jr. The Kidney. 3rd ed, Vols 1 and 2. Philadelphia, WB Saunders, 1986

Cogan MG and Garovoy MR. Introduction to Dialysis. New York, Churchill Livingstone, 1985

Corriere JN Jr (ed). Essentials of Urology. New York, Churchill Livingstone, 1986

Dalton JR and Berquist EJ. Urinary Tract Infections. London, Croom Helm, 1987

Garovoy MR and Guttman RD. Renal Transplantation. New York, Churchill Livingstone, 1986

Gillenwater JY et al. Adult and Pediatric Urology, Vols 1 and 2. Chicago, Year Book Medical Pub, 1987

Gillit D, Stover J and Spinozzi NS. A Clinical Guide to Nutrition Care in End-Stage Renal Disease. Chicago, American Dietetic Association, 1987

Javadpour N (ed). Principles and Management of Testicular Cancer. New York, Thieme, 1986

Kandel LB, Harrison LH and McCullough DL. Extracorporeal Shock Wave

Lithotripsy. Mount Kisco, Futura Publishing, 1987

Kaufman JJ. Current Urologic Therapy. Philadelphia, WB Saunders, 1986

King LR, Stone A and Webster GD. Bladder Reconstruction and Continent Urinary Diversion. Chicago, Year Book Medical Pub, 1987

Kunin CM. Detection, Prevention and Management of Urinary Tract Infections. 4th ed. Philadelphia, Lea and Febiger, 1987

Mandal DK and Jennette JC. Diagnosis and Management of Renal Disease and Hypertension. Philadelphia, Lea and Febiger, 1988

Marshall FF. Urologic Complications. Chicago, Year Book Medical Pub, 1986

Mitch WE and Klahr S. Nutrition and the Kidney. Boston, Little, Brown & Co, 1988

Newman E, Price M and Magney J. Care of the Disabled Urinary Tract. Springfield, Charles C Thomas, 1986

Rous SN. Stone Disease. Orlando, Grune and Stratton, 1987

Schrier RW and Gottschalk CW. Diseases of the Kidney, Vols 1–3. Boston, Little, Brown & Co, 1988

Skinner DG and Lieskovsky G. Diagnosis and Management of Genitourinary Cancer. Philadelphia, WB Saunders, 1988

Smith DB and Johnson DE. Ostomy Care and the Cancer Patient: Surgical and Clinical Considerations. Orlando, Grune & Stratton, 1986

Smith JA Jr and Middleton RG. Clinical Management of Prostatic Cancer. Chicago, Year Book Medical Pub, 1987

Tanagho EA and McAninch JW. Smith's General Urology. 12th ed. Norwalk, Appleton and Lange, 1988

Walsh PC et al. Campbell's Urology, Vols 1–3, 5th ed. Philadelphia, WB Saunders, 1986

Whitfield HN and Hendry WF. Textbook of Genito-urinary Surgery, Vols 1 and 2. New York, Churchill Livingstone, 1985

Williams RD (ed). Advances in Urologic Oncology. New York, Macmillan, 1987

Yalla SV et al (eds). Neurourology and Urodynamics. New York, Macmillan, 1988

Journals

Cancer of the Bladder/Urinary Diversion

Broadwell DC. Rehabilitation needs of the patient with cancer. Cancer 1987 Aug 1; 60(3 Suppl):563–568

Brogna L and Lakaszawski M. Nursing management: The continent urostomy. J Enterostomal Ther 1986 Jul–Aug; 13(4):139–147

Cassileth BR and Steinfeld AD. Psychological preparation of the patient and family. Cancer 1987 Aug 1; 60(3 Suppl):547–552

Denis L et al (eds.) Developments in bladder cancer. Prog Clin Biol Res 1986; 221:1–238

Donohue JP (ed). Controversies in urologic oncology. Urol Clin North Am 1987 Nov; 14(4):657–804

Friedell GH. Urinary bladder cancer. Cancer 1987 Aug 1; 60(Suppl 3):496–501

Gray M. Treatment modalities for bladder cancer. Semin Oncol Nurs 1986 Nov; 2(4):260–264

Grieg BJ. Interventions of the ET nurse with the continent urinary Kock pouch patient. J Enterostomal Ther 1986 Nov–Dec; 13(6):226–231

Grunberg KJ. Sexual rehabilitation of the cancer patient undergoing ostomy surgery. J Enterostomal Ther 1986 Jul–Aug; 13(4):148–152

Hanson MJ. The challenge of home care. J Enterostomal Ther 1986 May–Jun; 13(3):118–120

Herr HW. Intravesical therapy: A critical review. Urol Clin North Am 1987 May; 14(2):399–401

Messing EM. Early stage bladder cancer. Wis Med J 1987 Feb; 86(2):14–17

Olson CA (ed). Continent urinary diversion. Semin Urol 1987 Feb; 5(1):1–79

Parry WL and Hemstreet GP III. Cancer detection by quantitative fluorescence image analysis. J Urol 1988 Feb; 139(2):270–274

Pontes JE and Smyth EM. Selection of the type of urinary diversion in conjunction with radical cystectomy. J Urol 1987 Jun; 137(6):1154–1155

Prout GR Jr et al. Photodynamic therapy with hematoporphyrin derivative in the treatment of superficial transitional-cell carcinoma of the bladder. N Engl J Med 1987 Nov 12; 317(20):1251–1255

Reddy PK and Lange PH. Bladder replacement with sigmoid colon after radical cystoprostatectomy. Urology 1987 Apr; 29(4):368–371

Schover LR. Sexuality and fertility in urologic cancer patients. Cancer 1987 Aug 1; 60(3 Suppl):553–558

Skinner DG et al (eds). Urinary diversion. Curr Probl Surg 1987; 24(7):407–471

Soloway MS. Introduction and overview of intravesical therapy for superficial bladder cancer. Urology 1988 Mar; 31(3 Suppl):5–16

Soloway MS. Selecting initial therapy for bladder cancer. Cancer 1987 Aug 1; 3(3 Suppl):502–513

Torrence RJ et al. Prognostic factors in patients treated with intravesical bacillus Calmette–Guerin for superficial bladder cancer. J Urol 1988 May; 139(5):941–944

Watt RC. Nursing management of a patient with a urinary diversion. Semin Oncol Nurs 1986 Nov; 2(4):265–269

Whitmore WF. Toward the rational management of bladder cancer: An overview. Urology 1988 Feb; 31(2 Suppl):5–8

Catheter Management

Bristoll SL et al. The mythical danger of rapid urinary drainage. Am J Nurs 1989 Mar; 89(3):344–345

Crow R, Mulhall A and Chapman R. Indwelling catheterization and related nursing practice. J Adv Nurs 1988 Jul; 13(4):489–495

Maynard FM and Glass J. Management of the neuropathic bladder by clean intermittent catheterisation: 5 year outcomes. Paraplegia 1987 Apr; 25(2):106–110

Schaeffer AJ. Catheter-associated bacteriuria. Urol Clin North Am 1986 Nov; 13(4):735–747

Wein AJ and Van Arsdalen KN. Nonsurgical management of neuropathic voiding dysfunction. Semin Urol 1985 Aug; 3(3):216–237

Dialysis/Transplantation

Carlson DM et al. Functional status of patients with end-stage renal disease. Mayo Clin Proc 1987 May; 62(5):338–344

Casati S et al. Benefits and risks of protracted treatment with human recombinant erythropoietin in patients having haemodialysis. Br Med J 1987 Oct 4; 295(6605):1017–1020

Cheesbrough JS, Finch RG and Burden RP. A prospective study of the mechanisms of infection associated with hemodialysis catheters. J Infect Dis 1986 Oct; 154(4):579–589

Ferrans CE, Powers MJ and Kasch CR. Satisfaction with health care of hemodialysis patients. Res Nurs Health 1987 Dec; 10(6):367–374

Glass CA et al. Factors related to sexual functioning in male patients undergoing hemodialysis with kidney transplants. Arch Sex Behav 1987 Jun; 16(3):189–207

Gokal R et al. Outcome in patients on continuous ambulatory peritoneal dialysis and haemodialysis: 4-year analysis of a prospective multicentre study. Lancet 1987 Nov 14; 2(8568):1105–1109

Hunter DW and So SK. Dialysis access: Radiographic evaluation and management. Radiol Clin North Am 1987 Mar; 25(2):249–260

Keown PA and Stiller CB. Kidney transplantation. Surg Clin North Am 1986 Jun; 66(3):517–539

Khanna R and Oreopoulos DG. Dialysis: Continuous ambulatory peritoneal dialysis and haemodialysis. Clin Endocrinol Metab 1986 Nov; 15(4):823–836

Kherlakian GM et al. Comparison of autogenous fistula versus expanded polytetrafluoroethylene graft fistula for angioaccess in hemodialysis. Am J Surg 1986 Aug; 152(2):238–243

Knudsen PKK. Diet and dialysis. Br Med J 1987 Sep 26; 295(6601):767–768

Koch KM et al. Advances in extracorporal blood treatment. Clin Nephrol 1986; 26(Suppl 1):S1–S83

Nelson EW. Venous access techniques. Urol Clin North Am 1986 Aug; 13(3):475–487

Nova G. Dialyzable drugs. Am J Nurs 1987 Jul; 87(7):933–942

Raju S. PTFE grafts for hemodialysis access. Ann Surg 1987 Nov; 206(5):666–673

Rizzuti RP, Hale JC and Burkart TE. Extended patency of expanded polytetrafluoroethylene grafts for vascular access using optimal configuration and revisions. Surg Gynecol Obstet 1988 Jan; 166(1):23–27

Infections

Andriole VT. Urinary tract infections: Recent developments. J Infect Dis 1987 Dec; 156(6):865–869

Fierer J. Acute pyelonephritis. Urol Clin North Am 1987 May; 14(2):251–256

Fowler JE Jr. Urinary tract infections in women. Urol Clin North Am 1986 Nov; 13(4):673–683

Glockner WM et al. Plasma exchange and immunosuppression in rapidly progressive glomerulonephritis: A controlled, multi-center study. Clin Nephrol 1988 Jan; 29(1):1–8

Johnson JR and Stamm WE. Diagnosis and treatment of acute urinary tract infections. Infect Dis Clin North Am 1987 Dec; 1(4):773–801

Nicolle LE and Ronald AR. Recurrent urinary tract infection in adult women: Diagnosis and treatment. Infect Dis Clin North Am 1987 Dec; 1(4):793–806

Roberts JD. Pyelonephritis, cortical abscess and perinephric abscess. Urol Clin North Am 1986 Nov; 13(4):637–645

Shalom R. Problem areas in the management of urinary tract infections. J Am Coll Health 1987 Nov; 36(3):165–170

Shea DJ. Pyelonephritis and female urinary tract infection. Emerg Med Clin North Am 1988 Aug; 6(3):403–417

Stein GE et al. A multicenter comparative trial of three-day norfloxacin vs ten-day sulfamethoxazole and trimethoprim for the treatment of uncomplicated urinary tract infections. Arch Intern Med 1987 Oct; 147(10):1760–1762

Wilhelm MP and Edson RS. Antimicrobial agents in urinary tract infections. Mayo Clin Proc 1987 Nov; 67(11):1025–1031

Prostatic Conditions

Consensus Conference. The management of clinically localized prostate cancer. JAMA 1987 Nov 20; 258(19):2727–2730

Editorial. Medical treatment of benign prostatic hyperplasia. Lancet 1988 May 14; 1(8594):1083–1084

Ercole CJ et al. Prostatic specific antigen and prostatic acid phosphatase in the monitoring and staging of patients with prostatic cancer. J Urol 1987 Nov; 138(5):1181–1184

Gaddipati J, Ahmed T and Friedland M. Prostatic and bladder cancer in the elderly. Clin Geriatr Med 1987 Nov; 3(4):649–667

Grayhack JT, Keeler TC and Kozlowski JM. Carcinoma of the prostate: Hormonal therapy. Cancer 1987 Aug 1; 60(3 Suppl):589–601

Guthrie TH Jr and Watson P. Prostate cancer. Am Fam Physician 1987 Oct; 36(4):217–224

Hilaris BS, Nori D and Batata M. Cancer of the prostate: Current perspectives. Cancer Invest 1987; 5(5):459–468

LaFollette SS. Radical retropubic prostatectomy. AORN J 1987 Jan; 45(1):57–63, 66–71

Loughlin KR and Whitmore WF. Managing prostate disorders in middle age and beyond. Geriatrics 1987 Jul; 42(7):45–56

Malone PR et al. Prostatectomy: Patients' perceptions and long-term follow-up. Br J Urol 1988 Mar; 61(3):234–238

Meares EM Jr. Acute and chronic prostatitis: Diagnosis and treatment. Infect Dis Clin North Am 1987 Dec; 1(4):855–873

Melamed AJ. Current concepts in the treatment of prostate cancer. Drug Intell Clin Pharm 1987 Mar; 21(3):247–254

Murphy GP et al. Prostate cancer. Part A: Research, endocrine treatment, and histopathology. Progr Clin Biol Res 1987; 243A:1–571

O'Brien WM and Lynch JH. Current approaches to prostate cancer. Hosp Pract (Off) 1988 Jan 15; 23(1):143–145, 149–150, 155 passim

Rifkin MD. Endorectal sonography of the prostate: Clinical implications. AJR 1987 Jun; 148(6):1137–1142

Schover LR. Sexuality and fertility in urologic cancer patients. Cancer 1987 Aug 1; 60(3 Suppl):553–558

Smith RA, Wake R and Soloway MS. Benign prostatic hyperplasia. Postgrad Med 1987 May 1; 83(6):79–85

Stamey TA et al. Prostate-specific antigen as a serum marker for adenocarcinoma of the prostate. N Engl J Med 1987 Oct 8; 317(15):909–916

Walsh PC and Lepor H. The role of radical prostatectomy in the management of prostatic cancer. Cancer 1987 Aug 1; 60(3 Suppl):526–537

Renal Failure: Acute and Chronic

Amerio A et al. Acute renal failure. Adv Exp Med Biol 1987; 212:1–324

Burke JF. The etiology and management of acute renal failure. Del Med J 1987 Apr; 59(4):273–278

Corwin HL and Bonventre JV. Acute renal failure in the intensive care unit. Part I. Intensive Care Med 1988; 14(1):10–16

Corwin HL and Bonventre JV. Acute renal failure in the intensive care unit. Part II. Intensive Care Med 1988; 14(2):86–96

Davis RF. Acute renal failure following traumatic injury or major operation. Int Anesthesiol Clin 1987 Spring; 25(1):117–142

El Nahas AM. Management of progressive renal failure: The role of dietary manipulations. Postgrad Med J 1987 Aug; 63(742):611–615

Eschbach JW. Correction of the anemia of end-stage renal disease with recombinant human erythropoietin: Results of a combined phase I and II clinical trial. N Engl J Med 1987 Jan 8; 316(2):73–78

Faubert PF and Porush JG. Managing hypertension in chronic renal disease. Geriatrics 1987 Jan; 42(1):49–51, 55–58

Goodship THJ and Mitch WE. Nutritional approaches to preserving renal function. Adv Intern Med 1988; 33:337–355

Hong BA et al. Depressive symptomatology and treatment in patients with end-stage renal disease. Psychol Med 1987 Feb; 17(1):185–190

House A. Psychosocial problems of patients on the renal unit and their relation to treatment outcome. J Psychosom Res 1987; 31(4):441–452

Hyneck ML. Current concepts in clinical therapeutics: Drug therapy in acute renal failure. 1986 Nov; 5(11):892–910

Johnson CA and Chester MIS. Pathophysiology and treatment of the anemia of renal failure. Clin Pharmacol 1988 Feb; 7(2):117–122

Lange HW, Aeppli DM and Brown DC. Survival of patients with acute renal failure requiring dialysis after open heart surgery: Early prognostic indicators. Am Heart J 1987 May; 113(5):1138–1143

Mault JR et al. Continuous arteriovenous filtration: An effective treatment for surgical acute renal failure. Surgery 1987 Apr; 101(4):478–484

Muschio G et al (eds). Hypertension in renal failure. Contrib Nephrol 1987; 54:144–230

Pattison ME, Lee SM and Ogden DA. Continuous arteriovenous hemodiafiltration: An aggressive approach to the management of acute renal failure. Am J Kidney Dis 1988 Jan; 11(1):43–47

Reed WE Jr and Sabatini S. The use of drugs in renal failure. Semin Nephrol 1986 Sep; 6(3):259–295

Rorer B, Tucker CM and Blake H. Long-term nurse-patient interactions: Factors in patient compliance or noncompliance to the dietary regimen. Health Psychol 1988; 7(1):35–46

Shen P-F and Zhang S-c. Acute renal failure and multiple organ system failure. Arch Surg 1987 Oct; 122(10):1131–1133

Siegal BR, Calsyn RJ and Cuddihee RM. The relationship of social support to psychological adjustment in end-stage renal disease patients. J Chronic Dis 1987; 40(4):337–344

Spiegel DM, Burnier M and Schrier RW. Acute renal failure. Postgrad Med 1987 Sep 15; 82(4):96–105

Van Duyn MAS. Acceptability of selected low-protein products for use in a potential diet therapy for chronic renal failure. J Am Diet Assoc 1987 Jul; 87(7):909–914

Zeller KR. Review: Effects of dietary protein and phosphorus restriction on the progression of chronic renal failure. Am J Med Sci 1987 Nov; 294(5):328–340

Renal Tumor

Bracken RB. Renal carcinoma. Semin Roentgenol 1987 Oct; 22(4):241–247

deKernion JB. Renal cell carcinoma. J Urol 1986 Oct; 136(4):882

Felson B and Wiot JF (eds). Renal neoplasms. Semin Roentgenol 1987 Oct; 22(4):233–391

Linehan WM. Renal cell carcinoma. J Urol 1988 Feb; 139(2):540–541

Newson GD and Vugrin D. Etiologic factors in renal cell adenocarcinoma. Semin Nephrol 1987 Jun; 7(2):109–116

Novick AC. Partial nephrectomy for renal cell carcinoma. Urol Clin North Am 1987 May; 14(2):419–423

Paulson DF. Treatment strategies in renal carcinoma. Semin Nephrol 1987 Jun; 7(2):140–151

Ritchie AWS and deKernion JB. The natural history and clinical features of renal carcinoma. Semin Nephrol 1987 Jun; 7(2):131–139

Rotolo JE, O'Brien WM and Lynch JH. Renal cell carcinoma. Hosp Pract (Off) 1987 Feb 15; 22(2):59–61, 64–67

Testes/Adjacent Structures/Penis

Babaian RJ and Zagars GK. Testicular seminoma: The MD Anderson experience. An analysis of pathological and patient characteristics, and treatment recommendations. J Urol 1988 Feb; 139(2):311–314

Bergman KA. Current concepts in clinical therapeutics: Testicular cancer. Clin Pharmacol 1987 Sep; 6(9):693–706

Blackmore C. The impact of orchiectomy upon the sexuality of the man with testicular cancer. Cancer Nurs 1988 Feb; 11(1):33–40

Donohue JP. Selecting initial therapy. Seminoma and nonseminoma. Cancer 1987 Aug 1; 60(3 Suppl):490–495

Editorial. Progress in management of epididymitis? Lancet 1987 Dec 5; 2(8571):1310–1311

Einhorn LH. Complicated problems in testicular cancer. Semin Oncol 1988 Jun; 15(3 Suppl 3):9–15

Ellis M and Sikora K. The current management of testicular cancer. Br J Urol 1987 Jan; 59(1):2–9

Grant JBF et al. The role of *Chlamydia trachomatis* in epididymitis. Br J Urol 1987 Oct; 60(4):355–359

Greenberg MJ. Vasectomy technique. Am Fam Physician 1989 Jan; 39(1):131–138

Gribetz ME and Fine EM. Inflammatory and neoplastic lesions of penile gland and periglandular regions. Clin Dermatol 1987 Apr–Jun; 5(2):77–86

Jordan GH and Devine PC. Management of urethral stricture disease. Urol Clin North Am 1988 May; 15(2):277–289

Kennedy BJ et al. National survey of patterns of care for testis cancer. Cancer 1987 Oct 15; 60(8):1921–1930

Krieger JN et al. Evaluation of chronic urethritis. Arch Intern Med 1988 Mar; 148(3):703–707

La Nasa JA and Lewis RW. Varicocele and its surgical management. Urol Clin North Am 1987 Feb; 14(1):127–136

Lucas LM and Smith D. Nongonococcal urethritis. J Gen Intern Med 1987 May–Jun; 2(3):199–203

Melekos MD and Asbach HW. Epididymitis: Aspects concerning etiology and treatment. J Urol 1987 Jul; 138(1):83–86

Mohammed SH and Wirima J. Balloon catheter dilatation of urethral strictures. AJR 1988 Feb; 150(2):327–330

Moynihan C. Testicular cancer: The psychosocial problems of patients and their relatives. Cancer Surv 1987; 6(3):477–510

Persky L and deKernion J. Carcinoma of the penis. CA 1986 Sep–Oct; 36(5):258–273

Schmidt SS. Vasectomy. Urol Clin North Am 1987 Feb; 14(1):149–154

Stanford JR. Testicular cancer. Nursing (Lond) 1988 Feb; 3(26):957–960

Weidner W, Schiefer HG and Barbe C. Acute nongonococcal epididymitis. Drugs 1987; 34(Suppl 1):111–117

Urolithiasis

Bagley DH. Pharmacologic treatment of infection stones. Urol Clin North Am 1987 May; 14(2):347–352

Coe FL and Parks JH. Pathophysiology of kidney stones and strategies for treatment. Hosp Pract (Off) 1988 Mar 15; 23(3):185–189, 193–195, 199–200 passim

Mulley AG, Carlson KJ and Dretler SP. Extracoporeal shock-wave lithotripsy: Slam-bang effects, silent side effects? AJR 1988 Feb; 150(2):316–318

National Institutes of Health Consensus Development Conference Statement. Prevention and treatment of kidney stones. 1988 Mar 30; 7(1):1–23

Newman DM et al. Extracorporeal shock-wave lithotripsy. Urol Clin North Am 1987 Feb; 14(1):63–71

O'Brien WM, Rotolo JE and Pahira JJ. New approaches in the treatment of renal calculi. Am Fam Physician 1987 Nov; 36(5):181–194

Poore CW and Graham BJ. Extracorporeal shock wave lithotripsy. AORN J 1988 Jan; 47(1):202–205, 208–209, 212

Preminger GM. Pharmacologic treatment of calcium calculi. Urol Clin North Am 1987 May; 14(2):325–333

Preminger GM. Pharmacologic treatment of uric acid calculi. Urol Clin North Am 1987 May; 14(2):335–338

Roth RA and Beckmann CF. Complications of extracorporeal shock-wave lithotripsy and percutaneous nephrolithotomy. Urol Clin North Am 1988 May; 15(2):155–166

Switters DSM. Teaching the patient to perform renacidin irrigation at home. J Urol Nurs 1987 Apr–Jun; 6(2):76–91

Wilbert DM et al. New generation shock wave lithotripsy. J Urol 1987 Sep; 138(3):563–565

Williams CM et al. Extracorporeal shock-wave lithotripsy: Long-term complications. AJR 1988 Feb; 150(2):311–315

Wilson JWL, Nickel JC and Nolan R. Percutaneous renal surgery. Can J Surg 1987 Nov; 30(6):389–391

28 Gynecologic Disorders

Disturbances of Menstruation

The Menstrual Cycle

Phases

1. *Menstrual or bleeding phase*—day 1 of cycle; endometrial sloughing and discharge
2. *Postmenstrual phase*—4–5 days after period ends; thin endometrium
3. *Proliferative phase*—estrogen increases thickness of endometrium; includes ovulation, the expulsion of ovum from ovary, approximately 14 days before onset of next menstrual period.
4. *Secretory phase*—approximately days 16–23; corpus luteum forms and then regresses unless pregnancy occurs; thick endometrium due to increased progesterone.
5. *Premenstrual phase*—days 24–28.

Menstruation

Characteristics	Range	Average
Menarche (onset)	9–17 years of age	12.5 years
Cycle length	24–32 days	29 days
Flow—duration	1–8 days	3–5 days
Flow—amount	10–75 ml.	35 ml.
Menopause—onset	45–55 years of age	47–50

Dysmenorrhea

Dysmenorrhea is painful menstruation; most common of gynecologic dysfunctions.

Types

1. Primary
   a. Absence of pelvic lesion; usually intrinsic to uterus.
   b. Current research supports increased prostaglandin production by the endometrium as the chief cause.
   c. May also be due to hormonal, obstructive, and psychological factors.
2. Secondary
   Due to lesion such as endometriosis, pelvic infection, congenital abnormality, uterine fibroids

Clinical Manifestations

1. Pain may be due to increased uterine contractility and decreased endometrial flow.
2. Characteristics of pain—colicky or dull, usually in lower midabdominal region, spasmodic or constant.
3. May also experience nausea, vomiting, diarrhea, headache, chills, tiredness, nervousness, and low backache.

Management

(of primary dysmenorrhea; treatment of secondary dysmenorrhea is aimed at underlying pathology)
1. Physical examination to rule out pathology
2. Local heat; such as heating pad to increase blood flow and decrease spasms
3. Exercise to increase endorphin release, which decreases pain perception; and to suppress prostaglandin release
4. Non-narcotic analgesics
5. Oral contraceptives to inhibit ovulation to decrease flow and contractility
6. Prostaglandin inhibitors, such as aspirin, indomethacin, and ibuprofen
7. Neurectomy for intractable pain; usually provides complete relief
8. Dilatation and curettage

Nursing Interventions

1. Explain to patient possible causes of dysmenorrhea.
2. Teach patient nonpharmacologic methods to reduce pain:
   a. Apply heating pad to lower midabdomen or take warm tub baths.
   b. Exercise regularly (30 minutes, 3 times a week).
3. Teach patient to use prescribed medications effectively by taking medication at beginning of discomfort and repeating as necessary, especially on first day of menses.
4. Teach patient side effects of medications.
5. Encourage patient to reduce stress through adequate sleep, good nutrition, exercise, and coping with stressors.
6. Discuss patient's feelings toward menstruation (hygienic issues, inconvenience, female identity).
7. Question patient after several consecutive menses to assess pain control.

Premenstrual Syndrome (PMS)

Premenstrual syndrome is a group of symptoms such as headache, irritability, depression, breast tenderness, and bloating that is clearly related to onset of menstruation.

Etiology

1. Linked to hormonal imbalances, prostaglandins, endorphins, psychological factors such as attitudes and beliefs related to menstruation, and environmental factors such as nutrition and pollution.
2. Most common in women in their 30s.
3. May occur in 25%–50% of menstruating women.

Clinical Manifestations

1. Symptoms may begin 7–14 days prior to the onset of menstrual flow; diminish 1 or 2 days after menses begins.
2. Physical—edema of extremities, abdominal fullness, breast swelling and tenderness, headache, vertigo, palpitations, acne, backache, constipation, thirst, weight gain.
3. Behavioral—irritability, fatigue, lethargy, depression, anxiety, crying spells

Management

1. Restrict sodium, caffeine, tobacco, alcohol, and refined sweets.
2. Promote aerobic exercise (to increase endorphins), good nutrition, and rest.
3. Vitamin B_6 supplements
4. Progesterone replacement therapy
5. Prostaglandin inhibitors
6. Diuretics to decrease fluid retention and weight gain
7. Anxiolytic agents
8. Refer for counseling if improvements are not seen.
9. *Oophorectomy* (removal of ovaries) for severe cases and for women who do not desire children

Nursing Interventions

1. Ask patient to describe symptoms and their onset and means of relief.
2. Encourage patient to keep a diary for several consecutive months including dates, cycle days, symptoms and their severity, and stress level.
3. Instruct patient in use and side effects of prescribed medications.
4. Teach patient possible causes of PMS and nonpharmacologic methods to alleviate distress, such as dietary modifications, exercise, and rest.
5. Provide emotional support to patient and family.
6. Teach stress reduction techniques such as imagery and deep breathing.
7. Refer for supportive services such as a support group to share problems and advice.
   Premenstrual Syndrome Action
   P.O. Box 16292
   Irvine, CA 92713

Amenorrhea

Amenorrhea is absence of menstrual flow.

Types

1. *Primary*
   a. Menarche does not occur by age 16
   b. Due to chromosomal, hormonal, nutritional, psychogenic disorders or pregnancy
2. *Secondary*
   a. Menstruation stops for three cycle intervals, or 6 months of amenorrhea in a woman who previously menstruated.
   b. May be due to normal pregnancy or lactation, menopause, psychogenic, hormonal, nutritional, or exercise-related disorders.
   c. Some medications, such as phenothiazines and oral contraceptives, also may induce amenorrhea.

Management

1. Progesterone challenge test
   a. Positive—bleeding occurs—chronic anovulation is most likely.
   b. Negative—no bleeding occurs—may indicate organ failure—other tests are needed.
2. Discontinue causative medications.
3. Nutritional or psychological counseling as indicated.
4. Hormonal replacement therapy
5. Treat systemic disease such as anemia.
6. Recommend decreased exercise in athletes to increase body fat and decrease stress.

Other Menstrual Disorders

A. **Oligomenorrhea**—markedly diminished menstrual flow; may also be irregular, but consistent periods with long intervals.

B. **Menorrhagia**—excessive bleeding during regular menstruation; can be increased in duration and/or amount.

C. **Metrorrhagia**—bleeding from uterus between regular menstrual periods; significant because it is usually a symptom of disease.

D. **Polymenorrhea**—frequent menstruation occurring at intervals of less than 3 weeks.

Menopause

Menopause is described as the physiologic cessation of menses associated with failing ovarian function and decreased estrogen production.

Climacteric is the transition period (perimenopausal) during which the woman's reproductive function gradually diminishes and disappears. It usually occurs at about the age of 50.

Artificial menopause may occur secondary to surgery or radiation involving the ovaries.

Clinical Manifestations

1. *Endocrine*—changes due to a lack of estrogen; some estrogen still comes from the conversion of androgens; menstrual flow gradually diminishes and then ceases.
2. *Genitalia*—atrophy of vulva, vagina, urethra results in dryness, bleeding, itching, burning, dysuria, thinning pubic hair, loss of labia minora, decreased lubrication.
3. *Sexual function*—dyspareunia, decreased intensity and duration of sexual response, but can still have active function.
4. *Vasomotor flushes*—60%–70% of women experience them; "hot flash," which may be preceded by an anxious feeling; sweating; occur irregularly.
5. *Osteoporosis*—decreased bone mass results in increased hip fractures, spinal compression fractures.
6. *Cardiovascular*—increased coronary artery disease, cholesterol level, and palpitations.
7. *Psychological*—insomnia, irritability, anxiety, memory loss, fear, and depression may be experienced.

Management

1. Estrogen replacement therapy
   a. Indicated for severe symptoms; some advocate its use for prevention of osteoporosis and coronary artery disease.
   b. Topical preparations may be used for atrophic vaginitis.
   c. May cause endometrial hyperplasia and cancer, breast cancer, gallbladder disease.
2. Progestins—if uterus intact, to prevent endometrial hyperplasia
3. Vaginal lubricants—to decrease vaginal dryness
4. Vitamin E and B supplements—to decrease hot flashes
5. Calcium supplements and weight-bearing activity—to prevent bone loss

Nursing Interventions

1. Assess genitalia for atrophy, lubrication, elasticity. Question patient about symptoms (and sexual functioning when appropriate).
2. Teach patient that menopause is a normal process resulting in decreased estrogen levels that account for many of the signs and symptoms.
3. Inform patient that sexual functioning does not decrease, but may even increase because of the loss of fear of pregnancy and increased time if children are grown.
4. Instruct patient to use a water-based lubricant for intercourse to decrease vaginal dryness and pain.
5. Provide patient with information related to estrogen replacement therapy if she so desires.

6. Review schedule, route, and side effects of drug if estrogen therapy is prescribed.
7. Instruct patient in sources of vitamins E, B, and calcium. Remind her of importance of weight-bearing activity to prevent osteoporosis.
8. Encourage patient to discuss her views about menopause.
9. Review stress management techniques such as adequate rest, exercise, diversional activities.

Diagnostic Studies for Gynecologic Conditions

Pelvic Examination

A *pelvic examination* includes inspection and palpation of the vulva, perineum, vagina, cervix, and palpation of the fundus, adnexa, and rectum. (For Guidelines: Pelvic Examination by the Nurse, see below.)

A. Patient Preparation

1. Provide psychological support
   a. The patient needs reassurance, understanding, and skillful consideration of her emotional as well as physical problems.
   b. In adolescents, important considerations include trust, need for control, increased self-consciousness, and fear of pain.
2. Instruct the patient to avoid douching for 24 hours before examination—cellular deposits might wash away.
3. Encourage the patient to void and evacuate the bowels before examination—provides more relaxation of perineal tissues.
4. Advise the patient to remove sufficient clothing to permit adequate exposure of genitalia and allow for examination of the abdomen.
5. Avoid undue exposure of the patient.

B. Lithotomy Positioning of Patient

1. Most common position used
2. On examination table
   a. Patient lies on back with knees and hips flexed, heels resting on footrests.
   b. Drape sheet diagonally over patient so that corner may be grasped and pulled upward to expose perineal area.
3. On Bed
   a. Patient is positioned across the bed with her hips extending slightly over the edge (dorsal supine).
   b. Feet are placed on the examiner's knees or on two chairs placed next to the bed.
4. Semi-sitting position
   a. Place patient in a position similar to lithotomy on examining table, but instead of lying supine, patient is in a semi-sitting position.
   b. Advantages: greater physical comfort, improves verbal communication and eye contact, easier bimanual examination for examiner, and patient can see anatomy with a hand-held mirror, resulting in more effective patient teaching.
5. Other positions, such as Sims' and knee–chest, may also be used.

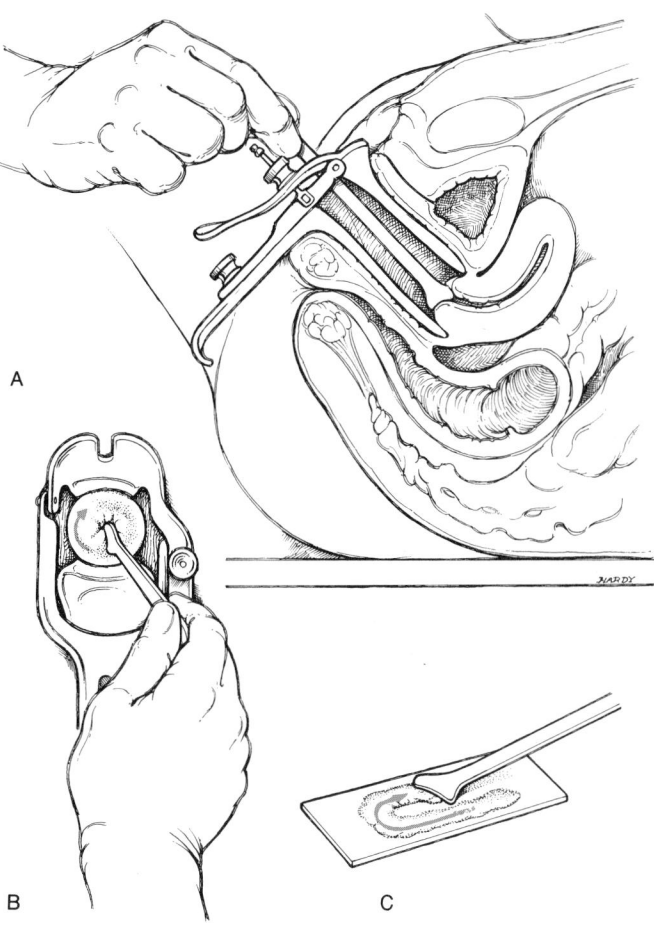

Figure 28-1. *A cervical scrape of secretions for cytology is obtained by using a wooden Ayre spatula. (A) Shows the speculum in place: the Ayre spatula is inserted so that the longer end is placed snugly in the os. (B) A representative sample of secretions is obtained by rotating the spatula. (C) Cervical secretions are gently smeared on a glass slide in a single circular motion. The slide is placed in the appropriate fixative immediately. Using a cotton-tipped applicator, also obtain a smear from the floor of the vagina below the cervix and preserve in the same manner.*

C. Procedure

1. Observe external genitalia for signs of inflammation, swelling, bleeding, discharge, or local skin and epithelial changes.
2. A speculum is inserted so that vaginal tissues and cervix can be visualized.
3. A cytology smear (Papanicolaou or ''Pap'') is made by scraping cervix (see Fig. 28-1).
4. A bimanual examination is done by inserting 1 or 2 gloved fingers of the left hand in the vagina and palpating the abdomen with the right hand. It is possible to further examine the uterus and adnexa for size, shape, mobility, masses, and tenderness and the cervix for cervical motion tenderness (Chandelier's sign). (See Fig. 28-2).
5. A rectal examination is done to detect abnormalities of contour, motility, and placement of adjacent structures; especially useful to feel the posterior uterus.

D. Nursing Interventions

1. Attend and support the patient by encouraging her to relax, by holding her hand, taking deep breaths, etc.
2. Focus the light and uncover examining tray with speculum, swabs, cytology necessities, etc.

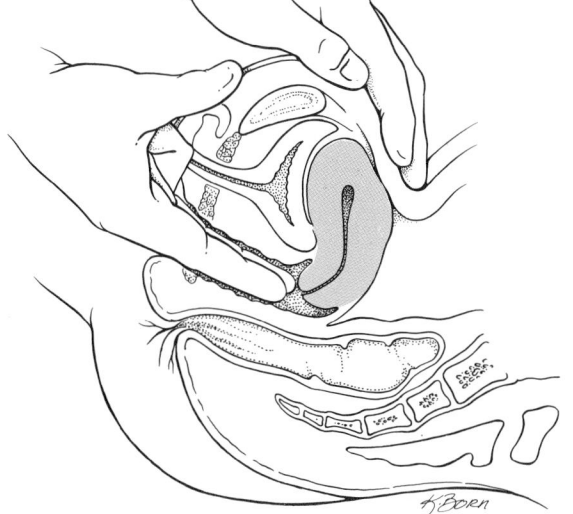

Figure 28-2. *Bimanual examination of the pelvic organs.*

3. Assist physician by providing gloves, lubricant, etc.
4. At conclusion of examination, wipe discharge from the patient before assisting her from the table.
5. Have the patient slide up on table before removing feet from stirrups.

6. Allow time for the older patient to adjust to sitting position before helping her off the table.
7. Answer any questions the patient may have; elaborate on physician's instructions.
8. Assist the patient with dressing if necessary.

Guidelines Vaginal Examination by the Nurse

Purposes
1. To inspect the vaginal canal and cervix
2. To obtain tissue specimen for cervical cytology and other tests

Equipment
Perineal drape
Vaginal specula
Water-soluble lubricant
Sterile gloves

Long swab sticks
Pap smear equipment
Adequate lighting

Procedure

Preparatory Phase

1. Have the patient void before assistant positions her on examining table.
2. Position the patient on examining table (slip may be kept on, but other clothing from waist to knees is removed).
    a. Have buttocks at edge of table.
    b. Position feet in stirrups to assume dorsal lithotomy position.
    c. Make the patient as comfortable as possible with a small pillow under her head.
    d. Drape the patient to permit minimal exposure (but adequate for examiner).
3. Encourage the patient to relax; tell her what you are doing and what she may feel.
4. Adjust light for maximum focus.
5. Offer the patient a mirror to watch the examination in order to teach vulvar self-examination and about contraceptives as appropriate.

Nursing Action	**Rationale/Amplification**

Performance Phase

1. Be gentle and take your time; wash hands; don sterile gloves; lubricate fingers.
2. Observe external genitalia for apparent abnormalities, gently separate labia and continue visual inspection.
3. To encourage relaxation in the patient, gently place the tip of 1 or 2 fingers into introitus.
4. Identify cervix manually and depress the perineum downward with your fingers.
5. Lubricate speculum with warm water.

6. Gently insert warm speculum horizontally, passing it over your fingers and aiming it toward the cervix.

7. Slowly open the speculum and lock into position. With slow manipulation, the speculum can be turned to permit visualization of the vaginal walls.
8. Inspect the cervix, which should be pink. Normally, the os is a dent, unless the woman has had children, in which case a slit is noted.

9. If Pap test is to be done, follow procedure in Figure 28-1. For a Schiller test, see page 719
10. When removing speculum, hold it open until cervix is cleared, then withdraw speculum, allowing it to close.
11. For palpation (bimanual examination), see Figure 28-2.

1. This promotes relaxation of the patient, making the procedure easier for both.
2. Note any evidence of irritation, infection, or abnormalities such as swelling, bleeding, erythema, discharge (other than clear and odorless)
3. Say to the patient, "Tighten your muscles and squeeze my fingers—try hard—then relax."
4. Downward pressure is away from the more sensitive anterior structures.
5. Any lubricant other than water may interfere with cytology results.
6. If it is preferred not to initially insert gloved fingers, the speculum is introduced vertically using a downward pressure; after entering the vestibule, the speculum is slowly rotated to the horizontal position.
7. Walls normally are pink and moist. A pale white secretion may be noted.

8. If woman is taking an oral contraceptive, the cervix may be deep pink to red. A thread coming out of the cervix would suggest presence of an intrauterine device (IUD). Abnormal cervical signs include erosion, lacerations, and polyps.

10. By the time speculum is completely withdrawn, it will be closed.

Nursing Action	Rationale/Amplification

Follow-Up Phase

1. Gently wipe the perineal area with soft tissue or gauze, using firm strokes from the pubic area back to beyond the rectum.
2. Instruct assistant in carefully helping the patient to remove feet from stirrups.
3. Elevate the lower third of the examining table to receive legs. Keep the patient covered with a sheet.
4. Assist the patient in sliding toward head end of table; provide a wide-based stool for her to step on as she gets off table.
5. Assist the patient in dressing if necessary. Answer any queries she may have.

1. This will remove secretions and liquid lubricant.

2. Both feet must be removed at the same time to reduce strain.
3. This permits the patient to assume dorsal recumbent position.
4. Do not rush the patient as she is getting off the table, as sudden shifting from recumbent to sitting position may cause a feeling of dizziness.

Other Diagnostic Tests

Cytology Tests for Cancer

A. Purpose—to screen for cervical dysplasia and/or cancer. May also detect endometrial cancer, infections, and endocrine status.

B. Procedure—See Figure 12-1; should not be performed during menses.

C. Classification

1. *Papanicolaou* (original classification system)
   Class 1—absence of atypical or abnormal cells
   Class 2—atypical cytology but no evidence of malignancy
   Class 3—cytology suggestive of, but not conclusive for, malignancy
   Class 4—cytology strongly suggestive of malignancy
   Class 5—cytology conclusive for malignancy
2. *Bethesda System* (descriptive diagnoses)
   Infection
   Reactive and Reparative Changes (i.e., inflammation)
   Epithelial cell abnormalities
       (including atypia, squamous intraepithelial lesion, and squamous cell carcinoma)
   Nonepithelial malignant neoplasm
   Hormonal Evaluation

D. Interpretation and Follow-up Care

1. Recently, a histologic description of the findings (such as the Bethesda System) appears to be preferred.
2. If the patient has an abnormal smear, explain that this is not always conclusive but requires further testing such as biopsy, conization, or colposcopy. *Encourage the patient to return for further testing.*

E. Screening Guidelines and Recommendations

1. *American Cancer Society*
   a. Every 3 years after two annual negative smears
   b. May stop at age 65 if not at high risk
2. *American College of Obstetricians and Gynecologists* and *Planned Parenthood*
   Annually
3. Post-hysterectomy
   a. Vaginal cytology every 3–5 years if hysterectomy was not for cancer.
   b. If it was, then annual cytology should be done.

> **GERONTOLOGIC ALERT:** Pap smears should continue beyond 65 years of age if a woman is considered high risk: has multiple partners, sexually transmitted disease history, is a smoker, or had early intercourse.

Schiller's Iodine Test

A. Purpose—To outline unhealthy epithelium

B. Rationale—Cancer epithelium contains no glycogen, whereas normal cervical epithelial cells do. Glycogen has the ability to absorb iodine.

Note: Schiller's test is unreliable for cancer and only suggests some epithelial change. It is infrequently used, as colposcopy is preferred.

C. Procedure—A long applicator stick is used to paint the cervix with Schiller's iodine solution.

1. Negative result—a mahogany brown color covering the entire surface indicates a reaction between iodine and glycogen of normal cells.
2. Positive result—tissues are not stained brown, indicating that immature cells are present and suggesting the need for a biopsy.

Cervical Biopsy

A. Purpose—To remove cervical tissue for laboratory study if there is a visible lesion.

B. Patient Preparation

1. To be done preferably at a time when cervix is least vascular (usually a week after the end of the menstrual flow).
2. Explain the nature of the procedure to the patient.
3. Place the patient in lithotomy position and drape her properly.
4. Explain to the patient that no anesthesia is required, as the cervix does not have pain receptors.
5. Provide emotional support for anxiety due to potential for cancer.

C. Procedure

1. After the speculum is positioned in the vagina and the cervix is properly exposed, the surgeon, under colposcopic guidance, uses biopsy forceps to obtain bits of cervical tissue.

2. Tissue is preserved in 10% formalin, labeled, and sent to the laboratory. Suturing and packing may be necessary if bleeding occurs.

D. Aftercare of the Patient

1. A brief rest after the procedure is usually necessary before the patient leaves.
2. Discharge instructions/patient education—instruct the patient as follows:
   a. Avoid heavy lifting for 24 hours.
   b. Packing will remain in place for 12–24 hours, depending on physician's preference.
   c. There may be some bleeding; however, more than that of a normal period must be reported to the physician.
   d. Obtain physician's instructions regarding douching and sexual relations.

Conization

Conization is the excision of a cone-shaped piece of tissue from the cervix, including the area where the squamous and columnar epithelial meet (transformation zone). The transformation zone is the site of most cervical cancers.

A. Patient Preparation—explain to the patient that the procedure requires anesthesia in ambulatory surgery setting or hospitalization.

B. Procedure

1. After colposcopy or Schiller's test is performed to outline the lesions, a cone-shaped specimen is excised with a laser or knife.
2. Bleeding is controlled by cauterization or suturing and packing.

C. Aftercare

1. Usually the patient stays for observation and is discharged the next day.
2. Avoid tampons, douching, or intercourse for 2 weeks.

Laparoscopy

Laparoscopy is the endoscopic visualization of the pelvic and abdominal cavities through a small incision. It is used to evaluate pelvic pain and infertility, treat endometriosis adhesions, and perform tubal sterilizations (the most common use).

A. Patient Preparation

1. Inform the patient that she will be NPO and may receive an enema prior to the procedure.
2. Inform patient that she may experience shoulder or abdominal discomfort after the procedure from the injection of carbon dioxide.

B. Procedure

1. Usually done in ambulatory surgery with general, local, or regional anesthesia.
2. Incision is made below the umbilicus.
3. A small needle is inserted and CO_2 is injected into it.
4. The patient's head is tilted down to displace the intestines for better visualization.
5. The scope is inserted to visualize and manipulate the pelvic organs.

C. Aftercare of Patient

1. Monitor bleeding, vital signs, and bowel movements.
2. Administer oral analgesics as prescribed.
3. Dressing may be applied.

4. Inform patient not to have intercourse or strenuous activity for 2–3 days. Tell patient to report bleeding, cramping, or fever to physician.

Culdoscopy

A *culdoscopy* is an uncommon operative, diagnostic procedure in which an incision is made into the posterior vaginal cul-de-sac so that a culdoscope can be inserted for the purpose of visualizing the uterus, tubes, broad ligaments, uterosacral ligaments, rectal wall, sigmoid, and even the small intestines.

1. The patient is prepared as for any vaginal operation.
2. Anesthesia may be local, general, or regional.
3. The knee–chest position is best for a culdoscopy.
4. Following the examination, the scope is withdrawn and sutures placed; the patient is returned to her room.

Hysteroscopy

Hysteroscopy is the endoscopic visualization of the uterine cavity by means of a hysteroscope. It is used to stage endometrial cancer, check tubal patency, determine the cause of uterine bleeding, remove polyps or fibroids, and observe the placement/appearance of IUDs.

A. Patient Preparation and Examination

1. Administer the prescribed sedative and mild tranquilizer prior to the examination. Explanation is similar to that for dilatation and curettage (D&C).
2. Place the patient in the lithotomy position as for a D&C.
3. Cleanse the perineum and vagina immediately prior to sterile draping.
4. The examiner performs a bimanual palpation of the uterus.
5. Local anesthesia is injected into the cervix, which is positioned with a tenaculum forceps.
6. Sounds are inserted into the cervical canal for dilatation prior to insertion of endoscope.
7. With endoscope in place, a concentrated solution of dextran is slowly infused into the endometrial cavity to distend it.
8. Uterine walls are viewed under magnification.

B. Follow-Up

1. Following removal of instruments, the patient is encouraged to rest.
2. The patient may be discharged later the same day.

Endometrial Biopsy

A. Purpose—to obtain cells from uterine lining to assist in the diagnosis of endometrial cancer, menstrual disorders, and infertility.

B. Patient Preparation

1. Usually done in doctor's office with local anesthesia.
2. Prostaglandin inhibitor administered to decrease uterine cramps postoperatively.
3. Place patient in dorsal lithotomy position.

C. Procedure (by physician)

1. A speculum is inserted after local anesthesia has been accomplished.
2. A uterine sound is introduced; if this cannot be accomplished, the cervix is dilated.
3. The specimen is withdrawn by curet or suction from 4 quadrants.
4. Specimen is placed in formalin and sent to the laboratory.

D. Patient Education

1. Inform patient that she may experience light bleeding and occasional cramping for a few days.
2. Instruct the patient to report fever, chills, and increased bleeding.
3. A D&C is done if there is positive pathology or further problems.

Hysterosalpingogram

A *hysterosalpingogram* is an x-ray study of the uterus and uterine (fallopian) tubes.

A. Purpose

1. To determine extent of tubal patency
2. To note the presence of pathology in the uterine cavity
3. To examine for intrapelvic disease
4. To examine for peritoneal adhesions

B. Patient Preparation

1. Administer enema to decrease intestinal gas.
2. Administer prescribed medication to decrease anxiety.
3. Determine last menstrual period—test is done a few days after menses ends, before ovulation. Pelvic examination also may be done to rule out pregnancy.

C. Procedure

1. The patient is placed in lithotomy position on a fluoroscopic x-ray table.
2. The bivalve speculum is introduced to expose cervix.
3. Contrast medium is injected into uterine cavity.
4. X-rays are taken to determine configuration of pelvic area.
5. If tubes are patent, contrast medium enters the peritoneum in 10–15 minutes.

D. Follow-Up Care and Patient Education

1. Apply perineal pad for drainage of contrast medium or blood.
2. Tell patient to inform physician if bloody drainage continues after 3 days or if any signs of infection are present.
3. Inform patient that she may have some shoulder discomfort due to dye irritation of the phrenic nerve.

Colposcopy

A *colposcopy* is an examination of the cervix with a bright light and under magnification of 10–40 times.

It is done to determine distribution of abnormal squamous epithelium and to pinpoint areas from which biopsy tissue can be taken.

Dilatation and Curettage (D&C)

Dilatation and curettage is a widening of the cervical canal with a dilator and the scraping of the uterine canal with a curette. The cervix is scraped first without dilatation.

It is the most common gynecologic surgery and is usually done on an outpatient basis.

A. Purpose

1. To control uterine bleeding
2. To secure endometrial and endocervical tissue for tissue study
3. To serve as a therapeutic measure for incomplete abortion
4. To provide temporary relief of dysmenorrhea after medical measures fail

B. Patient Preparation

1. Inform the patient of the nature of the operation to be done (usually done by a gynecologist).
2. Ascertain what the patient has been told about postoperative discomfort and drainage following the D&C.
3. Answer questions the patient has about the procedure and aftercare.
4. Request the patient to void.
5. Assist patient in the dorsal lithotomy position.

C. Complications

1. Perforation of uterus
2. Laceration of cervix

D. Aftercare of Patient

1. Immediately postoperatively, monitor vital signs at frequent intervals—potential for hemorrhage exists.
2. Monitor perineal pads/bed for amount of bleeding; report excessive bleeding.
3. Offer prescribed analgesics for low-back and pelvic pain; cramping may occur for 2–3 days due to dilatation of the cervix.
4. Instruct patient to maintain bedrest for remainder of day to decrease cramping and bleeding.
5. Instruct patient to use perineal pads at home and to report fever, heavy bleeding, and severe cramping.
6. Instruct patient to avoid strenuous activity until bleeding stops.
7. Discuss with patient that a D&C does not affect sexual functioning, but that she should refrain from sexual intercourse per physician's directive; usually 2–3 weeks.

Conditions of the External Genitalia and Vagina

Inflammatory Disorders

Vulvitis

Vulvitis is inflammation of the vulva.

A. Causative Factors (local)

1. Infections; trichomonas, bacterial, fungal, etc.
2. Irritants
   a. Urine, feces, vaginal discharge
   b. Close-fitting, synthetic fabrics
   c. Chemicals such as laundry detergents, vaginal sprays, deodorants, perfumes
3. Atrophy of vulva—due to decreased estrogen secondary to menopause
4. Carcinoma

B. Causative Factors (systemic)

1. Diabetes mellitus
2. Drug sensitivities or allergies
3. Vitamin deficiencies
4. Diseases: anemia, hepatitis, leukemia, psoriasis

C. Clinical Manifestations

1. Pruritus (itching)—more acute at night; aggravated by warmth
2. Reddened, edematous tissue
3. Pain, burning; worse with intercourse
4. Ulceration
5. Exudation—profuse, purulent

D. Diagnostic Evaluation

1. Physical examination and laboratory tests—to rule out diabetes and other systemic diseases
2. Cultures—to rule out infectious organisms
3. Biopsy of vulvar tissue

E. Management

1. Topical steroids; anti-infectives; sedatives as required
2. Treatment of underlying diseases, i.e., diabetes

F. Nursing Interventions and Patient Education

1. Examine external genitalia and lymph nodes.
2. Question patient regarding recent use of new laundry detergents, drug allergies.
3. Teach patient hygienic principles:
    a. Wipe from front to back after toilet use.
    b. Use cotton moistened with warm, bland soap solution; pat dry.
    c. Apply nonirritating powder such as cornstarch.
4. Teach patient to avoid chemical irritants such as sprays, perfumed soaps, new laundry detergents.
5. Teach patient to avoid mechanical irritants such as tight clothing, synthetic fabrics and undergarments; replace these with loose-fitting cotton undergarments.
6. Review prescribed pharmacologic agents, i.e., topical steroids.
7. Instruct patient to use cool compresses to area of itching.
8. Review diabetes management if appropriate.

Infection of the Greater Vestibular Gland
(Bartholinitis)

These glands lie on both sides of the vagina at the base of the labia minora; serve to lubricate the vagina.

1. If they become obstructed secondary to infection, abscess or cyst formation may occur (Fig. 28-3); may spontaneously rupture
2. Most commonly seen in sexual transmission

A. Clinical Manifestations

1. Asymptomatic cyst
2. Pain, erythema, tenderness, swelling
3. If abscess is present: pain, edema, cellulitis
4. Possible abscess

B. Diagnostic Evaluation

Culture of organisms

C. Consecutive Management

Warm soaks or sitz baths 3–4 times daily; antibiotics if cellulitis is present.

D. Surgical Intervention

1. Incision and drainage—provides immediate relief; can recur
2. Wound catheter
3. Marsupialization for recurrent abscesses
    a. Contents are opened and drained, then edges of abscess are sutured to edges of external incision to keep cavity open
    b. Healing occurs from within the area of the abscess.

E. Nursing Interventions

1. Inspect labia minora for erythema and swelling.
2. Describe to the patient how to take a sitz bath or use warm moist compresses.
3. Encourage patient to remain in bed as much as possible, as pain is exacerbated with activity.
4. Encourage patient to take prescribed antibiotics on schedule.
5. Instruct patient to take analgesic medication as prescribed.
6. Prepare patient for incision and drainage, which provides immediate relief.
7. For marsupialization: apply ice packs intermittently for 24 hours to reduce edema and provide comfort; thereafter warm sitz baths or a perineal heat lamp provide comfort.

F. Patient Education

1. Teach patient that infections, especially sexually transmitted infections, are the chief cause of bartholinitis.
2. Review principles of perineal hygiene with the patient.
3. Inform patient that infection and abscess may recur and require surgical treatment.

Vaginal Fistula

A *fistula* is an abnormal, tortuous opening between 2 internal hollow organs, or between an internal hollow organ and the exterior of the body.

Ureterovaginal fistula is an opening between the ureter and vagina.

Vesicovaginal fistula is an opening between the bladder and vagina.

Rectovaginal fistula is an opening between the rectum and vagina.

Causes

1. Obstetric injury, especially in long labors and in countries with inadequate obstetrical care

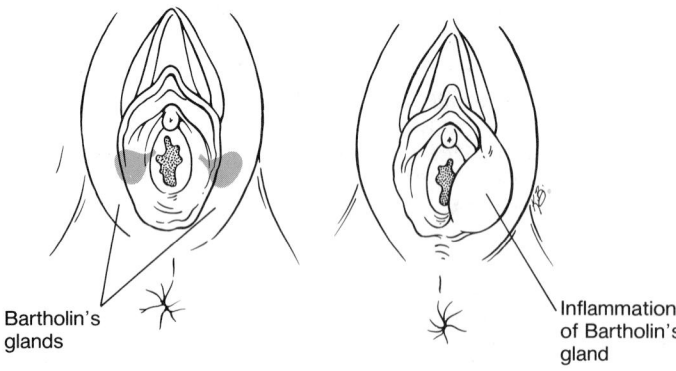

Bartholin's glands

Inflammation of Bartholin's gland

Figure 28-3. *Site and infection of vestibular gland.*

2. Pelvic surgery—hysterectomy or vaginal reconstructive procedures
3. Carcinoma—extensive disease or complication of treatment, i.e., radiation therapy

Clinical Manifestations

1. Vesicovaginal—most common type of fistula
   a. Constant trickling of urine into vagina
   b. Loss of urge to void, as bladder is continuously emptying
   c. May cause excoriation and inflammation of vulva
2. Rectovaginal
   a. Fecal incontinence and flatus through the vagina; malodorous
   b. May present as vulvar ulcer

Diagnostic Evaluation

1. Methylene blue test—following instillation of this dye in the bladder
   a. Methylene blue appears in vagina in vesicovaginal fistula.
   b. Methylene blue does not appear in vagina in ureterovaginal fistula.
2. Indigo carmine test—following a negative methylene blue test, indigo carmine is injected intravenously. If dye appears in vagina, this indicates a ureteral fistula.
3. Intravenous pyelogram—(see p. 660) a valuable test for determining presence of hydroureter or hydronephrosis, and position or location of the fistula
4. Cystoscopy—performed to determine number and location of fistulas

Management

1. Fistulas recognized at time of delivery should be corrected immediately.
2. Treatment of postoperative fistulas may be delayed for 2–3 months to allow treatment of infection.
3. Surgical closure of opening via vaginal or abdominal route (when patient's tissues are healthy)
4. Fecal or urinary diversion procedure may be required for large fistulas.
5. Rarely, a fistula may heal without surgical intervention.
6. Medical approach:
   a. Prosthesis to prevent incontinence and allow tissue to heal; done for patients who are not surgical candidates
   b. Prosthesis is inserted into vagina; it is connected to drainage tubing leading to a leg bag.

Nursing Interventions

A. General Measures

1. Encourage frequent sitz baths.
2. Suggest patient use perineal pads or other incontinence products.
3. Recommend the use of cornstarch to prevent excoriation.
4. Teach the use of vaginal irrigation as prescribed, page 739.

B. Preoperative Nursing Interventions

1. Encourage patient to take prescribed antibiotics to reduce pathogenic flora in intestinal tract.
2. Encourage taking prescribed oral estrogens if patient is postmenopausal—to promote healthier tissues.

C. Postoperative Nursing Interventions

1. Following vesicovaginal repair
   a. Maintain proper drainage from indwelling catheter to prevent pressure on newly sutured tissue.
   b. Administer vaginal or bladder irrigations gently because of tenderness at operative site.
   c. Maintain strict intake and output records.
2. Following rectovaginal repair
   a. Maintain patient on clear liquids as prescribed to limit bowel activity for several days.
   b. Encourage rest because of debilitation.
   c. Administer warm perineal irrigations to decrease healing time and increase comfort.
3. Allow patient to express feelings about her altered route of elimination, i.e., frustration, embarrassment, anger. Encourage her to share these feelings with significant others.
4. Encourage patient to use morale boosters such as manicure, facial, new hairstyle.

Vaginal Infections

Vaginal infections cause inflammation of the vagina due to the introduction of pathogens
1. Sexual transmission is the mode in the majority of patients.
2. More common in diabetes, pregnancy, and with stress
3. 90% due to bacterial vaginosis (nonspecific or *Gardnerella*), *Candida,* or trichomoniasis.

Normal Vaginal Condition

1. Sensitivity to estrogen
   a. Stimulates vaginal secretions
   b. Secretions are usually odorless and increase in amount at time of ovulation and just before menstruation
   c. In low estrogen conditions (before menarche and after menopause), secretions decrease due to inactive epithelium.
2. Acidic secretions
   a. *p*H 3.5–4.5 due to conversion of glycogen to lactic acid by Döderlein's bacilli, which normally inhabit the vagina.
   b. Acidity inhibits the growth of many pathogens.
   c. In low estrogen conditions, the *p*H is 6–7 due to lack of glycogen and lactobacilli

Types of Vaginitis *(Table 28-1)*

1. Simple
2. *Gardnerella*
3. *Trichomonas*
4. *Candida albicans*
5. Atrophic
6. Human papillomavirus

Clinical Manifestations

1. Itching, irritation, burning
2. Odor; increased vaginal discharge
3. Dyspareunia; pelvic pain; dysuria
4. May be asymptomatic

Diagnostic Evaluation

1. Laboratory tests, including wet smear for microscopic examination

Table 28-1. *Types of Vaginitis*

Description	Manifestations	Management
Simple Vaginitis (Contact Vaginitis)		
An inflammation of the vagina, with discharge; this may be due to invading organisms, irritation, poor hygiene. *Urethritis* often accompanies vaginitis because of the proximity of the urethra to the vagina. Predisposing factors: Contact allergens, excessive perspiration, synthetic underclothing, poor hygiene, foreign bodies (tampons, condoms, diaphragms that have been left in too long)	1. Increased vaginal discharge with itching, redness, burning, and edema. 2. Voiding and defecation aggravate the above symptoms.	1. Enhance the natural vaginal flora by administering a weak acid douche, 15 ml. of vinegar to 1,000 ml. water, (1 T. white vinegar to 1 qt. water). 2. Stimulate the growth of lactobacilli (Döderlein's bacilli) by administering beta-lactose vaginal suppository; this dissolves with body heat, and the sugar then acts. 3. Foster cleanliness by meticulous care after voiding and defecation. 4. Discontinue use of causative agent.
Gardnerella Vaginitis (Nonspecific or bacterial)		
An inflammation of the vagina heretofore referred to as "nonspecific vaginitis," since it is not caused by *Trichomonas, Candida,* or gonorrhea. It is considered a sexually transmitted disease.	1. Vaginal discharge with odor. 2. Itching and burning may suggest concomitant organisms present. 3. It is benign in that when the discharge is wiped away, underlying tissue is healthy and pink. 4. Vaginal pH is between 5.0 and 5.5 5. May be asymptomatic	1. Metronidazole (Flagyl) taken 3 times daily for 7 days. May also use tetracycline, ampicillin, or clindamycin. 2. Alcohol intake should be avoided during Flagyl treatment to avoid nausea and vertigo. Flagyl has been associated with teratogenic effects and should not be used in pregnant women. 3. Treating partners is controversial unless the condition is recurrent; if so, Flagyl is usually prescribed.
Trichomonas Vaginalis		
A condition produced by a protozoan, (pear-shaped and mobile), that thrives in an alkaline environment. Remissions may occur, but organism remains resistant to treatment in the urinary tract.	1. Copious malodorous discharge; may be frothy and yellow-green in color. 2. May have pruritus, dyspareunia, and spotting. 3. Red, speckled (strawberry) punctate hemorrhages on the cervix. 4. May also have vulvar edema, dysuria, and hyperemia secondary to irritation of discharge.	1. Destroy infective protozoa by taking metronidazole (Flagyl) for 10 days (orally). NOTE: Flagyl is contraindicated in the first trimester of pregnancy. 2. Prevent reinfection by treating male concurrently with Flagyl.
Candida Albicans		
A fungal infection caused by *Candida albicans.* *Incidence*—several factors have been found to be significantly associated with the incidence of *Candida albicans:* 1. Steroid therapy 2. Obesity 3. Pregnancy 4. Antibiotic therapy 5. Diabetes mellitus 6. Oral contraceptives 7. Frequent douching 8. Chronic debilitative diseases Characteristics 1. *Candida albicans* is a normal inhabitant of the intestinal tract and therefore a frequent contaminant of the vagina. 2. Since this fungus thrives in an environment rich in carbohydrates, it is seen commonly in patients with poorly controlled diabetes. 3. This infection is observed in patients who have been on antibiotic or steroid therapy for a while (reduces natural protective organisms in vagina).	1. Vaginal discharge is thick and irritating; white or yellow patchy, cheese-like particles adhere to vaginal walls. 2. Itching is the most common complaint. 3. May also experience burning, soreness, dyspareunia, frequency, and dysuria.	1. Eradicate the fungus by applying miconazole nitrate vaginal cream, 1 application daily at bedtime for 7 days; and clotrimazole (Gyne-Lotrimin Vaginal Cream) one applicator-full intravaginally nightly for 1 week. 2. Treat the symptomatic or uncircumcised partner by applying antifungal cream under the foreskin nightly for 7 nights.

(continued)

Table 28-1. *Types of Vaginitis (continued)*

Description	Manifestations	Management
Atrophic Vaginitis		
This is a common postmenopausal occurrence due to atrophy of the vaginal mucosa secondary to decreased estrogen levels; more susceptible to infection.	1. Vaginal itching, dryness, burning, dyspareunia, and vulvar irritation. 2. May also have vaginal bleeding. **NURSING ALERT:** In the postmenopausal woman, if vaginal bleeding occurs, encourage the patient to see her physician immediately, because cancer may be suspected.	Since this is a manifestation of general body estrogenic depletion, the patient should be treated with oral, water-soluble, natural, conjugated estrogen (Premarin). The condition reverses itself under treatment, which must be maintained. If infection is also present, this is treated. Estrogenic or cortisone vaginal cream or transdermal patch may be prescribed.
Human Papillomavirus		
Causes condyloma acuminatum (venereal warts). Implicated in intraepithelial neoplasia of the vulva, vagina, and cervix. Sexually transmitted; highly contagious. May spontaneously regress in one third of patients. Significant recurrence rate.	1. Vulvar or vaginal lumps or warty growths 2. Occasional bleeding 3. Asymptomatic lesions may be detected by Pap smear. 4. May have increased discharge, odor, or dyspareunia	Podophyllin (not for vaginal warts), Trichloroacetic acid, or topical 5-FU. May perform cryotherapy, electrocautery, laser treatment, or local excision for larger lesions (greater than 2 cm.) Should be treated during pregnancy due to risk of neonatal laryngeal papillomatosis. CO_2 laser and trichloroacetic acid have been used.

a. Saline slide—discharge mixed with saline; useful in detecting *Gardnerella* and *Trichomonas*
b. Potassium hydroxide (KOH)—discharge mixed with 10% KOH; useful in detecting *C. albicans.* If fishy odor is noted, suspect *Gardnerella.*
2. Culture—significant when purulent discharge is present; used to detect gonorrhea
3. Vaginal *p*H—use Nitrazine paper
   Normal *p*H—4.0–4.5
   Gardnerella—5.0–5.5
   Trichomonas—5.5+
4. Pap test

Management

1. Antibiotics (oral, creams, suppositories). See Table 28-1, page 724.
2. Douches may be prescribed.

Nursing Assessment

1. Health history including questions specific to the condition:
   a. Nature of discharge: Cheeselike, frothy, puslike, thick or thin, scant? When was it first noticed? Character, color, odor? Other symptoms: dysuria, itching, dyspareunia?
   b. Menstrual history: Age at menarche, menopause; length of cycles, duration and amount of flow, dysmenorrhea, amenorrhea, dysfunctional bleeding?
   c. Disease history: Presence of diabetes mellitus in patient or family? Other debilitating diseases? Control of these? Previous vaginal infections? Sexually transmitted diseases?
   d. Pregnancy history
   e. Sexual history: Partner(s), how active sexually? Its nature? Urogenital infections in partner? Nature of contraceptives?
   f. Medications being taken: Purpose?
   g. Vaginal hygiene: Use of douches, deodorants, sprays, ointments; type of tampons, bubble bath, shower/bath, nature of clothing (tight-fitting)?
   h. Concerns, stresses, anxieties, any questions?
2. Physical examination, including vaginal examination

Nursing Diagnoses

1. Pain related to vaginal irritation
2. Impaired tissue integrity related to vaginal infection
3. Sexual dysfunction related to abstinence secondary to treatment
4. Knowledge deficit of prevention and treatment of vaginitis

Nursing Interventions

A. Increasing Comfort

1. Instruct patient to discontinue use of irritating agents, i.e., bubble baths, etc., if appropriate.
2. Suggest patient take cool baths or sitz baths and pat dry or dry with hair dryer on low setting.
3. Encourage patient to wear loose cotton undergarments.
4. Encourage patient to take prescribed steroids and analgesics.
5. Provide emotional support.

B. Restoring Healthy Vaginal Tissues

1. Teach patient to cleanse perineum before applying medication.

2. Demonstrate application of prescribed medications.
3. Emphasize importance of schedule and length of time medication is to be applied, not just until she feels better.
4. Stress importance of follow-up visits.
5. Teach side effects of medications (i.e., Teach patient to avoid alcohol when taking Flagyl until 24 hours after treatment ends.).
6. Instruct patient on the technique of douching.

C. Improving Sexual Functioning

1. Discuss alternative sexual practices during active vaginal infection.
2. Recommend the use of a condom by partner if intercourse is resumed before completion of treatment.
3. Instruct in the use of a water-soluble lubricant if vagina is dry or atrophic.
4. Recommend that partner be examined if he is symptomatic.

Patient Education

1. Teach causes of vaginitis; usually sexually transmitted, especially if multiple partners; inadequate perineal hygiene.
2. Teach measures to prevent vaginitis.
   a. Wipe from front to back after toilet use.
   b. Keep area clean and dry.
   c. Avoid sharing towels.
   d. Wear loose cotton clothing—to absorb moisture and provide good circulation.
   e. Change sanitary pads/tampons frequently so they do not become saturated.
   f. Avoid bubble baths, vaginal deodorants, sprays, and douches.
   g. If insist on using douches, use a mild vinegar solution (2 tsp. white vinegar to 1 qt. water).
3. Teach nutritional modifications as appropriate (i.e., diabetes).

Assist patient to eliminate foods from diet that are conducive to vaginal *p*H change, such as high carbohydrates.

Evaluation

1. Verbalizes relief of pain
2. Vaginal mucosa appears pink with normal amount and color of secretions.
3. Reports adequate sexual functioning
4. States preventive measures and treatment of vaginitis

Herpes Genitalis *(Herpes Simplex Virus Type 2)*

Herpes genitalis is a viral infection that causes lesions on the cervix, vagina, and external genitalia.

Etiology and Course

1. May be dormant and reactivate periodically
2. Has an affinity for skin, mucous membranes, and central nervous system
3. Sexually transmitted disease, with about 500,000 new cases/year (10–20 million Americans are infected.)
4. Attributed to higher incidence of cervical cancer
5. May infect babies delivered vaginally of herpetic mothers. Also responsible for increased incidence of spontaneous abortions

6. A chronic illness; recurrence rate of 50%–60%; precipitated by stress, fever, heat

Clinical Manifestations

1. Lesions occur 2–10 days (average, 6 days) after initial exposure and last 3–6 weeks. First exposure is the most severe and prolonged.
2. Lesions may proceed from macules to papules to vesicles to pustules to ulcers, which may crust and heal with scars. Usually present as multiple vesicles with a clear, shiny, or red base.
3. Lesions are usually located on the vagina, vulva, cervix, perineal area, or buttocks, thighs, or penis.
4. Erythema, pruritus, painful lesions, watery discharge from vagina or urethra, lymphadenopathy, inguinal tenderness are most common symptoms.
5. May also experience dysuria, dyspareunia, bleeding, fever, malaise, and headaches.
6. May lead to meningitis, neuralgia, and transverse myelitis
7. May be asymptomatic

Diagnostic Evaluation

1. Usually can be made by inspection.
2. To determine true causative agent, cell cultures are taken; 1–3 days required for results.
3. Pap smear—if herpes infection is present, multinucleated giant cells are noted.
4. Tzanck smear
   a. Scrapings from base of a vesicle are obtained.
   b. If herpetic, multinucleated giant cells containing viral inclusion bodies are noted.
   c. Note: Other herpetic disease such as "shingles" or chickenpox will also yield positive findings.
5. Enzyme immunoassay (EIA) test detects antibody to herpes virus; used for diagnosis and screening.

Management

1. Acyclovir (Zovirax)—suppresses virus by inhibiting viral DNA polymerase to prevent virus replication. Decreases length of infection, pain, and healing time.
   a. Topical—for initial symptoms; not recurrences
   b. Oral—for recurrences, especially first 48 hours. Also need for prophylaxis—continuous administration for 4–6 months; long-term effects unknown.
   c. Intravenous—for severe cases and immunocompromised patients.
2. Lidocaine jelly—topical anesthetic
3. Bedrest—for severe symptoms
4. Condoms and spermicidal cream—to prevent transmission

Nursing Assessment

1. Question patient about frequency and type of sexual activity; discomfort noted.
2. Question patient about pruritus, burning, tenderness, urinary symptoms, unusual discharge.
3. Assess patient's view of herpes; stigmas, misconceptions, fears.
4. Inspect genitalia for lesions, erythema, edema. Use speculum to examine vagina and cervix. Perform diagnostic tests as above.

Nursing Diagnoses

1. Pain related to vesicular lesions
2. Impaired skin integrity related to herpetic lesions

3. Self-esteem disturbance related to stigma attached to herpes
4. Altered sexuality patterns related to potential transmission of herpes
5. Knowledge deficit of manifestations and management of herpes

Nursing Interventions

A. Increasing Comfort

1. Demonstrate and encourage the use of warm sitz baths to increase blood supply to the area and facilitate healing.
2. Instruct patient to keep the area clean and dry. Pat dry with a clean towel or use blow dryer. Wear loose cotton undergarments and loose clothing.
3. Encourage bedrest if disease is severe.
4. Administer pain medications as prescribed.
5. Encourage patient to void in a warm sitz bath if painful urination.
6. Insert indwelling catheter if urination is very painful or retention occurs.
7. Encourage fluid intake.

B. Restoring Skin Integrity

1. Teach patient appropriate application of acyclovir cream—apply as soon as lesions appear and reapply frequently.
2. Keep lesions clean and dry.
3. Teach patient not to rub or scratch lesions.

C. Improving Self-Esteem

1. Explore with patient her feelings about being "herpetic."
2. Reiterate that when she is feeling better physically, her feelings about herself and others will improve.
3. Discuss effects of stress on future outbreaks. Assist patient to identify stressors in her life.
4. Review stress reduction methods: relaxation, imagery, distraction.
5. Encourage patient to discuss her feelings with family and significant others.
6. Refer for support groups such as HELP for long-term emotional support and information.

Patient Education

A. General Points

1. Inform patient that initial outbreak is more severe than recurrences.
2. Review method of transmission: contact with lesions or shedded viral particles.
3. Assist the patient to recognize precipitating factors such as heat, stress, and fever.
4. Discuss signs and symptoms with patient and means to alleviate them.
5. Review various treatments with patient, especially acyclovir route and administration.
6. Emphasize the importance of Pap smears to detect cervical transformation.
7. Remind patient of the effects on a neonate and the importance of notifying her health care provider if she becomes pregnant.

B. Resuming Satisfying Sexual Activity

1. Teach patient to avoid intercourse when lesions are active and painful.
2. Inform patient that partner should use condoms for intercourse, but that they are not fully protective.

3. Explore possibility of noncoital aspects of sexual relationship.

Evaluation

1. Verbalizes decreased pain
2. Skin appears intact, without sign of secondary infection.
3. Verbalizes improved self-esteem
4. Reports satisfying sexual activity
5. States manifestations and treatment of herpes genitalis

Problems Resulting From Relaxed Pelvic Muscles

Cystocele and Urethrocele

Cystocele is a downward displacement (protrusion) of the bladder into the vagina.

Urethrocele is a downward displacement of the urethra into the vagina.

A. Etiology

1. Associated with obstetrical trauma to fascia, muscle, and ligaments during childbirth (results in poor support).
2. Often becomes apparent years later, when genital atrophy associated with aging occurs.
3. May also be due to congenital defect or posthysterectomy.

B. Clinical Manifestations

1. May be asymptomatic in early stages
2. Later, complains of pelvic pressure or heaviness ("like sitting on a ball"), backache, nervousness, fatigue
3. Urinary symptoms—urgency, frequency, incontinence, incomplete emptying
4. Aggravated by coughing, sneezing, standing for long periods, and obesity, which increase intra-abdominal pressure
5. Relieved by resting or lying down

C. Diagnostic Evaluation

1. Clean-catch urine specimen for culture and sensitivity
2. Urinalysis
3. Observation of patient in upright position for bulge in the vagina
4. Check for residual urine if signs and symptoms indicate

D. Management

1. Vaginal pessary—temporary treatment to support pelvic organs
   a. Prolonged use may lead to necrosis and ulceration.
   b. Should be removed and cleaned every 1–2 months
2. Estrogen therapy after menopause to decrease genital atrophy
3. Surgery
   a. If cystocele is large and interferes with bladder functioning
   b. May do *anterior vaginal colporrhaphy* (repair of anterior vaginal wall).
   c. *Complications*
      (1) Urinary retention—place indwelling catheter for 2–5 days.
      (2) Bleeding—vaginal packing for hemostasis

E. Nursing Interventions

1. Encourage fluids to decrease bacterial flora in the bladder.
2. Catheterize patient if urinary retention is suspected.
3. Teach patient Kegel's pelvic floor exercises to regain muscle tone; especially postpartum.
   a. Tighten the vaginal muscles; hold for a count of 3 and then relax.
   b. Repeat 10 times several times daily.
4. Teach patient to practice stopping the flow of urine during micturition—simulates Kegel's exercises.
5. Postoperative care
   a. Encourage voiding every 4–8 hours to reduce pressure so that no more than 150 ml. will accumulate in bladder—catheterization or use of an indwelling catheter may be required.
   b. Administer perineal care to the patient after each voiding and defecation.
   c. Employ a heat lamp to help dry the incision line and enhance the healing process.
   d. Use available sprays for anesthetic and antiseptic effects.
   e. Apply an ice pack locally to relieve congestion and discomfort.
   f. Administer analgesics as prescribed for relief of pain.

Rectocele/Enterocele

Rectocele is displacement (protrusion) of the rectum into the vagina. *Enterocele* is displacement of intestine into vagina.

A. Etiology

Similar to cystocele; however, posterior vaginal wall is weakened in a rectocele.

B. Clinical Manifestations

1. Pelvic pressure or heaviness—"bearing down feeling"
2. Constipation—may have difficulty in fecal evacuation; patient may use fingers into vagina to push feces up so defecation may take place.
3. Incontinence of feces and flatus—if tear between rectum and vagina
4. Protrusion of rectum or bowels
5. Perineal burning
6. Backache
7. Aggravated by standing for long periods

C. Diagnostic Evaluation

1. Observe patient in upright position for bulge into vagina.
2. May use Sims' speculum to uplift cervix

D. Management

1. Surgery—if rectocele is large enough to interfere with bowel functioning—posterior colpoplasty (perineorrhaphy)—repair of posterior vaginal wall
2. Pessary
3. Estrogen therapy

E. Nursing Intervention

1. Teach patient to increase fluid and fiber intake.
2. Encourage use of stool softeners or bulk laxatives to make passage of stool easier.
3. Promote rest.

4. Suggest low Fowler's position to decrease edema and discomfort.
5. Postoperative care—see Cystocele.

Malposition of the Uterus

When the uterus is in a normal position, the cervix lies in the axis of the vagina with the corpus inclined forward on the bladder.

Twenty-five percent of women have, to some degree, the reverse position (retroversion).

A. Retroversion and Retroflexion

In *retroversion,* the cervix remains in the normal axis, but body is directed to hollow of the sacrum.

In *retroflexion,* angulation of the corpus on the cervix is extreme.

1. *Clinical manifestations*
   a. Absent in mild displacement
   b. Significant displacement—pelvic pain, backache, dysmenorrhea, possibly infertility
2. *Management*
   a. Uterine replacement with bimanual examination
   b. Pessary placement for temporary relief of symptoms
   c. Uterine suspension—surgical shortening of round ligament

B. Uterine Prolapse

1. Definition—herniation of the uterus through the pelvic floor with a resultant protrusion into the vagina (prolapse) and at times even beyond the introitus (procidentia).
2. Degrees
   1st degree—cervix, without straining or traction, is at the introitus (spread the labia and it is visible).
   2nd degree—the cervix extends over the perineum.
   3rd degree—the entire uterus (or most of it) protrudes.
3. *Etiology*—usually due to obstetrical trauma and overstretching of musculofascial supports
4. *Clinical manifestations*
   a. Backache and/or abdominal pain
   b. Pressure and heaviness in vaginal region
   c. Bloody discharge due to cervix rubbing against clothing or inner thighs
   d. Ulceration of cervix
   e. Symptoms aggravated by obesity, standing, straining, coughing, or lifting a heavy object, due to increased intra-abdominal pressure
5. *Diagnostic evaluation*
   Pelvic examination
6. *Management*
   a. Surgical correction is recommended treatment with an anterior and posterior repair; effective and permanent.
   b. Vaginal pessary—temporary or palliative if surgery cannot be done; should be removed and cleaned every 1–2 months.
   c. Abdominal sacropexy—to anchor vagina
   d. Estrogen cream—to decrease genital atrophy changes
7. *Nursing interventions*
   a. Teach pelvic floor exercises to increase muscle tone.
   b. Control pain with sitz baths, acetaminophen, and heating pad.
   c. Increase fluids to decrease bladder infections.

d. Postoperative care—see Cystocele and Hysterectomy.

Gynecologic Tumors

Cancer of the Vulva

Clinical Features

1. Most common in women over 60 years of age; number of new cases has increased due to increase in elderly population.
2. Represents 3%–4% of gynecologic cancers.
3. Associated with history of infections such as human papillomavirus and herpes simplex virus.
4. Spread primarily through lymphatic system. Rare distant metastases.

> **GERONTOLOGIC ALERT:** Delay in seeking treatment is common, possibly due to modesty in older women.

Clinical Manifestations

1. Lump or lesion
   a. May be reddened, pigmented, white, or slightly elevated or ulcerated
   b. May have been present for months
   c. Most common site is labia majora, mid-or-anterior portion, and then clitoris.
2. Pruritus (vulvar)
3. Discharge or bleeding; may be foul-smelling due to secondary infection.
4. Pain
5. Dysuria due to invasion of urethra with bacteria
6. Edema of tissues
7. Lymphadenopathy

Diagnostic Evaluation

1. Biopsy—may be guided by colposcope. If lesion is small, may be excised. Most lesions are squamous cell carcinoma.
2. Palpation of lymph nodes in the groin for metastases.
3. Pelvic examination to determine the extent of cancer and rule out other pelvic neoplastic disease

Management

1. Carcinoma in situ (noninvasive) is usually treated by simple vulvectomy. Laser therapy may also be used.
2. Invasive carcinoma—radical or modified radical vulvectomy with bilateral groin lymph node resection
   a. Pelvic nodes also may be removed if involvement is suspected.
   b. If cancer is confined to the vulva, there is a 90% 5-year survival rate after surgery.
3. Advanced carcinoma—pelvic exenteration or surgery and radiation as a palliative measure.
   a. Radiation has a limited role due to tumor insensitivity and complications such as severe vulvitis.
   b. Chemotherapy is primarily investigational. May shrink lesion so surgery can be less extensive.
4. *Complications* (vulvectomy)
   a. Wound breakdown—most common complication (50%) due to skin tension.
   b. Lymphedema—due to decreased flow secondary to lymph node removal. May wear elastic support hose for a year.
   c. Leg cellulitis—recurrent problem; may use prophylactic penicillin.
   d. Vaginal stenosis.

Preoperative Nursing Interventions

1. Shave a wide area to include perineal, pubic, and inguinal areas.
2. Cleanse the vulva the night before with hexachlorophene or povidone-iodine shower or scrub.
3. Administer an enema to evacuate intestinal tract before surgery; there will be no bowel movements for 2–3 days postoperatively.
4. Adhere to protocol for preoperative care as described on page 52.
5. Prepare patient for postoperative IV, urinary catheter, and wound drains (see Fig. 28-4).
6. Have the patient describe what her understanding is regarding her problem.
7. Emphasize the positive outcomes of the prescribed treatment plan; reinforce what the physician has discussed with her.
8. Answer her questions tactfully; use available resources for those questions about which assistance is needed.
9. Encourage her to talk about her concerns regarding fear of mutilation and loss of sexual function.

Postoperative Nursing Interventions

1. Maintain drainage and compression of tissues to remove fluid that could cause edema and prevent wound healing. Empty drains as prescribed (at least every 8 hours).
2. Keep wound clean and dry.
   a. Sterile dressing changes as prescribed.
   b. Apply heat lamp if prescribed to increase circulation and oxygen to tissues.
   c. Perform perineal care or sitz baths after each bowel movement or voiding (after catheter removed).
   d. Maintain patency of urinary catheter (about 10 days) to prevent wound contamination with urine.

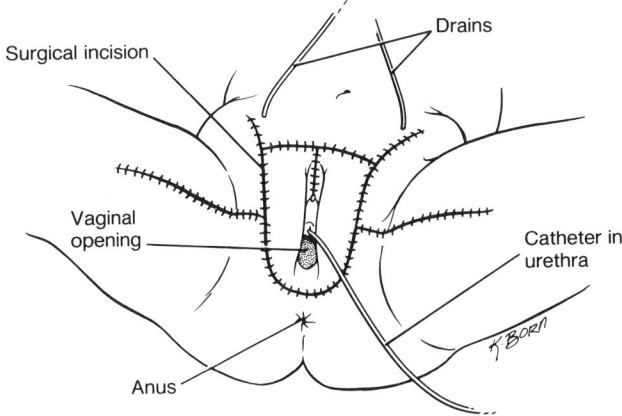

Figure 28-4. Postoperative appearance after radical vulvectomy.

3. Prevent cardiopulmonary complications (especially in older patient).
   a. Administer heparin subcutaneously as prescribed to prevent thrombus/embolus.
   b. Perform leg exercises and/or ambulate the day following surgery.
4. Promote comfort by placing patient in low Fowler's position with knees slightly elevated to decrease tension on sutures. Administer medication for pain as prescribed.
5. Prevent straining with defecation by providing a low-residue diet.
6. Encourage patient to ventilate feelings regarding altered body image and sexual functioning.

Patient Education

1. Teach patient that if vagina is still intact, intercourse and vaginal delivery are possible.
2. Inform patient of changes that may occur related to surgery (i.e., if clitoris is removed, may experience a loss of sensation).
3. Explore alternative means of increasing sexual satisfaction.

Cancer of the Cervix

Epidemiology

1. Most common between 35 and 55 years of age. 13,000 estimated new cases in 1989.
2. Early sexual activity, multiple sexual partners, and history of sexually transmitted diseases, especially human papillomavirus and herpes genitalis, are major risk factors.
3. Incidence is higher in lower socioeconomic status and blacks.
4. Decreased mortality rate in U.S., but most frequent malignancy among females in developing countries.

Types of Cervical Cancer

1. *Dysplasia*—atypical cells with some degree of surface maturation
2. *Carcinoma in situ* (CIS)—cytology similar to invasive carcinoma, but confined to epithelium
3. *Invasive carcinoma*—stroma is involved; 90% are of the squamous cell type. Spreads by local invasion and lymphatics

Clinical Manifestations

1. Early disease is usually asymptomatic.
2. Initial symptoms:
   a. Postcoital bleeding
   b. Irregular vaginal bleeding or spotting between periods or after menopause; as disease progresses becomes more constant and increases in amount
   c. Malodorous discharge
3. Pain is a large symptom—radiates to buttocks and legs.
4. Weight loss, anemia, fever—with advanced disease

Diagnostic Evaluation

1. Pelvic examination
2. Pap smear—routine screening measure; abnormal results warrant further diagnostic tests such as biopsy (with colposcopy or Schiller's test to visualize lesions) or conization.

3. Staging laparotomy—to evaluate metastasis outside the pelvis
4. Metastatic work-up—IVP, cystoscopy, sigmoidoscopy

Management

A. Radiotherapy—usual treatment for all stages
1. Intracavitary—radium via applicator
2. External—via linear accelerator or cobalt
3. *Complications:*
   a. Cystitis, proctitis, vaginal stenosis, uterine perforation (intracavitary)
   b. Nausea, vomiting, bone marrow depression, small bowel obstruction, fistula (external)

B. Surgery
1. Hysterectomy
   a. Done if childbearing no longer desired
   b. Usually combined with radiation therapy for CIS and invasive carcinoma
   c. May cause impaired bladder function
2. Pelvic exenteration
   a. Is the surgical removal of the vagina, uterus, uterine tubes, ovaries, bladder, rectum and supporting structures and the creation of an ileal conduit and fecal stoma.
   b. Is done for very advanced disease if radiation therapy cannot be used; also for recurrent cancer.
   c. Vaginal reconstruction may be done.
3. Conization—if childbearing is desired, depending on stage of cancer.

C. Laser Therapy—tissue destruction by vapors for dysplasia

D. Cryosurgery—destroy tissue by freezing it

E. Chemotherapy—adjuvant with surgery or radiation; radiosensitizer

Nursing Interventions

1. See p. 733 for hysterectomy nursing measures.
2. See p. 731 for radiotherapy nursing measures.
3. Provide emotional support for guilt, altered body image, and altered sexuality.
4. Assist patient to obtain information about the disease and treatment.

Patient Education

1. Stress importance of lifelong follow-up visits regardless of treatments:
   a. To determine response to treatment.
   b. To detect spread of cancer.
2. Inform patient that she should see a gynecologist, even following a hysterectomy.

Cancer of the Corpus Uteri

Epidemiology

1. Most common of gynecologic cancers
2. Ranks fourth in cancer incidence in women
3. Peaks about age 55, most common in postmenopausal women
4. Risk factors include obesity, late menopause, childlessness, estrogen therapy, and pelvic irradiation.

Clinical Manifestations

1. Irregular bleeding before menopause or postmenopausal bleeding
2. Vaginal discharge—watery, usually malodorous
3. Pain, fever, and bowel and bladder dysfunctions are late signs.
4. Anemia secondary to bleeding

Diagnostic Evaluation

1. Pelvic examination—enlarged uterus may be palpated.
2. Endocervical aspirate
3. Endometrial biopsy—positive results indicate cancer; whereas a negative result does not exclude cancer.
4. Fractional D&C—most accurate diagnostic tool
5. Hysteroscopy—to view lesion
6. Metastatic work-up—includes x-ray studies and cystoscopy

Management

1. Hysterectomy—primary therapy.
2. Radiation therapy—preoperative or postoperative; *complications* include hemorrhagic cystitis, rectal ulceration, or proctitis.
3. Hormonal therapy—progestational agents may alter receptor sites in endometrium for estrogen and thus decrease growth (for metastatic disease).
4. Chemotherapy—for metastatic and recurrent disease; low response rate of short duration

Nursing Interventions

In addition to interventions for Radiation Therapy (right-hand column) and Hysterectomy (p. 733):
1. Provide emotional support during diagnostic phase.
2. Explain types of diagnostic tests and what the patient can expect.
3. Explain the significance of postmenopausal bleeding.
4. Encourage the patient to keep follow-up visits with physician.

Myomas of the Uterus

Myomas of the uterus are benign tumors of the uterine myometrium (smooth muscle). Also called fibroids, leiomyomas, fibromyomas.

Incidence

1. Usually occur in women over 30 years old
2. Rarely develop after menopause; preexisting tumors may shrink.
3. Higher incidence in black women than white women
4. Responsible for one third of all hysterectomies

Clinical Manifestations

1. Small myomas do not cause symptoms.
2. After myomas (or myomata) grow, the first indication of the presence of a tumor is a palpable mass.
3. Excessive or prolonged menstruation is usually the chief symptom (with little or no change in the menstrual interval); intermenstrual or postmenopausal bleeding also may occur.
4. Pain comes from pressure on adjacent organs. As myomas grow, there may be a sensation of weight—a heavy feeling.

5. Secondary symptoms may be a feeling of lassitude, general weakness, anemia, and lower abdominal discomfort.
6. Unexplained infertility

Diagnostic Evaluation

1. Cytology, dilatation and curettage, cervical biopsy—done primarily to rule out cancer
2. Diagnosis is made by abdominal and bimanual palpation of the uterus.

Management

1. Myomectomy—if small tumor
2. Hysterectomy—for large tumor and/or symptomatic

Nursing Interventions

See Hysterectomy, page 733.

Nursing Care of the Patient Receiving Radiation Therapy to the Uterus

General Information

1. Applicators (tandems and ovoids) are positioned in the endocervical canal and vagina in the operating room with the patient under anesthesia. On recovery from anesthesia, x-rays are taken to check correct placement.
2. Radiologist inserts radioactive material (radium or cesium) into applicator.
3. Radiation source remains in place 24–72 hours.
4. Therapy is individualized according to the stage of disease and the patient's response to and tolerance of radiation.
5. Internal therapy may be supplemented with external radiation (supervoltage x-ray, telecobalt, or linear accelerator source) directed over the pelvis in an effort to eliminate cancer spread via lymphatic system.

Nursing Interventions

A. Patient Preparation

1. Prepare the patient for preliminary tests—blood studies, endometrium biopsies, chest x-ray, ECG, cystoscopy.
2. Instruct the patient regarding placement of applicator in the O.R. and anesthesia.
   a. Prepare the intestinal tract by enemas and the vagina by a cleansing douche per physician's directives.
   b. Insert an indwelling catheter if prescribed.
3. Encourage patient to bring diversional activities, as she will remain on bedrest during radiation treatment.
4. Instruct patient in radiation safety measures:
   a. Only source is radioactive (radium or cesium); neither patient nor secretions are radioactive.
      (1) DO NOT TOUCH SOURCE.
      (2) Notify someone IMMEDIATELY if source is dislodged.
   b. When needles or applicators are removed, there is no radioactivity remaining.
   c. Radioactivity is monitored by specially trained personnel.
   d. No pregnant visitors or children under 18 years old.

e. Lead shields may be used to decrease radiation emanating from the patient.

5. Reinforce that personnel are readily available.

B. During Radiation Treatment

1. Maintain patient on strict bedrest on her back with head of bed elevated 20–30 degrees. Patient may be "log rolled" 3–4 times per day. Use eggcrate mattress.
2. Have patient bathe upper body. Perineal care and linen changes are done only when absolutely necessary.
3. Maintain patient on a low-residue diet to prevent bowel movements, which could dislodge the apparatus. Encourage the patient to eat a variety of small rather than large servings.
4. Inspect indwelling catheter frequently to ensure proper drainage. A distended bladder may cause severe radiation burns.
5. Encourage fluids to prevent bladder infection.
6. Observe for signs and symptoms of radiation sickness—nausea, vomiting, fever, diarrhea, abdominal cramping.
7. Check applicator position every 8 hours, and monitor amount of bleeding and drainage (a small amount is normal).
8. Be supportive to patient to decrease anxiety and fear. Check on patient frequently, but minimize time spent at bedside to reduce radiation exposure.

C. During Radium Removal

1. Provide sterile gloves, long forceps, and lead container or "pig."
2. Check number of tubes removed against number applied; should be noted in chart.
3. Practice radium precautions in handling and returning source to radiation department.
4. Administer a cleansing enema and douche before the patient gets out of bed.
5. Provide assistance during ambulation because of postural hypotension resulting from prolonged bedrest.

Patient Education

Following radiation therapy:

1. Teach patient to maintain integrity of radiation-exposed skin: avoid soap, as it is irritating, pat dry, check with healthcare provider before using anything on skin (Usually cornstarch may be used to relieve itching and A&D ointment to relieve irritation.)
2. Discuss normal side effects such as fatigue and possibly nausea and vomiting.
3. Report signs and symptoms of radiation injury to the intestine—diarrhea, abdominal pain; or the bladder—dysuria, hematuria, or frequency.
4. Discuss effects of radiation on sexual function—dyspareunia may occur due to vaginal shortening and narrowing and vaginal dryness.
   a. Use water-soluble lubricant.
   b. Experiment with positions if experiencing discomfort.
   c. Increased foreplay may increase pain threshold.
   d. Use vaginal dilator for 5–10 minutes once or twice a day if do not have intercourse at least once a week.
   e. Condoms may decrease burning felt from contact with semen.
5. Provide emotional support—refer for support groups or counseling as needed.
6. Remind patient of the importance of follow-up visits to physician to assess radiation effects on cancer.

Ovarian Cancer

Characteristics

1. Second most common gynecologic cancer; most common cause of death from gynecologic cancers—due to frequent metastases as a result of failure to diagnose early.
2. Most common in postmenopausal women, aged 55–60 years. Associated with high-fat diet and nulliparity.
3. Direct spread intra-abdominally and through lymphatic channels.

Clinical Manifestations

1. No early manifestations
2. First manifestations—vague; related to GI tract
   a. Abdominal discomfort
   b. Indigestion
   c. Flatulence
   d. Anorexia
   e. Pelvic pressure
   f. Weight gain or loss
   g. Ovarian enlargement
3. Late manifestations—include abdominal pain, ascites, pleural effusion, intestinal obstruction

Diagnostic Evaluation

1. Pelvic examination—to detect enlargement, nodularity, immobility of the ovaries. A palpable ovary in a menopausal woman is abnormal.
2. Sonography and CT scan—useful to monitor therapy, but not helpful for early detection
3. Laparoscopy—to visualize mass
4. Paracentesis or thoracentesis—if signs and symptoms warrant
5. Laparotomy—to surgically stage disease
6. CA 125—an increase in this tumor marker signifies progression of disease.

Management

A. Surgery

1. Bilateral salpingo-oophorectomy and hysterectomy—most commonly performed to diagnose, stage, and debulk (remove as much of the tumor as possible)
2. Oophorectomy—if childbearing is desired and cancer is limited to one ovary with capsule intact.
3. "Second-look" laparotomy—performed after chemotherapy to reassess patients who have no clinical evidence of disease.
4. Palliative surgery—for bowel obstruction to resect or bypass

B. Other Treatment

1. Chemotherapy—more effective if tumor is optimally debulked; usually follows surgery due to frequency of advanced disease; may be given IV or intraperitoneal; usually cisplatin and cyclophosphamide are included in the combination.
2. Interferon—for recurrent disease after chemotherapy.
3. Radiation therapy—isotopes such as radioactive phosphorus.

Nursing Interventions

1. Provide preoperative and postoperative care (see Hysterectomy, p. 733).
2. Provide relief of chemotherapy side effects, especially

nausea and vomiting, with antiemetics such as meto-clopramide (a common problem with cisplatin and cyclophosphamide).
3. Assist patient to cope with change in body image, i.e., hair loss due to chemotherapy. Provide wigs, scarves, etc.
4. Assist patient to cope with fear and anxiety due to diagnosis of cancer and upcoming treatments. Spend time with patient. May need to refer for counseling and/or support groups as necessary.
5. Instruct patient in side effects of treatment and postoperative care—see Chemotherapy, page 103.
6. Instruct patient about the menopausal symptoms that may be experienced with oophorectomy (see Menopause, p. 716)

Hysterectomy

Hysterectomy is the surgical removal of the uterus.
Sixty-five percent of these procedures occur during the reproductive years.

Possible Indications

1. Malignant and nonmalignant growth on uterus, cervix, and adnexa that should be removed
2. Control of uterine bleeding and/or hemorrhage
3. Severe (life-threatening) pelvic infection
4. Correction of problems associated with pelvic floor relaxation—cystocele, rectocele
5. Treatment of endometriosis when conservative measures have failed
6. Irreparable rupture or perforation of uterus

Types of Hysterectomy *(See Table 28-2)*

A. Abdominal

1. *Subtotal hysterectomy*—corpus of uterus is removed, but cervical stump remains.
2. *Total hysterectomy*—entire uterus is removed, including cervix; tubes and ovaries remain.
3. *Total hysterectomy with bilateral salpingo-oophorectomy*—entire uterus, tubes, and ovaries are removed.

B. Vaginal

Nursing Assessment

1. Determine if patient knows reason for hysterectomy, what the procedure involves, and what to expect postoperatively.

2. Postoperatively assess:
   a. Wound appearance and drainage
   b. Vital signs, level of consciousness
   c. Level of pain
   d. Vaginal drainage
   e. Intake and output
   f. Urge to void, bladder distention, residual urine (if appropriate)
   g. Clarity, odor, and sediment of urine

Nursing Diagnoses

1. Pain related to surgical procedure
2. Altered pattern of urinary elimination related to decreased bladder sensation
3. Potential for infection related to surgical procedure
4. Potential for fluid volume deficit related to bleeding
5. Potential for altered tissue perfusion related to thrombus/embolus
6. Self-esteem disturbance related to alteration in female organs
7. Anxiety related to diagnosis and feelings of altered femininity.
8. Potential for sexual dysfunction related to alteration in reproductive organs and function

Nursing Interventions

A. Increasing Comfort

1. Assess pain location, level, and characteristics.
2. Administer prescribed pain medications.
3. Encourage patient to splint incision when moving.
4. Encourage patient to ambulate as soon as prescribed to decrease flatus and abdominal distention.
5. Institute sitz baths or ice packs as prescribed to alleviate perineal discomfort.

B. Maintaining Bladder Function

1. Monitor intake and output, bladder distention, signs and symptoms of bladder infection.
2. Maintain patency of indwelling catheter if one is in place.
3. Catheterize patient intermittently if uncomfortable or has not voided in 8 hours.
4. Check for residual urine after patient voids; should be less than 100 ml. Continue to check if more than 100 ml. or bladder infection may develop.
5. Encourage patient to empty bladder around the clock, not only when feeling the urge, due to loss of sensation of bladder fullness.
6. Encourage fluid intake to decrease risk of infection.

Table 28-2. *Abdominal vs. Vaginal Hysterectomy*

	Preferred for	Advantages	Disadvantages
Abdominal	Gynecologic malignancy Pelvic inflammatory disease Endometriosis	Thorough exploration of abdominal and pelvic cavities Decreased infection postoperatively	Abdominal scar Increased abdominal pain Longer hospitalization stay Slower recovery
Vaginal	Pelvic muscle relaxation High-risk patients, i.e., obesity	Fewer surgical complications No incision Shorter hospitalization stay Quicker recovery Less abdominal pain	Limited surgical field Increased rate of infection Increased bladder problems Vaginal shortening

C. Preventing Infection

1. Assess vaginal drainage for amount, color, and odor, incision site, and temperature.
2. Administer antibiotics as prescribed.
3. Assist patient to use incentive spirometer, coughing, deep breathing, and ambulation to decrease risk of pulmonary infection.

D. Preventing Fluid Volume Deficit

1. Monitor amount of bleeding—measure size of stains on vaginal pad or abdominal dressing. Weigh pad when removed—compare weight of saturated pad with that of a dry pad (the difference will be weight of blood loss).
2. Monitor vital signs, especially blood pressure and intake and output.
3. Report any increased bleeding or brightness (except small amount of serosanguineous discharge).
4. Encourage oral fluids or maintain intravenous fluids as required.

E. Preventing Thromboembolus

1. Assess for positive Homans's sign.
2. Administer prophylactic heparin as prescribed.
3. Apply antiembolism stockings.
4. Teach and encourage patient to exercise in bed and ambulate when permitted.
5. Tell patient to avoid placing pressure under knees or crossing legs.

F. Improving Self-Concept

1. Allow patient to discuss her feelings about herself as a woman.
2. Reassure patient she is still feminine.
3. Encourage her to discuss her feelings with her spouse or significant other.
4. Reassure her that she will not go through premature menopause if her ovaries were not removed.

G. Reducing Anxiety

1. Allow patient time to discuss fears and concerns related to surgery, pathology results.
2. Provide information to clarify misconceptions.
3. Offer emotional support.
4. Enlist spouse in discussion as appropriate.

H. Regaining Sexual Function

1. Discuss changes due to hysterectomy on sexual functioning (i.e., shortened vagina with a vaginal hysterectomy; dyspareunia due to dryness or with prolapse; loss of vaginal sensation).
2. Offer suggestions to improve sexual functioning:
   a. Water-soluble lubricants
   b. Change position—female dominant offers more control of depth of penetration.

Patient Education

1. A total hysterectomy produces a surgical menopause (if the adnexa were also removed).
2. Explain to the patient the importance of hormonal replacement (prescribed) if she has had a total hysterectomy with oophorectomy/salpingectomy.
3. Advise her against sitting too long at one time, as in driving long distances, because of the possibility of pooling of blood in the pelvis and of thromboembolism.
4. Suggest that the patient delay driving a car until the 3rd postoperative week, as even pressing the brake pedal may initiate slight discomfort in the lower abdomen.
5. Tell the patient to expect a "tired feeling" for the first few days at home and, therefore, not to plan too many activities for the first week.
6. Assist her in planning a flexible schedule so that she will be able to perform most of her usual household activities within a month; within 2 months, she will feel her "normal" self.
7. Stress that the patient should assume employment outside the home only when her physician indicates; this will depend on the type of work, etc.
8. Tell the patient not to feel discouraged if at times during convalescence she experiences depression, feels like crying, and seems unusually nervous. This is common, but will not last.
9. Remind her to ask her physician regarding resumption of various preferred physical activities; note that some of the most strenuous tasks are hanging clothes on a line and using the vacuum cleaner. These tasks should be delayed for several weeks. The patient should not lift heavy objects for at least a month to 6 weeks.
10. Determine what the physician has told the patient regarding resumption of intercourse; reinforce this and explain that too-enthusiastic genital sex may injure the incision site and produce bleeding. In other words, she is to "go easy" at first. Suggest coital position variation.

    Usually sexual relations, douching, or use of tampons is discouraged for 4–6 weeks, unless otherwise specified by the physician.
11. Showers are permitted, but tub bathing is deferred until the physician indicates that tissues are sufficiently healed.
12. Emphasize the importance of follow-up physical and gynecologic examinations, not only for peace of mind, but also to detect any beginning pathology. Temperature elevation over 37.8°C. (100°F.), heavy vaginal bleeding, drainage, and foul odor of discharge are reportable.

Evaluation

1. Verbalizes decreased pain
2. Voids every 8 hours of sufficient quantity
3. Absence of infection and bleeding
4. Maintains warmth and color of extremities
5. Presents an optimistic outlook
6. Exhibits minimal anxiety
7. Reports satisfying sexual function

Endometriosis

Endometriosis is a disease characterized by cells resembling the endometrium (uterine lining) growing outside the uterus.

Characteristics

1. May also be found outside the pelvic cavity; an intact uterus is not needed to have endometriosis.
2. Peaks in 25–45-year-old women; may occur at any age. Increased risk in siblings, women with shorter menstrual cycles and longer duration of flow. More common in whites than blacks, and in women who do not exercise and are obese.

3. Can lead to infertility
4. Responds to ovarian hormonal stimulation—estrogen increases it, progestins decrease it.
   a. Bleeds during uterine menstruation, resulting in accumulated blood and inflammation and subsequent adhesions and pain.
   b. Regresses during amenorrhea (i.e., pregnancy and menopause) and oral contraceptive and androgen use.

Theories of Origin

1. May be embryonic tissue remnants that differentiate as a result of hormonal stimulation and spread via lymphatic or venous channels
2. May be transferred via surgical instruments
3. May be due to retrograde menstruation through uterine (fallopian) tubes into peritoneal cavity.

Clinical Manifestations

1. Depends on sites of implantation; may be asymptomatic
2. Pelvic pain—especially during or before menstruation; or lower bilateral abdominal pain
3. Dyspareunia—especially if vaginal or uterosacral ligament is involved
4. Painful defecation—if implants are on sigmoid colon or rectum
5. Abnormal uterine bleeding
6. Persistent infertility
7. Hematuria, dysuria, flank pain—if bladder involvement
8. Ruptured cyst—mimics acute appendicitis or ruptured ectopic pregnancy

Diagnostic Evaluation

1. Pelvic and rectal examinations—tender, fixed nodules or ovarian mass or uterine retrodisplacement; nodules may not be palpable.
2. Laparoscopy—for definitive diagnosis to view implants and determine extent of disease
3. Other studies include ultrasound, CT, and barium enema to determine extent of organ involvement.

Management

Controversial due to uncertainty of cause. No treatment if pain-free and does not desire pregnancy.

A. Medical

1. Danazol—most commonly used drug; synthetic androgen suppresses endometrial growth. Do not administer during pregnancy.
2. Progestins—create a hypoestrogenic environment.
3. Gonadotropin-releasing hormone antagonists—create hypoestrogenic environment.
4. Oral contraceptives—use small amount of estrogen, maximum amount of progestin to decrease implant size.

B. Surgical

1. Laparoscopic surgery—preferred procedure to remove implants and lyse adhesions; not curative; high recurrence rate
2. CO_2 laser laparoscopy—for minimal to moderate disease; vaporizes tissue; may be done at same time as diagnosis; good pregnancy rate
3. Laparotomy—for severe endometriosis or persistent symptoms
4. Presacral neurectomy—to decrease central pelvic pain; preserves fertility
5. Hysterectomy—if fertility is not desired and symptoms are severe; ovaries are preserved if not affected.
6. In vitro fertilization—for recurrent endometriosis and infertility

Nursing Interventions

1. Assess pain—level, location, characteristics
2. Encourage use of heating pad and analgesics.
3. Encourage patient to try position changes for sexual intercourse if experiencing dyspareunia.
4. Encourage patient to obtain adequate rest.
5. Include the patient in the treatment plans so that she knows why a particular method of treatment has been selected.
6. Teach correct administration and side effects of prescribed medications.
7. Provide emotional support—allow patient to discuss feelings and concerns; include family or significant other as needed; refer to support groups as needed.
8. Prepare patient for surgery when indicated.

Patient Education

1. Review anatomy and physiology of reproductive system as needed.
2. Tell patient what to expect from diagnostic tests such as laparoscopy.
3. Instruct patient in the side effects of prescribed medications, i.e., Danazol may cause voice changes, increased facial hair, acne, weight gain, decreased breast size, and vasomotor reactions.

Pelvic Inflammatory Disease (PID)

Pelvic inflammatory disease is an infection that may involve the uterine tubes, ovaries, uterus, and/or peritoneum.

Clinical Features

1. Incidence of PID has increased dramatically. High recurrence rate due to reinfections.
2. Causative agents include *Neisseria gonorrhoeae; Chlamydia trachomatis,* and *Mycoplasma hominis.*
3. Predisposing factors include multiple sexual partners, early onset of sexual activity, use of intrauterine devices (wick serves to promote ascension of bacteria), and procedures such as therapeutic abortion, cesarian sections, and hysterosalpingograms.

Clinical Manifestations

1. More vague in chlamydia.
2. Pelvic pain—most common presenting symptom; usually dull and bilateral
3. Fever—especially seen with severe gonoccocal infections
4. Cervical discharge—mucopurulent
5. Cervical motion tenderness—especially with gonoccocal infections
6. Irregular bleeding
7. GI symptoms—nausea, vomiting, acute abdomen usually signifies abscess.
8. Urinary symptoms—dysuria, frequency

Diagnostic Evaluation

1. History—menstruation, contraception, sexual activity, including the number of partners, STD history, symptoms
2. Physical examination—including pelvic examination, especially alert to abdomen for tenderness, pain, rebound or mass.
3. Endocervical culture—to identify organisms
4. Complete blood count—shows increased leukocyte count and erythrocyte sedimentation rate.
5. Laparoscopy—provides direct visualization of the uterine tubes.

Management

A. Medical

1. Antibiotics—includes combinations such as tetracycline, doxycycline, cefoxitin, amoxicillin, and ampicillin.
2. Usually outpatient treatment. Inpatient therapy is warranted if uncertain diagnosis, abscess, pregnancy, severe infection, unable to maintain oral intake, prepubertal or more aggressive antibiotics required to preserve fertility.
3. Inpatient regimen—includes IV antibiotics for 4 days and 48 hours after patient improves, then orally on outpatient basis for 10 days.

B. Surgical

1. Salpingolysis or ovariolysis—to separate and remove adhesions from tubes or ovaries
2. Salpingostomy—reopen occluded end of uterine tube
3. Anastamosis of cornual occlusion—implant patent section of uterine tube into new opening in uterus.
4. Salpingo-oophorectomy—for ruptured or abscessed tube and ovary; may also need a hysterectomy
5. In vitro fertilization—if other methods fail

Complications

1. Infertility—due to adhesions of uterine tubes and ovaries
2. Ectopic pregnancy—due to inability of fertilized egg to pass stricture
3. Abscess rupture and sepsis

Nursing Interventions

1. Assist patient in comfort measures, i.e., pelvic rest (head and feet elevated with pelvis in dependent position), analgesics, and use of heating pad on abdomen or lower back to increase circulation.
2. Administer, or teach patient to administer, antibiotics on schedule and be alert for side effects.
3. Place patient in semi-Fowler's position to facilitate drainage of infection.
4. Follow procedures for infection control:
   a. Use gloves when handling contaminated items such as perineal pads or linens.
   b. Wash hands carefully before and after patient contact.
5. Monitor nutritional status, especially fluid intake.
6. Provide emotional support for feelings of guilt, fear, and anxiety.

Patient Education

1. Teach signs and symptoms of pelvic inflammatory disease to women at risk.
2. Assist patient in selection of contraceptive device: barrier types (diaphragm and condom) offer more protection from infections.
3. Review antibiotic schedule and possible side effects with patient.
4. Emphasize importance of follow-up visits to be certain that infection has cleared and the need to report fever and pain during treatment.
5. Reinforce need to have partner cultured and treated to prevent reinfection.
6. Teach patient to protect herself and others from reinfection by careful hand-washing and proper hygienic measures.
7. Remind patient to abstain from intercourse until infection subsides.
8. Tell patient to avoid use of tampons.

Toxic Shock Syndrome

Toxic shock syndrome is a condition caused by a bacterial toxin (*Staphylococcal aureus*) in the bloodstream; it can be life-threatening.

1. Found primarily in the U.S.
2. Origin is uncertain, but 70% of cases are associated with menstruation and tampon use.
3. Research studies suggest that magnesium-absorbing fibers in tampons may account for lower levels of magnesium in the body; this contributes to providing an ideal condition for toxin production by the bacteria.
4. TSS has been observed in nonmenstruating individuals with conditions such as cellulitis, surgical wound infection, vaginal infections, subcutaneous abscesses, and with the use of contraceptive sponge, diaphragm, and tubal ligation.
5. Oral contraceptives may be protective against toxic shock syndrome by increasing lactobacilli in vaginal flora.

Clinical Manifestations

1. Sudden onset of high fever >39°C. (102°F.)
2. Vomiting and profuse watery diarrhea
3. Rapid progression to hypotension and shock within 72 hours of onset
4. Mucous membrane hyperemia
5. Sometimes, sore throat, headache, and myalgia are experienced.
6. Rash (similar to sunburn) that develops 1–2 weeks after onset of illness and is followed by desquamation, particularly of the palms and soles

Diagnostic Evaluation

1. Determine whether the patient has used tampons recently.
2. Take blood and urine samples and throat cultures, and where appropriate, cerebrospinal fluid, vaginal, and/or cervical specimens.
3. Perform blood and urine studies.
4. Rule out other illnesses—sepsis, Rocky Mountain spotted fever, etc.
5. Determine whether there is a history of recent skin infection, childbirth, or surgery.

Management

1. Fluid and electrolyte replacement is instituted to increase blood pressure.
    a. Strict intake and output is maintained.
    b. Indwelling catheter is inserted if needed.
2. Monitor hemodynamic status as needed (i.e., arterial line.)
3. Medications administered to raise blood pressure (i.e., dopamine) as needed.
4. Antibiotics prescribed to control infection, such as penicillins or cephalosporins.
5. Nasogastric tube inserted if nausea and vomiting is a problem.
6. The use of steroids and immunoglobulins is controversial.

Complications

Respiratory distress syndrome—due to fluid overload from increased fluid replacement.
1. Monitor closely for signs and symptoms of fluid overload.
2. May require mechanical ventilation

Patient Education

A. For Individual Patient

1. May be fatigued and weak for months
2. May experience reversible hair loss 1–2 months after disease
3. Should not use tampons if she has had toxic shock syndrome
4. Requires close follow-up with pelvic examination and repeat cultures

B. General Population Education

1. Until more definitive research provides answers to this puzzling problem, women are advised to
    a. Alternate use of pads with tampons.
    b. Be alert to the symptoms of TSS.
    c. Change tampons frequently and not wear one longer than 8 hours; 4 hours is maximum for heavy discharge times.
    d. Be careful of vaginal abrasions that can be caused by some applicators.
    e. Avoid using super-absorbent tampons.

Fertility Control

Basic Principles

1. *Contraception* is the prevention of fertility on a temporary basis.
2. *Sterilization* is the permanent prevention of fertility.
3. Contraception effectiveness depends on motivation, which is a result of education, culture, religion, and personal situation. It is best to include both partners in any contraception decision.
4. Nurses should be familiar with contraceptive methods and educate patients without moral judgement.
5. Failure rate (pregnancy) is determined by the experience of 100 women for 1 year and is expressed as pregnancies per 100 woman-years.

Contraceptive Methods

See Table 28-3.

Future Directions

1. Injectable steroids (via IM): injection every 3 months of long-acting synthetic progestins.
2. Steroid capsules or rods implanted subdermally; may last as long as 5 years.
3. Vaginal contraceptive rings—silastic rings that release estrogen and progestin; left in place 3 out of 4 weeks; systemically absorbed.
4. Ombrelle 250 IUD—copper device; very flexible and adaptable to decrease risk of endometrial trauma and expulsion.
5. Birth control vaccines—antibodies are being developed to interfere with hormones and sperm antigens to prevent pregnancy.

Sterilization Procedures

A. Indications

1. Increasing numbers are performed annually in the U.S. for the purpose of birth control.
2. Other indications—illness, genetic abnormalities.

B. Legal Considerations

1. Informed consent needed
2. Waiting period between signing consent and procedure if federal funds used (30 days)

C. Tubal Sterilization

1. Approaches:
    a. Abdominal—most frequently used: may be postpartum laparotomy, minilaparotomy, or laparoscopy. Laparoscopy, with electrocoagulation, is the most frequently performed. It is a very safe and effective procedure.
    b. Vaginal—incision in posterior vagina (colpotomy) with the uterine tube pulled through it; higher rate of complications.
2. Techniques:
    a. Electrocoagulation—most common; burn section of tube with or without excision; low reversal rate.
    b. Pomeroy—tube tied in midsection and section removed; may be reversed.
    c. Fimbriectomy—fimbriated end removed and end tied; irreversible.
    d. Cornual resection—remove section of tube nearest uterus and suture cornual opening closed.
    e. Silastic bands—plastic or metal clips to occlude tube; may be reversed.
3. Complications:
    a. Tubal pregnancy
    b. Hemorrhage, infection, uterine perforation, damage to bowel or bladder
4. Nursing interventions:
    a. Assess motivation for sterilization. Remind patient procedure is irreversible for the most part.
    b. Teach patient that there is no effect on hormones and menstruation will continue.
    c. Teach patient there should not be any adverse effect on sexual response.
5. Vasectomy (see p. 709)
6. Hysterectomy (see p. 733)—not usually used for conception control.

Table 28-3. *Contraceptive Methods*

Methods	Definition	Procedure	Advantages	Disadvantages
Natural Methods				
1. Periodic abstinence	Abstain from intercourse during fertile period of each cycle.	Determine fertile period by: 1. Calendar method—ovulation occurs 14 days before next menstrual period. 2. Cervical mucus method—increase in mucus at time of ovulation; clear and stringy. 3. Basal body temperature—drops immediately before ovulation and rises 24–72 hours after ovulation. 4. Symptothermal method—combines 2 & 3.	1. No health hazards 2. Inexpensive 3. Religiously acceptable 4. Increased knowledge of cycles	1. 25% failure rate 2. Requires consistent record-keeping
2. Coitus interruptus	Withdrawal of penis from vagina when ejaculation is imminent.	Must withdraw before ejaculation so that ejaculation occurs away from female genitalia.	1. No cost 2. No health hazards 3. Always available	1. Failure rate of 35%–40%; pre-ejaculatory fluid may contain sperm. 2. Interruption of sexual act
3. Lactation	Breast-feeding has a contraceptive effect due to prolactin's inhibition of luteinizing hormone, which maintains menstruation.	Breast-feed on demand, around the clock, without formula supplementation.	1. No health hazards 2. No cost	1. Unreliable 2. Need to use other method such as spermicide or barrier, which have no effect on breast milk.
Barrier Methods				
1. Condom	Rubber or processed collagenous tissue sheaths, placed over erect penis to prevent semen from entering vagina	1. Place condom over erect penis. 2. Leave dead space at tip of condom (from which air has been expelled) to allow room for ejaculate. 3. Use spermicide agent to lubricate exterior for added protection. 4. Grasp ring around condom at time of withdrawal to avoid leaving condom in vagina.	1. Failure rate is low with proper application (2%–5%). 2. Prevention of sexually transmitted disease 3. Inexpensive 4. No health hazard 5. May help premature ejaculation by decreasing sensitivity 6. Increases male involvement in contraception	1. Decreased sensitivity 2. Interruption of sexual act 3. Sensitivity to rubber may be a problem.
2. Diaphragm	Rubber cap shaped like a dome with a flexible rim	1. Place spermicide inside dome. 2. Place diaphragm against and covering cervical opening, behind lower edge of pubic bone. 3. Leave in place for at least 6 hours after intercourse.	1. 80% effective; may be 98% with proper use 2. Protection against sexually transmitted diseases and possibly cervical neoplasia	1. Occasional toxic shock or allergic reactions 2. May experience pelvic discomfort
3. Contraceptive sponge	Polyurethane sponge that releases spermicide	1. Moisten with water and insert deep into the vagina prior to intercourse. 2. Leave in place 6 hours after intercourse.	1. 80%–90% effective 2. May decrease risk of sexually transmitted diseases	1. Risk of toxic shock syndrome 2. May produce local irritation and vaginal dryness 3. May be difficult to remove

(continued)

Table 28-3. *Contraceptive Methods (continued)*

Methods	Definition	Procedure	Advantages	Disadvantages
4. Cervical cap	Rubber cap, shaped like a cup with a tall dome and flexible rim.	Place spermicide inside cap and place cap over cervical opening prior to intercourse.	1. 80%–90% effective 2. May decrease risk of STDs	1. Not approved in U.S.; but are available 2. Risk of TSS, cervicitis, and PID
Spermicides	Nonoxynol-9 or octoxynol-9 available in a variety of forms: foam, jelly, cream, suppository, tablet	Place next to cervix prior to intercourse; better if used with a barrier method.	May kill STD agents	1. Less effective if not used with barrier method 2. Some patients are allergic. 3. May cause birth defects if pregnancy results
Intrauterine Devices	Small device made of plastic with exposed copper or progesterone-release system; acts to inhibit uterine wall implantation.	1. Physician inserts device; slowly and usually at time of menses. 2. Check IUD string regularly—at least once a month—or after each intercourse when it is first inserted.	1. 95% effective 2. Convenient; permits spontaneous intercourse 3. Replaced every 2–3 years	1. Risk of PID and resultant tubal damage and infertility 2. May cause spotting, bleeding, or pain 3. Risk of spontaneous abortion 4. Risk of uterine rupture
Hormones 1. Combination oral contraceptives	Tablets containing estrogen to inhibit ovulation and progestin to make cervical mucus impenetrable to sperm—lowest effective doses are used.	Take for 21 days with 7 days off or 28 days (if 7 days of placebos are included).	1. 98% effective 2. Decreased risk of endometriosis, ovarian cancer, benign breast disease 3. Possible decreased risk of PID 4. Aid in menstrual disorders 5. Improves acne	1. Increased risk of cardiovascular disease (higher in women who smoke) 2. Questionable risk of breast, cervical cancer 3. May experience nausea, vomiting, headache, weight gain
2. Progestin-only oral contraceptive (Mini-pill)	Smaller doses of progestins than in combined oral contraceptives	Take every day.	1. 96% effective 2. Avoids estrogen-related side effects and possibly cardiovascular risks 3. May offer protection against PID	1. May cause irregular menses, spotting, amenorrhea
3. Postcoital contraception (Morning-after pill)	May be combined estrogen and progestin, high-dose estrogen, or progestin	Must be started within 24–72 hours after intercourse.	1. Very effective	1. May be religiously opposed 2. Not FDA-approved for postcoital method 3. May cause birth defects

Procedures

Guidelines Vaginal Irrigation

Purpose
1. To cleanse or disinfect the vagina and adjacent tissues
2. To soothe inflamed tissue

Equipment
1. Sterile reservoir for irrigating fluid—can or bag.
2. Sterile irrigating fluid as prescribed (1,000–4,000 ml.) at 40.5°–43.3°C. (105°–110°F.)
3. Tubing, connecting tubes, and clamp (sterile)
4. Irrigating vaginal nozzle (sterile)

(continued)

Guidelines Vaginal Irrigation *(continued)*

Equipment
(continued)

5. Bedpan or douche pan
6. Waterproof pad
7. Sterile cotton balls, cleansing solution
8. Gloves

Procedure
(Fig. 28-5)

Nursing Action	**Rationale/Amplification**

Preparatory Phase

1. Check physician's directives for amount and temperature of irrigating fluid. Prepare equipment.
2. Identify patient and explain the procedure. Place patient in dorsal recumbent position with waterproof pad under her.
3. Wash hands.

    2. To permit gravity to assist in allowing fluid to reach distal areas of vagina.

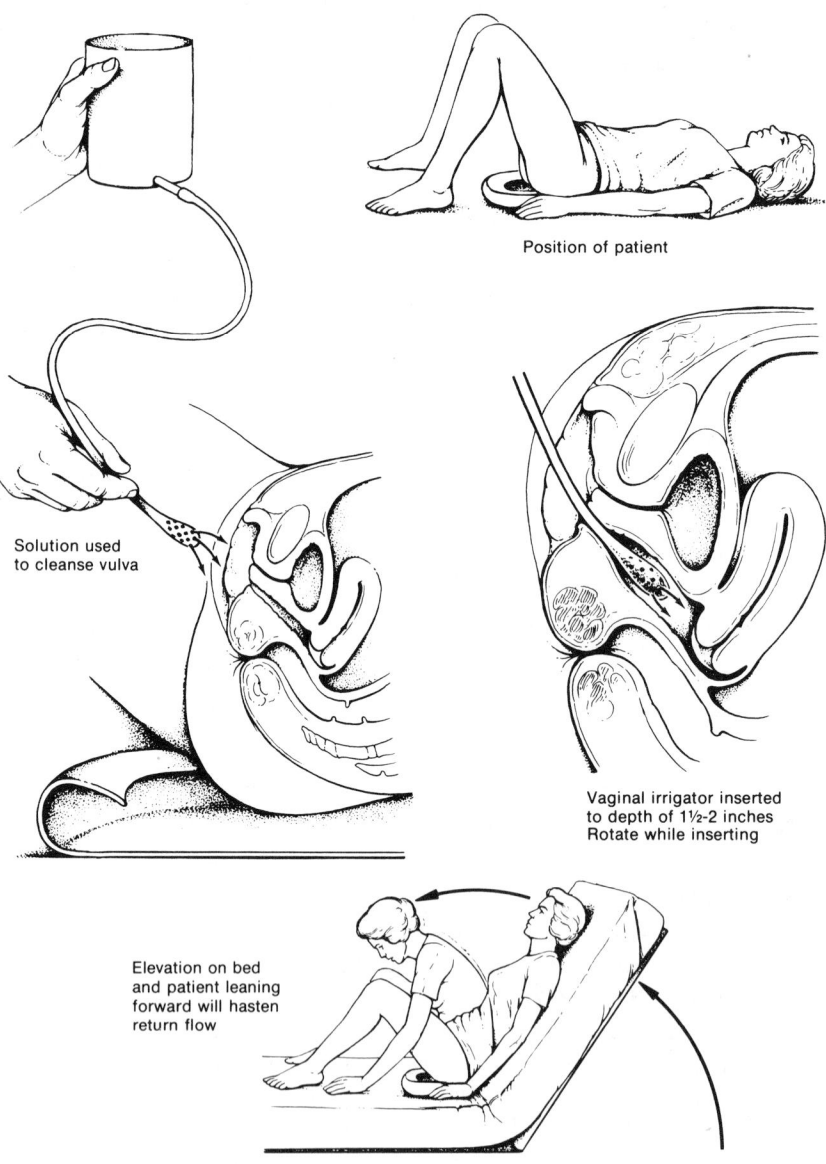

Position of patient

Solution used to cleanse vulva

Vaginal irrigator inserted to depth of 1½–2 inches Rotate while inserting

Elevation on bed and patient leaning forward will hasten return flow

Figure 28-5. *Vaginal irrigation. The nurse wears gloves while doing this procedure.*

Procedure
(Fig. 28-5)
(continued)

Nursing Action	Rationale/Amplification
4. Have the patient void before beginning irrigation.	4. A full bladder would prevent adequate distention of vagina by solution.
5. Drape the patient.	5. To prevent chilling and undue exposure.
6. Arrange irrigating receptacle at a level just above the patient's hips (not more than ½ meter, i.e., 18 inches above hips) so that fluid flows easily but gently.	6. The higher the fluid source, the greater the pressure.

Performance Phase

Nursing Action	Rationale/Amplification
1. Put on gloves	1. Clean gloves may be used, but sterile gloves should be used if there is an open wound.
2. Cleanse vulva by separating labia and allowing solution to flow over area; if insufficient, use cotton balls saturated in soap solution, cleanse from front toward anal area.	2. Materials found around vaginal meatus may be introduced into vagina and cervix. This is to be avoided.
3. Allow some solution to flow through tubing and out over nozzle to lubricate it.	3. Moisture provides lubrication and less resistance when one surface is moved against another.
4. Insert nozzle gently into vagina in a downward and backward direction, approximately 2 inches.	4. When the patient is in a dorsal recumbent position, the natural anatomical position of the vagina is in the downward-backward direction.
5. Rotate nozzle gently in the vagina during inflow.	5. All surfaces are irrigated when nozzle is rotated.
6. Clamp tubing when solution is almost all used, remove nozzle and permit the patient to sit on bedpan for return flow.	6. Gravity will assist in allowing return flow to drain from vaginal tract.

Follow-Up Phase

Nursing Action	Rationale/Amplification
1. Wipe the patient dry, using cotton balls in a front-to-back direction.	1. Drying the area prevents skin excoriation and promotes comfort.
2. Remove bedpan from the patient and apply sterile perineal pad.	
3. Remove gloves and wash hands.	
4. Document amount of returned fluid.	

Guidelines Vulvar Irrigation (Perineal Care)

Purpose To cleanse the perineal area after urination or a bowel movement in order to minimize infection.

Equipment

Sterile pitcher with irrigating fluid (300–500 ml.) 40.5°–43.3°C. (105°–110°F.)	Waterproof pad
Sterile sponge forceps and cotton pledgets	Paper bag for cotton pledget disposal
Bedpan	Gloves (optional)

Procedure
(Fig. 28-6)

Preparatory Phase

1. Wash hands. Prepare equipment.
2. Place waterproof pad under patient.
3. Place patient on bedpan in dorsal recumbent position with knees flexed and separated.
4. Drape patient with perineal area exposed.
5. Apply gloves (optional).

Nursing Action	Rationale/Amplification

Performance Phase

Nursing Action	Rationale/Amplification
1. Separate labia with nondominant hand. Pour warmed irrigating solution gently over vulva from a sterile pitcher.	1. Materials will be flushed from perineal area into bedpan.
2. Cleanse perineal area with cotton pledget held in a sponge holder, use a front-to-back direction and discard each sponge in a plastic or paper bag after one use.	2. Friction facilitates cleansing process and the removal of soil. Follow aseptic technique, cleanse urethral and vaginal areas first, then external labia, then anus.
3. Dry perineal area using dry cotton pledgets in same fashion as for cleansing.	3. Cleansing from front to back assists in preventing intestinal organisms from entering vaginal area.

(continued)

Guidelines Vulvar Irrigation (Perineal Care) *(continued)*

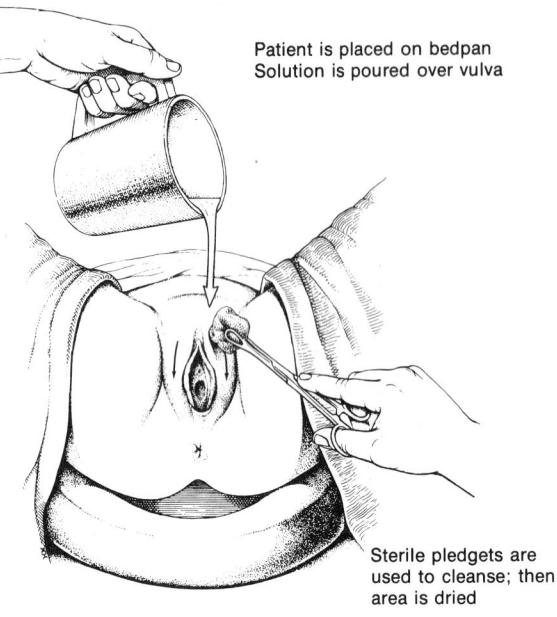
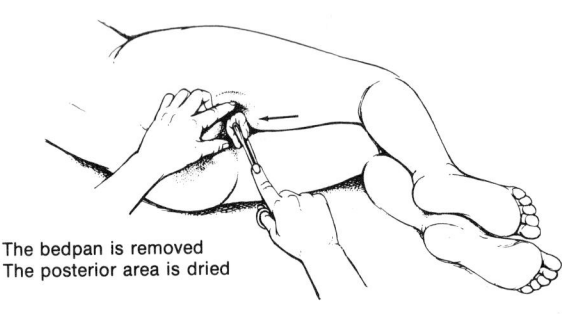

Figure 28-6. *Perineal care.*

Follow-up Phase

1. Apply sterile perineal pad.
2. Wash hands.

1. To maintain cleanliness and provide comfort for patient.

Bibliography

Gynecologic Conditions

Books

Barber HRK. Manual of Gynecologic Oncology. 2nd ed. Philadelphia, JB Lippincott, 1989

Bobak IM, Jensen MD and Zalar MK. Maternity and Gynecologic Care, The Nurse and The Family. 4th ed. St Louis, CV Mosby, 1989

Brush MG and Goudsmit EM (eds). Functional Disorders of the Menstrual Cycle. Chichester, John Wiley & Sons, 1988

Curtis LR, Curtis GB and Beard MK. My Body My Decision! What You Should Know about the Most Common Female Surgeries. Tucson, The Body Press, 1986

DiSaia PJ and Creasman WT. Clinical Gynecologic Oncology. 3rd ed. St Louis, CV Mosby, 1989

Dwyer JM. Manual of Gynecologic Nursing. Boston, Little, Brown & Co, 1986

Eskin BA (ed). The Menopause: Comprehensive Management. 2nd ed. New York, Mcmillan, 1988

Fioretti P et al (eds). Postmenopausal Hormonal Therapy—Benefits and Risks. New York, Raven Press, 1987

Fu YS and Reagan JW. Pathology of the Uterine Cervix, Vagina and Vulva. Philadelphia, WB Saunders, 1989

Glass RH (ed). Office Gynecology. 3rd ed. Baltimore, Williams & Wilkins, 1988

Gordon AG and Lewis BV. Gynecological Endoscopy. Philadelphia, JB Lippincott, 1988

Griffith-Kenney J. Contemporary Women's Health—A Nursing Advocacy Approach. Menlo Park, Addison-Wesley, 1986

Hatcher RA et al. Contraceptive Technology 1986–1987. 13th revised ed. New York, Irvington Publishers, 1986

Jones HW, Wentz AC and Burnett LS. Novak's Textbook of Gynecology. 11th ed. Baltimore, Williams & Wilkins, 1988

Jones JOM et al. Women's Health Management: Guidelines for Nurse Practitioners. Reston, Reston Publishing, 1984

Keye WR. The Premenstrual Syndrome. Philadelphia, WB Saunders, 1988

Kistner RW. Gynecology—Principles and Practice. 4th ed. Chicago, Yearbook Medical Pub, 1986

Kurman RJ (ed). Blaustein's Pathology of the Female Genital Tract. 3rd ed. New York, Springer-Verlag, 1987

Mittag H–C. Toxic Shock Syndrome and the Other Staphylococcal Toxicoses. Stuttgart–New York, Schattauer, 1988

Niswander KR (ed). Manual of Obstetrics—Diagnosis and Therapy.

3rd ed. Boston, Little, Brown & Co, 1987

O'Connor DT. Endometriosis. Current Reviews in Obstetrics and Gynecology. Edinburgh and New York, Churchill Livingstone, 1987

Ridley CM (ed). The Vulva. Edinburgh, Churchill Livingstone, 1988

Runnebaum B, Rabe T and Kiesel L (eds). Female Contraception—Updates and Trends. New York, Springer-Verlag, 1988

Sanz LE (ed). Gynecologic Surgery. Oradell, Medical Economics Books, 1988

Schencken RS. Endometriosis—Contemporary Concepts in Clinical Management. Philadelphia, JB Lippincott, 1989

Talwar GP (ed). Contraceptive Research for Today and the Nineties. New York, Springer-Verlag, 1988

Teoh E (ed). Endometriosis. Advances in Fertility and Sterility Series. Park Ridge, The Parthenon Publishing Group, 1986

Varma TR. Manual of Gynecology. Edinburgh, Churchill Livingstone, 1986

Wilson EA (ed). Endometriosis. New York, Alan R. Liss, 1987

General

Books

Kim MJ, McFarland GK and McLane AM. Pocket Guide to Nursing Diagnoses. 3rd ed. St. Louis, CV Mosby, 1989

Simon RR and Brenner BE. Emergency Procedures and Techniques. 2nd ed. Baltimore, Williams & Wilkins, 1987

Skidmore-Roth L and Jaffe M. Medical-Surgical Nursing Care Plans. Norwalk, Appleton-Century-Crofts, 1986

Wieck L, King E and Dyer M. Illustrated Manual of Nursing Techniques. 3rd ed. Philadelphia, JB Lippincott, 1986

Ziegfeld CR (ed). Core Curriculum for Oncology Nursing. Philadelphia, WB Saunders, 1987

Journals

General

Foley SF. Preventive gynecologic nursing in an inpatient setting. J Obstet Gynecol Neonatal Nurs 1987 May–Jun; 16(3):160–166

Kennedy AW, Flagg JS and Webster KD. Gynecologic cancer in the very elderly. Gynecol Oncol 1989 Jan; 32(1):49–54

Krouse HJ. A psychological model of adjustment in gynecologic cancer patients. Oncol Nurs Forum 1985 Nov–Dec; 12(6):45–49

Krzyston D. Nursing assessment and general care of the gynecological patient. Emerg Med Clin North Am 1987 Aug; 5(3):399–404

Moreland BJ. A nursing form for gynecology patient assessment. Oncol Nurs Forum 1987 Mar–Apr; 14(2):19–23

Silverberg E and Lubera JA. Cancer statistics, 1989. CA 1989 Jan–Feb; 39(1):3–20

Menstruation

Brown MA and Zimmer PA. Personal and family impact of premenstrual symptoms. J Obstet Gynecol Neonatal Nurs 1986 Jan–Feb; 15(1):31–38

Havens B and Swenson I. Menstrual perceptions and preparation among female adolescents. J Obstet Gynecol Neonatal Nurs 1986 Sep–Oct; 15(5): 406–411

Ouellette MD, MacVicar MG and Harlan J. Relationship between percent body fat and menstrual patterns in athletes and non-athletes. Nurs Res 1986 Nov–Dec; 35(6):330–333

Swenson I and Havens B. Menarche and menstruation: A review of the literature. J Commun Health Nurs 1987; 4(4):199–210

Treybig M. Primary dysmenorrhea or endometriosis? Nurse Pract 1989 May; 14(5):9–18

Walton J and Younkin E. The effect of a support group on self-esteem of women with premenstrual syndrome. J Obstet Gynecol Neonatal Nurs 1987 May–Jun; 16(3):174–178

Wickes SL. Premenstrual syndrome. Prim Care 1988 Sep; 15(3):473–487

Woods MF, Most A and Longenecker G. Major life events, daily stressors and perimenstrual symptoms. Nurs Res 1985 Sep–Oct; 34(5):263–267

Menopause

Bachman GA. Sexual dysfunction in postmenopausal women: The role of medical management. Geriatrics 1988 Nov; 43(11):79–83

Civitelli R et al. Bone turnover in postmenopausal osteoporosis. J Clin Invest 1988 Oct; 82(4):1268–1274

Cobb JO. Demystifying menopause. Can Nurse 1987 Aug; 83(7):17–20

Engel NS. Menopausal stage, current life change, attitude toward women's roles, and perceived health status. Nurs Res 1987 Nov–Dec; 36(6):353–357

Ernster VL et al. Benefits and risks of menopausal estrogen and/or progestin hormone use. Prev Med 1988 Mar; 17(2):201–223

Gibbons WE et al. Biochemical and histologic effects of sequential estrogen/progestin therapy on the endometrium of post-menopausal women. Am J Obstet Gynecol 1986 Feb; 154(2):456–461

Lam SY et al. Gynaecological disorders and risk factors in premenopausal women predisposing to osteoporosis. A review. Br J Obstet Gynaecol 1988 Oct; 95(10):963–972

Lindsay R. Estrogen therapy in the prevention and management of osteoporosis. Am J Obstet Gynecol 1987 May; 156(5):1347–1351

Lievertz RW. Pharmacology and pharmakinetics of estrogens. Am J Obstet Gynecol 1987 May; 156(5): 1289–1293

McKeon VA. Dispelling menopause myths. J Gerontol Nurs 1988 Aug; 14(8):26–29

Metzger DA and Hammond CB. Are estrogens indicated for the treatment of postmenopausal women? Drug Intell Clin Pharm 1988 Jun; 22(6):493–496

Nicoll JE. Estrogen replacement therapy. Nurse Pract 1986 Aug; 11(8):71, 75

Prough SG et al. Continuous estrogen/progestin therapy in menopause. Am J Obstet Gynecol 1987 Dec; 157(6): 1448–1453

Utian WH. Transderman estradiol overall safety profile. Am J Obstet Gynecol 1987 May; 156(5):1335–1338

Whitehead MI and Fraser D. Controversies concerning the safety of estrogen replacement therapy. Am J Obstet Gynecol 1987 May; 156(5): 1313–1322

Pelvic Examination and Diagnostic Assessment

Beal MW. Understanding cervical cytology. Nurse Pract 1987 Mar; 12(3): 8–10, 15, 18–22

Brown FH and Kammeyer SE. Office gynecologic procedures. Prim Care 1986 Sep; 13(3):493–511

Celentano DD. Updated approach to screening for cervical cancer in older women. Geriatrics 1988 Apr; 43(4):37–44

Goode RL, Degraw JR and Hildebrand WL. Abnormal pap smear: Colposcopy and cryosurgery. Am Fam Physician 1986 Dec; 34(6):99–105

Jones WB and Siago PE. The "atypical" Papanicolaou smear. CA 1986 Jul–Aug; 36(4):237–242

Lawhead RA. Vulvar self-examination. Am J Obstet Gynecol 1988 May; 158(5):1238

Loffer FD. Major ambulatory surgery of the gynecologic and obstetric patient. Surg Clin North Am 1987 Aug; 67(4): 791–804

Mandelblatt J, Gopaul I and Wistreich M. Gynecological care of elderly women—Another look at Papanicolaou smear testing. JAMA 1986 Jul 18; 256(3):367–371

Modica MM and Timor-Tritsch IE. Transvaginal sonography provides a sharper view into the pelvis. J Obstet Gynecol Neonatal Nurs 1988 Mar–Apr; 17(2):89–95

Noller KL. Cervical cytology and the evaluation of the abnormal Papanicolaou smear. Prim Care 1988 Sep; 15(3):461–471

Sandella J. Vulvar self examination (VSE). Oncol Nurs Forum 1987 Nov–Dec; 14(6):71–73

Szydlo VL. Approaching an adolescent about a pelvic exam. Am J Nurs 1988 Nov; 88(11):1502–1506

Willard MD, Heaberg GL and Pack JB. The educational pelvic examination—Women's responses to a new approach. J Obstet Gynecol Neonatal Nurs 1986 Mar–Apr; 15(2):135–140

Vulva and Vagina

Boronow RC et al. Combined therapy as an alternative to exenteration for locally advanced vulvovaginal cancer. II. Results, complications, and dosimetric and surgical considerations.

Am J Clin Oncol 1987 Apr; 10(2):171–181

Bouma J and Dankert J. Recurrent acute leg cellulitis in patients after radical vulvectomy. Gynecol Oncol 1988 Jan; 29(1):50–57

Burrell MO et al. The modified radical vulvectomy with groin dissection: An eight year experience. Am J Obstet Gynecol 1988 Sep; 159(3):715–722

Green DE and Phillips GL. Vaginal prosthesis for control of vesicovaginal fistula. Gynecol Oncol 1986 Jan; 23(1):119–123

Grunberg KJ. Sexual rehabilitation of the cancer patient undergoing ostomy surgery. J Enterostomal Ther 1986 Jul–Aug; 13(4):148–152

Josey WE. Anovaginal fistula presenting as a vulvar ulcer—A report of two cases in postmenopausal women. J Reprod Med 1988 Oct; 33(10):857–858

Kaufman RH et al. Human papillomavirus and herpes simplex virus in vulvar squamous cell carcinoma in situ. Am J Obstet Gynecol 1988 Apr; 158(4):862–871

Lacey CG et al. Vaginal reconstruction after exenteration with use of gracilis myocutaneous flaps: The University of California, San Francisco experience. Am J Obstet Gynecol 1988 Jun; 158(6):1278–1284

Lamb M. Vulvar cancer: Patient information booklet. Oncol Nurs Forum 1986 Nov–Dec; 13(6):79–82

Lamb M and Chu J. Invasive cancer of the vulva—Diagnosis, surgical management, and nursing care. AORN J 1988 Apr; 47(4):928–936

Levin W et al. The use of concomitant chemotherapy and radiotherapy prior to surgery in advanced stage carcinoma of the vulva. Gynecol Oncol 1986 Sep; 25(1):20–25

Rubin D. Gynecologic cancer: Cervical, vulvar, and vaginal malignancies. RN 1987 May; 50(5):56–63

Wright VC and Davies E. Laser surgery for vulvar intraepithelial neoplasia: Principles and results. Am J Obstet Gynecol 1987 Feb; 156(2):374–378

Infections and Herpes Genitalis

Baker DA et al. Clinical evaluation of a new herpes simplex virus ELISA: A rapid diagnostic test for herpes simplex virus. Obstet Gynecol 1989 Mar; 73(3):322–325

Bourcier KM and Seidler AJ. Chlamydia and condylomata acuminata: An update for the nurse practitioner. J Obstet Gynecol Neonatal Nurs 1987 Jan–Feb; 16(1):17–22

Breslin E. Genital herpes simplex. Nurs Clin North Am 1988 Dec; 23(4):907–915

Chantigian PDM. Vaginitis: A common malady. Prim Care 1988 Sep; 15(3):517–548

Enterline JA and Leonardo JP. Condylomata Acuminata (venereal warts). Nurse Pract 1989 Apr; 14(4):8–16

Gietl KA. Role of the nurse practitioner in the management of vaginitis. Am J

Obstet Gynecol 1988 Apr; 158(4):1009–1011

Hill LVH and Embil JA. Vaginitis: Current microbiologic and clinical concepts. Can Med Assoc J 1986 Feb; 134(4):321–331

Lafferty W. Genital herpes—recommendations for comprehensive care. Postgrad Med 1988 Feb; 83(2):157–160, 163–165

McLarnon LD and Kaloupek DG. Psychological investigation of genital herpes recurrence: Prospective assessment and cognitive behavioral intervention for a chronic physical disorder. Health Psychol 1988 Nov; 7(3):231–249

McQuiston CM. The relationship of risk factors for cervical cancer and HPV in college women. Nurse Pract 1989 Apr; 14(4):18–26

Schwartz DB et al. Genital condylomas in pregnancy: Use of trichloroacetic acid and laser therapy. Am J Obstet Gynecol 1988 Jun; 158(6):1407–1416

Steinmetz KS. Gardnerella vaginalis vaginitis—A guide to identification and management for the practitioner. J Nurse Midwifery 1986 Mar–Apr; 31(2):87–92

Swinker ML. Clinical aspects of genital herpes. Am Fam Physician 1986 Sep; 34(3):127–132

Thin RN. Management of genital herpes simplex infections. Am J Med 1988 Aug; 85(supp2A):3–6

Woolard DG, Larson J and Hudson L. Screening for *Chlamydia trachomatis* at a university health service. J Obstet Gynecol Neonatal Nurs 1989 Mar–Apr; 18(2):145–149

Toxic Shock Syndrome

Bartter T et al. 'Toxic Strep Syndrome'—A manifestation of group A streptococcl infection. Arch Intern Med 1988 Jun; 148(6):1421–1424

Faich G et al. Toxic shock syndrome and the vaginal contraceptive sponge. JAMA 1986 Jan 10; 255(2):216–218

Lanes SF et al. Toxic shock syndrome, contraceptive methods, and vaginitis. Am J Obstet Gynecol 1986 May; 154(5):989–991

Petitti DB and Reingold A. Tampon characteristics and menstrual toxic shock syndrome. JAMA 1988 Feb 5; 259(5):686–687

Wright SW and Trott AT. Toxic shock syndrome: A review. Ann Emerg Med 1988 Mar; 17(3):268–273

Ovary and Uterus

Barber HRK. Ovarian cancer. CA 1986 May–Jun; 36(3):149–184

Barter JF et al. Complications of combined radical hysterectomy—Postoperative radiation therapy in women with early stage cervical cancer. Gynecol Oncol 1989 Mar; 32(3):292–296

Cashavelly BJ. Cervical dysplasia—An overview of current concepts in epidemiology, diagnosis and treatments. Cancer Nurs 1987 Aug; 10(4):199–206

Chagares R. Intrathoracic endometriosis: A women's health issue. Heart Lung 1987 Mar; 16(2):183–187

Connell A. Abnormal uterine bleeding. Nurse Pract 1989 Apr; 14(4):40–57

Cramer DW et al. The relation of endometriosis to menstrual characteristics, smoking and exercise. JAMA 1986 Apr 11; 255(14):1904–1908

DiSaia PJ. Conservative management of the patient with early gynecologic cancer. CA 1989 May–Jun; 39(3):135–154

Drutz HP and Cha LS. Massive genital and vaginal vault prolapse treated by abdominal-vaginal sacropexy with use of Marlex mesh: Review of the literature. Am J Obstet Gynecol 1987 Feb: 156(2):387–392

Franks AL et al. Postmenopausal smoking, estrogen replacement therapy, and the risk of endometrial cancer. Am J Obstet Gynecol 1987 Jan; 156(1):20–23

Gusberg SB. Current concepts in the control of carcinoma of the endometrium. CA 1986 Jul–Aug; 36(4):245–253

Henderson JS and Taylor KH. Age as a variable in an exercise program for the treatment of simple urinary stress incontinence. J Obstet Gynecol Neonatal Nurs 1987 Jul–Aug; 16(4):266–272

Lilley LL. Human need fulfillment alteration in the client with uterine cancer—The registered nurse's perception versus the client's perception. Cancer Nurs 1987 Dec; 10(6):327–337

Lovejoy NC. Precancerous lesions of the cervix: Personal risk factors. Cancer Nurs 1987 Feb; 10(1):2–14

McDermott DF et al. The effect of surgical debulking on the response of patients with ovarian carcinoma to chemotherapy. Am J Clin Oncol 1988 Oct; 11(5):520–523

Nelson JH, Averette HE and Richart RM. Cervical intraepithelial neoplasia (dysplasia and carcinoma in situ) and early invasive cervical carcinoma. CA 1989 May–Jun; 39(3):157–178

O'Laughlin KM. Changes in bladder function in the woman undergoing radical hysterectomy for cervical cancer. J Obstet Gynecol Neonatal Nurs 1986 Sep–Oct; 15(5):380–385

Richards S and Hiratzka S. Vaginal dilatation post pelvic irradiation: A patient education tool. Oncol Nurs Forum 1986 Jul–Aug; 13(4):89–91

Rodau SK and Thomason JL. Vaginal eversion repair—Sacrospinous ligament fixation procedure. AORN J 1988 Feb; 47(2):539–552

Rubin SC. Ovarian cancer—Diagnosis and surgical treatment. AORN J 1988 Jun; 47(6):1427–1441

Shell JA and Carter J. The gynecological implant patient. Semin Oncol Nurs 1987 Feb; 3(1):54–66

Sonnendecker EWW. Is routine second look laparotomy for ovarian cancer justified? Gynecol Oncol 1988 Oct; 31(2):249–255

Webb C. Professional and lay support for hysterectomy patients. J Adv Nurs 1986 Mar; 11(2):167–177

Wells MP and Villano K. Total abdominal hysterectomy—Perioperative patient care. AORN J 1985 Sep; 42(3):368–373

Pelvic Inflammatory Disease

Hemsell DL. Acute pelvic inflammatory disease—Etiologic and therapeutic considerations. J Reprod Med 1988 Jan; 33(1 supp):119–123

Shattuck JC. Pelvic inflammatory disease—Education for maintaining fertility. Nurs Clin North Am 1988 Dec; 23(4):899–906

Torrington J. Pelvic inflammatory disease. J Obstet Gynecol Neonatal Nurs 1985 Nov–Dec; 14(6supp):21s–31s

Fertility Control

Boyers SP et al. The effects of Lubrin on sperm motility in vitro. Fertil Steril 1987 May; 47(5):882–884

Eichhorst BC. Contraception. Prim Care 1988 Sep; 15(3):437–459

Kugel C and Verson H. Relationship between weight change and diaphragm size change. J Obstet Gynecol Neonatal Nurs 1986 Mar–Apr; 15(2):123–129

Riedmann GL. The fertility history card—Clinical use in improving contraceptive efficacy. J Nurse Midwifery 1988 Jan–Feb; 33(1):15–24

Sexual Considerations

Glasgow M, Halfin V and Althausen AF. Sexual response and cancer. CA 1987 Nov–Dec; 37(6):322–333

Jenkins B. Sexual healing after pelvic irradiation. Am J Nurs 1986 Aug; 86(8): 920–922

Jenkins B. Patients' reports of sexual changes after treatment for gynecological cancer. Oncol Nurs Forum 1988 May–Jun; 15(3):349–354

Kaempfer SH and Major P. Fertility considerations in the gynecologic oncology patient. Oncol Nurs Forum 1986 Jan–Feb; 13(1):23–27

McKenzie F. Sexuality after total pelvic exenteration. Nurs Times 1988 May 18–24; 84(20):26–30

Assessment of the Breast

Physical Examination

1. Annual physical checkup should include breast examination and palpation.
2. Twice-a-year examination recommended for women with a family history of cancer.
3. Normal breast changes in the elderly include drooping, flaccid breasts due to decreased subcutaneous tissue from decreased estrogen levels. Nipple size and erection are also reduced.
4. For procedure for Breast Examination by the Nurse, see Guideline, page 749.
5. Breast self-examination is an essential first step in prevention of breast cancer.

Diagnostic Tests

A. Mammography

1. Roentgenography of breast without injection of contrast medium;
2. Two views are taken
   a. Caudal
   b. Mediolateral
3. *Dedicated mammography units*—include a compression device to improve the picture and decrease amount of radiation required. They also deliver a lower amount of radiation.
4. Indications
   a. Greatest value is in detecting minimal breast cancer, even before a lump is felt. It is the hallmark of breast cancer screening.
   b. May also be used for questionable lumps found on physical examination, lumpy or very large breasts, which are difficult to examine, and screening the opposite breast in a woman with a mass on one side.
5. Guidelines for mammography screening:
   a. Under 35—no mammography, because of increased effects of radiation on young tissue
   b. 35–39 years of age—baseline mammogram
   c. 40–50 years of age—every 1–2 years, recommended annually if family history of breast cancer
   d. Over age 50—annually
6. Needle localization of nonpalpable lumps may be done during mammography to allow the surgeon to do biopsies of abnormalities and reduce unnecessary tissue removal.

GERONTOLOGIC ALERT: Less than one third of women over age 50 have had a mammogram in the last year.

B. Ultrasonography

1. Sensitive to differentiating a solid from a cystic lesion
2. Most useful test after mammography, but not for screening purposes
3. Painless and noninvasive
4. Helpful if radiation contraindicated (i.e., pregnant or less than 35 years of age).

C. Thermography

1. Infrared photography gives a pictorial representation of heat patterns on the surface of the breast, which may indicate signs of abnormality.
2. Abnormality is recognized by either graphic or thermal asymmetry.
3. Very sensitive to infection or inflammation due to the heat generated by increased blood supply in these areas
4. Provides little information in addition to mammography and physical examination; not used for screening
5. Advantage of no radiation exposure

D. Diaphonography

1. A combination of transillumination, visual inspection, and documented film-recording with nonionizing radiation
2. Is similar in value to spot-filming in fluoroscopy
3. Not routinely used due to lack of studies

E. Computed Tomography

1. May be useful in detecting cancer in small, dense, breasts, which are difficult to examine by mammography.
2. It is unsuitable for routine screening and diagnostic studies.

F. Galactography

1. Injection of a water-soluble contrast medium into a duct for patient with persistent bloody nipple discharge.
2. May outline intraductal papilloma.

G. Summary

1. None of the above techniques are used as a substitute for mammography.
2. None eliminates the need for surgical biopsy or breast aspiration if clinically indicated

Biopsy

A. Fine Needle Aspiration (Fig. 29-1).

1. Usually done on outpatient basis, by gynecologist, with local anesthetic
2. Results within 24 hours
3. Inexpensive compared with surgical biopsies
4. Small risk of hematoma and infection
5. Solid benign lesions warrant an excisional biopsy. Cystic benign lesions (which disappear when aspirated) should be rechecked in a month; fluid should be sent for cytology if appears suspicious (bloody or cloudy).

B. Incisional (Surgical)

1. Incision is made along outer edge of areola if possible (circumareolar).
2. Tissue specimen is removed and sent for frozen section and receptor assay. If entire mass is removed, it is called an excisional biopsy or lumpectomy.
3. Pressure dressing is applied—should watch for bleeding.
4. Most accurate diagnostic tool.
5. May be one-step (followed immediately by a mastectomy; not done as often now) or two-step procedure.

Estrogen-Receptor and Progesterone-Receptor Assay

1. A test of tumor tissue to determine whether or not the cancer cells have receptor sites.
2. If such sites are present, the patient is more likely to respond to hormonal manipulation.
3. Determined from tissue biopsy
4. About two thirds are estrogen-receptor–positive—have better survival rates.

5. Positive results—if more than 10 fmol/mg. protein; the larger the value, the better the prognosis.

Breast Self-Examination (BSE)

A. Clinical Value

1. BSE is an inexpensive, risk-free method to detect cancer.
2. Experience has verified that 90% of breast cancers are found by women themselves.
3. When women discover lumps in their breasts at a very early stage, they have a better chance for long-term survival.
4. Do not neglect males when teaching BSE—1% of breast cancers are in men.

Patient Education

A. General Points to Emphasize

1. Examine your breasts once a month, just after the menstrual period, because breasts are less engorged at this time and a tumor is easier to detect, and at regular monthly intervals after the cessation of menses (Fig. 29-2).
2. It is most important to examine all of the breast. Use the most comfortable pattern: circular, vertical, wedge.
3. Apply enough pressure to palpate deeply.
4. Use the finger pads of the three middle fingers for increased sensitivity.
5. When in doubt, compare findings with the opposite breast.
6. Be aware that 80% of breast lumps are not cancer.

> **NURSING ALERT:** Nurses play an important role in promoting BSE. Women report increased frequency of BSE when taught by a nurse.

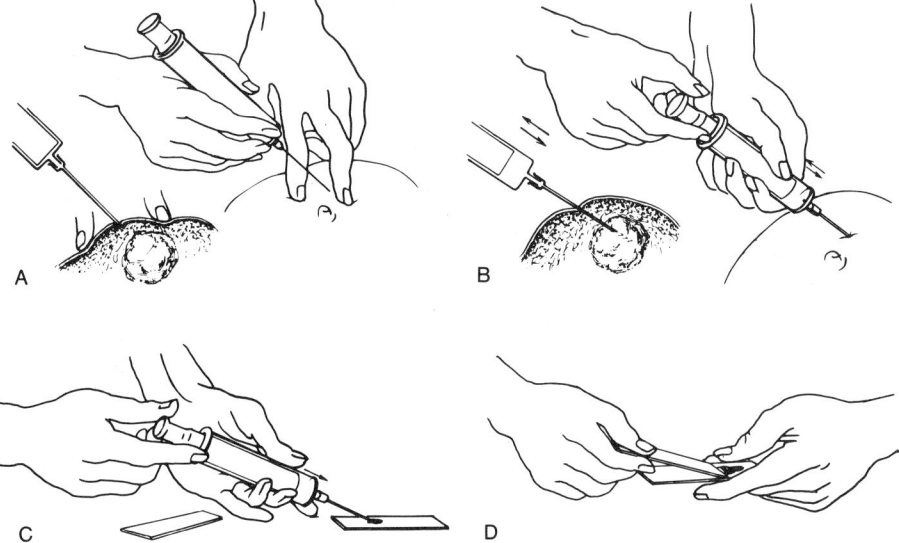

Figure 29-1. *Aspiration cytology. (A) Tumor is immobilized with two fingers before the needle is inserted. (B) A vacuum is created by withdrawing the plunger slowly but forcefully several times. Before the needle is removed, the pressure is allowed to equalize. (C) Contents of the needle are placed on a glass slide. (D) The smear is spread forward gently with a glass slide inclined at an angle of about 35°, with an up-and-down movement. (Zajdela A. The value of aspiration cytology in the diagnosis of breast cancer. Cancer 35)*

A   B   C   D

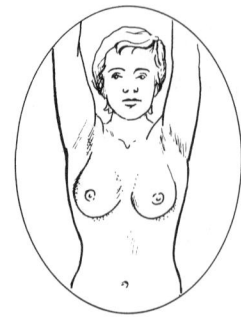
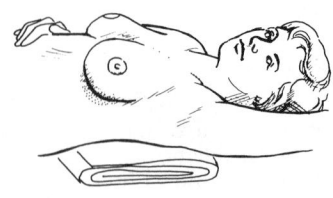
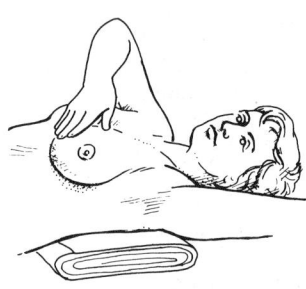

1. Careful examination of the breasts before a mirror for symmetry in size and shape, noting any puckering or dimpling of the skin or retraction of the nipple.

2. Arms raised over head, again studying the breasts in the mirror for the same signs.

3. Reclining on bed with flat pillow or folded bath towel under the shoulder on the same side as breast to be examined.

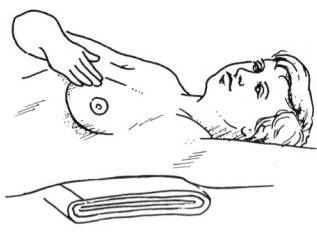
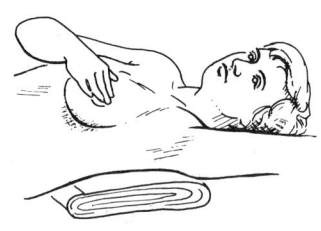

4. To examine the inner half of the breast, the arm is raised over the head. Beginning at the breastbone and, in a series of steps, the inner half of the breast is palpated.

5. The area over the nipple is carefully palpated with the finger pads of the three middle fingers.

6. Examination of the lower inner half of the breast is completed.

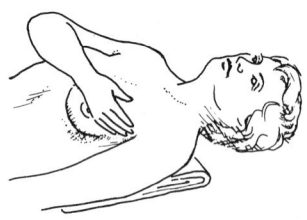
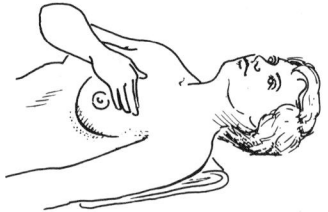
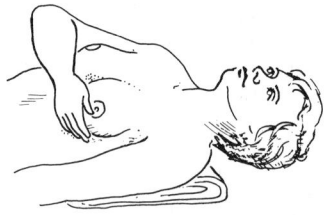

7. With arm down at side, self examination of breasts continues by carefully feeling the tissues that extend to the armpit.

8. The upper outer quadrant of the breast is examined with the finger pads of the three middle fingers.

9. The lower outer quadrant of the breast is examined in successive stages with the finger pads of the three middle fingers.

Figure 29-2. *Breast self-examination. (Courtesy American Cancer Society)*

B. Suggestions for Patients Who Find Self-Examination Difficult

1. Tenderness—gentle self-examination may be more effective and less painful than examination by someone else.
2. Cystic breasts—recommend professional examination annually and instruct patient to compare changes in breasts from one month to the next, and to compare breasts.
3. Large, pendulous breasts—encourage woman to support her breast with her hand to palpate thoroughly; lying down may help to flatten breasts.

C. Community Health Education

1. Recommend that women's organizations view film on breast self-examination. Pamphlets and breast models with "lumps" are also available from the American Cancer Society.
2. Reinforce that early detection may mean cure.
3. Know the resources within the community where medical help is available.

Guidelines | Examination of the Breast by the Nurse

Purpose
1. To detect abnormalities in the breasts
2. To teach a woman how to perform breast self-examination

Equipment   A good lamp and privacy

Procedure

Nursing Action	Rationale/Amplification

Sitting Position

1. Wash your hands under warm water and dry them. Apply powder if they feel "sticky."

2. Have the woman strip to her waist and sit comfortably facing the examiner. Observe breast for abnormalities.

1. The breast is sensitive to cold. Powder reduces friction.

2. This provides an opportunity to observe breasts visually for lack of symmetry and for gross signs such as redness, irritated nipple, dimpling, orange-peel skin.

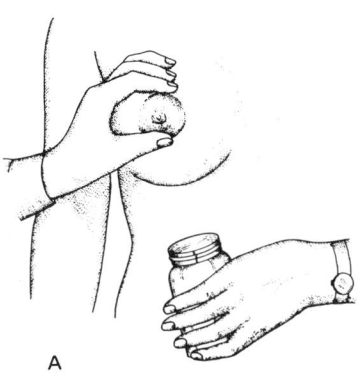

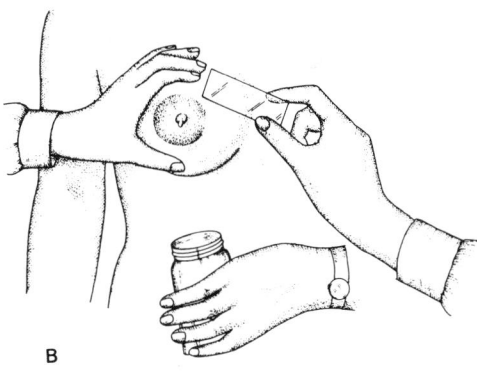

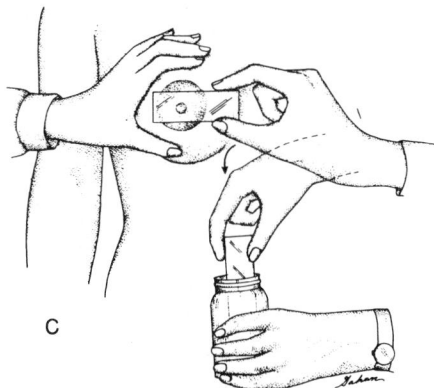

Figure 29-3. *Obtaining nipple discharge specimen for cytologic examination.*
1. *Wash nipple gently with cotton pledget, pat dry.*
2. *Gently strip duct and express fluid only until a small pea-sized drop appears on nipple.*
3. *Obtain assistance of the patient in holding container of fixative solution near breast to receive the prepared slide.*
4. *Stabilize breast with fingers and thumb of one hand (A).*
5. *Gently place one end of slide on nipple (B); rapidly draw slide across nipple and immediately drop into fixative solution or spray with fixative (C).*
6. *This may be repeated to secure additional specimens if necessary.*
NOTE: 1. Positive results are significant.
      2. Negative results may be "false-negatives." This test is never used alone but in conjunction with other diagnostic tests.

(continued)

Guidelines   Examination of the Breast by the Nurse *(continued)*

Procedure *(continued)*	Nursing Action	Rationale/Amplification
	3. Have patient raise arms overhead.	3. Changes in lower half of breast are more visible.
	4. Palpate supraclavicular area.	4. Note whether lymph nodes are enlarged, fixed, movable, or difficult to locate.
	5. Palpate axillary nodes; hold the woman's forearm in your left palm while you check nodes with your right fingertips. Repeat on other side.	5. Same as 4 above.
	Lying Position	
	1. Instruct the patient to lie down with her right arm under her head. Place a small pillow under the right shoulder.	1. This will spread breast tissue evenly over chest wall.
	2. With the finger pads of 2 or 3 fingers, gently palpate breast tissue, beginning at the upper outer quadrant.	2. The sensitive fingers, proceeding in a kneading fashion, can detect thickened, lumpy, or "buckshot" tissue between the patient's skin and chest wall. As the majority of breast lesions are in the upper outer quadrant, this segment is double checked.
	a. Proceed in an orderly pattern around the breast and repeat the first quarter examined.	
	b. Repeat procedure for other breast.	
	3. Recognize that there is a prolongation of the axillary extension of normal breast tissue, which may extend high into axilla.	3. This is normal if symmetrical and abnormal if asymmetrical.
	4. Check the areolar area for crustiness, nipple discharge, signs of infection.	4. Prepare to collect a discharge specimen for cytology if indicated (see Fig. 29-3).
	5. Record findings and report abnormalities to the physician.	
	6. Instruct the patient in performing self-examination on her own (Fig. 29-2). Encourage her to ask any questions; provide her with appropriate literature.	6. Ninety-five percent of women discover their own abnormalities.

Conditions of the Nipple

Fissures

A. Clinical Manifestations

A *fissure* of the nipple is a longitudinal type of ulcer that occasionally develops in the breast of a nursing mother.
1. Nipple appears sore and irritated.
2. Bleeding from nipple.

B. Causes

1. Lack of preparation of nipples in prenatal period.
2. Condition aggravated by sucking infant.

C. Treatment and Nursing Interventions

1. Wash nipples with sterile saline solution.
2. Use artificial nipple for nursing.
3. If above does not initiate healing process, stop nursing and use breast pump.

D. Patient Education

1. Teach proper breast-feeding techniques; make sure infant's mouth covers areola, not just the nipple.
2. Keep nipple clean by washing and drying after each nursing period.
3. May use lanolin cream to prevent cracking. Must remove before breast feeding.
4. In prenatal period, wash, dry, and lubricate nipples in preparation for nursing.

Bleeding from the Nipple

A. Clinical Manifestations

Bloody discharge—usually on edge of areola.

B. Causes

1. Most commonly due to wart-like papilloma in one of larger collecting ducts at edge of areola.
2. Occasionally a malignancy is responsible (Fig. 29-1, cytology examination).

C. Treatment

1. Surgery for palpable mass
   a. Duct is identified.
   b. Papilloma is excised (or a wedge of breast from area producing the bleeding is excised if no gross papilloma is identified) through a small periareolar incision—send for laboratory analysis.
   c. Sterile dressings applied
2. If no palpable mass, mammography and xerography

Inflammation of the Breast

Acute Mastitis

A. Incidence

Usually occurs at beginning of lactation in first-time breast-feeding mothers.

B. Source of Infection

1. Hands of patient
2. Personnel caring for patient
3. Baby's nose or throat
4. Blood-borne
5. Milk stasis—leads to obstruction, followed by noninfectious mastitis, then infectious mastitis

C. Clinical Manifestations

1. Redness, warmth, edema
2. Breast feels doughy and tough
3. Dull pain in affected area
4. May have nipple discharge

D. Management

1. May or may not have patient stop breast-feeding (controversial)
2. May apply heat to resolve tissue reaction; however, it may cause increased milk production and worsen symptoms.
3. May apply cold to decrease tissue metabolism and milk production
4. Administer medication as prescribed, such as antibiotics, hormones, and analgesics.
5. Have the patient wear firm breast support.
6. Encourage the patient to practice meticulous personal hygiene.

Mammary Abscess

A. Incidence

May follow acute mastitis if untreated

B. Clinical Manifestations

1. Affected area is sensitive, dusky red; may have palpable mass.
2. Pus may be expressed from nipple.
3. Fever, chills, malaise

C. Management

1. May perform needle aspiration if superficial mass
2. Incise and drain if deep
3. Administer antibiotics and other medications as prescribed.
4. Apply hot, wet dressings to increase drainage and hasten resolution.

Fibrocystic Disease

Fibrocystic disease is a general term that includes a variety of changes in the breast, namely fibrosis and cystic dilatation of the ducts. It is related to the cyclic stimulation of the breast by estrogen, but represents a departure from the normal stimulation and regression pattern of this process.

Incidence

1. The most common lesion of the female breast; 3 to 4 times more prevalent than cancer.
2. Occurs usually in women between 35 and 50 and is endocrine related.

Clinical Manifestations

1. Lumps or cysts—soft or firm, single or multiple, smooth, round, movable, may be bilateral and usually occur in upper, outer quadrant
2. Pain and tenderness—especially before menstrual period
3. Nipple discharge—may be present; clear, milky, yellow or greenish

Diagnostic Evaluation

1. Mammography
2. Aspiration—if single, palpable mass
3. Biopsy—if discrete, tender mass

Management

1. Aspiration
2. Excision—if recurrent cysts or cannot be aspirated
3. Hormonal treatment
   a. Danazol—to decrease hormonal stimulation of the breast by suppressing gonadotropins. Side effects include menstrual irregularities and weight gain.
   b. Tamoxifen—blocks estrogen stimulation; side effects are minimal—may have hot flashes.

Patient Education

1. Emphasize the importance of monthly BSE—cysts may mask underlying cancer.
2. Reinforce patient's confidence in BSE by rechecking her findings.
3. Offer suggestions for alternative methods if exam is difficult to do, i.e., tender breasts.
4. Encourage patient to see physician regularly for examinations.
5. Offer emotional support for her anxiety and fear of cancer.

Tumors of the Breast

Fibroadenomata

Fibroadenomata is a tumor composed of fibrous and ductal tissue; usually slow-growing.

Incidence

1. Is third most common tumor of the breast (after cysts and cancer).
2. Most common in 15–35-year-olds.

Clinical Manifestations

1. Firm, smooth, movable lumps
2. Usually painless
3. Size doesn't fluctuate with menstrual cycle changes.

Diagnostic Evaluation/Management

Surgical excision of lump

Cancer of the Breast

Epidemiology

1. Leading cause of cancer incidence in American women—142,900 estimated new cases yearly.
2. Second highest cause of deaths from cancer in American women (after lung cancer)
3. Survival rates:
   a. Overall 10-year survival is 50%.
   b. Five-year survival if localized to breast is 85%.
   c. Five-year survival if spread to nodes is 55%.
4. Most common sites of metastases are: axillary nodes, lung, bone, liver, and adrenal glands. Ten percent have distant metastases at time of diagnosis.

Major Types of Breast Cancer

A. Intraductal

1. Invasive
   a. Solitary, palpable hard mass; highest treatment failure
   b. Incidence—70%–80%; most common

2. Noninvasive
   a. May be palpable, half are centrally located, may have nipple discharge; good prognosis
   b. Incidence—1%–3%
3. Inflammatory
   a. Erythema, warmth, tenderness, edema (peau d'orange)
   b. Incidence—1%–4%

B. Lobular

1. Invasive
   a. Bilateral, multicentric, tends to spread to bone and meninges
   b. Incidence—12%
2. In situ (noninvasive)
   a. Bilateral and multicentric, nonpalpable, usually younger women, best survival rate—must follow closely or do bilateral mastectomies
   b. Incidence—10%

Risk Factors

1. Major
   Female over 45 years old, prior history of breast cancer, family history (especially mother, sisters), and premenopausal, from North America or Northern Europe
2. Probable
   Nulliparity, first child after 35 years old, late menopause, early menarche, fibrocystic disease, other female organ cancers, i.e., endometrial
3. Controversial
   Oral contraceptive use (estrogen and progestin may stimulate tumor growth with long-term use), estrogen replacement therapy, alcohol and tobacco use, radiation exposure, obesity and increased dietary fat intake, and stress (may alter immunity or hormonal environment, making one more susceptible to cancer).

Clinical Manifestations *(see Fig. 29-4)*

1. Mass
   a. Most common sign
   b. 50% located in upper outer quadrant of breast
   c. Usually painless
   d. May be an isolated lump or thickening
2. Nipple discharge—may be bloody or serous
3. Breast asymmetry—affected breast appears more elevated.
4. Nipple retraction or scaliness—especially in Paget's disease
5. Dimpling of the skin
6. Late signs—pain, ulceration, edema

Diagnostic Evaluation

1. Physical examination
2. Mammography—most accurate method to detect nonpalpable lesion
3. Biopsy or aspiration—conclusive for cancer diagnosis and to determine type of breast cancer
4. Metastatic workup—may include bone scan, liver scan, and liver function tests, chest x-rays, brain scan, and lab work.
5. Axillary node sampling or dissection
6. Estrogen and progesterone receptor assay

Management

Based on stage and type of breast cancer (see displayed material at top of opposite page) and status of nodes, receptors, and menopause (see Table 29-1).

A. Surgery

1. *Lumpectomy* (tylectomy, local excision, excisional biopsy)—removal of tumor; may also remove lymph nodes
2. *Quadrantectomy*—removal of a breast quadrant that includes the tumor area and overlying skin.

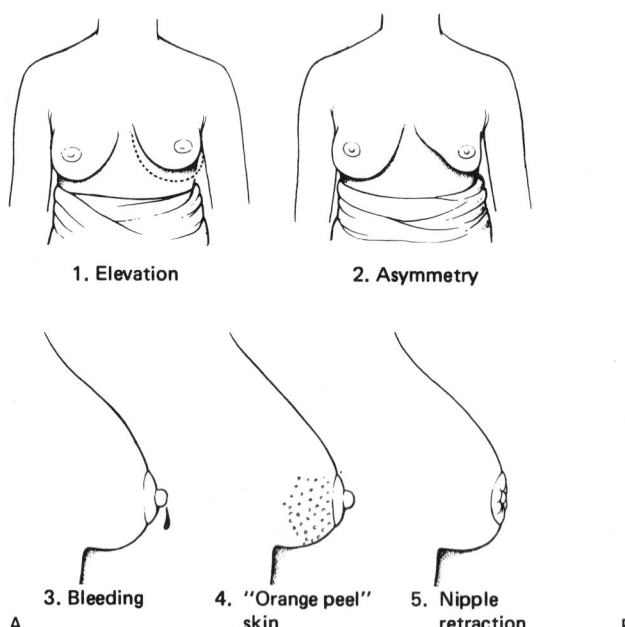

1. Elevation 2. Asymmetry

3. Bleeding 4. "Orange peel" skin 5. Nipple retraction

A

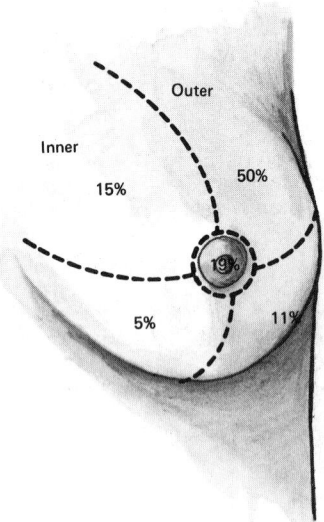

B

Figure 29-4. *(A) Signs of cancer of the breast. (B) Distribution of carcinomas in different areas of breast.*

Treatment of Breast Cancer Relative to Staging

Stage	Treatment Options
Tumor < 2 cm., negative nodes and no metastasis	Modified radical mastectomy Tumor excision, axillary dissection, and radiation Total mastectomy and axillary dissection
Tumor between 2 and 5 cm., 1–3 positive axillary nodes and no metastasis	Modified radical and/or radiation therapy Tumor excision, axillary dissection, and radiation (for tumors < 4 cm.)
Tumor may be > 5 cm., may involve axillary, supraclavicular, and internal mammary nodes, no metastasis	Modified radical and radiation or chemotherapy Primary radiation if tumor is fixed to pectoralis muscle or bulky lymph nodes (nonoperable) Chemotherapy, before or after radiation or surgery Hormonal therapy
Any size of tumor or node involvement, positive distant metastasis	Chemotherapy Hormonal therapy Surgery and radiation, palliative (usually for pain or bowel obstruction)

3. *Partial mastectomy* (segmental)—removal of tumor plus 2–3-cm. wedge of normal surrounding tissue
4. *Total mastectomy*—removal of entire breast
5. *Modified radical mastectomy*—removal of entire breast, pectoralis minor muscle, and axillary lymph nodes
6. *Radical mastectomy*—removal of entire breast, pectoral muscles, axillary nodes—rarely done today
7. *Prophylactic mastectomy*—removal of breast tissue (leaving skin and nipple area), followed by insertion of a mammary implant, in carefully selected patients who are high risk for developing breast cancer
8. *Mammaplasty*—reconstruction of the breast (see p. 757).
9. Surgical complications—infection, hematoma, lymphedema, nerve injury

B. Radiation Therapy

1. Radiation is effective in damaging and preventing cell reproduction.
2. Utilization in breast cancer:
   a. As adjuvant therapy with surgery or chemotherapy
   b. To shrink a large tumor to operable size
   c. To alleviate pain caused by metastasis
   d. As primary therapy
3. Method—following tumor and lymph node excision, a series of external radiation treatments are begun 3–4 weeks after incision is healed:
   a. Usually 4–5 treatments a week for 4–5 weeks
   b. Radiation directed to chest wall, remaining lymph nodes
   c. Side effects—mild fatigue, sore throat, nausea, anorexia; later, skin will look and feel sunburned and eventually the breast becomes more firm.
   d. A "booster" or second phase of treatment may be given: electron beam or radioactive implant.
4. Complications—include increased arm edema, decreased arm mobility, pneumonitis, brachial nerve damage, secondary cancers.

C. Cytotoxic Chemotherapy

1. Systemic treatment for patients who have positive lymph nodes or distant metastases; 50%–60% response rates.
2. Adjuvant
   a. With surgery or radiation

Table 29-1. *Treatment Relative to Menopausal, Nodal, and Receptor Status*

Menopausal Status	Node and Receptor Status	Treatment
Premenopausal	Node positive 1. Estrogen receptor positive 2. Estrogen receptor negative Node negative	 Oophorectomy Additive hormones Chemotherapy Chemotherapy for high risk
Postmenopausal	Node positive 1. Estrogen receptor positive 2. Estrogen receptor negative Node negative	 Tamoxifen Aminoglutethimide or Adrenalectomy as second line treatment Chemotherapy No treatment

b. Usually include combination of drugs—cyclophosphamide, methotrexate, 5-fluorouracil, doxorubicin;
c. Usually begin treatment 4 weeks after surgery (very stressful for patient who just finished major surgery)
d. Six months is optimal duration.
3. Primary—for inflammatory breast cancer
4. Palliative—for metastatic disease or recurrence
5. Side effects—include bone marrow suppression, nausea and vomiting, hair loss, weight gain, fatigue, stomatitis, anxiety, depression
6. Complications—infection, bleeding, sterility, secondary cancer, cardiotoxicity

D. Hormonal Therapy

1. Systemic therapy for estrogen and/or progesterone receptor-positive patients
   a. Most commonly used for metastases or recurrence
   b. Response is slower than with chemotherapy.
2. Anti-estrogens; Tamoxifen—binds estrogen receptors, thereby blocking estrogen
   a. First choice in postmenopausal women with positive nodes and receptors
   b. Given for at least 2 years; oral administration twice a day
3. Estrogens
   a. Most commonly used in women who are 5 or more years postmenopausal with recurrent breast cancer
   b. Diethylstilbestrol or ethinyl estradiol are the estrogens used.
   c. Remissions last 3 months to several years. Recurrence is usually treated with surgical ablation.
4. Progestins
   a. May decrease estrogen receptors
   b. Second choice of therapy for postmenopausal women
   c. Remissions less than 1 year.
5. Androgens
   a. May suppress FSH and estrogen production
   b. Remissions less than 1 year
   c. Used in postmenopausal women

6. Aminoglutethimide
   a. Suppresses estrogen production by blocking adrenal steroids; "medical adrenalectomy"
   b. Must be administered with hydrocortisone
   c. Especially useful for women with bone and soft tissue metastases (removal of ovaries)
7. Oophorectomy (removal of ovaries)
   a. Primary treatment for recurrent or metastatic estrogen receptor-positive premenopausal women
   b. Deprives tumor of primary estrogen source
   c. Remissions of 3 months to several years.
8. Adrenalectomy
   a. Removal of adrenal glands, which produces an androgen that converts to an estrogen
   b. Rarely done because of need for long-term steroid replacement therapy
   c. Remissions may last 6 months to several years.
9. For nursing intervention for hormonal therapy, see Table 29-2.

E. Immunotherapy

1. No role for routine use; no evidence of increased survival or decreased recurrence
2. BCG and levamisole have been tried.

F. Bone Marrow Transplant (see p. 292).

1. Autologous method after high-dose chemotherapy; may be curative because it allows for high doses of drugs.
2. Especially indicated for stage 3 disease

Nursing Assessment

A. Preoperative

1. Assess patient's knowledge of surgical procedure and postoperative course.
2. Assess level of anxiety.
3. Inquire about support systems.
4. Discuss patient's concerns and usual coping mechanisms.

B. Postoperative

1. Assess vital signs, level of consciousness, breath sounds, and urine output.

Table 29-2. *Nursing Interventions for Patients on Hormonal Therapy for Breast Cancer*

Hormonal Treatment	Side Effects	Intervening Measures
1. Estrogen	1. Nausea and vomiting	1. May need to change to another estrogen preparation. Take with meals or at bedtime.
	2. Edema	2. May need to restrict dietary sodium; diuretics. Wear a supportive bra for breast tenderness.
	3. Vaginal bleeding	
	4. Flare reaction (increased pain, swelling, erythema in soft tissue, increased bone pain, hypercalcemia.)	4. Inform patient that this is common and will diminish. Need to increase fluids and ambulation for hypercalcemia. May take analgesics.
2. Progestin	1. Weight gain	1. May need to consult nutritionist for dietary changes to accommodate increased appetite.
	2. Hot flashes	
	3. Vaginal bleeding	
3. Androgens	1. Virilization (male characteristics)	1. Report to physician.
	2. Weight gain	
	3. Fluid retention	3. Restrict sodium in diet. May need diuretics.
4. Tamoxifen	1. Nausea	1. Side effects are usually minimal; requiring no intervention.
	2. Hot flashes	
	3. Depression	
	4. Flare reaction	
5. Aminoglutethimide	1. Rash	1. Report rash to physician; dose may need to be reduced.
	2. Lethargy	2 & 3. Warn patient about symptoms; will usually subside in a few days.
	3. Dizziness	

2. Assess pain level (Level 1, designating minimum pain, to Level 10, designating maximum pain).
3. Assess dressing and wound (after dressing is removed) for redness, swelling, tenderness, odor, and drainage.
4. Assess knowledge of surgical outcome.
5. Assess knowledge of BSE.
6. Inquire about female relatives, especially sisters, daughters, and mother.

Nursing Diagnoses

A. Preoperative

1. Knowledge deficit of breast cancer and mastectomy
2. Anxiety related to diagnosis and treatment

B. Postoperative

1. Pain related to surgical incision
2. Ineffective breathing pattern related to pain, anesthetic, medication, and dressing
3. Impaired physical mobility related to impaired movement of arm on operative side
4. Self-care deficit related to restrictive arm movement and pain
5. Potential for physical injury related to interruption of lymph nodes and incision
6. Knowledge deficit of care of incision, arm, and performance of BSE
7. Body image disturbance related to loss of breast
8. Anxiety related to diagnosis of cancer
9. Potential for altered sexuality patterns related to loss of breast
10. Potential for altered family processes related to hospitalization of patient and fear of recurrence

Nursing Interventions

A. Increasing Comfort

1. Assess pain level and affected arm for malalignment and edema.
2. Administer pain medications as prescribed.
3. Use alternative pain relief measures such as back massage, heating pad, relaxation techniques to relieve muscle tension.
4. Position affected arm on pillows with hand elevated, in good alignment.
5. Discuss phantom limb pain, so patient is aware of phenomenon and realizes it is normal.

B. Improving Breathing Pattern

1. Encourage coughing and deep breathing every 4 hours. Teach patient to support incision.
2. Ambulate patient per prescription, usually within 24 hours.
3. Assess compression of dressing. Inform physician if it is too restrictive.
4. Monitor vital signs and breath sounds.
5. Teach use of incentive spirometer to decrease atelectasis.

C. Mobilizing Affected Arm

1. Instruct patient in arm exercises to prevent "frozen shoulder." (Initially, wrist and elbow flexion and extension)
2. Encourage use of arm for washing face, combing hair, applying lipstick, and brushing teeth.
3. Support arm in sling if prescribed to prevent strain on the incision.
4. Provide patient with arm and shoulder exercises to do when physician permits (See Table 29-3).

Table 29-3. *Exercises for the Rehabilitation of the Patient Following Mastectomy*

Exercise	Equivalent Daily Activities

1. Stand erect.
   Lean forward from waist.
   Allow arms to hang.
   Swing arms from side to side together: then in opposite direction.
   Next: swing arms from front to back together; then in opposite direction.
	Broom sweeping
	Vacuum cleaning
	Mopping floor
	Pulling out and pushing in drawers
	Weaving
	Playing golf

2. Stand erect facing wall with palms of hand flat against wall; arms extended.
   Relax arms and shoulders and allow upper part of body to lean forward against hands.
   Push away to original position; repeat.
	Pushing self out of bath tub
	Kneading bread
	Breast stroke—swimming
	Sawing or cutting types of crafts

3. Stand erect facing wall with palms of hands flat against wall. Climb the wall with the fingers; descend, repeat.	Raising windows Washing windows Hanging clothes on line Reaching to an upper shelf
4. Stand erect and clasp hands at small of back; raise hands; lower; repeat. Clasp hands back of neck; reach downward; upward; repeat.	Fastening brassiere Buttoning blouse or dress Pulling up a dress zipper Fastening beads Washing the back

5. Toss a rope over the shower curtain rod.
   Hold the ends of the rope (knotted) in each hand and alternately pull on each end.
   Using a see-saw motion and with arms outstretched, slide the rope up and down over the rod.
	Drying the back with a bath towel
	Raising and lowering a window blind
	Closing and opening window drapes

6. Flex and extend each finger in turn	Sewing, knitting, crocheting Typing, painting, playing piano or other musical instrument

---

Hand Care*

After a radical mastectomy, an arm may swell because lymph nodes and lymph vessels were necessarily removed and the body is therefore less able to combat infection in this extremity.

Make every effort to avoid all cuts, scratches, pin pricks, hangnails, insect bites, burns, and the use of strong detergents, as these can lead to serious infection with increased swelling.

Some "DO NOT'S":

DO NOT hold a cigarette in this hand

DO NOT carry your purse or anything heavy with this arm

DO NOT wear a wristwatch or other jewelry on this arm

DO NOT cut or pick at cuticles or hangnails on this hand

DO NOT work near thorny plants or dig in the garden

DO NOT reach into a hot oven with this arm

DO NOT permit injection in this arm

DO NOT permit blood to be drawn from this arm

DO NOT allow your blood pressure to be taken on this arm

Some "DO'S":

DO wear a loose rubber glove on this hand when washing dishes

DO wear a thimble when sewing

DO apply a good lanolin hand cream several times daily

DO wear your "Life-Guard Medical Aid" tag engraved with "CAUTION—LYMPHEDEMA ARM—NO TESTS—NO HYPOS"

DO contact your doctor if your arm gets red, warm, or unusually hard or swollen

DO return for a check-up and re-measurement for a new sleeve in two months

DO show this Hand Care Sheet to your surgeon

* Reprinted through the courtesy of the CLEVELAND CLINIC Department of Physical Medicine and Rehabilitation.

D. Increasing Self-Care Activities

1. Assess patient's ability to perform self-care and factors impeding performance.
2. Assist patient to perform personal hygiene she is unable to do herself.
3. Encourage patient to gradually increase own performance of self-care activities, especially with affected arm.

E. Preventing Infection of Affected Arm, Due to Obstructed Lymph Flow (Lymphedema), and Surgical Incision

1. Do not take blood pressure or inject medications or IVs in affected arm. Post sign over bed.
2. Inform patient not to wear constrictive clothing or jewelry on affected arm.
3. Assess incision for erythema, edema, drainage, and foul odor. Assess arm for edema, erythema, and pain.
4. Elevate affected arm on pillows, above level of heart, and hand above elbow to promote gravity drainage of fluid.
5. Provide patient with information on arm and hand care. (See chart, above).
6. Teach patient to massage affected arm if prescribed to increase circulation and decrease edema.
7. Administer antibiotics or diuretics as prescribed if lymphedema and/or infection occurs.
8. Monitor temperature and drainage.
9. Change dressing as prescribed.

F. Increasing Knowledge of Follow-up Care After Mastectomy (Patient Education)

1. Teach care of incision.
   a. Explain how wound will gradually change.
   b. Note that the newly healed wound may have less sensation because of severed nerves.
   c. Bathe gently and blot carefully to dry.
   d. Recognize signs of infection—pain, tenderness, redness, swelling; if these are present, report to physician.
   e. Massage gently the healed incision with cocoa butter to encourage circulation and increase skin elasticity. This is initiated with physician's approval.
2. Teach care of drains, if appropriate.
3. Teach importance of and procedure for monthly BSE and follow-up visits.
4. Teach care of affected arm. (See Hand Care chart, above.)

G. Enhancing Body Image

1. Discuss patient's views on how her body image has been altered.
2. Assess patient's knowledge of prosthesis and reconstruction options.
3. Provide information of above as desired by patient.
4. Suggest clothing adjustments to camouflage loss of breast.
5. Assist patient to obtain a temporary prosthesis (Reach to Recovery may provide).
   a. First prosthesis should be light and soft to allow incision to heal.
   b. May wear the heavier type usually after 4–8 weeks (Make sure physician's approval has been secured).
6. Encourage patient to discuss feelings with husband/significant other.
7. Encourage patient to allow herself to experience the grief process over the loss of her breast and to learn to cope with these feelings.

H. Reducing Anxiety

1. Familiarize patient with Reach to Recovery (an American Cancer Society program consisting of volunteers who have had mastectomies, who visit postoperatively in the hospital to provide support and information).
2. Arrange for patient to have a visitor from Reach to Recovery if she desires and physician approves.
3. Discuss patient's usual coping mechanisms.
4. Encourage and assist family to support patient.
5. Assist patient to maintain control by planning care with her and incorporating her usual routines.

6. Refer for post-mastectomy support group as needed and desired.
7. Offer list of community resources such as through the American Cancer Society and the YWCA-Encore program.
8. Remind patient that stress related to breast cancer and mastectomy may persist for 1 year or more and to seek help.

I. Maintaining Sexual Activity

1. Discuss effect of loss of breast on view of self as a woman.
2. Explore alternative means of sexual activity such as changing position during intercourse to decrease pressure on incision.
3. Encourage patient to discuss concerns with husband/significant other.
4. Assist patient and husband to look at incision when ready (progress from pictures to description to touching to looking).
5. Encourage her to wear nightgown and prosthesis to bed.

J. Maintaining Family Coping Skills

1. Inform patient and family that stress may persist for a long period, even up to a year.
2. Support husband and family of patient as well, as they tend to be left out.
3. Assist them to communicate with and care for patient.
4. Encourage them to attend support groups as needed.

Evaluation

1. Verbalizes increased comfort; ambulates in halls; performs self-care activities
2. Improves breathing pattern; normal respiratory rate and depth, absence of adventitious sounds
3. Moves affected arm within limits prescribed by surgeon
4. Performs self-care activities
5. Absence of infection or swelling in affected arm
6. States care of incision, drains. Performs BSE
7. Expresses positive body image
8. Exhibits minimal anxiety
9. Reports satisfactory sexual activity and/or sexuality
10. Reports adequate family coping

Breast Reconstruction (Mammaplasty)

Reconstruction of the breast using prosthetic implants or fashioning a flap from patient's own tissue
1. Usually performed 3 months to 1 year after mastectomy to allow for wound healing; however, may be done immediately or as long after surgery as desired.
2. Benefits include improved psychological coping due to improved body image, and self-esteem.
3. Contraindications include obesity, smoking, and possibly previous radiation therapy and radical mastectomy.

Types of Reconstruction

A. Implants

1. Usually made of silicone—feels hard
2. Placed in pocket under skin or pectoralis muscle (See Fig. 29-5)
3. Scar tissue usually forms around it, resulting in firmness; may be painful.
4. Complications—include infection, hematoma, capsular contraction (scar tissue around implant).

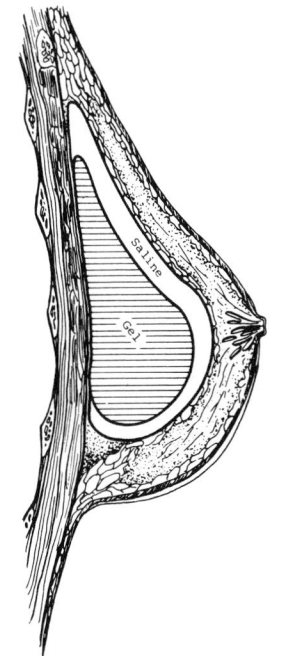

Figure 29-5. *The diagrammatic sketch shows the placement of a mammary implant—in this case, one featuring a sealed inner gel implant surrounded by an inflatable outer saline implant. (Courtesy American Heyer–Schulte Corporation, Goleta, CA 1980)*

5. Nursing interventions
   a. Teach signs and symptoms of infection, migration, and deflation.
   b. Teach patient to massage breast to decrease capsule formation around implant and keep it mobile; perform 3 times a day from sides to center and bottom to top.

B. Tissue Expanders

1. Inflatable silicone envelope placed under muscle or skin, usually after mastectomy.
2. Expander is filled with saline once incision is healed (about 4 weeks). Saline (30–200 ml.) is instilled every 1–3 weeks until the expander is beyond desired size.
3. Later, expander is removed and a permanent implant is placed. Some types of expanders may be left in permanently.
4. Indicated for patients with inadequate breast tissue and skin of good quality
5. Complications include infection, hematoma, skin necrosis, expander deflation, and arm paresthesias.
6. Advantages—no extra incision; less fibrosis. Disadvantage—may take months.
7. Nursing Interventions
   a. Teach signs and symptoms of infection, deflation. Teach patient to report paresthesias.
   b. Teach patient she will feel pressure but not pain with the expansions.
   c. Recommend patient use temporary prosthesis in between inflation procedures.

C. Flap Grafts

1. The transfer of skin, muscle, and subcutaneous tissue from another part of the body to the mastectomy site.

2. Indicated for patients who need additional tissue. Provides better cosmesis.
3. Disadvantages include cost, several hospitalizations required, slow process—done in stages, increased morbidity
4. Complications include flap loss, hematoma, infection, seroma, abdominal hernia.
5. Two types
   a. Latissimus dorsi—skin, fat, and muscles of back between shoulder blades are tunneled under skin to front chest; silicone implant placed under muscle.
   b. Rectus abdominus—abdominus muscles, fat, skin, and blood supply are tunneled to breast area; can be single-step procedure; can do if radiated skin.
6. Nursing Interventions
   a. Assess flap and donor site for color, temperature, and wound drainage.
   b. Control pain.

c. Provide support with bra or abdominal binder to maintain position of prosthesis.
d. Teach patient to bathe with warm, not hot, water so she does not increase oxygen demands of tissue.
e. Teach patient to massage implant if prescribed by surgeon, to soften the prosthesis and decrease capsule formation.
f. Tell patient to avoid vigorous exercise.
g. Teach patient to perform BSE monthly and that she may have some asymmetry, small ridges, and increased density.

D. Nipple–Areolar Reconstruction

1. Usually done at a separate time from breast reconstruction
2. Use skin and fat from reconstructed breast for nipple and upper thigh for areola; tanning or tatoo done to obtain appropriate color

---

Bibliography

Breast Conditions

Books

Bassett LW and Gold RH. Breast Cancer Detection: Mammography & Other Methods in Breast Imaging. 2nd ed. Orlando, Grune & Stratton, 1987

Cooper CL (ed). Stress and Breast Cancer. Chichester, John Wiley & Sons, 1988

Donegan WL and Spratt JS. Cancer of the Breast. 3rd ed. Philadelphia, WB Saunders, 1988

Haagensen CD. Diseases of the Breast. 3rd ed. Philadelphia, WB Saunders, 1986

Harris JR et al (eds). Breast Diseases. Philadelphia, JB Lippincott, 1987

Lippman ME, Lichter AS and Danforth DN. Diagnosis and Management of Breast Cancer. Philadelphia, WB Saunders, 1986

Marchant DJ (ed). Breast Disease— Contemporary Issues in Obstetrics and Gynecology. New York, Churchill Livingstone, 1986

Pfeiffer CH and Mulliken JB (eds). Caring for the Patient with Breast Cancer. Reston, Reston Publishing, 1984

Porrath S. A Multimodality Approach to Breast Imaging. Rockville, Aspen Publishers, Inc, 1986

Stoll BA (ed). Breast Cancer—Treatment and Prognosis. Oxford, Blackwell Scientific Publications, 1986

Uppenberger V and Goldhirsch A (eds). Recent Results in Cancer Research. Endocrine Therapy and Growth Regulation of Breast Cancer. Berlin, Springer-Verlag, 1989

US Department of Health and Human Services. The Breast Cancer Digest. 2nd ed. PHS. NIH Pub. #84-1691. National Cancer Institute, Bethesda, MD, 1984

Journals

Breast Self-Examination and Diagnostic Evaluation

Clarke DE and Sandler LS. Factors involved in nurses' teaching breast self-examination. Cancer Nurs 1989 Feb; 12(1):41–46

Fletcher SW. Internal medicine. JAMA 1989 May 19; 261(19):2853–2855

Guarda NP and Peterson JZ. If your patient must undergo fine-needle biopsy. RN 1986 Oct; 49(10):34–35

Habegger D and Ellerhorst-Ryan JM. Needle localization for nonpalpable breast lesions. Oncol Nurs Forum 1988 Mar–Apr; 15(2):192–194

Hayes H, Vandergrift J and Diner WC. Mammography and breast implants. Plast Reconstr Surg 1988 Jul; 82(1):1–6

Howard J. Using mammography for cancer control: An unrealized potential. CA 1987 Jan–Feb; 37(1):33–48

Kopans DB and Swann CA. Preoperative imaging—guided needle placement and localization of clinically occult breast lesions. AJR 1989 Jan; 152(1):1–9

Lee GF. Fine-needle aspiration of the breast: The outpatient management of breast lesions. Am J Obstet Gynecol 1987 Jun; 156(6):1532–1537

Lorenzen JR and Gravdal JA. Bloody nipple discharge. Am Fam Physician 1986 Jul; 34(1):151–154

Ludwick R. Breast examination in the older adult. Cancer Nurs 1988 Apr; 11(2):99–102

Massey V. Perceived susceptibility to breast cancer and practice of breast self-examination. Nurs Res 1986 May–Jun; 35(3):183–185

Paulus DD. Imaging in breast cancer. CA 1987 May–Jun; 37(3):133–150

Redeker NS. Health beliefs, health locus of control and the frequency of practice of breast self-examination in women. J Obstet Gynecol Neonatal Nurs 1989 Jan–Feb; 18(1):45–51

Rudolph A and McDermott R. Breast physical examination—Its value in early cancer detection. Cancer Nurs 1987 Apr; 10(2):100–106

Rutledge DN. Factors related to women's practice of breast self-examination. Nurs Res 1987 Mar–Apr; 36(2):117–121

Shamian J and Edgar L. Nurses as agents for change in teaching breast self-examination. Public Health Nurs 1987 Mar; 4(1):29–34

Welch-McCaffrey D and Dodge J. Planning breast self-examination programs for elderly women. Oncol Nurs Forum 1988 Nov–Dec; 15(6): 811–814

Winchester DP et al. The Early Detection and Diagnosis of Breast Cancer. Atlanta, American Cancer Society, 1988 (Pamphlet)

Benign Breast Disease

Davis JE. Major ambulatory surgery of the general surgical patient—Management of breast disease and hernias of the abdominal wall. Surg Clin North Am 1987 Aug; 67(4):733–760

Devitt JE. Benign disorders of the breast in older women. Surg Gynecol Obstet 1986 Apr; 162(4):340–342

Ellerhorst-Ryan JM, Turba EP and Stahl DL. Evaluating benign breast disease. Nurse Pract 1988 Sep; 13(9):13–28

Fentiman IS and Powles TJ. Tamoxifen and benign breast problems. Lancet 1987 Nov 7; 2(8567):1070–1072

Mitchell GW. Benign breast disease and cancer. Clin Obstet Gynecol 1986 Sep; 29(3):705–714

Breast Cancer—General

Jones RC. Oncology practice 1989: A perspective on breast cancer. Cope 1989 Apr–May; 34–37

Greifzu S. Breast cancer: The risks and the options. RN 1986 Oct; 49(10):26–32

Morrison AS, Brisson J and Khalid N. Breast cancer incidence and mortality in the breast cancer detection demonstration project. J Natl Cancer Inst 1988 Dec 7; 80(19):1540–1547

Northouse LL. A longitudinal study of the adjustment of patients and husbands to breast cancer. Oncol Nurs Forum 1989 Jul–Aug; 16(4):511–516

Northouse LL. Social support in patients' and husbands' adjustment to breast cancer. Nurs Res 1988 Mar–Apr; 37(2):91–95

Northouse LL and Swain MA. Adjustment of patients and husbands to the initial impact of breast cancer. Nurs Res 1987; Jul–Aug 36(4):221–225

Sinsheimer LM and Holland JC. Psychological issues in breast cancer. Semin Oncol 1987 Mar; 14(1):75–82

Swain SM. Lobular carcinoma in situ—Incidence, presentation, guidelines to treatment. Oncology 1989 Mar; 3(3):35–40

Breast Cancer—Etiology and Risk Factors

Baron JA et al. Cigarette smoking in women with cancers of the breast and reproductive organs. J Natl Cancer Inst 1986 Sep; 77(3):677–680

Goodwin PJ and Boyd NF. Critical appraisal of the evidence that dietary fat intake is related to breast cancer risk in humans. J Natl Cancer Inst 1987 Sep; 79(3):473–485

Harvey EB et al. Alcohol consumption and breast cancer. J Natl Cancer Inst 1987 Apr; 78(4):657–661

Hiatt RA and Fireman BH. Smoking, menopause and breast cancer. J Natl Cancer Inst 1986 May; 76(5):833–838

Lemon HM and Lynch HT. Breast cancer and the use of oral contraceptives. JAMA 1986 Nov 7; 256(17):2346

Lindsey AM, Dodd M and Kaempfer SH. Endocrine mechanisms and obesity: Influences in breast cancer. Oncol Nurs Forum 1987 Mar–Apr; 14(2):47–51

Lipnick RJ et al. Oral contraceptives and breast cancer—A prospective cohort study. JAMA 1986 Jan 3; 255(1):58–61

Longman SM and Buehring GC. Oral contraceptives and breast cancer—In vitro effect of contraceptive steroids on human mammary cell growth. Cancer 1987 Jan 15; 59(2):281–287

Lubin F, Wax Y and Modan B. Role of fat, animal protein, and dietary fiber in breast cancer etiology: A case-control study. J Natl Cancer Inst 1986 Sep; 77(3):605–612

Schatzkin A et al. Is alcohol consumption related to breast cancer? Results from the Framingham heart study. J Natl Cancer Inst 1989 Jan; 81(1):31–35

Willett WC et al. Dietary fat and the risk of breast cancer. N Engl J Med 1987 Jan 1; 316(1):22–28

Breast Cancer—Surgery

Bloom JR et al. Psychological response to mastectomy—A prospective comparison study. Cancer 1987 Jan 1; 59(1):189–196

Dietrick-Gallagher M and Hyzinski MM. Teaching patients to care for drains after breast surgery for malignancy. Oncol Nurs Forum 1989 Mar–Apr; 16(2):263–265

Lierman LM. Phantom breast experiences after mastectomy. Oncol Nurs Forum 1988 Jan–Feb; 15(1):41–44

Martin JK et al. Is modified radical mastectomy really equivalent to radical mastectomy in treatment of carcinoma of the breast? Cancer 1986 Feb 1; 57(3):510–518

Rice MA and Szopa TJ. Group intervention for reinforcing self-worth following mastectomy. Oncol Nurs Forum 1988 Jan–Feb; 15(1):33–37

Rutherford DE. Assessing psychosexual needs of women experiencing lumpectomy—A challenge for research. Cancer Nurs 1988 Jul–Aug; 11(4):244–249

Breast Cancer—Radiation Therapy

Harris JR, Hellman S and Kinne DW. Limited surgery and radiotherapy for early breast cancer. CA 1986 Mar–Apr; 36(2):120–125

McCarthy CP. The role of interstitial implantation in the treatment of primary breast cancer. Semin Oncol Nurs 1987 Feb; 3(1):47–53

Sheldon T et al. Primary radiation therapy for locally advanced breast cancer. Cancer 1987 Sep 15; 60(6):1219–1225

Breast Cancer—Chemotherapy

Andrykowski MA. Prevalence, predictors, and course of anticipatory nausea in women receiving adjuvant chemotherapy for breast cancer. Cancer 1988 Dec 15; 62(12):2607–2613

Bonadonna G and Valagussa P. Adjuvant chemoendocrine therapy in breast cancer. J Clin Oncol 1986 Apr; 4(4):451–453

Bonadonna G and Valagussa P. Current status of adjuvant chemotherapy for breast cancer. Semin Oncol 1987 Mar; 14(1):8–22

Carey RL and Jevne R. Development of an information package for post-mastectomy patients on adjuvant therapy. Oncol Nurs Forum 1986 May–Jun; 13(3):78–83

Coates A. Improving the quality of life during chemotherapy for advanced breast cancer. N Engl J Med 1987 Dec 10; 317(24):1490–1495

Doig B. Adjuvant chemotherapy in breast cancer—A review of the literature. Cancer Nurs 1988 Apr; 11(2):91–98

Falkson G et al. Treatment of metastatic breast cancer in premenopausal women using CAF with or without oophorectomy: An Eastern Cooperative Oncology Group Study. J Clin Oncol 1987 Jun; 5(6):881–889

Grindel CG, Cahill CA and Walker M. Food intake of women with breast cancer during their first six months of chemotherapy. Oncol Nurs Forum 1989 May–Jun; 16(3):401–407

Hopkins MB. Information-seeking and adaptational outcomes in women receiving chemotherapy for breast cancer. Cancer Nurs 1986 Oct; 9(5):256–262

Jacobsen PB et al. Nonpharmacologic factors in the development of posttreatment nausea with adjuvant chemotherapy for breast cancer. Cancer 1988 Jan 15; 61(2):379–385

Organ CH. Surgery. JAMA 1989 May 19; 261(19):2892–2894

Perloff M et al. Combination chemotherapy with mastectomy or radiotherapy for stage 3 breast carcinoma: A Cancer and Leukemia Group B Study. J Clin Oncol 1988 Feb; 6(2):261–269

Swain SM and Lippman ME. Systemic therapy of locally advanced breast cancer: Review and guidelines. Oncology 1989 Jan; 3(1):21–28

Breast Cancer—Hormonal Therapy

Dunne CF. Hormonal therapy for breast cancer. Cancer Nurs 1988 Oct; 11(5):288–294

Goodman M. Concepts of hormonal manipulation in the treatment of cancer. Oncol Nurs Forum 1988 Sep–Oct; 15(5):639–647

Yonemoto RE. Tamoxifen equivalent to oophorectomy in advanced breast cancer. Oncology 1989 Feb; 3(2):17–18

Breast Reconstruction

Becker H. Breast augmentation using the expander mammary prosthesis. Plast Reconstr Surg 1987 Feb; 79(2):194–199

Bostwick J. Breast reconstruction following mastectomy. CA 1989 Jan–Feb; 39(1):40–48

D'Angelo TM and Gorrell CR. Breast reconstruction using tissue expanders. Oncol Nurs Forum 1989 Jan–Feb; 16(1):23–27

Dinner MI and Coleman C. Breast reconstruction—Use of autogenous tissue. AORN J 1985 Oct; 42(4):490–496

Goldwyn RM. Breast reconstruction after mastectomy. N Engl J Med 1987 Dec; 317(27):1711–1713

Hartrampf CR and Bennett GK. Autogenous tissue reconstruction in the mastectomy patient. Ann Surg 1987 May; 205(5):508–519

Hutcheson HA. TAIF: New option for breast reconstruction. Nursing 1986 Feb; 16(2):52–53

Kramer AS. Immediate breast reconstruction. Plast Surg Nurs 1988 Winter; 8(4):150–154

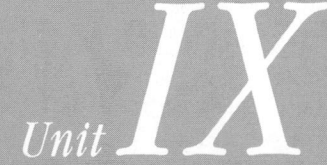

Unit *IX*

Musculoskeletal Disorders

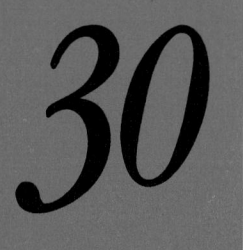

30 Musculoskeletal Trauma and Fractures

Diagnostic Evaluation of Musculoskeletal Problems

Physical Assessment

Data on current system condition and functional abilities are secured through inspection, palpation, and measurement. Always compare with contralateral side (one side of the body to the other).

A. Skeletal Component

1. Note deviations from structural normal—bony deformities, length discrepancies, alignment, amputations.
2. Identify abnormal motion and *crepitus* (grating sensation) as found with fractures.

B. Joint Component

1. Identify swelling that may be due to inflammation or effusion
2. Note deformity associated with contractures or dislocations
3. Evaluate stability, which may be altered
4. Estimate ROM (range of motion), both actively and passively

C. Muscle Component

1. Inspect for size and contour of muscles.
2. Assess coordination of movement.
3. Palpate for muscle tone.
4. Estimate strength through cursory evaluation (i.e., handshake) or scaled criteria (i.e., 0 = no palpable contraction to 5 = normal range of motion against gravity with full resistance).
5. Measure girth to note increases due to swelling or bleeding into muscle or decreases due to atrophy (difference of more than 1 cm. is significant).
6. Identify abnormal *clonus* (rhythmic contraction and relaxation) or *fasciculation* (contractions of isolated muscle fibers).

D. Neurovascular Component

1. Assess circulatory status of involved extremities by noting skin color and temperature, peripheral pulses, capillary refill response, pain.
2. Assess neurologic status of involved extremities by the patient's ability to move distal muscles and description of sensation (e.g., paresthesia).
3. Test reflexes of extremities.

E. Skin Component

1. Inspect traumatic injuries (e.g., cuts, bruises, etc.).
2. Assess chronic conditions (e.g., dermatitis, stasis ulcers, etc.).
3. Note hair distribution and nail condition.

F. Subjective Component

Elicit data from patient concerning presence of pain, tenderness, abnormal sensation, or tightness during physical examination.

Diagnostic Evaluation

A. Radiologic and Imaging Studies

1. *X-rays*
   a. Of bone—to determine bone density, texture, integrity, erosion, changes in bone relationships
   b. Of cortex—to detect any widening, narrowing, irregularity
   c. Of medullary cavity—to detect any alteration in density
   d. Of involved joint—to show fluid, irregularity, spur formation, narrowing, changes in joint contour
2. *Tomogram*—special x-ray technique for detailed view of specific plane of bone
3. *Computed tomogram*—to identify tumors of the soft tissues or injuries to ligaments or tendons; to identify location/extent of fractures in difficult-to-define areas; to identify disc herniation
4. *Bone scan*—parenteral injection of bone-seeking radiopharmaceutical; concentration of isotope uptake

revealed in primary skeletal disease (osteosarcoma), metastatic bone disease, inflammatory skeletal disease (osteomyelitis); fracture

5. *Arthrogram*—injection of radiopaque substance or air into joint cavity to outline soft tissue structures (e.g., meniscus) and contour of joint
6. *Myelogram*—injection of contrast medium into subarachnoid space at lumbar spine to determine level of disc herniation or site of tumor; see page 571
7. *Discogram*—injection of small amount of contrast medium into lumbar disc to visualize disc abnormalities
8. *MRI* (magnetic resonance imaging)—uses magnetic fields to demonstrate differences in hydrogen density of various tissues. Demonstrates tumors and soft tissue (muscle, ligament, tendon) abnormalities.

NURSING ALERT: Patients with metal implants, metal braces, pacemakers, or claustrophobia are not able to undergo MRI.

B. Joint Examinations

1. *Arthrocentesis*—insertion of needle into joint and aspiration of synovial fluid for purposes of examination.
2. *Arthroscopy*—endoscopic procedure that allows direct visualization of joint structures (synovium, articular surfaces, menisci, ligaments) through a large bore needle. May be combined with arthrography.

C. Muscle and Nerve Studies—to differentiate nerve root compression, muscle disease (dystrophy, myositis, etc.), peripheral neuropathies, central nervous system–anterior horn cell neuropathies, neuromuscular–junction problems.

1. *Electromyography* (EMG)—measures electrical potential generated by the muscle during relaxation and contraction
2. *Nerve conduction velocities* (NCVs)—measures the rate of potential generation along specific nerves (speed of impulse conduction)

D. Laboratory Studies—baseline hematology, serum chemistry, and urinalysis provide information on the general health of the patient. Few laboratory studies are specific for orthopedic conditions.

1. Clotting factors—evaluation prior to orthopedic surgery desirable; person with hemophilia prone to specific orthopedic problems; assessed in prophylactic and therapeutic anticoagulant regimens
2. Calcitonin—bone metabolism
3. Calcium—osteomalacia, parathyroid function, Paget's disease, prolonged immobilization
4. Creatine phosphokinase (CPK)—skeletal muscle disease
5. Parathyroid hormone (PTH)—bone metabolism
6. Hyperkalemia—trauma with massive tissue damage
7. Phosphatase, acid—cancer metastatized to bone, Paget's disease
8. Phosphatase, alkaline—bone metabolism (osteoblastic activity), bone tumors, Paget's disease
9. Phosphorus, inorganic—parathyroid problems
10. Thyroid studies—bone metabolism
11. Transaminase (SGPT)—skeletal muscle trauma
12. Vitamin D (1,25(OH)2D3)—bone metabolism
13. Urine: Bence–Jones protein—multiple myeloma
14. Urine: calcium—bone metabolism; parathyroid function
15. Urine: phosphorus—rickets

E. Special Studies—bone biopsy, densitometry, total body calcium, etc.

Nursing Process Overview: The Patient With a Musculoskeletal Problem

Assessment

A. General Observation—data on ability to move, existence of discomfort and gross abnormalities, and presence of involuntary movement

1. Observe gait and intentional movement for coordination and speed.
2. Note posture and body positions.
3. Identify use of assistive devices—canes, walker, prosthesis, etc.

B. Nursing History

The patient supplies data on primary problem and information indicating impact of problem on functional health and activities of daily living (ADLs).

1. Elicit information concerning chief complaint and how the patient has been handling the problem (coping–stress-tolerance pattern).
2. Assist the patient to describe symptoms such as pain, stiffness, and cramps and effect of these on sleep–rest pattern.
3. Identify concurrent health problems (including medications), health maintenance practices (nutritional–metabolic pattern; elimination pattern), and allergies.
4. Note impact of musculoskeletal disorder on activity–exercise pattern, role relationship patterns, self-perception—self-concept pattern; family economics, etc.
5. Assess the patient's perceptions and expectations related to health problems.
6. Estimate the patient's ability to learn (i.e., note language barriers).

Nursing Diagnoses

1. Pain related to skeletal or muscular dysfunction
2. Impaired physical mobility related to limitations imposed by underlying condition and treatment modalities such as casts, traction, or bed rest
3. Potential for injury (neuromuscular compromise such as compartment syndrome) related to constrictive dressings, crush injuries, ischemic swelling following arterial injury, increased tissue pressure, etc.
4. Ineffective coping related to enforced immobility and altered life-style.

Nursing Interventions

A. Relieving Pain

1. Secure data concerning pain.
   a. Have the patient describe the pain, location, characteristics (dull, sharp, continuous, throbbing, boring, radiating, aching, etc.)
   b. Ask the patient what causes the pain; makes the pain worse; relieves the pain, etc.

c. Evaluate the patient for proper body alignment, pressure from equipment (casts, traction, splints, appliances).

2. Initiate activities to prevent or modify pain.
   a. Assist the patient with pain-reduction techniques—cutaneous stimulation, distraction, guided imagery, transcutaneous electrical nerve stimulation (TENS), biofeedback, etc.
   b. Immobilize injured part.
   c. Position the patient in correct alignment.
   d. Move the patient slowly and steadily, providing adequate support to painful structure, and help of additional personnel as needed.
   e. Elevate painful extremity to diminish venous congestion.
   f. Apply heat or cold modalities as prescribed.
   g. Modify environment to facilitate rest and relaxation.

3. Administer prescribed pharmaceuticals (nonsteroidal anti-inflammatory drugs [NSAIDs]; narcotics) as indicated. Encourage use of less potent drugs as severity of discomfort decreases.

4. Establish a supportive relationship to assist patient to deal with discomfort.

5. Encourage the patient to become an active participant in rehabilitative plans.

B. Promoting Maximum Physical Mobility Within Limits of Musculoskeletal Problem and Therapeutic Regimen

1. Assess degree of physical mobility present.
   a. Identify use of mobility aids.
   b. Note ability to reposition self and ability to transfer from one place to another.
   c. Determine availability of assistants to facilitate mobility.
   d. Assess body systems (e.g., respiratory, gastrointestinal, etc.) for responses to limited activity.
   e. Evaluate short-term and long-term effects of chosen treatment modalities on mobility.

2. Identify true extent of imposed physical immobility.

3. Develop exercise regimen within prescribed physical activity limits.

4. Encourage weight-bearing and walking activities when possible.

5. Establish plan of range-of-motion and isometric exercises (e.g., quadriceps—setting exercise) as preparation for resumption of full mobility.

6. Encourage movement of all uninvolved bodily parts.

7. Teach proper and safe use of mobilization aids.

C. Avoiding Neuromuscular Compromise and Ensuring Optimum Circulation, Tissue Perfusion, and Nerve Function

1. Assess for clinical manifestations of neuromuscular compromise.
   a. Complaint of deep, throbbing pain with persistent pressure sensation.
   b. Abnormal sensory evaluation (e.g., paresthesia, hypesthesia, loss of sensation)
   c. Pain with stretch of involved muscle
   d. Tight, tense muscle mass on palpation
   e. Elevation of tissue pressure indicated by direct needle measurement (above 30 mm. Hg) (Fig. 30-1)
   f. Muscle paresis (weakness) or paralysis

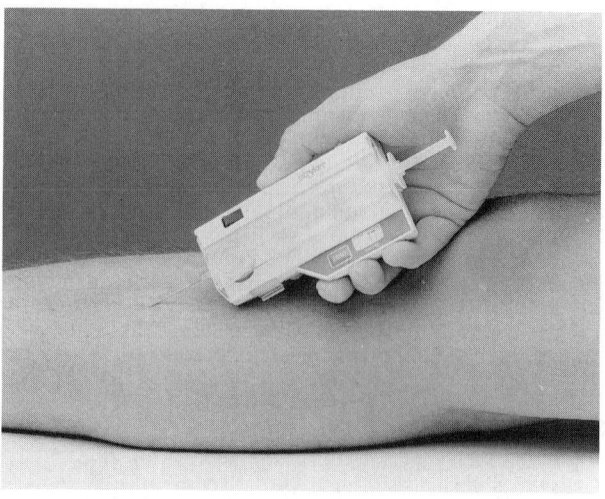

Figure 30-1. *Tissue pressure monitoring device. (Photo courtesy Stryker Surgical)*

NURSING ALERT: Pulse and capillary refill may be present with inadequate tissue perfusion and can contribute to a false sense of security concerning impending compartment syndrome.

2. Elevate injured extremity to minimize edema.

3. Apply ice pack to fresh injury if prescribed to control bleeding and swelling.

4. Inform the patient that frequent neurovascular assessments will be performed.

5. Have the patient move fingers or toes distal to injury.

6. Have the patient describe sensations in injured extremity.

7. Assess color, temperature, capillary refill, and pulses of involved extremity. Compare with contralateral extremity.

8. Notify physician immediately of compromised neurovascular status.

9. Release constrictive devices (e.g., bivalve cast).

10. If no improvement when external devices are released, a decompression fasciotomy (incision of tissue surrounding muscle) will be anticipated.

11. Give health education concerning preoperative and postoperative care.

12. Teach the patient to recognize and report increasing pain, tingling, and numbness.

D. Strengthening Coping Abilities

1. Nursing assessment
   a. Assess the patient and family for reactive behaviors of denial, anger, bargaining, depression, acceptance.
   b. Identify anxious behaviors.
   c. Note expressions of diminished self-worth and self-concept.
   d. Assess degree of independence in self-care activities.
   e. Identify social isolation behaviors.

2. Promote gradual acceptance of disabilities due to musculoskeletal problem.

a. Assist the patient to recognize the impact of the musculoskeletal problem.
b. Support the patient through the phases of acceptance.
c. Recognize that the patient and family may be at different phases of coping/acceptance process.
d. Accept the patient's behaviors as expressions of the coping process.
e. Encourage the patient to focus on current abilities (instead of losses).
3. Reduce anxiety related to impact of musculoskeletal problem on life-style.
   a. Explore the patient's understanding of musculoskeletal problem and its therapeutic regimen.
   b. Identify areas for additional teaching.
   c. Clarify misconceptions.
   d. Encourage the patient to participate actively in planning and implementation of therapeutic regimen.
   e. Facilitate acceptance of abilities by the patient and family.
   f. Assist the patient to identify stress-producing situations.
4. Initiate measures to cope with altered self-concept related to modified life role.
   a. Identify activities within treatment regimen where the patient can establish control.
   b. Provide genuine praise for self-care abilities.
   c. Encourage the patient to make own decisions within scheduled therapeutic regimen.
   d. Assist family in use of the patient's contributions to solve home problems.
   e. Promote feelings of independence.
5. Counter self-care deficits related to musculoskeletal problem or treatment modality.
   a. Assess residual abilities and use these in development of self-care regimens.
   b. Encourage the patient to assist in own care to fullest ability.
   c. Modify activities to facilitate maximum independence.
   d. Maximize time allotted for accomplishment of self-care activities.
   e. Integrate physical therapy, occupational therapy, and other therapeutic approaches into nursing care activities.
6. Minimize social isolation related to hospitalization and decreased mobility.
   a. Plan frequent periods of interaction with the patient.
   b. Encourage contacts with family and friends.
   c. Facilitate visits with children and other family members when feasible.
   d. Involve the patient in personal and therapeutic decision-making processes.
   e. Develop supportive relationships.

Evaluation

1. Achieves pain relief
   a. Participates in pain-reduction activities by elevating extremity, use of pain-reduction modality, accepting assistance in pain-producing situations
   b. Decreases use of pharmaceutical agents in the management of discomfort
2. Increases physical mobility
   a. Moves unaffected joints and extremities

b. Uses mobilization aids safely and effectively
c. Remains free of immobility complications
3. Maintains adequate circulation and nerve function
   a. Minimal discomfort, normal sensations, and normal movement of fingers or toes of involved extremity.
   b. No extremity contracture or evidence of loss of function of extremity due to compromised circulation
4. Exhibits effective coping
   a. Participates in rehabilitation activities
   b. States modifications in life-style necessary to accommodate musculoskeletal disability
   c. Increases participation in rehabilitation through self-care and mobilization activities
   d. Plans for continuing care needs

Contusions, Strains, and Sprains

A *contusion* is an injury to the soft tissue produced by a blunt force (blow, kick, or fall).

A *sprain* is an injury to ligamentous structures surrounding a joint; it is usually caused by a wrench or twist resulting in a decrease in the joint stability.

A *strain* is a microscopic tearing of the muscle caused by excessive force, stretching, or overuse.

Clinical Manifestations

A. Contusion
1. Hemorrhage into injured part (ecchymosis)—from rupture of small blood vessels; also associated with fractures
2. Pain, swelling, and discoloration
3. Hyperkalemia may be present with extensive contusions, resulting in destruction of body tissue and loss of blood

B. Strain
1. Hemorrhage into the muscle
2. Swelling
3. Tenderness
4. Pain with isometric contraction

C. Sprain
1. Rapid swelling—due to extravasation of blood within tissues
2. Pain on passive movement of joint
3. Increasing pain during first few hours due to continued swelling
4. X-ray of area reveals no bone injury.

Nursing Interventions

A. Relieving Discomfort
1. Elevate the affected part.
2. Apply cold compresses for the first 24 hours (20–30 minutes at a time)—to produce vasoconstriction, decrease edema, and reduce discomfort.
3. Apply heat to affected area after 24 hours (20–30 minutes at a time) 4 times a day—to promote circulation and absorption.
4. Apply pressure bandage—to control bleeding and swelling.
5. Assess neurovascular status of contused extremity every

hour to every 4 hours as the patient's condition indicates.
6. Instruct the patient on use of pain medication as prescribed.

B. Immobilizing Injured Part to Allow for Healing

1. Splint and immobilize injured part.
2. Elevate injured extremity to minimize swelling.
3. Use elastic compressive dressing to support weakened joint structures and to control edema.
4. Severe sprains may require surgical repair and/or cast immobilization.

C. Resuming Self-Care Activities

1. Assist the patient in use of self-care and mobility aids to maintain independence within activity restrictions.
2. Participate in patient teaching on need to rest injured part for about a month to allow for healing.
3. Teach the patient to resume activities gradually.
4. Teach the patient to avoid excessive exercise of injured part.
5. Teach the patient to avoid re-injury.

Traumatic Joint Dislocation

A *dislocation of a joint* occurs when the surfaces of the bones forming the joint are no longer in anatomic contact—this is a medical emergency because of associated disruption of surrounding blood and nerve supplies.

Clinical Manifestations

1. Pain
2. Deformity
3. Change in the length of the extremity
4. Loss of normal movement
5. X-ray confirmation of dislocation without associated fracture

Management

1. Immobilize part while the patient is transported to emergency department, x-ray department, or clinical unit.
2. Secure reduction of dislocation (bring displaced parts into normal position) as soon as possible; usually performed under anesthesia.
3. Stabilize reduction until joint structures are healed.
4. Monitor for development of sequelae (unstable joint, aseptic necrosis of bone, circulatory or nerve impairment).

Nursing Interventions

A. Promoting Comfort

1. Secure the patient's permission to undergo reduction of dislocation under anesthesia if necessary.
2. Give medication to relieve discomfort.
3. Immobilize reduced joint.

B. Resumption of Self-Care Activities

1. Assist the patient with activities of daily living as needed.
2. Initiate health teaching concerning need to comply with activity limitations, rehabilitation therapies, and long-term monitoring for sequelae.

Knee Injuries

Causes and Clinical Manifestations

1. Severe stresses are applied to the knee during many sport activities (e.g., soccer, skiing, running).
2. Injury to knee structures occur during rapid position changes involving flexing and twisting of the joint.
3. Torn cartilage (meniscus) causes pain, tenderness, joint effusion, clicking sensations, and decreased range of motion.
4. Knee ligaments may be torn, resulting in pain and joint instability. The patellar tendon may rupture.

Management

1. Arthroscopic meniscectomy
   Removal of cartilage fragments through operating arthroscope inserted through a small incision into the knee joint.
2. Open meniscectomy
   Direct surgical approach to knee joint structures for repair of disrupted structures.
3. Ligament injuries
   Treated with immobilization (i.e., elastic bandage, splint, cast) or suturing of ligament, depending on severity of injury.
4. Rupture of tendon
   Must be sutured and immobilized during healing.

Patient Education

1. Elevate leg to minimize swelling.
2. Quadricep setting exercises and straight leg raising
3. Weight-bearing and exercise program as prescribed

Fractures

A *fracture* is a break in the continuity of bone. A fracture occurs when the stress placed on a bone is greater than the bone can absorb. Muscles, blood vessels, nerves, tendons, joints, and other organs may be injured when fracture occurs.

Types of Fractures

1. *Complete*—involves the entire cross section on the bone, usually displaced (not normal position)
2. *Incomplete*—involves a portion of the cross section of the bone or may be longitudinal
3. *Closed (simple)*—skin (mucous membranes) not broken
4. *Open (compound)*—skin broken, leading directly to fracture
   Grade I—minimal soft tissue injury
   Grade II—laceration greater than 1 cm. without extensive soft tissue flaps
   Grade III—extensive soft tissue injury, including skin, muscle, neurovascular structure, with crushing
5. *Pathological*—through an area of diseased bone (osteoporosis, bone cyst, bone tumor, bony metastasis)

Patterns of Fracture (Fig. 30-2)

1. *Greenstick*—one side of a bone is broken and the other side is bent

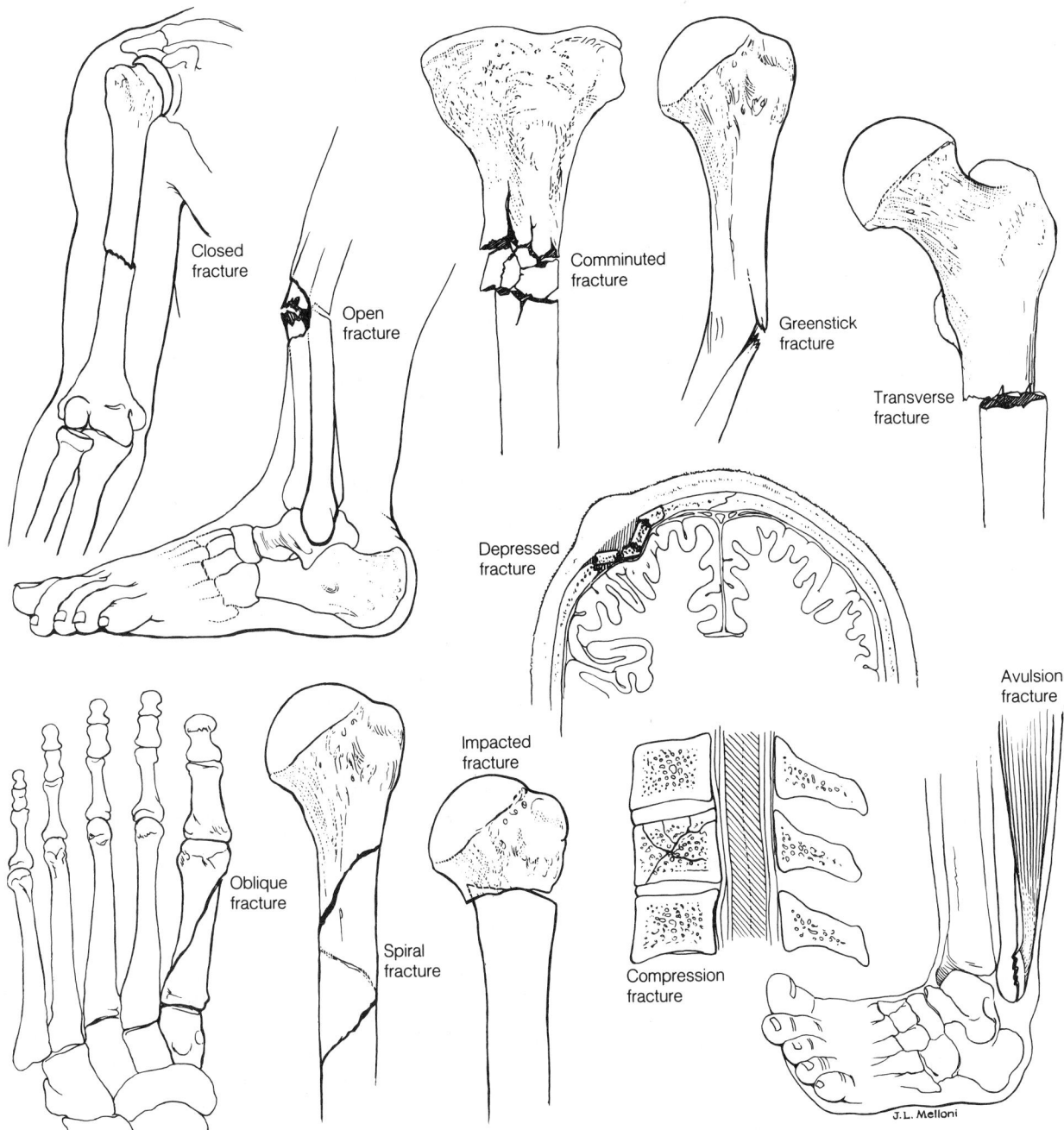

Figure 30-2. Patterns of fractures.

2. *Transverse*—straight across the bone
3. *Oblique*—at an angle across the bone
4. *Spiral*—twists around the shaft of the bone
5. *Comminuted*—bone splintered into several fragments
6. *Depressed*—fragment(s) indriven (seen in fractures of the skull and facial bones)

7. *Compression*—bone collapses in on itself (seen in vertebral fractures)
8. *Avulsion*—fragment of bone pulled off by ligament or tendon attachment
9. *Impacted*—fragment of bone wedged into other bone fragment

10. *Fracture–dislocation*—fracture complicated by the bone being out of the joint
11. *Other*—described according to anatomic location: epiphyseal, supracondylar, mid-shaft, intra-articular, etc.

Clinical Manifestations

A. Physical Findings

1. Pain at site of injury
2. Swelling
3. Tenderness
4. False motion and crepitus (grating sensation)
5. Deformity
6. Loss of function
7. Ecchymosis
8. Paresthesia

B. Altered Neurovascular Status

1. Injured muscle, blood vessels, nerves
2. Compression of structures resulting in ischemia
3. Findings
   a. Progressive uncontrollable pain
   b. Pain on passive movement
   c. Altered sensations (paresthesia)
   d. Loss of active motion
   e. Diminished capillary refill response
   f. Pallor

C. Shock

1. Bone is very vascular.
2. Overt hemorrhage through open wound
3. Covert hemorrhage into soft tissues (especially with femoral fracture) or body cavity, as with pelvic fracture
4. May be fatal if not detected

Diagnostic Evaluation

1. X-ray and other imaging studies to determine integrity of bone
2. Blood studies (CBC, electrolytes) with blood loss and extensive muscle damage
3. Arthroscopy with joint involvement
4. Angiography with blood vessel injury
5. Nerve conduction and electromyogram studies with nerve injury
6. Differential diagnostic studies with pathological fracture

Management

(Emergency management—see p. 946.)

A. Factors Influencing Choice of Fracture Management Approach

1. Type, location, and severity of fracture
2. Soft tissue damage
3. Age and health status of patient, including type and extent of other injuries

B. Goals

1. To regain and maintain correct position and alignment
2. To regain the function of the involved part
3. To return the patient to usual activities in the shortest time and at the least expense

C. Process

1. *Reduction*—setting the bone; refers to restoration of the fracture fragments into anatomic position and alignment

2. *Immobilization*—maintains reduction until bone healing occurs
3. *Rehabilitation*—regaining normal function of the affected part

Approaches

A. Closed Reduction

1. Bony fragments are brought into *apposition* (ends in contact) by manipulation and manual traction—restores alignment
2. May be done under anesthesia for pain relief and muscle relaxation
3. Cast or splint applied to immobilize extremity and maintain reduction (see Casts, p. 778)

B. Traction

1. Pulling force applied to accomplish and maintain reduction and alignment (see Traction, p. 784)
2. Used for fractures of long bones
3. Techniques
   a. *Skin traction*—force applied to the skin using foam rubber, tapes, etc.
   b. *Skeletal traction*—force applied to the bony skeleton directly, using wires, pins, or tongs placed into or through the bone

C. Open Reduction With Internal Fixation

1. Operative intervention to achieve reduction, alignment, and stabilization (see Orthopedic Surgery, Special Nursing Considerations, p. 794).
   a. Bone fragments are directly visualized.
   b. Internal fixation devices (metal pins, wires, screws, plates, nails, rods) used to hold bone fragments in position until solid bone healing occurs (may be removed when bone is healed).
   c. After closure of the wound, splints or casts may be used for additional stabilization and support.

D. Endoprosthetic Replacement

1. Replacement of a fracture fragment with an implanted metal device
2. Used when fracture disrupts nutrition of the bone or treatment of choice is bony replacement.

E. External Fixation Device

1. Stabilization of complex and open fracture with use of a metal frame and pin system
2. Permits active treatment of injured soft tissue.
   a. Wound may be left open (delayed primary wound closure).
   b. Repair of damage to blood vessels, soft tissue, muscles, nerves, and tendons as indicated.
   c. Reconstructive surgery may be necessary. (See External Fixation, p. 788)

Complications

A. Complications Associated With Immobility

1. Muscle atrophy
2. Loss of muscle strength and endurance
3. Loss of range of motion—joint contracture
4. Pressure sores at bony prominences or from immobilizing device pressing on skin
5. Diminished respiratory, cardiovascular, gastrointestinal function, resulting in possible pooling of respiratory secretions, orthostatic hypotension, anorexia, constipation

6. Altered interpersonal interactions, resulting in depression, altered emotions, and behavior

B. **Venous Stasis and Thromboembolism**—particularly with fractures of the hip and lower extremities

C. **Neurovascular Compromise**

D. **Infection**—especially with open fractures

E. **Shock**

F. **Pulmonary Emboli**

G. **Fat Emboli Syndrome**

1. Associated with embolization of marrow or tissue fat or platelets and free fatty acids to the pulmonary capillaries producing rapid onset of symptoms
2. *Clinical manifestations*
   a. *Respiratory distress*—tachypnea, hypoxemia, crackles, wheezes, acute pulmonary edema, interstitial pneumonitis
   b. *Mental disturbances*—irritability, restlessness, confusion, disorientation, stupor, coma due to systemic embolization, and severe hypoxia
   c. *Fever*
   d. *Petechiae* in buccal membranes, hard palate, conjunctival sacs, chest, anterior axillary folds due to occlusion of capillaries

NURSING ALERT: Restlessness, confusion, irritability, and disorientation may be the first signs of fat embolism syndrome. Confirm hypoxia with arterial blood gas analysis. Young adults (20–30 years old) and older adults (60–70 years old) with multiple fractures, fractures of long bones, and pelvis are particularly susceptible to development of fat emboli.

H. **Bone Union Problems**

1. *Delayed union* (takes longer to heal than average for type of fracture)
2. *Nonunion* (fractured bone fails to unite)
3. *Malunion* (union occurs but is faulty—misaligned)

Nursing Process Overview: The Patient With a Fracture

Assessment

1. Ask patient how the fracture occurred—mechanism of injury important in determining possible associated injuries.
2. Ask patient to describe location, character, and intensity of pain to help determine possible source of discomfort.
3. Ask patient to describe sensations in injured extremity—to aid in evaluation of neurovascular status.
4. Observe patient's ability to change position—to assess functional mobility.
5. Note patient's emotional status and behavior—indicators of ability to cope with stress of injury.

NURSING ALERT: Change in behavior and/or cerebral functioning may be an early indicator of cerebral anoxia from diminished cardiovascular function or pulmonary or fat emboli.

6. Assess patient's support system; identify present and potential sources of assistance/caregiving.
7. Review findings on past and present health status—to aid in formulating plan of care.
8. Conduct physical examination.
   a. Examine skin for lacerations, abrasions, ecchymosis; note areas of swelling and edema.
   b. Ascultate lungs to establish baseline assessment of respiratory function.
   c. Assess pulses and blood pressure; assess peripheral tissue perfusion, especially in injured extremity, to establish circulatory status baseline.
   d. Determine neurological status (sensations and movement) of extremity distal to injury.
   e. Note length, alignment, and immobilization of injured extremity.
   f. Evaluate behavior and cognitive functioning of patient to determine ability to participate in care planning and patient education activities.

GERONTOLOGIC ALERT: Assessment of patient's health, functional abilities prior to fracture, and available support system facilitate development of realistic rehabilitation and discharge goals.

Nursing Diagnoses

1. Altered tissue perfusion related to swelling, disrupted circulation, blood loss, compartment syndrome, thrombus formation, pulmonary emboli, fat emboli, orthostatic hypotension, impaired gas exchange
2. Potential impaired skin integrity related to trauma, surgery, pressure from immobility or immobilizing device
3. Potential for infection related to bacterial invasion of open fracture, surgical incision, pressure sore formation
4. Potential for injury: disruption of healing related to inadequate immobilization, disrupted circulation, infection, poor nutrition
5. Potential urinary retention related to unnatural voiding positions, anesthesia, pain, medications
6. Pain related to fracture, soft tissue damage, swelling, muscle spasms, nature of management approach
7. Self-care deficit related to fracture, soft tissue trauma, treatment modality (immobilization)
8. Altered physical mobility related to fracture, soft tissue trauma, treatment modality, muscle atrophy, joint contracture
9. Potential for disuse syndrome related to immobilizing device, reduced level of activity, immobility-induced bone demineralization
10. Altered post-trauma response related to situational and personal coping variables
11. Knowledge deficit of restorative regimen, self-care, and home care management approaches

Monitoring for Potential Complications

A. Evaluating for Hemorrhage and Shock

1. Monitor vital signs as frequently as clinical condition indicates, observing for hypotension, elevated pulse, cold clammy skin, restlessness, pallor.
2. Watch for evidence of hemorrhage on dressings or in drainage containers.
3. Review laboratory data; report abnormal values.

4. Administer prescribed fluids/blood to maintain circulating volume.

B. Monitoring for Impaired Gas Exchange

1. Evaluate changes in mental status and restlessness.
2. Review diagnostic evaluation data—especially arterial blood gas values and chest x-ray.
3. Position to enhance respiratory effort.
4. Encourage coughing and deep breathing to promote lung expansion and diminish pooling of pulmonary secretions.
5. Administer oxygen as prescribed.
6. See Management of Respiratory Insufficiency and Failure, page 208.

C. Promoting Tissue Perfusion

1. Monitor neurovascular status for compression of nerve, diminished circulation, development of compartment syndrome.
   a. *Pain*—progressive, localized, deep throbbing, persistent, unrelieved by immobilization and medications
   b. *Pain*—on passive stretch
   c. *Weakness* progressing to paralysis
   d. *Altered sensation,* hypothesis, anesthesia
   e. *Poor capillary refill response*
   f. *Skin color*—pale; cyanotic
   g. *Elevated compartment pressure*—palpable tightness of muscle compartment; elevated measured tissue pressure
   h. *Pulselessness*

> **NURSING ALERT:** Monitoring the neurovascular integrity of the injured extremity is essential. Development of *compartment syndrome* (increased tissue pressure causing anoxia)—leads to permanent loss of function in 6–8 hours. This situation must be identified and managed promptly.

   i. Review arteriogram and venogram results if procedures are done.
2. Reduce swelling.
   a. Elevate injured extremity.
   b. Apply cold to injury if prescribed.
3. Relieve pressure caused by immobilizing device as prescribed (such as bivalving cast, rewrapping elastic bandage, or splinting device).
4. Relieve pressure on skin to prevent development of pressure sore.
   a. Frequent repositioning
   b. Skin care
   c. Special mattresses

D. Preventing Development of Thromboembolism

> **GERONTOLOGY ALERT:** Older adults with fractures, trauma, immobility, obesity, or prior history of thrombophlebitis are at high risk for developing thromboembolism.

1. Encourage active and passive ankle exercises.
2. Use elastic stockings and sequential compression devices as prescribed.
3. Elevate legs to prevent stasis, avoiding pressure on blood vessels.
4. Encourage mobility; change position frequently; encourage ambulation.
5. Administer anticoagulants as prescribed.

6. Monitor for development of thrombophlebitis.
   a. Note complaint of pain and tenderness in calf.
   b. Report positive Homan's sign (p. 395).
   c. Report increased size and temperature of calf.

E. Monitoring for Development of Infection

1. Cleanse, debride, and irrigate open fracture wound as prescribed as soon as possible, to minimize chance of infection.
   a. Open fractures are contaminated.
   b. Begin prescribed antibiotic therapy promptly after wound culture obtained.
2. Use sterile technique during dressing changes to minimize infection of wound, soft tissues, and bone.
3. Evaluate patient for elevation of temperature at regular intervals.
4. Note elevated white blood counts.
5. Report areas of inflammation and swelling around incision or open wound.
6. Report purulent drainage.
7. Obtain specimens for culture and sensitivity to determine causative organism.
8. Administer antibiotic therapy as prescribed.

F. Monitoring Bone Healing

1. Review serial x-ray reports, noting callus formation and fracture healing.
2. Support patient during prolonged treatment periods.
3. Explain possible contributing factors to delayed union or nonunion.
   a. Inadequate immobilization
   b. Tissue interposed between bone fragments
   c. Infection
   d. Excessive distraction (too much space between bone fragments)
   e. Altered blood supply (avascular necrosis)
   f. Altered bone metabolism
4. Encourage adequate balanced diet to promote tissue healing.

G. Monitoring Urinary Retention

1. Assess urinary output.
2. Examine abdomen for evidence of bladder distention.
3. Encourage fluid intake.
4. Provide assistance in positioning to promote comfort.
5. Encourage out-of-bed toileting as soon as mobility restrictions permit, for more natural voiding posture.
6. Provide privacy during toileting.
7. If catheter is used, provide catheter care and use strict sterile technique during catheterization.

Nursing Interventions

A. Relieving Pain and Discomfort

1. See Nursing Interventions, Relieving Pain, page 763.
2. Immobilize bone fragments—movement of fragments causes pain.
3. Support splinted fracture above and below fracture when repositioning or moving the patient.
4. Reposition patient with slow and steady motion; use additional personnel as needed.

B. Promoting Self-Care Activities Within the Limits of Fracture Treatment

1. Encourage participation in care.
2. Arrange patient area and personal items for patient convenience to promote independence.
3. Modify activities to facilitate maximum independence.
4. Allow time for patient to accomplish task.
5. Teach safe use of mobility and other aids.

6. Assist with activities of daily living as needed.
7. Teach family how to assist patient while promoting independence in self-care.

C. Promoting Physical Mobility

1. Perform active and passive exercises to all nonimmobilized joints
2. Encourage patient participation in frequent position changes, maintaining supports to fracture during position changes.
3. Minimize prolonged periods of physical inactivity, encouraging ambulation when prescribed.
4. Administer prescribed analgesics judiciously to decrease pain associated with movement.

D. Preventing Development of Disuse Syndrome

1. Teach and encourage isometric exercises to diminish muscle atrophy
2. Encourage use of immobilized extremity within prescribed limits.

E. Promoting Positive Psychological Response to Trauma

1. Monitor patient for symptoms of post-trauma stress disorder
      Memory of event; anger, helplessness, vulnerability, mood swings, depression, cognitive impairment; sleep disturbance, increased dependency, social withdrawal
2. Assist patient to move through phases of post-traumatic stress (outcry; denial; intrusiveness; working through; completion).
3. Establish trusting therapeutic relationship with patient.
4. Encourage patient to express thoughts and feelings about traumatic event.
5. Encourage patient to participate in decision-making to reestablish control and overcome feelings of helplessness.
6. Teach relaxation techniques to decrease anxiety.
7. Encourage development of adaptive responses and participation in support groups.
8. Refer patient to psychiatric liaison nurse or refer for psychotherapy as needed.

Patient Education/Discharge Planning

1. Explain basis for fracture treatment and need for patient participation in therapeutic regimen.
2. Promote adjustment of usual life-style and responsibilities to accommodate limitations imposed by fracture.
3. Instruct the patient to actively exercise joints above and below the immobilized fracture at frequent intervals.
      a. Isometric exercises of muscles covered by cast—start exercise as soon as possible after cast application.
      b. Increase isometric exercises as fracture stabilizes.
4. After removal of immobilizing device (e.g., cast, splint), have the patient start active exercises and continue with isometric exercises.
5. Instruct the patient on exercises to strengthen upper extremity muscles if crutch walking is planned.
6. Instruct the patient in methods of safe ambulation—walker, crutches, cane.
7. Emphasize instructions concerning amount of weight bearing that will be permitted on fractured extremity.
8. Discuss prevention of recurrent fractures—safety considerations; avoidance of fatigue; proper footwear.
9. Discharge teaching—follow-up medical supervision; symptoms needing attention (e.g., numbness, decreased function, increased pain, elevated temperature); medication teaching

Evaluation

1. Achieves adequate tissue perfusion—reports absence of swelling, excessive blood loss, development of compartment syndrome, thrombophlebitis, pulmonary or fat emboli, orthostatic hypotension
2. Maintains normal sensation and use of extremity distal to injury
      a. Sensations normal
      b. Color normal
      c. Capillary refill normal
      d. Swelling minimal
      e. Movement normal
3. Achieves healing of traumatized skin—experiences no skin breakdown from immobilizing devices or from immobility
4. Is free of infection
      a. Demonstrates wound healing
      b. No signs of inflammation or evidence of purulent wound drainage
      c. Maintains vital signs within normal limits
5. Achieves bone union within normal length of time for type and location of fracture
      a. X-rays demonstrate callus formation and evidence of healing
      b. No motion at healed fracture site
      c. No pain at fracture site on weight-bearing
6. Achieves normal pattern of voiding—empties bladder
7. Is free of pain
8. Achieves self-care within limits of therapeutic regimen
      a. Participates in self-care and activities of daily living
      b. Uses assistive devices safely
9. Regains pre-fracture level of physical mobility
10. Demonstrates minimal disuse syndrome
      a. Minimal muscle atrophy
      b. Restores pre-fracture muscle strength
      c. Achieves pre-fracture range of motion
11. Demonstrates psychological adjustment to impact of trauma
      a. Participates in therapeutic-rehabilitation program
      b. Maintains interpersonal relationships
      c. Participates in support groups and uses psychological therapy as needed
12. Demonstrates compliance with restorative regimen
      a. Participates in self-care activities
      b. Maintains prescribed immobilization
      c. Exercises as directed
      d. Takes medications as prescribed
      e. Keeps follow-up appointments with health care providers

---

Fractures of Specific Sites*
Fractures of the Upper Extremity

Fracture of the Clavicle (Collar Bone)

A. Function of Clavicle

The clavicle helps to hold the shoulder upward, outward, and backward from the thorax.

* For fracture of the skull see page 581; fracture of the cervical spine, page 616; and rib fracture, page 194.

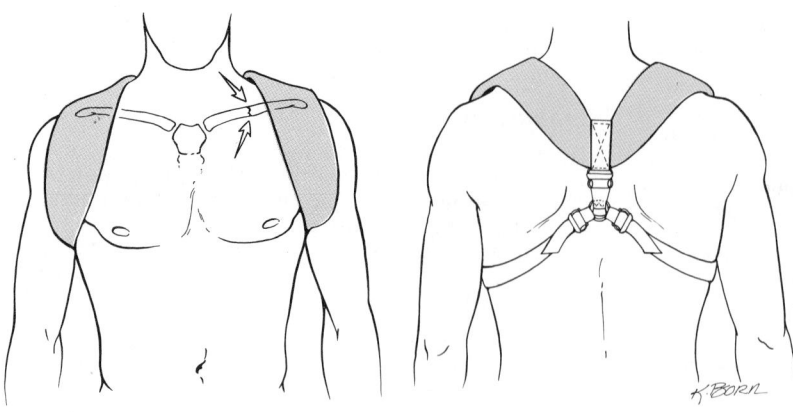

Figure 30-3. *Method for immobilizing a clavicular fracture with a clavicular strap.*

B. Management

1. Most fractures of the clavicle are treated by closed reduction and immobilization with a clavicular strap, figure 8 bandage, or sling (Fig. 30-3).
   a. Pad axilla to prevent nerve damage from pressure of the immobilizer.
   b. Assess the neurovascular status of the upper extremities.
2. Open reduction and internal fixation may be done for marked displacement, severely comminuted fracture, and extensive soft tissue injury.
   a. Patient's arm is kept in a sling.
   b. Assess the neurovascular status of the involved upper extremity.

C. Patient Education

1. Exercise elbow, wrist, and fingers as soon as possible.
2. Do shoulder exercises to obtain full shoulder motion as prescribed.

Fractures of the Surgical Neck of the Humerus
(Fractures of the Proximal Humerus)

A. Mechanism of Fracture

Most occur from falls in which the outstretched arm strikes the ground. Osteoporosis is a predisposing factor.

B. Management

1. Many impacted fractures of the surgical neck of the humerus do not require reduction. The weight of the arm helps to correct displacement.
   a. Place a soft pad under the axilla to prevent skin maceration.
   b. The arm is supported by a sling and swathe or Velpeau bandage for comfort (Fig. 30-4).
   c. Suggest sleeping in a semi-Fowler's position.
2. Displaced fractures are treated with reduction under x-ray control, open reduction, or replacement of humeral head with prosthesis.
3. A program of exercises is started after a specified period of immobilization, with emphasis on range of motion of the shoulder.

C. Patient Education

1. Start active motion of shoulder joint early—to prevent limitation of motion and stiffness of shoulder.
2. Instruct the patient to lean forward and allow affected arm to abduct and rotate.

Fractures of the Shaft of the Humerus

A. Mechanism of Fracture

1. Fractures of the shaft of the humerus are most frequently caused by direct violence—falls, blow to arm, auto injuries.
2. The radial nerve may be injured in this fracture because it lies immediately adjacent to the midportion of the humerus in the musculoskeletal groove.

B. Management

1. Sling and swathe, splints, or hanging casts may be used to immobilize the fracture.
2. Hanging cast is frequently applied to oblique, spiral, and displaced fractures with shortening of humeral shaft—the weight of the cast helps to correct displacement.

NURSING ALERT: A hanging cast must remain unsupported to provide traction force on the long axis of the arm. The patient must avoid supporting the elbow in the lap while seated.

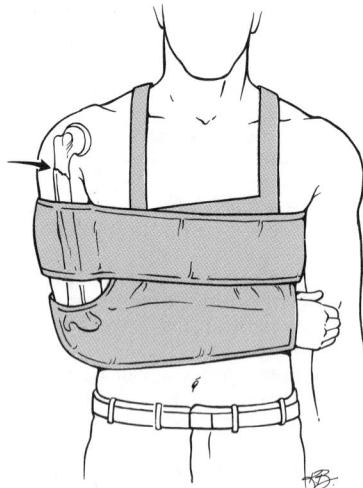

Figure 30-4. *Immobilization of fracture of upper humerus can be achieved with conventional sling and swathe.*

3. The patient sleeps in a fairly upright position to maintain uninterrupted 24-hour traction.
4. Exercise fingers immediately after the application of the cast.
5. Start pendulum exercises as directed—provides active exercise of shoulder to prevent adhesions of the shoulder joint capsule after cast removal.
6. Surgical reduction and internal fixation is used with associated vascular injury or pathological fracture. The arm is placed in a sling until the bone unites.

Fractures About the Elbow and Forearm

A. Mechanism of Fracture

Fractures about the elbow and forearm usually occur as the result of a fall on the elbow, on the outstretched hand, or from a direct blow (sideswipe injury).

B. Management

1. Options
   a. Nonoperative (cast immobilization)
   b. Operative (open reduction and internal fixation; arthroplasty)
   c. External fixation
   d. Treatment depends on the specific characteristics of the fracture.
2. Elbow is immobilized in flexion to prevent extension contracture.
3. A closed drainage system may be used to decrease possibility of hematoma and associated swelling.

C. Nursing Interventions

1. Watch for signs of neurovascular impairment of the forearm and hand.
   a. Observe hand for swelling, skin color (blueness or blanching of nailbeds), and temperature, comparing it with the unaffected hand.
   b. Evaluate radial pulse; if it weakens or disappears, call orthopedic surgeon *immediately,* as irreversible ischemia may develop.
   c. Assess for paresthesia (pricking and burning sensations) in the hand, inability to move fingers, pain on passive movement of fingers—indicate nerve injury or impending ischemia.
2. Elevate arm to control edema.
3. Encourage the patient to move his fingers and shoulder frequently.
4. Encourage prescribed exercises to increase range of motion.

Fracture of the Wrist

A. Mechanism of Fracture

1. *Colles' fracture* is a fracture of the radius 1.2–2.5 cm. (½–1 inch) above the wrist with dorsal displacement of the lower fragment.
2. This fracture is frequently seen in patients with osteoporosis.

B. Management

Usually consists of closed reduction with splint or cast support or percutaneous pins and external fixator or plaster cast.

C. Nursing Interventions

1. Elevate arm above level of heart for 48 hours after reduction.
2. Watch for swelling of fingers—indicates decreased venous and lymphatic return. Check for constricting bandages or cast.

D. Patient Education

Instruct the patient to do finger exercises to reduce swelling and prevent stiffness.
1. Hold hand above level of heart.
2. Move fingers from full extension to flexion (fist position). Hold and release.
3. Repeat at least 10 times every half hour when awake—as long as hand has a tendency to swell.
4. Encourage the patient to continue *daily* program of repetitive, progressive exercises (as prescribed). The exercise program is designed to restore full extension and supination.

Fractures of the Hand

1. Numerous injuries to the hand require extensive reconstructive surgery, which is beyond the scope of this book. The reader is referred to specialized texts on the hand.
2. Objective of treatment is to regain maximum function of the hand.
3. *Undisplaced fracture of the distal phalanx* (finger) Splinted (to adjoining finger or by a dorsal or volar splint)—to relieve pain and to protect finger tip from further trauma.
4. *Open fractures* may be handled by Kirschner wire fixation following debridement and irrigation.

Fractures of the Hip *(Proximal Femur)*

Hip (proximal femur) fractures frequently occur in older adults and contribute to their mortality. Occur more frequently in women, often after insignificant injuries, and are associated with osteoporosis.

Types of Hip Fractures

1. *Intracapsular fracture*—fracture of femoral neck occurring within the joint capsule
2. *Extracapsular fracture*—femoral neck fracture occurring outside the joint. Also called *intertrochanteric* (between the greater and lesser trochanter); femoral fracture occurs outside the joint.
3. *Subtrochanteric* femoral fracture occurs at or just below the level of the lesser trochanter.

Clinical Manifestations

1. Shortening and external rotation of the affected leg.
2. Pain in hip or in the knee.
3. Patient usually unable to move leg, but is able to wiggle toes.
4. Mental confusion may be present in the older adult due to underlying systemic illness, cardiopulmonary disease with inadequate cerebral oxygenation, stroke, etc.

Management

1. Surgical repair is accomplished as soon as medical stability is established. Prolonged bedrest is detrimental to the elderly.
2. The leg may be immobilized by Buck's extension traction until surgery.
3. Options
   a. Internal fixation (nail, nail–plate combination, multiple pins, screw, sliding nails)

b. Femoral prosthetic replacement
c. Total hip replacement (both femoral and acetabular components)
d. Choice depends on the location and character of the fractured proximal femur and multiple patient factors (age, health status, bone stock, mobility, etc.).

Complications

1. Pneumonia
2. Thrombophlebitis
3. Fat emboli
4. Dislocation of prosthesis
5. Infection
6. Pressure sores

Nursing Interventions

A. Preventing Complications Associated With Surgery and Immobility

1. Use anticipatory nursing techniques to avoid complications.
2. **Thrombophlebitis/Thromboembolism**
   a. Use antiembolism stockings as prescribed.
   b. Institute hourly ankle exercises.
   c. Promote venous drainage. Avoid positioning that contributes to venous stasis.
   d. Ensure adequate hydration.
   e. Early ambulation as prescribed.
   f. Prescribed warfarin, aspirin, or low doses of heparin given subcutaneously may be effective in reducing the incidence of venous thrombi.
3. Monitor neurovascular status of the leg.
4. Provide special skin care.
   a. Prepare bed with trapeze and special skin care mattress.
   b. Keep skin dry.
   c. Relieve pressure areas.
   d. Inspect the heel *daily*—a patient with a painful hip tends to let weight of leg press the heel against the bed; area loses sensation when blood supply diminishes and nerve endings necrose.
   e. Support leg with pillow if permitted—distributes pressure more evenly.
   f. Place a sheepskin pad under the leg.
5. Encourage the patient to move by herself as much as possible to decrease the likelihood of complications (thromboembolism, diminished cerebral perfusion, aspiration of secretions and pneumonia, gastrointestinal stasis, urinary problems, increase in bone mineral loss, pressure sores).
6. Use orienting activities to prevent confusion—clock, calendar, television, explanations and reassurance, same care-giver.
7. Prevent urinary tract infection.
   a. Avoid the routine use of an indwelling catheter—infection almost always follows the use of an indwelling catheter. (A urinary tract infection can cause a prolonged period of morbidity, incontinence, and confusion in the elderly.)
   b. Watch the color, odor, and volume of urinary output.
   c. Maintain a liberal fluid intake (within limits of cardiorenal function).

B. Promoting Comfort

1. Place a pillow between the legs—to keep affected leg in abduction.

2. With two nurses positioned on each side of the bed, use the draw sheet to lift and reposition the patient in bed.
3. Position the patient supine, placing a pillow under the affected leg from mid-thigh to ankle, keeping the leg in a neutral rotation.
4. Handle the affected extremity gently.
5. Give analgesics as the patient's condition indicates.

Patient Education

1. Teach the patient to assist with turning by having her grasp the trapeze or bedrails.
2. Encourage the patient to take deep breaths while turning.
3. Teach the use of incentive spirometer, coughing, deep-breathing, and exercises, especially quadriceps setting.
4. Clarify treatment plans and discuss the patient's participation.

Fractures of the Lower Extremity

Fracture of the Shaft of the Femur

A. Mechanism of Fracture

1. Fracture of the shaft of the femur may be accompanied by marked concealed blood loss.
2. Fractures of the femoral shaft occur most frequently in young and middle-aged adults.

B. Management

1. Closed reduction
   a. Fracture reduced and stabilized by means of balanced skeletal traction, such as Thomas leg splint with a Pearson attachment (see Fig. 30-9) may be treatment of choice.
   b. Skeletal traction in long axis of thigh is applied by means of a Kirschner wire or Steinman pin.
   c. Thomas splint suspends the thigh; Pearson attachment applied to the splint allows knee flexion and supports the leg below the knee.

> **NURSING ALERT:** Examine the skin under the ring of the Thomas splint for signs of pressure.

   d. After a period of traction, immobilization may be achieved by orthosis (cast–brace) (Fig. 30-5), which allows weight-bearing to enhance healing.
2. Open reduction
   a. With pins, plates, screws, and intramedullary (within the bone) rods.
   b. Bone grafting may be needed to fill bone gap or stimulate healing.
3. External fixator may be used.

C. Nursing Interventions

See nursing interventions under specific management modalities.

Fractures at the Knee

A. Mechanism of Fractures

1. Fractures at the knee may involve the distal shaft of femur (supracondylar fracture), the articular surfaces (femoral condyles and/or tibial plateau fracture), or the patella.
2. Joint and ligamentous injury occur with the fractures.

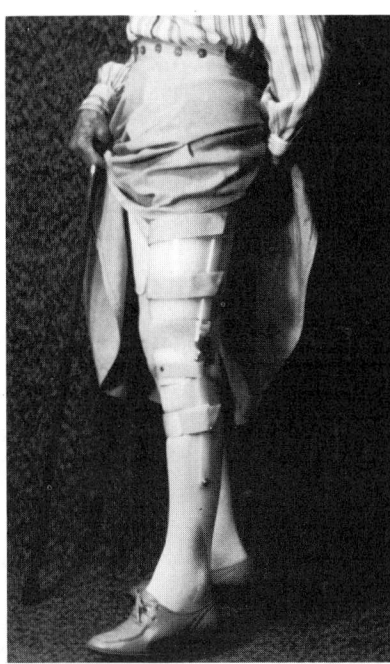

Figure 30-5. *Cast–brace provides circumferential support and immobilization to a fracture while allowing mobility of adjacent joints. The molded plastic cast–brace orthosis is removable for skin care. (Brunner LS and Suddarth DS. Textbook of Medical–Surgical Nursing. 6th ed. Philadelphia, JB Lippincott, 1988)*

B. Management

1. Management may include traction, internal fixation, and/or immobilization.
2. Knee mobility is a concern in the overall treatment of these fractures.

C. Nursing Interventions

1. Elevate extremity; raise the gatch of the foot of the bed.
2. Evaluate for effusion of the knee—produces marked pain.
   a. Cut pressure dressing and reapply if pain is severe. Report to physician.
   b. Support the patient undergoing aspiration of fluid from knee joint.
3. Encourage quadriceps exercise to prevent atrophy of the thigh muscles.
4. Progressive exercises (straight leg raising, progressive resistive exercises) usually follow.
5. Weight-bearing is according to prescription. (Generally, full weight-bearing is not advised until 3–4 months postinjury.)

Fractures of the Tibia and Fibula

A. Mechanism of Fracture

1. There is a high incidence of open infected fractures, as the tibia lies superficially beneath the skin.
2. These fractures may require prolonged immobilization, as union is slow. (Generally the tibia heals in 12–16 weeks; however, open and comminuted fractures take longer.)

B. Management

1. Treatment approach depends on the specific characteristic of the fracture.
2. Closed fractures
   a. May be managed by simple manipulation and the reduction maintained by application of plaster cast (toe to groin).
   b. In time, the long leg cast may be replaced with a short leg cast or brace orthosis, which allows knee joint motion and weight-bearing as prescribed.
3. Fracture may be treated by open reduction and fixation (plate, compression plate, intermedullary nails).
4. External fixator may be used with open fracture.

C. Nursing Interventions

1. Elevate lower extremity to control edema.
2. Assess neurovascular status of involved extremity.
3. Prepare the patient to anticipate a temporary stiff ankle joint following immobilization.

Fractures of the Ankle

A. Mechanism of Fracture

1. Fracture may occur in the distal tibia and/or fibula, medial or lateral malleoli, or superior talus, and include avulsion fracture.
2. The fracture is generally the result of forceful twisting of the ankle and is associated with ligament disruption.

B. Management

1. Treatment includes immobilization with cast or splint and possible open reduction and internal fixation to reestablish the joint.

C. Nursing Interventions

1. Elevate lower extremity to control edema.
2. Teach patient about weight-bearing according to prescription.

Fractures of the Foot

1. Fractures of the metatarsals and phalanges result from crush injuries of the foot.
2. Generally treated by immobilization with cast, splint, or strapping.
3. Partial weight-bearing is generally allowed.
4. Teach patient to elevate foot to control edema.

Rehabilitation and Patient Education After Fracture of Lower Extremity

A. During Immobilization

1. Apply elastic stockings to uninvolved leg to prevent stasis of blood, development of edema, and thrombophlebitis.
2. Avoid placing extremity in dependent positions for prolonged periods.
3. Elevate affected extremity to promote venous return and relieve pain.
   a. The early reestablishment of venous return helps absorb blood and tissue fluid (edema from bleeding is a common cause of disability following fractures).
   b. Chronic edema predisposes extremity to fibrosis and ulceration.
   c. *It is desirable for the patient to lie down when elevating a leg cast.*
4. Exercise regularly all joints that do not move the bone fragments.

5. Mobilize the patient as soon as possible, permitting weight-bearing as prescribed. Instruct regarding safe use of ambulatory/mobility aids (crutches, walker, cane, wheelchair).

B. After Immobilization Device Is Removed

1. Physical therapy procedures may be used (heat, cold, massage, exercise)—to restore joint mobility, increase muscle strength and endurance.
2. Instruct the patient to wear elastic stockings to support venous circulation and to reduce edema.
3. Advise the patient to move feet up and down (unless immobilized) in a pumping motion to exercise the calf muscles.
4. Recommend exercise in warm water, which supports the leg and relaxes muscles.
5. Encourage adherence to weight-bearing prescription limits.

Fractures of the Spine
(Thoracic and Lumbar)

(Fractures of the cervical spine are discussed on p. 616)

Mechanism of Fracture

1. May involve the vertebral body, lamina and articulating processes, and spinous or transverse processes.
2. Fracture is due to trauma sustained in falls or accidents (automobile, diving) or excessive loading (beyond physiologic limits).
3. Most fractures of the spine are stable compression fractures without neurological deficit.
4. Spinal cord or spinal nerve injury may occur with unstable fractures, displacement, or multiple bone fragments.
5. Compression fractures are most common and may involve several vertebrae.

GERONTOLOGIC ALERT: Osteoporosis is the most common cause of compression fractures, resulting in thoracic and lumbar discomfort and deformity.

Clinical Manifestations

1. Pain
   a. Present at the level of injury is related to both the fracture and muscle spasm. The area is tender to touch.
   b. The pain is worse with movement and coughing and may radiate to extremities, abdomen, or intercostal muscles.
2. Potential neurological deficits
   a. Includes paresthesia, radiating pain, paresis, paralysis, altered reflexes, paralytic ileus, bladder distention associated with spinal cord or nerve injury/compression
   b. The level of injury is reflected in the presenting neurological deficits.
3. Deformity of spine
4. Altered ability to preform activities of daily living

Diagnostic Evaluation

1. Physical examination
2. Diagnostic imaging, including x-rays, tomograms (CT scans), myelograms, and MRI.

Management

A. For Stable Fractures

1. Bedrest on a firm mattress until pain subsides
2. "Log roll" patient to change positions.

NURSING ALERT: Avoid twisting of spine or loading of spine, which occurs with sitting.

---

3. Symptomatic relief of pain
4. Progressive ambulation when pain subsides. Corset-type brace may be used when ambulating.
5. Exercise to increase or maintain the strength of back muscles (2–3 weeks after fracture).
   a. Exercises that strengthen spinal extensor muscles are prescribed.
   b. Exercises that encourage spinal flexion are contraindicated.

B. For Unstable Fractures/Displaced

1. The fracture may be reduced by postural positioning, protracted periods of immobilization, or open operation with internal fixation (Harrington rod).
2. The patient may then be placed in a body cast for immobilization.
3. Laminectomy with spinal fusion (see p. 621) when indicated.
4. "Log roll" patient to change position avoiding twisting or loading of spine.
5. Mobilize the patient when physical examinations and x-ray evaluations determine that there is no displacement or neurological deficit.

Complications

1. Potential spinal cord or nerve injury
2. Potential immobility-related complications
3. Nausea, vomiting, and constipation related to pain medications, paralytic ileus, and immobility

Nursing Interventions

A. Avoiding Spinal Cord Injury

1. Stabilize spine during diagnostic evaluation for fracture and displacement.
2. Monitor neurologic status (i.e., motion and sensations in extremities).
3. Provide nursing care according to the patient's condition and treatment regimen (e.g., laminectomy and fusion, internal fixation, casting).

B. Relieving Pain

1. Give analgesics and muscle relaxants as required, as pain may be severe.
2. Encourage the patient to roll from side to side; the patient should not sit up during acute stage.
3. Assist patient in application and removal of brace or back support if one is used.

C. Avoiding Complications Associated With Spinal Fracture and Immobility

1. Use measures to prevent risk of thromboembolic complications—apply elastic stockings, encourage active ankle motion, give anticoagulant therapy as prescribed for patient at high risk.
2. Monitor bowel and bladder function.
3. Assist the patient to ambulate (wearing shoes) when

discomfort subsides and when no neurologic deficits or vertebral displacement have been determined.
4. Encourage the patient to do the prescribed back exercises.

Discharge Planning/Patient Education

1. Teach body mechanics for back conservation.
2. Encourage weight reduction, if applicable.
3. Encourage compliance with prescribed exercise regimen.
4. Instruct patient in the use of analgesics and alternative pain management techniques.
5. Teach patient with osteoporosis to avoid falls.

Fractures of the Pelvis

Pelvic fractures include fractures of the sacrum, ilium, pubis, ischium, and coccyx.

Types of Pelvic Fractures

A. Stable Fractures—which do not involve the pelvic ring or result in minimal displacement (most common type)

B. Unstable Fractures
1. *Open book*
   a. Rotationally unstable
   b. Distraction occurs at the symphysis pubis.
2. *Lateral compression*—compression fractures at sacrum and symphysis pubis
3. *Vertical shear*
   a. Vertically unstable
   b. Sides of pelvis are displaced in opposite superior–inferior directions

Mechanism of Fracture

1. Auto accidents, crush injuries, and falls cause most pelvic fractures
2. Injury to internal organs (i.e., bladder, urethra, liver, spleen) and blood vessels (e.g., iliac arteries and veins) frequently accompany these fractures
3. Bleeding from bone fragments also occurs.

Clinical Manifestations

1. Pelvic fractures are frequently seen in patients with multiple trauma.
2. Shock from intraperitoneal hemorrhage
3. Pain with movement and tenderness over fracture site(s)—symphysis pubis, anterior iliac spines, iliac crest, sacrum, coccyx
4. Inability to bear weight because of pain
5. Back pain from fracture and/or sacroiliac joint disruption
6. Paralytic ileus

Diagnostic Evaluation

1. Evaluation for presence of shock (hypotension, tachycardia, tachypnea) due to intra-abdominal hemorrhage.
2. Physical examination
   a. Absence of peripheral pulses may indicate major vessel disruption (torn iliac artery).
   b. Determine rotational and vertical stability of pelvic ring.
3. Imaging of abdomen and pelvis (x-ray, CT scan, venogram, bone scan).

Possible Associated Injury

1. Neurological dysfunction—numbness, tingling, pain in spine, loss of function, and diminished rectal tone and perianal sensation
2. Genitourinary injury

NURSING ALERT
1. Do not attempt to insert an indwelling catheter until the status of the urethra is known.
2. Urethral injury is suspected in *male* patients with anterior fractured pelvis presenting with blood at the urethral meatus.
3. Voiding urethrogram should be done prior to attempting to pass catheter, to prevent further injury.
4. Female patients rarely have urethral lacerations.

---

3. Intra-abdominal injury
   Peritoneal lavage for intra-abdominal hemorrhage and perforation of bowel
4. Open perineal wounds

Management

A. Emergency Management of Hemorrhage and Shock
1. Pneumatic antishock garment allows compression of pelvic area—provides tamponade for bleeding and immobilizes fracture.
2. Angiographic visualization of pelvic vascular tree
   a. For localization of bleeding points
   b. Bleeding artery may be occluded by an injection of autologous clotted blood deposited proximal to bleeding vessel, by Gelfoam, or by balloon-tip catheter.
3. External skeletal frame or clamp to stabilize pelvic ring and reduce hemorrhage

B. Internal Organ Injury

Is determined and treated according to problem (e.g., ruptured bladder requires surgical intervention and repair.

C. Definitive Treatment—depends on the nature and characteristics of the fracture
1. *Stable fracture*
   a. Bedrest for several days
   b. Progressive weight-bearing as prescribed
2. *Unstable fracture*
   a. Bedrest
   b. External fixation
   c. Open reduction and internal fixation
   d. Skeletal traction
   e. Pelvic sling

Complications

1. Mortality is high because of intra-abdominal hemorrhage, infection, pulmonary complications, fat emboli, intravascular coagulation, thromboembolitic complications.
2. Complications associated with injured organs (gastrointestinal, genitourinary), pelvic vessels, peripheral nerves, and perineal wounds
3. Malunion and nonunion
4. Residual gait disturbances
5. Long-term discomfort (especially back pain) associated with ligament injury of displaced pelvic fracture.

Nursing Interventions

A. Promoting Adequate Tissue Perfusion
1. Monitor vital signs and level of consciousness.
2. Interpret laboratory data.
3. Support vital functions as needed and prescribed.

B. Ensuring Abdominal-Organ Functioning
1. Monitor urine output for blood.
2. Monitor bowel function.
3. Assist the patient with therapeutic regimen prescribed for management of injury.

C. Relieving Discomfort
See Pain related to musculoskeletal conditions, page 763.

D. Promoting Ambulation and Activities of Daily Living
1. Turn the patient as a unit.
2. Encourage exercises (e.g., leg, breathing, isometric) and activities to minimize development of immobility-related problems.
3. Assist the patient being treated with pelvic sling.
   a. Fold sling back over buttocks to enable the patient to use the bedpan.
   b. Reach under sling to give skin care—sheepskin may be used to line sling to prevent pressure sores.
   c. Loosen the sling only on physician request.
4. Assist the patient with gradual resumption of activity and ambulation.
   Mobilization and weight-bearing are determined by x-ray and the patient's reaction to mobility.

Discharge Planning/Patient Education
1. Instruct patient on care associated with external fixator.
2. Encourage gradual resumption of activities within rehabilitation regimen.
3. Assure safe use of ambulatory aids (walker, cane) as needed.

Casts

A *cast* is an immobilizing device made up of layers of plaster or "fiberglass" (water-activated polyurethane resin) bandages molded to the body part that it encases.

Purposes
1. To immobilize and hold bone fragments in reduction
2. To apply uniform compression of soft tissues

3. To permit early mobilization
4. To correct and prevent deformities
5. To support and stabilize weak joints

Types of Casts

A. **Short-arm Cast**—extends from below the elbow to the proximal palmar crease

B. **Gauntlet Cast**—extends from below the elbow to the proximal palmar crease, including the thumb (thumb spica)

C. **Long-arm Cast**—extends from upper level of axillary fold to proximal palmar crease; elbow usually immobilized at right angle

D. **Short-leg Cast**—extends from below knee to base of toes

E. **Long-leg Cast**—extends from upper thigh to the base of toes; foot is at right angle in a neutral position

F. **Body Cast**—encircles the trunk stabilizing the spine

G. **Spica Cast**—incorporates the trunk and an extremity
1. *Shoulder spica Cast*—a body jacket that encloses trunk, shoulder, and elbow
2. *Hip spica cast*—encloses trunk and a lower extremity
   a. Single hip spica—extends from nipple line to include pelvis and 1 thigh
   b. Double hip spica—extends from nipple line or upper abdomen to include pelvis and extends to include both thighs and lower legs
   c. One and a half hip spica—extends from upper abdomen, includes 1 entire leg, and extends to the knee of the other

H. **Cast-brace** (see Fig. 30-5)—external support about a fracture that is constructed with hinges to permit early motion of joints, early mobilization, and independence
1. Cast-bracing is based on the concept that some weight-bearing is physiologic and will promote the formation of bone and contain fluid within a tight compartment that compresses soft tissues, providing a distribution of forces across the fracture site.
2. Cast-brace is applied after initial edema and pain have subsided and there is evidence of fracture stability.

Cast Procedures
1. See Guidelines: Application of a Cast
2. See Guidelines: Removal of a Cast

Guidelines Application of a Cast

Equipment	Plaster or synthetic bandages in desired widths
	*Stockinette (tubular knitted material)
	*Cast padding (roll padding)
	Splints (for reinforcement)
	*Cotton, polyester, or polyurethane foam padding for bony prominences
	Cast knives, scissors
	Polyethylene sheeting or newspaper—to protect floor
	Disposable gloves—to protect hands of operator

* Material needs to be nonabsorbent if non-plaster cast is used.

Large, plastic-lined pail of water at room temperature—21°–24°C. (70°–75°F)—or as recommended by cast material manufacturer
Cast finishing hand cream for synthetic cast as needed

Underlying Considerations

1. The application of a cast requires 2–3 persons: one to apply the plaster (operator), one to dip and hand the plaster bandages to the operator, and a third person to hold the extremity in correct position. (Body spicas may require additional personnel.)
2. The time required for the cast to become rigid varies with the material used—generally 2–6 minutes.
3. There should be no movement of the extremity while the cast is being applied and set.
4. In general, the joints above and below the involved bone are immobilized.

Procedure

Action	Rationale/Amplification

Preparatory Phase

1. Spread polyethylene sheeting or newspaper on floor.
2. Explain to the patient that there will be a feeling of warmth as the plaster is applied.
3. Apply stockinette and roll cast padding on the extremity or part to be immobilized.
   a. Apply roll padding as smoothly and snugly as possible so that each turn overlaps the preceding turn by ½ the width of the roll.
   b. Extra pieces of padding may be placed over bony prominences: olecranon process, malleoli, patella.
4. While keeping the thumb under the forward edge of the bandage, submerge the plaster bandage vertically in water (room temperature) for a minute or so, or until bubbles cease to rise.
   Check directions on synthetic cast materials.
5. Expel excess water by squeezing (not wringing) toward the center of the bandage; hand bandage to operator with free end hanging loose.

2. Heat is produced by crystallization as plaster sets. The reaction of water with plaster of paris liberates heat.
3. Padding is used to pad the sharp cast margins for patient comfort and to prevent pressure areas, minimize circulatory problems, and facilitate cast removal. It is applied from the distal to the proximal end of the extremity. When too much padding is used, it may shift and produce pressure areas under the cast.

4. Water that is too warm will accelerate setting time, may cause a burn, and may result in excessive plaster loss by loosening the adhesive agents that bond the plaster to the fabric.

5. The cast will dry more quickly (and thus will acquire maximum strength sooner) if a well-squeezed plaster bandage is used.
   Maximum strength is achieved by synthetic casts through chemical reaction in about ½ hour.

Performance Phase (by operator)

1. Starting at the distal end, roll the bandage gently and evenly on the extremity, overlapping the preceding turn by ½ the width of the roll.
2. Keep the bandage moving and in constant contact with the surface of the extremity. Smooth and rub down successive layers or turns of each bandage into the layers below with the thumbs and thenar eminences (mound on the palm) in circumferential and longitudinal directions.
3. Take tucks in the lower border of the bandage by lifting the bandage off the surface (without tension) and overlapping it in a V-shaped fashion.
4. Trim the cast to size with a sharp knife. Fold stockinette over edges of cast and anchor with cast material.
5. Finish synthetic cast with cast hand cream as indicated.
6. Ask the patient if there is any discomfort or pain.

1. Roll inward toward the patient's body for ease of control.

2. This keeps the cast uniformly thick.
   Rubbing the plaster as it is applied will form a smooth, solid, and well-fused cast. Avoid indenting the cast with the fingertips, as this may produce pressure sores on underlying skin. Handle fresh casts with palms.
3. Tucking the bandage helps to contour the cast to the changing circumference of the extremity. Do not twist or reverse the bandage to change its direction, as this produces sharp cutting edges.
4. Stockinette produces smooth, comfortable edges on cast. Do not pull too vigorously on the stockinette, as this may cause pressure on bony prominences.
5. Smooths rough exterior surface.
6. If a patient complains of pain, it may be due to manipulation of fracture during setting; pain should subside rapidly. If it persists, the cast and encircling dressings are split to avoid constriction, circulatory problems, and pressure sores.

Follow-Up Phase

1. Support the cast with the palm of the hand while moving the patient. Avoid indentations from tips of fingers.
2. Expose the cast to warm, circulating, dry air. Or blow air over cast with a circulating fan to increase the evaporation of water.

1. Finger indentation on a fresh cast can produce pressure sores.
2. Avoid covering the cast when it is drying, as this delays drying time. Usually the plaster cast will reach its maximum temperature 5–15 minutes after it is applied and will then cool rapidly. The ultimate plaster cast strength is obtained after the cast is dry (up to 48 hours, depending on outside temperature and humidity).
   The synthetic cast strength is maximum within 30 minutes of application and not dependent on being dry.

3. Clean equipment and store ready for use.

Removal of a Cast

Equipment
Cast cutter—an electric saw with circular blade that oscillates and is connected to a vacuum collector
Cast spreader
Plaster knife
Scissors
Felt tip pen

Procedure

Nursing Action	**Rationale/Amplification**

Preparatory Phase

1. Describe to the patient how and where the cast cutter will be used and the expected sensations.
   Turn on the cutter and allow the patient to hear the motor.
2. Determine whether or not the cast is padded.

3. Determine where the cut will be made. Mark, with a felt pen, the area to be cut.

1. Reassures the patient that the cutter produces vibrations but not pain.

2. An electric plaster cast cutter should not be used on un-padded casts.
3. The line should be in front of the lateral malleolus and behind the medial malleolus on a lower extremity cast. An upper extremity cast is usually split along the ulnar or flexor surface.

Performance Phase

1. Inform the patient to shield eyes.
2. Grasp the electric cutter as illustrated (Fig. 30-6).
3. Rest the thumb on the cast.

4. Turn on the electric cutter. Push the blade firmly and gently through the cast while holding the thumb against the cast to steady the blade while cutting through the cast.
5. As the blade cuts through the plaster, a sudden lack of resistance is felt; plaster will "give" (or "dip") when the cut is completed.
6. Lift the cutting blade up a degree (but not out of the cutting groove) and advance the blade at a slightly higher or lower level. The cast is cut by a series of alternating pressure and linear movements along the line of the cut (Fig. 30-6).

1. Plaster dust may be irritating to the eyes.

3. The thumb serves as a depth gauge and acts as a guard in front of the blade.

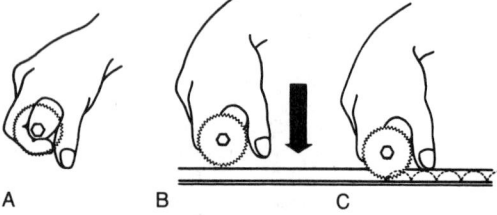

A   B   C

Figure 30-6. *Operating a cast cutter. (Photo courtesy Stryker Corporation)*

7. Avoid drawing the cutting blade along the extremity in a single motion.

8. Cut the cast on both sides. Then rock the anterior portion of the cast over the posterior portion.
9. Insert the blades of the cast spreader in the cut trough. Separate the 2 halves with the spreader at several sites along the cast split. Separate the cast with the hands.
10. Cut through the padding and stockinette with scissors, keeping the scissor blade that is closest to the skin parallel to the skin.
11. Lift the extremity carefully out of the posterior portion of the cast. Support the extremity so that it is maintained in the same position as when in the cast.

7. This will cut the skin. If saw blade is in contact with padding too long, the patient will feel burning sensation on skin from rapidly oscillating blade.
8. This maneuver allows the operator to determine if the cast is completely cut.

10. Use bandage scissors; place the flat blade closest to the skin.

11. When the support of the cast has been removed, stresses and strain are placed on parts that have been at rest.

Nursing Action	Rationale/Amplification
After Removal of Cast	
1. Cleanse the skin gently with mild soap and water. Blot dry. Apply a skin cream.	1. Explain to the patient that the skin will be scaly and the extremity will appear "thin" from disuse. Reassure him that it will take a few weeks to regain normal appearance and function.
2. Emphasize the importance of continuing the prescribed exercises, reporting for physical therapy, etc.	2. Exercises are necessary to redevelop and increase strength and function. Pain and stiffness may be expected after cast removal.

Nursing Process Overview: The Patient With a Cast

Assessing for Complications

A. Neurovascular Problems

1. Trauma or surgery affecting an extremity will produce swelling (result of hemorrhage from bone and surrounding tissue and of tissue edema). Vascular insufficiency and nerve compression due to unrelieved swelling can cause irreversible damage to an extremity.
2. Symptoms and signs
   a. Pain
   b. Swelling
   c. Discoloration—pale or blue
   d. Cool skin distal to injury
   e. Tingling or numbness (paresthesia)
   f. Pain on passive extension (muscle stretch)
   g. Slow capillary refill; diminished or absent pulse
   h. Paralysis

B. Necrosis, Pressure Sores, and Nerve Palsies

1. Pressure of cast on neurovascular and bony structures causes necrosis, pressure sores, and nerve palsies.
2. Symptoms and signs
   a. Severe initial pain over bony prominences; this is a warning symptom of an impending pressure sore. *Pain decreases when ulceration occurs.*
   b. Odor
   c. Drainage on cast
3. Pressure sites (See Fig. 30-7)
   a. *Lower extremity*—heel, malleoli, dorsum of foot, head of fibula, anterior surface of patella
   b. *Upper extremity*—medial epicondyle of humerus, ulnar styloid
   c. Plaster jackets or body spica casts—sacrum, anterior and superior iliac spines, vertebral borders of scapulae

> **NURSING ALERT:** Do not ignore the complaint of pain of the patient in a cast. Suspect circulatory complications or a pressure sore. Notify physician if symptoms persist. Cast may have to be split or removed.

C. Multisystem Complications

1. Immobility and confinement in a cast—particularly a body cast—can result in multi-system problems.
2. Symptoms/signs/causes
   a. *Nausea, vomiting,* and abdominal distension associated with *cast syndrome (superior mesenteric artery syndrome,* resulting in diminished blood flow to the bowel), adynamic ileus, and possible intestinal obstruction.
   b. *Acute anxiety* reaction symptoms (i.e., behavioral changes and autonomic responses—increased respiratory and heart rate, elevated blood pressure, diaphoresis) associated with confinement in a space
   c. *Thrombophlebitis* and possible pulmonary emboli associated with immobility and ineffective circulation (e.g., venous stasis)
   d. *Respiratory atelectasis* and pneumonia associated with ineffective respiratory effort
   e. *Urinary tract infection*
      Renal and bladder calculi associated with urinary stasis, low fluid intake, and calcium excretion associated with immobility
   f. *Anorexia and constipation* associated with decreased activity
   g. *Psychological reaction* (e.g., depression) associated with immobility, dependence, and loss of control

Nursing Diagnoses

1. Altered peripheral tissue perfusion related to trauma, bleeding into the tissues, associated edema, and constrictive bandage/cast.
2. Impaired physical mobility related to trauma, pathological condition, and treatment regimen.

Nursing Interventions

A. Maintaining Adequate Tissue Perfusion

1. Elevate the extremity on cloth-covered pillow above the level of the heart. Keep the heel off the mattress.
2. Avoid resting cast on hard surfaces or sharp edges that can cause denting or flattening of the cast and consequent pressure sores.
3. Handle moist cast with palms of hands.
4. Turn the patient every 2 hours while cast dries.
5. Assess neurovascular status hourly during the first 24 hours; then less frequently as condition warrants and swelling resolves.
6. If symptoms of neurovascular compromise occur:
   a. Notify physician immediately
   b. Bivalve the cast: split cast on each side over its full length into 2 halves.
   c. Cut the underlying padding—blood-soaked padding may shrink and cause constriction of circulation.
   d. Spread cast sufficiently to relieve constriction.
7. If symptoms of pressure area occur, cast may be "win-

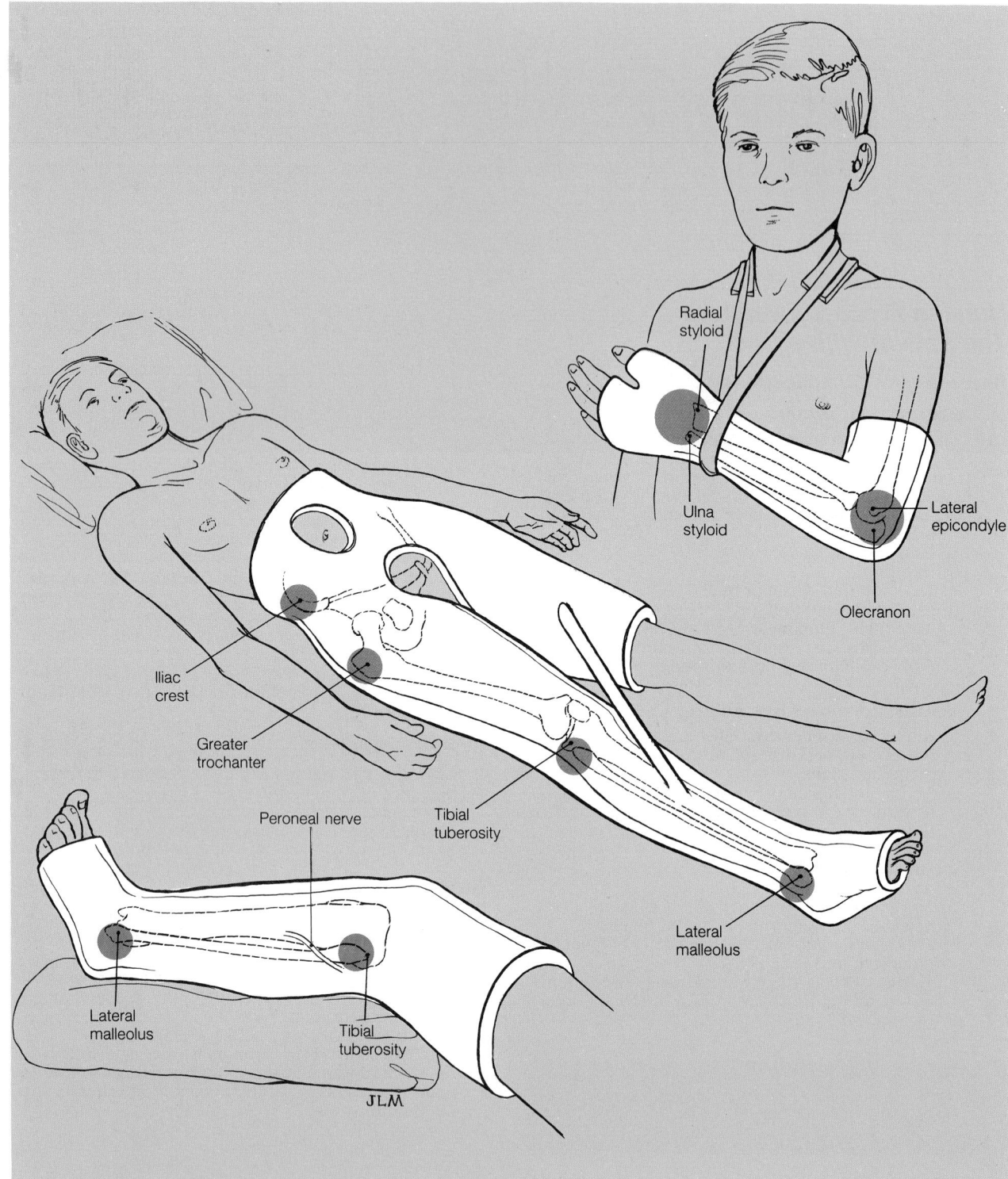

Figure 30-7. *Pressure areas in different types of casts.*

dowed" (hole cut in it) so that the skin at the pain point can be examined and treated. The window must be replaced so that the tissue does not swell and cause additional pressure problems at window edge.

B. Monitoring for Cast Syndrome and Adynamic Ileus.

1. Symptoms (nausea, vomiting, abdominal distention, abdominal pain, diminished bowel sounds) occur.
2. Notify physician promptly.
3. Place patient in a prone position, if tolerated, to relieve pressure symptoms.
4. Employ nasogastric suction as prescribed.
5. Maintain electrolyte balance by intravenous replacement of fluids as prescribed.
6. Physician may remove cast if condition does not improve.
7. Surgical intervention (duodenojejunostomy) may be necessary when conservative measures fail to relieve duodenal obstruction.
8. Encourage the patient to verbalize fears and concerns. Facilitate active participation in decision-making. Encourage family support.

C. Preventing Thromboembolic Complications

> **NURSING ALERT:** Individuals at high risk include older adults, previous thromboembolism, obesity, congestive heart failure, multiple trauma. They may require prophylaxis against thromboembolism.

1. Encourage the patient to move about as normally as possible.
2. Encourage compliance with prescribed exercises.
3. Have the patient exercise the parts of the body that are not immobilized by the cast at regular and frequent intervals.
4. Reposition and turn patient frequently.
5. Avoid pressure behind knees, which reduces venous return.
6. Use antiembolism stockings as prescribed.
7. Administer prophylactic anticoagulants as prescribed.

D. Implementing General Nursing Measures

1. Encourage deep-breathing exercises and coughing at regular intervals.
2. Encourage the patient to drink liberal quantities of fluid—to avoid urinary infection and calculi.
3. Encourage balanced nutritional intake
   a. Assess the patient's food preferences. Serve small meals
   b. Provide natural bowel stimulants (e.g., fiber)
   c. Monitor bowels and use a bowel program if necessary.
4. Facilitate patient participation in care planning and activities. Encourage mobility within limits of therapeutic regimen.

Specific Care for Patient in Spica/Body Cast

A. Positioning

1. Place a bedboard under the mattress for uniform support of the body.
2. Support the curves of the cast with cloth-covered flexible pillows—prevents cracking and flat spots while cast is drying.
   a. Place 3 pillows crosswise on bed for body cast.
   b. Place 1 pillow crosswise at the waist and 2 pillows

lengthwise for affected leg for spica cast. If both legs are involved, use 2 additional pillows.
3. Encourage the patient to maintain physiological position by:
   a. Using the overhead trapeze.
   b. Placing good foot flat on bed and pushing down while lifting himself up on the trapeze.
   c. Avoiding twisting motions.
   d. Avoiding positions that produce pressure on groin, back, chest, and abdomen.

B. Turning

1. Move the patient to the side of the bed, using a steady, even, pulling motion.
2. Place pillows along the other side of the bed; 1 for the chest and 2 (lengthwise) for the legs.
3. Instruct the patient to place his arms at his side or above his head.
4. Turn the patient as a unit. Avoid twisting the patient in the cast.
5. Turn the patient toward the leg not encased in plaster or toward the unoperated side if both legs are in plaster.
   a. One nurse stands at other side of bed to receive the patient's shoulders.
   b. Second nurse supports leg in plaster while the third nurse supports the patient's back as he is turned.
   c. *Do not grasp cross bar of spica cast to move the patient.* The purpose of the bar is to strengthen the cast.
   d. Turn the patient in body cast to a prone position twice daily—provides postural drainage of bronchial tree; relieves pressure on back.
6. Keep the cast level by elevating the lumbar sacral area with a small pillow when the head of the bed is elevated.

C. Hygienic Care

1. Provide hygienic care of the patient.
2. Protect cast from soiling.
   a. Cover perineum with a towel and apply spray (lacquer-type) to perineal area of cast. Tuck 10-cm. (4-inch) strips of thin polyethylene sheeting under perineal area of cast and tape to cast exterior. Replace when soiling occurs.
   b. Clean outside of cast with dry cleanser on almost-dry cloth.
3. Roll the patient onto fracture bedpan; use small pillow in lumbosacral area for support.

D. Skin Care

1. Inspect skin for signs of irritation:
   a. Around cast edge
   b. Under cast—pull skin taut and inspect under cast, using a flashlight for illumination.
2. Reach up under cast and massage accessible skin.
3. Protect the toes from the pressure of the bedding.

Discharge Planning/Patient Education

A. Neurovascular Status

1. Instruct patient to check neurovascular status and to control swelling.
2. Watch for signs and symptoms of circulatory disturbance including blueness or paleness of fingernails or toenails accompanied by pain and tightness, numbness, cold or tingling sensation.
3. Elevate affected extremity and wiggle fingers/toes.
4. Apply ice bags as prescribed ($\frac{1}{3}$–$\frac{1}{2}$ full) to each side

of the cast, making sure that they do not make indentations in plaster.

5. Call physician promptly if excessive swelling, paresthesia, persistent pain, pain on passive stretch, paralysis occur.

6. After the patient begins ambulation, encourage to elevate the cast when seated. Encourage the patient to lie down several times daily with cast elevated.

B. Skin Irritation

1. Prevent skin irritation at cast edge.
2. Pad edges of cast with moleskin or "petal" cast edges with strips of adhesive tape.

C. Exercise

1. Instruct patient to actively exercise every joint that is not immobilized and to perform isometric exercises (contract muscles without moving joint) of those immobilized to maintain muscle strength and to prevent atrophy.
2. Perform hourly when awake.
   a. Leg-cast—"Push down on the popliteal (knee) space, hold it, relax, repeat." Move toes back and forth; bend toes down, then pull them back.
   b. Arm cast—"Make a fist, hold it, relax, repeat." Move shoulders.

D. Cast Care

1. Avoid getting cast wet, especially padding under cast—causes skin breakdown as plaster casts become soft.
2. Do not cover a leg cast with plastic or rubber boots, as this causes condensation and wetting of the cast.
3. Avoid weight-bearing or stress on plaster cast for 24 hours.
4. Report to the physician if the cast cracks or breaks; instruct the patient not to try to fix it himself.
5. To clean the cast:
   a. Remove surface soil with slightly damp cloth.
   b. Rub soiled areas with household scouring powder.
   c. Wipe off residual moisture.

E. Safety

1. Avoid walking on wet floors or sidewalks, to prevent falls.
2. Do not place objects under the cast, to prevent pressure and injury to the skin.

F. After Cast Is Removed:

1. Cleanse skin with mild soap and water
2. Blot dry.
3. Apply emollient lotion to dry skin.
4. Avoid scratching the skin.
5. Continue prescribed exercises. Gradually resume activities.
6. Elevate extremity to control swelling.

Evaluation

1. Maintains adequate tissue perfusion
   a. Minimal edema—no swelling or pressure
   b. Intact neurovascular status—normal sensations, capillary refill, controllable discomfort, normal movement
   c. Intact skin over bony prominences
2. Demonstrates normal body system functioning
   a. Absence of nausea, vomiting, anorexia
   b. Normal bowel and urinary elimination patterns
   c. Absence of thrombophlebitis
   d. Vital signs normal
   e. Normal respiratory pattern
3. Demonstrates satisfactory psychological adjustment—expresses feelings and fears, but maintains positive outlook and expectations.
4. Participates in self-care activities and rehabilitation regimen

---

Traction

Traction is force applied in a specific direction. To apply the force needed to overcome the natural force or pull of

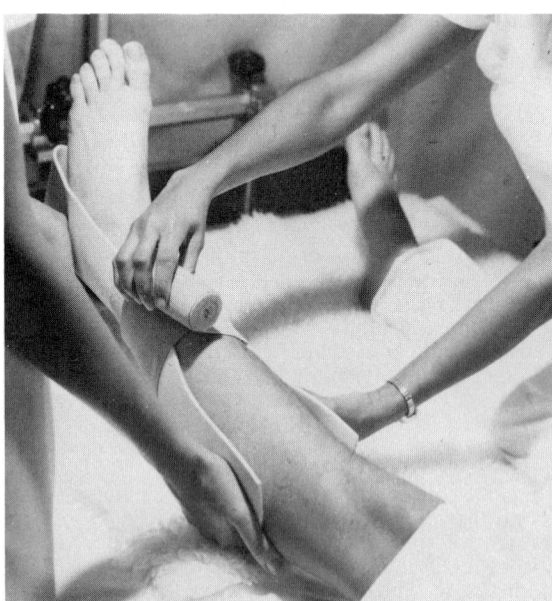
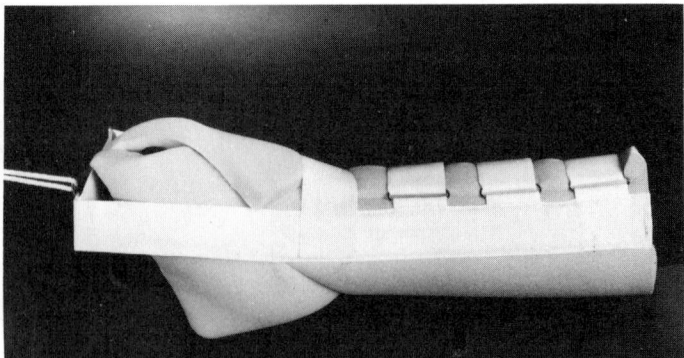

Figure 30-8. *(Left) Applying elastic bandage for Buck's extension traction. (Right) Prepadded boot that may be used in Buck's extension. (Photo of boot courtesy of All Orthopedic Appliances)*

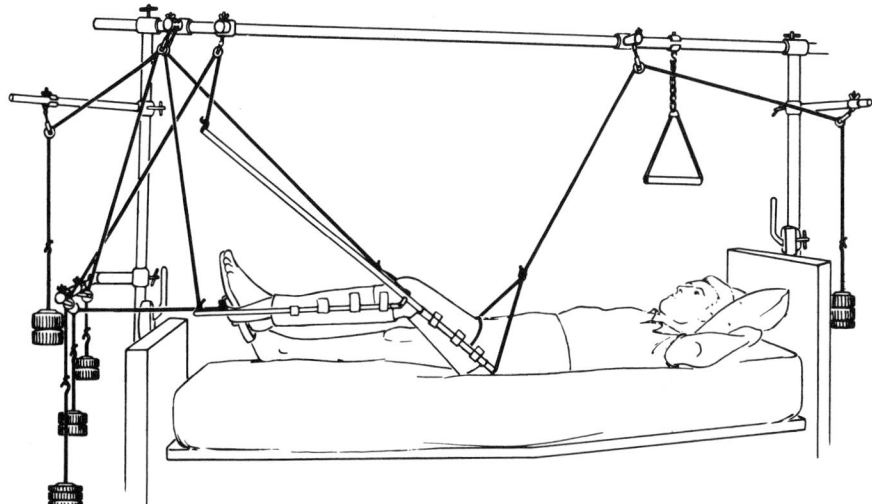

Figure 30-9. *Balanced skeletal traction using Thomas leg splint and Pearson attachment.*

muscle groups, a system of ropes, pulleys, and weights is used.

Purposes of Traction

1. To reduce and immobilize fracture
2. To regain normal length and alignment of an injured extremity
3. To lessen or eliminate muscle spasm
4. To prevent deformity
5. To give the patient freedom for "in-bed" activities
6. To reduce pain

Types of Traction

A. Running Traction

1. Is a form of traction in which the pull is exerted in one plane.

2. May use either skin or skeletal traction
3. Buck's extention traction (Fig. 30-8) is an example of running skin traction.

B. Balanced Suspension Traction

1. Uses additional weights to counterbalance the traction force and floats the extremity in the traction apparatus.
2. The line of pull on the extremity remains fairly constant despite changes in the patient's position (Figs. 30-9 and 30-10).

Application of Traction

Traction may be applied to the skin or to the skeletal system.

A. Skin Traction

1. Is accomplished by applying a light force that pulls on tape, sponge rubber, or special device (boot,

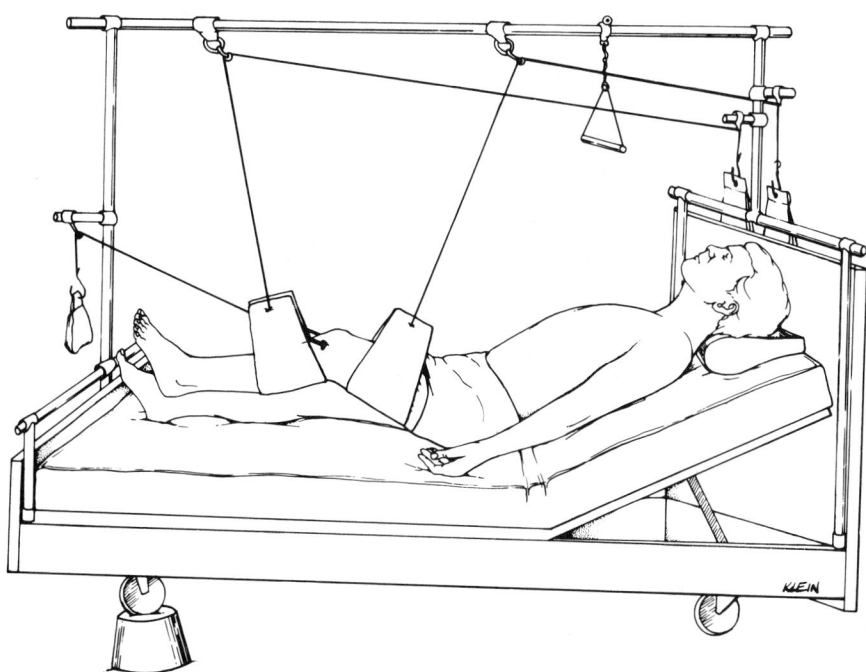

Figure 30-10. *Balanced skeletal traction using slings for support and suspension.*

cervical halter, pelvic belt) that is in contact with the skin.

2. The pulling force is transmitted to the musculoskeletal structures.
3. Skin traction is used as a temporary measure in adults to control muscle spasm and pain.
4. It is used prior to surgery in the treatment of hip fracture (Buck's extension, see Guidelines, below), and femoral shaft fractures (Russell's traction).
5. Pelvic and cervical traction are used for treatment of back disorders or injuries. Skin traction may be used definitively to treat fractures in children.

B. Skeletal Traction

1. Is traction applied by the orthopedic surgeon under aseptic conditions using wires, pins, or tongs placed through bones.
2. Skeletal traction is used most frequently in treating fractures of the femur, humerus (supracondylar fractures), tibia, and cervical spine.

Guidelines ## Application of Buck's Extension Traction

Buck's extension skin traction is used as a temporary measure to provide immobility, support, and comfort until definitive treatment is accomplished (see Fig. 30-8).

Equipment
Foam Buck's traction boot or traction tape and 10-cm. (4-inch) elastic bandage
Spreader block or metal spreader
Pulley, nylon rope, and weights (2.3–3.1 kg. [5–7 lbs.] is usual; (amount of weight is prescribed by physician)
Sheepskin pad
Shock blocks or adjustable bed for Trendelenburg's position.

Procedure

Nursing Action	Rationale/Amplification

Preparatory Phase

1. Place bedboard under the mattress.
   Bed position is flat or in Trendelenburg's position. This depends on the size of the patient and the weight applied.
2. Question the patient to determine previous skin conditions (contact dermatitis). Inspect skin for evidences of atrophy, abrasions, and circulatory disturbances.
3. Make sure that the skin of the extremity is clean and dry.
4. Document the neurovascular status of the extremity, any evidence of skin problems or varicosities.

1. Elevating the foot of the bed (countertraction) helps prevent the patient from sliding down toward the foot of the bed.

2. The skin must be in healthy condition to tolerate skin traction.

3. A clean, dry skin helps traction tape adherence.

Performance Phase

1. Position the patient in center of bed in good alignment.
If traction tape is used:
2. Apply continuous traction tape to medial and lateral aspects of lower leg (below knee and loosely around foot to allow for attachment of spreader).

3. Have a second person elevate and support the extremity under the ankle and knee while the elastic bandage is applied. Beginning at the ankle, wrap the elastic bandage snugly over the tape up to the tibial tubercle.
4. Attach a spreader block (or metal spreader) to the distal end of the tape. Attach a rope to the spreader block and pass it over a pulley fastened to the end of the bed and gently apply weights.
5. Place a sheepskin pad under the leg (or use a commercial heel protector).
If foam boot is used:
1. Apply antiembolitic stockings if prescribed.
2. Place leg in foam boot, adjusting it so that the heel is in the heel of the boot.
3. Secure Velcro bootstraps, avoiding excessive pressure on malleoli and fibular head.
4. Attach rope to built-in spreader plate, pass it over pulley, and apply weights gently.

1. For effective line of pull.

2. Avoid pressure over malleoli and head of fibula. Pressure sores develop rapidly over bony prominences. Pressure over the region of the fibular head and common peroneal nerve may produce peroneal palsy and footdrop.
3. The elastic bandage holds tape to the skin and helps prevent slipping.

4. The spreader block prevents pressure along the side of the foot. The spreader should not be too narrow (causes pressure sores on ankle) or too wide (pulls traction tape away from the heel).
5. Sheepskin is used to reduce friction of the heel against the bed.

1. Prophylactic measure in high-risk population.
2. Preventing sore heels is a primary concern.

3. Pressure over bony prominences causes skin breakdown, and pressure on peroneal nerve may result in footdrop.
4. The rope should move unobstructed and the weights should hang free of the bed and not touch the floor.

Procedure *(continued)*	**Nursing Action**	**Rationale/Amplification**
	Follow-Up Phase	
	1. Check traction system	1. Make sure knots are tied securely. Ropes move unobstructed. Weights hang free of bed and do not touch the floor. Effective traction is accomplished with unobstructed system. Reapply traction when ineffective.
	2. Ensure the patient is in proper alignment. Maintain extension in neutral position, avoiding external rotation.	2. The part of the body in traction should be in line with the pull of the weight.

	3. Assess neurovascular status.
	  a. Evaluate dorsum of foot for loss of sensation.
	  b. Assess for weakness of dorsiflexion of toes and foot.
	  c. Assess for complaints of itching and burning.
		3. Change in neurological status may indicate pressure on the peroneal nerve.

	4. Palpate over area of traction tapes daily; if tender to palpation, suspect skin irritation. Report immediately.	

	5. Unwrap elastic bandage/remove boot periodically to assess skin status. Have second person stabilize leg in position, applying manual traction when inspecting skin or when giving skin care. Provide skin care at regular intervals.	5. Inspect for skin irritation and pressure on
		  a. Achilles tendon
		  b. Heel (keep heel off bed)
		  c. Malleoli
		  d. Peroneal nerve (at head of fibula just below the knee)

	6. Assess patient position to maintain effective traction.	6. Maintain the extremity in a neutral position. Avoid external rotation.
	7. Check for slipping of traction tape/boot.	7. Slipping of dressing or boot causes pressure on bony prominences.

	8. Inspect and bathe back. To give back care, instruct the patient to:
	  a. Place hands on overhead trapeze.
	  b. Bend the knee of unaffected extremity and place foot flat on bed.
	  c. Push down on the uninvolved foot and at the same time pull up on the trapeze—allows the entire body and trunk to rise off the bed.
	  d. The shoulders, back, and buttocks must move as a single, straight unit.
		8. The patient may not turn from side to side because the position of the leg on the bed will cause the bony fragments to move against each other.

Nursing Process Overview:
The Patient in Traction

Nursing Assessment

A. Assess the Patient's Physiologic and Psychological Status

1. Pain
2. Deformity
3. Swelling
4. Neurovascular status—paralysis, paresthesia, pulse, color
5. Skin condition—examined frequently for evidence of pressure or friction over bony prominences
6. Emotional reactions
7. Understanding of treatment regimen

B. Examine Traction Equipment for Safety and Effectiveness

1. The patient is placed on a firm mattress, often with a hinged bedboard beneath it.
2. The ropes and the pulleys should be in alignment.
3. The pull should be in line with the long axis of the bone.
4. Any factor that might reduce the pull or alter its direction must be eliminated.

  a. Weights should hang freely.
  b. Ropes should be unobstructed and not in contact with the bed or equipment.
  c. Help the patient to pull himself up in bed at frequent intervals.

NURSING ALERT:
1. Traction is *not* accomplished if the knot in the rope or the footplate is touching the pulley or the foot of the bed, or if the weights are resting on the floor.
2. Never remove the weights when repositioning the patient who is in skeletal traction, as this will interrupt the line of pull.

5. The amount of weight applied in skin traction must not exceed the tolerance of the skin. The condition of the skin must be inspected frequently.
6. Cover exposed sharp ends of skeletal pins with cork or other pin covering to protect patient and caregivers from injury.

C. Monitor for Possible Complications

1. Evaluate the patient in skeletal traction for the possible development of infection.
2. Review body systems for possible immobility-related problems (e.g., pneumonia, constipation, thrombophlebitis, depression).

Nursing Diagnoses

1. Impaired physical mobility related to traction therapy and underlying pathology
2. Potential impaired skin integrity related to pressure on soft tissues
3. Potential for infection related to bacterial invasion at skeletal traction site
4. Potential altered tissue perfusion related to injury or traction therapy

Nursing Interventions

A. Monitoring Patient in Traction

1. Check traction apparatus at repeated intervals
   a. Direction of pull is correct.
   b. Ropes and pulleys are unobstructed and freely movable.
   c. Weight is correct.
   d. Counter-traction is maintained through adjustment of bed position.
   e. Patient is comfortable.
2. The traction must be continuous to be effective, unless prescribed as intermittent, as with pelvic traction.
3. *With running traction,* the patient may not be turned without disrupting the line of pull.
4. *With balanced suspension traction,* the patient may be elevated, turned slightly, and moved as desired.

NURSING ALERT: Every complaint of the patient in traction should be investigated immediately.

B. Monitoring Patient for Normal Body Systems Function

1. Encourage deep breathing hourly to facilitate expansion of lungs and movement of respiratory secretions.
2. Auscultate lung fields twice a day.
3. Encourage fluid intake of 2,000–2,500 ml. daily.
4. Provide balanced high-fiber diet rich in protein; avoid excessive calcium intake.
5. Establish bowel routine through use of diet and/or stool softeners, laxatives, and enemas as prescribed.

C. Promoting Physical Mobility

1. Encourage active exercise of uninvolved muscles and joints to maintain strength and function. Dorsiflex feet hourly to avoid development of footdrop and aid in venous return.
2. Encourage patient participation in planning and care activities.

D. Maintaining Intact Skin Without Development of Pressure Areas

1. Examine bony prominences frequently for evidence of pressure or friction irritation.
2. Observe for skin irritation around the traction bandage.
3. Observe for pressure at traction–skin contact points.
4. Report complaint of burning sensation under traction.
5. Relieve pressure without disrupting traction effectiveness.
6. Special care must be given to the back at regular intervals, because the patient maintains a supine position.

E. Avoiding Infection at Pin Site

1. Monitor vital signs.
2. Watch for signs of infection, especially around the pin tract.

a. The pin should be immobile in the bone and the skin wound should be dry. Small amount of serous oozing from pin site may occur.
b. If infection is suspected, percuss gently over the tibia; this may elicit pain if infection is developing.
c. Assess for other signs of infection: heat, redness, fever.

If directed, clean the pin tract with sterile applicators and prescribed solution/ointment—to clear drainage at the entrance of tract and around the pin, as plugging at this site can predispose to bacterial invasion of the tract and bone.

F. Monitoring Tissue Perfusion of Lower Extremities

1. See Neurovascular Compromise, page 764
2. Assess motor and sensory function of specific nerves that might be compromised.
   a. Peroneal nerve; have patient point great toe toward his nose; check sensation on dorsum of foot; presence of footdrop.
   b. Radial nerve; have patient extend thumb; check sensation in web between thumb and index finger.
   c. Median nerve; thumb–middle finger apposition; check sensation of index finger.
3. Determine adequacy of circulation (e.g., color, temperature, motion, capillary refill of peripheral fingers or toes).
   a. With Buck's traction, inspect the foot for circulatory difficulties within a few minutes and then periodically after the elastic bandage has been applied.
4. Notify physician promptly if change in neurovascular status is identified.
5. Examine the patient for development of thrombophlebitis (e.g., calf tenderness).

Patient Education

1. Teach the patient the purpose of traction therapy.
2. Delineate limitations of activity necessary to maintain effective traction.
3. Teach use of patient aids (e.g., trapeze).
4. Instruct the patient not to adjust or modify traction apparatus.
5. Instruct the patient in activities designed to minimize effects of immobility on body systems.
6. Teach the patient necessity for reporting changes in sensations, pain, movement, etc.

Expected Outcomes

1. Maintains muscular strength and joint mobility; participates in exercise program and activities of daily living
2. Achieves effective traction therapy, immobilization, and comfort
3. Shows no evidence of skin breakdown; no reddened skin from pressure
4. Experiences no infection at pin site—tissue at pin site is not inflamed, red, or tender; no fever.
5. Maintains normal neurovascular functioning—normal sensations, movement, and circulatory parameters
6. Maintains normal respiratory pattern; normal blood gases, vital signs, and lung sounds

---

External Fixation

External fixation is a technique of fracture immobilization in which a series of transfixing pins is inserted through bone and attached to a rigid external metal frame (Fig. 30-11). The method is used mainly in the management of open fractures with severe soft tissue damage.

Advantages

1. Permits rigid support of severely comminuted open fractures, infected nonunions, and infected unstable joints.
2. Facilitates wound care (frequent debridements, irrigations, dressing changes) and soft tissue reconstruction (delayed wound closure, muscle flaps, skin grafts)
3. Allows early function of muscles and joints
4. Allows early patient comfort

Ilizarov External Fixator

A. Purpose—May be used for limb lengthening, correction of angulation and rotation defects, and in treatment of nonunion.

B. Components

1. This fixator apparatus consists of through-the-bone tension wires placed above and below the treatment site.

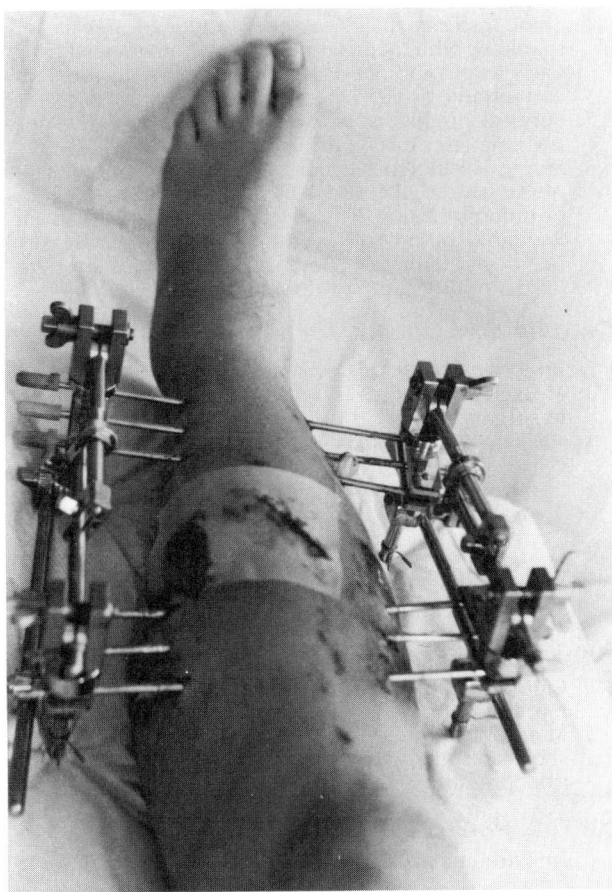

Figure 30-11. *External fixation device used for reduction and immobilization of complex fracture, allowing treatment of soft tissue wounds. (From Brunner LS and Suddarth DS. Textbook of Medical–Surgical Nursing. 6th ed. Philadelphia, JB Lippincott, 1988)*

2. The wires are attached to fixator rings surrounding the limb.
3. The rings are connected to one another by telescoping rods.

C. Management

1. Adjustments are made daily at about 1 mm. per day, stimulating callus and bone formation.
2. Patient compliance is essential.
3. Weight-bearing is encouraged.
4. When the desired length or correction is achieved, the fixator is left in place without further adjustment until bone healing occurs.

Application of External Fixator by Physician

1. Under general anesthesia, the skin is cleansed and transfixing pins are inserted into the bone through small incisions above and below the fracture.
2. Following reduction of the fracture, the appliance is stabilized by adjusting and tightening the bars connecting the sets of pins.
3. The sharp pin heads are covered with plastic, cork, or rubber covers to protect the other extremity and caregivers.

Nursing Assessment

1. Determine the patient's understanding of procedure and fixation device.
2. Evaluate neurovascular status of involved body part.
3. Inspect each pin site for redness, drainage, tenderness, pain, and loosening of the pin.
4. Inspect open wounds for healing, infection, or devitalized tissue.
5. Assess functioning of other body systems.

Nursing Diagnoses

1. Anxiety related to appearance of external fixation device and wound.
2. Potential altered tissue perfusion related to swelling, altered neurovascular status, and injury.
3. Potential for infection related to open injury and skeletal pin insertion.
4. Knowledge deficit of self-care related to altered mobility, external fixator device, and wound.

Nursing Interventions

A. Relieving Anxiety Related to the External Fixation Device

1. If possible before placement of the device, reassure the patient that although the fixator appears clumsy and cumbersome, it should not hurt once it is in place.
2. Emphasize the positive aspects of this device in treating complex musculoskeletal problems.
3. Encourage the patient to verbalize reaction to the device.
4. Inform the patient that he will achieve greater mobility with an external fixation device, thereby minimizing the development of other system problems.
5. Involve the patient in his care and in the management of external fixator.

B. Maintaining Intact Neurovascular Status

1. See Neurovascular Compromise, page 764.
2. Establish baseline of functioning for comparative monitoring. Complex musculoskeletal injuries frequently result in disruption of soft tissue functioning.

> **NURSING ALERT:** Assess neurovascular status frequently and *record findings.*

3. Elevate extremity to reduce swelling.
    a. Extremity can be suspended by hanging the fixator directly to the traction frame.
    b. Suspension is for control of edema and not for application of traction force.
4. Notify physician of change in neurovascular status.

C. Avoiding Infection

1. Pin site and fixator care:
    a. Cleanse pin sites and remove crusts with sterile cotton applicator, using solution and/or ointment as prescribed by physician or established standard of care.
        (1) Crusts formed by serous drainage can prevent fluid from draining and cause infection.
        (2) A small amount of serous drainage from the pin sites is normal.
    b. Note and report inflammation, swelling, tenderness, and purulent drainage at pin site.
    c. Note skin tension at pin site—tension can cause discomfort.
    d. Report loosened pins to physician.
    e. Cleanse fixator with clean cloth and water as needed.
2. Wound care:
    a. The open wounds at the fracture site are usually treated by daily dressing changes.
    b. Use sterile technique.
    c. Note wound appearance. Monitor healing. Report signs of infection.
3. Monitor for local and systemic indicators of infection.

D. Promoting Self-Care Activities

1. Encourage the patient to participate in care activities. Patient may become the "authority" for routine care activities (e.g., pin care).
2. Assure the patient that pain associated with injury will diminish as tissue reactions to injury and manipulation resolve and healing progresses.
3. Inform the patient that the external fixator maintains the fracture in a very stable position and that the extremity can be moved. Adjustment of the fixator is done by the physician. (Patient is taught how to adjust the Ilizarov fixator.)
4. To move the extremity, grasp the frame and assist the patient to move. Reassure the patient that the fixator can withstand normal movement.
5. Quadriceps exercises and range-of-motion for joints are usually started on first postoperative day.
6. Patient ambulates on crutches when soft tissue swelling has diminished; weight-bearing is as prescribed.

Discharge Planning/Patient Education

1. Inspect around each pin site daily for signs of infection and loosening of pins. Watch for pain, soft tissue swelling, and drainage.
2. Cleanse around each pin daily, using aseptic technique. *Do not touch wound with hands.*
3. Clean fixator regularly—to keep it free of dust and contamination.
4. *Do not tamper with clamps or nuts*—can alter compression and misalign fracture.

5. Review weight-bearing and other restrictions associated with injury and treatment regimen.
6. Encourage the patient to follow rehabilitation regimen.

Evaluation

1. Overcomes any anxiety about the external fixation device—does not appear worried about it; handles and cares for equipment with ease
2. Maintains adequate tissue perfusion; demonstrates normal sensations, movement, and circulation; exhibits minimal or no swelling
3. Is free of infection; demonstrates no signs of inflammation, tenderness, or purulent drainage at pin sites; wound healing progresses as anticipated; exhibits no signs of systemic infection (i.e., elevated temperature).
4. Performs self-care within limits of treatment regimen; when indicated uses ambulatory aids safely; complies with prescribed pin care, external fixator care, and wound care regimens; reports signs of infection, change in neurovascular status, and loosening of pins.

Internal Fixation

General Considerations

1. Some fractures may be reduced under anesthesia and stabilized with the surgical implantation of metal nails, nail–plate combinations, compression screw devices, and intramedullary nails.
2. Surgical procedure is usually carried out as soon as possible after full medical assessment.
3. Surgical fixation of a fracture permits early mobilization of the patient, thereby decreasing the adverse effects of immobilization. The metal hardware is not strong enough to permit full weight bearing on the extremity, but does facilitate maintenance of muscle strength, joint mobility, and development of bony union.

Gerontologic Considerations

1. Prolonged bedrest is detrimental to older adults.
2. Measures to prevent complications are instituted prior to surgery.
    a. Special skin care and use of therapeutic mattress—to prevent skin breakdown
    b. Deep breathing and coughing—to prevent respiratory depression
    c. Antiembolism stockings as prescribed—to prevent circulatory stasis
    d. Ankle exercises
    e. Adequate hydration

Nursing Assessment

1. Carry out neurovascular check of affected extremity.
2. Monitor drainage from portable suction.
3. Monitor for development of systemic complications—shock, respiratory problems, circulatory stasis, infection, pressure areas.

Nursing Diagnoses

1. Impaired physical mobility related to fracture and surgery
2. Self-care deficit related to injury, immobility, limited use of extremity with internal fixation of fracture
3. Pain related to fracture and surgical intervention

Nursing Interventions

A. Monitoring and Preventing Complications

1. Monitor drainage from surgical site, noting amount and character.
2. Maintain proper alignment of extremity, using pillows for support and/or elevation.
    For internal fixation of hip fracture, place pillow between legs to keep leg in mild abduction and to support leg when patient is turned on side.
3. Monitor incision for healing and signs of infection (induration, erythema, tenderness, drainage).
4. Assess pulmonary function and encourage deep breathing and coughing.
5. Assess for deep vein thrombosis. Encourage ankle exercise and use of antiembolism stockings as prescribed.

B. Promoting Physical Mobility as Soon as Possible

1. Reposition in bed, encouraging active participation.
2. Encourage quadriceps-setting and gluteal contraction exercises hourly to maintain muscle strength for ambulation.
3. If patient is to use an ambulatory aid, assist patient in use of trapeze and in performing arm-strengthening exercises to strengthen shoulder girdle and upper extremities.
4. Avoid positions contributing to flexion contracture. Assist with range-of-motion exercises.
5. Avoid positions that will place a stress on fractured area (e.g., internal fixation of hip fracture—sitting with leg in extension, adduction, or legs crossed).
6. Assist patient out of bed several times a day when prescribed, permitting prescribed amount of weight-bearing on injured extremity. Transfers and ambulation may need to be non–weight-bearing.

> **NURSING ALERT:** Internal fixation device is not strong enough to permit full weight-bearing.

1. Check with surgeon as to amount of weight-bearing permitted.
2. Remind patient of weight-bearing limitations.
3. Progression of weight-bearing depends on bony union.
4. Physician prescribes amount of weight-bearing.

C. Encouraging Self-Care

1. Encourage and support patient participation in activities of daily living.
2. Teach patient to use aids designed to assist in self-care.

> **GERONTOLOGIC ALERT:** Provide sufficient time for the patient to complete the task or to accomplish a position change.

Evaluation

1. Achieves bony union and wound healing without complications; achieves full function of injured extremity.
2. Participates in prescribed exercises; transfers out of bed independently; protects injured extremity from stress; provides support for healing fracture.
3. Achieves independence in self-care; understands weight-bearing and activity limitations; uses ambulation and self-care aids safely.

Bibliography

Books

Adams JC. Outline of Fractures. 9th ed. Edinburgh, Churchill Livingstone, 1987

Albright J and Brand R. (eds). The Scientific Basis of Orthopaedics. 2nd ed. Norwalk, Appleton and Lange, 1987

American Nurses' Association and National Association of Orthopaedic Nurses. Orthopaedic Nursing Practice. Kansas City, MO, American Nurses' Association, 1986

Apley AG and Solomon L. Concise System of Orthopaedics and Fractures. London, Butterworths, 1988

Birnbaum JS. The Musculoskeletal Manual. 2nd ed. Orlando, Grune & Stratton, 1989

Cittadine TJ. Orthopedic Terminology: Including Sports Medicine. Thorofare, NJ, Charles B Slack, 1988

Crenshaw AH (ed). Campbell's Operative Orthopaedics. 7th ed. St Louis, CV Mosby, 1987

Dandy DJ. Essential Orthopaedics and Trauma. Edinburgh, Churchill Livingstone, 1989

Dee R, Mango E and Hurst LC. (eds). Principles of Orthopaedic Practice. New York, McGraw–Hill, 1988

Farrell J. Illustrated Guide to Orthopedic Nursing. 3rd ed. Philadelphia, JB Lippincott, 1986

Footner A. Orthopaedic Nursing. London, Baillière Tindall, 1987

Gartland JJ. Fundamentals of Orthopaedics. 4th ed. Philadelphia, WB Saunders, 1987

Gates SJ and Mooar PA. Orthopaedics and Sports Medicine for Nurses. Baltimore, Williams & Wilkins, 1989

Gerhardt JJ, King P and Buyer WD (eds). Interdisciplinary Rehabilitation in Orthopedic Medicine. Toronto, Hans Huber Publisher, 1987

Hughes SPF and Fitzgerald RH. Musculoskeletal Infections. Chicago, Year Book Medical Pub, 1986

Hughes SPF, Benson MK and Colton CL (eds). Orthopaedics: The Principles and Practice of Musculoskeletal Surgery and Fractures. Edinburgh, Churchill Livingstone, 1987

Iversen LD and Clawson DK. Manual of Acute Orthopaedic Therapeutics. 3rd ed. Boston, Little, Brown & Co, 1987

Lewis MM and Weiner LS. Orthopaedics. Philadelphia, JB Lippincott, 1989

Magee DJ. Orthopedic Physical Assessment. Philadelphia, WB Saunders, 1987

Mears DC and Rubash HE. Pelvic and Acetabular Fractures. Thorofare, NJ, Charles B Slack, 1986

Mercies LR. Practical Orthopedics. 2nd ed. Chicago, Year Book Medical Pub, 1987

Miller TR. Evaluating Orthopedic Disability: A Commonsense Approach. 2nd ed. Oradell, NJ, Medical Economics Books, 1987

Mourad LA and Droste MM. The Nursing Process in the Care of Adults with Orthopaedic Conditions. 2nd ed., New York, John Wiley & Sons, 1988

Paton DF. Fractures and Orthopaedics. Edinburgh, Churchill Livingstone, 1988

Pellino T et al. (eds). Core Curriculum for Orthopaedic Nursing. Pitman, NY, National Association of Orthopaedic Nurses, 1986

Powell M (ed). Orthopaedic Nursing and Rehabilitation. 9th ed. Edinburgh, Churchill Livingstone, 1986

Schlossberg D. Orthopedic Infection. New York, Springer–Verlag, 1988

Schoen DC. The Nursing Process in

Orthopaedics. Norwalk, Appleton–Century–Crofts, 1986

Sikorski JM. Understanding Orthopaedics. Sydney, Butterworths, 1986

Smith C. Orthopaedic Nursing. London, William Heinemann Nursing, 1987

Stearns CM and Brunner NA. Opcare: Orthopaedic Patient Care. A Nursing Guide, Vols 1, 2, 3. Rutherford, NJ, Howmedica, 1987

Journals

Assessment/Diagnostic Procedures

Amadio PC. Pain dysfunction syndromes. J Bone Joint Surg (Am) 1988 Jul; 70(6):944–949

Chambers JK. Metabolic bone disorders. Imbalances in calcium and phosphorus. Nurs Clin North Am 1987 Dec; 22(4):861–972

Edeiken K and Karasick D. Imaging in bone cancer. CA 1987 Jul–Aug; 37(4): 239–245

Gavant ML. Digital subtraction angiography of the foot in atherosclerotic occlusive disease. South Med J 1989 Mar; 82(3):328–334

Hodges DL, McGuire TJ and Kumar VN. Diagnosis of hip pain: An anatomical approach. Orthop Rev 1987 Feb; 16(2):109–113

Zubay R. Understanding magnetic resonance imaging from a nursing perspective. Orthop Nurs 1988 Nov–Dec; 7(6):17–23

Psychological Response to Injury

Gustafson Y et al. Acute confusional states in elderly patients treated for femoral neck fracture. J Amer Geriatr Soc 1988 Jun; 36(6):525–530

Horowitz M. Stress response syndromes: A review of posttraumatic and adjustment disorders. Hosp Community Psychiatry 1986 Mar; 37(3):241–249

Moore K and Thompson D. Posttraumatic stress disorders in the orthopaedic patient. Orthop Nurs 1989 Jan–Feb; 8(1):11–19

Payne MB. Utilizing role theory to assist the family with sudden disability. Rehabil Nurs 1988 Jul–Aug; 13(4):191–194

Sports Injury

Cabot A. Tennis elbow: A curable affliction. Orthop Rev 1987 May; 16(5): 322–326

Folcik MA. Winter sports injuries: An overview. Orthop Nurs 1988 Nov–Dec; 7(6):25–28

Hoshowsky VM. Chronic lateral ligament instability of the ankle. Orthop Nurs 1988 May–Jun; 7(3):33–40

McInerney VR, Mailly KH and Paonessa KJ. Rehabilitation of the sports-injured patient. Orthop Clin North Am 1988 Oct; 19(4):725–735

Montgomery JB. Dislocation of the knee. Orthop Clin North Am 1987 Jan; 18(1): 149–156

Fractures

American Pain Society. Relieving pain: An analgesic guide. Am J Nurs 1988 Jun; 88(6):815–825

Antrum R and Solomkin J. A review of antibiotic prophylaxis of open fractures. Orthop Rev 1987 Apr; 16(4): 246–254

Bone L and Bucholz R. The management of fractures in the patient with multiple trauma. J Bone Joint Surg (Am) 1986 Jul; 68(6):845–949

Bray TJ et al. The displaced femoral neck fracture. Internal fixation versus bipolar endoprosthesis. Clin Orthop 1988 May; 230:127–140

Burgess AR et al. Management of open grade III tibial fractures. Orthop Clin North Am 1987 Jan; 18(1):85–93

Burgess AR et al. Pedestrian tibial injuries. J Trauma 1987 Jun; 27(6): 596–601

Carlson DC. Common fractures of the extremities. How to recognize and treat them. Postgrad Med 1988 Mar; 83(4):311–317

Christie J et al. Intramedullary locking nails in the management of femoral shaft fractures. J Bone Joint Surg (Br) 1988 Mar; 70(2):206–210

Cooke PH and Newman JH. Fractures of the femur in relation to cemented hip prosthesis. J Bone Joint Surg (Br) 1988 May; 70(3):366–369

Dellinger EP et al. Risk of infection after open fracture on the arm or leg. Arch Surg 1988 Nov; 123(11):1320–1327

Edwards CC et al. Severe open tibial fractures. Results treating 202 injuries with external fixation. Clin Orthop 1988 May; 230:98–115

Gabel GT et al. Intraarticular fractures of the distal humerus in the adult. Clin Orthop 1987 Mar; 216:99–108

Gershuni DH et al. Fracture of the tibia complicated by acute compartment syndrome. Clin Orthop 1987 Apr; 217: 221–227

Gamron R. Taking the pressure out of compartment syndrome. Am J Nurs 1988 Aug; 88(8):1076–1080

Hansel MJ. Fractures and the healing process. Orthop Nurs 1988 Jan–Feb; 7(1):43–50

Harper MC and Hardin G. Posterior malleolar fractures of the ankle associated with external rotation–abduction injuries. Results with and without external fixation. J Bone Joint Surg (Am) 1988 Oct; 70(9):1348–1356

Jones–Walton P. Effects of pin care on pin reactions in adults with extremity fractures treated with skeletal traction and external fixation. Orthop Nurs 1988 Jul–Aug; 7(4):29–33

Lapik S and Woodbury D. Volkmann's ischemic contracture: A case report. Orthop Rev 1988 Jun; 17(6):618–624

Liang QY and Wu JW. Fracture of the patella treated by open reduction and external compression skeletal fixation. J Bone Joint Surg (Am) 1987 Jan; 69(1):83–89

Lhowe DW and Hansen ST. Immediate nailing of open fractures of the femoral shaft. J Bone Joint Surg (Am) 1988 Jul; 70(6):812–820

Loder RT. The influence of diabetes mellitus on the healing of closed fractures. Clin Orthop 1988 Jul; 232: 210–216

Matta JM and Merritt PO. Displaced acetabular fractures. Clin Orthop 1988 May; 230:83–97

Mayo KA. Fractures of the acetabulum. Orthop Clin North Am 1987 Jan; 18(1): 43–51

Merritt K. Factors increasing the risk of infection in patients with open fractures. J Trauma 1988 Jun; 28(6): 823–827

Miller B and Eden–Kilgour S. Preventing peroneal nerve damage. Orthop Nurs 1987 Jul–Aug; 6(4):41–46

Mims BC. Fat embolism syndrome: A variant of ARDS. Orthop Nurs 1989 May–Jun; 8(3):22–27

Peimer C. Compression neuropathies of the upper extremity. Orthop Rev 1987 Jun; 16(6):379–385

Schuind F et al. External fixation of clavical fracture for non-union in adults. J Bone Joint Surg (Am) 1988 Jun; 70(5):692–695

Seyfer AE and Lower R. Late results of free-muscle flaps and delayed bone grafting in the secondary treatment of open distal tibial fractures. Plast Reconstr Surg 1989 Jan; 83(1):77–84

Szabo RM and Weber SC. Comminuted intraarticular fractures of the distal radius. Clin Orthop 1988 Mar; 230:39–48

tenDuis HJ et al. Fat embolism in patients with an isolated fracture of the femoral shaft. J Trauma 1988 Mar; 28(3):383–390

Waldrop J et al. Fractures of the posterolateral tibial plateau. Am J Sports Med 1988 Sep–Oct; 16(5):492–498

Zagorski JB et al. Diaphyseal fractures of the humerus. Treatment with prefabricated braces. J Bone Joint Surg (Am) 1988 Apr; 70(4):607–610

Hip Fractures

Billing N, Ahmed SW and Kenmore PL. Hip fracture. Depression cognitive impairment: A follow-up study. Orthop Rev 1988 Mar; 17(3):315–320

Felson DT. Prevention of hip fractures. Hosp Pract 1988 Sep; 23(9A):23–32, 37–38

Krug BM. The hip: Nursing fracture patients to full recovery. RN 1989 Apr; 52(4):56–61

Reinhard S. Case managing community services for hip fractured elders. Orthop Nurs 1988 Sep–Oct; 7(5):42–49, 71

Pelvic Fractures

Coyer HM et al. Pelvic fracture classification: Correlation with hemorrhage. J Trauma 1988 Jul; 28(7): 973–980

Denis F, Davis S and Comfort T. Sacral

fractures: An important problem. Clin Orthop 1988 Feb; 227:67–81

Kellam JF et al. The unstable pelvic fracture: Operative treatment. Orthop Clin North Am 1987 Jan; 18(1):25–41

Lin PS et al. Acute bowel entrapment and perforation following operative reduction of pelvic fracture. J Trauma 1987 Jun; 27(6):684–686

Lowe MA et al. Risk factors for urethral injuries in men with traumatic pelvic fractures. J Urol 1988 Sep; 140(3):506–507

Mucha P Jr and Welch JT. Hemorrhage in major pelvic fractures. Surg Clin North Am 1988 Aug; 68(4):757–773

Seibel RW and Flint L. Management of complicated pelvic fractures. Curr Surg 1986 Sep–Oct; 43(5):391–394

Spirnak JP. Pelvic fracture and injury to the lower urinary tract. Surg Clin North Am 1988 Oct; 68(5):1057–1069

Tile M. Pelvic ring fractures: Should they be fixed? J Bone Joint Surg (Br) 1988 Jan; 70(1):1–12

Ward EF et al. Open reduction and internal fixation of vertical shear pelvic fractures. J Trauma 1987 Mar; 27(3): 291–295

Other Management Modalities

American Pain Society. Relieving pain: An analgesic guide. Am J Nurs 1988 Jun; 88(6):815–825

Calhoun JH and Burke EE. Orthopedic rehabilitation at home. Phys Med Rehabil 1988 Aug; 2(3):415–459

Dunwoody CJ. Patient controlled analgesia: Rationale, attributes, and essential factors. Orthop Nurs 1987 Sep–Oct; 6(5):31–36

Hines NA and Bates MS. Discharging the patient in skeletal traction. Orthop Nurs 1987 Jul–Aug; 6(4):21–24

Holmes R et al. Nutrition know how: Combating pressure sores—nutritionally. Am J Nurs 1987 Oct; 87(10):1301–1303

Lavine LS and Grodzinsky AJ. Electrical stimulation in repair of bone. J Bone Joint Surg (Am) 1987 Apr; 69(4):626–630

Newschwander GE and Dunst RM. Limb lengthening with Ilizarov external fixator. Orthop Nurs 1989 May–Jun; 8(3):15–21

Osborne LJ and DiGiacomo I. Traction: A review with nursing diagnoses and interventions. Orthop Nurs 1987 Jul–Aug; 6(4):13–19

Paley D et al. Ilizarov treatment of tibial nonunions with bone loss. Clin Orthop 1989 Apr; 241:146–165

Rubin M. The physiology of bedrest. Am J Nurs 1988 Jan; 88(1):50–56

Wienke VK. Pressure sores: Prevention is the challenge. Orthop Nurs 1987 Jul–Aug; 6(4):26–30

Orthopedic Surgery

Special Nursing Considerations

Preoperative Nursing Interventions

1. Conduct nursing assessment according to standards for individuals undergoing surgery.
2. Assess nutritional status; hydration, protein and caloric intake. Elderly persons undergoing orthopedic surgery are at risk for undernutrition and poor healing.
3. Determine if person has had previous corticosteroid therapy—could contribute to current orthopedic condition (aseptic necrosis of the femoral head; osteoporosis), as well as affect the patient's response to anesthesia and the stress of surgery.
4. Determine if the person has an infection (cold, dental, skin, urinary tract infection)—could contribute to development of osteomyelitis following surgery.

Patient Education

1. Teach patient about the following: tests and routines, coughing and deep-breathing, and immediate postoperative activities.
2. Have the patient practice voiding in bedpan or urinal in recumbent position before surgery. This helps reduce the need for postoperative catheterization.
3. Acquaint the patient with traction apparatus and the need for splints and casts—to familiarize him with postoperative environment.

Postoperative Assessment and Nursing Interventions

A. Assess Cardiovascular Status

Evaluate the blood pressure and pulse rates frequently—rising pulse rate or slowly falling blood pressure indicates persistent bleeding or development of a state of shock.

B. Assess Respiratory Status and Maintain Sufficient Pulmonary Ventilation

1. Avoid or give respiratory depressant drugs in minimal doses.
2. Change position every 2 hours—mobilizes secretions and helps prevent bronchial obstruction.

C. Monitor Neurovascular Status (Nerve Function and Circulation) of Affected Extremity

1. Watch circulation distal to the part where cast, bandage, or splint has been applied.
2. Prevent constriction leading to interference with blood or nerve supply.
3. Elevate affected extremity and apply ice packs as directed.
4. Watch toes and fingers for healthy color.
5. Check pulses of affected extremity; compare with unaffected extremity.
6. Note skin temperature.
7. Document observations.

NURSING ALERT: If neurovascular problems are identified, notify surgeon and loosen cast or dressing at once.

D. Monitor for Hemorrhage—orthopedic wounds have a tendency to ooze more than other surgical wounds

1. Measure suction drainage if used.
2. Anticipate up to 200–500 ml. of drainage in the first 24 hours, decreasing to less than 30 ml. per 8 hours within 48 hours, depending on surgical procedure.

E. Assess Pain

1. Institute pain relief measures as prescribed.
2. Be aware that muscle spasms may contribute to pain experience.
3. Administer prescribed parenteral medications to control pain during the first few postoperative days.
    a. Avoid injection sites near operative site.
    b. Swelling and edema in operative area reduce absorption.
    c. Rotate injection sites.
4. Use patient-controlled analgesia (PCA) according to standards of care.

F. Prevent Venous Complications

1. Encourage the patient to exercise by himself with a planned program of exercise as soon as possible after surgery.
2. Have the patient flex his knee, extend the knee with hip still flexed, and then lower the extremity to the bed.

3. Encourage the patient to move fingers and toes periodically.
4. Advise the patient to move joints that are not fixed by traction or appliance through their range of motion as fully as possible.
5. Suggest muscle-setting exercises (quadriceps setting) if active motion is contraindicated.
6. Apply antiembolism stockings as prescribed.
7. Give prophylactic anticoagulants as directed (heparin, warfarin, aspirin, etc.).
8. Encourage early resumption of activity.

G. Watch for Signs and Symptoms of Anemia—especially after fracture of long bones

1. Fractures bleed into the adjacent tissues.
2. Blood loss from fracture and at time of surgery can result in anemia.
3. Hemoglobin and hematocrit determinations done in postoperative period indicate status and possible need for therapeutic intervention.
4. Report below-normal results to surgeon.

H. Provide a Balanced Diet

1. Increase fluids and fiber to reduce incidence of constipation associated with immobility.
2. Avoid giving large amounts of milk to orthopedic patients on bedrest—adds to calcium pool in the body and demands more calcium excretion by the kidneys, predisposing to the formation of urinary calculi.
3. Administer iron suppliment for anemia as prescribed.

I. Maintain Urinary Output by Maintaining Adequate Fluid Intake

Watch for urinary retention—elderly men with some degree of prostatism may have difficulty in voiding.

J. Monitor for Signs and Symptoms of Infection

1. Monitor vital signs.
2. Examine incision for redness, increased temperature, swelling, and induration.
3. Note character of drainage.
4. Evaluate complaints of recurrent or increasing pain.
5. Administer antibiotic therapy as prescribed.

Patient Education

1. Teach the patient activities that will minimize the development of complications (e.g., turning, coughing, and deep-breathing).
2. Instruct the patient in dietary considerations to facilitate healing and minimize development of constipation and renal calculi.
3. Inform the patient of techniques that facilitate moving while minimizing associated discomforts (e.g., supporting injured area and practicing smooth, gentle position changes).

Arthroplasty and Total Joint Replacement

Arthroplasty is reconstructive surgery to restore joint motion and function and to relieve pain. It generally involves replacement of bony joint structure by a prosthesis.

Total joint arthroplasty is the replacement of both articulating surfaces with metal or plastic components.

Types of Joint Replacement

Total hip replacement (total joint arthroplasty) is the replacement of a severely damaged hip with an artificial joint. Although a large number of implants are available, most consist of a metal femoral component topped by a spherical ball fitted into a plastic acetabular socket (Fig. 31-1).

A *total knee arthroplasty* is an implant procedure in which tibial, femoral, and patellar joint surfaces are replaced because of destroyed knee joint (Fig. 31-2).

Considerations

1. The prostheses are of various designs and may be fixed to the remaining bone by cement, press fit, or bone ingrowth.
2. Selection of the prosthesis and fixation technique depends on individual patient's bone structure, joint stability, and other individual characteristics including age, weight, and activity level.
3. Arthroplasty is an exacting and meticulous procedure. To reduce the risk of an infected prosthesis, special precautions are carried out in the OR (impermeable OR attire, clean air system) to reduce particulate matter and bacterial count of the air.

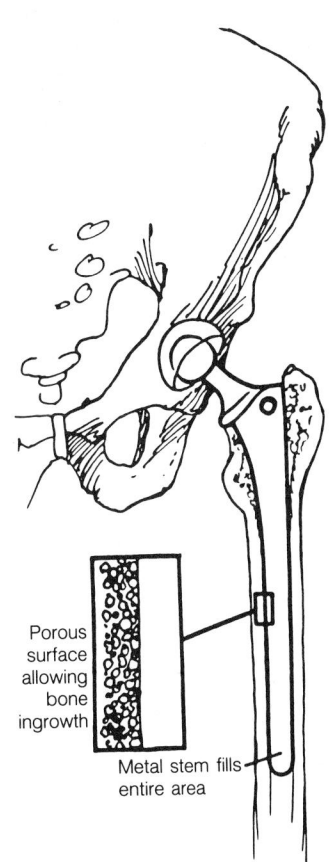

Porous surface allowing bone ingrowth

Metal stem fills entire area

Figure 31-1. *Total hip replacement using ingrowth porous-coated prosthesis. (Photo courtesy Charles Engh, M.D., Arlington, VA)*

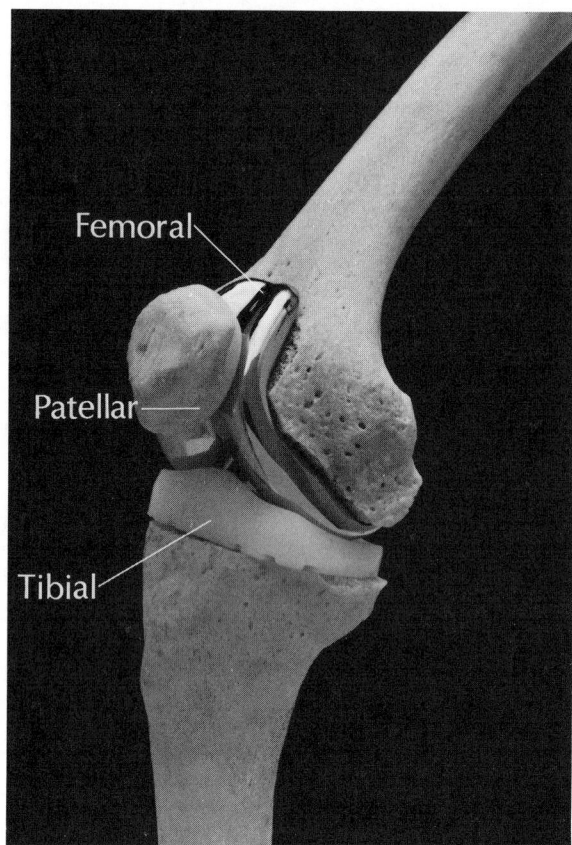

Figure 31-2. *Total knee replacement. (Photo courtesy Richards Manufacturing Co., Inc.)*

Clinical Indications

1. For patients with unremitting pain, irreversibly damaged joints
   Primary degenerative arthritis (osteoarthritis)
   Rheumatoid arthritis
2. Selected fractures (e.g., femoral neck fracture)
3. Failure of previous reconstructive surgery (osteotomy, cup arthroplasty, femoral neck fracture complications—nonunion, avascular necrosis)
4. Congenital hip disease
5. Pathologic fractures from metastatic cancer
6. Joint instability

Management

Reduce or eliminate pain.
Restore, improve, or maintain joint function.
Provide greater stability of the joint.

Preoperative Nursing Interventions

1. Assess patient for infections (bladder, dental, skin)—potential foci of infection for seeding prosthesis infection.
2. Provide preoperative patient teaching.
   a. Educate the patient concerning his postoperative regimen (e.g., extended exercise program will be carried out after surgery—atrophied muscles must be reeducated and strengthened).
   b. Teach isometric exercises (muscle setting) of quadriceps and gluteal muscles; teach active ankle motion.
   c. Teach bed-to-wheelchair transfer without going beyond the hip flexion limits (usually 45 degrees).
   d. Practice nonweight- and partial weight-bearing ambulation with ambulatory aid (walker, crutches) to facilitate postoperative ambulation.
   e. Demonstrate abduction splint, knee immobilizer, or continuous passive motion (CPM) if equipment will be used postoperatively (Fig. 31-3).
3. Use antiembolism stockings to minimize development of thrombophlebitis.
4. Give meticulous skin preparation with antimicrobial solution to reduce skin microorganisms, a potential source of infection.
5. Administer antibiotics as prescribed to assure therapeutic blood level during and immediately after surgery. Antimicrobials usually given immediately preoperatively, intraoperatively, and postoperatively to reduce incidence of infection.

Postoperative Nursing Interventions

1. Assess the patient's position for compliance with positioning prescription.
   Note: Numerous modifications are required in positioning these patients postoperatively.
   Following hip arthroplasty
   a. The patient is usually positioned supine in bed.
   b. The affected extremity is held in slight abduction by either an abduction splint or pillow or Buck's extension traction to prevent dislocation of the prosthesis.
   c. Avoid acute flexion of the hip.

NURSING ALERT: The patient must not adduct or flex operated hip—may produce dislocation. Signs of joint dislocation include shortened extremity, increasing discomfort, inability to move joints.

Following knee arthroplasty
   a. The knee may be immobilized in extension with a firm compression dressing and an adjustable soft extension splint or long-leg plaster cast.
   b. Leg is elevated on pillows to control swelling.
   c. Alternatively, continuous passive motion may be started.
2. Turn the patient to provide skin care and to prevent pressure sores.
   Following hip arthroplasty:
   a. Two nurses turn the patient on unoperated side while supporting operated hip securely in an abducted position; the entire length of leg is supported by pillows.
   Use pillows to keep the leg abducted; place pillow at back for comfort.
   b. Keep bed flat except during prescribed intervals to prevent hip flexion contracture.
   c. The bed is usually not elevated more than 45 degrees; placing the patient in an upright sitting position puts a strain on the hip joint and may cause dislocation.

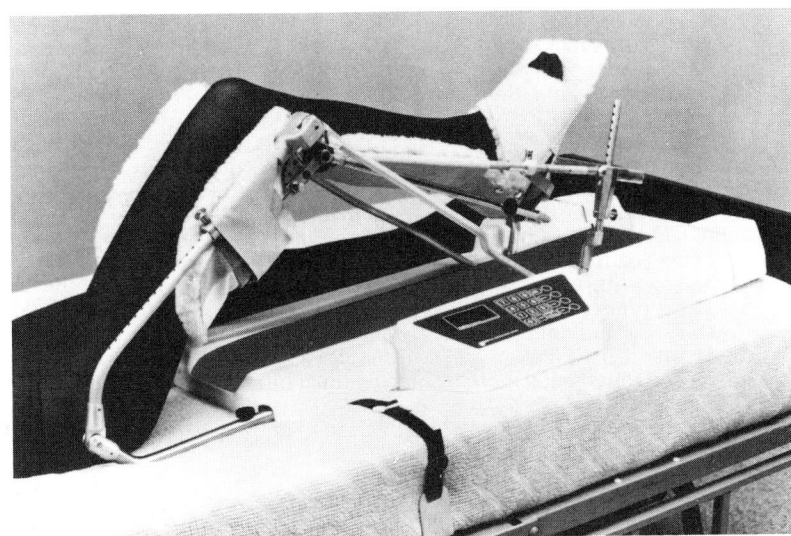

Figure 31-3. *Continuous passive motion device used for postoperative total knee arthroplasty patients to facilitate joint range of motion. (Courtesy of Sutter Biomedical Inc.)*

   d. Support the low back with a small pillow or towel when the patient is supine—to relieve strain placed on muscles by the flat position.

   e. As the patient becomes familiar with the turning routine, assist him to change position by using overhead trapeze.

3. Assist in use of the fracture bed pan
   a. Instruct the patient to flex the unoperated hip and knee and pull up on the trapeze to lift buttocks onto pan.
   b. Instruct the patient *NOT* to bear down on the operated hip in flexion when getting off the pan.

4. Assess the patient for development of early complications (hemorrhage, shock, nerve palsy, infection, and thromboembolic and respiratory complications).

Preventing Complications

1. Assess neurovascular status of operated extremity—check sensation, pulses, color, and skin temperature and compare with unoperated leg.

2. Monitor blood loss—portable suction is used to decrease incidence of wound hematoma, which is a possible focus of infection.

3. Thromboembolism (major threat following reconstructive hip operations).
   a. Continue to exercise ankles and legs—accelerates blood flow and prevents venous stasis.
   b. Antiembolic stockings for uninvolved extremity—to increase venous velocity; elastic stocking applied to operated extremity when elastic compression dressing is removed.
   c. Check for calf edema, tenderness, local pain.
   d. Heparin, warfarin, aspirin—may be used for thromboembolic prophylaxis.

4. Infection
   a. Give antimicrobials as directed.
   b. Watch for elevation of temperature and inspect wound at intervals.
   c. Infection may not become apparent until months or years after surgery.
   d. Deep infection almost always requires removal of implant.

5. Complicating medical conditions (cardiac, gastrointestinal, genitourinary).

6. Pain
Give narcotics as required the first 24 hours postoperatively and then taper to nonnarcotic analgesia thereafter.

7. Contractions
   a. Encourage the patient to carry out prescribed exercise program, usually under direction of physical therapist.
   b. Assist and encourage the patient during exercise.
   c. Assist the patient in use of continuous passive motion equipment. Early postoperative passive exercise of joint facilitates joint healing and restoration of joint range of motion.

Promoting Mobility

Following hip arthroplasty:
1. Use an abduction splint or pillows while assisting the patient to get out of bed.
   a. Keep the hip at maximum extension.
   b. Instruct the patient to pivot on unoperated extremity.
   c. Assess the patient for orthostatic hypotension.

2. When the patient is ready to ambulate, teach him to advance the walker and then advance the operated extremity to the walker permitting weight-bearing as prescribed.

3. With increased stability, patient progresses to use of crutches or cane as prescribed.

Following knee arthroplasty,
1. The patient may transfer out of bed into wheelchair with extension splint in place.

2. No weight-bearing is permitted until prescribed by the orthopedic surgeon.

Discharge Planning/Patient Education

Instruct the patient as follows:
1. Continue to wear elastic stockings after going home until full activities are resumed.

2. Avoid excessive hip adduction, flexion, and rotation.
   a. Avoid sitting in low chair/toilet seat.

    b. Keep knees apart; do *not* cross legs.
    c. Limit sitting to 30 minutes at a time—to minimize hip flexion and the risk of prosthetic dislocation and to prevent hip stiffness and flexion contracture.
3. Continue quadriceps setting and range-of-motion exercises as directed.
    a. Have a *daily* program of stretching, exercise, and rest throughout lifetime.
    b. Do not participate in any activity placing undue or sudden stress on joint (jogging, jumping, lifting heavy loads, becoming obese, excessive bending and twisting).
    c. Use a cane when taking fairly long walks.
4. Use self-help and energy-saving devices.
    a. Handrails by toilet
    b. Raised toilet seat if there is some residual hip flexion problem
    c. Bar-type stool for shower and kitchen work
5. Lie prone twice daily for 30 minutes.
6. Report for follow-up evaluation and testing.
7. Monitor for late complications—deep infection, increased pain and/or decreased function associated with loosening of prosthetic components, implant wear, dislocation, fracture of components, avascular necrosis or dead bone caused by loss of blood supply, heterotrophic ossification (formation of bone in periprosthetic space).
8. Use supportive equipment (crutches, canes, raised toilet seat) as prescribed.
9. Take prophylactic antibiotic if undergoing any procedure known to cause bacteremia (tooth extraction, manipulation of genitourinary tract).
10. Avoid MRI studies, because of implanted metal component.

Amputation

Amputation is the total or partial surgical removal of an extremity. Amputation is considered a surgical reconstructive procedure.

Conditions Warranting Amputation

1. Inadequate tissue perfusion such as results with diabetes mellitus or other peripheral vascular diseases
2. Severe trauma
3. Malignant tumor
4. Congenital deformity

Diagnostic Evaluation

1. Hemodynamic evaluation—angiography, arterial blood flow, xenon[133]—to determine optimal amputation level
2. Culture and sensitivity tests of draining wounds to assist in control of infection preoperatively
3. Evaluation of sound (contralateral) extremity
4. Evaluation of cardiovascular, respiratory, renal, and other body systems to determine preoperative condition of patient

NURSING ALERT: Amputation of the lower extremity can be a life-threatening procedure, especially in patients over the age of 60 with peripheral vascular disease. Significant morbidity accompanies above-knee amputations because of associated poor health and disease, as well as the complications of sepsis and malnutrition and the physiologic insult of amputation.

5. Evaluation of the patient's and family's emotional response to amputation
    a. Anticipation of relief of pain related to amputation is frequent.
    b. Distress at anticipated loss of body part exhibited by patient and family

Management

1. The surgeon considers possible limb salvage techniques.
    a. Revascularization
    b. Hyperbaric oxygenation
    c. Tumor resection with bone grafting
2. Determines level for amputation based on level of maximal viable tissue for wound healing
3. Develops a functional, nontender, pressure tolerant residual limb.

Types of Amputation

A. Open (Guillotine)

1. Used with infection and patients who are poor surgical risks
2. Wound heals by granulation or secondary closure in about a week.

B. Closed (Myoplastic)

1. Residual limb is covered by a flap of skin.
2. Flap of skin is sutured posteriorly.

Types of Dressings

A. Soft Dressing

1. Secured with elastic bandage
2. Permits wound inspection
3. Used with patients who should avoid early weight-bearing (e.g., those with peripheral vascular disease)

B. Closed, Rigid Plaster Dressing

1. Applied immediately after surgery
2. Controls edema
3. Support circulation, promoting healing
4. Minimizes pain on movement
5. Shapes residual limb
6. Permits attachment of prosthetic extension (pylon) and early ambulation

Preoperative Nursing Diagnoses

1. Anxiety related to proposed amputation
2. Pain related to primary condition requiring amputation
3. Altered physical mobility related to disfunctional limb and general muscle weakness
4. Altered health maintenance related to chronic health problem
5. Knowledge deficit of expected participation in projected rehabilitation program

Preoperative Nursing Interventions

A. Reducing Anxiety

1. Support concept of amputation as a surgical reconstructive procedure.
2. Explore patient's perception of procedure and impact on life-style.
3. Avoid unrealistic and misleading reassurance—management of prosthesis can be slow and painful.

4. Encourage the patient to attain his maximal physical and emotional state of health in preparation for rehabilitation.

B. Relieving Pain

1. Instruct patient on use of pain-modifying techniques.
2. Inform the patient of the availability of postoperative pain medication.
3. Explain to the patient that he will continue to "feel" (phantom sensations) the amputated body part for some time.

C. Increasing Mobility

1. Encourage the patient to reposition self every 1–2 hours.
2. Encourage good posture.
3. Teach exercises to strengthen muscles for use of ambulatory aids (lower limb amputee).
   a. Flex and extend arms while holding traction weights.
   b. Do push-ups from a prone position if feasible.
   c. Do sit-ups from a seated position if feasible.
4. Teach use of ambulatory aids.
   a. Instills confidence in ability
   b. Maintains mobility
   c. Prepares for postoperative mobility

D. Establishing Maximal Health Status Prior to Surgery

1. Evaluate each body system for adequacy of function.
2. Assess laboratory reports for optimal values (e.g., hematology, urinalysis, and blood chemistries are within normal limits).
3. Encourage balanced diet with adequate protein to enhance wound healing.

E. Patient Education

1. Clarify plans for management of perioperative and postoperative periods as outlined by the physician.
2. Teach postoperative routines (i.e., turn, cough, deep breathe, etc.).
3. Explain various phases of rehabilitation. Active participation in rehabilitation is essential for a successful outcome.
4. Introduce the patient to the physical therapist.
5. Discuss possible use of prostheses. Not all amputees can benefit from a prosthesis.
   a. Diabetes mellitus, heart disease, infection, stroke, COPD, peripheral vascular disease, and increasing age are factors limiting rehabilitation.
   b. Wound breakdown, infection, and delay in healing of residual limb delay rehabilitation.

Postoperative Nursing Diagnoses

1. Potential fluid volume deficit related to hemorrhage from disrupted surgical hemostasis
2. Altered tissue perfusion related to edema and tissue responses to surgery and prosthesis
3. Ineffective coping related to change in body image and self-care
4. Pain related to surgical procedure and phantom sensations
5. Altered physical mobility related to amputation, muscle weakness, change in body weight distribution
6. Knowledge deficit of management of residual limb (stump) and prosthesis

Postoperative Nursing Interventions

> **NURSING ALERT:** Prevention of complications associated with a major operation and facilitation of early rehabilitation are essential to prevent prolonged disability. Frequent monitoring of the patient's physiologic responses to anesthesia, surgery, and immobility are required.

A. Monitoring Fluid Balance

1. Monitor patient for systemic symptoms of excessive blood loss.
2. Watch for excessive wound drainage.
   a. Keep tourniquet (in view) attached to end of bed to apply to residual limb (stump) if excessive bleeding occurs.
   b. Reinforce dressing as required, using aseptic technique.
   c. Measure suction drainage.
   d. Maintain accurate record of bloody drainage on dressing and in drainage system.
3. Monitor intake and output for fluid balance.

B. Maintaining Adequate Tissue Perfusion

1. Control edema.
   a. Elevate residual limb to promote venous return.
   b. Use air splint if prescribed.
2. Maintain pressure dressing.
   a. Reapply if necessary, using sterile dressing secured with elastic bandage.
   b. Notify surgeon if rigid cast dressing comes off.

C. Supporting Effective Coping

1. Accept patient responses to loss of body part (i.e., depression, withdrawal, denial, frustration).
2. Encourage expression of fears and concerns.
3. Recognize that modification of body image takes time.
4. Encourage participation in rehabilitation planning and self-care.
5. Assist patient to adapt to changes in self-care activities.
   a. Upper extremity amputation—encourage independence in one-handed self-care activities using one-handed aids (e.g., one-handed knife) as needed.
   b. Lower extremity amputation—encourage mobility using transfer assistance and ambulatory aids as needed.

D. Controlling Pain

1. Surgical pain
   a. Assess the patient's pain experience.
   b. Administer prescribed medications as needed to control postoperative pain.
   c. Use nonpharmaceutical pain management techniques.
   d. Recognize that increasing discomfort may indicate presence of hematoma, infection, or necrosis.
2. Phantom sensations (pain)
   a. Anticipate complaint of pain and sensation located in the missing limb ("phantom pain").
   b. Use physical modalities (e.g., wrapping, temperature changes) and TENS, if prescribed, in relieving discomfort.
   c. Encourage patient activity to decrease awareness of phantom limb pain.
   d. Reassure the patient that phantom limb pain will diminish over time.

E. Promoting Physical Activity

1. Encourage frequent repositioning in bed.
2. Teach patient to avoid long periods in one position.
   a. Avoids dependent edema.
   b. Avoids flexion deformity.
   c. Avoids skin pressure areas.

3. Prevent deformities.
   a. Lower extremity amputations—hip flexion contracture (avoid placing residual limb on pillow; encourage prone position twice a day) and abduction deformity (use trochanter roll; avoid pillow between legs).

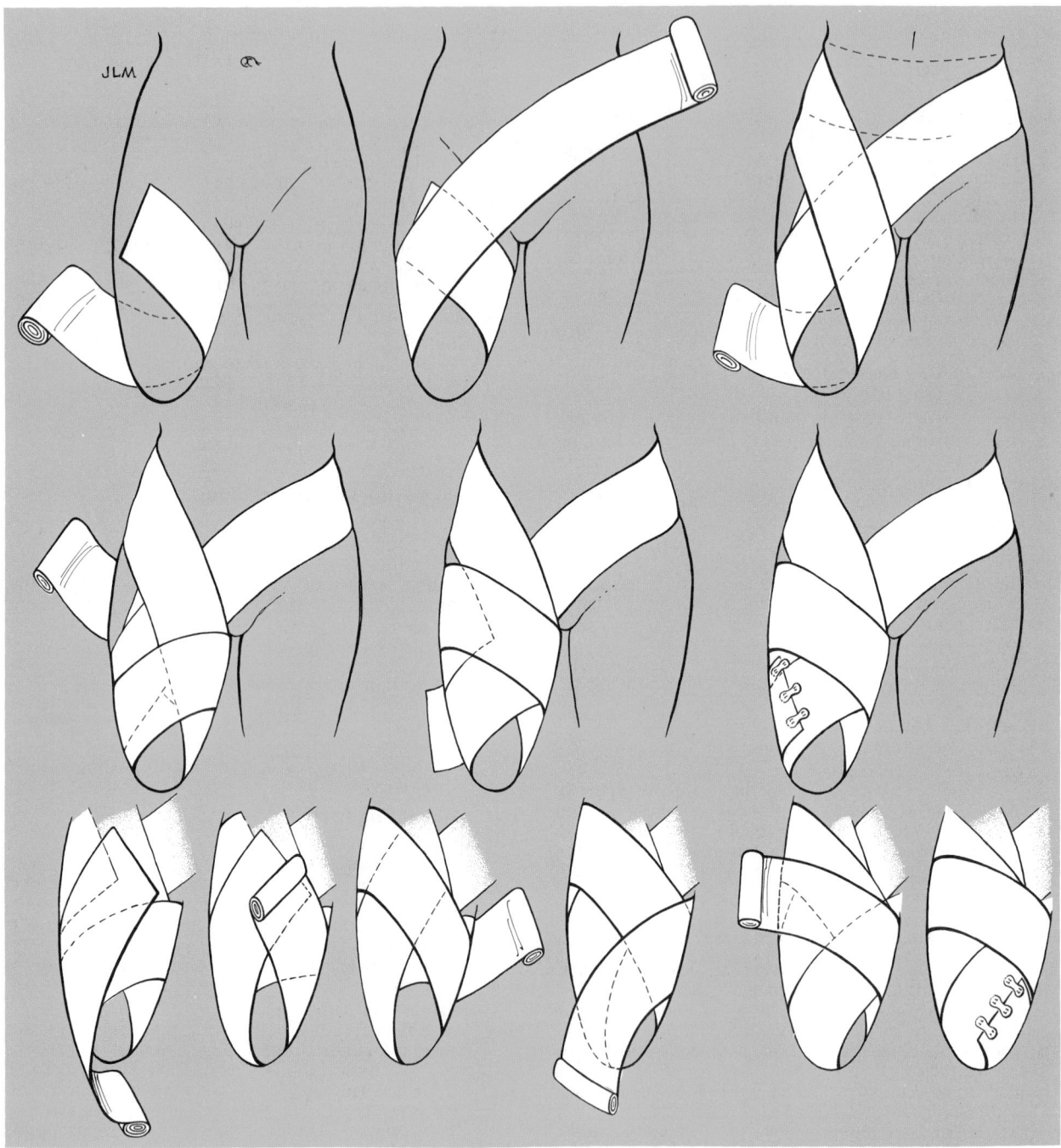

Figure 31-4. *Wrapping above-knee residual limb. Elastic bandaging reduces edema and shapes the residual limb in a firm conical form for the prosthesis.*

b. Upper extremity amputations—postural abnormalities (encourage good posture).
4. Encourage active range of motion and muscle-strengthening exercises when prescribed to:
    a. Minimize muscle atrophy.
    b. Increase muscle strength.
    c. Prepare residual limb for prosthesis.
5. Promote reestablishment of balance (amputation alters distribution of body weight).
    a. Transfer to chair within 48 hours of surgery.
    b. Instruct and guard lower limb amputee during balance exercises (i.e., arise from chair; stand on toes holding onto chair; bend knee holding onto chair; balance on one leg without support; hop on one foot while holding onto chair).
6. Supervise ambulation, use of wheelchair, and self-care activities.

Patient Education

1. Teach patient and family how to wrap residual limb with elastic bandage to control edema and to form a firm conical shape for prosthesis fitting (Figs. 31-4 and 31-5).
    a. Wrapping generally begins 1–3 days after surgery or after hard plaster dressing is removed.
    b. Use diagonal figure 8 bandaging technique.
    c. Wrap distal to proximal to maintain pressure gradient and to control edema.
    d. Begin wrapping with minimal tension and increase as wound heals and sutures are removed.
    e. Flatten skin at ends of incision to ensure conical stump shape.
    f. Rewrap residual limb a couple of times a day and as necessary to achieve a smooth, graded tension dressing.
    g. Rewrap if patient complains of more pain—dressing is probably too tight.
    h. Keep residual limb wrapped at all times except when bathing.
2. Teach patient residual limb-conditioning.
    a. Push the residual limb against a soft pillow.
    b. Gradually push residual limb against harder surfaces.
    c. Massage healed residual limb to soften scar, decrease tenderness, and improve vascularity.
3. Fitting of prosthesis

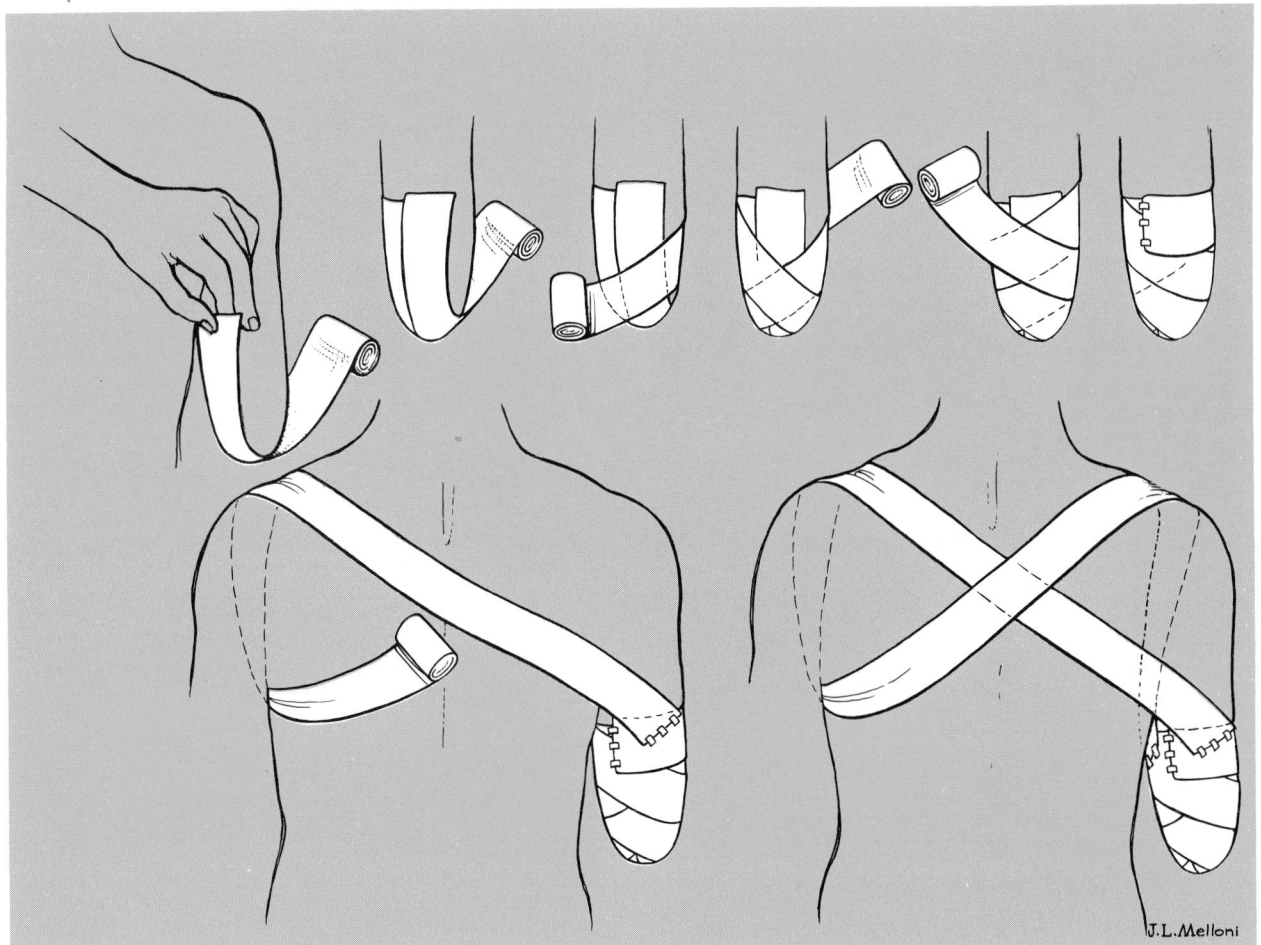

Figure 31-5. *Wrapping above-elbow residual limb. Elastic bandaging reduces edema and shapes the residual limb for the prosthesis. Bandage may need to be secured by wrapping across back and shoulders.*

a. Note residual limb contour.

b. Assess for residual limb contraction.

c. When maximum shrinkage occurs, the prosthetist measures and fits the prosthesis.

d. Adjustments are made by the prosthetist to minimize skin problems.

4. Continuing care of residual limb and prosthesis.

a. Instruct patient to wash and dry limb thoroughly at least twice a day, removing all soap residue, to prevent skin irritation and infection.

b. Avoid soaking residual limb because it results in edema.

c. Inspect residual limb and skin under prosthesis harness daily for pressure, irritation, and actual skin breakdown.

d. Wear residual limb sock/cotton underwear—to absorb perspiration and to avoid direct contact between prosthetic socket/harness and skin.

e. Avoid wrinkles in residual limb sock—potential pressure areas.

f. Wipe the socket of prosthesis with a damp cloth when prosthesis is removed for evening.

g. Have prosthesis checked periodically.

5. Teach patient to protect the remaining extremity from injury and to secure prompt treatment of problems.

Discharge Planning

1. The patient will require referral to rehabilitation services to achieve maximal level of independence.

2. Ongoing support is needed for adjustment to change in body image and independent functioning.

Evaluation

1. Maintains fluid balance: avoids excessive blood loss following surgery; maintains hematology values in normal range; avoids systemic symptoms of excess blood loss; maintains optimal hydration

2. Controls residual limb edema: elevates residual limb; maintains pressure dressing; achieves conical shape residual limb needs for prosthesis fitting

3. Exhibits behavior indicating effective coping and adjustment to altered body image; has realistic future orientation; participates in self-care activities; uses assistive devices effectively

4. Controls discomfort through variety of pain control modalities: describes decreasing frequency of phantom pain experiences

5. Increases physical mobility: repositions self in bed; avoids contractures and deformities; participates in active range of motion, muscle-strengthening, balance, postural, and other exercises as prescribed

6. Demonstrates ability to care for residual limb and prosthesis: washes residual limb daily; inspects residual limb and skin under harness for skin pressure, irritation, or breakdown; keeps residual limb wrapped at all times; works with physical therapist and prosthetist to obtain optimal fit and function; demonstrates ability to care for residual limb and prosthesis

Low Back Pain

Low back pain is characterized by an uncomfortable or acute pain in the lumbosacral area associated with severe spasm of the paraspinal muscles, often with radiating pain.

Muscle spasm is a condition in which muscles are painfully contracted.

Etiology

(Multiple causes)

1. Mechanical (joint, muscular, or ligamentous sprain)

2. Degenerative disc disease; acute herniation of disc(s)

3. Lack of physical activity and exercise; weakness of musculature of back

4. Arthritic conditions

5. Diseases of bone (osteoporosis, vertebral fracture, Paget's disease, metastatic carcinoma)

6. Congenital disorders

7. Systemic diseases

8. Infections of disc spaces or vertebrae

9. Spinal cord tumors

10. Referred pain from other areas

Diagnostic Evaluation

1. History—to determine when, where, and how the pain occurs, aggravating or relieving factors, relationship of pain to specific activities, presence of numbness or paresthesia.

2. Neurologic evaluation—to spot localized weakness of extremities and reflex and sensory loss; to exclude neurogenic disease.

3. Evaluation of muscular system—for changes in strength, tone, and flexibility of key posture muscles.

4. Diagnostic studies

a. X-rays of lumbar spine (anteroposterior, lateral, and oblique)

b. Computed tomography of spine.

Note: If patient has neurological deficit, intractable pain, loss of bowel and/or bladder control, chronic depression, or 7–10 days of conservative treatment without improvement, additional studies may be appropriate.

c. Electromyography—to record changes in electric potential of muscle and nerves leading to it

d. Magnetic resonance imaging

e. Myelography

f. Psychological testing (e.g., Minnesota Multiphasic Personality Inventory [MMPI]).

Management

1. Rest in bed in a semi-Fowler's position (hips and knees flexed)—to relieve painful muscle and ligament sprain, heal soft tissue injury, remove stress from lumbar sacral area, relieve tension on sciatic nerves, and open the posterior part of the intervertebral spaces

a. Acute spasm should subside in 3–7 days if there is no nerve involvement or other serious underlying disease.

b. Do prescribed isometric exercises hourly while on bed rest if possible.

2. Heat or ice used to relax muscle spasm and relieve discomfort. Follow heat by massage.

3. Medications

a. Oral pain medication and muscle relaxants.

b. Painful trigger points may be injected with hydrocortisone/xylocaine for pain relief (by physician).

c. Parenteral pain medication in acute severe pain syndromes.

4. Pelvic traction and manipulation may be used to relax muscles. (Fig. 31-6)

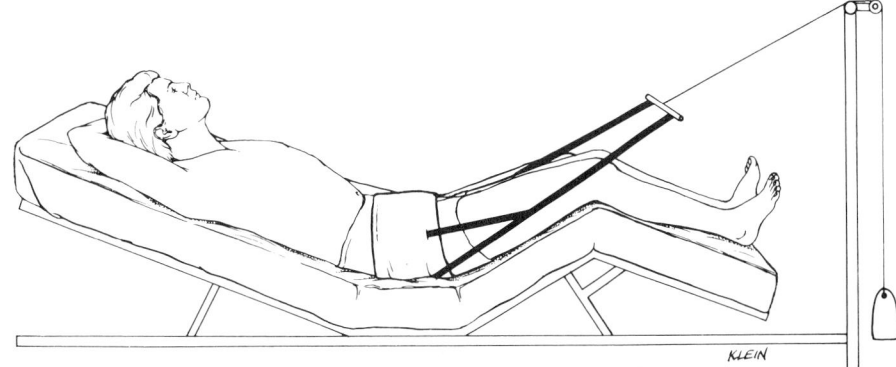

Figure 31-6. *Pelvic traction with lumbar flexion to alleviate low back pain. (From Brunner LS and Suddarth DS. Textbook of Medical–Surgical Nursing. 6th ed. Philadelphia, JB Lippincott, 1988)*

5. Lumbosacral support may be used—provides abdominal compression and decreases load on lumbar intervertebral discs.
6. Transcutaneous nerve stimulation (TENS) may be helpful in relieving pain.
7. Psychiatric intervention may be needed for the patient with chronic depression, anxiety, and low back syndrome.
    Psychotropic medication may be used for treatment of depression and anxiety, which potentiate pain.

Nursing Interventions

A. Relieving Discomfort

See Pain related to musculoskeletal disorders, page 763
1. Advise the patient to rest in bed. (Rest in bed may eliminate the need for pain medications.)
2. Keep pillow between flexed knees while in side-lying position—minimizes strain on back muscles.
3. Apply heat (moist towels; hydrocolator packs) or ice as prescribed.
4. Administer pain medications and muscle relaxants as prescribed.

B. Assisting With Resumption of Activities

1. Encourage range-of-motion of all uninvolved joints.
2. Suggest gradual increase of activities and alternating activities with rest in semi-Fowler's position.
3. Avoid prolonged periods of standing or sitting.
4. Encourage the patient to discuss problems that may be contributing to his backache.
5. Encourage the patient to do prescribed back exercises (Fig. 31-7). Exercise keeps postural muscles strong, helps recondition the back and abdominal musculature, and serves as an outlet for emotional tension.

Patient Education

Instruct the patient to avoid recurrences as follows:
1. Standing, sitting, lying, and lifting properly are necessary for a healthy back.
2. Alternate periods of activity with periods of rest.
    a. Avoid prolonged *sitting* (intradiscal pressure in lumbar spine is higher during sitting), standing, and driving.
    b. Change positions and rest at frequent intervals.
    c. Avoid assuming tense, cramped positions.
    d. Sit in a straight back, fairly high-seated chair. Sit

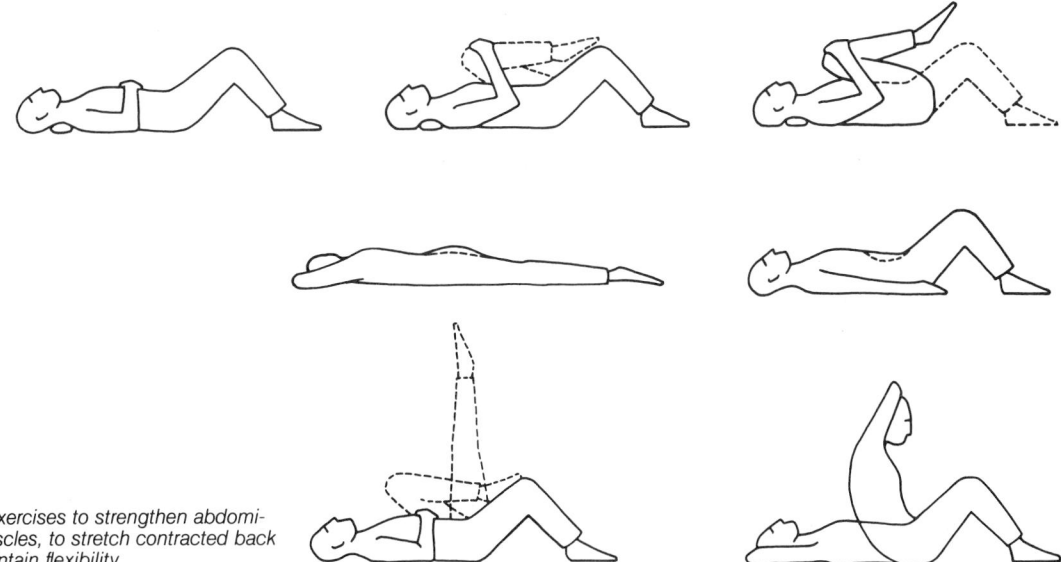

Figure 31-7. *Back exercises to strengthen abdominal and postural muscles, to stretch contracted back muscles, and to maintain flexibility.*

with the knees higher than the hips. Use a footstool.
   e. Flatten the hollow of the back by sitting with the buttocks "tucked under." Pelvic tilt (small of back is pressed against a flat surface)—decreases lordosis.
   f. Avoid knee and hip extension. When driving a car, have the seat pushed forward as necessary for comfort. Place a cushion in the small of the back for support.
3. When standing for any length of time, rest one foot on a small stool or wooden box to relieve lumbar lordosis.
4. Avoid fatigue, which contributes to spasm of back muscles.
   a. Sleep on a firm mattress
   b. Avoid sleeping in a prone position
   c. When lying on the side, place a pillow under the head and one between the flexed knees to reduce strain on the back muscles.
5. Pick up objects or loads correctly.
   a. Maintain a straight spine.
   b. Flex knees and hips while stooping.
   c. Keep load close to body.
   d. Lift with the legs.
   e. Avoid twisting trunk while lifting.
   f. Avoid lifting above waist level and reaching up for any length of time.
6. *Daily exercise is important in the prevention of back problems.*
   a. Do prescribed back exercises twice daily. Strengthens back, leg, and abdominal muscles.
   b. Walking outdoors (progressively increasing distance and pace) is recommended.
   c. Reduce weight if necessary. Decreases strain on back muscles.

Osteoporosis

Osteoporosis is a condition in which the bone matrix is lost, thereby weakening the bones and making them more susceptible to fracture.

Etiology

1. Occurs most frequently in postmenopausal women.
2. Other factors
   a. Age
   b. Inactivity
   c. Chronic illness
   d. Medications
   e. Calcium and vitamin D deficiency

Assessment

1. Identification of individuals at high risk (small, thin, white or Asian females; sedentary; nulliparity; early menopause; family history of osteoporosis; alcohol and/or cigarette use).
2. Review the patient's dietary pattern, assessing for adequate calcium and vitamin D intake.
3. Determine use of estrogens in menopausal and postmenopausal women.
4. Review x-ray reports for evidence of osteoporosis.
5. Assess symptoms associated with vertebral compression fracture—local back pain, loss of body height, kyphosis, respiratory (e.g., hypoventilation, episodic pneumonia) and abdominal (e.g., bloating, constipation) symptoms.

Clinical Manifestations

1. Demineralization is a silent process, causing no apparent problem until a fracture occurs following minor trauma.
2. Most frequent fractures associated with osteoporosis include fractures of the distal radius, vertebral bodies, proximal humerus, pelvis, and proximal femur (hip).

Management

A. Prevention

1. Adequate intake of calcium (RDA, 800 mg.)
2. Adequate intake of vitamin D (exposure to sunlight)
3. Weight-bearing exercise (walking) throughout life
4. Use of conjugated estrogen therapy for menopausal women, which is viewed as more effective than calcium supplements
5. Prevention of falls in the elderly

B. Patient Education

1. Encourage exercise for all. Teach the value of walking daily throughout life to provide stress required for strong bone remodeling.
2. Provide dietary education in relation to adequate daily intake of 800 mg. or more (1000–1500 mg.) of calcium. Anyone with a history of urinary tract stones should consult with the physician before increasing calcium intake.
3. Participate in dietary education related to vitamin D intake. Vitamin D is required for calcium absorption and utilization. Vitamin D requirements increase with age, especially when the person is not exposed to the sun.
4. Encourage young women at risk to maximize bone mass through nutrition and exercise.
5. Suggest perimenopausal women confer with the physician concerning need for calcium supplements and estrogen therapy.
6. Teach strategies to prevent falls. Assess home for hazards (e.g., scatter rugs, slippery floors, extension cords, adequate lighting). Encourage use of walking aids when balance is poor and muscle strength weakens.

Bone Tumors

Pathophysiology

A. Benign Bone Tumors

Osteoid osteoma, chondroma, and osteoclastoma (benign giant cell tumor) are examples of benign bone tumors. Malignant transformation occurs with some.

B. Malignant Bone Tumors

1. Chondrosarcoma and osteosarcoma are examples of primary malignant bone tumors. Hematogenous spread to the lung occurs.
2. Multiple myeloma is a malignant neoplasm arising from the bone marrow.

C. Metastatic Bone Tumors

1. Metastatic bone tumors are most frequently associated with cancers of the breast, the prostate, and the lung (primary malignancy site).
2. Bone metastasis most frequently occurs in the vertebrae and results in pathological fracture.

Clinical Manifestations

1. Pain in the involved bone—from effects of tumor (destruction, erosion, and expansion of tumor)
   a. Generally mild to constant pain, which may be worse at night or with activity.
   b. Pain will be acute with fracture.
   c. Neurological symptoms may present with nerve root compression.
2. Swelling and limitation of motion and joint effusion
3. *Physical findings*
   a. Palpable, tender, fixed bony mass
   b. Increase in skin temperature over mass
   c. Superficial veins dilated and prominent

Diagnostic Evaluation

1. X-ray will usually reveal bone tumor; may show increased or decreased bone density
2. Computed tomography and/or magnetic resonance imaging demonstrate soft tissue involvement and location of tumor(s)
3. Bone scan—helpful in detecting initial extent of malignancy, planning therapy, defining level of amputation, and following course of radiation/chemotherapy
4. Serum alkaline phosphatase—usually increased
5. Bence–Jones protein in urine with multiple myeloma
6. Biopsy of bone—to confirm suspected diagnosis
7. Chest x-ray and lung scan—to determine if metastases are present
8. Arteriography—to assess soft tissue involvement

Complications

1. Lack of tumor control and metastases
2. Pathological fracture
3. Hypercalcemia from bone destruction
4. Associated with treatment approaches
   a. Radiotherapy—poor wound healing, sloughing of tissue
   b. Chemotherapy—alopecia, nausea and vomiting, stomatitis, bone marrow depression, nephrotoxicity, ototoxicity, pulmonary fibrosis, peripheral neuropathy
   c. Surgery—fracture at biopsy site, delayed wound healing, neuroma and phantom pain with amputation, failure of limb salvage approach

Management

1. A multidisciplinary approach in a cancer center is often preferred.
2. The basic objective is to halt the progression of the tumor by destroying or removing the lesion.
3. Treatment depends on the type of tumor. Combinations of chemotherapy, surgery, and/or radiation may be indicated as most appropriate for specific type of tumor.
4. Surgery
   a. Tumor curettement or resection with bone grafting may be used.
   b. Limb-salvaging procedures involve resection of affected bone and surrounding normal muscle tissue and reconstruction using metallic prostheses or allografts for bone/joint replacement and skin grafting as needed.
5. Chemotherapy may be used as preoperative, adjunctive, and palliative treatment.
   a. Chemotherapy may be administered before (to shrink the tumor) and after (to destroy metastases) surgery.
   b. Chemotherapy used in combination to achieve a greater patient response at a lower toxicity rate and to minimize potential problems of drug resistance and may be given in varying courses separated by rest periods.
6. Radiotherapy
   a. Tumor irradiation may be used.
   b. Prophylactic lung irradiation may be carried out—to suppress metastases.
7. Immunotherapeutic approach may be selected.
8. Hormone therapy may be used with metastatic tumors of the breast and prostate.
9. If pathologic fracture occurs, the fracture is managed with open reduction and internal fixation or other fracture treatment method.

Nursing Interventions

A. Relieving Pain

1. Use multiple approaches to reduce discomfort.
2. Administer pain medications ½ hour before ambulation or other uncomfortable movement.
3. Support painful extremities on pillows.

B. Preventing Pathologic Fractures

1. Assist the patient in movement with gentleness and patience.
2. Avoid jarring the patient or bed.
3. Support joints when repositioning the patient.
4. Guard the patient to avoid falls.
5. Create a hazard-free environment.

C. Strengthening Coping Abilities

1. Create a supportive environment.
2. Use psychological support services as needed.

D. Promoting Self-Care Activities

1. Encourage the patient to help self.
2. Allow sufficient time for the patient to complete tasks.
3. Space activities to avoid fatigue.
4. Assist the patient as needed.

Bibliography

Books

Adams JC. Outline of Orthopaedics. 10th ed. Edinburgh, Churchill Livingstone, 1986

Albright J and Brand R (eds). The Scientific Basis of Orthopaedics. 2nd ed. Norwalk, Appleton & Lange, 1987

American Nurses' Association and National Association of Orthopaedic Nurses. Orthopaedic Nursing Practice. Kansas City, MO, American Nurses' Association, 1986

Avioli LV. The Osteoporotic Syndrome. 2nd ed. Orlando, Grune & Stratton, 1987

Bohne WHO. Atlas of Amputation Surgery. New York, Thieme Medical Publishers, 1987

Booth RE, Balderston RA and Rothman RH. Total Hip Arthroplasty. Philadelphia, WB Saunders, 1988

Borenstein DG and Wiesel SW. Low Back Pain. Philadelphia, WB Saunders, 1989

Brashear HR Jr and Raney RB. Handbook of Orthopaedic Surgery. 10th ed. St Louis, CV Mosby, 1986

Buckle P. Musculoskeletal Disorders at Work. London, Taylor and Francis, 1987

Cailliet R. Low Back Pain Syndrome. 4th ed. Philadelphia, FA Davis, 1988

Chapman MW (ed). Operative Orthopaedics. Philadelphia, JB Lippincott, 1988

Crenshaw AH (ed). Campbell's Operative Orthopaedics. 7th ed. St Louis, CV Mosby, 1987

Dahlin DC and Unni KK. Bone Tumors. 4th ed. Springfield, Il, Charles C Thomas, 1986

Dee R, Mango E and Hurst LC (eds). Principles of Orthopaedic Practice. New York, McGraw-Hill, 1988

Epps CH Jr. Complications in Orthopaedic Surgery. 2nd ed. Philadelphia, JB Lippincott, 1986

Farrell J. Illustrated Guide to Orthopedic Nursing. 3rd ed. Philadelphia, JB Lippincott, 1986

Gartland JJ. Fundamentals of Orthopaedics. 4th ed. Philadelphia, WB Saunders, 1987

Gerhardt JJ, King P and Guyer WD (eds). Interdisciplinary Rehabilitation in Orthopedic Medicine. Toronto, Hans Huber Publishers, 1987

Gerhardt JJ, King PS and Zettl JH. Immediate and Early Prosthetic Management. Toronto, Hans Huber Publishers, 1986

Hadler NM. Clinical Concepts in Regional Musculoskeletal Illness. Orlando, Grune & Stratton, 1987

Horowitz M. Stress Response Syndromes. Northvale, NJ, Aronson, 1986

Hughes SPF and Fitzgerald RH. Musculoskeletal Infections. Chicago, Year Book Medical Pub, 1986

Hughes SPF, Benson MK and Colton CL (eds). Orthopaedics: The Principles and Practice of Musculoskeletal Surgery and Fractures. Edinburgh, Churchill Livingstone, 1987

Iversen LD and Clawson DK. Manual of Acute Orthopaedic Therapeutics. 3rd ed. Boston, Little, Brown & Co, 1987

Kirkaldy-Willis WH (ed). Managing Low Back Pain. 2nd ed. New York, Churchill Livingstone, 1988

Laurin CA, Riley LH Jr. and Roy-Camille R (eds). Atlas of Orthopaedic Surgery. Chicago, Year Book Medical Pub, 1989

Lewis MM. Bone Tumor Surgery: Limb Sparing Techniques. Philadelphia, JB Lippincott, 1988

Lewis RC. Primary Care Orthopedics. New York, Churchill Livingstone, 1988

Mercies LR. Practical Orthopedics. 2nd ed. Chicago, Year Book Medical Pub, 1987

Mourad LA and Droste MM. The Nursing Process in the Care of Adults with Orthopaedic Conditions. 2nd ed. New York, John Wiley & Sons, 1988

Pellino T et al (eds). Core Curriculum for Orthopaedic Nursing. Pitman, NJ, National Association of Orthopaedic Nurses, 1986

Powell M (ed). Orthopaedic Nursing and Rehabilitation. 9th ed., Edinburgh, Churchill Livingstone, 1986

Reynolds D and Freeman M (eds). Osteoarthritis in the Young Adult Hip: Options for Surgical Management. Edinburgh, Churchill Livingstone, 1989

Rodrigo J. Orthopaedic Surgery: Basic Science and Clinical Science. Boston, Little, Brown & Co, 1986

Schlossberg D. Orthopedic Infection. New York, Springer-Verlag, 1988

Schoen DC. The Nursing Process in Orthopaedics. Norwalk, Appleton-Century-Crofts, 1986

Scott WN. Total Knee Revision Arthroplasty. Orlando, Grune & Stratton, 1987

Sikorski JM. Understanding Orthopaedics. Sydney, Butterworths, 1986

Sim FH. Diagnosis and Management of Metastatic Bone Disease. A Multidisciplinary Approach. New York, Raven Press, 1989

Smith C. Orthopaedic Nursing. London, Heinemann Nursing, 1987

Stearns CM and Brunner NA. Opcare: Orthopaedic Patient Care. A Nursing Guide, Vols 1-3. Rutherford, NJ, Howmedica, 1987

Tam CS, Heersche JNM and Murray TM. Metabolic Bone Disease: Cellular and Tissue Mechanisms. Boca Raton, CRC Press, 1989

Tollison CD and Kriegel ML (eds). Interdisciplinary Rehabilitation of Low Back Pain. Baltimore, Williams & Wilkins, 1989

Yaremchuk MJ, Burgess AR and Brumback RJ. Lower Extremity Salvage and Reconstruction. New York, Elsevier, 1989

Journals

Special Nursing Considerations

American Pain Society. Relieving pain: An analgesic guide. Am J Nurs 1988 Jun; 88(6):815-825

Calhoun JH and Burke EE. Orthopedic rehabilitation at home. Phys Med Rehabil 1988 Aug; 2(3):415-459

Dunwoody CJ. Patient controlled analgesia; rationale, attributes, and essential factors. Orthop Nurs 1987 Sep-Oct; 6(5):31-36

Rubin M. The physiology of bedrest. Am J Nurs 1988 Jan; 88(1):50-56

Management Modalities

Esterhai JL et al. Treatment of chronic refractory osteomyelitis with adjunctive hyperbaric oxygen. Orthop Rev 1988 Aug; 17(8):809-815

Friedlaender GE. Bone grafts. J Bone Joint Surg (Am) 1987 Jun; 69(5):786-790

Martin ME. Oral antibiotics for treatment of patients with chronic osteomyelitis. Orthop Nurs 1989 May-Jun; 8(3):35-38

Total Joint Replacement

A conversation with William L Bargar MD. Custom cementless total hip replacement. Orthop Rev 1987 Jan; 16(1):27-35

Apley AG. The prevention of deep sepsis in joint replacement. J Bone Joint Surg [Br] 1987 Aug; 69(4):517-518

Cushner FD and Friedman PJ. Osteonecrosis of the femoral head. Orthop Rev 1988 Jan; 17(1):29-32

Doheny M and Ceccio CM. Total shoulder replacement: Preparing patients for discharge. Orthop Nurs 1988 May-Jun; 7(3):13-21

Dunajcik LM. The hip: When the joint must be replaced. RN 1989 Apr; 52(4): 62-71

Figgie HE and Goldberg VM. Some success rates of revision total knee arthroplasty. Orthop Rev 1988 May; 17(5):464-466

Follman D. Nursing care concerns in total shoulder replacement. Orthop Nurs 1988 May-Jun; 7(3):29-31

Goldberg VM et al. Total elbow arthroplasty. J Bone Joint Surg [Am] 1988 Jun; 70(5):778-783

Haddad RJ, Cook SD and Thomas KA. Biological fixation of porous-coated implants. J Bone Joint Surg [Am] 1987 Dec; 69(9):1459-1466

Hughes SPF. The use of antibiotics in orthopaedic surgery: Total joint single v multiple dose prophylaxis. Orthop Rev 1987 Apr; 16(4):209-214

Nelson CL. Infected joint implants: principles of treatment. Orthop Rev 1987 Apr; 16(4):215-223

Radin EL. Loosening of total hip replacement prosthesis. Orthop Rev 1989 Mar; 16(3):134-136

Sculco T. Approaches to senior care. Orthop Rev 1988 Mar; 17(3):239-240

Amputation

Adler JC et al. Treadmill training program for a bilateral below-knee amputee patient with cardiopulmonary disease. Arch Phys Med Rehab 1987 Dec; 68(12):858-861

Barker-Stotts KA. Action STAT! Traumatic amputation. Nursing 1988 May; 18(5):51

Bild DE et al. Lower-extremity amputation in people with diabetes: Epidemiology and prevention. Diabetes Care 1989 Jan; 12(1):24-31

Ceccio CM et al. Teaching the elderly amputee to meet the world. RN 1988 Sep; 51(9):70-72, 74, 76-77

Finsen V et al. Transcutaneous electrical nerve stimulation after major amputation. J Bone Joint Surg [Br] 1988 Jan; 70(1):109-112

Huber PM et al. Prosthetic problem inventory scale. Rehabil Nurs 1988 Nov-Dec; 13(6):326-329

Miller RA et al. Immediate postop prosthesis. Am J Nurs 1987 Mar; 87(3): 310-311

Moore TJ et al. Prosthetic usage following major lower extremity amputation. Clin Orthop Related Res 1989 Jan; 238:219–242

Pinzur MS et al. Psychological testing in amputation rehabilitation. Clin Orthop Related Res 1988 Apr; 229:236–240

Low Back Pain

Anderson L. Educational approaches to management of low back pain. Orthop Nurs 1989 Jan–Feb; 8(1):43–46

Boachie-Adjei O. Conservative management of low back pain: An evaluation of current methods. Postgrad Med 1988 Sep; 84(3):127–133

Dwyer AP. Backache and its prevention. Clin Orthop 1987 Sep; 222:35–43

Fast A. Low back disorders: Conservative management. Arch Phys Med Rehab 1988 Oct; 69(10):880–891

Gottlieb H et al. Self management for medication reduction in chronic low back pain. Arch Phys Med Rehab 1988 Jun; 69(6):442–448

Jameson RN, Matt D and Parris W. Treatment outcome in low back pain patients: Do compensation benefits make a difference. Orthop Rev 1988 Dec; 17(12):1210–1215

Lanier DC and Stockton P. Clinical predictors of outcome of acute episodes of low back pain. J Fam Pract 1988 Nov; 27(5):483–489

Lee CK. Office management of low back pain. Orthop Clin North Am 1988 Oct; 19(4):797–804

Posner JB. Back pain and epidural spinal cord compression. Med Clin North Am 1987 Mar; 71(2):185–205

Rosen CD et al. A retrospective analysis of the efficacy of epidural steroid injections. Clin Orthop 1988 Mar; 228:270–272

Stauffer JD. Antidepressants and chronic pain. J Fam Pract 1987 Aug; 25(2):167–170

Swezey RL. Low back pain in the elderly: Practical management concerns. Geriatrics 1988 Feb; 43(2):39–44

Tollison CD and Kriegel ML. Physical exercise in treatment of low back pain. Part I. Orthop Rev 1988 Jul, 17(7):724–729; Part II. Orthop Rev 1988 Sep; 17(9):913–923; Part III. Orthop Rev 1988 Oct; 17(10):1002–1006

Warfield CA. Facet syndrome and the relief of low back pain. Hosp Pract 1988 Oct 30; 23(10A):41–42; 47–48

Osteoporosis

Barth RW and Lane JM. Osteoporosis. Orthop Clin North Am 1988 Oct; 19(4):845–858

Barzel US. Estrogens in prevention and treatment of postmenopausal osteoporosis: A review. Am J Med 1988 Dec; 85(6):847–850

Bellantioni MF and Blackman MR. Osteoporosis: Diagnostic screening and its place in current care. Geriatrics 1988 Feb; 43(2):63–66; 69–70

Carter LW. Calcium intake in young adult women: Implications for osteoporosis risk assessment. J Obstet Gynecol Neonatal Nurs 1987 Sep–Oct; 16(5):8301–8308

Chambers JK. Metabolic bone disorders. Imbalances of calcium and phosphorus. Nurs Clin North Am 1987 Dec; 22(4):861–872

Holm K and Dudas S. Osteoporosis: Implications for critical care. DCCN 1987 May–Jun; 6(3):158–164

Lamb K, Miller J and Nernandez M. Falls in the elderly: Causes and prevention. Orthop Nurs 1987 Mar–Apr; 6(2):45–49

Lane JM et al. Osteopenic syndromes. Orthop Rev 1988 Dec; 17(12):1231–1235

Lindsay R. Osteoporosis: An updated approach to prevention and management. Geriatrics 1989 Jan; 44(1):45–46; 51–52; 54

Lindsay R. Prevention of osteoporosis. Clin Orthop 1987 Sep; 222:44–59

Marcus R. Understanding and preventing osteoporosis. Hosp Pract 1989 Apr; 15; 24(4):189–204; 209–211; 215

Martin AD and Houstin CS. Osteoporosis, calcium, and physical activity. Can Med Assoc J 1987 Mar 15; 136(6):587–593

McKenna MJ and Frame B. Hormonal influences on osteoporosis. Am J Med 1987 Jun 26; 82(1B):61–67

Pak CYC et al. Safe and effective treatment of osteoporosis with intermittent slow-release sodium fluoride: Augmentation of vertebral bone mass and inhibition of fractures. J Clin Endocrinol Metab 1989 Jan; 68(1):150–159

Raisz LG. Local and systemic factors in the pathogenesis of osteoporosis. N Eng J Med 1988 Mar 31; 318(13):818–828

Resnick NM and Greenspan SL. 'Senile' osteoporosis reconsidered. JAMA 1989 Feb 17; 261(7):1025–1029

Rodysill KJ. Postmenopausal osteoporosis—intervention and prophylaxis. J Chronic Dis 1987; 40(8):743–760

Santora AC II. Role of nutrition and exercise in osteoporosis. Am J Med 1987 Jan 26; 82(1B):73–79

Silverberg SJ and Lindsay R.

Postmenopausal osteoporosis. Med Clin North Am 1987 Jan; 71(1):41–57

Sinak M. Exercise and osteoporosis. Arch Phys Med Rehab 1989 Mar; 70(3):220–229

Solomon DH et al. New issues in geriatric care. Ann Intern Med 1988 May; 108(5):718–732

Thorneycroft IH. The role of estrogen replacement therapy in the prevention of osteoporosis. Am J Obstet Gynecol 1989 May; 160(5 Suppl):1306–1310

Walden O. The relationship of dietary and supplemental calcium intake to bone loss and osteoporosis. J Am Diet Assoc 1989 Mar; 89(3):397–400

Watts NB. Osteoporosis. Am Fam Physician 1988 Nov; 38(5):193–207

Bone Tumors

Barker C. Is it drug toxicity—or something else? Nursing 1989 Apr; 19(4):84–86

Nicholson S. Femoral–tibial replacement for osteosarcoma. Nurs Times 1988 Feb 17–23; 84(7):34–37

Siegal RD, Ryan LM and Antman KH. Osteosarcoma in adults. Clin Orthop 1989 Mar; 240:261–269

Simon MA. Limb salvage for osteosarcoma. J Bone Joint Surg [Am] 1988 Feb; 70(2):307–310

Springfield DS et al. Surgical treatment for osteosarcoma. J Bone Joint Surg [Am] 1988 Sep; 70(8):1124–1130

Stine KC et al. Systemic doxorubicin and intraarterial cisplatin preoperative chemotherapy plus postoperative chemotherapy in patients with osteosarcoma. Cancer 1989 Mar 1; 63(5):848–53

Taylor WF et al. Prognostic variables in osteosarcoma: a multi institutional study. J Natl Cancer Inst 1989 Jan 4; 81(1):21–30

Limb Salvage

Colon LB. Limb salvage in the patient with severe peripheral vascular disease: The role of microsurgical free-tissue transfer. Plast Reconstr Surg 1987 Mar; 79(3):389–395

Lord CF et al. Infection in bone allografts. Incidence, nature, and treatment. J Bone Joint Surg [Am] 1988 Mar; 70(3):369–376

Raconlin, AA and Present D. Osteochondral allografts for limb salvage. Orthop Nurs 1989 Mar–Apr; 8(2):35–39

Sartoris D, Kusnick C and Resnick D. New concepts in bone grafting. Orthop Rev 1987 Mar; 16(3):154–164

Integumentary Problems

32 Dermatologic Conditions

Diagnostic Evaluation of Skin Lesions

Description of Skin Lesions (Fig. 32-1)

A. Primary Lesions (initial lesions)

1. *Macule*—a flat, circumscribed discoloration of the skin; may have any size or shape
2. *Papule*—a solid, elevated lesion less than 1 cm. (0.4 inch) in diameter
3. *Nodule*—a raised, solid lesion larger than 1 cm. (0.4 inch) in diameter
4. *Vesicle*—a circumscribed elevated lesion that contains fluid
5. *Bulla*—a large vesicle or blister larger than 1 cm. (0.4 inch) in diameter
6. *Pustule*—a circumscribed raised lesion that contains pus; may form as a result of purulent changes in a vesicle
7. *Wheal*—transient elevation of the skin caused by edema of the dermis and surrounding capillary dilatation
8. *Plaque*—a solid, elevated lesion on the skin or mucous membrane, larger than 1 cm. (0.4 inch) in its largest diameter; most commonly seen in psoriasis
9. *Cyst*—a sac that contains semisolid or liquid material

B. Secondary Lesions (changes that take place in primary lesions and possibly modify them)

1. *Scales*—heaped-up, horny layers of dead epidermis; may develop as a result of inflammatory changes
2. *Crusts*—a covering formed by the drying of serum, blood, or pus on the skin
3. *Excoriations*—linear scratch marks or traumatized area of skin
4. *Fissures*—cracks in the skin, usually from marked drying and long-standing inflammation
5. *Ulcer*—lesion formed by local destruction of the epidermis and part or all of the underlying dermis
6. *Lichenification*—thickening of skin accompanied by accentuation of skin markings
7. *Scar*—a fibrotic change in the skin following a destructive process
8. *Atrophy*—diminution in the size of a cell, tissue, organ, or part of the body

C. Shape and Configuration (Fig. 32-2)

After the type of lesion is identified, the shape, configuration or arrangement (in relation to each other), and their pattern of distribution is noted. The following are descriptions frequently used:

Annular—ring-shaped
Circinate—circular
Confluent—lesions run together or join
Discoid—disc-shaped
Discrete—lesions remain separate
Generalized—widespread eruption
Grouped—clustering of lesions
Guttate—droplike
Herpetiform—grouped vesicles
Iris—a ring or a series of concentric rings
Keratosis—horny thickening
Linear—in lines
Multiform—more than one kind of skin lesion
Nummular—coin-shaped
Polymorphous—occurring in several or many forms
Reticulated—lacelike network
Serpiginous—snakelike or creeping eruption
Telangiectasia—tiny, superficial, dilated cutaneous vessel; can be seen as a red thread or line

Primary Lesions

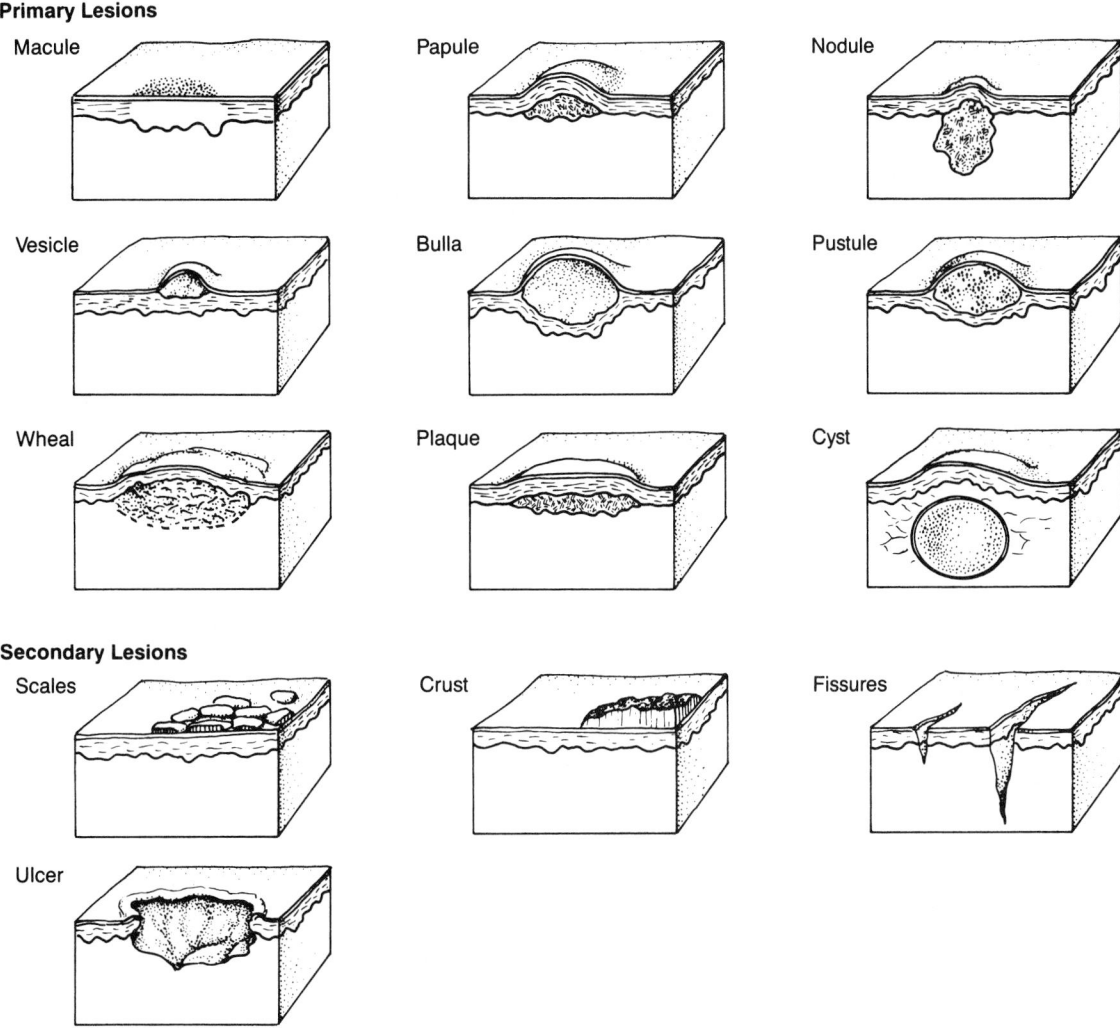

Figure 32-1. *Types of skin lesions. (From Brunner LS and Suddarth DS. Textbook of Medical–Surgical Nursing. 6th ed. Philadelphia, JB Lippincott, 1988).*

Zosteriform or *dermatomal*—bandlike distribution limited to one or more dermatomes of skin

Diagnostic Evaluation

Skin disease is diagnosed by a detailed examination of skin, hair, nails, and mucous membranes, the patient's history, the appearance of the lesions, and biopsy or culture to identify abnormal cells/causative organisms.

1. *Skin biopsy*—performed to obtain tissue for microscopic examination. May be obtained by scalpel excision or by a skin punch that removes a small core of tissue.
2. *Immunofluorescence (IF) testing*—an antigen or an antibody is combined with fluorochrome dye and used to localize the site of an immune reaction.
3. *Patch testing*—used to document contact sensitivity or allergy.
   a. Suspected allergens are placed on normal skin under occlusive patches.
   b. After about 48 hours, the patches are removed, and the underlying skin is inspected.
4. *Skin scrapings*—taken from suspected fungal skin lesions with a scalpel blade, transferred to a glass slide, and examined microscopically.
5. *Diascopy*—glass slide is pressed firmly against skin to permit observations of changes produced after the blood vessels are emptied and the skin is blanched.
6. *Tzanck smear*—used for cytologic evaluation of blistering diseases of the skin; suspected vesicle/pustule is opened and contents applied to a glass slide and examined after staining.
7. *Wood's light examination*—a special long-wave ultraviolet light produced by a Wood's lamp induces visible fluorescence in certain infectious agents (mostly fungal).
8. *Clinical photographs*—reveal nature and extent of skin condition and show progress or improvement of resulting treatment.

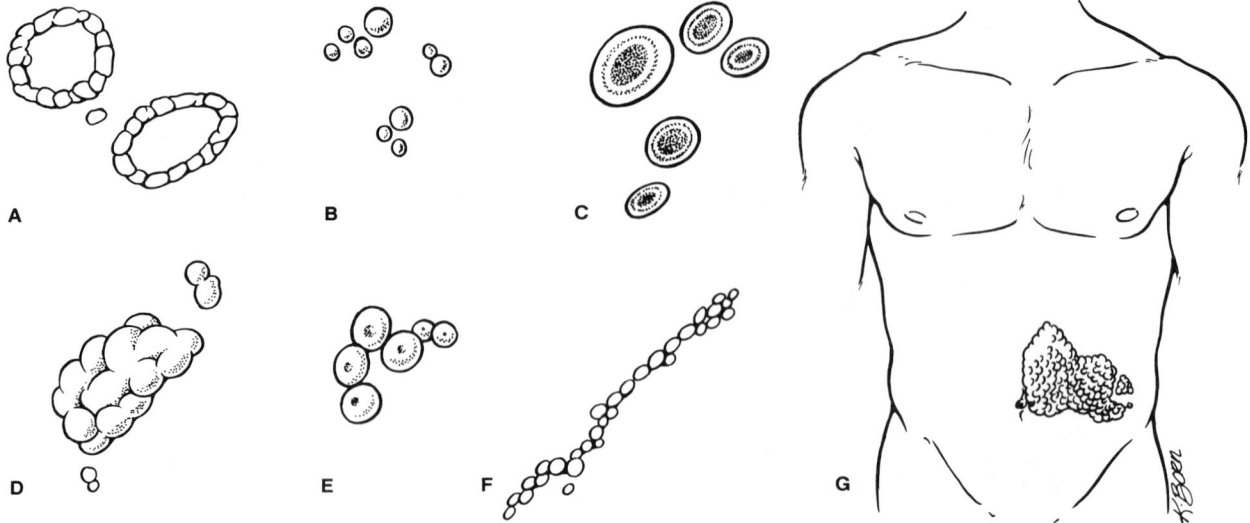

Figure 32-2. *Shape and arrangement of skin lesions: (A) annular; (B) grouped; (C) iris; (D) confluent; (E) herpetiform; (F) linear; (G) zosteriform.*

Nursing Approach to Patients With Dermatologic Conditions

Psychologic Considerations

1. Patients with dermatologic problems can see and feel their problems and are more disturbed by their complaints than many patients with other conditions.
2. Skin eruptions evoke feelings of shame, disgust, avoidance, withdrawal, and anger that compound the problems of management of patients with skin conditions. Touching the patient reduces his sense of isolation.
3. Irritation is a constant feature of skin disease and produces loss of sleep, anxiety, and depression, which in turn reinforce discomfort and fatigue.
4. Cosmetic needs constitute the underlying motive that brings the patient to treatment.
5. Nursing support requires understanding, unending patience, and continuing encouragement for these patients.

Nursing Process Overview:
The Patient With Dermatoses (Abnormal Skin Conditions)

Nursing Assessment

A. Nursing History

1. When did you first notice this skin problem? Onset? Duration? Intensity?
2. Has it occurred previously?
3. Are there any other symptoms?
4. What site(s) was first affected?
5. What did the rash/lesion look like when it first appeared?
6. Where and how fast did it spread?
7. Is there itching, burning, tingling, or a crawling sensation? Loss of sensation?
8. Is it worse at a particular time? Season?
9. Do you have any idea how it started?
10. Do you have a history of hay fever, asthma, hives, eczema, allergies?
11. Does anyone in your family have skin problems or rashes?
12. Did the eruptions appear after certain foods were eaten? Alcohol?
13. What medications are you taking?
14. What medication (ointment, cream, salve) have you put on the lesion? Include over-the-counter medications.
15. What skin products do you use? (soap, cream, make-up, etc.)
16. What is your occupation?
17. What in your immediate environment (plants, animals, chemicals, infections) might be precipitating this problem? Anything new/changes in the environment?
18. Does anything touching your skin cause a rash?
19. Is there anything you wish to talk about in regard to this problem?

B. Physical Assessment

1. Ask the patient to undress; the entire skin must be examined.
2. Have good lighting available. Use a hand magnifying lens to inspect for fine detail (altered skin markings, loss of skin lines, etc.).
3. Inspect the skin in an orderly sequence: hair, scalp, nails, buccal mucosa, skin surface.
4. Assess the general appearance of the skin, observing temperature, moisture, dryness, skin texture (rough or smooth).
5. Look at the distribution, arrangement, and grouping of the rash/lesions. Compare the left and right sides of the body.
6. Note the shape, border, color, texture, and surface of the lesion.
7. Palpate the shape, border, texture, and surface of the lesion.
8. Use a metric ruler to measure the size of lesions—to

compare extension of lesions from baseline measurements.

C. Assessment of Patients With Dark or Black Skin

1. Healthy dark skin has a reddish undertone; buccal mucosa, tongue, lips, and nails normally appear pink.
2. Lightening, darkening, or blotching of the skin are very noticeable and can cause emotional distress.
   a. Hyperpigmentation of the mouth is normal in some individuals.
   b. Some blacks have pigmented streaks on nails; usually normal.
3. The degree of pigmentation of the black patient may affect the appearance of a lesion; lesions may be black, purple, or gray (instead of tan or red color that is seen in the white patient).
4. Certain procedures (freezing, topical peeling and drying agents, or diseases) can cause hypopigmentation (loss or decrease in skin color) or hyperpigmentation (increase in color). These changes are more apparent in dark-skinned patients.
5. Have good lighting; look in mouth and nail beds as well as entire skin area.
6. Palpate all suspicious areas.
7. For rash:
   a. Ask the patient if any area itches.
   b. Stretch the skin gently to decrease the reddish tone and make the rash stand out.
   c. Palpate by running fingertips lightly over the skin—to feel the differences in skin temperature and to feel the borders of the rash.
   d. Palpate the lymph nodes; take the patient's temperature.
8. For erythema:
   a. Inspect for a purplish-grayish cast of skin.
   b. Palpate for increase in warmth and for signs of smoothness (edema) or hardness—to detect possible infection.
9. For cyanosis:
   a. Look for a gray cast of the skin.
   b. Inspect areas around the mouth, lips, over cheek bones, and earlobes.
   c. Evaluate for the usual signs of shock.

D. Documentation

Describe and document the dermatosis (abnormal condition of the skin) clearly and in detail.

1. What is (are) the color(s) of the lesion?
2. Is there redness, heat, pain, or swelling?
3. How large an area is involved; where is it?
4. Is the eruption macular, papular, scaling, oozing, discrete, confluent?
5. What is the distribution of the lesion—symmetrical, linear, circular?

Nursing Diagnoses

1. Potential impaired skin integrity related to change in barrier function of the skin
2. Pain (intolerable itching and discomfort) related to the primary skin disease, systemic disease (diabetes mellitus, blood disorders, cancer), medications, certain drugs, soaps and chemicals, dry skin, or psychologic factors
3. Disturbance in self-concept (body image) related to unsightly appearance of skin
4. Knowledge deficit of skin care
5. Knowledge deficit of the treatment regimen and lifestyle adjustment required

6. Other nursing diagnoses that could be applied include:
   • Potential fluid volume deficit related to loss of tissue fluids and serum from denuded skin (see p. 827)
   • Potential sexual dysfunction related to feelings of low self-worth and reactions of others.

Nursing Interventions

A. Maintaining Skin Integrity

1. Bathe in warm, *not* hot, water with minimal soaping; rinse well and dry by gently patting skin with a towel.
2. Apply an emollient to moist skin—to trap moisture.
3. Prevent and treat xerosis (dry skin).
   a. Keep environmental humidity above 40%; use a humidifier.
   b. Avoid excessive bathing.
   c. Use mild soaps.
   d. Avoid vasodilatation from hot foods, alcohol, and coffee.
4. For persons with hand irritations:
   a. Protect hands from contact with soaps, detergents, and other chemicals by wearing cotton-lined rubber or plastic gloves—the skin on the back of the hands is thin and sensitive with poor resistance to soaps and detergents.
   b. Keep hands out of water.
   c. Wear cotton gloves for dry housework.
5. Advise patient to use sunscreen to prevent sunburn and degenerative changes from sun (wrinkling, pigment alterations, actinic keratoses, skin cancer).

B. Relieving Discomfort

1. Bear in mind that many skin disorders cause discomfort and unbearable itching.
2. Control environmental and physical factors.
   a. Maintain cool, humid environment—itching is aggravated by heat, chemicals, and physical irritants.
   b. Keep cool, especially at night. Reduce excess bedding.
   c. Avoid taking hot baths and wearing woolen clothing.
   d. Avoid irritants and strong soaps.
   e. Use tepid cooling baths or cool wet dressings—gradual evaporation of water from dressings cools the skin and relieves pruritus.
   f. Protect healthy skin from maceration when applying wet dressings.
   g. Trim nails to decrease skin damage from scratching.
3. Keep skin hydrated and lubricated—to prevent skin breakdown.
4. Instruct the patient to refrain from self-medication with lotions and creams that are commercially advertised.
5. Be aware that the *sudden* onset of a generalized rash may indicate drug allergy.

C. Developing Self-Acceptance

1. Find out what concerns and fears the patient has—to neutralize undue anxiety and provide reassurance.
2. Listen in an open, nondefensive manner to expressions of anxiety and grief about changes in body image.
3. Help the patient to list personal strengths, enjoyable activities, and successful coping activities used in the past.
4. Encourage patient to mobilize support system.
5. Praise the patient's efforts to improve condition and appearance.

6. Advise of available cosmetic services to conceal disfiguring conditions.
7. Reinforce the therapeutic goals and nature of prescribed treatment. Help the patient to accept the prolonged treatment that some skin conditions require.
8. Encourage patient to use all available resources: educational materials, peer support groups, counseling, and community, educational, and recreational services.

D. Acquiring Knowledge and Understanding of Skin Care

1. Advise patient to keep skin moist and flexible with hydration and application of skin cream or lotion—the stratum corneum needs water for hydration, and the application of cream or lotion prevents dryness, scaling, and cracking.
2. Encourage a healthy, nutritious diet; skin changes may be a feature of abnormal nutrition.

E. Acquiring Knowledge of Treatment Regimen

1. Instruct the patient clearly and in detail to ensure that treatments are carried out as prescribed.
2. Teach patient the following:
   a. Use topical medications containing corticosteroids exactly as prescribed.
   b. Be aware of possible ill effects of long-term use of fluorinated topical steroids.
   c. Remove old medications, crusts, and scales before applying topical medications.
   d. Use tub baths to loosen exudates and scales.
   e. Use wet dressings on smaller areas to loosen exudate and scales and to reduce intensity of inflammation.
   f. Protect healthy skin from maceration (softening of skin by soaking) when applying wet dressings.
3. Observe the lesion periodically for changes in response to therapy.
4. Correct misconceptions and misinformation.

Evaluation

1. Attains/maintains skin integrity; absence of skin cracking
2. Achieves relief of discomfort and itching
3. Demonstrates increasing self-acceptance; shows interest in grooming
4. Acquires understanding of skin care
5. Demonstrates ability to perform treatments

Dermatologic Therapy
Baths and Wet Dressings

Therapeutic Baths (Balneotherapy)

A medicated bath is used to apply medication to the entire skin surface and is useful in treating widespread eruptions and general pruritus. Baths soothe, soften, reduce inflammation, and relieve itching and dryness.

A. Clinical Uses

1. Vesicular, bullous, and ulcerative disorders
2. Acute inflammatory conditions
3. Erosions and exudative, crusted surfaces

B. Types of Therapeutic Baths

See Table 32-1.

Open Wet Dressings

Wet dressings are wet compresses applied to skin areas. They may be either sterile or unsterile, depending on the condition being treated.

A. Purposes

1. To reduce inflammation by producing vasoconstriction—thus decreasing vasodilatation and the local blood flow present in inflammation.
2. To cleanse skin of exudates, crusts, and scales.
3. To maintain drainage of affected areas.

B. Types of Open Wet Dressings

See Table 32-2.

Medications for Skin Conditions

A. Types of Medications

See Table 32-3.

B. Patient Education

1. Use topical medication *only* as directed.
2. Wash hands thoroughly before applying.
3. Avoid reapplying prescribed topical agent at frequent intervals to improve appearance or for cosmetic purposes; may cause further irritation or impede healing.
4. Do not use over-the-counter hydrocortisone preparations indiscriminately because chronic abuse can produce steroid rosacea and thinning of the skin.

Table 32-1. *Therapeutic Baths*

Bath Solution and Medication	Desired Effect	Nursing Interventions
Water Saline	Same effects as wet dressings Used for widely disseminated lesions	• Fill the tub half full. • Keep the water at a comfortable temperature.
Colloidal—oatmeal or Aveeno Sodium bicarbonate Starch	Antipruritic and demulcent Cooling Soothing	• Do not allow the water to cool excessively. • Use a bath mat—*medications may cause tub to be slippery.*
Tar baths (follow package directions) Alma-Tar, Balnetar, Lavatar, Polytar	Tar baths are used for psoriasis and chronic eczematous conditions.	• Apply a lubricating agent to wet skin after bath if emollient action is desired—increases hydration. Because tars are volatile, the bath area should be well ventilated. • Dry by blotting with a towel.
Bath oils Alpha-Keri, Lubath, Nutraderm Bath Oil	Bath oils are used for antipruritic and emollient soothing properties Used for acute and subacute eczematous eruptions.	• Keep room warm to minimize temperature fluctuations. • May be applied to moist skin after bathing. • Encourage the patient to wear light, loose clothing after the bath.

Table 32-2. *Open Wet Dressings*

Solution and Material	Desired Effect	Nursing Interventions
Solution		
Room-temperature tapwater Physiologic saline solution Aluminum acetate solution Magnesium sulfate	Effective in treating oozing dermatosis or swollen, infected dermatitis (furunculitis, cellulitis) Relieves inflammation, burning, and itching Has cooling effect	Wash hands thoroughly before applying dressings Protect areas of normal skin with petrolatum jelly or a silicone oil or zinc oxide paste to avoid skin maceration. Keep dressing at room temperature. Moisten compress to the point of slight dripping. Compresses may be remoistened using an asepto syringe. Add ice cubes to solution if coolness is desired. Apply for 15 minutes 3–4 times daily unless otherwise indicated. Reapply every 5 minutes or so, as compresses reach body temperature rather quickly. Keep the patient warm if extensive areas are to have compresses. Do not treat more than ⅓ of the body at one time, because chilling and hypothermia may result. Discard dressing material daily. CAUTION: Avoid burns.
Material		
Soft toweling Diapers Soft cotton sheeting Kerlix (Bauer and Black)		

Dressings for Skin Conditions

A. **Occlusive Dressing**—an airtight plastic or vinyl film is applied to cover medicated skin (usually corticosteroid).
  1. Purposes
      a. Enhances absorption of topically applied medication
      b. Promotes moisture retention; prevents medication from evaporating.
  2. Patient instructions:
      a. Wash area and pat dry.
      b. Rub medication into lesion while skin is still moist.
      c. Cover with plastic wrap, vinyl gloves, plastic bag.
      d. Seal with paper tape at edges or cover with a dressing (see below).

> **NURSING ALERT:** Prolonged use of occlusive dressings may cause skin atrophy, striae, telangiectasia, folliculitis, nonhealing ulceration, erythema, and systemic absorption of corticosteroids. Dressings should be removed for 12 out of 24 hours to prevent some of these complications.

      e. Plastic surgical tape containing corticosteroid is available and can be cut to size.
B. **Other Dressings**
  1. Fingers and toes—gauze or cotton cloth; held in place with small size tubular material (Surgitube, Tubegauze)
  2. Hands—disposable polyethylene gloves; sealed at wrists
  3. Feet—cotton socks or disposable plastic bags covered with cotton socks
  4. Extremities (arms and legs)—cotton cloth covered with tubular material
  5. Groin, perineum—disposable diapers; cotton cloth folded in diaper fashion
  6. Axillae—cotton cloth taped in place or held by commercial dress shields
  7. Trunk—cotton or light flannel pajamas
  8. Scalp—turban or plastic shower cap
  9. Face—mask made from gauze with holes cut out for eyes, nose, mouth

Acne Vulgaris

Acne vulgaris is a common disorder of the sebaceous (oil) glands and their follicles (pilosebaceous follicles), characterized by the presence of closed comedones (whiteheads), open comedones (blackheads), papules, pustules, nodules, and cysts. The primary sites are the face, chest, upper back, and shoulders.

Predisposing Factors

1. Genetic predisposition—strong genetic overtones
2. Hormonal changes of adolescence—from androgenic stimulation of sebum production
3. Cutaneous flora—high concentration of *Propionibacterium acnes* found in acne-susceptible individuals
4. External irritants—climate, chemical, mechanical irritants, cosmetics, pharmacologic agents

Altered Physiology

Stimulation of androgenic hormones → increase in amount and thickness of oil secretion → lipids arising in the sebaceous glands → follicular bacteria (*P. acnes*) → obstruction of sebaceous glands by blackheads (comedones) → disruption of the follicular epithelium, allowing discharge of the follicular contents into the dermis → inflammatory reaction → papules → pustules → nodules → cysts.

Clinical Manifestations

1. Closed comedones (white heads); small whitish papules with minute follicular openings—from impacted lipids or oils and keratin that plug the dilated follicle
2. Open comedones (black heads)
3. Papules, pustules, nodules, cysts, or abscesses may subsequently develop.

Table 32-3. *Medications for Skin Conditions*

Type of Medication	Desired Effect	Nursing Interventions
Lotions Liquid vehicles for carrying medication	Cool through water evaporation May be protective antipruritic, and drying; may act as sunscreen.	May be applied with cotton gauze or soft paintbrush or by hand, using a firm stroke for a thin, even coat. Not usually washed off between applications.
Creams (suspensions of oil and water) Have greasy, nongreasy, or penetrating base, depending on nature of lesion and drug applied	For moisturizing and emollient effects Serve as vehicle for medications.	Creams are rubbed into the skin by hand. Teach the patient to apply his own cream.
Gels Transparent emulsions that liquefy on contact with skin	Dries as a thin, greaseless nonocclusive, nonstaining film; some topical steroids are prescribed in gel form.	See corticosteroid agents below.
Ointments Contain mineral or vegetable oils as the base	Usually used when inflammation becomes chronic and skin is dry, with scaling and lichenification (leathery thickening of the skin). Retard water loss and lubricate and protect the skin.	Applied by hand or wooden tongue depressor. Ointments may have to be covered with a dressing to prevent soiling of clothing.
Pastes Mixtures of a powder in an ointment base	Used in inflammatory conditions	May need to be removed with a cotton ball soaked in mineral oil or vegetable oil.
Topical corticosteroid agents (many preparations available)	Have anti-inflammatory action, thus relieving pain and itching. Fluorinated steroids may be associated with transient adrenocortical suppression when large areas of the body are being treated	Apply on hydrated skin sparingly; rub it into skin thoroughly Cover with occlusive dressing as directed—enhances penetration. Prolonged or excessive use may produce thinning of the skin, stretch marks, and susceptibility to bruising. Apply with caution around the eyes—chronic use around the eyes may cause glaucoma, cataracts, and viral and fungal infections.
Powders (usually with a talc, zinc oxide, bentonite or cornstarch base)	Act as hygroscopic agents (take up moisture). Reduce friction between skin surfaces and between skin and bedding	Be sure area is thoroughly dry to prevent caking. Dispense with shaker top. Avoid accumulating powder in intertriginous areas.
Other Skin Medications		
Intralesional therapy Injection of sterile suspension of medication (usually suspension of corticosteroid) into lesion	Has anti-inflammatory action. Skin lesions treated with intralesional therapy include psoriasis, keloids, and cystic acne.	Be aware that local atrophy may result if injection is made into subcutaneous fat.
Systemic medications Corticosteroids Antibiotics Antifungals Sedatives and tranquilizers Analgesics Antineoplastics		

Management and Nursing Interventions

A. Preventing Obstruction of the Oil Glands

1. Wash face gently 1–2 times daily with mild soap and water.
   Mild abrasive soaps and drying preparations may be used for mild involvement (mainly comedones)—to eliminate the oily feeling.
2. Shampoo scalp nightly or twice weekly with medicated shampoo.
3. Use bath brush if back is involved.
4. Advise the patient to have blackheads removed manually with a comedone extractor.
5. Removal of superficial skin cells may be done mechanically by use of a polyester sponge pad (Buf-Puf).

B. Applying Topical Agents for More Severe Involvement—to clear keratin plugs from follicular ducts and to suppress *P. acnes* in the follicles. The therapeutic regimen depends on the type of lesion (comedonal, papular, pustular, or cystic).

1. Topical benzoyl peroxide—exerts antibacterial effects, suppresses *P. acnes,* reduces concentration of surface free fatty acids, and is a comedolytic.
   a. Apply sparingly to completely dry skin; adjusted to point of tolerance.
   b. Advise patient that he may not see improvement for 1–2 or up to 6 weeks.
2. Topical retinoic acid (tretinoin [Retin-A])—speeds up the cellular turnover, which forces out the comedones

and prevents occurrence of new comedones. Instruct the patient as follows:

   a. The symptoms may worsen during the early weeks of treatment because of action of medication on previously unseen comedones; there is a possibility of some erythema and peeling. Improvement may take 6–12 weeks.

   b. Read the product-information brochure.

3. Topical antibiotic therapy—suppresses growth of *P. acnes* and produces decrease in comedones, papules, and pustules without systemic side effects.

     Topical clindamycin, erythromycin, tetracycline, and meclocycline are used alone or in combination with other agents.

C. Systemic Antibiotics

Systemic antibiotics appear to reduce *P. acnes* in pilosebaceous follicles and inhibit sebum production, and are used for the more inflammatory and extensive lesions.

1. Tetracycline, erythromycin, or minocycline is given and adjusted according to therapeutic response.
2. Long-term, low-dose antibiotic may be given
3. May take several weeks for effect of antibiotics to show.
4. Instruct the patient to take tetracycline at least 1 hour before or 2 hours after mealtime; avoid taking any dairy products (milk, ice cream) within 2 hours before or after taking medication—tetracycline is poorly absorbed with food.
5. Side effects of tetracycline include nausea, diarrhea, superinfection, and candidiasis (vaginitis in women; cutaneous infection in either sex, but more often in men).

D. Retinoid Therapy

D. Retinoid Therapy—oral isotretinoin (Accutane), a synthetic derivative of vitamin A used to treat severe disfiguring cystic acne that is unresponsive to standard therapies—appears to have an inhibitory effect on sebum production and sebaceous gland secretion.

1. *Adverse effects*
   a. Mucocutaneous effects—cheilitis, facial dermatitis, dry nose and mouth, dry eyes, conjunctivitis, pruritus, epistaxis.
   b. Systemic effects—headache, thirst, arthralgia, fatigue, elevation of triglyceride and cholesterol levels, and lowering of high-density lipoproteins.
   c. Headache is a serious symptom. It may be associated with increased intracranial pressure, papilledema, projectile vomiting, and other signs of pseudotumor cerebri. Persistent headache should be evaluated by a neurologist.
   d. Most serious side effect is its teratogenicity; major fetal abnormalities related to isotretinoin have been documented.

2. Patient education for patients receiving retinoid therapy
   a. Women of childbearing potential should be counseled about risks to the fetus.
   b. Determine what the patient actually knows about contraception and if she is capable of complying; effective contraception must be used at least 1 month before beginning therapy, during therapy, and 1 month following discontinuation of therapy.
   c. A serum pregnancy test is obtained within 2 weeks prior to beginning therapy.
   d. Avoid vitamin supplements containing vitamin A because of possible additive toxic effects.

E. Estrogen therapy—(usually in form of oral contraceptive)—suppresses the androgenic stimulation of sebum production.

Usually reserved for young women with severe cystic acne; not given to males because of undesirable side effects (symptoms and signs of feminization).

F. Surgical Interventions

1. Intralesional injection of steroids (triamcinolone acetonide). Diluted steroid suspension is injected into inflamed lesions—leads to rapid resolution.
2. Incision and drainage of cysts and pustular lesions—may be required in large, fluctuant, nodular–cystic lesions.
3. Cryosurgery (freezing with liquid nitrogen)—for nodular and cystic forms of acne.
4. Dermabrasion—surgical planing of skin to reduce surface configuration of old scars and give smooth appearance.
5. Collagen injected intradermally into scar to raise scar surface to the level of the surrounding skin.

Patient Education

1. Gain the patient's confidence. Outline the therapy—try to relieve unspoken fear and guilt.
   a. Acne is not caused by dirt and cannot be washed away; it is a chemical imbalance that causes the oil in the skin to form blackheads.
   b. Acne is *not* related to sexual activity.
2. Keep hands away from face.
3. Do not squeeze pimples or blackheads—squeezing the skin makes acne worse. The majority of blackheads are pushed down into the skin by squeezing and this increases the likelihood that the lesion will rupture into the dermis, causing more inflammation.
4. Eat a healthy well-balanced diet; eliminate any food that you believe worsens your acne.
5. Keep hair off the face; wash hair daily if necessary.
6. Avoid friction and trauma.
   a. Do not prop your hands against your face.
   b. Avoid overzealous washing of face, rubbing the face, pressure from tight collars/helmets.
   c. Avoid perspiration around the face.
7. Use water-based and hypoallergenic cosmetics; avoid oily cosmetics, including cleansing creams, shaving creams, and lotions.
8. Continue treatment even though your skin clears.
9. Talk over your problems with an understanding person; emotional stress may worsen acne.

Infections and Infestations of the Skin

Bacterial Infections (Pyodermas)

Bacterial infections of the skin may be primary, originating in previously normal-appearing skin and usually caused by a single organism, or secondary, arising from a preexisting skin disorder in which several microorganisms may be implicated. The most common primary bacterial skin infections are *impetigo* and *folliculitis*.

Impetigo

Impetigo is a superficial infection of the skin caused by streptococci, but staphylococci and streptococci or multiple bacteria can usually be recovered on routine culture. See page 1389.

   Bullous impetigo is a superficial infection of the skin caused by *S. aureus,* characterized by the formation of bullae from original vesicles, which rupture, leaving a raw area.

Folliculitis

Folliculitis is a bacterial infection that arises within the hair follicle.
1. Lesions may be superficial or deep; single or multiple papules or pustules appear close to the hair follicle.
2. Folliculitis commonly seen in the hair area of men who shave and on women's legs.
3. *Pseudofolliculitis barbae* (shaving bumps)—an inflammatory reaction on face of curly haired males caused by ingrowing hairs that pierce the skin, causing an irritative reaction.
   a. Common problems in black males.
   b. Management
      (1) Avoid shaving; grow a beard or use a hand-brush over facial area to mechanically dislodge hairs.
      (2) A depilatory cream may be used if the patient must shave.

Furuncle

Furuncle (boil) is an acute inflammation arising deep within one or more hair follicles and spreading into surrounding dermis (a deeper form of folliculitis); the causative agent is almost always *Staphylococcus aureus.*

Clinical Manifestations

1. Tenderness, pain, and surrounding cellulitis; after furuncle localizes, the center becomes boggy and fluctuant, and a soft yellow or white head appears on the surface.
2. Sites of predilection—back of neck, axillae, buttocks.

Management

1. Surrounding skin is cleansed with antibacterial soap or antiseptic (chlorhexidine), as auto-infectivity is possible in peripheral skin.
2. Warm wet compresses are applied to lesion—increases vascularization and hastens resolution.
3. Antibiotic therapy is prescribed ((floxacillin; erythromycin) (must be followed exactly and as long as prescribed).
4. Surgical drainage may be performed when furuncle has become localized and shows fluctuation (wave-like motion on palpation)—to relieve pressure and pain.

> **NURSING ALERT:** Take special precautions with boil on face, as the skin area drains directly into the cranial venous sinuses.

Patient Education

1. Instruct the patient to wash his hands after handling lesion/dressings and all clothing coming in contact with the lesion—to prevent further spread of bacteria.
2. In the event of recurrent furunculosis, the patient and his/her household contacts should be examined and treated as possible carriers (distributors of infection).
3. See Patient Education under "Carbuncles."

Carbuncles

Carbuncle is a group of boils (or very large boil) joined together by tunnels under the skin; usually caused by *Staphylococcus aureus.*

Clinical Manifestations

1. Fever, leukocytosis, and pain
2. Bacteremia is common because the extensive inflammation makes it difficult to completely wall off the infection, so that absorption of toxins takes place.
3. Seen most frequently within the thick, fibrous inelastic skin of the back of the neck and upper back.
4. More apt to occur in older and debilitated person, especially frequent in persons with diabetes mellitus.

> **NURSING ALERT:** Recurring carbuncles may be a sign of an underlying problem such as an immune disease or diabetes mellitus.

Management

1. Antibiotic (based on sensitivity studies)—continued until infection is controlled
2. Supportive management includes intravenous infusions, fever sponges, bedrest for the toxic patient.
3. Surgical incision and drainage when definite fluctuance occurs.
4. Search for an underlying disease condition (diabetes, hematologic or immune disease, etc.)

Patient Education

Instruct the patient as follows:
1. Wash hands thoroughly before and after caring for lesion.
2. Avoid excessive manipulation of the lesion, as this may cause dispersion of the bacteria.
3. Keep draining lesion covered with a dressing.
4. Wrap soiled dressings in paper and burn; discard razor blades after each use.
5. Use disposable tissues for wiping the nose—to reduce skin contamination.
6. A boil may be infectious; do not work in health-care facility or in food-service occupation until boil has healed.
7. If boil does not improve after treatment, report to the physician/clinic, as a different antibiotic or treatment is indicated.

Mycotic (Fungal) Infections

Fungi are plant-like organisms that feed on organic matter; they are responsible for a variety of common skin infections. The mycoses affecting primarily the skin may be divided into 3 groups: dermatophyte (*Trichophyton, Epidermophyton,* and *Microsporum* genera), candida (*Candida albicans*), and *Malassezia furfur.*

Tinea Pedis (Athlete's Foot) Or Ringworm of the Feet

Tinea pedis (*athlete's foot*) is a superficial fungal infection due to *Trichophyton rubrum, Trichophyton mentagrophytes,* or *Epidermophyton floccosum,* which may manifest itself as an acute, inflammatory, vesicular process or as a chronic rash involving the soles of the feet and the interdigital web spaces.

Clinical Features

1. Tinea pedis is the most common fungal infection
2. Causes intense itching, burning, and erythema
3. Lymphangitis and cellulitis may occur when bacterial superinfection is present

Diagnostic Evaluation

1. Direct examination of scrapings (skin, nails, hair)
2. Isolation of the organism in culture

Management of Cutaneous Mycotic Infections

A. Topical Agents—have antifungal and anticandidal activity
1. Clotrimazole
2. Miconazole
3. Econazole
4. Tolnaftate

B. Systemic Antifungal Therapy (griseofulvin; ketoconazole)—for failure of topical therapy or widespread infection.

Side effects of griseofulvin include headache, nausea, urticarial reactions, phototoxicity.

C. Other Management Instructions
1. Use tap water soaks (or prescribed solution) to remove scales, crusts, debris, and residual medications; also for mild anti-inflammatory effect.
2. For the vesicular–bullous type of painful infection, elevation of the feet is advised.
3. Apply topical antifungal agent to affected area; rub it in well.
4. Continue with topical therapy for several weeks—there is a high rate of recurrence.

Preventive Measures and Patient Education

Instruct the patient to keep feet dry—moisture encourages the growth of fungi.
1. Dry carefully between the toes.
2. Alternate shoes—to permit adequate drying of shoes between wearings.
3. Wear cotton socks or stockings with cotton feet—synthetic material does not absorb perspiration as well as cotton.
4. Change socks frequently; wash contaminated socks in hot water to avoid reinfection.
5. Wear perforated shoes if feet perspire excessively—to permit aeration of feet.
6. Apply talcum powder or antifungal powder twice daily—to keep feet dry and decrease moisture, which is needed to promote fungal growth.
7. Use small pieces of cotton between toes at night—to absorb moisture.
8. Avoid plastic or rubber-soled footwear, rubber boots, and tight shoes.

Tinea Corporis or Tinea Circinata

Tinea corporis or *tinea circinata* is ringworm of the body.

Clinical Manifestations

1. Intense itching
2. Appearance—begins as scaling erythematous lesions

advancing to rings of vesicles with central clearing; lesions appear in clusters.
3. Lesions usually appear on exposed areas of body; may extend to scalp, hair, or nails.

Management

1. Topical antifungal medication applied to small areas (clotrimazole, miconazole, tolnaftate, haloprogin; naftifine; bifonazole)
2. Griseofulvin may be used in very extensive cases in which the skin is broken, weeping, or oozing or for noninflammatory ringworm that is of the chronic, extensive, scaling type.
3. Ketoconazole (an alternate oral treatment) is effective in the griseofulvin-resistant patient.

Patient Education

Instruct the patient as follows:
1. Wear clean cotton clothing next to skin.
2. Use a clean towel daily; dry thoroughly all areas and skin folds that retain moisture, as fungi thrive in a warm, moist environment.
3. Use self-monitoring for signs of reinfection after a course of oral therapy for chronic tinea corporis.
4. An infected pet is a common source of infection and should be inspected and treated by a veterinarian.

Tinea Cruris

Tinea cruris ("jock itch") is a superficial fungal infection of the groin, which may extend to the inner thighs and buttock area and is commonly associated with tinea pedis.

Clinical Manifestations

1. Appears as a dull-red to red-brown eruption of the upper thighs; then advances outward from the crural (thigh) creases and extends to form circular plaques with elevated scaly or vesicular borders. Itching is usually present.
2. Seen most frequently in joggers, obese individuals, and those wearing tight underclothing.

Management

1. Topical therapy (miconazole cream or lotion; clotrimazole cream and lotion).
2. Griseofulvin (orally) for extensive eruption.
3. Treatment of concomitant tinea pedis to minimize reinfection.

Patient Education

1. Avoid excessive washing/scrubbing.
2. Avoid nylon underclothing, tight-fitting underwear, and prolonged wearing of a wet bathing suit.
3. Wear cotton underwear.

Tinea Capitis (Ringworm of the Scalp)

Tinea capitis (*ringworm of the scalp*) is a fungal disease of the scalp. See page 1390.

Parasitic Skin Diseases

Three varieties of lice infest humans; their itching bites are the cause of many skin problems. Lice bite the skin to obtain the blood on which they feed. They leave their eggs and excrement on the skin; lice are passed from person to person.

Pediculosis capitis is an infestation of the scalp by the head louse, *Pediculus humanus,* var. capitis. See page 1391.

Pediculosis Corporis

Pediculosis corporis is an infestation of the body by the body louse, *Pediculus humanus,* var. corporis.

Clinical Features and Clinical Manifestations

1. The body louse lives chiefly in the seams of undergarments and other clothing to which it clings.
2. Its bite causes characteristic minute hemorrhagic points.
   a. Purpuric macule at site of the bite is the primary lesion.
   b. Widespread excoriations may appear on the shoulders, trunk, and buttocks.
   c. May produce secondary lesions—hyperemia, parallel linear scratches, and hyperpigmentation in persistent cases.
3. Areas of skin involved are those that come in closest contact with the undergarments (axillae, neck, trunk, thighs).
4. The lice and nits may be seen in the seams of clothing. They move to the skin for blood feedings and then return to the clothing.

Management

Instruct the patient as follows:
1. Bathe with soap and water.
2. Put on clean clothing.
3. Machine wash clothing on hot cycle; dry on hot cycle; or after washing press with hot iron, paying special attention to the seams, as lice adhere to the seams; or dry-clean clothing.
4. Examine and treat all family members and contacts.
5. Report for additional health care if severe pruritus, dermatitis, or secondary bacterial infections develop.

Pediculosis Pubis

Pediculosis pubis is an infestation by *Phthirus pubis* (crab louse); it is transmitted chiefly by sexual contact and is generally localized to the genital region.

Clinical Manifestations

1. Chief symptom is itching.
2. Black or rust-colored dots clinging to the base of the hairs.
3. Lice may infest hairs of chest, axillary hair, beard, and eyelashes.
4. Gray-blue macules (1–3 cm. in diameter) may be seen on the trunk, thighs, and axillae as a result of the action of the insects' saliva on bilirubin—converts it to biliverdin.
5. Itching of eyelid margins, blepharitis, and conjunctival inflammation—associated with *Phthirus pubis* palpebrarum.

Management and Patient Education

1. Instruct the patient as follows:
   a. Bathe with soap and water.
   b. Apply lindane lotion or shampoo or pyrethrin

(RID®) to areas of involvement.
   (1) Leave on for specified period.
   (2) Do not apply lindane to eyebrows, eyelids, or eyelashes—may cause eye irritation.
      (a) Apply ophthalmic petrolatum to eyelashes and eyebrows—smothers the lice and allows easier removal of nits and lice.
      (b) Remove nits manually from eyelashes and eyebrows with cotton-tipped applicator, toothpick, or fine tweezers.
      (c) Physostigmine ophthalmic ointment may then be applied to lid margins as directed.
      (d) Discard eye cosmetics.
   c. Machine wash all clothing and bedding with hot water; a temperature of 50°C. (122°F.) kills both lice and eggs in 30 minutes.
2. Treat all sexual contacts, family members, and close companions.
3. Schedule the patient for workup for coexisting sexually transmitted disease.
4. Be sure to follow directions; do not misuse product. Persistent itching is not uncommon, even after infestation has been effectively controlled.

Scabies

Scabies is an infestation of the skin by *Sarcoptes scabiei* (itch mite). Scabies is transmitted by close personal contact.

Clinical Features

1. Adult female burrows into superficial layer of skin after fertilization has occurred on skin surface; burrows are short, wavy, brownish or blackish, thread-like lesions (Fig. 32-3).

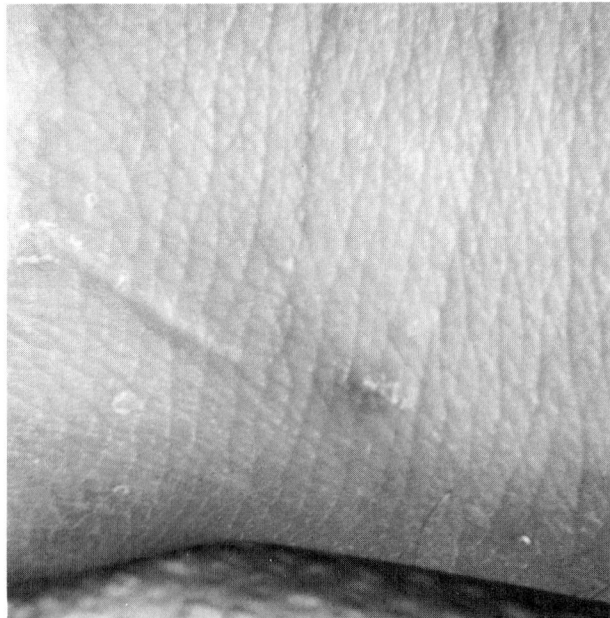

Figure 32-3. *Burrow in the epidermis made by the mite Sarcoptes scabiei. (Photo courtesy Michael Rosenbaum, M.D.)*

2. She extends the burrow, laying 2–3 eggs daily for up to 2 months, and then dies. The eggs progress through larval and nymphal stages to form adult mites in 10 days.
3. It takes about 4 weeks from time of contact for patient's symptoms to appear.

Clinical Manifestations

1. Symptoms: intense itching, more pronounced at night
2. Ask the patient where itch is most severe at the time you are examining him; look for burrows (short, wavy, dirty-appearing lines) with a magnifying glass (may or may not be visible). See below for procedure for obtaining skin scrapings for mite.

3. Look for small erythematous papules—scabies can imitate almost all pruritic dermatoses.
4. Secondary lesions include vesicles, papules, pustules, excoriations, and crusts; secondary bacterial infection of excoriated skin is frequent.
5. Sites—between fingers, on flexor surfaces of wrists and palms, around nipples, umbilicus, in axillary folds, under pendulous breasts, in or near groin or gluteal fold, penis, scrotum.

Diagnostic Evaluation

1. Examination of skin scrapings microscopically to confirm finding any stages of mites (adults, eggs, egg casings, larva, nymphs, fecal pellets).
2. See Guidelines: Skin Scrapings for Scabies, below.

Guidelines **Skin Scrapings for Scabies**

Purpose   To demonstrate the mite *Sarcoptes scabiei* (or ova or feces) in skin scrapings removed from burrows or papules.

Equipment   Hand lens
Mineral oil in dropper bottle
Scalpel and scalpel blade, No. 15
Glass slide/cover slip
Microscope

Procedure

Nursing Action	Rationale/Amplification
Preparatory Phase	
1. Place a small drop of oil in the middle of a glass slide.	
Performance Phase	
1. Inspect for the burrows of *Sarcoptes scabiei* on webs of fingers, lower abdomen, pubic and axillary areas, legs, arms.	1. The female scabies mite, ova, and fecal deposits may be found in burrows on the skin.
2. Apply a small amount of mineral oil on unexcoriated burrows or papule.	2. The mineral oil causes the mite to float and enhances visualization.
3. Scrape the involved skin with the scalpel blade.	
4. Transfer the scrapings to the prepared glass slide and apply coverslip; or pick out the mite with a disposable needle and transfer it to a glass slide.	4. To avoid air bubble.
5. Examine the slide with a scanning lens of the microscope.	5. Look for the mites, eggs, egg casings, and fecal pellets (which outnumber living organisms).

GERONTOLOGIC ALERT: Infestation with scabies can be a problem in nursing homes, particularly among debilitated patients who require extensive hands-on care.

Management/Patient Education

Instruct the patient as follows:
1. Take a warm soapy shower/bath to remove scaling debris from crusts. Dry thoroughly and allow skin to cool.

2. Apply prescribed scabicide such as lindane lotion or cream (Kwell) or crotamiton lotion or cream (Eurax).
   a. Apply thin layer from neck downward, with particular attention to hands, feet, and intertriginous areas; every inch of skin must be treated because mites are migrating. Apply to dry skin. (Wet skin allows more penetration and the possibility of toxicity.)
   b. Leave medication on for specified period but no longer, as this will irritate the skin. Then wash thoroughly. The patient is no longer able to transmit the disease 24 hours after effective treatment.

c. Machine wash and dry clothing and bed linens using the hot cycle.
d. A bland ointment may be applied to the skin for itching after the completion of treatment.
e. Avoid hot showers, as this dries the skin and produces more itching.

3. All family members and sexual contacts are treated simultaneously to eliminate the mites.
4. The animal with scabies is treated by a veterinarian.
5. Advise the patient that he may be uncomfortable and that itching may persist for days or weeks (this is from an allergic reaction to the mites); do *not* apply more mite-killing medicine, but go to clinic/physician for special treatment if itching and rash persist (postscabies pruritus).

Viral Infection: Herpes Zoster

Herpes zoster (shingles) is an inflammatory condition in which a virus produces a painful vesicular eruption along the distribution of the nerves from one or more posterior ganglia. The prevalence increases with age.

Etiology

Caused by a varicella-zoster virus, which is a member of a group of DNA viruses.

Virus appears to be identical to the causative agent of varicella (chickenpox). After the primary infection, the varicella-zoster virus may persist in a dormant state in the dorsal nerve root ganglia. The virus may emerge from this site in later years, either spontaneously or in association with immunosuppression, to cause herpes zoster.

Clinical Manifestations

1. Eruption usually accompanied or preceded by fever, malaise, headache, and pain; pain may be burning, lancinating, stabbing, or aching.
2. Inflammation is usually unilateral, involving the thoracic, cervical, or cranial nerves in a bandlike configuration.
3. Vesicles appear in 3–4 days.
   a. Characteristic patches of grouped vesicles appear on red and swollen skin.
   b. Early vesicles contain serum; later become pustular, rupture, and form crusts; scarring may occur.
   c. If ophthalmic nerve is involved, patient may have a painful eye.
   d. In normal host, lesions resolve in 2–3 weeks.
4. A susceptible person can acquire chickenpox if he comes in contact with the infective vesicular fluid of a zoster patient. A person with a previous history of chickenpox is immune and thus is not at risk from infection after exposure to zoster patients.

NURSING ALERT: Varicella–zoster virus may be a life-threatening condition to the patient who is immunosuppressed or is receiving cytotoxic chemotherapy or is a bone marrow transplant recipient.

Diagnostic Evaluation

Culture of varicella-zoster virus from lesions or detection by fluorescent antibody techniques, including viral detection using monoclonal antibodies (MicroTrak)

Management

A. Local Management of Skin Lesions

1. Open cool wet dressings to cool and dry areas by means of evaporation.
2. Lotions (calamine)—for cooling and soothing and drying effect of the powder that remains on skin after evaporation
3. Ointments (after acute stage) to soften and separate adherent crusts.

B. Pharmacotherapy

1. Antiviral drugs for treatment of immunosuppressed and/or debilitated patients (acyclovir)—interfere with viral replication.
2. Corticosteroids *early* in illness—given for severe herpes zoster if symptomatic measures fail; given for anti-inflammatory effect and relief of pain. Controversial.
3. Pain management; aspirin, acetaminophen, nonsteroidal anti-inflammatory drugs—useful during the acute stage, but not generally effective for postherpetic neuralgia.

C. Complications

1. Chronic pain syndrome (postherpetic neuralgia) characterized by constant aching and burning pain or intermittent lancinating pain or hyperesthesia of affected skin after it has healed.
2. Ophthalmic complications with involvement of ophthalmic branch of trigeminal nerve with keratitis, uveitis, corneal ulceration, and possibly blindness
3. Facial and auditory nerve involvement resulting in hearing deficits, vertigo, and facial weakness
4. Visceral dissemination—pneumonitis; esophagitis; enterocolitis; myocarditis; pancreatitis

Nursing Interventions and Patient Education

1. Assess patient's discomfort and response to pain medication; work collaboratively with physician to make necessary adjustments.
   a. Encourage diversional activities.
   b. Teach relaxation techniques.
2. Teach patient the following:
   a. Use proper handwashing techniques to avoid spreading herpes zoster virus.
   b. Apply wet dressings and topical medications to lesions.
   c. Do not open the blisters.
3. Reassure that shingles is a viral infection of the nerves; "nervousness" does not cause shingles.
4. A care-giver may be required to assist with dressings and meals. In older persons, the pain is more pronounced and incapacitating. Dysesthesia and skin hypersensitivity are distressing.

Contact Dermatitis

Contact dermatitis is a common inflammatory, often eczematous, condition caused by a skin reaction from contact with a variety of irritating or allergenic materials. There is damage to the epidermis by repeated physical and chemical insults.

1. *Primary irritant contact dermatitis* is a nonallergic reaction caused by exposure to an irritating substance.

2. *Allergic contact dermatitis* results from exposure of sensitized individuals to contact allergens.

Causes

1. Poison ivy
2. Cosmetics
3. Soaps, detergents, and scouring compounds
4. Hair dye, metals, rubber, chemicals

Predisposing Factors

1. Preexisting irritant dermatitis
2. Extremes of heat and cold—low humidity favors irritant contact dermatitis; high humidity favors allergic contact dermatitis
3. Frequent immersion in soap and water
4. Friction; occlusion

Clinical Manifestations

(Skin eruptions begin at point of contact with causative agent.)
1. Itching, burning, erythema, and vesiculation
2. Weeping, crusting, drying, fissuring, and peeling
3. Thickening of skin (lichenification) and pigmentation changes, if repeated reactions occur or if there is continual scratching by the patient.
4. Secondary bacterial invasion may occur—prevention of normal sweating produces vesicles, itching, and inflammation.

Diagnostic Evaluation

1. Inspect the entire body for a distribution pattern—helps to narrow down possible causes, which may be irritant or allergic.
2. Obtain a detailed history including the *site* of the initial eruption.

Management/Patient Education

Instruct the patient as follows:
1. Identify and remove the causative agent and contributing factors.
   a. Avoid heat, soap, rubbing—all are external irritants.
   b. Avoid exposing skin to the causative agent after recovery.
   c. Wear protective gloves (thin white cotton under rubber gloves) when using soap and water.
   d. Wash thoroughly immediately after exposure to antigens.
   e. Protect the skin from trauma, excessive sunlight, wind, and rapid temperature change while the dermatitis is active.
2. Topical treatment
   a. Use cool, wet dressings 15–20 minutes, 3–4 times daily for small areas of acute, vesicular dermatitis—for soothing and to help stop oozing.
   b. Cleanse away softened crusts and other debris.
   c. Apply a thin layer of cream or gel containing one of the steroids as prescribed.
   d. Use medicated baths at room temperature for larger areas of dermatitis.

Poison Ivy Dermatitis

Poison ivy dermatitis is an allergic reaction. Poison ivy grows in the form either of climbing vines or of upright shrubs; the leaves grow in clusters of 3, one at the end of the stalk and the other 2 opposite one another. Poison ivy has a sticky sap that contains an active ingredient known as *urushiol,* an oleoresin (a combination of plant resin and volatile oil). This urushiol can cause an allergic skin reaction (contact dermatitis).

Exposure to Urushiol

1. Urushiol must make contact with the skin—contact is usually made by touching the plant leaves or vines or roots.
2. Contact with urushiol may be made indirectly—clothing, tools, or fur of a pet, by the wind.
3. Smoke from burning plants carries droplets containing urushiol, which can get on the skin.

Clinical Manifestations

1. Eruption may develop in hours or days after contact.
   a. Reddened area will be noted, followed by rash and edema.
   b. Eruption occurs in a streak or line; it burns and itches.
   c. Small weeping areas may form (papules, vesicles, blisters)—in more severe cases, large blistered areas with inflammation and swelling may appear.
2. Secondary infection may give lesion the appearance of pyoderma (purulent skin disease) or plaque of eczema.

Management

A. Mild to Moderate Eruption

1. Cold or tepid compresses are prescribed for weeping lesions, or use tub baths if rash is diffuse.
2. Calamine lotion can be applied for soothing effect or
3. Topical cortisone cream may be prescribed.
   a. If applied before blistering, a gel steroid may stop or ease reaction.
   b. May also be helpful after vesicular stage has resolved to relieve itching, drying, and scaling.

B. Severe Eruption

Systemic corticosteroid (prednisone) may be prescribed.
1. Dosage is adjusted according to severity of reaction and then tapered off gradually.
2. The drug can be buffered with milk or antacid if there is a history of peptic ulcer.

Patient Education

1. Advise the patient as follows to recognize and avoid contact with urushiol (poison ivy, poison oak, or poison sumac).
   a. Do not pull, chop, or burn vines and brush—sap-carrying smoke may produce outbreak in a sensitive person.
   b. Wear protective clothing (long sleeves, gloves, slacks) in heavily wooded areas—to guard against exposure.
   c. Apply protective ointments before working in the vicinity of the plants.
   d. Take off contaminated clothing carefully and wash clothing immediately—urushiol on clothing can cause outbreak of poison ivy.
   e. Wash skin *immediately* with nonirritating soap and rinse well—to remove the plant oil; dermatitis may be prevented in most instances if done in 5–10 minutes after exposure.

2. Avoid overtreatment.
3. Be aware that poison ivy rash is not contagious; the blister fluid does not contain the oil and does not cause dermatitis if spread onto adjacent skin.
4. Report severe redness, local heat, swelling, red streaks, or pus or purulent drainage from eyes—signify secondary infection.

Noninfectious Inflammatory Dermatoses

Psoriasis

Psoriasis is a chronic inflammatory disease of the skin in which the production of epidermal cells occurs at a rate that is approximately 6–9 times faster than normal. There appears to be a loss of normal regulatory mechanisms of cell division.

A combination of specific genetic makeup and environmental stimuli may trigger the onset of the disease. There is some evidence that the cell proliferation is mediated by the immune system.

Pathophysiology

1. The cells in the basal layer of the skin divide too quickly; the newly formed cells move so rapidly to the skin surface that they become evident as profuse scales or plaques of epidermal tissue.
2. As a result of the increased number of basal cells and rapid cell passage, the normal events of cell maturation and growth cannot take place; this abnormal process does not allow formation of normal protective layers of the skin.

Clinical Manifestations

1. The lesions appear as red, raised patches of skin covered with silvery scales. In time the patches coalesce (fuse together), forming extensive, irregularly shaped patches (Fig. 32-4)
2. Sites (bilateral symmetry)
   a. Bony prominences (knees, elbows, sacrum), scalp, external ears, genitalia, perianal area, nails and dorsa of hands
   b. Psoriasis of the ears—scaling and dryness
   c. Psoriasis of palms and soles—scaly and pustular pruritic lesions
   d. Psoriasis of nails—thickening, discoloration, crumbling beneath free edges; pitting of nails
   e. Psoriasis between skin folds—smooth, shiny red lesions, easily fissured
3. The disease may range from a benign cosmetic source of annoyance to a physically disabling and disfiguring affliction with significant morbidity. It may be life-ruining—physically, emotionally, and economically.

Complications

1. Psoriasis may be coupled with arthritis of multiple joints (10% of patients), causing crippling disability.
2. Exfoliative psoriatic state that progresses to involve total body surface
3. Skin cancer when higher doses of ultraviolet are used

Management and Nursing Interventions

A. Daily Skin Care

Instruct patient to take daily tub bath—to help soak off scales.

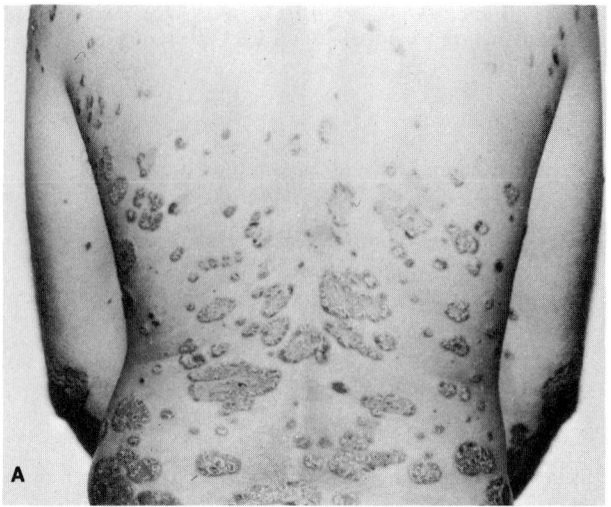

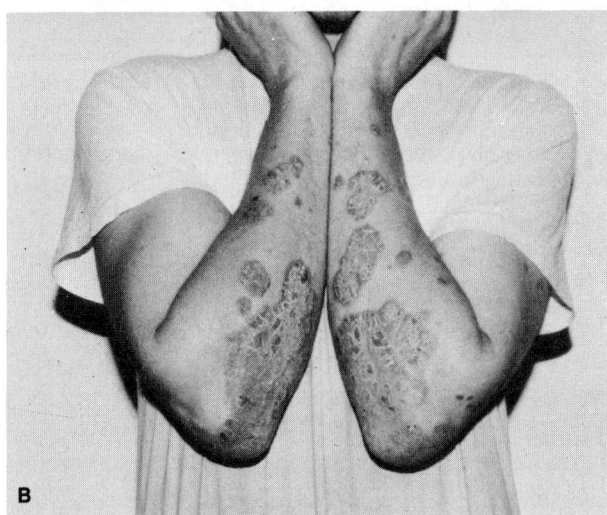

Figure 32-4. *The lesions of psoriasis appear as red raised patches of skin covered with silvery scales that, in time, coalesce, forming irregularly shaped patches. (Photos courtesy the National Psoriasis Foundation)*

1. Gently remove excess scales with a soft brush while bathing.
2. Apply prescribed ointment after removal of scales.

B. Topical Therapy

(includes coal tar, antralin, corticosteroids, etc.)
1. Coal tar preparations (lotions, ointments, pastes, creams, and shampoos)—retard and inhibit the rapid growth of psoriatic tissue.
   a. Preparation is applied for a period; may then be removed; this treatment is followed by carefully graded doses of ultraviolet radiation, which produces mild redness and slight desquamation (shedding).
   b. Advise the patient to wear goggles to protect the eyes and use a timer to prevent severe burns due to overexposure to the light rays.
   c. Daily tar shampoo followed by application of steroid lotion may be used for scalp lesions.
2. Anthralin preparations (a distillate of crude coal tar)—

useful for especially thick and resistant psoriatic plaques.

3. Topical steroids—may be applied for their anti-inflammatory activity. After the medication is applied, the area is covered with an occlusive plastic film dressing to enhance drug penetration and soften scaly plaques.

C. Intralesional Therapy (triamcinolone acetonide)—may be injected directly into psoriatic plaques.

D. Systemic Therapy (for severe psoriasis)

1. Methotrexate—inhibits DNA synthesis and hence has a marked suppressive effect on the reproduction of rapidly proliferating cells.
   a. Is hepatotoxic and requires pretreatment and follow-up liver tests and blood counts.
   b. Caution the patient to avoid alcohol intake while on methotrexate—increases possibility of liver damage.
   c. The drug is teratogenic (producing physical defects in the fetus) in pregnant women.
2. Oral retinoids (synthetic derivatives of vitamin A and its metabolite, vitamin A acid)—modulate the growth and differentiation of epithelial tissue; may be used with other forms of therapy; potentially teratogenic.
3. Hydroxyurea (Hydrea)—inhibits cell replication by affecting DNA synthesis
4. Cyclosporine

E. Photochemotherapy (PUVA therapy)—the use of psoralen plus ultraviolet radiation of long wavelength UVA; known as PUVA therapy.

1. Oral psoralen tablets (methoxsalen or 8-MOP, a photosensitizing chemical) followed by exposure to long-wave ultraviolet light (UVA)—in the presence of ultraviolet light, methoxsalen binds to DNA and leads to temporary inhibition of DNA synthesis (inhibits abnormally rapid multiplication of cells).
2. Long-term concerns include skin cancer, cataracts, aging effect, and systemic effects on other organs.
3. Methoxsalen capsules taken with milk or food 2 hours before scheduled UVA exposure in a UVA irradiation chamber; exposure is determined by the patient's skin type.
4. Patient teaching with PUVA therapy
   a. Because PUVA treatment produces photosensitization, the patient is sensitive to sunlight the entire day of treatment; must wear protective clothing and use a sunscreen on exposed areas of the body.
   b. Suitable protective wraparound gray- or green-tinted glasses must be worn for remainder of day of treatment when patient is out of doors or exposed to sunlight near window glass.
   c. Eye examinations are required at specified times.
   d. PUVA may cause irreversible or slowly reversible clinical and histologic skin changes—loss of elasticity, irreversible solar damage, cancer.

F. Combination Therapy (PUVA and retinoids; PUVA and methotrexate)

Patient Education

1. At this time there is no permanent cure of psoriasis, but it usually can be cleared and controlled.
2. Psoriasis is a disease of the entire skin, but it is not infectious or contagious.
3. Have an awareness of factors that may precipitate flare-ups.
   a. Know provoking factors—illness, certain drugs (beta blockers; indomethacin)

   b. Develop insight and determine what life events worsen the condition.
4. Avoid irritation and injury to the skin, as patches of psoriasis bleed after minor trauma.
   a. Do not rub or scratch your skin.
   b. Keep skin, especially on the hands, as pliable and soft as possible by applying appropriate creams.
   c. Wear heavy gloves when doing gardening, etc.
   d. Keep the skin from drying, as this worsens psoriasis.
      (1) Wash with warm water; pat the skin dry with a towel.
      (2) Apply an emollient, which allows trapped water to hydrate the stratum corneum.
   e. Report to the physician if severe injury to skin has occurred; injection of intralesional steroids may prevent untoward response.
5. Use a sunscreen. Try to schedule controlled exposure to sunlight on a regular basis but avoid sunburn, as it can cause a generalized flareup.
6. Secure prompt treatment for upper respiratory infections, which may cause a flareup.
7. Avoid overweight—seems to worsen psoriasis in many patients.
8. Join a support group to help come to terms with psoriasis.
   National Psoriasis Foundation
   6443 S.W. Beaverton Highway
   Suite 210
   Portland, OR 97221

Exfoliative Dermatitis
(Generalized Exfoliative Erythroderma)

Exfoliative dermatitis represents a cutaneous inflammation characterized by an initial erythema with the subsequent development of scaling or exfoliation arising from a variety of causes (see below).

Clinical Manifestations

A. Appearance

1. May start acutely, as either a patchy or a generalized erythema, accompanied by fever, shivering, and malaise.
2. The skin color changes from pink to dark red; then after a week, the characteristic exfoliation (scaling) begins, usually in the form of thin flakes that leave the underlying skin hot and red; new scales form as the older ones are cast off.
3. Severe pruritus; pain
4. Hair loss and nail shedding may accompany the disorder.

B. Systemic Effects

Exfoliative dermatitis has a marked effect on the entire body.
1. Profound loss of stratum corneum (outermost layer of the skin)—causes substantial fluid, electrolyte, and protein loss.
2. Lymphadenopathy; hepatomegaly
3. Invasion of bacteria and other organisms through the skin may lead to septicemia

C. Multiplicity of Causes

1. Preexisting skin disease (psoriasis; eczema)
2. Allergic reaction to drugs/other agents (penicillin; sulfonamides; phenytoin)

3. Underlying malignant disease (lymphoma; leukemia; mycosis fungoides)
4. Idiopathic

D. Complications

1. Heart failure
2. Pneumonia; sepsis

Management and Nursing Interventions

1. All offending drugs must be discontinued; early recognition of offending drug(s) will shorten duration of illness.
2. Underlying systemic disease is treated if known—to control erythroderma secondary to neoplastic process.
3. Patient is hospitalized and placed on bed rest.
   a. Maintain comfortable room temperature—patient does not have normal thermoregulatory control because of temperature fluctuations from vasodilatation and transepidermal water loss.
   b. Avoid cooling and overheating.
4. Fluids and electrolytes are monitored; any deficit is corrected.
5. Topical and/or systemic steroids are administered—prescribed for selected patients depending on underlying cause.
6. Soothing baths and lubrication with emollients are used—to give symptomatic relief.
7. Watch for symptoms of heart failure—hyperemia and increased cutaneous blood flow can produce a cardiac failure of high-output origin.
8. Nursing surveillance is maintained for intercurrent or cutaneous infection; the erythematous, moist skin is receptive to infection and becomes colonized with pathogenic organisms, which produce more inflammation.
9. See page 849 for management of the patient following a burn, as this patient has also lost normal barrier function of the skin.
10. Patient is advised to avoid all irritants, particularly drugs.

Pemphigus

Pemphigus is a serious autoimmune disease of the skin and mucous membranes characterized by the appearance of blisters (bullae) of various sizes on apparently normal skin and mucous membranes (mouth, esophagus, conjunctiva, vagina) (Fig. 32-5). The cause is unknown.

Familial benign chronic pemphigus (Hailey–Hailey disease) is a familial type of pemphigus appearing in adult life, affecting particularly the axillae and groin. There are other variants of the disease.

Clinical Manifestations

1. Initial lesions may appear in oral cavity; flaccid blisters (bullae) may arise on normal or erythematous skin.
   a. The bullae enlarge and rupture, forming painful raw and denuded areas that eventually become crusted.
   b. The eroded skin heals slowly; eventually, huge areas of the body are involved.
   c. In the mouth, the blisters are usually multiple, of varying size and irregular shape, painful, and persistent. Oral lesions may appear *initially;* may also affect mucous membranes of pharynx, esophagus, conjunctivae, larynx, urethra, cervix, and rectum.

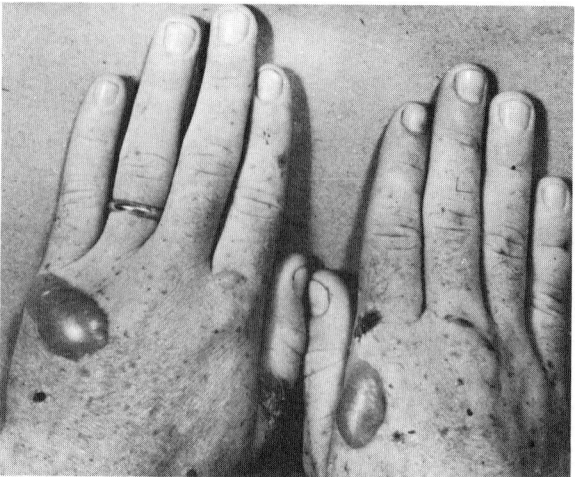

Figure 32-5. *Pemphigus—bullous dermatitis of hand (vesicles). (Photo courtesy Armed Forces Institute of Pathology)*

2. An offensive odor emanates from the bullae.
3. Positive Nikolsky's sign—separation of epidermis when minimal lateral pressure is applied to edge of blister or to normal-appearing skin.

Diagnostic Evaluation

1. Skin biopsies of blisters and surrounding skin—demonstrates *acantholysis* (separation of epidermal cells from each other)
2. Immunofluorescent studies of serum—reveal circulating antibodies (pemphigus antibodies)

Management

1. Corticosteroids (prednisone) in large doses to control the disease and keep skin free of blisters.
   a. High-dosage level is maintained until remission is apparent.
   b. Medication is given with or immediately after a meal; may be accompanied by an antacid as prophylaxis against gastric complications.
2. Immunosuppressive agents (cyclophosphamide, azathioprine [employed alone or in combination with steroids])—for immunosuppressive and steroid-sparing effect.
3. Plasmapheresis—reinfusion of specially treated plasma cells; temporarily decreases serum level of antibodies
4. Treatment of denuded skin

Complications

1. Infections (skin; pneumonia; septicemia)
2. Psychosis
3. Side effects from corticosteroids; gastrointestinal bleeding; CNS toxicity; hyperglycemia

Nursing Interventions

A. Relieving Oral Discomfort and Achieving Intact Oral Mucous Membranes

1. Inspect oral cavity daily; note and report any changes—oral lesions heal slowly.
2. Keep oral mucosa clean and allow regeneration of epithelium—secondary infection may be associated with

offensive odor from oral lesions. *Candida albicans* infection of the mouth frequently seen in patients on high-dose steroid therapy.

3. Give topical oral therapy as directed.
4. Offer prescribed mouth washes through a straw to rinse mouth of debris and to soothe ulcerative areas.
5. Teach patient to apply petrolatum to lips frequently.
6. Use cool mist therapy to humidify environmental air.

B. Attaining Skin Integrity and Relieving Skin Discomfort

1. Keep skin clean and eliminate debris and dead skin— the bullae will clear if epithelium at the base is clean and not infected.
2. Check skin cultures—most common organism is *Staphylococcus aureus.*
3. Administer cool, wet dressings and/or baths—patients with large areas of blistering have a characteristic odor that is lessened when secondary infection is under control.
   a. Potassium permanganate baths help keep areas from becoming infected and to some extent pre-cipitate some of the protein that oozes through open skin.
      (1) Dissolve potassium permanganate crystals thoroughly in small container; then pour into bathtub.
      (2) Undissolved crystals may be irritating if pa-tient sits on them.
   b. Following the bath, dry the patient and cover him with talcum powder as directed—enables the pa-tient to move more freely in bed. Fairly large amounts are necessary to keep patient from stick-ing to sheets.
4. The nursing management of patients with blistering or bullous skin conditions is similar to that of the pa-tient with a burn (see p. 846).

C. Achieving Fluid Balance

1. Evaluate for fluid and electrolyte imbalance—extensive denudation of the skin leads to fluid and electrolyte imbalance.
   a. Monitor serum albumin and protein levels.
   b. Monitor vital signs.
   c. Take measurements of body weight; test urine for glucose.
   d. Administer saline infusions as directed—signifi-cant loss of tissue fluids and therefore of sodium chloride occur through the skin.
   e. Encourage the patient to maintain hydration; offer cool nonirritating fluids (e.g., grape or apple juice).
   f. Give soft, high-protein, high-calorie fluids (En-sure®; Sustacal®; eggnogs, milk shakes)—patients with painful oral involvement have difficulty maintaining nutrition.
   g. See Nursing Process Overview: The Patient With a Burn, page 846, as large amounts of serum may be lost through denuded skin.

D. Attaining Resolution of Infection

1. Assess the patient for evidence of local and systemic infection—bullae are susceptible to infection, and septicemia may follow. Combinations of steroids and immunosuppressive drugs predispose the patient to severe infection.
2. Observe for psychiatric problems caused by high-dose steroids.

E. Achieving Reduction of Anxiety

1. Develop a trusting relationship with the patient.
2. Educate patient and family about the disease and its treatment—reduces uncertainty and enhances patient's ability to act on his own behalf.
3. Give expert nursing care.
4. Encourage free expression of anxieties, discomfort, and feelings of hopelessness.
5. Listen, interact, and demonstrate a warm, caring con-cern.
6. Arrange for "significant other" to spend more pro-longed periods with patient.

Patient Education

Instruct the patient as follows:
1. The disease may be characterized by relapses that re-quire continuing therapy to maintain control.
2. Long-term administration of immunosuppressive drugs is associated with increased risk of cancer; report for health care follow-up regularly.
3. Monitor skin/mouth for recurrence of pemphigus ac-tivity.

Toxic Epidermal Necrolysis (TEN)

Toxic epidermal necrolysis (TEN) is a severe, potentially fatal skin disease associated with erythema and epidermal sloughing. Its cause is unknown, but it is probably linked to the immune system as a reaction to drug ingestion or possibly secondary to a viral infection.

The drugs most commonly implicated are phenytoin, phenobarbital, the sulfonamides, and the penicillins.

Clinical Manifestations

1. Initial signs of conjunctival burning or itching; cuta-neous tenderness
2. Fever; extreme malaise; and myalgias
3. Erythema, involving much of skin surface
4. Appearance of large, flaccid bullae
5. Wide, sheet-like peeling and denudation of the skin— appearance is that of a second-degree burn with a moist, blistered, and tender surface
6. Skin necrosis; ulcerations of lips and oral pharynx
7. Positive Nikolsky's sign (desquamation of skin in sheets on light digital pressure)
8. Severe systemic toxic reactions

Diagnostic Evaluation

1. Cytodiagnosis of collections of cellular material from freshly denuded areas
2. Cultures taken of nasopharynx, eyes, ears, blood, urine, skin, and unruptured blisters—to determine presence of pathogenic organisms

Management

1. Treatment in intensive care unit or regional burn cen-ter, as TEN has similar pathophysiologic characteristics to those of extensive burns
2. Treatment of affected skin:
   a. Patient taken to operating room; anesthetized
   b. Wounds are washed; loose skin and blisters re-moved, areas of necrotic epidermis debrided— these may become the focus for infection.
   c. Temporary biological dressings (porcine cuta-neous xenographs, amnion, collagen-based skin

substitute [Bioderm], or plastic semipermeable dressings) applied—to prevent secondary skin infection while awaiting reepithelialization.
3. All nonessential drugs are stopped immediately
4. Fluid replacement therapy, depending on extent of epidermal necrolysis and severity of mucous membrane lesions
5. Enteral alimentation established through nasogastric tube
6. Daily examination of corneas by opthalmologist, with removal of synechiae (corneal adhesions)

Complications

1. Overwhelming infection; sepsis of denuded skin and/or lungs (mainly from *Staphylococcus aureus* and *Pseudomonas aeruginosa*)
2. Pneumonia secondary to aspiration of sloughed mucosa, shallow breathing from chest wall pain; atelectasis
3. Pulmonary embolism
4. Gastrointestinal bleeding
5. Poor vision/blindness, secondary to corneal ulceration and adhesions

Nursing Interventions

A. Achieving Skin and Oral Tissue Healing

1. Place patient on a warmed air–fluidized bed—to distribute weight with minimal shearing forces to an already denuded skin; also keeps xenograft dry.
2. Use extreme care in handling patient, as skin is very fragile. Secure services of several healthcare personnel to support an extremity evenly when patient moves.
3. Monitor vital signs (Indwelling arterial line with pressure transducer is used, giving a constant readout of blood pressure and pulse; avoid using a cuff sphygmomanometer because of skin trauma.).
4. Gently apply warm, wet compresses of prescribed antiseptic solution to reduce bacterial population of wound surface if skin is infected.
5. Inspect xenograft several times daily for dislodgment or purulence; these will require covering with new xenograft.
6. Watch for new areas of TEN; note and record progression of skin slough and compare with condition on admission.
7. Maintain a warm environment.
8. Employ meticulous oral hygiene:
   a. Inspect oral cavity daily; note any changes.
   b. Rinse mouth with prescribed solution to remove debris and soothe ulcerated area.
   c. Apply petrolatum or cover cracked, swollen lips with petrolatum-impregnated gauze.

B. Avoiding Infection

1. Use strict isolation precautions, including masking, sterile gloves (Patient placed in private room.).
2. Monitor for evidence of sepsis: hypothermia, fever, diminishing level of responsiveness, falling urine output, any *sudden* change in patient's condition.
3. Discontinue IV lines as soon as possible;
   a. Central venous lines and indwelling catheter should be avoided; sites may become infected and result in septicemia.
   b. Any intravascular catheter tips are cultured on removal.
4. Obtain samples for cultures from sputum, blood, skin, and mucous membranes.

5. Monitor urethral, vaginal, and anal regions for signs of infection/bleeding.

C. Attaining/Maintaining Fluid Balance

1. Monitor vital signs and sensorium for signs of hypovolemia.
2. Measure urinary output hourly—hypovolemia and renal damage are complications of TEN.
3. Evaluate results of laboratory tests (serum electrolytes); weigh patient on bed scale daily.
4. Give intravenous fluids as prescribed—daily evaporative losses may be high.
5. Start oral fluids as soon as patient demonstrates tolerance.

D. Achieving Relief of Pain

1. Assess and record evidence of pain and its characteristics, location, quality, frequency, and duration.
2. Maintain a regular, round-the-clock schedule of analgesic administration as prescribed, as a preventive approach to pain relief.
3. Assess patient's response to analgesic.
4. Assess for anxiety and depression.
5. Speak soothingly to patient during treatments to alleviate anxiety that may worsen pain.
6. Provide ongoing emotional support and reassurance.
7. Encourage patient to express feelings; listening to concerns and being available with skilled and compassionate care are anxiety-relieving interventions.

E. Other Nursing Interventions

1. Preventing ophthalmologic complications:
   a. Remove crusts from eyelid margins with sterile prescribed solution.
   b. Apply bland eyedrops/ointment as prescribed.
2. Pulmonary care:
   a. Monitor results of daily chest roentgenograms and blood gas measurements.
   b. Be aware that tracheostomy and mechanical ventilation may be necessary.
3. Nutritional care:
   a. Be aware that patient is in hypermetabolic state from evaporated water losses and increasing nitrogen losses from epidermal sloughing.
   b. Monitor nutritional status with measurement of nitrogen excretion—this provides a guide to adequacy of protein intake.
   c. Feed via nasogastric tube.

Patient Education

1. Recent exposure to drugs is implicated as the cause in most instances of TEN.
2. Any medication should be stopped if abnormal signs and symptoms develop.

Ulcers and Tumors of the Skin

Ulcers of the Skin

Ulceration is a superficial loss of surface tissue from the death of cells.

Causes

Ulcers of the skin usually arise from (1) infection or (2) an interference with the blood supply.

1. Infection as cause of skin ulcers.
   a. Usually develop from an infection with anaerobic streptococci or from combination of infections (hemolytic streptococci and staphylococci).
   b. Tend to progress peripherally—characterized by an overhanging edge.
2. Deficient arterial circulation as a cause of skin ulcers (See p. 399)
3. Pressure sores result from continuous pressure on an area (See p. 133).

Tumors of the Skin

Cysts

Epidermal cysts are common, slow-growing, firm, elevated tumors consisting of a mass of epidermal cells; frequently found on the back, neck, and upper chest.

Pilar cysts (trichilemmal cysts) are cysts that arise from the isthmus (middle) part of the hair follicle. They are common on the face and scalp.

Benign Tumors

A. Seborrheic Keratoses—tumors are benign wartlike lesions of varying size and color, ranging from light tan to black; most common skin tumors in middle-aged and elderly persons.

B. Actinic (solar) **Keratoses**—premalignant skin lesions appearing as rough, scaly patches with underlying erythema that develop as a consequence of prolonged exposure to ultraviolet rays.

1. Develop in chronic sun-exposed areas of body; may gradually transform into squamous cell cancer.
2. Many available treatments, including liquid nitrogen cryosurgery, curettage, etc.

C. Verrucae (warts)—common, benign skin tumors caused by viruses

1. Many times warts do not need treatment, as they tend to disappear spontaneously.
2. Treatment (remedies are legion)
   a. Freezing with liquid nitrogen—liquid nitrogen has a somewhat destructive action, although it tends to spare the epidermis.
   b. Area may be treated locally with salicylic acid plasters, electrodesiccation, application of cantharidin, topical fluorouracil, topical vitamin A acid, etc.

D. Angiomas (birthmarks)—benign vascular tumors involving the skin and subcutaneous tissues

1. May occur as flat, violet-red patches (port-wine angiomas) or as raised, bright-red nodular lesions (strawberry angiomas). Strawberry angiomas may involute spontaneously, whereas port-wine angiomas usually persist indefinitely.
2. Most patients use masking cosmetics (Covermark) to camouflage the defect.
3. Argon laser is being used with some success.

E. Pigmented Nevi (moles)—common skin tumors of various sizes and shapes, ranging from yellowish to brown to black.

1. May be flat, macular lesions or elevated papules or nodules that occasionally contain hair.
2. Majority of pigmented nevi are harmless; however, in rare cases, malignant changes supervene and a melanoma develops at the site of the nevus.
3. Treatment
   a. Nevi at sites subject to repeated irritation from clothing, etc., should be removed—for comfort.
   b. Nevi that show change in size or color, or become symptomatic (itch or bleed) or develop notched borders should be removed—to determine if malignant changes have occurred. This is especially true for nevi with irregular borders or variations of blue, red, and/or white color.

F. Keloids—benign overgrowths of fibrous tissue at site of scar or trauma in predisposed individuals.

1. More prevalent among black race
2. Usually asymptomatic—may cause disfigurement and cosmetic concern
3. Management—surgical excision, intralesional corticosteroid therapy, radiation

Cancer of the Skin

Clinical Features

1. Skin cancer is the most common malignancy; the number of cases is increasing yearly.
2. There is a 95% cure rate because of early diagnosis, the slow progression of most skin cancers, and the effective methods of treatment available.

Causes

1. Exposure to sun over a period of time. *Sun damage is cumulative.*
2. Persons who do not produce sufficient pigment to protect underlying tissue are susceptible to sun damage—fair, blue-eyed, red-haired persons of Celtic ancestry or those with ruddy or light complexions; those who sunburn and do not tan.
3. Outdoor workers; farmers, sailors, fishermen
4. Elderly with sun-damaged skin
5. Exposure to irradiation (history of x-ray treatment of benign skin lesions).
6. Exposure to certain chemical agents (arsenic, nitrates, tar and pitch, oils and paraffins).
7. Burn scars, areas of chronic osteomyelitis, fistulae of chronic nature
8. Immunosuppressive therapy
9. Genetic susceptibility

Types of Skin Cancer

A. Basal Cell Carcinoma

1. A malignant epithelial tumor of the skin that arises from the basal layer of the epidermis or the hair follicle; most common type of skin cancer
2. Lesions are small nodules with a rolled, pearly, translucent border with telangiectasia (dilatation of end blood vessels), crusting, and occasionally ulceration (Fig. 32-6).
3. These tumors may be pigmented, multiple, superficial or cystic.
   a. Lesions appear most frequently on sun-exposed skin, frequently on face between hair line and upper lip.
   b. A neglected basal cell carcinoma may cause local destruction, hemorrhage, and infection of adjacent tissues, producing severe functional and cosmetic disabilities.

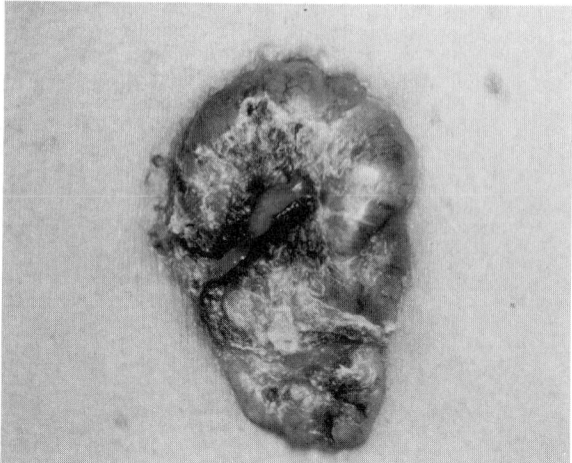

Figure 32-6. *Basal cell carcinoma. (Photo courtesy Mervyn L. Elgart, M.D.)*

B. Squamous Cell (Epidermoid) **Carcinoma**

1. A malignant proliferation arising from the epidermis; considered a truly invasive carcinoma.
2. Appears as a solitary rough, thickened, scaly tumor that may be asymptomatic or may involve bleeding; border of lesion may be wider, more infiltrated, and more inflammatory than that of basal cell carcinoma.
3. May be preceded by leukoplakia (premalignant lesion of mucous membrane), actinic keratoses, scarred or ulcerated lesions.
4. Seen most commonly on lower lip, rims of ears, head, neck, and dorsa of hands.
5. Requires more aggressive approach (wider margin of normal skin included in excision)—greater chance of metastases from squamous cell carcinoma and significantly lower cure rate.

NURSING ALERT: Any skin lesion that changes in size or color, bleeds, ulcerates, or becomes infected may be skin cancer.

Diagnostic Evaluation

1. Biopsy
2. Histologic evaluation

Management

Method of treatment depends on tumor location, cell type (location and depth), history of previous treatment, and whether or not it is invasive and metastatic nodes are present.

A. Curettage Followed by Electrodesiccation—usually done on small tumors (less than 1–2 cm.).

1. Curettage—excision of skin tumor by scraping with a curette; electrodesiccation (alternating high-frequency current, which results in death of cells) is used to achieve hemostasis and to destroy any viable malignant cells in margins or in base of wound.
2. Tumor is removed and the base cauterized; process is repeated a number of times.

B. Surgical Excision

1. Wide surgical excision—adequacy of excision verified by microscopic study of sections of the specimen.
2. May be followed by simple closure, flap or graft.

C. Microscopically Controlled Surgery (Chemosurgery)

1. Combined use of topically applied chemicals and serial excisions of tumors layer by layer.
2. Immediate microscopic examination is made of frozen section for evidence of cancer cells.
3. Procedure may be repeated until specimens are cancer-free.

D. Cryosurgery—deep freezing to destroy tumor tissue selectively.

1. Liquid nitrogen is applied by open spray or cryoprobe technique; tumor necrosis is achieved through freeze and thaw cycles.
2. Site thaws naturally and then becomes gelatinous and heals spontaneously.

E. Radiation Therapy—usually done for cancer of eyelid, tip of nose, in or near vital structures (facial nerve), where tissue sparing is difficult with other forms of treatment; used for extensive malignancies when goal is palliation or when other medical conditions contraindicate other forms of therapy.

1. Explain to the patient that he may experience skin reddening and swelling about the time of the third treatment; may progress to blistering.
2. Apply bland skin ointment as prescribed—to relieve discomfort.
3. Caution patient against exposure to the sun.

F. Other Therapeutic Regimens (used in certain cutaneous premalignancies and malignancies) include topical fluorouracil, combination chemotherapy, interferon, retinoids, and photoradiation therapy.

Patient Education

Instruct the patient as follows:

1. *Sunlight permanently damages the skin.* Most cancer can be prevented by avoidance of and protection from direct exposure to the sun.
2. Protective measures should be started in childhood and carried on throughout life.
3. Do not try to tan if your skin burns easily, never tans, or tans poorly.
4. *Do not become sunburned.*
5. Avoid unnecessary exposure to the sun, especially during times when ultraviolet radiation is most intense (10:00 A.M.–2:00 P.M.).
6. Apply a protective sunscreen if you must be in the sun; sunscreens block out harmful rays.
   a. Sunscreens with a sun protection factor (SPF) of 15 or greater, which are combinations of PABA and a benzophenone, offer good protection.
   b. Use a sunscreen with SPF 15 *routinely* applied evenly to all exposed areas of the body.
   c. Sunscreen should not come off easily. Periodically reapply more sunscreen, especially after swimming/bathing.
   d. Protect your lips; use a lip balm that contains a sunscreen with the highest SPF factor.
7. Wear protective clothing (long sleeves, broad-brimmed hat, etc.)—however, clothing does not pro-

vide complete protection, as up to 50% of sun's damaging rays can go through clothes.

8. Do not use sun lamps for indoor tanning; avoid commercial tanning salons.
9. Have moles removed that are accessible to repeated friction and irritation.
10. Watch for indications of potential malignancy in moles (e.g., change in color, increase in size, ulceration, bleeding, or serious exudation).
11. Have follow-up evaluation throughout lifetime. A person with one basal cell cancer has an increasing chance of having new skin cancers. (There is also an incidence of internal malignancy associated with squamous cell cancer.)
12. For information about patient education materials, contact:
    The Skin Cancer Foundation
    245 Fifth Avenue, Suite 2402
    New York, New York 10016.

Malignant Melanoma

A *malignant melanoma* is a malignant tumor occurring primarily in the skin in which atypical melanocytes (pigment cells) are present in both the epidermis and the dermis (and sometimes into cutaneous fat), from which sites they may metastasize. They occur in several forms (See Classification, below). The incidence is rising rapidly.

Malignant melanoma may arise in apparently normal skin or may arise in association with preexisting acquired and congenital melanocytic nevi.

Risk Factors

1. Sun exposure
2. History of melanoma in past; family history of melanoma, have giant congenital nevi or a significant history of severe sunburn
3. Skin pigmentation—fair-skinned, light-colored eyes; light-colored hair; persons who sunburn readily and do not tan.
4. Dysplastic nevi—acquired abnormal moles present both in general population and in certain melanoma-prone families.
   a. Have unusual moles, larger and more numerous, of irregular shape and variable colors (tan, brown, dark brown, pink)
5. Congenital nevi (a melanocytic nevus present at birth)

Classification *(Fig. 32-7)*

A. Superficial Spreading Melanoma (most common)

1. Occurs anywhere on body; usually affects middle-aged persons.
2. Tends to be circular, with irregular outer portions; the margins of the lesion may be flat or elevated and palpable.
3. Has combination of colors—hues of tan, brown, and black admixed with gray, bluish-black, or white.
4. May be dull pink-rose color in a small area within the lesion.

B. Lentigo-maligna Melanoma

1. Slowly evolving pigment lesions; occur on exposed skin surfaces of persons in the 5th or 6th decade.
2. First appears as tan, flat macule—malignant degeneration is manifested by changes in size, color, and topography.

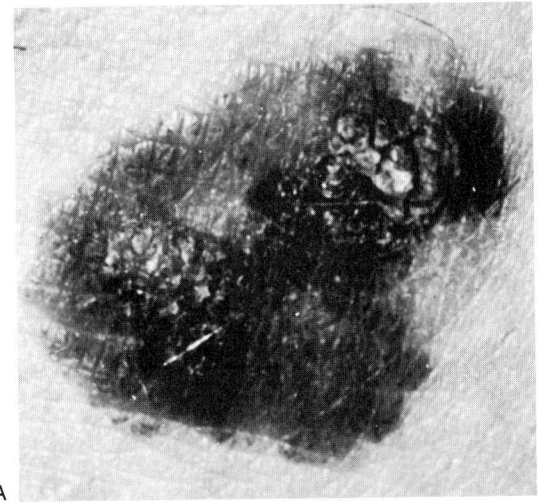

A

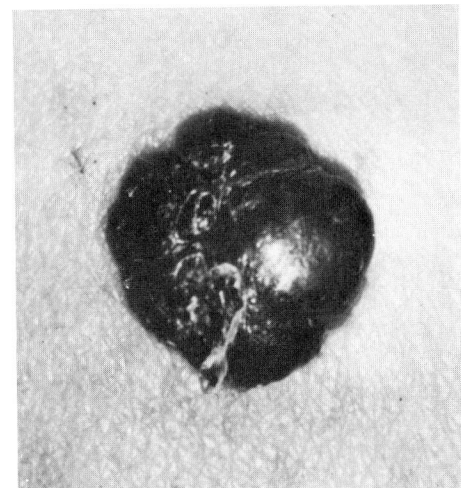

B

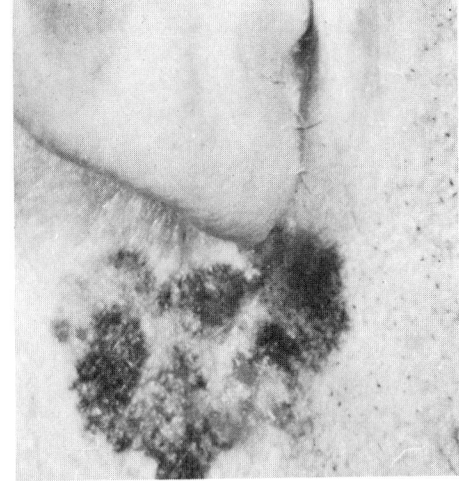

C

Figure 32-7. *(A) Superficial spreading melanoma; note irregular border. (B) Nodular melanoma. (C) Lentigo-maligna melanoma; note irregular pigment pattern. (Photos courtesy Arthur J. Sober, M.D.)*

C. Nodular Melanoma

1. Spherical blueberry-like nodule with relatively smooth surface and relatively uniform blue-black, blue-gray, or reddish-blue color; occurs commonly on back, head, and neck.
2. May be polypoidal, with smooth surface of rose-gray or black color; may be present as elevated, irregular plaque.
3. Invades directly into the subjacent dermis (vertical growth) and hence has a poorer prognosis.

D. Acral-lentiginous Melanoma

1. A tumor predominantly seen in blacks and dark-skinned persons; common sites are the palms, soles, nail beds, and mucous membranes.
2. Appear as irregular pigmented macules, which develop nodules; may become invasive early.

Clinical Manifestations

Signs that suggest malignant change
1. *Variegated color*
   a. Colors that may indicate malignancy in a brown or black lesion are shades of red, white, and blue; shades of blue are considered ominous.
   b. White areas within a pigmented lesion are suspicious.
   c. Some malignant melanomas are not variegated, but are uniformly colored (bluish-black, bluish-gray, bluish-red).
2. *Irregular border*—look for angular indentation or notch or scalloped edging in the border of the mole
3. *Irregular surface and elevation*
   a. Run your fingers lightly over surface and feel for uneven elevations of the surface; irregular topography may be palpable or visible; change in the surface (smooth to scaly).
   b. Some nodular melanomas have a smooth surface.
4. *Change in color, size, symmetry, surface characteristics, symptoms (itching, tingling, tenderness, pain), and shape.*
5. Common sites of melanoma—skin of back, legs

Diagnostic Evaluation

1. Appearance of lesion (see above) with consideration of history of recent changes within lesion.

2. Excision biopsy (for histopathologic diagnosis) and microstaging determination of thickness and level of invasion (Fig. 32-8)

Management

The therapeutic approach depends on the type, level, thickness, and location of the lesion, and the stage of disease.
1. Surgical excision of cutaneous melanoma ranging from simple to a wide excision, sometimes followed by plastic repair or skin grafting. The role of regional node dissection is in dispute.
2. Regional perfusion of an extremity as an adjuvant to surgery; anatomic region is isolated by mechanically controlling its arterial inflow and venous outflow. A chemotherapeutic agent is perfused directly into the area that contains the melanoma, allowing a higher concentration of cytotoxic drug to be delivered to cancer-bearing sites, with less systemic toxicity.
3. Immunotherapy—interferons (cellular proteins with a broad range of immunomodulatory and antiproliferative effects).
4. Chemotherapy—generally used for recurrence of metastasis or as palliation; may be combined with autologous bone marrow transplantation.
   Combination chemotherapy (DTIC; BCNU, cis-platin with tamoxifin) is showing some success.

Complications

Recurrence; regional metastases; systemic metastases
   CNS metastasis—headache, impaired mentation, motor deficits, seizures, cerebellar dysfunction

Nursing Assessment

1. Have a high index of suspicion for persons at risk.
2. Ask about sunbathing habits. Question patient about pruritus, tenderness, and pain, which are not features of a benign nevus.
3. Ask about changes in preexisting moles or development of a new pigmented lesion.
4. Use a magnifying lens in a brightly lit room to look for variegated color, irregular border, etc. in the mole. (See Clinical Manifestations) Use side lighting to assess for subtle elevation.

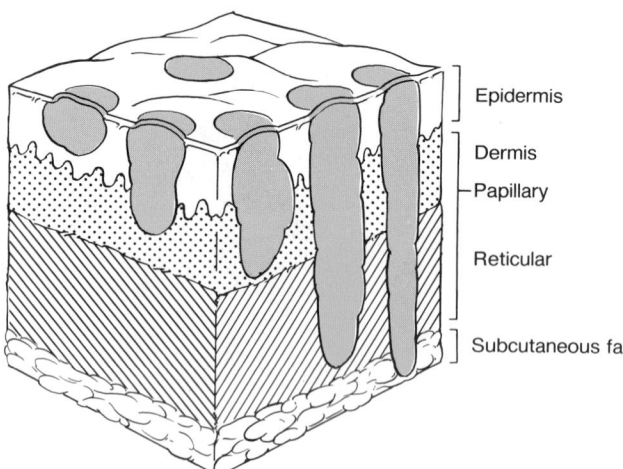

Epidermis

Dermis

Papillary

Reticular

Subcutaneous fat

Figure 32-8. *Vertical growth (dermal invasion) of malignant melanoma. The prognosis of the patient depends on the thickness of the melanoma and the depth of the dermal invasion.*

5. Examine entire skin surface, including scalp, genital area, gluteal folds, and soles of the feet. In black persons, look on less pigmented sites; palms, soles, subungual areas, mucous membranes.
6. Examine diameter of the mole; melanomas are often larger than 6 mm (greater than a pencil eraser); look for lesions situated near the mole.

Nursing Interventions

A. Achieving Reduction of Anxiety

1. Allow patient to express feelings about the seriousness of diagnosis.
2. Answer questions; clarify information and correct misconceptions.
3. Point out successes with past life experiences, including coping with difficulties.
4. Encourage patient to draw on social support system as a resource.

Discharge Planning/Patient Education

Instruct the patient as follows:
1. Examine your skin monthly in an orderly manner; include scalp examination.
   a. Use a full-length mirror and a small hand mirror to aid in examination.
   b. Learn where moles/birthmarks are located.
   c. Inspect all moles and other pigmented lesions; report to the physician/clinic immediately moles that change colors, enlarge, become raised or thicker, itch, or bleed.
   d. Have physician examine your skin at least twice yearly. A patient with malignant melanoma should have lifelong follow-up.
2. A key factor in development of malignant melanoma is exposure to sunlight. See page 830 for preventive aspects.
3. Use a sunscreen with a sun protection factor of at least 15; *never become sunburned*
4. Congenital moles are recognized as precursors of melanoma and should be carefully monitored and probably removed.
5. Be aware that nevi may change during puberty and pregnancy.

Dermatologic and Plastic Reconstructive Surgery

Reconstructive (plastic) surgery is performed to reconstruct or alter congenital or acquired defects to restore or improve the body's appearance and function.

Wound Coverage: Grafts and Flaps:

Definitions

1. *Skin graft*—a section of skin tissue that is separated from its blood supply and transferred as free tissue to a distant (recipient) site; it must obtain nourishment from capillary healing at the recipient site.
   In dermatology, skin grafting is used to repair defects resulting from excision of skin tumors and to cover areas of denuded skin.

2. *Autografts*—grafts done with tissue transplanted from the patient's own skin
3. *Allografts*—involve the transplant of tissue from one individual of the same species; these grafts are also called *allogenic* or *homografts*.
4. *Xenograft* or *heterograft*—involves the transfer of tissue from another species.

Classification by Thickness

1. *Split thickness* (thin, intermediate, or thick)—graft that is cut at varying thicknesses and is used to cover large wounds or defects for which a full thickness graft or application is impractical.
2. *Full thickness*—graft consists of epidermis and all of the dermis without the underlying fat; used to cover wounds that are too large to close primarily. They are used frequently to cover facial defects, for these grafts neither contract nor develop unsightly pigmentation.

Graft Application

1. Graft obtained by razor blade, skin grafting knife, electric or air-powered dermatome/drum dermatome.
2. Skin is taken from the "donor" or "host" site and applied to the wound/defect site, called the "recipient site" or "graft bed."
3. Process of revascularization and reattachment of the skin graft to the recipient bed is referred to as a "take."
4. Patient Education
   a. Keep the affected part immobilized as much as possible.
   b. Keep an affected extremity elevated, as the new capillary connections are fragile and excess venous pressure may cause rupture. Wear an elastic stocking to counteract venous pressure.
   c. Inspect the dressing daily. Report unusual drainage or signs of an inflammatory reaction.
   d. After 2–3 weeks, mineral oil or a lanolin cream may be massaged around the wound to stimulate circulation.
   e. Expect some loss of feeling/sensation in the grafted area for a time.

Flaps

1. A *flap* is a segment of tissue that has been left attached at one end (called a *base* or *pedicle*), while the other end has been moved to a recipient area. It is dependent for its survival on functioning arterial and venous blood supplies and lymphatic drainage in its pedicle or base.
   a. Flaps may consist of skin, mucosa, muscle, adipose tissue, omentum, and bone.
   b. Used for wound coverage and to provide bulk, especially when bone, tendon, blood vessels, or nerve tissue are exposed.
   c. Flaps offer the best aesthetic solution, because a flap retains the color and texture of the donor area.
   d. Series of operations usually required to move a flap.
2. *Free flap* or free-tissue transfer—one that is completely severed from the body and is transferred to another site; receives early vascular supply from microvascular anastomosis with vessels at recipient site.
3. Flaps are classified according to the method of movement, their composition, location, or function.

Selected Aesthetic (Cosmetic) Procedures

Rhytidectomy

Rhytidectomy (face lift) is the surgical procedure designed to lessen skin folds and wrinkles and to improve the appearance of the aging face. There are numerous techniques and various incisions, depending on the procedure. Rhytidectomy may be combined with liposuction to remove fat from the neck, chin, and jowls and/or with chemical face peeling.

A. Complications

1. Hematoma
2. Necrosis of skin flaps
3. Partial facial paralysis

B. Patient Education

1. Expect the face to be swollen, bruised and numb—due to pressure created by surgery and newly tightened muscles, fascia, and skin.
2. Rest quietly for 24 hours with head elevation. Minimize head motion and avoid neck flexion.
3. Take clear liquids through a straw; advance to full liquids and a soft diet when chewing becomes more comfortable.
4. Cleanse skin and use prescribed cream as directed after bandage removal.
5. Call the physician/clinic if sudden pain occurs—suggests hematoma.
6. Avoid lifting or bending—may increase edema and provoke bleeding.
7. Usually makeup may be applied in about 1 week; pat the makeup on and avoid stretching the skin.
8. Use a sunscreen and wide-brimmed hat for 3 months or more—to prevent sunburn and facial swelling.
9. Keep hair dryer on cool setting while in use, as the scalp may be numb after surgery for a varying period.

Blepharoplasty

Blepharoplasty—is an operation to remove excess skin or fat from the upper and lower eyelids. CO_2 laser excision surgery also is being used for this procedure.

A. Complications

1. Bleeding; hematoma
2. Dry eye
3. Eyelid retraction

B. Patient Education

1. Expect considerable eyelid swelling and ecchymosis, especially in lower eyelids, which may persist for 2 weeks.
2. Sleep with head elevated for first 2 weeks after surgery.
3. Use ice compresses almost continuously or intermittently as directed over eyes to reduce edema and ecchymosis.
4. Apply warm compresses as directed after 24 hours to hasten resolution.
5. Use a sunscreen after healing.
6. Some tingling or crawling sensations may be expected under the lower lashes for a time.
7. Instill artificial tears to combat feeling of burning, itching, and drying of eyes.

Rhinoplasty

Rhinoplasty involves reduction or augmentation, or both, of the nose. If the function of the nose is altered, the term *nasal reconstruction,* is used. Complications include bleeding and hematoma.

Patient Education

1. Expect to have symptoms of a head cold, swelling, and bruising, which will dissipate with time. Expect some oozing of blood for 24–48 hours.
2. Rest while sitting upright. Do not touch, pick, or blow nose—to avoid bleeding.
3. Apply cold compresses intermittently—to minimize swelling, ecchymosis, and discomfort.
4. Some type of splint (aluminum, plaster of Paris, molded plastic or gauze dressing) may be used to maintain nasal bones in desired position and protect the nose.
5. Packing may or may not be in place—acts as counterpressure to shape and mold nose.
6. Reduce physical activity; strenuous activity may not be undertaken for 6 weeks.
7. If sneezing is necessary, open the mouth while doing so.

Dermabrasion

Dermabrasion (skin planing) is a form of skin abrasion with a special instrument to remove the epidermis and superficial layers of the dermis to improve the appearance.

Management

1. The procedure is usually done as an outpatient procedure in the Ambulatory Surgery Center/office under local or general anesthesia.
2. After the procedure, the patient's face may be covered with wet dressings or emollient gauze to absorb oozing of blood and serum.

Patient Education

1. At the time specified by the surgeon, the patient is instructed to wash her face with her fingers and then apply a thin layer of cream; or an emollient may be used without washing the face.
2. Erythema (redness) is expected for 2 weeks and then will gradually fade.
3. Edema is inevitable and usually resolves in several weeks.
4. Elevate the head at night to lessen facial swelling.
5. Do not pluck at the crusts; this will injure new epithelium.
6. Avoid sunlight for at least 2 months—blotchy hyperpigmentation to dermabraded areas can occur.
7. After healing occurs, protect the face with a sunscreen; use hypoallergenic moisturizers and cosmetics.
8. Avoid exposure to heat, cold, wind, emotional upsets—will cause skin to become intensely pink due to increased blood flow.
9. Corrective cosmetics (Dermablend®) can effectively even skin tone and conceal skin blemishes, making them difficult to detect, even at close range.

Chemical Face Peeling (Chemoexfoliation; Chemosurgery)

Chemical face peeling involves the application of a chemical mixture to the face for the purpose of causing superficial destruction of the epidermis and the upper layers of the dermis.

It is used to remove fine wrinkling and irregularly pigmented areas of the skin.

Complications

1. Excessive skin bleaching or splotchy hyperpigmentation
2. Prolonged erythema
3. Scars

Procedure/Patient Education

1. A phenol-based chemical in solution is applied in a systematic manner to the face with cotton-tipped applicators. At this time the patient will experience a burning sensation.
2. A mask of waterproof tape is applied to the skin—provides an occlusive dressing that increases chemical penetration and action. (Not all dermatologic surgeons use tape).
3. The patient is kept comfortable with analgesics.
4. The patient is advised to refrain from talking and perioral movement—to avoid dislodging the tape.
5. After 48 hours the mask is removed, exposing edematous, weeping surface resembling a second degree burn.
6. Sometimes a powder is applied to the area to encourage crust formation. Within a specified period, the face is washed and lubricated several times a day.
7. It may take 6–8 weeks for normalization of color and skin texture.
8. Avoid the sun; use a sunscreen—to avoid hyperpigmentation.

Body Contouring Surgery: Liposuction

Liposuction is a technique of reducing localized deposits of fat with a cannula aided by suction. More recently, syringes combined with special fitting cannulae are being used.

1. Liposuction is used to remove localized deposits of fat that are genetically determined and cannot be lost by dieting. It is not a treatment for obesity and will not remove cellulite (dimples/irregularities in the skin).
2. This procedure may be done on the face, neck, breasts, abdomen, flanks, hips, buttocks, and extremities.

Procedure

1. Under local or general anesthesia, chilled diluted solution of lidocaine (for anesthesia) and epinephrine (for vasoconstriction) is infiltrated into the subcutaneous space.
2. The cannula is introduced through a skin puncture/incision; the suction apparatus is started and the cannula is passed into the deep fat and moved in and out of previously marked areas.
3. The removed fat contains blood, tissue fluids, and electrolytes; usually less than 2000 ml of fat is removed in one session.
4. Following the procedure, an elastic dressing is applied to provide hemostasis, and prevent edema and shifting of fluid into the third space. The compression dressing also helps to redrape the skin and its subcutaneous fat into proper position to give the desired cosmetic effect.

Complications

1. Excessive blood loss
2. Persistent skin irregularities
3. Hematoma; seroma (localized accumulation of serous fluid caused by traumatized lymphatic vessels)

Patient Education

1. Expected sequelae include ecchymosis, temporary skin irregularity, temporary paresthesias, and edema.
2. Do not take any aspirin or aspirin-containing medication or alcoholic beverages at least 1 week before and after surgery.
3. Rest in bed for 24–48 hours following the liposuction.
4. Drink liberal amounts of fluids.
5. The bandages will be removed in 4–7 days; a support garment will be then applied and is to be worn 4–6 weeks.
6. The physician will advise when to start gentle fingertip massage or manual kneeding of the area—to soften developing scar tissue.

Bibliography

Books

Arndt KA. Manual of Dermatologic Therapeutics. 4th ed. Boston, Little, Brown & Co, 1989

Asken S. Liposuction Surgery and Autologous Fat Transplantation. Norwalk, Appleton and Lange, 1988

Bennett RG. Fundamentals of Cutaneous Surgery. St Louis, CV Mosby, 1988

Bork K and Bräuninger W. Diagnosis and Treatment of Common Skin Diseases. Philadelphia, WB Saunders, 1988

Buxton PK. ABC of Dermatology. London, British Medical Association, 1988

Epstein E and Epstein E Jr. Skin Surgery. 6th ed. Philadelphia, WB Saunders, 1987

Findlay GH. The Dermatology of

Bacterial Infections. Boston, Blackwell Scientific Publications, 1987

Fitzpatrick TB et al. Dermatology in General Medicine. 3rd ed., Vols 1 and 2. New York, McGraw-Hill, 1987

Georgiade NG et al (eds). Essentials of Plastic, Maxillofacial, and Reconstructive Surgery. Baltimore, Williams & Wilkins, 1987

Greer KE. Common Problems in Dermatology. Chicago, Year Book Medical Pub, 1988

Koblenzer CS. Psychocutaneous Disease. Orlando, Grune & Stratton, 1987

Krusinski PA and Flowers FP. Life-Threatening Dermatoses. Chicago, Year Book Medical Pub, 1987

Lowe NJ. Practical Psoriasis Therapy. Chicago, Year Book Medical Pub, 1986

Maibach HI. Occupational and Industrial

Dermatology. Chicago, Year Book Medical Pub, 1987

Maize JC and Ackerman AB. Pigmented Lesions of the Skin. Philadelphia, Lea and Febiger, 1987

Marks R. Skin Disease in Old Age. London, Martin Dunitz Ltd., 1987

McCollough EG and Langsdon P. Dermabrasion and Chemical Peel. New York, Thieme Medical Publishers, 1988

Mier PD and van de Kerkhof PCM. Textbook of Psoriasis. New York, Churchill Livingstone, 1986

Provost TT and Farmer ER. Current Therapy in Dermatology. Philadelphia, BC Decker, 1988

Rook A et al (eds). Textbook of Dermatology. 4th ed, Vols 1–3. Boston, Blackwell Scientific Publications, 1986

Schwartz RA. Skin Cancer. New York, Springer–Verlag, 1988

Sheen JH and Sheen AP. Aesthetic Rhinoplasty. Vols 1 and 2. St Louis, CV Mosby, 1987

Shupack JL et al. Dermatologic Formulary. New York, McGraw-Hill, 1989

Sohn SA. Fundamentals of Aesthetic Plastic Surgery. Baltimore, Williams & Wilkins, 1987

Stark RB (ed). Plastic Surgery of the Head and Neck. Vols 1–2. New York, Churchill Livingstone, 1987

Teimourian B. Suction Lipectomy & Body Sculpturing. St Louis, CV Mosby, 1987

Thomas JR and Holt GR. Facial Scars: Incision, Revision & Camouflage. St Louis, CV Mosby, 1989

Tromovitch TA, Stegman SJ and Glogau RG. Flaps and Grafts in Dermatologic Surgery. Chicago, Year Book Medical Pub, 1989

Verbow JL. Current Concepts in Contact Dermatitis. Boston, MTP Press, 1987

Verbow J (ed). Treatment in Dermatology. Boston, MTP Press, 1987

Journals

Cancer of the Skin; Malignant Melanoma

Becker JK, Goldberg LH and Tschen JA. Differential diagnosis of malignant melanoma. Am Fam Physician 1989 May; 39(5):203–214

Boyce JA and Bernhard JD. Routine total skin examination to detect malignant melanoma. J Gen Intern Med 1987 Jan–Feb; 2(1):59–61

Costanzi JJ. Malignant melanoma. Why early diagnosis and treatment are crucial. Postgrad Med 1988 Nov 1; 84(6):159–160; 163–167

Das Gupta TK. Current status of surgical treatment of melanoma. Semin Oncol 1988 Dec; 15(6):566–568

Deleo VA. Prevention of skin cancer. J Dermatol Surg Oncol 1988 Aug; 14(8):902–906

Elwood JM. Malignant melanoma and naevi. Pigment Cell 1988; 9:1–152 (entire issue)

Goldberg LH and Rubin HA. Management of basal cell carcinoma. Postgrad Med 1989 Jan; 85(1):57–58; 61–63

Kopf AW. Prevention and early detection of skin cancer/melanoma. Cancer 1988 Oct 15; 62(8 Suppl):1791–1795

Lippman SM, Shimm DS and Meyskens FL. Nonsurgical treatments for skin cancer: Retinoids and α-interferon. J Dermatol Surg Oncol 1988 Aug; 14(8):862–869

Malignant melanoma of the skin. Drug Ther Bull 1988 Sep 19; 26(19):73–75

Marks R, Rennie G and Selwood T. The relationship of basal cell carcinomas and squamous cell carcinomas to solar keratoses. Arch Dermatol 1988 Jul; 124(7):1039–1042

McClay EF and Mastrangelo MJ. Systemic chemotherapy for metastatic melanoma. Semin Oncol 1988 Dec; 15(6):569–577

Morison WL. Skin cancer and artificial sources of UV radiation. J Dermatol Surg Oncol 1988 Aug; 14(8):893–896

Novick NL, Kest E and Gordon M. Advances in the biology and carcinogenesis of basal cell carcinoma. NY State J Med 1988 Jul; 88(7):367–370

Olweny CLM. Malignant melanoma: A clinical perspective. Med J Aust 1988 Jun 20; 148(12):638–646

Parnes R, Safai B and Myskowski PL. Basal cell carcinomas and lymphoma: Biologic behavior and associated factors in sixty-three patients. J Am Acad Dermatol 1988 Dec; 19(6):1017–1023

Peck GL et al. Treatment and prevention of basal cell carcinoma with oral isotretinoin. J Am Acad Dermatol 1988 Jul; 19(1 Pt 2):176–185

Pritchard GA, Zhang LJ and Hughes LE. Suture or graft? Changing trends in melanoma wound closure. Eur J Surg Oncol 1988 Oct; 14(5):371–377

Rhodes AR et al. Risk factors for cutaneous melanoma. JAMA 1987 Dec 4; 258(21):3146–3154

Stal S, Loeb T and Spira M. Melanoma of the head and neck. Update and perspective. Otolaryngol Clin North Am 1986 Aug; 19(3):549–564

Tucker MA and Bale SJ. Clinical aspects of familial cutaneous malignant melanoma. Semin Oncol 1988 Dec; 15(6):524–528

Dermatologic Surgery

Asken S. Facial liposuction and microlipoinjection. J Dermatol Surg Oncol 1988 Mar; 14(3):297–305

David LM. The laser approach to blepharoplasty. J Dermatol Surg Oncol 1988 Jul; 14(7):741–746

Fournier PF and Coleman EP III (eds). Special issue: Liposuction. J Dermatol Surg Oncol 1988 Oct; 14(10):1055–1172

Goodman T. Grafts and flaps in plastic surgery. AORN J 1988 Oct; 48(4):650–663

Grossman JA. Body contouring. AORN J 1988 Oct; 48(4):713–725

Hanke C. Liposuction under local anesthesia. J Dermatol Surg Oncol 1989 Jan; 15(1):12

Hetter GP. Closed suction lipoplasty on 1078 patients; Illouz told the truth. Aesthetic Plast Surg 1988 Aug; 12(3):183–185

General

Eaglstein WH, Mertz PM and Falanga V. Occlusive dressings. Am Fam Physician 1987 Mar; 35(3):211–216

Estlander T and Jolanki R. How to protect the hands. Dermatol Clin 1988 Jan; 6(1):105–114

Fisher AA. Recent developments in contact dermatitis and occupational dermatology. Cutis 1988 Sep; 42(3):169–172

Gayer KD and Burnett JW. Toxicodendron dermatitis. Cutis 1988 Aug; 42(2):99–100

Guidelines for prescribing isotretinoin (Accutane) in the treatment of female acne patients of childbearing potential. J Am Acad Dermatol 1988 Nov; 19(5 Part 1):920

Korman N. Pemphigus. J Am Acad Dermatol 1988 Jun; 18(6):1219–1238

Litt JZ. Alternative topical therapy. Dermatol Clin 1989 Jan; 7(1):43–52

Quan M and Strick RA. Management of acne vulgaris. Am Fam Physician 1988 Aug; 38(2):207–218

Thestrup-Pedersen K et al. The red man syndrome. J Am Acad Dermatol 1988 Jun; 18(6):1307–1312

Herpes Zoster

Balfour HH Jr. Varicella zoster virus infections in immunocompromised hosts: A review of the natural history and management. Am J Med 1988 Aug 29; 85(2A):68–73

Bryson YJ. Promising new antiviral drugs. J Am Acad Dermatol 1988 Jan; 18(1 Part 2):212–218

Post BT and Philbrick JT. Do corticosteroids prevent postherpetic neuralgia? J Am Acad Dermatol 1988 Mar; 18(3):605–610

Solomon AR. New diagnostic tests for herpes simplex and varicella zoster infections. J Am Acad Dermatol 1988 Jan; 18(1 Part 2):218–221

Straus SE et al. Varicella-zoster virus infections. Ann Intern Med 1988 Feb; 108(2):221–237

Strommen GL et al. Human infection with herpes zoster: Etiology, pathophysiology, diagnosis, clinical course and treatment. Pharmacotherapy 1988; 8(1):52–68

Infections/Infestations

Baig A, Grillage MG and Welch RB. A comparison of erythromycin and flucloxacillin in the treatment of infected skin lesions in general practice. Br J Clin Pract 1988 Mar; 42(3):110–115

Halder RM. Pseudofolliculitis barbae and related disorders. Dermatol Clin 1988 Jul; 6(3):407–412

Millikan LE et al. Naftifine cream 1% versus econazole cream 1% in the treatment of tinea cruris and tinea corporis. J Am Acad Dermatol 1988 Jan; 18(1 Part 1):52–56

Wheatley D, Richardson MD and Scott EM. Tinea infections treated with bifonazole gel. Mycoses 1988 Sep; 31(9):471–475

Psoriasis

Biren CA and Barr RJ. Dermatologic applications of cyclosporine. Arch Dermatol 1986 Sep; 122(9):1028–1032

Boyd AS. Scalp psoriasis. Am Fam Physician 1988 Oct; 38(4):163–170

Champion RH. Psoriasis. Br Med J 1986 Jun 28; 292(6537):1693–1696

Ginsburg IH and Link BG. Feelings of stigmatization in patients with psoriasis. J Am Acad Dermatol 1989 Jan; 20(1):53–63

Gupta AK and Anderson TF. Psoralen photochemotherapy. J Am Acad Dermatol 1987 Nov; 17(5 Part 1):703–734

Lowe NJ, Roenigk H and Voorhees JJ.

Etretinate. Arch Dermatol 1988 Apr; 124(4):527–5

Payne CME. Psoriatic science. Br Med J 1987 Nov 7; 295(6607):1158–1160

Scabies

Arlian LG, Estes SA and Vyszenski-Moher DL. Prevalence of *Sarcoptes scabiei* in the homes and nursing homes of scabietic patients. J Am Acad Dermatol 1988 Nov; 19(5 Part 1):806–811

Meyers LN. Clinical presentation of scabies in a nursing home population. J Am Acad Dermatol 1988 Feb; 18(2 Part 1):396–397

Rasmussen JE. Lindane: A prudent approach. Arch Dermatol 1987 Aug; 123(8):1008–1010

Rosenbaum M. Pruritus of unknown origin. Hosp Pract (Off) 1988 Oct 30; 23(10A):19–22, 24, 26

Treating scabies. Drug Ther Bull 1988 Mar 7; 26(5):19–20

Van Neste DJJ. Human scabies in perspective. Int J Dermatol 1988 Jan–Feb; 27(1):10–15

Toxic Epidermal Necrolysis

Editorial. Burn treatment for the unburned. JAMA 1987 Apr 24; 257(16): 2207–2208

Guillaume J-C et al. The culprit drugs in 87 cases of toxic epidermal necrolysis (Lyell's syndrome). Arch Dermatol 1987 Sep; 123(9):1166–1168

Halebian PH et al. Improved burn center survival of patients with toxic epidermal necrolysis managed without corticosteroids. Ann Surg 1986 Nov; 204(5):503–512

Heimbach DM et al. Toxic epidermal necrolysis. JAMA 1987 Apr 24; 257(16): 2171–2175

Prasad JK, Feller I and Thomson PD. Use of amnion for the treatment of Stevens–Johnson syndrome. J Trauma 1986 Oct; 26(10):945–946

Rayle RT. 5 nursing lessons from a patient with T.E.N. Am J Nurs 1986 Mar; 86(3):300–302

Revuz J et al. Toxic epidermal necrolysis. Arch Dermatol 1987 Sep; 123(9):1160–1165

Etiology and Physiology of Burns

Burns are a form of traumatic injury caused by thermal, electrical, chemical, or radioactive agents.

Inhalation injury and associated pulmonary complications are a significant factor in mortality and morbidity from burn injury (50%–60% of fire deaths are secondary to inhalation injury).

Etiology and Incidence

1. Over 2 million injuries and 7000–9000 deaths occur as a result of fire and burns each year in the US.
2. The home is most frequently the place where burn injuries occur.
3. Smoking, often combined with alcohol intake, is associated with at least half of major fire injuries and deaths.
4. The very young and the elderly are at greatest risk for burn injuries.
5. Infants and toddlers are especially prone to scald injuries.
6. School-age children may incur flame burns as a result of playing with matches and gasoline.
7. Teenage boys have a high incidence of electrical injuries.
8. Males are more commonly injured by burns than are females.

Severity

Severity of burn injury is related to:
1. Depth
2. Extent (percentage of body surface burned)
3. Age (the elderly and the very young have a poorer prognosis)
4. Parts of body burned
5. Past medical history
6. Concomitant injuries and illnesses
7. Presence of inhalation injury

Pathophysiology

A. Burn Injury

Burn injury usually results from energy transfer from a heat source to the body. It can occur by direct conduction or electromagnetic radiation. Many factors alter the response of body tissues to these sources of heat:
1. Conductivity of local tissues—nerves and blood vessels conduct heat with greatest ease, whereas bone is most resistant

2. Peripheral circulation
3. Surface pigmentation; presence of insulating material or clothing
4. Water content of tissue

B. Inhalation Injury

1. Types of pulmonary injury in burns
   a. Carbon monoxide poisoning
   b. Smoke toxicity
   c. Upper airway trauma
   d. Restrictive defects
2. Carbon monoxide (CO) is a colorless, odorless, tasteless, and nonirritating gas produced from incomplete combustion of carbon-containing materials.
3. Affinity of hemoglobin for CO is 200 times greater than for oxygen.
4. Toxicity will depend on concentration of CO in inspired air and the length of time of exposure.
5. Inhalation of hot, dry air (148.9°C. [300°F.] or higher) appears not to have much effect on the lower respiratory tract because a sudden closing of the glottis and reflex apnea occur.
6. From fire in a closed space, most particles of soot are filtered through upper airway, but they may be superheated and may cause direct damage to mucosa.
7. Sulfur dioxide (SO_2) and nitrous oxide (N_2O) (toxic agents) most likely are clinging to soot; in the presence of water, they form corrosive acids and alkalies that are extremely toxic.
8. Toxic fumes from burning plastic are more dangerous than smoke; noxious gases include hydrogen cyanide, hydrochloric acid, sulfuric acid, halogens, and perhaps phosgene.
9. Upper airway obstruction may occur during the first 48 hours postburn due to pharyngeal and laryngeal edema resulting from superficial burn of the upper airway. Edema of the neck may also decrease tracheal patency.
10. Restrictive pulmonary complications can occur because of the tourniquet effect of edema seen with circumferential chest burns. Lung compliance and alveolar gas exchange can also be decreased because of noncardiogenic pulmonary edema.

Local Effects of Burns

A. Burn Depth

1. The depth of injury is directly related to the temperature of the burning agent and the duration of contact with body tissue.
2. Below 44°C. (112°F.), no local damage occurs unless exposure is for a protracted period.

3. Between 44°C. (112°F.) and 51°C. (124°F.), the rate of cellular destruction doubles with each 1-degree rise in temperature. Only limited exposure is necessary for tissue destruction.

B. Partial Thickness and Full-Thickness Burns

A full-thickness burn may occur in as little as 1 second of exposure at 70°C. (158°F.).

1. *Partial-thickness* burn injuries involve the epidermis and upper portions of the dermis. Some of the dermal appendages remain, from which the wound can spontaneously re-epithelialize.
2. In *full-thickness* injuries, all layers of the skin and sometimes underlying tissues are destroyed. Grafting usually is required to close the wound (see Table 33-1 and Fig. 33-1).

C. Physiologic Reaction

1. When skin is burned, adjacent intact vessels dilate.
2. Platelets and leukocytes begin to adhere to the vascular endothelium as an early event in the inflammatory process.
3. Increased capillary permeability produces wound edema.
4. An influx of polymorphonuclear leukocytes and monocytes occurs at the injury site.
5. Eventually, new capillaries, immature fibroblasts, and newly formed collagen fibrils appear within the wound. This supports the regenerating epithelium or forms a granulating tissue bed to accept a skin graft.

Systemic Changes in Major Burn

A. Fluid Shifts

1. In addition to changes in the local burned area, there are alterations and disruptions in the vascular and other systems of the body.
2. The water-vapor barrier for the body is the outermost layer of epidermis. When it is rendered nonfunctioning, severe systemic reactions from fluid losses can occur.
3. Blanching of the skin following burn injury is caused by contraction of skin capillaries; redness occurs when arterioles and capillaries dilate.
4. Fluid volume deficit is directly proportional to extent and depth of burn injury.
5. Capillary permeability increases, permitting fluid and protein to move from vascular to interstitial spaces (edema results). Protein-rich fluid is lost in blebs of the burned tissues, as well as by weeping of second-degree wounds and surface of full-thickness wounds. With reduced vascular volume, the patient will go into shock if untreated.
6. Vascular fluid loss occurs rapidly and peaks at 12 hours postburn.
7. Capillary permeability returns to near normal in about 48 hours—but protein lost in interstitial spaces may remain there for 5 days to 2 weeks, before returning to the vascular system.
   a. When fluid mobilizes (moves from interstitial spaces back to vascular compartment), patients with good cardiac and renal function will diurese.
   b. Observe carefully for fluid overload and pulmonary edema; patient requires decreased fluid intake, frequent observation of vital signs, CVP, and urine output.
8. Red cell mass is also diminished, because of thrombosis sludging and red cell death from thermal injury; as fluid escapes from capillary walls, blood concentrates, and the flow is sluggish—hematocrit rises.
9. Capillary stasis may cause ischemia and even necrosis.
10. The body attempts to compensate for losses of plasma volume.
   a. Constriction of vessels
   b. Withdrawal of fluid from undamaged extracellular space

Table 33-1. *Assessment of Burn Injury*

Extent or Degree	Assessment of Extent	Reparative Process
Superficial partial thickness (first degree)	Pink to red: slight edema, which subsides quickly. Pain may last up to 48 hours; relieved by cooling.	In about 5 days, epidermis peels, heals spontaneously. Itching and pink skin persist for about a week. No scarring. Heals spontaneously if it does not become infected within 10 days–2 weeks.
Deep partial thickness (second degree)	*Superficial:* Pink or red; blisters form (vesicles); weeping, edematous, elastic. Superficial layers of skin are destroyed; wound moist and painful.	Takes several weeks to heal. Scarring may occur.
	Deep dermal: Mottled white and red; edematous reddened areas blanch on pressure. May be yellowish but soft and elastic—may or may not be sensitive to touch; sensitive to cold air. Hair does not pull out easily.	Takes several weeks to heal. Scarring may occur.
Full thickness (third degree)	Destruction of epithelial cells—epidermis and dermis destroyed. Reddened areas do not blanch with pressure. Not painful; inelastic; coloration varies from waxy white to brown; leathery devitalized tissue is called *eschar.*	Eschar must be removed. Granulation tissue forms to nearest epithelium from wound margins or support graft. For areas larger than 3–5 cm., grafting is required. Expect scarring and loss of skin function
Fourth degree	Destruction of epithelium, fat, muscles, and bone.	Area requires debridement, formation of granulation tissue, and grafting.

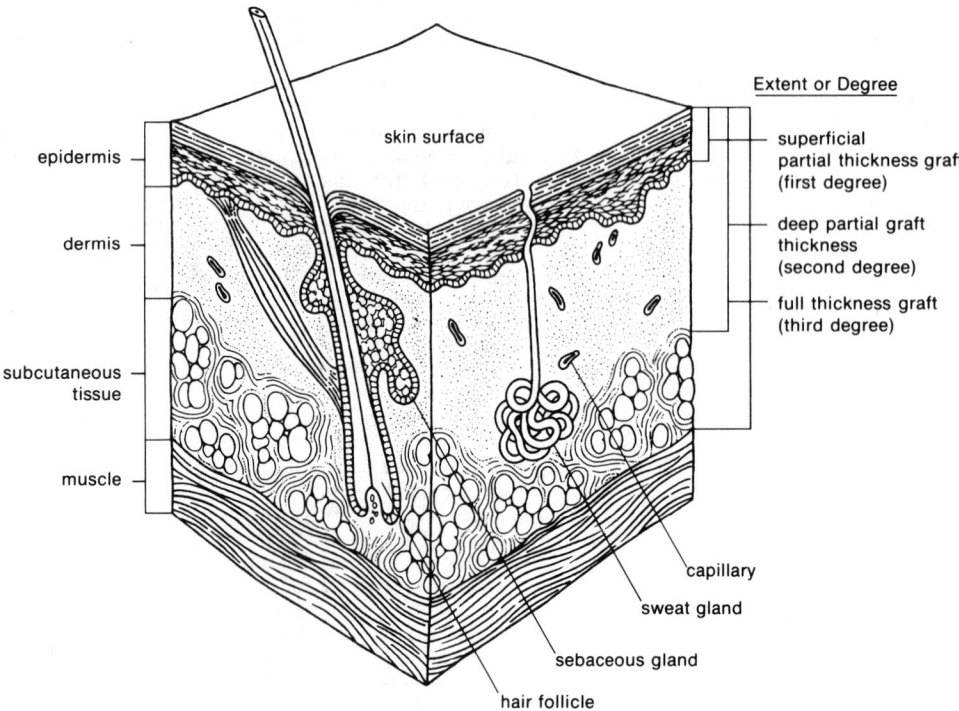

Figure 33-1. *Cross section of skin depicting blood supply, depth of burn, and relative thickness of skin grafts. (From The Burn Patient, Ethicon)*

  c. Patient is thirsty. (Oral fluids are not given until bowel sounds are heard.)

Fluid Loss

Adult	Amount per Hour per Square Meter of Body Surface
Normal unburned individual	15–20 ml.
Average adult with a flame burn of 40% of his body	100 ml.

B. Hemodynamics

1. Lessened circulating blood volume results in decreased cardiac output initially and increased pulse rate.
2. There is a decreased stroke volume, as well as a marked rise in peripheral resistance (due to constriction of arterioles and increased hemo-viscosity).
3. This results in inadequate tissue perfusion, which may in turn cause acidosis, renal failure, and irreversible burn shock.
4. A burn injury often upsets the acid–base balance; therefore, careful monitoring of arterial blood gases, serum electrolytes, and urine volume is needed for proper fluid therapy—this will allow one to replace fluid loss and prevent dilatation and paralytic ileus.

C. Metabolic Demands

1. Catecholamine release appears to be the major mediator of the hypermetabolic response to burn injury.

This results in cell breakdown (catabolism) and a marked outpouring of potassium and nitrogen.
2. Core body temperature increases by 1°–2°C.
3. Healing a large surface area requires much energy; glucose is the primary metabolic fuel.
4. Because total body glucose stores are limited and liver and muscle glycogen is exhausted within the first few days postburn, hepatic glucose synthesis increases.
5. Insulin levels decrease early postburn and patients develop hyperglycemia. They continue to be hyperglycemic when insulin levels increase, probably due to increased gluconeogenesis.
6. Skeletal and visceral protein is mobilized to meet increased nutritional demands.
7. When adequately treated, an extensively burned patient will probably increase his weight the first 3–4 days, because of collection of fluid in the interstitial spaces; thereafter, weight loss will be progressive, at the rate of about 1 pound a day in a young adult, for about a month, depending on nutritional support. *Adequate nutritional therapy* can reduce this loss to no more than 5%–10% of preburn body weight before weight stabilizes.
8. In spite of all nutritional support, it is almost impossible to counteract a negative nitrogen balance; the sooner a burn wound is closed, the more rapidly a positive nitrogen balance is reached.
9. The resting metabolic expenditure increases linearly with amount of burn surface area (BSA); a burn of 40%–50% BSA has a metabolic rate almost twice normal.
10. The postburn adult may require 3000–5000 calories a day; high calories, high protein may be given orally and in some instances by intravenous hyperalimenta-

tion or by nasogastric feeding along with normal meals and snacks.

D. Renal Activity

1. Glomerular filtration may be decreased in extensive injury.
2. Without resuscitation or with delay, decreased renal blood flow may lead to high output or oliguric renal failure and decreased creatinine clearance.
3. Hemoglobin and myoglobin, present in the urine of patients with deep muscle damage often associated with electrical injury, may cause acute tubular necrosis and call for a greater amount of initial fluid therapy and osmotic diuresis.

E. Pulmonary Changes

1. Hyperventilation and increased oxygen consumption are associated with major burns.
2. The majority of deaths from fire are due to smoke inhalation. See page 846 for discussion of inhalation injury.
3. Overzealous fluid resuscitation and the effects of burn shock on cell membrane potential may cause pulmonary edema, contributing to decreased alveolar exchange.
4. Initial respiratory alkalosis resulting from hyperventilation may change to respiratory acidosis associated with pulmonary insufficiency as a result of major burn trauma.

F. Hematologic Changes

1. Thrombocytopenia, abnormal platelet function, depressed fibrinogen levels, inhibition of fibrinolysis, and a deficit in several plasma clotting factors occur postburn.
2. Anemia results from the direct effect of destruction of erythrocytes due to burn injury, reduced life span of surviving red cells, overt or (more commonly) occult blood loss from duodenal or gastric ulcers, and blood loss during diagnostic and therapeutic procedures.

G. Immunologic Activity

1. The loss of the skin barrier and presence of eschar favor bacterial growth.
2. Granulation tissue, richly vascular, resists bacteria.
3. Abnormal inflammatory response after burn injury causes a decreased delivery of antibodies, white blood cells, and oxygen to the injured area.
4. Hypoxia, acidosis, and thrombosis of vessels in the wound area impair host resistance to pathogenic bacteria.
5. Several major immunoglobulins, complement, and serum albumin are decreased soon after the burn occurs.
6. Depressed cellular immunity is reflected by lymphocytopenia, impaired delayed skin sensitivity, decreased allograft rejection potential, depletion of thymus-dependent lymphoid tissue, and increased susceptibility to fungi, viruses, and gram-negative organisms.
7. Burn wound sepsis
   a. Following colonization of the burn wound surface by bacteria, subeschar and intrafollicular colonization develop. Intraeschar and subeschar colonization may progress to invasion of subadjacent, nonburned, previously viable tissue.
   b. A bacterial count of 10^5/gram of tissue as determined by burn wound biopsy indicates burn wound sepsis.

8. Seeding of bacteria from the wound may give rise to systemic septicemia.

H. Gastrointestinal

1. As a result of sympathetic nervous system response to trauma, peristalsis decreases and gastric distention, nausea, vomiting, and paralytic ileus may occur.
2. Ischemia of the gastric mucosa and other etiologic factors put the burn patient at risk for duodenal and gastric ulcer manifested by occult bleeding and, in some cases, life-threatening hemorrhage.

Methods of Treating Burns

Overview

1. Management of burn injury includes hemodynamic stabilization, metabolic support, wound debridement, use of topical antibacterial therapy and biologic dressings, and wound closure.
2. Prevention and treatment of complications, including infection and pulmonary damage, and rehabilitation are also of major importance.

Intravenous Therapy

Hemodynamic Stabilization; Prevention of Burn Shock

A. Intravenous Fluid Therapy

1. Immediate intravenous fluid resuscitation is indicated for:
   a. Adults with burns over greater than 15%–20% of body surface area.
   b. Children with burns involving more than 10% of body surface area.
   c. Patients with electrical injury, the elderly, or anyone with cardiac or pulmonary disease and compromised response to burn injury.
2. The goal is to give sufficient fluid to allow perfusion of vital organs without overhydrating the patient and risking later complications and circulatory overload.
3. Generally, a crystalloid (electrolyte) solution is used initially.
   a. Usually, 2–4 ml./kg./% burn surface area is required in the first 24 hours postinjury.
   b. One-half of the total calculated amount should be given in the first 8 hours postburn, and the other half over the next 16 hours.
   c. Colloids are usually added to the fluid regimen in the second 24 hours after injury. This has proven effective in restoring plasma volume and maintaining cardiac output.
4. Use formula as a guide only—Patient parameters, including urine output, vital signs, central venous pressure, and hematocrit, are the best indicators of fluid requirements and response.
5. A large-bore central venous catheter is recommended for large-volume replacement.
6. Fluids may be titrated to achieve a urine output of 30–50 ml./hour (0.5 ml./kg./hour) in an adult and 1 ml./kg./hour in a child.
7. An indwelling urinary catheter is needed to monitor response to fluid therapy.

8. Weigh the patient on admission and then daily.
9. Elevate extremities.
10. Monitor peripheral pulses.
11. Administer humidified oxygen.

Metabolic Support

1. Initially, keep the patient NPO until bowel sounds return (1–2 days).
2. Reduce metabolic stress by allaying pain, fear, and anxiety and maintaining a warm environment.
3. Nutritional management must be aggressive to combat acute nutritional deficiency and weight loss; a positive nitrogen balance should be the goal throughout the postburn course.
4. When bowel sounds return, administer oral fluids and advance diet as tolerated.
5. Offer more solid food after 2–3 days postburn as tolerance for food improves.
   a. Build up daily caloric intake to match daily caloric expenditure.
   b. Provide 3 gm. protein/kg. body weight; 20% of needed calories in form of fats; remainder in carbohydrates.
6. When caloric requirements cannot be met by enteral feedings, it may be necessary to initiate intravenous hyperalimentation (amino acids, carbohydrates) and fat emulsions.
7. Provide potassium and vitamin supplements.

Wound Care—Conservative Treatment

Wound Cleansing and Debridement

Conservative treatment of the burn wound includes daily or twice daily wound cleansing or hydrotherapy and dressing changes. After the burn eschar sloughs, usually within 2 weeks, autografting is performed for full-thickness burns.
1. Burn wounds must be cleansed initially and usually daily with a mild antibacterial cleansing agent and saline solution or water.
   a. This may be done in the hydrotherapy tub, in the bath tub, or at the bedside.
   b. See Hydrotherapy, below.
2. Nonviable tissue (eschar) may be removed through natural, enzymatic, mechanical, and/or surgical debridement.
3. Burn eschar will begin to separate from the underlying viable tissue by a natural process of bacterial growth, which causes a lysis of protein at viable–nonviable tissue interface.
4. Eschar can be removed through daily or twice-daily dressing changes and use of forceps and scissors at time of wound cleansing.
5. Enzymatic agents applied to the burn wound may be used for more rapid debridement of eschar.
6. In surgical excision, primary or tangential, all nonviable tissue is removed down to a viable base, which is covered with biologic dressings: heterograft, homograft (both temporary), or autograft.

Hydrotherapy

Hydrotherapy ("tubbing" or "tanking") is the bathing of the burn patient in a tub or tank of water to facilitate cleansing of the burn area (removal of dead tissue and topical medications).

A. Advantages
1. Topical medications, adherent dressings, and eschar are more easily removed.
2. Provides an opportunity for the patient to practice range-of-motion exercises.
3. Total assessment of the burn area is facilitated; total body cleansing can be achieved.

B. Disadvantages
1. Loss of body heat; sodium loss also occurs in tub water.
2. Uncomfortable to the patient and at times painful.
3. Maintenance of IV lines, ventilator care may be difficult during tubbing.

C. Nursing Interventions
1. Describe the procedure to the patient who is experiencing hydrotherapy for the first time.
2. Select the time for future tubbings in collaboration with the patient; administer a pain-control medication, if prescribed, before the treatment so that maximum benefit is realized. Use nursing activities to assist patient with his pain experience.
3. If the patient has an indwelling catheter, drain and plug it, or maintain a closed system to avoid contamination.
4. Isolation and aseptic technique are adhered to as closely as possible in preparing the patient for hydrotherapy, during hydrotherapy, and then in redressing wounds of the patient following therapy.
5. During hydrotherapy, following cleansing of the wounds, debride wound, shave adjacent areas at physician's direction, shampoo hair, and gently wash normal skin.
6. Limit therapy to no more than 30 minutes.
7. Never leave the patient unattended in the tub.
8. Respect the patient's feelings and expressions of stress, pain, cold, and fatigue.
9. Following treatment, the patient may be weighed before being carefully dressed and returned to his unit.
10. Document significant data, including status of the wound.

Topical Antimicrobials

Topical medications are used to cover burn areas and to reduce the number of organisms.

Principles

1. They are applied directly to the burn area as ointments, creams, or solutions, or they may be incorporated in single-layer dressings that do not stick to the wound but permit drainage.
2. During the early postburn period when eschar is softening and wound debridement is a goal, coarse mesh gauze is used to permit drainage and removal of exudate and eschar that are caught in the gauze interstices. Fine mesh gauze is used to protect granulation tissue and re-epithelializing wound.
3. Usually, these dressings are held in place by a single layer of stretch bandage or by net tube dressings (Surgifix).

4. When wet dressings are used, 20-ply gauze will help retain solution at the proper concentration if rewet every 4 hours. A dry top layer of stockinette or a cotton bath blanket prevents evaporative heat loss.
5. Desired characteristics in a topical antimicrobial
   a. Demonstrates action against a broad spectrum of bacteria.
   b. Has the ability to diffuse through the wound and penetrate the eschar.
   c. Nontoxic and noninjurious to body tissue.
   d. Inexpensive, pleasant to use, odorless or has pleasant odor; will not stain skin or clothing.
   e. Will not cause resistant strains of pathogenic organisms to develop.
6. Generally, all of the previously applied topical cream should be removed and the wound gently cleansed before applying new cream with each dressing change. Extremity dressings should be wrapped distally to proximally, taking care to avoid circulatory compromise when edema occurs or dressing is too tight.
7. To date there is no "ideal" topical antimicrobial.

Types of Topical Antimicrobial Agents
(Table 33-2)

1. Silver sulfadiazine
2. Mafenide acetate
3. Silver nitrate

Surgical Management

Increasingly common is the more aggressive approach of early excision and grafting.

A. Tangential Excision—performed between 2 and 5 days postburn.

1. A special blade is used to slice off thin layers of damaged skin until live tissue is evidenced by capillary bleeding.
2. Commonly used with deep partial-thickness burns and is followed with immediate coverage with a biosynthetic or biologic dressing or an autograft.

B. Primary Excision—excision of full-thickness burn down to fascia.

1. Performed 3 to 5 days postburn.
2. The skin, lymphatics, and subcutaneous tissue are removed, down to fascia, with either immediate autografting or temporary coverage with biologic or biosynthetic dressings.
3. This is repeated until all the deep burn areas are removed.

C. General Considerations.

1. Early surgical intervention reduces the potential for wound infection and speeds the course of hospital care.
2. Operative excision is very stressful metabolically and incurs heavy blood loss; therefore, more conservative measures may be indicated for some patients.

Burn Wound Coverings

Types of Burn Wound Coverings

For a comprehensive listing of burn wound coverings, see Table 33-3.

Biologic Dressings

Biologic dressings are used to cover large denuded surfaces of the body. Usually they are split-thickness grafts harvested either from human cadavers or other mammalian donors such as pigs. Human amnion may also be used.

An *allograft* is a graft of skin taken from a person other than the burn victim and applied to a burn wound temporarily (a cadaver is the most common source).

A *xenograft* or *heterograft* is a segment of skin taken from an animal such as a pig. It is useful in preparing debrided area for grafting and is really a biologic dressing (see p. 833 for skin grafting).

A. Donor Criteria

1. Skin color unimportant, since it is only a temporary graft.
2. Donor should be an adult free of infection.

B. Purpose and Benefits

1. Decreases heat, fluid, and protein losses
2. Reduces bacterial proliferation
3. Closes wound temporarily; enhances production and protection of granulation tissue
4. Protects exposed neurovascular and muscle tissue as well as tendons
5. Reduces pain and facilitates patient comfort
6. Acts as a test-graft to determine when granulating wounds will accept autograft successfully
7. Provides an effective donor-site dressing

C. Clinical Procedure

1. Porcine skin grafts (xenografts) are the most popular temporary biologic dressings.
2. Devitalized tissue is first removed surgically or enzymatically.
3. Porcine graft is applied directly (epidermis side up) to the denuded area; it may be trimmed to adhere to wound contour. Before applying, it may be dipped in saline solution.
4. Grafts are usually left exposed except when applied to circumferential wounds; stretch gauze (Surgifix) is applied to prevent adherence to and malpositioning by bed sheets.
5. The first xenograft dressing may have to be changed in 24 hours to permit more intimate adherence to granulating wound bed.
6. Thereafter, grafts may be left in place 2–5 days between changes; inspect wound daily to detect early signs of suppuration.
7. After good xenograft adherence is achieved, the wound is ready for autografting.

Biosynthetic Dressings

1. Temporary biosynthetic dressings that help prevent bacterial contamination.
2. Used when permanent autograft is unavailable or not necessary (as when partial-thickness wounds will heal spontaneously over time).
3. Biobrane (Woodruff Laboratories) consists of a custom-knit nylon fabric, mechanically bonded to an ultrathin silicone rubber membrane, to which collagenous peptides of porcine skin are covalently bonded.
   a. Has a longer shelf life and lower cost than biologic dressings such as pigskin.

Table 33-2. *Topical Antimicrobial Agents for Burns*

Topical Agent	Description and Indications	Disadvantages	Nursing Implications
Silver sulfadiazine 1% Silvadene (Marion Laboratories) SSD (Boots–Flint, Inc.)	A white, crystalline, highly insoluble compound in an opaque, odorless, water-miscible cream Exerts antimicrobial effect at level of cell membrane and cell wall against gram-negative and gram-positive bacteria and yeasts Penetration of silver sulfadiazine into wound is intermediate between silver nitrate and mafenide Systemic toxicity is rare Most widely used agent and least common incidence of side effects	May cause transient leukopenia that disappears after 2–3 days of treatment May increase possibility of kernicterus and should not be used in pregnant women approaching term, premature infants, or neonates < 2 months Impairment of hepatic and renal function that results in decreased excretion of drug constituents may preclude therapeutic benefits of continued silver sulfadiazine administration Exposure to sunlight produces gray discoloration Crystalluria and methemoglobinemia are rare toxic effects Protracted use may be associated with emergence of sulfadiazine resistance	Use with either open treatment, light or occlusive dressings Apply with sterile gloved hand directly to wound or applied to gauze dressing 0.16 cm. (1/16th inch) thick, once or twice daily after thorough wound cleansing
Mafenide acetate 10% cream or 5% solution Sulfamylon	Usually supplied in water-miscible, hydroscopic cream base Active against most gram-positive organisms and particularly, *Clostridia* sp. Active against common gram-negative burn wound pathogens but has little antifungal activity. Not significantly bound by protein and wound exudate Good penetrating power and useful for control of established invasive burn wound infection	Painful during and for awhile after application. A potent carbonic anhydrase inhibitor resulting in metabolic acidoses Brisk alkaline diuresis and inappropriate polyuria may result when used on patients with a large burn surface area. Compensatory hyperventilation and pulmonary failure may ensue if mafenide is not discontinued Hemolytic anemia is a rare complication	Cream is applied with or without dressing. Must be reapplied every 12 hours to maintain therapeutic effectiveness Therapeutic solution concentration is maintained with bulky wet dressings, rewet every 2–4 hours Application is associated with significant pain. Hypersensitivity evidenced by maculopapular rash; is treated with antihistamines and/or discontinuing use. Requires careful monitoring of pulmonary status and acid–base and fluid balance
Silver nitrate (0.5% solution)	Clear solution with low toxicity and significant antimicrobial effect against common burn wound pathogens Minimal absorption occurs because of the insolubility of its chloride and other salts Nonallergenic and not usually painful on application Best use is prophylaxis against infection	Can cause electrolyte abnormalities by depleting serum sodium, chloride, potassium, and magnesium Methemoglobinemia is a rare complication Stains everything (including normal skin) brown or black	Monitor electrolyte balance carefully; supplementation with sodium and potassium salts is routinely needed for patients with extensive burns Use bulky dressings, rewet every 2–4 hours, to maintain therapeutic concentration Maintain patient warmth and minimize transcutaneous evaporative water loss with dry top layer such as stockinette or bath blanket
Other topical agents Cerium nitrate (1.74% solution) Cerium nitrate combined with silver sulfadiazine cream Povidone-iodine (1% cream; also in foam and solution forms) (Betadine) Gentamicin (0.1% ointment) (Garamycin) Nitrofurazone (0.2% ointment) (Furacin) Polymixin B-bacitracin ointment (Polysporin)			

Table 33-3. Burn Wound Coverings

Description	Indications	Source or Form	Nursing Considerations
Amnion			
Amnionic and chorionic membranes collected from human placentas under sterile conditions	To protect partial-thickness burns To temporarily cover granulation tissue awaiting autograft	Obstetric department frees membranes from placenta and processes for short-term storage	Apply to clean wounds Change every 48 hours; wound may be left open to air or redressed immediately
Allograft Homograft			
Human cadaver skin, about 0.015-inch thick Preferred biologic dressing	To debride untidy wounds To protect granulation tissue after escharotomy To cover excised wound immediately To serve as test graft before autograft	Fresh, cryopreserved homografts available from tissue banks throughout US	Remember that length of time dressing is left in place varies greatly Observe for exudate; also, watch for local and systemic signs of infection and rejection
Xenograft Heterograft			
Pigskin similar to human skin, harvested after slaughter, then cryopreserved or lyophilized for long-term storage	Same as for homograft To cover meshed autografts To protect exposed tendons To cover partial-thickness burns that are eschar-free and clean or only slightly contaminated	Available in fresh, frozen, or lyophilized form, in rolls or sheets; also available meshed and impregnated with silver sulfadiazine	Change every 2–5 days; wound may be dressed or left open Observe for signs of infection
Biobrane			
Nylon fabric bonded to silicon rubber membrane, containing collagenous porcine peptides Elastic and durable; adheres to wound surface until removed or sloughed by spontaneous reepithelization	To cover donor graft sites To protect clean, superficial, partial-thickness burns and excised wounds awaiting autografts To cover meshed autografts	Individually packaged sterile sheets of various sizes; also in glove-shaped form for hand burns	Remember that Biobrane is useful for wounds awaiting autograft because it can be left in place 3–14 days or longer; and it is permeable to antimicrobials, which can be applied over it
Duo-Derm			
Hydroactive dressing that interacts with moisture on skin, creating bond that makes it adhere Interacts with wound exudate to produce soft, moist gel, facilitating removal	To cover small, partial-thickness burns To prevent bacterial contamination	Individual, peelable, "blister" packages containing sheets of various sizes (from 3 × 3 to 8 × 12 inches)	Use size that allows dressing to extend beyond wound onto healthy skin Be careful to distinguish pus from liquefied material that normally remains in wound
Op-Site			
Thin, transparent elastic film that adheres to dry surfaces, conforms to body contours, and stretches with movement Occlusive and waterproof; permeable to moisture, vapor, and air	To cover clean, partial-thickness burns and clean donor sites and to reduce pain from these wounds To provide moist environment for reepithelization	Individual, sterile, peelable packages of sheets in various sizes	Maintain closed dressing; if exudate forms, drain aseptically with needle and syringe; seal hole with Op-Site patch Check for pooling of exudate in dependent areas
N-terface			
Surface material used between burn and outer dressing Translucent, nonabsorbent, and nonreactive; permeable to air and fluid	To cover partial-thickness burns and newly applied autografts To eliminate shearing of epithelium and protect healing tissue	Sterile, individually packaged strips, sheets, or rolls of various sizes	Remember that N-terface will shorten time it normally takes to change dressing, eliminating soaking and other steps required with conventional gauze dressing
Vigilon			
Colloidal suspension on a polyethylene mesh support Permeable to gases and water vapor; provides moist environment Compatible with topical preparations	To clean small, partial-thickness burns	Individual sterile or nonsterile sheets in various sizes	For occlusive use, remove one polyethylene film backing and place uncovered side on wound; for nonocclusive use remove both backings and secure over wound with gauze or tape Change daily

Reprinted with permission. Bayley E and Smith G. The three degrees of burn care. Nursing 87 1987 Mar; 17(3): 34–41. Copyright ©1987, Springhouse Corporation, Springhouse, PA. All rights reserved.

b. Is widely used for coverage of: shallow wounds awaiting epithelialization; temporarily, excised wounds awaiting autografts; widely meshed autografts until closure of interstices; and, donor sites awaiting healing.

Artificial Dermis

1. Method being studied in selected burn centers to improve survival of patients with massive burns and little donor skin available.
2. Composed of a porous collagen-chondroitin 6-sulfate fibrillar mat covered with a thin Silastic sheet.
3. Used with an epidermal graft to provide a permanent cover that is at least as satisfactory as other available grafting techniques.
4. Used with donor sites that are thinner and that heal faster; seems to result in less hypertrophic scarring than the usual grafting methods.

Wound Closure

1. Skin grafting is usually required or preferred with full-thickness burns greater than 2 cm. in diameter or in deep partial-thickness wounds.
2. Following gradual eschar removal and development of a base of granulating tissue, or in the presence of viable tissue following excision, grafts of the patient's own skin (autografts) are applied.
3. Sheet grafts or meshed grafts, providing wider expansion from donor sites, may be used.
4. Blood flow is established by the 3rd or 4th day, and by the 7th–10th day postgrafting, vascular continuity and wound closure have been established.
5. Cultured epithelial autografts (CEAs) may be used for patients with large burns and little available donor skin.
   a. Biopsies of unburned skin are cultured in a specialized laboratory to yield confluent sheets of epithelial cells suitable for grafting in about 3 weeks.
   b. Available donor sites can be used for coverage of the most functional or posterior surfaces and the more delicate CEAs can be used to cover other large areas.
   c. Additional experience is needed to determine the long-term durability of CEAs, which may be life-saving treatment for the severely burned.
6. Many partial-thickness burn wounds will heal spontaneously within a few weeks, provided they are protected from infection.

Prevention and Treatment of Complications

Primary causes of morbidity and mortality in burn victims are those related to infection and pulmonary problems.
1. Intravenous antibiotics may be given prophylactically to prevent gram-positive infection.
2. Topical antibacterial agents help to retard the proliferation of pathogenic organisms until wound closure occurs spontaneously or through surgical intervention.
3. Broad-spectrum antibiotics may be necessary to treat systemic gram-positive and gram-negative infections and sometimes fungal infection.
4. Critical diagnostic parameters include observing for signs of burn-wound sepsis, including quantitative and qualitative wound biopsy, and for signs of systemic septicemia and taking blood for cultures.

Nursing Process Overview: The Patient With a Burn

Assessment

Note: As with all trauma victims, a primary and secondary trauma survey, including assessment of airway, breathing, and circulation as well as vital signs, is done. Other assessment parameters specific to the burn injury are included in the following:

A. Assessment for Inhalation Injury

1. If victim was burned in closed area, there should be a high index of suspicion that smoke inhalation has occurred (Fig. 33-2).
2. Evaluate all patients in closed space fires for presence of symptoms of carbon monoxide poisoning: headache, visual changes, confusion, irritability, decreased judgment, nausea, ataxia, collapse.
3. Question the patient about types of things that burned in this room—type of carpet, vinyl articles, synthetics.
4. Observe for upper body burns, erythema or blistering of lips, buccal mucosa, or pharynx, singed nares hair, soot in oropharynx, dark gray or black sputum.
5. Listen for hoarseness and crackles.
6. Obtain blood gases and carboxyhemoglobin levels.
7. Prepare the patient for bronchoscopy to confirm presence of mucosal erythema, hemorrhage, ulceration, edema, carbonaceous particles.
8. Obtain chest x-ray for baseline data.

B. Signs and Symptoms of Toxicity From Carbon Monoxide

CO Blood Level	Manifestations
0–10%	None
	Smokers may normally have 10% CO level
10%–20%	Headache, visual disturbance, angina in patients with cardiovascular disease, slowed mental function
20%–40%	Tight feeling in head, rapid fatigue from muscular effort, decreased muscular coordination, confusion, irritability, ataxia, nausea, vomiting, increased pulse rate, decreased blood pressure, dysrhythmias
40%–60%	Pulmonary and cardiac dysfunction, collapse, coma, convulsions
Over 60%	Often fatal

C. Extent of Body Surface Burned

1. Anatomic location—burns affecting hands, feet, face, and perineum require specialized care.
2. Determination is based on the use of tables for this purpose, such as the "rule of nines" chart (Fig. 33-3) and the burn evaluation chart (Fig. 33-4). Calculation of the percent of burn surface area also serves as a guide for fluid therapy.
3. Repeat assessment on 2nd and 3rd day to verify demarcation of burned areas.

D. Depth of Burn and Triage Criteria

1. See Figure 33-1 (Assessment of Burn Injury).
2. It may be difficult to differentiate between partial- and

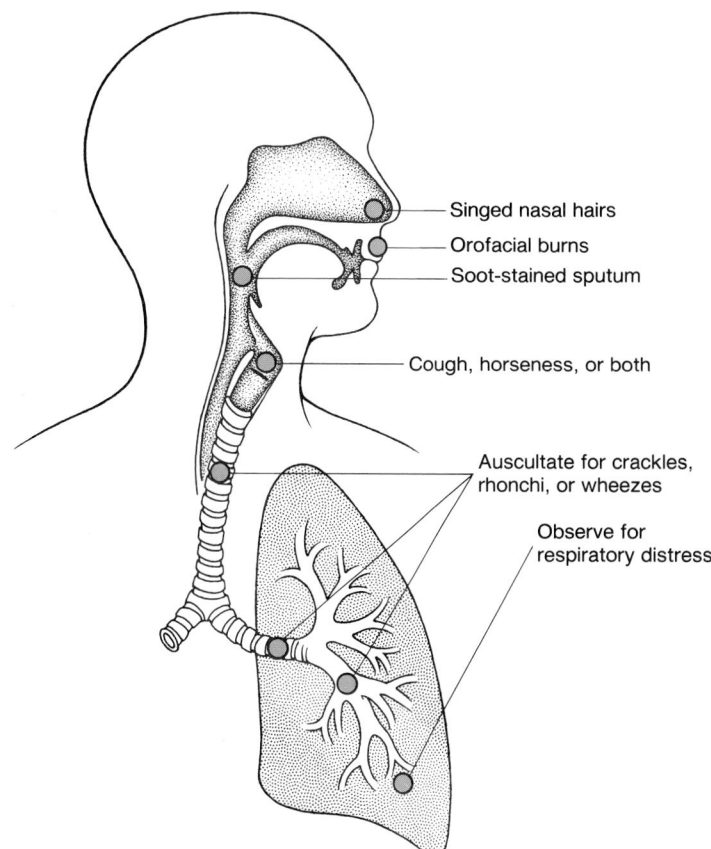

Singed nasal hairs
Orofacial burns
Soot-stained sputum

Cough, horseness, or both

Auscultate for crackles, rhonchi, or wheezes

Observe for respiratory distress

Figure 33-2. *In the nursing history, determine whether the victim was in a closed area during the fire and whether he lost consciousness. If any of the above physical findings are noted in addition to the nursing history data, the victim should be taken to a health center for further evaluation. Baseline arterial blood gas measurements (to detect hypoxemia) should be taken immediately upon admission.*

full-thickness wounds initially; if hair can be pulled out easily, there is likelihood of full-thickness injury.
3. Cleanse wounds and reassess daily for first several days.
4. Triage criteria—Table 33-4 presents triage criteria for determining when it is advisable to transfer a patient to a burn center.

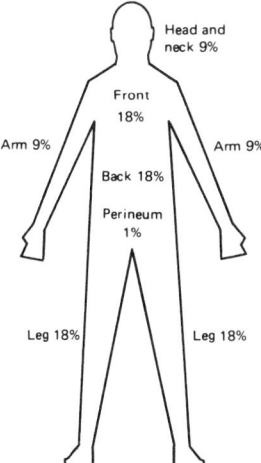

Head and neck 9%

Front 18%

Arm 9%   Arm 9%

Back 18%

Perineum 1%

Leg 18%   Leg 18%

Figure 33-3. *"Rule of nines" chart.*

E. Other Factors to Assess

1. Causative agent—hot water, chemical, gasoline, flame, etc.
2. Duration of exposure
3. Circumstances of injury, including whether in closed or open space
4. Age
5. Initial treatment, including first aid
6. Preexisting medical problems—heart disease, diabetes, ulcers, alcoholism, COPD, epilepsy, psychosis
7. Current medications
8. Concomitant injuries (e.g., from fall or explosion)
9. Evidence of inhalation injury (p. 846)
10. Allergies
11. Tetanus immunization status
12. Height and weight
13. Take photograph of burned area (with patient permission) for medical record of extent of burn

Nursing Diagnoses

1. Impaired gas exchange related to carbon monoxide poisoning, upper airway obstruction, smoke inhalation, and/or edema of lung parenchyma
2. Impaired ventilation related to circumferential edema of chest
3. Decreased cardiac output related to fluid shifts and hypovolemic shock
4. Inadequate peripheral tissue perfusion related to pe-

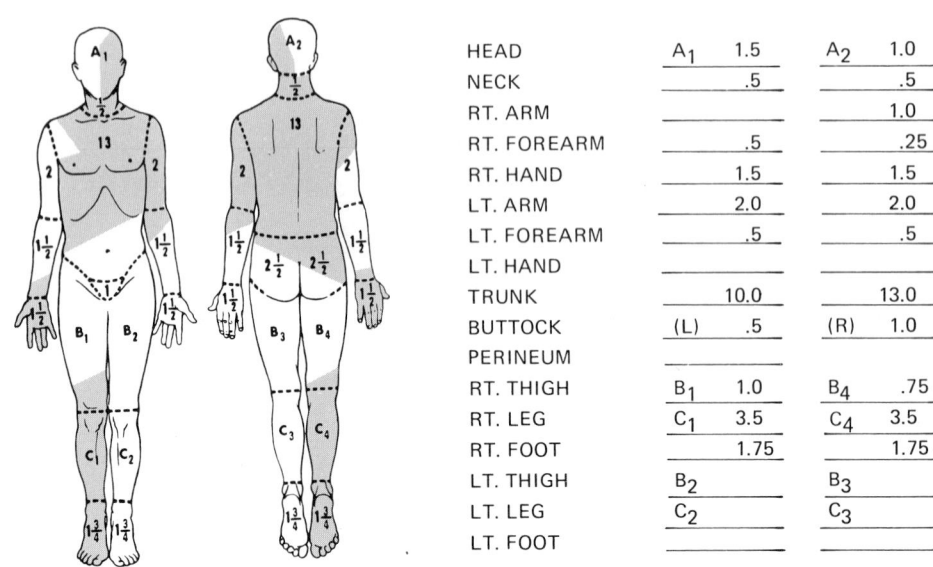

	ANTERIOR		POSTERIOR	
HEAD	A$_1$	1.5	A$_2$	1.0
NECK		.5		.5
RT. ARM				1.0
RT. FOREARM		.5		.25
RT. HAND		1.5		1.5
LT. ARM		2.0		2.0
LT. FOREARM		.5		.5
LT. HAND				
TRUNK		10.0		13.0
BUTTOCK	(L)	.5	(R)	1.0
PERINEUM				
RT. THIGH	B$_1$	1.0	B$_4$	.75
RT. LEG	C$_1$	3.5	C$_4$	3.5
RT. FOOT		1.75		1.75
LT. THIGH	B$_2$		B$_3$	
LT. LEG	C$_2$		C$_3$	
LT. FOOT				

PERCENT OF AREAS AFFECTED BY GROWTH:

		0	1	5	10	15	ADULT
A = ½	HEAD	9½	8½	6½	5½	4½	3½
B = ½	ONE THIGH	2¾	3¼	4	4¼	4½	4¾
C = ½	ONE LEG	2½	2½	2¾	3	3¼	3½

Mixed □   % PARTIAL THICKNESS _____

■   % FULL THICKNESS _____

TOTAL ___50%___

Figure 33-4. *Burn evaluation chart—estimation of percent of body burns. (Chart courtesy Crozer–Chester Medical Center)*

ripheral burn-wound edema, generalized edema, and circumferential full-thickness burn

5. Fluid volume deficit related to increased capillary permeability and evaporative fluid loss from burn wound
6. Potential for fluid volume excess related to fluid mobilization 3–5 days postburn
7. Impaired skin integrity related to burn injury and surgical interventions (donor sites)
8. Altered urinary elimination related to indwelling catheter

Table 33-4. *Triage Criteria for Determining When It Is Advisable to Transfer a Patient to a Burn Center*

Burn Center Triage Criteria

Burned area 2° and 3° (age <10 or >50): 10%
Burned area 2° and 3° (age >10 or <50): 20%
Burned area 3°: >5% at any age
Chemical burn
Electrical injury
Burn of face, hands, feet, or perineum
Burn accompanied by:
  Significant associated injury or pre-existing disease
  Airway or inhalation injury
  Suspected child abuse

Courtesy of the Burn Foundation, Philadelphia, PA.

9. Ineffective thermoregulation related to loss of skin microcirculatory regulation and hypothalamic response to burn injury
10. Potential for infection related to loss of skin barrier and altered immune response
11. Impaired physical mobility related to edema, pain, skin and joint contractures
12. Sleep pattern disturbance related to burn wound discomfort and treatment priorities
13. Activity intolerance related to long periods of immobility
14. Altered nutrition—less than body requirements—related to hypermetabolic response to burn injury
15. Impaired tissue integrity of gastric mucosa related to stress response
16. Pain related to injured nerves in burn wound and skin tightness.
17. Ineffective individual coping related to fear and anxiety
18. Knowledge deficit (burn wound care) related to inexperience with burn injury and subsequent related health-care needs
19. Potential (feeding, bathing, toileting, and/or dressing/grooming) self-care deficit related to functional sequelae of burn injury
20. Body image disturbance related to cosmetic and functional sequelae of burn wound.
21. Anticipatory/dysfunctional grieving related to biologic, psychological, and social losses resulting from burn injury

Nursing Interventions

A. Establishing Adequate Tissue Oxygenation and Respiratory Function

1. Provide humidified 100% oxygen until carbon monoxide level is known. (CAUTION: Adjust oxygen flow rate for patient with COPD as prescribed.)
2. Assess for signs of hypoxemia and differentiate this from pain.
3. Note history of injury; suspect respiratory injury if burn occurred in an enclosed space.
4. Observe for erythema or blistering of buccal mucosa, singed nares, burns of lips, face, or neck, increasing hoarseness.
5. Monitor respiratory rate, depth, rhythm, cough.
6. Auscultate chest and note breath sounds.
7. Note character and amount of respiratory secretions. Report carbonaceous sputum, tracheal tissue.
8. Observe for signs of inadequate ventilation and include monitoring of arterial blood gases and oxygen saturation.
9. Provide mechanical ventilation, continuous positive airway pressure or positive end-expiratory pressure if requested.
10. Keep intubation equipment at bedside and be alert for signs of respiratory obstruction.
11. In mild inhalation injury:
    a. Provide humidification of inspired air.
    b. Encourage coughing and deep breathing.
    c. Maintain pulmonary toilet.
12. In moderate to severe inhalation injury:
    a. Initiate more frequent bronchial suctioning.
    b. Monitor vital signs, urinary output, and blood gases.
    c. Judiciously administer bronchodilators.
    d. For additional respiratory problems, it may be necessary to have patient intubated and placed on mechanical ventilation.

B. Maintaining Adequate Tidal Volume and Unrestricted Chest Movement

1. Observe rate and quality of breathing; if progressively more rapid and shallow, notify physician.
2. Assess tidal volume; report decreasing volume to physician.
3. Encourage deep-breathing and incentive spirometry (or hyperinflation with Ambu-bag for artificial airway) hourly.
4. Place patient in semi-Fowler's position to permit maximal chest excursion.
5. Ensure that chest dressings are not constricting.
6. Document and report respiratory changes, including dyspnea, shortness of breath.
7. Prepare the patient for escharotomy and assist physician as indicated.

C. Restoration of Normal Hemodynamic Status With Slightly Elevated Cardiac Output

1. Position the patient to increase venous return.
2. Give digoxin per physician's request.
3. Give fluids as prescribed.
4. Monitor vital signs, including apical pulse, respirations, central venous pressure, pulmonary artery pressures, and urine output, at least hourly.
5. Determine cardiac output as requested.
6. Monitor sensorium.
7. Document all observations and particularly note trends in vital-sign changes.

D. Maintaining Adequate Circulation to All Areas, Including Extremities

1. Monitor peripheral pulses hourly.
2. Elevate extremities.
3. Remove all constricting jewelry and clothing. Loosen dressings if necessary.
4. Prepare the patient for escharotomy (surgical procedure to relieve constricting effect of edematous circumferential burns and permit adequate circulation to underlying tissues).
5. Monitor tissue pressure.
6. Monitor other signs of adequate tissue perfusion including urine output and mentation.

E. Maintaining Fluid and Electrolyte Balance Within a Normal Range

1. Titrate fluid intake as prescribed.
2. Maintain accurate intake and output records.
3. Weigh the patient daily.
4. Monitor serum potassium and provide potassium replacement as indicated and prescribed.
5. Be alert to signs of fluid overload and congestive heart failure during period of fluid mobilization, 3–5 days postburn.

F. Reestablishing Skin Integrity

1. Cleanse wounds daily with antibacterial solution or mild soap and water; pat dry. This may be done in the hydrotherapy tank, in the bath tub, or at bedside.
2. Debride eschar using scissors and forceps. Limit time to 20 minutes; stop if there is pain or bleeding.
3. Apply topical bacteriostatic agents as directed (see p. 842).
4. Dress wounds with coarse mesh gauze for new wounds requiring debridement; use fine-mesh gauze on granulating and healing wounds. (Many commercial dressings are available for special wound situations and may be used in consultation with the physician.)
5. For grafted areas, use extreme caution in removing dressings; observe for serous or sanguineous blebs or purulent drainage; report to physician. Redress grafted areas per physician's protocol.
6. Observe all wounds daily and document wound status on the patient's record.
7. Promote healing of donor sites by:
    a. Preventing contamination of donor sites that are clean wounds.
    b. Opening to air for drying 24 hours postoperatively if gauze or impregnated gauze dressing is used.
    c. Following physician's or manufacturer's instructions for care of sites dressed with synthetic materials.
    d. Allowing dressing to peel off spontaneously.
    e. Cleansing healing donor site with mild soap and water once dressings are removed; lubricating site twice daily when healed.

G. Avoiding Bladder Infection

1. Maintain closed urinary drainage system.
2. Ensure a patent urinary catheter.
3. Observe color, quality, amount of urine every 8 hours.
4. Empty drainage bag frequently.
5. Provide catheter-care protocol.
6. Encourage removal of catheter and use of urinal, bedpan, or commode as soon as frequent urine-output determinations are not required.

H. Maintaining Normal or Only Slightly Elevated Body Temperature

1. Be efficient in care; do not expose wounds unnecessarily.
2. Maintain warm ambient temperature.
3. Use heat lamps, radiant warmers, space blankets to keep the patient warm.
4. Provide a dry top layer for wet dressings to reduce evaporative heat loss.
5. Warm wound cleansing and dressing solutions to body temperature.
6. Use dry dressings and blankets in transporting patient outside of hospital.
7. Administer antipyretics as prescribed.

I. Avoiding Wound or Systemic Infection

1. Wash hands with antibacterial cleansing agent before and after all patient contact.
2. Use barrier garments—isolation gown or plastic apron—for all care requiring contact with the patient or the patient's bed.
3. Cover hair and wear mask when wounds are exposed or when performing a sterile procedure.
4. Use clean examination gloves for all care involving patient contact.
5. Maintain proper concentration of topical antibacterial agents used in wound care.
6. Be alert for reservoirs of infection and sources of cross-contamination in equipment, assignment of personnel, etc.
7. Check history of tetanus immunization and provide passive and/or active tetanus prophylaxis as prescribed.
8. Change intravenous tubing and lines according to CDC recommendations.
9. Administer antibiotics as prescribed and be alert for toxic effects and incompatibilities.
10. Assess wounds daily for local signs of infection—swelling and redness around wound edges, purulent drainage, discoloration, loss of grafts, etc.
11. Be alert for early signs of septicemia, including changes in mentation, tachypnea, and decreased peristalsis, as well as later signs, such as increased pulse, decreased blood pressure, increased or decreased urine output, facial flushing, increased temperature, malaise; report promptly to physician.
12. Promote optimal personal hygiene for the patient, including daily cleansing of unburned areas, meticulous care of teeth and mouth, shampooing of hair every other day, shaving of hair in or near burned areas, meticulous care of IV and urinary catheter sites.
13. Inspect skin carefully for signs of pressure and breakdown.
14. Observe for and report signs of thrombophlebitis or catheter-induced infections.
15. Prevent atelectasis and pneumonia through physical therapy, postural drainage, meticulous pulmonary technique, and, if indicated, tracheostomy care.

J. Enhancing Range of Joint Motion and Ability to Perform Activities of Daily Living

1. Obtain consultation from physical and occupational therapists.
2. Assist the patient with prescribed exercise regimen, passive and active range-of-motion exercises, ambulation (Fig. 33-5).
3. Maintain splints in proper position as prescribed by occupational therapist; remove splints on regular schedule and observe for signs of skin irritation before reapplying.
4. Position the patient to decrease edema and avoid flexion of burned joints.
5. Coordinate pain management and other care to allow optimal effort during periods of physical exercise.

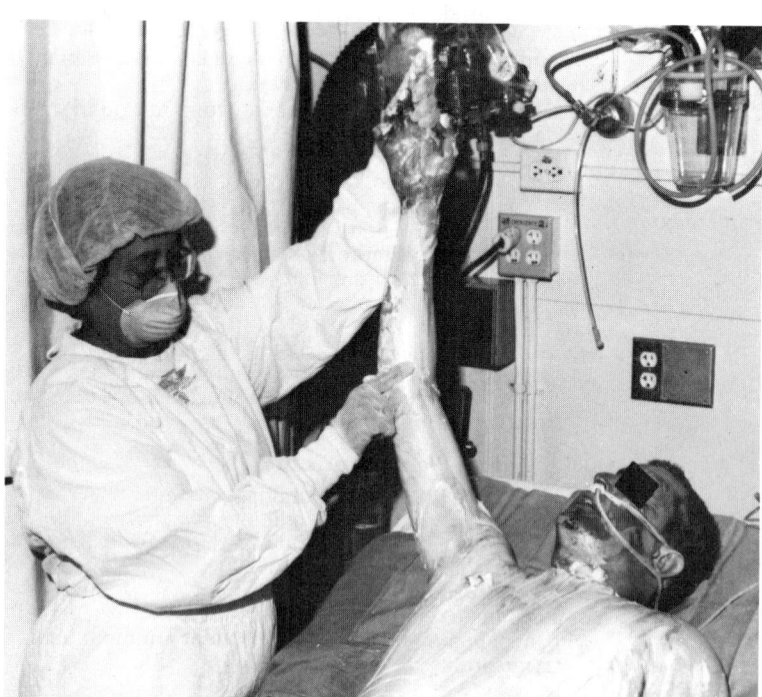

Figure 33-5. *The patient is put through full range-of-motion exercises at least twice daily to prevent contractures following application of topical antibacterial cream. (Photo courtesy U.S. Army Institute of Surgical Research, Fort Sam Houston, TX)*

6. Encourage independence in activities that afford motion of burned joints.
7. Initiate passive and active range-of-motion and breathing exercises during early postburn period.
8. Plan with physical, occupational, and respiratory therapists for a conditioning regimen that gradually increases energy expenditure and tolerance for activity.
9. Coordinate plan for rest, nutritional intake, and pain minimization to maximize physical and mental energy available for increasing activities.
10. Contract with the patient to assist him to meet goals for type and level of activity desired.
11. Act as advocate for the patient's need for rest by coordinating the patient's therapeutic and social activities and prioritizing interventions and visits.
12. Assess preburn sleep pattern and determine what helps the patient achieve relaxation and sleep; implement to the extent possible.
13. Provide sleep medication as prescribed.

K. Augmenting Nutritional Intake

1. Weigh the patient daily with dressings removed.
2. Obtain consultation from dietitian for calculation of nutritional needs based on age, weight, height, and burn size.
3. Administer vitamins and mineral supplements as prescribed.
4. Minimize metabolic stress by allaying fears, pain, and anxiety and by maintaining a warm environmental temperature.
5. When bowel sounds return, administer oral fluids slowly, so that patient tolerance can be observed. If there are no problems, advance diet to the patient's usual diet, as tolerated.
6. Provide nasogastric tube feedings as prescribed, using caution to prevent aspiration by checking tube placement prior to each feeding and checking amount of gastric aspirate.
7. Administer IV hyperalimentation and fat emulsions prescribed with usual nursing precautions (see p. 450).
8. Keep record of caloric intake.
9. Encourage the patient to feed self.
10. Supplement meals with between-meal high-protein, high-caloric snacks, including appropriate foods brought from home.

L. Resumption of Normal Gastric Motility and Function

1. Keep NPO until bowel sounds resume.
2. Assess bowel sounds every 2–4 hours while acutely ill. (Decreased peristalsis may be an early sign of septicemia.)
3. Decompress stomach with nasogastric tube on low intermittent suction until bowel sounds resume.
4. Check amount and pH of gastric drainage or aspirate and report as requested.
5. Administer antacids as prescribed.
6. Heed complaints of nausea while intubated by checking for abdominal distention, tube placement.
7. Provide mouth care every 4 hours while intubated.
8. Test stools for occult bleeding.

M. Reducing Pain and Enhancing Relaxation

1. Assess the patient for pain periodically.
2. Teach relaxation, imagery, breathing exercises, or other techniques to help the patient cope with pain.
3. Determine previous experience with pain, the patient's response and coping mechanisms.
4. Offer analgesics prior to wound care or before particularly painful treatments.
5. Change the patient's position when possible, supporting extremities with pillows.
6. Reduce anxiety by approaches such as sensory-oriented explanations of procedures.

N. Care of Concomitant Illnesses and Injuries

1. Obtain complete nursing data base, including history of events surrounding the burn injury, past health/illness, physical assessment, and laboratory results.
2. Observe for fractures, spinal, head, or internal organ damage in victims of electrical burns, explosions, or history of falling or jumping from a fire.
3. Obtain ophthalmologic consultation if face is burned.
4. Observe for signs and symptoms of chronic illness heightened by stress of burn injury.
5. Implement appropriate independent and dependent nursing activities related to above findings.

O. Promoting an Understanding of Consequences of Burn Injury, Required Therapy, and Rationale

1. Develop an individualized teaching plan that includes explanations of pathophysiologic changes resulting from burn injury (both immediate and long-term), treatments, and rationale.
2. Include aspects of care provided by all burn-team members.
3. Periodically "test" the patient's understanding.
4. Provide time for and encouragement of questions related to care, both in hospital and projected home setting.

P. Enhancing Coping Strategies

1. Assess the patient's coping mechanisms from past history and current behavior.
2. Provide opportunities for the patient to express his thoughts and feelings, and fears and anxieties regarding his injury.
3. Explore with the patient alternative mechanisms for coping with the burn injury and its consequences.
4. Assure the patient of the normality of his responses and the effect that time and healing will likely have on his current concerns.
5. Interpret patient behavior to concerned family and significant others.
6. Respect current coping mechanisms and remove them only when an appropriate alternative can be provided.
7. Support family and friends' communications and visits if this is noted to help the patient.
8. Assess need for psychiatric nursing consultation/medical (psychiatric) intervention.
9. Offer antianxiety medications as prescribed.
10. Assist the patient to adapt to altered body image or life-style resulting from burn injury.
    a. Gather data on the patient's preburn self-image and life-style.
    b. When the patient is ready, encourage him to express his concerns regarding changes in self-image or life-style that may result from burn injury.
    c. Be honest, but positive, in responding to the patient and family.
    d. Positively reinforce appropriate, effective coping mechanisms.
    e. Utilize hospital and community resources, including psychologists, counselors, teachers, clergy, and significant others to provide support for the patient.

11. Assist the patient to resolve grief related to burn injury in an appropriate manner.
    a. Recognize the patient's need to grieve over losses related to the burn injury.
    b. Support the patient and significant others through the grieving process, recognizing that each individual may move through this at a different pace.
    c. Differentiate between normal depression following traumatic injury and depression that requires medication or psychiatric intervention for amelioration.
    d. Arrange for the patient to talk with other patients who have had a similar injury and are progressing satisfactorily.
    e. Help the patient set short-term goals and reflect on progress in small steps.

Patient Education

Health education is closely related to the rehabilitation of the burn patient as he prepares to return to a productive place in society. Functional and cosmetic reconstruction is accomplished, and the patient attempts to integrate a new self-concept into social realities. Broadly viewed, health education focuses on biologic, psychological, and social parameters.
1. Assist the patient in transition from dependence on the health team to independence by helping him develop methods of communicating his needs and functioning abilities to others.
2. Guide the patient in thinking positively about himself. Promote ability to redirect others' attention from the scarred body to the self within.
3. Demonstrate and explain wound care procedures to be continued after discharge:
    a. Wash hands.
    b. Cleanse small open wounds with mild soap in tub or shower.
    c. Rinse well with tap water.
    d. Pat dry with clean towel.
    e. Apply prescribed topical agent and/or dressing.
4. Observe for local signs of wound infection:
    a. Increased redness of normal skin around burn area
    b. Increased cloudy yellow pus or drainage
    c. Increased pain, foul odor in burn area
    d. Elevated body temperature
5. Instruct the patient in measures to lubricate and enhance comfort of healing skin:
    a. Cleanse skin with mild soap and rinse well daily.
    b. Apply lubricant such as cocoa butter or Nivea to healed areas twice daily.
    c. Wear clean, white underwear and clothing free of irritating dyes.
    d. Take antipruritics as prescribed.
    e. Stay in a cool environment if itching occurs.
    f. Protect skin from further trauma, including sunburn (use sunblock containing PABA).
6. Develop a schedule to incorporate exercise regimen as prescribed by physical therapist.
    a. Assist the patient and family to practice exercises.

b. Suggest scheduling exercises immediately after wound cleansing and application of topical agent, since skin may be more pliable and less sensitive to stretching then.
7. Instruct the patient in use and care of splints and pressure garments.
    a. Cleanse with mild soap and rinse well daily.
    b. Keep away from heat; dry garment by laying it flat on towels.
    c. Wear garment on schedule prescribed by therapist.
    d. Pad open wounds with light dressing under splints or pressure garments.
    e. Observe for signs of skin breakdown.
    f. Wear/bring splints and pressure garments to follow-up visits to be checked for proper fit.
8. Acquaint patient and family with resources, including support groups for recovering burn victims, family group meetings in burn center, community resources as required.
9. Review with the patient and family common emotional responses during convalescence (depression, withdrawal, grieving, dreaming, anxiety, guilt, excessive sensitivity, emotional lability, insomnia, fear of future) and discuss usual temporary nature of these and effective coping mechanisms.
10. Arrange for return visit for follow-up care and home health-care services, as needed in interim.
11. Provide written instructions regarding all care required on discharge.

Evaluation

1. Achieves normal respiratory function (e.g., CO < 10, ABGs within normal limits, respiratory rate 12–20)
2. Achieves normal cardiovascular function (e.g., pulse 60–100, peripheral tissues adequately perfused)
3. Maintains fluid and electrolyte parameters in healthy balance
4. Demonstrates adequate wound healing—small open wound areas are clean
5. Skin is soft, comfortable; scars flat
6. Has normal urinary elimination
7. Demonstrates normal body temperature
8. Is free of pathogenic organisms
9. Achieves normal range of motion and can perform activities of daily living with necessary endurance
10. Achieves positive nitrogen balance; regains optimal weight
11. Regains normal integrity and function of gastrointestinal system
12. Reports minimal pain in burn area and joints; explains use of analgesics and other pain-reduction techniques
13. Uses appropriate coping mechanisms to deal with stress of burn injury and its sequelae
14. Adapts to losses and alterations in body image and to life-style resulting from the burn injury
15. Explains rationale of required self-care related to burn injury. Demonstrates ability to carry out wound and skin care, exercises, splint and pressure garment application

Bibliography

Books

Achauer BM (ed). Management of the Burned Patient. Norwalk, CT, Appleton & Lange, 1987

Bernstein N and Robson M. Comprehensive Approaches to the Burned Person. New York, Medical Examination Publishing, 1983
Boswick JA (ed). The Art and Science of

Burn Care. Rockville, MD, Aspen Publishers, Inc., 1987
Dressler DP, Hozid JL and Nathan P. Thermal Injury. St Louis, CV Mosby, 1988

Hummel RP (ed). Clinical Burn Therapy: A Management and Prevention Guide. Boston, John Wright-PSP, 1982

McLaughlin EG (ed). Critical Care of the Burn Patient: A Case Study Approach. Rockville, MD, Aspen Publishers, Inc., 1989

Salisbury RE, Newman NM and Dingeldein GP. Manual of Burn Therapeutics: An Interdisciplinary Approach. Boston, Little, Brown & Co, 1983

Trofino RM (ed). Burn Nursing: A Comprehensive Approach. Philadelphia, FA Davis (in press)

Journals

Abshagen D. Topical agents and emergency care for minor burn injuries. J Emerg Nurs 1984 Nov–Dec; 10(6):325–331

Arturson MG. The pathophysiology of severe thermal injury. J Burn Care Rehabil 1985 Mar–Apr; 6(2):124–146

Bayley DW and Smith GA. The three degrees of burn care. Nursing 1987 Mar; 17(3):34–41

Boswick JA (ed). Burn care. Surg Clin North Am 1987 Feb; 67(1):entire issue

Dailey MA. Carbon monoxide poisoning. J Emerg Nurs 1988 Mar–Apr; 15(2):120–123

DiGregorio VR (ed). Rehabilitation of the burn patient. Clin Phys Ther 1984; 4:entire issue

Doherty D and Austin EV. Effective management of cultured epithelial cells—Two case reports. J Burn Care Rehabil 1986 Jan–Feb; 7(1):33–34

Freeman J. Nursing care of the patient with a burn injury. Crit Care Nurse 1984 Nov–Dec; 4(6):52–68

Gallico GG and O'Connor NE. Cultured epithelium as a skin substitute. Clin Plast Surg 1985 Apr; 12(2):149–157

Gordon M (ed). Burn care protocols: Infection control in the burn unit. J Burn Care Rehabil 1987 Jan–Feb; 8(1):67–71

Gordon M. (ed). Synthetic and biosynthetic skin substitutes. J Burn Care Rehabil 1988 Mar–Apr; 9(2):209–217

Gordon M (ed). Burn wound care: Silver sulfadiazine application. J Burn Care Rehabil 1987 Sep–Oct; 8(5):429–433

Heimbach D et al. Artificial dermis for major burns. Ann Surg 1988 Sep; 208(3):313–320

Herndon DN et al. Postgraduate course: Respiratory injury. Part I. Incidence, mortality, pathogenesis, and treatment of pulmonary injury. J Burn Care Rehabil 1986 Mar–Apr; 7(2):184–191

Klein DG and O'Malley P. Topical injury from chemical agents: Initial treatment. Heart Lung 1987 Jan; 16(1):49–54

Marvin J et al. Pain management of the burn patient. J Burn Care Rehabil 1987 Jul–Aug; 8(4):307–318

McHugh TP et al. Therapeutic efficacy of Biobrane in partial and full-thickness thermal injury. Surgery 1986 Oct; 100(4):661–664

Monograph on cultured epithelial autografts. 1989 Mar; BioSurface Technology, Inc., One Kendall Square, Building 200, Cambridge, MA 02139; (617) 494-8484

Nichter LS et al. Injuries due to commercial electric current. J Burn Care Rehabil 1984 Mar–Apr; 5(2):124–137

Pelias ME and Parry SW. Thermal injuries. Curr Concepts Wound Care 1987 Fall; 10(3):5–10

Robertson K. Burn care: The crucial first days. Am J Nurs 1985 Jan; 85(1):29–45

Ruberg RL (ed). Advances in burn care. Clin Plast Surg 1986 Jan; 13(1):entire issue.

Smith GA and Savinski–Bozinko G. Giving emergency care for burns. Nursing 1989 Sep; 19(9):55–62

Watkins PN et al. Psychological stages in adaptation following burn injury: A method for facilitating psychological recovery of burn victims. J Burn Care Rehabil 1988 Jul–Aug; 9(4):376–384

Winkler JB (ed). Burn care update. Crit Care Q 1984 Dec; 7(3):entire issue.

Zawacki BE. Temporary wound closure after burn excision. J Burn Care Rehabil 1986 Mar–Apr; 7(2):138–143

Immune and Autoimmune-Related Disorders

Acquired immunodeficiency syndrome (AIDS) is defined as the most severe form of a continuum of illnesses associated with human immunodeficiency virus (HIV) infection. It causes a slow degeneration of the immune system with the development of opportunistic infections, malignancies, and, frequently, impairment of the central nervous system.

Management Considerations

Etiology

1. The causative agent is a retrovirus that damages the immune system by infecting and depleting the T4 helper lymphocytes. (These T4 cells play a central role in the regulation of the immune system.)
2. There are also abnormalities in the function of the B cells, T8 cells, NK cells, monocytes, and macrophages.
3. With loss of the immune function, the disease becomes clinically manifested.
4. HIV is transmitted by sexual contact, through exposure to blood and blood components, and perinatally from an infected mother to the child.

Risk Factors for HIV Transmission

1. Homosexual or bisexual men
2. Intravenous drug abusers
3. Transfusion and blood product recipients (prior to 1985)*
4. Heterosexual contacts of HIV-positive individuals
5. Newborn babies of mothers who are seropositive

Clinical Manifestations

A. Following Exposure to HIV Infection

1. Shortly following exposure (6 days to 7 weeks), there is an acute flulike illness lasting 2–4 weeks.
2. Manifested by fever, sweats, myalgia, arthralgias, malaise, sore throat, general lymphadenopathy, maculopapular rash, and fungal and viral infections of the mouth.

B. Development of AIDS-Related Diseases

1. Appears months to years after exposure

* Risk of infection to recipients of blood/blood products has gradually declined, although persons in this group already infected may progress to disease.

2. *Pulmonary manifestations*
   a. Persistent cough, shortness of breath, chest pain, fever
   b. From *Pneumocystis carinii* pneumonia (most common), disseminated *Mycobacterium avium*, Cytomegalovirus, Legionella, and other pathogens
3. *Gastrointestinal manifestations*
   a. Diarrhea, weight loss, anorexia, abdominal cramping, rectal urgency (tenesmus)
   b. From enteric pathogens including Salmonella, Shigella, Campylobacter, *Entamoeba histolytica*, Cytomegalovirus, Herpes simplex, Strongyloides, Giardia, Cryptosporidium, *Isospora belli*, Chlamydia, and others
4. *Oral manifestations*
   a. Appearance of oral lesions, white plaques on oral mucosa and angular cheilitis from *Candida albicans* of mouth and esophagus
   b. Vesicles with ulceration from viruses
   c. White lesions on margins of tongue from hairy leukoplakia
   d. Oral warts and associated gingivitis
   e. Peridontitis progressing to gingival necrosis and exposure of bone
5. *Central nervous system manifestations*
   a. Cognitive, motor, and behavioral symptoms (AIDS dementia complex)
   b. Demonstrated by mental slowing, impaired memory and concentration, loss of balance, lower extremity weakness, ataxia, apathy, and social withdrawal
   c. From CNS toxoplasmosis, cryptococcal meningitis, herpes virus infections, Cytomegalovirus (causing retinopathy and blindness), and CNS lymphoma
6. *Malignancies* (Fig. 34-1)
   a. Kaposi's sarcoma (rare and aggressive tumor involving skin, lymph nodes, gastrointestinal tract, and lungs)
   b. Non-Hodgkin's lymphoma (p. 274) and lymphomas (p. 272)
   c. Cloacogenic cancer (an unusual cancer of the anal area)

Diagnostic Evaluation

1. History of risk factors/high-risk behaviors
2. Positive blood test for HIV
   a. Enzyme immunoassay (EIA)—serologic test for detecting antibody to HIV
   b. Western blot test—used to confirm a positive result on EIA test

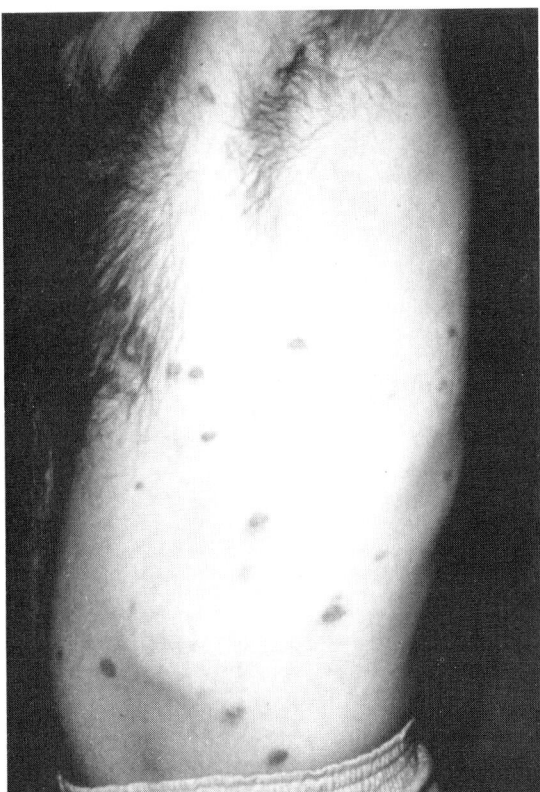

Figure 34-1. *Lesions from Kaposi's sarcoma of a patient with acquired immunodeficiency syndrome. In light-skinned persons the lesions appear blue to violet in color, while in darker individuals the lesions may appear nearly black. (Photo courtesy Henry Masur, M.D., Clinical Center, National Institutes of Health)*

3. Presence of indicator disease (e.g., *Pneumocystis carinii* pneumonia, candidiasis of esophagus, Kaposi's sarcoma, etc.)
4. Diagnostic procedures (biopsies, imaging procedures, etc.) of the organ system involved
5. Neuropsychological test—to identify cognitive deficits associated with AIDS dementia complex

Complications

1. Repeated overwhelming opportunistic infections
2. Respiratory failure

Management

A. Underlying Considerations

1. There are no treatments available at this time for the underlying immunodeficiencies.
2. Treatment is available for some opportunistic infections and other diseases associated with AIDS.
3. Management requires the expertise of many specialties: pulmonary medicine, infectious disease, gastroenterology, neurology, surgery, psychiatry, dental, nursing, social work.

B. Specific Treatment

1. Zidovudine (antiviral therapy)
   a. Appears to halt viral replication

b. May prolong survival time
   c. Considerable morbidity associated with its use.
2. Treatment of opportunistic infections or organ-specific symptoms
   a. Use of antifungal drugs (clotrimazole, amphotericin, ketoconazole); ganciclovir for Cytomegalovirus disease; acyclovir for viral infections; metronidazole for amebiasis/giardiasis
   b. Radiation and chemotherapy for management of malignancies
   c. Trimethoprim–sulfamethoxazole or pentamidine for *Pneumocystis carinii* pneumonia, etc.

C. Supportive Care

1. Treatment of reversible illnesses
2. Nutritional support
3. Palliation of pain
4. Dental management
5. Evaluation and management of psychologic and social aspects of AIDS
6. Treatment to relieve symptoms (cough, diarrhea)
7. Antidepressant drugs; psychiatric interventions

Universal Precautions*

1. Use appropriate barrier precautions to prevent skin and mucous membrane exposure when contact with blood or body fluids is anticipated.
2. Wear gloves when touching blood and body fluids, mucous membranes, or nonintact skin of all patients, when handling items or surfaces soiled with blood or body fluids, and when performing venipuncture and other vascular access procedures.
3. Change gloves after contact with each patient. Wash hands immediately after glove removal.
4. Wear masks and protective eyewear/face shields during procedures that are likely to generate droplets of blood or other body fluids to prevent exposure of mucous membranes of the mouth, nose, and eyes.
5. Wear gloves during procedures likely to generate splashes of blood or other body fluids.
6. Take precautions to prevent injuries caused by needles, scalpels, and other sharp instruments or devices; do not recap, bend, or break needles by hand. Place used disposable syringes, needles, or other sharp items in puncture-resistant containers for disposal.

Nursing Process Overview: *The Patient With AIDS*

Nursing Assessment

1. Review record for history of risk factors, constitutional signs and symptoms, recent infections, positive blood test for HIV antibodies.
2. Review record for patient's present complaint(s): cough, shortness of breath, diarrhea.
3. Review record to determine nutritional status; record of weight loss, body mass depletion, decreased skinfold thickness and mid-arm muscle circumference, hypoalbuminemia, decreased iron-binding capacity, and selenium deficiency.

* Recommendations for Prevention of HIV Transmission in Health-Care Settings. MMWR 1987 Aug 21; 36(Suppl No. 25).

4. Assess respiratory rate, depth, and auscultate lungs for breath sounds; assess for skin color and temperature, palpable lymph nodes, and evidence of fever.
5. Inspect mouth for lesions; examine skin for rash, sores, Kaposi's sarcoma lesions. Record number, size, and locations.
6. Ask about bowel patterns, changes in habits, constipation, abdominal cramping, number and volume of stools, presence of perianal pain and ulceration.
7. Is patient oriented to time, place, and person? Affect? Any problem with memory and concentration? Headaches? Seizures?
8. How much does the patient know about AIDS? Etiology? Signs and symptoms? Mode of transmission? Methods for limiting exposure?
9. Find out as much as possible about patient's premorbid personality, experience and skills, social support system.

Nursing Diagnoses

1. Fear (of disease progression, of infecting and reactions of others, treatment effects, isolation and abandonment, cognitive, physical and social losses) related to reality of having AIDS.
2. Potential for infection related to immunodeficiency, neutropenia secondary to medications/treatment.
3. Altered nutrition (less than body requirements) related to anorexia secondary to infection, catabolic state, impaired swallowing from oral and esophageal pain, side effects of drugs, malabsorption, dementia and impaired motor ability, extreme fatigue.
4. Altered oral mucous membranes related to opportunistic infections secondary to reduced immune function.
5. Altered bowel elimination (diarrhea) related to enteric pathogens and/or HIV infection, medication reactions, tube feeding intolerance.
6. Altered thought processes (impaired cognition and dementia) related to cortical atrophy, ventricular dilatation secondary to HIV cerebral infection and effects of AIDS dementia complex.
7. Altered body temperature (low grade or high fever) related to HIV infection, concurrent infection or infection by bacteria, virus, fungus, or parasite; lymphadenopathy, visceral involvement by Kaposi's sarcoma.
8. Altered breathing pattern related to lung involvement secondary to opportunistic infection and to noninfectious disorder (Kaposi's sarcoma of the lung).
9. Knowledge deficit of managing AIDS and of educational, social, and regional helping resources.
10. Other nursing diagnoses could include:
    a. Fatigue related to underlying HIV infection and reactive depression
    b. Disturbances in body image related to rapid body changes from debilitating disease
    c. Helplessness related to inexperience with illness, sense of loss of control, depression, and vulnerability associated with AIDS
    d. Pain related to infection, peripheral neuropathies, nodules of Kaposi's sarcoma, diarrhea
    e. Anticipatory grieving related to awareness of implications of AIDS, dying and death, unfinished business, multiple bereavements, and changes in life-style
    f. Social isolation related to attitudes of others, multiple losses

g. Ineffective family coping related to crisis created by AIDS, guilt, fear, overwhelming care-taking responsibilities.

Nursing Interventions

A. Coping With Fear

1. Maintain nonjudgmental attitude and nonprejudicial approach.
2. Anticipate that the patient may pass through series of stages: initial crisis, transitional stage, acceptance state, and preparation for death.
3. Allow patient to use denial as a protective mechanism—gives some control over when and how patient will control mortality.
    a. Expect some displaced anger; avoid being personally affronted by patient's anger.
    b. Allow patient to acknowledge reality of his situation without false reassurance.
4. Explain that symptoms of anxiety and depression are common initially but generally improve with time and support.
5. Anticipate that drug abusers may exhibit antisocial behaviors, feelings of alienation and isolation.
6. Provide careful discussion and clarification of treatment options.
7. Help patient set realistic goals and expectations.
8. Offer counseling services, especially when AIDS is initially diagnosed and as patient enters terminal phase of HIV illness.
9. Obtain social service referral for available resources and services: housekeeping, food shopping, community support services, cancer counseling agencies, Social Security Administration, etc.
10. Use all resources to identify and reduce stress load: perceived control, positive coping skills, stress reduction techniques, promotion of social support, making conscious effort to live each day fully.
11. Encourage patient to join a support group—helpful in defusing stressful issues and in developing strategies to cope with the disease.
12. Observe for emerging psychiatric problems, especially in persons who are socially isolated, those with guilt about sexuality and life-style, and those with poor accommodation.
13. Give patient opportunity to arrange personal business: power of attorney to delegate health care decisions, will, etc.—cognitive deterioration may make it impossible for patient to act on his own behalf at a later date.
14. Allow discussion of nature and management of death—minimizes negative impact of ever-present threat of death.
    a. Assure patient of palliative care, pain control, and help with anxiety and depression.
    b. Respect the right of the patient to participate in treatment decisions, i.e., to limit therapy and life-prolonging interventions.

B. Controlling and Preventing Infection

1. Have a high index of suspicion for infection even when clinical manifestations are subtle or absent—opportunistic infections may be reactivated at any time during the course of the disease.
2. Follow universal precautions for all patients. See page 857.
3. Administer prescribed pharmacologic agents; some

infections are not treatable with currently available regimens.

4. Administer and teach patient/family good skin care—a break in the skin is a source of secondary infection; use position changes, emollient lotions, special pads and beds, and attend to hydration and nutrition.
5. Maintain cleanliness of environment.
6. Employ aseptic techniques when performing invasive procedures.
7. Teach patient to make the most of what remains of his immune system by minimizing the risk of disease.
   a. Avoid exposure to persons with infections—may activate HIV.
   b. Turn, cough, and do breathing exercises, especially when confined to bed.
   c. Avoid continuing drug abuse and repeated exposure to HIV.
   d. Instruct visitors about hand washing before entering and leaving the room.

C. Improving Nutritional Status

1. Monitor nutritional status by weighing, dietary intake and calorie count, anthropometric measurement, and evaluation of serum albumin, BUN, protein, and transferrin levels.
2. Monitor for sore throat that progresses to dysphagia or odynaphagia (pain upon swallowing) or persistent heartburn—suggestive of oral candidiasis.
3. Consult with dietitian to develop strategies for nutrition care including additional calories and nutritional supplements to maintain strength, comfort, and level of functioning.
4. Include patient in decision making regarding his nutrition care.
5. Alter timing of drug administration to improve intake with meals.
   a. Give prescribed antiemetic 30 minutes before meals.
   b. Try to give drug infusions after meals.
6. For patient with oral/esophageal pain from candida esophagitis, herpetic esophagitis, endotracheal Kaposi's sarcoma:
   a. Administer prescribed antifungal therapy.
   b. Avoid highly seasoned or acidic foods.
   c. Offer fluids and blenderized foods to minimize chewing and ease swallowing.
   d. Suggest nutrition-dense supplements: instant breakfast drinks, protein-fortified juices for home care.
7. Encourage patient to maximize intake during periods he is feeling better.
8. Discourage excessive alcohol intake—has immunosuppressive effect.
9. Keep in mind that elemental diets/nutritional supplements may become intolerable to patient as anorexia progresses.
10. Prepare patient for enteral or parenteral feedings (see p. 446).
11. Make appropriate community referral if patient is unable to shop or prepare meals.
12. Encourage small, frequent meals as these may make best use of limited absorptive capacity.
13. For patients with neurologic involvement and dementia:
    a. Consult with occupational therapist for selection of eating utensils for patients with impaired motor ability.
    b. Monitor and encourage patient to eat; feed when appropriate.
14. Continue to monitor weight—chronic weight loss implies malnutrition, which has adverse effects on immune function.

D. Achieving Relief of Oral Discomfort

1. Ask about persistent sore throat, dysphagia, heart burn—all these symptoms are suggestive of oral/esophageal candidiasis.
2. Examine mouth for oral candidiasis, a harbinger of AIDS in HIV seropositive persons.
   a. Pseudomembranous candidiasis (thrush)—reveals removable white plaques on oral surface.
   b. Herpes simplex—recurrent intraoral lesions with small crops of painful vesicles that ulcerate.
   c. Hairy leukoplakia—white thickening of oral mucosa.
   d. Angular cheilitis—cracking and erythema at the corners of the mouth.
3. Offer prescribed nystatin mouth rinses and antifungal agents; acyclovir may be prescribed for herpes simplex.

E. Coping with Diarrhea

1. Keep in mind that gastrointestinal infections and diarrhea decrease absorptive efficiency.
2. Tell patient to monitor stools for blood and try to determine if bleeding is before, with, or after bowel movement.
3. Monitor intake and output; assess skin and mucous membranes for turgor and dryness.
4. Administer fluids and electrolytes as prescribed.
5. Advise patient to rest to achieve bowel rest.
6. Use enteric precautions.
7. Plan regimen of skin care including cleansing/blotting/drying of the anal area, application of ointment or skin barrier cream.
8. Eliminate caffeine, alcohol, dairy products, food high in fats, fresh juices, and acidic juices if diarrhea persists. Drink liquids at room temperature.
9. Avoid foods that increase intestinal motility and distention.
10. Report symptoms and signs of increased weakness, dizziness, and continuing weight loss.

F. Coping With Altered Thought Processes

1. Remember that the brain is a critical target organ for HIV infection.
2. Provide daily assessment of mental status; monitor for changes in behavior, memory, concentration ability, and motor system dysfunction—patient may become vegetative and unable to ambulate.
   Onset of dementia is usually insidious but may be abrupt, precipitated by acute infection.
3. Reorient patient frequently; use calendar, clock, family/friends' pictures, lists, structured plan of care.
4. Provide for patient safety: bedrails up; call signal available; things within patient's reach.
5. Give repeated reassurance.
6. Assess for depressive or suicidal symptoms—AIDS represents a significant risk for suicide.
7. Anticipate necessity of guardianship, durable power of attorney for health care, informed consent, etc., if patient has AIDS dementia complex, as patient may have poor insight and become indifferent to his illness.

G. Becoming Afebrile and Comfortable

1. Assess for chills, shortness of breath, cough, dyspnea, and changes in mental status.

2. Teach patient/care-giver to keep a temperature chart.
3. Encourage high fluid intake to replace insensible water losses incurred by fever/diaphoresis.
4. See page 894 for promotion of comfort of patient with elevated temperature.

H. Achieving Improved Breathing

1. Maintain adequate oxygenation and perfusion.
2. Watch for *sudden* change in respiratory function—patient may be developing a secondary infection.
3. Administer prescribed narcotic for postinfectious cough, a complication of *Pneumocystis carinii* pneumonia and viral pneumonia.
4. Encourage smoking cessation to enhance pulmonary ciliary defense.
5. Assist in securing induced sputum using saline delivered via a nebulizer—to obtain specific infecting organisms.
   a. Wear mask and gloves during sputum collection.
   b. Instruct patient to brush tongue, buccal surfaces, teeth, and palate with water before sputum induction—to remove superficial squamous epithelial cells and their adherent bacteria and foreign material.
   c. Instruct patient to gargle and rinse mouth with tap water.
6. Keep in mind that patient has the option of refusing mechanical ventilation.

Discharge Planning/Patient Education

1. Indicate that patient is a source of infection to others and should take actions that may reduce the progress of disease (use of safer sex, avoiding other infections, seeking prompt medical attention).
2. Teach patient to recognize and report important symptoms.

a. Change in pattern/magnitude of temperature elevation.
b. Development of a new focal complaint: skin spots, sore mouth, diarrhea.
3. Emphasize to drug users that continued use may expose them to additional infection and such infections may activate viral replication.
4. Encourage patient to modify sexual behaviors for safer sex.
   a. Use latex condoms supplemented by creams and jelly containing a viricidal agent.
   b. Refrain from oral and anal sex.
   c. Encourage patient to read literature from various AIDS action groups on "safe sex" techniques.
5. If a drug abuser:
   a. Enroll in a treatment program.
   b. Do not share needles ("works").
6. Teach patient to optimize immune system function by sound dietary practices, exercise, and regular periods of sleep; promote changes in the direction of more healthful living.
7. Emphasize positive aspects of patient's relatively good health.
8. *Resources*
   National AIDS Hotline—1-800-342-AIDS
   Operates 24 hours a day, 7 days a week; offers information on transmission, prevention, testing, and local referrals.
   National AIDS Information Clearinghouse
   P.O. Box 6003
   Rockville, MD 20850

   On-line Databases
   MEDLINE/AIDS Line
   National Library of Medicine
   8600 Rockville Pike
   Bethesda, MD 20894

Bibliography

Books

Blanchet KD. AIDS: A Health Care Management Response. Rockville, Aspen Publishers Inc, 1988

Corless IB and Pittman–Lindeman M. AIDS: Principles, Practices & Politics. Washington, DC, Hemisphere, 1988

DeVita VTJ, Hellman S and Rosenberg SA (eds). AIDS: Etiology, Diagnosis, and Prevention. 2nd ed. Philadelphia, JB Lippincott, 1988

Durham JD and Cohen FL (eds). The Person with AIDS: Nursing Perspectives. New York, Springer, 1987

Flaskerud JH. AIDS/HIV Infection: A Reference Guide for Nursing Professionals. Philadelphia, WB Saunders, 1989

Galea RP, Lewis BJ and Baker LA. AIDS and IV Drug Abusers. Owings Mills, MD, National Health Publishing, 1988

Halleron TA and Pisaneschi JI. AIDS Information Resources Directory. New York, American Foundation for AIDS Research, 1988

Harawi SJ and O'Hara CJ. Pathology and Pathophysiology of AIDS and HIV-Related Disease. St Louis, CV Mosby, 1989

Institute of Medicine, National Academy of Sciences. Confronting AIDS. Washington, DC, National Academy Press, 1988

Kaslow RA and Francis DP. The Epidemiology of AIDS. New York, Oxford University Press, 1989

Kübler–Ross E. AIDS: The Ultimate Challenge. New York, Macmillan, 1987

Lechtenberg R and Sher JH. AIDS in the Nervous System. New York, Churchill Livingstone, 1988

Leukefeld CG and Fimbres M (eds). Responding to AIDS: Psychosocial Initiatives. Silver Spring, MD, National Association of Social Workers, 1987

Madhok R, Forbes CD and Evatt BL (eds). Blood, Blood Products and AIDS. Baltimore, Johns Hopkins University Press, 1987

Malinowsky HR and Perry GJ (eds). AIDS Information Source Book. Phoenix, Oryx Press, 1988

Meisenhelder JB and LaCharite CL. Comfort in Caring: Nursing the Patient with HIV Infection. Glenview, IL, Scott, Foresman, 1989

Parrillo JE and Masur H (eds). The Critically Ill Immunosuppressed

Patient. Rockville, Aspen Publishers Inc, 1987

Robertson PB and Greenspan JS. Perspectives on Oral Manifestations of AIDS. Littleton, MA, PSG Publishing, 1988

Rosenblum ML, Levy RM and Bredesen DE. AIDS and the Nervous System. New York, Raven Press, 1988

Roth JS. All About AIDS. New York, Harwood Academic Publishers, 1989

Rubin RH and Young LS (eds). Clinical Approach to Infection in the Compromised Host. 2nd ed. New York, Plenum, 1988

Sande MA and Volberding PA (eds). The Medical Management of AIDS. Philadelphia, WB Saunders, 1988

Tuohey JF. Caring for Persons with AIDS and Cancer. St Louis, Catholic Health Association of the US, 1988

Journals

American Academy of Neurology AIDS Task Force. Human immunodeficiency virus (HIV) infection and the nervous system: Report from the American Academy of Neurology AIDS Task

Force. Neurology 1989 Jan; 39(1):119–122

American Academy of Neurology. Position of the American Academy of Neurology on certain aspects of the care and management of the persistent vegetative state patient. Neurology 1989 Jan; 39(1):125–126

Brew BJ, Rosenblum M and Price RW. AIDS dementia complex and primary HIV brain infection. J Neuroimmunol 1988 Dec; 20(2–3):133–140

Brock RB (ed). Caring for patients with AIDS: We've only just begun. J Adv Med Surg Nurs 1988 Dec; 1(1):1–84

Centers for Disease Control. Interpretation and use of the Western blot assay for serodiagnosis of human immunodeficiency virus Type 1 infections. MMWR 1989 Jul 21; 38(S-7):1–7

Centers for Disease Control. Recommendations for prevention of HIV transmission in health-care settings. MMWR 1987 Aug 21; 36(Suppl 2-S):3S–18S

Crowe M. The I.V. nurse and the I.V. drug abuser: Medical and psychosocial implications. J Intraven Nurs 1989 Nov–Dec; 12(6):405–408

Delakas M, Wichman A and Sever J. AIDS and the nervous system. JAMA 1989 Apr 28; 261(16):2396–2399

Epstein JB. Oral and pharyngeal candidiasis. Postgrad Med 1989 Apr; 85(5):257–269

Friedlander AH and Arthur RJ. A diagnosis of AIDS: Understanding the psychosocial impact. Oral Surg Oral Med Oral Pathol 1988 Jun; 65(6):680–684

Friedman SL (ed). Gastrointestinal manifestations of AIDS. Gastroenterol Clin North Am 1988 Sep; 17(3):451–468

Frierson RL and Lippman SB. Psychologic implications of AIDS. Am Fam Physician 1987 Mar; 35(3):109–116

Gallagher D (ed). Special focus: Nursing and the AIDS challenge. Imprint 1989 Feb–Mar; 36(1):40–56

Gallo RC. HIV—the cause of AIDS: An overview on its biology, mechanisms of disease induction, and our attempts

to control it. J Acquir Immune Defic Syndr 1988; 1(6):521–535

Grady C (ed). AIDS. Nurs Clin North Am 1988 Dec; 23(4):683–862

Grady C. Ethical issues in providing nursing care to human immunodeficiency virus-infected populations. Nurs Clin North Am 1989 Jun; 24(2):523–534

Groopman JE and Scadden DT. Interferon therapy for Kaposi sarcoma associated with the acquired immunodeficiency syndrome (AIDS). Ann Intern Med 1989 Mar 1; 110(5):335–337

Hilton G. AIDS dementia. J Neurosci Nurs 1989 Feb; 21(1):24–29

Houseman C and Pheifer WG. Potential for unresolved grief in survivors of persons with AIDS. Arch Psychiatr Nurs 1988 Oct; 2(5):296–301

Jacobson MA and Mills J. Serious cytomegalovirus disease in the acquired immunodeficiency syndrome (AIDS). Ann Intern Med 1988 Apr; 108(4):585–591

Kendall J et al. Doing well with AIDS: Three case illustrations. Arch Psychiatr Nurs 1989 Jun; 3(3):159–165

Kiecolt–Glaser JK and Glaser R. Psychological influences on immunity: Implications for AIDS. Am Psychol 1988 Nov; 43(11):892–898

Kotler DP. Intestinal and hepatic manifestations of AIDS. Adv Intern Med 1989; 34:43–71

Krown SE. AIDS-associated Kaposi's sarcoma: Pathogenesis, clinical course and treatment. AIDS 1988 Apr 2; 2(2):71–80

Lasher AT and Ragsdale D. The significant other's role in improving quality of life in persons with AIDS dementia complex. J Neurosci Nurs 1989 Aug; 21(4):250–255

Lovejoy NC. The pathophysiology of AIDS. Oncol Nurs Forum 1988 Sep–Oct; 15(5):563–571

Millar AB. Respiratory manifestations of AIDS. Br J Hosp Med 1988 Mar; 39(3):204–215

Mills J et al. Treatment of cytomegalovirus retinitis in patients with AIDS. Rev Infect Dis 1988 Jul–Aug; 10(Suppl 3):S522–524

Mitsuyasu RT. AIDS-related Kaposi's sarcoma: A review of its pathogenesis and treatment. Blood Rev 1988 Dec; 2(4):221–231

Moran TA. AIDS: Current implications and impact on nursing. J Intraven Nurs 1989 Jul–Aug; 12(4):220–226

Moss RJ and Miles SH. AIDS dementia. Clin Geriatr Med 1988 Nov; 4(4):889–895

Nyamathi A and van Servellen G. Maladaptive coping in the critically ill population with acquired immunodeficiency syndrome: Nursing assessment and treatment. Heart Lung 1989 Mar; 18(2):113–120

Ostrow D, Grant I and Atkinson H. Assessment and management of the AIDS patient with neuropsychiatric disturbances. J Clin Psychiatry 1988 May; 49(Suppl):14–22

Pinching AJ. Current issues in the management of AIDS patients. J Acquir Immune Defic Syndr 1988; 1(6):583–592

Price RW and Brew BJ. The AIDS dementia complex. J Infect Dis 1988 Nov; 158(5):1079–1083

Reeder JM. Ethical dilemmas in the care of patients with the human immunodeficiency virus. AORN J 1989 May; 49(5):1439, 1442–1443, 1446

Resler SS. Nutrition care of AIDS patients. J Am Diet Assoc 1988 Jul; 88(7):828–832

Rosenblum ML et al. Neurosurgical implications of the acquired immunodeficiency syndrome. Clin Neurosurg 1988; 34(1):419–445

Sande MA and Volberding PA. Medical management of AIDS. Infect Dis Clin North Am 1988 Jun; 2(2):285–550

Saunders JM (ed). The spectrum of HIV infection in adults. Semin Oncol Nurs 1989 Nov; 5(4):225–312

Scherer P. How AIDS attacks the brain. Am J Nurs 1990 Jan; 90(1):44–52

Whipple B and Scura KW. HIV and the older adult: Taking the necessary precautions. J Gerontol Nurs 1989 Sep; 15(9):15–19

White DA and Stover DE (eds). Pulmonary effects of AIDS. Clin Chest Med 1988 Sep; 9(3):363–505

Worth C. Handle with care. Am J Nurs 1989 Feb; 89(2):196–198

Connective Tissue Disorders

Rheumatoid Arthritis*

Rheumatoid arthritis is a chronic, systemic, progressive disease of unknown cause, characterized most prominently by recurrent inflammation involving the synovium or lining of the joints, leading to destructive changes in the joints (Fig. 35-1). Any or every organ or system may be involved by the connective tissue disease, which occurs most often in women (3:1).

Pathophysiology Underlying Joint Destruction

Inflammation of joint (synovitis) → synovial effusion → granulation tissue covering articular cartilage (pannus) → joint capsular and subchondral bone destruction → pain → loss of mobility of joint → muscular weakness about the joint → damage to tendons and ligaments → joint instability and deformity → joint malfunction and disuse → muscular atrophy and contracture deformity.

Clinical Manifestations

1. Morning stiffness; fatigue
2. Joint pain, stiffness, swelling, heat, redness, and limitation of motion
3. Subcutaneous nodules over bony prominences, bursae, and tendon sheaths
   a. May appear in myocardium, aorta, lung
   b. May involve deeper connective tissue structures
4. Anemia; weight loss; fever; depression
5. Late or severe stage symptoms: ocular features; Sjögren's syndrome (dry eyes and mouth); vasculitis (blood vessel inflammation); pulmonary, cardiac, and neurologic manifestations

Diagnostic Evaluation

1. History (onset of symptoms, areas and patterns of involvement, associated constitutional symptoms) and physical examination
2. Laboratory tests
   a. Complete blood tests—most patients have mild anemia
   b. Erythrocyte sedimentation rate—elevated during periods of active arthritis

* Arthritis is not one disease but a family of more than 100 separate rheumatic diseases and disorders. These diseases affect not only the joints but also other connective tissues of the body, including several supporting structures such as muscles, tendons, and ligaments, and the protective coverings of some internal organs.

   c. Tests for rheumatoid factor in the serum—positive in 70%–80% of patients with rheumatoid arthritis
   d. Documentation of presence of antinuclear antibodies
3. Roentgenograms of involved joints—to determine extent, rate of progress, and structural changes within bones; reveals swelling of soft tissue, erosion of bone at articular margins, narrowing of joint space
4. Synovial fluid analysis—to distinguish between inflammatory, traumatic, or degenerative arthritis
5. Arthroscopy—endoscopic examination of knee joint; allows observation of synovial lining, articular cartilage, and minisci; permits examination of knee during passive movements and allows biopsy under direct vision; detects pathology earlier than other methods

Management

1. Patient education about disease, medications, coping strategies, and optimizing health
2. Rest
   a. Systemic rest for extensive upper- and lower-extremity involvement and for generalized inflammation
   b. Joint rest, including splinting, to allow inflammation to subside and to relieve pain
3. Drug therapy (Table 35-1)
4. Pain-relieving modalities: analgesics, intra-articular injections of steroids; behavioral modification, desensitization and relaxation exercises to reduce muscle tension and pain
5. Surgical interventions, including synovectomy, arthrodesis, and total joint replacements (see Chapter 31)

Nursing Assessment

1. Study patient's record.
   a. Review the results of clinical examination, joints involved, pain score, laboratory and x-ray evaluations.
   b. Review the disability score of the Health Assessment Questionnaire (HAQ) and total health scores of Arthritis Impact Measurement Scales (AIMS), if done.
2. If appropriate, palpate each joint anteriorly, posteriorly, and laterally for skin temperature, joint swelling, tenderness, and irregularity.
   a. Ask what actions cause the most pain.
   b. Is pain persistent? Remittent?
   c. Quality and duration of morning stiffness?
3. Look for classic deformities of rheumatoid arthritis.
   a. Ulnar deviation with Swan neck or boutonnière fingers.

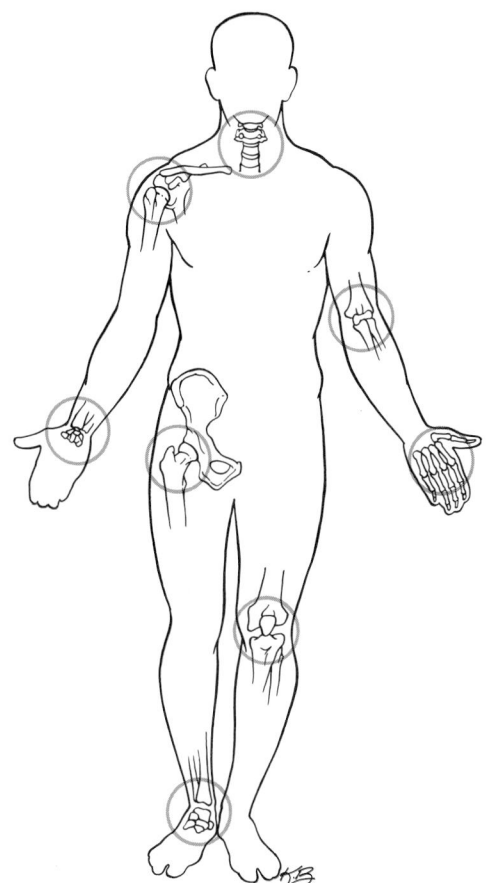

Figure 35-1. *Rheumatoid arthritis characteristically involves the joints of the hands, wrists, feet, ankles, knees, elbows, and the glenohumeral and acromioclavicular joints and the hips. The articulations of the cervical spine are also affected.*

    b. In osteoarthritis, Heberden's nodes or Bouchard's nodes may be present.

4. Evaluate muscle strength and neuromuscular status; observe the patient reaching overhead, arising from chair, negotiating stairs, walking—these are indications of patient's strength and ability.
5. Elicit patient's understanding of the disease: what does he see as the major problem?
6. Ask about patient's support system: Whom he lives with? Who gives assistance?

Nursing Diagnoses

1. Pain related to joint and muscle inflammation, stiffness, degeneration, and deformity
2. Impaired physical mobility related to pain, deformity, weakness, muscle atrophy, and disability
3. Self-care deficits (feeding, bathing/hygiene, dressing, grooming, toileting) related to stiffness, pain, deformity, and fatigue
4. Altered nutrition (less than body requirements) related to altered ability to self-feed secondary to small joint dysfunction, temporomandibular joint syndrome, and increased metabolic rate from inflammatory process.
5. Disturbance in self concept related to deformity and loss of independence.

6. Knowledge deficit of disease, its effects, and living within limits imposed.
7. Other possible nursing diagnoses:
   a. Fatigue related to inflammatory condition, coping with pain, medications, and depression
   b. Impaired home maintenance related to stiffness, pain, weakness, and instability of joints
   c. Sexual dysfunction related to pain, decreased range of motion, depression, fatigue, and diminished self-worth

Nursing Interventions

A. Achieving Relief of Pain and Discomfort

1. Schedule regular rest periods to relieve pain and control fatigue—arthritis affects the entire body.
   a. Complete bedrest for patients with active widespread inflammatory disease.
   b. Have the patient rest in a recumbent position (one pillow under head) on a firm mattress—to take the weight off the joints.
   c. Advise the patient to establish one or more daytime rest periods of 30–60 minutes.
   d. Encourage the patient to rest in bed 8–9 hours at night.
   e. Instruct the patient to lie in prone position twice daily to prevent hip flexion and knee contractures.
   f. Pillows should not be placed under painful joints—promotes flexion contractures.
2. Encourage the patient to use prescribed splint.
   a. Painful, inflamed joints may be rested with splints locally to decrease synovitis, reduce pain, stiffness, and swelling (in fingers and wrist) and to rest inflamed joints in optimum position and to prevent/correct deformities (Fig. 35-2).
   b. Use correctly designed splints: a "working" splint (Fig. 35-3) for daytime to allow continuing function despite a painful joint, and a "resting" splint for nighttime may be indicated.
   c. Metatarsal bars or pads (for shoes), inserts, or custom-made shoes may be used to decrease pressure on painful arthritic feet.
3. Teach patient to apply hot and/or cold applications to reduce joint pain and stiffness.
   a. Apply moist heat (15–30 minutes) to reduce muscle spasm and postrest stiffness; provide as much relief from pain as possible so that exercise program can be carried out.
      (1) Take warm bath or shower upon arising—shortens period of morning stiffness.
      (2) Use hot paraffin baths for fingers, hands.
   b. Use cold packs or ice when indicated for hot, swollen, acutely inflamed joints; heat is sometimes contraindicated when a joint is acutely inflamed. Cold will relieve swelling and pain and help restore function. (Keep commercial cold packs in freezer.)
   c. Employ gentle massage to relax muscles.
   d. Take joints through range of motion after heat treatments.
4. Emphasize the importance of taking anti-inflammatory and analgesic medications as prescribed.

B. Increasing Muscle Strength and Physical Mobility

1. Stress the importance of regular exercise to maintain function of all joints, to strengthen muscles that support the joints, to improve circulation, and to promote endurance.

Table 35-1. *Drugs Used in Arthritis and Related Disorders*

Drug	Action	Adverse Effects
Anti-Inflammatory Agents		
Salicylates Aspirin (may be buffered or enteric coated)	Anti-inflammatory, antipyretic, and analgesic effects	Tinnitus, gastric intolerance or gastrointestinal bleeding, and purpuric tendencies
Nonsteroidal anti-inflammatory drugs (NSAIDs) Ibuprofen (Motrin) Fenoprofen (Nalfon) Naproxen (Naprosyn) Tolmetin (Tolectin) Sulindac (Clinoril) Meclofenamole (Meclomen) Ketroprofen (Orudis) Salsalate (Disalcid) Diclofenac (Voltaren)	Anti-inflammatory and analgesic effects Mechanism of action may be related to inhibition of prostaglandin synthesis (prostaglandins have a role in inflammatory process, pain, and fever) Nonsteroidal antirheumatic agents for adjunctive treatment of rheumatoid arthritis Sometimes remarkably effective in control of articular symptoms	Gastrointestinal irritation: Nausea, vomiting, epigastric distress, precipitation and reactivation of peptic ulcer Hematologic: Bone marrow depression, anemia, leukopenia, thrombocytopenia purpura Sodium and water retention
Other Anti-Inflammatory Agents		
Indomethacin (Indocin)	Used for short-term treatment of active synovitis	Can produce significant side effects: gastrointestinal, CNS
Phenylbutazone (Butazolidin)	Nonsteroidal antirheumatic agents for adjunctive treatment of rheumatoid arthritis	Gastrointestinal: Nausea, vomiting, epigastric distress, precipitation and reactivation of peptic ulcer
Oxyphenbutazone (Tandearil)	Exerts analgesic, antipyretic, anti-inflammatory action Sometimes remarkably effective in control of articular symptoms Patient should be under close medical supervision Can cause salt and water retention Usually used only for short periods	Hematologic: Bone marrow depression, anemia, leukopenia, agranulocytosis, thrombocytopenia purpura Irreversible blood element depression may occur rapidly despite careful supervision and frequent testing.
Disease-Modifying Agents		
Gold Compounds (chrysotherapy) Oral: Auranofin (Ridaura) Injectable: Gold sodium thiomalate (Myochristine) Aurothioglucose (Solganal)	Mechanism of action unclear Anti-inflammatory, antiarthritic and immunomodulating effects	Cutaneous reactions ranging from dermatitis to life-threatening exfoliative dermatitis Renal toxicity Thrombocytopenia and marrow aplasia
Antimalarial Agents Hydroxychoroquine sulfate (Plaquenil) Chloroquine phosphate (Aralen)	Remission-inducing agents for rheumatoid arthritis Used also in certain forms of lupus	*Ocular toxicity* (retinopathy) that can result in permanent loss of vision; blurred vision, night blindness, scatoma
Penicillamine (Cuprimine; Depen)	Mechanism of action poorly understood Used in active progressive rheumatoid arthritis	Can cause severe toxic reactions: Mucocutaneous, renal, gastrointestinal, hepatic, and hematologic toxicities
Cytotoxic Drugs Methotrexate Azathioprine (Imuran)	Exert anti-inflammatory effect by inhibition of cellular replication Used in patients with inflammatory synovitis refractory to other therapy	Bone marrow suppression, hepatic and pulmonary toxicity reduce resistance to infection Possibility of a malignancy occurring many years after initiating therapy
Corticosteroids Prednisone Prednisolone	Potent anti-inflammatory drugs May also reduce immune response Usually used for *short-term* management of patients with severe limitations	Osteoporosis, fractures, avascular necrosis Gastric ulcers, psychiatric problems, infection susceptibility Hirsutism, acne, moon facies, abnormal fat deposition, edema, emotional disorders, menstrual disorders Hyperglycemia, hypokalemia Hypertension Cataracts and glaucoma

a. Encourage the patient to follow a prescribed *daily* program of exercise.
b. Encourage isometric exercises—to help prevent muscle atrophy, which contributes to joint instability.
c. Have patient move joints through full range of motion 1–2 times daily to maintain normal joint range, to prevent joint stiffness, and to increase joint range.
d. Have the patient do progressive resistive exercises—for muscle building, after joint inflammation has been controlled.

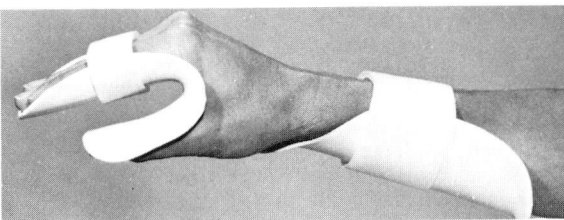

Figure 35-2. *Rest splint for the hand. Rest of the hand is important when soft tissues are acutely inflamed. Instruct the patient to maintain full range of motion of all joints and maintain tendon excursion while wearing a rest splint to prevent loss of important hand function. (Courtesy of The Western Pennsylvania Hospital, Pittsburgh, PA)*

2. Teach the patient to be aware of proper positioning to prevent flexion contractures of hips, knees, and neck.
3. Encourage the patient to use prescribed mobility aids (canes, crutches, walker) to reduce stress on inflamed hips, knees, ankles, or feet.

C. Working Toward Independence in Activities of Daily Living (ADLs)

1. Work cooperatively with occupational therapist to devise/obtain assistive devices to help with daily activities.
2. Allow extra time for patient to perform activities, assisting only if necessary.

D. Improving Nutritional Intake

1. Review feeding evaluation by occupational therapist/dietitian to assess impact of patient's disability on food preparation and self-feeding.
2. Encourage a well-balanced diet that includes foods high in protein, iron, and vitamin C.
3. Suggest nutrient-dense foods to maximize intake in patients with chewing and swallowing limitations (temporomandibular joint involvement).
4. Encourage weight loss, if the patient is obese, to prevent excess stress on weight-bearing joints.

E. Enhancing Self-Concept

1. Maintain a supportive relationship—successful management usually requires a long period of treatment.

2. Discuss nature of disease and positive expectations of treatment; encourage the patient to set goals.
3. Adopt a positive but realistic attitude.
4. Emphasize that something can and will be done to relieve the patient's pain and mobilize his joints.
5. Try to modify or adapt to stress-producing situations.
6. Promote independence in ADLs (see above).
7. Encourage the patient to participate in social activities, hobbies, and family activities.
8. Allow the patient to participate in decision-making concerning treatment plan.

Patient Education

A. Understanding About Disease

1. Learn the nature of the disease and its treatment: the role of rest, exercise, joint protection, and energy conservation.
2. Have confidence in your physician and treatment program.
3. Avoid "miracle cures," dietary fads, drugs not prescribed by your physician, and other forms of "quackery."
4. Report to the physician or clinic *regularly* for evaluation; have regular medical and functional reevaluation to determine if there is any loss of joint function.

B. Maintaining Independence

1. Rely on your own capabilities.
2. Participate in as many activities as possible without producing fatigue.
3. Conserve energy and simplify daily activities using self-help devices, work simplification methods, and energy-saving methods.
4. Work at an even pace.
5. Alternate periods of work, exercise, and rest. Avoid overdoing on good days.
6. Alternate sitting and standing tasks; do not remain seated too long.

C. Adhering to Medication Schedule

1. Aspirin may be prescribed for its anti-inflammatory effects. It must be taken over a long period and at high doses to achieve desired response. Long-term use does *not* lead to addiction.
2. Report ringing in the ears or decreased hearing, since this is a guide in controlling dosage.

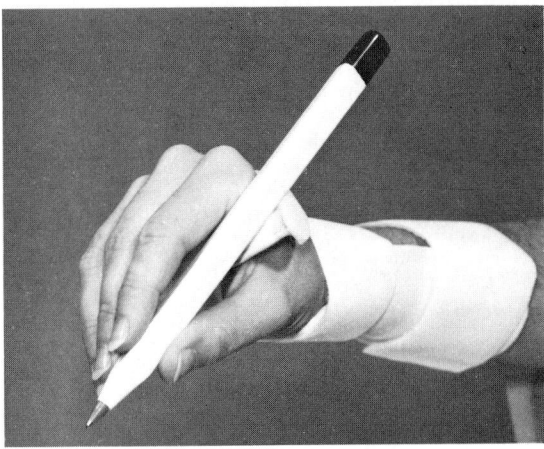
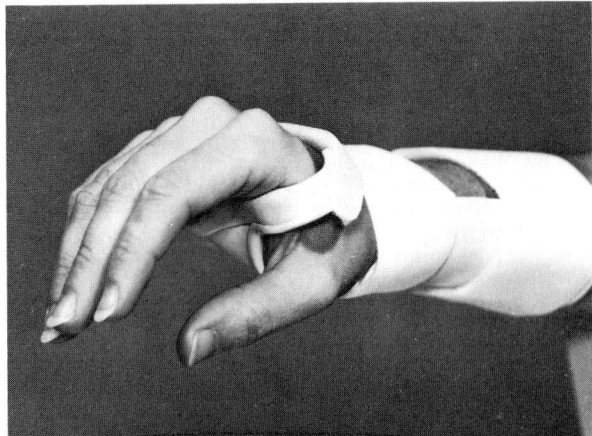

Figure 35-3. *Arthritic cock-up splint is a type of working splint that allows continuing function despite a painful joint. (Courtesy of The Western Pennsylvania Hospital, Pittsburgh, PA)*

3. Watch for symptoms of gastric irritation.
4. Take with food (a buffering agent).
5. Do not substitute acetaminophen (Tylenol), etc., for aspirin—this drug possesses no anti-inflammatory properties but is a pain reliever.

D. Using Heat and Cold Treatments—for muscle relaxation and relief of pain.

1. Take a warm shower or tub bath upon arising to relieve morning stiffness; rest in bed 20–30 minutes after warm bath.
2. If heat or cold treatment intensifies pain, discontinue and notify physician.
3. Try an electric blanket to ascertain its usefulness in relieving morning stiffness.

E. Doing Exercises

1. Do the prescribed exercises to preserve joint motion and to gain muscular strength and coordination.
2. Exercise also in water (pool; bathtub)—water provides buoyancy, support, and relaxation; muscles are exercised while joints are supported by water.
3. Exercise every joint *gently* and slowly without causing pain.
4. Space the individual exercises throughout the day; pain indicates that the joint is overstressed.

F. Conserving Energy

1. Pace yourself when doing activities.
2. Delegate jobs to others when possible.
3. Avoid rushing.
4. Organize and arrange materials, utensils, and tools.
5. Simplify all activities.
6. Perform any activity lasting more than 10 minutes in a seated position.

G. Protecting Joints From Further Damage

1. Consciously maintain correct posture—pain and swelling cause one to assume a position of deformity which makes muscles work harder.
2. Lower yourself gently into a chair, using the sidearms. Collapsing into a chair produces knee and hip joint trauma.
3. Use an elevated chair if knee and hip joints are affected.
4. Straighten up before walking.
5. Avoid tension and stress on fingers and thumb joints.
6. Avoid obesity, which places greater strain on weight-bearing joints.
7. Use a cane—to reduce load and impact on diseased joint.
8. Always use large joints to perform activities.
9. Slide objects instead of lifting them.
10. Respect pain—do on "good" days, don't do on "bad" days.

H. Other Teaching Points

1. Seek sexual counseling (position and techniques) if arthritic involvement is a barrier to sexual performance.
2. Surgical procedures are available for relief of pain and deformity (when recommended by physician).
   a. Osteotomy
   b. Synovectomy
   c. Total joint replacement (see pp. 795–798 for discussion).
3. The therapeutic program must be maintained for a lifetime; there is no cure at this time.
4. For informative booklets and audiovisual programs, sources of assistance and agencies, contact:
   The Arthritis Foundation
   1314 Spring Street, N.W.
   Atlanta, GA 30309

Evaluation

1. Achieves relief of joint pain and stiffness; no overt evidence of joint inflammation; moving joints more freely
2. Demonstrates increased mobility and muscle strength; ambulates without manual assistance
3. Achieves independence in self-care activities, including transporting self outside of home environment
4. Maintains optimal nutrition, keeping body weight between ideal and 10% over ideal body weight
5. Develops a more positive self-concept, expressing feelings and socializing with family and friends.
6. Describes disease and treatment plan, adhering to plan as prescribed

---

Osteoarthritis

Osteoarthritis (degenerative joint disease), the most common of all joint diseases, is the degeneration of the articular cartilage in the joints. It is characterized by bony spur formation at the edges of the joint surfaces, thickening of the capsule and the synovial membrane, and thinning of articular cartilage.

Although the exact underlying mechanism is not known, there appears to be a biochemical abnormality of cartilage.

Predisposing Factors

1. Aging
2. Anatomic abnormality; malalignment
3. Trauma (acute or repetitive)
4. Excessive joint use/abuse; obesity
5. Systemic diseases
6. Genetic factors; developmental disorders

Clinical Manifestations

1. Pain and swelling in one, two, or more joints, particularly after activity
2. Stiffness (occurs less frequently than in rheumatoid arthritis)
3. Enlargement of joint with limitation of joint motion and muscle spasm; particularly in weight-bearing and finger joints—from ossification of cartilage and ligaments
4. Heberden's nodes—nodular bony enlargements (spurs) that form on the distal joints of some or all of the fingers (Fig. 35-4)
5. Bouchard's nodes—nodular bony enlargements that form on the proximal joints of some or all of the fingers (Fig. 35-4)
6. Crepitus—audible grating sound (or a grinding sensation as the joint is moved) produced by bony irregularities within joint
7. Primary joints involved—hips, knees, vertebrae, and fingers

Diagnostic Evaluation

Radiographic examination demonstrates narrowing of joint space, bony hypertrophy, spur formation, and cartilage disruption.

Management

1. Patient education including self-management and joint protection
2. Pain relief: analgesics, nonsteroidal anti-inflammatory

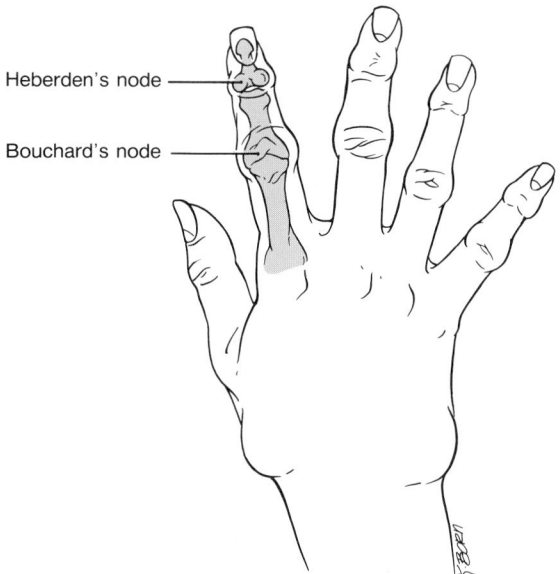

Heberden's node

Bouchard's node

Figure 35-4. *Hand deformities of osteoarthritis. Heberden's nodes (large osteophytes are due to synovial, capsular, and bony enlargement of the distal interphalangeal joints [DIPs]). Bouchard's nodes are cartilaginous and bony enlargements of the proximal interphalangeal of the fingers.*

drugs (NSAIDs), intra-articular (into the joint) injections of steroids, applications of heat (for muscle relaxation) and/or cold (analgesia), splinting of joints
3. Exercise program to improve muscle strength and to maintain and increase joint range of motion
4. Surgical interventions including total joint arthroplasty (surgical replacement of destroyed joint)

Nursing Assessment

See Nursing Assessment, Rheumatoid Arthritis, page 862.

Nursing Diagnoses

1. Pain, related to joint degeneration and muscle spasm
2. Impaired physical mobility related to pain and limited joint motion
3. Self-care deficits (feeding, bathing/hygiene, dressing, grooming, toileting) related to pain and limited joint movement
4. Other possible nursing diagnoses:
   a. Fear (of falling) related to decreased flexibility and instability of knees, pain, and diminishing strength
   b. Sleep-pattern disturbance related to spontaneous pain that worsens at night
   c. Hopelessness related to impact of arthritis (physical, socioeconomic, psychological)

Nursing Interventions

A. Attaining and Maintaining Relief of Pain and Discomfort
1. Advise patient to take prescribed anti-inflammatory drugs (see Table 35-1) when synovial inflammation is present; also used for analgesic effect.
2. Take prescribed analgesic drugs for pain control.
3. Provide rest for involved joints—excessive use aggravates the symptoms and accelerates degeneration.

a. Use splints, braces, cervical collars, traction, lumbosacral corsets as necessary.
   b. Have prescribed rest periods in recumbent position.
4. Avoid activities that precipitate pain.
5. Use heat as prescribed—relieves muscle spasm and stiffness; avoid prolonged application of heat—may cause increased swelling and flare of symptoms.
6. Use correct posture and body mechanics—postural alterations lead to chronic muscle tension and pain.
7. Sleep with a rolled terry towel under the neck—for relief of cervical osteoarthritis.
8. Use crutches, braces, or cane when indicated—to reduce weight-bearing stress on hips and knees.
9. Hold cane in hand on side opposite that of involved hip/knee.
10. Wear corrective shoes and metatarsal supports for foot disorders—also help in the treatment of arthritis of the knee.
11. Maintain proper weight—to decrease stress on weight-bearing joints.
12. Support the patient undergoing orthopedic surgery for unremitting pain and disabling arthritis of joints.
    a. Repair of joint-supporting structures (tendon repairs)
    b. Debridement of loose bodies (cartilage, bone, large spurs)
    c. Osteotomy to redistribute joint forces; arthrodesis (fusion of joint)
    d. Joint replacement (hip, knee, ankle, shoulder, elbow)

B. Increasing Physical Mobility
1. Keep active as much as possible without causing pain. (Fig. 35-5 shows the effect of inactivity on mobility.)
2. Use range-of-motion exercises to maintain joint mobility and muscle tone for joint support, to prevent capsular and tendon tightening, and to prevent deformities.
3. Avoid flexion and adduction deformities—if deformities are avoided, pain is more likely to disappear.
4. Use isometric exercises and graded exercises to improve muscle strength around the involved joint.
5. Put joints through range of motion following periods of inactivity (e.g., automobile ride).

C. Promoting Independence in Activities of Daily Living (ADLs)
See Rheumatoid Arthritis, pages 862–866.

Evaluation

1. Achieves relief of joint pain; takes fewer analgesics
2. Demonstrates increased mobility; ambulates without manual assistance
3. Achieves independence in self-care activities, including transporting self outside of home environment

Gout

Gout is a disease manifested by joint inflammation caused by the deposit of monosodium urate (MSU) crystals in the joints and connective tissues. In some patients uric acid lithiasis and/or renal disease involving glomerular, tubular, and interstitial tissues may occur.

1. *Uric acid*—end-product of purine metabolism derived from both dietary sources and endogenous synthesis.
2. *Hyperuricemia*—persistent elevation of uric acid in

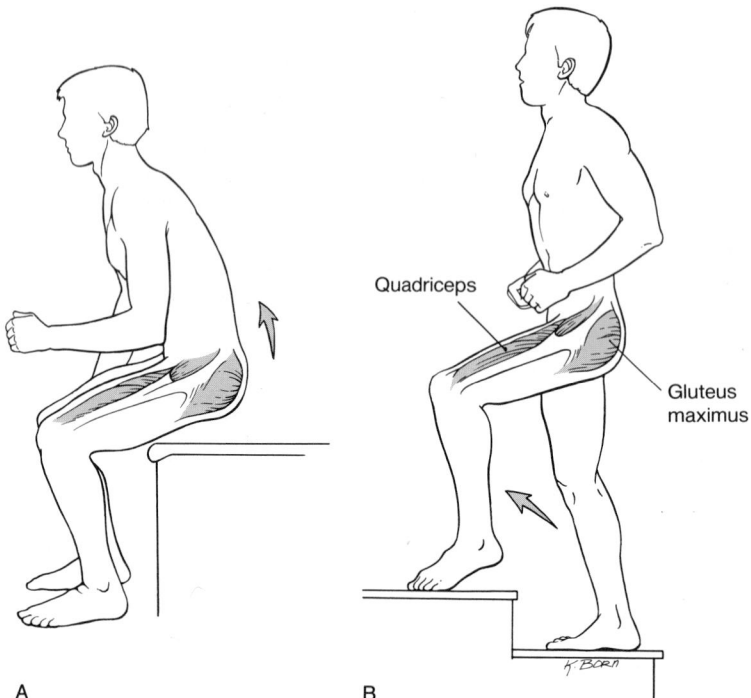

Quadriceps

Gluteus maximus

A   B

Figure 35-5. *The patient with painful knees has a tendency to become inactive, which produces weakness and muscle atrophy. Weakness of the hip and knee extensors (glutei and quadriceps femoris) leads to difficulty in arising from a chair and in climbing and descending stairs.*

the blood, usually found in gout. It is caused by overproduction or underexcretion of uric acid.
3. *Tophi*—deposits of urate crystals occurring in and around joints, cartilage (ear), soft tissue, and bone; development of tophi related to duration of disease, degree of hyperuricemia, and severity of renal involvement.

Types of Gout

1. *Primary gout*—due to an imbalance in uric acid metabolism; occurs most often in men over 40 years of age.
2. *Secondary gout* (an acquired disease)
   a. Hyperuricemia occurs in conditions in which there is an increase in cell turnover (leukemia, multiple myeloma, psoriasis) and in cell breakdown, or because of impaired renal excretion of uric acid.
   b. May be precipitated by prolonged ingestion of diuretic agents, aspirin, trauma, treatment of myeloproliferative diseases, alcohol.

Clinical Manifestations

A. Acute Gout
1. Sudden onset of severe pain in one or more peripheral joints—affected joint appears dusky red, hot, swollen, and *exquisitely tender.*
   a. First joint of great toe is susceptible.
   b. Other sites of involvement include instep, ankle, heel, knee, wrist, fingers, and elbow.
   c. Tissues surrounding joint become edematous and inflamed; intense itching may occur after swelling subsides.

d. Attacks involving the same joints tend to recur; variable lengths of time between attacks.

B. Chronic Gout
1. Occurs from repeated attacks and development of periarticular erosions and tophi.
2. Renal impairment (gouty nephropathy)
3. Joint deformity

Diagnostic Evaluation

Identification of monosodium urate crystals in synovial fluid—obtained by arthrocentesis (aspiration of fluid from a joint cavity)

Management

A. Immediate Control of Acute Attack
1. Early administration of anti-inflammatory agent (nonsteroidal anti-inflammatory drug, see Table 35-1) or colchicine
2. Rest in bed/chair with affected extremity elevated and protected
3. Analgesics for pain; intra-articular (into the joint) injection of steroids—may provide dramatic relief in acute gout limited to a single joint.

B. Long-Term Management
1. Dietary restriction of purine and alcohol—to reduce urinary uric acid
2. Uricosuric drugs (probenecid; sulfinpyrazone)—increase renal clearance of uric acid by inhibiting the renal tubular reabsorption of uric acid
3. Or allopurinol, a xanthine oxidase inhibitor—impairs the conversion of hyoxanthine to xanthine and xanthine to uric acid; used in patients with history of kid-

ney stones or renal insufficiency and in those known to be overproducers of uric acid.

Complications

1. Renal involvement with stone formation
2. Secondary degenerative arthritis

Nursing Interventions

A. Achieving Relief of Joint Pain

1. Immobilize and elevate affected joint(s); encourage the patient to rest, since early ambulation may precipitate a recurrence.
2. Instruct patient to take anti-inflammatory drug *early* when the attack starts.
   a. NSAIDs (see Table 35-1).
   b. Colchicine—suppresses inflammatory manifestations of acute gout; useful in establishing diagnosis since it gives dramatic relief if patient has gout.
3. Provide reassurance that initial attack is usually self-limited.

B. Ensuring Adequate Urinary Elimination

1. Encourage high fluid intake (at least 3000 ml./day) to maintain high urinary volume and dilute the uric acid urinary concentration.
2. Monitor intake and output.
3. Maintain an alkaline urine to prevent uric acid precipitation in the urinary system, if prescribed.

Patient Education

1. Take prescribed medication for chronic gout to lower uric acid level, even if asymptomatic.
   Review side-effects of prescribed drugs.
2. Maintain a high fluid intake to sustain a high urinary volume—promotes uric acid excretion and reduces danger of crystal formation in the kidney or ureter.
3. Avoid foods rich in purine content (sardines, anchovies, shell fish, organ meats)—to lessen the burden of uric acid excretion.
4. Avoid beer, ale, wine, and excessive alcohol use—may precipitate an attack.
5. Avoid fasting (to lose weight or when on alcoholic spree)—fasting has been found to increase the serum uric acid level.
6. Avoid crash diets—rapid reduction of weight may increase the serum uric acid level; slow weight reduction reduces the serum urate level without inducing an acute attack.
7. Avoid aspirin, diuretics, and other drugs that interfere with uric acid excretion.
8. Avoid trauma to susceptible joints and tophaceous areas.
9. Instruct patient to cover draining tophi and apply topical antibiotic ointment as directed.
10. Begin *prompt* treatment at first symptom—to abort an acute attack. Repeated attacks lead to joint deformity.

Systemic Lupus Erythematosus

Systemic lupus erythematosus (*SLE*) is a chronic, inflammatory, autoimmune disease involving multiple organ systems and producing widespread damage to connective tissues, blood vessels, serosal surfaces, and mucous membranes.

Discoid lupus erythematosus (DLE) is a chronic eruption of the skin, which, although often disfiguring, does not pose a threat to life. DLE may later become systemic.

Clinical Features

1. Etiology is not understood—genetic, hormonal, and environmental factors thought to play a role.
2. A lupus-like syndrome can be brought on by certain drugs (procainamide).
3. Most frequently found in young women with signs and symptoms referable to the joints and skin.
4. Is characterized by spontaneous remissions and exacerbations.

Clinical Manifestations

(Multiple organ involvement is explained by the deposit of antigen–antibody complexes throughout the body—kidneys, skin, brain, heart, and joints.)

1. *Joint involvement*—pain on motion, tenderness, effusion, or periarticular soft-tissue swelling; fatigue, fever, weight loss
2. *Skin involvement:*
   a. Erythematous flat or raised rash over malar eminences (butterfly rash)
   b. Nonspecific erythematous rash (resembling drug eruption) may be located anywhere on body but most often on face and chest
   c. Brittleness or loss of scalp hair
   d. Photosensitivity with rashes developing after sun exposure
   e. Oral ulcers
3. *Hematologic abnormalities*—hemolytic anemia, or leukopenia, or lymphopenia, or thrombocytopenia
4. *Cardiopulmonary involvement*—pleuritis, pleural effusion, pericarditis, cardiac tamponade
5. *Renal involvement*—proteinuria, hematuria, renal insufficiency, and renal failure
6. *Central nervous system (CNS) involvement*—psychosis, seizures, cognitive impairment, movement disorders, neuropathy, organic brain syndromes

Diagnostic Evaluation

1. Clinically documented multisystem disease
2. Abnormal titer of antinuclear antibodies; many other autoantibodies have been associated with SLE
3. Positive lupus erythematosus (LE) cell preparation
4. Serum complement levels usually decreased
5. Erythrocyte sedimentation rate—elevated during exacerbations of disease activity
6. Renal function studies

Management

1. Provision of emotional support
2. Patient education: rest, stress management, avoidance of sun exposure, exercise
3. Drug therapy
   a. See Table 35-1 for drugs used to suppress anti-inflammatory and abnormal immune responses
   b. Corticosteroids—used topically for skin manifestations and systemically in low doses for minor disease activity and in high doses for major disease activity (hematologic manifestations; pulmonary disease; lupus nephritis)
   c. Alternative therapies include antimalarial drugs, immunosuppressive drugs (mechlorethamine; cyclophosphamide; chlorambucil; azathioprine)

for life-threatening disease or intolerable corticosteroid toxicities

Complications

1. Death from underlying disease: renal failure, CNS involvement
2. Complications of long-term use of corticosteroids; cataracts, infections, aseptic necrosis of bone

Nursing Assessment

1. Review patient's record and determine what organ systems are involved; results of laboratory tests.
2. Review findings of mental status examination.
3. See Nursing Assessment, Rheumatoid Arthritis, page 862.

Nursing Diagnoses

1. Pain related to joint and muscle inflammation
2. Impaired skin integrity related to rash, vasculitis, and photosensitivity
3. Fatigue related to chronic inflammatory process, secondary to sleep/wake disturbances, chronicity of illness
4. Disturbance in self-concept related to appearance (cushingoid appearance, rash, alopecia) and/or joint deformity
5. Altered thought processes related to central nervous system involvement, systemic complications, and adjustment to chronic and unpredictable illness
6. Other possible nursing diagnoses:
   a. Altered nutrition (less than body requirements) related to anorexia, anemia, and weight loss
   b. Self-care deficits related to fatigue, weakness, pain, and joint deformity
   c. Anticipatory grieving related to unpredictability of chronic potentially fatal disease
   d. Impaired home maintenance related to severity of disease
   e. Potential altered parenting related to chronicity, uncertainty, and severity of the disease

Nursing Interventions

A. Relieving Joint Pain and Discomfort

1. Encourage patient to take prescribed anti-inflammatory drugs/analgesics for pain relief.
2. Reinforce the importance of adequate sleep and daily rest periods balanced with moderate activity—fatigue increases vulnerability to pain.
3. Teach stress reduction techniques—SLE is chronic, unpredictable, and multisystemic, all of which place psychological demands on the patient.
4. Include other pain-relieving modalities: muscle relaxation techniques, guided imagery; other forms of distraction.
5. Involve family in therapeutic program—to prevent buildup of pressure and to promote an environment that reduces stress.

B. Maintaining Skin Integrity

1. Keep skin clean; avoid irritants.
2. Avoid sunlight and ultraviolet lighting by wearing hat, sunglasses, and long-sleeved clothing; use sunscreen agents—sun can precipitate exacerbations and cause actinic damage.
3. Avoid trauma to skin.
4. Apply topical corticosteroid creams as prescribed.

5. Teach patient the importance of meticulous oral hygiene to prevent and care for oral and mucous lesions.

C. Coping With Fatigue

1. Plan for frequent rest periods combined with a 10–12-hour sleep period each night.
2. Use principles of energy conservation (see discussion under Rheumatoid Arthritis, p. 866).
3. Participate in a moderate exercise program to increase endurance, strengthen some muscle groups, improve activity tolerance, and enhance well-being.

D. Promoting a More Positive Self-Concept

1. Provide emotional support—use realistic but optimistic approach.
2. Refer to cosmetologist for skin make-up to cover lesions.
3. Encourage patient to join a support group.
4. Facilitate referral to mental health professional to facilitate adaptation to the disease and its consequences and for depression when appropriate.

E. Dealing With Altered Thought Processes

1. Be aware of mental changes, psychiatric manifestations, and psychological factors related to CNS involvement, the effects of systemic disease (fever, septicemia, azotemia, metabolic imbalance) and psychosocial stresses of SLE.
2. Emphasize the potential benefits of available treatment.
3. Educate patient about SLE; place emphasis on wide variability of disease. Explain that symptoms are usually time-limited and manageable.
4. Listen; help patient understand that she is not personally responsible for recurrences.
5. Help family engage patient in activities that are in keeping with patient's mental capabilities—to prevent undue anxiety.
6. Consult with mental health professional for assistance and direction for managing psychiatric problems related to organic etiology.

Patient Education

1. Obtain physical and emotional rest; fatigue and depression are fairly common.
2. Eat a well-balanced diet.
3. Avoid whatever you know may aggravate the condition.
   a. Avoid sun exposure—sunlight may worsen dermal lesions and precipitate a flare-up of the disease. Use a sunscreen when exposure to sun is necessary.
   b. Avoid any drugs except those prescribed by physician; avoid using sensitizing agents, such as hair dyes, insecticide sprays, etc.
   c. Avoid taking contraceptive pills—anovulatory drugs may precipitate lupus syndrome in susceptible person.
   d. However, pregnancy is to be avoided at times of major disease activity and when taking immunosuppressive drugs.
4. Use positive coping mechanisms or seek counseling to deal with stress—emotional turmoil may precipitate a flare-up.
5. Make-up such as Covermark or Dermablend may conceal facial lesions and scarring.
6. Report to the physician immediately any worsening of symptoms: fever, cough, skin rash, increasing joint pain, etc.—SLE also compromises the ability to fight infection.

7. Report onset of new signs and symptoms that may indicate additional complications of nephritis, congestive heart failure, central nervous system involvement, etc.
8. Seek medical attention for any concurrent illness (e.g., upper respiratory infection, urinary tract infection, etc.). Any illness, surgery, pregnancy, trauma may precipitate an exacerbation.
9. Observe for and report side effects of drugs.
10. See also Patient Education, Rheumatoid Arthritis, page 865.
11. Support groups:
    Arthritis Foundation
    1314 Spring Street
    Atlanta, GA 30309

    Lupus Foundation of America
    1717 Massachusetts Ave.
    Suite 203
    Washington, DC 20036

    American Lupus Society
    23751 Madison Street
    Torrance, CA 90505

Evaluation

1. Achieves relief of joint pain and discomfort
2. Maintains skin integrity; absence of skin breakdown and scarring
3. Reports lessening of fatigue
4. Expressing a more positive self-concept
5. Family making adaptations to patient's altered thought processes

---

Systemic Sclerosis

Systemic sclerosis is a generalized disorder of connective tissue characterized by hardening and/or thickening of the skin (scleroderma) and fibrotic degenerative and inflammatory changes with vascular insufficiency resulting in joint changes and dysfunction of certain internal organs (gastrointestinal tract, heart, lungs, kidneys). There are several forms of localized scleroderma.

Clinical Features

1. Thought to be an autoimmune disease.
2. Affects women more often than men, usually between the ages of 30 and 50.
3. Has a variable course, with spontaneous remissions and exacerbations.
4. Prognosis not as good as for lupus or other connective tissue diseases.

Clinical Manifestations

A. Hands and Face

1. The disease usually starts insidiously on hands and face:
2. Painless pitting edema of fingers, hands, feet, legs, face; edema gradually replaced by thickening and tightening of skin, which acquires a tense, wrinkle-free, bound-down appearance.
3. Wrinkles and lines are obliterated.
4. Skin is dry—sweat secretion over involved area is suppressed.
5. Face appears mask-like, immobile, and expressionless; mouth becomes rigid ("bird mouth").

6. Condition spreads slowly; extremities become stiff and immobile; the fingers, semiflexed, immobile, and useless, and the hands, claw-like.
7. Cutaneous manifestations may be accompanied or preceded by Raynaud's phenomenon.

B. Internal Effects

1. Detectable clinical changes may occur in the internal organs (treated symptomatically).
2. Heart becomes fibrotic—causing congestive heart failure, dysrhythmias and conduction disturbances, angina.
3. Esophagus is hardened, with disruption of normal esophageal peristalsis—gastroesophageal reflux, with heartburn and dysphagia.
4. Pulmonary fibrosis/pulmonary hypertension.
5. Intestines become hardened—digestive disturbances.
6. Progressive renal failure may occur (leading cause of death).
7. Variety of other disturbances develop, including Raynaud's phenomenon, arthritis, and polymyositis (inflammation of skeletal muscle).

C. C-R-E-S-T syndrome

Calcinosis
Raynaud's phenomenon
Esophagitis
Sclerodactyly
Telangiectasias

Diagnostic Evaluation

1. Physical examination to detect fibrotic changes in skin, lungs, heart, esophagus.
2. Circulating antibodies against antinuclear antibodies are found.

Management

1. Treated symptomatically; NSAIDs, (Table 35-1) to treat joint and muscle pain; vasodilating drugs for Raynaud's phenomenon
2. Care of sclerodermatous skin; topical preparations to replace natural oils
3. Surgical treatment of esophageal stricture
4. Management of renal failure, pulmonary fibrosis, pericarditis

Nursing Interventions

A. Improving Nutritional Intake

1. Encourage mouth stretching exercises to maintain oral opening; maintain adequate oral hygiene.
2. Maintain upright posture during and after eating; raise head of bed on blocks at night—to minimize reflux esophagitis.
3. Inform patient to eat foods that are soft, yet form a bolus (e.g., mashed potatoes, puddings).
4. Encourage intake of a well-balanced diet with supplement of protein and vitamin C.
5. Provide nutritional counseling if severe bowel involvement or evidence of malabsorption is present.

B. Maintaining Skin Integrity

1. Teach the patient to lubricate skin with topical creams and prescribed lubricants to prevent fissuring and ulceration.
2. Avoid detergents and other drying agents.
3. Monitor body temperature carefully as sweat secretion is decreased.

C. Optimizing Tissue Perfusion to Skin and Body Organs

1. Keep environment warm.
2. Instruct patient to use warm baths and massage to maintain joint mobility and reduce edema.
3. Avoid exposure to cold, trauma to hands, and smoking, which aggravates Raynaud's phenomenon.

D. Other Nursing Interventions

1. See also nursing interventions under Systemic Lupus Erythematosus, page 870.
2. Encourage verbalization of feelings—low self-esteem often accompanies living with chronic illness.
3. Talk to patient about joining a support group:
   United Scleroderma Foundation
   P.O. Box 350
   Watsonville, CA 95077

Polyarteritis Nodosa

Polyarteritis nodosa (periarteritis nodosa or PAN) is a disease of unknown cause (probably autoimmune) characterized by inflammation and necrosis of medium-sized and small vessels, especially arteries, which results in altered function of the organ system in which the arterial supply has been impaired.

Clinical Features

1. The walls of the vessels are involved; spotty inflammation causes changes in circulation and tissue damage.
2. Occurs most often in men.

Clinical Manifestations

Clinical manifestations vary according to organ(s) involved and amount of necrosis produced by obstructing vascular lesion.

1. Prolonged fever; weight loss and malaise can precede specific organ involvement.
2. Arteritis of intraparenchymal vessels leads to renal failure.
3. Vasculitis of gastrointestinal tract—abdominal pain, nausea, vomiting, diarrhea leading to necrotizing enterocolitis, bowel infarction/perforation.
4. Coronary insufficiency; myocardial infarction.
5. Ocular manifestations (retinal exudates and hemorrhages) are fairly common.
6. Skin lesions are usually in the form of painful nodules that may ulcerate.

Complications

1. Polyarteritis is apt to run a few years' duration.
2. Death may ensue from renal failure, cardiovascular disease, or gastrointestinal complications.

Management

1. Corticosteroids (prednisone)
2. Immunosuppressive drugs (cyclophosphamide) alone or with prednisone
3. Surgical intervention for intestinal perforation/obstruction

Diagnostic Evaluation

1. Biopsy (skin, muscle, kidney)—may confirm presence of small and medium vessel vasculitis
2. Selective angiography—for small aneurysms in renal, hepatic, and celiac vessels

Patient Education

1. Counsel about side effects of cyclophosphamide and prednisone.
2. Seek health care immediately in the event of developing a fever or any signs of infection.

Bibliography

Books

Beary JF, Christian CL and Johanson NA. Manual of Rheumatology and Outpatient Orthopedic Disorders. 2nd ed. Boston, Little, Brown, 1987

Blau SP. Emergencies in Rheumatoid Arthritis. New York, Futura Publishing, 1986

Brattström M. Joint Protection and Rehabilitation in Chronic Rheumatic Disorders. Somerset, Wolfe Medical Publications, 1987

Brown TM and Scammell H. The Road Back: Rheumatoid Arthritis—Its Causes and Its Treatment. London, Macmillan, 1988

Cailliet R. Soft Tissue Pain and Disability. 2nd ed. Philadelphia, FA Davis, 1988

DiPiro JT et al. Pharmacotherapy: A Pathophysiologic Approach. New York, Elsevier, 1989

Lahita RG. Systemic Lupus Erythematosus. New York, John Wiley & Sons, 1987

Lanyi VF. Rehabilitation management in arthritis and related disorders. In Goodgold J (ed). Rehabilitation Medicine, pp 206–216. St Louis, CV Mosby, 1988

Karpman RR and Baum J. Aging and Clinical Practice: Musculoskeletal Disorders. New York, Igaku–Shoin, 1988

Katz WA. Diagnosis and Management of Rheumatic Diseases. 2nd ed. Philadelphia, JB Lippincott, 1988

Kelley WN (ed). Textbook of Rheumatology. 3rd ed. Philadelphia, WB Saunders, 1989

Krusinski PA and Flowers FP. Life-Threatening Dermatoses. Chicago, Year Book Medical Pub, 1987

McCaffery M and Beebe A. Pain: Clinical Manual for Nursing Practice. St Louis, CV Mosby, 1989

McCarty DJ. Arthritis and Allied Conditions. 11th ed. Philadelphia, Lea & Febiger, 1989

Moll JMH. Rheumatology in Clinical Practice. Boston, Blackwell Scientific Publications, 1987

O'Sullivan SB and Schmitz TJ. Physical Rehabilitation: Assessment and Treatment. Philadelphia, FA Davis, 1988

Paulus HE, Furst DE and Dromgoole SH. Drugs for Rheumatic Disease. New York, Churchill Livingstone, 1987

Post M (ed). Physical Examination of the Musculoskeletal System. Chicago, Year Book Medical Pub, 1987

Sands JK and Matthews JH (eds). A Guide to Arthritis Home Health Care. New York, John Wiley & Sons, 1988

Schumacher HR, Klippel JH and Robinson DR. Primer on the Rheumatic Diseases. 9th ed. Atlanta, Arthritis Foundation, 1988

Schumacher HR and Gall EP. Rheumatoid Arthritis: An Illustrated Guide to Pathology, Diagnosis and Management. Philadelphia, JB Lippincott, 1988

Scott JT (ed). Copeman's Textbook of

the Rheumatic Diseases. 6th ed, Vols 1 and 2. New York, Churchill Livingstone, 1986

Trombly CA (ed). Occupational Therapy for Physical Dysfunction. 3rd ed. Baltimore, Williams & Wilkins, 1989

Wolfram G (ed). Genetic and Therapeutic Aspects of Lipid and Purine Metabolism. New York, Springer-Verlag, 1989

Journals

Arthritis

Altman RD. Salicylates in the treatment of arthritic disease. Postgrad Med 1988 Nov 1; 84(6):206–221

Arnett FC et al. The American Rheumatism Association revised criteria for the classification of rheumatoid arthritis. Arthritis Rheum 1988 Mar; 31(3):315–324

Banwell BF and Gall V (eds). Physical therapy management of arthritis. Clin Phys Ther 1988; 16:1–157

Bell CL. Rheumatoid arthritis: Current practices and rehabilitation. Top Geriatr Rehabil 1989 Apr; 4(3):10–22

Brassel MP. Pharmacologic management of rheumatic diseases. Orthop Nurs 1988 Mar–Apr; 7(2):43–51

Brooker DS. Rheumatoid arthritis: Otorhinolaryngological manifestations. Clin Otolaryngol 1988 Jun; 13(3):239–246

Felson DT. Epidemiology of hip and knee osteoarthritis. Epidemiol Rev 1988; 10:1–28

Fries JF. Advances in management of rheumatic disease, 1965–1985. Arch Intern Med 1989 May; 149(5):1002–1011

Goeppinger J et al. A nursing perspective on the assessment of function in persons with arthritis. Res Nurs Health 1988 Oct; 11(5):321–331

Gold RH, Bassett LW and Seeger LL. The other arthritides. Radiol Clin North Am 1988 Nov; 26(6):1195–1212

Halla JT et al. Involvement of the cervical spine in rheumatoid arthritis. Arthritis Rheum 1989 May; 32(5):652–659

Hicks JE et al. Prosthetics, orthotics, and assistive devices. 4. Orthotic management of selected disorders. Arch Phys Med Rehabil 1989 May; 70(5-S):S210–S217

Jaffe IA. Drug therapy of rheumatoid arthritis. Compr Ther 1989 Jan; 15(1):20–26

Kroop SF and Simon LS. Current pharmacologic therapy of arthritis. Compr Ther 1989 Jan; 15(1):55–66

Lipson SJ. Rheumatoid arthritis in the cervical spine. Clin Orthop 1989 Feb; 239:121–127

Moncur C and Williams HJ. Cervical spine management in patients with rheumatoid arthritis. Phys Ther 1988 Apr; 68(4):509–515

Oral gold in rheumatoid arthritis. Drug Ther Bull 1988 Sep 5; 26(18):69–72

Parker J et al. Coping strategies in rheumatoid arthritis. J Rheumatol 1988 Sep; 15(9):1383–1385

Schoen DC. Assessment for arthritis. Orthop Nurs 1988 Mar–Apr; 7(2):31–39

Touger-Decker R. Nutritional considerations in rheumatoid arthritis. J Am Diet Assoc 1988 Mar; 88(3):327–331

Tugwell P et al. Methotrexate in rheumatoid arthritis. Ann Intern Med 1989 Apr 15; 110(8):581–583

Ward JR. Role of disease-modifying antirheumatic drugs versus cytotoxic agents in the therapy of rheumatoid arthritis. Am J Med 1988 Oct 14; 85(4A):39–44

Whitwam L. Arthritis: Social problems and practical solutions. Nurs Times 1989 Feb 1–7; 85(5):36–39

Wilder RL. Treatment of the patient with rheumatoid arthritis refractory to standard therapy. JAMA 1988 Apr 22–29; 259(16):2446–2449

Gout

Campbell SM. Gout: How presentation, diagnosis, and treatment differ in the elderly. Geriatrics 1988 Nov; 43(11):71–77

Cornelius R and Schneider HJ. Gouty arthritis in the adult. Radiol Clin North Am 1988 Nov; 26(6):1267–1276

Elion GB. The purine path to chemotherapy. Science 1989 Apr 7; 244(4900):41–47

Reginato AJ and Schumacher HR. Crystal-associated arthropathies. Clin Geriatr Med 1988 May; 4(2):295–322

Wallace SL and Singer JZ. Therapy in gout. Rheum Dis Clin North Am 1988 Aug; 14(2):441–457

Polyarteritis

Albert DA, Rimon D and Silverstein MD. The diagnosis of polyarteritis nodosa. Arthritis Rheum 1988 Sep; 31(9):1117–1127

Bradley JP, Brandt KD and Katz BP. Infectious complication of cyclophosphamide treatment for vasculitis. Arthritis Rheum 1989 Jan; 32(1):45–33

Canoso JJ and Fienberg R. A 51-year-old man with fever, painful legs, and a rash. N Engl J Med 1988 Aug 4; 319(5):292–301

Guillevin L et al. Clinical findings and prognosis of polyarteritis nodosa and Churg-Strauss angiitis: A study of 165 patients. Br J Rheumatol 1988 Aug; 27(4):258–264

Karp DR et al. Successful management of catastrophic gastrointestinal involvement in polyarteritis nodosa. Arthritis Rheum 1988 May; 31(5):683–687

Scott DGI. Classification and treatment of systemic vasculitis. Br J Rheumatol 1988 Aug; 27(4):251–253

Systemic Sclerosis

Barnett AJ, Miller M and Littlejohn GO. The diagnosis and classification of scleroderma (systemic sclerosis). Postgrad Med J 1988 Feb; 64(748):121–125

Black CM and Stevens WM. Scleroderma. Rheum Dis Clin North Am 1989 May; 15(2):193–212

Krieg T and Meurer M. Systemic scleroderma. J Am Acad Dermatol 1988 Mar; 18(3):457–481

Merlo A and Cohen S. Swallowing disorders. Annu Rev Med 1988; 39:17–28

Oliver GF and Winkelmann RK. The current treatment of scleroderma. Drugs 1989 Jan; 37(1):87–96

Systemic Lupus Erythematosus

Harmon KR and Leatherman JW. Respiratory manifestations of connective tissue disease. Semin Respir Inf 1988 Sep; 3(3):258–273

Hughes GRV. Systemic lupus erythematosus. Postgrad Med J 1988 Jul; 64(753):517–521

Kimberly RP. Treatment: Corticosteroids and anti-inflammatory drugs. Rheum Dis Clin North Am 1988 Apr; 14(1):203–221

Lieberman JD and Schatten S. Treatment: Disease-modifying therapies. Rheum Dis Clin North Am 1988 Apr; 14(1):223–243

Mandell BF. Cardiovascular involvement in systemic lupus erythematosus. Semin Arthritis Rheum 1987 Nov; 17(2):126–141

The Allergic Reaction

Definitions

1. *Antigen*—a substance that stimulates an immune re-action causing the production of antibodies
2. *Antibody*—a globulin (protein) produced by B cells as a defense mechanism against foreign materials
3. *Atopy*—a term referring to a genetic predisposition to develop allergic disease
4. *Allergic reaction*—results from antigen–antibody re-action on a sensitized mast cell causing the release of chemical mediators
5. *Immunity*
   a. *Humoral*—the process by which B lymphocytes produce circulating antibodies to act against an-tigens
   b. *Cell-mediated*—that portion of the immune sys-tem in which the participation of T lymphocytes and macrophages is predominant
6. *Mast cell:*—a tissue cell that resembles a peripheral blood basophil and contains granules with chemical mediators

Immunoglobulins

Antibodies that are formed by lymphocytes and plasma cells in response to an immunogenic stimulus comprise a group of serum proteins called *immunoglobulins.*
1. The abbreviation for immunoglobulin is "Ig."
2. Antibodies combine with antigens in very special ways (lock-and-key style).
3. There are five major classes of immunoglobulins.
   a. *IgM*—comprises 10% of immunoglobulin pool; found mostly in intravascular fluid and is primarily engaged in initial defense.
   b. *IgG*—major immunoglobulin accounting for 70%–75% of secondary immune responses and in com-bating tissue infection.
   c. *IgA*—15%–20% of immunoglobulins; predomi-nantly found in seromucous secretions (such as saliva, tears) where it provides a primary defense mechanism.

   d. *IgD*—less than 1% of immunoglobulin pool; found on many circulating B lymphocytes, but function is unknown.
   e. *IgE*—only a trace found in serum; attaches to sur-face membrane of basophils and mast cells; re-sponsible for immediate types of allergic reac-tions.

Immunologic Reactions *(Fig. 36-1)*

A. Immediate Hypersensitivity (Type 1)

1. Characterized by:
   a. An allergic reaction
   b. Occurs immediately following contact with the antigen
   c. Causes release of chemical mediators
2. Example—anaphylaxis

B. Products of Immediate Hypersensitivity (Chemical Mediators)

1. *Histamine*—a bioactive amine stored in granules of mast cells and basophils
2. *Serotonin*—an amine released at the same time as his-tamine
3. *Bradykinin*—acts chiefly by increasing capillary per-meability and contractility of smooth muscle
4. *PAF—Platelet Activating Factor* has many properties; causes the aggregation of platelets
5. *SRS-A*—a slow-reacting substance of anaphylaxis
6. *Prostaglandins*—potent vasodilators as well as potent bronchoconstrictors
7. *ECF-A*—causes an influx of eosinophils into the area of allergic inflammation

C. Effects of Chemical Mediators and Their Manifestations

1. Generalized vasodilation, hypotension, flushing
2. Increased permeability
   a. Capillaries of the skin—edema
   b. Mucous membranes—edema
3. Smooth muscle contraction
   a. Bronchioles—bronchospasm
   b. Intestines—abdominal cramps, diarrhea
4. Increased secretions
   a. Nasal mucous glands—rhinorrhea
   b. Bronchioles—increased mucus in airways
   c. Gastrointestinal—increased gastric secretions
   d. Lacrimal—tearing
   e. Salivary—salivation
5. Pruritus (itching)

---

* The views expressed in this chapter are those of the authors and do not reflect the official policy or position of the Department of the Navy, Department of Defense, or the US Government.

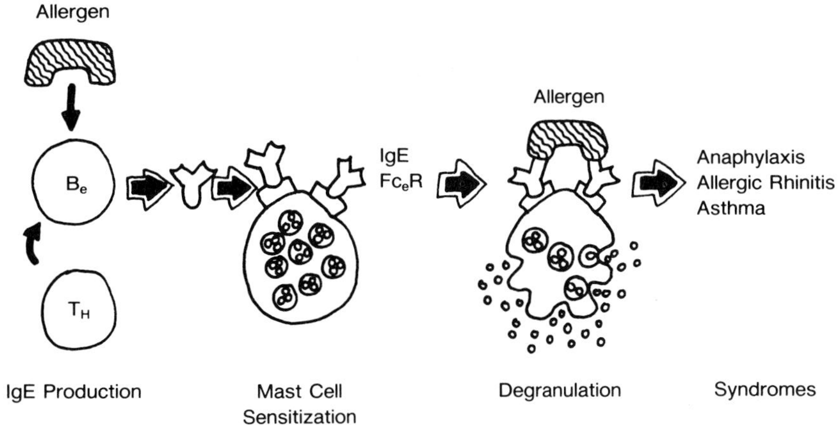

Figure 36-1. *Type I immediate hypersensitivity. Specific IgE is produced by B cells with T cell help as a result of allergen stimulation. The next step in sensitization is the attachment of the IgE antibody to the mast cell by the F_c receptor. When specific allergen reaches the sensitized mast cell and combines with the two adjacent antibody molecules on the surface of the cell, degranulation occurs, releasing chemical mediators that cause the symptoms associated with Type I hypersensitivity.*

a. Skin
b. Mucous membrane

D. Delayed Hypersensitivity (Type IV)

1. Characterized by a cell-mediated reaction between antigens and antigen-responsive T lymphocytes.
2. Maximal intensity occurs between 24 to 48 hours.
3. Usually consists of erythema and induration.
4. Examples—tuberculin skin test; contact dermatitis such as poison ivy.

Evaluation of the Patient for Allergy

Evaluation includes:

1. The allergy history (Allergy Survey, below).
2. Physical examination (Chapter 3).
3. Skin testing, page 876.
4. Other tests are indicated under specific allergic conditions.

Allergy Survey

Name _____ Age _____ Sex _____ Date _____

1. Reason for visit:
2. Do you have any of the following problems?

   _____ Hay Fever   _____ Sinus problems   _____ Eczema
   _____ Asthma   _____ Drug allergy   Other: (please specify)
   _____ Hives   _____ Insect allergy   _____
   _____ Food allergy   _____ Skin rash   _____

3. Does anyone in your family have allergies? _____
4. Have you ever been tested for allergies? _____
   When? _____ Results _____
5. Do you smoke? _____ How much? _____ No. of years _____
6. Exercise habits: _____
7. Other significant past medical history _____

8. Current symptoms: (Circle one(s) that applies)

   Nasal stuffiness/congestion   Mouth breathing   Shortness of breath
   Sneezing   Snoring   Diminished sense of
   Runny nose   Itching/irritation/redness/   smell
   Itching   tearing of eyes
   Postnasal drip   Cough
   Sinus headaches   Chest tightness
   Sinus infections   Wheezing

9. Do symptoms occur year 'round? _____
10. If not, during what seasons do your symptoms occur?

    Summer   Fall   Winter   Spring

(continued)

Allergy Survey (continued)

11. Where do symptoms occur? _____

    Home   Office   School   Outdoors   Basement   Bedroom

12. Are symptoms made worse by:

    Smoke   Heat   Humidity   Cold   Pollen   Pollution
    Dust   Exposure to strong odors—ammonia, paint, perfume
    Pets   Exercise   Eating   Drinking   Emotional stress

13. Have you had symptoms after eating? If so, list the foods:
14. Do you have pets? _____ Dog _____ Cat   Other: _____
15. List any medications that you are currently taking, including over-the-counter drugs:

    Do you know what they are for?

    Are you aware of possible side effects?

16. Can you take aspirin without any adverse reactions?

17. In what way(s) has your health problem affected your life-style?

Guidelines   Skin Testing

Skin testing has been used to diagnose allergic disease for over a century. The types of skin tests used in clinical allergy are: 1) epicutaneous (prick, puncture, or scratch) and 2) intradermal methods. The skin test remains unequalled as a sensitive and cost-effective test for the diagnosis of allergies.

Purpose   To identify antigens responsible for immediate hypersensitivity and to determine the level of sensitivity in an individual.

Epicutaneous (Prick) Method (Fig. 36-2)

Advantages

1. Safe—less chance for anaphylaxis due to minimal systemic absorption.
2. Efficient—results within 15 minutes.
3. Little discomfort to the patient.

Disadvantages

1. Less sensitive than the intradermal method.
2. Old or thick, leathery skin decreases reactivity.
3. Drops have a tendency to run together, which would effect the accuracy of the test.

Equipment   Antigens for testing
Controls
    Positive—histamine 1 mg./ml.
    Negative—glycerol saline
Pricking device (sterile needle or lancet)
Alcohol swabs
Paper tissues
Skin marking pencil
Millimeter ruler
Tourniquet
Epinephrine 1:1000 aqueous solution for injection for emergency use.

Procedure	**Nursing Action**	**Rationale**

1. Explain the procedure to the patient. Ask patient if he has taken antihistamines in the past 48–72 hours.
2. Prepare the site (volar surface of forearm or back) by cleansing with alcohol.

3. Mark the test sites with a skin marking pencil approximately 3–4 cm. apart.

4. Apply positive (histamine) and negative (glycerol saline) controls next to the appropriate markings. Introduce the tip of the pricking device at a 15–20-degree angle through each drop, lifting up and tenting the skin until the point pops loose without causing any bleeding. The pricking device must be wiped thoroughly with a paper tissue after each puncture.
5. Apply small drops of antigens next to the skin markings and prick the drops as described above. Blot (do not rub) skin surface with paper tissue (Fig. 36-2A).

1. Oral antihistamines taken 48–72 hours before skin testing are likely to prevent a reaction from occurring.
2. The forearm is usually preferable because in the event of a significant local or systemic reaction, a tourniquet may be placed proximal to the skin test to slow the diffusion of the antigen into the circulation.
3. Sites need to be spaced appropriately so that reactions will remain distinct from one another, thus allowing an accurate reading.
4. Because of interpatient variability in cutaneous reactivity, it is necessary to include positive and negative controls whenever skin testing is performed. A response to the positive control confirms an immunologic ability to react. A response to the negative control indicates reactivity to the diluting solution and/or mechanical trauma. Care must be taken to prevent cross-contamination between antigens.
5. Rubbing may cause redness and cross-contamination of antigens.

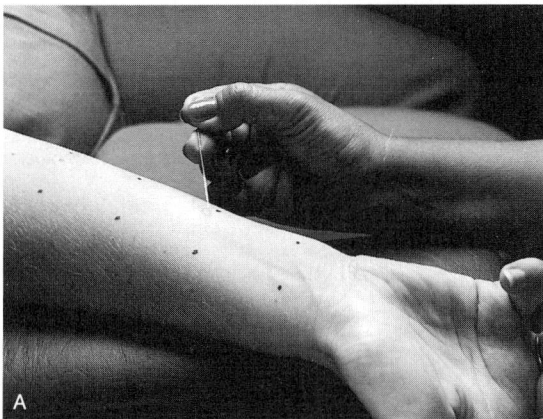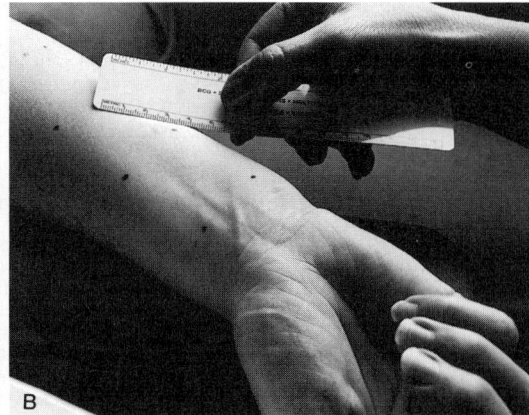

Figure 36-2. *Skin testing—epicutaneous (prick) method. (A) The volar surface of the forearm is marked and drops of antigen are applied 3–4 cm. apart. The skin is penetrated through the antigen with a pricking device. (B) The wheal-and-flare reaction is measured with a millimeter ruler.*

6. Instruct the patient not to scratch the test area during the 15-minute waiting interval before the reactions are graded.

7. Observe the patient closely for signs of impending anaphylaxis (such as itching, flushing, lump in throat).

8. Fifteen minutes after pricking the antigens, measure the extent of induration (wheal) and erythema (flare) in two perpendicular axes through the center of the reaction; record in millimeters (Fig. 36-2B).
9. Document the procedure, test results, patient tolerance, and any other pertinent observations.

6. It is normal for sensitive individuals to have a pruritic sensation at the testing site because of the histamine released by the mast cells.
7. General systemic or anaphylactic reactions are rare, but do occur. If suspected, apply tourniquet above test site and administer 0.3 ml. epinephrine 1:1000 subcutaneously.

Intradermal Method

Advantages

1. More sensitive than prick testing

Disadvantages

1. Increased possibility for anaphylactic reactions
2. Requires more time and skill to perform

(continued)

Guidelines Skin Testing *(continued)*

3. Increased discomfort to the patient
4. Less specific than prick testing

Equipment

Antigens for testing
Controls
    Positive—histamine 0.1 mg./ml.
    Negative—human serum albumin
1 mm. tuberculin syringes with 26- or 27-gauge intradermal needle
Alcohol swabs
Paper tissues
Skin marking pencil
Millimeter ruler
Tourniquet
Gloves
Epinephrine for emergency use

Procedure

Nursing Action	Rationale
1. Explain the procedure to the patient. Ask the patient if he has taken antihistamines in past 48–72 hours.	1. Oral antihistamines taken 48–72 hours before skin testing are likely to prevent a reaction from occurring.
2. Prepare the site (volar surface of forearm or upper arm) by cleansing with alcohol. Allow to dry.	
3. Mark the test sites with a skin marking pencil approximately 3–4 cm. apart.	3. Sites need to be spaced appropriately so that reactions will remain distinct from one another, thus allowing an accurate reading.
4. Using sterile technique, draw up testing materials. All bubbles must be carefully expelled to avoid "splash reactions," which reduce precision. While wearing gloves, place syringe at a 45-degree angle to the skin with the bevel up. Stretch the skin taut and insert 0.02 ml. of the positive and negative controls. The bevel should penetrate the skin entirely and end between the layers of skin. A bleb approximately 2 mm. in diameter should be produced.	4. Gloves should be worn when there is any possibility of exposure to blood or body fluids.
5. Inject 0.02 ml. of test antigens intradermally next to the skin markings. A different syringe and needle must be used for each antigen.	5. To avoid antigen and microbial contamination.
6. Blot skin surfaces dry with paper tissue. Do not rub.	6. Rubbing may cause redness and cross-contamination of antigens.
7. Instruct the patient not to scratch the test area during the 15-minute waiting interval before the reaction is graded.	7. It is normal for sensitive individuals to have a pruritic sensation at the testing site because of the histamine released by the mast cells.
8. Observe the patient closely for signs of impending anaphylaxis (itching, flushing, lump in throat).	8. There is an increased possibility of anaphylactic reactions with intradermal skin testing. If suspected, apply tourniquet above test site, and administer 0.3 ml. of epinephrine 1:1000 subcutaneously.

9. Fifteen minutes after applying antigens, measure the extent of induration (wheal) and erythema (flare) in two perpendicular axes through the center of the reaction and record in millimeters.
    Reactions are graded according to the following:
    0   2 mm. or less
    1+ 3–5 mm. wheal with erythema
    2+ 6–10 mm. wheal with erythema
    3+ over 11–15 mm. wheal without pseudopods*
    4+ wheal over 15 mm. with pseudopods
10. Document the procedure, test results, patient tolerance, and any other pertinent observations.

Complications

Local Reactions—unusually large 4+ reactions
1. Apply prescribed steroid cream to affected area.
2. If no relief, administer prescribed oral antihistamine.

* Pseudopods—asymmetric extensions of wheal that indicate increased sensitivity.

Procedure *(continued)*	**Nursing Action**	**Rationale**

Vasovagal Reactions—fainting episode
1. Monitor vital signs.
2. Reassure the patient.
3. Finish skin testing if possible.

Systemic Anaphylaxis
1. Stop testing and apply tourniquet above skin testing site.
2. Administer epinephrine subcutaneously.

Allergic Conditions

Anaphylaxis

Anaphylaxis is an immediate, life-threatening systemic reaction that can occur upon exposure to a particular substance. It is a result of a Type I hypersensitivity reaction in which chemical mediators released from mast cells affect many types of tissue and organ systems.

> **NURSING ALERT:** With immunotherapy (allergy shots), the risk of systemic reaction is always present. Skin testing can also result in systemic reactions. Have epinephrine 1:1000 available during these procedures (with syringe and tourniquet).

Causes

1. Immunotherapy
2. Stinging insects
3. Skin testing
4. Medications
5. Contrast media infusion
6. Foods
7. Exercise

Clinical Manifestations

1. *Respiratory*—laryngeal edema, bronchospasm, cough, wheezing, lump in throat
2. *Cardiovascular*—hypotension, tachycardia, palpitations, syncope
3. *Cutaneous*—urticaria (hives), angioedema, pruritus, erythema (flushing)
4. *Gastrointestinal*—nausea, vomiting, diarrhea, abdominal pain, bloating

Management

Prompt identification of signs and symptoms and immediate intervention is essential; the more quickly a reaction occurs, the more severe it tends to be.

A. Immediate Treatment

1. A tourniquet is applied above site of antigen injection (allergy injection, insect sting, etc.) or skin test site—to slow the absorption of antigen into the system.
2. Epinephrine is injected into opposite arm; may be repeated every 15–20 minutes if necessary—causes vasoconstriction, decreases capillary permeability, relaxes airway smooth muscle, and inhibits mast cell mediator release.

B. Simultaneous and Subsequent Treatment

1. Laryngeal edema
   a. An adequate airway is established.
   b. Epinephrine is administered by inhalation as directed.
   c. Insertion of endotracheal tube or tracheostomy.
2. Hypotension and shock
   a. Monitoring of vital signs
   b. Administration of H_1 and H_2 antihistamines intravenously (slowly) in an attempt to counteract hypotension by blocking histamine release
   c. Rapid infusion of intravenous fluids for maintenance of blood pressure and fluid replacement
   d. Vasopressors to raise blood pressure and cardiac output
3. Bronchospasm
   a. Administration of oxygen by nasal cannula at 2–5 L./minute.
   b. Nebulization treatment with bronchodilator.
   c. Administration of aminophylline intravenously (relaxes bronchial smooth muscle).
4. Urticaria and angioedema
   a. H_1 antihistamines, such as diphenhydramine hydrochloride (Benadryl), are usually sufficient—blocks the effect of histamine on the bronchioles, gastrointestinal tract, and blood vessels.
   b. In severe anaphylaxis, both H_1 and H_2 antihistamines, such as ranitidine (Zantac), are given by injection.
   c. Corticosteroids decrease vascular permeability and diminish the migration of inflammatory cells; may be helpful in preventing late phase responses.

Prevention

1. Carefully identify and document patient's allergies.
2. Instruct patients to wear a Medic Alert bracelet or tag at all times.
3. Ask patients, before administering any potentially harmful drug or other agent, if they have ever had a reaction to it. Do not rely on the chart alone.
4. Instruct patients receiving injections in an office or clinic to remain for at least 30 minutes after administration.
5. Instruct any patient predisposed to or with a history of anaphylaxis to carry epinephrine for self-injection at all times.

Patient Education

Instruct patients as follows:
1. Read labels and be familiar with the scientific name of the drug thought to cause a reaction.
2. Discard all unused drugs. Make sure any drug kept in the medicine cabinet is clearly labeled.

3. Familiarize yourself with drugs that may cross-react with a drug to which you are allergic.
4. Always know the names of every drug that you take.
5. Be extremely careful about everything you eat if you have a known sensitivity to a food product—allergic compounds are often hidden in a preparation (such as monosodium glutamate).
6. Teach the patient at risk for anaphylaxis about the potential seriousness of these reactions.
7. Educate patients to recognize the early signs and symptoms of anaphylaxis.
8. Persons allergic to bee stings should avoid wearing brightly colored or black clothes, perfumes, and hairspray. Shoes should be worn at all times.
9. For exercise-induced anaphylaxis, patients should exercise in moderation, preferably with another person, and in a controlled setting where assistance is readily available.
10. If food is associated with exercise-induced anaphylaxis, wait at least 2 hours after eating to exercise.
11. Instruct the patient in the self-injection technique for the administration of epinephrine.
12. Provide the patient with information on epinephrine (Epi-Pen; Ana-Kit), including the action of the drug, possible side effects, and the importance of prompt administration at the first sign of a systemic reaction.

Allergic Rhinitis

Allergic rhinitis is an inflammation of the nasal mucosa caused by an allergen.

Classification

1. Seasonal—offending allergen is a pollen or mold; symptoms are episodic.
2. Perennial—offending allergen is dust, dust mites, mold, or animal dander; symptoms occur year round.

Clinical Manifestations

1. Nasal—mucous membrane congestion, edema, itching, rhinorrhea with clear secretions, sneezing
2. Eyes—edema, itching, burning, tearing, redness
3. Ears—itching, fullness
4. Other—palatal itching, throat itching

Diagnostic Tests

1. *History*—essential for making a diagnosis, since there is no test that objectively determines allergic rhinitis
2. *Nasal smear*—the presence of an increased number of eosinophils suggests allergic disease
3. *Skin testing*—confirms a hypersensitivity to certain allergens
4. *Radioallergosorbent test (RAST)*—a test used to identify IgE antibodies in serum
5. *Sinus x-rays*—a high percentage of allergic patients will have concomitant sinus infections
6. *Rhinoscopy*—allows better visualization of the nasopharynx; useful to rule out physical obstruction (septal deviation, nasal polyps)

Management

A. Avoidance
Patients should minimize contact with offending allergens, regardless of other treatment.

B. Medications: Acute Phase

1. *H₁ antihistamines*—block the effects of histamine on smooth muscle and blood vessels by blocking histamine receptor sites, thereby relieving the symptoms of allergic rhinitis.
2. *Decongestants*—shrink nasal mucous membrane by vasoconstriction
3. *Anticholinergic agents*—inhibit mucus secretions

C. Medications: Preventive Therapy

1. *Cromolyn* (intranasal)—mast cell stabilizer; hinders the release of chemical mediators
2. *Corticosteroids* (oral and intranasal)
   a. Reduce inflammation of nasal mucosa
   b. Prevent mediator release
   c. Only given systemically for a short course during a disabling attack

D. Immunotherapy

1. Regimen consists of administering subcutaneous injections of increasing amounts of an allergen to which the patient is sensitive in an attempt to decrease sensitivity and reduce the severity of symptoms.
2. Immunotherapy produces the following immunologic changes:
   a. An increase in IgG blocking antibody that combines with antigen before it reacts with IgE antibodies.
   b. May decrease IgE antibodies against specific antigens.
   c. Decreases mast cell sensitivity.
3. Possible adverse reactions of immunotherapy
   a. Systemic reactions—anaphylaxis is rare, but potentially fatal.
   b. Local reactions—consist of erythema and induration at the site of injection.

Note: Immunotherapy should not be given to patients receiving beta-adrenergic blocking agents. It would be very difficult to reverse a systemic reaction, should one occur.

Patient Education

A. Information on Medications

1. Include the action, correct dosage, and possible side effects of prescribed drugs.
2. Instruct patients on proper use of nasal inhalers.
3. Avoid driving or other situations that require alertness if antihistamines have been prescribed.
4. Do not use nasal decongestants for more than 2–3 days because their effect is short-lived and a "rebound" effect causing nasal mucosal edema often occurs.

B. Immunotherapy

1. Provide information on the purpose, method of administration, time frame of expected results, and the possible risks involved (local reactions, anaphylaxis).
2. Inform the patient that close observation for 30 minutes is essential after each injection.
3. Alert patient to the possibility of a delayed reaction, which needs to be reported to the nurse and/or physician.

C. Self-Responsibility

1. Provide compliance counseling with a focus on self-responsibility.
2. Compliance is an important factor for immunotherapy due to requirements of frequent office visits and a long-term commitment (may take up to 1 year to obtain optimum results).

D. Environmental Control

Modification of the patient's environment will help to relieve symptoms.

1. Use nonallergic materials for bedding (pillows, blankets).
2. Keep clothing in a closet with door shut.
3. Avoid venetian blinds—use washable curtains.
4. Avoid stuffed animals and other dust collectors.
5. Encase mattress and boxsprings in zippered plastic covers.
6. Use synthetic pillows that can be washed and replaced frequently; bed linens should be washed in hot water (more than 130°F.).
7. Damp-dust daily and wear a mask while doing it.
8. Eliminate upholstered furniture, shag carpets, and draperies.
9. Use air conditioning to reduce antigen load indoors.
10. Change furnace filters frequently.
11. Using a high-efficiency air filtering system may help.
12. Avoid smoking and smoke-filled areas.
13. Avoid rapid changes in temperature.
14. Patients allergic to animal danders should not have household pets—or at least keep them out of the bedroom.
15. Avoid mold growth by using a fungicide in bathrooms, damp basements, food storage areas, and garbage containers.
16. Keep windows closed during high pollen season.
17. Avoid outdoor activities when high pollen/pollutants are in the air.

Bronchial Asthma

Bronchial asthma is a disease characterized by variable, recurrent, reversible airway obstruction clinically manifested by intermittent episodes of wheezing and dyspnea. It is associated with hyperresponsiveness of the bronchi to various stimuli that may be antigen-mediated (allergic).

Pathophysiology

The basic defect appears to be an abnormality in the host, which intermittently leads to an increased constriction of smooth muscle, hypersecretion of mucus in the bronchial tree, and mucosal edema.

A. Neuromechanisms (Autonomic Nervous System)

1. Stimulation of the vagus nerve (which is responsible for bronchomotor tone) by viral respiratory infections, air pollutants, and other stimuli causes bronchoconstriction, increased secretion of mucus, and dilation of the pulmonary vessels.
2. Beta-adrenergic receptor cells that line the airways are also responsible for bronchomotor tone. Abnormal functioning of these cells predisposes patients to bronchoconstriction.

B. Antigen–Antibody Reaction

1. Susceptible individuals form abnormally large amounts of IgE when exposed to certain allergens.
2. This immunoglobulin (IgE) fixes itself to the mast cells of the bronchial mucosa.
3. When the individual is exposed to certain allergens, the resulting antigen combines with the cell-bound IgE molecules, causing the mast cell to degranulate and release chemical mediators.
4. These chemical mediators act on bronchial smooth muscle to cause bronchoconstriction, on dilated epithelium to reduce mucociliary clearance, on bronchial glands to cause mucus secretion, on blood vessels to cause vasodilation and increased permeability, and on leukocytes to cause a cellular infiltration and inflammation.
5. Late-phase reactions (occurring 4–8 hours after the initial response) include the influx of neutrophils, eosinophils, lymphocytes, and monocytes.

C. Bronchial Inflammation

1. Occurs in both the immediate and late-phase reactions caused by antigen–antibody response.
2. Factors other than allergens (such as noxious environmental stimuli) cause bronchial inflammation and hyperreactivity by mast cell activation.

Classification

A. Extrinsic Asthma

1. Hypersensitivity reaction to inhalant allergens (dust, dust mites, mold, pollens, feathers, and animal dander are the major ones).
2. Mediated by immunoglobin E (IgE mediated).

B. Intrinsic Asthma

1. No inciting allergen
2. Infection, often viral
3. Environmental stimuli (such as air pollution)

C. Mixed Asthma

Immediate Type I reactivity appears to be combined with intrinsic factors.

D. Aspirin-Induced Asthma

1. Induced by ingestion of aspirin and related compounds.
2. "Triad" has been described as a combination of aspirin-induced asthma, nasal polyposis, and sinusitis.

E. Exercise-Induced Asthma

Symptoms vary from slight chest tightness and cough to severe wheezing/cough and shortness of breath that usually occur within 5–20 minutes after exercise.

F. Occupational Asthma

1. Caused by inhalation of industrial fumes, dust, and gases.
2. Cough without associated wheezing is a more common symptom than in other forms of asthma.

Triggers of Asthma

1. Allergens
2. Respiratory infections
3. Inhalation of irritating substances (dust, fumes, gases)
4. Environmental factors (weather, air pollution, and humidity)
5. Exercise, particularly in cold weather
6. Aspirin and its derivatives
7. Sulfiting agents used as food preservatives
8. Emotional factors

Clinical Manifestations

1. Episodes of coughing
2. Wheezing
3. Dyspnea
4. Feeling of chest tightness

Diagnostic Evaluation

1. History—family history of allergies and asthma, history of recent infections

2. Physical examination—include nasal examination, assessment of forced expiration/inspiration
3. Laboratory—increased levels of IgE are usually seen in atopic asthma
4. Pulmonary function testing
5. Bronchial methacholine challenge—demonstrates airway hyperreactivity by the inhalation of a cholinergic agent in serial concentrations delivered by nebulization; a positive response is indicated by a 20% greater decrease in the FEV_1 from the control value.
6. Skin testing to identify causative allergens
7. Sputum and nasal cytology (increased eosinophilia)
8. Chest x-ray to exclude other lung diseases

Management

The goal is to allow the person with asthma to live a normal life. It is important that the approach to management is structured and that the treatment is unique to the patient and his condition.

A. Medications

1. Include bronchodilators, corticosteroids, cromolyn sodium, antihistamines, and anticholinergics.
2. Aerosol therapy with beta-adrenoceptor agonists, cromolyn sodium, and inhaled steroids form the basis of asthma treatment.
3. The most convenient and inexpensive method of aerosol delivery to patients is the metered dose inhaler.

Note: Beta-blocking agents such as propranolol (Inderal) should not be given to patients with asthma because of its potential to cause bronchoconstriction.

B. Other Measures

1. Environmental control (see allergic rhinitis, p. 881)
2. Immunotherapy (see allergic rhinitis, p. 880)
3. Dietary control
   Foods that contain tartrazine (yellow dye #5) may cause asthma in aspirin-sensitive patients and should be avoided.
4. Exercise
   a. Regular aerobic exercise should be encouraged.
   b. Use of an inhaled beta-agonist or cromolyn taken 15–20 minutes prior to exercise will decrease postexercise bronchospasm.
5. Psychotherapy—if psychosocial functioning of the patient and/or family is affected, appropriate referral should be made.

Nursing Assessment

1. Review patient's record: ask about coughing, dyspnea, exertional changes, and increased mucus production.
2. Observe the patient and assess the rate, depth, and character of respirations, especially on expiration; observe for hyperinflation.
3. Auscultate the chest for breath sounds/wheezing.
4. After acute episode subsides, attempt to determine patient's degree of compliance with medications/management regimen.
5. Observe for level of anxiety and restlessness.
6. Determine patient's level of knowledge of condition and its management.

Nursing Diagnoses

1. Ineffective breathing pattern related to bronchospasm.
2. Anxiety related to fear of suffocating, difficulty in breathing, death.
3. Knowledge deficit of disease, triggering factors, medications, use of peak flow meter, inhaler and nebulizer.

Nursing Interventions

A. Attaining Relief of Dyspneic Breathing

1. Monitor vital signs, skin color, and degree of restlessness.
2. Provide nebulization therapy as prescribed.
3. Monitor airway functioning through peak flow meter or pulmonary function testing to assess effectiveness of treatment.
4. Encourage intake of fluids to liquefy secretions.
5. Instruct patient on positioning to facilitate breathing: sitting upright (leaning forward on a table).
6. Employ chest physical therapy/postural drainage—to mobilize secretions.
7. Encourage patient to use adaptive breathing techniques (pursed-lip breathing, etc.) to decrease the work of breathing.

B. Relieving Anxiety

1. Explain rationale for interventions to gain patient's cooperation.
2. Help patient clarify source(s) of anxiety; suggest measures to reduce anxiety.
3. Encourage and support efforts to comply with self-management plan.

Patient Education

1. Provide information on the nature of asthma and methods of treatment.
2. Provide information regarding medications, including proper use of inhaler devices; stress avoiding overuse of inhalers/nebulizers.
3. Demonstrate the use of peak flow meters and recording of peak flow measurements.
4. Help patient to identify what triggers his asthma, early warning signs of an impending attack, and intervention strategies for preventing an attack.
5. Teach adaptive breathing techniques and breathing exercises, such as pursed-lip breathing, positioning for comfort (see p. 172).
6. Discuss environmental control
   a. Avoid persons with respiratory infections.
   b. Avoid substances and situations known to precipitate bronchospasm, such as irritants, gases, fumes, and smoke.
   c. Wear a mask if cold weather precipitates bronchospasm.
   d. Stay inside when air pollution is high.
   e. See Patient Education, Allergic Rhinitis, page 880.
7. Promote optimal health practices, including nutrition, rest, and exercise.
   a. Encourage regular exercise to improve cardiorespiratory and musculoskeletal conditioning.
   b. Drink liberal amounts of fluids to keep secretions thin.
   c. Avoid taking sleeping pills after an asthmatic attack as these medications slow respirations and may make breathing more difficult.
   d. Try to avoid upsetting situations.
   e. Use relaxation techniques, biofeedback, stress management.
   f. Use community resources for smoking cessation classes, stress management, exercises for relaxation, etc.
8. Provide information on asthma self-management pro-

grams such as Airwise, Mothers of Asthmatics, Air Power (addresses at end of chapter).

Evaluation

1. Demonstrates adequate rate, depth, and character of respirations; absence of dyspnea and cyanosis.
2. Verbalizes lessening of anxiety; identifies methods of managing stress factors.
3. Demonstrates compliance with management plan; identifies triggers; demonstrates self-monitoring with peak flow meter; knows reasons for taking medications; demonstrates proper technique of use of inhaler/nebulizer.

Status Asthmaticus

Status asthmaticus is a severe form of asthma in which the airway obstruction is unresponsive to conventional drug therapy and lasts longer than 24 hours.

Contributing Factors

1. Infection
2. Overuse of tranquilizers
3. Nebulizer abuse
4. Dehydration
5. Inhalation of air pollutants
6. Noncompliance in taking medications
7. Sudden reduction in corticosteroids
8. Ingestion of aspirin and/or related drugs in aspirin-sensitive patient

Clinical Manifestations

1. Labored respirations, with increased effort on exhalation.
2. Distended neck and face veins.
3. Fatigue, headache, irritability, dizziness, impaired mental functioning—from hypoxia.
4. Muscle twitching, somnolence, diaphoresis—from continued carbon dioxide retention.
5. Tachycardia, elevated blood pressure.
6. Heart failure and death from suffocation.

Management and Nursing Interventions

1. Continuous monitoring of arterial blood gases, blood pressure, ECG, and respiratory rate.

> **NURSING ALERT:** In status asthmaticus, the return to a normal or increasing PCO_2 does not necessarily mean that the asthmatic patient is improving—it may indicate a fatigue state that develops just before the patient slips into respiratory failure.

2. Repeated aerosol treatments with bronchodilators (albuterol, terbutaline) as prescribed—may perpetuate intractability—administer with caution until the metabolic and respiratory acidosis and hypoxemia have been corrected.
3. Intravenous therapy
   a. When intravenous fluids are administered, aminophylline may be prescribed and administered *slowly* by constant infusion; the clinician must be constantly alert for signs of theophylline toxicity.
   b. Many physicians administer corticosteroids; since these act slowly, their beneficial effects may not be apparent for several hours.

4. Continuous humidified oxygen via nasal cannula as prescribed. (Patients with associated chronic obstructive pulmonary disease or emphysema are at risk for depressing hypoxemia ventilatory drive, thus compounding respiratory insufficiency.)
5. Mechanical ventilation, if necessary.
6. Mobilization of obstructing bronchial mucus.
   a. Chest physiotherapy (chest wall percussion and vibration).
   b. Administer expectorant and mucolytic drugs as prescribed.
   c. Remove secretions by suctioning or bronchoscopy.
   d. Provide adequate hydration.
7. Alleviate the patient's anxiety and fear by acting calmly and reassuring the patient during an attack. Stay with the patient until the attack subsides.

Food Allergies

Food allergies result when the body's immune system overreacts to certain otherwise harmless substances. Food allergies occur in 4%–6% of children and less than 1% of adults, although the perceived prevalence is much higher due to other existing adverse food reactions that cause similar symptoms.

Common Food Allergens

1. Cow's milk
2. Eggs
3. Shellfish
4. Peanuts
5. Soybean
6. Wheat

Classification of Adverse Food Reactions

1. *Food hypersensitivity*—a true food allergy is an IgE-mediated response to a food allergen (protein).
2. *Food intolerance*—an abnormal physical response to a food or additive and is *not* immunologic.
   a. Toxicity (poisoning)—caused by toxins contained in foods, microorganisms, or parasites
   b. Pharmacologic (chemical)—such as caffeine
   c. Idiosyncratic—etiology unknown

Clinical Manifestations of Food Allergies

1. *Respiratory*—rhinoconjunctivitis, sneezing, laryngeal edema, wheezing
2. *Cutaneous*—urticaria, angioedema, atopic dermatitis
3. *Gastroenteritis*—lip swelling, palatal itching, nausea, abdominal cramping, diarrhea
4. *Neurologic*—migraine headaches occur in some patients.

Diagnostic Tests

1. *History*—ascertain the symptoms associated with ingestion of foods in addition to the timing, severity and reproducibility of symptoms.
2. *Skin testing*
   a. Limit to those foods suspected of provoking symptoms based on history.
   b. Only epicutaneous testing is done.
   c. Intradermal testing has not been demonstrated to have a high degree of clinical correlation.
3. *RAST* (radioallergosorbent test)

a. An *in vitro* assay for determination of circulating antigen-specific IgE.
b. Is no more effective than skin testing.
c. Useful if food reactions have been so severe as to suggest that skin testing would be a risk to the patient.

4. *Oral challenge*
   a. Procedure in which the suspected food is given to the patient in an attempt to identify the allergen by reproducing the symptoms caused by the initial reaction.
   b. *Open*—may be used if the suspected food skin test is negative; suspected food is openly administered and the patient is monitored for a reaction.
   c. *Single-blind*—the suspected food is disguised in capsules, liquids, or other foods and administered to the patient in increasing doses at intervals determined by history and may be interspersed with placebo; may be used when the objectivity of the observer (nurse) is assured, otherwise some bias usually exists.
   d. *Double-blind, placebo-controlled*—the most definitive technique to confirm or refute histories of food allergies. The suspected food is administered in capsules or other vehicle that masks its identity and is interspersed with placebo so neither the doctor/nurse nor patient know whether the suspected food or placebo is being ingested.

5. *Diet diary*—an attempt to determine the offending food through a daily diary kept by the patient.

6. *Elimination diet*
   a. To determine if the patient's symptoms will stop when certain foods are avoided.
   b. Restrict 1–2 foods at a time if certain foods are suspected.
   c. If no particular food is suspected, a highly restricted diet for 7–14 days is preferable.

Management

1. Avoidance of specific foods is the only way of effectively preventing food allergy reactions.
2. Medications
   a. Antihistamines—may modify IgE symptoms but will not eliminate them.
   b. Corticosteroids—only used in the treatment of food allergy if associated with eosinophilic gastroenteritis or gastroenteropathy.
   c. Epinephrine—if history of anaphylaxis, patient should carry it at all times (Epi-Pen; Ana-Kit)

Patient Education

1. Provide the patient with information on epinephrine, including the action of the drug, possible side effects, and the importance of prompt administration at the first sign of a systemic reaction.
2. Instruct the patient in self-injection technique for the administration of epinephrine.
3. Dietary counseling by the nurse and/or dietitian should be done.
4. Hidden sources of foods must be explained to the patient to decrease the risk of unexpected exposure to an offending allergen.
5. Discuss alternative food preparation techniques and methods of substitution (such as using extra baking powder in place of eggs).
6. Provide patients with listings for telephone hot lines and written resource information.
7. Encourage and offer support for creativity and experimentation in the diet.
8. Caution highly allergic patients about restaurant food; when eating out, patients should request ingredient information—such brochures are now available in many restaurants, including fast food establishments.

Urticaria and Angioedema

Urticaria (hives) may affect 10% of the population at some time during their lives. *Angioedema* is a similar lesion but involves deep dermis and subcutaneous tissues. Urticaria and angioedema can occur individually or in combination.

Classification

1. Acute urticaria
   a. Hives lasting less than 6 weeks.
   b. A detectable cause is usually determined.
2. Chronic urticaria
   a. Hives lasting 6 weeks or longer.
   b. The cause is undetermined in 75%–90% of patients.

Causes

1. Ingested substances—food, food additives, drugs
2. Infections—viral, bacterial, parasitic
3. Physical factors—heat, sun, cold, pressure, emotional stress

Clinical Manifestations

1. Raised, dime-to-saucer–sized red edematous wheals
2. May affect any body region
3. Intense pruritus

Diagnosis

1. History to determine possible exposure to an offending agent.
2. Laboratory—erythrocyte sedimentation rate is often elevated.
3. Skin biopsy to rule out urticaria pigmentosa.
4. Challenge testing to determine physical cause
   a. Exercise challenge.
   b. Ice cube challenge.
   c. Heat challenge.
   d. Pressure challenge.

Management

A. Acute Urticaria

1. Identification and elimination of causative factors
2. Medications
   a. H_1 antihistamine (terfenadine)
   b. Epinephrine 1:1000 (0.3–0.5 ml. subcutaneously) for extensive urticaria, angioedema
   c. Corticosteroids—limited to severe cases unresponsive to antihistamines

B. Chronic Urticaria

1. Elimination diet
2. Medications
   a. H_1 antihistamines (terfenadine)
   b. H_1 and H_2 antihistamines (hydroxyzine and ranitidine)
   c. Tricyclic antidepressants (doxepin)—given for antihistaminic effect
   d. Topical agents to relieve itching (Lubriderm)

Patient Education

1. Avoid exposure to heat, exercise, sunburn, fever, anxiety, and alcohol—factors that may aggravate reactions due to vasodilation.

2. Avoid triggers of exacerbation if identified.
3. Inform patients of action of medications prescribed, correct dosage, and possible side effects.
4. Instruct patients in self-administration of epinephrine if there is a history of laryngeal edema.

Bibliography

Books

Ames SW and Kneisl CR. Essentials of Adult Health Nursing. Menlo Park, CA, Addison-Wesley, 1988

Brunner LS and Suddarth DS. Textbook of Medical–Surgical Nursing. Philadelphia, JB Lippincott, 1988

Graziano FM and Lemanske RF. Clinical Immunology. Baltimore, Williams & Wilkins, 1989

Kaplan A. Allergy. New York, Churchill Livingstone, 1985

Lockey RF and Bukantz SC. Fundamentals of Immunology and Allergy. Philadelphia, WB Saunders, 1987

Lockey RF and Bukantz SC, Principles of Immunology and Allergy. Philadelphia, WB Saunders, 1987

Middleton E Jr et al. Allergy: Principles and Practice. St Louis, CV Mosby, 1988

Patterson R. Allergic Diseases. Philadelphia, JB Lippincott, 1985

Roitt I et al. Immunology. St Louis, CV Mosby, 1985

Schwartz GR et al. Emergency Medicine. Philadelphia, WB Saunders, 1989

Stites DP. Basic and Clinical Immunology. Norwalk, CT, Appleton & Lange, 1987

Journals

Allergy

Alderman C. Starting from scratch. Nurs Stand 1988 May 28; 2(34):36–37

Bernstein IL. Proceedings of the task force on guidelines for standardizing old and new technologies used for the diagnosis and treatment of allergic diseases. J Allergy Clin Immunol 1988 Sep; 82(3):487–526

Blumenthal MN et al. Preventive allergy: Genetics of IgE-mediated diseases. J Allergy Clin Immunol 1986 Nov; 78(5 Part 1):962–968

Bock SA et al. Double-blind placebo-controlled food challenge as an office procedure: A manual. J Allergy Clin Immunol 1988 Dec; 82(6):986–997

Carlson RW et al. Anaphylactic, anaphylactoid, and related forms of shock. Crit Care Clin 1986 Apr; 2(2):347–372

Dawson M. Immunology. Nurs Times 1988 Apr 27–May 3; 84(17):75–78

Dawson M. Specific immunity. Nurs Times 1988 May 4; 84(18):73–76

Dawson M. Specific immunity. Nurs Times 1988 May 11; 84(19):69–72

Fineman SM. Urticaria and angioedema. Immunol Allergy Clin North Am 1987 Aug; 7(2):265–275

Frank G. Scratching the surface. Nurs Times 1987 Sep 30; 83(39):66–68

Guerin B and Watson RD. Skin tests. Clin Rev Allergy 1988 Summer; 6(2):211–227

Guill MF. Allergy emergencies. Immunol Allergy Clin North Am 1987 Dec; 7(3):485–500

Kaliner MA. Late phase reactions. N Engl Reg Allergy Proc 1986 May–Jun; 7(3):236–240

Klein GL et al. The miseries of hay fever. Postgrad Med 1989 May; 85(6):163–172

Lehmann P. More than you ever thought you would know about food additives. FDA Consumer HEW Publication No (FDA) 79-2119 US Department of Health, Education, and Welfare. Reprinted from Jun 1979

Leinhas JL et al. Food allergy challenges: Guidelines and implications. J Am Diet Assoc 1987 May; 87(5):604–608

Lockey RF and Bukantz SC. Allergy and immunology. JAMA 1989 May 19; 261(19):2824–2825

Marone G et al. Pathophysiology of human basophils and mast cells in allergic disorders. Clin Immunol Immunopathol 1989 Jan; 50:(1 Part II):S24–S40

Paller AS. Allergy and atopic dermatitis. Immun Allergy Clin North Am 1987 Aug; 7(2):255–264

Pepper GA. OTCs vs Rx for allergic rhinitis. Nurse Pract 1987 Jun; 12(6):58–62

Randall BJ. Reacting to anaphylaxis. Nursing 1986 Mar; 16(3):34–39

Reckling JB and Neuberger GB. Understanding immune system dysfunction. Nursing 1987 Sep; 17(9):34–41

Regan C. The foodservice industry's responsibility toward the food-sensitive patient. Ann Allergy 1988 Dec; 61(6 Part 2):88–90

Shapiro GG. Understanding allergic rhinitis: Differential diagnosis and management. Pediatrics Rev 1986 Jan; 7(7):212–218

Van Arsdal P Jr and Larson EB. Allergy testing. Ann Intern Med 1989 Feb; 110(4):317–320

Van Arsdal P Jr and Larson EB. Diagnostic tests for patients with suspected allergic disease. Ann Intern Med 1989 Feb; 110(4):304–312

Wiggins CA et al. Idiopathic anaphylaxis: A review. Ann Allergy 1989 Jan; 62(1):1–5

Wilson NM. Bronchial hyperreactivity in food and drink intolerance. Ann Allergy 1988 Dec; 61(6 Part 2):75–79

Asthma

Alexander JS et al. Effectiveness of a nurse-managed program for children with chronic asthma. J Pediatr Nurs 1988 Oct; 3(5):312–317

Barger LW et al. Further investigation into the recent increase in asthma death rates: A review of 41 asthma deaths in Oregon in 1982. Ann Allergy 1988 Jan; 60(1):31–39

Barnes G. Asthma: Latest developments in care. Prof Nurse 1988 Jan; 3(9):364–367

Barnes PJ. Airway receptors and asthma. N Engl Reg Allergy Proc 1986 May–Jun; 7(3):219–227

Barnes PJ. Asthma management—A new dimension. J Int Med Res 1987 Nov–Dec; 15(6):397–400

Burr ML. Is asthma increasing? J Epidemiol Community Health 1987 Sep; 41(3):185–189

Connolly CK et al. The influence of social factors on the control of asthma. Postgrad Med J 1989 May; 65(763):282–285

Holgate ST and Finnerty JP. Recent advances in understanding the pathogenesis of asthma and its clinical implications. Q J Med 1988 Jan; 66(249):5–19

Kaliner M. Asthma and mast cell activation. J Allergy Clin Immunol 1989 Feb; 83(2):510–519

Klingelhofer EL and Gershwin ME. Asthma self-management programs: Premises, not promises. J Asthma 1988 Apr; 25(2):89–101

Morris HG. An update on treatment of asthma with inhaled steroids. N Engl Reg Allergy Proc 1987 Mar–Apr; 8(2):85–94

Norn S and Clementsen P. Bronchial asthma: Pathophysiological mechanisms and corticosteroids. Allergy 1988 Aug; 43(6):401–405

Palma-Carlos AG. Prevention of asthma. Allerg Immunol (Paris) 1986 Apr; 18(4):27–29

Parker SR. The future role of asthma self-management. J Allergy Clin Immunol 1987 Sep; 80(3):511–514

Pollart SM et al. Epidemiology of acute asthma: IgE antibodies to common inhalant allergens as a risk factor for emergency room visits. J Allergy Clin Immunol 1989 May; 83(5):875–881

Sears MR. Increasing asthma mortality—Fact or artifact? J Allergy Clin Immunol 1988 Dec; 82(6):957–960

Shekelton ME. Coping with chronic respiratory difficulty. Nurs Clin North Am 1987 Sep; 22(3):569–581

Taggart VS et al. Adapting a self-management education program for asthma for use in an outpatient clinic. Ann Allergy 1987 Mar; 58(3):173–178

Tobin DL et al. The asthma self-efficacy scale. Ann Allergy 1987 Oct; 59(4): 273–277

Wilson–Pessano SR and Mellins RB. Workshop on asthma self-management. J Allergy Clin Immunol 1987 Sep; 80(3):487–491

Wissing DR et al. Use of respiratory care procedures in the management of hospitalized asthmatics. Ann Allergy 1988 Dec; 61:407–415

Agencies

American Academy of Allergy and
  Immunology
611 East Wells St.
Milwaukee, WI 53202

Asthma and Allergy Foundation of
  America
1717 Massachusetts Ave.
Suite 305
Washington, DC 20036

Mothers of Asthmatics
10875 Main Street
Suite 210
Fairfax, VA 22030

National Institute of Allergy and
  Infectious Diseases
National Institutes of Health
Bethesda, MD 20892

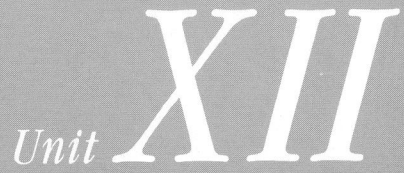

Unit *XII*

Acute Problems

37 Infectious Diseases

The Infection Process

The transmission of an infectious agent is accomplished by an infectious source, a vector of spread, and a susceptible host.

Causative Agent

Type: bacterium, virus, fungus, parasite, rickettsia, helminth, etc.
1. Pathogenicity (ability to cause disease)
2. Virulence (disease severity) and invasiveness (ability to enter and move through tissue)
3. Infective dose (number of organisms needed to initiate infection)
4. Organism specificity (host preference), antigenic variations
5. Elaboration of toxins

Reservoir

(The environment in which the agent is found)
1. Human—man is the reservoir of diseases that are more dangerous to humans than to other species
2. Animal—responsible for infestations with trophozoites, worms, etc.
3. Nonanimal—street dust, garden soil, lint from bedding

Mode of Escape from Reservoir

1. Respiratory tract (most common in human)
2. Gastrointestinal tract
3. Genitourinary tract
4. Open lesions
5. From bloodstream or tissues by insect bites, hypodermic needles, or surgical instruments

Mode of Transmission

There are 4 main routes of transmission.

A. By Contact Transmission
1. Direct contact (person to person)
2. Indirect contact (usually an inanimate object)
3. Droplet contact (from coughing, sneezing, or talking by an infected person)

B. By Vehicle Route (through contaminated items)
1. Food—salmonellosis
2. Water—shigellosis, legionellosis
3. Drugs—bacteremia resulting from infusion of a contaminated infusion product
4. Blood—hepatitis B

C. Airborne Transmission
1. Droplet nuclei (residue of evaporated droplets that remain suspended in air)
2. Dust particles in the air containing the infectious agent
3. Organisms shed into environment from skin, hair, wounds, or perineal area

D. Vectorborne Transmission

Via contaminated or infected arthropods, such as flies, mosquitoes, ticks, and others

Mode of Entry of Organisms Into Human Body

1. Respiratory tract
2. Gastrointestinal tract
3. Genitourinary tract
4. Direct infection of mucous membranes/break in skin

Host Factors

Illness following entrance of infection into the body depends on:
1. Number of organisms to which host is exposed; duration of exposure

2. Age, genetic constitution of host, and general physical, mental, and emotional health and nutritional status of host
3. Status of hematopoietic system; efficacy of reticulo-endothelial system
4. Absent or abnormal immunoglobulins
5. The number of T lymphocytes and their ability to function

Changing Patterns of Infectious Diseases
(Fig. 37-1)

1. Changing world with acceleration of speed and extent in number of ideas, objects, people
2. Life style changes including sexual practices, abuse of illicit substances, dietary trends, ready availability of travel, immigration
3. Impact of medical progress: infectious disease complications of transplant recipients/immunosuppressed hosts, foreign implants (prosthetic joints; heart valves), hemodialysis, indwelling lines, use of blood and blood products for therapeutic purposes, fungemia, bacteremia, atypical mycobacterial abscesses, etc.
4. Acute gastroenterologic problems are a major source of morbidity and mortality in most Third World countries, causing a cycle of infection–malabsorption–malnutrition.

Epidemiology, Therapy, and Control of Communicable Infections

See Table 37-1, pages 890–892.

Control and Management of Infectious Disease

Immunization

Immunity is the resistance that an individual has against disease.

1. Specific immunity to a particular organism implies that an individual has either generated the appropriate antibody in his own body or received ready-made antibodies from another source.
2. Immunity may be natural (not acquired through previous contact with the infectious agent) or acquired (resistance acquired by the host as a result of previous exposure to the disease).
3. Acquired immunity may be *passive* or *active*.

Active Immunization

Active immunization is immunization that has been produced by natural or acquired stimulation so that the body produces its own antibodies.

1. It may result from clinical or subclinical infection (the person gets the disease); by vaccination with live or killed microorganisms or their antigens; or by inactivated vaccines and toxoids.
2. The organisms have been treated by heating or by chemical inactivation to destroy their harmful properties without destroying their ability to stimulate antibody protection.
3. Depending on age and health status, adults may be immunized against tetanus, diphtheria, measles, and rubella and high-risk groups (those over 65, and those with chronic heart, lung, and metabolic diseases) may be immunized against influenza, pneumococcal pneumonia, and hepatitis B.
4. Current recommendations for the administration of vaccines and other biologicals are available from the Advisory Committee on Immunization Practices of the US Public Health Service, Centers for Disease Control, Atlanta, GA 30333.

Passive Immunity

Passive immunity to a disease is a state of relatively short-lived immunity produced by the injection of serum containing antibodies that have been formed in another host. Types of preparations for passive immunity:

1. Nonspecific immune globulin—used for immune maintenance of selected immunodeficient persons as

(Text continues on p. 893)

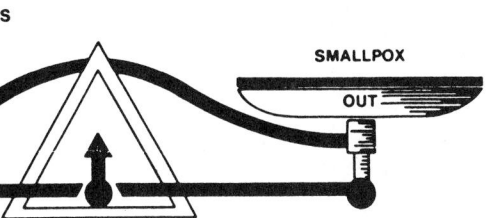

AIDS
BABESIOSIS
LASSA FEVER
TOXIC SHOCK
LYME DISEASE
INFANT BOTULISM
CRYPTOSPORIDIOSIS
KAWASAKI DISEASE
NON A, NON B HEPATITIS
ROTAVIRUS DIARRHEA
LEGIONNAIRES' DISEASE
DELTA VIRUS HEPATITIS
CHLAMYDIA PNEUMONIA
INVASIVE EXTERNAL OTITIS
CAMPYLOBACTER ENTERITIS
PSEUDOMONAS FOLLICULITIS
AMEBIC MENINGOENCEPHALITIS
VIBRIO PARAHEMOLYTICUS ENTERITIS
CLOSTRIDIUM DIFFICILE DIARRHEA
AND OTHERS

IN

SMALLPOX

OUT

Figure 37-1. *Changing patterns of infectious diseases: The last 20 years. None of the new infectious diseases on the left-hand side of the balance was part of our health care vocabulary 20 years ago. While acquiring many new afflictions, we rid ourselves of one very old one—smallpox. (From Lorber B: Changing patterns of infectious diseases. Am J Med 1988 Mar; 84 [3, part 2]:571)*

Table 37-1. *Epidemiology and Control of Selected Communicable Infections*

Disease	Infective Organism	Infectious Sources	Entry Site	Method of Spread	Incubation Period	Prophylaxis
Amebiasis	*Entamoeba histolytica*	Contaminated water and food	Gastrointestinal tract	Patients and carriers; fecal–oral route; oral and sexual contact	Variable	Detection of carriers and their removal from food handling; plumbing safeguards
Bacillary dysentery (shigellosis)	*Shigella* group	Contaminated water and food	Gastrointestinal tract	Patients and carriers; fecal–oral route	24–48 hours	Detection and control of carriers; inspection of food handlers, decontamination of water supplies
Brucellosis	*Brucella melitensis* and related organisms	Milk, meat, tissues, blood, and absorbed fetuses and placentas from infected cattle, goats, horses, and pigs	Gastrointestinal tract	Ingestion of or contact with infective material	5–30 days (variable)	Milk pasteurization; control of infection in animals
Chancroid	*Haemophilus ducreyi*	Human cases and carriers	Genitalia	Direct sexual contact	3–5 days	Effective case-finding and treatment of infection
Chickenpox (varicella)	Varicella-zoster (V-Z) virus	Human cases	Probably nasopharynx	Probably respiratory droplets	13–17 days	Varicella-zoster immune globulin (VZIG) primarily for immunocompromised children and certain neonates exposed *in utero*
Diphtheria	*Corynebacterium diphtheriae*	Human cases and carriers; fomites; raw milk	Nasopharynx	Nasal and oral secretions; respiratory droplets	2–5 days	Active immunization with diphtheria toxoid
Encephalitis, epidemic (eastern and western equine)	Viruses	Chicken and wild-bird mites; horses	Skin	Mosquitoes	Variable	Destroy larvae; eliminate breeding of mosquitoes Eastern equine encephalitis vaccine for those under continued and intensive exposure
Gonorrhea	*Neisseria gonorrhoeae*	Urethral and vaginal secretions	Urethral or vaginal mucosa; pharynx; rectum	Sexual activity	2–7 days	Examination culture; treatment of sexual partners
Granuloma inguinale	*Calymmatobacterium granulomatis*	Infectious exudate	External genitalia; inguinal and anal region	Direct contact with lesions during sexual activity	Unknown, presumably 8–80 days	Chemotherapy of carriers and contacts; case-finding and treatment of patients
Infectious mononucleosis	Epstein–Barr virus	Human cases and carriers	Mouth	Probably oral–pharyngeal route; via blood transfusion in susceptible recipients	2–6 weeks	None
Influenza	Virus	Human cases	Respiratory tract	Respiratory	24–72 hours	Influenza virus vaccine
Lymphogranuloma venereum	*Chlamydia trachomatis*	Human cases	External genitalia; urethral or vaginal mucosa	Sexual intercourse; indirect contact with contaminated articles/clothing	5–21 days	Case-finding and treatment of infection

Disease	Causative organism	Reservoir/Source	Portal of entry	Mode of transmission	Incubation period	Control measures
Malaria	*Plasmodium vivax, P. falciparum, P. malariae, and P. ovale*	Human cases	Skin	Mosquitoes (*Anopheles*)	Variable, depending on strain	Coordinated measures for wide-scale mosquito control; prompt detection and effective treatment of cases; suppressive drugs in malarious areas
Measles	Virus	Human cases	Respiratory mucosa	Nasopharyngeal secretions	8–13 days	Measles vaccine
Meningococcal meningitis	*Neisseria meningitidis*	Human cases and carriers	Nasopharynx; tonsils	Respiratory droplets	2–10 days	Meningococcal polysaccharide vaccine for persons at risk; rifampin for carriers or contacts
Mumps	Virus	Human cases (early)	Upper respiratory tract	Respiratory droplets	2–3 weeks (avg. 18 days)	Live mumps vaccine
Paratyphoid fever	*Salmonella paratyphi* A, B, and C, and related organisms	Contaminated food, milk, water	Gastrointestinal tract	Infected feces or rarely urine	7–21 days	Control of public water sources, food vendors, food handlers; treatment of carriers
Pneumococcal pneumonia	*Streptococcus pneumoniae*	Human carriers; patient's own pharynx	Respiratory mucosa	Respiratory droplets	Variable	Polyvalent pneumococcal vaccine; control of upper respiratory infections; avoidance of alcoholic intoxication
Poliomyelitis	Polioviruses (types I, II, III)	Human cases and carriers	Gastrointestinal tract	Pharyngeal secretions; fecal–oral	7–14 days	Oral polio vaccine (OPV), the live attenuated vaccine containing all three strains of poliovirus—produces long-lasting immunity in most recipients
Rocky Mountain spotted fever	*Rickettsia rickettsii*	Infected wild rodents, dogs, wood ticks, dog ticks	Skin	Tick bites	3–14 days	Avoidance of tick-infested areas, or wearing of protective clothing in such areas; frequent search for, and prompt removal of, ticks from body; specific vaccination of exposed persons
Rubella (German measles)	Virus	Human cases	Respiratory mucosa	Nasopharyngeal secretions	14–23 days	Rubella virus vaccine; immune globulin (human) given to contacts of rubella; rubella in early stages of pregnancy legally recognized as indication for abortion

(continued)

Table 37-1. Epidemiology and Control of Selected Communicable Infections (continued)

Disease	Infective Organism	Infectious Sources	Entry Site	Method of Spread	Incubation Period	Prophylaxis
Syphilis	*Treponema pallidum*	Infected exudates, body fluids, and secretions (saliva, semen, blood, vaginal secretions)	External genitalia; cervix; mucosal surfaces; placenta	Sexual activity; contact with open lesions; blood transfusion; transplacental inoculation	10–70 days	Case-finding by means of routine serologic testing and other methods; adequate treatment of infected individuals
Tetanus	*Clostridium tetani*	Contaminated soil	Penetrating and crush wounds	Horse and cattle feces	4–21 days (avg, 10 days)	Wound debridement; toxoid booster injections for patients previously immunized; tetanus toxoid and tetanus immune globulin (separate sites and separate syringes) for nonimmune persons
Trichinosis	*Trichinella spiralis*	Infected pigs	Gastrointestinal tract	Ingestion of infected pork, undercooked	2–28 days	Regulation of hog breeders; adequate meat inspection; thorough cooking of pork
Tuberculosis	*Mycobacterium tuberculosis*	Sputum from human cases; milk from infected cows (rare in US)	Respiratory mucosa	Sputum; respiratory droplets	Variable	Early discovery and adequate treatment of active cases; milk pasteurization
Tularemia	*Francisella tularensis*	Wild rodents and rabbits	Eyes; skin; gastrointestinal tract	Handling infected animals; ingestion of undercooked, infected meat; drinking contaminated water; bites from infected flies, ticks	1–10 days	Use of rubber gloves when skinning/handling potentially infectious wild animals; avoidance of contact with potentially infected rodents; adequate cooking of wild rabbit dishes; vaccination of hunters, butchers, laboratory workers risking heavy exposure
Typhoid fever	*Salmonella typhi*	Contaminated food and water	Gastrointestinal tract	Infected urine and feces	1–3 weeks	Decontamination of water sources; milk pasteurization; individual vaccination of high-risk persons; control of carriers.
Typhus, endemic	*Rickettsia typhi (mooseri)*	Infected rodents	Skin	Flea bites	1–2 weeks	Delousing procedures; case quarantine
Whooping cough (pertussis)	*Bordetella pertussis*	Human cases	Respiratory tract	Infected bronchial secretions	Commonly 7 days	Active immunization with vaccine; case isolation

well as for passive immunization against hepatitis A and possibly measles.

2. Specific immune globulins—contain high levels of antibody against specific pathogens that include hepatitis B, rabies, varicella-zoster, and tetanus.
3. Animal serum or antitoxins—may cause an anaphylaxis-like reaction or serum sickness.

Controlling Infectious Diseases in Health Care Facilities

General Measures

1. *Wash hands immediately after contact with each patient and after every contact with material that may be contaminated and potentially infectious.*
   a. Wash hands even if sterile gloves are used.
   b. Wear gloves for direct exposure to blood, drainage, or secretions.
2. Plan what you are going to do *before* the initial patient contact.
3. Carry out isolation precautions as required to prevent spread of microorganisms among patients, personnel, and visitors.
4. Observe asepsis as indicated.
5. Use gown when clothing is likely to become soiled with infective secretions or excretions.
   a. Use gown once and discard in appropriate receptacle.
   b. Use sterile gown in certain instances (extensive burns; wounds).
   c. Collect linen in water-soluble bags; double-bag and mark "Isolation."
6. Use gloves when indicated by the patient's condition (e.g., when excretions, secretions, blood, or body fluids are considered to be infective material).
   a. Disposable, single-use gloves should be worn.
   b. Use once and discard in appropriate receptacle.
7. Handle needles and syringes with *extreme* care because it is usually not known which patient's blood is contaminated with hepatitis virus or human immunodeficiency virus (HIV).
   a. Place used needles in a labeled, puncture-resistant container; do not bend or break by hand.
   b. Blood spills should be cleaned up promptly with a solution of 5.25% sodium hypochlorite solution diluted 1:10 with water.
8. Disinfect and handle wastes with all due precautions.
9. Handle bed linens and fomites with care.
10. Carry out concurrent disinfection of fomites.
11. Control dissemination of infectious droplets.
    a. Encourage the patient to cover nose and mouth when coughing or sneezing.
    b. Wrap contaminated tissues and articles in paper before disposal.
12. Control dust and maintain environmental cleanliness.
13. Ventilate the patient's room properly with a system that directs room air to the outside.
14. Keep the door to the room closed.

Isolation Techniques

1. *Isolation precautions* may be used to prevent the spread of infectious agents among patients, personnel, and visitors.
   a. Isolation precautions are used to isolate the infection rather than the patient.
   b. Appropriate types of isolation are selected according to the mode of transmission and pathogenesis of the infection. There are several systems for isolation:
      (1) Category-specific isolation precautions
      (2) Disease-specific isolation precautions
      (3) One designed by the individual health agency
2. The Infection Control Committee of the health agency makes the decision regarding which of the alternative systems of isolation precautions is to be used.
3. Standards of practice are evaluated in the face of new information and changing situations and are revised periodically. The Centers for Disease Control publishes an updated guideline for isolation precautions for health care facilities.

Nursing Process: The Patient With an Infectious Disease

Nursing Assessment and Clinical Manifestations

The following questions are important when taking the nursing history:

1. History of fever? Chills? (an abrupt onset of fever is usually associated with chills) Night sweats?
2. Back pain? General myalgias? Arthralgias? Headache?
3. Sore throat?
4. Diarrhea? Vomiting? Abdominal pain? Anyone in the family with these symptoms?
5. Urinary symptoms: Dysuria? Frequency? Purulent discharge?
6. Evidence of local infection: Redness? Heat? Swelling? Pain?
7. Any contact with an ill person's secretions/excretions?
8. Insect bite? Animal bite? Cat scratch? Exposure to rodents or birds?
9. History of illness that may compromise the body's defenses?
10. Medications, especially antibiotics, taken? Alcohol intake?
11. Sexual practices?
12. Travel to or from a developing country? Vaccination history?

Physical Examination

1. Look for manifestations common to many infectious diseases: breaks in skin; skin rashes; lesions in mucous membranes and skin; productive cough; breathing difficulties; purulent drainage from any site; lymph node enlargement.
2. Review results of physical examination and try to determine if patient is at risk for infecting himself or others.
3. Evaluate the nutritional status of the patient.

Management

1. The specific organism is identified, and specific therapy is instituted when available.
   a. Drug of choice is usually the most active drug against the pathogenic organism or the least toxic alternative
   b. Choice of therapy also depends on the susceptibility of the organism in the patient's environment.
2. Supportive therapy includes monitoring the patient's response to therapy, ensuring hydration, fluid balance,

and oxygenation, and maintaining watchfulness for complications.

Nursing Diagnoses

1. Ineffective breathing pattern related to infectious process; impaired host defenses secondary to immune diseases and malignancies
2. Altered body temperature (fever) related to infection
3. Potential fluid volume deficit related to excessive fever, diaphoresis, diarrhea, inability to ingest fluids
4. Altered oral mucous membranes related to fever, inability to ingest fluids, presence of oral lesions
5. Altered bowel elimination (diarrhea) related to enteric diseases secondary to bacterial, parasitic, and viral agents; altered bowel flora secondary to antibiotics
6. Altered nutrition (less than body requirements) related to prolonged infection and increased basal metabolic rate from fever
7. Potential for infection (spread to others)
8. Social isolation related to nature of disease, physiologic and organic dysfunction secondary to disease, underlying emotional state, negative interactions with others
9. Knowledge deficit of specific disease, therapeutic regimen, prevention of spread of disease, sanitation, etc.

Nursing Interventions

A. Attaining a Normal Breathing Pattern

1. Identify those at-risk for pulmonary infection and subsequent ineffective breathing patterns.
   a. Pre-existing illness (impaired immune defenses; alcoholism)—tend to cause impaired lung clearance
   b. Viral infections—cause peripheral small airway obstruction and hyperreactivity.
   c. Aging patients—have decreased pulmonary compliance
   d. Patients with endotracheal intubation/mechanical ventilation—have impaired mucociliary clearance and transport
2. Monitor for cough, sputum production, dyspnea, pleuritic pain, and changes in skin and mucous membrane color.
3. Evaluate respiratory rate, depth, and pattern; auscultate chest for breath sounds.
4. Turn the patient frequently to drain secretions; encourage the taking of deep breaths, yawning, and coughing—to expand alveolar sacs.
5. Suction when indicated.
6. Encourage a high fluid intake—to thin secretions.
7. Humidify air—to loosen secretions and improve ventilation.
8. Encourage ambulation—helps mobilize secretions and expand the lungs.

B. Attaining Normal Body Temperature

1. Take patient's temperature on a regular basis to determine magnitude of temperature elevation, duration, analysis of fever curve (intermittent, remittent, recurrent/relapsing, continuous).
   a. Most infectious diseases produce temperatures between 37° and 41°C. (99°–106°F.).
   b. Hypothermia in the presence of an infectious disease may be considered a poor prognostic indicator as fever indicates ability to respond to infection and is considered a beneficial response.
   c. Patients who are immunocompromised, those

with chronic renal insufficiency, patients with alcoholism, and the elderly may be afebrile.

> **GERONTOLOGIC ALERT:** The elderly person with an infectious disease may be afebrile. A history of sudden mental confusion in the elderly suggests an infectious cause.

2. Measure pulse rate simultaneously while taking temperature—to determine if patient's cardiovascular response is appropriate to degree of fever.
3. Assess for other manifestations of infection—headache, joint pain, muscle aches, back pain, cough, diarrhea, enlarged lymph nodes, chills, perspiration.
4. Increase fluid intake—water, Gatorade, juices, popsicles, ice chips.
5. Monitor for procedures related to bacteremia
   a. Suctioning of endotracheal tube
   b. Catheter or wound irrigation
   c. Probing or manipulating wounds
   d. These may cause single spikes of temperature.
6. Use appropriate nursing interventions to combat generalized discomfort that accompanies fever.
   a. Rest—to lower metabolic activity
   b. Intermittent cool compresses to head
   c. Oral hygiene
   d. Massage when indicated
   e. Humidification of air to relieve dry cough
7. Use tepid water sponging for reduction of fever only when appropriate as fever is an important host defense mechanism—sponging cools body by evaporation of water.

C. Attaining Fluid Balance

1. Assess for signs of dehydration—thirst, weakness and malaise, dry mucous membranes, decreased skin turgor, decreased sweating, orthostatic changes in pulse and blood pressure, weight loss.
2. Note serum electrolyte values—dehydration produces a deficit of some electrolytes.
3. Maintain input and output record; monitor urine specific gravity.
4. Administer prescribed intravenous (IV) fluids—to restore volume deficits.
5. Vary the type and temperature of oral fluids when patient is able to ingest fluids.

D. Achieving Healthy Oral Mucous Membranes

1. Inspect oral cavity daily for color, signs of infection, bleeding, and presence of cracks, lesions, or coatings.
2. Reinforce the importance and techniques of oral hygiene.
3. Use normal saline or warm-water mouth rinses—to remove debris and keep mucosa clean and moist; avoid strong mouthwashes.
4. Apply petrolatum to dry, cracked lips.
5. Encourage a high fluid intake.

E. Achieving Satisfactory Bowel Elimination

1. Ask about the number, color, form of stools. Blood or mucus present?
2. Determine if there is nausea, vomiting, abdominal pain. Fever?
3. Assess for signs and symptoms of dehydration.
4. Monitor and record intake, output, and weight.
5. Use enteric precautions for collecting stool specimens and for hospitalized patients with infectious diarrhea.
6. Give prescribed oral glucose/rehydration solution;

advise clear liquids such as gingerale, Gatorade, or broth taken in small amounts every 30 minutes when there are prolonged symptoms.

7. Administer prescribed IV fluids for severe dehydration.

8. Inspect perianal area for signs of skin breakdown. Instruct patient to cleanse area with mild soap and water and blot dry after each bowel movement.

9. Use meticulous handwashing technique.

F. Improving Nutritional Status

1. Take a food history to determine what the patient is actually eating.

2. Monitor weight.

3. Assess food intake—a high-calorie, high-protein diet is usually prescribed for patients with fever to replenish energy used by increased metabolism.

G. Preventing the Spread of Infection

1. Follow the general measures described under Controlling Infectious Diseases in Health Care Facilities, page 893.

2. Implement appropriate isolation techniques according to institutional protocols.

H. Promoting Social Participation

1. Develop a trusting relationship with the patient and family.
   a. Spend unhurried time with the patient.
   b. Show sensitivity to the patient's feelings; avoid showing repulsion.
   c. Employ a nonjudgmental approach to the patient with sexually transmitted disease.
   d. Lend encouragement to the patient faced with prospect of prolonged convalescence.

2. Relieve anxiety and depression of patient/family.
   a. Recognize loneliness of the isolated patient.
   b. Employ active listening without interruption; accept the patient's feelings and thoughts without judgment.
   c. Give appropriate feedback.
   d. Include the patient in decision making.
   e. Encourage family to communicate feelings, expressions of support and affection.

Patient Education

1. Give brief and focused information about the organism and its spread and how the illness is treated—help the patient to become an active participant.

2. Correct any misunderstandings.

3. Give the patient/family instruction in handwashing and personal hygiene measures as well as in isolation precautions.

4. Educate the public with respect to:
   a. Availability and importance of prophylactic immunization
   b. Manner in which infectious illnesses are spread, methods of avoiding spread, and the importance of available immunizations
   c. Importance of seeking health care promptly in the event of a febrile illness or skin eruption
   d. Importance of environmental cleanliness and personal hygiene
   e. Importance of adequate housing and nutrition
   f. Means of preventing the contamination of food and water supplies
   g. Knowledge of insect, rodent, and other animal vectors and reservoirs of human infections and the importance of eliminating them

Evaluation

1. Attains/maintains normal breathing pattern

2. Demonstrates absence of elevated body temperature

3. Attains fluid balance; normal skin turgor

4. Attains/maintains intact and and healthy-appearing oral mucous membranes

5. Regains a more normal elimination pattern.

6. Achieves improved nutritional status; appears to have more energy

7. Protects self and others from spread of infection

8. Achieves some social participation; shares feelings and anxieties of alienation

9. Becomes informed of infectious disease process; knows measures to take when symptoms appear

---

Sexually Transmitted Diseases (STDs)

Sexually transmitted diseases are transmitted by sexual activity and include the traditional venereal diseases as well as nonspecific urethral and genital infections, enteric infections, and parasitic infestations (Table 37-2).

1. More than 30 etiologic agents are transmitted by sexual activity; most cases arise in sexually active adolescents and young adults.

2. Patients present with multisystem manifestations, urethritis, urethral and vaginal discharge, lesions and rashes.

3. Coinfection with two or more STDs is fairly common.

4. Persons at risk are heterosexuals and homosexuals who change partners frequently.

Basic Facts About STD

1. Sexually transmitted disease is acquired by sexual contact (vaginal sexual intercourse, anal intercourse, oral intercourse) and by close and direct contact with an infected person.

2. A person who thinks that he may have a sexually transmitted disease or who has been exposed to someone who might have it should have a checkup. Immediate treatment should be sought if symptoms develop.

3. Anyone who is sexually active with a number of sexual partners should have regular checkups.

4. Washing the sex organs (before and after sexual contact) and the use of a condom may give limited protection against sexually transmitted disease.

5. Birth control pills and IUDs give no protection against sexually transmitted disease.

6. Gonorrhea and syphilis are different diseases, caused by different organisms.
   a. They attack the body in different ways but are spread in the same manner.
   b. A person may have both gonorrhea and syphilis as well as other sexually transmitted diseases at the same time.

7. There appears to be no natural or acquired immunity to gonorrhea and syphilis. A person can get gonorrhea and syphilis again and again.

8. Pregnant women may pass infection of syphilis to the unborn child. Pregnant women may pass gonorrhea to the baby during the birthing process.

9. Bacteria from gonorrhea may enter the bloodstream and affect joints, joint linings, heart valves, etc.

(Text continues on p. 902)

Table 37-2. Sexually Transmitted Disease Summary—1986 *

Disease and Etiologic Agents	Typical Clinical Presentation	Presumptive Diagnosis (warrants full treatment and follow-up)	Definitive Diagnosis
CHLAMYDIAL INFECTIONS			
Nongonococcal Urethritis (NGU)			
Chlamydia trachomatis A human mycoplasma of the T-strain. Other sexually transmissible agents can cause NGU; these include *Ureaplasma urealyticum, Trichomonas vaginalis, Candida albicans,* Herpes simplex virus.	Men usually have dysuria, frequency, and mucoid to purulent urethral discharge. Some men have asymptomatic infections. Steady female sexual partners of men with chlamydial NGU are likely to have chlamydial endocervicitis.	Men with typical clinical symptoms are presumed to have NGU when their gonorrhea tests are negative and they have either WBCs on Gram stain of urethral discharge or sexual exposure to an agent known to cause NGU. Asymptomatic men with negative gonorrhea tests are also presumed to have NGU if they have at least 4 WBCs per oil immersion field on an intraurethral smear.	An agent etiologically associated with NGU is recovered from the male urethra. **NOTE:** Gonococcal and nongonococcal urethritis may coexist in the same patient.
Mucopurulent Cervicitis (MPC)			
Chlamydia trachomatis is the principal pathogen, although *Neisseria gonorrhoeae,* herpes simplex virus, *Candida albicans,* and *Trichomonas vaginalis* can also produce cervicitis (see relevant panels).	The patient may be symptomatic or asymptomatic, and a yellow mucopurulent endocervical exudate may be present. Cervical ectopy appears to be correlated with cervical infection with this agent.	The presence of yellow mucopurulent endocervical exudate or the finding of this exudate on a white cotton-tipped swab of endocervical secretions suggests infection with *C. trachomatis.* In women without visible mucopus, the presence of greater than or equal to 10 PMN leukocytes per × 1000 field on a Gram-stained specimen of endocervical mucus (without contamination by vaginal cells) also allows a presumptive diagnosis.	Definitive diagnosis is made by growth of *C. trachomatis* on cycloheximide-treated McCoy cells. If confirmatory tests are not available or affordable, empirical therapy can be given on clinical grounds.
GONORRHEA			
Neisseria gonorrhoeae A gram-negative diplococcus.	When symptomatic, men usually have dysuria, frequency, and purulent urethral discharge. Women may have abnormal vaginal discharge, abnormal menses, dysuria, or be asymptomatic. Anorectal and pharyngeal infections are common. These may be symptomatic or asymptomatic.	Microscopic identification of typical gram-negative intracellular diplococci on smear of urethral exudate (men) or endocervical material (women). Cervical specimens that are Gram stain tested should also be cultured for *N. gonorrhoeae.* OR Growth on selective medium demonstrating typical colonial morphology, positive oxidase reaction, and typical Gram stain morphology.	Growth on selective medium demonstrating typical colonial morphology, positive oxidase reaction, typical Gram stain morphology, and confirmed by sugar utilization, coagglutination or antigonococcal fluorescent antibody (FA) testing. A definitive diagnosis is required if specimen is extragenital, from a child, or medico–legally significant.
PELVIC INFLAMMATORY DISEASE (PID)			
Neisseria gonorrhoeae *Chlamydia trachomatis* An obligate intracellular organism of immunotypes A through K. Other microorganisms cause PID. Most of these have not been associated with sexual transmission.	The patient may present with pain and tenderness involving the lower abdomen, cervix, uterus, and adnexae, possibly combined with fever, chills, and elevated white blood cell (WBC) count and erythrocyte sedimentation rate (ESR). The diagnosis is more likely if the patient has multiple sexual partners, a history of PID, uses an intrauterine device (IUD), or is in the first 5–10 days of her menstrual cycle.	Women who have the typical clinical presentation are presumed to have PID if other serious conditions such as acute appendicitis or ectopic pregnancy can be excluded. **Hospitalization and Inpatient Treatment** Hospitalization of patients with acute PID should be strongly considered when: (1) The diagnosis is uncertain; (2) surgical emergencies such as appendicitis and ectopic pregnancy can-	Direct visualization of inflamed (edema, hyperemia, or tubal exudate) fallopian tube(s) at laparoscopy or laparotomy makes the diagnosis of PID definitive. A culture of tubal exudate establishes the etiology.

Tetracycline hydrochloride (HCl) 500 mg., by mouth, 4 times daily for 7 days; OR

Doxycycline 100 mg., by mouth, twice daily for 7 days

Alternative Regimens

(for patients in whom tetracyclines are contraindicated or not tolerated)

Erythromycin base or stearate: 500 mg., by mouth, 4 times daily for 7 days; OR

Erythromycin ethylsuccinate 800 mg., by mouth, 4 times daily for 7 days.

NOTE: Patients with persistent or recurrent objective signs of urethritis after adequate treatment of themselves and their partners warrant further evaluation for less common causes of urethritis.

Urethral strictures

Prostatitis

Epididymitis

Chlamydial NGU may be transmitted to female sexual partners resulting in mucopurulent endocervicitis, PID, and other adverse outcomes. (See below.)

Understand how to take any prescribed oral medications. If tetracycline is prescribed, take it 1 hour before or 2 hours after meals and avoid dairy products, antacids, iron or other mineral-containing preparations, and sunlight.

Return for test-of-cure or evaluation 4–7 days after completion of therapy, or earlier if symptoms persist or recur.

Refer sexual partner(s) for examination and treatment.

Avoid sex until patient and partner(s) are cured.

Use condoms to prevent future infections.

If *N. gonorrhoeae* is not found, treatment should be given as noted above for NGU.

Special considerations should be given in the following cases:

Treatment During Pregnancy

Erythromycin base or stearate: 500 mg., by mouth, 4 times daily for 7 days on an empty stomach; OR

Erythromycin ethylsuccinate 800 mg., by mouth, 4 times daily for 7 days.

Alternative Regimen (for women who cannot tolerate these regimens)

Erythromycin base or stearate: 250 mg., by mouth, 4 times daily for at least 14 days; OR

Erythromycin ethylsuccinate 400 mg., by mouth, 4 times daily for at least 14 days.

NOTE: The optimal dose and duration of antibiotic therapy for pregnant women has not been established.

If *N. gonorrhoeae* is found on Gram stain or culture of endocervical or urethral discharge, treatment should be given as recommended for uncomplicated gonorrhea in adults. (See immediately below.)

Ascending infections may lead to symptomatic or asymptomatic endometritis and salpingitis and subsequent infertility. Ascending infection during pregnancy may lead to adverse obstetric outcomes, conjunctivitis, or pneumonia in the infant, and puerperal infection.

Understand how to take any prescribed oral medications. If tetracycline is given, take it 1 hour before or 2 hours after meals, and avoid dairy products, antacids, iron or other mineral-containing preparations, and sunlight.

Return for reevaluation 4–7 days after completion of therapy, or earlier if symptoms persist or recur.

Refer sexual partner(s) for examination and treatment.

Avoid sex until patient and partner(s) are cured.

Use condoms to prevent future infections.

Amoxicillin 3.0 g. by mouth; OR

Ampicillin 3.5 g. by mouth; OR

Aqueous procaine penicillin G (APPG) 4.8 million units IM; OR

Ceftriaxone 250 mg. IM

NOTE: Amoxicillin, ampicillin, and penicillin (but not ceftriaxone) are accompanied by probenecid 1 g by mouth

PLUS

Tetracycline HCl 500 mg., by mouth, 4 times daily for 7 days; OR

Doxycycline 100 mg., by mouth, twice daily for 7 days.

In patients in whom tetracyclines are contraindicated or not tolerated, the single dose regimen may be followed by:

Erythromycin base or stearate: 500 mg., by mouth, 4 times daily for 7 days; OR

Erythromycin ethylsuccinate 800 mg., by mouth, 4 times daily for 7 days.

Special Considerations

In women with rectal infection, the above regimens are effective.

Homosexual men with rectal gonococcal infection should be treated with ceftriaxone 250 mg. IM or aqueous procaine penicillin G 4.8 million units IM plus probenecid 1.0 g. by mouth. For those allergic to penicillin, use spectinomycin 2.0 g IM.

Patients allergic to penicillins, cephalosporins, or probenecid should be treated with tetracycline 500 mg. by mouth 4 times daily for 7 days or doxycycline 100 mg. by mouth twice daily for 7 days

Those patients who cannot tolerate tetracyclines may be treated with spectinomycin 2.0 g. IM followed by erythromycin (except for homosexual men)

NOTE: Spectinomycin, 2.0 g. IM, is indicated for patients with uncomplicated penicillin resistant *N. gonorrhoeae* (PPNG and CMRNG) infections, treatment failures and patients unable to tolerate both penicillin and tetracycline.

10%–20% of women develop pelvic inflammatory disease (PID) and are at risk for its sequelae (see below).

Men are at risk for epididymitis, sterility, urethral stricture, and infertility.

Newborns are at risk for ophthalmia neonatorum, scalp abscess at the site of fetal monitors, rhinitis, pneumonia, or anorectal infections.

All infected, untreated persons are at risk for disseminated gonococcal infection (includes septicemia, arthritis, dermatitis, meningitis, and endocarditis).

Understand how to take any prescribed oral medications. If tetracycline is prescribed, take it 1 hour before or 2 hours after meals and avoid dairy products, antacids, iron or other mineral-containing preparations, and sunlight.

Return for test-of-cure 4–7 days after completing therapy.

Refer sexual partners for examination and treatment.

Avoid sex until patient and partner(s) are cured.

Return early if symptoms persist or recur.

Use condoms to prevent future infections.

Regimen A

Doxycycline 100 mg. IV twice daily; PLUS

Cefoxitin 2.0 g. IV 4 times daily

Regimen B

Clindamycin 600 mg. IV 4 times daily; PLUS

Gentamicin 2.0 mg./kg. IV followed by 1.5 mg./kg. 3 times daily in patients with normal renal function.

NOTE: Continue drugs IV at least 4 days and at least 48 hours after patient improves. Then continue doxycycline 100 mg. by mouth twice a day (Regimen A) OR clindamycin 450 mg. by mouth 4 times daily (Regimen B), to complete 10–14 days total therapy.

Potentially life-threatening complications include ectopic pregnancy and pelvic abscess. Other complications are involuntary infertility, recurrent PID, chronic PID, chronic abdominal pain, pelvic adhesions, premature hysterectomy, and depression.

Understand how to take any prescribed oral medications. If tetracycline is given, take it 1 hour before or 2 hours after meals and avoid dairy products, antacids, iron or other mineral-containing preparations, and sunlight.

Return 2–3 days after initiation of therapy for progress evaluation.

Return for test-of-cure 4–7 days after completing therapy.

Refer sexual partner(s) for evaluation and treatment.

Avoid sexual activity until patient and partner(s) are cured.

(continued)

Table 37-2. Sexually Transmitted Disease Summary—1986 * (continued)

Disease and Etiologic Agents	Typical Clinical Presentation	Presumptive Diagnosis (warrants full treatment and follow-up)	Definitive Diagnosis
		not be excluded; (3) a pelvic abscess is suspected; (4) severe illness precludes outpatient management; (5) the patient is pregnant; (6) the patient is unable to follow or tolerate an outpatient regimen; (7) the patient has failed to respond to outpatient therapy; or, (8) the clinical follow-up after 48–72 hours of starting antibiotic treatment cannot be arranged. Many experts recommend that all patients with PID be hospitalized for treatment.	

VAGINITIS

Trichomonas vaginalis vaginitis A motile protozoan with an undulating membrane and four flagella. *Bacterial vaginosis* (also called nonspecific vaginitis or *Gardnerella vaginalis*-associated vaginitis). An infection of uncertain etiology: *Gardnerella vaginalis* (a small gram-negative pleomorphic coccobacillus), *Mobiluncus* spp. (motile, curved anaerobic rods), and other anaerobes have been implicated. Fungal vaginitis (predominantly *Candida albicans*) Dimorphic fungi which grow as oval budding yeast cells and as chains of cells (hyphae). Other vaginitides Other infectious, chemical, allergenic, and physical agents can cause vaginitis.	Presentations vary from no signs or symptoms to erythema, edema, and pruritus of the external genitalia. Excessive and/or malodorous discharge are common findings. Male sexual partners may develop urethritis, balanitis, or cutaneous lesions on penis.	*Trichomonas vaginalis vaginitis* There are no presumptive criteria for this diagnosis. *Bacterial vaginosis* The presumptive criteria including three of the following: • A homogenous gray or white, adherent discharge • Vaginal pH greater than 4.5 • Release of a fishy amine odor from vaginal fluid mixed with 10% KOH • Presence of "clue cells" Fungal vaginitis The presumptive criteria are the typical symptoms of vaginitis or vulvitis and microscopic identification of yeast forms (budding cells or hyphae) in Gram stain or KOH wet mount preparation of vaginal discharge.	*Trichomonas vaginalis vaginitis* A vaginal culture is positive for *T. vaginalis* OR typical motile trichomonads are identified in a saline wet mount of vaginal discharge. *Bacterial vaginosis* The most practical confirmatory microbiological test is the demonstration of characteristic changes in vaginal flora by Gram stain of vaginal fluid; few or no lactobacilli, with predominance of *G. vaginalis* plus other organisms resembling gram-negative Bacteroides sp., anaerobic gram-positive cocci, and/or curved rods. Fungal vaginitis Culture may be useful when signs and symptoms are suggestive but when the fungus cannot be identified by direct microscopy.

GENITAL WARTS

Human papilloma virus A small slowly growing DNA virus belonging to the papovavirus group.	Presents as single or multiple soft, fleshy, papillary or sessile, painless growths around the anus, vulvovaginal area, penis, urethra, or perineum.	A diagnosis may be made on the basis of the typical clinical presentation. Colposcopy may also aid in the diagnosis of certain cervical lesions. Exclude the possibility of condylomata lata by obtaining a darkfield and/or serologic test for syphilis.	A biopsy, although usually unnecessary, is required to make a definitive diagnosis. Very atypical lesions, where neoplasia is a consideration, should be biopsied before initiating therapy. A Pap smear of cervical lesions shows typical or cytologic changes.

HERPES GENITALIS

Herpes simplex virus (HSV) types 1 and 2 DNA viruses that cannot be distinguished clinically.	Single or multiple vesicles appear anywhere on the genitalia. Vesicles spontaneously rupture to form shallow ulcers that may be very painful. Lesions resolve spontaneously without scarring. The first occurrence is termed *initial infection* (mean duration 12 days). Subsequent, usually milder, occurrences are termed *recurrent infections* (mean duration 4.5 days). The interval between clinical episodes is termed *latency*. Viral shedding occurs intermittently during latency.	When typical genital lesions are present or a pattern of recurrence has developed, herpes infection is likely. A presumptive diagnosis is further supported by direct identification of multinucleated giant cells with intranuclear inclusions in a clinical specimen prepared by Papanicolaou or other histochemical stain; OR typical HSV morphology by electron microscopy; OR detection of HSV antigens by monoclonal or polyclonal antibody detection systems. (**NOTE:** Antibody detection systems may detect biologically inactive viral particles.) Primary HSV infection is presumed if an initially negative serologic titer becomes significantly detectable in convalescent serum.	An HSV virus tissue culture demonstrates the characteristic cytopathogenic effect (CPE) following inoculation of a specimen from the cervix, the urethra or the base of a genital lesion. The isolates can be identified as type 1 or type 2 by fluorescent antibody, neutralization, or other serological techniques.

Therapy	Complications and Sequelae	Behavioral Messages to Emphasize

Ambulatory Treatment

Cefoxitin 2.0 g. IM; OR amoxicillin 3.0 g. by mouth; OR ampicillin 3.5 g. by mouth; OR aqueous procaine penicillin G 4.8 million units IM at 2 sites; OR ceftriaxone 250 mg. IM.

NOTE: Each of these regimens, except ceftriaxone, is accompanied by probenecid 1.0 g. by mouth.
FOLLOWED BY
Doxycycline 100 mg. by mouth twice daily for 10–14 days.

NOTE: Tetracycline HCl 500 mg. 4 times daily may be substituted for doxycycline but is less active against certain anaerobes and requires more frequent dosing; these are potentially important drawbacks in the treatment of PID.

If an IUD is used, consult with family planning physician.

Use condoms to prevent future infections.

Trichomonas vaginalis vaginitis

Metronidazole 2.0 g., by mouth, in a single dose.

Alternative Regimen

Metronidazole 250 mg., by mouth, 3 times daily for 7 days.

Bacterial vaginosis

Metronidazole 500 mg., by mouth, twice daily for 7 days.

Alternative Regimen

Ampicillin or amoxicillin 500 mg., by mouth, 4 times daily for 7 days is less effective but may be used for pregnant patients or individuals for whom metronidazole is contraindicated.

NOTE: Treatment is not recommended for male or female asymptomatic carriers of *Gardnerella vaginalis*.

Fungal vaginitis

Miconazole nitrate or clotrimazole 100 mg. intravaginally daily for 7 days. The medication is available as cream or tablets, and the forms are equally effective; OR miconazole nitrate or clotrimazole 200 mg. intravaginally daily for 3 days; clotrimazole 500 mg. tablet intravaginally as a single dose; OR nystatin 100,000 unit tablets, 1 tablet intravaginally daily for 2 weeks.

Secondary excoriations.

Recurrent infections are common.

Bacterial vaginosis may be associated with infectious complications of pregnancy, such as chorioamnionitis and puerperal infection, and with polymicrobial upper genital tract infections in nonpregnant women, such as endometritis and salpingitis.

Fungal vaginitis in pregnancy increases the risk of neonatal oral thrush.

Understand how to take or use any prescribed medications.

Avoid alcohol until 3 days following completion of metronidazole therapy.

Continue taking vaginally-administered medications even during menses.

Return if problem not cured or if it recurs.

Use condoms to prevent trichomonas infections.

Cryotherapy, e.g., liquid nitrogen or carbon dioxide (dry ice);
OR
Podophyllin, 10% in compound tincture of benzoin.
Apply carefully to each wart avoiding normal tissue.
Wash off thoroughly in 1–4 hours. Some consultants use a longer period, but this must be individualized after patient tolerance and compliance have been established. Repeat once or twice weekly. If warts do not regress after 4 applications of podophyllin, alternative treatments are indicated.

Alternative Regimen

Electrosurgery, surgical removal

NOTE: No treatment is completely satisfactory. Podophyllin should not be used during pregnancy or with oral warts. Some consultants recommend against its use for vaginal/cervical warts.

Lesions may enlarge and produce tissue destruction. Giant condyloma, while histologically benign, may simulate carcinoma. Cervical lesions have been associated with neoplasia.

In pregnancy, warts enlarge, are extremely vascular, and may obstruct the birth canal necessitating cesarean section.

Return for weekly or biweekly treatment and follow-up until lesions have resolved.

Partners should be examined for warts.

Abstain from sex or use condoms during therapy.

There is no known cure.

First Clinical Episode

To reduce the signs and symptoms, use Acyclovir 200 mg., by mouth, 5 times daily for 7 to 10 days, initiated within 6 days of onset of lesion.

For patients who have severe symptoms or complications that necessitate hospitalization, an alternative regimen is Acyclovir 5 mg./kg. of body weight IV every 8 hours for 5 to 7 days.

Recurrent Genital Herpes

Acyclovir 200 mg., by mouth, 5 times daily for 5 days initiated within 2 days of onset.

Suppression of Recurrent Genital Herpes Infection

Continuous treatment with acyclovir 200 mg., by mouth, 2 to 5 times daily reduces the frequency of active disease by at least 75% among patients with frequent (at least 6 per year) recurrences.

NOTE: Intravenous and topical acyclovir are not indicated for recurrences, and the safety of systemic acyclovir for the treatment of pregnant women has not been established. Topical acyclovir ointment has marginal benefit in decreasing virus shedding but has no significant effect on symptoms or healing time.

Males and females: Neuralgia, meningitis ascending myelitis, urethral strictures, and lymphatic suppuration may occur.

Females: There is possibly an increased risk for cervical cancer and fetal wastage.

Neonates: Virus from an active genital infection may be transmitted during vaginal delivery causing neonatal herpes infection. Neonatal herpes ranges in severity from clinically inapparent infections to local infections of the eyes, skin, or mucous membranes to severe disseminated infection that may involve the central nervous system. The infection has a high case fatality rate and many survivors have ocular or neurologic sequelae.

Keep involved area clean and dry.

Since both initial and recurrent lesions shed high concentrations of virus, patients should abstain from sex while symptomatic.

An undetermined but presumably small risk of transmission also exists during asymptomatic intervals. Condoms may offer some protection.

Annual Pap smears are recommended. Pregnant women should make their obstetricians aware of any history of herpes.

(continued)

Table 37-2. *Sexually Transmitted Disease Summary—1986 * (continued)*

Disease and Etiologic Agents	Typical Clinical Presentation	Presumptive Diagnosis (warrants full treatment and follow-up)	Definitive Diagnosis
SYPHILIS			
Treponema pallidum A spirochete with 6–14 regular spirals and characteristic motility.	*Primary:* The classical chancre is painless, indurated, and located at the site of exposure. All genital lesions should be suspected to be syphilitic. *Secondary:* Patients may have a highly variable skin rash, mucous patches, condylomata lata, lymphadenopathy, or other signs. *Latent:* Patients are without clinical signs.	*Primary:* Patients have typical lesion(s) and either a newly positive serologic test for syphilis (STS) or their present STS titer is at least fourfold greater than the last, or there has been syphilis exposure within 90 days of lesion onset. *Secondary:* Patients have the typical clinical presentation and a strongly reactive STS. *Latent:* Patients have serologic evidence of untreated syphilis without clinical signs.	Primary and secondary syphilis are definitively diagnosed by demonstrating *T. pallidum* with darkfield microscopy of FA techniques in material from a chancre, regional lymph node, or other lesion. A definitive diagnosis of latent syphilis cannot be made under usual circumstances.
CHANCROID			
Haemophilis ducreyi A pleomorphic gram-negative bacillus commonly observed in small clusters along strands of mucus. On culture, the organism tends to form straight or tangled chains.	Usually a single (but sometimes multiple), superficial, painful ulcer appears and is surrounded by an erythematous halo. Ulcers may also be necrotic or severely erosive with ragged serpiginous borders. Accompanying adenopathy is usually unilateral. A characteristic inguinal bubo occurs in 25%–60% of cases.	A clinical presentation consistent with chancroid involving the genitalia. Since many STD cause genital ulcers, it is crucial to differentiate them. All should be examined with darkfield microscopy. Gram-stained smears of ulcer exudate are unreliable.	The diagnosis is definitive when *H. ducreyi* is recovered by culture. Vancomycin containing selective media facilitate culture and subsequent identification by x and v factor tests.
PEDICULOSIS PUBIS			
Phthirus pubis (pubic or crab louse) A grayish ectoparasite that is 1–4 mm. long with segmented tarsi and claws for clinging to hairs.	Symptoms range from slight discomfort to intolerable itching. Erythematous papules, nits, or adult lice clinging to pubic, perineal, or perianal hairs are present and often noticed by patients.	A presumptive diagnosis is made when a patient with a history of recent exposure to pubic lice has pruritic, erythematous macules, papules, or secondary excoriations in the genital region.	A definitive diagnosis is made by finding lice or nits attached to genital hairs.
SCABIES			
Sarcoptes scabiei The female mite is 0.3–0.4 mm: the male is somewhat smaller. The female burrows under the skin to deposit eggs.	Symptoms include itching, often worse at night, and the presence of erythematous, papular eruptions. Excoriations and secondary infections are common. Reddish-brown nodules are caused by hypersensitivity and develop 1 or more months after infection has occurred. The primary lesion is the burrow. When not obliterated by excoriations, it is most often seen on the fingers, penis, and wrists.	The diagnosis is often made on clinical grounds alone. A history of exposure to a patient with scabies within the previous 2 months supports the diagnosis.	Definitive diagnosis is made by microscopic identification of the mite or its eggs, larvae, or feces in scrapings from an elevated papule or burrow.
HEPATITIS B			
Hepatitis B Virus (HBV) A DNA virus with multiple antigenic components.	Hepatitis B is clinically indistinguishable from other forms of hepatitis. Most infections are clinically inapparent. Clinical symptoms and signs include various combinations of anorexia, malaise, nausea, vomiting, abdominal pain and jaundice. Skin rashes, arthralgias, and arthritis can also occur.	HBV infection is clinically indistinguishable from other forms of viral hepatitis and many times from hepatitis caused by toxins or drugs. The diagnosis should be considered in a symptomatic patient with symptoms suggestive of an acute viral illness and with an occupational exposure or sexual history that places the patient in a high risk group. Groups at high risk of acquiring infection include: Immigrants/refugees from areas of high HBV endemicity; patients in institutions for the mentally retarded; users of illicit parenteral drugs; homosexually active men; household contacts of HBV carriers; and patients of hemodialysis units.	Serodiagnosis of HBV infection is the only method for clinicians to reach a definitive diagnosis. A positive result for hepatitis B surface antigen (HBsAg) indicates active infection with HBV, either acute HB or the chronic carrier state. **NOTE:** HBsAg was previously termed hepatitis associated antigen (HAA) and Australia antigen. Hepatitis B e antigen (HBeAg)—Correlates with infectivity. Anti-HBsAg—Usually indicates past infection with present immunity. Anti-HB core antigen—Past or current infection.

Therapy	Complications and Sequelae	Behavioral Messages to Emphasize
Primary, secondary, or early syphilis of less than 1 year's duration: Benzathine penicillin G, 2.4 million units IM. Syphilis of indeterminate length or of more than 1 year's duration: Benzathine penicillin G, 7.2 million units total; 2.4 million units IM, weekly, for 3 successive weeks. Patients allergic to penicillin: Tetracycline HCl 500 mg., by mouth, 4 times daily† For penicillin-allergic pregnant patients or tetracycline-intolerant patients only: Erythromycin (stearate, ethylsuccinate or base) 500 mg., by mouth, 4 times daily† **NOTE:** Infants who are born to mothers treated with erythromycin for early syphilis during pregnancy should be treated with penicillin. † Duration of therapy depends upon estimated duration of infection. If less than 1 year, treat for 15 days; otherwise, treat for 30 days.	Both late syphilis and congenital syphilis are complications since they are preventable with prompt diagnosis and treatment of early syphilis. Sequelae of late syphilis include neurosyphilis (general paresis, tabes dorsalis and focal neurologic signs), cardiovascular syphilis (thoracic aortic aneurysm, aortic insufficiency), and localized gumma formation.	Understand how to take any prescribed oral medications. If tetracycline is given, take it 1 hour before or 2 hours after meals, and avoid dairy products, antacids, iron or other mineral-containing preparations, and sunlight. Return for follow-up serologies 3, 6, 12, and 24 months after therapy. Refer sexual partner(s) for evaluation and treatment. Avoid sexual activity until patient and partner(s) are cured. Use condoms to prevent future infections.
The susceptibility of *H. ducreyi* to antimicrobial agents differs among geographic regions and this should be taken into account when selecting therapy. Erythromycin 500 mg., by mouth, 4 times a day for 7 days; OR Ceftriaxone 250 mg., IM in a single dose. **Alternative Regimens** Trimethoprim/sulfamethoxazole one double-strength tablet (160/800 mg.) by mouth twice daily for a minimum of 7 days; OR Trimethoprim/sufamethoxazole 640 mg./3200 mg. (4 double-dose or 8 single-dose tablets) by mouth in a single dose; OR amoxicillin 500 mg. plus clavulanic acid 125 mg. 3 times daily for 7 days. **NOTE:** The ceftriaxone, amoxicillin, and trimethoprim/sulfamethoxazole 640 mg./3200 mg. regimens have not been evaluated in the United States. The trimethoprim/sulfamethoxazole combination should be limited to areas where favorable susceptibility patterns have been established. Successfully treated ulcers are almost invariably clinically improved by 7 days after institution of therapy. If they are not, use of an alternative regimen should be considered. Antimicrobial susceptibility testing should be performed on *H. ducreyi* isolated from patients who do not respond to recommended therapies. For persistent treatment failures, consultation with an expert is recommended.	Systemic spread is not known to occur. Lesions may become secondarily infected and necrotic. Buboes may rupture and suppurate, resulting in fistulae. Ulcers on the prepuce may cause paraphimosis or phimosis.	Assure examination and treatment of sexual partner(s) as soon as possible. Return weekly or biweekly for evaluation until the infection is entirely healed. Use condoms to prevent future infections.
Lindane (1%) lotion or cream applied in a thin layer to the infested and adjacent hairy areas and thoroughly washed off after 8 hours; or Lindane (1%) shampoo applied for 4 minutes and then thoroughly washed off (not recommended for pregnant or lactating women); OR Pyrethrins and piperonyl butoxide applied to the infested and adjacent hairy area and washed off after 10 minutes. **NOTE:** Retreatment is indicated after 7 days if lice are found or eggs are observed at the hair–skin junction.	Secondary excoriations. Lymphadenitis. Pyoderma.	Clothing and linen should be disinfested by washing them in hot water, by dry cleaning them, or by removing them from human exposure for 1–2 weeks. Avoid sexual or close physical contact until after treatment. Assure examination of sexual partners as soon as possible. Return if problem is not cured or recurs.
Lindane (1%), 1 oz. of lotion or 30 g. of cream applied thinly to all areas of the body from the neck down and washed off thoroughly after 8 hours. Not recommended for pregnant or lactating women, or infants and young children. **Alternative Regimens** Crotamiton (10%), applied to the entire body nightly for two nights and washed off thoroughly 24 hours after the second application; OR Sulfur (6%) in petrolatum, applied to the entire body nightly for 3 nights. Patients may bathe before each application.	Secondary bacterial infection occurs, particularly with nephritogenic strains of streptococci. Norwegian or crusted scabies (with up to 2 million adult mites in the crusts) is a risk for patients with neurologic defects and the immunologically incompetent.	Clothing and linen should be disinfested by washing them in hot water, by dry cleaning them, or by removing them from human exposure for 1–2 weeks. Avoid sexual or close physical contact until after treatment. Assure examination of sexual partners as soon as possible. Return if problem is not cured or recurs.
No specific therapy is available for the various types of acute hepatitis whether sexually transmitted or not. See "Recommendations for Protection Against Viral Hepatitis," Immunization Practices Advisory Committee, Morbidity and Mortality Weekly Report 1985; 34(22):313–335.	Long-term sequelae include chronic persistent and chronic active hepatitis, cirrhosis, hepatocellular carcinoma, hepatic failure, and death. Rarely, the course may be fulminant with hepatic failure, resulting in early death. Infectious chronic carriers may be completely asymptomatic.	The frequency of clinical follow-up is determined by symptomatology and the results of liver function tests. Hepatitis B immune globulin (HBIG) and hepatitis B vaccine are available. Both are protective against hepatitis B infection.

(continued)

Table 37-2. *Sexually Transmitted Disease Summary—1986 * (continued)*

Disease and Etiologic Agents	Typical Clinical Presentation	Presumptive Diagnosis (warrants full treatment and follow-up)	Definitive Diagnosis
ENTERIC INFECTIONS			
Shigella, hepatitis A virus, *Giardia lamblia*, *Entamoeba histolytica* and a variety of other organisms that produce enteric disease are sexually transmissible, particularly among male homosexuals.	Infections are frequently asymptomatic or minimally symptomatic. Symptoms include abdominal pain and cramping, diarrhea, fever, tenesmus, nausea, and vomiting; all in highly variable degrees of severity. Many cases give a history of frequent oral–genital and oral–anal contact, and/or a history of enteric illness in a recent sex partner.	The typical clinical findings suggest enteric infection. Examination of a fresh stool specimen can be helpful. The finding of white cells on direct microscopy of a suspension of fresh stool, or the finding of guaiac-positive or grossly bloody stools support the diagnosis.	Definitive diagnostic tests vary according to the agent involved: Microscopic examination for ova and parasites (amebiasis, giardiasis); cultures (shigellosis); or serologic tests (hepatitis A).
AIDS (ACQUIRED IMMUNODEFICIENCY SYNDROME) AND HTLV-III/LAV INFECTIONS			
Human T-lymphotropic virus type III/ lymphadenopathy associated virus and AIDS-related retrovirus. (All are agreed to be the same virus that contains RNA and is in the retrovirus family.)	The range of symptoms associated with HTLV-III/LAV may extend from minimal to the full clinical syndrome of AIDS. Patients with the clinical syndrome of AIDS often give a history of nonspecific symptoms for months prior to diagnosis. These symptoms may include easy fatigue, poor appetite, weight loss, lymphadenopathy, diarrhea, fever and night sweats. Other symptoms specific to opportunistic diseases occur in patients with AIDS, such as purple to bluish skin lesions associated with Kaposi's sarcoma (KS) or shortness of breath and nonproductive cough resulting from *Pneumocystis carinii* pneumonia (PCP).	Presumptive diagnosis of HTLV-III/LAV infection is made usually on clinical evidence, supported by serologic tests for antibodies to HTLV-III/LAV. Once an individual is infected, current research suggests the individual remains infected indefinitely and may transmit the infection to others. As yet unidentified factors may influence which infected individuals develop AIDS and which particular opportunistic illness may occur.	Currently, isolation of the virus from body fluids is the most highly specific means to make a definitive diagnosis of HTLV-III/LAV infection. Only a very few research laboratories have the technology to perform viral isolation. Viral antigen detection techniques are not generally available. Results from repeatably reactive ELISA tests, Western Blots, and other confirmatory tests, and repeat serology when combined with a careful history and physical examination can usually resolve questionable cases. Diagnosis of the clinical syndrome AIDS requires that an illness predictive of cellular immune deficiency be reliably diagnosed (such as KS or PCP) in the absence of any known cause of immune deficiency.

Nursing History

1. Foster a nonjudgmental attitude and atmosphere because this is an emotionally laden area.
   a. Convey an attitude of acceptance
   b. Explain why the following questions are relevant.
2. Ask or discuss the following:
   a. The patient's sexual orientation (heterosexual, bisexual, homosexual). Use nongender terms (i.e., "person," "individual").
   b. Is the patient involved primarily with one individual or different individuals?
   c. How many sexual contacts over a defined length of time?
   d. Where is the place of sexual encounter? Singles bars? Gay bars? Bath house? (Risk of disease transmission is higher in certain places.)
   e. Sexual practices? What orifices are used for sexual activities?
   f. What other sexual behaviors are practiced? (Behaviors that cause trauma, abrasions, etc., increase risk of systemic access to infection.)
3. Permit the patient to carry discussion further.
4. Know the disease spectrum in the area; there are geographic differences in incidence and types of STDs.
5. Identify the patient's chief complaint.
   a. When?
   b. Character of complaint? Location?
   c. Related to sexual activity?
   d. Any previous episode of STD? What was the treatment?
   e. Have you a sex partner with a known STD?
   f. Any history of drug allergies?
   g. For women: Any abortions? Miscarriages?

6. Inform the patient that the major STDs are reportable; the health department is notified when the diagnosis is confirmed.
   a. All test results are held in strictest confidence.
   b. Local health departments in most communities have a Disease Intervention Specialist who is a public health professional trained in the management of sex partner referral.

Prevention and Patient Education

1. Sexually transmitted disease is acquired by sexual contact (vaginal sexual intercourse, anal intercourse, oral intercourse) and by close and direct contact with an infected person.
2. The only effective way to prevent acquiring an STD is to abstain from all forms of sexual contact.
3. To reduce the risk of STD:
   a. Avoid multiple partners, anonymous partners, prostitutes, and other persons with multiple sex partners.
   b. Avoid sexual contact with persons who have a genital discharge, genital warts, genital herpes lesions or other suspicious genital lesions, or laboratory evidence of infection.
   c. Avoid oral–anal sex to prevent enteric infections.
   d. Avoid genital contact with oral "cold sores."
   e. Use condoms in combination with spermicides.
   f. Have periodic examination for sexually transmitted diseases if at high risk.
4. Secure active and passive hepatitis B virus immunization.
5. Know the signs and symptoms of STDs.

Therapy	Complications and Sequelae	Behavioral Messages to Emphasize
Treatment of proctitis and enterocolitis should be based on etiologic diagnosis. Some asymptomatic, infected individuals for whom anal–oral contact is a sexual practice should be treated in accordance with recommendations for symptomatic individuals, as should persons whose work or social situation is associated with a likelihood of transmission (e.g., food handlers, hospital workers, day care center employees, etc.) For disease-specific treatment recommendations see appropriate references.*	Complications and sequelae vary with the disease agent, health of the host, therapy, and other factors. Spontaneous cures are common. Morbidity may be severe, requiring hospitalization and intravenous hydration. Infections may become systemic (such as gram-negative septicemia) or distantly localized (amebic hepatic cyst). Some infections may rarely be fatal (hepatitis A, disseminated bacterial disease).	Follow dietary and medical regimens. Avoid oral–anal contact at least until infection is cleared. Refer sexual partner(s) for examination. Avoid sex until patient and partner(s) are cured. Return early if symptoms persist or recur.
To date, no treatment has been identified to eradicate the virus or reverse the immunologic dysfunction associated with HTLV-III/LAV infection. Standard therapy consists of treating opportunistic diseases aggressively as they occur.	The outcome in patients with HTLV-III/LAV infection is not completely understood. Studies in a cohort of gay men whose serum contained antibody to HTLV-III/LAV showed about 5%–10% of these patients were subsequently diagnosed with the clinical syndrome AIDS within 2–5 years, and another 25% had genealized lymphadenopathy or other AIDS-related conditions. The other two thirds of the men were clinically well after 5 years.	Sexual contact with individuals who have had sex with multiple or anonymous partners increases risk of infection and should be avoided. For individuals who choose to initiate a new sexual relationship with a person at increased risk for HTLV-III/LAV infection or who maintain casual sexual relationships, sexual practices should be limited to those that do not permit any exchange of blood or bodily secretions. Condoms should be used consistently. Fisting is strongly discouraged. Do not inject illicit drugs. If such practices continue, do not share needles and syringes. Do not use inhalant nitrates ("poppers"). These have been implicated as a cofactor for Kaposi's sarcoma.

* Based upon STD treatment guidelines, 1985, "Quality Assurance Guidelines for STD Clinics—1986" and subsequent updates; Contact Technical Information Services, Center for Prevention Services, Centers for Disease Control, Atlanta, GA 30333.

6. Seek early diagnosis and treatment if you acquire an STD.
7. Secure written instructions on taking medication, including dosage, timing, and length of regimen. Prescribed medication must be taken for the full course.
8. STD National Hotline: 800-227-8922 or 8923 (nationwide); and 800-982-5883 (California)—provides toll-free information and referral services for sexually transmitted diseases.

AIDS

See Chapter 34.

Syphilis

Syphilis is a chronic infectious multisystem disease caused by *Treponema pallidum* (a spirochete). It is acquired by sexual contact, contaminated blood products, and transplacentally.

Clinical Manifestations

Syphilis is capable of destroying tissue in almost any organ in the body; it thus produces a wide variety of clinical manifestations. Syphilis is divided into chronological stages:

Stages of Untreated Syphilis

A. Incubation Period

1. 10–90 days; average 21 days
2. No symptoms or lesions
3. Spirochetemia is present; the patient's blood is infective

B. Primary (early) Syphilis

1. Most infectious stage; lasting 1–6 weeks
2. Manifestations include:
   a. Chancre or primary sore, a painless ulcer, appears at the site where the treponema enter the body (genitalia, anorectal area, lips, oral cavity, fingers), which is generally related to the pattern of sexual activity.
   b. Chancre becomes eroded and heals after 4–6 weeks, leaving a small scar; in some patients, no primary sore can be found.
   c. Enlargement of regional lymph nodes.

NURSING ALERT: Syphilis should be suspected when an indolent, painless ulceration appears on the body.

C. Secondary Syphilis

1. Secondary stage follows onset of chancre by 9–90 days; this is the stage of systemic involvement as treponema spread throughout body.
2. Signs and symptoms of secondary syphilis:
   a. Influenza-like syndrome—headaches, lacrimation, nasal discharge, sore throat, generalized arthralgia
      (1) Rise in temperature
      (2) *Generalized lymphadenopathy*
   b. Generalized skin eruption—maculopapular rash, etc.; bilaterally symmetric in distribution, polymorphous (macular, papular, follicular, pustular)
   c. Moist papules occur most frequently in anogenital region (condylomata) and in mouth.
   d. Lesions of mouth, throat, and cervix (mucous

patches) frequently occur in secondary stage; lesions are highly infectious.
  e. Generalized patchy hair loss on scalp.

D. Late Syphilis (clinically destructive stage after latent period)—manifestations may occur 10–30 years after exposure; recovery unpredictable.
  1. Granulomatous lesions appear in skin, bones, liver, cardiovascular system, and central nervous system.
  2. Syphilis will mainly affect cardiovascular system (aneurysm of ascending aorta, aortic insufficiency), central nervous system, and skeletal system.

Diagnostic Evaluation

  1. Dark-field examinations and direct fluorescent antibody tests on lesions or tissue—definitive methods
  2. Presumptive diagnosis is possible by using two types of serologic tests for syphilis.
      a. Treponemal (fluorescent treponemal antibody absorbed [FTA-ABS], microhemagglutination assay for antibody to *T. pallidum* [MHATP])
      b. Nontreponemal (Venereal Disease Research Laboratory [VDRL], rapid plasma reagin [RPR])

Management*

  1. Benzathine penicillin G (intramuscularly [IM]) at a single session.
  2. Other treatment schedules are available for persons with penicillin allergies, those who are pregnant, patients with syphilis of more than 1 year's duration, etc.
  3. Post-treatment follow-up is essential.
  4. *Jarisch–Herxheimer reaction* is an acute febrile reaction often accompanied by headache, myalgia, and other symptoms that may occur after any therapy for syphilis. The patient should be forewarned.

Patient Education

  1. Treatment failures can occur with any regimen; patients should be reexamined at 3 and 6 months.
  2. Early treatment is essential for pregnant woman—treatment begun later in pregnancy may cause infant to demonstrate some of the stigmata of congenital syphilis.
  3. See Prevention and Patient Education in Sexually Transmitted Diseases, page 902.

Gonorrhea

Gonorrhea is an infection involving the mucosal surface of the genitourinary tract, rectum, and pharynx; it is caused by the gonococcus *Neisseria gonorrhoeae.* It is an infectious disease that is transmitted sexually, the exception being gonococcal ophthalmia of the newborn. It may be acquired by sexual intercourse, orogenital, and/or anogenital contacts between members of opposite sexes as well as between members of the same sex.

Clinical Problems

  1. Gonorrhea is the most frequently reported bacterial infection in the US; peak incidence in the US is 20–24 years in men and 18–24 years in women.

---

* 1989 Sexually Transmitted Diseases Treatment Guidelines. Public Health Service, Centers for Disease Control.

  2. Gonorrhea has a short incubation period, which permits rapid spread; a high percentage of infected women are symptom-free.
  3. There is a high frequency of coexisting chlamydial and gonococcal infections.
  4. There is an increasing incidence of infections due to both penicillinase-producing *N. gonorrhoeae* (PPNG) and chromosomally mediated resistant *N. gonorrhoeae.*

Clinical Manifestations

A. Men
  1. Incubation period of 2–7 days
  2. Urethral discharge or dysuria
  3. Spread of infection to posterior urethra, prostate, seminal vesicles, and epididymis
  4. Complications
      a. Postgonococcal urethritis; urethral stricture
      b. Epididymitis
      c. Prostatitis

B. Women
  1. Symptoms less specific; majority of women are asymptomatic and attend STD Clinic following referral as a contact.
  2. Vaginal discharge
  3. Urinary frequency and pain
  4. Abnormal uterine bleeding
  5. Complications
      a. Pelvic infection (endometritis; salpingitis; peritonitis)
      b. Infertility; ectopic pregnancy

C. Anorectal Manifestations

Anal and rectal burning, itching, bleeding, mucopurulent discharge, or painful defecation; may be asymptomatic

D. Pharyngeal Manifestations

Sore throat, but may be asymptomatic

E. Adult Gonococcal Conjunctivitis

Gonococci usually reach the eye via the fingers.

F. Disseminated Gonococcal Infection

Produces joint inflammation, tenosynovitis, skin lesions, and/or endocarditis

Diagnostic Evaluation

  1. Diagnosis is made by identification of organism on gram-stained smears, by culture, or by antigen detection of enzyme immunoassay test. See Guidelines: Obtaining Culture Specimen for Diagnosis of Gonorrhea, opposite page.
  2. Serologic test for syphilis

Management* (of Uncomplicated Urethral, Endocervical, or Rectal Infections)

  1. Ceftriaxone (IM) once *plus* doxycycline orally for 7 days. (Other alternative antimicrobial regimens are available.)
  2. Re-examination with culture 1–2 months after treatment.
  3. Examination, culture, and treatment of sexual partners.

Note: The susceptibility of *N. gonorrhoeae* to antibiotics is likely to change over time in any locality.

Principles of Control

1. Gonorrhea is a reportable disease; public health authorities are notified so that sexual contacts can be found and treated.
2. Each patient is interviewed for names of contacts. Contacts of known gonorrhea cases are investigated and treated.

3. The patient is instructed to avoid reinfection by sexual activity with untreated previous sexual partners until they have been tested and treated.

Patient Education

See Patient Education, Sexually Transmitted Diseases, page 902.

Guidelines Obtaining Culture Specimen for the Diagnosis of Gonorrhea*

Purpose	To obtain specimens from the cervix (women), anal canal (men and women), urethral specimen (men), or oropharynx specimen (men and women) for culture for *N. gonorrhoeae*.

Equipment	Vaginal speculum
	Ring forceps
	Cotton balls
	Sterile, calcium alginate swabs (Calgiswab)
	Sterile wire loop
	Sterile disposable gloves
	Thayer-Martin or other compatible medium

Procedure

Nursing Action	Rationale/Amplification

Preparatory Phase

1. Place patient in dorsal lithotomy position with adequate draping.
2. Put on sterile disposable gloves.

Performance Phase

For Female Patient

Cervical Culture

1. Moisten vaginal speculum with warm water. Do not use any other lubricant.
2. Separate labia. Depress the perineum and posterior vaginal wall with the finger of one hand.
3. Gently insert a bivalve vaginal speculum.

 2. This maneuver helps avoid uncomfortable pressure against the more sensitive anteriorly placed structures.
 3. The speculum is made self-retaining by adjusting one or more screws. The short blade should be uppermost. The tip of the posterior blade is pushed down into the posterior fornix.

4. Remove excessive cervical mucus with a cotton ball held in ring forceps.
5. Insert sterile swab into endocervical canal (Fig. 37-2A).
   a. Move from side to side in cervix.
   b. Allow 30 seconds for absorption of organisms by the swab.

 5. The endocervical canal is considered the best culture site. Movement of the cotton swab ensures adequate sampling.

Anal Canal Culture (Rectal Culture)

1. Obtain anal specimen *after* getting cervical specimen.

2. Insert sterile swab approximately 2.5 cm. (1 inch) into the anal canal (Fig. 37-2B).
3. Move swab from side to side in anal canal.

4. Allow 20–30 seconds for absorption of organism by the swab.

 1. The anal canal is the most likely site to be positive when the cervix is negative.
 2. Use another swab to obtain specimen if swab contains feces.
 3. Movement of the swab in anal canal permits specimen to be secured from anal crypts.

Oropharynx Culture

1. Swab the posterior pharynx and tonsillar crypts with a calcium alginate swab.

 1. Oropharyngeal specimens should be obtained from patients suspected of having disseminated gonococcal infection.

(continued)

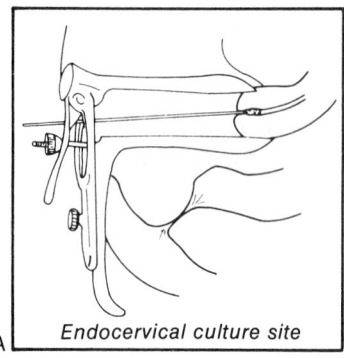

A *Endocervical culture site*

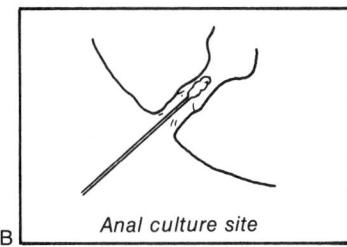

B *Anal culture site*

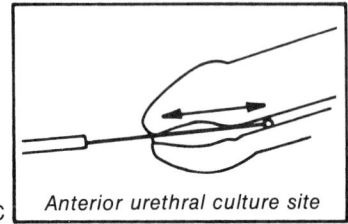

C *Anterior urethral culture site*

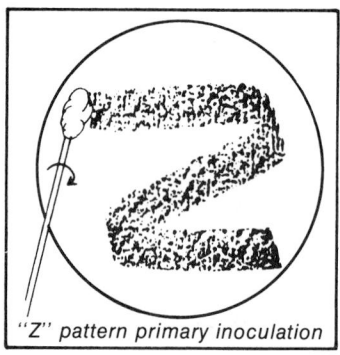

D *"Z" pattern primary inoculation*

Figure 37-2. *Obtaining culture for specimen in diagnosis of gonorrhea. (From Criteria and Techniques for the Diagnosis of Gonorrhea. US Public Health Service, Centers for Disease Control)*

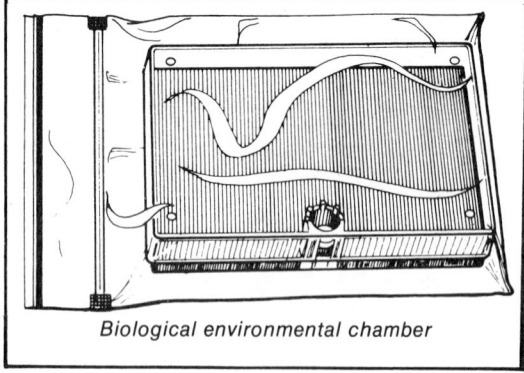

Biological environmental chamber

E

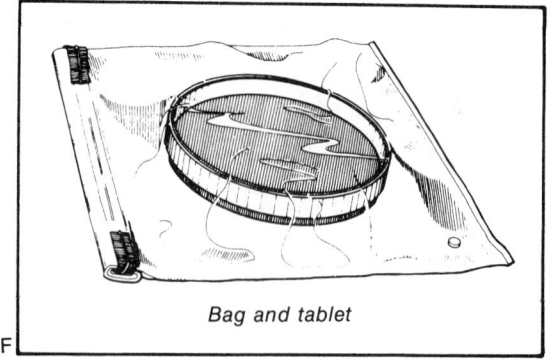

Bag and tablet

F

Procedure (continued)	Nursing Action	Rationale

For Male Patient

Urethral Culture

1. Use sterile bacteriologic wire loop or a sterile calcium alginate urethral swab to obtain a specimen from the anterior urethra by gently scraping the mucosa (Fig. 37-2C). Do not insert loop or swab more than 2 cm. into urethra.

Anal Canal Culture
(Same as in women)

Oropharynx Culture
(Same as in women)

To Inoculate Selective Medium in Plates:

Candle Jar System

1. Roll swab in a large "Z" pattern, exposing all surfaces of the swab on selective medium (Fig. 37-2D). If a second specimen is collected, inoculate on a separate part of medium.

2. Cross streak immediately with a sterile wire loop or tip of swab (in the clinical facility).

3. Place the culture plate in a CO_2-enriched atmosphere (candle jar) within 15 minutes of inoculation.

4. Incubate plates within 1–2 hours at 35°–36°C. (95°–96.8°F.).

CO_2 Tablet/Plastic Bag System

1. After the medium is inoculated, place the CO_2-generating tablet in a special well of the plate (biologic environmental chamber), *not* on the medium surface (Fig. 37-2E). Use forceps to handle the tablets. Secure the top of the plate tightly.

2. Another method is to drop a CO_2-generating tablet into the plastic bag (Fig. 37-2F).

3. Place plate in plastic bag. Expel excess air from the bag and seal it tightly. No portion of the bag is to be left open.

4. Incubate plates within 1–2 hours at 35°–36°C. (95°–96.8°F.).

Rationale column:

1. An urethral culture of the male is indicated when the Gram stain of urethral exudate is not positive, in tests-of-cure, or as a test for asymptomatic urethral infection. Avoid using a standard cotton-tipped swab because it is too large.

1. This pattern provides adequate exposure of swab to plate for transfer of organisms.

2. Streaking with a wire loop isolates colonies of *N. gonorrhoeae* from the few contaminants that occasionally grow on selective medium.

3. Successful recovery of *N. gonorrhoeae* requires an atmosphere enriched with carbon dioxide.

1. Read the package inserts on the handling and storing of CO_2 tablets.

2. The tablet and plastic bag system is easy to use, safe, and economical.

3. Moisture from the medium will activate the CO_2-generating tablet.

---

* Adapted from Criteria and Techniques for the Diagnosis of Gonorrhea, U.S. Public Health Service, Centers for Disease Control.

Bacterial Infections

Nosocomial (Hospital-Associated) Infections

Nosocomial infections are infections acquired in a health care facility during hospitalization; infection is neither present nor incubating at the time of admission unless it is related to a previous hospitalization. The major cause of hospital-associated infections in the United States is gram-negative bacteria, although in other countries, gram-positive pathogens are on the rise.

Gram-Negative Infections

1. Gram-negative infections are bacterial infections caused most frequently by *Escherichia coli*.

2. Other frequent pathogens are *Enterobacter, Serratia,* and *Proteus.*

3. *Bacteremia*—is a general term meaning the presence of bacteria in the bloodstream. Approximately 75% of bacteremias are nosocomial.

Predisposing Events

1. Most gram-negative bacilli are not invasive in normal hosts; they are opportunistic bacteria that become invasive in persons with diminishing defense mechanisms or serious underlying disorders.

2. Diagnostic and treatment procedures (tubes, catheters, etc.) disrupt usual protective barriers provided by the skin and mucous membranes.

3. Potent immunosuppressive drugs, cytotoxic drugs, steroids, radiation therapy, and previous splenectomy diminish defense mechanisms.

NURSING ALERT: Persons over 70 years of age are at high risk of acquiring a nosocomial infection.

4. Patients in intensive care units (ICUs) are at risk.
   a. Underlying conditions compromise host defenses.
   b. Frequent exposure to invasive procedures.
   c. Close proximity to other susceptible/at-risk patients that allows opportunity for cross-infection.
   d. Resistant microorganisms in ICU environment.

Other Contributing Factors

1. Genitourinary tract—indwelling catheters, instrumentation, urinary obstruction
2. Gastrointestinal tract—from obstruction, perforation, neoplasia, abscesses, diverticuli
3. Biliary tract—cholangitis, obstruction (stones), surgical procedures
4. Extensive use of antimicrobial agents—alters flora of gastrointestinal tract and pharynx and the types of organisms likely to produce bacteremia
5. Emergence of antibiotic–resistant bacteria
6. Reproductive system—abortion, instrumentation, postpartum period
7. Vascular system—venous cutdowns, intravenous catheters, intracardiac pacemakers, prosthetic heart valves, total parenteral nutrition, indwelling arterial lines, pressure-monitoring devices, surgical procedures
8. Skin—wound infections, burns, pressure sores
9. Respiratory tract—aspiration, tracheostomy, mechanical ventilation, contaminated inhalation therapy equipment

Prevention

1. *Handwashing by personnel and patient—fundamental to the control of all infections.*
2. Identify patients at risk and use every opportunity to reduce their exposure to pathogenic organisms.
3. Institute isolation precautions for immunosuppressed patients.
4. Practice strict aseptic technique for all diagnostic/therapeutic procedures—wounds, tracheostomies, tube drainage, catheters, intravenous therapy, cardiac pacing, ventilatory equipment.
   a. Avoid invasive procedures as much as possible.
   b. Anchor IV catheter securely to prevent movement in vein; avoid prolonged IV therapy.
5. Be alert for factors that affect catheter-related sepsis.
   a. Catheter size, type, and duration.
   b. Use closed urinary drainage system if an indwelling catheter is required.
   c. Regard outside of catheter and drainage bag as highly contaminated.
   d. Avoid housing 2 patients with indwelling catheters in the same room.
6. Monitor sterilization procedures and practices.
7. Use nursing surveillance to prevent cross-contamination.

Septic Shock

Septic shock is the systemic response to sepsis (presence of microorganisms or their toxins in the bloodstream) and is characterized by hemodynamic, metabolic, and cellular abnormalities.

Clinical Features

1. Septic shock usually develops as a complication of overwhelming infection in hospitalized patients with predisposing factors: elderly, immunosuppressed, diabetic, etc.).
2. It is usually caused by gram-negative enteric bacilli (*Escherichia coli, Klebsiella, Enterobacter, Proteus, Pseudomonas, Bacteroides, Salmonella*).
   a. Other organisms may initiate the syndrome, including gram-positive bacteria, spirochetes, viruses, fungi and rickettsiae.
   b. Some cases of septic shock involve more than one organism.
3. The hemodynamic responses of septic shock result in many physiologic alterations. When vital organs are inadequately perfused and cells cannot maintain a steady metabolic status, multiple organ systems failure ensues.

Clinical Manifestations

1. Fever; often chills
2. Tachypnea
3. Warm, dry, flushed skin during early stage (warm shock)
4. Altered mental state; confusion, agitation, lethargy (due to reduced cerebral blood flow)
5. *Hypotension* and *shock*
   a. Tachycardia/tachypnea
   b. Cool clammy skin/peripheral cyanosis (cold shock)
   c. Oliguria
   d. Vascular collapse
6. Intravascular coagulation

Diagnostic Evaluation

1. Cultures of blood, urine, sputum, and other appropriate specimens
2. Arterial blood gas measurements
3. Baseline coagulation studies

Management

(Septic shock is a medical emergency and treatment is carried out in an intensive care unit).
1. Volume replacement (fluids; blood) guided by pulmonary artery catheterization for assessment of cardiac function and volume status to maintain cardiovascular function.
2. Mechanical ventilatory support—to ensure adequate oxygen delivery to tissues
3. Surgical debridement/drainage of infected tissues/abscesses and removal of foreign bodies (tubes, catheters)
4. Administration of antibiotic(s) after cultures are obtained.
5. Maintenance of arterial blood pressure with supportive care, parenteral fluids, and pharmacologic agents
6. Nutritional and metabolic support
7. Monitoring of hemodynamic parameters
8. Optimization of cardiac output with positive inotropic agents and antidysrhythmic drugs
9. Treatment of disseminated intravascular coagulation with factor replacement and platelets

Complications

1. Sepsis-induced lung failure
2. Multiple systems organ failure

Nursing Interventions

A. Establishing Tissue Oxygenation and Organ Perfusion to Promote Recovery from Shock

1. Monitor the state of responsiveness.
   a. Skin temperature, moisture, color, turgor
   b. Appearance of mucous membranes and nails
   c. Pulse and respiration
   d. Input and output
   e. Blood pressure, heart and lung sounds
   f. Peripheral pulses
   g. Focus assessment on *trends* and patterns of change.
2. Monitor fluid and blood replacement.
   a. Follow central venous pressure measurements and measurements of left ventricular filling pressures.
   b. Monitor serum electrolytes every several hours.
3. Auscultate lung fields when fluid is being administered—to detect inspiratory and expiratory wheezes, moist, fine crackles and rhonchi—may indicate impending pulmonary edema.

B. Promoting Adequate Breathing

1. Administer oxygen as prescribed to keep arterial PO_2 at desired level.
   a. Follow blood gas and pH measurements to assess the patient's need for assisted ventilation.
   b. Inadequate respiratory exchange is a frequent cause of death.
2. Instruct the patient to cough, turn, change positions, and breathe deeply at intervals—to reduce potential for retention of secretions.

C. Monitoring Urinary Output

1. Monitor urinary output
   a. Kidney function deteriorates with septic shock.
   b. An increase in urine (greater than 30 ml./hour) usually means that tissue perfusion and, hence, renal perfusion are improving.
2. Measure specific gravity at prescribed intervals—increases when oliguria is developing.

Staphylococcal Infections

Staphylococci are gram-positive cocci that are responsible for a variety of infections. The most common pathogenic strain, *Staphylococcus aureus,* produces a wide range of infections due to its ability to produce a number of enzymes (coagulase, catalase, lipolytic) and toxins (hemolytic, endotoxins, exotoxins, exfoliatins).

Examples of Staphylococcal Disease

1. *Skin and soft tissue infections*—furuncles (boils), impetigo, carbuncles, cellulitis, abscesses, infected lacerations
2. *Invasion of lymphatics*—axillary, cervical, mediastinal, retroperitoneal, and subdiaphragmatic abscesses
3. *Invasion of bloodstream*—endocarditis, pneumonitis, empyema, perinephritic abscess, hepatic abscess, splenic abscess, staphylococcal enteritis, septic arthritis, meningitis, osteomyelitis, generalized septicemia

Modes of Transmission

1. Direct hand transfer
2. Ingestion of contaminated food
3. Nasal secretions, draining wound, asymptomatic carrier
4. Break in skin/mucous membrane

5. Aerosolization during dressing changes
6. Vascular access sites (intravenous lines, drug abusers)

Diagnostic Evaluation

1. Gram stain of involved tissues, body fluids, or purulent material.
2. Blood culture—to determine if bacteremia has occurred.

Management

1. Penicillinase-resistant penicillins (methicillin, nafcillin, oxacillin, cloxacillin, dicloxacillin) and the cephalosporins (cephalothin), etc., are antistaphylococcal drugs and are selected according to site of infection, severity of illness, and sensitivity of the organism.
   a. Serious staphylococcal infections may require a prolonged course of treatment.
   b. Intravenous administration is usually selected because of the large doses of drug required.
2. Supportive care—surgical measures, pain relief, treatment of fever, etc.

Nursing Interventions

1. Monitor patient's response to prescribed therapy.
2. Suspect drug resistance, drug allergy, or superinfection (a second organism resistant to the antibiotic in use) if the patient experiences continuing or recurring fever.
3. See page 894 for Nursing Interventions for the patient with a fever.
4. Encourage meticulous handwashing techniques among personnel/patient/visitors.

Preventive Measures and Patient Education

1. Public should be educated concerning personal hygiene.
2. Persons with draining lesions should be isolated from their group and treated.

Streptococcal Infections

Most *streptococcal infections* in humans are caused by group A streptococci. Streptococci gain entrance to the body primarily through the upper respiratory tract or skin; transmission is by persons with streptococcal infections or by asymptomatic carriers.

Beta Hemolytic Streptococcal Infections

1. Streptococcal pharyngitis ("strep" sore throat, p. 151)
2. Wound and skin infections—impetigo, puerperal infections, cellulitis, erysipelas
3. Scarlet fever (streptococcal throat with a rash that occurs if infectious agent produces erythrogenic toxin to which patient is not immune)
4. Sinusitis, otitis media, mastoiditis, peritonsillar abscess
5. Pericarditis, arthritis, peritonitis, meningitis
6. Pneumonia and empyema

Poststreptococcal Diseases
(Sequelae of Hemolytic Streptococci)

1. Rheumatic fever
2. Acute glomerulonephritis

Diagnostic Evaluation

Isolation of etiologic agent from throat or skin lesion

Management

1. Penicillin is the drug of choice in streptococcal infections (except enterococcal streptococci group D infections).
   a. Therapy should be continued for at least 10 days—to eliminate the organism, reduce frequency of suppurative complications, prevent the majority of cases of rheumatic fever and help prevent further spread of streptococci.
   b. Erythromycin for penicillin-allergic patient
2. Make sure that the patient understands the importance of *completing* the course of antimicrobial treatment.

Preventive Measures and Patient Education

1. Public should be educated concerning the relationship of streptococcal infections to heart disease and glomerulonephritis.
2. Long-term penicillin prophylaxis may be used for high-risk individuals (rheumatic heart disease)—to prevent a repeat attack.
3. Obstetric patients should be protected from personnel or visitors with respiratory or skin infections.
4. Food handlers should be instructed about and monitored for hygienic procedures.

Pulmonary Tuberculosis

Tuberculosis is an infectious disease caused by bacteria (*Mycobacterium tuberculosis*) that are usually spread from person to person through the air. It usually infects the lung, but can occur at virtually any site in the body.

Transmission

1. The term *mycobacterium* is descriptive of the organism, which is a bacterium that resembles a fungus. The organisms multiply slowly and are characterized as acid-fast aerobic organisms that can be killed by heat, sunshine, drying, and ultraviolet light.
2. Tuberculosis is an airborne disease transmitted by droplet nuclei, usually from within the respiratory tract of an infected person who exhales them during coughing, talking, sneezing, or singing.
3. When an uninfected susceptible person inhales the droplet-containing air, the organism is carried into the lung to the pulmonary alveoli.
4. Most individuals who become infected do not develop clinical illness, because the body's immune system brings the infection under control.

Pathology

1. Tubercle bacilli infect the lung, forming a tubercle (lesion).
2. The tubercle
   a. May heal, leaving scar tissue.
   b. May continue as a granuloma:
      (1) May heal.
      (2) May be reactivated.
   c. May eventually proceed to necrosis, liquefaction, sloughing, and cavitation.
3. The initial lesion may disseminate tubercle bacilli:
   a. By extension to adjacent tissues
   b. Via bloodstream
   c. Via lymphatic system
   d. Through the bronchi

Risk Factors for Activation of Tuberculosis

Persons at risk:
1. Adults whose initial infection was acquired many years previously; these persons harbor live dormant bacilli that at any time may reactivate and spread disease.
2. Persons in close contact with someone who has infectious tuberculosis.
3. Persons whose tuberculin skin tests have recently converted to a significant reaction.
4. Persons with declining immunity; those infected with HIV.
5. Elderly persons, particularly those living in extended care facilities who have healed dormant lesions.
6. Certain minority groups, recent immigrants, and the homeless.
7. Medical risk factors include silicosis, gastrectomy, immunosuppressive therapy.

Clinical Manifestations

Patient may be asymptomatic or may have insidious symptoms that are ignored.
1. Generalized systemic signs and symptoms
   a. Fatigue, anorexia, weight loss, low-grade fever, night sweats, indigestion
   b. Some patients have acute febrile illness, chills, generalized influenza-like symptoms
2. Pulmonary signs and symptoms
   a. Cough (insidious onset) progressing in frequency and producing mucoid or mucopurulent sputum
   b. Hemoptysis; chest pain; dyspnea (indicates extensive involvement)
3. Extrapulmonary tuberculosis: *Mycobacterium* can infect any organ in the body (pleurae, lymph nodes, genitourinary tract, bones/joints, peritoneum, central nervous system)

Diagnostic Evaluation

1. Sputum smear and culture—diagnosis made by finding the acid-fast bacilli in sputum obtained by coughing and expectoration, induced by inhaled aerosols, bronchoscopic aspiration, transtracheal aspiration.
2. Chest x-ray—to determine presence and extent of disease.
3. Tuberculin skin test (Mantoux test)—inoculation of tubercle bacillus extract (tuberculin) into the intradermal layer of the inner aspect of the forearm (see p. 912).
4. Screening tests—multiple puncture tests—introduce either dried or liquid tuberculin into skin by puncturing the skin with an applicator (e.g., tine test; Mono-Vac test).
   a. Used for screening large groups since there is no way to standardize the amount of tuberculin introduced, which does not allow precise interpretation of test results.
   b. All significant reactors to multiple puncture tests must be confirmed with the Mantoux test.

Management: Chemotherapy (Table 37-3)

1. A combination of drugs to which the organisms are susceptible is given to destroy viable microbial organisms as rapidly as possible and to protect against the emergence of drug-resistant organisms.
2. Current recommended regimen of uncomplicated pulmonary tuberculosis is 2 months of bactericidal drugs isoniazid (INH), rifampin (RIF), and pyrazin-

Table 37-3. *Recommended Drugs for the Initial Treatment of Tuberculosis in Adults*

Drug	Dosage Forms	Daily Dose*	Twice Weekly Dose	Major Adverse Reactions
Isoniazid	Tablets: 100 mg., 300 mg.[†‡] Syrup: 50 mg./5 ml. Vials: 1 g.	5 mg./kg. PO or IM	15 mg./kg. Maximum 900 mg.	Hepatic enzyme elevation, peripheral neuropathy, hepatitis, hypersensitivity
Rifampin	Capsules: 150 mg., 300 mg.[†‡] Syrup: formulated from capsules, 10 mg./ml.[‡]	10 mg./kg. PO	10 mg./kg. Maximum 600 mg.	Orange discoloration of secretions and urine; nausea, vomiting, hepatitis, febrile reaction, purpura (rare)
Pyrazinamide	Tablets: 500 mg.[‡]	15–30 mg./kg. PO	50–70 mg./kg.	Hepatotoxicity, hyperuricemia, arthralgias, skin rash, gastrointestinal upset
Streptomycin	Vials: 1 g., 4 g.	15 mg./kg.[§] IM	25–30 mg./kg. IM	Ototoxicity, nephrotoxicity
Ethambutol	Tablets: 100 mg., 400 mg.	15–25 mg./kg. PO	50 mg./kg.	Optic neuritis (decreased red-green color discrimination, decreased visual acuity), skin rash

Adapted from the Joint Statement of the American Thoracic Society and the Centers for Disease Control. Treatment of tuberculosis and tuberculosis infection in adults and children. Am Rev Respir Dis 1986 Aug; 134(2): 355–363.

* Doses based on weight should be adjusted as weight changes.

[†] Isoniazid and rifampin are available as a combination capsule containing 150 mg. of isoniazid and 300 mg. of rifampin.

[‡] A combination of isoniazid, rifampin, and pyrazinamide in a single capsule is being introduced.

[§] In persons older than 60 years of age the daily dose of streptomycin should be limited to 10 mg./kg. with a maximal dose of 750 mg.

amide (PYZ) followed by 4 months of isoniazid and rifampin.

3. Six months of therapy is usually effective for killing the three populations of bacilli: those rapidly dividing, those slowly dividing, and those only intermittently dividing.

4. Sputum smears may be obtained every 2 weeks until they are negative; sputum cultures do not become negative for 3–5 months.

5. Second-line drugs (capreomycin, kanamycin, ethionamide, para-aminosalicylic acid, and cycloserine) are used in patients with resistance, for retreatment, and in those with intolerance to other agents. Patients taking these drugs should be monitored by health providers experienced in their use.

Nursing Interventions and Patient Education

1. The patient usually ceases to be infectious 2–4 weeks after initiation of chemotherapy.

2. Educate the patient about the disease. Stress the importance of continuing to take medicine for the prescribed time.

3. Review the side effects of the drug therapy (Table 37-3). Question the patient specifically about common toxicities of drugs being used and emphasize immediate reporting to the clinic should these occur.

4. Review possible complications with the patient and family: hemorrhage, pleurisy, symptoms of recurrence (persistent cough, fever, or hemoptysis).

5. Educate the patient to control propagation of secretions while coughing.
   a. Cover mouth and nose with double-ply tissue when coughing/sneezing. Do not sneeze into bare hand.
   b. Wash hands after coughing/sneezing.

6. Encourage the patient to eat a nutritious diet.

7. Patients with problems of alcoholism should be referred to an alcoholic clinic or other appropriate health agency.

8. Avoid job-related exposure to excessive amounts of silicone (working in foundry, rock quarry, sand blasting).

9. Encourage the patient to report to clinic/physician at specified intervals for bacteriologic (smear) examination of sputum to monitor therapeutic response and patient compliance.

NURSING ALERT: Patient compliance remains a major problem in eradicating tuberculosis.

Preventive Treatment *(Chemoprophylaxis)*

1. Prevention of tuberculosis by prophylactic treatment with isoniazid.

2. Most tuberculosis cases occur in persons known to be significant tuberculin reactors.

3. These patients are the source of infection in 80%–90% of future cases of active tuberculosis disease.

A. Isoniazid Prophylaxis

1. Isoniazid therapy is given to persons infected with the tubercle bacillus without the disease—to prevent disease from occurring or to individuals at high risk of becoming infected.

2. Recommended for the following groups*:
   a. Household members and other close associates of potentially infectious tuberculosis cases
   b. Newly infected persons
   c. Persons with past tuberculosis
   d. Persons with significant reactions to tuberculin skin test and who are in special clinical situations
   e. Tuberculin skin test reactors under 35 years of age with none of the aforementioned skin risk factors

* Official Statement of the American Thoracic Society and the Centers for Disease Control. Am Rev Respir Dis 1986 Aug; 134(2): 355–363.

B. Complications of Isoniazid Therapy

1. Liver dysfunction and progressive liver damage.
2. Question the patient about loss of appetite, fatigue, joint pain, fever, and dark urine.
3. Monitor for fever, right upper quadrant abdominal tenderness, nausea, vomiting, rash, persistent paresthesias of hands and feet.
4. Encourage patient to report for liver function studies at prescribed intervals.

Guidelines | Tuberculin Skin Test

The *tuberculosis intradermal skin test* is used to detect tuberculosis infection.

Purposes
1. To detect infection, either past or present, with *Mycobacterium tuberculosis*.
2. To serve as a diagnostic procedure in selected patients.

Equipment
Purified protein derivative (PPD) tuberculin antigen; intermediate strength
Tuberculin syringe
Short 1.25 cm. (½ inch) 26- or 27-gauge steel needle
Alcohol sponge

Procedure

Nursing Action	Rationale/Amplification
1. Determine if the patient has ever had BCG vaccine, recent viral disease, immunosuppression by disease, drugs, or steroids.	
2. Draw up PPD-tuberculin into tuberculin syringe.	2. Follow the manufacturer's directions. Each 0.1-ml. dose should contain 5 tuberculin units (TU of PPD-tuberculin). Use the antigen immediately to avoid absorption onto the plastic/glass syringe.
3. Cleanse the skin of the inner aspect of forearm with alcohol. Allow to dry.	
4. Stretch the skin taut.	
5. Hold the tuberculin syringe close to the skin so that the hub of the needle touches it as the needle is introduced, bevel up.	5. This reduces the needle angle at the skin surface and facilitates the injection of tuberculin just beneath the surface of the skin.
6. Inject the tuberculin into the superficial layer of the skin to form a wheal 6 mm. to 10 mm. in diameter.	6. If no wheal appears (because the injection was made too deep), inject again at another site at least 5 cm. (2 inches) away.

To Read the Test

1. Read the test within 48–72 hours when the induration is most evident.	1. Tuberculin skin tests are tests of *delayed hypersensitivity*.
2. Have a good light available. Flex the forearm slightly at the elbow.	
3. Inspect for the presence of *induration:* inspect from a side view against the light; inspect by direct light.	3. Induration refers to hardening or thickening of tissues.
4. Palpate: Lightly rub the finger across the injection site from the area of normal skin to the area of induration. Outline the diameter of induration.	4. Erythema (redness) without induration is generally considered to be of no significance.
5. Measure the maximum transverse diameter of induration (not erythema) in millimeters with a flexible ruler.	5. The extent of induration is measured in two diameters and recorded

Interpretation

1. Significant reaction: Induration 10 mm. or more in diameter.	1. A significant reaction indicates that a patient has had contact with tubercle bacillus. It does not necessarily mean that active disease is present in the body.
2. Insignificant reaction: Induration less than 10 mm. in diameter.	2. This is considered ''not significant'' in persons who are not tuberculosis suspects or who are not close contacts of someone whose sputum is or was recently positive for *M. tuberculosis*.

Note: A tuberculin converter is a person whose tuberculin reaction changes from less than 10 mm. in diameter to 10 mm. or more in diameter, with the increase measuring at least 6 mm. (American Lung Association).

Follow-up Phase

1. Size of induration.
2. Name of antigen, strength of antigen, lot number, date of testing, date of reading.

Salmonella Infections (Salmonellosis)

Salmonellosis refers to infections caused by bacteria of the genus *Salmonella.* Salmonellosis is seen in several forms, each with its own symptoms: gastroenteritis, enteric fever (typhoid fever, p. 914), bacteremia with and without metastatic disease, and the asymptomatic carrier state.

Although there are over 200 serotypes known, *Salmonella typhimurium* is the most commonly reported in the US.

The patient is infected by ingesting the organism in food contaminated by infected feces of humans or animals, in eggs/egg products, in meat/meat products, in poultry, and in pharmaceuticals of animal origin.

Clinical Manifestations

(Usually 8–48 hours after ingestion of contaminated food)
1. Sudden onset of colicky abdominal pain and loose watery diarrhea
2. Fever to 38°–39°C. (100.4°–102.2°F.); may be accompanied by a chill
3. Nausea and vomiting
4. Symptoms usually subside in 2–5 days
5. Other manifestations due to infectious agent localizing in any body tissue—abscesses, cholecystitis, arthritis, endocarditis, meningitis, pericarditis, pneumonia, etc.

Diagnostic Evaluation

Isolation of organism from stool or ingested food

Management

1. Treatment is supportive, with emphasis on prevention of dehydration.
   a. Restrict food until nausea and vomiting subside.
   b. Offer clear liquids as soon as tolerated; the emphasis is on fluid replacement.
   c. Instruct the patient to avoid beverages with caffeine because these increase intestinal motility.
   d. Advise the patient to avoid taking antimotility drugs (anticholinergics; paregoric) since a slowed peristaltic activity may extend the period of diarrhea by interfering with the cleansing mechanism of diarrhea.
2. For patients with moderate to severe illness:
   a. Intravenous therapy may be necessary if symptoms are prolonged.
   b. Trimethoprim–sulfamethoxazole or chloramphenicol may be given for bacteremia or a prolonged febrile course.

Prevention and Patient Education

1. Prevent the contamination of food and water with fecal material.
2. The patient must wash hands after using toilet, particularly during illness and carrier state—to prevent infection of others.
3. Raw eggs or egg drinks should not be ingested, nor should cracked or dirty eggs be used.
4. All foods from animal sources, especially fowl, egg products, and meat dishes, should be thoroughly cooked.
5. Foods should be refrigerated during storage and should be protected against insects and rodents.
6. Chicks, ducklings, and turtles (as well as other domestic animals and pets) are regarded as sources of infection.
7. Food service workers should be instructed on an on-going basis about foodborne illnesses, avoidance of food contamination, food storage methods, cleaning of food preparation and service areas, and maintenance of good personal hygiene, including *handwashing.*

Shigellosis (Bacillary Dysentery)

Shigellosis, an acute bacterial disease of the intestinal tract, includes a group of enteric infections caused by bacilli of the *Shigella* group of which there are 4 types: *S. sonnei, S. flexneri, S. boydii,* and *S. dysenteriae.* The source of infection is feces from an infected person. The route of spread is fecal–oral. Foodborne outbreaks can almost always be traced to contamination of food by a food handler. Shigellosis may also be of sexual origin (anal–oral contact).

Clinical Manifestations

(The rectosigmoid colon is predominantly affected)
1. Fever and headache
2. Cramping and abdominal pain
3. Mild diarrhea to a severe dysenteric syndrome with blood, mucus, and pus in the stools—from impaired absorption of water and electrolytes by the inflamed colon
4. Rectal pain and tenesmus
5. Profound prostration

Diagnostic Evaluation

1. Stool culture
2. Fecal leukocyte examination

Management

1. Antibiotic therapy (trimethoprim-sulfamethoxazole; ampicillin; nalidixic acid)
   a. Initial therapy is guided by susceptibility pattern of *Shigella* species in the community—there is increasing resistance to antibiotic therapy being seen.
   b. Antibiotics are indicated as they shorten duration of illness and decrease duration of excretion of shigellae.
2. Maintenance of fluid and electrolyte balance—to prevent dehydration and correct signs of saline depletion.
   a. Intravenous fluids
   b. Oral rehydration solutions
3. Notification of local and state health authorities

Complications

1. Dehydration—may be fatal in elderly
2. Postdysenteric syndromes: arthritis, urethritis, conjunctivitis

Nursing Interventions

1. Assess patient for dehydration—weight loss, skin turgor, dryness of mucous membranes, altered vital signs (weak rapid pulse; postural hypotension), decreased urinary volume.
2. Offer clear caffeine-free liquids during acute stage of illness—supplement with bouillon broth.
3. Instruct the patient to avoid taking antimotility agents—may prolong duration of illness, presumably by retarding intestinal clearance of microorganisms.
4. Assist in carrying out epidemiology studies of every patient in whom organism is found.

a. Question the patient about travel to underdeveloped countries, exposure to crowded institutions, swimming in contaminated rivers. Inquire about water supplies, food eaten at home/restaurant.
b. Inform the patient that infected individuals for whom anal–oral contact is a sexual practice should be treated.

Preventive Measures and Patient Education

1. Stress *handwashing* and good personal hygiene.
2. See Patient Education for typhoid fever, page 915.
3. The following are essential:
   a. Program of fly control
   b. Surveillance of water sanitation
   c. Adequate sewage disposal
   d. Detection and treatment of carriers
4. Untreated sexual partners, particularly those of homosexual men, may reinfect the patient.

Typhoid Fever

Typhoid fever is a systemic bacterial infection transmitted by contaminated water, milk, shellfish, or other foods. It is caused by *Salmonella typhi,* which is harbored in human excreta. Today it is spread chiefly by carriers, patients who have recovered from the fever, but whose stools or urine may spread these bacilli for years. The ingestion of infected oysters or shellfish taken from waters contaminated by off-shore sewage disposal depots is another common source of infection. There is an increased incidence of typhoid acquired during foreign travel (certain areas of the developing world) and in microbiology laboratories.

Altered Physiology

The organism enters the body via the gastrointestinal tract; it invades the walls of the gastrointestinal tract, leading to bacteremia that localizes in mesenteric lymph nodes, in the masses of lymphatic tissue in the mucous membrane of the intestinal wall (Peyer's patches), and in small, solitary lymph follicles in the ileum and colon; ulceration of the intestines may ensue.

Clinical Manifestations

A. Gradual Onset

1. Severe headache, malaise, muscle pains, nonproductive cough.
2. Chills and fever; temperature rises slowly, reaching highest level in 3–7 days (40°–41°C. [104°–105°F.]).
3. Pulse is full and slow in comparison to height of fever.
4. Skin eruption—irregularly spaced small rose spots on abdomen, chest, back. Each spot fades over a period of 3–4 days.

B. Second Week

1. Fever remains consistently high.
2. Abdominal distention and tenderness; constipation or diarrhea.
3. Intense prostration
4. Delirium in severe infections—from severe toxemia.

C. Third Week

Gradual decline in fever and subsidence of symptoms

NURSING ALERT: Typhoid fever runs an aggressive course in patients with AIDS.

Diagnostic Evaluation

1. White blood cell count—leukopenia is a distinctive hematologic feature, but is not always present.
2. Blood or bone marrow culture.
3. Urine and stool cultures become positive in later stage of illness.
4. Blood serum agglutination test usually becomes positive by end of second week.

Management

1. Specific treatment to eradicate *S. typhi*
   a. Chloramphenicol; ampicillin; trimethoprim and sulfamethoxazole; furazolidone.
   b. Drug resistance is a recognized problem in infections acquired in some foreign countries.
2. High-dose dexamethasone—for patients with delirium, coma, or shock (in addition to antibiotics)
3. Intravenous infusions for correction of electrolyte and acid–base disturbances—for treatment of dehydration and diarrhea

Complications

1. *Perforation of intestine*—from erosion of one of the ulcers; most common during the third week.
   a. Clinical manifestations
      (1) Sudden, sharp abdominal pain—may stop suddenly
      (2) Abdominal rigidity
      (3) Shock
   b. Management
      Prepare for intestinal decompression procedure, intravenous fluids, and surgical intervention if conservative measures do not produce clinical improvement.
2. *Intestinal hemorrhage*—from erosion of blood vessel in ulcerated small intestine.
   a. Clinical manifestations
      (1) Apprehension, sweating, pallor
      (2) Weak, rapid pulse; narrowing pulse pressure
      (3) Hypotension
      (4) Bloody or tarry stools
   b. Management
      (1) Withhold food
      (2) Blood transfusions
      (3) Bowel resection is sometimes necessary
3. Relapse
4. Other complications: thrombophlebitis, urinary infections, cholecystitis, meningitis, osteomyelitis

Nursing Interventions

A. Giving Supportive Care

1. Support the patient during period of toxemia—the patient may be drowsy, partially incontinent, or delirious.
2. Awaken patient for medications, fluids, nourishment, and position changes.
3. Position the patient to prevent aspiration.
4. Use enteric precautions—patient may be incontinent, have diarrhea or retention of feces.
5. Give tepid water fever sponge for temperature of 40°C. (104°F.) or higher.
6. Encourage a high fluid intake—the patient may become dehydrated from high insensible water loss, vomiting, and/or diarrhea and poor oral intake.
7. Watch for bladder distention—the patient may lose the urge to void during toxic state. Keep input and output record.

B. Monitoring for Complications

See preceding discussion.

Prevention and Patient Education

1. Live oral typhoid vaccine for *Salmonella typhi* (Ty21a) has been successfully used as an effective public health tool for control of typhoid in developing countries.
2. The patient must be followed with routine stool culture after recovery to detect the development of the carrier state.
   a. Approximately 1%–3% of typhoid patients become chronic carriers, harboring the organism and excreting it in their urine and stools.
   b. Carriers may be given ampicillin or amoxicillin—to attempt to abolish carrier state.
   c. Positive chronic carrier state—documented evidence of *S. typhi* in stool or urine for 1 year or more.
   d. Carriers must not become food or milk handlers.
3. Environmental hygiene should be established in endemic areas.
   a. Protection and purification of water supplies
   b. Sanitary waste disposal techniques
   c. Pasteurization of milk and dairy products; should be refrigerated when being transported
   d. Avoidance of eating fresh, uncooked vegetables or unpeeled fruits (in endemic areas) that have not been washed in iodinated or chlorinated water
   e. Proper use of handwashing facilities by food handlers

Bacterial Meningitis
(Meningococcal Meningitis)

Meningitis is an inflammation of the membranes surrounding the brain and spinal cord. Any microorganism (bacteria, virus, fungus, protozoa) can cause a meningitis.

Bacterial meningitis is most frequently caused by *Neisseria meningitidis, Streptococcus pneumoniae* (in adults), and *Haemophilus influenzae* (in young children). It starts as an infection of the nasopharynx and is followed by meningococcal septicemia, which extends to the meninges of the brain and the upper region of the spinal cord. There are several distinct immunologic strains of the meningococcus, but groups A, B, C, and Y cause the majority of cases of bacterial meningitis.

Clinical Features

1. The mode of transmission is by direct contact, including droplets and discharges from the nose and throat of carriers (most often) or infected persons.
2. Meningococcus may localize in the brain, skin, or joint synovia.
3. Predisposing factors include alcoholism, malignant disorders, immunodeficiency states, diabetes mellitus, renal disease, sickle cell anemia, pneumonia, splenectomy, recent neurosurgical procedures, head trauma.
4. The disease occurs in winter and spring months; epidemics are most apt to occur when people live in crowded quarters.

Clinical Manifestations

Symptoms result first from infection and then from increased intracranial pressure.

1. *Severe headache*
2. Fever; nausea and vomiting
3. Neck, shoulder, and back pain and stiffness—from spasm of extensor muscles due to meningeal irritation
4. Petechial rash
5. Altered mental status: irritability, confusion, delirium, convulsions
6. Focal neurologic deficits
7. Signs of meningeal irritation
   a. Positive Kernig's signs—when lying with the thigh flexed on the abdomen, patient cannot completely extend his leg.
   b. Positive Brudzinski's sign—passive neck flexion produces flexion of knees and hips.

Diagnostic Evaluation

Organism usually demonstrated by smear and culture of cerebrospinal fluid and blood.

Complications

1. Shock; metabolic acidosis, "shock" lung
2. Increased intracranial pressure with brain herniation/brain stem injury
3. Cranial nerve palsies
4. Disseminated intravascular coagulation; congestive heart failure

Management

Management is carried out in intensive care—considered a medical emergency

1. Specific drug therapy initiated within shortest time possible
   a. Intravenous penicillin G (drug of choice); ampicillin; cefotaxime; ceftriaxone, depending on culture and sensitivity tests.
   b. Antibiotics given in larger doses and more frequent intervals—to ensure penetration across blood–brain barrier.
2. Management of shock
   a. Intravenous therapy to provide volume expansion
   b. Cardiovascular monitoring
   c. Correction of metabolic imbalances
   d. Monitor urinary output (maintain at 40–50 ml./hour)
3. Management of airway
   a. Arterial blood gas determinations
   b. Cuffed endotracheal tube/tracheostomy
   c. Oxygen to maintain arterial PO_2 at desired levels
4. Monitor for increased intracranial pressure.
5. Management of intracranial hypertension—in part due to cerebral edema and altered spinal fluid absorption. (See page 578.)
6. Management of fever
   a. Fever increases the brain's metabolic demands and cerebral blood flow
   b. Fever managed with antipyretic agents; cooling blankets
7. Control of seizures with diazepam, phenytoin

Prevention and Patient Education

1. Antimicrobial (rifampin) prophylaxis is indicated for persons who have intensive direct contact with the infected patient.
2. A quadrivalent vaccine consisting of types A, C, Y, and W-135 is available for use in the event of an outbreak of meningeal disease.

3. Close contacts should be observed and immediately evaluated if fever or other signs and symptoms of meningococcal meningitis develop.
4. Prevent overcrowding of living quarters and poor air hygiene; increase ventilation.
5. Improve practices of personal hygiene, particularly control of droplet infection.

Tetanus (Lockjaw)

Tetanus is an acute disease caused by the tetanus bacillus *Clostridium tetani,* whose spores are introduced into the body when an injury becomes contaminated with soil, street dust, or animal or human feces. The bacillus is an anaerobe (cannot live in presence of oxygen).

Clinical Manifestations

(Caused by potent neurotoxins elaborated by *C. tetani,* which have a special affinity for nervous tissue.)
1. Hyperirritability; restlessness, headache, low-grade fever
2. Rigidity of muscles, muscle spasms of both flexor and extensor muscle groups
   a. *Trismus*–painful spasms of masticatory muscles; difficulty in opening the mouth (lockjaw); neck rigidity, stiffness, dysphagia
   b. *Risus sardonicus*—distorted grin produced by spasm of facial muscles
   c. Recurrent painful reflex spasms of almost every muscle group in body—involvement of respiratory muscles may lead to respiratory failure; fractures of the vertebral bodies can occur during severe spasms.
   d. *Opisthotonus*—arching of the trunk (from spasms)

> **NURSING ALERT:** In recent years, approximately two thirds of the patients with tetanus have been over 50 years old. This may be the result of inadequate or absent immunization or of waning immunity. Parenteral drug abusers are at risk due to contaminated drugs or equipment.

Management

A. Wound and Systemic Care
1. Tetanus immune globulin (human) (TIG)
   a. Usually given 1–2 hours before wound debridement—to neutralize the toxins and ensure appropriate circulating levels when the wound is debrided.
   b. Prevents neurotoxins released into circulation during debridement from being attached to nerve endings.
2. Effective wound care includes cleaning, irrigation, debridement, and removal of all foreign bodies.
3. Active immunization with tetanus toxoid (according to immune status of the patient) is started—clinical tetanus does not produce immunity.
   a. Depends on patient's immune status.
   b. Separate syringes and separate sites are used when tetanus toxoid and TIG are given concurrently.
4. Antimicrobial therapy (penicillin or an alternate antibiotic)—to eradicate persistent *C. tetani* and other pathogens from wound.

Management of Tetanus
1. Sedatives and muscle relaxant medications (diazepam; chlorpromazine)—large doses may be necessary.
2. Neuromuscular blockade (vecuronium; pancuronium)—for treatment of severe, uncontrolled general spasms.
3. Cardiac monitoring.
4. Sympathetic blocking agents for management of persistent hypertension and tachycardia due to autonomic nervous system dysfunction.

Complications
1. Cardiac arrest
2. Autonomic disturbances; dysrhythmias
3. Bacterial shock

Nursing Interventions

(In ICU)

A. Preventing Respiratory and Cardiovascular Complications
1. Monitor for dysphagia—may warn of risk of asphyxiation and aspiration.
2. Initiate intubation and mechanical ventilation as quickly as possible if spasms are interfering with respiratory function.
3. Maintain an adequate airway—tetanic spasms of larynx, pharynx, and respiratory muscles usually occur during convulsions and may lead to hypoxia, asphyxia, and death.
4. Provide cardiac monitoring—overactivity of sympathetic nervous system may lead to ''sympathetic crisis'' and death.
   a. Watch for isolated unexplained tachycardia, temporary hypertension, premature ventricular contractions, sweating.
   b. Keep a vein open for infusions and in event of respiratory/cardiac arrest.

B. Providing Ongoing Assessment and Support
1. Support the patient during tetanic spasm and convulsions—caused by the action of toxins in the cells of central nervous system; mortality rate of patients with frequent and severe spasms is high.
   a. Spasms are *painful* and may cause hypoxia and vertebral fractures.
   b. Give diazepam as directed, and sedatives to treat muscle rigidity and reflex spasms.
2. Plan nursing management during periods when sedation has maximum effect for minimal patient disturbance—spasms occur in response to a stimulus.
   a. Place the patient in a quiet, semi-dark environment—to avoid stimulating reflex spasms.
   b. Avoid sudden stimuli and light—slightest stimulation may trigger paroxysmal spasms.

> **NURSING ALERT:** The hearing of the patient with respiratory paralysis may be acute. Do not make unguarded comments in his presence.

3. Maintain fluid and electrolyte balance. Parenteral nutrition may be required—aspiration is a constant threat.
4. Avoid contractures and pressure sores—from prolonged immobility.
5. Watch for urinary retention—occurs when perineal muscles are affected.

6. Be alert for the development of fractures of the long bones and vertebral bodies that may occur with severe spasm.
7. Monitor for fecal impaction.
8. See page 583 for management of the patient with convulsive seizures and page 575 for management of the unconscious patient.

Prevention and Patient Education

1. Tetanus has occurred almost exclusively in persons who are unimmunized or inadequately immunized, or whose immunization history is unknown.
2. The primary immunization series for tetanus consists of a combination of tetanus and diphtheria toxoids, adult type (Td)
   a. Three doses given IM
   b. The second dose is given 4–8 weeks after the first
   c. The third dose is given 6–12 months after the second
   d. Booster immunization with Td every 10 years is recommended
3. Consider every break in the skin as a potential portal of entry for *C. tetani*
   a. Tetanus-prone wounds—compound fractures; gunshot injuries; burns; foreign bodies; wounds contaminated with soil or feces; wounds neglected for more than 24 hours; puncture wounds; wounds infected with other microorganisms; wounds from induced abortions; wounds made by dirty hypodermic needles (drug abusers).

> **NURSING ALERT:** Tetanus-prone wounds are those in which there has been an invasion of soil or feces or those involving a severe traumatic injury. Tetanus may develop from an insignificant wound contaminated by soil. Deep necrotic pressure sores are tetanus-prone.

4. The most important step in the prevention of tetanus is the thorough washing and cleansing of the wound, with removal of all foreign material and devitalized tissue—helps eliminate tetanus bacilli from wounds and removes the material that forms a focus in which tetanus spores can develop.
5. Following injury, the immunization status of the patient will determine whether or not to provide active immunization with tetanus toxoid and/or passive immunization with tetanus immune globulin; the nature and age of the wound, the conditions under which it was incurred, and the treatment are considered on an individual basis.
6. Encourage the patient to keep an up-to-date record of his immunization status.

Clostridial Myonecrosis (Gas Gangrene)

Gas gangrene is a severe soft tissue infection with muscle necrosis, gas production, and systemic toxicity caused by gram-positive clostridia, which may complicate compound fractures, wounds, or following surgical procedures producing exotoxins that destroy tissue. Several species of clostridia (*C. perfringens, C. septicum, C. histolyticum, C. novyi,* and others) may produce gas gangrene. These organisms are putrefactive, gram-positive, spore-forming encapsulated bacilli. They are found widely in soil and naturally inhabit the gastrointestinal tract, respiratory tract and female genital tract.

> **NURSING ALERT:** Nontraumatic metastatic clostridial infections are being seen with increasing frequency, presumably from bacteremic spread of organisms from the bowel to skeletal muscle.

Clinical Manifestations

1. Sensation of heaviness in involved region followed by severe *pain*—caused by gas and edema in the tissues
2. Apprehension; tachycardia; prostration; altered mental status—from systemic toxicity
3. Appearance of wound
   a. Skin is white and tense initially; then progresses to bronze, brown, or black color.
   b. Soft tissue crepitus (crackling)—produced by gas in the tissue.
   c. Vesicles appear; are filled with red, watery fluid.
   d. Muscle is dark red or black and edematous, contains red, watery, foul-smelling fluid.
   e. Gas bubbles seen emanating from tissues—toxins ferment muscle sugar; produce acid and gas, which digest muscle protein. (Obvious gangrene is present.)
4. Anemia and jaundice—from hemolysis

Diagnostic Evaluation

Gram stain of exudate/muscle tissues—shows gram-positive rods

Management and Nursing Interventions

1. Volume expansion and blood transfusion—to counteract shock and replenish red blood cells lost to hemolysis.
2. Antimicrobial therapy (penicillin; chloramphenicol)—for treatment of gas gangrene and bacteremia
3. Surgical exploration and debridement of necrotic tissue—preventive as well as curative
   a. Early excision of all devitalized and infected tissue with wide incisions will render wound unsuitable for growth of clostridium; also diminishes intracompartmental pressure, thereby reducing muscular necrosis.
   b. Extensive incisions (once infection has developed) in affected part allow air to inhibit growth of anaerobic organisms.
4. Hyperbaric oxygen therapy—increases the dissolved oxygen in the arterial system by increasing the partial pressure of the oxygen breathed by the patient; stops toxin production
5. Administration of tetanus prophylaxis
6. Ongoing assessment for patient with toxemic manifestations
   a. Central venous pressure, pulmonary capillary wedge pressure; and urinary output (patient at risk for developing renal failure).
   b. Potassium levels—hemolysis and tissue destruction may lead to hyperkalemia.

Prevention and Patient Education

1. All wounds should be treated promptly.
2. Patients with infection from *C. septicum* should have a diagnostic work-up for occult malignancy following acute treatment.

3. Persons with diabetes are prone to opportunistic infections with *C. septicum.*

Botulism*

Botulism is a type of poisoning that affects the central nervous system; it is caused by eating food in which *Clostridium botulinum* has grown and produced toxins. The organism is widely distributed in soil. Human intoxication usually follows ingestion of contaminated foods: home-canned, dried, or smoked foods; or poorly processed foods.

Course

1. Variable; illness may be prolonged with a high risk of superinfection and fatal outcome.
2. Recovery in survivors may be prolonged.

Clinical Manifestations

(Usually begin 12–36 hours after ingestion of contaminated food)

The toxins elaborated by *C. botulinum* are extremely potent and are rapidly absorbed by the gastrointestinal tract; they become bound to neural tissues and produce a neuroparalytic syndrome.

1. Descending flaccid paralysis beginning with muscles innervated by cranial nerves
   a. Blurred vision; inability to open eyes
   b. Difficulty in speaking and swallowing
   c. Severe dryness of mouth and throat
2. Gastrointestinal symptoms: nausea, vomiting, abdominal pain
3. Descending involvement of motor neurons to peripheral muscles including muscles of respiration—weakness and paralysis with normal mental status

Diagnostic Evaluation

1. Suspected cases should be reported to public health authorities in order to identify and treat patients *early* in the course of illness
2. Examination of fecal samples, serum, incriminated food—for botulinal toxins
3. Electromyography—to document electrophysiologic abnormalities
4. Mouse-toxin neutralization test—for detection of botulinal toxin; the patient's serum is sent to a laboratory that has capacity for performing this test.

Management

A. **Intensive Supportive Care**—death is frequently due to onset of respiratory failure

1. Measurement of vital capacity and inspiratory force—for indication of ventilatory impairment.
   a. Arterial blood gas evaluations—may show only minor abnormalities despite substantial loss of ventilatory reserve.
   b. Monitoring for aspiration pneumonia.
   c. Endotracheal intubation and mechanical ventilation.
2. *Early* administration of ABE botulinal antitoxin—to neutralize unbound toxin in the circulation.

---

* Botulism is an intoxication, not an infection. The Centers for Disease Control, Atlanta, GA 30333, offer diagnostic consultation and laboratory testing services and support for epidemiologic studies of botulism.

a. Ascertain patient's history of allergies or previous exposure to horse serum—to minimize risk of adverse reaction to antitoxin.
   b. Perform a skin test for sensitivity; read package insert.
   c. Have ventilatory equipment and emergency drugs ready in event of life-threatening reaction.
3. Early administration of cathartics, enemas, and gastric lavage (when these can be safely administered)—to eliminate unabsorbed toxin from gastrointestinal tract; in event of respiratory paralysis or an ileus, these procedures may not be prescribed.
4. ECG monitoring—to detect signs of cardiac arrest.
5. Family teaching (during convalescence).
   a. High prevalence of persistent symptoms (tiredness, weakness, dyspnea) 1 year or more after onset of illness
   b. Recovery requires regeneration of the nerve endings that have been poisoned with toxin.

Complications

1. Respiratory or bulbar paralysis
2. Infectious complications

Prevention and Patient Education

1. Home canners should be taught how to prevent botulism—use proper containers and adhere to time and temperature guidelines for processing.
2. Home-canned foods should be inspected before being eaten—foods contaminated with *Clostridium botulinum* may look soft, contain gas bubbles, and give off an odor of decay. However, contaminated food items may have a normal appearance and taste.
3. Discard any rusty or swollen canned food; do not taste contents.
4. Canned foods should be heated at temperature over 80°C. (176°F.) for 30 minutes or boiled for 10 minutes—toxins are heat-labile and destroyed by proper cooking of foods.
5. Be careful in preparing food for canning at high altitudes since it is difficult to provide a temperature high enough to destroy the spores of *Clostridium botulinum.* Use pressure cooker method of canning at high altitudes.
6. Do not use punctured or swollen cans or jars with defective seals.

Viral Infections

Influenza

Influenza is an acute infectious disease caused by an RNA-containing myxovirus. It is characterized by respiratory and constitutional symptoms. Epidemics of influenza develop rapidly; there is a fairly high mortality rate among the elderly and those debilitated by chronic disease.

Etiology

1. The primary factor in the etiology of influenza is a filterable virus of which three major strains have been isolated, designated types A, B, and C.
2. The numerous variants within a given type are called subtypes.
3. Three subtypes of hemagglutin (H_1, H_2, H_3) and two subtypes of neuraminidase (N_1, N_2) are among influ-

enza A viruses that have caused widespread human disease.
4. Influenza appears to become epidemic when new strains appear against which most of the population lacks immunity.
5. Transmission is by close contact or by droplets from the respiratory tract of an infected person.

Clinical Course

1. The virus is airborne and multiplies in the upper respiratory tract—selected invasion of nasal, tracheal, and bronchial mucosal cells.
2. Influenza virus damages the ciliated epithelium of the tracheobronchial tree, rendering the patient vulnerable to the development of secondary invaders such as pneumococci or staphylococci, *Haemophilus influenzae,* streptococci, and other organisms.

Clinical Manifestations

1. Sudden onset of fever (39°–40°C. [102°–104°F.]), malaise, sore throat, cough, rhinorrhea, headache, myalgia
2. Prostration

Management

1. Patient usually treated at home with bedrest, fluids, analgesics, nasal spray, cough syrup, and vaporizer.

> **NURSING ALERT:** Aspirin should not be used for those under 16 years of age because of its possible association with the occurrence of Reye's syndrome.

2. Specific antiviral therapy (amantadine hydrochloride [Symmetrel])
   a. Appears to interfere with the uncoating step in the virus replication cycle and also reduces virus shedding—shortens duration of fever and other symptoms.
   b. Used for therapy and prevention.

Complications

1. Pulmonary complications (viral pneumonia, secondary bacterial pneumonia, mixed viral and bacterial pneumonia)
2. Exacerbation of chronic obstructive pulmonary disease
3. Neurologic complications—meningoencephalitis
4. Reye's syndrome, in adolescents

Prevention

A. Vaccination With Inactivated Virus Vaccine

1. Immunization consists of a single dose of vaccine (influenza virus vaccine) for either primary or annual booster vaccination.
2. Influenza vaccine should be given in late fall (mid-October through mid-November) to render optimal protection during peak influenza months of January and February.
3. Annual vaccination with inactivated influenza vaccine decreases incidence of complications, hospitalization, and deaths, especially in elderly. Recommended for the following:
   a. Persons at high risk (i.e., the elderly, persons with chronic disorders of cardiovascular, pulmonary,

and/or renal system, metabolic disease, severe anemia, and/or compromised immune function).
   b. Residents of nursing homes and chronic care facilities.
   c. Health care workers and others who administer care to high-risk populations.

B. Antiviral therapy

1. Amantadine hydrochloride (Symmetrel)—used for *prevention and treatment* of respiratory tract infection caused by influenza A viruses.
   a. Chemoprophylaxis for unvaccinated high-risk persons exposed to influenza—used immediately after exposure to influenza because virus replication occurs early in disease.
   b. Amantadine shortens duration of fever and systemic and respiratory symptoms.
   c. Side effects—dizziness, nervousness, irritability, and insomnia.

Patient Education

1. The risk of developing influenza is related to crowding and close contact of groups of individuals.
2. Restrict visiting privileges within health care facilities during epidemics—to minimize chance of introducing influenza.
3. It appears wise to humidify home and office air and to discourage cigarette smoking for high-risk persons.
4. The Immunization Practices Advisory Committee of the Centers for Disease Control publishes recommendations for influenza vaccinations annually.

Infectious Mononucleosis

Infectious mononucleosis ("mono") is an acute infectious disease of the lymphatic system caused by the Epstein–Barr virus (EBV), a DNA virus of the herpes virus group. Cytomegalovirus infection can produce a clinical picture closely resembling that of infectious mononucleosis. Infectious mononucleosis occurs in individuals without antibodies to EBV.

Incidence and Transmission

1. Occurs mainly between ages of 15 and 25; high frequency of occurrence in college students and military population.
2. The virus is excreted in the saliva of patients with active disease or of those who are carriers, and is spread by intimate personal contact. It can also be transmitted by blood transfusion.

Clinical Manifestations

(May be vague and masquerade as those of leukemia, streptococcal sore throat, hepatitis, drug rash)
1. Sore throat, fever, lymphadenopathy (particularly in posterior cervical lymph nodes, producing neck pain)
2. Edema of upper eyelids, headache, malaise, muscle aches
3. Generalized fatigue
4. Skin rash, petechiae on palate
5. Enlargement of spleen

Diagnostic Evaluation

1. Blood smears—show lymphocytosis and atypical lymphocytes

2. Heterophil antibody agglutination test—increase in titer
3. EBV specific antibody test (positive)
4. Abnormal liver function tests

Complications

1. Splenic rupture, usually secondary to trauma
2. Chronic fatigue syndrome
3. Hemolytic anemia and/or immune thrombocytopenia
4. Neurologic events—Guillain–Barré syndrome; encephalitis
5. Cardiac disease: heart block, dysrhythmia, pericarditis
6. Hepatitis

Management

1. The treatment is symptomatic and supportive.
   a. Bedrest during febrile period.
   b. Increase activity to individual tolerance.
   c. Acetaminophen—for headache and muscle pains.
2. Steroids may be used for impending airway obstruction or severe thrombocytopenia.

Patient Education

Inform the patient as follows:
1. Avoid constipation and straining—increases pressure on an enlarged spleen.
2. Avoid heavy lifting, strenuous exercise, and contact sports until recovery is complete—exertion or trauma may cause rupture of the spleen.
3. The need for increased sleep and rest may continue for a period of time; prolonged fatigue is not uncommon.
4. Observe for abdominal and upper quadrant pain radiating to shoulder—evidence of splenic rupture.

Rabies *(Hydrophobia)*

Rabies is a severe viral infection of the central nervous system that is communicated to humans in the saliva of infected animals, especially wildlife (bats, skunks, raccoons, foxes) and cattle. The infection is transmitted by a bite or by contact of the animal's saliva with mucous membranes or with open wounds such as cuts, scratches, or abrasions.

Incubation Period

1. Varies from 10 days–1 year (average 31–60 days).
2. Influenced by species of the animal vector, location and severity of the wound, and host response; severe bites on the face and neck are most dangerous.

Prevention

Rabies in humans can be prevented by eliminating exposure to rabid animals and by promptly treating local wounds and immunizing when exposed.

Prophylactic Management of the Patient

A. Local Treatment of Wound

1. Immediately wash wound and surrounding skin area with soap and water—to remove saliva from area. This may be crucial for survival irrespective of subsequent immunization.
2. Take victim to emergency department for further cleansing and flushing of wound.

3. Provide tetanus prophylaxis and antibacterial therapy as required.

B. Rabies Postexposure Prophylaxis of the Patient

1. Postexposure rabies prophylaxis includes *both* active and passive immunization and thorough local treatment (soap and water cleansing) in previously nonimmunized individuals.
2. Rabies vaccine—used to promote active immunity to rabies in individuals exposed to the virus; promotes production of rabies antibody.
   a. Human diploid cell vaccine (HDCV) is given at the same time as a single injection of rabies immune globulin is given.
   b. Vaccine is administered IM in the deltoid area as soon as possible after exposure, and the remaining doses are administered 3, 7, 14, and 28 days after the first dose (see product information sheet).
   c. Antirabies treatment is discontinued if fluorescent antibody tests of the animal's brain are negative.
3. Rabies immune globulin (RIG) (passive immunization) provides antibody until the patient starts producing antibody in response to vaccine.
   a. Part of the RIG is infiltrated around the wound and the rest is administered IM into the deltoid muscle or anterolateral aspect of the thigh.
   b. RIG and rabies vaccine should *not* be given in the same syringe nor injected at the same site since neutralization of the vaccine may occur.
4. Alternative low-cost immunization regimens with new purified rabies vaccines are being used in less-developed countries where rabies is endemic.

Management of the Biting Animal

1. A healthy domestic dog or cat that bites a human is confined under veterinary or animal control surveillance; this may enable the bitten person to avoid undergoing rabies vaccination unnecessarily.
   a. If animal remains healthy for 10 days, it is assumed that it was not infected with rabies.
   b. If the animal becomes ill (or dies), the animal is humanely killed and the brain examined for the characteristic Negri bodies. The local health department is notified.
2. Any wild animal that bites or scratches a human should be killed at once and the brain examined for evidence of rabies.
3. If the biting animal escapes or is unknown, determination of the degree of risk is judged by the following factors:
   a. Prevalence of rabies in the area
   b. Species of biting animal
   c. Severity of wound(s)
   d. Whether attack was provoked or unprovoked; circumstances of the biting incident
   e. Consultation with local or state public health authorities
4. Any domestic animal that is bitten or scratched by a bat or by a wild carniverous mammal that is not available for testing should be regarded as having been exposed to a rabid animal.

Clinical Course and Clinical Manifestations of Rabies in Humans

A. Prodromal Stage

1. Headache and nausea
2. Fever

3. Malaise; loss of appetite; mental depression
4. Sore throat
5. Pain and paresthesia of bitten areas
6. Unusual sensitivity to sound, light, and changes in temperature
7. Dilation of pupils; increased salivation

B. Stage of Excitement

1. Episodes of irrational excitement alternating with periods of alert calm
2. Convulsions
3. Severe and painful throat spasms when the patient attempts to swallow (or even views) liquids (hydrophobia); violent spasms of inspiratory muscles
4. Death usually occurs in this stage from cardiac or respiratory failure.

C. Paralytic Stage

Fatal progressive paralysis

Diagnostic Evaluation

1. History of exposure and development of characteristic symptoms
2. Demonstration of rabies antibodies in the patient's blood
3. Demonstration of characteristic *Negri bodies* in samples of brain tissue of infected animal

Management of Rabies in Humans

No specific treatment; the care of the patient is symptomatic and supportive in the intensive care unit.

NURSING ALERT: The rabies virus is contained in the saliva of patient with this disease, constituting a distinct hazard to personnel caring for him.

Spirochetal Infections

Lyme Disease

Lyme disease (lyme borreliosis) is a multisystem infectious syndrome commonly affecting the skin, nervous system, heart, and joints, which is caused by a spirochete, *Borrelia burgdorferi*. It is introduced by the bites of Ixodid ticks, which have a wide range of hosts including deer, mice, sheep, and cattle.

In the US, Lyme disease is endemic along the northern Atlantic coast (Massachusetts, Rhode Island, Connecticut, New York), in the northern Midwest (Minnesota, Wisconsin), and the Pacific Northwest (California, Oregon, Utah, and Nevada).

Clinical Manifestations

A. Stage I

1. Usually occurs within 1 month after tick bite
2. Characterized by red papule or macule at site of tick bite expanding to form an erythematous lesion with bright red border and partial central clearing (erythema chronicum migrans [ECM]; Fig. 37-3).
3. ECMs range in size from 3–68 cm. and may last several months.

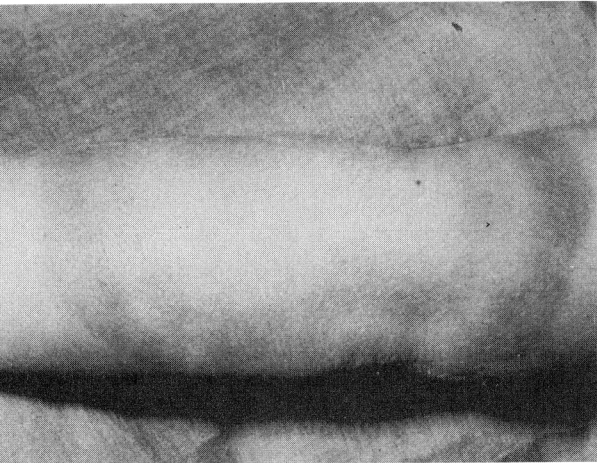

Figure 37-3. *The tick bite in Lyme disease is characterized by an expanding erythematous lesion with bright red border and partial central clearing (erythema chronicum migrans). (Courtesy Rocky Mountain Laboratories, The National Institute of Allergy and Infectious Diseases, The National Institutes of Health)*

4. Accompanied by fatigue, fever, headache, arthralgias, and myalgias.

B. Stage II

1. Occurs 2–3 months after onset of ECM.
2. Neurologic abnormalities—symptoms of meningitis (stiff neck, headache), difficulty with memory and concentration, cranial nerve dysfunction (Bell's palsy) or peripheral neuropathies.
3. Cardiac abnormalities—syncope, dizziness, shortness of breath, substernal chest pain, dysrhythmias, atrioventricular block, myopericarditis.

C. Stage III

1. May manifest months to years after initial infection.
2. Arthritis, especially in knees
3. Chronic neurologic and neuropsychiatric syndromes

Diagnostic Evaluation

1. History; recognition of ECM
2. Serologic tests—may not become positive until later stages of disease

Management

1. Varying regimens of antibiotic therapy: tetracycline; doxycycline; penicillin; amoxicillin—given *early* generally shorten duration of symptoms and prevent/ameliorate complications
2. Ceftriaxone—may be drug of choice with CNS manifestations

Prevention and Patient Education

Instruct people living or visiting an endemic area as follows:
1. Conduct systematic searches over entire body surface for ticks.
2. Apply insect repellant (with active ingredient, permethrin) to clothing.
3. Tuck pants into boots or socks; ticks are easier to see

on light-colored clothing as unengorged nymphs appear as 1–2 mm. dark specks.
4. Remove tick with forceps, exerting slow, steady upward pull; avoid squeezing the tick.
5. Clean site of attachment with soap and water; wash hands immediately with soap and water—salivation may last several minutes after the tick has been removed.
6. Shampoo pets routinely.
7. See Prevention and Patient Education, Rocky Mountain Spotted Fever, below.

Rickettsial Infections

Rocky Mountain Spotted Fever

Rocky Mountain spotted fever (typhus fever, tick-borne) is a severe infection caused by *Rickettsia rickettsii* transmitted to human by various species of ticks. It is caused by the bite of an infected tick, by crushing an infected tick on the skin, or via conjunctival contamination with infected tick secretions.

Etiology

1. The wood tick, *Dermatocenter andersonii,* is the primary carrier of *R. rickettsii* in the western US, and the dog tick, *D. variablis,* is the major vector in the eastern US.

Clinical Manifestations

During infection, *R. rickettsii* localize and proliferate in the vascular endothelium of small- and medium-sized blood vessels, producing widespread swelling and degeneration. This generalized vasculitis accounts for the manifestations of the disease and may involve virtually every organ.

The symptoms usually begin within 2 weeks after the tick bite.
1. Severe headache, malaise, prostration, photophobia, muscle pain involving the back and legs.
2. High fever—up to 42°C. (107°F.) in severe cases—subsides by lysis.
3. Rash—appears in 3–7 days (discrete maculopapular rose lesions appearing on distal parts of body (wrists, ankles, soles, and palms) and spreading to central parts of the body; may progress to petechial or purpuric stages; large subcutaneous hemorrhages may appear. *The rash is sometimes absent.*
   a. Areas of skin necrosis may appear as a result of endarteritis—necrosis may involve ear lobes, fingers, toes, and scrotum.
   b. Generalized edema—from generalized vascular involvement and resultant escape of serum.
4. Abdominal pain, rigidity, rebound tenderness—from vasculitis in the small abdominal vessels.
5. Restlessness, insomnia, hyperesthesia, and stupor and delirium
6. Thrombocytopenia

Diagnostic Evaluation

1. History of possible tick exposure; typical clinical picture
2. Immunofluorescence studies performed on tissue from a punch biopsy of involved skin lesion
3. Serologic testing

Management

1. Administration of antibiotic agents (tetracycline or chloramphenicol)—effective if given *early* before irreversible tissue damage occurs
2. Fluid and electrolyte replacement
3. Treatment of coagulation disturbances

Complications

1. Vasculitis leading to microthrombi, luminal occlusion, and microinfarction of virtually any organ.
2. Gangrene of digit or pressure point—from vascular thrombosis and poor circulation

Nursing Interventions

1. Use supportive nursing measures for combating fever and promoting patient comfort.
   a. Turn frequently and give skin care; position patient carefully—disease can cause vasculitis (inflammation of a vessel) with severe edema and necrosis.
2. Measure circumference of abdomen, arms, and legs—to determine extent of edema.
3. Keep input and output records for determination of oliguria—the patient may develop renal failure because of poor tissue perfusion from vascular degeneration.
4. Watch for signs and symptoms of disseminated intravascular coagulation, circulatory collapse, hypotension, oliguria, azotemia, hypoproteinemia, myocarditis, and pulmonary complications—Rocky Mountain spotted fever is an infectious vasculitis and can produce marked physiologic disturbances.
   a. Support vital functions.
   b. Central venous pressure measurements are used to guide fluid and electrolyte replacement because myocarditis is present in some patients and there is a risk of congestive heart failure.

Prevention and Patient Education

1. Clean weeds and cut brush and grass in recreational areas. Spray heavily infested areas (chemical control of recreation sites).
2. Exterminate rodents—serve as hosts for immature ticks.
3. Avoid sitting on grass or logs in infested areas.
   a. Wear clothing tucked in at wrists and ankles.
   b. Apply tick repellent to clothing and exposed parts of body.
4. Remove tick by grasping with tweezers as close as possible to the point of attachment and by steadily pulling upward with even pressure until removal. If tweezers are not available, protect hands with paper towel/tissue or rubber gloves. *Bare fingers should not be used.*
   a. Do not crush, squeeze, or puncture the tick—to avoid contamination of the broken skin with infectious tick secretions.
   b. Disinfect the attachment site and inspect site for remaining foreign material. Wash hands with soap and water immediately.
   c. Discard the tick immediately in a container of alcohol or flush down the toilet; if in the field, bury it.
5. Examine household pets and their sleeping areas daily for ticks; if infested, shampoo or dust with an appro-

priate agent. Do not crush the tick when deticking a pet.
6. Instruct the patient/family to advise the physician/clinic of history of tick bite if systemic symptoms occur.

Protozoan Infections

Malaria

Malaria is an acute and chronic infectious disease caused by protozoa plasmodia. Transmission is by way of an intermediate host (the bite of an infective female *Anopheles* mosquito). Malaria has also been transmitted via blood transfusions and from the use of shared contaminated needles and syringes by drug abusers.

Etiology

1. Four species of malaria parasites—grouped under genus *Plasmodium,* each causing a different type of malaria: *P. falciparum, P. vivax, P. malariae, P. ovale.*
2. The parasite has a complicated life cycle. Not all patients demonstrate classical cycles of fever and chills.
3. *P. falciparum* causes the most serious type of malaria because of the development of high parasitic densities in blood; infected red blood cells tend to agglutinate and form microemboli.

Clinical Problems

1. It is estimated that over 50% of the world's population is at risk to malaria, with an estimated 1–2 million deaths every year.
2. Malaria control is difficult due to emergence of widespread multidrug-resistant *P. falciparum* malaria, adaptation and resistance of anopheline mosquitoes to insecticides, and socioeconomic realities.
3. There has been an increased number of cases imported into the US since millions of Americans each year are traveling to tropical countries.

Clinical Manifestations

1. Malaise, headache, muscular pain, nausea, and dizziness.
2. Paroxysms of shaking chills; rapidly rising fever followed by profuse sweating; fever is often continuous.
3. Splenomegaly, hepatomegaly, orthostatic hypotension, anemia.
4. Paroxysms may last about 12 hours, after which the cycle may be repeated daily, every other day, or every third day.

Diagnostic Evaluation

1. Demonstration of malaria parasites in blood smears by microscopic examination—confirms presence, species, and density of parasites.
2. Travel in an endemic area is an important diagnostic clue.

Management

Specific therapy depends on species of parasite involved; malarial parasites can evolve drug-resistant forms.

A. For *P. vivax, P. malariae,* and *P. ovale* Malaria

1. Chloroquine: agent of choice
2. Daily monitoring of blood for parasitemia

B. For *P. falciparum* Malaria

1. Intensive care monitoring, as this is considered a medical emergency.
2. Quinine (or quinidine), usually IV—used to reduce parasitemia; a second drug may be added to aid in eliminating remaining parasites. For quinine-resistant *P. falciparum,* pyrimethamine-sulfadoxine (Fansidar).
3. Blood levels for parasites are monitored every 12 hours—to make sure parasite load is reduced.
4. Exchange blood transfusion—may be done for rapid reduction of high levels of parasites.
5. Hemodynamic and cardiac monitoring.
6. Maintaining renal function
   a. Monitor intake and output—to monitor for development of renal failure and pulmonary edema.
   b. Dopamine and furosemide—to maintain renal blood flow and urinary output.
   c. Hemodialysis—for renal failure; may be lifesaving.
7. Watch for jaundice—related to density of the falciparum parasitemia (presence of malarial parasites in the blood); abnormalities of hepatic function are also common in falciparum malaria.
8. Evaluate degree of anemia—related to severity of infection.
9. Watch for abnormal bleeding (nose bleeds, oozing of blood from venipuncture sites, passage of blood in the stool)—may be due either to decreased production of clotting factors by a damaged liver or to disseminated intravascular coagulation (DIC).

Prevention and Patient Education

1. Exposure to malaria can be reduced either by destroying the vector mosquitoes or by preventing human–mosquito contact.
2. Advise travelers of risk in areas where malaria is endemic—Centers for Disease Control (CDC) booklet, *Health Information for International Travel,* annually updates the current status of malaria in each country and advises of the most recent prophylactic recommendations.
   a. Limit dusk-to-dawn outdoor exposure, wear protective clothing, live in screened quarters, sleep under mosquito netting impregnated with safe insecticide, and use insect repellent on skin and clothing (mosquitoes can penetrate cloth).
   b. Advise malaria chemoprophylaxis when traveling to areas where malaria is endemic. Malaria prophylaxis should start *before* a person enters the area and for 4 weeks after leaving the area.
   c. No single advocated regimen of chemoprophylaxis can guarantee 100% protection. Symptoms may appear up to 1 year after the trip.
   d. Advise the traveler to seek prompt health care if he develops fever after stopping prophylaxis.

Amebiasis (Amebic Dysentery)

Amebiasis is a worldwide parasitic disease that is responsible for multiple medical–surgical problems. It is caused by the protozoa *Entamoeba histolytica* and is acquired by ingestion of the cyst stage of *E. histolytica* in food or water contaminated by infected human feces. It is also acquired by person-to-person transmission of enteric pathogens by orogenital, oroanal, or proctogenital sexual activity, particularly among homosexuals.

Incidence

1. An estimated 10% of the world's population is infected; commonly found in tropical and subtropical countries.
2. Risk for carriage of *E. histolytica* includes low socio-economic status, inadequate water supply, poor sanitation, poor hygiene, crowded circumstances, and poor education.
3. In the US, found in rural areas; in patients who have lived or traveled in the tropics. Institutionalized individuals or those in communal living settings are at increased risk.

Pathologic Insights

1. *E. histolytica* lives in the large intestine and feeds mainly on bacteria.
2. Amebas may be located in the bowel lumen and intestinal wall or outside the gastrointestinal tract.
   a. Trophozoites develop from viable cysts in the small intestine.
   b. Trophozoites may erode intestinal mucosa, invade the bloodstream, and travel to the liver via the portal circulation.
   c. Amebas can produce abscesses and other serious complications.

Clinical Manifestations

(May be symptomatic or asymptomatic)
1. Colicky abdominal pain
2. Frequent bloody stools

Diagnostic Evaluation

1. Demonstration of trophozoites and/or cysts in stool samples; multiple stool samples may have to be examined as the parasite is excreted intermittently.
2. Scraping of lesions obtained during endoscopy examination.
3. Finding specific antibodies in patient's serum.

Complications

1. Liver abscess; peritonitis due to liver abscess rupture or intestinal perforation or obstruction.
2. Thoracic amebiasis (from hematogenous spread of amebae from liver or intestine or by direct penetration of liver abscess into chest cavity).
3. Ameboma (amebic granuloma found in cecum, rectum, transverse and sigmoid colon).

Management

1. Treatment consists of a systemic drug plus a lumen amebicide: metronidazole (Flagyl) followed by iodoquinol or diloxanide furoate—produces cessation of diarrhea and eradicates encysted organisms in most patients.
   a. Caution the patient not to drink alcohol when taking Flagyl; may cause severe reaction.
   b. Serial follow-up of stools is necessary—relapses are common.
2. Place the patient on enteric precautions.
3. Keep the patient on bed rest if diarrhea is acute.
4. Give intravenous infusions as indicated to correct fluid and electrolyte imbalance resulting from severe diarrhea.
5. Prepare for aspiration of liver abscess.

Prevention and Patient Education

1. Prevent contamination of food and water with human feces.
2. Carry out health education in personal hygiene—hand washing after defecation, before food preparation and eating.
3. Avoid ground-grown vegetables (lettuce, etc.) and local water supply when traveling in areas where amebiasis is endemic.
4. Boil water to ensure elimination of amebae; avoid ice cubes, etc., in endemic areas.
5. Examine contacts of recently diagnosed patients.
6. Advise male homosexuals of person-to-person transmission of enteric pathogens by sexual activity.

Giardiasis

Giardiasis is a protozoan infection of the small intestine caused by the flagellate *Giardia lamblia.* This water-borne parasite is found in two forms: cysts and trophozoites.

Transmission is by ingestion of cysts that are excreted in the feces of a human or animal host. It is transmitted to humans by person-to-person contact or from fecal contamination of food or water.

At Risk

1. Persons living in residential facilities and day care centers
2. Homosexual men engaging in anal–oral sexual practices
3. Campers/skiers drinking untreated surface water (in uninhabited mountain areas)

Clinical Manifestations

1. Bloated feeling/abdominal pain; symptomatic disease is not a constant feature
2. Protracted diarrhea with loose, watery, foul-smelling stools; abdominal cramping, weight loss
3. Malabsorption of fats (steatorrhea) accompanied by weight loss, general debility, and fatigue—indicative of chronic infection

Diagnostic Evaluation

1. Stool specimen to detect cysts or trophozoites of *Giardia lamblia*
2. Enterotest—swallowing of small gelatin capsule lined with silicon rubber and suspended on a nylon string—to retrieve duodenal mucus for parisitologic examination
3. Small bowel biopsy

Management

1. Quinacrine; side effects are dizziness, headache, nausea and vomiting, and yellow staining of skin.
2. Alternative drugs are metronidazole or furazolidone.

Prevention and Patient Education

1. Travelers and hikers should boil water in endemic areas.
2. Avoid raw, unpeeled fruits and vegetables in areas where giardiasis is endemic.
3. Use careful handwashing and personal cleanliness to prevent person-to-person transmission.

4. Proper disposal of feces and maintenance of community water supplies are essential.

Systemic Mycotic Infections
(Fungal Infections)
Mycoses and Histoplasmosis

Fungi are primitive organisms that take their nourishment from living plants and animals and from decaying organic material. The three main types of mycoses (fungal infections), determined by the tissue level at which the fungus settles, are:

1. Systemic or deep mycoses—primarily involve the internal organs, usually centering in the lungs.
2. Subcutaneous mycoses—involve the skin, subcutaneous tissue, and sometimes the bone.
3. Superficial or cutaneous mycoses—grow in outer layer of skin (epidermis), in hair, and in nails.

Histoplasmosis is a chronic systemic fungus infection caused by a spore-bearing mold called *Histoplasma capsulatum.* It is found in soil, particularly soil enriched with bird or bat excrement. This highly infectious mycosis is acquired by inhalation of spores, typically after the disturbance of contaminated soil.

The two major forms of clinical disease due to *H. capsulatum* are pulmonary and disseminated infection.

Clinical Manifestations

1. Clinical features are usually nonspecific; fungal infections mimic other diseases.
2. Acute pulmonary histoplasmosis may manifest as an acute flu-like illness with fever, headache, cough, and pleuritic pain.
3. Chronic pulmonary histoplasmosis (usually in patients with history of COPD) produces interstitial pneumonia, necrosis, and cavity formation, with symptoms of cough, sputum production, weight loss, and hemoptysis.
4. Disseminated histoplasmosis is characterized by constitutional symptoms (fever, chills, anorexia, weight loss) along with evidence of extrapulmonary disease to one or multiple organ systems: oropharynx, lymph nodes, liver, bone marrow.

Diagnostic Evaluation

1. Cultures of blood, bone marrow, and other tissues/body fluids
2. Serologic tests for histoplasma

Management

1. Patients with acute pulmonary histoplasmosis usually do not require treatment as antifungal treatment is reserved for more severe forms.
2. Amphotericin B is the mainstay of therapy for disseminated disease.
   a. Dosage is controlled by blood level studies. (The patient is assessed for renal toxicity, manifested by rising blood urea nitrogen, decreased creatinine clearance, and other laboratory tests.)
   b. Severe toxic reactions to amphotericin B include nausea and vomiting, chills, fever, headache, phlebitis.

3. Ketoconazole is an alternate therapy; may be drug of choice in immunocompetent patient with nonlifethreatening disease. Adverse effects include nausea, vomiting, anorexia, and hepatomegaly.
4. Surgical intervention may be advised for persistent lung cavitation or for acute emergency with gastrointestinal histoplasmosis (bowel perforation).

Patient Education

1. Avoid stirring up dust around bird-roosting sites (raking and sweeping, etc.) Exposure to *Histoplasma capsulatum* is associated with spelunking (cave exploration).
2. Minimize exposure to dust in a contained closed environment; spray area with water to reduce dust.
3. Disseminated histoplasmosis is being seen with increasing frequency in patients with AIDS. The disease is often more severe and the clinical manifestations are not specific.

Helminthic Infestations
Hookworm Disease

Hookworm disease (ancylostomiasis; "ground itch") is the result of infestation of the small intestine by quite similar hookworms about 1.2 cm. (½ inch) long. Two species of hookworms infect humans:

Necator americanus (predominant species in US)
Ancylostoma duodenale

The infection is usually contracted by penetration of the skin or oral mucosa by infected larvae in the soil.

Incidence

1. Southeastern US
2. Endemic in tropical and subtropical countries

Clinical Course

1. Hookworm eggs are passed in human feces onto the ground (indiscriminate defecation habits). Eggs develop into infective larvae.
2. The larvae *bore through the skin of bare feet* ("ground itch") or penetrate subcutaneous tissues, usually through a hair follicle or an abraded area. Infection with *Ancylostoma duodenale* can be by both percutaneous and oral route (eating contaminated vegetables).
3. After gaining access to the blood or lymph vessels, they are carried via the blood to the lungs, migrate from the pulmonary capillaries into the alveoli, reach the pharynx, and are swallowed, maturing to adult worms in the small intestine.

Clinical Manifestations

1. *Dermatitis* ("ground itch")—occurs at site where larvae penetrate skin.
2. Coryza, pharyngitis, laryngitis, sensation of obstruction in throat, cough—from larval migration to upper respiratory tract.
3. *Gastrointestinal symptoms*—maturation of worms in the intestine is usually marked by epigastric/abdominal pain, diarrhea, and other gastrointestinal symptoms.
4. Low-grade fever and malaise.

5. *Severe anemia* and hypoproteinemia—the worms attach to intestinal mucosa and suck blood; a single adult worm can extract 0.03 ml. of blood daily. The patient's iron stores become depleted. A low level of serum protein develops (protein malnutrition).

Diagnostic Evaluation

1. History of anemia and malnutrition
2. Recovery and identification of the eggs in the stool

Management

1. Pyrantel pamoate (single dose) or mebendazole (multiple dose usually required).
2. Ensure that the patient is eating a nutritious diet—hookworm disease occurs in persons suffering from malnutrition.
3. Give protein and iron supplementation—to aid in correction of anemia.

Prevention and Patient Education

1. The sanitary disposal of human feces is the single most effective control measure in preventing the spread of hookworm infection.
2. Instruct the patient to wear shoes at all times; however, poverty often precludes buying shoes.
3. Treat infected individuals: an estimated one fourth of the world's people are hookworm-infected.
4. "Night soil" (human excrement used as fertilizer) and sewage effluents should not be used for fertilizer as they place large segments of the population at risk.

Trichinosis (Trichinellosis)

Trichinosis is infestation by the parasite *Trichinella spiralis,* one of the roundworms. It is acquired by consuming infected meat, usually pork.

Clinical Course

1. Tiny embryos of the parasite *Trichinella spiralis* become encysted in the muscle fibers of an infected pig.
2. These calcified cysts appear in meat (chiefly pork); resemble tiny grains of sand.
3. If insufficiently cooked pork is eaten, the embryos are set free by the gastric juice and develop in the intestine during the following week, becoming adult worms 3–4 mm. long.
4. These worms make their way into the mucous membranes and there produce myriad embryos (larvae) (period of invasion).
5. The larvae, carried by the bloodstream and their own activity, migrate to all parts of the body (period of migration).
6. The larvae gradually become encysted in striated skeletal muscle.

Clinical Manifestations

A. **Intestinal Stage** (Begins in 24 Hours and May Last 1–7 Days)

1. May be asymptomatic
2. Gastrointestinal complaints: diarrhea, abdominal pain, nausea and vomiting
3. Mild fever—progresses to high and spiking by third week

B. **Muscular Invasion** (Symptoms Derive From Inflammatory Process Developing in the Muscles)

1. Edema of the eyelids; scleral hemorrhages; pain on eye motion
2. Generalized pain and soreness in the muscles (myalgia)
3. Cardiac irregularities (occasional)—from trichinae in the heart muscle; may be fatal
4. Difficulty in breathing, masticating, swallowing, speaking
5. Evidence of myocardial and CNS involvement

Diagnostic Evaluation

1. Biopsy specimen of painful muscle—provides direct detection of parasites.
2. Positive serologic tests—demonstrable titers 3–4 weeks after infection
3. Rising eosinophil count

Management

1. Pyrantel or mebendazole are used to eradicate mature Trichinella forms.
2. Corticosteroid agents may suppress allergic and inflammatory reaction during acute stage.
3. Analgesics—to relieve muscle pain.
4. ECG evaluations—to determine evidence of myocarditis
5. Bed rest for symptom relief

Complications

1. Myocarditis
2. Neurologic abnormalities (encephalitis; meningitis)

Prevention and Patient Education

1. The public should be educated about the importance of thoroughly cooking all pork and pork products, especially sausage. There should be no trace of pink in cooked pork.
2. Smoking, pickling, seasoning, and spicing do not make pork safe unless it is thoroughly cooked (especially homemade sausage).
3. Beef hamburger may be contaminated by a meat grinder that has been used for pork.
4. Garbage intended for feed for hogs should be cooked.
5. Stringent rodent control is necessary.

Bibliography

Books

Christie AB. Infectious Diseases: Epidemiology and Clinical Practice, Vols 1 and 2. 4th ed. New York, Churchill Livingstone, 1987

Cook GC. Communicable and Tropical Diseases. London, Heinemann Medical Books, 1988

Cunha BA (ed). Infectious Diseases in the Elderly. Littleton, MA, PSG Publishing, 1988

Gantz NM et al. Manual of Clinical Problems in Infectious Disease. 2nd ed. Boston, Little, Brown & Co, 1986

Gear JHS. Handbook of Viral and Rickettsial Hemorrhagic Fevers. Boca Raton, FL, CRC Press, 1988

Gee G and Moran TA. AIDS: Concepts in Nursing Practice. Baltimore, Williams & Wilkins, 1988

George WL and Finegold SM. Clostridial myonecrosis. In Balows A et al. Laboratory Diagnosis of Infectious Diseases, Vol 1. Bacterial, Mycotic, and Parasitic Diseases. New York, Springer–Verlag, 1988

Gleckman RA, Gantz NM and Brown RB. Infections in Outpatient Practice. New York, Plenum, 1988

Grange JM. Mycobacteria and Human Disease. London, Edward Arnold Publisher, 1988

Hatheway CL. Botulism. In Balows A et al. Laboratory Diagnosis of Infectious Diseases, Vol 1. Bacterial, Mycotic and Parasitic Diseases. New York, Springer–Verlag, 1988

Heffernan JJ, Witzburg RA and Cohen AS. Clinical Problems in Acute Care Medicine. Philadelphia, WB Saunders, 1989

Hobbs BC and Roberts D. Food Poisoning and Food Hygiene. 5th ed. Baltimore, Edward Arnold Publishers, 1987

Hoeprich PD and Jordan MC. Infectious Diseases: A Modern Treatise of Infectious Processes. Philadelphia, JB Lippincott, 1989

Katz M, Despommier DD and Dwadz R. Parasitic Diseases. 2nd ed. New York, Springer–Verlag, 1989

Kilbourne ED. Influenza, New York, Plenum, 1987

Levin S et al. The Clinician's Guide to Sexually Transmitted Diseases. Chicago, Year Book Medical Pub, 1987

Manson–Bahr PEC and Bell DR. Manson's Tropical Diseases. 19th ed. Philadelphia, Bailliere Tindall, 1987

Parrillo JE and Masur H (eds). The Critically Ill Immunosuppressed Patient. Rockville, Aspen Publishers, 1987

Ravdin JI (ed). Amebiasis. New York, John Wiley & Sons, 1988

Rippon JW. Medical Mycology. 3rd ed. Philadelphia, WB Saunders, 1988

Rubin RH and Young LS (eds). Clinical Approach to Infection in the Compromised Host. 2nd ed. New York, Plenum, 1988

Strand CL and Shulman JA. Bloodstream Infections. Chicago, ASCP Press, 1988

Sun T. Color Atlas and Textbook of Diagnostic Parasitology. New York, Igaku–Shoin, 1988

Vedrus NA (ed). Evolution of Meningococcal Disease, Vol 1 and 2. Boca Raton, CRC Press, 1987

Wyngaarden JB et al. Cecil Textbook of Medicine. 18th ed. Philadelphia, WB Saunders, 1988

Journals

Control of Infectious Diseases

Cunha BA. Clinical implications of fever. Postgrad Med 1989 Apr; 85(5):188–200

Forrest BD. The development of a bivalent vaccine against diarrhoeal disease. Southeast Asian J Trop Med Public Health 1988 Sep; 19(3):449–457

Korn JE and Poland GA. Adult immunization. Primary Care 1989 Mar; 16(1):177–196

Lorber B. Changing patterns of infectious diseases. Am J Med 1988 Mar; 84(3, Pt 2):569–578

Mostow SR. Influenza: A controllable disease? J Am Geriatr Soc 1988 Mar; 36(3):281–283

Neu HC. Quinolones: A new class of antimicrobial agents with wide potential uses. Med Clin North Am 1988 May; 72(3):623–636

Sexually Transmitted Diseases

Cates W Jr. Epidemiology and control of sexually transmitted diseases: Strategic evolution. Infect Dis Clin North Am 1987 Mar; 1(1):1–23

Centers for Disease Control. 1989 Sexually Transmitted Diseases: Treatment Guidelines. Public Health Service, 1989

Centers for Disease Control. Division of Sexually Transmitted Disease. *Chlamydia trachomatis* infections: Policy guidelines for prevention and control. MMWR 1985 Aug 23; 34(3S): 53S–74S

Dallabetta G and Hook EW. Gonococcal infections. Infect Dis Clin North Am 1987 Mar; 1(1):25–54

Feder HM and Manthous C. The asymptomatic patient with a positive VDRL test. Am Fam Physician 1988 Jan; 37(1):185–190

Fraiz J and Jones RB. Chlamydial infections. Annu Rev Med 1988; 39: 357–370

Kraus SJ, Reynolds GS and Rolfs RT Jr. Therapy of uncomplicated gonorrhea due to antibiotic-resistant *Neisseria gonorrhoeae*. Sex Tran Dis 1988 Oct–Dec; 15(4):234–243

Larson RE and Shapiro M. Sexually transmitted urogenital diseases. Emerg Med Clin North Am 1988 May; 6(3): 487–508

McGregor JA, French JI and Spencer NE. Prevention of sexually transmitted diseases in women. J Reprod Med 1988 Jan; 33(1 Suppl):109–118

Paavonen J and Wolner–Hanssen P. *Chlamydia trachomatis*: A major threat to reproduction. Human Reprod 1989 Feb; 4(2):111–124

Rosen T et al. Vesicular Jarisch-Herxheimer reaction. Arch Dermatol 1989 Jan; 125(1):77–81

Stamm WE. Diagnosis of *Chlamydia trachomatis* genitourinary infections. Ann Intern Med 1988 May; 108(5): 710–717

Whelan M. Nursing management of the patient with *Chlamydia trachomatis* infection. Nurs Clin North Am 1988 Dec; 23(4):877–883

Wilson D. An overview of sexually transmissible diseases in the perinatal period. J Nurse Midwifery 1988 May–Jun; 33(3):115–128

Bacterial Infections

A strategic plan for the elimination of tuberculosis in the United States.

MMWR Suppl 1989 Apr 21; 38(S3):1–21

Arenas RB et al. *Clostridium septicum* myonecrosis in association with colonic malignancy. Conn Med 1988 Dec; 52(12):709–710

Balk RA and Bone RC (eds). Septic shock. Crit Care Clin 1989 Jan; 5(1):1–189

Buckley D and Kudsk K. Occult gastrointestinal carcinoma causing metastatic clostridial soft-tissue infection. Dis Colon Rectum 1988 Apr; 31(4):306–310

Calva E, Puente JL and Calva JJ. Research opportunities in typhoid fever: Epidemiology and molecular biology. Bioessays 1988 Nov; 9(5):173–177

Cohen JI, Bartlee JA and Corey GR. Extra-intestinal manifestations of *Salmonella* infections. Medicine 1987 Sep; 66(4):349–388

DuPont HL. Shigella. Infect Dis Clin North Am 1988 Sep; 2(3):599–605

Goldberg MB and Rubin RH. The spectrum of *Salmonella* infection. Infect Dis Clin North Am 1988 Sep; 2(3):571–598

Harris RL et al. Manifestations of sepsis. Arch Intern Med 1987 Nov; 147(11): 1895–1906

Iverson RL. Septic shock: A clinical perspective. Crit Care Clin 1988 Apr; 4(2):215–228

Jones LV and Rodriguez RS. Bacterial-induced diarrhoea. Drugs 1988; 36(Suppl 4):6–17

Keusch GT. Antimicrobial therapy for enteric infections and typhoid fever: State of the art. Rev Infect Dis 1988; Jan–Feb; 10(Suppl 1):S199–S205

Kornbluth AA, Danzig JB and Bernstein LH. *Clostridium septicum* infection and associated malignancy. Medicine 1989 Jan; 68(1):30–37

Luce JM. Pathogenesis and management of septic shock. Chest 1987 Jun; 91(6): 883–888

Macho JR and Luce JM. Rational approach to the management of multiple systems organ failure. Crit Care Clin 1989 Apr; 5(2):379–392

Mandal BK. Typhoid fever and other salmonellae. Current Opinion Infect Dis 1989 Feb; 2(1):101–105

Musher DM. The gram-positive cocci. II. Staphylococci. Hosp Pract 1988 Apr 15; 23(4):179–193

Oz MC et al. Review of Salmonella mycotic aneurysms of the thoracic aorta. J Cardiovasc Surg 1989 Jan–Feb; 30(1):99–103

Pickett JB. Botulism. Muscle Nerve 1988 Dec; 11(12):1201–1205

Rice V. Septic shock: Nursing implications of current medical research. NITA 1987 Sep–Oct; 10(5): 326–333

Roos KL and Scheld WM. The management of fulminant meningitis in the intensive care unit. Crit Care Clin 1988 Apr; 4(2):375–392

Scholz DG et al. Tetanus: An uncommon cause of dysphagia. Mayo Clin Proc 1989 Mar; 64(3):335–338

Wahl S. Septic shock—How to detect it early. Nursing 1989 Jan; 19(1):52–59

Woodson CE and Sachs GA. Prevention, diagnosis, and management of infection in the nursing home. Clin Geriatr Med 1988 Aug; 4(3):507–525

Viral Infections

Benson CA and Kessler HA. Update: Epstein-Barr virus-related disease. Compr Ther 1988 Mar; 14(3):58–64

Cheeseman SH. Infectious mononucleosis. Semin Hematol 1988 Jul; 25(3):261–268

D'Angelo LJ. Common infectious disease problems in adolescents and young adults. Compr Ther 1988 Dec; 14(12): 15–20

Ershler WB. Influenza vaccination in the elderly: Can efficacy be enhanced? Geriatrics 1988 Sep; 43(9):79–83

Fishbein DB and Baer GM. Animal rabies: Implications for diagnosis and human treatment. Ann Intern Med 1988 Dec 15; 109(12):935–937

Prevention and control of influenza. 1. Vaccines. JAMA 1989 Jun 9; 261(22): 3220–3227

Rabies vaccine failures. Lancet 1988 Apr 23; 1(8591):917–918

Robinson RG. Abdominal complications of infectious mononucleosis. J Am Board Fam Pract 1988 Jul–Sep; 1(3): 207–210

Thurn JR and Henry K. Influenza A pneumonitis in a patient infected with human immunodeficiency virus (HIV). Chest 1989 Apr; 95(4):807–810

Tominack RL and Hayden FG. Rimantadine hydrochloride and amantadine hydrochloride use in influenza A virus infections. Infect Dis Clin North Am 1987 Jun; 1(2):459–478

Vodopija I. Current issues in human rabies immunization. Rev Infect Dis 1988 Nov–Dec; 10(Suppl 4):S758–S763

Welliver RC and Pearay LO. Immunology of respiratory viral infections. Annu Rev Med 1988; 39:147–162

Rickettsial Infections

Halpern JS. Tick removal. J Emerg Nurs 1988 Sep–Oct; 14(5):307

Kamper CA, Chessman KH and Phelps SJ. Rocky Mountain spotted fever. Clin Pharmacol 1988 Feb; 7(2):109–116

Petri WA Jr. Tick-borne diseases. Am Fam Physician 1988 Jun; 37(6):95–104

Walker DH. Diagnosis of rickettsial diseases. Pathol Annu 1988; 23(Part 2): 69–96

Protozoan Infections

Bruce–Shwatt LJ. Malaria and its control: Present situation and future prospects. Annu Rev Public Health 1987; 8:75–110

Cattani JA. Malaria vaccines: Results of human trials and directions of current research. Exp Parasitol 1989 Feb; 68(2):242–247

Cook GC. The great malaria problem: Where is the light at the end of the tunnel? J Infect 1989 Jan; 18(1):1–10

Gilles HM. Malaria—An overview. J Infect 1989 Jan; 18(1):11–23

Krogstad DJ et al. Antimalarial agents: Specific treatment regimens. Antimicrob Agents Chemother 1988 Jul; 32(7):957–961

Mahajan RC, Sehgal R and Ganguly NK. Applications of ELISA in amoebiasis. Trop Gastroenterol 1988 Jul–Aug; 9(3):123–126

Malaria, mosquito control, and primary health care. Lancet 1988 Mar 5; 1(8584):511–512

Masley SC and Weiss BD. Malaria: Chemoprophylaxis and therapy. Am Fam Physician 1988 Aug; 38(2):109–118

Sitprija V. Nephropathy in falciparum malaria. Kidney Int 1988 Dec; 34(6): 867–877

Spirochetal Infections

Duffy J. Lyme disease. Infect Dis Clin North Am 1987 Sep; 1(3):511–527

Hamilton DR. Lyme disease: The hidden pandemic. Postgrad Med 1989 Apr; 85(5):303–308; 313–314

McAlister HF et al. Lyme carditis: An important cause of reversible heart

block. Ann Intern Med 1989 Mar 1; 110(5):339–345

McKenna DF. Lyme disease: A review for primary health care providers. Nurse Pract 1989 Mar; 14(3):18, 20, 22, passim

Sigal LH. Lyme disease: A world-wide borreliosis. Clin Exp Rheumatol 1988 Oct–Dec; 6(4):411–421

Sigal LH. Lyme disease, 1988: Immunologic manifestations and possible immunopathogenetic mechanisms. Semin Arthritis Rheum 1989 Feb; 18(3):151–167

Wright SW and Trott AT. North American tick-borne diseases. Ann Emerg Med 1988 Sep; 17(9):964–972

Fungal Infections

Cappell MS et al. Gastrointestinal hisoplasmosis. Dig Dis Sci 1988 Mar; 33(3):353–360

Davies SF. Diagnosis of pulmonary fungal infections. Semin Respir Infect 1988 Jun; 3(2):162–171

Greenfield RA. Pulmonary infections due to higher bacteria and fungi in the immunocompromised host. Semin Respir Med 1989 Jan; 10(1):68–77

Kauffman CA and Terpenning MS. Deep fungal infections in the elderly. J Am Geriatr Soc 1988 Jun; 36(6):548–557

Saag MS and Dismukes WE. Treatment of histoplasmosis and blastomycosis. Chest 1988 Apr; 93(4):848–851

Wheat LJ. Histoplasmosis. Infect Dis Clin North Am 1988 Dec; 2(4):841–859

Parasitic/Helminthic Infections

Drugs for parasitic infections. Med Lett Drugs Ther 1988 Feb 12; 30(759):15–24

Ivanoska D et al. Comparative efficacy of antigen and antibody detection tests for human trichinellosis. J Parasitol 1989 Feb; 75(1):38–41

Mandell WF and Neu HC. Parasitic infections. Med Clin North Am 1988 May; 72(3):669–690

Emergency Management*

Emergency management has traditionally referred to the care given to patients with urgent and critical needs. However, the philosophy of emergency care has broadened to include the concept that an emergency is whatever the patient or his family considers it to be.

Principles of Assessment and Emergency Management†

Underlying consideration: Injuries or conditions interfering with vital physiologic function take precedence.

(It is assumed that all treatment is given under the direction of a physician.)

A. Treat the Potentially Life-threatening Problems First

Goals:
Preserve life.
Prevent deterioration before more definitive treatment can be given.
Restore patient to useful living.

---

* This section will deal mainly with emergency management of trauma and other conditions not found elsewhere in this book. Management of acute heart conditions is found on page 297 and management of acute respiratory problems, on page 208.

† Resuscitation, stabilization, and evaluation of the patient are carried out simultaneously by the Emergency Department team.

B. Stabilize the Pulmonary, Cardiovascular, and Central Nervous Systems

1. Maintain a patent airway and provide adequate ventilation, employing resuscitation measures when necessary.
   Assess for chest injuries with subsequent airway obstruction.
2. Evaluate and restore cardiac output.
3. Control external hemorrhage and its consequences.
4. Prevent and treat shock; maintain or restore effective circulation.
5. Carry out a rapid initial and ongoing physical examination; the clinical course of the injured or seriously ill patient is not static, and assessment must be ongoing.
6. Assess whether or not the patient can follow commands; evaluate the size and reactivity of the pupils and motor responses.
7. Start ECG monitoring if appropriate.
8. Splint suspected fractures, including fractures of cervical spine in patients with head injuries.
9. Protect wounds with sterile dressings.
10. Check to see if patient has a Medic Alert or similar identification designating allergies, etc.
11. Start a flow sheet of the patient's vital signs, blood pressure, neurologic status, etc., to guide decision making.

Obtaining Data *(History)*

If possible, a brief history of the accident/illness is taken from the patient or the person accompanying him—relative, emergency medical technician.

1. What were the circumstances, forces, location, and time of injury?
2. When did the symptoms appear?
3. Was the patient unconscious after the accident?
4. How did the patient reach the hospital?
5. What was the health status of the patient before the accident or illness?
6. Is there a past history of illness? Of past admissions?
7. Is the patient currently taking any medications—especially hormones, insulin, digitalis, anticoagulants?
8. Does the patient have any allergies?
9. Does the patient have any bleeding tendencies?
10. Is the patient under a physician's care? (Name of physician)
11. When was the last meal eaten? (Important if an anesthetic is to be given.)
12. What was the date of the patient's most recent tetanus immunization?

Psychological Management of Patients and Families in Emergencies

Underlying consideration: Body trauma is an insult to physiologic and psychological homeostasis; it requires both physiologic and psychological healing.

A. Approach to the Patient

1. Understand and accept the basic anxieties of the acutely traumatized patient. Be aware of the patient's fear of death, mutilation, and isolation.
    a. Personalize the situation as much as possible—speak, react, and respond in a warm manner.
    b. Give explanations on a level that the patient can grasp—an informed patient can cope with psychological/physiologic stress in a more positive manner.
    c. Accept the rights of the patient and family to have and display their own feelings.
    d. Maintain a calm and reassuring manner—helps the emotionally distressed patient or family to mobilize their psychological resources.
2. Understand and support the patient's feelings concerning his loss of control (emotional, physical, and intellectual).
3. Treat the unconscious patient as if he were conscious—touch him, call him by name, and explain every procedure that is done. Avoid making negative comments about the patient's condition.
    a. Orient the patient to person, time, and place as soon as he is conscious; reinforce by repeating this information.
    b. Bring the patient back to reality in a calm and reassuring way.
    c. Encourage the family, when possible, to orient the patient to reality.
4. Be prepared to handle all aspects of acute trauma; know what to expect and what to do—alleviates the nurse's anxieties and increases the patient's confidence.

B. Approach to the Family

1. Inform the family where the patient is and give as much information as possible about the treatment he is receiving.
2. Recognize the anxiety of the family and allow them to talk about their feelings—allow expressions of remorse, anger, guilt, and criticism.
3. Allow the family to relive the events, actions, and feelings preceding admission to the emergency department.
4. Deal with reality as gently and quickly as possible; avoid encouraging and supporting denial.
5. Assist the family to cope with sudden and unexpected death. Some helpful measures include the following:
    a. Take the family to a private place.
    b. Talk to all of the family together—so that they can mourn together.
    c. Assure family that everything possible was done; inform them of the treatment rendered.
    d. Avoid using euphemisms such as "passed on," etc. Show the family that you care by touching, offering coffee, etc.
    e. Allow family to talk about the deceased and what he meant to them—permits ventilation of feelings of loss. Encourage family to talk about events preceding admission to the emergency department.
    f. Encourage family to support each other and to express emotions freely: grief, loss, anger, helplessness, tears, disbelief.
    g. Avoid volunteering unnecessary information (patient was drinking, etc.).
    h. Avoid giving sedation to family members—may mask or delay the grieving process, which is necessary to achieve emotional equilibrium and prevent prolonged depression.
    i. Encourage family members to view the body if they wish to do so—helps to integrate the loss (cover mutilated areas).
        (1) Go with family to see the body.
        (2) Show acceptance of the body—by touching—to give family "permission" to touch, talk to, etc., the body.
        (3) Spend a few minutes with the family, listening to them.
6. Encourage the emergency department staff to discuss among themselves their reaction to the event—to share intense feelings, for review, and for group support.

Cardiopulmonary Resuscitation and Airway Management

The provision of oxygenation and ventilation via a secure airway is the highest priority in emergency resuscitation.

Cardiopulmonary resuscitation is described in the Guidelines that follow. Artificial ventilation is also accomplished by a bag–mask unit (p. 224) or endotracheal intubation (p. 233). Cricothyroidotomy (p. 934) and esophageal obturator airway (p. 935) are used in certain emergencies for resuscitation. The management of foreign-body obstruction is included on page 933. Airway management and artificial ventilation are discussed in detail under Respiratory Failure and Insufficiency, Chapter 11, page 208.

Guidelines Cardiopulmonary Resuscitation for Cardiac or Respiratory Arrest*

Cardiac arrest is a sudden and unexpected cessation of the heartbeat and effective circulation that results in inadequate delivery of oxygenated blood to vital organs.

Causes

1. Cardiac arrest
   Ventricular fibrillation
   Ventricular tachycardia; asystole
   Electromechanical dissociation

2. Respiratory arrest
   Drowning
   Stroke
   Foreign-body airway obstruction
   Smoke inhalation
   Drug overdose
   Electrocution/injury by lightning
   Suffocation
   Accident/injury
   Coma

Signs and Symptoms

1. Absence of palpable carotid or femoral pulse; pulselessness in large arteries
2. Immediate loss of consciousness
3. Absence of breath sounds or air movement through nose or mouth
4. Ashen gray color

Purpose

To provide oxygen to the brain, heart, and other vital organs until appropriate definitive medical treatment can restore the heart and ventilatory function

Equipment

Trained personnel
Arrest board
Oral airway
Bag and mask device

Intravenous (IV) setup
Defibrillator
Emergency cardiac drugs
ECG machine

ABCs of CPR*

1. Airway
   Open the airway
   Determine whether patient is breathing (look, listen, feel)
2. Breathing
   Rescue breathing (mouth to mouth)
   Foreign-body airway obstruction
3. Circulation
   Establish presence or absence of pulse
   Active emergency medical services (EMS)
   Begin chest compression (if pulse absent)

Procedure

Action	Rationale/Amplification

Assessment

1. Determine unresponsiveness: tap or gently shake patient while shouting, "Are you OK?"
2. Call for help.
3. Place patient supine on a firm, flat surface. Kneel at the level of the patient's shoulders.
4. Open the airway.
   a. *Head-tilt/Chin-lift Maneuver:*
   Place one hand on the patient's forehead and apply firm backward pressure with the palm to tilt the head back.
   Then, place the fingers of the other hand under the bony part of the lower jaw near the chin and lift up to bring the jaw forward and the teeth almost to occlusion.
   b. *Jaw-thrust Maneuver:*
   Grasp the angles of the patient's lower jaw and lifting with both hands, one on each side, displace the mandible forward while tilting the head backward.

1. This will prevent injury from attempted resuscitation on a person who is not unconscious.

3. This enables the rescuer to perform rescue breathing and chest compression without moving the knees.

   a. In the absence of sufficient muscle tone, the tongue and/or epiglottis will obstruct the pharynx and larynx.

   This supports the jaw and helps tilt the head back.

---

* Adapted from: Standards and guidelines for cardiopulmonary resuscitation (CPR) and emergency cardiac care (ECC). JAMA 1986 Jun 6; 255(1):2905–2954.

(continued)

Procedure (continued)	Action	Rationale/Amplification

Breathing

Assessment

Determine presence or absence of spontaneous breathing.

1. Place ear over patient's mouth and nose while observing the chest, *look* for the chest to rise and fall, *listen* for air escaping during exhalation, and *feel* for the flow of air.

   Rationale: 1. Keep maintaining an open airway.

2. Perform rescue breathing—Mouth-to-mouth: While keeping the airway open, pinch the nostrils closed using the thumb and index finger of the hand that is on the forehead. Take a deep breath, open mouth wide, and place it outside of the patient's mouth, creating an airtight seal.

   Rationale: 2. This prevents air from escaping from the patient's nose.

   Ventilate the patient with two full breaths (1–1½ seconds each breath), taking a breath after each ventilation.

   If the initial ventilation attempt is unsuccessful, reposition the patient's head and repeat rescue breathing.

   Rationale: Adequate ventilation is indicated by seeing the chest rise and fall, feeling the air escape during ventilation and hearing the air escape during exhalation.

Circulation

Assessment

Determine pulselessness.

1. While maintaining head-tilt with one hand on the forehead, palpate the carotid or femoral pulse. If pulse is not palpable, start external chest compressions.

   Rationale: 1. Cardiac arrest is recognized by pulselessness in the large arteries of the unconscious, breathless patient. If there is a palpable pulse, but no breathing present, initiate rescue breathing at rate of 12 × per minute (once every 5 seconds) after initial two breaths.

External Chest Compressions

Consist of serial, rhythmic applications of pressure over the lower half of the sternum.

1. Kneel as close to side of patient's chest as possible. Place the heel of one hand on the lower half of the sternum, 3.8 cm. (1½ inches) from the tip of the xiphoid. The fingers may either be extended or interlaced but must be kept off the chest.

   Rationale: 1. The long axis of the heel of the rescuer's hand should be placed on the long axis of the sternum; thus the main force of the compression will be on the sternum and decrease the chance of rib fracture.

2. While keeping your arms straight, elbows locked, and shoulders positioned directly over your hands, quickly and forcefully depress the lower half of the patient's sternum straight down, 3.8–5 cm. (1½–2 inches).

3. Release the external chest compression completely and allow the chest to return to its normal position after each compression. The time allowed for release should equal the time required for compression. Do not lift the hands off the chest or change position.

   Rationale: 3. Release of the external chest compression allows blood flow into the heart.

4. Use 80 compressions per minute (100 if possible). For one rescuer, do 15 compressions at a rate of 80–100 per minute and then perform two ventilations; re-evaluate the patient.

   Rationale: 4. Rescue breathing and external chest compressions must be combined. Check for return of carotid pulse. If absent, resume CPR with 2 ventilations followed by compressions. For CPR performed by health professionals, mouth-to-mask ventilation is an acceptable alternative for rescue breathing.

5. For CPR performed by two rescuers, the compression rate is 80–100 per minute. The compression–ventilation ratio is 15:1 with a pause for ventilation (1–1½ seconds)

6. While resuscitation proceeds, simultaneous efforts are made to obtain and use special resuscitation equipment to manage breathing and circulation and provide definitive care.

   Rationale: 6. Definitive care includes defibrillation, pharmacotherapy for dysrhythmias and acid–base disturbances, and ongoing monitoring and skilled care in an intensive care unit.

Complications

Postresuscitation distress syndrome (secondary derangements in multiple organs)

Neurologic impairment; brain damage

NURSING ALERT: The patient who has been resuscitated is at risk for another episode of cardiac arrest.

Guidelines Management of Foreign-Body Airway Obstruction*

Foreign-body obstruction of the airway may be either partial or complete.

Clinical Manifestations
Weak, ineffective cough; high-pitched noises on inspiration
Respiratory distress
Inability to speak or breathe
Cyanosis; collapse

The *Heimlich maneuver* (subdiaphragmatic–abdominal thrusts) is recommended for relieving foreign-body airway obstruction in the adult.

Emergency Action	Rationale/Amplification

Heimlich Maneuver With Conscious Patient Sitting or Standing

1. Stand behind the patient; wrap your arms around his waist and proceed as follows:
   a. Make a fist with one hand, placing the thumb side of the fist against the patient's abdomen in the midline, slightly above the navel and well below the xiphoid process. Grasp the fist with the other hand.
   b. Press your fist into the patient's abdomen with a quick upward thrust. Each new thrust should be a separate and distinct maneuver.

b. A subdiaphragmatic abdominal thrust, by elevating the diaphragm, can force air from the lungs to create an artificial cough intended to move and expel an obstructing foreign body in the airway.

Heimlich Maneuver With Unconscious Patient Lying Down

1. Position patient supine with face up.
2. Kneel astride the patient's thighs, facing his head.
3. Place the heel of one hand against the patient's abdomen in the midline slightly above the navel and well below the tip of the xiphoid; place the second hand directly on top of the first.
4. Press into the abdomen with a quick upward thrust.

Finger Sweep

1. Open patient's mouth by grasping both the tongue and lower jaw between the thumb and fingers and lift the mandible (tongue–jaw lift).
2. Insert the index finger of the other hand down along the inside of the cheek and deeply into the throat to the base of the tongue.
3. Use a hooking action to dislodge the foreign body and maneuver it into the mouth for removal.

1. This maneuver is to be used only in the unconscious patient. This action draws the tongue away from the foreign body that may be lodged there.

3. Take care not to force the object deeper into the throat.

Chest Thrust With Conscious Patient Standing or Sitting

1. Stand behind the patient with arms under his axillae to encircle the patient's chest.
2. Place thumb side of your fist on middle of patient's sternum, taking care to avoid xiphoid process and rib cage margins.
3. Grasp your fist with the other hand and perform backward thrusts until the foreign body is expelled or patient becomes unconscious.

1. This technique is to be used only in advanced stages of pregnancy or in markedly obese person.

3. Each thrust is administered with the intent of relieving the obstruction.

Chest Thrust With Unconscious Patient Lying

1. Place the patient on his back and kneel close to the side of his body.
2. Place the heel of your hand on the lower half of the sternum.
3. Deliver each chest thrust slowly and distinctly with the intent of relieving the obstruction.

This maneuver is used only in the advanced stages of pregnancy or when the rescuer cannot apply the Heimlich maneuver effectively to the unconscious, markedly obese person.

---

* Adapted from: Standards and guidelines for cardiopulmonary resuscitation (CPR). II. Adult basic life support. JAMA 1986 Jun 6; 255(1): 2915–2932.

Guidelines Cricothyroidotomy

Cricothyroidotomy is the puncture or incision of the cricothyroid membrane to establish an emergency airway in certain emergency situations when endotracheal intubation or tracheostomy are not possible or contraindicated.

Equipment   No. 11 gauge needle or scalpel with No. 11 scalpel blade

Procedure

Nursing Action	Rationale/Amplification
1. Extend the neck. Place a towel roll beneath the shoulders.	1. So that the cricothyroid membrane can be palpated readily.
2. Identify the prominent thyroid cartilage (Adam's apple) and allow your finger to descend in the midline to the depression between the lower border of the thyroid cartilage and the upper border of the cricoid cartilage (Fig. 38-1).	2. This depression represents the cricothyroid membrane.

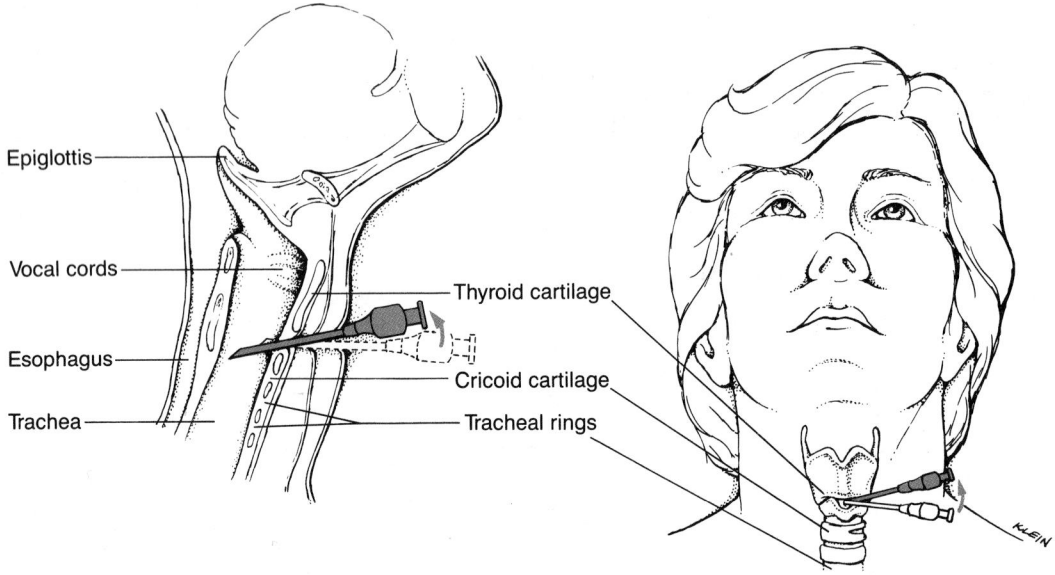

Figure 38-1. *Cricothyroidotomy, or cricothyroid membrane puncture.*

Nursing Action	Rationale/Amplification
3. Insert a needle or any sharp instrument at a 10- to 30-degree caudal direction in the midline just above the upper part of the cricoid cartilage.	
4. Listen for air passing back and forth through the needle synchronously with the patient's respirations.	
5. Direct the needle downward and posteriorly.	5. To avoid injury to the vocal cords (located cephalad to the cricothyroid membrane).
6. Tape the needle with adhesive for stability.	6. To prevent laceration or perforation of the posterior tracheal wall.
7. An alternate method is to make a transverse incision overlying the cricothyroid membrane and a similar incision through the membrane itself. The membrane incision is spread and a tracheostomy tube is inserted and directed into the trachea.	
8. Prepare for endotracheal intubation/tracheostomy.	8. After the patient is stabilized, a more permanent means of ventilatory support is implemented.
9. Potential complications: bleeding, aspiration.	

Guidelines Esophageal Obturator Airway (EOA) or Esophageal Gastric Tube Airway (EGTA)

The *esophageal obturator airway* (EOA) is a ventilatory device used in respiratory emergencies for resuscitation. It consists of (1) a face mask—to seal off the nose and mouth and anchor the airway; (2) a flexible tube with openings at the level of the pharynx—to permit ventilation of the lungs; and (3) a balloon (cuff) on the distal end of the tube—to block the esophagus, thus reducing the possibility of aspirating gastric contents. The *esophageal gastric tube airway* (EGTA) is a modification of the esophageal airway in that it has a central lumen that permits passage of a nasogastric tube for suctioning and decompression of the stomach without interfering with ventilation (Fig. 38-2).

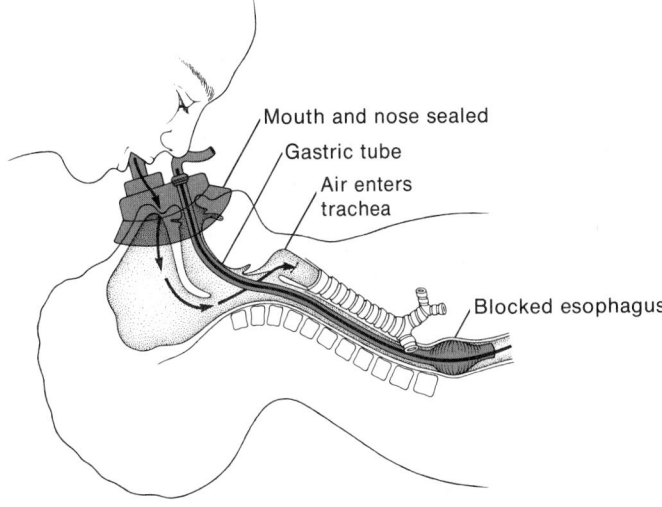

Mouth and nose sealed
Gastric tube
Air enters trachea
Blocked esophagus

Figure 38-2. *The Esophageal (Gastric Tube) Airway®. (Courtesy of Brunswick Mfg. Co., Inc. [Redrawn])*

Purpose   To ventilate an apneic, unconscious patient when endotracheal intubation is not feasible.

Equipment
Esophageal obturator airway   Water-soluble gel
50-ml. syringe   Bag and mask unit

Procedure

Nursing Action	Rationale/Amplification
Preparatory Phase	
1. Lubricate the tube and attach the mask to the tube by the snap lock.	1. This procedure is contraindicated in conscious or semi-conscious patients or in those with corrosive poisoning, esophageal disease, or a foreign body in the trachea.
2. Place patient's head in a neutral position.	
Performance Phase	
1. Using the left hand, insert the thumb as deeply as possible over the patient's tongue, pulling on it while using the fingers to lift the jaw upward and away from the posterior pharyngeal wall.	
2. Insert the esophageal obturator airway into the mouth, carefully guiding the tube over the tongue and past the pharynx; rotate the tube 180 degrees into the esophagus.	2. Maintain the patient's head in a neutral position.
3. Stop advancing the tube when the mask reaches the face; press the mask firmly against the face.	3. Proper positioning of the face mask with a good seal is essential for adequate ventilation.
4. Ventilate the patient by blowing a few breaths through the tube or by attaching a bag mask to it.	4. *If the tube is in the esophagus, the chest will rise.*
If the chest does not rise or no breath sounds are heard, withdraw the tube immediately.	Inadvertent tracheal intubation is a complication associated with the use of the EOA.
Continue ventilating the patient (by bag–mask ventilation) and prepare for and proceed with second attempt at insertion.	
5. Auscultate over both lung fields to check that *both* lungs are receiving adequate ventilation and that the airway is in the esophagus and *not* in the trachea.	5. Proper placement of the device is confirmed by auscultation of breath sounds and visualization of chest wall motion with ventilation.

(continued)

Procedure *(continued)*	**Nursing Action**	**Rationale/Amplification**
	6. Inflate the balloon (cuff) with approximately 30 ml. of air.	6. Inflating the balloon results in occlusion of the esophagus, minimizes the incidence of regurgitation, and prevents air leakage.
	7. Connect the end of the esophageal obturator to a bag–mask or mechanical ventilator, or continue mouth-to-tube ventilation.	7. Air or oxygen is blown into the sealed mask and exits through the holes at the hypopharynx, passing into the trachea and lungs.
	8. Do not remove the EOA until the patient regains consciousness or has a gag reflex *OR* until endotracheal intubation has been accomplished.	8. If the tube is taken out prematurely, regurgitation and aspiration are almost inevitable. The EOA tube must be deflated before it is removed.
	a. To remove tube: Have suction available. Turn the patient on to his side; deflate balloon and remove.	

Complication

Inadvertent insertion of EOA into trachea

Hemorrhage

Goals:
Control bleeding.
Maintain an adequate circulating blood volume for tissue oxygenation.
Prevent shock.

Assessment

(Signs and symptoms of shock occur.)
1. Increasing pulse rate
2. Cool, moist skin—from poor peripheral perfusion
3. Falling blood pressure
4. Decreasing urine volume

Emergency Management

A. Immediate Measures
1. Cut the patient's clothing away quickly and carry out a rapid physical examination.
2. Apply firm pressure over the bleeding area or the artery involved (Fig. 38-3); almost all bleeding can be stopped by direct pressure. Unchecked arterial bleeding results in death.
3. Apply a firm pressure dressing. Elevate the injured part to stop venous and capillary bleeding. Immobilize an injured extremity to control blood loss.

B. Fluid Replacement
1. Insert intravenous cannula to provide means of blood replacement.
2. Withdraw blood samples for analysis, typing, and cross-matching.
3. Give replacement fluids, including balanced electrolyte solution (lactated Ringer's solution) and blood, depending on clinical estimate of volume of blood loss—to correct intravascular deficit and interstitial fluid space deficit.
4. Fresh whole blood is infused when there is massive blood loss.
5. Additional platelets and coagulation factors are given when large amounts of blood are needed since replacement blood is deficient in clotting factors.
6. Warm the blood (commercial warmer or basin of warm water)—massive blood replacement has a cooling effect that can cause cardiac arrest.
7. Rate of infusion depends on severity of blood loss and clinical evidence of hypovolemia.

C. Measures for Internal Bleeding
1. Suspect internal bleeding in patients with hypovolemic shock with no external signs of bleeding: rising pulse rate; falling blood pressure; thirst; apprehension; cool, moist skin.
2. Give whole blood or plasma expanders at the rate of blood loss.
3. Prepare the patient immediately for surgical intervention to identify and control source of bleeding.
4. Apply pneumatic antishock garment if available—to control internal bleeding and to facilitate blood flow to vital areas (Fig. 38-4). (Its primary use is for hypovolemic shock secondary to bleeding in the lower part of the body.)
5. Monitor the patient's hemodynamic responses.
6. Obtain blood gas determinations; establish central venous pressure monitoring as an index of the amount of replacement fluid the patient can tolerate.
7. Maintain patient in supine position until hemodynamic/circulatory parameters begin to improve.

D. Measures for Oxygenation and Cardiac Function
1. Administer humidified oxygen.
2. Watch for cardiac arrest; patients who hemorrhage are candidates for cardiac arrest caused by hypovolemia with secondary anoxia.
3. Assess with ECG monitoring for dysrhythmias.

Control of Hypovolemic Shock

Shock is a condition in which there is loss of effective circulating blood volume; inadequate organ and tissue perfusion result, ultimately causing cellular metabolic derangements.

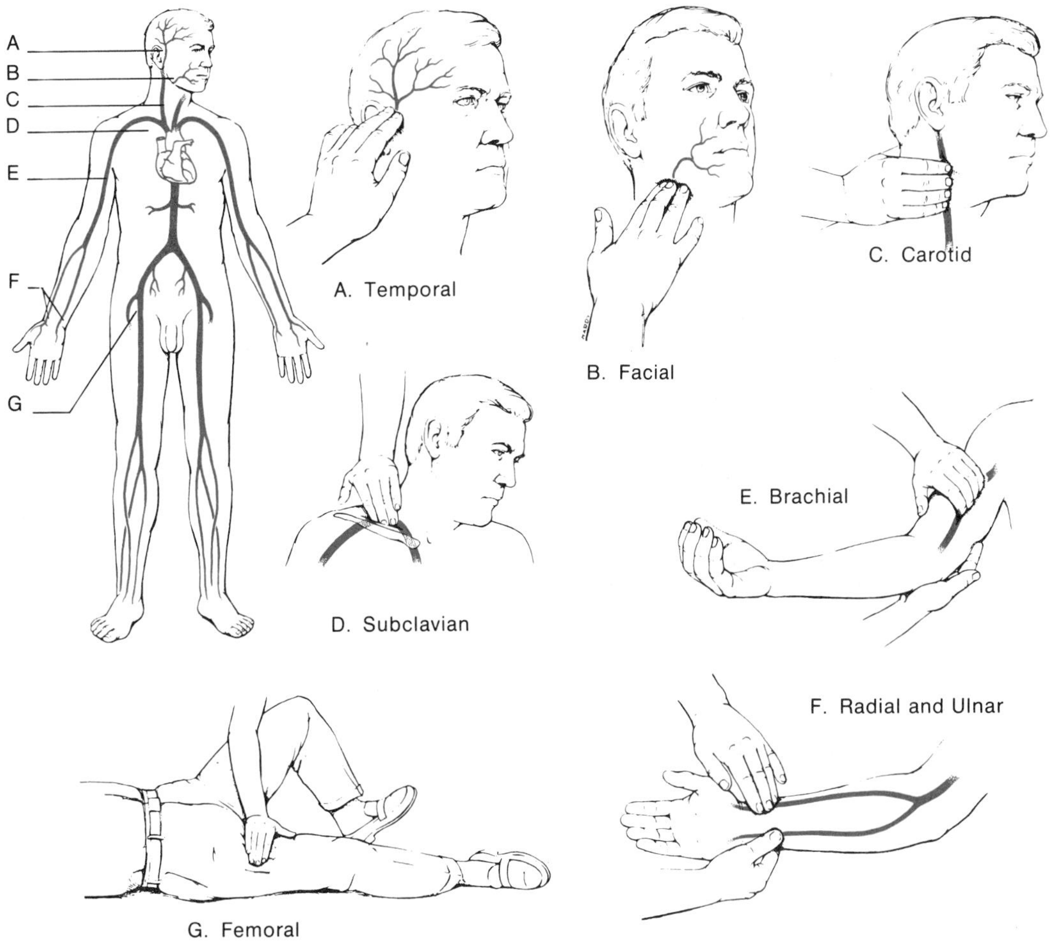

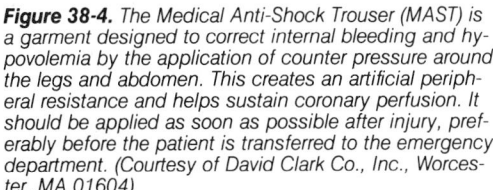

Figure 38-3. *Pressure points for control of hemorrhage.*

Clinical Manifestations

1. Decrease in systolic blood pressure
2. Increasing pulse rate; tachycardia
3. Cold, clammy skin; prostration
4. Pallor; circumoral pallor
5. Thirst
6. Alterations of mental status
7. Decrease in urine output

Emergency Management

Goal:

Restore hemodynamic stability and maintain tissue perfusion

A. Immediate Resuscitation Measures

1. Establish and maintain airway, breathing, and circulation; start resuscitation procedures as necessary.

Figure 38-4. *The Medical Anti-Shock Trouser (MAST) is a garment designed to correct internal bleeding and hypovolemia by the application of counter pressure around the legs and abdomen. This creates an artificial peripheral resistance and helps sustain coronary perfusion. It should be applied as soon as possible after injury, preferably before the patient is transferred to the emergency department. (Courtesy of David Clark Co., Inc., Worcester, MA 01604)*

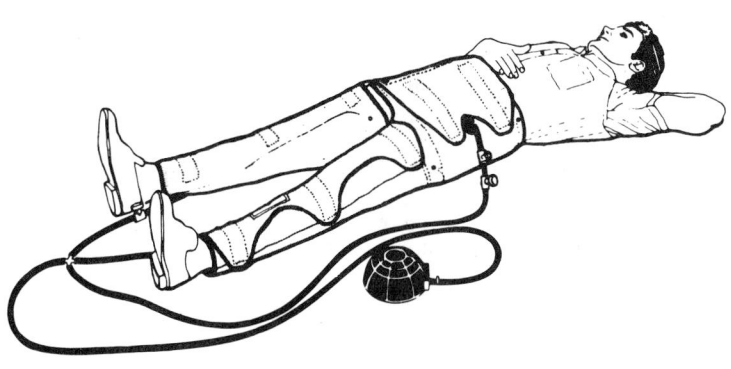

2. Administer oxygen to augment oxygen-carrying capacity of arterial blood.
3. Start ECG monitoring—dysrhythmias may contribute to shock.
4. Control hemorrhage—compounds shock state.

B. Fluid Replacement

1. Restore circulating blood volume with rapid intravenous fluid and blood replacement to optimize cardiac preload, correct hypotension, and maintain tissue perfusion.
2. Insert large-gauge needle/catheter into peripheral vein(s); two or more intravenous catheters may be necessary for rapid volume replacement and reversal of hemodynamic instability. The emphasis is on volume replacement.
3. Withdraw blood for specimens.
4. Start with electrolyte solution (lactated Ringer's)—to restore circulation. Amount given depends on results of volume administration including return of arterial pressure and urine output.
5. Start transfusion of blood component therapy, especially when blood loss has been severe or when patient continues to hemorrhage.
6. Carry out serial hematocrit examinations if continued bleeding is suspected. Hemorrhage will compound the shock state.

C. Ensuring Urinary Function

1. Insert an indwelling urinary catheter.
2. Record urinary output every 15–30 minutes.
3. Urinary volume reveals adequacy of kidney and visceral perfusion.

D. Insert Nasogastric Tube

E. Carry Out a Rapid Physical Assessment to Determine Cause of Shock

F. Monitoring

1. Maintain ongoing nursing surveillance of *total patient*—blood pressure, heart, and respiratory rates; skin temperature, color; central venous pressure (CVP), arterial blood gases, urinary output, ECG, hematocrit, hemoglobin, coagulation profiles, and electrolytes—to assess patient response to treatment. Keep a flow sheet of these parameters.
2. Trend analysis reveals improvement or deterioration of patient.
3. Elevate both legs, while maintaining the trunk and remainder of body in supine position. *(This position is contraindicated in patients with head injuries.)*

G. Pharmacotherapy

Give specific pharmacologic agents (inotropic drugs, etc.) as prescribed when indicated by the patient's condition.

H. Support the Defense Mechanisms of the Body

1. Reassure and comfort the patient; sedation may be necessary to relieve apprehension.
2. Relieve pain by *cautious* use of analgesics or narcotics.

I. Maintain Body Temperature

1. Too much heat produces vasodilatation, which counteracts the body's compensatory mechanism of vasoconstriction and also increases fluid loss by perspiration.
2. A patient who is in septic shock should be kept cool, since high fever will increase the cellular metabolic effects of shock.

Wounds

Wounds (injury to tissues) vary from minor lacerations to severe crushing injuries.
Underlying considerations: The problems of ensuring ventilation and oxygenation, maintaining cardiac output, and controlling bleeding are dealt with before wound is treated.

Emergency Management

Goals:
Preservation of tissue
Prevention of infection
Maintenance of function

A. Conduct Initial Assessment

1. Ask the patient *when* as well as *how* the wound occurred as well as about the environment, present medications, allergies, associated illnesses, and tetanus immunization status.
2. Inspect the wound using aseptic technique (sterile gloves; masks) to determine extent of damage to underlying structures.
3. Clip hair around wound (with exception of eyebrows) only if directed—this is done when it is anticipated that hairs will interfere with wound closure.

B. Cleanse and Debride the Wound

1. Irrigate gently and copiously with isotonic sterile saline solution—to remove dirt and debris.
2. Cleanse skin around wound with nontoxic topical antiseptic solution. Do not allow cleansing solution to get into wound, since it may be injurious to exposed tissues.
3. The wound is infiltrated with local anesthetic intradermally through the wound margins or by regional nerve block.
4. Devitalized tissue and foreign matter are removed—devitalized tissue inhibits wound healing and enhances chance of bacterial infection.

C. Wound Closure

1. Closure by *primary intent*
   a. Wound is repaired without delay following the injury; yields the fastest healing.
   b. Primary closure may be with sutures, skin tapes, staples, or tissue adhesives.
2. Closure by *secondary intent*
   a. Wound is allowed to granulate on its own without surgical closure.
   b. Wound is cleansed and covered with a sterile dressing.
3. Closure by *tertiary intent* or *delayed primary closure*
   a. Wound is cleansed and dressed.
   b. Patient returns in 3–4 days for definitive closure.

D. Wound Care

1. Apply nonadherent dressing—to protect the wound. Currently it is thought that the best environment for wound healing is a moist environment.
2. Immobilize the site—lymphatic flow decreases and this minimizes spread of wound microflora.
3. Elevate site of injury above level of heart—limits accumulation of fluid in the wound's interstitial spaces.

E. Pharmacotherapy

1. Give antimicrobial treatment as directed, depending on how injury occurred, age of wound, presence of soil-infection potential, etc.

2. Give tetanus prophylaxis as indicated, based on patient's immunization status and wound. For inadequate primary immunization, both tetanus toxoid and tetanus immune globulin are given.
3. Check current recommendations from Centers for Disease Control for updates in recommendations for tetanus prophylaxis or guidelines recommended by Committee on Trauma of the American College of Surgeons.
4. See Prevention and Patient Education, page 917.

Patient Education

1. Inform the patient that pain should subside in 24 hours.
   a. Acetaminophen (or prescribed drug) to be taken for the first 24 hours following a simple laceration.
   b. If pain reappears, a wound infection may be suspected.
2. Recommend that wound be elevated to limit accumulation of fluid in wound's interstitial spaces.
   a. Elevate extremity for first 48 hours.
   b. Sleep with the head elevated if facial lacerations are present.
3. Advise that physician/clinic be contacted if there is sudden or persistent onset of pain, fever/chills, bleeding, rapid swelling, foul odor, purulent fluid or redness surrounding the wound.
4. Recommend sunscreen (about 2 weeks after injury) for 3–6 months for sun-exposed wounds and surrounding skin—to avoid differential pigmentation of the healing region.
5. Recommend a reasonably priced bandage that is best suited for the injury.
6. Make arrangements to return for wound check as directed.

Intra-abdominal Injuries

Intra-abdominal injuries may be either penetrating or blunt.

Penetrating Abdominal Injuries

Persons with *penetrating abdominal injuries* (gunshot wounds, stab wounds, etc.) should be treated like critically ill patients.
High-velocity missiles (bullets) create extensive tissue and visceral damage; such damage usually requires surgical exploration.
Stab wounds may be managed more conservatively.

Assessment

1. Obtain a history of the mechanism of the injury, type of weapon, and estimated amount of blood loss.
2. Inspect the abdomen for obvious signs of injury (penetrating injury, bruises).
3. Assess the patient for progression of distention, tenderness, pain, muscular rigidity or rebound tenderness, diminished bowel sounds, hypotension, and shock.
4. Auscultate for bowel sounds because the absence of bowel sounds is an early sign of intraperitoneal involvement. If signs of peritoneal irritation are present, an immediate exploratory celiotomy (surgical incision into the abdominal cavity) is usually performed.

5. Look for chest injuries, which frequently accompany intra-abdominal injuries.

Emergency Management

Goals:
Control of bleeding and maintenance of blood volume
Prevention of infection of wounds that disrupt the gastrointestinal tract

A. Institute Immediate Measures

1. Keep the patient on the stretcher, since movement may fragment or dislodge a clot in a large vessel and produce massive hemorrhage.
2. Ensure patency of the airway and stability of the respiratory, circulatory, and nervous systems.
3. Cut the clothing away from the wound.
4. Tabulate the number of wounds.
5. Look for entrance and exit wounds.
6. If the patient is comatose, splint the neck until after cervical films are made.

B. Assess for Signs and Symptoms of Hemorrhage

Hemorrhage frequently accompanies abdominal injury, especially if the liver and spleen have been traumatized.

C. Control the Bleeding and Maintain the Blood Volume Until Surgery Can Be Performed

1. Apply compression to external bleeding wounds and occlusion of chest wounds.
2. Insert indwelling intravenous catheter(s) for rapid fluid replacement to restore circulatory dynamics.
3. Watch for occurrence of shock after an initial positive response to transfusion therapy—this is often the first sign of internal hemorrhage.

D. Aspirate the Stomach Contents With a Nasogastric Tube

Also helps detect gastric wounds and prevents lung complications from aspiration.

E. Cover Protruding Abdominal Viscera

1. Use sterile saline dressings to protect viscera from drying.
2. Flex the patient's knees, since this position will prevent further protrusion.
3. Withhold oral fluids to prevent increased peristalsis and vomiting.

F. Insert Indwelling Urethral Catheter

1. To ascertain the presence of hematuria and to monitor urinary output—serves as an index of tissue perfusion.

G. Pharmacotherapy

1. Carry out tetanus prophylaxis as directed.
2. Give broad-spectrum antimicrobial as directed to prevent infection, since bacterial contamination is a frequent complication (depending on history and nature of wound).

H. Other Measures

1. Keep an ongoing flow sheet of the patient's vital signs, urinary output, central venous pressure readings, hematocrit values, and neurologic status.
2. Prepare peritoneal lavage (see p. 941) when there is uncertainty about intraperitoneal bleeding.
3. For stab wounds, prepare for direct wound exploration under local anesthesia in the Emergency Department.
4. Prepare for surgery if the patient shows evidence of unexplained shock, unstable vital signs, peritoneal ir-

ritation, bowel protrusion or evisceration, significant penetrating injury, significant gastrointestinal bleeding, peritoneal air, etc.

Blunt Abdominal Trauma

Underlying Considerations

1. Trauma to the abdomen is frequently associated with extra-abdominal injuries, e.g., chest, head, and extremities, and severe concomitant trauma to multiple intraperitoneal organs.
2. The incidence of delayed trauma-related complications is greater than that associated with penetrating injuries; this is especially true of blunt injuries involving the liver, spleen, or blood vessels, which can lead to substantial blood loss into the peritoneal cavity.

Clinical Manifestations

1. Pain; pain on movement
2. Rebound and maximal point tenderness
3. Muscle guarding
4. Diminishing or absent bowel sounds; distention
5. Bruises on abdominal wall

Emergency Management

A. Immediate Measures

1. Begin resuscitation procedures and evaluation of the patient simultaneously.
2. Take a detailed history (frequently unobtainable, inaccurate, and misleading); obtain all possible data about the following:
   a. Method of injury
   b. Time of onset of symptoms
   c. Passenger location (driver frequently sustains spleen/liver rupture)
   d. Time of last food/fluid intake
   e. Bleeding tendencies
   f. Concurrent disease
   g. Immunization history, with attention to tetanus
   h. Allergies

B. Ongoing Assessment

1. Carry out ongoing examination (inspection, palpation, auscultation, and percussion of the abdomen). The changes noted in subsequent examinations may reveal an undetected abdominal injury.
2. Avoid moving the patient until initial assessment is done—movement may fragment a clot in a large vessel and produce massive hemorrhage.
3. Look for chest injuries, especially fracture of lower ribs.
4. Inspect the front, flanks, and back for bluish discoloration, asymmetry, abrasions, contusions.
5. Evaluate for signs and symptoms of hemorrhage—fre-

quently accompanies abdominal injury, especially if the liver and spleen have been traumatized.
6. Note tenderness, rebound tenderness, guarding, rigidity, and spasm.
   a. Press the area of maximal tenderness (let the patient point to the area).
   b. Remove the fingers quickly; pain at suspected point indicates peritoneal irritation.
7. Ask about referred pain: pain in left shoulder may be encountered in patient bleeding from ruptured spleen; pain in right shoulder can result from laceration of liver.
8. Look for increasing abdominal distention.
   Measure abdominal girth at umbilical level upon admission—serves as a baseline from which changes can be determined.
9. Auscultate for bowel sounds—a silent abdomen accompanies peritoneal irritation.
10. Note loss of dullness over solid organs (liver; spleen)—indicates presence of free air; dullness over regions normally containing gas may indicate presence of blood.
11. Assist with rectal examination/vaginal examination—for diagnosis of injury to pelvis, bladder, and intestinal wall.
12. Avoid giving narcotics during observation period—may mask clinical picture.
13. Monitor vital signs frequently and carefully—tachypnea, tachycardia, and hypotension may be clues to intra-abdominal bleeding.

C. Prepare the Patient for Diagnostic Procedures

1. Urinalysis—as a guide to possible urinary tract injury; to monitor urine output.
2. Serial hemoglobin and hematocrit levels—their trend reflects presence or absence of bleeding.
3. Complete blood count (CBC)—white blood cell count is generally elevated with trauma.
4. Serum amylase—elevation usually indicates pancreatic injury or perforations of gastrointestinal tract.
5. Computed tomography (CT) scans—permit detailed evaluation of abdominal and retroperitoneal injuries.
6. Abdominal and chest x-rays—may reveal free air beneath diaphragm, indicating ruptured hollow viscus.

D. Other Measures

1. Assist with peritoneal lavage—to test for intraperitoneal bleeding—organ laceration or bleeding may be diagnosed by gross and microscopic examination of fluid returned after peritoneal lavage.
2. Assist with insertion of a nasogastric tube—to prevent vomiting and subsequent aspiration; helpful in decompressing (removing fluid/air) from gastrointestinal tract.
3. Patient may be admitted for observation or exploratory laparotomy.

Guidelines   Peritoneal Lavage

Peritoneal lavage is a technique of irrigation of the peritoneal cavity and examination of the irrigating fluid to evaluate the effects of trauma to the abdomen (Fig. 38-5).

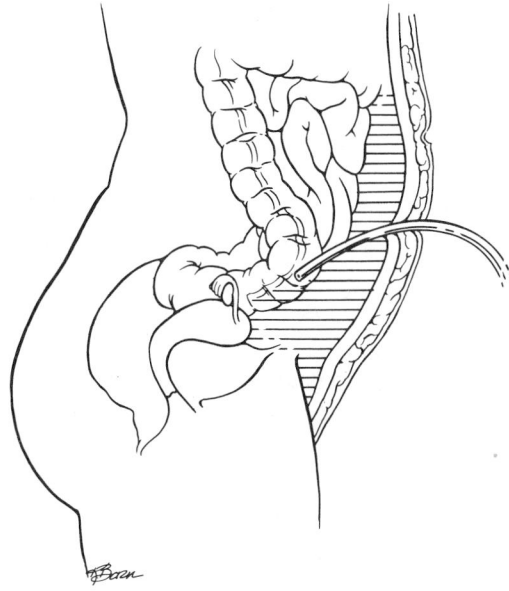

Figure 38-5. *Peritoneal lavage.*

Purposes
1. To test for intra-abdominal bleeding.
2. To test patients with equivocal abdominal findings.
3. To avoid unnecessary surgical exploration, especially in patients with altered states of consciousness (from head injuries, drugs, alcohol) and when physical findings are unreliable (spinal cord injuries).

Equipment
Peritoneal dialysis tray
Sterile solution (lactated Ringer's solution)
IV tubing; IV pole
Peritoneal dialysis catheter (multiple perforations)
Local skin anesthetic; sterile gloves

Procedure

Nursing Action	Rationale/Amplification

Preparatory Phase

1. Explain the procedure to the patient; see that the consent form has been signed.
2. Insert indwelling catheter into the bladder.
3. Prepare the abdomen as for surgery.

4. Place the patient in a supine position.
5. Fill the IV tubing with solution using aseptic technique.

2. To prevent puncture of urinary bladder.
3. To minimize or eliminate surface bacteria and decrease the possibility of wound contamination and infection.

Performance Phase (by the physician)

1. The skin is infiltrated 2–3 cm. (0.7–1.2 inches) below the umbilicus in the midline with local anesthetic.

2. A small vertical incision is made at the chosen site.
3. Bleeding vessels are carefully ligated.
4. The peritoneum is opened under direct vision and the peritoneal catheter is inserted into the peritoneal cavity, *OR*
5. A needle is passed intra-abdominally, a flexible wire is passed through the needle, and a catheter is guided over the wire.

1. The midline area is relatively avascular. Epinephrine may be injected with local anesthetic to produce capillary constriction and prevent a false-positive tap.

3. Ligation of vessels helps avoid a false-positive lavage.
4. There are various methods (open or percutaneous) of introducing the catheter into the peritoneal space.

(continued)

Guidelines   Peritoneal Lavage *(continued)*

Procedure *(continued)*	Nursing Action	Rationale/Amplification
	6. A syringe is attached to the catheter, and the peritoneal cavity is aspirated.	6. If more than 10 ml. of blood is obtained or the fluid contains bile, feces, or particulate matter, the test is considered positive and the patient is prepared for immediate celiotomy (incision into abdominal cavity).
	7. If no blood (or less than 10 ml.) is present, the catheter is attached to the IV tubing; 500–1000 ml. of solution is infused into the peritoneal cavity through the intravenous tubing attached to the dialysis catheter.	7. If not contraindicated by the patient's condition, he may be turned from side to side to ensure that the solution reaches all parts of the abdominal cavity.
	8. After the solution is infused, the empty IV bag is removed from the pole and lowered below the abdominal level (near the floor).	8. Lowering the bag creates a siphon effect to drain the excess fluid. As much of the fluid as possible is siphoned out of the peritoneal cavity by gravity.
	9. The peritoneal dialysis catheter is removed, and the wound is closed (unless laparotomy is necessary).	
	10. The fluid recovered from the peritoneal cavity is examined visually and is usually sent to the laboratory for cell counts and microscopic inspection of spun-down sediment.	

Interpretation of Lavage Fluid

Clear fluid indicates a lack of significant intraperitoneal bleeding.
Criteria for positive results:
    Aspiration of free blood from peritoneal cavity
    RBCs > 100,000 per mm^3
    WBCs > 500 per mm^3
    Amylase > 110 IU/dl.
    Presence of bile, bacteria, fecal or food particles in lavage fluid

This indicates a negative test.
If the test is positive, a laparotomy is usually done. Indeterminate or equivocal results merit monitoring and investigation.

Follow-up Phase

1. Assess the patient for complications.

1. Complications include visceral perforation, wound hematoma, perforated bowel, puncture of bladder, laceration of major vessels, infection.

2. Watch the patient closely for any type of deterioration.

2. Repeated physical examinations of the abdomen should be carried out when intra-abdominal injury is suspected.

Head Injuries

Head injuries are classified as open or closed injuries. About 15%–20% of all patients who come to Emergency Departments for treatment have some form of head trauma.

A severe head injury is one in which the patient is unable to open his eyes, talk, or move purposefully to painful stimuli. It may also be indicated by a total score on the Glasgow Coma Scale of 8 or less, persisting for 6 hours or more.

Emergency Management

NURSING ALERT: A fracture of the cervical spine frequently accompanies a head injury. The cervical spine should be immobilized immediately until a fracture is ruled out.

A. Immediate Measures

1. Continue to ensure adequate protection of the airway and ventilation—hypoxia and hypercapnia can increase brain swelling and cell damage and can convert a reversible brain injury to an irreversible injury.
2. Keep the patient with his neck in a neutral position with the cervical spine immobilized.
3. Clear the respiratory passages by careful suctioning.
4. Ensure adequate oxygenation and ventilation. The brain is very susceptible to lack of oxygen. Hypoxia of the brain leads to increased intracranial pressure, the most frequent cause of death following head injury.
5. Insert arterial pressure line—knowledge of arterial pressure is essential for clinical assessment of brain perfusion.
6. Assist with endotracheal intubation after the possibility of cervical fracture has been ruled out. Assisted ventilation with hyperventilation decreases intracranial pressure by causing cerebral vasoconstriction, thus decreasing cerebral blood flow.

B. Restore Blood Pressure and Other Body Functions

1. Hypotension can depress neurologic function—profound hypotension is usually due to extracranial injuries.

2. Provide IV fluid resuscitation as directed; usually guided by central venous pressure monitoring.
3. Look for an extracranial source of bleeding—thoracic, abdominal, retroperitoneal hemorrhage, bleeding into soft tissues surrounding long bone fracture.
4. Insert nasogastric tube—to decompress stomach and prevent aspiration.
5. Insert an indwelling catheter—to monitor urine output, an indicator of tissue perfusion and shock.

C. Neurologic Assessment

1. Carry out rapid neurologic assessment to estimate the severity of head injury and its clinical management; estimate prognosis for survival/neurologic outcome.
2. Make repeated examinations to determine if the patient is stable, improving, or deteriorating.
3. Assess level of responsiveness (consciousness), the most important parameter. Record exactly what the patient does on command to verbal and painful stimuli (see Glasgow Coma Scale, p. 579).
4. Evaluate pupil size, shape, reactivity to light, and ocular movements.
5. Note motor responses; movement and strength of extremities, purposeful or abnormal flexor or extensor posturing; note reflexes.
6. Evaluate for signs of rising intracranial pressure—deterioration in level of responsiveness, slowing of pulse, rising systolic pressure, increasing pulse pressure, changes in pattern of respiration, dilating, nonreacting pupils.
7. Ask the conscious patient about headache, double vision, nausea.
8. Look for presence of scalp laceration, cerebrospinal fluid (CSF) leak, and hemorrhagic exudation into the middle ear (hematotympanum).

D. Other Measures

1. Assess for injuries to other organ systems.
2. Continue to evaluate for changes in the patient's condition. *A change in the level of responsiveness is the most sensitive sign of improvement or deterioration.*
3. Prepare for computed tomography or angiography as soon as patient is stabilized to diagnose type of pathology and plan definitive care.
4. Prepare for immediate surgical intervention if patient shows evidence of neurologic deterioration.
5. Carry out specific therapy based on assessment of injury: hyperventilation, corticosteroids, hyperosmolar therapy, etc. See page 581 for definitive therapy of head trauma.

Cervical Spine Injuries

Injuries to the cervical spine are serious because the crushing, stretching, and rotational sheer forces exerted on the cord at the time of trauma can produce severe neurologic deficits. Edema and cord swelling contribute further to the loss of spinal cord function.

Any person with a head, neck, or back injury should be suspected of having a potential spinal cord injury until the suspicion is proved groundless.

Clinical Manifestations

1. Neck and/or back pain/extremity pain
2. History of unconsciousness
3. Intercostal paralysis with diaphragmatic breathing—indicates cervical spinal cord injury.

4. Total sensory loss and motor paralysis below level of injury.
5. Loss of bowel and bladder control; usually urinary retention and bladder distention.
6. Loss of sweating and vasomotor tone below level of cord lesion.
7. Marked reduction of blood pressure—from loss of peripheral and vascular resistance.
8. Priapism—persistent erection of penis.

Emergency Management

A. Immediate Measures

1. Keep patient immobilized on the transfer board until airway is managed, cardiovascular system is stable, imaging procedures are carried out, and transfer can be accomplished to a Stryker frame/proper bed surface.

> **NURSING ALERT:** A spinal cord injury can be made worse during the acute phase of injury, resulting in permanent neurologic damage. Proper handling is an immediate priority.

B. Implement ABC Measures

1. Assess and manage airway, breathing, and circulation and cervical spine while immobilization of the spine is maintained. (Immobilization of the cervical spine is maintained by immobilization of the head.)
2. Keep the head and neck in a straight line with the long axis of the body.
   a. Do not move the spine.
   b. Avoid flexion, extension, or rotation of the head and neck or flexing, extending, or twisting the spine.

C. Assess Respiratory Function

1. Continue to evaluate the patient's respiratory function—lesions from the fifth cervical vertebra to midthoracic area interfere with intercostal and abdominal breathing; lesions above C3 level cause immediate respiratory paralysis.
2. In conscious patient, observe for increased respiratory rate and difficulty in speaking due to shortness of breath.
3. Monitor blood gas values serially.
4. Prepare for nasotracheal intubation.

D. Ensure Stabilization of Physiologic Functioning

1. Initiate intravenous access—for volume resuscitation
2. Nasogastric intubation—to prevent regurgitation and aspiration from gastric dilation and ileus
3. Insertion of an indwelling urinary catheter to avoid bladder distention; indwelling system is converted to an intermittent catheterization schedule as soon as possible
4. Monitor for hypotension (may worsen neurologic damage), hypothermia, and bradycardia—associated with fracture of cervical spine and neurologic injury above level of T6.

E. Assess Level of Injury

1. Evaluate and examine the patient for level of spinal cord injury and associated injuries; the presence of spinal shock (p. 614) may make assessment difficult.
2. Test upper and lower extremity motor function, sensation to light, touch, and pin prick.
3. Observe the pattern of respirations—intercostal muscle paralysis causes paradoxical movement of chest and abdomen.

4. Observe for priapism (persistent erection of penis)—a sign of spinal cord injury.
5. Test the biceps, triceps, quadriceps, and Achilles reflexes.
6. Evaluate vital signs.
7. Assist with rectal examination to evaluate sphincter function.

F. Other Measures

1. Look for the presence of associated injuries.
2. Continue with repeated neurologic examinations to determine if there is deterioration in the spinal cord lesion; continue to evaluate respiratory status.
3. Administer dexamethasone, if prescribed.
4. After patient is stabilized, prepare for imaging studies (CT), cervical traction or surgical decompression, or surgical fixation of unstable fracture.
5. Give continuing explanations of what is being done—patient is usually very anxious.
6. See page 614 for definitive management of the patient with spinal cord injury.

Crush Injuries

Crush injuries occur when a person is crushed beneath debris, run over, or compressed by machinery.
   Crush syndrome refers to the edema, oliguria, and other symptoms of renal failure that follow crushing of a part, particularly a large muscle mass.

Clinical Manifestations

1. Oligemic shock—due to extravasation of blood and plasma into injured tissues after compression has been released.
2. Erythema and blistering of skin; paralysis of part.
3. Damaged part (usually an extremity) becomes swollen, tense, and hard due to extravasation of red blood cells and plasma through damaged vessels and capillaries.
4. Renal dysfunction—prolonged hypotension causes kidney damage and acute renal insufficiency.

Emergency Management

1. Control shock.
2. Provide prompt restoration of blood volume with blood, plasma, and electrolyte solution in sufficient volume to maintain adequate urine output.
3. Monitor urine output; urine may be colored from pigments of myoglobin or hemoglobin that have leaked into circulation following injury.
4. Observe carefully for acute renal insufficiency.
5. Splint major soft tissue injuries to control bleeding and pain.
6. Elevate the extremity; fasciotomy (surgical incision of fascia) of muscle compartments may be required.
7. Administer prescribed medication for pain and anxiety.

Multiple Injuries

Underlying Considerations

1. The patient with multiple injuries requires a team approach with one person responsible for coordinating the treatment.

2. *Evidence of gross trauma* may be slight or may be completely absent. The injury regarded as the least significant may be the most lethal.
3. Any injury interfering with a vital physiologic function is an immediate threat to life and has highest priority for immediate treatment (obstructed airway, hemorrhage).
4. After the patient is resuscitated, the clothing is usually cut off and a rapid physical assessment made. Critically traumatized patients should not be removed from the stretcher.
5. Treatment in a trauma center is appropriate for patients with major trauma.

Emergency Management *(Fig. 38-6)*

Goals:
Determine the extent of injuries.
Establish priorities of treatment.

A. Immediate Assessment

1. Carry out a *rapid* physical examination to determine if patient is breathing, bleeding, or in shock.*
2. Determine the status of his responsiveness and if he has severe wounds or fracture deformities.

B. Resuscitation Measures

1. Start resuscitation procedures (airway, breathing, circulation) simultaneously while another team member is conducting physical assessment.*
2. Note the character and symmetry of chest wall motion and pattern of breathing. Auscultate the lungs.
3. Ask the conscious patient if he is having difficulty in breathing. Ask if he has chest pain.
4. Apply suction to clear the trachea and bronchial tree.
5. Insert oropharyngeal airway—to prevent occlusion by tongue.
6. Ventilate the patient (bag–mask system) to alleviate hypoxia.
7. Prepare for endotracheal intubation if adequate airway cannot be maintained.
8. Suspect serious intrathoracic injuries if respiratory distress continues after adequate airway has been established. See pages 193–198 for management of chest injuries.

C. Cardiac Function

1. Assess cardiac function and treat cardiac arrest—hypoxia, metabolic acidosis, and chest trauma may precipitate cardiac arrest.*
2. For cardiac arrest, start closed chest compression and ventilation.
3. If chest wall is unstable (flail chest), emergency thoracotomy and manual compression may be necessary.
4. Be prepared to give sodium bicarbonate (IV) to compensate for acidosis if indicated—severely traumatized patients with respiratory and circulatory embarrassment will have some degree of metabolic acidosis.

D. Control Hemorrhage*

1. Apply pressure over bleeding points if hemorrhage is overt.
2. Expect significant blood loss in patient with fracture of shaft of femur, with multiple fractures, or with major pelvic trauma.
3. Use tourniquet(s) for massive arterial bleeding from extremities that cannot be halted with pressure.

* Imperative lifesaving procedures are performed simultaneously by the emergency team.

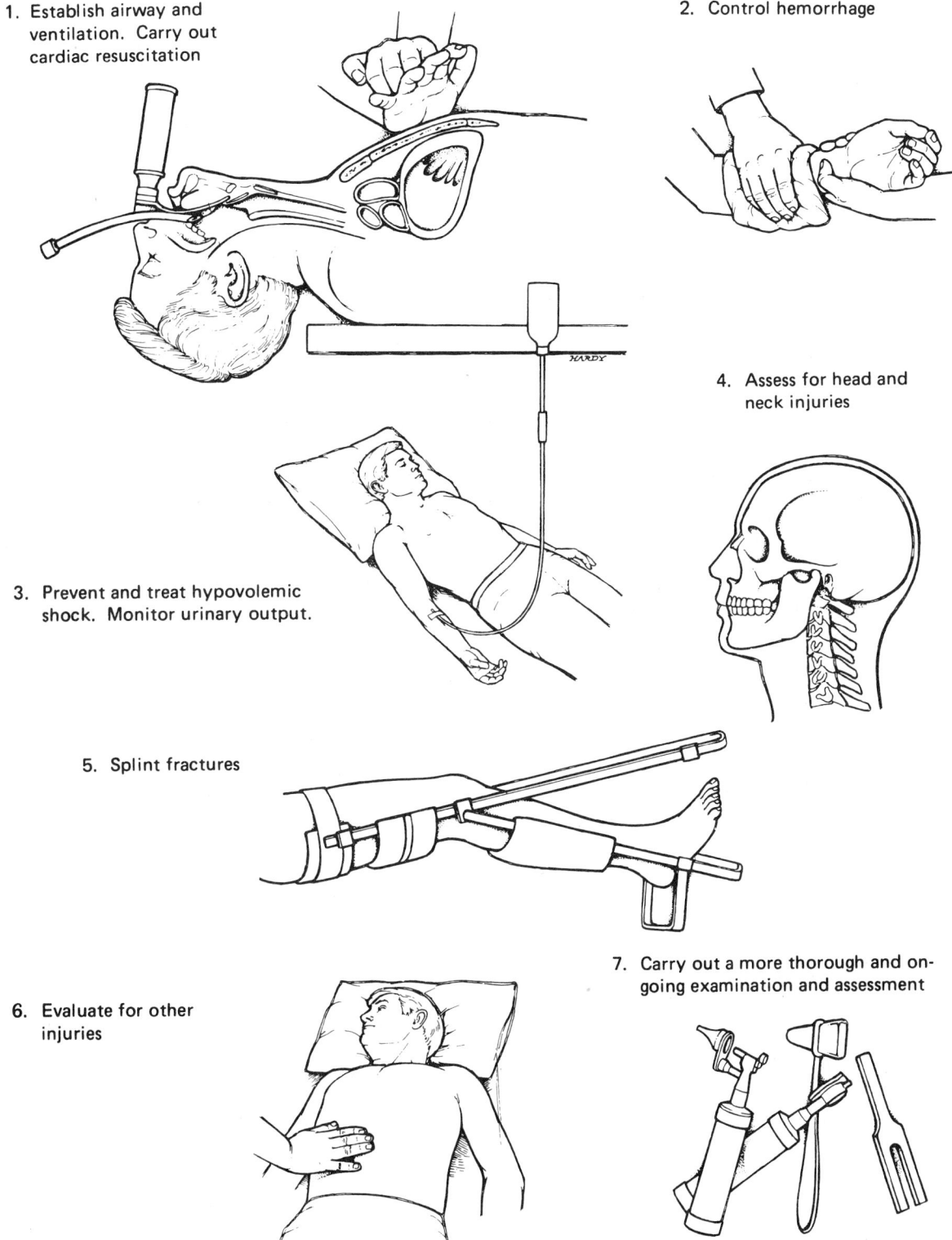

1. Establish airway and ventilation. Carry out cardiac resuscitation

2. Control hemorrhage

3. Prevent and treat hypovolemic shock. Monitor urinary output.

4. Assess for head and neck injuries

5. Splint fractures

6. Evaluate for other injuries

7. Carry out a more thorough and on-going examination and assessment

Figure 38-6. The patient with multiple injuries. Any injury that interferes with vital physiologic function and poses an immediate threat to life takes priority for immediate treatment. Imperative lifesaving procedures are performed simultaneously by the emergency team.

4. Prepare for immediate surgical intervention if patient is bleeding internally.

E. Prevent and Treat Hypovolemic Shock*

1. Insert at least two (sometimes four) IV lines, one above diaphragm and one below. Use venous cutdown if necessary.
2. Draw blood for laboratory studies as directed (typing and cross-matching, baseline CBC, electrolytes, blood urea nitrogen, glucose, prothrombin time).
3. Introduce central venous catheter to monitor the patient's response to fluid infusion—to prevent fluid overload and as a route for fluid infusion.
4. Start intravenous infusions.
   a. Balanced saline solution (lactated Ringer's solution) is given for volume replacement until blood is available.
   b. Give blood as directed—massive transfusions have a cooling effect that can cause cardiac irritability and arrest; blood should be warmed.
   c. Give intravenous infusions rapidly enough to keep central venous pressure readings at 5–15 cm. H_2O (see p. 307); monitor rate and direction of change (important parameters).

F. Evaluate Other Parameters

1. Insert indwelling urethral catheter and monitor urinary output to aid in diagnosis of shock and monitor effectiveness of therapy. Do not force the catheter—the patient may have a ruptured urethra.
2. Monitor ECG—to detect life-threatening dysrhythmias.
3. Carry out ongoing clinical evaluation to observe for improvement or deterioration: changes in vital signs, improvement in level of responsiveness, skin warmth, speed of capillary filling, etc., shows reversal of shock state.
4. Prepare for immediate surgical intervention if the patient does not respond to fluids or blood—inability to restore blood pressure and circulatory volume in the patient usually indicates major internal bleeding.

G. Assess for Head and Neck Injuries

1. Make definite statements concerning baseline neurologic status of the patient (level of responsiveness, size and reactivity of pupils, motor power, reflexes).
2. Neck (and chest) films may be taken; apply rigid cervical collar until x-rays preclude possibility of cervical spine injury.
3. Intracranial pressure monitoring may be instituted.

H. Pharmacotherapy

1. Administer dexamethasone as directed.
2. Corticosteroids appear to protect pulmonary function in patients with multiple injuries and help prevent posttraumatic pulmonary insufficiency. (However, this is considered a controversial issue.)

I. For Fractures

1. Splint fractures to prevent further trauma to soft tissues and blood vessels and to relieve pain.
2. Note presence or absence of pulses in fractured extremities.

J. Assess for Gastrointestinal Injuries

1. Examine the patient repeatedly for abdominal pain, muscular rigidity, tenderness, rebound tenderness, diminished bowel sounds, hypotension, and shock.
2. Prepare for peritoneal lavage to assess for intraperitoneal bleeding.

3. Assist with insertion of nasogastric tube for prevention of vomiting and aspiration.
4. Prepare for laparotomy if the patient shows continuing signs of hemorrhage and deterioration.

K. Ongoing Evaluation

1. Continue to monitor urinary output hourly—reflects cardiac output and state of perfusion of visceral organs.
   a. Assess for hematuria and oliguria.
   b. Record measurements on a flow sheet.
2. Evaluate the patient for other injuries and institute appropriate treatment including tetanus immunization.
3. Carry out a more thorough physical examination after resuscitation and management of the aforementioned priorities.

Fractures

A *fracture* is a break in the continuity of the bone.

Emergency Management*

A. Initiate Resuscitation Measures

1. Examine patient with attention given to airway, breathing, and circulation. Ensure oxygenation and ventilation.
2. Evaluate for respiratory difficulties—caused by edema due to facial and neck injuries, accumulation of secretions in respiratory tract, etc.
3. Examine chest for evidences of sucking chest wounds, pneumothorax, flail chest, etc.
4. Prepare for tracheal intubation or emergency tracheostomy.

B. Control Shock—usually the result of blood loss in patients with fractures.

1. Assess for falling blood pressure, cold and clammy skin, and rapid, thready pulse.
2. Keep in mind that a large amount of blood loss may accompany fractures of the femur and pelvis.
3. Maintain the blood pressure with intravenous infusions.
4. Give blood transfusion(s) or blood component therapy as soon as blood is available.
5. Administer oxygen—cardiopulmonary embarrassment produces decreased oxygen supply to the tissues and circulatory collapse.
6. Give analgesic to control pain. (Splinting the extremity and controlling pain are essential in treating shock accompanying fractures.)
7. Look for evidence of head, chest, and other injuries—patients with multiple fractures may have other serious injuries.

C. Control Hemorrhage

1. Control venous bleeding by direct pressure along with digital pressure over artery closest to bleeding area.
2. Suspect internal hemorrhage (pleural, pericardial, or abdominal) in the event of continuing shock and in the presence of injuries to chest and abdomen.

D. Inspect the Fractured Part(s)

1. Cut away clothing if necessary.
2. Observe the entire body using a methodical head-to-

---

*Imperative lifesaving procedures are performed simultaneously by the emergency team.

toe physical examination—inspect for lacerations, swelling, deformities, bruising, and loss of function.

3. Look for *angulation* (bending), *shortening,* and *rotation.*
4. Feel the pulse distal to the extremity fracture. Check all peripheral pulses.
5. Assess for coolness, blanching, decreased sensation and motor function, diminished or absent pulses—indicate injury to the blood supply.
6. Handle the part gently and as little as possible.

E. Apply Splint

1. Apply splint before the patient is moved since splinting prevents further injury to both bone and soft tissues, diminishes pain, and allows easier transportation.
2. Immobilize the joint above and below the fracture; place one hand distal to the fracture and apply some traction while placing the other hand beneath the fracture for support.
3. Extend the splints well beyond the joints adjacent to the fracture.
   a. Use the patient's clothing for padding (tie, shirt) if nothing else is available.
   b. Use newspapers, magazines, pillows, tree limbs, and boards for splints if necessary. (Specialized splints and traction are used in the hospital.)
   c. Splint joints in functional positions.
4. Check the vascular status of the extremity after splinting; check color, temperature, pulse, capillary refill.

F. Other Measures

1. Evaluate for neurologic deficits caused by the fracture.
2. Apply a sterile dressing if the fracture is an open one.
3. Investigate any complaint of pain or pressure.
4. Transport the patient gently and carefully.
5. See Chapter 30 for a complete discussion of the treatment of fractures at specific sites.

Temperature Emergencies

Heat Stroke

Heat stroke is a medical emergency caused by failure of the heat-regulating mechanisms of the body during extended heat waves, especially with high humidity.

Risk Factors

1. Persons who are not acclimatized to heat exposure
2. Those who are unable to care for themselves
3. Those with chronic and debilitating diseases
4. Those who are taking certain medications (tranquilizers, anticholinergics, diuretics, beta blockers)

GERONTOLOGIC ALERT: The majority of heat-related deaths occur in the aged because their cardiovascular systems are unable to compensate for stresses imposed by heat.

5. *Exertional heat stroke* occurs in healthy individuals during sports or work when heat loss is inadequate to prevent hyperthermia. It is a leading cause of death in athletes in this country.

Clinical Manifestations

1. History of exposure to elevated ambient temperature and/or excessive exercise

2. Body temperature 40.6°C. (105°F.) and above
3. Hot, dry skin; usually absence of sweating
4. Tachypnea
5. Central nervous system dysfunction manifested by confusion, bizarre behavior, delirium, coma

Emergency Management

A. Initial Measures

1. Remove patient's clothing.
2. Administer oxygen.

B. Temperature Reduction Measures

1. Reduce the core (internal) temperature to 39°C. (102°F.) as rapidly as possible (controversy surrounds body cooling techniques).
2. One or more of the following may be used to reduce stored body heat (as directed):
   a. Spray tepid water on skin while patient lies in a net hammock with fans turned to evaporate spray.
   b. Apply ice packs to neck, groin, axillae, and scalp (areas of maximal heat transfer); keep skin saturated with tepid water and direct fans on patient.
   c. Soak sheets/towels in ice water and place on patient using fans to accelerate evaporation/cooling rate.
   d. Wet the body with water and rub the body surface briskly with plastic bags containing ice.
   e. Immerse patient in cold water (controversial).
   f. Iced saline lavage of stomach or colon may be prescribed if temperature fails to come down.
3. Place electric fans to blow on the patient to augment heat dissipation by evaporation.
4. Massage the patient, especially the torso to neck and extremities, to promote circulation and maintain cutaneous vasodilation during cooling process.

C. Monitoring Parameters

1. Monitor and record the core temperature continually during cooling process to avoid hypothermia; also, hyperthermia may recur spontaneously within 3–4 hours.
2. Monitor the patient carefully—vital signs, ECG, CVP, and level of responsiveness change with rapid alterations in body temperature.

NURSING ALERT: A seizure may be followed by recurrence of hyperthermia.

3. Continue to oxygenate patient to supply tissue needs exaggerated by hypermetabolic condition. Intubate the patient with a cuffed endotracheal tube and attach to a ventilator if necessary to support failing cardiorespiratory systems.

D. Fluid Replacement

1. Start intravenous infusion as directed to replace fluid losses, maintain adequate circulation, and facilitate cooling.
2. Fluid replacement is based on patient's response and laboratory results.

E. Other Measures

1. Give supportive care as directed.
   a. Dialysis for renal failure
   b. Diuretics (mannitol) to promote diuresis
   c. Anticonvulsant agents to control seizures
   d. Potassium for hypokalemia and sodium bicarbonate to correct metabolic acidosis, depending on laboratory results

2. Measure urinary output—acute tubular necrosis is a complication of heat stroke.
3. Continue to monitor ECG for possible ischemia, infarction, dysrhythmias.
4. Carry out serial testing for bleeding diatheses (disseminated intravascular coagulation) and serum enzymes to estimate thermal hypoxic injury to the liver and muscle.
5. Admit the patient to intensive care unit; permanent liver, cardiac, and central nervous system damage may occur.

Patient Education

1. Advise the patient to avoid immediate reexposure to high temperatures; the patient may remain hypersensitive to high temperatures for a considerable length of time.
2. Emphasize the importance of maintaining an adequate fluid intake, wearing loose clothing, and reducing activity in hot weather.
3. Athletes should monitor fluid losses, replace fluids, and use a gradual approach to physical conditioning, allowing sufficient time for acclimatization.

Cold Injuries to Extremities (Frostbite)

Frostbite is trauma due to exposure to freezing temperatures that cause actual freezing of the tissue fluids in the cell and intracellular spaces, resulting in vascular damage.

Underlying Considerations

1. The extent of injury from exposure to cold is not always known when the patient is seen initially.
2. A frozen extremity may be hard, cold, and insensitive to touch and appear white or mottled blue–white.
3. The body parts most frequently affected by frostbite are the nose, ears, and distal extremities.

Emergency Management

Goal:
Restore normal body temperature

A. Rewarming Measures

1. Remove all constricting clothing that can impair circulation, including watchbands and rings.
2. Rewarm the extremity by controlled and rapid rewarming, 37–40°C. (98.6°–104°F.), in a fairly large water bath until the tips of the injured part flush (about 30 minutes)
   a. Flush indicates that circulatory flow is reestablished.
   b. Early rewarming reverses ice crystal formation in tissues.

B. Protection of Frostbitten Body Part

1. Handle the part gently to avoid further mechanical injury.
2. Administer an analgesic for pain; the thawing process may be very painful.
3. Protect the thawed part; do not rupture large blisters that develop in 1 hour to a few days after rewarming—to reduce the risk of infection.
4. Place sterile gauze or cotton between affected fingers/toes to absorb moisture.
5. Use strict aseptic technique during dressing changes—frostbite injuries make the patient susceptible to infection.

6. Elevate the part to help control swelling.
7. Use a foot cradle to prevent contact with bedding if the feet are involved—prevents further tissue injury.

C. Supportive Measures

1. Carry out physical assessment to look for concomitant injury (soft tissue injury, dehydration, alcohol coma, fat embolism).
2. Restore electrolyte balance; dehydration and hypovolemia occur frequently in frostbite victims.
3. Give tetanus prophylaxis if indicated by associated trauma.
4. The following may be carried out when appropriate:
   a. Whirlpool bath for the affected extremity—to aid circulation, debride dead tissue, and help prevent infection.
   b. Escharotomy (incision through the eschar)—to prevent further tissue damage, allow for normal circulation, and permit joint motion.
   c. Fasciotomy (incision in fascia to release pressure on the muscles, nerves, blood vessels)—to treat compartment syndrome.
5. Encourage hourly active motion of the affected digits to promote maximum restoration of function and to prevent contractures.
6. Advise patient not to use tobacco because of the vasoconstrictive effects of nicotine, which further reduce the already deficient blood supply to injured tissues.

Accidental Hypothermia

Accidental hypothermia is a condition in which the core (internal) temperature of the body is less than 35°C. (95°F.) as a result of exposure to cold.

Underlying Considerations and Clinical Manifestations

1. There is progressive deterioration marked by apathy, poor judgment, ataxia, dysarthria, drowsiness, and eventually coma. Shivering may be suppressed below a temperature of 32.2°C. (90°F.).
2. Below this temperature, the body's self-warming mechanisms become ineffective.
   a. The heartbeat and the blood pressure may be so weak that the peripheral pulsations become undetectable.
   b. Cardiac irregularities also may occur.
   c. Other physiologic abnormalities include hypoxemia and acidosis.
3. Those at risk include the *elderly,* the very young, and persons with concurrent illnesses.

GERONTOLOGIC ALERT: Impaired thermoregulation in old age is related to reduced activity, lack of thermogenic nutrients in the diet, and loss of lean body and muscle mass.

Emergency Management

(Management consists of continuing monitoring, rewarming, and supportive care carried out simultaneously.)

A. Ongoing Monitoring

1. Handle the patient *carefully and gently*—to avoid triggering ventricular fibrillation.
2. Monitor the patient: vital signs, CVP, urinary output, arterial blood gas values, blood chemistry determinations.

3. Monitor core body temperature with an esophageal or rectal thermistor probe.
4. Employ continuous ECG monitoring—cold-induced myocardial irritability leads to conduction disturbances, especially ventricular fibrillation.
5. Maintain an arterial line for recording blood pressure and to facilitate blood sampling—allows rapid detection of acid–base disturbances and assessment of adequacy of ventilation and oxygenation.

B. Rewarming Measures

1. The optimal method has not been determined.
2. Rewarming methods include active core (internal) rewarming, active external rewarming, and passive or spontaneous rewarming.

C. Supportive Care

1. Constant monitoring of core temperature, cardiac rhythm, and urine output
2. Ongoing cardiovascular support
3. Warmed intravenous fluids—to expand circulation, correct hypotension, and maintain urinary output
4. Delivery of heated, humidified oxygen
5. Indwelling urethral catheter to monitor output
6. Correction of acid–base imbalances
7. Specific drug therapy: antidysrhythmic agents, steroids, antibiotics

---

Poisoning

Poison is any substance that when ingested, inhaled, absorbed, applied to the skin, injected into or developed within the body, in relatively small amounts, produces injury to the body by its chemical action.

Swallowed Poisons

Goals of Emergency Management

1. Remove or inactivate the poison before it is absorbed.
2. Give supportive care to maintain vital organ systems.
3. Use the specific antidote to neutralize the poison.
4. Give treatment to hasten the elimination of the absorbed poison.

Emergency Management*

A. Resuscitative and Other Measures.

1. Attain control of the airway, ventilation, and oxygenation; in the absence of cerebral or renal damage, the patient's prognosis depends largely on successful management and support of vital functions.
2. Assess adequacy of ventilation by observing ventilatory effort, through blood gas analysis, or by the use of Wright's spirometer.
3. Assess cardiovascular function by measurement of pulse, blood pressure, central venous pressure, and temperature (core and peripheral).
4. Give artificial respiration if respiration is depressed—positive expiratory pressure applied to the airway (bag–mask) may help keep the alveoli inflated.
5. Administer oxygen for respiratory depression, unconsciousness, cyanosis, and shock.

* Many of these measures are done simultaneously by the Emergency Department team.

6. Treat shock.
7. Prevent aspiration of gastric contents by positioning (on side with head down), use of oropharyngeal airway, and suctioning.
8. Stabilize cardiovascular function. Take ECG.
9. Insert an indwelling urinary catheter to monitor kidney function.
10. Obtain blood to test for concentration of drug or poison.
11. Monitor neurologic status, including mentation; monitor the course of vital signs and neurologic status over time.
12. Conduct a rapid physical examination.

B. Identifying the Poison

1. Try to determine the product taken: where, when, why, how much, who witnessed event, time since ingestion, symptoms, age and weight of patient, and pertinent health history.
2. Call the poison control center in the area if an unknown toxic agent has been taken, or if it is necessary to identify an antidote for a known toxic agent.

C. Reducing Absorption of Poison

1. Give appropriate treatment to reduce absorption.
2. Gastric-emptying procedures.
   a. Induction of emesis with syrup of ipecac if the patient is conscious and has a good gag reflex; most effective within 30 minutes of ingestion of poison.

   Note: Do not induce emesis after ingestions of caustic substances or petroleum distillates.

   b. Administration of oral activated charcoal—adsorbs the poison on the surface of its particles and allows it to pass with the stool. Multiple doses may be administered.
   c. Gastric lavage (see Guidelines, p. 950) for the obtunded patient. Save gastric aspirate for toxicology screens.
   d. Administration of cathartic when appropriate to remove unabsorbed material from intestine.
3. Procedures to enhance the removal of the ingested substance if the patient is deteriorating.
   a. Forced diuresis with urine *p*H alteration—to enhance renal clearance.
   b. Hemoperfusion (process of passing blood through an extracorporeal circuit and a cartridge containing an adsorbent [such as charcoal], after which the detoxified blood is returned to patient).
   c. Hemodialysis—used in selected patients to purify blood and accelerate the elimination of circulating toxins.
   d. Repeated doses of charcoal—for binding nonabsorbed drugs/toxins.
4. Give specific antidotal therapy (available for only a few toxins). Administer the specific chemical antagonist or physiologic antagonist as early as possible to reverse or diminish effects of the toxin.

D. Supportive Measures

1. Support the patient having seizures; many poisons excite the central nervous system or the patient may convulse from oxygen deprivation.
2. Assist with supportive therapy, which includes intensive care and a multidisciplinary approach for the management of respiration, circulation, and other vital functions.

3. Monitor for fluid and electrolyte imbalance.
4. Reduce elevated temperature.
5. Give analgesics for pain cautiously—severe pain causes vasomotor collapse and reflex inhibition of normal physiologic functions.
6. Assist in securing specimens of blood, urine, stomach contents.
7. Provide constant nursing surveillance and attention to the patient in a coma—coma from poisoning results from interference with brain cell function or metabolism.

8. Monitor and treat for complications: hypotension, cardiac dysrhythmias, seizures.

E. Discharge Teaching

1. If the patient is discharged, give written instructions of signs and symptoms of potential problems and procedures for call-back or return.
2. Refer for psychiatric evaluation if poisoning was a suicide attempt.
3. Give poison prevention and home poison-proofing instructions to a patient with accidental ingestion.

Guidelines Assisting With Gastric Lavage

Gastric lavage is the aspiration of the stomach contents and washing out of the stomach by means of a gastric tube (Fig. 38-7).

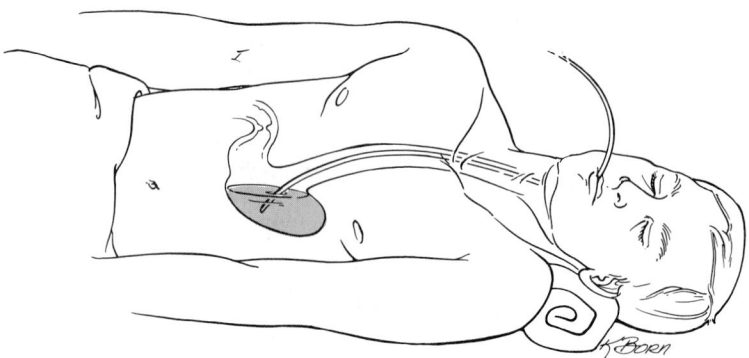

Figure 38-7. *Gastric lavage.*

Purposes
1. To remove unabsorbed poison after poison ingestion.
2. To diagnose gastric hemorrhage and for the arrest of hemorrhage.
3. To cleanse the stomach before endoscopic procedures.
4. To remove liquid or small particles of material from the stomach.

> **NURSING ALERT:** Gastric lavage may be dangerous (1) after the ingestion of acids, alkalis, hydrocarbons, or petroleum distillates and (2) in the presence of convulsions. It is dangerous after the ingestion of strong corrosive agents.

Equipment
Large-bore orogastric tubes or large-bore Ewald tube
Large irrigating syringe with adapter
Large plastic funnel with adapter to fit stomach tube
Water-soluble lubricant
Lavage fluid (warm saline or other prescribed solution)
Bucket for aspirate
Mouth gag; nasotracheal or endotracheal tubes with inflatable cuffs
Containers for specimens

Procedure

Emergency Department/Team Action	Rationale/Amplification
1. Remove dental appliances and inspect oral cavity for loose teeth.	1. To prevent accidental aspiration
2. Measure the distance on the lavage tube between the bridge of the nose and the xiphoid process. Mark with indelible pencil or tape.	2. This is a rule-of-thumb measurement of the distance the tube is passed to reach the stomach; avoids curling/kinking of excess tubing.
3. Lubricate the tube with water-soluble lubricant.	
4. If the patient is comatose, he is intubated with a cuffed nasotracheal or endotracheal tube.	4. A cuffed endotracheal tube prevents aspiration of gastric contents.
5. Place the unconscious patient in a left lateral position with the head (lowered approximately 15° downward), neck and trunk forming a straight line.	5. This position decreases passage of gastric contents into the duodenum during lavage and minimizes the possibility of aspiration into lungs.

Procedure *(continued)*	Emergency Department/Team Action	Rationale/Amplification
	6. Pass the tube via the oral (or nasal) route while keeping the head in a neutral position. Pass the tube to the adhesive marking or about 50 cm. (20 inches). After the lavage tube is passed, the head of the table is lowered. Have standby suction available.	6. The depth of insertion of the tube will vary with the height of the patient. If the tube enters the larynx instead of the esophagus, the patient will experience coughing and dyspnea.
	7. Submerge free end of tube below water level at the moment of the patient's exhalation or auscultate the stomach during injection of air with a syringe to confirm gastric location.	7. If tube is inadvertently in the lungs, the water will bubble with each exhalation.
	8. Aspirate the stomach contents with syringe attached to the tube before instilling water or antidote. Save the specimen for analysis.	8. Aspiration is carried out to remove the stomach contents. Initial gastric aspirates are saved for toxicologic analysis.
	9. Remove syringe. Attach funnel to the stomach tube or use 50-ml. syringe to put lavage solution in gastric tube. Volume of fluid placed in the stomach should be small.	9. Overfilling of the stomach may cause regurgitation and aspiration, or force the stomach contents through the pylorus.
	10. Elevate funnel above the patient's head and pour approximately 150–200 ml. of solution into funnel.	10. The lavage fluid is left in place about 1 minute and then allowed to drain.
	11. Lower the funnel and siphon the gastric contents into the bucket.	11. The fluid should flow in freely and drain by gravity.
	12. Save samples of first 2 washings.	12. Keep track of fluid input/output to be sure that most of fluid is being removed.
	13. Repeat lavage procedure until the returns are relatively clear and no particulate matter is seen.	13. This usually requires a total volume of at least 2 liters; some clinicians advocate 5–20 liters.

	14. At the completion of lavage:
	  a. Stomach may be left empty.
	  b. An adsorbent (powder form of activated charcoal mixed with water to form a slurry, the consistency of thick soup) may be instilled in the tube and allowed to remain in the stomach.
	
	  c. A saline cathartic may be instilled in the tube.
		
		b. Activated charcoal adsorbs a variety of drugs and toxic agents onto its surface and is used to prevent the gastrointestinal absorption of various substances. It renders the poison inaccessible to the circulation, thereby reducing its toxicity.
		c. A cathartic facilitates the transit of the charcoal and remains of the ingested substance through the intestinal tract.

	15. Pinch off tube during removal or maintain suction while tube is being withdrawn.	15. Pinching off the tube prevents aspiration and the initiation of the gag reflex. Keeping the patient's head lower than the body also gives this protection.
	16. Give the patient a cathartic if prescribed. Warn the patient that his stools will turn black from the charcoal.	16. A cathartic may be given if the poison has no corrosive action on the bowel. The cathartic will help remove unabsorbed material from the intestine.

Complications

Aspiration pneumonia
Esophageal trauma
Cardiorespiratory dysfunction

---

* Activated charcoal adsorbs (binds) many drugs in the gastrointestinal tract and prevents their absorption in the bloodstream.

Inhaled Poisons:
Carbon Monoxide Poisoning

May occur as an industrial or household accident or as an attempted suicide.

Underlying Principles

1. Carbon monoxide exerts its toxic effect by binding to circulating hemoglobin to reduce the oxygen-carrying capacity of the blood.
2. The affinity between carbon monoxide and hemoglobin is 200–300 times that between oxygen and hemoglobin. (Carbon monoxide combines with hemoglobin to form carboxyhemoglobin.) As a result, tissue anoxia occurs.

Clinical Manifestations

1. The patient may appear intoxicated from cerebral hypoxia.
2. Headache, muscular weakness, palpitation, dizziness, mental confusion—may progress rapidly to coma.
3. Skin may be pink, cherry red, or cyanotic and pale—*skin color is not a reliable sign.*
4. History of exposure to carbon monoxide justifies immediate treatment.

Emergency Management

Goals:
Reverse cerebral and myocardial hypoxia.
Hasten carbon monoxide elimination.

1. Give 100% oxygen at atmospheric or hyperbaric pressures to reverse hypoxia and accelerate elimination of carbon monoxide.
2. Draw blood for carboxyhemoglobin levels.
3. Employ continuous ECG monitoring; treat dysrhythmias and correct acid–base and electrolyte abnormalities.
4. Observe the patient constantly—psychoses, spastic paralysis, visual disturbances, and deterioration of personality may persist following resuscitation and may be symptoms of permanent central nervous system damage.

NURSING ALERT: Late neurologic sequelae may occur 3 days to 3 weeks after apparent recovery from carbon monoxide poisoning.

Patient Education

When unintentional carbon monoxide poisoning occurs, the health department should be contacted and the dwelling or building in question should be inspected.

Injected Poisons: Stinging Insects

(Bee, yellow jacket, hornet, wasp)

NURSING ALERT: A patient may have an extreme sensitivity to *Hymenoptera* stings (yellow jackets, bees, hornets, wasps, and some ants). This constitutes an acute emergency. Stings on the head and neck are especially serious, although stings in any area of the body can result in anaphylaxis.

Clinical Manifestations

Anaphylactic reaction (p. 879)
1. Severe fall in blood pressure
2. Difficult breathing
3. Edema of face, lips
4. Urticaria
5. Itching
6. Bronchial constriction
7. Diarrhea, abdominal cramps

Emergency Management

1. Give epinephrine as requested. Massage the site to hasten absorption.
2. If sting is on an extremity, apply a tourniquet with sufficient compression to occlude venous and lymphatic flow.
3. See page 879 for treatment of an anaphylactic reaction.

Patient Education

A. General Instruction
1. Always have epinephrine on hand (Ana Kit; EpiPen)
2. Wear medical emergency bracelets indicating hyposensitivity.

B. Instructions When Sting Occurs
1. Take epinephrine immediately if stung.
2. Remove stinger with one quick scrape of fingernail.
3. Do not squeeze venom sac—may cause additional venom to be injected.
4. Report to nearest health care facility for observation.

C. Avoiding Exposure
1. Avoid locales with stinging insects (camp and picnic sites).
2. Stay away from insect feeding areas—flower beds, ripe fruit orchards, garbage, fields of clover.
3. Avoid going barefoot outdoors—yellow jackets may nest on ground.
4. Avoid perfumes, scented soaps, bright colors—attract bees.
5. Keep car windows closed.
6. Spray garbage cans with rapid-acting insecticide, and keep areas meticulously clean.
7. Secure a professional exterminator to dispose of wasp/hornet nests or bee hives in home area.
8. Remain motionless if an insect is buzzing around; motion, especially running, increases the likelihood of being stung.

D. Follow-Up
Hyposensitization therapy should be given to persons who have had systemic or large local reactions.

Skin Contamination Poisons: Chemical Burns

Emergency Management

1. Drench skin with running water from a shower, hose, faucet—burning continues as long as agent is on the skin.
2. Continue to apply a stream of water on skin while removing clothing—damage is related to both concentration and duration of exposure.
3. Continue to irrigate skin thoroughly with water for at least 15–30 minutes (or longer, depending on agent).
   a. Personnel should wear impermeable gloves, goggles, gowns, and masks to avoid contamination with a toxic substance.
   b. After irrigation is complete, appropriate wound care is given (standard burn treatment; tetanus prophylaxis)—the identity and characteristics of chemical agent determine treatment.
4. Instruct the patient to have affected area reexamined at 24 and 72 hours and 7 days—there is a significant risk of underestimating these types of injuries.

Food Poisoning *

Food poisoning is an acute-onset illness that occurs after ingestion of food or drink contaminated by bacterial toxins or organisms, by chemical substances, or by naturally occurring organic substances.

---

* Botulism is discussed on page 918 since the treatment differs.

Emergency Management

1. Determine the source and type of food poisoning.
   a. Have family bring suspected food to medical facility.
   b. Take the history:
      (1) How soon after eating did the symptoms occur? Immediate onset suggests chemical, plant, or animal poisoning.
      (2) What was eaten in the previous meal? Did the food have any unusual odor or taste? Most foods causing bacterial poisoning do not have unusual odor or taste.
      (3) Did anyone else eating the same food become ill?
      (4) Did vomiting occur? What was the appearance of the vomitus?
      (5) Did diarrhea occur? Diarrhea is usually absent with botulism or with shell-fish or other fish poisoning.
      (6) Are any neurologic symptoms present? These occur in botulism, chemical, plant, and animal poisoning.
      (7) Does the patient have a fever? Fever is seen in salmonella, favism (ingestion of fava beans), and some fish poisoning.
      (8) What is the patient's appearance?
2. Collect food, gastric contents, vomitus, serum, and feces for examination.
3. Monitor vital signs on a continuing basis.
   a. Assess respiration, blood pressure, sensorium, central venous pressure (if indicated), and muscular activity.
   b. Weigh the patient for future comparisons.
4. Support the respiratory system. Death from respiratory paralysis can occur with botulism, fish poisoning, etc.
5. Maintain fluid and electrolyte balance; severe vomiting produces alkalosis and severe diarrhea produces acidosis. Large amounts of electrolytes and water are lost by vomiting and diarrhea.
   a. Watch for oligemic shock from severe fluid and electrolyte losses.
   b. Evaluate for apathy, rapid pulse, fever, oliguria, anuria, hypotension, and delirium.
   c. Carry out blood electrolyte studies.
6. Correct and control hypoglycemia.
7. Control the nausea.
   a. Give antiemetic drug parenterally if the patient cannot tolerate fluids or medications by mouth.
   b. Give sips of weak tea, carbonated drinks, and tap water for mild nausea.
   c. Give clear liquids 12–24 hours after nausea and vomiting subside.
   d. Graduate to a low-residue, bland diet.

Substance Abuse

Substance abuse includes the use of specific substances that are intended to alter mood or behavior.

Drug Abuse

Drug abuse is the use of drugs for other than legitimate medical purposes. There is a growing tendency among drug users to take a variety of drugs simultaneously, including alcohol, sedatives, hypnotics, and marijuana, which may have additive effects. The clinical manifestations may vary with the drug used, but the underlying principles of management are essentially the same.

Emergency Management of Acute Drug Reaction

Goals:
Support the respiratory and cardiovascular functions.
Give definitive treatment for drug overdose.
Prevent further absorption, enhance drug elimination, and reduce its toxicity.

A. Respiratory Measures

1. Assess the presence and adequacy of respirations. Attain control of the airway, ventilation, and oxygenation.
2. Use a cuffed endotracheal tube and provide assisted ventilation in a severely depressed patient lacking gag or cough reflexes.
3. Measure arterial blood gases—for hypoxia due to hypoventilation, acid–base derangements, etc.
4. Administer oxygen.

B. Cardiovascular Measures

1. Stabilize the cardiovascular system (this is done simultaneously with airway management).
2. Begin external cardiac compression and ventilation in the absence of heartbeat.
3. Start ECG monitoring.
4. Draw blood samples for testing glucose, electrolytes, BUN, creatinine, and appropriate toxicologic screen.
5. Start intravenous fluids.

C. Pharmacotherapy

1. Give specific drug antagonist if drug is known.
2. Naloxone hydrochloride (Narcan) is frequently used.
3. Fifty-percent glucose in water is also used.

D. Gastric Emptying

1. Remove the drug from the stomach as soon as possible (if drug has been ingested).
2. Induce vomiting if the patient is seen *early* after ingestion; save vomitus for toxicologic study.
3. Use gastric lavage if the patient is unconscious or if there is no way to determine when the drug was ingested; save gastric aspirate.

   Note: In patients lacking gag or cough reflexes, carry out this procedure only after intubation with cuffed endotracheal tube to prevent aspiration of stomach contents.

4. Activated charcoal may be a useful adjunct to therapy and is used after emesis or lavage.
5. Save gastric aspirate for toxicologic analysis.

E. Supportive Care

1. Take rectal temperature—extremes of thermoregulation (hyperthermia/hypothermia) must be recognized and treated.
2. Treat convulsions.
3. Assist with hemodialysis/peritoneal dialysis for potentially lethal poisoning.
4. Try to maintain a free urine flow since the drug or metabolites are excreted by the urine.

F. Physical Assessment

1. Do a thorough physical examination to rule out insulin shock, meningitis, subdural hematoma, stroke, trauma.
2. Look for needle marks and external evidence of trauma.
3. Carry out a rapid neurologic survey (level of respon-

siveness [depressed or stimulated], pupil size and reactivity, reflexes, focal neurologic findings).
4. Keep in mind that many drug abusers take multiple drugs simultaneously.
5. Be aware that there is a high incidence of acquired immunodeficiency syndrome (AIDS) and infectious hepatitis among drug users, which is thought to be the result of communal use of unsterile needles and syringes.
6. Examine the patient's breath for characteristic odor of alcohol, acetone, etc.
7. Try to obtain a history of the drug experiences (from the person accompanying the patient or from the patient himself).
    a. Adapt a supportive, empathetic, and realistic relationship with the patient.
    b. Do not leave the patient alone; there is a potential for the patient to harm himself or emergency department staff.

G. Follow-Up

1. Admit the patient to the intensive care unit if he remains unconscious; if the patient has deliberately taken a drug overdose, psychiatric consultation is necessary.
2. Make every effort to enroll the patient in a drug treatment program (detoxification and rehabilitation) to intervene in a life-style that fosters addiction.
3. Arrange consultation with a psychiatrist/social worker to explore the intent of poisoning (suicide?).

Acute Cocaine Toxicity

Cocaine is an alkaloid derived from the coca plant. It is now the most abused major stimulant in the US and has potentially fatal effects. When absorbed systemically, co-caine causes excessive adrenergic stimulation of the heart (Fig. 38-8), central nervous system, and respiratory system.

Routes of Administration

1. Smoking ("freebasing"); distributors sell cocaine in ready-to-smoke form ("crack," "rock") and a large quantity of cocaine is delivered to the vascular bed of the lung with *rapid* and profound effects.
2. Inhalation by nasal insufflation ("snorting")
3. Injection ("shooting"): subcutaneously, intramuscularly, intravenously

Clinical Manifestations

1. Forceful cardiac palpitations with feeling of impending doom, tachycardia, hypertension, dysrhythmia, myocardial ischemia/infarction
2. Cocaine euphoria, agitation, combativeness, confusion, seizures
3. Hallucinations, paranoia, aggressive behavior, suicidal attempts
4. Hyperpyrexia

Emergency Management of Acute Cocaine Intoxication

1. Secure airway, breathing, and circulation.
2. Assist with the treatment of specific problems.
    a. Ventricular dysrhythmias—IV lidocaine; propranolol
    b. CNS depression—naloxone
    c. Altered mental status—diazepam; haloperidol
    d. Hyperpyrexia—rapid cooling methods
    e. Seizures—diazepam, intubation, general anesthesia
    f. Hypotension—vigorous fluid replacement; hemodynamic monitoring

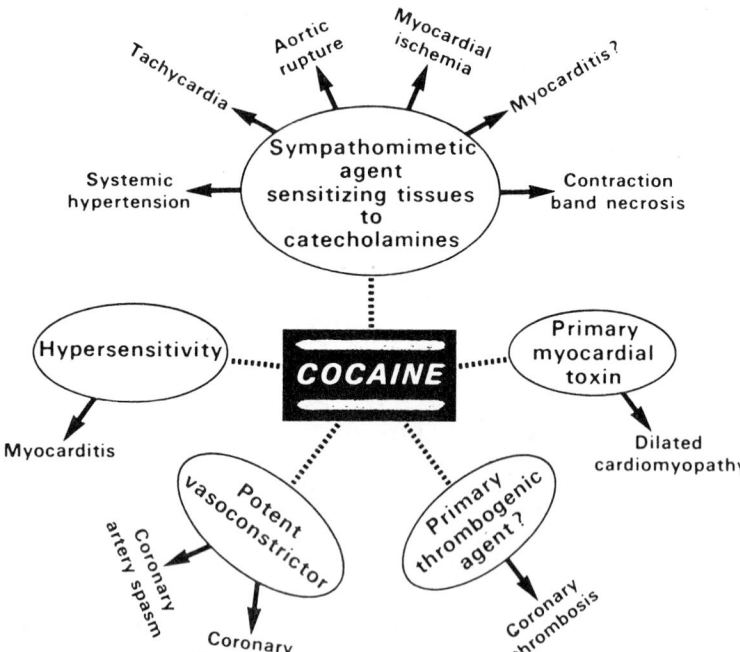

Figure 38-8. *Diagram showing the effects of cocaine on the heart. (From Indiana Med 1988 Nov; 81[11]: 957)*

3. Anticipate complications—sudden death from cerebral hypoxia, dysrhythmias, seizures, respiratory arrest, myocardial infarction.
4. See Emergency Management of Acute Drug Reaction, page 953.
5. See Emergency Management of Violent Patient, page 956.
6. Facilitate referral for psychiatric evaluation and for continuance of care and assessment of psychiatric disorders.

Hallucinogens or Psychedelic-Type Drugs

Common Forms

1. Lysergic acid diethylamide (LSD)
2. Phencyclidine HCl (PCP)
3. Mescaline, psilocybin
4. Jimson weed seeds

Clinical Manifestations

1. Marked anxiety bordering on panic
2. Confusion, incoherence, hyperactivity
3. Hallucinations
4. Hazardous behavior (delirium, mania, self-injury)
5. Flashback (return of the drug experience after acute effects have worn off—can occur months or even years after initial drug use)
6. Convulsions, coma, circulatory collapse, death

Emergency Management

1. Evaluate patient's airway, breathing, and circulation.
2. Determine if the patient has ingested a hallucinogenic drug or has a toxic psychosis.
3. Try to communicate with the patient—use "vocal anesthesia" to reassure him (except for PCP abusers).
   a. "Talking down" involves understanding the process through which the patient is proceeding and helping him overcome his fears while establishing contact with reality.
   b. Remind the patient that fear is common with this problem.
   c. Reassure the patient that he is not losing his mind; that he is experiencing effect of drugs and that this will wear off.
   d. Instruct the patient to keep his eyes open—reduces intensity of reaction.
   e. *Reduce sensory stimuli*—minimize noise, lights, movement, tactile stimulation.
   f. Do not leave the patient alone.
4. Sedate the patient if his hyperactivity cannot be controlled, as directed.
5. Search for evidences of trauma—hallucinogenic users have a tendency to "act out" their hallucinations.
6. Manage convulsions; place the patient in the intensive care unit.
7. Watch the patient closely and do not leave him unobserved—his behavior may become hazardous.
8. Monitor for hypertensive crisis if the patient has prolonged psychosis due to drug ingestion.
9. Place the patient in a protected environment under proper medical supervision to prevent self-inflicted bodily harm.

Management for Phencyclidine Abusers

1. Protect from self-injury—patients frequently have recurrent delusions of superhuman strength.
2. Place the patient in a calm, supportive environment to minimize stimuli.
3. Approach with great caution.
4. Avoid "talking down"—may increase agitation and belligerence.
5. Treat symptoms as they occur.
   a. Drug effects are unpredictable and prolonged.
   b. Symptoms are likely to exacerbate; the patient becomes out of control.
6. Refer the patient for psychiatric evaluation.

Alcohol Abuse
Alcohol Intoxication

Ethanol (alcohol) is a direct multisystem toxin and central nervous system depressant.

Clinical Manifestations

1. Slurred speech, incoordination, ataxia—*OR*
2. Belligerency, grandiosity, uninhibited behavior
3. Odor of alcohol on breath or clothing
4. Stupor and coma, potentially resulting in respiratory depression/death

Emergency Management

The treatment involves (1) detoxification of acute poisoning: (2) recovery, or "drying out"; and (3) rehabilitation.

A. General Approach

1. Approach the patient in a nonjudgmental manner. (Alcoholic patients have a tendency to stimulate rejecting behavior in health care personnel.)
2. Expect the patient to use mechanisms of denial and defensiveness.
3. Adapt a firm, consistent, accepting, and reasonable attitude.
4. Speak calmly and slowly—alcohol interferes with the thought processes.
5. If the patient appears intoxicated, he probably is even though he denies alcohol intake.
6. Draw blood for ethanol concentration, glucose, electrolytes, drug toxicologic screen; use nonalcohol swab to avoid falsely high blood–alcohol reading.
7. Allow the drowsy patient to "sleep off" the state of alcoholic intoxication; it takes time for the liver to metabolize the excess alcohol.
   a. Observe for symptoms of CNS depression; keep the patient under observation.
   b. Protect the airway.
   c. Undress the patient and cover him with a blanket.

B. Ongoing Monitoring

1. Examine the patient for injuries and organic disease that can easily be masked by alcoholic intoxication; chronic alcohol abusers suffer more injuries and illnesses than the general population.
2. Look for symptoms of head injury. Assess the neurologic status of the patient.
3. Assess for alcoholic coma—a medical emergency.

4. Evaluate for pulmonary infection.
5. Watch for hypoglycemia.

C. Supportive Measures

1. Sedate the belligerent, noisy patient as directed.
2. Monitor the patient carefully.
3. Check vital signs and monitor heart rate and blood pressure.
4. If patient is severely agitated or violent, restraints may be required for protection of patient/staff.
5. Provide reality orientation.
6. Assist the patient to the bathroom when necessary.
7. Continue to examine patient in the Emergency Department until he is sober.
8. Hospitalize if necessary, or admit to detoxification center; an effort should be made to examine the problems underlying substance abuse.

Alcohol Withdrawal Delirium

Alcohol withdrawal delirium (delirium tremens; alcoholic hallucinosis) is an acute toxic state that follows a prolonged bout of steady drinking or sudden withdrawal from prolonged intake of alcohol. It may be precipitated by acute injury or infection.

NURSING ALERT: Alcohol withdrawal delirium is a serious complication and is life threatening.

Clinical Manifestations

(Usually begin within 6–8 hours after last drink or reduction of alcohol intake)
1. Tremors, nausea and vomiting, malaise or weakness
2. Anxiety, uncontrollable fear, restlessness, agitation
3. Talkativeness; preoccupation
4. Visual, tactile, and auditory hallucinations, usually of a frightening nature.
5. Autonomic hyper-reactivity—tachycardia, diaphoresis, elevation of temperature, dilated but reactive pupils

Emergency Management

A. Assessment Parameters

1. Take the blood pressure since the patient's subsequent medication may depend on his blood pressure readings.
2. Try to obtain history of ethanol intake, determine severity of past withdrawal episodes, other drug intake.
3. Carry out physical examination to identify potential coexisting illnesses or injuries (head injury, pneumonia, metabolic disturbances)
4. Take a breath analyzer reading—indicates where patient is in the withdrawal process.
5. Using a nonalcohol swab, draw blood for measurement of ethanol concentration, toxicology screen for other drugs of abuse, and other tests as directed.

B. Pharmacotherapy

1. Sedate the patient with sufficient dosage of medication to produce adequate relaxation—to reduce agitation, prevent exhaustion, and promote sleep.
2. A variety of drugs and combinations of drugs are used—the benzodiazepines (diazepam; chlordiazepoxide) or haloperidol and others.

3. The dosage is titrated according to the patient's symptoms and blood pressure response; large doses may be required.
4. Monitor vital signs every 30 minutes.
5. Place the patient in a private room where he can be observed closely.

C. Supportive Measures

1. Maintain electrolyte balance and hydration via oral or intravenous route—fluid losses may be extreme because of profuse perspiration and agitation.
2. Administer prescribed anticonvulsant medication to prevent or control alcoholic or epileptic seizures—alcohol withdrawal is a common cause of adult-onset seizure disorder.
3. Assess respiratory, hepatic, and cardiovascular status of patient—pneumonia, liver disease, and cardiac failure are complications.
   a. Hypoglycemia may accompany alcoholic withdrawal because alcohol depletes liver glycogen stores and impairs gluconeogenesis; many patients also suffer from malnutrition.
   b. Administer thiamine followed by parenteral dextrose if liver glycogen is depleted.
   c. Give orange juice, Gatorade, or other carbohydrates to stabilize blood sugar and to counteract tremulousness.
4. Give supplemental vitamin therapy and a high-carbohydrate diet; these patients are usually vitamin deficient.
5. Refer to alcoholic treatment center for subsequent follow-up and rehabilitation.

Psychiatric Emergencies

A *psychiatric emergency* is an urgent, serious disturbance of behavior, affect, or thought that makes the patient unable to cope with his life situation and interpersonal relationships.

A patient presenting with a psychiatric emergency may be overactive or violent, depressed, or suicidal.

Violent Patients

Approach to the Violent Patient

Violent and aggressive behavior is usually episodic and is a means of expressing feelings of anger, fear, or hopelessness about a situation.

Persons with propensity for violence include:
1. Those intoxicated with drugs/alcohol
2. Those going through drug or alcohol withdrawal
3. Those with acute paranoid schizophrenic states, acute organic brain syndrome, acute psychosis, paranoia, borderline personality.

Emergency Management

Goals:
Bring violence under control
Protect patient and staff from harm

A. Establishing Control

1. Keep the door of the room open, and be in clear view of the staff.

2. Help the patient bring his violence under control.
   a. Give the patient space. Do not make any sudden movement.
   b. Avoid touching an agitated patient or standing too close.
   c. Ask if he has a weapon. Request that it be placed in a neutral area.
   d. If the patient will not surrender weapon, leave the room and allow security personnel/police to handle the situation.
3. Try not to leave the patient alone; this may be interpreted as rejection or the patient may try to harm himself.
4. Adopt a calm nonconfrontational approach and remain in control of the situation—external calm and structure may help the patient gain control.

B. Emotional Support

1. Talk and listen to the patient.
2. Crisis intervention is best done with an attitude of interest in the patient's well-being and with an attempt to "tune in" to the patient while at the same time remaining firm.
3. Acknowledge the patient's state of agitation, for example, "I want to work with you to relieve your distress."
4. Give the patient the opportunity to ventilate his anger verbally; avoid challenging the delusional state.
5. Try to hear what the patient is saying.
6. Convey the expectation of appropriate behavior and make the patient aware that help is available for him to gain control.
7. Administer prescribed tranquilizer if verbal management techniques fail to attenuate the patient's tension—to reduce anxiety, hyperactivity.
8. Offer protection of hospitalization; may be welcomed by the person who fears loss of control.

C. Securing Assistance

1. Allow security personnel/police to intervene if patient does not become calm.
2. Use restraints when absolutely necessary but with minimum of force.
3. Have a specific plan and enough well-trained personnel available when applying restraints; if patient is intoxicated, restrain him in a left lateral position and monitor closely for aspiration.
4. Talk reassuringly while applying restraints; use empathetic, supportive verbal interactions.
5. Monitor patient continuously after restraints are applied; check circulation of restrained extremities.
6. Refer for immediate psychiatric consultation/hospitalization.

Depressed Patients

Depression in the Emergency Department may be seen as the primary condition bringing the patient to the facility, or depression may be masked by anxiety and somatic complaints.

Assessment

1. Observe for sadness, apathy, feelings of worthlessness, self-blame, suicidal thoughts, desire to escape, worsening of mood in morning, anorexia, weight loss, sleeplessness, lessening interest in sex, reduction of activity or ceaseless activity.

2. The agitated depressed individual may exhibit motor restlessness and severe anxiety.

Emergency Management

A. Emotional Support

1. Listen to the patient in a calm, unhurried manner.
2. The patient will benefit from ventilation of feelings.
3. Give the patient an opportunity to talk about his problems.
4. Anticipate that the patient may be suicidal.
5. Attempt to find out if the patient has thought about or attempted suicide.
   a. "Have you ever thought about taking your own life?"
   b. The patient is generally relieved because of the opportunity to discuss his feelings.
6. Find out if there is an illness, perceived or real.
7. Assess whether there has been sudden worsening of depression.
8. Notify relatives about a seriously depressed patient. Do not leave the patient alone since suicide is usually an act committed in solitude.

B. Supportive Measures

1. Give antidepressant and antianxiety agents as prescribed.
2. Point out to the patient that depression is treatable.
3. Be aware of crisis and supportive services in the community: telephone counseling and referral, suicide prevention centers, group therapy, marital and family counseling, drug/alcohol counseling, adolescent counseling, befriending programs.
4. Refer for psychiatric consultation or to psychiatric unit.

Suicidal Patients

Suicide is the eighth leading cause of death in the US and the second lethal killer of young people.

Persons at Risk

1. Associated psychiatric illness (affective disorders and substance abuse in adults; conduct disorders and depression in young people).
2. Personality traits related to suicide: aggression, impulsivity, depression, hopelessness, borderline personality disorder, antisocial personality
3. Persons who have experienced early loss, decreased social support, chronic illness, recent divorce.
4. Genetic and familial factors: family history of suicide, certain psychiatric disorders or alcoholism; alcohol and substance abuse.

Assessment and Prevention

1. Be aware of persons at risk.
2. Determine whether patient has communicated *suicidal intent* such as preoccupation with death or talking of someone else's suicide.
3. Determine whether patient has ever attempted suicide—the risk is much greater in these persons.
4. Is there a family history of suicide?
5. Was there loss of a parent at an early age?
6. Does he have a specific plan for suicide? A means to carry out the plan?

Emergency Management

1. Treat the consequences of the suicide attempt (gunshot wound, drug overdose, etc.).
2. Prevent further self-injury—a patient who has made a suicide gesture may do so again.
3. Employ crisis intervention (a form of brief psychotherapy)—to determine suicide potential; discover areas of depression and conflict; find out about the patient's support system; and determine whether hospitalization, psychiatric referral, etc. is warranted.
4. Admit to intensive care unit (if condition warrants), arrange follow-up care, or admit to psychiatric unit, depending on assessment of suicide potential.

Sexual Assault

Rape is a legal term, defined as carnal knowledge of a female by force or the threat of force against her will. It is the fastest growing violent crime in this country. The patient should be seen immediately upon entrance to the Emergency Department.

Emergency Management

Note: Most emergency departments have commercially prepared rape evidence collection kits, as well as written protocols for treatment of injuries, legal documentation, and sexually transmitted disease and pregnancy prevention.

A. Initiating a Supportive Relationship

1. The manner in which the patient is received and treated in the Emergency Department is important to the future psychological well-being of the patient.
   a. Call the Rape-Crisis Intervention Counselor (if available), who will meet the patient/family in the Emergency Department.
   b. Do not leave patient alone. Accept the emotional reactions of the patient (hysteria, stoicism, overwhelmed feeling, etc.)
2. Emotional trauma may be present for weeks, months, years. Patient's reaction to rape has been called the "rape trauma syndrome." Patient may go through phases of psychological reactions:
   a. Acute phase (disorganization)—shock, disbelief, fear, anxiety, guilt, humiliation, suppression of feelings—may last for months to years.
   b. Phase of denial and unwillingness to talk about incident, followed by phase of heightened anxiety, fear, flashbacks, sleep disturbances, hyperalertness, and psychosomatic reactions.
   c. Phase of reorganization—putting incident into perspective.

NURSING ALERT: Some persons never fully recover and develop chronic stress disorders and phobias.

B. History-taking

1. Secure written, witnessed informed consent from the patient (or parent/guardian if patient is a minor) for examination and for the taking of photographs if necessary and for release of information to law enforcement agencies.
2. Take history *only* if the patient has not already talked to police officer, social worker, crisis intervention worker, etc. Do not ask the patient to repeat the history.
   a. Record history of event in the patient's own words.
3. Ask if the patient has bathed, douched, gargled or brushed teeth, changed clothes, urinated or defecated since attack—may alter interpretation of subsequent findings.
4. Record time of admission, time of examination, date and time of alleged rape, and the general appearance of the patient.
   a. Document any evidence of trauma—discoloration, bruises, lacerations, secretions, torn and bloody clothing.
   b. Record emotional state.

C. Preparing for Physical Examination

1. Assist the patient to undress over a sheet/large piece of paper to obtain debris.
2. Ask patient to place each item of clothing in a separate paper bag (plastic bags promote moisture retention, which may lead to formation of mold and mildew that can destroy evidence).
3. Label bags appropriately; give to appropriate law enforcement authority.

D. Physical Examination Findings

1. Examine the patient (from head to toe) for injuries, especially to the head, neck, breasts, thighs, back, and buttocks.
2. Assess for external evidence of trauma (bruises, contusions, lacerations, stab wounds).
3. Assess for dried semen stains (appearing as crusted, flaking areas) on the patient's body.
4. Inspect fingers for broken nails and tissue and foreign materials under nails.
5. Assist in conducting oral examination to determine secretion status of patient as compared with that of assailant
   a. Secure a specimen of saliva
   b. Take prescribed cultures of gum and tooth areas
6. Document evidence of trauma with body diagrams/photographs.

E. Assisting Patient Undergoing Pelvic and Rectal Examinations

1. Advise the patient of the nature and necessity of each procedure; give the rationale for each question asked.
2. Examine perineum and thighs with an ultraviolet light (Wood's lamp); areas that are found to fluoresce may indicate semen stains.
3. Note color and consistency of any discharge present.
4. Use water-moistened vaginal speculum for examination; do not use lubricant (contains chemicals that may interfere with later forensic testing of specimens and acid phosphatase determinations).

F. Assisting With Securing Laboratory Specimens

1. Collect vaginal aspirate, which is examined for presence or absence of motile/nonmotile sperm.
2. Use sterile swab to draw from vaginal pool for acid phosphatase, blood group antigen of semen, and precipitin test against human sperm and blood.
3. Obtain separate smears from the oral, vaginal, and anal areas.
4. Obtain culture of body orifices for gonorrhea.
5. Trim areas of pubic hair suspected of containing semen; obtain several pubic hairs with follicles; place in

separate containers and identify these as patient's pubic hairs.

6. Obtain blood serum for syphilis; a sample of serum may be frozen and saved for future testing.
7. Collect foreign material (leaves, grass, dirt) and place in appropriate container.
8. Examine rectum for signs of trauma, blood and semen stains.
9. Conduct a pregnancy test if there is possibility that patient may be pregnant.
10. Label all specimens with name of patient, date, time of collection, body area from which specimen was obtained, and names of personnel collecting specimens to preserve chain of evidence; give to designated person (crime laboratory, etc.) and obtain an itemized receipt.
11. Photographs are taken by designated person.

G. Treating Injuries and Preventing Sexually Transmitted Diseases

1. Protect against sexually transmitted disease(s) and pregnancy—usually defined by agency protocol.
2. Treat associated injuries.
3. Offer cleansing douche, mouthwash, fresh clothing.

H. Providing for Follow-up Services

1. Make an appointment for follow-up surveillance for pregnancy and sexually transmitted disease.
2. Inform the patient of counseling services to prevent long-term psychological effects; counseling services should be made available to the family.
3. Encourage the patient to return to previous level of functioning as soon as possible.
4. The patient should be accompanied by a family member or friend when leaving the health care facility.

Bibliography

Books

Burke JF, Boyn RJ and McCabe CJ. Trauma Management. Chicago, Year Book Medical Pub, 1988

Burnell GM and Burnell AL. Clinical Management of Bereavement. New York, Human Sciences Press, 1989

Cardonna VD et al. Trauma Nursing: From Resuscitation Through Rehabilitation. Philadelphia, WB Saunders, 1988

Callaham ML. Current Therapy in Emergency Medicine. Philadelphia, BC Decker, 1987

Cowley RA, Conn A and Dunham CM (eds). Trauma Care, Vols 1 and 2. Philadelphia, JB Lippincott, 1987

Ellenhorn MJ and Barceloux DG. Medical Toxicology: Diagnosis and Treatment of Human Poisoning. New York, Elsevier, 1988

Gilliland BE and James RK. Crisis Intervention Strategies. Pacific Grove, California, Brooks/Cole Publishing, 1988

Green WM. Rape: The Evidential Examination and Management of the Adult Female Victim. Lexington, MA, William M Green, 1988

Greenberg MD and Lieber JJ. Emergency Care: Medical and Trauma Scenarios. Philadelphia, JB Lippincott, 1989

Hales JRS and Richards DAB. Heat Stress: Physical Exertion. New York, Excerpta Medica, 1987

Hardaway RM (ed). Shock: The Reversible Stage of Dying. Littleton, MA, PSG Publishing, 1988

Heffernan JJ, Witzburg RA and Cohen AS. Clinical Problems in Acute Care Medicine. Philadelphia, WB Saunders, 1989

Hoff LA. People in Crisis: Understanding and Helping. 3rd ed. Redwood City, CA, Addison-Wesley, 1989

Howell E, Widra L and Hill MG. Comprehensive Trauma Nursing: Theory and Practice. Glenview, IL, Scott Foresman, 1988

Hyman SE. Manual of Psychiatric Emergencies. 2nd ed. Boston, Little, Brown & Co, 1988

Jaeger RW and deCastro FJ. Poisoning Emergencies: A Primer. St Louis, Catholic Health Association of United States, 1987

Koss MP and Harvey MR. The Rape Victim: Clinical and Community Approaches to Treatment. Lexington, MA, Stephen Greene Press, 1987

Lloyd EL. Hypothermia and Cold Stress. Rockville, Aspen Publishers, Inc., 1986

Lodge DW and Grant HD. Handbook of Emergency Care Procedures. Englewood Cliffs, NJ, Prentice-Hall, 1988

Mancini ME. Decision Making in Emergency Nursing. Philadelphia, BC Decker, 1987

Mattox KL, Moore EE and Feliciano DV (eds). Trauma. Norwalk, Appleton and Lange, 1988

McSwain NE Jr, Martinez JA and Timberlake GA. Cervical Spine Trauma: Evaluation and Acute Management. New York, Thieme Medical Publishers, 1989

Meyer PR. Surgery of Spine Trauma. New York, Churchill Livingstone, 1989

Mowad L and Ruhle DC. Handbook of Emergency Nursing: The Nursing Process Approach. Norwalk, Appleton and Lange, 1988

Pruitt BA Jr and Goodwin CW. Wound care. In Moylan JA (ed). Trauma Surgery, pp 361–374. Philadelphia, JB Lippincott, 1988

Persons CB. Critical Care Procedures and Protocols: A Nursing Process Approach. Philadelphia, JB Lippincott, 1987

Ropper AH and Kennedy SE. Neurological and Neurosurgical Intensive Care. 2nd ed. Rockville, Aspen Publishers, Inc., 1988

Rosen P et al. Emergency Medicine: Concepts and Clinical Practice. 2nd ed. St Louis, CV Mosby, 1988

Safar P and Bircher NG. Cardiopulmonary Cerebral Resuscitation: Basic and Advanced Cardiac and Trauma Life Support: An Introduction to Resuscitation

Medicine. Philadelphia, WB Saunders, 1988

Schwartz GR et al. Emergency Medicine: The Essential Update. Philadelphia, WB Saunders, 1989

Sheehy SB, Marvin JA and Jimmerson CL. Manual of Clinical Trauma Care: The First Hour. St Louis, CV Mosby, 1989

Shorvon SD. Neurological Emergencies. Boston, Butterworths, 1989

Siegel JH (ed). Trauma. Emergency Surgery and Critical Care. New York, Churchill Livingstone, 1987

Strange JM. Shock Trauma Care Plans. Springhouse, PA, Springhouse, 1987

Swearingen PL, Sommers MS and Miller K. Manual of Critical Care: Applying Nursing Diagnoses to Adult Critical Illness. St Louis, CV Mosby, 1988

Talbot L and Meyers–Marquardt M. Pocket Guide to Critical Care Assessment. St Louis, CV Mosby, 1989

Taylor P Jr. Substance Abuse: Pharmacologic and Developmental Perspectives. Springfield, Charles C Thomas, 1988

Tintinalli JE, Krome RL and Ruiz E. Emergency Medicine. 2nd ed. New York, McGraw-Hill, 1988

Westaby S. Trauma: Pathogenesis and Treatment. Oxford, William Heinemann, 1989

Wilkins EW Jr et al (eds). Emergency Medicine: Scientific Foundations and Current Practice. 3rd ed. Baltimore, Williams & Wilkins, 1989

Journals

Approach to Patient/Family

Bluhm J. Helping families in crisis hold on. Nursing 1987 Oct; 17(10):44–46

Coolican M, Vassar E and Grogan J. Helping survivors survive. Nursing 1989 Aug; 19(8):52–57

Trauma

Adelstein W. C1–C2 fractures and dislocations. J Neurosci Nurs 1989 Jun; 21(3):149–159

Asensio JA et al. Trauma: A systematic approach to management. Am Fam Physician 1988 Sep; 38(3):97–112

Coonan TJ. The management of acute severe head injury. Can J Anaesth 1989 May; 36(3 Pt 2):S26–30

Edwards CC. Management of open fractures in the multiply injured patient. Instr Course Lect 1988; 37:257–273

Evers BM, Cryer HM and Miller FB. Pelvic fracture hemorrhage: Priorities in management. Arch Surg 1989 Apr; 124(4):422–424

Feied CF. Diagnostic peritoneal lavage: Questions and answers. Postgrad Med 1989 Mar; 85(4):40–45, 49

Marx JA. Methods of diagnostic peritoneal lavage—better to be safe. Am J Emerg Med 1989 Jul; 7(4):452–453

Meredith JW and Trunkey DD. CT scanning in acute abdominal injuries. Surg Clin North Am 1988 Apr; 68(2):255–268

Mimc BC. Fat embolism syndrome: A variant of ARDS. Orthop Nurs 1989 May–Jun; 8(3):22–27

Mucha P Jr and Welch TJ. Hemorrhage in major pelvic fractures. Surg Clin North Am 1988 Aug; 68(4):757–773

Petersen LG. Acute response to trauma. Adv Psychosom Med 1986; 16:84–92

Perkins SB and Kennally KM. The hidden danger of internal hemorrhage. Nursing 1989 Jul; 19(7):34–42

Sinkinson CR and Zitelli JA. Maximizing a wound's potential for healing. Emerg Med Rep 1989 May 22; 10(11):83–90

Temperature Emergencies

Danzl DF. Hyperthermic syndromes. Am Fam Physician 1988 Jun; 37(6):157–162

Delaney KA et al. Assessment of acid-base disturbances in hypothermia and their physiologic consequences. Ann Emerg Med 1989 Jan; 18(1):72–78

Dunn MM. Guidelines for an effective personal fitness prescription. Nurse Pract 1987 Sep; 12(9):9–18, 23, 26

Knochel JP. Heat stroke and related heat stress disorders. Disease-A-Month 1989 May; 35(5):306–377

Kramer MR, Vandijk J and Rosin AJ. Mortality in elderly patients with thermoregulatory failure. Arch Intern Med 1989 Jul; 149(7):1521–1523

Moss J. Accidental severe hypothermia. Surg Gynecol Obstet 1986 May; 162(5):501–513

Patt A, McCroskey BL and Moore EE. Hypothermia-induced coagulopathies in trauma. Surg Clin North Am 1988 Aug; 68(4):775–785

Stewart CE and Dwyer BJ. Preventing progression of heat injury. Emerg Med Rep 1987 Aug 3; 8(16):121–128

Poisoning

Activated charcoal, emesis, and gastric lavage in aspirin overdose. Br Med J 1988 May 28; 296(6635):1507

Broome JR and Skrine H. Carbon monoxide poisoning: Forgotten not gone. Br J Hosp Med 1988 Apr; 39(4):298–305

Donovan JW. Activated charcoal in management of poisoning: A revitalized antidote. Postgrad Med 1987 Jul; 82(1):52–68

Garella S. Extracorporeal techniques in the treatment of exogenous intoxications. Kidney Int 1988 Mar; 33(3):735–754

Krenzelok EP. Selection of a gastric decontamination method for poisoning emergencies. Clin Pharmacol 1989 Apr; 8(4):294–295

Litovitz T and Greene AE. Health implications of petroleum distillate ingestion. State Art Rev Occup Med 1988 Jul–Sep; 3(3):555–568

Neuvonen PJ and Olkkola KT. Oral activated charcoal in the treatment of intoxications. Med Toxicol Adverse Drug Exp 1988 Jan–Dec; 3(1):33–38

Settipane GA and Boyd GK. Anaphylaxis from insect stings. Postgrad Med 1989 Aug; 86(2):273–281

Spyker DA and Minocha A. Toxicodynamic approach to the management of the poisoned patient. J Emerg Med 1988 Mar–Apr; 6(2):117–120

Treatment of carbon monoxide poisoning. Drug Ther Bull 1988 Oct 3; 26(20):77–79

Wason S and Karkal SS. Coping swiftly and effectively with caustic ingestions. Emerg Med Rep 1989 Feb 13; 10(4):25–32

Winchester JF. Poisoning: Is the role of the nephrologist diminishing? Am J Kidney Dis 1989 Mar; 13(3):171–183

Yarbrough BE. Current management of the poisoned patient. South Med J 1988 Jul; 81(7):892–901

Resuscitation

Erlandson MJ et al. Cricothyrotomy in the emergency department revisited. J Emerg Med 1989 Mar–Apr; 7(2):115–118

Jorden RC. Airway management. Emerg Med Clin North Am 1988 Nov; 6(4):671–686

Marsden AK. Emergency airway management. Acta Anaesthesiol 1988; 39(3 Suppl 2):139–145

Middaugh RE and Middaugh DJ. Current considerations in respiratory and acid-base management during cardiopulmonary resuscitation. Crit Care Nurs Q 1988 Mar; 10(4):25–33

Negovsky VA. Postresuscitation disease. Crit Care Med 1988 Oct; 16(10):942–946

Pons PT. Esophageal obturator airway. Emerg Med Clin North Am 1988 Nov; 6(4):693–698

Rolfsen ML and Davis WR. Cerebral function and preservation during cardiac arrest. Crit Care Med 1989 Mar; 17(3):283–292

Safar P. Resuscitation from clinical death: Pathophysiologic limits and therapeutic potentials. Crit Care Med 1988 Oct; 16(10):923–941

Standards and guidelines for cardiopulmonary resuscitation (CPR) and emergency cardiac care (ECC). JAMA 1986 Jun 6; 255(21):2905–2954

Walls RM. Cricothyroidotomy. Emerg Med Clin North Am 1988 Nov; 6(4):725–736

Willens JS and Copel LC. Performing CPR on adults. Nursing 1989 Jan; 19(1):34–43

Substance Abuse

Adinoff B, Bone GHA and Linnoila M. Acute ethal poisoning and the ethanol withdrawal syndrome. Med Toxicol Adverse Drug Exp 1988 May–Jun; 3(3):172–196

Brickner PW et al. Recommendations for control and prevention of human immunodeficiency virus (HIV) infection in intravenous drug users. Ann Intern Med 1989 May 15; 110(10):833–837

Brody SL and Slovis CM. Recognition and management of complications related to cocaine abuse. Emerg Med Rep 1988 May 14; 9(6):41–48

Chick J. Delirium tremens: Try to spot it early. Br Med J 1989 Jan 7; 298(6665):3–4

Choi YS and Pearl WR. Cardiovascular effects of adolescent drug abuse. J Adolesc Health Care 1989 Jul 10(4):332–337

Cregler LL. Adverse health consequences of cocaine abuse. J Natl Med Assoc 1989 Jan; 81(1):27–38

Cushman P Jr. Delirium tremens: Update on an old disorder. Postgrad Med 1987 Oct: 82(5):117–122

Derlet RW et al. Amphetamine toxicity: Experience with 127 cases. J Emerg Med 1989 Mar–Apr; 7(2):157–169

Derlet RW. Emergency department presentation of cocaine intoxication. Ann Emerg Med 1989 Feb; 18(2):182–186

DuPont RL (ed). Abuse of benzodiazepines: The problems and the solutions. Am J Drug Alcohol Abuse 1988; 14(Suppl 1):1–69

Easton C and MacKenzie FM. Sensory-perceptual alterations: Delirium in the intensive care unit. Heart Lung 1988 May; 17(3):229–235

Ellison DW and Pentel PR. Clinical features and consequences of seizures due to cyclic antidepressant overdose. Am J Emerg Med 1989 Jan; 7(1):5–10

Frishman WH, Karpenos A and Molloy TJ. Cocaine-induced coronary disease. Med Clin North Am 1989 Mar; 73(2):475–486

Gawin FH. Cocaine abuse and addiction. J Fam Pract 1989 Aug; 29(2):193–197

Kosten TR and Kleber HD. Rapid death during cocaine abuse: A variant of neuroleptic malignant syndrome? Am J Drug Alcohol Abuse 1988; 14(3):335–346

Li PKT and Lai KN. Active therapeutic approaches to drug intoxication. Adverse Drug React Acute Poisoning Rev 1988 Summer; 7(2):55–73

Menashe PI and Gottlieb JE. Hyperthermia, rhabdomyolysis, and myoglobinuric renal failure after recreational use of cocaine. South Med J 1988 Mar; 81(3):379–381

Nuckols CC and Greeson J. Cocaine addiction: Assessment and intervention. Nurs Clin North Am 1989 Mar; 24(1):33–43

Nutt D, Adinoff B and Linnoila M. Benzodiazepines in the treatment of alcohol. Recent Dev Alcohol 1989; 7: 283–313

Proudfoot AT. Clinical toxicology—Past, present and future. Hum Toxicol 1988 Sep; 7(5):481–487

Rich J. Action stat! Acute alcohol intoxication. Nursing 1989 Sep; 19(9): 33

Rosenbloom A. Emergency treatment options in the alcohol withdrawal syndrome. J Clin Psychiatry 1988 Dec; 49(Suppl):28–32

Roth D et al. Acute rhabdomyolysis associated with cocaine intoxication. N Engl J Med 1988 Sep 15; 319(11):673–677

US Preventive Services Task Force. Screening for alcohol and other drug abuse. Am Fam Physician 1989 Jul; 40(1):137–146

Vandegaer F. Cocaine—The deadliest addiction. Nursing 1989 Feb; 19(2): 72–73

Waller BF. Cocaine and the heart. Indiana Med 1988 Nov; 81(11):956–959

Psychiatric Emergencies

Blumenthal SJ. Suicide: A guide to risk factors, assessment and treatment. Med Clin North Am 1988 Jul; 72(4):937–971

Brizer DA. Psychopharmacology and the management of violent patients. Psychiatr Clin North Am 1988 Dec; 11(4):551–568

Dubin WR and Feld JA. Rapid tranquilization of the violent patient. Am J Emerg Med 1989 May; 7(3):313–320

Ellison JM, Hughes DH and White KA. An emergency psychiatry update. Hosp Community Psychiatry 1989 Mar; 40(3):250–260

Lande RG. The dangerous patient. J Fam Pract 1989 Jul; 29(1):74–78

Maltsberger JT. Suicide danger: Clinical estimation and decision. Suicide Life Threat Behav 1988 Spring; 18(1):47–54

Navis ES. Controlling violent patients before they control you. Nursing 1987 Sep; 17(9):52–54

Pary R, Lippmann S and Botias C. A preventive approach to the suicide patient. J Fam Pract 1988 Feb; 26(2): 185–189

Tardiff K. Management of the violent patient in an emergency situation.

Psychiatr Clin North Am 1988 Dec; 11(4):539–549

Sexual Assault

Damrosch SP et al. Nurses' attributions about rape victims. Res Nurs Health 1987 Aug; 10(4):245–251

Geist RF. Sexually related trauma. Emerg Med Clin North Am 1988 Aug; 6(3): 439–466

Gise LH and Paddison P. Rape, sexual abuse, and its victims. Psychiatr Clin North Am 1988 Dec; 11(4):629–648

Glaser JB, Hammerschlag MR and McCormack WM. Epidemiology of sexually transmitted diseases in rape victims. Rev Infect Dis 1989 Mar–Apr; 11(2):246–254

Heinrich LB. Care of the female rape victim. Nurse Pract 1987 Nov; 12(11): 9–27

Matheny J and Michels PJ. Office counseling of rape victims. J Fam Pract 1989 Jun; 28(6):657–660

Minden P. The victim care service: A program for victims of sexual assault. Arch Psychiatr Nurs 1989 Feb; 3(1):41–46

Neff JA, Osborn M and Bryan S. Evidentiary examination in sexual assault. JEN 1989 May–Jun; 15(3):284–290

Part *II*

Maternity Nursing

Introduction to Maternity Nursing

Providing care to childbearing families is aimed at the ideal of having every pregnancy result in a healthy mother, baby, and family unit. In the last 20 years, care provided to childbearing families has changed dramatically. Advances such as in vitro fertilization, embryo transplants, and intrauterine fetal surgery have just begun. Technological advances in fetal monitoring, sonography, and neonatal intensive care units are now providing the means to save fetuses and infants who would not have survived 20 years ago.

Regionalization of obstetric services so that childbearing families have access to the technological advances and skilled personnel capable of managing pregnancy or neonatal complications is being implemented. At the same time, childbearing families opposed to the use of advanced technology are demanding and receiving alternate types of care in birthing centers, birthing rooms in hospitals, home deliveries, alternate methods used during delivery, and changes in hospital policies such as 24-hour discharge following delivery and having children present during their mother's labor and delivery.

These changes in the delivery of care and advances in technology have also required changes in the delivery of nursing care, requiring advanced knowledge for nursing practice and additional educational preparation for many nurses. Currently *nurse–midwives,* nurses who have completed additional education in caring for childbearing women, normal newborns, and gynecologic problems of women, are providing more care to childbearing families. Other nurses specializing in the care of high-risk pregnant women and in the care of high-risk neonates are providing the link between advanced technology and more personal and human systems of health care.

Current Problems Affecting Maternal and Infant Morbidity and Mortality

1. Higher maternal and infant mortality among the nonwhite and rural populations
2. Higher mortality rate for fetuses of teenagers, women over 35 years of age, women in lower socioeconomic groups
3. Continued steady rate of low-birth-weight infants born annually
4. Infant deaths due to congenital malformations, sudden infant death syndrome, low birth weight and its resulting sequelae

Terminology

Gravida—a woman who is or has been pregnant, without regard to pregnancy outcome

Nulligravida—a woman who is not now and never has been pregnant

Primigravida—a woman pregnant for the first time

Multigravida—a woman who has been pregnant several times

Para—refers to past pregnancies that have reached viability

Nullipara—a woman who has never completed a pregnancy to the period of viability. The woman may or may not have experienced an abortion.

Primipara—refers to a woman who had completed 1 pregnancy to the period of viability regardless of the number of infants delivered and regardless of the infant being live or stillborn.

Multipara—refers to a woman who has completed 2 or more pregnancies to the stage of viability

A woman pregnant for the first time is a primigravida and is described as Gravida 1, Para 0.

A woman who delivered one fetus to the period of viability and who is pregnant again is described as Gravida 2, Para 1.

A woman with 2 abortions and no viable children is Gravida 2, Para 0.

In some obstetric services, a woman's past obstetric history is summarized by a series of 4 digits, such as 5-1-2-5. The first digit refers to the number of term infants, the second to the number of premature infants, the third to the number of abortions, and the fourth to the number of children currently alive.

The Expectant Mother

Manifestations of Pregnancy

Presumptive Signs and Symptoms

1. Cessation of menses—pregnancy is suspected if more than 10 days have elapsed since the time of the expected onset. Suggestive of pregnancy in a woman with a previously spontaneous, cyclic, and predictable menses.
2. Breast changes

a. Breasts enlarge and become tender. Veins in breast become increasingly visible.
b. Nipples become larger and more pigmented.
c. Colostrum, a thin, milky fluid, may be expressed in the second half of pregnancy.
d. Montgomery glands, small elevations on the areolae, may appear.
3. Vaginal color changes (*Chadwick's sign*)—a bluish discoloration and congestion of vaginal wall.
4. Abdominal striae (*striae gravidarum*)—sometimes appear on the breasts, abdomen, and thighs because of the stretching, rupture, and atrophy of the deep connective tissue of the skin.
5. Nausea and vomiting (morning sickness)—occurs mainly in the morning, but may occur at any time of the day, lasting a few hours. Usually disappears spontaneously near the end of the 1st trimester.
6. *Quickening* (sensations of fetal movement in the abdomen)—occurs between 16th and 20th week after the onset of the last menses.
7. Frequency of urination
   a. Caused by pressure of the expanding uterus on the bladder
   b. Decreases when the uterus rises out of the pelvis
   c. Reappears when the fetal head engages in the pelvis at the end of pregnancy
8. Fatigue—characteristic of early pregnancy.

Probable Signs and Symptoms

1. Enlargement of abdomen—at about 12 weeks' gestation, the uterus can be felt through the abdominal wall, just above the symphysis.
2. Changes in shape, size, and consistency of the uterus
   a. Uterus enlarges, elongates, and decreases in thickness as pregnancy progresses.
   b. *Hegar's sign*—lower uterine segment softens 6–8 weeks after the onset of the last menstrual period.
3. Changes in cervix
   a. At 6–8 weeks of gestation, the cervix often becomes considerably softened.
   b. *Goodell's sign*—softening of the cervix.
   c. With inflammation and carcinoma during pregnancy, the cervix may remain firm.
4. Intermittent contractions of the uterus (*Braxton Hicks contractions*)—painless, palpable contractions occurring at irregular intervals, more frequently felt after 28 weeks
5. *Ballottement*—a sinking and rebounding of the fetus in its surrounding amniotic fluid in response to a sudden tap on the uterus (occurs near midpregnancy).
6. Outlining of the fetal body through the maternal abdomen by palpation in the second half of pregnancy.
7. Positive hormonal tests for pregnancy (test reactions produced by the presence of gonadotropin in maternal plasma and urine).

Positive Signs and Symptoms

1. Fetal heartbeat (separate and distinct from that of the mother)—usually heard between 16th and 20th week of gestation with a fetoscope.
2. Fetal movements felt by the examiner (after about 20 weeks' gestation).
3. X-ray visualization of the fetus (after 16 weeks' gestation).
4. Sonographic evidence (after 8 weeks' gestation).

Maternal Physiology During Pregnancy

Duration of Pregnancy

1. Averages 280 days or 40 weeks from the first day of the last normal menstrual period.
2. Duration may also be divided into three equal parts, or trimesters, of slightly more than 13 weeks or 3 calendar months each.
3. *Estimated date of confinement* (EDC) is calculated by adding 7 days to the date of the 1st day of the last menstrual period and counting back 3 months (*Nägele's rule*).
   a. For example, if a woman's last menstrual period began on 9/10/91, her EDC would be 9/10/91 plus 7 days = 9/17/91, minus 3 months = 6/17/91.

Changes in Reproductive Tract

A. Uterus

1. Enlargement during pregnancy involves stretching and marked hypertrophy of existing muscle cells.
2. In addition to an increase in the size of the uterine muscle cells, there is an increase in fibrous tissue, elastic tissue, blood vessels, and lymphatics.
3. Enlargement and thickening of the uterine wall is most marked in the fundus.
4. By the end of the 3rd month (12 weeks), the uterus is too large to be contained wholly within the pelvic cavity—it can now be palpated suprapubically.
5. As the uterus rises out of the pelvis it rotates somewhat to the right because of the presence of the rectosigmoid on the left side of the pelvis.
6. By 20 weeks' gestation, the fundus has reached the level of the umbilicus.
7. By 36 weeks, the fundus has reached the xiphoid.
8. During the last 3 weeks, the uterus descends slightly—because of fetal descent into pelvis. Walls of uterus become thinner.
9. Changes in contractility occur—from the 1st trimester, irregular painless contractions occur (Braxton Hicks contractions). In latter weeks of pregnancy, these contractions become stronger and more regular.
10. There is a progressive increase in uteroplacental blood flow during pregnancy.

B. Cervix

1. Pronounced softening and cyanosis—due to increased vascularity, edema, hypertrophy, and hyperplasia of the cervical glands.
2. Clot of very thick mucus obstructs the cervical canal (cervical plug).
3. Erosions of cervix, common during pregnancy, represent an extension of proliferating endocervical glands and columnar endocervical epithelium.

C. Ovaries

1. Ovulation ceases during pregnancy; maturation of new follicles is suspended.
2. One corpus luteum functions during early pregnancy (first 8 weeks), producing mainly progesterone.

D. Vagina and Outlet

1. Increased vascularity, hyperemia, and softening of connective tissue in skin and muscles of perineum and vulva.

2. Chadwick's sign noted—characteristic violet color due to increased vascularity and hyperemia.
3. Vaginal walls prepare for labor: mucosa increases in thickness, connective tissue loosens, and small-muscle cells hypertrophy.
4. Vaginal secretions increase; pH is 3.5–6—because of increased production of lactic acid from glycogen in the vaginal epithelium by *Lactobacillus acidophilus.* (Acid pH probably aids in keeping vagina relatively free of pathogenic bacteria.)

Changes in the Abdominal Wall

1. Striae gravidarum often develop—reddish, slightly depressed streaks in the skin of abdomen, breast, and thighs (become glistening silvery lines after pregnancy).
2. *Linea nigra* may form a line of dark pigment extending from the umbilicus down the midline to the symphysis. Often during the first pregnancy the *linea nigra* occurs at the height of the uterus. During subsequent pregnancies the entire line may be present early in gestation.
3. *Diastasis recti* may occur as muscles (rectus) separate. If severe, a part of the anterior uterine wall may be covered only by a layer of skin, fascia, and peritoneum.

Breast Changes

1. Are tender and tingle in early weeks of pregnancy.
2. Increase in size by 2nd month—hypertrophy of mammary alveoli.
3. Nipples become larger, more deeply pigmented, and more erectile early in pregnancy.
4. Colostrum may be expressed by 2nd trimester.
5. Areolae become broader and more deeply pigmented. The depth of pigmentation varies with the individual's complexion.
6. Scattered through the areola are a number of small elevations (glands of Montgomery), which are hypertrophic sebaceous glands.

Metabolic Changes

Are numerous and intensive—response to rapidly growing fetus and placenta.

A. **Weight Gain Averages:** 11–13 kg. (24–28 lb.)

Area	gm. (lb.)
Fetus	3400 (7.5)
Placenta	450 (1)
Amniotic fluid	900 (2)
Uterus	1100 (2.5)
Breast tissue	1400 (3)
Blood volume	1800 (4)
Maternal stores	1800–3600 (4–8)

B. **Water Metabolism**

1. Average woman retains 6.5 liters of extra water during pregnancy.
2. Fetus, placenta, and amniotic fluid total 3.5 liters.
3. The uterus, maternal blood volume, and breast tissue total 3 liters.
4. Many pregnant women experience edema of the legs and ankles at the end of the day.

C. **Protein Metabolism**

1. Fetus, uterus, and maternal blood are rich in protein rather than in fat or carbohydrates.

2. At term, fetus and placenta contain 500 gm. of protein or approximately half of the total protein increase of pregnancy.
3. Approximately 500 gm. more of protein are added to the uterus, breasts, and maternal blood in the form of hemoglobin and plasma proteins.

D. **Carbohydrate Metabolism**

1. Pregnancy, potentially, can initiate diabetes.
2. Diabetes mellitus may be aggravated by pregnancy.
3. Clinical diabetes appears in some women only during pregnancy.
4. During pregnancy, there is a "sparing" of glucose used by maternal tissues and a shunting of glucose to the placenta for use by the fetus.
5. Human placental lactogen (placental hormone) promotes lipolysis, increases plasma free fatty acids, and thereby provides alternative fuel sources for the mother.
6. Human placental lactogen, estrogen, progesterone, and an insulinase produced by the placenta oppose the action of insulin during pregnancy.

E. **Fat Metabolism**

Fats are more completely absorbed during pregnancy; plasma lipid levels increase during the second half of pregnancy.

F. **Iron Metabolism**

1. Iron requirements increase to 20–40 mg. daily. This often exceeds amounts available.
2. Total circulating red blood cells increase about 40%–50% during pregnancy; therefore, iron requirements are increased.
3. During the last half of pregnancy, iron is transferred to fetus and stored in the fetal liver. This store lasts 3–6 months.
4. Supplemental iron is valuable during the latter half of pregnancy and for several weeks after pregnancy or lactation.

Changes in Cardiovascular System

A. **Heart**

1. Diaphragm is progressively elevated during pregnancy; heart is displaced to the left and upward, with the apex moved laterally.
2. Heart sounds—an exaggerated splitting of the first heart sound, a loud, easily heard 3rd sound.
3. Heart murmurs—systolic murmurs are common and usually disappear following delivery.

B. **Circulation**

1. Cardiac volume increases by 40%–50% from the beginning to the end of pregnancy, causing slight hypertrophy of the heart and increased cardiac output.
2. In the supine position, the large uterus compresses the venous return from the lower half of the body to the heart. This may cause arterial hypotension, referred to as the *supine hypotensive syndrome.* Cardiac output increases when the woman turns from her back to her left side.
3. Femoral venous pressure increases—because of retardation of blood flow from lower extremities as a result of pressure of enlarged uterus on pelvic veins and inferior vena cava.
4. Pulse rate usually increases 10–15 beats/minute during pregnancy.

5. Blood pressure—during the first half of pregnancy there is a slight decrease in systolic and diastolic blood pressure. During the last half of pregnancy the blood pressure gradually returns to prepregnancy levels.

6. Increased cutaneous blood flow dissipates excess heat caused by increased metabolism of pregnancy.

C. Hematologic Changes

1. Total volume of circulating red blood cells increases; hemoglobin concentration at term averages 12 gm./dl.

2. Leukocyte count is elevated to 25,000 or more during labor—cause unknown; probably represents the reappearance in the circulation of leukocytes previously shunted out of active circulation.

3. Blood coagulation—fibrinogen levels increase 50%. Other clotting factors that increase include: factor VII (proconvertin), factor VIII (antihemophiliac globulin), factor IX (plasma thromboplastin component), and factor X (Stuart factor). Factor II (prothrombin) increases slightly, while factors XI (plasma thromboplastin antecedent) and XIII (fibrin-stabilizing factor) are decreased during pregnancy. There is no significant change in the number, appearance, or function of platelets.

Changes in Respiratory Tract

1. Hyperventilation occurs—increase in respiratory rate, tidal volume (45%), and minute volume (40%).

2. Increased total volume lowers blood PCO_2, causing mild respiratory alkalosis that is compensated for by lowering of the bicarbonate concentration.

3. Increased respiratory rate and reduced PCO_2 are probably induced by progesterone and estrogen to a lesser degree on the respiratory center.

4. Diaphragm is elevated during pregnancy—chiefly by the enlarging uterus.

5. Thoracic cage expands by means of flaring of the ribs—result of increased mobility of rib attachments.

Changes in Urinary Tract

1. Ureters become dilated and elongated during pregnancy because of mechanical pressure and perhaps the effects of progesterone. When the uterus rises out of the uterine cavity, it rests on the ureters, compressing them at the pelvic brim. Dilation is greater on the right side—left side is cushioned by the sigmoid colon.

2. Glomerular filtration rate (GFR) increases early in pregnancy, and the increase persists almost to term. Renal plasma flow (RPF) increases early in pregnancy and decreases to nonpregnant levels in the 3rd trimester. These changes may be due to placental lactogen.

3. Glucosuria may be evident—because of the increase in glomerular filtration without increase in tubular resorptive capacity for filtered glucose.

4. Proteinuria does not occur normally, except for slight amounts during or just after vigorous labor.

5. Toward the end of pregnancy, pressure of the presenting part impedes drainage of blood and lymph from the bladder base, often leaving the area edematous, easily traumatized, and more susceptible to infection.

Changes in Gastrointestinal Tract

1. Gums may become hyperemic and softened and may bleed easily.

2. A localized vascular swelling of the gums may appear—called *epulis of pregnancy.*

3. Stomach and intestines are displaced upward and laterally by the enlarging uterus. Heartburn is common, caused by reflux of acid secretions in the lower esophagus.

4. Tone and motility of gastrointestinal tract decrease, leading to prolongation of gastric emptying due to large amount of progesterone produced by the placenta.

5. Hemorrhoids are common because of elevated pressure in veins below the level of the large uterus and constipation.

6. Distention of the gallbladder is common along with a decrease in emptying time and thickening of bile.

7. Liver function tests yield significantly different results during pregnancy.

Changes in Endocrine System

1. *Pituitary gland* enlarges slightly.

2. *Thyroid* is moderately enlarged because of hyperplasia of glandular tissue and increased vascularity.
   a. Basal metabolic rate increases progressively during normal pregnancy (as much as 25%)—because of metabolic activity of fetus.
   b. Level of protein-bound iodine and thyroxin rises sharply and is maintained until after delivery—because of increased circulatory estrogen.

3. *Adrenal* secretions considerably increased—amounts of aldosterone increase as early as 15th week.

4. *Pancreas:* Because of the fetal glucose needs for growth, there are alterations in maternal insulin production and usage.
   a. Estrogen, progesterone, cortisol, and hPL decrease maternal utilization of glucose.
   b. Cortisol also increases maternal insulin production.
   c. Insulinase, an enzyme produced by the placenta, deactivates maternal insulin.
   d. These changes result in an increased need for insulin, and the islets of Langerhans increase their production of insulin.

Changes in Integumentary System

1. Pigmentary changes occur because of melanocyte-stimulating hormone, the level of which is elevated from the 2nd month of pregnancy until term.

2. Striae gravidarum appear in later months of pregnancy as reddish, slightly depressed streaks in the skin of the abdomen and occasionally over the breasts and thighs.

3. A brownish black line of pigment is often formed in the midline of the abdominal skin—known as *linea nigra.*

4. Brownish patches of pigment may form on the face—known as *chloasma* or "mask of pregnancy."

5. Angiomas (vascular spiders), minute red elevations commonly on the skin of the face, neck, upper chest, and arms, may develop.

6. Reddening of the palms (*palmar erythema*) may also occur.

Changes in Musculoskeletal System

1. The increasing mobility of sacroiliac, sacrococcygeal, and pelvic joints during pregnancy is a result of hormonal changes.

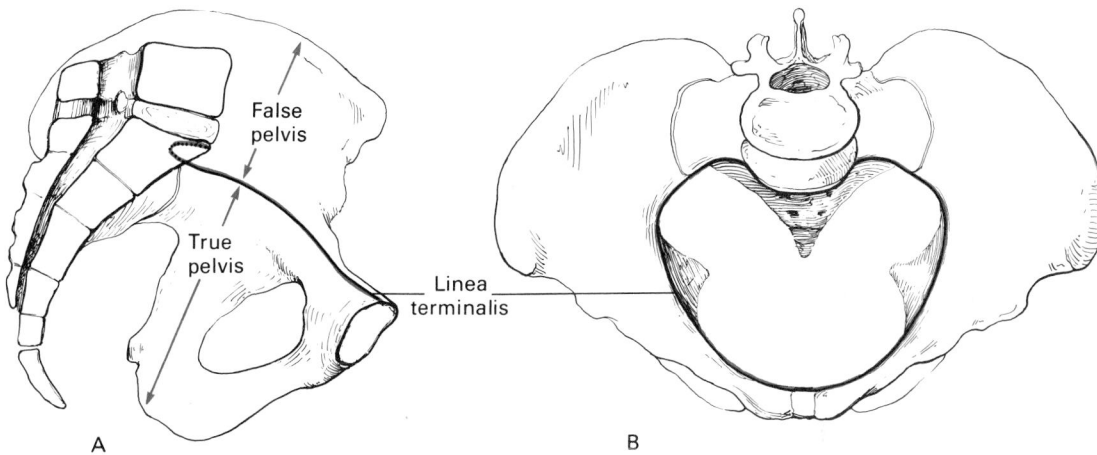

Figure 39-1. *(A) Side view of the true and false pelvis. (B) Front view showing linea terminalis (pelvic brim).*

2. This mobility contributes to alteration of maternal posture and to back pain.
3. Late in pregnancy, aching, numbness, and weakness in the upper extremities may occur because of lordosis, which ultimately produces traction on the ulnar and median nerves.
4. Separation of the rectus muscles due to pressure of the growing uterus creates a diastasis recti. If this is severe, a portion of the anterior uterine wall is covered by only a layer of skin, fascia, and peritoneum.

Pelvis

A. Bones of the Pelvis

Pelvis is composed of 4 bones:
1. Two innominate bones (hip bones) form sides and front
2. Sacrum and coccyx form the back

Pelvic bones are held together by fibrocartilage of the symphysis pubis and several ligaments.

B. Pelvis Is Divided Into Two Parts—false pelvis and true pelvis.

1. False pelvis—lies above an imaginary line called the *linea terminalis* (Fig. 39-1). Function of the false pelvis is to support the enlarged uterus.
2. True pelvis lies below the pelvic brim or linea terminalis; it is the bony canal through which the infant must pass. It is divided into three parts: the inlet, the midpelvis, and the outlet.

C. Inlet

1. Upper boundary of true pelvis—bounded by upper margin of symphysis pubis in front, linea terminalis on sides, and sacral promontory (1st sacral vertebra) in back.
2. Largest diameter of inlet is transverse (Fig. 39-2).
3. Smallest diameter of inlet is anteroposterior (AP).
4. AP diameter is most important diameter of inlet: measured clinically by *diagonal conjugate*—distance from lower margin of symphysis to the sacral promontory (usually 12.5 cm.) (Fig. 39-3).
5. *Obstetric conjugate*—distance between inner surface of symphysis and sacral promontory measured by subtracting 1.5–2 cm. (thickness of symphysis) from the diagonal conjugate. It is usually 11 cm.

D. Midpelvis

1. Bounded by inlet above and outlet below—the true bony cavity.
2. Diameters cannot be measured clinically.
3. Clinical evaluation of adequacy is made by noting the ischial spines. Prominent spines that protrude into the cavity indicate a contracted midpelvic space.

E. Outlet

1. Lowest boundary of the true pelvis.
2. Bounded by lower margin of symphysis in front, ischial tuberosities on sides, tip of sacrum posteriorly.
3. Most important diameter clinically is distance between the tuberosities (usually 9 cm.).

F. Pelvic Shapes

There are four main types of pelvic shapes (Fig. 39-4):
1. Gynecoid (normal female pelvis)
2. Android
3. Anthropoid
4. Platypelloid

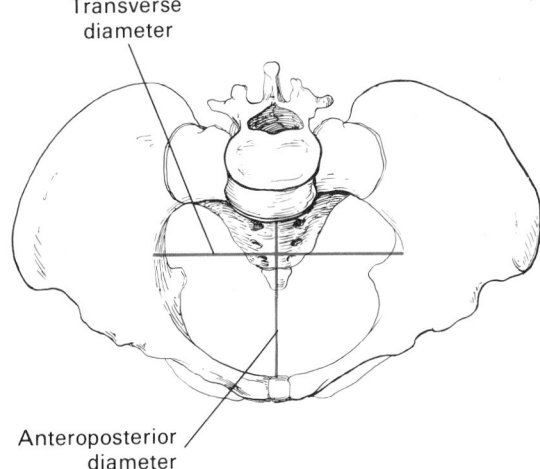

Figure 39-2. *Inlet of normal female pelvis showing transverse and anteroposterior diameters.*

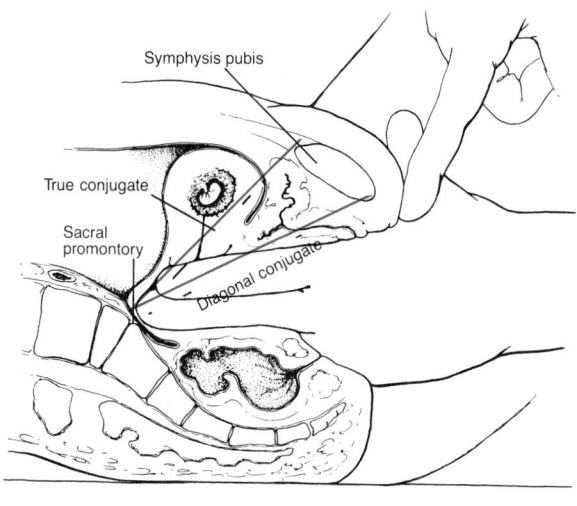

Figure 39-3. *Method of obtaining diagonal conjugate diameter.*

Assessment: Health History

A. Age

1. Adolescents have an increased incidence of anemia, pregnancy-induced hypertension, preterm labor, small-for-gestational-age infants, cephalopelvic disproportion, and dystocia.
2. Older women have an increased incidence of hypertension, pregnancies complicated by underlying medical problems, and infants with genetic abnormalities.

B. Family History

Congenital disorders; hereditary diseases; multiple pregnancies; diabetes; heart disease; hypertension; mental retardation.

C. Woman's Medical History

1. Childhood diseases, especially rubella
2. Major illnesses, surgery; blood transfusions
3. Drug, food, and environmental sensitivities
4. Urinary infections; heart disease; diabetes, hypertension, endocrine disorders; anemias
5. Use of oral or other contraceptives
6. History of sexually transmitted diseases
7. Menstrual history (menarche; length and regularity of menstrual cycle)
8. Use of medications, other drugs, alcohol, tobacco, and caffeine

D. Woman's Past Obstetric History

1. Problems of infertility, data of previous pregnancies and deliveries—dates; infant weights; length of labors; types of deliveries; multiple births; abortions; maternal, fetal, and neonatal complications.
2. Woman's perception of past pregnancy, labor, and delivery for herself and impact on her family.

E. Woman's Present Obstetric History

1. Gravidity; parity
2. Date of last menstrual period (LMP)
3. Estimated date of birth—expected date of confinement (EDC) is calculated by counting back 3 calendar months from the first day of the last menstrual period and adding 7 days.

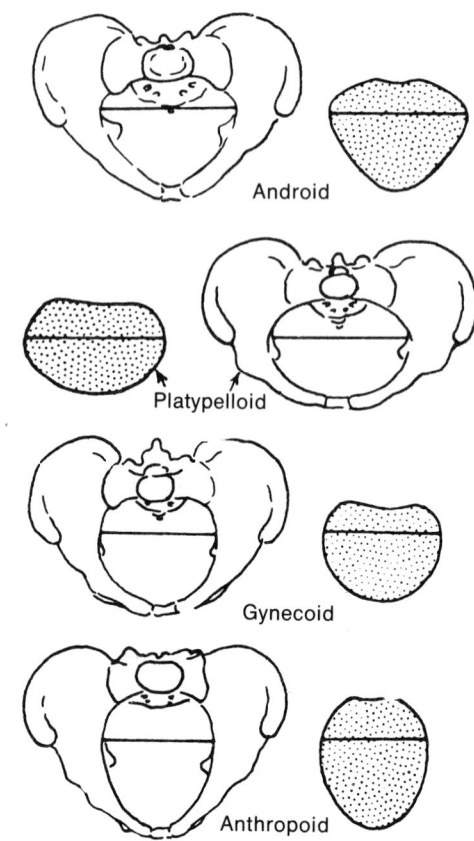

Figure 39-4. *The four types of female pelvis. Android—male-type pelvis. Platypelloid—broad pelvis with shortened anteroposterior diameter and flattened, oval, transverse shape. Gynecoid—typical female pelvis in which inlet is round instead of oval. Anthropoid—pelvis in which anteroposterior diameter is equal to or greater than the transverse diameter.*

4. Signs and symptoms of pregnancy—amenorrhea, breast changes, nausea and vomiting, fetal movement, fatigue, urinary frequency, skin pigmentary changes. For possible presumptive and positive signs of pregnancy, see pages 965–966. What are her expectations for her present pregnancy, labor, and delivery?
5. Rest and sleep patterns—length, quality, and regularity of rest and sleep.
6. Activity and employment—exercise patterns, type and hours of employment; plans for continued employment.
7. Sexual activity—sexual satisfaction; frequency and positions during intercourse; alternative practices used to achieve sexual satisfaction.
8. Diet history—weight gain; eating patterns (times and frequency of eating daily); social or cultural dietary habits; number of servings of food from 5 food groups (Table 39-1); calories, protein, vitamins, and minerals consumed daily.
9. Psychosocial status—emotional changes she is experiencing; woman's and family's reactions to present pregnancy; support system—family's and friends' willingness to provide support; woman's present coping with life-style changes caused by the pregnancy.

Table 39-1. *Recommended Dietary Allowances of Selected Nutrients for Pregnancy and Lactation*

Nutrient	11–14 Years (101 lb.—62 in.)	15–18 Years (120 lb.—64 in.)	19–22 Years (120 lb.—64 in.)	23–50 Years (120 lb.—64 in.)	Added for Pregnancy	Added for Lactation
Protein (gm.)	46	46	44	44	+30	+20
Fat-soluble vitamins						
Vitamin A (μg. RE)	800	800	800	800	+200	+400
Vitamin D (μg.)	10	10	7.5	5	+5	+5
Vitamin E (mg. αTE)	8	8	8	8	+2	+3
Water-soluble vitamins						
Vitamin C (mg.)	50	60	60	60	+20	+40
Thiamine (mg.)	1.1	1.1	1.1	1.0	+0.4	+0.5
Riboflavin (mg.)	1.3	1.3	1.3	1.2	+0.3	+0.5
Niacin mg NE	15	14	14	13	+2	+5
Vitamin B_6 (mg.)	1.8	2.0	2.0	2.0	+0.6	+0.5
Folacin (μg.)	400	400	400	400	+400	+100
Vitamin B_{12} (μg.)	3.0	3.0	3.0	3.0	+1.0	+1.0
Minerals						
Calcium (mg.)	1200	1200	800	800	+400	+400
Phosphorus (mg.)	1200	1200	800	800	+400	+400
Magnesium (mg.)	300	300	300	300	+150	+150
Iron (mg.)	18	18	18	18	30 to 60 mg. of supplemental iron is recommended	
Zinc (mg.)	15	15	15	15	+5	+10
Iodine (μg.)	150	150	150	150	+25	+50

(From Food and Nutrition Board, National Academy of Sciences—National Research Council.)

Laboratory Data

A. Urinalysis

1. Urine is tested for glucose and protein.
2. Glucose may be present in small amounts because the GFR is increased without the same increase in kidney tubular reabsorption.
3. Protein in the urine should be reported because it may be a sign of a hypertensive disorder of pregnancy or renal problems.
4. If the urine is cloudy and bacteria or leukocytes are present, a urine culture is done.

B. Blood

1. Determination of hematocrit and hemoglobin levels, and description of the morphology of the red blood cells are done to find evidence of anemias such as sickle cell or Mediterranean anemia.
2. Hemoglobin levels average 12 gm./dl.

C. Biochemical Determinations

Usually only glucose and urea nitrogen done; however, women with renal disorders may require estimation of total protein with albumin and globulin ratios.

D. Serologic Tests

1. Tests for syphilis (STS or VDRL) are usually done twice during pregnancy, on initial visit and at the beginning of the 3rd trimester.
2. Rubella titer—immunity can be measured by a positive hemagglutination inhibition test.
3. Blood type, Rh factor, and antibody screen—if the woman is found to be Rh negative or have a positive antibody screen, her partner is screened and a maternal antibody titer is drawn as indicated.

E. Cultures

1. *Gonorrhea*—cervical cultures are usually done at the initial visit and when symptoms are present.
2. *Herpes*—all possible lesions are cultured, and the cervix is cultured weekly beginning 4–8 weeks prior to delivery.
3. *Chlamydia*—done at the initial visit and when symptoms are present.

F. Alpha–Fetoprotein (AFP)

High maternal levels after 18 weeks may indicate a neural tube defect (NTD).

G. Human Immunodeficiency Virus (HIV)—screen is done on high-risk women.

Physical Assessment

A. General Approach

1. Ask the woman to empty her bladder before the examination so that during vaginal examination her uterus and pelvic organs may be readily palpated.
2. Evaluate the woman's weight gain and blood pressure.
3. Examination of eyes, ears, and nose—nasal congestion during pregnancy may occur as a result of peripheral vasodilation.
4. Examination of the mouth, teeth, throat, and thyroid—gums may be hyperemic and softened because of increased progesterone.
5. Inspection of breasts and nipples—breasts may be enlarged and tender; nipple and areolar pigment may be darkened.
6. Auscultation of heart
7. Auscultation and percussion of the lungs

B. Abdominal Examination

1. Examination for scars or striations, diastasis (separation of the rectus muscle), or umbilical hernia.
2. Palpation of the abdomen for height of the fundus (palpable after 13 weeks of pregnancy); measurement recorded and used as guideline for subsequent calculations (Fig. 39-5).
3. Palpation of the abdomen for fetal outline and position—3rd trimester (see Fig. 40-5, p. 991).

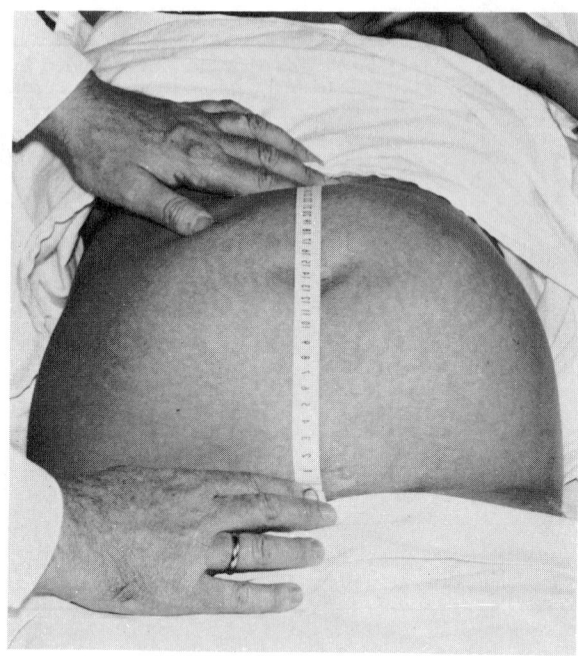

Figure 39-5. *Measuring fundus-to-symphysis distance by Mc-Donald's method. (From Danforth DN and Scott JR [eds]. Obstetrics and Gynecology. 5th ed. Philadelphia, JB Lippincott, 1986)*

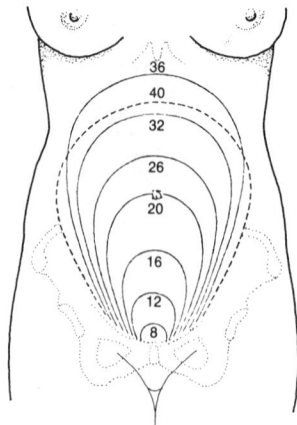

Figure 39-6. *Height of fundus. (From Danforth DN [ed]. Obstetrics and Gynecology. 5th ed. Philadelphia, JB Lippincott, 1986)*

4. Check of fetal heart tone (FHT)—FHTs are audible with a doptone after 12–13 weeks and at 18 weeks with a fetoscope.
5. Fetal position, presentation, and FHTs—are recorded.

C. Pelvic Examination

1. The woman is placed in lithotomy position.
2. Inspection of external genitalia.
3. Vaginal examination—done to rule out abnormalities of the birth canal and to obtain cytologic smear (Papanicolaou and, if indicated, smears for gonorrhea, vaginal trichomoniasis, candidiasis, herpes, and chlamydia).
4. Examination of the cervix for position, size, mobility, and consistency. Cervix is softened and bluish (increased vascularity) during pregnancy.
5. Identification of the ovaries (size, shape, and position).
6. Rectovaginal exploration to identify hemorrhoids, fissures, herniation, or masses.
7. Evaluation of pelvic inlet—anteroposterior diameter by measuring the diagonal conjugate (see Fig. 39-3).
8. Evaluation of midpelvis—prominence of the ischial spines.
9. Evaluation of pelvic outlet—distance between ischial tuberosities and mobility of coccyx.

Subsequent Prenatal Assessments

Monthly visits are made for the first 7 months, then every 2 weeks, and weekly during the last month, providing that the woman's pregnancy is healthy.

1. Uterine growth and estimated fetal growth (Fig. 39-6).
   a. Fundus at symphysis pubis = 12 weeks' gestation
   b. Fundus at umbilicus = 20 weeks' gestation
   c. Fundus 28 cm. from top of symphysis pubis = 28 weeks' gestation
   d. Fundus at lower border of rib cage = 36 weeks' gestation
   e. Uterus becomes globular and drops = 40 weeks' gestation
2. A greater fundal height suggests:
   a. Multiple pregnancy
   b. Miscalculated due date
   c. Polyhydramnios (excessive amniotic fluid)
   d. Hydatidiform mole (degeneration of villi into grapelike clusters; fetus does not usually develop)
3. A lesser fundal height suggests:
   a. Intrauterine fetal growth retardation
   b. Error in estimating gestation
   c. Fetal or amniotic fluid abnormalities
   d. Intrauterine fetal death
4. Fetal heart tones—palpate abdomen for fetal position
   a. Normal—120–160 beats/minute
5. Weight—major increase in weight occurs during 2nd half of pregnancy; usually between 0.22 kg. (0.5 lb.)/week and 0.44 kg. (1 lb.)/week. Greater weight gain may indicate fluid retention and hypertensive disorder.
6. Blood pressure—should remain near woman's normal baseline.
7. Hemoglobin—rechecked at beginning of the 3rd trimester and as indicated.
8. Culture smears for gonorrhea, chlamydia, and herpes, as indicated.
9. Urinalysis—for protein, glucose, blood, and nitrates.
10. Edema—check the lower legs, face, and hands.
11. Discomforts of pregnancy—fatigue, heartburn, hemorrhoids, constipation, and backache.
12. Evaluate eating and sleeping patterns, general adjustment and coping with the pregnancy.
13. Evaluate concerns of the woman and her family.
14. Evaluate preparation for labor, delivery, and parenting.
15. Unusual signs that should be reported at once
    a. Visual disturbances, blurring, spots or double vision
    b. Vaginal bleeding, new or old blood
    c. Edema of the face, fingers, or sacrum
    d. Headaches: frequent, severe, or continuous.
    e. Persistent vomiting or diarrhea
    f. Fluid discharge from the vagina
    g. Any abnormal or severe abdominal pain
    h. Chilling, fever, or burning on urination

i. Epigastric pain (severe stomachache)
j. Muscular irritability or convulsions

Patient Problems and Nursing Diagnoses

1. Pain (backache, hemorrhoids) related to body changes of pregnancy
2. Urinary elimination, altered patterns, (frequency) related to increased pressure from uterus
3. Bowel elimination, altered, constipation, related to physiologic changes of pregnancy
4. Knowledge deficit of nutritional needs, physical changes of pregnancy, psychosocial changes of pregnancy—related to lack of previous exposure or education.
5. Anxiety/fear related to lack of knowledge of labor process and infant care
6. Altered family process related to extra demands of pregnancy.

Nursing Interventions: Health Teaching

A. Dealing With Physical, Psychosocial, and Life-style Changes

1. Teach the woman reasons for fatigue and have her plan a schedule for adequate rest.
   a. Fatigue in the 1st trimester is due to increased progesterone and its effects on the sleep center.
   b. Fatigue in the last trimester is due mainly to carrying increased weight of the pregnancy.
   c. About 8 hours of rest is needed at night.
   d. Inability to sleep may be due to excessive fatigue during day.
   e. In the latter months of pregnancy, sleeping on the side with a small pillow under the abdomen may enhance comfort.
   f. Frequent 15–30-minute rest periods during the day are important to avoid overfatigue.
   g. Whenever possible, the woman should work while sitting with her legs elevated.
   h. The woman should avoid standing for prolonged periods of time, especially during the 3rd trimester.
   i. To promote placental perfusion, the woman should not lay flat on her back—the left lateral position provides the best placental perfusion.
2. Help the woman plan for adequate exercise.
   a. In general, exercise during pregnancy should be in keeping with the woman's prepregnancy pattern and type of exercise.
   b. Activities or sports that have a risk of bodily harm (skiing, snowmobiling, horseback riding) should be avoided.
   c. During pregnancy, endurance during exercise may be decreased.
   d. Exercise classes for pregnant women that concentrate on toning and stretching have resulted in enhanced physical condition, increased self-esteem, and greater social support as a result of being in the exercise group.
3. Teach the woman the importance of good nutrition for herself and her fetus; have her plan good daily nutrition.
   a. Pregnancy increases the need for protein, vitamins A, D, E, and B complex, calcium, phosphorus, and iron (see Table 39-1).
   b. Review Table 39-2 with the mother, emphasizing the important function of these nutrients for her body and the fetus during pregnancy.
   c. Daily calorie requirements are approximately 300 calories in addition to the prepregnancy maintenance calories.
   d. According to her life-style, culture, income, and eating patterns, have the woman plan daily menus that include the following:
      (1) 4 servings of protein foods
      (2) 4 servings of milk or milk products
      (3) 4 servings of grain products
      (4) 2 servings of vitamin C-rich fruits and vegetables
      (5) 2 servings of leafy green vegetables
      (6) 1 serving of other fruits and vegetables
   e. Average weight gain in pregnancy is 24 lb.: approximately 2 lb. in 1st trimester, 11 lbs. in 2nd trimester, and 11 lbs. in 3rd trimester.
   f. Women in their teens need additional nutrients to meet their own growth needs as well as those imposed by pregnancy.
   g. Carefully evaluate the dietary intake of overweight or underweight women, as well as those of vegetarian women.
   h. Caffeine intake should be limited to about 3 cups of coffee or its caffeine equivalent daily. Research on the association of caffeine intake and birth defects is inconclusive to date.
   i. Alcohol intake should be limited; no safe level of alcohol intake has been established; The March of Dimes recommends eliminating alcohol during pregnancy.
   j. Smoking should be eliminated or severely reduced during pregnancy; risk of spontaneous abortion, fetal death, birth of a low-birth-weight infant, and neonatal death increases directly with increasing levels of maternal smoking during pregnancy.
4. Discuss methods of achieving sexual satisfaction during pregnancy.
   a. There are no contraindications to intercourse or masturbation to orgasm, provided the woman's membranes are intact, there is no vaginal bleeding, and she has no current problems or history of premature labor.
   b. Sexual activity may change in frequency because of maternal fatigue, physical discomfort, loss of interest, or difficulty finding comfortable positions for intercourse. Some women experience heightened sexual activity during the second trimester.
   c. The woman may find deep penile penetration uncomfortable.
   d. Female superior or side-lying positions are often more comfortable in the latter half of pregnancy.
5. Assist the woman in her employment planning.
   a. Generally there is no reason to stop working unless complications arise or there are hazards to the fetus in the work place.
   b. It is desirable to avoid severe physical strain and get adequate periods of rest.
   c. Review use of good body mechanics.
   d. Avoid toxic substances such as chlorinated hydrocarbons, lead, benzene, toluene, pesticides, mercury, and radioactive substances.
   e. Investigate policy on pregnancy and childbirth furloughs and benefits.
   f. Begin childcare planning if employment after birth is planned.

Table 39-2. *Summary of Major Functions and Sources of Nutrients*

	Function	Source	

Protein	Growth of fetus and accessory tissues
	Production of breast milk
		Animal protein
		  Meat
		  Fish
		  Poultry
		  Eggs
		  Milk
		  Cheese
			Vegetable protein
			  Dried beans
			  Dried peas
			  Lentils
			  Nuts
			  Peanut butter

Iron	Maintains hemoglobin level of mother
	Maintains mother's stores of iron
	Provides iron for fetal development
	Furnishes infant with iron stores needed for blood formation during neonatal period before food sources of iron are added to diet
		Good sources
		  Pork liver
		  Kidney
		  Beef liver
		  Oysters
		  Clams
		  Canned dried beans
		  Prune juice
		  Liverwurst
		  Heart
		  Lean pork
		  Lean beef
		  Raisins
		  Cooked dried beans
		  Cooked dried peaches
		  Cooked dried apricots
		  Cooked dried prunes
		  Canned green peas
			Fair sources
			  Enriched pastas
			  Spinach
			  Canned mackerel
			  Enriched white bread
			  Kale
			  Mustard greens
			  Whole wheat bread
			  Canned string beans
			  Eggs
			  Brussels sprouts
			  Broccoli

Calcium	Skeletal structures of the fetus
	Production of breast milk
	Blood coagulation, neuromuscular irritability, and muscle contractility
		Good sources
		  Skim milk
		  Buttermilk
		  Whole milk
		  Nonfat dry milk
		  Cheese
		  Ice milk
		  Ice cream
			Fair sources
			  Dark-green leafy vegetables
			  Dried beans
			  Broccoli
			  Cottage cheese
			  Canned fish—including bones
			  Oranges

Vitamin A	Tooth formation
	Normal bone growth
	Healthy skin
	Vision—light/dark adaptation
		Vitamin A
		  Butter
		  Egg yolk
		  Fortified margarine
		  Kidney
		  Liver
		  Whole milk
		  Cream
			Carotenes
			  Dark-green and deep-yellow vegetables and a few fruits
			  Apricots
			  Broccoli
			  Cantaloupe
			  Carrots
			  Chard
			  Collards
			  Kale
			  Mustard greens
			  Persimmons
			  Spinach
			  Pumpkin
			  Sweet potatoes
			  Turnip greens
			  Winter squash

Riboflavin	Functions in number of enzyme systems in tissue respiration
	Metabolism of amino acids and carbohydrates
		Good sources
		  Heart
		  Kidney
		  Liver
		  Milk
		  Ice milk
			Fair sources
			  Broccoli
			  Cheese
			  Dark-green leafy vegetables
			  Eggs
			  Ice cream
			  Lean meat
			  Poultry

Thiamine	Maintains normal appetite and digestion
	Maintains health of nervous system
	Completion of carbohydrates
		Good sources
		  Whole grain and enriched bread
		  Whole grain and enriched cereals
		  Dried peas
		  Dried beans
		  Oranges
		  Liver
		  Heart
		  Kidney
		  Lean pork
		  Nuts
		  Potatoes
		  Peas
		  Wheat germ
			Fair sources
			  Eggs
			  Fish
			  Meat
			  Poultry
			  Milk
			  Many vegetables

(continued)

Table 39-2. *Summary of Major Functions and Sources of Nutrients (continued)*

	Function	Source	

Niacin	Helps translate sources of energy into usable form	Good sources
		  Fish
		  Heart
		  Lean meat
		  Liver
		  Peanuts
		  Peanut butter
		  Poultry
			Fair sources
			  Milk
			  Potatoes
			  Whole grain and enriched bread
			  Whole grain and enriched cereal

Ascorbic acid	Production of intercellular substances necessary for the development and maintenance of normal connective tissue in bones, cartilage, and muscles
	Improves health of bones and teeth
	Increases absorption of iron
		Good sources
		  Citrus fruits or juice
		  Broccoli
		  Brussels sprouts
		  Cantaloupe
		  Greens—collards, mustard, turnip
		  Peppers
			Fair sources
			  Asparagus
			  Cabbage, raw
			  Cauliflower
			  Chile, fresh or canned
			  Kale
			  Liver
			  Other melons
			  Potatoes or sweet potatoes in jackets
			  Spinach
			  Tomatoes or prunes

Vitamin D	Promotes absorption and retention of calcium and phosphorus necessary for growth and formation of bones and teeth	Good sources
		  Butter
		  Egg yolk
		  Fish oils
		  Liver
		  Milk fortified with vitamin D
		  Other foods may contain added
		    vitamin D—check labels	

(Cross AT and Walsh HE. Prenatal diet counseling. J Reproductive Med)

B. Minimizing Common Discomforts of Pregnancy

1. Morning sickness—nausea, sometimes accompanied by vomiting, occurs frequently in the morning but may occur at any time.
   a. Cause unknown—hormonal changes believed to be a causative factor. Duration of morning sickness mirrors duration of elevated human chorionic gonadotropin (HCG) production. Emotional upsets and hypoglycemia also seen as contributing factors; self-limited to 1st trimester.
   b. Eating dry carbohydrates such as toast or crackers often helps.
   c. Eating frequent, small meals is helpful.
   d. Avoid hard-to-digest, greasy, pungent foods and odors.
2. Urinary frequency
   a. Cause—pressure of enlarging uterus on bladder
   b. Course—usually subsides spontaneously by the end of the 1st trimester when the uterus rises into the abdominal cavity and returns in the last weeks of pregnancy when the vertex drops into the pelvic cavity.
3. Heartburn
   a. Cause—pressure on the stomach from enlarged uterus and decreased gastric motility result in a reflux of stomach contents in the lower esophagus.
   b. Smaller, more frequent meals of foods easy to digest are helpful.
   c. Local antacids such as aluminum hydroxide gels soothe the mucosa and neutralize acid reflux.
   d. Avoid sodium bicarbonate because it results in absorption of excessive sodium and fluid retention.
4. Backache
   a. Cause—pregnant woman's center of gravity changes; to compensate, she walks with head and shoulders backward, chest forward. This posture may produce lordosis and backache. Late in pregnancy, relaxation of pelvic joints exaggerates the problem.
   b. Standing tall, good posture, avoiding fatigue, and good body mechanics help.
   c. Wear comfortable, low-heeled shoes with good arch supports.
   d. Maternity girdle may help.
   e. Pelvic rocking exercises can provide relief.
5. Constipation
   a. Cause—decreased intestinal peristalsis due to pressure of gravid uterus and effects of progesterone.
   b. Additional fluid and dietary roughage will help.
   c. Adequate daily exercise is an aid.
   d. Establish regular patterns of elimination.
   e. If a laxative is necessary, prune juice, bulk-forming agents, stool softeners, or milk of magnesia are usually prescribed. Mineral oil interferes with absorption of fat-soluble vitamins.
6. Respiratory discomfort
   a. Cause—pressure of enlarged uterus on diaphragm.
   b. Spontaneous relief occurs with "lightening" (sensation of decreased abdominal distention caused by descent of fetus into pelvis) or with the birth of the baby.
   c. Provide relief by assuming semi-Fowler's position arranged with pillow.
   d. Some relief obtained with good posture and standing tall.
   e. Eating small, frequent meals prevents increased pressure from full stomach.
7. Varicose veins—may affect lower extremities, vulva, pelvis, and anus.
   a. Cause—hereditary predisposition, pressure of gravid uterus on large veins, prolonged standing may be contributing factors.

b. Rest frequently by sitting or lying with legs elevated.
c. For leg varicosities, wear support hose and avoid constricting clothing.
d. For vulvar varicosities, rest periodically with small pillow under buttocks to elevate pelvis.
e. For anal varicosities (hemorrhoids)
   (1) Avoid constipation
   (2) Apply cold compresses with or without witch hazel
   (3) Avoid standing or sitting for prolonged periods—rest lying down
f. Varicosities are totally or greatly resolved after delivery.

8. Leg cramps ("charley horse")
   a. Cause unknown—fatigue, impaired circulation because of gravid uterus, impaired calcium absorption.
   b. Frequent rest periods with legs elevated may be helpful.
   c. Adequate calcium intake may decrease the incidence.
   d. For immediate relief, dorsiflex the foot, push toes upward while applying pressure to the knee to straighten the leg.

9. Leg and ankle edema
   a. Cause—pressure of gravid uterus impeding venous and lymphatic return.
   b. Rest frequently with legs elevated in a side-lying position.
   c. Combined with facial and finger edema, may be a sign of hypertensive disorder of pregnancy.

10. Vaginal discharge
    a. Increased vaginal discharge is common in pregnancy. Increased hygiene (washing) is important.
    b. Green, yellow, foul-smelling, or bloody discharge may indicate infection or other complication—see midwife or physician.

11. Tender breasts and nipple irritation
    a. Wear well-fitting supporting brassiere.
    b. Wash breasts and nipples with water only.
    c. Nipple rolling 3 times a day (between thumb and forefingers) and drying nipples with a rough towel daily may toughen nipples for breastfeeding.
    d. Lanolin creams applied to nipples help minimize irritations from colostrum and clothing.

C. Reducing Anxiety and Preparing for Upcoming Labor and Delivery

1. Have the woman/couple discuss knowledge, perception, and expectations of labor and birth process.
   a. Have the woman/couple write a birth plan covering what they would like their birth experience to be.
2. Provide information on childbirth education, sibling education, and breast-feeding classes, and encourage them to attend.
3. Have the woman/couple tour labor and delivery area.
4. Discuss value of breathing exercises as another tool for coping with labor and encourage their practice and use.
5. Have the woman identify when to come to the birthing center or hospital (primigravida—when contractions are 5–10 minutes apart; multigravida—when contractions have established a regular pattern).
6. The woman also knows signs of complications during pregnancy (see p. 972).

D. Preparing for Parenthood

1. Have the woman/couple discuss perceptions and expectations of new parenthood.
   a. Perceptions of their "idealized child"
   b. Perceptions and expectations of infant's sleeping, eating, activity, and response patterns
   c. Expectations of returning to work and child-care arrangements when appropriate; babysitters for evenings or hours out.
2. Physical preparations for the newborn—crib or other place to sleep, clothing, blankets, bathing equipment, feeding equipment
3. Help the woman/couple plan for time for themselves and each other apart from the newborn.

Expected Outcomes

1. Understands reason for fatigue, establishes and follows a schedule for adequate rest, and avoids tiring activities such as standing for long periods
2. Engages in prescribed program of exercise
3. Understands the essentials of good nutrition during pregnancy; follows adequate diet for self and fetus, including proper intake of protein, milk products, grains, vegetables, and fruits
4. Avoids potentially harmful substances such as alcohol, cigarettes, and excessive caffeine
5. Is aware of impact of pregnancy on sexual functioning and becomes informed of methods of achieving sexual satisfaction
6. Learns and practices ways of dealing with physical discomforts of pregnancy—morning sickness, urinary frequency, backache, constipation, varicosities, leg cramps, edema, breast tenderness
7. Couple prepares for upcoming labor and delivery by discussing expectation of labor and delivery, attending childbirth classes, and preparing for life-style changes to result from presence of new baby in the home

Psychosocial Adaptation of Pregnancy

A. Rubin's Framework for Maternal Role Assumption

1. Attainment of motherhood role occurs with each pregnancy.
2. Involves a series of cognitive operations.
   a. Replication—involves mimicry of role play in which the woman begins modeling her behavior and trying on the maternal role.
   b. Fantasy—dreaming of how the motherhood role will be.
   c. Dedifferentiation—examination and evaluation of the goodness of fit with her current self-image.
3. Maternal task
   a. Safe passage—the mother seeks to ensure a safe passage for her fetus and self throughout her pregnancy. During the 1st trimester the focus is on self-safety, in the 3rd trimester the safety of the fetus is inseparable from self-safety.
   b. Acceptance by other—acceptance of this child by each family member.
   c. Binding-in to the child—maternal perception of the child as a real person.
   d. Giving of oneself—the most complex task, in which the mother is learning to give to the unborn child and placing the unborn child's need in relation to her own needs.

B. Ledermans's Conceptual Framework for Maternal Role Assumption

Seven personality dimensions—these are seven areas that change as the woman changes from a woman-without-child to a woman-with-child.

1. Acceptance and adaptation to pregnancy
2. Identification with motherhood role
3. Relationship to own mother
4. Relationship to husband
5. Preparation for labor
6. Fear of loss of control in labor
7. Fear of loss of self-esteem

The Fetus

In the past, methods used to determine how well the fetus was growing and maturing consisted of evaluating uterine growth and listening to fetal heart sounds. During the last 25 years, advances in knowledge and technology have provided newer methods for assessing fetal well-being, including ultrasound, amniocentesis, additional laboratory tests, and fetal monitoring. These advances have made possible the diagnosis of abnormalities and multiple pregnancies, and interventions such as intrauterine blood transfusions and fetal surgery.

Fetal Growth and Development (Fig. 39-7)

A. 1st Lunar Month (fertilization–2 weeks of embryonic growth)

1. Implantation is complete.
2. Primary chorionic villi forming.
3. Embryo develops into two cell layers (bilaminar embryonic disc).
4. Amniotic cavity appears.

B. 2nd Lunar Month (3–6 weeks of embryonic growth)

1. At the end of 6 weeks of growth, the embryo is approximately 12 mm. long.
2. Arm and leg buds are visible; arm buds are more developed with finger ridges beginning to appear.
3. Rudiments of the eyes, ears, and nose appear.
4. Lung buds are developing.
5. Primitive intestinal tract is developing.
6. Primitive cardiovascular system is functioning.
7. Neural tube, which forms the brain and spinal cord, closes by the 4th week.

C. 3rd Lunar Month (7–10 weeks of growth)

1. At the end of 10 weeks of growth, the fetus is 61 mm. from crown to rump and weighs 14 gm.
2. The middle of this period (8 weeks) marks the end of the embryonic period and the beginning of the fetal period.
3. Appearance of external genitalia.
4. By the middle of this month, all major organ systems have formed.
5. The membrane over the anus has broken down.
6. The heart has formed 4 chambers (by 7th week).
7. The fetus assumes a human appearance.
8. Bone ossification begins.
9. Rudimentary kidney begins to secrete urine.

D. 4th Lunar Month (11–14-week-old fetus)

1. At the end of 14 weeks of growth, the fetus is 120 mm. crown-rump length and 110 gm.
2. Head erect; lower extremities well developed.

3. Hard palate and nasal septum have fused.
4. External genitalia of male and female can now be differentiated.
5. Eyelids are sealed.

E. 5th Lunar Month (15–18-week-old fetus)

1. At the end of 18 weeks of growth, the fetus is 160 mm. crown-rump length and 320 gm.
2. Ossification of fetal skeleton can be seen on x-ray.
3. Ears stand out from head.
4. Meconium is present in the intestinal tract.
5. Fetus makes sucking motions and swallows amniotic fluid.
6. Fetal movements may be felt by the mother (end of month).

F. 6th Lunar Month (19–22-week-old fetus)

1. At the end of 22 weeks of growth, the fetus is 210 mm. crown-rump length and 630 gm.
2. Vernix caseosa covers the skin.
3. Head and body (lanugo) hair visible.
4. Skin is wrinkled and red.
5. Brown fat, an important site of heat production, is present in neck and sternal area.
6. Nipples are apparent on the breasts.

G. 7th Lunar Month (23–26-week-old fetus)

1. At the end of 26 weeks of growth, the fetus is 250 mm. crown-rump length and 1000 gm.
2. Fingernails present.
3. Lean body.
4. Eyes partially open; eyelashes present.
5. Bronchioles are present; primitive alveoli are forming.
6. Skin begins to thicken on hands and feet.
7. Startle reflex present; grasp reflex is strong.

H. 8th Lunar Month (27–30-week-old fetus)

1. At the end of 30 weeks of growth, the fetus is 280 mm. crown-rump length and 1700 gm.
2. Eyes open.
3. Ample hair on head; lanugo begins to fade.
4. Skin slightly wrinkled.
5. Toenails present.
6. Testes in inguinal canal, begin descent to scrotal sac.
7. Surfactant coats much of the alveolar epithelium.

I. 9th Lunar Month (31–34-week-old fetus)

1. At the end of 34 weeks of growth, the fetus is about 320 mm. crown-rump length and 2500 gm.
2. Fingernails reach fingertips.
3. Skin pink and smooth.
4. Testes in scrotal sac.

J. 10th Lunar Month (35–38-week-old fetus; end of this month is also 40 weeks from onset of last menstrual period)

1. End of 38 weeks of growth, fetus is about 360 mm. crown-rump length and 3400 gm.
2. Ample subcutaneous fat.
3. Lanugo almost absent.
4. Toenails reach toe tips.
5. Testes in scrotum.
6. Vernix caseosa mainly on the back.
7. Breasts are firm.

Alternate Methods of Fertilization

A. Artificial Insemination

1. Placing a semen specimen at the cervical os.
2. Used when the sperm has poor motility or quality.
3. The sperm may be from the husband or a donor.

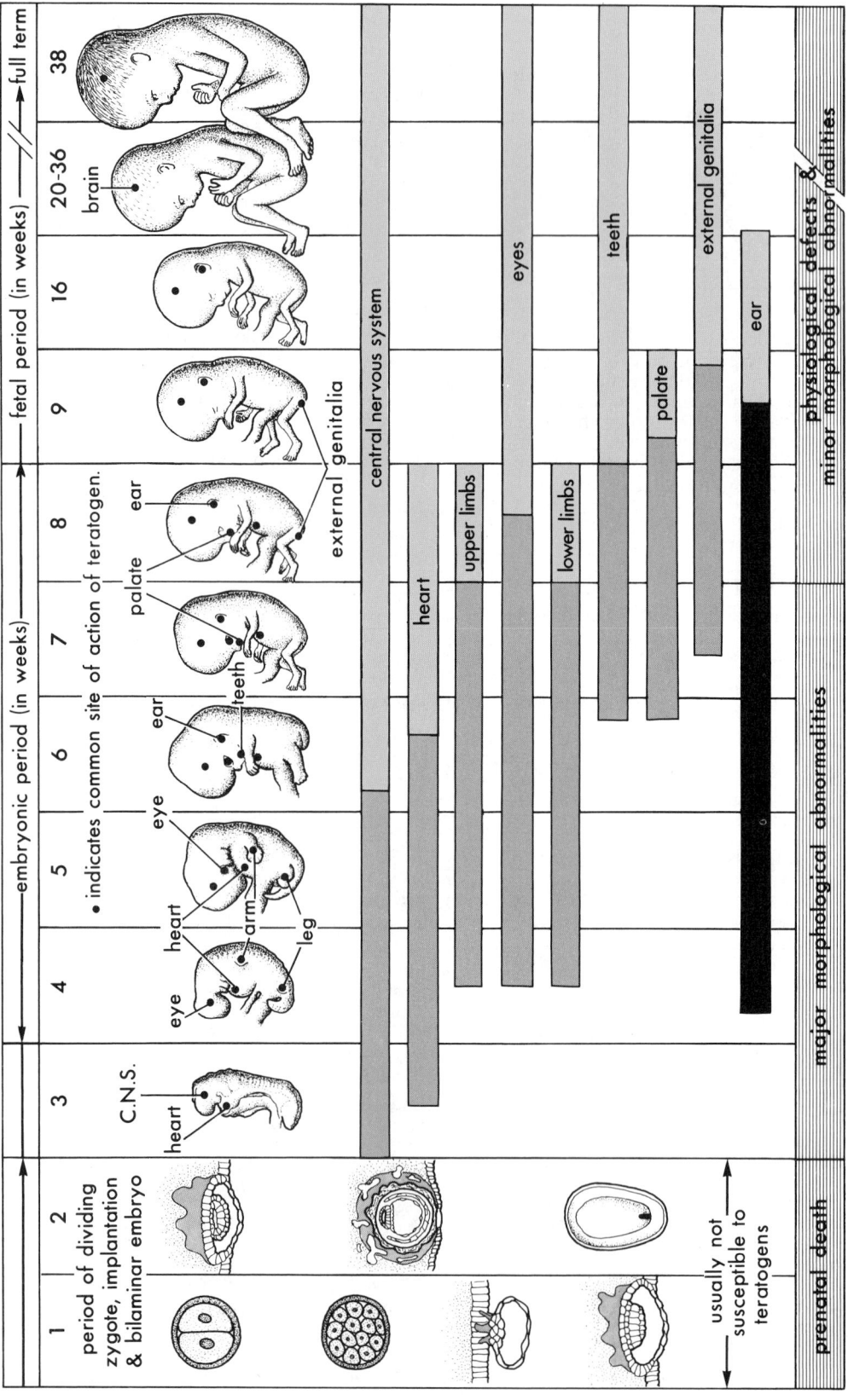

Figure 39-7. *Schematic illustration of the sensitive or critical periods in human development. During the first 2 weeks of development, the embryo is usually not susceptible to teratogens. During these predifferentiation stages, a substance either damages all or most of the cells of the embryo, resulting in its death, or damages only a few cells, allowing the embryo to recover without developing defects. The left (shaded) sides of the bars denote highly sensitive periods; the right sides indicate stages that are less sensitive to teratogens. (From Moore KL. The Developing Human: Clinically Oriented Embryology. 4th ed. Philadelphia, WB Saunders, 1988.)*

B. In Vitro Fertilization (IVF)

Used when a woman's uterine tubes are damaged or obstructed and transport of a fertilized egg to the uterus is not possible.
1. The woman is often given infertility drugs such as clomiphene citrate (Clomid) or menotropins (Pergonal) to stimulate ovulation.
2. The ovary is punctured via laparoscopy and mature follicles are removed by suction.
3. Each egg is placed in a mixture of salts, sugars, and proteins designed to simulate the maternal fluids found in the uterine tubes.
4. Following several hours of incubation to maturity, semen is added and the egg and fluids are again incubated for several hours. If the egg is fertilized, it is incubated further until it begins division. At this stage, the fertilized egg is deposited in the woman's uterus via a thin plastic catheter.

C. Embryo Transplants

Used when the woman is not capable of producing normal mature follicles, but the male partner is fertile.
1. Through hormonal therapy, the menstrual cycles of the donor woman and the recipient woman are synchronized.
2. Sperm of the fertile husband is artificially inseminated in a fertile donor woman following her normal ovulation.
3. If fertilization occurs, several days later the fertilized egg is washed from the donor woman's uterus.
4. The fertilized egg is then deposited in the uterus of the wife who was incapable of producing a normal mature follicle. If successful, implantation occurs soon afterward.

D. Gamete Intrafallopian Tube Transfer (GIFT)

Used when the tubes are patent. Ovulation is induced and the oocytes are removed. The oocytes and sperm are mixed in the laboratory and then transferred to the uterine tubes where natural fertilization occurs.

Fetal Circulation—Before and After Birth

(See Fig. 39-8)

Assessment of Fetal Maturity and Well-Being

Maternal History and Examination

A. History
1. The woman's general health
2. History of current pregnancy and identified risk factors
3. Health during previous pregnancies
4. Outcome of previous pregnancies

Estimation of Fundal Height

(see p. 972).

Fetal Heart Tones

1. Can be heard using a fetal stethoscope (fetoscope) after 20 weeks' fetal gestation
2. Can be heard using techniques that amplify sounds (Doppler) at approximately 10 weeks' fetal gestation
3. Rate—between 120 and 160 beats/minute
4. In latter months of pregnancy, fetal heart sounds found:
   a. Near the woman's midline in fetal occipitoanterior positions
   b. Lateral to midline in fetal occipitotransverse positions
   c. In the woman's flank in fetal occipitoposterior positions
   d. Below the woman's umbilicus in cephalic presentations
   e. At or above the woman's umbilicus in breech presentations
5. Failure to hear FHTs at the expected time may be due to maternal obesity, polyhydramnios, error in date calculation, or fetal death.

Ultrasound

1. Utilizes reflected soundwaves as they travel in tissue to produce a picture.
2. Pregnancy can be identified as early as 5 weeks' gestation, when the sac size is measured. At 8 weeks the fetus can be seen in the sac, and at 10 weeks fetal activity and cardiac activity can be seen.
3. Used also to detect multiple pregnancy, fetal abnormalities, hydatidiform mole, fetal death, fetal presentation, placental position, and fetal weight.
4. Measurements to determine gestational age use the biparietal diameter (BPD) and femur length (FM). These measurements must be compared with charts that are specific to the population. A BPD greater than 9 cm. correlates with a gestational age of 37 weeks.
5. Since fetal head growth can vary, ultrasound is used to determine BPD of fetal head and thoracic diameter; in times of stress, head growth is spared and body wasting occurs; therefore, abdominal transverse diameter or abdominal circumference is an important measure. Head/abdomen (H/A) ratios are also used. An H/A ratio below 1.0 has been correlated with gestations greater than 36 weeks.
6. Portable ultrasound (real-time imaging) can be used to visualize the fetus in motion (e.g., breathing movements, cardiac activity including activity of the heart valves and chambers, swallowing, and fetal motion).

Amniotic Fluid Studies (Amniocentesis)

Amniocentesis is a procedure in which amniotic fluid is removed from the uterine cavity by insertion of a needle through the abdominal and uterine walls and into the amniotic sac.

A. Determination of Fetal Maturity
1. Lecithin/sphingomyelin (L/S) ratio measures the maturity of the fetal lung.
   a. When the ratio of lecithin to sphingomyelin is 2:1 or greater, the fetal lung is considered mature and the incidence of respiratory distress syndrome in the newborn is low.
   b. May have false mature L/S ratios in some maternal conditions such as maternal diabetes.
   c. A rapid foam test, mixing amniotic fluid and ethanol, is also used to determine the presence of mature L/S ratios. Adequate amounts of lecithin are present when a stable foam ring forms and remains on top of the solution after vigorous shaking.
2. Presence of phosphatidyl glycerol (PG) indicates fetal lung maturity.
   a. PG is an important phospholipid that functions to stabilize lecithin in the fetal alveoli of the lung.

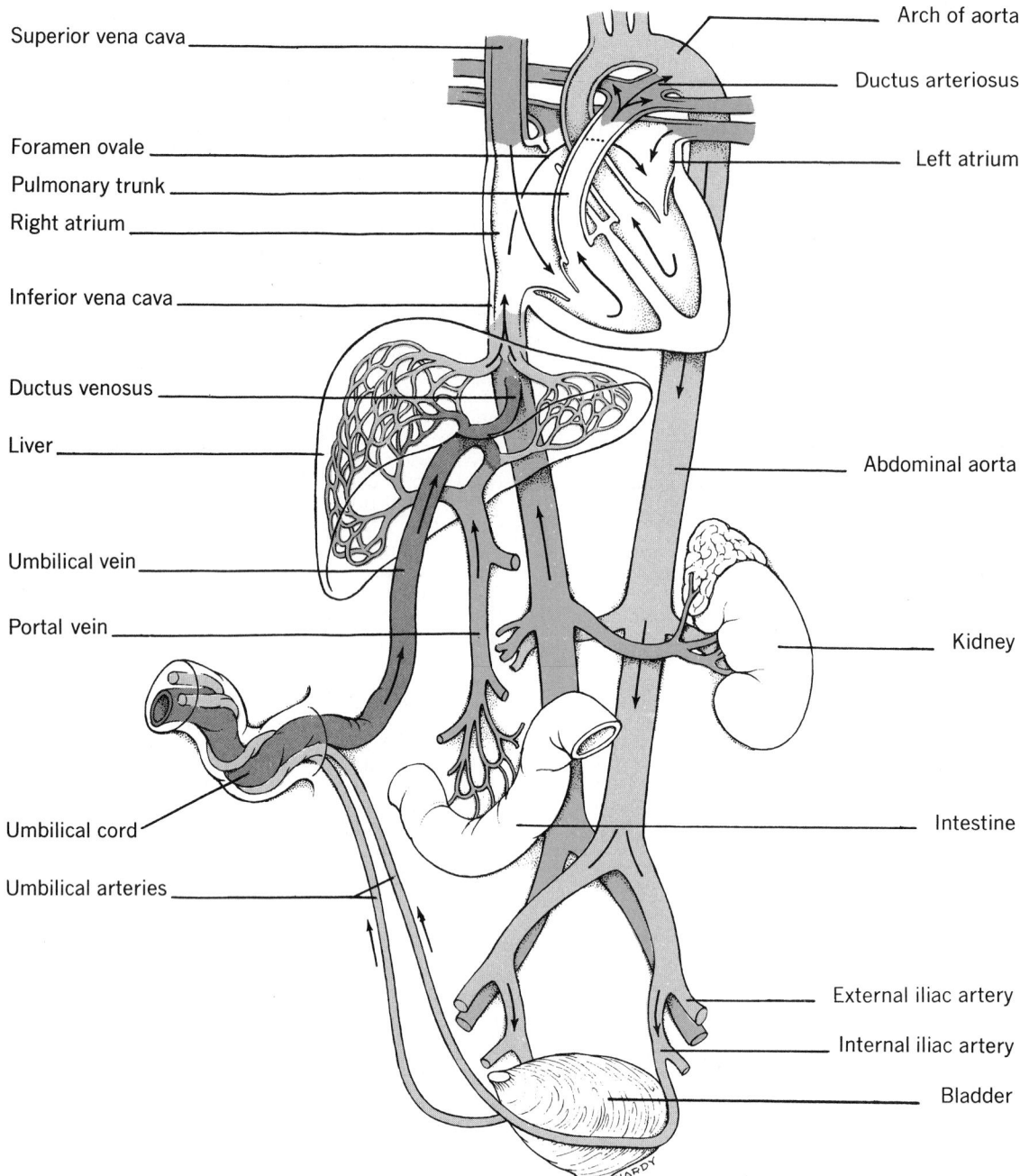

Superior vena cava

Arch of aorta

Ductus arteriosus

Foramen ovale

Left atrium

Pulmonary trunk

Right atrium

Inferior vena cava

Ductus venosus

Liver

Abdominal aorta

Umbilical vein

Portal vein

Kidney

Umbilical cord

Intestine

Umbilical arteries

External iliac artery

Internal iliac artery

Bladder

Figure 39-8. *Diagram of the fetal circulation shortly before birth. Arrows indicate course of blood.*

   b. The presence of PG may be a more accurate predictor of lung function than the L/S ratio.

3. Creatinine
   a. Used in conjunction with other measures such as L/S ratio to indicate fetal maturity.
   b. Levels increase after 34 weeks' gestation; levels in excess of 2 mg./100 ml. correlate with gestational ages over 37 weeks.

   c. Concentration depends on fetal muscle mass, kidney excretion, amniotic fluid volume, and maternal serum levels. Misleadingly high levels are found in women with impaired renal function.

4. Fat cells
A 20% fat cell count has been used to indicate fetal maturity. Fat cells increase in amniotic fluid after 36 weeks' gestation.

B. Determination of Fetal Well-Being

1. *Bilirubin*—generally very little bilirubin is found after 36 weeks' gestation. An increase in bilirubin levels occurs with hemolytic disease. When used to determine fetal maturity, optical density (OD) measure of OD 650 ≥ 0.15 have been correlated with mature fetuses and low incidence of respiratory distress syndrome.
2. *Alpha-fetoprotein*—major plasma protein of early fetuses; levels decrease rapidly in amniotic fluid after 13 weeks' gestation; increased levels are found in fetuses with spina bifida, anencephaly, and other neural tube defects.
3. *Estriol*—levels increase as pregnancy progresses. Levels that drop 40%–50% or more in 1 week signify danger to the fetus. Serum determination or 24-hour urinary levels can be used. Estriol level are used primarily in pregnancies complicated by diabetes.
4. *Karyotyping and cell enzyme studies*
   a. Used to determine sex of fetus, normalcy of the chromosomes, and presence or lack of enzymes found in some inherited disorders.
   b. Sex determination is important in sex-linked disorders such as hemophilia and severe immune deficiencies.
   c. Evaluation of chromosomes is important when trisomy 21 (Down's), trisomy 18 (Edwards'), trisomy 13 (Patau's), cri-du-chat, and other chromosomal problems are suspected.
   d. Enzyme evaluation can detect over 60 inborn errors of metabolism.

C. Nursing Interventions During Amniocentesis

1. Reduce anxiety related to the procedure.
   a. Reduce the parents' anxiety by determining their understanding of the procedure and the meaning it holds for them.
   b. Explain the procedure before it begins and answer any questions they have.
   c. Provide explanations during the procedure; correct misinformation they may have; make sure they know when the results will be available and how they may obtain the results as soon as possible.
2. Reduce pain and discomfort related to the procedure.
   a. Reduce discomfort by having the mother lie comfortably on her back with her hands and a pillow under her head. Relaxation breathing may help.
   b. Ensure adequate time between infiltration of local anesthetic and introduction of needle into the amniotic sac.
3. Reduce potential for traumatic injury to fetus, placenta, or maternal structures.
   a. Have the woman empty her bladder if the fetus is more than 20 weeks' gestation to avoid injury to the woman's bladder. If the fetus is less than 20 weeks' gestation, the woman's full bladder will hold the uterus steady and out of the pelvis. The placenta is localized via ultrasound.
   b. Obtain maternal vital signs, and a 20-minute fetal heart rate tracing to serve as a baseline to evaluate possible complications.
   c. Monitor the woman during and following the procedure for signs of premature labor or bleeding.
   d. Tell the woman to report signs of bleeding, unusual fetal activity or abdominal pain, cramping, or fever while at home following the procedure.

Chorionic Villus (CV) Biopsy

Used to obtain samples of CVs (tissue of fetal origin) to test for genetic disorders in the fetus.
1. Using an ultrasound picture, a catheter is passed vaginally into the woman's uterus, where a sample of CV tissue is snipped off or obtained by suction.
2. Samples can be obtained earlier in pregnancy than can fetal cells obtained via amniocentesis. Biopsy is performed between 8 and 12 weeks of pregnancy.
3. Results from CVs are available in 1–2 weeks.
4. Complications include rupture of membranes, intrauterine infection, spontaneous abortion, hematoma, fetal trauma, or maternal tissue contamination.
5. Incidence of fetal loss is about 5%.

Magnetic Resonance Imaging (MRI)

1. A noninvasive method of evaluating soft tissues.
2. Provides measurements of fetal development such as the amount of subcutaneous fat, along with assessing fetal blood flow, nutritional status, and organ anatomy.

Percutaneous Umbilical Cord Blood Sampling (PUBS)

1. Following an ultrasound scan, a needle is inserted into the fetal umbilical vein and a blood sample is obtained.
2. Used to identify fetal blood dyscrasias or intrauterine infections, and also for fetal karyotyping.
3. Complications include fetal loss, infections, and prematurity.
4. Future use may include intrauterine transfusion.

Computed Tomography (CT) Scanning

Used to assess pelvic diameters accurately and to note the exact degree of fetal head flexion.

Assay of Maternal Urine

1. Estriol levels (24-hour urine specimens)
   a. Provide information on fetal, placental, and maternal renal function. The biosynthesis of estriol by the placenta depends on precursor substances produced in the fetal adrenal gland.
   b. Levels found in a 24-hour urine specimen are influenced by length of gestation, fetal and placental size, multiple pregnancy, maternal renal function, and adequacy of urine collection.
   c. Since there is considerable variation in amount of excretion by different women, serial testing is done rather than a single 24-hour sample.
   d. Levels of estriol that drop between 40% and 50% within 1 week signify danger to the fetus.

Assay of Maternal Serum

1. Plasma estriol levels may be measured.
2. Maternal serum may be analyzed for alpha-fetoprotein levels. Increased levels are associated with Rh and ABO maternal immunization, fetoplacental dysfunction, and fetal neural tube defects.

Nonstress Test (NST)

1. Used to evaluate fetal heart rate accelerations that normally occur in response to fetal activity in a fetus in good condition.
2. Indications—pregnancy beyond 41 weeks, Rh sensi-

tization, suspected intrauterine growth retardation, older gravida, chronic renal disease, sickle cell disease, maternal diabetes, hyperthyroidism, collagen disease, hypertension, history of poor pregnancy outcome, and history of intrauterine fetal death.

3. Nursing interventions
   a. Place woman in semi-Fowler's position in bed; external fetal and uterine monitoring is performed.
   b. Make mark on monitoring paper each time fetal movement is felt.
   c. Evaluate response of fetal heart rate immediately following fetal activity.
   d. Monitor mother's blood pressure and uterine activity for deviations during procedure.
4. *Interpretation*—test period should be a minimum of 40 minutes to allow for fetal rest cycle patterns.
   a. *Reactive*—fetal heart rate increased by 15 beats/minute above baseline in response to fetal activity. To label fetal heart rate reactive, 5 such responses should be obtained during a 20-minute recording.
   b. *Nonreactive*—fetal heart rate does not increase with fetal movements, or fewer than 5 such responses are found within a 20-minute recording. Test period is usually extended to allow for fetal rest cycles.
   c. *Unsatisfactory*—fetal heart rate tracing is not adequate for interpretation.

Oxytocin Challenge Test *(OCT)*, **Stress Test** *(ST)*, or Contraction Stress Test *(CST)*

1. Used to evaluate the ability of the fetus to withstand the stress of uterine contractions as would occur during labor. The test is generally used after 34 weeks' gestation; used with decreasing frequency since it may stress an already stressed fetus.
2. *Indications*—usually used when a woman has a nonreactive nonstress test. In this situation, should a woman have a positive OCT, it indicates placental dysfunction placing the fetus at risk. Used with women who have diabetes, prolonged pregnancy, hypertensive disorders, history of previous stillbirth, abnormal estriol values, or other evidence of potential fetal distress.
3. *Contraindications*—women with previous cesarean birth, 3rd trimester bleeding, multiple gestations, incompetent cervix, or premature rupture of membranes.
4. Nursing interventions
   a. Have woman void.
   b. Place in semi-Fowler's or side-lying position.
   c. Obtain a 30-minute strip of the fetal heart rate and uterine activity for baseline data.
   d. Obtain maternal vital signs.
   e. Administer diluted oxytocin via an infusion pump.
   f. Increase oxytocin every 20–30 minutes until three contractions occur within 10 minutes.
5. *Interpretation*
   a. Negative test—three contractions of good quality and duration without late decelerations or other ominous responses of the fetal heart rate. Indicates adequate placental sufficiency.
   b. Positive test—occurrence of late or other ominous responses of the fetal heart rate in response to the uterine contraction; indicates placental insufficiency in response to the stress of a uterine contraction.
   c. Hyperstimulation—late decelerations with excessive uterine activity.

d. Suspicious—late decelerations with less than half of the contractions.
e. Unsatisfactory—inadequate contraction pattern or tracing too poor to interpret.

Biophysical Profile

1. Assessment of five biophysical variables to determine fetal wellness.
   a. If the criteria are met, a score of 2 is given.
   b. For an abnormal observation, a score of 0 is given.
   c. A total score of 8 or 10 is normal, 6 is equivocal, and 4 or less is abnormal.
   d. If there is decreased amniotic fluid, the infant is suspected of chronic asphyxia and should be delivered.
2. Nonstress test (NST)—looking for acceleration in relation to fetal movements
3. Amniotic fluid volume—assessing for one or more pockets of amniotic fluid measuring 1 cm. in two perpendicular planes.
4. Fetal breathing—one or more episodes lasting at least 30 seconds.
5. Gross body movements—three or more body or limb movements in 30 minutes.
6. Fetal tone—one or more episodes of active extension with return to flexion.

Acoustic Stimulation Test

1. A loud sound is used to stimulate the fetus and assess its reaction to the sound.
2. This test may be as good a screening tool as the NST because the loud noise stimulates the fetus and notes ability to respond to the noise by increasing heart rate.
3. One method of evaluation indicates that a reactive acoustic stimulation test will have at least one acceleration of at least 15 beats/minute lasting 2 minutes or two accelerations with an increase of 15 beats/minute lasting 15 seconds within 5 minutes of stimulation.

Fetoscopy

The insertion of a fiberoptic instrument into the uterine cavity to examine the fetus visually or to obtain blood, placental or tissue samples for identification and diagnosis of:

1. Congenital anomalies or teratogenic-induced malformations
2. Hemoglobinopathies such as sickle cell anemia and beta-thalassemia
3. Sex-linked autosomal abnormalities or neural tube disorders
4. Metabolic disorders

Other Studies

A. Amnioscopy

The insertion of a fiberoptic instrument into the woman's cervical canal to visualize the amniotic fluid for the presence of blood or meconium.

B. X-Ray

Has been used to determine fetal maturity based on epiphyseal centers of ossification, the size of the fetal skull, fetal length, multiple pregnancy, fetal death, hydrocephalus, and fetal edema found in hydrops fetalis. Currently the use of x-ray to determine fetal maturity has been largely replaced by the use of ultrasound, thus avoiding exposure to radiation for fetus and mother.

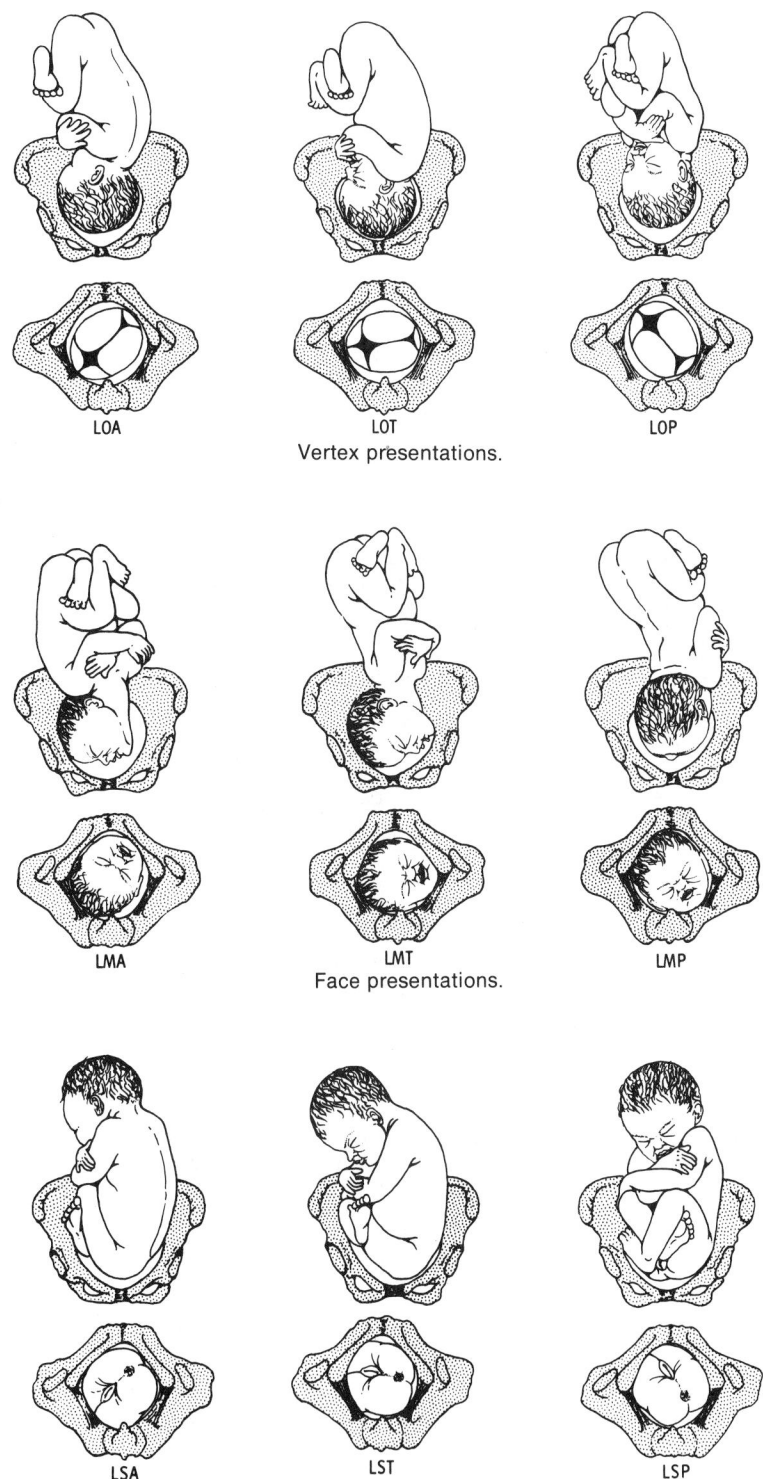

LOA

LOT

LOP

Vertex presentations.

LMA

LMT

LMP

Face presentations.

LSA

LST

LSP

Breech presentations.

Figure 39-9. Fetal presentations. See text, p 984, for definition of abbreviations. (From Benson RC. Handbook of Obstetrics and Gynecology. Los Altos, CA, Lange Medical Publication)

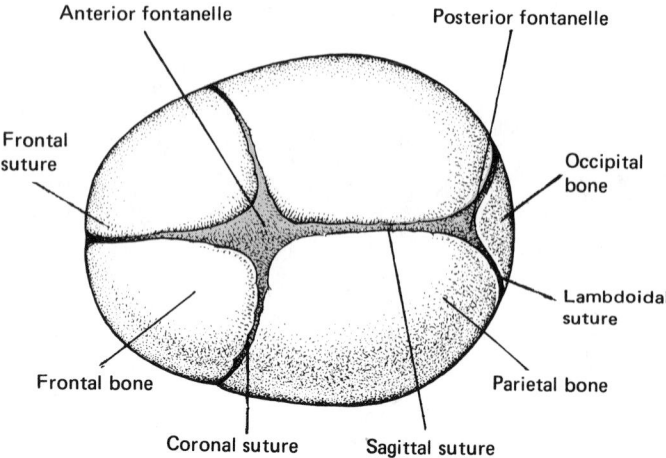

Figure 39-10. *Fetal skull.*

In Utero Fetal Surgery

1. Used to correct malformations through hysterotomy in which the fetus may be brought partially out of the uterus, operated upon, and replaced in the uterus, or through fetoscopy in utero.
2. Used to correct malformations such as congenital hydronephrosis, obstructive hydrocephalus, and neural tube defects.
3. Used when delivery of the fetus or other treatment is not yet possible and further normal growth and development are not possible.
4. Complications include uterine damage, hemorrhage, and premature delivery.

Assessment of Fetal Presentation and Position

As pregnancy progresses, it becomes important to determine the presentation and position of the fetus in relation to the mother's pelvis (Fig. 39-9). In approximately 95% of all births, the fetal head presents first, making its landmarks very important.

General Terms

1. *Lie*—a comparison of the long axis of the fetus with the long axis of the mother. Fetal lie is either longitudinal or transverse. In a longitudinal lie either the fetal head presents (cephalic) or the buttocks presents (breech). In a transverse lie, the shoulder presents.
2. *Presentation*—the part of the fetus deepest in the birth canal. Presentation may be vertex, face, brow, breech, or shoulder.
3. *Presenting part*—portion of the fetus deepest in the birth canal and felt on vaginal examination.

4. *Attitude*—relationship of fetal parts to each other.
5. *Position*—relationship of landmark on the fetal presenting part to the front (anterior = A), back (posterior = P), or side (transverse = T) of the mother's pelvis. Landmarks on the fetal presenting parts include head = occiput (O); buttocks = sacrum (S); shoulder = scapula or acromion (A); face = chin or mentum (M).

Fetal Head

(See Fig. 39-10)

A. Bones of the Fetal Skull

1. Occipital bone posteriorly
2. 2 Parietal bones on the sides
3. 2 Temporal bones anteriorly
4. 2 Frontal bones anteriorly

B. Sutures of the Fetal Skull—membranous spaces between the bones of the fetal skull

1. Frontal suture—between the 2 frontal bones
2. Sagittal—between the 2 parietal bones
3. Coronal—between the frontal and parietal bones
4. Lambdoid—between the back of the parietal bones and the margin of the occipital bone

C. Fontanelles—irregular spaces formed where 2 or more sutures meet. Sutures and fontanelles allow fetal skull bones to overlap in order to pass through the maternal pelvis.

1. Anterior fontanelle—junction of the sagittal, frontal, and coronal sutures—closes by 18 months of age.
2. Posterior fontanelle—located where the sagittal suture meets the lambdoidal (smaller than anterior)—closes at 6–8 weeks of age.

Bibliography

Books

Bobak I, Jensen M and Zalar M. Maternity and Gynecologic Care. 3rd ed. St. Louis, CV Mosby, 1989

Cunningham F, MacDonald P and Gant N. Williams Obstetrics. 17th ed.

Norwalk, CT, Appleton and Lange, 1989

Dickason EJ, Schult M and Silverman B. Maternal Infant Nursing Care. Philadelphia, JB Lippincott, 1990

Doenges M, Kenty J and Moorehouse M. Maternal/Newborn Care Plans:

Guideline for Client Care. Philadelphia, FA Davis, 1988

Gorrie TM. A Guide to the Nursing of Childbearing Families. Baltimore, Williams & Wilkins, 1989

Houldin A, Saltstein S and Ganley K. Nursing Diagnoses for Wellness

Supporting Strength. Philadelphia, JB Lippincott, 1987

Lederman R. Psychosocial Adaptation in Pregnancy. Englewood Cliffs, NJ, Prentice–Hall, 1984

May K and Mahlmeister L. Comprehensive Maternity Nursing: Nursing Process and the Childbearing Family. 2nd ed. Philadelphia, JB Lippincott, 1990

Neeson J. Clinical Manual of Maternity Nursing. Philadelphia, JB Lippincott, 1987

Olds S, London M and Ladewig P. Maternal Newborn Nursing: A Family-Centered Approach. 3rd ed. Menlo Park, CA, Addison–Wesley, 1988

Reeder S and Martin L. Maternity Nursing. 16th ed. Philadelphia, JB Lippincott, 1987

Rubin R. Maternal Identity and the Maternal Experience. New York, Springer, 1984

Sherwen L. Psychosocial Dimensions of the Pregnant Family. New York, Springer, 1987

Worthington–Roberts B and Williams S. Nutrition in Pregnancy and Lactation. 4th ed. St. Louis, Times Mirror/Mosby, 1989

Journals

Abrams B et al. Maternal weight gain and preterm delivery. Obstet Gynecol 1989; 74:577–583

Baskett T and Liston R. Fetal movement monitoring: Clinical application. Clin Perinatol 1989; 16:613–625

Bocking A. Observations of biophysical activities in the normal fetus. Clin Perinatol 1989; 16:583–594

Brar H, Platt L and Devore G. The biophysical profile. Clin Obstet Gynecol 1987; 30:936–947

Buerle J and Behamroun B. The fetal biophysical profile: Interpretation and nursing implications. Crit Care Nurse 1988; 8:52–55

Clark S, Sabey P and Jolley K. Nonstress testing with acoustic stimulation and amniotic fluid volume assessment: 5973 tests without unexpected fetal death. Am J Obstet Gynecol 1989; 160:694–697

Davis L. Daily fetal movement counting: A valuable assessment tool. J Nurse Midwif 1987; 32:11–19

Devoe L et al. The effects of biratory acoustic stimulation on baseline fetal heart rate in term pregnancy. Am J Obstet Gynecol 1989; 160:1086–1090

Druzin M. Fetal bradycardia during antepartum testing. Further observations. J Reprod Med 1989; 34:47–51

Druzin M. Antepartum fetal heart rate monitoring. State of the art. Clin Perinatol 1989; 16:627–642

Garite T. Fetal maturity testing. Clin Obstet Gynecol 1987; 30:985–991

Grant A et al. Routine formal fetal movement counting and risk of antepartum late death in normally formed singletons. Lancet 1989; 2 (8659):345–349

Guidetti D, Divon M, and Langer O. Postdate fetal surveillance: Is 41 weeks too early? Am J Obstet Gynecol 1989; 161:91–93

Hill A. Assessment of the fetus: Relevance to brain injury. Clin Perinatol 1989; 16:413–434

Judge N et al. Clinical associations of variable decelerations during reactive nonstress tests. Obstet Gynecol 1989; 74:351–356

Mattison D et al. Magnetic resonance imaging in maternal and fetal medicine. J Perinatol 1989; 9:411–419

Moore T and Piacquadio K. A prospective evaluation of fetal movement screening to reduce the incidence of antepartum fetal death. Am J Obstet Gynecol 1989; 160:1075–1080

Morgan C and Elias S. Prenatal diagnosis of genetic disorders. J Perinat Neonat Nurs 1989; 2:1–12

Myhre C, Richards T and Johnson J. Maternal serum fetoprotein screening: An assessment of fetal well being. J Perinat Neonat Nurs 1989; 2:12–20

Nagey D. The content of prenatal care. Obstet Gynecol 1989; 74:516–528

Owen J et al. A comparison of perinatal outcome in patients undergoing contraction stress testing performed by nipple stimulation versus spontaneously occurring contractions. Am J Obstet Gynecol 1989; 160:1081–1085

Porto M. Comparing and contrasting methods of fetal surveillance. Clin Obstet Gynecol 1987; 30:956–967

Ray D. Biochemical fetal assessment. Clin Obstet Gynecol 1987; 30:887–898

Rayburn W. Monitoring fetal body movement. Clin Obstet Gynecol 1987; 30:899–911

Salvador H and Koos B. Effects of regular and decaffeinated coffee on fetal breathing and heart rate. Am J Obstet Gynecol 1989; 1603:1043–1047

Stephenson J. Pregnancy testing and counseling. Pediatr Clin North Am 1989; 36:681–696

Stevens K. Nursing diagnoses in wellness childbearing settings. J Obstet Gynecol Neonat Nurs 1988; 17:329–336

Stole K. Nursing diagnosis and the childbearing woman. Am J Matern Child Nurs 1986; 11:13–15

Vintzileos A et al. Fetal biophysical profile scoring: Current status. Clin Perinatol 1989; 16:661–689

Witter F and Besinger R. The effects of maternal position on uterine artery flow during antepartum fetal heart rate testing. Am J Obstet Gynecol 1989; 160:379–380

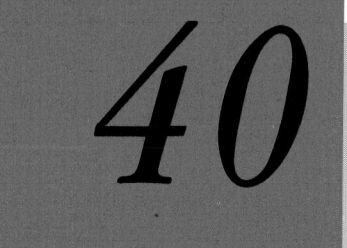

40

Nursing Management During Labor and Delivery

The Labor Process

Initiation of Labor

The exact mechanism that initiates labor is unknown. Theories include:
1. Uterine stretch theory—uterus becomes stretched and pressure increases, causing physiologic changes that initiate labor.
2. As pregnancy progresses, there is a gradual rise in the amount of circulating oxytocin.
3. As pregnancy advances, progesterone is less effective in controlling rhythmic uterine contractions that normally occur. In addition, there also may be an actual decrease in the amount of circulating progesterone.
4. There is increased production of prostaglandins by fetal membranes and uterine decidua as pregnancy advances.
5. In later pregnancy, the fetus produces increased levels of cortisol that inhibit progesterone production from the placenta.

Factors Affecting Labor

Successful labor and delivery depend on adequate pelvic dimensions, adequate fetal dimensions and presentation, and adequate uterine contractions.

A. Pelvic Dimensions

1. Adequate pelvic inlet (anteroposterior diameter; normal shape)
2. Adequate midpelvis (ischial spines do not protrude into bony canal)
3. Adequate outlet (adequate distance between tuberosities; mobile coccyx)
4. Adequacy of pelvic dimensions determined by pelvic examination during pregnancy (see p. 972) and again with the onset of labor

B. Fetal Dimensions—important fetal dimensions influenced by fetal size, posture, lie, and presentation. Fetal position is also an important factor in successful labor.

1. Fetal size—with excessive size, fetal skull bones may not be able to override enough to be accommodated in the bony pelvic cavity.
2. Fetal posture—fetus assumes a characteristic posture in later pregnancy to accommodate to the uterine cavity. The fetal head is flexed, back is bent, and extremities are flexed. Flexed head allows smallest diameter of fetal head to present and pass through the birth canal (Fig. 40-1).
3. Fetal lie—fetus assumes a lie (comparison of the fetal long axis to the long axis of the woman) that is either transverse or longitudinal. In a longitudinal lie (99% of all births), the fetal head will present (cephalic presentation) or the buttocks or feet will present (breech presentation). In a transverse lie, the shoulder presents.
4. Fetal presentation—whichever portion of the infant is deepest in the birth canal and is felt on vaginal examination is referred to as the presenting part; this determines fetal presentation.
5. Fetal position—designation of landmark of fetal presenting part (occiput, mentum, sacrum, acronium) to right or left, and anterior, posterior, or transverse portion of the woman's pelvis. For example, a fetus presenting by the vertex with his occiput on the left anterior part of the woman's pelvis would have his presentation and position described as LOA, or left occiput anterior (see Fig. 39-9, p. 983).

C. Uterine Contractions

Successful labor also depends on uterine contractions occurring at regular intervals and having adequate intensity.
1. Uterine contractions are involuntary.
2. During uterine contractions, the active upper portion of the uterus becomes thicker, while the lower uterine segment stretches and becomes thinner.
3. At the completion of a contraction, the upper uterine segment retains its shortened, thickened cell size and with each succeeding contraction becomes thicker and shorter. Cells of lower uterine segment become thinner and longer with each contraction. This mechanism is greatly responsible for the progress of the fetus through the birth canal.

Events Preliminary to Labor

1. Lightening (the settling of the fetus in the lower uterine segment) occurs 2–3 weeks before term in the primigravida and later, during labor, in the multigravida.
   a. The woman's breathing becomes easier as the fetus falls away from the diaphragm.
   b. Lordosis of the spine is increased for the woman as the fetus enters the pelvis and falls forward. Walking may become more difficult; leg cramping may increase.
   c. Urinary frequency occurs because of pressure on the bladder.

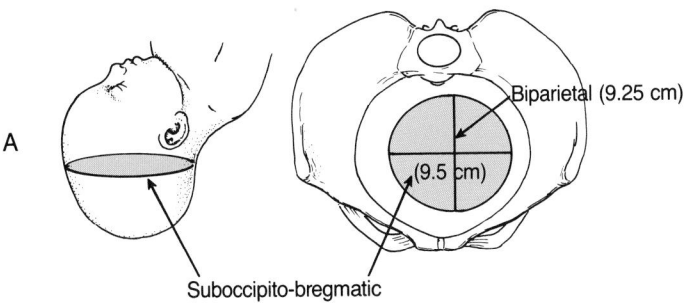

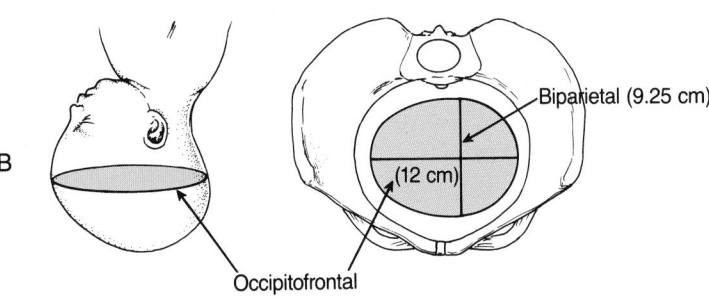

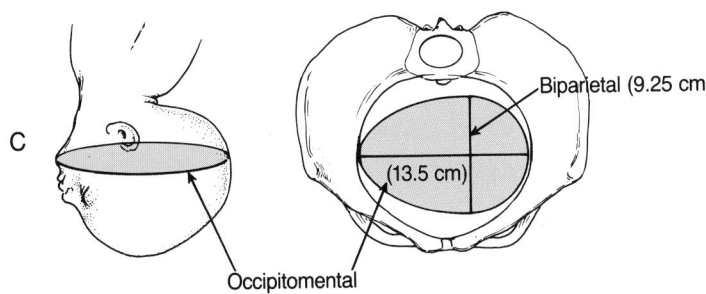

Figure 40-1. *(A) Complete flexion allows smallest diameter of head to enter pelvis. (B) Moderate extension causes larger diameter to enter pelvis. (C) Marked extension forces largest diameter against pelvic brim, but head is too large to enter pelvis.*

2. Vaginal secretions may increase.
3. Mucous plug is discharged from the cervix along with a small amount of blood from surrounding capillaries—referred to as "show" ("bloody show").
4. Cervix becomes soft and effaced (thinned).
5. Membranes may rupture.
6. False labor contractions may occur (Table 40-1).
7. Backache may increase.
8. Diarrhea may occur.
9. Weight loss of 1–3 lb.
10. Sudden burst of energy is experienced by some women.

Stages of Labor

A. First Stage of Labor (Stage of Cervical Dilation)

1. Begins with the first true labor contractions and ends with complete effacement and dilation of the cervix (10 cm. dilation)
2. *Latent phase (early)*
   a. Dilates from 0 to 4 cm.
   b. Contractions are usually every 5–10 minutes, lasting 20–40 seconds, and of mild intensity.

3. *Active phase* (includes acceleration phase and phase of maximum slope)
   a. Dilates from 4 to 7 cm.
   b. Contractions are usually every 2–5 minutes; lasting 30–50 seconds, and of mild to moderate intensity.
4. *Transitional phase* (deceleration phase)
   a. Dilates from 8 to 10 cm.
   b. Contractions are every 2–3 minutes, lasting 50–60 seconds, and of moderate to hard intensity.

B. Second Stage of Labor, or Stage of Expulsion

Begins with complete dilation and ends with birth of the baby.

C. Third Stage of Labor, or Placental Stage

Begins with delivery of the baby and ends with delivery of the placenta.

D. Fourth Stage

Lasts from delivery of the placenta until the postpartum condition of the woman has become stabilized (usually 1 hour after delivery).

Table 40-1. *True and False Labor Contractions*

True Labor Contractions	False Labor Contractions
Result in progressive cervical dilation and effacement	Do not result in progressive cervical dilation and effacement
Occur at regular intervals	Occur at irregular intervals
Interval between contractions decreases	Interval between contractions remains the same or increases
Intensity increases	Intensity decreases or remains the same
Located mainly in back and abdomen	Located mainly in lower abdomen and groin
Generally intensified by walking	Generally unaffected by walking
Not affected by mild sedation	Generally relieved by mild sedation

Mechanisms of Labor

1. If the woman's pelvis is adequate, size and position of the fetus are adequate, and uterine contractions are regular and of adequate intensity, the fetus will move through the birth canal.
2. The position and rotational changes of the fetus as he moves down the birth canal will be affected by resistance offered by the woman's bony pelvis, cervix, and surrounding tissues.
3. The events of engagement, descent, flexion, internal rotation, extension, external rotation, and expulsion overlap in time (Fig. 40-2).

A. Engagement

When biparietal diameter of fetal head has passed through pelvic inlet:
1. Primigravidas—occurs up to 2 weeks before onset of labor
2. Multigravidas—usually occurs with onset of labor
3. Since biparietal diameter is narrowest diameter of fetal head, and anteroposterior diameter is narrowest of pelvic inlet, the fetal head usually enters pelvis in a transverse position

B. Descent

Occurs throughout labor and is essential for fetal rotations prior to birth.
1. Accomplished by force of uterine contractions on fetal portion in fundus; during second stage of labor, bearing down increases intra-abdominal pressure, thus augmenting effects of uterine contractions.
2. Degree of descent described as:
   a. Floating—fetal presenting part is not engaged in pelvic inlet (Fig. 40-3).
   b. Fixed—fetal presenting part has entered pelvis.
   c. Engagement—fetal presenting part (usually biparietal diameter of fetal head) has passed through pelvic inlet
   d. Station—relation of the presenting part to the ischial spines.
   e. Stations that are −1, −2, −3, or −4 occur when the presenting part is 1, 2, 3, or 4 cm. above the level of the ischial spines (Fig. 40-4).
   f. Station 0 occurs when the presenting part is at the level of the ischial spine.
   g. Station +1, +2, +3, or +4, is when the presenting part is 1, 2, 3, or 4 cm. below the ischial spines. A station of +4 indicates that the presenting part is on the pelvic floor.

C. Flexion

Resistance to descent causes head to flex so that the chin is close to the chest; this causes the smallest fetal head diameter, the suboccipitobregmatic (9.5 cm.) to present through the canal.

D. Internal Rotation

In accommodating to the birth canal, the fetal occiput rotates anteriorly from its original position toward the symphysis. This movement results from the shape of the fetal head, space available in the midpelvis, and contour of the perineal muscles. The ischial spines project into the midpelvis causing the fetal head to rotate anteriorly to accommodate to the available space.

E. Extension

As the fetal head descends further, it meets resistance from the perineal muscles and is forced to extend. The fetal head becomes visible at the vulvovaginal ring; its largest diameter is encircled (*crowning*), and the head then emerges from the vagina.

F. External Rotation

When the head emerges, the shoulders are undergoing internal rotation as they turn in the midpelvis to accommodate to the projection of the ischial spines. The head, now born, rotates as the shoulders undergo this internal rotation.

G. Expulsion

Following delivery of the infant's head and internal rotation of the shoulders, the anterior shoulder rests beneath the symphysis pubis. The posterior shoulder is born, followed by the anterior shoulder and the rest of the body.

Assessment

When Labor Begins

History and Baseline Data

1. Introduce yourself; ask for name of woman's midwife or physician and if he or she has been notified that the woman was coming to the hospital or birth center.
2. Establish baseline information.
   a. Gravidity, parity, expected date of delivery or confinement (EDC)
   b. When did contractions begin? How far apart are they? How long do they last?
   c. Have the membranes ruptured? Color? Consistency? Amount of fluid?
   d. Is there any bloody show?
   e. How much discomfort is the woman experiencing?
   f. What, if any, problems has the woman had in this pregnancy? Problems in past pregnancies?
   g. Blood type and Rh?

Figure 40-2. *Mechanism of delivery for a vertex presentation. (From Whitley N. A Manual of Clinical Obstetrics. Philadelphia, JB Lippincott, 1985)*

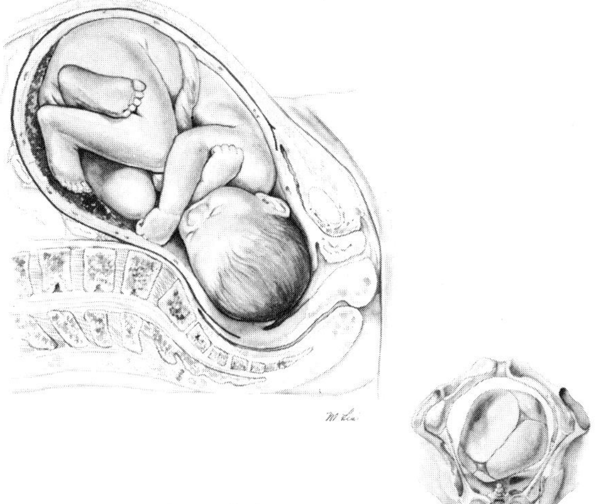

Engagement, descent flexion

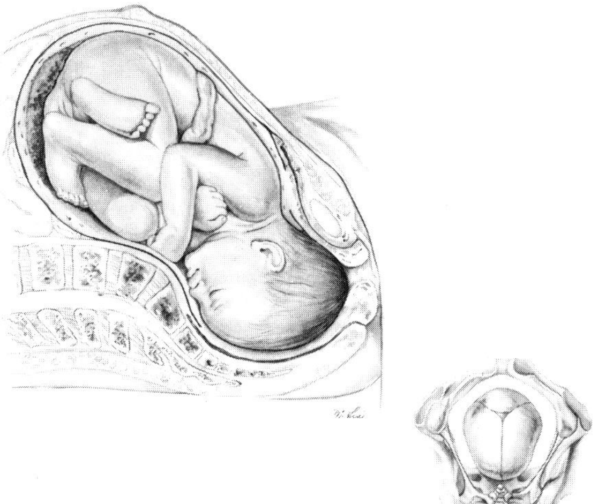

Internal rotation

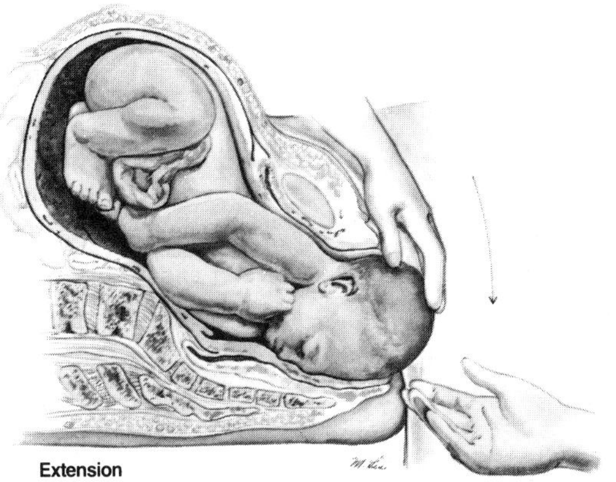

Extension

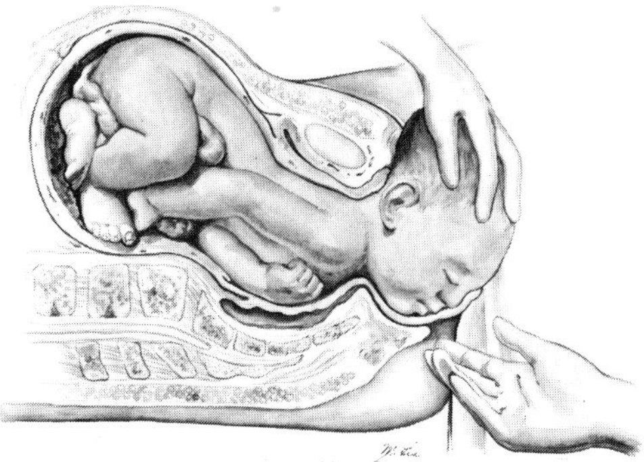

Extension complete (delivery of fetal head)

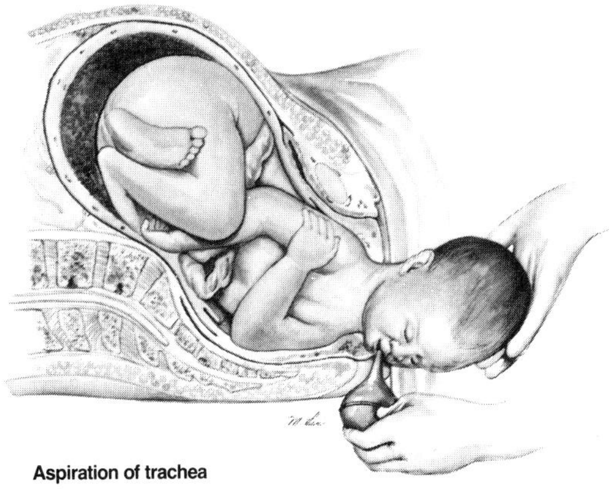

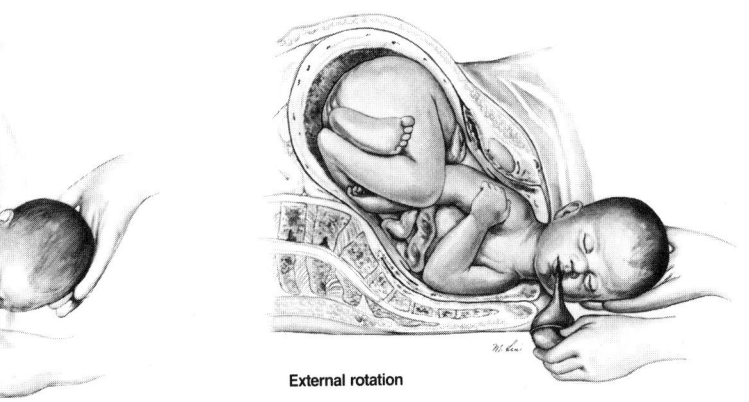

Aspiration of trachea

External rotation

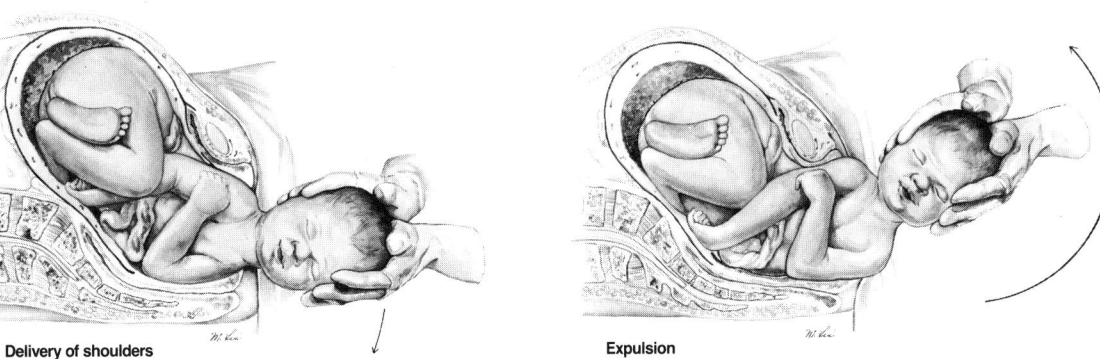

Delivery of shoulders

Expulsion

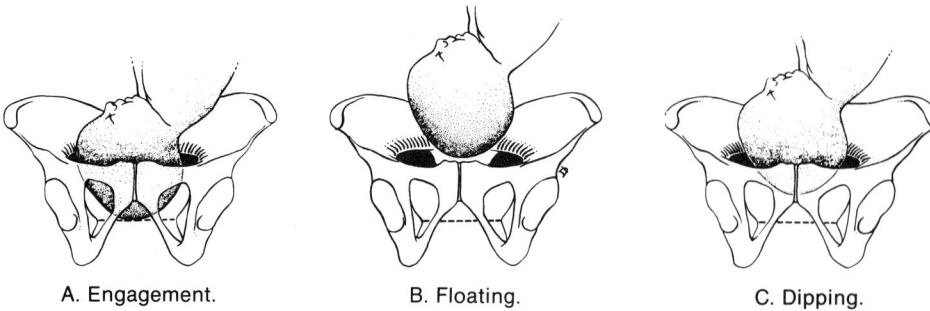

A. Engagement.   B. Floating.   C. Dipping.

Figure 40-3. *Engagement, floating, and dipping. (From Oxom H and Foote WR. Human Labor and Birth. New York, Appleton–Century–Crofts)*

3. Establish baseline maternal and fetal vital signs.
   a. Temperature—elevation suggests a possible infection or dehydration.
   b. Pulse—evaluate between contractions; may be slightly elevated over the resting rate.
   c. Respirations—evaluated between contractions.
   d. Blood pressure—evaluated between contractions.
      (1) A slight elevation over baseline may be attributed to anxiety.
      (2) A blood pressure with a systolic elevation of 30 mm. Hg, or greater than 140 mm. Hg, and a diastolic elevation of 15 mm. Hg, or greater that 90 mm. Hg suggest hypertension and require further evaluation.
   e. Assess the fetal heart rate; if a fetal monitor is to be used, run a 30-minute strip for baseline data.
4. Obtain a urine specimen—test the urine for glucose and protein. Protein may be positive if the membranes have ruptured.

Methods for Determining Fetal Presentation

A. Vaginal Examination and Determination of Fetal Landmarks Presenting

B. Leopold Maneuvers

Determined by abdominal palpitation (Leopold maneuvers; Fig. 40-5).

1. First maneuver (Fig. 40-5*A*)—to determine if fetal head or breech is in uterine fundus. Palpate sides of uterus and fundus. Head feels hard and round, freely movable and ballotable; breech feels large, nodular, softer.
2. Second maneuver (Fig. 40-5*B*)—to determine the position of the fetal extremities, the fetal back, and the anterior shoulder. Place hands on the sides of the abdomen to identify the location of the back and small parts. Palpate down sides of uterus applying gentle but deep pressure. On side of fetal back, a long continuous structure will be felt; side with fetal extremities will feel nodular, reflecting portions of fetal extremities.

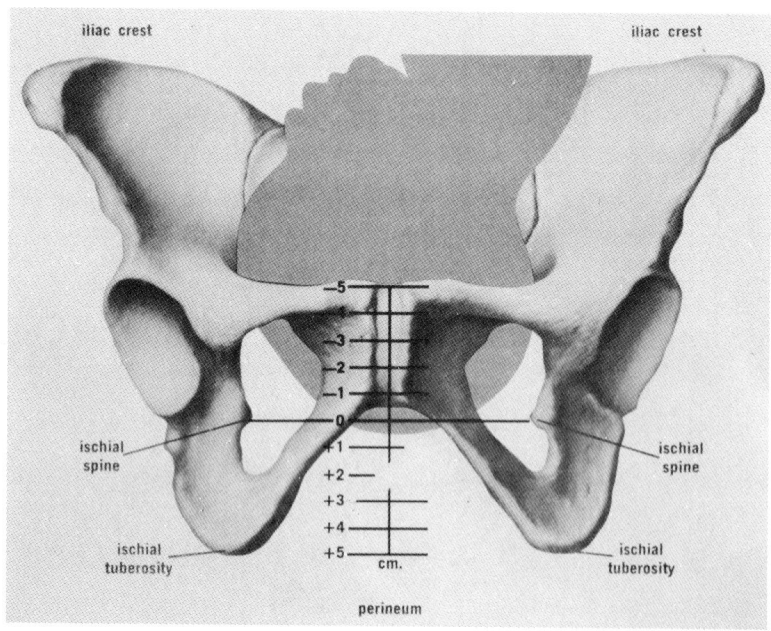

Figure 40-4. *Stations of presenting part. The location of the presenting part in relation to the level of the ischial spines is designated station and indicates the degree of advancement of the presenting part through the pelvis. Stations are expressed in centimeters above (minus) or below (plus) the level of the ischial spines (zero). (Courtesy of Ross Laboratories)*

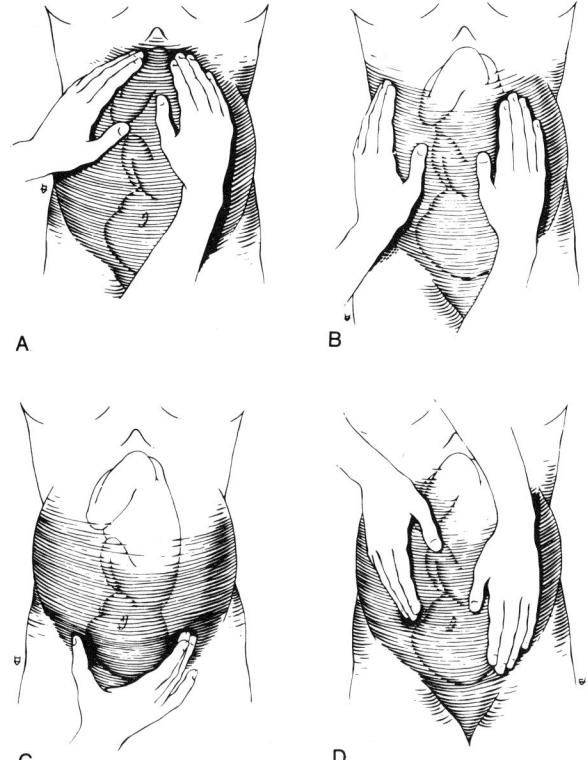

A   B

C   D

Figure 40-5. *Leopold's maneuvers.*

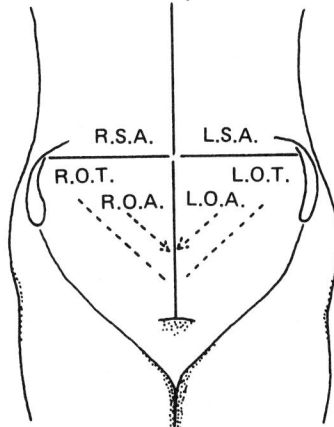

Figure 40-6. *Fetal heart tone locations on the abdominal wall indicating possible corresponding fetal positions and the effects of the internal rotation of the fetus.*

3. Third maneuver (Fig. 40-5*C*)—to determine the portion of the fetus that is presenting and if engagement has occurred. Grasp the lower uterine segment between the thumb and fingers of one hand to feel the presenting part. If presenting part is movable, engagement has not occurred; if engagement has occurred, fetal part feels fixed in the pelvis. The head is at inlet or in pelvis in 90% of women.
4. Fourth maneuver (Fig. 40-5*D*)—to confirm the findings of the third maneuver and to determine the flexion of the vertex. Turn and face the woman's feet. Gently move the fingers down the sides of the uterus. The cephalic prominence is felt on the side where there is greater resistance to the descent of the fingers into the pelvis.

C. Ultrasonography (see p. 979)

D. X-Ray—rarely used today; replaced by ultrasonography

Assessing Fetal Heart Tones

Fetal heart tones are auscultated with a DeLee–Hillis fetoscope, Leffscope, or doptone.
1. Determine the position, presentation, and lie of the fetus by palpation. As internal rotation and descent occur, the location of the fetal heart tones (FHT) changes, swinging gradually from the lateral to the medial area and dropping until immediately before birth, when it is above the pubic bone (Fig. 40-6).
2. Place the fetoscope or doptone on the abdomen over the back or chest of fetus. Avoid friction noises caused by fingers on the abdominal surface area (Fig. 40-7).
3. Differentiate between FHT and other abdominal sounds.
   a. *Fetal heart tone*—a rapid crisp or ticking sound.
   b. *Uterine bruit*—a soft murmur, caused by the passage of blood through dilated uterine vessels; is synchronous with maternal pulse.
   c. *Funic souffle (uterine souffle)*—a hissing sound produced by passage of blood through the umbilical arteries; it is synchronous with the fetal heart rate.
4. Listen and count the rate for 1 full minute; note the location and character when counting.
5. Check the rate before, during, and after a contraction to detect any slowing or irregularities.
6. Check the FHT immediately following the rupture of membranes; a sudden release of fluid may cause a prolapse of the umbilical cord.

Assessing Uterine Contractions

Intensity, frequency, duration:
1. Place fingertips gently on the fundus.
2. As contraction begins, tension will be felt under the fingertips. Uterus will become harder, then slowly soften.
3. The intensity may be described as follows:
   a. Mild—the uterine muscle is somewhat tense.
   b. Moderate—the uterine muscle is moderately firm.
   c. Strong (hard)—the uterine muscle is so firm that it seems almost board-like.
4. The frequency is measured in minutes—represents the time from the beginning of one contraction until the beginning of the next.
5. Duration of a contraction is timed from the moment the uterus first begins to tighten until it relaxes again.
6. As labor progresses, the character of the contractions changes and they last longer.
7. When the cervix becomes completely dilated (the transition stage), the contractions become very strong, last for 60 seconds, and occur at 2–3-minute intervals.

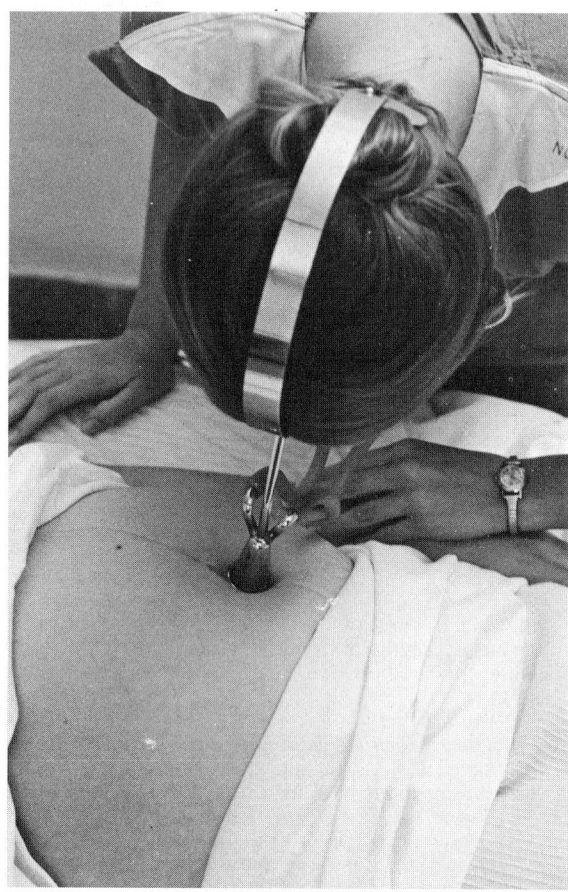

Figure 40-7. Auscultation of the fetal heart beat using the fetoscope.

NURSING ALERT: If any contraction lasts longer than 70 seconds and is not followed by a period of uterine muscle relaxation, notify the attending physician immediately. Uterine rupture and fetal hypoxia may occur.

Vaginal Examination *(Fig. 40-8)*

1. Place the woman in lithotomy position.
2. Conduct examination gently, under aseptic conditions.
3. Evaluate the following:
   a. Condition of cervix
      (1) Hard or soft (in labor cervix is soft)
      (2) Effaced and thin or thick and long (in labor cervix is thin and effaced)
      (3) Easily dilatable or resistant
      (4) Closed or open (dilated); degree of dilation
   b. Presentation
      (1) Breech, cephalic (head), or shoulder
      (2) Caput succedaneum (edema occurring in and under fetal scalp) present (small or large)
      (3) Station identified (see Fig. 40-4): engaged; floating
   c. Position
      (1) Cephalic presentation (identification of the sagittal suture and of its direction)
      (2) Location of posterior fontanelle
   d. Membranes
      (1) Intact
      (2) Ruptured
         (a) Drainage of fluid
         (b) Passage of meconium
      (3) Usually increases frequency and intensity of uterine contractions
      (4) Contraindicated in presence of vaginal bleeding, premature labor, or abnormal fetal presentation or position

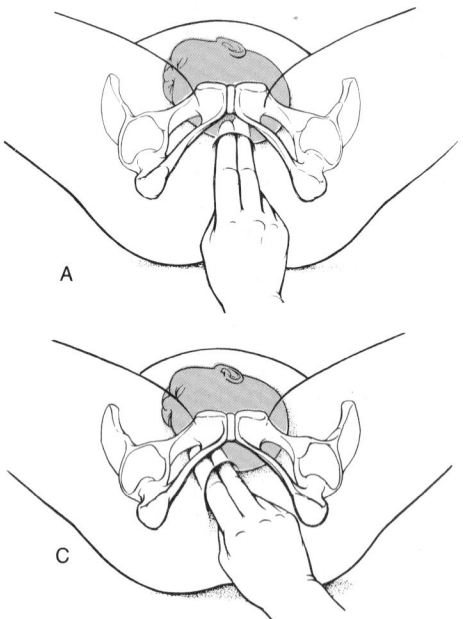

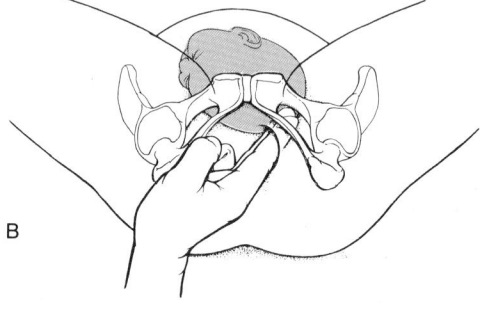

Figure 40-8. Vaginal examination. (A) Determining the station and palpating the sagittal suture. (B) Identifying the posterior fontanelle. (C) Identifying the anterior fontanelle.

Assessing Woman's/Couple's Expectations and Concerns

1. What are their concerns?
2. How anxious are they?
3. What has been their preparation for labor (type, by whom, and when)?
4. What is their understanding of the labor process?
5. What are their expectations of the labor and delivery process (prepared childbirth, anesthesia, analgesics, use of birthing room etc.)?
6. How well are they coping and how well are they communicating with each other?
7. Review written birth plan with the couple.

Fetal Monitoring

Purpose

The purposes of *continuous fetal monitoring* during labor are
1. To monitor the progress of a woman's contraction pattern
2. To monitor the condition of the fetus in response to the stress of uterine contractions

Reactions to Monitoring

Women's reactions to being monitored vary.
1. Some women are reassured by hearing the continuous fetal heart sounds.
2. Some women/couples use the printout of the contraction pattern to assist them in using breathing techniques since they can see when the contraction begins.
3. Some women experience discomfort because of the abdominal straps and their interference with effleurage, as well as difficulty assuming a comfortable position.

External Monitoring (Indirect Monitoring)

Separate transducers are secured to the woman's abdomen: a tokodynamometer (tocotransducer) measures abdominal tension, and an ultrasonic transducer transmits fetal heart sounds into electrical signals that record on a graph chart. The external monitoring of uterine contractions is not accurate for intensity. External monitoring of fetal heart rate is not accurate for variability.
1. The ultrasonic transducer device should be applied over the area of the abdomen where the sharpest fetal heart sound is heard. Lubricate the face of the transducer with a thin layer of ultrasonic gel to aid in the transmission of sounds.
2. The transducer will need to be readjusted when the fetus changes positions.
3. The tokodynamometer recording uterine contractions will need to be reapplied over the fundus as the fetus and uterus descend during labor.

Internal Monitoring (Direct Monitoring)

A method of recording intrauterine pressure and the fetal heart rate (FHR) through internal measurements, this method is more accurate than external monitoring.
1. Fetal electrocardiograph—obtained by screwing a small spiral electrode into the presenting part (the membranes must be ruptured, the cervix dilated at least 2–3 cm., the presenting part must be accessible and identifiable).
2. Uterine contractions are recorded by means of a water-filled catheter placed in the uterine cavity behind the presenting part.
   The catheter is filled with sterile water and is connected to an external pressure transducer that converts the pressure values into mm. Hg on the graph.
3. Monitor strips record the fetal heart and uterine contraction simultaneously.

Interpretation

A. Baseline Rate

1. Fetal heart rate is initially evaluated for the baseline rate.
2. Baseline rate is the FHR when the mother is not in labor, when the fetus is not moving, between contractions, and when the fetus is not being stimulated.
3. Fluctuations in the heart rate are either accelerations or decelerations.

B. Tachycardia

1. A sustained FHR of 160 or more or more than 30 beats/minute above the normal baseline rate.
2. *Etiology*
   Early fetal hypoxia, fetal immaturity, maternal fever, maternal hyperthyroidism, maternal ingestion of parasympatholytic and beta-sympathomimetic drugs, amnionitis, fetal anemia, fetal cardiac arrhythmias, and fetal heart failure.

C. Bradycardia

1. A baseline fetal heart rate below 120.
2. Fetal bradycardia above 90 beats/minute in the third stage of labor is not considered abnormal unless there is a loss of variability.
3. *Etiology*
   Late or profound fetal hypoxia, maternal hypotension, prolonged umbilical cord compression, hypothermia, maternal ingestion of beta-adrenergic blocking drugs, and anesthetics.

D. Variability

1. Beat-to-beat changes in FHR that result for the interplay between the sympathetic and parasympathetic nervous systems.
2. Variability indicates normal neurologic function in relation to heart rate and also fetal reserve.
3. *Short-term variability*—the beat-to-beat change in the FHR.
4. *Long-term variability*—the rhythmic changes in the hear rate, usually 3–5 cycles/minute.
5. Short- and long-term variability tend to increase and decrease together.
6. *Normal variability* is 6–25 beats/minute and is described according to the table below.
7. Overview of FHR variability

Beats/minute	Descriptive Term
0–2	No variability
3–5	Minimal variability
6–10	Average variability
11–25	Moderate variability
>25	Marked variability

E. Periodic FHR Changes

1. Acceleration or deceleration of the FHR are due to stress experienced by the fetus.
2. *Acceleration*—increases in the FHR
   a. *Etiology*—most often fetal movements or fetal stimulation; also seen with breech presentations,

occiput posterior presentations, and uterine contractions.
  b. *Shape*—may or may not resemble the shape of the uterine contraction.
  c. *Recovery*—varies, and if they occur with contractions, they may return to baseline as the uterine pressure decreases.
  d. *Treatment*—none other than observe the tracing for late or variable decelerations later in labor.
3. *Early decelerations*
  a. *Etiology*—head compression from uterine contractions, vaginal examination, scalp stimulation; also frequently seen in women who are completely dilated.
  b. *Shape*—mirror image of the contraction, and all look the same.
  c. *Onset*—early in the contraction, with the peak being at the acme of the contraction.
  d. *Recovery*—returns to baseline by the end of the contraction.
  e. *Treatment*—none.
4. *Late decelerations*
  a. *Etiology*—uteroplacental insufficiency.
  b. *Shape*—uniform in shape with a reverse mirror image of the contraction phase.
  c. *Onset*—late in the contraction, usually after the acme of the contraction with the low point of the deceleration occurring well after the acme.
  d. *Recovery*—returns to baseline after the end of the contraction.
  e. *Treatment*—is aimed at increasing uteroplacental perfusion.
    (1) Includes changing maternal position, with the left lateral being the position of choice, correcting any hypotension through increasing the maintenance intravenous (IV) fluids.
    (2) Oxytocin is stopped.
    (3) Oxygen is administered by face mask at 8–12 liters/minute.
5. *Variable decelerations*
  a. *Etiology*—cord compression that can result from maternal position, prolapsed cord, cord around a fetal part, a short cord, and a true knot in the cord.
  b. *Shape*—variable, and does not follow the uterine contraction; Frequently are shaped like a "U" or "W."
  c. *Onset*—variable, frequently preceded by an acceleration.
  d. *Recovery*—occurs rapidly, often followed by an acceleration.
  e. *Treatment*—involves changing of maternal position, observing that the return occurs quickly and that there is no loss of variability.
6. Combined deceleration patterns do occur and make identification of the patterns difficult.

Nursing Interventions for Fetal Monitoring

1. Provide explanations to the woman and her family; ideally these should be given in the prenatal period during tours of the labor and delivery rooms or by means of films.
  Information should include the following:
  a. Why the monitor is being used and the benefits derived from its use.
  b. What the monitor does and what causes the "bleeps."
  c. How the monitor is applied.
  d. What limitations of movement will be necessary, if any.

2. Provide comfort measures.
  a. Give back rubs.
  b. Assist the woman to change position; changes should be noted on graph since slight variations may occur.
  c. Reposition external monitors.
  d. Assist the woman with general hygiene; she may be concerned about disturbing the attachments.
3. Assist the woman to cope with anxieties and discomfort she may have.
  Use relaxation techniques and comfort measures.

Nursing Diagnoses and Interventions

Nursing Diagnoses

1. Anxiety related to uncertainties/misconceptions of the labor and birthing process, hospital environment, physical stressors, fear for self and baby
2. Pain and discomfort related to uterine contractions, passage of baby through birth canal, possible tearing of perineum
3. Potential for ineffective coping related to length and discomfort of labor process, fatigue, decreased energy
4. Potential for infection related to ruptured membranes
5. Potential complications: blood loss and related effects
6. Alterations in tissue perfusion, related to inadequate placental circulation

Nursing Interventions to Reduce Anxiety

1. Monitor the woman's/couple's concerns.
2. Keep the woman/couple informed of labor progress.
3. Answer questions the couple may have.
4. Explain any procedure and equipment that must be used.
5. Describe hospital policies and procedures.

Interventions During Stages of Labor

First Stage of Labor—Latent Phase *(0–4 cm.)*

A. Monitoring

1. Maternal vital signs as follows:
  a. Temperature, every 4 hours, unless elevated or membranes ruptured, then every 2 hours.
  b. Pulse and respiration every hour.
  c. Blood pressure should be evaluated every hour unless hypertension or hypotension exists, then evaluate more frequently based on findings.
2. Fetal heart rate
  a. If monitor not used, evaluate hourly.
  b. If monitor is used, evaluate the strip at least hourly.
  c. When the membranes rupture, evaluate the FHR immediately and then after each of the next 5 contractions.
3. Urine
  a. Encourage woman to void every hour or two.
  b. Evaluate protein and glucose in urine as indicated.

B. General Comfort Measures

1. Provide clear liquids and ice chips as allowed.
2. Ambulate as tolerated if membranes are not ruptured and the presenting part is engaged. (This may vary according to midwife or physician.)
3. Review birth plan and make any changes that need to be made.

4. Encourage diversional activities such as reading, watching TV, playing cards.

C. Breathing and Pushing Techniques

Review, evaluate, and teach proper techniques.

1. *Early first stage*
   Relax, take 1 deep breath and exhale slowly and completely. Breathe deeply, slowly, rhythmically throughout contraction. Follow with another deep, complete breath.
2. *Late first stage*
   Take 1 deep breath and exhale slowly and completely. Breathe regularly at more shallow level. When stronger contraction occurs, breathe more quickly with very light breaths. Then take deep breath and exhale slowly.
3. *Transition stage*
   Concentrate on breathing in controlled manner. Take a deep breath and exhale slowly and completely. At beginning of contraction, take a fairly deep breath. Then engage in shallow breathing. If there is an urge to push, puff out every 3rd, 4th, or 5th breath. Take deep breath at end of contraction.
4. *Second stage*
   When pushing (as directed), catch breath as needed. Relax pelvic floor and go limp between contractions. During contractions pant and push gently as directed.
5. Involve support person in the woman's care.
   a. Coach during breathing.
   b. Help with timing of contractions.
   c. Provide back massage.
   d. Provide woman with emotional support.
6. Provide privacy for the couple and family.

First Stage of Labor—Active Phase (4–7 cm.)

A. Monitoring

1. Maternal vital signs as follows:
   a. Temperature every 4 hours, unless elevated or membranes ruptured, then every 2 hours.
   b. Blood pressure, pulse, and respirations every 30 minutes.
2. FHR
   a. Evaluated every 30 minutes unless using continuous monitoring.
   b. If intermittent monitoring is used, run a 10-minute strip every hour.

B. Comfort Measures

1. Pain increases, and coping becomes more difficult, especially if the woman is tired. Provide encouragement, and support. Use back rubs and leg rubs, along with breathing and relaxation techniques.
2. Encourage comfortable position—side-lying position is usually more comfortable; removes pressure of uterus on the vena cava and increases blood flow to the placenta.
3. Provide sacral pressure, back rubs, and a backrest.
4. Change damp or soiled linen and clothing.
5. Provide and assist with mouth care.
6. Sponge-bathe face, neck, and back.
7. Provide encouragement and update on progress.
8. Administer prescribed analgesia as needed (Table 40-2).
9. Assist with regional anesthesia if needed.

Table 40-2. *Obstetric Analgesia and Anesthesia*

Method	Comment	Precautions
Obstetric Analgesia		
Prepared childbirth (Read, Lamaze methods)	Requires preparation and psychological support, controlled breathing, voluntary muscle relaxation	Requires commitment of woman and partner and support of obstetric staff
Hypnosis		Requires a willing woman, considerable prenatal training
Narcotics (such as meperidine and pentazocine)	Decrease fear and anxiety, promote physical relaxation and rest between contractions; may cause nausea and vomiting	
Tranquilizers (ataractics)	May be used in combination with narcotics; reduced dose of narcotic required; allay anxiety	
Barbiturates	Given in combination with analgesic; produce sedation and hypnosis	May depress infant for many hours after birth
Trichloroethylene (Trilene)—inhalation anesthetic agent	Usually is self-administered by cannister and face mask	For best results, the woman must be carefully instructed on how to use the equipment Prolonged use may cause confusion and overdose, eliminating protective mechanism; if vomiting occurs, respiratory obstruction and asphyxia may result
General Anesthesia		
Nitrous oxide with oxygen	Administered in low concentrations to allow fetal oxygenation	
Halothane	Produces good uterine relaxation quickly; useful in tetanic contractions; useful for intrauterine manipulations such as removal of retained placenta. Because of its potent relaxant effect, postpartum hemorrhage may be a problem.	
Thiopental (Pentothal sodium)	For rapid induction of anesthesia for cesarean deliveries	
Cyclopropane	Rapid induction and recovery and can be used with high concentrations of oxygen; disadvantage is its flammability; if deep anesthesia is required, can cause fetal and maternal respiratory depression	
Ether	Inexpensive and easy to administer; wide margin of safety; high incidence of nausea and vomiting; irritates respiratory tract	

C. Other Measures

1. Maintain hydration and glucose level of the woman—IV fluids may be needed.
2. Encourage the woman to void every hour or two.

First Stage of Labor—Transitional Phase (7–10 cm.)

A. Monitoring

1. Maternal vital signs as follows:
   a. Temperature—every 4 hours unless elevated or membranes ruptured, then every 2 hours.
   b. Blood pressure, pulse, and respirations—every 15 minutes.
2. FHR and contractions—every 15 minutes, unless using continuous monitoring.

B. Comfort Measures

1. During transition there is a decrease in coping skills; breathing techniques may need to be altered to cope with the increasing intensity of the contractions.
2. Frequently the woman experiences partial amnesia between contractions; she needs to be awakened prior to the beginning of each contraction in order that she may gain control of her breathing.
3. Nausea and vomiting are common
   a. Have an emesis basin ready.
   b. A cool washcloth on the forehead or neck may decrease nausea.
4. Diaphoresis increases—a cool cloth helps to promote comfort during this time, along with change of pads and linens as appropriate.
5. Comfort measures change quickly in the transition phase; during one contraction the woman may want her back rubbed and during the very next contraction may not want anyone to touch her.
   a. Comfort measures are directed by what the woman wants and may include back and leg rubs, cool cloth to face, neck, abdomen or back, ice chips to moisten the mouth
   b. Avoid any unnecessary talk or noise in the room.
6. Rectal pressure is often present during transition, and the women should be encouraged not to push until complete cervical dilatation has occurred.
7. Provide frequent, brief, positive encouragement to both the woman and her support person.
8. Encourage the woman to void so the presenting part will descend quicker.

C. Preparation for Delivery

1. Prepare to move to delivery room, or prepare birthing room for delivery.
   a. The primigravida is usually taken to the delivery room when the fetal head is crowning.
   b. The multigravida is taken earlier depending on fetal size and speed of fetal descent.
2. If the woman is moved to the delivery room, place all side rails up prior to moving, and move from the bed to the delivery table between contractions.

Second Stage of Labor

(From complete dilation of cervix to birth of the infant)

A. Monitoring

1. Maternal vital signs as follows:
   a. Blood pressure—every 5 minutes
   b. Pulse and respirations—every 15–30 minutes.
2. FHT and contractions
   a. Evaluated every 5 minutes.

   b. Some fetal bradycardia and early decelerations may occur due to head compression.
   c. Normally there is no loss of variability during the second stage.
   d. Contractions are still hard, but may space out some in frequency.

B. Comfort Measures

Assist the woman to a comfortable pushing position. (This may include left lateral position, squatting position, semi-Fowler's, or sitting.)
1. Having the woman pull her legs back will open up the birth canal.
2. If the woman is placed in a lithotomy position, place both legs in the stirrups at the same time to avoid ligament strain, backache, or injury.

C. Pushing Technique

Coach the woman and her support person on correct pushing technique. Use the abdominal muscles, push with the contractions, and take breaths every 10–20 seconds during pushing.

D. Other Measures Immediately Preceding Delivery

1. When delivery is near, place the mirror where both the coach and mother can see the presenting head.
2. Cleanse the vulva and perineal areas, cleanse from the mons to the lower abdomen, then the groin to the inner thigh of each side and then each labia, and finally the introitus.
3. Place equipment according to hospital policy.
4. Make sure infant resuscitation equipment is available, gather equipment for newborn care.
5. Evaluate bladder fullness—if full, catheterize.

E. Measures During Delivery

1. When the fetal head is encircled by the vulvovaginal ring, an episiotomy may be performed to prevent tearing.
2. When the head is delivered, mucus is wiped from the face and the mouth and nose are aspirated with a bulb syringe.
3. If loops of umbilical cord are found around the infant's neck, they are loosened and slipped from around the neck. If the cord cannot be slipped over the head, it is clamped with two clamps and cut between the two clamps.
4. Following this step the woman is asked to give a gentle push in order that the infant's body may be quickly delivered.
5. After delivery of the infant's body and cutting of the cord, the infant is shown to the parents and then placed on the maternal abdomen, or taken to the radiant warmer for inspection and identification procedures.

Third Stage of Labor (Placental Expulsion Stage)

Following the birth of the baby the uterus continues to contract and relax until the placenta is expelled.

A. Signs of Placental Separation

1. The uterus rises upward in the abdomen
2. The umbilical cord lengthens
3. Trickle or spurt of blood appears.
4. The uterus becomes globular in shape.

B. Placental Delivery

1. Following the signs of placental separation, the woman is usually asked to bear down gently, or fundal pressure may be applied to facilitate delivery of the placenta (Fig 40-9)

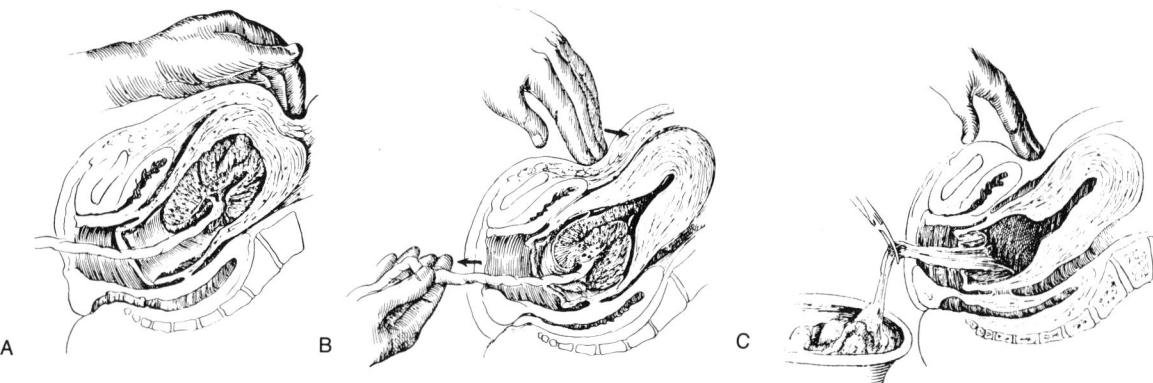

Figure 40-9. *Delivery of the placenta. (From Willson JR. Atlas of Obstetric Technic. 2nd ed. St. Louis, CV Mosby)*

2. This stage usually lasts 5–10 minutes; its maximum length is 30 minutes.
3. Following placental delivery, the placenta is evaluated for size, shape, and implantation of the cord site. The placenta and membranes are checked to see that they are complete.
4. The vagina and cervix are inspected for lacerations; any repairs are made at this time.

Fourth Stage of Labor

(From placental separation until postpartum condition is stable)

A. Monitoring
1. Maternal vital signs are taken as follows:
   a. Blood pressure, pulse, and respirations are taken every 15 minutes for the first 2 hours.
   b. Temperature is taken every 4 hours unless elevated.
2. Postpartum assessment also includes (1) the uterine fundus, (2) lochia (type and amount), and (3) perineal area for any edema, discoloration, or hematoma formation.
3. The episiotomy is evaluated for intactness and bleeding—every 15 minutes for the first 2 hours.
4. Maternal interaction with the newborn and family members is also evaluated.
5. Bladder and uterus are assessed—bladder distention can cause the uterus to be relaxed and displaced to the side.
6. Sensation is evaluated—the effects of anesthesia (if anesthetic agent used) are also evaluated.

B. Comfort Measures
1. If an episiotomy has been performed, or if there was perineal tearing, a covered ice bag can be applied to the perineal area.
2. Tremors are common during this time; a warm blanket often helps the woman feel better.
3. Privacy should be provided for the new family.
4. Partial bath and perineal care, with linen and pad changes, also help the woman feel better.
5. Allow for rest periods between the 15-minute checks.

Expected Outcomes

1. Manages anxiety and fear; pulse and blood pressure are within normal levels.
2. Copes with pain; utilizes breathing and relaxation techniques adequately in relation to contractions; fo-

cuses on just one contraction at a time; works with the labor process; does not fight the contractions; relaxes between contractions.
3. Remains in control; interacts with support person and health professionals; asks questions about progress of labor; listens to teaching and attempts to follow instructions.
4. Absence of untoward bleeding, vital signs within normal range.
5. No evidence of infection.

Immediate Care of the Newborn

The sequence of procedures may differ from one birth setting to another. In more traditional settings, the care is performed immediately after birth. In other settings, many aspects are performed after the parents have had an hour or more to become acquainted with their newborn.

Assessment and Interventions

A. Immediate Care
1. Immediately after delivery, dry the infant—a wet, small newborn loses up to 200 calories/kg./minute in the delivery room through evaporation, convection, and radiation. Drying the infant cuts this heat loss in half.
2. Aspirate mucus from the mouth and pharynx with suction catheter

B. Apgar Score
Evaluate infant's condition by Apgar scoring system (Table 40-3) at 1 and 5 minutes after birth.
1. Infants scoring 7–10 are free of immediate stress.
2. Infants scoring 4–6 are moderately depressed.
3. Infants scoring 0–3 are severely depressed.

C. Cord Care
1. The cord is clamped approximately 2.5 cm. (1 inch) from the abdominal wall with a plastic or metal cord clamp.
2. Count the number of vessels in the cord—fewer than 3 vessels have been associated with renal and cardiac anomalies.

D. Eye Care
1. Prophylactic treatment against ophthalmia neonatorum (gonorrheal or chlamydial) is mandatory in all states.
2. Treatment may be with an antibiotic ophthalmic oint-

Table 40-3. *Apgar Scoring Chart*

Sign	0	1	2
Heart rate	Absent	Slow (less than 100)	Over 100
Respiratory effort	Absent	Slow, irregular	Good, crying
Muscle tone	Flaccid	Some flexion of extremities	Active motion
Reflex irritability	No response	Cry	Vigorous cry
Color	Blue, pale	Body pink, extremities blue	Completely pink

ment such as erythromycin, tetracycline, or penicillin or with silver nitrate drops.

3. If the mother has a positive gonococcal or chlamydial culture, the baby will require further treatment.

E. Vitamin K

1. A prophylactic injection is given to prevent a neonatal hemorrhage during the first few days of life prior to the infant beginning to produce its own vitamin K.
2. There is some controversy over the routine administration in a nontraumatic birth, since it may predispose the infant to hyperbilirubinemia.

F. Identification

1. Identification bands or bracelets are placed on the infant's arms or legs.
2. Information includes: the mother's name, hospital number, infant's sex, race, and date and time of birth.
3. A similar bracelet is also placed on the mother.
4. Fingerprints of the mother and footprints of the infant also may be done. If footprints are to be done, remove all vernix from the foot prior to inking to improve the quality of the footprint.
5. All identification procedures are completed prior to the infant leaving the delivery room.

G. Other Assessment Measures

1. Weigh and measure the infant.
2. Assess the general well-being of the infant.

Newborn Resuscitation

This procedure is most effective when there is a simple, organized, and efficient system established in the birth area.

Goals

1. To maintain adequate oxygenation and ventilation.
2. To maintain adequate tissue perfusion through adequate cardiac output.
3. To maintain a normal body temperature.

Causes

Asphyxia is the main reason for newborn resuscitation.

A. Primary Apnea

1. Intrauterine asphyxia may result in passage of meconium, fetal tachycardia, loss of variability, late decelerations, or prolonged bradycardia.
2. Infants born with primary apnea will need sensory stimuli (tactile or positive-pressure ventilation) to initiate respirations.

B. Secondary Apnea

1. Secondary apnea occurs when primary apnea is unresolved. The heart rate drops and spontaneous gasps occur.

2. May occur in utero or following birth.
3. At birth these infants are pale, flaccid and bradycardic. Spontaneous respirations will not occur with sensory stimuli because of the biochemical, neurologic, and circulatory changes that have occurred.

Steps in Newborn Resuscitation

1. Place the infant in a warm radiant warmer in a Trendelenburg position.
2. Suction the nose and mouth with a bulb syringe or wall suction.
3. Dry off the trunk with warmed towels and attempt to keep the infant warm.
4. Assess respiratory and cardiac status.
5. Begin bag and mask ventilation.
   a. Use an inspiratory pressure of 20–30 cm. H_2O at a rate of 30–40 breaths/minute.
   b. Observe chest movement and auscultate for air-movement in all lung fields.
6. If needed, begin external cardiac massage at a rate of 100–120 compressions/minute.
7. Endotracheal intubation may be needed.
8. An umbilical venous line may be inserted for administration of medications and fluids.
9. Transport when stable.

Emergency Delivery

In delivery under emergency conditions, consider the woman and infant as a unit; work to prevent infection, injury, and hemorrhage in woman and infant and to establish respirations in the newborn.

Interventions

1. Have the woman assume a lithotomy position.
2. If time permits, the person attending the delivery should wash his/her hands and cleanse the mother's perineum.
3. Using a clean or sterile towel, exert gentle pressure against the head of the fetus to control its progress and prevent too rapid a delivery.
   a. Prevents undue stretching of the perineum
   b. Prevents sudden expulsion through the vulva with subsequent infant and maternal complications
4. Encourage the woman to pant at this time to prevent bearing down.
5. If membranes have not ruptured by the time the head is delivered, they must be removed immediately by tearing them at the nape of the infant's neck.
6. Wipe the infant's face and mouth with a clean towel. Suction the nose and mouth with a bulb syringe if available.
7. If the cord is looped around the infant's neck, gently slip it over the head. If the cord is too tight to permit

this, it must be clamped in 2 places and cut between the clamps before the rest of the body is delivered.

8. Holding the infant's head in both hands, gently exert downward pressure toward the floor, thus slipping the anterior shoulder under the symphysis pubis.
9. Support the infant's body and head as it is born.
10. Pick up the infant gently by feet, with head down to help drain mucus; wipe away excess mucus from mouth and nose; gentle rubbing of the back may stimulate breathing.
11. After the infant cries, place him gently on mother's abdomen where she can see him.
12. Avoid touching perineal area to prevent infection.
13. Avoid pulling on cord, which might break and cause hemorrhage.
14. Watch for signs of placental separation.
15. When placenta is delivered, do the following:
    a. Clamp cord with surgical clamp when cord stops pulsating. If clamp is not available, tie off cord with any suitable material several centimeters from the infant's abdomen
    b. Do not cut cord; the physician or midwife will cut it later under more sterile conditions.
    c. Wrap the infant and placenta in a blanket; keep the infant warm and close to the mother.
16. Check fundal contractions; massage if indicated. Putting the baby to breast may help the uterus to contract.
17. Place identification of some kind on mother and infant.
18. Give the woman fluids.
19. If the woman is not in bed or a place where she can lie down, she should be assisted to move to a more suitable environment.
20. Do not leave the woman alone.
21. Teach the woman to massage her fundus; explain why the cord has not been cut.
22. Record the time and date of birth.

Childbirth Approaches

Prepared Childbirth

In the past, the term *natural childbirth* was used to describe one approach to giving birth. To some, natural childbirth meant delivery without analgesic or anesthesia, whereas to those who had developed the approach it simply meant being prepared for childbirth through prenatal education and training. This preparation gave the woman a method of coping with the discomforts of labor and delivery. To avoid the suggestion that analgesia or anesthesia is unavailable to the woman during labor and delivery should she need it, the term "*prepared childbirth*" is now used instead of natural childbirth.

Method of Grantly Dick-Read

1. This method is based on the idea that fear and anticipation of pain arouse natural protective tensions in the body, both psychic and muscular.
2. Fear stimulates the sympathetic nervous system and causes the circular muscle of the cervix to contract.
3. The longitudinal muscles of the uterus then have to act against increased cervical resistance, causing tension and pain.
4. Tension and pain aggravate fear, which produces a vicious cycle of tension, pain, and fear.
5. A minor degree of pain, magnified by fear, becomes unbearable.

6. According to Dick-Read, prenatal courses and training reduce fear, overcome ignorance, and build a woman's self-confidence. Included in this method are:
    a. Explanations of fetal development and childbirth
    b. Descriptions of methods available to relieve pain
    c. Exercises that strengthen certain muscles and relax others
    d. Breathing techniques that will enable the woman to relax in the first stage of labor and work effectively with muscles used during delivery
    e. Explanations of the value of improved physical health and emotional stability for childbirth
    f. The woman is not told that labor and delivery will be painless; analgesia and anesthesia are available if needed or desired
    g. The woman is given empathetic understanding and support during labor by her partner, the nurse, and the physician

Psychoprophylactic or Lamaze Method

1. Psychoprophylactic childbirth has a rationale based on Pavlov's concept of pain perception and his theory of conditioned reflexes (the substitution of favorable conditioned reflexes for unfavorable ones). The Lamaze method is an example of this technique.
2. The woman is taught to replace responses of restlessness, fear, and the loss of control with more useful activity. A high level of activity can excite the cerebral cortex efficiently to inhibit other stimuli, such as pain in labor.
3. The mother-to-be is taught exercises that strengthen the abdominal muscles and relax the perineum.
4. Breathing techniques to help the process of labor are practiced.
5. The woman is conditioned to respond with respiratory activity and disassociation or relaxation of the uninvolved muscles, while controlling her perception of the stimuli associated with labor.
6. One method of control consists of breathing normally while silently mouthing the words to a song and simultaneously tapping the rhythm with the fingers.
7. Similarity between the Dick-Read and Lamaze methods:
    a. Fear, which enhances the perception of pain, may diminish or disappear when the woman understands the physiology of labor.
    b. Since psychic tension enhances perception of pain, relaxation is achieved more easily in a calm, agreeable atmosphere with supportive persons nearby.
    c. Muscular relaxation and a specific type of breathing diminish or abolish the pains of labor.

The Leboyer Method of Delivery

1. The *Leboyer method* is based on the premise that the infant suffers psychological shock at the time of delivery. An effort is made to reduce the contrast between the intrauterine environment and the outside world.
2. Gentle, controlled delivery—prenatal education, support from family and personnel to decrease anxiety, fear, and tension.
3. Emphasis on providing protection to the craniosacral axis by gently supporting the newborn infant's head, neck, and sacrum. The craniosacral axis is completely relaxed, and lost body heat restored in a warm water bath.
4. Avoiding overstimulation of the newborn sensorium—the infant is allowed to breathe spontaneously; cutting

the cord is delayed to permit placental blood transfusion for improved respiration.

5. Importance of maternal–infant bond—skin-to-skin contact with mother is provided, and infant is fondled and stroked.

Home Delivery

1. *Home delivery,* although controversial, has won increasing support in recent years.
2. Motivations for home delivery:
   a. Belief that home birth has significant advantages for the family and the newborn infant.
   b. Objection to the impersonal and authoritarian atmosphere of the hospital environment with enforced separation of woman and family.
   c. Desire to avoid such practices as routine cesarean delivery for breech presentation, episiotomy, forceps delivery, oxytocin stimulation, routine monitoring of the FHT, and other practices associated with hospitals.
   d. Risk of in-hospital infections; belief that infant is immune to own-home bacteria.
   e. Rising costs of hospitalization.
3. Contraindications
   a. High-risk indications for infant or mother.
   b. Patient with history of premature or postdate delivery in previous pregnancy.
   c. Woman with medical or emotional complications.
   d. Patient who cannot be quickly transported to a hospital.
4. Alternatives
   a. Alteration of hospital setting to a family-centered approach.
   b. Birthing centers for low-risk women with adequate facilities for emergency care.
   c. Properly educated and motivated support personnel.

Bibliography

Books

Bobak I, Jensen M and Zalar M. Maternity and Gynecologic Care. 3rd ed. St. Louis, CV Mosby, 1989

Cunningham F, MacDonald P and Gant N. Williams Obstetrics. 17th ed. Norwalk, CT, Appleton and Lange, 1989

Dickason EJ, Schulte M and Silverman B. Maternal–Infant Nursing Care. Philadelphia, JB Lippincott, 1990

Doenges M, Kenty J and Moorehouse M. Maternal/Newborn Care Plans: Guidelines for Client Care. Philadelphia, FA Davis, 1988

Gorrie TM. A Guide to the Nursing of Childbearing Families. Baltimore, Williams & Wilkins, 1989

Houldin A, Saltstein S and Ganley K. Nursing Diagnoses for Wellness Supporting Strength. Philadelphia, JB Lippincott, 1987

Malinowski J, Pedigo C and Phillips C. Nursing Care During the Labor Process. 3rd ed. Philadelphia, FA Davis, 1989

Murray M. Antepartal and Intrapartal Fetal Monitoring. Washington DC, NAACOG, 1988

Neeson J. Clinical Manual of Maternity Nursing. Philadelphia, JB Lippincott, 1987

Olds S, London M and Ladewig P. Maternal Newborn Nursing: A Family-Centered Approach. 3rd ed. Menlo Park, CA, Addison–Wesley, 1988

Reeder S and Martin L. Maternity Nursing. 16th ed. Philadelphia, JB Lippincott, 1987

Tucker S. Pocket Guide to Fetal Monitoring. St. Louis, CV Mosby, 1988

Journals

Crowe K and von Baeyer C. Predictors of a positive childbirth experience. Birth 1989; 16:59–63

Day T. Community use of paracervical block in labor. J Fam Pract 1989; 28: 545–550

Devoe L et al. Monitoring intrauterine pressure during active labor. A prospective comparison of two methods. J Reprod Med 1989; 34:811–814

Duchene P. Using biofeedback to ease the pain of childbirth. Am J Nurs 1989; 89:1070B–1070D

Fukushima T et al. A beltless tocodynamometer—a preliminary report. Obstet Gynecol 1989; 73:823

Galvan B et al. Using amnioinfusion for the relief of repetitive variable decelerations during labor. J Obstet Gynecol Neonatal Nurs 1989; 18:222–229

Geden F et al. Effects of music and imagery on physiologic and self-respect of analogued labor pain. Nursing Research 1989; 38:37–41

Harvey C. Interpreting the electronic fetal monitor: Strategies for management. J Nurse Midwif 1989; 34(2):75–84

Hodnett E and Osborn R. Effects of continuous intrapartum professional support on childbirth outcomes. Res Nurs Health 1989; 12:289–297

Holland R and Smith D. Management of the second stage of labor: A review. SD J Med 1989; 42(5):11–14

Johnson G et al. Alteration of maternal posture and its immediate effect on epidural pressure. Anaesthesia 1989; 44:750–752

Killien M and Shy K. A randomized trial of electronic fetal monitoring in preterm labor: Mother's views. Birth 1989; 16(1):7–12

Kilpatrick S and Laros R. Characteristics of normal labor. Obstet Gynecol 1989; 74:85–87

Knorr L. Relieving fetal distress with amnioinfusion. MCN 1989; 14:346–350

Lazebnik N et al. Intravenous, deltoid or gluteus administration of meperdine during labor. Am J Obstet Gynecol 1989; 160:1184–1189

Luiu Y. The effects of the upright position during childbirth. Image 1989; 21:13–18

Mansouri H et al. Relationship between fetal heart rate and umbilical blood flow velocity in term human fetuses during labor. Am J Obstet Gynecol 1989; 160:1007–1012

Newton E. The fetus as a patient. Med Clin North Am 1989; 73:517–540

Nicholson C and Ridolfo E. Avoiding the pitfalls of epidural anesthesia in obstetrics. J Am Assoc Nurse Anesth 1989; 57:220–230

Rayburn W et al. Randomized comparison of meperidine and fentanyl during labor. Obstet Gynecol 1989; 74:604–606

Reddy V and Careny J. Effect of umbilical vein oxytocin on puerperal blood loss and length of third stage of labor. Am J Obstet Gynecol 1989; 160:206–208

Roberts J. Managing fetal bradycardia during second stage of labor. MCN 1989; 14:394–398

Sequin et al. The components of women's satisfaction with maternity care. Birth 1989; 16:109–113

Sleutel M. An overview of vibroacoustic stimulation. J Obstet Gynecol Neonat Nurs 1989; 18:447–452

Strong T and Paul R. Intrapartum uterine activity evaluation of an intrauterine pressure transducer. Obstet Gynecol 1989; 73:431–434

Varrassi G et al. Effects of physical activity on maternal plasma beta-endorphin levels and perception of labor pain. Am J Obstet Gynecol 1989; 160:707–712

Wuitchik M et al. The clinical significance of pain and cognitive activity in latent labor. Obstet Gynecol 1989; 73:35–42

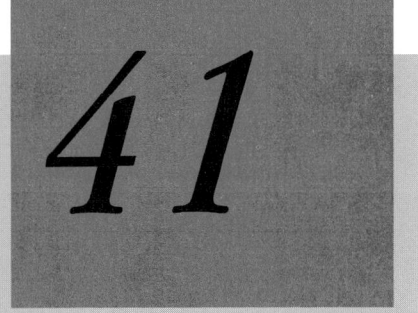

Care of the Mother and Newborn During the Postpartum Period

The Puerperium

Physiologic Changes of the Puerperium

The *puerperium* is the period beginning after delivery and ending when the woman's body has returned as closely as possible to its prepregnant state. The period lasts approximately 6 weeks.

1. Uterine changes
   a. The fundus is usually midline and about at the level of the woman's umbilicus after delivery. Within 12 hours of delivery the fundus may be 1 cm. above the umbilicus. After this, the level of the fundus descends about 1 finger breadth (or 1 cm.) each day until, by the 10th day, it has descended into the pelvic cavity and can no longer be palpated.
   b. Postdelivery, *lochia* (a vaginal discharge), consisting of fatty epithelial cells, shreds of membrane, decidua, and blood, is red (*lochia rubra*) for about 2–3 days. It then progresses to a paler or more brownish color (*lochia serosa*), followed by a whitish or yellowish color (*lochia alba*) in the 7th to 10th day. Lochia usually ceases by 3 weeks and the placental site is completely healed by the 6th week.
2. The vaginal walls, uterine ligaments, and muscles of the pelvic floor and abdominal wall regain most of their tone during the puerperium.
3. Postpartum diuresis occurs between the 2nd and 5th postpartum days, as extracellular water accumulated during pregnancy begins to be excreted. A diuresis may also occur shortly after delivery if urinary output was obstructed because of the pressure of the presenting part or if intravenous fluids were given to the woman during labor.
4. Breasts
   a. With loss of the placenta, circulating levels of estrogen and progesterone decrease while levels of prolactin increase, thus initiating lactation in the postpartum woman.
   b. *Colostrum,* a yellowish fluid containing more minerals and protein but less sugar and fat than mature breast milk and having a laxative effect on the infant, is secreted for the first 2 days postpartum.
   c. Mature milk secretion is usually present by the 3rd postpartum day but may be present earlier if a woman breast-feeds immediately following delivery.
   d. Breast engorgement with milk, venous and lymphatic stasis, and swollen, tense, and tender breast tissue may occur between days 3 and 5 postpartum.

Emotional and Behavioral Status

1. Following delivery, the woman may progress through Rubin's stages of "taking in" and "taking hold."
   a. "Taking in"
      (1) May begin with a refreshing sleep following delivery
      (2) Woman exhibits passive, dependent behavior
      (3) Woman is concerned with sleep and the intake of food, both for herself and for the infant
   b. "Taking hold"
      (1) Woman begins to initiate action and to function more independently
      (2) Woman may require more explanation and reassurance that she is functioning well, especially in caring for her infant
      (3) As the woman meets success in caring for the newborn, her concern extends to other family members and their activities
2. Some women may experience a euphoria in the first few days following delivery and set unrealistic goals for activities following discharge from the birthing place.
3. Many women may experience temporary mood swings during this period because of the discomfort, fatigue, and exhaustion following labor and delivery and because of hormonal changes following delivery.
4. Some mothers may experience "postpartum blues" about the third postpartum day and exhibit irritability, poor appetite, insomnia, tearfulness, or crying. This is a temporary situation. Severe or prolonged depression is usually a sign of a more serious condition.
5. Nursing research findings indicate that new mothers identified the following postpartum needs: Coping with
   a. The physical changes and discomforts of the puerperium, including a need to regain their prepregnancy figure.
   b. Changing family relationships and meeting the needs of family members including the infant.
   c. Fatigue, emotional stress, feelings of isolation, and being "tied down."
   d. A lack of time for personal needs and interests.

Immediate Postpartum Assessment

The first hour after delivery of the placenta ("4th stage of labor") is a critical period; postpartum hemorrhage is most likely to occur at this time.

1. Check fundus frequently and massage gently if fundus is not firm.
2. Inspect perineum frequently for visible signs of bleeding.
3. Evaluate vital signs at frequent intervals as determined by the woman's condition.
4. Assess bladder. Birth trauma, anesthesia, and pain from lacerations and episiotomy may reduce or alter the voiding reflex. Bladder distention may displace the uterus upward and to the side.
5. Avoid leaving the woman alone at this time since changes in condition can occur precipitously.

Subsequent Postpartum Assessment

1. Check firmness of the fundus at regular intervals.
2. Inspect the perineum regularly for frank bleeding.
   a. Note color, amount, and odor of the lochia (perineal discharge).
   b. Count the number of perineal pads that are saturated in each 8-hour period.
3. Assess vital signs at least once daily and more frequently if indicated.
4. Assess for bowel and bladder elimination.
5. Evaluate interaction and care skills of mother and family with infant.
6. Assess for breast engorgement and condition of nipples if breast-feeding.
7. Inspect legs for signs of thromboembolism, and assess Homans' sign.
8. Assess incisions for signs of infection and healing.

Patient Problems and Nursing Diagnoses

1. Potential complication: bleeding, related to vaginal delivery, uterine atony, cesarean delivery, episiotomy
2. Altered comfort (backache, uterine cramping, breast engorgement, edema of episiotomy, hemorrhoids) related to process of labor and delivery
3. Urinary retention related to bladder trauma
4. Constipation related to decrease in muscle tone of intestines, lack of food and fluid during labor, perineal tenderness, episiotomy, hemorrhoids
5. Infection related to prolonged labor, vaginal delivery, lacerations, anemia, inadequate hygiene
6. Knowledge deficit related to inadequate childbirth/parenting preparation, lack of self-confidence
7. Impaired maternal–infant bonding related to age of mother, marital status, socioeconomic factors, separation from infant
8. Anxiety related to inability to integrate labor experience, adapting to new family member, chronic fatigue, lack of experience with infant care
9. Positive adaptation could be identified as: adequate knowledge of self and infant care, related to previous teaching, experience, and exposure to infants; adequate family coping, related to integration of infant into family unit.

Nursing Interventions:
Immediate Postdelivery Care

A. First Hour After Delivery (4th Stage of Labor)

1. Provide a quiet environment for the woman and family to promote as much rest as possible
2. Evaluate the woman's vital signs every 15 minutes or less frequently, depending on her condition.
3. Evaluate fundal height and position when checking vital signs. Height should be at the umbilicus or below, and at the midline.
   a. If uterus is displaced to right or left, the woman's bladder may be full.
   b. If fundus is not firm, massage gently and express clots that may be collecting in the uterine cavity.
   c. Teach the woman to feel her fundus and explain the reasons for your actions as you proceed.
4. Inspect perineum for signs of bleeding, including hematoma formation. An ice pack on the perineum will promote comfort and help to reduce swelling of the tissue.
5. Evaluate the amount of vaginal bleeding.

Scant	Only blood on tissue when wiped, or less than 1-inch stain on peripad within 1 hour.
Small/Light	Less than 4-inch stain on peripad within 1 hour.
Moderate	Less than 6-inch stain on peripad within 1 hour.
Heavy	Saturated peripad within 1 hour.

Nursing Interventions:
Subsequent Postpartum Care

A. General Measures

1. Minimize interruptions; promote a quiet environment to allow frequent rest periods for the woman.
2. Assess height and firmness of the fundus and vital signs once daily or more frequently if indicated.
3. Inspect the woman's perineum daily for healing and signs of bleeding or infection.
4. Evaluate breasts daily.
5. Evaluate mother–infant interaction and interaction with other family members.
6. If a patient is Rh negative, evaluate the need for RhoGam. If indicated, administer the RhoGam within 72 hours of delivery.
7. If the woman is not rubella immune, a rubella vaccination may be given, and pregnancy must be avoided at least 3 months.

B. Perineal Care

1. Teach the woman to carry out perineal care—warm water over the perineum after each voiding and/or bowel movement and routinely several times a day to promote comfort, cleanliness, and healing.
2. Sitz baths may be used for the same purpose.
3. Teach the woman to apply perineal pads by touching the outside only, thus keeping clean the portion that will touch her perineum.
4. Teach the woman to use witch hazel compresses or anesthetic sprays or ointments for relief of perineal discomfort.
5. Teach the woman to contract her buttocks before sitting to reduce perineal discomfort while sitting in a chair.

C. Voiding

1. Check the woman's voiding pattern. Most women void in sufficient amounts within 8 hours of delivery.
2. If the woman's meatus or bladder has been traumatized during delivery, she may need to be catheterized until the urinary tract swelling has subsided.
3. Teach the woman to void every several hours to keep her bladder empty. This may help reduce uterine cramping and promote comfort.

D. Breast Care

1. Assess the condition of the woman's breasts and nipples. Inspect nipples for reddening, erosions, or fis-

sures. Reddened areas may be improved with A & D ointment, a lanolin cream, and air drying for 15 minutes several times a day.

2. Teach the woman to wash her breasts with warm water and NO soap—prevents the removal of the protective skin oils.

3. Teach the woman to wear a brassiere or breast binder that provides good support night and day.

4. Lactation suppressants such as bromocriptine mesylate may be given to bottle-feeding mothers to suppress milk production and breast engorgement.

> **NURSING ALERT: Patient education**—Bromocriptine mesylate (Parlodel) may increase fertility, so a form of contraception should be used when sexual activity is resumed.

5. Check the breasts for signs of engorgement (swollen, tender, tense, shiny breast tissue).
   a. If breasts are engorged and the woman is breast-feeding:
      (1) Allow warm to hot shower water to flow over the breasts to improve comfort.
      (2) Hot compresses on the breasts may improve comfort.
      (3) Express some milk manually or by breast pump to improve comfort and make nipple more available for infant feeding.
      (4) Nurse the infant.
      (5) A mild analgesic may be used to improve comfort.
   b. If breasts are engorged and the mother is bottle-feeding:
      (1) Teach the woman to wear a supportive breast binder night and day.
      (2) Teach the woman to avoid handling her breasts since this stimulates more milk production.
      (3) Suggest ice bags to the breasts to provide comfort.
      (4) Moderately strong analgesics may be needed to provide comfort.

E. Diet and Elimination

1. Review the woman's dietary intake with her.
2. Emphasize foods high in iron, protein, and vitamins to aid the healing process. Foods such as fresh fruits and vegetables with high fiber will help reestablish normal bowel habits.
3. Remind the woman that not all of her weight gain during pregnancy was lost at delivery; approximately 5 lb. will be lost during the puerperium.
4. If the woman is breast-feeding, she should add between 500 and 900 additional calories daily for milk production. She also needs 20 gm. more protein than before she was pregnant, and additional calcium, phosphorus, vitamins D, A, C, E, B_1 and B_2, niacin, zinc, and iodine.
5. Bowel activity is sluggish because of decreased abdominal muscle tone, anesthetic effects, effects of progesterone, decreased solid food intake during labor, and prelabor diarrhea.
6. Hemorrhoids and episiotomy and laceration pain may cause the woman to delay her first bowel movement.
7. Promoting frequent ambulation, ensuring adequate fluid intake, and providing a diet with fresh fruits and fiber encourage regular bowel elimination.

F. Exercise

1. Review postpartum exercises aimed at regaining muscle tone and body shape and promoting comfort (see Postpartum Exercises, p. 1004).

G. Rest and Ambulation

1. Most mothers ambulate within 8–12 hours after delivery or sooner.
2. When assisting the woman to ambulate for the first time, have her sit on the edge of the bed for 5 minutes, then ambulate only with assistance to avoid falling because of dizziness and fainting.
3. Counsel the woman to rest for at least 30 minutes after she arrives home from the hospital and to rest several times during the day for the first few weeks.
4. Counsel the woman to confine her activities to one floor if possible and avoid stair climbing as much as possible for the first several days at home.

H. Resumption of Sex

1. Intercourse may be resumed when perineal and uterine wounds have healed.
2. Healing occurs within 2–4 weeks; however, evaluation by the midwife or physician during the follow-up visit is necessary. Methods of contraception should be reviewed.
3. For women who are bottle-feeding, menstruation usually returns within 4–8 weeks.
4. For women who are breast-feeding, menstruation usually returns within 4 months, but may return between 2 and 18 months postpartum.

> **NURSING ALERT: Patient Education**—Nursing mothers may ovulate even if experiencing amenorrhea, and so a form of contraception should be used if pregnancy is to be avoided.

I. Personal Needs

1. Counsel the woman to provide quiet times for herself at home and help her establish realistic goals for resuming her own interests and activities.
2. Counsel the couple to provide times to reestablish their own relationship and to renew their social interests and relationships.

Expected Outcomes

1. Absence of untoward bleeding; uterus firm; decreasing color and amount of lochia; normal vital signs; normal hematocrit values; level of fundus at normal position; no clots/tissues passed vaginally
2. Reports decrease in discomfort; able to care for self and infant
3. Voids freely and without discomfort
4. Lack of constipation; eats high-fiber foods and uses stool softeners
5. Absence of infection; normal vital signs and laboratory values; no abnormal redness of perineum; no purulent discharge nor foul odor of lochia, no urinary complaints, no pain or swelling in legs
6. Demonstrates ability to perform infant care; shows confidence in caring for infant
7. Shows maternal–child bonding—maintains eye contact; calls infant by name; talks to infant; strokes infant and holds him close between feedings; shows she is moving into "taking hold" phase; participates in daily care of infant

8. Verbalizes diminishing anxiety; talks about labor and delivery experience; discusses infant's schedule; making plans for household help and for renewing some social activities

Postpartum Exercises

Exercises for the Immediate Postpartum Period

(can be performed in bed)

Toe Stretch (Tightens Calf Muscles)
While lying on your back, keep your legs straight and point your toes away from you, then pull your legs toward you and point your toes toward your chest. Repeat 10 times.

Pelvic Floor Exercise (Tightens Perineal Muscles)
Contract your buttocks for a count of 5 and relax. Contract your buttocks and press thighs together for a count of 7 and relax. Contract buttocks, press thighs together, and draw in anus for a count of 10 and relax.

Exercises for Later Recovery Period
(After First Postpartum Visit)

Bicycle (tightens thighs, stomach, waist)
Lie on your back on the floor, arms at sides, palms down. Begin rotating your legs as if you were riding a bicycle, bringing the knees all the way in toward the chest and stretching the legs out as long and straight as possible. Breathe deeply and evenly. Do the exercises at a moderate speed and do not tire yourself.
Buttocks Exercise (tightens buttocks)
Lie on your stomach and keep your legs straight. Raise your left leg in the air, then repeat with your right leg (feel the contraction in your buttocks). Keep your hips on the floor. Repeat 10 times.
Twist (tightens waist)
Stand with legs wide apart. Hold your arms at your sides, shoulder level, palms down. Twist your body from side to front and back again. Feel the twist in your waist.

Guidelines Breast-Feeding

Procedure	Action	Rationale/Amplification
	1. Have the mother wash her hands before breast-feeding.	1. Protects the infant and mother's breasts from infection.
	2. Have the mother breast-feed very soon after delivery.	2. Stimulates earlier milk production; gives the infant full benefit of colostrum; aids in contraction of the mother's uterus.
	3. Have the mother assume a comfortable position—lying on her side, sitting upright, tailor sitting, etc.—with the infant facing the mother (Fig. 41-1).	3. Enhances milk letdown, more complete emptying of the breasts, lessens nipple trauma.
	4. When beginning breast-feeding, have the mother "point up" the nipple by gently pressing the areola between two fingers.	4. Helps the infant get a firm grasp on the nipple and areola.
	5. Make sure the infant has both the areola and nipple in his mouth.	5. Sucking on only the nipple causes nipple pain and trauma.
	6. Make sure the infant's nasal pathway is open. If the infant's nose is flat against the mother's breast, have her indent her breast near the infant's nose to ensure an open breathing space.	6. An obstructed nasal pathway will cause the infant to stop breast-feeding
	7. Have the mother alternate the breast she begins breast-feeding with at each feeding.	7. The infant's sucking is most rigorous at the beginning of breast-feeding. Alternating the breast used first at each feeding will reduce nipple pain and trauma.
	8. Have the mother use each breast at each feeding. Begin with 5 minutes at each breast, then increase the time at each breast, allowing the infant to suck until he stops sucking actively. Pin a safety pin to the bra as a reminder of which breast to start with at the next feeding.	8. Empties each breast and maintains milk supply.
	9. Have the mother breast-feed frequently and on a demand schedule (every 2–4 hours).	9. Frequent feedings maintain the milk supply and prevent overly vigorous sucking on the nipple and nipple trauma.
	10. Have the mother break the infant's suction by placing her finger in the corner of his mouth.	10. Prevents nipple trauma.
	11. Have the mother air dry her nipples for 15–20 minutes after each feeding.	11. Prevents or reduces nipple trauma.
	12. Have the mother burp the infant at the end or midway through the feeding.	12. Releasing air in the infant's stomach will make him more satisfied and less fretful.
	13. Alert the mother that uterine cramping may occur, especially in multiparous women.	13. Nursing stimulates release of oxytocin causing uterine cramping, which can be worse in women with lessened uterine tone.
	14. Teach the mother to provide for adequate rest and to avoid tension, fatigue, and a stressful environment.	14. Maternal fatigue, stress, and tension inhibit the letdown reflex and makes breast milk less available to the infant at feeding.
	15. Avoid taking medications and drugs.	15. Many substances pass into breast milk and can reduce milk production or have a deleterious effect on the infant.

Procedure (continued)	Nursing Action	Rationale

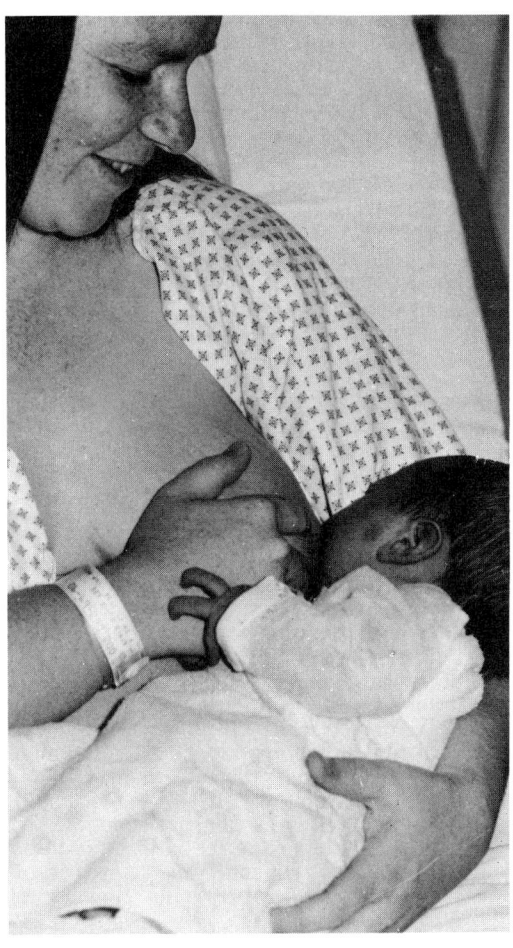

Figure 41-1. *The mother may prefer to assume a sitting position when nursing her infant.*

16. Provide a well-balanced diet with extra vitamins, calcium, and protein.

16. Extra nutrients are needed for milk production.

17. Provide 2–3 quarts of liquid per day.

17. Additional fluids are needed for milk production.

Physiology of the Newborn

Transitional Stages

The first 24 hours of life constitute a highly vulnerable time during which the infant must make several adjustments to extrauterine life. During this period of transition, 6 overlapping stages have been identified:

Stage 1. Receives stimulation (during labor) from the pressure of the uterine contractions and from changes in pressure when the membranes rupture.

Stage 2. Encounters a variety of foreign stimuli—light, cold, gravity, and sound.

Stage 3. Initiates breathing.

Stage 4. Changes from fetal to neonatal circulation.

Stage 5. Undergoes alteration in metabolic processes with activation of liver, and gastrointestinal tract for passage of meconium.

Stage 6. Achieves a steady level of equilibrium in metabolic processes (production of enzymes, increased blood oxygen saturation, decrease in acidosis associated with birth, and recovery of the neurologic tissues from the trauma of labor and delivery).

Respiratory Changes

A. Factors Initiating Respiration

1. *Physical*—Pressure changes from intrauterine to extrauterine life produce stimulation to initiate respirations.

2. *Chemical*—changes in the blood as a result of transitory asphyxia include:
   a. Lowered oxygen level
   b. Increased carbon dioxide level
   c. Lowered *p*H—if asphyxia is prolonged, depression of the respiratory center (rather than stimulation) occurs, and resuscitation is necessary
3. *Sensory*—Light, sound, and tactile stimulation when the infant is touched and dried contribute to the initiation of respiration.
4. *Thermal*—A drop in temperature from 37°C. (98.6°F.) to 21–24°C. (70–75°F.).
5. *First breath*—maximum effort is required to expand the lungs and fill the collapsed alveoli.
   a. Surface tension in the respiratory tract and resistance in the lung tissue, the thorax, the diaphragm, and the respiratory muscles must be overcome.
   b. First active inspiration comes from a strong contraction of the diaphragm, which creates a high negative intrathoracic pressure causing a marked retraction of the ribs and distention of the alveolar space. (Any remaining fluid is reabsorbed rapidly if the pulmonary capillary blood flow is adequate, since the fluid is hypotonic and passes easily into the capillaries.)

B. Character of Normal Respirations

1. The infant begins life with intense activity; diffuse, purposeless movements alternate with periods of relative immobility.
2. Respirations are rapid, as frequent as 80 breaths/minute, accompanied by tachycardia, 140–180 beats/minute.
3. Relaxation occurs and the infant usually sleeps; he then awakes to a second period of activity. Oral mucus may be a major problem during this period.
4. Respirations are reduced to 35–50 breaths/minute and become quiet and shallow; respiration is carried out by the diaphragm and abdominal muscles.
5. Period of dyspnea and cyanosis may occur suddenly in an infant who is breathing normally; this may indicate an anomaly or a pathologic condition.
6. Apnea is normal in the neonatal period and lasts 10–15 seconds.

Circulatory Changes

A. Anatomic Changes (see Chapter 39)

B. Blood Volume

85–100 ml./kg. at birth
Factors that influence blood volume:
1. Maternal blood volume (affected by maternal diseases and iron intake)
2. Placental function
3. Uterine contractions during labor
4. Amount of blood loss associated with delivery
5. Placental transfusion at birth—increase in blood volume of 60% if cord is clamped and cut after pulsation ceases

C. Peripheral Circulation

Residual cyanosis in hands and feet for 1–2 hours after birth because of sluggish circulation.

D. Pulse Rate

1. Generally follows pattern similar to that of respiration.
2. Apical pulse rate is more accurate.
3. Normal rate 120–150 beats/minute.
4. May rise to 180 beats/minute when the infant is crying or drop to 70 beats/minute during deep sleep.

E. Blood Pressure

1. 70/45 at birth; 100/50 by 10th day
2. Blood pressure rises with crying.
3. Blood pressure in the leg will be slightly higher.

F. Blood Coagulation

Coagulability is temporarily diminished because of lack of bacteria in the intestinal tract that contributes to the synthesis of vitamin K.
1. Coagulation time, 3–4 minutes
2. Bleeding time, 2–4 minutes
3. Prothrombin, 50% decreasing to 20%–30%

G. Blood Elements

Values for blood components in the neonate
1. Hemoglobin, 16–22 gm.
2. Reticulocytes, 2.5%–6.5%
3. Leukocytes, 15,000–20,000 cu. mm.
(See Appendix IV for detailed pediatric hematology table.)

Temperature Regulation

1. Mechanism not fully developed; heat production low.
2. Infant responds readily to environmental heat and cold stimuli.
3. Heat loss of 2°–3°C. may occur at birth by evaporation, convection, conduction, and radiation.
4. Infant develops mechanisms to counterbalance heat loss.
   a. Vasoconstriction—blood directed away from skin surfaces.
   b. Insulation—from subcutaneous adipose tissue.
   c. Heat production—by nonshivering thermogenesis elicited by the sympathetic nervous system's response to decreased temperatures; activated by adrenalin.
   d. Fetal position—by assuming a flexed position

Basal Metabolism

1. Surface area of infant is large in comparison with weight.
2. Basal metabolism per kg. of body weight is higher than that of adult.
3. Calorie requirements are high—117 calories per kilogram of body weight per day.

Renal Function

Low arterial blood pressure and increased renal vascular resistance lead to the following effects:
1. Decreased ability to concentrate urine because of low tubular reabsorption rate and low levels of antidiuretic hormone.
2. Limited ability to maintain water balance by excretion of excess water or retention of needed water.
3. Decreased ability to maintain acid–base mechanism; slower excretion of electrolytes, especially sodium and the hydrogen ions, results in accumulation of these substances, which predisposes the infant to dehydration, acidosis, and hyperkalemia.
4. Excretion of large amount of uric acid during newborn period—appears as "brick dust" stain on diaper.

Hepatic Function

Function limited because of lack of gastrointestinal tract activity and limited blood supply; consequences include the following:
1. Decreased ability to conjugate bilirubin (rationale for physiologic jaundice).

2. Decreased ability to regulate blood sugar concentration (rationale for neonatal hypoglycemia).
3. Deficient production of prothrombin and other coagulation factors that depend on vitamin K for synthesis (rationale for neonate's predisposition to hemorrhage).

Endocrine Function

Endocrine glands are better organized than other systems; disturbances are most often related to maternally provided hormones, which can cause the following:
1. Vaginal discharge (and/or bleeding) in female infants.
2. Enlargement of mammary glands in both sexes—related to increased estrogen, luteal, and prolactin activity. Milky secretions may be present.
3. Disturbances related to maternal endocrine pathology (e.g., diabetic mother or mother with inadequate iodine intake).

Gastrointestinal Changes

The newborn's intestinal tract is proportionately longer than the adult's; however, elastic tissue and musculature are not fully developed, and neurologic control is variable and inadequate.
1. Most digestive enzymes are present, with the exception of pancreatic amylase and lipase. Protein and carbohydrates are easily absorbed, but fat absorption is poor.
2. Limitations relate primarily to anatomic structures and neutrality of the gastric contents.
3. Imperfect control of the cardiac and pyloric sphincters and immaturity of neurologic control cause mild regurgitation or slight vomiting.
4. Irregularities in peristaltic motility slow stomach emptying.
5. Peristalsis increases in the lower ileum, resulting in stool frequency—1–6 stools per day. Absence of stool within 48 hours after birth is indicative of intestinal obstruction.

Neurologic Changes

Neurologic mechanisms are immature; they are not fully developed anatomically or physiologically, and as a result, uncoordinated movements, labile temperature regulation, and poor control over musculature are characteristic of the infant. Reflexes are important indices of infant neural development. (See Chapter 44, pages 1070–1072, for a detailed discussion of the pediatric neurologic examination. See also Chapter 45, pages 1080–1083, which describes reflexes of the newborn and traces appearance and disappearance of the various reflexes.)

Pertinent History

1. Mother's age, socioeconomic status, ethnic or cultural group, educational level, marital status
2. Mother's/family's past medical history
3. Mother's past obstetric history
4. Mother's prenatal history with this pregnancy
5. Labor and delivery

Physical Assessment Findings and Physiologic Functioning

A. Posture

1. Full-term newborn assumes symmetric posture; face turned to side, flexed extremities; hands tightly fisted with thumb covered by fingers.
2. Asymmetric posture may be caused by fractures of clavicle or humerus or by nerve injuries commonly of the brachial plexus.
3. Infants born in breech position may keep knees and legs straightened or in frog position depending on the type of breech birth.

B. Length

Average length of full-term newborn is 51 cm. (20 inches); range 46–56 cm. (18–22 inches).

C. Weight

Average weight of male infants is 3400 gm. (7½ lb.); female infants, 3200 gm. (7 lb.). Range of 80% of full-term newborns is 2900 to 4100 gm. (6 lb., 5 oz.–9 lb., 2 oz.).

D. Skin

Examine under natural light for:
1. Hair distribution—term infant will have some lanugo over back; most of the lanugo will have disappeared on extremities and other areas of the body.
2. Turgor—term infant should have good skin turgor.
3. Color
   a. Cyanosis—*acrocyanosis,* bluish color in hands and feet, is common due to immature peripheral circulation.
   b. Pallor—may indicate cold, stress, anemia, or cardiac failure.
   c. Plethora—reddish coloration may be due to excessive red blood cells from intrauterine intravascular transfusion (twins), cardiac disease, or diabetes in the mother.
   d. Jaundice—physiologic jaundice due to immaturity of liver is common beginning on day 2, peaking at 1 week and disappearing by the 2nd week. First appears in skin over face or upper body then progresses over larger area; can also be seen in conjunctivae of eyes.
   e. Meconium staining—staining of skin, fingernails, and umbilical cord indicates compromise in utero unless infant was in breech position.
4. Dryness/peeling—marked scaliness and desquamation are a sign of postmaturity.
5. Vernix—in full-term infants, most vernix is found in skin folds under the arms and in the groin.
6. Nails—should reach end of fingertips and be well-developed in the full-term infant.
7. Edema—some edema may be present over buttocks, back, and occiput if the infant has been supine; pitting edema may be due to erythroblastosis, heart failure, electrolyte imbalance.
8. Ecchymoses—may appear over the presenting part in a difficult delivery; may also indicate infection or bleeding problem.
9. Petechiae—pinpoint hemorrhages on skin due to increased intravascular pressure, infection or thrombocytopenia; regresses within 24–48 hours.
10. Erythema toxicum ("newborn rash")—pink to red papular rash appearing on trunk and diaper areas; regresses within 24–48 hours.
11. Hemangiomas—vascular lesions present at birth; some may fade, but others may be permanent.
12. Telangiectatic nevi (stork bites)—flat red or purple lesions most often found on back of neck, lower occiput, upper eyelid, and bridge of nose; regress by 2 years of age.
13. Milia—enlarged sebaceous glands found on nose, chin, cheeks, and forehead; regress in several days to a week or two.
14. Mongolian spots—blue pigmentation on lower back, sacrum and buttocks; common in Blacks, Asians, and

infants of Southern European heritage; regress by 4 years of age.

15. Café-au-lait spots—brown macules, usually not significant; large numbers may indicate underlying neurofibromatosis.

16. Harlequin color change—when on side, dependent half turns red, upper half pale; due to gravity and vasomotor instability.

17. Abrasions or lacerations can result from internal monitoring and instruments used at birth.

E. Head

1. Examine head and face for symmetry, paralysis, shape, swelling, movement.
    a. *Caput succedaneum*—swelling of soft tissues of the scalp because of pressure; swelling crosses suture lines.
    b. *Cephalohematoma*—subperiosteal hemorrhage with collection of blood between periosteum and bone; swelling does not cross suture lines.
    c. *Molding*—overlapping of skull bones caused by compression during labor and delivery (disappears in a few days).
    d. Examine symmetry of facial movements.

2. Measure head circumference—33–35 cm. (13–14 inches), approximately 2 cm. (1 inch) larger than chest. Measure just above the eyebrows and over the occiput.

3. Fontanelles—area where more than two skull bones meet; covered with strong band of connective tissue; also called "soft spot."
    a. Enlarged or bulging—may indicate increased intracranial pressure.
    b. Sunken—often indicates dehydration.
    c. Size—posterior may be obliterated because of molding—generally closes in 2–3 months; anterior is palpable—generally closes in 12–18 months.

4. Sutures—junctions of adjoining skull bones
    a. Overriding—due to molding during labor and delivery.
    b. Separation—extensive separation may be found in malnourished infants and with increased intracranial pressure.

F. Face

1. Eyes—examine the following:
    a. Color—sclerae in most full-term infants is white; eye color usually gray–blue in white infants, brown in dark-skinned infants; final eye color is evident by 6–12 months.
    b. Hemorrhagic areas—subconjunctival hemorrhages may appear as a red band from pressure during delivery; regresses within 2 weeks.
    c. Edema—of the eyelids may be due to pressure on the head and face during labor and delivery.
    d. Conjunctivitis or discharge—may be due to instillation of silver nitrate or infections from organisms such as staphylococcus or gonococcus.
    e. Jaundice—may be seen in sclera because of physiologic jaundice or, if severe, blood group incompatibility.
    f. Pupils—equal in size and should constrict equally in bright light.
    g. Infant can see and discriminate patterns; limited by imperfect oculomotor coordination and inability to accommodate for varying distances.
    h. Red reflex—red-orange color seen when light from an ophthalmoscope is reflected from the retina. Absence of the red reflex indicates cataracts.
    i. Brushfield's spots—white or yellow pinpoint areas on iris that may indicate trisomy 21.

2. Nose—examine the following:
    a. Patency—necessary since infants breathe through the nose, not the mouth.
    b. Nasal flaring—may indicate respiratory distress.
    c. Discharge—due to congestion or possibly infection.
    d. Sense of smell—infants will turn toward familiar odors and away from noxious odors.

3. Ears—examine the following:
    a. Formation—large, flabby ears that slant forward may indicate abnormalities of kidney or other parts of urinary tract.
    b. Position in relation to eye—helix (top of ear) on same plane as eye; low-set ears may indicate chromosomal or renal abnormalities.
    c. Cartilage—full-term infant has sufficient cartilage to make ear feel firm.
    d. Hearing—auditory canals may be congested for a day or two following birth; the infant should hear well in a few days.

4. Mouth—examine the following:
    a. Size—small mouth found in trisomy 18 and 21; corners of mouth turn down ("fish mouth") in fetal alcohol syndrome.
    b. Palate—examine hard and soft palate for closure.
    c. Size of tongue in relation to mouth—normally does not extend much past the margin of gums. Excessively large tongue seen in congenital anomalies such as cretinism and trisomy 21.
    d. Teeth—predeciduous teeth are found on rare occasion; if they interfere with feeding, they may be removed.
    e. Epstein's pearls—small white nodules found on sides of hard palate (often mistaken for teeth); regress in a few weeks.
    f. Frenulum linguae—thin ridge of tissue running from base of tongue along undersurface to tip of tongue; formerly believed to cause tongue tie; no treatment necessary.
    g. Sucking blisters (labial taberales)—thickened areas on midline of upper lip; no treatment necessary.
    h. Infections—thrush, caused by *Candida albicans,* may appear as white patches on tongue that do not wash away with fluids; treated with nystatin suspension.

G. Neck

Examine the following:
1. Mobility—infant can move head from side to side; palpate for lymph nodes; palpate clavicle for fractures, especially following a difficult delivery.
2. Torticollis—appears as a spasmodic, one-sided contraction of neck muscles; generally from hematoma of sternocleidomastoid muscle; usually no treatment required.
3. Excessive skin folds may be associated with congenital abnormalities such as trisomy 21.
4. Stiffness and hyperextension may be due to trauma or infection.
5. Clavicle—for intactness.

H. Chest

Examine the following:
1. Circumference and symmetry—average circumference is 30–33 cm. (12–13 inches), approximately 2 cm. smaller than head circumference.

2. Breast
   a. Engorgement—may occur at day 3 because of withdrawal of maternal hormones, especially estrogen; no treatment required—regresses in 2 weeks.
   b. Nipples and areolae—less formed and pronounced in preterm infants.

I. Respiratory System

1. Rate—normally between 40 and 60 breaths/minute; influenced by sleep–wake status, when last fed, drugs taken by mother.
2. Rhythm—respirations may be shallow with irregular rhythm.
   a. Respiratory movements are mainly diaphragmatic because of weak thoracic muscles.
   b. Periodic breathing—resumption of respiration after 5–15-second period without respiration; decreases over time; more common in preterm infant.
   c. Observe for abnormal respiratory signs.
3. Breath sounds—determined by auscultation
   a. Bronchial sounds are heard over most of the chest.
   b. Rales may be heard immediately after birth.

J. Cardiovascular System

1. *Rate*—ranges between 100 and 160 beats/minute; influenced by behavioral state, environmental temperature, medication; take apical count for 1 full minute.
2. *Rhythm*—common to find periods of deceleration followed by periods of acceleration.
3. *Heart sounds*—2nd sound higher in pitch and sharper than 1st; 3rd and 4th sounds rarely heard; murmurs common—great majority are transitory.
4. *Pulses*—examine for presence of brachial, radial, pedal, and femoral pulses; lack of femoral pulses indicative of inadequate aortic blood flow.
5. *Cyanosis*—examine for cyanosis—acrocyanosis of distal extremities is common; record location of any cyanosis, color changes over time, and when crying.
6. *Blood pressure*—newborns over 3 kg. have systolic blood pressure between 60 and 80 mm. Hg; diastolic, between 35 and 55 mm. Hg.

K. Abdomen

1. Shape—cylindrical, protrudes slightly, moves synchronously with chest in respiration.
2. Distention may be due to bowel obstruction, organ enlargement, or infection.
3. Palpate abdomen for masses; gap between rectus muscles is common; palpate liver and spleen.
   a. Liver has decreased ability to conjugate bilirubin (rationale for physiologic jaundice).
   b. Liver has decreased production of prothrombin and factors that depend on vitamin K for synthesis (rationale for neonate's predisposition to hemorrhage).
4. Auscultate abdomen for bowel sounds; usually bowel sounds are present an hour after delivery.
5. Kidneys—palpate kidneys for size and shape:
   a. Infant has decreased ability of kidney to concentrate urine, excrete a solute load, maintain water and electrolyte balance.
   b. Urine may contain uric acid crystals which appear on diaper as reddish blotches; uric acid crystals may yield false-positive result when the infant's urine is tested for protein.
6. Umbilical cord
   a. Normally contains 2 arteries, 1 vein; single artery

associated with renal and other congenital abnormalities.
   b. Signs of infection around insertion into abdominal wall—redness, discharge.
   c. Meconium staining—associated with intrauterine compromise or postmaturity.
   d. By 24 hours becomes yellowish brown; dries and falls off in about 7–10 days.
   e. Umbilical hernia—defect in abdominal wall.
7. Genitalia
   a. Female
      (1) Labia majora cover labia minora in full-term female infants.
      (2) Hymenal tag (tissue) may protrude from vagina—regresses within several weeks.
      (3) Vaginal discharge—white or pink discharge may be present because of the drop in maternal hormones; no treatment necessary.
   b. Male
      (1) Full-term—testes in scrotal sac; scrotal sac markedly wrinkled.
      (2) Edema may be present in scrotal sac if the infant was born in breech presentation; a frank collection of fluid in the scrotal sac is a *hydrocele*—regresses in about a month.
      (3) Examine glans penis for urethral opening—normally central; opening ventral (*hypospadias*); opening dorsally (*epispadias*); abnormally adherent foreskin (*phimosis*).

L. Back

1. Examine spinal column for normal curvature, closure, and presence of pilonidal dimple or sinus.
2. Examine anal area for anal opening, response of anal sphincter, fissures.

M. Musculoskeletal System

1. Examine extremities for fractures, paralysis, range of motion, irregular position.
2. Examine fingers and toes for number and separation: extra digits—*polydactyly;* fused digits—*syndactyly.*
3. Examine hips for dislocation—with the infant in supine position, flex knees and abduct hips to side and down to table surface; clicking sound indicates dislocation.

N. Neurologic System

1. Neurologic mechanisms are immature anatomically and physiologically; as a result, uncoordinated movements, labile temperature regulation, and lack of control over musculature are characteristic of the infant.
2. Examine muscle tone, head control, and reflexes.
3. Reflexes are important indices of infant neural development (see p. 1071).

Behavioral Assessment

A. Response to Stimulation

1. Newborns exhibit predictable, directed responses when in social interactions with nurturing adults or in response to attractive auditory or visual stimuli.
2. Newborn responses are influenced by states of consciousness such as:
   a. Quiet, deep sleep—no spontaneous activity, eyes closed, respirations regular
   b. Light, active sleep—random startles, eyes closed, rapid eye movements, frequent change of state with response to stimulation
   c. Drowsy awake—eyes open or closed, eyelids flut-

ter, variable activity level, mild startles periodically, delayed response to stimulation

 d. Quiet alert—eyes open, little motor activity, focuses on source of stimulation

 e. Alert active—eyes open, much motor activity, increase in startles in response to stimulation

 f. Crying—intense crying that is difficult to interrupt with stimulation

3. Behavioral examinations have been developed that test neurologic adequacy and behavioral responses to environmental stimuli (see Behavioral Assessment, below). Understanding how an infant responds can help the parents respond to and care for him, and alter the environment to be most helpful to him.

Behavioral Assessment

1. Response decrement to repeated visual stimuli
2. Response decrement to repeated auditory stimuli
3. Response decrement to pinprick
4. Orienting responses to inanimate visual and auditory stimuli
5. Quality and duration of alert periods
6. General muscle tone
7. Motor maturity
8. Traction responses as infant is pulled to sitting position
9. Responses to being cuddled by the examiner
10. Defensive reactions to a cloth over the face
11. Consolability with intervention by examiner
12. Attempts to control self and to control state behavior
13. Rapidity of buildup to crying state
14. Peak of excitement and capacity for self control
15. Irritability during the examination
16. General assessment of kind and degree of activity
17. Tremulousness
18. Amount of startling
19. Lability of skin color
20. Lability of states during the examination
21. Hand-to-mouth activity

Brazelton TB. Clin Obstet Gynecol 1973; 16:59

B. Sleeping Pattern

1. Length of sleep cycles (rapid eye movement [REM] active and quiet sleep) changes normally with maturation of the central nervous system.
2. Quiet sleep should increase over time in relation to REM sleep.
3. Newborns usually sleep 20 hours per day.

C. Feeding Pattern

1. Most newborns eat 6–8 times per day with 2–8 hours between feedings; establish fairly regular feeding patterns in about 2 weeks.
2. Calorie requirements are high—110–130 calories per kg. of body weight daily.
3. Most digestive enzymes are present at birth.
4. Imperfect control of cardiac and pyloric sphincters; immaturity results in regurgitation.

D. Pattern of Elimination

1. Stool
 a. Meconium is usually passed in 24 hours.
 b. Passage of meconium (tarry green–black stools) continues for 48 hours, followed by transitional stools (combination of meconium and yellow of milk stools). Milk stools (yellow) are passed by day 5.
 c. Newborn has up to 6 stools per day in the first weeks after birth.
2. Voiding
 a. Newborn voids within first 24 hours.
 b. After first few days, infant voids from 10 to 15 times a day

E. Temperature Regulation

1. Infant's body responds readily to changes in environmental temperature.
2. Heat loss at birth may occur via evaporation, convection, conduction, and radiation.
3. Physiologic mechanisms to avoid heat loss include:
 a. Vasoconstriction
 b. Nonshivering thermogenesis elicited by sympathetic nervous system in response to decreased temperature
 c. Adipose tissue and brown fat—the latter contains many small blood vessels, fat vacuoles, and mitochondria, and is a site of heat production. Brown fat is found between scapulae, around neck and thorax, behind sternum, and around kidneys and adrenals.
 d. Flexed position of full-term newborn

Metabolic Screening Tests

1. *Phenylketonuria* (*PKU*)—inability of the infant to metabolize phenylalanine; scheduled after 48 hours of protein feedings
2. *Galactosemia*—inborn error of carbohydrate metabolism, when galactose and lactose cannot be converted to glucose
3. *Hypothyroidism*—thyroid deficiency
4. *Maple sugar urine disease* (MSUD)—inability to metabolize leucine, isoleucine, and valine
5. *Homocystinuria*—inborn error of sulfur amino acid metabolism
6. *Sickle cell anemia*—abnormally shaped red blood cells with lower oxygen solubility

Guidelines Nursing Care of the Newborn

Purposes
1. To continue appraisal of the newborn by observing and recording vital signs, daily weight loss or gain, bowel and bladder function, activity or sleep.
2. To provide safeguards against infection.
3. To initiate feeding.
4. To provide health counseling to the parents.

Procedure

Nursing Action	Rationale/Amplification
General Considerations	
1. Carry out hospital policy for gowning and 3-minute scrub.	1. Utilizes basic principles of nursing care.
2. Never leave the infant alone.	2. Ensures safety factors.
3. Prevent undue exposure; provide warm environment (24°–27°C. [75°–80°F.]) and bath water (37°–38°C. [98°–100°F.]).	3. Prevents cold stress. Neonates have little adipose tissue to protect them.
Weight, Temperature, and Blood Pressure	
1. Weigh infant and record weight.	1. Infant may lose 5%–10% of birth weight because of minimal intake of nutrients and fluid and loss of excess fluid.
2. Take axillary temperature by placing thermometer in axilla and pressing infant's arm gently but firmly against it for 10 minutes.	2. Use of rectal thermometer predisposes to irritation of rectal mucosa.
3. Take blood pressure.	3. Hypotension may be present and require remedial action.
Bathing Technique	
1. Use cotton balls or soft, disposable wash cloths to wipe eyes, face, and outer ears. Eyes are wiped from inside corner outward.	1. Start from cleanest areas to most soiled.
2. Use a neutral soap—check *p*H. Clear water may be used if infant's skin is dry.	2. Prevents irritation of skin. The use of hexachlorophene to prevent staphylococcal infection is controversial. Hexachlorophene may cause brain damage if a sufficient quantity is absorbed through the skin.
3. Wash infant's head, using gentle circular motions.	3. Prevents cradle cap from forming, especially over the frontal areas.
4. Tilt head back to cleanse neck.	4. Exposes neck folds for more thorough cleansing.
5. Bathe torso and extremities quickly.	5. Prevents unnecessary exposure and chilling.
6. Inspect umbilical cord. Check area for bleeding or foul odor. A drying agent such as 70% alcohol or merthiolate is applied several times daily. Do not cover with diaper. Dressings are not used.	6. Minimizes colonization by bacteria.
7. Cleanse genital area of male infants.	
a. Retract foreskin gently for cleaning, and replace quickly.	a. Replacing foreskin quickly prevents edema.
b. Circumcision care—keep area clean. Place sterile petrolatum gauze over area for first 24 hours; change after voiding. Observe hourly for bleeding. Position infant and diaper to avoid friction.	b. Prevents infection and promotes healing. Bleeding can be controlled by pressure or by application of adrenalin solution. Prevents discomfort.
8. Cleanse genital area of female infants.	
a. Gently separate folds of the labia and remove secretions.	a. Vaginal discharge and smegma must be removed.
b. Wipe vaginal area with cotton ball, using 1 stroke in a front-to-back direction.	b. Front-to-back cleansing prevents contamination of vagina.
9. Bathe buttocks, using a gentle, patting motion. Keep area clean and dry.	9. Area is susceptible to skin breakdown because of acid reaction of urine and feces.
10. Prevent diaper rash. If rash does occur, protective ointment (zinc oxide or A & D) may be used. Exposure of buttocks to air or heat lamp is helpful.	
Stool Observation	
1. Observe stool pattern—meconium during first 2–3 days.	1. Material composed of epithelial and epidermal cells, lanugo, and bile pigments.

(continued)

Guidelines   Nursing Care of the Newborn *(continued)*

Procedure *(continued)*	Nursing Action	Rationale/Amplification
	2. Transitional stools—change from tarry black to greenish black, to greenish brown to brownish yellow to greenish yellow.	2. Changes reflect intake of milk—stools are composed of both meconium and milk stools.

	3. Number, color, and consistency are recorded daily.	3. For early identification of abnormalities.
		  a. No stool within 48 hours indicates an intestinal obstruction.
		  b. Passage of meconium only (without other stool) suggests obstruction in the ileum.
		  c. Thick, putty-like meconium may indicate cystic fibrosis.
		  d. Diarrhea may be caused by overfeeding or by gastroenteritis.
		  e. Blood in the stool is an indication of intestinal bleeding.

Nutritional Considerations

	1. Provide for nutritional intake.	1. Infants vary in their readiness to feed.
	2. Promote feeding method of choice. (See page 1004 for Guidelines for breast-feeding).	
	3. Test urine glucose using reagent strip test and blood glucose using enzymatic strip test.	3. Infant may be hypoglycemic and require feeding sooner than usual 4–6-hour wait.
	4. First feeding is sterile water. If retained, formula is given at next feeding.	4. Glucose water, if aspirated, is dangerous to lung tissue. Most hospitals use prepared milk mixture in disposable containers. Various formulas are available.

	5. Instruct the parent in technique of bottle-feeding.
	  a. Hold baby in semi-upright position.
	  b. Position bottle so that neck of bottle is filled.
	  c. Insert nipple into baby's mouth so that baby's tongue is under nipple.
	  d. Burp during feeding by holding infant upright.
		
		  a. Gravity assists flow of milk into stomach.
		  b. Prevents the baby from swallowing air.
		  c. Sucking and swallowing reflexes are used in feeding.
		  d. Allows air to escape from stomach, preventing distention or milk regurgitation.

	6. Metabolic screening is usually done 48 hours after birth; if discharged prior to this time, a repeat test will be needed. Testing is done for following diseases:
	  a. Phenylketonuria (PKU)
	  b. Galactosemia
	  c. Hypothyroidism
	  d. Sickle cell anemia
	  e. Maple sugar urine disease (MSUD)
	  f. Homocystinuria
		6. Most states require by law routine testing of newborn infants for metabolic disorders.

Discharge Planning

	1. Preparation for home care: instruction is given concerning infant bathing and care, preparation of formula, and infant feeding. Written formula with instructions for preparation is provided to parents.	1. Instruction for infant care is a combined responsibility of the medical and nursing staffs.
	2. Provide ample opportunity for parent contact.	2. Early attachment results in improved parent–child relationships.

Bibliography

Books

Bobak I, Jensen M and Zalar M. Maternity and Gynecologic Care. 4th ed. St. Louis, CV Mosby, 1989

Cunningham F, MacDonald P and Gant N. Williams Obstetrics. 18th ed.

Norwalk, CT, Appleton and Lange, 1989

Dickason EJ, Schult M and Silverman B. Maternal–Infant Nursing Care. Philadelphia, JB Lippincott, 1990

Doenges M, Kenty J and Moorehouse M. Maternal/Newborn Care Plans:

Guidelines for Client Care. Philadelphia, FA Davis, 1988

Gorrie T. A Guide to the Nursing of Childbearing Families. Baltimore, Williams & Wilkins, 1989

Houldin A, Saltstein S and Ganley K. Nursing Diagnoses for Wellness

Supporting Strength. Philadelphia: JB Lippincott, 1987

Lawrence R. Breast-feeding: A Guide for the Medical Profession. 3rd ed. St. Louis, CV Mosby, 1989

Merenstein G and Gardner S. Handbook of Neonatal Intensive Care. St. Louis, CV Mosby, 1989

Neeson J. Clinical Manual of Maternity Nursing. Philadelphia, JB Lippincott, 1987

Olds S, London M and Ladewig P. Maternal Newborn Nursing: A Family-Centered Approach. 3rd ed. Menlo Park, CA, Addison-Wesley, 1988

Reeder S and Martin L. Maternity Nursing. 16th ed. Philadelphia, JB Lippincott, 1987

Rubin R. Maternal Identity and the Maternal Experience. New York, Springer, 1984

Torgus J (ed). The Womanly Art of Breast-feeding. 4th ed. Franklin Park, IL, La Leche League International, 1987

Tully MR and Overfield M. Breastfeeding: A Handbook for Hospitals. Evansville, IL, Mead Johnson, 1989

Journals

Barness L and Gilbert–Barness E. What lies ahead in infant nutrition? Semin Perinatol 1989; 13(2):112–117

Drake M, Verhulst D and Fawcett J. Physical and psychological symptoms experienced by Canadian women and their husbands during pregnancy and the postpartum. J Adv Nurs 1988; 13:436–440

Eidelman A and Schimmel M. Phototherapy—1988: A green light for a new approach. J Perinatol 1988; 1:69–71

Frank D. Commercial discharge packs and breastfeeding counseling:

Summary of a study. Journal of Human Lactation 1989; 5:7–10

Halls A and Mcgahan M. Neonatal jaundice. Nebr Med J 1989; 74(4):83–84

Hampton S. Nursing interventions for the first three postpartum months. J Obstet Gynecol Neonat Nurs 1989; 18:116–122

Hartman G and Shochat S. Abdominal mass lesions in the newborn: Diagnosis and treatment. Clin Perinatol 1989; 16:123–135

Hiser P. Concerns of multiparas during the second postpartum week. J Obstet Gynecol Neonat Nurs 1987; 16:195–203

Houston M and Field P. Practices and policies in the initiation of breastfeeding. J Obstet Gynecol Neonat Nurs 1988; 17:418–424

Jacobson H. A standard for assessing lochia volume. Am J Matern Child Nurs 1985; 10:174–175

Kemper K et al. Jaundice, terminating breast-feeding, and the vulnerable child. Pediatrics 1989; 84:773–778

Kirshon B et al. Indirect blood pressure monitoring in the postpartum patient. Obstet Gynecol 1987; 70:799–801

Koutras A and Vigorita V. Fecal secretory immunoglobulin A in breast milk versus formula feeding in early infancy. J Pediatr Gastroenterol Nutr 1989; 9:58–61

Martone D and Nash B. Initial differences in postpartum attachment behavior in breastfeeding and bottle-feeding mothers. J Obstet Gynecol Neonat Nurs 1988; 17:212–213

Pascoe J and French J. Development of positive feelings in primiparous mothers toward their normal newborns. A descriptive study. Clin Pediatr 1989; 28:452–456

Pete J. Newborn infants' preference for sterile water versus five percent

glucose and water. J Pediatr Nurs 1989; 4:263–267

Phaosavasdi S et al. Effectiveness of benzathine penicillin regimen in the treatment of syphilis in pregnancy. J Med Assoc Thai 1989; 72(2):101–108

Ragan J and Weinfield A. VACNECCA—an eight point check for neonatal assessment. J Pract Nurs 1989; 39(2):39–43

Rutledge D and Pridham K. Postpartum mothers' perceptions of competence for infant care. J Obstet Gynecol Neonat Nurs 1987; 16:185–194

Sequin L et al. The components of women's satisfaction with maternity care. Birth 1989; 16:109–113

Stevens K. Nursing diagnosis in wellness childbearing settings. J Obstet Gynecol Neonat Nurs 1988; 17:329–336

Stewart L. A workable regime for managing maternal inability to produce adequate volumes of breastmilk. Journal of Human Lactation 1989; 5:16–18

Tontisirin K et al. Effect of phototherapy on nutrients utilization in newborn infants with jaundice. J Med Assoc Thai 1989; 72(Sup 1):177–182

Tribotti S et al. Nursing diagnoses for the postpartum woman. J Obstet Gynecol Neonat Nurs 1988; 17:410–416

Walker M and Driscoll J. Sore nipples: The new mother's nemesis. Am J Matern Child Nurs 1989; 14:260–265

Watson D et al. Bromocriptine mesylate for lactation suppression: A risk for postpartum hypertension. Obstet Gynecol 1989; 74:573–576

Wilkerson N. Treating hyperbilirubinemia. American Journal of Maternal Child Nursing 1989; 14:32–36

Wink D. Better breast milk for preemies. Am J Nurs 1989; 89:48–49

Ectopic Pregnancy

Ectopic pregnancy is any gestation located outside the uterine cavity. Although the majority of ectopic pregnancies are tubal implantations, other types include cervical, abdominal, or ovarian implantations. It is a major cause of maternal mortality because of rupture of the site and subsequent hemorrhage (Fig. 42-1).

Etiology

1. Structural factors that prevent or delay the passage of the fertilized ovum include adhesions of the tube, salpingitis, congenital and developmental anomalies of the fallopian or uterine tube, previous ectopic pregnancy, current use of an intrauterine device, and multiple induced abortions.
2. Functional factors include menstrual reflux and decreased tubal motility.

Pathophysiology

1. The fertilized ovum implants outside of the uterus.
   a. The most common site of implantation is the fallopian or uterine tube.
   b. Other sites include the abdomen and the ovaries.

Clinical Manifestations

1. Abdominal or pelvic pain is present in almost all ectopic pregnancies.
2. Amenorrhea is present in 75% of the cases.
3. Vaginal spotting or bleeding may be present—is usually scanty and dark in color.
4. Uterine size is usually similar to what it would be in a normally implanted pregnancy.
5. Abdominal tenderness is present upon palpation.
6. Nausea, vomiting, or faintness may also be present.
7. Pelvic examination reveals a pelvic mass, posterior or lateral to the uterus, and cervical pain on movement of the cervix.

Diagnostic Evaluation

1. *Culdocentesis*—aspiration of fluid from the cul-de-sac of Douglas. Presence of bloody fluid indicates intraperitoneal bleeding.
2. *Culdoscopy*—visualization of the pelvic organs through the punctured posterior fornix.
3. *Ultrasound*—identification of the gestational sac in the tube is difficult, but if a gestational sac is identified within the uterus, it is unlikely that one also coexists in the tube.

Medical Management

1. Preservation of maternal life, through removal of the pregnancy and reconstruction of the tube if possible.
2. Correction of maternal hemorrhage if it has occurred.

Nursing Assessment

A. Physical Assessment

1. Maternal vital signs
2. Amount of blood loss
3. Amount and type of pain
4. Presence of abdominal tenderness upon palpation
5. Date of last menstrual period
6. Presence of positive pregnancy test

B. Contributing Factors

1. Salpingitis
2. History of pelvic inflammatory disease
3. Endometriosis
4. Congenital anatomic irregularities

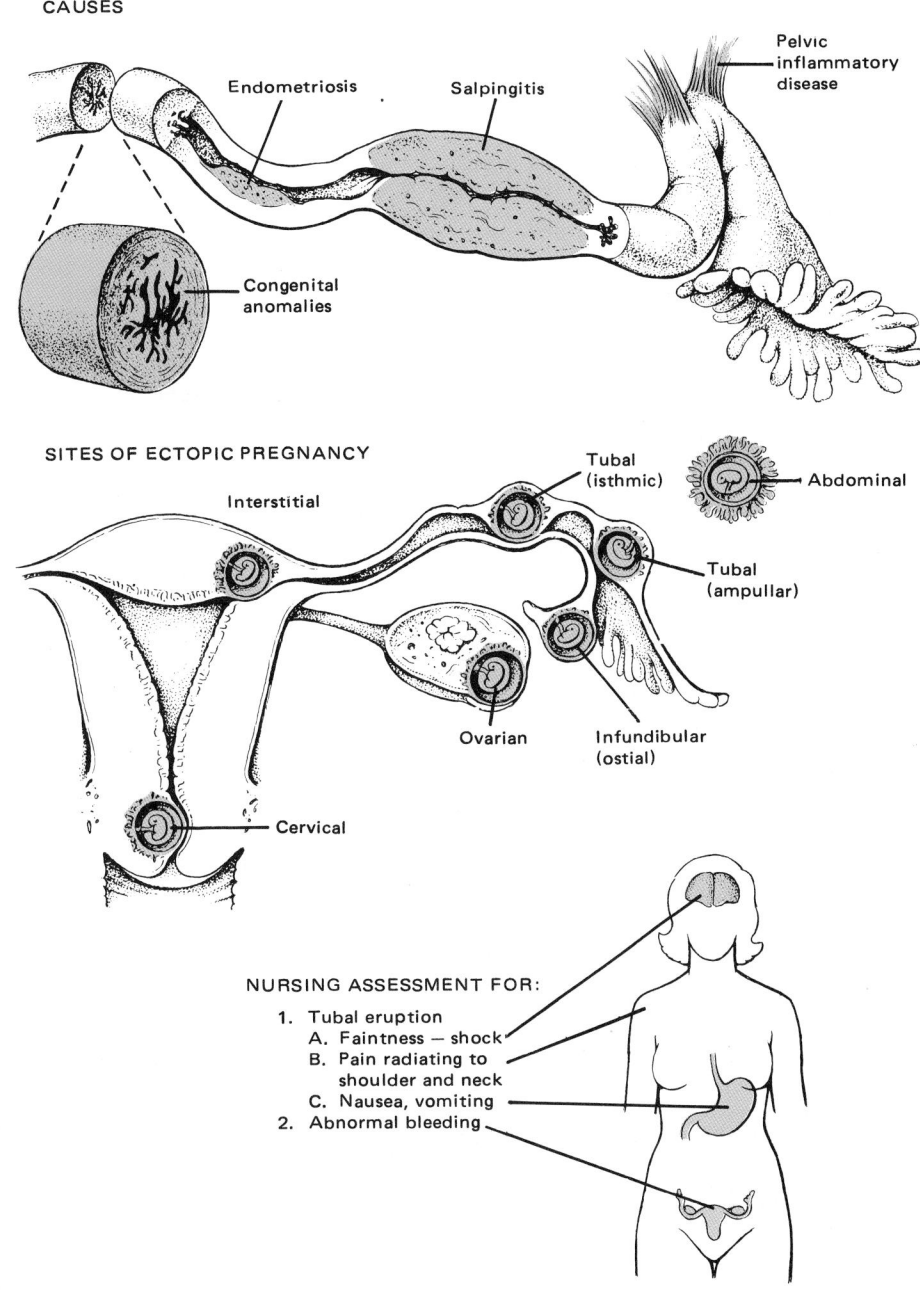

CAUSES

Endometriosis

Salpingitis

Pelvic inflammatory disease

Congenital anomalies

SITES OF ECTOPIC PREGNANCY

Tubal (isthmic)

Abdominal

Interstitial

Tubal (ampullar)

Ovarian

Infundibular (ostial)

Cervical

NURSING ASSESSMENT FOR:

1. Tubal eruption
   A. Faintness — shock
   B. Pain radiating to shoulder and neck
   C. Nausea, vomiting
2. Abnormal bleeding

Figure 42-1. *Ectopic pregnancy.*

5. Previous tubal surgery
6. Previous ectopic pregnancy
7. History of multiple induced abortions
8. Current use of intrauterine device

Nursing Diagnoses

1. Potential for fluid volume deficit related to blood loss from ruptured tube.
2. Pain related to rupture and outpouring of blood into the peritoneal cavity.
3. Anxiety related to uncertainty about condition and potential loss of childbearing capacity.

Nursing Interventions

A. **Replacing Fluid**

1. Establish an intravenous (IV) line with a large intracath and maintain the IV, as prescribed.
2. Type and screen woman for whole blood and administer as prescribed.

3. Monitor vital signs and bleeding frequently, depending on condition.

B. Relieving Pain and Anxiety

1. Remain with woman and provide psychosocial support.
2. Encourage the presence of a support person.
3. Administer analgesic as needed and as prescribed.
4. Encourage use of relaxation techniques.
5. Listen to what the patient and support person are saying regarding the childbearing.
6. Explain the need for the IV; reinforce the physician's explanation of surgery.
7. Realistically answer questions the patient and support person may have regarding further childbearing.
8. Do not provide false reassurance.

Evaluation

1. No signs of a fluid volume deficit, vital signs are stable
2. Verbalizes relief of pain
3. Discuss realistically childbearing capabilities

Hydatidiform Mole

Hydatidiform mole is a developmental anomaly of the placenta resulting in the conversion of the chorionic villi into a mass of clear vesicles. There may be no fetus, or a degenerating fetus may be present.

Etiology

1. It is believed to be derived from the paternal haploid, X-carrying set of chromosomes that reaches 46XX by its own duplication.
2. Not all moles have the 46XX chromosomal makeup.

Clinical Manifestations

1. Uterus that is large for gestational dates.
2. Persistent bleeding.
3. Signs of pregnancy-induced hypertension (PIH) prior to 20 weeks' gestation.

Diagnostic Evaluation

1. Bleeding and uterine size larger than expected for estimated date are suspicious of a hydatidiform mole.
2. Ultrasound will show a characteristic picture of the mole in most cases.
3. Symptoms of pregnancy-induced hypertension prior to 20 weeks' gestation may exist.

Management

1. Immediate evacuation of the mole
2. Follow-up for detection for malignant changes.

Nursing Assessment

1. Monitor maternal vital signs; note presence of hypertension.
2. Assess the amount and type of vaginal bleeding; note the presence of any other vaginal discharge.
3. Assess the urine for the presence of protein.
4. Palpate uterine height; if above the umbilicus, measure the fundal height.
5. Determine date of last menstrual period and date of positive pregnancy test.

Patient Problems/Nursing Diagnoses

1. Potential for fluid volume deficit related to maternal hemorrhage.
2. Anxiety related to loss of pregnancy, fear of impending procedures, fear of malignancy, and fear for future pregnancies.

Nursing Interventions

A. Ensuring Fluid Status

1. Type and screen the blood and have 2–4 units of whole blood available.
2. Establish and maintain IV line; start with a large needle.
3. Assess maternal vital signs and evaluate bleeding.
4. Observe for complications, e.g., recurrent hemorrhage

B. Reducing Anxiety

1. Prepare the patient for surgery (mole is removed by vacuum aspiration). Explain preoperative and postoperative care along with intraoperative procedures.
2. Educate patient and family on the disease process.
3. Allow the family to grieve over the loss of the pregnancy.
4. Allow the family to discuss their feelings regarding this diagnosis and implications.

Evaluation

1. Vital signs remain within a normal range, blood loss is minimal.
2. Anxiety is decreased; patient verbalizes understanding of disease process and is able to discuss openly feelings regarding loss of pregnancy and need for follow-up treatment.

Health Teaching

1. Advise the woman on the need for follow-up care and the importance of continuing the follow-up care.
2. Pregnancy to be avoided for a minimum of 1 year.
3. Biweekly measurement of chorionic gonadotropin levels is recommended.
4. A rise in chorionic gonadotropin levels or plateau requires further treatment.
5. When the chorionic gonadotropin levels have decreased to the lower level, testing is conducted monthly for 6 months and then every 2 months for a total of 1 year.

Abortion

Abortion is the termination of pregnancy at any time before the fetus has attained viability (20 weeks' gestation or fetal weight of 500 gm. [1.1 lb.]).

Types of Abortions

1. Spontaneous (Table 42-1)
   a. Threatened abortion
   b. Inevitable abortion
   c. Habitual abortion
   d. Incomplete abortion
   e. Missed abortion
2. Therapeutic/voluntary

Table 42-1. *Types of Spontaneous Abortions*

Classification	Clinical Manifestations	Management
1. Threatened	Vaginal bleeding or spotting Mild cramps Tenderness over uterus, simulates mild labor or persistent low backache with feeling of pelvic pressure Cervix closed or slightly dilated Symptoms subside or develop into an inevitable abortion	Vaginal examination Bedrest (some clinicians, citing the abnormal number of embryos that are aborted, will not limit activity in belief that the embryo will be aborted anyway) Pad count
2. Inevitable	Bleeding more profuse Cervix dilated Membranes rupture Painful uterine contractions	Embryo delivered, followed by D&C
3. Habitual	Spontaneous abortion occurs in successive pregnancies (3 or more)	D&C Treatment of possible causes: hormonal imbalance, tumors, thyroid dysfunction, abnormal uterus, incompetent cervix; with treatment, 70%–80% carry a pregnancy successfully Hysterogram to rule out uterine abnormalities, infections Surgical suturing of the cervix if incompetent cervix is a causative factor
4. Incomplete	Fetus usually expelled Placenta and membranes retained	D&C
5. Missed	Fetus dies in utero and is retained Maceration No symptoms of abortion, but symptoms of pregnancy regress (uterine size, breast changes)	Real time ultrasound, and if 2nd trimester, fetal monitoring to determine if fetus is dead If fetus is not passed after diagnosis, oxytocin induction may be used. Retained dead fetus may lead to development of disseminated intravascular coagulation (DIC) or infection Fibrinogen concentrations should be measured weekly

Spontaneous Abortion

Etiology

1. Frequently the cause of the spontaneous abortions is unknown.
2. 50% are due to chromosomal anomalies.
3. Incompetent cervix results in an increase in spontaneous abortions when the woman has had a voluntary or therapeutic abortion.

Contributing Factors

1. Exposure or contact with teratogenic agents
2. Poor maternal nutritional status
3. Maternal illness with virus such as rubella, cytomegalovirus (CMV), active herpes, and toxoplasmosis
4. Immunologic factor by which the mother and father are genetically similar, with similar major antigens, that cause the maternal immune system to reject the embryo.
5. Luteal phase defect
6. Postmature sperm or ova
7. Structural defect in the maternal reproductive system (including an incompetent cervix)
8. Imperfect sperm or ova

Incidence

1. Frequent complication of pregnancy
2. Actual rate is unknown, but thought to be between 10% and 60%, with an average of 43%
3. 80% occur in the first 12 weeks
4. 50% are due to chromosomal anomalies
5. Rate increase due to incompetent cervix after having a voluntary or therapeutic abortion

Clinical Manifestations

1. Vaginal bleeding usually begins as dark spotting, then progresses to frank bleeding as the embryo separates from the uterus.
2. Human chorionic gonadotropin (HCG) levels may be elevated for as long as 2 weeks after loss of the embryo.

Diagnostic Evaluation

1. Ultrasonic evaluation of the gestational sac or embryo is done.
2. Visualization of the cervix is done, and presence of dilation or tissue is evaluated.

Assessment

1. Monitor maternal vital signs
2. Evaluate the amount and color of blood that is present; determine the time the bleeding began and any precipitating factors
3. Evaluate any blood or clot tissue for the presence of fetal membranes, placenta, or fetus
4. Determine if a positive pregnancy test has previously been obtained, also the date of the last menstrual period.

Patient Problems/Nursing Diagnoses

1. Potential for fluid volume deficit related to maternal bleeding.

2. Anxiety related to loss of pregnancy, cause of the abortion, future childbearing.
3. Potential for infection related to dilated cervix and open uterine vessels.
4. Pain related to uterine cramping.

Nursing Interventions

A. Maintaining Adequate Fluid Volume

1. Evaluate bleeding, maternal vital signs, and length of time symptoms have been present.
2. Type and screen for blood administrations.
3. Establish and maintain an IV with large intracath.
4. Inspect all tissue passed for completeness.

B. Reducing Anxiety

1. Assess level of anxiety of patient and support person and provide information regarding current status as needed.
2. Encourage the patient to discuss her feelings about the loss of the baby and its effects on her and on her relationship with the father.
3. Do NOT give false reassurances regarding future childbearing
4. Provide time alone for the couple to discuss their feelings.
5. Discuss the prognosis of future pregnancies with the couple.
6. If the fetus is aborted intact, provide an opportunity for viewing if parents desire.
7. Refer to chaplain, if indicated or requested.

C. Preventing Infection

1. Evaluate temperature with a glass thermometer every 4 hours if normal, and every 2 hours if elevated.
2. Note odor of vaginal drainage.
3. Instruct on perineal care, and encourage to do perineal care following each urination.
4. Instruct on signs of infection and emphasize the need to report these signs to the physician if they develop following discharge from the hospital.

D. Increasing Comfort

1. Instruct patient on the cause of pain
2. Instruct and encourage the use of relaxation techniques.
3. Administer pain medications as needed and as prescribed.

Evaluation

1. Vital signs remain normal
2. Verbalizes feelings regarding the loss of the pregnancy
3. Temperature remains normal and no signs of infection appear
4. Verbalizes relief of pain

Health Teaching

1. Provide the names of local support groups for couples who have experienced an early pregnancy loss.
2. Discuss with the couple the methods of contraception to be used.
3. Explain the need to wait at least 3 months before trying for another pregnancy.

NURSING ALERT: If the woman is Rh negative, she needs to be evaluated for the need for RhoGAM.

Therapeutic or Voluntary Abortion

Therapeutic abortion is the termination of pregnancy before fetal viability for the purpose of safeguarding the woman's health. *Voluntary abortion* is the termination of a pregnancy before fetal viability as a choice of the woman.

Assessment

1. Review the woman's knowledge of her choice and the options that are available in regard to childbearing.
2. Discuss the woman's knowledge of the possible health benefits of a therapeutic abortion.

Patient Problems/Nursing Diagnoses

1. Grief over loss of pregnancy or baby
2. Potential for infection related to cervical dilation

Nursing Interventions

A. Providing Psychosocial Support

1. Allow the woman to discuss reason for choosing the abortion.
2. Encourage the woman to explore all options available regarding the pregnancy.
3. Do not provide false reassurance regarding future pregnancies.

B. Preventing Infection

1. Evaluate temperature with a glass thermometer every 4 hours if normal and every 2 hours if elevated.
2. Note odor of vaginal drainage.
3. Instruct on perineal care, and encourage doing perineal care following each urination.
4. Instruct on signs of infection and instruct to report these to physician if they develop following discharge.

Evaluation

1. Openly discusses feelings regarding the loss of pregnancy and/or baby
2. Does not develop symptoms of an infection

Hyperemesis Gravidarum

Hyperemesis gravidarum is exaggerated nausea and vomiting during pregnancy persisting past the first trimester. The persistent vomiting may result in fluid and electrolyte imbalances, dehydration, jaundice, elevation of serum transaminase, and retention of sulfobromophthalein.

Diagnostic Evaluation

Based on the presenting symptoms—persistent weight loss, dehydration, and signs of vitamin deficiency.

Medical Management

Control of dehydration, vomiting, weight loss, and nausea through use of medications and IV therapy.

Nursing Assessment

1. Evaluate weight gain or loss pattern.
2. Evaluate 24- or 48-hour dietary recall.
3. Evaluate environment for factors that may affect the woman's appetite.
4. Monitor vital signs.
5. Assess skin turgor and mucous membranes.

Patient Problems/Nursing Diagnoses

1. Potential for fluid volume deficit and electrolyte imbalance related to prolonged vomiting
2. Alterations in nutrition less than body requirements related to prolonged vomiting
3. Potential for ineffective coping related to stress

Nursing Interventions

A. Establishing Fluid Balance and Nutritional Needs

1. Establish and maintain an IV line as prescribed.
2. Monitor electrolyte status.
3. Medicate with antiemetics as prescribed.
4. Provide bland solid foods; serve hot foods hot and cold foods cold; do not serve lukewarm.
5. Avoid greasy, gassy, and spicy foods.
6. Provide liquids at times other than meal times.
7. Provide an environment conducive to eating.
8. Keep room cool and quiet before and after meals.
9. Keep emesis pan handy, yet out of sight.

B. Providing Psychosocial Support

1. Allow patient to verbalize feelings regarding this pregnancy.
2. Encourage patient to discuss any personal stress that could stir negative thoughts regarding this pregnancy.
3. Refer to social service and counseling services as needed.

Evaluation

1. Demonstrates proper hydration and electrolyte balance.
2. Maintains appropriate weight.
3. Openly discusses any current stressor.

Placenta Previa

Placenta previa is the development of the placenta in the lower uterine segment, partially or completely covering the internal cervical os (Fig. 42-2).

Clinical Manifestations

1. Characteristic sign is painless vaginal bleeding, which usually appears near the end of the second trimester or later.
2. Initial episode is rarely fatal and usually stops spontaneously, with subsequent bleeding episodes occurring spontaneously; each episode is more profuse than the previous one.
3. Bleeding from placenta previa may not occur until cervical dilation occurs and the placenta is loosened from the uterus.
4. With a total placenta previa the bleeding will occur earlier in the pregnancy and be more profuse.

Diagnostic Evaluation

1. Ultrasound will show the location of the placenta.
2. If the findings are questioned, transcervical ultrasound can improve the accuracy of the diagnosis.

Assessment

1. Determine the amount and type of bleeding; also, review any history of bleeding throughout this pregnancy.

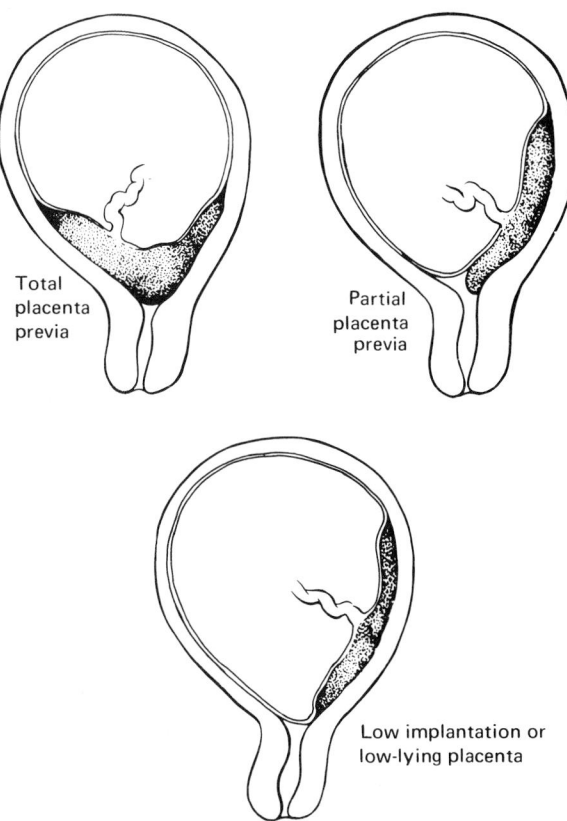

Figure 42-2. *Variations of placenta previa. (From Danforth DN and Scott JR. Obstetrics and Gynecology. 5th ed. Philadelphia, JB Lippincott, 1986)*

2. Record maternal and fetal vital signs.
3. Inquire as to the presence or absence of pain in association with the bleeding.
4. Palpate for the presence of uterine contractions.
5. Evaluate laboratory data on hemoglobin and hemocrit status.

Patient Problems/Nursing Diagnoses

1. Alterations in tissue perfusion: placental, related to excessive bleeding.
2. Fluid volume deficit related to excessive bleeding.
3. Potential for infection related to excessive blood loss and open blood vessels near cervix.
4. Fear or anxiety related to excessive bleeding and impending procedures.

Nursing Interventions

A. Improving Tissue Perfusion

1. Evaluate the amount of blood lost, length of time of bleeding, and history of previous bleeding episodes.
2. Monitor vital signs, fetal heart tones, and contractions if present.
3. Monitor hemoglobin and hematocrit.
4. Establish and maintain an IV line as prescribed. Establish with a large gauge needle in case a transfusion is needed.
5. Position on side to promote placental perfusion
6. Administer oxygen as indicated by face mask.

B. Ensuring Fluid Volume

1. Establish and maintain an IV line, as prescribed
2. Type and screen for blood replacement.
3. Position in a sitting position to allow the weight of fetus to compress the placenta and decrease bleeding.
4. Maintain strict bedrest during any bleeding episode.
5. If bleeding is profuse and delivery cannot be delayed, prepare the woman physically and emotionally for a cesarean delivery.

C. Preventing Infection

1. Use aseptic technique when providing care.
2. Evaluate temperature every 4 hours unless elevated; then, evaluate every 2 hours.
3. Evaluate white blood cell (WBC) and differential count.
4. Instruct on perineal care.
5. Assess odor of all vaginal bleeding or lochia.
6. Instruct on perineal care and handwashing techniques.

D. Reducing Fear and Anxiety

1. Explain all treatments and procedures and answer all related questions.
2. Encourage verbalization of feelings by patient and family.
3. Provide information on a cesarean delivery and prepare patient emotionally.
4. Discuss the effects of long-term hospitalization or prolonged bedrest.

Evaluation

1. Fetal condition is stable, infant is stable if born
2. Absence of shock, demonstrated by stable vital signs, and absence of bleeding
3. Does not develop any symptoms of an infection
4. Demonstrates an understanding of procedures and treatments

> **NURSING ALERT:** Never perform a vaginal examination on anyone who is bleeding. This may result in puncturing the placenta.

> **NURSING ALERT:** Women who have had a placenta previa are at risk for postpartum hemorrhage because of the decreased contractility of the lower uterine segment and the large space the placenta occupied.

Abruptio Placentae

Abruptio placentae is premature separation of the normally implanted placenta of an unknown etiology. There are two types of abruptio placentae: concealed hemorrhage and external hemorrhage. With a concealed hemorrhage the placenta separates centrally, and a large amount of blood is accumulated under the placenta. When an external hemorrhage is present, the separation is along the placental margin, and blood flows under the membranes and through the cervix (Fig. 42-3).

Etiology

Frequently, the etiology is unknown; however, those women at risk for development of abruptio placentae are

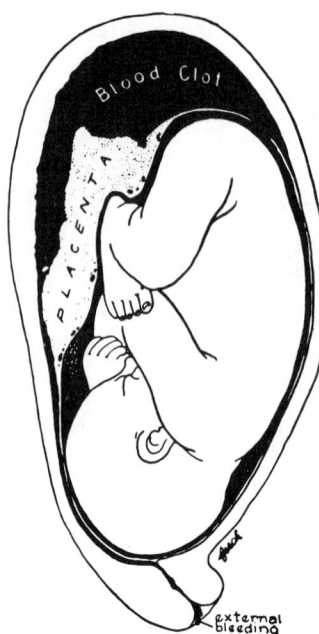

Figure 42-3. *Abruptio placentae with large blood clot between placenta and uterine wall.*

women with a history of hypertension or women who have rapid decompression of the uterine cavity, short umbilical cord, or presence of a uterine anomaly or tumor.

Contributing Factors

1. Pregnancies complicated by hypertension, trauma, previous history of abruptio placentae, and alcohol use increase the risk of abruptio placentae.

Incidence

1. The frequency varies based on the criteria used to make the diagnosis.
2. Incidence range from 1 in 75 to 1 in 90 deliveries.

Pathophysiology

1. Hemorrhage occurs into the decidua basalis.
2. The decidua basalis then forms a hematoma.
3. This hematoma can expand as the bleeding increases, causing the hematoma to increase in size and further detach the placenta from the uterine wall.

Clinical Manifestations

1. *Concealed hemorrhage*—results in a change in maternal vital signs, but no visible signs of hemorrhage are present
2. *External hemorrhage*—hemorrhage is evident along with a change in maternal vital signs.
3. Fetal heart rate may change, depending on the degree of hemorrhage.
4. Abdominal pain is often present.

Diagnostic Evaluation

1. Ultrasound is able to diagnose an abruptio placentae in less than 25% of the time.

2. Usually the woman is experiencing some uterine pain as a result of the blood collecting in the uterus.

Medical Management

1. Depends on extent of maternal hemorrhage.
2. Goal is to preserve the maternal life and fetus if possible.

Nursing Assessment

1. Determine the amount and type of bleeding and the presence or absence of pain.
2. Monitor maternal and fetal vital signs.
3. Palpate the abdomen.
   a. Note the presence of contractions and relaxation between contractions (if contractions are present).
   b. If contractions are not present, assess the abdomen for firmness.
4. Measure and record fundal height to evaluate the presence of concealed bleeding.

NURSING ALERT: External bleeding may seem out of proportion to symptoms displayed by the woman.

Patient Problems/Nursing Diagnoses

1. Alterations in tissue perfusion: placental related to excessive bleeding.
2. Fluid volume deficit related to excessive bleeding.

3. Potential for infection, related to excessive blood loss.
4. Fear or anxiety related to excessive bleeding and impending procedures.

Nursing Interventions

A. Improving Tissue Perfusion

1. Evaluate the amount of bleeding.
2. Position in the left lateral position, with the head elevated.
3. Administer oxygen through a face mask.
4. Establish an IV line with a large intracath, as prescribed, and maintain the IV site.
5. Evaluate fetal status with continuous external fetal monitoring.
6. Encourage relaxation techniques.

B. Ensuring Fluid Volume

1. Establish and maintain the IV line; replace with blood or blood products as prescribed.
2. Evaluate coagulation studies.
3. Monitor maternal vital signs; use continuous external fetal monitoring to evaluate the fetus.
4. Monitor vaginal bleeding, and evaluate fundal height to detect an increase in bleeding.

C. Preventing Infection

Use aseptic technique when doing invasive procedures.

D. Relieving Fear and Anxiety

1. Explain all procedures prior to carrying out, if possible; otherwise, explain each procedure as it is performed. Explain in calm manner using simple terms. Include the benefit to the woman and her fetus.

Characteristics of Abruptio Placentae and Placenta Previa

Characteristic	Abruptio Placentae	Placenta Previa
Onset	Third trimester	Third trimester (commonly in 8th month)
Bleeding	May be concealed, external dark hemorrhage, or bloody amniotic fluid	Mostly external, small to profuse in amount, bright red
Pain and uterine tenderness	Usually present; irritable uterus, progresses to board-like consistency	Usually absent; uterus soft
Fetal heart tone	May be irregular or absent	Usually normal
Presenting part	May or may not be engaged	Usually not engaged
Shock	Moderate to severe depending on extent of concealed and external hemorrhage	Usually not present unless bleeding is excessive
Delivery	Immediate delivery, usually by cesarean section	Delivery may be delayed, depending on size of fetus and amount of bleeding

2. Encourage the presence of support person.
3. When appropriate, encourage expression of feelings.

Evaluation

1. Fetal heart rate is within the normal range, without a loss of variability.
2. Absence of shock, demonstrated by stable maternal vital signs.
3. No signs of infection.
4. Decreasing anxiety, asking questions.

Pregnancy-Induced Hypertension

Pregnancy-induced hypertension (PIH, preeclampsia, toxemia of pregnancy) is a disorder occurring during pregnancy after the 20th week of gestation and involving edema, proteinuria, and hypertension. Eclampsia is diagnosed when convulsions occur in the absence of an underlying neurologic condition in the presence of hypertension, edema, and proteinuria.

Etiology

1. Actual cause is unknown.
2. Theories of the etiology include the exposure to chorionic villi for the first time, or in large amounts, along with immunologic, genetic, and endocrine factors.

Pathophysiology

1. Vasospasms occur and result in increased resistance in vascular flow, increasing the arterial blood pressure.
2. Increased sensitivity to angiotensin II prior to the onset of hypertension.
3. Hemoconcentration occurs related to the vasoconstriction or as a result of increased vascular permeability or a combination of both.

Contributing Factors

1. Primarily a disease of the nulligravida
2. Adolescents and women over 35 years of age
3. Multigravida with multiple gestations
4. Multigravidas with history of chronic hypertension, diabetes mellitus, and renal disease.

Incidence

1. Approximately 5% of all pregnancies are complicated by pregnancy-induced hypertension.
2. Approximately 20% of the nullipara develop the disease.

Clinical Manifestations

1. Hypertension, which is defined as a blood pressure of 140/90 mm. Hg or greater. (Some health professionals accept that an increase of 15 mm. Hg diastolic or 30 mm. Hg systolic at two readings at least 6 hours apart is hypertension).
2. Proteinuria—300 mg. or more of protein excreted in a 24-hour period.
3. Edema, nondependent, present after 8–12 hours of bedrest.
4. Weight gain of more than 2 lb. in 1 week or 6 lb. in 1 month.

Diagnostic Evaluation

1. Based on the presenting symptoms. Often the disease process has been slowly developing and affecting the renal and vascular system.
2. Frequently a sudden weight gain will occur, of 2 lb. or more in 1 week, or 6 or more lb. in 1 month. This often occurs before the edema is present.

Medical Management

1. Directed toward decreasing the maternal blood pressure through the use of bedrest and antihypertensive medications along with increase in dietary protein and an increase in calories, if indicated.
2. If symptoms increase or are not corrected, the woman may be hospitalized and started on magnesium sulfate.
3. If symptoms are uncontrollable, delivery is planned.

Assessment

1. Evaluate blood pressure in a sitting position and in the left lateral position.
2. Check the protein level of urine.
3. Evaluate edema, carefully noting the presence after 12 hours or more of bedrest.
4. Evaluate the presence of epigastric pain, visual changes, level of consciousness, and headaches.
5. Evaluate weight gain.
6. Evaluate for signs of placental separation, uterine rigidity, and vaginal bleeding.

Patient Problems/Nursing Diagnoses

1. Potential for fluid volume deficit, related to pregnancy-induced hypertension.
2. Potential of alterations in tissue perfusion: placental, related to pregnancy-induced hypertension.
3. Potential of injury, related to convulsions.
4. Potential for anxiety, related to diagnosis of pregnancy-induced hypertension
5. Potential of alterations in nutrition, less than body requirements, related to inadequate protein intake.
6. Potential for diversional activity deficit, related to prolonged bedrest or hospitalizations
7. Potential complications from side effects of medications.

Nursing Interventions

A. Maintaining Fluid Volume

1. Evaluate daily hematocrit levels to evaluate intravascular fluid status.
2. Evaluate urine output—should consist of 300 ml. or more with each voiding.
3. Encourage increased fluid intake (water and juice). Instruct to avoid carbonated beverages and other high-sodium fluids.
4. Evaluate skin turgor.

B. Ensuring Tissue Perfusion

1. Position on side, preferably the left side.
2. Monitor fetal activity.
3. Evaluate nonstress tests to determine fetal status.
4. Encourage increased fluid intake of juices and water.
5. Increase protein intake.

C. Protecting Against Convulsions

1. Instruct on the importance of reporting headaches, visual changes, dizziness, and epigastric pain.
2. Instruct to lay down on left side if symptoms are present.
3. Keep the environment quiet and as calm as possible.
4. If hospitalized, side rails should remain up and should be padded.
5. If hospitalized, oxygen and suction setup should be immediately available, along with a tongue blade and emergency medications.

D. Relieving Anxiety

1. Explain the disease process and treatment plan.
2. Explain that pregnancy-induced hypertension does not lead to chronic hypertension.
3. Explain that pregnancy-induced hypertension usually does not occur with subsequent pregnancies.
4. Discuss the effects of all medications on the mother and fetus.
5. Allow time to ask questions and discuss feelings regarding the diagnosis and treatment plan.

E. Promoting Adequate Nutrition

1. Evaluate nutritional adequacy of diet through a 24-hour recall or diet log.
2. Instruct on the need to increase protein intake and decrease the amount of processed foods and table salt in the diet.

3. Conduct daily weight and hematocrit to evaluate if weight gain is due to edema or nutritional causes.

F. Encouraging Diversional Activity

1. Evaluate feelings about bedrest or hospitalization.
2. Provide craft materials in bed. Be sure that materials are compatible with bedrest.
3. Provide information on childbirth and infant care.
4. Encourage visits from support persons.

Medication Side Effects

A. Magnesium Sulfate (MgSO₄)

1. Used to prevent and treat convulsions; its primary action is not to lower the blood pressure.
2. MgSO₄ decreases the neuromuscular irritability and depresses the central nervous system.
3. IV administration—MgSO₄ is administered intravenously with a loading dose of 3–4 gm., followed by hourly doses of 1–4 gm.
4. Intramuscular (IM) administration—MgSO₄ may also be administered intramuscularly.
   a. The usual dose is 5 gm. in each hip, every 4 hours.
   b. Must be given deep IM using the Z tract method.
   c. IM administration is painful and absorption is variable.
5. MgSO₄ is irritating to veins, so the infusion site must be closely monitored.
6. Because MgSO₄ is a central nervous system depressant, respiratory status must be monitored closely.
7. MgSO₄ is excreted through the kidneys, and urine output should be 30 ml. or more per hour to avoid toxicity.
8. Maintain strict hourly intake and output (I & O) records—if the patient is receiving a large dose, a Foley catheter may be inserted to evaluate the urine output accurately.
9. Evaluate deep tendon reflexes (DTR)—absence of DTR indicates an increase in the magnesium level.
10. Frequently evaluate the serum magnesium levels. A therapeutic level is 4–7.5 mEq/liter.
11. Maternal and fetal vital signs should be assessed at least hourly if receiving intravenous MgSO₄.
12. Calcium gluconate is the antidote of MgSO₄.

B. Antihypertensive Drug Therapy

1. Used when the diastolic pressure is above 110 mm. Hg or when cerebrovascular accident is impending.
2. Hydralazine (Apresoline) is the drug of choice. Hydralazine relaxes the arterioles and stimulates cardiac output.
3. Side effects include tachycardia, dizziness, faintness, headache, and palpations.

C. Other Drugs

1. Diazepam (Valium) and amobarbital sodium (Amytal Sodium) may be used if convulsions occur.
2. Beta-blockers are used by some to control acute hypertension. These drugs will rapidly lower the blood pressure; however further studies are needed on these drugs and their use in pregnancy.

Evaluation

1. Adequate fluid volume is maintained; hematocrit remains within normal range.
2. Fetal heart rate remains within normal range, and nonstress test is reactive.
3. Does not develop convulsions.
4. Is able to express fears and anxiety regarding the diagnosis and treatment.

5. Has a dietary intake of 100 gm. of protein per day.
6. Participates in diversional activities.
7. Does not develop any toxicity or side effects of medications used in treatment.
8. Does not develop any side effects or toxicity with drug therapy.

HELLP Syndrome

A severe complication of pregnancy-induced hypertension is the HELLP syndrome.

1. This syndrome is comprised of **H**emolysis, **E**levated **L**iver enzymes, and **L**ow **P**latelets.
2. These finding are frequently associated with disseminated intravascular coagulation (DIC) and may in fact be diagnosed as DIC.
3. The hemolysis of the red blood cells is seen in the abnormal morphology of the cells.
4. The elevated liver enzyme measurement is associated with the decreased blood flow to the liver as a result of fibrin thrombi.
5. The low platelet count is related to the vasospasm and platelet adhesions at the site, resulting in a low platelet count.
6. Treatment is similar to treatment for PIH with close monitoring of liver function and bleeding.
7. These women are especially prone to developing a postpartum hemorrhage.

Hydramnios (Polyhydramnios)

Hydramnios (polyhydramnios) is caused by an excessive amount of amniotic fluid. At 36 weeks of pregnancy there is usually about a liter of fluid present. The amount of amniotic fluid normally decreases after this time. The amount of amniotic fluid present is controlled in part by fetal urination, swallowing, and breathing. Two basic types are identified: chronic and acute. In the chronic type the fluid volume gradually increases; in the acute type the volume increases rapidly over a few days.

Etiology

1. Frequently related to an underlying fetal problem such as: esophageal atresia, neural tube defects, monozygotic twins, and hypoplastic lung disease.
2. Frequently seen in women with diabetes, the cause is unknown.
3. Prolactin levels in the amniotic fluid are elevated.

Contributing Factors

1. Infants with esophageal atresia
2. Infants with neural tube defects
3. Monozygotic twins
4. Maternal diabetes
5. Infants with hypoplastic lung disease
6. The placenta is usually extremely large, and the level of prolactin in the amniotic fluid is increased.

Incidence

1. Varies because the collection and measurement of amniotic fluid is difficult and often subjectively based.
2. Rates range from 1 in 60 to 1 in 750 deliveries.

Clinical Manifestations

Increased uterine size for gestational age usually accompanied by difficulty in palpating fetal parts and in auscultation of fetal heart.

Diagnostic Evaluation

1. A diagnosis is made based on the present symptoms and ultrasound evaluation.
2. Ultrasound evaluation will show large pockets of fluid between the fetus and uterine wall or placenta.

Management

1. If impairment of respiratory status occurs, an amniocentesis for removal of fluid may be performed.
   a. The amniocentesis is performed under ultrasound for location of the placenta and fetal parts.
   b. The fluid is then slowly removed.
   c. Rapid removal of the fluid can result in a premature separation of the placenta.
   d. Usually 1.5–2.5 liters of fluid are removed.
2. Occasionally the fluid is removed transcervically. The major disadvantage of this procedure is the potential for prolapse of the umbilical cord and premature separation of the placenta because decompression is usually very rapid.

Nursing Assessment

1. Evaluate uterine height and compare with previous findings.
2. Evaluate respiratory status.

Patient Problems/Nursing Diagnoses

1. Altered gas exchange related to pressure on the diaphragm
2. Altered tissue perfusion: placental related to pressure from the enlarged uterus
3. Altered comfort related to the edema and tightness experienced from the enlarged uterus.
4. Anxiety related to unknown (or known) fetal outcome.

Nursing Interventions

A. Promoting Gas Exchange

1. Position to promote chest expansion with head elevated.
2. Provide O_2 by face mask if indicated.
3. Limit activities, and plan for frequent rest periods.
4. Maintain an adequate intake and output.
5. Provide emotional support; discuss and explain all procedures.

B. Promoting Tissue Perfusion

1. Position on side if possible, with head elevated. If unable to position on side, use a wedge to displace the uterus to the left.
2. Encourage passive or active assisted range of motion to the lower extremities.
3. Provide for frequent rest periods throughout the day.
4. Provide a diet adequate in protein, iron, and fluids.

C. Promoting Comfort

1. Position for comfort.
2. Use diversional activities appropriately.
3. Provide for frequent rest periods.

D. Relieving Anxiety

1. Explain the cause of hydramnios, if known.
2. Encourage the patient and family to ask questions regarding any treatment or procedures.
3. Encourage to ventilate feelings.
4. Prepare for the type of delivery that is anticipated and for the expected finding at the time of delivery.

Evaluation

1. Respirations remain within normal limits and remain unlabored.
2. Fetal heart rate is within normal limits, and appropriate fetal growth occurs.
3. Does not complain of discomfort related to expanding uterus.
4. Is able to discuss realistically the pregnancy outcome; has no questions regarding self or fetal treatment.

NURSING ALERT: Following delivery, these women are at risk for developing a postpartum hemorrhage related to the gross distention of the uterus.

Oligohydramnios

Oligohydramnios is caused by a marked decrease in the amount of amniotic fluid. Usually the fluid is extremely concentrated. Cord compression and fetal distress frequently lead to a poor outcome. Often the infant will suffer from pulmonary hypoplasia due to a lack of fluid in the terminal air sacs.

Etiology

1. Frequently related to fetal problems such as obstruction in the urinary tract, renal agenesis, and intrauterine growth retardation (IUGR).
2. Frequently seen in postdate pregnancies.

Contributing Factors

1. Postdate pregnancy
2. Fetal obstruction of the urinary tract
3. Fetal renal agenesis
4. Intrauterine growth retardation

Clinical Manifestations

1. Prominent fetal parts on palpation of the abdomen.
2. Small-for-date uterine size.

Diagnostic Evaluation

1. Based on presenting symptoms.
2. Confirmed on ultrasound evaluation when amniotic pockets of 1 cm. in any vertical plane cannot be found.

Medical Management

1. Includes frequent evaluation of fetal status through nonstress test and stress test as indicated.
2. Ultrasound is also done to evaluate further fetal renal and urinary systems along with fetal growth.
3. Some experimental treatment includes instilling a saline solution into the amniotic sac during labor.

Nursing Assessment and Diagnosis

1. Evaluate fetal status
2. Anxiety related to unknown fetal outcome.

Nursing Interventions

A. Relieving Anxiety

1. Explain all diagnostic testing.
2. Answer questions patient and family have regarding testing and findings.
3. Encourage patient and family to discuss their feelings.
4. Provide tour of neonatal intensive care unit so parents will be aware of surroundings prior to birth.

Evaluation

1. Patient and family openly discuss their feelings regarding diagnosis and possible outcome.

Multiple Gestations
(Multifetal Pregnancy)

Multiple gestation results when two or more fetuses are present in the uterus at the same time.

Etiology

1. Types of twinning
   a. *Dizygotic*—occurs when two separate ovum are fertilized. Dizygotic twins do not have the same genetic makeup and are as similar as other brothers and sisters.
   b. *Monozygotic*—occurs when one ovum divides early in gestation and two embryos develop. Monozygotic twins are identical in genetic makeup.

Contributing Factors

1. Ovulation induced by gonadotropin or clomiphene increases the chance of multiple ovulation.
2. Twins are more common in the black race, least common in the Oriental race.
3. Twins are more common if the mother is herself a twin.
4. Increasing maternal age and parity also increase the chance of twinning.

Incidence

1. White women have a twin rate of 1 in 100 pregnancies.
2. Black women in the United States have a twin rate of 1 in 79 pregnancies.
3. Black women in Nigeria have a twin rate of 1 in 20 births.
4. Oriental women have a twin rate of 1 in 155 births.
5. Women who have used gonadotropin have a twin rate of 20%–40%.
6. In vitro fertilization has also increased the number of multiple births, because many institutions fertilize all collected ova and then return all to the uterus.

Clinical Manifestations and Diagnostic Evaluation

1. Usually the uterus is large for gestational age during the second trimester.
2. Ultrasound is able to identify separate gestation sacs early in pregnancy.
3. Separate fetal parts may be identified during the third trimester. Not always noted if the woman is obese, if one fetus is overlying the other, or if hydramnios is present.
4. Auscultation of two distinct and separate fetal hearts may occur with a doptone late in the first trimester or with a fetoscope after 20 weeks' gestation.

Nursing Assessment

1. Assess fundal height, if large for date; evaluate for the presence of more than one heart beat.
2. If greater than 13 weeks' gestation, attempt to palpate fetal parts.

Patient Problems/Nursing Diagnoses

1. Potential for ineffective family coping related to diagnosis of multiple pregnancy.
2. Potential for altered nutrition, less than body requirements, related to the increased needs of the multiple pregnancy.
3. Potential anxiety, related to diagnosis of multiple pregnancy.
4. Potential diversional activity deficit related to prolonged bedrest or hospitalization.

Nursing Interventions

A. Promoting Coping Abilities

1. Discuss the parents' feelings regarding the multiple birth.
2. Encourage the parents to discuss ways in which they will need help with child care prior to birth of the infants.
3. Provide names of resources for mothers of multiple births.

B. Promoting Proper Nutrition

1. Evaluate the nutritional adequacy of the diet through a 24-hour recall or a diet log.
2. Review the diet with the patient and family; note dietary strengths and weaknesses. Encourage the woman to increase her iron, protein, and folic acid intake.
3. Evaluate weight gain at each prenatal visit.
4. Monitor hemoglobin and hematocrit levels frequently.

C. Reducing Anxiety

1. Discuss realistically the effects a multiple pregnancy has on the woman and on her fetus.
2. Encourage the woman to discuss her feelings regarding a multiple pregnancy and all the limitations imposed on her.
3. Prepare for birth of twins, and eventual treatment and follow-up the infants may need.

D. Encouraging Diversional Activities

1. Evaluate woman's feelings about possible prolonged bedrest or hospitalization.
2. Provide craft materials. Be sure that the materials are compatible with bedrest.
3. Provide information on childbirth and infant care.
4. Encourage visits from support persons and children.

Evaluation

1. Parents are able to discuss their feelings regarding the multiple pregnancy and realistically discuss assistance that will be needed following the birth of the infants.

2. Hemoglobin and hematocrit levels will be within normal range. Adequate weight gain will occur.
3. Discusses realistically fears of multiple gestations.
4. Participates in diversional activities.

Medical Disorders Complicating Pregnancy

Cardiac Disease

Cardiac disease in pregnancy occurs as a complication in about 1% of all pregnancies. The outcome of the pregnancy depends on the functional capacity of the maternal heart, the complications that occur during the pregnancy and postpartum, financial and psychological resources, and medical care available.

Classification

Heart disease is classified by the New York Heart Association's functional classification of patients with cardiac disease:

Class 1. No limitation of physical activity; no symptoms of cardiac insufficiency or anginal pain

Class 2. Slight limitation of physical activity; comfortable at rest; excessive fatigue, palpitations, dyspnea, or anginal pain with ordinary physical activity

Class 3. Marked limitation of physical activity; comfortable at rest; excessive fatigue, palpitations, dyspnea, or anginal pain with less than ordinary physical activity

Class 4. Inability to perform any physical activity without discomfort; symptoms of cardiac insufficiency or anginal syndrome possible at rest; discomfort increased with physical activity

1. Most women in classes 1 and 2 are able to handle the physiologic demands of pregnancy
2. The cardiac status of women in all classifications should be evaluated very early in pregnancy if not before; examination should include chest x-ray, electrocardiogram, and tests for vital capacity.
3. Cardiac status and functional capacity are monitored carefully throughout pregnancy.
4. Monitor for signs of cardiac decompensation: crackles at the bases of lungs, cough, hemoptysis, dyspnea on exertion, cyanosis, labored respirations, increased pulse, edema of face, ankles, and hands.

Etiology

1. Most underlying cardiac disease is a result of congenital heart disease.
2. Rheumatic fever is no longer a major cause of cardiac problems.

Clinical Manifestations

1. Depend on the underlying disease. Many women progress through the pregnancy with little difficulty.
2. If complications do arise they usually appear in the last weeks of the pregnancy, during labor, or in the postpartum period and are usually in the form of cardiac failure with the following symptoms displayed in varying degrees:
   a. Severe dyspnea, with persistent rales at the base of the lungs
   b. Edema present after 12 hours of bedrest
   c. Distention of the jugular veins
   d. Palpations and tachycardia
   e. Hemoptysis and coughing

Diagnostic Evaluation

1. Based on the present symptoms and past medical history.
2. Invasive diagnostic procedures are not usually done.

Management

A. Classes I and II

1. Managed with 10 hours of rest each night, in addition to a 30-minute rest after each meal.
2. Weight gain is limited to 24 lb.; diet is high in iron and low in sodium.
3. Activities are limited to light work; no heavy work or lifting is permitted.
4. Medications are used as needed to control symptoms. Frequent dosage changes may be necessary as the blood volume increases throughout the pregnancy.
5. During labor relief of pain and anxiety is a primary goal.
6. Vaginal delivery is the delivery method of choice.
7. During the postpartum period, vital signs are closely evaluated for signs of congestive heart failure.
8. Other potential complications include: postpartum hemorrhage, infection, and thromboembolism.
9. Contraception is stressed during the postpartum period.

B. Class III

1. During the first trimester the woman should be counseled regarding a therapeutic abortion.
2. If the pregnancy continues, treatment is similar to care for a Class I or II patient but includes hospitalization with strict bedrest for most of the duration of the pregnancy.
3. A vaginal delivery is the preferred method because these women are poor surgical risks.
4. During the postpartum period these woman need to be monitored closely for congestive heart failure.

C. Class IV

1. Same care as listed for preceding classes.
2. This woman has congestive heart failure for most of the pregnancy and is treated as such.
3. The delivery and postpartum periods are especially critical for these women.

Assessment

1. Evaluation of cardiac status including pulse, respirations, lungs, jugular veins distention, cardiac auscultation
2. Evaluation of fetal growth pattern
3. Maternal weight gain pattern
4. Presence of dependent and nondependent edema
5. Psychosocial adaptation to the pregnancy, restrictions, and therapy

Patient Problems/Nursing Diagnoses

1. Altered tissue perfusion: placental, related to inadequate circulation
2. Activity intolerance related to dyspnea and tachycardia
3. Altered nutrition, less that body requirements, related to inadequate intake; or, altered nutrition, more than body requirements, related to excessive intake.

4. Diversion activity deficit related to prolonged bedrest.
5. Knowledge deficit of childbirth procedures and infant care.
6. Potential for family dysfunction, related to prolonged hospitalization or prolonged bedrest.

Nursing Interventions

A. Promoting Adequate Circulation

1. Position with head of bed elevated.
2. Position to the left side most of the time.
3. Evaluate fetal growth weekly by measuring the fundal height.
4. Evaluate fetal heart rate daily.
5. Begin nonstress test, as prescribed, after 28 weeks if maternal condition indicates.

B. Maintaining Comfort and Rest

1. Provide for frequent rest periods during the day. Allow for rest periods during activities of daily living. Do not interrupt rest periods if possible. Plan for 10 or more hours of rest at night.
2. Position of comfort

C. Providing Adequate Nutrition

1. Evaluate weight weekly; be sure to use the same scale each week.
2. Review dietary needs, stressing the need for protein and iron. Discuss the need to avoid excessive sodium intake.
3. If weight gain is excessive or inadequate do a 24-hour calorie count.

D. Promoting Activity

1. Discuss quiet activities that patient likes to do.
2. Discuss new activities that patient can learn while in bed.
3. Provide necessary instruction and supplies.
4. Encourage short visits from family and close friends.
5. Provide a quiet, uninterrupted time for visits and projects.

E. Providing Psychosocial Support

1. Allow patient and family member to discuss their feelings regarding hospitalization or home treatment.
2. Have family and patient discuss ways in which the patient can still be an active family member even if she is separated from the family.
3. Refer to social service if need for assistance with child and home responsibilities, and counseling as needed.

Patient Teaching

1. Provide information on normal changes of pregnancy, and relate to current disease problems.
2. Discuss birth options within the medical confines of patient's condition.
3. Involve patient and support person in planning for the birth experience.
4. Provide information on infant care, include written instructions and videos as available and when the patient is interested.

Evaluation

1. Will have minimal intolerance to necessary activities
2. Will have a weight gain of 24 lb.
3. Will participate in some diversional activities
4. Verbalizes understanding of the birth process and infant care

5. Family function is normal
6. Fetus will be appropriate size for gestation

Anemia

During pregnancy there is an increase in the amount of circulating plasma and red blood cells. The amount of plasma increase is greater than the red blood cell increase. This results in a hemodilution and drop in hemoglobin. During pregnancy or in the postpartum period the patient with a hemoglobin of 10 gm./dl. or hematocrit below 35% is considered anemic.

Clinical Manifestations

1. The clinical manifestations will depend on the type of anemia that is present.
2. Iron-deficiency anemia—is the most common hematologic disorder that occurs during pregnancy.
3. Symptoms frequently are not present; if they are present, the most common is fatigue.

Diagnostic Evaluation

1. Laboratory tests will show a hemoglobin level of 11 gm./dl. or a hematocrit of 35% or less.
2. Evaluation of the erythrocytes will show the cells to be microcytic and hypochromic.

Medical Management

1. Iron replacement therapy is the treatment. There is some disagreement over use of parenteral or oral therapy. Oral therapy is usually preferred; however, if the woman is not likely to comply with taking the iron, the parenteral therapy is used.
2. Daily doses of 200 mg. of elemental iron are the usual dosage of oral iron preparations.
3. Parenteral administration is often complicated by adverse reaction.
4. Transfusion of red blood cells or whole blood is rarely needed unless hypovolemia coexists.

Assessment

1. Evaluation of dietary intake of iron, folic acid, and ascorbic acid
2. Evaluation of oral iron preparation intake, and understanding of need for the medication.

Patient Problems/Nursing Diagnoses

1. Knowledge deficit of the need for increased iron intake related to lack of previous teaching
2. Altered nutrition, less than body requirements, of iron, related to lack of dietary intake

Patient Teaching

1. Review the purpose of iron in the pregnant woman's diet.
2. Explain the need for the woman to develop iron stores and fetal iron stores.
3. Review a list of foods that are high in iron.
4. Discuss how the woman can realistically incorporate these foods into her diet.
5. Have her keep a diet log for 3 days and then review the diet change at the next visit.
6. Review the importance of taking iron with a source of ascorbic acid.

Evaluation

1. Verbalizes an understanding for the increased need for iron, and incorporates iron into her diet.
2. Hemoglobin level increases to greater than 11 gm./dl. and hematocrit is greater than 35%.
3. Regularly takes iron as prescribed.

Sickle Cell Anemia

Sickle cell anemia is an autosomal recessive disorder that is manifested by sickle- or crescent-shaped red blood cells. The disease is a result of the substitution of the amino acid valine for glutamic acid in the sixth position of the beta chain. During pregnancy these women are at risk for urinary tract infections and fetal distress at the time of delivery. Symptoms displayed are because of a vasocclusion that leads to a decreased blood flow, causing pain.

Carriers of the sickle cell trait are rarely symptomatic except for exercise intolerance, particularly at high altitudes.

Diagnostic Evaluation

1. Diagnosis is based on red blood cell screening and identification of the sickle cells.
2. Frequent evaluations of the hemoglobin level are required. Rarely will symptoms of sickle cell crisis be evident unless the hemoglobin falls below 7 gm./dl. or in the presence of an infection or nutritional deficiency.
3. Evaluation for urinary tract infections

Medical Management

1. Supplementary folic acid of 1 mg. per day
2. Carefully assess for signs of infections and treat early symptoms of infections as they first appear
3. If the hemoglobin level falls below 6 gm./dl. or decreases at a rate of 2 gm./dl. or more in 24 hours, an exchange transfusion with only hemoglobin A blood is used.
4. When transfusions are done the goal is to obtain a hematocrit above 25% and the percentage of S red blood cells to be no greater than 60%.

Assessment

1. At the initial prenatal visit evaluate the woman's knowledge of the presence of sickle cell anemia in herself and her family. If her status is unknown, evaluate her for the presence of hemoglobin S (hemoglobin electrophoresis). If she is a carrier then evaluate the baby's father.
2. Evaluate nutritional intake of folic acid, protein, and iron.
3. Evaluate fetal growth patterns—these infants are prone to intrauterine growth retardation (IUGR) and prematurity.
4. Assess for infection—there is increased maternal risk for infections (especially urinary tract) due to an impaired immune response. In addition, sickle cell crisis, if it occurs, will result in acute pain in joints or bones, lungs, or abdominal organs.

Patient Problems/Nursing Diagnoses

1. Knowledge deficit of dietary needs related to lack of previous exposure
2. Potential altered tissue perfusion: placental, related to inadequate oxygenation
3. Potential for infection, related to impaired immune response

Nursing Interventions

A. Patient Teaching

1. Discuss the normal dietary need for pregnancy.
2. Discuss the role folic acid plays in the development of red blood cells.
3. Have the woman keep a diet log noting the sources of folic acid in her diet.
4. Discuss the need for supplemental folic acid and the importance of following through with this intake.

B. Promoting Tissue Perfusion

1. Encourage frequent rest periods during the day, and when resting the woman should lie in the left lateral position if possible.
2. Use oxygen as prescribed by the physician.

C. Avoiding Infection

1. Discuss the importance of early treatment of any infections that the woman develops, especially urinary tract infections.
2. Stress the importance of good handwashing technique and personal hygiene.
3. Encourage the woman to limit her exposure to large groups during peak cold and influenza seasons.

Evaluation

1. Ingests an adequate intake of folic acid
2. Fetus grows at the appropriate rate
3. Shows no signs of infections

Diabetes Mellitus

Diabetes mellitus is an endocrine disorder in which the body is unable to produce enough insulin to meet the needs for glucose metabolism. This failure to meet the glucose needs of the body results in metabolism of protein and fat. Pregnancy is a diabetogenic state and requires an increase in glucose by the body. Normally, during pregnancy, the body is able to adapt to *these* metabolic changes; however, in a woman who does not have diabetes, the symptoms of diabetes may occur during pregnancy as a result of the metabolic changes.

Contributing Factors

1. Previous history of stillbirth, infant with congenital anomalies, hydramnios, or infant weight greater than 9 lb.
2. Family history of diabetes, prior diagnosis of gestational diabetes
3. Obesity, hypertension, and maternal age over 35 years

Effects

A. Possible Effects of Diabetes

1. An increased risk of pregnancy-induced hypertension
2. Infections that may become severe
3. Birth trauma related to increased fetal size; postpartum hemorrhage.

B. Effects on Fetus

1. Hyperglycemia
   a. High glucose levels cross the placenta, without the needed insulin to metabolize.
   b. The increased glucose levels result in an increase in fetal production of insulin, which results in an increased rate of fetal growth.
   c. Chronic hyperglycemia may result in faulty DNA and RNA synthesis, which may result in congenital anomalies such as neural tube defects and congenital heart anomalies.
   d. In addition there will be decreased production of fetal cortisol and decreased lecithin production and, therefore, delayed lung maturity.
   e. Following birth there is an increase in neonatal insulin production without a glucose source, resulting in neonatal hypoglycemia.

Classification of Diabetes in Pregnancy
(Duration of Disease More Important Than Age at Onset)

Class A Gestational Diabetic (90% of All Patients With Diabetes Seen By the Obstetrician)

1. Normal fasting blood sugar
2. Abnormal glucose tolerance test
3. Usually controlled by diet
4. Infant may be large for gestational age (LGA)

Class B

1. Onset after age 20
2. Present less than 10 years
3. No vascular complications
4. May have been controlled by diet; now insulin-dependent
5. Infant may be LGA

Class C

1. Onset between ages 10 and 19
2. Present 10–19 years
3. No vascular complications
4. Insulin-dependent before pregnancy; now insulin requirements increase
5. Infant may be LGA

Class D

1. Onset before age 10
2. Present 20 years or more
3. Peripheral vascular disease
4. Retinal changes
5. Hypertension
6. Insulin-dependent
7. Infant may be small for gestational age (SGA)

Class F

1. Includes neuropathy with proteinuria and decreased creatinine clearance
2. Infant SGA

Class R

1. Proliferative retinopathy, which may intensify
2. Therapeutic abortion may be a consideration

Class G

1. When many failures have occurred in pregnancy; it is thus possible to have Class A–G

Class H

1. Includes patients with cardiopathy (may be symptomatic)
2. Classes may change during pregnancy!

Clinical Manifestations

1. If diabetes is present prior to the onset of pregnancy, glucose control and insulin need will change.
2. If diabetes is not present prior to pregnancy and gestational diabetes is present, blood glucose levels will be elevated (above 140 mg./dl.) in the routine screening done at 24–28 weeks of gestation.
3. If the glucose level is elevated in the glucose challenge test, a glucose tolerance test is performed—if gestational diabetes is present, this will also be elevated.
4. Cardinal symptoms of diabetes that may be present include polyuria, polydipsia, polyphagia, and weight loss.
5. In addition glyosuria (using Tes-Tape or Diastix), urine positive for ketones (using Ketostix), and a history of chronic monilial infections may be present in the gestational diabetic woman.

Diagnostic Evaluation

1. A glucose challenge test of 50 gm. of oral glucose is given at 24–28 weeks' gestation to all pregnant women. If the glucose level is 140 mg./dl. at 1 hour postglucose administration, a glucose challenge is administered.
2. The glucose challenge consists of giving 100 mg. of glucose to the fasting woman and then evaluating blood glucose levels at 1, 2, and 3 hours following administration.
3. If the woman has diabetes prior to pregnancy a hemoglobin A_1C test may be used to evaluate prior glucose control. Elevated hemoglobin levels may be associated with an increased incidence of congenital anomalies.

Medical Management

1. Aim of medical management is to control the glucose level and maintain a state of euglycemia.
2. Euglycemia is obtained through the use of diet, exercise, and insulin.
3. Dietary control includes caloric and glucose levels. The calories and glucose are spread throughout the day to provide the nutrients for fetal growth and maternal stores.
4. Consistent exercise is encouraged unless signs of uteroplacental insufficiency occur.
5. Human insulin is given in split doses in order to provide 24-hour coverage.
   a. Most of the insulin will be given in the morning, with a dose in late afternoon to cover the early morning hours.
   b. If glucose levels are difficult to control, injections of regular insulin may be given prior to each snack and meal, or an insulin pump may be used to provide continuous infusion of insulin into the body.
6. Blood glucose levels must be evaluated prior to mealtimes daily. These are then recorded and evaluated for patterns and adequacy of glucose control.

Nursing Assessment

1. Evaluate the urine at each prenatal visit for presence of glucose.

2. If blood glucose levels are being evaluated, review these findings, and look for patterns of elevated or decreased glucose levels.
3. Evaluate weight gain and diet control.

Patient Problems/Nursing Diagnoses

1. Knowledge deficit of diabetes and diabetic control measures related to lack of previous exposure
2. Potential altered nutrition, less than or more than body requirements, related to inadequate dietary intake.
3. Potential for urinary tract infection related to increased glucose in urine.
4. Potential for altered tissue perfusion, related to decreased maternal circulation
5. Potential for fear or anxiety of fetal outcome related to diagnosis of diabetes

Nursing Interventions

A. Patient Teaching

1. Develop a teaching plan that covers the basic pathophysiology of diabetes, effects of diabetes on the pregnancy, and methods of diabetic control during pregnancy.
2. Discuss the role of diet, exercise, and nutrition in the life of a diabetic.
3. Discuss the effects of the diagnosis of diabetes on the woman and her family.

B. Promoting Adequate Nutrition

1. Review the purpose of diet control in diabetes.
2. Explain the diabetic diet.
3. Have patient keep a diet log for 2 days and evaluate the log together.
4. Answer questions she may have regarding diet needs.

C. Preventing Infections

1. Explain that increased glucose levels in the urine increase the potential for a urinary tract infection.
2. Discuss the importance of increasing water intake to 8 glasses a day.
3. Explain that urination should occur each time the urge to urinate is felt.
4. Explain and demonstrate the importance of good handwashing technique.
5. Instruct the woman to wear cotton underwear and to wipe the perineal area from front to back only.
6. Educate woman to report any symptoms such as vaginal burning or itching, or burning or pain on urination.

D. Promoting Adequate Circulation

1. Encourage positioning to promote uteroplacental circulation. Also encourage frequent position changes.
2. Encourage adequate fluid intake and appropriate caloric intake.
3. Evaluate with a nonstress test or oxytocin challenge test after 37 weeks.

E. Reducing Anxiety and Fear

1. Allow the woman and her family to discuss the disease and treatment effects on the family.
2. Answer realistically any questions that the family has regarding current status and outcome.

Evaluation

1. Verbalizes understanding of the disease process, diet therapy, and glucose measurements methods.
2. Has an appropriate weight gain throughout the pregnancy.

3. Does not develop symptoms of a urinary tract or vaginal infection.
4. Fetus is active and has a reactive nonstress test when tested.
5. Openly discusses with health care providers and family the impact of the disease on self and fetus.
6. Verbalizes understanding of all antepartum testing, and keeps all appointments for antepartum testing.

Infections During Pregnancy

Sexually Transmitted Diseases (STDs)

A. Chlamydia

1. *Chlamydia* is a prevalent bacterial infection frequently seen with gonorrhea. It often presents as a yellow mucopurulent cervical discharge with cervicitis.
2. *Effects on pregnancy*
   a. Small-for-gestational-age (SGA) infants and low birth weight
   b. Ectopic pregnancies
   c. Premature rupture of the membranes
   d. Preterm labor
   e. Amnionitis
   f. Intrapartum fever
3. *Effects on fetus/newborn*
   a. Neonatal sepsis
   b. Conjunctivitis with possible conjunctival scarring and corneal vascularization
   c. Chlamydial pneumonia
4. *Treatment*
   a. During pregnancy both the woman and her partner are treated with erythromycin for 7 days.
   b. After delivery the neonate receives erythromycin ophthalmic ointment or tetracycline ophthalmic ointment to prevent chlamydial conjunctivitis.
   c. Neonatal pneumonia and conjunctivitis in the neonate may be treated with oral erythromycin syrup for 2 weeks.

B. Gonorrhea

1. *Gonorrhea* is the most common STD in the 15–24-year-old age group. Usually it is asymptomatic. Recently there has been an increase in a penicillinase-producing *Neisseria gonorrhoeae* (PPNG).
2. *Effects on pregnancy*
   a. Chorioamnionitis
   b. Preterm delivery
   c. Premature rupture of the membranes (PROM)
   d. Intrauterine growth retardation
3. *Effects on the fetus/newborn*
   a. The chance of contact with the bacteria during birth increases the longer the membranes are ruptured
   b. Bacterial contact can occur through ingestion of infected amniotic fluid.
   c. In addition to eye infections, the infants are also at risk for nasopharyngeal, vaginal, anal and ear infections and infections at the scalp electrode sites.
   d. Because these infants may be premature, a bacterial sepsis may occur.
   e. Ophthalmic infections are characterized by a thick, purulent drainage and conjunctival edema.
4. *Treatment*
   a. A pregnant woman and her partner(s) receive aqueous procaine penicillin G (IM) with oral

probenecid. If the woman is allergic to penicillin, spectinomycin is given.
  b. If PPNG is prevalent in the area, ceftriaxone IM is used.
  c. Preventive neonatal treatment includes topical application of silver nitrate, erythromycin, or tetracycline.
  d. Infants of mothers with gonorrhea infections are treated with crystalline penicillin G.

C. Syphilis

1. *Syphilis* is a bacterial infection caused by *Treponema pallidum.*
2. *Effects on pregnancy*
  a. During pregnancy the disease, at any stage, can be passed to the fetus. The effects on the fetus depend on the mother's stage of the disease.
3. *Effects on the fetus/newborn*
  If the mother has primary- or secondary-stage syphilis, there is a 50% chance that the fetus will die or that the infant will be premature or will die soon after birth. The other 50% will develop congenital syphilis.
4. *Treatment*
  a. Maternal prenatal syphilis is treated with benzathine penicillin G.
  b. For penicillin-allergic women erythromycin is given.
  c. The affected neonate is treated with penicillin.

D. Herpes

1. *Herpes simplex II* is the most common type of herpes virus infecting the female genital tract during pregnancy.
  a. A primary infection is usually symptomatic, with an incubation period of less than 1 week followed by eruption of the vesicles along with itching, tingling, and pain. Symptoms are gone in usually 2–4 weeks.
  b. Recurrent infections result in fewer, less tender vesicles, with viral shedding for less time.
  c. Diagnosis of the virus is by culture of a suspicious-looking vesicle.
2. *Effects on the fetus/newborn*
  a. Rarely is the disease transferred across the placenta.
  b. The fetus can contract the disease during labor with the rupture of membranes or through direct contact with the virus at the time of birth.
  c. Localized infections may result in vesicles on the skin, eye, or mouth.
  d. Disseminated disease is usually present in the premature infant and symptoms develop 9–11 days after birth.
3. *Treatment*
  a. Involves prevention of disease and/or spread of the disease.
  b. In the antepartal history, exposure to herpes is noted.
  c. If there is a positive history, any suspicious lesions should be cultured.
  d. In labor all women need an examination of the external genitalia and a speculum examination to determine the presence of lesions.
  e. If lesions or suggestive symptoms are present, a cesarean section is generally recommended.
  f. Women with only a history of herpes and no positive cultures or visual signs of herpes may deliver vaginally.

E. Cytomegalovirus

1. *Cytomegalovirus (CMV)* is a herpes virus that causes an infection with mononucleosislike symptoms. The infections are usually mild and may be asymptomatic.
2. *Effects on the pregnancy*
  a. A primary infection during pregnancy is thought to place the fetus at risk for congenital CMV.
  b. Most infections occurring during pregnancy are a reactivation of the infection.
3. *Effects on the fetus/neonate*
  a. Usually a result of a primary infection during the first trimester
  b. Neonatal infections vary from asymptomatic to profoundly symptomatic
  c. Congenital manifestations
    (1) Intrauterine growth retardation
    (2) Neonatal jaundice
    (3) Purpura
    (4) Microcephaly
    (5) Intracerebral calcification
    (6) Chorioretinitis
    (7) Progressive sensorineural hearing loss
4. *Treatment*—is symptomatic

F. AIDS

1. *Acquired immunodeficiency syndrome (AIDS)* is caused by the retrovirus human immunodeficiency virus (HIV).
2. Women who test positive for the HIV virus should be instructed as to the effects of the disease on her, her family, and the fetus/newborn. In addition the woman needs to be evaluated for opportunistic infections (e.g., herpes simplex and zoster, candidiasis, CMV, *Pneumocystis carinii,* and *Toxoplasma gondii*).
3. *Effects on the pregnancy*
  a. Premature rupture of the membranes (PROM)
  b. Preterm delivery
  c. The HIV virus is found in breast milk—it is recommended that a woman not breast-feed her infant
4. *Effects on the fetus/infant*
  a. Infant acquires the infection through intrauterine exposure.
  b. Usually the infant develops symptoms during the first 24 months of life.
  c. The infant may test positive from passive acquired immunity during the first year of life.

NURSING ALERT: Currently there are insufficient data to determine accurately maternal and fetal risk. Therefore any woman who is seropositive for the AIDS virus should be advised to delay pregnancy.

Substance Abuse

Substance abuse in pregnancy occurs in any pregnancy when a woman abuses alcohol or drugs in the antepartum period. These substances cross the placenta and enter fetal circulation.

Effects on Pregnancy

1. Spontaneous abortions
2. Premature separation of the placenta (abruptio placentae)
3. Breech presentation

4. Chorioamnionitis
5. Premature rupture of membranes (PROM)
6. Preterm labor
7. Placental insufficiency
8. Intrauterine death
9. Preeclampsia and eclampsia
10. Septic thrombophlebitis

Effects on Fetus/Neonate

1. Intrauterine growth retardation (IUGR)
2. Respiratory distress syndrome (RDS)
3. Hypoglycemia
4. Hypocalcemia
5. Hyperbilirubinemia
6. Intracranial hemorrhage
7. Meconium aspiration
8. Drug withdrawal

Treatment

1. Treatment programs for the pregnant woman are increasing in number throughout the United States. Many traditional drug programs do not accept pregnant women.
2. Treatment programs are directed toward long-term rehabilitation and prenatal care.

Complications of Labor

Preterm Labor

Preterm labor is uterine contractions occurring after 20 weeks' gestation and before 37 completed weeks of gestation. Contractions are less than 10 minutes apart, resulting in progressive cervical changes or cervical dilation of 2 cm. or effacement of 75%.

Clinical Manifestations

Regular uterine contractions that produce cervical changes

Diagnosis

Based on finding of a cervical examination and evaluation of uterine contraction pattern

Risk Factors

1. Multiple gestation
2. History of previous preterm labor and/or delivery
3. Abdominal surgery during current pregnancy
4. Uterine anomaly
5. History of cone biopsy
6. History of abortions—more than two 1st trimester abortions or more than one 2nd trimester abortion
7. Fetal and/or placental malformation
8. Diethylstilbestrol exposure
9. Bleeding after the 1st trimester
10. Maternal age of less than 18 or greater than 35 years
11. Poor nutritional status
12. Poor, irregular, or no prenatal care
13. Emotional stress
14. More than 10 cigarettes smoked in a day
15. Recreational drug use

Medical Management

A. Focus and Method

1. The focus of medical treatment is prevention of delivery of a preterm infant.
2. The method depends on the cervical dilatation and contraction pattern.
3. If contractions are detected early and treatment is begun early, there is a higher rate of labor stoppage.

B. Conservative Treatment

1. Treatment is begun early with the use of bedrest in a left lateral position.
2. Hydration with IV fluids and continuous monitoring of fetal status and uterine contraction pattern are instituted.
3. If this stops the contractions, tocolytic therapy is not needed.
4. Discharge planning includes
   a. Bedrest or limited activity
   b. Promotion of nutrition
   c. Stress management
   d. Increased fluid intake to 10 cups per day
   e. No sexual activity or breast preparation.

C. Tocolytic Therapy

1. If conservative therapy is not successful, tocolytic therapy is instituted.
2. Involves the use of beta-mimetic agents of ritodrine, isoxsuprine, and terbutaline (The only drug approved for tocolytic therapy by the Food and Drug Administration is ritodrine.)
   a. These drugs stimulate the $beta_2$-receptors, which causes uterine relaxation.
   b. Use of these drugs for a prolonged time can result in a decreased response to the medication.
   c. Initially the drugs are administered IV, then the woman is weaned either to subcutaneous or to oral administration.
3. Side effects
   a. Increased pulse
   b. Decreased blood pressure
   c. Increased plasma volume
   d. Decreased potassium concentration
   e. Hyperglycemia and hyperinsulinemia.
4. Diagnostic evaluation
   a. Prior to beginning administration of these medications the following laboratory tests should be done:
      (1) Complete blood count (CBC) with differential
      (2) Electrolytes
      (3) Glucose
      (4) Blood urea nitrogen (BUN)
      (5) Creatinine
      (6) Prothrombin time (PT), partial thromboplastin time (PTT)
   b. In addition a baseline electrocardiogram should be obtained.

Nursing Assessment

Nursing assessment during tocolytic therapy includes evaluation of
1. Fetal status
2. Contraction pattern
3. Respiratory status (pulmonary edema is a common side effect)

4. Muscular tremors
5. Palpations
6. Dizziness and or lightheadedness
7. Urinary output

Patient Problems/Nursing Diagnoses

1. Anxiety related to medication and fear of outcome of pregnancy
2. Knowledge deficit of treatment therapy and preterm labor
3. Diversional activity deficit related to prolonged bedrest
4. Disturbances in sleep pattern
5. Potential for ineffective coping

Nursing Interventions

A. Relieving Anxiety

1. Provide accurate information on the status of the fetus and labor (contraction pattern).
2. Answer question regarding woman's or fetus' status.
3. Allow the woman and her support person to verbalize their feelings regarding the episode of preterm labor and the treatment.
4. If a private room is not used do not place the woman in a room with an occupant who is in labor or who has lost an infant.
5. Encourage relationships with other patients who are also experiencing preterm labor.

B. Patient Teaching

1. Explain each step of the treatment prior to beginning any new therapy.
2. Answer all questions openly and honestly for the woman and her support system.
3. Provide information on preterm labor.

C. Promoting Suitable Activity

1. Determine quiet craft activities that can be done in bed.
2. Provide radio, books, and television.
3. Encourage visits from family, especially other children and friends. If possible encourage them to bring in favorite foods for the woman and to eat as a family.

D. Promoting Effective Sleep Patterns

1. Explain to the woman the need to maintain around-the-clock blood levels of the medication and evaluation of contraction and fetal status.
2. Plan to administer medications and to conduct assessments at the same time.
3. Plan for an afternoon nap and place a "Do Not Disturb" sign on the door during this daily rest period.

Evaluation

1. Demonstrate decreased anxiety
2. Verbalizes an understanding of preterm labor, its effects, and medications being administered
3. Maintains an interest in activities and surroundings
4. Achieves adequate rest and sleep

Preterm Rupture of Membranes (PROM)

Preterm labor may also be accompanied with preterm rupture of membranes (PROM). Most often PROM is seen in multiple gestations, chorioamnionitis, breech presentations, and fetal distress in labor.

Management

A. Nonintervention

The woman is watched and monitored for signs of infection and the beginning of spontaneous labor.

B. Tocolytics and Corticosteroids

1. Tocolytic therapy is used until fetal lungs have matured as a result of corticosteroid administration.
2. If this treatment is used two doses of betamethasone are given and delivery is delayed at least 24 hours.
3. If the infant is born within the next 7 days, the incidence of respiratory distress may be decreased.
4. If the infant is born after this time, there seems to be no effect on fetal lung maturation.
5. Studies are inconclusive in the effectiveness of corticosteroid therapy for fetal lung maturation. In addition the long-term effects of their use is unknown.

Nursing Assessment

1. Evaluate maternal temperature, pulse, respirations, and blood pressure every 4 hours.
2. Monitor the amount and type of amniotic fluid that is leaking
3. Evaluate daily CBC with differentials, noting any shift to the left.
4. Evaluate fetal status every 4 hours, noting fetal activity and heart rate.
5. Determine if uterine tenderness occurs on abdominal palpation

Patient Problems/Nursing Diagnoses

1. Same as preterm labor
2. Potential for infection

Nursing Interventions

A. Similar to Preterm Labor

B. Preventing Infection

1. Evaluate amount and odor of amniotic fluid leakage.
2. Do not perform vaginal examinations without consulting the primary health care provider.
3. Place patient on disposal pads to collect leaking fluid and change pads every 2 hours or more frequently as needed.
4. Review the need for good handwashing technique and hygiene following urination and defecation.
5. Monitor fetal heart rate and fetal activity every 4 hours.
6. Monitor maternal temperature, pulse respirations, blood pressure, and uterine tenderness every 4 hours.

Evaluation

1. Same as under Preterm Labor
2. Is free of any signs of infection

Induction of Labor

Induction of labor is the deliberate initiation of uterine contractions prior to their spontaneous onset.

Methods

1. *Amniotomy*
   a. Artificial rupture of the membranes
   b. Presenting part now puts greater pressure on cervix
   c. Contractions are stronger

2. *Stripping the membranes*
   a. Separating the membranes from the lower uterine segment without rupturing the membranes
   b. Usually done during vaginal examination
   c. Membranes and amniotic fluid now act as a wedge to dilate cervix
3. *Administration of oxytocin*
   a. Used to initiate and sustain uterine contractions
   b. Given IV
   c. Maternal and fetal vital signs and length, intensity, and frequency of contractions are monitored carefully
4. *Administration of prostaglandin*
   a. Used experimentally in the United States to induce and augment labor.
   b. The medication is administered as a vaginal suppository or gel with a diaphragm and will soften the cervix and stimulate uterine contractions.
   c. This medication is under investigation and is used only in limited research studies.
   d. Side effects of prostaglandin include fever, nausea, vomiting, and diarrhea.

Indications

When the woman's life or well-being is in danger or if the fetus may be compromised by remaining in the uterus any longer
1. Maternal hypertensive disease
2. Diabetes of mother
3. Premature rupture of membranes
4. Maternal renal disease
5. Fetal postmaturity
6. Erythroblastosis
7. Placental insufficiency
8. History of rapid labors and living a long distance from birth center
9. Intrauterine growth retardation (IUGR)
10. Intrauterine fetal death (IUFD)

Contraindications

1. Herpes outbreak in the genital area
2. Vaginal bleeding, known placenta previa
3. Abnormal fetal presentation
4. Previous uterine scar (is not considered by all to be a contraindication)
5. Know cephalopelvic disproportion (CPD)
6. Severe fetal distress

Medical Management

A. Amniotomy (Artificial Rupture of Membranes [AROM])
1. Baseline data on the mother and fetus are obtained.
2. Procedure is explained to the woman and her support person.
3. The supplies are gathered; the woman is positioned for a vaginal examination and the vulva is cleansed.
4. Amniohook is inserted through the cervix and membranes are ruptured after evaluation of fetal presentation.
5. The amount, color, and odor of the fluid are noted.
6. Fetal heart tones are assessed continually for at least the next 20 minutes.

B. Oxytocin
1. Oxytocin is administered after baseline fetal and maternal vital signs are obtained.
2. The woman is placed on the fetal monitor.

3. If membranes have ruptured, an intrauterine catheter and internal scalp electrode should be used.
4. An IV is mixed with 10 units of oxytocin and piggybacked into the primary IV at the port of entry nearest the skin insertion.
5. The oxytocin is given only with an infusion pump and when constant monitoring of maternal and fetal status is available.
6. The dose is increased every 20–30 minutes by 1 to 2 μU/minute. The total dose should not exceed 30 μU/minute.
7. The goal is to establish a regular labor pattern—contractions occurring every 2–3 minutes lasting 45 to 60 seconds and an intensity of 50 mm. Hg (moderate).

Nursing Assessment

A. Prior to Induction
1. Make sure that patient is aware of the procedures to be used and all questions have been answered.
2. Obtain a 30-minute strip for the fetal heart rate and uterine activity.
3. Evaluate maternal vital signs.
4. Evaluate the patency of the IV site.

B. Following the Administration of Oxytocin
1. Continuously monitor fetal heart rate and uterine activity.
2. Assess maternal vital signs every 15 minutes until a labor pattern is established, then every 30 minutes. Temperature is taken every 4 hours unless an amniotomy has been performed and then every 2 hours.
3. Limit vaginal examinations, especially after the membranes have ruptured.
4. Maintain intake and output records, and watch for signs of water intoxication.
5. Evaluate IV site for patency and rate control for correct rate at least hourly.

Patient Problems/Nursing Diagnoses

1. Knowledge deficit of labor induction
2. Anxiety
3. Disruption in uteroplacental circulation

Nursing Interventions

A. Patient Teaching
1. Explain the need for the induction to the woman and her family.
2. Explain how labor will be induced.
3. Show and explain all equipment that will be used during the induction.
4. Encourage the woman and her family to ask questions about the induction.

B. Reducing Anxiety
1. Instruct or review the use of relaxation and distraction techniques.
2. Prior to beginning any new procedure explain the procedure to the woman and her support person.
3. Answer questions that the family and woman may have.

C. Monitoring for Complications
1. Assess fetal status and uterine contractions continuously through the use of a monitor.
2. Position on the left side.
3. Have oxygen set up with a mask ready and administer as prescribed if decelerations occur.
4. If hyperstimulation of the uterus or fetal distress occurs,

discontinue the infusion, maintain the primary IV, and notify the physician

Evaluation

1. Verbalizes and understands the induction process
2. Does not appear anxious
3. Is free of complications

Precipitate Labor

Precipitous labor occurs when labor lasts less than 3 hours. It is most often seen in multigravida women with a large pelvis and small baby and little cervical or perineal resistance. The major problem with a precipitous labor is trauma to the fetus and mother, fetal hypoxia, and anxiety.

Assessment

1. Continuous evaluation of fetal status and uterine contractions
2. Evaluation of maternal anxiety

Patient Problems/Nursing Diagnoses

1. Anxiety
2. Altered comfort

Nursing Interventions

A. Reducing Anxiety

1. Maintain a calm atmosphere.
2. Encourage use of relaxation techniques; involve the support person.
3. Remain with the woman and her family at all times.
4. Explain procedures prior to performing, if possible.

B. Promoting Comfort

1. Encourage use of relaxation techniques.
2. Encourage support person to rub back and hold hand as needed.
3. Encourage frequent voiding.

Evaluation

1. Appears less anxious
2. Works *with* the contractions

> **NURSING ALERT:**
> 1. These woman are at risk for developing a postpartum hemorrhage because of the rapid labor they have experienced.
> 2. In addition the women are at risk for development of lacerations of soft tissue, of uterine rupture, and of amniotic fluid emboli.

Dystocia

Dystocia, or difficult labor, refers to abnormal progress in labor.

Causes

1. Problems with the force of labor will result in ineffective contractions and/or ineffective bearing down (pushing) during the second stage of labor.
2. Abnormalities in the passageway may be the result of problems in the pelvis or soft tissues of the reproductive tract.
3. Abnormal fetal presentation, position, size, or development result in a problem with the fetus.

4. Maternal psychological factors such as fear, anxiety, and exhaustion also may play a role in dystocia.
5. Often more than one cause exists at a time.

Underlying Mechanisms

A. Contraction Problems

1. Contractions that are not strong enough or frequent enough to produce a normal labor pattern will not result in dilatation and effacement within a normal time frame.
2. Using Freidman's curve, a prolonged latent phase in the primigravida is greater than 20 hours and in the multigravida it is greater than 14 hours.
3. During the active phase, the cervix of a primigravida will normally dilate at least 1.2 cm./hour, and the multigravida 1.5 cm. In addition, the fetus should be descending through the birth canal. In the primigravida the rate of descent is 1 cm./hour and 2 cm./hour for the multigravida.
4. Etiology of abnormalities in the force of labor include:
   a. Early or excessive use of analgesia
   b. Overdistention of the uterus
   c. Excessive cervical ridigity
   d. Grand multiparity
   e. Mild pelvic contraction
   f. Postmature and large infants
5. Medical treatment involves stimulation of labor through the use of oxytocin.

B. Passageway Problems

1. Most often problems with the passageway are a result of pelvic abnormalities that interfere with the engagement, descent, and expulsion of the fetus.
   a. Not only is the size of the pelvis important, but so is the shape of the pelvis.
   b. In addition, obstruction may result from problems of the soft tissue such as a uterine or ovarian fibromyoma.
2. *Etiology*
   a. Contractions of the inlet are noted when the anteroposterior diameter is less than 10 cm., or the greatest transverse diameter is less than 12 cm. Contracted inlets may be of genetic origin or a result of rickets.
   b. Midpelvic contractions occur when the distance between the ischial spines is less than 9 cm. Often this is not detected early in labor because the fetal head has engaged, and molding along with caput formation gives the suggestion that the head has descended further than it has.
   c. A contracted pelvic outlet is diagnosed when the distance between the ischial spines is less than 8 cm. When the pelvis is contracted and the fetus cannot fit through the pelvis, cephalopelvic disproportion exists (CPD).
3. *Medical treatment*
   a. Involves delivery in the safest manner for the mother and fetus.
   b. If the problem is related to the inlet or midpelvis, a cesarean delivery is indicated.
   c. If the size of the outlet is the problem, a forceps delivery is usually performed.

C. Fetal Problems

1. Normal fetal passage
   a. Normally the fetus enters the pelvic inlet transversely and then rotates to an occiput anterior po-

sition, allowing for the smallest diameter of the fetal head to pass through the pelvis.
   b. When the fetal head enters the pelvis posteriorly, it must rotate to the anterior position. This is done usually without problems if the fetus is of average size and well flexed and the contractions are a good quality.
2. If the fetus does not turn, then it remains in the posterior position and may slow down the progress of descent.
   a. If the pelvis is large enough, the baby can be born in the posterior position.
   b. If the pelvis is borderline and the contractions ineffective, a cesarean section may be necessary.
3. Breech presentations occur in approximately 3% of all deliveries.
   a. This presentation is more common in multiple gestations, increased parity, hydramnios, placenta previa, and preterm infants.
   b. Usually the method of choice for delivery is a cesarean section.
4. Shoulder presentation occurs when the infant lies crosswise in the uterus. The infant is delivered by cesarean section.
5. A large fetus has an increased risk of trauma in its attempt to fit through a normal-size pelvis. A large infant may not fit through the pelvis and cephalopelvic disproportion may result.

Assessment

1. Evaluation of fetal presentation, position, and size
2. Evaluation of progress of labor, noting dilations and effacement in relation to time of labor along with descent of the fetal head.
3. Fetal heart rate and contraction status at least every 30 minutes
4. Maternal vital signs at least every hour
5. Assess bladder fullness

Patient Problems/Nursing Diagnoses

1. Altered comfort
2. Anxiety
3. Ineffective coping

Nursing Interventions

A. Promoting Comfort

1. Review relaxation techniques
2. Encourage use of breathing techniques learned in prenatal classes
3. Encourage frequent change of position
4. Encourage voiding every hour
5. Provide back rubs and sacral pressure as needed
6. Offer ice chips as needed to combat a dry mouth
7. Provide a quiet, darkened room
8. Provide frequent encouragement to the woman and her support person

B. Reducing Anxiety

1. Instruct or review the use of relaxation and distraction techniques.
2. Prior to beginning any new procedure explain the procedure to the woman and her support person.
3. Answer questions that the family and woman may have.

Evaluation

1. Demonstrates effective coping ability with the pain of labor
2. Behaves in a calm nonanxious manner

Uterine Rupture

Uterine rupture is a spontaneous or traumatic rupture of the uterus.

Causes

1. Rupture of the scar from a previous cesarean delivery or hysterotomy
2. Prolonged or obstructed labor
3. Forced delivery of fetus with abnormalities (e.g., hydrocephalus)
4. Ill-advised podalic version
5. Application of forceps and extraction before cervical os has completely dilated
6. Injudicious use of oxytocin
7. Excessive manual pressure applied to the fundus during delivery

Clinical Manifestations

1. Complete rupture
   a. Sudden sharp abdominal pain during contractions
   b. Abdominal tenderness
   c. Cessation of contractions
   d. Bleeding into the abdominal cavity and sometimes into the vagina
   e. Fetus easily palpated; fetal heart tones cease
   f. Signs of shock—rapid, weak pulse; cold, clammy skin; pale color; flaring of nostrils due to air hunger
2. Incomplete rupture—develops over a period of a few hours
   a. Abdominal pain during contractions
   b. Contractions continue, but cervix fails to dilate
   c. Vaginal bleeding may be present
   d. Rising pulse rate and skin pallor
   e. Loss of fetal heart tones
3. Diagnosis is made based on the presenting symptoms

Medical Management

1. Preparation for surgery, including blood and fluid replacement
2. Following surgery, additional blood and fluid replacement is continued along with antibiotic therapy

Assessment

1. Continuous evaluation of maternal vital signs when there is an increase in rate and depth of respirations, an increase in pulse or a drop in blood pressure
2. Assessment of fetal status
3. Family understanding of the situation

Patient Problems/Nursing Diagnoses

1. Fluid volume deficit
2. Altered tissue perfusion
3. Anxiety

Nursing Interventions

A. Ensuring Proper Fluid Volume

1. Start or maintain an IV as prescribed. Use a large-gauge intracath when starting the IV
2. Maintain bedrest
3. Insert Foley catheter
4. Obtain and administer blood products as prescribed

B. Improving Tissue Perfusion

1. Start and maintain IV, as prescribed.
2. Administer oxygen using a face mask, as prescribed.

3. Elevate head of bed.
4. Continually monitor maternal and fetal vital signs.

C. Reducing Anxiety

1. Prior to beginning a procedure give a brief explanation to the woman and her support person.
2. Answer questions that the family and woman may have.
3. Maintain a quiet, calm atmosphere.
4. Remain with the woman until anesthesia has been administered.
5. Keep the family members aware of the situation while the woman is in surgery and allow them time to verbalize their feelings.

Evaluation

1. Vital signs and renal function remain normal
2. Maintains adequate tissue perfusion
3. Demonstrates effective coping techniques

Amniotic Fluid Embolism

Amniotic fluid embolism is the escape of amniotic fluid containing debris such as meconium, lanugo, and vernix caseosa into the maternal circulation, usually resulting in deposition of fluid or debris in the pulmonary arterioles; may also cause disseminated intravascular coagulation (DIC). Amniotic fluid embolism is rare and usually fatal.

Predisposing Conditions

Myometrial vessels are exposed, usually at placental site, and contractions are especially forceful.
1. Marginal placental separation
2. Uterine rupture
3. Hysterectomy

Clinical Manifestations

1. Sudden dyspnea and chest pain
2. Cyanosis
3. Tachycardia
4. Pulmonary edema
5. Profound shock due to:
   a. Anaphylaxis, which causes vascular collapse
   b. Uterine bleeding with development of hypofibrinogenemia

Medical Management

1. Mechanical ventilation
2. Blood replacement
3. Invasive cardiac monitoring
4. Treatment of infection

   Note: Maternal condition is guarded.

Prolapsed Umbilical Cord

Prolapsed umbilical cord—prolapses in front of or alongside the fetal presenting part.

Clinical Manifestations

1. Cord may be seen protruding from vagina.
2. Cord can be palpated in the vaginal canal or cervix.
3. Fetal distress may occur as the cord is compressed between the presenting part and the bony pelvis.
4. Fetal heart rate pattern may show variable decelerations with contractions or between contractions; often fetal bradycardia is present.
5. If the cord is exposed to the cold room air, there may be a reflex constriction of the umbilical blood vessels that further restricts the oxygen flow to the fetus.

Predisposing Factors

1. Rupture of membranes, when the presenting part is not engaged in the pelvis
2. More common in shoulder and foot presentations
3. Prematurity—small fetus allows more space around presenting part
4. Hydramnios—causes greater amount of fluid to be released with greater force when membranes rupture
5. Contracted pelvis
6. Placenta previa

Medical Management

Delivery of the fetus as soon as possible

Inverted Uterus

Inversion of the uterus—the uterus turns inside out during the third stage of delivery.

Usual Causes

1. Excessive traction on the cord while the placenta is still attached to the uterine wall
2. Lax or thin uterine walls
3. Fundal pressure
4. An inversion may also occur spontaneously

Clinical Manifestations

Maternal bleeding and shock, with symptoms often seeming out of proportion for the blood loss

Medical Management

1. Goal is to restore the uterus to its normal position.
2. Often involves the use of general anesthesia and tocolytic therapy (use of terbutaline, ritodrine or magnesium sulfate).
3. In addition, blood replacement therapy is instituted to correct the shock.
4. After the uterus has been restored to its normal position, oxytocin is given to contract the uterus.

Assessment

1. Assessment prior to correction
   a. Evaluation of blood loss
   b. Maternal vital signs
2. Assessment after correction
   a. Maternal vital signs
   b. Accurate intake and output
   c. Evaluation of uterine fundus for position and firmness
   d. Evaluation of lochia
   e. Evaluation for transfusion reactions

NURSING ALERT: Once the diagnosis of an inverted uterus has been made, begin an IV line with a large intracath as prescribed. If one line is in place, begin a second line. Do a type and crossmatch immediately for blood replacement.

Operative Obstetrics

Operative obstetrics refers to a number of procedures (episiotomy, forceps delivery, cesarean delivery) that may be used to assist the mother in labor and delivery.

Episiotomy

An *episiotomy* is an incision of the perineum during delivery to:
1. Substitute a straight surgical incision for the laceration that may otherwise occur.
2. Facilitate repair of laceration and promote healing.
3. Spare the infant's head from prolonged pressure and pushing against the rigid perineum, which may result in brain damage, especially in the premature infant
4. Shorten the 2nd stage of labor

Types of Episiotomies

A. Median
1. Incision is made in the middle of the perineum and directed toward the rectum (Fig. 42-4).
2. This method is believed to heal with few complications, is more comfortable for the woman during healing, and is easy to repair.
3. If a larger incision is needed during delivery, however, it may necessitate incision into anal sphincter.

B. Mediolateral (Midline)
1. Incision is made laterally in the perineum.
2. This method avoids the anal sphincter if enlargement is needed.
3. Women find it very uncomfortable during healing.

Assessment
1. Degree of healing
2. Edema
3. Infection
4. Redness
5. Hematoma formation
6. Bleeding

During the recovery period the episiotomy should be evaluated every 15 minutes, and 3 times a day after this.

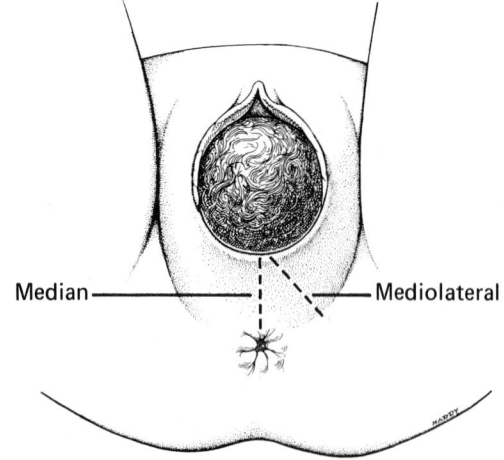

Median————————Mediolateral

Figure 42-4. *Types of episiotomies.*

Patient Problems/Nursing Diagnoses
1. Potential for infection, related to inadequate episiotomy care
2. Knowledge deficit of episiotomy care
3. Altered comfort related to episiotomy pain

Nursing Interventions

A. Preventing Infection
1. Instruct the woman to cleanse from the front to the back
2. Provide instructions on techniques used for perineal care.
3. Explain the importance of changing the perineal pad each time after urination and defecation and of not touching the inner surface of the pad.
4. Explain the importance of proper handwashing before and after perineal care.
5. Explain that perineal care should be carried out following urination and defecation and at least every 4 hours during the day.
6. Encourage a diet that is high in protein and vitamin C and encourage at least 2000 ml. of fluid each day

B. Promoting Comfort
1. Ice packs can be applied to the perineal area for the first 24 hours after delivery.
   The ice packs should not remain in place longer than 30 minutes at a time in order to get the maximum benefit for the treatment.
2. Sitz baths may be used with either warm or cool water. The warm water is soothing whereas the cool water helps to decrease pain sensation and edema.
3. Heat lamps may be used.
   a. The perineum should be thoroughly cleansed and dried prior to heat lamp treatment.
   b. The lamp is placed at least 18 inches from the perineum and is left on for no more than 20 minutes, two or three times a day.
4. Topical anesthetic agents may also be used following a sitz bath.
5. Perineal exercises are recommended—instruct the woman to tighten her buttocks and perineal muscles prior to sitting in a chair and to release the muscles once sealed.

Evaluation
1. Is free of any signs of episiotomy infection
2. Correctly performs perineal care
3. Verbalizes an increase in comfort

Forceps Delivery

The obstetric *forceps* consists of 2 pieces: a right blade, which is slipped into the right side of the mother's pelvis, and a left blade, which is slipped into the left side (Table 42-2). Forceps are designed for rotating or extracting the fetal head.

Types of Forceps Deliveries
1. Low forceps operation
   Forceps are applied after the head has reached the perineal floor with the sagittal suture in the anteroposterior diameter of the outlet.
2. Midforceps delivery
   a. Forceps are applied before the criteria for low forceps are met but after engagement has taken place.

Table 42-2. *Representative Types of Forceps**

Major Classifications	Use
1. Simpson—separated shanks (DeLee forcep is one example)	Extract fetus with elongated, molded head; commonly used with nulliparas who have long labors
2. Elliot—overlapping shanks (Tucker–McLean is one example)	Extract fetus with unmolded, rounder heads; commonly used with multiparas who have briefer labors
3. Specialized types	
a. Piper	Deliver aftercoming head in a breech presentation
b. Kielland	Rotate head from transverse or posterior position to an anterior position; used to deliver women with anthropoid pelves
c. Barton	Rotate head from transverse to an anterior position; designed for use in women with flat pelves

* There are more than 600 types of forceps.

b. Any forceps delivery requiring rotation, regardless of the station, is considered a midforcep delivery.
3. High forceps operation
Forceps are applied before engagement has taken place (has been replaced by cesarean delivery).

Indications for Forceps Delivery

A. Fetal Indications

1. Fetal distress ·
2. Cord prolapse
3. Excess pressure on the fetal head from arrested descent
4. Abruptio placentae

B. Maternal Indications

1. Heart disease
2. Acute pulmonary edema
3. Intrapartum infections
4. Maternal hemorrhage
5. Maternal exhaustion
6. Eclampsia
7. Epidural or spinal aneshesia

C. Other Conditions

1. Pelvis should be adequate, with no disproportion
2. Fetal head must be engaged—preferably deeply engaged
3. Cervix must be completely dilated
4. Accurate diagnosis of position and station must be made (see p. 984)
5. Membranes must be ruptured
6. Some form of anesthesia should be used
7. Rectum and bladder should be empty

Assessment

1. Following application of the forceps the fetal heart rate should be auscultated continuously or at least every 5 minutes for a full minute.
2. Evaluate maternal sensation.
3. Evaluate bladder fullness—bladder should be empty prior to the application of the forceps.

Patient Problems/Nursing Diagnoses

1. Anxiety
2. Altered comfort

Nursing Interventions

A. Relieving Anxiety

1. Explain how the forceps are applied.
2. Explain that a sensation of pressure will be felt but not much pain.
3. Answer any questions that the woman and her support person might have.

B. Promoting Comfort

1. Encourage use of breathing and relaxation techniques.
2. Make sure that bladder is completely empty.
3. Encourage relaxation between contractions and use of abdominal muscles and pushing with the contractions.

Evaluation

1. Appears less anxious
2. Is free of severe pain

NURSING ALERT
1. These women are at risk for a postpartum hemorrhage because of lacerations of the vagina and cervix.
2. Evaluate the baby for signs of facial paralysis, skin abrasions, bruising, and other injuries to the presenting part.

Vacuum Extraction

A *vacuum extractor* applies suction to the fetal head, creating an artificial caput within the suction cup, thus allowing adequate traction for delivery of the infant's head.

Uses

1. Dysfunctional labor
2. Fetal distress
3. Maternal cardiopulmonary disease
4. Hypertensive disorders of pregnancy
5. Abruptio placentae
6. Instances in which the thickness of forceps between the birth canal and presenting fetal head is to be avoided

Nursing Interventions

A. Explain Procedure to the Woman and Why It Is Needed

1. Help the woman relax during application of suction to fetal scalp.
2. Coach the mother to push with contraction when needed (time when traction is used with vacuum extractor to aid descent and delivery of fetal head).

B. Following Delivery

1. Examine the infant for scalp lacerations, cephalhematoma, or intracranial hemorrhage.
2. Examine the woman for cervical or vaginal lacerations.
3. Explain to the woman that fetal caput will regress in a few days.

Cesarean Delivery

Cesarean delivery is removal of the infant from the uterus through an incision made in the abdominal wall and in the uterus. This type of delivery is used in the following situations:

1. Cephalopelvic disproportion
2. Uterine dysfunction, inertia, inability of cervix to dilate
3. Neoplasm obstructing birth canal or pelvis
4. Malposition and malpresentation
5. Previous uterine surgery (cesarean delivery, myomectomy, hysterotomy) or cervical surgery
6. Complete or partial placenta previa
7. Premature separation of the placenta
8. Prolapse of the umbilical cord
9. Fetal distress
10. Active herpes outbreak

Types of Cesarean Delivery

A. Low Segment (Operation of Choice)

Incision made transversely in lower segment of uterus
1. Incision is made in thinnest portion so that blood loss is minimal and uterus is easier to open.
2. Lower segment is area of least uterine activity.
3. Postoperative convalescence is more comfortable.
4. Possibility of later rupture is lessened.
5. Peritoneal flap is brought over uterine incision, preventing lochia from entering peritoneal cavity.
6. Incidence of postoperative adhesions and danger of intestinal obstruction are reduced.

B. Classic

Vertical incision is made directly into the wall of the body of the uterus.
1. Useful when bladder and lower segment are involved in extensive adhesions
2. Selected when anterior placenta previa exists
3. Useful when fetus is in a transverse lie

Cesarean Hysterectomy

Cesarean delivery followed by removal of the uterus. Indications include:
1. Defective uterine scar
2. Ruptured uterus
3. Intrauterine infection
4. Hemorrhage due to uterine atony that does not respond to oxytocin, prostaglandin, or massage
5. Laceration of major uterine vessel
6. Severe dysplasia or carcinoma in situ of the cervix
7. Placenta increta or placenta accreta
8. Gross multiple fibromyomas

Assessment

A. Prior to Delivery

1. Knowledge of procedure
2. Maternal and fetal vital signs
3. Maternal blood type and Rh
4. Last time the woman ate
5. Maternal CBC and Coombs' test

B. After Delivery

1. Maternal vital signs every 15 minutes for the first 2 hours then hourly for at least 4 hours
2. Fundal position and firmness
3. Amount and type of lochia
4. Condition of the incision line or dressing
5. Urinary output—a Foley catheter will be in place in the immediate postoperative period
6. Level and presence of anesthesia or pain
7. Presence or absence of bowel sounds
8. Lung sounds
9. Maternal–infant bonding
10. Response to a surgical delivery

Patient Problems/Nursing Diagnoses

1. Knowledge deficit of cesarean delivery/birth
2. Altered comfort
3. Potential for infection
4. Potential for disturbance in self-concept

Nursing Interventions

A. Patient Teaching

1. Explain the reason for the cesarean delivery.
2. Answer any questions the woman and her support person may have regarding a cesarean delivery.
3. Explain all procedures prior to doing them, e.g., shaving of the abdomen, insertion of Foley catheter, grounding of cautery, placement of electrodes, and straps).
4. Allow the support person to attend the birth.
5. Explain that a sensation of pressure will be felt during the delivery, but that little pain will occur. Instruct that any pain should be reported to the nurse.
6. Explain that postdelivery pain may be experienced and that pain medication will be available if requested
7. Explain that Foley cather will prevent the need to void immediately.
8. Instruct about the need for frequent turning, coughing, and deep breathing.

B. Altered Comfort

1. Encourage use of relaxation techniques after medication has been given for pain.
2. Use a back rub and a quiet environment to promote the effectiveness of the medication.
3. Support/splint the abdominal incision when moving or coughing and deep breathing.
4. Encourage frequent rest periods, and plan for them after activities; also, place a "Do Not Disturb" sign on the door during rest and sleep periods.
5. To reduce pain caused by gas, encourage ambulation and the use of a rocking chair.

C. Preventing Infection

1. If skin preparation includes shaving, shave skin carefully, avoiding any nicks in the skin. Then, carry out surgical skin preparation correctly.
2. Postoperatively, use aseptic technique when changing dressings.
3. Provide perineal care every 4 hours.

4. Encourage frequent voiding once Foley catheter has been removed.
5. Encourage coughing and deep breathing every 2 hours during the day and every 4 hours at night.

D. Promoting a Positive Self-Concept

1. Prior to delivery encourage the woman and her support person to discuss their feelings regarding the cesarean birth. After the delivery discuss their feelings regarding the birth.
2. Encourage to ask questions regarding the birth
3. When talking of the birth, refer to it as a cesarean birth, to imply it is just another method of birth, not a surgical experience.

Evaluation

1. Verbalizes an understanding of the cesarean birth procedure and postdelivery care
2. Demonstrates relief of pain
3. Is free of any signs of an infection
4. Adapts to having had a cesarean birth

Postpartum Complications
Puerperal Infection

Puerperal infection is a postpartum infection of the genital tract, usually of the endometrium, that may remain localized or may extend to various parts of the body.

Causes

Bacterial organisms either are introduced from external sources or are normally present in the genital tract and are carried to the uterus.

Predisposing Factors

1. Prolonged labor
2. Prolonged rupture of membranes
3. Premature rupture of membranes
4. Number of vaginal (cervical) examinations
5. Infection elsewhere in the body
6. Anemia
7. Malnutrition
8. Size and number of perineal lacerations
9. Intrauterine manipulation
10. Retained placental fragments or membranes
11. Lapse in aseptic technique
12. Poor perineal hygiene

Diagnostic Evaluation

Diagnosis is made by sustained fever of 38°C. (100.4°F.) or higher occurring on any 2 of the first 10 days postpartum, excluding the first 24 hours. Symptoms depend on site and extension of infection.

Endometritis

Postpartum infection involving the endometrium

A. Clinical Manifestations

1. Uterus usually larger than expected for postdelivery day.
2. Lochia may be profuse, bloody, and foul smelling.
3. Woman may have chills and fever if lochial discharge is obstructed by clots.
4. Infection may spread to myometrium, parametrium, uterine (fallopian) tubes, peritoneum, and blood.

B. Diagnostic Evaluation

Diagnosis is made based on the presenting symptoms, review of labor record, complete physical examination, blood test results, cultures of lochia, and urinalysis.

C. Medical Management

1. Based on the causative agent, antibiotic therapy is instituted after cultures are obtained.
2. Supportive therapy is used to control pain and to maintain hydration and nutritional status.

D. Nursing Assessment

1. Postpartum assessment, noting uterine tenderness upon palpation and the color, amount, and odor of lochia
2. Evaluation of labor and delivery record
3. Evaluation of vital signs
4. Evaluation of nutritional and hydration status
5. Knowledge and skill of perineal hygiene

E. Nursing Interventions

1. Comfort measure
   a. Provide for adequate rest periods.
   b. Position in high-Fowler's position to promote drainage.
   c. Encourage verbalization of feelings regarding illness and treatment.
   d. Administer antibiotics as ordered.
   e. Offer pain medication.
2. Patient teaching
   a. Explain the pathophysiology of the disease.
   b. Explain the treatment and desired effects of the treatment.
   c. Explain the need for good handwashing technique.
   d. Explain how contamination of vagina from the rectum occurs.
   e. Discuss how to place perineal pads and medication, also the need to change pads with each voiding, bowel movement, or every 4 hours while awake.
   f. Explain the use of perineal washing or sitz baths.
3. Parenting measures
   a. Document the cause of the infection so that separation from the infant is not prolonged.
   b. Promote good handwashing technique for the mother prior to contact with the infant.
   c. Encourage her to hold the infant and provide care that she is able to.
   d. Provide care of the infant that the mother is unable to provide at the bedside.
   e. Encourage continuation of breastfeeding if this is the method of feeding.

Parametritis *(Pelvic Cellulitis)*

A. Characteristics

1. Infection of the pelvic connective tissue spread by the lymphatic system within the uterine wall.
2. Often a result of an infected wound in the cervix, vagina, perineum, or lower uterine segment.

B. Clinical Manifestations

1. Chills, fever (102–104°F.)
2. Tachycardia
3. Severe unilateral or bilateral pain in lower abdomen
4. Enlarged uterus—may be larger than expected for postdelivery day
5. Uterine tenderness

6. Uterine position may become fixed as it is displaced by the exudate along the broad ligament

C. Diagnostic Evaluation

Diagnosis is based on the presenting symptoms

D. Medical Management

1. If an abscess has developed, this is drained.
2. Antibiotic therapy is also begun.

E. Nursing Assessment

1. Postpartum assessment, noting uterine tenderness upon palpation and the color, amount, and odor of lochia.
2. Evaluation of labor and delivery record.
3. Evaluation of vital signs.
4. Evaluation of nutritional and hydration status.

F. Nursing Interventions

1. Comfort measures
   a. Provide for adequate rest periods.
   b. Position of comfort.
   c. Encourage verbalization of feelings regarding illness and treatment.
   d. Administer antibiotics as prescribed.
   e. Offer pain medication.
2. Patient teaching
   a. Explain the pathophysiology of the disease.
   b. Explain the treatment and desired effects of the treatment.
   c. Explain the need for good handwashing technique.
   d. Explain how contamination of vagina from the rectum occurs.
   e. Discuss how to place perineal pads and medication, also the need to change pads with each voiding, bowel movement, or every 4 hours while awake.
   f. Explain the use of perineal washing or sitz baths.

Thrombophlebitis

Inflammation of a venous wall with clot formation)—puerperal infection commonly spreads along the veins resulting in thrombophlebitis involving several sites

A. Femoral Thrombophlebitis

Infections of the endothelium with clot formation and attachment to the vein wall

1. Symptoms usually appear 10–20 days after delivery.
2. Pain and tenderness in the calf, positive Homans' sign.
3. The fever and chills are followed by stiffness and pain in the affected area.
4. The pain is followed by edema of the leg, giving the leg a shiny, tight appearance.
5. Symptoms may last for several weeks, with a gradual decrease in the pain.

B. Pelvic Thrombophlebitis

Infection of the veins of the uterine wall and broad ligament, usually involving an anaerobic streptococci

1. Symptoms usually appear about 2 weeks after delivery
2. Severe repeated chills, with a wide temperature change
3. Blood cultures may not isolate the causative organism

C. Predisposing Factors for Thrombophlebitis

1. Obesity
2. Increased maternal age and parity
3. Previous history of thrombophlebitis

4. Anemia
5. Heart disease
6. Vessel trauma during delivery
7. Venous stasis
8. Anesthesia during delivery

D. Diagnostic Evaluation

1. Review of medical history, including labor and delivery
2. Doppler flow studies
3. Blood cultures to isolate the organism

E. Medical Management

1. Strict bedrest.
2. Anticoagulant therapy, usually heparin is administered continuously for 7–10 days, with partial thromboplastin time to determine the effectiveness of the therapy. Heparin therapy is often followed by administration of dicumarol.
3. Antibiotics specific to the organism if the organism is isolated, or a wide-spectrum antibiotic.
4. Maintain adequate hydration.

F. Nursing Assessment

1. Evaluate hydration status.
2. Measure the area where the clot is if it is in the leg.
3. Evaluate for bleeding due to anticoagulant therapy.
4. Emotional status
5. Evaluate the extremities for symmetry in size, shape, color, and temperature
6. Frequent evaluation of vital signs

G. Nursing Interventions

1. Comfort measures
   a. Move the extremity carefully.
   b. Avoid pressure on the area related to positioning or bedcovers.
   c. Use ice or heat along the vein.
   d. Medicate as ordered for pain.
2. Patient teaching
   a. Explain the disease process and treatment to the patient and family.
   b. Explain how heparin and dicumarol work.
   c. Explain the side effects of anticoagulants, bleeding from gums, surgical sites, and injection sites. Explain that heparin does not pass into the breast milk and that dicumarol does no apparent harm to the infant.
   d. Explain the purpose of the laboratory testing and the need for follow-up.
   e. Explain injection technique if the woman is going home on heparin therapy.
3. Parenting measures
   a. If rehospitalized, provide opportunities for the infant to stay in the hospital with the mother or for extended visits with the mother.
   b. Allow pictures of the infant to be placed around the room.
   c. Encourage continuation of breast-feeding by providing a breast pump and time to pump each day.

> **NURSING ALERT:** Never give acetylsalicylic acid (aspirin) to women on anticoagulant therapy—it may cause bleeding.

> **NURSING ALERT:** While the woman is receiving heparin, have protamine sulfate available for administration. While the woman is receiving dicumarol, have vitamin K available for administration.

Postpartum Hemorrhage

Postpartum hemorrhage involves a loss of 500 ml. or more of blood; it occurs most frequently in the 1st hour following delivery.

Causes

1. Uterine atony—relaxation of the uterus secondary to:
   a. Multiple pregnancy—causes overdistention of uterus and a larger placental site
   b. Polyhydramnios (excessive amniotic fluid)
   c. High parity
   d. Prolonged labor with maternal exhaustion
   e. Deep anesthesia
   f. Fibromyomata—prevents uterus from contracting
   g. Retained placental fragments
2. Retained placental fragments—results from:
   a. Manual removal of placenta
   b. Succenturiate (additional) lobe
   c. Abnormal adherent placenta (placenta acreta)
3. Laceration of the vagina, cervix, or perineum secondary to:
   a. Forceps delivery, especially rotation forceps
   b. Large infant
   c. Multiple pregnancy

Clinical Manifestations

1. Uterine atony—uterus is soft or boggy, often difficult to palpate, and will not remain contracted; excessive vaginal bleeding.
2. Retained placental fragments—hemorrhage usually occurs about the 10th postpartum day.
3. Lacerations of the vagina, cervix, or perineum—bleeding is bright red, continuous, and often in spurts; the bleeding remains continuous even when the fundus is firm.

Diagnostic Evaluation

1. Based on the present symptoms
2. Evaluate hydration and fluid status

Medical Management

1. For uterine atony, oxytocin is prescribed.
2. Pain medication may be needed to counter uterine contractions.
3. If placental fragments have been retained, curettage of the uterus is indicated.
4. Lacerations may need to be repaired.

Nursing Assessment

1. Vital signs
2. Location and firmness of uterine fundus
3. Presence of bladder distention
4. Amount and type of bleeding, or lochia present and the presence of clots
5. Intactness of any perineal repair

Patient Problems/Nursing Diagnoses

1. Anxiety, related to unexpected blood loss
2. Fluid volume deficit
3. Potential for infection
4. Pain
5. Potential for altered parenting

Nursing Interventions

A. Relieving Anxiety
1. Maintain a quiet atmosphere.
2. Provide information about the situation and explain everything as it is done; answer questions that the woman and her family ask.
3. Encourage the presence of a support person.

B. Attending to Fluid Volume Needs
1. Maintain or start an IV line if vaginal bleeding becomes heavy; use an 18-gauge needle if possible.
2. Maintain IV fluids or blood administration at the desired rate.
3. Determine availability of crossmatched blood for the woman.
4. Monitor laboratory studies.
5. Evaluate urine output and specific gravity.
6. Maintain a quiet, calm atmosphere.
7. Keep woman NPO.

C. Avoiding Infection
1. Maintain aseptic technique.
2. Evaluate for symptoms of infection, chilling, and elevated temperature, changes in white blood cell count, uterine tenderness, and odor of lochia.
3. Administer antibiotics as prescribed.

D. Promoting Comfort
1. Administer pain medications as prescribed.
2. Position of comfort.
3. Encourage frequent voiding.
4. Provide comfort measures, back rubs, perineal care, and so forth.
5. Encourage use of same breathing techniques used during labor.

E. Encouraging Effective Parenting
1. Answer questions regarding infant's status.
2. Bring infant to parents when both mother and infant are stable and provide time to get to know the infant.

Evaluation

1. Anxiety and fears are minimized.
2. Vital signs and urinary output are normal.
3. Does not develop signs or symptoms of an infection.
4. Verbalizes relief of pain.
5. Beginning bonding behaviors are present.

Mastitis

Mastitis is inflammation of breast tissue. It may involve:
1. Formation of a subareolar abscess in the underlying milk glands
2. The lacteriferous tubules (parenchymatous of glandular mastitis)
3. Connective tissue and fat around the lobes and lobules (intramammary mastitis)

Cause

Usually due to *Staphylococcus aureus* derived from the nursing infant's nose and throat.

Clinical Manifestations

1. Symptoms may occur at the end of the 1st postpartum week but usually appear in 3rd to 4th week postpartum.
2. Marked breast engorgement
3. Chills

4. Elevated temperature
5. Increased pulse rate
6. Inflammation may be generalized or localized to one lobe of the breast; if localized, tenderness, warmth, and redness are present.

Diagnostic Evaluation

Diagnosis is made based on the presenting symptoms.

Medical Management

1. Milk cultures are done to determine the bacteria causing the infection.
2. Antibiotic therapy is then begun.
3. The best treatment is through prevention by use of good handwashing techniques, spacing of infants in the nursery, and encouragement of frequent nursing at the breast, long enough to empty the breast completely.

Assessment

1. Evaluate the breast for signs of engorgement and localized infection (redness, tenderness, warmth).
2. Evaluate the nipple, noting any cracks, fissures, or erosions of the nipple or areola.
3. Evaluate breast preparation and the infant at the breast for position, sucking, and duration of feeding.

Patient Problems/Nursing Diagnoses

1. Pain, related to infection
2. Potential knowledge deficit of breast care during lactation
3. Anxiety

Nursing Interventions

A. Promoting Comfort

1. Encourage wearing of a well-supportive bra or breast binder. Encourage wearing of the bra 24 hours a day.
2. Use ice bags to decrease the pain.
3. Support breast while in bed with towels and pillows.
4. If breast-feeding is continued, encourage frequent feeding to allow for emptying of the breast.
5. If abscess formation has occurred, use heat to the area to promote localization.
6. Mild analgesics may also be used.
7. Stress the importance of taking the prescribed antibiotic regularly and completely.

B. Breast Care Measures

1. Review the need for handwashing prior to breast-feeding and any time the breast will be touched.
2. Review use of massage prior to beginning breast-feeding.
3. Discuss correct placement of the infant at the breast, with the areola compressed and inserted well into the infant's mouth.
4. Discuss that breast should be alternated during the feeding after the infant has nursed for at least 8 minutes on one side, and to begin each feeding with the breast that was used last during the previous feeding.

C. Reducing Anxiety

1. Allow the mother to verbalize her feelings regarding the infection and breast-feeding.
2. Review breast-feeding techniques.

Evaluation

1. Verbalizes a decrease in the pain
2. Correctly performs breast care prior to breast-feeding and has the infant correctly positioned at the breast.

Postpartum Hematomas

Postpartum hematomas are localized collections of blood in loose connective tissue beneath the skin that covers the external genitalia, beneath the vaginal mucosa, or in the broad ligaments

A. Causes

1. Trauma during spontaneous labor
2. Trauma during forceps application or delivery
3. Inadequate suturing of an episiotomy

Clinical Manifestations

1. Complaints of pressure and pain, often noting that the pain is excruciating
2. Discolored skin that is tight, full feeling, and painful to touch

Diagnostic Evaluation

1. Made based on the presenting symptoms

Medical Management

1. Small hematomas are left to resolve on their own
2. Large hematomas may require evacuation of the blood and ligation of the bleeding vessel

Assessment

1. Inspect perineal and vulva area for signs of a hematoma when woman complains of pain or pressure following delivery.
2. If woman is unable to void after anesthesia has worn off, inspect the vaginal area for signs of a hematoma.
3. Evaluate for signs of shock.

Patient Problems/Nursing Diagnoses

1. Pain related to hematoma and inability to void
2. Fluid volume deficit

Nursing Interventions

A. Promoting Comfort

1. For hematoma
   a. Ice bag to perineal area
   b. Medicate with mild analgesics
   c. Position of comfort to decrease pressure on the affected area
2. For voiding problems
   a. Assist to bathroom to void if able to ambulate; if unable to ambulate, then assist to sit on bed pan and, if possible, to hang legs over side of bed.
   b. Provide privacy and run water while the woman is attempting to void.
   c. If unable to void, catheterize.

B. Maintaining Fluid Status

1. Evaluate vital signs, watching for a decrease in blood pressure.
2. Maintain or begin an IV line using an 18-gauge needle if signs of shock are present.
3. Keep NPO.
4. Evaluate hemoglobin and hematocrit.
5. If extensive blood is lost, type and crossmatch for a possible blood transfusion.

Evaluation

1. Verbalizes a decrease in pain.
2. Voids and states has had relief.

3. Maintains an adequate fluid balance and does not develop symptoms of shock.

Subinvolution

Subinvolution is a slowing or halting of the normal postpartum involution. The usual causes are pelvic infection, retention of placental fragments, and fibroid tumors.

Clinical Manifestations

1. Prolonged lochia discharge may be profuse at times.
2. Irregular uterine bleeding.
3. Prolonged leukorrhea.
4. Backache or a sense of fullness in the pelvis.

Diagnostic Evaluation

Diagnosis is usually made based on the presenting symptoms and bimanual examination findings of a uterus larger and softer than normal in the postdelivery period.

Medical Management

1. Treatment is based on the symptoms and may include antibiotic and oxytocin therapy.
2. Uterine curettage may be done for retained placental fragments.

Assessment

1. Evaluate maternal vital signs.
2. Assess uterine position, size, and firmness.
3. Assess lochia for amount, color, and odor.

Patient Teaching

1. Explain the process of involution.
2. Explain how alterations in the involutional process can occur.
3. Explain treatment, need, and purpose of medication and treatment to be used.
4. Instruct woman to call if lochia increases or is unchanged after 12 hours of medication, if there is an odor with the lochia, or if symptoms of hypertension occur.

Postpartum Depression

Postpartum depression may occur in the first 2 weeks after delivery and may be viewed as a normal developmental crisis related to the adjustments that are being made relative to the new role of parent, along with the added responsibilities, fatigue, and excitement that go with the birth. Many women experience this to some degree and will work through their feelings by the end of 2 weeks.

Postpartum psychosis is a severe form of depression that occurs in a small percentage of women giving birth.

Clinical Manifestations

1. Exaggerated and prolonged periods of irritability, moodiness, and hostility.
2. Ineffective coping.
3. Withdrawal and inappropriate response to the infant or family.

Medical Management

Counseling with a mental health professional

Bibliography

Books

Bobak I, Jensen M and Zalar M. Maternity and Gynecologic Care. 4th ed. St. Louis, CV Mosby, 1989

Cunningham F, MacDonald P and Gant N. Williams Obstetrics. 18th ed. Norwalk, CT, Appleton and Lange, 1989

Dickason EJ, Schult M and Silverman B. Maternal–Infant Nursing Care. Philadelphia, JB Lippincott, 1990

Doenges M, Kenty J and Moorehouse M. Maternal/Newborn Care Plans Guideline for Client Care. Philadelphia, FA Davis, 1988

Gilbert E and Harmon J. High Risk Pregnancy and Delivery. St. Louis, CV Mosby, 1986

Manlinowski J, Pedigo C and Phillips C. Nursing Care During the Labor Process. 3rd ed. Philadelphia, FA Davis, 1989

Neeson J. Clinical Manual of Maternity Nursing. Philadelphia, JB Lippincott, 1987

Olds S, London M and Ladewig P. Maternal Newborn Nursing: A Family-Centered Approach. 3rd ed. Menlo Park, CA, Addison–Wesley, 1988

Reeder S and Martin L. Maternity Nursing. 16th ed. Philadelphia, JB Lippincott, 1987

Tucker S. Pocket Guide to Fetal Monitoring. St. Louis, CV Mosby, 1988

Worthington–Roberts B and Williams S. Nutrition in Pregnancy and Lactation. 4th ed. St. Louis, Times Mirror/Mosby, 1989

Journals

Abrams B et al. Maternal weight gain and preterm delivery. Obstet Gynecol 1989; 74:577–583

Ales K et al. Early prediction of antepartum hypertension. Obstet Gynecol 1989; 73:928–933

Andolsek K. Ectopic pregnancy: "Classic" versus common presentation. J Fam Pract 1987; 24:481–485

Benoit J. Sexually transitted diseases in pregnancy. Nurs Clin North Am 1988; 23:937–945

Bracero L et al. Significance of umbilical and uterine artery velocimetry in the well-controlled pregnant diabetic. J Reprod Med 1989; 34:273–276

Brengman S and Burns M. Hypertensive crisis in L & D. Am J Nurs 1988; 88:325A–328L

Clark S et al. Central hemodynamic alterations in amniotic fluid embolism. Am J Obstet Gynecol 1988; 158:1124–1126

Cohn J. Virology, immunology, and natural history of HIV infection. J Nurse-Midwif 1989; 34:242–250

Cucco C et al. Maternal-fetal outcomes in prolonged pregnancy. Am J Obstet Gynecol 1989; 161:916–920

Davey D and MacGillivray I. The classification and definition of the hypertensive disorders of pregnancy. Am J Obstet Gynecol 1988; 158:892–898

Depue R et al. Hyperemesis gravidarum in relation to estradiol levels, pregnancy outcome and other maternal factors: A seroepidemiologic study. Am J Obstet Gynecol 1987; 156:1137–1141

Donner C and Cooper K. The critical difference: Ectopic pregnancy. Am J Nurs 1988; 88:843

Dorman K. Hemorrhagic emergencies in obstetrics. J Perinat Neonat Nurs 1989; 3:23–32

Dudley D et al. Long-term tocolysis with intravenous magnesium sulfate. Obstet Gynecol 1989; 73:373–378

Few B. Prostaglandin F2-alpha for treating severe postpartum hemorrhage. Am J Matern Child Nurs 1987; 12:168

Finley B. Acute coagulopathy in pregnancy. Med Clin North Am 1989; 73:723–743

Gill P, Smith M and McGregor C. Terbutaline by pump to prevent recurrent preterm labor. Am J Matern Child Nurs 1989; 14:163–167

Gilstrap L et al. Effect of type of anesthesia on blood loss at cesarean section. Obstet Gynecol 1987; 69:328–332

Ginsberg J et al. Heparin therapy during pregnancy. Risk to the fetus and mother. Arch Intern Med 1989; 149:2233–2236

Givens S. Update on tocolytic therapy in the management of preterm labor. J Perinat Neonat Nurs 1988; 2:21–32

Glazer G. Prostaglandin gel for cervical ripening. Am J Matern Child Nurs 1987; 12:28–31

Gross S, Librach C and Cecutti A. Maternal weight loss associated with hyperemesis gravidarum: A predictor of fetal outcome. Am J Obstet Gynecol 1989; 160:906–909

Helton D et al. Detection of glucose intolerance in pregnancy. J Perinatol 1989; 9:259–261

Holbrook RH. Evaluation of a risk scoring system for prediction of preterm labor. Am J Perinatol 1989; 6:62–68

Hovick T et al. Use of the fetal biophysical profile in severe oligohydramnios after preterm premature rupture of the membranes. J Reprod Med 1989; 34:353–356

Hunter L. Twin gestation: Antepartum management. J Perinat Neonat Nurs 1989; 3:1–13

Ismail A et al. Induction of labor by oral prostaglandin E_2 in protracted pregnancy. Intern J Gynecol Obstet 1989; 29:325–328

Johnson F. Assessment and education to prevent preterm labor. Am J Matern Child Nurs 1989; 14:157–160

Koniak-Griffine D and Dodgson J. Severe pregnancy-induced hypertension: Postpartum care of the critically ill patient. Heart Lung 1987; 16:661–669

Langer O et al. Gestational diabetes: Insulin requirements in pregnancy. Am J Obstet Gynecol 1987; 157:669–675

Lawrence R. Breastfeeding and medical disease. Med Clin North Am 1989; 73:583–603

Lee H et al. Postpartum hepatic hemorrhage in the syndrome of hemolysis, elevated liver enzymes, and low platelets: Diagnosis by radiocolloid scanning. Clin Nucl Med 1988; 13:635–637

Levine M and Esser D. Total parenteral nutrition for the treatment of severe hyperemesis gravidarum: Maternal nutrition effect and fetal outcome. Obstet Gynecol 1988; 72:102–107

Ljungstrom B et al. Indications for tocolytic therapy: Incidence of true preterm labor with uterine contractions as the sole deciding factor. Am J Perinatol 1989; 6:218–221

Lloyd T. Rh-factor incompatibility: A primer for prevention. J Nurse Midwif 1987; 32:297–306

Lopez Llera et al. Eclampsia in twin pregnancy. J Reprod Med 1989; 34:802–906

Martell L. Postpartum depression as a family problem. Am J Matern Child Nurs 1990; 15:90–93

Moleti C. Caring for socially high-risk pregnant women. Am J Matern Child Nurs 1988; 13:24–27

Montan S and Ingemarsson I. Intrapartum fetal heart rate patterns in pregnancies complicated by hypertension. Am J Obstet Gynecol 1989; 160:283–288

Morales W et al. Efficacy and safety of indomethacin versus ritodrine in the management of preterm labor: A randomized study. Obstet Gynecol 1989; 74:567–572

Neuhoff D et al. Cesarean birth for failed progress in labor. Obstet Gynecol 1989; 73:915–920

Newman R et al. Outpatient triplet management: A contemporary review. Am J Obstet Gynecol 1989; 161:547–553

Nurmberg H. An overview of somatic treatment of psychosis during pregnancy and postpartum. Gen Hosp Psychiatr 1989; 11:328–338

Ogle K and Davis S. Mastitis in lactating women. J Fam Pract 1988; 26:139–144

Ong B et al. Anesthesia for cesarean section—effects on neonates. Anesth Anal 1989; 68:270–275

Osguthorpe N. Ectopic pregnancy. J Obstet Gynecol Neonat Nurs 1987; 16:36–41

Osguthorpe N and Keating C. Ectopic pregnancy: Surgical intervention and perioperative nursing care. AORN 1988; 48:254–267

Owen J et al. Comparison of predelivery versus postdelivery Kleinhauer–Betke stains in cases of fetal death. Am J Obstet Gynecol 1989; 161:663–666

Peaceman A et al. The effect of magnesium sulfate tocolysis on the fetal biophysical profile. Am J Obstet Gynecol 1989; 161:771–774

Petrikovsky B et al. Electronic fetal heart rate monitoring during cesarean section in cases of fetal distress. Intern J Gynecol Obstet 1989; 29:215–218

Phaosavasdi S et al. Effectiveness of benzathine penicillin regimen in the treatment of syphilis in pregnancy. J Med Assoc Thai 1989; 72(2):101–108

Philipson E and Super D. Gestational diabetes mellitus: Does it recur in subsequent pregnancy? Am J Obstet Gynecol 1989; 160:1324–1329

Pircon R et al. Controlled trial of hydration and bed rest versus bed rest alone in the evaluation of preterm uterine contractions. Am J Obstet Gynecol 1989; 161:775–779

Poole J. Getting perspective on HELLP syndrome. Am J Matern Child Nurs 1988; 13:432–437

Quance D. Amniotic fluid embolism: Detection by pulse oximetry. Anesthesiology 1988; 68:951–952

Remich M. Factors associated with pregnancy-induced hypertension. Nurse Practitioner 1989; 14:20–24

Robertson C. When your pregnant patient has diabetes. RN 1987; 50(11):18–22

Robson S et al. Maternal hemodynamics after normal delivery and delivery complicated by postpartum hemorrhage. Obstet Gynecol 1989; 74:234–239

Rotmensch S et al. The impact of the acquired immunodeficiency syndrome epidemic on the philosophy of childbirth. Am J Obstet Gynecol 1989; 161:855–856

Russell J. The etiology of ectopic pregnancy. Clin Obstet Gynecol 1987; 30:181–190

Sala DJ and Moise K. The treatment of preterm labor using a portable subcutaneous terbutaline pump. J Obstet Gynecol Neonat Nurs 1990; 19:108–115

Schreyer P et al. The predictive value of fetal breathing movement and Bishop score in the diagnosis of "true" preterm labor. Am J Obstet Gynecol 1989; 161:886–889

Shannon D. HELLP Syndrome: A severe consequence of pregnancy-induced hypertension. J Obstet Gynecol Neonat Nurs 1987; 19:395–402

Siddiqi T et al. Biphasic intrauterine growth in insulin-dependent diabetic pregnancies. J Am Coll Nutr 1989; 8:225–234

Sperling R and Berkowitz R. Obstetric management of women with a history of recurrent genital herpes. Am J Perinatol 1989; 6:275–277

Taslimi M et al. A national survey on preterm labor. Am J Obstet Gynecol 1989; 160:1352–1357

Thorp J and Bowes W. Episiotomy: Can its routine use be defended? Am J Obstet Gynecol 1989; 160:1027–1030

Wasson C. Promoting wellness in the pregnant diabetic to improve fetal outcome. Nurs Admin Q 1987; 11:41

Weckstein L, Masserman J and Garite T. Placenta accreta: A problem of increasing clinical significance. Obstet Gynecol 1987; 69:480–482

Wilcox L et al. Episiotomy and its role in the incidence of perineal lacerations in a maternity center and a tertiary hospital obstetric service. Am J Obstet Gynecol 1989; 160:1047–1052

Wilson D. An overview of sexually transmissible diseases in the perinatal period. J Nurse Midwif 1988; 33:115–128

Zimmer E and Vadasz A. Influence of the fetal scalp electrode stimulation test on fetal heart rate and body movements in quiet and active behavioral states during labor. Am J Perinatol 1989; 6:24–29

Part III

Pediatric Nursing

Pediatric Assessment and Health Promotion

General Principles

A. Information About a Child Is Elicited for Several Reasons

1. To establish a relationship with the child and family
2. To assess what a family understands about their child's health
3. To formulate an individual plan of care
4. To correct any misinformation the family may have

B. Focus on Specific Topics in the History Depending on the Child's Age

1. Infant—stress prenatal and postnatal history
2. Toddler—home environment, safety issues
3. School age—school, friends, reaction to previous hospitalizations
4. Adolescent—alcohol, drugs, friends, sexual history

Identifying Information

A. Type of Information Needed

1. Date and time
2. Hospital name and telephone number, if known
3. Patient's name, address, telephone number, birth date
4. Referring health care source (e.g., physician, nurse practitioner, health care agency, etc.)
5. Insurance data

B. Method of Collecting Data

1. Identify the "care person" in charge of the patient by name and relationship to the patient; obtain relative's or care person's address, home and work telephone numbers, if different from those of the patient.
2. To make the informant feel more at ease, the questions should begin in a friendly, nonthreatening manner. Questions addressed to the parent should be phrased appropriately.
3. Casual, friendly responses or remarks on the part of the interviewer may also help break the ice.
   a. "Whoever takes care of this baby certainly does a good job."
   b. "That's a lovely outfit the baby is wearing." (Remember that families will often put a new dress or suit on a baby for a visit to a health care agency.)
4. Sometimes repeat the information in order to verify data. This will give you a better judgment of the care person's cooperation and reliability.

Chief Complaint

A. Method of Recording

1. Write an exact description of the complaint.
2. Use quotation marks to clearly indicate that the informant's words are being used. It is helpful to explain:
   a. "I'll write it down so there will be no mistake."
   b. "Let me read this back to you to be sure it is correct."
3. Quotation of the care person's exact words may give an indication of how he/she feels about the symptoms; may reflect fear, guilt, defensiveness, etc.

B. Method of Collecting Information

1. Begin with a helpful open-ended question. That is the first overture made to this patient.
   a. "How may I help you?"
   b. "Please tell me the reason for your coming here today."
   c. "What do you think is wrong with the baby?"
2. Avoid confusing questions that may elicit funny-sounding or "smart" answers.
   a. "What brings you here?" (Answer: "The bus.")
   b. "Why are you here?" ("That's what I came to find out.")

C. Duration of Complaint

1. The information obtained may indicate the natural history of the disease, if one is present, and its gradual evolution. Pursue the information with a series of probing questions.
   a. "How long has the baby (child) had this problem?"
   b. If the informant cannot remember, try another route:
      "When did he last act well?"
      "Do you remember last Christmas? Did the baby have the trouble then?"
2. Write down the responses; try to assess, as more questions are asked, how accurate the informant's answers may be.

History of Present Illness

A. Type of Information Needed

When the patient is an infant or a preverbal child, information will consist mainly of what the informant has been able to observe. Having established what the chief complaint is, identify further problems, if any. Obtain the following information for each problem:

1. Body location—of pain, itching, weakness, etc.
2. Quality of complaint—both type (a burning pain) and severity (knife-like, comes and goes).
3. Degree of symptom—(e.g., pain, how severe; cough, day and night; eye drainage, how much).
4. Chronology—indicate time sequence and whether problem is episodic (lasts for a while and then clears up completely).
5. Environment or setting—where and when the symptoms occur.
6. Aggravating and alleviating factors—what makes the pain worse or better?
7. Associated manifestations or symptoms—accompanied by vomiting, blurred vision, etc.

B. Importance of Detail

1. A carefully written description of a symptom will frequently be the source of a future diagnosis and will serve all who are involved in helping the patient.
2. Do not worry about large volume of notes at first.
3. You will be able to recheck this information when you do the review of systems.

Past History

A. Prenatal

1. Pregnancy—planned or not; source of care; date (approximately) of seeking care; birth order of this pregnancy, including miscarriages. This area of the history may be one of great sensitivity. Try to make the questions gentle and supportive.
   a. "Did you plan a baby around this time?"
   b. "When did you manage to get your first check-up for the pregnancy?"
   c. "Were there any unusual problems related to your pregnancy or delivery?"
2. Maternal health—includes illnesses and dates, abnormal symptoms (e.g., fever, rash, vaginal bleeding, edema, hypertension, urine abnormalities, sexually transmitted disease). Avoid technical words, if possible.
   a. "Did you have trouble with swollen feet?"
   b. "Were your rings tight?"
   c. "Do you know if your blood pressure went up?"
   d. "Did you have trouble with your urine?"
3. Weight gain—validate by trying to get a figure for nonpregnant weight and weight at delivery.
4. Medicines taken—(e.g., vitamins, iron, calcium, aspirin, cold preparations, tranquilizers ["nerve medicine"], antibiotics; use of ointments, hormones, injections during pregnancy, special or unusual diet; radiation exposure, sonography, amniocentesis.
5. Quality of the fetal movements: when felt, how brisk?

B. Natal

1. Expected date of delivery and approximate duration of pregnancy.
2. Place of delivery and who conducted the delivery.
3. Labor—spontaneous or induced; duration and intensity.
4. Analgesia or anesthesia.
5. Presentation—vaginal, breech, or vertex; cesarean delivery, forceps.
6. Episiotomy
7. Complications (e.g., need for blood transfusion, delay in delivery, etc.)

C. Neonatal

1. Condition of infant
2. Color (if seen) at delivery
3. Activity of infant
4. Crying heard
5. Breathing abnormality
6. Birth weight and length
7. Problems occurring immediately at birth

D. Postnatal

1. Duration of hospitalization of the mother and infant
2. Problems with baby's breathing or feeding
3. Need of supportive care (e.g., oxygen, incubator, special care nursery, isolation, medications)
4. Weight changes, weight at discharge if known
5. Color—cyanosis or jaundice
6. Bowel movements—when
7. Problems—seizures, deformities identified, consultation required
8. Mother's contact with the baby and her first impression
   a. "How did the baby look to you?"
   b. "What did the baby do when you were first together?"

E. Nutrition

1. Breast- or bottle-fed; what formula? how prepared?
2. Amounts offered and consumed
3. Frequency of feeding; weight gain
4. Addition of juice and/or solid foods
5. Food preferences or allergies
6. Feeding problems—variations in appetite
7. Age of weaning
8. Vitamins—type, amount, regularity
9. Pattern of weight gain
10. Current diet; frequency and content of meals

F. Growth and Development

1. Past weights and lengths if available
2. Milestones—sat alone unsupported; walked alone; used words, then sentences
3. Teeth—eruption, difficulty, cavities
4. Toilet training
5. Current motor, social, and language skills
6. Sexual development
   a. Infant—swollen breast tissue, vaginal discharge, hypertrophy of the labia
   b. Toddler or school-aged child—early development of breasts or pubic hair
   c. Prepubertal or pubertal child—in females, time of development of breasts, pubic hair; onset of menstruation. In males, time of enlargement of testes, penis; development of pubic and facial hair; voice changes; acne

G. Health Maintenance

1. Immunizations—smallpox, rubella, rubeola, mumps, polio, diphtheria, pertussis, tetanus toxoid, BCG, influenza
   Indicate number and dates.
2. Screening procedures—hematocrit, tuberculin testing, visual and auditory acuity; rubella antibodies; syphilis testing; gonorrhea screen, Papanicolaou smear
3. Dental care—source and frequency of care, dental hygienist visits, fillings or extractions

H. Acute Infectious Diseases

Rubella, rubeola, mumps, chickenpox, scarlet fever, rheumatic fever, hepatitis, infectious mononucleosis, sexually transmitted disease, tuberculosis. Recent exposure to communicable disease.

I. Hospitalizations and Operations

1. Dates, hospital, physician
2. Indications, diagnosis, procedures
3. Complications
4. Reactions to previous hospitalizations

J. Injuries

1. Emergency Department visits—frequency and diagnosis
2. Fractures—location and treatment
3. Trauma, burns, bruises
4. Ingestions

K. Medications

1. For general use such as vitamins, antihistamines, laxatives
2. Special or fad diets
3. Recent antibiotics
4. Routine use of aspirin
5. Oral contraceptives—types and dose, duration
6. Drugs, narcotics, marijuana, hallucinogens, mood elevators, tranquilizers, alcohol
7. Determine when last dose of medication was taken; is medication with patient? How does the child take the medication?

L. Radiation

1. Diagnosis requiring; number and occasion of exposures
2. Accidental exposure
3. Routine x-rays (chest, dental)
4. For injury, follow-up of fracture, etc.

Personal History

A. Type of Information Needed

1. Hygiene, exercise
2. Activities and hobbies, special talents
3. Friends
4. Sibling and parent relationships
5. Expression of emotions
   a. Blows up easily
   b. Rather quiet
6. Idiosyncratic behavior and habits (e.g., thumb sucking, nail biting, temper tantrums, head banging, pica, breath holding, rituals, tics, etc.)

B. Method of Collecting Data

1. Straightforward questions to a child (e.g., "What grade are you in?" "Who are your friends?")
2. Three wishes offered to the child:
   a. "If Christmas were here, what would you ask for?"
   b. "If you had your way, who would you like to be?"
   c. "What would be the best thing that could happen to you?"
3. "Who's your best friend?"
4. Adolescents—may want to interview without parents present

School History

A. Type of Information Needed

1. Present and past schooling, grade, and performance
2. Favored and least favored subjects
3. School-related behavior—anxious to go, anxious to stay home
4. General attitude toward school and any career plans

B. Method of Collecting Data

Emphasize the positive (e.g., "What's your best subject?" "Have you repeated a grade?" "Do you see your friends after school?")

Social History

A. Type of Information Needed

1. Environment—rural, urban
2. Housing—type, location, heating, sewage, water supply, family pets, other animal exposure
3. Parents' occupations (employment) and marital status
4. Number of individuals living in home, sleeping arrangements
5. Any religious affiliations
6. Utilization of social agencies previously
7. Health insurance and usual source of care

B. Method of Collecting Data

Parents are proud, so be careful with some of the questions. Ask permission.
1. "Can you tell me a little bit about your home?"
2. "I need to know more about how you live in order to help you with your child's problem."

Review of Systems

A. Type of Information Needed

1. General—activity, appetite, affect, sleep patterns, weight changes, edema, fever
2. Allergy—eczema, hay fever, asthma, hives, food or drug allergy, sinus disorders
3. Skin—rash or eruption, nodules, pigmentation or texture change, sweating or dryness, infection, hair growth, itching
4. Head—headache, head trauma, dizziness
5. Eyes—visual acuity, corrective lenses, strabismus, lacrimation, discharge, itching, redness, photophobia
6. Ears—auditory acuity, earaches (frequency), infection, drainage
7. Nose—colds and runny nose (frequency), infection, drainage
8. Teeth—hygiene practices, general condition
9. Throat—sore throat, tonsillitis, difficulty swallowing
10. Speech—peculiarity of or change in voice; hoarseness, clarity, enunciation, stammering
11. Respiratory—difficulty breathing, shortness of breath, chest pain, cough, wheezing, croup, pneumonia, tuberculosis or exposure
12. Cardiovascular—cyanosis, fainting, exercise intolerance, murmurs
13. Hematologic—pallor, anemia, tendency to bruise or bleed
14. Gastrointestinal—appetite (amount, frequency, cravings), nausea, vomiting, abdominal pain, abnormal size, bowel habits and nature of stools, parasites, encopresis (incontinence of feces), colic
15. Genitourinary—age of toilet training, frequency of urination, straining, dysuria, hematuria (or unusual color or odor of infant's soiled diaper), previous urinary tract infection, enuresis; urethral or vaginal discharge. Females: last menses, cramps, changes in interval and duration
16. Musculoskeletal—deformities, fractures, sprains, joint pains or swelling, limitation of motion, abnormality of nails
17. Neurologic—weakness or clumsiness, coordination, balance, gait, dominance, fatigability, tone, tremor. Seizures or paroxysmal behavior. Personality changes.

Bibliography

Books

Athreya BH, Silverman BK and Spitzer AR. Taking the history. In Pediatric Physical Diagnosis, pp 17–51. Norwalk, CT, Appleton–Century–Crofts, 1985

Bowers AC and Thompson JM. Clinical Manual of Health Assessment. 3rd ed. St Louis, CV Mosby, 1988

Engel J. Dimensions of a history. In Pocket Guide to Pediatric Assessment, pp 7–14. St Louis, CV Mosby, 1989

Gill D and O'Brien N. History taking. In Paediatric Clinical Examination, pp 10–21. New York, Churchill Livingstone, 1988

Guckian JC (ed). The pediatric patient. In The Clinical Interview and Physical Examination, pp 476–522. Philadelphia, JB Lippincott, 1987

Hoekelman RA et al. Communication with parents and patients. In Primary Pediatric Care, pp 48–51. St Louis, CV Mosby, 1987

James SR and Mott SR. Principles of assessment. In Child Health Nursing, pp 240–245. Reading, MA, Addison–Wesley, 1988

Kaye R, Oski FA and Barness LA. History and physical examination. In Principles and Practice of Pediatrics, pp 28–47. Philadelphia, JB Lippincott, 1990

Rudolph AM and Hoffman JIE. Assessment and care of child and adolescent. In Pediatrics. 18th ed, pp 17–34. Norwalk, Appleton and Lange, 1987

Schwartz MW et al. Interviewing hints. In Principles and Practice of Clinical Pediatrics, pp 14–16. Chicago, Year Book Medical Pub, 1987

Summitt RL. The pediatric history and physical examination. In Comprehensive Pediatrics, pp 253–261. St Louis, CV Mosby, 1990

Whaley LF and Wong DL. Communication and health assessment of the child and family. In Essentials of Pediatric Nursing, pp 100–128. St Louis, CV Mosby, 1989

Wood RA et al. The interview. In Pediatrics, pp 41–48. Philadelphia, JB Lippincott, 1989

Journals

Rankin WW. Listening with the heart. J Pediatr Nurs 1988 Apr; 3(2):127–129

Schneider E. Parent questionnaires: A useful tool to pediatric practice. Pediatr Nurs 1987 May–Jun; 13(3):193

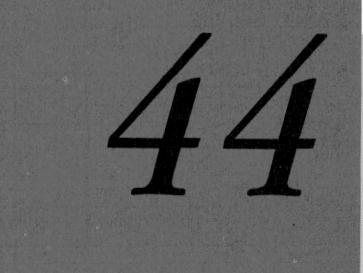

44 Pediatric Physical Examination

General Principles

1. Establish the order of all data collection according to the needs of the patients. For example:
   a. An exhausted parent with a screaming baby will not give a careful, comprehensive history.
   b. Alternative care may not be available for preschoolers when the newborn comes in for the first checkup.
2. If the parent has come in with more than 1 child, try to organize some supervision of the other children so that you can have a little time with the parent alone.
3. Remember that the safest place for any child is on the parent's knee. Privacy may not be possible because of the presence of other children.
4. Attempt to develop rapport with the young patient from the moment you first see or meet him or her.
5. Explain to the teenager what you are looking for as you proceed with the examination.

Approach to the Patient

1. Begin the examination with the patient on the parent's knee.
2. To evaluate the chest properly, you need to listen through 10 heartbeats when the child is not screaming; therefore, the chest is a good place to begin the examination.
3. The part to be examined should be completely exposed, but if an apprehensive child objects to having his clothes removed, slip your stethoscope under the shirt.
4. Forget the orderly and systematic approach, but remember to examine everything. Fortunately, children are small and one can check several systems very quickly over a small area.
5. As you examine each region, be aware that everything is confined to a small space.
6. Gradually remove the child's clothes, if you can; look for asymmetry very carefully in the bodies of all children.
7. Develop a pattern appropriate to the patient's age.
   a. Whistling is a great distraction.
   b. Keep a small music box or toy readily available.
8. Using a cold stethoscope may result in a frightened and screaming child, so warm the stethoscope before bringing it into contact with the child.
9. Some children are less frightened if able to hold the examining equipment first.
10. Show the child the procedure by demonstrating on the parent first.

Equipment

1. Have equipment ready and in working order before beginning.
2. Equipment is similar to that used in the adult physical examination:

   Thermometer
   Oto-ophthalmoscope
   Flashlight
   Tongue depressor
   Cotton applicator stick

   Stethoscope
   Reflex hammer
   Tuning fork
   Disposable gloves
   Lubricant

3. Additional equipment:
   Sphygmomanometer cuffs in different sizes
   Denver Developmental Test materials (see Appendix B, p. 1075)
   Items for distraction—music box, toys

Vital Signs

Refer to Chapter 47, Pediatric Techniques—Measuring vital signs in children.

Technique	Findings

Standing Height, Head Circumference, and Chest Circumference

1. Use tape measure to obtain accurate head circumference. Measure widest part of head.

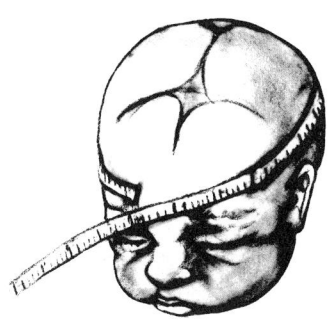

2. Record height and weight at each visit. Plot on growth chart.
3. Trends in growth are as important as the basic measurements.

Head and Chest Circumference

Age	Head Circumference		Chest Circumference	
Yr. Mo.	Inch	Cm.	Inch	Cm.
Birth	13.8	35.0	13.0	33.0
3	15.9	40.4	15.8	40.2
6	17.1	43.4	17.1	43.4
9	17.8	45.3	18.0	45.7
1–0	18.3	46.6	18.6	47.3
1–6	18.9	47.9	19.4	49.2
2–0	19.3	48.9	19.8	50.4
3–0	19.6	49.8	20.6	52.5
3–6	—	—	20.8	52.8
4–0	19.8	50.4	21.0	53.4
5–0	20.0	50.8	21.5	54.6

(From Studies at Harvard School of Public Health.)

General Appearance

1. Begin observations with the first contact with the patient, taking into account that there are at least 2 people to observe (child and parent).
2. The patient's interaction with the caretaker, whether it be the mother, a babysitter, an older sibling, or a friend of the family, is vital in the assessment of the child.

   As you observe for race, sex, general physical development, nutritional state, mental alertness, evidence of pain, restlessness, body position, clothes, apparent age, hygiene, and grooming, remember that many of these things are part of the parent's caretaking.

1. If the child is easily distracted or sleepy, it may be naptime.

2. Careful observation of the general state of the child will provide many clues about the child's relationship to the family and their response to the child.

Skin

Examine as you move through each body region. (Include hair as well as skin.)

Inspection

Inspection of the skin is the same as for the adult (see p. 20).

1. Observe for skin color, pigmentation, lesions, jaundice, cyanosis, scars, superficial vascularity, moisture, edema, color of mucous membranes, hair distribution.
2. Describe any variation in color, particularly in children with increased pigmentation. Absence of pigment, or vitiligo, in darker children can be noted.
3. Birthmarks of any type are recorded. (May change as child grows older.)
4. Bruises or unusual marks of any kind, wounds or insect bites, scratch marks, scars, etc., may have particular significance.

1. In young babies, the skin is soft, smooth, and velvety in texture.

2. Pigmentations vary in children, depending on race, and will change as the child gets older.

3. A suntan, freckles, small, light-brown patches or café-au-lait spots may occur.

4. Bruises are particularly important because of the possibility of child abuse.

Technique	**Findings**

5. Draw a picture of anything unusual like a scar, and measure the dimensions of the lesion when recording the findings.

6. To ascertain suspected jaundice, take the child to the window to get a true picture of the color of the skin. (A room with yellow walls and artificial lighting may create a wrong impression when jaundice is suspected.)

7. The skin of newborn infants will still be covered with vernix caseosa, the oily material that covers the fetus's body while in utero.

8. Postmature infants may have scaliness that persists for several weeks after birth, particularly around the feet. The color of the skin may change as the child gets a little older.

9. Note the presence of striae.

Palpation

1. Use the tips of the fingers to palpate—fingertips are more sensitive.

2. Feel the tension of the skin by pinching up a fold of skin—normal skin quickly falls back, but dehydrated skin remains in pinched position.

3. Feel the skin for texture, moisture, temperature, turgor, elasticity, masses, tenderness.

Nails

1. Observe for color, shape, irregularities in surface, and general nail care: cleanliness, evidence of biting, etc.

2. Palpate the skin around the fingernails for firmness. Palpate any part that appears inflamed.

Hair

1. Observe for color and distribution.
   a. Note according to the age of the child and race.
   b. Be aware that tufts of hair over the spine or sacral area may mark an underlying abnormality.

2. Note any change in pigmentation.

3. Palpate the hair for texture and thickness.

4. Examine to see if there are any patches where hair is missing on the head.

5. Separate thick hair on the head to get a good view of the scalp. Check for dandruff or scaliness in older children.

6. Check scalp for any signs of lice infestation.

7. Inspect in the axillae and over the pubis as well as the extremities for the presence and quantity of hair, to gauge the development and level of puberty.

---

5. If you have difficulty in describing something, use ordinary words rather than inaccurate technical terms.

6. Carotenemia, which causes the nose and palms of the hands to have a yellowish tinge, may lead the parents to suspect jaundice; however, carotenemia is due to eating an excessive amount of yellow vegetables (carrots, sweet potatoes, squash, etc.). In carotenemia, the sclerae are clear; this is not so in jaundice.

7. Swollen sebaceous glands over the nose and chin are frequently seen right after birth and are called *milia*.

8. The blotchy, pink patches over the eyelid, bridge of the nose, and the back of the neck may persist until the child is almost 2 years of age.

9. May indicate rapid weight gain.

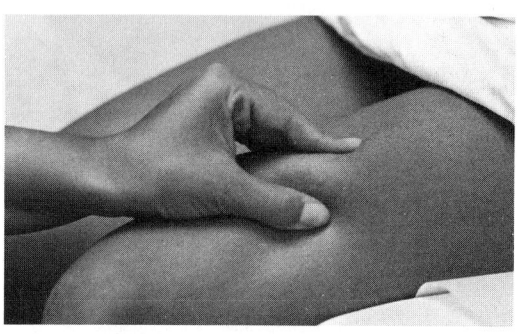

3. Skin that is rough and dry in texture may actually have a discrete rash that can be felt but not seen.

1. The nailbeds should be pink, the nails convex.

2. General care of the child is frequently reflected in good care of the nails.

1. *Newborn:* Normally varies from no hair to a thick bush.
   Infant: Consists of lanugo, a soft, downy covering frequently seen over the shoulders, back, arms, face, and sacral area, especially in dark-skinned children.
   Race: Variations in hairiness.

2. Remember, children frequently experiment with mother's hair dye or rinse.

3. Texture may be thick or thin, coarse or fine, straight or curly.

4. May denote underlying skin infection; however, some children pull their hair out; sometimes the hair is braided so tightly that it falls out.

5. Look carefully for broken hairs, for scaliness on the scalp or cradle cap in infants.

6. Nits (louse eggs) appear on the hair as little white dots. Lice may be seen on the scalp; they move quickly and may jump.

7. The child need not be totally undressed; a prepubertal child will usually be embarrassed if all of his or her clothes are removed.

(continued)

Technique	Findings

Head and Neck

1. Unless specifically requested to do otherwise, examine the eyes and ears at the very last, especially in the younger child.
2. Also, examine the throat toward the last, unless the child exhibits concern about the "throat stick." It is then best to examine the throat right away in order to "get it over with."
3. To avoid frightening the child when palpating the head, make a game out of it—ask, "Where's your nose?" "Where are your eyes?"

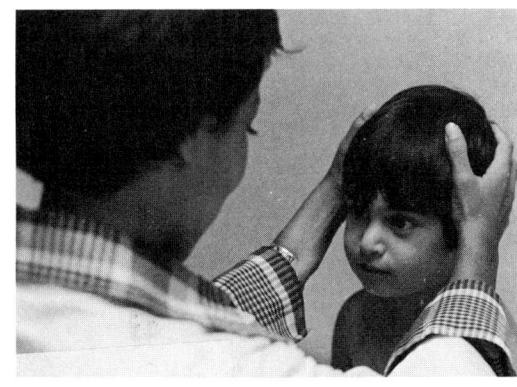

Inspection

1. Observe the face and skull for asymmetry, deformity, and abnormal or limited movements.

2. Closely observe facial expressions, blinking, etc., if the child is not crying. This may be one of your few moments to see the child when he is not crying.

    If you are examining a crying baby, watch particularly for asymmetry of the face.
3. Observe the movement of the head on the neck as the baby looks around. When turning an infant over, observe the head for control, position, and movement.
4. Since an infant's neck is often short and there are often several folds of skin under the chin, it is necessary to lift the chin a little to observe the skin completely—to see that it is clear and free of perspiration rash or irritation.

Palpation

1. Palpate the skull for the suture lines. Feel the face for any masses, noting size, consistency, surface, temperature, and tenderness.

2. Palpate the anterior and posterior fontanelles.

1. A baby's head may be asymmetrical because of pressure during pregnancy and delivery. The rounded head of the baby born by breech delivery contrasts with the long, pointed head of a baby who is a firstborn and whose head was moulded during a prolonged labor.
2. In a baby born by forceps delivery, there may be signs of weakness of the facial nerve caused by pressure of the forceps over the front of the ear where the facial nerve emerges. When the baby cries, the involved side will show weakness and downturning of the mouth.
3. There should be very little head lag beyond the age of 3 months.
4. In the back, the neck should be free of webbing or extra folds of skin extending from just beneath the ear toward the shoulder.

1. The suture lines of the skull may be felt to override as a result of the pressure applied when contractions occurred during labor. This is usually most marked between the frontal and the parietal bone where the coronal suture is located.
2. The fontanelles are soft and flat. Tense or bulging fontanelles may indicate hydrocephalus. Depressed fontanelles are often a sign of dehydration. The fontanelles usually close by 18 months.

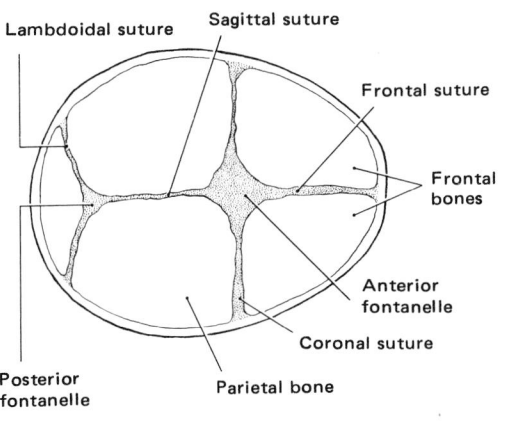

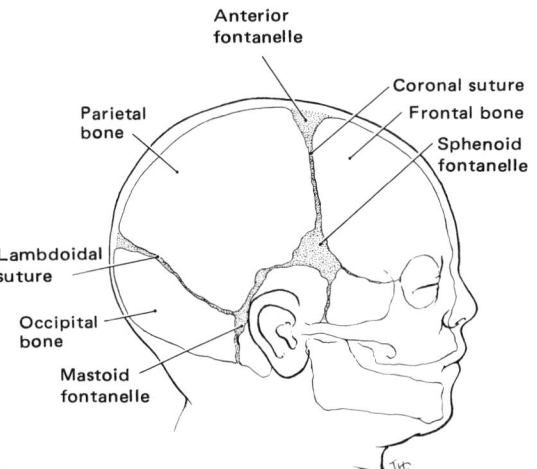

Technique	Findings

3. Palpate along the lambdoidal suture at the back of the head between the parietal bones and the occipital bone.

4. Palpate the neck for swollen lymph nodes, noting tenderness, mobility, location, and consistency.

4. Palpation of the lymph nodes may reveal slightly enlarged nodes in the anterior cervical chain secondary to sore throat.

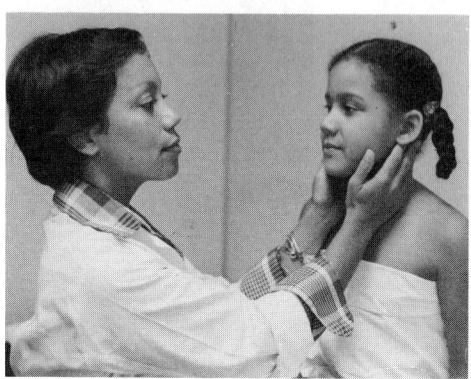

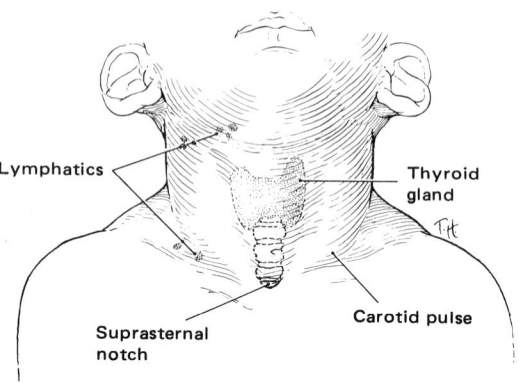

5. Note that there are other nodes, which are normally not palpable.

5. These include the pre- and postauricular, the posterior cervical (behind the sternomastoid), the submental and submandibular (under the jaw), and the occipital nodes (along the prominence of the occiput).

6. Feel the pulses in the neck for location, strength, and equality.
7. Check the thyroid for enlargement, position, texture, and tenderness.
8. Locate the trachea in the suprasternal notch for position in the center of the neck.

Percussion

1. Percussion of the face may elicit tenderness over the sinuses.

1. Tenderness may be due to a tooth cavity.

2. Percuss over the head and neck directly with the fingertips, usually the middle finger of the right hand.

2. Gentle tapping over the skull elicits a typical noise when the sutures are open and a different sound when the sutures are closed.

3. Percuss over the forehead for tenderness in the sinuses and across the zygoma, or cheekbone.

3. This is to determine underlying tenderness in the maxillary sinus.

Auscultation

Auscultate the skull and carotid arteries in the neck.

To determine presence of bruits.

Eyes and Vision

Equipment

Ophthalmoscope and penlight. Be sure batteries are new and lights are bright.

Inspection

(Similar to adult examination; p. 21)

1. Pay particular attention to the lacrimal duct.

1. Discharge from the eyes along the lower lid or from the lacrimal duct can occur as a result of infection or reaction to silver nitrate administered to the neonate.

2. Note the distance between the eyes and the distribution of the eyebrows.

2. Hypertelorism denotes a wider area between the eyes than normal. Excessively long and full eyebrows that meet in the midline and extra-long eyelashes may signify a developmental abnormality.

3. Test the eyes for light perception.

3. It is difficult to prevent children from blinking their eyes or closing them when testing light response.

Palpation

If the child is old enough, have him squeeze his eyes tightly (not possible in younger children).

Weakness of the muscles around the eyes is difficult to demonstrate in the young child. Muscle strength or weakness can be evaluated when the child cries.

(continued)

Technique	Findings

Fundoscopic Examination

1. Check to see that the child's eyes move in conjugate fashion.

   Ask the mother if she has noticed any signs of squinting, especially when the child is tired.

2. This is a difficult examination to conduct since children tend to watch the light and stare directly at you, which constricts their pupils. If the child cannot cooperate, it may be necessary to dilate the pupil to see the fundus.

3. Start your examination at about ⅓ meter (1 foot) from the patient. Look for the red reflex, which should be readily observable.

4. Look for any opacities and then slowly approach the patient, turning the ophthalmoscopic dial to the smaller plus (+) numbers. Start originally at +8 to +10.

   (Wearing glasses or contact lenses may make a difference in the type of lens you use in the ophthalmoscope.)

5. To help guide your gaze, put your hand on top of the child's head, with your thumb at the corner of the eye at the outer edge. If you lose the fundus, you can return to your thumb and get your bearings by directing your gaze medial to the tip of your thumbnail.

1. Loss of vision can occur if the eyes are not working together properly. Squinting can indicate vision problems.

2. A picture can be pinned to the wall opposite the child, who is then instructed to look at the picture during the examination. If the child is examined while lying down, a picture can be placed on the ceiling.

4. The red reflex is diminished if there is something obstructing your view. A cataract or an opacity in the retina can cause this, as would a tumor filling the posterior chamber. If there is any paleness in the red reflex or difficulty in identifying it, a consultation should be sought immediately.

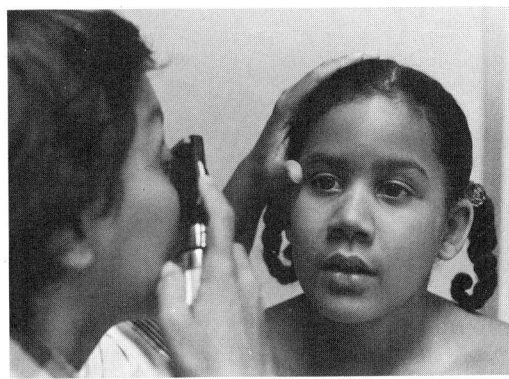

Ears and Hearing

Equipment

Tuning fork and otoscope
Small speculum for child's ear

Fresh batteries to ensure a bright light

Inspection

1. When examining the external ear, the auricle, or the pinna, be sure to note the position of the ear.

   The top of the ear should cross an imaginary line drawn between the edge of the eye and the back of the occiput. If the ear is positioned more obliquely or is low-set, some underlying abnormality, particularly of the genitourinary system, may be present.

2. If you cannot get the child to cooperate by offering an explanation or by playing a game, the child will have to be restrained.

   a. The child can be seated on the parent's knee with the child's legs wedged between the parent's knees and the head held firmly with one hand while the baby's hands are controlled with the other hand.

   b. An older child may be held in a supine position, with the parent holding the child's arms above the head and controlling the head.

   c. If the child is very restless and apprehensive, examine the child from the top while the parent leans over the child's body, holds the arms down with her elbows, and at the same time grasps the child's head with her hands.

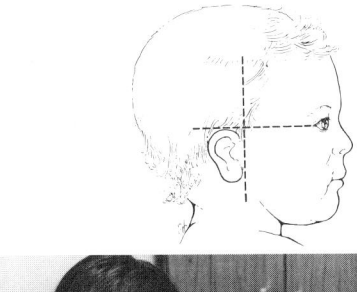

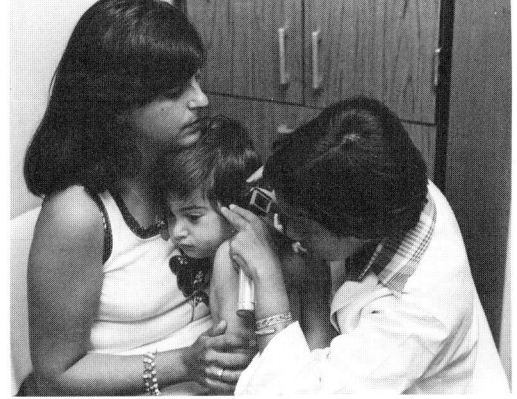

If the child is in a supine position, be sure to remove the shoes, because some children will kick when frightened.

Technique	**Findings**

Inspection with Otoscope

1. Hold the otoscope gently with the handle between the thumb and forefinger. This will enable you to control the head of the otoscope while keeping your hand steady on the child's head.

1. Small children will jerk about, so be careful not to push the speculum into the eardrum.

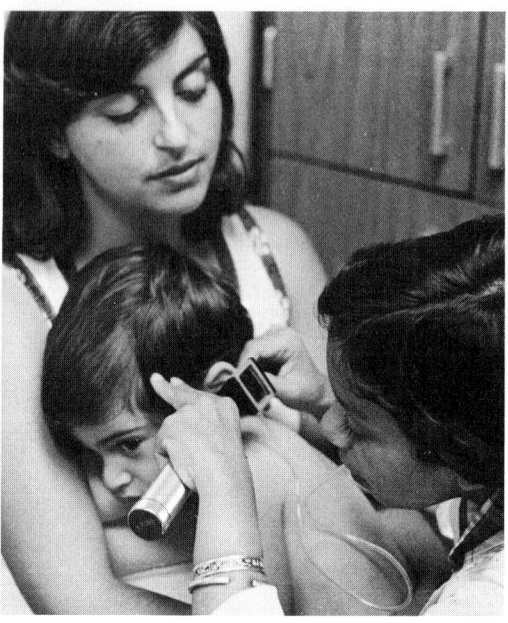

2. With your free hand, pull the pinna back and slightly upward to straighten the canal. Examine the canal.
3. Inspect the eardrum and test for mobility by means of the pneumatoscope (the tube attachment of the otoscope).
   a. Attach one end of the tube to the otoscope and place the other end in your mouth.
   b. Blow gently through the tube.
      By blowing through plastic tubing it is possible to see the normal eardrum move back and forth. If the eardrum does not move, this may be indicative of infection behind the drum (serous otitis media).
   c. This method is preferred to the squeeze bulb because it allows for greater control of the force with which the air is introduced into the ear.

2. Cerumen or wax may interfere with your view of the eardrum.
3. The normal eardrum moves slightly when a soft breath is blown into the ear canal.

Palpation

Palpate behind the ear over the mastoid process.

Tenderness behind the ear denotes infection.
Sometimes a lymph node can be felt in this area.

Mechanical

1. Most children will be able to respond to a test of gross hearing.

1. A small bell, such as the kind found in the Denver kit, can be used to determine hearing ability by noting if the child stops moving when the bell is rung and turns his head toward the sound.

2. More specific tests using an electric screening device are used prior to school age.

Nose and Sinuses

Equipment

Nasoscope, small speculum

Inspection

1. Observe for general deformity.
2. With nasoscope, examine nasal septum, mucous membranes and turbinates, and for discharge and nasal obstruction (see Adult Physical Examination, p. 24).

2. Dry mucous membranes may bleed and cause clots of blood to form in the nares. Scratches may also occur if child picks at nose or scratches when itching occurs.

(continued)

Technique	Findings

3. Check for presence of any foreign body. Always remember that any child who has a "strange" odor may have a foreign body in the nose or ear. (In a female child, do not forget the vagina.)

3. A foreign body in the nose will cause a foul odor, purulent discharge, and may possibly cause bleeding.

Palpation

Palpate the sinuses, remembering the order of development.

Sinuses develop in a set order; the ethmoid and maxillary sinuses are present at birth; the frontal sinus develops at around 7 years of age, and the sphenoid after puberty.

Mouth and Throat

Equipment

Penlight, Tongue Depressor

1. Shining the light into the mouth or around the lips and teeth is not a threatening gesture.
2. However, the tongue blade, which is used to press against the inside of the cheek to allow for examination of the mucous membranes and which is also used to push the tongue out of the way, is a threatening instrument.
3. When the tongue depressor is placed on the tongue, it can have the unpleasant effect of making the child gag.
4. To avoid this unpleasant occurrence, encourage the child to stick out his tongue, breathe deeply, and say "ah." This may allow for easy visualization of the palate and uvula, without need for the "stick."

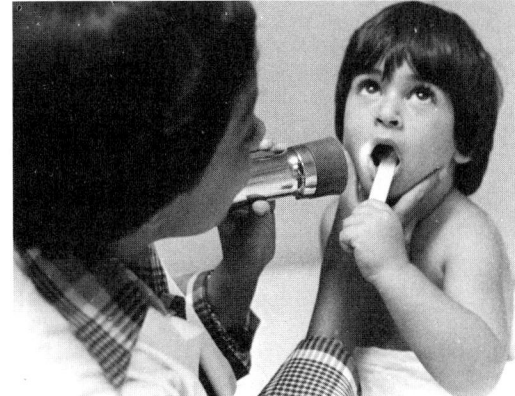

5. If these steps are not feasible, then the child may need to be restrained. If such is the case, examining the throat should be left to last, so as not to frighten the child.

A child may also be allowed to place the tongue blade directly on his own tongue while you guide him with your hand.

Inspection

1. Observe the lips, noting the color. (Remember that cyanosis is difficult to detect in a black child.)

1. *Infants:* There may be a protuberance on the upper lip, the so-called "sucking blister."
   Children: May have dry lips and redness around the lips due to an allergy or to some such activity as blowing bubble gum.

2. Count the teeth (see page 1062) and note any extra or missing teeth, and any evidence of caries, staining, tartar, and malocclusion.
3. Check the gums for swelling and signs of easy bleeding. Also note mouth odor.
4. Check the tongue for movement, color, and the presence of taste buds on the surface. Check to see that the frenulum under the tongue is of the proper length.

4. If the frenulum is too short, the child may be tongue-tied (meaning that the baby cannot advance the tip of the tongue beyond the lips), although this is not thought to interfere with sucking or speech.

5. As the gag reflex is elicited, note how the palate moves upward and the uvula springs into view.
6. Examine the roof of the mouth.

5. It should be midline and single, although occasionally it will be divided or bifid.
6. The roof of the mouth at the junction of the hard and soft palate will frequently reveal whitish lesions, or Epstein's pearls, which persist through infancy.

7. Inspect the height of the arch of the palate.

7. With experience, an unusually high arch is easily recognizable.

8. Note the tonsils on each side of the uvula and immediately posterior to it for position, surface, size, equality, and color.
9. As the baby cries, note the odor of the breath and any hoarseness of the voice; note difficulty on inspiration, as in croup, or wheezing on expiration.

8. Any coating with pus or ulcers or a pocket or cryptic appearance should be recorded.
9. These signs may indicate throat and chest disturbances.

Palpation

1. Palpate the lips and cheeks manually using a finger cot or glove.
2. Note any evidence of swelling.

1. By comparing one side with the other, differences due to abnormality can be detected.

Technique	Findings

Time of eruption of deciduous teeth

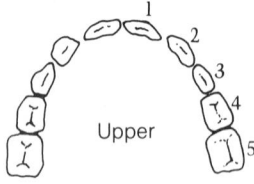

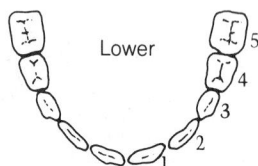

		(Upper)	(Lower)
1	Central incisor	8–12 mos.	5–9 mos.
2	Lateral incisor	8–12 mos.	12–18 mos.
3	Cuspid		18–24 mos.
4	First molar		12–18 mos.
5	Second molar		24–30 mos.

Time of eruption of permanent teeth

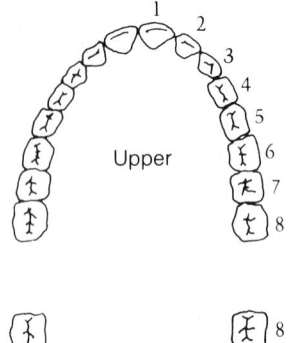

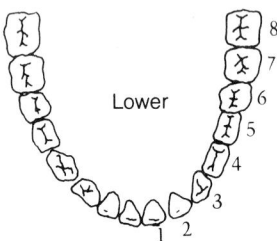

		(Upper)	(Lower)
1	Central incisor	6–7 yr.	7–8 yr.
2	Lateral incisor	7–8 yr.	8–9 yr.
3	Cuspid	9–10 yr.	11–12 yr.
4	First bicuspid	10–11 yr.	10–11 yr.
5	Second bicuspid	11–12 yr.	10–12 yr.
6	First molar	6–7 yr.	6–7 yr.
7	Second molar	11–13 yr.	12–13 yr.
8	Third molar	17 yr.	17–18 yr.

Breast and Thorax

1. Sometimes young children object to having their clothes removed.
2. The following approaches may overcome this problem:
   a. Distract the child by having him listen to a few heartbeats.
   b. Have the parent (while the child is on his or her knee) remove the underclothing while you stand by.
   c. For an older child entering puberty, provide an examining sheet, but stay in the room while the child puts on the gown, provided he or she is not embarrassed by your presence. During such preparation, you are able to make a superficial appraisal of the chest.

Breast

1. Check to see if there are any small extra nipples present.

2. In the newborn infant, the nipples appear a little darker than normal, and breast tissue underneath may form a small knot with occasional leakage of milk.
3. In the older child, a lump found under the nipple in either male or female may cause some concern for cancer.
4. Occasionally, the breasts begin to develop earlier than normal, at around 5 or 6 years.

1. These would appear along a line extending from the anterior axillary line through the normal nipple down toward the symphysis pubis.
2. This leakage is a secondary effect of the hormone level in the mother; instruct the mother not to try to express the milk, because of the danger of infection.
3. Such lumps are usually secondary to hormone stimulation and occur toward puberty.
4. This should be a reason for referral to a physician.

Thorax

Inspection

1. Observe the entire thorax as the child breathes; note symmetry and equal expansion of both sides as the lungs inflate.

1. In babies and young children (especially an infant lying on the parent's knee), diaphragm excursion is more marked than intercostal expansion. Thus the abdomen goes up and down more than the chest expands.

(continued)

Technique	Findings

2. Confirm the respiratory rate as you observe the child with his shirt off.

Percussion

Percussion of the child's chest is difficult. Because the underlying structures are crowded, not too much is elicited.
The heart edge is difficult to outline, and percussing the chest may be frightening to the child.

Very light percussion is necessary; a hyperresonant note may be elicited over air, particularly of a stomach bubble that projects up into the left side of the chest.

Palpation

1. Use warmed hands as you palpate the shape and angle of the sternum. Note if there is any sinking in of the sternum.

2. Palpate the costochondral junctions for tenderness and enlargement.
3. As you palpate, hoarse sounds (as in bronchitis) may be felt through your hands.
4. Vocal fremitus is difficult to elicit in the smaller child since it is difficult to have him make repetitive sounds on command.

1. The shape of the sternum may vary, although there may be a sinking in of the sternum (funnel sternum) that may cause subsequent trouble because of pressure on underlying structures. This should be referred to the pediatrician.
2. May suggest an underlying inflammatory response.

3. Normal inspiration and expiration do not give a sensation under the fingers, except for the expansion of the chest.
4. In the older child, it is worth trying, in order to obtain transmission of sound through the lung tissue.

Auscultation

The difficulty with examining a child is that everything sounds muddled and mixed. The examiner has to sort out breathing that is rapid from a heart rate that is also rapid, and must also differentiate between inspiration and expiration and the 1st and 2nd heart sounds.

1. Try to examine a baby before he begins crying.
2. Warm the stethoscope before using by rubbing it between your hands.
3. Be aware that breathing is louder in younger children with slightly increased length of inspiration, almost to the point of bronchovesicular breathing in the adult.
4. Crackles (discontinuous; interrupted, explosive sounds) may be heard more easily in children.

1. Note, however, that crying increases lung expansion.
2. A cold stethoscope will startle the child.

3. Bronchial breathing with equal inspiration and expiration is very loud and easy to hear if the patient has pneumonia.

4. Added coarse-quality sounds in the chest are commonly associated with mucus in the trachea or even in the back of the nose.

Heart

Inspection

In thin children, the apical beat or the point of maximal impulse (PMI) can easily be seen, particularly if you look obliquely across the chest wall.

As in all areas of the pediatric examination, measurement and documentation of the distance from the midline and the exact rib space are worth noting.

Palpation

The apical beat may be felt in the 6th intercostal space about 5 cm. (2 inches) from the midline in the school-aged child. It is more difficult to feel in the baby, particularly a plump child, and would not be so far out towards the anterior axillary line.

The apical beat will be deviated to the left with cardiac enlargement or a collapsed lung on that side.
The apical pulse could be pushed toward the right by a tumor or a collapsed lung on the right. Pneumothorax under tension will push the heart away from the side of the increased pressure.

Auscultation

1. Identify the 1st heart sound (S_1) (occurs during systole).
   a. Locate the apical beat (closing of the mitral valve) by placing the stethoscope over the maximum impulse area, concentrating on the first heart sound. (As the ventricle on the left contracts, pushing the blood up into the aorta, the sound of the mitral valve closing is heard.)
   b. That sound can be identified by placing the thumb on the carotid pulse of the neck, which will coincide very closely with the heart sounds.

1. Consists of the "lub" portion of the "lub-dub" heart sound.

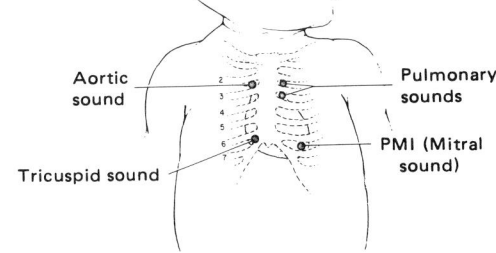

2. Identify the 2nd heart sound (S_2).
   a. Move the stethoscope up toward the sternum and to the left.
   b. At the base of the heart, both over the aortic and pulmonic areas, S_2 is louder than S_1.

2. Represents the "dub" portion of the "lub-dub" heart sound.

   b. In a child, S_2 can be heard as 2 heart sounds, since the 2 valves in the aorta and pulmonary vessels do not close at quite the same time. The "dub-dub" will disappear if you can get the child to cooperate and breathe deeply.

Technique	Findings

3. Move the stethoscope in small jumps from the apical area medially towards the sternum. Go up to the left side of the sternum, listening at each interspace next to the sternum.

3. This represents the area of maximum intensity of sound of the pulmonary vessels.

4. Move next to the patient's right second intercostal space—again next to the sternum.

4. It is at this area that you will hear the aortic sound best.

5. Descend down the right side of the sternum to the lower end where you will hear best the tricuspid valve from the right of the heart.

6. Listen to only 1 sound; concentrate on that to the exclusion of all others. Can you identify this sound? Is it clear? Compare it with your own heart sound or that of the parent.

6. The child will enjoy this comparison if he is allowed to listen.

7. If there is any question of a heart murmur or added sounds, refer to the physician.

8. As you listen to the heart sounds, you are also listening to the rhythm to confirm your findings on pulse.
   a. If he breathes in and out deeply, the sinus arrhythmia will be obvious.
   b. If a child holds his breath, the sinus arrhythmia will disappear.

8. The typical rhythm of a child is called *sinus arrhythmia*. As the heart speeds up, the child is breathing in; the heart slows down on expiration.

9. Be sure to count a rapid heart that is heard even when the child is quiet.

9. This may be indicative of a tachycardia that requires further investigation.

10. In the infant, heart sounds are just a series of taps; they occur so fast that it is impossible to make out which sound is the 1st heart sound.

10. In the infant, the 1st and 2nd heart sounds are equal in intensity.

Abdomen

1. For examination of the abdomen, the child should be lying down, relaxed, and not crying. Placing a small child, particularly around the age of 1–3 years, on a high table on cold paper can be very frightening; as a result, the abdomen will not be relaxed.
2. Babies up to about 1 year do not seem to be perturbed and will often lie down and play very nicely as long as they can see the parent, who should be stationed at the head of the child while you examine the abdomen.
3. Having the child lie across the parent's knees with the legs dangling on one side and the head cradled in his or her arms, will enable you to feel the abdomen quite well.
   a. You may find that with the baby's head in the parent's left arm, you can use your left hand to examine the baby's abdomen on the right, feeling up under the right costal margin and into the right hypochondrium.
   b. You may need to turn the baby around and use your right hand to examine the left side of the child's abdomen.
4. Do not discard the idea of using the floor.
   a. If the child is young, ask the parent if he or she minds putting the child on the floor on a sheet.
   b. The toddler will usually enjoy crawling around the floor and has probably been doing so while the history was being taken.

Inspection

1. Observe the abdomen for contour and any markings both while the child is standing and when he is lying down.

   As you inspect, you may see some abdominal movement with respiration. (Remember that the diaphragm, as it goes up and down, will move the contents of the abdomen.)

1. Sometimes superficial veins are seen on the abdomen, particularly in a very blond infant. Striae are often noticed on the flank following rapid loss or gain of weight.

2. Check for early signs of puberty as evidenced by pubic hair over the symphysis pubis.

2. Early pubic hair in younger children (8–10 years) may appear long and silky. This will ultimately become curly toward the onset of puberty.

3. Carefully inspect the umbilicus for cleanliness and the presence of any scar tissue.

3. A deep umbilicus may be difficult to keep clean.

   Immediately after the cord has dropped off, scar tissue or a granuloma may occur.

Auscultation

1. Since percussion and palpation will stimulate the small bowel and increase bowel sounds, auscultation should precede these 2 techniques.

1. Bowel sounds are heard as tinkling, irregular sounds that indicate that fluid is moving from one section of the bowel to the next.

2. To obtain the child's cooperation, you can conduct a running commentary as you listen, saying such things as, ''I can hear the Cheerios in there.''

2. In a quiet baby who has just eaten, not many bowel sounds will be heard. In a hungry child, noisy bowel sounds can be heard, even without a stethoscope.

Percussion

1. On the right side, percuss for the liver. Confirm on palpation.

1. Liver dullness can frequently be outlined.

2. Percuss over the left upper quadrant.

2. Percussion over a gas-filled bowel or stomach gives a high-pitched, hollow sound.

(continued)

Technique	Findings

3. Percuss the lower abdomen, particularly above the symphysis pubis.

3. Above the symphysis pubis, a filled bladder can produce a confusing sound, as does a pregnant uterus. (A mass in the abdomen of a girl over 10 years of age may be a fetus.)

Palpation

1. Divide the abdomen into imaginary quadrants, palpating each with the fingertips.
2. In the right upper quadrant, palpate for the liver edge.
   a. Although the liver is easily palpable in most children, you may have to press quite firmly.
   b. The liver is frequently felt about 1 cm. (⅜ inch) below the right costal margin and in some instances as low as 2 cm. (¾ inch). This is a common finding in the newborn and through the early school-age years.

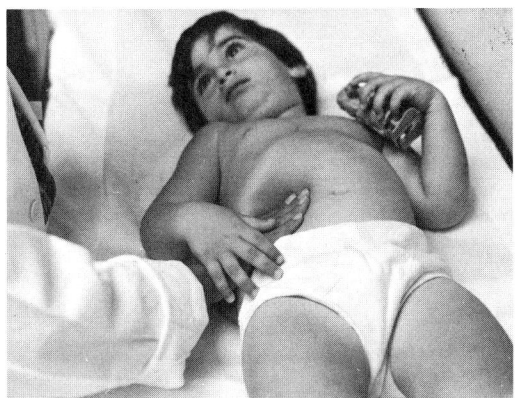

3. In the left upper quadrant, palpate for the spleen. Less resistance is encountered as you feel up under the left costal margin.
4. In the upper quadrants also try to palpate for the kidneys. Deep palpation for both kidneys should routinely be a part of the examination to make sure there is no enlargement of the kidney. Normally, the kidney is not palpable.

5. In the iliac fossa or the left lower quadrant, palpate for the descending bowel.

6. Palpate on the right lower quadrant (RLQ) where the appendix is located.

7. If the child has pain in any area or has pointed to the umbilicus when asked to show where the pain is, avoid the area demonstrated and leave it until last.
8. Palpate around the umbilicus for any masses that may indicate a hernia, especially in black children.
   As you press over the protruding hernia you can feel the sensation of gurgling under your fingers as the bowel returns to the abdomen.

3. Only the tip of the spleen can be felt in the upper outer left quadrant, in the early months of life and in very thin children of preschool age.
4. Kidney palpation is difficult, but during the newborn period, the lower pole of the right kidney can frequently be felt and sometimes the left as well. (This applies to the period immediately following delivery, when the infant's abdomen is relaxed and the bowel is not distended.)
5. The descending colon can be felt, particularly if filled with firm stool. It may be slightly tender, but it should not cause severe pain on gentle palpation.
6. In the RLQ, usually the only sensation is that of gas-filled bowel. Tenderness in this area could be related to an inflamed appendix.
7. If the painful area is palpated first, the child may tense up when the other areas of the abdomen are examined.

8. Most of these hernias heal naturally by the age of 6 years.
   A hernia above the umbilicus can be revealed by asking the child to lift his head from the table. (Widening of the muscles above the umbilicus is called *diastasis recti*.)

Rectum and Anus

1. Rectal examinations are rarely necessary in infants and young children.
2. If the child will be examined by a physician who will examine the rectum, it is not necessary to duplicate this part of the examination.
3. Rectal examinations are embarrassing and uncomfortable for most children. Explain the procedure before performing the examination.
4. Positioning for a rectal examination:
   a. Infants can be placed on their abdomens, sides, or backs with the legs raised to the chest.
   b. Young children and teenagers can be positioned on their sides.

Inspection

1. When examining a baby or toddler, place the child on a flat surface so that the weight is evenly distributed on the front of the pelvis. As the baby moves about on his abdomen, observe the entire back, the lower back, the upper thigh, and the tightening of the buttocks.

2. Notice particularly the lower part of the back for hairiness.

1. If one buttock is larger than the other, you will see that side projected above the other. Weakness of one side will be obvious as the baby moves around, although a child in the early stages of crawling will normally tend to use one knee as a predominant leader, dragging the other behind.
2. This may indicate an underlying abnormality of the vertebrae.

Technique	Findings
3. As the child moves away, part the buttocks and look at the cleft between them.	3. A pilonidal dimple or sinus may be seen over the lip of the coccyx at the superior end of the internatal cleft. This is a common finding, but parents should be told about it for cleaning purposes.
4. Pay careful attention to the outer appearance of the anus and the perineal body, the underside of the scrotum in the male, and the labia majora in the female. (Male genitalia, below, and pp. 1067–1068) (Female genitalia, pp. 1068–1069)	4. The anus is inspected for blood, fissures, or splitting in the external tissue, redness, swelling, or pads of extra flesh. On occasion, small white pinworms may be seen adhering to the anal skin.

Palpation

1. Take into consideration the child's age and feelings; ask the mother to assist if need be.	
2. Start by parting the buttocks with the left hand and introducing a well-lubricated finger (with finger cot) into the anus.	2. When an infant is being examined, the small finger should be used.
3. Gently apply pressure on the anal sphincter to allow the muscles to relax and the fingertip to slide into the rectum.	3. Apply pressure with pulp of the finger rather than jab at the anus with the fingertip.
4. Gently palpate the inner ring, feeling for areas of thickening and tenderness and simultaneously judging the sphincter tone.	4. As the perianal area is pressed upon from the inside, tenderness will be elicited if a deep fissure exists or if an infection has occurred around a fissure.
5. If the rectum is full of feces, it will be impossible to feel any other mass.	5. In the young child, particularly the infant, dilatation provided by the finger will result in a bowel movement. In the older child, a suppository or even an enema may be required.
6. Palpate the walls of the rectum.	6. Within the rectum, the mucosal walls should be smooth, and deep palpation should elicit mild tenderness and no acute pain.
7. As the finger reaches up from the rectum towards the right iliac fossa, place your other hand over the right iliac fossa, trying in effect to roll the appendix between your hands.	7. With an acutely inflamed appendix, this will elicit a great deal of pain and thus constitutes a significant finding.
8. In the male, gently turn your finger through 180 degrees and feel the posterior surface of the prostate. Note size, consistency, tenderness, and contour.	
9. In the female, perform a bimanual examination and palpate the cervix.	

Male Genitalia

1. This part of the examination requires a direct, matter-of-fact approach. Acknowledge that it is normal to feel embarrassed during an examination of the genitals. Explain what you are looking for as you proceed through the examination with a teenager.
2. Reassure the child after the examination that his genitals are normal. This decreases anxiety.

Scrotum and Testes

Inspection

1. Before touching the child, determine by observation of the testes whether they are in the scrotum.	1. Retraction of the testes into the abdomen occurs very frequently in young children; the development of the scrotum depends on the presence of the testes.
2. Observe the skin over the scrotum for color and surface appearance, noting the presence of wrinkles, or rugae.	2. The skin over the scrotum varies in color, being a darker brown to black in the more pigmented races and reddish in the fair-skinned. The wrinkles, or rugae, are more developed as the child grows older.

Palpation

1. Check the scrotum wall for swelling or sensitivity. Gently feel the testes, palpating across the upper pole and feeling for the epididymis. (Remember the scrotum is extremely sensitive to pressure.)	1. The epididymis is a ridge of soft, bumpy tissue extending from the superior pole and running down and behind the testis.
2. Estimate the size of the testes and identify the spermatic cord, tracing it from the testis up toward the groin.	2. The spermatic cord, with the vas deferens, feels firm and is accompanied by softer nerves, arteries, veins, and a few muscle fibers.
3. Make a special effort to locate the testis in a young child whose testes may be retracted into the abdomen via a hyperactive cremasteric reflex.	3. The presence of the testes in the scrotum is vital in the preschool or early school-age child. Nondescent of the testes requires that the child be referred to a physician.

(continued)

Technique	Findings

a. If the testes cannot be felt in the scrotum, gently run the skin of the upper scrotum between your fingers, moving superiorly and approaching the external inguinal ring.

b. Try to milk the testis down towards the scrotum from above with your hand.

c. If this fails, have the child sit cross-legged to abolish the reflex of the cremaster muscle.

4. When examining a boy in the early stages of puberty, it is important to note the size of the testis as well as the greater number of rugae on the scrotum and the appearance of pubic hair around the penis.

During this period the testis is about 1.5–2 cm. (½–¾ inch) in length.

In the quiescent period prior to puberty, the male genitalia remain fairly infantile.

4. In early puberty, the testes start to grow. Onset of puberty varies, occurring in some boys by age 10 and in others as late as age 14. In most teenagers, the findings are similar to those in adults.

Penis

1. Evaluate the penis on all sides by lifting up the shaft.

2. If the child is not circumcised, partially retract the foreskin to observe the glans and meatus.

3. Observe the position of the meatus and evert the lips of the meatus to reveal an adequate orifice.

4. In the older child, inspect the penis for ulcers, sores, or discharge from the meatus.

1. The shaft of the penis contains the urethra on the under, or ventral surface and is easily palpable.

2. The foreskin may adhere to the glans for the first few years of life. It is not necessary for the parent to "stretch" the foreskin by retraction.

Whitish discharge around the glans under the foreskin is normal and not a sign of infection. The foreskin should completely encircle the glans.

3. The meatus may be positioned off center. Refer the child to a physician if the meatus is located on the dorsal or ventral surface of the shaft.

4. Consider sexually transmitted diseases in the older child and teenager.

Inguinal Area

1. Palpate for hernia over the external inguinal ring. Have the child cough to enhance your observation.

1. Having the child stand either with the parent holding him or placing him against his or her knee will help you in locating a hernia in the inguinal area.

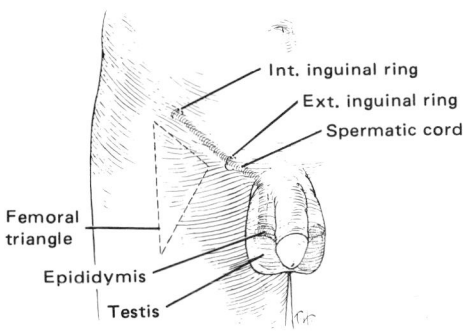

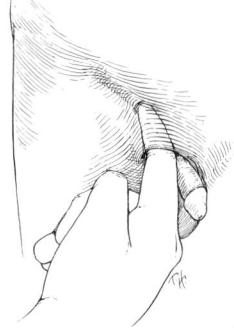

2. An increased cough reflex or swelling in the area should be checked by carefully placing the finger on the scrotal skin and invaginating the skin over your fingers toward the external ring. You are trying to follow the course of a hernia that would descend into the scrotum while you feel the external ring from below. A hernia in the inguinal region presents as a bulge that can be either seen or felt from below by placing the finger in the scrotum pointing up toward the external inguinal ring.

3. Also palpate for the inguinal lymph nodes.

3. The inguinal lymph nodes in an infant are palpable as small and "shotty." Anything more than this should alert you to possible infection, since the perianal area drains into the superficial inguinal lymph nodes. Thus, any signs of diaper rash will explain enlargement of the lymph nodes, which should be noted and reported.

Femoral Area

Palpate the femoral triangle carefully for a hernia and for lymph nodes.

In the femoral area, a swelling that can be reduced with a gurgling sound is an unusual finding.

Technique	Findings

Auscultation

If you are trying to reduce a mass, listen over the scrotum to see if there is a gurgling sound.

This will locate the bowel for you and confirm the presence of a hernia.

Transillumination

1. To locate the testis, darken the room and shine a bright light from behind the scrotum. In a normal child, the testis will stand out as the darker area.
2. Transilluminate any suspicious mass to help locate a hernia.

1. Testes that are swollen by fluid (hydrocele) will transilluminate. Fluid around the testes or cord must be differentiated from a hernia.
2. Any mass in this area must be reported to a physician immediately.

Female Genitalia

1. If the child will be examined by a physician who will examine the genitalia, it is not necessary to duplicate this part of the examination.
2. Place the infant or toddler on the table or on the parent's knee while he or she holds the knees in an abducted and flexed position.
3. A preschool child can be allowed to lean over her parent's knee. However, remember that the structures are being visualized upside down.
4. The older child or teenager should be draped as an adult would and should be placed in a lithotomy position with the aid of stirrups.

Equipment

Disposable gloves, speculum, light source

1. Carefully inspect the perineal area for cleanliness, inflammation, and abnormality.
2. Fold back the labia majora and note the labia minora.

3. Part the labia and note the clitoris and the meatus at the anterior end. (The clitoris is a hook-like structure that extends over the opening of the urethral meatus.)

    The meatus appears as a slit that is slightly darker in color against the pink of the mucosa about 2 cm. (¾ inch) posterior to the clitoris.
4. Having parted the labia, check for any signs of inflammation, discharge, tenderness, or infection. Include the urethral meatus, periurethral glands, the vagina, and the greater vestibular glands (Bartholin's). (Tenderness of these glands is unusual in young children, but may occur in adolescents.)

1. This includes the mons pubis, clitoris, labia, urethra, and perineal body.
2. The labia minora are seen as 2 slender folds of tissue inside the labia majora.
3. In some instances, adhesions of the labia minora occur because of the lack of natural hormones. The opening of the vagina is obscured by the two lateral flaps, which stick together, sometimes to the degree that urination is difficult because the urethral meatus is covered. This should be referred to a physician.
4. Inflammation and pus-like discharge from the urethra may be noted on palpation. The periurethral glands may be tender because of infection—possibly due to gonococci. If discharge is collected from the vagina, it should be cultured.

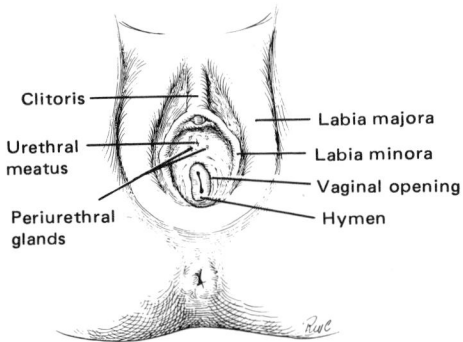

5. If the mother of a newborn infant has noted a bloody discharge from the infant's vagina during the first few days of life, reassure her that this is not an uncommon occurrence; the discharge will disappear, as will any swelling of the labia majora and clitoris and any enlargement of the infant's breasts.
6. Note the vaginal opening, which may vary in size because of the presence of a thin membrane, the hymen.

    The hymen varies in appearance according to the age of the child.

5. Hormone stimulation from the mother's body accounts for this occurrence. The discharge usually stops once the hormones are excreted. The bloody appearance on the diaper may be confused with the presence of urates, which are also orange-red and which appear quite normally in the urine.
6. The lack of an opening into the vagina may result in the retention of menstrual fluid when the child reaches puberty. In the sexually active adolescent, vestigial remains of the hymen may appear as small particles (caruncles) at the fringe of the vagina.

(continued)

Technique	Findings

7. In the young child, it is usually unnecessary to examine inside the vagina. Should you suspect the presence of a foreign body, insert a finger into the rectum and milk anteriorly to allow you to feel the lower part of the cervix and any firm foreign body within the vagina.

8. In an older child, the little finger can be inserted gently into the vagina and anterior pressure applied.

9. Turn the finger gradually, sweeping down the right side of the vagina, back over the rectum, and up on the left side of the vagina. Turn your finger, arm, and wrist so that undue pressure is not made on the child's tissues.

10. Once the genitalia are examined, lower the child's legs somewhat so that the femoral and inguinal areas can be palpated the same way as in the male.

7. A foreign body may be suspected if there is vaginal discharge (of any quantity) that is blood-tinged or has an odor. In the older child, vaginal discharge of this type may be due to gonorrhea.

8. Anterior pressure and milking downwards palpates the urethra towards the meatus. The periurethral glands are located on each side of the urethra.

10. Enlargement of the lymph nodes in the presence of a hernia in the femoral triangle may be found. Similarly, enlargement of the inguinal nodes may occur.

Musculoskeletal System

1. Evaluation of the musculoskeletal system can be done both in an informal manner while watching the child at rest and at play and in a formal manner as specific findings are methodically checked.
2. In the newborn, observe the position of the extremities during sleep and the quality of movement when the infant is awake.
3. Various aspects of size, shape, and movement are evaluated as the baby is observed pushing up on his arms and turning his head towards his mother.
4. The infant in the early stages of walking offers many opportunities for evaluation of muscle strength and movement.

   At the same time, rapport with the mother can be reinforced by your admiring the baby's ability and by inquiring if she is concerned about the manner in which the baby is walking.
5. A more mobile child can be evaluated as you watch him play and explore the room.
6. Having the older child reach for crayons, run after a ball, or walk around the room enables you to evaluate the musculoskeletal system and the child's sense of balance.

Upper Extremities

1. In the infant, evaluate the status of the clavicles when examining the skull and neck.

2. Carefully examine the hands to note shape of the hand, shape and length of the fingers, changes in the nails, and the presence of creases on the palms.

1. During a difficult delivery, the clavicle that has been exposed to traction may snap. A lump can be felt on the bone at about 3 weeks of age.

2. Any variation in the hands or unusual length of the fingers should be noted. An incurved little finger or low-set thumb with the single simian crease may reflect Down's syndrome, or mongolism.

Lower Extremities

1. Examine the appearance of the infant's foot, noting arch formation.

2. Inspect the angle of the foot and lower leg and then manipulate the ankle to evaluate the range of motion.

3. Place the knees together and see how far the ankles are separated.

4. Evaluate the baby's ability to walk, noting the appearance of the legs and foot placement. Remember to look at the child's shoes and see which side of the sole is worn down.

1. The foot of an infant is usually flat and appears broad since the arch on the inside of the foot is covered by a fat pad. Parents may need reassurance in this regard.

2. Full flexibility of the foot (plantar flexion) rules out underlying abnormality. The foot should return to the neutral position after manipulation. Frequently, the foot will turn in, or adduct. Such a finding should be recorded.

3. Normally there is only a small space between the ankles when the knees are held together. Marked bowing of the legs will be demonstrated by a wide distance between the ankles. This is particularly important following assumption of the upright position.

4. When babies first start to walk, their legs appear bow-legged. The feet are kept wide apart and turn slightly in, so that the ankles seem curved when viewed from behind.

Hip

1. When examining children under 1 year of age, check to see if there are signs of hip dislocation. (See illustration at top of page 70.) Refer to Chapter 59, Children With Orthopedic Conditions, Congenital Dislocation of the Hip, page 1468.

1. Any difficulties with hip examination call for immediate medical consultation because of possible congenital dislocation of the hip.

   In the normal infant, the lateral aspect of each knee will touch the examining table without difficulty.

Technique	Findings

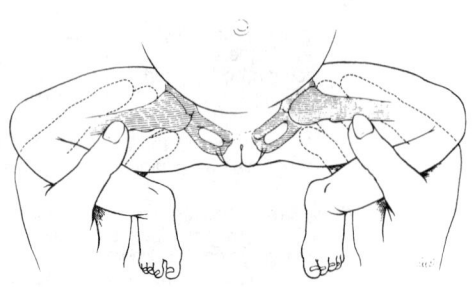

Spine

1. Check the spine for any signs of abnormal curvature.

1. The normal child has a curve inward at the lumbar region (lordosis), but this should not be exaggerated.
Abnormal curvatures include the following:
Kyphosis: Forward curvature of the shoulders.
Scoliosis: Side-to-side curvature of the spine.

2. Observe the child from the side and back in the standing position to see forward curving of the shoulders.
3. Have the child bend forward with the arms hanging down. A unilateral rib prominence will be seen in children with scoliosis.

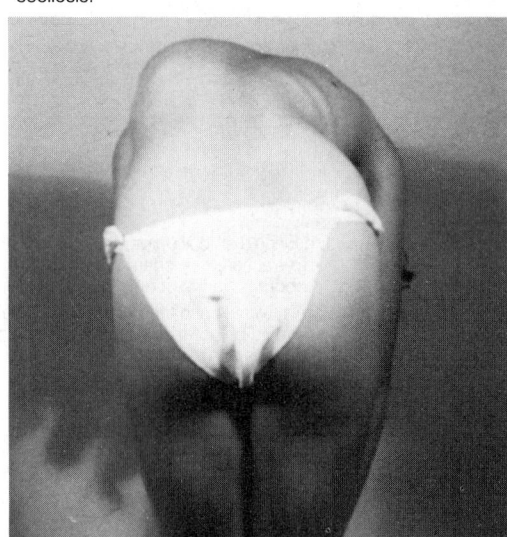

(O'Connor BJ. Scoliosis: Classification and diagnosis in pediatric orthopedics. ONA J 3:84, Mar 1976)

Neurologic Examination

1. The neurologic system at birth is different from that of the baby of a few months. There is an even greater contrast between the baby on the one hand and children and adults on the other.
2. The central nervous system at birth is underdeveloped and the functions tested are below the level of the cortex.

Equipment

Flashlight, noisemaker, ophthalmoscope, tongue depressor, tuning fork

Procedure for the Newborn and Young Infant

(See Guidelines: Nursing Care of the Newborn, pp. 1011–1012.)

1. Observe the newborn for general appearance, positioning, activity, crying, and alertness. Take note of the posture—including head, neck, and extremities.

1. Stiffness of the neck or marked attraction of the head will cause a position of opisthotonos.

(continued)

Technique	Findings

2. Note the pitch, volume, and character of the cry.

3. Observe the infant's facial expression and the symmetry of the face when crying or sucking.

4. Most of the cranial nerves are difficult to check at this early age.

Automatic Reflexes

1. *Blinking reflex due to loud noise*
   Clap your hands or produce a loud clicking noise, being careful not to clap near the baby so that a wave of air passes over his eyes and causes him to blink them anyway.

2. *Blinking reflex due to bright light*
   Shine a bright light into the infant's eyes to elicit blinking reflex.
   a. Cranial nerve 10 can be checked by using a tongue depressor to gag the infant.
   b. Cranial nerve 12 (hypoglossal) can be tested by pinching the nose closed as the baby sucks.

3. *Palmar grasp reflex*
   Place your fingers across the baby's palm from the ulnar side. The baby needs to be in a relaxed position with his head in a central position. Reinforcement may be offered by having the baby suck on the bottle at the same time.

4. *Rooting reflex*
   Touch the edge of the baby's mouth.

5. *Incurving of the trunk*
   Hold the baby horizontally and prone in one arm while using the other hand to stimulate 1 side of the infant's back from the shoulders to the buttocks.
   The trunk curves toward the stimulated side as the shoulders and pelvis move toward the stroking hand (persists until infant is about 2 months old).

6. *Vertical suspension position*
   Place your hands under the baby's axillae with thumbs supporting the back of the head and hold the baby upright.

7. *Stepping response*
   Hold the baby under its axillae with thumbs supporting the back of the head. Allow baby's foot to touch firm surface.

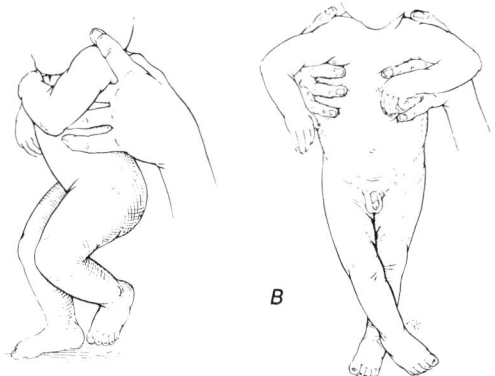

A   B

---

2. The high-pitched cry of the infant who has intracranial irritation is very distinctive.

3. Poor sucking, with dribbling, is abnormal. Transient weakness of the mouth due to 7th cranial nerve paralysis is frequently seen as a result of a forceps delivery in which the forceps is pressed on the facial nerve where it emerges from the ear.

1. Lack of a blink in response to a loud noise may indicate deafness.

2. Failure to blink may indicate blindness.

   a. Palate moves.

   b. The infant opens the mouth and raises the tip of the tongue reflexly.

3. Both hands will flex and can be compared for strength. Weakness on 1 side may be indicated by a failure to grasp when the palm is stimulated.

4. The baby's mouth will open, and the head will turn toward the side stimulated. This reflex is marked during the early weeks of life. (Persistence time varies.)

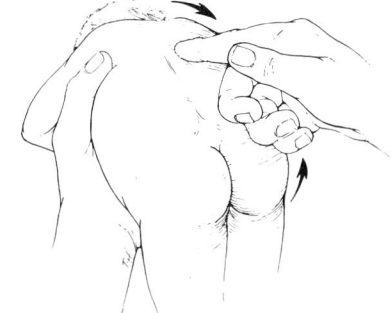

6. The legs flex at the hips and knees (persists for about 4 months).

7. Normally the baby responds by lifting 1 knee and hip into a flexed position and moving the opposite leg forward—making a series of stepping movements (*A*).
   a. Difficulty with the stepping reflex and stiffness or spasticity connected with crossing of the feet and scissoring (*B*) is indicative of spastic paraplegia or diplegia.
   b. It should be noted that the stepping response may be affected by breech delivery. (It may also be affected by weakness.)
   c. The stepping response is evident toward the end of the 1st week and persists for a variable time.

Technique	Findings

8. *Tonic neck reflex*
   Hold the baby in a supine position with the head turned to one side and the jaw held in place over the shoulder.

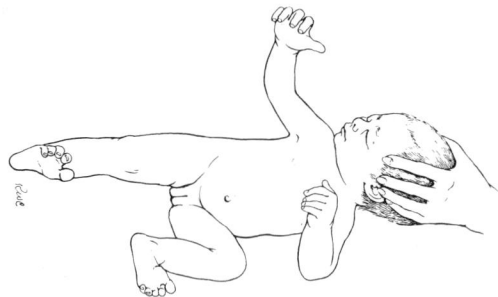

8. a. The arm and leg on the side to which the head is turned will extend, whereas those on the other side will flex (the so-called "bow and arrow position").
   b. This reflex persists for about 6 months; it may be present at birth or delayed until the baby is 6 or 8 weeks old.
   c. Persistence beyond 6 months suggests major cerebral damage.

9. *Mass reflexes (Moro or startle reflex)*
   Hold the baby along your arm with the other hand below the lower legs. Lower the feet and body in a sudden motion.

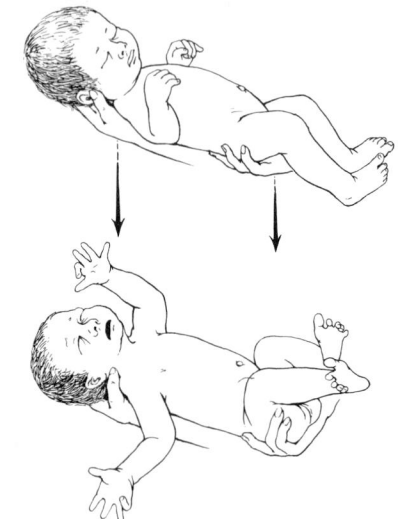

9. The arms will spring up and out, abducting and extending; the fingers are also extended. The arms then return forward over the body with a clasping motion. At the same time, the legs flex slightly and the hips abduct.

   a. The Moro reflex is present at birth and disappears at about the end of the 3rd month. Persistence beyond 6 months is significant.
   b. Asymmetric response may be due to paralysis of the arm following a difficult delivery, tension and injury to the brachial plexus, or a fracture of the clavicle or humerus. A dislocated hip would produce an asymmetrical response in the lower extremities.

10. *Perez reflex*
    Hold the baby in a prone position along your arm; place the thumb of the other hand on the sacrum and move it firmly toward the head, along the entire length of the spine.

10. The head and spine will extend and the knees will flex upward.

Summary
1. Some of the jerking and shaking movements seen in infants are normal, but they should be rechecked frequently during the first few weeks of life.
2. Plantar stimulation will elicit a Babinski response (toes curl upward) in most children until the age of 2; this is a normal finding.
3. Variants in the findings due to the baby's sleepiness or hunger should be taken into account and reevaluations should be carried out under different conditions.
4. Severe neurologic damage may be completely asymptomatic and impossible to detect during the first few weeks of life.

Neurologic Examination of the Toddler and Early School-Age Child
1. The neurologic examination for the toddler and the early school-age child is very similar to that for the adult.
2. The Draw-A-Person Test* and the Denver Developmental Assessment[†] are both excellent methods for testing areas in the development of the child.
3. Beyond the newborn period, specific gross and fine motor coordination testing, accompanied by appropriate evaluation of the Denver test, will assist in assessing the child's level of development.
4. These tests also assess social and language development and are important screening devices.
5. Interview techniques[‡] can also be useful in assessing development in the preschool child.

---

* See Appendix A, page 1074.
† See Appendix B, page 1075.
‡ See Appendix C, page 1077.

Bibliography

Books

Athreya BH, Silverman BK and Spitzer AR. Pediatric Physical Diagnosis. Norwalk, CT, Appleton–Century–Crofts, 1985

Avery ME and First LR (eds). Overview of the well child care. In Pediatric Medicine, pp 3–22. Baltimore, Williams & Wilkins, 1989

Bates BA. A Guide to Physical Examination. 5th ed. Philadelphia, JB Lippincott, 1991

Behrman RE and Kliegman R. Developmental and behavioral pediatrics. In Nelson Essentials of Pediatrics, pp 1–56. Philadelphia, WB Saunders, 1990

Bowers AC and Thompson JM. Clinical Manual of Health Assessment. 3rd ed. St Louis, CV Mosby, 1988

Engel J. Pocket Guide to Pediatric Assessment. St Louis, CV Mosby, 1989

Foster RLM, Hunsberger MM and Anderston JJT. Family-Centered Nursing Care of Children. Philadelphia, WB Saunders, 1989

Gill D and O'Brien N. Paediatric Clinical Examination. New York, Churchill Livingstone, 1988

Green M. Pediatric Diagnosis. 4th ed. Philadelphia, WB Saunders, 1986

Guckian JC (ed). The pediatric patient. In The Clinical Interview and Physical Examination, pp 476–522. Philadelphia, JB Lippincott, 1987

Kaye R, Oski FA and Barness LA. History and physical examination. In Core Textbook of Pediatrics, pp 1–7. Philadelphia, JB Lippincott, 1988

Hoekelman RA et al. The pediatric physical examination. In Primary Pediatrics, pp 63–109. St Louis, CV Mosby, 1987

James SR and Mott SR. Physical assessment. In Child Health Nursing, pp 249–291. Reading, MA, Addison–Wesley, 1988

Lingam S and Harvey DR. Manual of Child Development. New York, Churchill Livingstone, 1988

Marlow DR and Reading BA. Physical assessment. In Textbook of Pediatric Nursing, 6th ed, pp 84–162. Philadelphia, WB Saunders, 1988

Oski FA et al. The pediatric history and physical examination. In Principles and Practice of Pediatrics, pp 28–47. Philadelphia, JB Lippincott, 1990

Pillitteri A. Health assessment of children. In Child Health Nursing. Care of the Growing Family, pp 113–177. Boston, Little, Brown & Co, 1987

Rudolph AM and Hoffman JIE. Assessment and care of child and adolescent. In Pediatrics, 18th ed, pp 17–34. Norwalk, Appleton & Lange, 1987

Rudy EB and Gray VR. The pediatric patient. In Handbook of Health Assessment, pp 193–246. Norwalk, CT, Appleton–Century–Crofts, 1986

Schwartz MW et al. Principles and Practice of Clinical Pediatrics. Chicago, Year Book Medical Pub, 1987

Servonsky J and Opas SR. Assessment of the child's health status. In Nursing Management of Children, pp 66–108. Boston, Jones and Bartlett Pub., Inc., 1987

Smith MJ, Goodman JA and Ramsey NL. Children: Assessment, maintenance and promotion of health. In Child and Family. Concepts of Nursing Practice. 2nd ed, pp 313–351. New York, McGraw–Hill, 1987

Summitt RL. The pediatric history and physical examination. In Comprehensive Pediatrics, pp 253–261. St Louis, CV Mosby, 1990

Whaley LF and Wong DL. Physical and developmental assessment of the child. In Essentials of Pediatric Nursing, pp 129–175. St Louis, CV Mosby, 1989

Wood RA et al. The pediatric physical examination. In Pediatrics, pp 49–62. Philadelphia, JB Lippincott, 1989

Zitelli BJ and Davis HW (eds). Atlas of Pediatric Physical Diagnosis. St Louis, CV Mosby, 1987

Journals

Cohen KA and Byrne SM. The role of the nurse is assisting with eye examinations on premature infants. Neonatal Netw 1989 Oct; 8(2):31–35

Harris JA. Pediatric abdominal assessment. Pediatr Nurs 1986 Sep–Oct; 12(5):355–362

Paparella MM, Fox RY and Schachern PA. Diagnosis and treatment of sensorineural loss in children. Otolaryngol Clin North Am 1989 Feb; 22(1):51–74

Saal HM and Rosenbaum KN. Screening the newborn for anatomic and metabolic defects. Pediatr Ann 1988 Jul; 17(7):467, 470–472, 474–476

South–Paul JE. The well-baby examination. Am Fam Physician 1988 Jan; 37(1):167–172

Szydlo VL. Approaching an adolescent about a pelvic exam. Am J Nurs 1988 Nov; 88(11):1502–1506

U.S. Preventive Services Task Force. The periodic health examination: Age-specific charts. Am Fam Physician 1990 Jan; 41(1):189–204

Appendix A:

Goodenough–Harris Draw-a-Person Test

This test provides one of the methods of measuring the level of mental development of children between 3 and 10 years of age. It was originally described in 1926 and appears to be a sound one; there is a significant degree of correlation in the results of this test and IQ. Subsequently Harris brought the test up-to-date with specific scoring for drawings of a man or a woman.

1. *Procedure:* The child is supplied with a pencil (preferably a No. 2 with eraser) and a sheet of blank paper and instructed to "Draw a person," "Draw the best person you can." No additional directions are necessary. Encouragement may be supplied if necessary. Under no condition should the examiner suggest that the child's production needs to be supplemented or changed in any way—the only exception being the drawing of the stick figure. In this case the examiner is permitted to encourage the child to "draw a whole person."

2. *Scoring:* The child receives one point for each detail present according to the following scoring guides:

Drawing of a Woman

1. Head present
2. Neck present
3. Neck, 2 dimensions
4. Eyes present
5. Eye detail: brow or lashes
6. Eye detail: pupil
7. Nose present (not round ball)
8. Nose, 2 dimensions
9. Bridge of nose (straight to eyes, narrower than base)
10. Nostrils shown
11. Mouth present
12. Lips, 2 dimensions
13. Both nose and lips in 2 dimensions
14. Both chin and forehead shown
15. Hair I (any scribble)
16. Hair II (more detail)
17. Necklace or earrings
18. Arms present
19. Fingers present
20. Correct number of fingers shown
21. Opposition of thumb shown (must include fingers)
22. Hands present
23. Legs present
24. Feet (any indication)
25. Show "feminine" (any attempt such as high heels, open toe, strap)
26. Attachment of arms and legs I (to trunk anywhere)
27. Attachment of arms and legs II (to trunk at correct point)
28. Clothing indicated (any)
29. Sleeve
30. Neckline (any indication)
31. Trunk present
32. Trunk in proportion, 2 dimensions (length greater than breadth)

Drawing of a Man

1. Head present
2. Neck present
3. Neck, 2 dimensions
4. Eyes present
5. Eye detail: brow or lashes
6. Eye detail: pupil
7. Nose present
8. Nose, 2 dimensions (not round ball)
9. Mouth present
10. Lips, 2 dimensions
11. Both nose and lips in 2 dimensions
12. Both chin and forehead shown
13. Bridge of nose (straight to eyes; narrower than base)
14. Hair I (any scribble)
15. Hair II (more detail)
16. Ears present
17. Fingers present
18. Correct number of fingers shown
19. Opposition of thumb shown (must include fingers)
20. Hands present
21. Arms present
22. Arms at side or engaged in activity
23. Feet; any indication
24. Attachment of arms and legs I (to trunk anywhere)
25. Attachment of arms and legs II (at correct point of trunk)
26. Trunk present
27. Trunk in proportion, 2 dimensions (length greater than breadth)
28. Clothing I (anything)
29. Clothing II (2 articles of clothing)

3. *Norms:* Minimum score for child to be within one standard deviation of age-appropriate mean.

Age	Drawing of Man		Drawing of Woman	
---	By Boys	By Girls	By Boys	By Girls
3	4	5	4	6
4	7	7	7	8
5	11	12	11	14
6	13	14	13	16
7	16	17	16	19
8	18	20	20	23

Appendix B:

Denver Developmental Screening Test

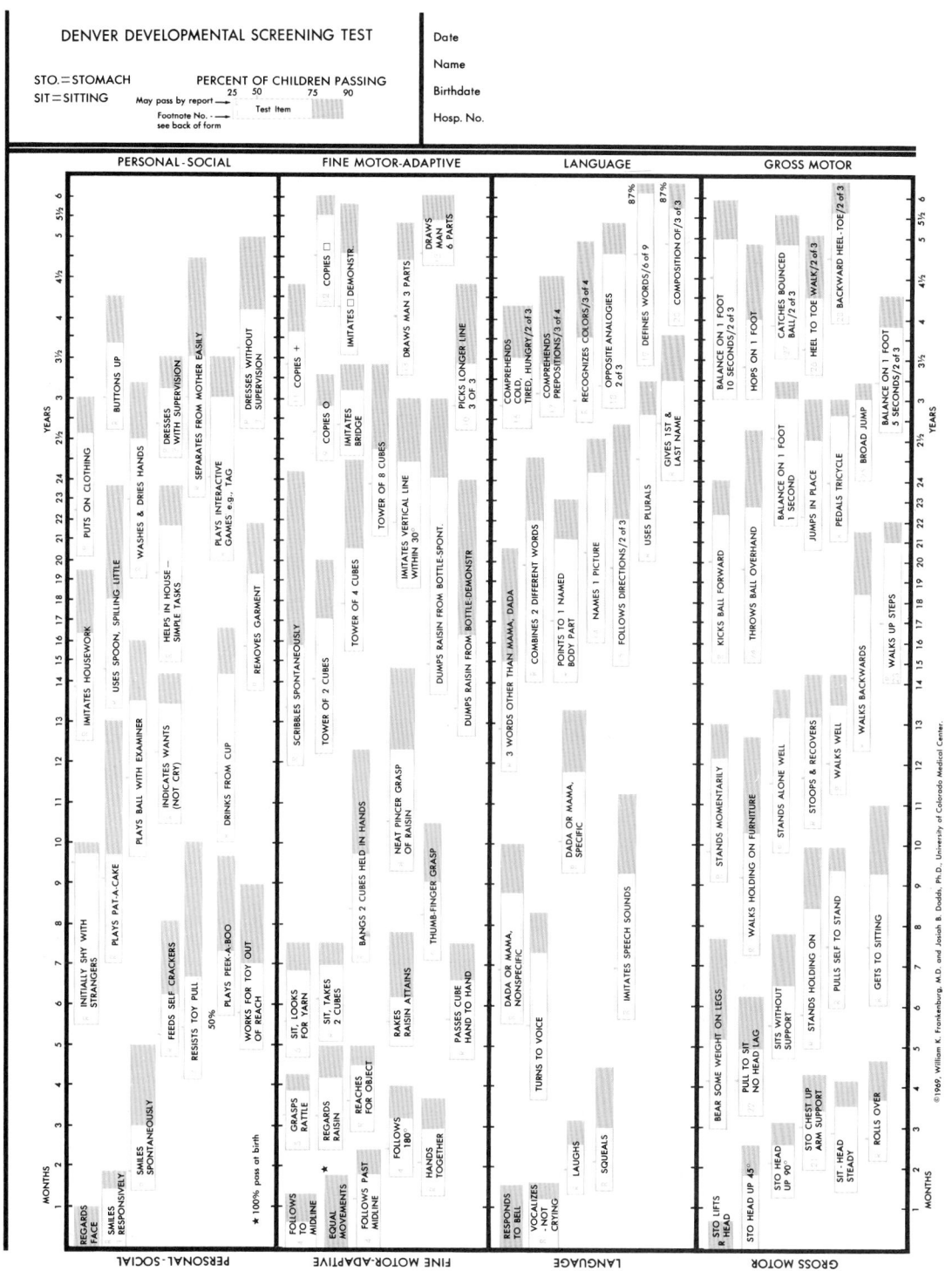

The Denver Developmental Assessment method developed by William K. Frankenburg, M.D., and his colleagues, is presented in a manual called Denver Developmental Screening Test. The test materials can be ordered from: Lodaco Project & Publishing Foundation, Inc., East 51st Avenue and Lincoln Street, Denver, Colorado 80216.

DATE
NAME
DIRECTIONS   BIRTHDATE
HOSP. NO.

1. Try to get child to smile by smiling, talking or waving to him. Do not touch him.
2. When child is playing with toy, pull it away from him. Pass if he resists.
3. Child does not have to be able to tie shoes or button in the back.
4. Move yarn slowly in an arc from one side to the other, about 6″ above child's face. Pass if eyes follow 90° to midline. (Past midline; 180°)
5. Pass if child grasps rattle when it is touched to the backs or tips of fingers.
6. Pass if child continues to look where yarn disappeared or tries to see where it went. Yarn should be dropped quickly from sight from tester's hand without arm movement.
7. Pass if child picks up raisin with any part of thumb and a finger.
8. Pass if child picks up raisin with the ends of thumb and index finger using an over hand approach.

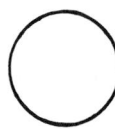   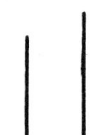   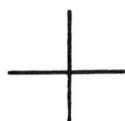   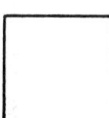

9. Pass any enclosed form. Fail continuous round motions.
10. Which line is longer? (Not bigger.) Turn paper upside down and repeat. (3/3 or 5/6)
11. Pass any crossing lines.
12. Have child copy first. If failed, demonstrate

When giving items 9, 11 and 12, do not name the forms. Do not demonstrate 9 and 11.

13. When scoring, each pair (2 arms, 2 legs, etc.) counts as one part.
14. Point to picture and have child name it. (No credit is given for sounds only.)

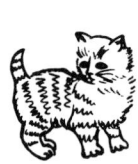 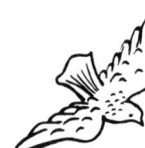 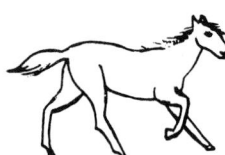 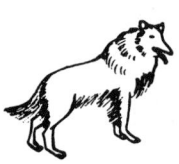 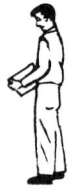

15. Tell child to: Give block to Mommie; put block on table; put block on floor. Pass 2 of 3. (Do not help child by pointing, moving head or eyes.)
16. Ask child: What do you do when you are cold? . . hungry? . . tired? . . Pass 2 of 3.
17. Tell child to: Put block <u>on</u> table; <u>under</u> table; <u>in front</u> of chair, <u>behind</u> chair. Pass 3 of 4. (Do not help child by pointing, moving head or eyes.)
18. Ask child: If fire is hot, ice is ?; Mother is a woman, Dad is a ?; a horse is big, a mouse is ?. Pass 2 of 3.
19. Ask child: What is a ball? . . lake? . . desk? . . house? . . banana? . . curtain? . . ceiling? . . hedge? . . pavement? Pass if defined in terms of use, shape, what it is made of or general category (such as banana is fruit, not just yellow). Pass 6 of 9.
20. Ask child: What is a spoon made of? . . a shoe made of? . . a door made of? (No other objects may be substituted.) Pass 3 of 3.
21. When placed on stomach, child lifts chest off table with support of forearms and/or hands.
22. When child is on back, grasp his hands and pull him to sitting. Pass if head does not hang back.
23. Child may use wall or rail only, not person. May not crawl.
24. Child must throw ball overhand 3 feet to within arm's reach of tester.
25. Child must perform standing broad jump over width of test sheet. (8½ inches)
26. Tell child to walk forward, heel within 1 inch of toe. Tester may demonstrate. Child must walk 4 consecutive steps, 2 out of 3 trials.
27. Bounce ball to child who should stand 3 feet away from tester. Child must catch ball with hands, not arms, 2 out of 3 trials.
28. Tell child to walk backward, 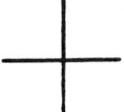 toe within 1 inch of heel. Tester may demonstrate. Child must walk 4 consecutive steps, 2 out of 3 trials.

<u>DATE AND BEHAVIORAL OBSERVATIONS</u> (how child feels at time of test, relation to tester, attention span, verbal behavior, self-confidence, etc.):

Appendix C:

Developmental Assessment by Interview

A method of evaluation has been developed by utilizing an interview technique asking parents a list of questions regarding milestones in achievements that most will remember. Developed by Drs. Capute and Biehl, it has been very successful in its use at the John F. Kennedy Institute for the Habilitation of Handicapped Children at John Hopkins Hospital.

Age	Gross Motor	Fine Motor	Language	Social
3 mo.	A. Does he support himself on forearms when lying?	A. Are his hands usually open at rest?	A. Does he laugh or make happy noises?	A. Does he smile at you?
	B. Does he hold his head up steadily while on his stomach?	B. Does he pull at his clothing?	B. Does he turn his head to sounds?	B. Does he reach for familiar people or objects?
6 mo.	A. Does he lift his head when lying on his back?	A. Does he transfer a toy from one hand to the other?	A. Does he "babble," repeat sounds together (i.e., mum-mum-mum)?	A. Does he stretch his arms out to be picked up?
	B. Does he roll from back to front?	B. Does he pick up small objects	B. Is he frightened by angry noise?	B. Does he show his likes and dislikes?
9 mo.	A. Does he sit for long periods without support?	A. Does he pick up objects with his thumb and one finger?	A. Does he understand "no-no," "bye-bye"?	A. Does he hold his own bottle?
	B. Does he pull up on furniture?	B. Does he finger-feed any foods?	B. Will he imitate any sounds or words if you make them first?	B. Does he play any nursery games ("peek-a-boo," "bye-bye")?
12 mo.	A. Is he walking (alone or with hand held)?	A. Does he throw toys (objects)?	A. Does he have at least one meaningful word other than "mama," "dada"?	A. Does he cooperate in dressing?
	B. Does he pivot when sitting?	B. Does he give you toys (let go) easily?	B. Does he shake his head for "no"?	B. Does he come when you call him?
18 mo.	A. Does he walk upstairs with help?	A. Does he turn book pages (2 or 3 at a time)?	A. Does he have at least 6 real words besides his "jargon"?	A. Does he copy you in routine tasks (sweeping, dusting, etc.)?
	B. Can he throw a toy while standing without falling?	B. Does he fill spoon and feed self?	B. Does he point at what he wants?	B. Does he play in the company of other children?
2 yr.	A. Does he run well without falling?	A. Does he turn book pages one at a time?	A. Does he talk in short (2–3 word) sentences?	A. Does he ask to be taken to the toilet?
	B. Does he walk up and down stairs alone?	B. Does he remove his own shoes, pants?	B. Does he use pronouns ("me," "you," "mine")?	B. Does he play in company of other children?
2½ yr.	A. Does he jump, getting both feet off the floor?	A. Does he unbutton any buttons?	A. Does he use plurals or past tense?	A. Does he tell his first and last name if asked?
	B. Does he throw a ball overhand?	B. Does he hold a pencil or crayon adult fashion?	B. Does he use the word "I" correctly most of the time?	B. Does he get himself a drink without help?
3 yr.	A. Does he pedal a tricycle?	A. Does he dry his hands (if reminded)?	A. Does he tell little stories about his experiences?	A. Does he share his toys?
	B. Does he alternate feet (one stair per step) going upstairs?	B. Does he dress and undress fully including front buttons?	B. Does he know his sex?	B. Does he play well with another child? Take turns?
4 yr.	A. Does he attempt to hop or skip?	A. Does he button clothes fully?	A. Does he say a song or a poem from memory?	A. Does he tell "tall tales" or "show off"?
	B. Does he alternate feet going downstairs?	B. Does he catch a ball?	B. Does he know all his colors?	B. Does he play cooperatively with a small group of children?
5 yr.	A. Does he skip, alternating feet?	A. Does he tie his own shoes?	A. Can he print his first name?	A. Is he a "mother's helper"—likes to do things for you?
	B. Does he jump rope or jump over low obstacles?	B. Does he spread with a knife?	B. Does he ever ask what a word means?	B. Does he play competitive games and abide by the rules?

(From Johns Hopkins Hospital: The Harriet Lane Handbook. 8th ed. Dennis L. Headings (ed). Copyright © 1978 by Year Book Medical Pub, Chicago. Used with permission.)

Pediatric Health Maintenance

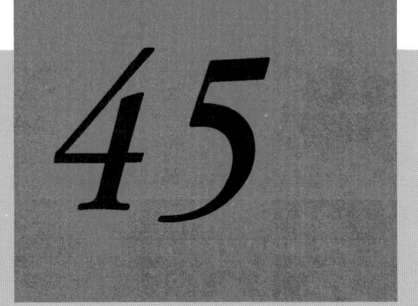

45

Growth and Development

Reflexes of the Newborn

1. *Pupillary reflexes*—ipsilateral (pertaining to the same side) constriction to light.
2. *Rooting*—when corner of mouth is touched and object is moved toward cheek, infant will turn head toward object and open mouth.
3. *Palmar grasp*—pressure on palm of hand will elicit grasp.
4. *Plantar grasp*—pressure on the sole of foot behind toes will cause flexion of toes.
5. *Tonic neck reflex*—sudden jolt will cause head to turn to one side with leg and arm on that side extended, while the extremities on the other side flex.
6. *Neck righting*—when head is turned to one side, the shoulder and trunk, followed by the pelvis, will turn to that side.
7. *Moro reflex*—response to sudden loud noise, causing body to stiffen and arms to go up and out, then forward and toward each other. Thumb and index finger will assume C-shape.
8. *Positive-supporting reflex*—when held in an erect position, baby will stiffen lower extremities and support his weight.
9. *Babinski's sign*—scratching sole of foot causes great toe to flex and toes to fan.
10. *Crossed extensor reflex*—when one leg is extended and the knee is held straight, while the sole of foot is stimulated, the opposite leg will flex.
11. *Landau's sign*—when baby is suspended horizontally with head depressed against trunk and neck flexed, legs will flex and be drawn up to trunk.
12. *Optical blink reflex*—when light is suddenly shone into open eyes, the eyes will close quickly with a quick dorsal flexion of head.
13. *Auditory blink reflex*—eyes quickly close if examiner loudly claps her hands about 30 cm. (11.5 inches) from infant's head.
14. *Recoil of arm*—when both arms are extended simultaneously by pulling outward and grasping wrists, both arms will flex at elbows when released.
15. *Withdrawal reflex*—pricking sole of foot will result in the baby's leg being flexed at hip, knee, and ankle.
16. *Stepping reflex*—when infant is held upright with dorsum of foot gently touching edge of table, he will bend his hips and knees and put foot on table. This will elicit stepping response in the opposite foot. Series of alternating stepping actions will result when infant is moved forward so that 1 foot at a time touches the firm surface.
17. *Parachute reflex*—while the infant is held prone and lowered quickly toward a surface, he will extend arms and legs.
18. *Side-turning*—placing baby prone with head in midline will elicit the baby's turning his head to the side.
19. Other characteristics of the newborn:
    a. Cries
    b. Sucks
    c. Has extremely sensitive skin
    d. Makes discriminating sounds
    e. Sleeps for long intervals
    f. Has little head control (head lag)

Infant to Adolescent

See table on pages 1080–1093.

Childhood Diseases

See table on pages 1094–1101.

Nutrition of Pediatric Patients

See table on pages 1102–1106.

Infant to Adolescent: Growth and Development

Age and Physical Characteristics	Behavior Patterns	Nursing Implications/ Parental Guidance
Birth–4 weeks (1 month)	***Motor Development*** Momentary visual fixation on objects and adult face. Eyes follow bright moving objects. Lies awake on back with head averted. Immediately drops objects placed in hands. Responds to sounds of bell and other similar noises. Keeps hands fisted. ***Socialization and Vocalization*** Mews and makes throaty noises. Shows interest in human face. ***Cognitive and Emotional Development*** Reflexive. External stimuli are meaningless. Responses are generally limited to tension states or discomfort. Gains satisfaction from feeding and being held, rocked, fondled, and cuddled. Has an intense need for sucking pleasure. Quiets when picked up.	***Play Stimulation*** Use human face—smile and talk. Dangle bright and moving object in field of vision (mobile). Hold, touch, caress, fondle, kiss. Rock, pat, change position. Play soft music or have infant listen to ticking clock, sing. Talk to infant, call him by name. ***Parental Guidance*** Begin to expose infant to different household sounds. Change crib location in room. Use bright-colored clothing and linen. Keep infant nearby. Allow him to sleep. Play with him when he is awake. Hold him during feeding.
8 weeks (2 months) Crossed extensor reflex disappears.	***Motor Development*** Reflexive behavior is slowly being replaced by voluntary movements. Turns from side to back. Begins to lift head momentarily from prone position. Shows eye coordination to light and objects. If bell is sounded near him, he will stop activity and listen. Eyes follow better, both vertically and horizontally. Focuses well. ***Socialization and Vocalization*** Begins vocalization—coos, especially to a voice. Crying becomes differentiated. Visually looks for sounds. May squeal with delight when stimulated by touching, talking, or singing. Begins social smile. Eyes follow person or object more intently. ***Cognitive and Emotional Development*** Recognizes familiar face. Becomes more aware and interested in environment. Anticipates being fed when in feeding position. Enjoys sucking—puts hand in mouth.	***Play Stimulation*** Arrange mobile over crib so infant's movement will set it in motion. Hang wind chimes near infant. Hang bright-colored pictures on wall (yellow and red-colored stripes, for example). Use cradle gym and infant seat. Use rattles. Hold infant and walk around room. Allow freedom of kicking with clothes off. ***Parental Guidance*** Talk to him and smile; get excited when he coos. Place infant seat near mother's activities but where he cannot fall off or tip over. Put in prone position in bed or on floor. Expose infant to different textures. Exercise infant's arms and legs. Sing to infant. Provide tactile experience during bathing, diapering, feeding. First DTP and TOPV immunization should be given.

(continued)

Age and Physical Characteristics	Behavior Patterns	Nursing Implications/ Parental Guidance
12 weeks (3 months) Landau reflex appears at 3–4 months; stepping reflex disappears. Positive support reflex disappears. Posterior fontanelle closes.	**Motor Development** When prone, he will rest on forearms and keep head in midline—makes crawling movements with legs, arches back, and holds head high; he may get chest off surface. Indicates preference for prone or supine position. Discovers hands—strikes at objects while watching hands. Holds objects in hands and brings to mouth. Has fairly good head control. **Socialization and Vocalization** Smiles more readily. Babbles and coos. Stops crying when mother enters room or when he is caressed. Enjoys playing during feeding. Stays awake longer without crying. Turns head to follow familiar person. **Cognitive and Emotional Development** Shows active interest in environment. Recognizes familiar faces and objects. Focuses and follows objects. Shows repetitiveness in play activity. Is aware of strange situations. Derives pleasure from sucking—purposefully gets hand to mouth. Begins to establish routine preceding sleep.	**Play Stimulation** Encourage socialization, smiling, laughing. Place on mat on floor. Continue to introduce new sounds. **Parental Guidance** Take on daily outing as weather permits. Bounce on bed. Play with infant during feeding. Rattles can be used effectively for visual following and for hand play.
16 weeks (4 months) Stepping reflex disappears. Rooting reflex disappears. By 4–5 months infant's weight approximately doubles birth weight. Birth to 6 months Average weekly weight gain, 140–200 gm. (4–7 ounces). Average monthly height gain, 2.5 cm. (1 inch). End of first year weighs three times birth weight. Pulse rate slows to 100–140 Respirations, 20–40/minute	**Motor Development** Eyes focus on small objects; he may pick a dangling ring. Holds head up (when being pulled to sitting position). Becomes more interested in environment. Hand comes to meet rattle. Listens—turns head to familiar sound. Sits with minimal support. Intentional rolling over, back to side. Reaches for offered objects. Grasps objects with both hands, and everything goes into mouth. **Socialization and Vocalization** Laughs and chuckles socially. Demands social attention by fussing. Recognizes mother.	**Play Stimulation** Encourage mirror play. Provide soft squeeze toys in vivid colors of varying texture. Allow infant to splash in bath. Infant still enjoys holding and playing with rattles. Enjoys old-fashioned clothespins and playing pat-a-cake, peek-a-boo. **Parental Guidance** Be certain button eyes on toys and other small objects cannot be pulled off. Hold rattle for him and let him reach and grasp it. When baby is in highchair, strap in. Let him play with food; give finger foods. Move mobile out of reach—he may grab it and cause injury.

(continued)

Infant to Adolescent:
Growth and Development *(continued)*

Age and Physical Characteristics	Behavior Patterns	Nursing Implications/ Parental Guidance
	Socialization and Vocalization *(continued)* Begins to respond to "No, no." Enjoys being propped in sitting position. ***Cognitive and Emotional Development*** Actively interested in environment. Enjoys attention; becomes bored when alone for long periods of time. Recognizes bottle. More interested in mother. Indicates increasing trust and security. Sleeps through night; has defined nap time.	***Parental Guidance*** *(continued)* Repeat child's sounds to him. Talk in varying degrees of loudness. Begin looking at and naming pictures in book. Begin roughhousing play by both parents. Second DTP and TOPV immunization should be given. Give space in playpen or on sheet on floor to practice rolling over.
26 weeks (7 months) By 5–6 months, tonic neck reflex disappears. By 6–7 months, palmar grasp disappears. By 7–9 months, develops eye-to-eye contact while talking; engages in social games. 2 central lower incisors erupt.	***Motor Development*** Shows momentary sitting, with hand support. Bounces and bears some weight when held in standing position. Transfers and mouths objects in one hand. Discovers feet. Bangs objects together. Rolls over well. May begin some form of mobility. ***Socialization and Vocalization*** Discriminates between strangers and familiar figures. Crows and squeals. Starts to say "Ma," "Da." Self-play is self-contained. Laughs out loud. Makes "talking" sounds in response to others' talking. Begins fear of strangers, 8½–10 months ***Cognitive and Emotional Development*** Secures objects by pulling on string. Searches for lost objects that are out of sight. Inspects objects; localizes sounds. Likes to sit in highchair. Drops and picks up objects. Displays exploratory behavior with food. Exhibits beginning fear of strangers. Becomes fretful when mother leaves. Shows much mouthing and biting.	***Play Stimulation*** Enjoys social games, hide-and-seek with adult, toys, large blocks. Likes to bang objects. Plays in bounce chair, walker. Enjoys large nesting toys (round rather than square). Likes to drop and retrieve things. Likes metal cups, wooden spoons, and things to bang with. Loves crumpled paper. Enjoys squeeze toys in bath. Likes peek-a-boo, bye-bye, and pat-a-cake. ***Parental Guidance*** Will play as long as you can. Tie toys to chair with short string. Let play with extra spoon at feeding. Give soft finger foods. Since infant puts everything in mouth, *use safety precautions.* Keep small items away from him; he could choke on them. Show excitement at his achievements. Supply kichen items for toys. Third DTP and TOPV immunization at 6 months.
40 weeks (10 months) 4 upper incisors erupt around 7–9 months. By 9–12 months, plantar reflex disappears.	***Motor Development*** Sits without support. Recovers balance. Manipulates objects with hands. Unwraps objects.	***Play Stimulation*** Encourage use of motion toys—rocking horse, stroller. Water play. Imitate animal sounds.

(continued)

Age and Physical Characteristics	Behavior Patterns	Nursing Implications/ Parental Guidance
By 9–12 months, neck-righting reflex disappears. 6–12 months Average weekly weight gain, 85–140 gm. (3–5 ounces). Average monthly height gain, 1.25 cm. (½ inch).	***Motor Development*** *(continued)* Creeps. Pulls self upright at crib rails. Uses index finger and thumb to hold objects. Rings a bell. Can feed himself a cracker and can hold bottle. Can control lips around cup. Does not like supine position. Can hold index finger and thumb in opposition. ***Socialization and Verbalization*** Claps hands on request. Responds to own name. Is very aware of social environment. Imitates gestures, facial expressions, and sounds. Smiles at image in mirror. Offers toy to adult, but does not release it. Begins to test parental reaction during feeding and at bedtime. Will entertain self for long periods of time. ***Cognitive and Emotional Development*** Begins to imitate. Shows more interest in picture books. Enjoys achievements. Has strong urge toward independence—locomotion, feeding, dressing.	***Play Stimulation*** *(continued)* Allow exploration outdoors. Provide for learning by imitation. Offer new objects (blocks). Child likes freedom of creeping and walking, but closeness of family is important. Good toys: milk carton; bean bag for tossing; fabric books; things to move around, fill up, empty out; pile-up and knock-down toys. ***Parental Guidance*** Do things with him. Protect him from dangerous objects—cover electrical outlets, block stairs, remove breakable objects from tables. Use plastic bottle. Have child with family at mealtime. Offer cup.

12 months (1 year)
By 12–18 months, Babinski sign disappears.
By 12–24 months, Landau reflex disappears.
By 10–14 months, anterior fontanelle closes.
Weight should approximately triple birth weight.
2 lower lateral incisors appear.
4 first molars appear by 14 months.
Child Development Theories
Freudian: Behavior
  Birth–1 year—Oral Stage
Eriksonian: Emotion/Personality
  Birth–1 year—Sense of Trust vs. Mistrust
Piagetian: Intellectual Activity (Thought Process)
  Birth–2 years—Sensorimotor Period
	Motor Development
	Cruises around furniture.
	Beginning to stand alone and toddle.
	Turns pages in book.
	Tries tossing object.
	Shows hand dominance.
	Navigates stairs; climbs on chairs.
	Builds a tower of 2 blocks.
	Puts balls in box.
	May use spoon.
	Can release objects at will.
	Has regular bowel movements.
	
	Socialization and Verbalization
	Uses jargon.
	Points to indicate wants.
	Loves give-and-take game.
	Responds to music.
	Enjoys being center of attention and will repeat laughed-at activities.
	
	Cognitive and Emotional Development
	Shows fear, anger, affection, jealousy, anxiety, and sympathy.
		Play Stimulation
		Ball play
		Cloth doll
		Motion objects and toys
		Transporting objects
		Name and point to body parts.
		"Put-in" and "take-out" toys
		Sand box with spoons and other similar objects.
		Blocks
		Music
		
		Parental Guidance
		Allow self-directed play rather than adult-directed play.
		Continue to expose to foods of different textures, taste, smell, substance.
		Offer cup.
		Show affection and encourage child to return affection.
		Tuberculin test as well as measles, mumps, and rubella immunization should be given at 15 months.

(continued)

Infant to Adolescent:
Growth and Development *(continued)*

Age and Physical Characteristics	Behavior Patterns	Nursing Implications/ Parental Guidance
	Cognitive and Emotional Development *(continued)* Experiments to reach new goals. Displays intense determination to remove barriers to action. Begins to develop concepts of space, time, and causality. Has increased attention span.	
18 months NOTE: Between 1 and 3 years the child is called a "toddler." Anterior fontanelle closes. Abdomen protrudes, arms and legs lengthen. Big muscles become well developed. 4 cuspids appear by 18 months. Fine muscle coordination begins to develop. Toddler Average yearly weight gain, 2–3 kg. (4½–6½ lbs.). Average height gain during second year, 12 cm. (4¾ inches).	***Motor Development*** Walks up stairs with help, creeps downstairs. Walks without support and with balance. Falls less frequently. Throws ball. Stoops to pick up toys, look at bug. Turns pages of book. Holds and lifts cup. Builds 3-block tower. Picks up and places small beads in container. Begins to use spoon. ***Cognitive and Emotional Development*** Has vocabulary of 10 words that have meanings. Uses phrases, imitates words. Points to objects named by adult. Follows directions and requests. Imitates adult behavior. Retrieves toy from several hiding places. Is beginning to develop symbolic thought. ***Psychosocial Development*** Develops new awareness of strangers. Wants to explore everything in reach. Plays alone, but near others. Is dependent upon parents, but begins to reach out for autonomy. Finds security in a blanket, toy, or thumbsucking.	***Play Stimulation*** Allow unrestricted motor activity (within safety limits). Offer push-pull toys. Child selects favorite toy. Child likes blocks, pyramid toys, teddy bears, dolls, pots and pans, cloth picture books with colorful large pictures, telephone, musical top, nested blocks. ***Parental Guidance*** Begin to teach tooth brushing to establish good dental habits. Safety teaching: Child gets into everything within his reach. Place medications in safe, locked place. Create a safe environment for child. DTP and TOPV booster immunization. Limits need to be set that give toddler sense of security, yet encourage exploration. Identify behavior changes common in toddler.
2 years Protruding abdomen less noticeable. Landau reflex disappears. During first 2 years 35 cm. (14–15 inches) are added to height.	***Motor Development*** Walks up and down stairs. Opens doors; turns knobs. Has steady gait. Holds drinking cup well with 1 hand. Uses spoon without spilling food (may prefer fingers). Kicks a ball in front of him without support. Builds a tower of 4–6 blocks. Scribbles.	***Play Stimulation*** Shows parallel play, although he enjoys having other children around him. Has very short attention span. Enjoys same toys as child of 18 months. Likes doll play, ball. Imitates parents in domestic activities. Likes swing, hammering, paper, large crayons.

(continued)

Age and Physical Characteristics	Behavior Patterns	Nursing Implications/ Parental Guidance
	Motor Development (continued) Rides tricycle or kiddie car (without pedals). ***Cognitive Development*** Has 200–300 words in vocabulary. Begins to use short sentences. Refers to self by pronoun. Obeys simple commands. Does not know right from wrong. Begins to learn about time sequences. ***Psychosocial Development*** Uses word "mine" constantly. Is possessive with toys. Displays negativism—uses "no" as assertion of self. Routine and rituals are important. Begins cooperation in toilet training. Resists restrictions on freedom. Has fear of parents' leaving. Shows parallel play. Dawdles. Resists bedtime—uses transitional objects (blanket, toy). Vacillates between dependence and independence.	***Parental Guidance*** Has need for peer companionship, although he displays his immaturity by his inability to share and take turns. A decrease in appetite normally occurs at this stage. Toilet training should be started (each child follows his own pattern). Begin to have child eat his meals with family if he has not already done so. Begin to read to child; child likes storybooks with large pictures.
2–3 years Height approximates half his adult height. Legs are about 34% of body length. Begins 2+ kg. (5 lbs.) weight gain per year until 5 years old. At 2½ years has full set (20) of baby teeth. 4 second molars appear by 2½ years. Height gain, 6–8 cm. (2⅜–3¼ inches). Lordosis and protuberant abdomen of toddler disappear	***Motor Development*** Throws objects overhead. Pedals tricycle. Walks backward. Washes and dries hands. Begins to use scissors. Can string large beads. Can undress himself. Feeds himself well. Tries to dance. Jumps in place. Builds tower of 8 blocks. Balances on one foot. Swings and climbs. Can eat an ice cream cone. Drinks from a straw. Chews gum without swallowing it. ***Cognitive Development*** Shows increased attention span. Gives first and last name. Begins to ask "why." Is egocentric in thought and behavior. Beginning ability to reflect on own behavior. Talks in short sentences. Uses plurals. May attempt to sing simple songs. Has vocabulary of 900 words.	***Play Stimulation*** Plays simple games with other children. Enjoys story-telling and dress-up play. Plays "house." Colors. Uses scissors and paper. Rides tricycle. Read simple books to him. Will assist in developing memory skills, visual discrimination skills, and language. ***Parental Guidance*** From 2–3 years, the child develops a seeming maturity; do not expect more of him than he is able to do. Arrange first visit to the dentist to have teeth checked. Be aware that negativistic and ritualistic behavior is normal. Be consistent in discipline. Control temper tantrums. Begin to teach traffic safety. Supervise outdoor play. Screening for serum cholesterol should be done if child at risk because of family history.

(continued)

Infant to Adolescent:
Growth and Development (continued)

Age and Physical Characteristics	Behavior Patterns	Nursing Implications/ Parental Guidance
	Cognitive Development (continued) Begins fantasy. Begins to understand what it means to take turns. Can repeat 3 numbers. Shows interest in colors.	

Child Development Theories
Freudian:
   1–3 years—Anal Stage
Eriksonian:
   1–3 years—Sense of Autonomy vs. Shame and Doubt
Piagetian:
   2–7 years—Preoperational Period; shows egocentrism and centering
	Psychosocial Development
	Negativism grows out of child's sense of developing independence—says "no" to every command.
	Ritualism is important to toddler for his security (follows certain pattern, especially at bedtime).
	Temper tantrums may result from toddler's frustration in wanting to do everything himself.
	Shows parallel play as well as beginning interaction with others.
	Engages in associative play.
	Fears become pronounced.
	Continues to react to separation from parents but shows increasing ability to handle short periods of separation.
	Has daytime bladder control and is beginning to develop nighttime bladder control.
	Becomes more independent.
	Begins to identify sex (gender) roles.
	Explores environment outside the home.
	Can create different ways of getting desired outcome.	

3–4 years NOTE: Between 3 and 5 years, the child is called a "pre-schooler."	***Motor Development*** Drawings have form and meaning, not detail. Copies a circle and a cross. Buttons front and side of clothes. Laces shoes. Bathes self, but needs direction. Brushes teeth. Shows continuous movement going up and down stairs. Climbs and jumps well. Attempts to print letters. ***Cognitive Development*** Awareness of body is more stable; child becomes more aware of own vulnerability. Is less negativistic. Learns some number concepts. Begins naming colors. Can identify longer of 2 lines. Has vocabulary of 1500 words. Uses mild profanities and name-calling.	***Play Stimulation*** Plays and interacts with other children. Shows creativity. Likes ring-around-the rosy. "Helps" adults. Likes costumes and enjoys dramatic play. Toys and games: record player, nursery rhymes, housekeeping toys, transportation toys (tricycle, trucks, cars, wagon), blocks, hammer and peg bench, floor trains, blackboard and chalk, easel and brushes, clay, crayon and finger paints, outside toys (sandbox, swing, small slide), books (short stories, action stories), drum, scrapbook. ***Parental Guidance*** Base your expectations within child's limitations. Provide limited frustrations from

(continued)

Age and Physical Characteristics	Behavior Patterns	Nursing Implications/ Parental Guidance
	Cognitive Development *(continued)* Uses language aggressively. Asks many questions. Can be given simple explanation as to cause and effect. Thinks very concretely; demonstrates irreversibility of thought. Has beginning understanding of past and future. Is egocentric in thought. ***Psychosocial Development*** Is more active with peers and engages in cooperative play. Performs simple tasks. Frequently has imaginary companion. Dramatizes experiences. Is proud of accomplishments. Exaggerates, boasts, and tattles on others. Can tolerate separation from mother longer without feeling anxiety. Is keen observer. Has good sense of "mine" and "yours." Behavior still frequently ritualistic. Becomes curious about life and sex. Often indulges in masturbation.	***Parental Guidance*** *(continued)* environment to assist him in coping. Give small errands to do around the house (putting silverware on table, drying a dish). Expand child's world with trips to the zoo, to the supermarket, to restaurant, etc. Prevent accidents. Provide for brief nonthreatening separation from parents and home. Reinforce correct use of language. Utilize opportunities for simple sexual education as child's needs arise. Accept masturbation as a normal phenomenon to be discouraged in public. Provide consistent discipline, motivated by love not anger. Prepare child for nursery school.

4–5 years
By 2–5 years adds 25 cm. (9–10 inches) to height.
At age 4, legs comprise about 44% of body length.
 	
Child Development Theories
Freudian:
   3–6 years—Phallic Stage
Eriksonian:
   3–6 years—Sense of Initiative vs. Guilt
Piagetian:
   2–7 years—Preoperational Period; shows egocentrism and centering
	Motor Development
	Hops 2 or more times.
	Dresses without supervision.
	Has good motor control—climbs and jumps well.
	Walks up stairs without grasping handrail.
	Walks backwards.
	Washes self without wetting clothes.
	Prints first name and other words.
	Adds 3 or more details in drawings.
	Draws a square.
	
	Cognitive Development
	Has 2100-word vocabulary.
	Talks constantly.
	Uses adult speech forms.
	Participates in conversations.
	Asks for definitions.
	Knows age and residence.
	Identifies heavier of two objects.
	Knows weeks as time units.
	Names days of week.
	Begins to understand kinship.
	Knows primary colors.
	Can count to 10.
	Can copy a triangle.
	Has high degree of imagination.
	Questioning is at a peak.
	Begins to develop power of reasoning.
		Play Stimulation
		Demonstrates gross motor activity—likes to jump rope, skip, climb on jungle gyms, etc.
		Prefers group play and cooperates in projects.
		Plays simple letter, number, form, and picture games.
		Plays with cars and trucks.
		Still likes being read to.
		Continues to enjoy fantasy play.
		
		Parental Guidance
		Child no longer takes an afternoon nap.
		Prepare child for kindergarten.
		Tell him stories.
		Provide opportunities and reassurance for group play; have his friends visit for lunch and an afternoon of playing.
		Prevent accidents.
		Between 4 and 6 years DTP and TOPV booster immunizations are needed.
		Encourage child's participation in household activities.

(continued)

Infant to Adolescent:
Growth and Development *(continued)*

Age and Physical Characteristics	Behavior Patterns	Nursing Implications/ Parental Guidance
	Psychosocial Development May have an imaginary companion. Has a sense of order (likes to finish what he has started). Is obedient and reliable. Is protective toward younger children. Begins to develop an elementary conscience with some influence in governing his behavior. Has increased self-confidence. Accepts responsibility for acts. Is less rebellious. Has dreams and nightmares. Is cooperative and sympathetic. Shows generosity with toys. Begins to question parents' thinking. Identifies strongly with parent of same sex.	
Middle Childhood (5–9 years) Growth rate is slow and steady. Child gains an average of 3.18 kg. (7 lbs.) per year. Height increases approximately 6.25 cm. (2½ inches) per year. Among children there is considerable variation in height and weight. Child appears taller and slimmer. Early lordosis disappears. Child begins to lose baby teeth; permanent teeth appear at a rate of about 4 teeth per year from 7–14 years. Neuromuscular and skeletal development allows improved coordination. Eyes become fully developed; vision approaches 20/20. ***Child Development Theories*** Freudian: 5–9 years—Beginning of Latency Period Eriksonian: 5–9 years—Industry vs. Inferiority Piagetian: 5–9 years—Enters stage of concrete operations	***Motor Development*** 6 years Is active and impulsive. Balance improves. Uses hands as manipulative tools in cutting, pasting, hammering. Can draw large letters or figures. 7 years Has lower activity level. Capable of fine hand movements; can print sentences. Nervous habits such as nail biting are common. Muscular skills such as ball throwing have improved. 8 years Moves with less restlessness. Has developed grace and balance, even in active sports. Has developed coordination of fine muscles, allowing him to write in script. 9 years Uses both hands independently Has become skillful in manual activities because of improved eye–hand coordination. ***Cognitive Development*** 6 years Begins to learn to read. Defines objects in terms of use. Time sense is as much in past as present. Is interested in relationship between home and neighborhood; knows some streets. Uses sentences well; uses language to share others' experiences; may swear or use slang.	Family atmosphere continues to have impact on child's emotional development and his future response within the family. The child needs ongoing guidance in an open, inviting atmosphere. Limits should be set with conviction. Deal with only one incident at a time. When punishment is necessary, the child should not be humiliated. He should know that it was the *act* that the adult found undesirable, not the child. Needs assistance in adjusting to new experiences and demands of school. Should be able to share experiences with family. Parents need to have communication with the teacher in order to work together for the health of the child. Convey love and caring in communication. The child understands language directed at feelings better than at intellect. Get down to eye level with the child. Focus attention on child's abilities and accomplishments rather than his shortcomings and limitations. Child is sex-conscious. He should be able to discuss his questions at home rather than with his friends. Requires simple, honest answers to questions. Common problems include teasing, quarreling, nail-biting, enuresis, whining, poor manners, swearing. These are usually fleeting phases and should not be han-

(continued)

Age and Physical Characteristics	Behavior Patterns	Nursing Implications/ Parental Guidance
	Cognitive Development *(continued)*	***Parental Guidance*** *(continued)*

Cognitive Development (continued)

Distinguishes morning from afternoon.

7 years

More reflective and has deeper understanding of meanings.

Interested in conclusions and logical endings. Begins to have scientific interests in cause and effect.

More responsible in relation to time, is more punctual. Sense of space is more realistic; child wants some space of own.

Knows value of coins.

8 years

Thinking is less animistic. Is aware of impersonal forces of nature. Begins to understand logical reasoning, conclusions, implications.

Less self-centered in thinking. Personal space is expanding; goes places on own. Aware of time; plans events of day. Understands right from left.

9 years

Intellectually energetic and curious. Realistic; reasonable in thinking. Able to plan in advance. Breaks complex activities into steps.

Focuses on detail.

Sense of space includes the entire earth.

Participates in family discussions. Likes to have secrets.

Psychosocial Development

(The following characteristics apply to the child in the 5–9-year group.)

Still requires parental support, but pulls away from overt signs of affection.

Peer groups provide companionship in widening circle of persons outside the home. Child learns more about self as he learns about others.

"Chum" stage occurs at about 9–10 years of age. Child chooses a special friend of same sex and age in whom to confide. This is usually child's first love relationship outside of home, when someone becomes as important to him as himself.

Play teaches the child new ideas and independence. He progres-

Parental Guidance (continued)

dled negatively. The causes for such behavior should be investigated and dealt with constructively.

The child needs order and consistency in his life to help him cope with doubts, fears, unacceptable impulses, and unfamiliar experiences.

Encourage peer activities as well as home responsibilities and give recognition to child's accomplishments and unique talents.

Television may stimulate learning in several spheres, but should be monitored.

Accidents are a major cause of disability and death. Safety practices should be continued. (Refer to section on safety, pp. 1111–1114

Exercise is essential to promote motor and psychosocial development. The child should have a safe place to play and simple pieces of equipment.

A school health program should be available and concerned with the child's physical, emotional, mental, and social health. This should be augmented by information and example at home.

Medical supervision should continue with yearly examination to detect developmental delay, disease. Appropriate immunizations should be administered.

Child frequently has "quiet days"— periods of shyness, which should be tolerated as part of growing up and deciding who he is.

Child may be subject to nightmares, a situation that requires reassurance and understanding.

Parents, teachers, and health professionals should be available and able to provide information and answer questions about the physical changes that occur.

(continued)

Infant to Adolescent: Growth and Development *(continued)*

Age and Physical Characteristics	Behavior Patterns	Nursing Implications/ Parental Guidance
	Psychosocial Development (continued) sively utilizes tools of competition, compromise, cooperation, and beginning collaboration. Body image and self-concept are quite fluid because of rapid physical, emotional, social changes. Latency-stage sexual drive is controlled and repressed. Emphasis is on the development of skills and talent. ***Patterns of Play*** 6–7 years Child acts out ideas of family and occupational groups with which he has contact. Painting, pasting, reading, simple games, watching television, digging, running games, skating, riding bicycle, and swimming are all enjoyed activities. 8 years Child enjoys collections; loosely formed, short-lived clubs; table games; card games; books; television; records.	
Late Childhood (9–12 years) Vital signs approach adult values. Loses childish appearance of face and takes on features that will characterize him as an adult. Growth spurt occurs, and some secondary sex characteristics appear: in females, at age 10–12 years; in males, at age 12–14 years. Physical changes of puberty: Increased height and weight, increased perspiration and activity of sebaceous glands; vasomotor instability; increased fat deposition. Physical changes in female: Pelvis increases in transverse diameter; hips broaden; tenderness in developing breast tissue; enlargement of areola diameter; appearance of pubic hair. Physical changes in male: Size of testes increases; scrotum color changes; breasts enlarge, temporarily; height and shoulder breadth increase Appearance of lightly pigmented hair at base of penis.	***Motor Development*** Energetic, restless, active movements such as finger-drumming or foot-tapping appear. Has skillful manipulative movements nearly equal to those of adults. Works hard to perfect physical skills. ***Cognitive Development*** 10 years Likes to reason, enjoys learning. Thinking is concrete, matter of fact. Wants to measure up to challenge. Likes to memorize, identify facts. Attention span may be short. Space is rather specific (i.e., where things are). Can write for relatively long time with speed. 11 years Likes action in learning. Concentrates well when working competitively. Can understand relational terms such as weight and size. Perceives space as nothingness that goes on forever. Able to discuss problems.	Continue appropriate nursing interventions related to early childhood. Continue sex education and preparation for adolescent body changes. Understanding is important. Encourage participation in organized clubs, youth groups. Democratic guidance is essential as child works through a conflict between dependence (on his parents) and independence. Child needs realistic limits set. Needs help channeling energy in proper direction—work and sports. Requires adequate explanation of body changes. Special understanding required for the child who lags in physical development. Continue consistent disciplinary style.

(continued)

Age and Physical Characteristics	Behavior Patterns	Nursing Implications/ Parental Guidance

Increase in length and width of penis.
Child Development Theories
Freudian:
  9–12 years—Latency Period continues
Eriksonian:
  9–12 years—Industry vs. Inferiority continues
Piagetian:
  9–12 years—Stage of concrete operations continues
	Cognitive Development (continued)
	Can describe some abstract terms.
	12 years
	  Enjoys learning.
	  Considers all aspects of a situation.
	  Motivated more by inner drive than by competition.
	  Able to classify, arrange, generalize.
	  Likes to discuss and debate.
	  Begins conceptual thinking.
	  Verbal, formal reasoning now possible.
	  Can recognize moral of a story.
	  Defines time as duration; likes to plan ahead.
	  Understands that space is abstract.
	  Can be critical of own work.
	
	Psychosocial Development
	Gang becomes important, and gang code takes precedence over nearly everything. Often gang codes are characterized by collective action against the mores of the adult world. Here, children begin to work out own social patterns without adult interference. Early gangs may include both sexes; later gangs are separated by sex.
	May strive for unreasonable independence from adult control.
	Often interested in religion, morality.
	Has increased interest in sexuality.
	May reach puberty; resurgence of sexual drives causes recapitulation of oedipal struggle.
	
	Patterns of Play
	Continues to enjoy reading, T.V., table games.
	More interested in active sports as a means to improve skills.
	Creative talents may appear; may enjoy drawing, modeling clay. By age 10, sex differences in play become profound.
	Occasional privacy is important.
	Begins to have vocational aspirations.	

Early Adolescence (females: 12–14 years; males: 14–18 years) Phase of development begins when reproductive organs become functionally operative; phase ends when physical growth is completed.	***Motor Development*** Often uncoordinated; has poor posture. Tires easily. ***Cognitive Development.*** Mind has great ability to acquire and utilize knowledge.	Stresses frequently result from conflicting value systems between generations. Parents may need help to see that the adolescent is a product of the times and that his actions reflect what is happening around him.

(continued)

Infant to Adolescent:
Growth and Development (continued)

Age and Physical Characteristics	Behavior Patterns	Nursing Implications/ Parental Guidance

Skeletal system grows faster than supporting muscles.
Hands and feet grow proportionately faster than rest of body.
Large muscles develop more quickly than small muscles.
Females:
    Physical changes include appearance of menarche; growth of axillary and perineal hair; deepened voice; ovulation; further development of breasts.
Male:
    Physical changes include growth of axillary, perineal, facial, chest hair; deepening of voice; production of spermatozoa; nocturnal emissions.
Child Development Theories
Freudian:
    12–14 years—Begins stage of sexuality
Eriksonian:
    12–14 years—Identity vs. Role Diffusion
Piagetian:
    12–14 years—Begins stage of formal operations
	Cognitive Development (continued)
	Categorizes thoughts into usable forms.
	May project thinking into the future.
	Is capable of highly imaginative thinking.
	Psychosocial Development
	Interest in opposite sex increases.
	Often revolts from adult authority to conform to peer-group standards.
	Continues to rework feelings for parent of opposite sex and unravel the ambivalence toward parent of same sex.
	Affection may turn temporarily to an adult outside of the family (for example, crush on family friend, neighbor, or teacher).
	Utilizes peer-group dialect—highly informal language or specially coined terminology.
	Peer groups are especially important and help adolescent to define own identity, to adapt to changing body image, to establish more mature relationships with others, and to deal with heightened sexual feelings. Cliques may develop.
	Dating generally progresses from groups of couples to double dates and finally single couples.
	Teenage "hangouts" become important centers of activity.
	Begins questioning existing moral values.
		Parents' limits and rules should be realistic and consistent. They should convey the love and concern of parents and should be a source of comfort and reassurance, protecting the child from activities for which he is not ready.
		The home should be an accepting, emotionally stable environment.
		Continue sex education, including discussion of ovulation, fertilization, menstruation, pregnancy, contraception, masturbation, nocturnal emissions, and hygiene.
		Adolescents have an increased need for rest and sleep, because they are expending large amounts of energy and are functioning with an inadequate oxygen supply.
		Recreational interests should be fostered. Favorite activities include sports, dating, dancing, reading, hobbies, and television. Talking on the telephone, listening to records are favorite pastimes.
		Adolescent health problems that require preventive education are accidents, obesity, acne, pregnancy, sexually transmitted disease, drug abuse.
		Allow adolescent to handle his own affairs as much as possible, but be aware of physical and psychosocial problems with which he will need help. Encourage independence but allow child to lean on parents for support when frightened or unable to attain his goals.
		Adolescents with special problems should have access to specialists such as adolescent clinics, and psychologists.
		Requires reassurance and help in accepting his changing body image. Parents should make the most of his positive qualities.
		Give gentle encouragement and guidance regarding dating. Avoid strong pressures in either direction.
		Understand his conflicts as he attempts to deal with social, moral, and intellectual issues.

(continued)

Age and Physical Characteristics	Behavior Patterns	Nursing Implications/ Parental Guidance
		Provide opportunities for adolescents to earn their own money; allow some financial independence. Provide safety education—especially regarding driving. Provide assistance to develop good attitudes toward health—smoking, drinking, drugs, nutrition, etc.

Late Adolescence
  Begins when physical growth is complete and extends from age 15–18 years for females and from 18–20 for males.
  Wisdom teeth erupt.
Males:
Genitals and pubic hair are adult in appearance. Physique is that of mature male.
Females:
  Breasts and pubic hair are adult in appearance.
 	
Child Development Theories
Freudian:
  15–18 years—Stage of Adult Sexuality
Eriksonian:
  15–18 years—May begin Intimacy vs. Isolation
Piagetian:
  15–18 years—Stage of Formal Operations
	Motor Development
	Energy is increased as growth spurt ends.
	Muscular ability and coordination increase.
	
	Cognitive Development
	Spends large amount of time in abstract and analytical thinking.
	Begins to develop workable philosophy of life.
	May accept or reject the family religion.
	
	Psychosocial Development
	Tasks include achievement of ego identity, establishment of heterosexual relationships, planning for the future and for occupational and marital choices.
	Dating emphasis shifts to sharing and to intimate relationship.
	Sexual experimentation is common in various forms—masturbation, necking, petting, intercourse.
	May seek alternatives to marriage—"living together," communes, etc.
	Ability to love becomes a major concern.
	Values include fidelity, friendship, cooperation.
	Ability to work is the culmination of the developmental life that began with play.
	Achieves emotional independence from parents and other adults.
		Continue appropriate nursing interventions related to early adolescence.
		
		Provide guidance in selection of and preparation for a vocation.
		
		Encourage discussion regarding mate selection and alternatives to marriage.
		
		Parents themselves may require assistance facing the loss of a child once dependent on them.

Childhood Diseases

Disease: *a.* Agent. *b.* Mode of transmission. *c.* Age when most common	Incubation (*I*) and Communicability (*C*) Periods	Symptoms
Rubella (German/3-day measles) a. Rubella virus, RNA togavirus b. Droplets or direct contact with infected persons or articles freshly contaminated with nasopharyngeal secretions, feces, urine c. School age, young adult; winter, spring *Diagnostic tests:* Tissue culture of throat, blood or urine; serologic studies (hemagglutination inhibition and complement fixation). ELISA antibody study on serum 1–2 weeks apart *Passive immunity:* Birth to about 1 year of age if mother is immune prior to pregnancy)	*I:* 14–21 days after exposure *C:* Virus can be passed from 7 days before to 5 days after rash appears.	a. Rash—enlarged lymph nodes in postauricular, suboccipital, and cervical areas b. In adolescents—headache, anorexia, low-grade fever, sore throat, coryza, conjunctivitis, generalized malaise 1–5 days before rash appears *Duration:* 3–5 days *Rash characteristics:* Pinpoint (or larger) red spots on soft palate (Forchheimer's spots) spread to face and downward toward the feet, covering entire body at end of first day; maculopapular eruption. Rash begins to subside on 2nd day in same order
Roseola infantum (exanthema subitum) a. Presumably caused by virus. May be syndrome due to many different viruses, not specifically roseola virus. b. Transmission not known c. 6 months–2 years; late fall–early spring	*I:* 5–15 days *C:* Not known—believed not to be highly contagious	a. Fever of 40°–40.5°C. (104°–105°F.), either intermittent or sustained 3–4 days; decrease in appetite; slightly irritable b. Fever suddenly drops and rash of red measles or maculopapules 2–3 mm. appears *Duration:* 1–2 days Rash fades on pressure. It appears first on trunk and spreads upward and downward.
Rubeola (hard, red, 7-day measles) a. Measles virus, RNA-containing paramyxovirus b. Direct contact with droplets from infected persons, respiratory route *Diagnostic tests:* Serologic procedures *Passive immunity:* Birth to about 1 year of age if mother is immune prior to pregnancy c. Over 10 years, adolescent, adult; spring/winter	*I:* 10–12 days *C:* 5th day of incubation to first 5–7 days of rash	a. Fever, lethargy, cough, coryza, conjunctivitis b. 48 hours—Koplik's spots on buccal mucosa (spots are reddened areas with grayish-blue center) c. 2 days later, rash appears at hairline and spreads to feet in one day, maculopapular eruption which begins to clear after 3–4 days d. Lymphadenopathy e. Anorexia f. Pruritus
Mumps a. Mumps virus, paramyxovirus b. Urine, blood, and saliva by direct contact or droplets; respiratory route *Diagnostic tests:* Complement fixation; cell culture from throat, urine, spinal fluid *Passive immunity:* Birth to 3–4 months of age if mother had antibodies against mumps prior to pregnancy c. School-age; late winter/early spring	*I:* 14–21 days *C:* 5 days before to 9 days after swelling appears; virus in saliva greatest just before and after parotitis onset	a. Headache, anorexia, generalized malaise; fever 1 day before glandular swelling; fever lasts 1–6 days. b. Glandular swelling, usually of parotid—one side or bilaterally c. Enlargement and reddening of Wharton's duct and Stensen's duct d. Subclinical infection may occur

(continued)

Treatment	Complications	Special Considerations

Symptomatic—Isolation	In adolescent and adult:
	  Arthritis; arthralgias
	  Encephalitis
	  Thrombocytopenia
		Exposure of nonimmune pregnant women in first trimester results in high percentage of affected fetuses and infants born with various birth defects: cataracts, heart murmur, deafness

Symptomatic—Antipyretic	Convulsions due to high fever Encephalitis (rare)	

Symptomatic
  Bed rest: isolation from onset of catarrh through 3rd day of rash
  Encourage fluid intake
Treatment of itching: Cornstarch bath, mitt hands, application of calamine lotion to lesions, keeping fingernails trimmed
	Otitis media, pneumonia, laryngitis, mastoiditis, encephalitis, appendicitis	

Isolation until swelling has subsided
Symptomatic
  Analgesics
  Hydration
  Alimentation
  Antipyretics
  Rest
	Meningoencephalitis
	Auditory nerve involvement, resulting in deafness
	Orchitis (if disease occurs after puberty)
		Passive immunization (immune globulin—human)—should be administered (0.25 mg./kg.) within 5 days; when susceptible child under 1 year has known exposure; especially important when child not immunized because of contraindications.
		0.5 ml./kg. IG for immunocompromised child, not to exceed 15 ml. of IG

(continued)

Childhood Diseases *(continued)*

Disease: *a.* Agent. *b.* Mode of transmission. *c.* Age when most common	Incubation (*I*) and Communicability (*C*) Periods	Symptoms
Chickenpox a. Varicella-zoster b. Highly communicable; acquired via direct contact, indirect contact, droplet spread, airborne transmission c. 2–8 years *Diagnostic tests:* Scrapings from vesicle; staining reveals multinucleated giant cells *Passive immunity:* Best accomplished by varicella-zoster immune globulin	*I:* 14–21 days after exposure *C:* Onset of fever (1 day prior to first lesion) until last vesicle is dried (5–7 days)	a. General malaise and fever for 24 hours b. Rash—macules to papules and vesicles to crusts within several hours c. Itching of lesions may be severe, and scratching may cause scarring *Rash characteristics:* Rash appears first on head and mucous membranes, then becomes concentrated on body and sparse on extremities, papulovesicular eruption
Diphtheria a. *Corynebacterium diphtheriae* b. Acquired through secretions of carrier or infected individual by direct contact with contaminated articles and environment c. Incidence increased in autumn and winter *Diagnostic tests:* Cultures of nose and throat	*I:* 2–6 days *C:* 2–4 weeks untreated; 1–2 days with antibiotic treatment	a. Pharyngeal and tonsillar diphtheria: (1) General malaise, low-grade fever, anorexia (2) 1–2 days later, whitish-gray membranous patch on tonsils, soft palate, and uvula (3) Lymph node swelling, fever, rapid pulse b. Nasal diphtheria: (1) Coryza with increasing viscosity, possibly epistaxis, low-grade fever (2) Whitish-gray membrane may appear over nasal septum c. Laryngeal diphtheria: (1) Usually spread from pharynx to larynx (2) Fever, harsh voice, barking cough; respiratory difficulty with inspiratory retraction d. Nonrespiratory diphtheria: affects eye, ear, genitals, or, rarely, skin
Pertussis (whooping cough) a. *Bordetella pertussis* b. Direct contact, droplet spread; indirect contact with contaminated articles c. Infants and young children; incidence higher in spring and summer *Diagnostic test*—culture of nasopharyngeal mucus	*I:* 5–21 days *C:* 7 days after exposure (greatest just before catarrhal stage) to 3 weeks after onset of paroxysms	a. Stage I (catarrhal stage) (1) Lasts 1–2 weeks (2) Coryza, sneezing, tearing, tickling/dry cough, fever, loss of appetite b. Stage II (paroxysmal stage) (1) Lasts 2–6 weeks (2) Severe, violent coughing attacks occurring in clusters leading to vomiting, cyanosis, and exhaustion c. Stage III (convalescent stage) (1) Lasts 2 weeks–several months (2) Coughing attacks decrease, but return with each respiratory infection *Duration:* 9 months–2 years

(continued)

Treatment	Complications	Special Considerations
Symptomatic: Short fingernails to prevent scratching Oral antihistamines to decrease pruritus Isolation until all lesions have crusted—about 5–6 days Treatment of itching: Mix baking soda (sodium bicarbonate) with warm water and pat on lesions drying lotion (i.e., calamine) *DO NOT GIVE* salicylates	Complications are rare in normal children Hemorrhagic varicella, encephalitis, pneumonia, and bacterial skin infection are not common, but they can occur Reye's syndrome	Severe in neonate and pregnant women Varicella-zoster immune globulin (VZIG) is available from Centers for Disease Control (Atlanta, GA) for high-risk susceptible children who have been exposed to varicella zoster. This should be given within 72 hours of exposure to varicella-zoster. If VZIG is unavailable, immune globulin at a dose of 0.6–1.2 ml./kg. body weight; promptly given, may modify varicella
Diphtheria antitoxin Antibiotic therapy (penicillin, erythromycin) Supportive treatment Respiratory support Isolation until 2–3 cultures are negative after antibiotic therapy is completed	Myocarditis Neuritis Paralysis	

Supportive:
  Bed rest
  Suctioning
  Antipyretics
  Antibiotics: erythromcyin, ampicillin
  Increase fluids; nutrition and electrolyte balance
  Place in an environment with reduced stimuli to reduce coughing
  Sedation
  Isolation 4 weeks after coughing begins and continued for 7 days after onset of therapy with erythromycin
	Respiratory: pneumonia, atelectasis, emphysema, bronchopneumonia
	Neurologic: brain damage	

NURSING ALERT: Before administering EACH DTP immunization, the parent or guardian should be questioned about possible adverse events following the previous dose.

(continued)

Childhood Diseases *(continued)*

Disease: *a.* Agent. *b.* Mode of transmission. *c.* Age when most common	Incubation (*I*) and Communicability (*C*) Periods	Symptoms
Tetanus (lockjaw) a. *Clostridium tetani*—prevalence in soil and animal feces; can be introduced into body through any break in skin or intestinal tract b. Direct or indirect contact with wound c. All ages *Diagnostic tests:* Wound culture anaerobically for *Clostridium tetani*	*I:* 3 days–3 weeks; 8 days average *C:* None	a. Stiffening of striated muscles, usually the jaw. b. 1–2 days later, stiffening leads to spastic rigidity and spreads down body to the extremities
Poliomyelitis (polio) a. Virus serotypes 1, 2, and 3; incidence is higher in summer and fall b. Virus is harbored in GI tract and is transmitted through saliva, vomitus, and feces c. Predisposing factors that increase risk of disease: recent tonsillectomy, tooth extraction or DTP injections, pregnancy, physical exhaustion *Diagnostic tests:* Isolation of polio virus from feces and throat	*I:* 7–14 days, paralytic or nonparalytic; 3–5 days for prodromal or minor illness *C:* Increases around onset when virus is in throat and is excreted in feces; virus is present in throat 1 week after onset, in stool 4–6 weeks after	a. Nonparalytic polio: (1) Headache, lethargy, anorexia, vomiting, fever (2) Muscle pain and stiffness b. Paralytic polio: (1) Same as nonparalytic type, lasting about 1 week (2) Then 1–2 days of CNS symptoms: loss of deep tendon reflexes, positive Kernig's and Brudzinski's signs, lethargy (3) 1–2 days later, weakening of muscles and paralysis
Streptococcal pharyngitis ("strep throat") a. Beta hemolytic streptococcus—group A strain b. Direct or indirect contact with nasopharyngeal secretion of infected person or recently established carrier c. Not under 3 years of age; 5–16 years; incidence higher in winter and spring *Diagnostic tests:* nasopharyngeal (throat) culture; rapid diagnostic test	*I:* 2–5 days *C:* Greatest during acute phase of illness	a. Onset is generally acute: high fever, headache, vomiting, scarlatina rash b. After 12–24 hours—sore throat of varying degrees of severity, dryness of throat, cervical lymphadenopathy, white tongue coating that gives way to strawberry-red tongue
Impetigo a. Group A streptococcus (more common in older children); *Staphylococcus aureus* (more common in younger children) b. Usually direct contact often initiated by abrasions/insect bites; streptococcal skin lesions often precede URI colonization *Diagnostic tests:* Lesions cleansed; culture on blood agar fluid from intact bleb or base of crusted lesion, no active or passive immunity. Diagnosis is generally made on typical appearance of lesions.	*I:* 7–10 days *C:* Until lesions healed	Lesions: Vesicular, become confluent and rapidly progress to pustular and crusting stage; do not appear in crops. Commonly involve nasolabial area and others easily scratched; typical lesion is a thick, adherent amber-colored crust Bullous impetigo usually caused by staphylococci—superficial bullae 0.5–3 cm., flaccid, thin margin of erythema surrounds bullae Purulent crusting lesions caused by hemolytic streptococci or staphylococci

(continued)

Treatment	Complications	Special Considerations
Tetanus antitoxin Surgical removal of wound site Reduce muscular spasm with medication, quiet, dark room Antibiotics: penicillin G or tetracycline* Tetanus immune globulin Human—(TIG), preferred to equine tetanus antitoxoid (TAT) Debridement of wound Fluid and nutrition	Convulsion with laryngospasms leading to death Asphyxia from dysphagia and secretions	

Nonparalytic:
Supportive (i.e., relief of pain)
Analgesics, heat
Enteric isolation
Bed rest
With muscle weakness:
    Hospitalize
    Fluid and electrolytes
    Rest
    Relief of muscle pain and spasms
    Respiratory support
	Respiratory paralysis
	Hypertension	

Isolation for 1 day while starting prescription
Antibiotic therapy:
    Penicillin G—IM
    Penicillin V—PO
Erythromycin—if allergic to penicillin
	Acute glomerulonephritis, 1–2 weeks after acute stage
	Rheumatic fever, 2–3 weeks after acute stage
	Peritonsillar abscess, cervical adenitis
	Pneumonia, otitis media, meningitis
		Throat cultures are considered for entire household when: others are symptomatic concurrently or within past 3 weeks; frequent or relapsing infections. Repeat throat cultures are recommended after treatment if child has clinical relapse or at high risk for rheumatic fever.

Specific: Systemic antimicrobial therapy for extensive impetigo—oral Pen V or penicillin G for injection; others as indicated Symptomatic: Careful cleansing of lesions with soap and water; short fingernails to prevent scratching	Glomerulonephritis	Isolation necessary for hospitalized child; observe for skin lesions and treat promptly

(continued)

Childhood Diseases *(continued)*

Disease: *a.* Agent. *b.* Mode of transmission. *c.* Age when most common	Incubation (*I*) and Communicability (*C*) Periods	Symptoms

Rabies
a. Rabies virus—a rhabdovirus
b. Saliva via a bite of an infected animal (most common)
c. All ages
Diagnostic tests:
  Infected animal—specific fluorescence in brain tissue
  Human—fluorescence of corneal smear
	I: 9 days–several months; 20–60 days most common	a. During incubation—signs of inflammation and wound healing
		b. Prodrome—2–10 days nonspecific (i.e., malaise, anorexia, fatigue, fever, headache, apprehension, anxiety, agitation, irritability, depression, insomnia)
		c. Acute neurologic (excitation stage)—2–7 days; objective signs of CNS involvement (i.e., hydrophobia, hyperactivity, aphasia, disorientation, hallucinations, seizures, bizarre behavior, nucal rigidity, increased deep tendon reflexes, progressive paralysis [paralysis stage], coma, and/or sudden death)

Rocky Mountain Spotted Fever a. *Rickettsia rickettsii* b. Bite of infected wood tick, American dog tick or Lone Star tick c. All ages; spring and summer *Diagnostic tests:* 1. Immunofluorescent identified virus in skin lesion by punch biopsy 2. Indirect fluorescent antibody 3. Complement fixation to specific antibody formation	*I:* 1–10 days, usually 1 week	a. 3–7 days after exposure: headache, decreased appetite, sore throat, photophobia, nausea, abdominal pain, joint pain b. 3–4 days after illness begins: high spiking fever, nonpitting edema, rash *Rash characteristics:* Rash appears 1–5 days after fever, macular with light rosy hue, blanching with pressure—concentrated on distal extremities, especially wrist and ankles. Rash becomes papular, frequently petechial, dark red, or dusky and slowly moves to trunk and head.

(continued)

Treatment	Complications	Special Considerations
Immediate and thorough cleansing of wound with 20% tincture of green soap with subsequent use of 70% alcohol Debridement as necessary Tetanus immunization Antibiotics *Immediate postexposure prophylaxis:* Concurrent use of active and passive immunity (human products preferable) There is no evidence that treatment of established illness with RIG is effective Isolation Supportive Airway Fluids Temperature control Staff protection—especially of respiratory secretions	Coma Death due to vascular collapse and respiratory arrest Disease may be severe in children with prominent CNS disorders, cardiac symptoms, splenomegaly Local reaction to antirabies treatment; systemic and allergic reactions	Passive Immunity: Human rabies immune globulin (HRIG) 20 IU/kg.; ½ injected around wound and ½ given intermuscular Active immunity: Human diploid cell vaccine (HDCV) five 1-ml. injections over 28 days: 0-3-7-14-28 with booster at 90 days. Duck embryo vaccine (DEV): use only if HDCV unavailable, check sensitivity to duck or chicken protein, given subcutaneous in abdomen—1 ml./dose. Injection every day for 21 days if wound is below waist, or injection two times a day for 7 days, then every day for 7 days if wound is above waist. Booster #1 in 10 days. Booster #2 in 20 days after completion of primary course
Early recognition (fever, rash, edema) Antibiotics—chloramphenicol and tetracyclines (not used for child under 9 years old) Supportive Bed rest Adequate fluid High-protein diet Antipyretics Public education—prevention is best treatment	When treatment is delayed: Brain damage Heart impairments Thrombocytopenia Death	During tick season, care should be given to frequent inspection of body of child for ticks twice daily. Prompt removal is important. To remove tick, use tweezers or fingers covered with tissue to prevent contamination and disease transmission. Grasp tick close to the site of its attachment to skin. Using firm, steady traction, pull tick away. Wash site with soap and water and apply antiseptic or antibiotic ointment, H_2O_2, or alcohol. DO NOT CRUSH TICK—dispose of in container of alcohol or flush down toilet

* Not given to children under 9 years old.
CDC, Atlanta, Georgia 30333; phone (404) 329-3727 days; 329-3644 nights.

Nutrition in Children*

Age and Developmental Influence on Nutritional Requirements and Feeding Patterns	Feeding Pattern/Diet	Nursing Implications/Parental Guidance

Neonate
(birth–4 weeks)
Newborn's rapid growth makes him especially vulnerable to dietary inadequacies, dehydration, and iron deficiency anemia.
Feeding process is basis for infant's first human relationship, his formation of trust. Feeding reinforces mother's sense of "motherliness."
Because of limited nutritional stores, neonates require vitamin and mineral supplements.
Neonates require more fluid relative to their size than do adults.
Sucking ability is influenced by individual neuromuscular maturity.
	Breast milk or formula is generally given in 6–8 feedings per day, spaced 3–4 hours apart.
	Feeding schedules should be individualized according to infant's needs.
		Provide information to help parents make decision concerning breast- or bottle-feeding.
		Support parents in their decision.
		Breast-fed infant (see p. 1004):
		1. Help mother assume comfortable and satisfying position for self and baby.
		2. Help mother to determine schedule, timing, and when infant is satisfied.
		3. Provide specific information about the following:
		  a. Feeding technique: position, "bubbling"
		  b. Care of breasts
		  c. Manual expression of milk from breast
		  d. Maternal diet
		Bottle-fed infant:
		1. Provide specific information concerning
		  a. Type of formula
		  b. Preparation of formula: measuring and sterilization
		  c. Equipment—types of bottles, nipples, etc.
		  d. Sterilization of equipment
		  e. Technique of feeding: position, "bubbling"
		2. Help mother to determine when infant is satisfied; develop schedule for feeding.
		Provide information concerning normal characteristics of stools, signs of dehydration, constipation, colic, milk allergy.
		Discuss need for vitamin supplements and how to administer.
		Discuss need for additional fluids during periods of hot weather, and with fever, diarrhea, and vomiting.
		Observe for evidence of common problems and intervene accordingly:
		1. Overfeeding
		2. Underfeeding
		3. Difficulty digesting formula because of its particular composition.
		4. Improper feeding technique; holes in nipples too large or too small; formula too hot or too cold; uncomfortable feeding position; failure to "bubble"; improper sterilization.
		5. Emotional problems in family may cause irritability, colic, and other similar disturbances.

Infant (3 months–1 year) Increased neuromuscular development allows infant to make transition from a totally liquid diet to a diet of milk and solid foods as well as to more active participation in the feeding process.	Number of feedings per day decreases through the first year. By 1 year of age, most infants are satisfied with 3 meals and additional fluids throughout the day.	New foods should be offered one at a time and early in the feeding while the infant is still hungry. The person feeding should be calm, gentle, relaxed, and patient in approach. When the child is first offered puréed foods with a spoon, he expects and wants to

(continued)

Age and Developmental Influence on Nutritional Requirements and Feeding Patterns	Feeding Pattern/Diet	Nursing Implications/Parental Guidance
Infant (continued) 3–6 months Sucking reflex becomes voluntary and chewing action begins; infant can approximate lips to rim of cup and may begin drinking from cup at 6 months. 6–12 months Eyes and hands can work together; infant is able to sit without support and has developed grasp; able to feed self a biscuit; bangs objects on table; able to hold own bottle at 9–12 months; has "pincher" approach to food; able to be weaned as child becomes developmentally able to take sufficient fluids from the cup. Food provides the infant with a variety of learning experiences; motor control and coordination in self-feeding; recognition of shape, texture, color; stimulation of speech movement through use of mouth muscles. Mealtime allows the infant to continue his development of trust in a consistent, loving atmosphere. The infant is forming his lifetime eating habits; it is therefore important to make mealtime a positive experience.	By 4–6 months of age, the infant is generally ready to begin eating strained foods. The usual sequence of foods is cereal followed by fruits, vegetables, and meats. This sequence may vary according to individual preferences of pediatrician and family. Mashed table foods or junior foods generally are started at 6–8 months, when infant begins chewing action. Infant begins to enjoy finger foods at 10–12 months. The transition from iron-fortified formula or breast milk to cow's milk is usually advised at about 12 months of age.	suck. The protrusion of his tongue, which is needed in sucking, makes it appear that he is pushing the food out of his mouth. This response should not be interpreted as dislike for the food; it is a result of immature muscle coordination and surprise at the taste and feel of the new food. The baby foods selected should be those that are high in nutrients without providing excessive calories. Personal and cultural preferences should be considered. Infants should be observed for allergic reactions when new foods are added. Common allergies are to citrus juices and egg white. Finger foods should be selected for their nutritional value. Good choices include teething biscuits, cooked vegetables, meat, cheese sticks, and enriched cereals. Avoid nuts, raisins and raw vegetables, which can cause choking. Parents can be taught to prepare their own strained or junior foods using a commercial baby food grinder or blender. Weaning is a gradual process. 1. Assist parents to recognize indications of readiness. 2. Do not expect the infant to completely drop his old pattern of behavior while learning a new one; allow overlap of old and new techniques. 3. Evening feedings usually the most difficult to eliminate, because the infant is tired and in need of sucking comfort. 4. During illness or household disorganization, the infant may regress and return to sucking to relieve his discomfort and frustration. SPECIAL CONSIDERATIONS: Hospitalized infant Obtain a thorough nursing history that includes the following: Feeding pattern and schedule; types of foods that have been introduced; likes and dislikes; breast- or bottle-fed, type of bottle; temperature at which infant prefers foods and fluids.
Toddler (1–3 years) Growth slows at the end of the first year. The slower growth rate is reflected in a decreased appetite. The toddler has a total of 14–16 teeth, making him more able to chew foods. Increased self-awareness causes	Appetite is sporadic, specific foods may be favored exclusively or refused from time to time. Child may be ritualistic concerning food preferences, schedule, manner of eating, etc. Diet should include a full	Provide foods with a variety of color, texture, and flavor. Toddlers need to experience the feel of foods. Offer small portions. It is fun for the child to ask for more. It is more effective to give small helpings than to insist that he eat a specific amount. Maintain a regular mealtime schedule. Provide appropriate mealtime equipment:

(continued)

Nutrition in Children* *(continued)*

Age and Developmental Influence on Nutritional Requirements and Feeding Patterns	Feeding Pattern/Diet	Nursing Implications/Parental Guidance
Toddler *(continued)*		
the toddler to want to do more for himself. Refusals of food or of assistance in feedings are common ways in which the toddler asserts himself. Since body tissues, especially muscles, continue to grow quite rapidly, protein needs are high.	range of foods: milk, meat, fruits, vegetables, breads, and cereals. Older toddler can be expected to consume about one-half the amount of food that an adult consumes.	1. Silverware scaled to size. 2. Dishes—colorful, unbreakable; shallow, round bowls are preferable to flat plates. 3. Plastic bibs, placemats, and floor coverings permit a relaxed attitude toward child's self-feeding attempts. 4. Comfortable seating at good height and distance from table. Adults who help toddlers at mealtime should be calm and relaxed. Avoid bribes or force feeding because this reinforces negative behavior and may lead to a dislike for mealtime. Encourage independence, but provide assistance when necessary. Do not be concerned about table manners. Avoid the use of soda or "sweets" as rewards or between-meal snacks. Instead, substitute fruit, juice, or cereal. Toddlers who show little interest in eggs, meat, or vegetables should not be permitted to appease their appetite with carbohydrates or milk because this may lead to iron-deficiency anemia (see p. 1299). SPECIAL CONSIDERATIONS: Hospitalized toddler Nursing history should include the following: Feeding pattern and schedule; food likes and dislikes; food allergies; special eating equipment and utensils; whether or not child is weaned and whether he takes bottle to bed; what child is fed when ill.
Preschooler (3–5 years of age) Increased manual dexterity enables child to have complete independence at mealtime. Psychosocially, this is a period of increased imitation and sex identification. The preschooler identifies with parents at the table and will enjoy what parents enjoy. Additional nutritional habits are developed that become part of the child's lifetime practices. Slower growth rate and increased interest in exploring his environment may decrease the preschooler's interest in eating. Eating assumes increasing social significance. Mealtime promotes socialization and provides the preschooler with opportunities to learn appropriate mealtime	Appetite tends to be sporadic. Child requires the same basic 4 food groups as the adult, but in smaller quantities. Generally likes to eat one food from plate at a time. Likes vegetables that are crisp, raw, and cut into finger-sized pieces. Often dislikes strong-tasting foods.	Emphasis should be placed on the quality rather than the amount of food ingested. Foods should be attractively served, mildly flavored, plain, as well as being separated and distinctly identifiable in flavor and appearance. Nutritional foods (e.g., crackers and cheese, yogurt, fruit) should be offered as snacks. Desserts should be nutritious and a natural part of the meal, not used as a reward for finishing the meal or omitted as punishment. Unless they persist, periods of overeating or not wanting to eat certain foods should not cause concern. The overall eating pattern from month to month is more pertinent to assess. Frequent causes of insufficient eating: 1. Unhappy atmosphere at mealtime 2. Overeating between meals 3. Parental example

(continued)

Age and Developmental Influence on Nutritional Requirements and Feeding Patterns	Feeding Pattern/Diet	Nursing Implications/Parental Guidance

Preschooler (continued)
behavior, language skills, and understanding of family rituals.

4. Attention-seeking
5. Excessive parental expectations
6. Inadequate variety or quantity of foods
7. Tooth decay
8. Physical illness
9. Fatigue
10. Emotional disturbance

Measures to increase food intake:
1. Allow child to help with preparations, planning menu, setting table, and other simple chores.
2. Maintain calm environment with no distractions.
3. Avoid between-meal snacks.
4. Provide rest period before meal.
5. Avoid coaxing, bribing, threatening.

SPECIAL CONSIDERATIONS: Hospitalized preschooler

Consider cultural differences.

Allow parents to bring in favorite foods or eating utensils from home.

Encourage family members to be present at mealtime.

Place children in small groups, preferably at tables during mealtime.

Provide simple foods in small portions. Peanut butter and jelly sandwiches are often favorites.

Allow and encourage children to feed themselves.

Utilize nursing histories as described for toddlers (see p. 1104).

Do not punish children who refuse to eat. Offer alternative foods.

School-Age Child

Slowed rate of growth during middle childhood results in gradual decline in food requirements per unit of body weight

The preadolescent growth spurt occurs about age 10 in girls and about age 12 in boys. At this time, energy needs increase and approach those of the adult. Intake is particularly important, since reserves are laid down for the demands of adolescence.

The child becomes dependent on peers for approval and makes food choices accordingly.

The child experiences increased socialization and independence through opportunities to eat away from home—for example, at school and homes of peers.

By this time, food practices are generally well-established, a product of the eating experiences of the toddler and preschool period.

Many children are too busy with other affairs to take time out to eat. Play readily takes priority unless a firm understanding is reached and mealtime is relaxed and enjoyable.

Nutrition education should help the child to select foods wisely and to begin to plan and prepare meals.

Parental attitudes continue to be important as the child copies parental behavior (e.g., skipping breakfast, not eating certain foods).

Most children require a nutritious breakfast to avoid lassitude in late morning.

Mealtime should continue to be relaxed and enjoyable. Diversions such as television and other children should be avoided.

Calcium and vitamin D intake warrant special consideration. They must be adequate to support the rapid enlargement of bones.

Parents and health professionals should be alert to signs of developing obesity. Intake should be altered accordingly.

Table manners should not be overemphasized. The young child often stuffs his mouth, spills foods, and chatters incessantly while eating. Time and experience will improve his habits.

(continued)

Nutrition in Children* *(continued)*

Age and Developmental Influence on Nutritional Requirements and Feeding Patterns	Feeding Pattern/Diet	Nursing Implications/Parental Guidance

School-Age Child (continued)

Provide some companionship and conversation at the child's level during meals. Peers should be invited occasionally for meals.

SPECIAL CONSIDERATIONS: Hospitalized child
Nursing history should include the following:

Food preferences; mealtime patterns and snacks; food allergies; food preferences when ill.

Provide opportunities for children to eat in small groups at tables.

Consider cultural differences.

Allow parents to bring in favorite foods from home.

Allow child to order his own meal.

Adolescent

(approximately 11–17 years of age)

Dietary requirements vary according to stage of sexual maturation, rate of physical growth, and extent of athletic and social activity.

When rapid growth of puberty appears, there is a corresponding increase in energy requirements and appetite.

Previously learned dietary patterns are difficult to change.

Food choices and eating habits may be quite unusual and are related to the adolescent's psychological and social milieu.

Generally, a significant percentage of the daily caloric intake of the adolescent comes from snacking.

Continue nutrition education, with special emphasis on the following:

1. Selecting nutritious foods.
2. Nutritional needs related to growth.
3. Preparing favorite "adolescent foods."
4. Kinds of foods that may aggravate acne.
5. Foods and physical fitness.

Informal sessions are generally more effective than lectures on nutrition.

Special problems requiring intervention:
Obesity
Excessive dieting
Extreme fads—eccentric and grossly restricted diets
Anorexia
Adolescent pregnancy

Provide nutritious foods relevant to the adolescent's life-style

Discourage cigarette smoking, which may contribute to poor nutritional status by decreasing appetite and increasing the body's metabolic rate.

SPECIAL CONSIDERATIONS: Hospitalized adolescent

Allow patient to choose own foods, especially if on a special diet.

Provide a refrigerator in the recreation room for snacks, or utilize a snack cart.

Serve foods that appeal to adolescents.

Utilize a nursing history similar to that for the school-age child.

* For recommended daily dietary allowances, refer to Appendix III.

Preventive Pediatrics

Immunization

General Considerations

A. Requirements of National Childhood Vaccine Injury Act (Effective 1988)

1. Childhood mandated vaccines (diphtheria-tetanus, toxoid, pertussis, polio, measles, mumps, and rubella vaccines—DTP, DT, Td, OPV, IPV, MMR, and any combination).
2. Health care provider must record in the patient's permanent record: date of administration of vaccine, manufacturer and lot number, name and address of person administering vaccine.
3. Reporting to the US Department of Health and Human Services (DHHS) selected events occurring after vaccination (see Table 45-1)

B. Immunization Schedules

1. Immunizations may be started at any age. If an immunization program is not begun in infancy, a slightly different schedule may be followed, depending upon the child's age and the prevalence of specific infections at the time.
2. An interrupted primary series of immunizations need not be restarted; it need only be continued, regardless of the length of time that has elapsed.
3. The recommended schedule for immunization is detailed in Tables 45-2 and 45-3.
4. The immunoresponse is limited in a significant proportion of young infants, and the recommended booster doses are designed to ensure and maintain immunity.

C. Contraindications

1. Immunizations should be deferred if child has an acute febrile infection or illness. The common cold, without fever, is not a contraindication to immunization.

Table 45-1. *Reportable Events Following Vaccination*

Vaccine/Toxoid	Event
DTP, P, DTP/Polio Combined	Anaphylaxis or anaphylactic shock Encephalopathy (or encephalitis) Shock-collapse or hypotonic–hyporesponsive collapse Residual seizure disorder Any acute complication or sequela (including death) of above events Events in vaccinees described in manufacturer's package insert as contraindication to additional doses of vaccine (such as convulsions)
Measles, Mumps, and Rubella; DT, Td, Tetanus Toxoid	Anaphylaxis or anaphylactic shock Encephalopathy (or encephalitis) Residual seizure disorder Any acute complication or sequela (including death) of above events Events in vaccinees described in manufacturer's package insert as contraindications to additional doses of vaccine

Oral Polio Vaccine	Paralytic poliomyelitis
	  • in a nonimmunodeficient recipient
	  • in an immunodeficient recipient
	  • in a vaccine-associated community case
	Any acute complication or sequela (including death) of above events
	Events in vaccinees described in manufacturer's package insert as contraindications to additional doses of vaccine

Inactivated Polio Vaccine	Anaphylaxis or anaphylactic shock Any acute complication or sequela (including death) of above event Events in vaccinees described in manufacturer's package insert as contraindications to additional doses of vaccine

From Centers for Disease Control: National Childhood Vaccine Injury Act: Requirements for permanent vaccination records and for reporting of selected events after vaccination. MMWR 1988;37:197–200.

Table 45-2. *Recommended Schedule for Active Immunization of Normal Infants and Children**

Recommended Age	Immunization(s)†	Comments
2 months	DTP, OPV	Can be initiated as early as age 2 weeks in areas of high endemicity or during epidemics
4 months	DTP, OPV	2 month interval desired for OPV to avoid interference from previous dose
6 months	DTP	A third dose of OPV is not indicated in the US but is desirable in geographic areas where polio is endemic
15 months	Measles, mumps, rubella (MMR)	MMR preferred to individual vaccines; tuberculin testing may be done at the same visit
18 months	DTP,†$ OPV,‖ PRP-D	See footnotes
4–6 years	DTP,¶ OPV	At or before school entry
14–16 years	Td	Repeat every 10 years throughout life

* For all products used, consult manufacturer's package insert for instructions for storage, handling, dosage, and administration. Biologics prepared by different manufacturers may vary, and package inserts of the same manufacturer may change from time to time. Therefore, the physician should be aware of the contents of the current package insert.

† DTP = diphtheria and tetanus toxoids with pertussis vaccine; OPV = oral poliovirus vaccine containing attenuated poliovirus types 1, 2, and 3; MMR = live measles, mumps, and rubella viruses in a combined vaccine; PRP-D = *Haemophilus* b diphtheria toxoid conjugate vaccine; Td = adult tetanus toxoid (full dose) and diphtheria toxoid (reduced dose) for adult use.

† Should be given 6–12 months after the third dose.

$ May be given simultaneously with MMR at age 15 months.

‖ May be given simultaneously with MMR at 15 months of age or at any time between 12 and 24 months of age.

¶ Up to the seventh birthday.

(From Report of the Committee on Infectious Diseases, 21st ed., Evanston, IL, American Academy of Pediatrics, 1988.)

Table 45-3. *Recommended Immunization Schedules for Children Not Immunized in First Year of Life*

Recommended Time	Immunization(s)	Comments
Less Than 7 Years Old		
First visit	DTP, OPV, MMR	MMR if child ≥15 months old; tuberculin testing may be done at same visit
Interval after first visit:		
1 month	PRP-D	For children aged 18–60 months; can be given concurrently with DTP (at separate sites) and other vaccines*
2 months	DTP, OPV	
4 months	DTP	A third dose of OPV is not indicated in the US but is desirable in geographic areas where polio is endemic
10–16 months	DTP, OPV	OPV is not given if third dose was given earlier
4–6 years (at or before school entry)	DTP, OPV	DTP is not necessary if the fourth dose was given after the fourth birthday; OPV is not necessary if recommended OPV dose at 10–16 months following first visit was given after the fourth birthday
10 years later	Td	Repeat every 10 years throughout life
7 Years Old and Older		
First visit	Td, OPV, MMR	
Interval after first visit:		
2 months	Td, OPV	
8–14 months	Td, OPV	
10 years later	Td	Repeat every 10 years throughout life

* The initial three doses of DTP can be given at 1- to 2-month intervals; so, for the child in whom immunization is initiated at age 24 months or older, one visit could be eliminated by giving DTP, OPV, and MMR at the first visit; DTP and PRP-D at the second visit (1 month later); and DTP and OPV at the third visit (2 months after the first visit). Subsequent DTP and OPV 10–16 months after the first visit are still indicated. PRP-D, MMR, DTP, and OPV can be given simultaneously at separate sites if return of vaccine recipient for future immunizations is doubtful.

(From Report of the Committee on Infectious Diseases, 21st ed, p 16. Evanston, IL, American Academy of Pediatrics, 1988).

2. Contraindications to receiving measles, mumps, and rubella vaccines include the following: pregnancy; generalized malignancy; cell-mediated immunodeficiency disorders; current immunodepressive therapy; sensitivity to animal species used in vaccine preparation; transfusion of immune globulin, plasma, or blood.

D. Preventive Considerations

1. A good nursing history will include determining whether or not the child has been exposed to any communicable disease or has experienced such. Surveillance in this area will prevent unnecessary disease and allow for proper immunization for the child and his family.
2. Strict adherence to the manufacturer's storage recommendations is vital. Failure to observe these precautions and recommendations may reduce the potency and effectiveness of the specific vaccine. Read manufacturer's package insert for volume of individual dose.

Specific Immunization

A. DTP

1. A time lapse of 8 weeks is recommended between the first 3 DTP injections for desirable maximum effects.
2. The combination of depot antigens is preferred, because it is more immunogenic.
3. Because of the increased risk of possible reactions to either diphtheria or pertussis antigen. Td (adult-type tetanus and diphtheria toxins) is recommended for children over 6 years of age.
4. For contaminated wounds, a booster dose of tetanus should be given if more than 5 years have elapsed since the last dose. No booster is needed for clean, minor wounds if immunizations are up to date and no more than 10 years have elapsed since last dose.

B. Pertussis

1. Protection of infants against pertussis should begin early.
2. In newborn infants, the best protection against pertussis is avoidance of household contacts by adequate immunization of older siblings.
3. Current vaccine available in the United States is a suspension of inactivated *Bordetella pertussis* cells combined with diphtheria and tetanus toxoids.
4. Mild adverse events are common and generally do not preclude subsequent doses.
   a. Redness, swelling, pain at site
   b. Fever
   c. Drowsiness, fretfulness
   d. Anorexia
   e. Vomiting
5. More severe adverse events have also been associated with the pertussis vaccine; however, less frequently
   a. High fever, above 40.5°C. (104.9°F.), convulsions, persistent or unusual crying (more than 3 hours) or screaming, collapse with a shock-like (hypotonic–hyporesponsive) state, encephalopathy, persistent neurologic damage, and death.
   b. These constitute contraindications to further administration of pertussis vaccine.
6. Other reasons to defer or omit pertussis vaccination in infants and children
   a. Underlying neurologic disorders or neurologic disorder characterized by progressive developmental delay or neurologic findings.
   b. Personal history of convulsions or suspicion of having neurologic conditions that predispose to either seizures or neurologic deterioration.
   c. Please refer to Report of Committee on Infectious Diseases, American Academy of Pediatrics, Red Book, 1988, for more specific and detailed information.

C. Tuberculin Test

1. It is recommended that the tuberculin test be given before measles vaccine.
   a. The measles vaccine may invalidate the tuberculin test, giving a false negative, if given within 6 weeks after measles immunization.
   b. Theoretically, measles vaccine could activate latent tuberculosis.
2. Frequency of repeated tuberculin testing depends upon the following:
   a. Risk of exposure of the child.
   b. Prevalence of tuberculosis in the population group.
   c. High-risk situations; intervals between routine testing should not exceed 6 months.

D. Measles Vaccine

1. Is most effective when given at 12–15 months of age. At this age, all maternal transplacental antibody has been catabolized.
2. Measles vaccine may be administered at 6 months of age when child is at a high risk of contact with natural measles. A second dose should be given at 12–16 months of age if the original vaccine was given prior to 1 year of age, since rate of seroconversion before 1 year of age is variable.
3. Live attenuated measles vaccine is used. Mild post-immunization symptoms: fever, malaise, faint rash.
4. Complications are rare but may include vaccine-induced neurologic disease, thrombocytopenic purpura, toxic epidermal necrosis.

E. Polio Vaccine

1. Live trivalent oral polio virus vaccine is preferred to the inactivated form, because administration is easier and the immunologic effects are broader and longer.
2. Inactivated polio virus vaccine can be used as follows:
   a. In those who refuse oral polio vaccine or have contraindications for its use.
   b. In adults as primary vaccination.
3. Live attenuated polio virus vaccine has some problems.
   a. Reduced seroconversion when given in the tropics.
   b. Viral interference from other enteroviruses.
   c. Vaccine-associated poliomyelitis.

F. Mumps Vaccine

1. All preadolescent or older males who have not had mumps should be immunized.
2. Live attenuated mumps virus results in life-long immunity.
3. No side effects.

G. Rubella Vaccine

1. Live vaccine is recommended for boys and girls between 1 year of age and puberty.
2. Immunity lasts 11–15 years.
3. Children in kindergarten should be given priority, because they are the major source of viral dissemination.
4. A history of rubella illness is not reliable enough to exclude children from immunization.
5. Adverse reactions
   a. Occasional rash, mild fever, lymphadenopathy, URI symptoms
   b. If any of these contraindications exist, immunizations may be temporarily deferred or an alternative vaccine preparation may be used.

H. Smallpox Vaccination

1. No longer recommended in US.
2. Where indicated (i.e., while traveling), initial smallpox vaccine may be given at any time between 12 and 24 months of age (after age 12, it may be given every 3–10 years).

Dental Care

Primary Teeth

A. Eruption

1. Two lower central incisors—appear by 6–7 months
2. Four upper incisors—appear by 9 months
3. Two lower lateral incisors—appear by 1 year
4. Four first molars—appear by 14 months
5. Four cuspids—appear by 18 months
6. Four second molars—appear by 2–2½ years

B. Dental Care for Primary Teeth

1. Toothbrushing and oral cleansing should be started early.
2. The infant's oral cavity can be cleansed by wiping area with a damp wash cloth daily to prevent plaque formation. In the very young child, parents should brush the teeth with plain water.
3. At about 2 years of age, toothbrushing should be started. At this age, most of the primary teeth have erupted, and the child's muscle coordination has developed enough to allow some form of brushing. The primary goal is to clean teeth.
4. By age 2–3 years the child should be examined by a dentist when all primary teeth have erupted; visits should be made every 6 months.
5. When decayed primary teeth are neglected, they endanger the child's health and may cause abscesses, fever, and excessive pain. The infected teeth may damage the permanent tooth that is forming within the jaw. A child with advanced tooth decay finds it difficult to chew some foods that are essential to a well-balanced diet.

C. Importance of Primary Teeth

1. Primary teeth act as a guide for the proper positioning of permanent teeth. Each primary tooth is holding the space for a permanent tooth that will replace it. If a primary tooth is lost prematurely, there will be a loss of space. This can result in crowding of permanent teeth, ultimately requiring orthodontic work when a child is older.
2. Primary teeth serve as a stimulus for growth of the jaws, aid in the development of speech, and serve a cosmetic function.
3. A young person can become very self-conscious when he loses a tooth in the front of his mouth and realizes that he looks different.
4. Indirectly, a child's speech may be affected if self-consciousness about his loss of teeth prevents him from opening his mouth for proper talking.
5. Ability to use the teeth for pronunciation is acquired entirely with the aid of the primary teeth. Early loss of front teeth may lead to difficulty in pronouncing "s," "f," "l," "z," and "th."
6. Even after the permanent teeth erupt, difficulty in pronouncing "s," "z," and "th" may persist to the point that the child requires speech correction.

Permanent Teeth

A. Eruption

1. Four "6-year molars" appear between the age of 6 and 7 years.
2. From this point onward, until 12–13 years of age, the primary teeth loosen, one by one, and each is replaced by a permanent tooth.
3. Four additional molars appear at 12–13 years of age.
4. Four molars ("wisdom teeth") appear at 17–21 years.

B. Importance of Early Dental Care

1. Care of teeth during infancy and childhood is necessary in order to:
   a. Promote proper development of the teeth.
   b. Prevent dental caries and periodontal disease.
   c. Establish good dental habits for optimal dental health.

Fluoridation

1. Fluoride supplements may be considered if the local drinking water supply does not contain fluoride.
2. Fluoride makes the tooth surface more resistant to disease.
3. Topical fluoride stimulates remineralization, the process by which calcium in the saliva is continually pushed back into the tooth.
4. Topical application of fluoride should be done twice a year.
5. Daily fluoride rinse after brushing is effective in decreasing dental caries in children. Rinse is not recommended for children under 6 years old because they swallow it.
6. Daily use of a dentifrice-containing fluoride is another source of protection.
7. Fluoride supplements are available in drops and chewable forms. If fluoride is not in drinking water, the recommended dose is 0.25 mg./day.
8. Sealant application (after age 4 when molars have erupted) can be applied professionally to high-risk children for dental caries in permanent teeth. The sealant is a form of acrylic, and decay cannot form underneath an intact sealant.

Health Maintenance

A. General Teaching

1. Take advantage of incidental opportunities to teach children and their parents information that will promote dental health.
2. Emphasize that inflammatory periodontal disease and dental caries are the results of dental plaque.
   a. *Dental plaque* is a mass composed primarily of microorganisms that adhere to the tooth surface.
   b. As these microorganisms grow, they form products that are destructive to the underlying tissue.
   c. Removal of this plaque and prevention of its collection is a major part of dental care.
3. Provide a well-balanced diet that is necessary for tooth development.
   a. Stress the importance of diet control in dental care.
   b. The microorganisms that form dental plaque need a sucrose substrate that comes from refined sugars for rapid growth.
   c. Therefore, decreasing the intake of such refined sugars is important.
4. Start child on the correct procedure by having a good attitude toward brushing. Parents serve as role models as well as assist the young child to care for his teeth.

5. Salivary tests are used to determine risk for cavities.
   a. Measure buffering capacity of saliva
   b. Measure salivatory lactobacillus bacterial colony count

B. Health Practices

1. Maintain the child's general health.
2. Encourage parents to arrange a dental visit when child is 2½–3 years old.
3. Teach child and parents good brushing technique and dental habits.
   a. Use soft-bristle nylon brush with polished ends. Brushes for small children should be ¼–⅓ smaller than adult brushes with a flat brushing surface, firm, resilient bristles, and head sufficiently small to allow access to all surfaces of the teeth.
   b. Place bristles at the gingival margin at a 45-degree angle to the tooth. The brush rotates from gingival toward occlusal surface. Occlusal surfaces are brushed with scrubbing motion with small strokes in every direction.
   c. Stress that the length of time and thoroughness of brushing are important.
   d. Disclosing tablets can be used during teaching program to show the location of dental plaque before and after brushing.
   e. Daily flossing should be started at age 8–9 years.

C. Adolescent Considerations

1. The adolescent needs special encouragement and attention to maintain good dental habits.
2. Stress importance of dietary control of refined sugars.
3. Encourage proper brushing technique. The circular motion method: the brush is carried up, back, and forward, then up again without twisting hand.
4. Encourage daily flossing in which floss is used correctly. (Improper use can cause traumatic injury to the gingiva.) Flossing is accomplished by passing the floss between the teeth with a back and forth motion. Place floss against tooth and move it up and down 6–7 times against the tooth as far as the gingiva permits. Repeat process on side of adjacent tooth. Repeat until all sides of all teeth are cleansed.

D. Practice Measures That Will Aid in Avoiding Cavities

1. Bottle-mouth syndrome
   a. High incidence of dental caries in child 18 months–3 years is the result of taking bottle of milk or juice to bed.
   b. The teeth become brown and rubbery; they crumble and cause painful infection and abscesses.
   c. This syndrome can be prevented.
   d. It is important that mothers, including nursing mothers, be made aware that this can happen and why it occurs, as well as ways to prevent it. Do not let child take a bottle to bed with him; if child does take a bottle, put plain water in it.
2. Have the child brush teeth after every meal and at bedtime. If brushing is not possible after meals, rinse mouth with water.
3. Reduce the amounts of sugar and sweets eaten by the child.
4. Beware of foods that contain large amounts of sugar:
   Bubble and chewing gum
   Cola drinks
   Peanut butter and jelly on white bread
   Candies, cookies, cakes
   Jelly, jam, honey
   Malted and sweet chocolate drinks

Synthetic orange juice (artificially sweetened)
White bread and raisin bread
Sugar-coated cereals

Safety

Incidence of Childhood Accidents

1. Accidents are the leading cause of death for children in the US.
2. Approximately 1 of every 3 children in the US is injured seriously enough each year to require medical treatment.

Role of the Nurse

1. Identify environmental hazards and take action to reduce or eliminate them.
2. Identify behavioral characteristics in individual children that may be related to accident liability and caution parents accordingly. Pay particular attention to children who show the following:
   a. Characteristics that increase exposure to hazards, such as excessive curiosity, inability to delay gratification, hyperactivity, and daring.
   b. Characteristics that reduce the child's ability to cope with hazards, such as aggressiveness, stubbornness, poor concentration, low frustration threshold, lack of self-control.
3. Provide anticipatory guidance about child development as it relates to accidents. Direct preventive teaching toward individuals or groups, toward children or adults.
4. Participate in policy-setting for accident prevention in institutions and communities.

Principles of Safety

1. The child's developmental stage influences the types of accidents that are likely to occur.
   Potential accident situations may be foreseen by parents who have knowledge of their own child's typical patterns of growth and development.
2. Children are naturally curious, impulsive, and impatient. The young child needs to touch, feel, and investigate.
   a. Patient adult supervision will enable the child to learn what he wants to know within the limits of safety for his stage of growth and development.
   b. Young children should never be left alone at home.
3. Children copy the behavior of their parents and absorb parental attitudes. Parents and other adults should be certain that their ways of doing things are safe.
4. Children become less careful and less willing to listen to warnings and to observe routine safety precautions when they are tired or hungry.
5. An estimated 90% of all accidents are preventable.

General Areas of Adult Safety Responsibility

A. Motor Vehicle

1. All automobiles should be maintained in good mechanical condition.
2. Seat belts should be worn at all times.
3. Driver should look carefully in front of and in back of the car before accelerating.
4. All car doors should be locked when a child travels in the vehicle.

5. Young children should never be left alone in a car.
6. Heavy or sharp objects should not be placed on the same seat with a child.

B. Sports and Recreation

1. Keep equipment in good condition and proper working order.
2. Wear appropriate clothing for the activity.
3. Do not attempt activities beyond one's physical endurance.
4. Keep firearms and ammunition locked up.

C. Electrical and Mechanical Equipment

1. Only underwriter-approved devices should be installed; they should be inspected periodically.
2. Dry hands before touching appliances. Keep radios, fans, portable heaters, and hair dryers out of the bathroom.
3. Disconnect appliances after use and before attempting minor repairs.
4. Keep garden equipment and machinery in a restricted area. Teach proper use of the equipment as soon as the child is old enough.
5. Avoid overloading electrical circuits.
6. Discourage children from playing with or being in area where appliances or power tools (e.g., washing machine, clothes dryer, saw, lawn mower) are in operation.

D. Prevention of Falls

1. Keep stairs well-lighted and free from clutter.
2. Provide sturdy railings.
3. Anchor small rugs securely.
4. Use rubber mats in the bathtub and shower.
5. Use only sturdy ladders for climbing.

E. Poisonings and Ingestions

1. Do not mix bleaches with ammonia, vinegar, and other household cleaners.
2. See section on ingested poisons, page 949; poisoning (pediatric), page 1511.

F. Fire

1. Maintain an adequate fire escape plan and routinely conduct home fire drills. Teach the child escape routes as soon as he is old enough.
2. Keep a pressure-type hand fire extinguisher on each floor. Instruct all family members who are old enough in its use.
3. Fit fireplaces with snug fireplace screens.
4. Store gasoline and other flammable fluids in tightly covered containers that are clearly labeled and away from heat and sparks.
5. Dispose of paint- and oil-soaked cloth quickly.
6. Utilize flame-retardant sleepwear.
7. Mark children's rooms so that they are obvious to firemen.
8. Teach children about the danger of smoke inhalation.

G. Swimming Pools

1. Completely enclose pool with a fence that complies with local regulations. The gate should be self-closing and have a lock.
2. Indicate water depth with numbers on the edge of the pool. Place a safety float line where the bottom slope begins to deepen.
3. Install at least 1 ladder at each end of the pool. Ladders should have handrails on both sides, and the diameter of the rails should be small enough for a child to grasp.
4. Use nonslip materials on ladders, deck, and diving boards.

5. Install underwater lighting as well as outdoor lights if the pool is used at night. A ground fault circuit interrupter should be installed on the pool circuit to cut off electrical power and thus prevent electrocutions should electrical fault occur.
6. Instruct children about safety rules such as not swimming alone, and not running around the pool or pushing others. Avoid using radios or other electrical appliances near the pool.
7. Keep essential rescue devices and first-aid equipment close to the pool.

H. Emergency Precautions

1. Record emergency telephone numbers in an obvious and easily accessible place.
2. Keep a well-stocked first-aid kit immediately available for emergencies.
3. Give instruction in principles of first aid to all family members who are old enough.
    a. Responsible adults should enroll in first-aid courses offered by the Red Cross, adult education programs, etc.
    b. Be aware of first-aid procedures for:
        Burns
        Electric shock
        Poisoning
        Bites and stings
        Cuts, scrapes, and punctures
        Drowning
        Fractures
        Cardiopulmonary arrest
    c. Teach children safety precautions concerning bicycles, telephone, door, strangers outside the home, being a pedestrian.
4. Know the location of gas, water, and electrical switches and how to turn them off in an emergency.

I. Miscellaneous

1. Take advantage of preventive health care.
    a. Obtain recommended immunizations.
    b. Have regular physical examinations.
2. Seek immediate treatment of all diseases and health problems.
3. Balance periods of work, rest, and exercise in daily living.

Specific Safety Concerns Related to Growth and Development

A. Infants

1. Newborn babies are helpless and need absolute protection. When they begin to move about they need close supervision.
2. Crib safety
    a. The crib should conform to the requirements of the Consumer Product Safety Commission.
    b. The sides of the crib should be kept up at all times.
    c. The crib should not be placed near a radiator or heating unit.
    d. The crib should be away from windows with blinds or draperies, to prevent the infant from becoming fatally entangled in a dangling cord.
3. Babies should not be left unattended on anything from which they might fall. Infant seats should not be left on tables, beds, or other furniture.
4. Infants should be strapped carefully in feeding chairs, infant seats, etc. A means should be provided to prevent the child from slipping down and being strangled by his waist strap.

5. No strings should be placed around the infant's neck.
6. Travel safety
    a. *For all children under 4 years of age or weighing less than 40 pounds, the standard seat belt is not safe.* Special restraint devices should be used, beginning with the ride home from the nursery.
    b. Infant car seats and car beds should meet the vehicle safety standards of the Department of Transportation for child-seating systems.
    c. There should be a means of anchoring the device to the seat of the vehicle with the standard lap belt.
    d. A harness should keep the child contained within the device.
    e. The device should include a head support to minimize the danger of whiplash injury.
    f. For older infants and toddlers, special devices are available that dispense with the harness and instead surround the child with a protective shield, thus distributing collision forces evenly.
    g. Adults should be aware of state laws regarding infant restraint during travel.
7. Infants may start to suck on toys, crib slats, and other objects.
    a. Paints containing lead should not be used on toys, furniture, or any other objects that the child is likely to put into his mouth.
    b. Stuffed toys should be checked carefully to be certain that button eyes and other small, attached parts cannot be pulled off and eaten by the child.
    c. Small objects should not be left within the reach of the infant.
    d. All plastic bags should be tied in knots and discarded to avoid danger of suffocation. Under no circumstances should mattresses be covered with thin plastic.
8. Children are still helpless in water for several years following infancy.
    a. The temperature of the bath water should be checked carefully to avoid scalding.
    b. The child should never be left unattended in the bathtub for any reason.
9. Infants are frequently victims of rats in highly populated metropolitan areas.
    a. The rats should be exterminated before the baby is discharged from the hospital.
    b. Infant beds should be high above the floor.
10. Infants should be carried from one place to another.
    a. The adult who carries the infant should avoid walking on slippery floors or where toys or other small objects have been scattered.
    b. *Hospitalized infants* should always be transported in cribs or strollers and never carried from place to place in the arms of the nurse.

B. Toddlers

Toddlers are adventurous and are eager to explore everything around them. Although they sometimes seem very mature and independent, they still require close adult supervision.

1. Toddlers want to roam all over the house.
    a. Gates should be used at the head and foot of stairways to prevent falls.
    b. Fireplaces should be screened.
    c. Radiators should be enclosed or covered.
    d. Cords on blinds or draperies should be tied or cut so that children cannot get their heads through the loops.

2. Toddlers poke and probe with their index fingers.
   a. Sharp objects such as scissors, and nail files should be kept out of reach.
   b. Bureau drawers and cabinets with anything potentially dangerous in them should be locked.
   c. Unused light sockets should be taped or capped.
   d. Electric fans or heaters should be out of reach.
   e. Electrical cords should be kept in good repair.
3. Toddlers are curious about many things, especially those things higher than their eye level.
   a. They should be lifted occasionally to satisfy their curiosity.
   b. Furniture should be balanced to prevent the child from pulling it over on himself.
   c. Hot, scalding foods should be kept out of the reach of the children.
   d. All handles of pots and pans should be turned to the back of the stove.
   e. Tablecloths should not hang over the edge of the table.
   f. A small child should never be left alone in the kitchen. Appliances such as hot ovens, toasters, coffee pots, and irons pose a special threat to small children.
4. A toddler puts almost anything into his mouth.
   a. Medicines, lye, and household cleaning products should be locked up out of the reach of children.
   b. Pins, buttons, and needles should be put away.
   c. Unbreakable toys that have no small, removable parts should be used.
   d. The child should be closely supervised if he plays with a balloon. Aspiration of rubber from broken balloons can be fatal.
   e. Foods such as popcorn and peanuts should not be offered to toddlers because of the danger of aspiration.
   f. Poisonous plants should be removed from the home.
5. Toddlers climb onto things.
   a. Toddlers should be protected from falls.
      (1) Windows should have guards on them.
      (2) Screens should be firm and securely fastened.
   b. Car doors should be locked.
   c. Special equipment for climbing (e.g., small wooden crates) should be provided, and climbing should be done under adult supervision.
6. They like to play outside and in water.
   a. The toddler must have close supervision while playing outside.
   b. His play yard should be fenced.
   c. Ponds, pools, wells, and other similar outdoor structures should be fenced or covered. Wading pools should be emptied immediately after use.
   d. The child should never be left alone in a wading pool.
   e. Caution should be used in allowing the toddler to play with older children. He may easily be injured by bats, hard balls, bicycles, and rough play.

C. Preschool Children

Preschool children are very active and inquisitive. They begin to develop increased self-control, but still have an immature understanding of danger. They are at an ideal age to learn simple safety routines.

1. Preschoolers can reach doorknobs and are eager to explore the world beyond.
   a. Doors that open to potential danger should be locked.
   b. Bathroom doors should have locks that can be opened from the outside to prevent the child from locking himself in the room.
   c. Unused refrigerators, freezers, and trunks should have doors, handles and/or hinges removed to prevent small children from climbing into them and becoming trapped inside.
2. Preschoolers enjoy taking things apart, putting them together again, and experimenting with their use.
   a. Dangerous items such as knives and electrical equipment should be put away.
   b. Matches and lighters should be kept well out of the child's reach.
3. Preschoolers are nimble on their feet and usually in a hurry.
   a. The child should not be allowed to walk or run while eating a lollipop.
   b. Stairs should have strong railings. They should be clear of objects or defective coverings on which a child can trip.
   c. Stairs and floors should not be highly waxed.
   d. Area rugs should be fixed.
4. Preschoolers often enjoy cooperative play with others.
   a. Toy trucks or wagons should be strong enough to bear their weight as well as that of their playmates.
   b. They should be taught to ride tricycles on the sidewalk and to watch for cars in driveways.
   c. They should be cautioned not to run after the ball if it rolls into the street or driveway.
   d. Clothes should allow the child freedom of action and shoes should be suitable for running and climbing.
   e. The play area should be checked for such hazards as old refrigerators, deep holes, construction, broken glass, and trash heaps.
   f. Swings and other equipment should be properly installed and maintained.
5. Preschoolers are proud to run simple errands. They should not be asked to do anything hazardous such as crossing the street or carrying a knife or glass container.
6. Preschoolers can take verbal directions, and their attention span is lengthening. They can be instructed in the following areas:
   a. Personal safety
      (1) To supply information such as their name, address, and telephone number.
      (2) To identify firemen, policemen, and other safety officials.
      (3) Not to accept gifts or rides from strangers.
   b. Home safety
      (1) The reasons for various safety measures such as keeping the floor clear of their toys.
      (2) The safe way to use tools.
      (3) Kitchen safety
      (4) The danger of matches, open flames, hot objects, and gas and electric equipment.
   c. Recreational safety
      Swimming instructions
   d. Motor vehicle and pedestrian safety
      (1) Safety rules and the dangers of traffic.
      (2) Obedience to the rules.
      (3) Appropriate use of automobile restraint systems.

D. School-Age Children

School-age children are usually fairly independent. They still need discipline and rules, but they also need to know *why* precautions are necessary and what the consequences are for failing to follow the rules.

1. School-age children are eager to make things and participate in household activities.
   a. They should be taught the proper use and storage of equipment such as those listed below:
      (1) Saws
      (2) Nails and hammer
      (3) Kitchen implements
      (4) Sewing machines
      (5) Gas and electric appliances
   b. They should be taught to wear protective devices over their eyes when doing anything potentially dangerous to their vision.
2. School-age children enjoy holding and attending parties, carnivals, and other similar gatherings. Party costumes and equipment should be checked to be certain that they are flameproof.
3. School-age children enjoy sports and outdoor play.
   a. Their whereabouts should be known at all times.
   b. The play areas should be inspected for broken glass, rusty nails, etc.
   c. They should be instructed regarding the dangers of playing in sand pits, old refrigerators, excavations, rickety shacks, and deserted buildings.
   d. They must learn the rules of the sports that they play. They should have the proper equipment and keep it in good working condition.
   e. Ice skating and other water sports should always be closely supervised.
   f. They should be taught how to climb a tree safely. Tree houses that are sturdily constructed under adult supervision may help prevent falls from trees.
4. Areas for teaching:
   a. The rules of cycling safety should be emphasized. A child with a bicycle must learn the rules of the road as well as respect for the traffic officers and their directions.
   b. Pedestrian safety rules should also be stressed because motor accidents are the most common cause of accidental injury in this age-group.
   c. Swimming instruction should be continued.

   d. The older child should be taught respect for fire, its uses, and its dangers.
   e. Safety with firearms should be discussed.
   f. Children should be taught to read labels and recognize symbols indicating poisons.

E. Adolescents

Adolescents are increasingly independent. They should be able to build on their past experiences and accept responsibility for their own safety. Limits must still be set, and direction given by adults because adolescents may lack emotional maturity.

1. Adolescents may obtain driving licenses.
   a. They should learn to maintain their automobiles in good mechanical condition.
   b. Seat belts should be worn at all times.
   c. They must be aware of traffic regulations and the penalty for not obeying them.
   d. They should be encouraged to participate in driver education and safety programs at school.
   e. Proper clothes should be worn while riding on motorcycles, motor scooters, or motorbikes. A safety helmet is essential.
2. Adolescents enjoy competing in competitive sports. Safeguards should be taken to prevent physical trauma when they want to do something beyond their physical endurance.
3. The values and habits of adolescents are greatly influenced by their peer groups and cliques.
   a. Parents should be aware of their child's activities.
   b. Constructive group activities should be encouraged.
   c. Formal instructions should be continued in the areas of sex education, drug and alcohol abuse, and smoking.
      Open discussions with responsible adults should be encouraged.
4. Older adolescents are capable of assuming some responsibility for family safety measures.
   a. They should be included in safety planning.
   b. Their opinions and suggestions should be considered.
   c. Specific areas of responsibility may be delegated to them.

Bibliography

Books

Anthony E and Chiland C (eds). The Child in His Family: Children and Their Parents in a Changing World. New York, John Wiley & Sons, 1978

Anthony E and Chiland C (eds). The Child in His Family: Children in Turmoil: Tomorrow's Parents. New York, John Wiley & Sons, 1982

Anthony E and Chiland C (eds). The Child in His Family: Perilous Development: Child Raising and Identity Formation Under Stress. New York, John Wiley & Sons, 1988

Arena J and Bachar M. Child Safety is No Accident. Chapel Hill, Duke University Press, 1978

Arneil GC and Metcoff J. Pediatric Nutrition. Boston, Butterworth, 1985

Alten M and McAnarney E. A Behavioral Approach to the Care of Adolescents. St. Louis, CV Mosby, 1981

Avery ME and First LR (eds). Pediatric Medicine. Baltimore, Williams & Wilkins, 1989

Baraff LJ. Pertussis vaccine. In Moss AJ (ed). Pediatrics Update. New York, Elsevier, 1987

Bolger N, Caspi A, Downey G and Moorehouse M. Persons in Context: Developmental Processes. New York, Cambridge University Press, 1988

Boynton R, Dunn E and Stephens G. Manual of Ambulatory Pediatrics. Boston, Little, Brown & Co, 1984

Chinn P. Child Health Maintenance: Concepts in Family Centered Care. 2nd ed. St. Louis, CV Mosby, 1979

Emond RT and Rowland HA. A Colour Atlas of Infectious Diseases. 2nd ed. London, Wolfe Medical Publications, 1987

Epanchin BC and Paul JL. Emotional Problems of Childhood and Adolescence. Columbus, Charles E Merrill, 1988

Evans J. Adolescent and Pre-Adolescent Psychiatry. New York, Academic Press, Grune & Stratton, 1982

Feigin RD and Cherry JD. Textbook of Pediatric Infectious Diseases, vols I and II. Philadelphia, WB Saunders, 1987

Ginsburg H and Opper S. Piaget's Theory of Intellectual Development. 2nd ed. Englewood Cliffs, Prentice-Hall, 1979

Grand RJ, Sutphen JL and Deitz WH (eds). Pediatric Nutrition. Boston, Butterworths, 1987

Greenspan S. The Clinical Interview of the Child. New York, McGraw–Hill, 1981

Harvey D. Parent–Infant relationships. In Perinatal Practice, vol 4. New York, John Wiley & Sons, 1987

Horowitz J, Hughes C and Perdue B. Parenting Reassessed: A Nursing Perspective. Englewood Cliffs, Prentice–Hall, 1982

Hymovich DP (ed). Child and Family Development: Implications for Primary Health Care. New York, McGraw–Hill, 1980

Illingsworth RS. The Development of the Infant and Young Child: Normal and Abnormal. 9th ed. New York, Churchill Livingstone, 1987

Johnson SH. High-Risk Parenting: Nursing Assessment and Strategies for the Family at Risk. Philadelphia, JB Lippincott, 1979

Karoly P (ed). Handbook of Child Health Assessment. New York, John Wiley & Sons, 1988

Kleinberg S. Educating the Chronically Ill Child. Rockville, MD, Aspen Publisher, Inc, 1982

Krasnegor NA, Arasteh JD and Cataldo MF. Child Health Behavior. New York, John Wiley & Sons, 1986

Krugman S and Katz SL. Infectious Diseases in Children. 7th ed. St. Louis, CV Mosby, 1985

Levine MO et al. Developmental–Behavioral Pediatrics. Philadelphia, WB Saunders, 1983

Levine MD (ed). Early Adolescent Transitions. Lexington, MA, Lexington Books, 1988

Lingam S and Harvey DR. Manual of Child Development. New York, Churchill Livingstone, 1988

McDonald RE and Avery DR. Dentistry for the Child and Adolescent. 5th ed. St. Louis, CV Mosby, 1987

Nelson JD. Current Therapy in Pediatric Infectious Diseases. St. Louis, CV Mosby, 1986

Peter G (ed). Report of the Committee of Infectious Diseases. Elk Grove Village, IL, American Academy of Pediatrics, 1988

Pringle SM and Ramsey BE. Promoting the Health of Children: A Guide for Caretakers and Health Care Professionals. St. Louis, CV Mosby, 1982

Prugh D. Psychosocial Aspects of Pediatrics. Philadelphia, Lea & Febiger, 1983

Rallison ML. Growth Disorders in Infants, Children, and Adolescents. New York, John Wiley & Sons, 1986

Rathus SA. Understanding Child Development. New York, Holt, Rinehart & Winston, 1988

Salkind NJ and Ambron SR. Child

Development. 5th ed. New York, Holt, Rinehart & Winston, 1987

Stewart RE and Troutman KC. Pediatric dentistry in the hospital. In Hooley JR and Daun LG (eds.) Hospital Dental Practice. St. Louis, CV Mosby, 1980

Skolnick A and Skolnick J. Family in Transition. Boston, Little, Brown & Co, 1986

Stone LJ et al. Childhood and Adolescence: A Psychology of the Growing Person. New York, Random House, 1984

Sutterly D and Donnelly G. Perspectives in Human Development. 2nd ed. Philadelphia, JB Lippincott, 1980

Trad PV. Psychosocial Scenarios for Pediatrics. New York, Springer–Verlag, 1988

Thompson CL and Rudolph LB. Counseling Children. 2nd ed. Pacific Grove, CA, Brooks & Cole Publishing, 1988

Vietze PM and Vaughan HG. Early Identification of Infants With Developmental Disabilities. Orlando, Grune & Stratton, 1988

Whaley LF and Wong DL. Nursing Care of Children. 2nd ed. St. Louis, CV Mosby, 1987

Wharton BA. Nutrition and Feeding of Preterm Infants. Boston, Blackwell Scientific Publications, 1987

Wilkinson SR. The Child's World of Illness. New York, Cambridge University Press, 1988

Zelter L and Jones LA. Amenorrhea in the adolescent. In Moss AJ (ed). Pediatric Update. New York, Elsevier, 1987

Journals

Asano Y et al. Immunoglobulin subclass antibodies to varicella-zoster virus. Pediatrics 1987 Dec; 80(6):933–936

Barton LL, Friedman AD and Portilla MG. Impetigo contagiosa: A comparison of erythromycin and dicloxacillin therapy. Pediatr Dermatol 1988 May; 5(2):88–91

Baraff LJ et al. Infants and children with convulsions and hypotonic-hyporesponsive episodes following diphtheria-tetanus-pertussis immunization: Follow-up evaluation. Pediatrics 1988 June; 81(66):789–794

Bausell RB and Solken KL. Results of the pediatric nursing survey on the importance of pediatric preventive behaviors. Pediatrics Nurs 1987 Nov–Dec; 13(6):421–423

Bearinger L and Gephart J. Priorities for adolescent health: Recommendations of a national conference. MCN 1987 May–June; 12(3):161–162, 164

Berwick DM et al. Impact of rapid antigen tests for Group A streptococcal pharyngitis on physician use of antibiotics and throat cultures. Pediatr Infect Dis J 1987 Dec; 6(7):1095–1102

Bigler–Doughten S and Jenkins RM. Adolescent snacks: Nutrient density and nutritional contribution of total intake. J Am Diet Assoc 1987 Dec; 87(12):1678–1679

Brauer H. Are we sweeping DTP contraindications under the rug? Am J Dis Child 1988 Jul; 142(7):698

Brooks–Gunn J and Warren MP. Biological and social contributions to negative affects in young adolescent girls. Child Dev 1989 Feb; 60(1):40–55

Brunell PA. Measles vaccine—one or two doses. Pediatrics 1988 May; 81(5):722–724

Bullock M and Lütkenhaus P. The development of volitional behavior in the toddler years. Child Dev 1988 Jun; 59(3):664–674

Burpo RH. A step beyond "Just Say NO." MCN 1988 Nov–Dec; 13(6):428–431

Cassidy J. Child–mother attachment and the self in six-year-olds. Child Dev 1988 Feb; 59(1):121–134

Court JM. Nutrition and adolescents: An overview of concerns in Western society. Med J Aust 1988 Feb; 148(Supp 1):S2–7

Crockett SJ, Mullis RM and Perry CL. Parent nutrition education: A conceptual model. J Sch Health 1988 Feb; 58(2):53–57

Crowe TK, Deitz JC and Bennett FC. The relationship between the Bayley Scales of infant development and preschool gross motor and cognitive performance. Am J Occup Ther 1987 Jun; 41(6):374–378

Davis JH. Pet care during preadolescence: Developmental considerations. Child Care Health Dev 1987 Jul–Aug; 13(4):269–276

Denny FW. Current problems in managing streptococcal pharyngitis. J Pediatr 1987 Dec; 111(6, pt 1):797–806

Dubowitz H, Newberger CM, Melnicoe LH and Newberger EI. The changing American family. Pediatr Clin North Am 1988 Dec; 35(6):1291–1311

DuRant RH, Pierce KL, Powell BJ and Sanders JM. Dentists' professional satisfaction with adolescent dentistry and its association with adolescent dental behavior. J Adolesc Health Care 1989 Jan; 10(1):46–50

Feldman S. Varicella zoster infections of the fetus, neonate, and immunocompromised child. Adv Pediatr Infect Dis 1986 1:99–115

Forney PD, Forney MA and Ripley WK. Alcohol and adolescents. J Adolesc Health Care 1988 May; 9(2):194–202

Foss RD. Sociocultural perspective on child occupant protection. Pediatrics 1987 Dec; 80(6):886–893

French DC. Heterogeneity of peer-rejected boys: Aggressive and nonaggressive subtypes. Child Dev 1988 Aug; 59(4):976–985

Fuller SA. Care of the postpartum adolescents. MCN 1986 Nov–Dec; 11(6):398–403

Gelbier S and Cushing A. Dental care in day nurseries. Commun Dent Health 1987 Sep; 4(3):251–256

Goldberg B, Rosenthal PP, Robertson LS and Nicholes JA. Injuries in youth football. Pediatrics 1988 Feb; 81(2):255–261

Grant LM and Demetriou E. Adolescent

sexuality. Pediatr Clin North Am 1988 Dec; 35(6):1271–1311

Greenberg MA and Birx DL. Safe administration of mumps-measles-rubella vaccine in egg-allergic children. J Pediatr 1988 Sep; 113(3): 504–506

Health Futures of Youth. J Adolesc Health Care 1988 Nov; 9(6 Supp):1s–69s

Heath RB. Prevention of varicella by vaccination. J Hosp Infect 1988 Feb; 11(Supp A):90–95

Hletko PJ, Rubin SS, Hletko JD and Stone M. Infant safety seat use. Am J Dis Child 1987 Dec; 141(12):1301–1304

Honig JC. Preparing preschool-aged children to be siblings. MCN 1986 Jan–Feb; 11(1):37–43

Immunization of children infected with human immunodeficiency virus: supplementary ACIP statement. Am J Dis Child 1988 Aug; 142(8):822

Johnson PA and Gaines SK. Helping families to help themselves. MCN 1988 Sep–Oct; 13(5):336–339

Joshi N and Scott M. Drug use, depression, and adolescents. Pediatr Clin North Am 1988 Dec; 35(6):1349–1364

Kamper CA, Chessman KH and Phelps SJ. Rocky mountain spotted fever. Clin Pharmacol 1988 Feb; 7(2):109–116

Kaplan EL and Johnson DR. Eradication of group A streptococci from upper respiratory tract by amoxicillin with clavulanate after oral penicillin V treatment failure. J Pediatr 1988 Aug; 113(2):400–403

Keener MA, Zeanah CH and Anders TF. Infant temperament, sleep organization, and nighttime parental interventions. Pediatrics 1988 Jun; 81(6):762–771

Kidwell-Udin P and Jacobson D. It's never too soon to teach car safety. MCN 1987 Sep–Oct; 12(5):344–345

Killam P and Smith K. Getting kids into car seats. MCN 1988 Mar–Apr; 13(2):124–126

King AC et al. Promoting dietary change in adolescents: A school-based approach for modifying and maintaining healthful behavior. Am J Prev Med 1988 Mar–Apr; 4(2):68–74

Klerman LV. School absence—A health perspective. Pediatr Clin North Am 1988 Dec; 35(6):1253–1269

Koniak-Griffin D and Ludington-Hoe SM. Developmental and temperament outcomes of sensory stimulation in healthy infants. Nurs Res 1988 Mar–Apr; 37(2):70–76

Lamont JH. Children's toys. Wis Med J 1988 Feb; 87(2):8–9

Lewis K et al. The effect of prophylactic acetaminophen administration on reactions to DTP vaccination. Am J Dis Child 1988 Jan; 142(1):62–65

Lewis T et al. Influence of parental knowledge and opinions on 12-month diphtheria, tetanus, and pertussis vaccination rates. Am J Dis Child 1988 Mar; 142(3):283–286

Liebovici L et al. An outbreak of measles among young adults. J Adolesc Health Care 1988 May; 9(2):203–207

Lott JW. Development care of the preterm infant. Neonatal Network 1989 Feb; 7(4):21–28

Lutzker JR, Touchette PE and Campbell RV. Parental positive reinforcement might make a difference: A rejoinder to forehand. Child Fam Ther 1988; 10(4):25–33

Macknin MC, Gustafson C, Gassman G and Barich D. Office education by pediatricians to increase seat belt use. Am J Dis Child 1987 Dec; 141(12):1305–1307

MacWhinney K, Cermak SA and Fisher A. Body part identification in 1- to 4-year-old children. Am J Occup Ther 1987 Jul; 41(7):454–459

Marino RV, Bomze K, Scholl TO and Anhalt H. Nursing bottle caries: Characteristics of children at risk. Clin Pediatr 1989 Mar; 28(3):129–131

Mauer AM. Dietary cholesterol recommendations for children. J Dent Child 1987 Nov–Dec; 54(6):454–457

McBean AM and Modlin JF. Rationale for the sequential use of inactivated polio virus vaccine and live attenuated polio virus vaccine for routine poliomyelitis immunization in the United States. Pediatr Infec Dis J 1987 Oct; 6(10):881–887

Middleton DB, D'Amico F and Merenstein JH. Standardized symptomatic treatment versus penicillin as initial therapy for streptococcal pharyngitis. J Pediatr 1988 Dec; 113(6):1089–1094

Miller SK and Slap GB. Adolescent smoking. J Adolesc Health Care 1989 Mar; 10(2):129–135

Moss SJ. Preventive techniques in infant dental care. Nurs Practit 1988 Jul; 134(7):37–38

National Children's Dental Health Month 1987. J Am Dent Assoc 1987 Oct; 115(4):625–629

National Child Health Vaccine Injury Act: Requirements for permanent vaccination records and for reporting of selected events after vaccination. Am J Dis Child 1988 Aug; 142(8):821

Ninio A and Rinott N. Fathers' involvement in the care of their infants and their attributions of cognitive competence to infants. Child Dev 1988 Jun; 59(3):652–663

Parker S, Greer S and Zuckerman B. Double jeopardy: The impact of poverty on early child development. Pediatr Clin North Am 1988 Dec; 35(6):1227–1240

Peter G. The child with group A streptococcal pharyngitis. Adv Pediatr Infect Dis 1986 1:1–18

Peterson L and Thiele C. Home safety at school. Child Fam Ther 1988, 10(1):1–8

Phillips MG and Stubbs PE. Head start combats baby bottle tooth decay. Children Today 1987 Sep–Oct; 16(5):25–28

Pipkin NL, Walker LG and Thomason MH. Alcohol and vehicular injuries in adolescents. J Adolesc Health Care 1989 Mar; 10(2):119–121

Prins PJM. Efficacy of self-instructional training for reducing children's dental fears. Child Fam Ther 1988 10(2/3):49–67

Read MH, Harveywebster M and Usinger-Lesquereux J. Adolescent compliance with dietary guidelines: Health and education implications. Adolescence 1988 Fall; 23(91):567–575

Restel M. Baby walkers. Pediatrics 1987 May; 79(5):839

Reutter L and Strang V. Yours, mine, and ours: Stepparents and their children. MCN 1986 Jul–Aug; 11(4):264–266

Rice ML and Woodsmall L. Lessons from television: Children's word learning when viewing. Child Dev 1988 Apr; 59(2):420–429

Rieder MJ, Schwartz C and Newman J. Patterns of walker use and walker injury. Pediatrics 1986 Sep; 78(3):488–493

Rolls BJ. Food beliefs and food choices in adolescents. Med J Aust 1988 Feb; 148(Suppl 1):s9–13

Rubenstein LK and Avent MA. Frequency of undesirable side-effects following professionally applied topical fluoride. J Dent Child 1987 Jul–Aug; 54(4):245–247

Rush D et al. Study of infants and children. National WIC evaluations: Evaluation of the special supplemental food program for women, infants and children. Am J Clin Nutrit 1988 Sep; 48(3 Suppl):811–818

Rushton CH. Promoting normal growth and development in the hospital environment. Neonatal Network 1986 Jun; 4(6):21–30

Siegal M. Children's knowledge of contagion and contamination as causes of illness. Child Dev 1988 Oct; 59(5):1353–1359

Schor EL. Foster care. Pediatr Clin North Am 1988 Dec; 35(6):1241–1252

Simoes EA, Balraj V, Selvakumar R and John J. Antibody response of children to measles vaccine mixed with diphtheria-pertussis-tetanus or diphtheria-pertussis-tetanus-poliomyelitis vaccine. Am J Dis Child 1988 Mar; 142(3):309–311

Smetana JG. Adolescents' and parents' conceptions of parental authority. Child Dev 1988 Apr; 59(2):321–335

Sparkman AF et al. Tools to measure sensory appeal of menus planned for children. J Am Diet Assoc 1988 Apr; 88(4):488–491

Spivak H, Prothrow-Stith D and Housman AJ. Dying is no accident. Pediatr Clin North Am 1988 Dec; 35(6):1339–1348

Starr RM and Gravitz RF. Pit and fissure sealants in the prevention of tooth decay. Pediatr Nurs 1985 Jul–Aug; 11(4):289–291

Stevens JH. Social support, locus of control, and parenting in three low-income groups of mothers: Black teenagers, black adults, and white adults. Child Dev 1988 Jun; 59(3):635–642

Thompson MK. Needling doubts about

where to vaccinate. Br Med J 1988 24 Sep; 297(6651):779–780

Taitz LS. Foods, fads and fats in under fives. Nutr Health 1987; 5(3/4):203–209

Taras HL et al. Early childhood diet: Recommendations of pediatric health care providers. J Am Diet Assoc 1988 Nov; 88(11):1417–1421

Taylor M. Conceptual perspective taking: Children's ability to distinguish what they know from what they see. Child Dev 1988 Jun; 59(3):703–718

Wald ER. Management of pharyngitis revisited. J Fam Pract 1988 Apr; 26(4):367–368

Wald ER et al. Acute rheumatic fever in western Pennsylvania and the tristate area. Pediatrics 1987 Sep; 80(3):371–374

Walker AM et al. Neurologic events following diphtheria-tetanus-pertussis immunization. Pediatrics 1988 Mar; 81(3):345–349

Walker ARP and Cleaton-Jones PE. Sugar intake and dental caries—Where do we stand? J Dent Child 1989 Jan–Feb; 56(1):30–35

Weinstein LB, Abrams RA and Ayers CS. A school program to reduce dental caries. J Sch Health 1988 Jan; 58(1):32–33

White CB et al. Streptococcal pharyngitis: Comparison of latex agglutination and throat culture. Clin Pediatr 1988 Sep; 27(9):431–434

Wintemute GJ, Teret SP and Kraus JF. Plastic handguns that resemble toy guns: New technology creates a uniquely hazardous product. Pediatrics 1988 Feb; 81(2):316–317

Wise PH and Meyers A. Poverty and child health. Pediatr Clin North Am 1988 Dec; 35(6):1169–1186

Wright SW and Trott AT. North American tick-born diseases. Ann Emerg Med 1988 Sep; 17(9):964–972

Unit *II*

Special Pediatric Considerations

46 | The Hospitalized Child

General Principles of Care

Emotional and Social Needs

1. The child has the same basic emotional and social needs during hospitalization as he does at home.
   a. He needs a chance to develop the following:
      (1) Motor skills
      (2) Social skills
      (3) Language skills
      (4) Psychological strengths
         (a) A sense of autonomy
         (b) Ego strength
         (c) A sense of identity
      (5) Patterns of behavior
   b. To help him accomplish these skills and strengths, he needs:
      (1) The continuing and reliable presence of someone who is important to him.
      (2) An appropriately stimulating environment.
      (3) Opportunities to explore and play.
      (4) Information and explanations concerning the hospital, illness and how sick people get better, treatments, procedures, routines, people, and expectations of him both before and during hospitalization. The child needs to know and to be able to predict how he will interact with his environment. Thus when he knows what to expect in an unfamiliar situation, he will be better able to cope and not feel so helpless.
2. The hospitalized child has special needs—to deal with the many new problems that confront him.
   a. Separation from home—implying loss of:
      (1) Consistent person who nurtures
      (2) Family associations
      (3) Familiar environment
      (4) Daily activities and routines
      (5) Peer associations
      (6) Independence
   b. Problems concerning the illness itself
   c. Hospital rules and regulations
   d. Surgery
   e. Death

Essential Elements

1. Parents must be closely involved with the child's hospitalization and the plan for his care. Parent participation is to be encouraged.

2. Nursing care should allow the child dependence, thus helping him to develop confidence and trust in the situation and at the same time assisting him to develop independence (refer to Chap. 45).
3. Nursing history should be taken when the child is admitted to the hospital. Specific questions should be asked to obtain information related to the following:
   a. Family home situation; parental anxieties
   b. Toilet habits and means of communicating
   c. Dietary habits
   d. Home routines and rituals
   e. Schooling
   f. Friends, peers
   g. Experience with illness
   h. Preparation for hospitalization
   i. Favorite toy, object, etc.
   j. How child handles frustration or stressful situations; his pattern for coping with strange situations and fears that arise
   k. Disciplinary practices at home
   l. Comforting practices at home
   m. Parental plans for visiting
4. Attempt to maintain home ties. Continuation of the ties within the existing family unit is a critical aspect of meeting the psychological needs of the child (refer to Family-Centered Care, p. 1125).
   a. Continue established rituals—rocking and story before bedtime.
   b. Have family photograph at the child's bedside.
   c. Use tape recorder to listen to tapes made of family conversations.
   d. Encourage use of the telephone, sending letters and pictures home, incoming cards.
   e. Talk about the people at home with the child.
   f. For the adolescent: assign roommate of same age, encourage use of telephone, encourage socialization with communal mealtimes and recreation periods.
5. Thorough explanations of the treatment plan and preparation for special tests, procedures, and surgery are essential. Unless the child is prepared for these experiences, he has minimal chance to mobilize his coping mechanisms to help him through his hospital experience.
   a. Listen to him repeat descriptions of his experience and continue to correct any misconceptions with factual information. Negative preparation of the child results in chaos, panic, doubt or fear, or fantasy.
   b. Make sure preparation is appropriate to:

(1) The child's age and personality
(2) Level of comprehension and developmental norms
(3) The child's attempt to cope with his frustrations and problems

c. Be creative; avoid using terminology that may have unintended alternate meanings to the child and that may cause him undue stress because of an inability to understand what is being said.
d. Use metaphors appropriate for cognitive age.
e. Include parents in the preparation process. Children through age 6 are dependent on their parents for identity and a sense of well-being, and will need their support. The parents know their child better than anyone and can serve as interpreters for child and health care personnel.

6. Play is a natural part of nursing care. It is a means to help the child cope with an unpleasant experience; it allows him to project his fears to the outside world, and it helps him to attain a feeling of independence and control of the situation. It is important for the child's physical, emotional, and social development. Therapeutic play allows the child to explore real and simulated equipment that will be used during procedures. It will allow the child to learn to cope with his fears, concerns, and fantasies.

7. Nursing care should relate illness to the child's personality, individual reaction, and previous experiences. Recognition must be given to:
   a. What the child comes from
   b. What he is returning to
   c. What he is experiencing during his hospitalization

8. The ultimate goal in pediatric nursing is directed toward:
   a. Reduction of stress
   b. Increasing the child's feeling of well-being and a sense of mastery about the situation

9. Postprocedural sessions and support should be part of the total nursing care of the child. This allows the child to
   a. Acquire a less stressful and more realistic perspective of what has happened
   b. Develop appropriate coping behaviors
   c. Develop a sense of mastery over the situation

10. Nursing care is successful when its outcome is therapeutic and encompasses growth.

Parental Support

1. Parental presence and involvement with the hospitalized child will decrease anxieties of the child. Parents, however, need encouragement, support, and education to be of the greatest help possible to their hospitalized child. Parental reactions to hospitalization affect the child's reaction.
   a. Identify anxieties the parents may have regarding hospitalization of the child.
      (1) Relinquishing their child's care to others
      (2) Preparation for surgery or surgical outcome
      (3) Opinions they feel others have of their child
      (4) Guilt feelings regarding disciplining the sick and hospitalized child
      (5) Dealing with the child upon return to the home
   b. Establish at an early stage the degree to which parents are able and want to participate in the care of their child. Reassess this periodically, and provide opportunities for parents to give continuity of care, thus promoting continued close parent–

child relationships (refer to Family-Centered Care, p. 1125).
      (1) Keep the family informed regarding the condition of the child.
      (2) Reassure parents that someone is available to help them.
      (3) Answer questions regarding hospital policy, procedures, or other concerns.

2. Begin early preparation and education of parents for possible posthospital behavior of their child.
   a. Frequently there are behavioral changes following hospitalization, especially in the child 18 months through 6 years of age. Behavioral changes may include increased demands for attention, withdrawal, violent reactions to temporary separation, changes in sleep patterns, shyness, increased clinging, bedwetting, temper tantrums, new fears, and changes in eating habits.
   b. Assist parents in anticipating these changes in their child's behavior. Help them to feel more adequate in coping with and responding to these temporary changes. Parents' reactions to posthospital behavior can either help to reinforce, prolong, and perpetuate these behaviors or gradually diminish these behaviors. Aid parents in identifying their reactions and feelings towards any posthospital alterations in their child's behavior.
   Include parents in postprocedural sessions.
      (1) Establish a parent–teacher, anticipatory-guidance program for parents.
      (2) Provide staff support to parents during and following hospitalization.

3. Consider effects of child's illness and hospitalization on siblings. They, too, need a plan of care and support, both by hospital staff and parents.
   a. Periodic visitation to sick child
   b. Evaluate the response of well siblings to illness of the sister or brother. Identify siblings at risk or who are not coping well, determine their needs, and initiate a plan of action that will help them with their coping and adjustment.

Impact of Hospitalization on the Child's Stage of Development

Neonate

Birth–1 Month

A. Primary Concern

1. Bonding—hospitalization interrupts the early stages of the development of a healthy mother–child relationship, thus early stages of the development of trust are missing.
2. Sensory–motor deprivation—tactile, visual, auditory, kinesthetic
3. Sensory bombardment

B. Reactions

1. Impairment of maternal–child attachment.
2. Impairment of mother's ability to love and care for her baby.
3. Risking of infant's emotional and physical well-being.

C. Nursing Interventions

1. Provide for continual contact between baby and his parents (eye contact and touch).

2. Minimize isolation and strangeness by explaining and reexplaining equipment, procedures, etc., to parents.
3. Actively involve parents in caring for their baby—provide for rooming in.
4. Foster good neonate–sibling relationships as appropriate.
5. Identify areas of infant deprivation and/or overstimulation. Plan a schedule of appropriate stimulation (i.e., hold and rock every 3–4 hours, eye contact).
6. Provide sensory–motor stimulation as appropriate.
7. Allow individuality to begin to emerge.
8. Provide consistent caretaker.

Infant

1–4 Months

A. Primary Concern

1. Separation—mother is learning to identify and meet the needs of her infant. Infant is learning to make his needs known and to trust his mother to meet them.
2. Sensory–motor deprivation
3. Needs—security, motor activity, comforting measures

B. Reactions

Separation anxiety is different from that of older child, because for the infant, his mother seems to be a part of him. Development of trust is disturbed when infant is separated from mother.

C. Nursing Interventions

1. Encourage mother to stay and care for her baby, thus minimizing separation. When mother is absent, give infant attention and frequent handling from a limited number of personnel.
2. Provide opportunity for sensory stimulation, motor development, and social responsiveness.
3. Help parents to work through their anxieties. Remember, a mother's touch communicates her comfort or discomfort to her infant.

4–8 Months

A. Primary Concern

Separation from mother—infant now recognizes his mother as a separate person from himself. He rejects strangers.

B. Reactions

Separation anxiety—crying, terror, somatic upset, blank facial expression, extreme preoccupation.

C. Nursing Interventions

1. Encourage mother to stay and care for her baby.
2. Attempt to adjust schedule to home routines.
3. Become friends with the infant through the mother.
4. The infant is beginning to develop purposeful activities and to strive toward independence. Provide opportunities and encouragement for this development to continue and provide ways for him to use newly acquired skills.

8–12 Months

A. Primary Concern

Separation—infant becomes more possessive of mother and clings to her at the time of separation.

B. Reactions

Separation anxiety—tolerance is very limited; fear of strangers, excessive crying, clinging, and overdependence on mother.

C. Nursing Interventions

1. Have the mother stay and care for her child.
2. Relieve some of his tensions and loneliness with "transference" object (i.e., blanket, toy).
3. Prepare the child for procedures—allow him to become familiar with simple equipment. Have the mother comfort child during procedures.
4. Provide for sensory stimulation and motor development appropriate for age. Provide opportunities for child to continue using skills he has acquired, such as feeding himself and drinking from cup.
   Child needs opportunity to foster increased independence, curiosity and exploration, locomotion, and language skills. Use infant seats, swing; give him room to move around in crib, playpen, or floor; use color, texture, and sound; physical stroking, rocking, and talking.

Toddler (1–3 years)

A. Primary Concerns

1. Separation anxiety—relationship with mother is intense. Separation represents the loss of family and familiar surroundings, resulting in feelings of insecurity, grief, anxiety, and abandonment. The toddler's emotional needs are intensified by his mother's absence.
2. Changes in rituals and routines, all of which are important to his sense of security, become a source of concern.
3. Inability to communicate—beginning use and understanding of language affords him limited communication between himself and the world. Limited capacity to understand reality, passage of time.
4. Loss of autonomy and independence—his egocentric view of life helps him develop a sense of autonomy. He expresses himself as a separate being with some potential control of his body and environment.
5. Body integrity—incomplete and inaccurate understanding of the body results in fear, anxiety, frustration, and anger.
6. Decrease in mobility—restricting his mobility causes frustration. He wants to keep moving for the pleasure it gives him as well as for the feeling of independence, the opportunity to learn about his world, and the route it provides for coping with frustrations that cannot be verbally expressed. Physical interference with this freedom results in a sense of helplessness.

B. Reactions

1. Protest:
   a. Has urgent desire to find mother.
   b. Expects that she will answer his cries, "I want mommy."
   c. Frequently cries and shakes crib.
   d. Rejects attention of nurses.
   e. When with mother, child shows signs of distrust with anger and/or tears.
2. Despair:
   a. Feels increasingly hopeless about finding his mother.
   b. Becomes apathetic, anorectic, listless; looks sad.
   c. May cry continuously or intermittently.
   d. Uses comfort measures—thumbsucking, fingering lip, tightly clutching a toy.
3. Denial:
   a. Represses all feelings and images of his mother.
   b. Does not cry when she leaves.

c. May seem more attached to nurses—will go to anyone.

d. Finds little satisfaction in relationships with people.

e. Accepts care without protest.

f. Regresses to an earlier state of development.

4. Regression:
Temporarily ceases use of newly acquired skills in an attempt to retain or regain control of a stressful situation.

C. Nursing Interventions

1. Rooming-in, unlimited visiting.
Parental visits provide:
   a. Opportunity for child to express some of his feelings about his situation.
   b. Assurance that his parents are not abandoning him or punishing him.
   c. Periods of comfort and reassurance that allow for the reestablishment of family bonds.

2. Attempt to continue routines used at home, especially with regard to sleeping, eating, and bathing. Reestablish trust through body contact and comfort.

3. Set limits.

4. Obtain from parents key words in communicating with child. Find out about his nonverbal behavior as well.

5. Allow child to make choices when possible. Arrange physical setting to encourage independence. Allow child to explore the environment.

6. A Band-Aid may give the child security of wholeness after an injection.

7. Replace lost mobility with another form of motion: moving about in a wheelchair, cart, or bed. Exercise restrained extremity. Provide opportunity for the child to release energy suppressed by decreased mobility (i.e., by pounding, throwing). Provide opportunity to continue learning about world through sensory modalities such as water play and diversional play.

8. Discharge:
If rooming-in has not occurred during hospitalization, parents must be prepared for the possible posthospital behavior of their toddler. They will need support in understanding and handling these behaviors. The child may do any of the following:
   a. Show lack of affection or resist close physical contact. Parents may interpret this as rejection.
   b. Regress to an earlier stage of development.
   c. Cling to mother, unable to tolerate any separation from her. Show excessive need for love and affection.

9. Appropriate parental response to the child's behavior is vital if relationships are to be reestablished.
   a. Extra love and understanding will help restore the child's trust.
   b. Hostility and withdrawal of love will cause the child further loss of trust, self-esteem, and independence.

Preschool Child (3–5 years)

A. Primary Concerns

1. Separation—although cognitive and coping capabilities have increased and the child responds less violently to separation from parents, separation and hospitalization represent stress beyond the coping mechanisms and adaptive capabilities of the preschool child. Loneliness and insecurities are experienced.

Language is important; although the child may not verbally express what he is feeling, there is an attempt at this in the 4- or 5-year-old.

2. Unfamiliar environment—this requires coping with a change in daily routine and represents a loss of control and security.

3. Abandonment and punishment—fantasies and thought may contain vengeful wishes for other persons, for which the child expects retribution. Illness may be interpreted as punishment for thoughts. Enforced parental separation may be interpreted as loss of parental love and represents abandonment by them.

4. Body image and integrity—hospitalization and intrusive procedures provide a multitude of threats of both bodily mutilation and loss of identity, which are just beginning to develop along with the acquisition of autonomy.

5. Immobility—mobility is the child's dominant form of self-expression and adaptation to the environment. He has a great urge for locomotion and exercise of large muscles. It represents his main expression of emotion and release of tension.

6. Loss of control—this influences the preschooler's perception of and reaction to separation, pain, and illness.

B. Reactions

1. *Regression*—child temporarily stops using newly acquired skills in an attempt to retain or regain control of a stressful situation. Preschooler may return to behavior of the infant or toddler.

2. *Repression*—child may attempt to exclude the undesirable and unpleasant stresses from consciousness.

3. *Projection*—preschooler may transfer his own emotional state, motives, and desires to others in his environment.

4. *Displacement/sublimation*—emotions are permitted to be redirected and expressed in other situations such as art or play.

5. *Identification*—the child assumes characteristics of the aggressor in an attempt to reduce fear and anxiety and to feel that he is in control of the situation.

6. *Aggression*—hostility is direct and intentional; physical expression takes precedence over verbal expression.

7. *Denial and withdrawal*—the child is able to ignore interruptions and disavow any thought or feeling that would result in a painful experience.

8. *Fantasy*—a mental activity to help the child to bridge the gap between reality and fantasy through imagination. The child has difficulty separating reality from fantasy because of lack of experience.

9. The preschooler may simply show similar behaviors (protest, despair, denial) to those of the toddler, although the stage of protest is usually less aggressive and direct.

C. Nursing Interventions

1. Minimize stress of separation by providing for parental presence and participation in care. Strive to shorten the hospital stay. Help parents understand what hospitalization means to the child.

2. Identify defense mechanisms apparent in the child and help him through the stressful situation by accepting him, showing him love and concern, and being alert to his readiness to relinquish them.

3. Set limits for the child. Let him know that someone is there. Help the child become master of something in the situation.

4. Provide opportunity and encouragement for child to verbalize.
5. Careful preparation for all procedures should be done on the child's level of development and comprehension.
6. Be sure the child has opportunities for play. Play is one important medium through which the child can overcome his fear and anxiety. A body outline, doll, and simple visual aids are appropriate teaching tools. Provide for self-expression; role reversal through puppets, dolls, drawings.
7. Encourage activities with other children.
8. Provide consistency in nursing personnel and approach to care.
9. Encourage the child to participate in his care and self-hygiene as appropriate.
10. Deal specifically with castration and mutilation fears. If the child is having surgery, describe exactly which body part will be repaired, and provide reassurance that nothing else will be removed or repaired.
11. Whenever appropriate, reassure the child that no one is to blame for his illness or hospitalization.

School-Aged Child *(5–12 years)*

A. Concerns

1. Many fear loss of recently mastered skills.
2. Many worry about separation from school and peers. They may fear loss of former roles.
3. Mutilation fantasies are common.
4. Some may believe that they or their parents magically caused the illness merely by thinking that the event would occur.
5. Often they have increased concerns related to modesty, privacy.
6. The imposed passivity may be interpreted as punishment.
7. Children may feel their body no longer is their own, but rather is controlled by doctors and nurses.

B. Reactions

1. Regression
2. Separation anxiety—especially early school-age period
3. Negativism
4. Depression
5. Tendency to be phobic (normal)
   a. Fears include that of the dark, doctors, hospitals, medication, and death.
   b. Unrealistic fears are commonly attached to needles, x-ray procedures, and blood.
6. Conscious attempts at mature behavior
7. Suppression or denial of symptoms

C. Nursing Interventions

1. Help parents to prepare the child for elective hospitalizations.
2. Obtain a thorough nursing history, including information regarding health and physical development, hospitalizations, social–cultural background, and normal daily activities. Utilize this information to plan care.
3. Provide for continuity of nursing personnel.
4. Provide order and consistency in the environment whenever possible.
5. Establish and enforce reasonable policies to protect the child and to increase his sense of security in his environment.
6. Arrange the environment to allow for as much mobility as possible (i.e., make sure articles are appropriately placed: move the bed if the child is immobilized).
7. Respect the child's need for privacy and respect modesty during examinations, bathing, etc.
8. Utilize treatment rooms whenever possible when performing painful or intrusive procedures.
9. Help young children identify problems and questions (often through play). Then help them find the answers.
10. Provide information about the illness and hospitalization based on assessment of what facts the child needs and wants and how this information can be made readily understandable to him.
11. View all nursing care activities as teaching situations. Explain the function of equipment and allow the child to handle it. Teach scientific terminology for body parts, procedures, etc.
12. When explaining a procedure, make sure that the child knows its purpose, what will be done, and what will be expected of him. Reassure the child during the procedure by continuing the explanations and support.
13. Reassure the child having surgery; explain where the organ to be removed or repaired is located, and that no other body part will be removed.
14. Carefully assess pain and provide appropriate relief.
15. Utilize play whenever appropriate to provide information about the hospital experience and to identify and decrease the child's fantasies and fears.
16. Reassure the child that he or his parents are not to blame for his illness.
17. Facilitate discharge of energy and aggression through appropriate play activities or through sharing aspects of ward management.
18. Encourage the child's participation in his care and self-hygiene.
19. Support intellectual potential through the use of games, books, puzzles, school work, and drawings.
20. Assist the child's family to understand his reactions to illness and hospitalization so that family members can facilitate positive coping patterns.
21. Let the child know that his normal status as a family member remains intact during his hospitalization. Encourage a consistent visiting pattern and allow sibling visits.
22. Help parents to deal with their own anxieties about hospitalization and assist them to help their child cope with the situation.
23. Encourage parental participation in the child's care when appropriate.
24. Encourage written communication with peers, and allow peer visiting when appropriate.
25. Begin discharge planning early, including plans for physical and emotional needs. Alert families to possible behavioral changes, including phobias, nightmares, regression, negativism, and disturbances in eating and learning.

Adolescent

A. Concerns

1. Physical illness, exposure, and lack of privacy may cause increased concern about body image and sexuality.
2. Separation from security of peers, family, and school may cause anxiety.
3. Interference with his struggle for independence and emancipation from his parents is a concern.
4. The adolescent may be very threatened by helpless-

ness. He may see illness as a punishment for feelings not mastered or for breaking rules imposed by his parents or physician.

B. Reactions

1. Anxiety or embarrassment related to loss of control
2. Insecurity in strange environment
3. Intellectualization about disease details in order to avoid addressing actual concerns
4. Rejection of treatment measures, even if previously accepted
5. Anger (may be directed toward parents or staff), because goals are being thwarted
6. Depression
7. Increased dependency on parents, staff
8. Denial or withdrawal
9. Demanding or uncooperative behavior (usually an attempt to assert control)
10. Capitalization on gains from illness or pain

C. Nursing Interventions

1. Help parents to prepare the adolescent for elective hospitalizations.
2. Assess the impact of illness on the adolescent by considering factors such as timing, nature of illness, new experiences imposed, changes in body image, and expectations for the future.
3. Introduce the adolescent to the hospital staff and to regular routines soon after admission.
4. Obtain a thorough nursing history that includes information about hobbies, school, family, illness, hospitalization, food habits, and recreation.
5. Encourage adolescents to wear their own clothes, and allow them to decorate their beds or rooms to express themselves.
6. Have drawers and closets available to store personal items.
7. Allow the adolescent access to a telephone.
8. Allow adolescents control over appropriate matters (i.e., timing of bath, selection of food, etc.).
9. Respect their need for periodic isolation and privacy.
10. Have a well-supervised recreational and activities program available that is planned by a professional child care worker.
11. Accept adolescent's level of performance. Allow regression with expectation of growth.
12. Involve the adolescent in planning his care so that he will be more accepting of restrictions and receptive to health teaching. He should be accepted as a vital member of the health-care team. His consent should be obtained for procedures and surgery.
13. Explain clearly all procedures, routines, expectations, and restrictions imposed by illness. If necessary, clarify the adolescent's interpretation of illness and hospitalization. Plan separate teaching sessions for parents.
14. Facilitate verbal rejection of treatment measures to protect the adolescent from harming himself physically by stopping treatment.
15. Assess the adolescent's intellectual skills and provide him with the necessary information to allow him to use problem-solving to deal with his illness and hospitalization.
16. Recognize positive and negative coping behaviors as attempts to adjust to a threatening situation. Attempt to deal with the feeling that caused the behavior as well as with the behavior itself.
17. Be a good listener. Maintain a sense of humor.
18. Provide opportunities such as writing, art work, and recreational activities to allow nonverbal adolescents to express themselves.
19. Foster interaction with other hospitalized adolescents and continuation of peer relationships with outside friends.
20. Establish regular group meetings to allow patients to meet with staff members and with each other to comment and to ask questions about their hospital experiences.
21. Set necessary limits to encourage self-control and ensure the rights of others.
22. Help adolescents work through sexual feelings. Avoid behavior that could be interpreted as provocative or flirtatious. Masturbation, unless excessive, may be considered a psychologically healthy way to discharge sexual tension.
23. Interpret the needs and reactions of hospitalized adolescents to parents. Emphasize the adolescent's need to be respected as a unique individual, separate from his parents.
24. Assist parents to cope with the illness and hospitalization as well as to deal effectively with the adolescent's response to related stress.
25. Encourage continuation of education.
26. Stress the confidential nature of conversations between nurse and patient, and physician and patient.

Family-Centered Care

Family-centered care provides an opportunity for the family to care for the hospitalized child with nursing support.

The *goal* of family-centered care is to maintain or strengthen the roles and ties of the family with the hospitalized child in order to promote normality of the family unit.

Benefits for Parents and Child

1. Continued close family interactions during stress
2. Absence of separation anxiety
3. Reactions of protest, denial, and despair are decreased or nonexistent
4. Greater sense of security for the child
5. Opportunity for family to fulfill their needs to care for their child physically and emotionally.
6. Allows parents to feel useful and important rather than making them dependent and destroying their confidence.
7. Lessening of parental guilt feelings.
8. Opportunities for parents to increase their competence and confidence in caring for the sick child.
9. Comfort for the family provided by other families.
10. Greater absorption of staff teaching by the family.
11. Posthospitalization reactions are diminished.

Implementation Strategies

Implementation of family-centered care will depend on regulations of the particular health care setting as well as the capabilities of the individual family unit. Examples of activities that can facilitate and strengthen family ties include:

1. Rooming-in for parents of young children
2. Parent participation in the child's physical care
3. Flexible visiting regulations for family members, including siblings

4. Having pictures of family members available at the hospital
5. Encouraging telephone contact
6. Use of family tape recordings

General Principles of Family-Centered Care

1. The nurse must be equipped with a broad knowledge base from the physical and behavioral sciences. Special emphasis is required in such areas as growth and development, family dynamics, socialization, and communication. Continuing education programs must be designed to support and improve family-centered care.
2. Staff must realize that parents are not time savers for nurses when they are participating in their child's care. The parents are not there to relieve the nurse of her routines and care.
   Additional nursing time is necessary to answer questions, to orient parents to the unit, to teach child care, and to comfort parents.
3. Family-centered care places a great deal of responsibility on the nurse and offers an opportunity to administer total patient care to the child and his family.
4. Family-centered care units should present a relaxed, comfortable atmosphere.
   a. Do not require parents to stay, but allow them to stay if they desire.
      (1) Some mothers may feel too anxious or guilty to participate.
      (2) Outside responsibilities may prohibit parents' staying.
   b. Provide physical comfort for participating parents.
      (1) Folding chair or bed in child's room
      (2) Comfortable lounge or waiting room
      (3) Eating facilities
      (4) Bathroom facilities, including showers
   c. Encourage parent(s) to take appropriate breaks from attending to the child.
      (1) Provides rest for the parent.
      (2) Helps child learn parent(s) will return and not abandon him.
5. When parents are active participants in their child's care, they too have certain needs, because they are concerned about their ill child.
   a. They want to care for their child as they would do at home.
   b. They are interested in working with the staff and learning from the staff how they can help their child.
   c. They like to have something to do for the child while visiting. This lessens their feeling of helplessness.
   d. Supports should be available (e.g., parent advocates, child care for well siblings, parent surrogates for times when parents cannot stay).
6. If parents know what is expected of them and what they can expect of the staff, many problems can be avoided. It helps parents feel more comfortable.
   a. Nursing and medical observations and care will be continued with or without the parents (or mother) present.
   b. Parents should be encouraged to assume a nurturing, comforting role. They should also be allowed to participate in the child's physical care to the extent that they desire or that will be necessary after the child's discharge. This requires encouragement, support, and education from the nurse.

c. Parents should allow child to become involved with peers on the unit.
   d. Parents should not ask for personal services.
7. Families of hospitalized children can offer a great deal of support to one another. Many times they have similar problems.
   a. Allow families to gather in groups—informal or formally planned group meetings.

Role of Parents

1. To serve as the child's primary resource of security and support so that he will be better able to tolerate unfamiliarity and discomfort and will be able to emerge from the experience with less likelihood of posthospitalization reactions.
2. To serve as the child's advocate in order to ensure that his basic human rights will be respected.
3. To teach nurses specific ways in which they can support the child.
4. To serve as role models and to support other families who may be dealing with similar problems.

Role of Nurse

1. To create an environment conducive to maintaining family integrity and unity. The nurse should:
   a. Help to maintain a healthy parent–child relationship. (Parents should not feel threatened by the nurse.)
   b. Facilitate a supportive marital relationship.
   c. Include siblings in planning and intervention as appropriate.
   d. Supplement the family in the common goal of the child's welfare.
2. To assist parents to make decisions about when to stay with their child.
   a. Parents' presence is especially important if the child is 5 years or younger, is especially anxious or upset, or is in medical crisis.
   b. The parents' decision is influenced by needs of other family members, as well as by job and home responsibilities.
   c. The nurse should try to alleviate guilty feelings of parents who are unable to stay with their child.
3. To develop trusting, goal-directed relationship with families.
   a. Obtain a thorough nursing history that provides information to assess strengths, relationships, and concerns.
   b. Plan with the family toward mutual, realistic goals.
   c. Recognize good care that the child receives from parents.
4. To observe the parent–child relationship in order to do the following:
   a. Evaluate the degree of participation of the parents in physical and emotional care.
   b. Observe parents' attitudes, skills, and techniques and the child's behavior and response to them.
   c. Assess what teaching needs to be done.
   d. Detect problems in parent–child relationships.
5. To teach parents knowledge, understanding, and skills necessary to function effectively with the hospitalized child. The nurse should:
   a. Perform nursing techniques safely and efficiently.
   b. Interpret the behavior of the hospitalized child to parents so that they can understand it and intervene appropriately (refer to the section, Impact

of Hospitalization on the Child's Stage of Development).

c. Interpret and reinforce what physician has told parents. Answer questions thoroughly and honestly as knowledge permits.

d. Interpret medical procedures and diagnostic tests.

e. Provide health teaching.

f. Offer anticipatory guidance.

6. To help parents adapt to the situation and to develop their own feeling of value by coping with the child's illness.

a. Be aware of common parental reactions to the stress experienced by families of children who have severe or chronic illness.

b. Be aware that defense mechanisms, if employed in moderation, are constructive and may facilitate optimal coping.

c. Help parents recognize their own feelings.

d. Identify parental support systems as well as adaptive and maladaptive coping.

e. Be perceptive of parents' physical and emotional needs and limitations.

(1) Do not allow parents to become fatigued.

(2) Allow parents to leave, take a break.

7. To assist families as appropriate in dealing with normal family developmental tasks.

a. Be aware that the child's hospitalization is often only one of many stresses a family experiences at a given time. Others frequently include:

(1) Interpersonal problems

(2) Debt, unemployment, job change

(3) Recent changes in dwelling place and consequent disruption

(4) Problems associated with child care and discipline

(5) Concurrent illness of other family members

8. To ensure continuity of family-centered care between the hospital and home.

Pediatric Intensive Care Unit

Nursing Role and Responsibilities in a Pediatric Intensive Care Unit

1. To provide continuing, comprehensive physical care and supportive treatment required to maintain life and to aid recovery of acutely ill children.

2. To provide emotionally supportive care to acutely ill children.

3. To provide empathetic support to parents and families of children in the intensive care unit (ICU).

4. To act as an integral and essential member of the health care team by assessing patient needs as well as by planning care and evaluating its effectiveness.

5. To act as child advocate by ensuring that basic human rights are respected.

6. To serve as nursing care consultants when children who require some intensive care nursing skills are admitted to regular pediatric units.

7. To serve as members of appropriate hospital committees (e.g., committees that decide policy on emergency care, protocol for admission to the pediatric ICU, etc.).

8. To teach intensive care nursing principles and skills to appropriate groups (e.g., nursing students, resident physicians, persons in continuing education programs).

9. To function effectively and safely, the ICU nurse should demonstrate the following capabilities:

a. Good physical and emotional health required to withstand the strain of continually nursing critically ill patients

b. Understanding of pathophysiology underlying disease

c. Knowledge and understanding of sophisticated monitoring equipment and special apparatus

d. Ability to reason objectively and to judge and be aware of rapidly changing situations

e. Ability to interpret data and to take rapid, decisive action

f. Ability to perform complex technical skills correctly and in an organized manner

g. Understanding of the impact of illness and hospitalization on the life of the child

h. Understanding of parental responses and ways of coping with the stress of a critically ill child

i. Ability to record data concisely, accurately, and thoroughly

Physical Care of the Child

1. Apply understanding of the pathogenesis of the disease in assessing patient needs and in planning care.

2. Perform complex technical skills to monitor and support the child (see text for specific procedures). These may include:

a. Cardiac, respiratory, and blood pressure monitoring

b. Basic interpretation of electrocardiogram (ECG) tracing

c. Endotracheal suctioning

d. Oxygen administration and monitoring

e. Tracheostomy care

f. Ventilator management

g. Monitoring central venous pressure

h. Monitoring intracranial pressure

i. Measuring arterial pressure

j. Hyperalimentation

k. Collection of specimens

l. Chest drainage

3. Perform nursing activities related to life support of the child (see text for specific procedures). These activities include the following:

a. Cardiopulmonary support

b. Respiratory management

c. Observation of neurologic signs

d. Fluid and nutritional assessment and management

e. Observations for complications and changing status

4. Apply general nursing measures for patient comfort and prevention of complications:

a. Positioning—to prevent contractures, to drain secretions from the lungs, and to minimize pressure effects on skin

b. Monitoring and regulation of body temperature

c. Skin care—to prevent breakdown

d. Eye care—to prevent conjunctivitis and injury to the cornea in unconscious children

e. Fluid balance—record daily fluid intake by all routes and losses of urine, stool, vomit, blood, and other drainage; be sensitive to weight loss and gain

f. Mouth care—to cleanse mouth of secretions, vomitus, especially in unconscious patient or patient with endotracheal tube

g. Control of infection

5. Provide careful, continuous clinical observations of the child.

Emotional Support of Child

1. Refer to the section on the impact of hospitalization on the developmental stage of the child, page 1121.
   In addition to the stress of hospitalization and the illness itself, the child must deal with the noxious environment: high noise level, loss of sleep, bright lights, random and unpredictable procedures, and the drastic change from his normal routine.
2. If possible, familiarize the child with the unit before admission.
3. Provide immediate physical care that communicates strength and facilitates trust.
4. Be alert to behavioral changes that may indicate physical distress.
5. Facilitate parent–child interaction—allow frequent family visits.
6. Question parents concerning the child's own way of responding to emotional stress. Utilize particular comforts that are most soothing to the child.
7. Support parents so that they will be best able to support their child.
8. Time activities; dim lights to allow for adequate sleep whenever possible—cluster care-giving activities.
9. Do everything possible to reduce the amount of pain that the child must endure; provide comfort measures.
10. Provide age-appropriate stimulation when indicated by the child's condition (TV, games, books, toys, etc.).
11. Provide opportunities for the child to express his fears and concerns.
12. If possible, avoid exposing an alert child to the death or resuscitation of another child. If the child is exposed, provide adequate explanation. The child must also be helped to express his feelings and work through the experience.
13. Prepare the child for transfer from the intensive care unit by implementing a nursing care plan similar to that which the child will experience on a regular unit (e.g., decrease frequency of monitoring of vital signs, encourage independence). Give a thorough report to the receiving nurse during transfer.

Emotional Support to Family

The parental role changes, once their child is admitted to the intensive care unit, from that of parents of a well child to one of parents of a critically ill child. To ease this transition parents have the need to be informed about their child's current condition, plan of care, and the future. They also have the need to feel needed and vital in their child's recovery.

1. Orient parents to the unit and its waiting areas. Clarify visiting policies and hospital expectations.
2. Encourage liberal visiting hours and unlimited phone calls from parents to the intensive care unit.
3. Assure parents that everything possible is being done for their child. Whenever possible, allow them to see child receiving treatment.
4. Make certain that parents are informed of important changes in the child's clinical status. Reinforce medical interpretations.
5. Explain special equipment and changes in nursing management.
6. Provide opportunities for parents to ask questions and have them answered.
7. Encourage parents to interact verbally and physically with their child. Support them in this endeavor.
8. Facilitate expressions of parental grief.
9. Provide opportunities for parents to talk to a person with whom they can share their concerns and fears. Be sure this person can see them as often as they require.
10. Provide opportunities for parents to meet together to share experiences and offer mutual support.
11. Be sensitive to parents' additional commitments to family and home as well as to their need to remain with their child. Whenever possible, allow visiting at a mutually convenient time.
12. Help parents provide anticipatory guidance for siblings and extended family members.
13. Refer parents to appropriate community resources for help with financial, environmental, or psychological problems.
14. Offer follow-up contact to parents if appropriate.
15. Refer to section on Family-Centered Care.

Child Life Programs

Many hospitals have established programs with a specially trained staff whose job it is to concern themselves solely with the social and emotional welfare of every pediatric patient. Such programs are called by a variety of names, including "Child Life," "Children's Activities," "Recreational Therapy," "Play Therapy," and others.

Rationale for Child Life Programs

1. Hospitalization separates a child from his home, family, and all that is familiar, and places him in an institution where he may experience intrusive, embarrassing, painful, and mutilating invasion of his body.
2. The short-term and long-term effects of illness and hospitalization on the intellectual, social, and emotional development of children have been documented by observations and research.
3. A separate child life department to meet the social and emotional needs of patients is justified, because such work requires the following:
   a. Special expertise and training.
   b. Adequate time that is free of other responsibilities.
   c. A special role definition of the staff member so that the child knows that this person will not become involved in his medical care.

Staffing of Child Life Programs

1. Staffing of child life departments differs among institutions according to their needs and resources. In most settings, they are staffed entirely by professionals who work with aides and volunteers.
2. Most child life workers have bachelor's or master's degrees in child-related professions such as preschool, kindergarten, and elementary education; nursing; social work; child development; and recreational therapy.
   a. Various educational institutions offer courses and areas of concentration in "The Hospitalized Child."
   b. Most child life departments offer their own in-service training programs so that the staff may learn to work with the hospitalized child.

Goals of Child Life Programs

1. To prevent some of the emotional pain and fear associated with illness and hospitalization.
   a. Child life workers may assume primary responsibility or a supportive role in the preparation of patients for hospitalization, surgery, and/or particular procedures.
   b. In many hospitals, child life workers arrange preadmission tours, puppet shows, and similar activities to which all children who are planned pediatric admissions are invited.
2. To provide a comfortable, accepting, and nonthreatening environment where the child may play and interact with other children and with an adult who is not involved with his health care.
   a. Ideally, there is a separate child life playroom in every unit. However, there may be only an open area at the end of a corridor or in the middle of the ward.
   b. Generally, there is a specific regulation that no medical procedures (even relatively benign ones such as taking a child's temperature) are to be carried out in the play area.
   c. In many settings, children are encouraged to have their meals in the playroom. Generally, they not only enjoy the opportunity to eat with others but also seem to eat better.
3. To provide the child with an opportunity for choice.
   a. The child may choose whether or not he wishes to come to the playroom. Once there, he may choose what to do.
   b. A variety of craft and play materials, including real and miniature medical equipment, is available.
   c. Should the child choose to sit and watch or be held and rocked, these activities are seen as acceptable choices.
4. To provide a continuing educational program.
   a. In some settings, teachers are paid by the hospital and are an integral part of the child life program. In others, teachers are provided by the local public schools, and they work in close cooperation with the child life department.
   b. In most hospitals, the educational program includes special activities for preschoolers and toddlers as well as a program of infant stimulation.

Role and Responsibilities of the Child Life Worker

1. To serve as advocate for the child.
   a. The worker serves as spokesperson for the child in his interaction with the health care delivery system.
   b. Serves as an instrument of change when the delivery system does not seem to be in the best interests of a large group of children.
2. To alleviate distress.
   a. Supports and tries to help children who have already been traumatized by their illness, surgery, and hospitalization.
   b. Is available for immediate crisis intervention such as comforting children during painful or frightening procedures, consoling children when expected visits from parents do not occur, and in other similar situations.
3. To provide therapeutic and recreational activity programs.

   a. The worker provides programs on the unit—both for individuals (at bedside) and for groups of children able to come to the play area.
   b. Utilizes play to allow the child to do the following:
      (1) Master his fears about an anticipated procedure or one that he has already experienced.
      (2) Express his feelings.
      (3) Give life to his fantasies and clarify misconceptions.
      (4) Try other roles (particularly those of doctor and nurse).
      (5) Distract himself.
      (6) Relieve boredom and simply have fun.
   c. The nature of such programs, the facilities for them, and the time allowed will necessarily vary from one hospital to the next.
4. To serve as a diagnostic observer.
   a. As a trained observer of the development and behavior of children, the child life worker acts as a member of the diagnostic team.
   b. Records observations and shares them with other members of the health team.
5. To participate in patient planning.
   Acts as a member of the health team to ensure that consideration is given to the child's social and emotional needs during and after hospitalization.
6. To serve as a source of support for parents.
   a. Is available to parents as needed to help them deal with their own anxieties as well as those of their children.
   b. In most settings, parents are encouraged to join their children in the play area.
7. To serve as teacher to physicians, nurses, and other hospital personnel.
   Teaches others in the areas of child development and behavior and the reactions of children to illness and hospitalization.

Shared Goals and Responsibilities

1. A child life department can exist only as one part of a hospital's total commitment to the social and emotional welfare of all children who enter the hospital.
2. Child life staff and nursing staff must work closely together and must complement each other's efforts.

Intensive Care Nursery

Nurse's Role and Responsibilities in an Intensive Care Nursery

1. The nurse is an active, integral part of the essential nurse–physician team in caring for the sick newborn.
   a. The nurse has a major responsibility in caring for the sick newborn. Much credibility is given to her observations because of continual contact with and care of the infant and past experience in making similar observations.
   b. It is not enough to follow the written prescription of the physician. The nurse must use initiative (i.e., must employ independent nursing judgment) in evaluating the infant's condition and must make changes in therapy when there are signs of deterioration or be able to handle a medical emergency. Subtle changes in behavior or condition of

the infant detected early by the nurse and related to the physician often result in treating the infant before he is critically ill or beyond the point where permanent damage may have occurred.

2. The nurse must have an understanding of pathogenesis of diseases of the newborn in order to program nursing activities in caring for the infant. The nurse must be informed about the following:
   a. Specific diseases of the newborn
   b. The treatment of their problems
   c. The uses of the equipment employed in caring for these infants
3. In addition, the nurse must possess the following qualities:
   a. Improved clinical awareness
   b. Increased diagnostic skills
   c. Ability to make nursing assessments
   d. Skills in performing special procedures
4. Working with the critically ill infant requires technical skills in several areas. Some of these include:
   a. Respiratory care
      (1) Endotracheal suctioning
      (2) Oxygen administration and monitoring
      (3) Ventilatory management
   b. Cardiac and vascular monitoring
      (1) Blood pressure assessment
      (2) Exchange transfusion and blood administration
      (3) Umbilical catheterization
      (4) Blood gas monitoring
   c. Other treatment and assessment modalities
      (1) Laboratory and roentgen studies
      (2) Phototherapy
      (3) Temperature control
   d. Equipment control
      Equipment working properly, etc.
5. The knowledge acquired in caring for the critically ill newborn will equip the nurse to compare signs such as respiration, fluctuating blood pressure, heart rate, subtle movement or lack of movement, and provide:
   a. Cardiopulmonary support
   b. Respiratory management
   c. Fluid and nutritional assessment and management
   d. Observation for complications and other illnesses
6. Infection control is within the realm of nursing responsibilities. Constant surveillance and strict adherence to procedures directed toward preventing infection must be practiced.
   a. Good handwashing technique:
      (1) 2- to 3-minute scrub with a brush and hexachlorophene or iodophor at the start of each tour of duty
      (2) 15-second scrub before and between infants
   b. Consider contact with Isolette or bassinet the same as contact with the infant himself.
   c. Nonhuman areas of contact and sources of possible contamination might be scales, examining table, and washing areas.
   d. Need for adequate and appropriate nurse–baby ratio.
   e. Surveillance of infant to recognize evidence of illness and source of infection to others.
   f. Removal from the area of individuals experiencing viral or bacterial illness.
   g. Effective cord care of the newborn—application of antiseptic dye (triple dye) or neomycin-polymyxin-bacitracin ointment.

h. If staphylococcal or streptococcal infection develops in the area, the following procedures should be followed:
   (1) Periodic bathing of infants with a 0.1N dilution (0.3%) of hexachlorophene solution is effective in controlling infection by these organisms. Blood levels of hexachlorophene are lower if this solution is used rather than the 3% solution.

NURSING ALERT: Hexachlorophene should be used cautiously and under strict and specific medical supervision in order to prevent neurotoxicity in the infant.

   (2) The Isolette and incubator serve as effective isolation when good handwashing is practiced.
   i. Invasive monitoring devices and procedures and ventilatory support bypass local defenses and can allow for bacteria to colonize, resulting in infection.
7. The nurse must begin to help form a bond between infant and his mother as well as to build cohesiveness of the family immediately upon the infant's admission to the intensive care unit (see Caring for Parents of Infant in Intensive Care Nursery).
8. Research indicates that to enhance the quality of the life saved and to provide the best chance for the child to achieve his potential, early environmental, emotional, and psychosocial stimulation is essential. By virtue of involvement, the nurse has a tremendous responsibility and opportunity in this area (see p. 1131).
9. It is vitally important that the nurse practice meticulous recording and documentation for the protection of the infant as well as the nurse:
   a. Always record routine procedures (i.e., hourly ventilator care).
   b. Record physician visits to infant and any contact by nurse with physician.
   c. Never erase. Errors should be crossed out with a single line, marked "error," and initialed.
   d. Record events accurately (e.g., emergency treatment).

Classification of High-Risk Neonate Requiring Intensive Care

1. *Premature*—problems are related to general immaturity: feeding, respiratory distress and/or apneic spells, hyperbilirubinemia.
2. *Small for gestational age*—problems include hypoglycemia, poor temperature control, and high susceptibility to infection.
3. *Medical problems*—these include respiratory distress, hypoglycemia, hyperbilirubinemia, erythroblastosis, sepsis neonatorum, hypocalcemia, infant of diabetic mother (IDM), drug withdrawal, and neurologic conditions.
4. *Surgical problems*—these include tracheoesophageal fistula, myelomeningocele, cleft palate, imperforate anus, and distended abdomen.
5. *Congenital malformations*—these include cardiac problems, genetic defects.

Caring for Parents of Infant in Intensive Care Nursery

Research has documented that infant–mother bonding is significantly influenced by events before and immediately after delivery and may greatly influence later maternal behavior and the infant–mother relationship. The mother's attachment to her infant is critical for his optimal growth and development, since he depends entirely on his mother to satisfy his needs.

A. Barriers to Healthy Mother–Infant Bonding

1. Grief, guilt, anger, fear, and anxiety felt by the mother at the birth of a child she expected to be perfect.
   a. Mother may mourn over loss of this child.
   b. The mother may also experience depression, powerlessness, hopelessness, isolation, and confusion.
2. Maternal background factors—socioeconomic status, educational training, own childhood experiences, emotional stability.
3. Expectations and attitudes of the mother toward her infant.
4. Separation of mother and her infant at a time when her sensitivity may be at a maximum for attachment to her infant.
5. Anticipatory grieving for possible loss of this infant and emotional withdrawal from infant.
6. Maternal attitude about herself—her lack of self-confidence in her ability to care for her infant; her negative feelings about her inability to carry her infant to term or to produce a normal child.
7. Disruption of care-eliciting behaviors by the infant; the infant serves as a stimulus for mother in helping her identify her offspring and promote her caretaking behaviors.
8. Stress elicited by physical presence of infant in intensive care nursery (i.e., realization of severity of illness of infant, emergency atmosphere, sensory deprivation)—all tend to diminish the mother's self-confidence—since she cannot give her own infant the special care he needs.
9. Maternal behaviors give clues to an altered relationship with her infant (i.e., lack of early claiming behavior and attachment, repulsion at infant's medical diagnosis or unrealistic view of infant's problems, infrequent visiting, anger towards staff, or inability to discuss problems).

B. Nursing Intervention to Help Foster Mother–Infant Bonding As Well As Eventual Appropriate Parenting Behaviors

1. Allow mother to see and touch her infant immediately after delivery and again as soon and as often as possible. This minimizes any fantasies that may develop.
2. Describe in detail all the equipment surrounding the infant in the intensive care nursery, prior to the mother's seeing the infant and again when she is near him.
3. Talk with mother on a personal basis; call her by name; make personal comments. Encourage parents to name their baby and refer to him by that name.
4. Encourage mother to enter the intensive care nursery as soon as possible and allow unlimited visiting except during specialized procedures. If daily visits are not always possible, encourage phone contact with nursery staff. The nurse should also call the mother.

5. Carefully consider the mother's concerns and feelings. Being the parent of a critically ill infant is emotionally devastating. Communicate to her your caring concern.
6. Encourage mother to touch her infant.
   a. This will help her to see him as real and will decrease some of her fears.
   b. Touching is the first step in the mother's developing her own self-confidence.
   c. Show mother how she can gradually assume more of infant's care and how she is better at mothering than the nurse.
7. Open communication channels with parents early.
   a. Meet parents in hospital of origin.
   b. Reinforce information given.
   c. Share good news—first feeding, physical activity, less oxygen needed, etc.
   d. Support them when discouraging news (e.g., discontinued feedings, increased apneic spells) is given.
   e. Often there develops a closeness between the mother and nurse that allows the mother to participate knowledgeably and confidently with the nurse in evaluating the infant's progress.
8. Observe the intensive care nursery physical setting in terms of parental needs (i.e., need for rocking chairs, bright pictures on the walls, parents' visiting area inside the nursery, pictures of past intensive care nursery babies who are growing and thriving).
9. Encourage active participation by the mother in the care of her infant (as the infant's condition permits). For example, instruct the mother on how to enter the Isolette; allow her to visit during feeding and to do something in connection with feeding.
   a. Explain how her visits and contact will benefit the baby.
   b. Assist her in touching and talking to her infant as necessary.
   c. Show her that increasing her physical contact with the infant will increase her involvement and confidence in caring for the child. Foster a sense of mastery and coping and of accomplishment within the mother. As the infant improves, the parents should become increasingly involved and ultimately competent and comfortable in caring for their infant.
   d. Continually assess the parents' (the mother's, in particular) ability to be involved; be sensitive to their tolerance for handling the infant and their degree of emotional tolerance.
10. There should be continuous focus on the family. Parents and infant must be treated as a unit.
    a. Priorities for this are:
       (1) Crisis intervention
       (2) Continual parent contact
       (3) Encouragement of parenting behaviors
    b. Goals are:
       (1) To develop mother's self-confidence and ability to rely on her own instincts and common sense in caring for her infant.
       (2) To assist the father in becoming involved emotionally and in developing competence in taking care of his family after discharge as well as in taking pleasure in his infant.
11. There is a necessity to decrease the social isolation that is often inherent in the birth of a critically ill baby.
    a. Initiate social service and community health nurse support early.

b. Provide mother (parents) with an opportunity to talk with other mothers (or parents) of infants with similar conditions, thus affording them the opportunity to express their feelings and concerns and to realize that they are not alone in feelings of guilt, failure, and fear.

c. Permit visits to infant and parents by others who will be a support to them.

d. The stress on older siblings of the birth of a sick infant can be overwhelming, and this affects parents and their fantasies of the child. Sibling visits can often help reduce these fantasies, fears, and anxieties with the support of parents and staff.

12. Provide some mechanism by which information concerning parents can be evaluated and trouble areas can be recognized early. Document information such as the following:

a. Parental involvement (phone calls, visits, handling and caring for infant).

b. Specific or special procedures observed by, taught to, and performed by parents.

c. Specific information discussed with parents—by whom and when.

d. Discharge teaching and plans.

13. Some interventions that may help parents become attached to their sick infant include transporting mother to be near infant, rooming-in, parent groups, transporting healthier infant to mother's room or to a hospital closer to her residence.

Stimulation: The Infant in Intensive Care Nursery

Every infant has the emotional need and right to recognize his mother's face, touch, and voice. The sick infant or premature infant is forced to accept less. Research documents that problems can arise from early sensory deprivation. The intensive care nursery is devoid of much sensory and perceptual stimuli—a situation that is harmful to the infant, the mother, and the mother–infant interactions. To maximize the potential to which the infant can develop, an early stimulation program should be planned.

1. Each stimulation program should be individualized for the specific infant–parent unit, based on:

a. Familiarization with the infant's physical condition and limitations.

b. Assessment of the infant's behavioral skills, developmental status, areas of deprivation or overstimulation.

c. Assessment of the parents' abilities to be involved in stimulating their child.

d. A program of infant stimulation adds specific sensory–motor activities and techniques to daily care activities for a specific area of development. It is not random activity meant to excite the infant.

2. Some general guidelines for establishing a psychosocial stimulation environment to be adapted for each infant include the following:

a. Provide for the continuity of the same caretaker each day, tour of duty. This will benefit both infant and parents.

b. Make the baby as attractive as possible—clean, colorful linen, lotion on skin, ribbon in hair. The general appearance of a "preemie" or sick infant makes it difficult for mother to relate to her infant.

c. Help infant establish a day/night cycle. Dim lights or cover infant's eyes.

d. Place an active mobile or colorful object in baby's line of vision, and adjust as his vision accommodation changes with age—about 23 cm. (9 inches) for newborn. This will increase visually directed reaching.

e. Encourage personnel to talk to and touch infant when caring for him. Hold him at feedings as well as between feedings when infant's condition allows this. Have personnel attempt to have infant focus upon their face and follow their head movement with his eyes.

f. Encourage personnel to follow specific procedure when feeding if infant is able to tolerate it.

(1) Hold infant in nursing position to aid in establishing en face.

(2) Rock, talk to, fondle, and pat infant before, during, and after feeding. Hold infant in upright position when burping to aid in this visual orientation.

g. Encourage parent participation in this program.

(1) Assist the parents so that they become emotionally involved with the baby.

(2) Point out specific responses and behavior of the infant they can look for and what these responses mean. This will help them learn to pay attention to the baby's behavior and to respond to his needs. Talk about this behavior and the parents' feelings about it.

(3) Encourage parents to visit during feeding time and to participate in the procedure. Even if gavage feedings are done, parents can hold infant, give him a pacifier, fondle him, and relate to him in many ways.

h. Be aware of specific sensory stimulation for the infant.

(1) Olfactory—mother's article of clothing near infant.

(2) Visual—change position of infant; change location of Isolette; use of mobiles or bright objects; imitate infant's movements.

(3) Auditory—music box, tape of mother's voice; imitate infant's sounds.

i. Attempt to minimize noxious environment to which the infant is subjected: monitor beeping, bright lights, voices, banging, physical restraint, etc.

Discharge Planning Begins Early

1. Maternal behaviors are learned. In order to provide the mother with an opportunity to build self-confidence and to develop to her potential, active participation with her infant during the infant's hospitalization is essential. Mother–infant bonding must be started and allowed to grow during this time for the well-being of both infant and mother.

2. Detailed preparation for home care is essential and must be given in advance.

a. Specific or special procedures and medications.

b. Information concerning routine baby care.

c. Crying pattern of the newborn.

3. Initiate social service and/or community nurse referrals long before discharge.

a. This provides parents with continual support by someone they know.

b. Initiating these referrals also gives the nurse feedback about the home situation and possible areas where problems can be averted.

c. Continual support by the community health nurse is important. Follow-up care can be directed also at assessing family interaction and parenting behaviors as well as development of the baby.
4. Evaluate the parents' willingness and ability to accept the child into their total care.
   Permit the mother a special nesting period when she can have close physical contact with her infant in privacy and can provide complete care for her infant. Nursing support and help are readily available for the mother to call on if needed.
   a. Instructions, demonstrations, and practice of procedures should have occurred prior to this time.
   b. It is possible that this period may enhance normal maternal attachment behaviors days or weeks after birth.
5. Encourage parents to continue psychosocial and intellectual stimulation of their infant at home. Provide a resource for parents so that they can assess child's readiness for the next step and promote it.

Realities of Nursing in the Intensive Care Nursery

Nursing in an intensive care nursery can be an emotionally draining experience; it can be difficult and depressing as well as hopeful and rewarding. Nurses frequently become surrogate mothers, grieving and rejoicing as the infant's condition changes. To minimize the personal agony frequently encountered, certain areas should be explored and opened to discussion.
1. Each nurse working in the intensive care nursery setting must be completely and totally educated to work in the area.
2. Discussions on grief and grieving should be open and frequent to allow each nurse to explore her own feelings.
3. Patient-centered discussions should be part of the routine to allow the nurse to express feelings about a particular patient.
4. Parent-centered discussions should focus on the parent's coping behaviors and stages of grief.
5. Each nurse must explore and acknowledge her feelings about the work in which she is involved.

The Child Undergoing Surgery

Preoperative Care

1. Provide emotional support, psychological preparation, and preoperative teaching appropriate for the age of the child. Such preparation and support will minimize stress and will help the child cope with his fears.
   a. Potential threats for the hospitalized child anticipating surgery are:
      (1) Physical harm—bodily injury, pain, mutilation, death
      (2) Separation from parents
      (3) The strange and unknown—possibility of surprise
      (4) Confusion and uncertainty about his limits and expected behavior
      (5) Relative loss of control of his world, his autonomy
      (6) Fear of anesthesia
      (7) Fear of the surgical procedure itself

   b. All preparation and support must be based on the child's age, developmental stage, and level; personality; past history and experience with health professionals and hospitals; background—including religion, socioeconomic group, culture, and family attitudes.
      (1) Know what information the child has already received.
      (2) Determine from the child what he knows or expects.
      (3) Additional guidelines in preparation include the following: Use illustration of a child's body, concrete examples and simple terms (not medical jargon); identify changes that may occur as a result of the procedure, both body and routine; give the explanation slowly and clearly, saving anxiety-producing aspects until the end.
         Make use of child's creative ability and logical thinking powers to aid in preparation for procedures.
   c. Orient patient and family to the unit, room, location of playroom, operating room, and recovery room and introduce them to other children, parents, and some of the personnel.*
      Make arrangements for the child to meet anesthesiologist as well as the operating room nurse and recovery room nurse.
   d. Allow and encourage questions. Give honest answers.*
      (1) Such questions will give the nurse a better understanding of the child's fears and perceptions of what is happening to him.
      (2) Infants and young children need to form a trusting relationship with those who care for them.
      (3) The older child tends to be reassured by the information he receives.
   e. Provide opportunity for child and parent to work out concerns and feelings (play, talk).
      Such supportive care should result in less upset behavior and more cooperation.
   f. Prepare child for what to expect postoperatively (i.e., equipment to be used or attached to child, different location, how he will feel, what he will be expected to do, diet, new health caretakers).*
2. Assist in physical preparation of patient for surgery.
   a. Assist with necessary laboratory studies. Explain to child what is going to happen prior to procedure and how he can respond. Give continual support during procedure.
   b. See that patient has nothing by mouth (NPO) (from Latin *nil per os*).
      Explain to child and parents what NPO means.
   c. Assist with fever reduction.
      (1) Fever will result from some surgical diseases (i.e., intestinal obstruction).
      (2) Fever increases risk of anesthesia and need for fluids and calories.
   d. Administer appropriate medications as prescribed. Sedatives and drugs to dry the secretions are often given on the unit.
   e. Establish good hydration.

* Other aspects of preparation for procedures to be emphasized.

Parenteral therapy may be necessary to hydrate the child, especially if he is NPO, vomiting, or febrile.

3. Support parents during this time of crisis. The attitudes of the parents toward hospitalization and surgery largely determine the attitudes of their child.
   a. The experience may be emotionally distressing.
   b. Parents may have feelings of fear or guilt.
   c. The preparation and support should be integrated for parent and child.
   d. Give individual attention to parents; explore and clarify their feelings and thoughts; provide accurate information and appropriate reassurance.
   e. Stress parents' importance to the child. Help mother understand how she can care for her child.

4. Special considerations should be made for the mentally retarded child requiring surgery. (See section on the mentally retarded child.)
   a. Remember that the parents know their child and his behaviors best and should be encouraged to share this knowledge with staff. Continue to work closely with parents throughout the hospitalization.
   b. Encourage parent(s) to remain with child to help him maintain a sense of security and to decrease his fears.
   c. Do not isolate the child. When placing him with others, explain his behavior to his peers in preparation for this social contact.
   d. Design play activities for his behavioral age.
   e. Communicate your knowledge of his behaviors, handicaps, etc., to others who will care for him.

Postoperative Care

A. Immediate

1. Maintain a patent airway and prevent aspiration.
   a. Position the child on his side or abdomen to allow secretions to drain and prevent tongue from obstructing pharynx.
   b. Suction any secretions present.
2. Make frequent observations of general condition and vital signs.
   a. Take vital signs every 15 minutes until child is awake and his condition is stable.
   b. Note respiratory rate and quality, pulse rate and quality, blood pressure, skin color.
   c. Watch for signs of shock.
      (1) All children in shock have signs of pallor, coldness, increased pulse, and irregular respirations.
      (2) Older children have decreased blood pressure and perspiration.
   d. Change in vital signs may indicate airway obstruction, hemorrhage, or atelectasis.
   e. Restlessness may indicate pain or hypoxia.
      Medication for pain is not usually given until anesthesia has worn off.
   f. Check dressings for drainage or constriction and pressure.
3. See that all drainage tubes are connected and functioning properly.
   Gastric decompression relieves abdominal distention and decreases the possibility of respiratory embarrassment.
4. Monitor parenteral fluids as prescribed (see p. 1167).
5. Be physically near the child as he awakens to offer

soothing words and a gentle touch. Reunite parents and child as soon as possible after the child recovers from anesthesia.
If a language barrier exists, the parents should be with the child as he recovers from anesthesia.

B. After Recovery From Anesthesia

After undergoing simple surgery and receiving a small amount of anesthesia, the child may be ready to play and eat in a few hours. More complicated and extensive surgery debilitates the child for a longer period of time.

1. Continue to make frequent and astute observations in regard to behavior, vital signs, dressings or operative site, and special apparatus (IV, chest tubes, oxygen).
   a. Note signs of dehydration.
      (1) Dry skin and membranes
      (2) Sunken eyes
      (3) Poor skin turgor
      (4) Sunken fontanelle in infant
   b. Record any passage of flatus or stool, bowel sounds.
      Observe for intestinal ileus, since crying children swallow air and even a minimal amount of ileus may cause gastric distention.
   c. Record voiding time, amount, characteristics.
2. Record intake and output accurately.
   a. Parenteral fluids and oral intake.
   b. Drainage from gastric tubes or chest tubes, colostomy, wound, and urinary output.
      Dressing may need to be weighed for more accurate estimate of output.
   c. Parenteral fluid is evaluated and prescribed by considering output and intake.
      Parenteral fluid is usually maintained until the child is taking adequate oral fluids.
3. Advance diet as tolerated, according to the child's age and the physician's directions.
   a. First feedings are usually clear fluids; if tolerated, advance slowly to full diet for age.
      Note any vomiting or abdominal distention.
   b. Since anorexia may occur, offer the child what he likes in small amounts and in an attractive manner.
4. Prevent infection.
   a. Keep the child away from other children or personnel with respiratory or other infections.
   b. Change the child's position every 2–3 hours—prop infants with a blanket roll.
   c. Encourage the child to cough and breathe deeply—let the infant cry for short periods of time, unless contraindicated.
   d. Keep operative site clean.
      (1) Change dressing as needed.
      (2) Keep diaper away from wound.
5. Provide good general hygiene.
   a. Good skin care will increase circulation and prevent pressure sores.
   b. Provide proper rest and sleep periods.
   c. Allow child exercise and movement out of bed when he feels better.
      Advance gradually.
   d. Allow diversional activity at intervals appropriate for age.
6. Offer the child measures of comfort.
   a. See that the child is warm and changes position as needed.
   b. Provide mouth care.

c. Allow the child to have and hold favorite toy or object.
d. Anticipate his needs.
e. Holding and rocking the infant or young child may be comforting.
f. Relief of pain—narcotics and other pain medications should be given as prescribed. Do not undermedicate. Develop methods for assessing pain even in the youngest child and allowing the child to assess his own pain, i.e., "Expressive Face," a tool to assess severity of pain.*
7. Provide emotional support and psychological security.
    a. Encourage the child to talk about his operation.
    b. Allow the child to play out his feelings.
    c. Return often to see and talk to the child.
    d. Reassure him that things are going well. Talk about going home, if appropriate.
8. Continue to offer support to the parents.
    a. Help to maintain healthy family relationships. (Encourage parents to care for their child.)
    b. Encourage parents to talk about their concerns.
    c. Begin early to prepare for discharge.
        (1) Teach any special procedures to be continued at home. Provide written instructions.
        (2) Arrange for community nurse referral.
        (3) Determine limits of activity for the child.
        (4) Make follow-up appointments.
        (5) Anticipate reactions of the child as a result of the hospitalization.
9. Do a follow-up evaluation of the hospitalization with telephone contact or letter–questionnaire.

Transcultural Nursing in Pediatrics
(Cross-Cultural Knowledge of Health–Illness Behavior)

General Principles

1. Comprehensive nursing should include being alert and responsive to the many cultural cues present in daily nursing situations. A conscious effort should be made to become knowledgeable about cultural diversity, and distinctiveness and similarities of the culture most likely to be served in nursing practice so that cues will be more meaningful and will be incorporated into patient assessment and care.
2. The nurse should be aware that cultural beliefs affect how a family perceives, experiences, and copes with health and illness. Culture influences how a family communicates about its health problems, the manner in which symptoms are presented, when and to whom members go for care, how long they remain in care, and how the care is evaluated.
3. It is possible that some health behaviors generated from cultural beliefs may be anxiety-producing and threatening to the nurse. Knowledge of and sensitivity to cultural diversity will decrease these anxieties, thus facilitating effective interactions and relationships with the child and his family.
4. The nurse should be aware of the beliefs of the popular

(family, community) and folk (nonprofessional healers) domains of health care available to her client as well as the accepted views of the medical profession so that discrepancies can be discussed and resolved. This folk health system can work with the professional health system to provide meaningful and therapeutic health services.
5. Knowledge of the cultural beliefs of the patient will assist the nurse in understanding behaviors that may seem negative, confusing, illogical, or primitive, and help in producing a response that is more appropriate for the client's condition.
6. Because of cultural influences, the patient may experience fear, anxiety, and loneliness, and have lack of knowledge regarding routine and inability to communicate with the nurse.

Assessment

Cultural background determines issues nurses should be aware of when caring for a child and his family.
1. Areas to consider when involved in cultural assessment*:
    a. Patterns or life-style of an individual or cultural group
    b. Specific cultural values, norms, and experiences of the client regarding health and illness
    c. Cultural taboos and myths
    d. The world view or ethnocentric tendencies
    e. The extent of assimilation into the mainstream cultural group
    f. Health and life-care rituals or rights of passage to maintain health and avoid illness
    g. Folk and professional approaches to healing
    h. Objectives and methods of caring for self and others
    i. Indicators of cultural change or adaptive behavior
2. In an attempt to become knowledgeable about cultural beliefs relating to pediatric nursing, the nurse must determine the following by talking with the patient and family about health values, beliefs, and practices*:
    a. What is the meaning of children in the culture?
    b. Do cultural patterns determine infant or child care? What are these patterns?
    c. Do cultural patterns determine parental responses to behaviors and appearances of the infant or child?
    d. What meaning does language or nonverbal communication have in the culture?
3. The acceptance of health care by a family or subculture may depend on the nurse's knowledge of the cultural beliefs and behaviors and her attempt to understand their values while working within given guidelines. It is essential to know how the family unit is culturally defined, the family's functions, and the functions of the child in order to work effectively with that unit.
4. The following questions may be helpful in eliciting the family's perception of the illness and related cultural beliefs[†]:
    a. What do you think caused the problem?
    b. Why do you think it started when it did?

---

* Young MR and Fu VR. Influence of play and temperament on the young child's response to pain. Child Health Care 1988 Winter; 16(3):209–215.

* Leininger M. Transcultural Nursing: Concepts, Theories and Practices, p. 88+. New York, John Wiley & Sons, 1978.
† Kleinman A, Eisenberg L and Good B. Culture, illness and care. Ann Intern Med 1978 Feb; 88(1):251–258.

c. What do you think your child's illness does to him?
d. How severe is your child's illness? Will it have a short or long course?
e. What kind of treatment do you think your child should receive?
f. What results do you hope to receive from this treatment?
g. What are the major problems your child's illness has caused you?
h. What do you fear most about your child's illness?
5. In addition to health care, cultural patterns and bereavement behaviors must also be understood in order to provide effective psychological services and support for family.

Bibliography

Books

Anthony EJ and Chiland C (eds). The Child in His Family. Perilous Development: Child Raising and Identity Formation Under Stress. New York, John Wiley & Sons, 1988

Avery G. Neonatology. 2nd ed. Philadelphia, JB Lippincott, 1987

Azarnoff P and Hardgrove C. The Family in Child Health Care. New York, John Wiley & Sons, 1981

Boyle JS and Andruos MM. Transcultural Concepts in Nursing Care. Glenview, IL, Scott, Foresman, 1989

Copeland DR, Pfefferbaum B and Stovall AJ (eds). The Mind of the Child Who Is Said to Be Sick. Springfield, IL, Charles C Thomas, 1983

Goodnow J. Children Drawing. Cambridge, Harvard University Press, 1977

Gottfried AW and Gaiter JR. Infant Stress Under Intensive Care. Baltimore, University Park Press, 1985

Hardgrove C and Dawson RB. Parents and Children in the Hospital. Boston, Little, Brown & Co, 1972

Harvey D. Parent–infant relationships. In Perinatal Practice, vol 4. New York, John Wiley & Sons, 1987

Hazinski M. Nursing Care of the Critically Ill Child. St. Louis, CV Mosby, 1984

Henning J (ed). The Rights of Children: Legal and Psychological Perspectives. 2nd ed. Springfield, IL, Charles C Thomas, 1982

Hofman A (ed). Adolescent Medicine. Menlo Park, CA, Addison–Wesley, 1988

Howe J. Nursing Care of Adolescents. New York, McGraw–Hill, 1980

Hymovich DP and Barnard M. Family Health Care. Developmental and Situational Crises, vol 2. New York, McGraw–Hill, 1979

Hymovich DP and Chamberlin RW. Child and Family Development: Implications for Family Health Care. New York, McGraw–Hill, 1980

Johnson SH. High Risk Parenting: Nursing Assessment and Strategies for the Family at Risk. Philadelphia, JB Lippincott, 1979

Karoly P (ed). Handbook of Child Health Assessment. New York, John Wiley & Sons, 1988

Klaus MH and Fanaroff A. Care of the High-Risk Neonate. Philadelphia, WB Saunders, 1986

Klaus MH and Icenell JH. Maternal–Infant Bonding. St. Louis, CV Mosby, 1983

Klepsch M and Logie L. Children Draw and Tell: An Introduction to the Projective Uses of Children's Human Figure Drawings. New York, Brunner/Mazel, 1982

Knones SB. High-Risk Newborn Infant: The Basis for Intensive Nursing Care. 3rd ed. St. Louis, CV Mosby, 1986

Krulik T, Holaday B and Martinson IM. The Child and Family Facing Life-threatening Illness. Philadelphia, JB Lippincott, 1987

Leape LL. Patient Care in Pediatric Surgery. Boston, Little, Brown & Co, 1987

Leininger M. Transcultural Nursing: Concepts, Theories and Practices. 2nd ed. New York, John Wiley & Sons, 1988

Lesner PA. Pediatric Nursing, Albany, Delmar, 1983

Levin D, Morriss F and Moore G. A Practical Guide to Pediatric Intensive Care. St. Louis, CV Mosby, 1984

McFadden EA. Case Studies in the Nursing of Children and Families. Baltimore, Williams & Wilkins, 1989

Melton G. Child Advocacy: Psychological Issues and Interventions. New York, Plenum, 1983

Miller J and Janosik E. Family Focused Care. New York, McGraw–Hill, 1980

Oremland E and Oremland J (eds). The Effects of Hospitalization on Children. Springfield, IL, Charles C Thomas, 1974

Petrillo M and Sanger M. Emotional Care of Hospitalized Children. Philadelphia, JB Lippincott, 1980

Robinson G and Clarke H. The Hospital Care of Children—A Review of Contemporary Issues. New York, Oxford University Press, 1980

Rubin J. Child Art Therapy: Understanding and Helping Children Grow Through Art. New York, Van Nostrand Reinhold, 1984

Schaefer C and O'Connor K. Handbook of Play Therapy. New York, John Wiley & Sons, 1983

Scipien G et al. Comprehensive Pediatric Nursing. New York, McGraw–Hill, 1985

Smith J. Pediatric Critical Care. New York, John Wiley & Sons, 1983

Smith M. Child and Family: Concepts of Nursing Practice. New York, McGraw–Hill, 1982

Smith M (ed). Chronic Disorders in Adolescence. Boston, John Wright & Sons, 1983

Steele S. Health Promotions of the Child with Long-Term Illness. 3rd ed.

Norwalk, CT, Appleton–Century–Crofts, 1983

Tackett J and Hunsberger M. Family Centered Care of Children and Adolescents. Philadelphia, WB Saunders, 1981

Whaley L and Wong D. Nursing Care of Infants and Children. 3rd ed. St. Louis, CV Mosby, 1987

Wilkinson SR. The Child's World of Illness. New York, Cambridge University Press, 1988

Journals

Impact of Hospitalization on the Child's Stage of Development

Azarnoff P. Preparing well children for possible hospitalization. Pediatr Nurs 1985 Jan–Feb; 11(1):53–56

Beyer JE and Aradine CR. Convergent and discriminant validity of a self-report measure of pain intensity for children. Child Health Care 1988 Spring; 16(4):274–281

Bolig R and Weddle KD. Resiliency and hospitalization of children. Child Health Care 1988 Spring; 16(4):255–260

Bosworth TL. Inside the bedrails: One child's view. MCN 1985 Jul–Aug; 10(4):243–245

Broome ME. The relationship between children's fears and behavior during a painful event. Child Health Care 1986 Winter; 14(3):142–145

Burke SO, Costello EA and Handley-Derry M. Maternal stress and repeated hospitalizations of children who are physically disabled. Child Health Care 1989 Winter; 18(2):82–90

Deatrick JA and Knafl KA. Developing programs for hospitalized children: Clinical significance of qualitative research. J Pediatr Nurs 1988 Apr; 3(2):123–126

Delpo E and Frick SB. Directed and nondirected play as therapeutic modalities. Child Health Care 1988 Spring; 16(4):261–282

Denholm CJ. Hospitalization and the adolescent patient: A review and some critical questions. Child Health Care 1985 Winter; 13(3):109–116

Erlen JA. The child's choice: An essential component in treatment decisions. Child Health Care 1987 Winter; 15(3):156–160

Facing Pain: How much does a child hurt? Am J Nurs 1988 Feb; 88(2):155–156

Faller HS. A child's perception of the hospital. MCN 1988 Jan–Feb; 13(1):38

Flint NS and Walsh M. Visiting policies in pediatrics: Parents' perceptions and preferences. J Pediatr Nurs 1988 Aug; 3(4):237–246

Fowler MD. Pediatric informed consent. Heart Lung 1988 Sep; 17(5):584–585

Francis S, Myers–Gordon K and Pyper C. Design of an adolescent activity room. Child Health Care 1988 Spring; 16(4):268–273

Gedaly–Duff V. Preparing young children for painful procedures. J Pediatr Nurs 1988 Jun; 3(3):169–179

Gill KM. Nurses' attitudes toward parent participation. Personal and professional characteristics. Child Health Care 1987 Winter; 15(3):149–151

Goodman S. Hospital teachers: Medical interpreters or raffia mafia? Arch Dis Child 1988 Mar; 63(3):333–338

Gross S. Pediatric tours of hospitals—Positive or negative? MCN 1986 Sep–Oct; 11(5):336–338

Hall D. Social and psychological care before and during hospitalization. Soc Sci Med 1987; 25(6):721–732

Haslum MN. Length of preschool hospitalization, multiple admissions and later educational attainment and behavior. Child Care Health Dev 1988 Jul–Aug; 14(4):275–291

Laine L et al. An educational booklet diminishes anxiety in parents whose children receive total parenteral nutrition. Am J Dis Child 1988 Mar; 143(3):374–377

LaMontagne LL. Adopting a process approach to assess children's coping. J Pediatr Nurs 1988 Jun; 3(3):159–163

Ledbetter B. Needle play must reflect current public health issues. Child Health Care 1988 Winter; 16(3):216–217

Lee EJ and Jacobson JM. Accident reports: Survey of high school injuries. 1987 May–Jun; 13(3):151–154

Levett J. Pediatric nursing: Lessening the emotional trauma. Del Med J 1988 Mar; 60(3):196–198

Ludman L, Lansdown R and Spitz L. Factors associated with developmental progress of full term neonates who require intensive care. Arch Dis Child 1989 Mar; 64(3):333–337

McCue K. Medical play: An expanded perspective. Child Health Care 1988 Winter; 16(3):157–161

McClowry SG. A review of the literature pertaining to the psychosocial responses of school-age children to hospitalization. J Pediatr Nurs 1988 Oct; 3(5):296–311

Melamed BG and Ridley–Johnson R. Psychological preparation of families for hospitalization. J Dev Behav Pediatr 1988 Apr; 9(2):96–102

Oldo AR. Designing for play: Beautiful spaces are playful places. Child Health Care 1988 Winter; 16(3):218–222

Ollendick TH, King NJ and Frary RB. Fears in children and adolescents: Reliability and generalizability across gender, age and nationality. Behav Res Ther 1989 27(1):19–26

Pazola KJ and Gerberg AK. Teen group: A forum for the hospitalized adolescent. MCN 1985 Jul–Aug; 10(4):265–269

Pidgeon V. Compliance with chronic illness regimens: School-aged children and adolescents. J Pediatr Nurs 1989 Feb; 4(1):36–47

Piersma HL and Van Wingen S. A hospital-based crisis service for adolescents: A program description. Adolescence 1988 Summer; 23(90):491–500

Pruitt DB and Strickland M. Psychological factors affecting children's response to medical procedures: A guideline for clinicians. Psychiatr Med 1987; 5(3):199–209

Reynolds EA and Ramenofsky ML. The emotional impact of trauma on toddlers. MCN 1988 Mar–Apr; 13(2):106–109

Rifkin L, Wolf MH, Lewis CC and Pantell RH. Children's perceptions of physicians and medical care: True measures. J Pediatr Psychol 1988 Jun; 13(2):247–254

Robinson CA. Roadblocks to family centered care when a chronically ill child is hospitalized. Modern Child Nurs J 1987 Fall; 16(3):181–191

Saunders RB, Miller BB and Cates KM. Pediatric family care: An interdisciplinary team approach. Child Health Care 1989 Winter; 18(1):53–58

Savedra MC and Highley BC. Photography: Is it useful in learning how adolescents view hospitalization? J Adolesc Health Care 1988 May; 9(3):219–224

Schlomann P. Developmental gaps of children with a chronic condition and their impact on the family. J Pediatr Nurs 1988 Jun; 3(3):180–187

Siegal M. Children's knowledge of contagion and contamination as causes of illness. Child Dev 1988 Oct; 59(5):1353–1359

Smith DP. Using humor to help children with pain. Child Health Care 1986 Winter; 14(3):187–188

Strickland MP, Leeper JD, Jessee P and Hudson C. Children's adjustment to the hospital: A rural/urban comparison. Modern Child Nurs J 1987 Fall; 16(3):251–259

Terry DG. The needs of parents of hospitalized children. Child Health Care 1987 Summer; 16(1):18–20

Vulcan BM and Nikulich-Barrett M. The effect of selected information on mother's anxiety levels during their children's hospitalization. J Pediatr Nurs 1988 Apr; 3(2):97–102

Wiles PM. The schoolteacher on the hospital ward. J Adv Nurs 1987 Sep; 12(5):631–640

Wilson CJ. Comparison of two methods of preparation for hospitalization. Child Health Care 1987 Summer; 16(1):24–27

Winkelstein ML and Carson VJ. Adolescents and rooming-in. Modern Child Nurs J 1987 Spring; 16(1):75–88

Wolfer J et al. An experimental evaluation of a model child life program. Child Health Care 1988 Spring; 16(4):244–254

Wyckoff PM and Erickson MT. Mediating factors of stress on mothers of seriously ill, hospitalized children. Child Health Care 1987 Summer; 16(1):4–12

Young MR and Fu VR. Influence of play and temperament on the young child's response to pain. Child Health Care 1988 Winter; 16(3):209–215

Zurlinden JK. Minimizing the impact of hospitalization for children and their families. MCN 1985 May; 10(3):178–182

Zweig CD. Reducing stress when a child is admitted to the hospital. MCN 1986 Jan–Feb; 11(1):24–26

Neonatal Intensive Care Unit

Aisenstein C. The psychiatrist in neonatology: A new frontier. Child Psychiatr Human Devel 1987 Fall; 18(1):3–12

Carter BS and Carter CA. The NICU experience in retrospect. Clin Pediatr 1988 Sep; 27(9):450

Cagon J. Weaning parents from intensive care unit care. MCN 1988 Jul–Aug; 13(4):275–277

Daga SR and Shinde SB. Mothers' participation in neonatal intensive care and its impact. J Trop Pediatr 1987 Oct; 33(5):274–277

Eikner S. Dealing with long-term problems: A parent's perspective. Neonatal Network 1986 Oct; 5(2):45–49

Field T. Alleviating stress in intensive-care unit neonates. J Am Osteopath Assoc 1987 Sep; 87(9):646–650

Fletcher AB and Sarin AV. Communicating with parents of high risk infants. Pediatr Ann 1988 Jul; 17(7):477–480

Franck LS. A national survey of the assessment and treatment of pain and agitation in the neonatal intensive care unit. J Obstet Gynecol Neonatal Nurs 1987 Nov–Dec; 16(6):387–393

Jenkins RL and Tock MK. Helping parents bond to their premature infant. MCN 1986 Jan–Feb; 11(1):32–34

Kelting S. Supporting parents in the NICU. Neonatal Network 1986 Jun; 4(6):14–18

Steele KH. Caring for parents of critically ill neonates during hospitalization: Strategies for health care professionals. MCN 1987 Spring; 16(1):13–27

Weibley TT. Inside the incubator. MCN 1989 Mar–Apr; 14(2):96–100

Pediatric Intensive Care Unit

Curley MA. Effects of the nursing mutual participation model of care on parental stress in the pediatric intensive care unit. Heart Lung 1988 Nov; 17(6):682–688

Jansen MT et al. Meeting psychosocial and developmental needs of children during prolonged intensive care unit hospitalization. Child Health Care 1989 Winter; 18(2):91–95

Kasper JW and Nyamathi AM. Parents of children in the pediatric intensive care unit: What are their needs? Heart Lung 1988 Sep; 17(5):574–581

Orsuto J and Corbo BH. Approaches of health caregivers to young children in a pediatric intensive care unit. MCN 1987 Summer; 16(2):157–175

Pollack MM, Ruttimann UE and Getson PR. Pediatric risk of mortality (PRISM) Score. Crit Care Med 1988 Nov; 16(1): 1110–1116

Pollack MM, Wilkinson JD and Glass NL. Long-stay pediatric intensive care unit patients: Outcome and resource utilization. Pediatr 1987 Dec; 80(6): 855–860

Proctor DL. Relationship between visitation policy in a pediatric intensive unit and parental anxiety. Child Health Care 1987 Summer; 16(1):13–17

Child Undergoing Surgery

Butler NC. The ethical issues involved in the practice of surgery in unanesthetized infants. AORN J 1987 Dec; 46(6):1138+

Byers ML. Same day surgery: A preschooler's experience. MCN 1987 Fall; 16(3):277–284

Campbell IR, Scaife JM and Johnstone JM. Psychological effects of day surgery compared with inpatient surgery. Arch Dis Child 1988 Apr; 63(4):415–417

Doroshaw ML and London DL. Surgery and children: A colorful way to introduce children to surgery. AORN J 1988 Mar; 47(3):696–697, 700

Ellis JA. Using pain scales to prevent undermedication. MCN 1988 May–Jun; 13(3):180–182

O'Brien SW and Konsler GK. Alleviating children's postoperative pain. MCN 1988 May–Jun; 13(3):183–186

Siaw SN, Stephens LR and Holmes SS. Knowledge about medical instruments and reported anxiety in pediatric surgery patients. Child Health Care 1986 Winter; 14(3):134–141

Transcultural Nursing in Pediatrics

Baker TL. The black american. Birth Defects 1987; 23(6):181–182

Colburn V. Behavior during childbearing: A cultural potpourri. Birth Defects 1987; 23(6):226–238

DeSantis L. The relevance of transcultural nursing to international nursing. Int Nurs Rev 1988 Jul–Aug; 35(4):110–112, 116

DeSantis L. Cultural factors affecting newborn and infant diarrhea. J Pediatr Nurs 1988 Dec; 3(6):391–398

DeSantis L and Thomas JT. Parental attitudes towards adolescent sexuality? Transcultural perspective. Nurse Pract 1987 Aug; 17(8):43–48

Diaz V. Caribbean Hispanics. Birth Defects 1987; 23(6):174–176

Fineman RM, Meier G, Nye G and Vetrano MA. The religious influences in the genetic counseling process: A round table discussion. Birth Defects 1987; 23(6):154–161

Flaherty MJ, Facteau L and Garver P. Grandmother functions in multigenerational families: An exploratory study of black adolescent mothers and their infants. MCN 1987 Spring; 16(1):61–73

Joyner M. Hair care in the black patient. J Pediatr Health Care 1988 Nov–Dec; 2(6):281–287

Kennell JH. The human and health significance of parent–infant contact. J Am Osteopath Assoc 1987 Sep; 87(9): 638–641+

Lum RG. The patient–counselor relationship in a cross-culture context. Birth Defects 1987; 23(6):133–143

Lum RG and Whipperman L. Practical methods in reaching and counseling the new American. Birth Defects 1987; 23(6):188–205

Manis EB and Hall RR. Asian family traditions and their influence in transcultural health care delivery. Child Health Care 1987 Winter; 15(3): 172–177

Norbeck JS and Tilden VP. International nursing research in social support: Theoretical and methodological issues. J Adv Nurs 1988 Mar; 13(2):173–178

Rankin WW. A child of poverty, a child of dignity. J Pediatr Nurs 1988 Jun; 3(3): 200–201

Rankin WW. The homes in their minds. J Pediatr Nurs 1988 Aug; 3(4):273–274

Richardson AG. Differences in adolescents' self-esteem across cultures. Psychol Rep 1987 Aug; 61(1): 19–22

Roberts RN. Welcoming our baby: An early intervention program for Hawaiian families. Child Today 1988 Jul–Aug; 17(4):6–10

Rowe P. Generations: Celebrating a cultural mosaic. Child Today 1988 Mar–Apr; 17(2):16–21

Sanchez GA. Hispanic Americans: Birth Defects 1987; 23(6):171–173

Smith G. Central America: The state of psychosocial care in pediatrics. Child Health Care 1986 Summer; 15(1):32–39

Smith SC. Barriers to cross-cultural counseling: The American Black perspective. Birth Defects 1987; 23(6): 183–187

Vargas MO. Tradition of nontradition— Our cultural blind spot. Birth Defects 1987; 23(6):122–132

Vavasseur JW. Psychosocial aspects of chronic disease: Cultural and ethnic implications. Birth Defects 1987; 23(6):144–153

Weisz JR. Epidemiology of behavioral and emotional problems among Thai and American children: Parent reports for ages 6 to 11. J Am Acad Child Adolesc Psychiatry 1987 Nov; 26(6): 890–897

Weisz JR et al. Thai and American perspectives in over- and undercontrolled child behavior problems: Exploring the threshold model among parents, teachers, and psychologists. J Consult Clin Psychol 1988 Aug; 56(4):601–609

Wilkerson LA. Black Americans: Birth Defects 1987; 203(6):177–180

Yamamoto K, Soliman A, Parsons J and Davies OL. Voices in unison: Stressful events in the lives of children in six countries. J Child Psychol Psychiatry 1987 Nov; 28(6):855–864

Yuen J. Asian Americans: Birth Defects 1987; 23(6):164–170

Additional Reading for Staff and Parents

Books

Azarnoff P and Flegal S. A Pediatric Play Program: Developing a Therapeutic Play Program For Children in Medical Settings. Springfield, IL, Charles C Thomas, 1980

Azarnoff P and Lindquist P (eds). Psychological Abuse of Children in Health Care: The Issues, Monograph no. 2. Santa Monica, CA, Pediatric Projects, 1985

Cohn AR and Leach LA (eds). Generations: A Universal Family Album. Washington, DC, Pantheon Books

Edelman MW. Families in Peril. Cambridge, MA, Harvard University Press, 1987

Goldfarb LA et al. Meeting the Challenge of Disability or Chronic Illness—A Family Guide. Baltimore, Paul H Brookes, 1986

Guillemin JH and Holmstrom LL. Mixed Blessings: Intensive Care for Newborns. New York, Oxford University Press, 1986

Harel S and Anastasiow NJ (eds). The At-risk Infant: Psycho/Socio/Medical Aspects. Baltimore, Paul H Brookes, 1985

Hobbs N, Perrin JM and Ireys HT. Chronically Ill Children and Their Families. San Francisco, Jossey–Bass, 1985

Krulik T, Haladay B and Martinson I. The Care of Families Facing Life-Threatening Illness. Philadelphia, JB Lippincott, 1987

Schaefer CE et al. Techniques for Problem Behaviors of Children and Teenagers. San Francisco, Jossey–Bass, 1984

Trad PV. Psychosocial Scenarios for Pediatrics. New York, Springer–Verlag, 1988

Journals

Croxton TA, Churchill SR and Fellin P. Counseling minors without parental consent. Child Welfare 1988 Jan–Feb; 67(1):3–14

Denholm CJ and Ferguson RV. Strategies to promote the developmental needs of hospitalized adolescents. Child Health Care 1987 Winter; 15(3):183–187

Harrison L et al. Establishing and evaluating a children's sick room program. MCN 1987 May–Jun; 12(3): 204–206

Vadasy PF. Grandparents of children with special needs: Supports especially for grandparents. Child Health Care 1987 Summer; 16(1):21–23

Wilson AL, Munson DP, Koel D and Hitterdahn M. Mothers and their children look at baby pictures: The NICU experience in retrospect. Clin Pediatr 1987 Nov; 26(11):576–580

Films and Videos

The following are from:
Association for the Care of Children's Health
3615 Wisconsin Ave, NW
Washington DC 20016

Family-Centered Care. 38-minute color documentary. Presents some of the ways in which family-centered care is being implemented in urban, suburban, and rural areas; in tertiary as well as community-based health care settings; and by a range of families and health care professionals. The accompanying study guide introduces the main characters of the film and suggests questions and issues for discussion. 1988

A Quiet Revolution . . . The First Twenty Years. Highlights key areas of progress in psychosocial care over the past 20 years, and presents an agenda for future action to improve the quality of child health care. 23 minute, color videotape in VHS ½″ or ¾″ format.

Seasons of Caring. 40-minute color film or videotape. Reveals the strengths and needs of families caring for children with special health needs. Addresses many issues encountered by parents, teachers, social workers, school administrators, physicians, nurses, and others who care for children with special needs and their families.

Seasons of Caring: Curriculum Guide. Discussion questions and activities that address the issues raised in the film.

Separate sections geared toward health professionals, parents, and teachers. J. Hanson and E. Jeppson, 1986, 225 pp.

A Space for Care. 28-minute color documentary developed for hospital design teams. Addresses key design issues and highlights specific innovative approaches used by hospitals throughout the U.S. and Canada. VHS ½″ or ¾″ format, 1987

For Children

Becky's Story. A book that encourages siblings of hospitalized children to explore and understand their own reactions, needs, and emotions. Line drawings illustrate the simple text. D. Baznik, 1981, 32 pp.

Family Medical Kit. Contains health care supplies, a book for children and guidelines to help families play, learn about, and prepare for health care experience.

Going to the Hospital. Booklet for children about going to the hospital. Each page provides simple, honest information illustrated by expressive and detailed photographs of children involved in hospital experiences.

The Hospital Book. Large photographs of children, staff, places, and procedures in the hospital illustrate the detailed information presented. Addresses the feelings and questions of the school-age child and family.

The Hospital Game. A board game for children to have fun and gain information about hospitals. E. Crocker, 1983

A Hospital Story. Photographs and a very simple child's text tell the story of a 5-year-old hospitalized for a tonsillectomy. Parallel text for parents encourages open discussion and suggests ways to help their child cope with hospitalization. S. Stein, 1974 (softcover), 48 pp.

School Kit: *"Learning about Hospitals"* Guidelines, booklets for children, a board game, casting materials and other medical supplies (including surgical masks, caps, and gloves for 30 children). Ideal for classroom use, health fairs, and library programs.

Special Care Babies. A warm and personal look at a young child's experience with the hospitalization of a sibling born prematurely. Soft, realistic drawings illustrate the informative text. Althea, 1986 softcover, 23 pp.

When You Visit the ICU. A coloring book to assist in preparing children for cardiac catheterization. J. Phillips and J. Bowen, 1983, 24 pp.

Additional Resource Films

Young Children's Reaction to Hospitalization. 14-minute video about children's ranges of hospital behaviors. From
American Journal of Nursing
555 W. 57th St.
New York, NY 10019-2961
212/582-8820

Elliott IG. Hospital Roadmap: A Book to Help Explain the Hospital Experience to Young Children. Belmont MA, Resources for Children in Hospitals, 1981

Rogers F. Going to the Doctor. New York, GP Putnam, 1986

47 Pediatric Techniques

Measuring Vital Signs in Children

Normal Vital Sign Ranges in Children

Temperature
  Oral 36.4°–37.4°C. (97.6°–99.3°F.)
  Rectal 36.2°–37.8°C. (97°–100°F.)
  Axillary 35.9°–36.7°C. (96.6°–98°F.)

Pulse and Respiratory Rates

Age	Pulse	Respirations
Newborn	70–170	30–50
11 months	80–160	26–40
2 years	80–130	20–30
4 years	80–120	20–30
6 years	75–115	20–26
8 years	70–110	18–24
10 years	70–110	18–24
Adolescence	60–110	12–20

General Considerations for Measuring Vital Signs

1. Vital sign values provide the nurse with only rough estimates of physiologic activity. It is important to identify trends, sudden discrepancies, and wide deviations from normal.
2. Vital signs should be taken as often as the nurse thinks necessary. They should not be delayed until the next scheduled time if it is suspected that a trend is developing.

Temperature

1. Normal body temperature represents a balance between the body heat produced and body heat lost.
2. The mode for taking the temperature should be kept as constant as possible. (Refer to Table 47-1 for methods of measuring body temperature in infants and children.)
3. Never leave the child alone when taking his temperature.
4. For security, safety, and accuracy, keep one hand on the thermometer when it is in place.
5. Record the temperature value and method used.
6. Report an elevated or subnormal temperature and initiate whatever nursing measures are indicated by the child's condition.
7. If using an electronic thermometer, follow manufacturer's directions explicitly.
8. Question the accuracy of any temperature reading that does not correlate with the child's signs and symptoms.
9. Wear gloves when taking a rectal temperature.

Table 47-1. *Methods of Measuring Body Temperature in Infants and Children*

Method	Advantages	Disadvantages	Length of Time Required for Accurate Measurement With Mercury-in-glass Thermometer
Rectal	1. Safe for children who are unable to co-operate and who may bite the thermom-eter 2. Not directly influenced by the ingestion of hot or cold fluids, smoking. 3. Method of choice if child has seizures or breathing difficulties; has had oral sur-gery.	1. Values may be altered by the presence of stool. 2. Emotional response may be negative. 3. Damage to rectal mucosa may occur. 4. Replication of the thermometer placement is difficult. 5. Contraindicated when child has diarrhea and following rectal surgery.	3–5 min.*
Oral	1. Easily accesible. 2. Replication of thermometer placement is easy. 3. Responds more quickly and regularly to changes in arterial temperature than does rectal method. 4. More aesthetically pleasing.	1. Value is readily influenced by ingestion of hot or cold fluids. 2. Requires child's cooperation to keep mouth closed and not to bite the thermometer. 3. Contraindicated if child has had oral injuries or surgery.	6–9 min.*
Axillary	1. Safe and easily accessible. 2. Avoids the danger of rectal or colon per-foration. 3. Avoids initiating defecation stimulus. 4. Often recommended for infants under 1 year.	1. Value is more readily influenced by environ-mental temperature and airflow. 2. Requires a relatively long period of time to obtain accurate reading.	9–11 min.*

* Time is generally decreased if an electronic thermometer is used.

Pulse

1. Take apical rate on an infant.
   a. Place stethoscope between left nipple and sternum.
   b. Take heart rate for 1 full minute.
2. With an older child, the pulse rate may be obtained at the radial, temporal, or carotid locations. (The pulse may be taken for 30 seconds and multiplied by 2.)
3. Take pulse rate prior to taking temperature because child may cry when temperature is taken; this increases the pulse rate and makes it more difficult to hear the apical rate.
4. Record accurately the following:
   a. Rate
   b. Rhythm (regular or irregular)
   c. Strength of beat (full, bounding, weak, faint)
   d. Activity of child at time pulse is taken (sleeping, crying, etc.)
5. Report immediately any changes in pulse character-istics, and initiate whatever nursing measures are in-dicated by the child's condition.

Respirations

1. Count respirations on an infant for 1 full minute. Ob-serve chest movement as well as abdominal move-ments.
2. Respirations may be counted for 30 seconds and mul-tiplied by 2 in the older child.
3. Obtain respiratory rate prior to taking temperature and pulse since the child may cry during these procedures.
4. Note and record accurately the following:
   a. Respiratory rate
   b. Depth of respirations
      (1) Feel exhaled air to estimate adequacy of tidal volume.
      (2) Observe excursions of the chest and dia-phragm.
   c. Quality of respirations
      (1) Determine if respirations are predominantly costal or abdominal. Dyspnea should be sus-pected in a school-age child who is breathing primarily with the abdomen.
      (2) Listen for unusual noises such as expiratory grunts, crowing noises, wheezing, or inspi-ratory stridor.
      (3) Observe for signs of dyspnea:
         (a) Restlessness
         (b) Retractions—sternal or intercostal
         (c) Nasal flaring
         (d) Cyanosis
   d. Activity of the child during the procedure.
5. Report immediately any change in respiratory status. Initiate whatever nursing measures are indicated by the child's condition.

Blood Pressure

Generally, the technique for taking the blood pressure of a child is the same as for the adult. The following principles are important to observe when dealing with the pediatric patient.

A. General Considerations

1. The cuff should cover no less than ½ and no more than ⅔ the length of the upper arm or leg. Even small vari-ations in cuff size may produce significant differences in blood pressure reading.

a. A cuff that is too narrow will produce an apparent increase in blood pressure.
b. A cuff that is too wide will produce an apparent decrease in blood pressure.
c. Using a flexible blood pressure cuff that can be folded to the correct size is frequently easier and more effective for the nurse than choosing among several assorted premeasured cuffs.
d. The cuff should be of consistent width each time that a child's blood pressure is measured during hospitalization.

2. If the child is excited or uncomfortable or if he distrusts the person taking the blood pressure, the systolic pressure may rise significantly.
    a. The blood pressure should be taken when the child is at rest and in a consistent position.
    b. The procedure should be explained to the child before it is done.
        (1) He should know that it will not hurt.
        (2) He should be allowed to handle the equipment, pump the cuff, etc.
        (3) It may be helpful for the child to use the equipment on his parents, the nurse, or a doll in order for him to overcome his fears and understand its use.

B. Methods Used in Obtaining Blood Pressure Measurements in Pediatrics

1. *Auscultatory method* (method of choice whenever possible)
    a. Center the bladder of the cuff over the artery.
    b. Apply the cuff evenly and snugly over the bare arm with the lower edge about 1.25 cm. (½ inch) above the antecubital space.
    c. Support the arm in a slightly flexed and abducted position at the level of the child's heart.
    d. Palpate the brachial artery and inflate the cuff until the palpated pulse is lost. Then pump for an additional 20–30 mm. Hg beyond that.
    e. Deflate the cuff slowly at a rate of about 5 mm. Hg/second.
    f. Deflate the cuff rapidly and completely when all sounds disappear.
    g. Record the reading and compare it with previous values.
        There continues to be a controversy as to what best indicates diastolic pressure. Therefore, it is good practice to record all 3 readings:
        (1) Systolic—point at which pulse becomes audible
        (2) Diastolic—point of muffling of sound
        (3) Point of disappearance of sounds
    h. The blood pressure may be obtained by the same method in the leg, using the popliteal artery.

2. *Palpatory method* (this method provides only an approximate mean pressure that lies between the systolic and diastolic pressures obtained by the auscultatory method)
    a. Follow steps 1–3 of the auscultatory method.
    b. Inflate the cuff to about 200 mm. Hg.
    c. Take the reading when the pulse distal to the cuff becomes palpable in the course of deflation.

3. *Flush method* (This method is especially useful with infants, but also has the disadvantage of providing only an approximate mean pressure.)
    a. The infant should be quiet and in the supine position.

b. Apply a blood pressure cuff to the upper or lower extremity, just above the wrist or ankle.
c. Squeeze the extremity distal to the cuff with a hand or firm wrapping to force blood into the upper extremity. This will blanch the child's arm or leg below the cuff.
d. Pump the manometer to 120–140 mm. Hg.
e. Release the hand or the wrapping.
f. Slowly deflate the cuff.
g. Take the reading at the point at which blood reenters the hand or foot, causing a sudden flushing.

4. *Electronic and ultrasonic methods*
    a. Equipment utilizes electronic circuitry or reflected sound to detect blood flow or movement of an arterial wall under an occluding cuff.
    b. Sophisticated equipment is available that can inflate and deflate the cuff and either hold or automatically record the measurement.
    c. Advantages
        (1) Especially useful in infants when the Korotkoff sounds may be inaudible by ordinary methods.
        (2) The child is subjected to minimal handling despite frequent monitoring of the blood pressure.
        (3) Observer bias is minimized since pressures are analyzed electronically rather than by the human ear. Therefore, blood pressure readings are more consistent.
        (4) Ultrasonic measurements correlate closely with intra-arterial pressures.
    d. Nursing considerations
        (1) Read specific instructions before operating the device.
        (2) Note specifically what sounds are being measured, and whether the equipment measures muffling or silence, or both as the diastolic pressure.

C. Principles Related to Pediatric Blood Pressure Values
(See Figs. 47-1 and 47-2)

1. The blood pressure varies with the age of the child and is closely related to his height and weight.
2. Variability of blood pressure among children of approximately the same age and body build is normal.
3. When the cuff technique is used, the pressure measurement in the legs may be slightly higher than that in the arms in children over 1 year of age.

Nursing Management of the Child With Fever

Fever is any abnormal elevation of body temperature. Prolonged elevation of temperature above 40°C. (104°F.) may produce dehydration and harmful effects on the central nervous system.

Causes

1. Infection
2. Inflammatory disease
3. Dehydration
4. Tumors
5. Disturbance of temperature regulating center
6. Extravasation of blood in the tissues
7. Drugs or toxins

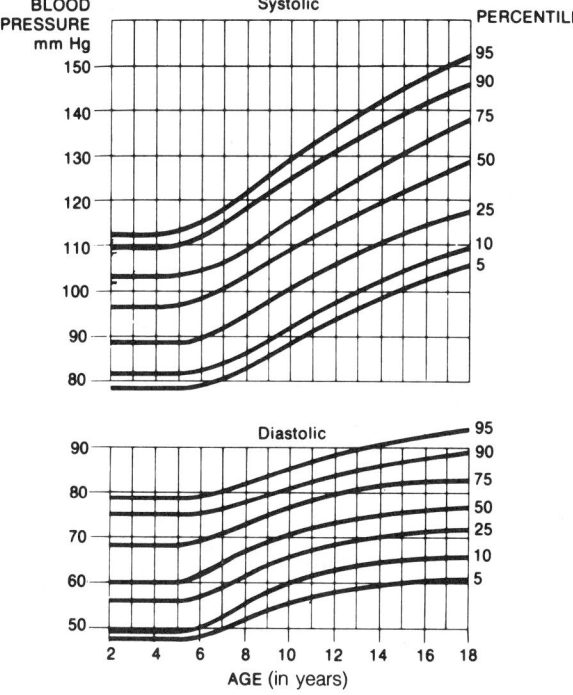

Figure 47-1. *Percentiles of blood pressure measurements in boys (right arm, seated).*

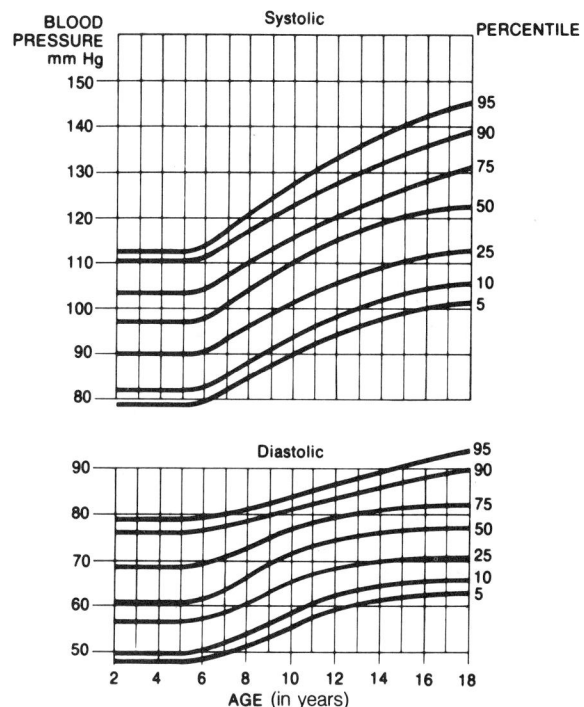

Figure 47-2. *Percentage of blood pressure measurements in girls (right arm, seated).*

Assessment

1. Consider basic principles related to temperature regulation in pediatric patients.
   a. Usually an infant's temperature does not stabilize before he is 1 week old. A newborn's temperature varies with the temperature of his environment.
   b. The degree of fever does not always reflect the severity of the disease. A child may have a very serious illness with a normal or subnormal temperature.
   c. Fever, itself, may cause convulsions in some children when the temperature goes very high, very quickly.
   d. The range for normal temperature varies widely in children. A common explanation for "fever" is misinterpretation of a normal temperature reading (refer to Measuring Vital Signs in Children, p. 1140).
   e. The child's temperature is influenced by activity and by time of day; temperatures are highest in late afternoon.
2. Be certain that accurate technique is used for temperature measurement. The mode should be appropriate for the child's age and condition, and the thermometer should be left in place for the required period of time (refer to Measuring Vital Signs in Children, p. 1140).
3. Assist the physician in determining the cause of the illness.
   a. History
      Information should be elicited regarding:
      Age of the child
      Pattern of the fever
      Length of the illness
      Change in normal patterns of eating, elimination, recreation, etc.
      Other symptoms
      Exposure to any illnesses
      Recent immunizations or drugs
      Treatment of the fever and effectiveness of treatment
      Previous experiences with fever and its control
   b. Physical examination
      Of special significance are:
      General appearance of the child
      Inspection of the skin for rashes, sores, flushed appearance
      Inspection of eyes, ears, nose, and throat for redness and/or drainage
      Auscultation of lungs for abnormal sounds
      Neurologic observation for changes in state of consciousness, pupillary reaction, strength of grip, abnormal muscle movement or lack of movement
      Inspection of the external genitals for redness and/or drainage
      Presence of abdominal or flank pain
      (Refer to Pediatric Physical Examination, p. 1054)
   c. Laboratory tests
      Initial tests frequently include complete blood count, urinalysis, cultures of the throat, nasopharynx, urine, blood, and spinal fluid, and x-ray of the chest.
4. Attempt to identify the pattern of the fever. Take the child's temperature by the same method every hour until stable, then every 2 hours until normal, then every 4 hours for 24 hours.

Nursing Measures to Reduce Fever

Fever itself does not necessarily require treatment. The presence of fever should not be obscured by the indiscrim-inate use of antipyretic measures. However, if the child is uncomfortable or appears toxic because of fever, an attempt should be made to reduce it by any of the following nursing measures or by a combination of these measures.

Nursing Action	Rationale/Amplification
1. Increase the child's fluid intake to prevent dehydration.	1. Fever increases the child's fluid requirements by increasing the metabolic rate.
2. Expose the skin to the air by leaving the child lightly dressed in an absorbent material. Avoid warm, binding clothing and blankets.	2. Loss of heat from the skin by radiation is the main temperature regulating mechanism available to the infant or small child.
3. Administer a tepid sponge bath (see Guidelines: Administering a Tepid Water Sponge for Fever, below.)	3. The temperature is lowered by evaporation of water from the surface of the skin.
4. Administer antipyretic drugs.	4. Although effective in reducing fever, antipyretic drugs may obscure the clinical picture and cause numerous side effects including diaphoresis, skin eruptions, nausea, vomiting, hematologic changes, and fever.
5. Use tub or a hypothermia blanket.	5. A tub bath is less frightening and is the preferred method for reducing fever if the child is able to cooperate.
6. Use ice bags for local comfort.	6. These should not be used for infants since they may produce chilling.

Guidelines Administering a Tepid Water Sponge for Fever

A *tepid water sponge* is bathing of the body for a period of time to reduce fever.

Equipment
Basin of tepid water (21.1°–27°C. or 70°–80°F.)
Plastic sheet
2 bath blankets
Hot water bottle with cover
Towels
6 washcloths

> **NURSING ALERT:** Cold water or alcohol sponges should not be administered to pediatric patients. Cold water may produce vaso-constriction and shivering, which raise central body temperature. Alcohol sponges may reduce the temperature too rapidly, leading to convulsions in small children. In addition, the fumes may be toxic.

Procedure

Nursing Action	Rationale/Amplification
Preparatory Phase	
1. Secure the child's cooperation.	1. This helps to increase the effectiveness of the procedure. A tub bath in tepid water is less frightening and is the preferred method for reducing a fever if the child is able to cooperate. When using this technique, it is best to start with warm water and gradually add cool water to the tub. This prevents sudden chilling of the child.
a. Explain the procedure to the child in language he can understand.	
b. A small infant may be held during sponging.	
c. Allow the child or his parent to participate in the procedure.	
d. Discontinue sponging if the child is extremely upset and uncooperative.	
2. Take temperature, pulse, and respiration before starting the sponge.	2. This serves as a baseline for comparison to determine the effectiveness of treatment.
3. Give antipyretic medication as prescribed 15–20 minutes before starting the sponge.	3. There is a more rapid reduction of fever when sponging is combined with administration of antipyretic medication.

Procedure
(continued)

Nursing Action	Rationale/Amplification

Performance Phase

1. Place a plastic sheet covered with a bath blanket under the child.
2. Place a bath blanket over the child, and remove top bedding.
3. Place cold moist cloths in each axilla and groin and on the forehead.
4. Expose the body area to be sponged. Place a towel under the area.
5. Slowly stroke the extremities with long, soothing strokes of the washcloth.
   a. Stroke each arm from the neck to the axilla and down to the palm of the hand.
   b. Stroke each leg from the groin to the foot.
   c. Bathe the back and buttocks.
6. Use gentle friction to bring the blood to the surface.
7. Change the water as often as necessary to maintain a water temperature of 21.1°–27°C. (70°–80°F.).
8. Continue this procedure until temperature is adequately reduced, more drastic measures are prescribed, or the child's condition indicates that it should be discontinued.

9. Pat dry with towel.

Follow-Up Phase

1. Remove bath blankets and plastic sheet. Place a dry gown on the child.
2. Record vital signs 30 minutes after the sponge is finished.

Rationale/Amplification:

3. This aids in lowering body temperature. The cloths should be changed as they become warm.

6. This increases the effectiveness of the treatment and prevents chilling.

8. Generally, the sponge should not last more than 30 minutes. Observe for shivering. If this occurs, cover the child and wait a few minutes before proceeding. Stop the sponge if cyanosis, mottling, or chilling do not stop when friction is applied to the skin. These symptoms indicate a change in vasomotor tone.

2. Postsponge values indicate whether or not treatment has been effective.

Administering Medications to Children

Purpose

To safely administer medications to the child as prescribed by the physician.

Important Considerations

1. The nurse's manner of approach should indicate that she firmly expects the child to take the medication. This manner often convinces the child of the necessity of the procedure. Establishing a positive relationship with the child will allow him to express feelings, concerns, and fantasies regarding medications.
2. Explanation about the medication should appeal to the child's level of understanding (i.e., color, comparison to something familiar).
3. The nurse must mask her own feelings regarding the medication.
4. Always be truthful when the child asks, "Does it taste bad?" or "Will it hurt?" Respond by saying, "The medicine does not taste good, but I will give you some juice as soon as you swallow it," or "It will hurt for just a minute, like a mosquito bite."
5. It is often necessary to mix distasteful medications or crushed pills with a small amount of carbonated drink or cherry syrup, honey, or applesauce.

6. Never threaten a child with an injection if he refuses an oral medication.
7. Medications should not be mixed with large quantities of food or with any food that is taken regularly (e.g., milk).
8. Medications should not be given at mealtime unless specifically prescribed.
9. The nurse must know the following about each medication she is administering: common usages and dosages, contraindications, side effects, and toxic effects.
10. When preparing intramuscular injections, draw in 0.2 ml. of air after the correct amount of solution is in the syringe. This serves to clear all medication from the needle upon injection and prevents backflow and the depositing of medication in subcutaneous fat upon withdrawal of the needle.

Calculating the Pediatric Dosage

Although it is not the nurse's responsibility to determine the dosage of a drug, it *is* her responsibility to know the safe dosage range of any medication administered to children.

1. Know what factors determine the amount of drug prescribed.
   a. Action of the drug, absorption, detoxification, excretion are related to the maturity and metabolic rate of the child.

b. The neonate and premature infants require a reduced dosage because of:
   (1) Deficient or absent detoxifying enzymes
   (2) Decreased effective renal function
   (3) Altered blood–brain barrier and protein-binding capacity

c. Dosages recommended according to age-groups are not satisfactory since a child may be much smaller or larger than the average child in his age-group.

d. Dosage calculations based on weight have limitations.

2. Be alert to a prescription that would be inappropriate for a child.

3. Consult drug literature for recommended dosage and other information.

Body Surface Area

The following formulas are used to estimate the pediatric dosage based on the child's body surface area. Body surface area (BSA) calculations are generally preferred because many physiologic processes in the child (i.e., blood volume, glomerular filtration) are related to BSA.

1. Surface area in sq. meters × Dose per sq. meter

$$= \text{Approximate child dose}$$

2. $\dfrac{\text{Surface area of child}}{\text{Surface area of adult}} \times \text{Dose of adult}$

$$= \text{Approximate child dose}$$

3. $\dfrac{\text{Surface area of child in sq. meters}}{1.75}$

$$\times \text{Adult dose} = \text{Child dose}$$

Clark's Rule

The following rule may be used as an estimate of the pediatric dosage based on the child's weight in respect to the adult dose of the drug.

$$\dfrac{\text{Child's weight in pounds}}{150} \times \text{Adult dose}$$

$$= \text{Approximate dose for child}$$

Identifying the Patient

Always check a child's identification bracelet with medication card before administering a medication. Ask the older child his name.

Oral Medications

A. Infants

1. Draw up medication in a plastic dropper or disposable syringe.
2. Elevate infant's head and shoulders; depress chin with thumb to open mouth.
3. Place dropper or syringe on the middle of the tongue and slowly drop the medication on the tongue.
4. Release thumb and allow child to swallow.
5. Once the correct amount of medication has been measured, it can be placed in a nipple and the infant can suck the medication through the nipple.
6. If the nurse feels comfortable managing the infant in her lap, it is acceptable to hold him for medication administration.

B. Toddlers

1. Draw up liquid medication in syringe or measure into medicine cup. Medications may be placed in medicine cup or spoon after being measured accurately in a syringe.
2. Elevate the child's head and shoulders.
3. Squeeze cup and put it to the child's lips; or place the syringe (without the needle) in the child's mouth, positioning the syringe tip in space between cheek mucosa and gum, and slowly expel the medicine. Child may prefer using the familiar teaspoon.
4. Allow the child time to swallow.
5. Allow the child to hold the medicine cup by himself, if he is able, and to drink it at his own pace. (This may be a more agreeable method.) Offer his favorite drink as a "chaser," if not contraindicated.
6. The small, safe, disposable medicine cups can be given to the child for play.

C. School-Age Children

1. When a child is old enough to take medicine in pill or capsule form, he should be taught to place the pill near the back of his tongue and immediately swallow fluid such as water or fruit juice. If the swallowing of the fluid is emphasized, the child will no longer think about the pill.
2. Always praise a child after he has taken his medication.
3. If the child finds it particularly difficult to take oral medications, the nurse must let him know that she understands some of his fear and displeasure and that she wants to help him.

Intramuscular Medications

A. General Considerations for IM Injections

1. After medication is drawn from vial, draw up an additional 0.2–0.3 ml. of air into syringe, thus clearing needle of medication and preventing medication seepage from injection site.
2. When injecting less than 1 ml. of medication, use a tuberculin syringe for accuracy.
3. Cleanse site thoroughly, using friction with an antiseptic solution; let site dry.
4. Establish anatomic landmarks (Fig. 47-3). Alternate injection site and keep record at bedside or on medication card.
5. After penetrating site, aspirate to check for blood vessel puncture. If this occurs, withdraw needle, discard medication, and start again.
6. Following injection, massage site (unless contraindicated). The complication of fibrosis and contracture of the muscle can be diminished by massage, warm soaks, and range-of-motion exercises to disrupt and stretch immature scar tissue when multiple injections are being administered.

B. Infants

1. Acceptable site selection:
   Rectus femoris (mid-anterior thigh)
   Vastus lateralis (middle third)
   Ventrogluteal—these areas are relatively free of major nerves and blood vessels.
   The gluteus maximus and deltoid muscles are underdeveloped in the infant and use of these sites can result in nerve damage.
2. Administration
   a. *Rectus femoris*
      (1) Place the child in a secure position to prevent movement of the extremity.

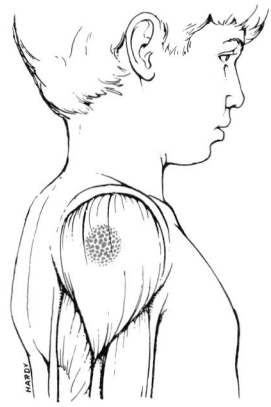
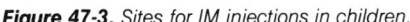
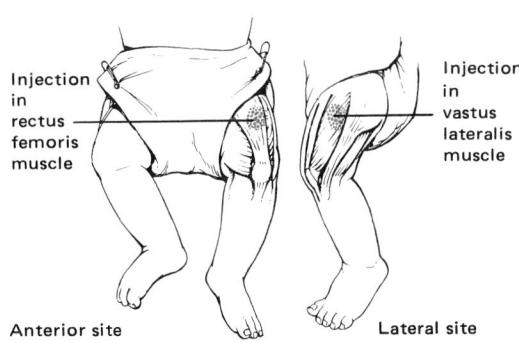

Arm for older child

Leg for small infant

Figure 47-3. *Sites for IM injections in children.*

(2) Do not use a needle longer than 2.5 cm. (1 inch).
(3) Use upper outer quadrant of the thigh.
(4) Insert needle at a 45-degree angle in a downward direction, toward the knee.

b. *Vastus lateralis*
(1) Place the child in prone or supine position.
(2) Area is a narrow strip of muscle extending along a line from the greater trochanter to lateral femoral condyle below.
(3) Insert needle perpendicular to skin 2–4 cm. deep—needle parallel to floor.

c. *Ventrogluteal*—see below.

Following administration of medication, hold and cuddle infant. This site is also used on the older child who may be difficult to restrain.

C. Toddlers and School-Age Children

1. Site selection
   a. *Posterogluteal-upper outer quadrant*
   (1) Gluteal muscles do not develop until the child begins to walk; they should be used only when the child has been walking for 1 year or more.
   Complications include sciatic nerve injury or subcutaneous injury due to medication being injected and poor absorption.
   (2) Upper outer quadrant of the young child's buttock is smaller in diameter than that of an adult; thus accuracy in determining the area comprising the upper outer quadrant is essential.
   (3) Administration
   (a) Do not use a needle longer than 2.5 cm. (1 inch).
   (b) Position the child in a prone position.
   (c) Place thumb on the trochanter.
   (d) Place middle finger on the iliac crest.
   (e) Let index finger drop at a point midway between the thumb and middle finger to the upper outer quadrant of the buttock. This is the injection site.
   (f) Insert needle perpendicular to the surface on which the child is lying, not perpendicular to the skin.

b. *Ventrogluteal*
(1) This site provides a dense muscle mass that is relatively free of the danger of injuring the nervous and vascular systems.
(2) The disadvantage is that the injection site is visible to the child.
(3) Administration
(a) Place the child on his back.
(b) Place index finger on the anterosuperior spine.
(c) With the middle finger moving dorsally, locate the iliac crest; drop finger below the crest. The triangle formed by the iliac crest, index finger, and middle finger is the injection site.
(d) Inject needle perpendicular to the surface on which the child is lying.

c. *Deltoid*
(1) May be used for older, larger children.
(2) Determine injection site as with an adult.
(3) Inject needle perpendicular to skin 2–3 cm. deep.

d. *Lateral and anterior aspect of the thigh*
(1) Do not use a needle longer than 2.5 cm. (1 inch).
(2) Use the upper outer quadrant of the thigh.
(3) Insert needle at a 45-degree angle in a downward direction, toward the knee.

2. Nursing support
   a. Explain to the child where you are going to give him the injection (site) and why he must receive the injection.
   b. Allow the child to express his fears.
   c. Carry out procedure quickly and gently. Have needle and syringe completely prepared and ready prior to contact with child.
   d. Numb site of injection by rubbing skin firmly with cleansing swab or with ice (older child may assist with this), and change needle after drawing medication through rubber stopper on medicine vial. Minimize pain of intramuscular injection by injecting needle into muscle with a quick, darting motion.
   e. Always secure the assistance of a second nurse to help immobilize the child and divert his attention as well as to offer him support and comfort.

f. Praise the child for his behavior after the injection. Often, allowing him to assist with applying a Band-Aid will give him some feeling of comfort.

g. Also encourage activity that will use the muscle site of injection—promotes dispersal of medication and decreases soreness. This can also be done by firmly massaging muscle following injection, unless contraindicated.

h. Record accurately the injection site to ensure proper site rotation.

Intravenous Medications

(See intravenous infusions, p. 1167)

A. Intravenous Drip

1. Selecting the proper site for injecting medication into an intravenous line depends on the correct dilution for the drug, the rate of fluid administration, and the amount of intravenous fluid tolerated by the child.

    a. *Piggyback*—a second container holding the drug and a relatively small volume of fluid and an administration set are attached at the injection site of the primary administration set tubing, and allowed to flow over a period of time from 20 minutes to 2 hours. This method maintains fluid schedule without fluid overload.

    b. *Bolus*—a rapid injection of a small volume of drug directly into the intravenous tubing or cannula by means of a syringe and needle.

    c. *Volume-control*—inject drug into gum-rubber injection port of volume control administration set. This allows for further dilution of drug with primary fluid or separate fluid reservoir. Then administer total fluid containing the drug in 30–60 minutes.

2. Prepare mixtures aseptically (laminar-flow hood) and use sterile technique when violating the line. (Sepsis is a constant threat when a child is receiving intravenous medications.)

3. Be aware that an exaggerated pharmacologic effect may exist with intravenous medications. As with any medication, know the use, side effects, and toxic effects of the drug, as well as the pharmacologic effect on the body.

4. Dilute intravenous medications and inject slowly—never less than 1 minute (this allows peripheral blood flow through the entire circulating system to dilute the medication and prevent high concentrations of the drug from reaching the brain and heart).

5. Be knowledgeable regarding compatibilities of drugs, electrolytes in IV solutions, and the fluid itself.

6. Observe IV site frequently. Restrain child, as needed, to prevent infiltration. Infiltration of fluids containing medications can cause rapid and severe tissue necrosis.

B. Heparin Lock (See Adult, p. 91).

Venipuncture setup with 3½-inch tubing ending in a re-sealing rubber diaphragm, creating a closed system.

1. The use of a heparin lock allows children who need repeated doses of chemotherapeutic agents or antibiotics to be fully mobile while reducing the trauma of repeated injections.

2. Heparin solution (0.25 ml. heparin, 1000 USP/ml. to 10 ml. sterile water) is administered prior to and following instillation of medication, and regular heparin flushing is done every 8 hours to maintain patency.

3. The heparin lock can be connected to standard pediatric administration sets so that larger volumes of vehicle solutions can be used for dilution of medications.

4. The heparin lock should be securely taped in place to prevent dislodgement. Patency of vein must be determined prior to administration of fluids or medications.

Enema

An *enema* is the insertion of fluid into the rectum for the purpose of cleansing the lower bowel, or cooling to reduce temperature. An enema for an infant or a young child is based on the same principles as for an adult and is essentially the same, except that *less fluid and pressure are used than in an adult.*

Guidelines   Administering an Enema to a Child

Equipment

Solution measurements:
   Soapsuds enema—add 8 ml. (2 drams) soap jelly to 500 ml. (1 pint) water
   Saline enema—add 4 ml. (1 dram) salt to 500 ml. (1 pint) water or 1 teaspoon salt to 500 ml. water
   Gloves

Procedure

Nursing Action	Rationale/Amplification
Preparatory Phase	
1. Explain procedure to the child according to his level of understanding.	1. Even though the child may not fully understand, an explanation will soothe him and build his trust in you.
2. Position	
a. *Older child:* Have him lie on his left side with his upper leg flexed.	a. This position places the descending colon at the lowest point.
b. *Infant:* Place infant in supine position, with a pillow under his head and back and a small bedpan under his buttocks. Gentle restraint may be needed—diaper placed under the bedpan, brought over thighs, and then pinned.	b. Infants and small children cannot retain enema fluid. Properly placed pillows promote body alignment.

Procedure (continued)	Nursing Action	Rationale/Amplification

Performance Phase

1. Wear gloves.
2. Insert rectal tube 3.7–10 cm. (1½–4 inches) into the rectum just within the anal sphincter.
3. Hang solution reservoir no higher than 25 cm. (10 inches) above the rectum.
4. Do not administer more than 300 ml. (10 oz.) of solution to infant unless otherwise prescribed.

5. Once the rectal tube is removed, the abdomen can be gently massaged, if there are no contraindications.
6. If young child is "potty trained," have a small potty chair available for his use.

7. When a retention enema is administered, the buttocks may be held or taped together to assist retention of fluid. Keep child as quiet as possible.

1. Universal precautions.

3. This allows the solution to run slowly with minimal pressure.

4. Fluid volume may range from 30–300 ml. (1–10 oz.) depending on the size of the child.
   Suggested amounts:
   Birth to 3 months: 30–100 ml.
   Infant: 150–250 ml.
   Child: 200–500 ml.
   Older child: 500–1000 ml.

5. This gentle massage will help relax the infant and assist in expelling the solution.
6. The familiarity of a potty chair will provide great comfort for the child and eliminate the possible embarrassment of a soiled bed or pants.

Protective Measures to Limit Movement *(Restraints)*

Protective measures to limit movement are mechanisms for restraining children (Fig. 47-4).

Purpose

1. To maintain the child's safety and protect him from injury.
2. To facilitate examination and minimize the child's discomfort during special tests, procedures, and specimen collections.

Underlying Principles

1. Protective devices should be used only when necessary and never as a substitute for careful observation of the child.
2. The reason for using the protective device should be explained to the child and his parents to prevent misinterpretation and to ensure their cooperation with the procedure. Restraints are often interpreted as punishment by children.
3. Any protective device should be checked frequently to make sure that it is effective. It should be removed periodically to prevent skin irritation or circulation impairment.
4. Protective devices should always be applied in a manner that maintains proper body alignment and ensures the child's comfort.
5. Any protective device that requires attachment to the child's bed should be secured to the bed springs or frame, *never* the mattress or side rails. This allows the side rails to be adjusted without removing the restraint or injuring the child's extremity.
6. Any knots that are required should be tied in a manner that permits their quick release. This is a safety precaution.
7. When a child must be immobilized, an attempt should

be made to replace the lost activity with another form of motion. For example, even though restrained, a child can be moved in a stroller, wheelchair, or in his bed. When arms are restrained, the child may be allowed to play kicking games. Water play, mirrors, body games, and blowing bubbles are helpful replacements.

Mummy Device

The *mummy device* involves securing a sheet or blanket around the child's body in such a way that his arms are held to his sides and his leg movements are restricted (see Fig. 47-4).

A. Purpose

To restrain infants and small children during treatments and examinations involving the head and neck.

B. Equipment

Small sheet or blanket
Several large safety pins

C. Nursing Action

1. Place the blanket or sheet flat on the bed.
2. Fold over one corner of the blanket.
3. Place the child on the blanket with his neck at the edge of the fold.
4. Pull the right side of the blanket firmly over the child's right shoulder.
5. Tuck the remainder of the right side of the blanket under the left side of the child's body.
6. Repeat the procedure with the left side of the blanket.
7. Separate the corners of the bottom portion of the sheet, and fold it up toward the child's neck.
8. Tuck both sides of the sheet under the infant's body.
9. Secure by crossing one side over the other in the back and tucking in the excess, or by pinning the blanket in place.

D. Special Precautions

Make certain that the child's extremities are in a comfortable position during this procedure.

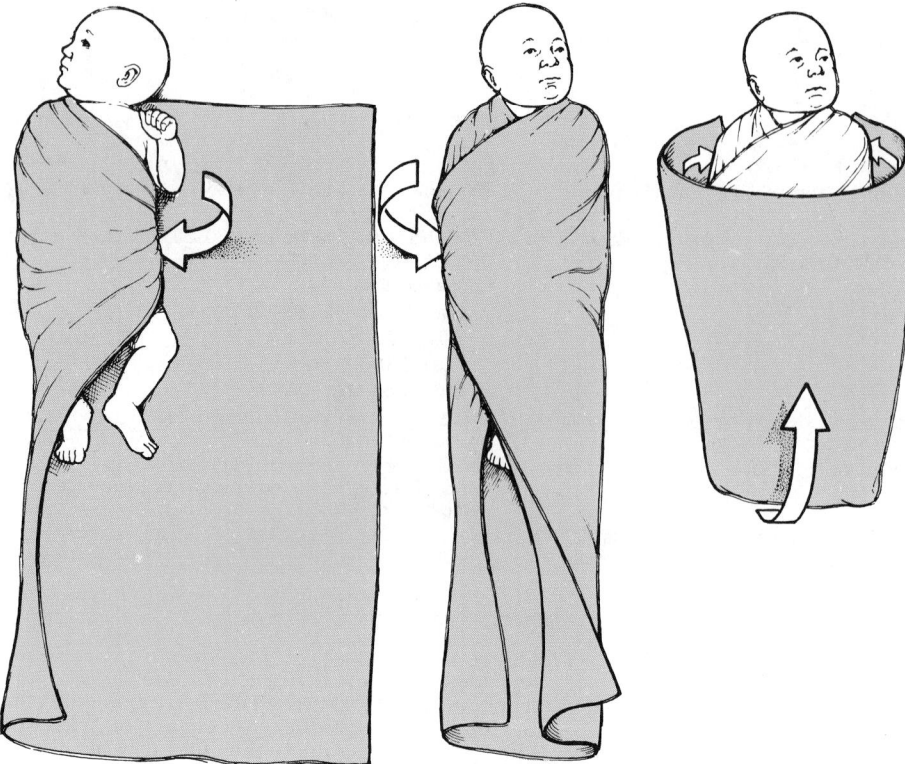

Mummy device

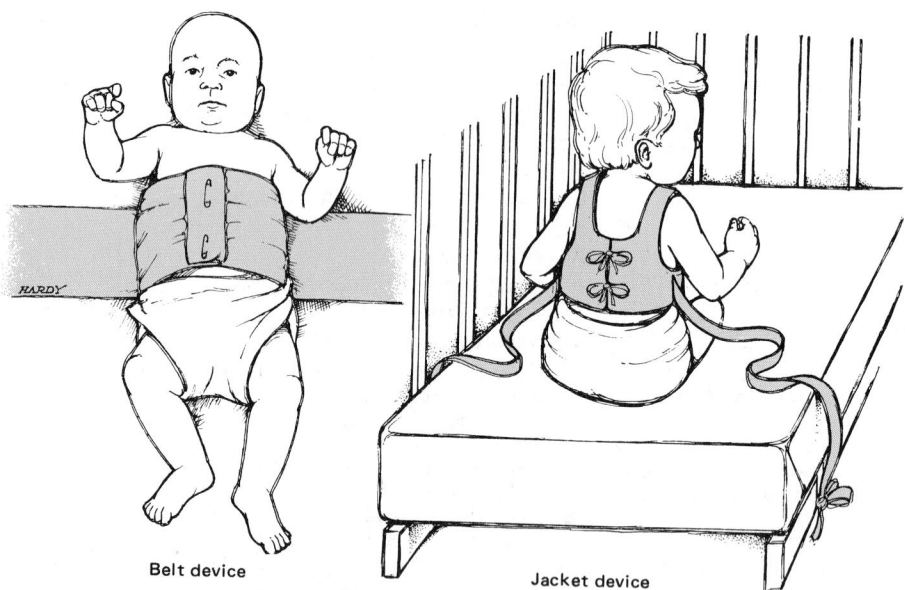

Belt device

Jacket device

Figure 47-4. *Types of restraints.*

Jacket Device

The *jacket device* is a piece of material that fits the child like a jacket or halter. Long tapes are attached to the sides of the jacket (see Fig. 47-4).

A. Purpose

To keep the child in his wheelchair, highchair, or crib.

B. Nursing Action

1. Put the jacket on the child so that the opening is in the back.
2. Tie the strings securely.
3. Position the child in his highchair, wheelchair, or crib.
4. Secure the long tapes appropriately:
   a. Under the arm supports of a chair.

b. Around the back of the wheelchair or highchair.

c. To the springs or frame of the crib.

C. Special Precautions

The child in a crib must be observed frequently to make certain that he does not entangle himself in the long tapes of the jacket device.

Belt Device

The *belt device* is exactly like the jacket method of restraining, except that the material fits the child like a wide belt and buckles in the back (see Fig. 47-4).

Elbow Device

The *elbow device* consists of a piece of material into which tongue depressors have been inserted at regular intervals. It is especially useful for infants receiving a scalp-vein infusion, those with eczema or cleft lip repair, and children having eye surgery.

A. Purpose

To prevent flexion of the elbow.

B. Equipment

Elbow cuff
Tongue depressors
Safety pins, tapes, or string

C. Nursing Action

1. Insert tongue depressors into the appropriate places in the elbow cuff.
2. Place the child's arm in the center of the elbow cuff.
3. Wrap the cuff around the child's arm.
4. Secure the cuff with pins, tapes, or string.

D. Special Precautions

1. The tongue depressors should be cut to about 10 cm. (4 inches) in length if the elbow cuff is to be used for an infant—for greatest comfort.
2. Additional security may be provided by dressing the child in a long-sleeved shirt prior to the application of the elbow cuff. The ends of the shirt can then be turned back over the cuff and pinned securely.

Devices to Limit Movement of the Extremities

There are many different kinds of devices to limit motion of one or more extremities. One commercial variety consists of a piece of material with tapes on both ends to be secured to the frame of the crib. The material also has two small flaps sewn to it for securing the child's ankles or wrists. Similar devices are available that use sheepskin flaps. These should be used when the device will be necessary over a prolonged period, or for children with very sensitive skin.

A. Purpose

To restrain infants and young children for such procedures as intravenous therapy and urine collection.

B. Equipment

Extremity restraint of appropriate size for the child (small, medium, or large)
Several safety pins
Cotton wadding covered with gauze

C. Nursing Action

1. Secure the device to the crib frame.
2. Pad the extremities to be restrained with cotton wadding covered with gauze or other suitable material.

3. Pin the small flaps securely around the child's ankles or wrists.
4. Adjust the device by pinning a tuck in the center of the material, if it is too large.

D. Special Precautions

1. The infant's fingers or toes should be observed frequently for coldness or discoloration and the skin under the device checked for signs of irritation.
2. The device should be removed periodically to provide skin care and range-of-motion exercises.

Abdominal Device

The *abdominal device* is used for restraining a small child in his crib. It operates exactly like the method described for limiting the movement of the extremities. However, the strip of material is wider and has only one wide flap sewn in the center for fastening around the child's abdomen.

Clove-Hitch Device

The *clove-hitch device* is a mechanism for restraining an extremity by tying gauze strips or a diaper in a special way.

A. Equipment

Cotton wadding covered with gauze
Gauze bandage cut in lengths of 1.37 meters (1½ yards)

B. Nursing Action

1. Pad the extremity to be restrained with cotton wadding that is covered with gauze or other suitable material.
2. Spread out the gauze strip on the bed.
3. Make a figure-8 loop in the center of the gauze strip.
4. Place the child's wrist or ankle in the loop of the device.
5. Pull the ends of the device to the desired tightness.
6. Tie the ends to the crib springs or frame.
7. Check the device to make certain that it does not tighten when both ends are pulled taut or slip over the child's hand or foot.

Mitts

Mitts are used to prevent a child from injuring himself with his hands. They are especially useful for children with dermatologic conditions, such as eczema or burns. Mitts can be purchased commercially or made by wrapping the child's hands in Kling gauze.

Special Precaution

Mitts should be removed at least twice during each tour of duty to permit skin care and to allow the child to exercise his fingers.

Crib Top Device

A *crib top device* is used to prevent an infant or small child from climbing over the crib sides. Several types of commercial devices are available, including nets, plastic tops, and domes. A crib top device should be applied to the crib of any infant capable of climbing over the crib sides.

Special Precaution

In all instances, it is essential to be certain that the crib sides are kept all of the way up and latched securely. There should be no space between the top of the crib sides and the bottom of the crib top device.

Feeding and Nutrition

Guidelines   Breast-Feeding the Ill or Hospitalized Infant*

Breast-feeding is suckling of an infant at the mother's breast to provide him with nourishment.

Purposes
1. To provide psychological and emotional satisfaction for the infant and the mother.
2. To feed the infant a natural and ideal food that will supply him with adequate nutrition as well as immunologic and anti-infection advantages.
3. To have milk always available at the right temperature.
4. To prevent chance of gastrointestinal disturbances and development of allergies.
5. To provide physical closeness of baby to mother during feeding.
6. To provide comfort after a frightening or painful procedure.

Points to Consider
1. The breast-fed infant up to 6 months of age may not have been started on solid foods.
2. The mother (at home) may give other liquids only by spoon or cup, not by bottle and nipple.
3. The infant may nurse frequently if mother is available.
4. Because breast milk is more easily and quickly digested, shorter periods of NPO both preoperatively and postoperatively may be used with the breast-fed infant.
5. Stress of child's hospitalization and illness experienced by the mother may decrease her milk supply and inhibit her "let down" reflex, as well as increase or decrease the infant's desire to suckle.
6. The infant in time of stress may cope with breast-feeding better than with bottle-feeding. Do not attempt to wean if avoidable.

Procedure

Nursing Action	Rationale/Amplification

Preparatory Phase

1. When an infant who is nursing is hospitalized, it is the nurse's responsibility to encourage the mother to continue breast-feeding if the infant's condition does not contraindicate it. Explain to the mother that: a. Supplemental artificial formula can be given to the infant if she is not available; or b. She can pump her breasts and bring in her milk to be given to the infant via bottle when she is not available.	1. Some mothers have very strong feelings about wanting to nurse their baby. It gives them an emotional satisfaction that is vitally important to the mother–child relationship since it is an integral part of the total mothering process. The nurse must help to foster this relationship as much as she can.
2. When nursing is to be done in the hospital pediatric setting, the physical surroundings may need to be altered somewhat. Provide the mother and infant with a relatively quiet area that is as private as possible and free from interruption.	2. This will provide the mother and infant with an opportunity to continue to develop their relationship during the crisis of illness and hospitalization.
3. Provide the mother with a comfortable armchair or pillow so that she can assume a comfortable position during the feeding. A footstool should also be available so that she can support her feet and the infant.	3. Proper and comfortable position of the mother will enable her to hold the baby correctly and support him while he is at the breast.
4. The infant should be awake and dry before the feeding is started.	4. If the infant is awake and comfortable, he will settle down and feed better.
5. Dress the infant appropriately so that he is not too warm or too cool during the feeding. The infant should also be hungry.	5. If he is too warm, he may fall asleep after the first few sucks of milk. A sleepy baby will not nurse well. If he is too cool, he may be fussy and restless.
6. Position the baby at breast. Put him in a semi-sitting position with his face close to the breast and supported by one arm and hand. A pillow may be used under the baby to support him. The breast may need to be supported by mother's other hand.	6. Proper positioning will provide the infant with comfort and security and make it easier for him to suck and swallow. This makes the nipple more easily accessible to the infant's mouth and prevents obstruction of nasal breathing.

Performance Phase

1. When the feeding is to start, let the breast touch the infant's cheek. Do not hold his cheek and try to help him find the nipple.	1. The rooting reflex will take over and the infant will turn his head toward the breast with his mouth open. If his cheek is touched with a hand, he will become confused, perhaps turning toward the hand.
2. The infant's lips should be out over the areola and not just around the nipple before he begins to suck.	2. Since the nipple is so small, suction cannot be achieved merely by grasping it. The areola must be in the infant's mouth in order to establish suction and make the suck effective.
3. Note the presence or absence of the "let-down" reflex during the nursing period.	3. Milk flowing from the other breast during nursing is quite normal. It is not usually present when the mother is worried.

Procedure *(continued)*	**Nursing Action**	**Rationale/Amplification**
	4. The length of feeding time may vary from 5 to 30 minutes. Let the infant nurse until he is satisfied.	4. When the infant is satisfied and has nursed well, he is relaxed and usually falls asleep. He will stop sucking.
	5. Instruct the mother to burp the baby during and at the end of the feeding.	5. When the infant is sucking, he swallows some air. Burping will help prevent abdominal distention and discomfort as well as regurgitation.
	6. One or both breasts may be used at each feeding. It makes no difference as long as (a) baby is satisfied at the end of the feeding and (b) 1 breast is completely emptied at the feeding.	6. Regular and complete emptying of the breast is the only stimulation for the production of milk.
	7. Once the infant has stopped sucking, he likes to cling to the breast. To break this suction, instruct mother to put her finger to the corner of the baby's mouth and gently pull.	7. Gentle pulling will not hurt mother or infant.

Follow-Up Phase

	Nursing Action	**Rationale/Amplification**
	1. When the infant has finished feeding, change his diaper if it is wet or soiled.	1. To provide comfort for a restful sleep and to prevent diaper rash.
	2. Position infant on his right side or on his abdomen in his bed.	2. This facilitates emptying of the stomach and decreases the possibility of regurgitation.
	3. Note if baby appears satisfied or still seems to be hungry.	3. Mother may not have enough milk to satisfy the baby. Supplemental formula may be necessary.

	4. Record descriptively and accurately:
	  a. How baby fed
	  b. How baby went to breast
	  c. Satiety or hunger after feeding
	  d. Breast or breasts used; which breast was emptied and which breast was nursed from thereafter.
		d. If both breasts were used, the second breast is not usually emptied and should be used first at the next feeding.

	5. For the new mother–infant nursing team:
	  a. Provide the mother with anticipatory guidance for possible problems (i.e., breast engorgement).
	  b. Promote maternal confidence in handling and nursing her infant.
	  c. Increase mother's knowledge about the mechanics of breast-feeding.
	  d. Provide mother with literature and resources.
	    The Womanly Art of Breast Feeding, 4th ed. LaLeche League International, 9616 Minneapolis Avenue, Franklin Park, IL 60131
		5. To help establish and maintain successful breast-feeding that will be continued following discharge. Encourage mother to continue to get adequate rest and nutrition during and following infant's discharge.

* See page 1004 for breast-feeding the newborn.

Guidelines	Artificial or Nipple Feeding

Artificial or *nipple feeding* is a method of supplying nutrition to the infant by oral feedings, using a bottle and nipple set-up.

Purposes
1. To provide the baby adequate fluid and calorie intake for appropriate growth.
2. To supplement breast-feeding with formula or water.
3. To provide additional fluid intake between feedings.

Equipment
Sterile nipple and bottle
Sterile formula or feeding fluid

Procedure	**Nursing Action**	**Rationale/Amplification**

Preparatory Phase

	Nursing Action	**Rationale/Amplification**
	1. Baby should be awake and hungry. Change wet or soiled diaper.	1. A sleepy baby will not feed well. A dry diaper will provide comfort so that the baby will settle down and eat more easily.
	2. Check formula for correct type and amount.	2. To prevent error.

(continued)

Guidelines   Artificial or Nipple Feeding *(continued)*

Procedure *(continued)*	Nursing Action	Rationale/Amplification
	3. Sit in a comfortable chair. Cradle baby with one hand and arm, while supporting baby against your body or lap.	3. Proper position will provide the baby with comfort and security and will make it easier for him to suck and swallow. Holding infant will enhance trust-building and provide sensory stimulation.

Performance Phase

Nursing Action	Rationale/Amplification
1. Let the baby root for the nipple by touching the corner of his mouth with the nipple. When he opens his mouth, insert the nipple.	1. Place the nipple on top of the tongue and far enough in his mouth so suction can be created when he sucks.
2. Hold the bottle at an angle to completely fill the nipple with fluid.	2. This prevents the baby from sucking and swallowing excessive amounts of air.
3. NEVER prop the bottle or leave the baby unattended during feeding.	3. This is unsafe. Should vomiting occur, aspiration is more likely.
4. The bottle should be handled so as not to contaminate the nipple or fluid.	4. Contamination will increase the chances of gastrointestinal disturbances.
5. Baby's feeding time will vary from 10 to 25 minutes. Position baby so eye contact can be established (en face) during feeding. Soothing talk and fondling can provide additional comfort to the baby.	5. The length of time will depend on the age of the baby and how vigorously he sucks.
6. Burp the baby at least once during the feeding and at the end of the feeding.	6. Most babies swallow some air during feeding. These positions aid in expelling air and thus prevent abdominal distention, discomfort, and regurgitation. Vigorous handling or patting may result in the infant spitting up or regurgitating feeding.
a. Place the baby in sitting position in nurse's lap, tilt him slightly forward, and gently rub or pat his back or abdomen.	
b. Place the baby in prone position on nurse's shoulder and gently pat or rub his back.	
c. Place the baby in prone position on nurse's lap and gently rub or pat his back.	

Follow-Up Phase

Nursing Action	Rationale/Amplification
1. After final burping, change wet or soiled diaper and place baby in crib on his abdomen or right side.	1. This position aids in emptying the stomach and prevents regurgitation.
2. Check baby in a few minutes. If he is restless, pick him up and burp him. Note if any spitting-up has occurred.	2. Some babies relieve themselves of air when in the crib and also bring up small amounts of formula at the same time.
3. Accurate and descriptive recording:	
a. What was fed and amount	
b. How feeding was tolerated	
c. Any regurgitation or emesis—amount and material	
d. Length of time of feeding	
e. How baby sucked and took the feeding; behavior before, during, and following feeding.	

Note: When feeding a premature infant, the same principles apply. The premature infant, however, will tire more easily and fall asleep. Allow him frequent rest periods and use a soft nipple so that less energy is needed to suck. To stimulate this infant to suck, the nurse can brush the infant's cheek with her finger, place thumb or finger under the infant's chin, or move the nipple slowly back and forth in his mouth. Feeding time should not exceed 30 minutes. Keep the infant warm during feeding.

Guidelines   Gavage Feeding

Gavage feeding is a means of providing food via a catheter passed through the nares or mouth, past the pharynx, down the esophagus, and into the stomach, slightly beyond the cardiac sphincter.

Purposes
1. To provide a method of feeding or administering medications that requires minimal patient effort, when the infant is unable to suck or swallow (i.e., infant under 32 weeks' gestation or under 1650 gm.).
2. To provide a route that allows adequate calorie or fluid intake.
3. To prevent fatigue or cyanosis that is apt to occur from nipple feeding.
4. To provide a safe method of feeding a limp and listless patient.

Equipment   Sterile rubber or plastic catheter, rounded-tip, size 5–10 (French Argyle feeding tube)
Clear, calibrated reservoir for feeding fluid
Syringe
Stethoscope
Water for lubrication
Tape—hypoallergenic
Feeding fluid, room temperature
Pacifier

Procedure

Nursing Action	Rationale/Amplification

Preparatory Phase

1. Position the infant on his side or back with a diaper roll placed under his shoulders. A mummy restraint may be necessary to help maintain this position.
2. Measure feeding catheter and mark with tape; measure distance from tip of nose to ear to xiphisternum.
3. Have suction apparatus readily available.

1. This position allows for easy passage of the catheter, facilitates observation, and helps avoid obstruction of the airway.
2. Premeasuring the catheter provides a guideline as to how far to insert catheter.
3. Suctioning clears the airway and prevents aspiration if vomiting occurs.

Performance Phase

1. Lubricate catheter with sterile water or saline.
2. Stabilize the patient's head with one hand; use the other hand to insert catheter.
   Push nose up to widen nostril.
   a. *Insertion through nares:* slip the catheter into nostril and direct toward the occiput in a horizontal plane along floor of nasal cavity.
   b. *Insertion through the mouth:* pass the catheter through the mouth toward the back of the throat. Depress anterior portion of tongue with forefinger, insert catheter along forefinger, and tilt head slightly forward.
3. If the patient swallows, passage of the catheter may be synchronized with the swallowing.
   Do not push against resistance.
4. If there is no swallowing, insert the catheter smoothly and quickly.
5. In the infant, especially, observe for vagal stimulation (i.e., bradycardia [slow heart rate] and apnea).

6. Once the catheter has been inserted to the premeasured length, tape the catheter to the patient's face (Fig. 47-5).

1. Do not use oil because of danger of aspiration.

   a. This direction will follow the nares passageway into the pharynx. Do not direct the catheter upward. Positioning in nares may cause partial airway obstruction; therefore, observe for respiratory distress. Avoid this route if there is critical airway compromise.

3. Swallowing motions will cause esophageal peristalsis, which opens the cardiac sphincter and facilitates passage of the catheter.
   Perforation occurs with very little pressure.
4. Because of cardiac sphincter spasm, resistance may be met at this point. Pause a few seconds, then proceed.
5. The vagus nerve pathway lies from the medulla through the neck and thorax to the abdomen. Above the stomach, the left and right branches unite to form the esophageal plexus. Stimulation of these nerve branches with the catheter will directly affect the cardiac and pulmonary plexus.
6. This prevents movement of catheter from the premeasured, preestablished correct position. Alternative method: loop narrow cloth tape around tube just below nostril, then secure it above lip or nose with tape. Some movement of tube may be seen with swallowing.

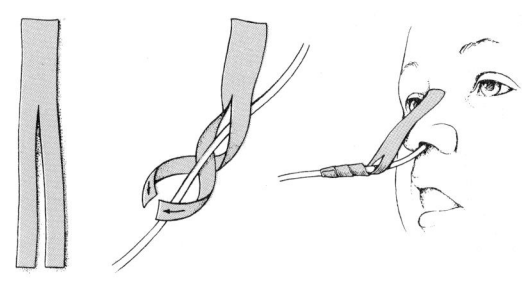

Steps in preparing adhesive tape to retain gavage tube

Gavage tube in jejunum

Figure 47-5. *Gavage feeding.*

(continued)

Guidelines Gavage Feeding *(continued)*

Procedure *(continued)*	Nursing Action	Rationale/Amplification
	7. Test for correct position of the catheter in the stomach:	
	a. Inject 0.5–5 ml. air into the catheter and stomach. At the same time listen to the typical growling stomach sound with a stethoscope placed over the epigastric region.	a. Aids in ensuring proper location of catheter.
	b. Aspirate injected air from the stomach.	b. This prevents abdominal distention.
	c. Aspirate small amount of stomach content and test acidity by pH tape.	c. Failure to obtain aspirate does not indicate improper placement; there may not be any stomach content or the catheter may not be in contact with the fluid.
	d. Observe and gently palpate abdomen for tip of catheter. Avoid inserting catheter into the infant's trachea. (An infant's anatomy makes it relatively difficult to enter the trachea since esophagus is behind the trachea.)	d. If improper placement occurs and the catheter enters the trachea, the patient may cough, fight, and become cyanotic. Remove the catheter immediately and allow the patient to rest before attempting intubation again.
	8. The feeding position should be right–side-lying, with head and chest slightly elevated. Attach reservoir to catheter and fill with feeding fluid. Allow infant to suck on pacifier during feeding. Hold infant when possible.	8. This position allows the flow of fluid to be aided by gravity. The use of the pacifier will relax the infant, allowing for easier flow of fluid as well as provide for normal sucking needs. Sucking will help develop muscles and provide a positive association between sucking and relief of hunger.
	9. Aspirate tube before feeding begins.	9. This is done to monitor for appropriate fluid intake, digestion time, and overfeeding that can cause distention. Note an increase in gastric residual contents.
	a. If over ½ the previous feeding is obtained, withhold the feeding.	
	b. If small residual of formula is obtained, return it to stomach and subtract that amount from the total amount of formula to be given.	
	10. The flow of the feeding should be slow. Do not apply pressure. Elevate reservoir 15–20 cm. (6–8 inches) above the patient's head.	10. The rate of flow is controlled by the size of the feeding catheter; the smaller the size, the slower the flow. If the reservoir is too high, the pressure of the fluid itself increases the rate of flow.
	11. Food taken too rapidly will interfere with peristalsis, causing abdominal distention and regurgitation.	11. The presence of food in the stomach stimulates peristalsis and causes the digestive process to begin. Also, when tube is in place, incompetence of the esophageal–cardiac sphincter may result in regurgitation.
	12. Feeding time should last approximately as long as when a corresponding amount is given by nipple, 5 ml./5–10 minutes or 15–20 minutes total time.	
	13. When the feeding is completed, the catheter may be irrigated with clear water. Before the fluid reaches the end of the catheter, clamp it off and withdraw it quickly.	13. Clamp the catheter before air enters the stomach and causes abdominal distention. Clamping also prevents fluid from dripping from the catheter into the pharynx, causing the patient to gag and aspirate.
	14. Discard feeding tube and any leftover solution.	

Note: Intermittent gavage feeding is often preferred to indwelling gavage feeding. An indwelling catheter may coil and knot, perforate the stomach, and cause nasal airway obstruction, ulceration, irritation of the mucous membranes, incompetence of esophageal–cardiac sphincter, and epistaxis. However, if intermittent intubation is not well tolerated and the indwelling method is used, the catheter should be clamped to prevent loss of feeding or entry of air and changed every 48–72 hours. (Use alternate sides of the nares.) Constant alertness to the above problems should be stressed. Indwelling method may be preferred with older infant or child.

Follow-Up Phase

	1. Burp the patient.	1. Adequate expulsion of air swallowed or ingested during feeding will decrease abdominal distention and allow for better tolerance of the feeding.
	2. Place the patient on right side or on abdomen for at least 1 hour.	2. To facilitate gastric emptying and minimize regurgitation and aspiration.
	3. Observe condition after feeding; bradycardia and apnea may still occur.	3. Because of vagal stimulation as mentioned above.
	4. Note any vomiting or abdominal distention.	4. Due to overfeeding or too rapid feeding. Regurgitation of 1–2 ml. may occur in the premature infant as the musculature of the sphincter of the gastrointestinal tract is relaxed and allows for easy reflux.
	5. Note infant's activity.	5. Fatigue or peaceful sleep.

Procedure *(continued)*	**Nursing Action**	**Rationale/Amplification**
	6. Accurately describe and record procedure, including time of feeding, type of gavage feeding, type and amount of feeding fluid given, amount retained or vomited, how the patient tolerated feeding, and activity before, during, and following feeding.	6. Observe for readiness of the infant to feed by nipple—note sucking activity and sleep–wake cycle in relation to feeding.

Guidelines · Gastrostomy Feeding

Gastrostomy feeding is a means of providing nourishment and fluids via a tube that has been surgically inserted via a stab wound through the abdominal wall into the stomach.

Purposes

1. To provide a method of nutrition and fluids that requires minimal effort when the patient is unable to suck or swallow for long periods of time.
2. To allow for better decompression of stomach (because of large tube size) following a surgical procedure.
3. To provide a safe method of feeding a hypotonic patient or one who cannot tolerate alternative methods. Specific indications may include duodenal atresia, tracheal esophageal fistula, and omphalocele.
4. To provide a route that allows adequate calorie and/or fluid intake in a child with chronic lung disease or in one who does not have continuity of the gastrointestinal tract (i.e., esophageal atresia).

Equipment

Warm feeding fluid
Pacifier
Reservoir syringe or funnel
Syringe for aspirating

Procedure

Nursing Action	**Rationale/Amplification**
Preparatory Phase	
1. Gastrostomy tube may be in one of 3 positions between feedings:	
a. Lowered and open to start drainage.	a. Constant decompression.
b. Open, connected to reservoir (funnel, syringe) that is elevated 10–12 cm. (4–4¾ inches).	b. To serve as safety valve outlet to prevent esophageal reflux and increased stomach pressure.
c. Clamped.	c. Most "normal" physiologic set-up, preparation for home care or tube removal.
2. The nurse may be directed to check residual stomach contents prior to any feeding.	2. This is done to monitor for appropriate fluid intake, digestion time, and overfeeding that can cause distention.
a. Attach syringe and aspirate stomach contents.	
b. Measure.	
c. Residual fluid may be returned to stomach or discarded, depending on amount.	
3. A Y-tube that is connected at the point where reservoir and gastrostomy tube join may be used during feeding.	3. To provide simultaneous decompression during feeding.
4. When feeding is about to begin, infant/child should be placed in comfortable position in bed—either flat or with head slightly elevated. If condition permits, the nurse should hold the infant. A pacifier can be given to him.	4. When the infant/child is comfortable and relaxed, feeding fluid will flow more easily into stomach. Pacifier will satisfy normal sucking activity, provide exercise for jaw muscles, and relax musculature as well as provide pleasure normally associated with feeding.
Note: *Gastrostomy tube feeding button:* The child may have a gastrostomy tube feeding button, in which case insert the special tube into the button and follow the feeding procedure in the Performance Phase.	
Performance Phase	
1. Attach reservoir syringe to tube (if not already open to continuous elevation) and fill reservoir with feeding fluid prior to unclamping tube.	1. Prevents air from entering tube (and then stomach), which may cause distention.
2. Elevate tube and reservoir to 10–12 cm. (4–4¾ inches) above abdominal wall. Do not apply any pressure to start flow.	2. This elevation level will allow for slow, gravity-induced flow. Pressure may cause a backflow of fluid into the esophagus.

(continued)

Guidelines   Gastrostomy Feeding *(continued)*

Procedure *(continued)*	Nursing Action	Rationale/Amplification
	3. Feed slowly, taking 20–45 minutes. Fill reservoir with remaining fluid before it is empty to avoid instillation of air.	3. Too rapid a feeding will interfere with normal peristalsis and will cause abdominal distention and backflow into reservoir or esophagus.
	4. Continue to provide infant with pleasant feelings associated with feeding.	
	5. When feeding is completed:	
	a. Instill clear water (10–30 ml., or 0.3–1 oz.) if tube is to be clamped. Apply clamp before water level reaches end of reservoir.	a. This rinses tubing and will prevent clogging.
	b. Leave tube unclamped and open to continuous elevation.	b. Feeding fluid is allowed to return to reservoir if infant cries or changes position, and thus decreases pressure on the stomach.
	6. Often when oral feedings are started, they are given simultaneously with gastrostomy feedings.	6. This allows the infant to learn or reestablish the sucking-swallowing process as well as to build up tolerance to eating without compromising nutritional intake.

Follow-Up Phase

	Nursing Action	Rationale/Amplification
	1. Check dressing and skin around point of tube entry for wetness. Clean skin and apply skin barrier (petrolatum, Maalox, aluminum paste, etc.). See that there is no pull on tube.	1. Skin breakdown is caused by continued exposure to stomach contents that may be leaking out around tube causing excoriation and infection. Constant pulling on tube can cause widening of skin opening and subsequent leakage.
	2. Leave the infant dry and comfortable. If unable to hold him during feeding, this may be a good time to hold, fondle, and provide him with warmth and love. Place him on right side or in Fowler's position.	2. To promote relaxation and improved digestion of feeding.
	3. Accurately describe and record procedure, including time of feeding, type and amount of feeding fluid given, amount and characteristics of residual (if any) and what was done with it, how the patient tolerated feeding, any abdominal distention, and activity following feeding.	

Note: Should infant pull out gastrostomy tube, cover ostomy site with sterile dressing and tape, notify physician, and accurately record events.

Guidelines   Nasojejunal Feeding

Nasojejunal (N-J) feeding is a means of providing full enteral feeding via a catheter passed through the nares, past the pharynx, down the esophagus, bypassing the stomach through the pylorus into the jejunum.

Purposes

1. To provide a method of feeding that requires minimal patient effort when the infant is unable to tolerate alternative feeding methods (i.e., low birth weight, persistent respiratory distress).
2. To provide a route that allows for adequate calorie or fluid intake (a full enteral feeding) via intermittent or continuous drip.
3. To provide a method of feeding a critically ill infant that minimizes regurgitation, aspiration, and gastric distention.
4. To provide a route for administration of oral medications (controversial).

Equipment

* Sterile radiopaque silicone or polyvinyl nasojejunal (N-J) tube, 1 meter (39 inches), No. 19, No. 21, or No. 23—may or may not have weighted tip
Tape
pH paper
Reservoir for feeding
Possibly an infusion pump
3-way stopcock
Syringe—0.5 ml. normal saline or sterile water
Equipment for nasogastric (N-G) tube insertion; introducer catheter

* See Gavage Feeding, page 1154.

Procedure	**Nursing Action**	**Rationale/Amplification**

Preparatory Phase

1. Attach cardiac monitor to infant.

1. To allow for continuous monitoring of heart rate and rhythm. The vagus nerve pathway lies from the medulla through the neck and thorax to the abdomen. Above the stomach, the left and right branches unite to form the esophageal plexus. Stimulation of these nerve branches with the catheter will directly affect the cardiac and pulmonary plexus.

2. Tube is generally inserted by a physician.
   a. Measure from glabella (prominent point between eyebrows) to the heel for estimated length.
   b. Measure and mark the remaining length of tubing and record.

   b. This serves as a double check to ensure that tube has not advanced farther than intended.

3. Place the infant on his right side with hips slightly elevated. Gentle restraint or soft mittens may have to be applied.

3. Facilitates passage of tube. Restraints prevent infant from pulling out tube before the tip passes the pylorus. Do not place on left side.

4. Tube is inserted by threading the N-J vinyl catheter into a No. 10 French feeding catheter and introducing both through the nostril into the stomach. The feeding tube is then withdrawn, and the N-J feeding tube is allowed to advance through the pylorus.

4. Oral insertion may cause increased salivation, air swallowing, and regurgitation.

5. Check intestinal aspirate for pH every 1–2 hours. Infant may be positioned on right side, back, or abdomen. Once the tube is past the pylorus, abdominal posteroanterior and lateral x-rays are taken to confirm that tip of catheter is at the ligament of Treitz.

5. When aspiration fluid reaches a pH of 5–7 or bile-colored fluid is obtained, the tip of the tube has passed the pylorus and duodenum into the jejunum.

6. A No. 5 French N-G feeding tube may be passed through the other nostril at this time and left indwelling. This is used to check stomach for residual fluid and regurgitation through the pylorus.

6. If gastric residual is significant, it will interfere with prescribed feeding. Notify physician. (4 ml/kg [0.12 oz/2.21 lbs] reflux in stomach is usually tolerated.) Do not remove N-G tube since it will adhere to N-J tube during withdrawal and pull out N-J tube also.

7. N-J feedings can generally be started following this progression:
   a. D_5W for 6–12 hours
   b. ½ strength formula with low osmolality for 6–12 hours.

   c. Full strength low osmolality formula.

   b. Low solute formulas include SMA, Similac, Enfamil (20 calories/30 ml., or 20 calories/1 oz.).
   c. Low osmolality formula is used to prevent loss of fluid into intestine and possible necrotizing enterocolitis.

   d. The volume of feeding is increased 2 ml. (0.06 oz.) at a time until infant's daily calorie and fluid requirements are being administered.

   d. 150 ml./kg. (4.5 oz./2.2 lbs.) fluid requirement is generally used (130–150 cal./kg.).

   e. Medications may be given via the N-J tube if prescribed. A 3-way stopcock will have to be placed at the connection of the N-J tube and the line from the feeding fluid. Alternative method for administering oral medications is by passing an oral–gastric or nasogastric feeding tube; in this way the stomach and process of digestion and absorption are not bypassed.

   e. Flush tubing with 0.5 ml. (.015 oz.) normal saline solution or sterile water after medication is administered to ensure that infant receives entire dosage prescribed and to prevent any sediment from remaining in tubing.

Performance Phase

1. N-J feedings can be given as follows:
   a. Intermittently (i.e., every 1–3 hours)
   b. In a continuous slow drip.

   b. Generally the preferred method to minimize the satiety–hunger cycle and large-volume instillation.

2. If intermittent feeding is the method used, the feeding techniques are the same as for nasogastric (gavage) feeding.

2. Feeding is given at room temperature. Avoid cold fluid, which may cause infant discomfort. If breast milk is used, gently rotate reservoir periodically to mix settled-out fat content.

3. If slow continuous drip method is used, the set-up used is similar to the pediatric IV infusion using an infusion pump and small (100–250 ml., or 3.0–7.5 oz.) closed chamber for reservoir.
   a. Reservoir chamber and tubing should be changed every 8–24 hours.
   b. Record input every hour. Fill reservoir as needed, with no more than 3 hours worth of feeding fluid.

   a. To prevent growth of bacteria.

   b. To ensure a constant flow and minimize overinfusion directly into the jejunum.

(continued)

Guidelines Nasojejunal Feeding *(continued)*

Procedure *(continued)*	**Nursing Action**	**Rationale/Amplification**

Follow-Up Phase

1. Be constantly alert for mechanical problems:
  a. Check for abdominal distention resulting from the infant's inability to handle ingested amount of fluid:
    • Palpate abdomen
    • Observe for ripple of intestines
    • Measure abdominal girth every 3–8 hours
    • Check residual formula in jejunum every 3–8 hours
    • Discard or refeed residual formula as prescribed.
  b. Check stools for occult blood, pH, and sugar every voiding or 4–8 hours to determine tolerance of feeding fluid.
  c. Check emesis for blood and report to physician immediately—may be a sign of necrotizing enterocolitis.
2. Position infant in recumbent position.
3. Observe infant closely to avoid potential dangers as tube passes the pylorus.
  a. Close attention to amount, type, concentration, and osmolality of feeding fluid is stressed.
  b. Check heart rate and blood pressure.
4. Hold, fondle, and give positive stimulation to the infant if conditions permit (see Premature Infant, p. 1235).
5. Accurately describe and record condition of infant and procedure, including type and amount of feeding given, amount of residual and characteristics, any signs of impending infant distress or problems.
	1. Tube clogging due to inadequate rinsing. Tube advancing too far into jejunum; check protruding tube measurement. Fluid overload, causing aspiration.
	
	2. Less likely for "dumping syndrome" to occur.
	3. Diarrhea; as the tube passes through the pylorus, it (the tube) becomes stiff because of the change in pH. A stiff tube has been reported to cause intestinal perforation. If tube becomes clogged or dislodged, it must be removed.
	
	4. This procedure limits the normal pleasures associated with feeding. Infant needs some attention to his psychological needs in order to thrive.

Specimen Collection

Guidelines Assisting With Blood Collection

Blood collection from a venous puncture in the extremity of an infant or young child is the same as for an adult, with the exceptions or additions noted below.

Equipment No. 23–19 gauge short needle or scalp-vein needle
Smaller volume or micro blood-collecting tubes
Smaller tourniquet (rubber band may be used with infant)
Gloves

Procedure	**Nursing Action**	**Rationale/Amplification**

Preparatory Phase

1. Immobilize the child by placing him in a mummy restraint if necessary (see p. 1149). 2. Position the patient. a. *Femoral venipuncture:* place the child on his back with legs in frog-like position. Nurse places her hands on child's knees (see position for bladder puncture, p. 1163).	1. Infants and young children squirm. Immobilizing them allows easier access to the venipuncture site. It also helps keep the infant warm. 2. These positions allow for optimal visualization and stabilization of the patient. Cover perineum to protect site and operator should infant void.

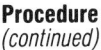

Procedure
(continued)

| Nursing Action | Rationale/Amplification |

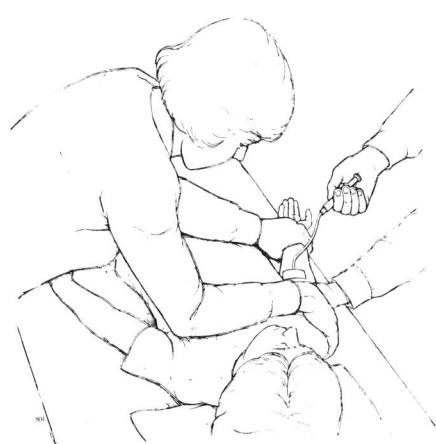

b. *External jugular venipuncture:* place the child in mummy restraint and lower his head over the side of the bed or table. Turn head to side and stabilize. Crying will make external jugular vein visible and causes blood to flow more readily.

c. *Antecubital fossa venipuncture:* place the child in a supine position. The nurse stands on the side opposite the site to be used (across from the person drawing the specimen). The nurse positions her right arm across the upper part of the child's chest and grasps the shoulder at the axilla position. Her left arm is placed across the lower part of the child's chest and is used to extend the child's arm at the wrist.

d. *Infant—heel, toe, or digital puncture:* warm area with warm compress for 5–10 minutes.

d. This dilates vessels allowing blood to flow more freely.

Performance Phase

1. Both persons holding the infant and drawing the blood should wear gloves.
2. After the specimen is collected and the needle is removed, apply pressure to the site with dry gauze for 3–5 minutes.
   a. *Jugular venipuncture:* while applying pressure to the site, place the patient in an upright sitting position. Do not apply excessive pressure that may compromise circulation or respiration.
   b. *Capillary:* clean area with antiseptic and dry with dry sterile 2 × 2 gauze. Hold heel firmly and with free hand quickly puncture with microlancet or sterile No. 21 gauge needle on most medial or lateral part of plantar surface. Puncture deeply enough to get free-flowing blood—never deeper than 2.4 mm. Discard first drop of blood; rapidly collect specimen in proper capillary tube.
3. When the bleeding has been stopped, soothe and comfort the child before leaving him.

1. Universal precautions.

2. Both the femoral and jugular veins are large vessels. Since respiratory pressure is great, bleeding, oozing, and hematoma formation may result. External pressure prevents this from happening.

3. Crying and thrashing about may initiate bleeding.

Follow-Up Phase

1. Check the patient frequently for 1 hour after the procedure for oozing, bleeding, or evidence of a hematoma.
2. Record carefully and accurately:
   a. Site of venipuncture
   b. How the patient tolerated procedure
   c. Bleeding stopped or continued and for how long
   d. For what test the specimen was collected

1. Reapply pressure and report if oozing continues.

Guidelines ## Collecting a Urine Specimen From the Infant or Young Child

Urine collection is a safe method of obtaining urine for a specified purpose.

Purposes
1. To check urine for presence of sugar, acetone, bacteria, and other urinary products.
2. To aid in diagnosis.
3. To determine the condition of the patient.
4. To determine effectiveness of therapy.

(continued)

Guidelines   Collecting a Urine Specimen From the Infant or Young Child *(continued)*

Equipment   Collecting device—plastic, disposable urine bag or collector (Hollister, U-Bag, double chamber)
Cleansing agent
Wiping material—4 × 4s or cotton balls
Clean or sterile water
Containers for solutions
Specimen container
Gloves

Procedure

Nursing Action	Rationale/Amplification
Preparatory Phase	
1. Offer the young child fluids he likes to drink 30–60 minutes prior to procedure, if no contraindications.	
2. Position the patient so that genitalia are exposed by placing him on his back with legs in frog-like position. Assistance may be needed to hold the legs of the young child in proper position.	2. Proper positioning will facilitate cleansing and allow for proper placement of collection device.
3. When small samples of urine are needed for pH, Clinitest, etc., to be done by the nurse, urine can be extracted from the diaper using a syringe or dropper.	
Performance Phase	
1. Wear gloves.	1. Universal precautions.
2. Cleanse genital area.	2. This method of cleansing the female will prevent contamination of the genitalia from the anus, and will prevent contamination of the urine specimen obtained. During the cleansing be gentle to avoid any injury or possible stimulation of urination.
a. *Female:* using cotton balls, dip into cleansing agent, wipe labia majora from top to bottom (clitoris to anus) only once with each cotton ball. Repeat this once more. Wipe again with clear water. Then spread labia apart with one hand while wiping the labia minora in the same manner with other hand. Wipe area dry.	
b. *Male:* wipe tip of penis in circular motion down towards the scrotum. Be certain to retract foreskin if present. Wipe first with cleansing agent 2–3 times, then clear water. Dry the area.	
3. Apply collecting bag firmly so that the opening is exposed to receive urine.	3. If collecting bag is properly and securely placed, the procedure will not have to be repeated.
a. *Female:* stretch perineum taut during application. Attach bag to perineum first, then proceed up to symphysis.	a. This should ensure leak-proof contact.
Elevate head of bed or place the child in an infant seat, if appropriate.	To aid flow of urine by gravity.
b. *Male (small boys):* place penis inside bag.	
4. Apply diaper to patient and comfort him; possibly give him additional clear fluids.	
5. Check the patient frequently (30–45 minutes) to see if he has voided. When the patient has voided, remove bag gently. Cleanse area and reapply diaper to the child. If child has not voided within 45 minutes, procedure must be repeated.	5. The adhesive on the collecting bag may tend to be sticky. Careful removal of the bag will prevent skin injury on and around genitalia. Also avoid spilling urine out of the bag during removal. Reapplication of bag will decrease the possibility of unreliable test results.
Follow-Up Phase	
1. Pour specimen into proper collecting container. Send specimen to the laboratory within 30 minutes or refrigerate.	1. Prompt delivery of specimen to the laboratory will prevent growth of organisms in an uncontrolled environment and distortion of the test results.
2. Accurately chart and describe the following in the nurse's notes:	2. Guideline for weighing diaper, excluding weight of dry diaper, 1 gm. = 1 ml. urine.
a. Time specimen collection was started and ended	
b. Amount of urine voided	
c. Color of urine (cloudy, clear, any sediment)	
d. Type of test to be done	
e. Condition of skin of perineal area	

Note: If 24-hour urine collection is needed, use a collection bag that has a long tube attachment to facilitate frequent emptying of urine every 1–2 hours. Place urine in receptacle in refrigerator. Adherence of bag to skin can be improved by applying a thin coating of tincture of benzoin to skin and allowing this to dry before attaching collection bag.

Guidelines Assisting With a Percutaneous Suprapubic Bladder Aspiration

Percutaneous bladder aspiration is an aseptic method of entering the bladder in the suprapubic location with a needle to obtain a urine specimen.

Purposes
1. To obtain urine in an aseptic manner for culture.
2. To aid in diagnostic workup.
3. To determine condition of the patient and aid in treatment.

Equipment
Antiseptic skin cleansing solution
Band-Aid
Sterile 4 × 4s
Gloves
Needle, No. 20–22 gauge, 3.7 cm. (1½ inches) long
Syringe, 20 ml.
Specimen container

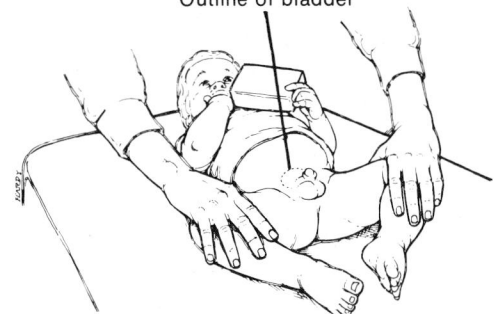
Outline of bladder

Procedure

Nursing Action	Rationale/Amplification

Preparatory Phase

1. Check diaper for wetness. If the child has just voided, report this to the physician or report last voiding time. At least 1 hour should pass without voiding.
2. Position the child on his back on the examining table. His head should be toward nurse, his feet toward the physician. Spread his legs apart in a frog-like position. Place hands on his knees and thumbs along his sides at the hip level.
3. Ensure that the skin over the puncture site is cleansed in an antiseptic manner.

1. In order to perform a successful bladder aspiration, enough urine must be present to distend the bladder up above the pubic symphysis—so that bladder is accessible.
2. This position allows the nurse to stabilize the child. It also gives a full view of the child, making it easier to observe him, talk to him, and soothe him.
3. To prevent infection from being introduced into the bladder by inserting the needle through unclean skin, which would contaminate the specimen.

Performance Phase

1. Both the physician and nurse should wear gloves.
2. While the procedure is being performed, note the condition of the patient and any signs of distress. Comfort him by talking to him and smiling at him.

3. To prevent urination during procedure, compress the infant's urethra:
   a. *Male:* pressure on penis.
   b. *Female:* digital pressure upward on urethra from rectum.
4. When urine has been obtained or the procedure is discontinued and the needle is removed, apply pressure over the puncture site with a 4 × 4 and fingers.
5. Apply a Band-Aid if necessary. Reapply diaper. Hold and comfort him for a few minutes.

1. Universal precautions.
2. Report any changes in color or respiration rate or other signs. Soothing the child will help him to relax so that he will not move about so much. Crying increases the muscle tone of the lower abdomen, making it more difficult to insert the needle.

4. This prevents any bleeding from occurring either internally or externally. Pressure should be maintained about 3 minutes or until oozing ceases and coagulation has taken place.
5. Holding the child will help to restore and maintain a good nurse–patient relationship and will help the child to relax after a frightening and painful procedure.

Follow-Up Phase

1. Check the child periodically for 1 hour after procedure to see that bleeding or oozing has not occurred.

1. This is not likely if pressure was applied properly after procedure and the patient was left quiet.

(continued)

Guidelines Assisting With a Percutaneous Suprapubic Bladder Aspiration *(continued)*

Procedure *(continued)*	Nursing Action	Rationale/Amplification

	2. Note time of first voiding after procedure. Note color of urine (it may be pink). Bloody urine should be reported to the physician.
	
	3. Accurately describe and chart the procedure, including:
	  a. Time of procedure
	  b. Whether or not a specimen was obtained
	  c. How the patient tolerated the procedure
	  d. Description and amount of urine obtained
	  e. Patient's condition and activity following the procedure
		2. It is important to note any changes in voiding pattern following the procedure since change might indicate injury. The first voided urine may be bloody because of a small amount of local capillary bleeding at the time of the procedure.

Guidelines Collecting a Stool Specimen

Stool collection is a method of obtaining a stool specimen from the patient.

Purposes
1. To check stool for presence of specific material (i.e., blood, ova, and parasites or bacteria).
2. To aid in diagnosis.
3. To determine condition or status of the patient.
4. To determine effectiveness of therapy.

Equipment
Diaper
Cellophane or plastic liner (used when stool is loose or watery)
Tongue blade
Specimen container
Gloves

Note: Collecting a stool specimen from an older child who is toilet-trained is the same as collecting such a specimen from an adult.

Procedure	Nursing Action	Rationale/Amplification
	Preparatory Phase 1. If a specimen is needed from a patient whose stools are loose or watery enough to be absorbed in the diaper, line the diaper with a piece of cellophane or plastic. Place this liner between the diaper and the skin. Then apply diaper to the child and position him so that his head is slightly elevated. If stools are soft or formed, apply diaper. **Performance Phase** 1. Wear gloves. 2. Check the child frequently to see if stooling has occurred. 3. Remove soiled diaper from child. Clean perineal area, apply clean diaper, and leave the child comfortable. 4. Remove small amount of stool from diaper with the tongue blade and place it in the specimen container. 5. Send labeled specimen to the laboratory promptly.	1. The liner and position will allow the loose stool specimen to collect in the liner and not be absorbed by the diaper. 1. Universal precautions. 2. A fresh specimen should be obtained so that test results will not be distorted by time-lapse. This will also decrease the chance of contamination of the stool with urine and will prevent skin irritation from the stool. 5. Prompt delivery to the laboratory will prevent changes from taking place in the specimen that could alter the test results.

Procedure *(continued)*	**Nursing Action**	**Rationale/Amplification**

Follow-Up Phase

1. Accurately describe and record the following:
   a. Time specimen was collected
   b. Color, amount, and consistency of stool (note any foul smell.)
   c. Type of specimen collected
   d. Nature of test for which the specimen was collected
   e. Condition of the skin

Guidelines Assisting With a Spinal Tap—Lumbar Puncture

A *spinal tap* in an infant or young child is based on the same principles and is essentially the same as for an adult, with the exceptions noted below.

Equipment No. 21 or 20 gauge, 3.5-cm. (1½-inch) long spinal needle
Sterile lumbar puncture tray

Procedure	**Nursing Action**	**Rationale/Amplification**

Preparatory Phase

1. Position the patient.
   a. *Side position* (similar to the adult): wrap the lower extremities in a sheet; if an older child, place the patient on his side facing the nurse; flex knees and neck by placing one hand on his shoulders and head and the other hand on buttocks and upper thigh.
   b. *Sitting position:* this position is primarily used with small infants. Place infant in sitting position; extend legs and arms in front of the infant; flex his neck so chin is almost resting on chest; back is rounded by placing thumbs on his shoulders and hands along side of his hips.

1. In either position the patient may squirm. Hold him securely to prevent him from moving and causing injury to himself or causing the spinal needle to be inserted too far, resulting in a traumatic tap.

NURSING ALERT: Observe for signs of respiratory distress. Because the trachea in the infant is so soft, it can kink very easily when the neck is flexed. If this happens and the airway is obstructed, the infant will stop breathing. This is an emergency situation.

Follow-Up Phase

1. It is not usually necessary to keep the infant or young child flat in bed following the procedure unless there are contraindications to his being up and physician has prescribed that he be kept in bed. It may be helpful to institute play activity and offer fluids to the child.

Fluid and Electrolyte Balance in Children

Basic Principles

1. Infants and small children have different proportions of body water (Table 47-2) and body fat than do adults.
   a. The body water of a newborn infant approaches 80% of his body weight, compared to that of an average adult male, which approaches 60%.

Table 47-2. *Body Fluids Expressed as Percentage of Body Weight*

Fluid	**Adult**		**Infant (%)**
	Male (%)	*Female (%)*	
Total Body Fluids	60	54	75
Intracellular	40	36	40
Extracellular	20	18	35

b. The normal infant demonstrates a rapid physiologic decline in the ratio of body weight to body water during the immediate postpartum period.

c. Proportion of body water declines more slowly throughout infancy and reaches the characteristic value for adults by approximately 2 years of age.

2. Compared with adults, a greater percentage of the body water of infants and small children is contained in the extracellular compartment.

   a. Infants—approximately ½ of the body water is contained in the cell.

   b. Adults—approximately ⅔ of the body water is contained in the cell.

3. Compared with adults, the water turnover rate per unit

Table 47-3. *Common Abnormalities of Fluid and Electrolyte Metabolism*

Substance	Major Function	Abnormality	Cause	Clinical Manifestation	Laboratory Data
Water	Medium of body fluids, chemical changes, body temperature, lubricant	Volume deficit	1. Primary—inadequate water intake 2. Secondary—loss following vomiting, diarrhea, excessive gastrointestinal obstruction, etc.	Oliguria, weight loss, signs of dehydration including dry skin and mucous membranes, lassitude, sunken fontanelles, lack of tear formation, increased pulse rate, decreased blood pressure	Concentrated urine, azotemia, elevated hematocrit, hemoglobin and erythrocyte count
		Volume excess	1. Failure to excrete water in presence of normal intake such as in congestive heart failure, renal disease 2. Water intake in excess of output	Weight gain, peripheral edema, signs of pulmonary congestion	Variable urine volume, low specific gravity of urine, decreased hematocrit
Potassium	Intracellular fluid balance, regular heart rhythm, muscle and nerve irritability	Potassium deficit	1. Excessive loss of potassium due to vomiting, diarrhea, prolonged cortisone, ACTH or diuretic therapy, diabetic acidosis 2. Shift of potassium into the cells such as occurs with the healing phase of burns, recovery from diabetic acidosis	Signs and symptoms variable, including weakness, lethargy, irritability, abdominal distention, and eventually cardiac arrhythmias	Low plasma K^+ level (may be normal in some situations); hypochloremic alkalosis; ECG changes
		Potassium excess	Excessive administration of potassium-containing solutions, excessive release of potassium due to burns, severe kidney disease, adrenal insufficiency	Variable, including listlessness, confusion, heaviness of the legs, nausea, diarrhea, ECG changes, ultimately paralysis and cardiac arrest	Elevated potassium plasma level
Sodium	Osmotic pressure, muscle and nerve irritability	Sodium deficit	Water intake in excess of excretory capacity, replacement of fluid loss without sufficient sodium; excessive sodium losses	Headache, nausea, abdominal cramps, confusion alternating with stupor, diarrhea, lacrimation, salivation, later hypotension; early polyuria, later oliguria	Sodium plasma level may be high, low, or normal
		Sodium excess	Inadequate water intake especially in the presence of fever or sweating; increased intake without increased output; decreased output	Thirst, oliguria, weakness muscular pain, excitement, dry mucous membranes, hypotension, tachycardia, fever	Elevated Na^+ plasma level, high plasma volume
Bicarbonate	Acid–base balance	Primary bicarbonate deficit	Diarrhea (especially in infants), diabetes mellitus, starvation, infectious disease, shock or congestive heart failure producing tissue anoxia	Progressively increasing rate and depth of respiration—ultimately becoming Kussmaul respiration, flushed, warm skin, weakness, disorientation progressive to coma	Urine pH usually less than 6 Plasma bicarbonate less than 20 mEq./liter Plasma pH less than 7.35
		Primary bicarbonate excess	Loss of chloride through vomiting, gastric suction, or the use of excessive diuretics, excessive ingestion of alkali.	Depressed respiration, muscle hypertonicity, hyperactive reflexes, tetany and sometimes convulsions	Urine pH usually above 7, plasma bicarbonate above 25 mEq./liter (30 mEq./liter in adults), plasma pH above 7.45

of body weight is 3 or more times greater in infants and small children.

   a. The child's metabolic rate is about 3 times that of an adult.

   b. The child has more body surface in relation to weight.

   c. The immaturity of kidney function in infants may impair their ability to conserve water.

4. Electrolyte balance is dependent on fluid balance and cardiovascular, renal, adrenal, pituitary, parathyroid, and pulmonary regulatory mechanisms.

5. Infants and children are more vulnerable to disorders of hydration than are adults.

   a. The basic principles relating to fluid balance in children make the magnitude of fluid losses considerably greater in children than in adults.

   b. Children are prone to severe disturbances of the gastrointestinal tract that result in diarrhea and vomiting.

   c. Young children cannot independently respond to increased losses by increased intake. They depend on others to provide them with adequate fluid.

Common Fluid and Electrolyte Abnormalities

See Table 47-3, opposite page.

General Goals of Fluid and Electrolyte Therapy

1. Repair of preexisting deficits that may occur with prolonged or severe diarrhea or vomiting.

   a. Deficits are estimated and corrected as soon and as safely as possible.

     (1) Initial therapy is aimed at restoring blood and extracellular fluid volume in order to relieve or prevent shock and restore renal function.

     (2) Intracellular deficits are replaced slowly over 8–12-hour period after the circulatory status is improved.

2. Provision of maintenance requirements

   a. Maintenance requirements occur as a result of normal expenditures of water and electrolytes due to metabolism.

   b. Maintenance requirements bear a close relationship to metabolic rate and are ideally formulated in terms of caloric expenditure.

3. Correction of concurrent losses that may occur via the gastrointestinal tract as a result of vomiting, diarrhea, or drainage of secretions.

   Replacement should be similar in type and amount to the fluid being lost.

   Replacement is usually formulated as ml. of fluid and mEq. of electrolytes replaced per ml. of fluid and mEq. of electrolytes lost.

Guidelines   Intravenous Fluid Therapy

Intravenous therapy refers to the infusion of fluids directly into the venous system. This may be accomplished through the use of a needle or by venous cutdown and insertion of a small catheter directly into the vein (Fig. 47-6).

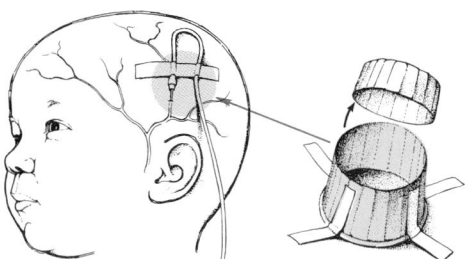

Venipuncture of scalp vein

Paper cup taped over venipuncture site for protection. A clear plastic cup may also be used.

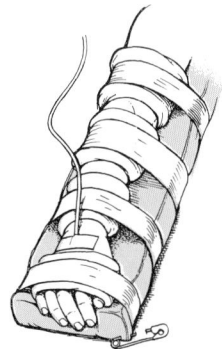

Restraint of arm when hand is site of infusion

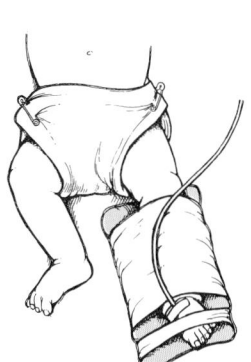

Infant's leg taped to sandbag for immobilization

Figure 47-6. *IV fluid therapy.*

(continued)

Guidelines Intravenous Fluid Therapy *(continued)*

Purpose   To restore and maintain the child's fluid and electrolyte balance and body homeostasis when his oral intake is inadequate to serve this purpose.

Equipment   A. Needle Method

IV solution
  The kind of solution is specified by the physician
  For small children, 250-ml. bottles should be used for purposes of safety
IV pole
IV administration set
The set should include a closed reservoir with a minidropper to ensure that the child will not receive an excessive amount of fluid in a brief period of time
Micropore filter
Syringe, 5 or 10 ml.—approximately ½–⅔ filled with normal saline
Butterfly needle or catheter of appropriate gauge
  The size of the needle depends on the age and size of the child and the type of fluid to be administered
Alcohol sponges, dry sponges
Betadine or other antibacterial cleansing solution
Normal saline
Small tourniquet or rubber band
Hypoallergenic tape, 1.2 cm. (½ inch), 2.5 cm. (1 inch), 5 cm. (2 inches)
Padded armboard
Gauze bandage for securing the extremity to the armboard
Restraining devices—bath blanket, extremity restraint, covered sandbags
  The type of restraint depends on the child's age, his level of cooperation, and the kind of IV to be started.
Safety razor (if scalp vein is to be used)

B. Cutdown Method

IV solution, IV pole, IV administration set
Alcohol sponges
Hypoallergenic tape, 1.2 cm. (½ inch), 2.5 cm. (1 inch), 5 cm. (2 inches)
Padded armboard
Dry sponges
Gauze bandage
Sterile cutdown tray
  The tray should include the following equipment: medicine cups, treatment towels, wound towel, syringe, No. 1-25 gauge 1.5-cm. (⅝-inch) needle, No. 1-20 gauge 2.5-cm. (1-inch) needle, knife handle and No. 15 blade, forceps, scissors, gauze sponges, 4–0 black silk suture, needle holder
Assorted sizes of sterile polyethylene tubing and Luer adapters
5–0 black silk suture with a straight eye needle
1%–2% procaine
Normal saline
Tourniquet
Sterile gloves
Restraining devices

Procedure

Nursing Action	Rationale/Amplification
Preparatory Phase	
1. Obtain the IV solution.	1. Although the type of solution and the rate of flow are prescribed by the physician, the nurse should be aware of the composition of common parenteral solutions and should know how to calculate maintenance therapy (Table 47-4).
2. Check the IV fluid for sediment or contaminant by holding the container up to the light.	2. Contaminant is most easily identified with the container in this position. If sediment is observed, the solution should be discarded.
3. Check the container for cracks.	3. If a flash of light can be seen through the bottle, it has a razor-thin crack and should be discarded.

Table 47-4. *Composition of Frequently Used Parenteral Fluids*

Liquid	CHO	Prot.*	Cal/liter	Na	K	Cl	HCO†	Ca	P‡
	gm./100 ml.				*mEq./liter*			*mg./dl.*	
D₅W	5	—	170	—	—	—	—	—	—
D₁₀W	10	—	340	—	—	—	—	—	—
Normal saline (0.9% NaCl)	—	—	—	154	—	154	—	—	—
½ Normal saline (0.45% NaCl)	—	—	—	77	—	77	—	—	—
D5 (0.2% NaCl)	5	—	170	34	—	34	—	—	—
3% Saline	—	—	—	513	—	513	—	—	—
8.4% Sodium bicarbonate (1 mEq./ml.)	—	—	—	1000	—	—	1000	—	—
Ringer's	0–10	—	0–340	147	4	155.5	—	4.5	—
Ringer's lactate	0–10	—	0–340	130	4	109	28	3	—
Amino acid 8.5% (Travasol)	—	8.5	340	3	—	34	52	—	—
Plasmanate	—	5	200	110	2	50	29	—	—
Albumin 25% (salt poor)	—	25	1000	100–160	<1	<120	—	—	—
Intralipid (Cutter)‖	2.25	—	1100	2.5	0.5	4.0	—	—	0.8

* Protein or amino acid equivalent.

† Bicarbonate or equivalent (citrate, acetate, lactate).

‡ Approximate values: actual values may vary somewhat in various localities depending on electrolyte composition of water supply used to reconstitute solution.

‖ Values are approximate—may vary from lot to lot.

From Johns Hopkins Hospital. The Harriet Lane Handbook. Chicago, Year Book Medical Pub 1987.

Procedure (continued)	**Nursing Action**	**Rationale/Amplification**
	4. Attach a micropore filter to the end of the infusion tubing that attaches to the needle. Use aseptic technique.	4. A 0.45-micron filter prevents entry into the vein of larger particles, air emboli, and most bacterial and fungal organisms except some pseudomonas organisms. A 0.22-micron filter prevents entry of any organisms but requires the use of an IV pump.
	5. Remove the metal seal from the IV container without touching the rubber top.	5. Do not use the solution if the seal has been broken. It is not necessary to cleanse the sterile, rubber top with alcohol unless it has been accidentally contaminated.
	6. Following product information, insert the end of the administration set into the container's opening. Fill the tubing with solution.	
	7. Promote the cooperation of the child. a. *Infant:* provide with a pacifier. b. *Older child:* explain the procedure and its purpose.	7. The procedure will be least traumatic for the child if he is able to cooperate and is not frightened or resistant.
	8. Position the child so that he is comfortable.	
	9. Restrain the child as necessary. a. *Infant or young child:* restraints may include mummy wrappings, jacket or elbow restraints, or small sandbags. b. *Older child:* the extremity to be used should be comfortably restrained on the armboard. Free extremities may also require light restraints to remind the child not to move.	9. Protective devices may be necessary to prevent the child from dislodging the IV needle. The type and size of such devices should be appropriate for the child's age and the position of the IV. b. Toes and fingers should be visible to avoid compromising blood flow. The restraint board must be padded and the main pressure points (heel, palm) padded with gauze. Before strapping an extremity to the armboard, back the adhesive with tape or gauze wherever it touches the skin (see Fig. 47-6).

Performance Phase

	Nursing Action	Rationale/Amplification
	1. The persons starting the IV and holding the infant should wear gloves.	1. Universal precautions.
	2. Assist the physician as necessary.	2. The nurse may insert the IV.
	3. When applying the tourniquet, a second rubber band is placed crosswise under it. To remove the tourniquet, grasp the unstretched rubber band, pull up, and cut the tourniquet.	

(continued)

Guidelines   Intravenous Fluid Therapy *(continued)*

Procedure *(continued)*	**Nursing Action**	**Rationale/Amplification**

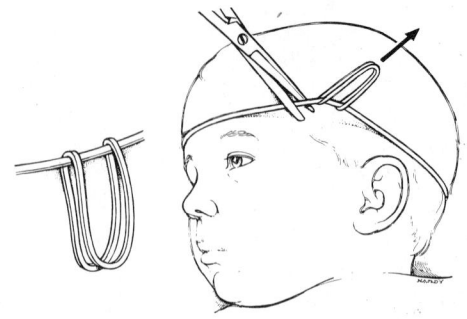

4. Check the restraints at intervals and adjust them as necessary.

4. The restraints may become loose after a period of time and must be secured to ensure the child's safety. They may also become too tight and require loosening to maintain adequate circulation.

5. Comfort and reassure the child.

5. The procedure is usually disturbing for the child. This should be acknowledged. If crying and upset, the child should be reassured that his behavior is acceptable.

6. Regulate the IV flow at the designated rate.
7. Record:
   Type of solution being used
   Reading on the container or reservoir
   Rate of flow
   Time that the infusion began
   Name of the physician or nurse who started the IV
   Site of administration
   Reaction of the child to the procedure
8. Return the child to his room.

Follow-Up Phase

1. Check the child at least hourly.
   a. Note the location of the IV.
   b. Note the color of the skin at the needle point.
   c. Check for swelling of the skin at the needle point.
      (1) If in a hand or foot, compare with the opposite extremity.
      (2) If in the head, look at the face to determine asymmetry.
   d. Feel the area around the IV site for sponginess or leakage.
   e. Check for blood return into the tube when the flow of fluid is stopped.
   f. Make certain that the child is adequately restrained.
2. Observe closely for complications.
   a. *Local reactions:*
      (1) Compromised circulation
      (2) Pressure sores
      (3) Thrombophlebitis
   b. *Fluid and/or electrolyte disturbances:*
      (1) Maintain an accurate record of intake and output.
         (a) Total the intake and output every 8 hours.
         (b) Describe carefully the amount and consistency of all stools and vomitus.
         (c) Collect all urine and weigh diapers if more accurate measurement of the child's output is necessary.
      (2) Weigh the child at regular intervals, using the same scales each time.

1. The child must be observed frequently to make certain that the IV is not infiltrating and is functioning properly. Report any swelling, discoloration, or leakage.

2. Complications associated with the administration of intravenous fluids to infants and children are very serious and may have fatal consequences. Any signs of complications must be reported immediately.

   b. Refer to Table 47-3.

   (2) An increase or decrease of 5% within a relatively brief period of time is usually significant and should be reported.

Procedure (continued)	Nursing Action	Rationale/Amplification

Nursing Action

    (3) Report:
        (a) Decreased skin turgor
        (b) Marked increase or decrease in urination
        (c) Fever
        (d) Sunken or bulging fontanelles in an infant
        (e) Sudden change in weight or vital signs
        (f) Diarrhea
        (g) Weakness, apathy, or lethargy
  c. Pyrogenic reactions

3. Record essential information.
  a. Reading on the container or reservoir
  b. Amount of fluid absorbed in the hour
  c. Total amount of fluid absorbed (compare with the total amount of fluid intended to have been absorbed)
  d. Rate of flow
  e. Apparent condition of the child
4. Regulate the rate of flow as necessary by any of the following methods:
  a. Raising the height of the container
  b. Adjusting the flow regulator
  c. Adjusting the position of the extremity
  d. Removing excess tubing or coiling it on the bed

  e. Adjusting the restraint

5. Irrigate the IV as necessary.
  a. Gather equipment:
    (1) Syringe with 1–3 ml. of normal saline solution
    (2) Several alcohol wipes
  b. Clamp off the IV solution.
  c. Disconnect the IV tubing at the needle insertion site. Keep it sterile.
  d. Remove the needle from the syringe.
  e. Connect the syringe to the tubing at the needle insertion site.
  f. Slowly inject the normal saline solution.

  g. Disconnect the syringe and reconnect the IV tubing to the needle insertion site.
  h. Unclamp the IV and regulate the flow of the solution.
  i. Check frequently to make certain that the IV is functioning properly.
6. Change the IV container and tubing every 24 hours.

7. If a catheter is used, check the dressing every tour of duty and change according to policy.
8. Disconnect the IV when prescribed or if it has obviously infiltrated
  a. Gather equipment
    (1) Scissors
    (2) 4 × 4 gauze square
    (3) Band-Aid
  b. Explain the procedure to the child, depending on his age.
  c. Clamp off the flow of the IV fluid.
  d. Determine the location of the needle.
  e. Loosen the tape around the needle, holding the needle firmly in position so that it does not slip out.

Rationale/Amplification

c. If severe, the IV should be discontinued. The solution should be saved for possible analysis.

d. If excess tubing falls below the level of the bed, the flow is slowed because the fluid must run uphill.
e. If an extremity is restrained too snugly, the restraint acts as a tourniquet, and the flow of solution will be slowed or stopped.
5. Irrigation may be required to dislodge small clots in the needle or to maintain the infusion rate of a sluggish IV.

f. Great force of injector should be avoided because this may cause the vein to rupture or the needle to become dislodged from the vein.

6. The IV set-up should be changed daily to maintain sterility and prevent contamination of the IV fluid during IV therapy.
7. This reduces the incidence of infection and other local complications.

(continued)

Guidelines   Intravenous Fluid Therapy *(continued)*

Procedure *(continued)*	Nursing Action	Rationale/Amplification
	f. Hold the 4 × 4 lightly over the insertion site and remove the needle quickly and carefully.	f. Inspect an Intracath or plastic needle to ensure that no portion has been left in the vein. If this is suspected, notify the physician. Alcohol sponges should not be used for removing IV needles because the stinging of alcohol on the puncture site causes unnecessary discomfort.
	g. Apply pressure to the site immediately and hold until bleeding stops.	
	h. Apply Band-Aid.	h. The Band-Aid should not be applied until all bleeding has stopped to minimize the possibility of prolonged or unnoticed bleeding.
	i. Remove the tape and armboard from the extremity.	
	j. Comfort the child as required.	
	k. Note the fluid level on the container or reservoir and complete recordings.	
	l. Record that the IV was discontinued.	

For additional information relating to intravenous therapy, including criteria for selecting a suitable vein for venipuncture, guidelines for administering an infusion using the antecubital fossa, and complications of intravenous therapy, refer to Chapter 5, IV Therapy.

Infusion Pumps

Infusion pumps are often used in pediatrics to provide a constant, slow rate of infusion. Several units are available and can be used with standard, commercial IV administration sets.

Types of Pumps

1. Peristaltic pumps—move fluid by compressing IV tubing.
2. Piston and cylinder pumps—move fluid by pushing it through a cylinder.

Indications for Use

1. When a constant rate of infusion is necessary, such as for administration of medication with a short half-life (e.g., insulin, lidocaine, catecholamines)
2. When a constant volume must be ensured per unit of time (e.g., prevention of volume overload in small infants, administration of parenteral hyperalimentation)
3. When patency of a vessel, usually an artery, must be preserved

Nursing Responsibilities

1. All nurses who operate a pump should be educated to do so correctly. Manufacturers' operating manuals and instruction sheets should be available.
2. Follow manufacturer's recommendations:
   a. In assembling equipment, initiating and maintaining infusion
   b. Before using an IV filter; some filters will blot out at infusion pump pressures, others can cause rate inaccuracies
   c. Before using a pump to infuse blood; some models can cause hemolysis
   d. In checking all parts of the pump frequently
3. Every hour, check:
   a. Delivery rate
   b. For infiltration, since many pumps will continue to infuse solution even if infiltration has occurred
4. Restart the pump promptly after it has been turned off to prevent the catheter from becoming clogged.
5. Turn off pump as soon as the infusion is completed. Failure to do so may damage some machines.
6. Be certain that the pump is tested for current leakage at least every 6 months to reduce electrical hazard.

Guidelines   Total Parenteral Nutrition (Hyperalimentation)

Hyperalimentation is a method of providing complete nutrition entirely by the intravenous route. It involves the infusion of hypertonic solutions of glucose, a nitrogen source, water, vitamins, minerals, and electrolytes at a constant rate (Fig. 47-7).

Types of Hyperalimentation

1. *Central line total parenteral nutrition (TPN):* Infusion occurs through an indwelling catheter placed in a central vein, usually the superior vena cava. It is the method of choice for long-term therapy or if a high concentration of infused glucose (20–25 gm./100 ml.) is necessary.
2. *Peripheral line TPN:* Infusion occurs through a single needle set, catheter, or cutdown into a peripheral vein, usually in the scalp or extremities. It is the method of choice for intralipid infusion, but generally restricts infused glucose concentrations to 10 gm./100 ml.

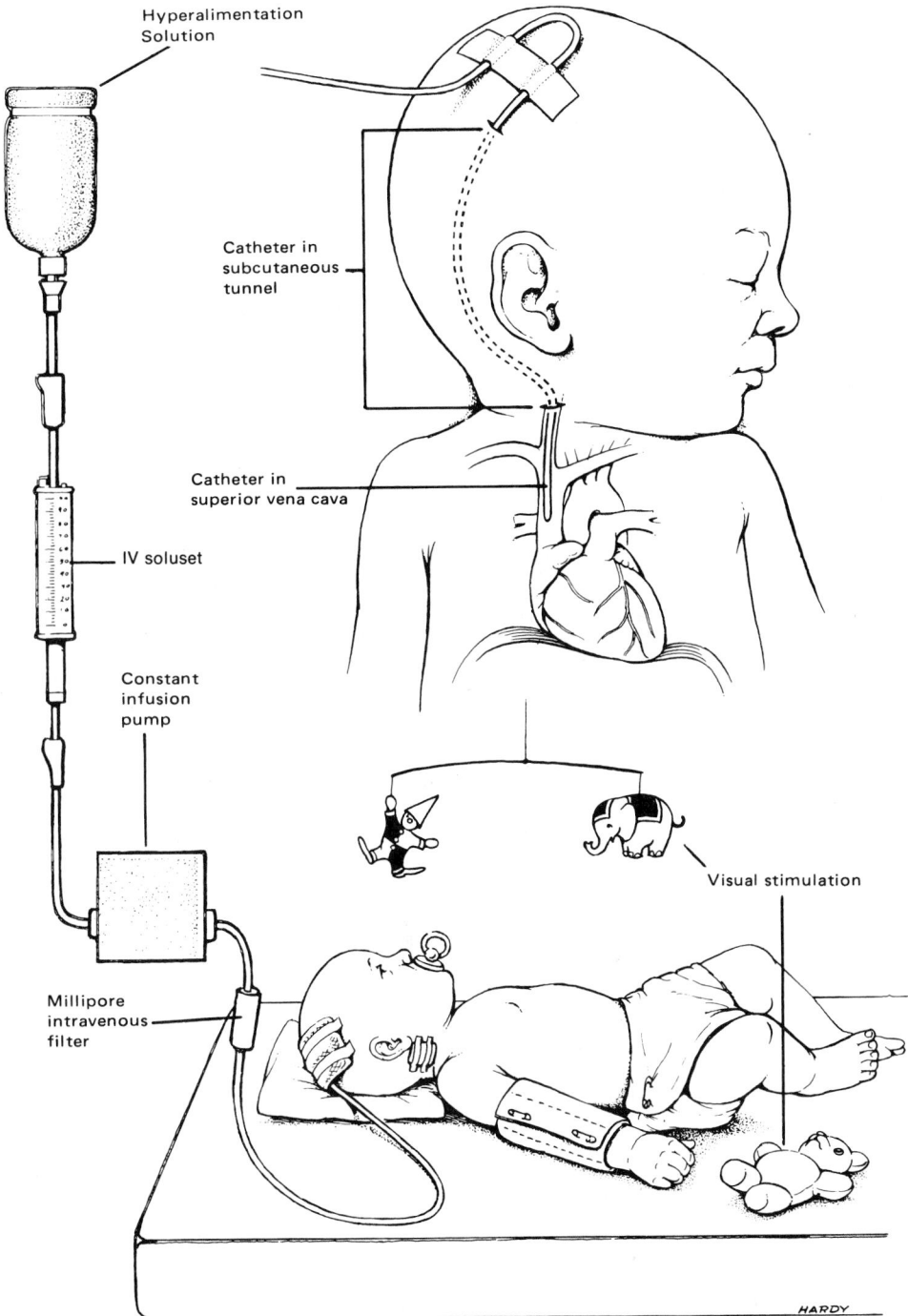

Figure 47-7. *Hyperalimentation.*

Purpose   To sustain life and promote growth in patients when oral or gastrointestinal tube intake is either impossible, potentially hazardous, or insufficient for an extended period of time.

1. The procedure has been used successfully in children with gastrointestinal diseases such as chronic diarrhea, malabsorption syndrome, bowel fistulas, esophageal atresia or obstruction, and omphalocele.

2. It is also useful when a child's condition produces excessive nutritional needs, as in the case of burns, neurosurgical procedures, major trauma, large wound infections, and cancer.

(continued)

Guidelines Total Parenteral Nutrition (Hyperalimantation) *(continued)*

Purpose *(continued)*	**Nursing Action**	**Rationale/Amplification**

3. Hyperalimentation has been successful in the treatment of premature infants of very low weights and infants with malnutrition or failure to thrive.

Equipment

Hyperalimentation solution:

The type, amount, and composition of the solution is prescribed by the physician.

The initial solution provides adequate daily fluid and minerals but less than optimal calories and nitrogen. The concentrations of caloric substances are increased daily over 3–5 days as the child tolerates higher glucose loads.

Micropore filter

IV extension tubing

Silastic catheter of appropriate size

Constant infusion pump

Alcohol wipes

Betadine

Benzoin

Antibacterial ointment

All of the equipment listed in the procedure for intravenous fluid therapy by cutdown method; see IV Fluid Therapy, cutdown method, page 1168.

Nursing activities for all phases of the administration of hyperalimentation solution are the same as those specified in the procedure for intravenous fluid therapy, with the following additions:

Procedure—Central Line TPN

Nursing Action	**Rationale/Amplification**

Preparatory Phase

1. Prepare the child and family for the procedure.
2. Administer preliminary medication, if prescribed.
3. Assemble necessary equipment.

Performance Phase

1. Assist the physician with the insertion of the hyperalimentation catheter. This may involve obtaining equipment, positioning and restraining the child, etc.

   a. The hyperalimentation catheter should be inserted under sterile surgical conditions. It is often inserted in the operating room.

       a. Violation of aseptic techniques at the time of insertion may result in overwhelming septicemia and death.

   b. In infants and small children, the vena cava is usually approached through one of the common facial, internal jugular, or (usually) external jugular veins.

Follow-Up Phase

1. Until x-ray confirmation of the location of the catheter tip, infuse only isotonic solutions at a slow, "keep open" rate.

   1. A chest x-ray confirms proper placement of the line and rules out complications such as pneumothorax or hemothorax that may be associated with catheter insertion. Infusing an isotonic solution minimizes the possibility of complications arising from the infusion of solution through a misplaced catheter.

2. Before hanging the solution, check:

   a. Content label against the physician's request

   b. Expiration date and time

   c. Container for defects

   d. Solution for cloudiness or separation

   2. Preparation of the solution should be done in the pharmacy using a closed system such as the laminar flow filtered air hood. Solutions should be prepared every 24 hours and refrigerated until used. Fat emulsions do not require refrigeration.

3. Check the infusion rate every ½–1 hour to make certain that the solution is infused continuously and at a constant rate.

   3. Continuous infusion is necessary to prevent such metabolic complications as osmotic diuresis, hypoglycemia, and pulmonary edema.

   a. Use a constant-infusion pump.

   b. Reset the rate to that prescribed by the physician as necessary, but do not slow or increase the drip to make up for an excess or deficit without consulting the physician.

       b. Increasing the rate may cause hyperglycemia with osmotic diuresis. Slowing the rate may cause hypoglycemia.

Procedure— Central Line TPN *(continued)*	Nursing Action	Rationale/Amplification

4. Change the container, tubing, and filter at least once each day.
   a. Remove the tape that secures the filter to the dressing.
   b. Attach a new infusion set to the new container.
   c. Prime tubing and tap the end gently.
   d. Connect the infusion set to the new filter housing carefully.
   e. Hang the new container on the pole.
   f. Remove the protective covering from the distal end of the filter and discard.
   g. Hold the filter parallel to the floor and run solution through the entire line.
   h. Gently tap the filter housing to dispel air and tap the end to free glucose droplets. Be careful not to contaminate the end of the filter.
   i. Change the IV line at the catheter union rapidly, with the patient flat in bed or in low Fowler's position. Instruct the patient to perform Valsalva's maneuver. Use a sterile Kelly clamp to grasp the catheter hub for leverage during the tubing change.
   j. Anchor the filter to the dressing.
   k. Cleanse all connection sites with Betadine; allow to dry, and wrap with sterile 2 × 2 gauze pads.
   l. Secure all IV tubing joints with adhesive tape.

   m. Readjust flow rate.
   n. Write time and date on new tubing.
   o. Culture the filter each time it is changed (optional).

4. This is another attempt to prevent contamination and reduce the possibility that the child will develop infection.

   b. Cleanse each connecting point with Betadine.
   c. This dislodges any glucose droplets.
   d. Avoid contamination of the filter.

   g. This position allows for complete filling of the filter housing.
   h. Air bubbles will cause difficulty in maintaining constant flow.

   i. This technique minimizes the danger of air embolism. Using a Kelly clamp helps reduce traction on the catheter and the chance of dislocation.

   j. This prevents tension on the catheter.

   l. This prevents accidental separation of the tubing from the catheter and prevents air embolus.

   o. It is possible, by culturing the filter, to detect microbial contamination prior to the development of clinical signs. Cultures should include fungal studies since a special danger of hyperalimentation is fungal septicemia.

5. Change the dressing around the catheter three times a week using sterile technique. Face masks should be worn by all persons at the head of the bed to prevent airborne contamination at the insertion site by nasopharyngeal organisms. The child should also wear a mask and turn his head away from the dressing.
   a. Remove the dressing carefully.

   b. Using an alcohol wipe, cleanse a large area surrounding the insertion site. Move in a circular motion from the center to the periphery.
   c. Paint the skin with Betadine solution and allow to dry.
   d. Apply a prescribed antibacterial ointment directly to the catheter insertion site and 2–3 cm. down the catheter.
   e. Cover site with transparent dressing such as Op-site.
   f. Tape looped tubing to the skin.
   g. Label dressing with date, time, and initials.
   h. Record the dressing change, how the child tolerated the procedure, and any relevant condition.

5. This reduces the possibility of infection at the catheter site. The dressing should be changed immediately if it becomes soiled or wet. Most health care agencies have established policies for catheter care.

   a. Extreme care is necessary to avoid dislodging the catheter.
   b. This removes surface skin fats that might harbor organisms and removes remaining traces of adhesive tape that have adhered to the skin.

   e. This allows for observation of the insertion site.
   f. This prevents tension on the catheter.

   h. Consider condition of the skin, drainage, catheter placement, placement of needle guard, and presence of suture.

6. Monitor fractional urine specimens for glucose, acetone, pH, blood, protein, and specific gravity every 2–8 hours.

6. Some children require supplemental parenteral insulin to utilize the required amount of infused glucose. Children receiving certain drugs may show false-positive results. Positive urine sugars are confirmed by blood glucose levels.

7. Keep an accurate record of the child's total intake and output, including bowel movements, emesis, and gastric drainage. If the child is allowed oral intake, a calorie count should be kept.

7. This helps to provide a clear picture of the child's fluid and electrolyte balance.

8. Monitor the child's weight daily. Weigh at the same time each day, with the same amount of clothing, and on the same scales.

8. Weight gain is one of the most reliable indications of a positive response to therapy.

(continued)

Guidelines   Total Parenteral Nutrition (Hyperalimantation) *(continued)*

Procedure—Central Line TPN *(continued)*	Nursing Action	Rationale/Amplification
	9. In infants, measure length and head circumference weekly.	9. Hyperalimentation promotes growth in these dimensions.
	10. Observe for signs of complications resulting from therapy.	10.
	a. Complications related to the catheter	a. Three fourths of the major complications of therapy are of this variety. Sepsis accounts for more than half of these problems.
	(1) Septicemia	
	(2) Thrombosis of a major blood vessel	
	(3) Plugging or dislodging of the catheter	
	(4) Local skin infection	
	(5) Cardiac arrhythmia	
	(6) Leak around catheter or hole in catheter	
	(7) Air embolism	
	b. Metabolic complications	b. Careful clinical and chemical monitoring, especially during the initial period of hyperalimentation, can greatly reduce the incidence of these types of complications.
	(1) Hyperglycemia	
	(2) Hypoglycemia	
	(3) Dehydration	
	(4) Metabolic acidosis	
	(5) Electrolyte imbalances	
	(6) Amino acid imbalance	
	(7) Postinfusion hypoglycemia	
	11. Provide mouth care.	11. In patients who are NPO, the tongue, throat, and mouth tend to become dry, inflamed and uncomfortable. The total absence of taste is unpleasant for older children.
	a. If allowed, use a variety of mouthwashes to provide some change in taste.	
	b. Apply lip balm flavored with fruit or mint.	
	c. Offer crushed ice flavored with juice or syrup.	
	12. Provide the infant with a pacifier.	12. It is especially important to meet the sucking needs of the infant since hyperalimentation therapy may be necessary for several weeks or months.
	13. Discontinue the infusion when directed to do so by the physician. (In many hospitals this is the responsibility of the physician.)	13. The child is gradually tapered off from hyperalimentation to allow for adjustment to decreased levels of glucose. Final cessation is often followed by isotonic glucose infusion for at least 12 hours to protect against rebound hypoglycemia from still high insulin levels. During the weaning process, the child's oral intake is gradually increased as the hyperalimentation solution is proportionally decreased.
	a. Turn the flow rate off.	
	b. Remove the dressings.	
	c. Cut and remove the stay suture.	
	d. Pull out the catheter.	
	e. Apply pressure with a sterile 4 × 4 gauze for 5–10 minutes.	
	f. Cleanse the site with Betadine and apply a sterile dressing.	
	g. Record time and date procedure was discontinued, by whom, cultures sent, and child's condition.	
	h. Send the tip of the catheter, the filter, and the fluid in the tubing to the laboratory for culture.	

Procedure—Peripheral Line TPN	Nursing activities are essentially the same as for central line TPN although dressing changes are not indicated. However, peripheral sites should be checked and cared for at regular intervals to avoid infiltration and vascular inflammation. For additional information, refer to the following procedure for the administration of intralipids.

Guidelines   Intralipids—Intravenous Fat Emulsion

(See adult, p. 454.)

Purpose	Used in conjunction with partial parenteral (peripheral) nutrition (PPN) as an additional source of calories and essential fatty acids.
Equipment	Intralipid 10% fat emulsion—isotonic emulsion composed of 10% soybean oil (a triglyceride), 1.2% egg yolk phospholipids, 2.2% glycerin and water for injection. Total caloric value is 1.1 calorie/ml.

Equipment
(continued)

Antiseptic wipe
IV tubing and sterile needle
Complete infusion IV line
Constant infusion pump
Tape

Procedure

Nursing activities for the administration of Intralipid 10% are the same as those specified in the procedure for intravenous fluid therapy and total parenteral nutrition, with the following exceptions.

Nursing Action	Rationale/Amplification

Preparatory Phase

1. Prior to therapeutic administration of Intralipid 10%, a test dose of 0.1 ml./minute (10 mg.) is given in 10–15 minutes; afterwards, the rate is increased to permit 1 gm./kg. to run over 4 hours.
   a. Observe for immediate reactions of dyspnea, flushing, rash, sweating, sleepiness, headache, tachycardia, bradycardia, acidosis in infants.
   b. Should any of these signs appear, stop infusion and notify physician.

1. To identify any sensitivity the child may have to the emulsion.

2. Ensure that prescribed laboratory studies are done prior to commencement of test dose (i.e., cholesterol, triglycerides, platelets). Once testing has been accomplished, Intralipid 10% is administered as part of PPN, 1–4 gm./kg./24 hours based on age and size of the child.

2. To serve as baseline before test dose.

3. Ensure that nothing is added to emulsion (i.e., drugs, electrolytes, vitamins, or other nutrients).

3. May cause lipid to separate or cause a fat embolus.

4. Be aware of conditions that may contraindicate the use of Intralipid 10%—sepsis, hyperbilirubinemia, severe respiratory distress.

4. Prevents further compromise of the child: fat is taken up by the reticuloendothelial system; it displaces bilirubin from albumin and can plug small vessels in the lungs.

Performance Phase

1. Once the IV lines have been purged with the emulsion, connect the line to the existing peripheral or central line via piggyback or Y-connector just proximal to the infusion site. Tape connection. Do not pass solution through a bacterial filter because this can clog filter and break down emulsion. Peripheral line administration can be used.

1. Infuse emulsion as a separate line that is added into the existing IV. The emulsion is administered in the self-contained solution container from manufacturer, syringe, and tubing or pediatric infusion set. The emulsion is not added to the TPN solution bottle to avoid disturbing the stability of the emulsion. It is administered with another fluid to decrease the high concentration of fat. (Intralipid is isotonic.)

2. Administer emulsion using continuous flow pump separate from that of PPN. (Pumps with electric eye may not be effective because of the opaque solution.)

2. Allows flow rate of each solution to be controlled independently.

3. Monitor hourly the amount of emulsion infused.

3. To control fluid intake. Emulsion can be infused continuously or in 4 or 5 separate doses over 2–6-hour time periods.

4. Change bottle and tubing:
   a. Intermittent administration—each administration
   b. Continuous administration—every 8 hours

4. To assist in preventing infection.

Follow-Up Phase

1. Once prescribed emulsion has been infused, discontinue. Flush line with normal saline solution.
   Check to be sure there is no leaking at point where connection was made.

1. To prevent infection and inaccurate account of fluid intake as a result of the line being violated. Prevents coagulation of Intralipid in IV line.

2. Record time procedure was discontinued, by whom, amount given, and the child's condition.

3. Ensure that prescribed laboratory studies are done at designated times—usually 2–6 hours after emulsion is discontinued or weekly (i.e., lipid and triglyceride levels).

3. To see if fat has been metabolized and utilized and to detect any early signs of complications.

4. Continue to observe the child for any delayed adverse reactions: hepatomegaly, splenomegaly, thrombocytopenia, transient increase in liver function tests, system overload.

4. To detect any early signs of complications. In addition to physical assessment of the child, serum studies may include liver function, bilirubin, alkaline phosphatase, CBC or platelet count.

Pediatric Home Hyperalimentation

Home hyperalimentation programs have been developed to provide an alternative to hospitalization for children who require long-term TPN.

Benefits of Home Hyperalimentation

1. The child is able to maintain a more normal life-style in his home environment.
2. Stress is reduced for the child and his family.
3. Cost is greatly reduced.

Resources Necessary for an Effective Program

1. A pharmacy to prepare the solution
2. A physician available to deal with problems
3. A reliable microchemistry laboratory
4. Someone to deal with equipment procurement, maintenance, and problems
5. An insurance agency willing to cooperate with such a program
6. Effective community health nursing support

Criteria for Determining Family Readiness and Ability to Cope With Home TPN

1. Does the family comfortably participate in the technical procedures in the hospital?
2. Do the parents state a desire to perform the TPN procedure in the home?
3. Do the parents respond to cues from the child and deal with them appropriately?
4. Do the parents interact effectively with the child by providing nurturing care and comfort measures, which they will have to continue at home?
5. Do parents have support from the nuclear and extended family in conducting home TPN?
6. Are community support systems available?

Health Education

1. Explain the principles and concepts of TPN.
2. Instruct the parents concerning the methods, procedures, and prevention of complications of TPN administration.
3. Demonstrate TPN procedures to the parents.
4. Have parents demonstrate their ability to perform TPN procedures.
5. Encourage parents to carry out complete management of TPN until the child is discharged.
6. Provide means for continued education and problem solving during home TPN.
7. Evaluate treatment and follow-up.

Guidelines Assisting With Exchange Transfusion

Exchange transfusion is replacement of circulating blood by withdrawing blood and injecting donor's blood in equal amounts.

Purposes
1. To prevent accumulation of bilirubin in the blood above a dangerous level.
2. To prevent kernicterus (brain damage—occurs when there is yellow staining of brain tissue from deposits of indirect bilirubin).
3. To prevent accumulation of other by-products of hemolysis from hemolytic disease (i.e., ABO incompatibility).
4. To raise a very low hemoglobin.
5. To replace red blood cells that have poor oxygen-releasing capacity and poor carbonic anhydrase activity (i.e., as in a premature infant).
6. To remove toxic metabolites.
7. To treat irreversible acidosis, overwhelming neonatal septicemia, disseminated intravascular coagulation (DIC).

Equipment
Fresh donor blood—with hematocrit 50% ± 5%
Monitoring equipment
Sterile disposable exchange transfusion set containing:
    Stopcock with extension tubing
    Extra extension tubing
    Umbilical catheters sizes No. 5 and 8, French
    2 20-ml. syringes
    1 5-ml. syringe and No. 23 gauge needle
    Gauze sponges
Transfusion record
Cleansing solution
Means of warming infant
Means of warming blood
Calcium gluconate in 5-ml. syringe
50% glucose solution in 10-ml. syringe
Sodium bicarbonate in 10-ml. syringe
Waste-blood container
Blood administration set
Sterile gown and gloves for physician
Resuscitative equipment

General Considerations

1. Volume of blood given is 160–180 ml./kg. infant weight (2-volume exchange, replacing approximately 85% of the infant's blood).
2. The infant's blood volume is 80–90 ml./kg. body weight
3. Blood type used:
   Rh sensitivity = Rh-negative blood used (typed and cross-matched to mother's serum).
   ABO disease—group O blood used.

Procedure

Nursing Action	Rationale/Amplification

Preparatory Phase

1. Place the infant under heat lamps or radiant heating unit to keep his temperature within the thermoneutral zone. Environment temperature of 32°C. (86°F.) will usually maintain correct infant body temperature, depending on size of infant.

2. If the infant has not been NPO for 3–4 hours, it may be necessary to empty stomach contents via stomach tube.

3. Albumin (1 gm./kg.) may be given 1–2 hours prior to exchange transfusion.

4. Attach electronic cardiac monitoring device to infant if available. Otherwise place stethoscope over apex of heart. Also attach temperature-monitoring device. Monitor continuously.

5. Place infant on his back. Restrain all four extremities.

6. Have resuscitative equipment ready for immediate use: oxygen supply, mask, intubation equipment, laryngoscope, breathing bag, suction, sodium bicarbonate, and 50% glucose solution.

7. Check donor blood for type, age, and other identifying data. Check blood pH. It should be corrected to pH 7.1 or as specified by physician.

8. Assist the physician in setting up blood and exchange equipment. Blood should be run through a coil of tubing through a water bath at 38°C., (100°F.). Ensure that lines and connections are securely closed.

---

1. Chilling of the infant during the procedure can result in apnea and in increased caloric need and oxygen consumption, which can be exhausting to a baby with already limited amount of energy. Abnormal decrease in blood pH leading to acidosis can result from the stress of prolonged chilling. Hypothermia may also hinder albumin and bilirubin binding capacity. Hyperthermia may cause destruction of erythrocytes of donor blood.

2. To prevent aspiration, should vomiting occur during the procedure.

3. The albumin may increase the effectiveness of the transfusion by yielding more bilirubin binding sites.

4. Apnea, bradycardia, and cardiac arrest are complications of an exchange transfusion. Close monitoring will allow for immediate observation of signs of trouble.

5. This will prevent the infant from moving and inadvertently pulling out the exchange catheter.

6. Should the infant develop bradycardia, hypoglycemia, or cyanosis during procedure, these items will be necessary for immediate and supportive treatment.

7. Heparinized blood must be used within 24 hours of collection. Optimal age of ACD (heparin, acid-citrate-dextrose) or CPD (citrate-phosphate-dextrose) blood is less than 3 days old. CPD lasts longer—has better carbonic anhydrase level. Acidemia may result when fresh blood is not used because of the acid metabolites. Cardiac arrest may also occur from elevated potassium in donor blood.

8. Although hypothermia (i.e., rapid chilling of the infant) is a primary concern, increased blood viscosity and ventricular fibrillation can also result from administering cold blood.

Performance Phase

1. The infant's skin is cleansed with soap and water followed by an antiseptic solution. Sterile drapes are applied by the physician who is gowned and gloved. Strict attention should be paid to maintaining aseptic technique.

2. Once the umbilical catheter is in place in the umbilical vein, the initial venous pressure is measured (although it is not usually accurate) and the exchange is begun. (Preferred site is the umbilical vein; jugular or femoral vessels may be used.)

3. Note and record the time the exchange started. Record each successive withdrawal and infusion of blood stating exact amount and time. Report to the physician when each 100 ml. of blood is exchanged (see Record Chart, next page). This will prevent system overload from excessive infusion—resulting in cardiac failure and shock from too-rapid removal of infant's blood.

4. After each 100 ml. of blood is exchanged, 0.5–1.0 ml./kg. 10% calcium gluconate may be injected to prevent hypocalcemia. Blood-bank donor blood is calcium-deficient. Monitor cardiac rate very carefully during the injection.

---

1. To prevent infection or sepsis. A foreign body introduced into the blood vessel is always a potential for infection due to an infected cord stump or contaminated equipment.
   The umbilicus can be grossly contaminated and is impossible to sterilize.

2. Record the venous pressure. This will be maintained at about 10–12 cm. by equal volume exchanges. An increase in pressure during the procedure is an indication to stop and assess the infant.

3. Blood is exchanged slowly in amounts of 5–20 ml., depending on the infant's size and condition. The total amount exchanged is about 170 ml. of blood/kg. of body weight (80 ml./pound). About 75%–93% of the infant's total blood volume is exchanged. The exchange should take about 1 hour. Rapid exchange can aggravate cardiovascular changes and prevent normal metabolism of infused acid and citrate.

4. Calcium decreases the irritability and irregularity of the heart. Too rapid an injection will cause bradycardia. Especially important when CPD donor blood is used.

(continued)

Guidelines Assisting With Exchange Transfusion *(continued)*

EXCHANGE TRANSFUSION RECORD

HOSPITAL NO. _____

DATE OF DELIVERY:	*1/18/91*
NAME OF BABY: *Johnson, Clarence David*	TIME: *4:10 am*
NAME OF MOTHER: *Marsha Johnson*	APGAR SCORE AT DELIVERY: *8 at 1 min / 9 at 5 min*
BIRTH WEIGHT: *3580 grams*	INITIAL HEMOGLOBIN: *42*
BLOOD GROUP: *O neg.*	BILIRUBIN: *16.3*
TIME COMMENCING EXCHANGE: *3:45 pm*	POST-EXCHANGE BILIRUBIN: *11.8*
TIME FINISHING EXCHANGE: *4:17 pm*	AGE OF BABY IN HOURS: *30*

TIME	OUT Amount	OUT Total	IN Amount	IN Total	PULSE	RESPI-RATION	VENOUS PRESSURE	MEDI-CATION	COMMENTS
3:45	*20*	*20*	*20*	*20*			*10 cm*		
3:48	*20*	*40*	*20*	*40*					
3:51	*20*	*60*	*20*	*60*					
3:55	*20*	*80*	*20*	*80*					
3:58	*20*	*100*	*20*	*100*	*150*	*48*		*Ca 1ml*	
4:02	*20*	*120*	*20*	*120*			*10 cm*		
4:06	*20*	*140*	*20*	*140*					
4:10	*20*	*160*	*20*	*160*					
4:13	*20*	*180*	*20*	*180*					
4:17	*20*	*200*	*20*	*200*	*160*	*56*			

Procedure *(continued)*

Nursing Action	Rationale/Amplification
5. Constant monitoring of the cardiac rate is imperative. Also note respirations, skin color, and color of withdrawn blood. Keep transfusion lines tightly secured to prevent air embolus or exsanguination.	5. Observation and monitoring will allow immediate treatment if untoward signs appear. Bradycardia may occur at any time during the procedure due to a low pH of donor blood or old blood.
6. Protamine sulfate may be given after the transfusion is completed.	6. Because heparinized blood will affect the coagulation potential of the infant from 4–6 hours postexchange.

Procedure *(continued)*	Nursing Action	Rationale/Amplification

Follow-Up Phase

1. When transfusion is completed, umbilical catheter may be:
   a. Left in place with an IV plug or intravenous infusion or

   b. Removed

   a. If catheter is left in place, it is usually done for future exchange transfusions, easy withdrawal of blood for blood studies, administration of intravenous fluids and medications. Keep infant restrained.
   b. If catheter is removed, apply small pressure dressing and observe for any bleeding. Check the area every hour for 3 hours, then every 3 hours for 24 hours.

2. Record:
   a. Time transfusion was completed
   b. Total amount blood withdrawn and infused
   c. Any changes in vital signs
   d. Medications administered during exchange
   e. Infant's color and current vital signs
   f. Catheter removed or left indwelling
   g. How infant tolerated the procedure
   h. Any blood samples taken before or after exchange
3. Monitor infant for any signs of postexchange transfusion complications:
   a. Hypoglycemia—Dextrostix test every hour × 4

   b. Hemolytic reaction
   c. Thrombocytopenia and hemorrhage—check for bleeding at catheter site and petechiae.
   d. Intestinal perforation—observe for bloody stools, bile-stained vomitus, abdominal distention, respiratory distress, pallor.
   e. Metabolic acidosis—observe for deep, increased respirations; decreased consciousness; acid urine.
   f. Hyperkalemia

   a. Hypoglycemia frequently occurs with erythroblastosis fetalis. Incidence is also increased because of fasting prior to and during procedure.
   b. Reaction from donor blood.
   c. This results from overheparinized blood or when citrated blood is given without calcium replacement.
   d. Ischemia of bowel.

   e. Resulting from old donor blood.

   f. From donor blood

The Child Undergoing Dialysis

Dialysis refers to the process of separating substances in solution by movement through a semipermeable membrane.

Purpose

To preserve life by acting as a substitute for kidney function during renal failure.
1. Aids in the removal of toxic substances and metabolic wastes.
2. Removes excessive body fluid.
3. Assists in regulating the body's fluid and electrolyte balance.

Types of Dialysis

A. Peritoneal Dialysis

1. Mechanism
   a. The peritoneal lining is used as the semipermeable membrane.
   b. A catheter is inserted through the anterior abdominal wall, and the dialysis is instilled into the abdominal cavity.
   c. After an equilibration time (about 30 minutes), the fluid is drained by gravity and fresh dialysate is instilled.

2. Major uses
   a. Acute, reversible uremic episodes such as those due to sudden illness, trauma, poisoning, or drug intoxication.
   b. In terminal illness, to keep the child comfortable for as long as possible.
   c. Prior to acceptance in a long-term hemodialysis and transplantation program.
   d. In selected cases of chronic renal failure.
      (1) The child may be dialyzed at night through a semi-permanently implanted abdominal cannula by an automatic, continually recycling machine.
      (2) Continuous ambulatory peritoneal dialysis, (see p. 679) has been used successfully by many children.
3. Advantage
   Relatively safe and readily available.
4. Disadvantages
   a. Long periods of time required to effectively remove waste products.
   b. May cause abdominal pain and discomfort.
   c. Sterile dialysate is required.
   d. Complications
      (1) Peritonitis
      (2) Bowel perforation during insertion of the catheter
      (3) Respiratory distress caused by upward dis-

placement of the diaphragm by fluid in the peritoneal cavity

(4) Shock due to excessive fluid loss

(5) Protein loss because serum proteins pass through the peritoneal membrane during dialysis

(6) Bleeding and leakage at the catheter insertion site

(7) Inadequate fluid return

(8) Nausea, vomiting, diarrhea

B. Hemodialysis

1. Mechanism

  a. The semipermeable membrane is located in a machine through which the child's blood is directed.

  b. Access to the circulation is provided via a Teflon–Silastic arteriovenous shunt or a subcutaneously implanted arteriovenous fistula.

  c. The child's blood is diverted through the machine adjacent to the semipermeable membrane to equilibrate with dialysate on the other side of the membrane.

  d. Selection of the dialyzer depends on the size of the child. Considerations include:

    (1) Amount of blood the machine holds relative to the amount that the child can safely spare from the body at one time.

    (2) Efficiency of the machine relative to the child's weight.

(3) Speed with which fluid can be removed by the machine.

Note: Dialysis can be dangerous if it is too rapid.

2. Major uses

  a. Long-term therapy for chronic renal failure.

  b. Holding procedure prior to kidney transplant.

3. Advantages

  a. Shorter period of time required to effectively remove waste products.

  b. Does not require sterile dialysate.

  c. Is less traumatic to initiate once access to the circulation is made.

  d. Home dialysis is available in selected situations.

4. Disadvantages

  a. It is costly.

  b. There are inherent moral, legal, logistical, and technical problems.

  c. Complications

    (1) Clotting, infection, accidental separation of shunt

    (2) Anemia—because a small amount of blood remains behind in the machine with each run

    (3) Malaise, headache, nausea, and vomiting during dialysis

    (4) Hepatitis due to transfusions necessitated by uremic anemia

    (5) Seizures—possibly related to large changes in sodium osmolarity

Guidelines Caring for the Child Undergoing Dialysis

Nursing Care	Nursing Action	Rationale/Amplification
	1. Prepare the child for the procedure.	1. Dialysis is threatening to most children and may evoke fears of pain, mutilation, immobilization, helplessness, and dependency. Many children have fears of losing all of their blood in this process. A child who is well-prepared will be less frightened and better able to cooperate during the procedure.
	a. Explain the procedure to the child in terms that he can understand.	
	(1) Allow the child to handle equipment similar to that which will be used during dialysis.	
	(2) Encourage the child to express his fears so that misinterpretations can be corrected.	
	(3) Provide simple pictures and diagrams, if appropriate.	
	(4) Allow the child to talk with peers who have undergone dialysis.	
	b. Explain the procedure to the family and answer questions so that they will be in the best position to support their child.	
	2. Protect the child from infection.	2. These children are prone to infection because of their general debilitated state and because of protein loss and anemia.
	a. Keep the dressings and area around the catheter or shunt clean and dry.	
	b. Use aseptic technique throughout the dialysis procedure.	
	c. Avoid exposure to children or adults with infection.	
	d. Provide supplemental vitamins since a protein-restricted diet is poor in vitamins.	
	e. Provide meticulous daily hygiene.	
	3. Provide a high calorie diet that is low in sodium, potassium, and protein. Restrict fluids. Since the child often experiences anorexia, it may be helpful to allow him to choose foods from his allowances and offer small, frequent meals.	3. Fluids and sodium are restricted to prevent fluid overload. Potassium is limited to prevent complications related to hyperkalemia. Protein restriction reduces elevated BUN. The child may see dietary restrictions as punishment and must be helped to realize the purpose of the restrictions.
	4. Maintain careful records of intake and output, vital signs, blood pressure, and daily weights.	4. These provide valuable information about the effectiveness of the therapy.

Procedure	Nursing Action	Rationale/Amplification

1. Support the child during the dialysis procedure.
   a. Provide symptomatic relief of nausea, vomiting, malaise, or headache.
      Notify the physician if these symptoms are severe.
   b. Be alert to clues from the child for helpful methods of offering support.
      (1) Young children often cling to stuffed toys or blankets or depend on parents' presence at the bedside.
      (2) Older children may benefit from radio, television, magazines, or contact with peers.

2. Provide an environment that is as normal as possible.
   a. Encourage the family to bring in articles that will make the child's room appear more home-like (i.e., pictures, posters, etc.).
   b. Encourage the child to be as independent as possible in his daily care.
   c. Provide for age-appropriate recreation and/or diversion.
   d. Help the child to keep up with his school work by initiating a referral to a tutor, providing study times, etc.

2. Although life is preserved, it is by no means normal during the time on dialysis or between dialyses. These measures may increase the child's feeling of self-esteem and diminish regression and social isolation. By serving as role models, health professionals may encourage parents to recognize and foster the normal, healthy aspects of the child's daily life.

3. Offer appropriate support to the family.
   a. Provide opportunity for family members to discuss their feelings, fears, and frustrations and to ask questions.
   b. Allow family members to become involved in the child's care to the extent that they wish and that is helpful for the child and family.
   c. Provide for continuity of personnel.
   d. Initiate appropriate referrals. These may include referrals to a social worker, psychiatrist, dietitian, community health agency, other families who are coping with dialysis.

3. Families often need extensive support from many health professionals to cope with the physical, psychological, financial, and logistical aspects of renal failure and dialysis. Attention must be focused on siblings as well as parents since sibling relationships are often strained and difficult.

4. Teach the child and family about all of the important aspects of renal failure and dialysis, including:
   a. Signs and symptoms of uremia
   b. Shunt care and protection
   c. Protection from infection
   d. Dietary restrictions and recommendations; ways of incorporating the special diet into the family meal plan
   e. Dialysis schedule
   f. Medications
   g. Emergency procedures

4. The family should be prepared to care for the child at home well before the day of discharge. Learning about the child's care also helps restore some sense of control in a frightening situation.

Peritoneal Dialysis: Specific Nursing Responsibilities

Refer to Guidelines: Assisting the Patient Undergoing Peritoneal Dialysis, page 677. In addition, the following principles should be considered by the nurse working with pediatric patients.

1. Because of the child's smaller size, the volume of dialysate required is less.
2. Because the child may be unable to hold still, it may be necessary to apply protective measures to limit motion in order to avoid contamination of the sterile field or injury to the child (see p. 1149).
3. Because of the possibility of nausea and vomiting, oral intake should be limited to ice chips and small amounts of fluids during the first 12–24 hours of dialysis. Frequent mouth care should be provided.
4. Because the child may develop fears and fantasies about the equipment, it should be stored out of sight when not in use.

Hemodialysis: Specific Nursing Responsibilities

1. Care for the arteriovenous shunt (refer to Guidelines, below).
2. Assist in teaching the child and/or family proper care and protection of the shunt.
3. When possible, avoid giving subcutaneous or intramuscular injections because the child is anticoagulated with heparin at least twice weekly during dialysis, and extensive bleeding could occur as a result of such injections.
4. Care for the child during dialysis. (This aspect of nursing care is not presented because it is generally provided by specially trained personnel in a dialysis unit.)

Guidelines Care of the Arteriovenous Shunt

Purpose   To preserve shunt function and prevent separation of the cannulas.

Equipment   2 shunt clips
Dressing tray with:
    2 sterile plastic basins
    Sterile 2 × 2-inch sponges
    Sterile 4 × 3-inch sponges
    Kling bandage
    Hydrogen peroxide
    Betadine
    Normal saline solution
    Sterile applicators
    Sterile scissors
    Mask
    Sterile gloves

Procedure

Nursing Action	Rationale/Amplification
1. Place shunt clips on the dressing and keep with the child at all times.	1. The clamps are used to close the shunt in case it separates at its connection.
2. Use another extremity for:	2. Disturbing the shunt in any way can encourage clotting and infection.
a. Taking blood pressure	a. Inflation of blood pressure cuff may precipitate clotting by slowing the flow of blood through the tubing.
b. Giving medications	b., c. Injections in the extremity increase the possibility of thrombosis of the vein.
c. Giving infusions	
d. Taking blood samples	d. A rubber puncture site may be added to the shunt. This can be punctured with a needle to obtain blood specimens.

Note: The Silastic tubing should never be punctured since it will not seal.

Nursing Action	Rationale/Amplification
3. Cleanse the area around the shunt and change the dressing with each dialysis treatment, or p.r.n.	
a. Remove old dressing.	a. Never use scissors to remove the dressing to avoid accidentally cutting the cannulas.
b. Observe the shunt for malalignment or kinks.	b. These factors increase the possibility of clot formation and must be corrected.
c. Observe the area around the cannula insertion sites for signs of inflammation (redness, swelling, drainage).	c. If noted, report signs of inflammation, and take culture before cleansing the area.
d. Using aseptic technique, clean the venous insertion site first with hydrogen peroxide and then with Betadine. Take new swabs and clean the arterial site in the same manner.	d. Do not use the same swabs to clean both sites as this may cause cross-infection. When cleaning, begin at the insertion site and move outward in a circular motion.
e. Allow to dry. Rinse well with normal saline solution and dry with a sterile 4 × 4 gauze pad.	e. Avoid leaving Betadine on the cannula because this could make connections slippery.
f. Apply dry, sterile dressing to the areas of cannula insertion.	f. A 2 × 2 gauze pad under the cannula at each insertion site will lessen tension at the site and increase comfort.
g. Wrap arm with compression bandage firmly, but not tightly, leaving a small section of the shunt in view.	g. Leave a section small enough that it cannot be pulled out by the child. If protective devices to limit movement are indicated, apply below the shunt.
h. Retape shunt clips to outer dressing in full view.	
4. Check frequently for shunt obstruction.	
a. Use stethoscope or place fingertips on area between cannula insertion points to detect bruit.	a. Presence of bruit indicates free flow of blood through shunt.
b. Observe child for signs of pain in the extremity.	
c. Observe color of blood in tubing.	c. Blood should appear smooth and should be of uniform color. Fibrin may appear as white specks along the cannula wall.
d. Report clotting immediately to the physician.	d. Clotting is indicated by separation of blood (i.e., presence of a darkened clot and clear serum). The shunt feels cool rather than warm to the touch. Delay in declotting may necessitate replacement of the entire shunt.

Procedure *(continued)*	**Nursing Action**	**Rationale/Amplification**

	5. Be prepared for emergency action if the shunt should separate or the cannula should become dislodged.
	  a. Identify source of bleeding by unwrapping bandage.
	  b. Separation of shunt:
	    (1) Clamp tubes with shunt clips and rejoin shunt, or
	    (2) Pinch off tubes with fingers and rejoin shunt.
	  c. Dislodgment of arterial or venous cannula:
	    (1) Apply firm pressure over bleeding cannula site and clamp remaining cannula.
	    (2) Notify physician.
	6. Teach the child and parents how to care for the shunt.
	  a. Dressing changes and cleansing of area around shunt.
	  b. Observation for signs of inflammation, infection, obstruction.
	  c. Bathing
	    (1) Some children are permitted to bathe the shunted extremity, soaping the area at the beginning and at the end of the shower or bath.
	    (2) Swimming may be permitted if the extremity is completely protected with a waterproof covering.
	  d. Prevention of clotting
	    (1) Avoid constricting clothing that may impair blood flow through the shunt.
	    (2) Avoid keeping the extremity acutely flexed for long periods of time.
	    (3) Avoid sleeping on the shunted arm.
	  e. Emergency measures in case of accidental separation or dislodging of the cannula.
		5. These are emergency situations that may result in severe hemorrhage and possible exsanguination.
		
		c. These activities are allowed at the discretion of the individual physician.

Chest Physical Therapy and Respiratory Measures

Guidelines Promoting Postural Drainage in the Pediatric Patient

Postural drainage is the positioning of the patient so that gravity will assist in the movement of secretions from the smaller bronchial airways to the main bronchus and trachea, from which the secretions can be removed by coughing or suctioning.

Procedure	**Nursing Action**	**Rationale/Amplification**

	Preparatory Phase
	1. Assess the child's respiratory status.
	  a. Obtain a baseline respiratory rate.
	  b. Observe for respiratory distress, retractions, nasal flaring, etc.
	2. Identify the involved portion(s) of the lung by auscultation, percussion, and/or examination of the x-ray report.
	3. Explain the procedure to the child and/or the parent.
	
	4. Make the child comfortable.
	  a. Remove constricting clothes.
	  b. Flex the child's knees and hips.
	
	  c. Have tissues and an emesis basin available.
	  d. Have several pillows available.
	5. Provide bronchodilator and/or nebulization therapy if indicated.
		1. This is necessary in order to evaluate the effectiveness of the therapy.
		
		2. The positions selected for drainage will depend on what portion of the lung is involved.
		3. This allays anxiety and helps to secure the child's cooperation.
		
		b. To assist in relaxing and decreasing strain on the abdominal muscles during coughing.
		c. To collect mucus.
		d. To facilitate positioning.
		5. It is easier to raise mucus mechanically after the bronchi are dilated and the secretions are thinned.

(continued)

Guidelines Promoting Postural Drainage in the Pediatric Patient *(continued)*

Procedure *(continued)*	**Nursing Action**	**Rationale/Amplification**

Performance Phase

1. Place the child in a series of appropriate positions.
   a. The area to be drained should be elevated and its respective bronchus placed in a vertical position. (Specific drainage positions are described in Table 47-5, below.)
   b. The spine should be as straight as possible to permit optimal expansion of the rib cage.
2. Unless contraindicated, cup the chest wall for 1–2 minutes. (Description of cupping and vibration can be found below.)
3. Have the child inhale deeply; then, as he exhales, vibrate the chest wall during 3–5 exhalations.
4. Encourage the child to cough.
5. Allow the child to rest for a minute, then repeat cupping, vibration, and coughing until no more mucus is produced or the child's condition indicates that the procedure should be stopped.

1. The positions are selected and modified according to the lung area involved, the child's age and general condition, and equipment such as IV, tracheostomies, monitors, ventilators, etc.
   b. Infants are positioned on the nurse's lap, in the Isolette, or in the crib; older children may be treated on a tilt board or in bed.
2. More secretions can be raised in a shorter period of time when cupping and vibration are added to posturing.

4. Infants and young children may require suctioning.
5. Total treatment time should generally not exceed 20–30 minutes.
   a. In acute conditions such as atelectasis, postural drainage may be done for 5 minutes out of every hour.
   b. In chronic conditions such as cystic fibrosis, postural drainage may be done 2–5 times per day for 15–30 minutes.

NURSING ALERT: Postural drainage should not be done immediately after meals since it may induce vomiting.

6. Provide for patient safety.

6. Stay with the child during the procedure, especially when he is in a head-down position.

Table 47-5. *Postural Drainage Positions*

Area of Lung to be Drained	Position	Area of Percussion
Upper lobes, left and right anterior apical segments	Child sitting, leaning slightly backward	Percuss over the top of shoulder and anterior thorax. Hand, in cupped position, should be over the clavicle
Upper lobes, left and right posterior apical segments	Child sitting, leaning slightly forward	Percuss over the upper posterior thorax. Fingers should be contoured over the top of the child's shoulders
Upper lobes, left posterior segment	Child sitting, slightly reclined and rotated to the right. (Infant may be positioned on stomach with left shoulder elevated on therapist's arm.)	Percuss over the left scapula
Upper lobes, right posterior segment	Child lying flat and rotated onto the left side. (Infant may be positioned on stomach with right shoulder elevated on therapist's arm.)	Percuss over the right scapula
Upper lobes, left and right anterior segments	Child lying flat on back	Percuss the anterior chest directly under the clavicles. Avoid direct pressure on the sternum
Upper lobes, lingular segment	Child lying on right side, rotated back one-quarter turn and tilted 30 degrees	Percuss over the left breast
Right middle lobe	Child rotated one-quarter turn from supine position onto the left side and tilted 30 degrees	Percuss over the right breast
Lower lobes, left and right apical segments	Child lying flat in prone position	Percuss below the inferior angle of the scapula
Lower lobes, left and right anterior basal segments	Child lying on back, tilted about 45 degrees	Percuss slightly above the lower ribs
Lower lobe, left lateral basal segment	Child lying on right side, tilted about 45 degrees	Percuss the left lateral thorax at the level of the 8th rib
Lower lobe, right lateral basal segment	Child lying on left side, tilted about 45 degrees	Percuss the right lateral thorax at the level of the 8th rib
Lower lobes, left and right posterior basal segment	Child lying on stomach, tilted about 45 degrees	Percuss just above the 11th and 12th ribs

Procedure
(continued)

Nursing Action	Rationale/Amplification

Follow-Up Phase

1. Assist the child to slowly resume a normal position.

2. Provide oral hygiene.

3. Assess and record the effectiveness of the procedure and how well it was tolerated by the child.

1. It may take a few minutes for the child to regain his equilibrium.

2. This removes residual mucus from the child's mouth and promotes comfort.

Cupping and Vibrating the Pediatric Patient

1. Cupping, or percussion, should be performed with a cupped hand, contoured to the thorax. For infants, it may be more effective to use cupped fingers or a small face mask from a self-inflating bag. (If this method is used, the rim should be filled with air so that it is firm.)
2. Light clothing or a single-thickness diaper may be used between the therapist's hand and the child's chest to minimize discomfort during the procedure.
3. A hollow sound should be produced by the trapped air between the cupped hand and the patient. A slapping sound indicates that the hand is not cupped enough.
4. Cupping should not be performed directly over recent incisions, open wounds, or drainage tubes.
5. Cupping should be discontinued immediately if the percussion site is noted to be reddened.
6. To do vibration, the nurse must first observe the child for exhalation. With the upper arm stiffened, gently shake the child's chest; keep upper arm stiff and extend wrist. The older the child, the more force should be applied.
7. For infants who are breathing rapidly it is usually easier to vibrate with every second or third exhalation rather than with each exhalation. Hand electric vibrators may be easier to use with small infants.
8. For additional information, including the purpose, indications, contraindications, and procedure for administering cupping and vibration, refer to Guidelines: Percussion and Vibration, page 171.

Guidelines Assisting the Patient to Cough

Coughing is the process of expelling air suddenly and noisily from the lungs through the glottis.

Purpose To clear secretions from the airways.

Procedure

Nursing Action	Rationale/Amplification

Preparatory Phase

1. Position the child to help loosen and drain secretions.

2. Administer appropriate medications and allow time for them to take effect.
3. Explain the procedure to the child and/or parents.
4. Position the child for optimal chest expansion.

1. a. Turn from side to side.
   b. Position for postural drainage as indicated (see Table 47-5).
2. Medications may be utilized to loosen secretions or decrease pain awareness.
3. This helps to secure the child's cooperation.
4. The head should be elevated as high as possible.

Performance Phase

1. If the child has had surgery, splint the operative area with a pillow or by placing your hands on either side of the operative site.
2. Have the child take 3 or 4 deep breaths with emphasis on complete exhalation. Have him attempt to cough at the end of a series of deep breaths.
3. Repeat the procedure according to the child's tolerance until the airways are cleared.
4. Additional techniques for stimulating a cough in pediatric patients:
   a. Offer cold fluids or ice chips.
   b. Have the child swallow several times in sequence.
   c. Apply manual pressure by using an up-and-down movement of the finger with firm, steady pressure over the trachea above the manubrial arch.

1. This decreases the pain associated with the procedure by decreasing movement in the area.

2. This helps to stimulate the cough reflex. Full exhalation causes secretions to be moved into the larger airways where mechanical cough receptors are present.
3. Suctioning may be indicated if the child is unable to produce an effective cough.
4. These techniques cause an irritating sensation in the trachea, triggering the cough reflex.

(continued)

Guidelines Assisting the Patient to Cough *(continued)*

Procedure *(continued)*	Nursing Action	Rationale/Amplification
	d. Pass a sterile suction catheter to produce endotracheal stimulation.	d. The catheter is introduced through the child's nose and advances until coughing occurs (refer to the procedure for suctioning, below).
	Follow-Up Phase	
	1. Provide oral hygiene.	1. This removes residual mucus from the child's mouth and promotes comfort.
	2. Assess and record the effectiveness of the cough, the amount and nature of the secretions, and successful techniques for stimulating the child to cough.	
	3. Auscultate the lungs.	3. This helps determine the extent of airway clearing.

Assisting the Pediatric Patient With Breathing Exercises

Nursing Considerations*

1. Breathing exercises must be performed routinely and diligently to be effective. Whenever possible, the same nurse should instruct and work with the child.
2. The respiratory tract should be free of secretions. If indicated, aerosol treatments, postural drainage, coughing, or suctioning should be done prior to deep breathing exercises.
3. The child should be relatively free of pain. If necessary, pain medication should be administered and time allowed for it to take effect before breathing exercises are initiated. Operative incisions should be splinted.
4. The nurse should be relaxed and unhurried. Her tone of voice, approach, and mannerisms affect the child's ability to relax.
5. The child should be positioned to eliminate excessive muscular activity.
   a. Flexion of the hips and knees reduces tension of the abdominal muscles, aiding inspiration.

   b. Supporting the upper extremities on pillows relieves the thorax of this additional weight during inspiration.
   c. The position for breathing exercises depends on the specific pulmonary problem and its severity as well as on the child's age and general condition.
6. Techniques to facilitate diaphragmatic breathing
   a. Have the child place a book on his abdomen.
   b. Instruct him to make the book fall off as he takes air in and makes his abdomen round.
   c. Have him watch his abdomen get flat as he blows all the air out.
   d. The chest should move as little as possible.
7. Techniques to facilitate pursed-lip breathing
   a. Blow cotton balls or ping-pong balls across a bedside table.
   b. Blow bubbles.
   c. Blow a harmonica or party favor.
   d. Blow a pinwheel.
   e. Suspend a ping-pong ball on a string from a doorframe. Have the patient see how long he can keep it propelled away before he needs to inhale. He should attempt to increase his time.
8. Techniques to facilitate deep breathing
   a. Rebreathing tube
   b. Incentive spirometry (see p. 229)
   c. Blowing up balloons or examining gloves
   d. Blowing bubbles

* For additional information, including the purpose of and instruction for diaphragmatic and pursed-lips breathing, refer to pages 172–173.

Guidelines Suctioning

Suctioning is a method for removing excessive secretions from the airway. Suction may be applied to the oral, nasopharyngeal, or tracheal passages.

Purpose To provide a patent airway by keeping it clear of excessive secretions.

Equipment
Suction source
Suction catheter with vent
Connecting tube
Sterile basin (for tracheal and tracheostomy suctioning)
Sterile distilled water
Tissues
Sterile towel
Sterile gloves (for tracheal and tracheostomy suctioning)

Equipment
(continued)

Collection bottle
Manometer to measure amount of vacuum applied
Padded tongue blades, p.r.n.
Goggles

Procedure

Nursing Action	Rationale/Amplification

Oral Suctioning

Preparatory Phase

1. Gather equipment, including extra catheters of the appropriate size. Connect collection bottle and tubing to vacuum source.
2. Establish the need for suctioning by observing respirations and auscultating lungs.

3. Wash hands thoroughly.
4. Turn on suction to check system and regulate pressure if indicated and if equipment makes it possible.

5. Fill basin with sterile distilled water.
6. Position the child on his side, with his head slightly lowered. If necessary, seek an assistant to help maintain the child in this position.
7. Attach catheter to suction tubing; use a glove when handling catheter. Wear goggles or protective eye wear.
8. Place catheter tip in the basin and draw sterile distilled water through it.

1. Since suctioning is often done on an emergency basis, it is mandatory that the nurse keep the necessary equipment at the bedside.
2. The frequency of suctioning will vary with each patient. The need will be evidenced by noisy, moist respirations in a child who is unable to cough adequately.

4. Recommendations for *negative pressure wall suction:*
   Infants   60–100 mm. Hg
   Children   100–120 mm. Hg

6. This position aids in pooling and draining secretions.

7. Wear a glove to keep the catheter and the nurse's hand clean and to protect nurse from secretions.
8. This checks the patency of the system, lubricates catheter, and allows some water in the collection bottle that will prevent aspirated secretions from sticking to it.

Performance Phase

1. Use padded tongue blades to separate upper from lower teeth, if necessary.
2. Leave vent open to air and introduce catheter into the area to be suctioned.

3. Occlude vent with thumb and slowly withdraw catheter while rotating it between the thumb and finger. If catheter "grabs," remove thumb to stop suction.
4. Dip catheter in and out of the basin, drawing sterile distilled water through it to clean it.

5. Repeat steps 1–4 as necessary, suctioning no longer than 10 seconds at a time and allowing 1–3 minutes between suctioning periods (unless abundance of secretions makes this impossible).

1. This prevents the child from biting the catheter.

2. Area may include cheeks, beneath the tongue, and back of mouth. Avoid overstimulation of the gag reflex to prevent vomiting.
3. If catheter is allowed to remain in one place, the mucous membrane will be drawn against it. This will occlude the catheter and injure the tissues.
4. Use 50–100 ml. of water to adequately clean catheter. The bubbles created by the interrupted flow of water through the catheter increase the mechanical cleansing action.
5. Prolonged suctioning can produce laryngospasm, profound bradycardia and/or cardiac arrhythmias from vagal stimulation and loss of oxygen.

Follow-Up Phase

1. Turn off suction source, detach catheter from tubing, and wrap tubing in sterile towel. Discard disposable catheter.

2. Make the child comfortable and give mouth care.
3. Assess effectiveness by observing respirations and auscultating lungs.
4. Record the following:
   a. Amount, color, and consistency of secretions
   b. Coughing
   c. Dyspnea
   d. Cyanosis
   e. Frequency of suctioning
   f. Any bleeding
   g. Response of child to suctioning
5. Empty and rinse collection bottle before it fills completely and at the end of each tour of duty.

1. Preferably, a new catheter is used each time suctioning is required. The connecting tube should be changed at the end of each tour of duty, or more often if necessary.

3. Respirations should be quiet and occur with less effort.

(continued)

Guidelines Suctioning *(continued)*

Procedure
(continued)

Nursing Action	Rationale/Amplification

Nasopharyngeal Suctioning

Preparatory Phase

This is the same as for oral suctioning.
In addition, the nurse should:
    Measure the distance between the tip of the child's nose and the tragus of the ear to determine how far to insert catheter.

The catheter tip will reach the nasopharynx.

Performance Phase

1. Leaving the vent in the catheter open, elevate the tip of the nose, and introduce the catheter along the floor of the nose (with the patient facing straight ahead).
2. If obstruction is encountered, do not force, but remove and insert at another angle or try the other nostril.
3. Follow steps 3–5 of the procedure for oral suctioning. Alternate nostrils when introducing the catheter.

1. This position will facilitate introduction of the catheter.
2. Some resistance should be expected when the catheter reaches the nasopharynx.
3. Alternating nostrils will ensure cleaning of both nasal passages and will minimize trauma to either side

Follow-up Phase

This is the same as for oral suctioning.

Tracheostomy Suctioning

1. See pages 241–243.
2. Additional considerations for the pediatric patient include:
    a. Wall suction should be set at 50–95 mm. Hg for infants or at 90–115 mm. Hg for children.
    b. If sodium chloride solution is used to dilute secretions, the amount should be less (generally 1 ml. for infants and 1–5 ml. for children).
    c. The infant or young child should not be suctioned for more than 5 seconds at a time.
    d. The child's heart rate and color should be monitored throughout the procedure. In the event of irregularity, suctioning should be discontinued and oxygen or assisted ventilation administered.

Nasotracheal Suctioning

Preparatory Phase

1. Follow steps 1–4 of the Guidelines for oral suctioning.
2. Set wall suction at 50–95 mm. Hg for infants and 95–115 mm. Hg for children.
3. Make certain that an oxygen source is available.

4. Using aseptic technique, fill a sterile basin with sterile distilled water.
5. Position the child facing straight ahead with his head slightly tilted back. The infant should be placed in the "sniffing" position with chin up, head tipped slightly backward.
6. Open the package containing the sterile catheter. Wear a sterile glove on the hand that will handle the catheter. Attach the catheter to the suction tubing.
7. Place catheter tip in the basin and draw sterile distilled water through it.

3. This procedure may produce hypoxia and necessitate oxygen therapy.
4. Tracheal suctioning should be done with sterile equipment to minimize the danger of infection.
5. This position facilitates introduction of the catheter.

6. From now until termination of the procedure, this hand should touch only the catheter.

7. This checks the patency of the system, lubricates catheter, and allows some water in the collection bottle that will prevent aspirated secretions from sticking to it.

Performance Phase

1. Leaving the vent in the catheter open, elevate the tip of the nose and introduce the catheter along the floor of the nose (with the patient facing straight ahead).
2. If obstruction is encountered, do not force, but remove and insert at another angle or try the other nostril.
3. Move catheter forward slowly until it enters the trachea— when the following may happen:
    a. Child may cough.
    b. Air will be felt from vent in catheter on expiration.

1. This position will facilitate introduction of the catheter.

2. Some resistance should be expected when the catheter reaches the nasopharynx.

3. Attempt to enter the trachea carefully and on inspiration only. Tracheal tickle may be applied to stimulate coughing and ease the passage of the catheter into the trachea. Gentle pressure at the level of the vocal cords may also be helpful.

Procedure (continued)	**Nursing Action**	**Rationale/Amplification**

c. Voice or cry may change.
d. Child may show marked anxiety.

4. When catheter is in the trachea, occlude vent with the thumb of the ungloved hand and slowly withdraw catheter while rotating it between the thumb and finger.

5. Remove thumb from vent for several seconds between inspirations.

6. Dip catheter in and out of the basin, drawing sterile distilled water through it to clean it.

7. Repeat steps 1–6 as required, suctioning no longer than 5 seconds at one time and allowing 1–3 minutes between suctioning periods (unless the secretions are too abundant).

8. Monitor the child's heart rate and color throughout the procedure.

4. If catheter grabs, remove thumb from vent to stop suction.

5. Suctioning must be stopped at intervals to prevent hypoxia. During normal suction, 4 liters of air will be pulled out of the lungs in 15 seconds. *Never suction for longer than 5 seconds.*

6. Use 50–100 ml. of water to adequately clean catheter. The bubbles created by the interrupted flow of water through the catheter increase the mechanical cleansing action.

7. If child is receiving oxygen, provide oxygen during these rest periods.

8. Discontinue suctioning and administer oxygen or assisted ventilation in the event of any irregularity.

> **NURSING ALERT:** Tracheal suction can result in laryngospasm. This may be recognized as obstructed respiration (rapid and labored with inspiratory stridor) and may rapidly progress to complete apnea. The nurse should call for assistance; she should straighten the airway by hyperextending the patient's neck and pulling his jaw forward and should administer oxygen.

Follow-Up Phase

1. Follow the same procedure as for oral suctioning.
2. Administer oxygen if it is required by the patient's condition.

Guidelines	## Care of a Child With a Tracheostomy

For information concerning purposes for tracheostomy, kinds of tracheostomy tubes, techniques for performing a tracheostomy, and nursing management, refer to the section on tracheostomy in adults, pages 231–243.

Kinds of Tracheostomy Tubes for Pediatric Patients

1. Plastic (polyvinyl chloride or Silastic) tubes, usually without an inner cannula (most common).
2. Silver tubes consisting of 3 parts: obturator, inner cannula, and outer cannula.
3. Cuffs are not generally used for infants and small children since the tracheostomy tube itself is big enough relative to the size of the trachea to act as its own sealer.

Common Reasons for Performing Tracheostomies in Pediatric Patients

1. Laryngotracheal bronchitis
2. Congenital abnormalities such as laryngeal stenosis, choanal atresia, and various anomalies of the heart and lung
3. Foreign bodies lodged in the hypopharynx or larynx
4. Severe chest trauma
5. Burns of the head and neck
6. Laryngeal edema from prolonged intubation
7. Management of secretions and provision of assisted ventilation postoperatively
8. Problems requiring ventilatory support

Nursing Management

	Nursing Action	**Rationale/Amplification**

Physical Care of the Patient

1. Provide adequate humidity, usually via a ventilator, humidifier, or tent.

2. Aspirate secretions (using sterile technique) whenever indicated by noisy respiration, retractions, poor color, or change in vital signs (refer to procedure for aspirating a tracheostomy, pp. 241–243).

3. Suction the child after he has had nebulization therapy, chest therapy, and postural drainage.

1. The natural humidifying pathway of the oropharynx is no longer used. Mist will loosen mucus and secretions and reduce the chances of a mucous plug.

2. It takes a very small amount of secretions to obstruct a small tube.

3. The secretions will be more liquid, more copious, and more easily removed following these procedures.

(continued)

Guidelines Care of a Child With a Tracheostomy *(continued)*

Nursing Management *(continued)*	Nursing Action	Rationale/Amplification
	4. Observe closely for rising pulse rate and restlessness.	4. These are the first clinical signs of respiratory insufficiency and should be followed by careful tracheobronchial toilet.
	5. Monitor respirations frequently and observe for unequal chest expansion.	5. This might indicate the development of a pneumothorax.
	6. Keep the area around the tube clean and dry:	6. To minimize irritation and the risk of infection.
	a. Cleanse area with an applicator dipped in hydrogen peroxide.	
	b. Observe the site for bleeding and irritation.	
	c. Place an unfrayed sterile dressing around the tube and under the tapes that hold the tube in position.	
	7. Observe the child closely to prevent accidental removal of the tube. Arm restraints may be necessary.	7. These are safety precautions.
	a. Have necessary equipment available at the bedside: Duplicate tracheostomy tubes with tapes attached Tracheostomy set for emergency tracheostomy Materials for suctioning and cleansing tubes Materials for cleansing stomal site	
	b. Never immerse the child in a full bath.	b. To prevent fluids from entering the airway.
	8. Make certain that the tapes that hold the tube in place are tied securely with the proper amount of tension.	8. This prevents the tube from slipping out of place as the child becomes distressed or frightened or moves about.
	9. Change ties as needed.	9. The knot should be at the side of the neck to prevent pressure while the child is lying on his back. Old ties should remain in place until the new ties are secured.
	10. If an inner cannula is used it should be removed and cleaned of debris as needed, about every 4 hours.	

Special Considerations for the Infant

	1. Position the infant with his neck extended by placing a small roll under his shoulders.	1. An infant has a tendency to occlude the tube with his chin when his neck is flexed.
	2. Support the infant's head when moving him.	2. Sudden movements of the head and neck can cause the tube to slip out.
	3. When feeding, cover the tracheostomy with a moist piece of gauze. A bib may be used for older infants and young children.	3. This prevents food particles from dropping into the tube.

Psychosocial Care of Patients

	1. Explain, at the level of the child's understanding, the reasons for the tracheostomy and for all procedures and treatments.	1. The child's fantasies about what is happening and why may be more frightening than the truth. He may need reassurance that his voice will return once he is able to breathe normally again.
	2. Allay fears and anxieties of parents by explanations and support.	2. Parental attitudes are conveyed to the child.
	3. Provide some means of communication such as gestures, lip reading, magic slate, pad and pencil. An older child may enjoy alphabet letters or a word board.	3. The child is unable to communicate verbally.
	4. Make sure that a call bell is within easy reach of the child, and answer it promptly.	4. The child is dependent on others to meet even his most basic needs. Prompt attention to his needs will help the child build trust in the nursing personnel.

Nursing Considerations if the Child is Discharged With a Tracheostomy Tube in Place

1. Involve the parents with the child's care as soon as possible. First, explain procedures and their rationale, and have them observe. Gradually turn more of the procedure over to them under nursing supervision.
2. Teach at the parents' level and pace of understanding.
3. Help parents to obtain necessary equipment. Make sure that they have a very specific list of the equipment (and the amounts needed).
4. Be alert to financial difficulties associated with securing equipment or nursing services. Refer to social worker if appropriate.
5. Make certain that parents know what to do and where to go in an emergency.
6. If possible, put parents in contact with other families who have managed children at home with tracheostomies.
7. If appropriate, initiate a community health nursing referral for nursing intervention after discharge.
8. Provide the parents with a written procedure to study and take home.
9. Assist parents to appreciate the normalcy of their child and to recognize his needs for an environment that will support developmental potentials.

Guidelines Oxygen Therapy for Children

For additional information concerning the purpose, general considerations, and procedures for administering oxygen therapy, refer to Oxygen Delivery, pages 210–225.

General Nursing Responsibilities

Nursing Action	Rationale/Amplification
1. Explain the procedure to the child and allow him to feel the equipment and the oxygen flowing through the tube, mask, etc.	1. The child will be reassured if he understands the procedure and knows what to expect.
2. Maintain a clear airway by suctioning, if necessary.	2. The delivery of oxygen requires a clear airway.
3. Provide a source of humidification.	3. Oxygen is a dry gas and requires the addition of moisture to prevent drying of the tracheobronchial tree and thickening and consolidation of secretions.

4. Measure oxygen concentrations every 1–2 hours when a child is receiving oxygen via incubator hood, tent, or Croupette.
  a. Measure when the oxygen environment is closed.
  b. Measure the concentration close to the child's airway.
  c. Record oxygen concentrations and simultaneous measurements of the pulse and respirations.
	4. It is desirable to keep the oxygen concentration as low as possible while still providing for physiologic requirements. This minimizes the danger of the child's developing retrolental fibroplasia or pulmonary oxygen toxicity. (Desired oxygen concentrations are determined by the arterial oxygen tension measurement.) The oxygen analyzer itself should be calibrated daily on both room air and 100% oxygen. The concentration of oxygen within the space is determined by the liter flow, the efficiency of the equipment, and the frequency with which it is opened to the external environment.

5. Observe the child's response to oxygen.	5. Desired response includes:
	  a. Decreased restlessness
	  b. Decreased respiratory distress
	  c. Improved color
	  d. Improved vital sign values

6. Organize nursing care so that interruption of therapy is minimal.	6. Interruption of therapy may result in the return of anoxia and defeat the goals of therapy.
7. Periodically check all equipment during each tour of duty.	7. For optimal functioning, the equipment should be clean, undamaged, and in good working order.
8. Clean equipment daily and change it at least once each week. (Tubing and nebulizer jars should be changed daily.)	8. Unclean equipment may be a source of contamination.

9. Keep combustible materials and potential sources of fire away from oxygen equipment.
  a. Avoid using oil or grease around oxygen connections.
  b. Do not use alcohol or oils on a child in an oxygen tent.
  c. Do not permit any electrical devices in or near an oxygen tent.
  d. Avoid the use of wool blankets and those made from some synthetic fibers because of the hazards resulting from static electricity.
  e. Prohibit smoking in areas where oxygen is being used.
  f. Have a fire extinguisher available.
	9. Oxygen supports combustion.

10. Terminate oxygen therapy gradually.
  a. Slowly reduce liter flow.
  b. Open air vents in incubators.
  c. Open zippers or flip a section of the canopy over the top of the tent.
	10. This allows the child to adjust to normal atmospheric oxygen concentrations.

11. Continually monitor the child's response during weaning. Observe for restlessness, increased pulse rate, respiratory distress, cyanosis.	11. These are indications that the child is unable to tolerate reduced oxygen concentration.

(continued)

Guidelines   Oxygen Therapy for Children *(continued)*

Specific Methods for Administering Oxygen to Pediatric Patients	Nursing Action	Rationale/Amplification
	Oxygen by Nasal Cannula or Catheter	
	1. Refer to Guidelines: Administering Oxygen by Nasal Cannula or Catheter, pages 212 and 214.	
	Oxygen by Mask	
	1. Choose an appropriate size mask that covers the mouth and nose but not the eyes.	1. Extra space under the mask and around the face is added dead space and decreases the effectiveness of the therapy.
	2. Use a mask that is capable of delivering the desired oxygen concentration.	2. Venturi masks, available for use in pediatrics, deliver low to moderate concentrations of oxygen: 24%, 28%, 35%, or 40%.
	3. Place the mask over the child's mouth and nose so that it fits securely. Secure the mask with an elastic head grip.	3. Make sure that the mask is adjusted properly over the mouth and nose. Do not allow the oxygen to blow in child's eyes. Small pieces of cotton may be placed above the ears to help relieve pressure and discomfort caused by the head strap.
	4. Remove the oxygen mask at hourly intervals; wash the face and dry.	4. Makes the patient feel more comfortable.
	5. Do not use masks for comatose infants or children.	5. Such children are more likely to vomit. The risk of aspiration may be increased with mask therapy because of obstruction of the flow of vomitus.
	6. For additional information, refer to Guidelines: Administering Oxygen by Venturi Mask (p. 215) and by Face Mask (p. 217).	
	Face Tent	
	1. Face tents are available in the adult size only. They can be used effectively in pediatric patients if inverted to create a smaller reservoir and better fit.	1. Face tents combine the positive qualities of aerosol masks and mist tents. The child is accessible and may continue to play without feeling confined.
	2. A flow of 8–10 liters should be used to flush the system and provide a stable oxygen concentration.	2. Larger children will require higher flows.
	T-Bars and Tracheostomy Masks	
	1. These devices are used to deliver oxygen to intubated patients.	
	2. The flow rate must be set to meet the minute volume requirements of the child and to provide a 100% source of gas.	2. T-bars require a short, flexible tube on the distal end to act as a reservoir and prevent room-air entrapment.
	Oxygen Tent	
	1. Select the smallest tent and canopy that will achieve the desired concentration of oxygen and maintain patient comfort.	1. This increases the efficiency of the unit.
	2. Pad the metal frame that supports the canopy.	2. This protects the child from injury.
	3. Analyze and record the tent atmosphere every 1–2 hours. Concentrations of 30%–50% can be achieved in well-maintained tents.	3. The concentration varies with the efficiency of the tent, the rate of flow of oxygen, and the frequency with which the tent is opened to the outside environment.
	4. Maintain a tight-fitting canopy. Whenever possible, provide nursing care through the sleeves or pockets of the tent.	4. This prevents oxygen leakage and disruption of the tent atmosphere. a. If the child is extremely restless or uncooperative, it may be useful to permit a parent to hold the child's hand through a small opening in the zipper of the canopy.
	5. Make certain that the crib sides are up.	5. The canopy, when tucked into the mattress, often gives the illusion of a safe, confined environment.
	6. Select toys that retard absorption, are washable, and will not produce static electricity.	6. The child needs toys for stimulation and diversion. They should be safe and practical.
	Croupette	
	1. This is an oxygen tent equipped with a high-humidification system (refer to procedure under "Oxygen Tent" above).	1. If the child's condition requires high humidity but not oxygen, the unit can be operated with compressed air.
	2. Change the child's clothing and bed linen when damp. Cover the child with a cotton blanket.	2. This prevents chilling in an environment of cooled, supersaturated, aerated mist.
	3. Check the child frequently.	3. Condensation on the canopy may make it difficult to see the child.
	4. If possible, remove the child from the mist periodically.	4. This prevents maceration of the skin. Mist may be delivered via nebulizer tubing or mask during these periods.

Nursing Action	Rationale/Amplification
5. Promote postural drainage and suction the child as necessary.	5. Rapid mobilization of secretions may follow initiation of mist tent therapy.
6. Observe the small infant for signs of overhydration.	6. This occasionally results from intensive use of an ultrasonic nebulizer especially if a saline solution is nebulized.

Closed Incubators/Isolettes

Nursing Action	Rationale/Amplification
1. The incubator is used to provide a controlled environment for the neonate.	1. The unit is able to provide precise environmental control of temperature, oxygen, humidity, and isolation.
2. Adjust the oxygen flow to achieve the desired oxygen concentration.	2. Refer to Table 47-6, below.
a. An oxygen limiter prevents the oxygen concentration inside the incubator from exceeding 40%.	a. This is desirable because it reduces the hazard of the child's developing retrolental fibroplasia.
b. Higher concentrations (up to 85%) may be obtained by placing the red reminder flag in the vertical position.	b. This operates by reducing the air intake.

Table 47-6. *Incubator Oxygen Therapy*

Red Flag in Horizontal Position		Red Flag in Vertical Position	
Flow of Oxygen (L/minute)	*Concentration of Oxygen (%)*	*Flow of Oxygen (L/minute)*	*Concentration of Oxygen (%)*
4	28–31	4	Flow not sufficient for high concentration
6	32–36	8	70–75
8	37–40	10	75–80
		12	80–85

From Lough MD and Doershuk CF. Oxygen therapy. In Lough MD, Doershuk CF and Stern RC. Pediatric Respiratory Therapy. Chicago, Year Book Medical Pub. Used with Permission.

Nursing Action	Rationale/Amplification
3. Secure a nebulizer to the inside wall of the incubator if mist therapy is desired.	3. This should be cleaned and autoclaved daily. Sterile solutions are used to keep the bacteria count at a minimum.
4. Keep sleeves of incubator closed to prevent loss of oxygen	4. When incubator or sleeves are opened, supply supplemental oxygen with oxygen mask to face and nose.
5. Periodically analyze the incubator atmosphere.	5. To be certain that the child is receiving the desired concentration of oxygen.

Oxygen Hood

Nursing Action	Rationale/Amplification
1. Warmed, humidified oxygen is supplied via a plastic container that fits over the child's head (Fig. 47-8).	1. This is especially useful when high concentrations of oxygen are desired. The hood may be used in an incubator or with a warming unit. Oxygen should not be allowed to blow directly into the infant's face.

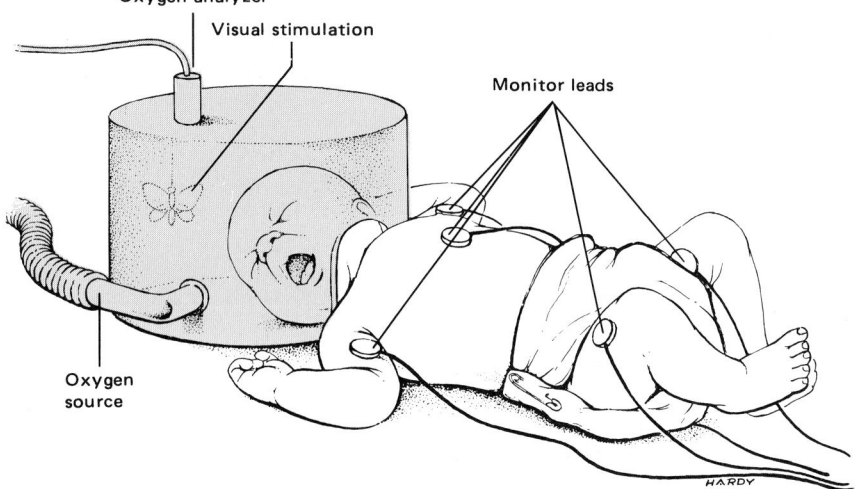

Figure 47-8. *Oxygen hood.*

(continued)

Guidelines Oxygen Therapy for Children *(continued)*

Nursing Action	Rationale/Amplification
2. Continuously monitor the oxygen concentration, temperature, and humidity inside the hood.	2. Oxygen should be warmed to 31°–34°C. (87.8°–93.2°F.) to prevent a neonatal response to cold stress—including oxygen deprivation, metabolic acidosis, rapid depletion of glycogen stores, and reduction of blood glucose levels.
3. Open the hood or remove the baby from it as infrequently as possible.	3. This prevents fluctuations of heat and oxygen, which may further debilitate the young infant.
4. Several different designs are available for use. The manufacturer's directions should be carefully followed.	4. This is a safety consideration.

Nursing Care of the Child Requiring Mechanical Ventilation

Characteristics of the Ventilator

Available ventilators have a wide range of capabilities, versatility, and clinical application. Some are more suitable for use with infants, others with children. It is wise for the nurse to be well-acquainted with the characteristics of the machine that is being used and to be able to answer the following questions.

A. Rate Control
1. How is the rate controlled?
2. Can the patient initiate the cycle (assisted ventilation)?
3. What is the response time (time elapsed between the initiation of respiration and response of the ventilator)? This must be rapid in infants.
4. Is there a sensitivity control that allows the machine to be more or less sensitive to the patient's efforts to initiate respiration?
5. Is an IMV (intermittent mandatory ventilation) feature present? This allows the patient to breathe on his own and, at certain intervals, a mandatory inspiration is provided by the ventilator.

B. Volume Control
1. How is the volume controlled?
   a. Automatically preset
   b. Variable, with a preset pressure
2. What is the range of inspiratory flow rate capability? A very low flow rate is required by neonates; the rate will increase with the size of the child.

C. Cycling
1. What controls the cycle of the machine?
   a. Time cycle—inspiration is terminated at the end of a preset period that is controlled by a timing device. The volume delivered is usually a function of flow per unit of time.
   b. Volume cycle—the inspiratory phase is terminated after the predetermined volume of gas has been delivered. The pressure generated is dependent on the characteristics of the lung.
   c. Pressure cycle—the inspiratory phase ceases when a preset pressure is achieved. The volume of gas delivered and the time required to achieve the preset pressure are dependent on the characteristics of the lungs.

d. Mixed cycle—many ventilators have two or more cycling modes.

D. Humidification
1. How is moisture added to the inspired air?
   a. Humidification
   b. Nebulization
2. Is there a means of controlling the temperature of the inspired air?
   Many models provide an adjustable thermostat on the humidifier controls.

E. Oxygen Control
1. What is the oxygen source?
2. How is the oxygen concentration controlled?

F. Pressure Control
1. How is the pressure controlled?
   a. Automatically preset
   b. Variable, with a preset volume
2. What do the pressure gauges indicate and how are they read?
   a. Airway pressure indicator
   b. Machine pressure indicator
3. What is the peak effective pressure capability?

G. Ratio of Inspiration to Expiration (I/E Ratio)
1. Is this variable?
2. How is it controlled?

H. PEEP (Positive End-Expiratory Pressure)
Does the ventilator have this feature? How is it controlled?
1. PEEP refers to positive airway at end expiration.
2. This helps minimize alveolar volume loss during expiratory pauses and thus decreases the tendency toward atelectasis.

I. CPAP (continuous positive airway pressure)
Does the ventilator have this feature? How is it controlled?
Refer to pages 1198–1200.

J. Sigh
Does the ventilator have this feature? How is it regulated?
1. Works by adding additional volume to the established tidal volume.
2. Has the effect of taking a deep breath and may expand alveoli, which tend to be collapsed at low volume ventilation.

K. Alarm Systems
What are the alarm systems to warn of possible problems?
1. Low pressure or disconnect alarm system.

2. High pressure alarm system to indicate rising pressures within the lung.
3. Electrical failure alarm system.
4. Volume and rate monitor
   a. Acceptable low and high rates and tidal volumes are set for the alarm.
   b. If either rate or tidal volume are outside acceptable parameters, an alarm sounds.

Nursing Management

Refer to Guidelines for Managing the Patient Requiring Mechanical Ventilation, pages 248–251. In addition, the following considerations should be kept in mind by the nurse who is caring for a pediatric patient.

A. Setting Controls

In setting controls, inspiratory flow rate will be less, and the respiratory rate will be greater than in the adult patient. These depend on the patient's size and condition and are determined by the physician and/or respiratory therapist.

B. Humidification

1. Because of their small diameters, pediatric endotracheal tubes easily become obstructed by thickened secretions. Therefore, adequate humidification must be maintained to keep secretions loose.
2. During ventilation of an infant in an incubator, the amount of ventilator tubing outside the incubator should be kept to a minimum. The warm temperature inside the incubator helps decrease the amount of condensation in the tubing and thus provides higher water content in the inspired gas.

C. Oxygen Concentration

1. Inspired concentrations of oxygen should always be kept as low as possible (while still providing for physiologic requirements), to prevent the development of retrolental fibroplasia or pulmonary O_2 toxicity.
2. The oxygen concentration should be checked periodically with an analyzer.

D. Blood Gases

1. The arterialized capillary sample method is inaccurate for infants in respiratory distress because the constricted peripheral circulation may not reflect the arterial blood gases accurately.
2. An umbilical artery catheter is most frequently used to obtain arterial blood samples.

E. Sterile Precautions

The newborn has only those antibodies transferred across the placenta from the mother. Therefore, sterile precautions are essential.
1. Ventilator tubing should be changed every 24 hours.
2. Routine cultures should be taken after intubation; there should be daily gram-staining of secretions.
3. Suctioning requires aseptic technique.

F. Tubing Support

1. Special frames are available to support ventilator tubing; this helps to prevent accidental decannulation in infants and small children.
2. Infants may require folded diapers or padding on either side and at the top of their heads to decrease mobility and take up space between the head and the frame.

G. Monitoring the Ventilator

1. Pressure gauges should be checked at frequent intervals since this gives an indication of changing compliance or increased airway resistance.
2. Volume measurements are difficult to obtain in infants since most spirometers incorporated into ventilators and meters (such as the Wright respirometer) do not read accurately at low volumes and flows. However, they are helpful with older children.
3. Measure respiratory rates of the machine and the patient at least every hour.

Weaning the Pediatric Patient From the Ventilator

A. Method 1—Permits the patient to breathe spontaneously for short periods of time:

1. Often used when ventilation has been solely for apnea.
2. The length of time without ventilator assistance is gradually increased, while observing that the infant does not become fatigued.
3. This method is often facilitated by applying continuous positive pressure to the airway when the infant is off the ventilator.
4. The CPAP (continuous positive airway pressure) can then be gradually decreased until the infant can breathe without assistance (see pp. 1198–1200).
5. A T-piece is generally attached to the child's artificial airway during this process to provide oxygen enrichment and humidification.

B. Method 2—Switches from the "control" to the "assist" mode to permit the child to trigger respiration by his own effort.

1. This method is preferred for children with lung disease.
2. The ventilator is switched to the "assist" mode.
3. The trigger sensitivity is gradually decreased as the patient is encouraged to provide greater effort until he is able to ventilate adequately without the assistance of the machine.
4. The patient is then taken off the ventilator for progressively longer periods until use of the ventilator can be discontinued completely.
5. CPAP can be used with this method during the periods that the patient is off the ventilator.

C. Nursing Management

1. Weaning children from a ventilator is frequently a long and tedious process. The child and/or his parents may need a lot of support and encouragement.
2. Frequent blood gas determinations are necessary to determine if the child is maintaining adequate oxygenation.
3. The child should be observed closely for signs of respiratory difficulty including fatigue, nasal flaring, increased pulse rate, sweating, facial pallor and cyanosis, and rising blood pressure.
4. A calm atmosphere should be maintained.
5. Whenever possible, the ventilator should remain at the bedside until the child is satisfied that he can breathe without it.

Guidelines CPAP (Continuous Positive Airway Pressure)

CPAP is a system of applying a constant distending or gas pressure that is greater than atmospheric pressure to the airway during spontaneous breathing. This system is also referred to as CPPB (continuous positive pressure breathing).

Purposes
1. To prevent alveolar collapse during expiration by keeping the alveoli open with pressure while avoiding overdistending already-expanded alveoli.
2. To prevent intrapulmonary right-to-left shunting.
3. To increase the oxygenation of the lungs, which in turn decreases potential for hypoxia, bradycardia, or apnea.
4. To decrease the work of breathing on the part of the infant.
5. To increase FRC (functional residual capacity).

Procedure

Nursing Action	Rationale/Amplification
Preparatory Phase	

1. The CPAP system is generally set up by the physician and/or respiratory therapist. The accepted early criteria for initiating CPAP are:
  a. Infant breathing spontaneously
  b. PaO_2 (arterial O_2 tension) < 60 mm. Hg (breathing) in 60%–65% oxygen less than 24 hours of age
  c. F_iO_2 (inspired oxygen) > 80% at any time
	1. The nurse must be in attendance to monitor the infant during application and must know and understand the workings of the CPAP system.

Endotracheal Tube	
1. Lubricate endotracheal tube with hydrocortisone cream prior to insertion. 2. Set up sterile suction equipment.	
Performance Phase	

1. The infant's status can change quickly. Carefully observe the condition of infant:
  a. Skin color–cyanotic, dusky, or too pink.
	1. CPAP can cause overdistention of lung alveoli leading to complications.
	  a. Changes may be signs of pneumothorax, reduced cardiac output, low PaO_2, too much O_2 administration, infant too hot or cold.

b. Respiratory pattern—rate, retractions, grunting, apnea, decreased breath sounds.	b. Change in respirations may indicate that the patient is not tolerating CPAP or that pneumothorax has occurred.
c. Cardiac pattern—rate, especially bradycardia, blood pressure, femoral pulses.	c. Hypocalcemia, hypoglycemia, or opening of ductus arteriosus should be suspected when changes occur.
d. Activity—sudden increase or decrease in movement.	d. Check for hypocalcemia, hypoglycemia, respiratory obstruction.
2. Observe closely for problems or malfunctions connected with CPAP system. a. Check inspired O_2 levels being delivered to the infant.	a. O_2 needs are determined by the PaO_2 values and the infant's condition. Allowing elevated levels is detrimental to the infant.
b. Blood gases are checked frequently and always 20 minutes after any change is made in the system. O_2 changes are usually made in 5% increments unless the PaO_2 is >100 mg./dl.	
c. Pressure levels should be maintained as prescribed. Check all lines and connections.	c. Any change in the pressure should be observed immediately and the cause determined. Increase in pressure indicates an obstruction in the baby or in the system tubing. Decrease in pressure indicates a leak in the system. CPAP levels are usually increased or decreased by 1–2-cm. H_2O increments.

d. Maintain O_2 humidification and temperature.	d. The air O_2 mixture must be properly humidified for the following reasons:
	    (1) To prevent drying of mucous membranes and thick secretions caused by too little moisture.
	    (2) Possible aspiration or water intoxication can occur from a collection of droplets accumulating on walls of tubing and flowing to infant.
	  Proper humidification is present when the tubing is evenly fogged with a fine mist.

Procedure (continued)	**Nursing Action**	**Rationale/Amplification**

NURSING ALERT: Improper temperature of the air–oxygen mixture can lead to hypothermia or hyperthermia and can increase oxygen consumption, resulting in acidosis and apnea. Proper temperature is just below body temperature and is not warm or cold when passing over one's skin.

3. Observe for signs of complications inherent with a premature infant (see p. 1221), respiratory distress syndrome (see p. 1284), and ventilation
   a. Spontaneous tension pneumothorax

   b. Metabolic acidosis

   c. Hyperbilirubinemia
   d. Infection, systemic

   e. Cardiac output reduction

   f. Hypocalcemia (blood calcium < 8 mg./100 ml.)
      Hypoglycemia (blood sugar < 20 mg./100 ml.)
   g. Hypovolemia
      (1) Accurate records should be kept of blood removed.
      (2) Monitor blood pressure.
   h. Abdominal distention—caused by inflation of air.

      (1) To decompress stomach use an NG (nasogastric) tube or aspirate air prior to NG (gavage) feedings.
      (2) Elevate the infant's head if possible during feeding and attempt to burp him.
      (3) NG tube may be kept in place and connected to elevated open reservoir between feedings to serve as overflow safety valve.
4. Additional nursing care responsibilities to consider when caring for infant being treated with CPAP:
   a. Provide and maintain thermal stability of infant (p. 1223).
   b. Provide adequate fluid and caloric intake to meet the infant's needs via intravenous fluids and/or nasojejunal (N-J), gavage, or other methods.
   c. Administer proper and adequate physical therapy to infant to help reduce the potential for pneumonia.

   d. Mechanical ventilation with anesthesia bag may be administered at specific times.
   e. Assist in obtaining blood gases at appropriate times.
      (1) Observe the infant for signs that would indicate need for special blood gas studies (also done after CPAP settings are changed and to monitor the infant's progress and condition).
      (2) When drawing blood, use a needle and syringe that have been rinsed with heparin. Avoid too much heparin since it will alter pH value. Store blood sample on ice while transporting to laboratory. Know normal blood gas values as well as the patient's "normal" values.
   f. Avoid irritation and drying of mouth and nares. The mouth should be cleansed frequently with lemon-glycerin or normal saline swabs.

a. Presenting signs include decreased chest movements and breath sounds on affected side, tachypnea, cyanosis, bradycardia, inspiratory pressure elevated on manometer, decrease in systolic blood pressure.
b. The blood pH is less than 7.3. This occurs because of tissue hypoxia and anaerobic metabolism.
c. See page 1244.
d. Temperature instability may be first indication of infection. Apnea, irritability, vomiting, diarrhea, change in status should be reported immediately.
e. Results from CPAP set at too-high levels for improving compliance of lungs. CPAP is transmitted through the lungs to the large vessels of mediastinum. The increasing pressure may cause the vessels to partially collapse, affecting the return of blood to the heart; this causes a decrease in cardiac output.
f. Symptoms are nonspecific: jitteriness, sweating, tachypnea or apnea, lethargy, convulsions, cyanosis.
g. This occurs from placenta previa or abruptio placentae, loss of blood into the placenta due to rapid clamping, or iatrogenically from too much sampling without replacement.
h. Most common when using nasal, mask, or hood CPAP. Abdominal distention and increasing gastric residuals may be first sign of necrotizing enterocolitis.

c. Physical therapy includes percussion or vibrating, postural drainage, suctioning, and position change. This prevents airway obstruction as a result of the presence of mucus anywhere along the respiratory tract.
d. To help decrease PCO_2, assist a tiring infant, increase O_2 levels prior to any CPAP change or suctioning.
e. Blood gases are always taken 20–30 minutes after CPAP settings are changed—this allows infant to stabilize with new settings. Arterial capillary blood is obtained from warmed heel blood. Arterial blood is drawn from umbilical artery indwelling catheter, radial or temporal artery puncture.

f. Prevents crust formation, which can lead to breakdown, by using an antibiotic ointment.

(continued)

Guidelines   CPAP (Continuous Positive Airway Pressure) *(continued)*

Procedure *(continued)*	**Nursing Action**	**Rationale/Amplification**
	g. Keep skin clean and dry. Massage reddened areas gently. Change position every 1–2 hours. Avoid using large quantities of tape.	g. Give good skin care to prevent breakdown and eventual ulceration and infection.
	h. Provide the infant with pleasant stimulation and love.	h. Colorful objects or pictures can be placed around the infant. Small musical toys and a pleasant, soothing voice combined with gentle touching can provide the necessary stimulation.

Follow-Up Phase

1. When the infant can maintain adequate arterial oxygenation with CPAP at 1–2 cm. H_2O for 2–4 hours, he is ready to come off CPAP.
2. Once CPAP is discontinued, the infant is placed in an environment that provides 10%–20% more oxygen than he was breathing while on CPAP. Blood gases are checked as O_2 concentration is decreased as tolerated (see Respiratory Distress Syndrome [RDS], p. 1284, for further in-depth discussion).

Cardiac and Respiratory Monitoring

Cardiac and respiratory monitoring refers to electrical surveillance of heart and respiratory rates and patterns. It is indicated in all patients whose conditions are unstable or potentially unstable.

Nursing Management

1. Select a monitor that is appropriate for the child's needs. This will depend on the child's age, ability to cooperate, purpose for monitoring, information desired, and equipment available.
2. Stabilize the device to reduce the amount of mechanical noise and for safety considerations.
3. Reduce the child's anxiety:
   a. Provide age-appropriate explanations of the equipment.
   b. When possible, involve the child in his own care, including change of electrodes.
4. Select lead placement sites according to equipment specifications:
   a. Cardiac monitors frequently employ three leads located at:
      (1) Right upper lateral chest wall below clavicle
      (2) Left lower chest wall in the anterior axillary line
      (3) Upper left chest wall
   b. Respiratory monitors frequently employ three electrodes located:
      (1) On either side of the chest (anterior axillary line in fourth or fifth intercostal space)
      (2) At a reference electrode placed on the manubrium or other suitable distal point
5. Apply electrodes by:
   a. Cleaning the appropriate areas on the chest with alcohol
   b. Placing a small amount of conductive gel at each area of contact unless pre-gelled, disposable electrodes are used
   c. Applying the electrode firmly to completely dry skin
6. Plug the leads into the lead cable at appropriate insertion points.
7. Be certain that the monitor alarms are in the "on" position. High and low alarm limits should be set according to the child's age and condition so that apnea, tachypnea, bradycardia, and tachycardia can be readily detected.
8. Avoid skin breakdown by changing lead placement sites as needed. Clean and dry old sites and expose them to the air.
9. Check integrity of the entire system at least once each tour of duty.
   a. Carefully inspect lead wires and cable for breaks and proper attachment.
   b. If malfunction is suspected, change equipment and notify the engineering department immediately.
10. Continue to count respiratory and apical rates at frequent intervals.
    a. Compare with monitor rates to verify accuracy of equipment.
    b. It must be remembered that monitors cannot substitute for close observation of the child.
11. Apnea mattresses or pads that employ sensing devices may be used for infants, eliminating the need for electrodes.
    a. Although less susceptible to cardiovascular artifact, these devices may record physical impact, vibrations, or body movements as breaths.
    b. In addition, older infants can easily roll or crawl off the pad.

Cardiopulmonary Resuscitation

Cardiopulmonary resuscitation involves measures instituted to provide effective ventilation and circulation when the patient's respiration and heart have ceased to function.

Underlying Considerations

A. Cardiac Arrest

1. Signs—absence of heartbeat and absence of carotid and femoral pulses.
2. Causes—asystole, ventricular fibrillation, or cardiovascular collapse related to arterial hypotension.

B. Respiratory Arrest

1. Signs—apnea and cyanosis
2. Causes—obstructed airway, depression of the central nervous system, neuromuscular paralysis

C. Emergency Preparation

1. Every hospital should have a well-defined and organized plan to be carried out in the event of cardiac or respiratory arrest.
2. Emergency carts should be placed in strategic locations in the hospital and checked daily to ensure that all equipment is available.

Equipment

Emergency cart—assembled and ready for use:
    Positive pressure breathing bag with nonrebreathing valve and universal 15-mm. adapter
    Masks (premature infant, infant, child, adult sizes)
    Oropharyngeal airways, sizes No. 0 to No. 4
    Laryngoscope with blades of various sizes
    Extra batteries and light bulbs for laryngoscope
    Endotracheal tubes with connectors (complete sterile set, 2.5–8.0 mm. I.D.)
    Portable suction equipment and sterile catheters of various sizes
    Bulb syringe, DeLee trap
    Oxygen source—portable supply gauge and tubing, masks of various sizes
    Cardiac board (30 by 50 cm.)
    Emergency drugs

Sodium bicarbonate	Calcium chloride 10%
Epinephrine	Dextrose 50%
Isoproterenol	Lidocaine (Xylocaine)
Dextrose	Atropine
Saline solution (for dilution)	Phenytoin sodium (Dilantin)
Diphenhydramine hydrochloride (Benadryl)	Insulin
	Procainamide (Pronestyl)
Diazepam (Valium)	Propranolol (Inderal)
Hydrocortisone sodium succinate	Dopamine
Digoxin	
Naloxone (Narcan)	
Calcium gluconate	

Intracardiac needles, No. 20 and 22 gauge, 6–8 cm. (2⅜–3⅛ inches long)
IV equipment

Fluids	Longdwell catheters of various sizes
Infusion set	
Tourniquet	3-way stopcock
Armboards	Cutdown set
Tape	Pole
Scalp-vein needles of various sizes	Labels

Nasogastric tubes of various sizes
Other equipment
    Syringes of various sizes
    Needles of various sizes

Alcohol wipes
Tongue blades
Sterile 4×4 gauze sponges
Sterile hemostat
Sterile scissors
Blood specimen tubes
Electrocardiograph and monitor
Lubricating jelly
Defibrillator and paddles (pediatric and adult)

Artificial Ventilation

Technique for Artificial Ventilation

A. Mouth to Mouth

1. *Infants*
   a. Slightly extend neck by gently pulling chin up and forward and the head back. Place a rolled towel or diaper under the infant's shoulders, or use one hand to support the neck in an extended position. Do not hyperextend the neck since this narrows the airway.
   b. Check the mouth and throat and clear mucus or vomitus with finger or suction, if necessary.
   c. Take a breath.
   d. Make a tight seal with your mouth over the infant's mouth and nose.
   e. Gently blow air from the cheeks and observe for chest expansion.
   f. Remove your mouth from infant's mouth and nose and allow the infant to exhale.
   g. If spontaneous respirations do not return, continue breathing at a rate and volume appropriate for the size of the infant (usually 20 times per minute or 1 breath every 3 seconds).

2. *Older children and adolescents*
   a. Clear mouth of mucus or vomitus with finger or suction.
   b. Hyperextend neck with one hand or a rolled towel.
   c. Clamp the nostrils with the fingers of one hand, which also continues to exert pressure on the forehead to maintain the neck extension.
   d. Take a deep breath.
   e. Make a tight seal with your mouth over the child's mouth.
   f. Force air into the lungs until chest expansion is observed.
   g. Release your mouth from the child's mouth and release nostrils to allow the child to exhale passively.
   h. Repeat approximately 12–15 times/minute or 1 breath every 4–5 seconds.

B. Hand-Operated Ventilation Devices

1. Remove secretions from mouth and throat and move mandible forward.
2. Appropriately extend the neck with one hand or place a diaper roll behind the neck.
3. Select an appropriate size mask to obtain an adequate seal, and connect mask to the bag.
4. Hold the mask snugly over the mouth and nose, holding the chin forward and the neck in extension.
5. Squeeze the bag, noting inflation of the lungs by chest expansion.
6. Release the bag, which will expand spontaneously. The child will exhale and the chest will fall.

7. Repeat 12–20 times per minute (depending on size of the child).
8. Since this technique is often difficult to master, it should be practiced in advance, under supervision.

Indications of Effective Technique

1. Victim's chest rises and falls.
2. Rescuer can feel in his own airway the resistance and compliance of the victim's lungs as they expand.
3. Rescuer can hear and feel the air escape during exhalation.
4. Victim's color improves.

Management of Complications

1. Gastric distention (occurs frequently if excessive pressures are used for inflation)
   a. Turn victim's head and shoulders to one side.
   b. Exert moderate pressure over the epigastrium between the umbilicus and the rib cage.
   c. A nasogastric tube may be used to decompress the stomach.

2. Vomiting
   a. Turn patient on side for drainage.
   b. Clear the airway with fingers or suction.
   c. Resume ventilations.

Artificial Circulation

General Principles Related to Artificial Circulation

See Table 47-7 and Fig. 47-9.
1. A backward tilt of the head lifts the back in infants and small children. A firm support beneath the back is therefore essential if external cardiac compression is to be effective.
2. A supine position on a firm surface is mandatory. Only in this position can chest compression squeeze the heart against the immobile spine enough to force blood into the systemic circulation.
3. External cardiac compression must always be accom-

Table 47-7. *Technique of Artificial Circulation*

Size of Child	Preparatory Phase	Action Phase	Distance of Compression	Rate
Neonate, premature, or small infant	1. Place in supine position 2. Encircle the chest with the hands, with thumbs over the midsternum *or* Use method for a larger infant, at a rate of 100–120/min.	1. Compress midsternum with both thumbs, gently but firmly	2/3 distance to the spine or 1.3–1.8 cm. (½–¾ inch)	100–120/minute
Larger infant	1. Place on a firm, flat surface 2. Support the back with one hand or use a small blanket under the shoulders 3. Place the tips of the index and middle fingers of one hand over the midsternum	Compress the midsternum with the tips of the index and middle fingers	1.3–2.5 cm. (½–1 inch)	>100/minute
Small child	1. Place on a firm, flat surface 2. Support the back by slipping one hand beneath it, or use a small blanket 3. Place the heel of one hand over the midsternum, parallel with the long axis of the body	1. Apply a rapid downward thrust to the midsternum, keeping the elbow straight 2. Hold for approximately 0.4 second 3. Instantly and completely release the pressure so the chest wall can recoil 4. Do not remove the heel of the hand from the chest	2.5–3.8 cm. (1–1½ inches)	80–100/minute
Larger child, adolescent	1. Place on a flat, firm surface or place a board under the thorax 2. Place the heel of one hand on the lower half of the sternum, about 2.5–3.8 cm. (1–1½ inches) from the tip of the xiphoid process and parallel with the long axis of the body 3. Place the other hand on top of the first one (may interlock fingers) 4. Place shoulders directly over child's sternum, in order to use own weight in application of pressure	1. Exert pressure vertically downward to depress lower sternum, keeping elbows straight 2. Hold for approximately 0.4 second 3. Instantly and completely release the pressure so the chest wall can recoil 4. Do not remove the hands from the chest	3.8–5 cm. (1½–2 inches)	80–100/minute

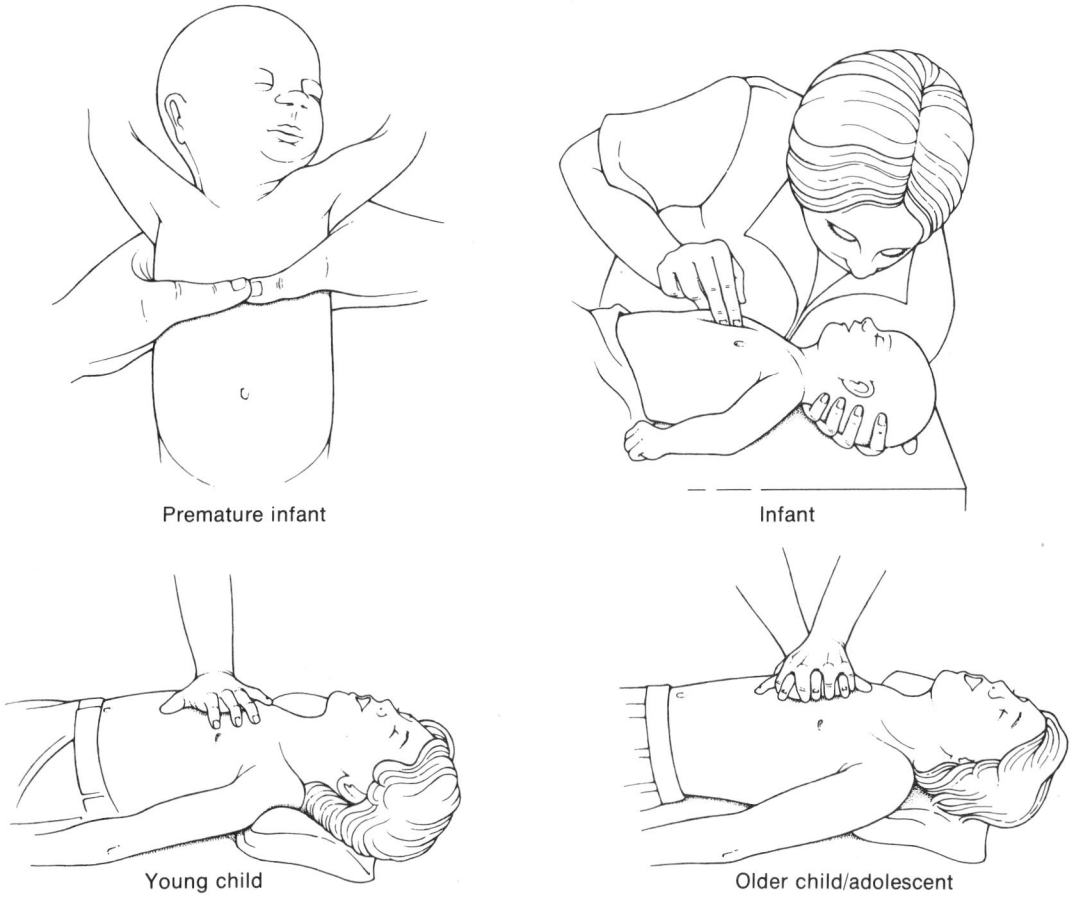

Premature infant

Infant

Young child

Older child/adolescent

Figure 47-9. *Cardiopulmonary resuscitation in children. In the young child, the heel of the hand is placed over the lower sternum. In older children and adolescents, both hands are used.*

panied by artificial ventilation for adequate oxygenation of the blood.
4. Compressions must be regular, smooth, and uninterrupted. Avoid sudden or jerking movements.
5. Relaxation must immediately follow compression; relaxation and compression must be of equal duration.
6. Between compressions, the fingers or heel of the hand must completely release their pressure but should remain in constant contact with the chest.
7. Fingers should not rest on the patient's ribs during compression. Pressure with fingers on the ribs or lateral pressure increases the possibility of fractured ribs and costochondral separation.
8. Never compress the xiphoid process at the tip of the sternum. Pressure on it may cause laceration of the liver.
9. Indications of effective technique include:
    a. A palpable femoral or carotid pulse
    b. Decrease in size of pupils
    c. Improvement in the patient's color

Nursing Management in Cardiopulmonary Resuscitation

1. Recognize cardiac and/or respiratory arrest.
2. Send for assistance and note time.
3. If alone:

a. First ventilate the child's lungs rapidly 4 times, using appropriate technique (p. 1201), then palpate the carotid or brachial pulse. If a pulse is palpated, continue ventilatory support.
    b. If no pulse is felt, institute artificial circulation using appropriate technique (p. 1202).
    c. For an infant or child, interpose 1 breath after each series of 5 compressions. For an adolescent, interpose 2 breaths after each series of 15 compressions.
    d. Continue repeating this cycle until help arrives.
4. When help arrives:
    a. One rescuer performs mouth-to-mouth resuscitation or institutes bag breathing.
    b. Another rescuer performs cardiac compressions.
    c. A ratio of 5 compressions to 1 breath is maintained for both infants and children.
    d. Cardiac compression should not be stopped for respiration. Breaths should be interposed on the upstroke of each fifth cardiac compression.
5. Anticipate and assist with emergency procedures and medications.
    a. Assist with intubation, monitoring, placement of cutdown, administration of intravenous fluids, defibrillation, and other definitive measures.
    b. Prepare and administer emergency medications as prescribed. Record dose and time.

6. After resuscitation:
    a. Care for the child as required.
    b. Determine if family members have been notified and are being cared for.
    c. Record all events.
    d. Restock emergency cart.

Traction

Traction refers to the extension of an injured extremity in the direction and position that will promote healing and optimal functioning. It is accomplished by the use of weights that pull a part in the desired direction in the presence of countertraction.

Purposes

1. To foster and/or maintain the realignment of fractured segments of a bone.
2. To prevent deformities from resulting in the presence of injury or inflammation.
    a. Fractures
    b. Arthritis
    c. Trauma
3. To correct existing deformities.
    a. Congenital dislocation of the hip
    b. Flexion contractures of the knees

4. To lessen muscle spasm.
5. To immobilize a part.
6. To reduce dislocation.

Types of Traction

1. Skin traction
    a. Used for younger children when the condition of the skin is good and mild forces of traction are sufficient.
    b. Traction is applied to the skin of the affected body part:
        (1) Moleskin, adhesive, or foam rubber extensions are fastened firmly to the skin.
        (2) Elastic bandages are applied to hold them in place.
        (3) Weights are attached to the extensions by cords that pass over one or more pulleys.
2. Skeletal traction
    a. Used in children when greater traction force is required or if the skin is damaged.
    b. Force is exerted against the bone by means of a metallic device such as a pin, wire, or Crutchfield tongs.
3. Traction may be continuous or intermittent, depending on its purpose.
    a. Continuous traction cannot be interrupted for dressing or other activities.
    b. Intermittent traction may be temporarily disconnected as specified by the physician.

Guidelines   Care of a Child in Traction

Equipment

Strips of moleskin
Adhesive tape
Elastic bandages
Square wooden blocks
Ropes, weights, pulleys
Traction bars
Slings

Procedure

Nursing Action	Rationale/Amplification
1. Explain the procedure to the child and his parents.	1. If the traction is to be effective, it is essential that the parents understand the procedure and cooperate while the child is in traction.
2. Maintain even, constant traction: a. Do not add or remove weights. b. Allow the weights to hang free at all times. Do not allow them to touch the floor or bed. c. Be certain that the ropes are in the wheel grooves of the pulleys. d. Keep the weights out of the child's reach. e. Wrap knotted areas of the ropes with adhesive tape to prevent slipping. f. Do not elevate the head or foot of the bed without consulting the physician. g. Supervise the child's position so that the purpose of the traction is accomplished.	2. Traction must be kept constant in order to achieve the desired results. Any change in the amount of weights or countertraction affects the entire traction system.
3. Check for disturbance of circulation by observing: a. Skin color—for redness, pallor, cyanosis b. Joint motion c. Skin temperature d. Tingling, numbness e. Swelling	3. Compare the affected extremity with the unaffected one.

Procedure (continued)	**Nursing Action**	**Rationale/Amplification**

Nursing Action

4. Provide skin care.

   a. Pad bony prominences (ankles) with cotton padding before wrapping with elastic bandages.
   b. Wash and dry all exposed areas thoroughly.
   c. Massage the child's back and sacral area at least 2–3 times daily. If indicated, apply cornstarch.
   d. Inspect the heels, ankles, popliteal space, and top of the foot for signs of pressure from elastic bandages.
   e. Keep the linen clean, and free from wrinkles and crumbs.

   f. Do not allow any traction cords to dig into the child's skin.
   g. Utilize a fracture bedpan.
5. Plan for short periods of muscle exercise every day.
   a. Encourage the child to move and exercise his unaffected extremities.
   b. Provide diversional therapy that requires the use of these muscles.
   c. Assist the child to exercise his toes.
6. Have the child breathe deeply at intervals. Provide him with soap bubbles, whistles, or party favors to make this more fun. An older child may use blow bottles.
7. Keep a record of the child's intake and output and do periodic urinalyses.
8. Provide a diet high in fiber and fluids (especially fruit juices) and low in calcium.
9. Provide daily diversion and encourage the child's family to visit frequently.

   a. Attempt to replace the lost activity with another form of motion.
   b. Suspend toys over the child's head so he can reach them. (Punching bag can help child relieve hostility.)
   c. Provide continuing education for the school-age child.
   d. Encourage projects that will allow child a feeling of accomplishment: painting, puzzles, knitting, ceramics.
   e. Patients who are immobilized in traction or casts should be grouped together.
10. If not contraindicated, supply the child with an overhead trapeze.
11. Record:
    a. Color, temperature, and appearance of the affected extremity
    b. Skin condition
    c. Evidence of local edema
    d. Body alignment
    e. Functioning of traction ropes, weights, and pulley
    f. Response of the child to therapy
12. Make certain that countertraction is provided.

    a. The foot of the child's bed may have to be raised or placed on shock blocks to counteract the traction weight and prevent the child from being pulled to the end of the bed.
13. Never disturb the traction device.
14. Avoid jarring the bed or swinging the weights.
15. Do not allow the weights to hang directly over the child's body.

Rationale/Amplification

4. Immobilized children readily develop areas of pressure unless meticulous skin care is provided.
   a. Protects skin from injury.

   c. Cornstarch absorbs moisture and prevents maceration of the skin.
   d. These are the areas most prone to breakdown.

   e. When a large bed is used, two folded sheets are often more easily managed than one large sheet. One is used to cover the upper half of the bed, and one to cover the lower half. This facilitates changing the bed and makes the procedure less uncomfortable for the child.

   g. This is less awkward and more comfortable for the child.
5. Disuse of muscles can result in atrophy and deformities.

6. Prolonged periods of immobilization may cause the child to develop hypostatic pneumonia.

7. Immobilization renders the child prone to developing urinary retention and renal calculi.
8. This helps to prevent constipation and the development of renal calculi.
9. Enforced bed rest makes time pass very slowly and can be very traumatic for a small child.

   a. Water play, mirrors, body games are helpful replacements. Often the child can be moved in his bed into the playroom or hall.

10. This will facilitate movement and self-help.

12. Usually, the patient's body acts as the counterweight that keeps the extremity aligned and immobilized.
    a. The child's weight is often insufficient to provide countertraction.

13. If it appears to need adjustment, notify the physician.
14. This may cause pain and is upsetting to the child.
15. This is a safety precaution.

(continued)

Guidelines   Care of a Child in Traction *(continued)*

Procedure *(continued)*	**Nursing Action**	**Rationale/Amplification**

Skin Traction

1. Shave the area if hair is present and paint the skin with tincture of benzoin.

1. This allows the adhesive to grasp the skin more firmly. Benzoin also disinfects the skin, allays itching, and prevents skin breakdown under the tape.

Skeletal Traction

1. Treat all entry sites, pins, wires, or tongs as surgical wounds.
   a. Wipe the insertion site with Betadine and apply an antibiotic ointment at least daily. Cover with a sterile 4 × 4 gauze *or*
   b. Dress the insertion site with a 4 × 4 sterile gauze treated with an antiseptic prescribed by the physician.
   c. Check the entry site regularly for any signs of infection and to be certain that the pin has not slipped through the bone.
2. Place corks or plastic guards over the exposed ends of the pins

a. This is an attempt to reduce the hazard of infection along the track of the pin. Some physicians prefer to let these areas crust over or cover them with plaster.

c. Notify the physician of either of these conditions.

2. This is a safety precaution to prevent injury to the nurse or patient.

Bryant's Traction (Fig. 47-10)

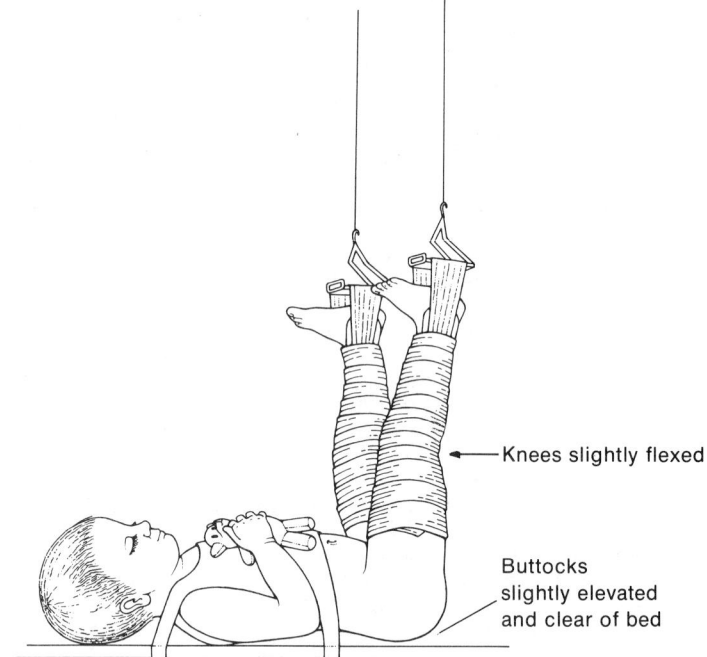

Knees slightly flexed

Buttocks slightly elevated and clear of bed

Figure 47-10. Bryant's traction.

Purpose

Used to reduce fractured femurs in small children.

Mechanism of Action

Involves bilateral, vertical extension of the child's legs. The child's weight serves as countertraction to the vertical pull of the weights. Skin traction is applied to both legs in order to minimize potential trauma to the affected leg and maintain the stability of the position.

1. Maintain the child in the appropriate position.
   a. The legs are extended at right angles to the body.
   b. The hips are elevated slightly from the bed.
   c. The buttocks are elevated and clear of the bed.
   d. The heels and ankles are free from pressure.

1. This position is essential in order to achieve the desired results.

Procedure *(continued)*	**Nursing Action**	**Rationale/Amplification**
	e. The child is flat in bed and unable to turn from side to side.	e. A jacket or abdominal restraint is usually necessary.
	2. Check the position of the elastic bandages and rewrap if necessary and permitted by the physician.	2. The bandages should be wrapped snugly around the legs without compromising circulation. They should not slip and cause pressure on the dorsa of the feet. If rewrapping is necessary, traction must be maintained by a second person during the procedure.

Russell's Traction (Fig. 47-11)

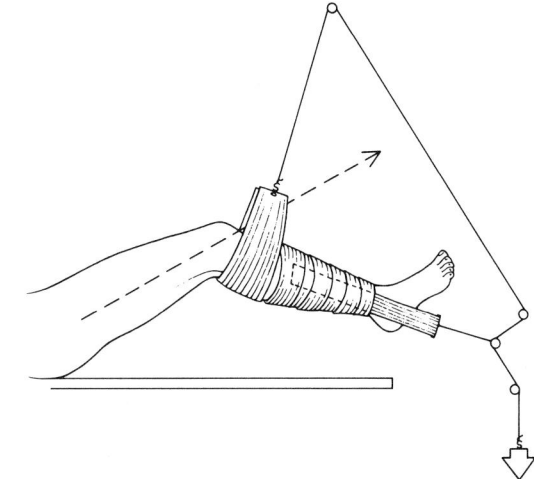

Figure 47-11. *Russell's traction.*

Purpose

To reduce contractures of the knee or hip, reduce dislocated hips, immobilize the knee or hip postoperatively, or reduce fractures of the femoral shaft.

Mechanism of Action

Force is exerted on the long axis of the lower leg, and a knee sling is used under the distal thigh to provide flexion of the knee and hip.

1. Application of elastic bandages:
   a. Wrap bandages from the ankle to the thigh on patients under 18 months of age.
   b. Wrap bandages from the ankle to the knee on patients over 18 months of age.
2. Place foot supports against the soles of both feet.
3. If necessary, place a small pillow under the thigh to maintain hip flexion at approximately 20 degrees.
4. Keep the heel free of the bed.
5. Carefully check the popliteal space for pressure sores. Make certain that the knee sling is positioned so that it does not exert pressure on the popliteal space.
6. Make certain that the bandages do not exert pressure over the dorsalis pedis artery (inside of top of foot) or the Achilles tendon (back of heel).
7. Make certain that the footplate or spreader is wide enough to prevent irritation of the skin but not so wide that the tapes tend to pull from the skin

a. The length of the leg from the knee to the foot is usually not long enough to maintain traction.
b. This length in an older child is sufficient to maintain traction.
2. Prevents foot drop.
3. Prevents hip contractures.

4. Prevents pressure sore of the heel.
5. Line the knee sling with a piece of felt or sheepskin for additional protection against pressure.

6. Prevents discomfort, pressure sores, and circulatory complications.

90-Degree–90-Degree Traction (90–90 Traction) (Fig. 47-12)

Purpose

Used to reduce a fractured femur when skin traction is not adequate.

(continued)

Guidelines   Care of a Child in Traction *(continued)*

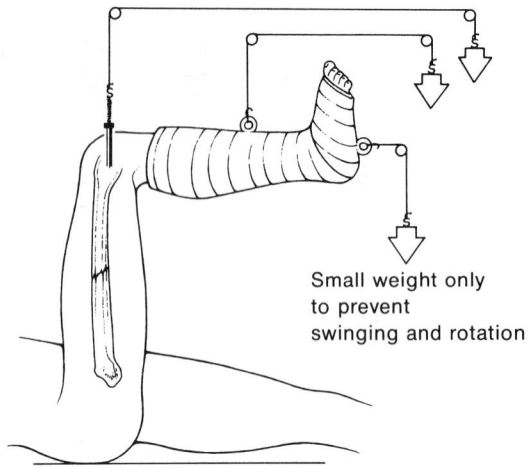

Small weight only
to prevent
swinging and rotation

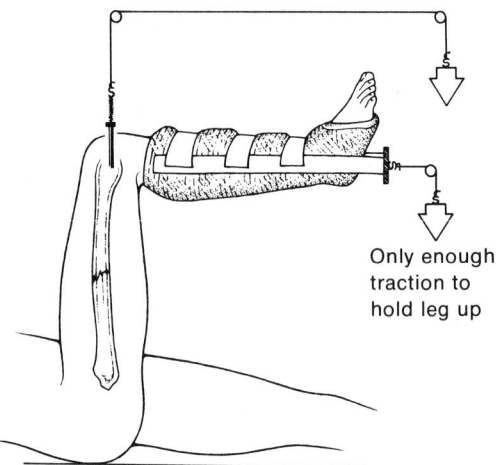

Only enough
traction to
hold leg up

Figure 47-12. *90–90 traction.*

Mechanism of Action

Both the affected knee and hip are flexed at a 90-degree angle. Traction is applied by a skeletal pin drilled through the distal femur. A short leg cast or polyfoam boot is used to suspend the lower leg.

Buck's Extension

Purposes

Used to correct knee and hip contractures, to rest the leg, and for other short-term immobilization. For additional information, refer to Guidelines: Application of Buck's Extension Traction, page 786.

Balanced Traction With Thomas Splint and Pearson Attachment

Purposes

Used in older children and adolescents for fractured femurs, to rest the hip and knee, or to immobilize the hip and knee postoperatively. Refer to Fracture of the Femur, page 774.

Dunlop's Traction (Fig. 47-13)

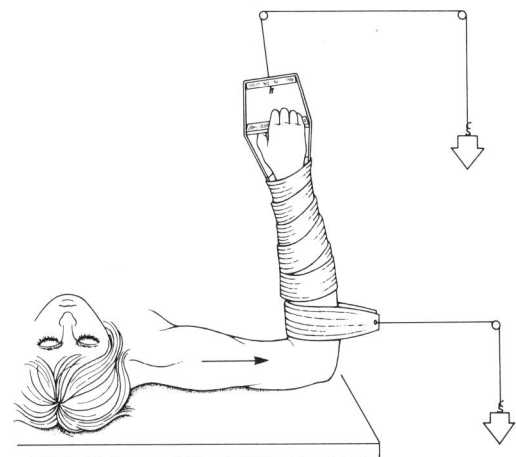

Figure 47-13. *Dunlop's traction.*

Purpose

Used to treat fractures or injuries of the humerus, shoulder, or shoulder girdle.

Mechanism of Action

Longitudinal traction on the humerus is applied using a soft sling to pull against the forearm or using a pin drilled through the olecranon. A suspension apparatus is applied to the forearm with traction straps and an elastic bandage, using only enough weight to hold the forearm upright and the elbow just touching the bed. The elbow is kept flexed at slightly more than 90 degrees.

1. Be certain that the sling at the proximal forearm is well padded and that the margin does not create a ridge at the bend of the elbow.
2. Check the child's fingers frequently for signs of circulatory impairment. Immediately report any coldness, pallor, cyanosis, swelling, pain, or limited sensation.

1. This is a precaution to avoid pressure on the ulnar nerve.
2. Prolonged circulatory impairment may lead to ischemia and Volkmann's contraction (clawhand) and flexion at the wrist and elbow.

Cervical Traction

Purposes

Used for children with spinal fractures, muscle spasms, or spinal injuries to provide immobilization in a neutral position that causes the least pressure on the spinal cord.

Mechanism of Action

Applied directly to the skull bone by a device such as the Crutchfield tong, or indirectly by using a head halter.

Cervical Skin (Head Halter)Traction (Fig. 47-14)

1. Check the position of the head halter frequently:
   a. The halter should not press on the ears.
   b. The rope should not rest against the skin.
   c. The chin piece should not press on the throat.
   d. Protect the chin halter when feeding the child.
2. Keep the position of the bed flat unless otherwise prescribed by the physician. Avoid lifting the child's head or flexing the neck.
3. Keep the child flat on his back.
4. Diversion
   a. Position an adjustable mirror at the head of the bed so that the child can see around the room.
   b. Encourage companionship:
   (1) Place the child in a room with other children his age.
   (2) Allow liberal visiting by parents, older siblings and friends.

1. It is important to prevent continuous pressure and rubbing on these areas in order to avoid skin breakdown.

2. Raising the head increases countertraction, which may be undesirable.

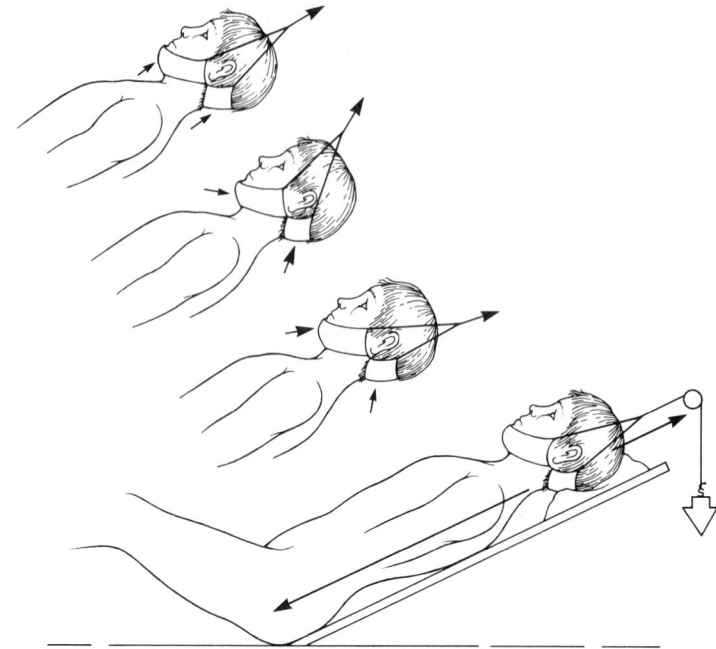

Figure 47-14. *Cervical traction.*

Procedure
(continued)

Nursing Action	Rationale/Amplification
c. Place colorful objects, cards, pictures, etc. within sight of the child. d. Utilize audiovisual stimulation—records, radio, television, etc. e. Provide for continuing education for the child of school age.	

Cervical Skeletal Traction

Nursing Action	Rationale/Amplification
1. If possible, place the child on a Stryker frame or CircOlectric bed.	1. Allows the child to be turned in one motion.
2. Make certain that the neck is held in steady longitudinal traction. When the child is lying on his abdomen, support his arms on pillows at his sides and at the level of the bed.	2. The neck should never be flexed because this may cause permanent spinal cord injury. The head should be in a neutral position in relation to the spine. The arms should not droop and the shoulders should not be hunched.
3. Do not allow the patient to reach for objects.	3. Reaching can disrupt spinal alignment.
4. Provide the child with adjustable mirrors at the head of the bed, and with prism glasses.	4. These aids enable the child to look around the room, watch television, or read while on his back.
5. Brush the child's teeth and frequently rinse his mouth with an antiseptic mouthwash. a. Instruct the child to try not to breathe through his mouth since this may cause dryness of the mucosa. b. Apply lemon-glycerin or a lip balm to his lips to prevent dryness and cracking.	5. This prevents mouth sores and is refreshing.

Cotrel's Traction

Purpose

To provide traction to the spine prior to surgery or to the application of a scoliotic brace.

Procedure *(continued)*	**Nursing Action**	**Rationale/Amplification**

Mechanism of Action

Traction is applied primarily to the occipital bone by means of a head harness that fits onto the chin and reaches around to the occiput. Pelvic straps maintain the pelvis in a fixed position.

Nursing Action	**Rationale/Amplification**

1. Check the head halter for proper placement.
  a. The chin pad should not compress the child's throat.
  b. The hair should be free from entanglement.
  c. The halter should not pinch the ears.
	1. This helps to ensure effectiveness of the treatment and prevents skin breakdown.

2. Check the facial skin, chin, occiput, and iliac crests for possible irritation and breakdown.	
3. Check the child frequently for maintenance of alignment.	3. It is relatively easy for the child to become malaligned in this type of traction.

Halo–Femoral Traction

Purposes

Utilized to correct severe and resistant spinal curvatures, and for treatment of vertebral fractures.

Mechanism of Action

An aluminum halo is fixed to the cranium with four threaded pins, and Steinman pins are placed in the distal ends of the femur. Upward traction is applied to the halo and downward traction to the femurs to pull the spine into alignment. Frequently, a suspension assembly is attached to the halo by threaded traction rods, the entire assembly being supported by a hoop attached to the pelvic pins. This apparatus allows control of position in all three planes plus progressive traction application. Femoral pins may be removed and countertraction applied by securing the halo device to a body jacket cast. This allows the child to be ambulatory.

Nursing Action	**Rationale/Amplification**

1. Prepare the child and the parents for the procedure.
  a. Explain the purpose, method of application, and approximate time required for the therapy. The child should know that the treatment is relatively pain-free and that the device does not penetrate the brain.
  b. If possible, introduce the child to other patients in the apparatus or those who have previously experienced it.
  c. Emphasize that this will provide optimal correction of the deformity and allow the child to appear more normal
	1. The appearance of the apparatus may be overwhelming and frightening. Diagrams and visual aids will enhance comprehension and allay fear.
	
	c. These children are often very sensitive about their body image, and will develop a more positive attitude if they realize that the deformity is being improved.

2. Observe the child carefully while traction is being increased for:
  a. Neck pain
  b. Respiratory distress
  c. Nerve injury
	2. Alteration of neurologic or respiratory status is regarded as a warning sign and a release of several turns on the extension bars may be carried out by the physician as an emergency measure. Neck pain is a less serious sign. The amount of traction is usually not increased until the pain disappears.

3. *Symptoms of injury*
  a. Spinal cord
  (1) Weakness, numbness in legs
  (2) Loss of bladder function
  (3) Upturning or downturning of toes
  (4) Clonus of ankles or knees
  b. Cranial nerves
  (1) Double vision
  (2) Difficulty in swallowing
  (3) Difficulty in coughing
  (4) Voice changes
  (5) Tongue weakness
  c. Upper extremities
  (1) Difficulty in moving hand, shoulder, or arm
  (2) Numbness or weakness in hand (check grip)	

4. Make certain that all of the fixtures on the apparatus are tightened.	4. Looseness and excessive movement of the apparatus may cause pain and infection. The physician should be notified.

(continued)

Guidelines   Care of a Child in Traction *(continued)*

Procedure *(continued)*	Nursing Action	Rationale/Amplification
	5. Report complaints of pain or drainage at the pin sites.	5. Most children have mild pain and headache for the first few days. Thereafter, pain at the pin site usually means that the pin is loose or infected, and it may be necessary to change the pin.
	6. Have an Allen wrench and torque wrench available.	6. The Allen wrench is used to release vest bolts quickly if CPR is necessary. The torque wrench is used to adjust the amount of traction on the bars.

Guidelines   Assisting the Child on a Bradford Frame

A *Bradford frame* is a piece of equipment that facilitates the nursing of young children who must be immobilized for extensive periods of time. It is frequently used for young infants with meningoceles, children in hip-spica casts, and children with extensive burns.

Purposes
1. To ensure correct positioning.
2. To facilitate the collection of urine and stools.
3. To protect the child from injury.

Equipment
Frame of appropriate size for the child
2 pieces of canvas of appropriate size to cover the head and foot of the frame
Plastic sheeting
2 crib sheets or draw sheets
Bedboard
Linen for the bed
Plastic drawsheet
Heavy blocks for supporting the frame
Material such as canvas strips for attaching the frame to the bed
Protective device to limit the child's movement

Procedure	Nursing Action	Rationale/Amplification
	Preparatory Phase	
	1. Select frame according to the size of the child.	1. Frame should be approximately 15 cm. (6 inches) longer and 5 cm. (2 inches) wider than the patient.
	2. Cover the head and foot areas with canvas.	
	a. Leave an open area between the head and foot sections for the drainage of urine and feces.	a. Make sure that the size of the opening is adequate for the size of the child.
	b. Stretch the canvas tightly over the frame.	b. If the canvas is not tight, it will stretch.
	3. Cover the top and bottom sections of the canvas with heavy plastic sheeting.	3. This protects the canvas from becoming soiled.
	4. Place a small sheet tightly over each section of the frame.	
	Performance Phase	
	1. Place a bedboard on the mattress.	1. A firm base is required for proper use of the frame.
	2. Place two draw sheets on the bed, one at each end.	2. The entire bed will not require changing when only one part is soiled.
	3. Place a plastic draw sheet under the center opening of the frame.	3. This is the area most likely to become soiled by urine or feces.
	4. Place blocks on the bed. Place the frame on the blocks.	4. The position of the blocks and frame will be prescribed by the physician. The blocks should always be placed under the child's shoulders, never directly under his head if the head of the frame is to be elevated.
	5. Secure the frame to the bed at the head and foot.	5. This is a safety precaution to prevent slipping.
	6. Place the bedpan below the center opening.	

Procedure (continued)	Nursing Action	Rationale/Amplification

	a. Plastic sheeting may be draped over the top and bottom edges of the opening of the frame.	a. This permits urine and feces to drain into the bedpan if the child is incontinent.
	b. Place diapers over the plastic.	b. This prevents irritation of the skin.
	7. Place the child on the frame.	
	a. Maintain his position by use of a jacket restraint (see procedure for protective measures to limit movement).	
	8. Place pillows at the sides of the frame to support the child's arms.	8. It is important to maintain proper body alignment.

Follow-Up Phase

1. Check the following frequently:	1. These are principles of safety (see procedure for protective devices to limit movement, p. 1149).
a. Position of the frame on the blocks.	
b. Security of all knots and materials that are used to fasten the frame to the bed.	
c. Position of the child on the frame.	
2. Provide meticulous general hygiene:	2. See procedure for traction and for care of a child in a spica cast.
a. Empty the bedpan frequently.	
b. Check the linen for soiling by urine or feces and change it if necessary.	
c. Cleanse the buttocks after each bowel movement and apply lotion or cornstarch.	
d. Bathe daily and provide skin care frequently.	
3. Provide for the prevention of contractures, muscle wasting, and the development of hypostatic pneumonia.	3. See procedure for traction.
4. Provide diversion. Move the child's bed from room to room for a change of scenery or out into the hall so that he can watch unit activities.	4. See procedures for traction and care of a child in a spica cast.
5. Reconstruct the child's frame as necessary.	
a. The child can usually be placed on a firm bed or stretcher while his frame is being changed.	a. Special care must be taken to ensure correct body alignment during this procedure.
b. If a second frame is available, this can be prepared and placed on another bed. The child can then be easily transferred from one frame to another.	

Casts

Nursing Considerations

Nursing activities related to the application and care of casts are essentially the same for pediatric and adult patients. The following points of consideration are important.

1. The child is usually more troubled by immobilization than the adult. A special attempt should be made to ensure that his activities are as normal as possible and that full use is made of his unaffected joints and muscles.
2. The younger child may not be able to understand why the cast is necessary. He may attempt to remove it, put pieces of toys or food under it, etc.
   a. An attempt should be made to allow the child to work through his questions and feelings via play (e.g., give him a doll with a cast).
   b. Close supervision is necessary to prevent the child from destroying the cast or injuring himself.
3. There is danger of soiling a long-leg or hip-spica cast with feces or urine. (The area of the cast near the buttocks and genitalia should be protected with waterproof material.)
4. Children may be especially frightened by removal of the cast. They often think of the cast as part of their body and may be helped by analogies of having fingernails or hair cut. Age-appropriate explanations and demonstration should be provided (refer to adult section, p. 781).
5. Parents should be instructed in care following cast removal. Daily soaking of the area may be necessary to remove desquamated skin and secretions. Oil or lotion may provide comfort. Exercises should be done as prescribed to increase strength and function.
6. For additional information, including types of casts, methods of application, complications, etc., refer to pages 778–784.

Guidelines Care of a Child in a Spica Cast

Procedure	Nursing Action	Rationale/Amplification
	1. If possible, prepare the child for the application of the cast.	1. This can best be accomplished by allowing the child to put a cast on a doll. Older children should see a picture of the cast that is going to be applied and receive an explanation of the method of application.
	2. Facilitate drying and accurate molding of the cast	2. About 24–48 hours are required for a cast to dry completely. A cast dries from the outside to the inside. It may feel dry to the touch but still be wet on the inside.
	a. Place a bedboard under the mattress.	a. Prevents sagging of the bed from pressure of the cast.
	b. Support the curves of the cast with small, plastic-covered pillows.	b. Prevents cracking while the cast is drying.
	c. Avoid placing a pillow under the head and shoulders.	c. Causes pressure on the chest by thrusting it forward in the cast.
	d. Keep the cast uncovered and turn the child every 1–2 hours.	d. Allows moisture to evaporate from the surface.
	e. Handle moist cast with the palms of hands.	e. Fingers may cause indentation in the moist plaster.
	3. Observe for complications resulting from pressure of the cast.	3. Vascular insufficiency due to unrelieved swelling can cause necrosis and pressure sores. It may be necessary to bivalve the cast.
	a. Impaired circulation to the toes	
	(1) Discoloration or cyanosis	
	(2) Impaired movement	
	(3) Loss of sensation	
	(4) Edema	
	(5) Temperature change	
	(6) Absent pedal pulses	
	b. Complaints of pain or pressure in any area where the cast fits closely over the body.	
	4. Provide good skin care.	4. Prevents the development of pressure sores.
	a. Bathe accessible skin and massage with emolient lotion. Pay special attention to the buttocks and genital area.	
	b. Massage the skin underneath the cast with alcohol.	
	c. Inspect the skin for signs of irritation:	
	(1) Around cast edge.	
	(2) Under the cast—pull skin taut and inspect under the cast, using a flashlight for illumination.	
	d. Investigate complaints of pain or burning or an offensive odor from the inside of the cast.	d. These may indicate that a pressure sore is forming or has become infected. It may be necessary to create a "window" in the cast.
	e. Relieve itching by blowing cool air through the cast with an asepto syringe or hair dryer.	e. Some physicians insert a strip of gauze through the cast which can be used to gently massage the skin. Do not use sharp objects such as coat hangers or knitting needles.
	f. Do not allow a small child to put objects inside his cast.	f. A small hand vacuum cleaner may be used to remove crumbs from inside the cast.
	(1) Keep small toys away from the child.	
	(2) Pad the edges of the cast with cotton padding or cover cast with a towel to prevent food particles and foreign objects from being inserted by the child.	
	5. Prevent the skin around the edge of the cast from becoming excoriated.	
	a. Smooth the edges of the cast and petal it with waterproof adhesive tape.	a. This prevents flakes of plaster from breaking off and slipping under the cast. It also facilitates cleansing of the cast.
	b. Do not lift infants by their legs to change diapers.	
	6. Prevent urine and feces from soiling the cast.	6. A soiled cast will cause skin irritation, become odorous, and may mildew or partially disintegrate.
	a. Offer the bedpan frequently.	
	(1) Elevate the child's head slightly higher than his feet to prevent urine from running under the cast.	
	(2) Place a sheet of plastic under the front and back edges of the cast opening for the buttocks and genitalia.	
	(3) Slip the fracture pan beneath the buttocks.	

Procedure (continued)	**Nursing Action**	**Rationale/Amplification**

Nursing Action

    (4) Allow the ends of the plastic strips to hang into the pan.

  b. Place the child who is not toilet-trained on a Bradford frame.

    (1) See procedure for care of the child on a Bradford frame, page 1212.

    (2) Line the edges of the cast with waterproof material such as plastic or cellophane.

    (3) Tuck a folded diaper or perineal pad under the cast edges and change it frequently.

  c. Keep the perineum clean

    (1) Wash the skin under the edge of the cast whenever necessary and dry it thoroughly.

    (2) Change diapers immediately after they become soiled.

  d. Clean the cast by rubbing it with a small amount of scouring agent on a damp cloth, then dry it promptly.

7. Plan for short periods of muscle exercise every day.

  a. Encourage the child to move and exercise his unaffected extremities. Provide diversional therapy that requires the use of these muscles.

  b. Exercise the child's toes.

8. Have the child breathe deeply at intervals. Provide him with soap bubbles, whistles, or party favors to make this more fun. An older child may use blow bottles.

9. Turn the child at least every 4 hours.

  a. Move the child to the side of the bed, using a steady, pulling motion.

  b. Place one hand under the head and back and one hand under the leg portion of the cast, and turn the child on his side.

  c. Second nurse accepts support of the child and cast as he is turned completely.

10. Assess the child's bowel and bladder function.

  a. Provide an adequate fluid intake, especially fruit juices.

  b. Check the urine for signs of infection.

11. Maintain correct position of the cast.

  a. Support the contour of the cast with pillows. Allow the heel to extend beyond the pillow to avoid pressure sores.

12. Provide as normal an environment as possible.

  a. Place the child on a cart or a stretcher so that he may leave his room. The child may be taken outdoors if the weather is suitable.

  b. Allow the child to be dressed. (Wide, flared pants are especially suitable.)

  c. Encourage contact with peers.

  d. Provide for play activities.

    (1) Provide the young child with large toys that he cannot put into his cast.

    (2) Television is a good method of diversion if used with discretion.

    (3) Older children often enjoy checkers, sewing, art work, building models, etc.

  e. Provide for education.

    (1) Refer the child to a visiting teacher service.

    (2) Provide for study time during each day.

13. Evaluate the home situation for feasibility of home care.

  a. The child's place in the family and the number of siblings.

  b. Additional needs of the parents, such as pursuing their vocations.

  c. Physical setup of the home

Rationale/Amplification

d. A solution of zephiran chloride 1:750 may be used sparingly to eliminate odor-causing bacteria from cast.

7. Disuse of muscles can result in atrophy and deformities.

8. Prolonged periods of immobilization may cause the child to develop hypostatic pneumonia.

9. Do not use the supporting bar between the legs as a lever when turning the child.

10. Immobilization may cause constipation and poor urinary drainage. Suppositories or mild laxatives may be necessary for the constipated child.

11. This prevents cracking or flattening of the cast.

12. Enforced immobility is often traumatic for the child and may cause regression.

(continued)

Guidelines	Care of a Child in a Spica Cast *(continued)*

Procedure *(continued)*	**Nursing Action**	**Rationale/Amplification**
	d. Financial situation	
	e. Ability of the family to keep follow-up appointments	
	14. Assist the family in caring for the child after discharge.	
	a. Initiate the appropriate referrals.	
	(1) Community health nurse	
	(2) Social service agency	
	(3) Home tutoring service	
	(4) Physical therapy	
	b. Begin teaching early.	
	(1) Instruct the parent on all aspects of the child's care.	(1) Teach only a few aspects of care each day. Have the parent(s) participate in the child's care until capable of providing total nursing care under supervision.
	(2) Emphasize safety measures such as elevating the child's head during meals to prevent choking; preventing the small child from dropping objects into his cast; using good body mechanics when lifting and transporting the child, etc.	
	(3) Provide with detailed, written instructions.	
	15. Assist with cast removal.	15. Children often believe that the saw will cut off an extremity, and are frightened by the loud noise.
	a. Prepare the child for the procedure.	
	(1) Describe the sensations that the child will feel (warmth, vibration, etc.) as well as the procedure itself.	
	(2) Allow the child to observe as the saw is lightly touched to the operator's palm.	
	b. Immobilize the child as necessary so that the procedure can be carried out quickly and safely.	
	16. Care for the child after cast removal.	
	a. Support the part with pillows	a. Maintain the same position that existed in the cast.
	b. Move the extremity gently.	b. It will be very weak and stiff.
	c. Wash the skin gently with mild soap and apply oil or lanolin.	c. An accumulation of sebaceous material and dead skin causes the skin to appear brown and flaky. Vigorous rubbing will cause skin trauma.
	d. Encourage the child to do prescribed exercises.	d. These will strengthen muscles and relieve joint stiffness.
	e. Elevate the extremity when sitting.	e. Minimizes the development of edema.

Bibliography

Books

Avery ME and First LR. Pediatric Medicine. Baltimore, Williams & Wilkins, 1989

Barkin RM and Rosen P. Procedures. In Emergency Pediatrics: A Guide to Ambulatory Care, pp 671–686. St Louis, CV Mosby, 1990

Behrman RE and Kliegman R (eds). Nelson Essentials of Pediatrics. Philadelphia, WB Saunders, 1990

Bentley D and Lawson M. Clinical Nutrition in Paediatric Disorders. London, Bailliere Tindall, 1988

Brown PA et al. Pulmonary system. In Quick Reference to Pediatric Intensive Care Nursing, pp 83–121. Rockville, MD, Aspen Publishers, 1989

Eichenwald HF, Stroder J and Mietens C. Principles of pediatric therapy. In Current Therapy in Pediatrics—2, pp 1–25. Philadelphia, BC Decker, 1989

Fitzgerald JF and Clark JH. Parenteral nutrition. In Manual of Pediatric Gastroenterology, pp 171–187. New York, Churchill Livingstone, 1988

Fleisher GR. Resuscitation—Pediatric basic and advanced life support. In Textbook of Pediatric Emergency Medicine, pp 1–30. Baltimore, Williams & Wilkins, 1988

Ford DC, Leist ER and Phelps SJ. Guidelines for Administration of Intravenous Medications to Pediatric Patients. Bethesda, American Society of Hospital Pharmacists, 1988

Graef JW (ed). Manual of Pediatric Therapeutics. 4th edition. Boston, Little, Brown & Co, 1988

Kaye R, Oski FA and Barness LA. Fever. In Core Textbook of Pediatrics. 3rd ed, pp 56–60. Philadelphia, JB Lippincott, 1988

Koff PB, Eitzman DV and Neu J (eds). Neonatal and Pediatric Respiratory Care. St Louis, CV Mosby, 1988

Morray JP. Fluids, electrolytes and nutrition. In Pediatric Intensive Care, pp 1–42. Norwalk, Appleton & Lange, 1987

Oski FA et al (eds). Principles and Practice of Pediatrics. Philadelphia, JB Lippincott, 1990

Raffensperger JG (ed). Critical care. In Swenson's Pediatric Surgery. 5th ed, pp 65–101. Norwalk, Appleton & Lange, 1990

Ross Laboratories. Enteral Feeding. Columbus, OH, Ross Laboratories, 1988

Wood RA et al. Pediatrics. Philadelphia, JB Lippincott, 1989

Journals

Vital Signs

Ingelfinger SR. Noninvasive evaluation of pediatric hypertension. Pediatr Ann 1989 Sep; 18(9):551–552, 554–555, 558–560

Park MK and Lee DH. Normative arm and calf blood pressure values in the newborn. Pediatrics 1989 Feb; 83(2): 240–243

Park MK and Menard SM. Normative oscillometric blood pressure values in the first 5 years in an office setting. Am J Dis Child 1989 Jul; 143(7):860–864

Fever

Doyle M and Pickering LK. Is this child's fever a worry? Postgrad Med 1989 Apr; 85(5):207–214, 219, 222

Kilmon CA. Home management of children's fevers. J Pediatr Nurs 1987 Dec; 2(6):400–404

Medications/Intravenous Infusions

Anderson LJ and Anderson JM. An assistive device for toddlers ambulating with an intravenous pole. Am J Occup Ther 1988 Oct; 42(10): 671–672

Beecroft PC and Redick S. Possible complications of intramuscular injection on the pediatric unit. Pediatr Nurs 1989 Jul–Aug; 15(4):333–336, 376

Morrow JC. Simplifying nursing management of pediatric airways and intravenous infusions. JEN 1988 Mar–Apr; 14(2):103–106

Rahman O et al. Rapid intravenous rehydration by means of a single polyelectrolyte solution with or without glucose. J Pediatr 1988 Oct; 113(4):654–660

Ross P Jr et al. Thrombus associated with central venous catheters in infants and children. J Pediatr Surg 1989 Mar; 24(3):253–256

Specimen Collection

Patel H, Ryan SW and McLain B. Sources of error in neonatal blood sampling. Arch Dis Child 1988 Jul; 63(7 Spec No):752–753

Rutledge JC. Pediatric specimen collection for chemical analysis. Pediatr Clin North Am 1989 Feb; 36(1):37–47

Suri S. Simplifying urine collection from infants and children without losing accuracy. MCN 1988 Nov–Dec; 13(6): 438–441

Varnier OE et al. Whole blood collection on filter paper is an effective means of obtaining samples for human immunodeficiency virus antibody. AIDS Res Hum Retroviruses 1988 Apr; 4(2):131–136

Fluid and Electrolyte Balance

Costarino AT and Baumgart S. Controversies in fluid and electrolyte therapy for the premature infant. Clin Perinatol 1988 Dec; 15(4):863–878

Hazinski MF. Understanding fluid balance in the seriously ill child. Pediatr Nurs 1988 May–Jun; 14(3):231–236

Penatzer M et al. Common pediatric IV meds at a glance. Pediatr Nurs 1988 Jan–Feb; 14(1):56–58

Rimar J. Guidelines for the intravenous administration of medications used in pediatrics. MCN 1987 Sep–Oct; 12(5): 322–340

Wildblood R and Strezo P. The how-to's of home IV therapy. Pediatr Nurs 1987 Jan–Feb; 13(1):42–46, 48

Parenteral Nutrition/Gastrostomy

Berry R and Jorgensen S. Growing with home parenteral nutrition: Adjusting to family life and child development. Pediatr Nurs 1988 Jan–Feb; 14(1):43–45

Berry R and Jorgensen S. Growing with home parenteral nutrition: Maintaining a safe environment. Pediatr Nurs 1988 Mar–Apr; 14(2):155–157

Cory DA, Fitzgerald JF and Cohen MD. Percutaneous nonendoscopic gastrostomy in children. Am J Roentgenol 1988 Nov; 151(5):995–997

deAngelis GL et al. Gastrin pepsin and acid secretion during total parenteral nutrition and constant rate nutrition in infancy. J Parenter Enter Nutr 1988 Sep–Oct; 12(5):505–508

Garvin G and Franck LS. Preventing delivery of enteral formula via parenteral route. Pediatr Nurs 1989 Jan–Feb; 15(1):17–18

Gottschlich MM et al. Diarrhea in tube-fed burn patients: Incidence, etiology, nutritional impact, and prevention. J Parenter Enter Nutr 1988 Jul–Aug; 12(4):338–345

Haas-Beckert B. Removing the mysteries of parenteral nutrition. Pediatr Nurs 1987 Jan–Feb; 13(1):37–41

Heird WC et al. Pediatric parenteral amino acid mixture in low birth weight infants. Pediatrics 1988 Jan; 81(1):41–50

Huddleston K et al. MIC or Foley: Comparing gastrostomy tubes. MCN 1989 Jan–Feb; 14(1):20–23

Huth M and O'Brien M. The gastrostomy feeding button. Pediatr Nurs 1987 Jul–Aug; 13(4):241–245

Laine L et al. An educational booklet diminishes anxiety in parents whose children receive total parenteral nutrition. Am J Dis Child 1989 Mar; 143(3):374–377

Koo WK et al. Minimal vitamin D and high calcium and phosphorus needs of preterm infants receiving parenteral nutrition. J Pediatr Gastroenterol Nutr 1989 Feb; 8(2):225–233

Pineault M. Total parenteral nutrition in the newborn: Impact of the quality of infused energy on nitrogen metabolism. Am J Clin Nutr 1988 Feb; 47(2):298–304

Sangster W, Cuddington GD and Bachulis BL. Percutaneous endoscopic gastrostomy. Am J Surg 1988 May; 155(5):677–679

Spear ML et al. Effect of heparin dose and infusion rate on lipid clearance and bilirubin binding in premature infants receiving intravenous fat emulsions. J Pediatr 1988 Jan; 112(1): 94–98

Dialysis

Goodenough GK, Lutz LJ and Gregory MC. Home-based renal dialysis. Am Fam Physician 1988 Feb; 37(2):203–214

Lopez–Herce J et al. Continuous arteriovenous haemofiltration in children. Intensive Care Med 1989;15(4):224–227

Mattern WD, Morris CR and Heffley DL. A three-year experience with CCPD in a university-based dialysis and transplantation program. Clin Nephrol 1988; 30(Suppl 1):S49–S52

McFarland K. Pediatric peritoneal dialysis. Pediatr Nurs 1988 Sep-Oct; 14(5):426

Neff EJA. Nursing the child undergoing dialysis. Issues Compr Pediatr Nurs 1987; 10(3):173–185

Wong SN and Geary DI. Comparison of temporary and permanent catheters for acute peritoneal dialysis. Arch Dis Child 1988 Jul; 63(7):827–831

Suctioning

Cunningham AS et al. Tracheal suction and meconium: A proposed standard of care. J Pediatr 1990 Jan; 116(1):153–154

Stone KS and Turner B. Endotracheal suctioning. Annu Rev Nurs Res 1989; 7: 27–49

Tracheostomy

Black TL, Fernandes ET and Carr MP. Preventing accidental decannulations following tracheostomy. J Pediatr Surg 1988 Feb; 23(2):143

Calhoun KH et al. Long-term airway sequelae in a pediatric burn population. Laryngoscope 1988 Jul; 98(7):721–725

Campbell JB, Morgan DW and Pearman K. Experience with the home-care of tracheotomised paediatric patients. Arch Otorhinolaryngol 1989; 246(5): 345–348

Hall SS and Weatherly KS. Using sign language with tracheotomized infants and children. Pediatr Nurs 1989 Jul–Aug; 15(4):362–367

Hazinski M. Pediatric home tracheostomy care: A parent's guide. Pediatr Nurs 1986 Jan–Feb; 12(1):41–48

Piotrowski JJ and Moore EE. Emergency department tracheostomy. Emerg Med Clin North Am 1988 Nov; 6(4):737–744

Oxygen Therapy

Bancalari E and Flynn JT. Respiratory physiology, oxygen therapy and monitoring: Report of a clinical trial of constant monitoring. Birth Defects 1988; 24(1):41–52

Brown M and Vender JS. Noninvasive oxygen monitoring. Crit Care Clin 1988 Jul; 4(3):493–509

Cheng M and Williams PD. Oxygenation during chest physiotherapy of very-low-birth-weight infants: Relations among fraction of inspired oxygen levels, number of hand ventilations, and transcutaneous oxygen pressure. J Pediatr Nurs 1989 Dec; 4(6):411–418

Dudell G, Cornish JD and Bartlett RH. What constitutes adequate oxygenation? Pediatrics 1990 Jan; 85(1):39–41

Fanconi S and Sigrist H. Transcutaneous carbon dioxide oxygen tension in newborn infants: Reliability of a combined monitor of oxygen tension and carbon dioxide tension. J Clin Monit 1988 Apr; 4(2):103–106

Hader CF and Sorense ER. The effects of body position on transcutaneous oxygen tension. Pediatr Nurs 1988 Nov–Dec; 14(6):469–473

Shann F, Gatchalian S and Hutchinson R. Nasopharyngeal oxygen in children. Lancet 1988 Nov 26; 3(8622):1238–1240

Short BL and Lotze A. Extracorporeal membrane oxygenation therapy. Pediatr Ann 1988 Aug; 17(8):516–518, 220, 522–523

Stine MJ, Gladieux G and Tetrick L. Neonatal oxygen monitoring. Indiana Med 1988 Jun; 81(6):517–518

Vain NE et al. Regulation of oxygen concentration delivered to infants via nasal cannulas. Am J Dis Child 1989 Dec; 143(12):1458–1460

Vyas H, Helms P and Cheriyan G. Transcutaneous oxygen monitoring beyond the neonatal period. Crit Care Med 1988 Sep; 16(9):844–847

Ventilatory Support and Monitoring

Andrews M and Nielson D. Technology dependent children in the home. Pediatr Nurs 1988 Mar–Apr; 14(2):111–113, 151

Barkin RM. Pediatric airway management. Emerg Med Clin North Am 1988 Nov; 6(4):687–692

Cunningham MD. Intensive care monitoring of pulmonary mechanics for preterm infants undergoing mechanical ventilation. J Perinatol 1989 Mar; 9(1):56–59

Dixon M and Holmes RB. The care of a ventilator-dependent child on a general pediatric unit. J Pediatr Nurs 1987 Jun; 2(3):184–192

Greenough H and Pool J. Neonatal patient triggered ventilation. Arch Dis Child 1988 Apr; 63(4):394–397

Harrison L. Teaching parents to provide home care for ventilator-dependent children. MCN 1989 Jul–Aug; 14(4):281

HFI Study Group. High-frequency oscillatory ventilation compared with conventional mechanical ventilation in the treatment of respiratory failure in preterm infants. N Engl J Med 1989 Jan 12; 320(2):88–93

Kim EH. Successful extubation of newborn infants without preextubation trial of continuous positive airway pressure. J Perinatol 1989 Mar; 9(1):72–76

McCarthy M. A home discharge program for ventilator-assisted children. Pediatr Nurs 1986 Sep–Oct; 12(5):331–335, 380

Millette SW. High frequency oscillatory ventilator: Neonatal application. Dimens Crit Care Nurs 1988 Jul–Aug; 7(4):220–225

Mitchell A, Greenough A and Hird M. Limitations of patient triggered ventilation in neonates. Arch Dis Child 1989 Jul; 64(7):924–929

Norton LC et al. Common problems and state of the art in nursing care of the mechanically ventilated patient. Am Rev Respir Dis 1988 Oct; 138(4):1055–1056

Posch CM and Edwards PA. The ventilator-dependent child: Challenge and opportunity. Rehabil Nurs 1988 Jan–Feb; 13(1):15–18

Scharer K and Dixon MM. Managing chronic illness: Parents with a ventilator-dependent child. J Pediatr Nurs 1989 Aug; 4(4):236–247

Wegener D and Aday L. Home care for ventilator-assisted children: Predicting family stress. Pediatr Nurs 1989 Jul–Aug; 15(4):371–376

Whitford KM. Health care needs of ventilator-dependent children. Pediatr Nurs 1988 May–Jun; 14(3):216–219

Cardiopulmonary Resuscitation

Brunette DD and Fischer R. Intravascular access in pediatric cardiac arrest. Am J Emerg Med 1988 Nov; 6(6):577–579

Carter JH. CPR: Breathing life back into a child. Nursing 1986 Oct; 16(10):52–57

Curley MAQ and Vaughan SM. Assessment and resuscitation of the pediatric patient. Crit Care Nurs 1987 May–Jun; 7(3):26–45

Fredrickson JM. Basic pediatric cardiopulmonary resuscitation (CPR) update. JEN 1988 Mar–Apr; 14(2):76–81

Goodwin BA. Pediatric resuscitation. Crit Care Nurs Q 1988 Mar; 10(4):69–79

Goodwin R. Critical care: Cardiopulmonary resuscitation in children. Nurs Times 1988 Aug 31–Sep 6; 84(35):48–51

Hazinski MF. New guidelines for pediatric and neonatal cardiopulmonary resuscitation and advanced life support. III: Neonatal advanced life support. Pediatr Nurs 1987 Jan–Feb; 13(1):57–59

Zaritsky A. Selected concepts and controversies in pediatric cardiopulmonary resuscitation. Crit Care Clin 1988 Oct; 4(4):735–754

Supporting Children Undergoing Procedures

Forlini J, Morin DM and Treacy S. Painless peds procedures. Am J Nurs 1987 Mar; 87(3):321–323

Gedaly–Duff V. Preparing young children for painful procedures. J Pediatr Nurs 1988 Jun; 3(3):169–179

Pridham KF, Adelson F and Hansen MF. Helping children deal with procedures in a clinic setting: A developmental approach. J Pediatr Nurs 1987 Feb; 2(1):13–22

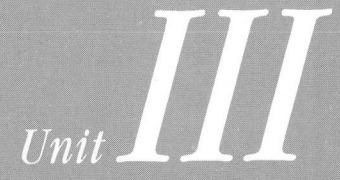

Nursing Care of Children With Specific Health Problems

Management of the Premature Infant

The *premature infant* is a viable infant born before the completion of 37 weeks' gestation.

A *low-birth-weight (LBW)* infant is one whose birth weight is 1501–2500 gm. (3 lbs. 5 oz.–5 lbs. 8 oz.) without regard to gestational age.

A *very low birth weight (VLBW)* infant is one whose birth weight is below 1500 gm. without regard to gestational age.

Etiology

1. Unknown
2. Maternal factors associated with prematurity:
   a. Chronic poor nutrition
   b. Diabetes
   c. Multiple births
   d. Drug abuse
   e. (IUD) in gravid uterus
   f. Chronic disease
      (1) Heart disease
      (2) Kidney disease
      (3) Infection
   g. Complications of pregnancy
      (1) Pre-eclampsia–eclampsia
      (2) Bleeding
      (3) Placenta previa or abruptio placentae
      (4) Incompetent cervix
      (5) Premature rupture of membranes
      (6) Polyhydramnios
      (7) Chorioamnionitis
   h. Multigravida under 18 years of age; primigravida over 35 years of age
   i. Idiopathic premature labor
3. Fetal factors associated with prematurity:
   a. Chromosomal abnormalities
   b. Anatomic abnormalities
      (1) Tracheoesophageal atresia or fistula
      (2) Intestinal obstruction
   c. Fetoplacental unit dysfunction

Altered Physiology

The premature infant has altered physiology due to immature and often poorly developed systems. The severity of any problem that occurs depends on the gestational age of the infant.

A. Respiratory System*

1. Alveoli begin to form at 26–28 weeks' gestation; therefore, lungs are poorly developed.
2. Respiratory muscles are poorly developed.
3. Chest wall lacks stability.
4. Production of surfactant is reduced.
5. There is reduced compliance and low functional residual capacity of the lung.
6. Breathing may be labored and irregular with periods of apnea and cyanosis.
7. Infant is prone to atelectasis.
8. Gag and cough reflexes are poor; thus, aspiration may be a problem.

B. Digestive System*

1. The stomach is small, and vomiting is likely to occur because of poor muscle tone at the cardiac sphincter. It is difficult to provide caloric requirement in early days.
2. Tolerance is decreased related to decreased enzymes.
3. Lacks bile salts that aid digestion of fats and absorption of vitamin D and other fat-soluble vitamins.
4. Limited ability to convert glucose to glycogen and break down glycogen to glucose.
5. Limited and immature ability to release insulin in response to glucose.
6. Lacks coordinated sucking–swallowing reflex before 32–34 weeks' gestational age. Immature esophageal motility.

C. Poor Thermal Stability*

1. Has very little subcutaneous fat; thus, there is no heat storage or insulation; poor glycogen and lipid stores.
2. Limited ability to shiver; has poor vasomotor control of blood flow to skin capillaries.
3. There is a relatively large surface area in comparison to body weight.
4. Sweat glands are decreased; infant cannot perspire under 32 weeks' gestation.
5. Has reduced muscle and fat deposits that restrict metabolic rate and heat production.
   Brown fat is deposited after 28 weeks' gestation in adipose tissue around axillae, kidneys, scapula, neck, and adrenal glands.

---

* Systems and situations that are most likely to cause problems in the premature infant.

6. Usually is less active.
7. Posture flaccid—increasing surface area exposed.

D. Renal Function

1. Sodium excretion is probably increased, which may lead to hyponatremia; there is difficulty in excreting potassium.
2. Ability to concentrate urine decreases; thus, when vomiting or diarrhea occurs, dehydration is likely to follow. Decreased ability to conserve or excrete fluid.
3. Ability to acidify urine decreases.
4. Glomerular tubular imbalance accounts for sugar, protein, amino acids, and sodium present in urine.

E. Nervous System

1. Response to stimulation is slow.
2. Suck, swallow, and gag reflexes are poor; feeding and possible aspiration, therefore, are problems.
3. Cough reflex is weak or absent.
4. Centers that control respirations, temperature, and other vital functions are poorly developed.

F. Infection* (see p. 1251, Septicemia Neonatorum)

1. Actively formed antibodies are lacking at birth (active immunity).
2. No IgM is present at birth.
3. Limited chemotaxis (reaction of cell to chemical stimuli).
4. Decreased opsonization (preparation of cells for phagocytosis).
5. Limited phagocytosis (digestion of bacteria by cells).
6. Hypofunctioning adrenal gland contributes to a decreased anti-inflammatory response.

G. Liver Function

1. Does not have good ability to handle and conjugate bilirubin.
2. Does not store or release sugar well; thus, there is a tendency toward hypoglycemia.
3. There is a steady decrease in hemoglobin after birth and in the production of blood; therefore, anemia may occur.
4. Does not make or store vitamin K; thus, infant is susceptible to hemorrhagic disease.

H. Eyes

1. Oxygen may cause retinal arteries to constrict, resulting in anoxic damage.
2. The retinae detach from the surface of posterior chambers, and a fibrous mass forms, resulting in an inability to receive visual stimulation. This is *retrolental fibroplasia* (RLF).
3. There are many stages of RLF.
4. The exact amount and level of oxygen needed to produce RLF is unknown. An infant under 1000 gm. is at high risk for RLF. It is also related to sepsis, transfusions, chronic disease, hypoxia, etc.

I. Skin

1. Sensitive because of permeability and collagen instability.
2. Decreased cohesion between epidermis and dermis.
3. Decreased thickness of stratus corneum (outer layer of epidermis).
4. Delayed skin pH recovery to acidity following washing with alkaline-base soap, creams, and emollients.

* Systems and situations that are most likely to cause problems in the premature infant.

5. Increased risk of toxicity from topical application and percutaneous absorption of drugs and substances.

Complications in Premature Infants

1. The severity of any problem that occurs in the premature infant depends on the gestational age of that infant.
   a. Hyaline membrane disease (respiratory distress syndrome)
   b. Aspiration
   c. Infection
   d. Hypoglycemia
   e. Hypocalcemia
   f. Patent ductus arteriosus
   g. Apnea
   h. Feeding intolerance
   i. Intracranial hemorrhage
   j. Hyperbilirubinemia
2. Major complications related to low-birth-weight infants include:
   a. Hypoxia, hyperoxia
   b. Hypoglycemia, hyperglycemia
   c. Difficulty feeding with malnutrition
   d. Dehydration
   e. Chronic lung disease—bronchopulmonary dysplasia
   f. Retrolental fibroplasia
   g. Hearing loss
   h. Psychological and behavioral problems
   i. Psychomotor retardation

Clinical Manifestations

1. Physical appearance
   Hair—lanugo, fluffy
   Poor ear cartilage
   Skin—very thin; capillaries are visible (may be red and wrinkled)
   Lack of subcutaneous fat
   Sole of foot is smooth
       (36 weeks' gestation—anterior ⅓ of foot is creased)
       (38 weeks' gestation—⅔ of foot is creased)
   Breast buds 5 mm.
       (36 weeks' gestation—none)
       (38 weeks' gestation—3 mm.)
   Testes—undescended
   Labia minora—undeveloped
   Rugae of scrotum—very fine
   Fingernails—soft
   Abdomen—relative large
   Thorax—relatively small
   Head—appears disproportionately large
   Facies resembles "an old man"
   Muscle tone poor—reflexes weak
2. Generally, maturation and growth rate increase after birth.

Assessment

A. Accurate Body Measurements (Fig. 48-1)—including:

1. Head circumference—frontal–occipital circumference (FOC) one finger above eyebrows, using parallel lines of tape around head.
2. Chest circumference—at nipple line.

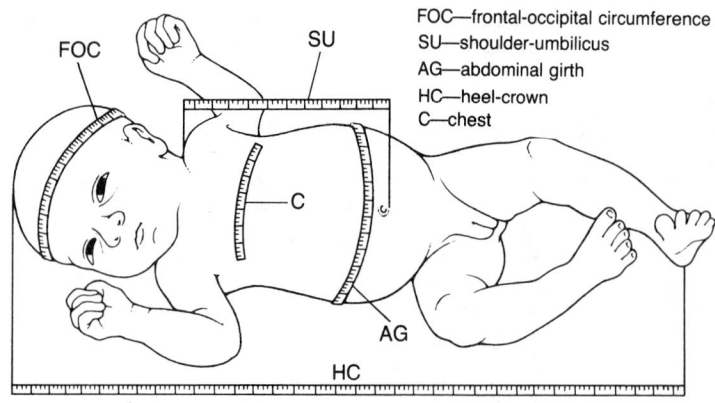

FOC—frontal-occipital circumference
SU—shoulder-umbilicus
AG—abdominal girth
HC—heel-crown
C—chest

Figure 48-1. *Infant measurements. (Adapted from Levin DC, Morriss FC and Moore GC. A Practical Guide to Pediatric Intensive Care. St. Louis, CV Mosby)*

3. Abdominal girth—one finger above umbilicus, mark location.
4. Heel–crown—used to calculate nasotracheal tube length.
5. Shoulder to umbilicus—used to calculate proper length of catheter for umbilical arterial catheter placement.
6. Weight

B. Assessment to Determine Gestational Age (Table 48-1)

Ballard scoring system (recommended by Committee of Fetus and Newborn of American Academy of Pediatrics): Observation of physical and neurologic characteristics that change predictably with growth and maturation. Ideally done at 1–2 hours after birth and repeated after 48 hours of life.

1. Physical assessment of maturity (i.e., sole creasing, presence of lanugo, skin transparency)
2. Neurologic assessment
   a. Maturation of the nervous system progresses at its own pace, and its rate is not increased by birth.
   b. The value of a neurologic evaluation increases after 48 hours of life.
   c. This examination is used primarily to estimate the infant's gestational age.
   d. The examination should be done when the infant is awake and quiet.
   e. Examination includes evaluation of muscle tone and evaluation of reflexes and reactions.
   f. In the LBW infant, the physical criteria may be more accurate than the neurologic criteria, which can be affected by birth trauma and breech delivery, chronic stress, maternal hypertension, or chronic malnutrition that can accelerate neurologic development; inaccurate for infant under 28 weeks' gestation.
3. Assessment for appropriateness of size for gestational age—Colorado Intrauterine Growth Chart acknowledges that maturation is based on age, not size.
   a. Once weight, length, head circumference, and gestational age have been determined, these criteria are plotted on the intrauterine growth curve to determine if the infant is small, appropriate, or large for his gestational age.
   b. This knowledge will aid in anticipating potential problems that may occur in the infant.
   c. Brazelton Neonatal Assessment Scale—can assist in identifying interactive capabilities of the infant and in assessing the impact of these capabilities

on the parents. Use of this information can enhance parent–infant interactions and relationships. Tool used from 3–30 days of age on full-term infant.
   d. Adjusted or corrected age:
      Once the infant reaches term (40 weeks after conception), his chronologic age is adjusted for prematurity by taking gestational age minus 40 plus chronologic age = developmental or corrected age; this is the age the infant would have been if he had been born at 40 weeks' gestation.
   e. Laboratory data as appropriate:
      (1) Blood gases
      (2) Blood sugar or Dextrostix
      (3) CBC or Hb and Hct
      (4) Lecithin/sphingomyelin ratio (L/S ratio) assessment of lung maturity
      (5) Electrolytes
      (6) Bilirubin
      (7) Calcium, potassium
      (8) Albumin

Potential Problems and Nursing Diagnoses

1. Potential complications related to immature development of systems: Respiratory distress, apnea, aspiration, hypoglycemia, intracranial hemorrhage, hyperbilirubinemia, fluid and electrolyte imbalance, altered cardiac status (patent ductus arteriosus), hypocalcemia, and hyponatremia
2. Sensory perception alteration related to hospitalization and altered nurturing activities
3. Infiltrated intravenous infusions
4. Potential for infection
5. Potential impaired skin integrity
6. Breastfeeding, ineffective
7. Nutrition, altered, less than body requirements
8. Hypothermia
9. Alteration in parenting activities and parent–infant bonding related to illness, parental feelings, hospitalization and separation
10. Parental anxiety related to lack of understanding of infant's condition; infant's small size and physical appearance; presence of tubes, monitors, and other equipment

Expected Outcomes

1. Premature infant progresses to wellness with no or minimal complications; respirations within expected

range; gaining weight; demonstrates thermal stability; absence of infection, jaundice, etc.
2. Responds to auditory, visual, and tactile input; stroking, cuddling, verbal stimulation, and eye contact
3. Absence of injury and complications from treatment protocols
4. Parents demonstrate appropriate parent–infant bonding; interact with the infant; maintain eye contact while feeding
5. Parents demonstrate diminishing anxiety, make frequent visits to the nursery to see the infant, participate in care, handle the infant gently and firmly

Admission to the Nursery

Nursing Interventions

A. Observe for any Gross Abnormalities as in the Case of a Full-Term Infant on Admission, and Pay Special Attention to Respirations, Heart Rate, Blood Pressure, Muscle Tone, and Activity

1. Respirations above 40/minute over a period of time may be indicative of respiratory difficulty.
   a. Expiratory grunting, retractions, chest lag, or nasal flaring should be reported immediately (Retractions chart, Fig. 48-2).
   b. Cyanosis (other than acrocyanosis—coldness and cyanosis of hands and feet) should be watched for along with other signs of respiratory distress.
2. Increased (above 180/minute) or irregular heart rate may indicate cardiac or circulatory difficulties.
3. Muscle tone and activity should be evaluated.
4. Hypotension, indicated by blood pressure measurement, may be due to hypovolemia.

B. Maintain a Patent Airway

1. Have oxygen, suction, and resuscitation equipment readily available.

2. Suction mouth and pharynx if mucus is present—to prevent aspiration. Premature infants often have an excess amount of mucus as well as poor cough, swallow, and gag reflexes.
3. Position infant in Isolette or radiant heater to allow for easy drainage of mucus from his mouth.
   a. Very small premature infants—place on side.
   b. Larger premature infants—place on abdomen.
   c. Head may be tilted down—this may be contraindicated because of increased intracranial pressure or increased respiratory distress due to liver pushing against diaphragm decreasing lung expansion, especially in the asphyxiated infant.
4. Obtain blood gas values.
5. Administer emergency oxygen to just barely relieve cyanosis.

C. Provide and Maintain Thermal Neutrality of the Premature Infant

1. Obtain weight and temperature; then attach cardiac monitor leads quickly and place infant in warm environment (Isolette, radiant heater). Omit bath until infant's temperature has stabilized.
2. The premature infant's ability to control his own body temperature is inhibited by many factors related to his immaturity (see p. 1220).

D. Ensure That Prophylactic Measures Have Been Administered Against Ophthalmia Neonatorum and That Vitamin K_1 has Been Administered

Since the premature infant is frequently taken from the delivery room as soon as possible after birth, prophylactic measures may have been omitted.

E. Be Aware of Early Complications That May Arise as a Result of Complications of the Pregnancy, Labor, or Delivery

1. Maternal medication
   a. Drugs pass quickly from mother's blood, across the placenta into the infant's blood.

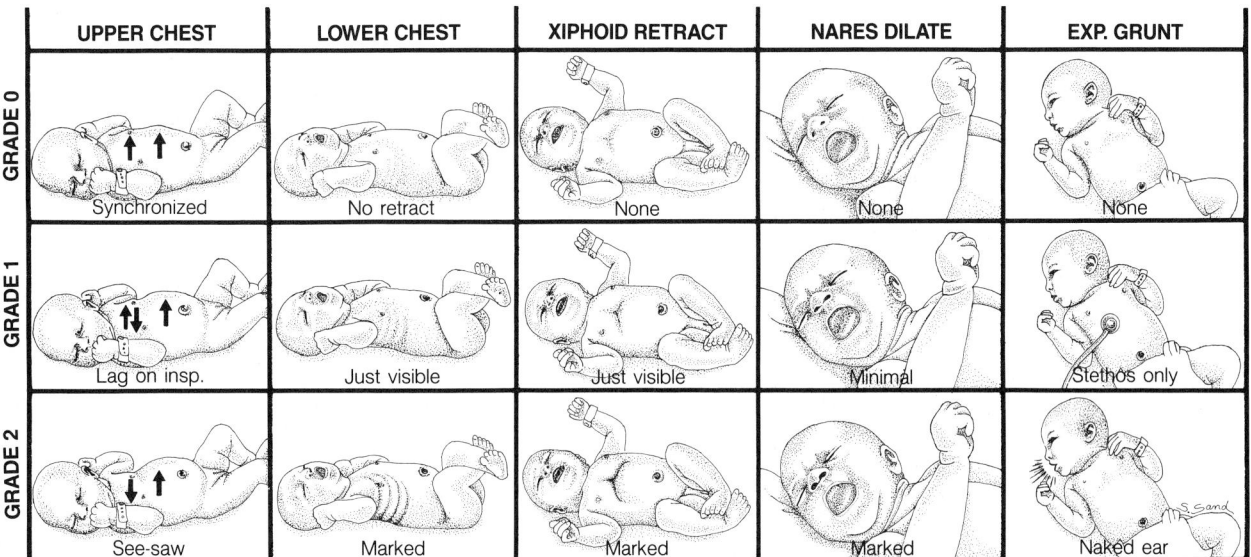

	UPPER CHEST	LOWER CHEST	XIPHOID RETRACT	NARES DILATE	EXP. GRUNT
GRADE 0	Synchronized	No retract	None	None	None
GRADE 1	Lag on insp.	Just visible	Just visible	Minimal	Stethos only
GRADE 2	See-saw	Marked	Marked	Marked	Naked ear

Figure 48-2. *Observation of retractions. An index of respiratory distress is determined by grading each of five arbitrary criteria. Grade 0 indicates no difficulty; grade 1 indicates moderate difficulty; and grade 2 indicates maximum respiratory difficulty. The retraction score is the sum of these values; a total score of 0 indicates no dyspnea, whereas a total score of 10 denotes maximal respiratory distress.*

Table 48-1. *Clinical Estimation of Gestational Age*

Examination First Hours

PHYSICAL FINDINGS		20–23	24–26	27–29	30–32	33–35	36–37	38–39	40–41	42–44	45–48
Vernix		Appears	Covers body, thick layer					On back, scalp, in creases	Scant, in creases	No vernix	Scant, in creases
Breast tissue and areola			Areola and nipple barely visible, no palpable breast tissue			Areola raised	1–2 mm nodule	3–5 mm	5–6 mm / 7–10 mm	?12 mm	
Ear	Form	Flat, shapeless				Beginning incurving superior	Incurving upper 2/3 pinnae	Well-defined incurving to lobe			
	Cartilage	Pinna soft, stays folded			Cartilage scant, returns slowly from folding		Thin cartilage, springs back from folding	Thin cartilage, springs back from folding	Pinna firm, remains erect from head		
Sole creases		Smooth soles without creases				1–2 anterior creases	2–3 anterior creases	Creases anterior 2/3 sole	Creases involving heel	Deeper creases over entire sole	
Skin	Thickness & appearance	Thin, translucent skin, plethoric, venules over abdomen, edema				Smooth, thicker, no edema		Few vessels	Some desquamation pale pink	Thick, pale, desquamation over entire body	
	Nail plates	Appear		Nails to finger tips						Nails extend well beyond finger tips	
Hair		Appears on head	Eye brows and lashes	Fine, woolly, bunches out from head				Silky, single strands, lays flat		?Receding hairline or loss of baby hair, short, fine underneath	
Lanugo		Covers entire body				Vanishes from face		Present on shoulders		No lanugo	
Genitalia	Testes			Testes palpable in inguinal canal				In upper scrotum	In lower scrotum		
	Scrotum			Few rugae			Rugae, anterior portion		Rugae cover	Pendulous	
	Labia & clitoris			Prominent clitoris, labia majora small, widely separated		Prominent clitoris, labia majora small, widely separated	Labia majora larger, nearly cover clitoris		Labia minora and clitoris covered		
Skull firmness		Bones are soft		Soft to 1″ from anterior fontanelle		Spongy at edges of fontanelle, center firm		Bones hard, sutures easily displaced		Bones hard, cannot be displaced	
Posture	Resting	Hypotonic, lateral decubitus	Hypotonic		Beginning flexion, thigh	Stronger hip flexion	Frog-like	Flexion, all limbs	Hypertonic	Very hypertonic	
	Recoil - leg	No recoil					Partial recoil		Prompt recoil		
	Arm	No recoil				Begin flexion, no recoil		Prompt recoil, may be inhibited		Prompt recoil after 30″ inhibition	

Confirmatory Neurologic Examination To Be Done After 24 Hours

Weeks Gestation: 20 21 22 23 24 25 26 27 28 29 30 31 32 33 34 35 36 37 38 39 40 41 42 43 44 45 46 47 48

Category	Physical Findings	Progression (by weeks gestation)
Tone	Heel to ear	No resistance (~26) → Some resistance (~30) → Impossible (~35)
	Scarf sign	No resistance (~21) → Elbow passes midline (~31) → Elbow at midline (~37) → Elbow does not reach midline (~44)
	Neck flexors (head lag)	Absent (~21) → Head in plane of body (~40) → Holds head (~44)
	Neck extensors	Head begins to right itself from flexed position (~34) → Good righting cannot hold it (~37) → Holds head few seconds (~39) → Keeps head in line with trunk >40″ (~42) → Turns head from side to side (~45)
	Body extensors	Straightening of legs (~34) → Straightening of trunk (~37) → Straightening of head and trunk together (~43)
	Vertical positions	When held under arms, body slips through hands (~29) → Arms hold baby, legs extended? (~35) → Legs flexed, good support with arms (~38) → Head above back (~44)
	Horizontal positions	Hypotonic, arms and legs straight (~29) → Arms and legs flexed (~37) → Head and back even, flexed extremities (~40)
Flexion angles	Popliteal	No resistance (~21) → $150°$ (~28) → $110°$ (~33) → $100°$ (~35) → $90°$ (~39) → $80°$ (~41)
	Ankle	$45°$ (~33) → $20°$ (~37) → $0°$ (~41); A pre-term who has reached 40 weeks still has a $40°$ angle
	Wrist (square window)	$90°$ (~29) → $60°$ (~33) → $45°$ (~37) → $30°$ (~39) → $0°$ (~41)
Reflexes	Sucking	Weak, not synchronized with swallowing (~27) → Stronger, synchronized (~33) → Perfect (~35)
	Rooting	Long latency period slow, imperfect (~27) → Hand to mouth (~31) → Brisk, complete, durable (~36) → Perfect, hand to mouth (~39) → Complete (~44)
	Grasp	Finger grasp is good, strength is poor (~27) → Stronger (~33) → Can lift baby off bed, involves arms (~39) → Hands open (~46)
	Moro	Barely apparent (~22) → Weak, not elicited every time (~27) → Stronger (~34) → Complete with arm extension, open fingers, cry (~35) → Arm adduction added (~39) → ?Begins to lose Moro (~46)
	Crossed extension	Flexion and extension in a random, purposeless pattern (~27) → Extension, no adduction (~33) → Still incomplete (~36) → Extension, adduction, fanning of toes (~40) → Complete (~44)
	Automatic walk	Minimal (~31) → Begins tiptoeing, good support on sole (~33) → Fast tiptoeing (~37) → Heel-toe progression, whole sole of foot (~40) → A pre-term who has reached 40 weeks walks on toes (~45) → ?Begins to lose automatic walk (~47)
	Pupillary reflex	Absent (~21) → Appears (~30)
	Glabellar tap	Absent (~21) → Appears (~33)
	Tonic neck reflex	Absent (~21) → Appears (~29)
	Neck-righting	Absent (~21) → Appears (~35) → Present after 37 weeks

(Reproduced with permission from Kempe CH, Silver HK and O'Brien D (eds). Current Pediatric Diagnosis and Treatment. 4th ed. Los Altos, Lange Medical Publications)

b. Infant may be drowsy and have slowed respirations.

c. Because of poor development, respiratory difficulty may occur.

2. Blood incompatibility of mother and infant
   a. Premature infant is more susceptible to jaundice, even without incompatibilities.
   b. Observe closely for early signs of jaundice (see p. 1244, Hyperbilirubinemia).

3. Maternal conditions that may predispose to infant problems.
   a. Infection or illness
   b. Diabetes
   c. Drugs

4. Perinatal asphyxia
   a. Apgar score of less than 5 at 1 minute and less than 7 at 5 minutes
   b. *Asphyxia* is lack of oxygen.
      Secondary problems:
      (1) Hypoxia (reduced oxygen available)
      (2) Anoxia (total lack of oxygen)
      (3) Hypercapnia (inability to eliminate CO_2)
      (4) Acidosis
      (5) Hypotension
      (6) Hypoglycemia
   c. Causes of asphyxia or hypoxia can originate in the mother, the placenta, or the infant, or may be a result of the delivery.

The First 24–48 Hours of Life

This period after birth is the most critical time for the premature infant.

Nursing Assessment

A. Be Constantly Aware of the Infant's Condition and Make Frequent Observations

1. This poorly developed, immature infant is prone to sudden and rapid changes in condition.

2. Early recognition of symptoms and reporting observations to the physician are the most valuable contributions the nurse can make in caring for and saving the premature infant's life.

3. Note bleeding from the umbilical cord.
   a. Should bleeding occur, apply pressure.
   b. Estimate amount of bleeding and record.
   c. Notify the physician immediately—replacement transfusion may be necessary.

4. Note first voiding.
   a. This may occur up to 36 hours after birth, but it usually occurs within the first 24 hours. Report any 4–6-hour period when voiding does not occur.
   b. Note amount, color, and frequency of voidings; 2–3 ml./kg./hour; specific gravity 1.003–1.010.
   c. Lack of voiding may indicate renal system anomalies, shock, or poor circulation.

5. Note stools.
   a. Note when first stool occurred and its characteristics.
   b. Abdominal distention and lack of stool may indicate intestinal obstruction or other intestinal tract anomalies. Measure abdominal girth at regular intervals.

6. Note activity and behavior.
   a. Note amount of lethargy or activity or need for stimulation.

b. Look for sucking movement, hand-to-mouth maneuver. This can help to determine oral feeding initiation.

c. Note quality of cry.

7. Observe for a tense and bulging fontanelle; feel suture lines noting separation or overriding.
   a. Full fontanelle may indicate intracranial hemorrhage.
   b. Be alert to twitching and seizures.
   c. Intracranial pressure monitor for fontanelle pressure may be used.

8. Note color of skin.
   a. Cyanosis
      (1) Circulatory or cardiac difficulties may be present.
      (2) Respiratory effort may be ineffective.
   b. Jaundice may indicate:
      (1) Infection
      (2) Enclosed hemorrhage; bruising

9. Carefully monitor, record, and report vital signs.

Nursing Interventions to Maintain Respirations

A. Emergency Measures

1. Immediate emergency support may be necessary, since respiratory system is poorly developed and ability to control respirations is often barely sufficient.

2. Have available resuscitative equipment, oxygen, and suction apparatus.
   a. Mucus may not be handled well, because of poor gag, cough, and swallowing reflexes.
      (1) Clearing the airway is of major importance.
      (2) A rubber ear bulb syringe is often all that is necessary for clearing the mouth.
      (3) Frequent suctioning of the pharynx may not be necessary.

B. Positioning

1. Position infant to allow for easy ventilation.

2. Supine position permits free expansion of the thoracic cage (infant's body weight is on the chest and abdomen when he is prone).

3. Elevate head and trunk to decrease pressure on diaphragm from abdominal organs.

4. Slight neck extension affords opening of trachea; place small roll under shoulders.

5. Do not constrict abdominal area, since abdominal muscles are used to aid respiratory effort.

6. Flex and abduct arms to enhance chest expansion.

7. Change position from side to side. Perform postural drainage every 2 hours to aid in draining fluid accumulation in thoracic cavity.

C. Oxygen Therapy

1. Use only the percentage of oxygen necessary to maintain appropriate blood gas values.

2. Oxygen is used with moisture to prevent mucous membranes from drying and becoming irritated.

3. Monitor oxygen with analyzer every hour to ensure consistency in percentage used.

4. Transcutaneous PO_2 monitor may be used ($TcPO_2$)—values should correlate with blood gases.
   a. Ensure that site of probe is changed every 2–6 hours; probe placement is on chest, abdomen, back (depending on size of infant).
   b. Monitor is calibrated according to manufacturer's directions.
   c. Complication of transcutaneous monitor probe is

in a skin reaction: red marks at site of electrode placement; burn.

    d. Skin can be protected by spraying a thin layer of copolymer acrylic dressing (Op-site) on area where probe is to be placed, allowing to dry before applying probe. Be sure to remove dressing after use to prevent build-up.

5. Pulse oximeter correlates well with oxygenation (O_2 saturation of arterial hemoglobin) of the blood.

    a. The sensor probe wraps around the infant's hand or foot; it is not heated or adherent.

    b. It displays changes in oxygenation instantaneously.

    c. It is most sensitive to hypoxemia, less accurate to hyeroxemia.

D. Ongoing Monitoring

1. Note any changes in respiratory effort and report these to the physician.

    a. Note quality and rate particularly.

    b. Use retractions score for continual, consistent assessment of the respiratory status (see Fig. 48-2).

    c. Hyaline membrane disease or respiratory distress syndrome occurs during the first 24 hours of life. Observe for and report immediately any signs and symptoms of respiratory difficulty:

        (1) Increased respiratory rate (usually above 60/minute)

        (2) Thoracic retractions

        (3) Nasal flaring

        (4) Cyanosis

        (5) Expiratory grunting

        (6) Developing exhaustion

        (7) Periods of apnea

2. Hypoxemia is associated with birth asphyxia and recurrent apneic episodes. Serum PaO_2 less than 40 mm. Hg.

3. Hypoventilation—tendency to retain CO_2 because of irregular breathing, poor respiratory muscle activity, and flexible thoracic cage. PCO_2 greater than 50 mm. Hg.

E. Periodic Breathing Versus Apneic Episodes

1. *Periodic breathing*—regular repetition of breathing pauses of less than 10-second duration alternating with breaths of regularly increasing and then decreasing amplitude for 10–15 seconds.

2. *Apneic episodes*

    a. Nonbreathing periods of more than 20-second duration may be accompanied by bradycardia (heart rate below 100) and cyanosis; related to immature respiratory center. Infant is hypotonic and unresponsive.

    b. Stimulation or resuscitation is required to restart breathing and increase heart rate.

F. Apnea

1. Provocative conditions that increase apneic spells include:

Hyperthermia, hypothermia
Hypoglycemia
Hypocalcemia
Acidosis
Hyperbilirubinemia
CNS disease—intraventricular hemorrhage
Pulmonary insufficiency
Infection
Patent ductus arteriosus (PDA)
Sodium disturbances

Hypoxemia
Congenital anomalies
Gastroesophageal reflux
Pneumonia/sepsis
Respiratory distress syndrome (RDS)
Low hematocrit
Airway obstruction

2. Apnea may cause hypoxemia (decreased oxygen in blood) leading to hypoxia (decreased oxygen in tissues), which may result in complications (i.e., intracranial hemorrhage, PDA, atelectasis and hypoglycemia).

3. Theophylline or aminophylline may be given to reduce the frequency of apneic episodes.

    a. The drug acts centrally by increasing the respiratory center activity and increasing the infant's sensitivity to CO_2.

    b. Is a CNS stimulant that improves the respiratory drive and rate and $PaCO_2$ sensitivity.

4. *Nursing management* following administration of pharmacotherapy.

    a. Observe for tachycardia (heart rate of 180–190/min)—cardiac contractility, cardiac output, and stroke volume increase with this drug.

    b. Monitor serial weights, urine output, and serum electrolytes because of mild diuretic action and increased sodium loss; strict intake and output.

    c. Check urine Chemstix and glucose—serum glucose levels increase along with early rise in insulin. The LBW infant is at risk for hyperglycemia.

    d. When given orally, medication should be given with feeding to reduce gastric side effects, even though the absorption time may be slower.

    e. Administer intravenously over 20–30 minutes to prevent acute toxic reaction.

    f. Monitor the quality of respirations—decreased apnea, improved breath sounds, decreased wheezing.

    g. The metabolism rate of the drug may be changed by the presence of infection or other drugs.

    h. Note appearance of side effects

        Tachycardia

        Gastrointestinal irritability—vomiting, restlessness, agitation, sleeplessness

    i. Toxic effects

        Pronounced manifestation of side effects
            Prolonged diuresis; hypotension; cardiac tachycardia, dysrythmias, tachypnea; respiratory arrest; hyperglycemia, ketonuria, glucosuria

    j. Gastroesophageal reflux may be exaggerated when theophylline is used.

    k. Waterbed or tactile stimulation schedule every hour may help decrease frequency of apnea.

    l. Keep infant's temperature close to the low range of the thermal neutral zone.

Other Nursing Interventions

A. Conserve the Infant's Energy While Providing Necessary Care

1. Be organized in caring for the infant.

    Collect all equipment before starting care, do what needs to be done, and then let the infant rest. Infant's position will affect his ability to rest.

2. Premature infants tire very easily.

    a. Any activity increases oxygen need, thus increasing respiratory rate, taxing already limited energy.

Holding the infant, suctioning, linen change, chest physical therapy, repositioning often cause significant lowering of PaO_2. Recovery to adequate PaO_2 depends upon the drop in PaO_2.

b. Watch TcO_2 monitor—stop procedure if necessary or possible if TcO_2 levels fall.

c. Adjust the infant's environment so that rest and sleep are not hindered—decreases the risk of causing hypoxia.

d. Interventions must be evaluated for their relative value versus the trauma they entail.

B. Provide and Maintain Thermal Neutrality of the Premature Infant

1. Maintain infant's temperature at the thermoneutral zone (i.e., at the environmental temperature in which the resting infant maintains normal body temperature and still utilizes minimum energy–oxygen consumption and calories).

   a. Infant's core temperature (rectal temperature) should be maintained at 36.5–37.2°C. (98.6°F.). Axillary and abdominal skin temperature should be 36.0–36.8°C. (96.8–97.2°F.).

   b. Keep environmental (ambient) temperature ranges from 32°–35.5°C. (89.6–95.0°F.). Smaller premature infants may need higher temperature, 35°C. (95°F.); larger premature infants, around 32°C. (89.6°F.).

      Generally, ambient temperature is 1°–1.5°C. warmer than abdominal skin temperature; thus oxygen consumption is minimal.

2. Be aware that the infant loses heat by radiation, conduction, convection, and evaporation; thus, the nurse must be alert to conditions that influence heat loss or gain by the infant.

   a. Note location of warming unit in relation to air conditioners, direct sunlight, and drafts. Move the unit, if necessary.

   b. Minimize porthole entrance activities into Isolette; keep portholes tightly closed when they are not in use or tightly fitting around arm when entering Isolette.

   c. Infant should be undressed to allow direct body contact with warm air.

   d. To minimize heat loss by radiation, consider the possibility of partially lining the Isolette with foil, being careful not to obstruct view of infant. Covering infant from shoulders to feet with a plastic (kitchen plastic material) bubble may also aid in maintaining a stable temperature. Commercial products are also available.

3. Avoid constant or drastic changing of temperature-control dial (decreases risk of missing infection).

   a. If ambient temperature rises, skin and core temperature of the infant will rise resulting in increased metabolic rate and insensible water loss. The infant may exhibit weight loss, abdominal distention, regurgitation of feeding, and irritability.

   b. Decrease in ambient temperature will result in a decrease of the infant's skin temperature and an increase in metabolic rate in an attempt to increase heat production. Skin temperature reflects thermal stress first.

      (1) If the infant cannot compensate for the increased heat loss, his body temperature will drop.

(2) Hypothermia results in tachycardia, hypoglycemia, metabolic acidosis, apnea, and inactivity.

4. Skin temperature probe should be placed on the trunk of the infant rather than extremities which are more susceptible to changes in peripheral circulation.

   a. Prevent the infant from lying on thermistor.

   b. Cover skin probe with a heat-reflecting material (foil) to decrease influence of ambient temperature on sensor.

   c. Skin receptors are sensitive to environmental temperature. When stimulated by cold, norepinephrine is released into brown fat, which in turn leads to lipolysis and brown fat oxidation. Heat is released into the circulating blood—this is nonshivering thermogenesis.

5. Monitor both the infant's temperature and Isolette or radiant warmer temperature. Temperature-control centers are poorly developed in the premature infant, and his temperature is easily influenced by his environment. Hypermetabolic state and inadequate peripheral circulation predispose the premature infant to hyperthermia. Infant must be naked. When caring for the premature infant under the radiant warmer:

   a. Use white linen to increase efficiency of the unit.

   b. Monitor temperature every 30–60 minutes to determine specific temperature needed to keep the infant at correct temperature. Start unit setting at 37°–37.5°C. and adjust slowly. Increase temperature only 0.5°C. per hour (1.5°C. warmer than skin temperature) until the infant's temperature is stable. Then monitor every 1–4 hours.

   c. Keep alarm for overheating in operation.

   d. Be aware of the complications associated with the use of radiant warmer:

      (1) Overheating—increase in the infant's oxygen consumption

      (2) Flash burns—avoid oil on the infant's skin

      (3) Cataracts—observe closure of eye lids

      (4) Excess drying of skin and tissue breakdown

6. When assessing temperature regulation of the premature infant, consider the following:

   a. Note if the infant's body or extremities are cool to touch—possibly due to underheated incubator or heat loss from radiation.

   b. Note activity—restlessness or hyperactivity may indicate inappropriate temperature for comfort.

   c. Be aware of reasons for increased temperature of infant—overheated incubator, early sign of illness, incorrect placement of sensor.

   d. Be aware of causes for drop in temperature of infant—underheated incubator, infection, faulty sensor-skin contact from feces or bony prominence, vasoconstriction, iatrogenic (cold O_2).

7. When humidity is increased in the incubator, it will reduce infant heat loss and insensible water loss.

8. Avoid measuring rectal temperature.

   a. Stimulates defecation, resulting in fluid and caloric loss.

   b. Rectal perforation—at a depth of 3 cm., infant's colon changes from an anterior to posterior angle.

   c. Axillary temperature reflects heat/cold stress sooner than rectal, which is the core temperature, and decreases after the skin temperature drops. Generally there is less disturbance of the infant when taking an axillary temperature.

9. Insensible water loss is increased with use of radiant warmer by evaporation. Monitor fluid volume, urine

output, and specific gravity. Transcutaneous fluid loss can be reduced by stretching a layer of plastic wrap over but not touching the infant.

10. Rocker bed and tactile and auditory stimulation may contribute to maintaining thermal neutrality in the infant.

C. Prevent Infection in This Very Susceptible Premature Infant

1. The premature infant is particularly susceptible to viral, fungal, and gram-negative and gram-positive bacterial infections. Septicemia, meningitis, and urinary tract infections are a constant hazard postnatally.
2. Specific techniques should be employed to ensure the control of infection (see pp. 1252–1254).
    a. Scrupulous handwashing must be practiced by all personnel handling the infant and entering the nursery.
    b. Use gown and mask technique as prescribed by the health agency. Short-sleeved gowns allow for proper handwashing up to the elbows.
    c. Minimize the infant's contact with unsterile equipment; equipment should be individualized.
    d. Minimize the number of persons who come in contact with the infant.
    e. Exclude from nursery any person who is febrile, has draining lesions, or has acute respiratory or gastrointestinal infections.

> **NURSING ALERT:** Routine use of hexachlorophene for infant bathing is to be avoided. Data indicate a marked association between its use and neuropathologic lesions.

3. Early symptoms of infection may include (see p. 1252):
    a. Hypothermia or hyperthermia
    b. Jaundice
    c. Lethargy
    d. Poor eating
    e. Apneic spells
4. Factors predisposing to infection
    a. Maternal infection
    b. Difficult and prolonged labor
    c. Prolonged rupture of membranes
    d. Manipulative measures—resuscitation, umbilical catheterization, surgery

D. Maintain Fluid Balance

1. Monitor fluid intake and output and urine specific gravity.
2. Increased fluid may result in pulmonary edema, congestive heart failure, and 2nd-degree PDA, and may increase risk of bronchopulmonary dysplasia (BPD) and possibly intraventricular hemorrhage.
3. Too little fluid may lead to dehydration, hypotension, acidosis, or electrolyte imbalance.

E. Provide Appropriate Skin Care to Protect Skin Integrity

1. Skin provides important functions: protects internal organs; intact skin provides protection against foreign substances and organisms, helps regulate body temperature, stores fats, discharges electrolytes and water, and provides for tactile stimulation.
2. Specific techniques should be employed to ensure skin integrity.
    a. Avoid use of alkaline-base soaps which may cause alteration of skin pH (acid pH skin surface provides bacteriocidal quality).

    b. Increased permeability and large surface area put infant at risk of toxicity from topical application of drugs, lotions, etc.
    c. Lubrication of dry, flaky skin is not recommended. If cracking or fissures occur, a thin layer of non-perfumed emollient may be used.
    d. Avoid the use of adhesive—epidermis may be pulled off upon removal, increasing the risk of infection.
    e. Remove adhesive substances with cotton balls soaked in water or soapy solution while gently pulling edges back, or use commercial adhesive remover with care and rinse skin with clear water following use.
    f. Evaluate skin-care techniques used (e.g., tincture of Benzoin, Hollihesive, Op-site, Skin-gel).
    g. Zinc deficiencies may result in skin breakdown, especially around the mouth, buttocks, fingers, toes, and creases.

F. Prevent Nonintentional Cranial Deformity ("preemie head")

1. Premature infants develop dolichocephalic head shape, which is a flattened calvorium without rounded shape (convexity) at the temporal/parietal area that is longer from front to back than it is broad. This occurs as a result of head positioning from side to side on a firm mattress.
2. Preventive measures include:
    Water mattress
    Donut-shaped head pillow
    Turn head every 2 hours including supine with occiput resting on bed
    Upright infant seat
    Hold infant as much as possible

G. Protect the Infant's Eyes From Injury

1. Protect eyes from too much light, especially when eyes are dilated.
    a. During procedures and from bright sunlight
    b. Intensive light may contribute to RLF or other retinal damage.
2. Corneas need protection when the infant's eyes remain open, (i.e., when the infant is receiving Pavulon).

Complications

A. Hypoglycemia

1. Hypoglycemia—serum sugar levels are less than 40 mg./100 ml.; whole blood level, 20 mg./100 ml., under 30 mg./100 ml. if infant under 3 days of age.
2. Hypoglycemia is most likely to occur in first 12 hours after birth and as late as 48 hours after birth.
3. Hypoglycemia is likely to occur in the premature infant because of the reduced glycogen storage he has at birth and his limited carbohydrate tolerance.
4. *Symptoms* are nonspecific. Many infants with clinical hypoglycemia may be asymptomatic.
    a. Jitteriness
    b. Tachypnea or apnea
    c. Lethargy, listlessness
    d. Cyanosis
    e. Convulsions
    f. High-pitched or weak cry
    g. Pallor
    h. Temperature instability
    i. Sweating
    j. Tachycardia
    k. Poor feeding

5. *Predisposing factors*
   a. Infant of diabetic mother—2–72 hours
   b. Erythroblastosis fetalis—4–72 hours
   c. Sepsis
   d. Intrauterine malnutrition—2 hours–1 week
   e. Development defects
   f. Asphyxia
   g. Respiratory distress
   h. Hypothermia
6. Blood sugar levels should be accurately monitored. Dextrostix screening can be done by the nurse.
   a. When a blood specimen is collected, ideally a capillary tube should be used to prevent the reactive tip from coming in contact with the skin, which may give a false reading.
   b. Specimen should remain on reactive tip for 60 seconds, then forcefully rinsed with clear running water.
   When Dextrostix* values are below 40 mg./dl., a blood glucose should be done. Chemstrip bG† and Dextrometer should be used when available for more accurate values.
   c. Check urine for excess levels of sugar.
7. *Treatment* is to increase blood sugar intake by oral feeding or intravenously. If IV glucose is given too rapidly, hyperglycemia may occur because of poor insulin response. Maintain blood sugar at greater than 45 mg./100 ml.

B. Hyperglycemia

1. Hyperglycemia (blood sugar above 125 mg./dl.) is not uncommon in the infant weighing less than 1000 gm.
2. This infant often requires use of insulin to ensure adequate calories and has reduced ability to absorb adequate amounts.
3. Hyperglycemia and resultant glycosuria lead to dehydration secondary to osmotic diuresis.

C. Hypocalcemia

1. Hypocalcemia—serum calcium levels are less than 7 mg./100 ml. (3.5 mEq./liter).
2. Low blood calcium is reached the first day of life.
3. *Symptoms* are nonspecific:
   a. Twitching
   b. Convulsions (late sign)
   c. Hypotonia
   d. Lethargy
   e. High-pitched cry
   f. Increased apneic spells
   g. Abdominal distention with ileus
4. Hypocalcemia occurs in the premature infant because of reduced calcium storage at birth and reduced ability to absorb adequate amounts
5. Predisposing factors
   a. Hypoglycemia
   b. Previous maternal abortion
   c. Low infant Apgar rating—asphyxia
   d. Hyaline membrane disease
   e. Lack of intake
   f. Treatment of acidosis with bicarbonate
   g. Decreased renal capacity for phosphorus excretion
6. Try to maintain serum calcium above 8 mg./100 ml.
7. *Treatment* is to give calcium intravenously or orally.

---

* Dextrostix: Ames Laboratory, Elkhart, IN 46514

† Chemstrip: Bio-Dynamics, 9115 Hague Road, Indianapolis, IN 46250

Intravenous calcium given too rapidly will cause bradycardia.

D. Hypoxia or Anoxia at Birth

1. The degree of asphyxia is judged immediately after delivery by Apgar scores and blood gas changes.
2. Specific problems to be anticipated include:
   a. Hyaline membrane disease
   b. Profound acidosis
   c. Hypoglycemia
   d. Abnormal clotting function
   e. Hyperbilirubinemia
   f. Apneic episodes
   g. Poor temperature control
   h. Intracranial hemorrhage
   i. Cardiac failure

E. Patent Ductus Arteriosus (PDA)

1. PDA occurs frequently in premature infants with respiratory distress syndrome and in less mature infants (24–30 weeks' gestation) with associated congestive pulmonary failure.
2. A majority of very low birth weight infants recovering from respiratory distress syndrome develop serious signs of this disease.
3. The preterm infant is at risk for left-to-right shunting of blood through the patent ductus.
4. *Clinical signs*
   a. Bounding peripheral pulses
   b. Chest retractions with mild cyanosis
   c. Diminished breath sounds on auscultation
   d. Moist crackles
   e. Elevated PCO_2
   f. Apneic periods
   g. Systolic murmur—clicking sound, low-pitched, coarse, rumbling murmur, mid and late systolic, left sternal border, intensity increases during pauses in breathing.
   h. Tachypnea
   i. Deterioration of general condition
   j. Inability to wean from ventilator
5. Medical Treatment:
   a. Fluid restriction, maintenance of normal blood *p*H, oxygen as needed, maintenance of adequate hemoglobin levels, digitalization, when congestive heart failure is present, diuretics, indomethacin for closure.
   b. Blood transfusion to maintain normal hemoglobin (12 g./dl.)
   c. When indomethacin is used, the nurse should observe for diminished urine output, azotemia, and creatinemia. Contraindications: if the infant has bilirubin levels greater than 10 mg. (drug binds to albumin), bleeding tendencies (may alter platelet formation), renal problems, or necrotizing enterocolitis.
6. Surgical
   1. Ligation of ductus arteriosus
   2. Complications: pneumothorax, pleural effusion, nerve injury
7. Spontaneous closure of the PDA in the premature infant is likely to occur 2–6 weeks after birth.

F. Sodium Disturbances

1. Hypernatremia
   a. Serum sodium level above 150 mEq./liter; generally occurs because of inadequate hydration

and/or insensible water loss or overuse of Na-HCO$_3$ for acidosis.

   b. Hypernatremia occurs frequently in the very low birth weight infant regardless of sodium intake.

2. Hyponatremia—serum sodium level below 125–130 mEq./liter is generally secondary to loss of sodium in urine and inadequate intake.

G. Intracranial Hemorrhage (most likely to occur in sick premature infants)

1. Intracranial hemorrhage is a common cause of death in extremely premature infants.

2. Factors predisposing infant to CNS bleeding
   a. Immaturity
   b. Respiratory distress syndrome
   c. Hypoxia in fetus or neonate
   d. Pneumothorax or any air leak
   e. Hypercapnia
   f. Acidosis
   g. Sudden rise in blood pressure
   h. Administration of sodium bicarbonate, rapid blood volume expansion, PDA, disturbances in hemostasis.

3. *Clinical signs*
Signs may be slow and subtle in appearance, or sudden, catastrophic neurologic deterioration may take place.
   a. Labored respirations
   b. Hypoventilation
   c. Cyanosis
   d. Apnea
   e. High-pitched cry
   f. Convulsions
   g. Bulging fontanelle
   h. Clinical deterioration; shock-like appearance

4. *Classification*—describes location of hemorrhage and size of ventricles
   a. Grade I—subependymal, germinal matrix hemorrhage
   b. Grade II—intraventricular extension, no ventricular dilatation
   c. Grade III—intraventricular extension with ventricular dilatation
   d. Grade IV—intraventricular hemorrhage and intraparenchymal hemorrhage

5. Intracranial hemorrhage occurs more frequently in the preterm under 1500 gm. and 35 weeks' gestation. Generally occurs 1–7 days after birth with a peak at 12–36 hours.

6. *Prevention* of intraventricular hemorrhage is the best treatment, because once bleeding begins, it is difficult to control.
   a. Keep the infant adequately oxygenated. Prevent asphyxia and hypercapnia.
Stabilize PaO$_2$ early (low PaO$_2$ increases risks).
   b. Maintain thermoneutral environment.
   c. Maintain normal acid–base balance.
   d. Maintain normal blood volume
   e. Avoid fluctuations of arterial and venous blood pressure.

H. Hypertension

1. Hypertension may occur in infants with a history of indwelling artery catheter, patent ductus arteriosus, or perinatal hypoxia. These conditions put infant at risk for renal artery thrombosis and hypertension.

2. *Signs*
   a. Increasing blood pressure and considerable fluctuation in blood pressure

   b. Tachypnea and cyanosis
   c. Lethargy
   d. Tremors
   e. Apnea

3. *Treatment*
Diuretics and/or antihypertensive medications

I. Hypotension—indicative of hypovolemia, sepsis, abdominal or intracranial hemorrhage, shock

J. Hypothermia—cold stress

1. Temperature instability in the premature infant may result in hypothermia. Cold stress results when norepinephrine is released to activate brown fat metabolism (nonshivering thermogenesis).

2. This hypermetabolic state requires increased oxygen and calories in the already compromised infant.

3. By-products of brown fat metabolism are heat production and acidosis from ketones and lactic acid. Hypoglycemia also occurs because of rapid depletion of stored glucose.

4. As this state continues, the infant is at risk for apnea, intracranial hemorrhage, acidosis, and hypoglycemia.

K. Hyperthermia

1. Results when the infant attempts to dissipate heat.

2. Skin vessels dilate, metabolic rate increases, oxygen and caloric consumption increases, and respiratory effort is increased.

3. The infant is at risk for intracranial hemorrhage.

L. Retinopathy of Prematurity (ROP) (retrolental fibroplasia)

1. ROP is ocular underdevelopment resulting from interruption of the normal progression of newly forming retinal vessels.

2. Usually a state of hyperoxia is associated with retinal changes.

3. However, many other factors also seem to be associated with the disease such as extreme prematurity, low birth weight (especially <1000 gm.), apnea, sepsis, hypercapnia, hypocapnia, vitamin E deficiency, IVH, anemia, hypoxia, lactic acidosis, bright lights, exchange transfusion, PDA and indomethacin, and maternal complications.
   a. Newly developed capillaries constrict permanently and become necrotic, resulting in vaso-obliteration.
   b. Remaining normal vessels go through a phase of vasoproliferation in an attempt to reestablish retinal circulation.
   c. These new vessels may extend into the vitreous, causing leakage or hemorrhage.
   d. Fibrosis occurs; scar tissue shrinks and causes tension on the retina, resulting in detachment of retina.
   e. In most cases, reversal of this process is possible before fibrosis occurs. In severe cases or advanced stages, permanent blindness may occur.

4. *International classification of ROP*
   a. Describes staging of active disease based on description of location of disease on retina, extent of vasculature involved, and grading of disease
   b. Stage I—a thin line of demarcation develops between vascularized region of retina and avascular zone.
   c. Stage II—line develops into a ridge protruding into vitreous where there is histologic evidence of arteriovenous shunt.

d. Stage III—extraretinal fibrovascular proliferation with the ridge; neovascular areas may be noted posterior to ridge.

e. Stage IV—fibrosis and scarring as vascularization extends into vitreous with traction on the retina resulting in detached retina.

5. *Diagnosis*—made by ophthalmologic examination at 6–8 weeks of age and repeat examinations every 2–3 weeks until disease shows resolution, or every 3–4 weeks in absence of disease until retina is mature.

6. Nursing must use continuous with judicious monitoring and administration of oxygen, monitor FiO_2 as well as SaO_2 and blood gases. Be particularly aware of hyperoxia.

a. When eye drops are administered for dilation, this can be stressful to the infant, causing increase in blood pressure, bradycardia, and apnea from vagal stimulation due to pressure on the globe of the eye. The infant's eyes may become reddened with swollen lids.

b. Strive to decrease light intensity, particularly around infants at risk for ROP.

c. Vitamin E administration for ROP is controversial. Should it be ordered, serum levels should be monitored.

7. *Treatment*—consists of attempting to prevent long-term sequela, i.e., blindness.

a. Laser therapy—reattaches gaping or detached retina.

b. Cryotherapy—freezing of selected retinal tissue in an attempt to prevent abnormal vasoproliferation.

c. Cryotherapy and sclera buckling—involves encircling the globe of the eye with a band that reduces eye diameter and increases the chance of retinal reattachment.

8. Parents need to be aware of the risks relating to ROP. Help them understand the disease, why examinations need to be repeated, the reason their infant has red, swollen eyes.

M. Iatrogenic Complications

Procedures performed on the preterm infant to assist him through the clinical course may result in additional problems related to noise, tape altering skin integrity, radiation exposure, burns, intravenous infiltration with tissue sloughing, sensory deprivation, etc.

N. Psychosocial Support

1. Offer support to the parents of the premature infant during this crucial period.

2. Most parents, particularly mothers, are physically and emotionally unprepared for the early arrival of their baby.

3. Allow the parents to see their infant and touch him if this is feasible, and they are able to cope with doing so.

4. Listen to the parents talk and express their concerns. Encourage them, but do not give them false hope.

a. Assess where they are in their grief, in coping, and in accepting their infant.

b. Be alert to the father who may be overwhelmed with concern for the infant and mother (who also is hospitalized) and who may not know how to help or meet the needs of the mother at this time. Provide appropriate support.

c. Refer to social worker as necessary.

5. If this pregnancy occurred outside of marriage, the premature birth may precipitate other feelings of guilt or punishment in the parents. The parents may need help in identifying and working through these feelings in order to progress towards a healthier attitude.

Preparing Infant for Transport

A. Anticipatory Consideration

1. Assist in the preparation of the neonate for transport to another institution/regional perinatal center.

2. Anticipation and early decision to transport a sick neonate to a regional center should be made before the infant deteriorates critically. Conditions that may require transport: LBW <1500 gm., severe asphyxia, RDS, sepsis/meningitis, metabolic abnormalities, multiple congenital anomalies, surgical emergencies.

3. The infant's condition must be stabilized before transport. The more stable the infant at the time of transport, the more favorable the outcome.

B. Nursing Responsibilities

1. Continuous observation and assessment. Obtain initial vital signs immediately.

   Initiate procedures for assessment—electronic cardiopulmonary monitoring, thermal warming equipment, etc.

2. Assist in respiratory support and oxygenation.

a. Suction mouth, nasopharynx (trachea)—use bulb syringe, DeLee mucus trap, or mechanical suction as appropriate.

b. Maintain airway—artificial ventilation by bag and mask or endotracheal tube.

c. Position for optimal air exchange.

d. Ventilator assistance: continuous positive airway pressure (CPAP), positive pressure

3. Establish and maintain thermal neutrality. This is CRITICAL—overhead radiant warmer, Isolette, heat lamp, chemically heated mattress; have heated transport unit in delivery room, heated blankets.

4. Assist in establishment of IV access—immediate access is essential in preventing dehydration, acidosis, and hypoglycemia, and for providing a route for medications and calories.

a. Almost always $D_{10}W$ infusion is started. D_5W might be used in the VLBW infant whose glucose tolerance is low and electrolyte free because of minimal urine output and serum sodium and potassium rise after birth.

b. Provide necessary equipment: IV catheters, scalp vein needles, microdrip set-up, volumetric infusion pump, record sheet.

c. Veins in the dorsum or scalp are used. Umbilical venous catheter may also be used. Ensure that line is securely taped.

5. Assist in diagnostic procedures: obtaining specimens, positioning infant for x-rays.

a. Screen for hypoglycemia with Dextrostix or Chemstrip.

b. Urine specific gravity, pH, etc.

6. Nasogastric tube placement. Use No. 5 or 8 French orogastric tube. Enables removal of gastric secretions and stomach decompression.

7. Assess circulatory status—check pulses, blood pressure, capillary refil, skin color. Apical pulse should be auscultated for rate, rhythm, and quality.

8. Ensure that routine measures are done:

a. Eye prophylaxis

b. Vitamin K administered

9. Help prepare the family for the transfer of their infant.
   a. Gently answer questions.
   b. Take a picture of the infant, which will be given to the mother.
   c. Facilitate the process of the mother seeing and touching her infant prior to transfer.
   d. Following the transfer, provide support to the mother who may be feeling very frightened and lonely. Encourage her to establish phone contact with the unit to which the infant has transferred.
   e. Don't forget the father who is experiencing concern for both mother and infant.
10. Accurate and descriptive charting is essential to assist the transporting team.

The Growing or Older Premature Infant

Complications

After the first few days have passed without any complications, the premature infant is very busy growing. During this time, however, it must be remembered that other complications can occur. Be constantly alert to signs and symptoms of complications. The areas of concern mentioned above are still important, along with the following:

A. Aspiration

1. The growing premature infant may still have poor gag and cough reflexes.
2. The premature infant will show signs of respiratory distress.
   Suction mouth and pharynx immediately and get medical assistance.

B. Latent Acidosis of Prematurity (developing after 3 days of life). This is less common when new infant formulas are used.

1. Metabolic acidosis occurring during first few weeks (*p*H and bicarbonate or base excess drops) is associated with immaturity of the kidneys and is unrelated to major cardiovascular or respiratory problems.
   a. Infant may hyperventilate to blow off excess CO_2.
   b. Urine *p*H varies from 6.0–7.5; blood *p*H ranges from 7.25–7.30 with base deficit.
2. *Symptoms*
   a. Infant begins to feed poorly and takes longer to eat. He is sleepy and needs stimulation to keep awake; he displays lethargy.
   b. The infant shows increased frequency and severity of apneic spells.
   c. The infant may remain vigorous and take adequate fluid and calories, yet fail to gain weight.
   d. Inadequate weight gain or loss when there is large caloric intake.
   e. Stools become watery.
   f. Skin may take on a gray pallor.
3. *Treatment*—consists of replacing bicarbonate lost through excretion and adjusting the intake via formula to decrease in amount of protein load and total calories.

C. Fluid Retention

1. Abnormal fluid retention results from the infant's inability to excrete solutes or to excrete water.
2. *Symptoms*
   a. Excessive weight gain
   b. Pitting edema of feet, then body
   c. Chest retractions

   d. Inspired air diminished on auscultation with possible crackles
   e. Increase in oxygen need; increase in PCO_2
3. *Treatment*—consists of giving diuretic agent and possibly decreasing fluid intake.
4. *Predisposing factors* that lead to fluid retention include:
   a. Patent ductus arteriosus with borderline heart failure
   b. Bronchopulmonary dysplasia
   c. Low total serum proteins

D. Wilson–Mikity Syndrome

1. Chronic form of respiratory distress. Infant may or may not have had respiratory distress syndrome.
2. *Insidious symptoms*
   a. Gradual increase in chest retractions
   b. Decrease in inspired air on auscultation
   c. Slowly increasing need for oxygen to about 30%–40%
   d. Characteristic streaky pattern of lungs, progressing to soap-bubble appearance on x-ray

E. Hyperbilirubinemia (see p. 1244)

1. Bilirubin concentrations are generally higher in the premature infant because of the impaired ability to conjugate bile in the liver.
2. If infant is bruised from delivery or is plethoric, the risk of hyperbilirubinemia is increased.
3. Hypoproteinemia and acidemia increase risk of low bilirubin kernicterus.

F. Necrotizing Enterocolitis (NEC)

1. A disease of the neonate, particularly the premature, that is multifactorial of uncertain etiology; the immature intestine reacts to injury and mucosal damage resulting in patches of necrotic mucosa and intramural gas.
2. *Possible risk factors*
   a. Hypoxic–ischemic asphyxia, RDS, umbilical catheterization, exchange transfusion, shock, PDA, congenital heart disease, polycythemia, thrombocytopenia, anemia
   b. Feeding—hypertonic formula, hypertonic medication, medication toxicity, overfeeding, early feeding, nonbreast milk feeding, nasojejunal feeding, milk allergy
   c. Pathogens—rotavirus type A and non-type A, coronavirus, anaerobic bacteria, new enteric pathogens
   d. Prematurity and low birth weight
   e. 10% to 30% of the infants that develop NEC have no identifiable risk factors other than being premature.
3. *Signs and symptoms*
   a. Onset of symptoms occurs between 1–14 days of life, most often between 3–7 days of life
   b. Can occur several weeks after birth and may recur.
   c. May present as benign gastrointestinal abnormality with mild abdominal distention and increased gastric residual volumes.
      Nonspecific signs include apnea/bradycardia, acidosis, lethargy, temperature instability, cyanosis, jaundice, decreased urine output with increased specific gravity.
   d. *Rapid onset*—marked abdominal distention and tenderness, frank and occult blood in stool, bilious emesis, gastric aspirates in larger volumes, abdominal wall erythema, right lower quadrant mass, diarrhea, signs of peritonitis, shock.

e. *X-ray findings* show pneumatosis intestinalis—appears as cystic lesions in a linear pattern along outside of bowel in varying lengths, usually along the terminal ileum and proximal colon. Hepatic portal venous gas appears as gas within the portal venous system of the liver.

4. *Diagnostic work-up*
   a. Electrolytes
   b. Platelet count
   c. Bleeding times
   d. Blood gases
   e. Bilirubin
   f. Blood sugar
   g. X-ray of abdomen
   h. Cultures to determine causative agent, if any.
   i. Liver ultrasonogram
   j. Breath hydrogen excretion analysis

5. *Supportive treatment*
   a. Gastric decompression with nasogastric tube; NPO
   b. Antibiotic therapy—intravenously and orally to treat sepsis
   c. IV hyperalimentation, intralipids
   d. Fluids and electrolyte balance
   e. Proper thermal and environmental factors
   f. Respiratory support
   g. Surgery—resection of gangrenous bowel

6. *Prevention*
   a. Caution with enteral feeding; NPO first week of life; introduce and advance feedings slowly.
   b. Use iso-osmolar milk at start of feedings; MCT may be added for calories.
   c. Feed via nasogastric or orogastric tube to allow amount of gastric residual to be monitored.
   d. Prevent gastric distention from high-volume feedings.
   e. Monitor abdominal girth.
   f. Check stool for reducing substance (sugar).
   g. Breast milk may be used, since it contains living macrophages that combat infection, has a high *p*H which inhibits growth of *E. coli, Shigella,* and yeasts, and contents limit growth of *E. coli* and *Salmonella,* and has a high content of IgA which may protect against intestinal infection.
   h. Enteral antibiotics to combat proliferation of intestinal bacteria resulting from feeding (controversial).
   i. Good handwashing and infection control

7. *Nursing responsibilities*
   a. Acute, constant observations—place the infant in an Isolette or a radiant warmer.
   b. Close monitoring of vital signs and general condition; report even minute changes in the infant.
      (1) Stop oral feeding.
      (2) Abdominal girth measurement; note distention or rigidity, redness or shininess, erythema, observable bowel loops.
      (3) Check bowel sounds with stethoscope with minimal abdominal palpation.
      (4) Check stools for occult blood and reducing substance; save specimen as appropriate for examination by physician.
   c. Prevent additional stress to infant by maintaining stability in environment, IV intake, and gastric decompression.
   d. Minimize handling and trauma to abdomen—x-rays may be taken frequently to evaluate status. Place the infant in a supine position; undress to decrease pressure on abdomen.
   e. Do not take rectal temperatures.

f. Provide meticulous skin care when diarrhea and vomiting are present.
g. Prevent dehydration and electrolyte imbalance by monitoring fluids.
h. Prevent acute respiratory distress with positioning, temperature control, etc.

G. Bronchopulmonary Dysplasia (BPD)

1. Chronic lung disorder characterized by coarse cystic-appearing lungs with hyperinfiltration, obstructive bronchiolitis, and pulmonary fibrosis from respiratory distress syndrome with high concentrations of oxygen and positive-pressure ventilation.

2. Other factors associated with BPD include:
   a. Endotracheal tube
   b. Patent ductus arteriosus
   c. Pulmonary edema from increased fluid loads in first days of life
   d. Smaller premature infant with severe respiratory distress syndrome

3. *Signs and symptoms*
   a. Tachycardia
   b. Difficulty weaning from oxygen or ventilator
   c. Respiratory distress
   d. Cyanosis
   e. CO_2 retention
   f. Increased apnea
   g. Pulmonary hypertension; right heart failure
   h. Generalized edema associated with low serum protein

4. *Treatment*—supportive
   a. Respiratory support—O_2, ventilator
   b. Sodium-free albumin
   c. Diuretics and digitalization as indicated
   d. Maintain nutritional support and fluid and electrolyte balance.
   e. Vitamin E—may help protect retina and lungs from toxic effects of oxygen, although this has not been proved.

5. *Nursing responsibilities*
   a. Support respiratory effort with gentle airway suctioning, chest physical therapy, and positioning.
   b. Observe and record frequency of persistent apnea, cyanotic episodes, tachypnea, retractions, and crackles.
   c. Allow infant to rest during feeding regardless of method used (nipple or gavage). He will tire easily and respond with apnea.
   d. Exercise constant vigilance to avoid respiratory infection in the infant, which could lead to death.
   e. Help to maintain a meaningful parent-infant relationship through the long duration of treatment.

Providing Adequate Nutrition

A. Growth and Development Considerations

1. The growth rate of the premature infant should parallel the expected in utero growth rate: about 20 gm./24 hours after 30 weeks' gestation and 30 gm./24 hours as the infant approaches term.
   a. From birth to 5–10 days of age there will be a 5%–10% weight loss; then the infant should begin to gain weight.
   b. The smaller the infant, the greater the percentage of weight loss.

B. Caloric Needs

1. The premature infant has a small gastric capacity but a great need for calories.

2. 110–140 Kcal./kg./24 hours (40%–45% of total calorie intake) should be provided by carbohydrates
3. Caloric intake is dependent on age and birthweight of the premature infant. RDS and metabolic stress may also require caloric manipulation

> 120–150 ml./kg./24 hours of fluid
> 70 ml./kg./24 hours at birth
> 100 ml./kg./24 hours at 1 week
> 140–150 ml./kg./24 hours at 2 weeks
> This, however, depends on the size of the infant.
> 2–4 gm. protein/kg./24 hours

C. Gastric Capacity

1. If more than 4 gm./kg./24 hours of protein is given, the premature infant may present with signs of acidosis, azotemia, and other problems leading to neurologic abnormalities.
2. Generally, the premature infant (except the very low birth weight infant) has adequate gastric capacity, intestinal motility, and absorption to tolerate small, frequent feedings.
3. The gastric capacity expands during the first few weeks of life; this enables the infant to tolerate larger feedings.
4. Overfeeding increases the risk of vomiting. Vomiting can lead to dehydration, loss of hydrochloric acid, alkalosis, and aspiration.
5. The premature infant regurgitates feedings easily because of poor muscle tone at the cardiac sphincter. Expect small amount after feeding, especially with burping.
6. Bubble the infant frequently during feeding.
7. Formula should be adequate in calories, fluid, electrolytes, iron, and vitamins to meet the needs of the infant.

D. Considerations for Enteral Feeding

1. *Breast milk of the preterm-delivered mother*
   a. Appears to have higher protein and mineral content than milk from the term-delivered mother; provides protein and fat that is more easily metabolized and provides immunologic and anti-infective factors.
   b. Is low in calcium and phosphorus and has a low renal solute load. Supplemental vitamins are always given.
   c. Human milk fortifiers are also sometimes given.
   d. Involve mother in planning for breast milk feeding.
   e. Avoid breast milk if mother is taking certain drugs: chlorammphenicol, tetracycline, metronidazole, sulfonamide, some anticoagulants, anticancer agents, antithyroid drugs, Diazepam, meprobamate, recreational drugs.
2. Special premature formulas are available that provide appropriate concentrations of protein, CHO, sodium, and phosphorus with an osmolality of 300 mOsm./kg./water.
3. Diluted formula should be used for early feedings to decrease stress and test the infant's tolerance.
4. Vitamins E and D may be supplemented, as well as calcium for the low-birth-weight infant.
5. Zinc is also given.

E. Inappropriate Weight Gain—in relation to caloric intake can indicate problems.

1. Unusually large weight gain for caloric intake may indicate excessive fluid retention.
2. No weight gain or a loss with adequate caloric intake may indicate acidosis, sepsis, or malabsorption.

F. Other Measures

1. Allow the infant to rest prior to feeding. The premature infant tires easily from procedures and will eat better if rested.
2. Gavage is indicated for very small premature infant who does not demonstrate good sucking or synchronized sucking and swallowing. Diarrhea may result from malabsorption if feeding is advanced too rapidly.
3. Pacifier sucking (non-nutritive) during feeding may decrease feeding time, stimulate gastric motor function, and reduce gastric retention, thus facilitating digestive process.
4. Dropper or nipple feeding is indicated for a vigorous premature infant with good suck, gag, and swallowing reflexes.
5. Breast-feeding might be considered when the infant is ≧1300 gm.
6. Consider demand feeding for the growing premature above 1800 gm and over 5 days of age. Use cues from the infant regarding his sleep–wake cycle.
7. Constant drip feeding may be best for the very low birth weight or chronically ill infant.

G. Anemia

1. Hemoglobin less than 8–10 gm./100 ml.
2. Reasons
   a. Total body iron content is less.
   b. There is a proportionally larger blood loss from sampling.
   c. Relative body growth is more rapid, and there is an expanding blood volume.
3. Supplemental iron is needed to supply new iron stores. The iron is generally started when the infant is 2 months of age.
   Folic acid and vitamin B_{12} may also be supplemented.
4. Blood transfusions are indicated to replace sampling blood in the sick preterm infant. Keep accurate records of blood output.
5. Symptomatic O_2 deficiency with anemia may present as minimal weight gain, decreased activity, temperature instability, poor feeding, apnea, tachycardia, tachypnea, PDA, pallor, or poor perfusion.

Psychosocial Interventions

A. Meet the Psychological Needs of the Premature Infant, Who Is an Individual in His Own Right

1. At first, even though handling is minimal, the nurse should talk to and caress the infant while performing procedures.
   a. Stroking and gentle handling will provide necessary sensory stimulation, especially after feeding.
   b. A pacifier can be used during feeding if the infant is fed by gavage.
   c. A soft musical sound may also be comforting.
2. Once the premature infant is able to leave the Isolette even for short periods of time, he should be held for feedings.
   a. Carefully observe the infant to learn his reactions and tolerance to stress.
   b. While holding him, stroke him and talk to him.
   c. Keep him warmly wrapped; this will also give him a feeling of security.
3. If the infant is restless in his incubator, he may be calmed by propping him against a blanket or diaper roll.
   The freedom of movement, restrained only by the mattress, cannot offer much security to the infant.

4. Remember that the infant's ability to hear, see, smell, and touch are intact. Give him the opportunities to develop these capabilities and encourage the development of his interaction potential by providing sensory input.
   a. Use the infant's cues to initiate visual and auditory stimulation.
   b. Recognize signs of infant stress and respond appropriately: Changes in vital signs, reflex withdrawal, crying, irritability, grimacing, frowning, gagging, spitting up, finger splaying, and arching.
   c. Positive signs include infant sounds, tongue extension, finger folding, sucking, grasping.
   d. Be aware of noxious environmental stresses: lighting, temperature of unit and Isolette, noise level, kinesthetic factors, tactile and visual stimuli. Seek to reduce these extraneous stimuli.
5. Physical contact is important for a sense of security.
   a. Arrange environment so eye-to-eye contact can be established between caretaker or mother and infant.
   b. Allow the infant freedom of movement for self-stimulation.
   c. Change the infant's position and location of Isolette to encourage him to see his environment. Avoid sudden position changes; be slow and gentle. Avoid bumping into the Isolette.
   d. Encourage flexion
   e. Facilitate development of head control
   f. Increase social awareness
   g. Consider using waterbeds, propping with supports and special infant seats
   h. Involve physical and occupational therapy resources
6. Include parents in this activity to help them get to know their infant and incorporate these activities into their behavior so they will continue this at home.

B. Provide the Premature Infant With an Environment That Helps Him to Merge Successfully Into a State of Well-being and to Become a Healthy Growing Baby

1. Conserve his energy.
   a. Promote rest and sleep by the following:
      (1) Appropriate handling
      (2) Organizing and controlling interruptions
      (3) Proper positioning of infant
   b. Support physiologic functions and provide assistance as necessary (i.e., monitor respiration, temperature, and nutrition).
2. Assess stress of infant caused by medical procedures, response to stimuli and environment.
3. Change position every 2 hours. This does the following:
   a. Stimulates circulation
   b. Facilitates respirations
   c. Prevents stasis of accumulated secretions
   d. Minimizes skin irritation
   e. Provides infant with opportunity for different stimulation input
4. Provide for physical safety and comfort.
   a. Bathing—gives nurse opportunity to observe infant thoroughly.
   b. Protect infant from self-inflicted injury by own random movements.
   c. Protect from injury by equipment.
   d. Use protective devices as necessary but allow the infant some unrestricted self-stimulation.
   e. Keep portholes of Isolette closed.

f. Keep the infant warm when out of the Isolette—wrap with blanket and cover head with bonnet.

C. Foster Healthy Family Relationships With the Premature Baby

1. Encourage the parents to make frequent visits to the nursery so they can become familiar with all aspects of care of their infant.
   a. When they visit, explain the equipment and procedures that may be foreign to them.
   b. Help them to feel comfortable and confident in handling their infant.
   c. Parents may lose interest in the infant if the hospitalization is long. If parents cannot visit daily, encourage them to call, or call them at predetermined times.
   d. Involve parents in planning care for the infant.
   e. Give parents concrete suggestions as to how they can participate in the care of their infant.
   f. Encourage then to bring in appropriate clothing, toys, baby articles, mobiles, music boxes, etc.
2. Help the mother to see her infant as an individual and to develop mothering behaviors based on the infant's behavior.
   a. The infant's size and physical characteristics are generally unexpected and are different from those of the expected full-term baby.
   b. The premature infant's reflexes and responses to his environment are immature. The mother's expectations of his responses are based on those of a full-term baby.
   c. Explain these discrepancies between expectations and reality. The mother may associate her infant's responses with her inadequacies rather than those of the baby.
   d. Be aware of reflexes and responses that may elicit reactions in the mother. For example:
      (1) Uncoordinated sucking and swallowing—the mother experiences disappointment in not being able to feed, especially if she wanted to breast-feed her infant.
      (2) Gag reflex—the mother fears choking of the infant.
      (3) Respiratory immaturity—periodic breathing frightens the mother.
      (4) Grasp reflex—the mother is disappointed if her infant does not grasp her finger.
      (5) Moro reflex—exaggerated Moro reflex may make the mother feel she has frightened her infant.
   e. Reassure the mother that as the infant matures, he will change his response and reflex behaviors.
3. The support and help given to parents during hospitalization will make home care easier.
   a. Observe and assess behaviors as an aid to assessing attachment or bonding relationships and ability to relate to the infant.
   b. Teach the mother how to care for her infant. Thorough and careful preparation of the mother in feeding and caring for her infant often results in earlier discharge.
   c. The small size of the infant often is the single factor that frightens parents the most.
4. Family centered care should be integrated into the parent–newborn relationships. Allow and encourage sibling visitation as appropriate.
   a. Screen all children for communicable illness. They must not have a fever or upper resitatory tract infection.

b. Age-appropriate preparation of the siblings should be done in advance of the visit.

c. Provide appropriate coloring books and written material.

d. Visiting siblings should be supervised by parent or responsible adult.

5. Initiate community-nurse referral if the parents seem anxious about caring for their baby at home.

a. If this premature infant is the first baby, the referral may be particularly helpful to the mother.

b. Home follow-up will enable the nurse to assess family interactions, parenting behaviors, and infant developmental screening.

6. Encourage parents to talk about their feelings or fears concerning their infant and how they will care for him.

a. By listening, the nurse can gain some insight as to what to talk about or to teach the parents.

b. Parents' feelings can frequently interfere with appropriate home care.

c. Parents often treat the "preemie" as if he were fragile and more prone to illness. Overconcern is potentially harmful.

d. Parents worry about how to feed and protect the infant.

7. Help the family prepare for the time when their new baby will arrive home.

a. Because of the early, unexpected arrival of the infant, things such as clothing, bed, and bottles may not be ready.

b. If there are other children at home, they need to be prepared for the homecoming of the premature infant. This preparation should begin early—using, for example, pictures of the infant and conversations about him.

c. The readiness for the premature infant to go home is evaluated and assessed in terms of the following:
   (1) The infant's weight and progress
   (2) Maternal attachment to the infant
   (3) Maternal competence in caring for the infant

8. Consider transfer to community hospital once the infant is stable and growing.

9. Some regional centers have available to their families a transitional infant care facility. This provides a homelike environment that serves as a bridge between the neonatal intensive care unit (NICU) and home. When infants no longer need intensive care but are not quite ready to go home, the transitional unit offers the family a supportive environment where they can learn to become independent of the NICU. They assume care and planning of care of their infant.

Health Education

1. Help the family to understand that caring for the premature infant at home should not be any different from caring for a full-term infant.

a. Special treatment may lead to behavior problems later.

b. At first a little extra caution should be practiced. Cyanotic spells and severe infection are major concerns for the premature infant during first few weeks at home.
   (1) Keep room temperature fairly constant.
   (2) Sponge-bathe the infant instead of bathing in tub and keep him warm during procedure.
   (3) Feed the infant the recommended amount of formula to be certain he receives the necessary calories for continual growth. Maintain iron therapy.

(4) Keep the infant away from crowds and people who have colds.

2. Spend enough time with the mother teaching her how to feed and care for her infant.
Show her how, then watch her and help her improve and gain confidence.

a. The infant needs gentle, firm handling.

b. The infant needs to be mothered and kept comfortable with minimal tension.

c. A soothing voice can be comforting.

d. Sucking provides a pleasant experience.

3. Stress the importance of medical follow-up for the baby after discharge from the hospital.
Anemia and failure to thrive are common long-term side effects of prematurity.

4. Help mother understand the importance of good, early prenatal care for subsequent pregnancies.
Once a woman has had one premature infant, this classifies her as high-risk for another premature delivery with future pregnancies.

5. Discharge planning implemented long before discharge of the high-risk infant should include:

a. Assessing and reassessing needs of the infant

b. Assessing and reassessing needs of the caretaker

c. Establishing and implementing a teaching plan

d. Identifying and acquiring equipment needed at home

e. Initiating a community-agency referral as necessary

f. Verbalizing and demonstrating an understanding of teaching plan by caretaker

6. Discharge plans should include:

a. Follow-up phone call within 48 hours of discharge to assess how the mother and family are coping with the infant being home, etc.

b. Parenting classes that specifically address the premature infant and the parents.

c. Assist the parents in identifying and developing a support system within the community.

d. Nurse-facilitated parent discussion groups should be continued after discharge and be given at times and places that are accessible to parents.

e. Follow-up contact should be made at least 2 months and 1 year after discharge.

Small-for-Gestational-Age Infant

The *"small-for-gestational-age infant" (SGA)* is a newborn who shows a discrepancy between growth and gestational age or whose weight is 2 standard deviations below expected weight for duration of gestation, or is plotted below the 10th percentile on intrauterine growth chart.

Intrauterine growth retarded (IUGR) is used interchangeably with SGA.

Etiology

IUGR may be due to reduction of total number of cells in the body (hypoplastic), to a reduction in cell size (hypotrophic), or to both.

While the etiologic factors are unknown in many cases, other cases may result from the following causes.

A. Maternal Factors

1. Undernutrition

2. Diminished uterine blood flow
   a. Preeclampsia
   b. Toxemia

c. Chronic hypertensive vascular disease
  d. Diabetes mellitus
3. Small stature
4. Smoking
5. Inadequate prenatal care
6. Low socioeconomic class
7. Heart disease
8. Low maternal age
9. Primiparity
10. Grand multiparity
11. Low prepregnant weight
12. Substance abuse
13. Hemoglobinopathy (sickle cell disease)
14. Phenylketonuria

B. Environmental Factors

1. High altitude
2. Teratogens
3. Irradiation

C. Placental Lesions

1. Infarcts
2. Premature placental separation
3. Hemangiomas
4. Thrombosis of fetal vessels
5. Single umbilical artery
6. Avascular terminal villi
7. Twin-to-twin transfusion

D. Fetal Causes

1. Genetic dwarfs
2. Anencephaly
3. Infections (rubella, cytomegalovirus, toxoplasmosis, herpes simplex)
4. Chromosomal aberrations
    a. Turner's syndrome
    b. Down's syndrome
    c. Trisomy syndromes
    d. Cri-du-chat syndrome
5. Congenital anomalies
    a. Osteogenesis imperfecta
    b. De Lange's syndrome
    c. Cystic fibrosis
    d. Galactosemia
    e. Pierre Robin syndrome
    f. GI tract malformations
6. Cardiovascular abnormalies
7. Inborn errors of metabolism

Altered Physiology

Although, in general, the physiologic maturity of fetal organs develops according to gestational age, there are exceptions to organ maturation being consistent with gestational age that result in problems (conditions) associated with IUGR.

1. Poor glucose control
    a. Hyperglycemia related to severe intrauterine fetal growth retardation (IUGR).
        (1) Transient diabetes mellitus may be seen related to immaturity of insulin releasing mechanism and endogenous insulin levels are low. High glucose levels are found in the absence of ketones.
        (2) Symptoms include weight loss, dehydration, fever, and glucosuria.
    b. Hypoglycemia is probably due to rapid depletion of hepatic glycogen stores and to ineffective functioning of hepatic enzyme system responsible for gluconeogenesis.

2. Limited temperature control
    a. The infant has relatively large surface area per unit of body weight.
    b. The infant lacks energy stores and subcutaneous fat insulation; decreased brown fat stores.
    c. The infant can assume position of flexion of extremities—reduces surface area exposed to environment and decreased heat loss by radiation and convection.
    d. Has vasomotor control over peripheral circulation to dilate or constrict capillaries as needed.
    e. Sweating mechanism is intact.
3. High hemoglobin, increased plasma volume, and enlarged extracellular fluid volume per kilogram of body weight, putting the infant at risk for respiratory distress, cardiac and circulatory problems, and hyperbilirubinemia.
4. Minimal weight loss with rapid initial weight gain
    a. Weight gain is not maintained throughout first year.
    b. Rapid initial weight gain may suggest rehydration as well as tissue growth.
5. Late anemia
    Secondary to rapid weight gain and poor iron stores present at birth, especially in the premature infant.
6. Elevated immunoglobulin (IgM) in infants with intrauterine infection.
7. High nonprotein nitrogen levels, possibly due to:
    a. Increase in fetal catabolism—or
    b. Impaired placental excretion of fetal waste products
8. Prone to postasphyxial problems
    a. The asphyxial process of normal labor is associated with metabolic acidosis.
    b. Fetal malnutrition, in addition to the birth process, predisposes the infant to asphyxia neonatorum.
9. Limited fat and glycogen reserves due to intrauterine growth retardation
10. X-ray findings:
    a. Atrophy of thymus
    b. Thin ribs

Complications

1. Problems associated with asphyxia neonatorum and meconium aspiration syndrome
2. Hypoglycemia and hypocalcemia
3. Polycythemia
4. Pulmonary hemorrhage
5. Prematurity with intrauterine growth retardation
6. Infection associated with maternal conditions
7. Hypothermia
8. Late anemia
9. Future growth retardation (depends on cause of IUGR)
10. Delays in developmental and motor skills; difficult behavior styles (depends on cause of IUGR)
11. Congenital malformations

Clinical Manifestations

Clinical manifestations of the SGA infant are related to the duration, intensity, and time of onset of the influence (factors) causing intrauterine growth retardation.

1. Chronic IUGR—growth of the fetus has been curtailed by insult for weeks or months prior to birth. Note the following characteristics (hypoplastic stage):
    a. Body proportions remain unaltered—weight, length, and possibly head circumference are below normal for gestational age.
    b. Creases on soles of feet

c. Coarse, straight, silky hair
d. Well-developed ear cartilage
e. Firm skull bones
2. Subacute IUGR—growth of fetus has been curtailed by insult only a few days or weeks prior to birth (hypotrophic stage).
   a. Weight is diminished; length of body and head circumference may be normal.
   b. Wasted look with loose, thin skin
   c. Long, thin appearance
   d. Face has look of "worried little old man"
   e. Scaphoid abdomen
   f. Skin dry, cracked, and peeling
   g. Thin umbilical cord that dries and hardens rapidly
   h. Widened skull sutures

Diagnostic Evaluation

1. Evaluate general appearance of the infant.
2. Determine gestational age using physical characteristics and neurologic examination (see Table 48-1, pp. 1224–1225).
3. The infant can be SGA and preterm, SGA and term, or SGA and post-term.
4. Measure weight, length, and head circumference; plot on Colorado intrauterine growth chart and compare relative percentiles.
5. Determine blood sugar.
6. Obtain hematocrit (Hct) and hemoglobin to determine polycythemia and hyperviscosity (venous Hct over 65%).

Potential Problems and Nursing Diagnoses

The small-for-gestational-age infant is prone to complications and should be considered at-risk.
1. Complications related to SGA: pulmonary hemorrhage and infection
2. Problems associated with asphyxia neonatorum or meconium aspiration related to fetal distress
3. Hypoglycemia related to rapid depletion of glycogen stores
4. Hypothermia related to lack of energy stores and subcutaneous fat
5. Problems related to polycythemia (i.e., jaundice, tachypnea, tachycardia, respiratory distress)
6. Nutrition, altered, less than body requirements
7. Other problems related to hospitalized premature infant (see Preterm, Potential Problems, p. 1222)

Nursing Interventions

The nursing management of the SGA infant in many aspects is similar to that for the premature infant (see p. 1223). The following are major interventions of the nurse caring for the SGA neonate:

A. Observe for Any Gross and Less Obvious Congenital Anomalies as in the Case of Any Infant Upon Admission to the Nursery

1. Congenital anomalies are often associated with intrauterine growth retardation.
   Genitourinary, cardiovascular and skeletal complications and syndromes are common problems.
2. Certain types of intrauterine infection account for intrauterine growth retardation and may present signs of skin rash, petechiae and ecchymoses, hepatomegaly, splenomegaly, early-onset of obstructive jaundice, chorioretinitis, lethargy, and irritability.
3. Report any suspicious findings and observations to the physician immediately.

B. Observe for Problems Associated With Asphyxia Neonatorum

The SGA neonate has an increased incidence of asphyxia neonatorum. His lessened metabolic stores of carbohydrates lower his ability to handle the stresses of delivery. Acidosis may develop quickly.
1. Be aware of the Apgar scores which will help in determining degree of asphyxia (Apgar less than 5 at 1 minute or less than 7 at 5 minutes).
2. See that blood gas studies are done to confirm adequate oxygenation and acidosis. Frequent monitoring should be continued.
3. Observe for signs of respiratory distress.
   a. Adequate oxygenation is imperative for improving prognosis.
   b. Suction and oxygen equipment should be available and ready for immediate use.
   c. Aspiration pneumonia and pulmonary hemorrhage are postasphyxiation problems.
4. Check vital signs frequently and note behavior (i.e., reflex responses, irritability; cardiac function can be affected and CNS damage can occur with severe asphyxia.
5. Check and record intake and output. Renal damage is a common sequel of severe asphyxia.
6. Observe for abnormal clotting function and hyperbilirubinemia.
7. Postasphyxial hypocalcemia may occur.
8. Record and report all observations appropriately.

C. Screen for Hypoglycemia, Beginning Soon After Birth

1. The SGA infant has reduced carbohydrate stores at birth. Glycogen reserves are depleted almost immediately after birth. Gluconeogenesis is inadequate because of reduced stores of muscle protein and fat tissue, as well as reduced hyperglycemic response to norepinephrine and glucagon, which activate the gluconeogenesis process.
2. Hypoglycemia is most likely to occur from 12–72 hours after birth.
   Severely hypoxic, hypothermic SGA infants can become hypoglycemic as early as 6 hours after birth.
3. Blood sugars should be monitored frequently (every 30–60 minutes) by Dextrostix during the first few hours after birth and during IV glucose therapy.
   a. If Dextrostix evaluation is below 40 mg./100 ml., report this to physician immediately because measurement of serum glucose should be done.
   b. Keep Dextrostix bottle tightly covered and out of direct sunlight to avoid false reading on Dextrostix.
4. When IV infusion of glucose is used to prevent or treat hypoglycemia, particular care must be given to prevent infiltration and subsequent slough and necrosis of tissue.
5. With the infant at risk for hypoglycemia, oral feeding should be started as early as 2 hours after birth (if there are no contraindications).
6. Signs of hypoglycemia include:
   a. Jitteriness
   b. Sweating
   c. Tachypnea or apnea
   d. Cyanosis
   e. Convulsions
   f. Respiratory distress
7. Report all observations to the physician and record accurately.

D. Prevent Hypothermia and Maintain Thermal Stability of the SGA Neonate (see pp. 1227–1229).

1. Ensure that adequate environmental heat is provided to maintain the infant's abdominal skin temperature at 36.0°–36.5°C. (96.8°F.), thus decreasing calories needed for heat production, which would slow growth rate.
2. Prevent the infant from lying on the thermistor. Environmental temperature needs may be less than those of normally grown infants of comparable weight due to metabolic mass.

E. Take Measures to Deal With Polycythemia

Polycythemia, which is increased red blood cell volume, is frequently seen in SGA infants when growth retardation is due to placental insufficiency.

1. Polycythemia is identified by a high hematocrit or hemoglobin level (i.e., venous blood Hct over 65%); Hb of 20–22 gm./100 ml.). Hyperviscosity can result from this condition.
2. Signs and symptoms of viscosity include:
   a. Plethora
   b. Jaundice
   c. Tachypnea
   d. Tachycardia
   e. Peripheral cyanosis
   f. Grunting
   g. Nasal flaring, intercostal retractions
   h. Scrotal edema
   i. Priapism (persistent, abnormal erection of penis)
   j. Tremors, irritability, possibly seizures
3. Ensure that the Hct or Hb is monitored during the first 6–12 hours after birth in the high-risk infant.
4. Treatment for Hct above 70% usually consists of partial exchange transfusion. The nurse must be prepared to assist with this by using fresh frozen plasma or whole blood.

F. Provide Adequate Nutrition for Growth

1. Parenteral nutrition may be considered if the infant cannot tolerate enteral feedings by 3rd day of life.
2. Synchronized suck–swallow reflex does not become effective until 32–34 weeks' gestational age.
   Alternate gavage and nipple feeding are used when weight is above 1800 gm. and the infant is of 34 weeks' gestation or more.
3. The SGA infant can be difficult to feed because of being less relaxed and responsive. This may lead to failure to thrive.
4. Because these infants have a greater number of cells per unit mass, their metabolic expenditures and caloric needs are great.
5. Fluid requirements per kg. may be less than those of normally grown infant of the same weight.

G. Prevent Spread of Infection to Personnel and Other Neonates if Infant IUGR Is Due to Congenital Infection

1. Initiate isolation precautions according to health agency policy.

H. Accurately Measure and Record Daily Weights and Monitor Length and Head Circumference

Rapid weight gain is expected the first few days and weeks.

I. Support the Parents of the Infant (see pp. 1236–1237).

1. The long-term outcome of the SGA infant often represents an increase in long-range sequelae frequently manifested in lowered intellectual achievement resulting from malnutrition during peak intrauterine brain growth (depends on cause of IUGR).
2. Long-term prognosis depends on adequate treatment of problems encountered immediately after birth, etiology of problems, and subsequent home environment.
3. Teach parents about their infant: temperament, behavior styles, what comforts or irritates the infant, corrected gestational age as a criterion for developmental expectations.
4. Establish parent–infant bonding.
5. Emphasize importance of follow-up medical care.

Evaluation

1. Absence of complications; no evidence of pulmonary hemorrhage; normal breathing pattern for gestational age; no temperature elevation
2. Maintains normal respiratory status and adequate oxygenation; absence of respiratory distress; appropriate PaO_2.
3. Shows no signs of hypoglycemia; normal serum glucose
4. Maintains temperature stability; avoids fever and infections
5. Shows no signs of polycythemia; normal hematocrit and hemoglobin values
6. Receives adequate nutrition; gaining weight

Postmature Infant

The *postmature infant* is one whose gestation is 42 weeks or longer and who may show signs of weight loss with placental insufficiency.

Etiology

1. Not known in many cases.
2. Maternal factors associated with postmaturity:
   a. Primigravida and high-parity mother at any given age.
   b. Prolonged gestation in preceding pregnancies.

Altered Physiology

1. The postmature infant appears to have suffered from intrauterine malnutrition and hypoxia.
   Before the termination of the pregnancy, but at the point when the birth should have occurred, the placental function begins to diminish, resulting in impaired oxygen exchange and inadequate nutrient transfer to the fetus.
2. There are stages of postmaturity—severity of associated problems is determined by length of gestation (i.e., the longer the gestation, the more severe the problems).

Clinical Manifestations

Physical appearance—the following characteristics are most often seen in infant of 44 weeks' gestation or more:

1. Reduced subcutaneous tissue—loose skin, especially of buttocks and thighs
2. Long, curved fingernails and toenails
3. Reduced amount of vernix caseosa
4. Abundant scalp hair
5. Wrinkled, macerated skin; possibly pale, cracked, parchment-like skin.

6. Having the alert appearance of a 2–3-week old infant following delivery
7. Greenish-yellow staining of skin, indicating fetal distress

Diagnostic Evaluation

1. Evaluate general appearance.
2. Determine gestational age—give neurologic examination.
3. Measure weight, length, and head circumference, and plot on Colorado intrauterine growth chart. Compare percentiles.
4. Determine blood sugar. In hypoglycemia, the serum sugar level is below 40 mg./100 ml.
5. Assessment of asphyxia neonatorum.
   a. Apgar score
   b. Blood gas analysis

Potential Problems and Nursing Diagnoses

1. Asperation, potential for
2. Respiratory distress related to meconium aspiration, asphyxia neonatorum, pulmonary hemorrhage, pneumonia or pneumothorax, polycythemia
3. Hypoglycemia related to decreased glycogen stores and malnutrition due to placental dysfunction
4. Birth injury related to large size
5. Other complications related to sick infant and hospitalization (see Premature Infant, pp. 1223 and 1226)

Complications

1. Meconium aspiration
2. Hypoglycemia and hypocalcemia
3. Polycythemia
4. Pulmonary hemorrhage
5. Problems associated with asphyxia neonatorum
6. Pneumonia
7. Pneumothorax
8. Long-term pulmonary sequelae

Nursing Interventions

Problems and nursing care encountered in the postmature infant may include the metabolic disturbances of the SGA infant and complications of asphyxia neonatorum as well as polycythemia (see SGA, pp. 1239–1240). Massive meconium aspiration causes specific problems for the postmature infant (refer to nursing objectives for the premature infant, p. 1223 and SGA, p. 1239).

A. Meconium Aspiration and Respiratory Distress

1. The stage is set for meconium aspiration when placental function diminishes and oxygen transport to the fetus decreases, leading to cerebral hypoxia.
   a. The anal sphincter relaxes and meconium passes into the surrounding amniotic fluid.
   b. The asphyxiated fetus gasps and aspiration occurs.
2. Signs and symptoms of meconium aspiration—severity depends on amount and thickness of meconium aspirated, as well as the location of the aspirate in the respiratory tract.
   a. Tachypnea, increasing signs of cyanosis; difficulty breathing, with need for ventilation
   b. Tachycardia
   c. Inspiratory nasal flaring and retraction of chest
   d. Expiratory grunting
   e. Increased anteroposterior diameter of the chest
   f. Palpable liver

g. Crackles and rhonchi on chest auscultation
h. Concomitant cerebral irritation—jitteriness, hypotonia, seizures
i. X-ray—classic coarse, patchy, irregular pulmonary infiltrates ranging in severity
j. Additional signs: metabolic acidosis, hypotension, hypoglycemia, hypocalcemia

3. Mainly supportive treatment
   a. Warmth—maintain thermally neutral environment so the infant uses fewer calories and less oxygen
   b. Adequate oxygenation and humidification to maintain PaO_2 at 50–70 mm. Hg.
   c. Respiratory support with ventilator
      (1) Be aware that metabolic disturbances often accompany respiratory problems.
      (2) Ensure that monitoring of blood gases and pH is done.
      (3) Carefully record blood sampling.
   d. Adequate administration of calories and fluid Accurately record intake and output—assess possible alteration in kidney function due to hypoxia.
   e. Antibiotics
      (1) Prophylactically—meconium may lead to a chemical pneumonia and the growth of gram-negative bacteria. Therefore, antibiotics specifically for gram-negative bacteria may be used.
      (2) Treatment—antibiotics used only when clinical evidence indicates infection.
   f. Pulmonary physical therapy—every 30–60 minutes first few hours
      (1) Postural drainage (p. 1185)
      (2) Pulmonary lavage—using nonirritating solution and immediate suctioning of mouth, pharynx, and trachea; bag ventilate using high concentrations of oxygen between lavage procedures
      (3) Change position from side to side frequently and elevate head by adjusting the mattress to a 20-degree angle
      (4) Complications of meconium aspiration
         (a) Pneumothorax and/or pneumomediastinum
         (b) Secondary pneumonia
         (c) Pulmonary hypertension with persistent fetal circulation
         (d) Respiratory failure
         (e) Death
      (5) Prevention
         Most cases of meconium aspiration can be prevented if meconium is removed from the mouth and trachea by proper suctioning, prior to the infant's taking his first breath.

Note: If ventilator management is indicated, treatment is similar to that of the infant with hyaline membrane disease (pp. 1284–1289).

B. Hypoglycemia (see SGA, p. 1239).

1. Oral feeding or IV glucose is usually initiated soon after birth. If oral feedings are not contraindicated, they can begin 1–2 hours after birth.
2. Close and careful monitoring of blood sugar should be done with Dextrostix every hour until condition stabilizes.
3. Persistent hypoglycemia may contribute to CNS problems.
4. Be alert to signs and symptoms of hypoglycemia and report to physician.

C. Persistent Pulmonary Hypertension of the Newborn (PPHN).

1. *Pathophysiology*
   a. Physiologic disorder characterized by severe, labile cyanosis arising from persistent or return to suprasystemic pulmonary vascular resistance and pressure normally found in the fetus.
   b. The increase in pulmonary pressures cause right-to-left shunting of blood through the ductus arteriosus and/or the foramen ovale.
   c. Unsaturated venous blood is mixed with saturated arterial blood resulting in hypoxemia and metabolic acidosis, which results in further vasoconstriction, resulting in the cycle of shunting–hypoxia–acidosis.

2. *Causes*
   a. PPHN may be idiopathic or associated with pathologic conditions.
   b. Possible causes include: sepsis, acidosis, hypothermia, hypoxemia, postmature, meconium aspiration syndrome, hypoglycemia, shock, hypocalcemia, polycythemia, congenital heart disease, RDS, congenital diaphragmatic hernia, pulmonary hypoplasia, renal agenesis and dysplasia, Rh isoimmunization, maternal ingestion of prostaglandin inhibitors, or genetic.

3. *Signs and symptoms*
   a. Cyanosis—may be differential
   b. Pronounced respiratory distress
   c. Presence of murmur and/or congestive heart failure

4. *Diagnosis*
   a. Difficult to diagnose because it can occur in conjunction with other conditions including pulmonary, cardiovascular, or more generalized disorders
   b. CBC
   c. Acid-base studies
   d. Platelet count
   e. Electrolytes
   f. Serum glucose levels
   g. Serum cultures
   h. Pre- and postductal arterial blood gases or TcPO$_2$
   i. Chest x-ray, ECG, echocardiogram—may or may not be helpful
   j. Hyperoxic test—profound hypocapnia and respiratory alkalosis will produce dramatic rise in postductal oxygen tension
   k. Cardiac catheterization

5. *Treatment*
   a. Is directed at reducing pulmonary vascular resistance
   b. Specific therapy related to cause
   c. Supportive therapy—IV fluids, oxygen administration, correct acid–base imbalances
   d. Antibiotics—infection may be the cause or can aggravate the condition
   e. Achieve normal pH and PaCO$_2$–NaHCO$_3$ and mechanical (hyper) ventilation
   f. Vasodilators—Tolazoline
   g. Transfer to a tertiary NICU
      Nondepolarizing muscle relaxant
      Extracorporeal membrane oxygenation (ECMO)

6. *Nursing responsibilities*
   a. On-going observations and assessments; close monitoring of vital signs and general condition.
      (1) Obtain blood gases as indicated
      (2) Respiratory status—support respiratory effort, i.e., ventilator, position, temperature control, etc.
   b. Ensure that infant experiences minimal stress
      (1) Continuous monitoring
      (2) Quiet environment
      (3) No percussion or postural drainage
      (4) No heel sticks
      (5) Minimal suctioning
      (6) Minimal handling and disturbance
   c. Prevent dehydration and electrolyte inbalance by monitoring fluids
   d. Provide care specific to pharmacologic agents used in treatment
      (1) Cardiopulmonary monitor
      (2) Suction as necessary
      (3) Mechanical ventilation
      (4) Monitor blood pressure
      (5) Credé bladder
      (6) Careful control of fluid balance
      (7) Nasogastric tube to straight drainage
      (8) Urine specific gravity, Hematest urine, gastric aspirates, and stools
   e. Assist with transfer of infant to tertiary NICU. Help parents through this stressful time. (See Transport, pp. 1232–1233)

D. Psychosocial Support of Parents (see Premature Infant, p. 1232).

The long-term sequelae common in the postmature infant are associated with central nervous system (neurologic) problems.

Evaluation

1. Maintains adequate oxygen–carbon dioxide exchange; no evidence of respiratory distress
2. Shows no signs of hypoglycemia; taking oral feedings; maintaining appropriate serum glucose levels
3. Demonstrates no signs of birth injuries
4. No signs of complications related to hospitalization (see premature infant, pp. 1236–1237)

Infant of Diabetic Mother

The *infant of a diabetic mother (IDM)* is the infant born to a mother with diabetes. The mother may be an overt diabetic or gestational diabetic. The severity of infant problems depends on the severity of the maternal diabetes (Table 48-2).

Altered Physiology

Hyperinsulinemia in utero secondary to decreased epinephrine and glucose response result in the following in the infant:

1. Increased amount of body fat, not edema.
   a. Total body water is somewhat reduced at birth.
   b. High urinary output during first 2 days of life, probably from freeing of intracellular water.
2. Hypoglycemia
   a. Occurs within first 2–12 hours of life; may occur within minutes after birth.
   b. The infant's response to glucose is excessive (i.e., insulin blood level will have a slight elevation, will drop and then peak within 1 hour). This is probably due to maternal hyperglycemia.
   c. The infant's cord insulin levels may not be higher

Table 48-2. *White's Classification of Diabetes in Pregnancy*

Class A	Highest probability of fetal survival No insulin, little dietary regulation Includes gestational diabetes and prediabetes
Class B	Onset at age 20 or older Duration less than 10 years before pregnancy No vascular disease
Class C	Onset between 10 and 19 years of age Duration between 10 and 19 years Minimal vascular disease (retinal arteriosclerosis, calcification of vessels in the legs only)
Class D	Onset before age 10 years Duration 20 years or more Moderately advanced vascular disease (diabetic retinopathy, transient albuminuria, and hypertension)
Class E	Characteristics of class D plus calcification of pelvic vessels
Class F	Characteristics of class D plus nephritis
Class R	Active retinitis

(Krones SB. High-Risk Newborn Infant: The Basis for Intensive Nursing Care. 3rd ed, p. 307. St Louis, CV Mosby, 1981)

than in a normal infant unless a large amount of glucose is given.
  d. IDM may be symptomatic or asymptomatic with blood sugars below 20 mg./100 ml.
3. Hypocalcemia
  a. Associated with prematurity, difficult labor and delivery, asphyxia at birth, and/or decreased functioning of parathyroid glands.
  b. Generally occurs during first 24–72 hours of life.
  c. Levels below 7 mg./dl. with symptoms or 6 mg./dl. without symptoms.
4. Hyperbilirubinemia
  a. Most likely to occur within 48–72 hours after birth.
  b. Immature liver results in inability to conjugate bilirubin.
  c. Hct is higher on the 3rd day after birth and extracellular volume is decreased.
  d. Because of large size, birth trauma may increase risk of enclosed hemorrhage.
5. Prematurity
  a. May be premature or small for gestational age when associated with placental insufficiency in classes D–F mothers (Table 48-1).
  b. Respiratory function is similar to that of other premature infants—thus the infant is prone to hyaline membrane disease.
6. Polycythemia
  a. Venous hematocrit greater than 65% or venous hemoglobin 22 gm./100 ml.
  b. Polycythemia increases the risks of occurrence of renal vein thrombosis, respiratory distress, hypoglycemia, and hypocalcemia.
7. Congenital anomalies
  a. Increased incidence of congenital anomalies may be due to:
    (1) Divergent gene pattern
    (2) Glucose homeostasis in utero
  b. Most common anomalies are skeletal and cardiac.
8. Infection
  a. Prematurity and lowered passive immunity

  b. Possible maternal urinary tract infection and bacteria crossing the placenta

Diagnostic Evaluation

1. Maternal history of diabetes
2. Physical assessment of infant and determination of gestational age
3. Blood studies
  a. Glucose
  b. Calcium, phosphorus
  c. Hct and Hb
  d. Blood gas analysis
  e. Magnesium (if indicated)
  f. Electrolytes
  g. Bilirubin

Clinical Manifestations

1. Macrosomia
2. Cardiomegaly
3. Hepatomegaly
4. Large umbilical cord and placenta
5. Plethora
6. Full-face
7. Tendency to be large for gestational age; some may be normal weight or SGA; IUGR when mother has had long-standing insulin dependency
8. Abundant fat, hair, and vernix caseosa
9. Hypertrichosis pinnae

Complications

1. Hypoglycemia
2. Hypocalcemia
3. Hyaline membrane disease
4. Polycythemia and renal vein thrombosis
5. Infection
6. Hyperbilirubinemia
7. Hypermagnesemia or hypomagnesemia
8. Congenital anomalies
9. Birth injuries—cephalohematomas, facial nerve paralysis, fractured clavicles, brachial nerve plexus
10. Prematurity
11. Congestive heart failure secondary to congenital heart disease, subaortic stenosis, asymmetrical ventricular septal hypertrophy
12. Asphyxia neonatorum
13. Organomegaly
14. Neurologic instability
15. RDS or other respiratory illness

Potential Problems and Nursing Diagnoses

1. Respiratory distress and infection related to prematurity
2. Hypoglycemia and hypocalcemia related to prematurity
3. Birth injuries related to large size
4. Potential for other problems related to hospitalization of premature infant (see preterm infant, p. 1222)

Nursing Assessment and Interventions

Except for specific considerations discussed below, the nursing care of the infant of a diabetic mother (IDM) is the same as for the premature infant (pp. 1226–1229).

A. Observe Closely for Hypoglycemia.

Report any irregularities immediately to physician.
1. Monitor serum glucose levels every 30–60 minutes beginning immediately after birth for 24 hours or every

4–8 hours until stabilized. Glucose levels are lowest 1–2 hours after birth; at 2–6 hours, glucose levels even off and gradually increase. Warm the extremity prior to capillary sampling to prevent false-low value resulting from stasis.

2. The infant with hypoglycemia (premature infant: below 20 mg./100 ml.; term infant: below 30 mg./100 ml.) may be symptomatic or asymptomatic. Signs include:
   a. Jitteriness
   b. Tremors
   c. Convulsions
   d. Sweating
   e. Cyanosis
   f. Weak or high-pitched cry
   g. Refusal to eat
   h. Hypotonia (reduced muscle tone)
   i. Apnea
   j. Temperature instability
   k. Rotating eye movements
3. Hypoglycemia may be prevented or treated by early feedings of 10%–20% glucose or formula by nipple or gavage.
   a. IV glucose, 10%–15%, may be given for very low serum glucose levels or when infant's condition prevents oral feeding.
   b. Glucose levels should be maintained in the low-normal range.
   c. Overfeeding or excessive IV infusion of glucose may result in a rebound effect causing insulin levels to increase and hypoglycemia to reappear.
   d. IV glucose must not be discontinued abruptly in order to prevent rebound hypoglycemia.

B. Monitor Infant Closely for Changes in Acid–Base Status, Respiratory Distress, Temperature, Hypocalcemia, and Sepsis.

C. Observe for Hyperbilirubinemia.

1. Infants of diabetic mothers have a higher incidence of hyperbilirubinemia.
   Levels will be elevated 48–72 hours after birth.
   Other predisposing factors include prematurity and polycythemia, which increases the load of bilirubin from the natural process of RBC breakdown to be cleared, decreased extracellular fluid, and birth trauma related to increased birth weight.
2. The infant may need an exchange transfusion at relatively lower bilirubin levels (as in the premature infant) to prevent kernicterus. Phototherapy may need to be initiated early.
3. The blood sugar must be monitored during and following exchange transfusion.
   CPD (citrate phosphate dextrose) contains large amounts of dextrose which may subsequently cause rebound hypoglycemia.

D. Assist in the Prevention of Dehydration and Maintenance of Fluid and Electrolyte Balance.

1. Because of the increase in fatty tissue and decrease in total amount of body water, the freeing of intracellular water after birth will increase urinary output. This, along with inability to concentrate urine, increases the risk of dehydration. Dehydration increases risk of polycythemia.
2. Accurately record intake and output; administer prescribed fluids and evaluate laboratory studies to determine current status.

E. Be Aware of the Infant Who is Predisposed to Hypomagnesemia or Hypermagnesemia and Observe for Signs and Symptoms of Each.

1. Hypermagnesemia may occur when the preeclamptic mother was treated with magnesium sulfate.
   a. Signs and symptoms may include:
      (1) Hypotonia
      (2) Weak or absent cry
      (3) Severe respiratory distress with apnea or cyanosis
   b. Treatment is an exchange transfusion.
2. Hypomagnesemia may accompany hypocalcemia or follow an exchange transfusion.
   a. Severe neuromuscular excitability may be the presenting symptom.
   b. IM magnesium sulfate is the treatment.

F. Be Alert for Development of Renal Vein Thrombosis in the Infant During the First Few Days of Life.

1. Polycythemia, transient dehydration, and decreased extracellular fluid may be causes.
2. Observe for hematuria and proteinuria.
3. Flank masses may be palpable.

G. Observe the Infant for Possible Cardiac Anomalies (see p. 1311).

Monitor cardiac and respiratory rates.

H. Support the Mother Who May Have Feelings of Severe Guilt or Inadequacy, Since She Is Directly Related to the Problems Her Infant May be Having.

1. Encourage and allow the mother to talk about these feelings.
2. Encourage her, when appropriate, to have close obstetrical care for subsequent pregnancies.
3. Stress importance of a periodic evaluation for diabetes in her child.

Evaluation

1. Reveals no signs of respiratory distress; normal vital signs; laboratory values within acceptable ranges
2. Achieves physiologic balance soon after birth; normal serum glucose values; absence of tremors, convulsions, etc.
3. Has no evidence of birth injury
4. Shows no evidence of other complications related to prematurity

Jaundice in the Newborn (Hyperbilirubinemia)

Hyperbilirubinemia (jaundice) in the newborn is an accumulation of serum bilirubin above normal levels.

Etiology

1. Increased bilirubin load
   a. Hemolytic disease—Rh and ABO incompatibility
   b. Morphologic abnormalities of red blood cells
   c. Red blood cell enzyme defects
   d. Physiologic jaundice (see later discussion of "physiologic jaundice")
2. Extravascular blood
   a. Cephalohematoma

b. Pulmonary or cerebral hemorrhage

c. Any enclosed occult blood

3. Decrease or inhibition of bilirubin conjugation

    a. Inherited bilirubin conjugation defect: Crigler-Najjar syndrome (deficiency of glucuronyl transferase).

    b. Acquired bilirubin conjugation defect: breast-milk jaundice, Lucey-Driscoll syndrome, infant of diabetic mother, asphyxiated infant with respiratory distress

4. Increased extrahepatic circulation

    Intestinal obstruction

5. Polycythemia

    a. Twin–twin transfusion

    b. Maternofetal transfusion

    c. Infant of diabetic mother

    d. Small-for-gestational-age infant

6. Mixed jaundice—increased bilirubin load and decreased clearance resulting in elevated indirect and direct bilirubin levels

    a. Sepsis

    b. Severe hemolytic disease

    c. Intrauterine transfusion

    d. Galactosemia

    e. Biliary atresia—absence of extrahepatic ducts or presence of cordlike structures without a lumen

7. Hypothyroidism

8. Familial, transient—associated with inhibiting factor in plasma

9. Unknown

Altered Physiology

A. Bilirubin Production

1. 75% of the bilirubin present in the newborn is from red blood cell breakdown.

    a. The red blood cell is broken down into protein and globin is combined with heme, which is an iron–porphyrin complex.

    b. In the presence of the enzyme called heme oxygenase:

        (1) Globin is reduced to amino acids.

        (2) Iron is broken off and stored.

        (3) Porphyrin moiety is broken into biliverdin, which is reduced to bilirubin.

    c. This bilirubin is unconjugated or indirect; "free" bilirubin moves across the blood–brain barrier, binds to tissues, and damages cells of the CNS.

    d. Indirect bilirubin, bound to albumin, is present in circulating blood and tissues.

    e. The liver selectively removes this albumin-bound bilirubin from the blood.

    f. Once the unconjugated bilirubin is in the liver, it is converted to direct or conjugated water-soluble bilirubin with the aid of enzymes, one of which is glucuronyl transferase.

    g. From the liver, conjugated bilirubin is excreted via the bile into the intestine and is excreted in the stool or is hydrolyzed to unconjugated bilirubin in the intestine and reabsorbed across the intestinal mucosa into the circulation (enterohepatic circulation).

    h. Meconium has a high concentration of bilirubin. When the sterile intestine is colonized with normal flora after birth, bacterial enzymes convert the bilirubin to urobilinogen, most of which is excreted in the stool.

2. 25% of the bilirubin present in the newborn is from nonerythrocyte-containing heme proteins.

B. Physiologic Jaundice

1. Increased load of bilirubin on liver cells.

    a. Increased bilirubin production—more rapid hemolysis because of higher level of circulating RBCs per kg. (2.2 lbs.) of body weight and a shorter RBC life span.

    b. Enterohepatic circulation—reabsorption of unconjugated bilirubin.

2. Decreased clearance of bilirubin from plasma.

    a. Predominant bilirubin-binding protein in liver cells may be deficient the first days of life.

    b. Glucuronyl transferase enzyme activity may be decreased, resulting in impaired conjugation of bilirubin.

    c. Liver may show decreased ability to excrete large amounts of conjugated bilirubin.

    d. Poor portal blood supply may decrease the liver's capacity to act effectively.

    e. Open ductus venosus may allow blood to bypass liver.

C. Erythrocyte Destruction

1. Erythroblastosis fetalis (isoimmunization due to Rh factor or ABO incompatibility)

    a. Immune hemolysis or Rh/ABO blood group incompatibility; the mother's and fetus's blood are different.

    Rh factor; different ABO blood groups (see Coombs' test, below).

    b. Mother produces antibodies against the antigen of the fetus's blood. Fetal cells frequently cross the placenta.

    c. Antibodies of the mother's blood are present in the infant's blood at birth, causing the following conditions:

        (1) There is hemolysis of the infant's red blood cells.

        (2) Hemolysis leads to a rising level of indirect bilirubin.

2. Glucose-6-phosphate dehydrogenase deficiency (G-6-PD)—nonimmune hemolytic disease (erythrocyte biochemical factor)

    a. Deficiency results in reduced stability to oxidative destruction from substances that act as oxidizing agents (i.e., vitamin K, naphthalene, salicylates).

    b. X-linked recessive disease that affects primarily Black and Mediterranean–Oriental groups.

    c. Screen maternal blood for carrier state and screen neonate blood in high-risk groups.

3. Other conditions associated with increased erythrocyte destruction:

    a. Infection—bacterial, viral, and/or protozoan

    b. Structural abnormal erythrocyte

    c. Sequestered blood (i.e., cephalohematoma, ecchymoses)

D. Other Considerations

1. Each gram of hemoglobin breakdown forms 35 mg. of bilirubin (1 molecule hemoglobin breaks down into 4 molecules bilirubin).

2. An unmeasurable amount of bilirubin does not bind to albumin. Free indirect bilirubin is very toxic to the cells of the CNS.

3. The enzyme system responsible for conjugation of bilirubin is oxygen-dependent and altered by infant's pH,

temperature, etc. Thus infants who are acidotic, hypoxic, or hypothermic tend to present with higher levels of bilirubin.

Clinical Manifestations

1. Onset of clinical jaundice seen when serum bilirubin levels are 5–7 mg./100 dl.
2. Physiologic jaundice—occurs 3–5 days after birth.
   a. Increase in unconjugated bilirubin levels; levels must not exceed 5 mg./100 dl. per day.
   b. Peak bilirubin levels not to exceed 12 mg./100 dl. in full-term infant and 15 mg./100 dl. in premature infant.
   c. Full-term peak levels (6 mg./100 dl.) are reached by 48–72 hours after birth; clinical jaundice declines in 1 week, and normal bilirubin levels are reached in 2 weeks.
   d. Premature peak levels (10–15 gm./100 dl.) are reached by 4–6 days of age; clinical jaundice declines in 2 weeks and normal bilirubin levels are reached in 3–4 weeks.
3. Erythroblastosis—may occur within 24 hours after birth.
4. Signs and symptoms
   a. Sclerae appearing yellow before skin appears yellow
   b. Skin appearing light to bright yellow
   c. Lethargy
   d. Dark amber, concentrated urine
   e. Poor feeding
   f. Dark stools

Diagnostic Evaluation

1. All infants who have clinical signs of hyperbilirubinemia should be given the following work-up:
   a. Serum bilirubin levels—total and direct
   b. Peripheral smear—for evidence of red blood cell morphology and reticulocyte count
   c. Reticulocyte count—to determine rate of hemolysis
   d. Coombs' test—to check for Rh and ABO or other group incompatibility between the mother and infant—direct Coombs' test on infant serum
   e. Blood typing of mother and infant
   f. Total serum protein—to measure binding capacity
   g. Hematocrit or hemoglobin
   h. Acid–base status
   i. Albumin-binding test—to measure reserve binding sites (if available)
2. Measuring the bilirubin–albumin binding capacity of the plasma can also be valuable in determining the risk of kernicterus (see below) and the need for an exchange transfusion. This test defines the upper limits to which serum bilirubin is allowed to rise when an exchange transfusion is done.
   a. $\dfrac{\text{Total bilirubin}}{\text{Total serum protein}} =$
      (1) If less than 3.7—no danger of kernicterus
      (2) If greater than 3.7—treatment by exchange transfusion is indicated.
   b. Total serum protein × 3.7 = level of bilirubin at which to do exchange transfusion.
3. The level of bilirubin at which the infant is at risk for brain damage depends on the degree of prematurity, presence of acidosis, hypoxia, or drugs which bind albumin indirect bilirubin (20 mg. of bilirubin/100 ml. of blood in term infant is not necessarily the upper limit of bilirubin as formerly thought).
4. Appropriate cultures when infection is suspected.
5. Serum glucose levels.
6. Urine for reducing substances.
7. Thyroid screen.

Complications—Kernicterus

Kernicterus is a yellow discoloration of specific areas of brain tissue by unconjugated bilirubin; can be confirmed only by death and autopsy.

Bilirubin encephalopathy best describes the occurrence of the syndrome and the accompanying neurologic sequelae in neonates.

1. Early signs of kernicterus
   a. Poor feeding
   b. Vomiting
   c. Lethargy
   d. High-pitched cry
   e. Hypotonia
   f. Decrease of normal reflexes, Moro reflex
2. Later signs
   a. Opisthotonus; spasticity
   b. Apnea
   c. Irritability
   d. Seizures
   e. Deafness to high-pitched sounds
3. Occurrence of kernicterus at low levels of bilirubin may be seen in infants with
   a. Previous asphyxia (acidosis)
   b. Respiratory distress
   c. Sepsis
   d. Hypothermia
   e. Prematurity; especially low birth weight
   f. Hypoglycemia
4. Bilirubin is nephrotoxic and especially compromises renal concentrating capacity.
5. Bilirubin increases affinity of RBC for oxygen.
6. Controversy exists as to the actual mechanics and causes involved with the development of kernicterus and the serum bilirubin levels at which exchange transfusions are done.

Treatment

1. Exchange transfusion—to mechanically remove bilirubin.
2. Phototherapy—to allow for utilization of alternate pathways for bilirubin excretion.
3. Enzyme induction agent—to reduce bilirubin levels by inducing hepatic enzyme system involved in bilirubin clearance (i.e., phenobarbital, ethanol).

Potential Problems and Nursing Diagnoses

1. Alteration in fluid and electrolyte balance related to decreased oral fluid intake and hyperthermia
2. Potential behavioral changes in the infant (i.e., poor sucking, irritability) related to increased serum bilirubin
3. Altered comfort to the infant related to procedures (i.e., blood drawing, phototherapy, exchange transfusion)
4. Alteration in skin integrity related to prolonged pressure, diarrhea
5. Sensory perceptual alteration related to phototherapy treatment
6. Altered parenting related to hospitalization and separation from infant
7. Parental anxiety related to uncertainty about outcome

Nursing Assessment and Interventions

A. Observe the Infant's Skin for Appearance of or Increase in Jaundice

1. Make observations in daylight, sunlight, or white fluorescent light.
2. Blanch the skin during the observation to clear away capillary coloration: forehead, cheeks and clavicle sites allow for clear view. Record findings at least twice daily.
3. Transcutaneous measurements:
   a. Quantifies skin color in relation to total serum bilirubin level.
   b. The procedure is a noninvasive screening test for significant jaundice.
   c. A number of transcutaneous bilirubinometers are being evaluated.
4. Be aware of any blood incompatibility between the infant's and mother's blood.
5. Be alert to the infant's age in connection with the appearance of jaundice.

B. Note any Changes in Urine Pigmentation and Frequency of Urination

Careful notation of frequency, amount, and color of urine should be made so changes will be noticed immediately. Test for presence of bilirubin (urobilinogen).

C. Maintain Adequate Fluid Intake

1. Be aware of feeding history and amount of fluid taken.
2. If the infant is a slow eater, feed small amounts frequently.
3. The amount of fluid intake determines the amount of hydration and in turn determines the excretion of bilirubin. Early feeding is a good preventive prescription for hyperbilirubinemia.
4. If the infant is receiving intravenous fluid, keep an accurate hourly record of fluid intake. Do not allow intake to fall behind prescribed rate. Observe IV site for infiltration so IV can be discontinued and restarted immediately.

D. Be Alert for any Behavior Changes and Report Them to the Physician

Note particularly increasing lethargy, change in sucking activity or quality, or vomiting.

E. Be Alert to Signs of Kernicterus (bilirubin encephalopathy) and Report Them to the Physician

Observe for signs of decreased muscle tone, no sucking, no hand grasp, or regurgitation of feedings not previously observed. In time, the infant becomes opisthotonic and irritable.

F. Administer the Treatment of Phototherapy Safely and Properly, Should It Be Prescribed

1. Phototherapy is a mechanism for detoxifying bilirubin—involves shining daylight fluorescent bulbs or blue light directly on the exposed skin of the infant
2. The *irradiance* or *flux,* which is the unit of measurement of energy output of lamps, at 425–475 nm. is important in bilirubin degradation.
3. The distance of the infant from the light should be 45–60 cm.
4. Check light intensity for therapeutic range daily. Use commercial Bililight.
5. Effectiveness of phototherapy depends on: intensity of illumination; area of skin exposed; initial phototherapy effect on bilirubin in skin appears to have greater influence.
6. The physician will determine the length of time the infant is to be under the lights based on serum bilirubin levels and clinical condition of the infant.

Nursing Care Related to Phototherapy

A. General Measures

1. Have the infant completely undressed so entire skin surface is exposed to light.
2. Keep the infant's eyes covered to protect them from the constant exposure to high-intensity light which may cause retinal injury.
   a. Do not apply pressure when the eyes are covered because this may cause corneal ulceration.
   b. Be certain both eyes are occluded with protective cover and that eyelids are closed.
   c. Change protective covers routinely and check for conjunctivitis.
   d. Make sure nose is not occluded and respiratory distress does not occur.
   e. Shield gonads.
3. Develop a systematic schedule of turning infant so all surfaces are exposed (i.e., every 2 hours).
4. Maintain thermo-neutrality
   a. Measure incubator or Isolette temperature as well as that of the infant.
   b. Light affects the ambient temperature.
   c. There is an increase in skin blood flow, temperature, respiratory and heart rate.
   d. Use servocontrol to prevent rise in skin temperature.
   e. Do not expose the thermistor probe to the lights without the probe's being covered with an opaque tape.
   f. Avoid hyperthermia. Monitor temperature every 2–4 hours.
5. Adequate fluid intake should be provided either orally or intravenously.
   a. Vasodilatation increases insensible water loss, and there is excess stool loss from occasional diarrhea.
   b. Keep urine specific gravity below 1.015.
   c. Monitor intake and output. Check for signs of dehydration.
6. The infant should be shielded (by Plexiglas) from direct exposure of the lights to filter out and protect him from the ultraviolet radiation of daylight and cool white fluorescent lights. This shield will also protect the infant from injury should the lights break.
7. Ensure that serum bilirubin levels are obtained as prescribed. The diminishing icterus (i.e., the lowering of unconjugated bilirubin from cutaneous tissue) does not reflect the serum bilirubin concentration.
   a. Lights should be turned off when blood is being collected to eliminate false-low bilirubin levels.
   b. When phototherapy has been discontinued, check serum bilirubin levels within 4 hours to determine rebound.
8. If possible, remove the infant from under the lights, remove eye covers, and hold the infant for feedings. This will allow for some human contact and pleasure during feeding and a chance to open his eyes and look around, and perhaps will encourage parental involvement in the infant's care.
9. Note sleeping and eating patterns.
   a. The feeding schedule may need to be adjusted to the infant's pattern for better feeding.
   b. Obtain daily weight. Increased metabolic rate may increase caloric needs.

10. Develop a schedule for changing light bulbs.
    a. The effectiveness of light of this wavelength decreases after 800 hours of use; thus, the bulbs should be changed at that time.
    b. A record of hours of use will be helpful.
    c. Measure effective light life with light meter.

B. Side Effects of Phototherapy

1. Lethargy
2. Loose, green stools
3. Dark urine
4. Temperature elevation
5. Skin changes—rash due to capillary dilatation; Black infant skin may darken
6. Priapism—turn the infant on his abdomen for short periods of time, and this will cease.
7. Dehydration from increased insensible water loss
8. Possible damage to photo receptors of retinae when eyes not shielded
9. Airway obstruction from slippage of eye shield
10. Possible decreased ability of albumin binding to bilirubin.
11. Possible effect on biological rhythm
12. Obscures diagnosis of other problems
13. Increased platelet turnover
14. Once phototherapy has been discontinued, serum bilirubin level may show a rise or rebound of approximately 2 mg./dl. then slowly decline.
15. Bronze baby—dark coloration of skin seen when infant has cholestatic jaundice, probably due to retention of the products of phototherapy.

Other Measures

A. Be Aware of Drugs That May Compete With Bilirubin for Binding to Albumin Free Fatty Acids (sulfonamides, chloramphenicol, salicylates, caffeine, novobiocin)

Their administration will result in increasing serum level of "free" unconjugated bilirubin.

B. Observe for Hypoglycemia in the Infant With Erythroblastosis Resulting From Islet Cell Hyperplasia, and Increased Insulin Secretion

1. Hypoglycemia may occur because of hyperplasia of beta cells in the pancreatic islet of Langerhans causing secondary hyperinsulinism.
2. Other complications may occur:
    a. Respiratory compromise related to hydrops or fluid in lungs or ascites.
    b. Persistent fetal circulation—resulting in intense pulmonary vasoconstriction secondary to hypoxemia, acidosis, or hypertension.
    c. Anemia—depends on rate of hemolysis; observe for associated edema, ascites, pleural effusion, petechia, and tachycardia.
    d. Pulmonary, intracranial, and gastrointestinal hemorrhage; thrombocytopenia (especially following exchange transfusion), and increased platelet count should also be watched for in the infant.
3. Hyperbilirubinemia is generally absent at birth; however, postnatal destruction of red blood cells contribute to rapid increase in serum bilirubin levels. Hepatosplenomegaly may be evident as a result of increased activity of these organs to compensate for increasing hemolysis of erythrocytes.
4. Hydrops fetalis is the severest form of erythroblastosis fetalis.

a. Progressive hemolysis of erythrocytes causes hypoxia, pleural, pericardial, and peritoneal effusion and cardiac failure.
    b. Mortality rate is high.
5. Continuous and careful observations, monitoring, and interventions are essential components of nursing care.

C. Assist in Treatment of Exchange Transfusion.

1. Used to stop hemolytic process (erythroblastosis fetalis), correct anemia, and treat potential/actual bilirubinemia.
2. Complications: hypoglycemia, necrotizing enterocolitis.

D. Support the Mother Should Jaundice in Her Infant Be Related to Breast-Feeding or Breast Milk

1. Breast milk jaundice syndrome
    a. Unconjugated hyperbilirubinemia in healthy newborn.
    b. Jaundice appears after 5 days of life and peak bilirubin levels occur 5–15 days.
    c. If breast-feeding is interrupted 24–48 hours, serum bilirubin levels drop within 24 hours, often to half the original level.
    d. When breast-feeding resumes, bilirubin levels increase 1–3 mg./dl. within 48 hours. Levels plateau for several days, then slowly decline, reaching normal levels in 3–12 weeks.
    e. This will also happen if breast-feeding is not interrupted. It should also be noted that many physicians do not recommend interruption of breast-feeding as treatment.
    f. Cause is an unknown factor in human milk. May be:
       (1) Glucuronyl transfer activity inhibitor in the breast milk.
       (2) High lipoprotein lipase activity of breast milk that results in increased amount of unsaturated fatty acid, which inhibits conjugation.
    g. Treatment is not usually necessary if serum levels remain below 20 mg./dl.
2. Breast-feeding-associated jaundice
    a. Onset early—within first week of life.
    b. Contributing factors include poor past birth weight recovery; smaller, less vigorous infant who doesn't feed well, therefore has caloric deprivation and increased enterohepatic circulation of bilirubin.
    c. Treatment consists of stimulation of early milk production and infant intake, lowering serum bilirubin levels by phototherapy or exchange transfusion.
3. Help mother learn appropriate methods for expressing breast milk during the time of feeding interruption.
4. Help mother express her concerns and work through her feelings.

E. Foster a Healthy Family–Child Relationship

1. Encourage parents to visit infant as much as possible during hospitalization.
2. Allow the parents to fondle, care for, hold, and feed the infant as much as possible or as his condition permits.
3. Initiate a community-nursing referral if the parents are particularly anxious about caring for their infant at home after discharge.
4. If breast-feeding is temporarily discontinued, encourage the mother to pump her breasts; be supportive.

5. If the mother is still a patient on the obstetric unit, and there are no contraindications, consider treating infant in mother's room.

Health Education

1. Help the family to understand what is wrong with their baby. Explain in simple terms what the doctor has already told them. Allow them to ask questions about the baby and treatment.
2. If the baby has erythroblastosis fetalis, help the parents understand the importance of prenatal care and monitoring should another pregnancy occur.
3. Stress the importance of close follow-up of the baby after hospital discharge. Anemia is a common long-term side effect of red blood cell hemolysis and exchange transfusion. The baby's hemoglobin level should be monitored for some time after illness so appropriate treatment can be initiated if necessary.
4. Unsensitized Rh-negative mother, after delivery of an Rh-positive infant, should receive Rho immune globulin (RhoGAM) to prevent isoimmunization with subsequent pregnancies.

Expected Outcomes

1. Achieves and maintains fluid and electrolyte balance; adequate urine output and specific gravity; gaining weight; shows adequate serum electrolyte values
2. Demonstrates minimal behavioral changes; achieves normalization of serum bilirubin levels
3. Experiences minimal trauma and discomfort; normal vital signs; no abnormal crying; comforted when held and cuddled
4. Maintains skin integrity; no signs of skin breakdown
5. Demonstrates normal developmental behavior; no evidence of sensory or psychological deprivation while in nursery
6. Parent-infant bonding observed; parents show willingness to visit child, hold him, and participate in his care
7. Parents show lessening of anxiety; ask appropriate questions; verbalize that they understand treatment protocols

---

Failure to Thrive

"Failure to thrive" syndrome is a term used to identify infants characterized by growth and developmental failure along with psychosocial disruption.

Etiology

1. Unknown
2. Organic
   a. Central nervous system
   b. Cardiovascular
   c. Renal
   d. Gastrointestinal
   e. Respiratory
   f. Endocrine
   g. Metabolic
3. Nonorganic
   a. Inadequate caloric intake; disturbed feeding patterns
   b. Maternal deprivation or faulty mother–child relationship
   c. Family problems (socioeconomic problems)
   d. Environmental deprivation

Clinical Manifestations

1. Weight measurement falls below 2 standard deviations from mean for age (weight and length fall below that expected for gestational and postnatal age).
2. Infant fails to gain weight or loses subcutaneous fat and muscle mass.
3. Possible presenting manifestations that are associated with maternal deprivation:
   a. Developmental retardation
   b. Disturbed psychosocial development
      (1) Inappropriate response for age to strangers
      (2) Avoidance of eye contact with another person
      (3) Exaggerated self-comfort measures
      (4) Withdrawn—no interest in environment
4. Somatic manifestations
   a. Gastrointestinal
      (1) Anorexia
      (2) Vomiting
      (3) Diarrhea
      (4) Rumination
      (5) Dehydration
   b. Respiratory—coughing
5. Most frequently seen at age 6–16 months

Diagnostic Evaluation

1. Detailed history—including dietary and family (social)
2. Physical examination—accurate measurements of length, weight, and head circumference—general condition
3. Laboratory data—preliminary tests should be minimal, unless history or examination indicates a specific line of inquiry. Include the following tests:
   a. Complete blood count
   b. Urinalysis and culture
   c. Stool for fat, occult blood, ovum and parasites, and pH, trypsin
   d. Levels of serum sodium, potassium, CO_2, chlorides, creatinine, calcium
   e. Tine test
4. Observe systematic behavioral distortions.

Treatment

(When no organic reasons have been found)
1. Adequate caloric intake for weight gain (120–150 cal./kg./day based on appropriate weight for gestational and postnatal age). Significant weight gain will usually occur within 7–10 days.
2. Appropriate "mothering"—nurturing activities and environmental stimulation. Investigation has suggested that weight gain will occur when adequate nutrition is taken independent of nurturing activities; however, one is also dealing with a hospitalized child who is subjected to parental separation or deprivation.
3. If, after a trial of adequate caloric ingestion, the infant does not gain weight, intensive investigation is done. Trial period may have to be 7–10 days in some instances.
4. Provide a nurturing environment that will enhance positive patterns of behavior toward interaction of the family unit.

Prognosis

1. Prognosis generally depends on the etiology, severity, and duration of the condition, as well as on the home situation to which the child returns.

2. Long-term—continued impaired growth rate and failure to thrive, lowered intelligence, and emotional disorders.

Potential Problems and Nursing Diagnoses

1. Nutrition, altered, less than body requirements related to fatigue during feeding
2. Altered growth and development related to inappropriate nutrition
3. Potential for aspiration
4. Parental anxiety related to lack of knowledge, guilt, or concern for child
5. Altered parenting (mother–infant bonding/relationship) related to lack of understanding, frustration, and anxiety

Nursing Interventions

A. Make an Assessment of the Infant's General Condition, Level of Development, Coping Mechanisms, and Behavior

1. Carefully note what behaviors need attention and/or modifying.
2. Accurately record findings in nursing notes.
3. Obtain and record accurate height, weight, and head circumference.

B. Develop a Detailed Nursing Care Plan That Is Workable Based on:

1. The infant's physical condition and limitations
2. Medical management
3. Nursing history
4. Input from other multidiscipline team members

C. Understand That the Reason for This Child's Condition May Not Totally Be the Mother's Fault

1. Lack of food availability may be a result of socioeconomic situation.
2. Disturbed feeding patterns may have continued despite attempts by mother to correct them.
3. Disturbed mother–infant relationship resulting from separation at neonatal period.

D. Provide and Maintain Nutritional Intake That Will Allow for Weight Gain

1. Determine if a feeding problem does exist. Document feeding behaviors (i.e., sleep/wake cycle related to eating, clues of hunger, response to offered food).
2. Infant may need to be taught to eat appropriately for his age (i.e., cup, solids, spoon, finger food).
3. If the child vomits, then smaller, more frequent feedings may be necessary; prop him up in sitting position for feeding.
   a. Assess what effect environment, position, and other factors have on vomiting and feeding behavior.
   b. Prevent ruminating or self-induced vomiting.
   c. Daily weights and accurate input and output are necessary to evaluate progress.

E. Gently and Warmly Provide Nurturing to This Infant

1. Assess what the infant can tolerate and base activities on this, slowly increasing TLC and physical contact as infant can accept it.
2. Encourage the development of a trusting relationship between 1 or 2 persons and the infant.

3. Use each opportunity presented by daily care to develop the relationship, help the infant become interested in and enjoy his environment and eventually reach out to explore himself and people and things around him.
4. Part of nurturing activities include the therapeutic use of tactile, visual, and auditory stimulation through play. Do not force this on child if he is unable to tolerate it. Have items within reach, occasionally showing infant how they operate.
5. Talk to the infant, use his name; slowly help him to tolerate eye-to-eye contact.
6. Document the infant's reactions and responses to handling, playing, etc.

F. Establish a Relationship With the Mother (parents) That Will Allow for Open Communication and Cooperative Efforts

1. Accept the mother as a person, one who may have problems with which she cannot cope. She may be young and inexperienced or have doubts about her ability to be a mother, as well as socioeconomic problems.
2. A trusting relationship between the nurse and mother will enhance identifying infant-care problems the mother may be experiencing as well as make her more receptive to any teaching or information the nurse may offer.
3. The mother (parents) must be allowed to express her (their) feelings.

G. Work as a Contributing Integral Part of the Multidiscipline Team Caring for This Infant and Family

1. The physician—responsible for medical diagnosis and management of the family with regard to the child's illness.
2. The social worker—helps the parents handle the stress that prevents them from assuming their parenting roles.
3. The nurse—coordinates infant care and participates in teaching infant care to the mother.
4. The parents—must be included in the team because the plan of approach must be acceptable and understood in order to be used by them.
5. Other members of the team may include a psychiatrist, child-life worker, physical therapist, occupational therapist.

H. Help the Mother and Infant Establish a Healthy Relationship That Will Continue to Grow When the Infant Is Discharged (see also ICN, p. 1129).

1. Encourage the mother to be active in the plan of treatment. Identify areas of involvement in the nursing care plan.
2. Praise the mother's positive efforts; gradually redirect negative aspects.
3. Identify and interpret the infant's behavior pattern for the mother.
   a. Help her to understand the discrepancies between her expectations and reality.
   b. Teach her expected growth and development.
4. Help the mother to understand her importance to the infant and that the relationship is based on reciprocal needs and responses between the mother and infant.
5. Observe and document mother–infant interactions.
   a. Mother—holding, interest in infant, comforting activities

b. Infant—response to mother (i.e., looking at the mother, squirming, cuddling, crying, cooing).
6. The mother may actually need to be taught "mother craft"—how to cuddle, feed, play, and react to her child.

I. Initiate Community-Nurse Referral Before Discharge and/or Communicate With Community Nurse Already Involved.

1. Provides the parents with continual support by someone they know.
2. Gives feedback as to the home situation and possible areas where problems can be avoided.

J. Help the Mother (parents) **Understand and Accept the Need for Continual Follow-Up Care of Her** (their) **Infant.**

1. Be certain the mother knows where and when to obtain this care.
2. Encourage the mother to seek support from appropriate resources as necessary.

Expected Outcomes

1. Demonstrates improved nutritional status; eating; gaining weight
2. Shows advances in developmental level; shows appropriate behavior for age; reaching out; accepts physical contact
3. Responds to nurturing; tolerates eye-to-eye contact; shows evidence of establishing trusting relationship; accepts comforting
4. Parents demonstrate an understanding of the causes of the child's illness; express their feelings and concerns
5. Mother begins to establish infant-mother bonding; holds and comforts the infant; is reading materials on growth and development

---

Septicemia Neonatorum

Septicemia neonatorum (sepsis) is a generalized infection that may occur in the neonate and is characterized by the proliferation of bacteria in the bloodstream and frequently involves the meninges (as distinguished from simple bacteremia, congenital infection, septicemia following major diseases or surgery, or major congenital anomalies).

Etiology

1. The distribution of etiologic agents varies from year to year and from institution to institution.
2. Gram-negative organisms:
   E. coli
   Klebsiella (enterobacteriaceae)
   Pseudomonas
   Proteus
   Salmonella
   H. influenzae
3. Gram-positive organisms:
   Group B beta-hemolytic *Streptococcus*
   Listeria monocytogenes
   Staphylococcus aureus—coagulase-negative and coagulase-positive
   Staphylococcus epidermidis
   Streptococcus pneumoniae
   Streptococcus faecalis

4. It should be noted that fungal infections from the organism *Candida albicans* is increasing in incidence, especially in the low-birth-weight infant.
5. Predisposing factors
   a. Sex—male predominance
   b. Perinatal factors
      (1) Maternal complications
         Prolonged rupture of membranes
         Prolonged and difficult labor; precipitous delivery
         Chorioamnionitis
         Endometritis
         Urinary tract infection
         Toxemia
         Abruptio placentae
         Maternal illness
         Cardiovascular disease
         Colonization of organisms in genital tract
      (2) Infant complications
         Prematurity or low birth weight
         Congenital heart disease
         Intracranial bleeding
         Respiratory distress syndrome
         Skin infections
         Difficult/traumatic labor or delivery; asphyxia
   c. Iatrogenic or environmental factors
      (1) Related to type of equipment used in caring for infant
         Catheters
         Oxygen and humidity
         Resuscitative
      (2) Defective or unclean equipment
      (3) Obstetric and nursery practices
      (4) Surgical procedures
6. Mode of entry
   a. Infection may gain access into the amniotic sac either prior to or after rupture of the membranes; the fetus may aspirate some of this infected fluid.
   b. Bacteria may enter the fetal circulation following invasion of the decidua from the amniotic cavity.
   c. After birth, bacteria may enter the infant's circulation by a variety of routes. Infection may originate in the skin, umbilical stump, or mucous membranes of the eyes, nose, pharynx, and ear as well as the respiratory, gastrointestinal, and genitourinary tracts.
   d. Iatrogenic—equipment, resuscitation.

Altered Physiology

1. Temporary breakdown or depression of the infant's defense mechanisms for unknown reason
   a. Possibly due to stress of labor and delivery
   b. Predisposing factors (see under Etiology)
2. The defense systems of the newborn, especially the low-birth-weight infant, are ineffective with regard to:
   a. Active immunity
      (1) Significant formation of IgG (immunoglobulin G) begins at 1–3 months of age
      (2) Significant formation of IgM (immunoglobulin M) begins at birth to 7 days
   b. Passive immunity
      Born without IgM antibodies and bactericidal protection against gram-negative organisms
   c. Phagocytosis and minimal inflammatory response
      Neutrophils are less active in response to

chemotactic stimuli and migrate more slowly to areas of inflammation

d. Unknown factors

Complications

1. Meningitis—very common complication
2. Shock
3. Adrenal hemorrhage
4. Disseminated intravascular coagulation
5. Metabolic derangements
6. Pneumonia
7. Urinary tract infection
8. Congestive heart failure
9. High mortality rate

Clinical Manifestations

1. The early signs of sepsis are usually vague and subtle. The infant is often described as not doing well. The signs often include:
   a. Poor feeding; gastric retention; weak sucking
   b. Lethargy, limpness; weak crying
   c. Temperature alteration—generally hypothermia, but infant may have hyperthermia
2. Additional signs and symptoms may include any of the following:
   a. Pallor, cyanosis or apneic episodes, respiratory distress
   b. Jaundice
   c. Abdominal distention
   d. Vomiting and/or diarrhea
   e. Paronychia
   f. Petechiae or purpura
   g. Vesicles or pustules
   h. Hepatosplenomegaly
   i. Irritability, convulsion
   j. Bulging fontanelles
   k. Hypotonia
   l. Bradycardia/tachycardia

Diagnostic Evaluation

1. History of predisposing factors
2. Physical findings
3. Laboratory—recovery of organism from blood cultures must be obtained for a diagnosis of sepsis neonatorum
   a. Cultures to detect specific organism
      (1) Blood
      (2) Urine
      (3) Spinal fluid—delay in unstable infant
      (4) Umbilical stump
      (5) Skin lesions
      (6) Nose, throat, rectal
      (7) External auditory canal
      (8) Gastric fluid
   b. WBC and differential—nonspecific test; may be difficult to interpret; thrombocytopenia
   c. Hemoglobin, hematocrit—red blood cell counts may hemolyze with some bacteria
   d. Blood chemistries—sugar, calcium, pH, electrolytes
   e. C-reactive protein and erythrocyte sedimentation rate
   f. Acid–base studies (acidosis)
   g. Bilirubin
   h. TORCH (toxoplasmosis–rubella–cytomegalic inclusion virus–herpes–other)—detect antibodies

against common intrauterine-infective agents or specific IgMs and cultures for cytomegalovirus
      i. Arterial blood gases
4. Chest x-ray—may demonstrate pulmonary infection
5. Urinalysis

Treatment

A. Antibacterial Therapy—Based on the Identified Organism

1. Before the specific organism is identified, and after cultures have been obtained, the antibacterial therapy is based on the more common causative agents and their anticipated susceptibilities.
   a. Knowledge of particular nursery offenders and their antibiotic susceptibilities is needed for proper drug selection for both gram-negative and gram-positive organisms.
   b. Therapy duration is generally 5–10 days after clinical improvement, but may be as long as 3–4 weeks with complicated infections.
   c. Serum levels

B. Supportive Therapy

1. Observation
2. Isolation, if indicated
3. Fluid and caloric maintenance
4. Oxygen therapy
5. Regulation of thermal environment
6. Blood transfusion to correct anemia, shock
7. Others, as indicated
8. Exchange transfusion (controversial)
9. Protect from further infection

Potential Problems and Nursing Diagnoses

1. Complications related to infection and its systemic effects: meningitis, shock, disseminated intravascular coagulation, congestive heart failure, apnea, jaundice
2. Hypothermia related to unstable central temperature control and stress of infection
3. Nutrition, altered, less than body requirements, related to fatigue and disinterest
4. Other complications related to hospitalized infant (see premature infant, p. 1221)

Nursing Interventions

(See also ICN, p. 1129)

A. Review Maternal History. Identify Infants at Risk for Infection

B. Practice Measures That Will Prevent the Transmission of Infection in the Nursery

1. Practice careful handwashing technique and serve as a model of good technique.
2. Personnel with infection should avoid contact with infants.
   a. Seek health care for infection. (Cultures should be done.)
   b. Remain out of the nursery.
   c. Wear a mask when it is necessary to enter the nursery.
3. Teach parents and other persons entering the nursery proper handwashing and gown techniques.
4. Maintain sterile technique when procedures demanding this technique are performed.
5. Promote general cleanliness of the nursery environment.

Infected equipment and stagnant water provide excellent conditions for bacterial growth.

C. Observe Infants for the Vague Symptoms That Appear Early in the Course of Sepsis.

1. Observe for the following:
   a. Lethargy, decreased activity, and loss of muscle tone
   b. Poor feeding or refusal to feed
   c. Temperature alterations, especially hypothermia
   d. Alteration in vital signs
   e. Skin color and condition
   f. Intake and output
   g. Examine each body system
2. Be consistent in planning for the care of infants to provide a means whereby these early symptoms may be detected.
   a. Accurate charting of the infant's previous behavior
   b. Assigning the same nurse to care for an infant on successive days
3. Report to the physician the symptoms observed.
4. When neonatal sepsis is caused by B group streptococci, the disease may take one of two courses:
   a. Early onset—within 12–24 hours after birth and within 3 days of age.
      (1) Acute septicemia with fulminant clinical course; high mortality and severe neurologic sequelae in survivors.
      (2) There is generally a history of obstetric complications, and the serotypes of streptococci from the mother's birth canal and the infant are the same.
      (3) Signs and symptoms include respiratory symptoms—in particular, acute respiratory distress, hypoxia, leading to shock.
   b. Delayed onset—occurs 10 days to 6–12 weeks after birth
      (1) Illness is severe and associated with meningitis.
      (2) Normal obstetric history; probably acquired infection from environment.
      (3) Disease is characterized by meningeal symptoms, including bulging fontanelle and seizures.
5. Observe for signs of complications—meningitis, urinary tract infection, pneumonia.

D. Observe for Episodes of Apnea and Initiate Measures to Stimulate Respiration

1. Observe the infant closely for apnea or place the infant on a respiratory monitor.
2. Stimulate the infant when apnea does occur.
3. Report frequent periods of apnea to physician.
4. Report length of apneic episode and response to stimulation.

E. Observe the Infant for Convulsions That May Occur With Sepsis

1. Immediately report to the physician any twitching or convulsive activity.
   a. Remain with the infant.
   b. Suction mouth and nose if the infant has secretions or vomitus in his mouth.
   c. Turn head to side.
   d. Protect the infant from banging against side of Isolette or incubator or falling from radiant warmer.
   e. Provide oxygen if cyanosis or respiratory distress occurs.
   f. Administer any medication prescribed to control the convulsions.
2. Record the length of and the type of convulsion, the parts of the body involved, the infant's general appearance before and following the convulsion, and response to any therapy given.

F. Ensure That Evaluation and Diagnostic Tests Be Initiated Promptly and Correctly to Avoid Altered Results From Contamination

1. Tests should be completed prior to starting antibiotics.
2. Since the infective organism must be recovered in blood cultures, strict antiseptic technique in obtaining cultures is vital.
   a. Peripheral venipuncture is the site of choice (the umbilical vessels are already contaminated, and the femoral vein offers possible contamination from perineum).
   b. Cleanse skin with an antiseptic solution (e.g., iodine solution). For maximal aseptic effect, allow the solution to dry.

G. Provide for the Nutritional Needs of the Infant

1. During the acute phase of the illness, the infant may not be able to take or tolerate oral feedings.
   a. Monitor the administration of intravenous fluids. Nasogastric tube may be in place to aid in preventing abdominal distention.
   b. Provide for the sucking needs of the infant by giving him a pacifier.
   c. Gavage feedings may be given to the infant.
2. Initiate oral feedings of formula as soon as the infant's condition improves.
   a. Begin by offering small feedings and observe following responses:
      Vomiting
      Abdominal distention
      The infant's interest in feeding and ability to suck
      Whether the infant tires with feeding
   b. Nipple feedings may be supplemented with gavage feedings.
   c. Gradually increase amount of feeding. Do not force feedings—vomiting associated with diarrhea may result, leading to dehydration.
   d. Resume regular feeding schedule based on the infant's ability to tolerate feeding.
3. Hold the infant for feedings as soon as his condition warrants it.

H. Provide Measures to Maintain the Infant's Temperature Within Normal Range

1. Take the infant's temperature at hourly intervals.
2. Adjust the Isolette temperature to maintain the infant's temperature between 36° and 37°C. (96.8° and 98.6°F.).
3. When the infant is placed in an open crib, maintain temperature and cover the infant appropriately.
4. Report hypothermia or hyperthermia to the physician.

I. Administer the Prescribed Antibiotic Therapy to Control the Infection

Common antibiotics used in the infant include cefotaxime, vancomycin, penicillin G, kanamycin, methicillin, and nafcillin.

1. Administer the prescribed medications.
   a. Be aware of the action and side effects of the specific medications.

    b. Be aware of the route of excretion.
    c. Be aware of drug incompatibilities.
2. Observe the infant's apparent response to therapy.
    a. Note the child's activity, feeding behavior, and weight.
    b. Observe for the development of new symptoms.

J. Be Prepared to Assist With Blood Transfusions Used to Correct Anemia and Shock (see Exchange Transfusions, p. 1178)

Adult whole blood also provides specific factors that enhance the phagocytic abilities of neonate leukocytes.

K. Observe for the Occurrence of Septic Shock and Report Immediately.

Early phase—associated with peripheral vasodilatation and hypotension with metabolic acidosis.

    Later phase—peripheral vasoconstriction occurs with deterioration of heart and lung function. Decrease in cardiac output and arterial blood pressure is associated with increased central venous pressure.
1. Monitor blood pressure.
2. Check peripheral resistance in pulses in all extremities; note color and temperature.
3. Monitor hourly urine output for evaluation of renal function.

L. Provide for the Emotional Needs of the Infant
1. Place bright, colorful objects in the crib or Isolette.
2. Talk gently and quietly while caring for the infant.
3. Touch and gently stroke the infant.
4. Encourage the parents to visit and allow them to hold the infant as soon as possible.

M. Involve the Parents in the Infant's Care in the Hospital and Prepare Them for the Infant's Discharge
1. Encourage the parents to visit the infant.
    a. Allow them to hold and feed the baby.
    b. Answer questions they may have regarding the infant's progress and care.
    c. Provide them with an opportunity to explain their concerns.
2. Discuss symptoms of complications that may occur and should be watched for following discharge.
3. Give specific instruction regarding medications to be given at home.

Expected Outcomes

1. No complication as evidenced by stable function of body systems.
2. The infant maintains stable temperature.
3. The infant achieves and maintains appropriate nutrition as evidenced by weight gain.
4. The parents and infant experience no other complications related to their hospitalization experience.

Infant of Addicted Mother

An *infant of an addicted mother* is one who is born to a mother who is narcotic- or methadone-dependent and who takes the drug or drugs in varying dosages for varying periods during her pregnancy.

Etiology

A. Maternal Use of Narcotics or Methadone or Both Drugs During Pregnancy
1. The drugs cross the placental barrier and enter the fetal circulation.
2. The supply to the infant is abruptly terminated at delivery.
3. Other agents (i.e., phenobarbital, alcohol, propoxyphene) are capable of causing withdrawal symptoms.

B. Fetal Alcohol Syndrome—etiology
1. Direct ethanol toxicity to developing fetus
2. Maternal malnutrition—vitamin deficiency
3. Hypoglycemia, maternal
4. Concurrent drug abuse
5. Smoking
6. Alcohol-induced illness (i.e., gastric hemorrhage, cirrhosis of liver)
7. Alcohol freely crosses placenta and is found in amniotic fluid and cord blood.
8. Maturity of infant's metabolic and excretory mechanism is important.

C. Maternal Use of Cocaine During Pregnancy
1. Cocaine is a CNS stimulant
    a. Acts peripherally to inhibit nerve conduction by blocking reuptake of norepinephrine at nerve endings.
    b. Result is increased norepinephrine levels, which leads to vasoconstriction, tachycardia, hypertension, and uterine contractions.
2. The low molecular weight and lipophilic characteristics allow drug to cross the placenta and fetal blood–brain barrier.
3. Vasoconstriction of placental vessels with simultaneous abrupt increase in blood pressure may lead to abruptio placenta.
4. Tachycardia and hypertension in infant may cause cerebral infarction.
5. Chronic maternal anorexia results in fetal malnutrition.

Prognosis

A. For Drug Addiction
1. The long-term biologic effects on the infant of a drug-dependent mother are not fully known. These children may have:
    a. Abnormal psychomotor development associated with intrauterine growth retardation
    b. Behavioral disturbances such as hyperactivity, brief attention spans, temper tantrums
2. The unstable environment that the drug-addicted mother (or parents) may provide is a major threat to the child's health and development.

B. For Fetal Alcohol Syndrome
1. Intellectual impairment
2. Poor fine motor control
3. Difficulty feeding
4. Hyperactive
5. Developmental delay of gross motor skills
6. Minimal brain dysfunction
7. Slow postnatal catching up

C. For Cocaine Abuse
1. Spontaneous abortion
2. Premature labor

3. Abruptio placenta
4. Meconium staining

Complications

A. For Drug Addiction

1. Prematurity
2. Intrauterine growth retarded infant (IUGR); small-for-gestational-age infant (SGA)
3. Fetal anoxia with meconium aspiration
4. Infection-associated maternal sexually transmitted disease or hepatitis
5. Hypoglycemia
6. Hypocalcemia
7. Respiratory complications—RDS related to prematurity, aspiration pneumonia, transient tachypnea
8. Septicemia
9. Hyperbilirubinemia, especially with methadone-addicted mother
10. Electrolyte imbalance
11. Seizures
12. Temperature instability and fever
13. Cardiovascular collapse
14. AIDS (HIV)

B. For Fetal Alcohol Syndrome

1. Metabolic imbalance
2. Hypoglycemia
3. Respiratory distress
4. Neurologic pathology
5. Craniofacial anomalies
6. Congenital heart disease
7. Renal malformations

C. For Cocaine Abuse

1. Teratogenic effects are unknown
2. Disordered neurobehavioral functions—Brazelton Score shows significant depression of organizational response to environmental stimuli.
3. Prematurity
4. Intrauterine growth retardation
5. Renal and urinary tract abnormalities
6. Cerebral infarction
7. Visual dysfunction
8. EEG abnormalities
9. Hypertension
10. Increased risk for SIDS
11. Congenital malformations
12. AIDS (HIV)
13. Ischemic infarction of bowel
14. Seizures

Clinical Manifestations *(of Neonatal Withdrawal)*

A. Drug Addiction

1. The degree of withdrawal symptoms the infant manifests may be related to the duration of the mother's drug habit, the type and dosage requirements of her addiction, and her drug level immediately prior to her delivery.
    a. The closer to delivery the mother received her last dose, the longer her addiction and the higher her dose need, the longer the delay of withdrawal symptoms, and the more severe the symptoms will be in the infant.
    b. Although heroin and methadone produce similar withdrawal symptoms in the infant, those same symptoms are generally more severe with methadone withdrawal—probably because of the high level of the mother's dose, the pharmacologic characteristics of the drug itself, and the use by the mother of other drugs simultaneously.
2. Onset of symptoms
    a. Heroin—several hours after birth to 3–4 days of life
    b. Methadone—7–10 days after birth to several weeks of life
3. Cardinal signs of neonatal narcotic withdrawal
    a. Coarse, flapping tremors
    b. Irritability; hyperactivity; hypertonicity
    c. Prolonged, persistent, high-pitched cry
    d. Restlessness; sleepiness
4. Other signs and symptoms of acute withdrawal:
    a. Vigorous, ineffective sucking; poor feeding
    b. Excessive tearing; excessive sweating
    c. Increased salivation
    d. Sneezing, nasal stuffiness
    e. Vomiting and/or diarrhea
    f. Muscle rigidity
    g. Yawning
    h. Convulsions—with methadone withdrawal
    i. Tachypnea with associated respiratory alkalosis
    j. Exaggerated reflexes
    k. Hyperpyrexia
    l. Hiccoughs
5. Prematurity
    High incidence of infants born to addicted mothers are premature and/or small for gestational age.

B. Fetal Alcohol Syndrome

(Develop within first 24 hours of life)
1. Difficulty establishing respirations
2. Metabolic problems
3. Irritability
4. Increased muscle tone, tremulousness
5. Lethargy
6. Opisthotonus
7. Poor sucking reflex
8. Abdominal distention
9. Seizure activity

C. Cocaine Abuse

1. Does not appear to experience classic neonatal abstinence syndrome
2. Mild tremulousness
3. Increased irritability and startle response
4. Muscular rigidity
5. Difficult to console
6. Pronounced state of lability
7. Tachycardia and tachypnea
8. Poor tolerance for oral feedings, diarrhea
9. Disturbed sleep pattern

Diagnosis

1. Thorough maternal history, including drug habits
2. Physical assessment; Kahn's criteria of tremulousness and irritability:*
    a. Grade I—signs recognizable but mild
    b. Grade II—signs marked but only when the infant is disturbed

* Kahn EJ et al. The course of heroin withdrawal syndrome in newborn infants treated with phenobarbital or chlorpromazine. J Pediatr 75:495

c. Grade III—signs marked and occurring at frequent intervals, even when the infant is undisturbed
3. Laboratory studies
   a. Urine for toxicologic studies
      (1) Will detect maternal cocaine exposure within past 6–9 days.
      (2) Consider cocaine intoxication from breast milk of mother exposed to the drug.
   b. Blood glucose
   c. Serum calcium, magnesium, sodium, and total protein
   d. Hematocrit
   e. Platelets
   f. Blood gases—respiratory alkalosis
   g. Serologic studies for syphilis
   h. Appropriate cultures if systemic bacterial infection is suspected
4. Many of the clinical signs of neonatal narcotic withdrawal are nonspecific and may indicate other problems: hypoglycemia, hypocalcemia, CNS disorders or hemorrhage, infection, other, nonnarcotic drug withdrawal

Treatment

A. Drug Addiction

1. Narcotic antagonist for narcotic-induced respiratory depression at birth (morphine addiction)
2. Drug therapy for alleviation of signs of narcotic withdrawal. Duration of therapy using decreasing dosages may be from 4–40 days
   a. Paregoric (camphorated tincture of opium) orally
   b. Phenobarbital, orally
   c. Chlorpromazine (Thorazine) orally
   d. Diazepam (Valium) intramuscularly
   e. Methadone
3. Supportive therapy as appropriate

B. Fetal Alcohol Syndrome

1. Quiet environment with minimized auditory and sensory stimulation
2. Drug therapy to control seizures
3. Intravenous therapy for dehydration that accompanies alcohol withdrawal
4. Supportive therapy as appropriate

Potential Problems and Nursing Diagnoses

1. Hypoglycemia related to prematurity or SGA
2. Nutrition, altered, less than body requirements
3. Withdrawal symptoms (complications) related to maternal substance abuse
4. Respiratory distress related to prematurity, SGA, meconium aspiration
5. Potential for infection related to maternal disease
6. Parenting, altered related to maternal addiction and status as well as infant behaviors.

Nursing Interventions

A. Be Familiar With Withdrawal Symptoms in Order to Facilitate Early Diagnosis, Which in Turn Will Decrease Incidence of Morbidity and Mortality of High-Risk Infants

1. Recognize cardinal as well as other symptoms.
2. Identify infants likely to have symptoms.
3. Report to physician any suspicious behavior.

B. Ensure That Prophylactic Measures Have Been Administered Against Ophthalmia Neonatorum

There is a high incidence of gonococcal infection in drug-addicted pregnant women.

C. Ensure That Diagnostic Measures Are Carried Out

Collect urine for toxicologic studies within 24 hours after birth, since narcotic metabolites disappear rapidly.

D. Administer Nursing Care Appropriate for the Symptoms of Withdrawal the Infant Is Experiencing

1. Irritability and restlessness, high-pitched crying
   a. Loosely swaddle (be aware that this may increase the infant's temperature).
   b. Minimize handling—holding may aggravate irritability; some infants respond well to close contact and body movement.
   c. Decrease environmental stimuli (i.e., light, noise).
   d. Organize care to allow for periods of uninterrupted sleep.
   e. Prone positioning may help the infant organize his motor movements.
   f. Give medications with meals unless there is vomiting; then 30 minutes before.
   g. Nonoscillating water bed
2. Floppy tremors
   a. Protect skin from irritation and abrasions:
      (1) Use sheepskin.
      (2) Change position frequently.
      (3) Give good frequent skin care—keep the infant clean and dry.
3. Frantic sucking
   a. Give pacifier between feedings.
   b. Protect the infant's hands from excoriation.
4. Poor feeding—similar to the premature infant's inability to take an adequate amount at feedings
   a. Give small, frequent feedings.
   b. Maintain caloric and fluid intake requirement for the infant's desired weight.
5. Vomiting/diarrhea
   a. Position the infant to prevent aspiration.
   b. Provide good skin care to areas exposed to vomitus or stool.
6. Muscle rigidity—hypertonicity
   a. Change position frequently to minimize development of pressure areas.
   b. Use sheepskin.
   c. Skin care.
7. Increased salivation and/or nasal stuffiness
   a. Aspirate nasopharynx; suction tracheal mucus.
   b. Provide frequent nose and mouth care.
   c. Note respiration rate and characteristics and the infant's color.
8. Tachypnea
   a. Note onset and severity of accompanying signs of respiratory distress; place the infant on respiratory monitor.
   b. Position the infant for easier ventilation—semi-Fowler's position; tilt head back slightly.
   c. Minimize handling.
   d. Have resuscitative equipment available.
9. Tachycardia and hypertension—monitor vital signs closely; Cardiopulmonary monitor may be indicated.

E. Record Accurately and in Detail All Symptoms, Including the Following:

1. Time of onset
2. Duration and frequency

3. Severity
4. Treatment initiated and the infant's response
   Example: extent of irritability, changes in feeding behavior, tolerance of handling, characteristics and frequency of stool
5. Vital signs

F. Maintain Caloric and Fluid Requirements and Balance

1. Keep accurate intake and output records to prevent dehydration.
2. Maintain IV fluids as appropriate when the infant experiences vomiting or diarrhea.
3. The infant may feed better on a demand schedule.
4. The infant may need increased calories because of increased activity.

G. Support Drug Therapy When Used to Control Symptoms of Withdrawal

1. When diazepam (Valium) is used, be alert for the appearance of jaundice.
   Sodium benzoate is used as a preservative in preparation and interferes with binding of albumin with unconjugated bilirubin.
   Hepatic and cerebral complications may be related to propylene-glycol and ethyl-alcohol contents in diazepam.
2. Methadone withdrawal symptoms are frequently more difficult to control than those of heroin withdrawal.
3. Chlorpromazine may cause adverse effects on the CNS, endocrine glands, and the autonomic nervous system.
4. Paregoric may be associated with CNS depression or stimulation, acidosis, respiratory distress, renal failure.
5. Phenobarbital is a CNS depressant and impairs sucking reflex and bonding behaviors. There may be an increased risk of seizures with its use. Serum levels should be monitored carefully.
6. Note appearance of side effects of depression from oversedation:
   a. Respiratory distress
   b. Lethargy
   c. Decreased sucking activity
   d. Hypotonia

H. Protect the Infant From Pathophysiologic Processes to Which He Is Predisposed Because of Prematurity or Being Small for Gestational Age

1. Hypoglycemia
2. Hypocalcemia
3. Hypothermia
4. Hypoxia
5. Sepsis

I. Encourage Multidisciplinary Conferences in an Attempt to Treat the Whole Family

1. Initiate early referrals as needed to social services, child welfare agency, and/or community nurse to provide for continuity of care after discharge.
   a. The unstable environment into which the infant may be discharged offers a threat to the child's future well-being and development.
      Discharge to a foster home may be considered.
2. Evaluate the mother's attitude toward her infant.
   a. She may be able to accept the responsibility of her child and to accept help offered her.
   b. She may become nonfunctioning as a result of the birth of her infant; she may feel inadequate, angry, guilty or see the infant as an added economic burden.

J. Encourage Parental Involvement in the Care of This Infant

Frequently the infant may not be discharged with the mother. Promote early mother–infant attachment and foster their relationship.

1. Encourage frequent mother–infant contact.
2. Help the mother understand the behaviors she sees in her infant. She should be taught how to handle her infant, who may cry hysterically at her touch or stiffen when she is trying to cuddle him.
3. Have the mother feed the infant.
4. Pace the growth of the relationship between the infant and mother based on the infant's progress and the mother's positive reactions.
5. Keep in mind that cocaine, methadone, and heroin can be detected in breast milk and may lead to permanent addiction of the infant should the mother breastfeed.

Health Education

1. Carefully planned follow-up care for the infant is essential.
   a. Explain to the mother the need for consistent follow-up care of her infant.
   b. Infants of drug-dependent mothers are at risk; they may show failure to thrive, experience battering, succumb to sudden infant death syndrome, and may be at risk for AIDS.
   c. Involve the community health nurse in the planning early in hospitalization. This early involvement may offer mother some security.
   d. Social work involvement may be indicated to determine ability of the parents to care for the child at home.
   e. It is often difficult to maintain contact for follow-up.
2. The mother may be accepting of rehabilitation during the postpartum period. Contact appropriate people or provide appropriate information for her; incorporate her into total care of the infant prior to discharge
3. Help the mother understand what she should expect in the infant's behavior upon discharge.
   a. Many infants are irritable and restless for several months after birth.
   b. Discuss with the mother the feelings she may have as a result of a strained mother–child relationship.

Expected Outcomes

1. The infant maintains normal metabolic status: normal serum glucose levels.
2. Achieves adequate intake as evidenced by weight gain.
3. The infant proceeds through withdrawal with minimal complications as evidenced by calm behavior, weight gain, and stable vital signs.
4. The infant maintains adequate oxygenation and does not experience respiratory distress.
5. The infant is free of infection as demonstrated by normal vital signs and laboratory values.
6. Maternal–infant bonding is established and demonstrated during hospitalization.

Resources

Perinatal Center for Chemical Dependence
215 E. Chicago Avenue, Suite 501
Chicago, IL 60611
(312) 908-0867

March of Dimes Birth Defects Foundation
Community Services Department
1275 Mamaroneck Avenue
White Plains, NY 10605
(914) 428-7100

March of Dimes has available a brochure, "Drugs, Alcohol, and Tobacco Abuse During Pregnancy," and a 10-minute videotape, "Cocaine's Children."

Acquired Immunodeficiency Syndrome (AIDS) in the Infant

Risk Factors

1. High-risk mother
   a. Mother infected with HIV
   b. Mother IV drug user
   c. Hemophiliac
   d. Spouse of bisexual man
   e. Geographic location with prevalence of disease in heterosexuals
   f. Spouse of hemophiliac
2. Blood transfusion recipient of infected blood or blood products.
3. Breast milk—may be mode of transmission to infant from infected mother.
4. The precise mode of transmission from mother to infant is not known. Possibilities include:
   a. In utero transplacental transmission
   b. Perinatal transmission may occur at the time of delivery through contact with maternal blood
   c. Postnatal transmission may be possible by intimate nonsexual contact with parents with AIDS or ARC (AIDS-related complex)

Clinical Manifestations

1. The mean age of onset in the infant is 4 months after exposure.
   The shorter incubation period is compatible with in utero transfusion and possibly to the immature cellular immune system of the neonate.
2. The infant may present asymptomatic.
3. *Signs and symptoms*
   a. Low birth weight, premature, IUGR, and failure to thrive
   b. Weight loss
   c. Recurrent bacterial infections
   d. Lymphadenopathy
   e. Hepatosplenomegaly
   f. Diarrhea—chronic or recurring
   g. Persistent candidiasis
   h. Neutropenia
   i. Thrombocytopenia
   j. Interstitial pneumonitis
   k. Recurrent enlargement of parotid glands
   l. Recurrent otitis media
4. Infants with ARC present with:
   a. Generalized lymphadenopathy
   b. Recurrent fevers
   c. Mild immune dysfunction
   d. No opportunistic infections
5. Dysmorphic syndrome associated with AIDS has been identified by some clinicians; however, there is some controversy about this.
   a. Growth failure

b. Craniofacial abnormalities
   (1) Microcephaly
   (2) Prominent boxlike ears
   (3) Flattened nasal bridge that appears scooped-out in profile
   (4) Mild upward or downward obliquity of the eyes
   (5) Prominent palpebral fissures, with blue scleras
   (6) Ocular hypertelorism
   (7) Short nose with flattened columella
   (8) Well-formed triangular philtrum with petulous lips
6. Most common opportunistic infections:
   a. Cytomegalovirus
   b. *Pneumocystis carinii*
   c. Herpes virus
   d. *Candida albicans*
   e. Epstein–Barr virus

Diagnostic Evaluation

1. Exclusion of all other causes of immunodeficiency:
   a. Primary immunodeficiency disease—DiGeorge syndrome, Wiskott–Aldrich syndrome, agammaglobulinemia
   b. Secondary immunodeficiency associated with immunosuppressive therapy, starvation, lymphoreticular malignancy.
   c. Congenital infections that result in immunodeficiency such as cytomegalovirus, rubella virus, Epstein–Barr virus. The onset, however, is usually prenatal/perinatal and immunodeficiency is mild and transient.
2. Laboratory
Diagnosis of HIV (human immunodeficiency syndrome) in newborns is difficult because of transplacental passage of maternal antibody to HIV in infants born to seropositive mothers. A seropositive result in the infant may not be an indication for HIV infection. Some infants fail to elaborate HIV antibody and will be HIV antibody negative, but will be identified as HIV infected by viral culture or antigen detection.
   Frequently, laboratory evidence of immunodeficiency precedes clinical manifestations of AIDS.
   a. CBC–Hct–Hbg
      (1) Serum immunoglobulins—elevated
      (2) Lymphocyte ratio reversed—T4/T8
      (3) Abnormal lymphocyte response to mitogens and antigens
      (4) Hypergammaglobulinemia with T-cell dysfunction and depletion; antibody deficient
      (5) Increased circulating immune complexes—show failure of appropriate antibody response to antigen
      (6) Thrombocytopenia
      (7) Anemia
   b. HIV antibody identification
      (1) ELISA-positive may indicate passive transfer of antibody from mother
      (2) Western blot antibody analysis—may need serial testing
3. Presence of "marker" disease

Treatment

Treatment is directed at the prevention of transmission of the infection, treating infection in the infant, and alleviating existing symptoms and preventing further complications.

1. Irradiate all blood and blood products given to the infant to prevent Graft-versus-host disease.
2. Prophylactic gamma globulin—to compensate for deficiency of B lymphocytes.
   a. Given specifically to reduce risk of bacterial sepsis and meningitis.
   b. Controversy over this practice.
3. Prophylactic trimethoprim-sulfa—to reduce risk of pneumocystis—controversial.
4. Corticosteroids—for lymphoid interstitial pneumonia before irreversible pulmonary fibrosis occurs.
5. Optimal nutrition—preferably high-caloric oral feeding since parenteral feeding increases risk of infection.
6. Antibiotic therapy specific for active infections.

Complications

1. Respiratory infections
2. Oral candidiasis and diaper rash
3. Bacterial infections
4. Fluid and electrolyte imbalance
5. Failure to thrive
6. Bleeding disorders
7. Sensory deprivation
8. Death

Potential Problems and Nursing Diagnoses

1. Potential for infection related to altered or immature immune system.
2. Hemorrhage related to hemopoietic changes.
3. Breathing pattern, ineffective, related to infection.
4. Altered skin integrity related to diarrhea and/or candida infection.
5. Sensory perception alteration related to isolation.
6. Growth and development, impaired, related to limited contact with others.
7. Altered parenting related to anxiety and fear.

Nursing Interventions

A. Identify Any Infant at Risk for HIV (AIDS)

1. Offspring of at-risk mother
2. Recurrent infections
3. Failure to thrive

B. Prevent Transmission of Virus

1. Universal precautions
2. American Academy of Pediatrics Task Force on AIDS recommended guidelines:
   a. Newborn infants should be handled with gloves until blood and amniotic fluid have been removed from skin.
   b. Use mechanical suction equipment when assisting with resuscitation. In emergency when mouth suction of airway is performed, an inline trap should be used.
   c. Infants of known seropositive mothers may be cared for in normal nursery and do not require isolation in private room or cubicle. Gloves should be worn for contact with blood or blood-containing fluids as well as for procedures that involve exposure to blood.
   d. HIV-infected mothers should be advised not to breast-feed their infants.
   e. The woman who is seropositive or at increased risk should receive counseling and guidance regarding the implications of current or future pregnancy to herself and her baby.

3. It is suggested that gloves be worn when changing diapers.
4. Proper handwashing is essential.
5. The policy "No pregnant caregivers" may be appropriate.

C. Be Aware of the Complications That Can Occur in the Infant With AIDS.

Note: Remember that many of these infants are born premature and/or SGA and are also at risk for problems related to those conditions.

1. *Respiratory infections*
   a. Ongoing clinical assessment of vital signs, respiratory status, breath sounds, etc.
   b. Ventilatory support may be necessary. Monitor blood gases; pulmonary toilet as needed.
   c. Administer antibiotics promptly and carefully. Serum antibiotic levels may be ordered. Correct timing is important.
   d. Keeping the infant well hydrated will aid in keeping secretions liquified and mobilized.
2. *Other infections*
   a. Oral infection from *Candida albicans* is common. Treatment—oral nystatin
   b. Diaper rash related to diarrhea. Treatment—topical nystatin and open-air exposure
   c. Fungal and bacterial invasion via peripheral and central lines.
   d. Meticulous skin care, position changes should help keep the infant comfortable.
3. *Dehydration*—generally resulting from diarrhea
   a. Strict recording of intake and output. Maintain fluid balance and monitor electrolytes.
   b. Check urine specific gravity and Dipstix frequently.
   c. Monitor for other signs of dehydration, skin turgor, vital signs, etc.
4. *Hemorrhage*
   a. Provide safe environment, handle infant gently; pad bed to prevent bruising.
   b. Check urine, stool, stomach content for occult blood.
   c. Observe for bruising, bleeding from heel sticks, umbilical cord, etc.
   d. Ensure that lab work is done on time and results reported to physician—prothrombin time, partial prothrombin, platelet count. Keep accurate record of sampling blood count.
   e. Replacement transfusions may be necessary.
5. *Failure to thrive*
   a. Adequate nutrition is essential for normal growth and healing—high-caloric formula.
   b. Oral lesions from Candida can interfere with sucking and oral feeding may be difficult. Nasogastric or orogastric feeding tube will facilitate giving infant nutrition.
   c. If adequate calories cannot be given orally, parenteral nutrition will be instituted. This increases the risk of infection. Monitor site carefully. Observe for signs of infection.
6. *Sensory deprivation and unmet developmental needs*
   a. Sensory stimulation is necessary for normal development. The nurse, the primary provider of care in the nursery, can serve as a role model for others in caring for this infant. Hold and rock infant during and after feeding, talk softly to him during procedures, play soft music or tapes of par-

ent voices, place him on a water bed, have objects and pictures for infant to look at.

b. Encourage parents to visit and participate in the care of their baby as much as possible. They should be active participants in making plans concerning the care.

c. Protect the infant from noxious stimuli.

d. Provide for periods of uninterrupted rest.

D. Provide Emotional Support to the Family

1. This family will be experiencing the same feelings and fears as any other parent of a seriously ill infant.

2. They may also be experiencing fears and emotions related to the specific diagnosis, the guilt, perceived social stigma of AIDS. They may need help expressing their feelings.

3. Help parents deal with the poor prognosis of the infant's illness. Assist them in establishing a support network that will help them through the crisis.

E. Provide Essential Discharge Planning for Family Taking Home Infant With AIDS

1. Teach essentials of care—procedures necessary to be carried out at home, medications, feeding, enteric precautions, signs and symptoms of infection, skin care, etc.

2. Initiate home care services or community nurse referral. Social work referral as indicated.

Health Education

1. Educate the parents about AIDS. Fear of caring for the infant should be reduced and effective bonding and parenting behaviors should be seen.

2. Stress the importance of close follow-up of the infant after hospital discharge.

3. Help the family understand ongoing developmental needs of the infant.

Expected Outcomes

1. No evidence of infection will be seen.

2. Hemorrhage resulting from hemopoietic changes will not occur.

3. Achieves stable respiratory status. Demonstrates normal vital signs.

4. Maintains skin integrity; no signs of skin breakdown.

5. Demonstrates normal developmental behavior; no evidence of sensory or physiologic deprivation while in the nursery.

6. Parent–infant bonding observed; parents show willingness to visit infant, hold him, and participate in his care.

Neonatal or Prolonged Sleep Apnea of Infancy *(Near-miss SIDS)*

1. *Apnea of infancy* is the cessation of breathing for more than 20 seconds, or a shorter episode associated with bradycardia, cyanosis, or pallor; frequently identified as an infant, usually between 2 weeks and 6 months of age, who is brought to medical attention because of an unexplained frightening respiratory or cardiac event, usually occurring while the infant is asleep.

2. Sudden infant death syndrome (SIDS)
   The sudden death of any infant or young child, which is unexplained by history, and in which a thorough postmortem examination fails to demonstrate an adequate cause of death.

Etiology

1. Unknown—may result from many different pathologic processes.

2. Apnea related to organic disorders:
   a. Seizure disorders
   b. Gastroesophageal reflux
   c. Significant anemia
   d. Sepsis, severe infection
   e. Hypoglycemia
   f. Impaired regulation of breathing
   g. Maternal cocaine abuse

3. Current theories relating to the cause of SIDS:
   a. Prolonged sleep apnea
   b. Chronic oxygen deficiency
   c. Enzyme abnormalities
   Although many feel that some infants with prolonged sleep apnea are at risk for SIDS, a definitive causal relation between the two has not been scientifically established.

4. Characteristics that may identify infants at risk for SIDS include:
   a. Prematurity
   b. Neonatal conditions with apnea
   c. History of apnea
   d. History of SIDS in family

5. Characteristics of SIDS pattern include:
   a. Prematurity
   b. Preceding cold or URI
   c. Peak age, 2–4 months
   d. Occurs in males in a ratio of 3:2

Management

1. Cardiopulmonary monitoring—is critical

2. Specific treatment of any underlying cause

3. Consultation with infant apnea team

4. Theophylline—may be used to decrease apneic spells

5. Long-term follow-up for physiologic and neurologic behavioral functions

Prognosis

1. Infants who have experienced infant apnea may be at risk for recurrent apnea, hypoxia, and sudden death.

2. Because of hypoxemia that may have occurred, child should be assessed for learning difficulties (hearing, eyesight), discrete neurologic impairments, personality disorders, etc.

Clinical Manifestations

1. The infant is usually found by parents or caretaker to be:
   a. Limp
   b. Cyanotic
   c. Pale
   d. No respiration
   e. Cool to touch
   f. Normal muscle tone

2. Some form of resuscitation may be required—mouth-to-mouth respiration or cardiopulmonary assistance.

3. The infant usually exhibits symptoms when asleep, although the syndrome may occur during waking hours.

4. Types of sleep apnea include:
   a. Central or diaphragmatic—chest movement ceases, absence of airflow

b. Obstructive—chest and diaphragm move but there is no air-exchange.
c. Mixed—cessation of airflow and chest movement, followed by respiratory effort without airflow.

Diagnostic Evaluation

It must be established that a primary life-threatening failure in physiologic homeostasis has occurred, ruling out other medical problems that could result in respiratory failure as a secondary cause. To accomplish this the following procedures are generally included:

1. Detailed history of the event including information concerning what happened, appearance of infant, type of intervention, how the infant responded, conditions prior to the event, special past medical history, special family history
2. Medical evaluation of the infant (physical examination)
3. Laboratory data—generally minimal unless history or examination indicates a specific line of inquiry
   a. Complete blood count with differential
   b. Serum glucose
   c. Electrolytes
   d. Calcium and phosphate
   e. Magnesium
   f. Blood gases, as indicated
4. Chest x-ray
5. Electrocardiogram
6. Electroencephalogram (may not be routine) and neurologic examination
7. Respiratory studies—a pneumogram 12–24-hour tape recording of small changes in electrical resistance with each breath or respiratory pattern; multichannel sleep test with continuous print-out
8. Continuous cardiac and apnea monitoring for recurrence of event, prolonged apnea, or bradycardia
9. Barium swallow for gastroesophageal reflux

Potential Problems and Nursing Diagnoses

1. Breathing pattern, ineffectual, related to alteration/cessation of respirations
2. Parental knowledge deficit as to cause and explanation of what is happening
3. Parental anxiety related to frightening episode of infant apnea
4. Alterated parenting related to parental anxieties and fears

Nursing Interventions

A. Be Prepared for the Infant's Admission.

Have all equipment, including apnea monitor, ready for use.

1. Select a room that is clearly visible from the nursing station; the room should be quiet in order to reduce sensory stimulation, which may reduce the likelihood of a recurring episode.
2. The family has just experienced the extreme stress of feeling that their infant has almost died. Professional efficiency and empathy at the time of admission is reassuring and builds parental confidence in nursing care.

B. Obtain a Nursing History With Special Attention to:

1. The parents' description of the events that preceded hospitalization, and their understanding of prolonged apnea.

a. This information may provide clues for factors to observe during hospitalization and provides data for the development of a teaching plan.
b. It also allows for the correction of misinformation and misconceptions.
2. Have the parents describe sleep patterns, feeding habits, prior health problems, immunizations, and medications; this information may provide data regarding possible influencing factors or causes of the condition.
3. Have the parents describe a typical day in the life of the infant and the family unit. This provides important data on how home-monitoring may affect family life, and contributes to the effective development of home management and family teaching plans; it also provides a basis for continuity of care for the infant.

C. Orient the Parents to the Unit and the Equipment Used in the Infant's Care.

Explain the visiting policy and encourage the parents to visit as much as possible.

1. The parents must be willing and available for comprehensive instruction in their infant's condition and necessary interventions so that they feel competent in the infant's care prior to discharge.
2. Assignment of consistent nursing (primary nurse) is helpful so that families can develop a trusting relationship that will help them deal with the emotional aspects of the diagnosis and the complexities of the treatment plan.
3. Preparing the parents for all diagnostic tests that will be performed helps reduce the fear surrounding these procedures.

D. Monitor Constantly, and Document any Apneic Event the Infant May Experience.

1. Condition of the infant
   a. Awake/asleep
   b. Respirations—none, normal, shallow; color of infant
   c. Monitor reading—apnea, bradycardia and rate
   d. Position of infant—limp, vomited, etc.
2. Intervention
   a. Nothing—infant all right or self-corrected
   b. Gentle stimulation
   c. Vigorously shaken
   d. Resuscitation

E. Serve as a Role Model for the Family in the Following Areas of Infant Care.

1. Use of the infant monitor (i.e., electrode placement, operation of controls, care of lead wires to prevent damage, etc.). Discussion of home-monitoring should not take place until it has been determined that this procedure will be used.
2. Methods of responding to alarms. Respond to all alarms immediately according to established procedures (i.e., observation and assessment of infant, stimulation, resuscitation, etc.).
3. Recording procedure—complete documentation of any apneic episode; record each time alarm sounds.
4. Administration of theophylline, if prescribed.
   a. Observe for signs of toxicity: apical rate above 200, vomiting, and agitation.
   b. Although the mechanism by which theophylline reduces or prevents apnea in some infants is not understood, research indicates it may act by:
      (1) Inducing rapid shallow breathing
      (2) Increasing metabolic rate with an increase in

alveolar ventilation in proportion to increased CO_2 production.

5. Continue the infant's normal activities whenever possible (i.e., holding him for feedings, playing with him, disconnecting him from monitor for bathing); allow for continuation of usual eating or sleeping patterns. Simulating the home environment as much as possible will encourage deep-sleep patterns, which may stimulate apnea in some infants (valuable diagnostic information).

F. Effectively Prepare Parents for Eventual Discharge of Infant.

Since the parents have experienced at least one apneic episode prior to hospitalization, the fear of their infant's sudden death has been heightened. When discharged, the parents have direct and full responsibility for appropriate action should the infant's breathing cease.

1. Assess what parents know and understand about apnea. Correct any misconceptions and provide accurate information.
2. Make sure parents know about feeding precautions—frequent burping, no bottle in bed, upright position after feeding, elevation of the head of the bed, position on abdomen for sleep.
3. Have parents contact local emergency service to discuss prolonged apnea of infancy and CPR, and to be certain they have infant resuscitation equipment. It may be possible to arrange for the power company to notify the parents if power supply is to go off.
4. Instruct the parents in the administration of any medications (i.e., theophylline).
5. Teach CPR to the parents as well as to another responsible person, relative, or friend, to provide some relief for the parents from infant care.

G. Teach and Prepare the Parents for Home-Monitoring, if Necessary.

1. Show the parents how to operate and maintain the monitor. Reinforce teaching by equipment supplier. Be sure they know how to contact a monitor technician.
2. Describe apnea recording procedure to be used (see D).
3. Teach methods of responding to alarms—what to observe (i.e., color, presence or absence of breathing) and how to respond (gentle and vigorous stimulation, CPR).
4. Discuss adjustments in daily living that will be necessary. Start by identifying a typical family day, then discuss anticipated changes.
   a. Emphasize that this responsibility must be shared by both parents.
   b. Discuss the possible impact on siblings.
   c. Caution the parents to eliminate noises that would interfere with their ability to hear the alarm (i.e., showering, vacuum cleaning) when only one parent is present. Someone must always be available to hear and respond to the alarm.
   d. Avoid traveling long distances alone with infant.
   e. Encourage the parents to maintain their relationship with one another by using another person trained in CPR to assume infant care occasionally.
5. Use anticipatory guidance in preparing parents for complication of home monitoring:
   a. Increased anxiety and tension
   b. Constant worry about the alarm—even when it does not go off
   c. Fatigue
   d. The financial and emotional burdens encountered by the entire family

e. Loss of "normal, healthy child"—parents then grieve when given the diagnosis

6. Emphasize the healthy aspects of the infant. Encourage the parents to continue as many usual routines as possible. Provide specific things parents can do to encourage normal development and a healthy parent–child relationship.
7. Encourage the parents to provide total care for their infant for 24 hours prior to discharge.

H. Continue to Observe Family Dynamics.

1. Assess for family conflicts or problems that can be alleviated.
2. Families who are overly stressed or demonstrate a maladaptive response may require social service or psychiatric consultation.
3. Modification of the management plan may be indicated.

I. Document Patient/Family Progress in Order to Facilitate Comprehensive Care and Discharge Planning.

Daily notes should include:
1. Frequency and type of monitor alarms; intervention required
2. Teaching
3. Family dynamics
   a. Who visited and for how long
   b. Description of parent–child interaction
   c. Description of parent interaction
   d. Amount of care done by parents
   e. Assessment of parental competence in providing care

J. Ensure Adequate Follow-Up Support.

Most families are frightened by the responsibility of home-monitoring and will require support after discharge.
1. Some may need a community health nurse—homemaker/home health aide.
2. Instruct the parents regarding when and how to obtain assistance for medical, technical, and psychosocial problems.
3. Facilitate contact with other parents of infants with prolonged apnea.
4. Assist the parents with arrangements for competent babysitting help.

K. Be Aware that Successful Outcome for Every Baby With Prolonged Apnea Cannot Be Certain, Despite Continuous Surveillance With or Without Monitors and Appropriate Intervention.

L. Participate in Community Education Regarding Prolonged Apnea and SIDS.

Expected Outcomes

1. Infant regains normal breathing pattern; does not experience recurring apnea; vital signs stable
2. Parents verbalize some understanding of the apnea event
3. Parents recall what to observe in infant; demonstrate appropriate interventions (CPR; use of apnea monitoring equipment) when apnea occurs
4. Parents appear to reestablish and maintain normal parenting relationship with the infant

Available Resources

National Sudden Infant Death Syndrome Foundation (NSIDF), Dept. NB3, 2 Metro Plaza, Suite 205, 8240 Professional Plaza, Landover, MD 20785: 1-800-221-SIDS

The International Guild for Infant Survival, Inc., 1515 Reistertown Road, Suite 300, Baltimore, MD 21208; (301) 484-0111.

National Foundation for Sudden Infant Death, 1501 Broadway, New York, NY 10036.

Guidelines for Home Apnea Use*

1. Monitor high-risk infants, who include:
   a. Symptomatic premature infant with pathologic apnea beyond normal time of discharge

* Adapted from Home Apnea Use Guidelines: Consensus Development Conference on Infantile Apnea and Home Monitoring, October 1986, National Institutes of Health, Washington, DC.

   b. Infant with significant acute life-threatening life event
   c. Infant with two or more siblings with SIDS.
2. Parents and clinicians must agree on the use of home monitoring. The issues of social, emotional, and financial impact must be addressed.
3. There must be available comprehensive community supportive services and ongoing follow-up.
4. Pneumograms not suggested for use as a screening tool for SIDS or severe apnea.
5. Routine monitoring of asymptomatic infant not suggested.
6. Routine monitoring of normal infant not indicated.
7. Improve monitor safety.

Bibliography

Books

Avery GB. Neonatology. 3rd ed. Philadelphia, JB Lippincott, 1987

Bergman AB. The "Discovery" of Sudden Infant Death Syndrome. New York, Praeger, 1986

Brazelton TB et al. Neonatal Behavioral Assessment Scale. 2nd ed. Philadelphia, JB Lippincott, 1984

Daddy: NICU: A Conversation with Fathers of Intensive Care Infants. Omaha, NE, Centering Corp, 1988

Fanaroff AA and Martin RJ (eds). Neonatal–Perinatal Medicine. 4th ed. St Louis, CV Mosby, 1987

Gellis SG and Kagan BM. Current Pediatric Therapy, vol. 12. Philadelphia, WB Saunders, 1986

Gomella TL (ed). Neonatalogy: Basic Management, On Call Problems, Diseases, Drugs. Norwalk, CT, Appleton and Lange, 1988

Gottfried AW and Gaiter JL. Infant Stress under Intensive Care. Baltimore, University Park Press, 1985

Hodson WA and Truog WE. Critical Care of the Newborn. Philadelphia, WB Saunders, 1989

Johnson SH. High-Risk Parenting: Nursing Assessment and Strategies for the Family at Risk. 2nd ed. Philadelphia, JB Lippincott, 1986

Klaus MH and Kennell JH. Maternal–Infant Bonding. St Louis, CV Mosby, 1983

Klaus MH and Fanaroff AA. Care of the High-Risk Neonate. Philadelphia, WB Saunders, 1986

Krones SB. High-Risk Newborn Infant: The Basis for Intensive Nursing Care. 3rd ed. St Louis, CV Mosby, 1986

MacDonald MG (ed). Emergency Transport of Perinatal Patient. Boston, Little, Brown & Co, 1989

Merenstein GB and Gardner SL. Handbook of Neonatal Intensive Care. St Louis, CV Mosby, 1989

Nugent JK. Using the NBAS with Infants and Their Families. White Plains, NY, March of Dimes Birth Defects Foundation, 1985

Sammons WH and Lewis JM. Premature babies—A Different Beginning. St Louis, CV Mosby, 1985

Schreiner RL and Bradburn NC (eds). Care of the Newborn. 2nd ed. New York, Raven Press, 1988

Simpson H and McFayden UM. Near-Miss for Sudden Infant Death Syndrome: A Clinical Approach. In Meadow R (ed). Recent Advances in Paediatrics; pp 201–216. New York, Churchill Livingstone, 1986

Stern L. Feeding the Sick Infant. New York, Raven Press, 1987

Stern L and Vert P. Neonatal Medicine. New York, Mosson Publishing, 1987

Streeter NS. High-Risk Neonatal Care. Rockville, MD, Aspen Publications, 1986

Taelusch HW and Yogman MW (eds). Follow-up Management of the High-Risk Infant. Boston, Little, Brown & Co, 1987

Vidyasagar D and Sarnaik AP (eds). Neonatal and Pediatric Intensive Care. Littleton, MA, PSG Publishing, 1985

Whaley LE and Wong DL. Essentials of Pediatric Nursing. St Louis, CV Mosby, 1989

Journals

Ammann AJ. Immunopathogenesis of pediatric acquired immunodeficiency syndrome. J Perinatal 1988 8(2):154–159

Amon E et al. Factors responsible for preterm delivery of the immature newborn infant (<1000 gm). Am J Obstet Gynecol 1987 May; 156(5): 1143–1148

An international classification of retinopathy of prematurity. Pediatrics 1988 Jul; 82(1):37–43

Arenson J. Discharge teaching in the NICU: The changing needs of NICU graduates and their families. Neonatal Network 1988 Feb; 6(4):29–30, 47–52

Asselin BL and Lawrence RA. Maternal disease as a consideration in lactation management. Clin Perinat 1987 Mar; 14(1):71–88

Auerbach KG. Infant formula samples and breast feeding. J Obstet Gynecol Neonatal Nurs 1987 Mar–Apr; 16(2):86

Auerbach KG and Gartner LM. Breastfeeding and human milk: Their association with jaundice in the neonate. Clin Perinat 1987 Mar; 14(1):89–107

Bauchner H, Brown E and Peskin J. Premature graduates of the newborn intensive care unit: A guide to follow-up. Pediar Clinic North Am 1988 Dec; 35(6):1207–1227

Beaver PK. Premature infants' response to touch and pain: Can nurses make a difference? Neonatal Network 1987 Dec; 6(3):13–17

Bergman AB. Twenty-fifth anniversary of the National Sudden Infant Death Syndrome Foundation. Pediatrics 1988 Aug; 272–273

Berry RK. Home care of the child with AIDS. Pediatr Nurs 1988 Jul–Aug; 14(4):341–344

Bengol N et al. Teratogenicity of cocaine in humans. J Pediatr 1987 Jan; 110(1): 93–96

Black VD. Neonatal hyperviscosity syndromes. Curr Probl Pediatr 1987 Feb; 17(2):73–130

Boyes SM. AIDS virus in breast milk: A new threat to neonates and donor breast milk banks. Neonatal Network 1987 Apr; 5(5):37–39

Brady MT and Ng A. Protection of neonates from transfusion-associated AIDS by the use of CMV-seronegative blood before availability of specific serologic tests for HTLV-111 (HIV). J Perinatol 1987 Oct; 4(4):305–307

Brown DR, Milley JR, Ripepl UG and Biglan AW. Retinopathy of prematurity. Am J Dis Child 1987 Feb; 141(2):154–160

Brown L. Physiologic responses to cutaneous pain in neonates. Neonatal Network 1987 Dec; 6(3):18–22

Brown MS, Nelson S and Stewart BJ. Detection of neonatal hypoglycemia—A comparison of three reagent strips. Nurs Pract. 1988 Oct; 13(10):15–16, 18, 23–4

Budreau GK. Postnatal cranial molding and infant attractiveness: Implications for nursery. Neonatal Network 1987 Apr; 5(5):13–19

Burns EA, House JD and Ankenbauer MR. Sibling grief in reaction to sudden infant death syndrome. Pediatrics 1986 Sep; 78(3):485–487

Butler KM and Baker CJ. Candida: An increasing important pathogen in the nursery. Pediatr Clin North Am 1988 Jun; 35(3):543–563

Butts PA et al. Concerns of parents of low birth weight infants following hospital discharge: A report of parental-initiated telephone calls. Neonatal Network. 1988 Oct; 7(2):37–42

Chan MM. Sudden infant death syndrome and families at risk. Pediatr Nurs 1987 May–Jun; 13(3):166–168

Chasnoff DJ, Burns KA and Burns WJ. Cocaine use in pregnancy: Perinatal morbidity and mortality. Neurotoxicol Teratol 1987 Jan–Feb; 9(4):291–293

Chasnoff IJ, Lewis DE and Squires L. Cocaine intoxication in breast-fed infant. Pediatrics 1987 Dec; 80(6):836–838

Chessex P, Blouet S and Vaucher J. Environmental temperature control in very low birth weight infants (less than 1000 grams) cared for in double-walled incubators. J Pediatr 1988 Aug; 113(2):373–380

Cheu HW, Brown DR and Rowe MI. Breath hydrogen excretion as a screening test for the early diagnosis of necrotizing enterocolitis. Am J Dis Child 1989 Feb; 143(2):156–159

Church MW and Gerkin KP. Hearing disorders in children with fetal alcohol syndrome: Findings from case reports. Pediatrics 1988 Aug; 82(2):147–154

Cohen–Addad NE et al. Congenital acquired immunodeficiency syndrome and congenital toxoplasmosis: Pathologic support for a chemology of events. J Perinatol 8(4):328–331

Colditz PB, Williams GL, Berry AB and Symonds PJ. Fontanelle pressure and cerebral perfusion pressure: Continuous measurement in neonates. Crit Care Med 1988 Sep; 16(9):876–879

Consolvo CA. Siblings in the NICU. Neonatal Network 1987 Apr; 5(5):7–12

Constantine NA et al. Use of physical and neurologic observations in assessment of gestational age in low birth weight infants. J Pediatr 1987 Jun; 110(6):921–928

Crouse DT and Philips JB. Persistent pulmonary hypertension of the newborn. Perinatal Neonatology 1987 Sep–Oct; 11(5):12–14, 16–20

Currao WJ, Cox C and Shapiro DL. Dilute formula for beginning the feeding of premature infants. Am J Dis Child 1988 Jul; 142(7):730–731

Dachman RS. Development and evaluation of an infant-care training program with first-time fathers. J Appl Behav Anal 1986 Fall; 19(3):221–230

Daily DK. Home oxygen therapy for infants with bronchopulmonary dysplasia. Perinatal Neonatology 1987 Jun; 11(3):26, 30, 32, 35

Davidson SL et al. Sudden infant death syndrome in infants evaluated by apnea programs in California. Pediatrics 1986 Apr; 77(4):451–458

DeCurtis M, McIntosh N, Ventura V and Brooke U. Effect of nonnutritive sucking in nutrient retention in preterm infants. J Pediatr 1986 Nov; 109(6):888–890

Dincsoy MY et al. Intracranial hemorrhage in low-birth weight twins during neonatal period. Am J Perinatol 1987 Jul; 4(3):220–224

Dixon AG. Think zinc. Neonatal Network 1987 Feb; 5(4):29–33

Dodman N. Newborn temperature control. Neonatal Network 1987 Jun; 5(6):19–23

Dorm SM. Interteriary neonatal transport. Neonatal Perinatology 1987 Nov–Dec; 11(6):35–36, 50

Dortch E and Spottiswoode P. New light on phototherapy: Home use. Neonatal Network 1986 Feb; 4(4):30–34

Dunn PA, Bhutani V, Weiner S and Ludomirski A. Care of the Neonate with erythroblastosis fetalis. J Obstet Gynecol Neonatal Nurs 1988 Nov–Dec; 17(6):382–386

Dutton EB, West DL and Brano YW. Medium-chain triglycerides in neonatal nutrition. Am J Perinatol 1987 Jan; 4(1):5–7

Eckburg JJ, Bell EF, Rios GR and Wilmoth PK. Effects of formula temperature on postprandial thermogenesis and body temperature of premature infants. Pediatrics 1987 Oct; 111(4):588–592

Eden RD, Seifert LS, Winegar A and Spellacy WN. Postdate pregnancies: A review of 46 perinatal deaths. Am J Perinatol 1987 Oct; 4(4):284–287

Edwards KA and Allen ME. Nursing management of the human response to the premature with experience. Neonatal Network 1988 Apr; 82–86

Edmondson KS. Acquired immune deficiency syndrome in the neonate. Neonatal Network 1988 Feb; 6(4):7–12

Evans NJ and Rutter N. Reduction of skin damage from transcutaneous oxygen electrodes using a spray on dressing. Arch Dis Child 1986 Sep; 61(9):881–884

Everett AD, Koch WC and Saulsbury FT. Failure to thrive due to obstructive sleep apnea. Clin Pediatr 1987 Feb; 26(2):90–92

Fajardo B. Brief intervention with parents in the special care nursery. Neonatal Network 1988 Jun; 6(6):23–30

Fay MJ. The positive effects of positioning. Neonatal Network 1988 Apr; 5(6):23–28

Field T, Scafidi F and Schanberg S. Massage of preterm newborns to improve growth and development. Pediatr Nurs 1987 Nov–Dec; 13(6):385–387

Flandermeyer AA. A comparison of the effects of heroin and cocaine abuse upon the neonate. Neonatal Network 1987 Dec; 6(3):42–48

Fraley AM. Chronic sorrows in parents of premature children. Child Health Care 1986 Fall; 15(2):114–116

Franck LS. A national survey of the assessment and treatment of pain and agitation in the neonatal intensive care unit. J Obstet Gynecol Neonatal Nurs 1987 Nov–Dec; 16(6):387–393

Frank DA et al. Cocaine use during pregnancy: Prevalence and correlates. Pediatrics 1988 Dec; 82(6):888–895

Frank DA and Zeisel SH. Failure to thrive. Pediatr Clin North Am 1988 Dec; 35(6):1187–1206

Frank M. Theophylline: A closer look. Neonatal Network 1987 Oct; 6(2):7–13

Friesen RH, Honda AT and Thieme RE. Changes in anterior fontanel pressure in preterm neonates during tracheal intubation. Anesth Analg 1987 Sep; 66(9):874–878

Garza C, Schanler RJ, Beetle NF and Motil KJ. Special properties of human milk. Clin Perinatol 1987 Mar; 14(1):11–32

George DS, Stephen S, Fellows KR and Bremer DC. The latest on retinopathy of prematurity. MCN 1988 Jul–Aug; 13(4):254–258

Ginoza GW, Strass AA, Iskra MK and Modanlou HD. Potential treatment of theophylline toxicity by high surface area activated charcoal. J Pediatr 1987 Jul; 111(11):140–142

Givens S. Nonimmune hydrops fetalis. Neonatal Network 1988 Oct; 7(2):15–27

Glass SM and Giacoia GP. Intravenous drug therapy in premature infants: Practical aspects. JOGNN 1987 Oct; 16(5):310–318

Goldberg SJ. Response of the patent ductus arteriosus to indomethacin treatment. Am J Dis Child 1987 Mar; 141(3):250

Gozal D, Colin AA, Iaskaloric YI and Jaffe M. Environmental overheating as a cause of transient respiratory chemoreceptor dysfunction in an infant. Pediatrics 1988 Nov; 82(5):738–740

Greer FR and McCormick A. Bone mineral content and growth in very-low-birth weight premature infants. Am J Dis Child 1987 Feb; 141(2):179–183

Grippi C, Ward L and Roncoli M. The case of baby Alice: AIDS/ARC in infancy. Neonatal Network 1988 Apr; 6(5):9–15

Gunderson LP and Kenner C. Neonatal stress: Physiologic adaptation and nursing implications. Neonatal Network 1987 Aug; 6(1):37–42

Gunderson LP and Kenner C. Transcutaneous oxygen monitoring: Description and clinical application. Neonatal Network 1988 Jun; 6(6):7–14

Haddock BJ, Merrow DC and Vincent PA. Comparison of axillary and rectal temperatures in the preterm infant. Neonatal Network 1988 Apr; 6(5):67–71

Hader CF and Sorensen ER. The effects of body position on transcutaneous oxygen tension. Pediatr Nurs 1988 Nov–Dec; 14(6):469–473

Hanigan WC et al. Administration of indomethacin for the prevention of periventricular-intraventricular hemorrhage in high-risk neonates. J Pediatr 1988 Jun; 112(6):941–947

Hargrove C. Administration of IV medications in the NICU: The development of a procedure. MCN 1987 Oct; 6(2):41–49

Heiser CA. Home phototherapy. Pediatr Nur 1987 Nov–Dec; 13(6):425–427

Henneberry C. Candida sepsis in the very low birthweight infant. Neonatal Network 1987 Jun; 5(6):39–45

Hermansen MC, Hasan S, Hoppin J and Cunningham MD. A validation of a scoring system to evaluate the condition of transported very-low-birthweight neonates. Am J Perinatol 1988 Jan; 5(1):74–78

Houston MR. A cautionary note. J Obstet Gynecol Neonatal Nurs 1987 Mar–Apr; 16(2):87–88

Houston MJR and Field PA. Practices and policies in the initiation of breast feeding. J Obstet Gynecol Neonatal Nurs 1988 Nov–Dec; 17(6):418–424

Inglis AD and Loranzo M. AIDS and the neonatal ICU. Neonatal Network 1986 Dec; 5(3):39–43

Jain L, Sivieri E, Abbasi S and Bhutani V. Energetics and mechanics of nutritive sucking in the preterm and term neonate. J Pediatr 1987 Dec; 111(6 pt 1):894–901

Jenkins RL and Lock MKS. Helping parents bond to their premature infant. MCN 1986 Jan–Feb; 11(1):32–33

Jennis MD and Peabody JL. Pulse oximetry: An alternative method for the assessment of Oxygenation in newborn infants. Pediatrics 1987 Apr; 79(4):524–527

Kanto WP et al. Perinatal events and necrotizing enterocolitis in premature infants. Am J Dis Child 1987 Feb; 141(2):167–169

Karp WB and Robertown AF. Vitamin E in neonatology. Adv Pediatr 1986 33: 127–148

Kaufmann RC, Amankwak KS, Colliver JA and Arbuthnot J. Diabetic pregnancy. Am J Perinatol 1987 Jan; 4(1):72–74

Kliegman RM and Walsh MC. Neonatal necrotizing enterocolitis: Pathogenesis, classification and spectrum of illness. Curr Prob Pediatr 1987 Apr; 17(4):217–288

Kliegman RM and Walsh MC. The incidence of meningitis in neonates with necrotizing enterocolitis. Am J Perinatol 1987 Jul; 4(3):245–252

Koldovsky O. Perinatal adaptation of gastrointestinal tract function in man. Perinatal Neonatology 1987 Jan–Feb; 11(1):31–32, 37–39

Koniski Y, Kuriyama M. Mikawa H and Suzuki J. Effect of body position on later postural and functional laterolities of preterm infants. Dev Med Child Neurol 1987 Dec; 29(6): 751–757

Krilov LR et al. Longitudinal serologic evaluation of an infant with acquired immunodeficiency syndrome. Pediatr Infect Dis J 1987 Nov; 6(11):1066–1067

Kramer MS. Intrauterine growth and gestational duration determinants. Pediatrics 1987 Oct; 80(4):502–511

Krener PG. Impact of the diagnosis of AIDS in hospital care of an infant. Clin Pediatr 1987 Jan; 26(1):30–34

Kretzer FL and Hittner HM. Retinopathy of prematurity: Clinical implications of retinal development. Arch Dis Child 1988 Oct; 63(10):1151–1167

Kuban KC et al. Respiratory complications in low-birth-weight infants who receive phenobarbital. Am J Dis Child 1987 Sep; 141(9):996–999

Larson E. Rituals in infection control: What works in the newborn nursery. J Obstet Gynecol Neonatal Nurs 1987 Nov–Dec; 16(6):411–416

Lucas A and Baker BA. Breast milk jaundice in premature infants. Arch Dis Child 1986 Oct; 61(10):1063–1067

Lawrence RA. The management of lactation as a physiologic process. Clin Perinatol 1987 Mar; 14(1):1–10

Lawson M. Persistent pulmonary hypertension of the newborn: Current trends in classification and diagnosis. Neonatal Network 1987 Aug; 6(1):27–35

Loisel DB. Methylxanthines in the NICU. Neonatal Network 1987 Dec; 6(3):23–28

Loisel DB, Smith MM and MacDonald MG. Plasma theophylline levels as related to toxicity in infancy with severe chronic lung disease. MCN 1987 Oct; 6(2):15–19

Lott JW. Developmental care of the preterm infant. Neonatal Network 1989 Feb; 7(4):21–28

Luginbuhl LM et al. Neonatal enterococcal sepsis: Case-control study and description of an outbreak. Pediatr Infect Dis J 1987 Nov; 6(11):1022–1026

Lynch TM, Jung AL and Bose CL. Neonatal back transport: Clinical outcome. Pediatrics 1988 Dec; 82(6): 845–851

Madden JD, Payne TF and Miller S. Maternal cocaine abuse and effect on the newborn. Pediatrics 1986 Feb; 77(2):209–211

Maisels MJ, Gifford K, Antle CE and Leib GR. Jaundice in the healthy newborn infant: A new approach to an old problem. Pediatrics 1988 Apr; 81(4): 505–511

Marcey TJ, Harmon RJ and Easterbrooks MA. Impact of premature birth on the development of the infant in the family. J Consult Clin Psychol 1987 Dec; 55(6):846–852

Marcus M, Paneth N, Kiely JL and Susser MW. Determinants of interhospital transfer of low-birth-weight newborns. Med Care 1988 May; 26(5):462–473

Marion RW et al. Fetal AIDS syndrome score. Am J Dis Child 1987 Apr; 141: 429–431

Martin RJ et al. Effect of head position on distribution of nasal airflow in preterm infants. J Pediatr 1988 Jan; 112(1):99–103

Martin RJ, Miller MJ and Carlo WA. Pathogenesis of apnea in preterm infants. J Pediatr 1986 Nov; 109(5): 733–741

Masterson J, Zucker C and Schulze K. Prone and supine positioning effects on energy expenditure and behavior of

low birth weight neonates. Pediatrics 1987 Nov; 80(5):689–692

Mathew OP. Nipple units for newborn infants: A functional comparison. Pediatrics 1988 May; 81(5):688–691

McBride MC and Danner SC. Sucking disorders in neurologically impaired infants: Assessment and facilitation of breast feeding. Clin Perinatol 1987 Mar; 14(1):109–130

McCormick MC. Long-term follow-up of infants discharged from neonatal intensive care units. JAMA 1989 Mar 24–30; 261(12):1767–1772

Meier P and Anderson GC. Responses of small preterm infants to bottle- and breast-feeding. MCN 1987 Mar–Apr; 12(2):97–105

Meis PJ, Ernest JM and Moore ML. Causes of low birth weight births in public and private patients. Am J Obstet Gynecol 1987 May; 156(5): 1165–1168

Merber L, Higgins P and Kinnard E. Assessing narcotic addiction in neonates. Pediatr Nurs 1985 May–Jun; 11(3):177–181

Miodovnik M et al. Management of the insulin dependent diabetic during labor and delivery. Am J Perinatol 1987 Apr; 4(2):106–114

Moen JE et al. Axillary versus rectal temperatures in preterm infants under radiant warmers. J Obstet Gynecol Neonatal Nurs 1987 Oct; 16(5):348–352

Moore MC. Total parenteral nutrition for infants. MCN 1987 Oct; 6(2):33–40

Morett LA and Ortega R. Pulmonary hypertension in the fetus, the newborn, and the child. Clin Perinatol 1987 Mar; 14(1):227–242

Morgan MEI and Durbin GM. Pulse oximetry in neonatal care. Arch Dis Child 1986 Dec; 61(12):1247

Morriss FH, Moore M, Weisbrodt NW and West S. Otogenic development of gastrointestinal motility: IV. Duodenal contractions in preterm infants. Pediatrics 1986 Dec; 78(6):1106–1113

Moser J. Examining the issue of tactile stimulation for preterm infants. Neonatal Network 1985 Dec; 4(3):25–32

Mullen MK et al. Mother–infant feeding interaction in full-term small-for-gestational-age infants. J Pediatr 1988 Jan; 112(1):143–148

Muttitt SC et al. Neonatal apnea: Diagnosis by nurse versus computer. Pediatrics 1988 Nov; 82(5):713–720

Myers SA, Paton JB and Fisher DE. The effects of initial Apgar score on the birthweight-specific survival of the very low-birth-weight infant. Am J Perinatol 1987 Oct; 4(4):288–292

Naylor A and Wester R. Providing professional lactation management consultation. Clin Perinatol 1987 Mar; 14(1):33–38

Nelson M. Forecast for neonatal monitors. Perinatal Neonatology 1987 Jul–Aug; 11(4):23–24, 26–27

Ohlsson A and Cumming WA. Candidiasis in very low birthweight infants. Am J Perinatol 1986 Jan; 3(1): 13–15

Oro AS and Dixon SD. Perinatal cocaine and methamphetamine exposure: Maternal and neonatal correlates. J Pediatr 1987 Oct; 111(4):571–578

Oro AS and Dixon SD. Waterbed care of narcotic-exposed neonates. Am J Dis Child 1988 Feb; 142(2):186–188

Osborn LM. Management of neonatal jaundice. Nurs Pract 1986 Apr; 11(4): 41, 44, 49–51, 52

Paton JY, Macfadyln UM and Simpson H. Sleep phase and gastroesophageal reflux in infants at possible risk for SIDS. Arch Dis Child 1989 Feb; 64(2): 264–269

Pediatric guidelines for infection control of human immunodeficiency virus (acquired immunodeficiency virus) in hospitals, medical offices, schools and other settings. Pediatrics 1988 Nov; 82(5):801–807

Perlman M and Frank JW. Bilirubin beyond the blood–brain barrier. Pediatrics 1988 Feb; 81(2):304–315

Pinelli J and Ferguson MK. Transporting high-risk newborns: The importance of communication. Neonatal Network 1985; 3(6):23–26

Pugh EJ, Statham R and Jarvis S. Cot deaths, stillbirths, and the probation service: A potentially recognisable at risk group. Arch Dis Child 1987 Feb; 62(2):146–147

Ramsay JM et al. Response of the patent ductus arteriosus to indomethacin treatment. Am J Dis Child 1987 Mar; 141(3):294–297

Rice BR and Feeg VD. First-year developmental outcomes for multiple-risk premature infants. Pediatr Nurs 1985 Jan–Feb; 11(1):30–35

Rivera–Calimlim L. The significance of drugs in breast milk. Clin Perinatol 1987 Mar; 14(1):51–70

Rochefort MJ and Wilkinson AR. New fontanometer for continuous estimation of intracranial pressure in the newborn. Arch Dis Child 1987 Feb; 62(2):152–155

Rushton CH. Promoting normal growth and development in the hospital environment. Neonatal Network 1986 Jun; 4(6):21–30

Ryan L, Ehrlich S and Finnegan L. Cocaine abuse in pregnancy: Effects on fetus and newborn. Neurotoxicol Teratol 1987 Jul–Aug; 9(4):295–299

Salitros PH. Transitional infant care: A bridge to home for high-risk infants. Neonatal Network 1986 Feb; 4(4):35–41

Satariano HJ, Briggs NJ and O'Neal C. Discharge from neonatal intensive care: How satisfied are parents? Pediatr Nurs 1987 Sep–Oct; 13(5):352–353, 357

Sauve RS et al. Home oxygen therapy: Outcome of infants discharged from NICU on continuous treatment. Clin Pediatr 1989 Mar; 28(3):113–118

Shannon LF. Insulin usage in the neonate. Neonatal Network 1988 Apr; 5(6):31–39

Shapiro C. Retrolental fibroplasia: What we know and what we don't know.

Neonatal Network 1986 Jun; 4(6):33–44

Sherwin L. Nursing interventions: Caring for parents of a newborn transferred to a regional intensive care nursery—a challenge for low risk obstetric specialists. J Perinatol 1988 8(3):271–275

Shonkoff JP and Hauser–Cram P. Early intervention for disabled infants and their families: A quantitative analysis. Pediatrics 1987 Nov; 80(5):650–658

Shuckla H. Postnatal overestimation of gestational age in preterm infants. Am J Dis Child 1986 Oct; 140(10):1106–1107

Sims–Jones N. Back to the theories: Another way to view mothers of prematures. MCN 1986 Nov–Dec; 11(6):394–397

Sims ME et al. Prophylactic oral nystatin and fungal infections in very-low-birthweight infants. Am J Perinatol 1988 Jan; 5(1):33–36

Smith J. The dangers of prenatal cocaine use. MCN 1988 May–Jun; 13(3):174–179

Snydman DR, Greer C, Meissner HC and McIntosh K. Prevention of nosocomial transmission of respiratory syncytial virus in a newborn nursery. Infect Contr Hosp Epidemiol 1988 Mar; 9(3):105–108

Stap LJ and Reinhart PA. A seat for premature infants. Am J Occup Ther 1987 Oct; 41(10):667–671

Steichen JJ, Krug–Wispé SK and Lsang RC. Breast feeding the low birth weight premature infant. Clin Perinatol 1987 Mar; 14(1):131–171

Stierman ED. Emotional aspects of perinatal death. Clin Obstet Gynecol 1987 Jun; 30(2):352–361

Stockman JA. APNEA and SIDS: Issues clarified. Perinatal Neonatology 1987 Jul–Aug; 11(4):8, 10

Swaminathan S et al. Long-term pulmonary sequelae of meconium aspiration syndrome. J Pediatr 1989 Mar; 114(3):356–361

Task Force on Pediatriac AIDS. Perinatal human immunodeficiency virus infection. Pediatrics 1988 Dec; 82(6):941–944

Tan KL. Blood pressure in full-term healthy neonates. Clin Pediatr 1987 Jan; 26(1):21–24

Taylor RL et al. Operative closure of patent ductus arteriosus in premature infants in the neonatal intensive care unit. Am J Surg 1986 Dec; 152(6):704–708

Telsey AM, Merritt TA and Dixon SD. Cocaine exposure in a term neonate: Necrotizing enterocolitis as a complication. Clin Pediatr 1988 Nov; 27(11):547–550

Tenorio GM, Nazvi M, Bickers GH and Hubbird RH. Intrauterine stroke and maternal polydrug abuse. Clin Pediatr 1988 Nov; 27(11):565–567

Trouy MB. Sibling grief. Neonatal Network 1988 Feb; 5(4):35–40

Troy P, Wilkinson–Faulk D, Smith AB and Alexander DA. Sibling visiting in the NICU. Am J Nurs 1988 Jan; 88(1):68–70

Updike C et al. Positional support for premature infants. Am J Occup Ther 1986 Oct; 40(10):712–715

VanBaar AL et al. Neonatal behavior after drug dependent pregnancy. Arch Dis Child 1989 Feb; 64(2):235–240

Van Baar AL, Fleury P and Ultee CA. Behavior in first year after drug dependent pregnancy. Arch Dis Child 1989 Feb; 64(2):241–245

Van De Bor M, Van Bell F, Lineman R and Ruys JH. Perinatal factors and periventricular-intraventricular hemorrhage in PT. Am J Dis Child 1986 Nov; 140(11):1125–1130

VanZoeren–Grobben D, Schrijver J, Van Den Berg H and Berger HM. Human milk vitamin content after pasteurisation, storage, or tube feeding. Arch Dis Child 1987 Feb; 62(2):161–165

Wagner P and Segall ML. The NICU graduate. Perinatal Neonatology 1987 Jul–Aug; 11(4):12, 14, 17–18

Walsh MC, Noble LM, Carlo WA and Martin RJ. Relationship of pulse oximetry to arterial oxygen tension in infants. Crit Care Med 1987 Dec; 15(12):1102–1105

Walther FJ, Sims ME, Siassi B and Wu PYK. Cardiac output changes secondary to throphyline therapy in preterm infants. J Pediatr 1986 Nov; 109(5):874–876

Walther FJ, Wu PYK and Siassi B. Cardiovascular changes in preterm infants nursed under radiant warmers. Pediatrics 1987 Aug; 80(2):235–239

Wareham JA, Haugh LD, Yeager SB and Hobur JD. Prediction of arterial blood pressure in the premature neonate using the oscillometric method. Am J Dis Child 1986 Oct; 140(10):1108–1110

Weaver KA and Anderson GC. Relationship between integrated sucking pressures and first bottle-feeding scores in premature infants. J Obstet Gynecol Neonatal Nurs 1988 Mar–Apr; 17(2):113–1120

West DL and Brans YW. Maternal diabetes and neonatal macrosomia. Am J Perinatol 1986 Jan; 3(1):9–14

Weibley TT. Inside the incubator. MCN 1989 Mar–Apr; 14(2):96–100

Whitehouse H. How infants achieve self-organization and self-confidence: Implications for health care professionals and parents. I. MCN Curr 1987; 34(5):17–21

Whitehouse H. How infants achieve self-organization and self-confidence: Implications for health care professionals and parents. II. MCN Curr 1988; 35(1):1–5

Whitelaw A et al. Skin to skin contact for very low birthweight infants and their mothers. Arch Dis Child 1988 Nov; 63(11):1377–1381

White–Traut RC and Goldman MBC. Premature infant massage: Is it safe? Pediatr Nurs 1988 Jul–Aug; 14(4):285–289

White–Traut RC and Pabst MK. Parenting of hospitalized infants by adolescent mothers. Pediatr Nurs 1987 Mar–Apr; 13(2):97–100

Whitford KM. Health care needs of ventilator-dependent children. Pediatr Nurs 1988 May–Jun; 14(3):216–219

Widstrom AM et al. Nonnutritive sucking in tube-fed preterm infants: Effects on gastric motility and gastric contents of somatostatin. J Pediatr Gastroenter Nutr 1988 Jul–Aug; 7(4):517–523

Wilks S and Meier P. Helping mothers express milk suitable for preterm and high-risk infant feeding. MCN 1988 Mar–Apr; 13(2):121–123

Wilkerson NN. A comprehensive look at hyperbilirubinemia. MCN 1988 Sep–Oct; 13(5):360–364

Wilkerson NN. Treating hyperbilirubinemia. MCN 1989 Jan–Feb; 14(1):32–36

Weibley TT et al. Gavage tube insertion in the premature infant. MCN 1987 Jan–Feb; 12(1):21–27

Wood AF. Sequelae of perinatal asphysia. Neonatal Network 1987 Apr; 5(5):21–23

Wright S, Norton C and Kestin K. Retention of infant CPR instruction by parents. Pediatr Nurs 1989 Jan–Feb; 15(1):37–41

Yazdari M et al. Phenobarbital increases the theophylline requirement of premature infants being treated for apnea. Am J Dis Child 1987 Jan; 141(1):97–99

Additional Pertinent References

Caring for your Hospitalized Baby. Washington, DC, Association for the Care of Children's Health, 1984

Henig RM and Fletcher AB. Your Premature Baby. New York, Rawson Associates, 1983

Metcalf SC. Getting to Know Your Premature Baby. Louisville, KY, National Foundation March of Dimes.

Nance S. Premature Babies: A Handbook for Parents. New York, Arbor House, 1982

National SIDS Foundation, Two Metro Plaza #205, 8240 Professional Pl, Landover, MD 20785; 1-800-221-5103

Reukauf DM and Trause MA. Common Sense Breast Feeding. New York, Atheneum, 1988

Woessner C, Lauwers J and Bernard B. Breast Feeding Today. Garden City Park, NY, Avery Publishing Group, 1987

Overview of Childhood Respiratory Disorders

Common Types of Respiratory Disorders

Examples of common childhood respiratory disorders can be found in Table 49-1. The following disorders are included:
1. Bacterial pneumonia
2. Viral pneumonia
3. *Pneumocystis carinii* pneumonia
4. Mycoplasma pneumonia
5. Bronchiolitis
6. Croup

Note: Children, aged 18 months to 4 years, in day care centers, are at risk for *Haemophilus influenzae,* type B.

Assessment

Determine the severity of the respiratory distress that the child is experiencing. Make an initial nursing assessment.
1. Observe the respiratory rate and pattern.
   a. Count the respirations for 1 full minute.
   b. Observe the child for retractions, and note severity and location.
   c. Listen to the chest with a stethoscope to determine if crackles are present and to evaluate the breath sounds.
2. Observe the child's color, and note any presence of cyanosis.
3. Observe for nasal flaring.
4. Evaluate the child's degree of restlessness, apprehension, and motor tone.
5. Note any wheezing, stridor, or hoarseness.

Potential Problems and Nursing Diagnoses

1. Breathing pattern, ineffectual, related to impaired oxygen–carbon dioxide exchange
2. Comfort, altered, related to respiratory distress, infectious process, and treatments
3. Fluid volume deficit related to increased respiratory effort, nausea and vomiting, and decreased appetite
4. Potential for infection related to underlying disease condition
5. Anxiety related to respiratory distress and hospitalization
6. Parental anxiety related to uncertainty about the child's well-being

Nursing Interventions

A. Provide a Humidified Environment Enriched With Oxygen to Combat Anoxia and to Liquefy Secretions.

1. Place the child in a Croupette with cool mist or use ultrasonic mist in tent (see Oxygen Therapy, p. 1193): Moistens airway, minimizes fluid loss from lungs, liquefies and facilitates mobilization of respiratory secretions, allows for oxygen therapy up to 40% concentration, and cool environment aids in fever reduction.

> **NURSING ALERT:** At no time should the mist be allowed to become so dense that it obscures clear visualization of the patient's respiratory pattern.

2. Observe the child's response to this environment.
   a. Child may experience fear of confinement or suffocation.
   b. Vision is distorted through the plastic.
   c. The environment is noisy and damp.
   d. There are restricted physical and diversional activities—boredom.
   e. Decreased parental contact
   f. Interrupted sleep
3. Place the child in a comfortable position to promote easier ventilation.
   a. Semi-Fowler's—use pillows, infant seat, or elevate head of bed.
   b. Side or abdominal position will aid drainage of liquified secretions.
4. Frequent changing of clothing and bed linen will prevent chilling and will provide comfort.
   a. Temperature in mist tent is usually 6°–15°F. below room temperature.
   b. Socks, booties, stockinette cap will help keep child warm.
5. Reduce stress and keep child as calm as possible, which in turn will reduce pulmonary workload and oxygen consumption.
6. Help parents understand the purpose of the mist tent and how to work with it
   a. Discuss their fears and concerns about the tent.
   b. Parental anxiety may influence the way their child responds to the tent.
7. Compressed air or oxygen concentration is always supplied when using the mist tent to avoid excess CO_2 concentrations.

B. Provide the Child With Adequate Hydration.

1. Maintain the administration of intravenous fluids at the prescribed rate.
2. When the child is in severe respiratory distress, he is given nothing by mouth because of the danger of aspiration.
3. Offer the child small sips of clear fluid when the respiratory status improves.
   a. Note any vomiting or abdominal distention after the oral fluid is given.
   b. As the child begins to take more fluid by mouth, notify the physician so that intravenous fluid rate may be adjusted to prevent fluid overload.
   c. Do not force the child to take fluids orally that he does not want, since this may cause increased distress and possibly vomiting. Anorexia often accompanies acute febrile infection. Generally, do not awaken a sleeping child just to give frequent fluids.
4. Record the child's intake and output.
   a. Measure urinary output and record.
   b. Check specific gravity of urine.

C. Provide the Child With Both Physical and Psychological Rest.

1. Disturb the child as little as possible by organizing nursing care, and protect him from unnecessary interruptions.
2. Be aware of the age of the child and be familiar with his level of growth and development as it applies to hospitalization.
3. The presence of the child's parents will alleviate some of his apprehension.
4. Provide opportunities for quiet play as the child's condition improves.
5. Explain procedures and hospital routine to the child as appropriate for his age.
6. Reduce anxiety and apprehension to aid in decreasing psychological distress, which will help the child relax and ease respiratory effort.

D. Provide Good Skin Care to Prevent Skin Excoriation From Secretions, Accompanying Diarrhea, and Skin Breakdown From Confinement to Bed.

E. Provide Measures to Improve Ventilation of Affected Portion of the Lung.

1. Change position frequently.
2. Provide postural drainage if prescribed.
3. Relieve nasal obstruction that contributes to breathing difficulty.
   Instill saline solution or prescribed nose drops and apply nasal suctioning.
4. Crying can be an effective method for ventilating the lungs.
5. Coughing is a normal tracheobronchial cleansing procedure. Constant coughing can be relieved temporarily by allowing the child to sip water; use extreme caution to prevent aspiration.
6. Abdominal distention frequently accompanies respiratory infection and can be painful and a hindrance to respiration.
   a. Place in semi-Fowler's position.
   b. Rectal tube, small enema, or suppository may give relief.
   c. Nasogastric tube may be prescribed to relieve distention.

F. Assist in the Control of Fever.

1. Give antipyretics as prescribed.
2. Increase evaporation from skin with cool sponges.

G. Provide for Adequate Nutrition to Meet the Growth and Development Needs of the Child.

1. Determine the child's food preferences.
2. Offer the child small meals.

H. Administer Appropriate Antibiotic Therapy.

1. Observe for drug sensitivity.
2. Observe the child's response to therapy.

I. Be Alert for the Appearance of Specific Complications That May Accompany Respiratory Infection and Notify Physician Immediately (see Table 49-1).

J. Include Parents in the Planning of Care and in Caring for the Child.

Recognize the parents' anxieties. The mother may be exhausted from caring for her sick child prior to his hospitalization.

> **NURSING ALERT:** To minimize spasm and sudden blockage of airway:
> *Avoid:*
>
> Making the child lie flat
> Forcing the child to drink
> Looking down the child's throat

Expected Outcomes

1. Shows no signs of complications of respiratory distress; stable vital signs; normal blood gas values
2. Experiences minimal respiratory distress as evidenced by stable vital signs, by statements that discomfort has subsided and appropriate age-related behaviors
3. Attains/maintains fluid and electrolyte balance; normal laboratory values; appropriate intake and output
4. Absence of infection; temperature normal; lessening of colored sputum; thinning of secretions
5. Experiences lessening of anxiety as evidenced by appropriate coping behaviors; appears relaxed and at ease
6. Parents verbalize understanding of illness; make appointment for follow-up care

Tonsillectomy and Adenoidectomy

Tonsillectomy and *adenoidectomy* are the surgical removal of the adenoidal and tonsillar structures, part of the lymphoid tissue that encircles the pharynx.

Function of Tonsils and Adenoids

1. Serve as a first line of defense against respiratory infections
2. Because the growth of the tonsils and adenoids in the first 10 years of life exceed general somatic growth, these structures appear especially large in the child.
3. The natural process of involution of tonsillar and adenoidal lymphoid tissue in prepubertal years is associated with decreased frequency of throat and ear infections.

(Text continues on p. 1274)

Table 49-1. *Respiratory Disorders*

Condition and Causative Agent	Age and Incidence	Clinical Manifestations
I. Bacterial Pneumonia		
A. Streptococcus pneumonia *Streptococcus pneumoniae* (gram-positive) This type of bacterial pneumonia is most frequent in children.	Birth–2 years Winter and spring (especially in patients with sickle cell disease and patients without spleens)	Mild upper respiratory infection (URI) with sudden symptoms Infants Refusal to eat Vomiting, diarrhea Hypo- or hyperthermia May be Tachypnea Grunting Retractions Nasal flaring Older child Prodromal upper respiratory infection Headache Anorexia Malaise Dry cough Fever Restlessness Pleuritic pain Grunting with shallow, rapid respirations Possibly abdominal pain
B. Streptococcal pneumonia Beta-hemolytic streptococcus Group A (gram-positive)	3–5 years	Commonly superimposed on febrile respiratory infection in a child already ill with a viral exanthem Shows sudden increased fever, worsening cough, chills, pleuritic pain, respiratory distress
C. Staphylococcal pneumonia Coagulase-positive *Staphylococcus aureus* (gram-positive)	Birth-2 years Oct–May	History of predisposing factors. Gradual onset with respiratory symptoms or sudden onset with systemic involvement (very toxic child) Presence of coarse, bubbly crepitations
D. *Haemophilus influenzae,* type B (less common in healthy child)	6 months–3 years	Similar to other lobar pneumonias and bronchopneumonia with spasmodic cough, "toxic" appearance Common associated infection: otitis media, meningitis, epiglottitis
II. Viral Pneumonia Respiratory syncytial virus (RSV) (most common) Parainfluenza virus, types 1-2-3 Adenoviruses Influenza viruses	Birth–2 years; higher incidence in females than in males Winter and early spring	Gradual onset following an upper respiratory infection RSV turns into extension of bronchiolitis Parainfluenza virus causes coryza, pharyngitis, cough may succeed pneumonia Adenovirus causes pharyngitis and cervical adenitis, may succeed pneumonia

Diagnostic Evaluation	Treatment and Nursing Management	Complications

X-ray—patchy area around bronchi
Positive cultures
    Sputum
    Nasopharyngeal secretions
    Blood
    Pronounced leukocytosis
	Penicillin G
	Symptomatic
	    Rest, with gradually increasing exercise
	    Fluids—input and output
	    Antipyretics
	    O_2 mist
	    Position change
	Bronchodilators
	Other: erythromycin, clindomycin, chlor-
	    amphenicol, cephalosporins, ampicil-
	    lin, trimethoprim-sulfamethoxazole
		Rare with antibiotic prescription
		May see
		    Otitis media
		    Sinusitis
		    Empyema
		    Bacteremia

X-ray—usually patchy, but may show
    disseminated infiltrate
WBC increased—polymorphic leu-
    kocytosis
Erthrocyte sedimentation rate (ESR)
    increased
Positive culture from:
    Respiratory secretions
    Empyema fluid
    Increased serum antistreptolysin
    titer
	Penicillin G
	Symptomatic
		Empyema
		Pneumatocele to pneumothorax
		Permanent pulmonary fibrosis and pleural
		    thickening (fibrothorax)

X-ray—patchy consolidation of one
    or more lobes; pneumatocele
    abscesses
Culture: sputum, or gastric aspirate,
    pulmonary fluid or lung aspirate
WBC—elevated in older child
Mild—moderate anemia is common
	Methicillin or penicillin G
	    Rapid treatment is important
	    Symptomatic special attention to fluid
	    balance, treatment of pleural compli-
	    cations, treatment of anemia; O_2 mist
	Be alert to signs of tension pneumothorax;
	    abrupt onset of pain; cyanosis, dysp-
	    nea, diminished chest movement on
	    one side
	Ampicillin—if organism is not resistant
	Other: penicillin G, chloramphenicol
		Empyema
		Pneumothorax
		Lung abscess
		Osteomyelitis
		Staphylococcal pericarditis
		Bronchiectasis
		All infants with staphylococcal pneumonia
		    should be tested for cystic fibrosis and
		    screened for immunodeficiency dis-
		    ease

Culture: blood, nasal secretions:
    WBC shows an increase—lym-
    phocytosis
X-ray—lobar consolidation (may
    also have pleural effusion)
	Symptomatic cough suppression
	Chloramphenicol
	Other: ampicillin, cephalosporins
		Empyema
		Respiratory isolation for 24 hours follow-
		    ing therapy initiation

X-ray—infiltration of one or more
    lobes is more extensive than
    clinical picture would suggest
Culture: nasopharyngeal
Increase titer of specific antibody
	Broad-spectrum antibiotic therapy (unit
	    confirmation of organism is estab-
	    lished)
	Symptomatic and supportive
	Aerosolized ribavirin if RSV is causative
	    organism	

(continued)

Table 49-1. *Respiratory Disorders (continued)*

Condition and Causative Agent	Age and Incidence	Clinical Manifestations
III. Pneumocystis carinii Pneumonia *Pneumocystis carinii*—parasite of uncertain systemic status; presumed to be a sporozoan	Predisposing factors: Prematurity, immature debilitated infant, infectious disease, especially cytomegalic inclusion disease; serious compromising disease (e.g., cystic fibrosis) Children receiving immunosuppressive medication for malignant diseases Immunodeficiency disease especially in children under 1 year of age AIDS (HIV)	Onset is generally slow, taking 3–6 weeks to peak, with increasing tachypnea, extreme grayish cyanosis and dyspnea at rest, cough, O_2 desaturation Presence of predisposing factors

IV. Mycoplasma Pneumonia
  Mycoplasma pneumoniae (pleuropneumonia-like organism)
Microorganisms with properties between bacteria and viruses
	10–15 years
	Late fall and winter
		Onset is insidious, 2–3 weeks incubation
		  Malaise, headache, low-grade fever, sore throat, irritating cough, vomiting, possible crepitation
		Subacute tracheobronchitis

V. Bronchiolitis Respiratory syncytial virus (RSV) Adenovirus Parainfluenza virus, types 1 and 3 Influenza virus *Mycoplasma pneumoniae*	Most common in infants and children under 6 months; may occur in child up to 2 years of age Greater incidence in males than in females Winter–spring Increased incidence in day care centers	Onset is often gradual and associated with exposure to respiratory infection Coryza of 1–3 days, tachypnea Intercostal and suprasternal retraction Expiratory rhonchi Dry cough; paroxysmal cough; may have wheezing Fever Cyanosis Possible dehydration Tachypnea

Diagnostic Evaluation	Treatment and Nursing Management	Complications

X-ray shows bilateral diffuse alveolar densities, especially perihilar overdistention
Observe cysts in special stained smear in material obtained from lung biopsy (not reliable)
Lung aspiration by needle
Endotracheal brush catheter biopsy
Elevated IgM—ELISA
Mild leukocytosis
Moderate eosinophilia
	Trimethroprim-sulfamethoxazole
	Supportive: maintain oxygen and respirations; administer immunoglobulins, possibly withhold immunosuppressive chemotherapy, maintain fluid, electrolyte, and acid–base balance, maintain nutrition
	Be alert to early signs and predisposing factors that will aid in early diagnosis
	Carefully observe for adverse effects of drug therapy: abscess formation and necrosis of injection site, if pentamide isethionate used
	   Hypoglycemia
	   Nephrotoxicity
	   Hypotension
	   Tachycardia
	   Hypocalcemia
	   Nausea and vomiting
	   Skin rash
	   Anemia
	   Hyperkalemia
	   Thrombocytopenia
	Isolate from immunosuppressed patients for 48 hours following therapy initiation
		Pneumothorax from diagnostic tests, concomitant bacterial pneumonia or sepsis
		Death

X-ray shows peribronchial infiltrate in lower lobes Increase in complement fixation test Positive sputum culture Cold agglutinins	Erythromycin Tetracycline may be used in child over 9 years Supportive antipyretic cough suppression Secretion precautions	Systemic or superimposed on chronic lung disease—death
X-ray demonstrates overinfiltration of lungs Virologic or serologic studies to isolate virus on throat swab PaO_2 decreases, PaO_2 increases (late finding)	Antibiotic therapy given to severely ill child until laboratory confirmation is established Humidified O_2 to relieve arterial hypoxemia Avoid high-density humidity that may cause bronchospasm Monitoring blood gasses and correction of acidosis Possible ventilatory assistance Maintain fluid–electrolyte–acid–base and nutritional balance Keep nasal airway open and clear of mucus to decrease respiratory difficulty, because infant is an obligatory nose breather Position baby in infant seat inside Croupette; it may provide some respiratory assistance Be alert to signs of impending respiratory acidosis and dehydration, and cardiac involvement Epinephrine theophylline or racemic epinephrine by intermittent positive-pressure breathing (IPPB) may relieve bronchospasm Ribavirin aerosol for RSV infection	Exhaustion and anoxia Secondary bacterial infection Pneumothorax and pneumomediastinum (occasional) Apneic spells Circulatory collapse Increase—predisposed to asthma

(continued)

Table 49-1. *Respiratory Disorders (continued)*

Condition and Causative Agent	Age and Incidence	Clinical Manifestations

VI. Croup and Epiglottitis
A. Croup (subglottic)
   Acute laryngotracheobronchitis (LTB); laryngotracheitis
   Parainfluenza virus 1-2-3 (most common virus)
   Respiratory syncytial virus (RSV)
   Influenza virus during epidemics
   Rhinovirus
   Adenovirus
	3 months–3 years
	Winter
	Greater incidence in males than females
		Generally onset is gradual and progresses slowly, following 1 to several days after an upper 24–72-hour respiratory infection
		Coryza
		Croupy cough, barking cough
		Inspiratory stridor
		Hoarseness
		Low-grade fever
		Increasing respiration and pulse rate
		Apprehension, restlessness, anxiety

B. Bacterial tracheitis (Pseudomembranous croup) (Structure—inflammation in subglottic region) *Staphylococcus aureus* Streptococci *Haemophilus influenzae*	Age variable Any season	Rapid onset, toxic appearing, high fever, progressive upper airway obstruction from copious production of purulent secretions and mucosal necrosis No drooling
C. Epiglottitis (Structure—supraglottis) (Fig. 49–1) Bacterial *Hemophilus influenzae* type B (most common) Pneumococci *Staphylococcus aureus* Beta-hemolytic streptococcus	3–10 years 1–5 years peak ages Seasonal variations Increases in winter	Onset and progression are rapid—6–24 hours, may follow short duration of coryza Severe inspiratory stridor with marked supraclavicular and intercostal refractions Sore throat–refusal to eat, dysphagia High fever 39°–40°C. (102°–104°F.) Tachycardia No cough Drooling, respirations may be shallow, hoarseness; paleness and exhausted appearance, may insist on sitting up—tripod position—sit erect flexed forward at waist with tripod placement of arms for support; condition worsens when lying down; cherry-red epiglottis; apprehension; restlessness; anxiety; cannot swallow; mouth open and chin thrust forward with tongue out

Clinical Manifestations

1. Acute or chronic infection of tonsils and adenoids
2. Hypertrophy produces obstruction to:
   a. Breathing
   b. Swallowing
   c. Auditory (eustachian) tube
3. Common childhood diseases of the tonsils and adenoids
   a. Acute and chronic infections
   b. Secondary extension of microorganisms or toxins into lymphatics
   c. Direct spread of infection into the nose, paranasal sinuses, eustachian tube, middle ear, or lower respiratory tract
   d. Enlargement of the tonsils and adenoids with airway obstruction
      (1) Adenoiditis (chronic) may occur in the child under 4 years without chronic tonsillitis—adenoidectomy is the treatment of choice
      (2) In children over 4 years, tonsillitis usually accompanies adenoiditis

Diagnostic Evaluation

Since bleeding is a likely complication of surgery in this highly vascular area, preoperative blood studies must be completed.
1. Clotting time
2. Smear for platelets
3. Prothrombin time
4. Partial prothrombin time
5. Others specific for general anesthesia

Complications

1. Hemorrhage—although unusual, it can occur
2. Emotional/psychological sequelae
3. Reactions to anesthesia

Diagnostic Evaluation	Treatment and Nursing Management	Complications
History and clinical evaluation—laboratory findings PCO_2 increased (late finding), PO_2 decreased Normal—mild leukocytosis X-ray of neck—subglottic edema (below vocal cords) narrowing Normal supraglottic structures	Supportive: high humidification with oxygen, as necessary; hydration; nebulized racemic epinephrine with or without IPPB, minimal handling; allow undisturbed sleep; monitor vital signs, SaO_2 monitor Teach parents home management of croup (see below) Syrup of ipecac may be beneficial in reducing coughing in spasmodic croup Severe obstruction—airway Edema severe—tracheostomy	Airway obstruction Anorexia
X-ray—severe narrowing of trachea Leukocytosis Culture tracheal aspirants	Supporting and symptomatic—endotracheal suctioning, nasotracheal tube, humidified oxygen IV ampicillin and flucloxacillin Other: cefuroxime, oxacillin, chloramphenicol	
History and clinical evaluation—laboratory findings PCO_2 increased (late finding); PO_2 decreased Leukocytosis X-ray of neck—epiglottic edema (above vocal cords); normal trachea and larynx	Medical emergency; endotracheal/nasotracheal intubation or tracheostomy; "cool humidified oxygen" Antibiotic therapy Chloramphenicol Fluids Rest Observe carefully for signs and symptoms of increasing respiratory distress; have in readiness equipment for intubation or tracheostomy (see p. 1191) Teach parents home care of tracheostomy Community health nurse referral	Airway obstruction Death Other: bacteremia, pneumothorax, mediastinal emphysema, interstitial bronchopneumonia Interval between onset and death may be as short as 4 hours Use of hemophilus type B vaccine should decrease incidence in child over age 2 years

4. Otitis media; bacteremia
5. Lung abscess; pneumonia; septicemia—all very rare

Treatment

Although tonsillectomy and adenoidectomy are separate procedures with separate indications, indications for combined operation occur frequently. Controversy exists among experts as to indications, necessity, and benefits of surgery.

A. Indications for Tonsillectomy

1. Conservative:
   a. Recurrent or persistent tonsillitis with documented streptococcal infection 4 times in 1 year
   b. Marked hypertrophy of tonsils, which distorts speech, causes swallowing difficulties, and causes subsequent weight loss
   c. Tonsilar malignancy
   d. Diphtheria carrier
   e. Cor pulmonale due to obstruction

2. Controversial:
   a. Peritonsillar abscess or retrotonsillar abscess
   b. Suppurative cervical adenitis with tonsillar focus
   c. Persistent hyperemia of anterior pillars
   d. Enlarged cervical nodes

B. Indications for Adenoidectomy

1. Conservative:
   a. Adenoid hypertrophy resulting in obstruction of airway leading to hypoxia, pulmonary hypertension, and cor pulmonale
   b. Hypertrophy with nasal obstruction accompanied by breathing difficulty and severe speech distortion
   c. Hypertrophy associated with chronic suppurative or serous otitis media and sensorineural or conductive hearing loss, chronic mastoiditis, or cholesteatoma
   d. Mouth-breathing due to hypertrophied adenoids

2. Controversial:
   a. Enlarged adenoids, chronic otitis media, and no evidence of complications

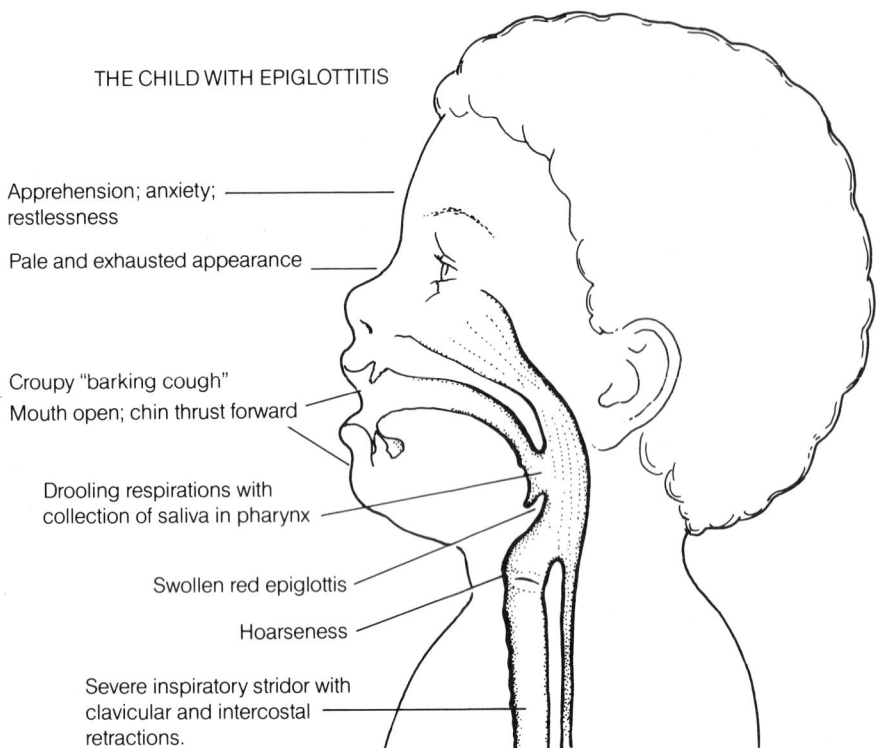

THE CHILD WITH EPIGLOTTITIS

Apprehension; anxiety; restlessness

Pale and exhausted appearance

Croupy "barking cough"

Mouth open; chin thrust forward

Drooling respirations with collection of saliva in pharynx

Swollen red epiglottis

Hoarseness

Severe inspiratory stridor with clavicular and intercostal retractions.

Figure 49-1. *Epiglottitis.*

Contraindications to Surgery

1. Bleeding or coagulation disorders
2. Uncontrolled systemic disorders (i.e., diabetes, rheumatic fever, cardiac, renal disease)
3. Child under the age of 5–6 years—unless life-threatening situation
4. Presence of upper respiratory infection in child or immediate family
5. Specific for adenoidectomy—certain palate abnormalities (i.e., cleft palate or submucus cleft palate)

Potential Problems and Nursing Diagnoses

1. Anxiety and fear of child related to surgery
2. Potential postoperative hemorrhage related to surgery in the highly vascular area of tonsils and adenoids
3. Potential for fluid volume deficit related to pre- and postoperative regimen and to poor oral intake postoperatively from reluctance to swallow because of pain
4. Comfort, altered, related to surgery
5. Parental anxiety related to surgical procedure

Preoperative Nursing Interventions

A. Assess Upon Admission the Psychological Preparation of the Child for Hospitalization and Surgery.

1. The child should know why he has been admitted to the hospital and what will happen to him.
2. When the parents have not told the child about hospitalization, it may be because they cannot.
   a. They do not know what will happen.
   b. They do not know how to tell the child because of their own anxieties.
   c. They do not understand the importance of telling the child the truth in order to perpetuate the child's trust in the parents.
3. Help the parents in preparing the child by talking at first in general terms about hospitalization.
4. The child may have preconceived ideas from parents and peers about what to expect. (These may pose a threat to the child.)
   a. Introduce the child to other children on the unit, especially those who have had and are recovering from surgery.
   b. Talk about and show the child the new things he will see.
   c. Correct any misunderstandings the child may have.
5. The preschool child is very vulnerable to psychological trauma as a result of this experience.
   a. Tell the child the truth.
   b. Include parents when helping the child.

B. Take Nursing History From Parents at the Time of Admission to Obtain Any Pertinent Information That Would Contraindicate Surgery.

1. Infection
   a. When was the most recent infection? It is desirable for the patient to be free of respiratory infection for at least 2–3 weeks.
   b. Has child been exposed to any communicable diseases?
2. Safety
   a. Does the child have any loose teeth?
   b. Are there any bleeding tendencies in child or family?

C. Maintain Adequate Hydration Prior to Surgery, Since Blood Loss May Be Extensive During Surgery.

1. Encourage the child to drink fluids the night before surgery.
2. The child usually is NPO a few hours prior to surgery.

D. Prepare the Child Specifically (appropriate for age) **for What to Expect Postoperatively.**

1. Where he will wake up
2. Sore throat, emesis of blood, position, foul taste and smell in mouth
3. Ice collar, medications
4. Fluid regimen

E. Encourage the Mother to Stay With Her Young Child the Day and Night of Surgery or at Least Before Surgery and When the Child Returns to His Room and Is Waking Up.

Prepare the mother as to what to expect when she sees the child postoperatively.

1. Vomiting
2. Skin color
3. Crying, angry, or frightened

F. Know If the Child Has a History of Chronic Infection or Rheumatic Fever so Antibiotics May be Given Pre- and Postoperatively.

G. Ensure That Preoperative Bleeding and Clotting Time Blood Studies Have Been Done.

Postoperative Nursing Interventions

A. Administer Good Postoperative Care Based on General Principles and Observe for Usual Postoperative Complications (see p. 1134).

Be particularly alert to adequate fluid intake.

B. Assist the Child in Maintaining a Patent Airway, by Draining Secretions and Preventing Aspiration of Vomitus.

1. Place the child prone or semiprone before he becomes alert with head turned to side.
2. Allow the child to assume position of comfort when he is alert. (Mother may hold the child.)
3. The child may vomit old blood initially. If suctioning is necessary, avoid trauma to oropharynx.
4. Remind the child not to cough or clear throat unless necessary.

C. Observe the Child Constantly Until He Is Awake, and Then Frequently Thereafter; Monitor Vital Signs and be Alert to Signs of Hemorrhage.

1. Indications of hemorrhage (the most frequent complication)
   a. Increasing rapid pulse
   b. Frequent swallowing
   c. Pallor
   d. Restlessness
   e. Clearing of throat and vomiting of blood
   f. Continuous slight oozing of blood over a number of hours postoperatively
   g. Check vomitus for any fresh bleeding
   h. Inspect throat for signs of oozing
2. Have emergency equipment readily available.
   a. Suction equipment
   b. Packing material

D. Offer Measures of Comfort to the Child.

1. Cool liquids offer some relief from sore throat, as well as prevent dehydration and temperature elevation.
   a. Give ice chips 1–2 hours after awakening.
   b. When vomiting has ceased, advance to clear liquids cautiously.
   c. Offer cool, synthetic fruit juices and milk at first since they are best tolerated; then offer Popsicles, cool water for first 12–24 hours.
2. Ice collar to neck may provide some comfort. (Remove ice collar if child becomes restless.)
3. Give analgesic, especially to older child.
4. Rinse mouth with cool water or alkaline solution.
5. Keep child and environment free from blood-tinged drainage to help decrease anxiety.
6. There is some controversy regarding intake of milk and ice cream the evening of surgery: it can be soothing and reduce swelling but it does coat the mouth and throat, causing child to clear throat more often and this may initiate bleeding.

E. Provide Opportunity For the Child to Have as Much Rest as Possible.

1. Encourage the mother to be with the child when he awakens since he is usually frightened. (The mother's presence can be very comforting.)
2. When mother must leave, reassure the child that she will return.
3. Keep the child in bed in a quiet room.

Health Education

1. Explain and write instructions as to the care of the child at home after discharge (usually the day after surgery).
   a. Diet should still consist of large amounts of fluids as well as soft, cool, nonirritating foods. (Supply list of suggestions.)
   b. Eating helps promote healing because it increases the blood supply to tissues.
   c. Bedrest should be maintained for a couple of days, then daily rest periods for about a week. Resume normal activities about 2 weeks following surgery.
   d. Avoid contact with persons with infections.
   e. Discourage the child from frequent coughing and clearing of throat.
   f. Avoid gargling. Mouth odor may be present for a few days after surgery; only mouth rinsing is acceptable.
   g. If signs and symptoms of impending trouble occur, the physician should be called immediately.
      (1) Earache accompanied by fever
      (2) Any bleeding, often indicated only by frequent swallowing; most common about 5th–10th day when membrane sloughs from surgical site
   h. How to give any medications the physician may prescribe
   i. The telephone number of the physician or emergency department if trouble occurs
2. Discuss with the mother (parents) what results they can expect from the surgery.
   a. Decreased number of sore throats
   b. Lessened evidence of obstructive symptoms
   c. Decreased incidence of cervical lymphadenitis
   d. Improvement in nutritional status
   e. Will not improve nasal allergies
   f. Will not improve secretory otitis media
3. Guide parents in helping the child think of the hospital experience as a positive one once he has returned home.

a. Talk about what happened.
b. Let the child play out his feelings.

Expected Outcomes

1. Experiences minimal anxiety and fear evidenced by appropriate coping behaviors
2. Achieves stabilized postoperative condition; vital signs normal; no unusual bleeding
3. Demonstrates appropriate fluid intake and output
4. Experiences minimal discomfort as evidenced by normal vital signs, ability to swallow, and relaxed behavior
5. Parents verbalize postoperative plan of care at home (i.e., diet, activities, follow-up)

Asthma

Asthma is a recurrent, reversible condition of the lungs characterized by increased responsiveness or irritability of the trachea and bronchi, in which there is spasm of the bronchial smooth muscle, edema of the mucosa, and increased mucus secretions in the bronchioles as a response to various stimuli that change in severity either spontaneously or with treatment.

Classification of Asthma

1. *Spasmodic*—sporadic in nature, with varying intervals of freedom from difficulty and with precipitating factors often readily defined
2. *Continuous*—no outward signs or symptoms of asthma, but some shortness of breath on occasion, transitory wheezing on strenuous exercise, and wheezy crackles heard during deep inspiration
3. *Intractable asthma*—persistent wheezing requiring regular, daily medication, for either the control of symptoms or the ability to function
4. *Status asthmaticus*—severe attack in which the patient deteriorates despite adequate treatment with sympathomimetic drugs

Etiology

1. Asthma is an inflammatory reaction that induces prolonged hypersecretion and bronchospasm or constriction in response to chemical mediators brought about by inhaled allergens for chemical sensitizers or viral infections.
2. Changing concepts related to asthma:
   a. Asthma is an inflammatory disease not simply bronchospasm.
   b. Airway changes are not always completely reversible.
   c. Frequent typical presentation includes cough and recurrent pneumonia.
   d. Bronchial hyperreactivity, asthma, often occurs with other diseases.
   e. Hyperreactivity can vary spontaneously and be affected by medications and removal of triggers.
3. The stimuli responsible for triggering attacks of asthma are as follows:
   a. Extrinsic—antigen–antibody reaction, a positive reaction to certain allergens. IgE or IgA antibodies are activated by allergens resulting in bronchospasm, edema, and increased secretions of mucus (allergy to pollen, animal dander, feathers, foods, house dust, and mites).
   b. Intrinsic—symptoms caused by other nonallergic factors—little evidence of IgE antibodies.
      (1) Infection—respiratory syncytial virus (RSV), parainfluenza virus (types I and II), mycoplasmal pneumonia
      (2) Physical factors
         (a) Cold
         (b) Meteorologic factors (i.e., humidity, sudden changes in temperature and barometric pressure)
      (3) Inheritable tendencies
      (4) Irritants
         (a) Chemicals
         (b) Air pollutants (e.g., sulfur dioxide, carbon monoxide, particulate matter)
      (5) Psychic or emotional factors (i.e., tension, fear, anxiety)
      (6) Physical stress—fatigue, excessive exercise
      (7) Endocrine—may worsen in relation to mensus or improve at puberty

Incidence

1. The incidence of asthma in infancy exists but increases in children 3 years and older.
   a. In younger children, the incidence is greater in males.
   b. Incidence is equal in males and females during adolescence.
   c. Infants with eczema are at increased risk for developing asthma after the age of 10 years.
2. Childhood asthma may decrease at puberty.
3. Approximately 3% of school-age children have symptoms of asthma.

Altered Physiology

1. The turbinates warm and moisten all air that passes into the lung.
2. Inspired air contains particulate matter which is removed by the blanket of mucus present in the tracheobronchial tree. This mucus is kept moistened by inspired moist air.
3. The blanket of mucus is moved constantly upward by the propelling action of the cilia, and if mucus becomes thickened or inspissated, it cannot be moved.
4. Increased local deposition and concentration of allergens occur.
5. This produces intrabronchial accumulation and stagnation of mucus which is the primary cause of the respiratory embarrassment.
6. Chemical mediators in asthma:
   a. Primarily involved are histamine and SRS-A (slow-reacting substance of anaphylaxis). SRS-A appears after histamine release, and persists for a longer period. It is not inhibited by the action of the antihistamines.
   b. These materials are primarily responsible for changes in the blood vessels and mucous membrane in the bronchi and bronchioles, as well as for the initiation of bronchospasm.
7. During an asthma attack, abnormal constriction of muscles surrounding the bronchioles (spasm) results in narrowed bronchiolar lumen and decreased oxygen supply in alveoli.
   a. In addition, edema, inflammation, and increased mucus production further compromise respirations.

b. Hyperresonance and decreased breath sounds may be observed (ominous sign).

8. There are bronchial smooth muscle hypertrophy, bronchial spasms, mucus gland hypertrophy, and edema of respiratory mucosa, and mucus plugging.

Complications

1. Infections—bronchiectasis, pneumonia, bronchiolitis
2. Status asthmaticus
3. Atelectasis
4. Pneumothorax
5. Emphysema
6. Cor pulmonale
7. Misuse of medications
8. Emotional and behavioral problems
9. Dehydration
10. Pneumomediastinum
11. Hypotension, hypertension
12. Cardiac arrhythmias
13. Infants (up to 2 years)—serious respiratory failure due to the stage of development of their anatomic structures and physiologic mechanisms that are unable to cope with the insult and compensatory demands of the disease

Clinical Manifestations

1. The onset of an asthmatic attack may be gradual, with nasal congestion, sneezing and a watery nasal discharge present before the attack.
2. Attacks may occur suddenly, often at night, when the child awakens with the following symptoms:
   a. Wheezing, which occurs primarily with expiration—may be reduced due to minimal air movement
   b. Anxiety and apprehension
   c. Diaphoresis
   d. Uncontrollable cough
   e. Dyspnea, with increased effort during expiration
3. With treatment, the attack may be controlled. The asthmatic attack may progress, however, and the child will develop the following symptoms:
   a. Increasing dyspnea
   b. Thick, tenacious mucus
   c. Coarse and fine musical crackles
   d. Flaring of the alae nasi
   e. Use of accessory muscles for respiration
   f. Cyanosis
   g. Hypoxemia
   h. Respiratory alkalosis leading to respiratory acidosis
   i. Hypercapnia
   j. Increased heart and respiratory rates
   k. Abdominal pain from severe coughing
   l. Vomiting
   m. Extreme anxiety and apprehension
4. Chronic cough relieved by bronchodilators
5. Nonspecific episodic dyspnea unrelated to exercise
6. Hypersecretions and recurrent lung infiltration and atelectasis
7. Frequent hospital admissions for acute symptoms
8. Physical characteristics
   a. May be smaller in size
   b. Anterior–posterior chest diameter may be increased
   c. Excessive nasal secretions

d. Mouth gaping
e. Inspiratory and expiratory wheeze

Diagnostic Evaluation

1. Eosinophilia in peripheral blood, nasal secretions, and sputum
2. Polymorphonuclear leukocytosis in the presence of infection
3. Pulmonary function studies—diminished maximal breathing capacity, tidal volume and timed vital capacity; spirometric picture of obstruction
4. Determination of blood gases and *p*H—respiratory acidosis and later metabolic acidosis
5. Gross and microscopic examination of sputum—bronchial casts and eosinophilia
6. Serum CBC
7. Chest x-ray—to exclude presence of other diseases; child may show hyperventilation during asthma attack; air trapping, atelectasis, pulmonary hypertension, edema
8. Routine skin testing may help determine allergic causes
   a. Serum IgE—elevated if allergic disease
   b. RAST (radioallergosorbent test)—assay for allergen-specific IgE

Treatment

A. Acute or Emergency Care

Relieve symptoms and increase ventilatory capacity.
1. Bronchodilators—intravenous aminophylline; subcutaneous epinephrine; inhalation sympathomimetics; metered inhalers used to deliver beta-agonists
2. Continual assessment of respiratory status, blood gas studies
3. Maintain patient airway and oxygenation; suction viscous secretion; ensure humidity and oxygenation; position correctly
4. Reestablish and maintain fluid and electrolyte balance
5. Cardiac monitoring—monitor for hypertension and right-sided heart failure and arrhythmias
6. Maintain rest and physical comfort
7. Give patient and parental reassurance
8. Anti-inflammatory agents; expectorants as indicated
9. Intubation and ventilation if necessary

B. Long-Term Care

Prevention of acute asthmatic episodes and school absences; maximum control of symptoms with minimal medications and treatments; participation in normal activities; normalization of pulmonary function tests; normal growth and development.

Education of the parents and family to understand, accept, and manage asthma that can accommodate the family's life-style.
1. Removal of suspected stimulus—allergen, irritant, exercise, emotional factors
2. Desensitization to build up the child's resistance to his allergens
3. Drug therapy to control symptoms
4. Chest physical therapy—bronchial drainage, breathing exercises
5. Supportive:
   a. Adequate hydration
   b. Adequate oxygenation
   c. Appropriate treatment of any existing infection

d. Correct acid-base imbalance
e. Relieve fatigue

Assessment

1. Make a baseline nursing assessment of the child's condition to determine the severity of the attack and the degree of respiratory distress.
   a. Observe the child's breathing pattern:
      (1) Determine whether the expiratory phase of respiration is increased.
      (2) Determine whether the child is wheezing. (In severe attacks, wheezing is audible at a distance from the child.)
         Assess for inspiratory as well as expiratory wheeze.
      (3) Determine whether the child is using accessory muscles for breathing.
   b. Listen to the child's chest with a stethoscope to determine whether crackles and wheezing are present and to determine whether all areas of the lung fields are being aerated.
   c. Assess the child's level of anxiety and apprehension.
   d. Observe for flaring of the alae nasi.
   e. Observe the child for the development of cyanosis, using adequate light.
2. Determine the heart and respiratory rates; record and report to the physician any significant change.
3. Identify what medications were administered at home and when.
4. Discuss with the physician the plan of medical care.

Potential Problems and Nursing Diagnoses

1. Breathing pattern, ineffective, related to impaired gas exchange
2. Fluid volume deficit related to hyperventilation and decreased oral intake
3. Potential complications of respiratory acidosis and hypoxemia
4. Comfort, altered, related to respiratory distress
5. Anxiety related to difficult breathing and hospitalization
6. Potential complications from medications
7. Potential for atelectasis or pneumothorax related to hyperinfiltration of lungs

Nursing Interventions

A. Provide Measures to Relieve the Respiratory Distress the Child Is Experiencing.

1. Position the child in high Fowler's position to allow maximum lung expansion.
   a. Raise the head of the bed to achieve high Fowler's position.
   b. Place an overbed table padded with a pillow in front of the child and have him extend his arms over the table—this provides a comfortable position and allows maximum utilization of accessory muscles for breathing.
2. Administer oxygen when signs of air hunger are present.
   a. Do not wait for the appearance of cyanosis before administering oxygen.
   b. Oxygen must be administered with caution because the child with severe respiratory distress may be dependent upon his low PO_2 to stimulate spontaneous respiration. In the face of a rising PCO_2 and a potential carbon dioxide narcosis, the administration of oxygen may remove the last stimulus to spontaneous respirations.
      Mild asthma attacks cause respiratory alkalosis, but as air flow obstruction worsens, the $PaCO_2$ rises causing respiratory acidosis. When there is bronchospasm, hypoxemia, and a normal $PaCO_2$, this a sign that the child is tiring. Blood gases should be monitored.
3. Humidity may be used with or without oxygen to help liquefy secretions and reduce mucosal inflammation and edema.
   If humidity is too high or droplets are present, further bronchospasm may be triggered.
4. Explain to the child the purpose of the oxygen equipment before oxygen is administered and allow the child to feel and touch the equipment.
5. Use aerosolized bronchodilators or inhaler with bronchodilators.

B. Relieve the Anxiety and Apprehension That Results From the Respiratory Embarrassment.

1. Place the child in a quiet, clean room, where he can be closely observed.
2. Provide the child with maximum reassurance.
   a. Allow the parents to remain with the child.
      (1) Keep the parents informed of the child's progress—what is being done and why—to relieve their apprehension. Parental anxiety is readily transmitted to the child.
      (2) Talk calmly and quietly to the child.
      (3) Assure the child that you will not leave him alone.
      (4) Allow the child to have his favorite security object.
3. Organize care so as to avoid disturbing the child any more than necessary.
4. Evaluate the need for sedation.
5. When the child falls asleep, allow him to continue to sleep and do not disturb him unless absolutely necessary.

C. Provide Adequate Hydration to Liquefy and Mobilize Bronchial Secretions and Maintain Electrolyte Balance.

Dehydration occurs secondary to decreased fluid intake, excessive perspiration, vomiting, increased respiration and infection; some bronchodilators may cause dehydration.
1. Observe for signs of dehydration.
   a. Lack of skin turgor
   b. Lack of tears
   c. Dry, parched lips
   d. Depressed fontanelle
   e. Decreased urinary output—high specific gravity; concentrated appearance
2. Maintain parenteral fluid administration.
3. Encourage oral fluid intake.
   a. Determine the child's fluid preferences.
   b. Offer small sips of fluid frequently, when respiratory effort improves.
   c. Avoid iced fluids which may provoke bronchospasm.
   d. Avoid carbonated beverages when the child is wheezing.
4. Allow the child to return to a regular diet as soon as possible.
5. Observe for signs of overhydration and pulmonary edema, related to high negative pleural pressure generated during bronchospasm and accumulation of interstitial fluids.

D. Be Aware of the Action and Side Effects of Drugs Used in the Treatment of Asthma.

1. *Aminophylline*—bronchodilator
   a. Toxic reaction may occur, but it is more likely to happen with prolonged overdose or when given in conjunction with epinephrine or ephedrine without reducing aminophylline dosage.
      (1) Serum drug levels should be done.
      (2) Toxic reactions include:
         Fever, restlessness, nausea and vomiting, hypotension, abdominal distention.
   b. Side effects—irritability, excitability, continued dehydration, vomiting, diuresis and tachycardia, hematemesis, proteinuria, stupor, convulsions, coma, death. Hypotension occurs with IV use. Avoid ingestion of stimulants.
   c. Occasionally cyanosis and syncope may appear after only a small amount of the prescribed dose. This is considered an idiosyncracy, and the drug should be discontinued.
   d. Use caution when other medications are also given to determine drug interaction.
2. *Epinephrine*—relaxes bronchial smooth muscle and constricts bronchial mucosal vessels, thereby reducing congestion and edema; acts as a bronchodilator.
   a. The smallest dose affording relief should be used.
   b. Side effects—insomnia, headache, nervousness, palpitations, precordial pain, hypertension, hypoxemia, tachycardia, nausea, sweating, urinary retention. (It may potentiate aminophylline toxicity.)
3. *Ephedrine*—relaxes bronchial smooth muscle and constricts bronchial mucosal vessels, thereby reducing congestion and edema. Acts as a bronchodilator.
   a. Has the advantage of prolonged action and oral administration
   b. Side effects—same as for epinephrine
   c. Do not allow child to drink cola, tea, or coffee, since they may increase nervousness.
4. *Pseudoephedrine*
   a. Has prolonged action and can be administered orally
   b. Side effects—relatively free
5. *Isoproterenol (Isuprel)*—bronchodilator
   a. Toxic reaction—headache, flushing, dizziness, tremors, nausea and vomiting
   b. Side effects—nervousness, palpitations, pink saliva or sputum if administered orally
   c. Do not use concurrently with epinephrine.
6. *Expectorants*—given as an adjunct to hydration; thins secretions and helps the child to cough productively (i.e., saturated solution of potassium iodide, Robitussin)
7. *Aerosolized bronchodilator*—Bronkosol
8. *Inhaled sympathomimetics*—(beta-adrenergic agonists): metaproterenol, isoetharine, isoproterenol
   a. Can use aerosol compressor/nebulizer system for the child under 6 or metered-dosed inhalers for the older child
   b. Side effects—may be shakiness and cardiac stimulation
9. *Corticosteroids*—beclomethasone dipropionate; antiinflammatory agents; diminish the inflammatory component of asthma, thus reducing airway obstruction.
   a. Produce beneficial effects only after several hours
   b. Used when other drugs fail to bring relief from an asthmatic attack

   c. Side effects—persistent use for mild attacks may lead to suppression of adrenal activity. Prolonged use may lead to growth retardation and steroid dependency, sodium retention, hypokalemia, immunosuppression, and infection.
   d. Corticosteroids by inhaler (Vanceril/Beclovent)—fewer side effects than with oral or IV administration; however, oral candidiasis is common.
10. *Cromolyn sodium prophylaxis*—adjunct to existing treatment, especially for steroid-dependent child. It inhibits the release of histamine and the SRS-A. It has prophylactic action; it should not be used in acute attack. This medication is used only as an inhalant. Side effects may include irritation of throat and trachea and a rash.
11. During the transition from intravenous to oral bronchodilators, respirations should be monitored carefully and frequently.
12. Nebulizer and metered-dose inhaler:
    a. Nebulizer is attached to compressed air source that delivers medication in moist air by a face mask.
    b. Metered-dose inhaler delivers premeasured dose of prescribed medication.
    c. Teach and have parents demonstrate their understanding of use and care of equipment.
    d. Instruct parents and child not to change or exceed prescribed medication dose.
    e. Ensure that parents and child know and report side effects of treatment and recognize improvement.
    f. Stress the importance of seeking medical attention for acute exacerbations.

E. Encourage the Child and His Parents to Practice Measures That Will Help to Maintain Optimal Health, to Prevent Acute Attacks, to Ameliorate Chronic Symptoms, and to Prevent Onset of Progression of Respiratory Disabilities.

1. General health measures
   a. Provide a well-balanced diet and increased fluid intake.
   b. Ensure sleep, rest, and reasonable exercise; avoid fatigue and chilling.
   c. Avoid known irritants.
2. Psychological measures
   a. Attempt to keep the child emotionally calm and at ease.
   b. Maintain optimistic attitude.
3. Regular medical follow-up
   a. Ensure strict adherence to medication regimen.
   b. Give prompt attention when infection is present and new or progressive respiratory symptoms appear.

F. Teach the Child and Involve the Parents in the Teaching of Proper Breathing Habits.

The exercises strengthen the diaphragm so that breathing will become much better and the total lung capacity will be increased. Breathing exercises used with postural drainage may lessen the need for continuous medication and contribute to increased expectoration of mucus that causes respiratory difficulty. Breathing exercises will also aid in promoting improved posture, physical training, and mental relaxation.

1. Instruct the child to clear his nasal passages before beginning exercises.
2. Each exercise should start with a short, gentle inspi-

ration through the nose, followed by a prolonged expiration through the mouth.

3. During inspiration, the upper portion of the thorax should be kept immobilized.

4. During expiration, abdominal muscles should be pulled in.

5. On no account should the child take a deep inspiration during the exercise, but instead he should see how long he can continue the expiration.

   a. *Exercise I—Abdominal Breathing*

     (1) Lie on back with knees drawn up, body relaxed, and hands resting on upper abdomen.

     (2) Exhale slowly (through mouth), gently sink the chest and then upper abdomen until retracted at end of expiration.

     (3) Relax upper abdomen (bulges forward) while taking brief inspiration through nose (chest is not raised).
     Repeat 8–16 times; rest 1 minute; repeat.

   b. *Exercise II—Side Expansion Breathing*

     (1) Sit relaxed in a chair and place palms of hands on each side of lower ribs.

     (2) Exhale slowly through mouth, contracting upper part of thorax, then lower ribs, then compress palms against ribs. (This expels air from base of lungs.)

     (3) Inhale, expanding lower ribs against slight pressure from hands.
     Repeat 8–16 times; rest 1 minute; repeat.

   c. *Exercise III—Forward Bending*

     (1) Sit with feet apart, arms relaxed at sides.

     (2) Exhale slowly, drop head forward and downward to knees, while retracting abdominal muscles.

     (3) Raise trunk slowly while inhaling and expand upper abdomen.

     (4) Exhale quickly, sinking chest and abdomen, but remain erect.

     (5) Inhale, expanding upper abdomen.

   d. *Exercise IV—Elbow Arching*
   (This exercise is performed between breathing exercises.)

     (1) Sit leaning slightly forward, back straight, and fingers on shoulders.

     (2) Move elbows in circles forward, upward, backward, and downward.
     Repeat 4–8 times; rest; repeat.

   e. *General Instructions*
   Perform exercises:

     (1) In the morning before breakfast when the child is feeling fresh

     (2) At night, before getting into bed to clear the lungs before sleep

     (3) At the first sign of an impending attack to prevent asthma from developing

6. Less complicated exercises using same principles can be blowing of a cotton ball or ping pong ball across a table top—keeping score of the distance achieved (make a game of activity), and blowing large soap bubbles.

7. Regular exercise not only improves the lung capacity but also the general physical and emotional well-being of the child.

8. Special exercise programs and camps have been developed throughout the United States to help children with asthma.

Note: Many patients can abort their attacks entirely by doing simple exercises gently. Should the child become short of breath or wheeze slightly, take single dose of whatever medication relieved him before beginning the exercises. Exercise may occasionally produce wheezing or coughing at the end of exercise. It may distress the child, but with perseverance the mucus in the bronchial tubes becomes loosened, and the patient may be able to cough it up with consequent relief of attack.

Health Education

A. Assist the Parents to Develop a Realistic Attitude Toward the Child's Illness.

1. Try to treat the child as a completely normal child who needs only a few additional restrictions imposed because of his illness.

   a. Accept him as a unique person with unique contributions to make.

   b. Let him know he is capable, loved, and respected.

   c. Set consistent behavior limits. Do not accept child triggering attack to gain secondary rewards.

2. Allow the child the same duties and rights as other children in the family.

3. Try to explain why he must watch for certain things and why he is restricted in some ways.

4. Teach the child the symptoms of an asthma attack and how to relax.

   a. Give explanations instead of orders and show him confidence and respect.

   b. Be honest with him and express empathy.

   c. Help him to express his feelings rather than use his illness as an excuse for physically aggressive hostility or manipulative behavior.

5. Avoid overprotection and unnecessary surveillance.

6. Teach the child to gradually manage for himself rather than depend on parents.

   a. Allow him to actively explore his limitations and capabilities.

   b. Teach him all the symptoms of asthma—will aid in early treatment.

   c. Encourage him to keep a daily diary of symptoms, activity, environment, etc., noting any changes.

   d. Explain to him what medications he is taking and why and when they are taken.

   e. Show him the importance of a regular exercise program.

   f. Teach him to recognize signs of respiratory infection and to seek medical attention when appropriate.

   g. Encourage him to become involved in hyposensitization (if used). Perhaps he can even administer his own medications.

   h. Teach him the importance of increasing fluid intake, especially during an asthma attack when fluid is needed to compensate for fluid loss resulting from dyspnea and diaphoresis.

   i. Teach him to keep records of activities, symptoms, weather, etc.

   j. Teach him when to seek medical help—when usual medication fails to provide relief, when asthma suddenly worsens, with onset of fever or other signs of infection.

   k. Teach proper use of airflow meter and inhaler as appropriate.

7. If the child is too much engrossed with his illness, he can be diverted with kindly scolding, friendly minimizing of his ailments, or by encouraging other interests, so that he forgets his troubles as much as possible.

a. Encourage him to build on his interests; help him to find activities that will not hurt him.
b. The child's ability to control his breathing problems, in addition to learning that he can participate in some way with his peers, will increase his self-confidence and self-value, and result in beneficial physical and attitudinal changes.
c. Involvement in physical activity should be encouraged, as should rest at signs of fatigue.

8. Do not talk about the child's illness any more than necessary—do not allow secrecy or whispering. Recognize the child's feelings about his illness and allow him to talk about them with parents and family.

9. Inform friends and relatives of problems so that the necessary consideration is given him.
a. Plan a team conference involving parent(s), school nurse, and teacher.
b. The school nurse should be provided with information relating to: child's activity, what to do during an attack, medications to be taken during school hours, especially inhaler, who to call for information or if problems arise that cannot be handled at school.

10. Create an atmosphere at home that is not provoking or upsetting—but is still not artificially calm.

11. Prepare the child for approaching events (if bursts of emotions have an effect on his illness).

12. Teach the child special skills.
a. Let him develop special hobbies and interests that can be combined with his illness.
b. Remember that accomplishments that develop respect and admiration in peers are particularly desirable and aid in building self-confidence and a feeling of security.

13. Both parents and child feel greater assurance if they are aware of how the child should be treated at certain stages of the disease.
a. Have special instructions and medications on hand.
b. An emergency plan should be developed by the nurse and family so that the child and parents will not panic during a crisis and will respond appropriately.

14. If the child takes medications for his allergy or specific symptoms, administer them in a matter-of-fact manner without making any fuss. Encourage taking medication when stomach is empty, drinking adequate amount of fluid.

15. Child needs security, self-confidence, and love. (Do not force these on the child.) Exaggeration is never beneficial.

16. Provide information and literature for the family. Encourage contact with the local chapter of the American Lung Association or Asthma and Allergy Foundation of America for information on existing programs in which other children with asthma and their parents come together.

B. Teach the Child and His Parents Protective Measures That Will Encourage Environmental Control and Help to Avoid the Offending Allergen, as Well as Practice Measures That Will Help Control Asthma Attacks.

1. Keep the child's bedroom as free from dust as possible.
a. Keep in bedroom only the furniture that is absolutely necessary.
b. Remove upholstered furniture, draperies, carpets, pictures, books, toys, and unnecessary dust-collecting objects.
c. Use washable curtains and cotton or synthetic rugs.
d. Use cotton or synthetic blankets and washable bedspreads (not chenille or tufted types).
e. Do not use insect or other sprays in the bedroom.
f. Do not store outer clothing or household articles in bedroom closets.
g. Enclose mattresses, box-springs, and pillows in dustproof covers (unless they are synthetic).
h. Blankets and clothing that have been stored should be thoroughly aired before use.

2. Avoid irritating odors such as paint, tobacco smoke, insect powders, pine oils, jellies, and irritating cooking odors.

3. If possible, use an exhaust fan in the kitchen to remove cooking odors.

4. Remove all overstuffed furniture and rugs.

5. Avoid sitting and playing on overstuffed furniture and down pillows.

6. Avoid carbonated drinks, such as ginger ale and colas (especially when wheezing).

7. Avoid any physical exertion that causes wheezing or excessive shortness of breath.

8. Avoid using irritating salves on chest or in nose.

9. Avoid dusty and musty places (basements, storerooms, etc.).

10. Avoid felt rug pads because of animal hair content.

11. Purchase foam furniture and foam rubber pads if possible when refurnishing the home.

12. If home is heated by a circulating hot-air system, shut it off in the bedroom (use electric heater if necessary). A central air filter in the furnace is desirable; clean or replace it frequently.

13. Take only drugs prescribed by the physician.

14. Report for treatment as directed by physician.

C. Help Foster a Healthy Mother–Child Relationship by Understanding the Feelings of Anxiety, Guilt, or Frustration the Mother May Have.

1. Remember that the mother's life-style may have changed with the diagnosis of asthma in her child, resulting in loss of sleep, constant care, etc.

2. Listen to her and provide appropriate support.

3. Initiate social service referral as indicated.

Expected Outcomes

1. Demonstrates improved respiratory function; rapid abatement of symptoms; normal blood gas values

2. Demonstrates adequate hydration; urine specific gravity and vital sign measurements within normal ranges; normal tissue turgor

3. Attains/maintains normal electrolyte balance and blood gas values

4. Experiences increasing comfort; improved respiratory status; normal vital signs and behavior

5. Shows minimal anxiety; has relaxed behavior and improved respiratory status

6. Reveals normal cardiac function; normal vital signs; ECG, heart auscultation, and chest x-ray results normal

7. Exhibits normal respiratory function; no atelectasis or pneumothorax; normal vital signs

8. Patient and parents demonstrate understanding of disease and care; demonstrate breathing exercises; verbalize information concerning medications, activities needed to remove trigger mechanisms, follow-up visits, etc.

Respiratory Distress Syndrome
(Hyaline Membrane Disease)

Respiratory distress syndrome (RDS) is a syndrome of immature infants that is characterized by a progressive and frequently fatal respiratory disorder resulting from atelectasis and immaturity of the lungs.

Etiology

The exact etiology of RDS is not clearly defined.
1. Adequate pulmonary function at birth depends on the following:
   a. Adequate amount of surfactant (a lipoprotein mixture) lining the alveolar cells, which allows for alveolar stability and prevents alveolar collapse at the end of expiration.
   b. Adequate surface area in air spaces to allow for gas exchange (i.e., sufficient pulmonary capillary bed in contact with this alveolar surface area).
2. RDS is the result of decreased pulmonary surfactant, incomplete structural development of lung, and highly compliant chest wall.
3. Contributing factors—any factor that decreases surfactant, such as
   a. Prematurity and immature alveolar lining cells
   b. Acidosis
   c. Hypothermia
   d. Hypoxia
   e. Hypovolemia
   f. Diabetes
   g. Elective cesarean section
   h. Unknown
   i. Some episode of fetal or intrapartum stress that compromises blood supply to fetal lung: vaginal bleeding, maternal hypertension, difficult resuscitation associated with birth asphyxia
      It should be noted that some situations result in the acceleration of surfactant (steroid therapy; heroin-addicted mother).

Incidence

RDS occurs most frequently in:
1. Premature infants (primarily weighing between 1000–1500 gm. [2.2–3.3 lbs.]) and between 28–37 weeks' gestation; incidence increases with increased degree of prematurity.
2. Infants of mothers who have diabetes
3. Infants delivered by cesarean section–probably related to underlying indication for surgery
4. Infants of mothers who have experienced intrauterine vaginal bleeding

Altered Physiology

It is thought that both a biochemical and an anatomic basis affect the susceptibility of immature lungs to hyaline membrane disease (HMD).
1. Immature lung—underdeveloped and uninflated alveoli, immature pulmonary capillary bed
2. Surfactant lowers surface tension at alveolar surface, giving alveoli stability; at end of expiration, some of the air remains in the lung (called the functional residual capacity or FRC), thus requiring less negative pressure and exertion to take next breath. When surfactant is deficient, surface tension is higher and alveoli are unstable and collapse at end of expiration. There is decreased FRC; thus, the next breath requires almost as much effort as the first breath after birth.
3. Sequence of events resulting in HMD:
   a. Deficient surfactant, by Type II alveolar cells (Although some surfactant may be present at birth, it may not be regenerated at a rate commensurate with disappearance.)
      (1) Alveoli inflate unequally on inspiration and collapse on expiration.
      (2) More oxygen and energy are required by the infant to expand the alveoli with each breath that he inhales, causing him to tire.
      (3) The number of alveoli that expand progressively decreases.
      (4) Surfactant production may be reduced due to:
         (a) Extreme immaturity of alveolar lining cells
         (b) Diminished or impaired production rate resulting from fetal or early neonatal stress
         (c) Impairment of release mechanism for surface-active phospholipid from limiting membrane within type II alveolar cells
         (d) Death of many of these cells responsible for decreased surfactant production
   b. Alveolar instability and atelectasis
      (1) Pulmonary vascular resistance increases—hypoperfusion of lung
      (2) Fetal circulation right-to-left shunt results, leading to hypoxemia and hypercapnia, which lead to respiratory and metabolic acidosis.
   c. Hypoxemia and pulmonary vascular pressure cause ischemia in the alveoli (Fig. 49-2).
      (1) Effusion of plasma through capillary walls (transudate) into alveoli
      (2) Necrotic cells and fibrin form a membranous layer in alveoli.
      (3) Gas exchange becomes inhibited.
      (4) Lungs become stiff (decreased compliance), requiring more pressure to expand them.
   d. Airway obstruction leads to increased asphyxia and vasoconstriction, and the cycle continues.
4. RDS is usually a self-limited disease and symptoms peak in about 3–4 days, at which time surfactant synthesis begins to accelerate and pulmonary function and clinical appearance begin to improve.
   a. Moderately ill infants or those who do not require assisted ventilation show the following:
      (1) Slow improvement by about 48 hours
      (2) Rapid recovery over next 3–4 days; few complications
   b. Severely ill and very immature infants who require some ventilatory assistance:
      (1) Demonstrate rapid deterioration (see Clinical Manifestations)
      (2) Ventilatory assistance may be required for several days; chronic lung disease is a frequent complication.
      (3) Iatrogenic harm more likely (i.e., infection, necrotizing enterocolitis, etc.)

Complications

1. Complications related to respiratory therapy:
   a. Air leak: pneumothorax—pneumomediastinum, pneumopericardium, and pneumoperitoneum

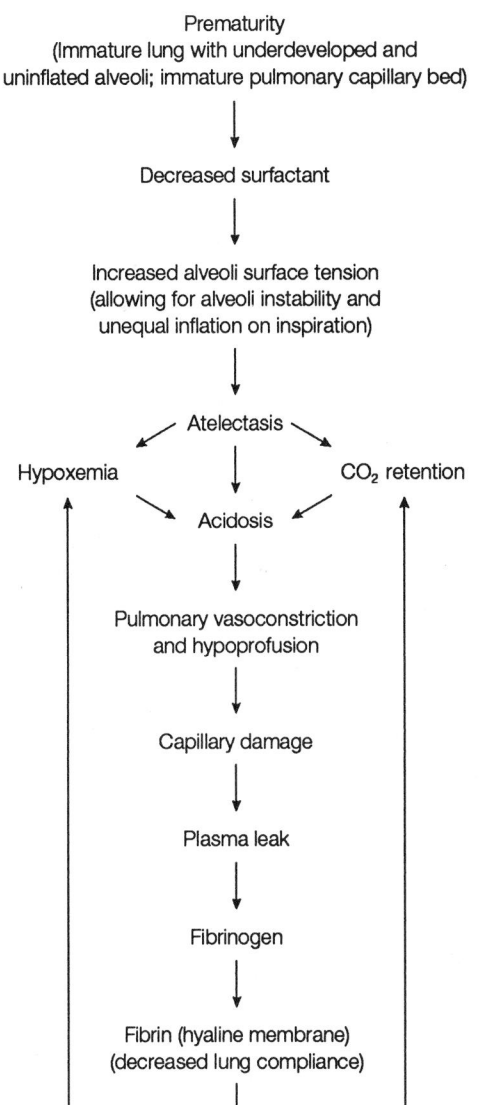

Prematurity
(Immature lung with underdeveloped and
uninflated alveoli; immature pulmonary capillary bed)

↓

Decreased surfactant

↓

Increased alveoli surface tension
(allowing for alveoli instability and
unequal inflation on inspiration)

↓

Atelectasis

Hypoxemia CO_2 retention

Acidosis

↓

Pulmonary vasoconstriction
and hypoprofusion

↓

Capillary damage

↓

Plasma leak

↓

Fibrinogen

↓

Fibrin (hyaline membrane)
(decreased lung compliance)

Figure 49-2. *Schematic outline of hyaline membrane disease.*

b. Pneumonia—especially gram-negative organisms
c. Pulmonary interstitial emphysema
2. Patent ductus arteriosus (PDA)
3. Intraventricular hemorrhage—especially in infant less than 1500 gm. (3.3 lbs.)
4. Disseminated intravascular coagulation (DIC)
5. Chronic problems associated with long-term use of oxygen:
   a. Bronchopulmonary dysplasia—lungs cystic-appearing with hyperinfiltration, obstructive bronchiolitis, dysplastic changes, and pulmonary fibrosis
   b. Chronic respiratory infections
6. Necrotizing enterocolitis
7. Tracheal stenosis
8. Retinopathy of prematurity (retrolental fibroplasia)
9. Other complications related to prematurity

Clinical Manifestations

Symptoms are usually observed soon after birth and may include:

A. Primary Signs and Symptoms

1. Expiratory grunting or whining (when infant is not crying)
2. Sternal, suprasternal, substernal, and intercostal retractions progressing to paradoxical seesaw respirations (see Observation of Retractions, Fig. 48-2)
3. Inspiratory nasal flaring
4. Tachypnea
5. Hypothermia
6. Cyanosis when child is in room air (infants with severe disease may be cyanotic even when given oxygen), increasing need for oxygen
7. Decreased breath sounds and dry "sandpaper" breath sounds—on auscultation of chest
8. As the disease progresses:
   a. Seesaw retractions become marked with marked abdominal protrusion on expiration.
   b. Peripheral edema increases.
   c. Muscle tone decreases.
   d. Cyanosis increases.
      (1) Body temperature drops.
      (2) Short periods of apnea occur.
      (3) Bradycardia may occur.
   e. Asphyxia becomes more severe.
      (1) Apneic episodes develop.
      (2) Changes in distribution of blood throughout body result in pale gray skin color.

B. Secondary Signs and Symptoms

1. Hypotension
2. Edema of hands and feet
3. Bowel sounds absent early in the illness
4. Urine output decreased

Diagnostic Evaluation

1. Laboratory tests
   a. PCO_2—elevated
   b. PO_2—low
   c. Blood pH—low due to metabolic acidosis
   d. Calcium—low
2. Chest x-ray—demonstrates a diffuse, fine granularity; air bronchograms show "ground glass" appearance with prominent air bronchogram extending into periphery of lung fields; "whiteout"—very heavy, uniform granularity reflecting fluid-filled alveoli representing atelectasis of some alveoli, surrounded by hyperdistended bronchioles.
3. Pulmonary function studies—demonstrate stiff lung with a reduced effective pulmonary blood flow.

Treatment

1. Early recognition is imperative so that treatment may be instituted immediately.
2. Transportation to a facility providing specialized care is desirable when possible.
3. The objectives of treatment include supportive measures:
   a. Maintenance of oxygenation—PaO_2 at 60–80 mm. Hg—to prevent hypoxia; frequent arterial pH and blood gases
   b. Maintenance of respiration with ventilatory support if necessary—intermittent positive pressure breathing (IPPB) + positive end-expiratory pres-

sure (PEEP), continuous positive airway pressure (CPAP)

   c. Maintenance of thermoneutral state—to prevent hypothermia

   d. Maintenance of fluid, electrolyte, and acid–base balance—buffer metabolic acidosis with $NaHCO_3$

   e. Maintenance of nutrition—IV 10%

   f. Antibiotics—pneumonia, catheters, etc.

   g. Constant observation for complications—pneumothorax, disseminated intravascular coagulation (DIC), PDA with heart failure, chronic lung disease

   h. Care appropriate for small premature infant

Assessment

A. Check the Birth History for Pertinent Information to Assist in Determining the Intensity of Observation and Care That the Infant May Require.

1. The Apgar score 1 minute after birth and 5 minutes after birth (see p. 998)
2. The type of resuscitation required
3. Any treatment or medication administered
4. Any medication or anesthesia the mother received during labor
5. Estimated gestational age
6. Maternal history—contributing factors or complications

B. Make a Generalized Nursing Assessment of the Infant's Condition Immediately Upon Admission.

Early diagnosis is critical to increasing survival rate.

1. Record and report any findings to physician immediately.
2. Determine the degree of respiratory distress.
   a. Observe the type of retraction.
     (1) Determine the type of retraction.
     (2) Determine the degree and severity of retractions.
   b. Count the respiratory rate for 1 full minute.
     (1) Observe and determine if respirations are regular or irregular.
     (2) Observe to determine if the infant experiences any periods of apnea.
       (a) Note the length of apnea.
       (b) Note what type of stimulation initiates breathing.
     (3) Note the infant's activity at the time respirations are recorded (e.g., crying, sleeping).
   c. Listen for expiratory grunting or whining sounds from the infant when he is not crying. This partial Valsalva maneuver is expiration against a partially closed glottis in an attempt to maintain PEEP and FRC to prevent alveoli from collapsing.
   d. Maintain clear airway, pulmonary toilet.
   e. Observe for nasal flaring.
   f. Observe for cyanosis.
     (1) Note location of cyanosis.
     (2) Note if cyanosis improves with oxygen administration.
   g. Listen to the chest with a stethoscope.
     (1) Note diminished breath sounds and location.
     (2) Note the presence of crackles.
3. Determine the infant's cardiac rate and rhythm.
   a. Count the apical pulse for 1 full minute.

   b. Note any irregularity in the heart rate; bounding pulses.

4. Observe the infant's general activity.
   a. Determine if the infant is lethargic or listless.
   b. Determine if the infant is active and responds to stimuli.
   c. Determine if the infant cries.
5. Observe the infant's skin color; note:
   a. Cyanosis as to degree and location
   b. Evidence of jaundice
   c. Skin mottling
   d. Paleness or grayness
6. Observe the general appearance of the infant's body.
   a. Note edema and location (face, hands, feet, etc.).
   b. Note any other abnormal appearance of body.
7. Check the infant's body temperature.
8. Listen to abdomen with a stethoscope to determine if bowel sounds are present. Note any stool passed and observe and record type of stool.
9. Note any urinary output—assess fluid balance.
   a. Apply urine collector to obtain sample of urine.
   b. Observe color of urine.
   c. Check specific gravity of urine and frequency.
   d. Record amount of urine and frequency.

Potential Problems and Nursing Diagnoses

(Refer to the Premature Infant, p. 1222 for potential problems related to prematurity.)

1. Hypoxia, acidosis, atelectasis, and insufficient oxygen–carbon dioxide exchange related to decreases in surfactant and immaturity of lungs
2. Breathing pattern, ineffective, related to pneumothorax, PDA, and later chronic lung disease
3. Cerebral hemorrhage related to hypoxia
4. Potential for necrotizing enterocolitis related to hypoxia
5. Nutrition, altered, less than body requirements, related to fatigue and prematurity
6. Parenting, altered, related to separation as a result of life-support equipment attached to infant

Nursing Interventions

The reader is referred to specific areas throughout this text for in-depth discussion of specific conditions.

A. Provide Measures to Relieve Respiratory Distress.

1. Have emergency equipment readily available for use in the event of cardiac or respiratory arrest.
2. Provide measures for monitoring ECG and respiratory rate.
3. Place the infant in an oxygen-rich environment.
   a. Incubator with oxygen at prescribed concentration
   b. Plastic hood with oxygen at prescribed concentration
   c. Plastic hood with oxygen at prescribed concentration when using radiant warmer
   d. Nasal CPAP
   e. Mechanical ventilation with endotracheal intubation
   f. Measure oxygen concentration every hour and record
   g. Monitor blood gases as appropriate
     (1) Direct sampling of infant's blood by indwelling catheter, arterial puncture or capillary puncture

(2) Pulse oximetry—provides continuous monitoring of oxygen saturation of arterial blood (SaO_2) beat by beat.

    (a) Noninvasive, nontraumatic sensor with a light source and photodetector on a flexible plastic that is placed around an extremity (finger, foot, or hand). The source and detector are placed opposite each other on either side of an arterial bed.

    (b) SaO_2 is determined by comparing the amount of light absorbed by the filled arterial blood with the light absorbed after blood leaves the arterial bed.

    (c) Unreliable determination when infant is hyperoxic, when oxygen saturation is 95%–100%.

    (d) The sensor is extremely sensitive to infant movement. False alarm when pulse impulse is lost due to activity and the placement of the sensor is dislodged, losing pulsation of the arterial blood field

    (e) It is often difficult to keep the proper placement of the sensor when the infant is active. Avoid using adhesive to secure the device. Wrap it snugly enough to reduce sensitivity to movement but not tight enough to constrict blood flow.

(3) Transcutaneous PO_2 monitor ($TcPO_2$) provides continuous measurement of blood partial pressure of oxygen (PO_2).

    (a) Superficial or severe burns may occur because, to achieve arterialization of skin, the sensor probe is heated to warm the skin.

    (b) The probe must be repositioned every 3–4 hours; therefore repeated trauma to the skin occurs by removing the adhesive that holds the probe in place, especially in the very low birth weight (VLBW) infant.

    (c) Accuracy depends on good perfusion.

    (d) PO_2 is underestimated when there is increased tissue density or skin thickness.

    (e) Monitor needs recalibration, a 15-minute process, about every 4 hours, leaving the infant's oxygenation status uncertain.

4. Observe the infant's response to oxygen.

  a. Observe for improvement in color, respiratory rate and pattern, and nasal flaring (see retraction score, p. 1223)

  b. Note response by improvement in pH, PO_2, PCO_2 (arterial), or capillary blood gas.

5. Observe closely for apnea.

  a. Stimulate infant if apnea occurs.

  b. If unable to produce spontaneous respiration with stimulation within 15–30 seconds:

    (1) Call for help.

    (2) Clear airway.

    (3) Tilt head back.

    (4) Apply hand resuscitator attached to an oxygen supply, or apply mouth-to-mouth resuscitation (see p. 1201).

    (5) Intubation may be necessary:

      (a) Obtain heart rate during intubation by physician.

      (b) Initiate cardiac massage if severe bradycardia or asystole occurs.

      (c) Listen to breath sounds after intubation; make sure that they are equal bilaterally and that x-ray for tube position is taken and checked.

      (d) Attach infant to appropriate ventilator. Secure endotracheal tube. Suction tube to maintain patency.

      (e) Continue to monitor vital signs.

  c. Record events.

6. Position the infant to allow for maximal lung expansion.

  a. Prone position provides for a larger lung volume because of the position of the diaphragm but may be contraindicated when umbilical artery catheter is in place.

  b. Change position frequently.

7. Suction as needed—because the gag reflex is weak and cough is ineffective.

B. Be Familiar With the Methods of Providing Assisted or Controlled Ventilation and the Nursing Implications for Each.

The objective of ventilation therapy is to ventilate the infant effectively, using the lowest possible F_1O_2 pressures and cycling frequency to eliminate oxygen toxicity and to minimize mechanical trauma, thus reducing complications of treatment.

1. PEEP
2. CPAP
3. Positive or negative pressure respirator
4. Face mask and bag

C. Continue the Administration of IV Fluids Necessary to Meet the Metabolic Demands of the Infant.

Hypovolemia can affect pulmonary perfusion by associated metabolic acidosis resulting in pulmonary vasoconstriction.

1. Monitor flow.
2. Observe site for infiltration or infection.
3. If umbilical artery catheter is in place, observe for bleeding.
4. Record the amount of blood drawn for laboratory analysis (small infants can become anemic from having large amounts of blood removed for samples).
5. Prepare and administer prescribed medications.

D. Provide Adequate Caloric Intake (80–120 kcal./kg./24 hours) **as indicated.**

1. Nasojejunal
2. Nasogastric
3. Parenteral nutrition
4. Monitor for hypoglycemia—especially common during stress

E. Maintain the Infant's Abdominal Skin Temperature Between 36.0° and 36.5°C. (97° and 98°F.), **Thus Minimizing Oxygen Consumption Rate.**

Hypothermia may result in vasoconstriction and acidosis, increasing complications in the already compromised infant.

1. Adjust Isolette or radiant warmer accordingly.

  a. For the infant under 1250 gm., the radiant warmer should be used with caution because of increase of water loss and potential for hyperglycemia.

2. Prevent frequent opening of Isolette.

3. Ensure that O_2 is warmed to 32°–34°C. (87.6°–93.2°F.) with 60%–80% humidity.

F. Constantly and Carefully Observe for Any Complications That May Occur From Ventilatory Assistance, Prematurity, or the Disease Itself.

Record and report observations to physician immediately.

G. Assist the Physician in Other Supportive Measures Used to Treat the Infant.

1. Ventilatory assistance, oxygen therapy
2. Endotracheal tube, suctioning, physical therapy
3. Monitoring blood values
4. Monitoring vital signs, including blood pressure, and general condition
5. Monitoring machines

H. Be Vigilant in Observing for Complications That May be Associated With RDS and Prematurity (see Premature Infant, p. 1222).

Bronchopulmonary dysplasia (BPD) is a complication of RDS, especially in the infant under 1500 gm.

1. BPD is a chronic lung disorder characterized by coarse cystic-appearing lungs with hyperinfiltration, obstructive bronchiolitis, and pulmonary fibrosis. Alveolar and bronchiolar epithelial damage is followed by bronchiolar metaplasia, peribronchial and interstitial fibrosis. There is diffuse scarring in the lungs and areas of bullous emphysema may be interspersed with the areas of pulmonary fibrosis.
2. BPD is radiologically divided into stages that are used for classification.
   * *Stage I*—(2–3 days) is a period of acute HMD indistinguishable from severe HMD without respirator therapy. The bronchiolar epithelium is intact except for early interstitial changes—"ground glass" appearance.
   Stage II—(4–10 days) is a period of regeneration. Necrosis with beginning and proliferation of bronchial epithelium is seen. There is opacification of the lung and air bronchogram.
   Stage III—(10–20 days) is a period of transition to chronic disease. Extensive repair with phagocytosis of membrane and advanced alveolar epithelial regeneration occurs. Bronchiolar metaplasia and interstitial fibrosis are seen in the same sections as residual membrane and cell proliferation. This stage is characterized by the presence of cystic infiltrates—small round areas of radiolucency distributed throughout lung.
   Stage IV—(beyond 1 month) is a period of chronic disease. The most prominent findings are obliterative bronchiolitis with interstitial fibrosis—pulmonary parenchymal density.
3. Other factors associated with BPD include:
   a. High ambient oxygen
   b. Positive pressure ventilator
   c. Endotracheal tube
   d. Abnormal or immature lungs
   e. Lung damage from HMD (RDS)
   f. Barotrauma—high peak airway pressures
   g. PDA

* Adapted from: Avery GB. Neonatology, 3rd ed, p 446. Philadelphia, JB Lippincott, 1987

h. Pulmonary edema from increased fluid loads in first days of life
   i. Smaller premature infant under 1500 gm., with severe RDS
4. Signs and symptoms include:
   a. Tachycardia
   b. Difficulty weaning from oxygen or ventilator, increasing oxygen requirement
   c. Respiratory distress
   d. Cyanosis
   e. CO_2 retention
   f. Increased apnea
   g. Pulmonary hypertension; right heart failure (cor pulmonale)
   h. Generalized edema associated with low serum protein
   i. Hypoxemia
   j. Poor weight gain
5. Treatment—supportive
   a. Respiratory support—O_2, ventilator
   b. Maintain fluid and electrolyte balance—fluid restriction first few days of life
   c. Chest physical therapy and tracheal toilet
   d. Maintain nutritional support—high caloric intake
   e. Bronchodilators (theophylline)
   f. Diuretics—to control increase in interstitial fluid
   g. Vitamin E—may help protect retina and lungs from toxic effects of oxygen, although this has not been proven. Vitamins A—as an antioxident
   h. Steroids—controversial—increase risk of infection
6. Long-term outcome
   a. Substantial mortality
   b. Growth retardation
   c. Recurrent pulmonary infections
   d. Recurrent hospitalization—possible reinstitution of ventilatory support
   e. Neurological abnormalities

See Premature Infant (pp. 1221–1222) for other complications—retinopathy of prematurity, necrotizing enterocolitis, PDA.

7. Nursing responsibilities include:
   a. Support respiratory effort with gentle airway suctioning, chest physical therapy, and positioning.
   b. Observe and record frequency of persistent apnea, cyanotic episodes, tachypnea, retractions, and crackles.
   c. Allow infant to rest during feeding regardless of method used (nipple or gavage). He will tire easily and respond with apnea.
   d. Exercise constant vigilance to avoid respiratory infection in the infant, which could lead to death.
   e. Help to maintain a meaningful parent–infant relationship through the long duration of treatment.

I. Provide an Environment That Allows Infant Rest and Minimal Disturbance Balanced With Necessary Procedures and Treatment Based on the Infant's Condition.

Infants undergoing multiple procedures lasting 45 minutes to 1 hour have shown a moderate decrease in PO_2 on continuous PO_2 measurement.

Position seems to have an effect on oxygenation. Prone may improve oxygenation, decrease energy expenditure and time spent awake, and increase time in quiet sleep. **Caution:** Turning head to side can compromise upper airway and increase air flow resistance; observation of chest is obstructed and retractions are more difficult to detect; abdominal distention is more difficult to recognize.

J. Assist in Preparations for Transfer of Infant to Another Hospital Where Current Approaches to Management May be Under Study. (See Transfer of the Premature pp. 1232.)

1. Administration of exogenous surfactant into the lungs of infant with HMD early in the disease. Appears to be especially beneficial in the VLBW infant.
2. High-frequency ventilation—mechanical ventilation that uses rapid rates (can be greater than 900 breaths/minute) and tidal volumes near and often less than anatomical dead spaces.
3. ECMO—extracorporeal membrane oxygenation—is the use of a modified heart-lung machine to which blood is diverted from the venous system of the infant, where oxygen is added and carbon dioxide removed with a membrane oxygenator, and the oxygenated blood is returned to the infant.

K. Provide for the Psychological Needs of the Infant With RDS.

Do not neglect his need for tactile, visual, and auditory stimulation.

L. Support the Parents of This Critically Ill Infant.

1. Help them work through their grief.
2. Assist them with psychological, emotional, and physical attachment to the infant as appropriate.

Health Education

A. Prepare the Family for Long-Term Follow-Up as Appropriate.

Infants with BPD (chronic lung disease) may eventually go home on oxygen therapy.

Note: The premature infant with respiratory difficulty should continue to be observed very closely and his therapy should be adjusted as his condition changes. When his condition stabilizes, resume care as for a premature infant (see p. 1223).

Expected Outcomes

1. The infant achieves adequate oxygenation as indicated by blood gas studies and stable respiratory status
2. The infant shows stable condition (no evidence of cerebral hemorrhage; stable vital signs and normal neurological status)
3. No signs of necrotizing enterocolitis: stable abdominal girth measurement, normal elimination pattern, tolerance of enteral feeding
4. Attains and maintains normal nutritional status as evidenced by weight gain
5. Begins appropriate infant-maternal bonding as demonstrated by parental behaviors and verbalization and response of infant

Cystic Fibrosis

Cystic fibrosis is a generalized multisystem disorder affecting the exocrine glands so that the substances they secrete are abnormally viscous, affecting primarily pulmonary and gastrointestinal function.

Etiology and Incidence

1. Condition is inherited as an autosomal mendelian recessive trait.
2. Underlying cause of the abnormal secretions is unknown.
3. Incidence is estimated to be 1:1600–1:2000 in predominantly white population
   a. About 4%–5% of Caucasian population are carriers.
   b. Male to female ratio is 3:1.

Altered Physiology

1. The secretions of the exocrine glands are thick and sticky rather than thin and slippery.
2. Pulmonary involvement
   a. Decreased ciliary action
   b. Metaplasia and hyperplasia of squamous cells of mucus-secreting cells leading to increased production of thick secretions (increased risk of infection)
   c. Bronchi and bronchioles become plugged, resulting in bronchiectasis and bronchiolitis.
   d. Atelectasis and hyperinfiltration of lungs results.
   e. Irreversible fibrotic changes occur in lungs.
3. Gastrointestinal and pancreatic involvement
   a. Acini and ducts of pancreas become filled with thick mucus and are obstructed.
   b. Trypsin, chymotrypsin, lipase, and amylase do not reach the small intestine.
   c. Digestion is impaired, especially protein, carbohydrates, and fat. Interruption of the enterohepatic circulation of bile acids probably results in interference with normal pancreatic lipolysis and fat absorption through intestinal wall.
   d. There is abnormality of stools, loss of foodstuff in feces (fat and nitrogen [protein])—malabsorption syndrome
   e. Meconium ileus in infant—bowel obstructed by thick intestinal secretions
   f. Biliary cirrhosis—intrahepatic biliary tract obstructed by thick secretions
4. Involvement of sweat glands
   Secretions contain excessive amount of sodium and chloride, leading to excessive loss of these substances—especially in hot weather, when child experiences fever or becomes overheated with activity. Saliva also contains an excess of sodium and chloride.

Complications

1. Pulmonary infections
   a. Most frequently caused by *Pseudomonas aeruginosa, Staphylococcus,* and *Haemophilus influenzae*
   b. Also bronchiectasis and bronchiolitis
2. Other lung complications
   a. Emphysema
   b. Atelectasis
   c. Pneumothorax
3. Biliary cirrhosis—portal hypertension, esophageal varices, splenomegaly
4. Pancreatic fibrosis; islets of Langerhans may be fibrotic, resulting in glucose intolerance; diabetes
5. Cor pulmonale
6. Enlarged and plugged mucus-secreting glands; chronic sinusitis
7. Rectal polyps (3 months–3 years)
8. Intussusception (under 2 years of age)
9. Pancreatitis
10. Nasal polyps
11. Heat prostration

12. Fibrosis of epididymis and vas deferens in male; aspermia
13. Hemoptysis
14. Growth retardation
15. Hypoelectrolytemia—sodium and chloride
16. Metabolic acidosis

Clinical Manifestations

1. Diagnosis is frequently made prior to 6 months of age—can be made at any age.
   Neonatal screening, diagnosis and treatment may result in prevention of serious deterioration and reduce the extent of early irreversible lung damage.
2. Meconium ileus is found in newborn.
3. Other presenting signs:
   a. Salty taste when skin is kissed
   b. Cough (dry and hacking to loose and productive); wheezing
   c. Failure to gain weight or grow in the presence of a good appetite
   d. Frequent, bulky, and foul-smelling stools; excessive flatus
   e. Protuberant abdomen—pot belly
   f. Wasted buttocks
   g. Vomiting following coughing
   h. Recurrent pulmonary infections
   i. Clubbing of fingers—in older child
   j. Increased anteroposterior chest diameter
   k. Decreased exertional endurance
   l. Maldigestion; steatorrhea (loss of lipid-soluble fat and vitamins in stool)
   m. Hyperglycemia, glucosuria with polyuria, and weight loss

Diagnostic Evaluation

1. Check for family history of cystic fibrosis, failure to thrive, and unexplained infant death; check the child's history and physical condition. Carefully listen for subtle information that may be suggestive of cystic fibrosis.
2. Measurement of sodium and cloride level in sweat—chloride level of more than 60 mEq./L. is virtually diagnostic.
   a. 40–60 mEq./L. is borderline and repeated.
   b. Sodium levels greater than 60 mEq./L. are diagnostic.
3. Measurement of trypsin concentration in duodenal secretions—absence of normal concentration is virtually diagnostic.
4. Analysis of digestive enzymes (trypsin and chymotrypsin) in stool
   Level is lower—used for initial screening for cystic fibrosis
5. Chest x-ray
   a. May be normal initially
   b. Later shows increased areas of infection, overinflation, bronchial thickening and plugging, atelectasis, and fibrosis
6. Analysis of stool for steatorrhea
7. BMC (Boehringer–Mannheim Corp.)—meconium strip test includes lactose and protein content, both present in babies with cystic fibrosis, used for screening
8. Pulmonary function studies (after 4 years old)
   a. Decreased vital capacity and flow rates
   b. Increased residual volume or increased total lung capacity or both

9. Diagnosis is made when a positive sweat test is seen in conjunction with one or more of the following:
   a. Positive family history for cystic fibrosis
   b. Typical chronic obstructive lung disease
   c. Documented exocrine pancreatic insufficiency

Treatment

A. Prevent and Control Pulmonary Infection.

1. Antimicrobial therapy as indicated for pulmonary infection
2. Bronchodilators and vasoconstrictors—for relief of bronchospasm
3. Aerosol, expectorants, and mucolytic agents—decrease viscosity of secretions
4. Antihistamines (controversial)—for hayfever-like symptoms
5. Physical therapy—bronchial drainage, especially during acute exacerbations
   a. Postural drainage
   b. Breathing exercises
6. Bronchopulmonary lavage—treatment of atelectasis and mucoid impaction, using large volumes of saline (used in some institutions in country)
7. Lobectomy—resection of symptomatic lobar bronchiectasis to retard progression of lesion to total pulmonary involvement

B. Establish and Maintain Good Nutrition.

1. Pancreatic enzyme supplement with each feeding
2. Enteric—coated, encapsulated microsphere preparation of pancreatic enzymes (Pancrease):
   a. Do not produce hyperuricosuria, therefore reduce the risk of renal injury
   b. Improve fat absorption
   c. Are not inactivated by acidic gastric content thus enzymes are present in an active form in the duodenum or jejunum
3. Others: Ilozyme (highest lipase activity)
   Cotazyme
   Viokase
4. Occasionally antacid is helpful to improve tolerance of enzymes.
5. Favorable response to enzymes is based on tolerance of fatty foods, stool frequency, presence of fatty foul stools, appetite, and abdominal pain.
6. High-energy diet by increasing carbohydrates, protein, and fat, possibly as high as 40%. Increases in dietary intake should consider growth and repair, infection, the work of breathing and energy expenditure for coughing, malabsorption, and physical activity.
7. Zinc and iron supplements
8. Daily intake of water-soluble vitamins
9. Supplementary fat-soluble vitamins
10. Adequte fluid and salt intake

C. Promote Normal Growth and Development.

1. Treat the child as a normal person.
2. Encourage normal relationships with peers and family.
3. Promote positive self-image.

Assessment

1. Characteristics of stool
2. Respiratory status
3. General behavior and activity
4. Compliance to test being done
5. The child's response to any treatments done

Potential Problems and Nursing Diagnoses

1. Impaired gas exchange related to thick pulmonary secretions
2. Comfort, altered, related to illness and treatments
3. Nutrition, altered, less than body requirements, related to decreased appetite and/or inadequate absorption
4. Potential for infection related to thick pulmonary secretion
5. Anxiety related to hospitalization and disease process
6. Parenting, altered, related to hospitalization, disease, and inappropriate coping behaviors
7. Knowledge deficit of appropriate home care

Nursing Interventions

A. Establish and Maintain Adequate Nutrition to Allow for Growth and Development.

1. Diet composed of foods high in calories, protein, and moderate to high in fat recommended since absorption of food is incomplete.
   a. Growth is demonstrated when the percent of energy intake that is absorbed exceeds 100%–110% RDA—thus the intake would be 120%–150% RDA since about 85%–90% intake is absorbed.
   b. Malnutrition affects growth and contributes to severity of pulmonary involvement and ultimately affects life span. With an improved diet, growth, and well-being, respiratory function may improve and pulmonary involvement may be reduced.
2. Fat-soluble vitamins in water-miscible solution are given in quantities that are 2–3 times the normal dose. (The child shows difficulty in absorption.)
   a. Vitamins A, D, and E are given daily.
   b. Vitamin K may be given when the child has infection and is being treated with antibiotics.
3. Absent pancreatic enzymes are replaced with extracts of animal pancreas to obtain normal stools, nutrition, and growth.
   a. Give with each meal and snacks.
   b. Mix capsule, granules, or powder with small portion of food for infant or small child (e.g., mashed banana, applesauce). Never mix in formula.
   c. Offer the older child capsules or tablets.
   d. May not be given if the child is taking only a clear liquid diet (e.g., postoperative vomiting).
4. Salt intake will need to be increased during hot weather or during excessive exercise when sweating increases, to prevent salt depletion and heat prostration and cardiovascular collapse. During periods of profuse sweating, infant may become hyponatremic and alkalotic.
5. Use patience when feeding the child.
   a. The child may be irritable and fussy.
   b. Breathing may be difficult; coughing and vomiting may be common.
6. Supplemental diet that is readily absorbed and requires a minimum of digestive enzymes may be prescribed.

B. Assist in Preventing or Treating Lung Infections and Support Respirations by Thinning Secretions and Clearing Them From the Respiratory Tract.

1. Intermittent aerosol therapy
   a. Usually done prior to postural drainage. (Treatment may also be done following drainage, or both.)
   b. Provides small amount of medication or water in droplet form to penetrate respiratory tract.
   c. Treatment is 3–4 times daily.

2. Mist tent (controversial)
   a. Frequently used only with patients who have already used mist; not started on newly diagnosed patients.
   b. High humidity loosens secretions.
   c. Used primarily at night or nap time.
   d. Check temperature often and maintain below 26.6°C. (80°F.).
   e. Mist inhalation therapy may be used when secretions are particularly thick or copious.

NURSING ALERT: Mist therapy may cause airway resistance to increase in some patients.

3. Chest physical therapy (see Chest Physical Therapy, p. 1185, and Fig. 49-3)
   a. Usually follows aerosol therapy 3–4 times per day for 20–30 minutes.
      (1) May need to be increased if infection is present.
   b. Treatment ideally done 1 hour after eating to prevent vomiting or discomfort.
   c. Place child in position that gives greatest access to affected lobes of lung and facilitates gravity drainage of mucus from specific lung area (Fig. 49-3). The following positions are useful:
      (1) Leaning over side of bed
      (2) Infant held in lap
      (3) Using pillow
   d. Clapping with cupped hands and vibrating for 1–2 minutes in each area loosens plugs of mucus. Clapping is usually done 20–30 minutes, 3–4 times a day; may need to be increased when infection is present.
   e. A relaxed patient will cough more easily; coughing should be encouraged after postural drainage. Suctioning of an infant or young child may be necessary when the child will not cough.
4. Breathing exercises
   Have the child exhale slowly with pursed lips to increase the duration of exhalation.

C. Understand What Medications Are Given in Treatment and Why They Are Given.

1. Antibiotics
   a. Frequently given when a child is not doing well generally
   b. Broad-spectrum antibiotics to treat specific organism causing infection
   c. Specific antibiotics to treat specific organism causing infection—often given intravenously
2. Expectorants are used to thin bronchial mucous secretions.
3. Bronchodilators are used to increase width of bronchial tubes, allowing free passage of air into lungs.

D. Give Meticulous Attention and Care in Hygiene to the Patient and Prevent Infection.

1. Provide good skin care and position changes to prevent skin breakdown of malnourished child.
2. See that diaper area is clean to reduce offensive odor from stool and to prevent diaper rash.
3. Because child may perspire freely, change clothing as often as necessary to keep him dry.
4. Mouth care is important, since mucus is present so frequently.

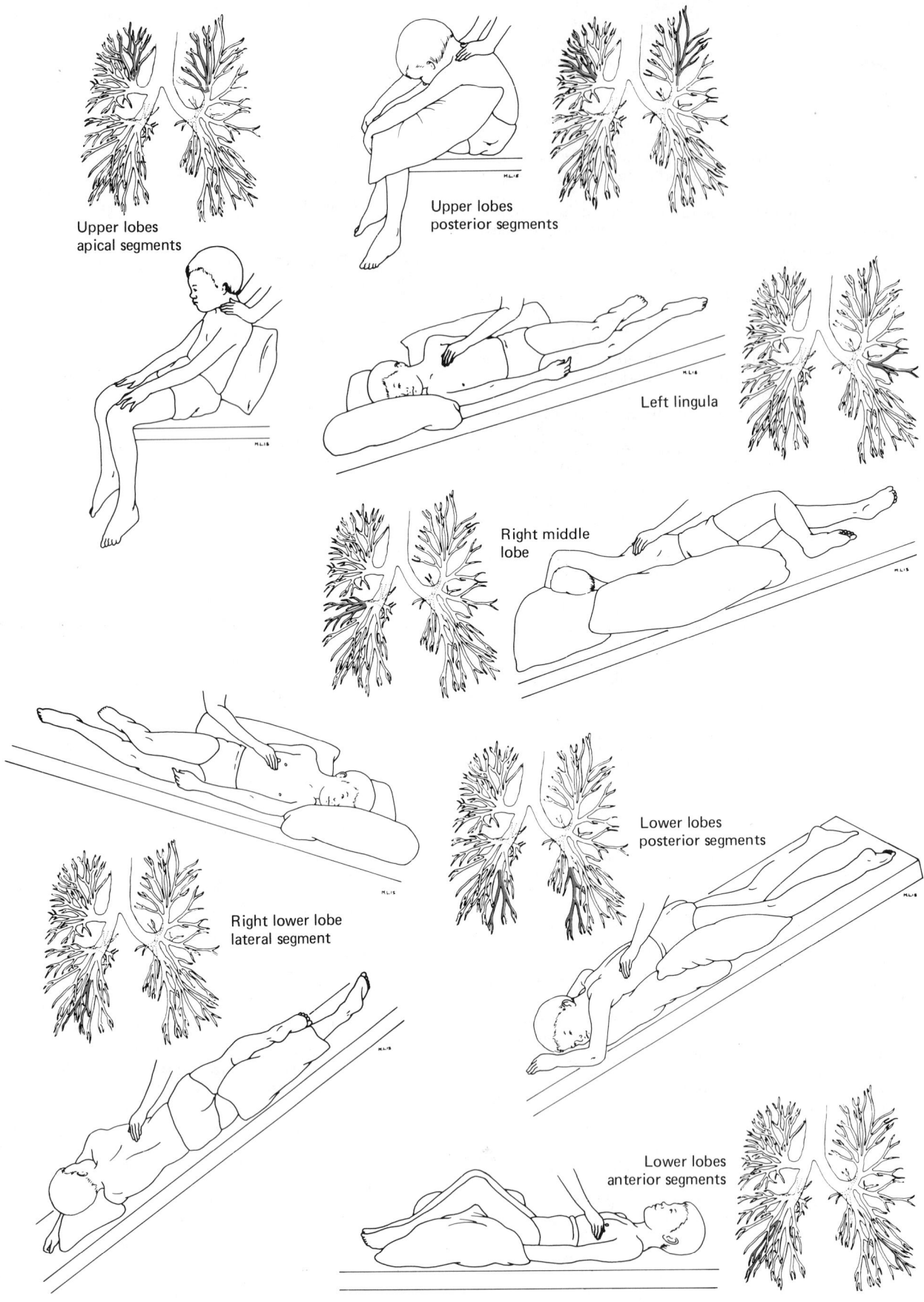

Upper lobes
apical segments

Upper lobes
posterior segments

Left lingula

Right middle
lobe

Right lower lobe
lateral segment

Lower lobes
posterior segments

Lower lobes
anterior segments

5. Shampooing and bathing will provide comfort by removing sticky residue from mist and aerosol therapy.
6. Restrict contact with person with respiratory infection.

E. Support the Child's Emotional, Psychological, and Intellectual Needs and Development.

1. Explain each procedure (new or routine), medications, etc. to the child in a manner that is appropriate for his age.
2. Allow the child to show his frustrations, fears, and feelings by talking, complaining, or crying.
   a. Support him during these times.
   b. Comfort him by talking to him and holding him.
3. Provide diversional activities appropriate for age, during or between treatments.
4. The older child may begin to take responsibility for treatments with minimal supervision.
   a. Teach him about his disease (i.e., food, medications, treatments, equipment).
   b. Help him identify his strengths and limitations, and to feel good about himself as a person.
   c. Foster independence.
   d. Nursing care of adolescents should be directed toward enhancing development:
      (1) Task of establishing self-identity can be severely affected by secondary effects of delayed sexual growth and maturation.
      (2) Task of establishing independence can be affected by treatments that force dependency on others.
      (3) Psychosocial maladaptive coping responses may be seen.
5. Frequently the child will manifest his anger, fear, and other emotions by resistance to chest physical therapy. Allowing child to engage in normal activities (e.g., swimming) within his physical tolerance can help to redirect these feelings as well as to improve respiratory function.

F. Make and Record Observations of the Child and His Condition and Behavior That Will Give Information Concerning His Condition.

1. Characteristics of stools: color, size, consistency, frequency
2. Eating habits
   a. Foods taken or refused
   b. Appetite—good or poor
3. Coughing and description of secretions produced
4. Daily weight to determine weight gain or loss
5. General behavior
   a. Irritability
   b. Cooperativeness
6. Conservation of energy—periods of rest, nonstrenuous activity

G. Encourage Parental Participation in Learning to Care for and Handle the Child and Foster Acceptance of the Child and His Illness by His Parents and Family.

1. Provide opportunities for the parents to learn all aspects of care of their child.
2. Note that all the support and help given the parents during hospitalization will make home care easier.

3. Initiate community nurse referral, which provides the following:
   a. Facilitates preparing the home for the child's entry, both emotionally and physically
   b. Can assist the family in properly carrying out treatments
4. Initiate social work referral. The social worker can help the parents to better understand their family situation and their feelings about their child and cystic fibrosis; she can arrange for financial assistance if appropriate. The worker can be an emotional support to the mother who may be physically and emotionally exhausted from caring for the child with cystic fibrosis.
5. Inform friends and relatives of the child's illness so that necessary consideration is given him. Plan a team conference including the parent(s), school nurse, teacher, and physical education teacher, as appropriate.
6. Assist with interpretation of the disease to family and patient. Help them to talk about their feelings and fears. Be honest with the parents and child; help them understand there may be gradual lung involvement.
7. Initiate a teaching program for the child and his family early. Offer them available literature and help them to become familiar with the Cystic Fibrosis Foundation* and the nearest chapter.
   a. Multidiscipline team approach and cooperation is vital.
   b. Incorporate teaching program into nursing care plan. Be consistent with information and methods.

Health Education

Education of the parents is important in preparing them to continue the child's care at home.

1. The parents must have a thorough understanding of the dietary regimen. Help them to know what types of foods the child is allowed to have and which foods are restricted. Talk about ways to make each meal or certain foods attractive. Discuss need for salt replacement—free access to salt; increase salt intake on hot summer days or when vomiting and diarrhea occur.
2. Help the parents to become thoroughly familiar with the pulmonary therapy regimen. Do not rush your explanation; take time to demonstrate and explain procedures. Then allow the parents to demonstrate all the treatments to be done at home.
3. Help the family to plan the most normal family pattern of living in relation to treatment of their child.
   a. Consider the marriage needs of the parents and the needs of other members of the family.

* Cystic Fibrosis Foundation
6000 Executive Blvd, Suite 309
Rockville, MD 20852
Publications from CF Foundation:

What everyone should know about Cystic Fibrosis

Cystic Fibrosis: A summary of symptoms, diagnosis and treatment

Your Child and Cystic Fibrosis

Living with Cystic Fibrosis—A Guide for the Young Adult.
A Teacher's Guide to Cystic Fibrosis
Listing of Publications and Educational Materials for Physicians and Scientists

Figure 49-3. *Postural drainage. Position for draining upper lobes, anterior segments is the same as the position for draining lower lobes, anterior segments.*

b. Encourage family activities, vacations, etc. during the child's remission of symptoms.

4. Help the parents to understand and to provide emotional support of their child. Explain that he will experience the usual problems of growing up as well as the problems of cystic fibrosis and hospitalizations. The child needs love, understanding, and security—not overprotection. He needs growing independence, peer relationships, and personal achievements.

5. Help the parents understand the rebellious and uncooperative behavior of their adolescent. It is a normal part of this age; however, it may be directed toward the illness and treatment. Be firm with the child—optimistic, yet realistic, understanding, and loving.

6. Help the parents understand the value of genetic counseling and support the information given to them through counseling.
   a. Diagnosis may cause family discord and anger.
   b. A period of grief and mourning is normal following diagnosis.

7. Impress upon the parents the importance of regular medical follow-up care:
   a. Routine immunizations—measles vaccine and influenza given early in infancy
   b. Continuing evaluation and supervision in home management
   c. New developments through research that may change therapy
   d. Detection or prevention of complications

8. Inform parents of the future of their child in society.

a. With the medical advancements that have occurred, there is every reason to believe that, depending on pulmonary involvement and complications, the child with cystic fibrosis may grow to adulthood. When the child grows up, he may be smaller and shorter than expected.

b. Play and school participation depends on severity of illness.

c. Have the parents discuss the child's problem with the school nurse, teacher, and other responsible adults who have close contact with the child.

d. Encourage the parents to allow the child to participate in as well as take additional responsibility for his own care and treatment as he gets older.

e. Support agency, see footnote.

Expected Outcomes

1. Child demonstrates improved oxygen–carbon dioxide gas exchange; improved general respiratory status; normal blood gas values

2. Experiences minimal discomfort; shows relaxed behavior; engages in play activities appropriate for age

3. Demonstrates improved nutritional status evidenced by weight gain

4. Experiences lessening anxiety; appropriate behavior for age; interacting with other children and personnel

5. Parent–child relationship appropriate as evidenced by verbalization and behavior

6. Parents show understanding of disease and can explain home care requirements

Bibliography

Books

Aloan CA. Respiratory Care of the Newborn. Philadelphia, JB Lippincott, 1987

Avery ME and First LR (eds). Pediatric Medicine. Baltimore, Williams & Wilkins, 1989

Avery GB (ed). Neonatology. 3rd ed. Philadelphia, JB Lippincott, 1987

Behrman RE and Vaughan VC. Nelson Textbook of Pediatrics. Philadelphia, WB Saunders, 1987

Carlo WA and Chatburn RL (eds). Neonatal Respiratory Care. 2nd ed. Chicago, Year Book Medical Pub, 1988

Catlin FI. Otolaryngologic Disorders. In Welch KJ et al (eds). Pediatric Surgery. 4th ed, pp 470–476. Chicago, Year Book Medical Pub, 1986

Committee on Infectious Diseases, American Academy of Pediatrics. Report of the Committee on Infectious Diseases. 21st ed. Elk Grove Village, IL, AAP, 1988

Ehrlich FE (ed). Pediatric Emergency Medicine. Rockville, MD, Aspen Publishers, Inc, 1987

Eigan H and Scott PH. Asthma and allergic rhinitis. In Green M and Haggerty RJ (eds). Ambulatory Pediatrics, pp 378–391. Philadelphia, WB Saunders, 1984

Falliers CJ. Asthma, eczema, and related allergies. In Levine MD (ed). Developmental–Behavioral Pediatrics, pp 474–482. Philadelphia, WB Saunders, 1983

Fleisher GR and Ludwig S. Textbook of Pediatric Emergency Medicine. 2nd ed. Baltimore, Williams & Wilkins, 1988

Hoeprich PD and Jordan MC. Infectious Diseases. 4th ed. Philadelphia, JB Lippincott, 1989

Koff PB, Eitzman DV and Neu J (eds). Neonatal and Pediatric Respiratory Care. St. Louis, CV Mosby, 1988

Krugman S and Katz SL. Infectious Diseases of Children. St. Louis, CV Mosby, 1985

Laraya–Cuasay LR and Hughes WT (eds). Interstitial Lung Diseases in Children, Vol I, II, III. Boca Raton, FL, CRC Press, 1988

Lloyd–Still JD. Textbook of Cystic Fibrosis. Boston, John Wright & Sons, 1983

Stern L and Vert P (eds). Neonatal Medicine. New York, Masson Publishing USA, 1987

Tinkelman DG, Falliers CJ and Naspitz CK (eds). Childhood Asthma. New York, Marcel Dekker, 1987

Whaley LF and Wong DL. Nursing Care of Infants and Children. St. Louis, CV Mosby, 1987

Journals

General

Brodsky L, Moore L and Stanievich J. The role of *Haemophilus influenzae* in the pathogenesis of tonsillar hypertrophy in children. J Pediatr Otorhinolaryngol 1988 Oct; 98(10):1055–1059

Clarke PH and Deeds NC. The child in a mist tent. Pediatr Nurs 1988 Nov–Dec; 14(6):446–450

Couriel JM. Management of croup. Arch Dis Child 1988 Nov; 63(11):1305–1308

Fulginiti VA. Acute supraglottitis (epiglottitis): To look or not? Am J Dis Child 1988 Jun; 142(6):597

Gilsdorf JR. Use of the *Haemophilus influenzae* type b vaccine among preschool attendees. Clin Pediatr 1988 Jun; 227(6):285–286

Isaacs D. Production of interferon in respiratory syncytial virus bronchiolitis. Arch Dis Child 1989 Jun; 64(1):92–95

Mauro RD, Poole SR and Lockhart CH. Differentiation of epiglottis from laryngotracheitis in the child with stridor. Am J Dis Child 1988 Jun; 142(6):679–682

Manning SC et al. An assessment of preoperative coagulation screening for tonsillectomy and adenoidectomy. Int J Pediatr Otorhinolaryngol 1988 Sep; 13(3):237–244

Palumbo FM. Pediatric considerations of infections and inflammations of Walduyer's ring. Otolaryngol Clin North Am 1987 May; 20(2):311–316

Pifer LL et al. *Pneumocystis carinii* serologic study in pediatric acquired immunodeficiency syndrome. Am J Dis Child 1988 Jan; 142(1):36–39

Ramsey KP et al. *Haemophilus* b polysaccharide vaccine. Am J Dis Child 1989 Jan; 143(1):128–133

Richmond KH, Wetmore RF and Baranak CC. Postoperative complications following tonsillectomy and adenoidectomy—who is at risk? Int J Pediatr Otorhinolaryngol 1987 Aug; 13(2):117–124

Shott SR, Myer CM and Cotton RT. Efficacy of tonsillectomy and adenoidectomy as an outpatient procedure: A preliminary report. Int J Pediatr Otorhinolaryngol 1987 Aug; 13(2):157–163

Tinker TD and Stacy TM. Ten caveats in the early management of acute epiglottis in children. J Okla State Med Assoc 1988 Aug; 81(8):503–509

When a child's symptoms suggest croup (based on interviews with Gershon AA et al.). Patient Care 1982 Nov 30; 16(20):15–18+

Asthma

Alexander JS et al. Effectiveness of a nurse-managed program for children with chronic asthma. J Pediatr Nurs 1988 Oct; 3(5):312–317

Amaro-Galvez R et al. Grading severity and treatment requirements control symptoms in asthmatic children and the relationship with airway hyperreactivity to methacholine. Ann Allergy 1987 Oct; 59(4):298–302

Baker MD. Pitfalls in the use of clinical asthma scoring. Am J Dis Child 1988 Feb; 142(2):183–185

Blessing-Moore J, Fritz G and Lewiston NJ. Self-management programs for childhood asthma. Chest 1985 Jan suppl; 87(1):107–110S

Carlsen KH et al. Nebulized beclomethasone dipropimate in recurrent obstruction episodes after acute bronchiolitis. Arch Dis Child 1988 Dec; 63(12):1428–1433

Christiaanse ME, Lavigne JV and Lerner CV. Psychosocial aspects of compliance in children and adolescents with asthma. J Dev Behav Pediatr 1989 Apr; 10(2):75–80

Duffy DM and Halloran MC. Effects of an educational program on parents of children with asthma. Child Health Care 1987 Fall; 16(2):76–81

Ellis EF. Asthma: Current therapeutic approach. Pediatr Clin North Am 1988 Oct; 35(5):1041–1052

Fourie PR and Joubert JR. Determination of airway hyper-reactivity in asthmatic children. A comparison among exercise, nebulized water and histamine challenge. Pediatr Pulmonol 1988 Jan–Feb; 4(1):2–7

Gleeson JG, Green S and Price JF. Air or oxygen as driving gas for nebulized salbutamol. Arch Dis Child 1988 Aug; 63(8):900–904

Hargreave FE. Lot-phase asthmatic response and airway inflammation. J Allergy Clin Immunol 1989 Feb; 82(2 pt 2):525–536

Hill RA, Standen PJ and Littersfield AE. Asthma, wheezing and school absence in primary asthma. Arch Dis Child 1989 Feb; 64(2):246–251

Koliner M. Asthma and mast cell activation. J Allergy Clin Immunol 1989 Feb; 82(2 pt 2):510–520

König P. Asthma: A pediatric pulmonary disease and a changing concept.

Pediatr Pulmonol 1987 Jul–Aug; 3(4): 264–275

Mendlowitz DR et al. Understanding respiration and digestion: A developmental comparison of healthy and asthmatic children. Child Health Care 1988 Summer; 17(1):45–49

Newcomb RW and Akhter J. Respiratory failure from asthma. Am J Dis Child 1988 Oct; 142(10):1041–1044

Pediatric asthma deaths continue to increase. Am Fam Physician 1988 Sep; 38(3):372, 376

Pool JB et al. Inhaled bronchodilator treatment via the nebulizer in young asthmatic patients. Arch Dis Child 1988 Mar; 63(3):288–291

Ramsey AM and Siroky AS. The use of puppets to teach school-age children with asthma. Pediatr Nurs 1988 May–Jun; 14(3):187–190

Rappaport L et al. Effects of theophylline on behavior and learning in children with asthma. Am J Dis Child 1989 Mar; 143(3):368–372

Reimers TM. Enhancing child compliance with nebulized respiratory treatment. Clin Pediatr 1988 Dec; 28(12):605–608

Ryan CA, Willan AR and Wherrett BA. Home nebulizers in childhood asthma. Clin Pediatr 1988 Sep; 27(9):420–424

Shohat M et al. Childhood asthma and growth outcome. Arch Dis Child 1987 Jan; 62(1):63–65

Shohat M et al. Transient tachypnea of the newborn and asthma. Arch Dis Child 1989 Feb; 64(2):277–279

Storr J, Barrell E and Lenney W. Rising asthma admissions and self referral. Arch Dis Child 1988 Jul; 63(7):774–779

Storr J and Lenney W. School holidays and admissions with asthma. Arch Dis Child 1989 Jan; 64(1):103–107

Strachan DP. Damp housing and childhood asthma: Validation of reporting of symptoms. Br Med J 1988 Nov 12; 297(6658):1223–1226

Traver GA and Martinez M. Asthma update. Part I. Mechanisms, pathophysiology, and diagnosis. Part II. Treatment. J Pediatr Health Care 1988 Sep–Oct; 2(5):221–233

Wasilewski Y et al. The effect of paternal social support on maternal disruption caused by childhood asthma. J Commun Health 1988 Spring; 13(1): 33–42

Wesolowski CA. Self-contracts for chronically ill children. MCN 1988 Jan–Feb; 13(1):20–23

Zahr LK, Connolly M and Page DR. Assessment and management of the child with asthma. Pediatr Nurs 1989 Mar–Apr; 15(2):109–114

Zimo DA, Gaspar M and Akhter J. The efficacy and safety of home nebulizer therapy for children with asthma. Am J Dis Child 1989 Feb; 143(2):208–211

Cystic Fibrosis

Ansaldi-Balocco N, Santini B and Sarchi C. Efficacy of pancreatic enzyme supplementation in children with cystic fibrosis: Comparison of two preparations by random crossover

study and a retrospective study of the same patients at two different ages. J Pediatr Gastroenterol Nutr 1988; 7(Suppl 1):S40–S45

Bouquet J, Sinaasappel M and Neijens HJ. Malabsorption in cystic fibrosis: Mechanisms and treatment. J Pediatr Gastroenterol Nutr 1988; 7(Suppl 1): S30–S35

Brown GA et al. Faecal chymotrypsin concentrations in neonates with cystic fibrosis and healthy controls. Arch Dis Child 1988 Oct; 63(10):1229–1233

Buchdahl RM et al. Energy and nutrient intakes in cystic fibrosis. Arch Dis Child 1989 Mar; 64(3):373–378

Coates AL. The efficacy of chest physical therapy in cystic fibrosis. Pediatr Pulmonol 1988; Suppl 2:51–52

Costantini D et al. The management of enzymatic therapy in cystic fibrosis patients by individualized approach. J Pediatr Gastroenterol Nutr 1988; 7(Suppl 1):S36–S39

Dankert-Roelse JE et al. Survival and clinical outcome in patients with cystic fibrosis, with and without neonatal screening. J Pediatr 1989 Mar; 114(3): 362–367

David ML and Kanga JF. Pneumoparotid in cystic fibrosis. Clin Pediatr 1988 Oct; 27(10):506–508

Dibble SL and Savedra MC. Cystic fibrosis in adolescence: A new challenge. Pediatr Nurs 1988 Jul–Aug; 14(4):299–303

Dodge JA. Nutritional requirements in cystic fibrosis: A review. J Pediatr Gastroenterol Nutr 1988; 7(Suppl 1): S8–S11

George DE and Mangos JA. Nutritional management and pancreatic enzyme therapy in cystic fibrosis patients: State of the art in 1987 and projections into the future. J Pediatr Gastroenterol Nutr 1988; 7(Suppl 1):S49–S57

Goldberg S. Risk factors in infant–mother attachment. Can J Psychol 1988 Jan; 42(2):173–188

Holsclaw DS and Daubee J. Efficacy of postural drainage and chest physical therapy. Pediatr Pulmonol 1988; Suppl 2:53–54

Johnson JP. Genetic counseling using linked DNA probes: Cystic fibrosis as a prototype. J Pediatr 1988 Dec; 113(6): 957–964

Myer PA. Parental acceptation to cystic fibrosis. J Pediatr Health Care 1988 Jan–Feb; 2(1):20–28

Orr HT et al. Cystic fibrosis: Chromosome 7 DNA genotyping. Clin Pediatr 1988 Dec; 27(12):591–595

Parsons HG. Supplemental calories improve essential fatty acid deficiency in cystic fibrosis patients. Pediatr Res 1988 Sep; 24(3):353–356

Patton AC, Ventura JN and Savedra M. Stress and coping responses of adolescents with cystic fibrosis. Child Health Care 1986 Winter; 14(3):153–156

Reismann JJ. Role of conventional physiotherapy in cystic fibrosis. J Pediatr 1988 Oct; 113(4):637–640

Roberts G et al. Screening for cystic fibrosis: A four year regional experience. Arch Dis Child 1988 Dec; 63(12):1438–1443

Rosenstein BJ and Langbaum TS. Misdiagnosis of cystic fibrosis. Clin Pediatr 1987 Feb; 26(2):78–82

Tepper RS et al. Infants with cystic fibrosis: Pulmonary function at diagnosis. Pediatr Pulmonol 1988; 5(1):15–18

Wells PW and Meghdadpour S. Research yields new clues to cystic fibrosis. MCN 1988 May/June; 13(3):787–790

Zinman R et al. Nocturnal home oxygen in the treatment of hypoxemic cystic fibrosis patients. J Pediatr 1989 Mar; 114(3):368–377

Respiratory Distress Syndrome

Alverson DC, Isken VM and Cohen RS. Effects of booster blood transfusions on oxygen utilization in infants with bronchopulmonary dysplasia. J Pediatr 1988 Oct; 113(4):722–726

Avery ME. Update on prenatal steroid for prevention of respiratory distress. J Obstet Gynecol 1986 Jul; 155(1):2–5

Avery ME et al. Is chronic lung disease in low birth weight preventable? A survey of eight centers. Pediatrics 1987 Jan; 79(1):26–30

Baley JE, Hancharik SM and Rivers A. Observations of a support group for parents of children with severe bronchopulmonary dysplasia. J Dev Behav Pediatr 1988 Feb; 9(1):19–24

Bancalari E and Gerhardt T. Bronchopulmonary dysplasia. Pediatr Clin North Am 1986 Feb; 33(1):1–24

Blanchard PW, Brown TM and Coates AL. Pharmacotherapy in bronchopulmonary dysplasia. Clin Perinatol 1987 Dec; 14(4):881–910

Boros SJ and Mammel MC. A practical guide to high-frequency ventilation. Pediatr Ann 1988 Aug; 17(8):508, 10, 12–15

Bozynski ME et al. Prolonged mechanical ventilation and intracranial hemorrhage: Impact on developmental progress through 18 months in infants weighing 1200 grams or less at birth. Pediatrics 1987 May; 79(5):670–676

Budreau G and Kleiber C. Nursing management of the infant with an intraoral appliance. J Obstet Gynecol Neonatal Nurs 1987 Jan–Feb; 16(1): 23–25

Clancy GT. Blood gas monitoring and management of neonates with respiratory distress. J Perinat Neonat Nurs 1987 Jul; 1(1):72–82

Daily DK. Home oxygen therapy for infants with bronchopulmonary dysplasia. Perinatol Neonatol 1987 May–Jun; 11(3):26+

D'Costa M, Dassin R and Bryan H. Lecithin/sphingomyelin ratios in tracheal aspirates from newborn infants. Pediatrics 1987 Aug; 22(2): 154–157

Doyle LW, Murton LJ and Kitchen WH. Mortality with increasing assisted ventilation of very-low-birth-weight infants. Am J Dis Child 1989 Feb; 143(2):223–227

Dunn MS et al. Two year follow-up of infants enrolled in a randomized trial of surfactant replacement therapy for prevention of neonatal respiratory distress syndrome. Pediatrics 1988 Oct; 82(4):543–547

Durand DJ et al. Theophylline treatment in the extubation of infants weighing less than 1250 grams: A control trial. Pediatrics 1987 Nov; 80(5):684–688

Eikner S. Dealing with long-term problems: A parent's perspective. Neonatal Netw 1986 Oct; 5(2):45–49

Few BJ. Corticosteroids and respiratory distress syndrome. MCN 1988 Jan–Feb; 13(1):17

Frank M. Theophylline: A closer look. Neonatal Netw 1987 Oct; 6(2):7–13

Grennough A and Greenall F. Observation of spontaneous respiratory interaction with artificial ventilation. Arch Dis Child 1988 Feb; 63(2):168–175

Greenspan JS, Abbasi S and Bhutani VK. Sequential changes in pulmonary mechanics in the very low birth weight (≤1000 grams) infant. J Pediatr 1988 Oct; 113(4):732–737

Gunderson LP and Kenner CA. Socializing of newborn intensive care unit nurses through the use of mentorship. Neonatal Netw 1988 Oct; 7(2):7–13

Hudak BB et al. Home oxygen therapy for chronic lung disease in extremely low-birth-weight infants. Am J Dis Child 1989 Mar; 143(3):357–360

Inwood S, Finley GA and Fitzhardinge PM. High-frequency oscillation: A new mode of ventilation for the neonate. Neonatal Netw 1986 Apr; 4(5):53–58

Jobe A and Ikegami M. Surfactant for the treatment of respiratory distress syndrome. Am Rev Respir Dis 1987 Nov; 136(5):1256–1275

Joshi A et al. Blood transfusion effect on the respiratory pattern of preterm infants. Pediatrics 1987 Jul; 80(1):79–84

Karp TB et al. High frequency jet ventilation: A neonatal nursing perspective. Neonatal Netw 1986 Apr; 4(5):42–50

Kling P. Respiratory distress syndrome in the tiny baby. Neonatal Netw 1986 Apr; 4(5):7–13

Lioy J and Manginello FP. A comparison of prone and supine positioning in the immediate post-extubation period of neonates. J Pediatr 1988 Jun; 112(6): 982–984

Loisel DB. Methylxathines in the NICU. Neonatal Netw 1987 Dec; 6(3):23–28

Loisel DB, Smith MM and MacDonald MG. Plasma theophylline levels as related to toxicity in infants with severe chronic lung disease. Neonatal Netw 1987 Oct; 6(2):15–19

Loper DL. Surfactant replacement therapy. Neonatal Netw 1986 Apr; 4(5):14–17

Ludman WL et al. Birth weight, respiratory distress syndrome and cognitive development. Am J Dis Child 1987 Jan; 141(1):79–83

McCord FB et al. Surfactant treatment and incidence of intraventricular haemorrhage in severe respiratory distress syndrome. Arch Dis Child 1988 Jan; 63(1):10–16

Merritt TA and Hallman M. Surfactant replacement. Am J Dis Child 1988 Dec; 142(12):1339

Milner AD and Hoskyns EW. High frequency positive pressure ventilation in neonates. Arch Dis Child 1989 Jan; 64(1):1–3

Moa G et al. A new device for administration of nasal continuous positive airway pressure in the newborn: An experimental study. Crit Care Med 1988 Dec; 16(12):1238–1242

Mok JY et al. Effect of age and state of wakefulness in transcutaneous oxygen values in preterm infants: A longitudinal study. J Pediatr 1988 Oct; 113(4):706–709

Monin P and Vert P. The management of bronchopulmonary dysplasia. Clin Perinatol 1987 Sep; 14(3):531–549

Nugent J. Extracorporeal membrane oxygenation in the neonate. Neonatal Netw 1986 Apr; 4(5):27–38

Ortega M et al. Early prediction of ultimate outcomes in newborn infants with severe respiratory failure. J Pediatr 1988 Oct; 113(4):744–747

Pearlman SA and Maisels MJ. Preductal and postductal transcutaneous oxygen tension measurements in premature newborns with hyaline membrane disease. Pediatrics 1989 Jan; 83(1):98–100

Polak MJ, Donnelly WH and Bucciarelli RL. Comparison of airway pathologic lesions after high-frequency jet or conventional ventilation. Am J Dis Child 1989 Feb; 143(2):228–232

Prendiville A, Thomson A and Silverman M. Effect of tracheobronchial suction on respiratory resistance in intubated preterm babies. Arch Dis Child 1986 Dec; 61(12):1178–1183

Prone or supine for preterm babies? Lancet 1988 26 Mar; 1(8587):688–689

Riedel K. Pulse oximetry: A new technology to assess patient oxygen needs in the neonatal intensive care unit. J Perinat Neonat Nurs 1987 Jul; 1(1):49–57

Rome ES et al. Effect of sleep state on chest wall movements and gas exchange in infants with resolving bronchopulmonary dysplasia. Pediatr Pulmonol 1987 Jul–Aug; 3(4):259–263

Saigal S and O'Brodovich H. Long-term outcome of preterm infants with respiratory distress. Clin Perinatol 1987 Sep; 14(3):635–650

Samuels MP and Warner JO. Bronchopulmonary dysplasia. Arch Dis Child 1987 Nov; 62(11):1099–1101

Sinkin RA and Phelps DL. New strategies for the prevention of bronchopulmonary dysplasia. Clin Perinatol 1987 Sep; 14(3):599–620

South M, Morley CJ and Hughes G. Expiratory muscle activity in preterm babies. Arch Dis Child 1987 Aug; 825–829

Stark AR and Frantz ID. Respiratory distress syndrome. Pediatr Clin North Am 1986 Jun; 33(3):533–544

Svenningsen N et al. Endotracheal administration of surfactant in very low birth weight infants with respiratory distress syndrome. Crit Care Med 1987 Oct; 15(10):918–922

Thoresen M, Cowan F and Whitelaw A. Effect of tilting on oxygenation in newborn infants. Arch Dis Child 1988 Mar; 63(3):315–317

Vaucher YE et al. Neurodevelopmental and respiratory outcome in early childhood after human surfactant treatment. Am J Dis Child 1988 Sep; 142(9):927–930

Vidyasagar D et al. Surfactant replacement therapy: Clinical and experimental studies. Clin Perinatol 1987 Sep; 14(3):713–736

Vidyasagar D and Shimada S. Pulmonary surfactant replacement in respiratory distress syndrome. Clin Perinatol 1987 Dec; 14(4):991–1015

Wiebicke W, Poynter A and Chernick V. Normal lung growth following antenatal dexamethasone treatment for respiratory distress syndrome. Pediatr Pulmonol 1988; 5(1):27–30

Additional Suggested Reading for Staff and Parents

You Have Cystic Fibrosis—You are not alone. CF Foundation, Metro Washington DC Chapter, 8401 Corporate DR, Landover, MD 20785, 301–459–8444

Goodfellow P. Cystic Fibrosis. New York, Oxford University Press, 1989

Hobbs N and Perrin JM (eds). Issues in the Care of Children With Chronic Illness. San Francisco, Jossey–Bass, 1985

Living with asthma: Manual for teaching parents and children the self-management of childhood asthma. (NIH–1986) NIH Publication no. 86–2364, Washington DC, US Govt Print Office

Merritt TA, Boynton BR and Northway WH Jr. Bronchopulmonary Dysplasia. Chicago, Blackwell Scientific Publications, 1988

Orenstein DM. Cystic Fibrosis: A Guide for Patients and Their Families. New York, Raven Press, 1989

Plant TF. Children with Asthma: A Manual for Parents. Amherst, MA, PediPress, 1983

Weinstein AM. Asthma. New York, McGraw–Hill, 1987

Anemia

Anemia refers to a deficit of red blood cells (RBC) or hemoglobin in the blood resulting in decreased oxygen-carrying capacity. It is the most frequent hematologic disorder encountered in children.

Etiology

A. Blood Loss Related to:

1. Trauma/ulceration
2. Decreased production of platelets
3. Increased destruction of platelets
4. Decreased number of clotting factors

B. Impairment of RBC Production

1. Nutritional deficiency
   a. Iron deficiency
   b. Folic acid deficiency
   c. Vitamin B_{12} deficiency
   d. Vitamin B_6 deficiency
2. Decreased erythrocyte production
   a. Pure RBC anemia
   b. Secondary hemolytic anemias associated with chronic infection, renal disease, and drugs
   c. Bone marrow depression
      (1) Leukemia
      (2) Aplastic anemias

C. Increased Erythrocyte Destruction

1. Extrinsic factors
   a. Drugs and chemicals
   b. Infections
   c. Antibody reactions
      (1) Passively acquired antibodies against Rh
      (2) A or B isoimmunization
      (3) Autoimmune hemolytic anemia
   d. Burns
   e. Poisons, including lead poisoning
2. Intrinsic factors
   a. Abnormalities of the RBC membrane
   b. Enzymatic defects—G6PD (glucose-6-phosphate dehydrogenase) deficiency
   c. Abnormal hemoglobin synthesis
      (1) Abnormal hemoglobins—sickle cell disease
      (2) Thalassemic syndromes

Altered Physiology

A. General Considerations

1. RBCs and hemoglobin are normally formed at the same rate at which they are destroyed.

2. Whenever formation of RBCs or hemoglobin is decreased or their destruction is increased, anemia results.
3. The ability of hemoglobin to carry oxygen to the tissues and remove carbon dioxide for excretion by the lungs is decreased.
4. Anemia of chronic infection and inflammation
   a. Life span of the RBC is moderately decreased.
   b. The ability of the bone marrow to produce RBCs is significantly decreased. (This is the principal factor in determining the degree of anemia.)
5. Hemolytic anemias
   a. The RBCs are destroyed at abnormally high rates primarily by the spleen.
   b. The activity of the bone marrow increases to compensate for the shortened survival time of the RBCs.
   c. Bone marrow hypertrophies and occupies a larger than normal share of the inner structure of bones.
   d. Products of RBC breakdown increase with hemolysis.
   e. Jaundice results when the liver is unable to clear the blood of the pigment resulting from the breakdown of hemoglobin from destroyed RBCs.
   f. Iron builds up (hemosiderosis) and may deposit on body tissues.
6. Sickle cell anemia (see p. 1300)

Clinical Manifestations

1. Condition may be acute or chronic
2. Early symptoms
   a. Listlessness
   b. Fatigability
   c. Anorexia related to decreased energy
3. Late symptoms
   a. Pallor
   b. Weakness
   c. Tachycardia
   d. Palpitations
   e. Tachypnea; shortness of breath on exertion
   f. Jaundice (with hemolytic anemias)
4. Eventual symptoms
   a. Mental sluggishness; decreased energy to carry out usual childhood activities; decreased attention span
   b. Growth retardation related to anorexia and decreased cellular metabolism; delayed motor development related to weakness and poor muscle tone
   c. Cardiac enlargement and symptoms of congestive

heart failure related to increased strain on the heart due to the demand for increased oxygen by tissues

   d. Osteoporosis in chronic anemia

5. Prognosis
   a. Varies with the type of anemia
   b. Death may result because of cardiac failure related to circulatory collapse and shock

Potential Problems and Nursing Diagnoses

1. Fatigue related to decreased ability of blood to transport oxygen to the tissues
2. Activity intolerance related to fatigue
3. Anxiety related to hospitalization and painful diagnostic procedures (venipunctures, finger sticks)
4. Altered nutritional intake related to less than body requirements of specific nutrients
5. Potential for infection related to generally debilitated state
6. Parental knowledge deficit regarding recommended dietary allowances and iron supplementation
7. Altered growth and development related to decreased energy

Nursing Interventions

A. Make a Baseline Assessment of the Child's Condition.

1. Examine skin and mucous membranes for evidence of pallor.
2. Estimate the child's current functional level, including exercise tolerance and level of frustration.
3. Question the parents regarding the child's normal level of activity, any symptoms that they have observed (pallor, decreased appetite, excessive fatigue, etc.), ways that their child indicates frustration, fatigue.
4. Obtain a history related to possible causative factors:
   a. Dietary habits
   b. Persistent infection, chronic disease
   c. Use of or exposure to drugs, poisons, etc.
   d. Check urine and stool for blood loss.

B. Prevent Infection and Assess for Signs of Infection.

1. See that the child maintains good general body hygiene (handwashing, mouth care)
2. Avoid exposure to other children with colds, infections, etc.
3. Always be sure to wash hands thoroughly and advise visitors to do the same.
4. Report any temperature elevation to the physician.

C. Ensure Adequate Rest; Decrease Oxygen Demands.

1. Plan nursing care to allow for lengthy periods when the child is not disturbed by hospital routines, procedures, treatments, etc; set priorities.
2. Observe for early signs of fatigue such as irritability, hyperactivity, etc.
3. Encourage sedentary rather than active projects.
4. Relieve dyspnea if present.
5. Do not always encourage self-care.
6. Provide foods that are easy to chew to conserve energy.

D. Provide a Diet High in Vitamins, Calories, and Iron.

1. Be aware of the child's food preferences and plan his diet accordingly.
2. Offer small amounts of food at frequent intervals.
3. Reward the child for positive attempts to eat.
4. Allow the child to participate in selection of foods and in preparation of his meal tray.
5. Avoid tiring activities and unpleasant procedures at mealtime.
6. Make mealtime as pleasurable as possible (refer to section on Nutrition, p. 1102).
7. Provide food supplements and vitamins when necessary.
8. If iron is ordered, give between meals and with orange juice.

E. Minimize the Child's Anxieties and Ensure His Cooperation During Hospitalization.

1. Allow the child to handle equipment used for tests and procedures (tourniquets, syringes, etc.).
2. Explain all procedures and the treatment plan to the child in a way that he can understand.
3. Allow the older child to look through a microscope at a blood smear.
4. Permit the child to cleanse the area for a venipuncture or finger stick and to choose the finger.

Nursing Management of Specific Anemias

A. Iron Deficiency Anemia

1. Administer iron as prescribed by the physician.
   a. Oral iron preparations
      (1) Administer between meals if tolerated.
      (2) Absorbed best in acidic environment; therefore administer with orange juice.
      (3) Administer with a dropper or straw, or dilute with water or fruit juice to prevent staining of teeth.
         Dental stains can be removed by brushing the teeth with sodium bicarbonate or hydrogen peroxide and then rinsing with water after each administration.
      (4) Observe for side effects.
         (a) Gastric distress
         (b) Colic pain
         (c) Diarrhea or constipation
      (5) Caution the mother that iron medication causes the child's stools to be dark green or black.
      (6) Stress to the parents the importance of continuing the iron therapy according to the physician's directions even though the child may not appear ill.

> **NURSING ALERT:** There is a great deal of variation in the elemental iron content of the commercially available liquid preparations containing iron. To avoid confusion, the dosage should be expressed in terms of elemental iron and then converted to the proper amount of the therapeutic agent selected.

   b. Intramuscular iron preparations
     (1) Dosage
       (a) Calculated by the physician
       (b) Depends on the child's weight and hemoglobin level
     (2) Special precautions
       (a) Should be injected into a large muscle, preferably the gluteus maximus (buttock).
       (b) Injection sites should be recorded and rotated.

(c) The injection site should not be massaged.
Any pressure on the site may force the medication out of the muscle into the subcutaneous tissue.
Walking will help absorption.
(d) Parenteral iron should be administered with discretion and only to those children whose anemia is not amenable to oral iron therapy.
(e) Parenteral iron is contraindicated in children sensitive to the preparation or in anemias other than iron deficiency anemia.
(3) Technique of administration
(a) Use a separate needle to withdraw the medication from the ampule and for injection.
(b) Use a needle which is 5 cm. (2 inches) long.
Medication must be injected deeply into the muscle to avoid staining the tissue.
(c) Allow 0.5 ml. of air in the syringe before injecting.
(d) Retract the skin over the muscle laterally before inserting the needle.
(e) Insert the needle and withdraw the plunger to check against entry into a blood vessel.
(f) Inject the medication and the 0.5 ml. of air following the injection—to clear the needle and prevent leakage of the medication along the injection track when needle is withdrawn.
(g) Wait 10 seconds after injection before removing the needle.
(4) Observe for side effects
(a) Local
Pain at the injection site
Skin discoloration
Local inflammation with lymphadenopathy
(b) Systemic toxicity (occurs within 10 minutes of injection)
Headache
Muscle and joint pain
Nausea and vomiting
Dizziness
Tachycardia
Bronchospasm with dyspnea
Circulatory collapse (rare)
Fever/chills
Urticaria

> **NURSING ALERT:** Because of the possibility of anaphylaxis, a test dose should be given before initiating parenteral iron therapy.

2. Initiate and reinforce good dietary habits.
   a. Determine from the parents the type and amount of foods customarily eaten, the feeding methods, and the child's reaction to eating.
   b. Introduce foods rich in iron such as dark green leafy vegetables, fortified cereals, dried fruits, nuts.
   c. Do not allow the child to drink excessive quantities of milk to the exclusion of other foods that contain more iron. Limit milk intake to 1 liter (1 quart) per day.

d. Provide vitamin supplements if necessary. Vitamin C appears to enhance the absorption of iron.
e. Explain the reasons for diet change to parents in language they can understand. Visual aids and pictures may be helpful.
f. Assist the parents to select iron-rich foods that are acceptable to the child, within the family's food budget, and culturally acceptable.
g. Make mealtime a pleasurable experience (refer to section on nutrition, p. 1102).
3. Investigate social, economic, and environmental problems that may contribute to the child's disease. Complete a referral to a community health nurse if it appears that the mother will need support in dealing with the child's chronic disease.

B. Megaloblastic Anemias

Administer folic acid or vitamin B_{12} as directed by the physician.
1. Folic acid (pteroylmonoglutamic acid)
   a. Dosage—must be determined by trial for each patient.
   b. Route
      (1) Oral route is preferred.
      (2) May be administered intramuscularly if malabsorption is suspected.
   c. Toxic effects—none
2. Vitamin B_{12} (cyanocobalamin)
   a. Dosage—regulated by individual trial for each patient
   b. Route
      (1) Intramuscular injection is preferred.
   c. Side effects—none
   d. Points of emphasis
      Regular administration of the medication is essential. Patients may be tempted to miss injections because they are not in distress before the injection or do not feel significantly better after it.

Health Education

1. Discuss general hygiene measures, including adequate rest, diet, sunshine, fresh air.
2. Encourage regular medical and dental evaluations.
3. Explain that infection may be prevented by dressing the child according to the weather and keeping him away from persons with colds, sore throats, and other infections.
4. Teach the parents how to administer medication.
5. Alert the parents to signs of disease progress.

Expected Outcomes

1. The child experiences less fatigue evidenced by increasing activity, improved appetite.
2. Indicates basic understanding of diagnostic tests either verbally or through play.
3. Remains free of infection; normal temperature.
4. Parents indicate understanding of anemia and its treatment through compliance with management recommendations; the child does not have a recurrence of anemia.

Sickle Cell Disease *(Sickle Cell Anemia)*

Sickle cell disease is a severe, chronic, hemolytic anemia occurring in persons who are homozygous for the sickle gene. The clinical course is characterized by episodes of pain due to the occlusion of small blood vessels by sickled RBCs. Persons heterozygous for the sickling gene are said to possess sickle cell trait, which is associated with a benign clinical course.

Etiology

1. Genetically determined, inherited disease.
2. Each person inherits 1 gene from each parent which governs the synthesis of hemoglobin (Table 50-1).

Incidence

1. Found almost entirely in American blacks and persons of northern Mediterranean ancestry.
2. Approximately 8% of black Americans have sickle cell trait. (Gene is received from only 1 parent.)
3. Approximately 1 of every 600 black infants born in the US has sickle cell anemia. (Gene is received from both parents.)

Altered Physiology

1. Each hemoglobin molecule consists of 4 molecules of heme folded into 1 molecule of globin.
2. Each globin molecule consists of 2 alpha chains and 2 beta chains.
3. The amino acid sequence on the beta chain is altered in sickle cell hemoglobin.
   Valine is substituted for glutamic acid in the 6th position of the 574 amino acids that make up the globin fraction of hemoglobin.
4. Sickle cell hemoglobin aggregates into elongated crystals under conditions of low oxygen concentration, acidosis, and dehydration.
5. This distorts the membrane of the RBC causing it to assume a crescent or sickle shape. The cells easily become entangled and enmeshed leading to increased blood viscosity, vessel occlusion, and tissue necrosis.
6. Sickled RBCs are fragile and are rapidly destroyed in the circulation; they live 6 to 20 days versus 120 days for normal RBCs.
7. Anemia results when the rate of destruction of RBCs is greater than the rate of production.

Prognosis

1. Variable; improving with new forms of treatment
2. Greatest risk of death is in children under 5 years of age, mainly from overwhelming sepsis or sequestration.
3. Crises usually become less frequent and severe as a child becomes older.

Preventive Measures

1. Every black child admitted to the hospital should be tested for sickle cell anemia.

Table 50-1. *Transmission of Sickle Cell Disease*

	Probability of Abnormal Hemoglobin in Offspring		
Genotype of Parents	*Normal*	*Trait*	*Disease*
1 parent with trait	50%	50%	0
Both parents with trait	25%	50%	25%
1 parent with trait; 1 parent with disease	0	50%	50%
Both parents with disease	0	0	100%

2. Parents at risk should be counseled regarding the genetic aspects of sickle cell anemia.
3. All siblings of any child who is admitted to the hospital with sickle cell anemia should be tested for the disease.
4. Education related to sickle cell disease and preventive treatment should be initiated as soon as a diagnosis is made.

Clinical Manifestations

A. Symptoms

1. Children are rarely symptomatic until late in the first year of life, related to increased amounts of fetal hemoglobin (HgF).
2. Clinical manifestations are sporadic.
   a. The child may be asymptomatic for several months.
   b. Periods of crisis occur at variable intervals.
   c. Precipitating factors of crisis include:
      (1) Dehydration
      (2) Infection
      (3) Trauma
      (4) Strenuous physical exertion
      (5) Extreme fatigue
      (6) Cold exposure
      (7) Hypoxia
      (8) Acidosis
   d. Symptoms may last 1–2 weeks and may subside spontaneously.
3. Signs of anemia
   a. Hemoglobin—6–9 gm./dl.
   b. Loss of appetite
   c. Paleness
   d. Weakness
   e. Fever
   f. Irritability
   g. Jaundice; increased hemolysis results in hemosiderosis (increased iron storage)

B. Vaso-occlusive Crisis

(Most common form of crisis)

1. Small blood vessels are occluded by the sickle-shaped cells, causing distal ischemia and infarction.
2. Extremities
   a. Bony destruction—related to erythroid hyperplasia of marrow leading to osteoporosis or ischemic necrosis
   b. Bone pain; painful and swollen large joints
   c. Dactylitis ("hand–foot" syndrome)
      (1) Often first vaso-occlusive crisis seen in infants and toddlers
      (2) Aseptic infarction of metacarpals and metatarsals
      (3) Symmetrical swelling and pain
3. Spleen
   a. Abdominal pain
   b. Splenomegaly
   c. Spleen initially increases in size due to increased activity as site of RBC hemolysis; increased size results in discomfort.
   d. Following multiple episodes of splenic vaso-occlusion, the spleen becomes fibrotic and atrophied.
   e. Decreased splenic function increases the risk of infection.
4. Cerebral occlusion
   a. Strokes
   b. Hemiplegia

c. Retinal damage leading to blindness
d. Seizures
5. Pulmonary infarction
6. Altered renal function: enuresis, hematuria
7. Impaired liver function
8. Priapism (abnormal, recurrent, prolonged, painful erection of the penis)

C. Splenic Sequestrian Crisis

1. Large amounts of blood become pooled in the spleen.
2. Spleen becomes massively enlarged as it "pools" blood.
3. Massive decrease in RBC mass within hours
4. Signs of circulatory collapse develop rapidly.
5. Frequent cause of death in infant with sickle cell disease

D. Aplastic Crisis

Bone marrow ceases production of RBCs.

E. Chronic Symptoms

Chronic organ damage results in organ dysfunction.
1. Jaundice
2. Gallstones
3. Progressive impairment of kidney function
4. Fibrotic spleen resulting in high susceptibility to *Haemophilus influenzae, Streptococcus pneumoniae,* osteomyelitis, and pneumococcal septicemia
5. Growth retardation; spinal deformities
6. Delayed puberty
7. Cardiac decompensation related to chronic anemia
8. Chronic, painful leg ulcers related to decreased peripheral circulation and unrelated to injury; take months to heal
9. Decreased life span

Diagnostic Evaluation

1. Sickle cell prep (Sickling Test)
   a. Done by finger stick
   b. Oxygen is removed from a drop of blood
   c. The blood is observed under the microscope for the presence of sickle-shaped cells
   d. Does not distinguish between persons with sickle cell trait and disease
2. Sickledex
   a. Done by finger stick
   b. A small amount of blood is placed in a solution containing a chemical reducing agent
   c. The presence of sickle hemoglobin is indicated if the solution turns cloudy
   d. Also does not distinguish between persons with sickle cell trait and disease
3. Hemoglobin electrophoresis
   a. Requires venipuncture
   b. Hemoglobin is subjected to an electric current that separates the various types and determines the amounts present
   c. Used to diagnose both sickle cell trait and sickle cell disease if 2 types of hemoglobin are demonstrated in approximately equal amounts.
   A person is diagnosed as having sickle cell anemia if the majority of his hemoglobin is sickle hemoglobin.
4. Antenatal diagnosis is available to the high-risk group through amniocentesis and gene mapping.

Potential Problems and Nursing Diagnoses

1. Altered comfort: pain related to agglutination of sickled cells within the small blood vessels

2. Altered tissue perfusion related to increased blood viscosity
3. Potential for infection related to fibrotic changes in the spleen
4. Potential for injury related to IV therapy
5. Family coping related to hereditary nature of the disease
6. Knowledge deficit regarding sickle cell anemia and its management
7. Activity intolerance related to anemia
8. Impaired gas exchange related to increased destruction of RBCs

Nursing Interventions

A. Dilute the Blood and Reverse the Agglutination of Sickled Cells Within the Small Blood Vessels.

1. Maintain IV therapy if indicated (see procedure for the administration of IV fluids, p. 1167).
2. Increase the amount and frequency of liquid intake to rehydrate cells.
   a. Offer fruit juice, water, milk, etc.
   b. Offer the child a choice in selection of fluids and method of drinking (straw, etc.).
3. Record the child's intake and output accurately.
4. Assist with a partial exchange transfusion if required. This technique is designed to remove some of the sickled cells and replace them with normal ones.
5. Reverse acidosis, if present.

B. Prevent Hypoxia; Decrease Energy Expenditure

1. Short-term oxygen therapy to prevent further sickling
2. Bedrest to decrease energy expenditure
3. Space activities to allow for maximal rest
4. Decrease emotional stress
5. Avoid low oxygen environment
6. Loosen clothing to avoid constriction on vessels
7. Keep extremities warm to enhance circulation

C. Reduce the Child's Fever, Which May Aggravate Dehydration.

1. Make frequent assessments of the child's temperature.
2. Administer antipyretic drugs as prescribed by the physician.
3. Refer to the section on fever, p. 1142.

D. Alleviate the Child's Pain During a Crisis.

1. Identify effective measures to alleviate pain by questioning parents and by personal trial and error. Consider any of the following measures:
   a. Carefully position and support painful areas.
   b. Hold or rock the infant; handle gently.
   c. Distract the child by singing to him, reading stories, providing play activities.
   d. Provide familiar objects; encourage visits by familiar persons.
   e. Bathe the child in warm water, applying local heat or massage.
   f. Give suitable medications. *DO NOT* give aspirin, as it enhances acidosis.
   g. Maintain bedrest.
2. Share effective methods of reducing pain with other nursing staff and family.

E. Prevent or Treat Associated or Precipitating Infections.

1. Treatment will depend on the specific nature of the infection.
2. Administer antibiotics as prescribed by the physician.
3. Give meticulous care to leg ulcers; use bed cradle.

F. Administer Blood in Cases of Severe Anemia.

1. Refer to information on blood transfusion, p. 1305.
2. Be especially alert for signs of transfusion reaction, which is a very serious problem.
3. *DO NOT* give anticoagulants; vaso-occlusion is *NOT* due to clotting problems.

G. Decrease Surgical Risk.

1. Administer preoperative blood transfusion(s) as prescribed.
   Preoperative blood is usually prescribed to suppress the formation of new sickle cells and to reduce the threat of anoxia.
2. Prepare the child emotionally for surgery.
3. Maintain adequate hydration before and after surgery.
4. Avoid sedatives and analgesics which depress the respiratory center.
5. Observe the child closely for evidence of infection, especially of the respiratory tract.
6. Inform anesthesia department of child's disease status.

H. Provide Emotional Support to the Child and His Parents.

1. Encourage parents to talk about their child, his disease, and how they feel about it.
   a. Expect such feelings as guilt, shock, frustration, depression, and resentment.
   b. Accept negative feelings.
   c. Counsel the parents concerning ways to recognize and alleviate their child's apprehension.
   d. Provide factual information so that parents are prepared to answer their child's questions.
      (1) The recessive nature of the inheritance should be explained.
      (2) Make certain that the parents understand the difference between sickle cell trait and sickle cell anemia.
2. Alleviate the child's anxieties concerning his illness.
   a. Role playing and play activities are useful in identifying his fears.
   b. Explain what is happening to him in a way that he can understand.
      Numerous teaching tools such as coloring books are available for this purpose.
   c. Adolescents should be assured that although sexual development is delayed, they will eventually catch up with their peers.
3. Stress the positive aspects of his disease.
   a. Sickle cell disease does not affect intelligence.
   b. Between periods of crisis the child can usually participate in peer group activities with the exception of some strenuous sports.
   c. Discuss the positive achievements of recent research and correct misconceptions.
4. Encourage quiet activities in which the child can excel—art, painting, leather work, metal and woodworking, chess, etc.
5. Plan for the child to continue his education.
   a. Encourage the parents to bring school work to the child during a lengthy hospitalization.
   b. Refer the child to a home teacher if necessary.
   c. Be certain that the child receives vocational guidance if appropriate.
6. Inform parents of community resources, such as the school nurse or groups for parents and children.

I. Make Certain That the Child Receives Coordinated and Continuous Care.

Send a nursing care summary to the community health nurse or school nurse who will work with the child after he is discharged from the hospital.

Health Education

1. Provide factual information about the disease and its cause. Encourage questions.
2. Discuss the genetic implications of sickle cell disease and offer genetic counseling to the family.
3. Instruct the parents in ways that they can help their child to avoid sickling episodes.
   a. Do not allow the child to become chilled or to wear tight clothing that might impede circulation.
   b. Maintain adequate hydration. Give the parents written instructions regarding the minimum amount of fluid required by their child each day. Discuss implications of abnormal fluid loss (i.e., vomiting, excessive sweating). Instruct parents how to recognize signs of dehydration.
   c. Instruct the child to avoid strenuous physical activity, especially in the presence of an enlarged spleen.
   d. Provide prompt treatment of cuts, sores, mosquito bites, etc. Notify the physician if the child is exposed to a communicable disease.
   e. Maintain good dental hygiene and be certain that the child receives frequent dental checkups.
   f. Be certain that the child receives regular medical supervision, including all the normal childhood immunizations and a PPD (purified protein derivative) test for tuberculosis every 2–3 years. In addition, children over 2 years of age should be immunized against pneumococcal infection and *Haemophilus,* type B, and children over 5 years of age should receive meningococcal vaccine.
   g. Teach the child to avoid undue emotional stress.
   h. Instruct the child to avoid areas of low oxygen concentration (i.e., high mountains and unpressurized airplanes).
   i. Encourage proper handwashing.
4. Teach the parents that the child has the same needs as a normal, healthy child for a balanced diet, good fluid intake, adequate rest, and daily exercise. The child will learn his own activity limitations and will rest when he becomes fatigued. He should not be pampered, but should receive the same love, discipline, privileges, and responsibilities of a normal child his age. Decrease guilt should enuresis be present.
5. Sexually active adolescents should receive contraceptive information, should be helped to make informed choices, and should receive genetic counseling.
6. Teach parents how to recognize the signs of mild crisis:
   a. Fever
   b. Decreased appetite
   c. Irritability
   d. Pain or swelling in abdomen, extremities, back
7. Instruct the parents regarding home management of mild crisis.
   a. Encourage adequate hydration. Teach techniques for increasing fluid intake.
   b. Administer antipyretic medications.
   c. Encourage rest.
   d. Keep the child warm.
   e. Apply warm compresses to the affected area.
   f. Hospitalize child if pain becomes severe or if IV hydration is required.
8. Teach the parents the signs of severe crises:
   a. Pallor
   b. Lethargy and listlessness
   c. Difficulty in awakening
   d. Irritability
   e. Severe pain

f. High fever or a moderate fever that persists for 2 days
9. Instruct the parents to have emergency information available to those involved in the child's care (school nurse, teacher, babysitter, family members, etc.).
   a. Name and phone number of physician and alternate physician
   b. Closest emergency facility and ambulance number
   c. Child's blood type, allergies, medications, and hospital chart number
   d. Name of informed neighbor or relative to be notified in an emergency
10. Stress the benefit of wearing a Medic Alert tag.

Teaching Aids

The following may be useful in providing information to the parents and child:
1. National Sickle Cell Disease Program, National Heart, Lung, & Blood Institute, 7550 Wisconsin Ave, Room 504, Bethesda, MD 20205
2. National Association for Sickle Cell Disease, Inc., 4221 Wilshire Blvd, Los Angeles, CA 90010
3. National Center for Education in Maternal and Child Health, 3520 Prospect Street, NW, Washington, DC 20007

Expected Outcomes

1. The child experiences relief of pain: appears more comfortable and does not cry or complain of pain
2. Does not become hypoxic, as demonstrated by normal laboratory evaluation
3. The child remains free of infection; temperature normal
4. The parents discuss their feelings and work out any sense of guilt.
5. The parents accurately describe sickle cell anemia and discuss the major management principles; the parents manage mild crises successfully at home.

Thalassemia Major (Cooley's Anemia)

Beta-thalassemia (β-thalassemia) refers to an inherited hemolytic anemia characterized by a reduction or absence of the beta globulin chain in hemoglobin synthesis.

This RBC has a decreased amount of hemoglobin resulting in a fragile RBC with a short life span.

Homozygous β-thalassemia is the most severe of the β-thalassemia syndromes and is also known as thalassemia major or Cooley's anemia.

Etiology

1. Genetically determined, inherited disease
2. Autosomal-recessive pattern of inheritance
3. Homozygous form of the disease

Incidence

1. Most prevalent in the Mediterranean basin, Middle East, Southeast Asia, and Africa.
2. In the United States, it is most common in children of Italian or Greek ancestry.

Altered Physiology

1. Insufficient beta globin chain synthesis allows large amounts of unstable alpha chains to accumulate.

2. The precipitates of alpha chains that form cause RBCs to be rigid and easily destroyed, leading to severe hemolytic anemia and resultant chronic hypoxia.
3. Erythroid activity is markedly increased in an attempt to overcome the increased rate of destruction, resulting in enormous expansion of bone marrow, thinning of bony cortex leading to:
   a. Skeletal deformities
   b. Growth retardation
   c. Pathological fractures
4. Rapid destruction of defective RBCs, decreased production of hemoglobin, and increased absorption of dietary iron due to the body's response to anemia result in an excess supply of available iron (hemosiderosis), which deposits iron on organ tissues resulting in decreased function (especially cardiac).
5. In response to the low level of adult hemoglobin, large concentrations of HgF, which does not contain beta chains, are produced; HgF does not hold oxygen well.

Prognosis

1. No known cure
2. Often fatal in late adolescence or early adulthood

Preventive Measures

1. Parents of a child with thalassemia should be tested for the trait, and referred for genetic counseling (refer to p. 1498).
2. Prenatal diagnosis is possible through fetal blood sampling early enough to allow the opportunity to terminate the pregnancy.

Clinical Manifestations: Anemia

1. Onset is usually insidious, with symptoms noted toward the end of the first year of life.
2. Symptoms are primarily related to the progressive anemia, expansion of the marrow cavities of the bone, and the development of hemosiderosis (excess iron storage in various body tissues).
3. Early symptoms often include progressive pallor, poor feeding, and lethargy.
4. Further signs of progressive anemia include headache, bone pain, exercise intolerance, jaundice, and protuberant abdomen due to hepatosplenomegaly.

Complications

A. Splenomegaly

1. Uniformly present because of extramedullary hemopoiesis and rapid destruction of defective RBCs
2. Causes abdominal discomfort, pressure on other organs, and increased transfusion requirements
3. Usually requires splenectomy for improved wellbeing and to decrease the need for transfusions
4. Overwhelming postsplenectomy infection seen in 25% of these patients

B. Growth and Endocrine Complications

1. Growth retardation in second decade
2. Delayed development of secondary sex characteristics
   a. The majority of males fail to undergo puberty.
   b. Most females experience alteration in menstruation.
3. Diabetes mellitus is often seen in older patients, related to iron deposits on the pancreas.
4. Hypermetabolic rate results in increased temperature and lethargy.

C. Skeletal Complications

1. Becoming less common because of early transfusion therapy and keeping hemoglobin levels > 10 gm./dl.
2. Excessive expansion of the erythroid marrow (hyperplastic marrow) may cause:
   a. Frontal and parietal bossing (enlarging)
   b. Maxillary hypertrophy leading to malocclusion
   c. Broad ribs
   d. Premature fusion of epiphyses of long bones
   e. Generalized skeletal osteoporosis
3. Pathological fractures of the long bones and vertebral collapse may occur.

D. Cardiac Complications

1. Fibrosis/hypertrophy resulting from iron deposits on heart muscle.
2. Pericarditis
3. Congestive heart failure
   This is the usual cause of death in thalassemic patients.

E. Liver Enlargement

1. This is initially due to extramedullary hemopoiesis.
2. Later, the liver becomes the main storage area for excess iron resulting in fibrosis and eventually cirrhosis.
3. May lead to coagulation abnormalities

F. Gallbladder Disease

1. Gallstones are common by late adolescence.
2. May require cholecystectomy

G. Megaloblastic Anemia

1. Folic acid deficiency may be sporadically present related to increased use by hyperplastic marrow.
2. Prevented by daily, oral supplementation

H. Skin

May have bronze pigmentation because of iron deposits in the dermis and jaundice (hematochromatosis).

I. Leg Ulcers

Uncommon in well-transfused patients

Diagnostic Evaluation

1. Hemoglobin level—decreased
2. RBC indices—microcytosis and hypochromia
3. Peripheral blood smear—many anisopoikilocytes, nucleated RBCs
4. Reticulocyte count—low, usually less than 10%
5. Hemoglobin electrophoresis—elevated levels of HgF and HgA_2; limited amount of HgA

Patient Problems and Nursing Diagnoses

1. Altered comfort: bone pain related to progression of disease in bone
2. Activity intolerance related to bone pain and anemia
3. Altered nutrition related to anemia and iron overload
4. Knowledge deficit regarding thalassemia and its management
5. Disturbance in self-concept related to endocrine and skeletal complications
6. Potential for infection related to progressive anemia and splenic malfunction
7. Anxiety related to the need for frequent transfusions
8. Parental guilt related to the hereditary nature of the disease
9. Ineffective coping related to presence of a potentially fatal diagnosis
10. Fear related to the costs of treatment

Management

1. Frequent and regular blood transfusions of packed RBCs to maintain hemoglobin levels above 10 gm./dl.
   a. Washed, packed RBCs are usually used to minimize the possibility of transfusion reactions.
   b. The frequency and amount of transfusions depend on the size of the child, with older children often reaching a peak requirement of 500 ml. of packed cells every 2–3 weeks.
2. Iron chelation therapy with deferoxamine to reduce the toxic side effects of excess iron
3. Supportive management of complications
4. Splenectomy due to its hemolytic response to altered RBCs and enlarged size resulting in increased abdominal pressure
5. Bone marrow transplants resulting in cure for some young patients and fatal to others

Nursing Interventions

A. Increase Circulating Hemoglobin and Prevent Tissue Hypoxia.

1. Administer blood transfusions (refer to care of the child with anemia, p. 1298).
   a. Because the chance of usual complications (sensitization, febrile reactions, hives, and hepatitis) is increased with the frequency of transfusions, it is essential to observe the child closely for signs indicative of a reaction.

B. Administer Blood and Maintain the Transfusion.

1. The procedure is similar to the administration of IV fluids (see p. 1167).
   The blood administration set contains a filter in the drip chamber. The blood level should cover the filter.
2. Packed cells are frequently administered to enable the child to receive a high concentration of erythrocytes in a small quantity of fluid.
   The bag should be squeezed every 20–30 minutes during the transfusion to prevent settling of the RBCs.
3. Take special precautions.
   a. The patient's name, physician's name, hospital number, and blood type must correspond with the information on the blood container from the blood bank.
   b. Identifying information such as donor type and number, patient's name on the blood label, kind of blood, and expiration date should always be checked by 2 people.
   c. The blood should be checked for abnormal cloudiness or color and for gas bubbles.
   d. The child's temperature and vital signs should be taken as a baseline measurement before the transfusion is begun.
   e. Normal saline should be hung so that the tubing can be flushed before and after blood is administered and when medications must be given (a separate infusion line for IV medications is preferable).

> **NURSING ALERT:** Medications should not be given in the infusing blood. Blood should never be given with a dextrose and water solution because hemolysis and clotting in the IV tubing can occur.

f. Blood should be run through new IV tubing, and after blood administration, the tubing should be changed before IV fluids are resumed.

g. The rate of flow should be carefully regulated to prevent circulatory overload, especially in those children receiving multiple transfusions. Blood is administered slowly at first as a precautionary measure in case of transfusion reaction, and to allow the blood to reach room temperature.

h. The same blood should not be left running over a long period of time (usually not over 4 hours).

i. Recommendations of the blood bank for storage and administration of blood should be followed explicitly.

4. Observe the child for signs of transfusion reaction.

a. Reaction usually occurs within 15–20 minutes from the start of the transfusion.
Stay with the patient during this time and take frequent vital signs.

b. Signs and symptoms:
  (1) Restlessness
  (2) Irritability
  (3) Chills
  (4) Elevation of temperature; decreased blood pressure
  (5) Sudden changes in pulse and respiration
  (6) Rash or change in the color of the skin; urticaria
  (7) Changes in the appearance or quantity of urine output
  (8) Hemorrhagic phenomena
  (9) Pain, sensation of tightness in the chest; flank pain
  (10) Discontinue the transfusion, but keep the intravenous line open with saline solution.

c. Notify the physician immediately if a transfusion reaction is suspected

5. For additional information, refer to Transfusion Therapy and Guidelines: Administering Blood (Adult), pp. 283 and 291.

C. Prevent Infection and Assess for Signs of Infection (refer to care of the child with anemia, p. 1298).

1. Splenectomy is often required to decrease hemolysis and increase RBC survival. It results in further increased susceptibility to infection.
  a. These children should be maintained on oral penicillin prophylaxis.
  b. Vaccination against *Haemophilus influenzae* and pneumococcal infections should be considered.
  c. Prompt medical attention is essential for fever or signs of infection.

D. Eliminate the Toxic Side Effects of Excess Iron.

1. Deferoxamine (Desferal) is used as a chelating agent to decrease iron deposits in tissues and to increase iron excretion through the urine and feces.
  a. Parents are usually taught to administer the drug subcutaneously during an overnight infusion.

> **NURSING ALERT:** Because of the excess iron deposition in children with thalassemia, dietary iron should be decreased as much as possible.

E. Prevent Megaloblastic Anemia.

1. Administer daily, oral folic acid supplementation.

F. Provide Supportive Care for the Child in Congestive Heart Failure (refer to care of the child with congestive heart failure, p. 1322).

G. Assist the Child to Cope With Thalassemia and Its Management.

1. Alleviate the child's anxieties about his illness.
  a. Role playing and play activities are useful in identifying concerns.
  b. Explain what is happening in a way that the child can understand.
  c. Explore the child's feelings about being different from other children.
  d. Adolescents may require counseling to deal with their feelings about delayed or absent sexual maturity.
  e. Discuss the positive achievements of recent research and correct misconceptions.

2. Plan treatment so that it interferes minimally with the child's regular activities and social interactions.

3. Encourage less strenuous activities in which the child can excel.

4. Encourage interaction with peers.

5. Plan for the child to continue his education.

6. Assist the child with vocational planning.

7. Include child in a support group of other children with thalassemia.

8. Provide supportive care to the dying child (refer to p. 1523).

H. Provide Emotional Support to the Parents.

1. Encourage the parents to express their thoughts about their child's disease.
  a. Feelings of guilt, shock, frustration, depression, and resentment are common.

2. Counsel parents regarding ways to recognize and alleviate their child's apprehension.

3. Inform parents of community resources that may provide financial, social, or other types of support.

4. Include parents in a support group if one is available.

5. Help the parents deal with the potentially fatal nature of the disease (refer to care of the dying child, p. 1523).

Parental Education

1. Provide factual information about thalassemia, including its etiology, usual course, and treatment.

2. Discuss the genetic implications of thalassemia and offer genetic counseling to the family (refer to p. 1498).

3. Explain that the child has the same developmental needs as any healthy child. He should be encouraged to participate in the usual activities of childhood to the extent that he is safely able to do so. The child should not be pampered, but should receive the same love, discipline, privileges, and responsibilities as a healthy child of his age.

4. Provide detailed instruction regarding:
  a. Prevention and prompt treatment of infections
  b. Medications
  c. Home chelation therapy
  d. Dietary modifications
  e. Activity restrictions including avoidance of activities that increase the risk of fractures
  f. Signs of complications

5. Encourage parents to provide information about the child's condition to significant adults who are involved with the child (teacher, school nurse, babysitter, scout leader, etc.).

Table 50-2. *Transmission of Hemophilia*

	Probability of Abnormality in Offspring				
	Female			**Male**	
Genotype of Parents	*Normal*	*Carrier*	*Hemophiliac*	*Normal*	*Hemophiliac*
Female carrier/normal male	50%	50%	0	50%	50%
Noncarrier female/hemophiliac male	0	100%	0	100%	0
Female carrier/hemophiliac male	0	50%	50%	50%	50%

Expected Outcomes

1. The child becomes more comfortable: does not cry in a distressed manner or complain of pain; engages in more activity; appears relaxed
2. Engages in age-related activity
3. Continues to develop in accordance with age
4. Increases and alters nutritional intake
5. Copes well with body-image problems
6. Avoids infection (temperature normal; improved blood counts)
7. The parents are able to express their feelings and concerns about their child's illness.
8. The parents gain an understanding of their child's illness and the necessary treatment.

Hemophilia

Hemophilia is usually an inherited, congenital blood dyscrasia that is characterized by a disturbance of blood clotting factors. It appears primarily in males but is transmitted by females.

Etiology

1. Hereditary (about 80% of patients)
   a. Sex-linked, recessive trait
      (1) Caused by a gene carried on the sex-linked X chromosome
      (2) Transmitted by asymptomatic females who carry the hemophilic gene on one of their X chromosomes
      (3) Appears in males who have the hemophilic gene on their only X chromosome
      (4) Affected males may pass the gene to female offspring making them a carrier.
      (5) May appear in females if a female carrier mates with a male hemophiliac
2. Spontaneous mutations may cause the condition when the family history is negative for the disease (about 20% of patients).

Transmission of Hemophilia

See Table 50-2.

Altered Physiology

1. Hemophilia results from the absence or malfunction of any one of the blood clotting factors from the plasma. The basic defect is in the intrinsic phase of the coagulation cascade.
2. The blood clotting factors are necessary for the formation of prothrombin activator, which acts as a catalyst in the conversion of prothrombin to thrombin.
   a. The rate of formation of thrombin from prothrombin is almost directly proportional to the amount of prothrombin activator available.
   b. The rapidity of the clotting process is proportional to the amount of thrombin formed.
3. The result is an unstable fibrin clot.
4. The most common types of hemophilia and the clotting factors involved are shown in the chart below.
5. **Note:** platelet number and function are normal; therefore external lacerations and small hemorrhages are usually not a problem.

Clinical Manifestations

A. General Considerations

1. Seldom diagnosed in infancy unless excessive bleeding is observed from the umbilical cord or after circumcision
2. Usually diagnosed after the child becomes active
3. Varies in severity depending on the plasma level of the coagulation factor involved
   a. Children with factor levels of less than 1% of normal are considered severe hemophiliacs and often demonstrate severe clinical bleeding with a tendency for spontaneous bleeds.
   b. Children with factor levels of 1%–5% of normal are considered moderately afflicted. These children may be free of spontaneous bleeding, and may not manifest the potentially severe bleeding disorder until after trauma.

Most Common Types of Hemophilia

Type of Hemophilia	Clotting Factor
Hemophilia A (classic hemophilia)	Factor VIII (antihemophilic factor)
Hemophilia B (Christmas disease)	Factor IX (plasma thromboplastin component)
Hemophilia C	Factor XI (plasma thromboplastin antecedent)

c. Children with factor levels of 6%–30% of normal are considered mildly afflicted. They usually lead normal lives and bleed only with severe injury or surgery.

d. Degree of severity tends to be constant within a given family.

B. Clinical Signs and Symptoms

1. History of prolonged bleeding episodes, such as after circumcision
2. Easily bruised
3. Prolonged bleeding from the mucous membranes of the nose and mouth or from lacerations
4. Spontaneous soft-tissue hematomas
5. Hemorrhages into the joints—especially elbows, knees, and ankles (hemarthrosis) causing pain, swelling, limitation of movement
6. Spontaneous hematuria
7. Gastrointestinal bleeding

C. Complications

1. Airway obstruction due to hemorrhage into the neck and pharynx
2. Repeated hemorrhages may produce degenerative joint changes with osteoporosis and muscle atrophy.
3. Contaminated cryoprecipitate can result in chronic active hepatitis and cirrhosis and/or AIDS.
4. Intestinal obstruction due to bleeding into intestinal walls or peritoneum
5. Compression of nerves with paralysis due to hemorrhaging into deep tissues
6. Intracranial bleeding

D. Prognosis

1. Uncertain—a normal life span is possible for many hemophiliacs because of advances in therapy.
2. Cycles may occur with periods of little bleeding followed by periods of severe bleeding.
3. Death may result from intracranial hemorrhage or from exsanguination following any serious hemorrhage.

Diagnostic Evaluation

1. Prothrombin time and bleeding time are normal for hemophilia A.
2. Partial thromboplastin time—prolonged
3. Prothrombin consumption—decreased
4. Thromboplastin generation—increased
5. Assays for specific clotting factors—abnormal
6. Testing to detect carrier state
7. Prenatal diagnosis now possible

Potential Problems and Nursing Diagnoses

1. Potential fluid volume deficit related to exsanguination related to inability of blood to clot
2. Potential for injury from disease complications related to inability of blood to clot
3. Altered comfort related to bleeding into joints
4. Anxiety related to the need for frequent transfusions
5. Activity intolerance related to painful joints
6. Maternal guilt related to hereditary nature of the disease
7. Altered parenting related to overprotection for fear of injury
8. Knowledge deficit regarding hemophilia and its management

Nursing Interventions

A. Provide Emergency Care for Bleeding Wounds.

1. Apply local measures for control of bleeding.
   a. Apply pressure and cold on the area for 10–15 minutes to allow clot formation.
   b. Place fibrin foam or absorbable gelatin foam in the wound.
   c. Suturing and cauterization should be avoided.
2. Cleanse wound thoroughly.
3. Immobilize the affected part and elevate above the level of the heart.
4. Administer cryoprecipitate or lyophilized factors VIII or IX containing the necessary factor (see procedure for the administration of intravenous fluid, p. 1167, and for blood transfusion, p. 1305).
   a. Avoid rapid administration to minimize the possibility of transfusion reaction.
   b. Stop the transfusion if hives, headaches, tingling, chills, flushing, or fever occur.
5. Apply fibrinolytic agents for mouth bleeds.
6. Keep the child quiet during treatment to decrease pulse and bleeding.
   a. Remain calm.
   b. Sedate the child if necessary.

B. Provide Supportive Care for the Child With Hemarthrosis.

1. Control bleeding.
   a. Immobilize the joint in a position of slight flexion.
   b. Elevate the affected part above the level of the heart.
   c. Apply ice packs.
   d. Administer plasma or therapeutic concentrate as directed by the physician.
2. Alleviate pain.
   a. Administer sedatives or narcotics as prescribed by the physician.
   b. Use a bed cradle to keep the weight of the bedcovers off the affected part.
3. Prevent further bleeding.
   a. Continue immobilization of the joint. (A bivalve plaster cast may be necessary.)
   b. Maintain the child on bedrest. (Careful handling of the child is essential.)
4. Prevent permanent deformities and crippling.
   a. Begin gentle, passive exercise 48 hours after the acute phase to prevent joint stiffness and fibrosis. Progress to active exercises.
   b. Refer the child for physical therapy on an outpatient basis if this is indicated by:
      (1) Presence of persistent deformity.
      (2) Need to use orthopedic devices such as crutches, braces, splints, etc.
      (3) Need for specialized programs such as whirlpool baths, electrical stimulation, increased physical exercises
   c. Reconstructive orthopedic surgery may be required.
5. Assess the child for evidence of disease progress:
   a. Increased pain
   b. Further swelling of joints
   c. Limitation of movement
   d. Flexion contractures

C. Prevent Hemorrhage During Nursing Procedures.

1. Temperature measurement
   Insert the thermometer gently axillary or orally

2. Injections (avoid if possible)
   a. Administer medications orally whenever possible.
   b. Choose injection sites carefully and rotate them. The subcutaneous route is preferred.
   c. Inject the medication slowly.
   d. Apply pressure to the area for 5 minutes.

> **NURSING ALERT:** Children with hemophilia should not receive aspirin or compounds containing aspirin because this medication affects platelet function and prolongs bleeding time.

D. Maintain a Safe Environment During Hospitalization.

1. Pad crib rails.
2. Inspect toys for sharp or rough edges.
3. Offer foods and fluids in plastic or paper containers.
4. Supervise small children when they are ambulatory.
5. Use protective devices which the child brings from home. (Many children wear helmets, knee pads).
6. Continually assess environment for potential hazards.

E. Provide Emotional Support to the Child and His Family.

1. Permit the child to participate in as many normal activities as possible within the realm of safety.
2. Allow the child to handle equipment used in his care. Use play to help the young child adjust to his illness by "transfusing" his teddy bear, etc.
3. Encourage the child's continuing education.
   a. Have parents bring assignments from the child's teacher.
   b. Refer to a home teacher if indicated.
   c. Investigate the possibility of a school-to-home telephone service.
4. Encourage parental participation in the child's care.
   a. Refer to section on family-centered care, page 1125.
   b. Assess the parents' attitudes and understanding about the disease. Clarify information if necessary.
   c. Teach the parents aspects of their child's care which must be continued after discharge. Have them practice appropriate techniques including IV administration of cryoprecipitate, if appropriate, with nursing supervision until they achieve competence and are comfortable in the situation (see Health Education, below).
5. Counsel the parents concerning:
   a. Financial problems caused by repeated hospitalizations and transfusions.
   b. Feelings of guilt at having given birth to the child or resentment at having to care for him.
   c. Refer the parents to a social worker or psychiatrist if indicated.
6. Introduce the child and his family to other hemophiliac families.
   a. Information concerning the location of parent groups may be obtained from the National Hemophilia Foundation, 19 West 34th Street, Room 1204, New York, NY, 10001.
   b. Numerous specialized hemophilia centers have been established in the United States.
7. Initiate a community health nursing referral if appropriate.

Health Education

1. Protecting the child from trauma
   a. Select toys that are soft and without rough edges.
   b. Pad the sides of cribs, playpens, etc.
   c. Offer food and liquids in plastic containers to avoid laceration.
   d. Guard against child's falling when he is learning how to stand and walk.
      (1) Remove potential sources of injury from furniture.
      (2) Pad the child's knees and buttocks.
      (3) Use a helmet for the child's head.
   e. Supervise play closely.
   f. Inform the child's teacher and playmates, the school nurse, and other adults of his condition so that they can be supportive of the child's needs and know what to do in an emergency.
   g. Have the child wear a Medic Alert bracelet.
   h. Do not administer aspirin to the child.
   i. Encourage physical therapy—as strong muscles protect joints.
2. Emergency treatment for hemorrhage
   a. Immobilize the part.
      This may be done with splints or an elastic compression bandage. (These materials should be immediately available in the home.)
   b. Apply ice packs.
      Parents should keep 2 or 3 plastic bags of ice immediately available in the freezer.
   c. Consult the child's physician and initiate additional recommended therapy.
3. Regular medical and dental supervision
   a. Preventive dental care is important. Soft-bristled or sponge-tipped toothbrushes should be used to prevent bleeding. Hospitalization may be necessary for extensive dental work and extractions.
   b. HBV vaccine to protect against hepatitis from blood transfusions.
4. Diet
   Modify diet to avoid overweight, which places additional strain on the child's weight-bearing joints and predisposes him to hemarthrosis.
5. Information concerning the disease itself
   a. The child should be helped to understand the exact nature of his illness as early as possible. Special attention should be given to the signs of hemorrhage, and the child should be told of the need to report even the slightest bleeding to an adult immediately.
   b. *Understanding Hemophilia—A Guide for Parents* (1979), Hemophilia Foundation of Illinois, 327 South LaSalle Street, Chicago, IL 60604
   c. National Center for Education in Maternal and Child Health, 3520 Prospect Street NW, Washington, DC 20007
6. Avoidance of overprotection—this can be more disabling than the disease itself.
   a. Promote a sense of independence and self-care within the patient's limitations.
   b. Encourage healthful activity and reasonably aggressive pursuits. Reinforce self-judgment of child or teenager in selection of safe physical activities.
   c. Participate in as many age-appropriate activities as possible.
   d. Help parents understand the importance of vocational guidance for their child—emphasis given to occupations using intellect or skills rather than physical effort.
7. Genetic counseling and family planning services
   These should be offered to the family and to the adolescent patient.

8. Home care program
   a. Home care programs teach the parents and children to administer infusion therapy at home when a hemorrhage episode begins.
   b. Advantages of home treatment:
      (1) Can be initiated immediately
      (2) Earlier recovery of joint functions
      (3) Greater self-sufficiency for patient and family
      (4) Fewer absences from school or work
      (5) Less anxiety related to traveling
      (6) Decrease in the cost of treatment
   c. General criteria for acceptance into program:
      (1) Adequate knowledge of the disease
      (2) Willingness to learn venipuncture technique
      (3) Demonstrated ability to follow directions
      (4) Acceptance of the necessity for follow-up care
      (5) Emotional stability sufficient to accept the responsibility
   d. Teaching is usually done by the nurse in the specialty clinic and includes instruction and practice in the following:
      (1) How to assess the child to determine if and what treatment is needed
      (2) Storage and preparation of replacement factors
      (3) Venipuncture technique
      (4) Transfusion management
      (5) Record keeping

   (6) Awareness of signs of transfusion reaction
   (7) Recognition of indications of need for subsequent transfusions
   e. Hospital nursing responsibilities:
      (1) Screen patients and families who may be eligible for home care programs.
      (2) Facilitate appropriate self-management by children and families enrolled in home care programs if hospitalization becomes necessary. Establish communication with the clinic nurse.

Expected Outcomes

1. The child or parents achieve prompt control of bleeding episodes by administration of adequate treatment
2. Appears more comfortable as joint pain is relieved, achieves improved range of motion and does not demonstrate permanent joint deformities
3. Is not unduly anxious about transfusions, evidenced by his verbal and nonverbal communication
4. Demonstrates an age-appropriate level of independence
5. The parents are able to talk about their concerns or guilt.
6. The family gains an understanding of hemophilia and its treatment.

Bibliography

Books

Behrman R and Vaughan V. Nelson's Textbook of Pediatrics. Philadelphia, WB Saunders, 1987
Buckner C, Gale R and Lucarelli G. Advances and Controversies in Thalassemia Therapy. New York, Alan Liss, 1989
DeMaeyer EM. Preventing and Controlling Iron Deficiency Anaemia through Primary Health Care. Geneva, World Health Organization, 1989
Hayman L and Sporing E (eds). Handbook of Pediatric Nursing. New York, John Wiley & Sons, 1985
Hilgartner M. Hemophilia in the Child and Adult. New York, Masson Publishing USA, 1989
Johnson SH. High Risk Parenting. Philadelphia, JB Lippincott, 1986
McKenzie S. Textbook of Hematology. Philadelphia, Lea & Febiger, 1988
Nathan D and Oski F. Hematology of Infancy and Childhood. 3rd ed. Philadelphia, WB Saunders, 1987

Simmons A. Hematology—A Combined Theoretical and Technical Approach. Philadelphia, WB Saunders, 1989
Whaley L and Wong D. Nursing Care of Infants and Children. St. Louis, CV Mosby, 1987
Whitten and Bertles J. Sickle Cell Disease, vol 565. Ann NY Acad Sci, 1989

Journals

CDC criteria for anemia in children and childbearing-aged women. MMWR 1989 Jun 9; 38(22):400–404
Festa R. Modern management of thallassemia. Pediatr Ann 1985; 14(9): 597–606
Golematis B et al. Overwhelming post-splenectomy infection in patients with thallassemia major. Mt Sinai J Med 1989; 56(2):97–98
Hernandez J, Gray D and Lineberger H. Social and economic indicators of well-being among hemophiliacs over a

5 year period. Gen Hosp Psychiatry 1989; 11:241–247
Kamani N. Marrow transplatation in pediatric hematologic disorders. Pediatr Ann 1985; 14(9):661–670
Karayalcin G. Current concepts in the management of hemophilia. Pediatr Ann 1985; 14(9):640–659
Lanzkowsky P. Problems in diagnosis of iron deficiency anemia. Pediatr Ann 1985; 14(9):618–636
Shende A. Idiopathic thrombocytopenic purpura in children. Pediatr Ann 1985; 14(9):609–616
Stehr–Green J, Holman R and Mahoney M. Survival analysis of hemophilia-associated AIDS cases in the U.S. Am J Public Health 1989 July; 79(7):832
Walter T et al. Iron deficiency anemia: Adverse effects on infant psychomotor development. Pediatrics 1989 July; 84(1):7–17
Zurlo M et al. Survival and causes of deaths in thalassemia major. Lancet 1987 July 1; 27–29

Children With Cardiovascular Disorders

51

Congenital Heart Disease

Congenital heart disease is a structural malformation of the heart or great vessels, present at birth but not necessarily detected at birth.

Etiology

1. Exact cause is unknown
2. Results from abnormal embryonic development or the persistence of fetal structure beyond the time of normal involution
3. Possible causes
   a. Fetal and maternal infection occurring during first trimester (primarily rubella)
   b. Teratogenic effects of drugs (i.e., lithium) and alcohol
   c. Maternal dietary deficiencies
   d. Genetic factors (trisomies)
   e. Maternal age greater than 40
   f. Maternal insulin-dependent diabetes
4. Frequently associated with other congenital defects

Incidence

1. Approximately 32,000 infants are born each year with congenital heart disease (4–8/1000 live births)
2. As a category, congenital heart disease is the most common congenital malformation.

Common Congenital Heart Malformations

(Table 51-1)

A. Acyanotic
1. Obstructive lesions
   a. Aortic valvular stenosis
   b. Pulmonic stenosis
   c. Coarctation of the aorta
2. Left-to-right shunts
   a. Patent ductus arteriosus
   b. Atrial septal defect
   c. Ventricular septal defect

B. Cyanotic
1. Right-to-left shunts
   a. Tetralogy of Fallot
   b. Tricuspid atresia
   c. Transposition of great arteries

Aortic Valvular Stenosis

Aortic valvular stenosis occurs when there is obstruction to the left ventricular outflow at the level of the valve. This is the most common form of aortic stenosis, others being hypertrophic subvalvular stenosis and supravalvular stenosis. This accounts for 6% of all congenital heart defects.

Pathophysiology

1. Blood flows from the left ventricle through the obstructed aortic valve into the aorta.
2. Left ventricular pressure increases to overcome the resistance of the obstructed valve.
3. Myocardial ischemia may occur as a result of an imbalance between the increased oxygen requirements of the hypertrophied left ventricle and the amount of oxygen that can be supplied to the myocardium.
4. Left ventricle may fail, resulting in pulmonary edema.

Clinical Manifestations

1. Rarely symptomatic during infancy; in severe cases, infants may demonstrate evidence of decreased cardiac output, such as faint peripheral pulses or exercise intolerance.
2. Older children may experience chest pain, dyspnea, fatigue, and shortness of breath with exertion.
3. Narrow pulse pressure
4. Weak peripheral pulses
5. Fatigue or fainting spells
6. Pale hands and feet related to decreased cardiac output

Diagnostic Evaluation

1. Auscultation:
   a. Harsh, low-pitched systolic ejection murmur, maximal at the second right intercostal space, radiates to apex, back, neck
   b. Ejection click at fourth interspace to the left of the sternum (mild or moderately severe cases)
   c. Single or narrowly split second heart sound

Table 51-1. Congenital Heart Abnormalities*

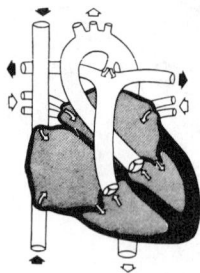

Patent Ductus Arteriosus (PDA)

The PDA is a vascular connection that, during fetal life, short circuits the pulmonary vascular bed and directs blood from the pulmonary artery to the aorta. Functional closure of the ductus normally occurs soon after birth. If the ductus remains patent after birth, the direction of blood flow in the ductus is reversed by the higher pressure in the aorta.

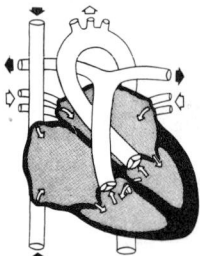

Ventricular Septal Defects (VSD)

A VSD is an abnormal opening between the right and left ventricle. VSDs vary in size and may occur in either the membranous or muscular portion of the ventricular septum. Due to higher pressure in the left ventricle, a shunting of blood from the left to right ventricle occurs during systole. If pulmonary vascular resistance produces pulmonary hypertension, the shunt of blood is then reversed from the right to the left ventricle, with cyanosis resulting.

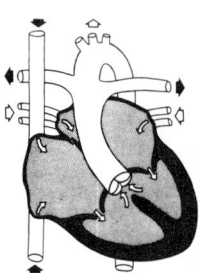

Truncus Arteriosus

Truncus arteriosus is a retention of the embryologic bulbar trunk. It results from the failure of normal septation and division of this trunk into an aorta and pulmonary artery. This single arterial trunk overrides the ventricles and receives blood from them through a ventricular septal defect. The entire pulmonary and systemic circulation is supplied from this common arterial trunk.

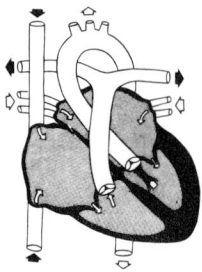

Subaortic Stenosis

In many instances, the stenosis is valvular with thickening and fusion of the cusps. Subaortic stenosis is caused by a fibrous ring below the aortic valve in the outflow tract of the left ventricle. At times, both valvular and subaortic stenosis exist in combination. The obstruction presents an increased work load for the normal output of the left ventricular blood and results in left ventricular enlargement.

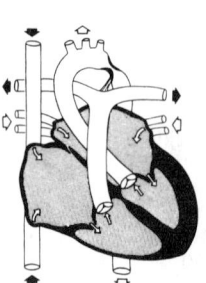

Coarctation of the Aorta

Coarctation of the aorta is characterized by a narrowed aortic lumen. It exists as a preductal or postductal obstruction, depending on the position of the obstruction in relation to the ductus arteriosus. Coarctations exist with great variation in anatomic features. The lesion produces an obstruction to the flow of blood through the aorta causing an increased left ventricular pressure and work load.

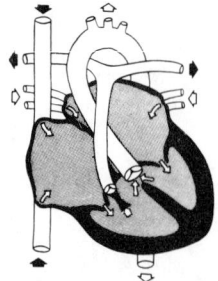

Tetralogy of Fallot

Tetralogy of Fallot is characterized by the combination of 4 defects: (1) pulmonary stenosis, (2) ventricular septal defects, (3) overriding aorta, (4) hypertrophy of right ventricle. It is the most common defect causing cyanosis in patients surviving beyond 2 years of age. The severity of symptoms depends on the degree of pulmonary stenosis, the size of the ventricular septal defect, and the degree to which the aorta overrides the septal defect.

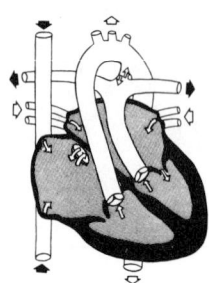

Complete Transposition of Great Vessels

This anomaly is an embryologic defect caused by a straight division of the bulbar trunk without normal spiraling. As a result, the aorta originates from the right ventricle, and the pulmonary artery from the left ventricle. An abnormal communication between the 2 circulations must be present to sustain life.

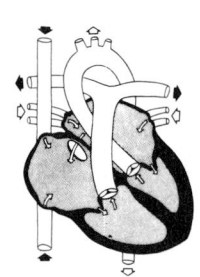

Atrial Septal Defects (ASD)

An ASD is an abnormal opening between the right and left atria. Basically, 3 types of abnormalities result from incorrect development of the atrial septum. An incompetent foramen ovale is the most common defect. The high ostium secundum defect results from abnormal development of the septum secundum. Improper development of the septum primum produces a basal opening known as an ostium primum defect, frequently involving the atrioventricular valves. In general, left-to-right shunting of blood occurs in all ASDs.

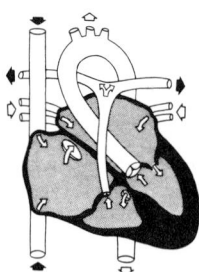

Tricuspid Atresia

Tricuspid valvular atresia is characterized by a small right ventricle, large left ventricle and usually a diminished pulmonary circulation. Blood from the right atrium passes through an ASD into the left atrium, mixes with oxygenated blood returning from the lungs, flows into the left ventricle and is propelled into the systemic circulation. The lungs may receive blood through 1 of 3 routes: (1) a small VSD, (2) PDA, (3) bronchial vessels.

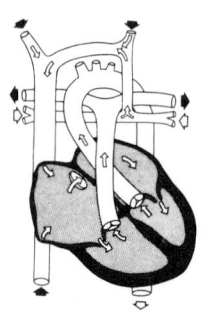

Anomalous Venous Return

Oxygenated blood returning from the lungs is carried abnormally to the right heart by one or more pulmonary veins emptying directly, or indirectly through venous channels, into the right atrium. Partial anomalous return of the pulmonary veins to the right atrium functions the same as an atrial septal defect. In complete anomalous return of the pulmonary veins, an interatrial communication is necessary for survival.

* Courtesy, Ross Laboratories.

2. Chest x-ray—dilated ascending aorta and varying degrees of left ventricular enlargement
3. Electrocardiogram (ECG)—normal or left ventricular hypertrophy. Strain pattern (T wave inversion) is evidence of severe stenosis. ST segment depression indicates myocardial ischemia.
4. Echocardiography and Doppler measurements of peak flow velocity
5. Cardiac catheterization
6. Angiography

Complications

1. Congestive heart failure
2. Syncope
3. Bacterial endocarditis (increased incidence with age)
4. Sudden death

Treatment

Aortic valvulotomy or prosthetic valve replacement (indicated for children who are symptomatic or have evidence of left ventricular strain on ECG).

Pulmonic Stenosis

Pulmonic stenosis refers to any lesion that obstructs the flow of blood from the right ventricle. It accounts for 8% of congenital heart defects.

Pathophysiology

1. Blood flows from the right ventricle through the obstructed pulmonary valve into the pulmonary artery.
2. Right ventricular pressure increases to maintain normal cardiac output.
3. Right ventricular hypertrophy develops.
4. Right-sided heart failure occurs in severe cases.

Clinical Manifestations

1. Generally asymptomatic; the child may have decreased exercise tolerance.
2. With severe obstruction, the child may have dyspnea, generalized cyanosis.
3. May complain of precordial pain.

Diagnostic Evaluation

1. Auscultation
   a. Systolic ejection murmur over pulmonic area
   b. Often will hear an ejection click and a widely split second sound
2. Chest x-ray—right ventricular enlargement, main pulmonary artery enlargement, normal pulmonary vascularity, and normal left side. In severe stenosis, right atrial hypertrophy is also observed.
3. ECG—moderate or severe cases demonstrate right ventricular hypertrophy.
4. Two-dimensional echocardiography and Doppler study
5. Cardiac catheterization
6. Angiocardiography

Complications

1. Anoxic spells in infants with severe lesions
2. Bacterial endocarditis
3. Sudden death at any age

Treatment

1. Surgery (valvulotomy) is generally indicated for all patients with severe stenosis and for symptomatic patients with moderate stenosis.
2. Asymptomatic children with moderate pulmonic stenosis should be evaluated at regular intervals for progression of the lesion.

Coarctation of the Aorta

Coarctation of the aorta is a narrowing or constriction of the vessel at any point. Most commonly, the constriction is located just distal to the origin of the left subclavian artery in the vicinity of the ductus arteriosus. It accounts for 6% of congenital heart defects.

Altered Physiology

1. The narrowing of the aorta obstructs blood flow through the constricted segment of the aorta, thus increasing left ventricular pressure and work load.
2. Collateral vessels develop, arising chiefly from the branches of the subclavian and intercostal arteries, bypassing the coarcted segment of the aorta and supplying circulation to the lower extremities.

Clinical Manifestations

1. Usually asymptomatic in childhood—growth and development are normal.
2. May demonstrate:
   a. Occasional fatigue
   b. Headache, dizziness
   c. Nose bleeds
   d. Leg cramps
   e. Cold feet
3. Absent or greatly reduced femoral pulsations; full bounding carotid pulses; wide pulse pressure
4. Hypertension in upper extremities and diminished blood pressure in lower extremities
5. Symptoms secondary to hypertension (rare in children)
6. Severe anomalies cause symptoms in infants, including growth failure, tachypnea, dyspnea, peripheral edema, and severe congestive heart failure.

Diagnostic Evaluation

1. Auscultation—nonspecific systolic murmur heard along the left sternal border
2. Chest x-ray:
   a. Prominent aorta
   b. Rib notching is a common finding in children over 10 years of age.
   c. Seriously ill infants demonstrate significant cardiomegaly with increased pulmonary vascularity.
3. ECG—normal or varying degrees of left ventricular hypertrophy
4. Ultrasound, echocardiogram, and Doppler studies
5. Barium esophagogram
6. Cardiac catheterization and angiography (frequently not needed)

Complications

1. Congestive heart failure
2. Cerebral hemorrhage
3. Infective endocarditis
4. Rupture of the aorta

Treatment

1. Infants—vigorous management of congestive heart failure and surgical correction is indicated for infants who present in the first 6 months of life with heart failure.
2. Asymptomatic older child—surgical resection is recommended for children between the ages of 2–4 years with significant coarctation.
3. Surgery—resection of the coarcted segment and end-to-end anastomosis or graft

Patent Ductus Arteriosus

Patent ductus arteriosus (PDA) is the persistence of a fetal connection (ductus arteriosus) between the pulmonary artery and the aorta, resulting in a left-to-right shunt. PDA accounts for 10% of congenital heart defects.

Altered Physiology

1. During fetal life, the ductus arteriosus allows most of the right ventricular blood to bypass the nonfunctioning lungs by directing blood from the pulmonary artery to the aorta.
   a. It is maintained open by endogenous production of prostaglandin E, which relaxes ductal smooth muscle in the low-oxygen intrauterine environment.
2. After birth, with the initiation of respiration, the ductus arteriosus is no longer necessary. It should functionally close within several hours after birth and anatomically close within several weeks after birth.
   a. The smooth muscle in the wall of the ductus arteriosus contracts to obliterate the lumen within 24 hours of birth.
   b. Within several weeks after birth, degenerative changes occur in the ductus arteriosus, and it becomes a cord of fibrous connective tissue (ligamentum arteriosum).
3. When the ductus arteriosus remains patent, oxygenated blood from the higher pressure systemic circuit (aorta) flows to the lower pressure pulmonary circuit (pulmonary artery) through the PDA.
4. The volume of blood that the heart must pump to meet the demands of the peripheral tissues is increased. A greater volume burden is placed on the lungs and eventually on the left heart.

Clinical Manifestations

1. Small PDA—usually asymptomatic
2. Large PDA—may develop symptoms in very early infancy
   a. Slow weight gain
   b. Feeding difficulties; decreased exercise tolerance
   c. Frequent respiratory infections
   d. Congestive heart failure; dyspnea

Diagnostic Evaluation

1. Auscultation—continuous machinery-like murmur at the left intraclavicular area is heard in most older children. Neonates with PDA have a variety of murmurs.
2. May have a wide pulse pressure and/or bounding posterior tibial and dorsalis pedis pulses
3. Chest x-ray:
   a. Normal with small PDA

   b. Large PDA shows left-sided hypertrophy, a prominent ascending aorta, and dilation of the proximal pulmonary arteries.
4. ECG—may be normal; may demonstrate left ventricular hypertrophy
5. Echocardiography and Doppler study
6. Cardiac catheterization—may not be necessary
7. Angiocardiography

Complications

1. Congestive heart failure
2. Infective endocarditis

Treatment

Note: Indomethacin appears to trigger the natural closing of the ductus. It is the treatment of choice for many preterm infants.

Surgical division of the PDA (closed heart surgery to ligate the ductus)
1. In early infancy if congestive heart failure develops and cannot be controlled
2. Electively by 1–2 years

Atrial Septal Defect

Atrial septal defect (ASD) is an abnormal opening in the septum between the left atrium and the right atrium. ASD accounts for 9% of congenital heart defects.
1. *Ostium secundum type*—located in the center of the atrial septum (most common)
2. *Ostium primum type*—large gap at the base of the atrial septum frequently associated with deformities of the mitral and tricuspid valves and/or a small, high ventricular septal defect (endocardial cushion defects).

Altered Physiology

1. The pressure in the left atrium is greater than the pressure in the right atrium and promotes the flow of oxygenated blood from the left atrium to the right atrium (a left-to-right shunt)
2. The oxygenated blood that flows through the defect enters the right atrium and mixes with the systemic venous blood returning to the lungs. The blood flow through the shunt recirculates through the lungs, thus increasing the total blood flow through the lungs.
3. The major hemodynamic abnormality is volume overload of the right ventricle resulting in hypertrophy of the right ventricle.
4. Eventually if the pulmonary resistance is great, this may increase right atrial pressure, thus causing a reversal of the shunt, with unoxygenated blood flowing from the right atrium to the left atrium. (This situation will produce cyanosis.)

Clinical Manifestations

1. *Ostium secundum type*—generally asymptomatic even when this defect is large.
2. *Ostium primum type*—generally asymptomatic, although the following may occur:
   a. Slow weight gain
   b. Fatigability
   c. Dyspnea with exertion
   d. History of frequent respiratory infections

e. Congestive heart failure
f. Hypertension related to pulmonary edema

Diagnostic Evaluation

1. Auscultation
   a. Systolic, medium-pitched ejection murmur heard best at the second left interspace
   b. Fixed widely split second sound
   c. May have mid-diastolic filling sound at the lower left sternal border
2. Chest x-ray—prominent main pulmonary artery, right atrial and right ventricular enlargement, increase in vascular markings of the lungs.
3. ECG may demonstrate right ventricular hypertrophy and right axis deviation (ostium secundum defect); left axis deviation, P wave changes indicating atrial enlargement, and prolonged P+R interval are common in ostium primum defects.
4. Two-dimensional echocardiogram and Doppler study
5. Cardiac catheterization
6. Angiocardiography
7. Magnetic resonance imaging (MRI)

Complications

(Rare in children)
1. Infective endocarditis
2. Cardiac failure
3. Pulmonary hypertension
4. Coronary artery disease
5. Atrial fibrillation
6. Mitral valve prolapse

Treatment

1. Spontaneous closure in a small percentage
2. Surgical closure with cardiopulmonary bypass by suture or patch
3. Treatment of any congestive heart failure that may occur
4. Complications of surgical repair
   a. Cardiac dysrhythmias
   b. Heart block
   c. Mitral insufficiency

Ventricular Septal Defect

Ventricular septal defect (VSD) is an abnormal opening in the septum between the right and left ventricles. It may vary in size from very small defects to very large defects, and may occur in either the membranous or muscular portion of the ventricular septum. VSD accounts for 25%–29% of all congenital heart defects.

Altered Physiology

1. The pressure in the left ventricle is greater than the pressure in the right ventricle and promotes the flow of oxygenated blood from the left ventricle to the right ventricle (a left-to-right shunt)
2. The oxygenated blood that flows through the defect mixes with the blood returning from the right atrium. The blood flow through the shunt recirculates through the lungs, thus increasing the total blood flow through the lungs.
3. The major hemodynamic abnormalities are:
   a. Increased right ventricular and pulmonary arterial pressure

   b. Increased blood flow to the right ventricle, pulmonary arteries and lungs
4. If the pulmonary vascular resistance is great, this may increase right ventricular pressure, thus causing a reversal of the shunt with unoxygenated blood flowing from the right ventricle to the left ventricle (this situation, termed *Eisenmenger's complex*, will produce cyanosis).

Clinical Manifestations

1. Small VSDs—usually asymptomatic (many close spontaneously)
2. Large VSDs—may develop symptoms as early as 1–2 months of age
   a. Slow weight gain, failure to thrive
   b. Feeding difficulties; increased fatigue
   c. Pale, delicate-looking, scrawny appearance
   d. Frequent respiratory infections
   e. Tachypnea
   f. Excessive sweating
   g. Congestive heart failure

Diagnostic Evaluation

1. Auscultation—harsh holosystolic murmur, heard best at the fourth interspace to the left of the sternum. Elevated pulmonary resistance is manifested by a loud, banging, pulmonic component of the second sound.
2. Chest x-ray—ranges from normal (small defect) to varying degrees of biventricular hypertrophy, left atrial enlargement, pulmonary artery enlargement, and increased pulmonary vascular markings.
3. ECG—normal or biventricular hypertrophy
4. Two-dimensional echocardiography and Doppler studies—identify presence, size, and location of defects and associated chamber enlargement
5. Cardiac catheterization
6. Angiocardiography

Complications

1. Infective endocarditis
2. Congestive heart failure

Treatment

1. Medical management of congestive heart failure if this occurs in infancy
2. If congestive heart failure is intractable to medical management, surgical patch closure is indicated.
3. Patients with pulmonary arterial hypertension require early surgery (before 2 years of age) to avoid irreversible pulmonary bed changes.
   a. This is pulmonary artery banding around the pulmonary artery to decrease pulmonary blood flow and control congestive heart failure and prevent pulmonary arteriolar disease.
   b. Later: deband and do patch closure.
4. Surgery is contraindicated in patients with Eisenmenger's complex.

Tetralogy of Fallot

Tetralogy of Fallot is a cyanotic heart defect consisting of four abnormalities (1) pulmonary valve stenosis; (2) ventricular septal defect; (3) overriding of the aorta (dextraposition of the aorta); and (4) right ventricular hypertrophy. It accounts for 6%–10% of all congenital heart defects.

Altered Physiology

1. Obstruction of the blood flow from the right ventricle to the pulmonary circulation is caused by obstruction at the pulmonary valve level or the infundibular area of the right ventricle below the pulmonary valve.
2. Unoxygenated blood is shunted from the right ventricle through the ventricular septal defect directly into the aorta (a right-to-left shunt)
3. The right ventricle is hypertrophied because of high right ventricular pressure.
4. Unoxygenated blood is shunted back through the body.

Clinical Manifestations

1. The clinical manifestations are variable and depend on the size of the ventricular septal defect and the degree of right ventricular outflow obstruction.
2. Cyanosis
   a. Initially, the shunt through the ventricular septal defect may be from left to right. Many infants with this defect are not cyanotic at birth, but they develop cyanosis as they grow and as the stenosis becomes relatively more severe.
   b. Cyanosis may at first be observed only with exertion and crying, but during the first few years of life, the child may become cyanotic even at rest.
   c. Infundibular stenosis may be minimal so that cyanosis never develops ("pink tetralogy").
   d. Polycythemia resulting in increased hematocrit
3. Clubbing of the fingers and toes
4. Squatting (a posture characteristically assumed by children with this defect once they have reached the walking stage)
   a. Used to deflect blood flow to extremities and keep oxygenated blood in the trunk and head
   b. Increases systemic resistance and aids in venous return
5. Slow weight gain; failure to thrive
6. Dyspnea on exertion
7. Hypoxic spells ("tet" spells); transient cerebral ischemia
   a. Common in children under age 2 years
   b. Especially initiated by crying

Diagnostic Evaluation

1. Auscultation
   a. Single second sound (aortic component)
   b. Systolic ejection murmur at the second and third interspaces to the left of the sternum
   c. Prominent ejection click heard immediately after the first heart sound
2. Chest x-ray
   a. Heart size normal
   b. Pulmonary segment small and concave ("boot-shaped heart")
   c. Diminished pulmonary vascular markings
3. ECG—right axis deviation; right ventricular hypertrophy
4. Cardiac catheterization
5. MRI
6. Two-dimensional echocardiography and Doppler study
7. Laboratory data
   a. Polycythemia
   b. Increased hematocrit

Complications

1. Congestive heart failure—may occur in newborn but is uncommon beyond infancy
2. Infective endocarditis
3. Cerebral vascular accident (due to thrombosis caused by increased blood viscosity or severe hypoxia)
4. Brain abscess

Treatment

Goal:
Improve oxygenation of arterial blood

1. Palliative (for some)
   a. Blalock–Taussig shunt—anastomosis between the right or left subclavian artery and the right pulmonary artery (preferred method). (Creates an artificial ductus arteriosus.)
   b. Waterston shunt—anastomosis between the posterior lateral aspect of the ascending aorta and the right pulmonary artery
2. Total correction (the first treatment of choice)
   a. Removal of shunt if previously performed
   b. With cardiopulmonary bypass, VSD is repaired with patch closure and right ventricular outflow obstruction is relieved.
   c. Total correction is increasingly being advocated for all infants in whom pulmonary arteries are of sufficient size.

Transposition of the Great Arteries

Transposition of the great arteries occurs when the pulmonary artery originates posteriorly from the left ventricle and the aorta originates anteriorly from the right ventricle. It accounts for 5%–10% of congenital heart defects.

Altered Physiology

1. This defect results in 2 separate circulations; the right heart manages the systemic circulation (unoxygenated) and the left heart manages the pulmonary circulation (oxygenated).
2. To sustain life, there must be an accompanying defect that provides for the mixing of oxygenated and unoxygenated blood between the 2 circulations.
3. The mixing of oxygenated and unoxygenated blood occurs through one or more of the following shunts:
   a. ASD
   b. VSD
   c. PDA
   d. Patent foramen ovale

Clinical Manifestations

Influenced predominantly by the extent of intercirculatory mixing:
1. Cyanosis, usually developing shortly after birth (degree depends on the type of associated malformations)
2. Low Apgar score at birth
3. Fatigability
4. Slow weight gain
5. Clubbing of the fingers and toes
6. Congestive heart failure may coexist, manifested by tachypnea, cardiomegaly, hepatomegaly

Diagnostic Evaluation

1. Auscultation—murmurs may be absent in infancy; may be a murmur of an associated defect
2. Chest x-ray—cardiomegaly, narrow mediastinum, egg-shaped cardiac silhouette, increased vascular markings (decreased vascular markings in children with associated pulmonary stenosis). Neonatal x-ray is often normal.
3. ECG—right axis deviation, right or biventricular hypertrophy. Variable findings depending on age and anatomic factors.
4. Two-dimensional echocardiogram and Doppler study
5. Laboratory tests
   a. Polycythemia
6. Cardiac catheterization
7. MRI
8. Radionuclide angiography

Complications

1. Congestive heart failure
2. Infective endocarditis
3. Brain abscess
4. Cerebral vascular accident (due to thrombosis or severe hypoxia)

Treatment

1. Vigorous medical management of congestive heart failure
2. Palliative procedures
   a. *Rashkind procedure*—the creation of an atrial septal defect with a balloon catheter during cardiac catheterization
   b. *Blalock–Hanlon procedure*—surgical creation of an ASD
   c. Medical use of prostaglandin E to keep PDA open
3. Complete correction
   a. *Mustard procedure*—with cardiopulmonary bypass, the atrial septum is removed and a baffle of Dacron velour and/or pericardium is sutured in place in such a way that the pulmonary venous blood is directed toward the right ventricle and the systemic venous blood is directed toward the left ventricle
   b. *Senning procedure*—with cardiopulmonary bypass, the systemic and pulmonary returns are rerouted by arranging flaps of the interatrial septum and right atrial free wall to form the new venous channels.
   c. *Rastelli procedure*
      (1) Surgery of choice for transposition with ventricular septal defect and left ventricular outflow tract obstruction
      (2) With cardiopulmonary bypass, the ventricular septal defect is closed in such a way that the left ventricle communicates with the aorta. The pulmonary artery is ligated, and the right ventricle is connected to the distal portion of the pulmonary artery by means of a valve-bearing tubular graft.
   d. Recent procedures have been developed for anatomic correction of transposition of the great arteries by direct contraposition of the transposed vessels. This may become the preferred treatment in the future.
   e. As with other types of congenital cardiac surgery, the question of optimum timing for surgery is controversial. Increasingly, total correction is recommended when feasible.

Tricuspid Atresia

Tricuspid atresia is a condition in which there is (1) atresia of the tricuspid valve so that there is no communication between the right atrium and right ventricle, (2) interatrial septal defect (or patent foramen ovale) and (3) a hypoplastic right ventricle.

Pathophysiology

1. Blood from the systemic circulation is shunted from the right atrium through an interatrial communication to the left atrium and then to the left ventricle.
2. Pulmonary blood flow is established either through a PDA, bronchial circulation, or a VSD.

Clinical Manifestations

1. Severe cyanosis in the neonatal period
2. Respiratory distress (exertional dyspnea)
3. Clubbing
4. Hypoxic spells
5. Delayed weight gain
6. Right heart failure (may occur)
7. Easy fatigability

Diagnostic Evaluation

1. Auscultation
   a. Pansystolic murmurs are audible along the left sternal border.
   b. The second heart sound is single.
2. Chest x-ray—patients with diminished pulmonary blood flow have a normal to mildly increased cardiac silhouette, concavity in the region of the main pulmonary artery, and diminished pulmonary vascular markings; those with increased pulmonary flow have cardiac enlargement and plethoric pulmonary vasculature (less common)
3. ECG—right atrial, left atrial, left ventricular hypertrophy, left axis deviation
4. Two-dimensional echocardiogram—demonstrates diminutive right ventricular chamber and no tricuspid valve
5. Cardiac catheterization
6. Angiocardiography
7. Laboratory assessment:
   a. Polycythemia

Complications

1. Cerebral vascular accident
2. Brain abscess
3. Bacterial endocarditis

Treatment

1. Palliative procedures to increase pulmonary blood flow:
   a. *Waterston shunt*—anastomosis between the ascending aorta and right pulmonary artery
   b. *Glenn procedure*—side-to-end anastomosis of the superior vena cava to the right pulmonary artery
   c. *Blalock–Taussig shunt*—subclavian to pulmonary artery anastomosis

d. Infusion of prostaglandin E to maintain patency of ductus arteriosus

2. Complete correction:
   a. *Fontan procedure*—involves placement of a tubular conduit with a valve between the right atrium and main pulmonary artery. The atrial defect is closed and the main pulmonary artery is ligated just above the pulmonary valve.
   b. Has been done successfully in a limited number of older, symptomatic patients with diminished blood flow

Aortic Valve/Hypoplastic Left Heart Syndrome

Hypoplastic left heart syndrome is a condition in which there is (1) mitral atresia or stenosis; (2) a diminutive or absent left ventricle; and (3) failure of the aortic valve to develop resulting in aortic atresia, a severe hypoplastic ascending aorta, and aortic arch.

Pathophysiology

1. The left ventricle is not functional.
2. The right ventricle has to pump blood through both pulmonary and systemic circulations.
3. A patent foramen ovale allows a left-to-right shunt, as blood is shunted from the left atrium back to the right atrium.
4. A PDA is the sole supply of blood to the system until it begins to close.

Clinical Manifestations

1. May appear normal at birth; signs increase shortly afterward
2. Congestive heart failure
3. Dyspnea
4. Hepatomegaly
5. Low cardiac output
   a. Pallor; mild to moderate cyanosis
   b. Weak peripheral pulses
   c. Decreased blood pressure

Diagnostic Evaluation

1. Auscultation
   a. Nondescript systolic murmur
   b. Single second sound representing closure of only the pulmonary valve
2. Chest x-ray—cardiomegaly and increased pulmonary vascularity
3. Echocardiography—increased right atrium and right ventricle, a diminutive left ventricle, and a poorly functioning or absent mitral valve

Complications

1. Shock
2. Death in over half of the cases in the first few months of life

Treatment

1. Prostaglandin E infusion to maintain patency of ductus arteriosus until surgery
2. Fontan surgical procedure
   (Right atrium is anastomosed to the pulmonary artery

and the left atrium communicates with the tricuspid valve)

3. Cardiac transplantation has been tried in a few infants.

Treatment and Nursing Management of the Child With a Congenital Heart Defect

Nursing Process Overview

Nursing Assessment

A. Become Informed About the Child's Symptomatology and the Plan of Medical Care.

1. Obtain a thorough nursing history to become familiar with the child and his family to recognize normal and abnormal patterns (color, respirations, murmur; feeding schedule, amount, and method; skin temperature of the extremities; exercise tolerance, etc.).
2. Discuss with the physician the plan for medical care.

B. Make a Baseline Nursing Assessment of the Child's Condition.

1. Observe and record information relevant to the child's growth and development (motor coordination, muscular development, cognitive abilities, psychosocial skills).
   a. Compare data with that for siblings, other family members, and children of the same chronological age.
   b. Plot appropriate information on growth chart.
2. Observe and record the child's level of exercise tolerance.
   a. Observe the child at play:
      Is play interrupted to rest?
      How does he play as compared with his peers?
      Does he squat during play? (Squatting is a characteristic position a cyanotic child assumes when resting after exertion.)
   b. Observe infants while feeding.
      Does the infant stop feeding to rest, or does he fall asleep during feeding? Assess pulse and respiratory rate of children during feedings.
3. Observe the child's skin and mucous membranes for color and temperature changes.
   a. Skin
      Color changes vary from pink, dusky, mottled, to cyanotic.
      Earlobes are good indicators of the degree of oxygen saturation.
      Circumoral cyanosis occurs with oxygen deprivation.
      Nailbeds are good indicators of color change.
   b. Mucous membranes
      Lips and tongue indicate color change because they are very vascular areas and contain superficial blood vessels; mucous membranes are the best places to observe for cyanosis.
   c. Extremities
      Are extremities cool? Is there a difference between upper and lower extremities?
      Check quality of pulses in all four extremities.
      Check edema in extremities.

d. Record where cyanosis was observed (localized or generalized), when it was observed and the duration (continuous or intermittent, whether variable with exercise).
4. Observe for clubbing (rounding) of the fingers, especially the thumbnails, with thickening and shininess of the terminal phalanges—may occur in cyanotic children by 2–3 months of age.
5. Observe for chest deformities.
   a. Visible pulsations
   b. Left- or right-sided prominence
6. Observe respiratory pattern.
   a. Remove any clothing or covers which obscure visualization of the chest.
   b. Count respirations for at least 30 seconds.
   c. Count respirations while a child is at rest; if unable to soothe the child, document that he is crying, irritable, etc.
   d. Observe for increased respiratory rate, grunting, retractions, nasal flaring, irregularity of respirations.
   e. Record all signs of respiratory distress including change from usual pattern, when it occurred, duration, etc.
   f. Ascultate for crackles, rhonchi, stridor, congestion, etc.
   g. Assess quality of the cry.
7. Palpate the child's pulses in all extremities.
   a. Radial or dorsalis pedis is difficult to feel in the newborn.
   b. Femoral pulsations are easily felt in the inguinal region and can be compared with brachial pulsations.
   c. Record the strength of the pulse (full, bounding, weak, or faint).
   d. When a pulse is difficult to locate, mark its location with a pen to facilitate locating it the next time.
8. Auscultate the child's heart:
   a. Count apical pulse rate for 1 full minute
   b. Determine cardiac rhythm or change in rhythm
   c. Become familiar with a known murmur
   d. Determine the presence of new murmurs
9. Record vital signs (apical pulse, blood pressure, respirations).
   a. Have child quiet for baseline vital signs
   b. Record quality and quantity of pulse and blood pressure in all extremities.
   c. Record which extremity is used for blood pressure measurement.
   d. Refer to vital sign procedure (see p. 1140).

Note: Make sure that blood pressure cuff is the appropriate size for the child—either 1.5 times the diameter of the extremity being used or "no less than ½ and no more than ⅔" of the part of the extremity being used.

Patient Problems and Nursing Diagnoses

1. Impaired gas exchange related to altered pulmonary blood flow or oxygen deprivation
2. Altered cardiac output related to the specific anatomic defect
3. Activity intolerance related to decreased oxygenation in blood and tissues
4. Fluid volume excess with congestive heart failure
5. Altered nutrition: less than body requirement related to the excessive energy demands required by increased cardiac workload

6. Increased potential for infection related to congestive heart failure and poor nutritional status
7. Anxiety related to diagnostic procedures and hospitalization
8. Developmental delay related to decreased energy, inadequate nutrition, physical limitations, and social isolation
9. Alteration in parenting, (overprotection, lack of discipline) related to parental perception of the child as vulnerable

Nursing Interventions

A. Provide Adequate Nutritional and Fluid Intake to Maintain the Growth and Developmental Needs of the Child.

1. Feed slowly in a semierect position; burp infants after each ounce to decrease compression of stomach on heart and lungs.
2. Use soft nipples with large holes which make it easier for the infant to suck.
3. Provide small, frequent feedings; provide foods easy to chew and digest.
4. Feeding should generally be completed within 45 minutes or sooner if the infant tires.
5. Provide foods that have high nutritional value.
   a. Add needed calories for healing.
   b. Check iron and potassium levels; provide foods high in iron and potassium if needed.
6. Determine the child's likes and dislikes and plan meals with the dietitian, taking into consideration the child's preferences.
7. Observe the child at mealtime; does a poor appetite represent a lack of interest in food, or does the child become fatigued while eating?
8. Report vomiting and specify the amount, type, and relationship to feeding or to medications.
9. Report diarrhea and specify type and amount.
10. Maintain adequate hydration in the cyanotic child when he is vomiting, has diarrhea or fever, or is exposed to high environmental temperatures since polycythemia predisposes him to thrombosis.
11. Dyspnea and tachycardia during feedings may result in the need for nasogastric feedings.
12. Strict intake and output
13. Maintain ordered low sodium and/or fluid restriction in children with congestive heart failure.
14. Daily weight (same scale, same time of day, same attire) to check fluid retention/diuresis or physical growth

B. Prevent Infection.

1. Prevent exposure to communicable disease, including exposure to children with upper respiratory infections, diarrhea, wound infections, etc.
2. Check with the parents to be certain the child's immunizations are up to date.
3. Practice careful handwashing technique and teach this to the child.
4. Report temperature elevation, diarrhea, vomiting, and upper respiratory symptoms promptly; use axillary temperature.
5. Be certain that the child receives prophylactic medication for infective endocarditis before genitourinary instrumentation or dental work (refer to American Heart Association recommendations).
6. Prevent cold stress.

C. Reduce the Work Load of the Heart Since Decreased Activity and Expenditure of Energy Will Decrease Oxygen Requirements.

1. Organize nursing care to provide periods of uninterrupted rest.
2. Avoid unnecessary activities such as frequent, complete baths and clothing changes; avoid excessive handling.
3. Prevent excessive crying; anticipate needs.
    a. Use pacifier.
    b. Hold the infant.
    c. Feed when hungry.
    d. Keep the infant comfortable.
4. Explain to the child the need for rest.
5. Provide diversional activities that require limited expenditures of energy; provide passive play.
6. Avoid discussing the child's condition or the condition of other children in the presence of the patient to prevent unnecessary anxiety.
7. Avoid temperature excesses; maintain warmth.
8. Prevent constipation.

D. Relieve the Respiratory Distress Associated With Increased Pulmonary Blood Flow or Oxygen Deprivation.

1. Determine the degree of respiratory distress.
    a. Infants—respirations greater than 60/minute are indicative of respiratory difficulty.
    b. Young children—respirations greater than 40/minute are indicative of respiratory difficulty.
    c. Observe the regularity of the respiratory pattern.
    d. Observe for retractions (drawing in of soft tissue in the rib interspaces, below the costal margin, or above and below the sternum with each inspiration; may be barely visible, mild or severe).
    e. Observe for nasal flaring; listen for grunting.
2. Include specific information in nursing record.
    a. Number of respirations per minute
    b. Regularity of respirations
    c. Type and severity of retractions
    d. Presence of nasal flaring, grunting
    e. Response to oxygen therapy
    f. Response to positioning
    g. Color changes
    h. Irritability or anxiety observed
3. Position the child at a 45° angle (orthopnic position) to decrease pressure of the viscera on the diaphragm and increase lung volume.
    a. Infant—(depends on the child) place in an infant seat or prone, propped on knees
    b. Children—elevate head of the bed and support the arms with pillows
4. Pin diapers loosely; provide loose-fitting pajamas for older children.
5. Feed slowly, allowing frequent rest periods.
    a. Rapid respirations and frequent coughing predispose the child to aspiration.
    b. May require gavage feeding
    c. Observe for abdominal distention which may increase respiratory difficulty.
6. Tilt the infant's or child's head back slightly.
7. Suction the nose and throat if the child is unable to adequately cough up secretions.
8. Provide oxygen therapy as indicated.

E. Improve Oxygenation so That Body Functions May be Maintained.

1. Provide a safe, effective oxygen environment (refer to procedure on oxygen therapy, p. 1193).

2. Explain to the child how oxygen will help; orient him to equipment before it is used on him (e.g., tent, mask).
3. Observe the child's response to oxygen therapy.
    a. Improvement of color
    b. Change in rate and character of respiration
    c. Change in anxiety level
4. Observe the child's response while he is being weaned from oxygen.
   Reduce liter flow gradually and observe response after each reduction.
   Measure oxygen saturation with pulse oximeter.
5. Measures that are directed to relieve respiratory distress will aid in improving oxygenation.

F. Relieve the Hypoxic Spells Associated With Cyanotic Types of Congenital Heart Disease (Primarily Tetralogy of Fallot).

1. Observe for hypoxic spells/"tet" spells (attacks of acute oxygen deprivation), characterized by:
    a. Increased rate and depth of respiration
    b. Increasing cyanosis
    c. Murmur that becomes less intense, may disappear
    d. Bradycardia
    e. Progressive limpness and syncope
    f. The possibility of convulsions
2. Be aware that these attacks frequently occur in the morning after awakening from sleep, during or after crying, during or after defecation, or during or immediately following feeding.
3. Once an attack is recognized, call for assistance and immediately:
    a. Place child in knee-chest position with head of bed elevated.
    b. Administer oxygen by mask.
    c. Be prepared to administer medications as prescribed.
       Morphine sulfate
       $NaHCO_3$ to correct acidosis
       Propranolol
    d. Assume a calm, reassuring attitude.
4. Observe the child closely following recovery from an attack. Encourage fluid intake.
5. Record observations in the following areas:
    a. Condition and activity before the attack
    b. Response to positioning and medication
    c. Vital signs during and after attack
6. Do not disturb a child who assumes a "squatting" position; if he does not appear to be in distress, merely observe and note his positioning.

G. Observe the Child for Symptoms of Congestive Heart Failure That Occur Frequently as a Complication of Congenital Heart Disease. (For nursing management, refer to section on congestive heart failure, p. 1322)

1. Respiratory distress (tachypnea, retractions, nasal flaring, grunting, voice changes)
2. Tachycardia, gallop heart rhythm
3. Fatigue (as evidenced by poor feeding in infants)
4. Edema
   Periorbital edema is often observed in infants; older children develop swelling of the hands and feet.
5. Weight gain
6. Irritability
7. Sweating
8. Liver enlargement
9. Splenomegaly

10. Orthopnea
11. Neck vein distention (rarely seen in infants)
12. Murmurs (may appear, or the characteristics of previously heard murmur may change)
13. Cyanosis (may occur)
14. Pulmonary crackles (may occur)

H. Observe for the Development of Symptoms of Infective Endocarditis That May Occur as a Complication of Congenital Heart Disease.

1. Be aware of the symptoms of infective endocarditis.
   a. Spiking fever
   b. Petechiae
   c. Anorexia
   d. Pallor
   e. Fatigue
2. Be aware of the need for infective endocarditis prophylaxis for selected children undergoing surgery, dental work, and laceration repair.
3. For nursing management, refer to section on infective endocarditis, p. 1330.

I. Observe for the Development of Thrombosis That may Occur as a Complication of Cyanotic Heart Disease.

1. Be aware of the signs and symptoms of thrombosis:
   a. Irritability and restlessness
   b. Convulsion, coma, neurological signs
   c. Paralysis
   d. Rapid onset of edema
   e. Anuria, oliguria, hematuria
2. Be aware that thrombosis is more likely to occur during phases of acute dehydration, fever, and vomiting.

J. Prepare the Child for Diagnostic and Treatment Procedures.

1. Explain to the child what is going to be done in simple terms (refer to section on hospitalized child, p. 1120).
2. Encourage the child to express his fears and fantasies verbally or through play.
3. Diagnostic procedures may include:
   a. ECG
   b. MRI
   c. Echocardiogram with Doppler probe
   d. Chest x-ray
   e. Barium swallow
   f. Cardiac catheterization and angiocardiography
   g. Complete blood count
   h. Platelet count
   i. Blood gases

K. Explain the Cardiac Problem to Child and Parents.

1. Discuss with the parents the importance of being truthful with the child about his heart condition.
2. The time to tell the child is generally when the child begins asking questions as to why he visits the doctor so frequently and why the doctor listens to his heart so closely.
3. The child's questions should be answered truthfully in a simple way.
4. Clarify misconceptions.
5. Support positive coping mechanisms.

L. Refer the Family to Appropriate Resources Concerned With the Financial and/or Emotional Aspects of Caring for a Child With Congenital Heart Disease.

1. Social worker
2. Crippled children's program
3. Parents and organized parent groups
4. American Heart Association

Health Education

1. Instruct the family in necessary measures to maintain the child's health:
   a. Complete immunization
   b. Adequate diet and rest
   c. Prevention and control of infections
   d. Regular medical and dental checkup
      The child should be protected against infective endocarditis when undergoing certain dental procedures (refer to American Heart Association Protocol).
   e. Regular cardiac checkups
2. Teach the family about the defect and its treatment.
   a. Pathophysiology and natural history
   b. Signs and symptoms of disease progress
   c. Signs and symptoms of complications
   d. Signs of infection, dehydration
   e. Medications and side effects
   f. Special diets
   g. Emergency precautions related to hypoxic attacks, pulmonary edema, cardiac arrest (if appropriate)
3. Encourage the parents and other persons (teachers, peers, etc.) to treat the child in as normal a manner as possible.
   a. Avoid overprotection and overindulgence.
   b. Avoid rejection.
   c. Promote growth and development with modifications.
      Facilitate performance of the usual developmental tasks within the limits of the child's physiologic state.
      With most congenital cardiac defects it is not necessary to restrict the child's activity; the child will rest when he becomes tired and then will resume his play.
   d. Prevent adults from projecting their fears and anxieties onto the child.
   e. Help family deal with their anger, guilt, and concerns related to their disabled child.
4. Initiate a community health nursing referral if indicated.

Expected Outcomes

1. The child breathes with little or no difficulty as evidenced by decreased respiratory rate, increased regularity of breathing, and decreased retractions and grunting.
2. Maintains adequate or improved oxygenation as evidenced by normal color, decreased cyanosis, and improved blood gases.
3. Demonstrates adequate weight gain according to his normal curve
4. Remains free of infections (normal temperature) or receives prompt treatment if fever occurs
5. Effectively expresses his thoughts and fears about his illness and hospitalizations either verbally or through play
6. Achieves age-appropriate developmental milestones
7. The parents encourage and promote the child's normal development.
8. The parents accurately explain the child's diagnosis and treatment, administer prescribed therapies, and recognize and report changes in the child's condition, signs of complications, and side effects of medications.

Congestive Heart Failure

Congestive heart failure occurs when the cardiac output is inadequate to meet the metabolic demands of the body and results in accumulation of excessive blood volume in the pulmonary and/or systemic venous system.

Etiology

1. Congenital heart disease, especially left-to-right shunts (primary cause in the first 3 years of life)
2. Acquired heart disease—rheumatic heart disease, endocarditis, myocarditis
3. Noncardiovascular causes—acidosis, pulmonary disease, various metabolic diseases

Altered Physiology

1. For any number of reasons, cardiac output is inadequate to meet the oxygenation and nutritional requirements of vital organs.
2. Various compensatory mechanisms occur.
   a. Stroke volume increases and cardiomegaly develops.
   b. Tachycardia occurs in an effort to maintain adequate stroke volume.
   c. Catecholamines are released by the sympathetic venous system that increase systemic vascular resistance and venous tone and decrease cutaneous, splanchnic, and renal blood flow.
   d. Glomerular filtration decreases, and tubular reabsorption increases, causing diminished urinary output and sodium retention.
   e. Diaphoresis occurs.
3. Cardiac output decreases further as compensatory mechanisms fail.
4. The pulmonary vascular bed is not emptied efficiently, causing engorgement of the pulmonic system with subsequent pulmonary hypertension and edema.
5. There is diminished blood return to the heart, with venous congestion and a rise in venous pressure.

Complications

1. Respiratory infections
2. Pulmonary edema
3. Intractable congestive heart failure
4. Myocardial failure

Assessment

1. Dyspnea and tachypnea
2. Tachycardia
3. Orthopnea
4. Nonproductive, irritative cough
5. Peripheral edema—often scrotal or periorbital related to rising venous pressure
6. Neck vein distention
7. Weight gain
8. Restlessness
9. Easy fatigability
10. Weak cry
11. Feeding difficulties, anorexia
12. Pallor
13. Diaphoresis or decreased urinary output
14. Growth failure
15. Hepatomegaly/abdominal discomfort

Diagnostic Evaluation

1. Palpation
   a. May have weak peripheral pulses
   b. Hepatomegaly (feature of right heart failure) related to blood backing up in venous system
   c. Abnormal precordial activity may occur.
2. Auscultation
   a. Gallop rhythm (frequent)
   b. Cardiac murmurs may or may not be present
   c. Crackles (infrequent in infants)
3. Chest x-rays—cardiomegaly; pulmonary congestion
4. Laboratory data:
   a. Dilutional hyponatremia
   b. Hypochloremia
   c. Hyperkalemia

Patient Problems and Nursing Diagnoses

1. Decreased cardiac output related to the specific anatomic defect
2. Fluid volume excess related to the inability of the heart to pump blood from the ventricle(s), and decreased blood flow to the kidney
3. Impaired gas exchange related to pulmonary engorgement
4. Activity intolerance related to fatigue
5. Growth failure related to general weakened state
6. Altered nutrition: less than body requirements related to decreased energy for feeding
7. Anxiety of child or parent related to their perception(s) of the child's condition and potential for death
8. Knowledge deficit about congestive heart failure and its treatment

Nursing Interventions

A. Improve Myocardial Efficiency.

1. Administer digoxin as prescribed by the physician.
   a. Carefully calculate dosage *DAILY* based on child's daily weight; digoxin is given to infants and children in very small amounts.
   b. Count apical pulse for 1 full minute before administering.
      Be aware of the heart rate at which the physician wants the medication withheld (usually 90–100 for infants and 70 for older children).
   c. Report vomiting, which may occur following administration of digoxin, to determine if physician desires dose to be repeated.
   d. Observe for the development of premature ventricular contractions when digoxin is initially started; report this to physician.
   e. Be aware of signs of digitalis intoxication.
      (1) Decreased appetite
      (2) Bradycardia
      (3) Dysrhythmias
      (4) Gastrointestinal symptoms
      (5) Altered emotional status, "digitalis blues" (not as evident in young children)

B. Reduce Energy Requirements.

1. Organize nursing care to provide periods of uninterrupted rest.
2. Avoid unnecessary activities such as frequent complete baths and clothing changes.
3. Prevent excessive crying; anticipate needs.
   a. Use pacifier.
   b. Hold baby.

c. Eliminate sources of distress (e.g., hunger, wet diapers).
4. Explain to the child the need for rest.
5. Provide diversional activities that require limited expenditure of energy.
6. Provide small frequent meals with foods easy to chew and digest.
7. Avoid constipation.

C. Remove Accumulated Sodium and Fluid.

1. Administer diuretics as prescribed by the physician.
   a. Be aware of the side effects of the prescribed medication.
   b. Weigh the child at least daily to observe response (same time of day, same scale, same attire).
   c. Maintain an accurate record of intake and output. Record urine specific gravity.
   d. Encourage foods such as bananas and orange juice that have a high potassium content to prevent potassium depletion associated with many diuretics.
      (1) Hypokalemia may cause weakened myocardial contractions and may precipitate digoxin toxicity.
      (2) Oral potassium supplements may be indicated when a child is on diuretics for an extended period of time.
2. Restrict sodium intake
   a. The child may be placed on a low-sodium diet.
   b. Be aware of the prescribed diet and the amount of sodium in foods and fluids offered to the child.
   c. Question the child about his likes and dislikes so that the diet can be made as appealing as possible.
   d. Interpret the diet and its purpose to the child and his parents.
   e. Infants may require low-sodium formulas.
3. Fluid restriction
   a. Check child's tray, as dietary does not measure fluids.
   b. Remember to count fluids used for medication administration in intake.
   c. Do not leave fluids at the bedside.
   d. Put fluids in small cups to make them appear more than they are.

D. Relieve the Respiratory Distress Associated With Pulmonary Engorgement.

Refer to section on Congenital Heart Disease, p. 1311.

E. Improve Tissue Oxygenation.

1. Administer oxygen therapy—refer to procedure, pp. 1193–1196.
2. Maintain the infant in a neutral thermal environment.
3. Elevate head of bed.
4. Do not use constricting clothing.

F. Provide Adequate Nutrition to Meet the Caloric Requirements of the Child.

1. Provide foods that the child enjoys in small amounts, because he may have a poor appetite due to liver enlargement.
2. Infant feeding:
   a. Feed frequently in small amounts.
   b. Feed slowly in a sitting position, allowing frequent rest periods.
   c. Supplement oral feedings with gavage feeding if the infant is unable to take an adequate amount of formula by mouth.
   d. Record the amount of formula taken.
   e. Place the child in an infant seat following feeding to prevent pressure of the viscera on the diaphragm.
   f. Observe for distention and vomiting following feeding.

G. Decrease the Danger of Infection.

1. Practice careful handwashing technique.
2. Avoid exposure to other children with upper respiratory infections, diarrhea, etc.
3. Report changes such as temperature elevation, diarrhea, vomiting, and upper respiratory symptoms promptly.

H. Observe for Signs of Disease Progress or Response to Treatment.

1. Record and report in detail presence or disappearance of signs and symptoms.
2. Monitor vital signs frequently and report any significant changes.

I. Explain the Condition and Treatment to the Child and Family.

1. Use terminology that the child and parents can understand.
2. Correct misinterpretations—parents and children frequently interpret congestive heart failure to be synonymous with myocardial infarction, or they may fear that the heart is about to stop beating.

Health Education

1. Describe symptoms to be aware of and to be reported.
2. Teach the family how to administer medications and about the side effects.
3. Explain dietary and/or activity restrictions.
4. Explain methods to prevent infection.
5. Initiate a community health nursing referral if indicated.

Expected Outcomes

1. The child achieves improved cardiac output, evidenced by his clinical condition and laboratory measurements.
2. Achieves and maintains fluid and electrolyte balance, evidenced by decreased edema and laboratory measurements
3. Maintains or improves oxygenation, evidenced by normal color, decreased cyanosis, and improved blood gas values
4. Conserves energy and rest in accordance with needs
5. Achieves normal growth pattern as evidenced by weight, height, and developmental tasks
6. Maintains adequate nutritional intake
7. The parents discuss their concerns about the child's condition with one another.
8. The parents accurately describe congestive heart failure and its treatment, correctly administer digoxin and diuretics, and recognize signs and symptoms of complications.

Nursing Care of the Child Undergoing Cardiac Catheterization

Cardiac catheterization involves introducing a radiopaque catheter into a vein or artery in the groin or in the arm, either percutaneously or by means of a cutdown. The catheter is advanced into the cardiac chambers and vessels, where pressures are measured and samples for oxygen concentration are obtained. The procedure is usually done in conjunction with angiography, the injection of radiopaque material into various chambers of the heart.

Purposes

1. To establish diagnosis of a cardiovascular defect
2. To identify the severity of the defect
3. To evaluate the effects of the defect on cardiovascular function

Complications

1. Dysrhythmias
2. Hemorrhage
3. Arterial blockage
4. Infection
5. Allergic reaction to the dye

Preoperative Nursing Interventions

A. Prepare the Child and Parents for the Procedure.

1. Reinforce explanations of the procedure to the child and parents.
   a. Provide specific information about:
      (1) Time of the test
      (2) Preparation for the procedure (NPO, sedation, etc.)
      (3) Site of the venipuncture (if known)
      (4) What the child will see (atmosphere of the catheterization room)
      (5) What will be expected of the child during the procedure
      (6) Routines after the procedure
   b. Detail, length, and timing of explanations should be appropriate to the child's age and level of cognitive development.
      (1) Photographs or a miniature replica of the cardiac laboratory and equipment may facilitate understanding of explanations.
      (2) Older children and parents may benefit from an opportunity to see the room where the procedure will be done.
      (3) It is helpful for some children to handle the mask and other equipment that will be used.
      (4) Describe sensations with careful choice of words and with appropriate timing based on the age of the child.
          With injection of the dye, child may experience warmth, nausea, headache, restlessness, and chest pains.
      (5) In preparing the child, do not use the word "dye" for the injectable substance; use "special medicine."
   c. Parents should be provided with an opportunity for private discussion of the anticipated procedure.
2. Maintain adequate hydration (especially important for children with cyanotic heart disease).
   Offer fluids just prior to NPO period.
3. Cleanse proposed catheterization site thoroughly. Clean fingernails and/or toenails.
4. Obtain baseline set of vital signs just prior to the time of catheterization.
   a. Blood pressure in all four extremities
   b. Color and temperature of all extremities
   c. Activity level of child
   d. Child's weight

   e. Quality of pulses in all extremities
   f. Baseline oximetry level
5. Administer sedation if prescribed.
   a. Raise and secure side rails after the child has been medicated.
   b. Observe the child closely for depressed respirations.

Postoperative Nursing Interventions

A. Observe for and Prevent Postoperative Complications.

1. Monitor vital signs frequently and report:
   a. Sudden drop in blood pressure
   b. Changes in pulse rate or rhythm
   c. Increased or depressed respirations
   d. Faintness, weakness
   e. Elevated temperature
   f. Decreased temperature in the extremity used for the catheterization
   g. Hemorrhage or hematoma at the injection site
   h. Inflammation at the site or other signs of infection
2. Observe for complications resulting from damage to the vessels through which the catheter was passed.
   a. Check the dressing or puncture site for bleeding.
   b. Observe site for redness, swelling, pain, or induration.
   c. Observe for numbness, pallor, decreased temperature, decreased motion, cyanosis, or mottling of affected extremity.
   d. Palpate pulses in affected extremity and compare with pulses in the opposite extremity.
3. Keep the child warm to avoid the risk of hypothermia. This is especially important for small infants and children who may already be hypoxic because of their cardiac condition.
4. Maintain the child in a reclining position for several hours after catheterization to avoid:
   a. Possibility of sudden drop in blood pressure that may accompany an abrupt assumption of an upright position
   b. Bleeding at the site of catheter entry
5. Offer fluids as soon as the child is able to take them to avoid dehydration.
   This is especially important for cyanotic children who are polycythemic and prone to thrombus formation.
6. Make security objects and favorite toys available to child in recovery room.

B. Prepare the Child and Parents for Discharge.

1. Reinforce discharge information. Parents should be informed about:
   a. Care of the incision, puncture site
   b. Dressing change (if any)
   c. Activity limitations (if any)
   d. Observation for and reporting of late complications (especially infection)
   e. Follow-up medical care
2. If the child is a candidate for surgery, use appropriate opportunities to prepare him and his family for the experience.
   a. Encourage contact with children who are convalescing from surgery.
   b. Answer immediate questions of the parents.

Cardiac Surgery

Generally, nursing care of children who require cardiac surgery is the same as that of adults (refer to pp. 353–358).

In addition, the following considerations should be kept in mind by the nurse who works with pediatric patients.

Preoperative Nursing Interventions

A. Prepare the Parents for the Experience Prior to the Day of Admission for Surgery.

1. Parents frequently ask questions about:
   a. What to tell the child
   b. When to begin preparation
   c. What to bring to the hospital
   d. Anticipated sequence of events
   e. Separation—rooming-in, whether or not to leave at night, etc.
2. Use opportunities for teaching—physician's office, catheterization episode, puppet shows, telephone calls, contact with other patients.
3. Teaching is based on the child's age: Be honest.
4. Encourage young children to bring special toys (e.g., baby blanket or stuffed toys) to the hospital with them.

B. Prepare the Child for What He Will Experience During Hospitalization.

1. Consult with the parents prior to beginning explanation. Their desires regarding how much information to give the child should be respected, and they should be active participants in preparation of the child.
2. Most children need information about:
   a. Preparation for surgery:
      (1) Diagnostic tests
      (2) Antibacterial skin preparation or baths
      (3) NPO period
      (4) Injections—antimicrobials and/or sedatives
      (5) Time of the surgery
      (6) Transportation to the operating room
      (7) Sensation in the operating room (sounds, temperature, colors, dress and masks worn by OR staff)
   b. Postoperative expectations:
      (1) Incision (location)
      (2) Chest tube
      (3) Dressings
      (4) Nasogastric tube
      (5) IVs
      (6) Monitors
      (7) Endotracheal tube, ventilator
      (8) Suctioning
      (9) Oxygen equipment
      (10) Pain (ability to relieve)
      (11) Restraints
      (12) Bed scale (may fantasize that it is a stretcher to return child to the OR)
      (13) Appearance of intensive care unit; visiting regulations for parents
3. Have the child practice coughing and deep-breathing exercises (see Procedure, p. 1187).
4. Detail, length, and time of explanations should be appropriate to the child's age and level of cognitive development.
   a. Photographs or a miniature replica of the intensive care unit may facilitate understanding of explanations.
   b. Older children and parents often benefit from an opportunity to see the intensive care unit.
   c. It is helpful for some children to have an opportunity to manipulate some of the equipment that will be used.
      (1) Try on mask, OR cap, sterile gloves, and scrub suit

      (2) Experience blood pressure cuff, oxygen mask, cardiac leads
   d. Use a model of the heart to explain what will be done.
   e. Demonstrate on a doll the site of the incision, dressings, and tubes.
5. Test the child's comprehension of teaching by asking him simple questions, having him place equipment on a doll, demonstrating coughing and deep breathing, and other similar activities.
6. Allow opportunity for the child to express his concerns, either verbally or in play situations.

C. Provide Opportunity for Private Discussions With the Parents About the Anticipated Surgery.

1. Parents need the same type of information as their child. They also need information about the following:
   a. Scheduled time of surgery
   b. Whether or not they can accompany their child to the operating room
   c. Waiting area
   d. Usual length of surgery
   e. Intensive care unit expectations and policies
2. Provide emotional support to the parents and answer their questions so that they are in the best position to support their child.
   a. The parents may need help dealing with guilt feelings that they had a role in causing the disease, that they did not seek medical advice soon enough, etc.
   b. Parents frequently have fears that the child will suffer excessive pain or die.
   c. Parents may ask technical questions relating to such matters as the heart–lung machine, and the type of material used for patching defects.

D. Make Baseline Assessments That are Essential in Planning Postoperative Care:

1. Height and weight
2. Vital signs
3. Sleep/wake patterns
4. Elimination patterns and toileting words
5. Normal intake and special feeding routines

E. Observe for Any Indications That Surgery May Need to be Cancelled.

1. Signs of infection or inflammation (upper respiratory infection, hoarseness, elevated temperature, vomiting, diarrhea, skin lesions, etc.).
2. Congestive heart failure (see p. 1322)
3. Anemia (see p. 1298)

F. Perform Appropriate Nursing Activities Associated With Congenital Heart Disease (see p. 1318).

Immediate Postoperative Nursing Interventions

A. Ensure Continuity of Care.

1. Send the nursing history and care plan to the intensive care unit and relay information about the child and family to appropriate personnel.

B. Provide Safe Physical Care to the Child.

C. Observe the Child for Complications and Implement Nursing Measures.

1. Be aware of general complications that may arise and implement appropriate nursing measures.
   a. Respiratory distress
      (1) Provide oxygen by nasal cannula or tent.

(2) Do chest percussion and postural drainage, if ordered.

(3) Assess chest tubes.

(4) Minimal deep suctioning to avoid vagal stimulation and laryngospasm

b. Overwork of the heart

(1) Provide rest; organize care.

(2) Decrease stress.

(3) Decrease pain; initially medicate on a regular schedule and not PRN.

(4) Provide passive stimulation.

c. Fluid overload

(1) Monitor intake and output.

(2) Monitor specific gravity and reducing substances in urine.

(3) Monitor chest tube drainage.

d. Hemorrhage related to increased anticoagulants used while on heart–lung machine

(1) Monitor blood loss from all orifices and wounds.

(2) Handle gently.

e. Acid–base imbalance

2. Be aware of specific complications that may occur following surgery for congenital heart disease.

a. PDA (rare)
Laryngeal nerve damage
Phrenic nerve damage
Diaphragmatic paralysis

b. Coarctation of the aorta
Paradoxical hypertension
Abdominal pain, distention
Aneurysm at synthetic patch site
Bacterial endocarditis

c. ASD
(1) Atrial dysrhythmias
(2) Transient or permanent heart block
(3) Left ventricular failure

d. VSD
(1) Conduction disturbance; complete heart block
(2) Residual VSD
(3) Impaired cardiac output

e. Tetralogy of Fallot
(1) Low cardiac output
(2) Rhythm disturbances
(3) Complete heart block
(4) Residual VSD

f. Transposition of great arteries (Mustard procedure)
(1) Dysrhythmias
(2) Low cardiac output
(3) Hemorrhage leading to cardiac tamponade

g. Aortic stenosis
Aortic insufficiency
Altered renal function
Endocarditis

h. Tricuspid atresia status post-Fontan procedure
(1) Increased pulmonary vascular resistance resulting in decreased pulmonary blood flow
(2) Systemic venous hypertension
(3) Dysrhythmias and heart block
(4) Left ventricular dysfunction

i. Hypoplastic left heart
(1) Altered pulmonary flow
(2) Hemorrhage

D. Provide Emotional Support to the Parents.

1. Support the parents during the time that the child is in the intensive care unit.

a. Accompany the parents when they first visit their child following surgery. Since this may be traumatic, do not force them to maintain lengthy contact with the child.

b. Address parental concerns and answer questions such as:

(1) How they should react to their child

(2) Amount of parental participation that is beneficial

(3) Fears and fantasies during lengthy periods when they are unable to visit child

(4) Concern for other children and families

(5) Technical questions

c. Provide the parents with the telephone number of the intensive care unit if they elect to leave.

d. Make certain that parents have a comfortable place to sleep if they elect to stay at the hospital.

e. Reassure the parents that it is normal for children to regress following such extensive surgery.

Convalescent Nursing Interventions

A. Observe for Late Complications.

1. Respiratory (atelectasis, pneumothorax, pulmonary edema)

a. Continue coughing and deep-breathing exercises.

b. Ambulate child as tolerated.

c. Note changes in the character of respirations, dyspnea, chest pain, tachycardia, and cyanosis.

2. Infection, especially bacterial endocarditis

a. Monitor temperature at regular intervals.

b. Observe incision(s) for redness, swelling, drainage.

c. Prophylactic antibiotics may be needed prior to dental procedures.

3. Congestive heart failure
See Nursing Interventions, pp. 1322–1323.

4. Hematologic

a. Anemia and thrombocytopenia related to hemorrhage and trauma by heart–lung machine

5. Infective endocarditis (see p. 1330)

B. Provide Emotional Support to the Child and Parents:

1. Explain procedures, medications, special diet to the child and parents.

2. Encourage the child to attend to his personal needs as he is able.

3. Allow the child to make some decisions to give him a feeling of control.

4. Provide the child with appropriate diversion and play materials.

5. Encourage parental participation in the child's care.

a. Teach the parents those aspects of the child's care that they can assume (e.g., coughing and breathing exercises).

b. Discuss usual convalescent expectations of patient with parents (e.g., fatigue, itching at incision, emotional reactions).

C. Prepare the Child and Parents for Discharge.

1. Active parental participation in the child's care facilitates discharge teaching.

2. Provide the family with oral and written discharge recommendations including:

a. Activity restrictions

b. Care of incision

c. Medications—exact amounts and times of administration

d. Special diet (low sodium is often indicated)
e. Emotional reactions—child may demonstrate:
  (1) Regression in toilet habits, feeding and other learned skills
  (2) Nightmares
  (3) Increased dependency
  (4) Decreased appetite
  (5) Demanding behavior—need to set limits
f. Observation for complications:
  (1) Fever
  (2) Increased heart rate
  (3) Chest pain
  (4) Shortness of breath
  (5) Problems with the incision
  (6) Vomiting or diarrhea
  (7) Rash
3. Provide the parents with the names and telephone numbers of persons to call for questions and emergencies.

Acute Rheumatic Fever

Acute rheumatic fever (ARF) is a systemic disease characterized by inflammatory lesions of connective tissue and endothelial tissue. It is a primary type of acquired heart disease.

Etiology

1. The pathogenesis is thought to be an autoimmune response to group A beta-hemolytic streptococcus.
2. Most first attacks of ARF are preceded by an untreated streptococcal infection of the throat or upper respiratory tract at an interval of 7–35 days.
3. ARF is *NOT* caused by direct infection by the organism.
4. Commonly seen in children 5–15 years of age, during winter months, and in poorer living conditions

Altered Physiology

1. There is a cross reactivity between cardiac tissue antigens and streptococcal cell wall components.
2. The streptococcus may no longer be present, but "self" antibodies attack one's heart (myocardium, pericardium, or valves).
3. The unique pathological lesion of rheumatic fever is the Aschoff body, a collection of reticuloendothelial cells surrounding a necrotic center on some structure of the heart.
4. The inflammatory process involves the heart, joints, and skin. The inflammation may involve the leaflets and/or chordae tendinae of the heart valves, most frequently the mitral and/or aortic valves, resulting in sclerosis and fusion of valve margins.
5. Valvular incompetence results.
6. There is a high recurrence rate.
7. 75% of those with ARF progress to rheumatic heart disease in adulthood.
8. ARF is a preventable condition with penicillin treatment of the primary infection.

Clinical Manifestations and Diagnostic Evaluation

No single clinical or laboratory finding is characteristic of ARF. The diagnosis is based on a combination of manifestations characteristic of this disease and in the absence of other diseases that may mimic it.

1. For this reason, the Jones Criteria, as established by a committee of the American Heart Association, are used.
2. The presence of 2 major criteria, or 1 major and 2 minor criteria, plus evidence of a preceding streptococcal infection are required to establish a diagnosis.

A. Major Manifestations

1. Carditis—manifested by significant murmurs, signs of pericarditis, cardiac enlargement, or congestive heart failure.
2. Polyarthritis—almost always migratory and manifested by swelling, heat, redness and tenderness, or by pain and limitation of motion of 2 or more joints. (The synovial fluid is sterile.)
3. Chorea, a CNS disorder that lasts 1–3 months—purposeless, involuntary, rapid movements often associated with muscle weakness.
4. Erythema marginatum—an evanescent nonpruritic, pink rash.
  a. The erythematous areas have pale centers and round or wavy margins.
  b. They vary greatly in size and occur mainly on the trunk and extremities.
  c. The erythema is transient, migrates from place to place, and may be brought out by the application of heat.
5. Subcutaneous nodules—firm, painless nodules seen or felt over the extensor surface of certain joints, particularly elbows, knees, and wrists, in the occipital region, or over the spinous processes of the thoracic and lumbar vertebrae; the skin overlying them moves freely and is not inflamed.

B. Minor Manifestations

1. *Clinical*
  a. History of previous rheumatic fever or evidence of preexisting rheumatic heart disease
  b. Arthralgia–pain in one or more joints without evidence of inflammation, tenderness to touch, or limitation of motion
  c. Fever–temperature in excess of 38°C. (100.4°F.)
2. *Laboratory*
  a. Erythrocyte sedimentation rate–elevated
  b. C-reactive protein–positive
  c. ECG changes—mainly PR interval prolongation
  d. Leukocytosis

C. Supporting Evidence of Streptococcal Infection

1. Increased titer of streptococcal antibodies (antistreptolysin O, or ASO titer)
2. Positive throat culture for group A beta-hemolytic streptococci
3. Recent scarlet fever

Patient Problems and Nursing Diagnoses

1. Altered comfort: pain related to polyarthritis
2. Decreased cardiac output related to heart damage
3. Disturbed body image related to chorea and/or steroid therapy
4. Potential for injury related to chorea
5. Activity intolerance related to muscle weakness and inflamed joints
6. Potential for infection related to steroid therapy and disease recurrence
7. Knowledge deficit about rheumatic fever and its treatment
8. Diversional activity deficit related to prolonged bedrest
9. Ineffective coping related to forced bedrest

Nursing Interventions

A. Become Informed About the Child's Symptomatology and the Medical Plan of Care.

1. Discuss with the physician the plan for medical treatment.
2. Make a baseline nursing assessment of the child's condition.
   a. Listen to the child's chest with a stethoscope to become familiar with the murmur or to determine the presence of a murmur not previously heard; listen for a friction rub.
   b. Determine from the child whether he is experiencing any pain or discomfort (also observe the child's facial expression as he moves since children may deny pain, thinking they will be able to go home) or resume activity.
   c. Describe the pain as to location, when it occurs, whether there is any heat, swelling, redness or tenderness.
   d. Examine the knees, elbows, wrists, occipital region and spine for nodules; describe location.
   e. Determine whether the child has any muscle weakness or rapid, purposeless movements.

B. Initiate Specific Preventive Teaching to Prevent a Recurrence or an Additional Case of Rheumatic Fever Within the Family.

1. Have all family members screened for streptococcus by referring them for throat cultures.
2. All persons with positive cultures should be treated.
3. Teach the specific symptoms of streptococcal infections and the need for antibiotics.

C. Treat the Precipitating Streptococcal Infection.

Administer antibiotics as prescribed by the physician (generally intramuscular penicillin G).

NURSING ALERT: Before administering penicillin, elicit a history for possible drug allergy.

D. Evaluate the Child for Evidence of Response to Treatment or Progression of Disease.

1. Observe for the development or disappearance of any major or minor manifestations of the disease.
2. Monitor carditis by careful documentation of the child's pulse, respirations, and blood pressure.
   a. The pulse should be counted for 1 full minute.
   b. The sleeping pulse is a good indicator of the extent of carditis.

E. Provide Symptomatic Management of the Child's Fever.

1. Refer to section on fever, p. 1142.
2. Antipyretic drugs are usually withheld during the diagnostic period.

F. Suppress the Rheumatic Inflammatory Process by Administering Appropriate Medications.

1. Salicylates (generally prescribed for patients with arthritis but *without* carditis)
   a. Observe for gastrointestinal upsets, ringing in the ears, headaches, bleeding, and disturbances in the mental state.
   b. Administer milk or antacids with salicylates.
   c. Report side effects promptly.
   d. Aspirin therapy should be monitored by salicylate levels in the blood.

2. Steroids (generally prescribed for patients *with* carditis; as steroids are tapered, administration of salicylates is begun)
   a. Prepare the child and his family for the expected side effects of steroid therapy.
      (1) Body appearance may change through rounding facial contour
      (2) Localized fat deposits
      (3) Appearance of acne or excessive hair
      (4) Weight gain with linear markings appearing in the stretched skin
   b. Mental and emotional disturbances may necessitate discontinuance of the medication.
   c. Hypertension and the tendency to retain water and sodium may result from steroid therapy.
      (1) Provide a low-sodium diet.
      (2) Weigh the child daily—report sudden weight increases.
   d. Steroids diminish the child's resistance to infection and may mask symptoms of infection.

NURSING ALERT: Do not place a child with an infectious disease in the room with the child with rheumatic fever.
Restrict visitors and personnel with infectious diseases from contact with the child on steroid therapy.

   e. A combination of steroid therapy and stress may lead to the development of gastric ulcers.
3. Administer medications punctually and at regular intervals to achieve constant therapeutic blood levels.
4. Report signs of increased rheumatic activity as salicylates or steroids are being tapered.

G. Alleviate the Child's Anxiety About the Functioning of His Heart, Because Anxiety Uses Energy and Produces Fatigue.

1. Give the child information about rheumatic fever in terms that he can understand, e.g., "Rheumatic fever is a hard thing to understand because you can't see it. When you scratch yourself, you can see the mark, and you can see the scratch heal. Rheumatic fever is something like that—only you can't see the healing because it happens to the tissue underneath the skin. (And sometimes it happens to the valves in the heart)"
2. Assure the child that physicians know how to treat rheumatic fever.
3. Communicate information about the child's reactions to all staff members to provide consistent information.
4. Children may be concerned that they have had a heart attack; reassure that their heart is functioning okay by letting them listen to it.

H. Decrease the Cardiac Workload Until the Acute Inflammatory Reaction Has Subsided.

1. Explain to the child the need for rest (usually prescribed for 4–12 weeks, depending on the severity of the disease and physician's preference).
2. Assure the child that bedrest will be imposed no longer than necessary. This is usually until the sedimentation rate returns to normal.
3. Organize nursing care to provide periods of uninterrupted rest.
4. Assure the child that his needs will be met.
   a. Give the child a bell to call the nurse.
   b. Answer his calls promptly.
5. Assist the child to resume activity very gradually once he is asymptomatic at rest and indicators of acute inflammation have become normal.

a. Allow the child to participate in decisions about such matters as timing his periods of activity.
b. Monitor the pulse rate carefully after periods of activity in order to assess the degree of cardiac compensation.

I. Provide Comfort Related to Arthritis and Bedrest.

1. Use bed cradle.
2. Reassure that arthritis is *NOT* destructive.
3. Change positions in bed often to decrease stiffness and decrease skin breakdown.
4. Support inflamed joints; handle gently.
5. Provide meticulous skin care.
6. Position the legs in good body alignment—use a footboard.
7. Elevate the back of the bed and support the arms with pillows when child is dyspneic.

J. Provide Nursing Care for the Child With Congestive Heart Failure.

Refer to section on congestive heart failure, p. 1322.

K. Provide Safe, Supportive Care for the Child With Chorea.

1. Place the child in a bed with padded side rails, especially if uncontrolled body movements are severe.
2. Feed the child slowly and carefully because of incoordinate movements of the head, mouth, and swallowing muscles. Avoid the use of sharp eating utensils and do not use straws.
3. Provide frequent feedings that are high in calories, protein, vitamins, and iron, because constant movements cause the child to burn calories at a rapid rate.
4. Spend time talking with the child even though his speech may be defective. If severe, use other methods of communication.
5. Administer sedation, if prescribed.
6. Reassure the child about the cause of his instability and tell him that his symptoms will subside.
7. Encourage positive parent–child relationships that may have been strained if the onset of symptoms was insidious (lack of concentration at school, mood swings, deteriorating handwriting, irritability, etc.).
8. Help the child regain his former skills once symptoms begin to subside.
   a. Support the child during periods of ambulation.
   b. Provide activities that require the use of large muscles and progress to materials that require fine coordination.
9. Keep the environment calm and provide increased periods of rest as movements increase with fatigue and increased excitement.

L. Assist the Child to Develop a Realistic Attitude Toward His Illness and Encourage Him to Discuss His Concerns.

1. Help the child to realize the restrictions he must face and the fact that progress is slow.
2. Attempt to avoid negative connotations related to activity restrictions. Emphasize what the child is allowed to do—that is, say, "You may be up in the chair for 2 hours every day," rather than "You have to stay in bed all day, except for 2 hours."
3. Alleviate the child's anxieties about keeping up with his class and school activities.
   a. Initiate a referral for a hospital-based school teacher to see him on a regular basis.
   b. When this service is not available, encourage the parents to contact his teacher, who will prepare lesson plans and short assignments for him—encourage the parents to maintain this contact with the teacher.
   c. Plan time each day on a regular basis for the child to complete his assignments.

M. Provide for Diversional Activity That Will Help the Child Feel a Sense of Achievement and Satisfaction.

1. Initiate some long-term projects.
2. Refer to section on the hospitalized child, p. 1120.

N. Assist the Family to Deal With the Emotional and Financial Stresses Caused by the Illness and Hospitalization.

1. Assess the family's needs in this area and initiate a referral to a social worker if indicated.
2. Refer to section on family-centered care, p. 1125.
3. Promote home care.

O. Prevent a Recurrent Attack of Rheumatic Fever by Reinforcing the Need for Prophylactic Antimicrobial Therapy.

1. Penicillin is the drug of choice—either intramuscular benzathine G every 28 days or oral penicillin V or G twice daily.
2. Continuous prophylaxis is recommended throughout the childhood years and well into adult life, often indefinitely.
3. Use creativity in recommending methods to remind families about administering the medication.
   a. The child should be taught to assume responsibility for his own medication at an early age so that it becomes habitual.
   b. Some children profit from the use of a calendar or special chart. Others find it useful to associate their medication schedule with other routine tasks, such as brushing their teeth.
4. Be certain that the child receives his prophylactic medication on schedule during his hospitalization and during subsequent hospitalizations (including hospitalization for treatment of other illnesses).
5. When indicated, additional prophylaxis should be used for prevention of infective endocarditis.
   The American Heart Association's recommendations for the prevention of endocarditis should be observed for children undergoing certain dental procedures as well as for surgery or instrumentation of the upper respiratory tract, genitourinary tract, or lower gastrointestinal tract.

P. Begin to Prepare for Discharge Early Enough With the Parents in Order That Sufficient Adjustments and Preparation May Be Made.

1. The child should have a bed of his own and, preferably, a room of his own.
2. A responsible adult must be in the home to care for him.
3. Provide information about:
   a. Activity restrictions
   b. Medications—dosage, schedule, side effects
   c. Dietary instruction
   d. Symptoms to report—pain, malaise, anorexia, tachycardia, tachypnea, weight gain
   e. Telephone number of physician
   f. Follow-up appointment
4. Initiate a community nursing referral—this may be done prior to discharge if a home evaluation is desired.

For nursing care of the adult patient with rheumatic heart disease, refer to page 340.

Expected Outcomes

1. The child experiences relief of pain evidenced by facial expressions.
2. Copes effectively with altered body-image evidenced by relaxed behavior
3. Conserves energy by resting and limiting activity
4. Engages in quiet activity that promotes cognitive development
5. Avoids injury during choreic movements
6. Avoids infection during treatment for rheumatic fever; or infections are recognized and treated promptly
7. Family accurately describes rheumatic fever and its treatment.
8. The child does not have a recurrent attack of rheumatic fever.

Infective Endocarditis

Infective endocarditis refers to infection of the endocardial surface of the heart or the intimal surface of certain arterial vessels especially valves, endocardium, or endothelium of the heart. It is a rare condition that is usually associated with preexisting cardiovascular disease (congenital or rheumatic) but may develop in a normal heart during a course of septicemia. It is usually due to bacterial or fungal agents.

Children with congenital heart defects are especially susceptible because of turbulent blood flow that results in tissue damage to areas of the heart. Bacteria are trapped in these damaged areas and proliferate. It is also referred to as *subacute bacterial endocarditis* and *acute bacterial endocarditis.*

For etiology, clinical manifestations, pathophysiology, treatment and nursing management, refer to discussion on adult, pages 337–340. In addition, the following points of management should be considered by the pediatric nurse.

Nursing Assessment

1. Although any child with heart disease is at risk for developing endocarditis, those most at risk are older (over 10 years of age) children with:
   a. Prosthetic valves
   b. Congenital heart defects and their repair
      (1) Tetralogy of Fallot
      (2) VSD
      (3) Coarctation of the aorta
      (4) PDA
      (5) Aortic stenosis
   c. Intrusive procedures (i.e., catheterizations)
   d. Rheumatic heart disease
   e. Bacteria are often introduced during dental procedures, upper respiratory infections, gastroenteritis, urinary tract infections, and skin infections.
2. Symptoms most commonly seen
   a. Fatigue; malaise
   b. Fever
   c. Nausea/vomiting; anorexia
   d. Weight loss
   e. Heart murmur
   f. Spenomegaly
   g. Positive blood culture
   h. Elevated erythrocyte sedimentation rate

Nursing Management

1. Long-term (usually at least 4–6 weeks) IV administration of antimicrobials is indicated in all cases.
   a. Careful management of IV therapy is essential.
      (1) Refer to Intravenous Therapy Procedure, p. 1167.
      (2) Drugs must be administered according to schedule to maintain constant therapeutic levels.
      (3) Notify appropriate personnel immediately if the IV infiltrates, so that it can be restarted.
      (4) Heparin locks may be used to allow the child freedom of movement between intervals of medication.
2. Monitor for fever.
3. Maintain bedrest.
4. Treat congestive heart failure, if present.
5. Prevent and monitor for emboli.
6. Appropriate measures should be initiated to help the child maintain his level of development during the lengthy hospitalization.
   a. Refer to The Hospitalized Child, p. 1120.
   b. Arrange for continuation of school work.
   c. Facilitate interaction with family, including siblings.
   d. Provide diversional activities that will help the child feel a sense of achievement and satisfaction.
   e. Facilitate contact with peers through written correspondence, telephone, or selected visiting.
7. Prevention is an important nursing responsibility.
   a. Procedures which increase the risk of bacteria gaining access to the bloodstream include:
      (1) Tooth extraction, oral surgery, and periodontal procedures
      (2) Tonsillectomy and adenoidectomy
      (3) Bronchoscopy
      (4) Instrumentation of the genitourinary tract
      (5) Surgery or instrumentation of the lower gastrointestinal tract
      (6) Childbirth
   b. Almost all children with congenital or rheumatic heart disease should receive prophylactic antibiotics in conjunction with these procedures to reduce bacteremia and prevent bacterial implantation. The current recommendations of the American Heart Association for chemoprophylaxis should be observed.
   c. The child and family should be instructed regarding the importance of good dental hygiene.
   d. Families of children with heart disease should be instructed about prevention of endocarditis, as well as about signs and symptoms of the disease.

Atherosclerosis

Atherosclerosis is a condition characterized by fatty deposits (plaques) on the walls of arteries. It may lead to narrowing and obstruction of major vessels such as the coronary arteries, the arteries of the neck and brain, and those of the lower extremities. It is a cause of coronary heart disease and cerebrovascular disease.

Although the major clinical manifestations of atherosclerosis occur in middle-age and older adults, the precursors of atherosclerosis may become established in childhood. Thus, the pediatric nurse should be aware of the following factors:

1. Although much is known about the pathology of atherosclerosis and its evolution in adults, there is still much to be learned about its earlier stages.
2. The atherosclerotic process is probably influenced by a variety of inheritance factors, including vascular structure and metabolism as well as environmental factors such as diet.
3. Data indicate that irreversible atherosclerotic changes may occur by 20 years of age. Therefore, the pediatric patient must be identified as being at risk in order for medical treatment to be instituted early enough to alter the course of the disease meaningfully.

Identified Risk Factors

1. Serum lipid disorders—may be genetically determined (e.g., inherited hypercholesterolemia) or acquired—probably resulting from an excess intake of saturated fat and cholesterol
2. Hypertension—probably caused by a hereditary predisposition, interacting with environmental factors such as obesity, increased sodium intake, and endogenous and exogenous vasoconstrictors
3. Impaired glucose tolerance
4. Obesity
5. Sedentary living habits, lack of regular exercise
6. Smoking
7. Renal conditions: nephroses, chronic renal failure, chronic hepatic disease
8. A chronic complication of diabetes

Nursing Interventions

A. Screen All Children at Risk for Lipid Abnormalities and Correct These by Diet or Other Procedures as Indicated.

1. Infants of families with any history of familial hypercholesterolemia or premature cardiovascular disease should be studied for lipid abnormality. If negative, these children should receive periodic reevaluation.
2. All siblings of hyperlipoproteinemic children should be tested.

B. Screen Children for Hypertension at Periodic Intervals, and Initiate Appropriate Treatment.

1. Refer to procedure for taking blood pressure, p. 1141 and normal vital sign values, p. 1140.

C. Initiate Diet Counseling.

1. Discourage the common habit of adding salt to childhood diets because the habit of adding salt to practically all foods is developed early in life.
2. Teach parents to read labels to learn the sodium content of commercial food products, including baby foods.
3. Counsel parents to provide meals that are low in cholesterol and saturated fats. Emphasize skimmed milk and dairy products derived from skimmed milk, legumes, fruits, whole grains, lean meats, poultry, and fish. Substitute margarine for butter. Deemphasize egg yolks, animal fat, and organ meats.
4. Discourage overeating and overfeeding.
5. Refer to section on Pediatric Nutrition, p. 1102.

D. Encourage Physical Activity.

1. Discuss the benefits of physical activity with parents and encourage them to set an example for their children.
2. Encourage participation in physically active games and sports; this helps to establish a pattern for a physically active way of life in adulthood.

E. Discourage Cigarette Smoking.

1. Discuss the dangers of smoking with parents and encourage them to set a positive example for their children.
2. Make children aware of the dangers of smoking at an early age so that they will be less inclined to develop the habit during adolescence or adult life.

Bibliography

Books

Adams F, Emmanovilides G and Riemenschneider T. Moss' Heart Disease in Infants, Children and Adolescents. Baltimore, Williams & Wilkins, 1989

American Heart Association. If Your Child has a Congenital Heart Defect: A Guide for Parents, 1987

Anderson R et al. Pediatric Cardiology. Edinburgh, Churchill Livingstone, 1987

Anderson et al. Perspectives in Pediatric Cardiology, vol 1. New York, Futura Publishing, 1988

Behrman R and Vaughan V. Nelson's Textbook of Pediatrics. Philadelphia, WB Saunders, 1987

Crupi G, Parenzan L and Anderson R. Perspectives in Pediatric Cardiology, vol 2. New York, Futura Publishing, 1988

Fink B. Congenital Heart Disease. Chicago, Year Book Medical Pub, 1985

Hallman G, Cooley D and Gutgesell H. Surgical Treatment of Congenital Heart Disease. Philadelphia, Lea & Febiger, 1987

Hazinski MF. Nursing Care of the Critically Ill Child. St. Louis, CV Mosby, 1986

Liberthson R. Congenital Heart Disease: Diagnosis and Management in Children and Adults. Boston, Little, Brown & Co, 1989

Magilligan D and Quinn E. Endocarditis. New York, Marcel Dekker, 1986

Mullins C and Mayer D. Congenital Heart Disease: A Diagrammatic Atlas. New York, Alan R. Liss, 1988

Whaley L and Wong D. Nursing Care of Infants and Children. St. Louis, CV Mosby, 1987

Journals

Callow L. Post-operative nursing care of the patient who has undergone the Fontan procedure. Focus Crit Care 1987; 14(4):24–31

Cogwill LD (ed). Cyanotic congenital heart disease. Cardiac Surgery 1989; 3(1):1–272

Fisk R. Management of the pediatric cardiovascular patient after surgery. Crit Care Nurs Q 1986; 9(2):75–82

Gerraughty A. Caring for patients with lesions obstructing systemic blood flow. Crit Care Nurs Clin North Am 1989; 1(2):231–243

Kron I (ed). Innovations in congenital heart surgery. Cardiac Surgery 1989; 3(2):279–443

Kulik L. Caring for patients with lesions decreasing pulmonary blood flow. Crit Care Nurs Clin North Am 1989; 1(2): 215–229

Malinowski P and Yablonski C. Congenital heart disease in infants: Nursing assessment. Crit Care Nurs Q 1986; 9:6–22

Mitiguy J. A surgical liaison program: Making the wait more bearable. Matern Child Care Nurs 1986; 11(6):388–392

Moynihan P and King R. Caring for patients with lesions increasing pulmonary blood flow. Crit Care Nurs Clin North Am 1989 Jun; 1(2):195–213

Myrer M. Respiratory care of the post operative cardiac surgery patient. Crit Care Nurs Q 1986; 9(2):64–74

Norwood W and Pigott J. Recent advances in cardiac surgery. Pediatr Clin North Am 1985; 32(5):1117–1124

O'Brien P and Boisvert J. Discharge planning for children with heart disease. Matern Child Care Nurs 1989; 11(6):297–305

Page G. Tetralogy of Fallot. Heart Lung 1986; 15(4):390–399

Rotondi P. Intensive care unit management of the post operative cardiac surgery patient. Crit Care Nurs Q 1986; 9(2):49–62

Smith P. Current diagnostic and therapeutic catheterization techniques. Crit Care Nurs Q 1986; 9(2):24–39

Shastry P et al. Persistance of heart reactive antibodies (HRA) in acute rheumatic fever (ARF) and rheumatic heart disease (RHD) patients. J Clin Lab Immunol 1988; 27:87–90

Scrima D. Infective endocarditis: Nursing considerations. Crit Care Nurs 1987; 1(2):47–56

Turina M et al. Long-term outlook after atrial correction of transposition of the great arteries. J Thorac Cardiovasc Surg 1988; 95(5):828–835

Vincent R and Collins G. Cardiac embryology and fetal cardiovascular physiology. Crit Care Nurs Q 1986; 9(2):1–5

Vincent R and Elixson E. Hemodynamic monitoring. Crit Care Nurs Q 1986; 9(2):40–48

Digestive Disorders, Pediatric Considerations

52

Dental Caries

Dental caries involves loss of tooth structure or the formation of a cavity as a result of bacterial attack—first on the enamel, which is the hard surface of the tooth, and then progressing inward toward the pulp.

Etiology and Altered Physiology

A. Bacteria

1. Acidogenic organisms—decalcify the hard tissue by producing acids on the tooth surface.
2. Proteolytic organisms—digest the product of tooth surface (decalcification thus produces odor and discoloration).
3. Leptotrichae organisms—form structures on the smooth tooth surface which houses acidogenic organisms.

B. Contributing Factors

1. Age—most susceptible age-groups are children, 4–8 years (primary teeth), and adolescents, 12–18 years (permanent teeth).
2. Diet—large intake of simple sugars between meals, milk-bottle caries in infants and toddlers
3. Familial tendency to tooth decay
4. Lack of proper oral hygiene
5. Poor state of health (illness alters the normal bacteriostatic quality of saliva), chronic disease

Complications

As a result of missing teeth or multiple caries, the child may experience many problems:
1. Poor nutrition
   a. Refusal to eat foods that need chewing
   b. Teeth drift and cause malocclusion
2. Faulty speech habits and articulation
   a. Weak jaw muscles
   b. Abnormal alveolar bone development
3. Psychological problems
   a. Embarrassment caused by appearance of teeth and oral odor
4. Oral foci of infection
   a. Subacute bacterial endocarditis may result in child with congenital heart disease.

Prevention

1. Regular frequent dental observation by dental professional
2. Decreased eating between meals
3. Fluoridation of water supply
4. Biannual topical application of fluoride to teeth
5. Decreased eating of sucrose-containing snacks
6. Removal of plaque and debris from tooth surface with brushing

Clinical Manifestations

1. Decay is acute and rapidly penetrates the tooth in children.
2. Caries occur where food debris collects.
   a. Pits and fissures
   b. Between teeth
   c. At neck of tooth
3. Discoloration of teeth
4. Decay odor
5. Pain, abscess, or infection

Treatment

1. Removal of decay and restoration of tooth surfaces involved
2. Removal of diseased tooth or teeth that are decayed beyond restoration

Patient Problems and Nursing Diagnoses

1. Anxiety related to hospitalization and surgery
2. Potential altered nutrition, less than body requirements, related to discomfort when eating as a result of long-standing caries or missing teeth and malocclusion
3. Communication, impaired, verbal, related to weak jaw muscles, abnormal alveolar bone development, and missing teeth
4. Potential for infection related to poor oral hygiene
5. Knowledge deficit of adequate nutrition and oral hygiene practices

Nursing Interventions

Hospitalization of a child for treatment of dental caries is likely only when special behavior difficulties are anticipated in treatment, when medical problems complicate dental treatment or when extensive repair is necessary.
   (See Preventive Pediatrics, Dental Care, p. 1109.)

A. Prevent Dental Caries in All Patients.

The nurse should be an active member on the dental health care team in preventive education by motivating the child and family toward good dental hygiene and nutritional practices.

B. Know That There is a Direct Relationship Between Incidence of Dental Caries in Children and Dental Health Education or Knowledge of Parents.

1. Assess parental knowledge and use opportunities to teach parents preventive care.
2. Encourage parental participation with the young child during teeth-brushing exercise.

C. Know the Principles of Good Oral Hygiene and Practice Them When Caring for Each Pediatric Patient.

1. Encourage mouth rinsing or teeth brushing after eating. Brush before bedtime to decrease bacteriogenic activity in the warm, undisturbed mouth during sleep.
2. Encourage proper brushing of teeth.
   a. Brush crosswise with a soft-bristled brush.
   b. Electric tooth brush cleans teeth and stimulates the gingivae.
3. Supervise brushing in young children. (Dentrifice is not necessary.)

D. Know the Value of Good Nutrition and Its Effect in Preventing Dental Caries.

1. No between-meal snacking with refined-sugar foods. No gum chewing, except of sugarless gum.
   a. Improves appetite at meals.
   b. Substitute fresh fruit for refined sugars. (No lollipops between meals; give after meal before brushing.)
2. Discourage a bottle, other than water, at bedtime or before sleep.
   Residue is left on teeth during long periods of sleep and results in rampant decay.

E. Know the Value of Periodic Dental Examination and Preventive Measures Used to Decrease Decay.

1. Encourage patient and parent to participate in regular dentist visits.
   a. Regular visits for cleaning and checking for decay; repair if necessary
      First visit is to familiarize the young child with the dentist and equipment.
      (1) Usually age 18–30 months—or when all primary teeth have erupted
      (2) Should not be when the child has a toothache
   b. During childhood and adolescence, visits are every 3–6 months.
      New decay appears suddenly in multiple areas and advances rapidly.
2. If fluoridation is not supplied in community water, topical application is advisable.
   a. Most effective when applied on newly erupted teeth
   b. Fluoride makes enamel more resistant to decay as it strengthens calcification of the developing dental tissue.

F. Keep the Adolescent Aware of His Diet and Its Effect on Dental Decay.

1. Keep in mind diet fads and peer-group pressure.
2. Have the patient keep a dietary record for 1 week. Then evaluate it against an example of a good, nutritious diet. Encourage the patient to make his own evaluation.

Health Education

1. After assessment of parental knowledge has been made, embark on a teaching program.

Main areas of concern:
   a. Proper technique of dental hygiene
   b. Value of good nutrition
   c. Value of fluoridation
   d. Importance of regular visits to the dentist every 3–6 months.
2. American Dental Association, 211 East Chicago Avenue, Chicago, IL 60611

Expected Outcomes

1. Experiences minimal anxiety; relaxed behavior; restful sleep; willingness to engage in play activities
2. Achieves improved nutritional status; alert appearance; weight gain
3. Demonstrates improved speech habits and articulation
4. Is free of infection as evidenced by normal vital signs and laboratory values
5. Patient and parents verbalize understanding of nutritional practices and demonstrate care of the child's teeth

Cleft Lip and Palate

Cleft lip and palate facial malformation results when fusion involving the first brachial arch fails to take place during embryonic development.

Etiology

1. Failure of embryonic development—cause not known
2. Hereditary factor
3. May be related to mutant genes, chromosomal abnormalities, teratogens

Incidence

1. Cleft lip—approximately 1:1000 births; more frequent in males (with or without cleft palate)
2. Cleft palate—approximately 1:2500 births; more frequent in females
3. Combination of cleft lip and palate account for about 50%, cleft lip about 25%, and cleft palate about 25%

Altered Physiology

A. Types of Defect

1. The lip and palate develop independently; thus, any combination of defects can occur.
2. Cleft lip—prealveolar cleft
   a. Varies from a notch in the lip to complete separation of the lip into the nose
   b. May be unilateral or bilateral
   c. Failure of maxillary process to fuse with nasal elevations on frontal prominence—normally occurs during 5th to 6th week of gestation
   d. Merging of upper lip at midline is complete between 7th and 8th week of gestation.
3. Isolated cleft palate—postalveolar cleft
   a. Cleft of uvula
   b. Cleft of soft palate
   c. Cleft of both soft and hard palate through roof of mouth
   d. Unilateral or bilateral
   e. Failure of mesodermal masses of lateral palatine process to meet and fuse—normally occurs between 7th and 12th week of gestation.
4. Cleft lip and palate combined
   Any degree of involvement

5. Submucous cleft
    a. Muscles of soft palate are not joined.
    b. Not recognized until child talks; cannot be seen at birth

B. Associated Problems
1. Eating
    a. Suction cannot be created for effective sucking
    b. Food returns through the nose
2. Nasal speech
3. Lack of normal dental function and appearance
4. Repeated bouts of otitis media with subsequent hearing loss

Complications

1. Associated problems:
    a. Pierre Robin syndrome
    b. Intellectual deficits
2. Long-term problems:
    a. Speech impairment
    b. Improper tooth placement
    c. Recurring otitis media
    d. Hearing impairment
    e. Faulty social adjustment related to poor self-concept and abnormal speech

Clinical Manifestations

Physical appearance of cleft lip or palate
1. Incompletely formed lip
2. Opening in roof of mouth felt with examiner's finger on palate

Treatment

1. General management is focused on closure of the cleft(s), prevention of complications, habilitation, and facilitation of normal growth and development of the child.
2. The cleft lip is generally repaired before the palate defect.
    a. Immediate repair—(Some surgeons may use an intraoral or extraoral appliance for several weeks before repair.)
    b. Later repair—when infant is 6–12 weeks of age, hemoglobin 10 gm./dl., steady weight gain seen—10 lbs and/or 10,000 mm³ WBC
3. Cleft palate repair may be done anytime between 6 months and 5 years—based on degree of deformity, width of oropharynx, neuromuscular function of palate and pharynx, and surgeon preference.

Patient Problems and Nursing Diagnoses

1. Nutrition altered, less than body requirements, related to eating difficulties from facial or oral deformity
2. Potential for infection related to open wound created by cleft palate
3. Communication, impaired, verbal, related to oral malformation
4. Self-concept, disturbance in body image, related to embarrassment from oral deformity and abnormal speech
5. Family process, altered, related to parents' reactions to child's appearance
6. Patient anxiety related to hospitalization and treatments

Nursing Interventions for the Newborn

A. Show Acceptance of the Baby.
1. The nurse must maintain composure and not show shock when handling the infant. The manner in which the nurse handles the baby can make a lasting impression on the parents.
    a. The baby with a cleft lip can be unattractive and can cause shock when first seen.
    b. When showing a newborn baby to parents for the first time, support them by accepting both the baby and the parents' feelings. Parents may be grieving about the perfect infant they did not have and may harbor ambivalent feelings about this baby.
    c. The sequence of normal parental responses may include shock and disbelief, sadness, anxiety and anger, and then proceed to a state of equilibrium and reorganization.
    d. Be supportive of the parents by reassuring them that reparative surgery can be done with much success.
        (1) The time when reparative surgery is done depends on the surgeon, the condition of the baby, and the degree to which the parents have accepted the baby.
        (2) Lip surgery may be done several hours after birth or when the infant is 2–3 months of age or has gained 4.54 kg. (10 lbs.), and hemoglobin is 10 gm./dl.
2. Reparative surgery of the palate is usually done between 12 and 24 months of age.
    a. At this age, speech patterns have not been set, yet growth of involved structures allows for improved surgical repair.
    b. If repair is delayed to age 4 or 5 years, a special denture palate is used to help occlude the cleft and aid in establishing speech patterns.

B. Establish and Maintain Adequate Nutrition for Growth and Development.
1. Some surgeons prefer to delay nipple feeding because sucking may spread cleft of lip.
2. Babies with just a cleft lip may feed well if a soft nipple with enlarged holes is used.
3. With certain types and combinations of cleft lips and palates, the baby is unable to create a vacuum and is thus unable to suck.
    a. Several types of nipples and feeding devices are available to make feedings easier.
    b. A soft base or disposable bottle can be helpful by applying gentle, constant pressure to maintain flow.
    c. Feeding devices include regular nipple with enlarged holes: Lamb's nipple, Duckey nipple, Brecht feeder, and Premi nipple.

Note: Lamb's nipple may evoke gagging.

    d. Rubber-tipped asepto syringe or dropper. (Rubber extension should be long enough to extend back into the mouth to prevent regurgitation through the nose.)
    Direct tip to side of mouth and give feeding slowly.
4. Feed baby in an upright, sitting position to decrease possibility of fluid being aspirated or returned through the nose, or back to the auditory canal.
    a. Feed slowly; place the nipple in the infant's mouth so it can be compressed between the existing palate and tongue.
    b. Bubble frequently during feeding, because these babies swallow a great deal of air.
    c. Avoid repeated removal of nipple from the infant's mouth because of fear of choking because this only frustrates the infant, causing him to cry and increasing chances of aspiration.

d. Smaller but more frequent feedings may be necessary if the infant tires or requires an extended period of time to eat.

5. Advance diet as appropriate for age and needs of the baby.
   Eating often improves when solids are introduced, since they are easier for the baby to manipulate.

6. Encourage the mother to begin feeding the infant herself as soon as possible. Use feeding time to help mother and infant develop their relationship.

C. Prevent Infection In the Child So That Surgery Will Not Have to Be Delayed.

1. Avoid patient contact with anyone who has an infection.
2. Change the baby's position frequently.
3. Clean the cleft after each feeding with clear water and a cotton-tipped applicator.

D. Support the Respiratory Efforts and the Feeding and Nutritional Needs of the Infant With Pierre Robin Syndrome. (Features of Pierre Robin syndrome are cleft palate, glossoptosis [tongue falls back on pharynx], and micrognathia [underdeveloped mandible].)

1. Prevent respiratory obstruction, especially on inspiration and when the infant is quiet.
   a. Place the infant in prone position so that tongue and jaw fall forward.
   b. Tilt head back as best tolerated by the infant and slightly elevate upper trunk.
   c. Stockinette cap securely attached to the infant's head and suspended from an overhead support may be of some benefit in assisting the infant to maintain a position for easy ventilation.
   d. Suction nasopharynx as needed.
   e. The tongue may be sutured to pull it forward; if this is done, observe for slipping, cut tongue, and infection.

2. When this infant is fed, consideration must be given to his respiratory effort, flaccid tongue, and cleft palate. Generally, feeding can be done with a nursing bottle (feeding techniques similar to those used for cleft palate).
   a. Use orthopneic position—vertical and slightly forward; this allows infant to push jaw forward to suck and also allows the feeder a clear view of the infant.
   b. Gentle finger pressure by feeder at mandibular attachment can aid in bringing jaw forward.
   c. Feed slowly.

3. By 3–4 months of age, the mandible has grown enough to accommodate the tongue, and respiratory difficulty is greatly diminished.

4. Additional complications associated with Pierre Robin syndrome are slow weight gain and ear infections.

E. Assist Parents In Preparing to Take the Newborn Home From the Nursery Before Lip and Palate Surgery Have Been Done.

Health Education

1. Prepare the mother for home feedings. She should have several days to practice feeding to become familiar with the baby's feeding pattern.
   a. Home equipment should be used in the hospital.
   b. The mother should be aware of difficulties with feeding and how to manage them.
      (1) Formula returning through the nose

(2) Respiratory distress
(3) Longer time necessary for feeding

c. Suggest that about a week or so prior to scheduled admission for surgery, the mother begin using feeding technique preferred by surgeon for postoperative feeding.
   (1) Side of spoon
   (2) Rubber-tipped dropper
   (3) Toddler cup

2. Encourage the parents to prepare siblings at home for the arrival of this baby. (Pictures of the new baby might be suggested.)

3. Initiate a community nurse referral to continue emotional support and teaching program at home.

4. Offer parents available literature about children with cleft lip and palate.*

5. Parents should know what plans have been started for surgical treatment.

6. Social work referral may be indicated.
   a. To listen to the mother express her concerns regarding management at home with a handicapped child
   b. To arrange financial assistance

F. Be Aware of the Complexity of Long-Range Care and the Importance of the Many Disciplines Involved In the Eventual Outcome. The nurse should know all the ramifications and potential problems for this child and his family.

1. The organization of trained professional people from the many disciplines that become involved include pediatrician, plastic surgeon, otologist, general dentist, orthodontist, prosthodontist, medical-social worker, nurse, speech therapist, and psychologist.

2. Long-term follow-up and reparative surgery:
   a. Chronic otitis media and hearing loss (The auditory canal is abnormally located.)
   b. Lip, palate, and orthodontic repair
   c. Speech therapy
   d. Psychological insult to the child

3. Financial burden on the family
   State programs for crippled children can offer relief.

4. Psychological trauma to the family

G. Emphasize the Importance of the Mother's Role In Caring for the Child During Outpatient Treatment and the Many Hospitalizations Required.

The mother can offer a great deal of security to the child when he is subjected to the trauma and frightening experiences of treatment.

Preoperative Care of the Child With a Cleft Lip

A. Prepare the Infant for Postoperative Care So That It Will Be Familiar to Him, Less Frightening, and Easier for Him to Accept After Surgery.

1. Practice the feeding method to be used as preferred by the surgeon

---

* Snyder GB et al. *Your Cleft Lip and Palate Child: A Guide for Parents.* Florida CP Association, Mead Johnson & Company Laboratories (ND)

The Child with a Cleft Palate, US Department of Health and Human Services, Social and Rehabilitation Service.

Booklets sponsored by Mead Johnson & Company Laboratories, Evansville, IN 47721:

Road to Normalcy for the Cleft Lip and Palate Child
Steps in Habilitation for the Cleft Lip and Palate Child

a. Rubber-tipped syringe or asepto syringe

b. Side of spoon

2. Elbow restraints may be used for short periods of time.

    a. Let the child play with them if he is old enough.

    b. Allow the mother to become involved in their use.

    c. Jacket restraint may be necessary in the older child to prevent him from rolling over, and rubbing against the sheets.

3. Help the infant get used to being on his back or propped on his side for long periods of time.

B. Prepare the Mother (parents) **As to What to Expect When She Sees the Child Postoperatively.**

1. Explain the use of the Logan bow (a curved metal wire that prevents stress on the suture line) and restraints.

2. Encourage the mother to be with the infant, especially when he wakes up from anesthesia, to offer him security and comfort.

Postoperative Care of the Child With a Cleft Lip

A. Administer Good Postoperative Care Based On General Principles and Observe for Usual Postoperative Complications.

B. Prevent Injury to the Suture Line of the Lip.

1. Elbow restraints are the most effective way to prevent busy hands from reaching the lip, yet still allow some freedom of movement.

    a. Pad restraint and place it from the axilla to inner aspect of the wrist.

    b. Remove restraints occasionally, one at a time, to exercise the arms.

    c. Restraints or cuff of shirt may need to be pinned to the bed to decrease chances of the infant rubbing his lip with his upper arm.

2. Logan bow, butterfly-type adhesive, or Band-Aid placed cheek-to-cheek across top of lip prevents lateral tension.

    Prevent wetting tape, or it will loosen.

3. Prevent the infant from crying, because crying also increases tension on the suture line.

    a. Encourage the mother to hold and cuddle the infant.

    b. Keep the infant dry, fed, and comfortable.

4. Position the infant on his back or propped on his side to keep him from rubbing his lip on the sheets. An infant seat may be useful for variation of position, comfort, and entertainment. Provide for appropriate diversional activity, hanging toys, mobiles, etc.

C. Maintain Adequate Nutrition and Fluid Intake for Weight Gain, Growth, and Prevention of Dehydration.

1. For several days postoperatively, feeding will have to be accomplished without tension on the suture line.

    a. Dropper or syringe with a rubber tip, inserted from the side to avoid suture line or to avoid stimulating sucking

    b. Side of spoon (Never put spoon into the mouth.)

    c. Nasogastric gavage—usually last treatment of choice

2. Advance slowly to nipple feeding as indicated by physician preference.

    The infant should be able to suck more efficiently with the lip repaired.

3. Encourage the mother to participate as much as possible in the care of the infant. It is good for both infant and mother to continue their relationship.

D. Keep the Suture Line Clean to Decrease Infection and Eliminate Crust Formation That Enlarges the Resulting Scar.

The sutures are removed from 3–14 days after surgery.

1. Clean suture line after every feeding.

    a. The cleansing solution used is usually the physician's choice.

        (1) Water

        (2) Hydrogen peroxide

        (3) Saline solution

    b. Gently and frequently wipe with a wet cotton-tipped applicator.

    c. Gently dry by patting.

        (1) May use antibiotic ointment or petrolatum after drying.

        (2) May be left open to the air.

    d. Water should be given after feeding to cleanse the mouth.

Preoperative Care of the Child With a Cleft Palate

(Repair may require several operations.)

A. Be Familiar With Growth and Development As Well As the Emotional and Psychological Needs of the Toddler, 12–18 Months Old. (This is the age most common for palate repair.)

1. Primary objectives for palate repair are to improve speech and to minimize maxillary growth retardation and dental alveolar deformity.

2. This toddler age is selected because the anatomic structures involved are still growing.

3. The toddler finds the hospital strange and frightening (see p. 1122).

    a. Encourage the mother to stay with the child if possible.

    b. Encourage play.

B. Prepare the Child for Postoperative Care; If He Is Familiar With the Procedures and Routines, He Will Be Less Frightened and More Likely to Cooperate.

1. Use elbow restraints frequently for short periods of time.

2. Do not allow the child to suck from a bottle. Ideally, he has been taught to drink from a cup. Feed him in the manner in which he will be fed postoperatively.

3. Practice frequent mouth irrigations using the same solution and equipment to be used postoperatively. Allow the child to handle and become familiar with equipment.

C. Prevent Infection By Keeping the Child Away From Anyone With Infection.

D. Prepare the Parents As to What to Expect When They See the Child Postoperatively.

Include the parents in the preparation of the child. Then, with the parents alone discuss in more depth what to expect.

Postoperative Care of the Child With a Cleft Palate

A. Administer Good Postoperative Care and Observe for Possible Postoperative Complications.

1. Breathing with a closed palate is different from the child's customary way of breathing; the child must also contend with increased mucous production.

2. Note respiratory effort.
3. Croup tent with mist decreases occurrence of respiratory problems and provides moisture to mucous membranes that may become dry because of mouth breathing.
4. Infant may lie on abdomen.

B. Prevent Injury to the Suture Line In the Mouth.

1. Use elbow restraints.
2. Do not put anything into the mouth. Do not allow the use of straws, eating utensils, fingers.
3. Prevent the child from crying. Blowing, sucking, talking, and laughing put strain on the suture line.

C. Keep the Suture Line and Mouth Clean to Prevent Infection.

1. Irrigate the mouth with normal saline solution or water.
   a. Direct a gentle stream over the suture line using an ear bulb syringe.
   b. Have the child in sitting position with his head forward.
2. Keep the mouth moist to promote healing and provide comfort.
3. Rinse the mouth after each feeding.

D. Maintain Adequate Nutrition for Growth and to Promote Healing.

1. Diet progresses from clear liquids to full liquids to soft foods.
   Soft foods are usually continued for about 1 month after surgery at which time a regular diet is started, excluding hard food.
2. Check weight periodically to see if adequate nutrition is being maintained.
3. Feed the child in the manner used preoperatively (cup, side of spoon, or rubber-tipped syringe). Never use straw, nipple, or plain syringe.

E. Administer Antibiotics As Prescribed.

The mouth and suture line are constantly contaminated.

F. Provide Opportunities for Social Relationships and Play As Soon As Possible.

1. While the child must be restrained, he especially needs to have some stimulation and diversional activity.
2. A satisfactory relationship with the mother or the nurse can minimize frustration and discomfort from surgery and restraints.

G. Continue Support of Parents Who Have Already Encountered Many Frustrations In Caring for the Child, and Foster Continual Parental Acceptance of the Child and His Handicap.

1. Solicit assistance of social worker if appropriate; the mother may talk about problems she is having rearing a handicapped child.
2. Sincerely compliment the parents for the good work they have already done with this child.
3. Help the parents understand that this child can live a normal life in the community.

H. Begin Discharge Planning and Health Teaching Soon After Admission So the Parents Can Learn How to Care for the Child At Home.

1. Continued protection of the mouth.
   a. May need to use elbow restraints
   b. A child this age will put everything into his mouth—restrict this.
   c. No sucking or blowing
2. Diet of soft foods will need to be continued. Do not give this child lollipops.

3. Infection must be prevented.
   Continue to cleanse his mouth after eating.

Health Education

1. There are 3 specific times when parental teaching is vitally important for continual, effective management of the child:
   a. Management of the child with cleft lip and palate not yet repaired
   b. Preparing for lip or palate surgery
   c. Preparing for the patient's discharge following surgery
2. In each case specific instructions need to be given in the following areas:
   a. Good nutrition and feeding techniques
   b. Proper oral hygiene
   c. Prevention of injury to operative site
   d. Prevention of infection
   e. Function of therapy; purpose of any appliances plus proper use and care
   f. Plan for follow-up, especially after surgery
   g. Psychological and social development of the child—including speech therapy, hearing tests, and understanding of the normal sounds at specific stages of growth and development
3. Other members of the family must be considered.
   a. The child with a cleft lip or palate should not be thought of as sick, but as a child who has special needs. It is important to promote his individual growth and development, but he does not require attention all the time.
   b. The family should be included in his care, but they also must have a life of their own.
   c. The parents need time to themselves.
4. Help the parents realize that even though rehabilitation of the child is long, drawn-out, and expensive, the child can live a normal life.
   a. Have the parents discuss the child's problem with the school nurse, the teacher and other responsible adults who will have close contact with the child.
   b. Long-range planning should include detailed communication between the family and various disciplines.
      (1) Collaborative effort between disciplines promotes the effectiveness of each discipline.
      (2) Parents may need help in understanding the value of each discipline for the future well-being of their child.
      Speech therapy is often one area where the value is not completely understood. This needs to be emphasized.

Support Agencies

Special Child Health Services, 2023 W. Ogden Avenue, Chicago, IL 60612
National Institute of Dental Research, Westwood Bldg, 5333 Westbard Avenue, Bethesda, MD 20205

Expected Outcomes

1. Demonstrates appropriate nutritional intake and status as evidenced by weight gain and eating habits
2. Is free of infection and aspiration as evidenced by normal vital signs and laboratory values
3. Parents show appropriate bonding and ability to care for child as evidenced by their actions, verbalization and demonstration of feeding and handling, etc., of child.

4. Develops a positive self-image and socialization as evidenced by play activity, interest in surroundings and outgoing behavior
5. Experiences minimal anxiety as evidenced by appropriate coping behaviors

Esophageal Atresia With Tracheoesophageal Fistula

Esophageal atresia is failure of the esophagus to form a continuous passage from the pharynx to the stomach during embryonic development. *Tracheoesophageal fistula* (TEF) is the abnormal connection between the trachea and esophagus.

Etiology

1. Failure of embryonic development
2. Cause unknown in most cases
   a. May have possible inheritable genetic factor
   b. Teratogen may have some influence
   c. Environmental factors

Altered Physiology

A. Basic Problem

Failure of proper separation of the embryonic channel into the esophagus and trachea occurring during the 4th and 5th weeks of gestation.

B. Classification of Esophageal Atresia (Fig. 52-1)

1. Type I—Proximal and distal segments of esophagus are blind; there is no connection to trachea—10%–15% of cases.
2. Type II—Proximal segment of esophagus opens into trachea by a fistula; distal segment is blind—very rare.
3. Type III—Proximal segment of esophagus has blind end: distal segment of esophagus connects into trachea by a fistula (most common; discussion is limited to this type—80%–90% of cases).
4. Type IV—Esophageal atresia with fistula between both proximal and distal ends of trachea and esophagus—very rare.
5. Type V—Both proximal and distal segments of esophagus open into trachea by a fistula; no esophageal atresia (H-type)—not usually diagnosed at birth.

C. Tracheoesophageal Fistula (TEF)—Type III

1. Child is unable to swallow effectively.
2. Saliva or formula accumulates in upper esophageal pouch and is aspirated into airway from spillover.
3. Regurgitation of gastric acid through distal fistula.
   a. Abdominal distention occurs as a result of air entering the lower esophagus through the fistula and passing into the stomach, especially when the child is crying.
   b. Gastric distention may be severe enough to cause respiratory distress by elevation of the diaphragm.

Complications Associated with TEF

1. Pneumonitis—secondary to
   a. Salivary aspiration
   b. Gastric acid reflux
2. Concomitant lesions
   a. Congenital heart disease
   b. Gastrointestinal anomalies, particularly imperforate anus

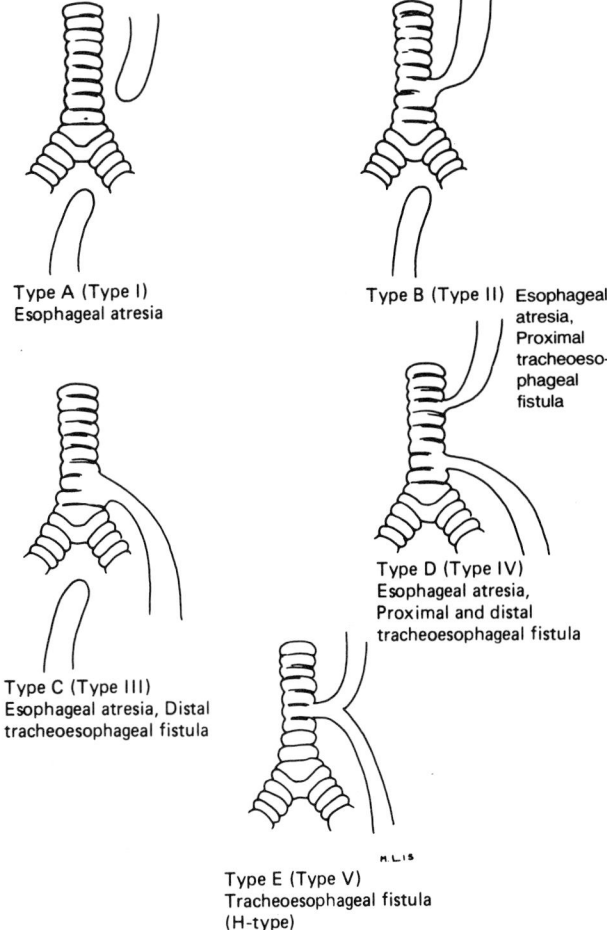

Type A (Type I)
Esophageal atresia

Type B (Type II) Esophageal atresia, Proximal tracheoesophageal fistula

Type C (Type III)
Esophageal atresia, Distal tracheoesophageal fistula

Type D (Type IV)
Esophageal atresia, Proximal and distal tracheoesophageal fistula

Type E (Type V)
Tracheoesophageal fistula (H-type)

Figure 52-1. *Types of esophageal atresia: Esophageal atresia and tracheoesophageal fistula (TEF).*

c. Skeletal and muscular deformities
   d. Renal anomalies
   e. Vertebral defects
3. Prematurity

Postoperative Complications

1. Leak at anastomosis site
2. Recurrent fistulas
3. Esophageal strictures
4. Abnormal function of distal esophagus sphincter (gastroesophageal reflux) and esophagitis
5. Tracheomalacia
6. Feeding problems with the older child

Clinical Manifestations

Appear soon after birth
1. Excessive amount of secretions
   a. Constant drooling
   b. Large amount of secretions from nose
2. Intermittent cyanosis—unexplained; laryngospasm caused by aspiration of accumulated saliva in blind pouch
3. Abdominal distention
   Inspired air from trachea passes through fistula into stomach.

4. If fed, the infant will respond violently after first or second swallow.
   a. The infant coughs and chokes.
   b. Fluid returns through nose and mouth.
   c. Cyanosis occurs.
   d. The infant struggles.
5. Inability to pass catheter through nose or mouth into stomach—tip of catheter will stop at blind pouch, or atresia.

Note: Be aware of coiling of catheter; coiling may make catheter *appear* to be descending into stomach.

Diagnostic Evaluation

1. Recognize infants at risk for TEF. Two major groups are at risk:
   a. Infants with polyhydramnios
   b. Premature infants
2. Observations of specific symptoms manifested by infant.
3. Inability to pass a stiff, radiopaque 10–14 Fr. catheter into stomach through nose or mouth.
4. X-ray, flat plate of abdomen and chest—reveals presence of gas in stomach and tip of catheter in blind pouch

Treatment

A. Immediate Treatment

1. Propping infant at 30° angle to prevent reflux of gastric content
2. Suctioning of upper esophageal pouch with Replogle tube or sump drain
3. Gastrostomy to decompress stomach and prevent aspiration; later used for feedings

B. Appropriate Treatment of Any Existing Pathological Processes—either acquired complications, such as pneumonitis, or complications from concomitant lesions, such as congestive heart failure.

C. Supportive Therapy—meeting nutritional requirements, IV fluids, antibiotics, respiratory support, maintaining thermally neutral environment

D. Surgery

1. Prompt primary repair—division of fistual followed by esophageal anastomosis of proximal and distal segments (infant is greater than 2000 gm. and is without pneumonia).
2. Short-term delay—subsequent primary repair—used to stabilize infant and to prevent deterioration when the patient's condition contraindicates immediate surgery.
3. Staging—initial fistula division and gastrostomy with later secondary esophageal anastomosis. Approach may be used with a very small premature infant or a very sick neonate, or when severe congenital anomalies exist.
4. Circular esophagomyotomy—on proximal pouch to gain length and allow for primary anastomosis at initial surgery.
5. Cervical esophagostomy—when ends of esophagus are too widely separated; esophageal replacement with segment of intestine is done at 18–24 months of age.

Patient Problems and Nursing Diagnoses

1. Impaired gas exchange related to excessive nasopharyngeal secretions and gastric secretions refluxing into the tracheobronchial tree

2. Nutrition, altered, less than body requirements, related to tracheal-esophageal reflux
3. Potential for alteration in electrolyte and fluid balance related to lack of oral nutrition and gastric fluid loss
4. Potential for complications (i.e., temperature instability) related to prematurity
5. Parental anxiety related to the child's illness and insecurity in caring for the child

Preoperative Nursing Intervention

A. Position the Infant With Head and Chest Elevated 20°–30° to Prevent or Decrease Reflux of Gastric Juices Into the Tracheobronchial Tree.

1. This position may also ease respiratory effort by dropping the distended intestines away from the diaphragm.
2. Prone position will allow gastric juices to pool anteriorly away from the esophagus. Turn frequently to prevent atelectasis and pneumonia.

B. Assist In Removing Nasopharyngeal Secretions From Esophageal Blind Pouch and Support the Infant's Respiration.

1. Intermittent nasopharyngeal suctioning or indwelling Replogle tube (double lumen tube) or sump tube with constant suction is used.
   a. Tip of tube is placed in the blind pouch.
   b. Replogle or sump tube allows air to be drawn in through a second lumen and prevents tube obstruction by mucous membrane of pouch.
   c. Maintain indwelling tube patency by irrigating with 1 ml. normal saline solution frequently.
   d. Change indwelling tube as needed and at least once every 12–24 hours (by the physician); alternate nostrils. Take care to prevent necrosis of nostrils from pressure by catheter.
2. Place the infant in an Isolette or under a radiant warmer with high humidity to aid in liquefying secretions and thick mucus. Give mouth care.
3. Administer oxygen as needed.
4. Suction mouth to keep clear of secretions and prevent aspiration.
5. Be alert for indications of respiratory distress:
   a. Retractions
   b. Circumoral cyanosis
   c. Restlessness
   d. Nasal flaring
   e. Increased respiration and heart rate
6. The infant is to receive nothing by mouth.

C. Administer Antibiotics and Other Medications Prescribed.

Give to prevent or treat associated pneumonitis.

D. Monitor Parenteral Fluids As Prescribed In Order to Prevent Dehydration and Electrolyte Imbalance (see p. 1165).

1. Supplies water and caloric and mineral requirements.
2. The infant does not receive oral feedings.

E. Observe Infant Carefully for Any Change In Condition; Report Changes Immediately.

1. Check vital signs, color, amount of secretions, abdominal distention, and respiratory distress.
2. Also be alert for complications that can occur in any neonate or premature infant.

F. Prevent Infection By Using the Principles of Isolation.

Isolette may be used for environmental isolation.

G. Be Available and Recognize Need for Emergency Care or Resuscitation.

Accompany the infant to the x-ray department or the operating room in Isolette with portable oxygen and suction equipment.

H. Administer Supportive Nursing Care That Will Prevent Any Deterioration of Infant's Condition and Will Assist In Preparation for Surgery.

1. Careful observations, recording and reporting of any signs or symptoms that may indicate additional congenital anomalies or complications.
2. Maintain the infant's temperature in thermoneutral zone.
3. Gastrostomy tube may be placed prior to definitive surgery to aid in gastric decompression and prevention of reflux. The gastrostomy tube is generally attached to straight gravity drainage, and irrigation is not done before surgery.

I. Ensure That Bougie Dilatation (should it be done) **Remains Undisturbed.**

Postoperative Nursing Interventions

There are 2 types of surgery considered for esophageal atresia with tracheoesophageal fistula: (1) fistula division and esophageal anastomosis (called *primary repair*) and (2) palliative surgery temporarily using a gastrostomy and cervical esophagostomy until the infant gains weight so that a bowel transplant or anastomosis can be done. Generally the nursing care is essentially the same for either procedure.

A. Administer Good Postoperative Care and Observe for Signs of Possible Complications.

B. Maintain a Patent Airway to Prevent Oxygen Starvation, Apnea, and Aspiration of Secretions.

1. Request that the physician mark a suction catheter, indicating how far the catheter can be safely inserted without disturbing the anastomosis.
   a. Suction frequently—every 5–10 minutes may be necessary; at least every 1–2 hours.
   b. Observe for signs of obstructed airway.
2. Administer chest physiotherapy as prescribed by physician.
   a. Change the infant's position by turning; stimulate him to cry so that he fully expands his lungs.
   b. Head and shoulders elevated 20°–30°.
   c. Mechanical vibrator (to minimize trauma to anastomosis) may be used 2–3 days postoperatively, followed by more vigorous physical therapy after the 3rd day. Care should be taken not to hyperextend the neck, causing stress to the operative site.
3. Continue use of Isolette or radiant warmer with humidity. Either device does the following:
   a. Provides an environment in which infant can maintain his temperature in thermoneutral zone.
   b. Provides humidity to liquefy secretions.
   c. Allows for observation of and easy access to infant.
4. Be prepared to function in an emergency.
   Have emergency equipment available:
     a. Suction machine, catheter
     b. Oxygen
     c. Laryngoscope, endotracheal tubes in varying sizes

C. Be Aware of Type of Chest Drainage Present, Which May Be Determined By Surgical Approach, and Provide Appropriate Care.

1. Retropleural—small tube in posterior mediastinum; may be left open for drainage.
2. Transthoracic—chest tube placed in pleural space and connected to suction.
   a. Keep tubing free from clots; keep it unkinked and without tension.
   b. If a break occurs in the closed drainage system, immediately clamp tubing close to the infant to prevent pneumothorax.

D. Assist In Maintaining Adequate Nutrition to Promote Healing, Growth, and Development.

Feedings may be given by mouth, by gastrostomy, or—rarely—by a feeding tube into the esophagus, depending on the type of operation performed and the infant's condition. The gastrostomy is generally attached to gravity drainage for 3 days postoperatively, then elevated and left open to allow for air escape and passage of gastric secretions into the duodenum for a period of time before feedings are begun.

1. Gastrostomy feeding
   a. Gastrostomy feeding can be started prior to esophageal healing—adequate nutrition is an important factor in healing. Give the infant a pacifier to suck during feedings, unless contraindicated.
   b. Gastrostomy feedings may be continued until the infant can tolerate full feedings orally.
   c. Care should be taken not to allow air to enter the stomach, thereby causing gastric distention and possible reflux.
   d. Check with the surgeon before allowing the infant to suck on a pacifier during gastrostomy feeding.
2. Oral feedings may begin 10–14 days postoperatively following anastomosis.
   a. Feed slowly to allow the infant time to swallow.
   b. Use upright sitting position.
   c. Burp frequently.
   d. Demand feeding may be more successful and pleasant for the infant than strictly scheduled feeding.
   e. Do not allow the infant to become overtired at feeding time. Note cardiac rate.
   f. Try to make each feeding a pleasant experience for the infant. Use a consistent approach and patience. Encourage parental involvement.

E. Care Appropriately for Cervical Esophagostomy (artificial opening in neck that allows for drainage of the upper esophagus).

1. Keep the area clean of saliva.
   a. Wash with clear water.
   b. Place an absorbent pad over the area.
2. As soon as possible, allow the infant to suck a few milliliters of milk at the same time gastrostomy feeding is being done. Advance the infant to solid foods as appropriate if esophagostomy is maintained for a few months.
   a. Encourage sucking and swallowing.
   b. Familiarize the infant with food, so that when he is able to eat orally, he will be used to it.

F. Be Aware of Impending Complications of Esophageal Repair.

1. Leak at the anastomosis (development of mediastinitis, pneumothorax, and saliva in chest tube)
   a. Hypothermia or hyperthermia
   b. Pneumothorax
      (1) Severe respiratory distress
      (2) Cyanosis
      (3) Restlessness
      (4) Weak pulses
2. Stricture at the anastomosis
   a. Difficulty in swallowing
   b. Vomiting or spitting up of ingested fluid
   c. Refusing to eat
   d. Fever—secondary to aspiration and pneumonia
3. Recurrent fistula
   a. Coughing, choking, and cyanosis associated with feeding
   b. Excessive salivation
   c. Difficulty in swallowing associated with abnormal distention
   d. Repeated episodes of pneumonitis
   e. General poor physical condition—no weight gain
4. Atelectasis or pneumonitis
   a. Aspiration
   b. Respiratory distress

G. Provide for the Infant's Emotional and Social Needs.

The extent of hospitalization and long-term care puts a strain on the normal opportunities in these areas (see ICN, p. 1129).

1. Hold and cuddle the infant for feedings and after feedings.
2. Encourage mother (parents) to cuddle and love the infant.
3. Provide for visual, auditory, and tactile stimulation as appropriate for the infant's physical condition and age.

H. Encourage Parental Participation In Learning to Care for and Handle the Infant and to Foster Acceptance of the Child By His Parents and Family.

1. Provide opportunities for the parents to learn all aspects of care of their infant.
2. Initiate a teaching program for the parents early. Offer them available literature and help them become familiar with community resources.
3. Initiate a community nurse referral for continuity of care in the home.
4. Encourage the parents to talk about their feelings, fears, and concerns.
5. Help to develop a healthy parent–child relationship.
   a. Frequent visiting
   b. Phone calls
   c. Physical contact of child and parents

Health Education

1. Teach carefully and thoroughly all procedures to be done at home. Show the parents how; then watch return demonstration of the following procedures:
   a. Gastrostomy feedings and care
   b. Esophagostomy care with feeding technique
   c. Suctioning
   d. Identifying signs of respiratory distress
2. Help the parents understand the psychological needs of the infant for sucking, warmth, comfort, stimulation, and love. Suggest that activity be appropriate for age.

3. Encourage the parents to continue close medical follow-up and help them learn to recognize possible problems.
   a. Dilatation of esophagus to treat stricture at the site of the anastomosis
   b. Raspy cough for 6–24 months
   c. Eating problems, especially when solids are introduced
   d. Repeated respiratory tract infection
   e. Occurrence of stricture at site of anastomosis weeks to months later—recognized by difficulty in swallowing; spitting of ingested fluid; fever
   f. Signs of fistula leakage: dusky or choking with feeding
4. Help the parents understand the need for good nutrition and the need to follow the diet regimen suggested by the physician.

Expected Outcomes

1. Shows no signs of respiratory distress; maintains adequate oxygen–carbon dioxide exchange; normal blood gas values; stable vital signs
2. Receives adequate nutritional intake; demonstrates willingness to eat; shows weight gain
3. Maintains normal fluid and electrolyte balance; has adequate intake and output; normal laboratory values
4. Experiences minimal complications of prematurity (i.e., thermal stability); laboratory values within normal range; stable vital signs; improved appearance
5. The parents verbalize an understanding of illness and follow-up care; becoming involved in child care and the bonding process

---

Gastroesophageal Reflux

Gastroesophageal reflux (GER) is a malfunction of the distal end of the esophagus, antireflux barrier, permitting return of acid stomach content into the esophagus.

Etiology

1. The cause is undetermined in most patients.
2. Possible causes:
   a. Neuromuscular imbalance; delayed development
   b. Cerebral defects
   c. Obstruction at or just below the pylorus
   d. Physiologic immaturity
3. Mechanisms of GER may involve an interplay of
   a. Esophageal motility
   b. Lower esophageal sphincter activity
   c. Gastric emptying
4. Associated conditions that cause reflux
   a. Coughing and wheezing from cystic fibrosis, bronchopulmonary dysplasia (BPD), asthma
   b. Indwelling oro–nasogastric feeding tube
   c. Medications—theophylline affects lower sphincter and increases gastric acidity
   d. Position—supine, chest physical therapy positions

Altered Physiology

1. The lower esophageal sphincter is a physiologic rather than an anatomic segment that forms an antireflux barrier
   a. The segment is 2–5 cm. in length.
   b. The segment is characterized by a pressure greater than that found proximally in the esophagus or distally in the stomach.

c. Constitutes an effective barrier to protect the esophageal mucosa from damage by gastric contents (acid, pepsin, bile salts).

2. GER—consequence of incompetence or malfunctioning of this lower esophageal sphincter
    a. Filling of the esophagus from the stomach upon inspiration, leading to vomiting
    b. Increased intra-abdominal pressure

Complications

Resulting from frequent and sustained reflux of gastric contents into lower esophagus:
1. Recurrent pulmonary disease; aspiration pneumonia
2. Chronic esophagitis
3. Failure to thrive
4. Anemia
5. Cyanotic episodes
6. Esophageal stricture from scarring; esophagitis
7. Asthma
8. Hiatal hernia frequently associated with chalasia

Clinical Manifestations

A. Infant

1. Vomiting (unexplained)
    a. Immediately after feeding, especially when the infant is placed in a prone position
    b. Usually regurgitation rather than projectile vomiting
2. Onset usually soon after birth
3. Weight loss or failure to gain weight; rumination
4. Dehydration
5. Recurrent pulmonary symptoms
6. Colic, excessive crying
7. Sleep disturbances

B. Older Child

1. Substernal burning
2. Upper abdominal discomfort; pressure or "squeezing" feeling
3. Persistent pulmonary problems
4. Dysphagia as evidenced by irritability during eating
5. Anemia

Diagnostic Evaluation

1. Upper GI barium x-ray with fluoroscope (barium esophagogram)
   Barium enters stomach but then is regurgitated back into the esophagus.
2. Monitor pH in esophagus
3. Serum studies
    a. Calcium level—may be lowered
    b. Alkalosis—pH greater than 7.45
    c. Hemoglobin and hematocrit

Treatment

A. Positioning

1. *Infant*—under 6 months
    a. Prone—elevated
    b. Position in harness at 60° angle, 60 minutes to constant 24 hours.
    c. Infant may also be held upright.
    d. When positioned in infant seat, infant will probably slump, causing increased intra-abdominal pressure and increased GER.
2. *Older child*—raise head of bed with 8-inch blocks

B. Antacid—between feedings if esophagitis is present (forms a floating barrier)

Infant—thickened feedings

C. Feeding

1. *Infant*
    a. Thickened feedings such as dry rice cereal or commercial thickening agent.
    b. May cause a decrease in the number of episodes; however, the duration of reflux episodes may increase, thus increasing the risk of complications.
2. *Older child*
    a. Nothing to eat 2 hours before bedtime
    b. Possible avoidance of certain foods
    c. Child should also stand or sit upright while awake.

D. Medication

1. Medication to stimulate lower esophageal sphincter pressure (tone) and increase peristaltic wave amplitude and clearance rate (metoclopramide)
2. Cimetidine when esophagitis has been documented

E. Surgery

Surgical reconstruction of esophagogastric junction—fundoplication—if conservative management does not improve condition or recurrent severe respiratory disease and apnea, or refractory esophagitis with stricture

Patient Problems and Nursing Diagnoses

1. Impaired gas exchange related to frequent and sustained reflux of gastric contents into tracheobronchial tree
2. Nutrition, altered, less than body requirements related to decreased oral intake
3. Potential fluid volume deficit related to frequent vomiting
4. Altered comfort related to nausea
5. Potential for infection related to malnourishment
6. Parental anxiety and concern related to the child's illness

Nursing Interventions

A. Assist In Treatment of Dehydration

1. Monitor intravenous therapy (see p. 1167).
2. Observe and record accurately urinary output.
    a. Amount, frequency, color, and concentration
    b. Specific gravity
3. Promote good skin care to prevent lesions of dry and delicate tissues.
    a. Change position frequently.
    b. Change soiled diapers often.
    c. Apply lotion and gently massage any reddened areas.

B. Maintain Adequate Nutrition and Prevent Likelihood of Vomiting.

1. Thicken formula for each feeding.
    a. May use cereal.
    b. Enlarge nipple hole so that formula can be more easily extracted.
2. Prop the infant in upright position.
    a. 60°, prone
    b. Suggested methods: elevate mattress, saddle
    c. Non-nutritive sucking on a pacifier may increase reflux when infant is prone, but not when infant is seated upright after eating.
3. Handle the infant gently, with minimal movement during and after feeding.

4. Bubble frequently during and at completion of feeding.
5. Record accurately activity of infant.
   a. Amount of feeding taken; whether retained
   b. Emesis, estimated amount, type, occurrence in relation to feeding
   c. Any change in behavior as a result of feeding technique

C. Support the Family, Especially the Mother, and Encourage Them to Participate In Care and Feeding of the Infant.

1. The mother may be overly concerned about the infant and blame herself and feeding technique for the infant's condition.
   a. Help the mother understand it is not her fault; she is not a "bad mother."
   b. Let her talk about her concerns.
2. Encourage the mother to take an active part in caring for the infant—provides a good opportunity to guide the mother in correct or preferred methods of handling baby with this condition.

Health Education

1. Plan a program of intensive parental teaching on how to handle and care for the infant. Be certain the parents understand why this is being done. Ensure they have proper equipment for propping the infant.
   a. Help the parents understand that it is not necessary to keep infant in infant seat or propped at all times.
      (1) Bathe or play with the infant *prior to feeding.*
      (2) Change position about 1 hour after feeding.
      (3) During the night after feeding, the infant can sleep in an upright position.
      (4) Expect occasional small amounts of vomiting.
2. Help parents to understand that chalasia is self-limited—symptoms usually disappear within 12 months.
3. If a temporary gastrostomy is done, ensure that the parents know how to use the tube, clear it, and replace it.
4. Help the parents understand the importance of follow-up of weight gain and development.

Expected Outcomes

1. Breathes more easily and shows minimal respiratory distress; normal blood gas values and vital signs; lungs clear on auscultation
2. Ingests adequate amount of food; shows willingness to eat; gaining weight
3. Maintains balanced fluid and electrolyte values
4. Experiences minimal discomfort; stable vital signs; shows calm behavior; engages in play activities
5. Absence of infection; stable vital signs; normal laboratory values
6. The parents have overcome their anxiety; appear more relaxed; express sense of relief; becoming involved in the child's care

Hypertrophic Pyloric Stenosis

Hypertrophic pyloric stenosis is congenital, progressive hypertrophy of the muscle of the pylorus, causing partial or total obstruction of the stomach outlet (pyloric sphincter).

Etiology

1. Unknown
2. Possibly, immature pyloric ganglion cells—environmental, partial genetic basis

Incidence

1. 1:800 whites; 1:2000 blacks
2. 4:1 ratio, with males predominating

Altered Physiology

1. Increase in size of the circular musculature of the pylorus with thickening (size and shape of an olive). The pylorus muscle becomes elongated and thickened and is enlarged—about twice the usual size.
2. Hypertrophy of the pylorus musculature occurs with narrowing of the pyloric lumen.
3. Constriction of the lumen of the pyloric canal (at the distal end of the stomach) causes the stomach to become dilated.
4. Gastric emptying is delayed; vomiting after feeding and obstruction also occur.

Clinical Manifestations

Onset is within the first 2 months after birth, usually about 3 weeks of age.
1. Vomiting—onset may be gradual and intermittent or sudden and forceful. The following characteristics may be noted:
   a. Occasional, nonprojectile vomiting at first, gradually increasing in frequency and intensity
   b. Projectile vomiting, not bile-stained
2. Constipation—decreased quantity of stools
3. Loss of weight or failure to gain weight
4. Visible gastric peristaltic waves, left to right
5. Excessive hunger—willingness to eat immediately after vomiting
6. Dehydration—electrolyte disturbance with alkalosis
7. Decreased urinary output
8. Palpable pyloric mass in upper right quadrant of abdomen, to the right of the umbilicus and best felt during feeding or immediately after vomiting

Diagnostic Evaluation

1. Palpation of pyloric mass ("olive") in conjunction with persistent, projectile vomiting with associated alkalosis
2. Tests for metabolic alkalosis—due to loss of hydrochloric acid and potassium from vomiting
   a. Serum sodium—decreases
   b. Serum chloride—decreases
   c. Serum potassium—decreases
   d. Serum pH—increases above 7
   e. Serum CO_2—increases
3. Urinalysis—urine becomes alkaline and concentrated
4. Blood hematocrit and hemoglobin—elevated due to hemoconcentration
5. Flat film of abdomen—dilated, air-filled stomach; nondilated pyloric canal
6. X-ray examination with barium
   a. Narrowing of pyloric canal
   b. Delayed gastric emptying time
   c. Enlarged stomach
   d. Increased peristaltic waves
   e. Gas distal to stomach

Treatment

1. Initial treatment:
   a. Rehydrate and correct electrolytes
   b. Correct alkalosis
2. Surgical—pyloromyotomy (Fredet–Ramstedt procedure)
   a. Hypertrophy of the pyloric muscle regresses to normal size by about 12 weeks postoperatively.

b. Gastroesophageal reflux may be a complication of surgery.

Patient Problems and Nursing Diagnoses

1. Potential fluid volume deficit related to frequent vomiting
2. Nutrition, altered, less than body requirements, (failure to thrive) related to vomiting
3. Comfort, altered, related to frequent hunger and/or surgical procedure
4. Parental anxiety related to the child's illness and insecurity in caring for child

Preoperative Nursing Interventions

A. Assist In Restoring Hydration and Electrolyte Balance.

1. IV therapy is usually initiated (see p. 1167). Corrects dehydration, metabolic alkalosis, and electrolyte deficiency
2. Careful observation of output, amount, and characteristics
    a. Urine (check specific gravity)
    b. Vomiting
    c. Stools
3. Accurate daily weight—serves as a guide for calculating need for parenteral fluid

B. Prevent or Decrease the Likelihood of Vomiting.

1. Patient may be NPO with indwelling nasogastric tube to remove any residual barium and retained formula. Ensure proper functioning of tube and note drainage.
2. Oral feedings may be continued.
    a. Feed small, frequent feedings, given slowly.
    b. Bubble frequently, before, during, and after feeding.
    c. Thickened formula may be prescribed.
3. Proper positioning (Fig. 52-2)
    a. Prop the patient in upright position.
       (1) Elevate head of bed, mattress, or infant seat at a 75° to 80° angle.
       (2) Place slightly on right side—to aid in gastric emptying.
       (3) Handle gently and minimally after feeding.

C. Make Frequent, Accurate Observations of the Infant's Condition.

1. Dehydration
2. Vomiting
3. Stools and urine output
4. Vital signs
5. Electrolyte imbalance

NURSING ALERT: Respiratory rate may be irregular with apnea when the patient is in severe alkalosis.

D. Provide Comfort for the Infant.

1. Mouth care—wet lips
   Let the infant suck on a pacifier.
2. Physical contact or nearness of the nurse or mother
3. Audio or visual stimulation may be soothing
4. Minimal palpation of pyloric "olive"—will decrease risk of postoperative wound infection from bruising abdominal wall and excoriation of tissue in operative site

E. Prevent Infection.

The infant is at increased risk for infection because of his decreased nutritional status.

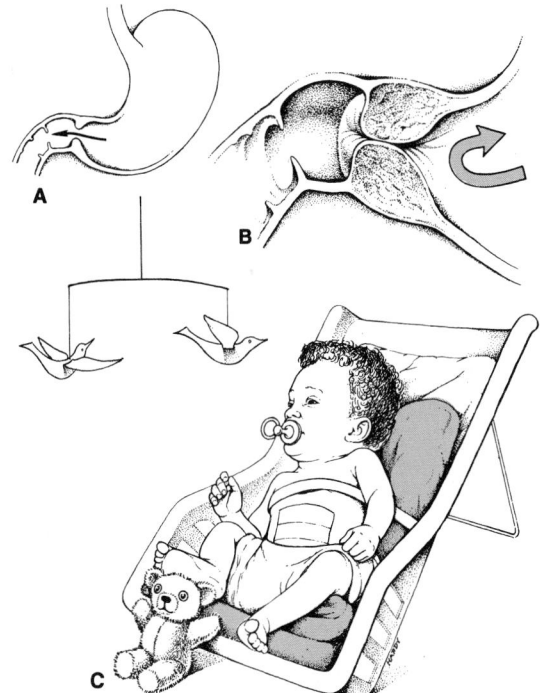

Figure 52-2. Pyloric stenosis. (A) Normal passage through pyloric sphincter. (B) Stoppage of flow due to stenotic sphincter. (C) Postoperative treatment: Child propped on right side after feeding to aid gastric emptying.

F. Support the Parents, Who Are Usually Very Concerned and Worried.

1. The mother may feel guilty (i.e., she may feel she has a poor feeding technique).
   Help her understand that she did not do anything to cause this deformity.
2. Prepare the parents for the surgery of their child.
    a. Be honest with them.
    b. Inform them of the expected postoperative appearance of the infant.
    c. Show them where the operating room and recovery room are located and where to wait during surgery.
3. Encourage the parents to maintain a good relationship with the infant. Allow them to hold the infant.
4. Encourage them to get some rest.
   The mother may be tired and frustrated because of the extensive care she has had to give to the child prior to hospitalization.

Postoperative Nursing Interventions

A. Give Good Postoperative Care and Observe for the Usual Postoperative Complications (see p. 1134).

B. Monitor Parenteral Fluids to Maintain Hydration.

IV therapy may be continued until adequate oral intake is obtained.

C. Assist In Resuming Oral Feedings.

1. Feeding is usually resumed 2–8 hours after surgery.
    a. Feedings usually start with small, frequent feedings of glucose water and slowly advance to full-strength formula and regular diet.

b. Report any vomiting—the amount and characteristics. Feeding schedule may be withheld 4 hours and then restarted.
c. Feed slowly and bubble frequently.
d. Note how feeding is taken and if it is retained.
e. The amount of feeding is increased as the time interval between feedings is lengthened.

2. Continue to elevate the infant's head and shoulders after feeding for 45–60 minutes for several feedings after surgery. Place on right side to aid gastric emptying.

3. Regurgitation may continue for a short period after surgery.

D. Encourage the Parents to Resume Care—Especially Feeding—of Their Infant.

1. This will help to restore their confidence in caring for their baby.

2. This activity provides an opportunity for the nurse to teach.

3. If the mother was breast-feeding, she should resume this as soon as possible.

Health Education

1. Help the parents to understand that surgery has corrected the pyloric stenosis.
   a. Discharge of baby may be from 2–5 days after surgery.
   b. Proper care of the operative site can be done by the mother.
   c. A modified method of feeding technique will be continued at home for only a short period of time.

2. Since this may be a new mother, and the infant may be under 6 weeks of age, the mother may need help with routine infant care.

Expected Outcomes

1. Attains/maintains fluid and electrolyte balance; appears well hydrated; experiences fewer vomiting episodes; normal skin turgor

2. Shows improved nutritional status; retains feedings; shows more alert appearance; has weight gain

3. Appears more comfortable; rests for longer periods; appears satisfied after feeding; no signs of excessive peristalsis or abdominal distinction

4. The parents participate in their child's care and express understanding of follow-up care of wound site and feeding

Celiac Disease

Celiac disease, also called gluten-sensitive enteropathy, is a disease of the small intestines characterized by a permanent inability to tolerate dietary gluten.

Etiology

1. Unknown. Although the relationship of gluten to mucosal abnormalities is established, the way in which these mucosal changes occur is not clear.

2. Genetics
   a. Familial incidence
   b. Mode of inheritance is not clear, probably autosomal recessive with incomplete penetrance

3. Environmental inference likely—role of other "allergens" unclear

4. Current theories being investigated include the following:
   a. Immunological (autoimmune vs. specific immune abnormality, aberrant immunological response to gluten)
   b. Search to identify deficient enzymes that digest gluten, or possible lack of intestinal enzymes that detoxify gluten
   c. Altered epithelial cell surfaces—allow gluten or gluten-fragment binding with resultant cellular toxicity

Altered Physiology

1. Characteristics of celiac disease include
   a. Impaired intestinal absorption
   b. Histologic abnormalities of the small intestine
   c. Clinical and histologic improvement with wheat- and rye-free (possibly also barley- and oat-free) diet
   d. Recurrence of clinical manifestations and histologic changes after reintroduction of dietary gluten

2. Histologic changes in mucosa of small bowel, especially duodenum and jejunum resulting from dietary gluten include
   a. Irregularity of epithelial cells
   b. Loss of normal villous pattern
   c. Obliteration of intervillous spaces which are infiltrated with plasma cells and eosinophils
   d. Loss of epithelial cell brush border

3. This mucosal damage results in
   a. Disaccharidase deficiency
   b. Depression of peptidase activity

4. Subsequent malabsorption probably results from
   a. Decreased area of absorption in small bowel
   b. Impaired enzyme activity

5. Inability to absorb fats, fat-soluble vitamins (A, D, K, and E), minerals, and some protein and carbohydrates. The severity of symptoms of the disease depends on the extent of intestine with histologic changes.
   a. The extent of affected intestine is variable.
   b. Generally, proximal small intestine mucosal damage is most severe and condition decreases in severity distally.

Complications

1. Recurrence of symptoms if diet is not followed

2. Possible predisposition to malignant lymphoma of small intestine at later age, if dietary restrictions are terminated

3. Refractory sprue

4. Associated disorders
   a. Dermatitis herpetiformis
   b. Insulin-dependent diabetes mellitus
   c. Cystic fibrosis

5. Manifestations secondary to malabsorption
   a. Anemia
   b. Hypoalbuminemia
   c. Hypocalcemia
   d. Hypoprothrombinemia
   e. Disaccharide intolerance

Clinical Manifestations

The age and mode of presenting signs and symptoms are extremely variable. Diagnosis is most commonly made by 6–24 months of age; however, it can be made in the adult.

A. 3–9 Months of Age

1. Acutely ill
2. Severe diarrhea and vomiting
3. Possibly failure to thrive

B. 9–18 Months of Age (age when "typical" celiac appearance is seen)

1. Impaired growth
   a. Normal growth during early months of life
   b. Slackening of weight and weight loss follow
2. Abnormal stools
   a. Pale
   b. Soft
   c. Bulky
   d. Having offensive odor
   e. Greasy—steatorrhea
   f. May increase in number
3. Abdominal distention
4. Anorexia
5. Muscle wasting—most obvious in buttocks and proximal parts of extremities
6. Hypotonia
7. Mood changes—ill humor, irritability, temper tantrums, shyness
8. Mild clubbing of fingers
9. Vomiting—often occurring in evening

C. Older Child

1. Signs and symptoms often related to nutritional or secondary deficiencies resulting from disease
2. May have abnormal stools and growth impairment
3. May have colicky abdominal pain with constipation and large, pale stools

D. Manifestations Secondary to Malabsorption

1. Anemia, vitamin deficiency
2. Hypoproteinemia with edema
3. Hypocalcemia
4. Hypoprothrombinemia—resulting from impaired vitamin K absorption
5. Disaccharide intolerance—with acid-sugar-containing stools (secondary to the altered small bowel mucosa)

E. Celiac Crisis—most often seen in very young child and toddler (although rare)

1. Profound anorexia
2. Severe vomiting and diarrhea
3. Weight loss
4. Marked dehydration and acidosis (secondary to intractable diarrhea and vomiting)
5. Immobility
6. Grossly distended abdomen
   a. Fluid rattle is present.
   b. Abdomen flattens with passage of large liquid stool.
   c. The patient appears shock-like.
7. Looks profoundly depressed

Diagnostic Evaluation

1. Thorough evaluation of history and general status of child
2. Small bowel biopsy—demonstrates abnormal mucosa Diagnostic criteria:
   a. Severely damaged or flat, villous lesions
   b. Clinical response to gluten elimination
   c. Histologic recovery following gluten elimination
   d. Histologic recurrence of villous injury within 2 years of gluten reintroduction
3. D-Xylose absorption—less 20–25 mg./dl. at 60 minutes
4. Red blood count smear—hypochromia
5. Serum iron and folate—folic acid reduced
6. Immunoglobulin determination—IgA may be increased in acute stage of disease
7. Determination of fat absorption—fecal fat excretion—24-hour collection 3 times
8. Measurement of hemoglobin levels—may be reduced
9. Prothrombin time—before intestinal biopsy
10. Radiologic studies—skeletal x-rays commonly show
    a. Demineralization
    b. Retarded bone age
11. Sweat test and pancreatic function studies to rule out cystic fibrosis

Treatment

1. *Lifelong* gluten-free diet
   a. Avoid *all* foods containing wheat or rye gluten. The exclusion of barley and oats is controversial; however, it is often wise to err on the safe side or to offer specific challenges and to test with biopsy.
   b. The small intestine mucosa will always respond abnormally to dietary gluten, even though clinical signs may not be immediately evident.
   c. Biopsy reverts to normal with appropriate diet.
   d. Clinical signs of improvement should be seen 1–4 weeks after proper diet is initiated.
2. Adequate caloric intake
3. Supplemental vitamins and minerals
   a. Folic acid for 1–2 months
   b. Vitamin D
   c. Iron for 1–2 months
4. Reduction of fat intake (rare)
5. Possible elimination of lactose from diet for 6–8 weeks—based on reduced disaccharidase activity
6. Treatment of celiac crisis
   a. IV restoration of electrolyte balance and fluids for replacement of blood volume
   b. Steroids
   c. Parenteral hyperalimentation with amino acids, medium chain triglycerides, and glucose—for short periods of time may be necessary
   d. Initial oral feedings may need to be disaccharide- or completely sugar-free

Patient Problems and Nursing Diagnoses

1. Nutrition altered, less than body requirements, related to malabsorption of nutrients, diarrhea, and vomiting
2. Infection related to malnourishment and anemia
3. Coping, ineffective, related to dietary restrictions
4. Potential for celiac crises related to vomiting and diarrhea
5. Anxiety and fear related to illness, hospitalization, treatments, and separation from parents
6. Parental anxiety related to the child's illness and lack of understanding of condition

Nursing Interventions

A. Assist With Diagnostic Evaluation.

1. Prepare the child for diagnostic tests appropriate for age. Assist him during the procedure to aid in compliance and reduce fear and anxiety.
2. Collect stool specimens for 3 days for fat analysis.
3. Ensure that the child is appropriately prepared for special blood studies (i.e., glucose tolerance test).

B. Follow Explicitly the Dietary Regimen That Has Been Calculated By the Physician and Dietitian to Include Enough Calories for Weight Gain Yet to Exclude Wheat, Rye, Barley, and Oat Glutens That Produce Enteropathy.

1. Initial diet is high in protein, relatively low in fat, and starch-free.
   a. Milk protein or skim milk is sweetened with sucrose or banana powder.
   b. Infants and young children may have a problem in intestinal fat absorption; therefore, fat intake may be reduced.
2. Proteins and sugars should be added gradually.
   a. Individual foods are added one at a time at several-day intervals. Foods included and added are lean meat, cottage cheese, egg white, and raw ground apple.
   b. Starchy foods are added to diet last.
   c. Wheat and rye are never added to diet.
3. The child is given nothing by mouth during the initial treatment of celiac crisis or during diagnostic testing.
4. If the child is ambulatory, take special precautions to ensure that he does not eat restricted foods.
5. The child may have anorexia; feeding him can be difficult.
   a. Make mealtime pleasant.
   b. Serve small, attractive portions.
   c. Do not force him to eat.
6. Note carefully the child's reaction to food. Close observation of the child's responses to food may reveal other intolerances. Note and record:
   a. Intake, foods refused
   b. Appetite
   c. Change in behavior after eating
   d. Characteristics and frequency of stools
   e. General disposition—behavior improvement often seen within 2–3 days after diet control is initiated
7. New foods may be temporarily eliminated if symptoms increase.

C. Prevent Infection In This Child Who Is Malnourished, Anemic, and Very Susceptible to Respiratory Infection, Which In Turn Will Increase Indigestion.

1. Avoid exposing the child to anyone with an infection of any kind.
2. The child usually perspires freely and has a subnormal temperature with cold extremities.
   a. Keep him dry.
   b. Cover the child lightly when the room is cool.
3. If the child remains quiet in bed, change his position frequently because he is prone to upper respiratory infections.
4. Promote good hygiene.

D. Be Aware of the Child's Behavior or Change In Behavior and Care for Him Accordingly.

1. Diet and eating have a direct effect on behavior. A hungry child may be irritable.
2. Behavior is indicative of how the child is feeling.
3. The child is prone to mood swings—from having temper tantrums to being very timid, nervous, or unstable.
   a. Allow the child to express his feelings freely. Provide different types of media for child to express himself.
      (1) An older child talks or complains.
      (2) A baby cries and whines.

b. The nurse must exhibit patience.
c. Socialize routine procedures.
4. Record changes in behavior, especially in relation to eating and diet.
5. Avoid conflicts or emotionally upsetting situations; these may precipitate diarrhea, vomiting, and celiac crisis.
6. Teach the older child how to adjust his diet. He can eat buckwheat, millet, corn (maize), and rice.

E. Meet the Child's Emotional and Psychological Needs and Provide Diversional Activities Appropriate for His Age and Severity of Disease.

1. This child may be withdrawn and indulge in self-play. Provide opportunity for play with other children, especially when the child begins to feel better.
2. Frequently, play is more passive than active. Activity may be very exhausting. Provide appropriate material for constructive activities.
3. The toddler may cling to infantile habits for security. Allow this behavior; it may disappear as his physical condition improves and he feels better.
4. The nurse must show the child she understands his mood swings and irritability by being patient with him. He needs a great deal of emotional satisfaction and support.
5. Offer the child other sensory stimulation to compensate for lack of eating pleasure.

F. Support the Parents and Foster Continuing Parental Acceptance of the Child, His Disease, and His Behavior.

Help the parents maintain a healthy relationship with their child. The most important aspect in working with parents and child is stressing health and family counseling.
1. Encourage the parents to visit and care for the child as much as possible. Comforting and holding the child can be very helpful. The child needs much love and understanding, especially from his parents.
2. Start teaching the parents early about the disease and how they should care for the child at home.
   a. Acquaint them with available literature, parent groups, and community resources.
   b. Initiate community-nurse referral to provide for continued support and teaching at home.
3. Listen to parental concerns and questions.
   a. Give simple, honest answers.
   b. Reinforce what the physician has told them.
4. Allow the parents to continue to maintain what other responsibilities they may have outside the hospital. Do not insist they stay at the hospital and attend only to this child.
5. Help the parents to understand that after initial rapid weight gain further improvement may be slow.

G. Be Aware of the Signs and Symptoms of Celiac Crisis and Attend to the Child's Care According to Medical Plans.

Initial treatment:
1. Replace fluids and electrolytes by parenteral therapy.
2. Give nothing by mouth, especially if child is vomiting. Nasogastric tube may be prescribed.
3. Observe the child carefully.

H. Be Familiar With the Medications Used In the Treatment of Celiac Disease and Their Implications.

1. Vitamins A and D—not absorbed well
2. Vitamin B complex and vitamin C—given if the child is receiving antibiotics

3. Iron—given if the child is anemic
4. Vitamin K—for hypothrombinemia and bleeding
5. Calcium lactate—given if milk is restricted from diet
6. Water-miscible vitamins and minerals should be used
7. When nutrients and drugs are essential, IV infusion may be used since absorption is poor

I. Assist With Gluten-Challenge Diet, If Used, to Evaluate Histologic and Clinical Response.

1. After an extended period of time on dietary regimen, the child may dislike gluten-containing foods.
2. The child and parents may be extremely apprehensive about the possible effects of gluten.
3. The child may have mild gastrointestinal symptoms (i.e., loose stools, vague abdominal pain, etc.). These may be related to anxiety.
4. Support the family and provide reassurance. The gluten-challenge diet may last 3–4 months before bowel biopsy is repeated.

Health Education

1. Help the parents to understand what celiac disease is and how it is controlled by diet.
    a. Provide a specific list of restricted foods as well as foods the child is allowed to eat.
    b. Teach the mother (parents) how to read labels on foods to identify those containing wheat and rye glutens, thus avoiding them.
    c. Grains—corn, rice, soybean flour and gluten-free starch are used as substitutes for wheat, rye, barley, and oats.
    d. Help the mother become comfortable and proficient in situation problem-solving (e.g., What can be done when her child is invited to a birthday party where cake will be served? Bake gluten-free cupcakes and take to party).
    e. Provide opportunity for mother, dietitian, and nurse to come together and talk about diet. At the same time, foster a positive feeling toward dietary controls.
    f. Be certain the parents understand the importance of the vitamin regimen.
    g. Help the parents understand the importance of continued adherence to diet, even though the child is feeling well, eating well, and has normal stools. Advancing diet too rapidly may result in a setback.
    h. Adolescent compliance may be variable. They need support and understanding. A break in avoidance diet may mean ill health.
    i. Alteration in diet may have significant cultural, ethnic, and religious implications. Help parents identify how adjustments can be made.
2. Impress upon the parents the importance of regular medical follow-up.
    a. Encourage the parents to seek prompt medical attention if the child has an upper respiratory infection that might trigger celiac crisis if untreated.
    b. Ensure that the parents understand measures to prevent celiac crisis—dietary control, dangers of prolonged fasting, inform unfamiliar physician of celiac disorder, and use of anticholinergic drugs.
3. Encourage the parents to practice good hygiene to prevent infection.
   This child is especially prone to infection because of malnutrition and anemia.
4. Help the parents to understand that the emotional climate in the home and around the child is vitally important in maintaining the child's medical and physical stability.
    a. The parents must exhibit patience with the child.
    b. Have the parents set defined limits of behavior for the child; everyone in the family should know what these limits are.
    c. Avoid conflicts or any emotional upsets in the child's presence.
    d. A social worker may need to become involved if there is domestic disharmony.
    e. Other children and their needs must also be considered in the total family picture.
5. Help the parents to understand that the child's physical condition and behavior problems are related to the disease.
    a. The parents may feel guilty or ambivalent toward the child.
    b. Show them how they may avoid becoming overprotective of the child.
6. Help the parents to understand that the disorder is lifelong; however, changes in the mucosal lining of the intestine and in general the clinical condition of their child are reversible when dietary gluten is avoided.
7. Offer parents available literature about the American Celiac Society; help them to become familiar with the society and the chapter nearest them.*

Expected Outcomes

1. Attains and maintains adequate nutritional status; appropriate weight gain; normal range of laboratory values
2. Is free of infection; has normal vital signs and laboratory values
3. Demonstrates normalization of behavior; absence of temper tantrums; becoming more social; adheres to diet
4. Absence of celiac crises
5. Experiences minimal anxiety and lessening of fear; normalization of behavior; engaging in play activities
6. Reduction in parental anxiety; verbalize understanding of illness, treatment, and follow-up care

---

Diarrhea

Diarrhea is an excessive loss of water and electrolytes that occurs with passage of one or more unformed stools. It is a symptom of many conditions and may be caused by many diseases (Table 52-1).

Etiology

Often the cause is difficult to determine; occasionally it is unknown. The numerous causes of diarrhea in infants and young children include:

A. Acute and Infectious Factors

1. Bacterial
    a. Enteropathogenic *Escherichia coli*
    b. *Salmonella*
    c. *Shigella*
    d. *Yersinia enterocolitica*
    e. *Campylobacter fetus*

---

* American Celiac Society, 45 Gifford Avenue, Jersey City, NJ 07304.

Table 52-1. *Some Malabsorption Syndromes—Based on Types of Stool*

Disease	Diagnostic Studies	Etiology
A. Watery Stools		

1. Disaccharide intolerance
   a. Lactose
      (lactose → glucose, galactose)
         ↑
      enzyme lactase
	1. Stool pH
	2. Stool reducing substances
	3. Lactose intolerance test
	4. Enzyme assay
		Primary—congenital absence of enzyme lactase
		Secondary—any disease that damages epithelium of small intestine (e.g., gastroenteritis, cow's milk sensitivity, celiac sprue)

b. Sucrose
      (sucrose → glucose, fructose)
         ↑
      enzyme sucrase
	1. Stool pH
	2. Stool reducing substances
	3. Sucrose tolerance
	4. Enzyme assay
		Primary—congenital absence of enzyme sucrase
		Secondary—any disease that damages epithelium of small intestine

2. Monosaccharide intolerance (glucose-galactose)	1. Stool pH 2. Stool-reducing substances 3. Glucose-galactose tolerance tests 4. Trial carbohydrate elimination, using fructose	Primary—congenital defect in glucose transport Secondary—damage to and decrease of epithelium of intestine from acute gastroenteritis or persistent diarrhea, showing intolerance to fructose, glucose, and galactose
3. Cow's milk protein sensitivity	1. Lactose tolerance test 2. Elimination of cow's milk from diet 3. Rechallenge with cow's milk will produce same symptoms	Unknown Sensitivity to cow's milk
B. Parasites		
Strongyloidiasis (roundworm)	Examination of intestinal content for rhabtidiform	*Strongyloides*
Giardia lamblia (protozoan)	Stool examination for *Giardia* cysts; duodenal aspirate for trophozoites	Protozoan *Giardia lamblia*
C. Fatty Stool		
Cystic fibrosis, celiac sprue (see above discussion) Pancreatic insufficiency and bone marrow failure (Schwachman syndrome) Short-bowel syndrome Biliary tract obstruction	Pancreatic enzymes abnormal; sweat test normal; neutropenia	Familial pancreatic enzymes are probably reduced Inadequate absorptive surfaces Extensive bowel resection, increase in gastric acidity and production rate (hypersecretion), which in turn may inactive pancreatic enzymes Biliary atresia Choledochal cyst Obstructive neonatal hepatitis
D. Normal Stools		
Juvenile pernicious anemia (vitamin B_{12} malabsorption)		Absence of intrinsic factor activity—cannot absorb vitamin B_{12}

2. Viral
   a. Enteroviruses—ECHO viruses
   b. Adenoviruses
   c. Human reovirus-like agent (HRVL)
   d. *Rotovirus*
3. Normal intestinal tract inhabitants act as pathogens in certain circumstances (i.e., after ingestion of antibiotics)
4. Fungal—*Candida* enteritis
5. Parasitic—*Giardia lamblia*
6. Protozoal

B. Noninfectious Factors

1. Allergy to certain foods—milk, wheat protein
2. Metabolic disorders
   a. Celiac disease
   b. Cystic fibrosis of pancreas
3. Disaccharidase deficiencies
4. Infant exposed to overfeeding; displaying emotional excitement and fatigue
5. Direct irritation of gastrointestinal tract by foods
6. Inappropriate use of laxatives and purgatives

C. Mechanical Disorders

1. Malrotation
2. Incomplete small bowel obstruction
3. Intermittent volvulus

D. Congenital Anomalies—Hirschsprung's disease

E. Day Care Center Diarrhea

Infants and young children in day care centers may be at increased risk for diarrhea due to *Shigella, Salmonella,* rotovirus, and endopathogenic *E. coli.*

Altered Physiology

1. The particular etiology of diarrhea does not influence the potentially dangerous cycle of events as much as does the virulence of the organism and the general condition of the child.
2. The effects of diarrhea present more of a threat to infants and young children than to the older child and adult.
   a. Extracellular fluid volume is proportionately larger in the infant and young child
   b. Nutritional reserves are relatively smaller in the young child
3. Major alterations in physiology
   a. Dehydration—extracellular fluid loss—results from the following:
      (1) Large loss of fluid and electrolytes in watery stools
      (2) Losses with repeated vomiting
      (3) Decreased fluid intake
      (4) Increased insensible fluid losses from skin and lungs resulting from fever and rapid respirations
      (5) Continued urine excretion
   b. Electrolyte imbalance
      (1) Potassium—varies
      (2) Chloride; sodium; hypotonic, isotonic, or hypertonic dehydration may occur
   c. Acid–base imbalance—metabolic acidosis may result from
      (1) Large losses of potassium, sodium, and bicarbonate in stools
      (2) Impairment of renal function

Complications

1. Direct disturbances caused by diarrhea itself
   a. Dehydration
   b. Acidosis
   c. Hypernatremia
   d. Alterations in potassium levels
   e. Monosaccharide intolerance
   f. Protein hypersensitivity
2. Infection
   a. Local (i.e., site of cutdown, injection site)
   b. Respiratory tract
   c. Middle ear (otitis media)
3. Nervous system, hemorrhage
4. Iatrogenic
   a. Potassium depletion—"washing out"
   b. Hypernatremia—sodium chloride overload
   c. Edema—excessive amount of parenteral fluids

Clinical Manifestations

A. Classification

1. Mild diarrhea—hospitalization may not be indicated.
2. Severe diarrhea with gradual onset
3. Severe diarrhea with sudden onset—incidence of death is high in infants.

B. Symptoms

All classifications have symptoms, the severity of which depends on the intensity of diarrhea and type of onset.
1. Fever—low-grade to 41.1°C. (100°F.)
2. Anorexia
3. Mild and intermittent to severe vomiting
4. Stools
   a. Appearance of diarrhea varies from a few hours to 3 days
   b. Loose and fluid in consistency
   c. Greenish or yellow–green color
   d. May contain mucus, pus, or blood
   e. Frequency varies from 2–20/day
   f. Expelled with force; may be preceded by pain
5. Behavior change
   a. Irritability and restlessness
   b. Weakness/pallor
   c. Extreme prostration
   d. Stupor and convulsions
   e. Flaccidity
6. Respirations
   a. Rapid
   b. Hyperpneic
7. Dehydration
   a. Little to extreme loss of subcutaneous fat
   b. Up to 50% total body weight loss
   c. Urinary output decreases or stops
   d. Poor skin turgor and dry skin
   e. Fontanelles and eyes sunken
   f. Collapse imminent, low blood pressure, high pulse

Diagnostic Evaluation

1. Thorough history of onset of diarrhea and cause
2. Evaluation of general physical appearance and condition of child, including weight
3. Studies to establish nature of the child's condition
   a. Electrolyte status and kidney function
      (1) Serum sodium
      (2) Serum chloride
      (3) Serum potassium
      (4) BUN (blood urea nitrogen)
   b. Acid–base imbalance
      (1) Serum pH (acidosis)
      (2) Serum CO_2 content or combining power
   c. Plasma volume by hematocrit and hemoglobin; also complete blood count, sedimentation rate, and culture
   d. Urinalysis
   e. Stool pH, reducing substances
4. Studies to determine cause of diarrhea
   a. Bacteriologic cultures of stool
   b. Bacteriologic cultures of rectal swab
   c. Serologic studies for viral pathogens or direct visualization under electron microscope (i.e., HRVL)

Treatment

1. Prevent spread of disease—suspect disease to be communicable until proven otherwise. Isolation; use enteric isolation precautions.
2. Supportive care—maintain hydration and electrolyte balance; record IV fluids, weights, fluid loss from diarrhea, urine, and vomiting.

3. Specific antimicrobial therapy
   a. Complications:
      (1) Dehydration
      (2) Protracted diarrheal state
      (3) Transient lactase deficiency—lactose intolerance

Patient Problems and Nursing Diagnoses

1. Potential fluid volume deficit related to diarrhea and extracellular fluid loss
2. Potential for additional infection related to debilitated state and altered nutritional status
3. Nutrition, altered, less than body requirements, related to malabsorption
4. Comfort, altered, related to effects of disease and treatments
5. Anxiety and fear related to hospitalization and illness
6. Parental anxiety related to the child's illness, hospitalization, and lack of understanding of the child's condition

Nursing Interventions

A. Monitor IV Fluid Therapy (Both Amount and Rate), Which Has Been Appropriately Calculated By the Physician.

1. Fluid prescribed as maintenance or replacement, depending on degree of patient's dehydration, must be checked.
2. Fluid is calculated carefully so as not to overload circulatory system.
   a. Check flow rate and amount absorbed hourly and totally.
   b. Check IV site for infiltration or improper flow so site can be changed as necessary.
3. Use appropriate protective devices to prevent the patient from moving and injuring himself or causing IV to malfunction.
4. When preparing solution for therapy, use sterile solution and equipment.
5. Weigh the patient daily to serve as a guide for specific fluid needs and current patient status.
6. When oral feedings are given in conjunction with IV fluid, careful adherence to prescribed volume is vital to prevent circulatory overload.

B. Provide Physical Comfort for the Patient.

1. If protective devices are used, passive range of motion may help to keep the patient's joints from stiffening.
2. While the patient is given nothing by mouth, special mouth care should be administered.
   An infant may find comfort in sucking a pacifier. Bubble him frequently to help expel air he has swallowed during sucking.
3. Change position and give good skin care to prevent lesions that may occur because of dehydration. Change soiled diapers quickly, because diarrheal stool will cause excoriation. Clean perineum thoroughly after each stool; application of ointment to skin may help protect it from contact with stool. Ointment must be completely removed after each stool. Leave diaper area exposed to air.

C. Make Frequent Observations and Be Constantly Alert to the Patient's Condition.

Record and report any changes immediately. Careful observations can give clues to improvement or deterioration in the patient's condition and can serve as a guide to medical care.

1. Note any changes in vital signs.
2. Note stool characteristics and number.
   a. Abnormal constituents
   b. Foul odor
   c. Test stool for pH, reducing substances (Clinitest tablets), and occult blood.
3. Note activity, level of consciousness, and neurological signs.
4. Note vomiting—frequency and characteristics.
5. Record urinary output—amount, frequency, and characteristics.
6. Check for presence of edema, and skin characteristics.
7. Assess the child's behavior to determine how he feels.
   a. Eating and restful sleep indicates he feels fairly good.
   b. Crying or legs drawn up to abdomen usually indicates pain.

D. Prevent Spread of Infection By Using Good Handwashing and Gown Techniques As Indicated By Hospital Policy.

1. Many hospitals use isolation technique for children admitted with diarrhea until the cause has been determined. (Infectious pathogens can spread rapidly and easily among infants and young children.)
2. Follow hospital policy as to care of diapers.

E. Meet the Emotional and Psychological Needs of the Patient.

1. Hospitalization is frightening—especially when it is sudden, as with diarrhea.
2. Many treatments and procedures are painful—give reassurance to the child before, during, and after treatment.
   a. Talk to the child.
   b. Hold him and comfort him after the procedure.
   c. Explain to him in language appropriate for his age what is to be done.
3. Provide some means of pleasant stimulation, entertainment, or diversion—especially while he must remain in bed.
   a. Infant—mobile, musical toy
   b. Young child—read to him, something appropriate for age
4. A hungry child is not easily comforted. Physical closeness may be helpful.
   a. Petting, stroking
   b. Holding and rocking

F. Provide and Assist In Resuming Adequate Caloric and Volume of Oral Intake.

1. If diarrhea is mild, oral electrolyte solution may be given. (Do not advance too quickly—base administration of solution on number of stools.)
2. After rehydration, lactose-free oral feeding may be given.
3. Fluid is usually advanced slowly from clear liquids, such as gelatin-flavored water, to half-strength formula, to regular diet
   a. Older child may advance more rapidly.
   b. If infant or young child is well hydrated, regular formula may not be omitted.
4. As diet is advanced, note any vomiting or increase in stools and report it immediately. Oral feedings should not be resumed too early or advanced too rapidly, because diarrhea may recur.

G. Provide Support for the Family, Especially the Mother.

1. Reassure the mother that she is not the cause of her child's illness.
2. Explain procedures and need for treatment in easy-to-understand language. Be sure family understands the following:
   a. Why the infant's hair was shaved off his head for an IV
   b. Reason for not giving the child anything to eat or drink
   c. Need for protective devices
3. Allow mother (parents) to care for and comfort the child as much as possible.
4. Allow her to leave the hospital and attend to other family members and matters. Invite the parents to call the hospital when they cannot be there.
5. Initiate a community-nurse referral, especially if other children at home are ill or if home conditions have precipitated the diarrhea.

Health Education

1. After the cause of the diarrhea is determined, it may be necessary to teach proper formula or food preparation, handling, and storage.
   It is especially important to be certain that the mother knows proper formula and bottle sterilization procedures.
2. Parents may need help in understanding the symptoms of a sick child.
3. Help the parents understand the importance of medical care and general good hygiene.

Expected Outcomes

1. Shows proper hydration; maintains acid–base and fluid and electrolyte balance; has normal laboratory values; demonstrates weight gain
2. Is free of secondary infection; normal vital signs and laboratory values
3. Reestablishes a more normal bowel elimination pattern; gains weight; eating more solid foods
4. Shows minimal discomfort; lessening of abdominal cramps; resting; fewer complaints; stable vital signs
5. Shows lessening of anxiety; more relaxed; willing to play; takes interest in surroundings
6. The parents gain an understanding of the child's treatment; verbalize the dietary protocol and measures to prevent recurrences

Hirschsprung's Disease

Hirschsprung's disease (congenital aganglionic megacolon) is a congenital absence of the parasympathetic ganglion nerve cells from within the muscle wall of the intestinal tract, usually at the distal end of the colon.

Etiology

1. An arrest in embryologic development affecting the migration of parasympathetic nerves (innervation) of the intestine, occurring prior to the 12th week of gestation
2. The cause is unknown—may be familial

Incidence

1. 1:500–1:3000; accounts for about 25% of all intestinal obstructions in the newborn
2. 4:1 male ratio

Altered Physiology

1. Absence or reduced number of the parasympathetic ganglion cells in Auerbach's plexus within the intestinal tract muscle wall, usually the distal end of the colon and the rectum. Most commonly affected site is the rectosigmoid colon.
2. No peristalsis occurs in the affected portion of intestine (i.e., spastic and contracted).
   a. This section is usually narrow; therefore, no fecal material passes through it.
   b. The intestine above the affected section has an accumulation of fecal material.
3. Proximal to the narrow affected section, the colon is dilated.
   a. Filled with fecal material and gas.
   b. Hypertrophy of muscular coating.
   c. In newborn, may see ulceration of mucosa.
4. The internal rectal sphincter fails to relax and evacuation of fecal material and gas is prevented. Abdominal distention and constipation result.

Complications

1. Prior to primary surgery
   a. Enterocolitis—a major cause of death
   b. Hydroureter or hydronephrosis
   c. Water intoxication from tap water enemas
   d. Cecal perforation
2. Postoperative
   a. Enterocolitis
   b. Leaking of anastomosis and pelvic abscess
   c. Temporary sudden inability to evacuate colon
   d. Long-term: intestinal obstruction from adhesions, volvulus, intussusception
3. Postoperative—colostomy
   a. Abdominal distention
   b. Respiratory distress
   c. Infection
   d. Hemorrhage, shock

Clinical Manifestations

Vary depending on degree of involved bowel
1. Appearing at birth or within first weeks of life
   a. No meconium passed
   b. Vomiting—bile-stained or fecal
   c. Abdominal distention
   d. Constipation
   e. Overflow-type diarrhea
   f. Anorexia
   g. Temporary relief of symptoms with enema
2. Older child—symptoms not prominent at birth
   a. History may reveal obstipation at birth
   b. Distention of abdomen—progressive enlarging
   c. Thin abdominal wall—superficial veins are visible
   d. Peristaltic activity observable
   e. Constipation
      (1) Never has fecal soiling
      (2) Relieved temporarily with enema
   f. Stool appears ribbon-like, fluid-like or in pellet form

g. Failure to grow
   (1) Loss of subcutaneous fat
   (2) Appears malnourished; perhaps has stunted growth

Diagnostic Evaluation

1. Rectal examination—exhibits absence of fecal material
2. Roentgen examination with barium enema
   a. Narrow segment of intestine proximal to anus
   b. Dilated intestine proximal to narrow segment
3. Rectal biopsy—absence or reduced number of ganglion nerve cells
4. Anorectal manometry—records the reflex response of sphincter
5. Ultrasonogram

Treatment

Definitive treatment is removal of the aganglionic, nonfunctioning, dilated segment of the bowel, followed by anastomosis, and improved functioning of internal rectal sphincter.

1. Initially a colostomy or ileostomy is performed to decompress intestine, divert fecal stream, and rest the normal bowel
2. Definitive surgery
   a. Abdominoperineal pull-through
   b. Endorectal pull-through, rectorectal pull-through
   c. May be delayed until age 9–12 months or until child is 6.8–9.0 kg. (15–20 lb.).
3. In older child when symptoms are chronic but not severe, treatment may consist of isotonic enemas, stool softeners, and low-residue diet.

Patient Problems and Nursing Diagnoses

1. Impaired gas exchange in infant related to abdominal distention
2. Nutrition, altered, less than body requirements, related to poor intake
3. Comfort, altered, pain related to abdominal distention
4. Acid–base imbalance and dehydration related to vomiting
5. Bowel elimination, altered, constipation related to decreased peristalsis in affected bowel
6. Potential alteration in skin integrity around colostomy stoma related to drainage and excoriation
7. Anxiety and fear, especially in older child, related to illness, hospitalization, and treatments
8. Family process, altered, related to family reaction to illness of child, hospitalization, and temporary colostomy

Preoperative Nursing Interventions

A. Assist In Emptying the Bowel and In Preparing for Surgery.

1. Give repeated enemas and colonic irrigations.

   a. Procedure for enema in an infant is similar to that in an adult, except that less fluid and pressure are used.
   b. Chemotherapeutic agents are used to reduce the bacterial flora.
   c. Physiologic saline solution (warmed) should be used for irrigations.
      Tap water may result in large quantities of water being absorbed and in water intoxication.

   d. Carefully note return from irrigation and degree of abdominal distention.
      Measure returned fluids; retained fluid may be absorbed and result in water intoxication and cerebral edema.
   e. If enema is not expelled, siphoning may be indicated.
   f. Continuous use of a rectal tube may be prescribed; ensure that it is properly located and remains in place.
2. Note and record frequency and characteristics of stools. (Obstipation is likely to occur.)
3. Prevent injury to mucosa by taking axillary temperature.

B. Observe for Abdominal Distention and Its Effect on the Patient's Condition.

1. Note any change in degree of distention before and after irrigation. Record if location of distention changes (i.e., upper or lower abdomen).
2. Respiratory embarrassment may result from abdominal distention.
   Elevate head and chest of infant by tilting mattress.
3. Note degree of abdominal tenderness.
   a. Legs of infant drawn up
   b. Chest breathing
4. Note color of abdomen and presence of gastric waves; take sequential measurements of abdominal girth.

C. Assist In Establishing and Maintaining Hydration and Adequate Nutrition So That Growth and Weight Gain May Take Place.

1. Monitor parenteral fluids appropriately. Measure all output.
2. Feeding may cause additional discomfort because of distention and nausea.
3. Offer small, frequent feedings. (Low-residue diet will aid in keeping stools soft.)
   a. Appetite is poor.
   b. The child must be fed slowly.
   c. Provide as comfortable a position as possible for child during feedings.

D. Obtain a Dietary History Regarding Food and Eating Habits.

1. This will contribute to planning dietary alterations.
2. Eating problems are common with Hirschsprung's disease.

E. Properly Care for the Patient When a Nasogastric Tube Is Used to Aid in Decreasing Abdominal Distention.

1. Note drainage from nasogastric tube and chart characteristics.
2. Check for patency.
   a. Saline irrigations may be requested.
   b. Carefully record input and output.
   c. Note increasing distention; measure abdominal girth.
3. Give adequate mouth care.
4. Alternate nares when changing nasogastric tube every 24 hours. (Use minimal amount of tape to prevent skin irritation.)

F. Provide Emotional and Psychological Support Needed By the Child.

1. Encourage the mother to visit, even for short periods.
2. Irritable child may be calmed with holding and rocking.
3. Provide suitable diversion appropriate for age.

Postoperative Nursing Interventions

One of 2 surgical procedures may be done in treatment of Hirschsprung's disease: (1) primary resection of aganglionic segment or (2) temporary colostomy above the narrowed section; when condition of child is stabilized or weight is obtained, resection is done and colostomy closed (most common).

A. Give Good Postoperative Care and Observe for Possible Postoperative Complications.

(see p. 1134).

B. Prevent Infection.

1. At the site of the surgical wound
   a. Dressing change, using sterile technique
   b. Prevent contamination from diaper.
      (1) Apply diaper below dressing.
      (2) Change frequently.
      (3) Prevent perianal and anal excoriation by frequent changing, thorough cleansing, and use of ointments.
   c. Use careful handwashing technique.
   d. Report any redness, swelling or drainage, evisceration, or dehiscence immediately.
2. Of the tracheobronchial tree and lungs
   a. Suction secretions frequently.
   b. Encourage frequent coughing and deep breathing. Allow the infant to cry for short periods.
   c. Change position frequently to increase circulation and allow for aeration of all lung areas.

C. Properly Care for Colostomy and Understand Its Purpose.

1. Proper functioning of colostomy
   a. Note drainage from colostomy—characteristics, frequency, fecal material, or liquid drainage.
   b. Note abdominal distention.
   c. Measure fluid loss from colostomy as the amount will affect fluid replacement.
2. Signs of obstruction from peritonitis, paralytic ileus, handling bowel, or swelling
   a. No output from colostomy
   b. Increased tenderness
   c. Irritability
   d. Vomiting
   e. Increased temperature
3. Good skin care to prevent breakdown around colostomy
   a. Change soiled dressing or diaper frequently.
   b. Wash skin with clear water.
   c. Use karaya gum, aluminum paste, Maalox, or other means to protect skin from contact with secretions.
   d. Keep area open to air occasionally.

D. Prevent Abdominal Distention.

1. Nasogastric tube may be used immediately postoperatively.
   a. Check patency.
   b. Watch for increasing abdominal distention; measure abdominal girth.
   c. Measure fluid loss because amount will affect fluid replacement.
2. Once oral feeding is begun, the nasogastric tube will be removed.
   a. Avoid overfeeding.
   b. Bubble frequently during feeding.
   c. Proper positioning after feeding.

E. Continue Taking Axillary Temperatures.

1. Avoids injury
2. Allows for more accurate reading

F. Continue to Provide Emotional Support to the Patient (see p. 1349, Diarrhea).

1. Recognize the effects of immobility, less handling, and less activity than is generally given the healthy infant.
2. Allow the infant to derive some satisfaction from using a pacifier. Hold him often during this time if condition permits.
3. Prepare the parents for what they will see postoperatively (i.e., equipment, dressings, stoma).

G. Help the Parents Understand and Accept the Child and the Disease, As Well As All That Has Happened.

1. Even a temporary colostomy can be a difficult procedure to accept and to learn to care for.
   a. Support the parents when teaching them to care for the colostomy. Include them, soon after surgery, in dressing changes.
   b. Try to help them treat the baby or child as normally as possible.
2. Encourage the parents to talk about their fears and anxieties.
   Anticipating future surgery for resection may be confusing and frightening.
3. Initiate community-nurse referral to help the parents care for the child at home away from the comfortable situation of the hospital, and obtain necessary equipment.

Ostomy Care

Colostomy and ileostomy care in the infant and young child is based on the same principles and is essentially the same as that for an adult (see pp. 483–493), with the following exceptions:

1. Colostomy irrigation is not part of management in small children. Irrigation is primarily for the purpose of regulating the colostomy to empty at regular intervals. Since children have bowel movements at more frequent intervals, this type of control is not feasible. Irrigation should only be done in preparation for tests or surgery and occasionally for the treatment of constipation.
2. Dehydration occurs quickly in the infant or small child; therefore, it is particularly important to observe drainage for amount and characteristics. It should be measured to provide an accurate basis for computation of fluid replacement.
3. Prevention and treatment of skin excoriation around the stoma is of primary concern and is a nursing challenge. With the advent of better skin shields and equipment that is designed especially for the pediatric patient, keeping an ostomy appliance in place is much less of a problem than it has been in the past. Through careful application and by trying different types of pouches until a proper fit is obtained, most children can be kept clean and dry for at least 24 hours between changes. This is a very significant factor in preventing skin breakdown and subsequent infections in the peristomal area. It is helpful to remember, however, that in the infant, dressings must be checked frequently:
   a. Dressings and collection bags may not adhere well or stay in place.

b. Skin breakdown is more frequent.

c. Infant elimination is more frequent than in the older child.

4. Helping agency for parents:
United Ostomy Association, 2001 W. Beverly Boulevard, Los Angeles, CA 90057

5. Some companies manufacturing pediatric size ostomy equipment:
United Surgical (Division of Howmedia, Inc.), Largo, FL 33540
Coloplast, C.R. Bard Inc., 713 Central Avenue, Murray Hill, NJ 07974
Hollister, Inc., 211 E. Chicago Avenue, Chicago, IL 60611

6. Suggested reading:
Jeter K. *These Special Children*. Palo Alto, CA, Bull Publishing Co, 1982; written specifically for parents of children with colostomies, ileostomies, and urostomies

Health Education

1. Begin early to teach thoroughly and carefully what the colostomy is for, how it works, and how to care for it and the child.
   a. Involve the whole family in teaching colostomy care to enhance acceptance of body change of the child.
   b. An older child should become totally responsible for his colostomy care.
   c. Procedures needed to be thoroughly understood and practiced include preparation of skin, application of collecting appliance, care of appliance, and control of odor.
   d. Signs of stomal complications: ribbon-like stool, diarrhea, failure of evacuation of stool or flatus, bleeding.
   e. Dilatation of stoma with finger may need to be taught and practiced.
   f. Increased fluid intake is needed because colon absorption is decreased; low-residue food is needed to decrease bulk of stool.
   g. Prepare parents and older child for colostomy closure as appropriate.

2. The parents may also need to know gastrostomy feeding techniques as well as procedures for care and dilation of anus.

3. Allow the parents to learn and practice these procedures long before the infant is to be discharged.

4. Emphasize the importance of treating the child as normally as possible to prevent behavior problems later.

5. Good nutrition and diet need to be understood by parents prior to discharge. Involve the dietitian as necessary.

6. Encourage close medical follow-up and general good health and hygiene.
   a. Nutrition
   b. General growth and development
   c. Immunizations

Expected Outcomes

1. Regains normal breathing pattern; shows relief of abdominal distention; stabilization of vital signs; blood gas values returning to normal

2. Takes small frequent feedings or receives parenteral feedings; shows weight gain

3. Achieves normal acid–base balance; has good skin turgor and moist mucous membranes; normal laboratory values

4. Demonstrates appropriate elimination pattern following surgery

5. Maintains skin integrity around colostomy site

6. Becomes less irritable when held and rocked

7. Parents express fears and anxieties about child's condition; engage in appropriate parent-child relationships

8. Parents demonstrate colostomy care; verbalize need for follow-up care

---

Intussusception

Intussusception is the invagination or telescoping of a portion of the intestine into an adjacent, more distal section of the intestine.

Etiology

1. Not usually known
   May be due to increased mobility of intestine and hyperperistalsis present in young children.

2. Possible contributing causes in older child
   a. Meckel's diverticulum
   b. Polyps, cysts in the bowel
   c. Malrotation of intestines
   d. Acute enteritis
   e. Abdominal injury
   f. Abdominal surgery; intestinal intubation
   g. Cystic fibrosis
   h. Celiac disease

Altered Physiology

1. Mesentery is pulled into intestine when invagination occurs.

2. Progression to obstruction
   a. Intestine becomes curved, sausage-like—blood supply is cut off.
   b. Bowel begins to swell—hemorrhage may occur.
   c. Complete intestinal obstruction results—necrosis of involved segment.

3. Classification of location.
   a. *Ileocecal* (most common)—ileum invaginates into ascending colon
   b. *Ileocolic*—ileum invaginates into colon
   c. *Colocolic*—colon invaginates into colon
   d. *Ileo-ileo*—(enteroenteric) small bowel invaginates into small bowel

Clinical Manifestations

A. Age

1. Incidence is rare in first month of life.

2. 4–10 months is most common age of onset (50%–70%), in well-nourished, otherwise healthy child

3. 1–2 years of age—frequency of occurrence is high.

B. Sudden Onset

1. Paroxysmal abdominal pain

2. Currant jelly-like stools
   a. Blood and mucus present in stool
   b. One or more stools with this characteristic
   c. Presence of bloody mucus on finger following rectal examination
   d. Hemoccult positive

3. Vomiting

4. Increasing absence of stools

5. Increasing abdominal distention and tenderness

6. Sausage-like mass palpable in abdomen

7. Dehydration and fever
8. Shock-like state
   a. Rapid pulse
   b. Pale skin
   c. Marked sweating

Diagnostic Evaluation

1. General condition and appearance of child; history
2. X-ray examination
   a. Flat plate of abdomen—reveals staircase pattern (invagination appears like stair steps on x-ray)—"coiled spring"
   b. Barium enema under fluoroscopy—coil-like appearance of bowel
3. Ultrasonogram

Treatment

1. Hydrostatic reduction of telescoped bowel with barium enema used during first 48 hours after onset.
2. Surgical reduction of intussusception; resection if bowel is gangrenous.

Patient Problems and Nursing Diagnoses

1. Comfort, altered, pain related to paroxysmal abdominal pain, fever, and treatments
2. Potential fluid volume deficit related to vomiting
3. Potential intestinal obstruction
4. Respiratory distress related to abdominal distention
5. Anxiety related to pain, hospitalization, and treatments
6. Parental anxiety related to suddenness of child's illness and lack of understanding of disease and its consequences

Preoperative Nursing Interventions

A. Assist in Maintaining or Restoring Hydration and Electrolyte Balance.

Monitor parenteral fluids (see Intravenous Fluid Therapy, p. 1167)

B. Prevent Vomiting and Aspiration.

1. Stomach may be deflated by insertion of nasogastric tube.
2. Maintain patency of nasogastric tube if one is inserted.
   a. Irrigate at frequent intervals.
   b. Note drainage and return from irrigation.
3. Patient is likely to be NPO.
   a. Wet lips and give mouth care.
   b. Give infant pacifier to suck.

C. Be Aware of the Patient's Condition By Frequent Observations, Thereby Contributing to the Total Care of the Patient.

1. Respirations are affected because of abdominal distention.
   a. Grunting
   b. Shallow and rapid if patient is in shock-like state
2. Abdominal distention and unusual appearance of anus—intussusception may look like rectal prolapse.

NURSING ALERT: When anus has an unusual appearance, take axillary temperatures to prevent injury.

3. Behavior
   a. Irritable—very sensitive to handling (Be gentle!)
   b. Lethargic or unresponsive
   c. Behavior indicative of presence or absence of pain

D. Prepare the Patient for Surgery When He Is Shock-like or Febrile.

1. Blood or plasma is given to restore circulating blood volume—observe for transfusion reactions.
2. Observe pulse rate carefully—safe range is below 140/minute.
3. Reduce temperature—fever increases metabolism and makes oxygenation during anesthesia more complicated.

E. Offer Support to the Parents During This Time of Crisis and Fear.

1. Encourage the parents to verbalize their concerns.
2. Reinforce what the physician has told them.
3. Encourage them to be with the child whenever possible.
4. Help them understand the basic defect and the reason for surgery.

Postoperative Nursing Interventions

A. Give Good Postoperative Care and Observe for Possible Postoperative Complications

(see p. 1134).
Care of the child following reduction of intussusception by hydrostatic barium enema involves careful monitoring of vital signs and general condition, especially abdominal tenderness, bowel sounds, lethargy, and tolerance to fluids.

B. Be Constantly Alert for Complications Arising From Surgery for Intussusception.

1. Fever is usually present.
   a. As a result of absorption of foreign protein
   b. From absorption of bacteria through the damaged intestinal wall
2. Diarrhea—from exposure to others who are infected
3. Shock
4. Dehydration
5. Toxicity
6. Peritonitis

C. Assist In Maintaining Stomach Decompression Until First Stool Is Passed.

1. See that indwelling nasogastric tube is functioning properly.
   a. Tube is usually connected to constant intermittent suction.
   b. Note returns from drainage and irrigation.
2. The patient is usually given nothing by mouth.
   Give mouth care.
3. Note passing of flatus or stool and report—indicates peristalsis has returned to normal activity.
   Oral feedings may start.

D. Gradually Resume Full Caloric Intake and Volume of Oral Intake Appropriate for Age and Weight.

Progression will vary with physician and will depend on whether bowel reduction or resection was the surgical procedure.
1. Oral fluid is usually begun after the first stool is passed—about 4–5 days after surgery. When only a reduction was performed, oral fluid may be resumed when abdominal peristaltic activity is audible.
2. Give frequent, small feedings.
   a. Start with glucose water or water.
   b. Note and report any abdominal distention or vomiting.

E. Provide Emotional Support and Meet the Psychological Needs of the Child.

(See Diarrhea, p. 1352)

F. Support the Parents and Help Them to Maintain a Good Relationship With Their Child.

1. Encourage them to visit and call. Allow the parents to become involved in caring for their child.
2. Help the parents to understand that recurrence is rare, but that certain short-term limits must be placed on the child's activity after discharge.

Expected Outcomes

1. Experiences increasing comfort; shows more normal breathing pattern; more restful behavior; decrease in distressed crying; has relaxed body posture
2. Attains/maintains fluid and electrolyte balance; normal laboratory values and skin turgor
3. Passes stool within 4–5 days following surgery; has audible abdominal peristaltic activity; ingests prescribed feedings without signs of abdominal distention or vomiting
4. Exhibits decrease in abdominal girth; absence of respiratory distress
5. Responds to comfort measures with more relaxed behavior
6. Parents participate in child's care; show an understanding of the treatment protocol

---

Imperforate Anus

The term *imperforate anus* is used to describe all congenital abnormalities of the anorectal canal or in the location of the anus within the perineum.

Etiology and Incidence

1. An arrest in embryologic development of the anus, lower rectum, and urogenital tract at the 8th week of embryonic life
2. Cause unknown
3. 1:4000–1:5000 incidence; slight male predominance
4. Closely associated with other congenital deviations, including:
   a. Congenital heart disease
   b. Esophageal atresia
   c. Spinal malformations
   d. Hydronephrosis
   e. Low birth weight
5. Increased incidence associated with Down syndrome

Types

1. Low imperforate anus (transelevator)—implies that the rectum has descended below the pubococcygeal line (puborectalis muscle) and is in normal anatomic relationship to levator sling and puborectus muscle (Fig. 52-3).
   a. Female
      (1) 90% of females with this condition present with low imperforate anus.
      (2) Fistula is present; rectum ends in fistula that presents in any location from low in vagina to normal position of anus.
   b. Male
      (1) 50% of males with imperforate anus present with this type.
      (2) Perineal fistula is present and is located from anterior or normal position of anus to ventral surface of penis (supraelevator).
2. High imperforate anus (supraelevator)—term implies that the rectal pouch is at or above the pubococcygeal line or the levator musculature (75%).
   a. Male
      (1) 50% of males with imperforate anus present with this type.
      (2) If fistula is present, it will usually communicate with the posterior urethra.
   b. Female
      (1) 10% of females with imperforate anus present with this type.
      (2) Fistula will end high in vagina.

Complications

1. Rectal stenosis or prolapse, usually confined to mucosa
2. Separation of anastomosis
3. Urethral injury or stricture
4. Urinary retention and infection
5. Recurrent urinary fistulas
6. Fecal impaction or incontinence
7. Small bowel obstruction
8. Postoperative colostomy complications
   a. Stenosis of colostomy with enterocolitis
   b. Urinary tract infection in presence of fistula from rectum to urinary tract
   c. Hyperchloremic acidosis in association with proximal colostomy
   d. Persistent diarrhea

Clinical Manifestations

Condition is usually discovered immediately after birth or within several hours.

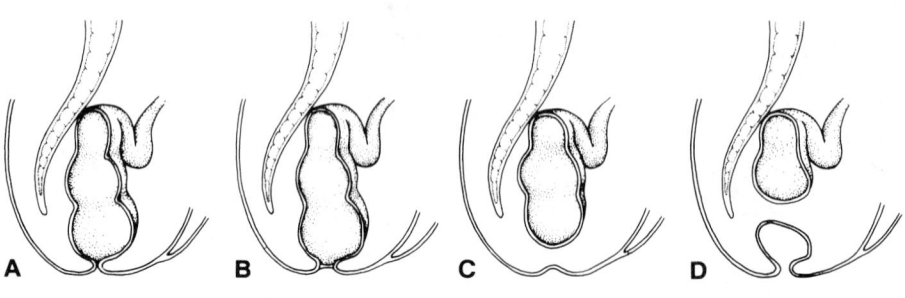

A	B	C	D
Anal stenosis	Imperforate anal membrane	Anal agenesis	Rectal agenesis

Figure 52-3. *Anorectal malformations.*

1. No anal opening
2. Thermometer or small finger cannot be inserted into rectum
3. Absence of meconium stool
4. Green-tinged urine—if fistula is present (high, male)
5. Progressive abdominal distention
6. Fistula is likely to be present
   a. Female—occurs between rectum and vagina or perineum.
   b. Male—occurs between rectum and urinary tract, scrotum, or perineum.

Diagnostic Evaluation

1. Visual examination
   a. Presence of perineal fistula
   b. Meconium coming from vagina or presence of meconium-stained urine
2. General examination or presence of other associated manifestations
3. Urine examination for presence of meconium and epithelial debris—indicates presence of fistula.
4. Voiding cystourethrogram
5. Wangensteen-Rice x-ray (upside-down position)
   a. Limited accuracy in locating rectal pouch
   b. Useful only after infant is 24 hours of age
6. Sonography
7. Neurologic examination

Treatment

1. Low—female
   a. Decompression of bowel with catheter irrigations
   b. Dilatation of fistula for 8–12 months thereafter
   c. Definitive repair
2. Low—male
   a. Rectal cutback anoplasty or Y–V plasty
   b. Local dilatation of fistula
3. High—male
   a. Colostomy for decompression
   b. Definitive pull-through surgery—deferred until about 1 year of age or when child attains 6.75–9 kg. (15–20 lbs.)
4. High—female
   a. Colostomy
   b. Definitive repair done when infant is 1 year of age or 6.75–9 kg. (15–20 lbs.)

Preoperative Nursing Interventions

A. Assist In Maintaining Stability In the Patient's General Condition Prior to Emergency Surgery.

1. Feedings are usually withheld. Note any vomiting, color and amount.
2. Nasogastric tube may be passed to decompress the stomach. Measure abdominal girth.
3. Observe the patient carefully for any signs of distress and report these to physician. Check vital signs frequently. Maintain temperature stability.

B. Observe the Infant Carefully for Any Other Anomalies or Changes In Condition.

1. Use an Isolette or radiant warmer.
2. Observe for stool coming from a fistula.
3. Note that urine may be green-tinged.
4. Keep area clean.

Postoperative Nursing Interventions

Depending on the location of the rectum (see types of imperforate anus), and sex of child, 1 of 3 surgical approaches may be used: (1) anoplasty, (2) temporary colostomy with definitive pull-through at a later time when the child is older and larger, or (3) abdominal or sacroperineal pull-through.

A. Give Good Postoperative Care and Observe for Possible Postoperative Complications.

(See p. 1134)
Especially note any vomiting or stooling.

B. Provide Appropriate Care for Perineal Anoplasty, Prevent Infection of Suture Line, and Promote Healing.

1. Do not put anything in rectum.
2. Expose perineum to air.
3. Position the infant for easy access to perineum for cleansing and minimal irritation to site (i.e., place the infant on abdomen, possibly with hips elevated, to prevent pressure on perineal surfaces; turn side-to-side).

C. Provide Good Colostomy Care and Prevent Skin Breakdown.

(See Hirschsprung's disease, p. 1355)

D. Provide Appropriate Care for Definitive Pull-Through Surgery.

1. Carry out perineal care as stated above.
2. Provide proper care of gastrostomy or nasogastric tube used to decompress the gastrointestinal tract until peristalsis returns.
3. Provide proper care of bladder catheter, if used, and measure urinary output accurately.
4. Observe carefully for abdominal distention, bleeding from perineum, and respiratory embarrassment.

E. Maintain Adequate Nutrition As Well As Caloric and Fluid Intake to Prevent Dehydration and Electrolyte Imbalance.

1. Oral feedings are usually started within hours after an anoplasty.
2. Oral feedings are usually withheld until peristalsis returns. When primary repair is done, nasogastric suction may be maintained until feedings are started.
3. Monitor parenteral fluids (see p. 1167).

F. Foster Acceptance of the Child and His Diagnosis By His Parents.

1. Assure the parents that colostomy is temporary.
2. Encourage the parents to become involved in care of the child and to give him the emotional security he needs.
3. Support teaching program of surgeon for special care needed at home.
   a. Colostomy care
   b. Anal dilatation to prevent a stricture at site of anastomosis from scar tissue after instructions by physician
4. Initiate referral to community nurse, especially if the parents are particularly anxious about caring for the child at home.
5. Encourage the parents to talk about their concerns.

Health Education

1. Provide careful, thorough teaching of special care and procedures to be continued at home—colostomy care, anal dilatation. Develop a plan for return demonstration by mother.

2. Help the parents to understand situations that may be encountered as a result of imperforate anus as the baby gets older:
   a. Fecal impaction due to lack of sensation to defecate
   b. Future surgery—if primary repair was not done
   c. Toilet training
   d. Inability to control fecal seepage from rectum
3. Some practical guidelines to help parents cope:
   a. Fecal control may not be achieved until age 10 years.
   b. Encourage patterning of defecation (i.e., after breakfast).
   c. Know foods that produce laxative effect—plums, prunes, chocolate, nuts, corn—and foods that have binding effect—peanut butter, hot cereal, cheese.
   d. Antidiarrheal medications may be effective, especially Immodium.
   e. Rectal inertia may cause fecal impaction in rectosigmoid colon with soiling from fluid overflow. Bisacodyl suppository or cleansing enema provide assistance in management.

Bibliography

GI Disorders

Books

Anderson CM, Burke V and Gracey M. Paediatric Gastroenterology. Boston, Blackwell Scientific Publications, 1987

Avery ME and First LR. Pediatric Medicine. Baltimore, Williams & Wilkins, 1989

Fleisher GR and Ludwig S. Textbook of Pediatric Emergency Medicine. Baltimore, Williams & Wilkins, 1988

Gryboski J and Walker WA. Gastrointestinal Problems in the Infant. Vol. 2: Gastrointestinal Disease and Nutritional Inadequacies. New York, Raven Press, 1981

Kenner C, Harjo J and Brueggemeyer A. Neonatal Surgery: A Nursing Perspective. Orlando, Grune & Stratton, 1988

Krulik T, Holaday B and Martinson I. The Child and Family Facing Life-Threatening Illness. Philadelphia, JB Lippincott, 1987

Silverberg M and Daum F (eds). Textbook of Pediatric Gastroenterology. Chicago, Yearbook Medical Pub, 1988

Whaley LF and Wong DL. Nursing Care of Infants and Children. St. Louis, CV Mosby, 1987

Journals

General

Mack JE. Ribavirin: An antiviral agent with promise. Pediatr Nurs 1988 May–Jun; 14(3):220

Shaw JH. Causes and control of dental caries. N Engl J Med 1987 Oct; 317(16):996–1004

Wood B et al. Sibling psychological status and style as related to the disease of their chronically ill brothers and sisters: Implications for models of biopsychosocial interactions. Develop Behav Pediatr 1988 Apr; 9(2):66–72

Diarrhea

Andres JM. Advances in understanding the pathogenesis of persistent diarrhea in young children. Adv Pediatr 1988; 30:483–498

Brown KH et al. Effect of continued oral feeding on clinical and nutritional outcomes of acute diarrhea in children. J Pediatr 1988 Feb; 112(2): 191–200

Conway SP and Ireson A. Acute gastroenteritis in well nourished infants: Comparison of four feeding regimens. Arch Dis Child 1989 Jan; 64(1):87–91

DeBenham BJ et al. Initial assessment of chronic diarrhea in toddlers. Pediatr Nurs 1985 Jul–Aug; 11(4):281–285

Ho MS et al. Diarrheal deaths in American children. JAMA 1988 Dec 9; 260(22):3281–3286

Rajah R et al. The effect of feeding four different formulas on stool weight in prolonged dehydrating infantile gastroenteritis. J Pediatr Gastroenterol Nutr 1988 Mar–Apr; 7(2):203–207

Tucker JA and Sussman–Karten K. Treating acute diarrhea and dehydration with an oral rehydration solution. Pediatr Nurs 1987 May–Jun; 13(3):169–174

Cleft Lip and Palate

Campbell AN and Tremouth MJ. New feeder for infants with cleft palate. Arch Dis Child 1987 Dec; 62(12):1292

Jones MC. Etiology of facial clefts: Prospective evaluation of 428 patients. Cleft Palate J 1988 Jan; 25(1):21–25

Jones WB. Weight gain and feeding in the neonate with cleft: A three-center study. Cleft Palate J 1988 Oct; 25(4): 379–384

Pannbacker M. Prevention of communication problems associated with cleft palate. J Commun Disord 1988 Sep; 21(5):401–408

Porterfield HW. Feeding infants with cleft lip, cleft palate, or both. Cleft Palate J 1988 Jan; 25(1):80

Pate CM. Care of the family following the birth of a child with a cleft lip and/or palate. Neonatal Netw 1987 Jun; 5(6): 30–37

Richman RA et al. Olfactory deficits in boys with cleft palate. Pediatrics 1988 Dec; (6):840–844

Seth AK and McWilliams BJ. Weight gain in children with cleft palate from birth to two years. Cleft Palate J 1988 Apr; 25(2):146–150

Strauss RP et al. Perceptions of appearance and speech by adolescent patients with cleft lip and palate and by their parents. Cleft Palate J 1988 Oct; 25(4):335–342

Wasserman GA et al. Maternal interaction and language development in children with and without speech-related anomalies. J Commun Disord 1988 Aug; 21(4):315–331

Pyloric Stenosis

Jedd MB et al. Factors associated with infantile hypertropic pyloric stenosis. Am J Dis Child 1988 Mar; 142(3):334–337

Okorie NM et al. What happens to the pyloris after pyloromyotomy? Arch Dis Child 1988 Nov; 63(11):1339–1341

Rollins MD et al. Pyloric stenosis: Congenital or acquired? Arch Dis Child 1989 Jan; 64(1):138–139

Zeidan B et al. Recent results of treatment of infantile hypertrophic pyloric stenosis. Arch Dis Child 1988 Sep; 63(9):1060–1064

Intussusception, Hirschsprung's Disease, Imperforate Anus

Bonadio WA. Intussusception reduced by barium enema. Clin Pediatr 1988 Dec; 27(12):601–604

Bruce J et al. Intussusception: Evolution of current management. J Pediatr Gastroenterol Nutr 1987 Sep–Oct; 6(5):663–674

Donaldson JS et al. Ultrasound of the distal pouch in infants with imperforate anus. J Pediatr Surg 1989 May; 24(5):465–468

West KW et al. Postoperative intussusception: Experience with 36 cases in children. Surgery 1988 Oct; 104(4):781–787

Franken EA. Nonsurgical treatment of intussusception. AJR 1988 Jun; 150(6): 1353–4

Phelan E, deCampo JF and Malecky G. Comparison of oxygen and barium reduction of ileocolic intussusception. AJR 1988 Jun; 150(6):1349–1352

Vane DW et al. Hirschsprung's disease: Current management. Perinat/Neonatol 1987 Nov–Dec; 11(6):26–33

West KW et al. Intussusception: Current management in infants and children. Surgery 1987 Oct; 102(4):704–710

Tracheoesophageal Atresia

Black CT and Sherman JO. The association of low imperforate anus and Down's Syndrome. J Pediatr Surg 1989 Jan; 24(1):92–94

Chetcuti P et al. Chest wall deformity in patients with repaired esophageal atresia. J Pediatr Surg 1989 Mar; 24(3): 244–247

Chittmittrapap S et al. Oesophageal atresia and associated anomalies. Arch Dis Child 1985 Mar; 64(3):364–368

Ohkawa H et al. Clinical experience with a sucking sump catheter in the treatment of esophageal atresia. J Pediatr Surg 1989 Apr; 24(4):333–335

Pohlson EC et al. Improved survival with primary anastomosis in the low birth weight neonate with esophageal atresia and tracheosophageal fistual. J Pediatr Surg 1988 May; 23(5):418–421

Celiac Disease

Bentley AC. A survey of celiac–sprue patients: Effect of dietary restrictions on religious practices. J Gen Psychol 1988 Jan; 115(1):7–14

Bitman J et al. Lipid composition of milk from mothers with cystic fibrosis. Pediatrics 1987 Dec; 80(6):927–932

Bonamico M et al. Iron deficiency in children with celiac disease. J Pediatr Gastroenterol Nutr 1987 Sep–Oct; 6(5):702–706

Goleano NF et al. Comparison of two special infant formulas designed for the treatment of protracted diarrhea. J Pediatr Gastroenterol Nutr 1988 Jan–Feb; 7(1):76–83

Greco L et al. Discriminant analysis for the diagnosis of childhood celiac disease. J Pediatr Gastroenterol Nutr 1987 Jul–Aug; 6(4):538–542

Kumar PJ et al. The teenage celiac: Follow-up study of 102 patients. Arch Dis Child 1988 Aug; 63(8):916–920

Walker-Smith JA. Relapses in celiac disease. J Pediatr Gastroenterol Nutr 1987 Mar–Apr; 6(2):314–315

Weizman Z et al. Treatment failure in celiac disease due to coexistent exocrine pancreatic insufficiency. Pediatrics 1987 Dec; 80(6):924–926

Gastroesophageal Reflux

Bailey DJ et al. Lack of efficacy of thickened feeding as treatment for gastroesophageal reflux. J Pediatr 1987 Feb; 110(2):187–189

Beasley SW and Myers NA. The diagnosis of congenital tracheosophageal fistula. J Pediatr Surg 1988 May; 23(5):415–417

Carre IJ. Treatment of gastroesophageal reflux. J Pediatr 1988 Mar; 112(3):502–503

Cucchiara S et al. Pathophysiology of gastroesophageal reflux and distal esophageal mobility in children with gastroesophageal reflux disease. J Pediatr Gastroenterol Nutr 1988 Nov–Dec; 7(6):830–836

Fann JI et al. "Waterseal" gastrostomy in the management of premature infants with tracheosophageal fistula and pulmonary insufficiency. J Pediatr Surg 1988 Jan; 23(1 pt 2):29–31

Mahony MJ et al. Motor disorders of the oesophagus in gastro-oesophageal reflux. Arch Dis Child 1988 Nov; 63(11):1333–1338

Nordstrom DG. Cloth sling for treatment of infant gastroesophageal reflux. Am J Occup Ther 1988 Jul; 42(7):465–468

Nussbaum E et al. Association of lipid-laden alveolar macrophages and gastroesophageal reflux in children. J Pediatr 1987 Feb; 110(2):190–193

Orenstein SR. Effect of nonnutritive sucking on infant gastroesophageal reflux. Pediatr Res 1988 Jul; 24(1):38–40

Orenstein SR and Orenstein DM. Gastroesophageal reflux and respiratory disease in children. J Pediatr 1988 Jun; 112(6):847–858

Orenstein SR et al. Thickening of infant feedings for therapy of gastroesophageal reflux. J Pediatr 1987 Feb; 181–186

Orenstein SR and Whitington PF. Positioning for prevention of infant gastroesophageal reflux. J Pediatr 1983; 103(4):534–537

Paton JY et al. Vomiting and gastrooesophageal reflux. Arch Dis Child 1988 Jul; 63(7):837–838

Shepherd RW et al. Gastroesophageal reflux in children. Clin Pediatr 1987 Feb; 26(2):55–60

Sutphen JL and Dillard VL. Effect of feeding volume on early postcibal gastroesophageal reflux. J Pediatr Gastroenterol Nutr 1988 Mar–Apr; 7(2):185–188

Ulshen MH. Treatment of gastroesophageal reflux: Is nothing sacred? J Pediatr 1987 Feb; 110(2): 254–255

Vandenplas Y et al. Incidence of gastroesophageal reflux in sleep, awake, footed, and postcibal periods in asymptomatic and symptomatic infants. J Pediatr Gastroenterol Nutr 1988 Mar–Apr; 7(2):177–180

Vandenplas Y and Sacre L. Mild-thickening agents as a treatment for gastroesophageal reflux. Clin Pediatr 1987 Feb; 26(2):66–68

Pediatric Ostomy Products

Educational material and educational puppet program
ConvaTec, CN 5254
Princeton, NJ 08543-5254

or

The Kids on the Block
9385 C Gerwig Lane
Columbia, MD 21046
Phone: 301/290-9095

or

1–800–368–KIDS (except in MD)

Acute Glomerulonephritis

Glomerulonephritis refers to inflammation of the kidneys caused by an antigen–antibody reaction following an infection in some part of the body. Acute glomerulonephritis is predominantly a disease of childhood and is the most common type of nephritis in children.

Etiology

1. Presumed cause—antigen–antibody reaction secondary to an infection elsewhere in the body
2. Initial infection
   a. Usually either an upper respiratory infection or a skin infection
   b. Most frequent causative agent—nephritogenic strains of group A beta hemolytic streptococcus

Incidence

1. Unknown—milder cases are not recognized
2. More common in males than females (2:1)
3. Most common in early school-age group
4. Rare in children under 2 years of age
5. Varies with the prevalence of nephritogenic strains of streptococci and the likelihood of cross-infection

Altered Physiology

1. The organisms responsible for nephritis contain antigens similar to those of the basement membrane of the renal glomeruli.
2. Antibodies produced to fight the invading organism also react against the glomerular tissue, forming immune complexes.
3. The immune complexes become trapped in the glomerular loop and cause an inflammatory reaction in the affected glomeruli.
4. Changes in the glomerular capillaries reduce the amount of the glomerular filtrate, allow passage of blood cells and protein into the filtrate, and reduce the amount of sodium and water that is passed to the tubules for reabsorption.
5. General vascular disturbances, including loss of capillary integrity and spasm of arterioles, are secondary to kidney changes and are responsible for much of the symptomatology of the disease.

Clinical Manifestations

A. Onset

1. Usually 1–2 weeks after the onset of the initiating infection
2. May be abrupt and severe, or mild and detected only by laboratory measures

B. Signs and Symptoms

1. Urinary symptoms
   a. Decreased urine output
   b. Bloody or brown-colored urine
2. Edema
   a. Present in most patients
   b. Usually mild
   c. Often manifested by periorbital edema in the morning
   d. May appear only as rapid weight gain
   e. May be generalized and influenced by posture
3. Hypertension
   a. Present in over 50% of patients
   b. Usually mild
   c. Rise in blood pressure may be sudden
   d. Usually appears during the first 4–5 days of the illness
4. Malaise
5. Mild headache
6. Gastrointestinal disturbances, especially anorexia and vomiting

Diagnostic Evaluation

1. Urinalysis
   a. Decreased output—may approach anuria
   b. Microscopic or gross hematuria
   c. Specific gravity—moderately elevated
   d. Proteinuria (3+ to 4+)
   e. Microscopic—red blood cells, leukocytes, epithelial cells, and casts
2. Serum complement level—usually reduced
3. BUN and creatinine—often mildly to moderately elevated

4. ASO or antistreptokinase titer—rarely elevated
5. DNase B antigen titer—elevated
6. Sedimentation rate—elevated
7. Chest x-ray—may show pulmonary congestion, cardiac enlargement
8. Renal function studies—normal in 50% of the patients

Prognosis

1. At least 95% of affected children recover completely.
   a. Acute symptoms usually disappear in 1–3 weeks.
   b. Blood chemistry is usually normal by the end of the 2nd week.
   c. Urine sediment may be abnormal for months or even years following the acute episode.
   d. Sedimentation rate may remain elevated for several months.
2. Death during the acute phase is very uncommon, but may occur due to the effects of hypertensive encephalopathy or heart failure.
3. There is no evidence that affected children develop chronic glomerulonephritis.

Complications

(Occur infrequently)

A. Hypertensive Encephalopathy

1. Manifestations
   a. Restlessness
   b. Stupor
   c. Convulsions
   d. Vomiting
   e. Severe headache
   f. Visual disturbances
2. Cause—probably ischemia secondary to vasospasm
3. No correlation with the degree of renal impairment or fluid retention
4. Duration
   a. Usually 1–2 days
   b. Ends spontaneously with decreased blood pressure

B. Congestive Heart Failure

1. Cardiac failure may occur because of persistent hypertension, hypervolemia, and peripheral vasoconstriction.
2. Manifestations
   a. Dyspnea
   b. Tachycardia
   c. Gallop rhythm
   d. Liver engorgement
3. Duration
   a. Variable
   b. Usually subsides rapidly with the onset of diuresis and the fall in blood pressure

C. Uremia (rare)

Manifestations
1. Evidence of acidosis
2. Drowsiness
3. Coma
4. Stupor
5. Muscular twitching
6. Convulsions

D. Anemia

Usually caused by hypervolemia rather than a loss of red blood cells in the urine

Patient Problems and Nursing Diagnoses

1. Development of life-threatening complications, including hypertensive encephalopathy, congestive heart failure, and acute renal failure
2. Reduced urinary elimination related to glomerular dysfunction
3. Fluid volume excess related to kidney failure
4. Headache and discomfort related to toxic buildup in blood
5. Nutrition, altered, less than body requirements, related to anorexia
6. Anxiety related to uncertain course of disease and hospitalization
7. Activity intolerance related to fatigue caused by underlying disease
8. Knowledge deficit regarding acute glomerulonephritis and its management
9. Noncompliance to dietary and fluid restrictions

Nursing Interventions

A. Promoting Healing and Preventing Disease Complications.

1. No specific measures have been demonstrated to modify the inflammatory process.
2. General measures
   a. Maintain bedrest during the acute phase of the illness, at least until gross hematuria has disappeared and child is no longer hypertensive.
      (1) Organize nursing activities to allow the child to have periods of uninterrupted rest.
      (2) Explain to the child why it is necessary for him to stay in bed. (Bedrest is often interpreted by the child as punishment.)
      (3) Administer sedation if required to keep the child quiet and at rest.
      (4) Provide diversion appropriate for the child's age.
      (5) Place the child's bed in a position where he can watch the activities of the unit and other children.
      (6) Provide alternative means of rest for children who are too young to understand the necessity of remaining in bed. (Such children can be held by the mother or nurse in a chair.)
      (7) Observe the child closely for fatigue once ambulation is begun.
   b. Protect the child from infection.
      (1) Avoid placing the child in a room with patients who have fevers, upper respiratory infections, or any other contagious disease.
      (2) Administer therapeutic doses of antibiotics as prescribed by the physician to eradicate existing infection.
         (a) A 10-day course of intramuscular penicillin is often prescribed.
         (b) Points of emphasis
            Inject the medication into a large muscle. Rotate the site of injection.
            Observe the child closely for adverse reactions such as skin rash, urticaria, serum sickness, and anaphylaxis.
      (3) Protect the child from chilling or overheating.
      (4) Provide scrupulous daily hygiene, including mouth care. Keep the skin clean and dry.
   c. Provide a diet in conformity with the child's age and the recommendation of his physician.

(1) A regular diet without added salt is usually prescribed during the acute phase in non-complicated cases.

(2) A diet restricted in protein and potassium is necessary for children who demonstrate some degree of renal failure.

(3) Fluids must be restricted in children with hypertension, edema, congestive failure, or renal failure.

(4) Explain all dietary restrictions to the child and his parents.

(5) Obtain a careful history of dietary preferences and patterns so that the child's meals can be as acceptable as possible.

(6) Place a sign indicating dietary restrictions on the child's bed so that anyone approaching him will be aware of his special needs.

(7) If the child is to be given a restricted amount of fluids, offer small amounts of fluids spaced at regular intervals throughout the day and evening.

Use a cup of appropriate size for the amount of fluid being offered.

(8) Refer to section on nutrition, page 1102.

B. Observing and Recording Disease Progress.

1. Maintain a complete record of the child's intake and output.
   a. Measure fluids accurately in graduated containers. Do not estimate fluid intake or output.
   b. Place a sign on the child's bed to ensure that no urine is accidentally discarded and that all intake is recorded.
   c. Total the intake and output every 8 hours.
      (1) Notify the physician if output does not appear adequate.
      (2) In children who are not toilet trained, a fairly accurate record of output can be obtained by weighing diapers before and after voiding.
   d. Record other causes of fluid loss such as the number of stools per day, perspiration, etc.
2. Weight the child daily.
   a. An increase in weight may indicate fluid retention.
   b. Weigh the child on the same scale and at the same time each day.
      (1) It is usually advantageous to weigh the child before breakfast.
      (2) The child should be weighed in a consistent manner, with minimal clothing.
3. Record the blood pressure at frequent intervals.
   a. Refer to the method for determining blood pressure, page 1141.
   b. A diastolic pressure of 100 mm. Hg is an indication of concern and should be reported to the physician immediately.

   Place the child into bed and observe him closely for cerebral changes.
4. Observe for signs of complications.
   a. Increased blood pressure
   b. Fluid retention or edema
   c. Changes in vital signs, especially more rapid pulse or respirations
   d. Changes in activity status, especially lethargy, restlessness, stupor, or coma
   e. Vomiting
   f. Visual disturbances
   g. Severe headache
   h. Convulsions

5. Record appearance of urine.
   Note the persistence of hematuria or whether the urine appears to be clearing.

C. Reducing Hypertension.

1. Limit the fluid intake according to the physician's recommendation.
2. Maintain bedrest.
3. Administer antihypertensive drugs as prescribed by the physician.
   a. Reserpine is the drug most frequently used.
      (1) Route of administration—intramuscular or intravenous
      (2) Side effects—nasal stuffiness, dryness of mouth, diarrhea
   b. Hydralazine (Apresoline) is often combined with reserpine in refractory cases.
      (1) Route of administration
         (a) Intramuscular
         (b) This drug may be given orally once initial control of hypertension is established.
      (2) Side effects
         (a) Nausea, vomiting, diarrhea, anorexia
         (b) Headache
         (c) Tachycardia

D. Providing Appropriate Nursing Care to the Child With Disease Complications.

1. Encephalopathy (see the section on care of the child with seizures, p. 1449)
2. Congestive heart failure
3. Anemia
4. Renal failure

E. Providing Emotional Support to the Child and His Family During Hospitalization.

1. Explain all aspects of the diagnostic tests and treatment in terms that the family can understand.
2. Formulate a nursing care plan that facilitates a consistent approach to the child's care.
3. Allow the child to make some decisions and to participate in his care. He may decide when he wants his bath and should be allowed to make some dietary choices, etc.
4. Maintain discipline. Establish and enforce appropriate limits for the child's behavior.
5. Provide diversion appropriate for the child's age.
6. Arrange for the continued education of the school-age child.

F. Preparing the Child and His Parents for Discharge.

1. Encourage as much family participation as possible during the child's hospitalization (see the section on family-centered care, p. 1125).
2. Help the family plan for adaptation of the child's nursing care to the home environment.
   a. Review the medication schedule.
   b. Suggest means of implementing a sodium-restricted diet.
      (1) Provide the family with a list of commercial foods and fluids that are normally high in sodium content, so that they can avoid these.
      (2) Help the parents to plan sample menus.
      (3) Provide suggestions for low-sodium cooking and baking.
   c. Discuss activity and fluid restrictions if appropriate.
3. Make certain that the family has an appointment for continued medical supervision.

4. Initiate appropriate referrals.
   a. Community health nurse
   b. Home tutor

Health Education

1. Medical explanation of the disease process should be reinforced.
   a. The need for medical evaluation and culture of all sore throats should be emphasized.
   b. The family should be made aware of signs and symptoms of disease recurrence.
2. Tonsillectomy or other oral surgery is not recommended for several months after the acute phase of glomerulonephritis.
   If this type of surgery is necessary later, penicillin may be recommended before and after the procedure to prevent bacterial infection.

Expected Outcomes

1. Absence of life-threatening complications
2. Demonstrates increasing urinary output
3. Adheres to prescribed fluid restriction; maintains weight within acceptable level for condition
4. Copes with discomfort; engages in diversional activities in accordance with age
5. Eats prescribed diet
6. Adheres to treatment protocol; parents gaining an understanding of child's illness as evidenced by their questions, conversation, and participation in child's care

---

Nephrotic Syndrome

Nephrotic syndrome refers to a symptom complex characterized by edema, marked proteinuria, hypoalbuminemia, and hypercholesterolemia. Although there are many types of the disease, minimal change nephrotic syndrome is the most common in children.

Etiology

1. The symptom complex results from large losses of protein in the urine, too great for the body to replenish by albumin synthesis.
2. The syndrome may be classified as primary (associated with a primary glomerular disease) or secondary (resulting from a wide variety of disease states or nephrotoxic agents).

Incidence

1. Annually afflicts about 2–3 children per 100,000 under the age of 8 years in the U.S.
2. More common in males than in females (2:1)
3. Most common age of onset—between 2 and 6 years

Altered Physiology

1. For unknown reasons, the glomerular membrane, usually impermeable to large proteins, becomes permeable.
2. Protein, especially albumin, leaks through the membrane and is lost in the urine.
3. Plasma proteins decrease as proteinuria increases.
4. The colloidal osmotic pressure that holds water in the vascular compartments is reduced because of the decrease in amount of serum albumin. This allows fluid to flow from the capillaries into the extracellular space, producing edema.
5. Accumulation of fluid in the interstitial spaces and peritoneal cavity is also increased by an overproduction of aldosterone, which causes retention of sodium.
6. There is increased susceptibility to infection.
7. Generalized edema is responsible for most of the physical characteristics of the disease, including respiratory distress, gastrointestinal symptoms, umbilical and inguinal hernias, rectal prolapse, decreased ambulation, loss of body tissue, and malnutrition.

Clinical Course and Prognosis

1. The severity and duration of the clinical course is variable and affects the prognosis.
2. Most children experience remission following the initial course of treatment.
   a. Of these responders, most will relapse once or not at all during the subsequent 6 months.
   b. About ⅓ of the responders experience multiple relapses following the initial remission.
3. The majority of affected children eventually have a complete recovery.
4. Death may occur from profound sepsis, progressive renal insufficiency, or congestive heart failure.

Clinical Manifestations

A. Onset

1. Insidious
2. Edema is often the presenting symptom.
   a. Initially, usually slight and inconstant
   b. Usually first apparent around the eyes

B. Signs and Symptoms

1. Irritability and depression
2. Gastrointestinal disturbances, including vomiting and diarrhea
3. Anorexia—malnutrition may become severe
4. Recurrent infections
5. Edema—may be minimal or massive
   a. Ascites may be severe.
   b. Intense scrotal edema is common.
   c. Peripheral edema is dependent and shifts with the child's position.
   d. Striae may appear on the skin from overstretching.
6. Profound weight gain; the child may actually double his normal weight.
7. Decreased urine output during the edematous phase
8. Wasting of skeletal muscles may occur because of the continuous drain of plasma protein nitrogen into the urine.
9. Nephrotic crisis
   a. Abdominal pain
   b. Fever
   c. Erysipeloid skin eruption possible
   d. Symptoms subside within a few days
   e. Often followed by spontaneous diuresis

Diagnostic Evaluation

1. Urinalysis
   a. Proteinuria—marked
   b. Casts—numerous
   c. Hematuria—absent or transient
2. Renal function tests—variable, often normal
3. Blood
   a. Total serum protein—reduced
   b. Serum albumin—reduced

c. Total serum globulin—normal or increased
   Gamma fraction—reduced
d. Cholesterol and lipoproteins—increased
e. Serum calcium—reduced

4. Blood pressure—usually normal, although mild hypertension may be present

Patient Problems and Nursing Diagnoses

1. Fluid volume excess related to glomerular dysfunction
2. Impaired skin integrity related to edema
3. Altered urinary pattern related to glomerular dysfunction
4. Increased potential for infection related to disease process and steroid therapy
5. Pain and discomfort
6. Altered body image (round face; hirsutism) related to side effects of medications
7. Nutrition, altered, less than body requirements, related to anorexia
8. Anxiety and frustration related to the up-and-down course of the disease
9. Knowledge deficit about nephrotic syndrome

Nursing Interventions

A. Relieving Edema and Other Manifestations of the Nephrotic State.

1. Administer steroids as recommended by the physician.
   a. Steroid therapy is the preferred approach to treatment because steroids appear to affect the basic disease process in addition to controlling edema.
   b. Prednisone is usually the drug of choice because it is less likely to induce salt retention and potassium loss and is the least expensive. There is no standard program of therapy, but most children receive 2–3 mg./kg. until complete remission occurs; this is followed by low-dose maintenance therapy or an intermittent schedule for several months.
   c. Children with nephrotic syndrome may respond to steroid therapy in several ways:
      (1) Steroid-sensitive—children respond to a single short course of steroids without evidence of relapse after cessation of therapy.
      (2) Steroid-dependent—children respond incompletely or tend to relapse on lowered dosages of steroids and require additional supportive treatment.
      (3) Steroid-resistant—children become resistant to steroid therapy or cannot be maintained in remission without developing serious side effects of treatment.
   d. Observe for evidence of side effects and complications of therapy.
      (1) Cushing's syndrome
         (a) Manifestations include increased body hair (hirsutism), rounding of the face ("moon face"), abdominal distention, striae, increased appetite with weight gain, and aggravation of adolescent acne.
         (b) The child should have access to a mirror so that he can observe gradual physical changes in his body.
         (c) The child and his parents should be provided with opportunities to discuss their feelings about the child's altered body image. Play therapy may be helpful for the young child.
         (d) It should be stressed that these physical changes are not harmful nor permanent, and will disappear after the steroid treatment is stopped.
      (2) Serious side effects and uncommon complications
         (a) Masking of infections
            The child should be observed very closely for signs of inflammation or infection.
         (b) Peptic ulceration
            Give medication with milk or an antacid. Test all stools with Hematest.
         (c) Growth suppression
         (d) Precipitation of diabetes mellitus
         (e) Increased intracranial pressure manifested by headache, anorexia, vomiting, diplopia, and seizures
         (f) Osteoporosis
         (g) Cataracts
         (h) Thromboembolism
         (i) Adrenal suppression and insufficiency

NURSING ALERT: No vaccinations or immunizations should be given during active episodes of nephrosis or while the child is receiving immunosuppressive therapy.

2. Administer immunosuppressive drugs as prescribed by the physician.
   a. Cyclophosphamide is the drug of choice.
   b. This therapy is generally reserved for children with steroid-dependent or steroid-resistant nephrosis because of severe side effects. It should be administered only with informed consent of the patient or parent.
   c. Observe for complications of therapy.
      (1) Decreased white blood count renders the child very susceptible to infection.
      (2) Hair loss—the child should be prepared for this complication and should be helped to deal with the change in body image. Head scarves or wigs may minimize the child's distress.
      (3) Cystitis—the drug should be given in the morning and large volumes of fluid given orally to prevent concentration of the drug in the urine.
      (4) Sterility may result in both sexes from long-term use.

3. Administer diuretics as recommended by the physician.
   a. Be aware of those diuretics that may cause potassium depletion.
      (1) Offer foods high in potassium, such as orange juice or bananas.
      (2) Supplemental potassium chloride may be administered orally if the urine output is adequate.

4. Maintain the child on bedrest during periods of severe edema.
   See the section on acute glomerulonephritis, page 1363.

5. Administer a diet low in sodium and high in potassium.
   a. Moderate sodium restriction is usually indicated. Excessively salty foods are excluded, and extra salt is eliminated.
   b. Potassium may be provided in juices, fruits (especially oranges, grapes, and bananas), and milk.

6. Restrict fluids as requested by the physician.
   a. Fluid restriction is usually imposed only during the extreme edematous phases.
   b. Restriction is carefully calculated at frequent intervals, based on the urine output of the previous day plus estimated insensible losses.
   c. Offer small amounts of fluids spaced at regular intervals throughout the day and evening.
      Use a cup of appropriate size for the amount of fluid being offered.
   d. Measure fluids accurately in graduated containers. Do not estimate fluid intake or output.
   e. Place a sign on the child's bed to ensure that no urine is accidentally discarded and that all intake is recorded.
   f. Determine total intake and output every 8 hours. In children who are not toilet trained, a fairly accurate record of output can be obtained by weighing diapers before and after voiding.
   g. Record other causes of fluid loss such as the number of stools per day, perspiration, etc.
7. Assist with abdominal paracentesis when this is required because of marked ascites (see Guidelines, p. 1368).

B. Protecting the Child from Infection.

1. Apply measures stated in the section on acute glomerulonephritis, page 1363.
2. Closely observe the child who is on steroids for signs of infection; as this medication masks such symptoms.
3. Provide meticulous skin care to the edematous areas of the body.
   a. Bathe the child frequently and apply powder. Areas of special concern are the moist parts of the body and edematous male genitalia. Support the scrotum with a cotton pad held in place by a T-binder, if necessary, for the child's comfort.
   b. Position the child so that edematous skin surfaces are not in contact.
      Place a pillow between the child's legs when he is lying on his side, etc.
   c. Irrigate swollen eyes and cleanse the surrounding area several times daily to remove exudate. Elevate the child's head to reduce edema.
4. If possible, avoid femoral venipunctures and intramuscular injections in the buttocks.
   In addition to the risk of infection, the child may be predisposed to thromboembolism because of hypovolemia, stasis, and increased plasma concentration of clotting factors.

C. Restoring Lost Plasma and Tissue Proteins.

1. Offer a high-protein, high-calorie diet.
   a. Salt restriction is usually not necessary, except during periods of edema and hypertension.
2. Obtain a complete history of dietary preferences and patterns so that the child's meals can be as acceptable as possible.
3. Place a sign on the child's bed indicating any dietary restrictions, so that anyone approaching him will be aware of his special needs.
4. Permit additional amounts of food at the child's discretion.
5. See the section on nutrition, page 1102.

D. Observing for Disease Progress.

1. Apply nursing measures outlined in intervention B in the section on acute glomerulonephritis, page 1364.
2. Observe the child's entire body at frequent intervals for edema.
   a. Record areas of transient edema.
   b. Measure abdominal girth.
3. Measure all urine and test for protein, blood, and specific gravity.
   Record findings. Report:
   a. Decreased urine output
   b. Increased amount of protein
   c. Cloudiness
   d. Hematuria
4. Observe for side effects of all medications.
5. Observe for indications of thrombosis and report these to the physician immediately.

E. Providing Emotional Support to the Child and His Family.

1. Encourage frequent visiting.
   a. Allow as much parental participation in the child's care as possible.
   b. See the section on family-centered care, page 1125.
2. Allow the child as much activity as he can tolerate.
   a. Bedrest should be enforced during periods of hypertension.
   b. Balance periods of rest, recreation, and quiet activities during the convalescent phase.
   c. Allow the child to eat his meals with other children.
3. Encourage the child to verbalize his fears.
   a. Young children frequently fear abandonment by their parents or loss of body integrity. (The boy who is unable to visualize his penis because of extensive edema may think that he has been castrated and needs reassurance that his body is intact.)
   b. See the section on the hospitalized child, page 1120.
4. Assist the parents to verbalize their fears, frustrations, and questions.
   a. Parents often express frustration regarding the uncertainties associated with the cause of the disease, the clinical course, and prognosis.
   b. Parents may question the difference between nephritis and nephrosis.

F. Preparing for the Child's Discharge.

1. Begin discharge planning early.
   a. Have the dietitian discuss special diets with the parents. Encourage them to plan sample menus.
   b. Encourage the parents to administer the child's medication prior to discharge.
   c. Instruct the parents about urine testing.
   d. Provide suggestions regarding activity restriction at home.
2. Provide written discharge instructions concerning:
   a. Diet
   b. Prevention of infection
   c. Skin care
   d. Administration of medications
   e. Activity restrictions, if any
   f. Urine testing
   g. Symptoms of relapse
   h. Appointment for continued medical supervision.
3. Initiate a community health nursing referral if necessary for reinforcement of teaching.

Health Education

1. Reinforce medical interpretation of the child's disease. Stress the importance of attention to the details of the child's care and continued medical supervision.

2. Discuss the problem of discipline with the parents. Encourage them to set consistent limits on and expectations of their child's behavior.
3. Emphasize the necessity of taking medication according to the prescribed schedule and for an extended time. Discuss complications encountered with steroid therapy.

Expected Outcomes

1. Shows reduction in edema and ascites; cooperates with prescribed reduced fluid intake; abdominal girth decreasing
2. No signs of skin breakdown
3. Demonstrates urine output within acceptable range; laboratory values indicate trend toward recovery; no signs of hematuria
4. Absence of infection; no elevation of temperature
5. Appears more comfortable; engaging in play activities
6. Adheres to prescribed drug therapy; verbalizes that side effects are result of medications
7. Consumes prescribed diet
8. Demonstrates improved coping ability through play, interaction with other children, and normalization of behavior
9. Parents able to describe nephrotic syndrome and treatment program; discuss feelings and frustration with personnel

---

Guidelines   Assisting With Pediatric Abdominal Paracentesis

Purpose   To withdraw fluid from the peritoneal cavity in order to relieve pressure symptoms and respiratory distress

Equipment

Sterile equipment
  Hypodermic syringe
  Hypodermic and aspiration needles
  Novocain
  Scalpel
  Cannula
  Trocar
  Rubber tubing
  Needle holder
  Hemostat
  Specimen containers
  Large collection container

Suture needles and sutures
Forceps
Gloves
Towels
Graduated receptacle
Cotton balls
Gauze squares
Abdominal dressing
Abdominal binder
Safety pins
Nonsterile equipment
  Preparation tray
  Tape measure

Procedure

Nursing Action	Rationale/Amplification
Preparatory Phase	
1. Explain the procedure to the child in terms he can understand. Stress that he will feel better after the procedure.	1. To allay his fears and ensure his cooperation.
2. Have the child void just prior to the procedure.	2. To avoid puncturing the bladder during the procedure.
3. Secure the help of a second person.	3. To observe the child and assist the physician during the procedure.
4. Position the child correctly:	
a. Place him close to the edge of the examining table	
b. Support his back with your body	
c. Hold his hands	
Performance Phase	
1. Maintain the child's position.	1. To avoid injury.
2. Talk to the child frequently and hold his hands. Praise him for his cooperation.	2. To offer emotional support.
3. Observe the child's color and respirations.	3. Symptoms of shock develop if too much fluid is removed.
Follow-Up Phase	
1. Apply abdominal binder snugly.	
2. Place the child in bed.	
3. Record the amount and character of the drainage and the child's condition.	
4. Observe frequently for signs of shock and note the drainage on the bandages.	

Urinary Tract Infection

Urinary tract infection refers to an infection within the urinary system. Either the lower urinary tract (urethra, bladder, or the lower portion of the ureters) or the upper urinary tract (upper portion of the ureters or kidney) or both may be involved.

Etiology

1. Causative organisms—*E. coli* (most common)
2. Route of entry
   a. Ascent from the urethra (most common)
   b. Circulating blood
3. Contributing causes
   a. Obstruction, usually congenital
   b. Vesicoureteral reflux
   c. Infections elsewhere in the body
      (1) Upper respiratory
      (2) Gastrointestinal: diarrhea
   d. Poor perineal hygiene
   e. Short female urethra
   f. Catheterization and instrumentation
   g. Entrance of an irritant into the bladder
   h. Inherent defect in the ability of the bladder mucosa to protect it from microbial invasion
   i. Chronic or intermittent constipation
   j. Local inflammation
   k. Antimicrobials

Incidence

1. Most common renal disease in children.
2. Almost 10 times more common in females than in males, except in the neonatal period.

Altered Physiology

1. Inflammatory changes occur in the affected portions of the urinary tract.
2. Clumps of bacteria may be present.
3. Inflammation results in urinary retention and stasis of urine in the bladder. There may be backflow of urine into the kidneys through the ureters.
4. There are inflammatory changes in the renal pelvis and throughout the kidney when this organ is involved.
5. Scarring of the kidney parenchyma occurs in chronic infection and interferes with kidney function, particularly with the ability to concentrate urine.
6. Eventually, the kidney becomes small, tissue is destroyed, and renal function fails.

Prognosis

1. Generally good in uncomplicated cases.
2. There is a tendency for recurrent infection.
3. Children with obstructive lesions of the urinary tract and those with severe vesicoureteral reflux are at highest risk for kidney damage.

Clinical Manifestations

A. Onset

1. May be abrupt or gradual
2. May be asymptomatic

B. Signs and Symptoms

1. Fever
   a. May be moderate or severe
   b. May fluctuate rapidly
   c. May be accompanied by chills or convulsions
2. Anorexia and general malaise
3. Urinary frequency, urgency, dysuria, dribbling
4. Daytime or nocturnal enuresis
5. Foul odor or change in the appearance of urine
6. Abdominal or suprapubic pain
7. Tenderness over one or both kidneys
8. Irritability
9. Vomiting
10. Failure to thrive in infancy

Diagnostic Evaluation

1. Urine culture
   a. Documentation of pathogenic organisms in the urine is the only means of definitive diagnosis.
   b. A urine culture demonstrating more than 100,000 bacteria per milliliter indicates significant bacteriuria.
2. Urinalysis
   a. Pus is present in abnormal amounts.
   b. Casts, especially white cell casts, may be present and are indicative of intrarenal infection.
   c. Hematuria—occurs occasionally
3. Renal concentrating ability—decreased
4. Urologic and radiologic studies:

A voiding cystourethrogram and IVP should be done after the initial infection subsides to identify abnormalities, which might contribute to the development of infection, and to identify existing kidney changes due to recurrent infection.

Patient Problems and Nursing Diagnoses

1. Urinary elimination, altered (frequency, burning, pain, dribbling, and/or enuresis), related to infection
2. Comfort, altered, pain related to inflammatory changes in urinary tract
3. Potential development of toxic effects of antimicrobial therapy
4. Self-concept, disturbance, related to exposure and manipulation of the genitourinary tract
5. Knowledge deficit about urinary tract infections and prevention

Nursing Interventions

A. Obtaining a Clean Urine Specimen for Examination or Culture.

1. A freshly voided early morning specimen is most accurate. (This urine is usually acid and concentrated, which tends to preserve the formed elements.)
2. See the procedure for the collection of urine specimens, page 1161.
3. Obtain a midstream specimen whenever possible.
4. Catheterization may be necessary to obtain a sterile specimen.
   Defer this procedure whenever possible in order to avoid emotional trauma and the accidental introduction of additional bacteria.
5. The urine should be sent to the laboratory immediately or refrigerated to avoid a falsely high bacterial count.

B. Eradicating Infective Organisms.

1. Administer antibiotics as prescribed by the physician (Table 53-1).
2. Antibiotic therapy is generally determined by the results of urine cultures and sensitivities, and by the child's response to therapy.

Table 53-1. *Antimicrobial Agents Commonly Used in the Management of Childhood Urinary Tract Infection*

Drug	Toxic Effects	Nursing Considerations
Amoxicillin	Occasional nausea, vomiting, diarrhea Hypersensitivity reactions of skin	Readily absorbed. May be taken with food.
Ampicillin	Diarrhea, urticaria Anaphylactic reaction	Contraindicated in penicillin-sensitive children. Package insert should be consulted regarding reconstitution, administration, and storage of intramuscular and intravenous preparations. Absorption of oral preparations may be decreased with food. Dose must be repeated every 6 hours to ensure therapeutic blood levels.
Cephalexin	Diarrhea, nausea, vomiting	May be taken with food. Dose should be reduced if renal function is impaired.
Gentamicin	Renal and auditory toxicity; respiratory paralysis	Toxic effects can be minimized by slow intravenous infusion (over 1 hour).
Kanamycin	Renal and auditory toxicity	Keep the child well hydrated to minimize renal irritation. Warm soaks may relieve pain at injection sites.
Nitrofurantoin	Fever, nausea, vomiting, peripheral neuropathy	Recommended for prolonged use. Give with food or milk to decrease GI side effects. May cause urine to be amber or brown in color. Contraindicated in renal failure and in infants under 3 months of age.
Sulfonamides	Nausea, vomiting, drug fever, rashes, photosensitivity	Keep the child well hydrated to avoid crystallization of the drug in the urine. Contraindicated if known drug sensitivity and in infants under 2 months of age.
Trimethoprim–sulfamethoxazole	Same as with other sulfonamides	Commonly used if bacterial resistance is anticipated or the child fails to respond to initial therapy.

C. Providing for Symptomatic Relief of the Child's Discomfort During the Febrile Period.

1. Maintain bed rest.
2. Administer analgesic and antipyretic drugs as recommended by the physician.
3. Encourage fluids to reduce the fever and dilute the concentration of the urine.
   a. Obtain a complete nursing history regarding the child's fluid preferences and method of taking them.
   b. Administer intravenous fluids if necessary (see Guidelines, p. 1167).
4. Refer to the section on care of the child with fever, page 1142.

D. Observing for Progress of Disease.

Nursing notes should include:
1. Frequent recording of the child's temperature
2. Accurate measurement of intake and output
3. Description of the color and odor of the urine, especially if it is abnormal
4. Presence of any of the following symptoms:
   a. Frequency of urination
   b. Burning or pain with voiding
   c. Enuresis
   d. Urinary retention
5. General behavior and activity status of the child
6. Signs of untoward or toxic effects of drugs
7. Pain, especially in the kidney area

E. Providing Emotional Support to the Child and His Parents.

1. Reinforce medical explanations of the disease and its therapy.
2. Explain all diagnostic tests and procedures to the child before they are carried out.
3. Encourage the verbal child to talk about his experience and how he feels about it. Correct any misconceptions he may have, and particularly address concerns that

the functioning of the urinary tract is separate from any sexual functions. The child should be reassured that the tests and treatment are for a problem that he did not cause.
4. Provide an environment that is as close to normal as possible during hospitalization. Include opportunities for the child to play.

F. Preparing the Child and His Family for Discharge.

1. Discuss any treatment that will be required at home. Provide written discharge instructions regarding:
   a. Rest
   b. Fluid intake
   c. Administration of medications
   d. Appointment for continued medical supervision
2. Communicate or have the parents communicate with the school nurse if it is necessary for the child to receive medications at school.
3. Complete a community nursing referral if reinforcement of discharge teaching appears necessary.

Health Education

1. Long-term therapy is often prescribed to prevent recurrence of urinary tract infections.
   Schedules for prolonged therapy vary from several months to continuous prophylaxis.
2. The child should be kept under continued medical surveillance because of the possibility of disease recurrence.
   a. Emphasis should be placed on the fact that even though this disease may have few symptoms, it can lead to very serious, permanent disability.
   b. Periodic urine cultures are indicated for 2 years following the acute infection.
3. Measures of prevention:
   a. Spread of bacteria from the anal and vaginal areas to the urethra can be minimized in female children

by cleansing the perianal area from the urethra back toward the anus.

b. Bubble baths should not be used because of the bladder-irritant effect of these solutions.

c. Encourage adequate fluid intake, especially water.

d. Avoid carbonated beverages, because of their irritative effect on bladder mucosa.

e. Encourage the child to void frequently and to empty the bladder completely with each voiding.

Expected Outcomes

1. Is asymptomatic within 24–48 hours after initiation of treatment; decrease/cessation of urinary frequency, urgency, dysuria, burning on urination, and fever

2. Absence of complaints of pain during/after voiding; adheres to program of bed rest

3. Takes food and fluid with antimicrobial medication to avoid nausea, gastrointestinal side effects, etc.

4. Shows less anxiety about hospitalization; appears more relaxed about appearance, body image, tests, etc.

5. Parents discuss home care needs: rest, fluid intake, medications, possibility of recurrence, prevention of infection; follow-up care

Abnormalities of the Genitourinary Tract That Require Surgery

Exstrophy of the Bladder

In *exstrophy of the bladder,* the anterior surface of the bladder lies open on the lower part of the abdomen, allowing constant passage of urine to the outside. There are usually associated defects, including separation of the pubic rami and epispadias in both sexes: cleft scrotum, undescended testes, and a shortened penis in males; cleft clitoris, separated labia, or shortened vaginal orifice in females.

Etiology

Results from failure of the abdominal wall and its underlying structures to fuse in utero.

Clinical Manifestations

1. Constant dribbling of urine excoriates the skin.
2. Infection and ulceration of the bladder mucosa may occur.
3. Genitalia may be ambiguous.
4. Affected children walk with a waddling or unsteady gait.

Management

1. Surgical closure of bladder within first 48 hours.
2. Complete correction by school age by means of staged reconstructive and orthopedic surgery
3. Urinary diversion may be necessary.

Patient Problems and Nursing Diagnoses

1. Urinary elimination, altered patterns, related to the nature of the defect
2. Self-concept disturbance in body image, related to the appearance of the abdomen and genitalia
3. Increased potential for urinary tract infection or trauma to the exposed bladder

Nursing Interventions

A. Preoperative Care

1. Protect the bladder area from trauma and irritation.
   a. Position the infant on his back or side.
   b. Cleanse the area frequently with mild soap and water. Pat the area dry or use a hair dryer on lowest setting.
   c. Keep infant in Isolette to avoid irritation from clothing/blankets.
   d. Expose the area to warm, dry air, sunlight, or artificial light at least once or twice each day.
   e. Cover the defect with sterile gauze to which a moisture barrier or skin sealant has been applied, or with a layer of silastic or plastic wrap directly over the bladder.
   f. Change the gauze covering and the infant's diaper frequently.

2. Observe the infant closely for signs of infection.

3. Collect urine specimens by holding the infant over an emesis basin in a position that allows urine to drip into the container.

4. Assist the parents to deal with their emotional reactions regarding the child's defect.

5. Teach the parents how to care for the child at home. Initiate a community nursing referral if reinforcement of teaching or maternal support appears necessary.

6. Prepare the child and his parents for the proposed surgery (see p. 1133).

B. Postoperative Care

1. Provide care for the ureteral and urethral catheters. Observe and record the amount of urinary drainage, catheter positions, and occurrence of bladder spasms.

2. The child may be placed in a body cast for several weeks (see Guidelines: Care of a Child in a Spica Cast, p. 1214) or a traction system.

3. An ileal conduit may be necessary (see p. 1374).

4. Observe for complications:
   a. Urinary or incisional infections
   b. Fistulae in the suprapubic or penile incisions

5. Long-term support will be necessary for many children and families to help them deal with such fears as appearance of genitalia, potential inability to procreate, and rejection by peers. Ongoing discussion groups for parents and children may be helpful.

C. Resource for Parents

Parents of Children with Exstrophy, Children's Health Center, 2525 Chicago Avenue, South, Minneapolis, MN 55403

Expected Outcomes

1. Demonstrates adequate absorption (by diaper) of continually draining urine; free of odor

2. Parents/child show acceptance of altered body image evidenced by their verbal and nonverbal communication

3. Absence of urinary tract infection; absence of trauma to bladder; parents verbalize signs and symptoms of complications

Patent Urachus

Patent urachus is persistence of the embryonic connection between the umbilicus and the bladder. In many patients only a cyst persists, located at the upper end of the tract, under the umbilicus.

Clinical Manifestations

1. Urine dribbles from the umbilicus when entire urachus is present.
2. Midline swelling is present in cases of a cyst.
3. Infection of urachal cysts is common.

Treatment

1. Eradication of infection
2. Removal of cysts
3. Surgical obliteration of the patent urachus

Obstructive Lesions of the Lower Urinary Tract

Types of Obstruction

1. Urethral valves
   a. Filamentous valves that obstruct urine flow
   b. Most commonly found in males
2. Congenital narrowing of the urethra
3. Bladder neck obstruction
   Most common site of lower urinary tract obstruction
4. Meatal stricture
5. Neuromuscular dysfunction (see the section on spina bifida, p. 1442)
6. Severe phimosis (rare)
7. Inflammatory Processes
8. Neoplasia
9. Calculi
10. Trauma

Clinical Manifestations

Abnormal urination
1. Dysuria
2. Frequency
3. Enuresis
4. Dribbling
5. Reduced force of urine stream
6. Difficulty starting urine stream
7. Straining during urination
8. Abrupt cessation during urination

Altered Physiology

1. Urinary tract becomes distended proximal to the point of obstruction.
2. The bladder dilates and hypertrophies.
3. Stasis of urine occurs.
4. The ureters become elongated, dilated, and tortuous.
5. Hydronephrosis and destruction of kidney tissue inevitably result.

Treatment

1. Prevention or eradication of infection (see the section on urinary tract infection, p. 1369)
2. Dilation of urethral stenosis or stricture
3. Surgical relief of the obstruction

Obstructive Lesions of the Upper Urinary Tract

Types of Obstruction

1. Stricture of a ureter
2. Congenital absence of one ureter
3. Duplication of the ureter of one kidney
4. Compression of a ureter by an aberrant blood vessel

Clinical Manifestations

1. Often asymptomatic (There is seldom any problem with voiding.)
2. Vague symptoms such as failure to thrive may be present.
3. Urinary tract infections may be frequent.
4. Hypertension may occur.

Treatment

Same as for obstructions of lower urinary tract.

Hypospadias

Hypospadias is malposition of the urethral opening.

Altered Physiology

A. Males
1. The urethra opens on the lower surface of the penis, proximal to its usual site.
2. In severe cases, the urethra may open on the shaft of the penis, at its base, or on the perineum.
3. Frequently associated with congenital chordee in males—cord-like defect that extends from the scrotum up the penis and deflects the penis downward.

B. Females
The urethra opens into the vagina (rare).

Clinical Manifestations

1. Inability to void with the penis in the normal elevated position.
2. Severe forms interfere with the ability to procreate.

Treatment

Plastic surgery

Cryptorchidism (Undescended Testis)

Cryptorchidism is the absence of one or both testes from the scrotum. The testes may be located in the abdominal cavity or inguinal canal.

Etiology

Caused by delayed descent, prevention of descent by some mechanical lesion, or endocrine disorders (rare).

Clinical Manifestations and Altered Physiology

1. Normal development of secondary sex characteristics.
2. Degeneration of the sperm-forming cells occurs after puberty because of the higher temperature of the abdomen compared with the normal location in the scrotum. Sterility results.
3. Emotional disturbances often occur when the child discovers that he is different from his peers.
4. Associated hernias are found in more than 50% of the patients.
5. Increased risk of testicular malignancy in the third or fourth decade of life.

Treatment

1. Orchiopexy (placement of the testes in the scrotum) Surgery should be performed between the ages of 1 and 3 to prevent damage to the tissues and to lessen emotional concerns related to body image.
2. Plastic surgery in patients with an absent testis
3. Administration of chorionic gonadotropin—has produced descent of the testes in some children. (Testes would probably have descended spontaneously in these cases.)

Nursing Management

A. Preoperative Care

1. Encourage the child and his parents to express their feelings about the condition.
   Expect anxieties regarding sterility and homosexuality and perceptions of the child as defective or inadequate.
2. Discuss the condition and surgery frankly, in terms the child can understand.
   a. Maintain a matter-of-fact attitude.
   b. Clarify any misconceptions the child may have.
3. Provide privacy for medical examinations.

B. Postoperative Care

1. Prevent contamination of the suture line.
   If a 2-stage repair is used—
2. Maintain traction.
   a. A suture is placed in the lower portion of the scrotum and is attached to a rubber band that is fastened to the upper aspect of the inner thigh by a piece of adhesive.
   b. This traction anchors the testis to the scrotum and is removed in approximately 5–7 days.
3. Administer antibiotics as prescribed to prevent infection.

Ambiguous Genitalia

Female Pseudohermaphroditism

1. Most common problem of sexual differentiation.
2. A deficiency of hydrocortisone results in adrenocortical hyperplasia and an overproduction of androgens.
3. *Manifestations*—masculinization of the external genitalia in the female infant.
4. *Treatment:*
   a. Close observation for adrenal crisis
   b. Administration of hydrocortisone in children with adrenal hyperplasia
   c. Corrective plastic surgery, if needed
      This should be undertaken as early as possible, before social adjustment becomes a severe problem.

Male Pseudohermaphroditism

1. Normal female genitalia with testes internally
   Treatment:
   a. Surgical removal of testes
   b. Administration of estrogens at puberty
   c. Child reared as female
2. Predominantly male genitalia with testes internally
   Treatment:
   a. Surgical removal of all nonmale structures
   b. Child reared as male
3. Ambiguous genitalia

Treatment:
   a. Plastic reconstruction
   b. Gender assignment based on internal and external anatomy

True Hermaphroditism

1. May be either genetic males or females.
2. Have both ovarian and testicular tissue.
3. Genitalia are usually ambiguous.
4. Gender choice is based on the infant's anatomy.

Diagnostic Evaluation

1. Buccal smear to determine the presence or absence of sex chromatin
2. Endoscopy and x-ray studies to reveal presence, absence, and nature of internal genital structures
3. Chromosomal analysis to identify genetic sex
4. Biochemical tests of urinary steroid excretion patterns
5. Laparotomy or gonad biopsy

Nursing Management

1. Recognize the situation as a social emergency.
   Support the parents while they wait for gender assignment for the infant. This should be done as soon as possible, but may require several days or weeks for results of studies.
2. Reinforce medical explanations of the anatomic problems and treatment. Approach the situation in a matter-of-fact manner.
3. Initiate appropriate referrals for family support and counseling. These may include:
   a. Social work
   b. Psychiatry
   c. Community health nursing
   d. Child guidance clinic
   e. Genetic counseling

Care of the Child Requiring Urologic Surgery

Patient Problems and Nursing Diagnoses

1. Potential alterations in urination related to the nature of disease, especially if ileal conduit is required
2. Body image concerns related to appearance of genitalia or presence of stones
3. Potential for infection related to catheterization and after-effects of surgery
4. Anxiety related to proposed surgery
5. Knowledge deficit about surgery
6. Increased danger of fluid and electrolye imbalance related to surgery

Preoperative Care

1. Determine the child's fantasies regarding his illness and hospitalization. Correct any misconceptions that he reveals.
2. Provide an explanation of the anatomy and physiology of the urinary system in terms that the child can understand.
   a. Use a body outline appropriate for the age of the child.
   b. Explain how the child differs from the normal. Relate his defect to his symptoms whenever possible.

3. Explain all diagnostic tests prior to their occurrence. These may include urinalysis, 24-hour urine collections, intravenous and retrograde pyelography, angiography, and cystoscopy.
   a. Descriptions should include such information as:
      (1) Preparation required—fasting, enemas, etc.
      (2) Location of the test—operating room, radiology department, etc.
      (3) Appearance and attire of personnel
      (4) Positioning
      (5) Anesthesia
      (6) Pain or discomfort
      (7) Expectations following the procedure—diet, rest, urine collections, etc.
   b. Determine the child's understanding of the procedure.
      (1) Ask him simple, direct questions.
      (2) Allow him to perform the procedure on a doll or demonstrate it on a diagram.
4. Explain the surgical procedure.
   a. Explanations should include:
      (1) Preparation required—fasting, enemas, etc.
      (2) Description of the operating room, including the appearance of the personnel
      (3) Anesthesia
      (4) Postoperative appearance
         (a) Urinary drainage tubing and collection devices
         (b) Appearance of urine
         (c) Sutures
         (d) Bandages
         (e) Intravenous infusion
   b. Determine the child's understanding of his surgery and reinforce teaching when necessary.
5. Points of emphasis during the preparation:
   a. The child is in no way to blame for his illness.
   b. No other part of the body will be operated on.

Postoperative Care

1. Care for all catheters and urinary tubes according to hospital procedure. Maintain appropriate position of tubes.
2. Observe and record:
   a. Amount and appearance of urinary drainage
   b. Occurrence of bladder spasms
   c. Symptoms of urinary or incisional infection

Care of the Child Who Has an Ileal Conduit (Ileoloop)

Ileal Conduit. One or both ureters are anastomosed to a segment of ileum, which then serves to carry urine to the external body surface of the abdomen.

Preoperative Care

1. Refer to the preceding section on the emotional preparation of the child and his family for urologic surgery.
2. Allow the child to try on the ileal conduit apparatus in order to become familiar with it.
   Observe for discomfort and skin reactions to the adhesive or cement.
3. Administer antimicrobials as prescribed by the physician.

Be aware of the action, side effects, and contraindications of the prescribed therapy.
4. Provide the child and his parents with opportunities to express their fears and ask questions about the procedure.
   Expect concerns related to sterility, location and appearance of the stoma, activity restrictions, clothing, and management.
5. Reassure the child and his parents that they will be taught to manage the conduit before leaving the hospital.
6. If appropriate, introduce the family to a rehabilitated individual who has had the same surgery.
   Trained volunteers from the United Ostomy Association may be able to provide valuable psychological support.

Postoperative Care

1. Maintain the urinary collection apparatus. (A temporary collection bag is usually worn in the immediate postoperative period and may be replaced by a permanent appliance once edema of the stoma subsides.)
   a. Cleanse the area around the stoma with mild soap and water and dry it well.
   b. Keep the skin around the stoma completely dry during application of the appliance to ensure that it will remain attached.
   c. Place the adhesive plate of the appliance securely around the stoma.
      The opening in the adhesive plate should be of a size that fits snugly over the stoma but does not compromise circulation.
   d. Empty the appliance every 2 hours or whenever it contains approximately 100 ml. of fluid. (During the night, the appliance may be attached via tubing to a collection bottle.)
   e. Nursing observations related to the appliance:
      (1) Leaking around the appliance
      (2) Skin irritation
      (3) Improper fit of the appliance
   f. Points of emphasis:
      (1) A properly applied apparatus should remain in place 3–5 days. It needs to be changed only when it begins to leak or becomes uncomfortable.
      (2) It is normal for the urine to contain some mucus; it may be blood tinged.
2. Offer generous amounts of fluids to maintain hydration and keep the urine dilute and clear.
3. Carefully monitor intake and output.
   Decreased urine output may indicate dehydration, obstruction of ureters, urine drainage into the peritoneal cavity, or compromised kidney function.
4. Observe for complications:
   a. Wound infection
   b. Leaking at the site of anastomosis
   c. Peritonitis
   d. Paralytic ileus
   e. Intestinal obstruction
   f. Stenosis of the stoma
   g. Fluid and electrolyte disturbances
5. Assist the child and his family with problems related to altered body image.
   a. Assume a calm, understanding, and matter-of-fact attitude.

b. Keep equipment used in the management of the conduit out of sight to avoid embarrassment when visitors appear.
c. Encourage the child to wear his own clothes so he is reassured that the appliance is invisible under clothing.
d. Take precautions to prevent or eliminate odors (e.g., immediate cleansing of used collection bags, etc.).
e. Help the child and family to achieve control by teaching them to manage the care as soon as possible.
f. Encourage early resumption of as many normal activities as possible.
6. Prepare the family for discharge.
   a. Provide written information regarding the equipment that the child is using and where to obtain it.
   b. Provide at least a 2-week supply of equipment for the family to take home.
      Advise the parents to order new supplies before the old ones are depleted.
   c. Initiate appropriate referrals.
      (1) Community nursing agency
      (2) Local "ostomy" clubs

Health Education

1. Involve the child and his family in his self-care as soon as possible.
   Teaching should include how to assemble, apply, empty, change, and cleanse the appliance.
2. Explain that appliances can be adapted to meet the individual patient's needs.
   Some experimentation will probably be necessary before the most suitable equipment can be identified.
3. Adequate fluid intake (approximately 125 ml./kg. [1.7 oz./lb.]) is essential for maintaining good urine flow.
4. Two appliances should be available, one in use and the other as a spare.
5. The appliance should be cleaned and aired regularly to avoid odor or crusting.
   a. A few drops of Lysol to a quart of water whitens and deodorizes the bags.
   b. Crusting can be removed by a solution of white vinegar and water (approximately 1 cup of white vinegar to a quarter of water).
   c. A mild soap and warm water should be used to clean the appliance.
6. New appliances should be purchased approximately every 6 months or whenever old ones begin to feel thin or worn.
7. Activity limitations are usually not necessary unless the child has associated physical problems.
8. Clothing may have to be altered slightly to fit over the pouch of the appliance.
9. References for Parents
   Norris C. *All About Jimmy*. Los Angeles, United Ostomy Association, 1973
   United Ostomy Association, 2001 West Beverly Blvd, Los Angeles, CA 90057

Expected Outcomes

1. The child/parents attain ability to care for stoma, ostomy appliance, equipment, etc.

2. Shows a positive self-image evidenced by verbal and nonverbal communication
3. Absence of infection; vital signs normal; urine clear
4. Attains/maintains fluid and electrolyte balance; taking fluids well; laboratory values within acceptable range
5. Shows reduction of anxiety; no distressful crying; playing with toys; interacts with personnel; makes his needs known
6. Child/parents demonstrate application of appliance; monitoring of urinary output, care of collecting pouch

---

Acute Renal Failure

Nursing care of the children with acute renal failure is generally the same as that of adults (see pp. 672–674). The following considerations are important for pediatric patients:

Causes of Acute Renal Failure in Children

1. Prerenal causes (resulting from decreased perfusion to a normal kidney and collecting system)
   a. Dehydration (the most common cause of acute renal failure in children)
   b. Surgical shock
   c. Trauma
   d. Burns
2. Postrenal causes
   a. Uncommon, except for obstructive uropathies in the first year of life
   b. Renal function is restored with relief of the obstruction
3. Renal causes (the largest group to require extended medical management)
   a. Disease of the kidney
   b. Tubular destruction secondary to nephrotoxins, transfusion reactions

Clinical Course

1. The length of the oliguric phase is highly variable.
   a. Shorter in infants, children, and milder cases (3–5 days)
   b. Longer in older children and adolescents (10–14 days)
2. The diuretic phase is also highly variable, from mild and lasting only a few days, to profound.
3. 75% of children with acute renal failure attain complete recovery.

Management

1. Fluids are restricted to an amount needed to maintain zero water balance, calculated on the basis of endogenous water formation and sensible and insensible losses.
2. The child is weighed at least once each day, and is expected to lose 10–20 gm. per kg. of original body weight per day.
3. A major nursing goal is to support parents who may feel anxious and/or guilty about the child's condition.
4. Refer to the following sections:
   a. Pediatric Intensive Care, page 1127
   b. Dialysis, page 1181
   c. The Dying Child, page 1523

Chronic Renal Failure

Nursing care of children with chronic renal failure is similar to that of adults (see pp. 674–676). The following considerations are important for pediatric patients.

Etiology of Chronic Renal Failure in Children

1. Congenital renal and urinary tract abnormalities (most common cause under 5 years of age)
2. Glomerular disease
3. Hereditary renal disease
4. Renal vascular disorders

Most common causes from 5–15 years

Clinical Manifestations (Usually Emerge Only Late in the Course of the Disease, Similar to Adults)

1. Decreased interest in usual activities such as school and play
2. Increased urinary output and fluid intake
3. Bone or joint pain
4. Delayed or absent sexual maturation
5. Secondary amenorrhea in girls past puberty
6. Growth retardation
7. Dryness and itching of skin

Management

1. Dietary restriction of phosphorus (principally cow's milk) and reduction of protein reduces the excretory load on the kidneys.
2. Rapid correction of acidosis may precipitate tetany in the hypocalcemic child. Therefore, correction of acidosis is most safely attempted after calcium levels are elevated.
3. When serum phosphate levels are in the normal range, vitamin D in increasing doses or dihydrotachysterol is administered to increase the absorption of calcium via the gastrointestinal tract.
4. Growth retardation may be reduced by the administration of the anabolic steroid, oxandrolone.
5. Intercurrent infections are common and must be treated immediately. The dosage of antimicrobials excreted through the kidneys is usually reduced and the interval between doses extended to avoid toxic effects.

Clinical Course and Prognosis

1. Once symptoms of uremia appear, the disease progresses rapidly and terminates in death unless end-stage renal care is initiated.
2. Children are regarded as having end-stage renal disease when the glomerular filtration rate falls below 10 ml./min./1.73 m.^{2}.
3. End-stage renal disease is treated by dialysis or transplantation.

Nursing Interventions

1. Numerous psychosocial issues may interfere with the child's psychological and social development and education. A major nursing goal is to help the child and family to cope with:
   a. Uncertainty regarding the course of the disease and ultimate prognosis
   b. Stress of repeated hospitalizations and recurring need for painful medical procedures
   c. Abnormal life-style necessitated by dialysis
   d. Burden of dialysis and continuous administration of medications
   e. Problems of adjustment related to growth failure
   f. Fear of death, present in most children and adolescents
   g. Need for urinary diversion and manipulation of the genital area in cases of urologic abnormalities
   h. Transplantation involving major surgery, prolonged hospitalization, followed by altered body image due to high doses of steroids and potential for rejection, which may threaten survival
2. Refer to:
   a. The Child Undergoing Dialysis, page 1181
   b. Pediatric Renal Transplantation, see below
   c. The Dying Child, page 1523

Pediatric Renal Transplantation

Kidney transplantation is the treatment of choice for end-stage renal failure in the pediatric age-group. With transplantation, there is a greater likelihood of complete rehabilitation and better growth than with dialysis, although post-transplantation growth is variable and related to caloric intake, corticosteroid dosage, bone age at transplantation, and rejection episodes. Nursing care of children experiencing kidney transplantation is similar to that of adults (see p. 681). The following special considerations apply to pediatric patients.

Donor Selection (in Order of Priority)

1. Identical twin sibling
2. Sibling
   It is important to note that siblings cannot be used as donors until they are of legal age to give consent for removal of a kidney.
3. Parent
4. Aunt or uncle
5. Unrelated live donor (seldom used) or cadaver donor

Operative Procedure

Small children may require placement within the abdomen with vessel anastomosis to the aorta and inferior vena cava.

Potential Emotional Concerns of Children With Transplants

1. The concept of a foreign body, especially a cadaver kidney, inside his own body may be disturbing.
2. Fear that the kidney may wear out sooner if it is from an older person.
3. Altered body image due to growth failure and the effects of steroid therapy.
4. Guilt feeling if a live-donor transplant fails.

Nursing Care

Refer to sections on:
1. Chronic Renal Failure, this page, left-hand column
2. Care of the Child Requiring Urologic Surgery, page 1373

Bibliography

Books

Behrman RE, Vaughan VC and Nelson WE. Nelson Textbook of Pediatrics. 13th ed. Philadelphia, WB Saunders, 1987

Gellis SS and Kagan BM (eds). Current Pediatric Therapy 12. Philadelphia, WB Saunders, 1986

Rakel RE (ed). Conn's Current Therapy. Philadelphia, WB Saunders, 1990

Rudolph AM and Hoffman JIE (eds). Pediatrics. 18th ed. Norwalk, Appleton & Lange

Walsh PC et al. Campbell's Urology, vol 3. 5th ed. Philadelphia, WB Saunders, 1986

Whaley L and Wong D. Nursing Care of Infants and Children. 3rd ed. St. Louis, CV Mosby, 1987

Zimmerman SS and Gildea JH. Critical Care Pediatrics. Philadelphia, WB Saunders, 1985

Journals

Anderson GF and Smey P. Current concepts in the management of common urologic problems in infants and children. Pediatr Clin North Am 1985; 32:1133–1149

Bellinger MF. The history of urinary diversion and undiversion. J Enterostomal Ther 1989 Jan–Feb; 16(1):39–41

Bellinger MF et al. Orchiopexy: An experimental study of the effect of surgical technique on testicular histology. J Urol 1989 Aug; 142(2-2): 553–555

Burns MN, Burns JL and Kreiger JN. Pediatric UTI: Dx, Classification, & significance. Pediatr Clin North Am 1987 Oct; 34(5):1111–1120

Cendron M et al. Cryptorchidism, orchiopexy and infertility: A critical long-term retrospective analysis. J Urol 1989 Aug; 142(2-2):559–562

Chmielewski C. Early recognition of infection after renal transplantation. ANNA J 1987 Dec; 14(6):389–391, 408

Coco P. When kidneys fail . . . Nursing management of acute renal failure. AD Nurse 1988 Jul–Aug; 3(4):16–18

Connor JP et al. Long term followup of 207 patients with bladder exstrophy: Evolution in treatment. J Urol 1989 Sep; 142(3):793–795

Conway J. Taking a look at lower UTI's . . . Urinary tract infection. J Urol Nurs 1989 Apr–Jun; 8(2):641–643

Danziger CH. Uremic neuropathy and treatment with renal transplantation. ANNA J 1989 Apr; 16(2):67–70

de Man P et al. Bacterial attachment as a predictor of renal abnormalities in boys with UTI. J Pediatr 1989 Dec; 115(6):915–922

DiBattista JM. Teaching Kock pouch catheterization and irrigation. AUAA J 1987 Jul–Sep; 8(1):17–20

Donahoe PK. The diagnosis and treatment of infants with intersex abnormalities. Pediatr Clin North Am 1987 Oct; 34(5):1333–1348

Earle DP. Poststreptococcal acute glomerulonephritis, Hosp Pract 1985; 20(7):48E–48J, 48O–P, 48U, 48Z, 48AA–BB

Engle WD. Evaluation of renal function and acute renal failure in the neonate. Pediatr Clin North Am 1986; 33: 129–151

Fonkalsrud EW. Testicular undescent and torsion. Pediatr Clin North Am 1987 Oct; 34(5):1305–1317

Gearhart JP and Jeffs RD. Bladder exstrophy: Increase in capacity following epispadias repair. J Urol 1989 Aug; 142(2-2):525–526

Greig BJ. You and your Kock pouch. AUAA J 1988 Apr–Jun; 8(4):13–14

Hahn K. The many signs of renal failure. Nursing 1987 Aug; 17(8):34–42

Husmann DA, McLorie GA and Churchill BM. Closure of exstrophic bladder: Evaluation of factors leading to its success and its importance on urinary continence. J Urol 1989 Aug; 142(2-2): 522–524

Jeffs LD. Exstrophy, epispadias, and cloacal and urogenital sinus abnormalities. Pediatr Clin North Am 1987 Oct; 34(5):1233–1257

Jones KR. Policy and research in end-stage renal disease. Image—J Nurs Scholar 1987 Fall; 19(3):126–129

Klauber GT. Genitourinary trauma in children. Emerg Care Q 1987 May; 3(1):51–56

Lewies S. Nursing management of urinary tract infection. Infection Control Canada 1988 Sep–Oct; 3(3): 18–19

Lohr JA. The foreskin and urinary tract infections. J Pediatr 1989 Mar; 114(3): 502–504

Macfarlane FJ. Getting ready for certification. Urol Nurs 1989 Jan–Mar; 9(3):23–24

McEnery PT et al. Convulsions in children undergoing renal transplantation. J Pediatr 1989 Oct; 115(4):532–536

Mitchell ME and Rink RC. Pediatric urinary diversion and undiversion. Pediatr Clin North Am 1987 Oct; 34(5):1319–1332

Pitt M. Fluid intake and urinary tract infection. Nurs Times 1989 Jan 4-10; 85(1):36–38

Radebaugh LC. Nursing care of the infant with bladder exstrophy. AUAA J 1986 Oct–Dec; 7(2):11, 14–15

Reimer LG. The diagnosis of urinary tract infections. J Med Technol 1985 Dec; 2(12):754–756, 769–770

Reinberg Y and Gonzalez R. Upper urinary tract obstruction in children: Current controversies in diagnosis. Pediatr Clin North Am 1987 Oct; 34(5):1291–1304

Rivers R. Nursing the kidney transplant patient. RN 1987 Aug; 50(8):46–53

Sheldon CA and Duckett JW. Hypospadias. Pediatr Clin North Am 1987 Oct; 34(5):1259–1272

Sheldon CA et al. Surgical considerations in childhood end-stage renal disease. Pediatr Clin North Am 1987 Oct; 34(5):1187–1207

Sheldon CA, McLorie GA and Churchill BM. Renal transplantation in children. Pediatr Clin North Am 1987 Oct; 34(5):1209–1232

Smaill F. Diagnosis of urinary tract infections. Infection Control Canada 1989 Mar–Apr; 4(1):20–21, 23

Spiegel DM, Burnier M and Schrier RW. Acute renal failure. Postgrad Med 1987 Sep; 82(4):96–105

Burns in Children

Burns are a frequent form of childhood injury. The following types are considered very serious:
1. Second-degree burn of 10% or more of the body surface; 5% or more full-thickness
2. Burns of face, hands, feet, perineum, or joint surfaces.
3. Electrical burns
4. Presence of other injuries
5. When home situation is not adequate for optimal care

The effects of burns are not limited to the burn area.

Incidence and Etiology

A. Incidence

1. Burns are the second most important cause of accidental deaths in childhood, with the highest incidence of burns occurring in children under 5 years of age.
2. Children at high risk are black, poor, and of single parents.

B. Causes of Burns in Children

1. Burns from hot liquid
   a. Child (left unsupervised in tub) turns on the hot water tap
   b. Tap water temperature above 130°F. (54.4°C.) puts the child at high risk for injury.
   c. Child placed in tub of hot water that has not been tested
   d. Spilling of hot coffee, tea on child; spilling occurs especially when pot handles stick out on top of stove; hot liquids and foods removed from microwave oven
   e. Microwave oven causes burns from ingestion and aspiration of hot foods and liquids, as well as scald burns to skin and palate from hot formula.
   f. Most common in children under 3 years

C. Burns From Open Flames

1. House fires
2. Child climbing up to stove—clothing catches fire
3. Child playing with matches, especially 5–10 years old
4. Playing/working with gasoline
5. Gas tank explosion during automobile accident

D. Electrical Burns

1. Child playing with electrical outlets or appliances
2. Child playing with extension cords
3. Child playing on railroad tracks; climbing trees and touching high tension wires, lightning
4. Most common in toddlers and adolescents

E. Other Causes

1. Caustic acid or alkali burns of mouth and esophagus—child ingesting strong household cleaning products
2. Chemical burns of the skin—child playing with gasoline that comes in contact with skin (often the gasoline ignites)
3. Burns inflicted on the child as a result of neglect or child abuse—

   16% of all burns—immersion and contact burns most common, and higher incidence in child 1–3 years of age

4. Smoke inhalation and inhalation from plastic combustion
5. Radiation burns—resulting from the sun and radiation secondary to cancer therapy
6. Contact burns from touching hot surfaces such as radiators or wood-burning stoves
7. Fireworks burns, often as a result of misuse and lack of adult supervision

Altered Physiology

See burns in adults, Chapter 33.

Complications

Depend on severity of burn injury and are usually the rule rather than the exception, especially with severe burn injury.

A. Acute

1. Infection
   a. Burn wound sepsis
   b. Pneumonia
   c. Urinary tract infection
   d. Phlebitis
   e. Toxic shock syndrome
2. Curling's ulcer, GI hemorrhage—most likely to occur in burns >20% body surface area
3. Acute gastric dilation, paralytic ileus
   a. Occurs especially in child under 2 years of age with greater than 20% injury
   b. Develops early in postburn period, lasting 2–3 days
4. Renal failure
5. Respiratory failure
6. Postburn seizures
7. Hypertension
8. CNS dysfunction
9. Vascular ischemia
10. Anema and malnutrition
11. Fecal impaction

12. Depression—secondary to hospitalization and changing body image
13. Malnutrition—may resolve once burned area is covered

B. Long-term

1. Malnutrition
2. Scarring
3. Contractures
4. Psychological trauma

Clinical Manifestations

A. Characteristics of Burn Wounds (Table 54-1):

1. *First-degree burns* (partial-thickness—epidermal)—involve superficial epidermis; the skin is pink or red in appearance and is painful to touch.
2. *Second-degree burns* (partial-thickness—superficial or deep dermal)
    a. Involve the entire epidermis
    b. Skin is red, blistered, moist with exudate, and painful to pinprick or touch.
    c. Deep dermal injury penetrates into corium and may be anesthetic for 1–2 days after burn injury.

3. *Third-degree burns* (full-thickness—subdermal)
    a. Involve the dermis or underlying fat, muscle, or bone;
    b. Skin appears white, dry, or charred and has little pain.
    c. Often it is difficult to tell the degree of burn, especially in the young child.
4. *Electrical burn*—
    a. Especially of mouth when child under 2 years of age chews or sucks on live wire
    b. Takes several days before injury becomes demarcated.

B. Symptoms of Shock—Appear Soon After the Burn:

1. Rapid pulse
2. Subnormal temperature
3. Pallor
4. Prostration
5. Low blood pressure

C. Symptoms of Toxemia—may develop within 1–2 days after the initial burn:

1. Prostration
2. Fever

Table 54-1. *Classification of Depth of Burns*

Degree (Depth)	Appearance of Burn	Sensitivity to Pain	Tissue Involvement	Healing Time and Prognosis
First-degree (superficial)	Erythema; no blister formation; slight edema (gradual onset)	Intense pain—hyperesthesia; sensitivity to pinprick	Outer layer of epidermis (stratum corneum)	7–10 days; no scarring
Second-degree (partial-thickness but superficial)	Blister formation with oozing; subcutaneous edema	Pain—hyperesthesia; sensitivity to pinprick	All of epidermis, parts of stratum geminativum intact	5–21 days; as scabs fall off, skin remains red for several weeks. Ability to regenerate epithelium is intact; can scar
Second-degree (partial-thickness but deep)	Blister formation moist; subcutaneous edema; mottled red or pink	Pain variable; may be insensitivity to pinprick because of depth in dermal layer of skin	Deep dermis; cutaneous nerve endings may be damaged	21–35 days; firm eschar formation; regeneration takes place from epithelial lining of hair follicles and sweat gland. Pigmentation rarely returns to normal. *Please note:* Deep dermal burns are hard to distinguish from third-degree burns. In case of infection, injury may progress to third-degree.
Third-degree (full-thickness)	Blistering is not usual. Blanched, reddish, black; hard and leathery to touch; rapid edema; mottled	No pain because of destruction of nerve endings and anesthesia	Dermis and corium; deep third-degree burns extend into subcutaneous fat, muscles, and bones	Prolonged hospitalization; scarring; requires grafting, because no regeneration of skin layers

3. Rapid pulse
4. Glucosuria
5. Vomiting
6. Edema

Note: These symptoms may progress to coma or death.

D. Burns of the Respiratory Tract—result in symptoms of upper airway obstruction from acute edema and inflammation of the glottis, vocal cords, and upper trachea.

1. Rapid breathing
2. Dyspnea
3. Stridor, hoarseness, substernal retraction, and intercostal breathing
4. Nasal flaring
5. Restlessness

E. Smoke Inhalation—may cause no initial symptoms other than mild bronchial obstruction during the initial phase following the burn. Within 6–48 hours the child may develop sudden onset of the following conditions:

1. Bronchiolitis
2. Pulmonary edema
3. Severe airway obstruction
4. Damage from smoke inhalation—can present up to 7 days after the burn injury

Assessment

A. Calculation of the Burn Area

1. "Rule of Nines" (used in assessment of extent of burns in adults) has proved quite inexact when applied to young children. May be acceptable to use in child over 10 years of age.
   a. During infancy and early childhood, the relative surface area of different parts of the body varies with age.
   b. The younger the child, the greater the proportion of the surface area constituted by the head and the lesser the proportion of the surface area constituted by the legs.
2. Calculation of percentage of burn surface area is based on Lund and Browder's design (Fig. 54-1). This design compensates for the changes in percentage of body surface resulting from growth.
3. A rough estimate can be obtained by using child's hand, which is equal to 1%.

B. Categorization of Seriousness of Burn—is based on

1. Total area injured
2. Depth of injury
3. Location of injury

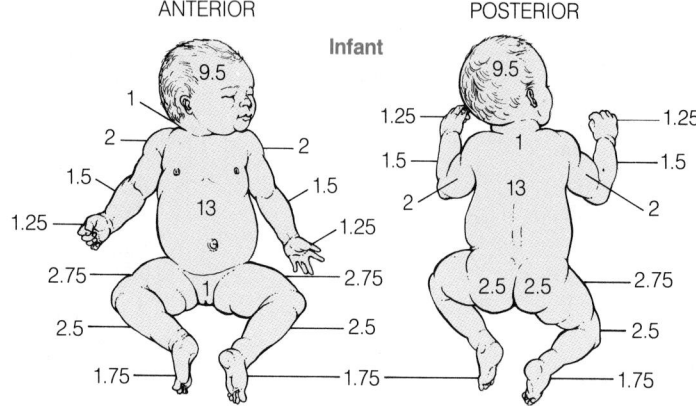

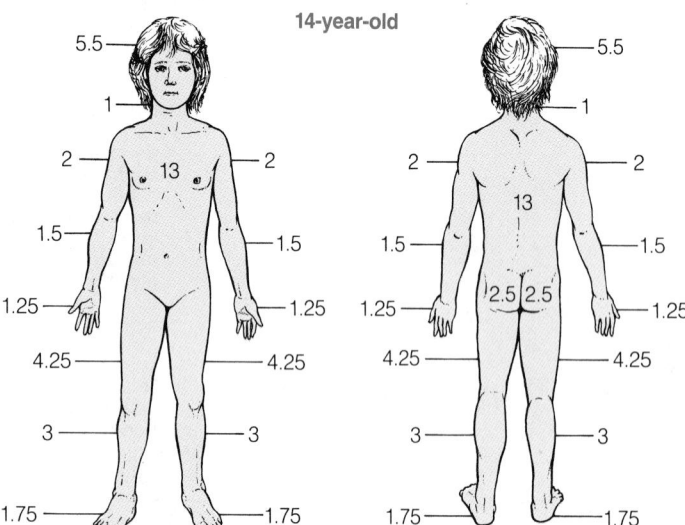

Figure 54-1. *Determination of extent of burns.*

4. Age of child
5. Condition of patient (i.e., level of consciousness)
6. Previous medical history (i.e., chronic disease)
7. Additional injuries

C. Schematic Classification of Burn Severity:*

1. Minor burn:
   10% Total body surface area, first- and second-degree burn
2. Moderate burn:
   a. 10%–20% Total body surface area, second-degree burn
   b. 2%–10% Total body surface area, third-degree burn not involving eyes, ears, face, or genitals
3. Major burn:
   a. 20% Total body surface area, second-degree burn
   b. All third-degree burns greater than 10%; depending on age of child, 5% is sometimes used
   c. All burns involving hands, face, eyes, ears, feet, and/or genitals
   d. All electrical burns
   e. Complicated burn injuries involving fracture or other major trauma
   f. All poor-risk patients (i.e., head injury, cancer, lung disease, diabetes)

Patient Problems and Nursing Diagnoses

(See burns in adults, p. 849–852)
1. Shock related to fluid loss, hypermetabolic state, and loss of skin integrity
2. Potential for infection related to injury, altered skin integrity, decreased circulation, etc.
3. Impaired gas exchange, related to inhalation injury or edema
4. Curling's ulcer, paralytic ileus related to stress
5. Nutrition, altered, less than body requirements, related to hypermetabolic state and poor appetite
6. Impaired mobility related to dressings, pain, and contractures
7. Comfort, altered, pain, related to dressing changes, physical therapy, itching, and treatments/procedures
8. Self-concept, self-esteem disturbance, related to pain, scarring, and disfigurement
9. Anxiety related to pain, treatments, procedures, and hospitalization
10. Altered parenting, related to crisis situation, prolonged hospitalization, and disfigurement
11. Parental anxiety related to fear, guilt, and lack of understanding of the treatment protocols

Nursing Interventions

A. Recognizing the Symptoms of Shock and Using Support Measures to Restore and Maintain Circulation.

1. Be alert to the symptoms of shock that occur very shortly after a severe burn.
   a. Tachycardia
   b. Hypothermia
   c. Hypotension
   d. Pallor
   e. Prostration
   f. Shallow respirations
   g. Anuria

* Cunningham G with Sand GX. *Never Quit.* Lincoln, VA, Chosen Books, 1981. *Never Quit* would be a valuable resource for adolescents facing a long illness or handicap resulting from burn injury.

2. Monitor the administration of intravenous fluid, as major burns are followed by a reduction in blood volume due to outflow of plasma into the tissues.
3. Maintain an accurate record of intake and output.
   a. Record time and amount of all fluids given.
   b. Measure accurate urinary output every ½ hour to 1 hour.
      (1) With severe burn injuries, an indwelling catheter may be used the first 3 days.
      (2) Urine flow is a most helpful clinical guide to fluid replacement and kidney function.
      (3) Estimate urine output: 1 ml./kg./hour or
         10–20 ml./hour under 2 years of age
         20–30 ml./hour 3–5 years of age
         30–50 ml./hour over 5 years of age
      (4) Check specific gravity.
      (5) Report diminishing urinary output.
   c. Monitor sensorium, pulse, pulse pressure, capillary filling, and blood gases.
4. Provide a rich oxygen environment in order to combat hypoxia, as necessary.
5. Provide sedation to relieve pain.
   a. Sedatives are given to children in very small amounts in order to prevent their depressant effect.
   b. In severe burn injury, sedation should be given intravenously because of lack of absorption of intramuscular medication during emergency phase and the possibility of the child receiving a large bolus once capillary integrity is restored. Morphine or meperidine are generally drugs of choice; however, their use is kept to a minimum in order to assess accurately brain perfusion by observation of sensorium. Serum titrate levels are closely monitored.
6. Provide a source of heat over the child's bed, as additional heat may be necessary to maintain body temperature.
7. Request laboratory results and record on special flow sheet.
   a. Hematocrit or RBC count serves as a rough guide to the adequacy of initial treatment, as the loss of plasma results in concentration of red blood cells.
   b. Electrolytes serve as a guide to fluid replacement.
8. Maintain close observation of vital signs in order to evaluate continuously the state of peripheral circulation; check for clear sensorium. Report immediately any significant changes.

B. Observing for Additional Complaints or Circumstances That Might Suggest Associated Injury.

1. Curling's ulcer and GI hemorrhage
   a. Symptoms of Curling's ulcer may be seen as early as 4 days if gastric, or 2–3 weeks if duodenal, postburn.
   b. Generally asymptomatic
   c. Abdominal discomfort
   d. Recurrent or intermittent bleeding—hematemesis
   e. Low hematocrit
   f. Altered vital signs
   g. Administer medications that may reduce development of Curling's ulcer.
      (1) Antacid to impair absorption of histamine and reduce acidity—aluminum hydroxide and/or magnesium hydroxide may be given separately or alternately to maintain gastric $pH \geq 7$. Common side effects include hypercalcemia, constipation, diarrhea, vomiting and aspiration, nephrolithiasis, osteomalacia.

(2) Histamine receptor antagonist to reduce gastric volume—cimetidine. May need to increase dose in the child because of increased renal clearance.

2. Acute gastric dilatation may occur, especially if the child has greater than 20% injury, associated injury, or tachypnea. Nasogastric tube may be inserted to prevent vomiting, aspiration, and paralytic ileus.

3. Ileus—associated with circulatory problems in small children; may be alleviated with insertion of nasogastric tube.

4. Determine need for tetanus inoculation.

C. Observing for Symptoms of Respiratory Distress and Initiating Measures to Alleviate Distress.

Most common form of airway obstruction in young child is from edema of the head and neck, and the glottic and subglottic areas.

1. Be alert for symptoms of respiratory distress:
   a. Dyspnea
   b. Stridor
   c. Rapid respirations
   d. Restlessness
   e. Cyanosis

2. Report these symptoms.

3. Provide an oxygen source in order to combat anoxia.

4. Monitor blood gases—serum dioxide (indicated only initially)

5. Intubation or tracheostomy may be performed.

D. Obtaining Medical History of the Child: Childhood Diseases, Immunizations, Current Medications, and Recent Infections.

E. Providing Scrupulous Skin Care in Order to Prevent Infection and Promote Healing.

Treatment

A. Fluid Resuscitation—IV Fluid Replacement

Note: Controversy exists regarding fluid resuscitation solution and amount.

1. Usually consists of Ringer's solution—an isotonic electrolyte solution

2. Formulas
   a. Many formulas are available to determine the fluid needed for resuscitation.
   b. The Parkland Formula:
      4 ml. × weight in kg. × % burn (resuscitation) plus maintenance fluid
   c. Resuscitation is based on: 5000 ml./m.^{2} of burned surface area and 2000 ml./m.^{2} of total body surface for maintenance, given over 24 hours, with half of the amount given in the first 8 hours postinjury.

3. Weight—this measurement is critical for accurate intravenous fluid volumes to be determined.
   Infants and small children: 4 ml./kg./% burn
   Older child: 2–3 ml./kg./% burn

4. Fluid loss from transcapillary leakage is greatest during the first 12 hours postinjury and diminishes to almost zero 12–24 hours postinjury. Fluid loss after 48 hours is due to vaporization of water from wound.

B. Burn Treatment

1. Exposure
   a. After cleansing, wound remains exposed to air:—maintains a dry surface, produces early formation of a protective eschar, and predisposes patient to less infection
   b. Usually combined with the use of antibacterial creams and daily soaking in Hubbard tank to remove cream and dead tissue
   c. Can allow for increased movement.

2. Occlusive dressing
   a. Burns are kept covered with dressings that have been soaked in a solution, or topical medication is applied followed by dressing.
   b. Dressings are changed every 8–24 hours.
   c. Burned areas are soaked daily in Hubbard tank.
   d. Children appear to be more mobile when burn injury is covered, as they are in less pain.

3. Primary excision of burn
   a. Necrotic eschar is immediately removed, allowing site to be grafted.
   b. Grafting may be postponed 24–48 hours with temporary cover of porcine xenograft or comparable biosynthetic material (i.e., Biobrane)

4. Escharotomy
   a. Incision through eschar to relieve severe constriction and compromised circulation, when burn eschar is circumferential.
   b. Is done within first 12–24 hours after injury.

5. Tangential debridement
   a. Slices of eschar are removed in full-thickness injury to expose subcutaneous fat or deeper structures.
   b. Primary excision is done 2–5 days postburn and repeated every 5–10 days until all necrotic tissue is removed and healthy granulation tissue develops to accept graft.

6. Tangential excision
   a. Necrotic surface of burn wound is excised to viable tissue in deep partial- or full-thickness injury that does not involve fat, and autogenous skin grafting
   b. Excision is done 3–5 days postburn.

7. Fascia excision: Criteria
   a. Burn wound sepsis
   b. Small local full-thickness injury
   c. Massive burns

8. Physicians have their own preferences as to which method is used. The goals remain the same—to prevent infection, to remove dead tissue, and to provide for early closure of wound.
   Sterility is maintained when working with the burn area, regardless of whether the open or closed method is used.

C. Cleansing the Wound and Changing the Dressing—is critical for preventing infection, preserving tissue, promoting early closure of the wound, and maintaining function.

1. Hubbard tank is treatment of choice for cleansing.

2. Use clean technique—gown, cap, mask, gloves, and plastic apron.

3. Limit tubbing to 20 minutes to prevent hypothermia, hyponatremia, and hemodilution.

4. Isotonic solution may be needed for large wounds and small children.

5. Gaining popularity is the use of a shower to facilitate the loosening and removal of sloughing tissue, eschar, exudate, and topical medications. The child is suspended over a tub in a fine-mesh nylon sling. The shower, water about 32°C. (90°F.), flows over the child; then debridement is done. The wound is air-dried before dressings are applied.

D. The Bradford Frame—may be used to facilitate skin care.

1. Provides a method for the collection of urine and feces and maintains cleanliness of the burn areas and dressings.

2. Contractures may be prevented by maintaining functional position of extremities and good body alignment.
3. Two Bradford frames may be used to change position of the child from back to stomach and vice versa without having to handle the severely burned child.

E. Other Skin Care Measures

1. Alternating water bed or sand bed may also be used.
2. Position the child and turn him frequently.
3. Apply protective devices to prevent the child from scratching the burn area, or give prescribed antipruritic drug when necessary.
4. Administer antibiotics as prescribed.
   Specific antibiotic therapy may be necessary for complicating infection.
5. Ensure that serial wound biopsy and quantitative cultures are done if prescribed.

F. Topical Antibiotic Therapy

1. Topical agents (antimicrobials) are the first line of defense against infection by delaying wound colonization. It is well to remember, however, that no single agent is totally effective against all burn wound microbes.
2. 1% silver sulfadiazine cream (Silvadene)—treatment of choice at present; especially for partial-thickness burn.
   a. Easy to apply—applied 1–2 times daily
   b. Does not hurt the child on application, but the child may complain of cold
   c. Allergic reactions occur very rarely
   d. Nontoxic
   e. Bactericidal for up to 48 hours
   f. Effective against gram-negative and gram-positive bacteria and *Candida albicans*
   g. Adverse reaction—transient leukopenia
3. Povidone-iodine (Betadine ointment)
   a. Allergic reaction fairly common
   b. Apparently nontoxic

   c. Effective against broad spectrum of organisms
   d. Associated with pain
   e. Eschar becomes stained and stiff
   f. Elevation of protein-bound iodine
4. 10% mafenide acetate (Sulfamylon) cream
   a. Allergic reaction (rash)—common
   b. Painful immediately after application where there is partial-thickness burn
   c. Metabolically active in kidney as carbonic anhydrase inhibitor resulting in metabolic acidosis and hyperventilation
   d. Most effective for extensive burns with thick eschar
   e. Easily applied
   f. Effective against many gram-positive and gram-negative organisms (i.e., *Pseudomonas* and *Clostridium*)
5. ½% silver nitrate soaks
   a. Solution is hypo-osmolar, leading to electrolyte deficiencies
   b. Soaks are continuous, messy, and turn everything they touch black
   c. Hypoallergenic
   d. Effective in controlling *Pseudomonas* and *Staphylococcus*.

G. Heterograft or Homografts (Table 54-2) are used to:

1. Restore water vapor barrier and decrease protein loss
2. Decrease pain
3. Decrease bacterial count at the wound as graft adheres to the site
4. Other fluid considerations
   a. Injury-induced fluid loss is greatest up to 48 hours postburn, at which time reabsorption of these fluids results in diuresis if renal function is intact; accurate urinary output measurement is critical during this time.
   b. Decreasing water loss by evaporation can be accomplished by keeping ambient air warm and moist, thus reducing high energy requirements and the chance of metabolic derangements. This,

Table 54-2. *Wound Closure*

Types of Coverage	Source
Permanent grafts	
Autograft	Tissue obtained from uninjured area on the child's own body.
Isograft	Histocompatible tissue obtained from genetically identical individual (i.e., child's identical twin).
Temporary grafts	
Homograft (allograft)	Tissue obtained from genetically different individual of same species—living or dead. Can be fresh or frozen.
Heterograft (xenograft)	Tissue obtained from other species—pigskin.
Human amnion	Material obtained by stripping the amniotic membrane from the placenta.
Biobrane (Woodroof Laboratories, Inc., Santa Ana, CA 92704)	Semisynthetic material consisting of knitted elastic, flexible, nylon fabric, which is bonded to silastic membrane.
Types of Grafts	***Methods of Covering Application***
Full-cover graft	Sheet of skin from donor site is applied as one piece on recipient site.
Postage-stamp graft	Donor site sheet of skin, cut into postage-stamp size and applied on recipient site with spaces between grafts, which allows for drainage.
Mesh, lace, or split graft	Donor site sheet of skin that has mechanically had splits made in it, which stretches to cover area about 3 times its size.

however, sets up an excellent environment for bacterial growth, especially of *Pseudomonas.*

   c. When parenteral hyperalimentation is used, there is increased risk of infection in the burned patient. Be alert to early signs and symptoms of infection.

   d. Fluid replacement after the first 24 hours remains fairly constant while the wound remains open.
     (1) Sodium requirements usually low—50 mEq/day
     (2) Potassium phosphate—20–30 mEq/day
     (3) D5 ⅓ normal saline usually used

   e. Transition to oral fluid from intravenous fluid may begin as early as second postburn day.

   f. Parenteral nutrition may be necessary when complications exist.

H. Providing a High-Protein, High-Calorie Diet in Order to Provide Nutrition Necessary for Healing and for the Growth and Developmental Needs of the Child.

1. Hypernutrition is important, because of the extreme hypermetabolism related to large burn injuries.
   a. Twice the predicted basal metabolic rate in calories, based on ideal weight, may be necessary.
   b. Hypermetabolic state generally subsides when the majority of the wounds are grafted or healed.
   c. High-caloric—to support hypermetabolic state; protein synthesis; calories should come from carbohydrates.
   d. High-protein—to replace protein lost by exudation; support synthesis of immunoglobulins and structural protein; prevent negative nitrogen balance
   e. Vitamin and mineral supplement—particularly vitamins B and C, and iron and zinc
   f. Caloric recommendation—1800 kcal/m² body surface for maintainance and 2000 kcal/m² burned surface area

2. Maintain ambient temperature 28–32°C.
   a. Minimizes metabolic expenditure by maintaining core temperature
   b. Also maximizes comfort

3. Anorexia is common in the burned child.
   a. Tell the child why eating is important.
   b. Offer small amounts of food, perhaps 4–5 feedings rather than 3 per day.
   c. Give him a choice of foods; determine his favorite foods.
   d. Offer high-protein, high-calorie dietary supplements.
   e. Make meals a pleasant time, unassociated with treatments or unpleasant interruptions.
   f. Nasogastric tube feedings may be necessary to supply high nutritive needs.

4. Monitor dietary compliance with dietary goals.

5. Hypoalbuminemia may occur when burn surface area exceeds 20% TBSA.
   a. Protein losses, as burn wound exudate continues until wounds are healed
   b. Protein replacement with human serum albumin or fresh frozen plasma

6. Monitor nutritional status
   a. Weight gain
   b. Wound healing
   c. Serum transferin
   d. Hypoalbuminemia may occur when burn injury exceeds 20% body surface. Protein losses continue as burn exudate until wounds as covered or healed.

I. Maintaining a Planned Physical Therapy Program to Achieve the Greatest Functional Capacity for the Child.

1. Carry out physical therapy procedures to minimize joint and skin complications:
   a. Position—position joint in opposite direction of expected contracture.
   b. Splints—aid joint positioning and decrease skin contractures and hypertrophy.
   c. Exercise—gain and maintain optimal range of motion.
   d. Pressure garment—aid circulation, protect newly healed skin, and prevent and treat hypertrophic scar formation by promoting dermal collagen fiber growth in parallel direction. It may be necessary to wear pressure garments 12–18 months after injury, at which time healed skin has matured and becomes supple.

2. Plan the time each day for the therapy to be carried out. Movement, a normal activity for a child, is now painful because of crusts, dressings, and pain from the burn area.

3. Use play opportunities to help the child accept the program (e.g., tricycle riding may be used as form of exercise).

4. Allow the child to be ambulatory as soon as he is able.

J. Preparing the Child for the Many Painful Surgical and Other Procedures That He Must Undergo.

1. Explain to the child what will happen before each procedure.

2. Explain to the child what will happen before he goes to the operating room, where he will wake up, and who will be there when he wakes up.

3. Explain and demonstrate what equipment will be used following surgery or other procedures.

4. Puppet or doll play, water play, clay or Play-Doh, and drawings can all be helpful in letting the child work through his feelings about all that is happening to him.

K. Providing Emotional Support for the Child Who Has Been Very Frightened and Traumatized by This Painful Experience.

1. The child may be suffering from all-encompassing physical pain for which he has no previous experience to prepare him; he becomes confused and frightened, and he may regress.
   a. Coupled with physical pain is psychological pain resulting from isolation, separation from parents, reliving the experience of being burned, fear of rejection, fear of death, immobilization, chronic pain, and repeated surgery.
   b. Prepare the child for dressing changes and debridement. Provide comfort after procedure.
   c. Use distraction, relaxation, imagery, and reinforcement to control pain, as well as medication. Patient-controlled analgesia also may be appropriate.

2. Encourage the child to talk about the way he feels.
   a. The child may feel guilty and think that the burn is punishment for some wrong deed.
   b. Allow the child opportunities at play where he may be able to begin to work out his feelings.

3. The child will be concerned about his appearance.
   a. Continually inform the child that you love him even though he has a bad burn.
   b. Encourage early contact with other children.
   c. Adjustment to disfigurement can be long and painful.

4. Psychiatric consultation is very frequently necessary to assist the child to work out his feelings.
   Signs may include:
   a. Persistent refusal to eat
   b. Resisting all nursing procedures
   c. Resisting socialization
5. Contact with the child's parents, siblings, and nurse will help him with his feelings of fear, isolation, and rejection.
6. Arrange for services of a schoolteacher for the school-age child as soon as his condition permits.

L. Supporting the Parents During This Very Difficult Time. They are Under Extreme Stress, Because a Burned Child Creates a Crisis.

1. Parents may react to the situation with depression and/or stress syndromes.
2. Use knowledge about the family's psychosocial status in planning care.
   a. A medical social worker may offer beneficial psychosocial support to the family.
   b. Be aware of siblings at home and that they may have needs that are being neglected as a result of this crisis.
3. Encourage the parents to visit their child often.
   a. Attempt to have them become actively involved in the child's care when they are ready to do so.
   b. Parental visits and involvement can have a direct impact on the child's survival and recovery.
   c. If the parents are unable to visit, telephone calls and family photographs are helpful.
4. Give the parents the opportunity to discuss their feelings.
   a. Parents frequently feel very guilty because they feel they did not give the child the appropriate supervision he should have had when the accident occurred.
   b. Frequently burn injury is associated with actual or perceived parental neglect. Remember this type of injury is sudden and acute, placing the family in a state of crisis.
5. Keep the parents informed of the child's progress.
   a. Begin initial teaching at admission with supportive words and limited technical information.
   b. Education and orientation to the facility and the burn injury will decrease some anxiety and begin to build rapport on which future support can be based.
   c. Parents' meetings can help the parents cope with trauma.
6. Psychiatric consultation is frequently required to assist the parents in coping with their feelings.

M. Preparing the Child and Family for Discharge With the Understanding That Rehabilitation Is Long-term.*

1. Separation from the hospital environment, caretakers, and other patients can produce excessive anxiety. Short-time home passes (overnight, weekend) are helpful prior to final discharge.
2. If the child is school age, prepare for school reentry—visit classroom and tell peers what to expect; at the same time teach how to prevent burn injuries.
3. Social reentry can be painful for the child, who may have to respond to questions and stares from strangers and rejection by friends.

* Adapted from Helm PA. Burn injury: Rehabilitation management: 1982. J Burn Care Rehabil 1983 Nov–Dec; 4(6):411

4. Hospitalization and future scar revisions may be necessary.
5. Special skin care is necessary following burn injury. Give written specific instructions to parents.
   a. Avoid exposure to sunlight.
   b. Use pressure garments to prevent hypertrophic scar and keloid formation.
   c. Use lotions and creams to prevent drying, cracking, and itching.
   d. Burn area has decreased sensation to touch, heat, and pressure; thus, precautions need to be practiced to prevent injury to area.
6. Psychological support of the child is necessary because of the trauma resulting from the burn injury, the actual event, and hospitalization.
7. Physical therapy must be continued.
8. Ensure that parents are able to:
   a. Discuss and demonstrate treatments, procedures, and dressing changes.
   b. Have obtained equipment necessary to perform treatments at home.
   c. Understand reason for and side effects of medications as well as dietary requirements.
   d. Have identified person(s) to contact to answer questions as well as community resources that can assist with adjustments and facilitate continuity of care.

N. Providing Educational Activities in the Community to Prevent Burn Injuries.

Health Education

1. Teach parents and children the prevention of burn injury. Parents can be taught common-sense safety measures as well as being aware of other fire hazards (i.e., turn pot handles toward stove rather than letting them extend over stove edge, avoid electrical cords hanging over table or counter edge, cover electrical outlets, do not leave small children alone in bathroom or kitchen, etc.).
2. Children can be taught the hazards of flame and other devices that can cause injury.
3. Parents can be taught first-aid emergency care for burn injury (i.e., cool burned area with cool water; remove clothing); parents should know when to seek medical assistance.
4. Children can be taught what to do in case of fire or if their clothes catch on fire (i.e., stop, drop, and roll, crawl to safety, etc.).
5. Community groups, media, clinics, and public areas can all be used for public education in prevention of burn injury.

Evaluation

(See Adult, p. 852)
1. Absence of shock; stabilization of vital signs; normal serum and electrolyte values
2. Absence of infection as demonstrated by normal laboratory values, clean wound, and normal vital signs
3. Is free of respiratory distress as demonstrated by stable vital signs, respiratory status, and blood gases
4. Shows no signs of gastrointestinal complications as evidenced by normal bowel sounds, normal elimination, stable vital signs
5. Maintains adequate nutritional status as demonstrated by weight gain and wound healing
6. Demonstrates improved mobility as evidenced by involvement in play and other activities
7. Experiences minimal discomfort as evidenced by sta-

ble vital signs, verbalization, involvement in play, and other activities
8. Develops a more positive self-image as evidenced by verbalization, socialization, and other behaviors
9. Experiences minimal anxiety as evidenced by appropriate coping behavior
10. Demonstrates appropriate parent/child relationships as evidenced by verbalization and other behaviors
11. Parents reveal lessening of anxiety and demonstrate behaviors of appropriate parent–child relationships, and understanding of illness, treatments, and follow-up care

Atopic Eczema
(Infantile and Childhood Eczema)

Atopic eczema is a term that describes any inflammatory dermatosis that is characterized by erythema, papulovesiculation, oozing, crusting, and scaling in various phases of resolution.

Etiology and Incidence

1. Infantile eczema usually manifests itself between the 2nd and 6th month of age, up to 2 years.
2. This type of dermatitis is the most common, earliest manifestation of allergy.
3. Atopic eczema is not a disease but, rather, a reaction state of the skin.
4. The exact etiology is not known. Many infants with eczema have a positive family history of allergy and later develop asthma or hay fever.
5. The following may be triggering factors affecting the day-to-day appearance of the lesions:
    a. Bacterial, viral, or fungal infections
    b. Particulate matter and contact irritants—clothing, soaps

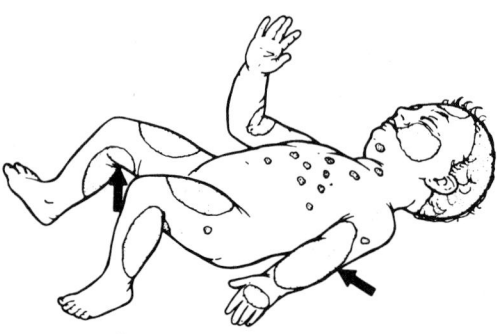

Diaper Area Usually Clear

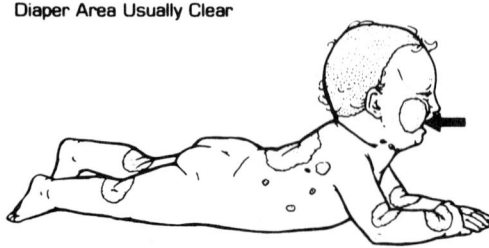

Figure 54-2. *Infantile atopic eczema. (From Sauer GC. Manual of Skin Diseases. 5th ed. Philadelphia, JB Lippincott, 1986)*

c. Environmental factors
    (1) Temperature and humidity—rapid changes
    (2) Inhalants
d. Foods
e. Emotional or physical stress
f. Drugs

Altered Physiology

1. The dermatitis involves the epidermis and the vascular layer of the cutis.
2. The dermatitis goes through a cycle involving areas of erythema, papules, vesicles, wheal reactions, and, ultimately, scaling eruption. There is no distinct primary cutaneous lesion. Pruritus followed by scratching and trauma leads to excoriation.
3. With superimposed infection, there is exudation, pustulation, and crust formation.
4. Various stages of the dermatoses can be present on different parts of the child's body.
5. The patient is subject to remissions and exacerbations.
6. Secondary infections may occur from scratching.

Complications

1. Acute infection—pyogenic infection may develop.
2. Long-term—eczema may progress to allergic rhinitis or asthma.

Clinical Manifestations

A. Infants—Lesions (2 mos.–2 years)

1. Erythematous, papular, and weeping lesions develop.
2. Oozing and crusting of the lesions occur, along with excoriation.
3. Cheeks, forehead, neck, behind ears, and the crawling surfaces of arms and legs are the areas most frequently involved.
4. Lesions are more concentrated on the head and body than on the extremities; however, they may progress to cover the body (Fig. 54-2).
5. May have dry skin that predisposes to itching and recurrent inflammation.

B. Older Children—Lesions (4–10 years)

1. Erythematous, papular, and weeping lesions develop.
2. Lesions are more scattered, less acute, and exudative.
3. Periorbital erythema and edema are common.
4. Oozing and crusting of the lesions occur.
5. The flexor surfaces of the upper and lower extremities, antecubital and popliteal fossae, in addition to the face and neck, are areas frequently involved.
6. As the disease becomes chronic, lichenification (leatheriness and hardening of skin) and hyperpigmentation develop.

C. General

1. Pruritus—may be mild or severe.
2. Excessive itching may cause restlessness, sleeplessness, and irritability.
3. Excessive scratching may result in an inflammatory reaction and excoriation, bleeding, and subsequent infection.
4. The color of lesions is red (possibly intense red).

Diagnoses

1. Family history of allergies
2. Positive dermal reaction
3. Presence of circulating Prausnitz–Küstner antibodies
4. Tendency to develop blood eosinophilia

5. Clearing of skin with removal of specific allergen and reappearance of dermal reaction on reexposure

Treatment

1. Symptomatic and supportive—to break itch–scratch cycle
   a. Trial period of hypoallergenic diet to eliminate any responsible food
   b. Avoidance by patient of any other known allergen; wool clothing, blankets, etc.
   c. Control of any complicating skin infection
   d. Relief of itching and irritability; sedation may be necessary
   e. Measures to improve condition of involved skin:
      (1) Prevent scratching
      (2) Cleansing
      (3) Topical steroid
      (4) Tar preparations
      (5) Lubricants
   f. Medications to relieve itching (chloral hydrate, diphenhydramine hydrochloride, Periactin)
   g. Antibiotics/antibacterials—as necessary to control infection
2. Preventive—teach the mother how to keep condition under control

Patient Problems and Nursing Diagnoses

1. Potential for infection, related to altered skin integrity and scratching
2. Comfort, altered, related to itching and crusted lesions
3. Anxiety related to discomfort and hospitalization
4. Impaired mobility related to discomfort on movement of crusted flexor surfaces of extremities

Nursing Interventions

A. Instituting Measures That Prevent the Child From Scratching Himself When He Experiences Severe Itching to Prevent Further Irritation and Possible Infection of the Skin.

1. Apply protective devices to prevent the child from scratching himself.
   a. Any one or combination of the following protective devices may be used (elbow cuff, ankle and wrist restraint, face mask, jacket restraint).
   b. Apply these protective devices only when absolutely necessary—when scratching cannot be controlled by other methods.
   c. Apply protective devices securely enough to prevent scratching, yet not so tight as to impair circulation. Check circulation frequently when protective devices are used.
   d. When protective devices are used, the device should be removed at frequent intervals.
      (1) Allow for free movement and active range of motion.
      (2) Allow the child to sit on the nurse's or mother's lap.
      (3) Attempt to divert the child's attention by playing with him and reading to him.
      (4) Allow the child to eat his meals free from protective devices; this requires direct supervision.
   e. When the child experiences severe itching and uncontrollable scratching, remove only one protective device at a time so that scratching can be controlled.

   f. Anger and frustration are frequently displayed in violent scratching.
      (1) Keep the child comfortable and anticipate his needs.
      (2) Provide as much personal contact and supervision as possible.
      (3) Allow play activities that afford the child the opportunity to act out his anger and frustrations.
      (4) Provide infants with a cradle gym and a pacifier.
2. Cotton hand mitts and booties may be applied to prevent the child from scratching himself.
3. Trim fingernails and toenails and keep them clean.
4. Provide safe toys that will not be used by the child to scratch himself. (Use soft playthings made of hypoallergenic material.)
5. Administer prescribed medications.
   a. Sedatives
   b. Antihistamines
   c. The use of local anesthetics to relieve itching is contraindicated because of their potential for skin sensitization.
   d. Antipruritics
   e. Topical steroids

B. Providing Measures that Will Improve the Condition of the Involved Skin.

1. Bathe the child by the prescribed method.
   a. Water and soap are often irritating.
   b. Starch baths may be used; oil baths may be soothing.
   c. Oil may be used if the skin is dry and crusted. (Apply oil with a soft cloth.)
   d. While giving the child a bath, keep him from scratching himself. (It may be necessary to maintain protective devices at this time.)
2. Local care of the skin is aimed at removing the debris and allaying the inflammatory reaction and pruritus.
   a. Wet soaks of Burow's solution may be applied to the affected areas.
      (1) These soaks are continuous and must be kept wet. Solution should be at room temperature.
      (2) These bulky, wet dressings may serve to immobilize the child sufficiently so that he does not require other protective devices.
   b. Lassar's paste or another hydrophilic preparation may be applied to the affected areas.
      (1) Local medications must be kept on the skin constantly.
      (2) Caution must be exercised to keep ointment out of the child's eyes.
         (a) Remove all old ointment before applying new ointment.
         (b) Starch bath may be used to remove ointment.
      (3) Routine urine examination should be done because of possible toxic effect of medications on kidneys.
      (4) Coal tar preparations should be used with caution during the summer when exposure to the sun is more likely, because they have a photosensitizing effect.
         Folliculitis and contact dermatitis may also occur.
3. Prevent skin irritation from bedding. Padding may be used.
4. Change diapers frequently to prevent skin excoriation.
5. Avoid extreme ambient temperatures.

C. Promoting Measures That Will Prevent Contact With Dietary and Environmental Allergens.

1. Review the child's chart and question the parents about known allergies.
   a. Note the known allergens on the Kardex and place a tag on the head of the bed to indicate that the child has an allergy.
   b. Inform the dietitian of the child's food allergies.
2. Avoid substances that have a high potential for sensitization.
   a. Foods such as milk, eggs, chocolate, wheat cereal, and orange juice are to be avoided.
   b. Wool and dust are to be avoided.
3. Observe the child's reactions when an elimination diet is prescribed.
   a. A minimal diet is prescribed. Trial diet may be composed of:
      (1) Milk substitute
      (2) Rice cereal
      (3) 2 fruits
      (4) 2 vegetables
      (5) Beef
      (6) Aqueous multivitamins
      (7) No egg products
   b. A new food is added to the diet every 3–5 days, during which time the response to that food is observed.
   c. An allergic response occurring during this 3- to 5-day period indicates sensitivity to that food; that particular food is then eliminated from the diet.
   d. If no response is apparent, that food is added to the child's diet.
   e. Another food substance is then added, and the child is observed for the following 3- to 5-day period. This method is followed until the food allergen is determined.
4. Provide a substitute for cow's milk when the child is allergic to it.
   a. Goat's milk may be used.
   b. Commercial formulas made from meat or vegetable protein substances are available.

D. Protecting the Child from Sources of Infection.

1. Protect the child from exposure to sources of infection known to cause exacerbations and severe infections.
   a. Contact with other children, visitors, and personnel who have the herpes simplex virus is to be avoided.
   b. Use single-patient rooms.

NURSING ALERT: If the child needs to be vaccinated against smallpox, it should not be done until his skin has been free from eczema for several months. Use caution with routine immunizations. Skin testing may be advisable.

   c. The child should not be exposed to individuals who have a fresh vaccine lesion.
2. When the child is immobilized, his position should be changed frequently to prevent respiratory complications.

E. Providing the Emotional Support Needed by Any Child His Age Who is Hospitalized; Providing Love and Attention, and Giving the Child Freedom to Express His Feelings.

Health Education

A. Assist the Parents in Providing for the Child's Care Following Hospitalization.

1. Explain to parents the usual causes of the problem.
   a. Help them to understand that eczema is chronic—that there is no cure—but that a therapeutic regimen can be followed that will control it.
   b. Home care is preferred, and a home care program is essential.
   c. Ensure that treatment for flare-up is understood, i.e., increasing number of baths per day (to decrease itching and preserve hydration) and applying topical medication immediately after bath (to increases penetration).
2. Demonstrate the application of topical medications and the application of dressings. Explain timing of application of medicine. Stress the importance of several thin applications rather than one thick layer.
   a. Weeping and moist areas—apply cream or lotion
   b. Drier areas—paste applied thickly or ointment
3. Give specific information about diet. Emphasize the foods that are allowed rather than foods to be avoided.
4. Demonstrate the application of protective devices and the precautions in using them.
5. Additional information in home management may include the following:
   a. Launder clothes with a neutral pH soap and double rinse.
   b. Control environment.
   c. Use apron to cover clothing when holding child.
   d. Avoid exposure of child to extreme heat or cold or to rapid changes in ambient temperature; have him avoid strenuous activity (can swim), soap, perfume, detergents, and stress.
   e. Keep the child's fingernails clean and cut short.
   f. Do not leave the child alone to entertain himself when itching is severe; prevent play with toys that can be injurious if used to scratch the skin.
   g. Baths may be effective in relieving itching—Alpha-Keri, Domol, Lubath; give bath using 2 cups cornstarch in tub of tepid water. Lubricate dry skin after bath.
6. Encourage the parents to hold and cuddle the child as much as possible to encourage the body contact that is frequently impossible because of protective devices and ointments.
7. Encourage the parents to discuss their feelings and concerns about the child's illness.
   a. The appearance of the child may be very disturbing to them.
   b. They need to feel adequate in caring for the child at home.
8. A community health nurse referral may be indicated to provide support to the family, especially during initial phases of adjustment.

Expected Outcomes

1. Absence of infection as evidenced by stable vital signs, normal laboratory values, and clean wound surfaces
2. Reveals minimal discomfort as evidenced by stable vital signs, behavior, and verbalization
3. Shows minimal anxiety demonstrated by appropriate behavior
4. Remains mobile and participates in activities of daily living

Common Skin Problems

Disorder/Organism	Clinical Manifestations	Treatment/Prevention	Specific Nursing Goals and Interventions*	Comments
Impetigo Bacterial infectious disease affecting the superficial layers of the skin and characterized by the formation of vesicles, crusts, or bullae. *Etiology and Incidence* 1. Bullous impetigo in neonate and infant—lesions are large, flaccid bullae containing pus and supernatant clear serum that rupture and leave raw edges. Lesions are more prominent in axillae and groin. 2. Impetigo contagiosa in the older child—lesions appear with thick, yellow crusts. 3. Impetigo is caused by staphylococci (bullous) or streptococci (crusted). 4. Occurs most frequently when personal hygiene is poor. 5. Occurs most frequently in children under 10 years of age. 6. Spread by contact—easily conveyed from person to person (using same handkershief, towels, napkins, pencils, toys, etc.); plastic wading pools in summer—when spilled water is replaced and no antiseptic	(Impetigo contagiosa) 1. Incubation period of 1–5 days. 2. Lesion first appears as pink-red macules that quickly change to vesicles that, in turn, enlarge, become pustular, develop crusts, and leave temporary superficial erythematous area a. Bullous (newborn and older child)—broken blisters form thin, light brown, liquorlike crust. b. Crusted (preschool-age—seen more often in summer on exposed body parts)—skin around crusts is red and weeping with satellite lesions. 3. Face, scalp, and hands are commonly involved, but other areas may be affected. 4. Regional lymphadenopathy—common with secondary infection of insect bites, eczema, poison ivy scabies.	Based on etiology and type of infection 1. Removal of undermined skin, crusts and debris: normal saline or 1:20 Burow's solution compresses to affected area. Remove crusts when softened. 2. Topical application of bactericidal medication (Bacitracin, Neomycin, Neosporin, or Garamycin, Betadine). 3. Systemic antibiotic—when severe, or recurrent (penicillin or erythromycin 4. Prevention—avoid contact with child and his siblings.	Be aware of the appearance of the characteristic lesion of impetigo. 1. Observe the condition of the child's skin on admission to the hospital. 2. Report any suspicious-appearing lesions. 3. Record the appearance and location of the lesion. 4. Initiate appropriate measures to prevent the spread of the infection. a. Place the child in a single room. b. Maintain medical aseptic technique. 5. Watch for the development of new lesions. Provide measures to prevent secondary infections. 1. Provide mittens or protective devices to prevent the child from scratching the lesions. 2. Trim the child's fingernails and toenails. 3. Maintain the cleanliness of fingernails and toenails. Provide measures to ensure the child's comfort until healing has occurred and the child is free from infection. 1. Hold the child frequently and release from any necessary protective device.	Practice good general health measures and provide teaching for the child and his parents that will be helpful in preventing spread and further infection. 1. General measures to improve personal cleanliness should be encouraged. 2. Minor wounds should be adequately cleansed and treated. 3. The child should be isolated if at home. 4. The child should be kept out of school until the lesions have healed. 5. Increased risk for acute glomerulonephritis

(continued)

* See Eczema for Patient Problems and Nursing Diagnoses, Interventions, and Expected Outcomes

Common Skin Problems *(continued)*

Disorder/Organism	Clinical Manifestations	Treatment/Prevention	Specific Nursing Goals and Interventions*	Comments
or disinfectant is used. Very contagious. 7. Any abrasion of skin may serve as portal of entry. *Diagnosis* 1. Aspiration and culture of bullae. 2. Culture after removal of crust.	5. Autoinoculation is major cause of spreading. 6. Pruritis may occur.		2. Provide diversional therapy. 3. Administer medication and treatment to relieve itching—local medications or packs that relieve itching and promote healing may be used. 4. Provide the child with a diet adequate to meet his growth and development needs.	
Ringworm of the Scalp (tinea capitis) A fungal infection of the scalp and hair follicles. *Etiology and Incidence* 1. Ringworm of the scalp is caused by different species of the *Microsporum canis, Trichophyton tonsurans* (most common). 2. Ringworm of the scalp is seen primarily in children before puberty. 3. Most commonly seen in ages 3–10 years. *Altered Physiology* 1. The fungal infection produces an inflammation of the scalp that causes alopecia and broken hairs. 2. The lesions of the scalp may have papulovesicular erythematous borders or may appear only as scaling with a few broken hairs. 3. *Kerion,* an acute inflammation that produces edema, pustules, and	1. Lesions usually develop in the occipital, temporal, and parietal areas of the scalp. 2. Pruritus usually occurs in the area. 3. The involved areas of the scalp appear as patches, rounded or oval in outline, covered by scales and lusterless, irregularly broken hairs. 4. Single patches or multiple patches may occur; alopecia. 5. Systemic manifestations are absent. 6. Evaluation a. Wood's lamp—a filtered ultraviolet radiation causes microsporon infections to fluoresce with a brilliant, greenish light.	1. Griseofulvin—an antifungal antibiotic that is administered orally, 5 mg./kg./dose b.i.d. × 6–8 weeks; 20 mg./kg./day for 7–14 days. 2. Topical agents—applied b.i.d. Antifungal—clotrimazole, haloprogin, or miconazole nitrate, Whitfield's ointment For *T. tonsurans*—selenium sulfide lotion, 2.5% (Selsun Brown, Exsel) 3. Keep head clean, and avoid scratching. Wear cap to prevent broken hair pieces from falling.	Recognize the characteristic lesions of ringworm of the scalp. 1. Observe the condition of the hair and scalp as a part of the routine assessment of the child on admission to the hospital and at daily bath. 2. Report suspicious-appearing lesions. 3. Record the appearance and location of the lesions. 4. Initiate the appropriate isolation techniques (as per hospital policy). Be aware of the side effects of the medications used in the treatment of ringworm of the scalp. 1. Griseofulvin may produce headache, heartburn, nausea, epigastric discomfort, diarrhea, and urticaria. 2. Record and report to the physician any side effects observed.	Teach the child and his family methods to prevent further episodes. 1. Teach general hygiene measures—regular shampooing and bathing. 2. Advise them to avoid the sharing of hats, combs, brushes, etc. 3. Stress the importance of wearing a cap continuously until the infection has been eliminated. 4. All lesions must be dry before child can return to school.

granulomatous swelling, may occur.

4. The painful infection may be spread through child-to-child contact, as well as through the common use of towels, combs, brushes, hats. Kittens and puppies may be the source of the infection.

b. Microscopic evaluation of infected hair follicles and fungal culture to identify *Tricbophyton*, which fluoresces poorly under Wood's lamp—spores coat hair in a visible way.

3. A diet high in fat may be prescribed to enhance intestinal absorption.

Be aware of the case-finding measures to prevent additional cases and to identify the earliest evidence of infection.

1. All family contacts should be screened.
2. The school should be notified so that appropriate case-finding techniques may be initiated.

Be aware of the psychological trauma associated with loss of hair, especially in a girl, and provide support as appropriate.

Use of wigs or scarves may provide some relief of embarrassment. Hair loss is usually temporary.

Pediculosis

The infestation of human beings by lice

Etiology

1. Three types of lice affect human beings.
   a. *Pediculosis capitis*—head louse
   b. *Pediculosis corporis*—body louse (rare in U.S.)
   c. *Phtbirus pubis*—pubic louse/crab louse (seldom found in children) can attach only to curly hair—pubes, axillae, eyebrows
2. Each type of louse generally remains in the area designated by its name, but it may occasionally be seen in other areas of the body

1. Severe itching in the area affected is the primary symptom of pediculosis; scratch marks will be evident in these areas.
2. In children, pubic lice are found most frequently in the eyelashes and eyebrows.
3. Infested scalp areas may become secondarily infected from scratching.
4. Crusts, pediculi, nits, and dirt may combine to cause a foul odor and matted hair.
5. Body lice may produce minute red lesions.

Eliminate and remove nits and pediculi (lice) and treat the irritated skin.

1. *Pediculosis capitis* may be treated with lindane 1% (Kwell), benzyl benzoate emulsion, or crotamiton (see package inserts).

Eggs are not killed by 5-minute wash; must repeat in 1 week when they hatch. Over-the-counter products (RID) appear to be safe and effective

Maintain technique that will prevent the spread of the infection.

Institute measures to carry out medical asepsis.

Perform the treatments prescribed to destroy and eliminate the parasite.

Observe and record the response to treatment.

1. Note the change in the degree of discomfort caused by itching.
2. Observe infected areas for changes in the characteristics of the lesions.
3. Observe for systemic manifestations of infection.

Provide measures to prevent the child from scratching himself.

1. Provide mittens or protec-

Provide appropriate teaching for the family to prevent recurrences.

1. Wash linens in water temperature above 52°C. (120°F.) for 10 minutes or store in a closed bag for 10 days.
2. Caution against using same hairbrush and comb. Do not wear one another's hats.
3. Screen the whole family for parasitic infection.

Nurses caring for affected child should wear gloves and protective cap during ex-

(continued)

Common Skin Problems (continued)

Disorder/Organism	Clinical Manifestations	Treatment/Prevention	Specific Nursing Goals and Interventions*	Comments
Lice are transmitted by personal contact with people harboring them or through contact with articles that temporarily harbor them (clothing, bed linen) *Altered Physiology* 1. The eggs of lice (nits) are attached to the hair or clothing by a sticky substance that hardens. The eggs hatch within 1 week—the lice reach maturity within 1 month and are then capable of reproducing. 2. The lice on the skin produce itching; the longer the infestation persists, the more severe the skin reaction becomes and the more severe the lesions appear. 3. The lice live on clothing and go to the body for feeding; thus, they produce visible scratch marks and points of puncture.		2. *Pediculosis corporis* may be treated with the above plus chlorophenothane powder.	tive devices to prevent the child from scratching. 2. Trim fingernails and toenails and keep them clean. 3. Provide the child with diversional therapy to distract him from itching. 4. Hold the child frequently and release him from the protective devices.	amination and treatment.
Scabies A disease of the skin produced by the burrowing action of a parasite mite resulting in irritation and the formation of vesicles or pustules. *Etiology* 1. Scabies is caused by the itch mite, *Sarcoptes scabiei.* 2. Scabies occurs most frequently in individuals	1. Itching, particularly at night, is the primary symptom. The itching is usually very severe. 2. Scratching frequently produces secondary skin infection. 3. Systemic manifestations are absent, unless they result from the secondary infec-	Destroy the parasite, to relieve itching, and to reduce skin irritation. 1. Scrubbing, soaking, use of soap and water bath to remove scaling and crusting debris. 2. Application of a	Same as for pediculosis (see above).	Nurses caring for affected children should wear gloves. All infected members of the family should be treated at the same time.

tion (i.e., fever, leukocytosis).

living in areas of poverty, where cleanliness is lacking.

3. Scabies occurs as a result of direct contact with infected persons or by indirect contact through soiled bed linen, clothing, etc.

Altered Physiology

1. Both the male and female parasite live on the skin.

2. The female parasite burrows into the superficial skin to deposit her eggs.

3. The burrow is seen most commonly between the fingers, but may occur in any natural fold of the skin or in pressure areas (e.g., heel of palm, axillary and buttock folds, male genitalia, female breasts).

4. The burrows may occur in any part of the body in infants and small children and are easily identifiable.

5. Pruritus occurs, and the scratching of the skin may produce secondary infection. Scattered follicular eruptions contain immature mites.

6. Inflammation may produce pustules and crusts.

7. Eggs hatch in 4 days. Larvae undergo a series of molts before becoming adult. The life cycle is complete in 1–2 weeks.

Diagnosis

Presence on skin of female mite, ova, and feces.

Skin scrapings.

scabicide:

a. Lindane 1% (Kwell)—cream or lotion. Apply topically from the neck down and remove with bath after 8–12 hours.

b. Crotamiton (Eurax) cream or lotion—recommended for use in infants, because Kwell may produce neurotoxic symptoms. Massage into skin nightly 2 times; 24 hours after second application, wash off thoroughly.

c. 6%–10% precipitate of sulfur in petrolatum.

3. Contagion unlikely 24 hours after treatment.

4. Launder all clothing and bedding with sufficient heat to kill mites.

5. Itching may continue 2–3 weeks after destruction of mites. This can be controlled by using a topical antipruritic.

(continued)

Common Skin Problems *(continued)*

Disorder/Organism	Clinical Manifestations	Treatment/Prevention	Specific Nursing Goals and Interventions*	Comments
Oral Candidiasis (Thrush)/Candidal Diaper Dermatitis	*Thrush*	*Thrush*	Recognize the appearance of thrush and be aware of the infant who is particularly susceptible to the development of the condition.	
Oral candidiasis is a mycotic stomatitis characterized by the appearance of white plaques on the oral mucous membrane, the gums, and the tongue.	1. The infant develops small plaques on the oral mucous membrane, tongue, or gums; these plaques appear like curds of milk but cannot be wiped out of the mouth.	1. Oral administration of nystatin in suspension 3–4 times daily (treatment of choice). Apply over affected surfaces of oral cavity after feeding, allowing the child to swallow any medication to treat any lesions along the gastrointestinal tract.	1. Newborns and infants who have particular susceptibility include: a. Sick, debilitated infants b. Infants who are on antibiotic therapy c. Infants with cleft lip and palate, hyperparathyroidism, and neoplasms	
Candidal diaper dermatitis is a rash characterized by red, scaly, sharply circumscribed but moist patches with pustular satellite lesions.	2. Thrush often appears to cause the infant no pain or discomfort, unless the case is severe and there is erosion and ulceration of the mucosa.		2. Inspect mouth *before* every feeding for presence of thrush.	
Etiology	3. The mouth may be dry.	2. Amphotericin B, clotrimazole, or miconazole is used for candidiasis resistant to nystatin.	3. Report the appearance of thrush to the physician and record this information on the nursing record.	
1. Caused by *Candida albicans.*	4. Occasionally, the infant may appear to have some difficulty in swallowing, or eat less vigorously.			
2. Most frequently seen in newborns, but may be seen in older infants, usually as a complication of antibiotic therapy or underlying disease (malignant neoplasm, immune deficiency disorders).	5. Enteric infection is frequently associated with oral thrust.	*Diaper dermatitis*	Practice measures that prevent the development and spread of thrush.	
3. Maternal vulvovaginal candidiasis is the primary source of neonatal thrush.	*Diaper dermatitis*	1. Keep dry and clean.	1. Practice careful hand-washing techniques.	
4. The growth of the organisms is favored by: a. Lack of cleanliness b. Malnutrition c. Diabetes d. Antibiotic treatment (destroys normal flora)	1. Buttock rash consisting of erythematous maculopapular eruption with perianal distribution.	2. Topical application of nystatin or miconazole nitrate cream or ointment.	2. Practice techniques that ensure that nipples, bottles, or any other object that comes into direct or indirect contact with the infant's mouth is clean.	
	2. Generally causes discomfort, especially	3. Nystatin may be given orally if rash is persistent.		

e. Neoplasms
f. Hyperparathyroidism
5. The infection may be acquired from:
   a. Contaminated hands
   b. Contaminated feeding equipment
   c. Contaminated bedding
   d. Another patient
6. Thrush frequently occurs in children with cleft lip and palate.

Altered Physiology Thrush:
1. Spores lodge between epithelial cells and gradually separate the layers.
2. The infection then spreads to the surface of the mucous membrane.
3. Growth usually begins in several discrete areas of the oral mucous membrane, with gradual spreading to the point where a continuous membrane may be formed.

with wetting and cleanings

Lesions last approximately 2 weeks, desquamate, and resolve without residual

4. Burrow's solution compress for severe inflammation or vesiculation.

Recognize the appearance of candidal diaper dermatitis and report to physician immediately.

Teach parents the general principles of preventing diaper dermatitis.
1. Change diaper as soon as possible after wetting or soiling. Check diaper every hour in newborn. Disposable diapers are useful.
2. Wash entire diaper area thoroughly and dry area before applying clean diaper.
3. Allow the infant to go without a diaper for short periods.
4. Use clean diapers that are soft to the touch and absorbent.
5. Use terminal aseptic rinse when washing diapers to neutralize ammonia produced when infant urinates; use vinegar, Borax, or Diaparene.
6. Avoid powder and oil, which tend to clog pores and cake on skin, retaining bacteria.
7. Avoid occlusive plastic coverings, tightly pinned or double diapers, all of which tend to increase production and retention of body heat and moisture.

Bibliography

Books

Arndt KA. Manual of Dermatologic Therapies. Boston, Little, Brown & Co, 1989

Boswick JA. The Art and Science of Burn Care. Rockville, Aspen Publishers, Inc., 1987

Carvajal HF and Parks DH. Burns in Children: Pediatric Burn Management. Chicago, Year Book Medical Pub, 1988

Green M and Haggerty RJ. Ambulatory Pediatrics. 3rd ed. Philadelphia, WB Saunders, 1984

Greer KE. Common Problems in Dermatology. Chicago, Yearbook Medical Pub, 1988

Provost TT and Farmer ER. Current Therapy in Dermatology—2. Philadelphia, BC Decker, 1988

Sauer GC. Manual of Skin Diseases. 5th ed. Philadelphia, JB Lippincott, 1985

Savedra MK. Passage through hospitalization of severely burned, isolated school-age children. In Krulik T, Holaday B, Martinson I, (eds). The Child and Family Facing Life-Threatening Illness, pp 279–292. Philadelphia, JB Lippincott, 1987

Whaley LF and Wong DL. Nursing Care of Infants and Children. St. Louis, CV Mosby, 1987

Journals

Bailey SL. Electrical injuries. AORN J 1989 Mar; 49(3):773–744+

Barton LL, Friedman AD and Portilla MG. Impetigo contagiosa: A comparison of erythromycin and dicloxacillin therapy. Pediatr Dermatol 1988 May 5; (2):88–91

Bell SJ et al. Weight maintenance in pediatric burn patients. J Am Diet Assoc 1986 Feb; 86(2):207–211

Benians RC. The influence of parental visiting on survival and recovery of extensively burned children. Burns Incl Therm Inj 1988 Feb; 14(1):31–34

Beyer JE and Levin CR. Issues and advances in pain control in children. Nurs Clin North Am 1987 Sep; 22(3):661–676

Bradshaw C et al. A study of childhood scalds. Burns Incl Therm Inj 1988 Feb; 14(1):21–24

Carrigan L, Heimbach DM and Marvin JA. Risk management in children with burn injuries. J Burn Care Rehabil 1988 Jan–Feb; 9(1):75–78

Cella DF et al. Depression and stress responses in parents of burned children. J Pediatr Psychol 1988 Mar; 13(1):87–99

Cheney J. Nutrition forum: Pediatric case studies. Burn Care Rehabil 1989 Jul–Aug; 10(4):379–380

Childs C. Fever in burned children. Burns Incl Therm Inj 1988 Feb; 14(1):1–6

Childs C and Little RA. Acetaminophen (paracetamol) in the management of burned children with fever. Burns Incl Therm Inj 1988 Oct; 14(5):343–348

Egan WC and Clark WR. The toxic shock syndrome in a burn victim. Burns Incl Therm Inj 1989 Apr; 14(2):135–138

Forshaw A. Aftercare for the burned child and his family—do they need it? Burns Incl Therm Inj 1987 Oct; 13(Suppl):S22–S24

Gurevitch AW. Scabies and lice. Pediatr Clin North Am 1985 Aug; 32(4):987–1018

Hammond JS, Hickman C and Ward CG. Burns in school-age children: Demographics and burn prevention. J Burn Care Rehabil 1987 Jul–Aug; 8(4):330–332

Hebert AA. Tinea capitis. Arch Dermatol 1988 Oct; 124(10):1554–1557

Helm PA et al. Burn injury: Rehabilitation management in 1982. J Burn Care Rehabil 1982 Nov–Dec; 4(6):411–422

Herndon DH et al. Treatment of burns in children. Pediatr Clin North Am 1985 Oct; 32(5):1311–1332

Hibbard RA and Blevins R. Palatal burn due to bottle warming in a microwave oven. Pediatrics 1988 Sep; 82(3):382–384

Katcher MC, Landry GL and Shapiro MM. Liquid-crystal thermometer use in pediatric office counseling about tap water burn prevention. Pediatrics 1989 May; 83(5):766–771

Kearse HL and Miller OF. Tinea pedis in prepubertal children: Does it occur? J Am Acad Dermatol 1988 Oct; 19(4):619–622

Love B et al. Adult psychosocial adjustment following childhood injury: The effects of disfigurement. J Burn Care Rehabil 1987 Jul–Aug; 8(4):280–285

Martyn JA. Cimetidine and/or antacid for the control of gastric acidity in pediatric burn patients. Crit Care Med 1985 Jan; 13(1):1–3

Maunder JW. Insecticides in pediculosis capitis. Arch Dis Child 1989 Jan; 64(1):69–70

McGrath PJ and Vair C. Psychological aspects of pain management of the burned child. Child Health 1984 Summer; 13(1):15–19

McLoughlin E and Crawford JD. Burns. Pediatr Clin North Am 1985 Feb; 32(1):61–75

Merrell SW et al. Fluid resuscitation in thermally injured children. Am J Surg 1986 Dec; 152(6):664–669

Montrey JS and Barcia PJ. Nonaccidental burns in child abuse. South Med J 1985 Nov; 78(11):1324–1326

Nichter LS et al. Scalp infections in black children: Think Kerion. Plast Reconstr Surg 1987 Nov; 80(5):717–719

Purdue GF, Hunt JL and Prescott PR. Child abuse by burning—An index of suspicion. J Trauma 1988 Feb; 28(2):221–224

Quay NB and Alexander LL. Preparation of burned children and their families for discharge. J Burn Care Rehabil 1983 Jul–Aug; 4(4):288–290

Reid WH et al. Hypertrophic scarring and pressure therapy. Burns Incl Thermal Inj 1987 Oct; 13(Suppl):S29–32

Roche J and Jackson D. Developing a patient/family burn unit information booklet. J Burn Care Rehabil 1983 Nov–Dec; 4(6):451–452

Rosenstein DL. A school reentry program for burned children. Part I: Development and implementation of a school reentry program. J Burn Care Rehabil 1987 Jul–Aug; 8(4):319–322

Sarov B et al. Evaluation of an intervention program for head lice infestation in school children. Pediatr Infect Dis J 1988 Mar; 7(3):176–179

Schachner L and Gonzalez A. Impetigo: A reassessment of etiology and therapy (Letter). Pediatr Dermatol 1988 May; 5(2):139

Showers J and Garrison KM. Burn abuse: A four-year study. J Trauma 1988 Nov; 28(11):1581–1583

Slater SJ, Slater H and Goldfarb IW. Burned children: A socioeconomic profile for focused prevention programs. J Burn Care Rehabil 1987 Nov–Dec; 8(6):566–567

Tanz RR, Hebert AA and Esterly NB. Treating tinea capitis: Should Ketoconazole replace griseofulvin? J Pediatr 1988 Jun; 112(6):987–991

Tweddell JS et al. Hematuria in the burned child. J Pediatr Surg 1987 Oct; 22(10):899–903

Varas R, Carbone R and Hammond JS. A one-hour burn prevention program for grade school children: Its approach and success. J Burn Care Rehabil 1988 Jan–Feb; 9(1):69–71

Veien NK et al. Oral challenge with food additives. Contact Dermatitis 1987 Aug; 17(2):100–103

Verbov J. Has impetigo in children disappeared? Practitioner 1987 May 8; 231(1429):645

Wilson GR, Fowler CA and Housden PL. A new burn assessment chart. Burns Incl Therm Inj 1987 Oct; 13(5):401–403

Zoberman-Saltiel E. Patchy alopecia in a young girl. Arch Dermatol 1989 Jan; 125(1):113, 116

Additional Reading

Neale HW et al. Complications of controlled tissue expansion in the pediatric burn patient. Plast Reconstr Surg 1988 Nov; 82(5):840–848

Youel L et al. Skeletal suspension in the management of severe burns in children. J Bone Joint Surg 1986 Dec; 68(9):1375–1379

Zambori WA, Cassidy M and Eriksson E. Hand burns in children under 5 years of age. Burns Incl Therm Inj 1987 Dec; 13(6):476–483

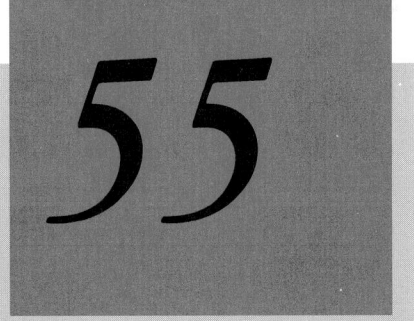

Major Endocrine Disorders of Childhood

Gland	Disorder	Etiology
Anterior pituitary	Growth retardation, dwarfism	Growth hormone deficiency
	Tall stature (Pituitary gigantism)	Growth hormone excess
Posterior pituitary	Diabetes insipidus (see p. 1402)	Vasopressin (antidiuretic hormone) deficiency
Thyroid	Hypothyroidism	Thyroxine (T_4) and triiodothyronine (T_3)
	Cretinism (see p. 535)	deficiency*
	Thyrotoxicosis (see p. 1405)	Thyroxine and triiodothyronine excess*
Parathyroid	Hypoparathyroidism (hypocalcemia, tetany, increased serum phosphorus)	Parathyroid hormone (PTH) deficiency
	Hyperparathyroidism (hypercalcemia, hypophosphatemia [rare in children])	Parathyroid hormone excess
Islets of Langerhans of pancreas	Diabetes mellitus (see below)	Insulin deficiency
Adrenal cortex	Adrenal insufficiency	Deficiency of adrenal hormones*
	Addison's disease (weakness, fatigue, weight loss, pigmentation of skin)	
	Cushing's syndrome (obesity of the face, trunk, and abdomen)	Cortisol excess*
	Adrenogenital syndrome	Androgen excess*
	Ambiguous genitalia (see p. 1373)	
Ovaries	Lack of or repressed female sexual development	Estrogen deficiency*
	Precocious puberty of female	Estrogen excess*
Testes	Delayed male sexual development	Testosterone deficiency*
	Eunuchoidism	
	Precocious puberty of male	Testosterone excess*

* May also result from deficiency or excess of appropriate stimulating hormones from the anterior pituitary (that is, thyrotropin [TSH], adrenocorticotropic hormone [ACTH], gonadotropins, follicle-stimulating hormone [FSH], luteinizing hormone [LH]).

Diabetes Mellitus

Diabetes mellitus is a disorder of carbohydrate metabolism resulting in high serum levels of glucose and the spilling of glucose in the urine. The disease is also associated with abnormal metabolism of fat and protein. With few exceptions, diabetes in children is of the type I insulin-dependent variety.

Etiology

1. Believed to be related to inheritance of certain HLA antigens that predispose an individual to autoimmune destruction of pancreatic islets.
2. Viral infection has been suggested as a triggering factor in individuals with a genetic predisposition for diabetes.

Incidence

1. Diabetes mellitus is the most common endocrine disorder of children.
2. Affects approximately 1.9 per 1,000 school-age children.
3. Age-related peaks of presentation occur among 5–7-year-olds and at puberty.

Altered Physiology

1. The pancreas produces an insufficient amount of insulin.
2. The body is unable to oxidize glucose properly.

3. Hyperglycemia results from the deficient oxidation of glucose and the inability of tissues to use glucose as fuel.
4. Glucosuria results when the serum level of glucose exceeds the renal threshold.
5. Diuresis is initiated and may progress to dehydration and impaired renal function.
6. Protein and fat are oxidized at abnormal rates.
7. Ketones accumulate in the blood when fat is oxidized at abnormal rates.
8. Ketones are excreted in the urine.
9. Acidosis occurs when ketosis is severe enough to lower the CO_2-combining power of the blood. Diabetic coma may result.

Clinical Manifestations

1. Rapid onset (usually over a period of a few weeks)
2. Major symptoms
   a. Increased thirst
   b. Increased urination, enuresis
   c. Increased food ingestion
   d. Weight loss
   e. Fatigue
3. Minor symptoms
   a. Skin infections
   b. Dry skin
   c. Monilial vaginitis in adolescent girls
4. Diabetic acidosis
   a. Precomatose state
   Drowsiness
   Dryness of skin
   Cherry red lips
   Increased respirations
   Nausea
   Vomiting
   Abdominal pain
   b. Comatose state
   Extreme hyperpnea (Kussmaul breathing)
   Soft, sunken eyeballs
   Rigid abdomen
   Rapid, weak pulse
   Decreased temperature
   Decreased blood pressure
   c. Circulatory collapse and renal failure may follow, resulting from the combination of lowered pH, electrolyte deficiency, and dehydration.
5. Side effects
   a. Stunting of growth

Complications

(Appear to be related to the degree of control of diabetes)
1. Retinopathy and cataracts
2. Neuropathy
3. Renal disease
4. Increased incidence of gangrene, myocardial infarction, and stroke

Patient Problems and Nursing Diagnoses

1. Potential complications: diabetic ketoacidosis and hypoglycemic reactions related to imbalances between insulin requirements and supply
2. Potential impaired skin integrity related to daily administration of insulin
3. Potential nutritional imbalance related to problems in following a regulated diet plan
4. Self-concept, disturbance in body image related to

limits imposed by treatment, stunting of growth, and delayed puberty
5. Growth and development, altered, related to prolonged dependence on parents because of treatment regimen
6. Knowledge deficit of parents and child regarding diabetes and its management

Nursing Interventions

A. Recognizing Signs of Diabetic Acidosis (see Clinical Manifestations) **and Providing Supportive Care to the Child Should This Develop.**

1. Be aware of common causes of diabetic acidosis
   a. Untreated diabetes
   b. Inadequate insulin coverage
   c. Failure to adhere to the prescribed diet
   d. Chronic or repeated infections
   e. Stress
   f. Vomiting
2. Apply the principles of nursing care of the comatose child (see Nursing the Unconscious Patient, p. 575).
3. Maintain intravenous therapy (see IV Procedure, p. 1167).
   a. Be prepared to administer intravenous sodium bicarbonate if $pH < 7.2$ (use somewhat controversial).
   b. Have intravenous glucose available should the child suddenly become hypoglycemic.
   Care is taken to avoid reducing the blood glucose to hypoglycemic levels.
   c. Parenteral fluids may need to be changed frequently because of continued polyuria and results of electrolyte determinations.
4. Be prepared to administer relatively large quantities of regular insulin.
   a. A variety of acceptable formulas are available for insulin therapy.
   b. A recent technique involves:
      (1) IV push injection of 0.1 unit of insulin per kg. body weight.
      (2) This is followed by a constant infusion of 0.1 unit of insulin per kg. body weight per hour until blood glucose reaches 300 mg./dl.
      (3) Insulin infusion is then discontinued, IV is changed to $D_{5\frac{1}{2}}NS$, and sliding-scale insulin therapy is begun.
5. Insert a nasogastric tube to relieve abdominal distention and prevent vomiting.
6. Monitor urine output exactly.
   Test each specimen for ketones.
7. Provide emotional support to the child and his family.
   a. Respond immediately to the child's needs for physical comfort.
   b. Discuss the child's treatment plan and expected response with his parents to alleviate their anxiety.
8. Reinstitute oral feedings when the child is sufficiently responsive and can tolerate them.
   a. This is usually after 12–16 hours of parenteral therapy.
   b. Begin with a low-fat, liquid diet.
   Observe closely for signs of insulin shock or recurrent acidosis once oral feedings are reinstituted.
9. Begin a teaching program with the child and family as soon as possible to allay their worries concerning physical status, prognosis, and treatment.
10. Documentation of all teaching sessions should include

the material presented, the child and family's responses, and further areas of need.

B. Providing a Diet Adequate for the Child's Normal Growth and Development and Sufficient to Satisfy His Appetite.

1. Nutritional requirements are determined by the child's symptomatology, family and cultural characteristics, and physician preference.
   a. Most prescribed diets are of the unmeasured type. The diet plan eliminates concentrated sweets, follows recommended allowances from all of the 4 basic food groups, but otherwise does not require measuring or rigidity.
   b. Occasionally a more rigid, strictly controlled diet is necessary.
   c. The diet should be composed of approximately 55% carbohydrate, 30% fat, and 15% protein.
      (1) Most diets are restricted in carbohydrates, saturated fats, and cholesterol, and may be based on the exchange method as recommended by the American Diabetes Association.
      (2) Approximately 70% of the carbohydrate content should be derived from complex carbohydrates such as starch.
      (3) Foods with high fiber content should be encouraged.
      (4) All diets must supply sufficient caloric intake for activity and growth, sufficient protein for growth, and the required vitamins and minerals.
   d. Foods are distributed throughout the day to accommodate varying peak action of insulin. Distribution may be adjusted for increased or decreased amounts of exercise.
2. Determine the child's usual dietary habits so that adherence to his controlled diet will be easier.
3. Include the child and his parents in his meal planning as soon as possible.
4. Allow the child normal activity while hospitalized so that the observed result of his dietary control will be valid. Because the child's activity level usually decreases during the hospital stay, the child and family must understand that the insulin and dietary needs will alter on discharge.
5. Allow the child to eat with other children.
6. Make certain that the child adheres to his prescribed diet and understands the rationale for this.

C. Administering Insulin in an Amount Adequate to Maintain the Child's Approximate Glycemic Equilibrium.

1. The dosage and kinds of insulin are determined from the results of blood glucose monitoring.
   a. Generally, a combination of about ⅓ short-acting insulin and ⅔ intermediate-acting insulin are prescribed, to be administered either once or twice daily.
2. Insulin should be given ½ hour before breakfast. If split-dose insulin is prescribed, it should be given ½ hour before breakfast and ½ hour before the evening meal.
3. Be aware of the major types of insulin and their effect (Table 55-1).
4. Develop a systematic plan for injections that emphasizes rotation of sites. In this way, it will be several weeks before it is necessary to return to the same site.

   a. The upper arms and thighs are the most acceptable sites for injection in children, but the outer areas of the abdomen or hips may also be used.
   b. A diagram showing injection sites should be used to maintain the rotation (Fig. 55-1).
      The sites can be checked off each day until the routine is familiar.
   c. Injections are begun at an upper corner of the area to be used.
   d. Subsequent injections are given about 2.5 cm. (1 inch) apart, working in rows.
   e. When all rows in one area are completed, injections are begun in the next area.
   f. Guidelines for site location:
      (1) *Arms*—Begin below the deltoid muscle and end one hand breadth above the elbow. Begin at the midline and progress outward laterally using the external surface only.
      (2) *Thighs*—Begin 1 hand breadth below the hip and end 1 hand breadth above the knee. Begin at the midline and progress outward laterally, using only the outer, anterior surface.
      (3) *Abdomen*—Avoid the beltline and 1 inch around the umbilicus.
      (4) *Buttocks*—Use the upper outer quadrant of the buttocks.
5. Be certain that the measuring scale of the syringe matches the unit strength on the bottle of insulin.
   a. Insulin is available in strengths of 40, 80, and 100 units per ml.
   b. U-100 insulin is preferred, as it allows the smallest possible amount to be given.
   c. New purified forms of insulin are available, but should not be used unless recommended by the physician because use may require a decrease in insulin dose.
6. Use insulin that is at room temperature.
   a. The bottle in use may be kept at room temperature without losing appreciable strength.
   b. Extra bottles should be stored in the refrigerator.
7. Mix the solution by rotating the vial between the hands. Do not shake vigorously.
8. Administer insulin subcutaneously to promote absorption.
9. Following injection, exert firm pressure with an alcohol sponge to prevent bleeding.
10. Observe the skin closely for signs of irritation. Avoid the injection site for several weeks if signs of local irritation are observed.
11. Observe the skin for a rash indicating an allergic reaction to the insulin. Notify the physician immediately if there is an allergic reaction.
12. Be aware of factors that vary the need for and utilization of insulin, particularly exercise and infection.

Table 55-1. *Types of Insulin and Their Effects*

Type of Insulin	Onset (hours)	Maximal Activity (hours)	Duration (hours)
Regular	½–1	2–4	6–8
Semi-Lente	½–1	2–4	10–12
NPH	2	4–12	24
Lente	2	8–10	24
Ultralente	4–8	14–20	36

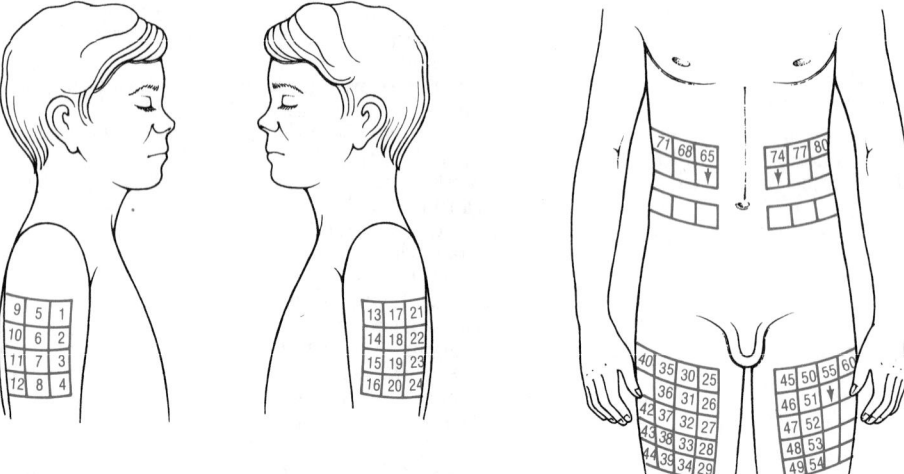

Figure 55-1. *Rotating injection sites for insulin in the pediatric patient.*

a. Exercise
  (1) Tends to lower the blood sugar level.
  (2) Encourage normal activity, regulated in amount and time.
b. Infection or illness
  (1) Increases the child's insulin requirement (Insulin is still administered during sick times.)
  (2) Be alert for signs of infection and dehydration.
13. Encourage the child to express his feelings about the injections.
  The child may be helped to master his fear of injections by gaining control of the situation through play and active participation in the procedure.
14. Insulin can also be administered by constant, subcutaneous infusion using a pump.
  a. The pump delivers fixed small amounts of insulin continuously.
  b. Before meals, the child (or parent) uses the pump to deliver a bolus dose of insulin.
  c. The amount of insulin is adjusted by the child (or parent) based on self-monitoring of blood glucose.
  d. Because of the expense and commitment required, pump therapy is most suited to older children and adolescents who have experienced control problems with conventional insulin therapy.
    Parents should be advised to determine if costs are covered by health insurance policy.

D. Being Aware of the Symptoms and Treatment of Hypoglycemic Reactions.

1. Common causes
  a. Overdose of insulin
  b. Reduction in diet or increased exercise without sufficient caloric coverage
2. Symptoms

Trembling	Drowsiness
Shaking	Odd behavior
Sweating	Mental confusion
Apprehension	Seizures
Tachycardia	Coma
Hunger	

3. Be prepared to give orange juice or other food containing readily available simple sugars.

4. Have glucose available for intravenous injection or glucagon available for intramuscular or subcutaneous injection.

E. Monitoring the Child's Blood Glucose Level to Evaluate Diabetic Control, and Adjusting Insulin Dosage and Nutritional Needs.

1. This method has become the means for monitoring control.
2. The procedure requires a drop of blood, obtained by finger stick, a reagent strip, and a reflectance meter.
3. Specific instructions for performing the procedure vary with the equipment being used and must be followed explicitly.
4. Blood glucose measurements are usually made 4 times per day, before meals and at bedtime.
5. Additional blood tests are helpful during episodes of hypoglycemic symptoms or other problem situations.
6. Urine tests for ketones should be continued if the child is ill or if blood glucose is greater than 240 mg./ 100 ml.
7. Record the results of blood glucose testing accurately.
  a. Use a standard form for recording so that the information will be clear and readily available.
  b. Help the child to understand how his disease is controlled by teaching him to test his own blood, record results, and report information to health care personnel or parents.

F. Preventing Infection.

1. Bathe daily.
2. Maintain meticulous skin care through such activities as frequent ambulation of the child and application of body lotion.
3. Keep fingernails and toenails clean and well trimmed.
4. Provide prompt treatment for any violations of the skin (bruises, abrasions, lacerations, etc.).

G. Fostering Acceptance on the Part of the Child That He is a Normal, Healthy Person and Able to Compete With His Peers.

1. Include the child and his parents in the treatment plan in its earliest stages.
2. Emphasize that daily management of his disease can become as routine as matters of personal hygiene.

3. Permit and encourage the development of the child's natural talents. Do not allow him to use his disease as a crutch.
4. Allow the child independence in his care as soon as possible, but provide the necessary direction.
5. Initiate a teaching program for the child and his parents early. Offer them available literature.
6. If appropriate, group diabetic children together on the unit. Initiate group discussions for diabetic adolescents.
7. Invite the parents to join a group of parents of diabetic children if such a group is available in the area.
8. Initiate a community nursing referral if the parents or the child appears apprehensive or seems to lack confidence.

Health Education

Patient or parental education is one of the most important aspects in the nursing care of the diabetic child. Thorough instruction is essential in the following areas:

1. Influence of exercise, emotional stress, and other illnesses on both insulin and diet needs.
2. Recognition of the symptoms of insulin shock and diabetic acidosis and knowledge of related emergency management
3. Prevention of infection
   a. Attend to regular body hygiene with special attention to foot care.
   b. Report any breaks in the skin. Treat them promptly.
   c. Use only properly fitted shoes; do not wear vinyl or plastic, which do not permit ventilation. Avoid calluses and blisters.
   d. Dress the child appropriately for the weather.
   e. See that the child receives regular dental checkups and maintenance every 6 months.
   f. Follow routine immunizations according to the recommended schedule.
4. Blood testing
   a. Demonstrate the procedure.
   b. Have the child and his parent demonstrate to the nurse.
   c. Allow the child to do the procedure under supervision until his accuracy is certain.
   d. Encourage the child to assume responsibility for his own blood testing.
   e. Help the child to develop an easy method of recording blood glucose results.
      A record should be used that includes blood test results, kind and amount of insulin given, and additional remarks, such as child's activity, insulin reactions, etc.
   f. Be certain the parents understand what results are desirable for the child and the appropriate action to take when test results are other than those desired.
5. Administration of insulin
   a. Both the child and his parents should be taught how to do this procedure and what effects the various forms of insulin have.
   b. Give parents an opportunity to express their feelings about the injection.
   c. Explain the procedure simply and demonstrate it.
   d. Discuss the procedure for rotation of sites and the rationale for this method.
   e. Allow the parent and child to practice by injecting normal saline into the nurse.
   f. Have the parent inject his child under supervision.
   g. Have the child inject himself.

(1) Most children over the age of 8 can be taught to give insulin to themselves.
(2) Generally, the earlier this responsibility is given to the child, the easier it is for him.
   h. Carefully check the dosage measured by the child and his parent until you are certain of their accuracy.
   i. Complete a community nursing referral for assistance with this procedure at home if indicated.
6. Diet
   a. Review the prescribed diet with the family.
   b. Discuss acceptable modifications of exchanges.
   c. Allow the child to manage his own diet as early as possible.
   d. Emphasize that the diet is based on normal household foods. The purchase of special, expensive dietetic foods is usually not necessary.
   e. Stress that food labels must be scrutinized. A label of "dietetic" or "low-calorie" does not necessarily mean that the food is acceptable for the child.
   f. Inform the parents and children of the exchange lists available from many of the national fast-food restaurants.
7. Precautionary measures
   a. Have the child carry with him an identifying card that states that he has diabetes and includes his name, address, telephone number, and his physician's name and telephone number.
   b. See that the child has orange juice, a lump of sugar, or a bar of candy available in case of an insulin reaction.
   c. Have the family discuss the child's disease with the school nurse and with other responsible adults who are in close contact with the child (teachers, scout leaders, etc.).
   d. Advise the parents that vials of insulin should be kept on one's person when traveling, because baggage may be subjected to extreme temperatures and pressures incompatible with the stability of insulin. If necessary, a thermos can be used to keep the insulin at the appropriate temperature.
8. Teaching materials and Resources for Children and Parents:
   Faro B et al. *Diabetic Teaching Manual for Children and Parents*. Unpublished manuscript. University of Rochester, School of Nursing, Rochester, NY 14642
   Kipnis L and Adler S. *You Can't Catch Diabetes From A Friend*. Gainesville, Triad Scientific Publishers, 1979
   Travis LB. *An Instructional Aid on Juvenile Diabetes Mellitus,* 6th ed. Galveston, Department of Pediatrics, University of Texas, Medical Branch, 1980
9. Agency:
   American Diabetes Association
   2 Park Avenue
   New York, NY 10020

Expected Outcomes

1. Blood glucose levels stay within normal range (no signs of ketoacidosis or hypoglycemia); carries identification stating diabetic condition; carries candy bar to offset potential insulin reaction
2. Child's skin remains intact without signs of irritation or infection
3. Child adheres to treatment regimen, demonstrates the proper method of insulin administration; adheres to diet restriction
4. Maintains healthy self-concept; participates in self-care, engages in normal activities for age; works toward independence

5. Assumes age-appropriate responsibility for his own care (A reasonable expectation is for total independence by the age of 12–13 years.)
6. The parents and child demonstrate understanding of the essentials of diabetes care; insulin administration; diet; infection control; signs of hypoglycemia; blood and urine testing; precautionary measures to avoid insulin reaction

Diabetes Insipidus

Diabetes insipidus is a disorder of water metabolism caused by a deficiency of vasopressin, the antidiuretic hormone (ADH) secreted by the posterior pituitary.

Etiology

1. Deficient secretion of vasopressin (antidiuretic hormone)
   a. Primary
      (1) Genetic transmission (autosomal dominant or X-linked inheritance)
      (2) Idiopathic (occurring without a known cause)
   b. Secondary
      (1) Brain tumors, especially those in the hypothalamic area (most frequent cause)
      (2) CNS malformation or degenerative disease
      (3) Head trauma or neurosurgery
      (4) General trauma—accidental or surgical
      (5) Infections of the central nervous system—i.e., meningitis or encephalitis
      (6) Vascular disease—aneurysm, thrombosis
      (7) Granulomatous disease
2. Failure of the renal tubules to respond to vasopressin (nephrogenic diabetes insipidus)
   a. Hereditary (X-linked) disease
   b. Found almost exclusively in males

Altered Physiology

1. Vasopressin normally acts on the distal tubules and collecting ducts of the kidney to facilitate reabsorption of water.
2. Pathology of the pituitary or hypothalamus results in a deficiency of vasopressin.
3. The kidney is unable to produce a concentrated urine without sufficient vasopressin.
4. Nephrogenic diabetes insipidus
   a. Vasopressin secretion is normal.
   b. The renal tubules do not respond to vasopressin.
   c. The kidney is unable to produce a concentrated urine.

Clinical Manifestations

1. Onset—usually sudden
2. Symptoms
   a. Depend on the age of the child, the extent of vasopressin deficiency, and the primary lesion
   b. Universal symptoms
      (1) Polydipsia (excessive thirst)
      (2) Polyuria (excessive urine output)
      (3) Inability to concentrate urine
   c. Symptoms in infants
      (1) Excessive crying (quieted with water rather than additional milk)
      (2) Hyperthermia
      (3) Vomiting
      (4) Constipation
      (5) Rapid weight loss
      (6) Dehydration
      (7) Growth failure
   d. Symptoms in older children
      (1) Excessive thirst, which may interfere with play and sleep
      (2) Enuresis, and/or nocturia
      (3) Anorexia
      (4) Pale and dry skin
      (5) Reduced sweating
      (6) Viscid saliva

Diagnostic Evaluation

A. Water Deprivation Test

1. After a 24-hour period of adequate hydration and stable weight, fluids are restricted for 6 hours.
2. Urine volumes and osmolality and the child's weights are recorded hourly.
3. Serum sodium and osmolality are measured at the beginning and end of the test.
4. Persistent excretion of dilute urine, a rise in serum sodium (>145 mEq./liter) and serum osmolality (>290 mOsm./kg.), and a weight loss of 3%–5% are suggestive of diabetes insipidus.

NURSING ALERT: The test should be terminated if weight loss approaches 5%, indicating moderate dehydration.

B. Vasopressin Sensitivity Test

1. A reduction of urine flow and an increase in urine concentration are observed following the administration of antidiuretic hormone.
2. This test should be used after it has been demonstrated that the child is unable to concentrate urine during the water deprivation test.

C. Skull X-Ray—To Detect a Tumor

D. Kidney Function Tests

E. Blood Electrolyte Levels—To Rule Out Renal Failure

F. Endocrine Studies

Nursing Interventions

A. Participating in the Diagnostic Evaluation of Diabetes Insipidus.

1. Explain the purpose of appropriate laboratory tests and the protocol that the child and family will be asked to follow.
2. Supervise the child closely to avoid surreptitious fluid intake during fasting periods.
3. Observe the child closely for evidence of fluid and electrolyte disturbances while the test is in progress.
   a. Dehydration and shock may occur in severely affected children during the water deprivation test.
   b. Overhydration may occur in patients with primary psychogenic polydipsia during the vasopressin sensitivity test.
4. Collect urine specimens as requested by the physician.

B. Preventing Dehydration and Restoring Electrolyte Balance.

1. Nursing actions when the disorder is caused by a deficiency of vasopressin.
   a. DDAVP (a synthetic analog of vasopressin), is the drug of choice for replacement therapy.

(1) Dosage-regulated by trial for each child; goal is to eliminate polyuria except for brief periods prior to the next dose
(2) Route of administration—nasal spray
(3) Duration—8–24 hours, depending on the child's state of hydration
(4) Special precautions
    (a) If the child is treated with a single, daily dose, it should be given in the evening, so that polyuria will not interfere with sleep or school.
    (b) Excess mucus such as occurs with upper respiratory infections or allergic rhinitis may interfere with hormone absorption.
  b. Pitressin tannate in oil may also be used as replacement therapy. It has the advantage of being much less expensive.
    (1) Dosage—regulated by trial for each child
    (2) Route of administration—intramuscular injection
    (3) Duration—approximately 48 hours
    (4) Special precautions
        (a) Careful attention must be given to adequate suspension of the pitressin tannate in oil.
        (b) Hold the ampule under hot water to reduce the viscosity of the suspending medium. (Immersion of the ampule in boiling water destroys the hormone.)
        (c) Shake the ampule vigorously until the active ingredient is smoothly dispersed.
        (d) Inject the medication with a 2.5-cm. (1-inch) No. 20-22 gauge needle.
        (e) Inject the medication deeply into the muscle.
        (f) Establish a pattern of systematic rotation of injection sites—maintain a daily record of these sites and teach the parents to document the rotation of the sites.

NURSING ALERT: Water intoxication is a dangerous complication if Pitressin is given too frequently.

---

  c. Aqueous vasopressin is available as a nasal spray, but the duration of action is so brief that administration is required every 3–4 hours.
2. Nursing actions when the disorder is caused by failure of the kidney to respond to vasopressin.
  a. Administration of Pitressin is ineffective.
    These children already produce a sufficient quantity of vasopressin.
  b. Administer water at frequent intervals and in sufficient volume to prevent dehydration.
  c. Administer a low-sodium, low-solute residue diet to reduce the osmolar load on the kidney.
  d. Administer thiazide therapy as prescribed by the physician.
    This causes sodium diuresis, which acts to promote proximal tubular sodium reabsorption.

C. Observing and Recording the Child's Response to Therapy.
1. Intake and output
  a. Total the intake and output record every 8 hours.
  b. Record daily weight
  c. Record the urine specific gravity of each voiding.
2. Temperature—be alert for the development of fever.

3. Skin turgor—decreased skin turgor is sign of dehydration.
4. Color
5. Appetite—record the child's intake accurately with each meal.

D. Providing Emotional Support to the Family.
Prognosis depends on the underlying condition.
1. Hereditary and idiopathic types—favorable with adequate treatment.
2. Trauma—spontaneous recovery often occurs.
3. Tumor
  a. Varies with the site of the lesion and type of tumor.
  b. Needs of the family accentuated by many problems including surgery and facing the death of the child.

Health Education

1. Explain the condition with specific clarification that diabetes insipidus and diabetes mellitus are very different disorders.
2. Teach the parents the correct procedure for preparation and administration of vasopressin.
3. Encourage the child to assume full responsibility for his care when he is old enough.
4. The child should wear a Medic-Alert tag that identifies his condition.
5. The older child should carry nasal spray for temporary relief of symptoms if necessary.
6. School personnel and other significant adults should be made aware of the child's problem.

Hypothyroidism

Hypothyroidism is an endocrine disease resulting from deficient production of thyroid hormone. It may be either congenital (cretinism) or acquired.

Etiology

A. Congenital
1. Embryonic defect with partial or complete absence of the thyroid gland
2. Defect in the synthesis of thyroid hormone
3. Destruction of fetal thyroid as a result of antigen–antibody reaction
4. Iodide deficiency (endemic cretinism)
5. Toxic substances encountered during pregnancy causing maldevelopment or atrophy of the fetal thyroid gland. These may rarely include some medications administered during pregnancy.

B. Acquired
1. Chronic lymphocytic thyroiditis
2. Subacute thyroiditis
3. Medications
  a. Iodides
  b. Thiouracil
4. Thyroidectomy
5. Hypothalamic or pituitary disease
6. Peripheral resistance to thyroid hormones
7. Congenital thyroid disorders that do not decompensate until later childhood, appearing acquired

Altered Physiology

Same as in the adult. (p. 535)

Clinical Manifestations

1. Depend on age at onset, the specific defect, the extent of thyroid deficiency, and its duration
2. Congenital hypothyroidism
   a. Clinical manifestations usually nonspecific and subtle
   b. Prolonged jaundice
   c. Lethargy
   d. Constipation
   e. Feeding problems
   f. Cool to touch
   g. Poor muscle tone—umbilical hernia
   h. Hoarse cry
   i. Hypotonia, slow reflexes
   j. Dry skin
3. Acquired hypothyroidism
   a. Decreased growth rate
   b. Goiter
   c. Increase in upper to lower body segment ratio
   d. Delayed dentition
   e. Mild obesity
   f. Delayed puberty
   g. Developmental delay
   h. Decreased school performance
4. Classic signs and symptoms of untreated hypothyroidism
   a. Generalized puffiness
   b. Skin—dry, thick, scaly, coarse, cool, and pale
   c. Facial characteristics
      (1) Bridge of nose—flat, broad, and undeveloped
      (2) Eyes—widely spaced with swollen eyelids
      (3) Anterior fontanelle widely open
      (4) Tongue—thick and protruding
   d. Hair—frequently dry, coarse, brittle, slow-growing
   e. Short stature
   f. Slow pulse and decreased blood pressure
   g. Protuberant abdomen and buttocks
   h. Delayed reflexes
   i. Dull, placid expression
   j. Poor appetite
   k. Constipation
   l. Lethargy
   m. Delayed motor and mental development
5. Clinical manifestations may be delayed in breast-fed infants until the child is weaned because of the thyroid hormone contained in breast milk.

Diagnostic Evaluation

1. X-ray shows retarded bone age.
2. Thyroid function test results are abnormal.
3. Thyroid scan reveals decreased uptake.
4. Neonatal screening is possible and is mandatory in most states.

Prognosis

1. Depends on the child's age at onset and the effectiveness of his therapy.
2. Congenital hypothyroidism is one of the most common preventable causes of mental retardation.
   a. If untreated, mentally deficient dwarf results.
   b. When treated:
      (1) Normal physical growth and development can occur.
      (2) Mental development can be normal.
         (a) The best results are obtained by giving continuous, full therapy as early as possible (within the first 3–6 weeks of life).

         (b) The best outlook is for children who have active thyroid tissue during the fetal life, have adequate treatment, and show a high family intelligence quotient.
3. Acquired hypothyroidism
   a. Risk of permanent intellectual impairment is small if hypothyroidism develops beyond age 2 or 3 years.
   b. All changes should be reversible.

Nursing Interventions

A. Administering Replacement Therapy for the Deficient Hormone.

1. Sodium-1-thyroxine is the most reliable replacement therapy.
2. Dosage
   a. Individualized for each child.
   b. Adjusted according to clinical response and results of thyroid function tests.
   c. Goal is to achieve normal growth and development.
3. Route of administration
   a. Always administer thyroid replacement orally.
   b. The tablet may be crushed and mixed with fruit for infants.
4. Special precautions
   a. The total daily requirement is given as a single dose.
   b. Administer the medication at the same time each day.
5. Observe for toxic effects.
   a. Excitability
   b. Nervousness
   c. Tachycardia
   d. Tremors
   e. Cramps

B. Providing a Complete, Well-Balanced Diet.

1. Special problems related to nutrition
   a. Increased skeletal development
      (1) Increases the need for additional vitamin D.
      (2) Encourage the child to drink 3–4 glasses of milk daily.
   b. Constipation
      Provide foods that are high in fiber such as raw fruits and vegetables.
2. Determine the child's dietary preferences and use this information to plan his menus.
   a. Include the child in menu planning when this is possible.
   b. See the section on nutrition, page 1102.

C. Providing Emotional Support to the Child and His Family.

1. Assess the child's capabilities and establish realistic expectations and limits.
2. Assist the parents to adjust to alterations in their child's behavior as he responds to treatment.
   The child may develop new enthusiasm for the naturally disturbing antics of childhood.
3. Allow the parents to discuss their feelings about the child's condition. Parents often feel guilty that they misinterpreted the child's symptoms, resulting in delayed treatment.

D. Providing Support to the Parents of a Mentally Retarded Child.

(See the section on mental retardation, p. 1502.)

Health Education

A. Medication

1. Give the medication at the same time every day.
2. Adjust the dosage (by the physician) to the needs of each individual child.
   a. Regular medical follow-up and frequent reevaluation are essential.
   b. Dose may have to be increased during puberty and the reproductive period.
3. Observe for signs of drug toxicity, especially rapid pulse, irritability, insomnia, fever, sweating, and weight loss. Teach parents how to measure the pulse and to consult the physician if the rate is above a certain value.
4. The medication must be continued throughout life.
5. Allow the parents to administer the medication during the child's hospitalization so that they will gain confidence in their ability to carry out the procedure.
6. Encourage parents to help the child accept increasing responsibility for his medications as he grows older.

Thyrotoxicosis *(Graves' Disease)*

Thyrotoxicosis is an endocrine disease resulting from an excessive secretion of thyroid hormone. It is frequently characterized by an enlarged thyroid gland (goiter) and prominent eyeballs (exophthalmos).

Etiology

1. Autoimmune process—most common
   a. Probable genetic basis
   b. Occasionally precipitated by stress
2. Tumors
3. Inappropriate secretion of thyroid-stimulating hormone (TSH)

Altered Physiology

Same as in the adult. (See Chapter 22.)

Clinical Manifestations

1. Rare and less severe in children as compared with adults.
2. More common in females than males.
3. Onset is usually between 10 and 15 years of age (usually gradual onset).
4. Signs and symptoms
   a. Enlarged thyroid gland (goiter)
   b. Exophthalmos accompanied by
      (1) Wide eye staring
      (2) Increased blinking
      (3) Drooping eyelids
      (4) Lack of convergence
      (5) Absence of wrinkling of forehead when looking up
   c. Nervousness and motor hyperactivity
      (1) Inability to sit still
      (2) Decreased attention span
      (3) Mood shifts
          Irritable
          Excitable
          Cries easily
      (4) Tremors
   d. Increased appetite and food intake
   e. Weight loss or no weight gain
   f. Heat intolerance
   g. Skin
      (1) Warm
      (2) Moist
      (3) Flushed
   h. Muscular weakness and fatigue
   i. Tachycardia, palpitation, and dyspnea
   j. Increased systolic blood pressure; increased pulse pressure
   k. Accelerated growth rate
   l. Delayed sexual maturation
   m. Possible amenorrhea in females
   n. Thyroid "crisis" or "storm" (very rare in children)
   o. Insomnia
   p. Vomiting
   q. Frequent bowel elimination
   r. Fine hair

Diagnostic Evaluation

1. High serum levels of T_4 and T_3
2. Radioactive iodine uptake—rapid
3. Thyroid antibody titers—increased

Treatment

1. Antithyroid drugs (recommended initial treatment)
2. Destruction of thyroid by radioiodine (not advocated until the child has reached maturity)
3. Subtotal thyroidectomy

Prognosis

1. Permanent remission using medical therapy is achieved in 36–61% of children.
2. Predictors of recurrence
   a. Noncompliance with medical therapy
   b. Long history of illness
   c. Large goiter
   d. Severe toxicity
   e. Strongly positive microsomal titer
3. Recurrences are generally treated surgically

Nursing Interventions

Nursing care of the child with hyperthyroidism is similar to that of the adult (see section on hyperthyroidism). The following objectives are of special importance in pediatrics:

A. Avoiding Excitement.

1. Provide a quiet environment.
   a. Avoid assigning the child to a large room with several other patients.
   b. Limit the number of playmates that the child has at any one time.
   c. Maintain a fairly constant schedule of daily activities
   d. Sedate the child if necessary.
      (1) Barbiturates or tranquilizers are the drugs of choice.
      (2) Sedation may be especially beneficial at bedtime.
2. Encourage quiet rather than strenuous activities. Interest the child in diversionary activities that do not require lengthy mental concentration.
3. Maintain constant but gentle discipline.

B. Providing a Diet High in Protein, Calories, and Vitamins.

1. Offer between-meal snacks such as milk shakes.
2. Vitamin supplements may be necessary.

3. Offer foods that can be easily swallowed if the child is experiencing dysphagia.

C. Administering Antithyroid Drugs.

1. Propylthiouracil (PTU) is the drug of choice
   a. Dosage
      (1) Must be individually regulated for each child.
      (2) It is essential to space the dose at regular intervals (every 6–8 hours) throughout a 24-hour period.
         Each dose is fully effective for only a few hours.
   b. Observe for
      (1) Clinical response
         (a) It is usually apparent in 2–3 weeks.
         (b) Exophthalmos may not reverse, but it should not advance.
         (c) Record disappearance of symptoms, including decreased enlargement of the thyroid gland.
2. Side effects
   a. Pruritus
   b. Skin rash
   c. Arthralgia (joint pain)
   d. Nausea and vomiting
3. Severe reaction—agranulocytosis
   a. Sudden onset of fever
   b. Skin rash
   c. Sore throat
4. Signs of overdose
   a. Lethargy
   b. Somnolence (sleepiness)
5. Signs of relapse when the drug is discontinued
   a. Usually discontinued after 2–3 years of administration if the child is euthyroid.
   b. Relapse usually occurs within 6 months of discontinuing the drug.

D. Demonstrating Understanding of the Child's Physical and Emotional Problems.

1. The disease frequently has its onset during adolescence when the child is very concerned with his body image.

2. Encourage the child to talk about his disease and how he feels about it.
   Correct misinformation and misinterpretations as necessary.
3. Assist the adolescent girl to apply make-up, which can significantly reduce the obviousness of her exophthalmos.
4. Discuss the child's disease and treatment with his parents and teachers so that their demands and expectations will be realistic.

E. Caring for the Child Who Requires Thyroidectomy.

(Refer to adult text, p. 541)
1. Indications for surgery in juvenile hyperthyroid patients include:
   a. Toxicity to antithyroid drugs
   b. Failure to cure after an adequate course of medical therapy
   c. Lack of parent or patient compliance
2. Psychological preparation for surgery is essential. The child may associate death with the thought of having his throat cut at the incisional site.

Health Education

A. Medication

1. Allow the parent to administer the child's medication under supervision during his hospitalization to ensure accuracy after discharge.
2. Points of emphasis
   a. The medication must be administered in the exact amount that was prescribed.
   b. Daily administration of the drug at regular intervals is essential.
   c. The child must be observed for signs and symptoms of drug toxicity.

B. Medical Supervision

Close medical follow-up is necessary to evaluate the child's progress and regulate his drug dosage.

Bibliography

Diabetes Mellitus
Books

Chase HP. Understanding Insulin Dependent Diabetes. 3rd ed. Colorado, United Artists, 1988
Saunders FM. Your Diabetic Child. New York, Bantam, 1987
Travis LB. An Instructional Aid on Insulin Dependent Diabetes Mellitus. 8th ed. Fort Worth, Stafford–Texas, 1988

Diabetes Mellitus
Journals

Atkin KL. Diabetes self-care involvement in children, age two to four: Case report. Diabetes Educ 1986 Winter; 12(1):40–42
Balik B, Broatch H and Moynihan PM. Diabetes and the school-aged child. The American Journal of Maternal/Child Nursing 1986 Sep–Oct; 11(5):324–330
Bannard JR. Children's concepts of illness and bodily function: Implications for health service providers caring for children with diabetes. Patient Education and Counseling 1987 Jun; 9(3):275–281
Edwards DL. Initial psychosocial impact of insulin dependent diabetes mellitus on the pediatric client and family. Issues Compr Pediatr Nurs 1987; 10(4):199–207
Harrigan JF. The application of locus of control to diabetes education in school-aged children. J Pediatr Nurs 1987 Aug; 2(4):236–243
Havenstein EJ et al. Stress in parents of children with diabetes mellitus. Diabetes Care 1989 Jan; 12(1):18–23

Hutchinson A and Pooley J. Diabetic control in adolescents. Nursing Mirror 1985 Oct 30; 161(18):26–27
Lipman TH et al. A developmental approach to diabetes in children: Birth through preschool. The American Journal of Maternal/Child Nursing 1989 Jul–Aug; 14(4):255–259
McKelvey J et al. Family support for diabetes: A pilot study for measuring disease specific behaviors. Child Health Care 1989 Winter; 18(1):37–41
Moldovanyi CP. Peer group support program for adolescents with diabetes. Diabetes Educ 1985; 11(3):50–52
Moran MM. Diabetes camps: Management guidelines. Pediatr Nurs 1985 May–Jun; 11(3):183–186
Moyer A. Caring for a child with diabetes: The effect of specialist nurse care on parents' needs and concerns. J Adv Nurs 1989 Jul; 14(7):536–545

Peck T and Cox M. A systems approach to home care of adolescent diabetes. Caring 1988 Nov; 7(11):49–50

Ryan CM. A team approach to the child with diabetes who is having academic difficulties. Diabetes Educ 1987 Winter; 13(1):58–60

Smith KE et al. Issues of managing diabetes in children and adolescents: A multifamily group approach. Child Health Care 1989 Winter; 18(1):49–52

Strang S. A spoonful of sugar . . . problems facing families with diabetic children. Community Outlook 1988 Apr; 19–21

Ward R. Meals for special children. Community Outlook 1984 Sep; 319–320

Diabetes Insipidus

Journals

Cunnah D et al. Management of cranial diabetes insipidus with oral desmopressin (ODAUP). Clin Endocrinol 1986 Mar; 24(3):253–257

Czernichow P et al. Diabetes insipidus in children. Anterior pituitary dysfunction in idiopathic types. J Pediatr 1985 Jan; 106(1):41–44

Doherty E and Copeland KC. Sweat tests in patients with diabetes insipidus. Clin Pediatr 1988 Jul; 27(7):330–332

German K. Fluid and electrolyte problems associated with diabetes insipidus and syndrome of inappropriate antidiuretic hormone. Nurs Clin North Am 1987 Dec; 22(4): 785–796

Littlefield LC. Interactions of drugs and antidiuretic hormone. J Pediatr Health Care 1988; 2(6):325–327

Lubani MM et al. Diabetes insipidus. Indian Pediatr 1987 Dec; 24(12):1150–1155

Mathewson MK. Antidiuretic hormone. Crit Care Nurse 1986 Sep–Oct; 6(5): 88–93

Stanhope R et al. Is diabetes insipidus during childhood ever idiopathic? Br J Hosp Med 1989 May; 41(5):490–491

Vokes TJ et al. Antibodies to vasopressin in patients with diabetes insipidus. Implications for diagnosis and therapy. Ann Intern Med 1988 Feb; 108(2): 190–195

Westgren U et al. Oral desmopressin in central diabetes insipidus. Arch Dis Child 1986 Mar; 61(3):247–250

Thyroid Disorders

Books

Hall R and Kobberling J. Thyroid Disorders Associated With Iodine Deficiency and Excess. New York, Raven Press, 1985

Hamburger JI (ed.) Diagnostic Methods in Clinical Thyroidology. New York, Springer–Verlag, 1988

Hypothyroidism

Journals

Allen DB et al. Screening programs for congenital hypothyroidism. How can they be improved? Am J Dis Child 1988 Feb; 142(2):232–236

Bamforth JS et al. Congenital anomalies associated with hypothyroidism. Arch Dis Child 1986 Jun; 61(6):608–609

Barnett SH et al. Redundancy of the skin of the neck as a sign of congenital hypothyroidism. Am J Dis Child 1987 May; 141(5):477

Cimino JA et al. Riboflavin metabolism in the hypothyroid newborn. Am J Clin Nutr 1988 Mar; 47(3):481–483

Chanoine JP et al. Increased recall rate at screening for congenital hypothyroidism in breast-fed infants born to iodine overloaded mothers. Arch Dis Child 1988 Oct; 63(10):1207–1210

Coody D. Congenital hypothyroidism . . . etiology, diagnosis, treatment and follow-up of infants. Pediatr Nurs 1984 Sep–Oct; 10(5):342–346

Delange F. Neonatal hypothyroidism: Recent development. Baillieres Clin Endocrinol Metab 1988; 2(3):637–652

DeZegher F et al. Congenital hypothyroidism and growth hormone deficiency. Lancet 1988 Dec; 2(8626–8627):1489–1490

Fernhoff PM et al. Congenital hypothyroidism: Increased risk of neonatal morbidity results in delayed treatment. Lancet 1987 Feb; 1(8531): 490–491

Fisher DA. Effectiveness of newborn screening programs for congenital hypothyroidism: Prevalence of missed cases. Pediatr Clin North Am 1987 Aug; 34(4):881–890

Frost GJ. Congenital hypothyroidism. Midwife Health Visit Community Nurse 1985 Oct; 21(10):358–359

Frost GJ and Parkin JM. Outcome for congenital hypothyroidism. Arch Dis Child 1985 Jan; 60(1):81

Grant DB. Neonatal screening with emphasis on congenital hypothyroidism. Midwives Chron 1985 Oct; 98(1173):9–11

Gravdal JA et al. Congenital hypothyroidism. J Fam Pract 1989 Jul; 29(1):47–50

Illig R et al. Mental development in congenital hypothyroidism after neonatal screening. Arch Dis Child 1987 Oct; 62(10):1050–1055

John R. Screening for congenital hypothyroidism. Ann Clin Biochem 1987 Jan; 24(Pt. 1):1–12

Kemper K and Bergman AB. Temperament problems and congenital hypothyroidism. J Pediatr 1989 Aug; 115(2):334–335

Klein RZ. Infantile hypothyroidism then and now: The results of neonatal

screening. Curr Probl Pediatr 1985 Jan; 15(1):1–58

La Franchi S. Diagnosis and treatment of hypothyroidism in children. Compr Ther 1987 Oct; 13(10):20–30

Leger J and Czernichow P. Congenital hypothyroidism: Decreased growth velocity in the first weeks of life. Biol Neonate 1989; 55(4–5):218–223

Rovet JF et al. Effect of thyroid hormone level on temperament in infants with congenital hypothyroidism detected by screening of neonates. J Pediatr 1989 Jan; 114(1):63–68

Sobel EH and Saenger P. Hypothyroidism in the newborn. Pediatrics in Review 1989 Jul; 11(1): 15–20

Tiwary CM. Neonatal screening for metabolic and endocrine diseases. Nurse Practitioner: The American Journal of Primary Health Care 1987 Sep; 12(9):28–31

Tymstra T. False positive results in screening tests: Experiences of parents of children screened for congenital hypothyroidism. Fam Pract 1986 Jun; 3(2):92–96

Virtanen M. Manifestations of congenital hypothyroidism during the 1st week of life. Eur J Pediatr 1988 Apr; 147(3): 270–274

Walfish PG. Neonatal screening. Diagnostic Medicine 1984 Feb; 7(2): 67–75

Graves' Disease

Journals

Alves C et al. Graves' disease presenting as painful thyroiditis. Eur J Pediatr 1989 Jun; 148(7):603–604

Foley TP et al. Juvenile Graves' disease: Usefulness and limitations of thyrotropin receptor antibody determinations. J Pediatr 1987 Mar; 110(3):378–386

Hoffman WH et al. Pharmacokinetics of propylthiouracil in children and adolescents with Graves' disease in the hyperthyroid and euthyroid states. Dev Pharmacol Ther 1988; 11(2):73–81

Levy WJ et al. Treatment of childhood Graves' disease. A review with emphasis on radioiodine treatment. Cleve Clin J Med 1988 Jul–Aug; 55(4): 373–382

McDougall IR and Bayer MF. Should a woman taking propylthiouracil breast-feed? Clin Nucl Med 1986 Apr; 11(4): 249–250

Shields CL et al. Neonatal Graves' disease. Br J Ophthalmol 1988 Jun; 72(6):424–427

Tamaki H et al. Universal predictive criteria for neonatal overt thyrotoxicosis requiring treatment. Am J Perinatol 1988 Apr; 5(2):152–158

Tan SH et al. Relapse markers in childhood thyrotoxicosis. Clin Pediatr 1987 Mar; 26(3):136–139

1: Conditions of the Eye

The Blind Child

Impaired vision (blindness) refers to insufficient or inadequate vision in varying degrees.

Etiology

1. Familial factors
   Genetic determination
2. Prenatal or intrauterine factors
   a. Rubella
   b. Toxoplasmosis
   c. Syphilis
3. Perinatal factors
   a. Prematurity
   b. Oxygen toxicity—Retinopathy of prematurity (ROP)
   c. Infections
4. Postnatal factors
   a. Injury or trauma
   b. Infections
   c. Inflammatory disease

Altered Physiology

1. Defective visual fields
2. Impaired color vision
3. Decreased visual acuity
4. No vision—or a small percentage of vision (may have light perception)

Complications

Developmental delays in motor, communication, ego, and behavior

Clinical Manifestations

A. Infant

1. No eye-to-eye contact, especially with the mother
2. Abnormal eye movements
3. Does not follow objects at 2 months of age
4. Failure to locate distant objects at 6–12 months of age
5. Mother senses "something is wrong"

B. Older Child

1. Squinting, frequent blinking
2. Bumping into things
3. Frequent rubbing of eyes

Diagnostic Evaluation

1. Legal definition—visual acuity 20/200 or less with correction
2. Tunnel vision—peripheral field of vision has an angular distance not greater than 20 degrees

Treatment

1. Surgical repair of defect
2. Glasses
3. Special training
   a. Language development and acquisition
   b. Mobility—perceptual motor training
   c. Early stimulation therapy

Patient Problems and Nursing Diagnoses

1. Anxiety and social isolation related to presence of strangers; fear of unknown
2. Sensory/perceptual alteration, related to inability to see items in surroundings
3. Altered parenting related to lack of eye contact and inadequate communication
4. Potential for injury related to falls and tendency to bump into things
5. Self-care deficit related to limitations imposed by visual impairment
6. Growth and development, altered, related to altered visual stimulation and possible overprotective behavior of parents

Nursing Interventions

The nurse may become involved with the blind child in the hospital in three critical situations: (1) before diagnosis has been made when she may detect a visual loss, usually in an infant, (2) at time of diagnosis, and (3) after diagnosis has been made and she is giving nursing care to the hospitalized child who is blind.

Detection; Early Care of the Blind Child After Diagnosis

A. Being Familiar With the Normal Pattern of Visual Development and Recognizing Deviations as Well as Manifestations of Visual Impairment.

1. Knowing the stages of growth and development can be helpful in recognizing or suspecting visual impairment in the individual child.
2. The appreciation of vision by the infant begins at about 3 months of age.
3. Be alert to and assess the child's response to visual stimulation.
   a. Does the infant follow the human face or bright object with his eyes according to his stage of development?
   b. Does the infant reach for objects?
   c. Does the 9- to 12-month-old child move around?

B. Being Familiar With the Causes of Visual Impairment and Blindness in Order to Recognize From the History Whether or Not the Child Is in a High-Risk Category.

1. Neonatal and perinatal factors
   a. Prematurity
   b. Oxygen therapy
   c. Infections
2. Past infections—inflammatory disease
3. Trauma

C. Recording Observations and Reporting Any Suspicious Behavior by the Infant or Child Indicating Visual Impairment.

1. Early diagnosis is the key to successful habilitation and optimal development of the child's capabilities.
2. The complication of complete withdrawal of the child can be avoided by early diagnosis and proper stimulation and emotional support.

D. Helping the Family of a Newly Diagnosed Visually Impaired Child.

1. Parents must be allowed time to understand and accept what has happened. The diagnosis can be a great shock.
2. They will experience guilt, anger, and depression. How they accept the child will depend on how they feel about having a handicapped child.
3. They may also feel they have a great burden of caring for this child.
4. Their life-style will have to change; they will need to find new ways to adjust socially and personally.

E. Working With Physician and Parents in Helping the Child Master Certain Developmental Tasks, Thus Aiding the Child in Achieving His Fullest Potential.

Parents need help in recognizing the clues the child presents indicating his need and readiness for new learning experiences. The child must also learn in his own natural way.

1. Continued communication must be fostered between parents, mother, and child.
   a. The mother must learn techniques of touching, handling, and talking to her child.
   b. Mother should make a special effort to help her baby associate her voice and body with receiving pleasure.
   c. Encourage touching by both mother and baby during feeding times, as well as other times. Touch is a good nonverbal form of communication.

2. *The child and parents must be helped to develop a discriminating relationship;* specific consistent clues of handling the child can be built into behavior. Parents need to become sensitive to the communication code of their infant to continue their relationship.
   a. Each parent shares some special, individualized activity with the child.
   b. Voice and touch bring parents and child together.
3. The child must be allowed and encouraged to use his hands for exploring his world. Child must also learn appropriate use of hands.
   a. Give the child objects of different shapes, sizes, and textures. Use toys that make noise and that are within reach and stay there.
   b. Give finger food to child during meals—when the child is about 8 months of age or when he sits up.
   c. Extra tactile opportunities provided for child will compensate to some extent for loss of visual input.
4. The child needs to learn to become mobile.
   a. The mother's voice can encourage child to move toward her.
   b. A favorite toy placed in front of child can encourage him to move toward it.
5. The child needs much help in learning to talk.
   a. Expose the child to sounds that have a specific function—cleaning equipment, dishes.
   b. Mother should talk a great deal to the child. The child cannot benefit from gestures and facial expression used in language.
6. The child needs social exposure to his peers. Nursery school can be very helpful.

F. Fostering Continuous Acceptance of the Child By His Parents and Providing Support for Them.

1. Evaluate the parents' emotional status and offer them reassurance and explanations.
   a. Parental acceptance and a healthy home atmosphere are vitally important in helping the visually impaired or blind child to accept and adjust to his limitations.
   b. The child can sense his parents' approval or disapproval and the degree to which they love and accept him.
2. Help the parents to understand and accept their responsibilities in the care of their child. Parents who have received appropriate information and guidance in handling their child can enrich the time spent with the child and prevent further handicapping and management problems. Indicate that they should do the following:
   a. Provide proper stimulation for the child to learn that which is ordinarily learned through vision. Frustration often occurs when the child gives little feedback. Efforts may decrease as a consequence.
   b. The voice is often used to protect the child.
   c. Reinforce that this child has the same needs for growth and development as any child.
3. Help parents understand how they can develop the child's skills in interpreting information through the senses of hearing, touch, smell, and taste. They can learn to understand their blind child.
   a. Hearing
      (1) Help the child to determine distance by ringing a bell.
      (2) Familiarize him with appliances, birds, voices.
      (3) Use voice—tone, expression, etc. because nonverbal cues go unnoticed.

(4) A tape recorder can be helpful in teaching the child to recognize different sounds.

b. Touch
  (1) Touch may serve as sense organizer.
  (2) Allow the child to handle different textured materials.

c. Smell
  Acquaint the child with flowers, perfume, kitchen odors.

d. Taste
  Help the child distinguish different kitchen substances.

e. Memory
  Have the child practice retelling stories, his telephone number, address, etc.

4. Initiate referral to the community nurse who can make home visits to reinforce and interpret what the mother has heard from the physician and to encourage the mother in her efforts.

5. Encourage the parents to discuss their feelings about caring for a handicapped child at home.
  Initiate a social worker referral. (The social worker can help parents deal with their feelings.)

6. Help the parents understand the problems the child faces and will face as he gets older.

  a. The child with probably be delayed in development. There can be a delay of up to 5 months in creeping and 7 months in walking, even though posture and balance for such activities are similar to those of sighted child.

  b. The child is likely to develop stereotypic behaviors, habits, or mannerisms of blind children; these are a manifestation of inadequate impulse control.

  c. The child may also show self-stimulatory behavior. These behaviors may be associated with excitement or arousal or withdrawal or boredom.

  d. Vision is the primary elicitor of the smile; thus, the infant will be late in development of the social smile. Subtle expressions used in communication will be missed by the infant, and skills will not be developed by imitation.

  e. Parents should help the child develop an awareness of self.
    (1) Child needs to know how the sighted world functions and
    (2) the unique contribution the child can make to society.
    (3) Help child develop the concept of different, not deficient

G. Being Familiar With the Community Resources and the Professional Team to be Involved in Habilitation of the Visually Impaired Child.

Several types of school programs are available to the child, depending on his confidence and coping abilities.

1. Residential schools.
  a. Used when nothing is available in the local community.
  b. Preferred when the home care of the child would be detrimental to his progress.

2. Day schools for the blind. (The child attends school during day but lives at home.)

3. Public school where the blind child is integrated with sighted child. (The child receives special training in braille.)

4. Vocational habilitation programs (training for some occupation.)

5. Public law 94-142 provides for public education of all handicapped children.

H. Evaluating How Well the Child Who Was Once Able to See Accepts Visual Impairment—In Terms of His Physical Abilities and Psychologic Dependence. (Vision helps to maintain contact with reality.)

1. A serious impairment in relationships with people can result when the child is unable to express his innermost sentiments.

2. Allow the child to express his feelings, especially those of fear and anger. Talk, play, and certain activities help the child express these feelings.

Hospital Care of the Visually Impaired or Blind Child

Many of the important areas discussed above must be considered when caring for the child in the hospital situation. In addition, emphasis must be placed on the following goals:

A. Interviewing the Parents at the Time of Admission to Learn as Much as Possible About the Child and His Care and Activities at Home.

1. Be aware of the child's schedule and activities during the day. Know what activities he can or cannot do, and what he likes to do.

2. Become familiar with how he is oriented to his new surroundings.
  a. How much does he ambulate?
  b. What precautions are necessary?

3. Be aware of how the parents comfort and discipline the child.
  a. How does he comfort himself or seek security?

4. What special care or treatment must be continued while the child is hospitalized?

5. Share this information with nursing staff in a nursing care plan so that continuity of care from home to hospital can minimize fear and frustration in the child.

B. Attending to the Child's Needs According to the Medical Problem That Required His Hospitalization.

C. Planning and Providing for the Appropriate Type of Play, Activities Program, and Stimulation for the Child.

1. Developmental lines of the sighted child need to be modified for the vision-impaired child.

2. Assess the child's level of growth and development and use the information obtained from parents.

3. Allow the child as much independence as possible in his care, but provide guidance as necessary.
  Orient the ambulatory child thoroughly to his room and surroundings.

4. Encourage the development of the child's abilities. Avoid overprotecting him.

5. Provide activities that will increase his learning and give him pleasure (e.g., talking records).

6. Provide emotional preparation for procedures and surgery, as appropriate.

D. Meeting the Psychological and Emotional Needs of the Visually Impaired or Blind Child for Protection and Security Against Harm.

1. The nurse should always speak to the child prior to touching him so as not to frighten or startle him.

2. Always use a warm and gentle touch.

3. Explain strange sounds that may be frightening. Tape recording of sounds he may hear helps put them into proper perspective.

4. Plan frequent nurse–patient interactions to increase the child's sense of security.

5. Place items he needs and uses within his reach.
   a. Familiar items that give the child security should also be close to him.
   b. Tell him if they are moved.
6. During any procedure, talk to the child the entire time. Explain what is going on around him.

E. Avoiding Overemphasizing the Child's Handicap and Being Unobtrusive About Meeting His Needs.

Allow the child to explore and learn about his new environment and the hospital.

Health Education

A. Provide Continual Parental Support.

1. Encourage the parents to become involved in the care of their child to help maintain or develop a healthy parent–child relationship.
   Separation from the parents can be extremely traumatic and has severe implications for the blind child.
2. Encourage the parents to talk about their fears and feelings concerning this child. Help them relax.
   The parents can be invaluable in increasing the security and decreasing the fear the child may have as a result of being in a strange place.
3. Discuss realistically long-term and short-term planning for the child (i.e., educational opportunities).
   a. Encourage the parents to tell teachers and adults responsible for his care about his special needs.
   b. Avoid overemphasis on educational achievements.
4. Help the parents understand that discipline, order, and consistency are necessary in the child's environment to give him security.
5. Emphasize that the parents' role is to give this child love and physical care as well as to stimulate and influence him so he may have satisfactory mental, social, and emotional growth.
6. Help the parents see that other members of the family also must be considered.
   a. Their handicapped child does need special attention, but he does not need all the attention all the time.
   b. Other members of the family should be included in his care, but they also have a life of their own and need as much attention from parents as they would have if the handicapped child were not present in the family.
   c. Parents need time to themselves. They should be encouraged to go out alone together and to give time to their marriage.
7. Help the parents realize that even though habilitation of their blind child is long, drawn out, and expensive, the child may be able to live a normal life in the community.
   a. Are the parents aware of and do they accept the short- and long-term goals?
   b. Many blind people are successful as technicians and professionals.

Expected Outcomes

1. Demonstrates lessening of anxiety; interacts with others in environment
2. Shows awareness of sensory stimulation; has access to auditory stimulation (records; radio; verbal communication); tactile stimulation, etc.
3. The parents demonstrate appropriate parenting behaviors; talking with child, touching, encouraging independence, establishing normal discipline, and order; exploring educational opportunities
4. Avoids injury through use of protective measures; accepts normal limits on behavior; adheres to social rules
5. Attempts to fulfill developmental tasks through age-related activities (within limits of visual impairment; tries to do things for himself)

Eye Defects Requiring Surgery

Eye defects requiring surgery are (1) structural manifestations of the eye present at birth or (2) acquired conditions of the eye. They can be extraocular or intraocular conditions.

Etiology

1. Congenital
   a. Hereditary tendencies
   b. Birth injury
   c. Innervational factors
   d. Intrauterine influences
2. Disease
   a. Metabolic
   b. Infection
3. Trauma to the eye

Strabismus

Strabismus is the inability to balance the extraocular muscles; thus the eyes cannot function together at the same time.

Altered Physiology

1. The visual axis of only 1 eye goes to the object being observed. The person appears to be looking in 2 directions at once.
2. Specific deviations
   a. Paralytic strabismus—muscles of 1 eye are underactive.
   b. Concomitant strabismus—both eyes move, but the deviation between the eyes is always the same.
   c. Hypertropia—eye deviation is upward.
   d. Hypotropia—eye deviation is downward.
   e. Vertical—vertical separation of visual axes.
   f. Esotropia—1 eye deviates toward other eye; convergent—"cross-eye."
   g. Exotropia—1 eye deviates away from the other eye; divergent—"wall-eye."

Complications

1. Amblyopia—poor vision in eye not used.
2. Emotional problems resulting from cosmetic aspect of deformity.
3. Repeated surgery may be necessary.
4. Diplopia

Clinical Manifestations

1. Deviations of the eye (constant or intermittent)
2. Squinting
3. Closing one eye to see
4. Tilting head
5. Stumbling or clumsy behavior
6. Inaccuracy in picking up objects
7. Double vision

Treatment

1. Corrective glasses (lenses)
2. Patching nondiverging eye
3. Surgery
   a. Lengthening or shortening of extraocular structures
   See right-hand column for nursing management.
4. Botulinum (limited use)
   a. Neurotoxin that produces temporary paralysis when injected into muscle
   b. Used as an alternative to extraocular muscle surgery

Cataract

Cataract is an opacification or milk-white appearance of the eye lens.

Altered Physiology

Inability of light to pass through the clouded lens in adequate amounts—loss of vision as lens becomes more opaque; loss of transparency.

Clinical Manifestations

1. Gradual diminution of visual acuity
2. Strabismus
3. Nystagmus
4. Gray opacities of lens

Diagnostic Evaluation

Ophthalmoscopic examination reveals opacification of the lens.

Treatment

1. Medication—dilation of pupil with mydriatic eye drops
2. Surgery
   a. Optical iridectomy
   b. Lens fragmentation, irrigation, and aspiration, or cutting and aspiration
   c. Intraocular lens implantation

Complications

A. Untreated Cataract

1. Bilateral cataract
   a. Nystagmus
   b. Stimulus-deprivation amblyopia
2. Unilateral cataract
   a. Strabismus
   b. Stimulus-deprivation amblyopia

B. Following Surgery for Congenital Cataract

1. Retinal detachment several years later
2. Average vision only 20/70
3. Need for glasses or contact lenses to replace refracting power of lens
   See below for nursing management.

Trauma

Trauma is injury to the globe, adnexa, and surrounding tissue of the eye as a result of blunt objects (baseball, rock) striking the eye area, or sharp items (scissors, knife) penetrating the eye area.

Altered Physiology

A. Blunt Injury

1. Subconjunctival hemorrhage and suffusion of blood into eyelid
2. Secondary hemorrhage occurring days after injury
   a. Accumulation of blood in anterior chamber and blocking of overflow channels
   b. Rapid rise of intraocular pressure (glaucoma)
3. Retinal edema, hemorrhages, and detachment
4. Maintain head of bed 30 degrees to avoid increased intraocular pressure
5. Protect eye from further damage by covering with perforated metal or plastic eye shield without pad.

B. Penetrating Injury

1. Loss of aqueous fluid, development of cataract
2. Bleeding into anterior chamber and vitreous
3. Retinal detachment
4. Keep child NPO in the event that surgery is necessary.
5. Do not apply pressure to eyeball.

C. Corneal Abrasions (i.e., from fingernail)

1. Common in young children
2. Treated for 24 hours with patching and antibiotic ointment

Complications

Sympathetic ophthalmia—inflammation of the uninjured eye probably due to an allergic reaction to pigment released from injured eye. This condition can lead to significant visual loss.

Nursing Management of the Child Undergoing Eye Surgery

Preoperative Nursing Interventions

A. Helping the Child and His Parents Know and Understand What the Surgery Entails. (Explanations should be appropriate for the age of the child.)

1. Take a trip to the operating and recovery rooms if the child is not on bedrest due to trauma.
2. Practice applying eye patches for short frequent periods.
   a. Allow the child to handle the equipment.
   b. Explain that the patches will only be temporary.
3. Help the child become familiar with the protective devices if they are to be used postoperatively.
4. Discuss and practice postoperative exercises if feasible.
5. Relieve the child's fears by telling him that there will be a little pain—as if something is in the eye.

B. Assessing the Child and His Needs According to Age and Specifically to His Eye Problem.

1. Can the child read or watch television?
2. Does the child wear glasses? When? Help him to learn to protect his glasses when not in use.

C. Providing as Much Comfort and Reassurance to the Child as Possible to Diminish His Fears, Especially Concerning Hospitalization and Impending Surgery.

1. Room assignment can be significant.
   a. A quiet room with subdued lighting can be more comfortable for trauma patients.
   b. Placement in a room with other children (without infection) may be comforting for elective surgery patients.

2. Allow the child to have familiar tactile and auditory stimulating objects around him.

Postoperative Nursing Interventions

A. Administering Effective Postoperative Care and Observing for Possible Postoperative Complications (see p. 1134).

Be alert to the care and considerations for specific eye defect.

1. Strabismus
   a. Frequently the child is discharged on the day of surgery, following recovery from anesthesia.
   b. Surgery is extraocular; no postoperative ocular rupture hazards exist.
   c. Activity is not restricted.
   d. Eye bandages may or may not be used.
   e. Eyes will probably be blood-tinged and will drain. Eyes may feel uncomfortable. Black eye is normal, as is postoperative swelling.
   f. Eyes may be difficult to open the morning after surgery. Gently separate lids from above and below. Do not force lids open. Tears will soften secretions.
   g. Child may have photosensitivity.
2. Cataract or intraocular surgery
   a. The child is generally positioned on his back; thus, prevention of aspiration is a concern.
   b. Avoid sudden head movement, crying, and vomiting, because these increase intraocular pressure; they cause strain on sutures and subsequent bleeding.
   c. Avoid surprising the patient and making him jump. Avoid loud noises. Speak gently before touching the child.
3. Emesis is a common complication following eye surgery.
   Note medications used during surgery and know the effects on the child postoperatively, i.e., lidocaine vs. droperidol (seems to reduce postoperative emesis)

B. Preventing the Child from Pulling Off the Dressing and Causing Injury or Contamination.

1. Sedation may be warranted until the child becomes accustomed to having his eye continually bandaged.
2. Protective devices may be used only if necessary. Rest is necessary during the immediate postoperative period, and a child struggling because of restraints can defeat their intended purpose.
3. Diet should be increased slowly to prevent vomiting; this could cause possible injury to the eye because of increased pressure.

C. Providing Emotional and Psychological Reassurance and Support to the Child Who Is Anxious Because His Eyes are Bandaged, Preventing Him From Seeing.

1. Encourage the parents to be with their child, especially when he is waking up from anesthesia. Someone should be with the child if the parents are unable to be present.
   a. Sit with child, stroke him, and speak gently and softly to him.
   b. Let him hold a familiar object.
   c. Hold him if there are no contraindications to his being lifted and held.
2. Always speak to child before touching him so as not to startle him.
   Explain what is going to be done to him before doing it.

3. Tell the child what foods are on his tray. Allow him to finger-feed himself.
4. Explain sounds. (Sounds in the world without sight can be very frightening.)
5. Reassure the child that patches will be removed soon, and he will be able to see again (if he is going to see).
6. Provide appropriate diversional activities for the child.
   a. Read him stories.
   b. Provide radio or phonograph.
   c. Talk with him.

D. Administering Appropriate Eye Medications and Changing Dressing as Prescribed.

1. First dressing change is usually done by the physician.
   a. Strabismus—dressing removed day after surgery.
   b. Cataract—dressing may be used for 5–10 days after surgery.
2. Be familiar with types of eye medications used.
   a. Mydriatic—used to dilate pupil.
   b. Miotic—constricts pupil and decreases increased intraocular pressure in early glaucoma.
   c. Anti-inflammatory drugs
   d. Antibiotics
3. Be familiar with the principles of instilling eye medications (drops, ointments, and irrigations).
   a. Have the room darkened—light may be uncomfortable.
   b. Try to gain the confidence and cooperation of the child and reassure him by talking to him during the procedure.
   c. Assistance may be necessary to stabilize the child's head and prevent injury. Have the child close his eye; drop medication onto the inner canthus; open the eye and the drop will roll in.
   d. Irrigate from the inner canthus outward.
   e. To instill drops, pull the lower lid down and drop the medication onto the conjunctiva from a dropper parallel to the lid. If drops are instilled on the conjunctiva and not on the cornea, the patient tolerates the medication better.
   f. Do not force the lid open.
   g. Blot away excess fluid with a paper tissue or cotton ball; do not rub the eye.
   h. Avoid contaminating the dressing.
   i. Always wash hands before and after contact with the eye for any procedure.

E. Involving the Parents and Child in Preparation for Discharge.

1. Teach the parents how to instill eye medications (see above).
2. Postoperative patches or glasses may be necessary. Help the parents and child understand the value and importance of the patching or glasses.
3. Encourage the parents to contact the school nurse and other adults responsible for child's care to explain special exercises or specific care for the child.
4. Encourage follow-up as advised by the physician.

Health Education

1. Help the parents understand what was wrong with the child, what was done to help correct the problem, and what the parental responsibilities are in continuing any recommended therapy with the child.
2. Be certain the parents understand what special care is to be given and how it is to be accomplished.
3. Prevention is the best treatment for eye injury.
   a. Eye-protective devices should be used during sports.

b. Street glasses are not a protection in contact sports; and special protectors (with built-in prescription) are advised.

c. Better education of parents, teachers, and coaches about potential for serious eye injury and ways to prevent such injuries

2: Conditions of the Ear

The Child With Impaired Hearing

Impaired hearing occurs when there is a hearing loss in speech frequencies of over 20 decibels, and the child does not learn to talk in the normal way. Speech essentially may have no meaning.

Etiology

1. Unknown
2. Familial factors—genetically transmitted; family history of hearing impairment*
3. Prenatal or intrauterine factors
   a. Rubella*
   b. Preeclampsia or eclampsia
   c. Drugs
   d. Congenital syphilis
4. Perinatal factors
   a. Prematurity*—especially <1,500 gm.
   b. Anoxia at birth—asphyxia with acidosis
   c. Hyperbilirubinemia*
   d. Erythroblastosis fetalis
   e. Neonatal sepsis,* meningitis
5. Postnatal factors
   a. Ototoxic drugs
   b. Acquired disorders of the central nervous system
   c. Acute infections, otitis media
   d. Injury
   e. Structural defects*
6. Chromosomal anomalies
   a. Trisomy 13-14-15
   b. Trisomy 18

Altered Physiology

A. Conductive Hearing Loss

1. Impairment in the mechanism of conducting sound waves to the cochlea; sound not transmitted well, distorted
   a. Blockage of sound waves from outer ear, external canal, or middle ear (lack of loudness)
   b. Tympanic membrane damage and scarring
   c. Dislocation or disturbance of tiny ossicular bones in the middle ear
2. Often recognized in the school-age child

B. Sensorineural Hearing Loss

1. Malfunction of inner ear apparatus or 8th cranial nerve—medically irreversible
   a. Lack of loudness
   b. Distorted sounds because of defect of cochlea or neural pathways to temporal lobe of the brain
   c. Problems with discrimination of sound

C. Mixed Hearing Loss

Both sensorineural and conductive hearing loss in some children

* Criteria for high risk of impaired hearing.

D. Central Hearing Loss

1. Middle ear transformer mechanics; the cochlea and nerves are probably functioning normally.
2. There is abnormal or inability to process auditory signals within the brain.

Complications

1. In childhood when there is a hearing disorder, there is a delay of speech and language development; thus, there is a loss of contact between the individual, his peers, and his environment.
2. Biological, behavioral, and social complications may result when there is a breakdown of the normal communicative process.
3. The seriousness of the total problem depends on the nature and extent of auditory involvement and on the age of onset and length of time before the hearing problem is detected.

Clinical Manifestations

A. Infant

1. Little or no interest in sounds of his environment
   a. Does not blink at loud noise
   b. Does not turn eyes toward sound of musical toy or mother's voice at 3 months of age
   c. Does not turn toward whispered voice within 1 meter (3 feet) at 8–12 months of age
   d. Hyperactivity or gesturing may increase
2. Lack of minimal vocalization
   a. Does not coo or gurgle
   b. May not smile
   c. Babbling decreases after 6–8 months of age
3. Lack of neonatal startle reflex to noise 1–2 meters (3–6 feet) away

B. Toddlers

1. Little or no vocalization
   a. Sounds produced poorly
   b. Will not repeat a word with single stimulus
   c. Uses gestures to express needs
2. Little interest in environmental sounds—does not respond to name, doorbell, or telephone

C. Preschool and School-age Child

1. Behavioral disturbances
   a. Intense, constant activity
   b. Temper tantrums
   c. Inattentiveness
   d. Slow learner
2. May show abrupt change in social or communicative behavior.

D. Sensorineural vs. Conductive Hearing Loss

1. Sensorineural
   a. The child may talk more loudly than necessary.
   b. The child may not respond to average loudness, but responds to loud sounds.
   c. When intensity of sound is increased above the threshold of sensitivity, the child shows some type of response.

2. Conductive
   a. The child has a tendency to talk in a relatively soft voice.
   b. The child hears better in a noisy environment.
   c. The child can hear loud speech and sounds.

Diagnostic Evaluation

1. Otolaryngologic examination (inspection of external ear and tympanic membrane)—to rule out involvement of conductive apparatus
2. Audiologic examination—to establish the extent of hearing loss and to determine type of hearing aid needed
   a. Observation of the child's response to sounds calibrated for intensity and frequency
   b. Objective measuring techniques of hearing loss, (i.e., cortical audiometry)
3. Hearing loss classification
   Pure tone audiometry hearing threshold level:
       0–20 db—Normal hearing
       21–40 db—Mild hearing impairment
       41–55 db—Moderate hearing loss
       56–70 db—Moderately severe hearing loss
       71–90 db—Severe hearing loss
       91+ db—Profound hearing loss
4. Limited high-risk register (to identify infants at high risk for hearing loss)
   a. Family history of child with hearing impairment
   b. Rubella or other nonbacterial infection
   c. Defects of ear, nose or throat, low-set or absent pinnae, cleft lip/palate
   d. Birth weight less than 1500 gm.
   e. Hyperbilirubinemia (greater than 20 mg./100 ml.)

Treatment

1. Conductive hearing loss
   a. Surgical correction of defect
   b. Hearing aid
2. Sensorineural hearing loss
   a. Hearing aid
   b. Special training
      (1) Language acquisition
      (2) Auditory training
      (3) Speech therapy
      (4) Perceptual motor training

Potential Problems and Nursing Diagnoses

1. Impaired communication related to inability to hear or express self through understandable speech pattern
2. Social isolation related to inability to interact verbally
3. Delayed developmental growth related to lack of auditory stimulation
4. Potential for injury related to failure to detect warning sounds
5. Parenting, altered related to inappropriate communication
6. Anxiety and ineffective coping related to reduced social interaction
7. Parental anxiety related to having a child with impaired hearing

Nursing Interventions

The nurse may become involved with the child with impaired hearing in the hospital in 3 situations: (1) before diagnosis has been made, when the nurse may detect a hearing loss, (2) at the time of diagnosis, and (3) after diagnosis has been made when giving nursing care to the hospitalized child.

Detection; Early Care After Diagnosis

A. Being Familiar With the Normal Pattern of Language and Learning Development and the Manifestations of Hearing Loss in the Infant and Child.

1. Knowing the stages of growth and development can be helpful in recognizing and suspecting hearing impairment in the individual child.
2. Be alert to and assess the child's response to auditory stimulation.
   a. Does the infant stop activity and listen to vocal sounds?
   b. Does the child respond to his name?
   c. Does the child have unusual visual alertness at age 1 year?
3. The critical period of learning or language development is from birth to 16 months.

B. Being Familiar With the Causes of Hearing Impairment and Recognizing From the History If the Child May Be in a High-Risk Category.

1. Ensure that follow-up hearing evaluation is planned.
2. Criteria for high risk of impaired hearing (see limited high-risk register, left-hand column)

C. Recording Observations and Reporting to Physician Any Suspicious Behavior by the Infant or Child That Indicates Possible Hearing Loss.

1. Early diagnosis is the key to successful habilitation and optimal development of the capabilities of the child. Early intervention is aimed toward the child's acquisition of heard and spoken language.
   a. After 16 months of age, habilitation is more difficult.
   b. If hearing loss occurs after the time of critical language development, rehabilitation is less difficult, as the groundwork for verbal communication has been established.
2. The impulse for learning spontaneous speech and acquiring most of the basic verbal skills, as well as the structure on which mature use of language and speech is built, is reached during the first 3–4 years of life.
3. A current screening device is the Crib-O-Gram*—an automated method of recording responses of the infant's motor activity before and after test sound.

D. Being Familiar With Community Resources and the Professional Team Involved in Habilitation.

1. Each child must be treated as an individual.
2. Knowing general philosophies and training techniques of the involved resource can be helpful.
   Help the child to capitalize on assets and minimize limitations.

E. Being Familiar With the Guidelines and Techniques of Educating a Child With Impaired Hearing.

1. The main mode of communication for the child with impaired hearing is visual, supplemented by auditory clues.

---

* Telesensory System, Inc., Palo Alto, CA.

a. Educational task is to develop the child's understanding and expression of language.
b. Speech can be learned through a multisensory approach, using visual, tactile, kinesthetic, and auditory stimulation.
2. The child with a less severe hearing loss uses auditory stimulation, supplemented by visual clues, as his main mode of communication.
The educational task is to develop adequate speech and language and the best use of residual hearing.
3. The 3 basic methods currently used in educating deaf children include:
a. *Oral Approach*—emphasizes verbal communication, speech reading, and auditory training.
Most useful when child has some hearing.
b. *Manual Communication*—sign language.
c. *Total Communication Approach*—combines sign language with auditory training and speech reading.
Language modes—child-devised gestures, sign, speech, speech reading, finger spelling, reading, and writing.
d. Binaural sensory aid—(sonar-aid)—used to encourage reaching
4. Cued speech, which visually pinpoints a single sound being spoken by using a manual supplement to lip reading of hand shapes used near the mouth to make language sounds look different on the lips or hand.
The tool is made up of 12 hand shapes and positions.
5. Whatever method of education and communication is used, it is *critical for parents* to enter the educational process so that they can establish communication with their child.

F. Being Familiar With Hearing Devices That Are Available and May Be Used by the Child.

1. Hearing aids
a. In the ear
b. Behind the ear
c. On the body or in the pocket
d. Eyeglass model
2. Technical aids—telecommunication device for the hearing impaired

G. Helping the Family Cope With and Accept a Newly Diagnosed Hearing Impairment in Their Child.

1. Encourage the physician to have both parents present when he tells them the diagnosis. This allows the parents to support each other.
2. Do not focus all your attention on the child. Show your concern for and interest in the parents.
3. Be aware that parents must be given time to adjust to this usually drastic and unexpected change in their lives before they can deal constructively with meeting the needs of the child.
4. At this time, parents need general information—good literature that is specific to their child's problem. Contact with other parents who have made successful adjustments to living with their hearing-impaired children can be helpful to parents. Acquaint them with organizations dealing with deafness (see below).

H. Being Aware of the Problems Facing the Parents (and Family) of a Hearing-Impaired Child.

Offer them specific guidance in handling and caring for the child.

1. Problems encountered
a. Lack of knowledge of principles of parenting methods that govern the child's development.
b. Unaware of cues from their child that are familiar to most parents.
c. Limited feedback from their child in speech (vocalization), emotional response, or achievement—all of which increase spontaneous parenting. Communication limitations tend to restrict early parent–child relationships.
Child is not equipped to show his attachment to his parents.
d. The parent must be in close contact with the child to control and regulate his behavior.
e. The child is lacking in impulse control and is unable to understand and order his world.
f. The parents may show embarrassment because of their child's behavior.
g. There is a possible tendency to neglect or deny common childhood conflicts and/or problems.
h. Frustration—they do not know how to help their child.
2. Specific guidance to offer parents:
a. Allow and encourage the parents to communicate with the child through mime, gestures, and body language. There is an increased need for stimulation and physical contact.
b. Optimize the auditory environment.
c. Teach the parents how to talk to their child—to use verbal and nonverbal reinforcement of behavior.
d. Help the baby develop "watching behavior" by rewarding him with pleasure and praise.
e. Encourage the parents to look directly into the child's eyes when they talk to him and to use appropriate facial expressions.
f. Help them to understand that their child is probably unable to express his anxieties; frustration leads to anger and sudden rage or temper tantrums. Help them to gain confidence in their own resourcefulness and care by anticipating the child's random behavior through their knowledge of its coincidence with certain situations.
g. Teach them the stages of language development.

Care of the Hospitalized Child With a Hearing Loss

A. Interviewing the Parents at the Time of Admission to Learn as Much as Possible About the Child and His Activities at Home.

1. What is the child's way of communicating his needs? How do the parents communicate with the child?
2. Be aware of the child's schedule and activities at home. Know what activities he can or cannot do and what he likes to do.
3. Be aware of how the parents discipline the child and how they comfort him.
4. Does the child wear a hearing aid? When? Any special exercises or training that needs to be continued?
5. Share this information with nursing staff in the nursing care plan to ensure continuity of care from home to hospital and to minimize fear and frustration in the child.

B. Attending to the Child's Needs According to the Medical or Surgical Problem That Required His Hospitalization.

Properly prepare the child for procedures, etc., using increased sense of touch and visual sense.

C. Planning and Providing for the Appropriate Type of Play Program and Stimulation for the Child.

1. Assess the child's level of development and growth and use information provided by parents.
2. Allow the child as much independence as possible in his care, but provide guidance as necessary—prevent boredom.
3. Encourage the development of the child's abilities.

D. Meeting the Emotional Needs of the Child With Impaired Hearing for Closeness and Belonging.

1. Place the child in a room with a friendly, outgoing child.
2. Plan frequent nurse–patient interactions.
   a. Gentle touch
   b. Games or activities he enjoys
3. Encourage the parents, especially the mother, to take an active part in his care, thus decreasing fear of desertion.
4. Be aware of coping behaviors seen in the child, including visual information gathering, avoidance, and comfort-seeking measures.
5. Adolescents may need special consideration, because at this developmental stage they normally may be experiencing a time of confusion.

Health Education

A. Foster Continuous Parental Acceptance of the Child and Provide Support for the Family.

1. Invite the parents to become involved in the care of their hospitalized child as much as possible.
2. Help the parents to understand the problems the child faces and will face as he gets older.
   a. Although hearing impairment does alter life experiences for the child, it does not limit intelligence or capacity for emotional response and normal growth and development.
   b. The child may not be able to participate in activities in which sounds and verbal commands are used.
   c. Often the referral agency will become very involved in supporting the family.
3. Help the parents become aware of their importance in the success of the habilitation of the child.
   a. Parents have the most important educational influence on their child.
   b. Opportunities to use effective ways of stimulating the child's awareness and understanding of speech occur daily in the home.
   c. The child needs the warmth and security of a family setting.
4. Help the parents to understand what can be accomplished in their child's education to enable him to be a contributing member of society.
5. Stress the importance of close follow-up by the specialists caring for the child.
6. Help the parents to understand the use and importance of the hearing aid their child is using.
   a. Most children with a hearing loss have enough residual hearing to respond to and/or recognize sounds with use of an aid.
   b. Use of the aid does not approximate normal hearing; the child receives sound differently.
   c. Parents must be convinced of the value of the aid but not pay too much attention to it.
   d. Young child does not have much difficulty in adjusting to the hearing aid if the ear mold is comfortable and the sound amplification is not too unpleasant. Place the aid on the child and have him wear it during waking hours.
   e. For the older child who has become used to the aid as a youngster, it is part of his body image and he is dependent on the sound.
   f. Parents should be sensitive to their child's reactions to the aid.
   g. Follow-up care is vital; a malfunctioning aid can cause the child to lose interest in its use.
7. Help shape healthy parental attitudes about their child and guide them through this difficult time.
   a. Prevent denial.
   b. Parents need sympathetic understanding during the time of diagnosis and immediately following when they are bewildered and grieving.
   c. Parental attitudes may be the primary factor in determining the success or failure of the child's progress.
8. Help the parents to maintain continued awareness of normal growth and development of their child and the normal stresses and needs during each stage.
9. Encourage the parents to write for literature from appropriate agencies.*

B. Offer Continuing Parental Support.

1. Help the parents to think of their child as a child first, then as a child with special needs.
2. Emphasize their importance in the habilitation of their child. Point out the value of the home environment in his development.
   a. Talk about the daily routines.
   b. Talk about mother's role in stimulating the child's interest in sounds and speech.
   c. Encourage the use of hearing aids and the learning program set up by specialists in hearing problems in children, as appropriate.
   d. Expose the child to other children his own age who have hearing impairment.
   e. An adult who is deaf (if parents are not) may also help the child.
   f. With the passage of Public Law 94-142, public education is provided for all handicapped children.
   g. Residential placement may be considered when local facilities are nonexistent or when the home environment would be detrimental to the child's progress.

---

* Organizations for parents concerned with hearing problems include the following:

1. Alexander Graham Bell Association for the Deaf, 3417 Volta Place NW, Washington, DC 20007
2. The John Tracy Clinic, 806 West Adams Blvd, Los Angeles, CA 90007. This clinic offers a free home correspondence course (in English and Spanish) for parents that provides them with information, guidance, and encouragement in training their child.
3. National Association of the Deaf, 814 Thayer Avenue, Silver Spring, MD 20910
4. National Easter Seal Society for Crippled Children and Adults, Inc., 2023 W. Ogden Avenue, Chicago, IL 60612
5. Bill Wilkerson Hearing and Speech Center, 1114 19th Avenue, South, Nashville, TN 37212
6. National Association for Hearing and Speech Action, 10801 Rockville Pike, Rockville, MD 20852
7. Gallaudet College, 800 Florida Avenue NE, Washington, DC 20002

3. Encourage the parents to talk about their fears, frustrations, and feelings in caring for the child at home. Initiate a social worker referral, if a social worker is not already involved from the special training center.

Expected Outcomes

1. Communicates through sign language, touch, eye contact, and visual clues
2. Interacts with people in the environment; uses assistive measures to communicate; undergoing auditory and speech training
3. Engages in play activities suitable for age; becoming less dependent
4. Practices safety measures; wears hearing aid
5. Interacts with parents; parents verbalize understanding of the child's stage of growth and development
6. Reveals lessening of anxiety; assumes a more confident manner; plays with other children; learning techniques to augment communication.
7. The parents are reinforcing tactile and visual methods of communication with the child; working out their own grief, anxiety and guilt feelings; exploring community resources; displaying an accepting, loving attitude toward child.

Otitis Media

Otitis media is an infection of the middle ear. It may or may not be infectious or be accompanied by effusion.

Classification

1. *Acute otitis media*—suppurative or purulent
2. *Chronic otitis media* with effusion (also called secretory, serous, nonsuppurative otitis media, and "glue ear." Chronic effusion may be serous, mucoid, or purulent)—Inflammatory process of the middle ear with effusion collection as a result of auditory canal blockage. Can occur with or without infection. Bacterial or viral agents cause purulent exudate to collect in the space of the middle ear behind the eardrum (tympanic membrane).

Etiology

A. Suppurative Otitis Media

1. Bacteriologic
   a. *Streptococcus pneumoniae*
   b. *Haemophilus influenzae*
   c. *Branhamella catarrhalis*
   d. *Streptococcus pyogenes* (group A)
2. Viruses
   a. *Mycoplasma pneumoniae*
   b. *Chlamydia trachomatis*
   c. Respiratory syncytial viruses:
      Influenza viruses
      Adenoviruses
3. Secondary
   a. Cold
   b. Measles
   c. Scarlet fever

B. Nonsuppurative Otitis Media

1. Allergy
2. Auditory canal dysfunction
   a. Obstruction
   b. Abnormal patency
3. Often unknown—nonsuppurative

C. Predisposing Factors

1. Auditory canal in children is shorter, wider, and more horizontal, thus making the middle ear more accessible to invasion of organisms.
2. Anatomic immaturity of tubal muscles and cartilage in children under 2 years of age.
3. Certain craniofacial congenital defects (i.e., cleft palate, Down syndrome).
4. URI, allergies

Incidence

1. Suppurative—children under 5 years of age, with highest incidence under 2 years of age
2. Nonsuppurative—school-age children
3. Increased incidence during winter and early spring

Altered Physiology

All related to alteration in function of auditory canal
1. Obstruction of the auditory canal by swelling of the mucous membranes.
   a. Air exchange does not take place between the pharynx and middle ear.
   b. Obstruction impedes drainage of secretions to the nasopharynx.
2. Secretions and bacteria becomes trapped in the middle ear (suppurative).
   a. Bacteria multiply rapidly in that environment, spread to mastoid bone or inner ear, and cause permanent damage.
   b. Examination reveals hyperemic, opaque, and bulging tympanic membrane with hypomobility, with or without effusion.
   c. Inadequate ventilation produces negative pressure in middle ear. The negative pressure eventually produces sterile transudate within the middle ear, which draws organisms from the nasopharynx into the middle ear.
3. Fluid and exudate replace air in the middle ear. Fluid changes from watery secretions to viscous glue-like substance (nonsuppurative).
   a. Examination reveals tympanic membrane that is opaque, but if translucent, an air fluid level or air bubbles may be seen. Amber or bluish fluid may be seen in the middle ear; hypomobility and tympanic membrane may be retracted or convex.
   b. Tympanic membrane may rupture.

Complications

From untreated or ineffective treatment of acute otitis media
1. Chronic otitis media
2. Mastoiditis
3. Septicemia
4. Meningitis and brain damage
5. Chronic otitis media with mastoiditis and perforated eardrum may lead to impaired hearing or deafness and retarded speech.
6. Transient or permanent hearing loss
7. Nonsuppurative otitis media (and tympanosclerosis; adhesive otitis media)
8. Mild to moderate conductive hearing loss
9. Cholesteatoma tympani

Clinical Manifestations

1. History of cold for several days
2. Fever
3. Older child
   a. Pain in affected ear; fullness, throbbing

b. Indistinct hearing
c. Headache
d. Vomiting
4. Infant
   a. May rub ear; (pain)
   b. Anorexia
   c. Turns head from side to side
   d. Diarrhea
5. Decrease in hearing

Diagnostic Evaluation

1. Examination will reveal bulging, red eardrum, partial or complete obstruction of bony landmarks, and lack of normal luster; ruptured drum may be obscured by secretions. Absence of light reflex, impaired mobility of eardrum when using pneumatic otoscope. Eardrum usually will be retracted.
2. Culture and sensitivity determination of drainage from ruptured drum or through myringotomy or needle tympanocentesis in order to select appropriate antibiotic therapy.
3. *Tympanometry*—the use of an electroacoustic impedance bridge with which a tympanogram can be obtained. The tympanograms produced show the dynamics of the tympanic membrane, middle ear, auditory canal system.
4. Acoustic emittance measurements—test for conductive hearing loss.
5. Radiography—especially useful with chronic otitis media

Medical Treatment

Goal:
to reduce fever and pain, accelerate resolution of middle ear fluid and hearing loss, and reduce complications, recurrence, and sequellae.

Identify etiology
1. Antibiotics—appropriate for organism
   a. Usually ampicillin or amoxicillin
   b. Alternatives:
      (1) Trimethoprim–sulfamethoxazole and erythromycin
      (2) Erythromycin and sulfisoxozole
2. Acetaminophen—for fever
3. Analgesic—local heat
4. Antihistamines and decongestant—to clear nasal pharyngitis and inflammation of auditory canals (controversial)
5. Follow-up hearing tests

Surgical Treatment

A. Myringotomy

1. Surgical incision of the tympanic membrane to allow drainage and relieve pressure.
2. Done when fluid remains in middle ear despite medical treatment, or performed for diagnostic reasons.
3. Heat probe may also be used.

B. Tympanostomy Ventilating Tube

1. Small plastic tube is inserted into the middle ear through a myringotomy incision, creating an artificial auditory canal to equalize pressure on both sides of the eardrum.
2. Indications for tubes insertion:
   a. Chronic otitis media with effusion
   b. Recurrent suppurative otitis media
   c. Primary or secondary tympanic membrane disease

3. The tube projects through the drum into the external auditory canal.
4. This tube is a substitute for the eustachian tube, allowing the following to occur:
   a. Continuous ventilation of the middle ear
   b. Drainage of fluid into the external auditory canal
   c. Promotion of healing of lining membranes
   d. Prevention of premature closing of incision
5. The tube may be left in place several weeks to several months. The perforation closes in about a week after the tubes are removed.
6. Hearing will improve in children with middle ear fluid
7. Most common age for treatment is between 2 and 7 years.
8. Complications of tympanostomy tube include:
   a. Recurring otitis media or suppurative otitis media
   b. Plugging of tube with blood, cerumen, or exudate
   c. Early spontaneous extrusion of tube
   d. Permanent perforations
   e. Tympanosclerosis
   f. Local or diffuse atrophy of tympanic membrane
   g. Otorrhea
9. Specific postoperative considerations
   Do not allow water to get into ears (during swimming or bathing) because of the infection potential. Emphasize the advantage—improvement of hearing

C. Tympanocentesis—aspiration of middle ear fluids

Patient Problems and Nursing Diagnoses

1. Potential complication: spread of infection to brain
2. Altered comfort: pain, related to alteration in eustachian tube function
3. Altered skin integrity related to drainage from ear
4. Anxiety related to procedures and treatment
5. Sensory alteration related to hearing impairment
6. Potential altered growth and development related to inability to react/relate to sounds in environment
7. Potential for knowledge deficit of parents

Nursing Interventions

A. Administering Medications and Treatments as Prescribed.

1. Give appropriate antibiotics according to sensitivity of organisms. Usual course of treatment is 10–14 days.
2. Instill nose drops and decongestant (controversial). May help to shrink mucous membranes and allow drainage from obstructed auditory canal.
3. Give ear irrigations and instill glycerin or oil for relief of pain.
   a. The child may need to be held, or "mummy" restraint used.
   b. For the child under 3 years old—pull auricle down and back.
   c. For the child over 3 years old—pull auricle up and back.
   d. Position the child so the affected ear is up—allows fluid to run onto the eardrum.

B. Preventing Mixed Infection and Reducing the Chances of Complications Arising From Present Infection.

1. Always wash hands prior to any treatment or contact with the ear.
2. Change position of the child as appropriate.
   a. Position affected ear up to instill medications or to irrigate ear.
   b. Position affected ear down to facilitate drainage when the child is resting.

3. Clean any exudate present from myringotomy or perforated drum.
   Prevents excoriation from drainage.

C. Providing Physical Comfort for the Child While Continuing Therapy.

1. Local heat
   a. Use hot water bottle containing water not over 38.9°C. (102°F.).
      Heating pad may be used with an older child (set on low).
   b. Place the child on his side, with affected ear on top of bottle to facilitate drainage.
   c. Ice pack may provide comfort by decreasing edema and pressure.
2. A mild analgesic may be necessary if the child is restless and indicates pain.
3. Myringotomy may be done in cases in which there is severe pain.
   Small incision of the tympanic membrane to relieve pressure and prevent a jagged opening from a spontaneous rupture. Prepare the child for procedure. Use model of ear anatomy for teaching. Show him and let him handle ventilating tubes.
4. If there is drainage, keep the external ear clean to prevent excoriation by using cotton pledgets soaked in hydrogen peroxide.
5. Encourage fluid intake to help maintain hydration, as the child may have a fever.
6. Give a soft diet; chewing may cause increased pain.

D. Observing for Signs of Complications and Reporting Them.

1. Mastoiditis
   a. Pain behind the affected ear
   b. Increasing irritability
   c. Onset or increase of fever
   d. Tenderness, redness, and swelling over mastoid area
2. Meningitis
   a. Sudden onset of high fever
   b. Stiffness of neck
   c. Irritability
   d. Headache
   e. Lethargy
3. Chronic otitis media with perforation of tympanic membrane
   Usually not observed until follow-up care by physician
4. Cholesteatoma—results from squamous epithelium of the external canal growing into the middle ear, to the mastoid antrum, and eroding the bone. It is seen as a shiny white mass. It is a complication of chronic suppurative otitis media and should be reported to the physician immediately.

E. Providing Emotional and Psychological Support Appropriate for Child's Age and Degree of Illness.

1. Encourage the child to participate in diversional activities.
2. Reassure the child.
   a. Talk to him gently.
   b. Allow the child to express his feelings, fears, and frustrations by talking, playing, and drawing.
   c. Hold and rock the younger child.
3. Encourage parental visits and involvement in the child's care.
   a. Ensure that the parents understand the diagnosis, pathology involved, and treatment.

b. Help them to understand the necessity for follow-up and return visit following the episode, and the possible complications.

F. Assessing for Signs of Hearing Loss and Social and Language Retardation.

1. Middle ear effusions remain in 60%–70% of these cases for about 2 weeks following diagnosis of otitis media. If this persists more than 3 months, tubes are recommended.

Health Education

A. Help the Parents Understand That Prevention of Recurring Otitis Media is Vitally Important for the Future Well-Being of the Child.

1. Explain the value of preventing and treating the common cold and preventing otitis media.
   a. Feed the child in a sitting or upright position.
   b. Teach the child to use gentle nose blowing during a cold.
   c. Replace air in the middle ear—bubble blowing, chewing sugarless gum, blowing up balloon, Valsalva's maneuver by forcing air into a closed mouth while holding nose.
2. Removal of hypertrophied and infected adenoid tissue may be necessary at a later date on the recommendation of the physician.
3. Explain that the child may have decreased hearing for several weeks following this episode of illness.
4. Help the parents learn what signs indicate recurrent otitis media and the need for immediate medical intervention.
   a. Prompt treatment can prevent permanent hearing loss.
   b. Identify the relationship between hearing and language development.
   c. Teach the parents signs of hearing loss and to monitor speech and language as well as social development.
5. Help the parents understand the necessity of continuing administration of antibiotics for the prescribed time even though the child may no longer appear sick.
6. Assess the need for community agency referral.

B. Help the Parents and Child Understand Treatment and Expectations Related to Ventilating Tubes.

1. Following surgery, antibiotic ear drops may be prescribed to aid in keeping tubes patent.
2. Hearing may not improve for 1–3 weeks postoperatively.
3. Tubes will remain in place from 2–10 months, and are designed to extrude into the external ear canal.
4. When tubes extrude, slight pain and a small amount of bloody drainage may occur. Physician should be notified that the tubes are out.
5. Controversial issue involves water and swimming:
   a. Water should be prevented from entering the external ear canal—use custom-made ear plugs, cottonballs coated with petroleum, etc.
      OR
   b. Rules about swimming—do not lower head below 6 inches from surface of water, no swimming in surf or wading pools, no diving or racing turns.
6. Prepare the parents and child for possible occurrence of otorrhea.
7. Stress the importance of regular medical follow-up to evaluate proper functioning of tubes.

Expected Outcomes

1. Shows recovery from infection; temperature returning to normal; taking prescribed antimicrobial medication
2. Experiences minimal discomfort; does not rub ear or have distressful cry; sleeping in a restful manner; no complaints of pain
3. Avoids skin breakdown in area of ear drainage
4. Shows reduced level of anxiety; complies with treatment; interacts with personnel; demonstrates appropriate age-related behaviors
5. Demonstrates improved hearing; responding to auditory stimulation
6. Parents demonstrate understanding by explaining illness, complications, and treatment

Bibliography

Books

Balkany TJ and Pashley NRT. Clinical Pediatric Otolaryngology. St. Louis, CV Mosby, 1986

Bluestone CD (ed). Pediatric Otolaryngology. Vol 1–2. Philadelphia, WB Saunders, 1983

Brodley JE, Brookhouser PE and Tucker GF. Ear, Nose, and Throat Disorders in Children. New York, Raven Press, 1986

Crawford JS et al. Pediatric Ophthalmology and Strabismus: Transactions of the New Orleans Academy of Ophthalmology. New York, Raven Press, 1985

Feigin RD, Kline MW and Spector G. Otitis Media In Feigin RD and Cherry JD (eds). Textbook of Pediatric Infectious Diseases. 2nd ed, pp 197–212. Philadelphia, WB Saunders, 1987

Fleisher G and Ludwig S. Textbook of Pediatric Emergency Medicine. 2nd ed. Baltimore, Williams & Wilkins, 1988

Giebink GS and Canafax DM. Controversies in the management of acute otitis media, pp. 47–64. In Aronoff SC (ed). Advances in Pediatric Infections, Vol 3, Diseases, pp 47–64. Chicago, Year Book Medical Pub

Harley RD (ed). Pediatric Ophthalmology. 2nd ed. Vol 1 and 2. Philadelphia, WB Saunders, 1983

Kelley SJ. Pediatric Emergency Nursing. Norwalk, Appleton & Lange, 1988

Nelson JD. Current Therapy in Pediatric Infectious Diseases. Philadelphia, BC Decker, 1986

Van Dyke RB, Desky AB and Daum RS. Infections of the eye and periorbital structures. In Aronoff SC (ed). Advances in Pediatric Infectious Diseases, Vol 3, pp 125–180. Chicago, Year Book Medical Pub, 1988

Whaley LF and Wong DL. Nursing Care of Infants and Children. St. Louis, CV Mosby, 1987

Wybar K and Taylor D. Pediatric Ophthalmology—Current Concepts. New York, Marcel Dekker, 1983

Journals

Ear

Adams JW and Tidwell R. Parents' perceptions regarding the discipline of their hearing-impaired child. Child Care Health Dev 1988 Jul–Aug; 14(4):265–273

Bernstein ME and Barta L. What do parents want in parent education? Am Ann Deaf 1988 Jul; 133(3):235–246

Butterfield SA and Ersing WF. Influence of age, sex, etiology, and hearing loss on balance performance by deaf children. Percept Mot Skills 1986 Apr; 62(2):659–663

del Bo M. Childhood deafness today. Adv Otorhinolaryngol 1987; 37:93–96

Drell MJ and Drell JM. Psychologic preparation of children for insertion of myringotomy tubes. Ear Nose Throat J 1988 Mar; 67(3):138+

Felder H. The use of tympanostomy tubes. Pediatr Ann 1988 Oct; 17(10):616, 618, 619

Humphrey GK et al. Can blind infants and children use sonar sensory aids? Can J Psychol 1988 Jun; 42(2):94–119

Loyer-Carlson VI and Sugarwara AI. Mothers' estimates of hearing family members' competence in sign language and the deaf child's loneliness. Percept Mot Skills 1988 Oct; 67(2):633–634

McCune N. Deaf in a hearing unit: Coping of staff and adolescents. J Adolesc 1988 Mar; 11(1):21–28

Musselman CR, Wilson AK and Lindsay PH. Effects of early intervention on hearing impaired children. Except Child 1988 Nov; 55(3):222–228

Pickett JM and Stark RE. Cochlear implants and sensory aids in deaf children. Int J Pediatr Otorhinolarygol 1987 Oct; 13(3):323–344

Rittenhouse RK and Kenyon PL. Educational and social language in deaf adolescent: TDD and school-produced comparisons. Am Ann Deaf 1987 Jul; 132(3):210–212

Ruben RJ. Diagnosis of deafness in infancy. Pediatr Rev 1987 Nov; 9(5):163–166

Watkins S. Long term effects of home intervention with hearing-impaired children. Am Ann Deaf 1987 Oct; 132(4):267–271

Eye

Agapitos PJ, Noel LP and Clarke WN. Traumatic hyphema in children. Ophthalmology 1987 Oct; 94(10):1238–1241

Buncic JR. The blind infant. Pediatr Clin North Am 1987 Dec; 34(6):1403–1413

Christenson GN and Rouse MN. Management of a young esotrope using vision therapy and prismatic prescriptions. J Am Optom Assoc 1987 Jul; 58(7):592–596

Christensen S, Farrow-Gillespie A and Lerman J. Incidence of emesis and postanesthetic recovery after strabismus surgery in children: A comparison of droperidol and lidocaine. Anesthesiology 1989 Feb; 70(2):251–254

Eustis S and Smith DR. Parental understanding of strabismus. J Pediatr Ophthalmol Strabismus 1989 Sep–Oct; 24(5):232–236

Fielder AR. The management of squint. Arch Dis Child 1989 Mar; 64(3):413–418

Freeman RD et al. Blind children's early emotional development: Do we know enough to help? Child Care Health Dev 1989 Jan–Feb; 15(1):3–28

Grin TR, Nelson LB and Jeffers JB. Eye injuries in childhood. Pediatrics 1987 Jul; 80(1):13–17

Kushner BJ and Meyers FL. Good visual outcome after endophthalmitis in an eye previously treated successfully for amblyopia. J Pediatr Ophthalmol Strabismus 1989 Mar–Apr; 26(2):69–71

Mokrohisky ST and Burchell MS. Toy balloons and eye injuries. Pediatrics 1988 Mar; 8(3):473

Phillips S and Hartley JT. Developmental differences and interventions for blind children. Pediatric Nurs 1988 May–Jun; 14(3):201–204

Robinson GC, Jan JE and Kinnis C. Congenital ocular blindness in children, 1945–1984. Am J Dis Child 1987 Dec; 14(12):1321–1324

Screening for squint and poor vision. Arch Dis Child 1987 Oct; 62(10):982–983

Sisson LA, Babeo TJ and Van Hasselt VB. Group training to increase social behaviors in young multihandicapped children. Behav Modif 1988 Oct; 12(4):497–524

Sonksen PM. Constraints upon parenting: Experience of a paediatrician. Child Care Health Dev 1989 Jan–Feb; 15(1):29–36

Thommessen M, Riis G and Kase BF. Nutrition and growth retardation in 10 children with congenital deaf-blindness. J Am Diet Assoc 1988 Jan; 89(1):69–73

Tobin MJ. Constraints upon parenting: Experience of a psychologist. Child Care Health Dev 1989 Jan–Feb; 15(1):37–43

Additional Reading for Nursing Staff

Bluestone CD and Klein JO. Otitis Media in Infants and Children (Major Problems in Clinical Pediatrics Series). Philadelphia, WB Saunders, 1987

Harley RK and Lawrence GA. Visual Impairment in the Schools. 2nd ed. Springfield, CC Thomas, 1984

Freeman RD, Goetz E and Richards DP. Thoughts from Canada: Starting school—emotional considerations. Child Care Health Dev 1989 Jan–Feb; 15(1):65–67

Jones H. Thoughts from England: Starting school—emotional considerations. Child Care Health Dev 1989 Jan–Feb; 15(1):59–64

Preisler G and Polmer C. Thoughts from Sweden: The blind child at nursery school with sighted children. Child Care Health Dev 1989 Jan–Feb; 15(1): 45–52

Programs and Services for the Deaf in the United States. Am Ann Deaf 1987 Apr; 132(2):57–172

Parent Reading

Tropp B. Thoughts from Scotland: Starting school—Emotional considerations. Child Care Health Dev 1989 Jan–Feb; 15(1):53–58

"Tubes for Davy" LSU Medical Center, Div Child Psychiatry, School of Medicine, New Orleans, 1542 Tulane Ave, New Orleans, LA 70112-2822 c/o Dr. Martin J. Drell

Corn AL, Cowan CM and Moses E. You Seem like a Regular Kid to Me. Publications & Information Services, American Foundation for the Blind, 15 W 16th St, New York, NY 10011

Seal BC. Working parents' dream: Instructional videotapes for their signing deaf child. Am Ann Deaf 1987 Dec; 132(6):386–388

Juvenile Rheumatoid Arthritis

Juvenile rheumatoid arthritis (JRA) is a chronic inflammatory, generalized, systemic disease that involves a wide spectrum of manifestations, including joint, connective tissue, and visceral lesions throughout the body.

Etiology and Incidence

1. The cause of juvenile rheumatoid arthritis is unknown.
2. Current hypotheses
   a. Infection from an unidentified organism
   b. Autoimmune process or hypersensitivity to unknown stimuli
   c. Genetic predisposition
3. Peak stages of onset
   a. 18 months–5 years of age
   b. 8½–12 years of age

Altered Physiology

1. In the early stages, one or many joints show signs of inflammation.
2. The inflammation is initially localized in a joint capsule, primarily in the synovium. The tissue becomes thickened from congestion and edema.
3. A characteristic inflammatory response develops in the form of a synovial proliferation that invades the interior of the joint.
4. The inflammatory tissue extends into the interior of the joint along the surface of the articular cartilage, to which it may be adherent, so that it deprives the cartilage of nutrition.
5. By starvation and invasion, this inflammatory tissue slowly destroys the articular cartilage.
6. Synovial tissue eventually frees the joint space, leading to narrowing, fibrous ankylosis, and bony fusion.
7. Growth centers next to inflamed joints may undergo either premature epiphyseal closure or accelerated epiphyseal growth.
8. Tendons and tendon sheaths may develop inflammatory changes similar to the synovial tissues.
9. Inflammation of muscle may occur.
10. Eventually there is deformity, subluxation, and fibrous or bony ankylosis (fusion) of joint(s).
11. The arthritis results from chronic synovial inflammation.
12. Rheumatoid nodules are uncommon in children.

Complications

1. Bony deformities—crippling from progressive polyarthritis
   a. Growth disturbance
   b. Failure to thrive—short stature
   c. Cervical spine and temporomandibular jaw problems
   d. Leg length discrepancies
2. Psychological and social reactions to this chronic illness
3. Iridocyclitis—leading to cataracts, glaucoma, or blindness
4. Pericarditis

Modes of Onset and Clinical Manifestations

A. Acute Febrile–Systemic Onset (Still's Disease)

1. Highest incidence of onset is in children under 7 years of age—can occur throughout childhood
2. Incidence slightly higher in males
3. Represents 20% of cases
4. Initially joint involvement is variable—from no joint pain to generalized florid arthritis
5. Systemic characteristics:
   a. Irritability, anorexia, and malaise
   b. Intermittent fever—1 or 2 spikes a day over 38.9°C. (102°F.); occurrence of subnormal temperature between elevations; possible seizures
   c. Rash consisting of small, discrete, pink macules with pale centers occurring on trunk and extremities; rash may be transient—occurring with elevated temperature
   d. Hepatosplenomegaly
   e. Generalized lymphadenopathy
   f. Anemia
   g. Periorbital edema
   h. Carditis—tachycardia (disproportionate to fever), tachypnea, pericarditis, myocarditis
   i. Pleuritis or pneumonitis independent of carditis
6. WBC count and sedimentation rate may be elevated
7. 20%–25% of those with systemic onset will progress to severe arthritis.

B. Polyarticular Onset

1. Higher incidence in females than males
2. Characterized by arthritis of more than 4 joints
   a. Acute onset is manifested by painful swelling of joints.
   b. Insidious onset—minimal or no joint pain; however, the child may wince on movement or may limp on walking.
   c. Large joints most often involved are knees, wrists, ankles, and elbows.
   d. Other areas are often involved.
      (1) Rheumatoid foot—metatarsophalangeal joints swollen and tender; pain in heel

(2) Cervical spine and hip—tenderness and restricted movement
3. Systemic manifestations occur less frequently than in acute febrile onset; may see low-grade fever and general lymphadenopathy

C. Negative Rheumatoid Factor

1. Represents 20%–25% of cases
2. Serum rheumatoid factor—negative; Antinuclear antibodies present in about 25% of cases
3. About 10% of the cases will progress to severe arthritis.
4. Age of onset can be throughout childhood.

D. Positive Rheumatoid Factor

1. Represents 5%–10% of cases
2. Serum rheumatoid factor present in all cases and antinuclear antibodies present in 75% of cases
3. More than 50% of the cases will progress to severe arthritis.
4. Age of onset is generally late childhood.

E. Pauciarticular Onset

1. Incidence
   a. Type I—onset in early childhood, 1–6 years; predominantly female. Represents 35%–40% of presenting cases
   b. Type II—onset in late childhood, over age 8 years; predominantly male—represents 10%–15% of presenting cases
2. Characterized by arthritis of 1 or up to 4 joints
   a. Type I
      (1) Child under 5 years may be listless and irritable, have low-grade fever, and fail to grow at normal rate.
      (2) Large joints, knee, ankle, and elbow
   b. Type II
      (1) Older child does not appear ill.
      (2) Large joints—hip girdle
3. Systemic manifestations are few.
   a. May see rash, low-grade fever, lymphadenopathy, and splenomegaly.
   b. There is increased incidence of iridocyclitis.
      (1) Type I—chronic iridocyclitis
      (2) Type II—acute iridocyclitis
4. Antinuclear antibodies test positive in about 90% of Type I pauciarticular onset
   a. HLA–B27—positive (human lymphocyte antigen)
5. Long-term complications
   a. Type I
      (1) Occular damage with iridocyclitis
      (2) Polyarthritis
   b. Type II
      Spondyloarthropathy—juvenile ankylosing spondylitis

Generalized Clinical Manifestations

A. Joints (changes may occur with or without systemic symptoms)

1. Symptoms may develop gradually with progressive stiffness, swelling, and impaired motion of a joint or joints.
2. Symptoms may develop rapidly with sudden appearance of symptomatic arthritis in one or more joints.
3. Knees, ankles, feet, wrists, or fingers are usually involved initially.
4. Joints are swollen and warm.
5. Pain and stiffness of joint may appear before objective changes develop.
6. Limitation of motion of inflamed joints occurs.

7. Characteristic posture is one of guarding joints from movement; an anxious pained expression (with polyarthritis) is common.
8. Morning stiffness of joints occurs following periods of inactivity.
9. Atrophy and weakness of muscles near the affected joints may develop.
10. Skin over inflamed joints may be pigmented.
11. Chronically affected joints may become dislocated, deformed, or fused.
12. Subcutaneous nodules may appear over pressure points (knees, elbows, etc.).
13. Condition may ultimately affect any joint in the body (knees, ankles, wrists, feet, fingers, toes, shoulders, elbows, neck, jaw, hips and sacroiliac joints are frequently involved).
14. Small, deformed feet result from foot involvement in early childhood.
15. Micrognathia (unusually small lower jaw), as a result of temporomandibular arthritis, is one hallmark of juvenile rheumatoid arthritis.
16. Spindling or fusiform changes of the fingers may occur.

B. Inflammation of the Eye (unilateral or bilateral uveitis; iridocyclitis)

Child may have no early symptoms. If symptoms occur late, child may develop irreversible eye damage, including scarring and adhesions of the iris and cataracts.
1. Redness
2. Pain
3. Photophobia
4. Decreased visual acuity
5. Nonreactive pupil

C. Generalized Growth Retardation

1. During periods of remission, growth spurts may occur.
2. Treatment with long-term steroid therapy as well as the disease process may contribute to growth failure.

Diagnostic Evaluation

(of limited value)
1. Elevated sedimentation rate (usually)
2. Leukocytosis
3. High total serum proteins
4. Positive creatine protein
5. High frequency of serum antinuclear antibodies with pauciarticular onset—Type I and polyarticular onset with positive rheumatoid factor
6. Possible alteration in serum proteins (increased alpha and gamma; decreased albumin)
7. Changes in bone, demonstrated by x-rays—initially nonspecific

Treatment

Goals:

Relieve joint inflammation and pain.
Maintain and increase joint range of motion, muscle strength, and tone, and prevent physical deformities.
Preserve total growth and development potential.
Support emotional outlook of patient and his family.

1. Although this is a painful disease of long duration, the outlook for remission is good.
2. There is no specific cure; treatment is supportive:
   a. Drug therapy to reduce inflammation; analgesia
   b. Exercise program to promote joint movement
3. Surgery
   a. Synovectomy—(to maintain function) when extensive synovitis develops, especially around wrists

b. Joint replacement—with severe destructive arthritis (ankylosing spondylitis)

Patient Problems and Nursing Diagnoses

1. Mobility, impaired, related to decreased joint range and muscle strength from the disease
2. Comfort, altered, pain related to joint inflammation
3. Noncompliance with treatment program related to psychological reactions to illness and/or lack of understanding
4. Anxiety related to hospitalization, pain, and treatments
5. Altered self-image and self-esteem related to decreased mobility and deformities
6. Potential complication: gastric upset or aspirin toxicity related to treatment doses

Nursing Interventions

A. Offering the Patient and His Parents Realistic Encouragement.

1. Although the response to medication is slow, the recovery is slow, and episodes of acute illness recur, the long-term outlook is generally good.
2. The child may be hospitalized during an acute attack and systemic illness, or to receive intensive physical therapy.

B. Discussing With the Parents and the Child What They Know About the Disease and What They Expect From Treatment.

1. Determine what information has been given to them by the physician.
2. The child and his family must understand the disease and treatment. This is a chronic disease and has an unpredictable course; however, compliance with prescribed treatment will minimize crippling from progressive polyarthritis and allow the child to grow and develop to his potential.

C. Being an Effective Member of the Special Team Caring for This Patient and His Family.

The team often includes pediatrician, rheumatologist, social worker, physical therapist, occupational therapist, psychologist/psychiatrist, ophthalmologist, hospital nurse, and community health nurse.

D. Assisting in the Program of Physical Therapy in Order to Maintain or Increase Joint Range of Motion and Muscle Strength and Tone (Figs. 57-1, 57-2, 57-3).

1. The parents and child are instructed in the exercises. Encourage development of program (with parental involvement) while patient remains in the hospital.

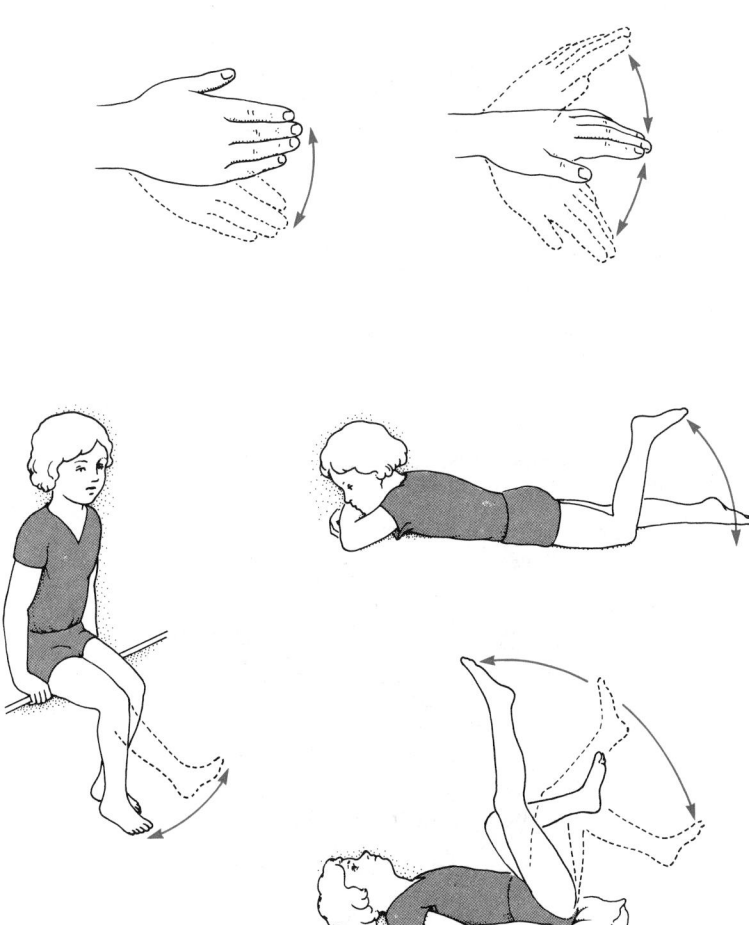

Figure 57-1. *Therapeutic exercise: active range of motion for wrists, knees, and hips.*

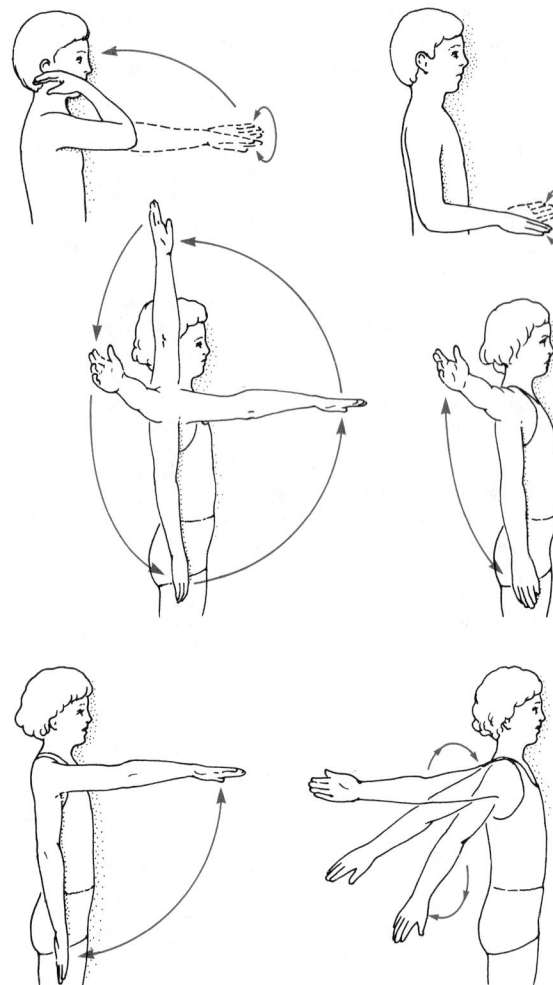

Figure 57-2. *Therapeutic exercise: active range of motion for wrists, elbows, and shoulders.*

2. Night splints for the wrists, knees, hip, and ankle may be prescribed to do the following:
   a. Give rest and relief of pain.
   b. Prevent or correct deformity.
   c. Maintain damaged joint in a functional position.
3. Know proper application of splint and help the patient to adjust to it.
4. A hot tub bath prior to the exercises and following long rest periods may make the exercises less painful. Whirlpool treatment will aid in decreasing stiffness.
5. Full range of motion exercises should be performed every day. Inactivity results in stiffness.
   a. Encourage the child to do his own exercises as soon as possible.
   b. Isometric exercise may be done when active free exercise may be too much strain for an arthritic joint, or when they are impractical because of physical location (riding in car, sitting at desk in school).
6. Orthopedic surgery may be required to correct some deformities.

E. Providing the Child With the Freedom to Engage in as Much Activity as He Is Able to Tolerate.
1. Children will limit their own activity. Play is an effective therapeutic modality.
2. Those activities that produce overtiring or cause joint pain should be avoided.
3. Diversional activities should encourage movement based on the child's tolerance.
4. Encourage the child to be as self-sufficient as possible.
5. Allow the child to make some decisions himself (e.g., when he prefers to do his exercises).
6. Limit the use of wheelchairs. Tricycles and pedal cars provide good modes of mobility and exercise.

F. Using the Principles of Proper Body Mechanics and Posture Whether the Child Is at Rest or Is Active.
1. Provide firm mattress to prevent sagging joints.
2. Use thin pillow (nor more than 5 cm. [2 inches] thick) to prevent dowager hump. Do not place pillows under joints.
3. The child may attempt to protect joints by assuming a position of flexion to ease discomfort.

G. Administering Medications Used to Treat JRA. Knowing Usage, Side Effects, and Screening Tests to Be Done During Therapy.
Drug classes include:
1. *Nonsteroid anti-inflammatory drugs*
   a. Aspirin is the drug of choice.
      (1) Therapeutic serum levels are 20–30 mg./dl.
      (2) Enteric-coated aspirin reduces incidence of gastrointestinal symptoms.
      (3) Salicylates
         (a) Anti-inflammatory, analgesic, antipyretic
         (b) See Salicylates and Steroids, under Rheumatic Fever, page 1327, for side effects.
      (4) Monitor liver enzymes for toxicity.
   b. Tolmetin
      (1) Used when aspirin is not effective or tolerated
      (2) Causes less gastric upset
      (3) May increase risk of anemia

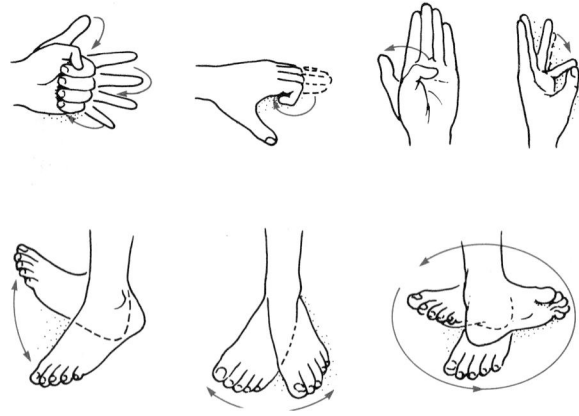

Figure 57-3. *Therapeutic exercise: active range of motion for fingers and ankles.*

(4) Excreted quickly; therefore, must be given 3–4 times daily

> **NURSING ALERT:** Because of the increased association of aspirin and Reye's syndrome, discontinue use of aspirin when the child has a viral illness.

2. *Analgesics*
   a. Aspirin
   b. Acetaminophen
3. *Corticosteroids*—Controversial because of side effects
   a. Used in addition to salicylates when salicylates alone are not effective. Their use does not prevent complications of severe arthritis or influence ultimate prognosis.
   b. See the reference to salicylates and steroids, under Rheumatic Fever.
   c. Tuberculin test should be done prior to starting steroid therapy.
   d. Monitor for glucosuria.
4. *Long-acting, disease-modifying agents*
   a. Water-soluble gold salts (sodium aurothiomalate)
      (1) Used in conjunction with salicylates when improvement is not apparent or progression is not halted after several months.
         Injection given weekly for several months.
      (2) Side effects include skin rash, nephritis with hematuria or proteinuria, thrombocytopenia, and neurotoxicity, gastric upset, leukopenia, anemia, and mucosal ulcers
      (3) Monitor urine for protein.
   b. *Antimalarial with anti-inflammatory activity* (hydroxychloroquine or chloroquine)
      (1) May cause gastric upset
      (2) Blindness—due to deposition of the compound in pigmented tissue, especially eyes; eye examination every 3–6 months is advocated
      (3) Used primarily with polyarticular disease

H. Assisting Child and Family in Learning Interventions That Promote Comfort.

1. Take morning medications as early as possible on waking and as prescribed throughout day
2. Warm bath or shower on arising
3. Limbering exercises in morning and as needed (see Fig. 57-1)
4. Maintain warmth during sleep by using sleeping bag, thermal underwear, footed pajamas, or leg warmers, heated waterbed.
5. Position changes during periods of sleep
6. Application of cool or warm packs to painful joint
7. Avoid activities that stress joints and avoid overdoing during periods of no or minimal pain.
8. Wear prescribed joint splints

I. Promoting General Good Health.

1. Well-balanced diet
2. Regular exercise and play appropriate for age
3. Avoid exposure to infections; seek medical treatment for infections
4. Ensure adequate rest
   Sleep may be difficult because of pain with movement—heated waterbed may be helpful.
5. Schedule regular medical and ophthalmologic examinations

Health Education

A. Educate and Motivate Parents and Child In Continuing Program of Treatment at Home.

Help parents to understand the needs of the child.
1. Extra rest—but not bed rest, which will contribute to contractures and muscle atrophy.
2. Program of daily exercise—this can be adjusted to fit in with the mother's or family's routine.
3. The child should attend school regularly and participate in regular school activities.
   a. This participation will allow the child to obtain social and scholastic achievement.
   b. Teachers should be informed of the child's condition and needs.
      (1) Child should get out of his seat and walk around room every hour.
      (2) Desk and chair should properly fit the child (i.e., when child is sitting with his back in the chair, his feet should be on the floor at right angles to legs; the seat should be deep enough to support thighs without pressure on popliteal arteries).
      (3) Individual educational plan (IEP)—deals with child's special needs—as mandated by PL 94-142: Education for all Handicapped Children Act.
   c. Recreation is important—swimming is a beneficial sport activity.
4. Compensate for activities of daily living—help the child understand he must do as much for himself as possible.
   Adapt items he uses to make their use easier (e.g., lift toilet seat several inches).
5. Provide nutritionally balanced diet to eliminate obesity that puts additional weight on joints.
6. Do not force unnecessary restrictions on the child that can produce acute behavioral upsets and interfere with his social development.
7. This disease affects the whole family. Remind parents to devote time to other members of the family and to their marriage. Various agencies can provide pertinent literature and can direct the family to helpful local resources.*
8. The child needs continual follow-up after hospitalization.
   a. Community health nurse can assist in home management of exercise program.
   b. Social worker can assist in helping parents work out their emotions and seek financial assistance.
   c. Ophthalmologist—must examine patient every 3–6 months for occurrence of iridocyclitis. Encourage the parents to report any eye symptoms that the child may develop.
   d. The physician must be consulted when any new symptoms occur, in an acute attack, or when progression is apparent, as well as for routine care.

Expected Outcomes

1. Demonstrates improved joint range of motion and muscle strength as evidenced by increased mobility, involvement in diversional activities, increased self-sufficiency, limited use of wheelchair or other assistive devices

* Contact the Arthritis Foundation, 1314 Spring Street, NW, Atlanta, GA 30309

2. Experiences minimal discomfort as evidenced by stable vital signs, increased mobility, play activity, interest in becoming involved with friends, use of proper body mechanics
3. Is free of complications related to aspirin use: absence of gastrointestinal upset and anemia
4. The patient/parents understand and can describe home-care measures to ensure rest, daily exercise, regular school attendance, maximum independence as able, proper diet

---

Systemic Lupus Erythematosus

Systemic lupus erythematosus (SLE) is a disease of the connective tissue with vascular and perivascular fibrinoid changes that may involve any organ or system.
Discoid lupus affects only the skin.

Incidence and Etiology

1. Incidence higher in females than in males; most common during the childbearing period (15–44 years of age). However, it can affect children 5–15 years of age.
2. Cause is unknown.
3. General theory of etiology is autoimmunity—believed to be an abnormal response of the body against its own connective tissue. Possible causes of this include the following:
   a. Genetic predisposition—genetic markers within HLA system have been demonstrated.
   b. Viral—nonspecific antibody rise as part of general immunologic hyperactivity
4. Possible factors that trigger or unmask initial symptoms:
   a. Exposure to sunlight; snow on bright day
   b. Injury
   c. Stress
   d. Radiation therapy
   e. Vaccination
   f. Antitoxins
   g. Other drugs (e.g., anticonvulsants, antibiotics)

Altered Physiology

1. Connective tissue in different organs develops nonspecific aberrations such as fibrinoid change in collagen and cellular infiltration, either in the walls of small blood vessels or elsewhere.
2. Alteration of collagen and subendothelial thickening of small blood vessels obstruct the flow of blood. These changes may be widespread or limited in distribution.

Complications

1. Sepsis—primarily resulting from steroid and immunosuppressive therapy
2. Renal involvement; chronic nephritis; renal failure
3. Cardiac complications
4. Neurologic involvement
5. Allergic reactions to drugs
6. Chronic fatigue
7. Pulmonary lupus and myocardial infarction
8. Growth retardation related to steroids and immunosuppressive therapy

Clinical Manifestations

1. General characteristic signs and symptoms may include:
   a. Malar erythema, which usually spreads over bridge of nose. (Butterfly rash may consist only of an erythematous blush or scaly erythematous papules; rash may be photosensitive.) Rash spreads from face and scalp to neck, chest, and extremities.
   b. Acute polyarthritis, arthralgia
   c. Fever
   d. Fatigue, malaise
   e. Anorexia, weight loss
   f. Cardiac involvement—pleurisy or pericarditis most diagnostic
   g. Nephritis—at onset or during course of disease
      (1) Hematuria
      (2) Proteinuria
   h. CNS involvement—during course of disease
      (1) Behavior disturbances
      (2) Convulsions
      (3) Coma
   i. Splenomegaly
   j. Hepatomegaly
   k. Lymphadenopathy
   l. Anemia, thrombocytopenia
   m. Hypoglobulinemia
   n. Raynaud's phenomenon
   o. Pulmonary involvement
      (1) Pleural effusion
      (2) Lupus pneumonitis
2. Onset may be gradual, with no specific signs and symptoms
   a. Aching joints
   b. Morning stiffness
   c. Butterfly rash
3. Onset may be abrupt, with the development of any of the following:
   a. High fever
   b. Dyspnea, chest pain
   c. Arthritis without severe deformities
   d. Abdominal pain

Diagnostic Evaluation

1. Thorough physical examination; patient and family history
2. Primary laboratory studies
   a. Fluorescent antinuclear antibody test (FANA) to detect antibodies that react with nucleus of cells—increased
   b. Lupus erythematosus (LE) cell test if FANA is positive—most diagnostic
   c. Serum sedimentation rate—elevated
   d. Serum complement studies—lowered
   e. CBC—leukopenia and mild to moderate anemia; can be hemolytic anemia thrombocytopenia
   f. Serum thrombotic accelerator (STA) (serology)—false-positive
   g. Blood chemistry—evaluate:
      (1) BUN—elevated
      (2) Blood sugar
      (3) Plasma protein—abnormal electrolytes
3. Kidney function studies
   a. Urine sediment—shows RBCs and granular casts, increased protein, leukocyturia
   b. Serum creatinine—elevated
   c. Urine protein—elevated
   d. Creatinine clearance
4. Presence of 4 or more of criteria for SLE proposed by American Rheumatism Association*

* Tan EM et al. The 1982 revised criteria for the classification of systemic lupus erythematosus. Arthritis Rheum 1982 Nov; 25(11): 1274

a. Malar rash
b. Discoid rash
c. Photosensitivity
d. Oral ulcers
e. Arthritis of two or more joints
f. Serositis—pleuritis or pericarditis
g. Renal disorder—persistent proteinuria or cellular casts
h. Neurologic disorder—seizures or psychosis
i. Hematologic disorder—hemolytic anemia, leukopenia, lymphopenia, or thrombocytopenia
j. Immunologic disorder—positive LE preparation or anti-DNA antibody or anti-Sm antibody or false-positive serologic test for syphilis
k. Antinuclear antibody

Treatment

1. Control of symptoms with medication
    a. Salicylates—relieve joint symptoms, fever, fatigue
    b. Antimalarials such as hydroxychloroquine sulfate (Plaquenil) to relieve joint symptoms and skin rash
    c. Steroids such as prednisone—used when there is renal or neurologic involvement or hemolytic anemia; TB test should be done prior to starting steroid therapy
    d. Immunosuppressive agents such as azathioprine and cyclophosphamide and chlorambucil—used in severe disease, especially with nephritis or steroid-resistant patients
    e. Topical steroid preparations—may help suppress cutaneous lesions
2. Careful and controlled monitoring of drug therapy and reassessment of clinical and laboratory picture
3. Supportive
    a. Rest
    b. Adequate nutrition
    c. Treatment of existing complications
    d. Early identification and treatment of opportunistic infection
    e. Patient education and counseling

Patient Problems and Nursing Diagnoses

1. Impaired mobility related to muscle weakness and joint pain
2. Altered nutrition, less than body requirements, related to loss of appetite from medication effects
3. Potential neurologic complications: excitability, headaches, seizures related to neurologic involvement
4. Potential respiratory complications related to inflamed serous lining of lungs, pleurisy, or pericarditis
5. Potential renal complications related to glomerular inflammation
6. Self-concept disturbance in body image, related to body changes from the disease and/or drugs
7. Noncompliance with treatment program related to lack of understanding

Nursing Interventions

A. Providing Opportunities for the Patient and the Parents to Discuss the Disease—Their Understanding of It and Their Expectations.

Assist the child and his family to adjust to the limitations and treatments of the disease.
1. Determine what information has been given to them by the physician.
2. Provide supportive care to help them work out feelings of fear, anxiety, and uncertainty.

3. Support them in accepting this condition as a long-term illness, with exacerbations and remissions.
    a. They will need continuing support. Initiate early referral to community health nurse and social worker.
    b. Provide available literature and encourage contact with the nearest chapter of the Lupus Erythematosus Foundation.*

B. Assisting the Child in Developing a Realistic Attitude About His Illness and Assisting Him in Expressing His Feelings About His Illness.

1. Provide the child with the opportunity to openly discuss his feelings about illness when he is able to verbalize these feelings.
2. Provide the child with the opportunity to express his feelings; use play as a method.
3. Arrange for a visiting teacher so that the child may have the opportunity to continue his education.
4. Encourage the child to continue contact with his peers (i.e., via telephone, letter-writing, etc.).
5. Allow the child to make some decisions and become involved in planning his own care.

C. Being Aware of the Action and Side Effects of Medications Used in the Treatment of Systemic Lupus Erythematosus.

Steroids and salicylates (see section on juvenile rheumatoid arthritis, p. 1423).

D. Observing Closely for the Development of Symptoms That May Indicate Development of Complications.

1. Observe for the development of renal symptoms. There is usually some degree of renal involvement.
    a. Record intake and output.
    b. Record specific gravity of urine.
    c. Observe the color and characteristics of urine, especially proteinuria.
    d. Observe for the development of edema.
2. Observe for the development of sepsis.
3. Report to the physician any abnormal findings.

E. Assisting the Child and Family in Understanding Ways to Prevent Exacerbations and Complications of the Disease.

1. Important "do's":
    a. Get enough rest.
    b. Avoid anxiety and tension.
    c. Follow treatment plan and medication schedule.
    d. Avoid contact with persons with infectious diseases.
    e. Follow prescribed diet, especially when receiving steroids.
    f. Seek medical attention at times of illness or stress.
    g. Recognize warning signs of exacerbation.
    h. Become knowledgeable about SLE.
2. Important "don'ts":
    a. Do not overexert.
    b. Do not alter prescribed medications.
    c. Do not use over-the-counter drugs.
    d. Do not ignore treatment plan.
    e. Do not expose self to sun and reflected sun through clouds, on snow, water, or white concrete, or fluorescent lighting.

* Lupus Foundation of America, 11921 Olive Blvd, St. Louis, MO 63141
National Lupus Erythematosus Foundation, 5430 Van Nuys Avenue, Van Nuys, CA 91401

F. Being Aware of the Special Situation When a Neonate is Born to a Known SLE Mother.

1. Positive ANA and LE factor transmitted transplacentally
   a. Infant may have clinical and/or nonclinical evidence of lupus erythematosus. Discoid lesions may be present.
   b. Other infants may have no clinical symptoms.
2. Symptoms usually resolve in 3–4 months; however, the child may develop SLE later in life.

Health Education

A. Inform the Parents About Requirements for Caring for the Child at Home.

1. Prevent direct exposure to the sun; if exposure to the sun cannot be avoided, a sunscreen lotion with PABA should be used.
   a. The child can go outside in early morning or late afternoon.
   b. The child should avoid snow on bright days, cement, and white buildings because of photosensitivity.
2. Discuss with the parents and be certain they are aware of and understand each of the following:
   a. Side effects of any medications being administered at home and what to do about these reactions
   b. Signs of worsening of the disease
   c. Factors that precipitate flare-up or early warning signs of flare-up: chills, fever, anorexia, and fatigue
   d. Problems that may be associated with the adolescent—i.e., body image, relationship with peers
3. Provide measures that will be helpful in preventing infection:
   a. Avoid exposure to individuals with infections.
   b. Practice general measures of personal hygiene.
   c. Provide a well-balanced diet.
4. Continual medical follow-up
   a. Disease progress needs reevaluation.
   b. Drug therapy must be strictly controlled, and it is based on the condition of the child as well as laboratory studies.
   c. Renal function specifically needs to constantly be evaluated.

Expected Outcomes

1. Demonstrates increased mobility and activity
2. Shows improved nutritional status as evidenced by appropriate intake and weight gain and laboratory values
3. Is free of neurologic complication such as headache or seizures
4. Maintains normal respiratory function and cardiac output as reflected by vital signs, behavior, and laboratory studies
5. Shows normal kidney function; normal urine output, specific gravity, color, and protein content
6. Avoids exposure to sunlight or sun glare
7. Demonstrates a self-confident attitude and improved self-image as reflected in play activity, willingness to interact with others, regular attendance at school, and eagerness to make decisions and to be independent
8. Adheres to the treatment regimen: gets rest, takes medication, follows diet
9. Parents understand and can explain home-care protocols for avoiding sunlight, side effects of medications, signs of exacerbation, the need for relaxed attitude, measures for maintaining social interactive skills

Schönlein–Henoch Purpura
(Anaphylactoid Purpura)

Schönlein–Henoch purpura is a diffuse disease resulting from inflammatory reaction around capillaries and arterioles involving the skin, intestines, joints, and kidneys.

Incidence and Etiology

1. Slightly higher incidence in males than in females. Increased incidence of onset is between ages 2 and 8 years.
2. Seen most often in winter and can occur in clusters.
3. Possible cause is an allergic reaction to a variety of antigenic stimuli such as infection (e.g., beta streptococci), allergens, insect bites, food, and drugs.
4. Cause is unknown.
5. Disease is usually self-limiting.

Altered Physiology

1. Acute vasculitis
   a. Swelling and edema of capillaries, small venules, and arterioles
   b. Fibrin is deposited in the glomeruli of the kidney
2. Vasculitis results in skin manifestations (purpura), arthritis, and gastrointestinal symptoms.

Complications

1. Acute nephritis or nephrosis that may lead to chronic nephritis (urinalysis should be done 6 and 12 months after episode).
2. Colicky abdominal pain, related to vasculitis and edema of the bowel; steroids may be used.
3. Intussusception

Clinical Manifestations

1. Rash—sudden onset may precede or follow other manifestations.
   a. Typical rash begins with itching, urticarial wheals, and then proceeds to maculopapular erythematous lesions.
   b. These lesions become less raised and more petechial or purpuric in character and do not fade with pressure. They blanch initially, then progress to ecchymotic areas until they fade.
   c. Several stages of the rash may be present at one time.
   d. Rash appears primarily on buttocks, lower back, extensor aspects of arms and legs, and face.
2. Arthritis of knee and ankle joints develops
   a. The condition is moderately severe, with painful swelling due to periarticular edema, migrating arthritis.
   b. Movement is limited.
3. Local edema—especially of scrotum.
4. Colicky abdominal pain—from submucosal hemorrhage.
5. Nausea and vomiting
6. Proteinuria
7. Microscopic hematuria
8. Symptoms may appear acutely or gradually.

Diagnostic Evaluation

1. Appearance of rash, frequently following URI
2. Blood studies—not diagnostic

a. Platelet count—normal
b. Erythrocyte sedimentation rate (ESR)—elevated
c. Anemia possible
d. Azotemia (with severe kidney involvement)
e. pH and prothromboplastin tests
3. Urine studies
   a. Proteinuria
   b. Microscopic hematuria
   c. Casts
4. Stool—shows occult or gross blood

Treatment

Treatment is primarily symptomatic and supportive.
1. Encourage bedrest until the child is able to ambulate and can do so without increasing edema of feet.
2. Remove allergen if it is known.
3. Give antibiotic therapy if acute episode was preceded by infection, especially streptococcal.
4. Manage complicating abdominal or renal involvement and arthritis
   a. Steroids (prednisone) may relieve abdominal symptoms and prevent intussusception.
   b. Immunosuppressive therapy (azathioprine or cyclophosphamide) may be given to stabilize persistent renal involvement.

Patient Problems and Nursing Diagnoses

1. Altered comfort, pain, related to arthritis, nausea, vomiting, and abdominal pain, and itching
2. Impaired mobility related to arthritis and edema
3. Potential for complications: intussusception and nephritis related to vasculitis and edema of gastrointestinal tract and glomeruli
4. Potential impaired skin integrity, related to erythematous lesions and itching
5. Anxiety and fear related to discomfort and hospitalization
6. Parental anxiety related to sudden onset of disease and lack of understanding

Nursing Interventions

A. Offering the Patient and His Parents Realistic Encouragement.

The long-term outlook is good when renal involvement is minimal.

B. Assisting the Child in Expressing His Feelings About Illness and Hospitalization.

1. Provide the child with an opportunity to openly discuss his feelings about illness and his situation when he is able to verbalize these feelings.
2. Provide the child with the opportunity to express his feelings; use play as a method.
3. Allow the child to make some decisions (appropriate for his age), and to become involved in planning his own care.
4. Consider his age and then allow and encourage parental participation.

C. Providing Physical Comfort for the Child's Painful and Swollen Joints.

Salicylates are found not to be particularly effective (see Juvenile Rheumatoid Arthritis, p. 1423).

D. Observing for Developing Signs and Symptoms of Complications.

1. Renal
   a. Record intake and output.

b. Record specific gravity of urine.
   c. Observe color and characteristics of urine.
   d. Observe development of or increase in edema.
2. Intussusception—sudden onset
   a. Paroxysmal abdominal pain
   b. Currant jelly-like stools
   c. Vomiting
   d. Increasing absence of stools
   e. Increasing abdominal distention and tenderness

E. Observing and Recording the Child's General Condition and the Current Status of the Rash.

F. Being Aware of the Action and Side Effects of Medications Used in the Treatment of Anaphylactoid Purpura.

See Juvenile Rheumatoid Arthritis, page 1423

Health Education

1. Reassure the parents that symptoms are self-limiting.
2. Ensure that parents understand treatment and signs and symptoms of complications.
3. Make community health nurse referral as needed.
4. Encourage the parents to return the child for follow-up urinalysis 6 and 12 months following acute episode.

Expected Outcomes

1. Shows relief of pain evidenced by verbalization and/or behavior
2. Increases mobility as arthritis and edema decrease
3. Maintains normal gastrointestinal function; shows no signs of intussusception: abdominal pain, vomiting, distention, failure to pass stool
4. Maintains normal urinary function: normal output, specific gravity; no edema
5. Demonstrates lessening anxiety; expresses feelings; engages in play activities; and has a more relaxed behavior
6. The parents gain an understanding of the child's illness, are supportive of the child, become involved in care, and follow through with home care in relation to medications and avoidance of complications

---

Kawasaki Disease (Mucocutaneous Lymph Node Syndrome)

Kawasaki disease is a multisystem vasculitis identified by a febrile illness with several distinguishing features that attack vital body systems.

Etiology and Prevalence

1. Cause is unknown.
2. Retrovirus has been suggested by some investigators.
3. Peak age of occurrence is between 1 and 2 years; half of the children are under 2 years and 80% are under 4. Seldom occurs in children over 8 years old. Boy:Girl ratio, 1.6:1.
4. Seasonal epidemics usually occur in spring and winter.

Altered Physiology

1. Although vasculitis is a multisystem disease, the cardiovascular system seems to be primarily involved.
2. Initially: stage I
   a. Perivasculitis of arterioles, venules, and capillaries
   b. Coronary arteries are included—pancarditis

3. As disease progresses: stages II and III
   a. Panvasculitis and perivasculitis of coronary arteries
   b. Aneurysm formation, pericarditis, myocarditis, endocarditis, and phlebitis may result.
4. Stage IV
   a. Coronary arterial scarring, stenosis, calcification
   b. Myocardial fibrosis and endocardial fibroelastosis
   c. Healing begins

Complications

1. Cardiac involvement during illness
2. Aspirin toxicity
3. Posthospital (postillness) cardiac involvement

Clinical Manifestations

A. **Acute Febrile Phase—Stage I:** The child appears severely ill and irritable (days 1–14).

*1. High, spiking fever, 5 or more days
*2. Bilateral conjunctival infection
*3. Oropharyngeal erythema, "strawberry" tongue, red and dry lips
*4. Indurative edema of hands and feet or erythema of palms and soles or general or periungual desquamation
*5. Erythematous rash
*6. Cervical lymphadenopathy
7. Carditis—pericarditis, myocarditis, cardiomegaly, congestive heart failure, coronary thrombosis

B. **Subacute Phase—Stage II:** Acute symptoms of stage I subside as temperature returns to normal. The child remains irritable and anorexic (days 10–25).

1. Dry, cracked lips with fissures (part of third criterion)
2. Desquamation of toes and fingers (part of fourth criterion)
3. Arthralgia, arthritis
4. Coronary thrombosis, aneurysms

C. **Convalescent Phase—Stage III:** The child appears well (days 25–60).

1. Transverse grooves of fingers and toenails (Beau's lines)
2. Coronary thrombosis; aneurysms (may occur)

Diagnostic Evaluation

A. **Demonstration of Criteria Seen Above**

B. **ECG and Echocardiographic Abnormalities**

C. **Although There Are No Specific Laboratory Tests, the Following May Help Support Diagnosis or Rule Out Other Diseases:**

1. White blood cell count—leukocytosis during acute stage
2. ESR—elevated during acute stage
3. Erythrocytes and hemoglobin—slight decrease
4. C-reactive protein—positive
5. Platelet count—increased during 2nd–4th week of illness
6. IgM, IgA, IgG, and IgF—transiently elevated
7. Urine—proteinuria and leukocytes present

Treatment *(controversial among authorities)*

1. Treatment goals: amelioration of symptoms and prevention of coronary thrombosis, coronary aneurysm, and death.

* Six major criteria—CDC requires that fever and four of the remaining symptoms be present for diagnosis. (Adapted from Advances in Pediatric Infectious Diseases, 1989; 4:176)

2. Immune globulin intravenous therapy (400 mg./kg./day) initiated within 10 days of onset of fever, in a 2-hour infusion for 4 consecutive days.*
3. Aspirin therapy*
   a. High dose (80–100 mg/kg./day) during acute stage of illness—given for anti-inflammatory and antipyretic effect
   b. Lower dose (3–5 mg./kg./day) after fever is controlled—used as platelet aggregation inhibitor in subacute phase and continued for 2 months postillness or until sedimentation rate and platelet count are normal, to reduce risk of spontaneous coronary thrombosis.
4. Supportive
   a. Maintain fluid and electrolyte balance; nutritional support.
   b. Provide comfort.
   c. Employ careful monitoring of cardiac status.
5. Cardiac follow-up by pediatric cardiologist and serial echocardiograms.*
6. Corticosteroids and anticoagulants are contraindicated. Antibiotics are not indicated.*

Patient Problems and Nursing Diagnoses

1. Parental anxiety and stress related to uncertainty about disease
2. Altered comfort, pain, related to fever, conjunctival inflammation, edematous and peeling skin, oral lesions and immobility
3. Altered skin integrity related to edema, dehydration
4. Cardiac complications from vasculitis
5. Potential aspirin toxicity from high-dose treatment
6. Fluid volume deficit related to hyperthermia and decreased fluid intake
7. Sensory/perceptual alteration related to presence of eye patches in treating conjunctivitis
8. Mobility impaired, related to joint pain and enforced bedrest
9. Anxiety and fear related to hospitalization, pain, and body changes that occur with the disease

Nursing Interventions

A. **Promoting Comfort and Rest of the Febrile Child, and Preventing Dehydration.**

1. Although aspirin is given in high doses in an attempt to control the quickly spiking temperature, it is often ineffective.
2. Give tepid sponge baths for temperature over 38.3°C. (101°F.), or a cooling blanket should be employed (see Child with Fever, p. 1142).
3. Monitor vital signs every 1–2 hours.
4. Offer clear liquids every hour when the child is awake (Popsicles are often accepted and may be soothing to sore oral mucous membranes).
5. Monitor urinary output and specific gravity.
6. Monitor intravenous infusion hourly.
7. Weigh daily in the morning.
8. Assess skin turgor, tears, etc. to aid in assessment of hydration status.
9. Pad side rails and have airway and suction available; seizures may occur because of rapid temperature rise.

B. **Carrying Out Continual Cardiac Monitoring and Assessment for Complications.**

1. Take vital signs and blood pressure every 2 hours; report abnormalities.

* Adopted from Report of the Committee of Infectious Diseases. American Academy of Pediatrics, 1988

2. Ensure proper functioning of cardiac monitor; observe for and report any arrhythmias.
3. Assess the child for signs of myocarditis: tachycardia, gallop rhythm, chest pain.
4. Monitor the child for congestive heart failure: dyspnea, nasal flaring, grunting, retractions, cyanosis, orthopnea, crackles, moist respirations, distended neck veins, and edema.

C. Monitoring the Child for Signs of Aspirin Toxicity When High-Dose Aspirin is Prescribed (see Rheumatic Fever, p. 1327)

(Serial aspirin serum levels are monitored.)

D. Providing Measures of Comfort for the Child With Altered Skin Integrity and Conjunctival Inflammation.

1. Comfort measures related to skin
   a. Cool, moist compresses to skin. Avoid use of soap because it tends to dry skin and make it more likely to break down.
   b. Elevate edematous extremities.
   c. Use sheepskin, egg crate mattress, and smooth sheets.
   d. If clothes are used, they should be of soft flannel or terry cloth.
2. Comfort measures related to eyes—conjunctivitis can cause photosensitivity
   a. Darken room; cover eyes with cool cloth or sunglasses.
   b. Instruct the child to avoid rubbing eyes.
   c. Consider using artificial tear drops to increase comfort.
3. Comfort measures related to altered oral mucous membranes
   a. Offer cool liquids—(ice chips and popsicles)
      (1) Progress to soft, bland foods.
      (2) Encourage the child to eat meats and snacks to prevent nutrition deficit.
      (3) Encourage the parents to participate in selecting food and feeding activities.
   b. Give mouth care every 1–4 hours—special mouth swabs; soft tooth brush only after healing has occurred.
   c. Apply petrolatum to dried, cracked lips.
   d. Observe the mouth frequently for signs of infection.
4. Comfort measures related to joint pain and tender lymph nodes
   a. Employ passive range of motion exercises every 4 hours while the child is awake because movement may be restricted.
   b. Allow and encourage the child to move about freely under supervision.
   c. Provide soft toys and quiet play and encourage use of hands and fingers.

E. Providing for Emotional Support and Diversional Activities Appropriate for Age.

1. The child is generally irritable, uncomfortable, and lethargic because of his illness and hospitalization.
2. Play therapy—both active and passive—can help the child express his feelings.
3. Explain procedures to the child.
4. Encourage the parents to be involved in care and help them offer support to their child.
5. Allow the child periods of uninterrupted rest—should decrease irritability.

F. Providing Emotional Support for the Parents Who Are Distressed and Concerned About Their Child.

1. Help the parents understand what is happening; they need to be told what changes they will see (i.e., fever spikes, eye changes, desquamation of hands and feet, irritable behavior, decreased appetite).
2. Encourage them appropriately; usually the disease is self-limiting, but there is potential for cardiac involvement.
3. Involve the parents in comforting and care of the child to help relieve some of their anxieties and feelings of helplessness.
4. Encourage the parents to verbalize their concerns, fears, and questions.

Health Education

1. Long-term care following discharge is critical because complications can occur during period of convalescence or months following acute illness. Medical observation, ECGs, and echocardiograms should be done every 3 months during the 1st year.
2. The parents should be given instructions (verbal and written) and demonstrate that they understand the specific information and instructions related to cardiac problems (i.e., color change, shortness of breath, chest pain, and lethargy).
3. The parents need to understand what medications are prescribed; dose, action, frequency of administration, and signs of toxic effects.
4. Anticipatory guidance is needed in terms of behavioral context.
   a. Do not overprotect the child.
   b. Allow him to be as active as he wants.
   c. Discuss regression that might occur as a result of hospitalization and how to deal with these changes.
5. Initiate community health nurse and/or social work referral as indicated.

Expected Outcomes

1. Child experiences increasing comfort as evidenced by appropriate behavior (i.e., less irritable, increased fluid intake, interest in diversional activities, ability to rest easily)
2. Maintains normal cardiac function as evidenced by normal echocardiogram, ECG, and vital signs; does not complain of chest pain
3. Shows no signs of aspirin toxicity, as evidenced by normal gastric function and appropriate serum aspirin levels
4. Remains well hydrated as evidenced by adequate intake and output, normal urine specific gravity and skin turgor
5. Engages in range of motion exercises and other activities to improve mobility
6. Skin remains intact; good turgor; no evidence of pressure
7. The parents comfort the child and participate in care when possible
8. The parents verbalize understanding of their homecare responsibilities in relation to detecting possible complications; administering medications, watching for side effects, and continuing with follow-up medical observation every 3 months for the 1st year

Bibliography

Books

Avery ME and First LR, (eds). Pediatric Medicine. Baltimore, Williams & Wilkins, 1989

Behrman RE and Vaughan VC (ed). Nelson Textbook of Pediatrics. 13th ed. Philadelphia, WB Saunders, 1987

Brewer EJ, Giannini EH and Person DA. Juvenile Rheumatoid Arthritis. 2nd ed. (Vol VI in series, Major Problems in Clinical Pediatrics). Philadelphia, WB Saunders, 1982

Provost TT and Farmer ER. Current Therapy in Dermatology—2. Philadelphia, BC Decker, 1988

Rudolph AM (ed). Pediatrics. 8th ed. Norwalk, Appleton & Lange, 1987

Whaley LF and Wong DL. Nursing Care of Infants and Children. St. Louis, CV Mosby, 1987

Journals

Baum J. Treatment of juvenile arthritis. Hosp Pract 1983 Sep; 18(9):121–124+

Brosius CL et al. Increased prevalence of atopic dermatitis in Kawasaki disease. Pediatr Infect Dis J 1988 Dec; 7(12): 863–866

Englund JA and Lucas RV. Cardiac complications in children with systemic lupus erythematosus. Pediatrics 1983 Nov; 72(5):724–729

Haugen MS and Lynch PA. Diagnostic tests in pediatric rheumatology: Application for nurses. Pediatr Nurs 1987 Nov–Dec; 13(6):389–393

McCowen C and Henderson DC. Sudden death in incomplete Kawasaki's disease. Arch Dis Child 1988 Oct; 63(10):1254–1256

Page–Goertz SS. Even children have arthritis. Pediatr Nurs 1989 Jan–Feb; 15(1):11–16

Peter G (ed). Report of the Committee of Infectious Diseases. Elk Grove Village, IL, American Academy of Pediatrics, 1988

Rauch AM. Kawasaki Syndrome: Issues in etiology and treatment. Adv Pediatr Infect Dis 1989; 4:163–182

Rauch AM. Kawasaki Syndrome: Review of new epidemiologic and laboratory developments. Pediatr Infect Dis J 1987 Nov; 6(11):1016–1021

Tan EM et al. The 1982 revised criteria for the classification of systemic lupus erythematosus. Arthritis Rheum 1982 Nov; 25(11):1271–1277

Update: Lupus Erythematosus Research Dept HHS—Public Health Service NIH, 1986

Urback AM et al. Kawasaki disease and perineal rash. Am J Dis Child 1988 Nov; 142(11):1174–1176

Vostrejs M and Hollister JR. Muscle atrophy and leg length discrepancies in pauciarticular juvenile rheumatoid arthritis. Am J Dis Child 1988 Mar; 142(3):343–345

Winkel MF. Juvenile rheumatoid arthritis—Parent support group: Do parents perceive a need? Pediatr Nurs 1988 Mar–Apr; 14(2):131

Suggested Reading for Parents/Patients

Rapuff MA. Helping children follow their medical treatment program: Guidelines for parents of children with rheumatic diseases. Kansas City, KS, Mid-America Pediatric Rheumatology Program, 1985

Rodnar GP, Schumacher HR and Vaifler NJ (ed). Primer on the Rheumatic Diseases. 8th ed. Atlanta, The Arthritis Foundation, 1983

Rose MH and Thomas RB. Children with Chronic Conditions: Nursing in a Family and Community Context. Orlando, Grune & Stratton, 1987

Patient, Family, and Teacher Education Materials

Arthritis Foundation and Arthritis Health Professions Association
1314 Spring Street, NW
Atlanta, GA 30309

Action for Childhood Arthritis Guide, 1985
Contains a reference list of materials about childhood arthritis

When Your Student Has Arthritis: A Guide for Teachers

American Juvenile Arthritis Organization
1314 Spring Street, NW
Atlanta, GA 30309

Arthritis Information Clearinghouse
PO Box 9782
Arlington, VA 22209
Provides bibliographies and listings of educational materials concerned with arthritis and related diseases

National Lupus Erythematosus Foundation
5430 Van Nuys Avenue
Van Nuys, CA 91401

Children With Neurologic and Neurosurgical Problems

58

Cerebral Palsy

Cerebral palsy is a comprehensive diagnostic term used to designate a group of nonprogressive disorders resulting from malfunction of the motor centers and pathways of the brain. Although there are varying degrees and clinical manifestations of cerebral palsy, it is generally characterized by paralysis, weakness, incoordination, and/or ataxia. Cerebral palsy is a major cause of disability among children in the US.

Etiology

A. Prenatal Factors

1. Infection, rubella, toxoplasmosis, herpes simplex, cytomegalic inclusions, and other viral or infectious agents
2. Maternal anoxia, anemia, placental infarcts, abruptio placentae
3. Prenatal cerebral hemorrhage, maternal bleeding, maternal toxemia, Rh or ABO incompatibility
4. Prenatal anoxia, twisting or kinking of the cord
5. Genetic factors
6. Miscellaneous—toxins, drugs

B. Perinatal Factors

1. Anoxia from any cause
   a. Anesthetic and analgesic drugs administered to the mother may cause anoxia in the infant's brain
   b. Prolonged labor
   c. Placenta previa or abruptio placentae
   d. Respiratory obstruction
2. Cerebral trauma during delivery
3. Complications of birth
   a. "Small for date" babies, prematurity, immaturity, postmaturity
   b. Hyperbilirubinemia
   c. Hemolytic disorders
   d. Respiratory distress
   e. Infections
   f. Electrolyte disturbances (hypoglycemia, hypocalcemia)

C. Postnatal Factors

1. Head trauma
2. Infections
   a. Meningitis
   b. Encephalitis
   c. Brain abscess
3. Vascular accidents
4. Anoxia
5. Neoplastic and late neurodevelopmental defects

Altered Physiology

A. Spastic Type

1. Defect in the cortical motor area or pyramidal tract causes abnormally strong tonus of certain muscle groups.
2. Attempt to move a joint causes muscles to contract and block the motion. Permanent contractures develop without muscle training.

B. Athetotic Type

Lesions of the extrapyramidal tract and basal ganglia cause involuntary, uncoordinated, uncontrollable movements of muscle groups.

C. Ataxia

Disturbances of balance result from cerebellar involvement.

Clinical Manifestations

A. Early Signs—may include one or more of the following:

1. Asymmetry in motion or contour
2. Listlessness or irritability
3. Difficulty in feeding, sucking, or swallowing
4. Excessive or feeble cry
5. Long, thin infants who are slow to gain weight

B. Late Signs—may include one or more of the following:

1. Failure to follow normal pattern of motor development. Delayed gross motor development is a universal manifestation of cerebral palsy.
2. Persistence of infantile reflexes
3. Weakness
4. Apparent preference for one hand before the infant is 12–15 months old
5. Abnormal postures
6. Delayed or defective speech
7. Evidence of mental retardation

C. Common Associated Findings

1. Seizures
2. Hearing deficiency
3. Visual defect
4. Perceptual disorders
5. Mental retardation
6. Language disorders

Diagnostic Evaluation

1. History, including prenatal and perinatal factors
2. Neurologic examination
3. Laboratory data (CT scan; blood testing—to rule out presence of toxins; infectious processes; neoplasms)
4. Psychological testing to determine cognitive functioning
5. Psychosocial assessment, including family adaptation

Classification of Cerebral Palsy

A. Clinical Type

1. Spasticity—in 50%–60% of patients
   a. Generally appears before 6 months of age.
   b. Characterized by hypertonicity, uneven tone distribution, persistent primitive reflexes, lack or delay of normal postural control, and spastic paresis.
   c. Motor activity is impaired because of disharmony of muscle movements.
      (1) Arms
         (a) The child often holds his arm pressed against his body with the forearm bent at right angles to the upper arm and the hand bent against the forearm. The fist may be clenched tightly.
         (b) The child with mild involvement may demonstrate an overextended appearance of the fingers and rotation of the wrists when he reaches for things.
      (2) Legs—may be more (usually) or less involved than arms.
         (a) Mild case may be evident only when the child walks, demonstrating wide-based gait (with arms outstretched). The fingers may be alternately clenched and extended.
         (b) The child with moderate involvement may demonstrate slow and labored movements. Walking is jerky and unrhythmic. Balance is poor.
         (c) The child with severe involvement may be unable to sit or walk unsupported.
         (d) When both legs are involved, bilateral contractures may cause "scissoring." (The child crosses his legs and points his toes.)
2. Dyskinesia—in 20%–25% of patients
   a. Characterized by involuntary, extraneous motor activity; accentuated by emotional stress.
   b. Athetosis is the most common manifestation of this group.
      (1) Characterized by uncontrollable, jerky, irregular, twisting movements of the extremities, especially the fingers and wrists, except when at rest or asleep.
      (2) Any or all extremities may be involved.
      (3) If legs are involved, the child may walk in a writhing, lurching, stumbling manner with noticeable incoordination of the arms. When calm and well-rested, he may walk well.
3. Ataxia—in 1%–10% of patients
   a. Characterized by inability to achieve balance or awkwardness in maintaining it, with associated gross and/or fine motor incoordination.
   b. Gait is often high-stepping, stumbling, or lurching.
   c. Nystagmus is common.
   d. Manifested in varying degrees depending on the pathology.

4. Mixed types—in 15%–40% of patients
   Consists of various combinations of the above types—most frequently, athetosis combined with spasticity.

B. Topographical Classification

1. *Hemiplegia*—findings are limited to 1 side of the body (35%–40% of patients); arm usually involved more than leg.
2. *Diplegia*—similar parts on both sides of the body involved (10%–20%), legs usually involved more than the arms.
3. *Paraplegia*—the legs only are involved (10%–20%).
4. *Quadriplegia*—all 4 extremities are involved (15%–20%); upper and lower extremities equally affected.
5. *Monoplegia*—only 1 extremity is involved (rare).
6. *Triplegia*—3 extremities are involved (rare).

C. Degree of Severity

1. Mild—impairment only of fine precision movement.
2. Moderate—gross and fine movements and speech are impaired, but the child is able to perform usual activities of living.
3. Severe—inability to perform adequately the usual activities of daily living (i.e., walking, using hands, communicating verbally).

Treatment

A. Goal—Normalization.
The aim is to help each child reach optimal functional ability in adulthood. Broad aims of therapy include:

1. To gain optimal appearance and integration of motor function.
2. To establish locomotion, communication, and self-help skills.
3. To correct associated defects.
4. To provide opportunities for education appropriate for the individual child's needs and capabilities.

B. Management

1. Requires comprehensive evaluation and intervention, including:
   a. General health care
   b. Correction or alleviation of specific neuromotor deficits and/or associated disabilities
   c. Developmental enrichment experiences
   d. Development of prevocational, vocational, and socialization skills
   e. Emotional, behavioral, and social adjustments
2. Requires coordination and integration of the contributions of numerous health care professionals as well as societal institutions.
3. The ability of the family to carry out both supportive and participant roles in rehabilitation is a key determinant of the success of any comprehensive management program.

Prognosis

Factors influencing the prognosis
1. Extent of the manifestations
2. Existence of associated defects, especially mental retardation
3. Ability of the family to cope and work with their child's strengths
4. Type and availability of community resources

Patient Problems and Nursing Diagnoses

1. Ineffective family coping: parental feelings of guilt, disappointment, grief, and/or anxiety at learning of the child's diagnosis

2. Altered growth and development, related to the nature and extent of the disorder
3. Self-care deficits related to the nature and extent of the disorder
4. Social isolation and ineffective coping related to the nature of the defect, the demands of daily management, and resultant changes in family life
5. Knowledge deficit of care requirements
6. Potential for injury related to deficit in motor activity

Nursing Interventions

Like other children, the child with cerebral palsy receives the bulk of his care at home and within his community. The nursing role is no longer confined to care within the hospital setting. Within the expanded role, nurses are involved in working with the family on household routines, integrating the child into the family unit, and helping to "mainstream" the child into regular schools, recreational activities, dating situations, etc.

However, the child with cerebral palsy may experience several hospitalizations for diagnostic evaluation, orthopedic management, and/or medical care. The nurse should consider the following guidelines when caring for the hospitalized child with cerebral palsy:

A. Assisting the Parents With Initial Coping and With Long-Range Adaptation to the Child's Disability.

1. Encourage the parents to express their feelings about the child and his diagnosis and help them to deal with these feelings.
2. Assist the parents to appraise the child's assets so that they may capitalize on these positive features.
   a. Early recognition of the extent of the child's disability and realistic direction for obtainable goals are essential.
   b. Help the parents to recognize immediate needs and identify short-term goals that can be integrated into the long-range plan.
3. Encourage the parents to care for the child during his hospitalization so that they will feel secure about meeting his daily physical needs (feeding, exercise, braces, etc.).
See Family-Centered Care, page 1125.
4. Introduce the parents to members of the health team who will be involved with the child's care and management.
5. Begin parental teaching about the disability.
   a. Provide the parents with appropriate reading material. Encourage their questions and provide them with the information they need.
   b. See Health Education, page 1438.
6. Assist the parents in interpreting the child's diagnosis and needs to other family members, teachers, and friends.
7. Initiate appropriate referrals.
   a. Community agencies for disabled children
   b. Community health nurse
   c. Day-care centers
   d. Clinics
   e. Local branch of the United Cerebral Palsy Association
   f. Parent groups

B. Promoting the Attainment of Developmental Milestones as Much as Possible.

1. Evaluate the child's developmental level and then assist him to build one skill on another. (Refer to sections on Growth and Development and the Hospitalized Child, pp. 1079 and 1120.)
2. Provide for continuity of care from home to hospital.
   a. Obtain a thorough history from the mother regarding the child's usual home routines, and use this in planning the child's care during hospitalization.
      (1) Feeding
      (2) Sleeping
      (3) Physical therapy
      (4) Stage of growth and development
      (5) Play
      (6) Special interests, security objects, etc.
   b. Ask the parents to bring to the hospital any special devices or equipment the child uses in his daily activities.
   c. Encourage the child's parents to participate in the child's care if they so desire and if it is medically feasible (See Family-Centered Care, p. 1125).
3. Be alert for associated defects that could be corrected.
   a. Hearing
   b. Speech
   c. Vision
      (1) Squinting
      (2) Failure to follow objects
      (3) Bringing objects very close to the face

C. Providing Emotional Support to the Parents.

1. Acknowledge the numerous challenges of daily management and the changes in family life associated with caring for a child with cerebral palsy.
2. Allow the parent(s) to express frustrations they may feel because of the many demands placed on them, with few rewards.
3. Acknowledge the parents' feelings of frustration and anger as legitimate and understandable.
4. Provide positive feedback for effective parenting skills and positive approaches to caring for the child.
5. Assist the parents to deal with siblings' responses to the disabled child.
6. Assist the parents to secure respite from the day-to-day care of the child, as appropriate.

D. Providing for the Child's Physical Care Needs.

1. Safety
   a. Evaluate the child's need for specific safety measures (suction machine, helmet, seizure precautions, etc.), and modify the environment as appropriate to ensure the child's safety.
   b. Select toys that are safe.
2. Nutrition
   a. Maintain a pleasant environment, free from distractions.
      (1) Provide a comfortable chair.
      (2) Serve the child alone, initially. After he begins to master the task of eating, he may enjoy eating with other children.
      (3) Do not attempt feedings if the child is very fatigued.
   b. Encourage independence, but do not force the child.
      (1) Find the eating position in which the child can do the most for himself.
      (2) Allow the child to hold the spoon even if he has to be fed with another one.
      (3) Stand behind the child and reach over his shoulder to guide the spoon from the plate to his mouth.
      (4) Serve foods that stick to the spoon, like thick applesauce, mashed potato, etc.

(5) Encourage finger foods that the child can handle alone.
(6) Provide appropriate special equipment for the child to use in feeding himself.
   (a) Spoon and fork with special handles
   (b) Plate and glass holders, etc.
   (c) Feeding chair
(7) Disregard "messy" eating.
   (a) Use a large plastic bib or towel to protect the child's clothes.
  c. If the child must be fed, do so slowly and carefully. The child may have difficulty sucking and swallowing because he cannot control the muscles of his throat.
   (1) Offer foods that the child likes.
   (2) Cut solid foods into small pieces.
   (3) Place the food back on the tongue for ease in swallowing.
3. Exercise
  a. Carry out appropriate exercises under the direction of the physical therapist.
  b. Use appropriate appliances to facilitate muscle control and improve body functioning.
   (1) Splints
   (2) Casts
   (3) Braces
  c. Encourage active motions that are functionally useful.
  d. Use play (games, peg boards, puzzles, etc.) as techniques to improve coordination.
  e. Maintain good body alignment to prevent contractures.
4. Rest
  a. Avoid exciting events before rest or bedtime.
  b. Administer tranquilizing agents or anticonvulsants, etc., as prescribed by the physician.
  c. Avoid stress and frustration during the child's program of physical therapy.

E. Ensuring Continuity of Care.

1. Communicate with representatives of all of the disciplines involved with the child's management.
2. Communicate with community agencies already involved with the child and his family (school, cerebral palsy center, community health nursing agency, etc.).
3. Formulate a consistent nursing care plan that is well coordinated with the plans and goals of related disciplines and meets the needs of the *entire* child and his family.
4. On discharge, send a report of the child's hospitalization, including a summary of nursing problems, to the appropriate community agencies.

Health Education

1. Instruct the parent in all areas of the child's physical care.
2. Reinforce teaching done by physical therapists. Assist the parents to integrate therapy into play activities.
3. Assist the parents to modify equipment and activities to facilitate home care.
4. Provide practical suggestions for feeding, holding, bathing, infant stimulation, etc.
5. The child needs regular medical and dental evaluations.
  a. The child should receive his childhood immunizations.
  b. He should be taken to the dentist every 6 months, starting at the age of 2 years.
  c. He may require some adaptations of his toothbrush to use it effectively.
   (1) The handle can be built up with a sponge or a more sophisticated enlarging device.
   (2) Brushes with specially bent handles are available.
6. The child needs discipline to feel secure and relaxed.
  a. He should have realistic limits set, within which he can function successfully.
  b. The parents should be firm but not rejecting.
7. References for Parents:
Brightman A. Hollis. New York, Scholastic Book Services, 1978.
Napear P. Brain Child, A Mother's Diary. New York, Harper & Row, 1974
Trevarton J. Amy Maura. Syracuse, Human Policy Press, 1975
United Cerebral Palsy Association, 66 E 34th Street, New York, NY 10016

Expected Outcomes

1. The parents discuss feelings with each other and with appropriate health care personnel
2. The child achieves sequential developmental milestones consistent with his condition
3. Achieves independence in feeding, dressing, and personal hygiene to the extent that is possible; develops realistic goals
4. The child/family participates in activities (school, church, etc.); seeks respite care on occasion
5. The parents take an active part in learning about child's condition; make plans for future; join a support group
6. Absence of injury; child wears helmet; plays with safe toys

---

Hydrocephalus

Hydrocephalus is a condition of altered production, flow, or absorption of cerebrospinal fluid. It is characterized by an abnormal increase in cerebrospinal fluid volume within the intracranial cavity and by enlargement of the head in infancy.

Etiology and Incidence

1. Obstruction in the system between the source of cerebrospinal fluid production and the area of its reabsorption (the obstruction may be partial, intermittent, or complete)
  a. The majority of cases are of this type.
  b. Causes:
   (1) Congenital—etiology largely unknown
   (2) Acquired
    (a) Infections
    (b) Trauma
    (c) Spontaneous intracranial bleeding
    (d) Neoplasms
2. Failure in the absorption system—cause unknown
3. Excessive production of cerebrospinal fluid—tumor or unknown causes (rare)
4. Approximately 3–4 cases per 1000 births, including those associated with spina bifida

Types of Hydrocephalus

A. Noncommunicating Hydrocephalus

An obstruction is located within or at the outlets of the ventricular system, preventing any or all of the cerebrospinal fluid from leaving the ventricles and entering the subarachnoid space.

B. Communicating Hydrocephalus

1. There is free communication between the ventricles and the subarachnoid space.
2. Abnormal reabsorption of the cerebrospinal fluid in the subarachnoid space occurs.
3. Excessive production of the cerebrospinal fluid

Altered Physiology

1. The ventricular system is greatly distended.
2. The increased ventricular pressure results in thinning of the cerebral cortex and cranial bones, especially in the frontal, parietal, and temporal areas.
3. The floor of the third ventricle commonly bulges downward, compresses the optic nerves, dilates the sella turcica, and often compresses the hypophysis cerebri.
4. The basal ganglia, brain stem, and cerebellum remain relatively normal but compressed.
5. The choroid plexus is usually atrophied to some degree.

Clinical Manifestations

1. May be rapid, slow and steadily advancing, or remittent.
2. Clinical signs depend on the age of the child, whether or not the anterior fontanelle has closed, whether the cranial sutures have fused, and the type and duration of hydrocephalus.
3. Infants
   a. Excessive head growth (may be seen up to 3 years of age)
   b. Delayed closure of the anterior fontanelle Fontanelle may become tense and elevated above the surface of the skull.
   c. Signs of increased intracranial pressure include:
      (1) Vomiting
      (2) Restlessness and irritability
      (3) High-pitched, shrill cry
      (4) Alteration in vital signs
         Increased systolic blood pressure
         Decreased pulse
         Decreased and irregular respirations
      (5) Pupillary changes
      (6) Seizures (possible)
      (7) Lethargy
      (8) Stupor
      (9) Coma
   d. Alteration of muscle tone of the extremities
   e. Later physical signs
      (1) Forehead becomes prominent.
      (2) Scalp appears shiny with prominent scalp veins.
      (3) Eyebrows and eyelids may be drawn upward, exposing the sclera above the iris.
      (4) Infant cannot gaze upward, causing "sunset eyes."
      (5) Strabismus, nystagmus, and optic atrophy may occur.
      (6) Infant has difficulty in holding head up.
      (7) Child may experience physical and/or mental developmental lag.
4. Older children who have closed sutures
   Signs of increased intracranial pressure include:
   a. Headache
   b. Vomiting

c. Lethargy, fatigue, apathy
d. Personality changes
e. Separation of cranial sutures (may be seen in children up to 10 years of age)
f. Double vision, constricted peripheral vision, sudden appearance of internal strabismus, pupillary changes
g. Alteration in vital signs similar to those seen in infants
h. Difficulty with gait
i. Stupor
j. Coma

Diagnostic Evaluation

1. Transillumination of the infant's head may show varying degrees of localized glowing indicative of abnormal fluid collection.
2. Percussion of the infant's skull may produce a typical "cracked pot" sound (Macewen's sign).
3. Ophthalmoscopy may reveal papilledema.
4. CT scan (computed tomography) provides a noninvasive means of diagnosing some types of hydrocephalus by computer analysis of x-ray transmission data. It is the diagnostic tool of choice.
5. Ventriculography (rarely used)—abnormalities are visualized in the ventricular system or the subarachnoid space.
6. Radiologic findings show the following:
   a. Widening of the fontanelle and sutures
   b. Erosion of intracranial bone

Surgical Treatment

A. General Techniques

1. Direct operation on the lesion causing the obstruction
2. Intracranial shunts—useful in selected cases of noncommunicating hydrocephalus to divert fluid from the obstructed segment of the ventricular system to the subarachnoid space beyond the block.
3. Extracranial shunts—divert fluid from the ventricular system to an extracranial compartment, frequently the peritoneum or right atrium. Preferred method for treating most cases of communicating hydrocephalus and cases of noncommunicating hydrocephalus not amenable to direct surgery or intracranial shunts.

B. Common Extracranial Shunt Procedures

1. Ventriculoperitoneal shunt (V–P shunt)
   a. Diverts cerebrospinal fluid from a lateral ventricle or the spinal subarachnoid space to the peritoneal cavity.
   b. A tube is passed from the lateral ventricle through an occipital burr hole subcutaneously through the posterior aspect of neck and paraspinal region to the peritoneal cavity through a small incision in the right lower quadrant.
2. Ventriculoatrial shunt (V–A shunt)
   a. A tube is passed from the dilated lateral ventricle through a burr hole in the parietal region of the skull.
   b. It then is passed under the skin behind the ear and into a vein down to a point where it discharges into the right atrium or superior vena cava.
   c. The tube passes at one point through a one-way pressure sensitive system.
   d. The valve or valves close to prevent reflux of blood into the ventricle and open as ventricular pressure rises, allowing fluid to pass from the ventricle into the bloodstream.

3. *Complications*
   a. Need for shunt revision frequently occurs because of occlusion, infection, or malfunction.
   b. Shunt revision may be necessary because of growth of the child. Newer models, however, include coiled tubing to allow the shunt to grow with the child.
   c. Shunt dependency frequently occurs. The child rapidly manifests symptoms of increased intracranial pressure if the shunt does not function properly.
   d. Children with ventriculoatrial shunts may experience endocardial contusions and clotting leading to bacterial endocarditis, bacteremia, and ventriculitis, or thromboembolism and cor pulmonale.
   e. Late complications occur with discouraging frequency the longer an operative series is followed.

Prognosis

1. Prognosis is dependent on early diagnosis and prompt therapy.
2. The outcome of treatment depends on the time it is begun, the success of the surgical procedure, good follow-up care, and the child's innate motor and intellectual capabilities.
   a. With improved diagnostic and management techniques, the prognosis is becoming considerably better. Many children experience normal motor and intellectual development.
   b. The severity of neurologic deficits is directly proportional to the interval between onset and the time of diagnosis.
3. Spontaneous arrest sometimes occurs as a result of natural compensatory mechanisms, persistent increased intracranial pressure, and herniation.
4. A child with postmeningitic hydrocephalus might also undergo spontaneous remission following gradual disappearance of adhesions.
5. Approximately two thirds of patients will die at an early age if they are not given surgical treatment.

Patient Problems and Nursing Diagnoses

1. Potential neurologic complications from increased intracranial pressure and shunt failure
2. Potential for infection related to bacterial infiltration of the shunt
3. Potential for altered skin integrity, related to immobility
4. Altered nutrition, less than body requirements, related to reduced oral intake and vomiting
5. Parental anxiety related to the diagnosis and surgery
6. Knowledge deficit about hydrocephalus and its treatment

Preoperative Nursing Interventions

A. Observing for and Recording Disease Progress.

1. Measure head.
   a. Measure at the occipitofrontal circumference (OFC)—point of largest measurement.
   b. Measure the head at approximately the same time each day.
   c. Use a centimeter measure for greatest accuracy.
2. Observe for evidence of increased intracranial pressure. Note especially:
   a. Change in level of consciousness
   b. Changes in vital signs
      (1) Increased systolic blood pressure
      (2) Decreased pulse rate
      (3) Decreased or irregular respirations
   c. Vomiting
   d. Pupillary changes
3. Note especially these changes in appearance:
   a. Increased head size, prominent forehead (noticeable over days or weeks)
   b. Full/bulging fontanelle
   c. "Sunset" eyes
   d. Opisthotonic positioning—occurs with brain stem herniation

B. Providing Adequate Nutrition.

1. Feeding is often a problem because the child may be listless, anorectic, and prone to vomiting.
2. Complete nursing care and treatments before feeding so that the child will not be disturbed after feeding.
3. Hold the infant in a semi-sitting position with head well supported during feeding. Allow ample time for bubbling.
4. Offer small, frequent feedings.
5. Place the child on his side with his head elevated after feeding to prevent aspiration.

C. Assisting With Diagnostic Procedures.

1. Be familiar with the procedure that is being performed (see Diagnostic Tests).
2. Explain the procedure to the child and his parents at their levels of comprehension.
   a. Make certain that they understand what will happen before and after as well as during the procedure.
   b. Play is frequently helpful for explaining the procedure to a young child.
3. Administer prescribed sedatives.
   a. Give the sedative exactly at the prescribed time to ensure its effectiveness.
   b. Organize activities so that the child is permitted to rest after administration of the medications.

NURSING ALERT: Sedatives are contraindicated in many cases because of increased intracranial pressure. If they are administered, the child should be observed very closely for evidence of respiratory depression.

4. Apply protective measures to limit motion as necessary (see section on pediatric techniques: restraints, p. 1149, and positioning for a lumbar puncture, p. 1165).
5. Observe the child closely following the procedure for:
   a. Leaking of cerebrospinal fluid from the sites of subdural or ventricular taps
      These tap holes should be covered with a small piece of gauze or cotton saturated with collodion.
   b. Reactions to the sedative, especially respiratory depression
   c. Changes in vital signs indicative of shock
   d. Signs of increased intracranial pressure, which may occur if air has been injected into the ventricles.

D. Providing Supportive Nursing Care as Indicated by the Child's Condition. (Without treatment, the child becomes more helpless as head size increases.)

1. Prevent pressure sores and the development of contractures.
   a. Place the child on a sponge rubber or lamb's wool pad or an alternating-pressure mattress to keep his weight evenly distributed.

b. Keep the scalp clean and dry.
c. Turn the child's head frequently; change his position at least every 2 hours.
   (1) When turning the child, rotate his head and body together to prevent strain on the neck.
   (2) A firm pillow may be placed under the head and shoulders for further support when lifting the child.
d. Provide meticulous skin care to all parts of the body.
   (1) Observe the skin for evidence of pressure sores.
   (2) Pressure sores on the head are a frequent problem.
e. Give passive range-of-motion exercises to the extremities, especially the legs.

2. Keep the eyes moistened if the child is unable to close his eyelids normally. This prevents corneal ulcerations and infections.
3. Provide for the child's emotional need for love and affection.
   a. Hold and cuddle the infant as much as possible.
   b. Play with the child according to his mental development.

E. Providing Emotional Support to the Parents.

1. Encourage the parents to visit and to participate in the child's care as much as possible.
2. Encourage the parents to talk about the child's condition and how they feel about it. Parents are generally fearful of any procedure involving the brain, and may have fears about mental retardation or brain damage.
3. Provide the parents with appropriate information concerning the defect. Answer their questions directly and honestly. Correct any misconceptions that they may have, such as fear that the child's head may burst.

Postoperative Nursing Interventions

A. Providing Immediate Supportive Nursing Care.

1. Monitor the child's temperature, pulse, respiration, blood pressure, and pupillary size and reaction every 15 minutes until fully reactive; then monitor every 1–2 hours.
2. Avoid hypothermia or hyperthermia.
   a. Provide appropriate blankets or covers as indicated by body temperature.
   b. An Isolette or warming cradle may be used for an infant.
   c. An older child may profit from use of the hypothermia blanket.
   d. Administer a tepid sponge bath or antipyretic medication for temperature elevation (see section on fever, p. 1144).
3. Aspirate mucus from the nose and throat as necessary to prevent respiratory difficulty.
4. Turn the child every 2 hours.
5. Use a nasogastric tube if necessary for abdominal distention.
   a. This is most frequently used when a ventriculoperitoneal shunt has been performed.
   b. Measure the drainage and record the amount and color.
6. Give frequent mouth care to prevent dryness of the mucous membranes.
7. Observe for pallor or mottled condition of the skin, coldness, or clamminess of the body and decreased level of consciousness.
8. Administer prescribed prophylactic antibiotics.

B. Allowing for Optimal Draining of Cerebrospinal Fluid Through the Shunt.

1. Pump the shunt and position the child as directed by the physician.
   a. If pumping is prescribed, carefully compress the valve the specified number of times at regularly scheduled intervals.
   b. Report any difficulties in pumping the shunt to the physician.
2. The height of child's bed may be elevated 30–45° to help shunt drain

C. Preventing the Development of Pressure Sores on the Skin Overlying the Shunt Reservoir.

1. Place cotton behind and over the ears under the head dressing.
2. Avoid positioning the child on the area of the valve or the incision until the wound is well healed.

D. Maintaining Fluid and Electrolyte Balance.

1. Accurately measure and record total fluid intake and output.
2. Administer intravenous fluids as prescribed (see procedure, p. 1167).
3. Begin oral feedings once the child is fully recovered from the anesthetic and displays interest.
   a. Begin with small amounts of 5% dextrose and water.
   b. Gradually introduce formula.
   c. Introduce solid foods suitable to the child's age and tolerance (see section on nutrition, p. 1102).
   d. Encourage a high-protein diet.

E. Observing for Signs of Complications

1. Increased intracranial pressure indicates shunt malfunction (see listing of symptoms under clinical manifestations).
   a. Older children should also be observed for changes in customary behavior, sleep patterns, and developmental capabilities.
2. Dehydration may be manifested in the following ways:
   a. Sunken fontanelle (Without additional signs of dehydration, this may indicate only a successful shunt.)
   b. Decreased urine output, increased specific gravity
   c. Diminished skin turgor and dryness of mucous membranes
   d. Lethargy
3. Infection may be manifested by:
   a. Fever (Temperature normally fluctuates during the first 24 hours after surgery.)
   b. Purulent drainage from the incision
   c. Swelling, redness, and tenderness along the shunt tract
4. Excessive drainage of fluid from the cranial cavity, manifested by
   a. Sunken fontanelle, agitation, restlessness (infant)
   b. Decreased level of consciousness (older child)

F. Providing Continued Emotional Support to the Parents.

1. Begin discharge planning early (see Health Education).
2. Accompany all instructions with reassurance necessary to prevent the parents from becoming anxious or fearful about assuming the care of the child.
3. Encourage the parents to treat the child as normally as possible, providing him with appropriate toys and love.

4. Help the parents with problems of assisting siblings and grandparents to deal with the child's needs.
5. Initiate appropriate referrals.
   a. Social worker
   b. Community health nurse
   c. Parent groups
   d. Community agencies
   e. Specialty clinics and schools

Health Education

1. Parents should be given complete explanations of the disease, the surgery, the changes that the surgery may produce, and the follow-up care that will be required.
2. Physical nursing care
   a. Special attention should be directed toward specific techniques of supportive nursing care, for example:
      (1) Turning
      (2) Skin care
      (3) Play
      (4) Exercises to strengthen the child's muscles
   b. Feeding techniques and patterns
   c. Pumping of shunt
3. Symptoms of increased intracranial pressure, shunt malfunction, infection, and dehydration must be treated. Parents should be taught not only to recognize these complications (see prior listing of signs of complications) but also to report them immediately to the physician.
4. Illnesses that cause vomiting and diarrhea or that prevent an adequate fluid intake are a great threat to the child who has had a shunt procedure. The parents should be instructed regarding:
   a. Prevention of such illnesses
   b. Early recognition of warning symptoms
   c. Necessity of seeking immediate medical care so that the child can receive intravenous therapy to replace fluid and electrolyte loss
5. The child's emotional needs should be stressed. Parents should be encouraged to treat the child as normally as possible. Generally, few restrictions need to be placed on his daily activities.
6. If appropriate, refer to the section on mental retardation for additional areas of parent teaching (see pp. 1504–1506).

Expected Outcomes

1. Avoids neurologic complications; no changes in vital signs or head size; parents recognize early signs of increased intracranial pressure
2. Shows no signs of developing infection; shunt site appears clean; vital signs stable
3. Maintains skin integrity and musculoskeletal function
4. Maintains adequate nutritional status; normal tissue turgor; normal serum electrolyte values; absence of vomiting
5. The parents discuss their feelings about hydrocephalus and surgery with one another and with appropriate health professionals
6. Parents verbalize an understanding of the cause and consequence of hydrocephalus and its treatment

---

Spina Bifida

Spina bifida refers to a malformation of the spine in which the posterior portion of the laminae of the vertebrae fails to close. Several types of spina bifida are recognized, of which the following 3 are most common (Fig. 58-1):
1. *Spina bifida occulta,* in which the defect is only in the vertebrae. The spinal cord and meninges are normal.
2. *Meningocele,* in which the meninges protrude through the opening in the spinal canal, forming a cyst filled with cerebrospinal fluid and covered with skin.
3. *Meningomyelocele* (or myelomeningocele), in which both the spinal cord and cord membranes protrude through the defect in the laminae of the spinal canal. Meningomyeloceles are covered by a thin membrane.

Etiology

1. Unknown but generally thought to result from genetic predisposition triggered by something in the environment.
2. Involves an arrest in the orderly formation of the vertebral arches and spinal cord that occurs between the 4th and 6th week of embryogenesis.
   Theories of causation:
   (a.) There is incomplete closure of the neural tube during the 4th week of embryonic life.
   (b.) The neural tube forms adequately but then ruptures.

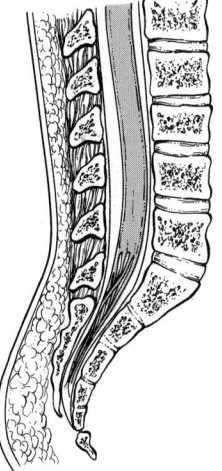 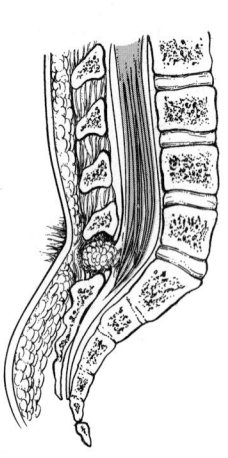 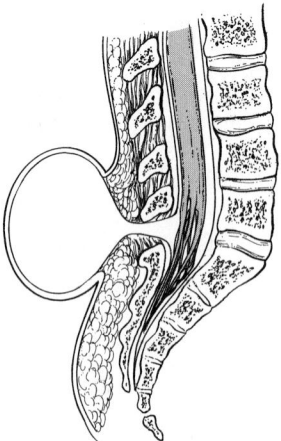 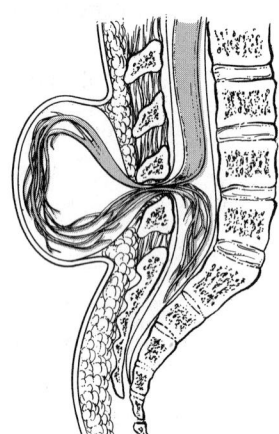

A   **B**   **C**   **D**

Figure 58-1. *Spina bifida. (A) Normal spine. (B) Spina bifida occulta. (C) Spina bifida with meningocele. (D) Spina bifida with myelomeningocele.*

Incidence

1. Geographical distribution and incidence vary widely.
2. Condition occurs in approximately 1 per 1000 live births in the U.S.
3. Most common developmental defect of the central nervous system.
4. More common in Caucasians than in nonwhite population.
5. Condition may have other congenital anomalies associated with it.
6. Women who have spina bifida and parents who have one affected child have an increased risk of producing children with neural tube defects.

Altered Physiology and Clinical Manifestations

A. Spina Bifida Occulta

1. Most common type; may occur in as many as 25% of otherwise normal children.
2. The bony defect may range from a very thin slit separating one lamina from the spinous process to a complete absence of the spines and laminae.
3. A thin, fibrous membrane sometimes covers the defect.
4. The spinal cord and its meninges may be connected with a fistulous tract extending to and opening onto the surface of the skin.
5. Most patients have no symptoms.
   a. They may have a dimple in the skin or a growth of hair over the malformed vertebra.
   b. There is no externally visible sac.
   c. With growth, the child may develop foot weakness or bowel and bladder sphincter disturbances.

B. Meningocele

1. An external cystic defect can be seen in the spinal cord, usually in the center line.
   a. The sac is composed only of meninges and is filled with cerebrospinal fluid.
   b. The cord and nerve roots are usually normal.
2. The defect may occur anywhere on the cord. Higher defects (from thorax and up) are usually meningoceles.
3. There is seldom evidence of weakness of the legs or lack of sphincter control.
4. Surgical correction is necessary to prevent rupture of the sac and subsequent infection.
5. Hydrocephalus may be an associated finding and may be aggravated after surgery for a meningocele.
   a. Occurs in about 9% of patients.
   b. Usually not associated with the Arnold–Chiari malformation.
6. Prognosis is good with surgical correction.

C. Meningomyelocele (Myelomeningocele)

1. Most common type of open spinal defect—occurs 4–5 times more frequently than meningocele.
2. A round, raised, and poorly epithelialized area may be noted at any level of the spinal column. However, the highest incidence of the lesion occurs in the lumbosacral area.
3. The lesion contains both the spinal cord and cord membranes. A bluish area may be evident on the top because of exposed neural tissue.
4. The sac may leak in utero or may rupture after birth, allowing free drainage of cerebrospinal fluid. This renders the child highly susceptible to meningitis.
5. Prognosis
   a. Influenced by the site of the lesion and the presence and degree of associated hydrocephalus. Generally, the higher the defect, the greater the extent of neurologic deficit and the greater the likelihood of hydrocephalus.
   b. In the absence of treatment, most infants with meningomyelocele die early in infancy.
   c. Surgical intervention is most effective if it is done early in the neonatal period, preferably within the first few days of life.
   d. Even with surgical intervention, infants can be expected to manifest associated neurosurgical, orthopedic, and/or urologic problems.
   e. New techniques of treatment, intensive research, and improved services have increased life expectancy and have greatly enhanced the quality of life for most children who receive treatment for the defect.

Clinical Problems Commonly Associated With Meningomyelocele

A. Neurologic Problems

1. Arnold–Chiari malformation
   a. Associated malformation involving the brain stem and cerebellum.
   b. Causes a block in the flow of cerebrospinal fluid through the ventricles and leads to failure in the reabsorption mechanism of cerebrospinal fluid.
   c. Produces significant hydrocephalus in approximately two-thirds of children with meningomyelocele.
2. Loss of motor control and sensation below the level of the lesion.
   These conditions are highly variable and depend on the size of the lesion and its position on the cord. For example:
   a. A low thoracic lesion may cause total flaccid paralysis below the waist.
   b. A small sacral lesion may cause only patchy spots of decreased sensation in the feet.

B. Mobility and Orthopedic Problems

1. Contractures may occur in the ankles, knees, and/or hips. Hips may be pulled out of the sockets.
   a. Nature and degree of involvement depends on size and location of lesion.
   b. Occurs because some threads of innervation do get through. One side of a hip, knee, or ankle may be innervated while the opposing side may not be. The unopposed side then becomes pulled out of position.
2. Clubfeet are a common accompanying anomaly.
   This anomaly is thought to be related to the position of paraplegic feet in the uterus.
3. Scoliosis is common in later years.
   a. Occurs in approximately 50% of patients.
   b. Caused by the congenital lesion in the spinal column.
4. Ambulation and ability to be upright are possible through various types of bracing and equipment. Extent of bracing will depend on extent of sensory and motor loss. Children with low sacral lesions can ambulate with small, short leg braces. Older children with significant loss may choose to use a wheelchair.

C. Urologic Problems

1. Almost all lesions affect the sacral nerves that innervate the bladder. The bladder fails to respond to normal messages that it is time to void, and simply fills and overflows. Usually, the bladder does not empty completely, causing two sets of problems:
   a. Susceptibility to urinary tract infections because of constant stasis
   b. Incontinence, because the bladder is never completely empty and fails to receive signals to void

2. Management
   a. Children must be followed routinely with IVP, voiding cystoureterogram, urine culture and sensitivity. BUN and creatinine levels must be measured to assess renal status.
   b. Continence management
      (1) Usually achieved with clean, intermittent self-catheterization.
         (a) Children can generally be taught to catheterize themselves by the age of 6–7 years.
         (b) Parents can catheterize younger children.
      (2) Surgically implanted mechanical urinary sphincters and bladder pacemakers are being used with increasing frequency.
      (3) Indwelling catheters or external collecting devices are used by some children.
      (4) Urinary diversion may be necessary in some cases.
   c. Medications
      (1) Antibiotics are used periodically or prophylactically to prevent urinary tract infections.
      (2) Medications such as imipramine hydrochloride (Tofranil) and ephedrine sulfate are used to help children retain their urine until it can be voided at one time (rather than to dribble continuously). When self-catheterization is used in conjunction with medication, many children can stay dry for 3–4 hours at a time.
   d. Dietary recommendations
      (1) Adequate fluid intake is essential to maintain good urinary flow.
      (2) Foods such as cranberry juice or medications such as vitamin C are often prescribed to acidify the urine, thus preventing stone formation.
   e. The ability to stay dry for reasonable time intervals is one of the greatest factors in enhancing self-esteem and positive body image.

D. Bowel Problems

1. Fecal incontinence and constipation are promoted by poor innervation of the anal sphincter and bowel musculature.
2. To compensate for decreased sensation, children are placed on a toileting schedule and are taught to push. Medications such as stool softeners, suppositories, or enemas may be used to help determine scheduling.
3. Remaining unconstipated is essential to any type of fecal control. High-bulk, high-fiber, and/or high-fluid diets as well as medications may be used to increase bulk or soften stool.

E. Skin Problems

1. Areas of decreased sensation have a tendency to break down. Braces and shoes should be checked frequently for rubbing.
2. During hospitalization, the nurse should be particularly watchful for areas of skin breakdown. The use of air mattresses, lamb's wool, and other similar materials may help to prevent skin breakdown in bedridden children.

F. Dietary Problems

1. Many children become overweight because of activity limitations.
2. Dietary control is necessary to prevent obesity.

G. Developmental Problems

1. Most children have average intellectual ability despite hydrocephalus.
   a. Most children are able to learn in a "mainstreamed" normal school, provided they are able to overcome other barriers (architectural and attitudinal).
2. The most significant problems are secondarily handicapping conditions that develop when a child has a disability of this degree.
3. Disabled children need exposure to all activities and to rules and regulations for the nondisabled.

Prevention and Treatment of Meningomyelocele

A. Prenatal Detection

Prenatal detection is now possible through amniocentesis and measurement of alphafetoprotein. This testing should be offered to all women at risk (women who are affected themselves or have had other affected children).

B. Surgical Intervention

1. Procedure
   Laminectomy and closure of the open lesion and/or removal of the sac usually can be done soon after birth.
2. Purpose
   a. To prevent further deterioration of neural function
   b. To minimize the danger of rupture and infection, especially meningitis
   c. To improve cosmetic effect
   d. To facilitate handling of the infant by parents and nurses

C. Multidisciplinary Follow-Up for Associated Problems

1. A coordinated team approach will help maximize the physical and mental potential of each affected child.
   a. A group of health care personnel (including a neurologist, neurosurgeon, orthopedic surgeon, urologist, pediatrician, nurse, social worker, and physical therapist) should be available to the child and family.
   b. A continuing, stable relationship with one person on the health care team who is coordinating efforts for the child is of great benefit.
2. Numerous neurosurgical, orthopedic, and urologic procedures and operations may be necessary to help the child achieve his maximum potential.

Patient Problems and Nursing Diagnoses

1. Altered parenting, related to the birth of a defective child
2. Potential for infection related to contamination of the meningomyelocele site or urinary stasis
3. Bowel elimination, altered, fecal incontinence/constipation related to impaired innervation of anal sphincter and bowel musculature
4. Potential altered skin integrity related to immobility and reduced sensation
5. Altered nutrition, greater than body requirements related to inactivity
6. Potential altered growth and development, related to neurologic deficits or locomotion restrictions
7. Self-concept, disturbance in body image, related to the child's appearance, difficulties with locomotion, and lack of control over excretory functions
8. Self-care deficit related to need for help in physical care and transportation
9. Ineffective family coping, related to long-term demands of caring for a disabled child

Preoperative Nursing Interventions for Initial Surgery in the Neonatal Period

A. Preventing Leakage of Cerebrospinal Fluid or Rupture of the Sac or Lesion.

1. Position the infant on his abdomen.
   a. Avoid placing the infant on his back, because this would cause pressure on the sac.
   b. A Bradford frame may be used to facilitate positioning (see procedure for the use of the Bradford frame, p. 1212).
   c. Check the position of the child at least once every hour.
2. Do not place a diaper or other covering directly over the sac.
3. Observe the sac frequently for evidence of irritation or leakage of cerebrospinal fluid.

B. Preventing Infection

1. Infection of the sac
   a. This is most commonly caused by contamination by urine and feces.
   b. Keep the buttocks and genitalia scrupulously clean.
      (1) Do not diaper the infant if the defect is in the lower portion of the spine.
      (2) Use a divided Bradford frame to allow urine and feces to drain away from the body (see technique, p. 1212).
      (3) A small plastic drape taped between the defect and the anus may help to prevent contamination.
   c. A sterile gauze pad or towel or a sterile, moistened dressing may be applied according to the physician's preference.
      (1) When the sterile covering is used, it should be changed frequently to keep the area free of exudate and to maintain sterility.
      (2) Care must be taken to prevent the covering from adhering to and damaging the sac.
2. Infection of the bladder and urinary tract
   a. Infection is frequently caused by stasis of urine.
   b. Use the Credé method for emptying the bladder if recommended by the physician.
      (1) Apply firm, gentle pressure to the abdomen, beginning in the umbilical area and progressing toward the symphysis pubis.
      (2) Continue the procedure as long as urine can be manually expressed.
      (3) This technique is often contraindicated for infants with vesicoureteral reflux.
   c. Encourage fluid intake to dilute the urine.
   d. Administer prescribed prophylactic antibiotics.

C. Preventing Deformities and Ulcerations of Lower Extremities.

1. Maintain the infant in the prone position with hips only slightly flexed to decrease tension on the sac.
2. Place a foam rubber pad covered with a soft cloth between the infant's legs to maintain the hips in abduction and to prevent or counteract subluxation. A diaper roll or small pillow may be used in place of the foam rubber pad.
3. Allow the baby's feet to hang freely over the pads or mattress edge to prevent aggravation of foot deformities.
4. Change the infant's position when permissible to relieve pressure.
5. Provide meticulous skin care to all areas of the body—especially ankles, knees, tip of nose, cheeks, and chin.

6. Provide passive range-of-motion exercises for those muscles and joints that the infant does not use spontaneously. Hip exercises should not be done unless recommended by the physician.
7. Use a foam or fleece pad to reduce pressure of the mattress against the infant's skin.

D. Providing Adequate Nutrition and Hydration.

1. Hold the infant for feedings if permissible. This provides the needed position change and affection and facilitates feeding.
   Position the infant in such a way that pressure on the back is eliminated. This may be accomplished by holding the infant in a normal feeding position with elbow rotated to avoid touching the sac. Alternatives include feeding the infant on his side or while he is prone on the nurse's lap.
2. The child who must be fed in the prone position should have his head turned to one side and tilted upward.
3. Stop the feeding frequently so that the baby can rest and air can be expelled.
   a. These infants cannot be bubbled in the same way as healthy babies.
   b. Small, frequent feedings may be necessary.
4. Monitor the infant's weight pattern to ensure adequate gain.

E. Providing Normal Infant Stimulation.

1. Establish eye contact with the infant by sitting at the crib with your face at the level of his.
2. Provide appropriate toys, such as bright mobiles or musical toys.
3. Refer to section on growth and development, page 1079.

F. Monitoring Neurologic Status and Observing for Signs of Complications.

1. Hydrocephalus
   a. Irritability
   b. Feeding difficulty, vomiting, decreased appetite
   c. Increased head circumference
   d. Tense fontanelle
   e. Temperature fluctuations
   f. Decreased alertness
2. Infection
   a. Oozing of fluid or pus from the sac
   b. Fever
   c. Irritability or listlessness
   d. Convulsions
   e. Concentrated or foul-smelling urine
3. Record the following:
   a. Frequent vital signs
   b. Behavior of the infant
   c. Movement of the legs
   d. Degree of continence
   e. Evidence of urine retention or fecal impaction
   f. Daily measurement of head circumference
   g. Evidence of complications

G. Providing Initial Emotional Support to the Family.

1. Encourage the parents to talk about their child and how they feel about the defect.
2. Provide them with basic information about the condition.
3. Encourage them to become involved with the child's care from the beginning.
   a. Demonstrate techniques for holding and feeding the child and for providing routine care.
   b. Emphasize the strengths of their infant.

4. Initiate communication with appropriate members of the multidisciplinary team that manages infants with these problems.

For nursing management of the infant with hydrocephalus or clubfoot, refer to Hydrocephalus, page 1438, and Clubfoot, page 1470, in the pediatric section.

Postoperative Nursing Interventions

A. Preventing Postoperative Complications.

1. Shock
   a. Keep the infant warm by placing him in an Isolette or infant warmer.
2. Respiratory problems
   a. Periodically change the infant's position if permitted by his condition and by the extent of surgery.
   b. Have oxygen available if necessary.
   c. Report abdominal distention, which may interfere with breathing and feeding.
3. Nutritional problems
   a. The infant may be fed intravenously for several days or may be fed via gavage if he is unable to take oral feedings (see procedures for intravenous therapy, p. 1167, and gavage feeding, p. 1154).
   b. Apply previously stated principles when bottle-feeding the infant.
4. Infection
   a. Keep the surgical dressing clean and dry.
   b. Observe the dressing frequently for drainage.
   c. Apply previously stated principles to prevent infection.
   d. Administer prescribed antibiotics.
5. Nursing observations—record the following:
   a. Frequent measurements of temperature, pulse, and respiration
   b. Color
   c. Neurologic status
   d. Evidence of abdominal distention
   e. Condition of dressing
   f. Evidence of infection
   g. Degree of continence (urine and stool)
   h. Behavior of the infant
   i. Evidence of hydrocephalus

B. Continuing Appropriate Preoperative Nursing Activities.

1. Once the infant's back is well healed, he may be placed in a supine position for brief periods, which are gradually increased as the skin tolerates it.
2. The infant also may be positioned on his side at no more than a 45-degree angle for brief periods. This position, however, has the disadvantage of placing the hips in flexion and reduces the desirable use of the arms.
3. Special positioning may be requested by the orthopedic surgeon or the physical therapist.
4. Diapers may be used "correctly" once the back is well healed.

C. Providing Continued Emotional Support to the Family.

1. Encourage continued participation by parents in the infant's care.
2. Facilitate communication and interaction with appropriate members of the multidisciplinary clinic for birth defects.
   It is essential that open lines of communication exist between clinic members and the staff that provides daily care for the infant. This ensures that families receive consistent information and facilitates continuity of care.
3. If a multidisciplinary team is not available, initiate appropriate individual referrals—to social worker, clergyman, community health nurse, physical therapist, etc.
4. Foster the goal of helping the child to become as independent as possible.
   a. Emphasize habilitation that makes use of the normal parts of the body and minimizes the disabilities.
   b. Focus on immediate planning in areas such as ambulating and bowel and bladder management.
5. Begin discharge teaching early (see below).
6. Provide support for dealing with the usual problems of a newborn baby. Answer questions related to formula, bath, problems of growth and development, and discipline.

Health Education

1. Prepare the parents to feed, hold, and stimulate their infant as normally as possible.
   Include information related to the management of the usual neonatal problems such as bathing, feeding, formula preparation, and sleeping (see section on growth and development, p. 1079).
2. Teach the parents any special techniques that may be required for the infant's physical care. Examples:
   a. Methods of holding and positioning the infant
   b. Techniques of feeding
   c. Care of the incision
   d. Provision for adequate elimination:
      (1) Procedure for bladder Credé method
      (2) Procedure for bladder catheterization
      (3) Administration of prescribed prophylactic antibiotics
      (4) Signs of constipation and alleviation of the problem through diet regulation
   e. Physical therapy exercises if prescribed
3. Infant stimulation
   Teach the parents ways to help the infant to accomplish developmental tasks of his age level within the limits imposed by his disabilities.
4. Safety
   The child with decreased sensation in the extremities should be protected from prolonged pressure, from burns or trauma due to bath water that is too warm, and from contact with hot or sharp objects.
5. Familiarize the parents with signs of associated problems, especially signs of increased intracranial pressure or shunt malfunction and signs of infection.
   Instruct the parents to notify the physician if a problem does occur.
6. Be certain that a mechanism is developed for the family to receive continued support and teaching following discharge.
   a. This is best provided through a birth defects center.
   b. A community health nursing referral is helpful for many families.

Expected Outcomes

1. The parents demonstrate bonding in their interaction with the infant
2. Avoids infection; signs of infection are recognized promptly and treatment is initiated

3. Adjusts to toileting schedule; eating diet high in fiber; maintains adequate fluid intake
4. Maintains skin integrity; avoids prolonged pressure; checks potential pressure areas from braces or prolonged sitting
5. Attains/maintains normal weight; adheres to dietary regimen
6. Accomplishes appropriate developmental tasks within limits imposed by disability
7. Attains/maintains a positive body image evidenced by verbal and nonverbal communication
8. Achieves maximum independence within limits imposed by his disability
9. The family discusses feelings associated with caring for disabled child; seeks help when necessary.

Bacterial Meningitis

Bacterial meningitis is an inflammation of the meninges that follows the invasion of the spinal fluid by a bacterial agent.

Etiology

1. The proportion of cases due to a specific organism varies from year to year; there is also considerable geographic difference.
2. The organisms most commonly causing bacterial meningitis in different age-groups are:
   a. Birth–2 months
      Escherichia coli
      Streptococcus, group B
   b. 2 months–3 years
      Haemophilus influenzae
      Streptococcus pneumoniae
      Neisseria meningitidis
   c. 3–16 years
      Streptococcus pneumoniae
      Neisseria meningitidis

Altered Physiology

1. Bacterial meningitis is almost always preceded by an upper respiratory infection, which is complicated by bacteremia.
2. Bacteria in the circulating blood then invade the spinal fluid.
3. Bacterial meningitis may occur as an extension of a local bacterial infection such as otitis media, mastoiditis, or sinusitis (less common).
4. Bacteria may also gain direct entry through a penetrating wound, spinal tap, surgery, or anatomic abnormalities.
5. The infective process results in inflammation, exudation, and varying degrees of tissue damage in the brain.

Clinical Manifestations

1. Signs and symptoms are variable, depending on the patient's age, the etiologic agent, and the duration of the illness when diagnosed.
   a. Infants less than 1 month of age display the following symptoms:
      (1) Irritability
      (2) Lethargy
      (3) Vomiting
      (4) Lack of appetite
      (5) Seizures
      (6) High-pitched cry
      (7) Fever
   b. Infants up to 2 years of age manifest symptoms similar to those of the young infant and in addition may have:
      (1) Fever
      (2) Tenseness of the fontanelle
      (3) Neck rigidity
      (4) Positive Kernig's and/or Brudzinski's signs
         (a) *Kernig's sign*
            With the child in the supine position and knees flexed, the leg is flexed at the hip so that the thigh is brought to a position perpendicular to the trunk. An attempt is then made to extend the knee. If meningeal irritation is present, this cannot be done and attempts to extend the knee result in pain.
         (b) *Brudzinski's sign*
            Spontaneous flexion of the lower limbs following passive flexion of the neck.
   c. Children over 2 years of age:
      (1) Common initial symptoms
         (a) Vomiting
         (b) Headache
         (c) Mental confusion
         (d) Lethargy
      (2) Later symptoms
         (a) Neck rigidity within 12–24 hours after onset
         (b) Positive Kernig's and/or Brudzinski's sign
         (c) Seizures
         (d) Progressive decline in responsiveness
2. Onset may be insidious or fulminant.
3. Petechiae or purpura may develop.
   a. Characteristic skin lesions are most often observed in cases of meningococcal or *Pseudomonas* infection.
   b. Hemorrhagic rashes may occur in any child with overwhelming bacterial sepsis because of disseminated intravascular coagulation.
4. Septic arthritis suggests either meningococcal or *Haemophilus influenzae* infection.

Diagnostic Evaluation

1. Diagnosis is usually established by performance of a lumbar puncture and examination of the cerebrospinal fluid.
   a. Cloudy or turbid appearance
   b. Elevated cerebrospinal fluid pressure
   c. High cell count with mostly polymorphonuclear cells
   d. Low glucose level
   e. Elevated protein level (may also be normal)
   f. Gram stain and cultures positive—to identify the causative organism
2. Additional laboratory studies
   a. Complete blood count (Total white blood cell count is often increased, with a preponderance of young neutrophils in the differential blood count.)
   b. Platelet count
   c. Urinalysis
   d. Blood, urine, and nasopharyngeal cultures
   e. Serum electrolytes—often demonstrate hyponatremia and hypochloremia

f. Serum glucose
g. Blood urea nitrogen (BUN) and creatinine
h. Tuberculin skin test
i. Skull and chest x-rays

Treatment

1. Intravenous administration of the appropriate antimicrobial agents to promote rapid destruction of the bacteria and to suppress the emergence of resistant strains
2. Recognition and treatment of hyponatremia
3. Supportive management of the comatose child or the child with seizures
4. Appropriate prophylactic treatment provided for contacts when indicated

Complications

1. Seizures
2. Cerebral edema
3. Subdural effusion
4. Hydrocephalus
5. Cerebral infarction or abscess
6. Diffuse residual effects, including slowed development

Patient Problems and Nursing Diagnoses

1. Potential complications: shock, peripheral circulatory collapse, disseminated intravascular coagulation, syndrome of inappropriate antidiuretic hormone secretion, seizures, and respiratory compromise
2. Altered comfort, pain, related to neurologic effects from the disease process
3. Altered nutrition, less than body requirements, related to inability to eat
4. Parental anxiety related to the life-threatening nature of the child's illness
5. Potential permanent sequelae, including impairment of learning or vision, paralysis, and behavioral defects

Nursing Interventions

A. Practicing Measures That Will Prevent the Transmission of Infection.

1. Place the child in isolation until at least 24 hours after initiation of antibiotic therapy.
2. Practice careful hand-washing technique.
3. Personnel with infection should avoid contact with infants.
   a. Seek medical care for infection. (Cultures should be taken.)
   b. Remain out of the nursery.
   c. Wear a mask when it is necessary to enter the nursery.
4. Teach parents and other visitors proper hand-washing and gown technique.
5. Maintain sterile technique when procedures demanding this technique are performed.
6. Identify close contacts or high-risk children who might benefit from meningococci vaccination.

B. Assessing the Child for Evidence of Disease Progression or Response to Therapy.

1. Determine baseline data at admission. Include the following information:
   a. Weight
   b. Head circumference
   c. Vital signs
   d. Blood pressure
   e. Neurologic status
   f. History related to present illness
   g. Usual behavior and feeding patterns

2. Monitor vital signs, blood pressure, and neurologic status at frequent intervals.
3. Monitor intake and output continuously.
4. Monitor weight and head circumference at least daily.
5. Observe for and report the appearance or disappearance of any of the previously listed clinical manifestations.
   a. Be especially alert for vague symptoms that appear early in the course of meningeal irritation in infants:
      (1) Lethargy
      (2) Irritability
      (3) Poor feeding or refusal to feed
      (4) Weight loss
      (5) Temperature changes
   b. Be consistent in planning for the care of infants to provide a means by which these early symptoms may be detected.
      (1) Accurate charting of the infant's previous behavior
      (2) Assigning the same nurse to care for an infant on successive days

C. Administering the Prescribed Antibiotic Therapy to Control the Infection.

1. Administer medications at the specified time to achieve optimal serum levels.
2. Because medications are generally administered intravenously for 2–3 weeks, restrain the child in a functional position that safeguards the integrity of the IV. Refer to sections on intravenous therapy, page 1167, and protective devices to limit movement, page 1149.
3. Observe medication sites for evidence of infiltration or development of tissue irritation.
4. Be aware of the actions, proper dilution, and side effects of specific medications.
5. Be aware of drug interactions and incompatibilities.

D. Observing for Evidence of Complications of the Disease.

Report the following:
1. Decreased respirations, decreased pulse rate, increased systolic blood pressure, visual disturbances, pupillary changes, or decreased responsiveness, which may indicate increased intracranial pressure.
2. Decreased urine volume and increased body weight, which may indicate inappropriate secretion of antidiuretic hormone.
3. Sudden appearance of a skin rash and bleeding from other sites, which may indicate disseminated intravascular coagulation.
4. Persistent or recurring fever, bulging fontanelle, signs of increased intracranial pressure, focal neurologic signs, seizures, or increased head circumference, which may indicate subdural effusion.
5. Hearing disturbances and apparent deafness.

E. Reducing Fever

1. Possible adverse effects of the increased cerebral metabolic rate associated with fever in the child with cerebral swelling and cerebral vascular compromise
2. Increased potential for seizures in the febrile child
3. Refer to section on management of fever, page 1142

F. Providing for the Nutritional Needs of the Patient.

1. During the acute phase of the illness, the patient may be unable to take or tolerate oral feedings.
   a. Carefully monitor the administration of intravenous fluids.

b. Provide nasogastric feedings if necessary (see section on feeding methods, p. 1152).

c. Provide for the sucking needs of the infant by offering a pacifier.

2. Initiate oral feedings as soon as the patient's condition improves.

a. Infants

  (1) Begin by offering small feedings and observe for the following responses:

    (a) Vomiting

    (b) Abdominal distention

    (c) The infant's interest in feeding and ability to suck

    (d) The infant tires with feeding

  (2) Supplement oral feedings with gavage feedings if necessary.

  (3) Gradually increase amount of feeding.

  (4) Resume regular feeding schedule based on the infant's ability to tolerate it.

  (5) Hold the infant for feedings as soon as his condition warrants it.

b. Older children—refer to section on nutrition, page 1102.

3. Carefully monitor the child's weight to ensure that caloric needs are being met.

G. Providing a Supportive Environment During the Stage of Irritability.

1. Reduce the general noise level around the child and shield child from sudden loud noises.

2. Organize nursing care to provide for periods of uninterrupted rest. Disturb only when necessary.

3. Keep general handling of the child at a minimum. When necessary, approach the child slowly and gently.

4. Maintain subdued lighting as much as possible.

5. Speak in a low, well-modulated tone of voice to reduce anxiety.

H. Providing Therapeutic Care for the Child Who Experiences Seizures.

(See section on seizures, below.)

I. Observing for Episodes of Apnea and Initiating Measures to Stimulate Respiration.

1. Observe the infant closely for apnea or have the infant placed on a respiratory monitor.

2. Stimulate the infant when apnea does occur.

a. Pinch feet and provide more vigorous stimulation if necessary.

b. When spontaneous respiration does not occur within 15–20 seconds, apply hand resuscitator or perform mouth-to-mouth resuscitation.

3. Report frequent periods of apnea to physician.

4. Record length of apnea episode and response to stimulation on nursing record.

J. Providing Supportive Care for the Child During the Convalescent Phase of Illness.

1. Record disappearance of symptoms and indications that the child is returning to his normal state.

2. Provide for the emotional needs of the child (see the section on the hospitalized child, p. 1120).

3. Encourage parental visiting and family-centered care.

4. Note any evidence that the child is developing sequelae of the illness, such as deafness, brain abnormality, or hydrocephalus.

Health Education

1. Encourage the parents to visit their child.

a. Encourage their participation in the child's care.

b. Provide them with an opportunity to express their concerns.

c. Answer questions they may have regarding the infant's progress and care.

2. Discuss symptoms the parents should watch for as signs of possible complications.

3. Give specific instruction regarding medications to be administered at home.

Expected Outcomes

1. Absence of serious complications; maintains normal respiratory, circulatory, and neurologic functions

2. Achieves pain relief; does not appear distressed

3. Receives adequate nutritional support; taking feedings; absence of vomiting and abdominal distention

4. The parents discuss their feelings about the child's illness with each other and with appropriate health care professionals

5. Recovers with no evidence of permanent sequelae of meningitis; no signs of visual or hearing impairment; no paralysis or developmental retardation noted

---

Convulsive Disorders
(Seizure Disorders, Epilepsy)

Convulsive disorder is a term used to encompass a number of varieties of episodic disturbances of brain function. Convulsions should not be regarded as one specific disease, but as a symptom of an underlying disorder. They are relatively common in children, being more prevalent during the first 2 years than at any other time in life.

Etiology

1. Idiopathic

2. Prenatal factors

a. Genetic predisposition

b. Congenital structural anomalies

c. Fetal infections

d. Maternal diseases

3. Perinatal factors

a. Trauma

b. Hypoxia

c. Jaundice

d. Infection

e. Prematurity

f. Drug withdrawal

4. Postnatal factors

a. Primary infection of the central nervous system

b. Infectious diseases of childhood with encephalopathy

c. Head trauma

d. Circulatory diseases

e. Toxic encephalopathy

f. Allergic encephalopathy

g. Metabolic encephalopathy

h. Degenerative diseases

i. Cerebral neoplasms

j. Renal disease

k. Anoxia

Altered Physiology

1. The basic mechanism for all seizures appears to be prolonged depolarization, causing brain cells to become overactive and to discharge in a sudden, violent, disorderly manner.

2. This paroxysmal burst of electrical energy spreads to adjacent areas or may jump to distant areas of the central nervous system. A seizure results.
3. The biochemical basis of seizures is incompletely understood.
4. Some seizures appear to occur under the influence of a triggering factor.
   a. Hormonal factors, such as those related to the menstrual period, menarche, and menopause
   b. Nonsensory factors, such as hyperthermia, hyperventilation, metabolic disorders, sleep deprivation, emotional disturbances, and physical stress
   c. Sensory factors, such as those related to vision, hearing, touch, the startle reaction, and those that are self-induced
5. For international classification of epileptic seizures refer to a neurology textbook.

Types of Seizures

A. Generalized Seizures (Convulsive and Nonconvulsive)
1. Onset
   a. Onset is abrupt.
   b. May occur at night.
   c. An aura (peculiar sensation, often dizziness) occurs in about ⅓ of epileptic children prior to a grand mal seizure.
2. Tonic spasm
   a. The child's entire body becomes stiff.
   b. He loses consciousness.
   c. The face may become pale and distorted.
   d. His eyes are frequently fixed in one position.
   e. His back may be arched with his head held backward or to one side.
   f. His arms are usually flexed and his hands clenched.
   g. If standing, the child falls to the ground.
   h. He may utter a peculiar, piercing cry.
   i. He is often unable to swallow his saliva.
   j. Breathing is ineffective and cyanosis results if spasm includes the muscles of respiration.
   k. The pulse may become weak and irregular.
3. Clonic phase
   a. Characterized by rhythmic, jerking movements that follow the tonic state.
   b. Usually start in one place and become generalized, including the muscles of the face.
   c. The child may be incontinent and may bite his tongue or cheek. (This occurs because of sudden forceful contraction of his jaw and abdominal muscles.)
4. Duration
   a. Varies, from a few seconds to 30 minutes or longer.
   b. Usually, convulsions cease after a few minutes.
5. Postconvulsive (postictal) state of child
   a. Usually is sleepy or exhausted
   b. May complain of headache
   c. May appear to be in a dazed state
   d. Often performs relatively automatic tasks without being able to recall the episode.
6. Secondary symptomatology
   a. Represents the patient's response over a long period of time to the injurious attitudes of other people toward the child and the diagnosis.
   b. The child develops a self-image consistent with his perception of how others view him.
7. Electroencephalogram (EEG)
   a. Definite abnormalities can usually be demonstrated in the interval between seizures.

(1) Random spike discharges
(2) Diffuse high-voltage slow waves
(3) Pattern abnormal for child's chronologic age
   b. Multiple high-voltage spike discharges are demonstrated during the seizure.
   c. Asymmetries between the 2 hemispheres and diffuse slowing may be observed after the seizure.

B. Status Epilepticus
1. State of continuing or recurring seizures that occur in series without the patient's regaining consciousness between attacks.
2. Transient postictal (i.e., period following seizures) signs and symptoms include ataxia, aphasia, and mental sluggishness.
3. Irreversible brain damage may occur secondary to prolonged cerebral hypoxia.
4. This condition should be treated as a medical emergency.

C. Petit Mal Epilepsy (Generalized Seizure)
1. Onset—rarely appears before 5 years of age.
   a. Absence seizure
2. Clinical signs
   a. Loss of contact with the environment for a few brief seconds:
      (1) The child may appear to be staring or daydreaming.
      (2) If reading or writing, the child will suddenly discontinue the activity and may resume it when the seizure has ended.
   b. Atypical absence seizure:
      Minor manifestations include rolling of the eyes, nodding of the head, slight hand movements, and smacking of the lips.
3. Duration—usually 5–10 seconds.
4. Frequency—varies from 1 or 2 per month to several hundred each day.
5. Precipitating factors may include hyperventilation, fatigue, hypoglycemia, and stress.
6. Postconvulsive state
   a. Child appears normal.
   b. Is not aware of having had a convulsion.
7. Electroencephalogram (EEG)
   Has characteristic 3-per-second spike and wave pattern during the seizure.

D. Partial Seizures
1. Psychomotor
   a. Occur most frequently in children from 3 years of age through adolescence.
   b. Seizure discharge usually originates in the temporal lobe and may be referred to as "temporal lobe seizures."
   c. Clinical signs:
      (1) Frequently experiences a sense of fullness rising from the abdomen to the thorax.
      (2) Aura, if present, often includes bad odor or taste.
      (3) May experience complex auditory or visual hallucinations, déjà vu feeling, or strong sense of fear and anxiety.
      (4) Perceptual alterations may occur.
      (5) Dysphagia or aphasia may be present.
      (6) Most common motor symptom is drawing or jerking of the mouth and face.
      (7) May perform coordinated but inappropriate movements repeatedly in a stereotyped manner (e.g., clutching, kicking, picking at clothes, walking in circles, chewing, licking, spitting).

(8) Consciousness may be impaired but is rarely completely lost.

d. Duration—brief, usually from 30 seconds to 5–10 minutes.

e. Postconvulsive state—the child is usually drowsy or sleeps after an attack. Confusion and amnesia are common.

2. Focal motor
   a. Clinical signs
      (1) Sudden jerking movements occur in a particular area of the body, such as the face, thumb, or toe.
      (2) Consciousness may or may not be disturbed.
      (3) Clonic movements occasionally begin in 1 area of the body and spread to adjacent areas on the same side in a fixed progression (Jacksonian seizures).
   b. Prognosis—seizures may become more extensive as the child matures, leading to grand mal seizures.

3. Focal sensory (rare in children)—sensations occur, such as numbness, tingling, and coldness in the part of the body controlled by the area of the brain cell overactivity.

E. Infantile Myoclonic Seizures (Massive Myoclonic Spasms)

1. These seizures are peculiar to infants; they are second in incidence only to grand mal seizures in this age-group.

2. Peak incidence is in children between 3 and 6 months; onset after 2 years of age is rare.

3. Clinical signs
   a. Sudden, forceful, myoclonic contractions involving the musculature of the trunk, neck, and extremities.
      (1) Flexor type—the infant adducts and flexes his extremities, drops his head, and doubles upon himself.
      (2) Extensor type—the infant extends neck, spreads arms out, and bends body backward in a position described as "spread eagle."
   b. A cry or grunt may accompany severe attacks.
   c. The infant may grimace, laugh, or appear fearful during or after the attack.

4. Duration—momentary (usually under 1 minute).

5. Frequency—varies from a few attacks per day to hundreds per day.

6. EEG—random, high-voltage slow waves and spikes suggestive of a diffuse disorganized state.

7. Prognosis
   a. Almost always associated with cerebral abnormalities.
   b. Usually this type of seizure disappears spontaneously by the time the child reaches 4 years of age.
   c. Subsequent grand mal or other types of seizures often develop.
   d. Mental retardation usually accompanies this disorder.

Chemotherapy

A. General Principles Related to the Administration of Medications

1. Selection of the most effective drug(s) depends on correct identification of the clinical seizure type.

2. A desirable drug level is one that will prevent attacks without producing undesirable side effects.

3. Dosages are adjusted according to blood level and clinical signs.

4. Accurate timing is essential to prevent seizures. This is especially true when there is a tendency for the child to have convulsions at a certain period each day.

5. Enteric-coated tablets, which have a delayed effect, should be used for children who are prone to attacks during sleep.

6. Most anticonvulsants are available in liquid form as well as in capsules or tablets.
   Tablets can be crushed and given to infants and small children in coke syrup or applesauce.

7. It may take several months to find the best combination of medications and the best dosages of each to control the child's seizures.

8. One hundred percent control of symptoms may not be achieved in every patient.

9. Dosage adjustment may be required from time to time because of the child's growth.

10. Blood counts, urinalyses, and liver-function studies are done at regular intervals in children receiving certain anticonvulsants.

11. Medication is often not discontinued until 2–3 years after the last attack.

12. Weaning from medication should always be gradual, with stepwise reduction of dosage and withdrawal of 1 drug at a time.

B. Drugs Commonly Used for the Control of Seizures in Children

1. Phenobarbital
   a. Dosage
      (1) An initial loading dose is usually given intramuscularly or intravenously for an acute, ongoing seizure, because it takes from days to weeks to achieve therapeutic blood levels by the oral route alone.
      (2) The dosage is reduced for maintenance therapy and is generally administered orally.
   b. Indications and advantages
      (1) Drug of choice for initial trial, except for petit mal seizures
      (2) One of the safest anticonvulsant drugs
      (3) Relatively inexpensive
   c. Untoward effects
      (1) Excitement, hyperactivity
      (2) Rash
      (3) Gastrointestinal symptoms
      (4) Dizziness, ataxia
      (5) Aggravated psychomotor seizures
      (6) Drowsiness
      (7) Irritability
      (8) Depression
   d. Toxic effects (rare, except in overdose, accidental ingestion)—respiratory, circulatory, or renal depression
   e. Contraindications
      (1) Severe hepatic or renal dysfunction
      (2) Hypersensitivity

2. Phenytoin (Dilantin)
   a. Route—oral
   b. Indications and advantages
      (1) Does not produce excessive drowsiness
      (2) Safest drug for the management of psychomotor epilepsy
      (3) Often used with phenobarbital
   c. Untoward effects
      (1) May accentuate petit mal seizures
      (2) Hypertrophy of the gums—daily gum massage is an important aspect of nursing care for a patient taking phenytoin
      (3) Hirsutism

    (4) Rickets
    (5) Nystagmus
    (6) Ataxia
    (7) Rash
    (8) Nausea and vomiting
    (9) Decreased alertness
    (10) Agitation
  d. Toxic effects—(rare, except in overdose, accidental ingestion)
    (1) Blood dyscrasia
    (2) Liver damage

3. Ethosuximide (Zarontin)
  a. Route—oral
  b. Indications and advantages
    (1) Used for petit mal seizures
    (2) Occurrence of blood dyscrasia is less common following administration of ethosuximide than with trimethadione (Tridione)—the other medication frequently used to control petit mal seizures.
  c. Untoward effects
    (1) Drowsiness
    (2) May increase grand mal seizures
    (3) Gastrointestinal symptoms—administer with food
    (4) Lethargy
    (5) Euphoria
  d. Toxic effects
    (1) Blood dyscrasias
    (2) Psychiatric symptoms
  e. Contraindications—hepatic or renal disease

4. Primidone (Mysoline)
  a. Route—oral
  b. Indications and advantages
    (1) Used alone or with other anticonvulsants to control mixed-type seizure patterns.
    (2) May control grand mal seizures not responsive to treatment by other anticonvulsant therapy.
  c. Untoward effects
    (1) More common
      (a) Ataxia
      (b) Vertigo
    (2) Occasional
      (a) GI symptoms
      (b) Fatigue
      (c) Diplopia
      (d) Nystagmus
      (e) Skin eruption
  d. Toxic effects
    (1) Megaloblastic anemia may occur as a rare idiosyncratic response to the drug.
    (2) Drowsiness in nursing newborns of primidone-treated mothers indicates that breast-feeding should be discontinued.
  e. Contraindications
    (1) Patients who are hypersensitive to phenobarbital
    (2) Patients with porphyria

5. Diazepam
  a. Route—oral, intravenous, or intramuscular
  b. Indications and advantages
    (1) Intravenous or intramuscular diazepam is indicated in the treatment of status epilepticus and severe recurrent convulsive seizures.
    (2) Oral diazepam may be used adjunctively in maintenance therapy for convulsive disorders.
  c. Special precautions
    (1) If administered intravenously, give slowly over 3 minutes. Avoid intra-arterial administration or extravasation.
    (2) Administer intravenously with caution to children with limited pulmonary reserve, because of the possibility that apnea and/or cardiac arrest may occur.
    (3) Tonic status epilepticus has been precipitated in patients treated with intravenous diazepam for petit mal seizures.
    (4) Concomitant use of barbiturates, alcohol, or other central nervous system depressants may potentiate the action of diazepam with increased risk of apnea.
    (5) Administer with caution to children with compromised renal function.
  d. Untoward effects
    (1) More common
      (a) Ataxia
      (b) Drowsiness
      (c) Fatigue
      (d) Venous thrombosis and phlebitis at injection site
    (2) Less common
      (a) GI symptoms
      (b) Confusion, depression
      (c) Headache
      (d) Tremor
      (e) Vertigo
      (f) Incontinence or urinary retention
      (g) Visual disturbances
      (h) Skin rash
      (i) Anxiety
      (j) Sleep disturbance
      (k) Neutropenia
      (l) Jaundice
  e. Toxic effects
    (1) Somnolence
    (2) Confusion
    (3) Diminished reflexes
    (4) Hypotension
    (5) Coma
    (6) Apnea
    (7) Cardiac arrest

6. Carbamazepine (Tegretol)
  a. Route—oral
  b. Indications and advantages—especially useful in treatment of major motor and psychomotor seizures.
  c. Special precautions—administration with phenytoin (Dilantin) reduces the half-life of phenytoin. The phenytoin dose may need to be increased when carbamazepine is added.
  d. Untoward effects (most likely to occur during the initial phases of therapy)
    (1) Dizziness
    (2) Drowsiness
    (3) Nausea and vomiting
  e. Toxic effects
    (1) Bone marrow depression (aplastic anemia, thrombocytopenia, agranulocytosis, and leukopenia)
    (2) Early toxic signs and symptoms
      (a) Fever
      (b) Sore throat
      (c) Ulcers in mouth
      (d) Easy bruising
      (e) Petechial or purpuric hemorrhage

f. Contraindications
(1) History of previous bone marrow depression
(2) Known hypersensitivity to the drug
(3) Used with caution in patients with cardiac, hepatic, or renal problems

Prognosis

1. General prognosis depends on type and severity of seizure disorder, coexisting mental retardation, organic disorders, and the type of medical management.
   a. Medically treated seizures—spontaneous cessation of seizures may occur. Drugs may be gradually discontinued when the child has been free from attacks for an extensive period and his EEG pattern has reverted to normal.
   b. Nontreated epilepsy—seizures tend to become more numerous.
2. Mental development
   a. Convulsive episodes do not in themselves usually cause irreversible brain damage.
   b. Hypoxia during seizures can cause mental retardation.
   c. Epileptic children with normal mentality can be expected to remain normal with proper control of seizures.

Patient Problems and Nursing Diagnoses

1. Potential for injury during a convulsive seizure
2. Potential ineffective breathing/cyanosis related to spasms of respiratory musculature
3. Thought processes, altered (disorientation), following seizure related to disruption of cerebral function
4. Possible noncompliance with treatment regimen (anticonvulsant medications)
5. Potential complication: undesirable/toxic effects from anticonvulsant medications
6. Anxiety related to hospitalization and the diagnostic procedures
7. Knowledge deficit about convulsive disorders and their management
8. Social isolation related to the child's feelings about his illness and/or public fears and misconceptions

Nursing Interventions

A. Controlling the Seizures.

Administer medications as prescribed.

B. Protecting the Child From Injury During a Convulsive Episode.

1. Preventive measures
   a. Remove hard toys from the bed.
   b. Pad the sides of the crib.
   c. Have a suction machine available to remove secretions during a seizure.
   d. Have an emergency oxygen source in the room in case of sudden respiratory difficulty.
2. Emergency actions
   a. Clear the area around the child if he is not in bed.
   b. Do not restrain him.
   c. Loosen the clothing around his neck.
   d. If the child is standing, ease him to his bed or the floor.
   e. Turn the child on his side so that saliva can flow out of his mouth.
   f. Place a small, folded blanket under the head to prevent trauma if the seizure occurs when the child is on the floor.

g. Suction the child and administer oxygen as necessary.
h. Do not give anything by mouth.
i. After the seizure, place the child on his side in bed, if he is not already there.

C. Accurately Recording the Seizures—including the following:

1. Significant preseizure events, such as noise, excitement, lethargy
2. Behavior before the seizure, aura
3. Types of movements observed
4. Time seizure began and ended
5. Site where twitching or contraction began
6. Areas of the body involved
7. Movements of the eyes and changes in pupil size
8. Incontinence
9. Amount of perspiration
10. Respiratory changes
11. Color change—pallor, cyanosis, flushing
12. Mouth—teeth clenched, movement, tongue bitten, foaming at the mouth
13. Apparent degree of consciousness during the seizure
14. Behavior after the seizure
    a. Degree of memory for recent events
    b. Types of speech
    c. Coordination
    d. Paralysis or weakness
    e. Sleeping after the attack
    f. Pupil reaction
    g. Vital signs
    h. Unusual sensations

D. Observing the Child for Recurrent Seizures.

1. Place the child where he can be watched closely.
2. Monitor vital signs and assess neurologic status frequently.
3. Check the child frequently. Report:
   a. Behavior changes
   b. Irritability
   c. Restlessness
   d. Listlessness

E. Providing Emotional Support to the Child's Parents.

1. Describe completely any examinations, evaluations, treatments that the child is receiving.
   a. EEG
   b. CT scan/MRI
   c. Blood studies
   d. Medications
2. Provide information regarding the disease itself.
   a. Epilepsy is *not* contagious, is seldom dangerous, and does *not* indicate insanity or mental retardation.
   b. Most children with epilepsy have infrequent seizures and with medications can completely control their convulsions.
   c. The child may have normal intelligence and can live a useful and productive life.
   d. The child's medication is not addicting when used as prescribed. It should in no way influence his mental ability or personality or cause him to become a drug addict.
   e. It is impossible to predict accurately the possibility of the convulsive disorder appearing in siblings or offspring of the affected child.
3. Observe the parent–child reaction for evidence of rejection or overprotection.

Offer reassurance and praise for achievements in dealing with the child's problem.
4. Prepare the parents for the fact that it may take several months of regulating drug dosages before adequate control is obtained.
5. Provide the parents with appropriate literature.
6. Refer the family to appropriate community resources and services.
   a. Social worker
   b. Community health nurse
   c. School nurse
   d. Psychiatrist
   e. Parent groups
   f. Voluntary agencies

F. Minimizing Anxiety During the Child's Hospitalization.

1. Rationale—the therapeutic value of anticonvulsant drugs is decreased if the child has more anxiety than he can handle
2. Explain the diagnostic and treatment plan to the child in a manner that he can understand.
3. Allow the child as much normal activity as possible. Allow him to be dressed if desired.
4. If the child does have a seizure, stay with him and remain calm.
   a. Stay with the child after a convulsion and reassure him and his parents that he is all right.
   b. Help the child to adjust to reality if he has difficulty remembering the episode.
   c. Older children may require intervention to deal with guilt and embarrassment secondary to incontinence and the loss of body control.
   d. Maintain a quiet environment if the child has had a long convulsive period.
5. Provide diversion appropriate for the child's age. Play equipment should be such that it will not cause injury during a seizure.
6. Avoid unnecessary stimulation.

Health Education

1. The child should be in an environment that is as normal as possible.
   a. Attendance at a regular school with healthy children should be encouraged.
      (1) Contact should be made with the school nurse, who can help the child's teacher understand his disease, emergency treatment of seizures, etc.
      (2) The child should be allowed to participate in organizations and outside activities with limited restrictions.
         (a) Each child must be treated individually; the kind of activity depends on the degree of control.
         (b) Generally, children with seizure disorders should not be allowed to climb in high places or to swim alone.
         (c) Responsible adults should be made aware of the child's disease.
      (3) The child should not be made to feel that he can never be left alone.
      (4) He needs to be disciplined as a normal child. He should not gain attention directly or indirectly by having seizures.
2. The child should be given appropriate information regarding his diagnosis and treatment. He is less confident of his body and his control over it and therefore less confident of himself.
   a. He should be included in conferences with the physician.
   b. He needs an opportunity to ask questions, which should be answered honestly.
   c. He should be aware of his restrictions and helped to deal with them.
   d. He should gradually be given responsibility for taking his own medications faithfully.
   e. He should be encouraged to wear a Medic Alert bracelet.
3. The older child or adolescent should be helped to achieve independence.
   a. He should be given the opportunity for privacy to discuss his diagnosis with his physician.
   b. He should be allowed to use his own judgment in his daily activities.
   c. He should be helped to develop realistic educational and career goals.
      (1) The assistance of a social worker or psychiatrist may be invaluable during this period.
      (2) Genetic counseling may be indicated in some cases.
         (a) People with epilepsy can marry and have children.
         (b) There is no proof that epilepsy is hereditary, although there may be a tendency to transmit a low convulsive threshold.
      (3) Counseling regarding matters such as securing a driver's license and obtaining life, health, and automobile insurance should be available.
   d. Fantasies that "there is nothing wrong with me" or the refusal to take medications requires prompt intervention.
4. Factors that may precipitate a convulsive episode should be avoided.
   a. The seizures should be treated matter of factly. A calm, reassuring attitude is essential during and after a seizure. The attitude of adults when the child has a seizure influences the attitude of other children toward him.
   b. The child should be kept in optimal physical condition with special attention to the status of his teeth and eyes and to the prevention of infection.
   c. Excessive-fatigue, overhydration, and hyperventilation should be avoided.
   d. Irregular, fluctuating schedules are detrimental. A routine of daily living should be encouraged.
5. Medical care and supervision to control convulsions are essential. Instructions regarding medical and nursing care should be stressed.
      (1) Administration of medications and side effects of prescribed drugs
      (2) Emergency care during a seizure
      (3) Observations
         (a) Signs of impending seizure
         (b) Behavior during and after the seizure
      (4) Diet—ketogenic diets are no longer widely used, except in difficult cases
6. Parents should be referred to appropriate support groups for help in dealing with their feelings, concerns, and problems related to their child.

Expected Outcomes

1. Avoids injury during a convulsive episode; takes protective measures; wears helmet
2. Regains normal breathing pattern following a seizure
3. Becomes oriented to time, place, and person after a seizure episode

4. Takes medications as prescribed
5. Does not experience untoward effects of his anticonvulsant medication; no dizziness, nausea, vomiting, mouth ulcers, fever
6. The child shows decreasing anxiety; asks appropriate questions; expresses his feelings through verbal and nonverbal communication and with play
7. The child and parents describe his disease; verbalize the importance of medication and follow-up
8. Participates in age-appropriate social activities

Febrile Convulsions

Febrile convulsions refer to seizures that occur in the context of a febrile illness in a previously normal child. The seizures are brief and generalized. They should be distinguished from focal or prolonged seizures, which occur in a child with an underlying seizure disorder that is exacerbated by fever.

Etiology

1. Accompany intercurrent infections—especially viral illness, tonsillitis, pharyngitis, and otitis.
2. Appear to occur in a familial pattern, although exact pattern of inheritance is incompletely understood.

Incidence

1. Febrile convulsions occur in approximately 3%–5% of all children.
2. The vast majority of first febrile seizures occur in children between the ages of 6 months and 3 years of age.
3. Febrile seizures are unusual after 5 years of age.

Clinical Manifestations

1. Most febrile convulsions consist of generalized tonic-clonic seizures.
2. Seizures generally last less than 15 minutes.
3. Fever is usually high—over 38.8°C. (101.8°F.) rectally.
4. Seizures usually occur near the onset of fever rather than after prolonged fever.

Diagnostic Evaluation

Measures are directed toward delineating the cause of any seizure as precisely as possible so that its implications and prognosis may be discussed with the parents. Diagnostic methods include:
1. Physical examination with special attention to neurologic status
2. Cerebrospinal fluid examination
3. Complete blood count and urinalysis
4. Cultures of nasopharynx, blood, or urine as appropriate to determine cause of fever
5. Blood sugar, calcium, and electrolyte levels
6. EEG
   a. Demonstrates mild, postictal slowing soon after the attack
   b. Pattern is generally normal after a few days

Prognosis

1. The likelihood of febrile seizure recurrence is about 40%–50% for a second febrile seizure.
2. Factors influencing recurrence rate
   a. The younger the child is at the time of the first seizure, the greater the risk for additional febrile seizures.

b. Children with a positive family history of febrile convulsions have a greater risk of recurrent febrile convulsions.
3. The risk for development of nonfebrile convulsions is relatively low (about 3%). At risk are those children who demonstrate the following characteristics:
   a. Multiple febrile seizures during 1 day
   b. Prolonged febrile seizures
   c. Persistent electroencephalographic abnormalities
   d. Central nervous system infections

Nursing Interventions

A. Assessing and Reducing Fever.
Refer to section on fever, page 1142.
B. Intervening Appropriately During and After the Seizure Episode(s).
See Nursing Interventions A–D in previous section, pages 1453–1454.

Health Education

1. Remain calm and efficient if the child has a seizure in the presence of his parents.
2. Reinforce realistic, reassuring information such as:
   a. A convulsion does not necessarily imply that the underlying disease is a serious one.
   b. Children rarely die in seizures.
   c. The prognosis depends on the cause of the convulsion.
      (1) A single febrile seizure is not indicative of later chronic epilepsy.
      (2) Children who have a tendency to develop febrile convulsions usually lose it as they grow older.
      (3) Occasional, brief convulsions have no adverse effects on the child's ultimate development.
3. Discuss and demonstrate emergency management of seizures.
4. Stress that medical evaluation is indicated as soon as the child develops a fever.
   a. Review technique of temperature measurement.
   b. Prompt administration of antipyretic measures is necessary when the child is febrile.
5. Reinforce medical instructions regarding anticonvulsant therapy.
   a. The advisability of long-term anticonvulsant medications in normal children with simple febrile convulsions is currently controversial. Recommendations vary among physicians from no medication to maintenance therapy with phenobarbital.
   b. Intermittent therapy with phenobarbital during febrile episodes is apparently of no value because of the length of time required to achieve therapeutic serum levels of the drug.

Subdural Hematoma

Subdural hematoma refers to an accumulation of fluid, blood, and its degradation products within the potential space between the dura and arachnoid (subdural space). Subdural hematomas are classified as acute, subacute, or chronic, depending on the time between injury and the onset of symptoms.

Etiology

1. Direct or indirect trauma to the head.
   a. Birth trauma
   b. Accidental causes
   c. Purposeful violence, as in the battered child syndrome (see p. 1518)
2. Meningitis

Classification*

A. Acute

Syndrome presents as an acute problem, closely related to the time of presumed injury.

B. Chronic

1. Signs and symptoms are nonlocalizing and subacute.
2. Most common type of subdural hematoma in children.
3. It is often difficult to delineate the exact time and type of injury, as the precipitating episode may appear relatively insignificant.

Altered Physiology

1. Trauma to the head causes tearing of the delicate subdural veins, resulting in small hemorrhages into the subdural space. (Bleeding may be of arterial origin in cases of acute subdural hematoma.)
2. As the blood breaks down, there is an increased capillary permeability and effusion of blood cells and protein into the subdural space.
3. The breakdown products of blood stimulate the growth of connective tissue and capillaries largely from the dura.
4. A membrane is formed that usually extends frontally and laterally over the hemispheres, surrounding the clot.
5. Fluid accumulates within the membrane and increases the width of the subdural space.
6. Further hemorrhages occur.
7. The lesion enlarges, expanding the skull, and, if unrelieved, ultimately causes cerebral atrophy or death from compression and herniation.
8. The lesion may arrest spontaneously at any point.
9. Further bleeding may occur into an already existing sac and may increase symptoms.
10. In long-standing subdural hematoma, the fluid may disappear, leaving a constricting membrane that prevents normal brain growth.

Clinical Manifestations

A. Acute

1. Often present with continuous unconsciousness from the time of injury, but child may present with a lucid interval.
2. Ensuing manifestations include deterioration of level of consciousness, evidence of progressive hemiplegia, focal seizures, and signs of brain stem herniation (pupillary enlargement, changes in vital signs, development of decerebrate state, and respiratory failure).

B. Chronic

1. Insidious onset
2. Symptoms are variable and are related to the age of the child.

* Classification does not imply any basic differences in the disease process, but refers only to the duration of the lesion before it becomes manifest. The classification varies slightly among several sources.

a. Infants
   (1) Early signs
      (a) Anorexia
      (b) Difficulty feeding
      (c) Vomiting
      (d) Irritability
      (e) Low-grade fever
      (f) Retinal hemorrhages
      (g) Failure to gain weight
   (2) Later signs
      (a) Enlargement of the head
      (b) Bulging and pulsation of the anterior fontanelle
      (c) Tight, glossy scalp with dilated scalp veins
      (d) Strabismus, pupillary inequality, ocular palsies (rare)
      (e) Hyperactive reflexes
      (f) Seizures
      (g) Retarded motor development
b. Older children
   (1) Early signs
      (a) Lethargy
      (b) Anorexia
      (c) Symptoms of increased intracranial pressure
         (1) Vomiting
         (2) Irritability
         (3) Increased blood pressure
         (4) Decreased pulse
         (5) Decreased or irregular respirations
         (6) Headache
   (2) Later signs (may occur immediately if bleeding takes place rapidly)
      (a) Convulsions
      (b) Coma

Diagnostic Evaluation

1. CT scan is the procedure of choice for diagnosing subdural hematomas.
2. Bilateral subdural taps may provide the diagnosis as well as immediate relief of increased intracranial pressure.

Complications

1. Mental retardation
2. Ocular abnormalities
3. Seizures
4. Spasticity
5. Paralysis

Treatment

1. Acute subdural hematoma—requires evacuation of the clot through a burr hole or craniotomy.
2. Chronic subdural hematoma
   a. Repeated subdural taps are done to remove the abnormal fluid.
      (1) In infants, the needle can be inserted through the fontanelle or suture line.
      (2) In older children, burr holes into the skull are necessary before the needle can be inserted.
      (3) The subdural taps may be the only treatment required if the fluid disappears entirely and symptoms do not recur.
      (4) Concurrently, treatment is instituted to correct anemia, electrolyte imbalance, and malnutrition.

b. Shunting procedure may be indicated if repeated taps fail to reduce significantly the volume or protein content of the subdural collections. Shunting is generally to the peritoneal cavity.

Prognosis

1. Treatment is usually successful when the diagnosis is made early—before cerebral atrophy and a fixed neurologic deficit have occurred. In such cases, subsequent development is normal.
2. Prognosis depends on the effect of the initial trauma on the brain as well as the effect of continued fluid collection.
3. Mortality in massive, acute subdural bleeding is very high, even if promptly diagnosed.

Nursing Interventions

A. Assessing the Child's Neurologic Status in Order to Help Evaluate the Effectiveness of Treatment or to Identify Disease Progress.

Observe for and document the following:
1. General behavior—especially irritability, lethargy, and evidence of personality changes.
   It is important to obtain a thorough history from the child's parents regarding his normal behavior and level of functioning so that abnormalities can be more easily recognized.
2. Appetite and feeding difficulties, including vomiting.
3. Signs of increased intracranial pressure.
   a. Vital signs, including pulse, respiration, and blood pressure should be monitored frequently.
   b. Be alert for:
      (1) Increased systolic blood pressure
      (2) Increased pulse pressure
      (3) Decreased pulse or irregularities
      (4) Changes in respiratory rate or difficulty breathing
4. Level of consciousness—describe findings explicitly. The following "levels" may be useful as guidelines:
   a. Alert and responds immediately and appropriately to visual, auditory, and tactile stimuli.
   b. Lethargic, drowsy, and inactive but can be aroused to an alert state.
   c. Lethargic and dull; responds with vigorous stimulation, but quickly returns to lethargic state.
   d. Can be aroused only to a very low level of response with vigorous stimulation.
   e. Moderate coma with rudimentary physiologic or psychomotor responses.
   f. Totally nonresponsive, even to deep pain stimuli.
5. Pupillary changes—especially dilated pupil, double vision, lack of response to light, alterations in visual acuity, and decreased integrity of eye movements.
6. Seizures
7. Motor function, including ability to move all extremities. The ability to grasp should be checked and compared bilaterally.
8. Drainage of cerebrospinal fluid from the nose or ears.

B. Observing for Signs of Complications.

1. Infection
   a. Record temperature frequently.
   b. Report purulent drainage from the site of the subdural tap.
2. Recurrent bleeding—note rapid changes in vital signs indicating shock or increased intracranial pressure.
3. Paralysis

C. Avoiding Additional Increase in Intracranial Pressure.

1. Maintain a quiet environment.
2. Avoid sudden changes in position.
3. Organize nursing activities to allow for long periods of uninterrupted rest.
4. Administer laxatives or suppositories to prevent straining during a bowel movement.

D. Assisting With Subdural Taps.

1. Wrap the infant or young child in a mummy restraint (see procedure on protective devices to limit movement, p. 1149).
2. Hold the child securely to avoid injury caused by sudden movement.
3. Apply firm pressure over the puncture site(s) for a few minutes after the tap has been completed to prevent fluid leakage along the needle tract.
4. Observe the child frequently after the procedure for:
   a. Shock
   b. Drainage from the site of the tap
      (1) Note whether this is serious drainage or frank blood.
      (2) Reinforce the dressing, if present, to prevent contamination of the wound.

E. Providing Adequate Nutrition.

Apply principles stated in the section on hydrocephalus, page 1438.

F. Providing Supportive Care to the Child in Coma.

1. Keep the child's eyes well lubricated to prevent corneal damage.
2. Suction the child as necessary to remove secretions in the mouth and nasopharynx.
3. Provide frequent mouth care.
4. Maintain adequate nutrition and hydration through nasogastric feedings (see procedure, p. 1158).
5. Carefully regulate fluid administration to avoid danger of rapidly increasing intracranial pressure.
6. Measure urine output and record specific gravity.
7. Administer suppositories or enemas as necessary to prevent constipation and impaction.
8. Change the child's position frequently and provide meticulous skin care to prevent hypostatic pneumonia and pressure sores.
9. Prevent contractures.
   a. Apply passive range of motion exercises to all extremities.
   b. Place pillows appropriately to support the child's body in good alignment.
   c. Use a footboard for the older child.
10. Have emergency equipment available for cardiopulmonary resuscitation, respiratory assistance, blood transfusion, subdural tap, etc.
11. Avoid discussing the child's condition near the bedside. Even though comatose, the child may be able to hear.
12. Observe for the development of the following complications:
    a. Respiratory problems (infection, aspiration, obstruction, atelectasis)
    b. Fluid and electrolyte imbalance
    c. Infection (urinary or central nervous system)
    d. Bladder and gastrointestinal distention

G. Caring for the Child With a Craniotomy.

See section on the postoperative care of the child with a brain tumor, page 1487.

H. Providing for the Child's Emotional Needs.

1. Hold and cuddle the infant as much as possible according to his condition.
2. Provide diversion according to the child's age.
   a. Infants—mobiles or musical toys
   b. Older children—quiet games, reading, etc.

I. Providing Emotional Support to the Parents.

1. Encourage as much parental participation in the child's care as possible.
2. Reassure the parents that the prognosis is favorable with adequate treatment.
3. Avoid blaming the parents for the child's injury
   a. Attempt to alleviate their guilt feelings if present.
   b. Refer the parents to a social worker or psychiatrist if this problem is severe.

Health Education

Reinforce explanations in the following areas:
1. The condition
2. The causes of the child's specific symptoms
3. The need and rationale for treatment
4. Postoperative and recovery expectations
5. Signs of recurrent bleeding
6. Safety measures to prevent accidents in the future

Reye's Syndrome

Reye's syndrome in children has been clinically characterized as a complex of signs and symptoms, including encephalopathy and fatty degeneration of the viscera, mainly affecting the liver, brain, and kidneys.

Etiology and Incidence

1. Unknown
2. Most consistent single factor is an antecedent viral infection
   a. Influenza B—clustered geographically, occurring in older children (mean age is 11 years)
   b. Varicella—sporadic occurrence in younger children (mean age is 6 years)
   c. Gastroenteritis
   d. Upper respiratory tract infection
3. Other related viruses include adenovirus, Coxsackie, ECHO, herpes simplex and zoster, reovirus, and polio type I.
4. Other controversial possibilities (contributors)
   a. Genetic make-up of individual child that increases his susceptibility, triggered by virus, toxins, drugs, or endogenous factors.
   b. Environmental factors—chemical toxins (i.e., pesticides or fertilizers).
   c. Clinical—salicylates and phenothiazines, acetaminophen.
5. Occurs more commonly in Caucasian children living in rural or suburban areas under the age of 16 years. Occurs more frequently in Black infants from lower socioeconomic urban areas than white infants.
6. Peak seasonal occurrences are in winter and spring.

Altered Physiology

1. Mitochondrial injury or change is primary in all tissues. Dysfunctioning mitochondri result in decreased enzymes for proper functioning of specific metabolic pathways.

2. Liver—enlarged and bright yellow; fatty infiltration in the form of small lipid droplets; mitochondria are large and swollen with some decrease of enzymatic activity, particularly for ammonia detoxification, thus hyperammoniemia.
   a. Liver function studies are elevated—SGOT, SGPT.
   b. Clotting disturbances result in decreased clotting factor and prolonged prothrombin time and partial prothrombin time.
   c. Dysfunction of gluconeogenetic enzymatic pathway and depleted supply of glycogen stores. Hypoglycemia leads to the increased production of ammonia and fatty acidemia. Hypoglycemia seen in younger children is related to less liver reserve of glycogen and a higher metabolic rate.
3. Brain—cerebral edema with small ventricles, possible neuronal necrosis, findings consistent with hypoxia, inflammatory reaction absent, grossly enlarged mitochondria; and pervasive watery blebs.
   a. Hypoxia and/or hypoglycemia are evidenced by neuronal degeneration.
   b. Cerebral spinal fluid is usually normal, except in later stages of disease when pressure is elevated.
4. Kidney—fatty degeneration of loop of Henle and proximal convoluted tubules with a few lipid droplets in distal tubular cells.
   Renal vasculature and glomeruli are normal.
   Renal insufficiency occurs. Edema, decreased urinary output, increased BUN and creatinine, and loss of autoregulation lead to decrease in cerebral blood flow, tissue hypoxia, and neuronal death.
5. Heart—fatty accumulation in fibers; bundle of His, and bundle branches.

Prognosis and Complications

1. Complete recovery
2. Recovery with brain damage—developmental delays, motor impairment, or mental retardation
3. Posthospital anxiety and apprehension

Clinical Manifestations

> **NURSING ALERT:** Early diagnosis is critical because of the rapidly fatal course of the disease.

1. Prodromal illness (see etiology) that may be improving
2. Sudden pernicious vomiting—fever usually not present
3. Irrational behavior
4. Altered sensorium—from mild lethargy to progressive stupor and coma
5. Hyperventilation, tachypnea
6. Hepatomegaly
7. Stages—children with Reye's syndrome advance through definite stages of progression. After diagnosis is made, the child should be categorized as fitting within one of the stages, with any progression noted. Generally, the more rapid the progression through these stages, the poorer the prognosis.
   Lovejoy's Stages of Progression follow:
   Stage I: Vomiting, lethargy, difficult to arouse, liver dysfunction, type I EEG
   Stage II: Disorientation, delirium, combativeness, hyperventilation, hyperactive reflexes, liver dysfunction, type II EEG
   Stage III: Decorticate positioning, obtundent, coma, hyperventilation, liver dysfunction,

presence of pupillary light reaction, type II EEG

Stage IV: Deepening coma, decerebrate rigidity, costal–caudal progression of brain stem dysfunction, loss of oculocephalic reflexes, fixed and dilated pupils, improvement of liver dysfunction, type III EEG

Stage V: Seizures, loss of reflexes, flaccidity, respiratory arrest, correction of liver dysfunction, isoelectric EEG

Diagnostic Evaluation

1. General condition and appearance of child:
   History of prodromal illness—mild upper respiratory infection or other infection with sudden development of pernicious vomiting, presence of other symptoms.
2. Differential diagnosis—acute toxic encephalopathy, hepatic coma, hepatitis, meningitis, or encephalitis. History to rule out ingestion of medications or toxic materials.
3. Laboratory data
   *a. Serum ammonia—elevated 48 μg./100 ml.
   *b. Liver enzymes (SGOT, SGPT)—elevated
   *c. Clotting factors (PT and PTT)—prolonged
   *d. Serum glucose—hypoglycemia
   e. Creatinine—elevated
   f. BUN—elevated
   g. Amino acid, free fatty acids—elevated
   h. Acid–base status—acidemia
   i. CBC
   *j. Serum bilirubin—mild, transient elevations to normal less than 3%
   k. Electrolytes
   l. Serum osmolality
   m. Serum levels of salicylates, acetaminophen, and phenothiazines
   n. Urine: analysis, electrolytes, and osmolality
4. Lumbar puncture—done if cerebrospinal fluid is needed to rule out other diagnoses. If symptoms of increased intracranial pressure exist, the performance of a lumbar puncture is to be avoided to prevent rapid decompression and herniation of the brain.
5. Liver biopsy—usually done; however, the biopsy may not be done unless evidence is insufficient to make a definite diagnosis (shows microvesicular fatty degeneration of liver).

Medical and Nursing Management

A. General Considerations

1. Because this is a multisystem disease, it must be emphasized that:
   a. Intracerebral integrity is of utmost priority, and if the brain can be supported through the course of the illness, the chances of the other organs running their course uneventfully are very high and are of less concern.
   b. The multidisciplinary team must have a leader who initiates, coordinates, and supervises *all* activities and medical planning. It may be the physician, neurosurgeon, endocrinologist, or the attending pediatrician. However, it should be the person with the knowledge and capability of monitoring and directing care 24 hours a day.

* Essential for diagnosis

2. Treatment is supportive by maintaining adequate levels of circulating glucose and cerebral perfusion while preventing or controlling IICP (increased intracranial pressure).
   Treatment is aimed toward normalizing organ function and protection of the brain from irreversible damage.

B. Supportive Interventions

1. Admission to an intensive care unit. Multisystem invasive monitoring: complex coordination of care (medical and nursing) of all systems is essential to control and reduce IICP.
   a. It takes many hours to several days after control of the disease process is achieved to begin to withdraw therapy or liberalize intervention without having recurring IICP symptoms.
   b. The nurse is the most constant and consistent person at the bedside in most institutions and must be alert to all aspects of this very complex critical-care problem.
   c. The nursing input may have a very significant impact on the morbidity of the patient; a knowledgeable nurse can make very important judgments concerning the timing of interventions and can anticipate problems and needs.
   d. Nursing responsibilities include assessment, reassessment, anticipation, and documentation of physical status, environmental impacts, and therapeutic interventions.
2. General supportive care includes:
   a. Correction of hypoglycemia
   b. Correction of fluid and electrolyte imbalance
   c. Correction of acidosis
   d. Prevention or correction of hypoxia
   e. Prevention of or treatment of increased intracranial pressure
   f. Correction of metabolic abnormalities
   g. Continuous monitoring of cardiopulmonary and neurologic status
   h. Evaluation of laboratory data
   i. Monitoring vital signs for signs of shock
3. Supportive care of the child in stage I or II (noncomatose):
   a. Hourly neurologic checks—see Glasgow Coma Scale (Table 58-1)
   b. Nothing by mouth
   c. Strict intake and output record
   d. Maintain serum glucose; 150–200 mg./dl. intravenous hypertonic glucose solution given
   e. Monitor body weight

Table 58-1. *Glasgow Coma Scale*

Eyes open	Spontaneously	4
	To speech	3
	To pain	2
	No response	1
Best verbal response	Oriented	5
	Confused	4
	Inappropriate words	3
	Incomprehensible sounds	2
	None	1
Best motor response	Obeys commands	5
	Localizes pain	4
	Flexion to pain	3
	Extension to pain	2
	None	1

f. Administer phytonadione—to combat coagulation defects

g. Sedation—to decrease anxiety and potential for IICP

4. Management of the child in stage III or IV (comatose):

a. Insert intraventricular pressure catheter or sub-arachnoid bolt with pressure monitoring and control of IICP. Goal is to maintain intracranial pressure within normal range of 10–15 torr.

b. Intubate (endo- or nasotracheal) and ventilate—to provide optimal cerebral blood flow. (Auto regulation − ↓ PCO_2 = ↓ size blood vessels = ↓ vol = ↓ ICP.)

Maintain $PaCO_2$ about 25 mm. torr and PaO_2 at 100–150 torr. Muscle relaxants and short-acting barbiturates are also used.

c. Establish arterial line for pressure monitoring and blood sampling.

d. Insert indwelling urethral catheter.

(1) Accurately record intake and output every 1–4 hours.

(2) Measure urine specific gravity.

e. Insert nasogastric tube and measure drainage. Give an antacid every 2–4 hours to maintain gastric pH above 4. Neomycin may be given via nasogastric tube to aid in reduction of ammonia accumulation.

f. Limit fluid intake—peripheral IV fluids given at a rate of ⅔ maintenance because of potential cerebral edema and IICP. Calculate administered medications as part of fluid intake.

g. Monitor blood glucose—give IV glucose to prevent any neurologic deterioration (hypertonic solution up to 15–20% IV drip through a central line). Keep serum glucose 200–300 mg./dl., serum osmolality 300–310 mOsm./liter.

5. Additional measures directed at controlling intracranial pressure:

a. Maintain core body temperature at 36.5°–37°C. (97.7°–98.6°F.). Moderate hypothermia (controversial) may be employed using a cooling blanket.

b. Position supine with head of bed elevated 30 degrees; keep head still—aids in intracranial venous drainage.

c. Provide chest physical therapy—to prevent infection and atelectasis, increased intrathoracic pressure, thus increasing intracranial pressure. The risk of increasing intracranial pressure must be weighed against the benefit of the procedure.

d. Observe for complications—cardiac arrhythmias, heme concentration, decreased urinary output, decreased mean arterial pressure, fluid overload (↑ CVP 6–8 cm. H_2O, urine output ↑ 2 ml./kg./hour, clinical edema), hypovolemia (mean arterial pressure ↓ 65 mm. Hg).

e. Monitor EEG continuously.

f. Monitor nursing activities that may cause an increase in intracranial pressure: suctioning, turning, chest physical therapy, painful (intrusive) procedures, conversation at bedside about diagnosis.

g. Prevent and control IICP with drugs.

(1) Muscle relaxation (pancuronium bromide) while on ventilator

(2) Sedation (diazepam, chloral hydrate)

(3) Osmotic diuretic (mannitol or glycerol)

(4) Barbiturate therapy (thiopental, phenobarbital)

h. Provide secondary infection coverage—especially staphylococcus (neurologic and lung).

6. When all intensive medical and nursing support has been exhausted and ICP is still uncontrollable or cardiovascular status is unstable, consideration for bilateral decompression craniectomies must be made by the medical team.

Patient Problems and Nursing Diagnoses

1. Potential respiratory complications: apnea, pulmonary congestion and obstruction, and coma

2. Potential cardiac complications from hypovolemia, dehydration/or fluid overload, altered electrolytes, cardiac instability, and impaired autoregulatory mechanism

3. Increased intracranial pressure from cerebral edema

4. Hypoglycemia from altered liver function

5. Potential complications from comotose state: skin breakdown, corneal injury

6. Anxiety and ineffective family coping related to lack of knowledge, fear, and/or guilt.

7. Anxiety related to acuteness of illness, procedures, hospitalization, and on recollection of events that occurred during critical phase of illness.

Nursing Interventions

A. Providing Acute and Intensive Nursing Care.

1. During the acute phase of the disease, the child should be cared for in an intensive care unit.

2. Refer to:
Respiratory measures, page 1185
Cardiopulmonary resuscitation, page 1200
Assisting with obtaining blood for gas analysis, page 164
Intensive care, page 1129
Intravenous therapy, page 1167
Increased intracranial pressure, page 1440
Care of the comatose patient, page 576
NG tube procedures, page 1158
Catheter procedure, page 665

B. Being Aware of the Medical Plan of Treatment and Being Alert to the Rapidity of the Course of the Disease. Particularly important factors:

1. Note and report immediately any changes in the child's status or stage of progression (see Clinical Manifestations).

2. Therapy is directed at maintaining normal intracranial pressure and adequate cerebral perfusion.

3. Protect the child from complications that may result from the comatose condition or life-saving medical intervention.

4. Maintain fluid and electrolyte balance.

5. Before any procedure is done for the child, consider the effects on his intracranial pressure.

C. Supporting Parents During the Time the Child May Be in the Intensive Care Unit.

1. Prior to the first visit, explain in detail what the child will look like. Accompany the parents when they first visit their child. Because this may be traumatic, do not force them to maintain lengthy contact with the child.

2. Address parental concerns and answer questions regarding:

a. How they should react to their child

b. Amount of parental participation that is beneficial

c. Fears and fantasies during lengthy periods when they are unable to visit child

d. Concerns for other children and other family members, and their reactions to the illness

e. Technical questions

3. Provide the parents with the telephone number of the intensive care unit.
4. Make sure the parents have a comfortable place to sleep if they elect to stay at the hospital.
5. Help the parents who request consultation—social service for ICU, chaplain, Reye's Syndrome Foundation parent group (if appropriate and available).
6. Help the family express their feelings about what has happened and how it is affecting them.
   a. Assess how they are coping; their family support systems.
   b. Initiate referrals to appropriate social agencies as needed.
   c. The lack of knowledge of the disease and rapid course from a mild to a critical illness may be difficult for parents to understand. They may have extreme feelings of guilt, and blame themselves or others for not recognizing the seriousness of the illness sooner. They may have other children at home with similar prodromal viral infections who may be experiencing guilty feelings about the ill sibling.

D. Providing Psychological and Emotional Support to the Child.

1. Although the child may be heavily sedated, comatose, or paralyzed from muscle relaxants, he perceives in varying degrees what is happening to him and to his environment.
2. Explain procedures to the child while they are being done.
3. Conversations about the child, his condition, or other children should take place away from the sick child.
4. Encourage parents to bring in a favorite toy or security object.
5. Show a constant awareness of any activity, noise, etc. that increases or changes intracranial pressure.
6. When a sedated or comatose child awakens, he may be disoriented and have no memory of previous events. Provide explanations and reassurance as appropriate.
7. Parental separation may increase anxiety; support as necessary.

E. Providing Continued Support of the Child and His Family When the Child is Transferred From the Critical Care Unit to the Pediatric Nursing Unit.

1. Once the child is alert, his condition stable, and he is recovering, he should be transferred to the regular pediatric unit.
2. The child recovering from Reye's syndrome without any neurologic sequelae should recover fairly rapidly. Provide support as needed.
3. When the child has experienced sequelae or complications, attention to his physical manifestations will be needed according to the child's specific deficit (e.g., physical therapy). A multidisciplinary team approach

to treatment will continue to provide for optimal functioning.
4. The child and his family will continue to need emotional support during this period.
5. A critical role of the nurse is to educate herself, other members of the staff, and the community about Reye's syndrome.*
   a. Learn to recognize the symptoms that may lead to a diagnosis of the illness.
   b. Be prepared for the course of the illness, from a mild disease to one that is life-threatening.
   c. Support parent groups and other community groups to educate parents about Reye's syndrome, and to seek medical consultation when symptoms may indicate the disease.

Health Education

1. Encourage the family to maintain a close physical and emotional relationship with the child during his illness
   a. Helps the child feel less disoriented
   b. Helps the family work through feelings of guilt and helplessness
2. Ensure that the parents understand the importance of medical follow-up, especially related to any complications associated with the illness
3. Become involved in community education to help caretakers recognize early signs and symptoms suggestive of Reye's syndrome

Expected Outcomes

1. Demonstrates adequate respiratory function, as evidenced by appropriate respiratory status, normal vital signs, and normal arterial blood gases
2. Achieves adequate circulatory function and cerebral perfusion, as evidenced by normal CVP values, normal urinary output, and normal sinus rhythm
3. Maintains integrity of cerebral blood flow and oxygenation and is free of neurologic deterioration, as evidenced by intracranial pressures ↓ <15 torr, absence of clinical signs of deterioration, and absence of hyperthermia
4. Shows no signs of hypoglycemia, as evidenced by appropriate serum glucose levels
5. Avoids complications of immobility and comatose state, as evidenced by intact skin, absence of secondary infections, etc.
6. Reveals minimal anxiety and disorientation, as evidenced by behaviors
7. The parents demonstrate and verbalize understanding of disease and events

* National Reye's Syndrome Foundation, 436 N. Lewis, Bryan, OH 43506
Reye's Syndrome Society, PO Box RS, 7045 Traverse Avenue, Benzonia, MI 49616

Bibliography

Books

American Association of Neuroscience Nurses. Core Curriculum for Neuroscience Nursing, Vol. I and II. 2nd ed. Park Ridge, AANN, 1984
Bell W and McCormick W. Neurologic Infections in Children. 2nd ed.

Volume XII in the Series, Major Problems in Clinical Pediatrics. Philadelphia, WB Saunders, 1981
Behrman RE and Vaughan VC. Nelson Textbook of Pediatrics. Philadelphia, WB Saunders, 1983
Chess S and Fernandez P. The Handicapped Child in School:

Behavior and Management. New York, Brunner/Mazel, 1981
Conway–Rutkowski B. Carini and Owen's Neurological and Neurosurgical Nursing. 8th ed. St Louis, CV Mosby, 1982
Danilova L. Methods of Improving the Cognitive and Verbal Development of

Children with Cerebral Palsy. New York, World Rehabilitation Fund, 1983

Darling R and Darling J. Children Who Are Different: Meeting the Challenges of Birth Defects in Society. St Louis, CV Mosby, 1981

Dobbing J (ed). Prevention of Spina Bifida and other Neural Tube Defects. New York, Academic Press, 1982

Downey J and Low N (eds). The Child with Disabling Illness: Principles of Rehabilitation. 2nd ed. New York, Raven Press, 1982

Farmer T (ed). Pediatric Neurology. 3rd ed. Philadelphia, Harper & Row, 1983

Fraser B and Hensinger R. Managing Physical Handicaps: A Practical Guide for Parents, Care Providers and Educators. Baltimore, Paul H Brookes, 1983

Hickey J. The Clinical Practice of Neurological and Neurosurgical Nursing. Philadelphia, JB Lippincott, 1986

Hicks DA. Cerebral edema. In Pierog JE and Pierog LJ (eds). Pediatric Critical Illness and Injury. Rockville, Aspen Publishers, Inc, 1984

Hoeprich PD (ed). Infectious Diseases. 3rd ed. Philadelphia, Harper & Row, 1983

Hopkins A. Epilepsy: The Facts. New York, Oxford University Press, 1981

Kaktis JV. An introduction to monitoring intracranial pressure in critically ill children. In Pierog JE and Pierog LJ (eds). Pediatric Critical Illness and Injury. Rockville, Aspen Publishers, Inc, 1984

Krugman S and Katz S. Infectious Diseases of Children. 7th ed. St Louis, CV Mosby, 1981

Levin D, Morriss F and Moore G (eds). A Practical Guide to Pediatric Intensive Care. 2nd ed. St Louis, CV Mosby, 1984

Levitt S. Treatment of Cerebral Palsy and Motor Delay. 2nd ed. London, Blackwell Scientific Publications, 1982

Oakes A (ed). Critical Care Nursing of Children and Adolescents. Philadelphia, WB Saunders, 1981

Pellock J and Myer E (eds). Neurologic Emergencies in Infancy and Childhood. Philadelphia, Harper & Row, 1984

Powell M. Assessment and Management of Developmental Changes and Problems in Children. 2nd ed. St Louis, CV Mosby, 1981

Roessler R and Bolton B. Psychosocial Adjustment to Disability. Baltimore, University Park Press, 1978

Rudy E. Advanced Neurological and Neurosurgical Nursing. St Louis, CV Mosby, 1984

Schafer M and Dias L. Myelomeningocele: Orthopedic Treatment. Baltimore, Williams & Wilkins, 1983

Scheiner A and Abrams I. The Practical Management of the Developmentally Disabled Child. St Louis, CV Mosby, 1980

Scherzer A and Tscharnuter I. Early Diagnosis and Therapy in Cerebral Palsy. New York, Marcel Dekker, 1982

Section of Pediatric Neurosurgery of the American Association of Neurological Surgeons (eds). Pediatric Neurosurgery: Surgery of the Developing Nervous System. New York, Grune & Stratton, 1982

Smith J (ed). Pediatric Critical Care. New York, John Wiley & Sons, 1983

Snyder M. A Guide to Neurological and Neurosurgical Nursing. New York, John Wiley & Sons, 1983

Swaiman K and Wright F. The Practice of Pediatric Neurology. St Louis, CV Mosby, 1982

Thompson G, Rubin I and Bilenker R. Comprehensive Management of Cerebral Palsy. New York, Grune & Stratton, 1982

Varni J. Clinical Behavioral Pediatrics. New York, Pergamon Press, 1983

Vestal K (ed). Pediatric Critical Care Nursing. New York, John Wiley & Sons, 1981

Wedgwood RJ et al. Infections in Children. Philadelphia, Harper & Row, 1982

Whaley L and Wong D. Nursing Care of Infants and Children. 2nd ed. St Louis, CV Mosby, 1983

Worcester CC. Reye's Syndrome. In Pierog JE and Pierog LJ (eds). Pediatric Critical Illness and Injury. Rockville, Aspen Publishers, Inc, 1984

Woodbury D, Penry J and Pippenger C. Antiepileptic Drugs. 2nd ed. New York, Raven Press, 1982

Zucman E. Childhood Disability in the Family. New York, World Rehabilitation Fund, 1982

Journals

Arcinue EL. Reye's syndrome: Contending with a mysterious and increasingly common disease. Consultant 1982 Nov; 22(11):165–167+

Aspirin and Reye's Syndrome. Am J Dis Child 1982 Nov; 136(11):971–972

Benjamin R and McKay R. Working with a brain-injured child. J Assoc Care Child Health 1980 Spring; 8(4):99–104

Berkowitz C and Jones C. The PNP's role in evaluation and management of febrile seizures. Pediatr Nurs 1983 Nov–Dec; 9(6):432–434

Boutros AR, et al. Reye syndrome: A predictable curable disease. Pediatr Clin North Am 1980 Aug; 27(3):539–552

Brink J, Imbus C and Woo-Sam J. Physical recovery after severe closed head trauma in children and adolescents. J Pediatr 1980 Nov; 97(5):721–727

Bruce D. The child's injured head: Trauma in the young. Emerg Med 1983 Aug 15; 15(14):45, 49–50, 55–56

Budd RA and Hobdell EF. Reye's syndrome. Crit Care Nurse 1983 Mar–Apr; 3(2):94–97

Budd RA and Rothwell R. Spotting Reye's syndrome while there's still time. RN 1983 Dec; 46(12):38–42+

Camfield P et al. The first febrile seizure—antipyretic instruction plus

either phenobarbital or placebo to prevent recurrence. J Pediatr 1980 Jul; 97(1):16–21

Cecconi C et al. Model instructional program for mainstreaming handicapped children . . . designed to teach normal children about cerebral palsy. Phys Ther 1980 Aug; 60(8):1022–1025

Charney EB et al. Management of the newborn with myelomeningocele: Time for a decision-making process. Pediatrics 1985 75:58–64

Chee D. Seizure disorders. Nurs Clin North Am 1980 Mar; 15(1):71–82

Clarke K et al. Reye's syndrome nursing protocol. J Nat Reye's Syn Found 1980 1(2):82–84

Clarkson J. Self-catheterization training of a child with myelomeningocele. AJOT 1982 Feb; 36(2):95–98

Coffey R. Pediatric neurological emergencies. Top Emerg Med 1982 Jul; 4(2):67–78

Colgan M. The child with spina bifida. Am J Dis Child 1981 Sep; 135(9):854–858

Consensus Development Panel. Febrile seizures: Long term management of children with fever-associated seizures. Pediatr Rev 1981 Jan; 2(1):209–212

Coulter D. The psychosocial impact of epilepsy in childhood. Child Health Care 1982 Fall; 11(2):48–53

Dalgas P. Reye's syndrome update. MCN 1983 Sep–Oct; 8(5):345–349

Dunne RS and Perez RC. Reye's syndrome: A challenge not limited to critical care nurses. Issues Compr Pediatr Nurs 1981 Jul–Aug; 5(4):253–263

Edwards M and Baker C. Complications and sequelae of meningococcal infections in children. J Pediatr 1981 Oct; 99(4):540–545

Ferry P. Computed cranial tomography in children. J Pediatr 1980 Jun; 96(6):961–967

Gaddy D. Meningitis in the pediatric population. Nurs Clin North Am 1980 Mar; 15(1):83–97

Graziani L et al. Ultrasound studies in preterm infants with hydrocephalus. J Pediatr 1980 Oct; 97(4):624–631

Griffiths S. Body image concerns of a four year old boy with meningitis. Matern Child Nurs J 1980 Summer; 9(2):127–136

Grow DH. Reye's syndrome. Nursing 1981 Nov; 11(11):156+

Gururaj V. Febrile seizures: Current concepts. Clin Pediatr 1980 Nov; 19(11):731–738

Hahn JF. Cerebral edema and neurointensive care. Pediatr Clin North Am 1980 Aug; 27(3):587–592

Haller J. Intracranial pressure monitoring in Reye's syndrome. Hosp Pract 1980 Feb; 15(2):101–108

Hausman KA. Critical care of the child with increased intracranial pressure. Nurs Clin North Am 1981 Dec; 16(4):647–656

Icenogle D and Kaplan A. A review of congenital neurologic malformations. Clin Pediatr 1981 Sep; 20(9):565–576

Jackson P. Increased intracranial pressure in infants and young children. Crit Care Q 1981 Mar; 3(4):47–59

Jackson P. Peritoneal shunting for hydrocephalus. Crit Care Update 1983 Apr; 10(4):33–39

Jackson P. Ventriculo-peritoneal shunts. Am J Nurs 1980 Jun; 80(6):1104–1109

Jamison-Smith P and Hamm P. Reye's syndrome. Crit Care Update 1983 Jul; 10(7):54–55

Jeffries J, Killam P and Varni J. Behavioral management of fecal incontinence in a child with myelomeningocele. Pediatr Nurs 1982 Jul–Aug; 8(4):267–270

Johnson LK. If your patient has increased intracranial pressure, your goal should be: No surprises. Nursing '83 1983 Jun; 13(6):58–63

Johnson M and Freeman J. Pharmacologic advances in seizure control. Pediatr Clin North Am 1981 Feb; 28(1):179–194

Kaplan S and Feigin. Treatment of meningitis in children. Pediatr Clin North Am 1983 Apr; 30(2):259–270

Killam P et al. Behavioral pediatric weight rehabilitation for children with myelomeningocele. MCN 1983 Jul–Aug; 8(4):280–286

Kolata GB. Reye's syndrome: A medical mystery. Science 1980 Mar 28; 207(4438):1453–1454

Kunkel J. Nursing management of the head injured patient. Crit Care Update 1981 Mar; 8(3):22–24+

Lovejoy FC et al. Clinical staging in Reye's syndrome. Am J Dis Child 1974 Jul; 128:36–41

Manella K and Varni J. Behavior therapy in a gait-training program for a child with myelomeningocele. Phys Ther 1981 Sep; 61(9):1284–1287

Martelli ME. Teaching parents about Reye's syndrome. Am J Nurs 1982 Feb; 82(2):260–263

McElroy D. Hydrocephalus in children. Nurs Clin North Am 1980 Mar; 15(1): 23–34

McGrath D. Video recording seizure activity in children. MCN 1983 May–Jun; 8(3):218–220

Meir E. Evaluating head trauma in infants and children. MCN 1983 Jan–Feb; 8(1):54–57

Miller J and Arsenault L. Reye's syndrome. J Neurosurg Nurs 1983 Jun; 15(3):154–164

Mills G. Preparing children and parents for cerebral computerized tomography. MCN 1980 Nov–Dec; 5(6):403–407

Mitchell PH, Ozuna J and Lipe HP. Moving the patient in bed: Effects on intracranial pressure. Nurs Res 1981 Jul–Aug; 30(4):212–218

Norman S. The pupil check. Am J Nurs 1982 Apr; 82(4):588–591

Norman S and Browne T. Seizure disorders. Am J Nurs 1981 May; 81(5): 985–994

Orlowski J, Rothner D and Lueders H. Submersion accidents in children with epilepsy. Am J Dis Child 1982 Sep; 136(9):777–780

Parrish MA. A comparison of behavioral side effects related to commonly used anticonvulsants. Pediatr Nurs 1984 Mar–Apr; 10(2):149–152

Passo S. Malformations of the neural tube. Nurs Clin North Am 1980 Mar; 15(1):5–21

Pinyerd B. Siblings of children with myelomeningocele: Examining their perceptions. Matern Child Nurs J 1983 Spring; 12(1):61–70

Pleasants D. Managing hydrocephalus with a ventricular shunt. AORN J 1982 Apr; 35(5):885–892

Pressman S. Myelomeningocele: A multidisciplinary problem. J Neurosurg Nurs 1981 Dec; 13(6):333–336

Raphaely R et al. Management of severe pediatric head trauma. Pediatr Clin North Am 1980 Aug; 27(3):715–727

Reye RD, Morgan G and Barae J. Encephalopathy and fatty degeneration of the viscera–a disease entity in children. Lancet 1963 Oct 12; 2(7310): 749–752

Reye Syndrome and aspirin use: The role of prodromal illness severity in the assessment of relative risk. Pediatrics 1982 Jun; 69(6):812–822

Rothner A and Erenberg G. Status epilepticus. Pediatr Clin North Am 1980 Aug; 27(3):593–602

Ruben F et al. Epidemiologic factors of Reye syndrome seen in southwestern Pennsylvania 1970–1980. AJPH 1983 Sep; 73(9):1063–1065

Santilli N and Tonelson S. Screening for seizures. Pediatr Nurs 1981 Mar–Apr; 7(2):11–15

Sasso S. Phenytoin for seizure disorders. MCN 1984 Jul–Aug; 9(4):279

Scarff T et al. Myelomeningocele: A review and update. Rehabil Nurs 1981 Nov–Dec; 6(6):26–29

Shaw L. A teaching plan for cerebroventricular shunting for hydrocephalus. AORN J 1982 Apr; 35(5):893–898

Shurtleff D. Myelodysplasia: Management and treatment. Curr Probl Pediatr 1980 Jan; 10(3):1–56

Smith EE. Reye's syndrome: Deadly threat to children. Am Lung Assoc Bull 1982 May; 68(4):11–12

Take two aspirin and call me in the morning: Salicylate use and Reye's syndrome. Am J Dis Child 1982 Nov; 136(11):973–974

Thurston J et al. Prognosis in childhood epilepsy: Additional follow-up of 148 children 15 to 23 years after withdrawal of anticonvulsant therapy. N Engl J Med 1982 Apr; 306(14):831–836

Trauner DA. Reye's syndrome. Curr Probl Pediatr 1982 May; 12(7):2–31

Tucker C. Complex partial seizures. Am J Nurs 1981 May; 81(5):996–1000

Vigliarolo D. Managing bowel incontinence in children with meningomyelocele. Am J Nurs 1980 Jan; 80(1):105–107

Waldman RJ et al. Aspirin as a risk factor in Reye's syndrome. JAMA 1982 Jun; 247(22):3089–3094

Wallack C. Head trauma in children. Nurs Clin North Am 1980 Mar; 15(1): 115–127

Walson P et al. Once daily doses of phenobarbital in children. J Pediatr 1980 Aug; 97(2):303–305

Wink D. Bacterial meningitis in children. Am J Nurs 1984 Apr; 84(4):456–460

Ziff S. The sexual concerns of the adolescent woman with cerebral palsy. Issues Health Care Women 1981 Jan–Feb; 3(1):55–63

Fractures

Generally, nursing care of the child with a fracture is similar to that of an adult. The child is usually hospitalized only for application of a cast (see procedure for cast care, p. 1213) or to be placed in traction (see procedure for traction, p. 1204). The nurse should be aware of the following principles concerning fractures in pediatrics.

General Considerations

1. Children's bones are softer and more pliable than adult's bones. They can tolerate a greater degree of deformity before breaking.
2. Greenstick fractures in normal bones are unique to children.
   a. The bone breaks at one cortex and bends at the other.
   b. There is no complete loss of bony continuity.
   c. The younger the child, the more likely he is to sustain a greenstick fracture.
   d. The radius, ulna, clavicle, or long bone in the hand are most likely to sustain a greenstick fracture.
3. Comminuted fractures are less common in pediatric patients.
4. Injuries of the epiphyseal plate are unique to children.
   a. The epiphyseal plate is weaker than normal tendons, ligaments, or the joint capsule.
   b. Injury resulting in a torn ligament or dislocation in the adult is more likely to produce a separation of the epiphysis in a child.
   c. The lower radial epiphysis is more frequently separated than any other.
   d. This type of injury may cause growth disturbance.
5. Fractures in pediatric patients heal more readily than those in adults.
   a. The younger the child, the more rapidly the fracture unites.
   b. The thick periosteum and abundant blood supply make nonunion rare.
6. End-to-end apposition of fracture surfaces is not essential in pediatric patients.
   a. The long bones may be allowed to unite with side-to-side apposition in children up to 11–12 years of age.
   b. Subsequent molding will produce a normal bone by the end of growth.
7. Following injury, the extremities in children are likely to swell much more rapidly and the swelling to disappear more quickly than in an adult.
8. Function is usually restored rapidly and sometimes spontaneously following injury in children.
9. Open fractures are an orthopedic emergency. Tetanus toxoid immunity must be checked.
10. Extremity ischemia is an important complication, especially in injuries around the elbow, knee, or fractures of forearm or lower leg. Observe for:
    a. Pain
       (1) Usually below splintage
       (2) Progressive pain after splintage with attempts to move toes/fingers distal to injury
    b. Paresthesia and paralysis distal to injury
    c. Cold, pallid, or cyanotic, pulseless—dependent on interruption of blood supply

Common Fractures in Children

Fracture of the Clavicle

A. Cause

1. Compression of the shoulders during delivery of a baby
2. Transmitted force caused by falling on an outstretched hand, elbow, or side of the shoulder
3. Direct force (rare)

B. Treatment

1. Immobilization in a figure 8 bandage or clavicle strap.
2. Closed reduction and use of a plaster figure 8 cast, or bed rest and side arm traction may be necessary in older children with displaced fractures.

C. Healing Time

1. Younger children: 3–4 weeks
2. Older children: 5–6 weeks

Fracture of the Neck of the Humerus

A. Cause

1. Indirect force from a fall on an outstretched hand
2. Direct force by blow or fall on the lateral aspect of the shoulder

B. Treatment

1. Minimal displacement—immobilization of the shoulder and upper extremity with stockinette collar and sling
2. Considerable displacement
   a. Reduction under anesthesia may be done.
   b. Immobilization of the shoulder and upper extremity in a collar and cuff sling or a shoulder spica.

c. Dunlop traction followed by use of a shoulder spica cast may be required in severe cases.

C. Healing Time

1. Minimal displacement: 3–4 weeks
2. Considerable displacement: 4–6 weeks

Fractures of the Shaft of the Humerus

A. Cause

1. Birth injury—most common long bone to be fractured at that time
2. Direct force, such as a fall on the side of the arm
3. Indirect force, such as the child throwing a ball, or a caretaker grabbing the child's arm to prevent a fall or pulling an arm in or out of a sleeve roughly

B. Treatment

1. Reduction of the fracture
2. Immobilization
   a. Infants and young children
      (1) A U-slab of plaster is used to keep the arm against the chest with the elbow at a 90- to 45-degree angle.
      (2) Skin traction may be necessary for 2–3 weeks if the fracture is unstable or oblique with much overriding of the fragments. The arm then is immobilized as described above until healing is complete.
   b. Older children or adolescents
      (1) A shoulder spica cast is used for an unstable fracture.
      (2) Skeletal traction and suspension of the forearm and hand are indicated if the local skin and soft tissue conditions do not permit skin traction.
      (3) A hanging cast may be used for an older adolescent.
         (a) This type of cast permits the child to be ambulatory and active.
         (b) Erect position should be maintained as much as possible during the day.
         (c) The child should sleep in a semirecumbent position.
         (d) There should be no support at the elbow.
         (e) Pressure from clothing or anything that might compress the arm against the body must be avoided, as it interferes with traction.

C. Healing Time

4–6 weeks

Supracondylar Fracture of the Humerus

A. Cause

Fall on an outstretched hand with hyperextension of the elbow (most common type of elbow fracture in children and adolescents)

B. Treatment

1. Should be managed as an acute emergency because of the danger of neurovascular complications.
2. Minimally displaced fractures—immobilization in a collar and cuff sling.
3. Moderately displaced fractures
   a. Closed reduction under anesthesia.
   b. Immobilization in a long arm cast or collar and cuff sling.

c. Need for Dunlop skin traction for a period of 5–7 days until swelling subsides and a long-arm cast can be applied. Circulation and neural function should be carefully assessed.

4. Severely displaced fractures
   a. Closed reduction under anesthesia.
   b. Skeletal traction with the shoulder abducted 60 degrees and the arm elevated 20 degrees above the horizontal until the fracture is stable. Circulation and neural function should be carefully assessed.
   c. Continued immobilization in a long-arm cast or collar and cuff sling.

C. Healing Time

1. 6–8 weeks
2. Several months may be required for complete restoration of function.

D. Complications

1. Malunion and changes in carrying angle.
2. Vascular complications—the extremity should be observed for pallor, pain, absent pulse, paresthesia, and paralysis.

Fractures of the Distal Third of the Radius and Ulna

A. Cause

1. Fracture may result from indirect force, such as falling on an outstretched hand.
2. Bones may break at different levels, and each fracture may be complete or greenstick.

B. Treatment

1. Greenstick fracture
   a. Closed reduction if the degree of angulation exceeds 30 degrees in infants or 15 degrees in children
   b. Immobilization in a long-arm cast
2. Complete fracture
   a. Reduction under anesthesia
   b. Immobilization in an above-elbow cast

C. Healing Time

4–6 weeks

Fractures Involving the Distal Radial Physis

A. Cause

1. Indirect force by falling on an outstretched hand
2. Most common physical injury

B. Treatment

1. Closed reduction
2. Immobilization in a long-arm cast

C. Healing Time

3–4 weeks

Fractures of the Phalanges

A. Cause

Direct force to the finger

B. Treatment

1. Distal phalanx
   a. Aluminum finger splint
   b. Splinting of adjoining finger
2. Middle phalanx
   a. Manual traction and flexion of the distal fragment

b. Immobilization in a below-elbow plaster cast with a padded aluminum splint
c. Unstable fractures—need for skeletal traction with a pin through the distal phalanx

C. Healing Time

2–5 weeks

Femoral Shaft Fracture

A. Cause

Major force, either direct or indirect, such as that sustained in automobile accidents or falls from a height

B. Treatment

1. Requires treatment as serious injury because of the blood loss and potential shock, which may accompany the primary trauma
2. Infants and children under 2 years of age
   a. Bryant's traction for 2–3 weeks until the fracture is stable
   b. Immobilization in a 1½ hip spica cast until solid union occurs
3. Older children and adolescents
   a. Undisplaced fracture—immobilization in a hip spica cast
   b. Displaced fracture
      (1) Reduction and traction until fracture is stable. Traction type depends on location and manner of displacement—usually Russell, split Russell, or balanced traction with Thomas splint and Pearson attachment.
      (2) Immobilization in a spica cast until bony union is firm.

C. Healing Time

3–12 weeks, depending on the child's age and the type of fracture

D. Complications

1. Discrepancy in extremity length
2. Angular deformities of the femoral shaft

Fracture of the Tibia or Fibula

A. Cause

1. Direct force
2. Indirect rotational twisting force

B. Treatment

1. Closed reduction
2. Immobilization in a long leg cast—during the final weeks of healing, partial weight-bearing in a walking cast may be permitted.
3. Careful evaluation of neurologic and vascular function is imperative.

C. Healing Time

3–6 weeks, depending on the age of the child and the type of fracture

---

Osteomyelitis

Osteomyelitis is an infection that may involve all parts of a bone.

Etiology

1. Pathogenic bacteria commonly associated with osteomyelitis

a. *Staphylococcus aureus*—responsible for the majority of cases (up to 90%)
b. Streptococcal organisms
c. *H. influenzae*
d. Pseudomonas
e. *E. coli*
2. Exogenous osteomyelitis—acquired by direct invasion of the bone by extension from the outside, as from a penetrating wound, fracture, etc.
3. Hematogenous osteomyelitis (more common)—
   a. Caused by hematogenous spread of organisms from another focus
   b. Frequently involves metaphysis of long bones in lower limbs.
4. Identifiable primary infections:
   a. Skin abscesses
   b. Otitis media
   c. Urinary tract infections
   d. Pneumonia
   e. Abscessed teeth
   f. In the infant under 1 year of age—process begins as hematogenous seeding of the metaphysis for the long bone, progression is more rapid, and joint infection often complicates neonatal and infantile osteomyelitis.
5. Preconditions favoring development of osteomyelitis in children
   a. Bone regions that have suffered trauma
   b. Bone that suffers from low oxygen tension of sickle cell anemia

Incidence

1. Most frequent occurrence between 5 and 14 years of age
2. More frequent in males than in females

Altered Physiology

1. Infection starts in the soft, medullary tissues.
2. This causes hyperemia, changes in the capillary permeability, and edema of the tissue.
3. Granulocytic leukocytes infiltrate the area and are destroyed by bacteria, liberating a proteolytic enzyme, which causes tissue necrosis.
4. The inflammatory reaction causes thrombosis of vessels, producing irregular areas of bone ischemia.
5. Pus forms and spreads toward the diaphysis and extends through the cortex of the bone.
6. A subperiosteal abscess is formed with elevation of the periosteum.
7. There is further interference of blood supply to the bone shaft.
   a. Vascular supply may remain sufficient to maintain life of bone tissue:
      (1) New bone is created.
      (2) Bone healing occurs.
   b. Vascular supply may be diminished below that necessary to maintain life of bone tissue:
      (1) Bone dies and becomes inert. Small pieces of dead bone may be completely destroyed by granulation tissue from contiguous living tissue.
      (2) Large pieces of dead bone cannot be completely destroyed.
         (a) Central residual remains as a sequestrum composed of cancellous or cortical bone or a combination.
         (b) New bone is laid down beneath the elevated periosteum and tends to form an

encasement (involucrum) around the sequestrum.

(c) The involucrum is punctured by numerous channels through which pus may escape from the inside.

(d) Pockets of infection are walled off in which organisms can lie dormant for long periods.

(e) Chronic sinuses may form, which eventually reach the surface and drain.

(f) Drainage continues until infection quiets once more.
Channels become plugged with granulations and remain closed until the pressure of the pus builds up and causes the sinuses to reopen or reach the surface via new channels (chronic osteomyelitis).

(g) Complete healing takes place only when all of the dead bone has been destroyed, discharged, or excised.

Clinical Manifestations

A. Onset
1. Usually abrupt
2. May be altered when osteomyelitis follows an infection that has been treated by antimicrobials.

B. Initial Symptoms
1. Pain in the involved area
2. Fever
3. Malaise

C. Later Symptoms
1. Swelling, redness, and warmth over the affected bone
2. Weakness
3. Irritability
4. Generalized signs of sepsis

D. Common Sites of Infection in Children
1. Large, cylindrical bones of the extremities
   a. Femur
   b. Tibia
   c. Humerus
   d. Radius

Diagnostic Evaluation

1. Leukocytosis
2. Blood culture—usually positive
3. Sedimentation rate usually elevated
4. Positive needle aspiration of the bone
5. X-ray data
   a. Progressive findings
      (1) Periosteal reaction
      (2) Areas of radiolucency secondary to bone destruction
      (3) Evidence of the formation of involucrum (reactive, living bone)
   b. Progress of the disease not seen on x-ray for at least 5 days in small children; as long as 8–10 days in older children
6. Bone scans—helpful in documenting the progress of the disease, but may be normal in the early period

Treatment

1. Intravenous administration of antimicrobial therapy—to achieve and maintain therapeutic serum levels for adequate amount of time.

2. Immobilization of the affected extremity
3. Surgical decompression of the infected bony area may be necessary with insertion of drains

Prognosis

1. Mortality rate markedly improved with the advent of modern antimicrobial agents
2. Depends on early institution of appropriate therapy and adequate continuation

Patient Problems and Nursing Diagnoses

1. Altered comfort, pain, related to the infectious process and required intravenous therapy
2. Impaired mobility related to pain and possible traction as part of treatment
3. Potential complication: adverse reaction to long-term antimicrobial therapy
4. Anxiety related to hospitalization and painful procedures
5. Social isolation related to possible isolation technique and long-term hospitalization
6. Parental knowledge deficit about osteomyelitis and its treatment
7. Ineffective family coping, related to feelings of guilt

Nursing Interventions

A. Treating the Infection With Antimicrobial Therapy.
1. Administer intravenous antimicrobials as prescribed by the physician.
   a. Administer medication exactly on schedule in order to maintain consistent blood levels.
   b. Monitor intravenous infusion carefully.
      (1) Notify the appropriate person if infiltration is suspected, so that the IV can be restarted.
      (2) A venous cutdown is often necessary, especially for a small child.
      (3) A constant infusion pump may be helpful if the infusion rate is slow.
      (4) A heparin lock may be useful because it allows the child to be more active between medication doses.
2. Perform irrigations of the infected area with antimicrobial solutions as prescribed by the physician.
3. Be alert for evidence of drug reactions.
4. Consider drug stability and compatability with other intravenous antibiotics when planning schedule for administration.

B. Increasing the Child's Comfort.
1. Administer analgesics as prescribed by the physician.
2. Rest the affected extremity.
   a. Traction or splints may be used to reduce pain and prevent contractures in the soft tissues.
   b. Avoid excessive handling of the infected extremity, because this is very painful and may spread infection.
      (1) Bed linens should be changed only when necessary.
      (2) When it is necessary to move the extremity, support the joints above and below the affected part as well as the area itself.
      (3) Move the extremity in a smooth, unhurried, and gentle manner.

C. Protecting Other Patients and Personnel From the Infectious Organism.
1. Isolate children with draining wounds.
2. Use careful hand-washing procedure.

3. Use strict aseptic technique when performing irrigations, changing dressings, and handling drainage.

D. Facilitating Wound Healing.

Maintain adequate nutrition and hydration.

1. Offer abundant fluids according to the child's preference.
2. Provide a diet rich in protein and vitamin C.
3. Allow the child to participate in selection of foods and preparation of his meal tray.
4. Refer to section on nutrition, p. 1102.

E. Observing for Evidence of Response to Treatment or Progress of Disease.

1. Monitor the child's temperature at frequent intervals and record the pattern. Notify the physician of a sudden increase in temperature.
2. Monitor and record the extent of swelling, redness, pain, and limitation of movement in the affected extremity.
3. Monitor and record the amount and nature of drainage if the infection has been drained.

F. Providing Emotional Support to the Parents.

1. Parents often feel guilty if they did not recognize early signs of the disease.
2. Assist the parents to express and deal with their feelings. Initiate a social service referral if appropriate.
3. See section on family-centered care, p. 1125.

G. Assisting the Child to Maintain Many of His Normal Activities During the Lengthy Hospitalization.

1. Allow the child to be dressed during the convalescent period.
2. Encourage the child to attend playroom activities, even if he must be moved in his bed.
3. Initiate plans for the child's continuing education, and provide time each day for his school work.
4. Encourage liberal visiting by family and friends.

H. Providing for Continuity of Care Following the Child's Discharge From the Hospital.

1. Encourage parents to participate in all aspects of the child's care during hospitalization.
   a. Parents should be instructed and should have an opportunity to practice (under nursing supervision) all procedures that will be required at home. (Procedures often include changes of dressing, application of a splint, or use of appliances such as crutches.)
   b. The child should not be discharged until both the parents and the nurse are satisfied with the parents' level of competency.
2. Instruct the parents to observe for evidence of complications, such as deformity, stiffness of joints, fracture, and disease recurrence.
3. Initiate a community health nursing referral if appropriate.

Expected Outcomes

1. Takes analgesics, rests extremity to relieve pain
2. Regains mobility function gradually
3. Adheres to drug therapy with no signs of adverse reaction to the drugs
4. Behaves in a less anxious manner
5. Participates in age-appropriate diversional and educational activities
6. Parents express an understanding of osteomyelitis and its treatment

7. Parents work out their guilt over the child's condition by talking about their feelings and realizing that they did not cause the problem

Congenital Dislocation of the Hip

Congenital dislocation of the hip refers to a malposition of the head of the femur in the acetabulum. The head of the femur is usually dislocated posterosuperiorly. Dislocation may be either partial or complete and may be either unilateral or bilateral.

Etiology

1. Unknown
2. Possible causes
   a. Abnormal development of the joint caused by:
      (1) Fetal position
      (2) Genetic factors
   b. Abnormal relaxation of the capsule and ligaments of the joint caused by hormonal factors
   c. Environmental factors such as breech delivery

Incidence

1. More common in female infants than in males.
2. Recurrence risk among siblings is greater when one child in the family has been affected.

Altered Physiology

1. Acetabulum tends to be shallow and extremely oblique.
2. Head of the femur tends to be smaller than normal.
3. Ossification centers are delayed in appearance.
4. Classification
   a. Dysplasia—shallow acetabulum, acetabular roof slants upward
   b. Sublaxation—acetabular surface of femoral head in contact with shallow dysplasic acetabular surface, but head slides laterally and superiorly
   c. Dislocation—articular cartilage of completely displaced femoral head does not contact acetabular articular cartilage

Clinical Manifestations *(Fig. 59-1)*

(May not be observed until 1–2 months of age)
1. Asymmetry of the gluteal folds with deeper creases apparent on the affected side.
2. Limited ability to abduct the hip when the infant is lying on his back with his knees and hips flexed to 90 degrees. Normally, the hips will abduct at least 65 degrees.
3. Trendelenburg's sign—pelvis drops on the normal side if the child stands on his abnormal leg.
4. Leg length inequality with unilateral complete dislocation.
5. Delayed walking
6. Limp
   a. Trunk dips when the child puts weight on his involved leg.
   b. Waddling gait is observed in children with bilateral dislocation.

Diagnostic Evaluation

1. *Barlow's maneuver*—performed first 6 months of age
   a. With the infant on a firm surface, the examiner grasps the symphysis pubis in front and the sacrum

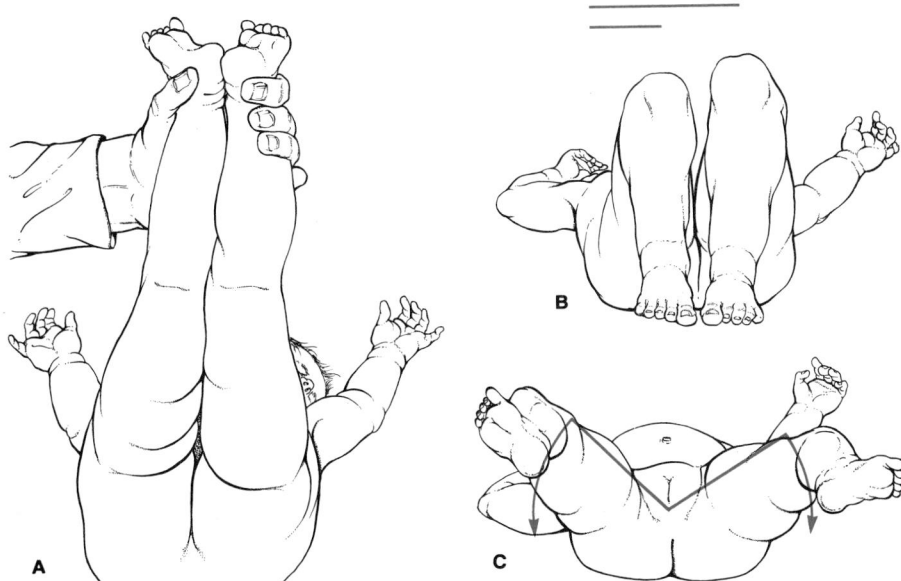

Figure 59-1. *Possible signs of congenital hip dislocation. (A) Asymmetry of thigh folds with extra fold noted on abnormal side. (B) Unequal leg lengths. (C) Limited hip abduction.*

in back with one hand. The second hand grasps the thigh on the side of the hip being tested.

  b. Slight outward pressure is applied over the proximal thigh by the thumb while longitudinal pressure is applied in an effort to dislocate the hip out of its socket.

  c. Sensation of abnormal movement indicates a dislocation.

2. *Ortolani's maneuver*

  a. The examiner positions his hands in the same manner as for Barlow's maneuver.

  b. The thigh is brought away from the midline of the body into a position of abduction.

  c. A sensation or sound of a clicking or jerking into place may be detected with reduction of the head into the socket.

3. X-ray data (helpful only after the age of 4–5 months, when the hip bones are sufficiently developed).

  a. Acetabular angle greater than 40 degrees

  b. Upward and outward displacement of the femoral head.

4. Ultrasonic examination

Treatment

Goal:

To restore as closely as possible anatomic alignment of hip while maintaining pain-free function. Early recognition is the key to successful treatment.

1. Varies with age and extent of the defect

2. Early stages (Birth–3 months)

  a. Reduction by gentle manipulation

  b. Splinting the hip in abduction by means of double or triple diapers, an abduction splint, or pillow or cloth harness, usually for 2–4 months continual and 2–6 months at night

3. Later stages (3–18 months)

  a. Preliminary traction

  b. Closed reduction

  c. Immobilization in a hip spica cast or splint or Pavlik harness (Fig. 59-2)

4. Older child (18 months–4 years)

  a. Preliminary traction

  b. Possible need for open reduction or osteotomy

  c. Immobilization in a hip spica cast

Prognosis

1. Depends on the age of the child when the condition is diagnosed.

2. Hips reduced up to 6 months of age have 98% success rate.

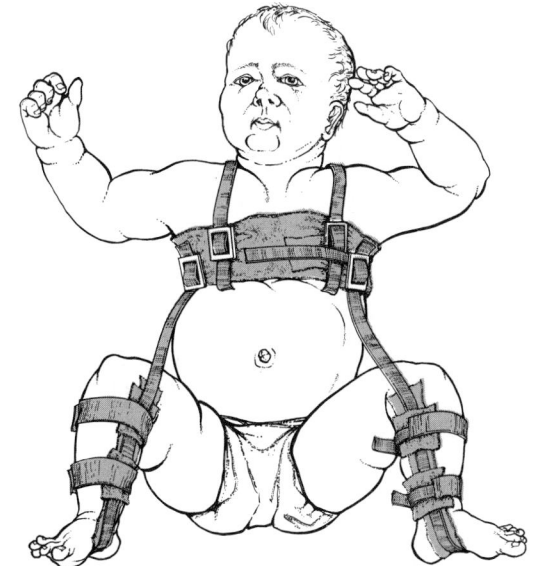

Figure 59-2. *Pavlik harness used in treating hip instability and dislocation in infant.*

3. After 1 year of age, some radiologic evidence of joint incongruity, which may lead to osteoarthritis in later life.
4. Delay in diagnosis prolongs treatment and may preclude formation of a normal hip.

Complications

Avascular necrosis of femoral head resulting from excessive abduction blocking perfusion to femoral head.

Nursing Interventions

Generally, nursing care of the child with congenital dislocation of the hip is provided at home. Nursing activities during hospitalization are those related to the child's care when he is in traction or after application of a hip spica cast (see p. 1214).

Health Education

1. If the child is to be treated with an abduction splint, explain its purpose and demonstrate its application to the parents.
   a. Allow the parents to practice application of the splint with nursing supervision.
   b. Clarify with parents the times that the splint is to be worn and if it can be removed for bathing, dressing, diaper changes, etc.
   c. Demonstrate handling of the child in such a way that the hips are kept abducted.

Congenital Clubfoot
(Talipes Equinovarus)

Congenital clubfoot refers to a deformity in which the affected foot and leg have a club-like appearance. Talipes equinovarus is one of the most common congenital deformities of the foot, occurring in approximately one in 1000 live births.

Etiology

1. Exact cause unknown.
2. Evidence indicates a mixed genetic and environmental causation.
3. Tends to recur in families already having 1 affected child.
4. Males are affected twice as often as females.

Altered Physiology

1. Pathologic anatomy
   a. Plantar flexion, adduction of the forepart of the foot
   b. Inversion of the heel
2. Soft tissue changes are adaptive in nature, conforming to the skeletal deformity. The soft tissues on the medial and posterior aspect of the foot and ankle are shortened.
3. Foot is often smaller in size

Clinical Manifestations

1. Varies in severity from a mild deformity to one in which the toes touch the medial side of the lower leg.
   a. Rigid type
      (1) Very severe deformity

(2) Corrected only minimally by passive manipulation
(3) Usually accompanied by moderate atrophy of the leg
   b. Flexible type—the condition can be readily corrected to neutral position by passive manipulation
2. Deformity increases progressively, and contractures become more rigid if the deformity is untreated.
   a. Child bears weight on the lateral border of the foot.
   b. Ambulation is difficult and gait is awkward.
   c. Callosities and bursae may develop over the lateral side of the foot.

Diagnostic Evaluation

1. Diagnosis is determined by clinical manifestations.
2. X-ray valuable for the following:
   a. Determination of the degree of varus and equinus deformity
   b. Demonstration of the deranged mechanics of the hindfoot
   c. Accurate assessment of the amount of correction obtained with treatment

Treatment

1. Manipulation of the foot into normal position, with or without serial casting.
2. Maintenance of correction until normal muscle balance is regained.
3. Surgical procedures may be necessary for some children.

Nursing Interventions

A. Manipulating Foot Into Normal Position.

1. Passive stretching exercises
   a. Technique of manipulation should be demonstrated to the nurse and parents by the physician, because there are many variations in the manner of performing the manipulation.
   b. Manipulation should be done before feedings, because it may cause some discomfort for the baby.
2. Manipulation and casting
   a. A plaster of paris cast is applied from the toes to the groin with the knee flexed. Casts are changed frequently; with each cast change, the foot is manipulated to obtain further correction.
   b. Once the deformity is fully corrected, the foot is held in an overcorrected position in a solid cast for 3–6 weeks.
      (1) The parents should be instructed in cast care (see p. 1213).
      (2) The parents should be alerted that if the foot portion of the cast becomes thin or worn, the cast should be reapplied.
      (3) The parents can be taught to soak off old casts prior to clinic visits by immersing the cast in a solution of 1 part vinegar to 4 parts water and then unwrapping the plaster.
3. Denis Browne splint
   a. The splint is composed of a flexible horizontal bar attached to a pair of footplates.
      (1) The infant's feet are attached to the footplates by means of special shoes or adhesive tape.
      (2) The desired position of the foot is controlled by positioning the abduction bar and the footplates.

(3) The infant provides his own corrective manipulation by his normal activity.
  b. Parents should be instructed in the following details of care:
    (1) Application and removal of the splint
    (2) Times the splint is to be worn
    (3) Protection of the feet by socks
    (4) Skin care
    (5) Use of splint key to tighten the shoes against the bar if they become loose
  4. Continued treatment
    a. Treatment is continued until the child is able to walk normally and until the wear on several pairs of shoes demonstrates that there has been no recurrence of deformity.
    b. Foot is held in an overcorrected position at night by means of bivalved casts or a Denis Browne splint.
    c. A prewalker clubfoot shoe with valgus strap may be prescribed for the infant's use during the day.
    d. An older child may require special shoes that promote walking in the overcorrected position.
    e. Passive stretching exercises are continued.
  5. Indications for surgical measures
    a. Failure of conservative methods to correct the deformity
    b. In older children, severe and rigid deformities that obviously will not respond to nonsurgical measures

B. Helping Family Understand the Terminology of Their Infant's Condition, Implications of the Treatment Regimen, and Potential Difficulties They may Encounter in Caring for Infant During Treatment.

The family needs to understand that the feet may never be normal, even with treatment, but that function may be restored to nearly normal.

Legg–Calvé–Perthes Disease
(Coxa Plana)

Legg–Calvé–Perthes disease is an aseptic necrosis of the capital femoral epiphysis secondary to ischemia to femoral head.

Etiology

Unknown

Incidence

1. Males between the ages of 4 and 10 years of age are most frequently affected.
2. Condition tends to recur in families.
3. White children are affected 10 times more frequently than black children.

Altered Physiology

The femoral head deformity occurs as a result of growth disturbance in the thickened articular cartilage and repaired fibrocartilage formed as result of the removal of crushed avascular trabeculae.

A. Stage I (Avascularity)

1. Spontaneous interruption of the blood supply to the upper femoral epiphysis occurs.

2. Bone-forming cells in the epiphysis die and bone ceases to grow.
3. Slight widening of the joint space occurs.
4. Swelling of the soft tissues around the hip occurs.

B. Stage II (Revascularization)

1. Growth of new vessels supplies the area of necrosis; both bone resorption and deposition take place.
2. The new bone is not strong, and pathologic fractures may occur.
3. Abnormal forces on the weakened epiphysis may produce progressive deformity.

C. Stage III (Reossification)

1. The head of the femur gradually reforms.
2. Nucleus of the epiphysis breaks up into a number of fragments with cyst-like spaces between them.
3. New bone starts to develop at the medial and lateral edges of the epiphysis, which becomes widened.
4. Dead bone is removed and is replaced with new bone, which gradually spreads to heal the lesion.

D. Stage IV (Postrecovery Period)

1. Without treatment
   a. Head of the femur flattens and becomes mushroom-shaped.
   b. Incongruity between the head of the femur and the acetabulum persists.
   c. Degenerative changes develop later in life.
2. Complete recovery
   a. Head of the femur remains spherical.
   b. Acetabulum appears normal.
   c. Width of the neck of the femur is normal.

Clinical Manifestations

(May be intermittent initially)
1. Synovitis causing limp and pain in the hip.
2. Referred pain to the knee, inner thigh, and groin
3. Limited abduction and internal rotation of the hip
4. Mild to moderate muscle spasm

Diagnostic Evaluation

1. X-ray findings are related to the stage of the disease, and may be normal early after its onset.
2. Bone scans—helpful in identifying those patients with extensive epiphyseal infarction early in the course of the disease.

Treatment

(Depends on type of involvement)
1. First goal—to restore full range of motion of the hip joint by alleviating synovitis and muscle spasm. Bed rest with or without traction.
2. Second goal—to locate the femoral head deep in the acetabulum, thereby protecting it while revascularization and growth occur.
   a. Non–weight-bearing abduction cast or brace.
   b. Weight-bearing abduction casts or braces, Atlantic Scottish Rite Hospital orthosis, may be used once full range of motion has been restored, except in older children with major femoral head involvement.
   c. Femoral osteotomy—indicated in cases of severe involvement of the femoral head.
3. Final goal—return to unassisted weight-bearing.
   a. Unassisted weight-bearing can be resumed once the increased density in the femoral head disappears, usually 6–15 months.

b. The child's time out of the brace is gradually increased, and his hip motion is evaluated frequently. Loss of motion is an indication that a longer period of bracing is necessary.

Prognosis

1. Appears to be directly related to the initial extent of femoral head involvement and age at time of healing.
2. Influenced by the stage at which the disease was diagnosed and treatment was instituted.
3. Limitation of motion and incongruity of joint surfaces may result if treatment is ineffective; condition may lead to degenerative joint disease in later life.
4. 60% of the cases will do well without treatment.

Nursing Interventions

A. Caring for the Child Requiring Traction or a Spica Cast.

See procedures, pages 1204 and 1214.

B. Evaluating the Home and Providing Guidance to the Family Regarding the Child's Home Care.

1. This guidance is important, because treatment may be continued in the home for an extended period.
2. Encourage family participation in the child's care so that members can become familiar with the details of his management (see section on family-centered care, p. 1125).
3. Appropriate referrals may include the following:
   a. Community health nurse
   b. Social service
   c. Home teacher
   d. Physical therapy
   e. Occupational therapy

C. Enabling the Child to Participate in as Many Normal Activities of Life as Possible.

1. Plans must be made for continuing education.
2. Diversion is an extremely important consideration.
3. Play should include exercise for uninvolved extremities.
4. Special activities with peers should be arranged.

D. Providing Emotional Support to the Child and His Family Because of the Long-Term Nature of the Illness.

1. Provide the family with frequent opportunities to express their feelings and concerns.
   Techniques of therapeutic play should be used with the child.
2. Point out even small indications of the recovery process.
3. Introduce the family to other families with similarly affected children, if possible.

Health Education

1. General techniques of home nursing
   a. Bathing and skin care
   b. Maintenance of good muscle tone, proper body alignment, and prevention of contractures
   c. Provision for elimination
   d. Nutritional considerations
   e. Bedmaking
   f. Special equipment (e.g., traction, casts)
2. Pathology of the disease and rationale of treatment
   a. Reinforce medical explanations and clarify interpretations as necessary.
   b. Allow the child to view his own x-rays with his parents, to increase his knowledge of the disease.

c. Emphasize that complete recovery can occur only with strict adherence to the treatment regimen.
3. Necessity of regular medical follow-up for evaluation of the child's progress.

Structural Scoliosis

Structural scoliosis is a lateral curvature of the spine of 10% or greater characterized by a defect in the bones and surrounding tissues of the spine.

Etiology

1. Idiopathic
   a. Accounts for 80% of cases
   b. Possible familial incidence
2. Congenital
   a. Failure of vertebral formation
   b. Failure of segmentation
3. Neuropathic—results from conditions such as poliomyelitis, cerebral palsy, paralysis, and neurofibromatosis
4. Myopathic—associated with conditions such as muscular dystrophy and myopathies
5. Osteopathic—results from conditions such as fractures, bone disease, arthritis, and infection
6. Trauma such as fractures, burns, thoracoplasty
7. Irritative phenomena such as spinal cord tumor or nerve root irritation
8. Miscellaneous—Marfan's syndrome, postirradiation, metabolic, nutritional, or endocrinic factors

Classification— *Idiopathic*

1. According to the spinal segment involved
   a. Thoracic
   b. Lumbar
   c. Thoracolumbar
2. According to age-group
   a. Infantile—birth-3 years—uncommon in the United States
   b. Juvenile—after 3 years of age, before puberty; boys outnumber girls with juvenile onset
   c. Adolescent—10 years to cessation of growth (usually found in females, with a right thoracic curve most common)

Represents 85%-90% of all cases of idiopathic scoliosis.

Altered Physiology

1. Lateral flexion of a scoliotic spine causes the trunk to shift away from the midline, altering the center of gravity and causing shortening of the spine.
2. Simultaneously, the spine rotates on its longitudinal axis, contributing to many of the clinical manifestations.
3. The vertebrae become permanently wedge-shaped.
4. The scoliosis is increased by additional factors:
   a. The weight of the trunk itself.
   b. The muscles on the concave side, being contracted, have a mechanical advantage over the lengthened muscles on the convex side.
   c. Disturbed forces on active growing vertebral elements bring about structural changes in the bone.
5. Changes occur in the shape of the rib cage.
   a. The thoracic cavity narrows.
   b. The ribs do not move in a plane that allows normal expansion of the lungs.

6. Untreated scoliosis may cause back pain, degenerative arthritis, and disturbances in cardiopulmonary function in later life.

   Psychogenic problems may be seen relating to body image and result in social problems.

Clinical Manifestations

1. Presenting complaints (see Pediatric Physical Examination, p. 1054)
   a. Poor posture
   b. One shoulder higher than the other
   c. Hemline hanging unevenly
   d. One hip that seems more prominent
   e. Crooked neck
   f. Lump on back
   g. Waistline uneven
   h. One breast appearing larger
2. Visualization of deformity
3. Back pain

Diagnostic Evaluation

1. Detailed history from patient, parent, and other family members
2. Thorough examination of the back with patient first in the forward bent position and then standing erect
3. Assessment of the neurologic status of the lower extremities
4. Inclusion of clinical photographs in the record for future reference
5. X-rays of the spine to identify and measure primary and compensating curves
6. Pulmonary function studies for children who require surgery to predict risk of postoperative respiratory complications
7. Intravenous pyelography for children with congenital scoliosis because of a high evidence of associated renal anomalies

Treatment

Goal:

To enable child to enter adult life with a balanced and stable spine, maximum flexibility, and acceptable residual deformity with the lowest possible morbidity.*

---

* From Scoles P. Pediatric Orthopedics in Clinical Practice. 1988, p 198.

A. Brace Management

1. Most effective for thoracic, thoracolumbar, and lumbar curves of less than 30–40 degrees, but greater than 20%, that are not associated with extreme deformity.
2. Goal is to prevent progression of the curve.
3. Brace programs usually last 4–6 years and require faithful compliance.
4. Types of braces (Figs. 59-3 and 59-4)
   a. Milwaukee brace—for thoracic curves or double major curves
   b. Cervical-thoraco-lumbo-sacral orthosis (CTLSO) —or thoraco-lumbar-sacral curve (TLSO)
   c. Boston brace—thoracic or thoracolumbar
   d. Wilmington plastic jacket
5. Recommended wearing time
   a. 23 hours a day
   b. Part-time—16 hours a day and no wearing during school for curvature < 35 degrees
6. Success is somewhat dependent on a cooperative patient who understands the need for orthosis and will comply with the regimen.

B. Surgery

1. Stabilization is the goal of surgery
   a. Strengthen spine within safe limits of neurologic toleration
   b. Balance spine over pelvis
   c. Stabilize spine in this position via bony fusion
2. Indications:
   a. Curve is too severe to be braced
   b. Progression occurs despite bracing, usually angle > 60%
   c. Brace management is not feasible
3. Preoperative casting or traction may be employed to increase curve flexibility prior to surgery
4. Types of surgery
   a. Harrington instrumentation and posterior spinal fusion
   b. Dwyer instrumentation and anterior spinal fusion
5. A protective cast is ordinarily required for 6 months–1 year following spinal fusion

C. Electrical Stimulation—via cutaneous electrodes over convexity of curvature.

1. Intermittant pulsations cause contractions of paraspinal musculature, especially curve between midthoracic and midlumbar.
2. Used only during periods while sleeping.

D. Exercise Program (controversial)—program to maintain flexibility of spine as well as to prevent para-

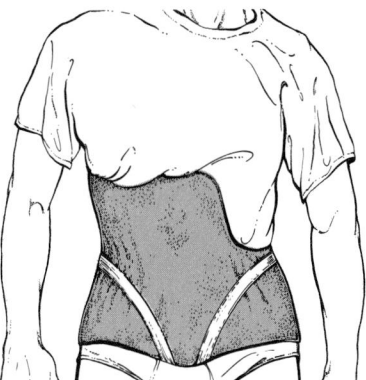

Figure 59-3. *Body brace. A short body brace may be used for small curves.*

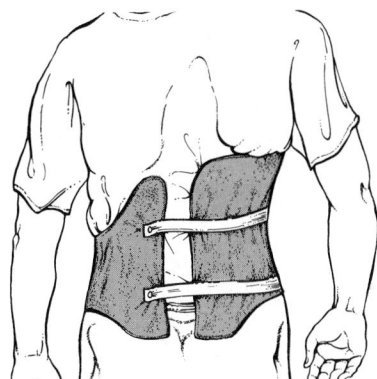

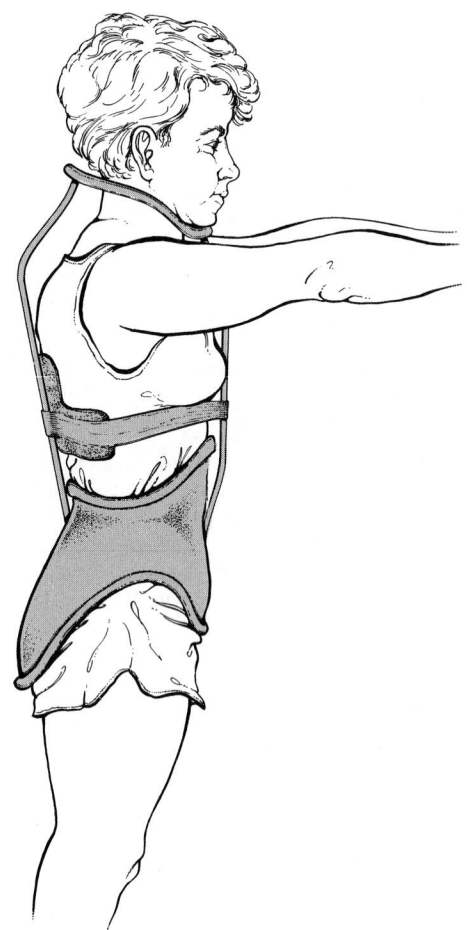

Figure 59-4. *Milwaukee brace: Used for upper thoracic curves.*

spinal muscle atrophy secondary to immobilizing effect of bracing (Fig. 59-5).

Prognosis

Best when curve is mild at the time of initial diagnosis and effective treatment is initiated early.

Complications

1. Decrease in vital lung capacity—with angle > 60%
2. Pulmonary hypertension—with angle > 80%
3. Back pain, chronic fatigue, spinal nerve root impingement

Patient Problems and Nursing Diagnoses

1. Self concept, disturbance in body image, related to the appearance of the deformity and/or immobilization in unattractive devices
2. Altered comfort, pain, related to the extent of the defect and/or surgery
3. Impaired skin integrity related to pressure from braces, traction, or casts
4. Potential serious postoperative complications: neurologic impairment, shock, infection, urinary retention, paralytic ileus

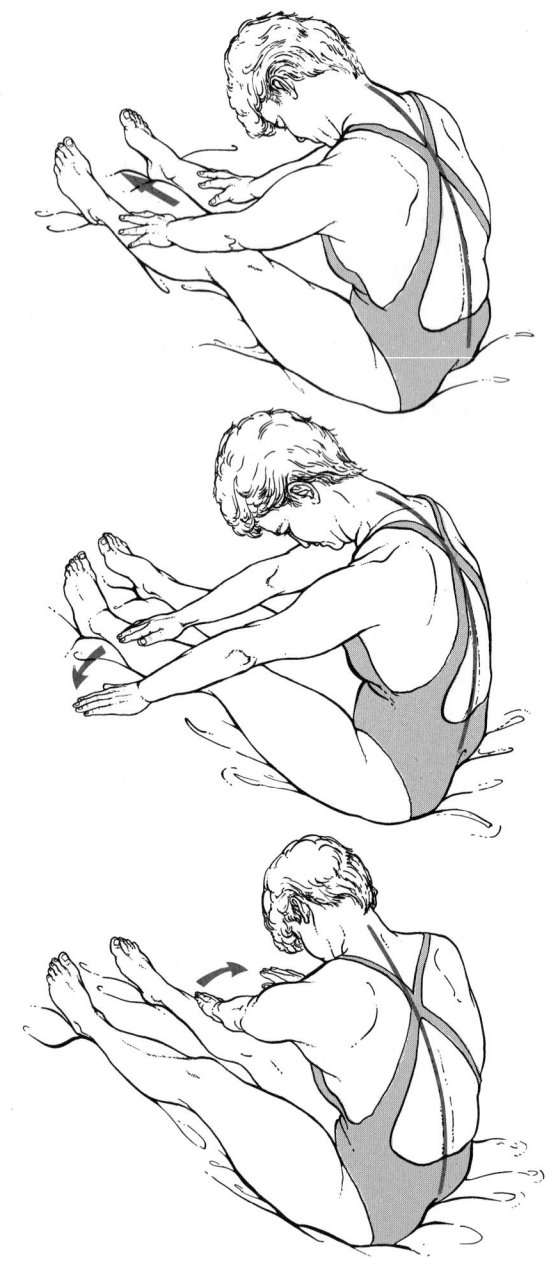

Figure 59-5. *Exercises for scoliosis.*

5. Anxiety related to hospitalization and surgery
6. Mobility impaired, related to brace
7. Social isolation and ineffective coping related to hospitalization and immobilization
8. Knowledge deficit regarding scoliosis and its management

Nursing Interventions

A. Caring for the Child Who Is Using a Brace.

1. Educate the child and parents concerning the brace and supplemental exercise program.

a. Clarify goals of therapy with the family.

b. Offer incentives for compliance with the recommended treatment program.

2. Prevent break in tissue integrity.

   a. Provide meticulous skin care to areas in contact with the brace.

   b. Use a smooth-fitting undershirt or stockinette under the brace to protect the skin.

   c. Examine skin surfaces for evidence of pressure areas.

   d. Have brace adjusted if skin breakdown occurs because of improper fit.

3. Assist the child and family to modify normal activities such as bathing and dressing to accommodate the brace.

   a. Clothing must be loose or must be purchased in larger sizes to fit over the outside of the appliance.

   b. Underpants should be worn over the brace to facilitate toileting.

4. Initial period associated with stress from soreness, skin irritation, uncertainty about fit, difficulty in breathing and eating, torn clothing and bed linens, discomfort while seated or during activity.

5. The child may experience emotional lability, anxiety, fear, isolation, and depression.

   a. Help child talk about these fears

   b. Assist child adapting to the brace-wearing

6. Encourage family and child to establish daily routines, as this facilitates coping with the bracewear.

7. Encourage child to be as active as possible

   a. Swimming, tennis, band, cheerleading are acceptable activities.

   b. Contact sports, trampoline are to be avoided.

B. Preparing the Child for Surgical Correction (spinal fusion).

1. Explain to the child and his parents the nature of the care immediately before surgery, the anesthesia, postoperative care, and appearance.

2. Introduce the child and his parents to a nurse from the intensive care unit if the child will be transferred there postoperatively.

3. Have the child practice aspects of the anticipated therapy, such as deep-breathing and other respiratory routines, leg exercises, logrolling, use of the Stryker frame or CircOlectric bed, and use of the fracture bedpan.

C. Providing Postoperative Care to the Child Following Spinal Fusion.

1. Observe for signs of hypotension.

   a. Monitor fluid balance.

   b. Maintain blood pressure at desired level; report changes.

2. Observe wound for bleeding, hematoma, or infection.

   a. Maintain aseptic technique when caring for the wound.

   b. Report any redness, swelling, drainage, or heat in the incisional area.

3. Relieve pain.

   a. Identify causes of pain through discussion with the child and through observation.

   b. Administer analgesic therapy as prescribed by the physician.

4. Maintain tissue integrity.

   a. Turn the child as prescribed (usually by logrolling at 2-hour intervals).

   b. Provide skin care with each turning maneuver.

   c. Use sheepskin under pressure areas.

5. Prevent respiratory complications—use breathing exercises, blow bottles, and/or intermittent positive pressure to increase respiratory exchange.

6. Observe for neurologic deficits.

   Assess neurologic status each tour of duty, including dorsiflexion, mobility of legs, perineal sensation, and bladder function.

7. Observe for evidence of urinary retention, which may develop as an effect of anesthesia, neurologic trauma, hypovolemia, or drugs.

   a. Maintain careful record of intake and output.

   b. Notify the physician if the child does not void within 8 hours following surgery.

   c. Care for the urethral catheter if present (see procedure, p. 665).

8. Observe for signs of paralytic ileus.

   Note hypoactive and hyperactive bowel sounds, nausea, vomiting, or abdominal pain as diet is gradually increased.

9. Prevent development of thrombophlebitis.

   a. Have the patient do leg exercises.

   b. Apply elastic stockings.

   c. Observe for leg swelling, redness, or pain on dorsiflexion; also note chest symptoms such as dyspnea, chest pain, or hemoptysis.

10. Prevent displacement of the rod or hook.

    a. Do not lift the child under the axillae.

    b. Use a turning sheet.

    c. Instruct the child not to lift hands over head.

11. Maintain adequate nutrition and hydration.

    a. Be aware of normal requirements for size and age.

    b. Evaluate nutritional value of diet and provide appropriate supplements.

12. Provide a safe environment for the patient.

    a. Place the bed so that it is not easily jolted.

    b. Be certain that all equipment is in good working order and that personnel are instructed in its use.

D. Caring for the Child Following Application of a Jacket Cast.

1. Stay with the child during the casting procedure to provide emotional support because of the unfamiliar, frightening, and embarrassing nature of the experience.

2. Observe for evidence of compromised circulation. Report changes in color, sensation, temperature of extremities, respiratory compromise, or abdominal distress.

3. Prevent potential trauma.

   a. Help the child to accept the realities of activity limitation by providing safe alternatives.

   b. Facilitate the child's getting in and out of bed by use of a hospital bed.

   c. Teach the child safe methods of becoming mobile.

4. Instruct the child/parents about how to arrange for cast changes as required either by growth of the child or by soiling of the cast.

5. For additional information related to cast care, see the section on casts, page 1213.

E. Providing Emotional Support for the Child.

1. Allow the child to continue as many of his normal activities as possible.

   a. Continue schooling.

   b. Encourage peer visiting or telephone contact.

2. Provide diversional activities.

   a. Assess the child's interests and provide things that he can do within the limits of his position.

b. Use prism glasses, mirrors, bedboards, and easels.
c. Bring others into the child's room and transport the child in his bed to the recreation room as soon as his condition allows.
d. Establish schedules and make each day meaningful.

3. Be sensitive to the child's concerns about body image and intervene appropriately.
   a. Many adolescent girls express concerns that the cast will prevent growth or change the shape of their breasts, or that menstruation will temporarily cease while they are in the cast.
   b. Children may feel vulnerable because of the restrictions imposed by casts or traction.
4. Provide as much privacy as possible, especially during bathing, toileting, and cast changing.
5. Refer to section on the hospitalized adolescent, page 1124.

Health Education

1. Have the child and family practice cast care during hospitalization.
2. Demonstrate techniques of personal hygiene, including matters such as special skin care and hair shampooing.
3. Assist the child to develop an exercise program within his limitations but adequate to maintain tonicity.
4. Provide dietary instructions, including basic nutritional needs for age and modifications necessary because of immobilization.
5. Provide assistive devices to facilitate physical care needs.
6. Arrange for home equipment with available services.
7. Provide continuity by referral to appropriate community agencies.

8. Arrange for transportation and/or social service assistance if needed.
9. Act as a liaison between the child and his school to encourage the school nurse to supervise patient compliance after the return to school and provide support for the child with adjustment problems.
10. References for patients and parents:
    Brower E. Children Should Be Seen . . . A Handbook for Teachers. University Youth Spine Center, 2074 Abington Road, Cleveland, OH 44106
    Scoliosis—A Handbook for Patients. Scoliosis Research Society, 444 N Michigan, Suite 1500, Chicago, IL 60611
    Schatzinger L. What if You Need An Operation for Scoliosis and Brace Yourself—Scoliosis and the Milwaukee Brace. University Youth Spine Center, 2074 Abington Road, Cleveland, OH 44106

Expected Outcomes

1. Maintains a positive body image, evidenced by verbal and nonverbal communication
2. Experiences relief of pain
3. Maintains skin integrity; wears undershirt under brace; adjusts brace when necessary
4. Recovers from surgery with no complications; vital signs within normal limits; moves extremities; incision healing
5. Appears less anxious about condition; discusses concerns about outcome
6. Engages in diversional activities and interacts with family and friends
7. Adjusts to immobilization; learns to use trapeze to turn, etc.; exercises within limits of enforced bedrest
8. The parents learn about cast care, special hygienic measures for skin care and washing hair, exercise, diet, assistive home equipment, and transportation needs.

Bibliography

Books

Chung SM. Handbook of Pediatric Orthopedics. New York, Van Nostrand Reinhold, 1986

Gillis SS and Kagan BM. Current Pediatric Therapy 12. Philadelphia, WB Saunders, 1986

Lovell WW and Winter RB. Pediatric Orthopaedics. 2nd ed. Philadelphia, JB Lippincott, 1986

Moe JH and Byrd JA. Idiopathic Scoliosis In Bradford DS et al (eds). Moe's Textbook of Scoliosis and Other Spinal Deformities. 2nd ed, pp 191–202. Philadelphia, WB Saunders, 1980

Rang M. Children's Fractures. 2nd ed. New York, Grune & Stratton, 1982

Renshaw TS. Pediatric Orthopedics. Philadelphia, WB Saunders, 1986

Scoles P. Pediatric Orthopedics in Clinical Practice. Chicago, Year Book Medical Pub 1988

Whaley L and Wong D. Nursing Care of Infants and Children. 2nd ed. St. Louis, CV Mosby, 1987

Journals

Asher MA. Scoliosis evaluation. Orthop Clin North Am 1988 Oct; 19(4):805–814

DeRosa GP and Fuller N. Treatment of congenital dislocation of the hip. Clin Orthop 1987 Dec; 225:77–85

Exner GU. Ultrasound screening for hip dysplasia in neonates. J Pediatr Orthop 1988 Nov–Dec; 8(6):656–660

Gentry LO. Home management of osteomyelitis. Bull NY Acad Med 1988 Jul–Aug; 64(6):565–569

Hadlow V. Neonatal screening for congenital dislocation of the hip. J Bone Joint Surg 1988 Nov; 70(5):740–743

Heikkila E. Comparison of the Frejka pillow and the Von Rosen splint in treatment of congenital dislocation of the hip. J Pediatr Orthop 1988 Jan–Feb; 8(1):20–21

Hensinger RN. Congenital dislocation of the hip. Orthop Clin North Am 1987 Oct; 18(4):597–616

Kehl DK and Morrissy RT. Brace treatment in adolescent idiopathic scoliosis. Clin Orthop 1988 Apr; 229: 34–43

Killam PE. Orthopedic assessment of young children: Developmental variations. Nurs Pract 1989 Jul; 14(7): 27–28+

Klisic P, Jankovic L and Basara V. Long-term results of combined operative reduction of the hip of older children. J Pediatr Orthop 1988 Sep–Oct; 8(5): 532–534

Koop SE. Infantile and juvenile ideopathic scoliosis. Orthop Clin North Am 1988 Apr; 19(2):331–337

Lieber MT and Taub AS. Common foot deformities and what they mean for parents. MCN 1988 Jan–Feb; 13(1):47–50

Lonstein JE and Winter RB. Adolescent idiopathic scoliosis: Nonoperative treatment. Orthop Clin North Am 1988 Apr; 19(2):239–246

MacEwen GD and Mason B. Evaluation and treatment of congenital dislocation of the hip. Orthop Clin North Am 1988 Oct; 19(4):815–820

MacLean WE et al. Stress and coping with scoliosis: Psychological effects on adolescents and their families. J Pediatr Orthop 1989 May–Jun; 9(3): 257–261

Miranda L et al. Prevention of congenital dislocation of the hip in the newborn. J Pediatr Orthop 1988 Nov–Dec; 8(6): 671–673

Perkins MD et al. Neonatal group B streptococcal osteomyelitis and suppurative arthritis. Clin Pediatr 1989 May; 28(5):229–230

Renshaw TS. Screening school children for scoliosis. Clin Orthop 1988 Apr; 229:26–33

Swagman A. Caring for limb-deficient children and their families. MCN 1986 Jan–Feb; 11(1):46–52

Szoke N, Kuhl L and Heinrichs J. Ultrasound examination of the diagnosis of congenital hip dysplasia of newborn. J Pediatr Orthop 1988 Jan–Feb; 8(1):12–16

Thompson GM and Salter RB. Legg–Calvé–Perthes disease. Orthop Clin North Am 1987 Oct; 18(4):617–635

Wise LB. A comparison of orthopedic casts: Breaking the mold. MCN 1986 May–Jun; 11(3):174–176

Additional Reading for Staff and Parents

Catterall A. Legg–Calvé–Perthes' Disease. London, Churchill Livingstone, 1982

Lonstein JE. Natural history and school screening for scoliosis. Orthop Clin North Am 1988 Apr; 19(2):227–237

Scoliosis: A handbook for patients. Scoliosis Research Society, 430 North Michigan Ave, Chicago, IL, 60611

Wojtys EM. Spots injuries in the immature athlete. Orthop Clin North Am 1987 Oct; 18(4):689–708

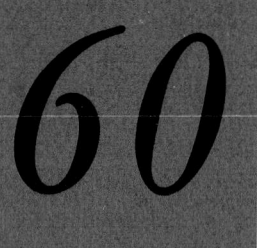

Pediatric Oncology

General Considerations

Incidence

1. Cancer is the leading cause of death from disease in children from 1–14 years of age.
2. Cancer affects approximately 10 per 100,000 children annually in the U.S.
3. The incidence of specific cancers is related to sex, age, and ethnic backgrounds.

Types

A. **Common Types of Cancer in Children** (in Order of Frequency)

1. Leukemia
2. Cancer of the central nervous system
3. Lymphoma
4. Neuroblastoma
5. Rhabdomyosarcoma
6. Wilms' tumor
7. Bone tumor
8. Retinoblastoma

Warning Signals of Cancer in Children

1. Chronic drainage from the ear
2. Recurrent fever with bone pain
3. Morning headache with vomiting
4. Presence of swelling, lump, or mass anywhere in the body
5. White dot in the eye
6. Any change in the size or appearance of moles or birthmarks
7. Unexplained stumbling in the child
8. Limping
9. Generally run-down condition
10. Paleness and fatigue
11. Unexplained pain or persistent crying of an infant or child
12. Bone pain
13. Weight loss
14. Bruising, petechiae

Treatment Modalities*

A. **Surgery**

B. **Radiation Therapy**

Nursing considerations:
1. Prepare the child and his family for the procedure.
2. Do not wash off any marks placed by the radiologist to indicate the area to be treated.
3. Initiate comfort and support measures when the child demonstrates any side effects of treatment.
   a. General malaise and headache
   b. Nausea and vomiting
   c. Diarrhea
   d. Anorexia
   e. Skin irritation and breakdown
   f. Lethargy
4. See the adult text, section on radiation in diagnosis and therapy, page 106.

C. **Chemotherapy**

Nursing considerations:
1. Be aware of the chemotherapeutic agents most frequently used to treat childhood cancer, their side effects, and precautions for administration. See Table 60-1, page 1479.
2. Care for the child who develops side effects of chemotherapy.
   a. Prepare the child and his family for the possible side effects of the chemotherapeutic agents he is receiving. Explain to the child that the medicine is to help him feel better, but that when he first begins to take the medicine he may feel sicker. If this is explained prior to the development of symptoms, the child will be more trusting and less frightened.
   b. Nausea and vomiting
      (1) Administer antiemetics as prescribed.
      (2) Plan activities and meals according to the medical schedule. Many children prefer to receive chemotherapeutic agents that cause nausea and vomiting during the evening so

* For additional information, see Chapter 6. Cancer Nursing, page 95.

Table 60-1. *Drugs Commonly Used in the Treatment of Childhood Cancer*

Drug Category	Administration	Side Effects/Toxicity	Specific Nursing Implications
Adriamycin (doxorubicin): antibiotic	IV	Nausea and vomiting, alopecia, stomatitis, myelosuppression, cardiotoxicity, red urine Causes chemical irritation on extravasation	1. Use the same precautions when administering this medication as with vincristine. 2. Observe for changes in heart rate or rhythm.
Bleomycin (Blenoxane): antibiotic	IV, IM, subcutaneous	Allergic reaction, anaphylaxis, nausea and vomiting, stomatitis, cumulative effects involving the skin and lung (pneumonitis, pulmonary fibrosis)	1. Administer test dose before giving a therapeutic dose. 2. Be prepared for allergic reaction, especially with first few doses.
Carmustine: (BiCNU)	IV	Facial burning and flushing on infusion, burning pain along IV infusion, nausea and vomiting, bone marrow depression	1. Avoid extravasation, as it can cause transient hyperpigmentation.
Chlorambucil (Leukeran): alkylating agent	PO	Nausea and vomiting, diarrhea, myelosuppression	1. Side effects usually related to high doses.
Cisplatin (Platinol)	IV	Severe renal toxicity, 8th nerve damage, severe nausea and vomiting, myelosuppression, neurotoxicity, anaphylactic reactions	1. Assess renal function before administration. 2. Maintain hydration before and during therapy. 3. Administer antiemetic. 4. Be prepared for allergic reaction. 5. Instruct the parents to report signs of hearing loss or neurotoxicity.
Cyclophosphamide (Cytoxan): alkylating agent	Oral or IV	Alopecia, nausea and vomiting, myelosuppression, hemorrhagic cystitis, mucous membrane ulceration, immunosuppression, infertility, hyperpigmentation	1. To prevent exposure of the bladder to chemical irritants, maintain liberal hydration for 48 hours after weekly dose and continuously when given daily. Have the child empty his bladder frequently after the drug is administered, including at least once during the night.
Cytarabine hydrochloride (Cytosar-U): antimetabolite; pyrimidine antagonist	IV, IM, subcutaneous, or intrathecal (IT)	Nausea and vomiting, myelosuppression, mucous membrane ulcerations, hepatotoxicity, immunosuppression	1. May require premedication with antiemetics. 2. Protect the child from infection. 3. Do not enter vial twice for IT use.
Dacarbazine	IV	Nausea and vomiting (especially after the first dose), flu-like syndrome, bone marrow depression Cause chemical irritation on extravasation	1. Used with caution in children with renal dysfunction. 2. Apply ice above injection site for local pain and/or burning.
Dactinomycin: antibiotic	IV	Myelosuppression, nausea and vomiting, mucositis. Causes chemical irritation on extravasation	1. Dose is calculated in micrograms. 2. Use preservative free diluent. 3. Use the same precautions when administering as with vincristine.
Daunorubicin: antibiotic	IV	Cardiotoxicity, myelosuppression, nausea and vomiting, abdominal pain, fever, skin rash, red urine Causes chemical irritation on extravasation	1. Use the same precautions when administering this medication as those followed with vincristine.
Etoposide (VP-16): plant alkaloid	IV	Myelosuppression, alopecia, nausea and vomiting, mucositis, mild neurotoxicity, hypotension, allergic reaction	1. Monitor BP. 2. Observe for hypersensitivity reactions.
5-Fluorouracil: antimetabolite	PO	Myelosuppression, mucositis, nausea and vomiting, diarrhea	1. Promote oral hygiene.
Ifosfamide: alkylating agent	IV	Myelosuppression, nausea and vomiting, alopecia, cystitis, neurotoxicity, renal toxicity	1. Same as for cyclophosphamide. 2. Mesna, a bladder uroprotector, is usually given in conjunction with this drug.
L-Asparaginase: enzyme	IV	Hypersensitivity reaction, nausea and vomiting, lethargy, somnolence, fever, hepatotoxicity, coagulopathy	1. Observe for hypersensitivity reaction. Have epinephrine and resuscitation equipment available.

(continued)

Table 60-1. *Drugs Commonly Used in the Treatment of Childhood Cancer (continued)*

Drug Category	Administration	Side Effects/Toxicity	Specific Nursing Implications
		Hyperglycemia Renal failure	2. Observe for confusion, irritability, convulsions, and other neurologic signs. 3. Do not shake vial. 4. Use clear solution only.
Lomustine: CCNU	PO	Nausea and vomiting, bone marrow depression	1. Administer 4 hours after meals on an empty stomach.
Mechlorethamine (nitrogen mustard): alkylating agent	IV, IT	Nausea and vomiting, myelosuppression, alopecia, local phlebitis	1. Use caution when mixing drug—wear eyeglasses or goggles. Rinse skin immediately if solution comes in contact with skin. 2. Use immediately after mixing. 3. Check patency of IV line before infusing and inject drug cautiously.
6-Mercaptopurine: antimetabolite—purine antagonist	Oral	Nausea and vomiting, myelosuppression, anorexia, dermatitis, mucous membrane ulceration, hepatotoxicity, abdominal pain	1. Dosage should be reduced to one-third of the usual dosage if a child is also receiving allopurinol, as this drug inhibits the degradation of 6-mercaptopurine.

Methotrexate: antimetabolite—folic acid antagonist	Oral, IV, IM, or IT	Nausea and vomiting, GI mucosal ulceration, myelosuppression, pneumonitis, osteoporosis, hepatotoxicity, hyperpigmentation
		Sensitivity to sun
			1. Avoid side effects of meningeal irritation during IT injection by diluting the drug in a preservative-free vehicle, bringing it to room temperature.
			2. Do not enter vial twice for IT use.
			3. Method of IT injection:
			  a. A lumbar puncture is performed.
			  b. A volume of spinal fluid equal to the volume of drug to be injected is removed.
			  c. Without aspiration, the medication is injected in a continuous infusion (15–30 seconds/10 ml. of solution.
			  d. The stylet is reinserted, and the needle is removed.
			  e. The child may be required to remain in the Trendelenburg position for 30 minutes after the injection to ensure optimal circulation of the medication throughout the central nervous system.
			  f. Use of an Ommaya reservoir may eliminate the need for repeated lumbar punctures.
			4. Avoid use of salicylates and sulfonamides, which increase toxicity of methotrexate.

Prednisone: adrenocorticosteroid	Oral	Increased appetite, weight gain, fluid retention, hypertension, Cushing's syndrome, immunosuppression, psychosis, GI tract ulceration	1. Avoid excessive sodium intake. 2. Observe for evidence of GI bleeding. 3. Protect from infection.
Procarbazine	PO	Severe nausea and vomiting, lethargy, dermatitis, arthralgia, bone marrow depression, stomatitis	1. Central nervous system depressants (phenothiazines and barbiturates) enhance CNS symptoms. 2. Acts as an MAO inhibitor—sympathomimetic drugs and natural foods such as yogurt, aged cheese, and bananas should be avoided.
Teneposide (VM-26): plant alkaloid	IV	Myelosuppression, alopecia, nausea and vomiting, mucositis, mild neurotoxicity, hypotension, allergic reaction	1. Same as for etoposide.

(continued)

Table 60-1. *Drugs Commonly Used in the Treatment of Childhood Cancer (continued)*

Drug Category	Administration	Side Effects/Toxicity	Specific Nursing Implications
6-Thioguanine: antimetabolite	PO	Myelosuppression, nausea and vomiting, mucositis, hepatic toxicity	1. Administer on an empty stomach.
Vincristine (Oncovin): periwinkle alkaloid	IV	Alopecia, constipation, peripheral neuropathy, mild myelosuppression. Causes chemical irritation on extravasation	1. Use different needles to withdraw and inject. Check patency of IV line with saline flush before injecting. Inject cautiously, observing for signs of infiltration. Follow injection with saline flush. 2. Observe for constipation; report condition promptly. Keep well hydrated. Administer laxatives or stool softeners as prescribed. 3. Alter activities appropriately if weakness of hands, feet, or legs occurs or if the child becomes easily fatigued. 4. Prepare children and parents for the possibility of numbness and tingling of fingers and toes.
Vinblastine (Velban): plant alkaloid	IV	Nausea and vomiting, alopecia, myelosuppression, neurotoxicity	1. Same as for vincristine.

that they can sleep through the hours of greatest nausea.
    (3) Carefully observe the sleeping child who is prone to vomiting. Position him in a manner that prevents aspiration.
    (4) Offer foods and fluids that are most appealing to the child (e.g., warm tea, carbonated beverages, soups).
    (5) Record the nature of the nausea and vomiting.
    (6) Report any prolonged or delayed nausea or vomiting, which may be an indication that the medication should be withheld or that the dosage should be reduced.
  c. Anorexia
    (1) Create a pleasant eating environment that is free of sights, sounds, and odors that cause nausea or that discourage or distract the child.
    (2) Encourage the child to eat in the playroom with other children.
    (3) Give good mouth care prior to eating.
    (4) Provide frequent, small meals.
  d. Extreme fluctuations in appetite—be aware that this is temporary and that eventually normal eating patterns will be established. Reassure the parents of this fact.
  e. Gastrointestinal mucosal cell damage causing stomatitis, gastrointestinal ulceration, rectal ulceration, diarrhea, or bleeding
    (1) Provide meticulous oral hygiene. Local anesthetics may be prescribed for painful mouth ulcers.
    (2) If diarrhea or rectal ulcers occur, keep the skin clean and dry to prevent maceration and secondary infection.
    (3) These signs of toxicity are generally indications for temporary discontinuation of therapy or a reduction of dosage.
  f. Alopecia
    (1) Assist the family in obtaining wigs or caps in preparation for hair loss.

    (2) Reassure the child and family that the hair will grow back, although it might be of a different color and texture.
  g. For side effects and nursing interventions associated with specific drugs, see Table 60-1, Drugs Commonly Used in the Treatment of Childhood Cancer.

Prevention

1. Children and adults should be educated about the hazards of known carcinogens, especially cigarette smoking, and excessive exposure to sunlight or radiation.
2. Female adolescents should be instructed concerning the method of breast self-examination. Males should be taught to do testicular self-examination. Periodic examinations should be encouraged for cancer screening.
3. Parents should be taught the warning signals of childhood cancer.

Acute Lymphocytic Leukemia

Acute lymphocytic leukemia (ALL) is a primary disorder of the bone marrow in which the normal marrow elements are replaced by immature or undifferentiated blast cells. When the quantity of normal marrow is depleted below the level necessary to maintain peripheral blood elements within normal ranges, anemia, neutropenia, and thrombocytopenia occur.

Etiology

1. The exact cause of acute leukemia is unknown.
2. Environmental causes, infectious agents (especially viruses), genetic factors, and chromosomal abnormalities are suspected in some cases.

Incidence and Classification

1. Acute leukemia is the most common malignancy in children, occurring in nearly 4 per 100,000 children under 15 years of age.
2. Acute leukemia is classified according to the cell type involved.
3. The incidence of ALL is more common among Caucasian children.
4. The incidence of ALL is higher in males than females, with the greatest difference during puberty.

Altered Physiology

1. Acute lymphocytic leukemia results from the growth of an abnormal type of nongranular, fragile leukocyte in the blood, forming tissues, particularly in the bone marrow, spleen, and lymph nodes.
2. The abnormal cell has little cytoplasm and a round, homogeneous nucleus, which resembles that of a lymphoblast.
3. Normal bone marrow elements may be displaced or replaced in this type of leukemia.
4. The changes in the blood and bone marrow result from the accumulation of leukemic cells and from the deficiency of normal cells.
   a. Red cell precursors and megakaryocytes from which platelets are formed are decreased, causing anemia, prolonged and unusual bleeding, and tendency to bruise easily.
   b. Normal white cells are markedly decreased, predisposing the child to infection.
   c. The bone marrow is hyperplastic with a uniform appearance due to the presence of leukemic cells.
5. Leukemic cells may infiltrate into lymph nodes, spleen, and liver, causing diffuse adenopathy and hepatosplenomegaly.
6. Expansion of marrow or infiltration of leukemic cells into bone results in bone or joint pain.
7. Invasion of the central nervous system by leukemic cells may cause headache, vomiting, cranial nerve palsies, convulsions, and coma.
8. Weight loss, muscle wasting, and fatigue may occur when the body cells are deprived of nutrients because of the immense metabolic needs of the proliferating leukemic cells.

Clinical Manifestations

1. Manifestations depend on the degree to which the bone marrow has been compromised and the location and extent of extramedullary infiltration.
2. Presenting symptoms
   a. Fatigability
   b. General malaise, listlessness
   c. Persistent fever of unknown cause
   d. Recurrent infection
   e. Prolonged bleeding following simple surgical procedures (e.g., dental extractions and tonsillectomy)
   f. Tendency to bruise easily
   g. Pallor
   h. Enlarged lymph nodes
   i. Abdominal pain due to organomegaly
   j. Bone and joint pain
   k. Headache and vomiting (with CNS involvement)
3. Presenting symptoms may be isolated or in any combination or sequence.

Diagnostic Evaluation

A. Physical Findings

1. Pallor, especially of the mucous membranes
2. Scattered petechiae and ecchymoses
3. Generalized lymphadenopathy
4. Enlarged liver and spleen
5. Unexplained bruising
6. Continued bone and joint pain
7. Fever

B. Laboratory Evaluation

1. May have altered peripheral blood counts. Blood studies may show the following:
   a. Low hemoglobin, red blood cell count, hematocrit, and platelet count
   b. Decreased, elevated, or normal white blood cell count
2. Stained peripheral smear and bone marrow examination show large numbers of lymphoblasts and lymphocytes.
3. Lumbar puncture—to determine if there is central nervous system involvement.
4. Renal and liver function studies—to determine any contraindications or precautions for chemotherapy.

Treatment

A. Supportive Therapy—to control disease complications such as hyperuricemia, infection, anemia, and bleeding

B. Specific Therapy—to eradicate malignant cells and to restore normal marrow function

1. Chemotherapy is used to achieve complete remission with restoration of normal peripheral blood and physical findings.
2. There is no universally accepted standard therapy for the treatment of children with acute leukemia, but most centers have similar protocols that use a combination of drugs (see Table 60-1).
3. Components of therapy
   a. Induction—course of therapy designed to achieve a complete remission
   b. Central nervous system prophylaxis—treatment begun early in the course of the illness to destroy leukemic cells that have infiltrated the central nervous system. It generally consists of intrathecal administration of methotrexate with or without cranial irradiation.
   c. Consolidation treatment—a period of intensified treatment immediately after remission induction to attempt total irradication of leukemic cells.
   d. Maintenance or continuation therapy—to prevent reappearance of the disease (usually continued for about 3 years)
   e. Reinduction therapy to reinduce remission if relapse occurs
   f. Extramedullary disease therapy
4. Research is continuing to determine the optimal method of inducing and maintaining remission with the least risk to the patient.
5. Bone marrow transplantation has been used successfully for treating children who fail to respond to conventional treatment.

Complications

1. Infection—most frequently occurs in the lungs, gastrointestinal tract, or skin

2. Hemorrhage—usually due to thrombocytopenia
3. Central nervous system involvement
4. Bony involvement
5. Testicular involvement
6. Urate nephropathy
7. Late effects of treatment

Prognosis

1. At least 95% of children with ALL can be expected to achieve an initial remission if treated in a specialized center.
2. At least 50% of children with ALL will survive more than 5 years.
3. Children with good prognostic features have a 70%–75% chance of long-term survival.
4. The prognosis becomes poorer with each relapse the child experiences.
5. The term "cure" is difficult to define because later relapses still occur after long remissions.
6. Prognosis appears to be related to the child's age and white blood cell count on diagnosis, and the exact cell type of the leukemia.

Patient Problems and Nursing Diagnoses

1. Parental anxiety/grief at learning of the diagnosis
2. Potential for infection related to decreased numbers of normal white blood cells
3. Potential complication: hemorrhage
4. Altered nutrition (less than body requirements), related to anemia and anorexia, nausea, and vomiting and mucosal ulceration secondary to chemotherapy and/or irradiation
5. Altered comfort, pain, related to the progress of the disease and to diagnostic and treatment procedures
6. Activity intolerance related to fatigue resulting from disease and treatment
7. Anxiety of the child related to hospitalization and to diagnostic and treatment procedures
8. Self-concept, disturbance in body image, related to alopecia associated with chemotherapy
9. Knowledge deficit about leukemia and its treatment

Nursing Interventions

A. Providing Emotional Support to the Parents When the Diagnosis of Leukemia Is Made Known to Them.

1. Be available to the parents when they feel that they want to discuss their feelings.
2. Kindness, concern, consideration, and sincerity toward the child and his parents help to serve as a source of consolation.
3. Contact the family's clergyman or the hospital chaplain if the parents desire this.
4. Use the services of a social worker as appropriate to help the family work out their feelings.
5. Avoid discussing life expectancy in terms of the time element—offer the hope that therapy will be effective and will prolong life.
6. Allow the parents to participate in the child's care so that they will feel that they are actually doing something for the child. This also helps the family feel more secure (see the section on family-centered care, p. 1125).
7. Assess family dynamics and coping mechanisms and plan intervention accordingly.

B. Giving Skillful, Supportive Care in the Early Stages of Treatment and Sustaining Life Until Antileukemic Agents Have Had a Chance to Become Effective.

1. Initiate nursing activities associated with anemia (see p. 1299).
2. Provide adequate hydration.
   a. Maintain parenteral fluid administration.
   b. Offer small amounts of oral fluids if tolerated.
   c. Record and report vomiting if this occurs.
3. Observe renal function carefully.
   a. Measure and record urinary output.
   b. Check specific gravity.
   c. Observe the urine for any evidence of gross bleeding.
4. Provide a highly nutritious diet if the child can tolerate it.
   a. Determine the child's likes and dislikes.
   b. Offer frequent, small meals.
   c. Offer supplemental feedings high in calories and protein.
   d. Encourage the parents to assist at mealtime.
   e. Allow the child to eat with a group at a table if his condition allows this.
5. Protect the child from sources of infection.
   a. Family, friends, personnel, and other patients who have infections should not visit or care for the child.
   b. Do not place a child with an infection in the room with a child with leukemia.
   c. Reverse isolation procedure may be used (a protective technique that provides the child with protection from those people with whom he has contact)—varies from good hand-washing to gowns and masks. Explain to both the child and his parents the purpose of this protective technique.
   d. Observe the child closely and be alert to signs of impending infection.
      (1) Observe any area of broken skin or mucous membrane for signs of infection.
      (2) Report any febrile incidents.
   e. Teach preventive measures at discharge (i.e., hand-washing, isolation from children with communicable disease).

C. Being Alert for the Symptoms of Hemorrhage That May Occur When the Platelet Count Is Diminished or May Appear as Side Effects of Antileukemic Therapy.

1. Record vital signs and report any changes that may indicate hemorrhage.
   a. Tachycardia
   b. Lowered blood pressure
   c. Pallor
   d. Diaphoresis
   e. Increasing anxiety and restlessness
2. Give careful oral hygiene, the gums and mucous membranes of the mouth bleed easily.
   a. Use a soft toothbrush.
   b. If the child's mouth is bleeding or painful, clean the teeth and mouth with a moistened cotton swab.
   c. Use a nonirritating rinse for the mouth (e.g., hydrogen peroxide).
   d. Apply petrolatum to cracked, dry lips.
3. Observe for gastrointestinal bleeding. Hematest all output.
   a. Hematemesis
   b. Tarry or bloodstained stools

4. Move and turn the child gently, as hemarthrosis may occur and cause movement to be very painful.
   a. Handle the child in a gentle manner.
   b. Turn frequently to prevent pressure sores.
   c. Place the child in proper body alignment, in a position comfortable for him.
   d. Allow the child to be out of bed in a chair if this position is more comfortable for him.
5. Avoid intramuscular injections if possible.
6. Handle catheters as well as drainage and suction tubes carefully to prevent mucosal bleeding.
7. Protect the child from injury by monitoring his activities and environmental hazards.
8. Be aware of emergency procedures for control of bleeding:
   a. Careful application of local pressure so as not to interfere with clot formation.
   b. Administration of blood and blood components (see the section on anemia, p. 1298).

D. Preparing the Child for Diagnostic and Treatment Procedures.

1. Use knowledge of growth and development to prepare the child for procedures such as bone marrow aspirations, blood transfusions, and chemotherapy (see the section on the hospitalized child, p. 1120).
2. Provide a means for talking about the experience. Play, storytelling, or role-playing may be helpful.
3. Convey to the child an acceptance of his fears and anger.

E. Controlling Hyperuricemia That May Occur Because of Rapid Cell Turnover and Tumor Lysis.

1. Administer allopurinal as prescribed to neutralize the effects of uric acid on the kidney.
2. Provide liberal oral and/or IV hydration.
3. Administer sodium bicarbonate or acetazolamide (Diamox) as prescribed to alkalize the urine.
4. Collect urine specimens to monitor urinary excretion of uric acid.

F. Being Aware of Chemotherapeutic Agents and the Side Effects of These Agents That Are Capable of Inducing Remissions in Children With Acute Leukemia.

1. Induction—usually includes a combination of vincristine and prednisone. A third drug, such as 6-mercaptopurine, L-asparaginase, daunorubicin, adriamycin, or cytosine arabinoside, may be added.
2. Maintenance—usually includes daily oral administration of 6-mercaptopurine and weekly oral administration of methotrexate with intermittent administration of other drugs such as vincristine, prednisone, cyclophosphamide, cytosine arabinoside, or daunorubicin.
3. Reinduction—remissions can often be reinduced using the same initial drugs or with other agents.
4. See Table 60-1, Drugs Commonly Used in the Treatment of Childhood Cancer.

G. Providing Symptomatic Care for the Child Who Develops the Side Effects of Chemotherapy.

See the section on chemotherapy, page 1478.

H. Observing for the Possibility of CNS Involvement.

Report changes in behavior or personality: persistent nausea and vomiting, headache, lethargy, irritability, dizziness, ataxia, convulsions, or alteration in state of consciousness.

I. Providing Supportive Nursing Care to the Child Receiving Cranial Irradiation.

Refer to section on radiation therapy, page 1478.

J. Providing Pain Relief.

1. Position the child so that he is most comfortable. Water beds and beanbag chairs are often helpful.
2. Administer medications on a preventive schedule before pain becomes severe. Individualize medication schedule for each patient.
3. Manipulate the environment as necessary to increase the child's comfort and minimize unnecessary exertion.

K. Providing Emotional Support to the Child.

1. Provide for continuity of care.
2. Encourage family-centered care (see p. 1125).
3. Prepare the child for potential changes in his body image (alopecia, weight loss, wasting, etc.) and help him cope with related feelings.
4. Facilitate play activities for the child and use opportunities to communicate with him through play.
5. Maintain some discipline, placing calm limitations on unacceptable behavior.
6. Provide appropriate diversional activities.
7. Encourage independence and provide opportunities that allow the child to control his environment.
8. Avoid exposing the child to activities that he will be unable to accomplish.

L. Providing Continued Emotional Support to the Parents Throughout the Course of Hospitalization.

1. Assist the parents to feel comfortable on the unit.
2. Provide guidelines concerning how parents and the treatment team can work together most profitably.
3. Encourage parental participation in care—to the extent that they feel comfortable.
4. Suggest tasks that the parents may do to reduce their feelings of helplessness and anxiety.
5. Provide for continuity of care so that the parents are able to establish trusting relationships with a few nurses.
6. Assist the parents to deal with anticipatory grief.
7. Assist the parents to deal with other family members, especially siblings and grandparents, and friends.
8. Encourage the parents to discuss concerns about limiting their child's activities, protecting him from infection, disciplining him, and having anxieties about the illness.
9. Answer parental questions related to such matters as home management, the purpose of periodic tests, treatments and clinic visits, side effects of medications, and indications for medical intervention.
10. Facilitate communication with the clinic nurse and/or clinical specialist who may interact with the child during the entire course of illness.
11. Initiate appropriate referrals (e.g., to social worker, parent group, clergy, and community health nurse).

M. Providing Supportive Care to the Terminally Ill or Dying Child.

See the section on care of the dying child, page 1523.

N. References for Children and Parents

Baker LS. You and Leukemia—A Day At A Time. Philadelphia, WB Saunders, 1988

Sherman M. The Leukemic Child, DHEW Pub No (NIH) 78-863 National Cancer Program, National Cancer Institute, Bethesda, MD 20892

Leukemia Society of America, 733 Third Avenue, New York, NY 10017

See the Bibliography, page 1494

Expected Outcomes

1. The parents discuss their feelings about the child's diagnosis
2. The child avoids infection
3. The child shows no signs of excessive bleeding—vital signs normal; no hematemesis or tarry stools
4. Eats at mealtime; takes between meal feedings
5. Experiences relief from pain (no crying or expression of pain)
6. Demonstrates lessened anxiety (talks about his feelings or shows them in play; participates in other age-appropriate activities
7. Maintains a positive body image; does not become overly self-conscious or shy about appearance
8. The parents indicate that they understand what leukemia is and how it is treated

Brain Tumors in Children

Brain tumors are expanding lesions within the skull. About 20% of the malignant tumors that occur in children are brain tumors.

Etiology

The etiology of brain tumors is unknown.

Clinical Manifestations

(Signs and symptoms are directly related to the location and size of the tumor.)
1. Headache
   a. Vague and nonspecific complaints of headache are more common than severe early morning headaches.
   b. May be intermittent and disappear for days or weeks—may be due to yielding of the sutures.
   c. Duration prior to diagnosis is usually less than 4–6 months.
2. Vomiting, usually without nausea
   a. May occur at any time, but frequently occurs in the early morning hours.
   b. Vomiting may be projectile.
3. Visual disturbances
   a. Nystagmus
   b. Diplopia
   c. Blurred vision
   d. Loss of peripheral vision
   e. Significant loss of visual acuity
4. Muscular problems
   a. Deficits of balance
   b. Poor coordination
   c. Deficits in muscle functioning—eyes, face, extremities
   d. Paralysis
   e. Spasticity
5. Behavioral changes
   a. Arrest or regression in development
   b. Irritability or lassitude
   c. Lack of attentiveness
   d. Deterioration in school performance
   e. Personality changes
   f. Loss of sphincter control
   g. Disturbances in sleep and eating patterns
6. Slow cerebration
   a. The child answers questions after a considerable delay.
   b. The child appears to talk slowly.
   c. The child responds to any stimulus in a slow manner.
7. Seizures—usually focal, psychomotor, or generalized

Diagnostic Evaluation

Determined by the type of tumor that is suspected; usually includes many or all of the following procedures:
1. Thorough neurologic examination
   a. Funduscopic examination
   b. Tests for cerebral function (level of consciousness, orientation, intellectual performance, mood, behavior, etc.)
   c. Assessment of cranial nerves
   d. Tests for cerebellar function (e.g., balance and coordination)
   e. Evaluation of the motor system—especially muscle size, tone, strength, and abnormal muscle movements
   f. Evaluation of the sensory system
   g. Assessment of reflexes
2. Electroencephalogram—of limited value, but possibly useful when seizures are manifested
3. Skull x-ray
4. CT–Computed tomography
   a. Safe, noninvasive procedure using a combination of sophisticated electronic and computer technology.
   b. Scanning of head by a slit x-ray beam passing through at a multitude of angles.
   c. Absorption values, varying with the density of tissues and fluids, are calculated and analyzed. This allows for differentiation of normal and abnormal brain tissue and ventricular sizes and configurations.
5. Isotopic brain scanning
6. Angiography
7. MRI–Magnetic Resonance Imaging
   a. No radiation exposure
   b. Does not require intravenous contrast agents.
   c. Images are obtained in multiple planes.
   d. Bone artifacts are avoided.
   e. May be more sensitive than CT scans for some brain tumors.
8. Myelogram
9. PET–Positron Emission Tomography
10. Lumbar puncture

Treatment

1. Surgery is performed to determine the type of the tumor, the extent of invasiveness, and to excise as much of the lesion as possible.
2. Radiation therapy is usually initiated as soon as the diagnosis is established and the surgical wound healed.
3. Chemotherapy is standard treatment for certain brain tumors, following surgery and radiation.

Prognosis

1. Prognosis is improved in cases involving early diagnosis and adequate therapy.
2. Prognosis is related to completeness of surgical removal, extent of invasion, and rate of tumor growth.
3. Five-year survivors are increasing, especially in children with low-grade astrocytomas or ependymomas.

Cerebellar Astrocytoma

Cerebellar astrocytoma is a slow-growing, often cystic type of tumor of the cerebellum that accounts for about 10%–20% of all pediatric brain tumors.

Clinical Manifestations

Insidious onset and slow course
1. Evidence of increased intracranial pressure—especially headache, visual disturbances, papilledema, and personality changes
2. Cerebellar signs—ataxia, dysmetria (inability to control the range of muscular movement), nystagmus
3. Behavioral changes

Pathophysiology

1. The tumor produces slowly increasing intracranial pressure.
2. Condition classified according to its malignancy—from grade I (least malignant) to grade IV (most malignant).

Treatment

Surgical removal—the tumor can often be removed with few sequelae.

Medulloblastoma (Primitive Neuroectodermal tumor—PNET)

Medulloblastoma is a highly malignant, rapidly growing tumor, usually found in the cerebellum.

Incidence

1. Medulloblastoma is the single most common tumor of the central nervous system in children.
2. About 65% of medulloblastomas occur in males.

Clinical Manifestations

1. Similar to manifestations of cerebellar astrocytoma, but condition develops more rapidly.
2. The child may present with unsteady gait, anorexia, vomiting, and early morning headache, and later develop ataxia, nystagmus, papilledema, and drowsiness.

Pathophysiology

1. The tumor grows rapidly and produces evidence of increased intracranial pressure progressing over a period of weeks.
2. As the tumor grows, it seeds along cerebrospinal fluid (CSF) pathways.

Treatment

1. Partial excision or decompression of the posterior fossa (complete removal is rarely possible)
2. Radiation of site and spinal canal

3. Chemotherapy
4. Shunt to relieve CSF obstruction

Brain Stem Glioma

Brain stem glioma is a tumor of the brain stem. It accounts for approximately 15% of brain tumors in children.

Clinical Manifestations

1. Cranial nerve palsies
   a. Strabismus
   b. Weakness, atrophy, and fasciculations of the tongue
   c. Swallowing difficulties
2. Hemiparesis
3. Cerebellar ataxia
4. Signs of increased intracranial pressure (rare)

Altered Physiology

Through its growth, this type of tumor interferes early with the function of cranial nerve nuclei, pyramidal tracts, and cerebellar pathways.

Treatment

1. Surgical removal is not possible
2. Radiation of site

Ependymoma of the Fourth Ventricle

Ependymoma is a tumor derived from the ependyma, or lining, of the central canal of the spinal cord and cerebral ventricles. It frequently arises on the floor of the fourth ventricle, causing obstruction of the flow of cerebrospinal fluid. Ependymomas represent about 5%–10% of all primary childhood CNS tumors.

Clinical Manifestations

1. Nausea or vomiting
2. Headache
3. Unsteady gait/ataxia; dysmetria
4. Signs of increased intracranial pressure

Altered Physiology

1. Tumors grow with varying speed.
2. Because of location, tumors can invade the cardiorespiratory center, cerebellum, and spinal cord.
3. Graded according to degree of differentiation, as are the astrocytomas.

Management

1. Partial surgical removal
2. Radiation therapy, including the entire craniospinal axis
3. Chemotherapy—Phase II and III trials.

Nursing Process Overview: Care of the Child Undergoing Surgery for Brain Tumor

Assessment

Assess the child's neurologic status to help locate the site of the tumor and the extent of involvement; identify signs of disease progress.

1. Obtain a thorough nursing history from the child and his parents—particularly data related to normal behavioral patterns and presenting symptoms.
2. Perform portions of the neurologic examination as appropriate. Assess muscle strength, coordination, gait, and posture.
3. Observe for the appearance or disappearance of any of the clinical manifestations previously described. Report these to the physician and record each of the following in detail:
   a. Headache—duration, location, severity
   b. Vomiting—time occurring, whether or not projectile
   c. Convulsions—activity prior to seizure; type of seizure; areas of body involved; behavior during and after seizure
4. Monitor vital signs frequently, including blood pressure and pupillary reaction.
5. Monitor ocular signs. Check pupils for size, equality, reaction to light, and accommodation.
6. Observe for signs of brain stem herniation—should be considered a neurosurgical emergency.
   a. Attacks of opisthotonos
   b. Tilting of the head; neck stiffness
   c. Poorly reactive pupils
   d. Increased blood pressure; widened pulse pressure
   e. Change in respiratory rate and nature of respirations
   f. Irregularity of pulse or lowered pulse rate
   g. Alterations of body temperature

Patient Problems and Nursing Diagnoses

1. Parental anxiety related to the nature of the diagnosis and usual need for surgery
2. Altered comfort, pain, related to increased intracranial pressure and surgery
3. Altered nutrition (less than body requirements), related to nausea and vomiting associated with increased intracranial pressure and to irradiation
4. Potential for postoperative complications: shock, increased intracranial pressure, respiratory arrest
5. Fatigue related to radiation therapy
6. Anxiety of the child related to hospitalization and to diagnostic and treatment procedures
7. Self-concept, disturbance in body image related to appearance of the incision, shaved head, and/or changes due to irradiation and/or chemotherapy.
8. Knowledge deficit regarding brain tumors and their treatment

Nursing Interventions

A. Providing the Parents and Child With Emotional Support During the Very Stressful Preoperative Period.

1. Assess the family unit and its coping mechanisms.
2. Allow parents to ask questions and encourage them to discuss their fears and concerns. Many parents feel guilty for not seeking help earlier because they either did not recognize or dismissed symptoms.
3. Deliver nursing care to the child in a manner that provides support.
   a. Assume a gentle, concerned attitude toward both parents and child.
   b. Make the child as comfortable as possible.

B. Providing Appropriate Nursing Care for the Child Undergoing Diagnostic Tests.

1. Prepare the child and parents for each procedure.
2. If prescribed, administer preliminary sedative on time. (If the child is not adequately sedated, completion of the test may be impossible.)
3. Refer to adult section, page 584, for nursing care related to specific procedures.

C. Preparing the Child and Parents for Surgery.

1. Refer to section on preparation for surgery, page 1133.
2. Determine physician's plans regarding shaving the head, bandages, and other procedures, and prepare the child accordingly.
   a. Encourage the child to express his feelings regarding the threat to his body image.
   b. Reassure the child that he will be able to wear a wig or hat after recovery.
   c. If the area is to be shaved, allow the child and parents the option of saving the hair.
3. Prepare the parents for the postoperative appearance of their child and for the fact that he might be comatose immediately following surgery.
4. If appropriate, introduce the child and his family to intensive care nursing personnel and arrange a tour of the unit.
5. Prepare the child for postoperative expectations (i.e., he may feel sleepy or have a headache and will need to remain quiet).

D. Providing an Adequate Diet for the Child Preoperatively.

1. Refeed the child when he vomits. (Vomiting is not usually associated with nausea.)
2. Allow the child to participate in the selection of foods and the preparation of his tray.
3. Maintain IV hydration if indicated.

E. Providing Care for the Child During the Immediate Postoperative Period. (This is usually provided in an intensive care unit).

1. Position the child according to physician's request—usually on his unaffected side with his head level.
   a. Raising the foot of the bed may increase intracranial pressure and bleeding.
   b. Post a sign above the bed noting the exact position of the head.
2. Check the dressing for bleeding and for drainage of cerebrospinal fluid.
3. Monitor the child's temperature closely.
   a. A marked rise in temperature may be due to trauma, to disturbance of the heat-regulating center, or to intracranial edema.
   b. If hyperthermia occurs, use appropriate measures to reduce it (see the section on fever, p. 1142). Temperature should not be reduced too rapidly.
4. Observe child closely for signs of shock, increased intracranial pressure, and alterations in level of consciousness.
5. Assess the child for edema of the head, face, and neck.
   a. Edema may inhibit respirations and impair circulation of lacrimal secretions.
   b. Apply cold compresses to the affected areas, being careful not to dampen the dressing.
   c. Instill prescribed ophthalmologic drops in the eyes to prevent corneal damage.

6. Carefully regulate fluid administration to prevent increased cerebral edema.
7. Change the child's position frequently and provide meticulous skin care to prevent hypostatic pneumonia and pressure sores.
   a. Move the child carefully and slowly, being certain to move the head in line with the body.
   b. Support paralyzed or spastic extremities with pillows, rolls, or other means.
8. Avoid discussing the child's condition in his presence, even if he appears to be unconscious.
9. Have equipment readily available for cardiopulmonary resuscitation, respiratory assistance, oxygen-inhalation, blood transfusion, ventricular tap, and other potential emergency situations.
10. Continue to support parents, who may be very frightened and upset by the appearance of their child and necessary emergency procedures.

F. Providing Care for the Child During the Convalescent Phase.

1. Maintain adequate nutrition and hydration.
   a. Encourage the child to eat increasingly larger meals.
   b. Provide tube feedings if the child is unable to eat.
2. Allow and encourage the child to regain his independence as his condition improves.
3. Facilitate the return of normal parent–child relationships.
   a. The parents may tend to be overprotective.
   b. Help the parents to see the child's increasing capabilities and encourage them to foster independence.
4. Make provisions for play activities.
   a. Allow the child to meet and play with other children.
   b. Provide the child with quiet play activities when it is necessary to encourage rest.
   c. Be careful that the child does not hit his head or fall until he is completely healed.
      A head dressing, football helmet, or wig may be used to prevent trauma should the child fall.
5. Assist the child to adjust to his altered body image.
   a. Use stocking caps, surgical caps, head scarves, hats, or wigs as appropriate.
   b. If the child's hair has not been totally shaved, it may be combed so that the area of baldness is not evident.
   c. Reassure the child that his hair will grow back.
6. For care of children with residual effects from surgery, refer to adult text, section on rehabilitation concepts, page 126.

G. Caring for the Child Receiving Radiation Therapy.

See the section on radiation therapy, page 1478.

H. Caring for the Child Receiving Chemotherapy.

Refer to section on chemotherapy, page 1478.

I. Preparing the Child and His Family for Discharge.

1. Provide parents with written information regarding the child's needs—medications, activity, care of incision, follow-up appointments, etc.
2. Initiate a referral to a community health nurse to reinforce teaching and to maintain therapeutic support for the family.

3. Encourage the parents to contact the child's teacher and the school nurse before the child returns to school so that they can prepare his classmates for his return and help them to deal with their feelings.
4. Provide the parents with the phone number of the clinic/nursing unit so that they may call if questions occur to them after discharge.
5. See the Bibliography, page 1496, for additional resources.

J. Providing Supportive Care to the Terminally Ill Child.

See the section on the dying child, page 1523.

Expected Outcomes

1. The parents discuss their feelings about the child's diagnosis and surgery
2. The child experiences relief from pain
3. Nutritional intake is adequate to meet body requirements
4. Does not develop life-threatening postoperative complications (shock, increased intracranial pressure, respiratory problems, edema)
5. Participates in age-appropriate activities within limitations imposed by fatigue
6. Demonstrates lessened anxiety through verbalization, play, or other age-appropriate activities
7. Maintains a positive body image, evidenced by his verbal and nonverbal communication
8. Parents accurately describe the brain tumor and its treatment

---

Neuroblastoma

Neuroblastoma refers to a malignant tumor arising from the sympathetic nervous system.

Etiology

Unknown

Incidence

1. Most common extracranial solid tumor of childhood
2. Occurs in approximately 1 per 10,000 live births
3. Primarily affects infants and young children
4. Occurs slightly more frequently in males.

Altered Physiology

1. Tumors arise from embryonic neural crest cells anywhere along the craniospinal axis.
2. Histologic picture varies greatly from tumor to tumor and even within the same tumor.
3. Tumors are staged primarily on the basis of the extent of disease.
   a. Evans Staging System
      (1) Stage I (tumor is confined to the organ or structure of origin) to stage IV (there is remote disease involving the skeleton, parenchymal organs, soft tissue, distant lymph glands, or bone marrow).
      (2) Stage IV-S refers to cases that would otherwise be stage I or II, but who have remote disease confined to 1 or more sites, either the liver, skin, or bone marrow, without evidence of skeletal metastasis.

b. Pediatric Oncology Group Staging
Stages A–D examine regional lymph nodes for presence of disease.
4. Neuroblastoma is one of the few tumors that may demonstrate spontaneous remission.

Clinical Manifestations

1. Symptoms depend on the location of the tumor and the stage of the disease.
2. Most tumors are located within the abdomen and present as firm, nontender, irregular masses that cross the midline.
3. Other common signs:
   a. Bowel or bladder dysfunction resulting from compression by a pelvic tumor
   b. Neurologic symptoms because of compression by the tumor on nerve roots or because of tumor extension
   c. Supraorbital ecchymosis, periorbital edema, and exophthalmos resulting from metastases to the skull bones and retrobulbar soft tissue
   d. Lymphadenopathy, especially in the cervical area
   e. Bone pain with skeletal involvement
   f. Swelling of the neck or face, and cough with thoracic masses
   g. General symptoms of pallor, anorexia, weight loss, and weakness with widespread metastasis

Diagnostic Evaluation

To document the extent of the disease:
1. X-rays of the chest, skull, abdomen, and long bones
2. Intravenous pyelogram
3. Bone marrow aspiration ± biopsy
4. CBC, platelet count, ferritin
5. 24-hour urine collection—elevated excretion of homovanillic acid (HVA) and vanillylmandelic acid (VMA)
6. Bone scan
7. Histologic confirmation
8. Additional studies
   a. CT scan
   b. Ultrasound examination
   c. Liver/spleen scan
   d. Inferior vena cavography
   e. Arteriography

Medical/Surgical Management

1. Surgery
   a. Role is both diagnostic and therapeutic.
   b. Either primary (prior to chemotherapy or radiation) or delayed/secondary (following therapy).
2. When complete surgical resection of a stage I tumor is possible, this may be the only treatment required.
3. Children with other than stage I disease generally receive a combination of surgery, radiation therapy, and chemotherapy.
   Drugs of choice include vincristine, dacarbazine, cyclophosphamide, doxorubicin, and cisplatin.

Prognosis

1. Overall survival rate is about 30%–35%, with almost all recurrences or deaths occurring within the first 2 years after diagnosis.
2. Influencing factors:
   a. Stage of disease—the earlier the stage, the better the prognosis.

b. Age—infants under 1 year of age demonstrate the best survival.
c. Pattern of metastasis—children with metastases to the bone marrow, liver, and skin have better prognoses than those with radiographic bone involvement.
d. Site of primary tumor–children with tumors of the thorax, pelvis, or neck appear to do better than children with abdominal tumors.
3. Neuroblastoma is one of few childhood tumors that has not responded dramatically to modern antitumor therapy.
4. The use of newer chemotherapy drugs and other techniques, such as immunotherapy and bone marrow transplant, may improve survival rates for these children.

Nursing Management

Nursing care for children with neuroblastoma is similar to that of children with other types of cancer.
Points of emphasis:
1. The child must be prepared for diagnostic tests and treatments in ways that are appropriate for his age and level of development.
2. General principles of preoperative and postoperative care should be applied for children who require abdominal, thoracic, or cranial surgery. See the sections on Wilms' tumor, cardiovascular surgery, page 1490, or brain tumor, page 1485.
3. For nursing care of the child receiving chemotherapy, see page 1478.
4. For nursing care of the child receiving radiation therapy, see page 1478.
5. Parents should be encouraged to express their feelings about the child's disease, and should be supported in their efforts to cope with the child's illness. Many parents feel guilty for not recognizing or reporting early signs of the illness. They may express anger toward health professionals or place blame on one another.
6. For nursing care of the terminally ill child, see page 1523.

Rhabdomyosarcoma

Rhabdomyosarcoma is a highly malignant soft tissue tumor that arises from the embryonic mesenchymal cells that form striated muscle.

Etiology

1. Unknown.
2. Genetic and environmental factors have been implicated.

Incidence

1. Most common soft tissue tumor in persons under age 21.
2. Accounts for 5%–8% of all malignant disease in children under 15 years of age.
3. Peak incidence is during the first decade of life.
4. Sixth most common form of cancer.

Altered Physiology

1. Classified in six pathologic categories based on histologic characteristics.

2. Tumor spreads either by local extension or by metastasis via the venous and lymphatic system.
3. Frequent sites of metastasis include the regional lymph nodes, lungs, bone marrow, bones, and brain.
4. Tumor staging is on the basis of the extent of the disease:
    a. Stage I: localized tumor, completely resected
    b. Stage II: regional disease, resected
    c. Stage III: localized disease, not completely resected
    d. Stage IV: metastatic disease at diagnosis

Clinical Manifestations

1. Often presents as an asymptomatic lump noted by the patient or parent.
2. Signs and symptoms variable and reflect the location of the tumor and metastases.
    a. Orbit—proptosis, chemosis, ocular paralysis
    b. Nasopharynx—epistaxis, pain, dysphagia, nasal voice, airway obstruction
    c. Sinuses—swelling, pain, discharge, sinusitis
    d. Middle ear—pain, chronic otitis, facial nerve palsy
    e. Neck—hoarseness, dysphagia
    f. Truncal, extremities, testicular areas—enlarging soft tissue masses
    g. Prostate, bladder—urinary tract symptoms
    h. Retroperitoneal tumors—gastrointestinal and urinary tract obstruction

Diagnostic Evaluation

To document the extent of the disease and provide objective criteria for measuring response to therapy
1. Complete blood count, liver and renal function tests, electrolytes, serum calcium and phosphorus, uric acid
2. Urinalysis
3. Chest x-ray
4. Bone scan and/or skeletal survey
5. Bone marrow aspiration and biopsy
6. Liver scan
7. CT scan of the chest and primary lesion
8. Skull x-ray, tomogram, CT scan and lumbar puncture—for children with cranial lesions
9. Lymph angiography and/or CT scan for patients with lower extremity and genitourinary lesions
10. Open biopsy of the primary tumor—definitive diagnostic procedure
11. Ultrasound
12. MRI

Treatment

1. Surgery—to biopsy the lesion, determine the stage of the disease, and completely remove or reduce the primary tumor—increasingly, chemotherapy/radiation therapy is used prior to surgery to avoid the disability associated with radical surgery for selected anatomic sites, (head, neck, and pelvis).
2. Radiation—high-dose radiation is generally recommended for the primary tumor and metastasis.
3. Chemotherapy
    a. Used for all patients, usually in combination with irradiation.
    b. Commonly used drugs include actinomycin D, vincristine, cyclophosphamide, doxorubicin, cisplatin, and VP-16.
    c. Other agents under investigation include ifosfamide and methotrexate.

Prognosis

1. Survival rates have improved considerably in recent years.
2. Overall survival rate is approximately 70%.
3. Prognosis is related to the stage of the disease at diagnosis and the location of the primary tumor.

Nursing Management

Nursing care is similar to that for a child with neuroblastoma (see p. 1489).

Wilms' Tumor

Wilms' tumor is a malignant renal tumor.

Etiology

1. The etiology of Wilms' tumor is not known.
2. Genetic inheritance has been documented in a small percentage of cases.

Incidence

1. Wilms' tumor is the most common neoplasm involving the retroperitoneal space in children.
2. It constitutes approximately 30% of all pediatric renal masses and 7% of all childhood tumors.
3. 75% of cases occur before the child is 5 years of age.
4. 1 child in 10,000 develops a Wilms' tumor.

Altered Physiology

1. Wilms' tumor has a capacity for very rapid growth and usually grows to a large size before it is diagnosed.
2. The effect of the tumor on the kidney depends on the site of the tumor.
3. In most cases, the tumor expands the renal parenchyma, and the kidney becomes stretched over the surface of the tumor.
4. The covering of the tumor may be very thin and easily torn.
5. The tumor is often exceedingly vascular, soft, mushy, or gelatinous in character.
6. Wilms' tumors present various histologic patterns from patient to patient.
7. The neoplasms metastasize early, either by direct extension or by way of the bloodstream. They may invade perirenal tissues, lymph nodes, the liver, the diaphragm, abdominal muscles, and the lungs. Invasions of bone and brain are less common.
8. Staging of Wilms' tumor is done on the basis of clinical and anatomical findings. It ranges from group I (tumor is limited to the kidney and is completely resected) to group IV (metastases are present in the liver, lung, bone, or brain). Group V includes those cases in which there is bilateral involvement either initially or subsequently.

Clinical Manifestations

1. A firm, nontender upper quadrant abdominal mass is usually the presenting sign; it may be on either side. (It is frequently observed by the parents.)
2. Abdominal pain, which is related to rapid growth of the tumor, may occur. As the tumor enlarges, pressure may cause constipation, vomiting, abdominal distress, anorexia, weight loss, and dyspnea.

3. Less common are hypertension, fever, hematuria, and anemia.
4. Associated anomalies:
   a. Hemihypertrophy
   b. Aniridia (absence of the iris)
   c. Genitourinary anomalies

Diagnostic Evaluation

1. IVP—to demonstrate the tumor and to assess the status of the opposite kidney
2. X-ray of chest and skeletal survey to identify metastases
3. CBC and peripheral smear
4. Urinalysis
5. Blood chemistries, especially serum electrolytes, uric acid, renal function tests (BUN and creatinine), and liver function tests (bilirubin, SGOT, SGPT, LDH, total protein, albumin, and alkaline phosphatase)
6. Coagulation studies—PT, PTT, and fibrinogen
7. Urinary VMA
8. Echograms to search for tumor extension
9. Ultrasonography to distinguish between a variety of renal masses
10. MRI
11. Radioisotope scans and tomography to rule out metastasis (often postponed until after surgery)

Treatment

1. Determined by the stage of the tumor
2. Includes a combination of surgery, radiation therapy, and chemotherapy

Prognosis

1. Overall survival rates for Wilms' tumor are the highest among all childhood cancers, greater than 85%.
2. High cure rate associated with early diagnosis and optimal treatment.
3. Prognosis best in children whose tumor is classified as group I or II and who receive multimodal therapy.
4. About 12% of children with Wilms' tumor have histologic features that are associated with a poor prognosis.

Nursing Interventions

A. Supporting the Family and the Child at the Time the Diagnosis Is Made.

1. Discuss with the physician what specific information has been given to the parents.
2. Provide the parents with the opportunity to express their concerns.
3. Provide the parents with a place where they may have some privacy when they wish to be alone.
4. Convey a compassionate attitude to the parents in talking with them, and assure them that their child's needs will be met.
5. See the section on family-centered care, page 1125.

B. Exercising Caution in the Manipulation of the Child in Order to Avoid Inadvertently Increasing the Danger of Metastasis.

1. Bathe the child carefully, avoiding manipulation of the abdomen.
2. Hold the child carefully to prevent abdominal pressure.
3. Communicate the need for this caution to all staff members.
4. Place a sign on the child's bed to reduce indiscriminate palpation.

C. Explaining to the Child and His Parents the Elements of Preoperative and Postoperative Care.

1. Use knowledge of growth and development to plan a teaching program for the child that will include diagnostic tests, preoperative care, and postoperative care (see the section on the hospitalized child, p. 1120).
2. Involve the parents in the teaching plan and encourage them to support the child at this time.
3. See the Bibliography, page 1494, for additional references.

D. Providing Preoperative and Postoperative Care for the Child.

1. See the section on the child undergoing surgery, page 1133.
2. Many children require gastric suction postoperatively to prevent distention or vomiting.
   a. See Guidelines: Nasogastric Intubation, page 464.
   b. Monitor gastric output accurately and replace it with appropriate IV fluids as prescribed by the physician.
   c. When oral feedings are resumed, begin with small amounts of clear fluids.
3. Continue to avoid abdominal manipulation, because cells may have escaped locally from the excised tumor.

E. Caring for the Child Receiving Radiation Therapy.

1. Radiation therapy is given to the tumor bed postoperatively to render nonviable all cells that have escaped locally from the excised tumor. It is usually indicated for all children with Wilms' tumor except those under 18 months of age with stage I disease.
2. Alterations in the growth and development of bones, joints, and musculature may occur as a result of radiation therapy.
3. Be aware that acute skin reactions occasionally occur when dactinomycin is given concomitantly with or following administration of radiation therapy.
4. See the section on radiation therapy, page 1478.

F. Caring for the Child Receiving Chemotherapy.

1. Chemotherapy is initiated postoperatively to achieve maximal killing of tumor cells.
2. The usual chemotherapeutic agents employed are actinomycin D, vincristine, and doxorubicin.
3. Prepare the child and his family for chemotherapy.
4. See the section on chemotherapy, page 1478.

G. Providing Diversional Therapy for the Child.

Provide the child with the opportunity for play as his condition permits.

H. Providing Supportive Care Appropriate for the Dying Child When the Tumor Metastasizes and the Child's Condition Deteriorates.

See the section on the dying child, page 1523.

Osteogenic Sarcoma

Osteogenic sarcoma is a malignant tumor of the bone.

Etiology

Unknown

Incidence

1. Most frequent malignant bone cancer in children.
2. Peak incidence between 10 and 25 years of age.
   a. Most common at the peak of the adolescent growth spurt.
   b. Males are affected more often than females, with a ratio of 1.5:1.
3. Common sites of occurrence—distal femur, proximal tibia, and proximal humerus. Less common sites include the pelvis, phalanges and jaw.

Altered Physiology

1. Presumably arises from bone-forming mesenchyme tissue.
2. Produces malignant spindle-cell stroma, which gives rise to malignant osteoid tissue.
3. Most osteogenic sarcomas are fully malignant, but may appear in relatively nonmalignant forms.
4. Most commonly metastasize to lungs and other bones.

Clinical Manifestations

1. Pain in the affected site, frequently causing limp or limitation of motion
2. Palpable, tender, fixed bony mass
3. Additional symptoms related to site of metastasis, if present

Diagnostic Evaluation

1. X-ray examination—to visualize the tumor
2. Serum alkaline phosphatase—often elevated but does not correlate reliably with extent of disease.
3. Bone scan—helpful in detecting initial extent of malignancy, planning therapy, and evaluating effects of treatment.
4. Biopsy of lesion—to confirm the diagnosis and provide histologic data for the selection of a treatment plan
5. Chest x-ray, tomography, or CT scan—to identify lung metastasis and to evaluate extent of primary tumor.
6. Renal and liver function tests—to screen for problems prior to initiating chemotherapy
7. MRI

Medical/Surgical Management

1. Radical amputation of the affected extremity, and often the joint proximal to the involved area, is required in most cases.
2. Newer techniques include transmedullary amputation and limb-salvaging surgery, such as total femur replacement.
3. Chemotherapy is advocated for 1–3 years following surgery. It is also used preoperatively for patients undergoing resectional surgery and for metastatic disease.

Prognosis

1. Survival has greatly improved with the aggressive use of multimodal therapy.
2. Approximately 50%–60% of patients who undergo surgery followed by chemotherapy can expect to be disease-free after 3 years.
3. Limb-saving surgery has improved the quality of life for many survivors.

Nursing Management

Nursing care of the child with osteogenic sarcoma is essentially the same as care of the adult. See page 805.

Points of emphasis:

1. The child must be prepared for diagnostic tests, surgery, and chemotherapy in ways that are appropriate for his age and level of development.
2. Radical body alterations caused by surgery and chemotherapy are especially upsetting for adolescents.
   a. They need time and support to accept the diagnosis and surgery, and to grieve for their lost body part.
   b. They can be helped to select clothing that camouflages the prosthesis yet is sexually appealing.
   c. Wigs, scarves, or hats are useful for children experiencing hair loss.
3. Discharge planning should be done to promote normalcy and resumption of appropriate presurgical activities.
   a. Accessibility of home and school should be assessed and environmental handicaps alleviated.
   b. The school nurse should be contacted to facilitate reentry into school.
   c. Visits by peers should be encouraged, and the child should be helped to deal with questions and reactions from peers.
   d. A tutor should be arranged for students who must remain out of school for lengthy periods.
   e. A community health nursing referral should be initiated if appropriate.
   f. See the Bibliography, page 1494, for additional references.
4. For nursing care of the hospitalized adolescent, see page 1124.
5. For nursing care of the child receiving chemotherapy, see page 1478.

Retinoblastoma

Retinoblastoma is a malignant, congenital tumor arising in the retina of one or both eyes.

Etiology

1. Unknown
2. Nonhereditary somatic mutations:
   a. Account for approximately 90% of all retinoblastomas.
   b. Always demonstrate unilateral involvement.
3. Hereditary germinal mutations:
   a. Account for approximately 10% of all retinoblastomas.
   b. May be bilateral or unilateral.
   c. Mode of inheritance is autosomal-dominant.
4. Can be associated with chromosomal aberrations.

Incidence

1. Relatively rare tumor, usually diagnosed in patients before 2 years of age.
2. Occurs in 1 in 18,000 live births, or approximately 200 children in the U.S. each year.
3. Incidence is increasing because of prolonged survival of affected children, with transmission of the tumor to their offspring, and increased exposure to mutagenic agents.

Altered Physiology

1. Retinoblastomas are malignant neuroblastic tumors that may arise in any of the nucleated retinal layers.

2. Usually arise in multiple foci rather than a single tumor.
3. Some tumors (endophytic type) arise in the internal nuclear layers of the retina and grow forward into the vitreous cavity.
4. Some tumors (exophytic type) arise in the external nuclear layer and grow into the subretinal space, with detachment of the retina.
5. Most tumors have a combination of endophytic and exophytic growth.
6. Extension of the tumor may occur into the choroid, the sclera, and optic nerve.
7. Hematogenous spread of the tumor may occur to the bone marrow, skeleton, lymph nodes, and liver.
8. Tumor staging reflects the extent of the disease and the probability of preserving useful vision in the affected eye, from group I = very favorable to group V = very unfavorable.

Clinical Manifestations

1. Signs and symptoms of an intraocular tumor depend on its size and position.
2. "Cat's eye reflex"—whitish appearance of the pupil, represents visualization of the tumor through the lens as light falls on the tumor mass—most common sign.
3. Strabismus—second most common presenting sign.
4. Other occasional presenting signs:
   a. Orbital inflammation
   b. Hyphema
   c. Fixed pupil
   d. Heterochromia iridis
5. Vision loss is not a symptom, as young children do not complain of unilaterally decreased vision.
6. Symptoms of distant metastasis—anorexia, weight loss, vomiting, headache

Diagnostic Evaluation

1. Careful history regarding visual changes and tumor occurrence in relatives
2. Bilateral indirect ophthalmoscopy under general anesthesia
3. Skull x-ray
4. CT scan
5. MRI
6. Determinations of lactic acid dehydrogenase (LDH) isoenzymes in the aqueous humor—not routinely done.
7. Bone marrow aspiration and lumbar puncture during ophthalmologic examination under anesthesia.

Treatment

1. Depends on the stage of the disease at the time of diagnosis.
2. Unilateral tumors in stages I, II, or III are usually treated with external beam irradiation.
   a. Goal of treatment is to eradicate the tumor(s) and preserve useful vision.
   b. Radiation is usually administered over a period of 3–4 weeks.
3. Surgery (enucleation) is the treatment of choice for advanced tumor growth, especially with optic nerve involvement.
4. Bilateral disease often requires enucleation of the severely diseased eye and irradiation of the least affected eye.
   a. Every attempt is made to salvage whatever vision there may be.
   b. Bilateral enucleation is indicated with extensive bilateral retinoblastoma where there is no hope of vision.
5. Radioactive applicators, light coagulation, and cryotherapy are sometimes used to treat small, localized tumors.
6. Chemotherapy is used for cases of extraocular disease: regional or distant metastases.
   Drugs commonly used include cyclophosphamide, vincristine, actinomycin D, doxorubicin, ifosfamide, cisplatin, and VM-26.

Prognosis

1. Overall survival rate is high (90%).
2. Heritable retinoblastoma and bilateral retinoblastoma are associated with a high incidence of spontaneous and radiation-related new tumors, particularly sarcomas.

Patient Problems and Nursing Diagnoses

1. Parental guilt related to the genetic implications of the diagnosis
2. Parental anxiety related to the nature of the diagnosis and treatment
3. Potential side effects of radiation (skin changes, loss of lashes, fat atrophy, impaired bone growth, dry eye)
4. Self-concept, disturbance in body image and ineffective coping, related to enucleation and need for an eye prosthesis
5. Anxiety of the child related to hospitalization and to diagnostic and treatment procedures
6. Parental knowledge deficit regarding retinoblastoma and its treatment

Nursing Interventions

A. Providing Emotional Support to the Parents at the Time the Diagnosis Is Made.

1. The parents often feel guilty about transmitting the disease to the child or because they did not notice the symptoms earlier.
2. The parents may exhibit anger toward one another or the physicians for ignoring parental remarks or postponing a thorough examination.

B. Caring for the Child Receiving Radiation Therapy.

1. Sedate the child as requested by the physician.
   a. Administer the medication in a timely manner so that sedation is adequate for current positioning of the child.
   b. Observe for possible side effects of irradiation and prepare the parents for their occurrence.
      (1) Skin changes at the temples
         (a) Use soap sparingly in these areas.
         (b) Avoid exposure to the sun.
         (c) Apply a nonirritating lubricant.
      (2) Loss of lashes
      (3) Fat atrophy with ptosis
      (4) Delayed wound healing
      (5) Dry eye
      (6) Permanent radiation dermatitis
      (7) Impaired bone growth

C. Providing Preoperative Care for the Child.

1. Encourage the parents to "room-in" and participate in the child's care to minimize separation anxiety.

2. Prepare the child and parents for all diagnostic procedures.
3. Describe the surgery and anticipated postoperative appearance of the child.
   a. The parents should be reassured that the operation is not extremely bloody or mutilating.
   b. All adnexal structures of the eye are left intact.
   c. A surgically implanted sphere maintains the shape of the eyeball.
   d. The child's face may be edematous and ecchymotic.
   e. A small dressing is used to cover the site.
4. Offer the family the opportunity to talk with another parent who has gone through the experience or to see pictures of another child with an artificial eye.
5. See nursing management of the child undergoing eye surgery, page 1412.

D. Providing Postoperative Care for the Child.

1. Change the dressing and cleanse the operative site as requested by the physician.
2. Encourage the parents to see the socket and participate in dressing changes soon after the surgery, as they will need to do this after discharge.
3. See nursing management of the child undergoing eye surgery, page 1412.

E. Caring for the Child Receiving Chemotherapy.

See the section on chemotherapy, page 1478.

F. Encouraging the Parents to Seek Genetic Counseling.

1. Discuss the benefit of consultation about the probability of having another affected child.
   a. Risk ranges from approximately 1%–10%, depending on family history and whether the affected child had unilateral or bilateral disease.
   b. The reportedly high lifelong cancer burden among retinoblastoma patients may also be important to parents in making informed decisions.
   c. Support parental decisions regarding future pregnancies.

2. Encourage the parents to seek genetic counseling for the affected child when he reaches puberty.
   a. The risk to his offspring is from 1%–50%, depending on family history and whether he had unilateral or bilateral disease.
   b. Among his affected offspring, there is a high probability (>50%) of bilateral disease.

Health Education

The parents should receive instruction concerning:
1. Care of the socket
2. Care of the prosthesis—initial instructions are provided by the ocularist and should be reinforced by the nurse.
3. Protection of the remaining eye from accidental injury.
4. Coping with limited vision, loss of peripheral vision, or blindness (see the section on childhood blindness, p. 1408)
5. Need to have subsequent children carefully evaluated for retinoblastoma.
   a. An ophthalmologic examination under anesthesia is usually recommended at about 2 months of age.
   b. The child should receive frequent examinations thereafter until he is judged safe from developing retinoblastoma, usually about age 3 years.

Expected Outcomes

1. The parents participate in genetic counseling.
2. The parents have an opportunity to discuss their feelings about retinoblastoma and its treatment and to express any sense of guilt they might have.
3. The child deals with side effects of radiation therapy—skin changes, possible ptosis, loss of lashes
4. Develops and maintains a positive body image—accepts the presence of the prosthesis and is not inhibited in his behavior
5. The child demonstrates lessened anxiety by his ability to participate in age-appropriate activities
6. The parents gain an understanding of retinoblastoma and its treatment, as reflected in their conversation and participation in the child's care.

Bibliography

Books

Chesler M and Barbarin O. Childhood Cancer and the Family. New York, Brunner/Mazel, 1987

DeVita V, Hellman S and Rosenberg S (eds). Cancer Principles and Practice of Oncology. Philadelphia, JB Lippincott, 1985

Fochtman D and Foley G (eds). Nursing Care of the Child with Cancer. Boston, Little, Brown & Co, 1984

Hockenberry M and Coody D. Pediatric Oncology and Hematology. St. Louis, CV Mosby, 1986

Johnson B and Gross J (eds). Handbook of Oncology Nursing. New York, John Wiley & Sons, 1985

Koocher G and O'Malley J. The Damocles Syndrome: Psychosocial Consequences of Surviving Childhood Cancer. New York, McGraw-Hill, 1981

Kubler-Ross E. On Children and Death. New York, Macmillan, 1983

Pizzo P and Poplack D (eds). Principles and Practice of Pediatric Oncology. Philadelphia, JB Lippincott, 1989

Schulman J and Kupst M. The Child with Cancer: Clinical Approaches to Psychosocial Care: Research in Psychosocial Aspects. Springfield, IL, Charles C Thomas, 1980

Spinetta J, Deasy-Spinetta P and Brandt S (eds). Living with Childhood Cancer. St Louis, CV Mosby, 1981

Tiffany R (ed). Oncology for Nurses and Health Care Professionals, Vol 1–3. London, Harper and Row, 1988

van Eys J. Cancer in the Very Young. Springfield, IL, Charles C Thomas, 1989

Journals

Barry S. Septic shock: Special needs of patients with cancer. Oncol Nurs Forum 1989 Jan–Feb; 16(1):31–35

Battista E. Educational needs of the adolescent with cancer and his family. Semin Oncol Nurs 1986; 2(2):123–125

Bellert J. Humor: A therapeutic approach in oncology nursing. Cancer Nurs 1989 Apr; 12(2):65–70

Blotcky A. Helping adolescents with cancer cope with their disease. Semin Oncol Nurs 1986; 2(2):117–122

Bonner K et al. Pathology, treatment and management of posterior fossa brain tumors in childhood. J Neurosci Nurs 1988 Apr; 20(2):84–93

Brown P. Families who have a child diagnosed with cancer: What the medical caregiver can do to help them and themselves. Issues Compre Pediatr Nurs 1989; 12(2–3):247–260

Buschsel P and Kelleher J. Bone marrow transplantation. Nurs Clin North Am 1989 Dec; 24(4):907–938

Burnham N and Betcher D. Pharmacology: Ifosfamide. J Pediatr Oncol Nurs 1987; 4(3–4):47–50

Cersosimo R. Update on acute leukemia. J Prac Nurs 1988; 38(3):49–59

Chekryn J et al. Normalizing the return

to school of the child with cancer. J Pediatr Oncol Nurs 1986; 3(2):20–24

Cogliano-Shutta N. Pediatric phase I clinical trials: Ethical issues and nursing considerations . . . Beneficence, autonomy and justice. Oncol Nurs Forum 1986 Mar–Apr; 13(2):29–32

Cohen D. Emergencies in the pediatric oncology patient. J Pediatr Oncol Nurs 1987; 4(3–4):5–6

Consalvo K et al. Winning the battle against Hodgkin's disease. RN 1986 Dec; 49(12):20–25

Coody D. High expectations: Nurses who work with children who might die. Nurs Clin North Am 1985 Mar; 20(1): 131–142

D'Angio G. Cure is not enough: Late consequences associated with radiation treatment. J Pediatr Oncol Nurs 1988; 5(4):20–23

Davis K. Educational needs of the terminally ill student. Issues Compre Pediatr Nurs 1989; 12(2–3):235–245

Dothage J et al. Use of a continuous intravenous morphine infusion for pain control in an infant with terminal malignancy. J Pediatr Oncol Nurs 1986; 3(4):22–24

Dreyer K. The special problems of childhood leukemia. RN 1986 Nov; 49(11):37

Dudjak L. Mouth care for mucositis due to radiation therapy. Cancer Nurs 1987 Jun; 10(3):131–140

Dunne C. Safe handling of antineoplastic agents: Self learning module. Cancer Nurs 1989 Apr; 12(2):120–127

Eland J. Pharmacologic management of acute and chronic pediatric pain. Issues Compre Pediatr Nurs 1988 Mar–Jun; 11(2–3):93–111

Fergusson J and Hobbie W. Home visits for the child with cancer. Nurs Clin North Am 1985 Mar; 20(1):109–115

Fergusson J et al. The effects of the treatment for cancer in childhood on growth and development. J Pediatr Oncol Nurs 1986; 3(4):13–21

Gallucci B. The immune system and cancer. Oncol Nurs Forum (suppl) 1987 Nov–Dec; 14(6):3–12

Gauvain-Piquard A et al. Pain in children aged 2–6 years: New observational rating scale elaborated in a pediatric oncology unit—Preliminary report. Pain 1987 Nov; 31(2):177–188

Gibbons M and Boren H. Stress reduction: A spectrum of strategies in pediatric oncology nursing. Nurs Clin North Am 1985 Mar; 20(1):83–103

Goodell A. Peer education in school for children with cancer. Issues Compre Pediatr Nurs 1984; 7:101–106

Gray E. The emotional and play needs of the dying child. Issues Compre Pediatr Nurs 1989; 12(2–3):207–224

Gyulay J. Grief responses. Issues Compre Pediatr Nurs 1989; 12(1):1–31

Gyulay J. Home care for the dying child. Issues Compre Pediatr Nurs 1989; 12(1):33–69

Hammond E. Anaphylactic reactions to chemotherapeutic agents. J Pediatr Oncol Nurs 1988; 5(3):16–19

Hammond E. Herpes-zoster infections in children with Hodgkin's disease. J Pediatr Oncol Nurs 1987; 4(1–2):23–29

Happ M. Life threatening hemorrhage in children with cancer. J Pediatr Oncol Nurs 1987; 4(3–4):36–40

Hathaway G et al. Autologous bone marrow transplantation in childhood cancer. Pediatr Nurs 1988 Nov–Dec; 14(6):454–456

Heiney S. Adolescents with cancer: Sexual and reproductive issues. Cancer Nurs 1989 Apr; 12(2):95–101

Heiney S et al. Effects of group on parents of children with cancer. J Pediatr Oncol Nurs 1989 Jul; 6(3):63–69

Hinds P et al. Nursing strategies to influence adolescent hopefulness during oncologic illness. J Pediatr Oncol Nurs 1987; 4(1–2):14–22

Hockenberry M and Contanch P. Hypnosis as adjuvant antiemetic therapy in childhood cancer. Nurs Clinics North Am 1985 Mar; 20(1):105–107

Hockenberry M. Relaxation techniques in children with cancer: The nurse's role. J Pediatr Oncol Nurs 1988; 5(1–2):7–11

Hockenberry M et al. Limb salvage procedures in children with osteosarcoma. Cancer Nurs 1988 Feb; 11(1):2–8

Kazak A. Psychological issues in childhood cancer survivors. J Pediatr Oncol Nurs 1989; 6(1):15–16

Kinrade L. Preparation of sibling donor for bone marrow transplant harvest procedure. Cancer Nurs 1987 Apr; 10(2):77–81

Klopovich P et al. Sexuality and the adolescent with cancer. Semin Oncol Nurs 1985; 1(1):42–48

Konradi D. A closeup look at leukemia. Nursing 1989 Jun; 19(6):34–42

Kramer R and Perin G. Patient education and pediatric oncology. Nurs Clin North Am 1985 Mar; 20(1):31–48

Lawson K. Oral–dental concerns of the pediatric oncology patient. Issues Compre Pediatr Nurs 1989; 12(2–3):199–206

Leahy N. Intraarterial cisplatin infusion: Nursing implications. J Neurosci Nurs 1986 Oct; 18(5):296–301

Leonard M et al. Late effects in adolescent survivors of childhood cancer. Semin Oncol Nurs; 2(2):126–132

Lydon J. Assessment of renal function in the patient receiving chemotherapy. Cancer Nurs 1989 Jun; 12(3):133–143

McCalla J. A multidisciplinary approach to identification and remedial intervention for adverse late effects of cancer therapy. Nurs Clin North Am 1985 Mar; 20(1):117–130

Mason C. Septic shock. J Pediatr Oncol Nurs 1987; 4(3–4):25–31

Meadows A. Second malignant neoplasms in childhood cancer survivors. J Pediatr Oncol Nurs 1989; 6(1):7–11

Meehan J. Pain control in the terminally

child at home. Issues Compre Pediatr Nurs 1989; 12(2–3):187–197

Meeske K et al. Cancer chemotherapy in children: Nursing issues and approaches. Semin Oncol Nurs 1987; 3(2):118–27

Metz E et al. Update on Hodgkin's disease. Hosp Med 1987 Apr; 23(4):78, 81, 85

Moore I et al. Late effects of central nervous system prophylactic leukemia therapy on cognitive functioning. Oncol Nurs Forum 1986; 13(4):45–51

Moore I et al. Care of the family with a child with cancer: Diagnoses and early stages of treatment: Part 1. Oncol Nurs Forum 1986 Sept–Oct; 13(5):60–66

Moshang T et al. Late effects: Disorders of growth and sexual maturation associated with the treatment of childhood cancer. J Pediatr Oncol Nurs 1988; 5(4):14–19

Niehaus C et al. Oral complications in children during cancer therapy. Cancer Nurs 1987 Feb; 10(1):15–20

Nirenberg A et al. Malignancies in adolescents. Semin Oncol Nurs 1986; 2(2):75–83

Olson R et al. Compliance with treatment regimens . . . adolescent cancer patients. Semin Oncol Nurs 1986; 2(2):104–111

Pack B et al. Neurological emergencies in pediatric oncology. J Pediatr Oncol Nurs 1987; 4(3–4):8–18

Patterson K et al. Metabolic emergencies in pediatric oncology: The acute tumor lysis syndrome. J Pediatr Oncol Nurs 1987; 4(3–4):19–24

Peakham V et al. Educational late effects in longterm survivors of childhood acute lymphocytic leukemia. Pediatrics 1988; 81(1):127–133

Peters C. Myths of antiemetic administration. Cancer Nurs 1989 Apr; 12(2):102–106

Pizzo P. Management of pediatric cancer. Hosp Pract 1986 Mar 15; 21(3):111–116, 118, 124–126

Poe C et al. Syndrome of IADH: Assessment and nursing implications. Oncol Nurs Forum 1989 May–Jun; 16(3):373–381

Pope N. Nursing care of patients receiving high dose Ara-C. Dimensions of Oncology Nursing 1988 Winter; 2(4):15–19

Riley-Lawless K. School reentry programs. J Pediatr Oncol Nurs 1989 Jul; 6(3):92–93

Rose M. Health promotion and risk prevention: Applications for cancer survivors. Oncol Nurs Forum 1989 May–Jun; 16(3):335–40

Sommer D. The spiritual needs of dying children. Issues Compre Pediatr Nurs 1989; 12(2–3):225–233

Stagner S. Congenital leukemia: An overview. J Pediatr Oncol Nurs 1986; 3(1):19–22

Sticklin L et al. Nursing care of the patient receiving subcutaneous low dose Ara-C therapy (teaching materials). Oncol Nurs Forum 1989 May–Jun; 16(3):365–369

Thurber W. Offspring of childhood cancer survivors. J Pediatr Oncol Nurs 1989; 6(1):17–19

Van der Wal R et al. Bone marrow transplant in children: Nursing management of late effects. Cancer Nurs 1988 Jun; 11(3):132–143

Walker E. Hyperglycemia: A complication of chemotherapy in children. Cancer Nurs 1988; 11(1):18–22

Waskerwitz M. Communication with the school teacher. J Pediatr Oncol Nurs 1987; 4(3–4):41–43

Waskerwitz M et al. Early detection of malignancy: From birth to 20 years. Oncol Nurs Forum 1986 Jan–Feb; 13(1):50–57

Weekes D et al. Adolescent cancer: Coping with treatment related pain. J Pediatr Oncol Nurs 1988 Oct; 3(5): 318–328

Welch-McCaffrey D. Metastatic bone cancer. Cancer Nurs 1988 Apr; 11(2): 103–111

Wickham R. Managing chemotherapy-related nausea and vomiting: The state of the art. Oncol Nurs Forum 1989 Jul–Aug; 16(4):563–574

Young J et al. Radiation treatment for the child with cancer. Issues in Comprehensive Pediatric Nursing 1989; 12(2–3):159–169

Additional References/Agencies

American Cancer Society
90 Park Avenue
New York, NY 10016

Association for Brain Tumor Research
3725 N. Talman Ave.
Chicago, IL 60618

Bombeck E. I want to grow hair, I want to grow up, I want to go to Boise. New York, Harper and Row, 1989

Candlelighters Foundation
2025 Eye Street, NW
Suite 1011
Washington, DC 20006

Center for Attitudinal Healing
19 Main Street
Tiburon, CA 94920

Copeland D, Copeland K and Pfferbaum B. The Andy Anderson Coloring Book. University of Texas System Cancer Center. M. D. Anderson Hospital and Tumor Institute, Parent Education Program, 6723 Bertner Avenue, Houston, TX 77030 (available in Spanish)

Gaes J. My Book for Kids with Cansur. Aberdeen, SD, Melius and Peterson, 1987

Standards of Oncology Nursing Practice. ANA Publication. 1987 #MS-16:1-28

US Department of Health and Human Services
Public Health Service
National Institutes of Health
Office of Cancer Communications
National Cancer Institute
Bethesda, MD 20892

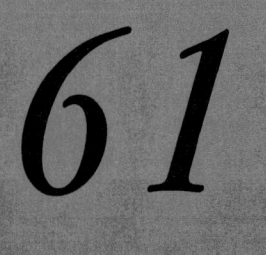

61 The Child at Risk—Special Pediatric Problems

Genetic Alterations

The term *genetic alterations* refers to disorders and chronic conditions resulting from genetic and chromosomal make-up, expression, and division. It encompasses the human concerns related to the risk and occurrence of the disorders.

Physiologic Principles

1. Chromosomes
   a. Occur in pairs: 22 pairs of autosomal and one pair of sex chromosomes.
   b. These 46 chromosomes are found in every cell nucleus and are in the shape of an "X."
   c. Each chromosome consists of DNA in a double helix.
   d. Segments of DNA are referred to as genes, which are the basic units of heredity.
2. Genes
   a. Each individual receives one gene from each parent for the same trait.
   b. *Homozygous* (alleles) refers to receiving the same gene from both parents (e.g., eye color); *heterozygous* refers to receiving different alleles for the same trait.
3. Genotype
   a. The genetic make-up of a chromosome; order and purpose/function of genes.
4. Karotype
   a. Quality and quantity of chromosomes; includes genotype.
5. Phenotype
   a. Physical, biochemical, and physiologic nature of an individual.
   b. Outward visible expression of genes.
   c. Genotype cannot be predicted from phenotype.
6. Normal cell division
   a. Mitosis occurs in all autosomal cells resulting in the formation of a cell identical to the original cell, with the same 46 chromosomes.
   b. Meiosis (reduction division) occurs in germ cells where each chromosomal pair provides only one chromosome, resulting in a gamete containing 23 chromosomes (one from each pair): one set in the egg and one set in the sperm.

Etiology

1. Genetic traits are passed to the child from one or both of the parents; traits are inherited by one or more genes
2. *Nondisjunction*
   a. Altered cell division resulting in failure of a pair of homologous chromosomes from either parent to separate during meiosis
   b. Results in the child receiving either 3 chromosomes on the same "pair" (total is 47 chromosomes) or receiving only one chromosome on a "pair" (total is 45 chromosomes and can only occur if a sex-linked chromosome is missing); three chromosomes on one pair is referred to as a *trisomy*
3. *Translocation*—altered cell division resulting from a chromosome breaking; parts of the chromosome break off and may attach to other chromosomes, or genes may switch their order or spacing
4. Many cases have no known cause

Classification

1. Autosomal dominant
   a. Only one parent has to pass the defective gene or set of genes
   b. If one parent carries the gene, the child has a 50% chance of receiving that gene (and the disorder) at conception
   c. Examples include Huntington's disease, Marfan's syndrome, osteogenesis imperfecta, neurofibromatosis
2. Autosomal recessive
   a. Both parents must carry the defective gene and both must pass it to the child
   b. With each pregnancy, the risk is a 25% chance the child will have the disease or condition, a 50% chance the child will be a carrier, and a 25% chance the child will not be affected
   c. Examples (and the chromosome that is affected) include cystic fibrosis (number 7), sickle cell disease (number 11), phenylketonuria (number 12), and Tay–Sachs disease (number 15)
3. Sex-linked (X-linked) disorders
   a. Are passed only on the X of the sex chromosome (the 23rd pair)
   b. Females have a second X and therefore are not affected by these conditions because the healthy

X prevails; the male Y is small and cannot oppose the affected X

c. These conditions are seen only in males
d. A father cannot pass the gene to his son, but he can pass it to all of his daughters, resulting in their being carriers
e. A carrier mother has a 50% chance of passing the gene to her sons, who will have the disease or condition and a 50% chance of making their daughter a carrier
f. Examples include color blindness, hemophilia A, Duchenne muscular dystrophy, glucose 6-phosphate dehydrogenase (G6PD) deficiency, and baldness

Indications for Prenatal Diagnosis of Genetic Disorders

1. Increased risk of chromosomal disorders
   a. Advanced maternal age—woman 35 years of age or older
   b. Parent known to be a carrier of chromosomal disorder
   c. Previous pregnancy resulting in child with chromosomal disorder
   d. Previous multiple congenital anomalies—when no cytogenetic analysis was done
   e. History of spontaneous abortions
2. Known risk for significant metabolic disorders
3. Known risk for significant sex-linked genetic disorders
4. Willingness to consider termination of the pregnancy if an abnormal fetus is detected

Prenatal Diagnosis of Genetic Disorders

Genetic screening provides information for identifying cases of treatable diseases before irreversible damage has taken place, provides reproductive options, and facilitates research.

A. Amniocentesis (see p. 979)

1. Method of obtaining amniotic fluid of a pregnant woman by inserting a needle transabdominally through the uterus.
2. Examination is made of amniotic fluid, amniotic fluid cells, and cultured amniotic fluid cells.
3. Procedure done at 12–16 weeks' gestation; results take 2–3 weeks
4. Useful in diagnosing some inborn errors of metabolism and chromosome abnormalities
5. Risk of miscarriage is less than 1%.

B. Chorionic Villus Sampling

1. Small piece of fetal portion of placenta is removed
2. Can be performed as early as 9 weeks; results take 24 hours
3. Can be tested for genetic and chromosomal conditions
4. Risk of miscarriage and post-test infection is 1% to 2%

C. Ultrasonography

1. Sound frequencies, when applied to the body, reflect back when they meet boundaries and between tissues of different densities, thus outlining anatomic structures.
2. Best performed at 16–18 weeks to check fetal structures.
3. Used to determine the size of the fetus and the fetal head; to locate the placenta and fetus prior to amniocentesis; to identify multiple gestation, neural tube defects (anencephaly, meningocele, hydrocephalus),

sternal agenesis, enlarged cystic kidneys, and some skeletal abnormalities; and to determine accurately gestational age.

D. Controversial Testing

1. Magnetic resonance imaging (MRI)
   a. A noninvasive procedure that provides quality pictures of soft-tissue structures
   b. No ionizing radiation is used
2. Amniography–Fetography
   a. A technique of intra-amniotic injection of a contrast material, which opacifies the fluid and adheres to fetal skin; is swallowed by fetus
   b. Useful in diagnosing, intrauterine growth retardation, and multiple gestation.
   c. This test uses ionizing radiation and is therefore a high-risk procedure.
3. Fetoscope
   a. Visualization of fetus in utero by endoscopic instruments
   b. Provides tissue sampling
      (1) Fetal blood for thalassemia, hemophilia, chronic granulomatous diseases, sickle cell anemia, and muscular dystrophy.
      (2) Fetal skin biopsy for ichthyosiform erythroderma and epidermolysis bullosa.
   c. Risks to the fetus (premature labor) range from 3% to 10%.

Genetic Counseling

Genetic counseling is the process of providing families with information about hereditary and congenital disorders. It involves determining the risk of occurrence or recurrence, interpreting the findings, and assisting the family in making a reasonable decision.

Parental Barriers to Counseling

1. Lack of knowledge or misinformation
2. Social and/or psychological implications
3. Cultural–religious beliefs
4. Financial

Goals of Genetic Counseling

1. To provide clients with information about the genetic defect in question. Identifies risks and provides information regarding severity of condition.
2. To communicate to clients the risk of transmitting the defect to subsequently conceived children.
3. To enable individuals and couples to make informed decisions regarding marriage and/or parenthood (e.g., having children, adopting children, continuing or terminating an existing pregnancy).
4. To provide psychological support to assist clients with their decision-making process and the necessary reordering of their lives.
5. To reduce the number of individuals affected by genetic disease.
6. To alert other health professionals involved with the family of the possibility of genetic disease in the family background.

Major Genetic Disorders

See Table 61-1.

Table 61-1. *Common Genetic Disorders*

Type	Incidence	Characteristics	Risk	Discussion
Chromosomal Disorders				
1. Autosomal abnormalities Down syndrome (trisomy 21) (see p. 1507)	1 in 600–800 live births; varies with maternal age; meiotic nondisjunction Young mother: 1 in 1000 live births Mother over 35: 1 in 300 live births	Brachycephalic skull; oblique palpebral fissures; epicanthal folds; Brushfield's spots; flat nasal bridge; protruding, fissured tongue; growth retardation; short extremities; dry, scaly skin; clinodactyly and simian line; mental retardation; congenital heart disease	Insufficient data Spontaneous abortion rates are high (10%–60%)	Chromosomal disorders result from: 1. Failure of a chromosome to separate at cell division (nondisjunction), causing loss or gain of genetic material 2. Results in 47 chromosomes
2. Sex chromosome abnormalities Klinefelter's syndrome (XXY abnormality)	1 in 500–1000 male live births	Diagnosis is rare before puberty; mentally retarded (mild); body may be tall, slim, and underweight; small testes; gynecomastia; pubertal development delayed; azoospermia and infertility; psychosocial, learning, or school adjustment problems		1. Due to nondisjunction 2. Results in 47 chromosomes
Turner's syndrome (X abnormality; also monosomy sex chromosome, applies to phenotype female with genotype 45; XO)	1 in 1500–3000 female live births	Low hairline; micrognathia; short stature; webbed neck; infantile external genitalia; underdeveloped breasts; widely spaced nipples; primary amenorrhea; lymphedema of hands and feet during infancy; learning disabled		Results in 45 chromosomes
Mendelian Disorders—Single Gene				
1. Autosomal dominant Achondroplasia, classic	1 in 10,000 live births	Brachycephaly; frontal bossing; depressed nasal bridge; dwarfism; short extremities; lumbar lordosis; bowed legs; pelvic tilt	Usually sporadic occurrence: affected parent has a 50% chance of having affected offspring with each pregnancy.	Mendelian inheritance: A single deleterious gene can cause multiple anomalies or isolated malformations.
Skeletal disorders (e.g., syndactyly)				

2. Autosomal recessive
    Sickle cell anemia*
    Cystic fibrosis*
	1 in 400 live births of blacks
	1 in 1800 live births (predominantly white)
			Risk of affected parent having affected offspring is 25% per pregnancy; 50% carrier state	

Tay–Sachs disease	50 live births per year (occurs mainly in Jewish children)	Lack of CNS maturation; impaired motor development; cherry-red spot on eyes; early death		Carrier can be identified.

(continued)

Table 61-1. *Common Genetic Disorders (continued)*

Type	Incidence	Characteristics	Risk	Discussion
3. Sex-linked recessive Glucose 6-phosphate dehydrogenase (G6PD)	10%–14% of male live births in blacks 24% of female live births in blacks		If affected male reproduces, offspring will be as follows: males are normal; females are carriers. Unaffected female carrier offspring: 50% male affected 50% male normal 50% female carrier 50% female normal	Sex-linked disorders occur mainly in males, although the female is the carrier. Most sex-linked disorders are recessive.
Duchenne's muscular dystrophy	1 in 7000 live births	Onset in early childhood; muscles seem well-developed but weak; slow to walk and climb—no gross motor milestones; Gower's sign (when in sitting position will climb up legs to stand)		
Multifactorial-Polygenic Disorders				
Neural tube defects* (myelomeningocele)	0.2–4.2 in 1000 live births		Risk varies with racial background. Recurrence risk is usually 2%–7% but is related to outcome of previous pregnancies	Polygenic disorders are probably the result of several deleterious genes combined with environmental factors.
Cleft lip and cleft palate*	1 in 1000 live births			These disorders are difficult to prove, because they are mainly the result of slight variation at multiple gene loci.
Pyloric stenosis*	1 in 200–300 male live births 1 in 1000 female live births			

* See text under the specific subject.

Nursing Interventions

A. Identifying Families Who Need Genetic Counseling and to Whom the Service Should Be Offered.

1. Be alert to information in the family history that would indicate referral for genetic counseling (e.g., exposure to environmental agents, multiple miscarriages, infertility)
2. Be aware of evidence of deviation from normal growth and development and of other abnormalities (e.g., a single umbilical artery, low-set ears, or defects of the genitalia) that may indicate genetic problems.
3. Offer the opportunity for counseling to any family that has a child with a known genetic problem.

B. Supporting Family Through the Process of Genetic Testing.

1. Use active listening.
2. Prepare parents for tests with knowledge about the procedure, what the test is for, how long it takes, how the test is done, and how long it takes until the results are ready.
3. Promote confidentiality of information.

4. Consider and be sensitive to the family's cultural beliefs—if the purpose of testing is to make a decision regarding termination of pregnancy and that is not part of the family's beliefs, other choices should be made.
5. Allay parental anxieties regarding testing.

C. Assisting Families to Acquire Sufficient and Correct Information About the Genetic Problem in Question.

1. Provide accurate and current information related to the identified problem.
2. Be knowledgeable about the types of genetic disorders and their probability of occurrence (see Table 61-1).
3. Inform parents of reproductive risk for future children.
4. Refer for genetic counseling.

D. Serving as a Liaison Between the Genetic Counselor and the Family.

Note: In some situations, the nurse acts as the counselor.

1. Prepare parents for the experience of counseling. Help them know what to anticipate to lower their anxiety level and to make the counseling sessions a better experience.

2. If possible, attend the counseling session. This facilitates reinforcement of information and makes it easier to answer questions adequately.
3. Assess the family's need for additional counseling sessions, and initiate these if the need is recognized.

E. Helping Families Handle the Information Received and Guiding Them in Coping With This Crisis in Their Lives.

1. Utilize interviewing skills to facilitate discussion regarding parental feelings.
   Consider factors such as timing and privacy.
2. Alleviate parental feelings of guilt and shame.
   a. If a recessive trait is involved, both parents may blame themselves. Parents who are carriers of a dominant anomaly may blame themselves, and the other parent may blame them as well even if she or he does not outwardly express these feelings.
   b. Emphasize that a person has no choice or responsibility in acquiring the genes that cause the problem. Assess whether parents view this child to be a curse from God or a result of their misdeeds or of their inability to produce a "perfect" child.
   c. Reassure the parents that information gathered is important for determining an accurate diagnosis and the nature of inheritance; assure them that it will be kept confidential.
   d. It may be helpful to inform the parents that many other people have hidden, recessive genes.
3. Anticipate parental questions and areas of difficulty and conflict.
   a. Many parents are afraid to ask questions. They may fear they will sound stupid or they may not know how or what to ask.
   b. Listen carefully for parental areas of unanswered or unasked questions.
   c. Help parents formulate questions. Use statements such as, "Many parents have questions about—."
   d. Be available to parents when they have something to ask.
4. Remain objective.
   a. Be aware of personal feelings about specific genetic disorders.
   b. Come to terms with your own emotional difficulty related to genetic disorders and issues such as abortion.
   c. Avoid letting personal reactions affect your attitude toward counseling and behavior toward the family.
      (1) If the nurse avoids the situation, parents are tacitly given professional sanction to do the same thing.
      (2) A nurse who conveys the impression that she cannot cope with the presence of genetic disease is unlikely to convey assurance that a family should be able to cope with the consequences of the disease.
5. Reinforce information about the genetic disorder: probability, possible interventions to correct the defect or minimize the disability, self-care goals, and limitations requiring adaptation.
   a. Frequently parents do not understand the meaning of the risk ratio quoted to them, or they may attach too much or too little importance to it.
   b. Be certain that parents understand specifically what the predictions imply.
   c. Provide information at the parents' cognitive level.
6. Clarify understanding of all family members. Have both parents present for discussions as frequently as possible to prevent misinterpretations and distortions from being passed from one to the other. Include grandparents and siblings as appropriate.
7. Assist the parents to evaluate the total situation and to see the ramifications of any decision they may make.
   a. Facilitate realistic assessment of the expected burden to the parents, the child, and society; have them evaluate their capacity for dealing with the situation and expected problems.
   b. Assure parents that they do not have to rush into a decision.
8. Provide psychological support to allow parents to make and carry out decisions.
   a. Parents who decide against having children should be given information about contraception and sterilization.
   b. Parents who elect pregnancy should be informed about appropriate techniques of prenatal diagnosis of genetic disorders.
   c. Parents who elect adoption should be given the opportunity for additional advice when the adoption is being undertaken.

F. Ensuring Continued and Comprehensive Nursing Care for the Affected Child and the Family.

1. Continue to educate parents about the defect the child may have. Even though they may have received genetic counseling, if they have a child with the defect they may not fully understand what it is and what it means.
2. To be more effective in supporting parents after the birth of an affected baby, it is important to understand the phases of adjustment they go through.
   a. Shock and disorganization—denial of the infant's defect while dealing with their own emotions
   b. Adjustment—partial acceptance along with anger
   c. Reintegration—resumption of effective and realistic functioning
3. Complete necessary referrals to appropriate professionals and to community resources. These may include infant stimulation programs, preschool programs, parent groups, social service agencies, and other similar resources.
4. Promote child's growth and development.
5. Reinforce family strengths.
6. Promote adaptation and autonomy of both the child and parents.
7. Enhance self-image and self-worth of both the child and parents.
8. Coordinate home care and therapy.
9. Parents need a resource readily available to help them in time of crisis.
   a. Supply information about community resources, providing telephone numbers and office hours.
   b. Written material should provide information regarding the clinical course of the genetic disorder, recurrent risk factors, etc.

Health Education

1. Provide information regarding known genetic risk factors to the general public.*

---

* Professional Education Department, March of Dimes Birth Defects Foundation, 1275 Mamaroneck Avenue, White Plains, NY 10605 (for information on location of genetic services)
National Clearinghouse for Maternal and Child Health, 3520 Prospect Street, NW, Suite 1, Washington, DC 20057 (centralized source of materials and information in the area of human genetics and child health)

a. Support the concept of premarital counseling.
b. Support prenatal counseling to increase awareness of potential hazards of infections such as rubella, of the impact of drugs on the fetus, and of pollution of water and foodstuffs by pesticides and fertilizers.
2. Encourage routine newborn screening.
3. Follow up on positive newborn screening results.
4. Test siblings, where appropriate.

Mental Retardation

Mental retardation refers to significantly subaverage general intellectual functioning existing concurrently with deficits in adaptive behavior and manifested during the developmental period.*

Etiology

A. General

1. There are over 250 causes of mental retardation.
2. General causes include:
   a. Congenital lack of brain cells
   b. Later destruction of cells originally present
   c. Altered neurologic pathways and structural development
   d. Altered metabolic processes

B. Prenatal Factors

1. Chromosomal/genetic abnormalities
2. Fetal irradiation
3. Infection—maternal or fetal (TORCH conditions: *t*oxoplasmosis, *o*ther [viruses], *r*ubella, *c*ytomegalovirus, *h*erpes [simplex viruses])
4. Anoxia
5. Cranial anomalies
   a. Hydrocephalus
   b. Craniosynostosis
   c. Microcephaly
6. Maternal nutrition
7. Maternal use or abuse of drugs/medications and alcohol
8. Maternal cigarette smoking
9. Parental age (debatable)

C. Natal Factors

1. Anoxia
   a. Maternal
   b. Placental
   c. Respiratory obstruction
   d. Breech delivery with delay in delivery of the head
2. Kernicterus due to Rh or ABO incompatibility
3. Cerebral injury
   a. Trauma
   b. Cephalopelvic disproportion
   c. Precipitate delivery
   d. Prematurity
   e. Intracranial hemorrhage
4. Infection (maternal herpes)
5. Hypoglycemia in the child
6. Congenital hypothyroidism
7. Maternal toxemia and eclampsia

D. Postnatal Factors

1. Central nervous system infection
2. Brain injury, hemorrhage, hydrocephalus, or tumor
3. Cerebral degenerative disease
4. Anoxia
5. Poisoning (lead)
6. Metabolic imbalance (inborn errors of metabolism)
   a. Phenylketonuria
   b. Galactosemia
   c. Tay–Sachs
7. Psychiatric disorders
   a. Autism
8. Nutritional deficiency
9. Emotional neglect

E. Other

1. No identifiable organic or biologic cause for 65%–75% of retardation in children
2. Suspected causes include sociocultural or environmental deprivation or poverty—85% of mild retardation is related to environmental conditions
3. Mental retardation can be secondary to an inferior education system, hearing and visual deficits, or prolonged hospitalization or chronic illness.

Incidence

1. Six million people, 3% of the US general population, is mentally retarded.
2. It is estimated that approximately 125,000 infants born each year in the US will at some time in their lives be classified as mentally retarded.
3. A decrease in infant deaths, a longer life span, and improved case finding have caused a rise in the total number of persons classified as mentally retarded.

Classification*

1. Mental retardation is most often classified according to the child's educational potential, based on the intelligence quotient (IQ) score (average IQ is 100)
   a. Mild (educable)—IQ of 50–55 to approximately 70 (represents 88% of all mental retardation)
   b. Moderate (trainable)—IQ of 35–40 to 50–55 (represents 7% of all mental retardation)
   c. Severe—IQ of 20–25 to 35–40 (represents 3.5% of all mental retardation)
   d. Profound (custodial)—IQ of below 20 or 25 (represents 1.5% of all mental retardation)
2. Although the IQ score may be helpful in assessing and planning for retarded children (it should be below 70), low IQ in itself is not sufficient to make a diagnosis of mental retardation.
3. Both intellectual level and a deficit in adaptive behavior (the effectiveness or degree with which the individual meets the standards of personal independence and social responsibility expected of his age and cultural group) should be considered.
4. Scales have been developed for measuring and classifying adaptive behavior based on the following expectations:
   a. *Infancy and early childhood*
      (1) Sensory–motor skills development
      (2) Communication skills (including speech and language)

---

* Definition of the American Association on Mental Deficiency. In Heber R (ed). A Manual on Terminology and Classification in Mental Retardation (monograph supplement). Am J Ment Defic 1958; 64:3.

* Grossman H (ed). Classification in Mental Retardation. Washington, DC, American Association on Mental Deficiency, 1983, pp. 11–26.

(3) Self-help skills
(4) Socialization
   b. *Childhood and early adolescence*
      (1) Application of basic academic skills in daily life activities
      (2) Application of appropriate reasoning and judgment in mastery of environment
      (3) Social skills, group activities
   c. *Late adolescence and adult life*
      (1) Vocational and social responsibilities and performances
5. Only those children or adults who demonstrate deficits in both intellectual level and adaptive behavior should be classified as mentally retarded.

Prognosis

1. Factors that influence the prognosis
   a. Degree of retardation
   b. Existence of additional physical defects
   c. Family and community resources available to help the child to use his mental resources
2. Factors that favor improvement in intelligence
   a. Modification of the environment to eliminate stress and deprivation
   b. Improvement in learning opportunities
   c. Increased social acceptance
   d. Early intervention
3. The prognosis is best for the mildly retarded child without a coexistent physical defect; mental retardation that is a function of environmental conditions or secondary to treatable conditions that have not yet received treatment can be partially or completely reversed if identified early in childhood and interventions are provided.
4. Prognosis is based on the degree of retardation.
   a. Mild: achieves self care; capable of independent living with some guidance; can assume family responsibilities
   b. Moderate: can learn self-care and some vocational skills; functions well in a sheltered environment, e.g., group home and sheltered workshop
   c. Severe: needs protective environment and supervision throughout life
   d. Profound: requires long-term total care

Clinical Manifestations

1. Developmental delay—failure to meet normal motor, mental, or social milestones for age
   a. Substantial functional limitations in areas of self-care, language, mobility, capacity for independent living, self-direction, and economic self-sufficiency
   b. Achieves at a slower pace
   c. Poor problem-solving ability
   d. A concrete thinker; limited or no abstract thought
   e. Decreased attention span
   f. Engages in self-stimulating behaviors (rocking, head banging)
   g. Altered ability to eat related to poor gross and fine muscle control, poor eye–hand coordination
2. Physical
   a. Approximately 75% of retarded individuals have no obvious physical stigma.
3. Associated conditions
   a. Seizures
   b. Cerebral palsy
   c. Behavioral disorders
   d. Speech and language defects
   e. Sensory defects
4. Manifestations—based on degree of retardation
   a. Mild: educable—reading and math abilities can reach a third to sixth grade level; mental age can reach 8–12 years
   b. Moderate: trainable—can function at first to third grade level; mental age can reach 3–7 years; can recognize important words and do basic counting
   c. Severe: marked delay—little or no communication; needs help with activities of daily living; minimal independent behavior; mental age can reach 1.5 years
   d. Profound: minimal capacity for functioning—cannot protect self; no communication; few walk

Diagnostic Evaluation

No single test can diagnose mental retardation; testing must be individualized
1. Diagnosis is difficult and is most reliable when the determination is made by a comprehensive team that offers medical, psychological, social, and educational examinations.
2. Care must be taken to ensure that no child is mislabeled as mentally retarded.
3. Intelligence tests (e.g., *WISC-R, Stanford–Binet, Peabody Picture Vocabulary*)—cognitive function should be at least two standard deviations below the mean
4. Developmental assessment (gross and fine motor, speech, personal–social)
5. Perinatal history, including maternal history of illness, drug and alcohol use, and trauma
6. Genetic screening/family history
7. Assessment of adaptive behavior
8. Psychological assessment
9. Physical assessment, including hearing and vision

Nursing Interventions

A. Supporting the Parents During the Initial Period of Diagnosis.

1. Provide time for the parents to comprehend the extent of their problem and to mobilize their resources to work on its solution.
   a. When the parents appear ready, offer counseling and verbal support at a slow pace, one step at a time.
   b. Be sensitive to clues concerning the type of support that is most helpful to each family.
2. Encourage both parents to talk about the diagnosis and how they feel about it.
   a. The parents' reaction will be determined individually by factors such as the nature of the diagnosis, the manner in which the family is told of the diagnosis, the perceived attitude of health professionals, and the parents' previous life experiences, their attitudes toward retardation, their marital relationship, and their personal aspirations.
   b. The culture of family may affect value judgment toward children with limited intellectual potential.
   c. Expect parent attitudes of guilt, shame, and self-pity; feelings of grief, hostility, and ambivalence; expressions of denial; thoughts that they might be unable to care for the child.
   d. Provide privacy for discussions.
   e. Express sympathetic understanding of the family's problems and show acceptance of their attitudes. Reassure them that many parents react to the di-

agnosis with grief and sorrow and mourn the loss of the "wished for" child.

3. Assure the family that their child has had the benefit of the best diagnostic procedures and will be given every treatment that is indicated.

4. If appropriate, initiate a referral to a social worker, a psychiatrist, or any other professional who may assist the family to deal with their immediate reactions. Many parents benefit from the continuous or intermittent support of a variety of health professionals.

5. Communicate a genuine concern for the parents as individuals and an understanding of the responsibilities that they have outside the hospital (i.e., care of other children, work, etc.).

B. Encouraging Parental Participation in Caring for and Handling the Infant and Fostering Acceptance of the Child by His Parents and Family.

1. Provide opportunities for the parents to learn all aspects of caring for their baby. The basic needs of the baby with mental retardation are the same as those of other infants.

   Emphasize the need for parents to appreciate the child for his unique attributes; he can be lovable and can be enjoyed as a person, but he requires special attention.

2. All the support and help given the parents during hospitalization will make home care easier. Early intervention and support should strengthen and support the parental role.

   a. Encourage the physician to have both parents present, possibly with the infant, when he tells them of the child's diagnosis. In this way, they can turn to one another for support.

   b. Make special efforts to involve the father. Respond to his needs—he may require special attention, support, and guidance.

   c. Adaptation by both parents is critical for the continual improvement of the child's functioning and to foster optimal growth and development.

   d. Help the parents to be honest in their thoughts and emotions concerning the baby.

3. Assist the parents in learning what mental retardation is and how it alters a child's mental and physical development.

   a. Provide appropriate literature (see the Bibliography, p. 1529, for some suggestions).

   b. Inform them of local or national organizations and encourage participation.

   c. If possible, provide an adjusted time table of development that takes into account the child's retardation.

   d. Answer parental questions sensitively but directly.

   e. Provide explanations in terms they can understand.

   f. Avoid vague generalities, such as "the child is slow," and demoralizing words, such as "moron" or "imbecile."

   g. Parents have the right to know what diagnostic tests have been done, what positive or negative conclusions have been reached, what uncertainties remain, and what general prognosis can be made.

4. Involve both parents in the child's care so that they may gain a realistic concept of his ability.

   a. Point out the child's areas of strengths and weaknesses and show how these can be considered in his management.

   b. Emphasize the *well* part of the child and that he

has the same needs as a normal child for love and security.

5. Be aware of problems that new parents may encounter when telling family and friends.

6. Emphasize the infant's need for love, affection, consideration, and individual attention.

7. Explore with parents their ability to carry out care activities versus the alternatives of adoption or institutionalization.

8. Serve as a role model by interacting with the child in a manner that conveys acceptance, respect, and love.

9. Clarify and support medical speculations regarding the cause of the retardation.

C. Planning Interventions to Promote Optimum Growth and Development With the Long-Range Goal of Developing Independent Behavior at the Highest Level Possible According to the Child's Potential.

1. Determine the child's care plan according to his individual areas of strengths and weaknesses and coordinate it with the plans of the related health professionals.

2. Because a retarded child has a limited attention span, present a smaller amount of material to him at a slower rate and over a longer period of time than to a normal child.

   a. Give simple, concrete, one-step directions.

   b. Give directions one at a time.

   c. Readjust goals to decrease frustration.

   d. Eliminate extraneous stimuli.

3. Break complex behaviors down into small steps that the child can easily achieve.

   a. This is important in the areas of feeding, dressing, and toilet training.

   b. Do not expect the child to transfer learning from one situation to another.

4. Provide organized, consistent, and repetitive experiences.

5. Employ techniques of positive reinforcement.

   a. Give rewards for positive responses so that the probability of recurrence of that response will be strengthened.

   Rewards should be given consistently and immediately after the approved response.

   b. Do not reward unacceptable behaviors.

6. Promote self-care behavior.

   a. Self-feeding: focus on gross and fine motor skills and hand–eye coordination.

   b. Toileting: focus on the child's ability to

   (1) Walk or at least sit alone with good balance

   (2) Sense and indicate need via some communication system; identify child's toileting pattern

   (3) Remove pants

   c. Dressing—provide easy-to-manipulate clothes

   d. Grooming—hygiene, dental care, and nutrition

   e. Provide speech therapy, if indicated

7. Promote normalization

   a. Develop normal routines

   b. Allow child to make choices

   c. Mainstream when appropriate

   d. Recognize the healthy aspects of the child's behavior

8. Promote safety

   a. Help child read words such as DANGER and STOP

   b. Teach child how to call and ask for help

   c. Teach child to say NO to strangers

d. Continuously check environment for safety needs for this child
e. Provide sex education at the child's level.
f. Infant may be very floppy because of poor muscle tone. When handling the infant, support him well with a firm grasp.
g. Position the infant so that if vomiting should occur he will not aspirate.
   (1) Prop him with a diaper roll so that position will be maintained.
   (2) This infant is not usually very active; thus, his position will need to be changed frequently.
9. Provide for physical needs
   a. For immobile children, physical, sensory, and psychosocial needs must be met—place a special emphasis on skin care
   b. Provide for adequate sleep, stimulation, and nutrition based on irregular sleep–wake rhythms and inability to maintain a sufficient intake or to control body weight
   c. Altered dentition may result in decreased ability to chew and speak; provide comprehensive dental care
   d. If the child is hypotonic or spastic, provide warmth
   e. Decreased muscle tone compromises respiratory expansion; frequently assess respiratory status
10. Base expectations for the child on his mental or developmental ability, *not* on his chronologic age.
11. Maintain a relaxed learning environment.
    a. Child needs to DO a task to learn it; watching is not as helpful
    b. Present learning in short segments
    c. Emphasize mastery rather than understanding of underlying principles
    d. Help to discriminate between stimuli by presenting the stimuli in an exaggerated form
12. The plan of intervention should be multimodal, directed toward cognitive, affective behavior, social, adaptive, and environment
13. Plan for all of the child's needs, not just his basic needs.

D. Providing Proper Stimulation According to the Child's Age.

1. Be aware that this child needs stimulation from the very start to begin to help him develop to his potential. Develop a plan of stimulation so that your activity and actions lead toward this goal.
   a. Infants with mental retardation who are quiet and undemanding tend to be understimulated, so they do not reach their full potential.
   b. Develop an early intervention/infant stimulation program with realistic goals.
      (1) Program should include exercises built around existing reflexes; these can reduce hypotonia.
      (2) Encourage exercises to develop eye–hand coordination and later finger–thumb grasp.
      (3) Place child in prone position to encourage development of head control

Note: Sensorimotor patterning is NOT approved by the American Academy of Pediatrics.

2. Offer positive and effective sensory stimulation. Hold and fondle the infant, especially during feeding and bath time; apply vibration to lips to stimulate sucking.
3. When the infant is awake, the adult face in his visual field is good stimulation and should interest him for a few seconds.

4. The gentle sound of talking or music can provide a pleasant auditory experience. The infant should stop activity and listen; older children like to move to the music.
5. Use art to help develop the child's image of self
   a. Trace body on paper
   b. Take pictures of the child and display them.

E. Reducing Destructive Behavior and Encouraging That Which is Socially Acceptable.

1. Establish a routine of daily living so that the child knows precisely what is expected of him.
2. Employ consistent discipline.
   a. Use language that the child understands so that he can comprehend his misdeed.
   b. When punishment is necessary, it should follow the misdeed immediately.
3. Provide immediate reinforcement for positive behaviors and ignore undesirable behaviors.

F. Fostering Continuing Family Acceptance of the Child and Providing Support for Them.

1. Help the parents to understand why the child behaves as he does.
2. Encourage the parents to talk about their feelings or problems they have with the child. Reemphasize the need for parents to appreciate their child for his unique attributes and special characteristics, such as sociability and sensitivity to the feelings of others.
3. Initiate a comprehensive and interdisciplinary teaching program for the child and his parents early. Continued educational experiences are vital. Offer the family available literature and help them to become familiar with community resources.
   a. Parents can provide positive and effective sensory training.
   b. Help the child to socialize with other children and provide an environment that will stimulate him mentally.
   c. The care plan should be based on the degree of the child's retardation, the reaction of the family to the diagnosis, and the availability of community resources.
   d. Promote the concept that this condition is not static; these children have the ability to learn and function, although they achieve at a slower pace.
4. Assist families in decision making.
   a. The family should be guided to make decisions for the child's care that will allow for maximum utilization of his capabilities.
   b. The family should be supported in the decisions they make.
5. Discuss with the parents their plans for dealing with the siblings of the retarded child.
   a. Adequate explanations and information should be given to siblings early to avoid any misconceptions later.
   b. Siblings often need help in explaining the retarded child's abnormality to their friends.
   c. Caution the parents to guard against intense sibling rivalry; the other children often feel neglected because of the amount of time devoted to the retarded child.
   d. Consider the emotional needs of siblings.
   e. Do not make nonretarded siblings responsible for the child who is retarded.
6. Address parental concerns.
   a. Guide them to avoid the extremes of overprotec-

tiveness and neglect related to the child's condition.

    b. Assist them in dealing with the question, "Who will care for this child after I die?"

7. If the child is hospitalized, allow the parents to continue to maintain other responsibilities they may have outside the hospital (i.e., other children, work). Do not insist that they stay at the hospital and attend only to this child.

    a. Obtain a thorough nursing history from the parent and/or child regarding the child's usual home routines.

    b. Counsel the mother that some regression can be anticipated even in normal children who require hospitalization.

    c. Know what activities the child can or cannot do and what he likes to do.

    d. Plan the child's day according to what he is used to as much as possible.

    e. Whenever possible, assign the same nursing personnel to care for the child.

    f. Explain procedures to the child using communication methods appropriate for his level of cognitive development.

      Share this information with nursing staff to ensure continuity of care from home to hospital to minimize fear and frustration in the child.

8. Parents need to know that they are important as people. They each should be encouraged to lead a normal life. They should be helped to feel that they are not their child's only resource, but that others care and are willing to help.

    Other members of the family must be considered.

    a. The child should not be thought of as a sick child, but as a child who needs special handling to promote his individual growth and development. But he does not need all the attention all the time.

    b. The family should be included in his care, but they also must have a life of their own and as much parental attention as they would receive if the child were not present in the family.

    c. Parents need time to themselves. They should be encouraged to go out alone together and to give time to their marriage.

    d. Encourage parents to be open with the family and to discuss concerns. Children are sensitive to parental distress. Lack of communication can create and increase parental isolation and can cause unrealistic concerns.

    e. Sibling reactions generally reflect the parents' reactions toward the child with mental retardation

    f. Assist parents to assess their family situation to promote healthy family relationships. Do the following situations exist?

      (1) Are older siblings frequent caretakers of the child with mental retardation?

      (2) Is there excessive parental attention to the afflicted child at expense of other siblings?

      (3) Do the parents show hostility toward the child?

      (4) Are there excessive expectations of other children?

      (5) Is the family dominated by the destructiveness or overactivity of child with mental retardation?

9. Parents should be made aware of community resources (see the Bibliography, pp. 1529).

    a. Community nursing agencies

    b. Day-care centers/nursery schools

    c. Foster grandparent programs, foster home

    d. Respite care

    e. Special schools

    f. Parent groups

    g. Volunteer organizations

    h. Specialized diagnostic facilities

    i. Recreational programs

    j. Vocational training

    k. Residential settings/group homes

    l. National associations

    m. Sheltered workshops

    n. Special camps

    o. Special Olympics

10. Reference for parents:
National Association of Retarded Citizens, 2501 Avenue J, Arlington, TX 76011

G. Preparing the Mentally Retarded Individual So That He May Cope Successfully (Within His Potential) With the Problems and Adjustments of Adult Life.

1. Help the parents identify areas of home responsibilities that may be delegated to the retarded child.

2. In the child's early learning activities, promote habits that are essential to his later vocational life.

    a. Getting to places on time

    b. Cooperating

    c. Focusing and holding attention on the task at hand

    d. Establishing acceptable interpersonal relationships

3. Help the child to develop a set of attitudes and behaviors that will motivate him to work.

4. Identify attainable occupational goals early in the child's educational experience.

    Early education should tie into later social and vocational programs.

5. Enhance the child's self-worth.

    a. Provide for a sense of accomplishment.

    b. Reinforce appropriate speech and behavior.

6. Provide for an optimal education.

    a. A free and appropriate education is mandated by law.

    b. Assist the family and school develop the Individualized Educational Plan, mandated by Public Law 94-142.

    c. Develop realistic goals.

7. The child should have the opportunity of participating in social, religious, and recreational activities.

    a. Organizations should be selected in which the probability of success is the highest.

    b. The parent should discuss the situation with the group leader and the leader should have an opportunity to meet the child so that both child and leader can assess each other.

H. Helping Modify Existing Social Attitudes Toward Retardation.

1. Assess and work through your own feelings about the retarded, including personal attitudes and defenses that are used to avoid personal involvement in the care of retarded children and their families.

2. Take advantage of opportunities to influence the attitudes of other hospitalized children and their families.

    a. Serve as a role model in your own interactions with retarded children.

    b. Encourage hospitalized children to socialize with the retarded child during play programs or other activities, and help them to understand and accept the child.

    c. Provide opportunities for other parents to discuss their feelings about retardation and to ask questions. Correct any misconceptions they may have.

    d. Team a normal child with a retarded child.

3. Initiate or support community educational and service programs.

4. Support federal legislation relating to funding for research and services for the mentally retarded.

I. Health Education

1. Prevent the occurrence of mental retardation.
    a. Encourage amniocentesis or chorionic villi sampling (CVS) for women over age 35.
    b. Provide genetic counselling.
    c. Encourage proper nutrition, routine prenatal care, and avoidance of drugs and alcohol during pregnancy.
    d. Remove lead from the environment (see Lead Poisoning, p. 1515)
    e. Treat infections promptly.
    f. Maintain proper immunization status.
2. Provide early identification and treatment.
    a. Provide early screening of infants for inborn errors of metabolism, thyroid function, phenylketonuria, galactosemia, and chromosomal defects.
    b. Identify infants who are
        (1) nonresponsive to contact.
        (2) have poor eye contact.
        (3) have decreased spontaneous activity.
        (4) have decreased alertness.
        (5) have feeding difficulties.
3. Minimize the long-term consequences
    a. Provide interventions to correct hearing, vision, metabolic conditions, and environmental deprivation
    b. Use educational and vocational resources available to all handicapped individuals.
4. The mentally retarded child may require more medical supervision than the normal child. Regular dental care is also essential.
    a. The child is often more susceptible to infections.
    b. He may eat poorly.
    c. He may be underweight or overweight.
    d. He may have poor motor coordination.
    e. He often has speech and language problems.
5. The child's environment has a greater influence on his behavior, growth, and development. It should provide experiences that contribute to a positive self-concept of a person who is loved, wanted, valued, and respected.
6. Parents need to be helped to recognize their child's method of communicating so that they can respond to his needs.
7. Parents should be assisted to identify learning readiness in their child in order to help him achieve his maximum level of development without subjecting him to unnecessary experiences of failure and frustration.
8. References for parents:
American Association on Mental Deficiency, 1719 Kalorama Road, NW, Washington, DC 20009
Association for Retarded Citizens, Inc., PO Box 6109, Arlington, TX 76011

National Association of Retarded Citizens, 2501 Avenue J, Arlington, TX 76011
National Information Center for Handicapped Children and Youth, PO Box 1492, Washington, DC 20013

Down Syndrome *(A Specific Cause of Mental Retardation)*

Down syndrome is a chromosomal abnormality involving an extra chromosome (number 21), characterized by a typical physical appearance and mental retardation.

Etiology

A. Trisomy 21

1. Primarily an error in meiotic cell division.
    a. Both number 21 chromosomes in the pair instead of just one of the pair migrate to one daughter cell during meiosis (nondisjunction); these two from one parent combine with the one from the other at conception on chromosome 21.
    b. There are three number 21 chromosomes (trisomy), thus extra genetic material.
    c. Every cell nucleus in the new individual has 47 chromosomes rather than the normal 46.
2. Occurrence is associated with advanced maternal age.
    a. Risk is increased after maternal age of 35.
    b. Occurrence in the same set of parents is rare but dependent on maternal age.
    c. Two-thirds are due to maternal nondisjunction; one third is due to nondisjunction by the father.
3. In 4% of cases, chromosome number 21 attaches to another chromosome, usually the 13–15 group (translocation).

Incidence

1. About 1 in 660–1000 live births each year will be diagnosed as having Down syndrome.
2. Down-syndrome children make up approximately 10% of the total mentally retarded population

Associated Problems

1. Congenital heart defects, especially septal defects (seen in up to 40% of Down-syndrome children)
2. Myelogenous leukemia (20 times more common in this population than in the general population)
3. Gastrointestinal anomalies (in 10%)
4. Recurrent infections, especially of upper respiratory tract and skin
5. Eye problems—strabismus; errors in refraction
6. Thyroid dysfunction
7. Premature aging
8. Males with Down syndrome are sterile
9. Dental misalignment

Clinical Manifestations

1. Physical stigmata recognized at birth
    a. Marked hypotonia and floppiness, including lax abdominal muscles
    b. Joint hyperextension or hyperflexibility
    c. Small oral cavity with tongue protruding; high, arched palate; furrowed tongue
    d. Brachycephaly with relatively flat occiput
    e. Eyes slant upward and outward with inner epicanthal folds; speckled iris (Brushfield spots)
    f. Excess skin on back of neck; short, broad neck
    g. Depressed nasal bridge and flat facial profile
    h. Small ears, often set low
    i. Broad hands; there is inward curving of distal phalanx of fifth finger; simian crease (transverse palmer crease)

    j. Short, broad feet; there is a wide separation between first and second toe (plantar furrow)

    k. Small male genitalia

    l. Weak or absent Moro reflex (response to sudden loud noise, causing body to stiffen and arms to go up and out, then forward and toward each other. Thumb and index finger will assume "C" shape.)

    m. Specific dermatoglyphics

2. Later findings in the child

    a. Slow intellectual development (moderate retardation)

    b. Delay in motor development, sexual development, dentition, and speech (also affected by protruding tongue)

3. Short limbs; short, stocky stature

4. Social age is 2–3 years higher than mental age

Diagnostic Evaluation

1. Chromosomal analysis (karyotyping) will usually show a third chromosome on number 21; or the results of translocation

Nursing Interventions

(See Section on Mental Retardation)

A. Supporting the Parents During the Initial Period of Diagnosis.

B. Helping the Parents to Accept the Fact That Their Child Has Down Syndrome and to Accept the Child for Himself.

1. Invite the parents to join a group of parents who have children with Down syndrome.

2. Parental education is one very important aspect in the nursing care of a child with Down syndrome, especially in the following areas:

    a. The environment has an influence on the rate of the child's progress in performance, behavior, growth, and development.

    b. The role of the parents is critical. A nurturing and loving environment gives the child the best chance to develop to his full potential.

    c. Encourage the entire family to be included in the child's care.

    d. The child will usually be lovable and quiet, affectionate, and socially responsive if he is loved and if individual attention is given to his specific needs.

    e. Patience and understanding must be developed by parents and family

3. Parents may be embarrassed by readily identifiable signs.

C. Planning Interventions to Promote Optimum Growth and Development.

1. See Section on moderate mental retardation.

2. Be alert that the small oral cavity may result in feeding and speech problems.

3. The child's motor development is slow. The degree of hypotonia probably greatly influences the early motor development; genetic potential and environmental stimulation of the child also influence motor development—encourage motor coordination. It will take time for the child to learn to sit.

D. Observing Carefully for Any Signs of Physical Complications That May Occur With Down Syndrome. Recording and Reporting Them Immediately.

1. Intestinal obstruction (duodenal stenosis)

    a. Observe for abdominal distention and its association with feeding.

    b. Note vomiting—what is vomited and when.

      (1) Bile-stained emesis indicates lower tract obstruction.

      (2) Partially digested milk indicates upper tract obstruction.

    c. Note absence of stools.

2. Congenital cardiac defect

    a. When taking vital signs, note any irregularity of the heart rate. Murmurs may not be evident to the untrained ear. Note any respiratory distress or labored respirations.

    b. Note any cyanosis and when it occurs—with crying, feeding, or all the time.

    c. Be particularly alert to the infant tiring easily during feeding.

3. Treat infections promptly.

4. Monitor blood for signs of leukemia.

5. Decrease involvement in sports involving stress on the head and neck related to the increased possibility of atlantoaxial instability.

E. Providing a Safe Environment for the Infant.

1. Infant is usually very floppy because of poor muscle tone. When handling the infant, support him well with a firm grasp.

2. Position the infant so that if vomiting should occur he will not aspirate.

    a. If he is on his abdomen, be certain that he can turn his head to the side.

    b. Prop him with a diaper roll so that position will be maintained.

    c. This infant is not usually very active; thus, his position will need to be changed frequently.

F. Establishing and Maintaining Adequate Nutrition to Allow for Growth and Development.

1. The diet is calculated according to the infant's needs.

2. Because of poor muscle tone and a protruding tongue, the infant may be a poor eater with a weak and ineffective suck.

    a. Provide the appropriate nipple so that minimal sucking effort is needed to feed.

    b. Allow adequate time for feeding. Do not allow the infant to become overly tired.

    c. Note and report poor eating and insufficient sucking.

G. Fostering Continuing Family Acceptance of the Child.

1. Help the parents to understand that in spite of signs of slow mental growth, the child can make steady progress. In early life, the child with Down syndrome should not be stereotyped in behavior. His behavior is similar to the norm when mental age is considered. Help parents not to lower their expectations.

    a. The child needs a great deal of repetition in all areas of learning.

    b. He usually has a good memory, can acquire a fairly large vocabulary and can learn to spell. Math may be more difficult for him.

    c. Speech may lag behind walking by 1–2 years. He may encounter trouble in pronouncing certain words. Stammering may occur if the child is under pressure.

    d. Parents need help in learning to recognize the child's readiness to learn these skills.

    e. A general decrease of IQ score occurs with increasing age and should be an expected occurrence because of the increasing verbal and abstract content of test materials at the higher mental age.

2. If appropriate, initiate a community health nursing referral for assistance with planning and implementing home care.

3. See information under mental retardation.

H. Preparing the Child for His Future.

1. The child with Down syndrome should go to school. He learns by copying. Have the parents discuss the child's problem with the school nurse, the teacher, and other adults who have close contact with the child.

2. Education enables the child with Down syndrome to be productive to some extent in society, to have a fuller life, and to take pride in his accomplishments. Such children can learn routine housework, gardening, or farming. They can run errands, learn to obey traffic rules, and ride buses.

3. Barring complications, these children have a normal life-span.

4. See related information under mental retardation.

5. References for parents:
National Down Syndrome Congress, 1640 W Roosevelt Road, Chicago, IL 60608 (publishes *Down's Syndrome News,* booklets, bibliographies for articles, etc.)

National Down Syndrome Society, 70 W 40th Street, New York, NY 10018

Parents of Down's Syndrome Children, % Montgomery County Association for Retarded Citizens, 11600 Nebel Street, Rockville, MD 20852

Learning Disabilities and Attention Deficit Hyperactivity Disorders

The term *learning disability* (*LD*) is defined as a "heterogeneous group of disorders manifested by significant difficulties in the acquisition and use of listening, speaking, reading, writing, reasoning, or mathematical abilities, or of social skills. . . . Even though a learning disability may occur concomitantly with other handicapping conditions (e.g., sensory impairment, mental retardation, social and emotional disturbance), with socioenvironmental influences (cultural differences, insufficient or inappropriate instruction, psychogenic factors), and especially with attention deficit disorder, all of which may cause learning problems, a learning disability is not the direct result of those conditions or influences"—Interagency Committee on Learning Disabilities, 1987.

The term *attention deficit hyperactivity disorder* (*ADHD*) is defined as "developmentally inappropriate degrees of inattention, impulsiveness, and hyperactivity"—*Diagnostic and Statistical Manual*-III-R, 1987).

Etiology

1. Intrinsic to the individual and presumed due to central nervous system dysfunction

2. Exact mechanisms are unknown

3. Multiple hypotheses
   a. Alteration in neurotransmitters, especially catecholamines
   b. Alteration in response–inhibition mechanism of the brain
   c. Structural anomaly of or damage to the brain
   d. Toxic substances (foods, chemicals)
   e. Allergic response
   f. Delayed cerebral maturation
   g. Genetic

4. Increased incidence in low-birth-weight infants and after cranial irradiation and intrathecal chemotherapy for brain cancer

Incidence

1. Estimated to occur in 5%–10% of children (range up to 30%)

2. Males are diagnosed twice as frequently as females.

3. Most prevalent cause of school underachievement.

Management

A multifaceted interdisciplinary approach involving some or all of the following aspects is necessary:

1. Family education and counseling concerning LD and ADHD

2. Involvement of nurses, physicians, psychologists, occupational and physical therapists, specialists in vision, speech and language, and educators

3. Environmental manipulation to decrease external stimuli and encourage desirable behavior patterns

4. Remedial education focused on the specific area(s) of deficit

5. For hyperactivity: central nervous system stimulants are effective in decreasing motor activity, increasing attention span and concentration, and letting child be more available for learning
   a. Medications are short acting
   b. Most common medications: methylphenidate (Ritalin), dextroamphetamine (Dexadrine), and pemoline (Cylert)
   c. Medications work for 70%–75% of ADHD children

6. Different strategies are needed at different ages

7. Treatment measures must be reevaluated every 2–3 years

Clinical Manifestations

The child usually demonstrates one or more of the following features:

1. Alteration in sensory/receptive intake
   a. Visual perceptual deficit
      (1) Dyslexia (letter or word reversals)
      (2) Poor visual memory
      (3) Misperceive distance
      (4) Difficulty copying
      (5) Difficulty reading across a line; jump from line to line
      (6) Difficulty with figure–ground perception
   b. Auditory perceptual deficit
      (1) Difficulty understanding verbal directions
      (2) Difficulty interpreting tone of voice
      (3) Difficulty differentiating sound of similar-sounding words
   c. Tactile/kinesthetic deficit
      (1) Unable to read body cues (e.g., the need to toilet or onset of menses)

2. Alteration in integrative processing
   a. Difficulty in retrieving and using information accurately
   b. Difficulty with
      (1) Sequencing data
      (2) Understanding concepts of time and space, part or whole, cause or effect

(3) Organization of thought and planning
(4) Analysis and abstract thought
3. Alteration in motor/expressive response
   a. Minor difficulty with gross and fine motor tasks, e.g., coordination, labeled as clumsy
   b. Speech disorder (stuttering; dysphasia)
   c. Poor handwriting
4. Hyperactivity
   a. Fidgets and squirms in seat
   b. Easily distracted; difficulty sustaining attention
   c. Difficulty remaining seated when required to do so
   d. Difficulty following through on instructions
   e. Talks excessively
   f. Loses things necessary for tasks
   g. Onset is before age 7
5. Soft neurologic signs
   a. Minor abnormalities in neurologic assessment
   b. Commonly found with LD/ADHD, but is of NO value in diagnosis and treatment

Diagnostic Evaluation

1. No single tool can diagnose LD or ADHD; multiple data sources are needed
2. Detailed medical, developmental, social, perinatal, and behavioral history
3. Current physical, behavioral, and social assessment; neurologic examination to detect abnormalities
4. Assessment of academic performance
5. Psychological testing to determine the exact nature of cognitive or perceptual dysfunctions that may be present as well as the child's intellectual potential
6. Additional testing depends on the child's symptomatology and frequently includes electroencephalographic vision and hearing evaluations
7. Detailed family history, especially related to problems of learning and behavior.

Nursing Interventions

A. Providing Patient and Classroom Teaching Geared to the Child's Special Needs

1. For visual perceptual deficit
   a. Present material verbally
   b. Use hands-on experience
   c. Tape record teaching sessions
2. For auditory perceptual deficit
   a. Provide materials in written form
   b. Use pictures
   c. Provide tactile learning
3. For integrative deficit
   a. Use multisensory approaches
   b. Print directions while you verbalize them
   c. Use calendars and lists to organize tasks and activities
4. For motor/expressive deficits
   a. Break down skills and projects into their multiple component parts
   b. Verbally describe the component parts
   c. Provide extra time to perform
   d. Allow child to type work rather than using cursive writing
5. For highly distractible child
   a. Provide a structured environment
   b. Have child sit in front of class
   c. Place child away from doors and windows
   d. Decrease clutter on desk

6. Additional suggestions for the classroom teacher
   a. Promote an environment conducive to learning.
   b. Utilize resource room and special education teachers.
   c. Participate in the development of the Individualized Education Plan.
   d. Provide untimed tests.
   e. Reinforce that the child may have failed a test/course but that the child is NOT a failure.
   f. Help child compensate for deficits.
   g. Help child stay focused on task.
   h. Provide printed and verbal instructions for tasks.
   i. Teach the steps of problem solving and decision making.
   j. Help the child pull new learning together.
   k. Encourage the child to participate actively in learning.
   l. Help the child set appropriate goals.
   m. Help the child organize and prioritize.

B. Providing Emotional Support to the Family.

1. Provide parents with opportunities to express their feelings and concerns about the diagnosis.
2. Expect such reactions as guilt, disbelief, relief, anger, and frustration. Reassure the parents that these feelings are normal and acceptable.
3. Provide factual information about the disorder and treatment plan.
4. Assist the parents to deal with identified problems, and provide them with positive feedback when appropriate.
5. Help the parents anticipate and deal with the reactions and needs of siblings, especially when younger siblings surpass the LD child or receive better grades.
6. Assist the family to find appropriate programs to meet the child's special needs.
7. Serve as coordinator of services between family, school, physician, and other agencies.
8. Refer to a parent support group if one is available.
9. They can be assured that there is no evidence that the drugs produce any euphoric effect or addiction in children.

C. Providing a Therapeutic Physical Home Environment.

1. Assist the parents to manipulate the home environment to reduce stimulation and stress.
   a. Maintain regular sleeping, eating, working, and playing routines.
   b. Provide a minimum of external stimuli and alternatives.
   c. Divide tasks and expectations into small, manageable parts. Give only one or two instructions at a time.
   d. Set firm but reasonable limits on behavior and carry through with consistent discipline.
   e. Avoid situations that cause excessive excitement, stimulation, or fatigue.
2. Evaluate the environment for safety hazards and eliminate them.
3. Provide for energy release.
   a. Plan for periods of physical activity, vocal outlet, and outdoor play.
   b. Channel need for movement into safe, appropriate activities.
4. Involve child in social activities.
5. Build self-esteem; recognize strengths and willingness to try.

D. Monitoring Stimulant Medication Administration

1. Administer before breakfast and lunch (sustained-release forms do not require a lunch dose).
2. Work with school system to insure lunch dose is given.
3. Recommend "drug holidays" during vacations and weekends to monitor effectiveness and the need for change; this is especially recommended at the start of each academic school year.
4. Stimulant medications are not usually given to children younger than 6 years of age.
5. The child is usually started on a small dose, which is gradually increased until the desired response is achieved.
6. Evaluate the child's response to medication by direct observation and consultation with others, such as parents and teachers.

E. Anticipating Side Effects of Stimulant Medications.

1. Insomnia may result from increased dosage or if administered too late in the day.
2. Anorexia and temporary growth retardation
   a. Measure height and weight at frequent intervals.
   b. Reassure that height will catch up after medications are discontinued.
3. Increased pulse and respiratory rates, nervousness, nausea, and stomachache.
4. Pemoline results in liver dysfunction—provide periodic liver function tests
5. Stimulant medications alter the effects of many anti-seizure drugs and tricyclic antidepressants.

F. Anticipating Associated Problems

1. Decreased self-esteem related to chronic failure
2. Inappropriate coping (behavior problems) related to multiple failures
3. Psychosomatic problems related to stress and fear of failure
4. Difficulty with peer relationships
5. Coping with the label "learning disabled"
6. Caution the parents about unproven approaches that profess a single solution to the problem of LD or ADHD.

G. Promoting Safety

1. Increased impulsiveness results in running into street and acting without thinking.
2. Decreased attention span and decreased ability to process auditory directions result in increased risk.
3. Decreased judgment of distance results in increased driving accidents among adolescents.

H. Caring for the Hospitalized Child Previously Diagnosed With LD or ADHD.

1. Elicit a detailed medical, developmental, and behavioral history emphasizing management techniques currently used by the family.
2. Continue home management techniques during the hospitalization as much as possible.
3. Manipulate the hospital environment to reduce unnecessary stimulation and decision making.
4. Eliminate any safety hazards.
5. Observe the child for response to hospitalization and his therapeutic regimen.
6. Provide continued support to parents.
7. Teach the child about his health problem.
   a. The teaching plan should be divided into short, concrete steps.

   b. Select a learning environment with minimal distraction. Limit interruptions.
   c. Use learning materials that are clear and specific. Avoid presenting too much equipment at one time.
   d. Select reading materials carefully, according to the reading ability of the child. Do not assume that the child understands the material simply because he can read it.
   e. Encourage eye-to-eye contact when talking with the child..

I. Making Appropriate Referrals.

1. Assist in identifying children who may be LD or AHDH and refer for appropriate screening.
2. If the LD is secondary to another condition, that condition needs to be addressed first.
3. Be familiar with Public Law 94-142
   a. Mandates free and appropriate education in the least restrictive environment for all handicapped children
   b. Requires development of Individualized Education Plan
4. Be familiar with Public Law 99-457
   a. Requires assessment of children in first 3 years of life for handicaps
5. Resource groups and information for parents:
   Children with Attention Deficit Disorders
   1859 N. Pine Island Road
   Suite 185
   Plantation, FL 33322

   Foundation for Children with Learning Disabilities
   99 Park Avenue
   New York, NY 10016

   Association for Children and Adults with Learning Disabilities
   4156 Library Road
   Pittsburgh, PA 15234

   Vocational rehabilitation services
   (available for learning disabled adults)

   Note: Remember—many learning disabled children grow up to be learning disabled adults.

Poisoning

Exposure to poisons can be by ingestion, inhalation, skin contact, or exposure can be ocular. This section will focus on ingested poisons.

Ingested Poisons

Poisoning by ingestion refers to the oral intake of a harmful substance that, even in a small amount, can damage tissues, disturb bodily functions, and cause possible death. In the pediatric population, poisoning is often caused by the ingestion of medications as well as toxic household substances such as furniture polish, plants, charcoal lighter, kerosene, paint remover, cleansers, and lye.
It is a major cause of death in children under 5 years of age and is most commonly seen during toddlerhood.

Etiology

1. Improper or dangerous storage
2. Poor lighting—causes errors in reading
3. Human factors
   a. Failure to read label properly
   b. Failure to return poison to its proper place
   c. Failure to recognize the material as poisonous

Clinical Manifestations

1. Gastrointestinal symptoms (common in metallic, acid, alkali, and bacterial poisonings)
   a. Anorexia
   b. Abdominal pain
   c. Nausea
   d. Vomiting (vomitus may contain undigested poison)
   e. Diarrhea or intestinal cramping
2. Central nervous system symptoms
   a. Convulsions—common in poisoning by central nervous system stimulants such as camphor and strychnine.
   b. Loss of consciousness/coma—common in poisoning by central nervous system depressants such as alcohol, atropine, chloral hydrate, chlorine components, and barbiturates.
      (1) Behavior change
      (2) Dizziness
      (3) Lethargy
      (4) Disorientation
      (5) Stupor
   c. Dilated pupils—common in poisoning by atropine, nicotine, cocaine, and ephedrine.
   d. Pinpoint pupils—common in poisoning by opiates.
3. Skin symptoms
   a. Rashes
   b. Burns/blisters to mouth, esophagus, and stomach
   c. Eye inflammation
   d. Skin irritation
   e. Stains around the mouth or lesions of the mucous membranes
   f. Cyanosis—cyanide and strychnine poisoning
4. Cardiopulmonary symptoms
   a. Dyspnea (especially related to aspiration of hydrocarbons)
   b. Cardiopulmonary depression or arrest
5. Other
   a. Odor around mouth

Diagnostic Evaluation

1. Analysis reveals presence of toxic substances in:
   a. Blood
   b. Urine
   c. Gastric washings
   d. Vomitus
   e. Stool
   f. Oral cavity
2. Assess liver and renal status

Nursing Interventions

A. Assisting the Family by Telephone Management.

1. Calmly obtain and record the following information:
   a. Name, address, and telephone number of caller
   b. Age, weight and signs/symptoms of the child, including neuro status
   c. Route of exposure
   d. Name of the ingested product, approximate amount ingested, and time of ingestion.
2. Instruct the caller regarding appropriate emergency actions (see below).
3. Direct the patient to the nearest emergency department. Dispatch an ambulance if necessary.
4. Instruct the caller to clear the child's mouth of any unswallowed poison.
5. Identify what treatments have already been initiated
6. Instruct the parents to save vomitus, unswallowed liquid or pills, and the container and to bring them to the hospital as aids in identifying the poison.
7. Identify whether other children were involved in the poisoning in order to initiate treatment for them also.

B. Intervening Related to the Patient's Condition.

1. Utilize vital signs and neuro assessment to determine a rough estimate of the child's status.
2. Provide emergency respiratory and circulatory support.
3. If needed, obtain venous access.
4. Maintain airway and safety during seizure activity.
5. Treat shock.

C. Identifying the Poison.

1. Determine the nature of the ingested substance from the child's history or by reading the label on the container.
2. If necessary, call the nearest poison control center or toxicology section of the medical examiner's office to identify the toxic ingredient and obtain recommendations for emergency treatment.
3. Save vomitus, stool, and urine for analysis once the child reaches the hospital.

D. Removing the Poison From the Body.

1. Dilute with 6–8 ounces of water if advised.
   a. For skin or eye contact, remove contaminated clothing and flush with water for 15–20 minutes.
   b. For inhalation poisons, remove from the exposure site.
2. Assess area (mouth, primarily) for burns.
3. Induce vomiting unless contraindicated.

NURSING ALERT: Do *not* induce vomiting if:
1. The child is convulsing, semiconscious, or comatose.
2. Poison is known to be a strong acid or alkali, strychnine, or a hydrocarbon (e.g., lighter fluid, gasoline, kerosene, paint remover, or fingernail polish remover). Strong acids or alkalis may damage the esophagus for a second time during emesis, and hydrocarbons can cause severe pneumonia if aspirated.

   a. For children over 1 year of age, administer syrup of ipecac according to the directions on the label. (The usual dose is 15 ml. [about 1 tablespoon] mixed in 6–8 ounces of warm water.)
   b. If no vomiting occurs after 20–30 minutes, repeat this process one time only.

NURSING ALERT: Do not use tincture of ipecac; it is much stronger than the syrup and is itself a poison.
Also, do not administer household neutralizing foods/products (unless physician recommended) because of the heat that is generated by the chemical reaction and the burn that could result (or exacerbation of the existing burn).

c. Position the child with his head down or on his side to prevent aspiration of vomitus.

4. Administer gastric lavage. (This is indicated when vomiting is impossible because of the child's condition or age, when induction of vomiting has been unsuccessful, or when the poison is one that is rapidly absorbed, e.g., cyanide). See *Guidelines,* page 950.
   a. A cuffed endotracheal tube may be inserted prior to lavage to protect the child from aspiration.
   b. Use the largest size tube that can be passed orally—preferably one with a double lumen.
   c. Ensure correct placement of the tube.
   d. Place the child on his left side with his head lower than his stomach.
   e. Aspirate the stomach.
   f. Lavage with small, repeated introductions and withdrawals of normal saline, ½ normal saline, or special lavage solution.
   g. Do not leave a large amount of water in the child's stomach.
   h. Follow lavage with a cathartic and activated charcoal to hasten removal of the poison from the gastrointestinal tract.
   i. Be aware of the dangers associated with lavage:
      (1) Esophageal perforation—may occur in corrosive poisoning
      (2) Gastric hemorrhage
      (3) Impaired pulmonary function resulting from aspiration
      (4) Cardiac arrest
      (5) Convulsions—may result from stimulation in strychnine ingestion

5. Administer cathartics, if ordered, to hasten emptying of gastrointestinal tract.
   a. Use cautiously with young children.

E. Reducing the Effect of the Poison by Administering an Antidote.

1. An antidote may either react with the poison to prevent its absorption or counteract the effects of the poison after its absorption.
2. Not all poisons have specific antidotes.
3. Information regarding appropriate antidotes for specific poisons is available through all poison control centers and in many pediatric textbooks.
   Antidotes for the most common poisons should be listed in the emergency department of the hospital.
4. Effectiveness of the antidote usually depends on the amount of time that elapses between ingestion of the poison and administration of the antidote.
5. Activated charcoal absorbs all poisons except cyanide, if given within 1 hour of poisoning and after the emetic. Administer orally, after vomiting has occurred, in a dose of 30–50 gm. in a child and 50–100 gm. in an adolescent in 177–237 ml. (6–8 oz.) of water with sweetener.

Note: Charcoal inactivates ipecac; therefore, administer charcoal only AFTER ipecac has induced vomiting.

F. Eliminating the Absorbed Poison.

1. Force diuresis.
   a. Administer large quantities of fluid either orally or intravenously.
   b. Carefully monitor intake and output.
2. Assist with kidney dialysis, which may be necessary if the child's own kidneys are not functioning effectively.
3. Assist with exchange transfusion if this method is indicated for removing the poison.

G. Observing the Child for Progression of Symptoms and Providing Supportive Care Should These Develop.

1. Central nervous system involvement
   a. Observe for restlessness, confusion, delirium, seizures, lethargy, stupor, or coma.
   b. Administer sedation with caution—in order to avoid depression and masking of symptoms.
   c. Avoid excessive manipulation of the child.
   d. See nursing care of the child with seizures, page 1453.
   e. See nursing care of the unconscious patient, page 576.
2. Respiratory involvement
   a. Observe for respiratory depression, obstruction, pulmonary edema, pneumonia, or tachypnea.
   b. Have an artificial airway and tracheostomy set available.
   c. Be prepared to administer oxygen and provide artificial respiration.
   d. Other nursing concerns:
      (1) Nursing care of the child on a ventilator, page 1196.
      (2) Procedures for administration of oxygen, page 1193.
      (3) Procedure for cardiopulmonary resuscitation, page 1200.
3. Cardiovascular involvement
   a. Observe for peripheral circulatory collapse, disturbances of heart rate and rhythm, or cardiac failure.
   b. Maintain intravenous therapy as directed to prevent shock. See procedure for the administration of intravenous fluids, page 1167.
      (1) Assess for complications of overhydration.
   c. Be prepared for cardiac arrest (see procedure for cardiopulmonary resuscitation, p. 1200).
4. Gastrointestinal involvement
   a. Observe for nausea, pain, abdominal distention, and difficulty in swallowing.
   b. Maintain intravenous therapy to replace water and electrolyte losses (see procedure for intravenous therapy, p. 1167).
   c. Offer a diet that is easily swallowed and digested.
      (1) Begin with clear liquids.
      (2) Progress to full liquids, soft foods, and then a regular diet as the child's condition improves.
5. Kidney involvement
   a. Observe the child for decreased urine output. Record oral and IV intake and urine output exactly.
   b. Observe for hypertension.
   c. Insert indwelling catheter if necessary for urinary retention.
   d. Administer appropriate amounts of fluids and electrolytes.
   e. See nursing care of the child with renal failure, page 1375.
   f. Correct and monitor acid–base balance.
6. General considerations
   a. Maintain adequate caloric, fluid, and vitamin intake. Oral fluids are preferable if they can be retained.
   b. Avoid hypothermia or hyperthermia.
      (1) Control of body temperature is impaired in many types of poisoning.
      (2) Monitor the child's temperature frequently.

c. Observe closely for inflammation and tissue irritation.
   (1) This is especially important in ingestion of kerosene or other hydrocarbons, which cause chemical pneumonitis.
   (2) Isolate the patient from other children, especially those with respiratory infections.
   (3) Administer antibiotics as prescribed by the physician.

H. Providing Emotional Support for the Child and His Family.

1. Remain calm and efficient while working rapidly.
2. Discourage anxious parents from handling, caressing, and overstimulating their child.
3. Counsel parents who often feel guilty about the accident.
   a. Encourage parents to talk about the poisoning.
   b. Emphasize how their quick action in getting treatment for the child has helped.
   c. Discuss ways that they can be supportive to their child during his hospitalization.
   d. Do not allow prolonged periods of self-incrimination to continue. Refer the parents to a psychologist for assistance in resolving these feelings if necessary.
4. Involve the young child in therapeutic play to determine how he views the situation.
   a. The child often sees nursing measures as punishments for his misdeed involving the poisoning.
   b. Explain the child's treatment and correct his misinterpretations in a manner appropriate for his age.

I. Preventing Further Poisoning Episodes.

1. Initiate patient and parental teaching only after the acute episode is over.
2. Initiate a community health nursing referral. A home assessment should be made so that underlying problems are recognized and appropriate help is provided.

Health Education

A. Prevention

1. Information concerning poison prevention should be available on every hospital pediatric unit and during every child health care visit.
   a. Many free booklets and home safety checklists are available from sources such as insurance companies and drug companies.
   b. Teaching may be done with any parent regardless of the reason for the child's hospitalization or office visit.
2. General precautions
   a. Keep medicines and poisons out of the reach of children.
   b. Provide locked storage for highly toxic substances; select cabinet that is higher than child can reach or climb.
   c. Do not store poisons in the same area as foods.
   d. Be certain all containers are properly marked and labeled. Keep medicines, drugs, and household chemicals in their original containers.
   e. Do not discard poisonous substances in receptacles where children can reach them, but *do* discard used containers of poisonous substances.
   f. Teach children not to taste or eat unfamiliar substances.
   g. Medications
      (1) Clean out medicine cabinets periodically.

(a) Dispose of old medications in containers out of the reach of children.
(b) Prescription medications should be discarded when the illness for which they were prescribed has run its course.
(c) Keep medications in "child-proof" containers that are securely closed.
   (2) Read all labels carefully before each use.
(a) Follow exact directions on the label.
(b) Never take a drug from an unlabeled bottle.
   (3) Do not give medicines prescribed for one child to another child.
   (4) Never refer to drugs as candy or bribe children with such inducements.
   (5) Never give or take medications in the dark.
   (6) Encourage parents not to take medication in front of young children, as children role-play adult behaviors.
   (7) Suggest that mothers NOT keep medications in their purses or on the kitchen table.
   (8) Keep baby creams and ointments away from young children.
h. Never puncture or burn aerosol containers.
i. Store lawn and garden pesticides in a separate place under lock and key outside of the house; do not store large quantities of cleaning products, pesticides, etc.
j. Keep a 30-ml. (1-ounce) bottle of ipecac syrup; be familiar with how to use it.
k. Keep a list of emergency telephone numbers including the poison control center, physician's number, nearest hospital, and ambulance service.
l. Be prepared to act in cases of poisoning. Keep a list of emergency actions readily available.
m. Remove plants from floors and low tables.
n. Reinforce the need for vigilance and consistent supervision for infants and young children due to their increased mobility, increased curiosity, and increased dexterity.

B. Emergency Actions to Teach Parents

1. Suspect poisoning with the occurrence of sudden, bizarre symptoms or peculiar behavior in toddlers and preschoolers.
2. Read the label on the ingested product or call the physician, hospital, or poison control center for instructions regarding treatment for the poisoning. Give all relevant information about the child, his condition, and the substance he took.
3. Maintain an adequate airway in a child who is convulsing or who is not fully conscious.
4. Dilute the poison with 6–8 ounces of water if advised.
5. Make the child vomit if so directed. Do not induce vomiting if any of the following occurs:
   a. The child is unconscious or convulsing.
   b. Ingested poison was a strong corrosive such as lye or drain cleaner.
   c. Ingested poison contains gasoline, kerosene, or other petroleum distillates.
6. Directions for making the child vomit:
   a. Administer 1 tablespoon of ipecac syrup with 250 ml. (about 1 cup) of warm water.
   b. If vomiting does not occur in 20 minutes, this dose may be repeated once only.
7. Transport the child promptly to the nearest medical facility.
   a. Wrap the child in a blanket to prevent chilling.

b. Bring the container and any vomitus or urine to the hospital with the child.
8. Avoid excessive manipulation of the child.
9. Act promptly but calmly.
10. Do not assume the child is safe simply because the emesis shows no trace of the poison or because the child appears well. The poison may produce a delayed reaction or may have reached the small intestine, where it is still being absorbed.

Poisoning With Acetaminophen

Acetaminophen is the most common drug poisoning agent in children.

A. Drug Action

1. Antipyretic
2. Analgesic

B. Diagnostic Measures

1. Serum acetaminophen level 4 hours after ingestion
   a. Toxicity occurs with ingestion of >140 mg./kg.
   b. Severe toxicity occurs when the blood level exceeds 150 μg./ml. 4 hours after ingestion
2. Liver and renal function studies

C. Clinical Manifestations

1. Acetaminophen is toxic to the liver, resulting in cell necrosis and possibly cell death.
2. First 24 hours after ingestion:
   a. May be asymptomatic
   b. Anorexia
   c. Nausea/vomiting
   d. Diaphoresis
   e. Malaise
   f. Pallor
3. Second 24 hours:
   a. Right upper quadrant pain due to liver damage
   b. Increased liver function tests
4. Days 3–8
   a. Jaundice
   b. Coagulation abnormalities
5. Mortality is 10%

D. Intervention

1. Administer syrup of ipecac, as recommended
2. Gastric lavage
3. Administration of charcoal
4. N-acetylcysteine (Mucomyst) as antidote—if charcoal is given, lavage it out before giving Mucomyst.

Poisoning With Aspirin (Acetylsalicylic Acid)

Aspirin is a major cause of childhood poisoning, but its incidence is decreasing as the use of acetaminophen is increasing.

A. Drug Action

1. Antipyretic
2. Analgesic
3. Anti-inflammatory
4. Inhibits platelet aggregation and prothrombin production

B. Diagnostic Measures

1. 2 gr./kg. results in mildly toxic ingestion
   a. For a toddler, approximately 24 baby aspirin tablets *or* 6 adult aspirin tablets *or* 3 extra-strength aspirin tablets would result in toxicity.
2. Toxicity is a blood salicylate level of 50–100 mg./ml.

C. Clinical Manifestations

The peak action of aspirin occurs 2–4 hours after ingestion
1. Nausea/vomiting
2. Tinnitus (ringing in the ears)
3. Prolonged bleeding time
4. Increased metabolic rate resulting in increased body temperature—often the parents think the child needs more aspirin.
5. Aspirin is an acid resulting in metabolic acidosis, which could lead to seizures, coma, and death.
6. Metabolic acidosis and increased metabolism result in an increased respiratory rate—this results in respiratory alkalosis.

D. Interventions

1. Treat acid–base imbalance.
2. Establish hydration and calories, related to increased metabolic rate.
3. Induce emesis and gastric lavage.
4. Provide activated charcoal and a cathartic, if ordered.
5. Treat fever with external measures.
6. Monitor salicylate level.
7. Assess kidney function and perform dialysis, if needed.
8. Assess bleeding tendencies and vitamin K level and provide vitamin K to decrease bleeding, if needed.

Lead Poisoning

Lead poisoning (plumbism) results from the consumption of lead in some form.
1. Each year, approximately 4% of children aged 6 months to 5 years in the US have evidence of excessive serum lead levels.
2. A small number of these victims die, and many are left with chronic neurologic handicaps, mental deficiency, and/or behavioral problems.

Etiology

1. Multiple episodes of ingestion of substances containing lead
   a. Toys, furniture, window sills, household fixtures, and plaster painted with lead-containing paint. (Legislation stipulates that toys, children's furniture, and the interior of homes be painted with lead-free paint; however, the problem may continue if the deeper layers of paint and plaster are contaminated with lead.)
      (1) It takes the body twice as long to secrete lead as it does to absorb it.
      (2) One paint chip contains much more lead than is considered safe.
   b. Lead toys
   c. Cigarette butts and ashes
   d. Acidic juices or foods served in lead-based earthenware pottery made with lead glazes
   e. Colored paints used in newspapers, magazines, children's books, matches, playing cards, and food wrappers
   f. Water from lead pipes
   g. Fruit covered with insecticides
   h. Dirt containing lead fallout from automobile exhaust
   i. Antique pewter, particularly when used to serve acidic juices or foods
   j. Lead weights (curtain weights, fishing sinkers)

2. Inhalation of fumes containing lead (less common cause in children)
   a. Leaded gasoline
   b. Burning storage batteries
   c. Dust-containing lead salts
   d. Dust in the air at shooting galleries and in enclosed firing ranges with poor ventilation
   e. Cigarette smoke

Altered Physiology

1. Lead salts are absorbed by the blood from the respiratory tract or the intestines; the body absorbs lead poorly.
2. Normally, lead is deposited in the bone, where it is stored in an inert form.
3. Excess lead is deposited in the soft tissues, causing damage primarily to the nervous system, red blood cells, and kidneys.
   a. Nervous system
      (1) Brain—increased capillary permeability results in edema, increased intracranial pressure, and vascular damage; destruction of brain cells causes seizures, mental retardation, paralysis, blindness, and learning disabilities.
      (2) Neurologic damage cannot be reversed.
   b. Blood
      (1) Lead attaches to red blood cells.
      (2) Inhibition of a number of steps in the biosynthesis of heme, thus reducing the number of red blood cells, increasing fragility, and reducing half-life.
      (3) The decreased production of hemoglobin results in anemia and respiratory distress.
   c. Kidneys—injury to the cells of the proximal tubules, causing increased excretion of amino acids, protein, glucose, and phosphate
4. Lead is slowly transferred from soft tissues to bone.
   a. It is deposited in insoluble form with calcium.
   b. The deposition causes increased thickness and density of long bones.
   c. Decalcification is associated with the release of lead from bone.
5. Lead is absorbed at a faster rate in children than in adults.

Epidemiologic Factors

1. Slums and old neighborhoods are high-risk areas because of old, deteriorating housing.
2. Pica (a habit of eating nonfood items such as paint chips, often involving a craving type of behavior) is a common precondition.
   a. Poisoning associated with pica is a chronic process.
   b. Clinical manifestations appear after 3–6 months of fairly steady lead ingestion.
3. Decreased parent–child interaction; decreased child supervision; decreased nutritional intake

Incidence

1. Highest in children between 1 and 6 years of age, especially those between 1 and 3 years
2. High in individuals living in old homes or slum areas
3. No significant difference in sex
4. High among siblings

5. Symptomatic lead poisoning most frequently occurs in the summer months
6. Recurrence rate is high

Clinical Manifestations

Symptoms may not develop until after 3 months of consistent ingestion
1. Gastrointestinal symptoms
   a. Vomiting
   b. Abdominal pain
   c. Colic
   d. Constipation
   e. Loss of appetite
   f. Weight loss
2. Central nervous system symptoms due to encephalopathy (common in children)
   a. Falling, clumsiness, loss of coordination (ataxia)
   b. Irritability or listlessness
   c. Seizures
   d. Local paralysis
   e. Drowsiness, coma
   f. Peripheral nerve palsies
   g. Learning disabilities
   h. Loss of newly acquired skills
3. Hematologic symptoms
   a. Anemia
   b. Pallor
   c. Respiratory distress
4. Cardiovascular symptoms
   a. Hypertension
   b. Bradycardia
5. Symptoms depend on the amount of lead in the soft tissues and blood
   a. Onset is insidious.
   b. Usually progresses from mild to severe manifestations as the lead slowly accumulates.
   c. Infants and toddlers may present severe manifestations initially.
   d. Symptoms may be intermittent for several months.

Diagnostic Evaluation

1. Detailed history with emphasis on the presence or absence of clinical symptoms, evidence of pica, family history of lead poisoning, possible source of exposure to lead, recent change in behavior, developmental delay, or behavior problems.
2. Erythrocyte protoporphyrin (EP) level—often used as the initial screening test. Children with values ≥ 50 μg./100 ml. should have a blood level determination done.
3. Blood lead level—values above 50 μg./100 ml. often indicate need for treatment, depending on the results of a more complete medical and laboratory examination of the individual child.
   a. A normal blood lead level is less than 20 μg./dL. Toxicity occurs at or above 34 μg./dL.
4. Hematologic evaluation for anemia.
5. Flat plate of abdomen—may reveal radiopaque material if lead has been ingested during the preceding 24–36 hours.
6. X-ray of long bones—may show increased density at the epiphyseal lines.
7. Calcium disodium edetate (EDTA) mobilization test—demonstrates increasing levels of lead in the urine over a 24-hour period following injection of calcium disodium edetate.

8. Urinary coproporphyrin (UCP) level—elevated with high blood lead levels greater than 150 μg./24 hours.
9. Urinary delta-aminolevulinic acid (ALA) level—20 μg./100 ml. is considered abnormal.

Prognosis

1. Improving, with increased emphasis on prevention and screening.
2. Children with central nervous system involvement have a poor prognosis for normal development. Residual effects on the nervous system are permanent. Late symptoms of learning disabilities may appear 3 or more years after treatment. Specific intellectual defect may interfere with the child's progress at school.

Nursing Interventions

A. Collecting a Urine Specimen as a Diagnostic Tool.

A 24-hour specimen is more accurate than a single voided specimen (see the section on specimen collection).

B. Increasing Excretion of Lead From the Body.

1. Administer cleansing enemas if radiopaque lead particles are observed on abdominal x-rays.
2. Administer appropriate chelating agents (edetate calcium disodium (EDTA) and British anti-Lewisite (BAL)
   a. Action—react with lead to form nontoxic compounds that are excreted by the bowel and kidney
      (1) BAL is given first to decrease the chance of seizures developing
      (2) EDTA with lead can be toxic to the kidneys
      (3) Initiated if serum lead level is greater than 25 μg/dL
   b. Dosage—depends on individual drug, the child's weight, severity of poisoning, prior history, and whether or not other chelating agents are being used simultaneously.
      (1) BAL is administered deep IM. This results in pain and tissue necrosis at the injection site.
      (2) EDTA is administered IV.
      (3) Chelating agents are given every 4 hours for 5 days.
      (4) Success is measured by the amount of lead excreted in the urine.
   c. Implement measures to decrease pain at injection site.
      (1) Rotate sites of injection.
      (2) Apply warm packs to site to decrease pain.
      (3) Move painful areas slowly.
   d. Appropriate play activities should be planned to prepare the child for the injections and as an outlet for the pain and anger he feels.

C. Treating Associated Problems.

1. Increase oral and IV fluids to enhance excretion, except if increased intracranial pressure is present.
2. Monitor
   a. Electrolytes
   b. Liver and kidney function BEFORE and AFTER chelation because lead excretion will increase the load on the kidneys
   c. Intake and output
3. Provide supplemental calcium, phosphorous, and vitamin D to help lead move from the blood (where it is toxic) to the bones (where it is nontoxic)
4. Treat anemia and any associated respiratory distress.

D. Providing Supportive Care to the Child With Encephalopathy.

1. Observe for:
   a. Rising blood pressure
   b. Papilledema
   c. Slow pulse
   d. Seizures
   e. Unconsciousness
2. See the section on pediatric neurologic problems, page 1435.
3. Maintain seizure precautions.

E. Observing for Factors Associated With Lead Poisoning.

1. Pica
   a. Observe and record the child's eating habits and food preferences.
   b. Report any attempted eating of nonfood substances.
   c. Provide regular meals and make mealtime a pleasurable time for the child.
   d. Discourage oral activity and substitute activity that contributes to play, social skills, and ego development.
   e. Refer the family for additional social or psychiatric casework if indicated to reduce the psychological or cultural factors that result in pica in the child.
2. Altered parent–child relationships—record when family members visit as well as the nature of their interaction with the child.

F. Providing the Child With Social and Motor Stimulation.

1. Assess the child's level of development. The DDST (Denver Developmental Screening Test) may be useful for this purpose (see pp. 1075–1076).
2. Provide and encourage activities that will help the child to learn and progress from his present developmental state (see the section on growth and development, p. 1079).
3. Initiate appropriate referrals in cases of obvious developmental delays or learning difficulties. Such referrals may be to such professionals as psychologists, psychiatrists, and specialists in early child education.
4. Share the results of developmental testing with the parent(s) and discuss ways to provide stimulation for the child at home.

G. Providing Emotional Support to the Parent(s) or Caretakers.

1. Use sensitivity in interviewing and teaching to avoid causing or increasing guilt feelings about the poisoning and to establish a positive, trusting relationship between the family and the health care facility.
2. Explain the treatment and its purpose because parents are frequently faced with putting an asymptomatic child through painful treatments.

H. Preventing Re-exposure of the Child to Lead.

1. Instruct the parents regarding the seriousness of repeated exposure to lead.
2. Initiate a referral to a community health nurse to determine if exposure to lead is continuing and to provide continuing support to the family; a home/environmental assessment should be done.
3. Advise the parents to require their landlord to professionally remove lead paint from the walls; assist them with this process.

a. Refer the parents to the housing authority.
b. Do not allow the child in the home while lead paint is being removed. Place the child temporarily in a convalescent home or foster home if necessary.

4. When it is impossible to eliminate lead hazards from the home:
   a. Scrape loose or chipped paint and plaster from the window sills, woodwork, moldings, etc., and tape the areas with contact paper; cover large problem areas with wood or paneling.
   b. Remove all crumbling plaster and replaster or cover the area with wallboard or contact paper.

5. Suggest periodic, focused household cleaning to remove the lead dust; use a wet mop.

6. Encourage handwashing before meals and at bedtime to eliminate lead consumption from normal hand-to-mouth activity.

7. Make certain that the family is able to provide close supervision of the child or assist them to make arrangements to ensure that the child is adequately supervised at home.

8. Make sure to assess the child's furniture and toys.

I. Preparing Parents for Long-Term Sequelae.

1. Long-term medical follow-up is essential.
   a. Residual lead is liberated gradually after treatment.
      (1) May result in the renewal of symptoms.
      (2) May increase serum lead to a dangerous level.
      (3) Additional damage to the central nervous system may become apparent for several months (after discharge from the hospital).
   b. Acute infections must be recognized and treated promptly. (These may reactivate the disease.)
   c. Some children are placed on D-penicillamine for long-term chelation only if current exposure to lead is definitely excluded. If this drug is used, it should be given on an empty stomach, 2 hours before breakfast.
   d. Many children require supplemental iron therapy. Parents should be instructed regarding its administration and side effects.

2. Reexposure to lead must be prevented.

J. Expanding Assessment and Intervention Beyond the Identified Client.

1. Inquire about the presence of pica in all children under 6 years of age.

2. Screen siblings and playmates of known cases immediately.

3. Screen all children from high-risk areas on a routine basis.

4. Provide follow-up to all children suffering from lead poisoning as well as to those in the early stage of undue lead absorption to prevent their becoming poisoned.

Health Education

1. Initiate and support educational campaigns through schools, day-care centers, and news media to alert parents and children to hazards and symptoms of lead poisoning.

2. Provide in clinics, waiting rooms, and other appropriate settings literature stressing the hazards of lead, sources of lead, and signs of lead intoxication.

3. Support legislation to study the nature and extent of the lead poisoning problem, to detect and treat such poisoning, and to eliminate the causes of lead poisoning.

4. Literature stressing the causes and prevention of lead poisoning should be provided.*

5. Nutritional teaching may be indicated (see the section on nutrition, p. 1102).

The Abused Child
(Child Abuse and Neglect)

Child abuse includes physical or emotional abuse/injury/trauma, neglect, or sexual abuse of a child that is intentional and nonaccidental. Abuse includes:

1. Battering—physical injury
2. Drug abuse—intentional administration of harmful drugs, especially during pregnancy
3. Sexual abuse
   a. Sexual assault or molestation (nonfamily offender)
   b. Incest (family offender)
4. Emotional abuse—scapegoating, belittling, humiliating, lack of mothering

Neglect is omission of certain appropriate behaviors, with such omission having detrimental physical or psychological effects on development. Neglect includes:

1. Child abandonment
2. Lack of providing the child with basic needs of survival: shelter, clothing, stimulation, medical care, food, love, supervision, education, attention, emotional nurturing, and safety

Etiology

Child abuse is not a uniform phenomenon with one set of causal factors, but a multidimensional phenomenon. The phenomenon may be related to the combined presence of three factors: special kind of child, special kind of parent or caretaker, special circumstances of crisis.

Contributing Factors *(Not Unicausal)*

1. Incidents of child abuse may develop as a result of disciplinary action taken by the abuser who responds in uncontrolled anger to real or perceived misconduct of the child. The parents may confuse punishment with discipline. "Good parenting" may be equated with physical contact to eradicate undesirable child behavior.
   The abuser may be a stern, authoritarian disciplinarian.

2. Incidents of child abuse may develop out of a quarrel between the caretakers. The child may come to the aid of one parent, may find himself in the midst of the quarrel, or may object to the quarrel; marital discord is common.

3. The abuser may be under a great deal of stress because of life circumstances (debt, poverty, illness) and may thus resort to child abuse. Crisis and stress may be ongoing. The abuser may have a low frustration tolerance level and may not have a well-developed means of coping with stress in general.

4. The abuser may be intoxicated with alcohol or drugs at the time of the abuse; only 10% of abusers have a history of mental illness.

5. Child abuse frequently occurs while the mother is away

* Literature is available from the Lead Industries Association, 292 Madison Avenue, New York, NY 10017 and from the US Department of Health and Human Services, Superintendent of Documents, US Government Printing Office, Washington, DC 20402.

from the home and the child is left in the care of a babysitter or boyfriend.

6. Lack of effective mothering, inappropriate mother–child bonding, and punitive treatment as a child may contribute to the parent becoming an abuser.

7. Specific characteristics evident in many abusing parents include:
   a. Low self-esteem—a sense of incompetence in role; unworthiness; unimportance
   b. Unrealistic attitudes and expectations of child; little regard for the child's own needs and age-appropriate abilities; lack of knowledge related to parenting skills
   c. Fear of rejection—a deep need to feel wanted and loved, but a feeling of rejection when love is not obvious; a crying infant may elicit a feeling of rejection
   d. Inability to accept help—isolation from the community; loneliness
   e. Unhappiness due to unsatisfactory relationships; may look to child for satisfaction of own emotional needs
   f. Child abusers are often the children of abuse.
   g. Abusers often have low self-esteem, have difficulty controlling aggressive impulses, and often live in social isolation.

8. Incidents of child abuse may develop from a general attitude of resentment or rejection on the part of the abuser toward the child.

9. Atypical child behavior (e.g., hyperactivity or a technology-dependent child who needs additional care may unintentionally provoke the abuser.

10. The degree of the family crisis is not usually in proportion to the degree of abuse.

Clinical Manifestations

A. Characteristics of the Child Utilized as an Index of Suspicion.

1. Child usually under 3 years of age. School-age children and adolescents are also subject to abuse. The average age of sexual abuse is 9.
2. General health of the child indicates neglect (diaper rash, poor hygiene, malnutrition).
3. Characteristic distribution of fractures (scattered over many different parts of body).
4. Disproportionate amount of soft-tissue injury.
5. Evidence that injuries occurred at different times (healed and new fractures, resolving and fresh bruises).
6. Cause of recent trauma in question.
7. History of similar episodes in past.
8. No new lesions occurring during the child's hospitalization.
9. May show a wide range of reactions—may be either very withdrawn or overactive. The child may be anxious, tense, or nervous.
10. May show unusual affection for strangers or may be overly fearful of adults and avoid any physical contact with them.
11. For sexual abuse: child may fear no one will believe them; may experience self-blame; most know their abuser.
12. Children may not "tell" about abuse from parents, fearing loss of security, i.e., "A bad parent is better than no parent at all."
13. Behavior problems, depression, and acting-out behaviors may result.

14. For abuse that occurs in school or day care, the child may exhibit fear of the teacher, have nightmares, decrease school attendance, or develop psychosomatic illnesses.

B. Injuries or Types of Abuse That May Occur:

1. Bruises, welts (linear or loop-like)
2. Abrasions, contusions, lacerations (most common)
3. Wounds, cuts, punctures
4. Burns (cigarette, radiator, etc.), scalding—stocking or glove distribution
5. Bone fractures (including skull)
6. Sprains, dislocations
7. Subdural hemorrhage or hematoma; "shaking baby syndrome"
8. Brain damage
9. Internal injuries
10. Drug intoxication
11. Malnutrition (deliberately inflicted)
12. Freezing, exposure
13. Whiplash-type injury
14. Eye injuries
15. Periorbital injuries; ear bruises
16. Dirty, infected wounds or rashes
17. Unexplained coma in infant
18. Failure to thrive
    a. Developmental delay
    b. Malnutrition with decreased muscle mass
    c. Decreased interaction with environment and with others
    d. Dental caries
    e. Listless, behavior problems
19. Sexually transmitted diseases
    a. Genital trauma

C. Identifying Behaviors Common in Abusing or Neglecting Parent(s):

(Be aware that not all abusing parents exhibit these behaviors.)

1. Anxiously volunteers information or withholds information.
2. Gives an explanation of the injury that does not fit the condition or gets story confused concerning the injury.
3. Shows inappropriate reaction or concern to severity of injury.
4. Becomes irritable about questions being asked.
5. Seldom touches or speaks to the child; does not respond to him. May be critical of the child or indicate unreal expectations of him (or may be over solicitous to him).
6. Delays seeking medical help; refuses to sign permit for diagnostic studies. Frequently changes hospitals or physicians.
7. Shows no involvement in care of the hospitalized child; does not inquire about the child.
8. The problem of abuse is a total family problem—family dysfunction is evident.
9. Little or no prenatal care.
10. Inappropriate response to newborn; disinterested or unhappy with child.

Incidence

1. 1–6 million children per year are abused.
2. 2000 children die each year from abuse.

Treatment

1. Prevention is the most critical aspect of treatment.
   a. Early recognition for potential abuse—identify family or child at risk: alcohol/drug abuser, ado-

lescent parent, low-income single-parent family, multiple births, or unwanted child; sickly and more demanding child or premature with long separation from mother at birth.

   b. Use community resources and special programs (i.e., "hot lines," crisis nurseries, self-help groups) to aid the parent in preventive support.

2. Once abuse or neglect is suspected:

   a. Public Law 94-247 (Child Abuse and Neglect Act—1973) requires that professionals report suspected abuse. Notify the appropriate officials.

   b. Since other children in the family may be involved, they should be examined by a physician as soon as possible.

   c. Establish and maintain a therapeutic relationship with the parents. Generally a team approach is recommended to assess family needs and determine the most effective use of community resources to protect the child and help the family. The parents are the focus of treatment. They are helped to develop a sense of self-esteem and confidence and to relinquish their abusive behavior.

   d. Specific counseling and/or psychiatric intervention for the abused child focusing on the emotional impact of the event(s).

Nursing Interventions

A. Inspecting Every Child's Body Upon Admission to the Hospital for Evidence of Possible Abuse.

1. Describe completely on nursing record all bruises, lacerations, etc., as to location and state of healing. Look carefully at areas generally covered with clothing (i.e., buttocks, underarms, behind knees, bottom of feet). Be alert for abuse of the school-age child. Most often the child's injury is not severe enough to require medical attention, but the child may be hospitalized for some other medical problem.

2. Quote descriptions of the injury, including the date, time, and place of the event. Describe old, healing injuries; assess developmental level.

3. Collect any necessary specimens for identification of organisms, sperm, or semen.

4. Take colored photographs.

5. Discuss with the physician the case of any child suspected of being abused.

   a. Every state (as well as the District of Columbia) has mandatory reporting laws. All states provide statutory immunity for those who report real or suspected child abuse. There is no immunity from civil or criminal liability for failure to report such.

   b. Every nurse is morally and legally responsible to report and provide protective services for the abused child.

   c. Become familiar with laws, procedures, and protective services in your community and state.

B. Providing Care to Meet the Physical Needs of the Child

1. Medical management depends on the injury.

2. Provide for nutritional, cleanliness, and safety needs.

C. Being Prepared to Care Effectively for the Child Who is the Victim of Sexual Assault or Incest.

1. Sexual abuse should be suspected when the young, prepubital child presents with:

   a. Trauma not readily explained

   b. Gonorrhea, syphilis, or other sexually transmitted organisms

   c. Blood in urine or stool

   d. Painful urination or defecation

   e. Penile or vaginal infection or itch

   f. Penile or vaginal discharge

   g. Report of increased, excessive masturbation

   h. Report of increased, unusual fears

2. Establish a relationship with the child based on mutual respect, empathy, and sensitivity.

   a. The child may be extremely calm or hysterical. She/he may verbally express a desire to talk about the incident. Take into consideration the different ways emotions are expressed by children at different developmental stages.

   b. Consideration of the child's emotions in conjunction with a good relationship may encourage the child to express his or her feelings either verbally or through drawings or play.

   c. Prepare the child both physically and psychologically for the necessary physical and pelvic examination.

   d. Talk with the child without the presence of the parents, especially when incest is possible.

   e. Prevent sexually transmitted disease, pregnancy, and tetanus. Prophylactic treatment should be given for penile penetration of any orifice.

D. Observing and Recording Pertinent Information Regarding the Parent–Child Relationship.

1. Do the parents visit the child? Do parents become involved in caring for child?

2. How do(es) the parent(s) respond to the child? Does the parent talk to the child, touch him, hold him, and play with him?

3. How does the child react to the parent? Is he excited when the parent arrives? Does he appear frightened and withdrawn? Does he cry when the parent leaves?

4. What does the parent expect of the child? Are his expectations appropriate for the child? Is there role reversal between parent and child?

E. Obtaining a Thorough Nursing History in Order to Establish a Nursing Care Plan That is Individualized to Meet Specific Needs of the Child.

1. Information should be obtained relating to the child's sleeping habits, toilet habits, favorite foods and eating habits, favorite toy or security objects, play habits and favorite playmate, names and ages of siblings, nickname, previous hospital experience, developmental assessment, and persons who will visit the child.

2. Care and good judgment must be used in obtaining this information from parents, because they undoubtedly have already been asked many questions by many people. Use chart information already obtained to eliminate repetition.

3. Obtaining a nursing history in a nonthreatening, nonjudgmental manner can convey to parents that you have a genuine interest in caring for their child, and that you respect the knowledge they have as parents of their child. Getting the history will also allow you to assess the parents' knowledge and expectations of their child and will set a positive atmosphere for a continued relationship.

F. Providing for the Child a Milieu to Reduce Trauma Similar to That of Any Hospitalized Child Placed in the Strange and Frightening Environment of the Hospital by Implementing the Principles of Emotional Support (see p. 1120).

The child must be treated as an individual. He may need extra help in the following areas:

1. Having ambivalent feelings toward his parent or parents or any adult caretaker
2. Overcoming his low self-image and the fear that something is wrong with him
3. Fearing future abuse upon his return home or for misbehavior in the hospital
4. Satisfying his strong need for attention, affection, and having a trusting relationship with an adult

   Note: Some of these children have never learned how to trust an adult; they are fearful of giving affection for fear of rejection.

5. Learning alternate ways of expressing his needs and feelings

G. Fostering a Trusting Relationship With the Child Who May be Fearful of Adults.

1. Assign one nurse to care for the child over a period of time.
2. Make no threatening moves toward the child. The child will indicate his readiness and awareness of the environment by his verbal or facial expressions.
3. Touch the child gently.
4. Provide nonthreatening physical contact (hold the child frequently and cuddle him). Pick him up and carry him around; encourage any exploration of your face, hair, etc.
5. Enlist the cooperation of volunteers to provide additional mothering.
6. Provide appropriate opportunities for play.
7. Set limits for him.
8. Provide therapeutic play to allow the child to express his fears and anger in a nonverbal manner; be nonjudgmental and supportive with his expression of feelings; correct misconceptions.

H. Fostering a Relationship With the Parents That Will Encourage Them to Accept Guidance and Will Help in Dealing With the Problem.

1. Assume a nonjudgmental attitude that is neither punitive nor threatening. The desire to help must be conveyed.
2. Refrain from questioning them about the incident of abuse. (The suspected abuser will be interviewed by the physician, the social worker, and the authority who investigates the case.)
3. Include the parents in the hospital experience (i.e., orient them to the unit and to any procedure to be done for the child). Serve as role model in the management of the child's behavior as well as their own. Try to give the parents as much information as possible about the care of their child. Listen to what they are saying.
4. Refrain from challenging all the information they may give.
5. Express appropriate concern and kindness. Remain objective yet empathetic. This will help foster the parents' self-respect and improve their self-image and dignity.
6. Discuss the reporting to the authorities with them because of the widespread nature of the problem and the need for education and assistance.
7. Support the parents who may have feelings of guilt, anger, and helplessness. Explain to them the extent of trauma and educate them. Allow them to ventilate their feelings. Support their parental role in handling the child (i.e., allow the child to talk about or play out the incident, but do not force it).

I. Fostering a Healthy Parent–Child Relationship.

1. Build a relationship by working with the parents' strengths rather than their weaknesses. Use compliments as positive reinforcement.
2. Serve as a role model of appropriate methods of child care in areas such as feeding, bathing, and play.
   a. Remember that many of these parents were abused as children and have no role models or personal experience with nurturing behaviors.
3. Assist parents to learn safe and appropriate parenting skills.
   a. Foster normal growth and development.
   b. Foster attachment between child and parents, not between child and nurse, when the parents are present; the latter would increase their feelings of incompetence in the parenting role.
   c. Correct their erroneous expectations as to what is appropriate behavior for a particular age group.
   d. Encourage parents to take time out from caring for their child in order to meet their own needs; assist them in identifying safe and appropriate resources for their child's care.
4. Provide the parent with psychological support and reinforcement for appropriate parenting behaviors that are exhibited.
5. Work with the parent in planning for the child's future care.
6. Determine in what areas the parent needs help: Does the baby cry a lot? How does this make her feel? How does she comfort him? When she is alone, is there someone she can call for help? Does she feel the child understands what she expects of him?
7. By forming a helping relationship with the parent, the nurse will strengthen the protective role of the parent and bind her to her child.

J. Coming to Terms With Your Own Feelings of Anger, Disgust, and Contempt for the Parents.

1. A critical part of working in this area is learning to recognize, examine, and work with these feelings. It may help to do the following:
   a. Realize that most abusing parents do love their child and want the best for him in spite of their ambivalent feelings for him.
   b. Understand the dynamics of child abuse and neglect. This crisis is due to the stress with which the parents are unable to cope and to the deprivations they have themselves suffered in their past.
   c. Focus on the needs of the parents rather than on the injuries of the child. Treatment is aimed at helping the parents reach their maximum potential as parents.
   d. Expect repeated rejection from the parents who lack self-esteem and trust.
   e. Understand that these parents are experiencing terror, guilt, and remorse; they are fearful and yet expect criticism and condemnation.
2. Before teaching or criticizing parenting behaviors, it is essential for the nurse to understand the culture of the client.

K. Being Aware of the Entire Scope of Nursing Responsibilities in Dealing With the Abused and Neglected Child.

1. Case finding—identify the potential (or suspected) abused and neglected child. Be a participating and contributing member of the multidisciplinary team in treating the abused child and his family.
   a. Recommend assessment of outside care facilities as a possible source of abuse.

b. If a teacher is suspected of being the abuser, the child may
   (1) Display increased fear of the teacher
   (2) Decrease school attendance
   (3) Develop psychosomatic symptoms during school days
   (4) Develop nightmares
   (5) Worry excessively over their school performance
c. Case finding involves an assessment of the parents, the child, and the environment.

2. Provide care for the physical, sexual, and psychosocial needs of the child.
3. Child advocacy
   a. Protect the child from further abuse.
   b. If necessary, recommend that the child be removed from an abusive environment to prevent further injury.
4. Nurse – parent relationship — develop therapeutic, trusting relationships that will help parents develop to their full potential.
5. Support community assistance programs to help parents overcome isolation—crisis nurseries, parent aids, Parents Anonymous, foster care facilities, and day-care centers.
6. Support public re-education to enhance the parenting capabilities of every man and woman: Education for Parenting, Home Start, and adolescent parenthood programs.

L. Being Aware That the Goal of Treatment of the Parents is to Ensure the Physical and Emotional Safety of the Child.

1. It is estimated that 90% of abusing parents can be rehabilitated.
2. The ideal approach is to return the child to his biologic parents.
3. Treatment is offered to help the parents do the following:
   a. Understand and redirect their anger.
   b. Develop an adequate parent–child relationship.
   c. See their child as an individual with his own needs and differences.
   d. Enjoy their child.
   e. Develop realistic expectations of their child.
   f. Decrease their use of criticism.
   g. Increase their own sense of self-esteem and confidence.
   h. Establish supportive relationships with others.
   i. Improve their economic situation (if appropriate).
   j. Show progress toward physical, emotional, and intellectual development of their child
4. Inform the parents of organizations designed to help them:
   a. Parents Anonymous, 7120 Franklin Avenue, Los Angeles, CA 90046 (1-800-421-0353). This is a private organization of self-help groups for parents who have abused or fear they might have abused their children. *Frontiers* is their publication.
   b. C. Henry Kempe National Center for the Prevention and Treatment of Child Abuse and Neglect, 1205 Oneida Street, Denver, CO 80220

M. Being Aware of the Child Who Has the Potential for Being Abused and Provide Anticipatory Guidance for Prevention of Abuse.

1. The premature infant, the hyperactive child, the chronically ill child, the retarded child, the child who requires a great deal of care and confines a parent to the home, the child involved in a disturbed mother–infant bond, all have the potential for being abused.
2. Encourage early participation of mother (parents) in the care of the child during hospitalization.
3. Prepare the parent for the fact that the child does require a great deal of care, but encourage her to find outlets for her frustrations.
4. Provide her with the name and telephone number of someone at the hospital to whom she can look for help (e.g., social worker).
5. Initiate a community nursing referral.

N. Supporting the Parent and the Child When a Decision is Made to Have the Child Removed From the Home.

1. The decision is made for the safety and protection of the child.
2. The parents are afforded the opportunity to have counseling to help them learn to deal with their problem.
3. The child must be prepared for his removal from the home and placement plans. He must be allowed time to work through his feelings.

Health Education

A. Teach the Parents About Normal Growth and Development.
(See the section on growth and development, p. 1079.)
1. Give specific information about and examples of the types of behavior to expect at the various stages of development. Point out in a nonthreatening way normal behavior exhibited by their child.
2. Give specific information on dealing with this behavior.
3. Serve as a role model and teacher; minimize intensity when the parents become threatened.

B. Teach the Parents How to Use Discipline Without Resorting to Physical Force.
1. Discipline must be consistent. Offer suggestions for alternative ways of handling undesirable behavior.
2. Rewards may be used for acceptable behavior (e.g., a trip to the zoo, staying up later than usual for a special television show, a special treat).
3. Rewards are withheld for unacceptable behavior.

C. Teach Children How to Avoid Being the Victim of Abuse.
1. Teach them about "good touch" and "bad touch."
2. Emphasize that they can say "no" to anyone who wants to touch their body.
3. Provide names or places where they can go if they feel they are being abused.
4. Assist them in dealing with their fears that their parents will be sent to jail or that they will be removed from the home.

D. Support the Parents and Child in Preparation for Discharge to Home.
1. Both parents and child (if age is appropriate) need to know and understand any specific instructions relative to injury and follow-up care.
2. The parents need to be made aware of the most common posthospitalization behavior children may have (see p. 1121).
3. Make known to parents your continued concern and your availability as a source of help. Stress the need for follow-up care. Help them to use community resources available (e.g., homemaker, community health nurse, therapy for parents, etc.).

Agencies and organizations dealing with abuse:
International Institute of Children's Nature and Their Rights, 1615 Myrtle Street, NW, Washington, DC 20012; (202) 726-3341; publishes journal

National Center on Child Abuse and Neglect, PO Box 1182, Washington, DC 20013

National Committee for Prevention of Child Abuse, 322 S Michigan Avenue, Suite 1250, Chicago, IL 60604; (312) 565-1100; publishes *Caring* (quarterly) and monographs

Society's League Against Molestation (SLAM), 524 S First Avenue, Arcadia, CA 91106; publishes *Guardian* (bimonthly) and a brochure; works to prevent sex abuse and molestation and to educate public through media

---

The Dying Child

Nursing Interventions

A. Analyzing One's Own Feelings About Death and Developing a Philosophy That Enables the Nurse to Support the Dying Child and His Family.

1. Become familiar with literature about death and dying and use it as a resource in planning nursing care.
2. Recognize that the goal is to assist the child and family to cope with the experience in such a way that it will promote growth rather than destroy family integrity and emotional well-being.

3. Share personal feelings about death and dying with colleagues. It is not unusual for the nurse to experience personal feelings of anger, frustration, helplessness, and guilt.

B. Recognizing the Stages of Dying as Identified by E. Kübler-Ross and Utilizing This Knowledge in Planning and Implementing Care (see below, Stages of Dying as Identified by Dr. Elizabeth Kübler-Ross).

1. Be aware that dying children, their families, and the staff will all progress through these stages, not necessarily at the same time.
2. Children experience the stages with much variation. They tend to pass more quickly through the stages and may merge some of these stages.
3. The nursing goal is to accept the child and family whatever stage they are experiencing, not to push them through the stages.

C. Understanding the Meaning of Illness and Death to the Child at the Various Stages of Growth and Development and Using This Information in Planning and Implementing Care.

1. See Stages in the Development of a Child's Concept of Death, page 1524.
2. Be aware of other factors that influence a child's personal concept of death. Of particular importance are:
   a. The amount and type of direct exposure a child has had to death.
   b. Cultural values, beliefs, and patterns of bereavement.
   c. Religious beliefs about death and an afterlife.

Stages of Dying as Identified by Dr. Elizabeth Kübler–Ross

Stage	Nursing Implications
I. Denial. Shock. Disbelief.	Accept denial, but function within a reality sphere. Do not tear down the child's (or family's) defenses.
	Be aware that denial usually breaks down in the early morning when it may be dark and lonely.
	Be certain that it is the child or family who is using denial, not the staff.
II. Anger. Rage. Hostility.	Accept anger and help the child express it through positive channels.
	Be aware that anger may be expressed toward other family members, nursing staff, physicians, and other persons involved.
	Help families to recognize that it is normal for children to express anger for what they are losing.
III. Bargaining (from "No, not me." to "Yes, me, but. . .")	Recognize this period as a time for the child and family to regain strength.
	Encourage the family to finish any unfinished business with the child. This is the time to do things such as take the promised trip or buy the promised toy.
IV. Depression. (The child and/or family experiences silent grief and mourns past and future losses.)	Recognize this as a normal reaction and expression of strength.
	Help families to accept the child who does not want to talk and excludes help. This is a usual pattern of behavior.
	Reassure the child that you can understand his feelings.
V. Acceptance.	Assist families to provide significant loving human contact with their child.

Stages in the Development of a Child's Concept of Death

Age of Child	Stage of Development
Child up to 3 years	At this stage, the child cannot comprehend the relationship of life to death, since he has not developed the concept of infinite time.
	The child fears separation from protecting and comforting adults.
	The child perceives death as a reversible fact.
Preschool-age child	At this age the child has no real understanding of the meaning of death; he feels safe and secure with his parents.
	The child may view death as something that happens to others.
	The child may interpret his illness as a type of punishment for real or imagined wrongdoing.
	The child may interpret the separation that occurs with hospitalization as punishment; the painful tests and procedures that he is subjected to support this idea.
	The child may become depressed because he is not able to correct these wrongdoings and regain the grace of adults.
	The concept may be connected with magical thoughts and mystery.
School-age child	The child at this age sees death as the cessation of life; he understands that he is alive and that he can become "not alive"; he fears dying.
	The child differentiates death from sleep. Unlike sleep, the horror of death is in pain, progressive mutilation, and mystery.
	The child is vulnerable to guilt feelings related to death because of difficulty in differentiating between death wishes and the actual event.
	The child learns the meaning of death from his own personal experiences.
	Pets
	Death of family members, political figures, etc.
	Television and movies have contributed to his concepts of death and understanding of the meaning of illness.
	Develops more knowledge in the meaning of diagnosis
	Death may occur violently
Adolescent	The adolescent comprehends the permanence of death much as the adult does, although he may not comprehend death as an event occurring to persons close to himself.
	He wants to live—he sees death as thwarting pursuit of his goals: independence, success, achievement, physical improvement, and self-image.
	He fears death before fulfillment.
	The adolescent may become depressed and resentful because of bodily changes that may occur, dependency, and the loss of social environment.
	The adolescent may feel isolated and rejected, since his own adolescent friends may withdraw when faced with his impending death.
	The adolescent may express rage, bitterness, and resentment. He especially resents the fact that he is fated to die.

D. Utilizing the Knowledge About Children's Interpretation of the Meaning of Death at the Various Stages of Growth and Development in Talking to the Child About His Illness and in Answering Questions Concerning Death.

1. Research indicates that children generally can cope with more than adults will allow, and that children appreciate the opportunity to know and understand what is happening to them.
2. It is important that the child's questions be answered simply, but truthfully, and that they be based on his particular level of understanding.
3. The following responses have been suggested by Eassom in *The Dying Child* and may be useful as a guide:

a. Preschool-age child
   (1) When the child at this age is comfortable enough to ask questions about his illness, his questions should be answered. When death is anticipated at some future time and the child asks, "Am I going to die?" a response might be, "We will all die someday, but you are not going to die today or tomorrow."
   (2) When death is imminent and the child asks, "Am I going to die?" the response might be, "Yes, you are going to die, but we will take care of you and stay with you."
   (3) The parents should be allowed to stay with

the child to provide him with protection and support.

(4) When the child asks, "Will it hurt?" the response should be truthful and factual. Death may be described as a form of sleep—a sleep where he will be secure in the love of those around him. (Some children may fear sleep as the result of this type of explanation.)

Note: Anesthesia is sometimes called a "special sleep" so it is NOT currently recommended to refer to death as "sleep."

(5) Parents can express to the child the fact that they do not want him to go and that they will miss him very much; they feel sad, too, that they are going to be separated.

b. School-age child

(1) Responses to the school-age child's questions about death should be answered truthfully. The child looks for support from those he trusts.

(2) The school-age child should be given a simple explanation of his diagnosis and its meaning; he should also receive an explanation of all treatments and procedures.

(3) The child should be given no specific time in terms of days or months, since each individual and each illness is different.

(4) When the school-age child asks, "Am I going to die?" and death is inevitable, he should be told the truth. The school-age child does have the emotional ability to look to his parents and those he trusts for comfort and support.

(5) The school-age child believes in his parents. He should be allowed to die in the comfort and security of his family.

(6) The school-age child knows death means final separation, and he knows what he will miss. He must be allowed to mourn this loss as he dies. He may be sad and bitter and demonstrate aggressive behavior. He must be allowed the opportunity to verbalize this if he is able to do so.

c. Adolescent

(1) The adolescent should be given an explanation of his illness and all necessary treatment procedures.

(2) The adolescent feels deprived and reasonably resentful regarding his illness because he wants to live and reach fulfillment.

(3) As death approaches, the adolescent becomes emotionally closer to his family.

(4) The adolescent should be allowed to maintain his emotional defenses—he may deny absolutely. The adolescent will indicate by his questions what kind of answer he wants.

(5) If the adolescent states, "I am not going to die," he is pleading for support. Be truthful and state, "No, you are not going to die right now."

(6) The adolescent may ask, "How long do I have to live?" He is able to face reality more directly and can tolerate more direct answers. No absolute time should be given since that blocks all hope. If an adolescent has what is felt to be a prognosis of approximately 3 months, the response might be, "People with an illness like yours may die in 3 to 6 months, but some may live much longer."

(7) The bitterness and resentment of the fact that he is fated to die may interrupt necessary procedures and treatments. This behavior must be appropriately handled.

E. Encouraging Parents to Discuss the Illness With the Child and Giving Them Information That Will Be Helpful in Allowing Them to Play a More Supportive Role.

1. Determine what information they have given the child about his illness, and how the child reacted to this information.

2. Determine what specific questions the child has asked about his illness and how the parents have responded.

3. Share with parents your assessment of what the child knows about his illness and what he wants to know.

4. Discuss with the parents how children of various age levels interpret the meaning of death and offer suggestions as to how children's questions regarding death may be answered.

5. Provide the parents with helpful literature about explaining death to children (see Bibliography, p. 1529).

6. Assist the parents to explain the child's illness to siblings and to answer their questions. If appropriate, help the parents to identify ways that siblings can share in the child's care.

7. Promote open and honest sharing between children and their parents.

F. Assisting the Parents in Dealing With Their Adaptation to Their Child's Illness and Anticipated Death.

1. Develop a plan of care that includes the following approach:
   a. The primary responsibility for communicating with the parents should be designated to one nurse.
   b. Information regarding the parents' concerns should be communicated to all staff members.

2. Accept parental feelings about the child's anticipated death and help parents deal with these feelings.
   a. It is not unusual for parents to reach the point of wishing the child dead and to experience guilt and self-blame because of this thought.
   b. The parents may withdraw emotional attachments to the child if the process of dying is lengthy. This occurs because the parents complete most of the mourning process before the child reaches biologic death. They may relate to the child as if he were already dead.

3. Provide anticipatory guidance regarding the child's actual death and immediate postdeath decisions and responsibilities.
   a. Describe what the death will probably be like and how to know when it is imminent. This is necessary to dispel the horrifying fantasies that many parents have.
   b. Clarify the parents' wishes about being present at the child's death and respect their desires.
   c. If appropriate, allow the parents to discuss their feelings about issues such as autopsy and transplant in order that they may make appropriate decisions.
   d. If necessary, assist the parents to think about funeral arrangements.

4. Be aware of factors that affect the family's capacity to cope with fatal illness, especially social and cultural features of the family system, previous experiences

with death, present stage of family development, and resources available to them.

5. Contact the appropriate clergy, if the family desires.
6. During the final hours, do not leave the family alone, unless they request it.
7. Encourage parents and siblings to share their thoughts with the dying child.

G. Performing the Nursing Measures That Provide the Child With Both Physical and Emotional Care During Illness.

1. Provide physical care that makes the child as comfortable as possible. Deliver care in a calm, assured, gentle manner.
2. Talk to the child and answer his questions truthfully.
3. Provide an atmosphere that offers the child the greatest security (e.g., room with another child, room near the nurses' station, etc.).
4. Provide opportunities for play therapy as the child's condition permits; allow the child to make items for family members and friends; older children may want to tape record messages to significant others.
5. Plan for consistency of assignment so that the child can experience continuity of contact with a few nurses who inspire confidence and trust.
6. Encourage active involvement in living to the extent that the child is able (e.g., participation in activities of daily living, play, schooling, socialization).
7. Observe children carefully during play for clues to their symbolic language. Watch carefully what they do and listen to what they say. Drawings and self portraits may also help the child to express his feelings.
8. Communicate caring through touch. The child is comforted by being held, especially by his parents.
9. Allow the child opportunity to direct activities and to let his wishes be known.
10. In the terminal stage, decrease emphasis on invasive procedures (lab studies, vital signs), and focus on comfort measures.
11. Set realistic limits for the child when necessary, and enforce them consistently.

H. Encouraging the Parents to Spend as Much Time as Possible With the Child and Participate in the Child's Care (see the section on Family-Centered Care, p. 1125).

1. Allow the parents to bathe the child and to do procedures within their ability and desire. This allows the parents the feeling that they are doing something for their child.
2. Teach the parents those aspects of the child's care with which they are not familiar.
3. Provide the parents with a place to stay and be comfortable. They should be told where they can find privacy when they want to be alone.
4. Assure the parents that their child will be well cared for in their absence.

I. Utilizing Appropriate Services and Resources in Planning the Care of the Child and Family.

1. Team members often include:
   a. Physician
   b. Nurse
   c. Child
   d. Family
   e. Social worker
   f. Psychiatrist
   g. Clergyman
   h. Community health nurse
   i. School nurse
   j. Parent groups
2. Teamwork is essential because:
   a. Terminally ill children and their families may require different kinds of assistance at different points in time.
   b. They face many problems that are nonmedical in nature.
   c. The child's need for assistance may be very different from that required by his family.
   d. Team members may support one another.
3. To be effective team members, nurses must:
   a. Communicate, collaborate, and cooperate with other members of the team.
   b. Accept responsibility for their contribution to the plan of care and be accountable for the outcome.

J. Providing Emotional Support to the Parents Following the Death of the Child.

1. Allow families who wish it the opportunity to spend some time alone with the child after death.
2. Provide privacy for parents to express their grief in whatever manner they choose.
3. If appropriate, compliment the parents on the excellent care they gave their child.
4. Be aware that your compassionate silence may be more helpful to families than small talk.
5. Assist families to contact other relatives and funeral home as appropriate.
6. Make certain that families have a safe and comfortable means to get home.
7. Invite the parents to call if they have lingering questions or concerns that they wish to discuss.
8. See the bibliography for additional resources.

Trauma—Prehospital Management of the Injured Child

Trauma is a physical or emotional wound or injury that compromises the functioning of major organ systems (i.e., burns, drowning, ingestion, blunt or penetrating injury). This section focuses on physical trauma that does not occur in a hospital.

Etiology

External forces—mechanical, chemical, electrical, or radiation in nature.

Incidence

A. Leading Causes of Death in Children—1 month through 14 years

1. Accidents
   a. Motor vehicle
   b. Fires, burns
   c. Drowning
   d. Ingestion of food or objects or poisons
   e. Firearms
   f. Falls
2. Congenital anomalies

B. Leading Causes of Death in Adolescents

1. Accidents (as above)
2. Homicide
3. Suicide

Immediate Intervention—Primary Survey

Perform the primary survey (initial assessment) in a systematic fashion to recognize and manage life-threatening injuries to the respiratory (airway and ventilation), circulatory (shock), and neurologic systems. Intervention also includes child and family crisis management.

Note: The nurse should provide for her own safety during any rescue or management initiatives.

As first responder, the nurse:

1. Notifies the emergency medical services via bystander, or self if feasible.
2. Does *not* move the child until the airway is patent and cervical spine immobilization is secured.
3. Provides airway management with cervical spine immobilization
   a. Clear the airway of any debris: blood, vomitus, or broken teeth.
   b. Relieve potential obstruction from the tongue falling into the posterior pharynx with a chin lift or jaw thrust maneuver. The chin lift maneuver is performed by placing the thumb into the mouth and the index finger on the chin and pulling outward to pull the tongue out of the posterior pharynx.
   The jaw thrust maneuver is performed by placing the finger at the temporal–mandibular joint and sliding the mandible forward to pull the tongue out of the posterior pharynx (Fig. 61-1*A*).
   c. In traumatic injury, always anticipate the possibility of a fractured cervical vertebra.
   d. Manually keep the head in midline by providing inline traction on the cervical spine. Inline traction is performed by placing the two middle fingers on the mastoid process of the occipital skull and pulling toward the rescuer who is at the child's head (Fig. 46-1*B*).
4. Respiratory
   a. Look, listen, and feel for spontaneous breathing if the airway is open.

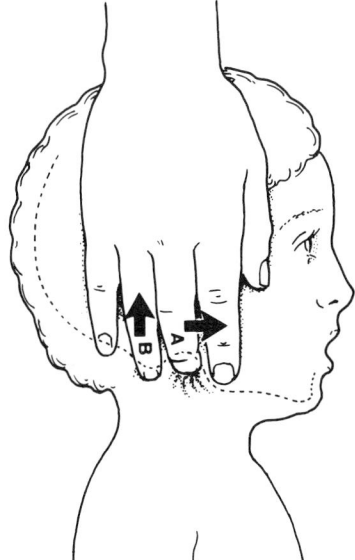

Figure 61-1. (A) Jaw thrust maneuver. (B) In-line manual traction.

   b. If the child is not breathing, initiate cardiopulmonary resuscitation (see CPR, p. 1200).
   c. If a chest wound is present, apply an airtight dressing to avoid spontaneous pneumothorax.
5. Circulation
   a. Apply direct pressure to the area of external bleeding.
   b. Apply direct pressure to the supplying artery to control the hemorrhage. (Children can bleed significantly from small wounds or lacerations.)
   c. Elevate the injured extremity.
   d. Place the child in Trendelenburg position if no head injury or respiratory difficulty is present.
   e. Apply a tourniquet as a last resort.
6. Neurologic
   a. Level of consciousness
      (1) Alert
      (2) Verbal response
      (3) Pain response
      (4) Unresponsive—comatose
   b. Pupil size
   c. Pupil reaction to light
   d. Symmetry of pupils
   e. Thermoregulation
      (1) Children have a larger surface area to body mass ratio. Their body temperature drops more rapidly than that of adults. If body temperature falls below 36° to 37°C. (98°–98.6°F.) resuscitative efforts are more difficult.
      (2) Prevent heat loss by applying any covering such as a blanket, jacket, or other clothing article.
   f. Head injury—elevate the patient to a semi-recumbent position. *Caution:* Do not bend head at neck; assume the existence of a cervical spine fracture.

Continued Intervention—Secondary Survey

Once life-threatening injuries are recognized and stabilized, the secondary survey is performed.

1. The secondary survey consists of a rapid head-to-toe evaluation for additional injuries.
   a. Head
      (1) Skull depression or deformities
      (2) Scalp, mouth, and facial lacerations
   b. Eyes
      (1) Foreign body or hemorrhage
      (2) Periorbital bruising around the eyes may indicate skull fracture (raccoon's sign)
   c. Ears
      (1) Ecchymotic area over the mastoid process may indicate a skull fracture (Battle's sign)
      (2) Clear fluid discharge may indicate a skull fracture
   d. Nose—clear fluid drainage may indicate a skull fracture
   e. Abdomen
      (1) Distention
      (2) Ecchymosis
      (3) Tenderness
   f. Extremities
      (1) Swelling
      (2) Deformity
      (3) Pain or tenderness
      (4) Loss of motion
      (5) Loss of sensation
      (6) Presence or absence of pulse
      (7) Color: pale or cyanotic
      (8) Bone protrusion

Diagnostic Evaluation

The nurse will not have access to diagnostic tools at the scene of the injury. She should use observational skills and understanding of the altered physiology caused by traumatic injury to help prevent death and disability at the scene by following the primary and secondary survey approach.

Nursing Assessments and Interventions

A. Performing a Cursory Physical Assessment.

1. Airway—obstructed, semi-obstructed, stridor
2. Respirations—tachypnea, dyspnea, cyanosis, nasal flaring, subclavicular or suprasternal retractions, paradoxical movement of the chest during inspiration and expiration
3. Circulation
   a. Signs and symptoms of shock occur after 20%–25% of the total blood volume has been depleted.
   b. Observe for tachycardia; pallor; cold, clammy skin surface; altered sensorium; delayed capillary refill.
      (1) Capillary refill is determined by depressing the thumb nailbed and observing the return blood flow.
      (2) Normal capillary refill returns within 2 seconds or the amount of time it takes to mentally say, "capillary refill." Anything greater than 2 seconds indicates that the child is in shock.
      (3) Assess pulses in extremities distal to the injury.
   c. Stop bleeding with direct pressure to wound or at pressure points
      (1) Elevate injured extremity.
4. Neurologic
   a. Eye opening
      (1) Spontaneous
      (2) To voice
      (3) To pain
      (4) None
   b. Verbal response
      (1) Oriented
      (2) Confused
      (3) Inappropriate words
      (4) Incomprehensible words
      (5) None
   c. Motor response
      (1) Obeys commands
      (2) Localizes pain
      (3) Withdraws (pain)
      (4) Flexion (pain)
      (5) Extension (pain)
      (6) None
   d. Check pupil size for equality and observe for any deviation of the eye(s) from normal center.
5. Extremity injury—immobilize injured or fractured extremity with minimal movement to prevent additional damage.
6. Child's and family's reactions—range from hysteria, indifference, shock, anger, controlled, or cooperative.
7. Child and family crisis intervention
   a. Identify the child
   b. Remain calm.
   c. Use a reassuring voice.
   d. Empathize with the child's pain and fear.
   e. Solicit the parents to aid and comfort the child if they are able.
   f. Reassure the child and family that everything possible is being done before and during transport to an emergency facility.
   g. If parents are not present, introduce child to person who will accompany him to hospital; promise to call parents to tell them where the child is.

B. Preventing Death.

Recognize life-threatening injuries and provide initial resuscitative efforts by:
1. Providing a patent airway
2. Covering open chest wounds
3. Control of obvious bleeding

C. Ensuring That the Child Avoids Further Disability or Complications.

1. Maintain adequate airway and ventilation for oxygen perfusion to the brain.
2. Prevent paralysis by providing cervical spine immobilization.
3. Keep the child calm through reassurance in an effort to avoid unnecessary movement.
4. Keep movement of possible extremity fractures to a minimum to avoid blood vessel, nerve, and tissue damage.
5. Provide warmth; prevent chilling.
6. Enhance asepsis as much as possible to decrease the chance of infection.
7. Do not apply salves or topical medications; removing them in the emergency department will result in additional trauma.

D. Assisting the Child to Achieve Psychological Homeostasis With Minimal Emotional Disruption.

1. Encourage the child to ventilate his feelings to avoid short- and long-term psychological maladjustment to the traumatic incident.
2. Permit the child to cry and verbalize discomfort at the scene.
3. Keep the parents at the child's side to give support at the scene of injury.

E. Ensuring That the Child Is Transported Rapidly to a Hospital Emergency Facility.

1. Notify the emergency medical services by telephoning 911 or its equivalent.
2. Enlist the family and bystanders to render assistance under the direction of the nurse while the child awaits emergency transport.
3. Transfer the child to the emergency medical services for rapid transport to a hospital emergency facility.

Health Education

1. Know the principles of safety for each developmental age group of children.
2. Be aware of potentially dangerous toys and products for children.
3. Keep matches, chemicals, medication, etc., out of the reach of children.
4. Teach children to respect traffic laws and look each way before crossing the street.
5. Be aware of infant and child automobile restraint laws.
6. Encourage children to play in designated areas.
7. Teach bicycle safety.
8. Encourage the use of protective sporting gear.
9. Teach the appropriate telephone number to access the emergency medical services of the community.
10. Teach CPR and first aid in the community.
11. Inform the nursing community of the Good Samaritan law.

Bibliography

Books

Genetic Alterations

Garver K and Marchese S. Genetic Counseling for Clinicians. Chicago, Year Book Medical Pub, 1986

Harper P. Practical Genetic Counseling. Boston, John Wright & Sons, 1988

Hollingsworth D and Resnik R. Medical Counseling Before Pregnancy. New York, Churchill Livingstone, 1988

Kelly T. Clinical Genetics and Genetic Counseling. Chicago, Year Book Medical Pub, 1986

Milunsky A. Genetic Disorders and the Fetus. New York, Plenum Press, 1986

Russell P. Essential Genetics. Boston, Blackwell Scientific Publications, 1987

Scriver C. The Metabolic Basis of Inherited Disease. New York, McGraw–Hill, 1989

Mental Retardation

Baroff G. Mental Retardation: Nature, Cause, and Management. Washington, DC, Hemisphere Publishing, 1986

Crump I. Nutrition and Feeding of the Handicapped Child. San Diego, College Hill Press, 1987

Gardner J and Chapman M. Program Issues in Developmental Disabilities. Baltimore, Brooks Publishing, 1990

Lane D and Startford B. Current Approaches to Down's Syndrome. New York, Praeger, 1985

Matson J. Handbook of Behavior Modification with the Mentally Retarded. New York, Plenum Press, 1990

Matson J and Marchetti A. Developmental Disabilities. Philadelphia, Grune & Stratton, 1988

McClurg E. Your Down's Syndrome Child. New York, Doubleday, 1986

Mental Retardation: Meeting the Challenge. Geneva, World Health Organization, 1985

Rubin IL and Crocker A. Developmental Disabilities. Philadelphia, Lea & Febiger, 1989

Sirrocco A. Characteristics of Facilities for the Mentally Retarded. Hyattsville, MD, US Department of Health and Human Services, 1989

Summers J. The Right to Grow Up. Baltimore, Brookes Publishing, 1986

Tingey C. Down Syndrome: A Resource Handbook. Boston, Little Brown, 1988

Van Hasselt V, Strain P and Hersen M. Handbook of Developmental and Physical Disabilities. New York, Pergamon Press, 1988

Wisniewski H and Snider D. Mental Retardation. New York, New York Academy of Sciences, 1986

Attention Deficit Disorders

Diagnostic and Statistical Manual of Mental Disorders (DSM-III-R) Washington, DC, American Psychiatric Association, 1987

Dworkin P. Learning and Behavior Problems of Schoolchildren. Philadelphia, WB Saunders, 1985

Gearheart B. Learning Disabilities: Educational Strategies. St. Louis, Times Mirror/Mosby, 1985

Interagency Committee on Learning Disabilities. Learning Disabilities: A Report to the US Congress. Washington, DC, US Department of Health and Human Services, 1987

Johnston R. Learning Disabilities, Medicine, and Myth. Boston, Little, Brown & Co, 1987

Nazum M. What Do Teens With Learning Disabilities Want to Know. A publication of the 92nd Street YM-YWHA: New York State Developmental Disabilities Planning Council and the Federation of Jewish Philanthropies, 1985

Wolraich M. The Practical Assessment and Management of Children with Disorders of Development and Learning. Chicago, Year Book Medical Pub, 1987

Poisonings

Goldfrank L. Toxicologic Emergencies: A Comprehensive Handbook in Problem Solving. 3rd ed. New York, Appleton–Century–Crofts, 1986

Hillman J. Initial Management of the Poison Patient. Secaucus, NJ, Network for Continuing Medical Education, 1989

Jaeger R. Poisoning Emergencies: A Primer. St. Louis, Catholic Health Association of the United States, 1987

Lead: Environmental Aspects. Geneva, World Health Organization, 1989

Preventing Lead Poisoning in Young Children. Atlanta: Centers for Disease Control, 1985

Child Abuse

A Report to the Congress: Joining Together to Fight Child Abuse. Washington, DC, US Government Printing Office, 1986

Brassard M, Germain R, and Hart S. Psychological Maltreatment of Children and Youth. New York, Pergamon Press, 1987

Browne K, Davies C and Stratton P. Early Prediction and Prevention of Child Abuse. New York, John Wiley & Sons, 1988

Daro D. Confronting Child Abuse. New York, Free Press, 1988

Goldman R and Gargiulo R. Children at Risk. Danville, IL, Interstate Printers and Publishers, 1990

Helfer R and Kempe R. The Battered Child. Chicago, University of Chicago Press, 1987

Holm M. Shall the Circle Be Unbroken? Longmont, CO: Bookmakers Guild, 1986

Oates K. Child Abuse and Neglect. New York, Brunner/Mazel, 1986

Walker CE. The Physically and Sexually Abused Child. New York, Pergamon Press, 1988

White K. Treating Family Violence in a Pediatric Hospital. Rockville, MD, US Department of Health and Human Services, 1987

Wissow L. Child Advocacy for the Clinician. Baltimore, Williams & Wilkins, 1990

The Dying Child

Kastenbaum R. Death, Society and Human Experience. 3rd ed. St. Louis, CV Mosby, 1986

Waechter E. The Child and Family Facing Life-Threatening Illness. Philadelphia, JB Lippincott, 1987

Journals

Genetic Alterations

Black R and Weiss J. Genetic support groups in the delivery of comprehensive genetic services. Am J Hum Genet 1989; 45(4):647–654

Butler W. Genetic counseling: Ethics and patients' rights. Consultant 1986; 26(4):87

Davidson R and Childs B. Perspectives in the teaching of human genetics. Adv Hum Genet 1986; 16:79–119

Evers-Kiebooms G. Genetic risk, risk perception, and decision making. Birth Defects 1987; 23(2)

Farrell C. Genetic counseling: The emerging reality. J Perinat Neonat Nurs 1989; 2(4):21–33

Gelehrter T. Genetic screening: What runs in the family? Emerg Med 1986; 18(16):84

Lamb C. Practical answers on prenatal genetics. Patient Care 1986; 20(12):108

Marks J. Genetic counseling principles in action. Birth Defects 1989; 25(5)

Morgan C and Elias S. Prenatal diagnosis of genetic disorders. J Perinat Neonat Nurs 1989; 2(4):1–12

Osband D. Multifactorial inheritance: Implications for perinatal and neonatal nurses. J Perinat Neonat Nurs 1989; 2(4):43–52

Rhodes A. Wrongful birth and wrongful life. MCN: 1989; 14(3):171

Stringer M. Chorionic villi sampling: A nursing perspective. J Obstet Gynecol Neonat Nurs 1989; 17(1):19–22

Weiss J. Genetic support groups. Birth Defects 1986; 22(2)

Williams J. Genetic counseling in pediatric nursing care. Pediatr Nurs 1986; 12(4):287–290

Williams J. Screening for genetic disorders. J Pediatr Health Care 1989; 3(3):115–121

Wilson G. Pediatric genetics. Pediatr Ann 1990; 19(2):

Mental Retardation

Abbott P and Sapsford R. Diverse reports: The load imposed on mothers who care for a mentally handicapped child at home. Nursing Times 1986; 82(10): 47–49

Cameron S and Orr R. Stress in families of school-aged children with delayed mental development. Can J Rehabil 1989; 2(3):137–144

Crocker A. Mental retardation. Pediatr Ann 1989; 18(10)

Feeg V. Developmental disabilities services and the territorial imperative. Pediatr Nurs 1987; 13(2):78

Gleeson S. Public sector perspective: Potential nursing services in mental retardation. Pediatr Nurs 1987; 13(2): 81–83

Green C. The importance of behaviour modification for the nursing process in mental handicap. Nurs Educ Today 1987; 7(2):59–62

Murphy D. Prehospitalization preparation for institutionalized people with mental retardation: A nursing approach. Ment Retard 1986; 24(5): 307–310

Rothery S. Understanding and supporting special siblings. J Pediatr Health Care 1987; 1(1):21–25

Savage T and Culbert C. Early intervention: The unique role of nursing. J Pediatr Nurs 1989; 4(5):339–345

Steele S. Deinstitutionalization of persons with mental retardation/developmental disabilities. Issues Compre Pediatr Nurs 1987; 10(4):235–250

Stone D. Professional perceptions of parental adaptation to a child with special needs. Child Health Care 1989; 18(3):174–177

Stravrakaki C. Psychiatric perspectives on mental retardation. Psychiatr Clin North Am 1986; 9(4)

Tarjan G. Mental retardation. Psychiatr Ann 1989; 19(4)

Tasch V. Parenting the mentally retarded adolescent: A framework for helping families. J Community Health Nurs 1988; 5(2):97–108

Taylor M. Teaching parents about their impaired adolescent's sexuality. MCN 1989; 14(2):109–112

Attention Deficit Disorders

Bond W. Recognition and treatment of attention deficit disorder. Clin Pharm 1987; 6(8):617–624

Coleman W and Levine M. Attention deficits in adolescence: Description, evaluation, and management. Pediatr Rev 1988; 9(9):287–297

Munoz–Millan R and Casteel CR. Attention deficit hyperactivity disorder: Recent literature. Hosp Community Psychiatry 1989; 40(7):699–706

Pelham W. What do we know about the use and effects of CNS stimulants in the treatment of ADD? J Child Contemp Soc 1987; 19(1–2):99–110

Selekman J. The learning disabled child: Another frontier for nursing. Holist Nurs Pract 1988; 2(2):1–10

Silver L. Controversial approaches to treating learning disabilities and attention deficit disorder. Am J Dis Child 1986; 140:1045–1051

Silver L. A review of the Federal Government's Interagency Committee on Learning Disabilities Report to the US Congress. Learning Disabilities Focus 1988; 3(2):73–80

Poisonings

Arena J. Poisoning in children. Pediatr Ann 1987; 16(11)

Blumer J and Reed M. Pediatric toxicology. Pediatr Clin North Am 1986; 33(2)

Curran A. Childhood lead poisoning: An overview. Hosp Med 1986; 22(12):40

Davidson L and Dierking B. Medical emergencies in the poisoning patient. J Emerg Med Serv 1989; 14(6):74–78

Gaudreault P, et al. Poisoning exposures and use of ipecac in children less than 1 year old. Ann Emerg Med 1986; 15(7), 808–810

Hilgartner M. Hematology. Pediatr Ann 1990; 19(3)

Leff K. Salicylate toxicity in the pediatric patient. Emerg Med Serv 1989; 18(5): 43–44

Needleman H. The persistent threat of lead: Medical and sociological issues. Curr Probl Pediatr 1988; 18(12)

Polin R and Fox W. The newborn. II. Pediatr Clin North Am 1986; 33(3)

Rudner N. Children with elevated lead levels. J Pediatr Health Care 1988; 2(1):46–49

Tenenbein M. Pediatric toxicology. Curr Probl Pediatr 1986; 16(4)

Throckmorton K and Throckmorton D. Pills, plants, and poisonings. Emergency 1988; 20(10):52–59

Trinkoff A and Baker S. Poisoning hospitalizations and deaths from solids and liquids among children and teenagers. Am J Public Health 1986; 76(6):657–660

Child Abuse

Brook U. Parental characteristics in cases of child-battering and abuse. Med Law 1988; 7(3):295–301

Bruce D and Zimmerman R. Shaken impact syndrome. Pediatr Ann 1989; 18(8):482

Carty H. Brittle or battered. Arch Dis Child 1988; 63(4):350–352

Dubowitz H. Prevention of child maltreatment: What is known. Pediatrics 1989; 83(4):570–577

Ewigman B and Kiviahan C. Child maltreatment fatalities. Pediatr Ann 1989; 18(8):476

Gill P. Caring for abused children in the emergency department. Holist Nurs Pract 1989; 4(1):37–43

Green A. Child maltreatment and its victims: Comparison of physical and sexual abuse. Psychiatr Clin North Am 1988; 11(4):591–610

Hobbs C. ABC of child abuse: Burns and scalds. Br Med J 1989; 298(6683): 1302–1305

Hobbs C. ABC of child abuse: Fractures. Br Med J 1989; 298(6679):1015–1018

Hobbs C. ABC of child abuse: Head injuries. Br Med J 1989; 298(6681): 1169–1170

Houck G and King M. Child maltreatment: Family characteristics and developmental consequences. Issues Ment Health Nurs 1989; 10(3–4):193–201

Kessler D and New M. Emerging trends in child abuse and neglect. Pediatr Ann 1989; 18(8):471

Malmquist C. Child abuse. Psychiatr Ann 1987; 17(4):222–283

Meadow R. ABC of child abuse: Epidemiology. Br Med J 1989; 298(6675):727–730

Meadow R. ABC of child abuse: Poisoning. Br Med J 1989; 298(6684): 1445–1446

Miles R and Burns R. Recognition of the subtle signs of child abuse. J Tenn Med Assoc 1990; 83(1):20–21

Newton R. Intracranial haemorrhage and non-accidental injury. Arch Dis Child 1989; 64(2):188–190

Nunno M and Motz J. The development of an effective response to the abuse of children in out-of-home care. Child Abuse Negl 1988; 12(4):521–528

Peters J. Criminal prosecution of child abuse: Recent trends. Pediatr Ann 1989; 18(8):505

Skuse D. ABC of child abuse: Emotional abuse and neglect. Br Med J 1989; 298(6689):1692–1694

Tammelleo A. If you suspect child abuse. RN 1988; 51(7):57–59

Widom C. Does violence beget violence? A critical examination of the literature. Psycholog Bull 1989; 106(1):3–28

Widom C. Sampling biases and implications for child abuse research. Am J Orthopsychiatry 1988; 58(2):260–270

Zeanah C and Zeanah P. Intergenerational transmission of maltreatment: Insights from attachment theory and research. Psychiatry 1989; 52(2):177–196

The Dying Child

Adam J. What about the relatives? Prof Nurse 1990; 5(5):260–262

Archer D and Smith A. Sorrow has many faces: Helping families cope with grief. Nursing 1988; 18(5):43–45

Bakke K and Pomietto M. Family care when a child has late stage cancer: A research review. Oncol Nurs Forum 1986; 13(6):71–76

Bluebond–Langner M. Worlds of dying children and their well siblings. Death Studies 1989; 13(1):1–16

Caruso–Herman D. Concerns for the dying patient and family. Semin Oncol Nurs 1989; 5(2):120–123

Castiglia P. Death of a sibling. J Pediatr Health Care 1988; 2(4):211–213

Coffel J. When a family loses a child. Issues Compr Pediatr Nurs 1989; 12(4):311–312

Davis K. Educational needs of the terminally ill student. Issues Compr Pediatr Nurs 1989; 12(2–3):235–245

Gray E. The emotional and play needs of the dying child. Issues Compr Pediatr Nurs 1989; 12(2–3):207–224

Gyulay J. Grief responses. Issues Compr Pediatr Nurs 1985; 12(1):1–31

Meehan J. Pain control in the terminally ill child at home. Issues Compr Pediatr Nurs 1989; 12(2–3):187–197

Pazola K and Gerberg A. Privileged communication—talking with a dying adolescent. MCN 1990; 15(1):16–21

Petix M. Explaining death to school-age children. Pediatr Nurs 1987; 13(6): 394–396

Rochester C. The child and family facing death. Issues Compr Pediatr Nurs 1989; 12(4):261–267

Sommer D. The spiritual needs of dying children. Issues Compr Pediatr Nurs 1989; 12(2–3):225–233

Trauma in Children

Mead D. The injured child. Nurs Times 1989; 85(36):28–32

Murphy R and Harris B. The art of accident scene care. Emergency Care Quarterly 1987; 3(1):7–13

Schwaitzbery S and Harris B. The epidemiology of pediatric trauma. Emergency Care Quarterly 1987; 3(1): 1–6

Appendixes and Index

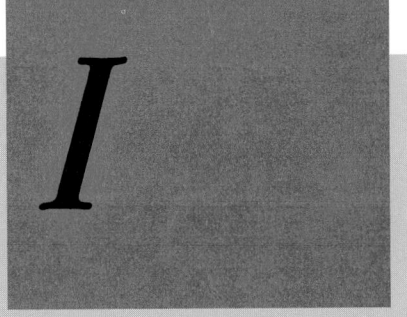
Abbreviations

Conventional Units

kg. = kilogram
gm. = gram
mg. = milligram
μg. = microgram
$\mu\mu$g. = micromicrogram
ng. = nanogram
pg. = picogram
dl. = 100 milliliters
ml. = milliliter

cu.mm. = cubic millimeter
fL. = femtoliter
mM. = millimole
nM. = nanomole
mOsm. = milliosmole
mm. = millimeter
μ. = micron or micrometer
mm.Hg = millimeters of mercury
U = unit
mU = milliunit
μU = microunit
mEq. = milliequivalent

IU = International Unit
mIU = milliInternational Unit

SI Units

g. = gram
L. = liter
d. = day
h. = hour
mol. = mole
mmol. = millimole
μmol. = micromole
nmol. = nanomole
pmol. = picomole

REFERENCE RANGES—HEMATOLOGY*

Determination	Reference Range		Clinical Significance
	Conventional Units	*SI Units*	
A$_2$ hemoglobin	1.5%–3.5% of total hemoglobin	Mass fraction: 0.015–0.035 of total hemoglobin	Increased in certain types of thalassemia
Bleeding time	2–8 min.	2–8 min.	Prolonged in thrombocytopenia, defective platelet function, and aspirin therapy
Factor V assay (proaccelerin factor)	60%–140%		
Factor VII assay (antihemophiliac factor)	50%–200%		Deficient in classical hemophilia
Factor IX assay (plasma thromboplastin component)	75%–125%		Deficient in Christmas disease (pseudohemophilia)
Factor X (Stuart factor)	60%–140%		Deficient in Stuart clotting defect
Fibrinogen	200–400 mg./dl.	2–4 g./dl.	Increased in pregnancy, infections accompanied by leukocytosis, nephrosis
Decreased in severe liver disease, abruptio placentae
Fibrin split products	Less than 10 mg./L.	Less than 10 mg./L.	Increased in disseminated intravascular coagulation
Fibrinolysins (whole blood clot lysis time)	No lysis in 24 h.		Increased activity associated with massive hemorrhage, extensive surgery, transfusion reactions

(continued)

REFERENCE RANGES—HEMATOLOGY (continued)

Determination	Reference Range		Clinical Significance
	Conventional Units	*SI Units*	
Partial thromboplastin time (activated)	20–45 sec.		Prolonged in deficiency of fibrinogen, factors II, V, VIII, IX, X, XI, and XII, and in heparin therapy
Prothrombin consumption	Over 20 sec.		Impaired in deficiency of factors VIII, IX, and X
Prothrombin time	9.5–12 sec.		Prolonged by deficiency of factors, I, II, V, VII, and X, fat malabsorption, severe liver disease, coumarin-anticoagulant therapy
Erythrocyte count	Males: 4,600,000–6,200,000/cu. mm.	$4.6–6.2 \times 10^{12}$/L.	Increased in severe diarrhea and dehydration, polycythemia, acute poisoning, pulmonary fibrosis
	Females: 4,200,000–5,400,000/cu. mm.	$4.2–5.4 \times 10^{12}$/L.	Decreased in all anemias, in leukemia, and after hemorrhage, when blood volume has been restored
Erythrocyte indices			
Mean corpuscular volume (MCV)	80–94 (cu. μ.)	80–94 fL.	Increased in macrocytic anemias; decreased in microcytic anemia
Mean corpuscular hemoglobin (MCH)	27–32 $\mu\mu$g./cell	27–32 pg.	Increased in macrocytic anemias; decreased in microcytic anemia
Mean corpuscular hemoglobin concentration (MCHC)	33%–38%	Concentration fraction: 0.33–0.38	Decreased in severe hypochromic anemia
Reticulocytes	0.5%–1.5% of red cells	Number fraction: 0.005–0.015	Increased with any condition stimulating increase in bone marrow activity (i.e., infection, blood loss [acute and chronic]); following iron therapy in iron deficiency anemia, polycythemia rubra vera. Decreased with any condition depressing bone marrow activity, acute leukemia, late stage of severe anemias
Erythrocyte sedimentation rate (ESR)—Westergren method	Males under 50 yr.: <15 mm./h. Males over 50 yr.: <20 mm./h. Females under 50 yr.: <20 mm./h. Females over 50 yr.: <30 mm./h.	<15 mm./h. <20 mm./h. <20 mm./h. <30 mm./h.	Increased in tissue destruction, whether inflammatory or degenerative; during menstruation and pregnancy; and in acute febrile diseases
Erythrocyte sedimentation ratio—Zeta centrifuge	41%–54% in both sexes	Fraction: 0.41–0.54	Significance similar to ESR
Hematocrit	Males: 42%–50%	Volume fraction: 0.42–0.5	Decreased in severe anemias, anemia of pregnancy, acute massive blood loss
	Females: 40%–48%	Volume fraction: 0.4–0.48	Increased in erythrocytosis of any cause, and in dehydration or hemoconcentration associated with shock
Hemoglobin	Males: 13–18 gm./dl. Females: 12–16 gm./dl.	2.02–2.79 mmol./L. 1.86–2.48 mmol./L.	Decreased in various anemias, pregnancy, severe or prolonged hemorrhage, and with excessive fluid intake. Increased in polycythemia, chronic obstructive pulmonary

(continued)

REFERENCE RANGES—HEMATOLOGY (continued)

Determination	Reference Range		Clinical Significance
	Conventional Units	*SI Units*	
			diseases, failure of oxygenation because of congestive heart failure, and normally in people living at high altitudes
Hemoglobin F	Less than 2% of total hemoglobin	Mass fraction: <0.02	Increased in infants and children, and in thalassemia and many anemias
Leukocyte alkaline phosphatase	Score of 40–100		Increased in polycythemia vera, myelofibrosis, and infections Decreased in chronic granulocytic leukemia, paroxysmal nocturnal hemoglobinuria, hypoplastic marrow, and viral infections, particularly infectious mononucleosis
Leukocyte count Neutrophils Eosinophils Basophils Lymphocytes Monocytes	Total: 5,000–10,000/cu. mm. 60%–70% 1%–4% 0%–0.5% 20%–30% 2%–6%	$5-10 \times 10^9$/L. Number fraction: 0.6–0.7 Number fraction: 0.01–0.04 Number fraction: 0.00–0.05 Number fraction: 0.2–0.3 Number fraction: 0.02–0.06	Elevated in acute infectious diseases, predominantly in the neutrophilic fraction with bacterial diseases, and in the lymphocytic and monocytic fractions in viral diseases Elevated in acute leukemia, following menstruation, and following surgery or trauma Depressed in aplastic anemia, agranulocytosis, and by toxic agents such as chemotherapeutic agents used in treating malignancy Eosinophils elevated in collagen disease, allergy, intestinal parasitosis
Osmotic fragility of red cells	Increased if hemolysis occurs in over 0.5% NaCl Decreased if hemolysis is incomplete in 0.3% NaCl		Increased in congenital spherocytosis, idiopathic acquired hemolytic anemia, isoimmune hemolytic disease, ABO hemolytic disease of newborn Decreased in sickle cell anemia, thalassemia
Platelet count	100,000–400,000/cu. mm.	$0.1-0.4 \times 10^{12}$/L.	Increased in malignancy, myeloproliferative disease, rheumatoid arthritis, and postoperatively; about 50% of patients with unexpected increase of platelet count will be found to have a malignancy Decreased in thrombocytopenic purpura, acute leukemia, aplastic anemia, and during cancer chemotherapy, infections, and drug reactions

* Laboratory values vary according to the techniques used in different laboratories.

REFERENCE RANGES—SERUM, PLASMA, AND WHOLE BLOOD CHEMISTRIES

| Determination | Normal Adult Reference Range | | Clinical Significance | |
	Conventional Units	*SI Units*	*Increased*	*Decreased*
Acetoacetate	0.2–1.0 mg./dl.	19.6–98 μmol./L.	Diabetic acidosis Fasting	
Acetone	0.3–2.0 mg./dl.	51.6–344.0 μmol./L.	Toxemia of pregnancy Carbohydrate-free diet High-fat diet	
Adrenocorticotropic hormone (ACTH) (plasma)—RIA*	Less than 50 pg./ml.	Less than 50 mg./L.	Pituitary-dependent Cushing's syndrome Ectopic ACTH syndrome Primary adrenal atrophy	Adrenocortical tumor Adrenal insufficiency secondary to hypopituitarism
Aldolase	3–8 Sibley-Lehninger U/dl. at 37°C.	22–59 mU/L. at 37°C.	Hepatic necrosis Granulocytic leukemia Myocardial infarction Skeletal muscle disease	
Aldosterone (plasma)—RIA	Supine: 3–10 ng./dl. Upright: 5–30 ng./dl. Adrenal vein: 200–800 ng./dl.	0.08–0.30 nmol./L. 0.14–0.90 nmol./L. 5.54–22.16 nmol./L.	Primary aldosteronism (Conn's syndrome) Secondary aldosteronism	Addison's disease
Alpha-1-antitrypsin	200–400 mg./dl.	2–4 g./L.		Certain forms of chronic lung and liver disease in young adults
Alpha-1-fetoprotein	None detected		Hepatocarcinoma Metastatic carcinoma of liver Germinal cell carcinoma of the testis or ovary Fetal neural tube defects—elevation in maternal serum	
Alpha-hydroxybutyric dehydrogenase	Up to 140 U/ml.	Up to 140 U/L.	Myocardial infarction Granulocytic leukemia Hemolytic anemias Muscular dystrophy	
Ammonia (plasma)	40–80 μg./dl. (enzymatic method); varies considerably with method	22.2–44.3 μmol./L.	Severe liver disease Hepatic decompensation	
Amylase	60–160 Somogyi U/dl.	111–296 U/L.	Acute pancreatitis Mumps Duodenal ulcer Carcinoma of head of pancreas Prolonged elevation with pseudocyst of pancreas Increased by drugs that constrict pancreatic duct sphincters: morphine, codeine, cholinergics	Chronic pancreatitis Pancreatic fibrosis and atrophy Cirrhosis of liver Pregnancy (2nd and 3rd trimesters)
Arsenic	6–20 μg./dl.; if 50 μg./dl., suspect toxicity	0.78–2.6 μmol./L.	Accidental or intentional poisoning Excessive occupational exposure	
Ascorbic acid (vitamin C)	0.4–1.5 mg./dl.	23–85 μmol./L.	Large doses of ascorbic acid as a prophylactic against the common cold	
Bilirubin	Total: 0.1–1.2 mg./dl. Direct: 0.1–0.2 mg./dl. Indirect: 0.1–1 mg./dl.	1.7–20.5 μmol./L. 1.7–3.4 μmol./L. 1.7–17.1 μmol./L.	Hemolytic anemia (indirect) Biliary obstruction and disease Hepatocellular damage (hepatitis) Pernicious anemia Hemolytic disease of newborn	

(continued)

REFERENCE RANGES—SERUM, PLASMA, AND WHOLE BLOOD CHEMISTRIES (continued)

	Normal Adult Reference Range		Clinical Significance	
Determination	Conventional Units	SI Units	Increased	Decreased
Blood gases				
Oxygen, arterial (whole blood):				
Partial pressure (PaO_2)	95–100 mm. Hg	12.64–13.30 kPa	Polycythemia	Anemia
Saturation (SaO_2)	94%–100%	Volume fraction: 0.94–1	Anhydremia	Cardiac decompensation Chronic obstructive pulmonary disease
Carbon dioxide, arterial (whole blood): partial pressure ($PaCO_2$)	35–45 mm. Hg	4.66–5.99 kPa	Respiratory acidosis Metabolic alkalosis	Respiratory alkalosis Metabolic acidosis
pH (whole blood, arterial)	7.35–7.45	7.35–7.45	Vomiting Hyperpnea Fever Intestinal obstruction	Uremia Diabetic acidosis Hemorrhage Nephritis
Calcitonin	Basal: nondetectable 400 pg./ml.	400 ng./L.	Medullary carcinoma of the thyroid Some nonthyroid tumors Zollinger-Ellison syndrome	
Calcium	8.5–10.5 mg./dl.	2.125–2.625 mmol./L.	Tumor or hyperplasia of parathyroid Hypervitaminosis D Multiple myeloma Nephritis with uremia Malignant tumors Sarcoidosis Hyperthyroidism Skeletal immobilization Excess calcium intake: milk-alkali syndrome	Hypoparathyroidism Diarrhea Celiac disease Vitamin D deficiency Acute pancreatitis Nephrosis After parathyroidectomy
CO_2, venous	Adults: 24–32 mEq./L. Infants: 18–24 mEq./L.	24–32 mmol./L. 18–24 mmol./L.	Tetany Respiratory disease Intestinal obstruction Vomiting	Acidosis Nephritis Eclampsia Diarrhea Anesthesia
Carcinoembryonic antigen (CEA)—RIA	0–2.5 ng./ml.	0–2.5 µg./L.	The repeatedly high incidence of this antigen in cancers of the colon, rectum, pancreas, and stomach suggests that CEA levels may be useful in the therapeutic monitoring of these conditions.	
Catecholamines (plasma)— RIA	Epinephrine, random: up to 90 pg./ml. Norepinephrine, random 100–550 pg./ml. Dopamine, random up to 130 pg./ml.	Up to 490 pmol./L. 590–3240 pmol./L. Up to 850 pmol./L.	Pheochromocytoma	
Ceruloplasmin	30–80 mg./dl.	300–800 mg./L.		Wilson's disease (hepatolenticular degeneration)
Chloride	95–105 mEq./L.	95–105 mmol./L.	Nephrosis Nephritis Urinary obstruction Cardiac decompensation Anemia	Diabetes Diarrhea Vomiting Pneumonia Heavy metal poisoning Cushing's syndrome Burns Intestinal obstruction Febrile conditions

(continued)

REFERENCE RANGES—SERUM, PLASMA, AND WHOLE BLOOD CHEMISTRIES (continued)

Determination	Normal Adult Reference Range		Clinical Significance	
	Conventional Units	*SI Units*	*Increased*	*Decreased*
Cholesterol	150–200 mg./dl.	3.9–5.2 mmol./L.	Lipemia Obstructive jaundice Diabetes Hypothyroidism	Pernicious anemia Hemolytic anemia Hyperthyroidism Severe infection Terminal states of debilitating disease
Cholesterol esters	60%–70% of total	Fraction of total cholesterol 0.6–0.7		The esterified fraction decreases in liver diseases
Cholinesterase	Serum: 0.6–1.6 delta pH Red cells: 0.6–1 delta pH	0.6–1.6 U 0.6–1 U	Nephrosis Exercise	Nerve gas intoxication (greater effect on red cell activity) Insecticides, organic phosphates (greater effect on plasma activity)
Chorionic gonadotropin, beta subunit— RIA	0–5 IU/L.	0–5 IU/L.	Pregnancy Hydatidiform mole Choriocarcinoma	
Complement, human C_3	Males: 88–252 mg./dl. Females: 88–206 mg./ dl.	880–2520 mg./L.	Some inflammatory diseases	Acute glomerulonephritis Disseminated lupus erythematosus with renal involvement
Complement C_4	14–51 mg./dl.	140–510 mg./L.	Some inflammatory diseases	Often decreased in immunologic disease, especially with active systemic lupus erythematosus Hereditary angioneurotic edema
Complement, total (hemolytic)	90%–94% complement		Some inflammatory diseases	Acute glomerulonephritis Epidemic meningitis Subacute bacterial endocarditis
Copper	70–165 µg./dl.	11–25.9 µmol./L.	Cirrhosis of liver Pregnancy	Wilson's disease
Cortisol—RIA	8 AM: 7–25 µg./dl. 4 PM: 2–9 µg./dl.	193–690 nmol./L. 55–248 nmol./L.	Stress: infectious disease, surgery, burns, *etc.* Pregnancy Cushing's syndrome Pancreatitis Eclampsia	Addison's disease Anterior pituitary hypofunction
C-peptide reactivity	1.5–10 ng./ml.	1.5–10 µg./L.	Insulinoma	Diabetes
Creatine	0.2–0.8 mg./ml.	15.3–61 µmol./L.	Pregnancy Skeletal muscle necrosis or atrophy Starvation Hyperthyroidism	
Creatine phosphokinase (CPK)	Males: 50–325 mU/ml. Females: 50–250 mU/ml.	50–325 U/L. 50–250 U/L.	Myocardial infarction Skeletal muscle diseases Intramuscular injections Crush syndrome Hypothyroidism Alcohol withdrawal delirium Alcoholic myopathy Cerebrovascular disease	
Creatine phosphokinase isoenzymes	MM band present (skeletal muscle); MB band absent (heart muscle)		MB band increased in myocardial infarction, ischemia	
Creatinine	0.7–1.4 mg./dl.	62–124 µmol./L.	Nephritis Chronic renal disease	Kidney diseases

(continued)

REFERENCE RANGES—SERUM, PLASMA, AND WHOLE BLOOD CHEMISTRIES (continued)

| | Normal Adult Reference Range | | Clinical Significance | |
Determination	Conventional Units	SI Units	Increased	Decreased
Creatinine clearance	100–150 ml. of blood cleared of creatinine per min.	1.67–2.5 ml./s.		
Cryoglobulins, qualitative	Negative		Multiple myeloma Chronic lymphocytic leukemia Lymphosarcoma Systemic lupus erythematosus Rheumatoid arthritis Infective subacute endocarditis Some malignancies Scleroderma	
11-Deoxycortisol	1 μg./dl.	<0.029 μmol./L.	Hypertensive form of virilizing adrenal hyperplasia due to an 11-β-hydroxylase defect	
Dibucaine number	Normal: 70%–85% inhibition Heterozygote: 50%–65% inhibition Homozygote: 16%–25% inhibition			Important in detecting carriers of abnormal cholinesterase activity who are susceptible to succinyldicholine anesthetic shock
Dihydrotestosterone	Males: 50–210 ng./dl. Females: none detectable	1.72–7.22 nmol./L.		Testicular feminization syndrome
Estradiol—RIA	Females: Follicular: 10–90 pg./ml. Midcycle: 100–500 pg./ml. Luteal: 50–240 pg./ml. Follicular phase: 2–20 ng./dl. Midcycle: 12–40 ng./dl. Luteal phase: 10–30 ng./dl. Postmenopausal: 1–5 ng./dl. Males: 0.5–5 ng./dl.	37–370 pmol./L. 367–1835 pmol./L. 184–881 pmol./L.	Pregnancy	Depressed or failure to peak—ovarian failure
Estriol—RIA	Nonpregnant females: <0.5 ng./ml. Pregnant females: 1st trimester: up to 1 ng./ml. 2nd trimester: 0.8–7 ng./ml. 3rd trimester: 5–25 ng./ml.	<1.75 nmol./L. Up to 3.5 nmol./L. 2.8–24.3 nmol./L. 17.4–86.8 nmol./L.	Pregnancy	Depressed or failure to peak—ovarian failure
Estrogens, total—RIA	Females: cycle days: Day 1–10: 61–394 pg./ml. Day 11–20: 122–437 pg./ml. Day 21–30: 156–350 pg./ml. Males: 40–115 pg./ml.	61–394 ng./L. 122–437 ng./L. 156–350 ng./L. 40–115 ng./L.	Pregnancy Measured on a daily basis, can be used to evaluate response of hypogonadotrophic, hypoestrogenic women to human menopausal or pituitary gonadotropin	Fetal distress Ovarian failure
Estrone—RIA	Females: Day 1–10: 4.3–18 ng./dl.	15.9–66.6 pmol./L.	Pregnancy	Depressed or failure to peak—ovarian failure

(continued)

REFERENCE RANGES—SERUM, PLASMA, AND WHOLE BLOOD CHEMISTRIES (continued)

| Determination | Normal Adult Reference Range | | Clinical Significance | |
	Conventional Units	SI Units	Increased	Decreased
Ferritin—RIA	Day 11–20: 7.5–19.6 ng./dl. Day 21–30: 13–20 ng./dl. Males: 2.5–7.5 ng./dl. Males: 10–270 ng./ml. Females: 5–100 ng./ml.	27.8–72.5 pmol./L. 48.1–74 pmol./L. 9.3–27.8 pmol./L. 10–270 µg./L. 5–100 µg./L.	Nephritis Hemochromatosis Certain neoplastic diseases Acute myelogenous leukemia Multiple myeloma	Iron deficiency
Folic acid—RIA	4–16 ng./ml.	9.1–36.3 nmol./L.		Megaloblastic anemias of infancy and pregnancy Inadequate diet Liver disease Malabsorption syndrome Severe hemolytic anemia
Follicle stimulating hormone (FSH)—RIA	Females: Follicular phase: 5–20 mIU/ml. Peak of middle cycle: 12–30 mIU/ml. Luteinic phase: 5–15 mIU/ml. Menopausal females: 40–200 mIU/ml.	5–20 IU/L. 12–30 IU/L. 5–15 IU/L. 40–200 IU/L.	Menopause and primary ovarian failure	Pituitary failure
Galactose	<5 mg./dl.	<0.28 mmol./L.		Galactosemia
Gamma glutamyl transpeptidase	Males: <45 IU/L. Females: <30 IU/L.	45 U/L. 30 U/L.	Hepatobiliary disease Anicteric alcoholics Drug therapy damage Myocardial infarction Renal infarction	
Gastrin—RIA	Fasting: 50–155 pg./ml. Postprandial: 80–170 pg./ml. Zollinger-Ellison syndrome: 200–over 2000 pg./ml. Pernicious anemia: 130–2260 pg./ml. (mean 912)	50–155 ng./L. 80–170 ng./L. 200-over 2000 ng./L. 130–2260 ng./L. (mean 912)	Zollinger-Ellison syndrome Peptic ulceration of the duodenum Pernicious anemia	
Glucose	Fasting: 60–110 mg./dl. Postprandial (2 h.): 65–140 mg./dl.	3.3–6.05 mmol./L. 3.58–7.7 mmol./L.	Diabetes Nephritis Hyperthyroidism Early hyperpituitarism Cerebral lesions Infections Pregnancy Uremia	Hyperinsulinism Hypothyroidism Late hyperpituitarism Pernicious vomiting Addison's disease Extensive hepatic damage
Glucose tolerance (oral)	Features of a normal response: 1. Normal fasting between 60–110 mg./dl. 2. No sugar in urine 3. Upper limits of normal: Fasting = 125 1 hour = 190 2 hours = 140 3 hours = 125	3.3–6.05 mmol./L. 6.88 mmol./L. 10.45 mmol./L. 7.70 mmol./L. 6.88 mmol./L.	(Flat or inverted curve) Hyperinsulinism Adrenal cortical insufficiency (Addison's disease) Anterior pituitary hypofunction Hypothyroidism Sprue and celiac diseases	(High or prolonged curve) Diabetes Hyperthyroidism Primary adrenal cortical tumor or hyperplasia Severe anemia Certain central nervous system disorders

(continued)

REFERENCE RANGES—SERUM, PLASMA, AND WHOLE BLOOD CHEMISTRIES (continued)

Determination	Normal Adult Reference Range		Clinical Significance	
	Conventional Units	*SI Units*	*Increased*	*Decreased*
Glucose-6-phosphate dehydrogenase (red cells)	Screening: Decolorization in 20–100 min. Quantitative: 1.86–2.5 IU/ml. RBC	1860–2500 U/L		Drug-induced hemolytic anemia Hemolytic disease of newborn
Glycoprotein (alpha-1-acid)	40–110 mg./dl.	400–1100 mg./L.	Neoplasm Tuberculosis Diabetes complicated by degenerative vascular disease Pregnancy Rheumatoid arthritis Rheumatic fever Infectious liver disease Lupus erythematosus	
Growth hormone—RIA	<10 ng./ml.	<10 mg./L.	Acromegaly	Failure to stimulate with arginine or insulin—hypopituitarism
Haptoglobin	50–250 mg./dl.	0.5–2.5 g./L.	Pregnancy Estrogen therapy Chronic infections Various inflammatory conditions	Hemolytic anemia Hemolytic blood transfusion reaction
Hemoglobin (plasma)	0.5–5 mg./dl.	5–50 mg./L.	Transfusion reactions Paroxysmal nocturnal hemoglobinuria Intravascular hemolysis	
Hemoglobin A1 (Glycohemoglobin)	Nondiabetics & diabetics whose control of glucose is: Good: 4.4%–8.2% Fair: 8.3%–9.2% Poor: >9.2%			
Hexosaminidase, total	Controls: 333–375 nM./ml./h. Heterozygotes: 288–644 nM./ml./h. Tay-Sachs disease: 284–1232 nM./ml./h. Diabetics: 567–3560 nM./ml./h.	333–375 μmol./L./h. 288–644 μmol./L./h. 284–1232 μmol./L./h. 567–3560 μmol./L./h.	Diabetes Tay–Sachs disease	
Hexosaminidase A	Controls: 49%–68% of total Heterozygotes: 26%–45% of total Tay-Sachs disease: 0%–4% of total Diabetics: 39%–59% of total	Fraction of total: 0.49–0.68 0.26–0.45 0–0.04 0.39–0.59		Tay-Sachs disease and heterozygotes
High-density lipoprotein cholesterol (HDL cholesterol)				HDL cholesterol is lower in patients with increased risk for coronary heart disease

Age (yr.)	Males (mg./dl.)	Females (mg./dl.)	Males (mmol./L.)	Females (mmol./L.)
0–19	30–65	30–70	0.78–1.68	0.78–1.81
20–29	35–70	35–75	0.91–1.81	0.91–1.94
30–39	30–65	35–80	0.78–1.68	0.91–2.07
40–49	30–65	40–85	0.78–1.68	1.04–2.2
50–59	30–65	35–85	0.78–1.68	0.91–2.2
60–69	30–65	35–85	0.78–1.68	0.91–2.2

(continued)

REFERENCE RANGES—SERUM, PLASMA, AND WHOLE BLOOD CHEMISTRIES (continued)

Determination	Normal Adult Reference Range		Clinical Significance	
	Conventional Units	*SI Units*	*Increased*	*Decreased*
17-Hydroxy-progesterone—RIA	Males: 0.4–4 ng./ml. Females: 0.1–3.3 ng./ml. Children: 0.1–0.5 ng./ml.	1.2–12 nmol./L. 0.3–10 nmol./L. 0.3–1.5 nmol./L.	Congenital adrenal hyperplasia Pregnancy Some cases of adrenal or ovarian adenomas	
Immunoglobulin A	Adults: 50–300 mg./dl. (in children the normals are lower and vary with age)	0.5–3 g./L.	Gamma A myeloma Wiskott-Aldrich syndrome Autoimmune disease Hepatic cirrhosis	Ataxia telangiectasis Agammaglobulinemia Hypogammaglobulinemia, transient Dysgammaglobulinemia Protein-losing enteropathies
Immunoglobulin D	0–30 mg./dl.	0–300 mg./L.	IgD multiple myeloma Some patients with chronic infectious diseases	
Immunoglobulin E	20–740 ng./ml.	20–740 µg./L.	Allergic patients and those with parasitic infestations	
Immunoglobulin G	Adults: 635–1400 mg./dl.	6.35–14 g./L.	IgG myeloma Following hyperimmunization Autoimmune disease states Chronic infections	Congenital and acquired hypogammaglobulinemia IgA myelomas, Waldenstrom's (IgM) macroglobulinemia Some malabsorption syndromes Extensive protein loss
Immunoglobulin M	Adults: 40–280 mg./dl.	0.4–2.8 g./L.	Waldenstrom's macroglobulinemia Parasitic infections Hepatitis	Agammaglobulinemias Some IgG and IgA myelomas Chronic lymphatic leukemia
Insulin—RIA	5–25 µU/ml.	0.2–1 µg./L.	Insulinoma Acromegaly	Diabetes mellitus
Iron	65–170 µg./dl.	11.6–30.4 µmol./L.	Pernicious anemia Aplastic anemia Hemolytic anemia Hepatitis Hemochromatosis	Iron deficiency anemia
Iron-binding capacity	IBC: 150–235 µg./dl. TIBC: 250–420 µg./dl. % Saturation: 20–50	26.9–42.1 µmol./L. 44.8–75.2 µmol./L. Fraction of total ironbinding capacity: 0.2–0.5	Iron deficiency anemia Acute and chronic blood loss Hepatitis	Chronic infectious diseases Cirrhosis
Isocitric dehydrogenase	50–180 U	0.83–3 U./L.	Hepatitis: cirrhosis Obstructive jaundice Metastatic carcinoma of the liver Megaloblastic anemia	
Lactic acid (whole blood)	Venous: 5–20 mg./dl. Arterial: 3–7 mg./dl.	0.6–2.2 mmol./L. 0.3–0.8 mmol./L.	Increased muscular activity Congestive heart failure Hemorrhage Shock Some varieties of metabolic acidosis Some febrile infections May be increased in severe liver disease	
Lactic dehydrogenase (LDH)	100–225 mU/ml.	100–225 U/L.	Untreated pernicious anemia Myocardial infarction Pulmonary infarction Liver disease	
Lactic dehydrogenase isoenzymes Total lactic dehydrogenase LDH-1 LDH-2	100–225 mU/ml. 20%–35% 25%–40%	100–225 U/L. Fraction of total LDH: 0.2–0.35 0.25–0.4	LDH-1 and LDH-2 are increased in myocardial infarction, megaloblastic anemia, and hemolytic	

(continued)

REFERENCE RANGES—SERUM, PLASMA, AND WHOLE BLOOD CHEMISTRIES (continued)

Determination	Normal Adult Reference Range		Clinical Significance	
	Conventional Units	*SI Units*	*Increased*	*Decreased*
LDH-3	20%–30%	0.2–0.3	anemia	
LDH-4	0–20%	0–0.2	LDH-4 and LDH-5 are	
LDH-5	0–25%	0–0.25	increased in pulmonary infarction, congestive heart failure, and liver disease	
Lead (whole blood)	Up to 40 μg./dl.	Up to 2 μmol./L.	Lead poisoning	
Leucine aminopeptidase	80–200 U/ml.	19.2–48 U/L.	Liver or biliary tract diseases Pancreatic disease Metastatic carcinoma of liver and pancreas Biliary obstruction	
Lipase	0.2–1.5 U/ml.	55–417 U/L.	Acute and chronic pancreatitis Biliary obstruction Cirrhosis Hepatitis Peptic ulcer	
Lipids, total	400–1000 mg./dl.	4–10 g./L.	Hypothyroidism Diabetes Nephrosis Glomerulonephritis Hyperlipoproteinemias	Hyperthyroidism

Lipoprotein Phenotype: Summary of Findings in the Primary Hyperlipoproteinemias

Type	Frequency	Appearance	Triglyceride	Cholesterol	Lipoprotein Staining				Secondary Causes
					Beta	*Pre-Beta*	*Alpha*	*Chylomicrons*	
Normal		Clear	Normal	Normal	Moderate	Zero to moderate	Moderate	Weak	
I	Very rare	Creamy	Markedly increased	Normal to moderately increased	Weak	Weak	Weak	Markedly increased	Dysglobulinemia
II	Common	Clear	Normal to slightly increased	Slightly to markedly increased	Strong	Zero to strong	Moderate	Weak	Hypothyroidism, myeloma, hepatic syndrome, macroglobulinemia, and high dietary cholesterol
III	Uncommon	Clear, cloudy, or milky	Increased	Increased	Broad intense band	Extends into beta	Moderate	Weak	
IV	Very common	Clear, cloudy, or milky	Slightly to markedly increased	Normal to slightly increased	Weak to moderate	Moderate to strong	Weak to moderate	Weak	Hypothyroidism, diabetes mellitus, pancreatitis, glycogen storage diseases, nephrotic syndrome, myeloma, pregnancy, and oral contraceptives
V	Rare	Cloudy to creamy	Markedly increased	Increased	Weak	Moderate	Weak	Strong	Diabetes mellitus, pancreatitis, and alcoholism

Types I and II are fat induced; types III and IV are carbohydrate induced; type V is fat and carbohydrate induced.

(continued)

REFERENCE RANGES—SERUM, PLASMA, AND WHOLE BLOOD CHEMISTRIES (continued)

Determination	Normal Adult Reference Range		Clinical Significance	
	Conventional Units	*SI Units*	*Increased*	*Decreased*
Lithium	Usual maintenance level: 0.5–1 mEq./L.	0.5–1 mmol./L.		
Low-density lipoprotein cholesterol (LDL cholesterol)	Age (yr.) mg./dl. 0–19 50–170 20–29 60–170 30–39 70–190 40–49 80–190 50–59 80–210	mmol./L. 1.30–4.40 1.55–4.40 1.80–4.92 2.07–4.92 2.07–5.44	LDL cholesterol is higher in patients with increased risk for coronary heart disease	
Luteinizing hormone—RIA	Males: 6–30 mIU/ml. Females: Follicular phase: 2–3 mIU/ml. Ovulatory peak: 40–200 mIU/ml. Luteal phase: 0–20 mIU/ml. Postmenopausal: 35–120 mIU/ml.	1.4–6.9 mg./L. 0.5–6.9 mg./L. 9.2–46 mg./L. 0–5 mg./L. 8–27.5 mg./L.	Pituitary tumor Ovarian failure	Depressed or failure to peak—pituitary failure
Lysozyme (muramidase)	2.8–8 µg./ml.	2.8–8 mg.	Certain types of leukemia (acute monocytic leukemia) Inflammatory states and infections	Acute lymphocytic leukemia
Magnesium	1.3–2.4 mEq./L.	0.7–1.2 mmol./L.	Excess ingestion of magnesium-containing antacids	Chronic alcoholism Severe renal disease Diarrhea Defective growth
Manganese	0.04–1.4 µg./dl.	72.9–255 nmol./L.		
Mercury	Up to 10 µg./dl.	Up to 0.5 µmol./L.	Mercury poisoning	
Myoglobin—RIA	Up to 85 ng./ml.	Up to 85 µg./ml.	Myocardial infarction Muscle necrosis	
5′ Nucleotidase	3.2–11.6 IU/L.	3.2–11.6 U/L.	Hepatobiliary disease	
Osmolality	280–300 mOsm./kg.	280–300 mmol./L.	Useful in the study of electrolyte and water balance	Inappropriate secretion of antidiuretic hormone
Parathyroid hormone	160–350 pg./ml.	160–350 ng./L.	Hyperparathyroidism	
Phenylalanine	1.2–3.5 mg./dl. 1st week 0.7–3.5 mg./dl. thereafter	0.07–0.21 mmol./L. 0.04–0.21 mmol./L.	Phenylketonuria	
Phosphatase, acid, total	0–11 U.L.	0–11 U.L.	Carcinoma of prostate Advanced Paget's disease Hyperparathyroidism Gaucher's disease	
Phosphatase, acid, prostatic—RIA	0–10 ng./ml. Borderline: 2.5–3.3 IU/L.	0–10 µg./L.	Carcinoma of prostate	
Phosphatase, alkaline	Adults: 30–115 mU/ml.	30–115 µ./L.	Conditions reflecting increased osteoblastic activity of bone Rickets Hyperparathyroidism Liver disease	
Phosphatase, alkaline, thermostable fraction	Thermostable fraction >35%: hepatic disease and combined disease with predominant hepatic component		Hepatic disease	

(continued)

REFERENCE RANGES—SERUM, PLASMA, AND WHOLE BLOOD CHEMISTRIES (continued)

| Determination | Normal Adult Reference Range | | Clinical Significance | |
	Conventional Units	*SI Units*	*Increased*	*Decreased*
	Thermostable fraction between 25% and 35%: combined hepatic and skeletal disease Thermostable fraction <25%: skeletal disease with increased osteoblastic activity			
Phosphohexose isomerase	20–90 IU/L.	20–90 U/L.	Malignancy Disease of heart, liver, and skeletal muscles	
Phospholipids	125–300 mg./dl.	1.25–3 g./L.	Diabetes Nephritis	
Phosphorus, inorganic	2.5–4.5 mg./dl.	0.8–1.45 mmol./L.	Chronic nephritis Hypoparathyroidism	Hyperparathyroidism Vitamin D deficiency
Potassium	3.8–5 mEq./L.	3.8–5 mmol./L.	Addison's disease Oliguria Anuria Tissue breakdown or hemolysis	Diabetic acidosis Diarrhea Vomiting
Progesterone—RIA	Follicular phase: up to 0.8 ng./ml. Luteal phase: 10–20 ng./ml. End of cycle: <1 ng./ ml. Pregnant: up to 50 ng./ml in 20th week	2.5 nmol./L. 31.8–63.6 nmol./L. <3 nmol./L. Up to 160 nmol./L.	Useful in evaluation of menstrual disorders and infertility and in the evaluation of placental function during pregnancies complicated by toxemia, diabetes mellitus, or threatened miscarriage	
Prolactin—RIA	6–24 ng./ml.	6–24 μg./L.	Pregnancy Functional or structural disorders of the hypothalamus Pituitary stalk section Pituitary tumors	
Protein, total Albumin Globulin	6–8 gm./dl. 3.5–5 gm./dl. 1.5–3 gm./dl.	60–80 g./L. 35–50 g./L. 15–30 g./L.	Hemoconcentration Shock Multiple myeloma (globulin fraction) Chronic infections (globulin fraction) Liver disease (globulin)	Malnutrition Hemorrhage Loss of plasma from burns Proteinuria
Electrophoresis (cellulose acetate) Albumin Alpha-1 globulin Alpha-2 globulin Beta globulin Gamma globulin	3.5–5 gm./dl. 0.2–0.4 gm./dl. 0.6–1 gm./dl. 0.6–1.2 gm./dl. 0.7–1.5 gm./dl.	35–50 g./L. 2–4 g./L. 6–10 g./L. 6–12 g./L. 7–15 g./L.		
Protoporphyrin erythrocyte (whole blood)	15–100 μg./dl.	0.27–1.80 μmol./L.	Lead toxicity Erythropoietic porphyria	
Pyridoxine	3.6–18 ng./ml.			A wide spectrum of clinical conditions such as mental depression, peripheral neuropathy,

(continued)

REFERENCE RANGES—SERUM, PLASMA, AND WHOLE BLOOD CHEMISTRIES (continued)

| Determination | Normal Adult Reference Range | | Clinical Significance | |
	Conventional Units	*SI Units*	*Increased*	*Decreased*
				anemia, neonatal seizures, and reactions to certain drug therapies
Pyruvic acid (whole blood)	0.3–0.7 mg./dl.	34–80 μmol./L.	Diabetes Severe thiamine deficiency Acute phase of some infections, possibly secondary to increased glycogenolysis and glycolysis	
Renin (plasma)—RIA	Normal diet: Supine: 0.3–1.9 ng./ml./h. Upright: 0.6–3.6 ng./ml./h. Low salt diet: Supine: 0.9–4.5 ng./ml./h. Upright: 4.1–9.1 ng./ml./h.	0.08–0.52 ng./L./S. 0.16–1.00 μg./L./S. 0.25–1.25 μg./L./S. 1.13–2.53 μg./L./S.	Renovascular hypertension Malignant hypertension Untreated Addison's disease Primary salt-losing nephropathy Low-salt diet Diuretic therapy Hemorrhage	Frank primary aldosteronism Increased salt intake Salt-retaining steroid therapy Antidiuretic hormone therapy Blood transfusion
Sodium	135–145 mEq./L.	135–145 mmol./L.	Hemoconcentration Nephritis Pyloric obstruction	Alkali deficit Addison's disease Myxedema
Sulfate (inorganic)	0.5–1.5 mg./dl.	0.05–0.15 mmol./L.	Nephritis Nitrogen retention	
Testosterone—RIA	Females: 25–100 ng./dl. Males: 300–800 ng./dl.	0.9–3.5 nmol./L. 10.5–28 nmol./L.	Females: Polycystic ovary Virilizing tumors	Males: Orchidectomy for neoplastic disease of the prostate or breast Estrogen therapy Klinefelter's syndrome Hypopituitarism Hypogonadism Hepatic cirrhosis
T_3 (triiodothyronine) uptake	25%–35%	Relative uptake fraction: 0.25–0.35	Hyperthyroidism TBG deficiency Androgens and anabolic steroids	Hypothyroidism Pregnancy TBG excess Estrogens and antiovulatory drugs
T_3, total circulating—RIA	75–200 ng./dl.	1.15–3.1 nmol./L.	Pregnancy Hyperthyroidism	Hypothyroidism
T_4 (thyroxine)—RIA	4.5–11.5 μg./dl.	58.5–150 nmol./L.	Hyperthyroidism Thyroiditis Elevated thyroxine-binding proteins caused by oral contraceptives Pregnancy	Primary and pituitary hypothyroidism Idiopathic involvement Cases of diminished thyroxine-binding proteins caused by androgenic and anabolic steroids Hypoproteinemia Nephrotic syndrome

(continued)

REFERENCE RANGES—SERUM, PLASMA, AND WHOLE BLOOD CHEMISTRIES (continued)

Determination	Normal Adult Reference Range		Clinical Significance	
	Conventional Units	*SI Units*	*Increased*	*Decreased*
T$_4$, free	1–2.2 ng./dl.	13–30 pmol./L.	Euthyroid patients with normal free thyroxine levels may have abnormal T$_3$ and T$_4$ levels caused by drug preparations	
Thyroid-stimulating hormone (TSH)—RIA		0.3–5 m/IU./L.	Hypothyroidism	Hyperthyroidism
Thyroid-binding globulin	10–26 μg./dl.	100–260 μg./L.	Hypothyroidism Pregnancy Estrogen therapy Oral contraceptives Genetic and idiopathic	Androgens and anabolic steroids Nephrotic syndrome Marked hypoproteinemia Hepatic disease
Transaminase, serum glutamic-oxaloacetate (SGOT, aspartate aminotransferase)	7–40 U/ml.	4–20 U/L.	Myocardial infarction Skeletal muscle disease Liver disease	
Transaminase, serum glutamic-oxaloacetate (SGPT, alanine aminotransferase)	10–40 U/ml.	5–20 U/L.	Same conditions as SGOT, but increase is more marked in liver disease than SGOT	
Transferrin	230–320 mg./dl.	2.3–3.2 g./L.	Pregnancy Iron-deficiency anemia due to hemorrhaging Acute hepatitis Polycythemia Oral contraceptives	Pernicious anemia in relapse Thalassemic and sickle cell anemia Chromatosis Neoplastic and hepatic diseases
Triglycerides	10–150 mg./dl.	0.10–1.65 mmol./L.	See *Lipoprotein Phenotype*	
Tryptophan	1.4–3 mg./dl.	68.6–147 nmol./L.		Tryptophan-specific malabsorption syndrome
Tyrosine	0.5–4 mg./dl.	27.6–220.8 mmol./L.	Tyrosinosis	
Urea nitrogen (BUN)	10–20 mg./dl.	3.6–7.2 mmol./L.	Acute glomerulonephritis Obstructive uropathy Mercury poisoning Nephrotic syndrome	Severe hepatic failure Pregnancy
Uric acid	2.5–8 mg./dl.	0.15–0.5 mmol./L.	Gouty arthritis Acute leukemia Lymphomas treated by chemotherapy Toxemia of pregnancy	Xanthinuria Defective tubular reabsorption
Viscosity	1.4–1.8 relative to water at 37°C. (98.6°F.)		Patients with marked increases of the gamma globulins	
Vitamin A	50–220 μg./dl.	1.75–7.7 μmol./L.	Hypervitaminosis A	Vitamin A deficiency Celiac disease Sprue Obstructive jaundice Giardiasis Parenchymal hepatic disease
Vitamin B$_1$ (thiamine)	1.6–4 μg./dl.	47.4–135.7 nmol./L.		Anorexia Beriberi Polyneuropathy Cardiomyopathies

(continued)

REFERENCE RANGES—SERUM, PLASMA, AND WHOLE BLOOD CHEMISTRIES (continued)

Determination	Normal Adult Reference Range		Clinical Significance	
	Conventional Units	*SI Units*	*Increased*	*Decreased*
Vitamin B_6 (pyridoxal phosphate)	3.6–18 ng./ml.	14.6–72.8 nmol./L.		Chronic alcoholism Malnutrition Uremia Neonatal seizures Malabsorption, such as celiac syndrome
Vitamin B_{12}—RIA	130–785 pg./ml.	100–580 pmol./L.	Hepatic cell damage and in association with the myeloproliferative disorders (the highest levels are encountered in myeloid leukemia)	Strict vegetarianism Alcoholism Pernicious anemia Total or partial gastrectomy Ileal resection Sprue and celiac disease Fish tapeworm infestation
Vitamin E	0.5–2 mg./dl.	11.6–46.4 μmol./L.		Vitamin E deficiency
Xylose absorption test	2 hr., 30–50 mg./dl.	2–3.35 mmol./L.		Malabsorption syndrome
Zinc	55–150 μg./dl.	7.65–22.95 μmol./L.	Zinc is essential for the growth and propagation of cell cultures and the functioning of several enzymes	

* By radioimmunoassay.

REFERENCE RANGES—URINE CHEMISTRY

Determination	Normal Adult Reference Range		Clinical Significance	
	Conventional Units	*SI Units*	*Increased*	*Decreased*
Acetone and acetoacetate	Zero		Uncontrolled diabetes Starvation	
Acid mucopolysaccharides	Negative		Hurler's syndrome Marfan's syndrome Morquio-Ulrich disease	
Aldosterone	Normal salt: Normal: 4–20 μg./24 h. Renovascular: 10–40 μg./24 h. Tumor: 20–100 μg./24 h.	11.1–55.5 nmol./24 h. 27.7–111 nmol./24 h. 55.4–277 nmol./24 h.	Primary aldosteronism (adrenocortical tumor) Secondary aldosteronism Salt depletion Potassium loading ACTH in large doses Cardiac failure Cirrhosis with ascites formation Nephrosis Pregnancy	
Alpha amino nitrogen	50–200 mg./24 h.	3.6–14.3 mmol./24 h.	Leukemia Diabetes Phenylketonuria Other metabolic diseases	
Amylase	35–260 units excreted per h.	6.5–48.1 U/h.	Acute pancreatitis	
Arylsulfatase A	>2.4 U/ml.			Metachromatic leukodystrophy
Bence-Jones protein	None detected		Myeloma	
Calcium	<150 mg./24 h.	<3.75 mmol./24 h.	Hyperparathyroidism Vitamin D intoxication Fanconi syndrome	Hypoparathyroidism Vitamin D deficiency

(continued)

REFERENCE RANGES—URINE CHEMISTRY (continued)

Determination	Normal Adult Reference Range		Clinical Significance	
	Conventional Units	*SI Units*	*Increased*	*Decreased*
Catecholamines	Total: 0–275 µg./24 h. Epinephrine: 10%–40% Norepinephrine: 60%–90%	0–275 µg./24 h. Fraction total: 0.10–8.4 Fraction total: 0.60–0.90	Pheochromocytoma Neuroblastoma	
Chorionic gonadotrophin, qualitative (pregnancy test)	Negative		Pregnancy Chorionepithelioma Hydatidiform mole	
Copper	20–70 µg./24 h.	0.32–1.12 µmol./24 h.	Wilson's disease Cirrhosis Nephrosis	
Coproporphyrin	50–300 µg./24 h.	0.075–0.45 µmol./24 h.	Poliomyelitis Lead poisoning Porphyria hepatica Porphyria erythropoietica Porphyria cutanea tarda	
Cortisol, free	20–90 µg./24 h.	55.2–248.4 nmol./d.	Cushing's syndrome	
Creatine	0–200 mg./24 h.	0–1.52 mmol./24 h.	Muscular dystrophy Fever Carcinoma of liver Pregnancy Hyperthyroidism Myositis	
Creatinine	0.8–2 gm./24 h.	7–17.6 mmol./24 h.	Typhoid fever Salmonella infections Tetanus	Muscular atrophy Anemia Advanced degeneration of kidneys Leukemia
Creatinine clearance	100–150 ml. of blood cleared of creatinine per min.	1.67–2.5 ml./s.		Measures glomerular filtration rate Renal diseases
Cystine and cysteine	10–100 mg./24 h.	0.08–0.83 mmol./24 h.	Cystinuria	
Delta aminolevulinic acid	0–0.54 mg./dl.	0–40 µmol./L.	Lead poisoning Porphyria hepatica Hepatitis Hepatic carcinoma	
11-Desoxycortisol	20–100 µg./24 h.	0.6–2.9 µmol./d.	Hypertensive form of virilizing adrenal hyperplasia due to an 11-beta hydroxylase defect	
Estriol (placental)	**Weeks of pregnancy µm./24 h. nmol./24 h.** 12 <1 <3.5 16 2–7 7–24.5 20 4–9 14–32 24 6–13 21–45.5 28 8–22 28–77 32 12–43 42–150 36 14–45 49–158 40 19–46 66.5–160			Decreased values occur with fetal distress of many conditions, including preeclampsia, placental insufficiency, and poorly controlled diabetes mellitus
Estrogens, total (fluorometric)	Females: Onset of menstruation: 4–25 µg./24 h. Ovulation peak: 28 µg./24 h. Luteal peak: 22–105 µg./24 h. Menopausal: 1.4–19.6 µg./24 h. Males: 5–18 µg./24 h.	4–25 µg./24 h. 28 µg./24 h. 22–105 µg./24 h. 1.4–19.6 µg./24 h. 5–18 µg./24 h.	Hyperestrogenism due to gonadal or adrenal neoplasm	Primary or secondary amenorrhea
Etiocholanolone	Males: 1.9–6 mg./24 h. Females: 0.5–4 mg./24 h.	6.5–20.6 µmol./24 h. 1.7–13.8 µmol./24 h.	Adrenogenital syndrome Idiopathic hirsutism	

(continued)

REFERENCE RANGES—URINE CHEMISTRY (continued)

Determination	Normal Adult Reference Range		Clinical Significance	
	Conventional Units	*SI Units*	*Increased*	*Decreased*
Follicle-stimulating hormone—RIA	Females: Follicular: 5–20 IU/24 h. Luteal: 5–15 IU/24 h. Midcycle: 15–60 IU/24 h. Menopausal: 50–100 IU/24 h. Males: 5–25 IU/24 h.	5–20 IU/d. 5–15 IU/d. 15–60 IU/d. 50–100 IU/d. 5–25 IU/d.	Menopause and primary ovarian failure	Pituitary failure
Glucose	Negative		Diabetes mellitus Pituitary disorders Intracranial pressure Lesion in floor of 4th ventricle	
Hemoglobin and myoglobin	Negative		Extensive burns Transfusion of incompatible blood Myoglobin increased in severe crushing injuries to muscles	
Homogentisic acid, qualitative	Negative		Alkaptonuria Ochronosis	
Homovanillic acid	Up to 15 mg./24 h.	Up to 82 μmol./d.	Neuroblastoma	
17-hydroxycorti-costeroids	2–10 mg./24 h.	5.5–27.5 μmol./d.	Cushing's disease	Addison's disease Anterior pituitary hypofunction
5-Hydroxyindoleacetic acid, qualitative	Negative		Malignant carcinoid tumors	
Hydroxyproline	15–43 mg./24 h.	0.11–0.33 μmol./d.	Paget's disease Fibrous dysplasia Osteomalacia Neoplastic bone disease Hyperparathyroidism	
17-ketosteroids, total	Males: 10–22 mg./24 h. Females: 6–16 mg./24 h.	35–76 μmol./d. 21–55 μmol./d.	Interstitial cell tumor of testes Simple hirsutism, occasionally Adrenal hyperplasia Cushing's syndrome Adrenal cancer, virilism Arrhenoblastoma	Thyrotoxicosis Female hypogonadism Diabetes mellitus Hypertension Debilitating disease of mild to moderate severity Eunuchoidism Addison's disease Panhypopituitarism Myxedema Nephrosis
Lead	Up to 150 μg./24 h.	Up to 60 μmol./24 h.	Lead poisoning	
Luteinizing hormone	Males: 5–18 IU/24 h. Females: Follicular phase: 2–25 IU/24 h. Ovulatory peak: 30–95 IU/24 h. Luteal phase: 2–20 IU/24 h. Postmenopausal: 40–110 IU/24 h.	2–25 IU/d. 30–95 IU/d. 2–20 IU/d. 40–110 IU/d.	Pituitary tumor Ovarian failure	Depressed or failure to peak—pituitary failure
Metanephrines, total	Less than 1.3 mg./24 h.	Less than 6.5 μmol./d.	Pheochromocytoma; a few patients with pheochromocytoma may have elevated urinary metanephrines but normal catecholamines and VMA	

(continued)

REFERENCE RANGES—URINE CHEMISTRY (continued)

Determination	Normal Adult Reference Range		Clinical Significance	
	Conventional Units	*SI Units*	*Increased*	*Decreased*
Osmolality	Males: 390–1090 mM./kg. Females: 300–1090 mM./kg.	390–1090 mmol./kg. 300–1090 mmol./kg.	Useful in the study of electrolyte and water balance	
Oxalate	Up to 40 mg./24 h.	Up to 456 µmol./d.	Primary hyperoxaluria	
Phenylpyruvic acid qualitative	Negative		Phenylketonuria	
Phosphorus, inorganic	0.8–1.3 gm./24 h.	26–42 mmol./24 h.	Hyperparathyroidism Vitamin D intoxication Paget's disease Metastatic neoplasm to bone Chronic lead poisoning	Hypoparathyroidism Vitamin D deficiency
Porphobilinogen, qualitative	Negative		Acute porphyria Liver disease	
Porphobilinogen, quantitative	0–1 mg./24 h.	0–4.4 µmol./24 h.	Acute porphyria Liver disease	
Porphyrins, qualitative	Negative		See porphyrins, quantitative	
Porphyrins, quantitative (coproporphyrin and uroporphyrin)	Coproporphyrin: 50–160 µg./24 h. Uroporphyrin: up to 50 µg./24 h.	0.075–0.24 µmol./24 h. Up to 0.06 µmol./24 h.	Porphyria hepatica Porphyria erythropoietica Porphyria cutanea tarda Lead poisoning (only coproporphyrin increased)	
Potassium	40–65 mEq./24 h.	40–65 mmol./24 h.	Hemolysis	
Pregnanediol	Females: Proliferative phase: 0.5–1.5 mg./24 h. Luteal phase: 2–7 mg./24 h. Menopause: 0.2–1 mg./24 h. Pregnancy:	 1.6–4.8 µmol./24 h. 6–22 µmol./24 h. 0.6–3.1 µmol./24 h.	Corpus luteum cysts When placental tissue remains in the uterus following parturition Some cases of adrenocortical tumors	Placental dysfunction Threatened abortion Intrauterine death

Weeks of gestation	**mg./24 h.**	**µmol./24 h.**
10–12	5–15	15.6–47
12–18	5–25	15.6–78.0
18–24	15–33	47.0–103.0
24–28	20–42	62.4–131.0
28–32	27–47	84.2–146.6

Determination	Conventional Units	SI Units	Increased	Decreased
	Males: 0.1–2 mg./24 h.	0.3–6.2 µmol/24 h.		
Pregnanetriol	0.4–2.4 mg./24 h.	1.2–7.1 µmol./24 h.	Congenital adrenal androgenic hyperplasia	
Protein	Up to 100 mg./24 h.	Up to 100 mg./24 h.	Nephritis Cardiac failure Mercury poisoning Bence-Jones protein in multiple myeloma Febrile states Hematuria	
Sodium	130–200 mEq./24 h.	130–200 mmol./24 h.	Useful in detecting gross changes in water and salt balance	
Titratable acidity	20–40 mEq./24 h.	20–40 mmol./24 h.	Metabolic acidosis	Metabolic alkalosis
Urea nitrogen	9–16 gm./24 h.	0.32–0.57 mol./L.	Excessive protein catabolism	Impaired kidney function
Uric acid	250–750 mg./24 h.	1.48–4.43 mmol./24 h.	Gout	Nephritis
Urobilinogen	Random urine: <0.25 mg./dl. 24-hour urine: up to 4 mg./24 h.	<0.42 mol./24 h. Up to 6.76 µmol./24 h.	Liver and biliary tract disease Hemolytic anemias	Complete or nearly complete biliary obstruction Diarrhea Renal insufficiency

(continued)

REFERENCE RANGES—URINE CHEMISTRY (continued)

Determination	Normal Adult Reference Range		Clinical Significance	
	Conventional Units	*SI Units*	*Increased*	*Decreased*
Uroporphyrins	Up to 50 μg./24 h.	Up to 0.06 μmol./24 h.	Porphyria	
Vanillylmandelic acid (VMA)	0.7–6.8 mg./24 h.	3.5–34.3 μmol./24 h.	Pheochromocytoma Neuroblastoma Coffee, tea, aspirin, bananas, and several different drugs	
Xylose absorption test (5 hour)	16%–33% of ingested xylose	Fraction absorbed: 0.16–0.33		Malabsorption syndromes
Zinc	0.15–1.2 mg./24 h.	2.3–18.4 μmol./24 h.	Zinc is an essential nutritional element	

REFERENCE RANGES—CEREBROSPINAL FLUID (CSF)

Determination	Normal Adult Reference Range		Clinical Significance	
	Conventional Units	*SI Units*	*Increased*	*Decreased*
Albumin	15–30 mg./dl.	150–300 mg./L.	Certain neurologic disorders Lesion in the choroid plexus or blockage of the flow of CSF Damage to the blood–CNS barrier	
Cell count	0–5 mononuclear cells per cu. mm.	$0–5 \times 10^6$/L.	Bacterial meningitis Neurosyphilis Anterior poliomyelitis Encephalitis lethargica	
Chloride	100–130 mEq./L.	100–300 mmol./L.	Uremia	Acute generalized meningitis Tuberculous meningitis
Glucose	50–75 mg./dl.	2.75–4.13 mmol./L.	Diabetes mellitus Diabetic coma Epidemic encephalitis Uremia	Acute meningitides Tuberculous meningitis Insulin shock
Glutamine	6–15 mg./dl.	0.41–1 mmol./L.	Hepatic encephalopathies, including Reye's syndrome Hepatic coma Cirrhosis	
IgG	0–6.6 mg./dl.	0–66 mg./L.	Damage to the blood–CNS barrier Multiple sclerosis Neurosyphilis Subacute sclerosing panencephalitis Chronic phases of CNS infections	
Lactic acid	<24 mg./dl.	<2.7 mmol./L.	Bacterial meningitis Hypocapnia Hydrocephalus Brain abscesses Cerebral ischemia	
Lactic dehydrogenase	1/10 that of serum	Activity fraction: 0.1 of serum	CNS disease	
Protein: Lumbar Cisternal Ventricular	15–45 mg./dl. 15–25 mg./dl. 5–15 mg./dl.	150–450 mg./L. 150–250 mg./L. 50–150 mg./L.	Acute meningitides Tubercular meningitis Neurosyphilis Poliomyelitis Guillain-Barre syndrome	

(continued)

REFERENCE RANGES—CEREBROSPINAL FLUID (CSF) (continued)

Determination	Normal Adult Reference Range		Clinical Significance	
	Conventional Units	SI Units	Increased	Decreased
Protein electrophoresis (cellulose acetate)	% of total:	Fraction:	An increase in the level of albumin alone can be the result of a lesion in the choroid plexus or a blockage of the flow of CSF. An elevated gamma globulin value with a normal albumin level has been reported in multiple sclerosis, neurosyphilis, subacute sclerosing panencephalitis, and the chronic phase of CNS infections. If the blood–CNS barrier has been damaged severely during the course of these diseases, the CSF albumin level may also be elevated.	
Prealbumin	3–7	0.03–0.07		
Albumin	56–74	0.56–0.74		
Alpha$_1$ globulin	2–6.5	0.02–0.065		
Alpha$_2$ globulin	3–12	0.03–0.12		
Beta globulin	8–18.5	0.08–0.185		
Gamma globulin	4–14	0.04–0.14		

GASTRIC ANALYSIS

Determination	Normal Adult Reference Range		Clinical Significance	
	Conventional Units	SI Units	Increased	Decreased
pH	<2	<2		Pernicious anemia
Basal acid output	0–6 mEq./h.	0–6 mmol./h.	Peptic ulcer	Gastric carcinoma
Maximum acid	5–40 mEq./h.	5–40 mmol./h.	Zollinger-Ellison syndrome	Chronic atrophic gastritis Decreased normally with age

MISCELLANEOUS VALUES

Determinations	Normal Value	Clinical Significance	
		Conventional Units	SI Units
Acetaminophen	Zero	Therapeutic level = 10–20 µg./ml.	10–20 mg./L.
Aminophylline (theophylline)	Zero	Therapeutic level = 10–20 µg./ml.	10–20 mg./L.
Bromide	Zero	Therapeutic level = 5–50 mg./dl.	50–500 mg./L.
Carbon monoxide	0%–2%	Symptoms with >20% saturation	
Chlordiazepoxide	Zero	Therapeutic level = 1–3 µg./ml.	1–3 mg./L.
Diazepam	Zero	Therapeutic level = 0.5–2.5 µg./dl.	5–25 µg./L.
Digitoxin	Zero	Therapeutic level = 5–30 ng./ml.	5–30 µg./L.
Digoxin	Zero	Therapeutic level = 0.5–2 ng./ml.	0.5–2 µg./L.
Ethanol	0%–0.01%	Legal intoxication level = 0.10% or above 0.3%–0.4% = marked intoxication 0.4%–0.5% = alcoholic stupor	
Gentamicin	Zero	Therapeutic level = 4–10 µg./ml.	4–10 mg./L.
Methanol	Zero	May be fatal in concentration as low as 10 mg./dl.	100 mg./L.

(continued)

MISCELLANEOUS VALUES (continued)

Determinations	Normal Value	Clinical Significance	
		Conventional Units	*SI Units*
Phenobarbital	Zero	Therapeutic level = 15–40 μg./ml.	10–20 mg./L.
Phenytoin	Zero	Therapeutic level = 10–20 μg./ml.	10–20 mg./L.
Primidone	Zero	Therapeutic level = 5–12 μg./ml.	5–12 mg./L.
Quinidine	Zero	Therapeutic level = 0.2–0.5 mg./dl.	2–5 mg./L.
Salicylate	Zero	Therapeutic level = 2–25 mg./dl.	20–250 mg./L.
		Toxic level = >30 mg./dl.	300 mg./L.
Sulfonamide	Zero	Therapeutic levels:	
		Sulfadiazine 8–15 mg./dl.	80–150 mg./L.
		Sulfaguanidine 3–5 mg./dl.	30–50 mg./L.
		Sulfamerazine 10–15 mg./dl.	100–150 mg./L.
		Sulfanilamide 10–15 mg./dl.	100–150 mg./L.

Appendix II: Conversion Tables

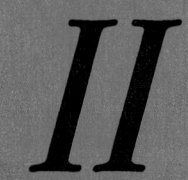

II

METRIC UNITS AND SYMBOLS

Quantity	Unit	Symbol	Equivalent
Length	millimeter	mm.	1000 mm. = 1 m.
	centimeter	cm.	100 cm. = 1 m.
	decimeter	dm.	10 dm. = 1 m.
	meter	m.	1000 m. = 1 km.
Volume	cubic centimeter	cc. or cm.^{3}	1000 $\dfrac{\text{cc or cm.}^3}{\text{ml.}}$ = 1 cm.^{3} or liter
	milliliter	ml.	
	cu. decimeter	dm.^{3}	1000 $\dfrac{\text{dm.}^3}{1}$ = 1 m.^{3}
	liter	L.	
Mass	microgram	μg.	1000 μg. = 1 mg.
	milligram	mg.	1000 mg. = 1 g.
	gram	g.	1000 g. = 1 kg.
	kilogram	kg.	1000 kg. = 1 metric ton (t)

TABLE OF METRIC AND APOTHECARIES' SYSTEMS

(Approved *approximate* dose equivalents are enclosed in parentheses. Use exact equivalents in calculations.)

Conversion Factors

Metric	Apothecaries	Metric	Apothecaries
1 milligram (mg.)	$^1/_{64}$ grain	3.888 cubic centimeters or grams	1 dram (4 cc. or grams)
64.79 milligrams	1 grain (65 mg.)	31.103 cubic centimeters or grams	1 ounce (30 cc. or grams)
1 gram	15.43 grains (15 grains)	473.167 cubic centimeters	1 pint (500 cc.)
1 cubic centimeter (cc.)	16 minims		

Weights

Metric	Apothecaries	Metric	Apothecaries
0.0001 gram—0.1 mg.—$^1/_{640}$ grain ($^1/_{600}$ grain)		0.057 gram —57 mg.—$^7/_8$ grain	
0.0002 gram—0.2 mg.—$^1/_{320}$ grain ($^1/_{300}$ grain)		0.06 gram —60 mg.—$^9/_{10}$ grain (1 grain)	
0.0003 gram—0.3 mg.—$^1/_{210}$ grain ($^1/_{200}$ grain)		0.065 gram —65 mg.—1 grain (60 mg.)	
0.0004 gram—0.4 mg.—$^1/_{150}$ grain		0.07 gram —70 mg.—$1^1/_{20}$ grains	
0.0005 gram—0.5 mg.—$^1/_{120}$ grain		0.08 gram —80 mg.—$1^1/_5$ grains	
0.0006 gram—0.6 mg.—$^1/_{100}$ grain		0.09 gram —90 mg.—$1^1/_3$ grains	
0.0007 gram—0.7 mg.—$^1/_{90}$ grain		0.097 gram —97 mg.—$1^1/_2$ grains (0.1 gram)	
0.0008 gram—0.8 mg.—$^1/_{80}$ grain		0.12 gram —120 mg.—2 grains	
0.0009 gram—0.9 mg.—$^1/_{75}$ grain		0.2 gram —200 mg.—3 grains	
0.001 gram—1 mg.—$^1/_{64}$ grain ($^1/_{60}$ grain)		0.24 gram —240 mg.—4 grains (0.25 gram)	
0.0011 gram—1.1 mg.—$^1/_{60}$ grain		0.3 gram —300 mg.—$4^1/_2$ grains	
0.0013 gram—1.3 mg.—$^1/_{50}$ grain (1.2 mg.)		0.33 gram —330 mg.—5 grains (0.3 gram)	
0.0014 gram—1.4 mg.—$^1/_{48}$ grain		0.4 gram —400 mg.—6 grains	
0.0016 gram—1.6 mg.—$^1/_{40}$ grain (1.5 mg.)		0.45 gram —450 mg.—7 grains	
0.0018 gram—1.8 mg.—$^1/_{36}$ grain		0.5 gram —500 mg.—$7^1/_2$ grains	
0.0020 gram—2 mg.—$^1/_{32}$ grain ($^1/_{30}$ grain)		0.53 gram —530 mg.—8 grains	
0.0022 gram—2.2 mg.—$^1/_{30}$ grain		0.6 gram —600 mg.—9 grains	
0.0026 gram—2.6 mg.—$^1/_{25}$ grain		0.65 gram —650 mg.—10 grains (0.6 gram)	
0.003 gram—3 mg.—$^1/_{20}$ grain		0.73 gram —730 mg.—11 grains	
0.004 gram—4 mg.—$^1/_{16}$ grain ($^1/_{15}$ grain)		0.80 gram —800 mg.—12 grains (0.75 gram)	
0.005 gram—5 mg.—$^1/_{12}$ grain		0.86 gram —860 mg.—13 grains	
0.006 gram—6 mg.—$^1/_{10}$ grain		0.93 gram —930 mg.—14 grains	
0.007 gram—7 mg.—$^1/_9$ grain		1.0 gram —1000 mg.—15 grains	
0.008 gram—8 mg.—$^1/_8$ grain		1.06 grams—1060 mg.—16 grains	
0.009 gram—9 mg.—$^1/_7$ grain		1.13 grams—1130 mg.—17 grains	
0.01 gram—10 mg.—$^1/_6$ grain		1.18 grams—1180 mg.—18 grains	
0.013 gram—13 mg.—$^1/_5$ grain (12 mg.)		1.26 grams—1260 mg.—19 grains	
0.016 gram—16 mg.—$^1/_4$ grain (15 mg.)		1.30 grams—1300 mg.—20 grains	
0.02 gram—20 mg.—$^1/_3$ grain		1.50 grams—1500 mg.—22 grains	
0.025 gram—25 mg.—$^3/_8$ grain		2 grams—2000 mg.—30 grains ($^1/_2$ dram)	
0.03 gram—30 mg.—$^2/_5$ grain ($^1/_2$ grain)		4 grams —1 dram (60 grains)	
0.032 gram—32 mg.—$^1/_2$ grain (30 mg.)		5 grams —75 grains	
0.04 gram—40 mg.—$^3/_5$ grain ($^2/_3$ grain)		8 grams —2 drams (7.5 grams)	
0.043 gram—43 mg.—$^2/_3$ grain (40 mg.)		10 grams —$2^1/_2$ drams	
0.05 gram—50 mg.—$^3/_4$ grain		15 grams —4 drams	
		30 grams —1 ounce	

Liquid Measures*

Metric	Apothecaries	Metric	Apothecaries
0.03 cubic centimeter —$^1/_2$	minim	8 cubic centimeters—2	fluid drams
0.05 cubic centimeter —$^3/_4$	minim	10 cubic centimeters—$2^1/_2$	fluid drams
0.06 cubic centimeter —1	minim	15 cubic centimeters—4	fluid drams
0.1 cubic centimeter —$1^1/_2$	minims	20 cubic centimeters—$5^1/_2$	fluid drams
0.2 cubic centimeter —3	minims	25 cubic centimeters—$^5/_6$	fluid ounce
0.25 cubic centimeter —4	minims	30 cubic centimeters—1	fluid ounce
0.3 cubic centimeter —5	minims	50 cubic centimeters—$1^3/_4$	fluid ounces
0.5 cubic centimeter —8	minims	60 cubic centimeters—2	fluid ounces
0.6 cubic centimeter —10	minims	100 cubic centimeters—$3^1/_2$	fluid ounces
0.75 cubic centimeter —12	minims	120 cubic centimeters—4	fluid ounces
1 cubic centimeter —15	minims	200 cubic centimeters—7	fluid ounces
2 cubic centimeters—30	minims	250 cubic centimeters—8	fluid ounces
3 cubic centimeters—45	minims	360 cubic centimeters—12	fluid ounces
4 cubic centimeters—1	fluid dram	500 cubic centimeters—1	pint
5 cubic centimeters—$1^1/_4$	fluid drams	1000 cubic centimeters—1	quart

* Note: A cubic centimeter (cc.) is the approximate equivalent of a milliliter (ml.). The terms are used interchangeably in general medicine.
(From Culver VM. Modern Bedside Nursing. Philadelphia, WB Saunders, 1969)

24-HOUR CLOCK

From midnight to noon—12-hour time⎫
24-hour time⎬ identical

From noon to midnight—Add 12 to P.M. time = 24-hour time

12-hour Time	24-hour Time
12:00 midnight	24:00
12:01 A.M.	00:01
12:59 A.M.	00:59
1:00 A.M.	01:00
12:00 noon	12:00
12:01 P.M.	12:01
1:00 P.M.	13:00
5:30 P.M.	17:30
10:08 P.M.	22:08
12:00 midnight	24:00

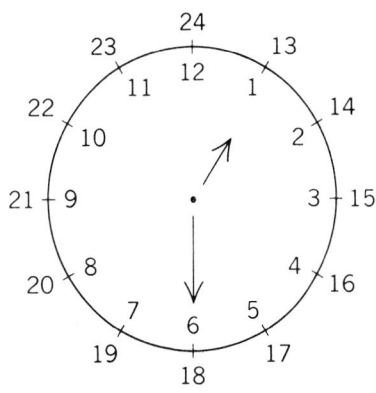

A useful clock for avoiding confusion about A.M. and P.M. designations

CELSIUS (CENTIGRADE) AND FAHRENHEIT TEMPERATURES

Celsius (Centigrade) 0°	Fahrenheit 32°
36.0	96.8
36.5	97.7
37.0	98.6
37.5	99.5
38.0	100.4
38.5	101.3
39.0	102.2
39.5	103.1
40.0	104.0
40.5	104.9
41.0	105.8
41.5	106.7
42.0	107.6

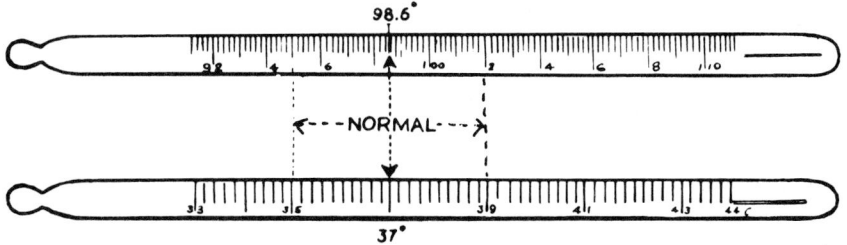

To convert degrees F. to degrees C.
Subtract 32, then multiply by 5/9
To convert degrees C. to degrees F.
Multiply by 9/5, then add 32

NOMOGRAM FOR ESTIMATING SURFACE AREA OF INFANTS AND YOUNG CHILDREN

HEIGHT		SURFACE AREA	WEIGHT	
feet	centimeters	in square meters	pounds	kilograms

```
HEIGHT                    SURFACE AREA              WEIGHT
feet    centimeters       in square meters     pounds      kilograms

                                                 65 ─┤    ┌─ 30
                                                 60 ─┤    │
                                                 55 ─┤    ┌─ 25
                                                 50 ─┤    │
                                   ─ .8          45 ─┤    ┌─ 20
        ┌─ 95                      ─ .7          40 ─┤    │
  3' ─┤ ┌─ 90
 34" ─┤ ┌─ 85                      ─ .6          35 ─┤    ┌─ 15
 32" ─┤ ┌─ 80
 30" ─┤ ┌─ 75                      ─ .5          30 ─┤    │
 28" ─┤ ┌─ 70
 26" ─┤ ┌─ 65                      ─ .4          25 ─┤    ┌─ 10
  2' ─┤ ┌─ 60                                    20 ─┤    │
 22" ─┤ ┌─ 55
 20" ─┤ ┌─ 50                      ─ .3          15 ─┤    │
 18" ─┤ ┌─ 45
 16" ─┤ ┌─ 40                      ─ .2          10 ─┤    ┌─ 5
 14" ─┤ ┌─ 35                                         │   ┌─ 4
  1' ─┤ ┌─ 30                                         │   ┌─ 3
 10" ─┤                                           5 ─┤    │
  9" ─┤ ┌─ 25                      ─ .1           4 ─┤    ┌─ 2
  8" ─┤
        └─ 20                                     3 ─┤
                                                      │   └─ 1
```

To determine the surface area of the patient, draw a straight line between the point representing the patient's height on the left vertical scale to the point representing the patient's weight on the right vertical scale. The point at which this line intersects the middle vertical scale represents the surface area in square meters. (Courtesy of Abbott Laboratories.)

NOMOGRAM FOR ESTIMATING SURFACE AREA OF OLDER CHILDREN AND ADULTS

HEIGHT		SURFACE AREA	WEIGHT	
feet	centimeters	in square meters	pounds	kilograms

```
HEIGHT                    SURFACE AREA          WEIGHT
feet    centimeters      in square meters    pounds   kilograms

                                              440 ── 200
                                              420 ── 190
                                              400 ── 180
                                              380 ── 170
                                              360 ── 160
                                              340 ── 150
          220              3.00               320
7' ──     215              2.90                     ── 140
10" ──    210              2.80               300
8" ──     205              2.70               290 ── 130
6" ──     200              2.60               280
4" ──     195              2.50               270 ── 120
2" ──     190              2.40               260
6' ──     185              2.30               250
          180              2.20               240 ── 110
10" ──    175              2.10               230
8" ──     170              2.00               220 ── 100
6" ──     165              1.95               210 ── 95
4" ──     160              1.90               200 ── 90
2" ──     155              1.85               190 ── 85
5' ──     150              1.80               180 ── 80
          145              1.75               170 ── 75
10" ──                     1.70               160
8" ──     140              1.65               150 ── 70
6" ──     135              1.60               140 ── 65
4" ──     130              1.55                   ── 60
2" ──     125              1.50               130
4' ──     120              1.45               120 ── 55
10" ──    115              1.40               110 ── 50
8" ──     110              1.35               100 ── 45
6" ──     105              1.30                90 ── 40
4" ──     100              1.25                80 ── 35
2" ──      95              1.20                70 ── 30
3' ──      90              1.15                60 ── 25
10" ──     85              1.10                50 ── 20
8" ──      80              1.05
6" ──      75              1.00
```

See Nomogram for Estimating Surface Area of Infants and Young Children for instructions on use. (Courtesy of Abbott Laboratories.)

COMPARATIVE SCALES OF MEASURES, WEIGHTS, AND TEMPERATURES*

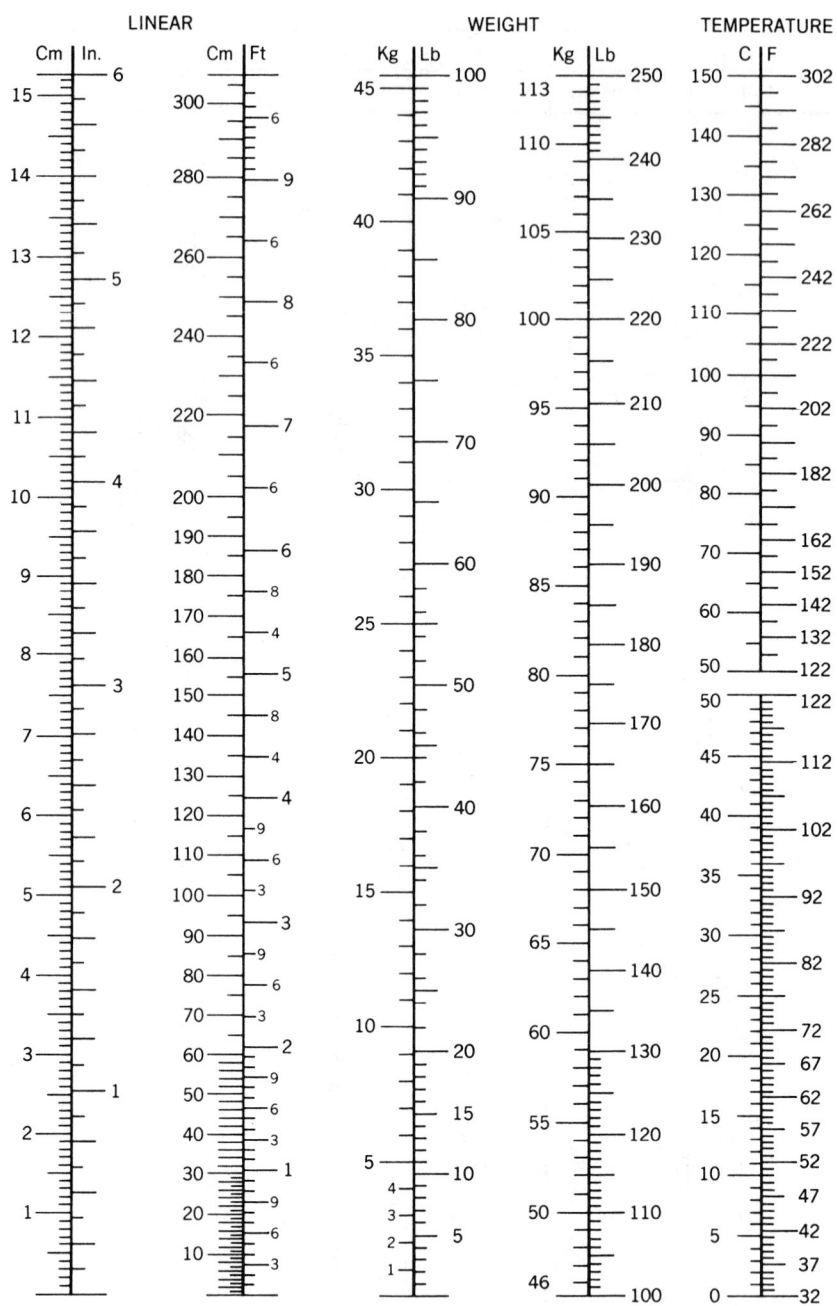

| LINEAR | WEIGHT | TEMPERATURE |

* 2.5 cm. = 1 inch   1 kg. = 2.2 lb.

Appendix III: Recommended Daily Dietary Allowances

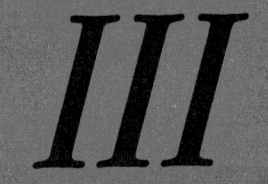

RECOMMENDED DIETARY ALLOWANCES*—REVISED 1989

From the Food and Nutrition Board National Academy of Sciences—National Research Council
Designed for the maintenance of good nutrition of practically all healthy people in the United States

Category	Age (yr.) or Condition	Weight[†] Kg.	Weight[†] Lb.	Height[†] Cm.	Height[†] In.	Pro-tein (gm.)	Fat-Soluble Vitamins Vitamin A (μg RE)[‡]	Fat-Soluble Vitamins Vitamin D (μg.)[§]	Fat-Soluble Vitamins Vitamin E (mg α-TE)[∥]	Fat-Soluble Vitamins Vitamin K (μg.)
Infants	0.0–0.5	6	13	60	24	13	375	7.5	3	5
	0.5–1.0	9	20	71	28	14	375	10	4	10
Children	1–3	13	29	90	35	16	400	10	6	15
	4–6	20	44	112	44	24	500	10	7	20
	7–10	28	62	132	52	28	700	10	7	30
Males	11–14	45	99	157	62	45	1000	10	10	45
	15–18	66	145	176	69	59	1000	10	10	65
	19–24	72	160	177	70	58	1000	10	10	70
	25–50	79	174	176	70	63	1000	5	10	80
	51+	77	170	173	68	63	1000	5	10	80
Females	11–14	46	101	157	62	46	800	10	8	45
	15–18	55	120	163	64	44	800	10	8	55
	19–24	58	128	164	65	46	800	10	8	60
	25–50	63	138	163	64	50	800	5	8	65
	51+	65	143	160	63	50	800	5	8	65
Pregnant						60	800	10	10	65
Lactating	1st 6 months					65	1300	10	12	65
	2nd 6 months					62	1200	10	11	65

* The allowances, expressed as average daily intakes over time, are intended to provide for individual variations among most normal persons as they live in the United States under usual environmental stresses. Diets should be based on a variety of common foods in order to provide other nutrients for which human requirements have been less well defined.

† Weights and heights of reference adults are actual medians for the US population of the designated age.

‡ 1 retinol equivalent (RE) = 1 μg. retinol or 6 μg. β-carotene.

§ As cholecalciferol; 10 μg. cholecalciferol = 400 IU vitamin D.

∥ 1 α-tocopherol equivalent (α-TE) = 1 mg. d-α tocopherol.

¶ 1 niacin equivalent (NE) = 1 mg. niacin or 60 mg. dietary tryptophan.

From the US National Research Council. Recommended Dietary Allowances. 10th ed. Washington, DC, National Academy Press, 1989.

Water-Soluble Vitamins							Minerals						
Vita- min C (mg.)	Thia- min (mg.)	Ribo- flavin (mg.)	Niacin (mg. NE)¶	Vita- min B₆ (mg.)	Fo- late (µg.)	Vita- min B₁₂ (µg.)	Cal- cium (mg.)	Phos- phorus (mg.)	Mag- nesium (mg.)	Iron (mg.)	Zinc (mg.)	Iodine (µg.)	Sele- nium (µg.)
30	0.3	0.4	5	0.3	25	0.3	400	300	40	6	5	40	10
35	0.4	0.5	6	0.6	35	0.5	600	500	60	10	5	50	15
40	0.7	0.8	9	1.0	50	0.7	800	800	80	10	10	70	20
45	0.9	1.1	12	1.1	75	1.0	800	800	120	10	10	90	20
45	1.0	1.2	13	1.4	100	1.4	800	800	170	10	10	120	30
50	1.3	1.5	17	1.7	150	2.0	1200	1200	270	12	15	150	40
60	1.5	1.8	20	2.0	200	2.0	1200	1200	400	12	15	150	50
60	1.5	1.7	19	2.0	200	2.0	1200	1200	350	10	15	150	70
60	1.5	1.7	19	2.0	200	2.0	800	800	350	10	15	150	70
60	1.2	1.4	15	2.0	200	2.0	800	800	350	10	15	150	70
50	1.1	1.3	15	1.4	150	2.0	1200	1200	280	15	12	150	45
60	1.1	1.3	15	1.5	180	2.0	1200	1200	300	15	12	150	50
60	1.1	1.3	15	1.6	180	2.0	1200	1200	280	15	12	150	55
60	1.1	1.3	15	1.6	180	2.0	800	800	280	15	12	150	55
60	1.0	1.2	13	1.6	180	2.0	800	800	280	10	12	150	55
70	1.5	1.6	17	2.2	400	2.2	1200	1200	320	30	15	175	65
95	1.6	1.8	20	2.1	280	2.6	1200	1200	355	15	19	200	75
90	1.6	1.7	20	2.1	260	2.6	1200	1200	340	15	16	200	75

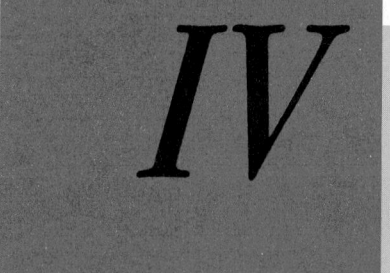

Appendix IV: Pediatric Laboratory Values

BLOOD CHEMISTRIES

These values are compiled from the published literature (Meites S [ed]. Pediatric Clinical Chemistry. 2nd ed. American Association for Clinical Chemistry, 1981; Tietz NW. Textbook of Clinical Chemistry. 1981; Lundberg GD et al. JAMA 1986; 255:2329–39; Scully RE et al. New Engl J Med 1986; 314:39–49) and from the Johns Hopkins Hospital Department of Laboratory Medicine. Normal values vary with the analytic method used. If any doubt exists, consult your laboratory for its analytical method and normal range of values.

Determination	Conventional Units	SI Units	Determination	Conventional Units	SI Units
Acid phosphatase			Bilirubin (total)		
Newborn	7.4–19.4 U/ml.	7.4–19.4 U/ml.	Cord	<1.8 mg./dl.	<30.6 µmol/L.
2–13 yrs	6.4–15.2 U/ml.	6.4–15.2 U/ml.	24 h.		
Adult	M: 0.5–11 U/ml.	0.5–11.0 U/ml.	Preterm	≤6 mg./dl.	≤103 µmol./L.
	F: 0.2–9.5 U/ml.	0.2–9.5 U/ml.	Term	≤6 mg./dl.	≤103 µmol./L.
Alanine Amino-			48 h.		
transferase			Preterm	<8 mg./dl.	<137 µmol./L.
(ALT)			Term	≤7 mg./dl.	≤120 µmol./L.
Infants	<54 U/L.	<54 U/L.	3–5 days		
Children/adults	1–30 U/L.	1–30 U/L.	Preterm	≤12 mg./dl.	≤205 µmol./L.
Aldolase			Term	≤12 mg./dl.	<205 µmol./L.
Adult	<8 U/L.	<8 U/L.	1 mo–Adult	≤1.5 mg./dl.	≤26 µmol./L.
Children	<16 U/L.	<16 U/L.	Conjugated	≤0.5 mg./dl.	≤9 µmol./L.
Newborn	<32 U/L.	<32 U/L.	Calcium (total)		
Alkaline phosphatase			Premature < 1 week	6–10 mg./dl.	1.5–2.5 mmol./L.
Infant	150–400 U/L.	150–400 U/L.	Full-term < 1 week	7–12 mg./dl.	1.75–3 mmol./L.
2–10 yr.	100–300 U/L.	100–300 U/L.	Child	8–10.5 mg./dl.	2–2.6 mmol./L.
11–18 yr.			Adult	8.5–10.5 mg./dl.	2.1–2.6 mmol./L.
Male	50–375 U/L.	50–375 U/L.	Calcium (ionized)	4.4–5.4 mg./dl.	0.1–1.35 mmol./L.
Female	30–300 U/L.	30–300 U/L.	Carbon dioxide (CO_2		
Adult	30–100 U/L.	30–100 U/L.	content)		
Alpha-1-antitrypsin	2.1–5 gm./L.		Cord blood	15–20 mmol./L.	15–20 mmol./L.
Alpha fetoprotein	<10 mg./dl.	<0.1 g./L.	Child	18–27 mmol./L.	18–27 mmol./L.
Ammonia nitrogen (ve-			Adult	24–35 mmol./L.	24–35 mmol./L.
nous sample:			Carbon monoxide		
heparinized			(carboxyhemo-		
specimen in			globin)		
ice water and			Nonsmoker	<2% of total hemoglobin	
analyzed			Smoker	<10% of total hemoglobin	
within 30 min.)			Lethal	>60% of total hemoglobin	
All ages	13–48 µg./dl.	9–34 µmol./L.	Carotenoids (carotenes)		
Amylase			Infant	20–70 µg./dl.	0.37–1.30 µmol./L.
Newborn	5–65 U/L.	5–65 U/L.	Child	40–130 µg./dl.	0.74–2.42 µmol./L.
>1 yr.	25–125 U/L.	25–125 U/L.	Adult	60–200 µg./dl.	1.12–3.72 µmol./L.
Arsenic	<30 µg/dl.	<0.4 mmol./L.	Ceruloplasmin	23–58 mg./dl.	1.32–3.83 µmol./L.
Aspartate aminotransfer-			Chloride	94–106 mEq./L.	94–106 mmol./L.
ase (AST)			Cholesterol	See Lipids	
Newborn/infant	25–75 U/L.	25–75 U/L.	Copper		
Child/adult	0–40 U/L.	0–40 U/L.	0–6 mo.	<70 µg./dl.	<11 µmol./L.
Bicarbonate			6 mo.–5 yr.	27–153 µg./dl.	4.2–24.1 µmol./L.
Premature	18–26 mEq./L.	18–26 mmol./L.	5–17 yr.	94–234 µg./dl.	14.2–36.8 µmol./L.
Infant	20–26 mEq./L.	20–26 mmol./L.	Adult	70–155 µg./dl.	11–24.4 µmol./L.
1–2 yr.	20–25 mEq./L.	20–25 mmol./L.			
>2 yr.	22–26 mEq./L.	22–26 mmol./L.			

(continued)

BLOOD CHEMISTRIES (continued)

Creatine Kinase (Creatine Phosphokinase)

	Upper 95th Percentile (U/L.)	
Age	*Males*	*Females*
1 d.	600	500
2–10 d.	440	440
<1 yr.	170	170
1–7 yr.	109	100
7–9 yr.	103	85
9–11 yr.	109	88
11–13 yr.	108	85
13–15 yr.	129	85
15–17 yr.	247	74
17–19 yr.	190	68

Creatinine (serum)

	Upper Limits, mg./dl. (μmol./L.)	
Age (yr.)	*Males*	*Females*
1	0.6 (53)	0.5 (44)
2–3	0.7 (62)	0.6 (53)
4–7	0.8 (71)	0.7 (62)
8–10	0.9 (80)	0.8 (71)
11–12	1.0 (88)	0.9 (80)
13–17	1.2 (106)	1.1 (97)
18–20	1.3 (115)	1.1 (97)
Adult	1.2 (106)	1.4 (124)

Ferritin		
Children	7–144 ng./ml.	7–144 μg./L.
Adult	F: 10–110 ng./ml.	10–110 μg./L.
	M: 30–265 ng./ml.	30–265 μg./L.
Fibrin degradation products		
Titer	1:50 = positive	
Fibrinogen	200–400 mg./dl.	2–4 g./L.
Folic acid (folate)	1.9–14 ng./L.	4.3–23.6 nmol./L.
Galactose		
Newborn	0–20 mg./dl.	0–1.11 mmol./L.
Thereafter	<5 mg./dl.	<0.28 mmol./L.
Gammaglutamyl transferase (GGT)		
Cord	19–270 U/L.	19–270 U/L.
Premature	56–233 U/L.	56–233 U/L.
0–3 wk.	0–130 U/L.	0–130 U/L.
3 wk.–3 mo.	4–120 U/L.	4–120 U/L.
>3 mo.		
M	5–65 U/L.	5–65 U/L.
F	5–35 U/L.	5–35 U/L.
1–15 yr.	0–23 U/L.	0–23 U/L.
16 yr.–Adult	0–35 U/L.	0–35 U/L.
Gastrin	<300 pg./ml.	<300 ng./L.
Glucose (serum)		
Premature	20–65 mg./dl.	1.1–3.6 mmol./L.
Full term	20–110 mg./dl.	1.1–6.4 mmol./L.
1 wk.–16 yr.	60–105 mg./dl.	3.3–5.8 nmol./L.
>16 yr.	70–115 mg./dl.	3.9–6.4 nmol./L.
Haptoglobin*	400–1800 mg./L.	0.4–1.8 g./L.

Iron

	Iron		Iron Binding Capacity		% Saturation
	(μg./dl.)	*(μmol./L.)*	*(μg./dl.)*	*(μmol./L.)*	**(μg./dl.)**
Newborn	110–270	19.7–48.3	59–175	10.6–31.3	65%
4–10 mo.	30–70	5.4–12.5	250–400	45–72	25%
3–10 yr.	53–119	9.5–27.0	250–400	45–72	30%
Adult	72–186	12.9–33.3	250–400	45–72	35%

Ketones		
Qualitative	Negative	
Quantitative	up to 3 mg%	
Lactate		
Capillary blood		
Newborn	≤30 mg./dl.	<3.0 mmol./L.
Child	5–20 mg./dl.	0.56–2.25 mmol./L.
Venous	5–18 mg./dl.	0.5–2.0 mmol./L.
Arterial	3–7 mg./dl.	0.3–0.8 mmol./L.
Lactate dehydrogenase (37°C.)		
Newborn	160–1500 U/L.	160–1500 U/L.
Infant	150–360 U/L.	150–360 U/L.
Child	150–300 U/L.	150–300 U/L.
Adult	100–250 U/L.	100–250 U/L.
Lactate dehydrogenase isoenzymes (% total)		
LD_1 Heart		24–34%
LD_2 Heart, erythrocytes		35–45%
LD_3 Muscle		15–25%
LD_4 Liver, trace muscle		4–10%
LD_5 Liver, muscle		1–9%
Lipase	20–180 U/L.	20–180 U/L.
Lipids		

	Normal Upper Limits			
	Total Serum Cholesterol mg./dl. (mmol./L.)		Serum Triglycerides mg./dl. (g./L.)	
Age	*Males*	*Females[†]*	*Males*	*Females**
0–4 yr.	203 (5.28)	200 (5.2)	99 (0.99)	112 (1.12)
5–9	203 (5.28)	205 (5.33)	101 (1.01)	105 (1.05)
10–14	202 (5.25)	201 (5.22)	125 (1.25)	131 (1.31)
15–19	197 (5.12)	200 (5.2)	148 (1.48)	124 (1.24)
20–24	218 (5.67)	216 (5.62)	201 (2.01)	131 (1.31)
25–29	244 (6.34)	222 (5.77)	249 (2.49)	144 (1.44)
30–34	254 (6.60)	230 (5.98)	266 (2.66)	150 (1.50)
35–39	270 (7.02)	242 (6.24)	321 (3.21)	176 (1.76)
40–44	268 (6.97)	252 (6.55)	320 (3.20)	191 (1.91)
45–49	276 (7.18)	265 (6.89)	327 (3.27)	214 (2.14)

* Detectable in only 10%–20% of newborns.
† Use of oral contraceptives significantly raises both total serum cholesterol and serum triglyceride levels.

(continued)

BLOOD CHEMISTRIES (continued)

	Normal Upper Limits					
HDL–Cholesterol mg./dl. (mmol./L.)		LDL mg./dl. (mmol./L.)		VLDL mg./dl. (mml./L.)		
Age	*Males*	*Females*	*Males*	*Females*	*Males*	*Females*
0–4	—	—	—	—	—	—
5–9	74 (1.91)	73 (1.89)	129 (3.34)	140 (3.62)	18 (0.47)	24 (0.62)
10–14	74 (1.91)	70 (1.81)	132 (3.41)	136 (3.52)	22 (0.57)	23 (0.59)
15–19	63 (1.63)	73 (1.89)	130 (3.36)	135 (3.49)	26 (0.67)	24 (0.62)
20–24	63 (1.63)	—	147 (3.80)	—	28 (0.72)	—
25–29	63 (1.63)	81 (2.09)	165 (4.27)	151 (3.90)	36 (0.93)	24 (0.65)
30–34	63 (1.63)	75 (1.94)	185 (4.78)	150 (3.88)	48 (1.24)	25 (0.65)
35–39	62 (1.60)	82 (2.12)	189 (4.89)	172 (4.45)	56 (1.49)	35 (0.91)
40–44	67 (1.73)	87 (2.25)	186 (4.81)	174 (4.50)	56 (1.49)	29 (0.75)
45–49	64 (1.66)	86 (2.22)	202 (5.22)	187 (4.84)	51 (1.32)	38 (0.98)

Magnesium	1.5–2 mEq./L.	0.75–1 mmol./L.
Manganese (blood)		
Newborn	2.4–9.6 µg./dl.	2.44–1.75 µmol./L.
2–18 yr.	0.8–2.1 µg./dl.	0.15–0.38 µmol./L.
Methemoglobin	<0.3 g./dl. or <3% of total Hb	<46.5 µmol./L.
5′ Nucleotidase	2.2–15 U/L.	2.2–15 U/L.
Osmolality	285–295 mOsm./kg.	270–285 mOsm./L. plasma
Phenylalanine		
Newborn	<4 mg./dl.	<0.24 mmol./L.
Child	<3 mg./dl.	<0.18 mmol./L.
Phosphorus		
Newborn	4.2–9.0 mg./dl.	1.36–2.91 mmol./L.
1 yr.	3.8–6.2 mg./dl.	1.23–2.0 mmol./L.
2–5 yr.	3.5–6.8 mg./dl.	1.13–2.2 mmol./L.
Adult	3.0–4.5 mg./dl.	0.97–1.45 mmol./L.
Porcelain	10–25 mg./dl.	No SI conversion factor
Potassium		
<10 days of age	3.5–6 mEq./L.	3.5–6 mmol./L.
>10 days of age	3.5–5 mEq./L.	3.5–5 mmol./L.
Prolactin		
Newborn	<200 ng./ml.	<200 µg./L.
Adult	<20 ng./ml.	<20 µg./L.

Proteins Average (Range) in gr./dl.

Age	Total	Albumin	Globulin	Gamma Globulin
Premature	5.5 (4.0–7.0)	3.7 (2.5–4.5)	1.8 (1.2–2.0)	0.7 (0.5–0.9)
FT newborn	6.4 (5.0–7.1)	3.4 (2.5–5.0)	3.1 (1.2–4.0)	0.8 (0.7–0.9)
1– mo.	6.6 (4.7–7.4)	3.8 (3.0–4.2)	2.5 (1.0–3.3)	0.3 (0.1–0.5)
3–12 mo.	6.8 (5.0–7.5)	3.9 (2.7–5.0)	2.6 (2.0–3.8)	0.6 (0.4–1.2)
1–15 yr.	7.4 (6.5–8.6)	4.0 (3.2–5.0)	3.1 (2.0–4.0)	0.9 (0.6–1.2)

Pyruvate		50–140 mmol./L.	
Sodium			
Premature	130-140 mEq./L.	130–140 mmol./L.	
Older	135–145 mEq./L.	135–145 mmol./L.	
Transaminase (SGOT)	*See Aspartate Aminotransferase (AST)*		
Transaminase (SGPT)	*See Alanine Aminotransferase (AT)*		
Triglycerides	*See Lipids*		
Urea nitrogen	5–25 mg./dl.	1.8–9 mmol./L.	
Uric acid			
0–2 yr.	2.0–7.0 mg./dl.	0.12–0.42 mmol./L.	
2–12 yr.	2.0–6.5 mg./dl.	0.12–0.39 mmol./L.	
12–14 yr.	2.0–7.0 mg./dl.	0.12–0.42 mmol./L.	
14–adult			
M	3.0–8.0 mg./dl.	0.18–0.48 mmol./L.	
F	2.0–7.0 mg./dl.	0.12–0.42 mmol./L.	
Vitamin A (retinol)			
0–1 yr.	20–90 µg./dl.	0.7–3.14 µmol./L.	
1–5 yr.	30–100 µg./dl.	1.05–3.50 µmol./L.	
5–16 yr.	60–100 µg./dl.	2.09–3.50 µmol./L.	
Adult	20–80 µg./dl.	0.70–2.79 µmol./L.	
Vitamin B$_1$ (thiamine)	5.3–7.9 µg./dl.	0.16–0.23 µmol./L.	
Vitamin B$_2$ (riboflavin)	3.7–13.7 µg./dl.	98–363 mmol./L.	
Vitamin B$_{12}$ (cobalamin)	130-785 pg./ml.	96–579 pmol./L.	
Vitamin C (ascorbic acid)	0.2–2 mg./dl.	11.4–113.6 µmol./L.	
Vitamin D (1.25 dihydroxy)			
Newborn	21 ± 2 pg./ml.	50 ± 4.8 nmol./L.	
Child	43 ± 3 pg./ml.	103 ± 7.2 nmol./L.	
Adult	29 ± 2 pg./ml.	69.6 ± 4.8 nmol./L.	
Vitamin E	5–20 µg./dl.	8.4–23 µmol./L.	
Zinc	55–150 µg./dl.	8.4–23 µmol./L.	

(From Johns Hopkins Hospital. The Harriet Lane Handbook. 11th ed. Chicago, Year Book Medical Pub, 1987)

TERM INFANTS—NORMAL BLOOD CHEMISTRY VALUES*

Determination	Sample Source	Cord	1–12 Hours	12–24 Hours	24–48 Hours	48–72 Hours
Sodium (mM./L.)	Capillary	147 (126–166)	143 (124–156)	145 (132–159)	148 (134–160)	149 (139–162)
Potassium (mM./L.)		7.8 (5.6–12)	6.4 (5.3–7.3)	6.3 (5.3–8.9)	6 (5.2–7.3)	5.9 (5–7.7)
Chloride (mM./L.)		103 (98–110)	101 (90–111)	103 (87–114)	102 (92–114)	103 (93–112)
Calcium (mg./dl.)		9.3 (8.2–11.1)	8.4 (7.3–9.2)	7.8 (6.9–9.4)	8 (6.1–9.9)	7.9 (5.9–9.7)
Phosphorus (mg./dl.)		5.6 (3.7–8.1)	6.1 (3.5–8.6)	5.7 (2.9–8.1)	5.9 (3–8.7)	5.8 (2.8–7.6)
Blood urea (mg./dl.)		29 (21–40)	27 (8–34)	33 (9–63)	32 (13–77)	31 (13–68)
Total protein (g./dl.)		6.1 (4.8–7.3)	6.6 (5.6–8.5)	6.6 (5.8–8.2)	6.9 (5.9–8.2)	7.2 (6–8.5)
Glucose (mg./dl.)		73 (45–96)	63 (40–97)	63 (42–104)	56 (30–91)	59 (40–90)
Lactic acid (mg./dl.)		19.5 (11–30)	14.6 (11–24)	14 (10–23)	14.3 (9–22)	13.5 (7–21)
Lactate (mM./L.)†		2–3	2			

(From Avery GB. Neonatology. 3rd ed. Philadelphia, JB Lippincott, 1987. Original data from: *Acharya PT and Payne WW. Arch Dis Child 40:430, 1965; † Daniel SS, Adamsons K Jr and James LS. Pediatrics 37:942, 1966)

LOW BIRTH WEIGHT INFANTS—NORMAL BLOOD CHEMISTRY VALUES (Capillary Blood, First Day)

Determination	<1000	1001–1500	1501–2000	2001–2500
Sodium (mM./L.)	138	133	135	134
Potassium (mM./L.)	6.4	6.0	5.4	5.6
Chloride (mM./L.)	100	101	105	104
Total CO$_2$ (mM./L.)	19	20	20	20
Urea (mg./dl.)	22	21	16	16
Total protein (g./dl.)	4.8	4.8	5.2	5.3

(From Avery GB. Neonatology. 3rd ed. Philadelphia, JB Lippincott, 1987)

NORMAL VALUES—HEMATOLOGY

Age	Hgb (gm %) Mean (−2SD)	Hct (%) Mean (−2SD)	MCV (fl.) Mean (−2SD)	MCHC (gm./% RBC) Mean (−2SD)	Retic (%)	WBC/mm³. × 100 Mean (−2SD)	Plts (10³/mm³) Mean (±2SD)
26–30 wk. gestation*	13.4 (11)	41.5 (34.9)	118.2 (106.7)	37.9 (30.6)	—	4.4 (2.7)	254 (180–327)
28 wk.	14.5	45	120	31	(5–10)	—	275
32 wk.	15.0	47	118	32	(3–10)	—	290
Term† (cord)	16.5 (13.5)	51 (42)	108 (98)	33 (30)	(3–7)	18.1 (9–30)†	290
1–3 days	18.5 (14.5)	56 (45)	108 (95)	33 (29)	(1.8–4.6)	18.9 (9.4–34)	192
2 wk.	16.6 (13.4)	53 (41)	105 (88)	31.4 (28.1)		11.4 (5–20)	252
1 mo.	13.9 (10.7)	44 (33)	101 (91)	31.8 (28.1)	(0.1–1.7)	10.8 (5–19.5)	
2 mo.	11.2 (9.4)	35 (28)	95 (84)	31.8 (28.3)			
6 mo.	12.6 (11.1)	36 (31)	76 (68)	35 (32.7)	(0.7–2.3)	11.9 (6–17.5)	
6 mo.–2 yr.	12 (10.5)	36 (33)	78 (70)	33 (30)		10.6 (6–17)	(150–350)
2–6 yr.	12.5 (11.5)	37 (34)	81 (75)	34 (31)	(0.5–1.0)	8.5 (5–15.5)	(150–350)
6–12 yr.	13.5 (11.5)	40 (35)	86 (77)	34 (31)	(0.5–1.0)	8.1 (4.5–13.5)	(150–350)
12–18 yr.							
Male	14.5 (13)	43 (36)	88 (78)	34 (31)	(0.5–1.0)	7.8 (4.5–13.5)	(150–350)
Female	14 (12)	41 (37)	90 (78)	34 (31)	(0.5–1.0)	7.8 (4.5–13.5)	(150–350)
Adult							
Male	15.5 (13.5)	47 (41)	90 (80)	34 (31)	(0.8–2.5)	7.4 (4.5–11)	(150–350)
Female	14 (12)	41 (36)	90 (80)	34 (31)	(0.8–4.1)	7.4 (4.5–11)	(150–350)

* Values are from fetal samplings.
† Under 1 month, capillary Hgb exceeds venous: 1 h–3.6 gm. difference; 5 days–2.2 gm. difference; 3 wks—1.1 gm. difference.
‡ Mean (95% confidence limits).

(From Johns Hopkins Hospital. The Harriet Lane Handbook. 11th ed. Chicago, Year Book Medical Pub, 1987)

URINE VALUES

Test	SI Reference Range	Conversion Factor	Conventional Units Reference Range
Aminolevulinic acid	8–53 μmol./d.	μmol./d. × 0.131 = mg./d.	1–7 mg./d.
Calcium	<0.1 mmol./kg./d.	mmol./d. × 40 = mg./d.	<4 mg./kg./d.
Copper	<0.6 μmol./d.	μmol./d. × 63.7 = μg./d.	<40 μg./d.
Coproporphyrin	<300 nmol./d.	nmol./d. × 1.527 = μg./d.	<200 μg./d.
Cortisol, free	70–340 nmol./d.	nmol./d. × 0.362 = μg./d.	25–125 μg./d.
Creatinine			
Infant	71–177 μmol./kg./d.	μmol./kg./d. × 0.0113 = mg./kg./d.	8–20 mg./kg./d.
Child	71–194		8–22
Adolescent	71–265		8–30
Cystine	40–260 μmol./d.	μmol./d. × 0.12 = mg./d.	5–31 mg./d.
Dehydroepiandrosterone (DHEA)			
<5 yr.	<0.3 μmol./d.	μmol./d. × 0.288 = mg./d.	<0.1 mg./d.
6–9 yr.	<0.7		<0.2
10–15 yr.	<1.4		<0.4
Adult (M)	<8.0		<2.3
Adult (F)	<4.2		<1.2
Epinephrine	<55 nmol./d.	nmol./d. × 0.183 = μg./d.	<10 μg./d.
Fluroide	<50 μmol./d.	μmol./d. × 0.019 = mg./d.	<1 mg./d.
	mmol./mol. Creatinine		**μg./mg. Creatinine**
Homovanillic acid (HVA)		mmol./mol. creatinine × 1.61 = μg./mg. creatinine	
1–12 mo.	0.75–21.7		1.2–35.0
1–2 yr.	2.5–14.3		4.0–23.0
2–5 yr.	0.43–8.4		0.7–13.5
5–10 yr.	0.31–5.6		0.5–9.0
10–15 yr.	0.15–7.4		0.25–12.0
15–18 yr.	0.31–1.24		0.5–2.0
	mmol./mol. Creatinine		**μg./mg. Creatinine**
Metanephrines		mmol./mol. creatinine × 1.74 = μg./mg. creatinine	
<1 yr.	0.001–2.64		0.001–4.6
1–2 yr.	0.15–3.09		0.27–5.38
2–5 yr.	0.20–1.72		0.35–2.99
5–10 yr.	0.25–1.55		0.43–2.70
10–15 yr.	0.001–0.38		0.001–1.87
15–18 yr.	0.03–0.69		0.001–0.67
Norepinephrine	<590 nmol./d.	nmol./d. × 0.169 = μg./d.	<100 μg./d.
Osmolality	50–1200 μmol./kg.		50–1200 mOsm./kg.
Oxalate	110–440 μmol./d.	μmol./d. × 0.088 = mg./d.	10–40 mg./d.
Porphobilinogen	0–8.8 μmol./d.	μmol./d. × 0.226 × mg./d.	0–2 mg./d.
Potassium	25–125 mmol./d.		25–125 mEq./d.
Pregnanetriol	(varies with diet)	μmol./d. × 0.3365 = mg./d.	<2.5 mg./d.
Protein	<7.4 μmol./d.		1–14 mg./dL.
	10–140 mg./L.		
Steroids			
17-hydroxycorticosteroid			
Prepubertal	2.76–15.5 μmol./d.	μmol./d. × 0.3625 = mg./d.	1–5.6 mg./d.
Adult (M)	11–33 μmol./d.		4–12 mg./d.
Adult (F)	11–22 μmol./d.		4–8 mg./d.
17-ketosteroids			
<1 mo.	≤6.9 μmol./d.	μmol./d. × 0.2884 = mg./d.	≤2 mg./d.
1 mo.–5 yr.	<1.73		<0.5
6–8 yr.	3.47–6.9		1–2
Adult (M)	21–62		6–18
Adult (F)	14–45		4–13
Uric acid	1.48–4.43 mmol./d.	mmol./d. × 169 = mg./d.	250–750 mg./d.
	mmol./mol. Creatinine		**μg./mg. Creatinine**
Vanilylmandelic acid (VMA)		mmol./mol. creatinine × 1.75 = μg./mg.	
1–6 mo.	1.71–9.71		3–7
6–12 mo.	1.14–8.57		2–15
1–5 yr.	1.14–5.71		2–10
5–10 yr.	0.86–4.00		1.5–7
10–15 yr.	0.57–3.43		1–6
>15 yr.	0.57–3.43		1–6

(From Oski FA et al. Principles and Practices of Pediatrics. Philadelphia, JB Lippincott, 1990)

NORMAL SEROLOGIC REFERENCE VALUES

Determination	Value
Antinuclear antibody	<1:160
Anti-streptolysin O Titer*	
Preschool	<1:85
School ages and adults	<1:170
Older adults	<1:85
Anti-hyaluronidase	<1:256
Anti-nuclear Antibody	<1:40
C-reactive Protein	Negative
C_1 esterase inhibitor	17.4–24 mg./dl.
C_3	
1–6 mo.	53–175 mg./dl.
7–12 mo.	75–180 mg./dl.
1–5 yr.	77–166 mg./dl.
6–10 yr.	88–199 mg./dl.
Adult	83–177 mg./dl.
C_4	
1–6 mo.	7–42 mg./dl.
7–12 mo.	9.5–39 mg./dl.
1–5 yr.	9–40 mg./dl.
6–10 yr.	12–40 mg./dl.
Adult	15–45 mg./dl.
C_{H50}	75–160 U/ml.
Rheumatoid factor	<20 negative
	20–40 suggestive
	≥80 positive
Rheumaton titer (modified Waaler-Rose slide test)	Negative
	≥10 may be significant
Total B cells	5%–20% of lymphocytes
Total T cells	50%–80% of lymphocytes
T helper cells	34%–56% of lymphocytes
T suppressor cells	18%–32% of lymphocytes
Helper/suppressor ratio	1.1–2.5

* Significant if rising titer can be demonstrated at weekly intervals.
(From Johns Hopkins Hospital. The Harriet Lane Handbook. 11th ed. Chicago, Year Book Medical Pub, 1987)

CEREBROSPINAL FLUID VALUES

Determination	Value
Cell Count	
Preterm mean	9.0 (0–25.4 WBC/mm.^{3}) (57% PMNs)
Term mean	8.2 (0–22.4 WBC/mm.^{3}) (61% PMNs)
>1 mo	0–7 (0% PMNs)
Glucose	
Preterm	24–63 mg./dl. (mean 50)
Term	34–119 mg./dl. (mean 52)
Child	40–80 mg./dl.
CSF Glucose/Blood Glucose (%)	
Preterm	55–105
Term	44–128
Child	50%
Lactic acid dehydrogenase	20 U/ml. (range 5–30 U/ml.)
Myelin basic protein	<4 ng./ml.
Pressure (initial lumbar puncture)	
Newborn	80–110 (<110) mm. H_2O
Infant/Child	<200 (lateral recumbent position) mm. H_2O
Respiratory movements	5–10 mm. H_2O
Protein	
Preterm	65–150 mg./dl. (mean 115)
Term	20–170 mg./dl. (mean 90)
Children	
Ventricular	5–15 mg./dl.
Cisternal	5–25 mg./dl.
Lumbar	5–40 mg./dl.

(From Johns Hopkins Hospital. The Harriet Lane Handbook. 11th ed. Chicago, Year Book Medical Pub, 1987)

SAMPLE CONVERSIONS OF POUNDS AND OUNCES TO GRAMS

Pounds	Ounces															
	0	1	2	3	4	5	6	7	8	9	10	11	12	13	14	15
0	—	28	57	85	113	142	170	198	227	255	283	312	340	369	397	425
1	454	482	510	539	567	595	624	652	680	709	737	765	794	822	850	879
2	907	936	964	992	1021	1049	1077	1106	1134	1162	1191	1219	1247	1276	1304	1332
3	1361	1389	1417	1446	1474	1503	1531	1559	1588	1616	1644	1673	1701	1729	1758	1786
4	1814	1843	1871	1899	1928	1956	1984	2013	2041	2070	2098	2126	2155	2183	2211	2240
5	2268	2296	2325	2353	2381	2410	2438	2466	2495	2532	2551	2580	2608	2637	2665	2693
6	2722	2750	2778	2807	2835	2863	2892	2920	2948	2977	3005	3033	3062	3090	3118	3147
7	3175	3203	3232	3260	3289	3317	3345	3374	3402	3430	3459	3487	3515	3544	3572	3600
8	3629	3657	3685	3714	3742	3770	3799	3827	3856	3884	3912	3941	3969	3997	4026	4054
9	4082	4111	4139	4167	4196	4224	4252	4281	4309	4337	4366	4394	4423	4451	4479	4508
10	4536	4564	4593	4621	4649	4678	4706	4734	4763	4791	4819	4848	4876	4904	4933	4961
11	4990	5018	5046	5075	5103	5131	5160	5188	5216	5245	5273	5301	5330	5358	5386	5415
12	5443	5471	5500	5528	5557	5585	5613	5642	5670	5698	5727	5755	5783	5812	5840	5868
13	5897	5925	5953	5982	6010	6038	6067	6095	6123	6152	6180	6209	6237	6265	6294	6322
14	6350	6379	6407	6435	6464	6492	6520	6549	6577	6605	6634	6662	6690	6719	6747	6776
15	6804	6832	6860	6889	6917	6945	6973	7002	7030	7059	7087	7115	7144	7172	7201	7228
16	7257	7286	7313	7342	7371	7399	7427	7456	7484	7512	7541	7569	7597	7626	7654	7682
17	7711	7739	7768	7796	7824	7853	7881	7909	7938	7966	7994	8023	8051	8079	8108	8136
18	8165	8192	8221	8249	8278	8306	8335	8363	8391	8420	8448	8476	8504	8533	8561	8590
19	8618	8646	8675	8703	8731	8760	8788	8816	8845	8873	8902	8930	8958	8987	9015	9043
20	9072	9100	9128	9157	9185	9213	9242	9270	9298	9327	9355	9383	9412	9440	9469	9497
21	9525	9554	9582	9610	9639	9667	9695	9724	9752	9780	9809	9837	9865	9894	9922	9950
22	9979	10007	10036	10064	10092	10120	10149	10177	10206	10234	10262	10291	10319	10347	10376	10404

(From Avery GB. Neonatology. 3rd ed. Philadelphia, JB Lippincott, 1987)

Index

Page numbers followed by *f* indicate illustrations;
t following a page number indicates tabular material.

ISBN 0-397-54787-0

90000

9 780397 547876